INTENSIVE CARE OF THE FETUS & NEONATE

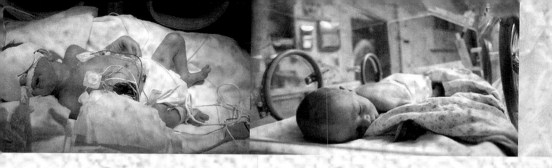
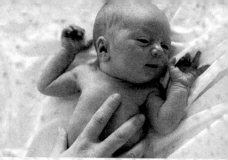

INTENSIVE CARE OF THE FETUS & NEONATE

SECOND EDITION

Alan R. Spitzer, MD
Senior Vice President and Director
The Center for Research and Education
Pediatrix Medical Group
Sunrise, Florida

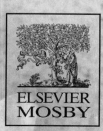

ELSEVIER
MOSBY

ELSEVIER
MOSBY

The Curtis Center
170 S Independence Mall W 300E
Philadelphia, Pennsylvania 19106

INTENSIVE CARE OF THE FETUS AND NEONATE, Second Edition   1–56053–512–1
Copyright © 2005, 1996 Elsevier, Inc.

NOTICE

Neonatology/Pediatrics is an ever-changing field. Standard safety precautions must be followed, but as new research and clinical experience broaden our knowledge, changes in treatment and drug therapy may become necessary or appropriate. Readers are advised to check the most current product information provided by the manufacturer of each drug to be administered to verify the recommended dose, the method and duration of administration, and contraindications. It is the responsibility of the licensed prescriber, relying on experience and knowledge of the patient, to determine dosages and the best treatment for each individual patient. Neither the publisher nor the authors assume any liability for any injury and/or damage to persons or property arising from this publication.

Library of Congress Cataloging-in-Publication Data

Intensive care of the fetus and neonate/edited by Alan R. Spitzer.—2nd ed.
    p. ; cm.
  Includes bibliographical references and index.
  ISBN 1-56053-512-1
    1. Perinatology. 2. Neonatology. I. Spitzer, Alan R.
  [DNLM: 1. Intensive Care, Neonatal. 2. Fetal Diseases—therapy. 3. Infant, Newborn, Diseases—therapy. 4. Perinatal Care. WS 421 I61 2005]
  RG600.I54 2005
  618.3′2—dc22   2004059708

Acquisitions Editor: Meghan Curry McAteer
Developmental Editor: Dana Lamparello
Senior Project Manager: Robin E. Davis
Marketing Manager: Theresa Dudas

Printed in the United States of America.

Last digit is the print number: 9   8   7   6   5   4   3   2   1

This book is dedicated to the great love of my life, my wife **Elaine,**
to my children and daughter-in-law, **Lauren, Sara, Steve,** and **Jen,**
and to my grandson, **Jacob Eli Spitzer,** whose premature birth
taught me more than I ever really wanted to know about neonatal medicine.

Contributors

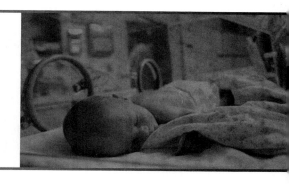

Steven H. Abman, MD
Professor, Department of Pediatrics, University of Colorado School of Medicine; Director, Pediatric Heart-Lung Center, Children's Hospital, Denver, Colorado
Bronchopulmonary Dysplasia

Raymond D. Adelman, MD
Pediatric Nephrologist, Phoenix Children's Hospital, Phoenix, Arizona
Acute Renal Failure

Antoun Al Khabbaz, MD
Attending Physician, Appalachian Regional Healthcare Daniel Boone Clinic, Harlan, Kentucky
Identification and Management of the Fetus at Risk for Acidosis

Carol E. Anderson, MD
Assistant Professor of Pediatrics, Drexel University College of Medicine; Director, Section of Clinical Genetics, St. Christopher's Hospital for Children, Philadelphia, Pennsylvania
The Genetics of Development

Paul Anisman, MD
Clinical Assistant Professor of Pediatrics, Jefferson Medical College of Thomas Jefferson University, Philadelphia, Pennsylvania; Pediatric Cardiologist, Nemours Cardiac Center, Alfred I. duPont Hospital for Children, Wilmington, Delaware
Diagnosis and Management of Cardiac Dysrhythmias

Jacob V. Aranda, MD, PhD, FRCPC, FAAP
Professor of Pediatrics, Pharmacology, and Pharmaceutical Sciences, Wayne State University; Chief, Division of Clinical Pharmacology and Toxicology; Attending Neonatologist; Director, Pediatric Pharmacology Research Unit Network, Children's Hospital of Michigan, Detroit, Michigan
Pharmacology in the Fetus and Newborn

L. Grier Arthur, MD
Surgical Resident, Department of General Surgery, Thomas Jefferson University Hospital, Philadelphia, Pennsylvania
Congenital Anomalies of the Gastrointestinal Tract

Kelly M. Axsom
Medical Student, Temple University School of Medicine; Research Coordinator, Division of Hematology, Children's Hospital of Philadelphia, Philadelphia, Pennsylvania
Transfusion Therapy

Stephen Baumgart, MD
Professor of Pediatrics, George Washington University School of Medicine and Health Sciences; Senior Staff Physician, Division of Neonatology, Children's Hospital National Medical Center, Washington, D.C.
Fetal and Neonatal Thermal Regulation; Modern Extracorporeal Membrane Oxygenation for the Human Newborn Infant

Tara Becker, MD
Clinical Instructor and Maternal-Fetal Medicine Fellow, University of Colorado Health Sciences Center, Denver, Colorado
Maternal Illness and the Effects on the Fetus

Richard M. Benoit, MD, MPH
Assistant Clinical Professor of Obstetrics and Gynecology, Division of Maternal-Fetal Medicine, Brown University School of Medicine; Women and Infants' Hospital, Providence, Rhode Island
Fetal Echocardiography in the Detection and Management of Fetal Heart Disease

Judy C. Bernbaum, MD
Professor of Pediatrics, University of Pennsylvania School of Medicine; Director, Neonatal Follow-up Program, Children's Hospital of Philadelphia, Philadelphia, Pennsylvania
Follow-up of the High-Risk Neonate

Vinod K. Bhutani, MD
Clinical Professor of Pediatrics, University of Pennsylvania School of Medicine; Adjunct Faculty, University of Pennsylvania School of Nursing, Philadelphia, Pennsylvania
Pulmonary Function Testing in the Sick Newborn

Ronald Bolognese, MD
Antenatal Testing Unit, Virtua West Jersey Hospital, Vorhees, New Jersey
Third-Trimester Hemorrhage

Richard E. Broth, MD
Attending Physician, Crozer-Chester Medical Center,
Upland, Pennsylvania
Third-Trimester Hemorrhage

Lawrence W. Brown, MD
Associate Professor of Neurology and Pediatrics,
University of Pennsylvania School of Medicine
and Children's Hospital of Philadelphia, Philadelphia,
Pennsylvania
Neurologic Examination

Vladamir Burdjalov, MD
Associate Staff, Department of Neonatology, Children's
Hospital at the Cleveland Clinic Foundation, Cleveland,
Ohio
Necrotizing Enterocolitis

M. Shannon Burke, MD
Assistant Professor, University of Colorado Health
Sciences Center, Denver, Colorado
Maternal Illness and the Effects on the Fetus

John Casey, MD, CM
Assistant Professor of Pediatrics, Division of
Neonatology, University of Connecticut Health Center,
Farmington, Connecticut
Prevention and Treatment of Neonatal Sepsis

Linda Chan, MD
Adjunct Associate Professor, Department of Obstetrics
and Gynecology, Uniformed Services University
of the Health Sciences, Bethesda, Maryland; Staff,
Maternal-Fetal Medicine, Department of Obstetrics
and Gynecology, Naval Medical Center San Diego,
San Diego, California
*Environmentally Induced Birth Defects; Premature Rupture
of Membranes: Diagnosis and Management*

See Wai Chan, MD, MPH
Assistant Professor, University of Pittsburgh; Assistant
Professor of Pediatrics, Magee-Womens Hospital
of University of Pittsburgh Medical Center, Pittsburgh,
Pennsylvania
Feeding the Critically Ill Neonate

Sudhish Chandra, MD
Assistant Professor of Pediatrics, Case Western Reserve
University School of Medicine; Attending Neonatologist,
Rainbow Babies and Children's Hospital, Cleveland,
Ohio
*Fetal and Neonatal Thermal Regulation; Modern
Extracorporeal Membrane Oxygenation for the Human
Newborn Infant*

Sylvain Chemtob, MD, PhD, FRCPC
Professor, Departments of Pediatrics, Pharmacology,
and Ophthalmology, University of Montreal Faculty
of Medicine; Staff Neonatologist, Hôpital Ste. Justine,
Montreal, Quebec, Canada
Pharmacology in the Fetus and Newborn

Frank A. Chervenak, MD
Professor and Chair, Department of Obstetrics and
Gynecology, Weill Medical College of Cornell University;
Obstetrician and Gynecologist-in-Chief, Department
of Obstetrics and Gynecology, New York–Presbyterian
Hospital, New York, New York
Management of Multiple Gestations

Reese H. Clark, MD
Consulting Associate Professor of Pediatrics,
Duke University School of Medicine, Durham,
North Carolina; Director of Research, Pediatrix Medical
Group, Inc., Fort Lauderdale, Florida
High-Frequency Oscillatory Ventilation

Mae M. Coleman, MD
Staff Neonatologist, St. Luke's Hospital, Jacksonville,
Florida
Intravenous Alimentation

Joshua A. Copel, MD
Professor of Obstetrics and Gynecology and Pediatrics,
Department of Obstetrics, Gynecology, and Reproductive
Sciences, Yale University School of Medicine,
New Haven, Connecticut
*Fetal Echocardiography in the Detection and Management of Fetal
Heart Disease*

C. Michael Cotten, MD
Assistant Clinical Professor of Pediatrics,
Duke University School of Medicine; Director, Neonatal
Clinical Research, Duke University Medical Center,
Durham, North Carolina
High-Frequency Oscillatory Ventilation; Air Leak Syndromes

David M. Coulter, MD
Associate Professor of Pediatrics, Division of Neonatology,
Department of Pediatrics, University of Utah School
of Medicine; Neonatologist, University of Utah Medical
Center, Primary Children's Medical Center,
and Latter-Day Saints Hospital, Salt Lake City, Utah
Hydrops Fetalis

Cynthia A. Cox, NNP
Alfred I. duPont Hospital for Children, Wilmington,
Delaware
Oxygen Therapy; Continuous Positive Airway Pressure

Jonathan M. Davis, MD
Professor of Pediatrics, State University of New York,
Stony Brook, School of Medicine, Stony Brook, New York;
Director of Neonatology and Director, Cardiopulmonary
Research Institute, Winthrop University Hospital,
Mineola, New York
Bronchopulmonary Dysplasia

Joseph D. DeCristofaro, MD
Associate Professor of Pediatrics, State University
of New York, Stony Brook, School of Medicine; Acting
Division Chief of Neonatology and Medical Director,
Infant Apnea Program, Stony Brook University Health
Sciences Center, Stony Brook, New York
Apnea of Prematurity and Apparent Life-Threatening Events

Maria Delivoria-Papadopoulos, MD
Professor Emeritus of Pediatrics and Physiology,
Department of Pediatrics, University of Pennsylvania
School of Medicine; Professor of Pediatrics and
Physiology, Department of Pediatrics, Drexel University
College of Medicine; Chief, Division of Neonatal-Perinatal
Medicine, Department of Pediatrics, St. Christopher's
Hospital for Children, Philadelphia, Pennsylvania
Differential Diagnosis of Neonatal Respiratory Disorders

Steven M. Donn, MD
Professor of Pediatrics, University of Michigan Medical
School; Director, Division of Neonatal-Perinatal
Medicine, Department of Pediatrics, C. S. Mott
Children's Hospital, University of Michigan Health
System, Ann Arbor, Michigan
Delivery Room Resuscitation

Willa H. Drummond, MD, MS
Professor of Pediatrics and Physiology, College
of Medicine; Professor of Large Animal Clinical
Sciences, College of Veterinary Medicine, University
of Florida; Attending Neonatologist, Shands Hospital
at the University of Florida, Gainesville, Florida
Ductus Arteriosus

Adre J. du Plessis, MBChB, MPH
Associate Professor, Harvard Medical School;
Associate in Neurology, Children's Hospital, Boston,
Massachusetts
*Perinatal Asphyxia and Hypoxic-Ischemic Brain Injury
in the Full-Term Infant*

Andrew Elimian, MD
Assistant Professor of Obstetrics and Gynecology,
State University of New York, Stony Brook,
School of Medicine, Stony Brook, New York
The Fetal Biophysical Profile

Mark I. Evans, MD
Professor of Obstetrics and Gynecology, Columbia
University College of Physicians and Surgeons;
Director, Institute for Genetics and Fetal Medicine,
St. Luke's–Roosevelt Hospital, New York, New York
The Fetus with a Treatable Endocrine and Metabolic Disorder

Roger G. Faix, MD
Professor of Pediatrics, University of Utah School
of Medicine; Attending Neonatologist, Primary
Children's Medical Center and Latter-Day Saints
Hospital, Salt Lake City, Utah
Delivery Room Resuscitation

Reinaldo Figueroa, MD
Associate Professor of Clinical Obstetrics, Gynecology,
and Reproductive Medicine, State University
of New York, Stony Brook, School of Medicine, Stony
Brook, New York; Attending Physician, Winthrop
University Hospital, Mineola, New York
*Ultrasound Evaluation of the Uncomplicated Pregnancy;
Identification and Management of the Fetus at Risk for Acidosis;
Preterm Labor*

T. Ernesto Figueroa, MD
Associate Clinical Professor of Urology,
Jefferson Medical College of Thomas Jefferson
University, Philadelphia, Pennsylvania;
Chief, Division of Pediatric Urology,
Alfred I. duPont Hospital for Children,
Wilmington, Delaware
Common Urologic Problems in the Fetus and Neonate

Neil N. Finer, MD
Professor of Pediatrics, University of California,
San Diego, School of Medicine, La Jolla, California;
Director of Neonatology, University of California,
San Diego, Medical Center, San Diego,
California
Neonatal Bronchoscopy

Richard L. Fischer, MD
Associate Professor of Obstetrics and Gynecology,
University of Medicine and Dentistry
of New Jersey, Robert Wood Johnson Medical School
at Camden; Co-Head, Division of Maternal-Fetal
Medicine, Cooper University Hospital, Camden,
New Jersey
Multifetal Pregnancy Reduction and Selective Termination

John W. Foreman, MD
Professor of Pediatrics, Duke University School
of Medicine; Chief of Pediatric Nephrology,
Department of Pediatrics, Duke University
Medical Center, Durham, North Carolina
Neonatal Hypertension

William W. Fox, MD
Professor of Pediatrics, University of Pennsylvania
School of Medicine; Neonatologist, Children's Hospital
of Philadelphia, Philadelphia, Pennsylvania
Oxygen Therapy; Continuous Positive Airway Pressure

Laura Frain, MD
The University of Chicago
*Neonatal Ethics and Epidemiology at the Dawn of a New
Millennium*

David F. Friedman, MD
Clinical Assistant Professor, University of
Pennsylvania School of Medicine; Associate Director
of the Transfusion Service, Children's Hospital
of Philadelphia, Philadelphia, Pennsylvania
Transfusion Therapy

Mamta Fuloria, MD
Assistant Professor of Pediatrics, Division
of Neonatology, Wake Forest University School
of Medicine, Winston-Salem, North Carolina
Meconium and the Compromised Fetus and Neonate

Jaya Ganesh, MD
Instructor in Pediatrics, Children's Hospital
of Philadelphia, Philadelphia, Pennsylvania
*Inborn Errors of Metabolism Manifesting as Catastrophic
Disease*

David J. Garry, DO
Assistant Professor, Department of Obstetrics,
Gynecology, and Reproductive Medicine, State
University of New York, Stony Brook, School
of Medicine, Stony Brook, New York
*Ultrasound Evaluation of the Uncomplicated Pregnancy;
Diabetes During Pregnancy*

Cara A. Geary, MD, PhD
Assistant Professor of Pediatrics, University of Texas
Medical Branch, Galveston, Texas
Amniotic Fluid Markers of Fetal Lung Maturity

Marsha Gerdes, PhD
Clinical Associate Professor, University of Pennsylvania
School of Medicine; Co-Director, Neonatal Follow-up
Program, Children's Hospital of Philadelphia,
Philadelphia, Pennsylvania
Follow-up of the High-Risk Neonate

Welton M. Gersony, MD
Alexander S. Nadas Professor of Pediatric Cardiology,
Columbia University College of Physicians
and Surgeons; Attending Physician, Children's Hospital
of New York–Presbyterian, New York, New York
Medical Management of Congenital Heart Disease

Ronald N. Goldberg, MD
Professor and Vice Chair, Department of Pediatrics, Duke
University School of Medicine; Chief, Neonatal-Perinatal
Medicine; Director, Neonatal Intensive Care Unit;
Director, Neonatal-Perinatal Research Institute,
Duke University Medical Center, Durham, North Carolina
Air Leak Syndromes

Leonard J. Graziani, MD
Professor of Pediatrics and Neurology, Jefferson Medical
College of Thomas Jefferson University; Attending
Pediatrician, Thomas Jefferson University Hospital,
Philadelphia, Pennsylvania
*Intracranial Hemorrhage and White Matter Injury in Preterm
Infants*

Jay S. Greenspan, MD
Professor of Pediatrics, Jefferson Medical College
of Thomas Jefferson University; Vice Chair of Pediatrics,
Director of Neonatology, Thomas Jefferson University
Hospital, Philadelphia, Pennsylvania; Nemours
Children's Clinic, The Nemours Foundation,
Wilmington, Delaware
Liquid Ventilation

Frank R. Greer, MD
Professor of Pediatrics, University of Wisconsin Medical
School, Madison, Wisconsin
Disorders of Calcium Homeostasis

George W. Gross, MD
Professor of Radiology, University of Maryland School
of Medicine; Director of Pediatric Radiology, University
of Maryland Medical Center, Baltimore, Maryland
Radiology in the Intensive Care Nursery

Louis P. Halamek, MD
Associate Professor of Pediatrics and Director,
Fellowship Training Program in Neonatal-Perinatal
Medicine, Stanford University School of Medicine;
Director, Center for Advanced Pediatric Education,
Palo Alto, California
Malformations of the Central Nervous System

John S. Hammes, MD
Assistant Clinical Professor, Department of Internal
Medicine, University of California, San Diego, School
of Medicine, La Jolla, California; Adjunct Assistant
Professor, Uniformed Services University of the Health
Sciences, Bethesda, Maryland; Head, Division
of Nephrology, Department of Internal Medicine,
Naval Medical Center San Diego, San Diego, California
Premature Rupture of Membranes: Diagnosis and Management

Laura S. Haneline, MD
Assistant Professor of Pediatrics and of Microbiology
and Immunology, Indiana University School
of Medicine, Indianapolis, Indiana
Stem Cells and Gene Therapy

Mary Catherine Harris, MD
Associate Professor of Pediatrics, University
of Pennsylvania School of Medicine; Senior Attending
Physician, Children's Hospital of Philadelphia
and the Hospital of the University of Pennsylvania,
Philadelphia, Pennsylvania
*Diagnosis of Neonatal Sepsis; Prevention and Treatment
of Neonatal Sepsis*

Michael R. Harrison, MD
Professor of Surgery, of Pediatrics, and of Obstetrics,
Gynecology, and Reproductive Sciences, University
of California, San Francisco, School of Medicine;
Director, Fetal Treatment Center, University of
California, San Francisco, Medical Center and Children's
Hospital, San Francisco, California
Surgery for Fetal Malformations

Claudia C. Herbert, RN, MS, CNNP
Clinical Instructor, State University of New York, Stony
Brook, School of Medicine; Neonatal Nurse Practitioner,
Stony Brook University Hospital, Stony Brook,
New York
Neonatal Nurse Practitioners in the Neonatal Intensive Care Unit

Michael D. Hnat, DO
Assistant Professor, Division of Maternal-Fetal Medicine,
Department of Obstetrics and Gynecology, University
of Texas Southwestern Medical School; Attending
Physician, Parkland Memorial Hospital, Dallas, Texas
Hypertensive Disorders in Pregnancy

Daphne T. Hsu, MD
Professor of Clinical Pediatrics, Columbia University
Medical Center; Attending Physician, Children's
Hospital of New York–Presbyterian, New York,
New York
Medical Management of Congenital Heart Disease

Carl E. Hunt, MD
Adjunct Professor of Pediatrics, Uniformed Services University of the Health Sciences; Director, National Center on Sleep Disorders Research, National Heart, Lung, and Blood Institute, National Institutes of Health, Bethesda, Maryland
Sudden Infant Death Syndrome

Hallam Hurt, MD
Associate Professor of Pediatrics, University of Pennsylvania School of Medicine; Attending Physician, Division of Neonatology, Hospital of the University of Pennsylvania and Children's Hospital of Philadelphia, Philadelphia, Pennsylvania
Substance Use During Pregnancy

Anthony Johnson, DO
Professor of Obstetrics and Gynecology and Director, Section of Reproductive Genetics and Prenatal Testing, Division of Maternal-Fetal Medicine, University of North Carolina School of Medicine, Chapel Hill, North Carolina
Amniocentesis

Kenneth Lyons Jones, MD
Professor of Pediatrics, Chief, Division of Dysmorphology, University of California, San Diego, School of Medicine, San Diego, California
Environmentally Induced Birth Defects

Bernard S. Kaplan, MBBCh
Professor of Pediatrics, University of Pennsylvania School of Medicine; Chief of Pediatric Nephrology, Children's Hospital of Philadelphia, Philadelphia, Pennsylvania
Chronic Renal Disease; Renal Tubular Disorders

Paige Kaplan, MBBCh
Professor of Pediatrics, University of Pennsylvania School of Medicine; Section Chief, Metabolic Diseases, Children's Hospital of Philadelphia, Philadelphia, Pennsylvania
Chronic Renal Disease; Renal Tubular Disorders

M. Gary Karlowicz, MD
Professor of Pediatrics, Eastern Virginia Medical School; Neonatologist, Children's Hospital of the King's Daughters, Norfolk, Virginia
Acute Renal Failure

Aviva L. Katz, MD
Assistant Professor of Surgery and Pediatrics, Jefferson Medical College of Thomas Jefferson University, Philadelphia, Pennsylvania; Attending Pediatric Surgeon, Alfred I. duPont Hospital for Children, Wilmington, Delaware
General Surgical Considerations

Lorraine Levitt Katz, MD
Assistant Professor of Pediatrics, University of Pennsylvania School of Medicine; Attending Physician, Children's Hospital of Philadelphia, Philadelphia, Pennsylvania
Disorders of Glucose and Other Sugars

Alfred P. Kennedy, Jr., MD
Assistant Professor of Surgery and Director of Pediatric Urology, University of Tennessee at Knoxville; Attending Physician, East Tennessee Children's Hospital, Knoxville, Tennessee
Common Urologic Problems in the Fetus and Neonate

Martin Keszler, MD
Professor of Pediatrics, Georgetown University School of Medicine; Director of Nurseries, Georgetown University Hospital, Washington, D.C.
High-Frequency Jet Ventilation

Meena Khandelwal, MD
Associate Professor, Division of Maternal-Fetal Medicine, Departments of Obstetrics/Gynecology and Internal Medicine, University of Medicine and Dentistry of New Jersey; Attending Physician, Cooper Hospital, Camden, New Jersey
Premature Rupture of Membranes: Diagnosis and Management

Joyce M. Koenig, MD
Associate Professor of Pediatrics, Division of Neonatology, University of Florida School of Medicine, Gainesville, Florida
White Blood Cell Disorders in the Neonate

Michael S. Kornhauser, MD
Clinical Assistant Professor of Pediatrics, Jefferson Medical College of Thomas Jefferson University, Philadelphia, Pennsylvania; Senior Vice President for Medical Affairs, ParadigmHealth Management Services, Paoli, Pennsylvania
Blood Gas Interpretation

Andrew H. Lane, MD
Assistant Professor, State University of New York, Stony Brook, School of Medicine, Stony Brook, New York
Neonatal Thyroid Disorders

John Lantos, MD
Professor of Pediatrics, Pritzker School of Medicine, The University of Chicago; MacLean Center for Clinical Medical Ethics, Chicago, Illinois
Neonatal Ethics and Epidemiology at the Dawn of a New Millennium

Grace Lee, BA
The University of Chicago
Neonatal Ethics and Epidemiology at the Dawn of a New Millennium

Hanmin Lee, MD
Assistant Professor in Residence of Surgery, Pediatrics, Obstetrics, Gynecology and Reproductive Sciences, University of California, San Francisco, School of Medicine; Attending Pediatric Surgeon, University of California, San Francisco, Medical Center, San Francisco, California
Surgery for Fetal Malformations

Dawnette Lewis, MD, MPH
Assistant Professor, North Shore–Long Island Jewish
Health System North Shore University Hospital,
Manhasset, New York
Third-Trimester Hemorrhage

Kathy Lin, BA
The University of Chicago
*Neonatal Ethics and Epidemiology at the Dawn
of a New Millennium*

Curtis L. Lowery, MD
Professor of Obstetrics and Gynecology, University of
Arkansas for Medical Sciences College of Medicine;
Section Head, Division of Maternal-Fetal Medicine,
Director, Obstetrics, UAMS Medical Center,
Little Rock, Arkansas
Diagnosis and Treatment of Preterm Labor

Catherine S. Manno, MD
Professor of Pediatrics, University of Pennsylvania
School of Medicine; Attending Physician, Division of
Hematology and Associate Chair for Clinical Activities,
Children's Hospital of Philadelphia, Philadelphia,
Pennsylvania
Transfusion Therapy

Steven McKenzie, MD, PhD
Professor of Pediatrics and Cardeza Professor
of Medicine, Jefferson Medical College of Thomas
Jefferson University, Philadelphia, Pennsylvania
Anemia

Alexander Meadow, BA
The University of Chicago
*Neonatal Ethics and Epidemiology at the Dawn
of a New Millennium*

William Meadow, MD, PhD
Professor of Pediatrics, Pritzker School of Medicine,
The University of Chicago; Associate Section Chief of
Neonatology, Department of Pediatrics, MacLean Center
for Clinical Medical Ethics, Chicago, Illinois
*Neonatal Ethics and Epidemiology at the Dawn
of a New Millennium*

Patricia C. Mele, RN, MS, CNNP
Clinical Assistant Professor, School of Nursing and
Clinical Instructor, School of Medicine, State University
of New York at Stony Brook; Neonatal Nurse
"Practitioner Coordinator, Stony Brook
University Hospital, Stony Brook,
New York
*Neonatal Nurse Practitioners in the Neonatal Intensive
Care Unit*

Kevin E. C. Meyers, MBBCh
Assistant Professor of Pediatrics, University of
Pennsylvania School of Medicine; Assistant Director
of Nephrology, Children's Hospital of Philadelphia,
Philadelphia, Pennsylvania
Chronic Renal Disease; Renal Tubular Disorders

Allison A. Murphy, MD
Fellow, Neonatal-Perinatal Medicine, Stanford
University School of Medicine, Palo Alto, California
Malformations of the Central Nervous System

Sharon A. Nachman, MD
Professor, Department of Pediatrics, State University of
New York, Stony Brook, School of Medicine; Director,
Division of Pediatric Infectious Diseases, Stony Brook
University Hospital, Stony Brook, New York
*Infection Control and Specific Bacterial, Viral, Fungal, and
Protozoan Infections of the Fetus and Neonate*

Paul L. Ogburn, Jr., MD
Professor, Department of Obstetrics, Gynecology, and
Reproductive Medicine, State University of New York,
Stony Brook, School of Medicine; Attending Physician
and Director, Maternal-Fetal Medicine, Stony Brook
University Hospital, Stony Brook, New York
Preterm Labor

Rees Oliver, MD
Assistant Professor of Pediatrics, Department of
Neonatal-Perinatal Medicine, University of Alabama
at Birmingham, Birmingham, Alabama
Liquid Ventilation

Robert I. Parker, MD
Professor of Pediatrics, State University of New York,
Stony Brook, School of Medicine; Director, Pediatric
Hematology, Stony Brook University Hospital,
Stony Brook, New York
Neonatal Thrombosis, Hemostasis, and Platelet Disorders

Patricia A. Parton, MD
Director, Division of Medical Genetics, State University
of New York, Stony Brook, School of Medicine,
Stony Brook, New York
The Genetics of Development

Irma Payan, MSN, CRNP
Pediatric Nurse Practitioner, Children's Hospital
of Philadelphia, Philadelphia, Pennsylvania
Inborn Errors of Metabolism Manifesting as Catastrophic Disease

Gilberto R. Pereira, MD
Professor of Pediatrics, University of Pennsylvania
School of Medicine; Neonatologist, Children's
Hospital of Philadelphia, Philadelphia,
Pennsylvania
Feeding the Critically Ill Neonate

Jeffrey P. Phelan, MD, JD
Chair and Director of Quality Assurance, Department
of Obstetrics/Gynecology, Citrus Valley Medical Center,
West Covina, California
Oligohydramnios and Polyhydramnios

Susan Plesha-Troyke, OTR
The University of Chicago
*Neonatal Ethics and Epidemiology at the Dawn
of a New Millennium*

Richard A. Polin, MD
Professor of Pediatrics, Columbia University College
of Physicians and Surgeons; Director, Division of
Neonatology, Children's Hospital of
New York–Presbyterian, New York, New York
Diagnosis of Neonatal Sepsis

Nicolas F. M. Porta, MD
Assistant Professor of Pediatrics, Northwestern
University Feinberg School of Medicine; Attending
Neonatologist, Children's Memorial Hospital, Chicago,
Illinois
Nitric Oxide and Alternative Pulmonary Vasodilators

Roy Proujansky, MD
Robert L. Brent Professor and Chair, Department of
Pediatrics, Associate Dean, Jefferson Medical College
of Thomas Jefferson University, Philadelphia,
Pennsylvania; Chief Executive, Physician Practice,
Nemours Children's Clinic, Alfred I. duPont Hospital
for Children, Wilmington, Delaware
Cholestatic Syndromes in Neonates

Graham E. Quinn, MD, MSCE
Professor of Ophthalmology, University of Pennsylvania
School of Medicine; Pediatric Ophthalmologist, Children's
Hospital of Philadelphia, Philadelphia, Pennsylvania
Retinopathy of Prematurity

J. Gerald Quirk, MD, PhD
Professor and Chair, Department of Obstetrics,
Gynecology, and Reproductive Medicine, State
University of New York, Stony Brook, School of
Medicine; Attending Physician, Stony Brook University
Hospital, Stony Brook, New York; Consultant,
St. Catherine of Siena Medical Center, Smithtown,
New York; Consultant, Mather Hospital and St. Charles
Hospital, Port Jefferson, New York
Identification and Management of the Fetus at Risk for Acidosis

E. Albert Reece, MD, PhD, MBA
Professor of Obstetrics and Gynecology, Medicine,
and Biochemistry; Vice Chancellor and Dean,
University of Arkansas College of Medicine, Little Rock,
Arkansas
Diagnosis and Treatment of Preterm Labor

Yaya Ren, PhD
The University of Chicago
Neonatal Ethics and Epidemiology at the Dawn of a New Millennium

Guy Rosner, MD
Faculty, Genetic Institute, Tel Aviv Sourasky Medical
Center, Tel Aviv, Israel.
The Fetus with a Treatable Endocrine and Metabolic Disorder

Judith L. Ross, MD
Professor, Department of Pediatrics, Jefferson Medical
College of Thomas Jefferson University, Philadelphia,
Pennsylvania
Disorders of the Adrenal in the Newborn

Joanne Giamboy Russo, RN
Nurse Clinician, Cardiothoracic Surgery, University
of Missouri, Columbia, Missouri
*Congenital Heart Defects in Newborns and Infants: Cardiothoracic
Repair*

Pierantonio Russo, MD
Chief of Pediatric Cardiac Surgery, Children's Hospital,
University of Missouri Health Care, Columbia,
Missouri
*Congenital Heart Defects in Newborns and Infants: Cardiothoracic
Repair*

Mark S. Scher, MD
Professor of Pediatrics and Neurology, Case Western
Reserve University School of Medicine; Director,
Pediatric Neurology and Residency Program Director,
Pediatric Neurology, Rainbow Babies and Children's
Hospital, Cleveland, Ohio
*Neonatal Seizures: Prenatal Contributions to a Neonatal Brain
Disorder*

Marshall Z. Schwartz, MD
Professor of Surgery and Pediatrics, Jefferson Medical
College of Thomas Jefferson University; Attending
Physician, St. Christopher's Hospital for Children,
Philadelphia, Pennsylvania
Congenital Anomalies of the Gastrointestinal Tract

Thomas H. Shaffer, PhD
Professor Emeritus of Physiology and Pediatrics,
Temple University School of Medicine; Professor
of Pediatrics, Jefferson Medical College of Thomas
Jefferson University, Philadelphia, Pennsylvania;
Associate Director of Biomedical Research; Director,
Nemours Research Lung Center; Director, Nemours
Office of Technology Transfer, The Nemours
Foundation, Wilmington, Delaware
Liquid Ventilation

Shai Ben Shahar
Genetic Consultant, Prenatal Diagnosis Unit, Genetic
Institute, The Tel Aviv Sourasky Medical Center,
Tel Aviv, Israel
The Fetus with a Treatable Endocrine and Metabolic Disorder

Baha M. Sibai, MD
Professor and Chair, Department of Obstetrics
and Gynecology, University of Cincinnati College
of Medicine; Attending Physician, Department of
Obstetrics and Gynecology, University Hospital,
Cincinnati, Ohio
Hypertensive Disorders in Pregnancy

Emidio M. Sivieri, MS
Biomedical Engineer, Children's Hospital of
Philadelphia Newborn Pediatrics, Philadelphia,
Pennsylvania
Pulmonary Function Testing in the Sick Newborn

Daniel W. Skupski, MD
Associate Professor of Obstetrics and Gynecology, Weill
Medical College of Cornell University, New York,
New York; Associate Director, Division of Maternal-Fetal
Medicine, New York–Presbyterian Hospital–Weill
Cornell Medical Center, New York, New York
Management of Multiple Gestations

Stephen J. Smith, MD
Clinical Assistant Professor, Department of Obstetrics
and Gynecology, Temple University School of Medicine,
Philadelphia, Pennsylvania; Associate Program Director,
Department of Obstetrics and Gynecology, Abington
Memorial Hospital, Abington, Pennsylvania
Maternal Fever and Chorioamnionitis

Kolawole O. Solarin, MD
Assistant Professor, Jefferson Medical College of
Thomas Jefferson University; Neonatologist, Alfred I.
duPont Hospital for Children, Wilmington, Delaware
Differential Diagnosis of Neonatal Respiratory Disorders

Samir Soneji, BA
The University of Chicago
*Neonatal Ethics and Epidemiology at the Dawn
of a New Millennium*

Michael L. Spear, MD
Clinical Professor of Pediatrics, Jefferson Medical
College of Thomas Jefferson University,
Philadelphia, Pennsylvania; Attending Neonatologist,
Christiana Care Health Services, Wilmington,
Delaware; Clinical Director, Neonatal Intensive Care
Unit, Alfred I. duPont Hospital for Children,
Wilmington, Delaware
Intravenous Alimentation

Alan R. Spitzer, MD
Senior Vice President and Director, The Center
for Research and Education, Pediatrix Medical Group,
Sunrise, Florida
*The Neonate as a Patient; Examination of the Critically
Ill Neonate; Positive-Pressure Ventilation: The Use of
Mechanical Ventilation in the Treatment of Neonatal
Lung Disease—General Principles of Care; Follow-up
of the High-Risk Neonate; Care of the Family in the Neonatal
Intensive Care Unit*

Pinchi Srinivasan, MBBS
Assistant Professor, Weill Medical College of Cornell
University, New York, New York; Attending Physician,
Wyckoff Heights Medical Center, Brooklyn, New York;
Neonatologist, New York Hospital Queens, Flushing,
New York
Necrotizing Enterocolitis

Charles A. Stanley, MD
Professor of Pediatrics, University of Pennsylvania
School of Medicine; Chief, Division of Endocrinology,
Children's Hospital of Philadelphia, Philadelphia,
Pennsylvania
Disorders of Glucose and Other Sugars

John L. Stefano, MD
Clinical Professor of Pediatrics, Jefferson Medical
College of Thomas Jefferson University, Philadelphia,
Pennsylvania; Director of Neonatology, Christiana Care
Health System, Wilmington, Delaware; Alfred I. duPont
Hospital for Children, Wilmington, Delaware;
St. Francis Hospital, Wilmington, Delaware; and
Bay Health Medical Center Kent General Hospital,
Dover, Delaware
Fluid and Electrolyte Physiology

Robin H. Steinhorn, MD
Professor of Pediatrics, Northwestern University Feinberg
School of Medicine; Head, Division of Neonatology,
Children's Memorial Hospital, Chicago, Illinois
Nitric Oxide and Alternative Pulmonary Vasodilators

David K. Stevenson, MD
Harold K. Faber Professor of Pediatrics and Senior
Associate Dean for Academic Affairs, Stanford
University School of Medicine; Director, Charles B. and
Ann L. Johnson Center for Pregnancy and Newborn
Services; Chief, Division of Neonatal and Developmental
Medicine, Stanford University Hospital and Clinics,
Palo Alto, California
Malformations of the Central Nervous System

Muhammad Subhani, MD, FAAP
Assistant Professor of Pediatrics, Neonatal Intensive
Care Unit, Good Samaritan Hospital, Rockland,
New York; Regional Neonatal Center, New York Medical
College Westchester Medical Center, Valhalla, New York
Intrauterine Growth Restriction

Sandra E. Sullivan, MD
Assistant Professor, Division of Neonatology,
Department of Pediatrics, University of Florida College
of Medicine, Gainesville, Florida
Ductus Arteriosus

Patrice M. L. Trauffer, MD
Associate Professor of Obstetrics and Gynecology, Drexel
University College of Medicine; Attending Physician,
Hahnemann Hospital, Philadelphia, Pennsylvania
Amniocentesis

John Tung, MBBS, MRCP
Assistant Professor, Department of Pediatrics, Jefferson
Medical College of Thomas Jefferson University,
Philadelphia, Pennsylvania; Attending Pediatric
Gastroenterologist, Alfred I. duPont Hospital
for Children, Wilmington, Delaware
Cholestatic Syndromes in Neonates

Keith K. Vaux, MD
Assistant Clinical Professor, Volunteer, Department
of Dysmorphology, Teratology, and Medical Genetics,
University of California, San Diego, School of Medicine,
La Jolla, California; Attending Physician, Department
of Pediatrics, Naval Medical Center San Diego,
San Diego, California
Environmentally Induced Birth Defects

Michael A. Vozzelli, MD
Assistant Professor, Department of Pediatrics, University of Vermont School of Medicine, Burlington, Vermont; Attending Neonatologist, Division of Neonatology, Maine Medical Center, Portland, Maine
Neonatal Hypertension

Ronald J. Wapner, MD
Professor and Chair, Department of Obstetrics and Gynecology, Drexel University College of Medicine
The Fetus as a Patient; Amniocentesis; Chorionic Villus Sampling; Multifetal Pregnancy Reduction and Selective Termination

Jon F. Watchko, MD
Professor of Pediatrics, Obstetrics, Gynecology, and Reproductive Sciences, Division of Neonatology and Developmental Biology, Department of Pediatrics, University of Pittsburgh School of Medicine; Senior Scientist, Magee-Womens Research Institute, Pittsburgh, Pennsylvania
Hyperbilirubinemia

Stuart Weiner, MD
Associate Professor, Department of Obstetrics and Gynecology, Jefferson Medical College of Thomas Jefferson University; Director, Division of Reproductive Imaging, Department of Obstetrics and Gynecology, Thomas Jefferson Hospital, Philadelphia, Pennsylvania
Maternal Fever and Chorioamnionitis

Carla M. Weis, MD
Assistant Professor of Pediatrics, Jefferson Medical College of Thomas Jefferson University; Neonatologist, Albert Einstein Medical Center, Philadelphia, Pennsylvania
Oxygen Therapy; Continuous Positive Airway Pressure

Jeffrey A. Whitsett, MD
Professor of Pediatrics, University of Cincinnati College of Medicine; Director of Pulmonary Biology and Neonatology, Cincinnati Children's Hospital Medical Center, Cincinnati, Ohio
Amniotic Fluid Markers of Fetal Lung Maturity

Thomas A. Wilson, MD
Professor of Clinical Pediatrics, State University of New York, Stony Brook, School of Medicine; Director of Pediatric Endocrinology, Stony Brook University Hospital, Stony Brook, New York
Neonatal Thyroid Disorders

Thomas E. Wiswell, MD
Professor of Pediatrics, Division of Neonatology, State University of New York, Stony Brook, School of Medicine; Attending Neonatologist and Director of Neonatal Research, Stony Brook University Hospital, Stony Brook, New York
Meconium and the Compromised Fetus and Neonate; Examination of the Critically Ill Neonate; Intracranial Hemorrhage and White Matter Injury in Preterm Infants

Marla R. Wolfson, PhD
Associate Professor of Physiology and Pediatrics, Temple University School of Medicine; Temple University Children's Medical Center, Philadelphia, Pennsylvania
Liquid Ventilation

Philip Wolfson, MD
Professor of Surgery, Jefferson Medical College of Thomas Jefferson University, Philadelphia, Pennsylvania; Attending Pediatric Surgeon, Alfred I. duPont Hospital for Children, Wilmington, Delaware
General Surgical Considerations

Yuval Yaron, MD
Senior Lecturer, Department of Obstetrics and Gynecology, Tel Aviv University; Director, Prenatal Diagnosis Unit, Genetic Institute, The Tel Aviv Sourasky Medical Center, Tel Aviv, Israel
The Fetus with a Treatable Endocrine and Metabolic Disorder

Mervin C. Yoder, MD
Professor of Biochemistry and Molecular Biology and Richard and Pauline Klingler Professor of Pediatrics, Indiana University School of Medicine, Indianapolis, Indiana
Stem Cells and Gene Therapy; White Blood Cell Disorders in the Neonate

Marc Yudkoff, MD
Professor of Pediatrics, University of Pennsylvania School of Medicine; Senior Physician, Children's Hospital of Philadelphia, Philadelphia, Pennsylvania
Inborn Errors of Metabolism Manifesting as Catastrophic Disease

Alan Zubrow, MD
Professor of Pediatrics, Drexel University College of Medicine; Attending Physician, St. Christopher's Hospital for Children, Philadelphia, Pennsylvania
Differential Diagnosis of Neonatal Respiratory Disorders

Preface

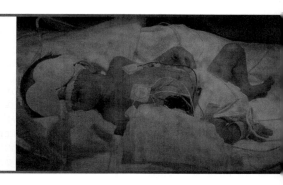

Since the first edition of this book, the world of neonatal-perinatal medicine has evolved in many ways that have continued to enrich and improve the care that we bring to the bedside in the intensive care nursery. Every time I begin to think that progress is slowing down, some new revelation—a brilliant research investigation or some new piece of equipment—illuminates another corner of the darkness, shedding a bit more light on some problem that previously seemed unfathomable. It has been this incredible excitement that has always fueled my fascination with neonatal intensive care and will continue to do so for the foreseeable future.

It is my hope that this book captures some of that excitement, through the remarkable words and achievements of the contributors, to whom I am most appreciative for the effort that they bring to each of their chapters. In a medical world in which time becomes more precious each day, their commitment to this book cannot be underestimated. I am deeply grateful to each of them.

With this edition, I have specifically tried to focus on the patient management of the fetus and neonate. There are several superb encyclopedic textbooks, such as Polin, Fox, and Abman's *Fetal and Neonatal Physiology,* and Fanaroff and Martin's *Neonatal-Perinatal Medicine,* to which the reader is referred for their illuminating and detailed descriptions of perinatal and neonatal problems. It is my hope, however, that when the clinician really needs to know how to attack a perplexing problem in the fetus or newborn, the current book will serve as the gold standard. In that respect, we have tried to keep the text within manageable size and to a single volume. Nothing frustrates me more than when I turn to a two-volume textbook, only to find that the volume I am looking for is somewhere else! In order to maintain the desired size, we have eliminated some chapters that seemed less directly relevant to fetal and neonatal decision making and patient management, while adding some new chapters that portend the future of neonatal-perinatal medicine. To the investigators whose research is paving the way to this future, many of whom have contributed to this book, all of us are deeply indebted. They have added immeasurably to our new insights into the care of the fetus and newborn and what lies ahead.

On a personal note, the past few years have been illuminating for me in different ways as well. Nearly two years ago, my first grandchild, Jacob, was born—an event for which my wife and I had been waiting for many years. Jacob, unfortunately, decided to show up more than 10 weeks early, had severe RDS, developed significant BPD, and had a grade 3 IVH. These events taught me more than I ever really wanted to know about the world of neonatal medicine as one experiences it from the other side. For everyone in the family, especially my son and my daughter-in-law, it was the most difficult time that we can recall, with some days seeming so grim that even the slightest effort was agonizingly painful. As I have often told many parents, however, most children, even those with these kinds of terrifying illnesses, do unbelievably well. Jacob was no exception, and his subsequent recovery has been startling, to say the least. By two years of age, one would not have known that he was a premie, and he continues to astound us every single day with his growing awareness and command of his world. Needless to say, he has become the light of our lives and serves as a constant reminder of why every child deserves the best possible neonatal care. It is for all critically ill children as Jacob once was that this book is intended, and I hope that it serves them well.

I am very grateful to my former colleagues at Stony Brook for their inspiration during the past five years. Stephen Baumgart, Thomas Wiswell, Joseph DeCristofaro, Rita Verma, Shanthy Sridhar, and Michael Friedman have been the best of friends, and I learned much from my years with them. I am also indebted to the Fellows, Residents, and Neonatal Nurse Practitioners whose daily questions and challenges always forced me to do my best. My new colleagues at Pediatrix Medical Group continue to provide the highest level of inspiration and support, constantly keeping me on my toes in our ongoing quest to define the best in neonatal and perinatal intensive care. I am especially grateful to Roger Medel, MD, for the kindness that he has shown me and his leadership qualities that have made Pediatrix into the most outstanding organization of its kind in maternal-fetal and newborn medicine.

The second edition of this book, like many infants I have cared for, has had a difficult, problem-filled gestation. With the ongoing changes that have occurred in the medical publishing world since the first edition, this textbook has been handed off to a series of publishers, finally winding up at Elsevier, whose efforts at putting the book together finally allowed this project to "give birth." I could not be more pleased with the final product, and am grateful to everyone at that company for their efforts. I am especially indebted to Meghan Curry McAteer, my primary editor at Elsevier, without whom there would be no book at all.

My two executive assistants, Caroline Lazzaruolo at Stony Brook and Janet Graff at Pediatrix Medical Group, have been invaluable in tracking down tardy authors, keeping manuscripts perfectly organized, and allowing me to finally put this book together. I cannot thank them enough for their assistance and their dedication to this project.

As always, I would be remiss if I did not acknowledge my greatest gifts, the love and companionship of my wife, Elaine, and the joys of watching my children, my son Steven and his wife Jennifer and my daughters Sara and Lauren, succeed in this difficult and often confusing world. Now I also have the thrill of experiencing the beginning of a new generation with Jacob, and the feeling is simply beyond words. Without my wonderful family, life would have far less purpose, and this book honors them as well.

Contents

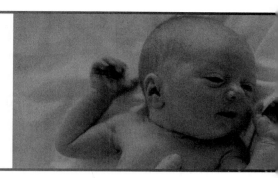

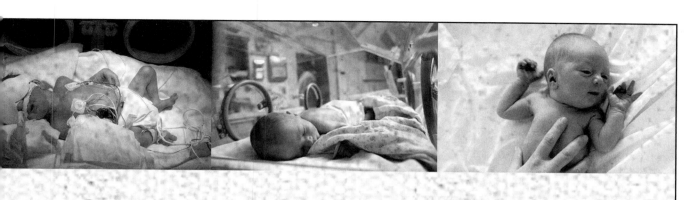

History of Fetal and Neonatal Intensive Care

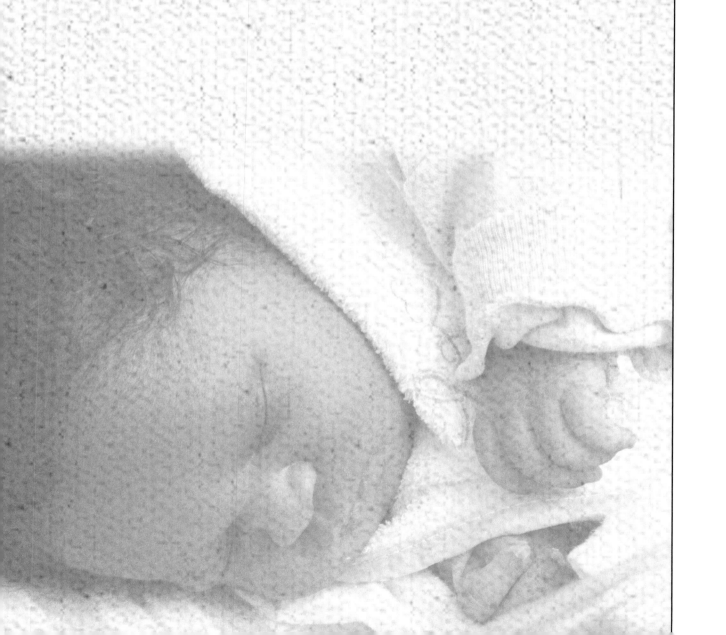

CHAPTER 1

The Fetus as a Patient

Ronald J. Wapner

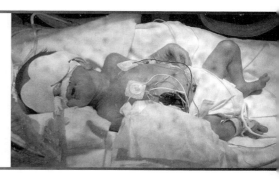

The concept of a fetal patient has evolved slowly over the past 400 years and has been driven by technologic advances that have allowed physicians to better explore the intrauterine environment. The fetus—once only a passive passenger whose care and treatment was entirely dictated by the medical needs of the mother—can now be independently visualized, monitored, measured, evaluated, and treated. With this emerging fetal status have come increasing responsibilities for the obstetric and perinatal physician.

Table 1-1 chronicles the historical evolution of fetal medicine. As early as the 1500s techniques such as cesarean section[1] and forceps delivery[2] were able to separate the maternal outcome from that of the fetus. However, these tools were predominately utilized as last resort modalities to save the life of the mother and rarely, if ever, used to improve the fetal condition. Not until the early 1800s was the fetal status independently explored when Mayor reported the ability to auscultate fetal heart tones[3] and Kennedy suggested that fetal bradycardia may represent fetal distress.[4] Another half century would pass without further improvement in fetal evaluation or treatment.

Amniocentesis was the first invasive fetal technique developed and in 1881 was used for the treatment of polyhydramnios.[5] Other uses followed, and in 1930 Menees and colleagues described the intraamniotic injection of contrast material to assist in the radiographic identification of placental location.[6] More than 20 years later, biochemical and genetic analyses of the amniotic fluid became clinically useful. In the early 1950s, the correlation between amniotic fluid nonheme iron levels and the severity of fetal anemia became recognized[7]; in the mid-1950s, fetal sex was determined by analysis of the Barr body in amniotic fluid cells.[8] Improvements in the analysis of amniotic fluid continued. In 1961, Liley presented his pioneering work, demonstrating that the optical density peak at 450 nm was an indirect measure of amniotic fluid bilirubin levels and could be used to predict the severity of fetal hemolysis in cases of rhesus sensitization.[9] Two years later, use of this diagnostic information led to the in utero treatment of fetal anemia by fluoroscopically guided intraperitoneal transfusion.[10] Almost simultaneously, tissue culture techniques of amniotic fluid were being investigated, and in 1966, Steele and Breg successfully cultured and karyotyped these cells,[11] which produced the first antenatal diagnosis of fetal chromosomal abnormalities.[12] In 1968, Nadler reported the first diagnosis of a fetal enzyme abnormality (galactosemia) by the analysis of amniotic fluid cells.[13] Amniocentesis continues to be the main invasive tool of the fetal diagnostician, and indications for its use have continued to expand, driven by the development of ultrasonography, which has improved its efficacy and safety.

Donald initially described the clinical potential of ultrasound imaging in 1955.[14,15] Since then, the sophistication of the technology has dramatically improved, and its use as a fetal diagnostic tool has continuously expanded. Ultrasound imaging is the technologic modality most responsible for establishing fetal medicine as a clinical reality. The clinical usefulness of early ultrasonography was limited by static images and poor resolution; however, by 1972, prenatal diagnosis was already possible for a small group of severe fetal abnormalities such as anencephaly and massive hydrocephalus.[16] Placental localization was also possible, twins could be detected (although not with 100% sensitivity), and gestational age could be estimated by measurement of the biparietal diameter of the fetal head. In more recent years, the introduction of gray scale imaging and real-time high-resolution equipment has allowed even subtle aspects of the fetal anatomy to be evaluated. The development of transvaginal scanning now enables detailed anatomic imaging of the first-trimester fetus, and many structural abnormalities can be diagnosed by 13 to 14 weeks. The introduction of Doppler flow analysis enables the perinatal physician to measure fetal and umbilical blood flow, allowing evaluation of the fetal biophysical status; for example, measurement of the flow velocity in the fetal middle cerebral artery is rapidly

Table 1–1. Evolution of the Fetus as a Patient

Year	Fetal Diagnostic Procedure	Fetal Therapeutic Procedure
1500		First recorded successful cesarean section was performed by Jacob Nufer, a swine gelder, on his wife
1500s		Peter the Elder of the Chamberlen family invented the obstetric forceps; used primarily to assist the mother
1588		First book on cesarean section was published
1600s	Marsac was the first to hear the fetal heartbeat	
1818	Mayor, a Swiss surgeon, reported the presence of fetal heart tones	
1833	Kennedy suggested FHR deceleration as an indicator of fetal distress	
1881		Amniocentesis for treatment of polyhydramnios was described
1933	Relationship between maternal urinary estriol excretion and fetal health was described	
1952	Bevis reported correlation between amniotic fluid nonheme iron and severity of fetal anemia	
1955	Ian Donald described the clinical potential of ultrasound imaging; Use of maternal urinary estriol excretion to evaluate fetal health became practical	
1956	Fetal sex determination was made by the presence of the Barr body in amniotic fluid	
1958	Hon reported method for continuous electronic recording of FHR and described early, late, and variable decelerations	
1961	Liley demonstrated that optical density peak at 450 nm reflects fetal hemolysis in Rh sensitization	
1963	Saling demonstrated fetal scalp sampling to evaluate fetal oxygenation during labor	Liley treated fetal anemia caused by Rh sensitization with fetal intraperitoneal transfusion
1965		Open fetal exchange transfusion was performed for severe fetal erythroblastosis; hysterotomy was used to expose fetus, and transfusion was done via peritoneal or internal jugular route
1966	Hammacher described lower Apgar scores and higher stillbirth rates when late decelerations are seen with spontaneous uterine contractions in the antepartum period; this set groundwork for fetal surveillance by antepartum FHR testing	
1967	Pose induced uterine contractions with oxytocin in antepartum period and confirmed Hammacher's work: first oxytocin challenge test; Intrauterine diagnosis of fetal genetic disorders by amniocentesis and culture and karyotype of amniotic fluid cells were described	

1972	Clinical value of the oxytocin challenge test was confirmed with blind prospective trial
	Elevated amniotic fluid AFP levels were reported with fetal neural tube defects
	Campbell described the in utero diagnosis of anencephaly by ultrasonography
	Liggins and Howie demonstrated that maternal administration of glucocorticoids prevents some cases of respiratory distress syndrome
1973	Detection of fetal neural tube defects by second-trimester maternal serum screening was reported
1974	American Board of Obstetrics and Gynecology developed certification for the Specialist in Maternal Fetal Medicine
	Fetal hemoglobinopathy was diagnosed by fetoscope-guided aspiration of fetal blood from placental vessels
1982	Chorionic villus sampling was performed for molecular diagnosis of fetal hemoglobinopathy
	Fetal hydronephrosis was treated by in utero drainage of fetal bladder
	Fetal hydrocephalus was treated by in utero insertion of one-way ventricular-amniotic shunt
1983	Ultrasonically guided percutaneous umbilical fetal blood sampling (PUBS) was described
	Trisomy 21 was first diagnosed by chorionic villus sampling
1984	Association of decreased maternal serum AFP levels with Down syndrome was reported
1986	Fetal stem cell transplantation was attempted for treatment of Rh disease, ADA deficiency, metachromatic leukodystrophy, and α-thalassemia
1987	Fetal percutaneous transfusion for severe anemia was developed
1988	Fetal alloimmune thrombocytopenia was treated with maternal immune globin and dexamethasone
1990	Maternal serum triple screen for Down syndrome risk assessment became standard of care
	Management of fetal erythroblastosis was improved by using Doppler evaluation of middle cerebral artery peak systolic velocity
	Successful in utero treatment of fetal diaphragmatic hernia was reported
	EXIT procedure (extrauterine maintenance of placental circulation) to maintain airway of fetus with tracheal obstruction was described
	Laser treatment of twin-twin transfusion was reported
	Fetal minimally invasive surgery included cord ligation of posterior urethral valves
2000	First-trimester Down syndrome screening was performed with biochemistry and measurement of the nuchal translucency
	Three- and four-dimensional ultrasound technology improved fetal imaging
	First randomized controlled trial evaluating the benefits of open fetal surgery for neural tube defects was conducted

ADA, adenosine deaminase; AFP, α-fetoprotein; FHR, fetal heart rate; Rh, rhesus factor.

replacing amniocentesis as the primary surveillance tool for the management of the Rh-sensitized pregnancy.[17] Three-dimensional ultrasound imaging represents the newest advance. The technology offers dramatic images of fetal anatomy (Fig. 1-1), and its clinical usefulness is just beginning to be appreciated. Although amniocentesis and fetal intraperitoneal transfusion were previously performed without continuous visualization, ultrasound guidance made these significantly safer. Direct imaging during invasive procedures also allowed more sophisticated fetal intervention. Techniques for shunting the fetal ventricles to treat hydrocephalus[18] (an approach that was subsequently found to be of only limited benefit) and for decompressing and shunting the fetal bladder to alleviate urinary tract obstruction[19] were introduced in the early 1980s. One of the most useful advances came in 1983 when Daffos and associates described ultrasonically guided percutaneous sampling of fetal umbilical blood.[20] Although sampling with a fetoscope had been possible since 1974,[21] the procedure was technically complex and carried a significant risk of miscarriage. Ultrasonically guided cordocentesis was both easier and safer, and the indications for its use expanded rapidly. In addition, cordocentesis provided a direct intravascular route for the administration of fetal therapies such as blood and platelet transfusions.

In addition to invasive therapy, the fetal patient is amenable to medical treatment administered to the mother and transferred across the placenta. The first major example of this approach occurred in the late 1970s after the demonstration by Liggins and Howie that maternal administration of glucocorticoids could accelerate fetal lung maturation and ameliorate or prevent many cases of respiratory distress syndrome.[22] Other examples include the treatment of fetal alloimmune thrombocytopenia with maternally administered gamma globulin and dexamethasone,[23] the treatment of fetal supraventricular tachyarrhythmias with digoxin and other cardiac medications,[24] and the prevention of ambiguous genitalia by the in utero treatment of congenital adrenal

hyperplasia secondary to 21-hydroxylase deficiency with dexamethasone.[25]

Fetal disease can occasionally be prevented by correcting a "fetotoxic" maternal milieu. For example, optimal periconceptional glucose control has been shown to reduce the incidence of congenital anomalies in the offspring of diabetic pregnant woman.[26] Similarly, rigorous prepregnancy dietary control of phenylalanine levels in potential mothers with phenylketonuria has been demonstrated to reduce the incidence of fetal anomalies, including microcephaly, heart defects, and mental retardation.[27] Another example of the prevention of fetal disease is the preconceptional administration of folic acid to reduce the risk of recurring fetal neural tube defects.[28] Vitamin administration can also reduce the frequency of neural tube defects in the general population,[29] and the fetal patient may soon benefit from public health measures that require the addition of folic acid to flour or bread.

The practice of fetal medicine is not limited to invasive procedures and treatment of fetal abnormalities; it also includes evaluation of fetal health. As mentioned, there was recognition more than a century ago that fetal compromise could be predicted in utero. Not until 1955, however, were the tools sensitive enough to be clinically useful. In the earliest modern evaluation of fetal health, maternal urinary estriol excretion was used to provide an indirect assessment of the function of the fetal-placental unit.[30] Although estriol proved helpful in the management of complicated pregnancies, its value was limited by the 24- to 48-hour delay necessary to collect and analyze the specimen and by the imprecise nature of the results. In 1958, Hon described continuous fetal heart rate monitoring and demonstrated specific fetal heart rate patterns predictive of a compromised fetus.[31] Initially, assessment was limited to intrapartum evaluation, but in 1966, Hammacher described lower Apgar scores and a higher stillborn rate when late decelerations were seen with spontaneous contractions in the antepartum period.[32] This observation set the groundwork for antepartum biophysical evaluation of the fetus and the subsequent development of the oxytocin challenge test, the nonstress test, and the biophysical profile.[33]

Since the late 1980s, two new technologies with significant implications for the fetal patient have developed. The first is open in utero surgery. The preliminary work has been accomplished: animal models have been developed to mimic the human fetal congenital abnormalities, the natural history of the defects has been investigated, and surgical techniques have been explored in the nonhuman primate. To date, human experience includes the treatment of fetal hydronephrosis by open-bladder marsupialization or ureterostomy, open treatment of fetal diaphragmatic hernia, removal of a sacrococcygeal teratoma, and resection of a cystic adenomatoid malformation of the fetal lung (see Chapter 16).[34,35] Most recently, repair of neural tube defects has been performed with improvement in fetal ventriculomegaly. Whether this will lead to an overall improvement in the long-term function is currently being evaluated. Although promising, this work has been hampered by difficulties with

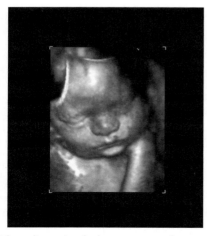

Figure 1–1. Three-dimensional ultrasonogram of a second-trimester fetus.

premature rupture of the membranes and preterm delivery. To minimize these complications, a few groups have begun to investigate performing minimally invasive fetal techniques through endoscopes inserted under ultrasound guidance. Through this approach, fetal posterior urethral valves have been ablated by laser,[36] and the umbilical cord of an acardiac twin can be either suture-ligated, cauterized, or laser-ablated to prevent the development of hydrops in the coexisting normal fetus.[37] Laser technology has also proved effective in the ablation of the vascular anastomosis that causes twin-twin transfusion syndrome.[38] Although encouraging, this work is preliminary, and further validation and investigation of the short- and long-term risks are awaited.

The second technology to have a significant implication for the fetal patient is the remarkable revolution in molecular genetics, which adds new dimension to the diagnosis of fetal disorders. Common diseases such as cystic fibrosis and thalassemia can now be diagnosed as early as the first trimester.[39] Determination of fetal attributes such as Rh or Kell type can be determined by analyzing fetal DNA obtained by chorionic villus sampling or amniocentesis, rather than retrieval of fetal blood.[40] In certain situations, these determinations are possible by analysis of free fetal DNA in the maternal plasma.[41] Equally important, molecular technologies are exceedingly sensitive and specific for investigating the transmission of viral infections from mother to fetus.[42] In addition to the diagnostic potentials of molecular biology, this also opens up an avenue for fetal therapy. Fetal bone marrow transplantation has been attempted in the human, and somatic cell gene therapy for genetic disorders will be possible.[43] The fetus may be the ideal patient because it is already prepared for engraftment and, in early gestation, is immunologically tolerant. Many questions remain about the safety and feasibility of this approach, but animal studies support its potential.

WHO IS THE FETAL PHYSICIAN?

Fetal disease can be complex and requires the expertise of multiple disciplines. Historically, the care of the pregnant mother has been within the domain of the obstetrician, whereas the newborn's care was provided by the pediatrician. Fetal care, however, transcends these classic divisions of responsibility and requires skills and knowledge of both disciplines. To address this void, the American Board of Obstetrics and Gynecology established the subspecialty of Maternal-Fetal Medicine in 1974 to train and certify physicians with the special expertise necessary to provide care to the fetal patient. Similarly, the American Board of Pediatrics recognizes neonatal-perinatal medicine as a pediatric subspecialty. In actuality, the care of the fetus is a continuum, starting at conception, progressing through the intrauterine stage, and then extending into the nursery. A collaborative approach is therefore ideal. It allows all disciplines to provide input into the therapy and introduces the neonatologist and the pediatric subspecialist to their ultimate patient early in the course of the disease process.

Although a team approach is required, one physician must be in charge of the care and ultimately dictate the treatment. While the fetus remains in utero, the perinatal obstetrician should assume this responsibility. He or she must utilize the expertise and accumulated knowledge of the other team members, including a geneticist, a neonatologist, pediatric subspecialists (e.g., surgeon, cardiologist, neurologist, urologist), and a radiologist with expertise in fetal imaging. All team members should meet the family before delivery to allow the family to become familiar with the physicians who will ultimately provide care to their newborn. This process allows the family ample opportunity to ask questions and to provide input in a more relaxed atmosphere than during the hectic period that often immediately follows birth.

In some aspects of fetal care, the pediatric subspecialist may actually assume primary management. For example, in the treatment of a resistant fetal supraventricular tachycardia, a pediatric cardiologist may be the physician most expert in the use of antiarrhythmia medications. Similarly, the treatment of fetal structural abnormalities amenable to fetal surgery requires the expertise of a pediatric surgeon. The ultimate goal must always be that the physician most skilled in the required therapy is the one to provide it.

PREREQUISITES FOR FETAL TREATMENT

Certain prerequisites must be achieved before fetal treatment is offered. First, an accurate diagnosis of the condition must be made. Second, a clear understanding of the pathophysiologic mechanism and natural history of the disorder is necessary. Because accurate prediction of the neonatal and long-term course is difficult, the spectrum of possible outcomes must be conveyed accurately. Third, the value of any intervention should be clearly known. To qualify for intervention, (1) the condition should have a severe effect on survival or long-term health, (2) there should be a major advantage to in utero treatment over treatment after delivery, and (3) the obstetric intervention should result in a reasonable expectation for a healthy newborn and an undamaged adult. Lastly, the risks to both the mother and the fetus should be known and discussed in detail. These tenets hold for all fetal treatments, including early delivery of the compromised fetus, medical treatment of the sick fetus, and invasive interventions for structural defects.

CONFLICTS IN THE CARE OF THE FETAL PATIENT

The recognition of the fetus as a patient provides a unique arrangement in medicine in that one physician is simultaneously providing care to two patients. In the majority of instances, the needs and requirements of both patients are the same. On occasion, however, conflict may develop between the needs or wishes of the mother and the potential consequences to the fetus. In an extreme example, a mother may be opposed to a fetal therapy that may benefit her offspring. If this were a pediatric situation, an established treatment could be mandated over the parents' wishes, because parental autonomy cannot ordinarily override the child's interest in life or health. When the child is still unborn, however, treatment will, by necessity, invade the mother's body, raising the issue of whether maternal autonomy should override the soon-to-be-born child's well-being. The situation is additionally complicated by the uncertainty and limitations of fetal diagnosis and treatment. Although there is precedent for a court-ordered mandate that a mother undergo therapy for the welfare of the child (usually a court-ordered cesarean section), there is strong sentiment that such power should only rarely, if ever, be used. The Ethics Committee of the American College of Obstetricians and Gynecologists warns that physicians should try *not* to resort to court actions for forced obstetric interventions. The committee recommends that in case of maternal refusal, the physician should obtain additional consultation for the pregnant woman to help her further consider the merits of the medical advice. Every effort should be made to resolve the conflict by using medical, mental health, and bioethical consultation. The courts should be relied on only after all attempts at conciliation have failed. The legal and ethical issues involved in such situations are quite complex and are reviewed in detail in Chapter 88 and elsewhere.[44,45]

SUMMARY

Before the 1960s, fetal care was provided by ensuring that the mother followed the accepted principles of antepartum care. Although this led to improvement in rates of overall perinatal morbidity and mortality, there was little ability to access and treat the problems of the individual fetus. Since the mid-1960s, the value of prenatal assessment has been enhanced and technologies that allow accessibility to the fetus are now available. The discipline of fetal medicine is only beginning. The natural history of relatively few fetal disorders is completely understood, and even less is known about the value of treatment. The causes of the most common fetal disorders such as fetal growth restriction, preterm labor, and intrauterine asphyxia still remain unknown.

REFERENCES

1. Douglass RG, Stromme WB: Operative Obstetrics. New York, Appleton-Century-Crofts, 1957, p 413.
2. Da KN: Obstetric Forceps: Its History and Evolution. St. Louis, CV Mosby, 1929.
3. Goodlin R: History of fetal monitoring. Am J Obstet Gynecol 33:325, 1979.
4. Kennedy E: Observations on obstetric auscultation. Dublin, Hodges and Smith, 1833.
5. Lambl D: Ein seltener fall von hydramnios. Zentrabl Gynaekol 5:329, 1881.
6. Menees TD, Miller JD, Holly LE: Amniography: Preliminary report. AJR Am J Roentgenol 24:363, 1930.
7. Bevis DC: The prenatal prediction of antenatal disease of the newborn. Lancet 1:395, 1952.
8. Fuchs F, Riis P: Antenatal sex determination. Nature 177:330, 1956.
9. Liley AW: Liquor amnio analysis in the management of the pregnancy complicated by rhesus sensitization. Am J Obstet Gynecol 82:1359, 1961.
10. Liley AW: Technique of fetal transfusion in treatment of severe hemolytic disease. Am J Obstet Gynecol 89:817, 1964.
11. Steele MW, Breg WR: Chromosome analysis and human amniotic fluid cells. Lancet 1:383, 1966.
12. Jacobson CB, Barter RH: Intrauterine diagnosis and management of genetic defects. Am J Obstet Gynecol 99:795, 1967.
13. Nadler HL: Antenatal detection of hereditary disorders. Pediatrics 42:912, 1968.
14. Donald I, MacVicar J, Brown TG: Investigation of abdominal masses by pulsed ultrasound. Lancet 1:1188, 1958.
15. Donald I: On launching a new diagnostic science. Am J Obstet Gynecol 103:609, 1969.
16. Campbell S, Johnstone FD, Holt EM, et al: Anencephaly: Early ultrasonic diagnosis and active management. Lancet 2:1226, 1972.
17. Mari G, Deter RL, Rahman F, et al: Non-invasive diagnosis by Doppler ultrasonography of fetal anemia due to maternal red cell immunization. N Engl J Med 342:9, 2000.
18. Clewell WH, Johnson ML, Meier PR, et al: A surgical approach to fetal hydrocephalus. N Engl J Med 306:1320, 1982.
19. Golbus MS, Harrison MR, Filly RA: Prenatal diagnosis and treatment of fetal hydronephrosis. Semin Perinatal 7:102, 1983.
20. Daffos F, Capella-Pavolsky M, Forestier F: Fetal blood sampling via the umbilical cord using a needle guided by ultrasound: Report of 66 cases. Prenat Diagn 3:217, 1983.
21. Hobbins JC, Mahoney MJ: In utero diagnosis of hemoglobinopathies: Technique for obtaining fetal blood. N Engl J Med 290:1065, 1974.
22. Liggins GC, Howie RN: A controlled trial of antepartum glucocorticoid treatment for prevention of the respiratory distress syndrome in premature infants. Pediatrics 50:515, 1972.
23. Bussel JB, Berkowitz RL, McFarland JG et al: Antenatal treatment of neonatal alloimmune thrombocytopenia. N Engl J Med 319:1374, 1988.
24. Kleinman CS, Copel JA, Weinstein EM, et al: Treatment of fetal supraventricular tachyarrhythmias. J Clin Ultrasound 13:265, 1985.
25. Evans MI, Chrousos GP, Mann DW, et al: Pharmacological suppression of the fetal adrenal gland in utero. Attempted prevention of abnormal external genital masculinization in suspected congenital adrenal hyperplastic inutero. JAMA 253:1015, 1985.
26. Miller E, Hare JW, Clohererty JP, et al: Elevated maternal hemoglobin. A1C in early pregnancy and major congenital anomalies in infants of diabetic mothers. N Engl J Med 304:1331, 1981.
27. Lenke RR, Levy HC: Maternal phenylketonuria and hyperphenylalaninemia. N Engl J Med 303:1202, 1980.
28. Laurence KM, James N, Miller MH, et al: Double-blind randomized controlled trial of folate treatment before conception to prevent recurrence of neural tube defects. BMJ 282:1509, 1981.
29. Mulinare J, Codero JF, Erickson JD, et al: Periconceptional use of multivitamins and occurrence of neural tube defects. JAMA 260:3141, 1989.
30. Brown JB: Chemical method for determination of estriol, oestrone, and oestradiol in human urine. Biochem J 60:185, 1955.
31. Hon EH: The electronic evaluation of the fetal heart rate (preliminary report). Am J Obstet Gynecol 75:1215, 1958.
32. Hammacher K: Fruherkennung intrauterineo gefahrenzustande durch electrophonocardiographie und focographie.

In Elert R, Hates KA (eds): Prophylaxe frund kinclicher hirnschaden. Stuttgart, Georg Thieme Verlag, 1966, p 120.

33. Ray M, Freeman RK, Pine S, et al: Clinical experience with the oxytocin challenge test. Am J Obstet Gynecol 114:12, 1972.

34. Crombleholme TM, Harrison MR, Langer JC, et al: Early experience with open fetal surgery for congenital hydronephrosis. J Pediatr Surg 23:1114, 1988.

35. Golbus MS, Fries MM: Surgical fetal therapy. In Lin CC, Verp MS, Sabbagha RE (eds): The High Risk Fetus. New York, Springer Verlag, 1993, pp 614-621.

36. Quintero RA, Romero R, Goncalves L, et al: Percutaneous fetal cystoscopy in the evaluation and management of the fetus with lower obstructive uropathy [abstract 616]. Am J Obstet Gynecol 172:427, 1995.

37. Quintero RA, Reich H, Puder KS, et al: Brief report: Umbilical cord ligation of an acardiac twin by fetoscopy at 19 weeks of gestation. N Engl J Med 330:56, 1994.

38. van Gemert MJ, Umer A, Tijssen JG, Ross MG: Twin-twin transfusion syndrome: Etiology, severity and rational management [review]. Curr Opin Obstet Gynecol 13:193, 2001.

39. Novelli G, Sangiuolo G, Dallapiccola B, et al: ΔF508 gene deletion and prenatal diagnosis of cystic fibrosis in Italian and Spanish families. Prenat Diagn 10:413, 1990.

40. Fisk N, Bennett P, Warwick M, et al: Clinical utility of fetal Rh D typing in alloimmunized pregnancies by means of polymerase chain reaction on amniocytes or chorionic villi. Am J Obstet Gynecol 171:50, 1994.

41. Bianchi DW: Prenatal exclusion of recessively inherited disorders: Should maternal plasma analysis precede invasive techniques? [comment]. Clin Chem 48:689, 2002.

42. Hogge WA, Buffone GJ, Hogge JS: Prenatal diagnosis of cytomegalovirus (CMV) infection: A preliminary report. Prenat Diagn 13:131, 1993.

43. Flake AW, Harrison MR, Adzick NS, et al: Transplantation of fetal hematopoietic stem cells in utero. The creation of hematopoietic chimeras. Science 133:776, 1986.

44. Evans MI, Robertson JA, Fletcher JC: Legal and ethical issues in fetal therapy. In Lin CC, Verp MS, Sabbagha RE (eds): The High Risk Fetus. New York, Springer Verlag, 1993, pp 627-639.

45. Fletcher JC, Jonsen AR: Ethical considerations in fetal treatment. In Harrison MR, Golbus MS, Filly RA (eds): The Unborn Patient, 2nd ed. Philadelphia, WB Saunders, 1991, pp 14-18.

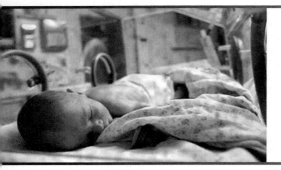

The Neonate as a Patient

Alan R. Spitzer

Consideration of the newborn with a life-threatening disease as a potentially treatable individual represents a relatively recent change in the practice of medicine. Historically, the probability of death during the neonatal period was so high that many traditional practices were postponed until after the first week of life, when the child's survival was more probable. Ritual circumcision of Jewish boys was performed on the eighth day of life for this reason, because it was thought that if the infant boy survived the first week of life, the chances of death were significantly diminished after that time. Furthermore, children who did die before this time were not mourned with a period of *shiva* (the Jewish time of mourning); they were, in fact, regarded as never having lived at all. Until recently, therefore, it was common for families to conceive numerous times, with the understanding that a certain percentage of pregnancies would not produce a viable child. In the modern era, in comparison, parents (and members of the legal profession) often expect even a 500-g infant to survive the neonatal period completely intact!

Perhaps the first movement toward attempting to assist the survival of small or ill infants occurred with the development of the neonatal incubator. Credit for the development of the modern incubator is usually given to Stephane Tarnier and Pierre Budin. In 1900, Budin reported the results of his studies on thermoregulation in premature neonates, which indicated that survival could be dramatically improved if rectal temperature was normalized in infants with birth weights less than 2000 g. Budin also designed an incubator that provided for heating of air by convection, addition of humidity, and temperature monitoring of the environment. Unfortunately, Budin's efforts to publicize the value of these techniques through demonstrations of his incubators and infants in the Berlin Exposition of 1896, as well as in subsequent exhibitions, served little more than to make the neonate into a sideshow freak. The medical treatment that Budin furnished to these premature infants was apparently quite remarkable for the time, however, and all the

premature infants in the Berlin Exhibition survived. The overall difficulty in caring for the preterm or sick infant, however, was demonstrated by the fact that even as recently as the New York World's Fair of 1939, Martin Couney, a disciple of Budin's, maintained a similar exhibition of premature babies. Couney apparently had a long and illustrious career as a showman of these infants, and it was estimated that he had cared for more than 80,000 premature infants in a series of exhibitions around the world that lasted more than 40 years, resulting in his reputation as the "incubator doctor."

The first significant medical trend that resulted in improved survival for newborns was the emergence of the hospital as the primary site of birth, with specialized areas within the nursery dedicated to the infirm infant. This change in practice, which began during the period from 1900 to 1920, resulted in a group of neonates housed together in a nursery setting, which mandated the attention of a physician dedicated to their care. Besides thermoregulation, much of the initial attention to care involved nutritional practices. Before this era, breast-feeding was essentially mandatory for neonates; if the mother was unable to comply, the use of a wet nurse was common. Artificial feeding, although it had stimulated much interest throughout history, was difficult. Not only was it a problem to match human milk, but also there were few, if any, satisfactory devices for the delivery of formula. In fact, it was not until 1894, when E. Allenbury and William Decker introduced two feeding devices that were the forerunners of the baby bottle, that artificial formula feeding became practical.

By the 1920s, the Pyrex company had developed a wide-mouth baby bottle and nipple that allowed the preparation, sterilization, and storage of formula with refrigeration. Although a variety of techniques was used to make a milk substitute for infants, it was the pioneering work of Thomas Morgan Rotch at the Boston Infant's Hospital that was the source of the term "formula." Rotch developed a milk substitute composed of 2% fat, 6% carbohydrate, and 2% protein for infant feeding, with the protein split equally between whey and casein. This composition was thus the "formula" for infant feeding. In 1915, H. J. Gerstenberger and his associates produced an artificial formula that added homogenized vegetable and animal fats to skimmed cow's milk to produce their Synthetic Milk Adapted (SMA). Of the other well-established modern formulas, Similac was introduced in 1923, whereas Enfamil was placed on the market much later, in 1959. The formulas for premature infants were introduced during the 1960s and 1970s and have been modified and refined numerous times, as have the standard formulas, because of research developments. The introduction of artificial formula, however, was critical to infant survival.

The other important development in infant feeding, which has enabled the survival of hundreds of thousands of critically ill infants (as well as children and adults), was the pioneering work of Douglas Wilmore and Stanley Dudrick at the University of Pennsylvania during the 1960s in the development of intravenous alimentation techniques. Because of the widespread application of this approach throughout medicine, health professionals often overlook the fact that these procedures were initially introduced for the treatment of short-bowel syndrome in neonates and infants. Their immediate value in the treatment of many other problems was readily apparent and led to the widespread proliferation of use in many branches of medical therapy.

Although the improvements in feeding and thermoregulation were of considerable importance to the sick neonate, few developments have been as critical as the ability to provide life support and critical care, particularly to the newborn with respiratory failure. The practices in this area in the modern era of neonatology are extensively covered in other chapters of this text. A few developments, however, should be cited. The first neonatal intensive care unit for neonates was started by Mildred T. Stahlman at Vanderbilt University in the early 1960s. This unit confirmed the concept that the neonate was indeed a "patient" and deserving of the best that medicine could offer. It appears that the "tipping point" event for the development of neonatal intensive care was the death of President John F. Kennedy's infant son, Patrick Bouvier Kennedy, in the summer of 1963. The President was faced with a most difficult dilemma at that time. He was aware that Swyer and Delivoria-Papadopoulos had successfully ventilated an infant with hyaline membrane disease in Canada but ultimately was advised that it would look bad for the President to fly his child outside the United States (personal communication, 1972, Maria Delivoria-Papadopoulos). Ultimately, the baby was flown to a hyperbaric oxygen chamber at Massachusetts General Hospital, where the baby died after 36 hours. This event made it painfully apparent that the neonate was deserving of better care than was obtainable in the United States at that time. Funding was soon made available, and the era of neonatal intensive care began. The proliferation of such units around the country (there are now more than 1000) are indicative of their success.

The problem that remained, however, was the fact that neonates still died from lung disease, particularly atelectasis neonatorum or hyaline membrane disease. Surfactant was isolated in 1957 by Clements, and Avery and Mead demonstrated 2 years later that neonates dying from hyaline membrane disease lacked pulmonary surfactant; these developments represented major steps forward in the understanding of this process. Three decades later, the administration of exogenous surfactant is commonplace in nurseries and has resulted in a significant decrease in mortality and morbidity from this disease. During this time, however, another development was progressing: namely, artificial life support.

Although attempts to artificially ventilate infants had been made periodically in the past (Alexander Graham Bell had, in fact, tried to develop an infant ventilator in 1899), the first significant progress was made during the early 1960s when a number of notable attempts to use negative-pressure ventilators were initiated. Using these devices, which were developed in part by Jack Emerson, Mildred T. Stahlman and James Sutherland at Vanderbilt University and L. Stanley James at Babies' Hospital in New York treated a number of patients who survived. Nearly simultaneously, Delivoria-Papadopoulos and Swyer in Toronto successfully applied the first positive-pressure ventilator to an infant with respiratory distress syndrome. The initial devices were modified adult units, which were soon followed by the introduction of ventilators specifically designed for neonates. Soon after, Gregory and colleagues introduced continuous positive airway pressure (CPAP), Kirby and associates developed a modified continuous flow circuit for ventilators, and the era of neonatal respiratory intensive care was launched. There has been a subsequent proliferation of neonatal ventilators, including high-frequency devices, capable of breathing for infants at hundreds of breaths per minute. Although all of these ventilatory devices have had a significant degree of success, they have not operated without problems. Bronchopulmonary dysplasia, or chronic lung disease from positive pressure ventilation, has remained a difficult issue throughout the period of neonatal intensive care, as has retinopathy of prematurity. The causes of both of these common afflictions remain only partly understood.

Other developments in the care of the newborn infant are too numerous to be fully recounted here. Exchange transfusion for Rh disease; the management of preterm labor; new imaging techniques, such as ultrasonography, computed tomography, and magnetic resonance imaging; the introduction of extracorporeal membrane oxygenation; the use of corticosteroids to help the fetal lung mature; and antibiotic therapy are but a few of the advances that have made the neonate truly a "patient."

More recently, the focus on the neonate as a patient has progressed. The eras of neonatal intensive care can probably be classified as follows:

The Era of Survival (1960 to 1975): Clinicians were simply attempting to find a way for the tiny, critically ill neonate to survive.

The Bronchopulmonary Dysplasia Era (1975 to 1990): The primary focus was on not only improving survival, but on reducing the incidence of chronic lung disease.

The Outcome Era (1990 to the present): The focus changed to examining the effects of neonatal intensive care unit intervention on long-term neurodevelopmental outcome.

In the modern period of neonatal care, quality-of-life issues have begun to predominate. No intervention can be successful unless the neurologic and developmental outcomes are successful or optimal as well. An example of this change can be seen in the debate over the use of postnatal glucocorticoids in the treatment of bronchopulmonary dysplasia. Although there is little question about the effectiveness of steroids to ameliorate the severity of bronchopulmonary dysplasia, the effects of these medications on somatic and brain growth have led to a drastic reduction in their use since 2000. It appears that quality of life and neurodevelopmental outcome will continue to gain in importance as this subspecialty evolves.

The advances in care that have occurred, however, have been expensive. There are few areas of medicine as costly as neonatal intensive care, and in this era of cost consciousness, people have begun to question the value of spending hundreds of thousands of dollars on a single life, when the same expenditure for preventive health care might be far more beneficial to society as a whole. Furthermore, increasingly available data indicate the striking degree of variation that exists in neonatal care around the country. For similar types of patients, hospital length of stay may vary dramatically from one community to another or from one hospital to another. Even in a single institution, the variation in practice among physician colleagues in a division of neonatology can be significant (any experienced neonatal nurse can attest to this fact). These variations in practice, however, can rarely be shown to affect outcome and can usually be traced back to the site at which an individual physician or group of physicians completed their fellowship training. The increasing awareness of this phenomenon has rightly led to an increasing emphasis on evidence-based medicine, or the process of decision making that is defined by information that can be gleaned from careful, thoughtful reviews of the medical literature, such as those in the Cochrane Neonatal Database. This healthy development is likely to assist in minimizing practice variation in the future, as the onus for accurate, evidence-based care continues to evolve. Nonetheless, stylistic mannerisms in neonatology continue to be noticeable, and efforts to reduce this trend are essential for the continued growth of neonatal care and reduction of health care costs.

One form of therapy that is likely to emerge as a substantial medical and ethical area for the fetus and neonate during the early 21st century is that of genetic intervention. Although initial forays into genetic treatment have had significant problems, there is little question that the genetic treatment of disease will become a major part of care. Because so many genetic diseases

seem to be amenable to therapy during the fetal or neonatal period, it appears that much treatment will be soon directed into this area. The human genome has now been catalogued, and, every day, new genetic errors that accompany many of the most common diseases, as well as some of the more obscure diseases, are described. Within the not-too-distant future, the genetic therapist is likely to perform as much "cutting and mending" as the pediatric surgeon. Unfortunately, it also seems probable that the ability to genetically diagnose diseases will be achieved before the ability to treat various diseases, and a particular genome will be found to produce certain problems in adulthood; both scenarios raise many ethical and moral dilemmas. As has been true for much of the 20th century, the fetus and neonate will continue to be a focus of much heated debate. Nevertheless, few areas of medicine are likely to be as rewarding, and the future promises to be incredibly exciting for the neonatal patient.

SUGGESTED READINGS

Avery ME, Mead J: Surface properties in relation to atelectasis and hyaline membrane disease. Am J Dis Child 97:517, 1959.

Budin P: "Le Nourrisson," Alimentation et Hygiene des Enfants Debiles—Enfants nes a Terme. Paris, Octave Doin, 1900.

Clements JA: Surface tension of lung extracts. Proc Soc Exp Biol Med 95:170, 1957.

Couzin J: Human genome. HapMap launched with pledges of $100 million. Science 298:941, 2002.

Delivoria-Papadopoulos M, Swyer PR: Assisted ventilation in terminal hyaline membrane disease. Arch Dis Child 39:481, 1964.

Gerstenberger MHJ: Studies in the adaptation of artificial food to human milk. Am J Dis Child 10:249, 1915.

Greenberg MH: Neonatal feeding. In Smith GF, Vidyasagar D (eds): Historical Review and Historical Advances in Neonatal and Perinatal Medicine. Evansville, Ind, Mead Johnson Nutritional Division, 1980, pp 55-78.

Gregory GA, Kitterman JA, Phibbs RH, et al: Treatment of the idiopathic respiratory distress syndrome with continuous positive airway pressure. N Engl J Med 284:1332, 1971.

Jobe AH, Ikegami M: Prevention of bronchopulmonary dysplasia. Curr Opin Pediatr 13:124, 2001.

Kirby R, Robinson EJ, Schulz J, et al: Continuous flow ventilation as an alternative to assisted or controlled ventilation in infants. Anesth Analg 51:871, 1971.

Libling AJ: Patron of the premies. New Yorker 15:19, 1939.

Touch SM, Greenspan JS, Kornhauser MS, et al: The timing of neonatal discharge: An example of unwarranted variation? Pediatrics 108:1240, 2001.

Touch SM, Greenspan JS, Kornhauser MS, Spitzer AR: Intensive care management of the term neonate: Are there regional differences in outcome? Clin Pediatr 41:587, 2002.

Wilmore DW, Dudrick SJ: Growth and development of an infant receiving all nutrients exclusively by vein. JAMA 203:860, 1968.

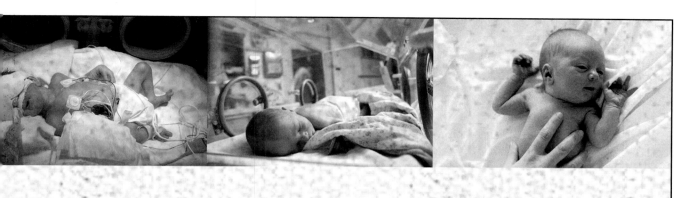

Fetal Development

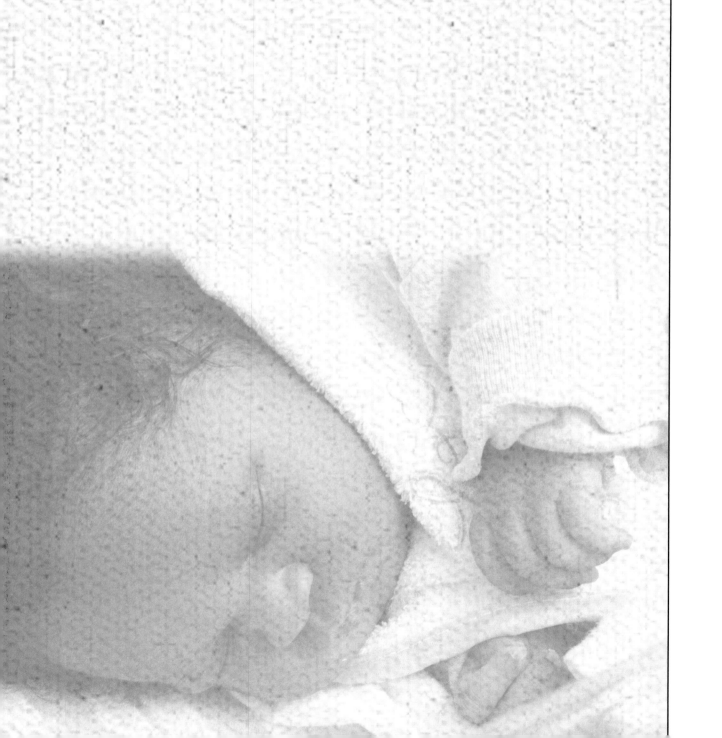

CHAPTER 3

The Genetics of Development

Patricia A. Parton and Carol E. Anderson

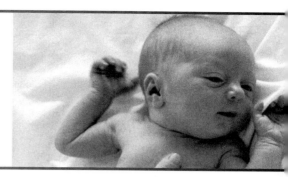

As treatment of infection, respiratory distress, and other problems related to prematurity has improved, congenital malformations and inborn errors of metabolism have begun to account for a greater proportion of the rates of neonatal mortality and morbidity.[1] Thus, an understanding of the genetic basis of development and application of that knowledge to identification, management, and support of newborns with congenital malformations and other genetic and metabolic conditions are important for clinicians involved in the care of the mother and newborn. Proliferation of knowledge of genetics is a relatively recent phenomenon. Although Gregor Mendel published his studies of genes in 1866, suggesting that discrete elements, or "genes," explained the inheritance of traits from generation to generation, it was only in the early 1900s that these concepts were found to apply to the inheritance of human characteristics. Since Watson and Crick's description of the double helical structure of deoxyribonucleic acid (DNA) in 1953,[2] evolving molecular genetic techniques based on the "one gene–one protein" model have allowed for localization, manipulation, and study of individual genes. It was only in 1956 that Tjio and Levan developed techniques to visualize human chromosomes, confirming that the normal human diploid number was 46.[3] Since then, special banding techniques and prometaphase preparations have enabled a more detailed analysis of smaller portions of those chromosomes. Somatic cell hybridization techniques in the 1970s allowed for localization of genes to particular chromosome segments, providing some of the first interface between the molecular techniques and cytogenetic techniques.

The Human Genome Project was formally started in 1990 and completed in 2003. The project's goals were to identify all the genes in human DNA, determine gene sequences, compose an international database, and improve investigative tools. This technologic advance has revolutionized the field of genetics and has led to the development of many new medical applications.[4] There now exist techniques that allow clinicians to identify extra or missing chromosome material that is too small for the microscope to detect, identify unknown extra chromosome material present in a karyotype, and determine whether each parent's chromosome contribution to their offspring has been processed correctly.

All this technology has been brought to bear on understanding the genetic contribution to development. Genetic contributions can be summarized in essentially four categories: single-gene inheritance, chromosomal inheritance, multifactorial inheritance, and nontraditional mechanisms of inheritance. This chapter is a review of examples of each of these mechanisms of inheritance, emphasizing developments and techniques. The latest developments in newborn screening used to identify presymptomatic neonates and the importance of early detection in symptomatic neonates are also discussed. This review is not encyclopedic; fortunately, there are references that are helpful in this regard.[5-10]

SINGLE-GENE DISORDERS

The single-gene disorder occurs when there is a mutation from the wild-type gene allele in either one or both members of a pair of genes that results in an observable phenotypic change. The inheritance of the phenotype follows mendelian rules for autosomal dominant, autosomal recessive, or X-linked inheritance. The number of genetic entries by mode of inheritance included in the most recent edition of *Online Mendelian Inheritance in Man*[11] is shown in Table 3-1.

Mendelian disorders are most likely to be recognized on the basis of family history. For any single category, however, a first example of the disorder may arise in the absence of family history. New mutations may produce an autosomal dominant or X-linked disorder. With an autosomal recessive disorder, the parents may be the first two carriers in either of their families to have an affected child. Thus, recognizing patterns in the family history may help in making the diagnosis of many of these disorders, but a family history is not required in order to make the diagnosis.

Table 3–1. Number of Genetic Disorders by Mode or Inheritance[11]

Pattern of Inheritance	Totals
Autosomal entries	13,467
X-linked entries	802
Y-linked entries	43
Mitochondrial entries	60
Total entries	14,372

Estimates based on population studies are that the incidence of single-gene disorders is between 2% and 3% by 1 year of age but closer to 5% by the age of 25. Obviously, such estimates do not include late-onset disorders such as familial polyposis or Huntington disease. The single-gene disorders that appear in the first year of life overlap the category of congenital malformations, estimated at 3% to 4% among newborns.[8] However, the two categories are also distinct in that most isolated major malformations are considered to be multifactorial in origin.

Autosomal Dominant Disorders

A dominant phenotype is defined to be one in which a single dose of the altered gene results in some degree of expression of the phenotype. Thus, an affected person with one dose of the altered gene has a 50% chance of passing the gene to an offspring, because genes come in pairs and the assortment is random. The gene can move in a vertical pattern, from generation to generation, affecting, on average, half the offspring of any affected individual. Boys and girls are affected in equal percentages. An important characteristic of dominant inheritance is male-to-male transmission. In instances of new mutations, the average age of the fathers is advanced, in comparison with that of the general population. Autosomal dominant phenotypes are notoriously variable, affecting different individuals in the family very differently.

Waardenburg syndrome[12] is an example of an autosomal dominant disorder defined by dystopia canthorum (the lateral displacement of medial canthi but normal interpupillary measurements), sensorineural deafness, pigmentary defects, and other developmental abnormalities such as Hirschsprung's disease (aganglionic megacolon) and cleft lip. Waardenburg syndrome illustrates heterogeneity, inasmuch as type I includes the dystopia canthorum, whereas type II does not. Type III includes both dystopia canthorum and limb abnormalities. A white forelock may be present at birth but may disappear with age in all three types of Waardenburg syndrome. Heterochromia of the irides and vitiligo are other examples of pigmentary abnormalities. Waardenburg syndrome demonstrates variability because some family members might show only one characteristic (such as the dystopia canthorum), whereas other family members might demonstrate only the deafness or the pigmentary abnormalities. As a consequence, all the first-degree relatives of

any affected person must be carefully examined and measured in order to confirm whether they carry the gene and are at risk to pass the gene on or to determine who might benefit from presymptomatic hearing evaluation to detect and treat the sensorineural hearing loss.

Through linkage techniques, the gene responsible for approximately half the type I families was found to be located on chromosome 2 at 2q37.[13] In the mouse, the Splotch locus maps to a homologous location. Heterozygotes in the mouse have white spots, and homozygotes have cochlear malformations causing hearing loss and neural tube defects. This homology aided in the identification of the human PAX3 mutations[14] in the families with Waardenburg syndrome, types I and III, which map to the 2q37 location. Expression of pax3, the mouse homologue, can be seen by immunohistochemical techniques in the developing neural crest cells that give rise to craniofacial mesectoderm and limb mesenchyme by the 10th to 12th day in the mouse embryo.[15] These changes subsequently give rise to the Splotch phenotype.

Autosomal Recessive Disorders

Although many structural disorders such as Marfan syndrome and neurofibromatosis are explained by autosomal dominant inheritance, the majority of metabolic disorders show autosomal recessive inheritance. An example of a recessive disorder in which the discovery of the gene has allowed an understanding of pathogenesis, improved carrier detection, and, it is hoped, improved treatment is cystic fibrosis. The cystic fibrosis transmembrane regulator (CFTR) gene was identified and mapped to chromosome 7, with the most common mutation identified as $\Delta F508$, resulting in a deletion of phenylalanine from the protein, which is usually 1480 amino acids in length.[16] The $\Delta F508$ accounts for 60% to 70% of the mutations in some patients, but the number of mutations described in the CFTR is now more than 600. There are some genotype-phenotype correlations. For example, homozygosity for $\Delta F508$ results in pancreatic insufficiency, whereas other "mild mutations" with mild effects on sweat electrolytes manifest mainly in pulmonary complications. The relationship between genotypic changes and recurrent bacterial infections of the lower respiratory tract, particularly with *Pseudomonas aeruginosa*, is still under investigation.

The course of pulmonary disease may vary strikingly among siblings with cystic fibrosis, although, in general, recessive disorders do not differ as much within families as do dominant disorders. Because early mortality (the mean life expectancy currently being approximately 30 years) is often secondary to respiratory failure, investigation into treatment is active. There are animal models: namely, mice with intestinal obstruction, reminiscent of the meconium ileus seen in the affected human infant. Therapeutic trials in which DNAase is used to thin secretions are in progress, and gene therapy, by introduction of the correct gene into the respiratory tree via an adenovirus vector, is currently being evaluated. In a family known to be at risk on the basis of a previous child affected with cystic fibrosis, an attempt can be made to identify the mutations in the parents by using molecular techniques to check for the most common mutations. With the advances from the Human Genome Project, the American College of Obstetricians and Gynecologists now recommends that DNA screening for cystic fibrosis be made available to all couples seeking preconception or prenatal care. If the prognosis of cystic fibrosis continues to improve, population screening to offer prenatal diagnosis to couples at risk may become less accepted. DNA direct mutation analysis might then be used to identify affected newborns before the onset of symptoms, so that the new treatments can be initiated immediately. Several states have already added cystic fibrosis to their newborn screening programs in the hopes that with earlier initiation of appropriate therapy, the long-term outcome may be improved.

X-Linked Recessive Disorders

An example of an X-linked disorder that can illustrate pleiotropism, lyonization, and progress in understanding the pathogenesis of the disorder is Alport syndrome. Although there is more than one form of inherited glomerulonephritis, the association of inherited nephritis with sensorineural deafness was appreciated as being more severe in affected boys and men than in affected girls and women. Because so many of these men developed renal failure early in adulthood, their reproductive disadvantage made it difficult to test for male-to-male transmission, the prerequisite for demonstrating dominant inheritance as opposed to X-linked inheritance. Microscopic hematuria could frequently be demonstrated in affected women, and nearly 7% of those women developed renal failure. Flinter and associates evaluated a group of 41 families for nephropathy, eye findings (lenticonus, speckled retina, and cataract), and sensorineural hearing impairment.[17] All of the families that met their clinical criteria for classic Alport syndrome showed inheritance consistent with X-linked recessivity. Subsequent linkage analysis confirmed X-linkage.[18] Mutations were first convincingly demonstrated in the 3′ or noncollagenous domain of a candidate gene: namely, that for the α-5 chain of type IV collagen (COL 4A5).[19] Type IV collagen is involved in the formation of basement membrane. The α-5 chain is peculiar to those in the glomerulus. The gene was localized to Xq22. The same novel collagen chain is present in the lens capsule and Descemet membrane, accounting for the pleiotropic effects of the mutation.

Interestingly, an association of the esophageal leiomyomatosis with Alport syndrome was reported.[20] The α-6 chain of type IV collagen was identified in a head-to-head arrangement and within 452 base pairs of the α-5 chain.[21] Patients with both Alport syndrome and diffuse leiomyomatosis were deleted for COL 4A5 and COL 4A6, suggesting that type VI collagen may be involved in smooth muscle differentiation. This process would represent an example of a contiguous gene syndrome detected on a molecular basis for a deletion of both genes. As additional mutations and type VI collagen are identified, additional phenotype-genotype correlations can be made. The molecular approach makes it possible to accurately identify female carriers in some families. It also creates the possibility of prenatal diagnosis or, at least, precise early

diagnosis in affected boys and men so that appropriate treatment can be offered.

CHROMOSOME ABNORMALITIES

Chromosomes are the structures in which genes are packaged. They are microscopically visible at the time of cell division, specifically at the metaphase stage of mitosis. The normal diploid number in humans is 46. Twenty-two pairs of chromosomes are called **autosomes** and the remaining pair (the X and the Y) are the **sex chromosomes.** In general, one member of each pair is inherited from each parent. Only when cells are dividing can chromosomes be visualized. Thus, culture techniques to grow cells are essential in order for chromosome analysis. For the sake of convenience, white blood cells from a heparinized blood sample are the easiest to culture. However, if blood is unavailable or if there is a need to evaluate other tissues, those tissues can be sampled to establish a fibroblast culture. This requires a longer time to achieve sufficient growth to analyze the chromosomes. Colchicine is used to stop the process of mitosis at the metaphase stage. Exposure to hypotonic solution lyses the nuclear and cell membranes, spreading the chromosomes from one cell just far enough apart that they can be stained and visualized. Initially, when human chromosomes were analyzed, they were stained homogeneously. A more detailed evaluation became possible in the 1970s when pretreatment of the chromosomes with a protease, usually trypsin, allowed for G (Giemsa) banding. Other stains allow for different banding patterns (Q, quinacrine bands, R, reverse bands, or C, centromeric bands) to study particular areas of interest. Preparing a karyotype for an individual means visualizing the chromosomes from one cell of that individual. Usually, at least 15 cells are analyzed, but more cells may be analyzed according to the clinical indication for the abnormality found. Cytogenetics is the study and analysis of chromosomes for structural abnormalities, because either excess or deficiency of chromosome material is usually what gives rise to a chromosome disorder. It is estimated that approximately 1 per 200 live newborns have a chromosome abnormality. The frequency of chromosome disorders is greater among infants who die in the perinatal period and is reported to vary between 5% and 10%. The frequency in first-trimester miscarriage is approximately 50%.

Abnormalities involving excess or deficiency can arise through either a change in chromosome number or a change in chromosome structure. Changes in chromosome number are of two types. One category is **polyploidy,** an abnormal multiple of the haploid number, such as triploidy, in which there are 69 chromosomes. The second type of error in chromosome number is **aneuploidy**, with a numeric deviation from normal as a deficiency or excess of a discrete number of chromosomes. Deficiency of one chromosome, **monosomy**, is most often lethal; the exception in live births is Turner syndrome (45,XO), in which there is only one sex chromosome. **Trisomy** refers to the presence of one extra member of one pair.

The report by John Langdon Down in 1866 gave rise to the eponym for this most common syndrome related to mental retardation detectable in the neonatal period. The biologic basis of Down syndrome was not recognized until 1959, when Jérôme Lejeune applied cytogenetics to a group of affected individuals, revealing trisomy 21 to be a common finding. The incidence among newborns is roughly 1 per 700 live births. The most constant feature is hypotonia, but even this is variable. Growth delay may not yet be evident at birth, although it is usually manifested later in life. There is increased joint laxity with characteristic facial features. The head tends to be small and round (brachycephalic) with flat facies. The bridge of the nose is related to epicanthal folds. There may be a slant to the palpebral fissure. The tongue may protrude, and the neck appears short with redundant skin folds. The ears tend to be small. There is an increased frequency of congenital heart disease (40%) as well as gastrointestinal malformations. The hands are relatively short (brachydactyly), and there is an increased frequency of clinodactyly. Dermatoglyphic features that are helpful in infancy include simian creases, a distal position of the palmar axial triradius, and an increased frequency of ulnar loop dermal ridge patterns on the fingers. Mental retardation varies widely and according to age. Improved medical care, particularly for congenital heart disease, as well as changed attitudes toward the medical care of persons with Down syndrome have resulted in increased life expectancy. Survival length is now estimated at 60 years of age.[22]

There are three categories of chromosome abnormalities as a basis for Down syndrome: (1) trisomy 21, usually arising from maternal nondisjunction; (2) translocation type or partial trisomy 21; and (3) mosaicism for trisomy 21. The most common of these three types is the trisomy 21, which is found in approximately 95% to 97% of affected individuals. With DNA markers, which represent an improvement over cytogenetic markers, it has been shown that the extra chromosome 21 is maternal in origin, in approximately 95% of cases. The association between advancing maternal age and the birth of a child with Down syndrome has been recognized since Lionel S. Penrose originally wrote about Down syndrome in 1933. Investigation into the maternal age relationship, as well as the basis for the empirically increased risk for a subsequent child with trisomy 21 (on the order of 1% to 2%), is active. Reduced chromosomal recombination with advanced age might contribute to nondisjunction in a substantial portion of cases with trisomy 21. The risk for recurrence in other categories is based on the chromosome findings in the affected individual. In fewer than 5% of cases, the trisomy 21 occurs as a result of an unbalanced translocation. In approximately half these cases, the translocation is de novo (i.e., not present in either parent) and therefore unlikely to recur (<1%). In the other half of the translocation cases, the balanced translocation is found in one of the parents. In these families, the estimated risk for another liveborn infant with partial trisomy depends on the chromosomes involved, as well as the sex of the parent carrying the balanced translocation. Evaluation of extended families starts with chromosome studies on first-degree relatives to define their risk of having a child with partial trisomy 21.

The final category, mosaicism for trisomy 21, is the rarest (<2%) and the most difficult to define. Chromosome studies are normally performed on blood because of its accessibility. However, the percentage of cells with trisomy 21 in that tissue is not necessarily predictive of the distribution of trisomic cells in other tissues. Objective measures in any group of children who are mosaic for trisomy 21 are closer to those of the mean of the general population than to those of a group of children in whom all the cells studied have the extra chromosome 21. It now appears that some portion of individuals who have more than one child with trisomy 21 may actually have either germline mosaicism for trisomy 21 or failure of spindle formation, which accounts for the recurrence in multiple children.

The advent of gene mapping, including both genetic as well as physical mapping of chromosome 21, has advanced genotype-phenotype correlation. For example, the association of partial trisomy 21 duplications in the critical chromosomal region, which correlates with features seen in the affected individual, allows for establishment of the relationship between the genotype and phenotype. For example, congenital heart disease was recorded in very few cases of partial duplication and in no cases in which the region 21q22 was not affected.[23] Therefore, it seems likely that the genes predisposing to congenital heart disease are found in that region.[24] In contrast, duplications over the entire length of the chromosome 21 critical region appear to contribute to the varying degree of mental retardation. The obvious goal would be to identify which genes in each area contribute to a given phenotypic feature and then assess how the genes gave rise to that feature at a cellular biologic level.

The Wolf-Hirschhorn syndrome (WHS) is a multiple malformation syndrome described by Wolf and Hirschhorn[25] in relation to a deletion of chromosomal material from the short arm of chromosome 4 (4p–). There is usually marked growth deficiency, microcephaly, and hypotonia, but the most characteristic feature is hypertelorism, with a prominent glabellar region that gives rise to the "Greek helmet" appearance. There may be clefting, with a short philtrum and a downturned "carplike" mouth, as well as preauricular pits and/or tags. A variety of other abnormalities may occur, such as cardiac or genital anomalies. Although the diagnosis has in the past depended on chromosome analysis, it is possible for a child to be affected with an apparently normal G-banded karyotype; that is, there may be a very small deletion, or there may have been an exchange with another similarly staining region. The parents' chromosomes should always be studied in order to rule out translocation as a basis of the deletion, although this is rarely the case. Fluorescent in situ hybridization (FISH) methods or molecular markers may be used to demonstrate very small deletions.[26]

The application of the techniques of molecular biology to cytogenetic preparations has opened up a whole new field of molecular cytogenetics. FISH is a physical DNA mapping technique in which a DNA probe labeled with a fluorescent marker is hybridized to a specific location on a chromosome and visualized under the microscope with ultraviolet light to study the structure and function of a very specific region. Telomeres, the physical ends of chromosomes, have the highest concentration of genes of any chromosomal region; therefore, submicroscopic deletions and duplications would have significant effects in these locations. Well-known examples of microdeletion syndromes include DiGeorge syndrome, velocardiofacial syndrome, and Williams syndrome, whereas Charcot-Marie-Tooth disease is an example of a microduplication syndrome. Cryptic, submicroscopic, telomeric rearrangements cannot be seen with conventional chromosome banding, and cryptic rearrangements have been implicated in a calculated 6% of unexplained cases of mental retardation.[27] Diagnostic studies involving telomeric probe assays are clinically useful in identifying rearrangements previously missed with older techniques. When absent or extra material is identified with these sensitive probes, comparative genomic hybridization (CGH) is used to detect global gains and losses of genomic material and to help identify break points.[28]

If a rearrangement is balanced (balanced translocation), in general, no clinical abnormality is observed. When there is an abnormal phenotype in such a case, there may be a disruption or conformational change of critical genes at the break point regions that are still too small to detect. CGH does not detect apparently balanced rearrangements, but multicolor FISH (M-FISH) does, as illustrated in Figure 3-1. Clinical applications of these new techniques include diagnosis of microdeletion and microduplication syndromes, detection of subtelomeric rearrangements in idiopathic mental retardation, identification of marker and derivative chromosomes, prenatal diagnosis of trisomy syndromes and gene rearrangements, and gene amplifications in tumors. It seems likely that the future of molecular cytogenetics will include the interaction of DNA chips, microarrays, and CGH techniques.[20]

Molecular cytogenetic methods have added new tools for investigation in order to provide more precise genetic diagnosis for clinical management and appropriate genetic counseling. Thus, the need for chromosome analysis in an affected infant might be clear; however, according to the list of indications indicated in Table 3-2, clinical input to the cytogenetics laboratory would be needed to justify the additional specialized studies of children whose karyotypes appear normal.

MULTIFACTORIAL INHERITANCE

The third category of genetic disorders grouped according to genetic mechanism is **multifactorial inheritance.** As the term implies, there are multiple contributing factors, including both genetic and environmental. There may be confusion with the term **polygenic**, which implies no environmental contribution and is strictly the result of the interaction of multiple genes. Another term sometimes applied to these disorders, **familial aggregation**, does not purport to separate genetic and environmental contributions but simply describes the patterns within families. Isolated congenital malformations represent one of the best characterized examples of multifactorial disorders.[29] These isolated malformations show familial patterns, but analysis of a large number of pedigrees does not support single-gene inheritance. Examples of the disorders tend to occur in the general population at a rate of 1 per 1000. Once there is an affected family member, first-degree relatives have a 3% to 5% risk of occurrence. The more closely related the family member, the higher the empirical risk of recurrence. More distantly related family members who share fewer genes in common have a lower risk of recurrence. The patterns vary slightly from malformation to malformation. In general, however, when more than one family member is affected, the recurrence

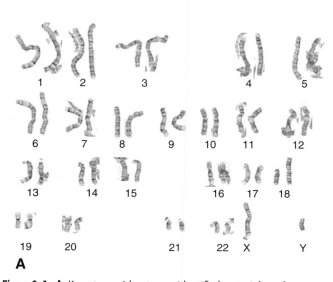

A

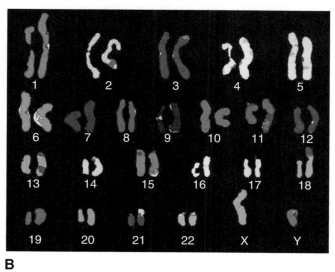

B

Figure 3–1. A, Karyotype with extra, unidentified material on chromosome 18 (18p). **B,** Multicolor fluorescent in situ hybridization (M-FISH) assay showing chromosomes that have been "painted," with a unique color representing each chromosome number (illustrated here in shades of grey). There is no banding pattern, but it is useful to identify translocations or extra material. In this case, the dark material on chromosome 18 looks like it was derived from chromosome 3.

Continued

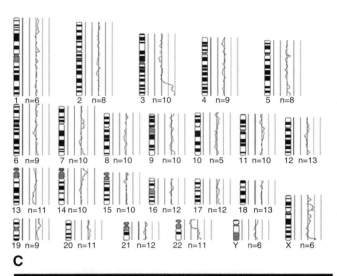

C

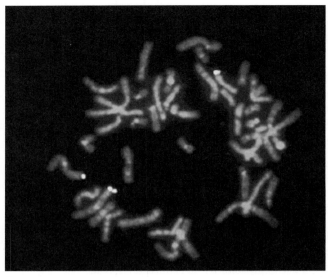

D

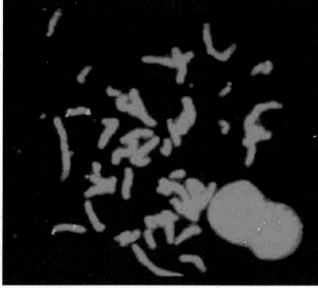

E

Figure 3–1, cont'd. C, Comparative genomic hybridization (CGH) study showing how a gain of duplicated material will scatter into the right columns or a loss of deleted material will scatter into the left columns. This study reveals that there is duplicated material from the long arm of chromosome 3 (dup 3q) and can provide break points. This technique is not useful if there is a balanced rearrangement. **D,** FISH study in which a telomere probe was used for 3q. In addition to the two normal signals, there is also a signal from chromosome 18. **E,** FISH study in which a telomere probe was used for 18p and 18q and confirmed that there is extra material beyond the telomeric area of 18p.

risk observed is higher. In conditions for which there is a marked sex ratio, such as pyloric stenosis, the risk is higher among the offspring of the less often affected sex. The idea is that there must have been more predisposing genes for the less affected sex to show the malformation in the first place. Hence, more of those predisposing genes are passed on to offspring. In general, the more severe the malformation, the higher the recurrence risk. Empirical risks should ideally be applied only to members of populations in which the observations were made in the first place.

One of the problems in the analysis of a defect or a group of defects, such as neural tube defects (NTDs), is etiologic heterogeneity. The apparent association of NTDs with maternal type I diabetes, chromosome abnormalities, prenatal valproic acid exposure, and the disruption of a normally developing fetus by amniotic bands suggests etiologic heterogeneity. Thus, before empirical risks are ever applied, a complete family history and physical examination are needed to try to rule out these other categories with different implications for family members of affected individuals.

The possibilities that nutritional factors could contribute to NTDs was supported by the observation in Great Britain that the recurrence risk appeared to be reduced by periconceptional folic acid supplementation.[30] Subsequently, a randomized trial in Britain confirmed the protective effect of folic acid supplementation: NTDs occurred in 6 (1%) of 593 infants or fetuses of women who received 4 mg of folic acid, in comparison with 21 (3.5%) of 602 infants or fetuses of women who did not receive the folic acid.[31] On the basis of these results, the Centers for Disease Control and Prevention in the United States recommended folic acid supplementation (4 mg/day) for

Table 3–2. List of Indications for Chromosome Analysis

Multiple malformations (or multisystem involvement)
Growth failure of unexplained origin
Developmental delay or mental retardation*
Stillbirth
Neonatal death, unknown cause
Family history of a previous child with a chromosome
  abnormality
Ambiguous genitalia/hypogonadism
Inguinal mass in a girl
Cryptorchidism or small testes
First-degree amenorrhea
Swollen dorsum of hands/feet
History of fetal cystic hygroma or hydrops,
  unknown cause
History of multiple miscarriages/stillbirths

*Regular chromosome analysis and, if indicated, DNA testing for fragile
X syndrome (FMR-1).

women who had previously had an affected infant or fetus with spina bifida, anencephaly, or encephalocele; this regimen was to start at least 4 weeks before conception and continue through the first 3 months of pregnancy. Physicians prescribing this level of folic acid must be careful to rule out a vitamin B$_{12}$ deficiency anemia before initiating therapy. The United States Public Health Service subsequently recommended that all women of childbearing age include at least 1 mg of folic acid in their daily diet. The fact that the folic acid supplementation does not prevent all recurrences of NTDs is probably related to etiologic heterogeneity. It is estimated that these levels of folic acid supplementation might prevent up to 60% of NTDs. There is also growing evidence of a possible role of folic acid supplementation in the prevention of other congenital anomalies, including cardiac defects and craniofacial malformations. Elevation of homocysteine levels has also been associated with these defects, and folic acid may protect against such rises.[32] There is still reason for families with affected children to receive genetic counseling and to include a review of prenatal diagnostic options such as amniocentesis, α-fetoprotein determination, and/or level II ultrasound evaluation, as well as the review of the limitations of prenatal diagnosis and other risk factors in the family history.

Another example of a multifactorial disorder is Wilms tumor (WT1). The incidence of this disorder is approximately 1 per 10,000 children in all ethnic groups. The age at onset is usually less than 6 years, with a median of 3.5 years. Of affected children, 5% to 10% have bilateral involvement. Familial patterns contributed to Knudson's two-hit hypothesis of oncogenesis (i.e., that somatic mutation allows for loss of tumor suppression) in 1972.[33] In the bilateral or familial form, Wilms tumor was more likely to be associated with such congenital anomalies as genitourinary abnormalities (5%), hemihypertrophy (approximately 3%), and aniridia (1% to 2%). Association with the congenital abnormalities led to the recognition

of the microdeletion syndrome of Wilms tumor, aniridia, genitourinary abnormality, and retardation (WAGR). In addition, approximately one fifth of sporadic Wilms tumors showed a loss of heterozygosity for 11p13 markers, which is consistent with a two-hit hypothesis. This finding suggested the presence of a tumor suppressor gene at this locus. After overlapping deletions suggested a critical area, the WT1 gene was identified as having zinc finger motifs. It is interesting that during embryonic development, the WT1 transcripts are found by immunohistochemical methods to be present not only in the developing kidney but also in the gonadal ridge and the mesothelial lining of the coelomic cavity, as well as several other organs.[34]

True genetic heterogeneity with regard to the Wilms tumor predisposition is seen from the second Wilms tumor locus on the short arm of chromosome 11 (11p15.5). This abnormality is associated with familial Beckwith-Wiedemann syndrome and possibly with other conditions.[35] Although the environmental factors that could predispose to a "second hit" have not been identified, environmental factors may have a role. Thus, Wilms tumor illustrates interaction between a transcription factor and nearby genes, the interaction of different gene products,[36] and the possibility of interaction with environmental factors. This situation represents a classic multifactorial condition in which predispositions may be used to predict which families have an increased risk of having another affected child, so that appropriate screening can be done.

NONTRADITIONAL MODES OF INHERITANCE

Some nonmendelian mechanisms of inheritance have been recognized and must be considered, because their manifestation may affect the counseling given to families (Table 3-3). One of these is maternal transmission of disorders through mitochondrial DNA (mtDNA) mutation. The discovery of maternal transmission of Leber hereditary optic atrophy first suggested that inheritance might be based on mtDNA, inasmuch as mtDNA is transmitted via the egg but not the sperm.[37] Subsequently, other neuromuscular and central nervous system abnormalities have been shown to be related to mtDNA

Table 3–3. Contiguous Gene Syndromes

Angelman syndrome (15q11)
Prader-Willi syndrome (15q11)
DiGeorge syndrome (22q11)
Wilms tumor, aniridia, genitalia anomalies, and
  retardation (WAGR) syndrome (11p13)
Retinoblastoma (13q14)
Langer-Giedion syndrome (8q24)
Miller-Dieker syndrome (17p13)
Smith-Magenis syndrome (17p11)
Williams syndrome (7q)

mutations; the syndrome of mitochondrial encephalomy-opathy, lactic acidosis, and stroke-like episodes (MELAS) and Leigh encephalomyopathy can affect young children. Myoclonic epilepsy with ragged red fibers (MERRF), Kearns-Sayre syndrome, and diabetes with sensorineural deafness are disorders of later onset. Human mtDNA is a small (16.5-kilobase), circular, double-stranded molecule coding for 13 structural genes of proteins involved in oxidative phosphorylation in the mitochondria. Other genes coded for proteins involved in oxidative phosphorylation also reside in the nucleus. Variability in phenotype is related to differences in the extent to which tissues depend on oxidative phosphorylation, as well as the proportion of mutant mtDNA in comparison with the wild-type mtDNA present in the tissue. Once a mitochondrial myopathy has been documented by muscle biopsy, characterization of mtDNA deletion may allow for appropriate genetic counseling. There are also some empirical therapies such as coenzyme Q and carnitine therapy, which may be tried in specific situations. Muscle biopsy in affected children, however, is necessary to document the disorder.

Another nonclassic mechanism of inheritance is imprinting, the inactivation or alteration of gene expression depending on the gamete of origin, whether it be maternal or paternal in origin. Prader-Willi syndrome and Angelman syndrome represent the best known illustrations of imprinting. Both syndromes involve genes located in the proximal long arm of chromosome 15 (15q11-q13) and can be the result of three shared genetic defects: microdeletion, uniparental disomy, and imprinting defects. Imprinting defects can be detected by abnormal methylation patterns. Prader-Willi syndrome was first recognized as a multiple malformation syndrome in infants with marked hypertonia and feeding difficulties. After the first year of life, hyperphagia results in obesity with secondary complications. Small hands and feet, mild mental retardation, genital abnormalities in the boy, and characteristic facies are noted. In 1981, a microdeletion of chromosome 15 (15q11-q13) was noted to be associated with more than half of the affected individuals.[38] Subsequently, with the availability of molecular markers, all the deletions were found to be in the chromosome 15 that was paternal in origin. Examples of uniparental disomy were found in nondeletion cases, such that two copies of the maternal chromosome 15, but no normal paternal chromosome 15, had been inherited.[38] An example of this inheritance occurred when trisomy for chromosome 15 was detected during chorionic villus sampling but only two chromosomes 15 were found on amniocentesis.[39] When the child demonstrated Prader-Willi syndrome, molecular studies showed that both the remaining chromosomes 15 were of maternal origin. This case suggested that a normal paternal contribution of genes in that particular region was required for normal development.

Angelman syndrome is a different multiple malformation syndrome, in which children have more severe mental retardation, microbrachycephaly, inappropriate laughter, puppet-like ataxic movements, and prognathism with tongue thrusting. Over half the patients affected with Angelman syndrome also have a deletion in the same critical region as for Prader-Willi syndrome, 15q11-q13.[40] In contrast to Prader-Willi syndrome, however, the de novo deletion occurs on the maternal chromosome 15. Uniparental disomy for paternal chromosome 15 has been shown.[41] Angelman syndrome can result from loss of function, by either imprinting or deficient expression or function of the maternally inherited UBE3A/E6-AP gene.[42] In summary, for the region 15q11-q13, normal development requires a contribution from both parents. It is important to determine which mechanism is responsible for the clinical phenotype, because imprinting mutations or UBE3A mutations may have a 50% recurrence risk, whereas uniparental disomy and microdeletions are generally sporadic events. There are nonetheless a limited number of disorders in which imprinting appears to influence counseling, but the true extent of imprinting remains to be defined.

The third and final example of a new mechanism that influences genetic counseling is the role of unstable trinucleotide repeat sequences, particularly in neurologic disorders. An example in which this might be relevant in the neonatal period is myotonic dystrophy. Myotonic dystrophy has a prevalence of approximately 1 per 3500 individuals. It is one of the most variable inherited disorders, in that one affected person might have only cataracts, whereas another person could develop a generalized muscle weakness in middle life. When it appears in the newborn as congenital myotonic dystrophy, most often the gene has been inherited from an affected mother. A cytosine-thymidine-guanine (CTG) repeat sequence is normally found in a nontranscribed region of the gene linked to myotonic dystrophy. The length of the CTG repeat sequence is correlated with the clinical symptoms.[43] The sequence in the range of 5 to 38 repeats is stable and without symptoms. There are no symptoms in the range of 42 to 180 repeats, but instability can occur with an increase into the range of 200 to 1000 repeats, in which the classic features of neuromuscular disorder occur. The more severely affected patients with early-onset congenital cases have a CTG repeat sequence 1000 to 2000 repeats long. Thus, the unstable DNA sequence seems to explain "anticipation," the apparent worsening with successive generations. This finding is comparable with the explanation of the Sherman paradox in the fragile X-linked mental retardation, in which a cytosine-cytosine-guanine (CCG) repeat sequence at the end of the FMR-1 gene seemed to correlate with worsening symptoms in successive generations.[44] The instability in that case resulted from maternal meiosis. In the more recently described Huntington chorea gene, the instability appears to pass through the paternal side.[45] Clinical observations had suggested that juvenile or early-onset cases were the offspring of fathers who carried the Huntington chorea gene. Several neurologic disorders have been discovered with repeat sequences; the extent and significance of these sequences remain to be seen.

GENETIC COUNSELING

The approach to genetic counseling is a team effort. It requires the cooperation of the clinician, possibly a clinical geneticist, to evaluate the family history, the physical examination, and any specialized test results in order to achieve a correct diagnosis to provide information to a family. The goal is to empower the family not only with information about the inheritance of the disorder but also with information about its natural history, prevention, treatment, and variability. With additional family members, a physical examination, review of records, or appropriate laboratory tests may be necessary to detect familial patterns. Chromosome analysis may be indicated in families with recurrent miscarriage, developmental delay, growth failure, fetal death, stillbirth, or unexplained death in infancy. An overall review of contributing medical conditions, pregnancy history, and possible teratogen exposure in instances of multiple malformations should be included.

A dysmorphologist is usually a pediatrician specially trained to evaluate patients for physical features that may give clues to the underlying cause of a multiple malformation syndrome or condition, as well as understanding etiopathogenesis. A dysmorphologist performs a more detailed physical examination, paying attention to details such as hair distribution, dermatoglyphics, skin texture, and joint laxity. Many relevant measurements are recorded, with comparisons made with appropriate growth standards for gestational age and racial background. Ethnic background may influence the assessment of the significance of a single finding such as hypertelorism. After complete lists of major malformations, minor malformations, and structural variations are made, these can be tabulated against a list of features with previously recognized syndromes. There exist computerized diagnostic assist programs[9,46,47] that are helpful in generating a list of differential diagnoses. Frequently, no single laboratory test is available to confirm a particular malformation syndrome. If that syndrome is considered, however, additional evaluations may be helpful in either verifying or ruling it out. It is necessary to determine whether there is sufficient evidence for a given diagnosis. Frequently, follow-up after the neonatal period is required in order to confirm the working diagnosis. No single genetic center may have extensive experience in all areas. Thus, clinical geneticists may confer with each other and present cases at meetings in order to get input not only from their colleagues but also from other subspecialists on whom they depend for information, including neurologists; pathologists; ophthalmologists; cardiologists; ear, nose, and throat specialists; physicians; neonatologists; and obstetricians.

Genetic counseling is a communication process by which information is conveyed to a family about a medical disorder. As the term implies, there must be an exchange of information. Counselors must be able to hear exactly what the family's questions are and where they are in the information-gathering process, and they must be able to assess the family's feelings and psychosocial situation. Genetic counselors are individuals who have gone through master's degree programs in order to receive training, supervised experience, and certification in the art of genetic counseling. The goal of genetic counseling is to be nondirective but accurate and complete with the information provided. The goal is to assist families in

their process of adjustment. Obviously, the timing of a counseling session can be critical in the situation in which a family is adjusting to the birth of a child with multiple malformations. In such situations, repeated sessions may be necessary so that the family is able to comprehend the information presented and reflect on possible future implications.

Clearly, a sensitive area for genetic counselors is the provision of information about prenatal diagnostic options. Optimally, for complicated problems, the options should be reviewed before the onset of a pregnancy, so that necessary studies are already completed to determine diagnostic options in advance. Realistically, most couples whose children are at risk for chromosome disorders on the basis of advancing maternal age do not actually seek counseling until they are in the midst of a pregnancy. Prenatal diagnostic procedures are described elsewhere in this text. Frequently, however, clinicians detect an abnormality for which a family requires as much information as possible about the natural history of the disorder before making a decision. These families need and deserve the same emotional support as a family adjusting to a presence of a developmental disorder in their newborn.

Neonatal Screening and Ethical Considerations

Technology has improved all aspects of genetics testing. The human genome project has identified many genes involved in clinical disease, thereby eliminating, in most situations, tedious tests such as linkage analysis and phase determination, which were dependent on key relatives to be both living and cooperative. The new techniques in molecular cytogenetics have enabled clinicians to determine microdeletions and cryptic rearrangements that were previously undetected. New theories such as imprinting and uniparental disomy have enhanced the understanding of inheritance patterns. New techniques are now available to lead to earlier and more accurate diagnosis of inborn errors of metabolism. Tandem mass spectrometry has become a key technology in the fields of biochemical genetics and neonatal screening.[48] The development of electrospray ionization with tandem mass spectrometry and associated automation of sample handling have enabled neonatal screening for an ever-growing number of disorders.[49] Every state in the United States has adopted a neonatal screening program, although the disorders screened vary from state to state. There have been numerous ethical debates over which disorders qualify for screening and what each state will offer. Every state in the union now tests for phenylketonuria (PKU), which was the first disorder to be tested with mass neonatal screening techniques. As successful as this program has been, however, new problems have been created. Women who have PKU must have strict metabolic control; otherwise, their children are at risk for congenital heart disease, microcephaly, and severe developmental delay. Clinicians have been very successful in identifying and treating newborns with PKU but less successful in helping these now-grown women maintain preconceptional and early gestational metabolic control. There is a generation of children with detrimental affects from maternal PKU even though they do not have PKU and their mothers were successfully treated. Depending on the birth state, one child may have the benefit of early treatment for a potentially devastating deficiency, whereas another child may suffer irreversible damage from lack of early diagnosis.

Fetuses who have specific fatty acid oxidation defects may cause their mothers to have life-threatening hepatic disorders (syndrome of hemolysis, elevated liver enzymes, and low platelet counts [HELLP]; acute fatty liver of pregnancy) during late pregnancy. These infants are also at risk for developing hypoketotic hypoglycemia, fatty liver, and cardiomyopathy. There is a 25% recurrence risk of those disorders with each pregnancy and clinical problems for the mother each time she carries an affected pregnancy. Genetic counseling, prenatal diagnosis or preimplantation diagnosis, and neonatal screening become important issues for these families.[50] New therapeutic techniques are also changing the profiles of which diseases should be considered for neonatal screening. Enzyme replacement therapy, cell replacement therapy, drug therapy, gene therapy, bone marrow transplantation, and, especially, hematopoietic stem cell transplantation, including that with umbilical cord stem cells, have yielded favorable clinical outcomes. Disorders such as adrenoleukodystrophy, metachromatic leukodystrophy, Hurler syndrome, Hunter syndrome, and Krabbe disease are now under investigation for mass screening programs.[51]

In the past, families of these affected infants were offered symptomatic support, genetic counseling, and the option of prenatal diagnosis. Now, if treatment can be started and finished before the onset of symptoms, these infants may have a potentially favorable outcome.[51] Currently, the siblings of patients with these nontraditional spectra of disorders are benefiting from these new treatment protocols. In most other infants, a workup is initiated only after the manifestation of clinical symptoms, at which point the disease is too far advanced to be treatable. These are devastating diseases that could potentially be treated successfully, but outside of familial cases, there is no effective way to identify potential candidates. Except for cases with a family history of the disease, the presymptomatic detection of these diseases is possible only through early diagnosis, as with a neonatal screening program. Much research is currently being aimed at developing mass screening programs for disease.

Because these are extremely difficult situations even with potentially favorable treatment protocols, there has been great interest in developing preimplantation genetic diagnosis. During the process of in vitro fertilization, sequential polar body analysis, along with embryo biopsy at the blastocyst stage, is conducted to identify the disorder for which the fetus is at risk. Only if the developing embryo is free of the disorder would it be introduced into the uterus for implantation. This approach has been used for many of the inborn errors.[52] Any single-gene disorder for which a gene has been identified and confirmed with a DNA diagnosis has the potential to be identified with this technique as long as a very unique short section can be sequenced in order to construct a disease-specific probe.

Using unique FISH probes, preimplantation genetic diagnosis has also been used to help couples who may carry familial chromosome rearrangements.[53] Because there are some disorders that still must be confirmed with linkage studies, strategies are being devised so that preimplantation genetic diagnosis techniques may be able to benefit families affected with disorders such as neonatal polycystic kidney disease.

With all of this new technology, this chapter does not even attempt to address topics such as genetic engineering or cloning. Research since the early 1980s has proved exciting in genetics, in which there were more new discoveries made than in any other era of recorded mankind. The next century continues to have the greatest potential for many new and exciting challenges and discoveries.

REFERENCES

1. National Institute of Child Health and Human Development: Antenatal diagnosis. Sponsored by the National Institute of Child Health and Human Development, March 5-7, 1979. Natl Inst Health Consens Dev Conf Summ 2:11, 1979,
2. Watson JD, Crick FHC: The molecular structure of nucleic acids: A structure of deoxyribose nucleic acid. Nature 171:737, 1953.
3. Tjio JS, Levan A: The chromosome number of man. Hereditas 42:1, 1956.
4. Austin CP: The impact of the completed human genome sequence on the development of novel therapeutics for human disease. Annu Rev Med 55:1, 2004.
5. Buyse ML (ed): Encyclopedia of Birth Defects, 2nd ed. Dover, Mass, Center of Birth Defects Information Services, 1992.
6. Gorlin RJ, Cohen MM, Levin LS: Syndromes of the Head and Neck, 3rd ed. London, Oxford University Press, 1990.
7. Jones KL: Smith's Recognizable Patterns of Human Malformations, 4th ed. Philadelphia, WB Saunders, 1988.
8. Stevenson RE, Hall JG, Goodman RM: Oxford Monographs on Medical Genetics, No. 27: Human Malformations and Related Anomalies. New York, Oxford University Press, 1993.
9. Winter RM, Baraitser M, Douglas JM: A computerized data base for the diagnosis of rare dysmorphic syndromes. J Med Genet 21:121, 1984.
10. Winter RM, Knowles, SAS, Bieber, FR, et al: The Malformed Fetus and Stillbirth: A Diagnostic Approach. Chichester, UK, John Wiley, 1988.
11. Online Mendelian Inheritance in Man, OMIM: Available at http://www.ncbi.nlm.nih.gov/omim/
12. Waardenburg PJ: A new syndrome combining developmental anomalies of the eyelids, eyebrows, and nose root with congenital deafness. Am J Hum Genet 3:195, 1951.
13. Foy C, Newton V, Wellesley D, et al: Assignment of the locus for Waardenburg type I to human chromosome 2q37 and possible homology to the Splotch mouse. Am J Hum Genet 46:1017, 1990.
14. Hoth CF, Milunsky A, Lipsky N, et al: Mutations in the paired domain of the human PAX3 gene cause Klein-Waardenburg syndrome (WS-III) as well as Waardenburg's syndrome type I (WS-I). Am J Hum Genet 52:455, 1993.
15. Goulding M, Chalepakis G, Deutsch U, et al: Pax-3, a novel murine DNA binding protein expressed during early neurogenesis. EMBO J 10:1135, 1991.

16. Kerem B, Rommens JM, Buchanan JA, et al: Identification of the cystic fibrosis gene: Genetic analysis. Science 245:1073, 1989.

17. Flinter FA, Cameron JS, Chantler C, et al: Genetics of classic Alport's syndrome. Lancet 2:1005, 1988.

18. Flinter FA, Abbs S, Bobrow M: Localization of the gene for classic Alport's syndrome. Genomics 4:335, 1989.

19. Barker DF, Hostikka SL, Zhou J, et al: Identification of mutations in the COL4A5 collagen gene for Alport's syndrome. Science 248:1224, 1990.

20. Clark J, Edwards S, Feber A, et al: Genome-wide screening for complete genetic loss in prostrate cancer by comparative hybridization onto cDNA microarrays. Oncogene 22:1247, 2003.

21. Zhou J, Mochizuki T, Sweets H, et al: Deletion of the paired alpha 5 (IV) and alpha 6 (IV) collagen genes in inherited smooth muscle tumors. Science 261:1167, 1993.

22. Fryers T: Survival in Down syndrome. J Ment Deficiency Res 30:101, 1986.

23. Korenberg JR, Kawashima H, Pulst SM, et al: Down syndrome: Toward a molecular definition of the phenotype. Am J Med Genet Suppl 7:91, 1990.

24. Korenberg JR, Bradley C, Disteche CM, et al: Down syndrome: Molecular mapping of the congenital heart disease and duodenal stenosis. Am J Hum Genet 50:294, 1992.

25. Wolf U, Reinwein H: Klinische und cytogenetische differential diagnose der defizienzen an den Kurzen Armen der B-chromosomen. Z Kinderheilkd 98:235, 1967.

26. Altherr MR, Bengtsson U, Elder FFB, et al: Molecular confirmation of Wolf-Hirschhorn syndrome with a subtle translocation of chromosome 4. Am J Hum Genet 49:1235, 1991.

27. Flint J, Wilkie AO, Buckle VJ, et al: The detection of subtelomeric chromosomal rearrangements in idiopathic mental retardation. Nat Genet 9:132, 1995.

28. Joly G, Lapierre JM, Ozilou C, et al: Comparative genomic hybridization in mentally retarded patients with dysmorphic features and a normal karyotype. Clin Genet 60:212, 2001.

29. Carter CO: Genetics of common single malformations. Br Med Bull 32:21, 1976.

30. Prevention of neural tube defects: Results of the Medical Research Council Vitamin Study. MRC Vitamin Study Research Group. Lancet 338:131, 1991.

31. Use of folic acid for prevention of spina bifida and other neural tube defects—1983-1991. MMWR Morb Mortal Wkly Rep 40:513, 1991.

32. Rosenquist TH, Ratashak SA, Selhub J: Homocysteine induces congenital defects of the heart and neural tube: Effect of folic acid. Proc Natl Acad Sci U S A 93:15227, 1996.

33. Knudson AG Jr, Strong LC: Mutations and cancer: A model for Wilms' tumor of the kidney. J Natl Cancer Inst 48:313, 1972.

34. Rauscher FJ III: The WT1 Wilms' tumor gene product: A developmentally regulated transcription factor in the kidney that functions as a tumor suppressor. FASEB J 7:896, 1993.

35. Koufos A, Grundy P, Morgan K, et al: Familial Wiedemann-Beckwith syndrome and a second Wilms' tumor locus both mapped to 11p15. Am J Hum Genet 44:711, 1989.

36. Maheswaran S, Park S, Bernard A, et al: Interaction between the p53 and Wilms' tumor (WT1) gene products: Physical association and functional cooperation. Proc Natl Acad Sci U S A 90:5100, 1993.

37. Wallace DC: Mitochondrial DNA mutations and neuromuscular disease. Trends Genet 5:9, 1989.

38. Nicholls RD, Knoll JH, Butler MG, et al: Genetic imprinting suggested by maternal uniparental heterodisomy in non-deletion Prader-Willi syndrome. Nature 342:281, 1989.

39. Cassidy SB, Lai L, Erickson RP, et al: Trisomy 15 with loss of the paternal 15 as a cause of Prader-Willi syndrome due to maternal disomy. Am J Hum Genet 51:7001, 1992.

40. Magenis RE, Brown MG, Lacy DA, et al: Is Angelman syndrome an alternate result of del (15) (q11q13)? Am J Med Genet 28:829, 1987.

41. Malcolm S, Clayton-Smith J, Nichols M, et al: Uniparental disomy in Angelman syndrome. Lancet 337:694, 1991.

42. Kishino T, Lalande M, Wagstaff S: UBE3A/E6-AP mutations cause Angelman syndrome. Nat Genet 15:70, 1997.

43. Hunter A, Tsilfidis C, Mettler G, et al: The correlation of age of onset with CTG trinucleotide repeat amplification in myotonic dystrophy. J Med Genet 29:774, 1992.

44. Fu Y-H, Kuhl DPA, Pizzuti A, et al: Variation of the CGG repeat at the fragile X site results in genetic instability: Resolution of the Sherman paradox. Cell 67:1047, 1991.

45. MacDonald ME, Ambrose CM, Duyao MP, et al: A novel gene containing a trinucleotide repeat that is expanded and unstable on Huntington's disease chromosomes. Cell 72:971, 1993.

46. Buyse ML: Center for Birth Defects Information Services. Birth Defects Orig Artic Ser 16(5):83, 1980.

47. Murdoch Children's Research Institute: POSSUM (Picture of Standard Syndromes and Undiagnosed Malformations). Available at http://www.possum.net.au/

48. Millington DS, Kodo N, Norwood DL, Roe CR: Tandem mass spectrometry: A new method for acylcarnitine profiling with potential for neonatal screening for inborn errors of metabolism. J Inherit Metab Dis 13:321, 1990.

49. Rashed MS, Ozand PT, Bucknall MP, Little D: Diagnosis of inborn errors of metabolism from blood spots by acylcarnitines and amino acids profiling using automated electrospray tandem mass spectrometry. Pediatr Res 38:324, 1995.

50. Ibdah JA, Bennett MJ, Rinaldo P, et al: A fetal fatty-acid oxidation disorder as a cause of liver disease in pregnant women. N Engl J Med 340:1723, 1999.

51. Krivit W, Lockman LA, Watkins PA, et al: The future for treatment by bone marrow transplantation for adreno-leukodystrophy, metachromatic leukodystrophy, globoid cell leukodystrophy and Hurler syndrome. J Inherit Metab Dis 18:398, 1995.

52. Galvin-Parton P, Godoy R, Weiss J, et al: Community follow-up of two infants delivered following a pregnancy involving preimplantation genetic diagnosis. Paper presented at the Annual Meeting of the American College of Medical Genetics, 2002. Rockville, Md.

53. Verlinsky Y, Cieslak J, Ivakhnenko V, et al: Prevention of age-related aneuploidies by polar body testing of oocytes. J Assist Reprod Genet 16:165, 1999.

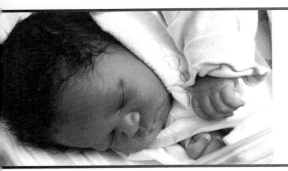

Environmentally Induced Birth Defects

Keith K. Vaux, Linda Chan, and Kenneth Lyons Jones

Environmentally induced fetal malformations are an important and potentially preventable cause of birth defects. **Teratogens** include any agent that alters form or function of a fetus or embryo and are thought to account for approximately 10% of all congenital defects identified at birth.[1] Before the 1960s, it was thought that most birth defects were genetic in origin and that the fetus was protected from environmental agents within the uterus. Although the effect of maternal rubella on the fetus had been described in 1941, it was not until 20 years later that prenatal exposure to a drug, thalidomide, was associated with severe defects in prenatal development.[2] The thalidomide incident led to extensive lay press coverage and heightened concern about environmental exposures and the association with congenital defects.

Because the testing of new medications on pregnant women is fraught with ethical and legal concerns, most new medications are not labeled for use in pregnancy, carrying instead the disclaimer "Use in pregnancy is not recommended unless potential benefits justify the potential risk to the fetus." However, with half of all pregnancies in North America unplanned, and with more than 3 billion drug prescriptions written in 2002, thousands of women are inadvertently exposed to medications before pregnancy recognition, about which there is no adequate information. These numbers do not even include the countless over-the-counter medications and herbal products used. Therefore, knowledge of the methods used to determine the teratogenicity of prenatal exposure to medications and environmental agents is essential to clinicians who care for pregnant women and for infants.

The purpose of this chapter is to provide an introduction to teratology and a discussion of specific human teratogens. Table 4-1 outlines the basic principles of teratology, followed by a discussion of other topics of interest to those who care for pregnant women and for infants. Table 4-2 outlines known teratogens, including common maternal medical conditions, as well as therapeutic, diagnostic, and environmental agents. The relatively short list may appear reassuring; unfortunately, it more probably reflects an overall lack of information about exposures during pregnancy, especially in terms of knowledge about the effects of agents on neurodevelopmental outcomes.

ASSESSING TERATOGEN RISK

A determination of human teratogenicity relies on evaluation of the agent in question through multiple methods, summarized in Table 4-1. The birth of a child with a structural defect who was prenatally exposed to an agent frequently arouses the parents' and physicians' suspicion that the agent may have caused or contributed to the defect. Causality assigned to an agent, or dismissed without adequate study, may deny the caregiver and the family essential information needed for the health of the mother, the fetus, and the neonate.

Unfortunately, the identification of prenatal effects of a particular pharmaceutical or environmental agent results from an accumulation of cases, leading to the eventual recognition of a causal relationship. Because the prenatal effect of a medication most commonly results in subtle minor malformations, it may take many years to identify an association. For instance it was 20 years between the marketing of warfarin (Coumadin) and its recognition as a human teratogen.[3-5] The study of environmental agents, particularly medications, therefore relies on two main sources of information: premarketing and postmarketing studies. Because randomized premarketing trials are designed to evaluate drug safety or efficacy, pregnant women are typically excluded. Thus, the premarketing sources include animal studies and coincidental pregnancies occurring during randomized premarketing trials. Although it is difficult to extrapolate from animal data to human clinical application because of species differences in susceptibility/sensitivity, as well as the differences in the dosage and route of administration, there are clearly important implications relative to adverse outcomes in experimental animal studies.

Postmarketing sources include retrospective and prospective studies. Retrospective sources include

Table 4–1.   Human Teratogenesis

Exposure to agent documented or verified during
   critical period of prenatal development
Consistent findings in at least two epidemiologic
   studies
Delineation of clinical cases
Rare environmental exposures are associated with rare
   defects in three or more cases
Teratogenicity in experimental animals
Biologic plausibility
Proof that agent acts in unaltered state

Adapted from Shepard TD: Dose response in human teratology. Teratology 65:199, 2001; and Brent RL: Evaluating the alleged teratogenicity of environmental agents. Clin Perinatol 13:609, 1986.

adverse outcomes reported to the U.S. Food and Drug Administration, case reports published in the literature, birth defect monitoring programs that attempt to document trends in major malformations, and case-control studies evaluating an association between a specific major malformation and a specific prenatal drug exposure. For most of these studies, identification of a single major malformation is the primary outcome. However, with few exceptions, the teratogenic effect of most drugs and other environmental agents is manifested in a pattern of malformations, as opposed to a single major malformation. Thus, time-honored retrospective approaches, in isolation, are frequently not sufficient to determine the teratogenic potential of a particular agent.

Prospective postmarketing studies include manufacturer's registries; large database linkage studies, in which pharmacy records are linked with birth records; and cohort studies. The strength of a cohort study that includes a specialized physical examination is its ability to identify patterns of malformation by individual physical examination, as well as identifying spontaneous abortion, intrauterine growth restriction, prematurity, and, potentially, neurobehavioral deficits.

The major criticism of cohort studies is that insufficient power is available to evaluate a potential increased risk for a single major malformation. Thus, complementary approaches are necessary to determine the potential safety of a drug during human pregnancy. For example, although the case-control method would have identified the structural defects attributable to prenatal exposure to thalidomide, the pattern of minor malformations plus developmental delay associated with prenatal exposure to carbamazepine would probably escape detection.[6] Furthermore, prenatal exposure to certain drugs is associated with an increased risk of both a pattern of minor malformation and a specific major malformation. Thus, a case-control study was ideal for documenting the increased risk of meningomyelocele in babies born to women taking valproic acid[7,8]; however, this approach was incapable of identifying the pattern of minor malformations characteristic of prenatal exposure to that drug.[7] Similarly, a combination of the cohort and case-control

approaches has been used to identify and clarify the risks associated with hyperthermia.[9-11]

No single method is sufficient to document the reproductive effects of all drugs or to delineate the complete spectrum of defects associated with prenatal exposure. This fact emphasizes the importance of embracing various postmarketing surveillance strategies in order to optimally characterize the reproductive effects of drugs taken by women during pregnancy.

OTHER CONCEPTS IMPORTANT TO THE STUDY OF TERATOGENS

Several other concepts, briefly discussed as follows, are important in considering whether an agent is teratogenic.

Placental Passage

For many years, the placenta was thought to protect the developing fetus from toxins. The placenta is able to metabolize many substances and contains enzymes, including cytochrome P-450.[12] For instance, aspartame, a common artificial sweeter, is metabolized by the mother into aspartic acid, which cannot cross the placenta and therefore does not present a risk to the developing fetus.[13] Agents that are teratogenic either must cross the placenta in sufficient doses to directly affect the fetus, interfere with placental function, and thereby indirectly affect the fetus or must affect maternal physiology to an extent that placental activity is also affected.

Timing of Exposure

The **timing of exposure** refers to the embryonic stage in development when the exposure occurred. The embryo appears to be protected from effects of teratogens during the first 2 weeks after conception, before the development of organs. During this "all-or-none" period, a toxic substance may lead to improper implantation, and therefore spontaneous abortion, but is not thought to cause damage to the embryo. However, the 14th to approximately 60th days, during which organogenesis occurs, is the critical period in which the embryo is at highest risk for malformation. Once an organ develops, a teratogen cannot cause a malformation, defined as a primary defect in development. However, the organ can be damaged by a disruption, defined as further inhibition of normal growth. For instance, alcohol is thought to be a teratogen throughout gestation because of its effect on central nervous system development and growth, and angiotensin-converting enzyme (ACE) inhibitor use is associated with oligohydramnios, renal tubular dysgenesis, and delayed development of the calvaria, but only when exposure occurs in the second or third trimester.[14]

Clinical Consistency

A common misconception is that teratogenic agents that produce specific malformations can produce any malformation. In fact, teratogenic agents produce a clinically consistent pattern of abnormalities when given during the critical period. Much of the confusion has arisen because for each and any pregnancy, regardless of exposures, there is a background risk for malformation of

Table 4–2. Known Human Teratogens

Teratogen	Adverse Effects	Critical Period
Maternal Conditions		
Diabetes	Holoprosencephaly	First trimester
	Porencephalic cysts	
	Cardiac defects	
	Sacral agenesis	
	Caudal regression	
	Laterality defects	
	Limb anomalies, including preaxial polydactyly	
	Facial clefts	
	Renal anomalies	
Hypothyroidism/hyperthyroidism	Mental retardation	Entire pregnancy
	Growth retardation	
Phenylketonuria (PKU)	Mental retardation	
	Microcephaly	
	Craniofacial	
Hyperthermia	Anencephaly and neural tube defects	2-4 weeks
Systemic lupus erythematosus	Neonatal SLE	
	IUGR	
	Prematurity	
	Congenital heart block	
Nonprescription Substance Use		
Alcohol	Short palpebral fissures	Entire pregnancy
	Postnatal-onset growth deficiency	
	Mild/moderate MR	
	Prenatal and postnatal growth deficiency	
	Microcephaly	
Tobacco	Low birth weight	Unknown
	Miscarriage	
Toluene	CNS (developmental delay)	Unknown
	Microcephaly	
	IUGR	
Medications		
Aminopterin/methotrexate	CNS defects	14-60 days
	Limb defects	
	Skeletal defects	
Amiodarone	Neonatal thyroid dysfunction	Second-third trimester
ACE inhibitors	Oligohydramnios	Second-third trimester
	Renal dysplasia/failure	
	IUGR	
	Joint contractures	
	Prenatal death	
Carbamazepine	Spina bifida	14-60 days
	Hypoplasia of distal phalanges	
	IUGR	
Cyclophosphamide	CNS defects	14-60 days
	Skeletal defects, especially cranial and digits	
	IUGR	
	Cleft palate	
	Neonatal death	
Fluconazole	Brachycephaly	First trimester
(Risk thought only to be with high doses, especially parenteral)	Abnormal facies	
	Abnormal calvarial development	
	Cleft palate	
	Cardiac defects	
	Skeletal defects (thinning)	
Indomethacin	Oligohydramnios	Second-third trimester
	Anuria	
	Necrotizing enterocolitis	
	Premature ductus areteriosus closure	
Lithium	Cardiac defects (Ebstein anomaly)	14-60 days

Table 4–2. Known Human Teratogens—cont'd

Teratogen	Adverse Effects	Critical Period
Medications—cont'd		
Methylene blue	Jejunal atresia	Second trimester
Misoprostol	Möbius anomaly	First-second trimester
	Terminal transverse limb deficiency	
	Arthrogryposis multiplex congenita	
	Talipes equinovarus	
Penicillamine	Connective tissue abnormalities	Unknown
Phenobarbital	CNS (structural and developmental delay)	14-60 days
	Facial clefting	
	Midface hypoplasia	
	Cardiac defects	
	Digital nail hypoplasia	
Retinoids: oral	CNS defects	Unknown
	Ocular defects	
	Cardiac defects	
	Great vessel defects	
	Microtia	
	Micrognathia	
	Cleft lip/palate	
	Limb defects	
	Thymic deficiency	
Selective serotonin reuptake inhibitors (SSRIs)	Prenatal complications	Third trimester
	Increase in minor anomalies	
Tetracycline	Staining of primary dentition	Second-third trimester
Thalidomide	Cranial nerve abnormalities	27-40 days
	Ocular defects	
	Cardiac defects	
	Oral/facial anomalies	
	Renal and urogenital defects	
Trimethoprim	Neural tube defects	First trimester
	Oral clefts	
	Hypospadias	
	Cardiovascular defects	
Trimethadione	CNS (developmental delay)	14-60 days
	Microcephaly	
	Cleft lip and/or palate	
	Broad nasal bridge	
	Genitourinary and gastrointestinal defects	
	Cardiac defects	
Valproic acid	CNS defects (including developmental delay, autism)	14-60 days
	Brachycephaly	
	Craniosynostosis	
	Microcephaly	
	Ocular hypertelorism	
	Midface hypoplasia	
	Septooptic dysplasia	
	Cleft lip/palate	
	Limb anomalies	
	Spina bifida	
Warfarin	CNS defects	6-9 weeks
	Ocular defects	After 9 weeks,
	IUGR	CNS, ocular, and
	Neonatal hemorrhage	disruptive defects
	Nasal hypoplasia	
	Vertebral abnormalities	
	Stippled epiphysis	
Infections		
Rubella	CNS defects (developmental delay)	0-16 weeks
	Deafness	
	Ocular defects (e.g., cataracts)	

Continued

Table 4–2. Known Human Teratogens—cont'd

Teratogen	Adverse Effects	Critical Period
Infections—cont'd		
Rubella—cont'd	IUGR	
	Microcephaly	
	Cardiac defects	
	Delayed skeletal development	
Cytomegalovirus	CNS defects (developmental delay, hydrocephaly)	Before 27 weeks
	Microcephaly	
	IUGR	
	Gastrointestinal defects	
	Hearing loss	
Parvovirus	Fetal death	10-25 weeks
	Fetal hydrops	
Syphilis	CNS defects (developmental delay)	10 weeks through neonatal period
	Ocular defects	
	Microcephaly	
	Cutaneous lesions	
	Nephrosis	
	Dental abnormalities	
Toxoplasmosis	CNS defects (developmental delay, hydrocephalus)	10-24 weeks
	Microcephaly	
	Blindness	
Varicella zoster	CNS defects (developmental delay)	Up to 20 weeks
	Ocular anomalies	
	Microcephaly	
	Neurogenic muscular atrophy	
	IUGR	
	Skin scarring	

ACE, angiotensin-converting enzyme; CNS, central nervous system; IUGR, intrauterine growth restriction; MR, mental retardation; SLE, systemic lupus erythematosus.

3% to 4%. Therefore, it is essential to compare exposed pregnancies with matched controls.

One area of increasing concern has been the effect of exposures on the central nervous system, especially agents whose primary mode of action is to modify the central nervous system in the mother. Longitudinal and developmental outcome studies are now required components of the evaluation of potential teratogens.

Species Specificity

In order to be considered teratogenic, an agent should produce an increase in defects in animals in comparison with unexposed controls.[1] However, an agent that is teratogenic in one species may have no effect on another species; therefore, safety during human pregnancy cannot be ensured by animal data. For instance, thalidomide had been tested in several animal species and was not found teratogenic, a fact that most likely delayed identification of the association.

Genetics

The role of the fetal and maternal genotype has become an increasingly important element in the study of teratology. For example, fetuses with a rare variation, or polymorphism, in the transforming growth factor α_1 have a threefold to sixfold increased risk of cleft palate if the mother smokes during pregnancy.[15,16] The extent to which prenatal effects of other agents are dependent on specific maternal and/or fetal polymorphisms has not been extensively evaluated.

Similarly, the ADH 2*3 allele has been noted in two separate studies to be protective against, as opposed to a risk factor for, neurodevelopmental problems in women who drink alcohol during their pregnancy. By virtue of the fact that ADH 2*3 is associated with more rapid metabolism of alcohol, it is likely that its protective effect is the consequence of decreased drinking by pregnant women with the ADH 2*3 allele.[17]

SELECTED TERATOGENS OF IMPORTANCE TO THE PERINATAL AND NEONATAL PRACTITIONER

Maternal Conditions

Diabetes

One of the most significant human teratogens is maternal diabetes. Multiple studies have demonstrated a twofold to threefold increase in malformations and pregnancy loss in women with insulin-dependent diabetes.[18] Poorly controlled or unrecognized gestational diabetes is associated with a lower, but still increased, risk of malformation.[19] Maternal diabetes causes specific defects in the fetus, including sacral agenesis, laterality defects, and holoprosencephaly, but it is also known to affect cardiovascular and genitourinary systems, as well as the ears, eyes, vertebrae, and limbs.[20]

Hyperthermia

Hyperthermia has long been recognized as a teratogen in animals, leading to adverse pregnancy outcomes in guinea pigs and a variety of other animals.[11] Retrospective studies have suggested that maternal hyperthermia is also a human teratogen, producing a recognizable pattern of malformation, as well as growth deficiency; central nervous system defects, including microcephaly, hypotonia, and microphthalmia; and variable malformations of the first and second brachial arches, resulting in midface hypoplasia, micrognathia, cleft lip with or without cleft palate, and malformed ears. Chambers and associates, in a prospective study, documented a 10-fold increase in anencephaly, as well as an association with minor malformations of the digits, short palpebral fissures, and cleft uvula.[10] The development of these features appears to be dependent on time of exposure; the susceptible period is between weeks 4 and 16 at a maternal body temperature of at least 39.8 °C.[21]

Phenylketonuria

The treatment of phenylketonuria in infancy and childhood has been a success story for public health screening programs. However, many women who avoided mental handicap as a result of strict dietary restrictions as children have relaxed those restrictions on reaching adulthood and childbearing age. Untreated phenylketonuria has been shown to cause increases in spontaneous abortions as well as increased risk of intrauterine growth restriction, microcephaly, congenital heart disease, and mental retardation.[22] Outcome is correlated with maternal phenylalanine levels in the first trimester, and maternal treatment later in pregnancy does not significantly improve outcome.

Recreational Drug Use

Maternal Alcohol Use

From a public health standpoint, perhaps the most significant human teratogen is alcohol; the fetal alcohol syndrome is the most common recognizable cause of mental retardation and growth deficiency in children.[23] There does not appear to be a safe period for alcohol exposure during pregnancy. The diagnosis of fetal alcohol syndrome in neonates requires a history of maternal alcohol intake during the pregnancy, characteristic growth and physical features of the exposed children, and the children's problems in intellectual performance. Longitudinal follow-up is required for the diagnosis in most neonates. It is important to recognize that many more children are affected by alcohol but do not have fetal alcohol syndrome.

Cocaine

Cocaine is a potent vasoconstrictor and has been associated with vascular disruptions, such as gastroschisis and small intestinal atresia, as well as terminal transverse limb deficiencies.[24-27] Much attention has been directed toward the negative effect of cocaine on fetal outcomes. Although there is an increased risk of miscarriage, abruptio placentae, and intracranial hemorrhage, several studies have not demonstrated any long-term effects on neurodevelopmental outcomes. The defects caused by in utero exposure to cocaine are disruptions, not malformations.

Tobacco

Smoking during pregnancy has been associated with decreased fetal growth and increased pregnancy loss.[28] Genetic risk factors have been identified that increase risk, especially for facial clefting and clubfoot.[29,30]

Diagnostic Techniques

Chorionic Villus Sampling

Early chorionic villus sampling has been associated with an increase in the prevalence of vascular disruption defects, including terminal transverse limb reduction defects, cleft palate, and Möbius sequence. Because these defects were not seen in association with later chorionic villus sampling, the cause may be bleeding in the chorion, which leads to hypoperfusion in the embryo. A consensus statement in 1993 recommended that chorionic villus sampling be performed after 10 weeks' gestation.

Radiation

Diagnostic radiation consisting of less than 5 rad in the first trimester is not considered teratogenic. Although concerns have been raised for exposures between 5 and 10 rad, serious risk to the fetus does not occur until the dose is 10 rad or more. Exposure to more than 10 rad of radiation during the 8th to 15th weeks of gestation has been associated with microcephaly, mental handicap, and optic abnormalities. Of particular concern is fetal exposure to the large doses of therapeutic radiation.

Therapeutic Agents

Angiotensin-Converting Enzyme Inhibitors

Prenatal exposure to ACE inhibitors has been associated with renal tubular dysplasia and the resulting oligohydramnios sequence.[31,32] ACE inhibitors are thought to act by reducing uterine blood flow and causing fetal hypotension through decreased placental flow, as well as blocking fetal ACE activity. ACE inhibitors affect fetal development only during the second and third trimesters.

Aminopterin and Methotrexate

Aminopterin and its methyl derivative, methotrexate, are folic acid antagonists that produce a specific pattern of malformation, including growth deficiency, microcephaly, cranial dysplasia, severe midface hypoplasia, limb defects, and other folate-related abnormalities such as cleft palate and neural tube closure defects. The critical period for exposure is thought to be the sixth to ninth gestional weeks.[33]

Anticonvulsant Embryopathy

Infants exposed to a variety of anticonvulsants in utero have similar patterns of malformation, growth deficiency, and mental deficiency, known as anticonvulsant embryopathy. Anticonvulsant embryopathy has been identified in association with prenatal exposure to hydantoin, carbamazepine, valproic acid, primidone, and phenobarbital. Some of these agents have been used for bipolar disorders, expanding the potential exposure during gestation. Specific malformations include hypoplasia of the midface, clefts of the lip with or without clefts of the palate, and hypoplasia of the nails and digits. Holmes and colleagues demonstrated that infants exposed to one anticonvulsant agent had higher frequencies of anticonvulsant embryopathy than did those in a control group, whereas offspring of women who had a history of seizures but were not on medications did not have a higher frequency.[34,35]

Diethylstilbestrol

Diethylstilbestrol was widely used to support high-risk pregnancies and was given to millions of pregnant women from 1941 to 1971. Diethylstilbestrol affects normal development of müllerian-derived structures if given before 18 weeks and also has been shown to lead to increased risk of carcinoma in girls and women.[36] Boys exposed to diethylstilbestrol in utero are at increased risk for microphallus, cryptorchidism, and testicular hypoplasia.[37]

Retinoic Acid Embryopathy

This widely used treatment for cystic acne was identified as leading to high rates of fetal loss and malformation.[38,39] There does not seem to be any safe period of exposure during the first trimester or any safe dosage or length of exposure. It is highly recommended that women of childbearing age undergo a pregnancy test and use highly effective or multiple methods of contraception. Etretinate, which is used to treat psoriasis, is highly lipophilic and may be detected in the serum years after the drug is discontinued, and therefore it should be avoided by women who have not completed their childbearing years. Topically administered retinoids such as tretinoin are metabolized by the skin and are thought not to result in increased malformations.

Warfarin

Prenatal exposure to warfarin causes increased pregnancy loss and fetal malformations if given during the sixth to ninth week of pregnancy. Warfarin embryopathy is characterized by nasal hypoplasia and stippled epiphyses. If given in the second and third trimesters, disruptions occur, thought to be a result of hemorrhage and disharmonic growth and scarring, especially of central nervous tissue.

SUMMARY

Although the current list of known human teratogens is relatively small, a number of factors make it essential that the neonatal practitioner be familiar with the principles of teratology. First, many pregnancies are unplanned. Second, there has been a dramatic increase in the number of medications available for use, including those that require a prescription and those that are available over the counter. Third, with improved medical care,

many women with medical conditions that have teratogenic potential, such as diabetes, are now able to conceive. In summary, although most agents are not teratogens, it is essential that the practitioner who cares for the fetus and neonate understand that most agents have not been adequately studied. The practitioner is not alone in that there are many resources available, including teratogen information services and online references. By utilizing these resources, the practitioner can be assured of receiving the most up-to-date and scientific data available.

ADDITIONAL RESOURCES

- Organization of Teratogen Information Services (OTIS)
  www.otispregnancy.org
  866-626-OTIS or 866-626-6847
- The Teratology Society
  www.teratology.org
- Find the nearest Teratogen Information Service
  www.otis.org

REFERENCES

1. Shepard TH: Catalog of Teratogenic Agents, 10th ed. Baltimore, Johns Hopkins University Press, 2001.
2. Briggs GG, Freeman RK, Yaffe SJ: Drugs in Lactation, 2nd ed. Baltimore, Williams & Wilkins, 1997.
3. Smith MF, Cameron MD: Warfarin as teratogen. Lancet 1:727, 1979.
4. Holmes LB: Teratogen-induced limb defects. Am J Med Genet 112:297, 2002.
5. Chernoff GF, Jones KL. Fetal preventive medicine: Teratogens and the unborn baby. Pediatr Ann 10:210, 1981.
6. Jones KL, Lacro RV, Johnson KA, Adams J: Pattern of malformations in the children of women treated with carbamazepine during pregnancy. N Engl J Med 320:1661, 1989.
7. DiLiberti JH, Farndon PA, Dennis NR, Curry CJ: The fetal valproate syndrome. Am J Med Genet 19:473, 1984.
8. Robert E, Rosa F: Valproate and birth defects. Lancet 2:1142, 1983.
9. Lynberg MC, Khoury MJ, Lu X, Cocian T: Maternal flu, fever, and the risk of neural tube defects: A population-based case-control study. Am J Epidemiol 140:244, 1994.
10. Chambers CD, Johnson KA, Dick LM, et al: Maternal fever and birth outcome: A prospective study. Teratology 58:251, 1998.
11. Edwards MJ, Shiota K, Smith MS, Walsh DA: Hyperthermia and birth defects. Reprod Toxicol 9:411, 1995.
12. Benirschke K, Kaufmann P: Pathology of the Human Placenta, 3rd ed. New York, Springer-Verlag, 1995.
13. Sturtevant FM: Use of aspartame in pregnancy. Int J Fertil 30:85, 1985.
14. Cunniff C, Jones KL, Phillipson J, et al: Oligohydramnios sequence and renal tubular malformation associated with maternal enalapril use. Am J Obstet Gynecol 162:187, 1990.
15. Shaw GM, Wasserman CR, Lammer EJ, et al: Orofacial clefts, parental cigarette smoking, and transforming growth factor–alpha gene variants. Am J Hum Genet 58:551, 1996.
16. Shaw GM, Wasserman CR, Murray JC, Lammer EJ: Infant TGF-alpha genotype, orofacial clefts, and maternal periconceptional multivitamin use. Cleft Palate Craniofac J 35:366, 1998.

17. McCarver DG, Thomasson HR, Martier SS, et al: Alcohol dehydrogenase-2*3 allele protects against alcohol-related birth defects among African Americans. J Pharmacol Exp Ther 283:1095, 1997.

18. Martinez-Frias ML: Epidemiological analysis of outcomes of pregnancy in diabetic mothers: Identification of the most characteristic and most frequent congenital anomalies. Am J Med Genet 51:108, 1994.

19. Sheffield JS, Butler-Koster EL, Casey BM, et al: Maternal diabetes mellitus and infant malformations. Obstet Gynecol 100:925, 2002.

20. Jones KL, Smith DW: Smith's Recognizable Patterns of Human Malformation, 5th ed. Philadelphia, WB Saunders, 1997.

21. Pleet H, Graham JM Jr, Smith DW: Central nervous system and facial defects associated with maternal hyperthermia at four to 14 weeks' gestation. Pediatrics 67:785, 1981.

22. Lenke RR, Levy HL: Maternal phenylketonuria and hyper-phenylalaninemia. An international survey of the outcome of untreated and treated pregnancies. N Engl J Med 303:1202, 1980.

23. Jones KL: The fetal alcohol syndrome. Addict Dis 2:79, 1975.

24. Hoyme HE, Jones KL, Dixon SD, et al: Prenatal cocaine exposure and fetal vascular disruption. Pediatrics 85:743, 1990.

25. Finnell RH, Toloyan S, van Waes M, Kalivas PW: Preliminary evidence for a cocaine-induced embryopathy in mice. Toxicol Appl Pharmacol 103:228, 1990.

26. Abdeljaber M, Nolan BM, Schork MA: Maternal cocaine use during pregnancy: Effect on the newborn infant. Pediatrics 85:630, 1990.

27. Cordero JF: Effect of environmental agents on pregnancy outcomes: Disturbances of prenatal growth and development. Med Clin North Am 74:279, 1990.

28. Shepard TH: Dose response in human teratology. Teratology 65:199, 2002.

29. Skelly AC, Holt VL, Mosca VS, Alderman BW: Talipes equinovarus and maternal smoking: A population-based case-control study in Washington state. Teratology 66:91, 2002.

30. Honein MA, Paulozzi LJ, Moore CA: Family history, maternal smoking, and clubfoot: An indication of a gene-environment interaction. Am J Epidemiol 152:658, 2000.

31. Brent RL, Beckman DA: Angiotensin-converting enzyme inhibitors, an embryopathic class of drugs with unique properties: Information for clinical teratology counselors. Teratology 43:543, 1991.

32. Beckman DA, Brent RL: Teratogenesis: Alcohol, angiotensin-converting-enzyme inhibitors, and cocaine. Curr Opin Obstet Gynecol 2:236, 1990.

33. Feldkamp M, Carey JC: Clinical teratology counseling and consultation case report: Low dose methotrexate exposure in the early weeks of pregnancy. Teratology 47:533, 1993.

34. Holmes LB, Harvey EA, Coull BA, et al: The teratogenicity of anticonvulsant drugs. N Engl J Med 344:1132, 2001.

35. Holmes LB: The teratogenicity of anticonvulsant drugs: A progress report. J Med Genet 39:245, 2002.

36. Herbst AL, Ulfelder H, Poskanzer DC: Adenocarcinoma of the vagina. Association of maternal stilbestrol therapy with tumor appearance in young women. N Engl J Med 284:878, 1971.

37. Stillman RJ: In utero exposure to diethylstilbestrol: Adverse effects on the reproductive tract and reproductive performance and male and female offspring. Am J Obstet Gynecol 142:905, 1982.

38. Lammer EJ, Chen DT, Hoar RM, et al: Retinoic acid embryopathy. N Engl J Med 313:837, 1985.

39. Lammer EJ, Flannery DB, Barr M: Does isotretinoin cause limb reduction defects? Lancet 2:328, 1985.

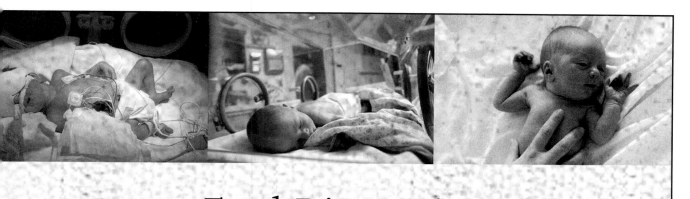

Fetal Diagnosis

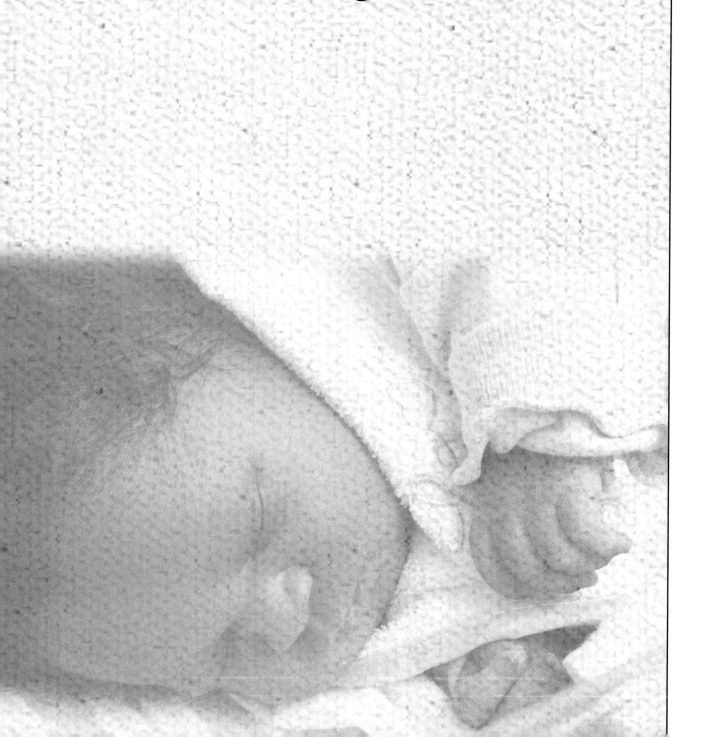

CHAPTER 5

Ultrasound Evaluation of the Uncomplicated Pregnancy

David J. Garry and Reinaldo Figueroa

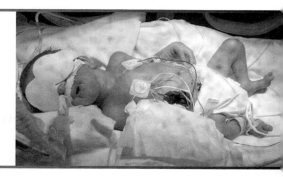

Since the early 1970s, the use of ultrasonography in pregnancy has become a mainstay of care. With continued improvement in technology, ultrasonography is the primary method for determining gestational age and fetal viability and number, assessing fetal anatomic structure, and evaluating the fetal surroundings.

Television commercials have raised public awareness of newer ultrasound advances related to three-dimensional imaging. Ongoing studies of first-trimester fetal evaluation and associated management protocols are pending in the United States and worldwide. Technologic advances, availability of ultrasonography, and commercialization have raised many issues. The concerns include the safety of the examination, timing of the examination, how often ultrasonography should be performed, who should perform the examination, and the accuracy of the examination.

SAFETY

The two major biologic effects of ultrasonography are related to thermal changes. One change results in an increase in temperature secondary to absorption, or sound wave energies lost by conversion into heat, and the other is cavitation, the production and subsequent collapse of small gas-filled bubbles.[1] With modern ultrasound machines, the rise in temperature is minimal (less than 1° C) and remains well below levels of 1.5° to 2° C over a maternal core temperature at which possible developmental effects are seen. The World Federation for Ultrasound in Medicine and Biology stated that an in situ maximum temperature increase that remained less than 1.5° C above physiologic levels may be used without reservation.[2] The organization also stated that fetal in situ temperatures above 41° C for 5 minutes should be considered potentially harmful.[2] Attention to the acoustic output, the duration of the examination, and the maintenance of machine settings as low as can be reasonably achieved is recommended.[3]

In an ultrasound safety review, Reece and associates reported that epidemiologic data in humans revealed no adverse effects with exposure during diagnostic ultrasonography use.[4] In 1984, Stark and colleagues evaluated a cohort of children exposed to ultrasonography in utero and another group that had no exposure.[5] At the ages of 7 to 12 years, children exposed to ultrasonography had an increased risk of dyslexia in compared to the unexposed children. All other aspects were similar in both groups. Multiple subsequent studies of the neurologic aspects of exposure to ultrasonography in utero have demonstrated no clinically relevant data of adverse outcomes.[6] A statistically significant association between left-handedness and ultrasound exposure was noted in some of these epidemiologic studies. The relevance of this association remains controversial.[7]

EQUIPMENT, DOCUMENTATION, AND TERMINOLOGY

Ultrasound evaluations should be conducted with real-time equipment through a transabdominal, translabial, or transvaginal approach. Transducer frequency choice is a balance between penetration and resolution.[8] Most newer transducers are multifrequency, with capabilities to maintain low temperatures.

Adequate documentation is an important part of all obstetric ultrasound examinations and should include a permanent record of the ultrasound images and incorporate the measurements and anatomic findings described in the guidelines. Images should be appropriately labeled with the examination date, patient identification, and, if needed, image orientation. A written report of the ultrasound findings should be included in the mother's medical record. Length of retention of images should be based on the clinical and legal requirements in the locality of the facility performing or interpreting the examination.

Gestational age, or the age of the fetus from conception to the time of evaluation, has been referred to synonymously with menstrual age, which spans the first day of the last menstrual cycle as day one to the time of evaluation. The true age of the conceptus, the fetal age, is the time from point of conception to the time of evaluation and has been arbitrarily determined by subtracting 2 weeks from the menstrual age. The conceptus is called an *embryo* up to the 10th week after the last menstrual period and is referred to as a *fetus* thereafter.

FIRST-TRIMESTER SONOGRAPHY

Early Gestation

The most common reasons for early evaluation of a gestation are vaginal bleeding, fetal viability, and pregnancy location. With high-resolution equipment, a gestational sac can almost always be identified by transabdominal scanning 5 weeks after the last menstrual period and by transvaginal imaging slightly earlier. It may be necessary to differentiate a normal intrauterine gestational sac from either an abnormal intrauterine pregnancy or, more important, from a decidual endometrial cast associated with an ectopic pregnancy. This distinction is often necessary in the time interval before an embryo is expected to be visualized, and the double decidual sac sign can be used in most cases to make this differentiation.[9] The normal gestational sac is an anechoic space surrounded by a hyperechoic rim. This rim is made up of the trophoblastic reaction of the embryo and the decidual reaction of the endometrium. At the implantation site, the hyperechoic rim is a single hyperechoic layer, termed the **chorion frondosum–decidua basalis complex.** On the opposite side, where the sac impinges on a closed endometrium, the hypoechoic line of the endometrial canal interrupts the normal hyperechoic line. This creates the double decidual sac sign and is quite specific for an early intrauterine pregnancy.[10] In contrast, a continuous hyperechoic ring of an abnormal intrauterine pregnancy and of a decidual cast (or pseudogestational sac) of an ectopic pregnancy is composed of only a single hyperechoic decidual layer.[9]

The identification of a yolk sac or embryo within the gestational sac is diagnostic for an intrauterine pregnancy (Fig. 5-1A). The yolk sac is normally the first structure seen and should be visualized transvaginally as a mean gestational sac diameter of 8 mm or, later, transabdominally as a mean gestational sac diameter of 20 mm.[9,11] Several authors have hypothesized that abnormal sonographic yolk sac structure may be predictive of abnormal fetal outcome. In a study of patients between 8 and 12 weeks' menstrual age, yolk sacs 2 mm or smaller and solid hyperechoic yolk sacs were associated with poor fetal outcomes.[12] In another study, yolk sacs with an internal diameter of more than 5.6 mm and subjectively "thin" yolk sac walls were also associated with an abnormal outcome.[13]

The amnion first becomes visible at 5.5 weeks by transvaginal ultrasonography. The developing embryo, termed the **prochordal plate** at this stage of development,

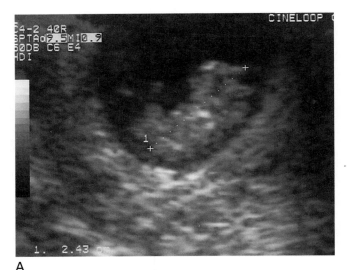

A

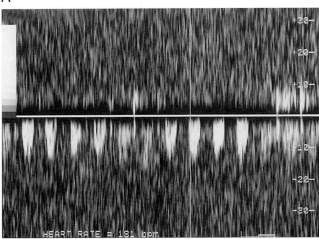

B

Figure 5–1. A, First-trimester sonographic examination demonstrating an embryo. The markers (*dotted line* bounded by plus signs) denote a crown-to-rump length (CRL), the longest axis of the embryo, measuring 2.43 cm, which is consistent with a gestational age of 9 weeks, 0 days. **B,** Pulsed Doppler examination demonstrating a fetal heart rate of 131 beats per minute.

is centered between the amniotic cavity and the secondary yolk sac. This configuration, the "double-bleb" sign, is surrounded by the chorionic sac.[14] The amnion continues to grow, filling the chorionic cavity and typically fusing with the chorion by 14 to 16 weeks. On occasion, fusion is still incomplete at 16 weeks.[15] Separation of the amnion from the chorion is therefore normal before this time.

The embryo is first visualized within the gestational sac at 5 to 6 weeks by transvaginal ultrasonography and at 6 to 7 weeks on transabdominal imaging. In a normal pregnancy, the embryo should be imaged when the average transvaginal sac is larger than 12 mm (5.3 weeks' gestational age) and when the average transabdominal gestational sac size is larger than 27 mm (7.5 weeks' gestational age).[16] For evaluating the long axis of the embryo, the crown-to-rump length (CRL) is measured to determine the gestational age (Table 5-1; see Fig. 5-1A).[17] The accuracy of the CRL measurement is ±5 to 7 days and is a measurement primarily up to 12 weeks; after 12 weeks, fetal flexion and extension make the CRL less reliable.[18]

Real-time observation of embryonic cardiac activity is necessary to determine embryonic life (see Fig. 5-1B).

Table 5–1. Crown-to-Rump Length (CRL) Measurement for Prediction of Gestational Age

Mean CRL (mm)	Gestational Age (Weeks)
6.7	6.3
7.4	6.4
8.0	6.6
8.7	6.7
9.5	6.9
10.2	7.0
11.0	7.1
11.8	7.3
12.6	7.4
13.5	7.6
14.4	7.7
15.3	7.9
16.3	8.0
17.3	8.1
18.3	8.3
19.3	8.4
20.4	8.6
21.5	8.7
22.6	8.9
23.8	9.0
25.0	9.1
26.2	9.3
27.4	9.4
28.7	9.6
30.0	9.7
31.3	9.9
32.7	10.0
34.0	10.1
35.5	10.3
36.9	10.4
38.4	10.6
39.9	10.7
41.4	10.9
43.0	11.0
44.6	11.1
46.2	11.3
47.8	11.4
49.5	11.6
51.2	11.7
52.9	11.9
54.7	12.0
56.5	12.1
58.3	12.3
60.1	12.4
62.0	12.6
63.9	12.7
65.9	12.9

Modified from Robinson HP, Fleming JE: A critical evaluation of sonar "crown-rump length" measurements. Br J Obstet Gynecol 82: 702, 1975.

Cardiac activity should be present in all embryos with a transvaginal CRL larger than 5 mm (≥6.2 weeks' gestational age) and a transabdominal CRL of 9 mm or more (≥6.9 weeks' gestational age).[16] If cardiac activity is not present, embryonic demise can be diagnosed, and an ultrasound follow-up study is unnecessary. In smaller fetuses (<5 mm by transvaginal measurement), failure to detect cardiac activity may not imply abnormality, and a follow-up examination is indicated.[13] Conversely, in smaller embryos, the presence of heart motion may be misleading, because embryonic demise can still occur spontaneously, estimated at a rate of 20% to 25% even in asymptomatic women.[13]

Fetal cardiac rate increases through the first trimester; the earliest activity is seen at 6 to 6.5 weeks' gestational age. The mean heart rate at 6 to 6.5 weeks is 111 ± 14 beats per minute (bpm) and increases to 157 ± 13 bpm at 7.6 to 8 weeks.[19,20] Fetal heart rates below 85 bpm at 6 to 8 weeks' gestation are associated with spontaneous pregnancy loss.[19] The fetal cardiac rate in early gestation has demonstrated an association with aneuploidy (trisomy 21, trisomy 13, and monosomy 45X [Turner syndrome] with tachycardia, and trisomy 18 and triploidy with bradycardia), although the utilization of a single measurement has not proved useful for screening purposes.[21,22]

Multiple Gestations

Twins can be detected sonographically at the time of visualization of the chorion, amnion, yolk sac, or embryo.[23] Three types of twinning can be diagnosed, all types with two embryos and, when identified, two yolk sacs. If each embryo is surrounded by its own chorion and amnion, then a **dichorionic, diamniotic** pregnancy can be identified by a thick interposed membrane (>2 mm) and/or two separate placentas (Fig. 5-2).[24,25] This thick membrane may appear thinner later in the gestation, and this appearance can overlap the next category. In a **monochorionic, diamniotic** twin pregnancy, the two amniotic sacs are contained within one chorionic sac. A thin membrane, composed of only two amnions, separates the embryos.[24,25] **Monochorionic, monoamniotic** twins have one sac surrounded by one amnion and one chorion with no interposed membrane. Monochorionic twins (monoamniotic or diamniotic) share a common placenta, whereas dichorionic twins (even when only one placental site can be identified) do not (Table 5-2).

The numbers of amniotic sacs and chorions of a twin pregnancy have an important bearing on prognosis. Perinatal mortality rates approximate 9% for dichorionic, diamniotic twins and can approach 50% for monochorionic, monoamniotic twins.[24] Because monochorionic twins share a common placenta, they are at risk for vascular placental anastomoses, which can lead to the twin-twin transfusion syndrome and, in rare cases, an acardiac twin anomaly. Monoamniotic twins have the additional risks of cord entanglement (which can cut off blood supply to one or both twins) and conjoined anomalies.

Uterus and Adnexa

The uterus, cervix, and adnexa should be evaluated throughout pregnancy. Size and location of uterine

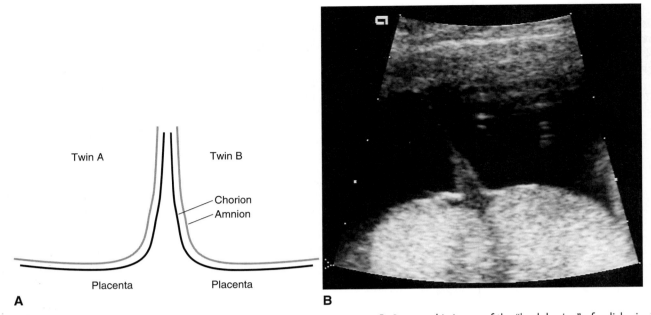

Figure 5–2. A, Schematic representation of dichorionic, diamniotic twin gestation. **B,** Sonographic image of the "lambda sign" of a dichorionic, diamniotic twin gestation.

myomas should be monitored closely, because they often enlarge during pregnancy and occasionally obstruct vaginal delivery or cause fetal malposition.

Adnexal structures are best visualized in the first trimester. The most common is the corpus luteum cyst, which secretes progesterone during the first trimester and supports the pregnancy until the placenta can take over its hormonal function.[26] Corpus luteum cysts tend to be less than 3 cm and resolve by the middle of the second trimester.[27] Lesions that are not typical for a corpus luteum cyst should be evaluated carefully and monitored. Although malignant ovarian neoplasms associated with pregnancy are rare, surgical removal may be necessary for any large adnexal masses, even when benign, because they can lead to torsion, rupture, and distortion of the birth canal.[28,29] If needed, surgery for an adnexal mass is typically performed early in the second trimester.

Prenatal Diagnosis in the First Trimester

First-trimester sonography of the gestation was initially limited to evaluation of gestational age and confirmation of viability. In 1998, Snijders and colleagues reported the measurement of the nuchal translucency, posterior sub-cutaneous edema of the neck region, and related the

results to fetal aneuploidy.[30,31] At a gestational age of 10 to 14 weeks, an increased nuchal translucency revealed 77% of affected aneuploid fetuses, specifically those with trisomy 21, with a false-positive rate of 5%. In addition to sonographic evaluation of the fetus, the use of first-trimester maternal biochemical markers, free β–human chorionic gonadotropin and pregnancy-associated plasma protein A can increase the detection rate of trisomy 21 to 85%, with a 3.3% false-positive rate.[32] An increased nuchal translucency in the euploid fetus has revealed congenital cardiac defects with a prevalence increased from 3%, when the nuchal translucency is 3.5 to 5.4 mm, to 15%, when the measurement is more than 5.5 mm.[33] An increased thickness nuchal translucency has also been related to other chromosomal abnormalities, including trisomy 18, trisomy 13, and monosomy 45X. Several syndromes have been identified through an increased nuchal thickness in the first trimester; they include pentalogy of Cantrell, Noonan syndrome, Jarcho-Levin syndrome, Fanconi anemia, achondrogenesis, and spinal muscle atrophy (Fig. 5-3).[34]

Another independent first-trimester sonographic marker of fetal aneuploidy has been identified. Cicero and associates described absence of the fetal nasal bone at

Table 5–2. Chorionicity and Amnionicity in Twin Gestations

Type	Frequency	No. of Gestational Sacs	No. of Placentas	No. of Amniotic Cavities
DC, DA	88%	2	2	2
MC, DA	11%	1	1	2
MC, MA	1%	1	1	1

DA, diamniotic; DC, dichorionic; MA, monoamniotic; MC, monochorionic.

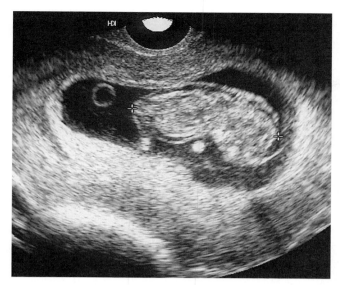

Figure 5–3. Longitudinal transvaginal image of a triploid (69,XXX) hydropic embryo at 11 weeks, 1 day. The patient subsequently miscarried.

11 to 14 weeks' gestation in 73% of fetuses with trisomy 21.[35] The absence or delayed ossification of the nasal bone appears unrelated to nuchal translucency. It therefore has potential to be used in combination with nuchal thickness or biochemical markers for increased detection of trisomy 21 in the first trimester (Fig. 5-4).

SECOND- AND THIRD-TRIMESTER SONOGRAPHY

In the second and third trimesters, the following are routine parts of the ultrasound examination:

1. Documentation of fetal life, number, and presentation.
2. Estimation of amniotic fluid volume.
3. Evaluation of the placenta.

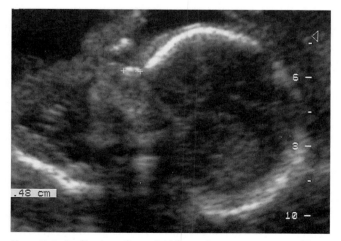

Figure 5–4. Profile view of a euploid fetus, demonstrating a nasal bone (*dotted line* bounded by plus signs) measuring 0.48 cm at the gestational age of 20 weeks.

4. Assessment of fetal size and gestational age.
5. Evaluation of fetal structure in detail.

Fetal Life, Number, and Presentation

As in the first trimester, real-time observation of cardiac activity is used to document fetal life. Abnormal heart rate or rhythm should be reported.[8] The normal fetal heart rate is 140 ± 20 bpm at 20 weeks' gestation and 130 ± 20 bpm near term.[36] Although not fully studied, a heart rate of less than 80 or more than 180 bpm is generally considered abnormal at any time during pregnancy.[37,38] An M-mode tracing may be needed to document the rate, particularly when the rate is abnormal.

It is also important to document fetal number in the second and third trimesters. If two separate placentas are identified, or if the fetuses are of different gender (different external genitalia), then the pregnancy is dichorionic, diamniotic.[27] A single placentation site does not reliably indicate monochorionic status because two separate but apposed dichorionic placentas may appear as one. Membrane analysis is important but may not be exact. Visualization of a membrane excludes a monoamniotic gestation; a thin membrane may be either dichorionic or monochorionic. Nonvisualization of a membrane is not always diagnostic for a monoamniotic gestation, because it is occasionally difficult to visualize a thin monochorionic, diamniotic membrane.[23]

Fetal presentation, or lie, should be recorded. At term, fetal position is a critical factor in obstetric management and can dictate the mode of delivery. The most common fetal presentation is cephalic (head closest to the internal os). Breech presentation and transverse lie, although frequent in the first and second trimesters, are relatively uncommon at term (3% to 4% and 0.25% to 0.5%, respectively).[39]

Amniotic Fluid Volume

Estimation of the amount of amniotic fluid is an important part of the routine obstetric ultrasound examination. Excessive fluid (polyhydramnios or hydramnios) and diminished fluid (oligohydramnios) are occasionally associated with specific structural abnormalities. During most of the first trimester, amniotic fluid is a filtrate of maternal plasma.[40] During the second trimester, multiple fluid pathways develop between the fetus and amniotic fluid.[41] The routes of fluid exchange include the fetal urinary tract, respiratory tract, gastrointestinal tract, and skin, as well as the placenta, membranes, and umbilical cord.[40] The stage of pregnancy must be taken into account because amniotic fluid volume peaks at 32 weeks and then decreases toward term.[42]

Amniotic fluid volume is most frequently assessed by subjective analysis. Such estimates have excellent intraobserver and interobserver agreement when made by experienced technicians.[43] With oligohydramnios, there is subjective crowding of fetal parts, poor definition of fetal interfaces, and obvious lack of fluid.[44] With polyhydramnios, the fetus appears less prominent because of increased amniotic fluid.[45,46] In the dependent position, the fetal anterior abdominal wall, which usually contacts the uterine wall in the third trimester, is separated from that structure by the fluid.[40] Several semiquantitative methods, of which the amniotic fluid index is most frequently used, have been devised to standardize the description and measurement of amniotic fluid.

The Placenta

The placenta is first visualized at 8 to 9 weeks as focal thickening at the site of the chorion frondosum–decidua basalis complex. The sonographic appearance of the placenta is uniformly hyperechoic with a thin, bright chorionic layer separating the placenta from the amniotic fluid. The placenta should be less than 4 cm in thickness.[47] It is separated from the myometrium by a thin hypoechoic layer (basilar plate) that frequently contains blood vessels.

As pregnancy progresses, calcifications are normally deposited in the perivillous and subchorionic spaces and along the basal plate and septa. These deposits become sonographically visible in approximately 60% of women in the third trimester as strong intraplacental echoes without prominent acoustic shadowing.[48-50] Some authors have suggested that their appearance before 30 weeks can be associated with placental dysmaturity and might lead to fetal growth restriction.[51] Others maintain that placental calcification has no proven clinical or pathologic significance.[52,53]

Throughout the second and third trimesters, hypoechoic to anechoic areas may be observed within the subchorionic space, within the space between the chorionic layer and the placenta, or within the placental parenchyma. These subchorionic collections are always benign, representing either flowing or pooled blood. The pooled blood may clot and eventually contracts, leaving subchorionic fibrin deposition.[54] The parenchymal lesions usually represent septated cysts or intervillous blood, which may be flowing or thrombosed,[49,55-57] and both are of no clinical significance. If placental infarctions occur, however, they may have significance if more than 30% of the placental substance is involved. Infarctions are generally not visible sonographically unless complicated by hemorrhage, when they typically appear hypoechoic with thick hyperechoic rims.[55]

The placental attachment (basilar plate) should be examined carefully for possible abruption, especially in the clinical setting of pain and/or vaginal bleeding. Blood collections between the placenta and myometrium may have variable echogenicity, from anechoic to hyperechoic or mixed. If the echogenicity is the same as the placenta, it may falsely give the appearance of placental thickening.[58,59] In all cases, if the abruption is large, blood supply to the fetus may be significantly impaired.

Absence of the basilar plate should also be sought. Although at times this finding may be technical, failure to identify the basilar plate is suggestive of a significant placental abnormality, growth of the placenta either into (accreta or increta) or through (percreta) the myometrium.[60-62]

The placental location and its relationship to the internal cervical os should be documented to rule out or to detect a placenta previa. Placenta previa is excluded if the placenta is completely free of the internal cervical os. If the placenta appears to cover the os during standard transabdominal imaging with a full urinary bladder, the patient should void and the scan should be repeated with one of three techniques: transabdominal, transvaginal, or translabial. A distended bladder may elongate the lower uterine segment and give the false impression that the placenta covers the cervical os.[27] Placenta previa can be subcategorized as partial (marginal) and complete. Marginal previa, when discovered early in the second trimester, frequently resolves, possibly as a result of differential growth of the lower uterine segment. Complete previa does not change.

The cervix should also be evaluated. The normal cervical length with a nondistended bladder is, on average, 2.9 to 3.2 cm; the lower limit of normal is 2.3 to 2.5 cm.[63,64] Foreshortening of the cervix has been described in cervical effacement and in cervical incompetence.[64-66] Widening of the internal os can also occur in cervical incompetence.[65,66]

Fetal Size and Gestational Age

If a first-trimester ultrasound study has not been performed, gestational age can be assessed in the second and third trimesters with the biparietal diameter (BPD) measurement. The BPD is obtained on a transaxial view of the head, perpendicular to the thalami or midbrain, and is measured from the outer hyperechoic calvarial margin, close to the transducer, to the inner calvarial margin, farther from the transducer. An established table is used to correlate the obtained BPD with a gestational age estimate (Fig. 5-5A; Table 5-3).[67] If the fetal head is unusually rounded (brachycephalic) or elongated (dolichocephalic), the BPD can either overestimate or underestimate gestational age. When this occurs, the BPD can be either area-corrected[68] or replaced by a head circumference measurement. A head circumference is obtained either by tracing the perimeter of the calvaria with a map reader or by using the formula for the circumference of a circle. A standard head circumference table can then be consulted (Table 5-4).[69] The accuracy of the gestational age estimate obtained from the corrected BPD and head circumference in the second trimester (up to 20 weeks) is ±5 to 7 days, similar to the first-trimester CRL.[70-72] In the third trimester, particularly after 30 weeks, the BPD accuracy decreases to ±2 weeks and approaches ±4 weeks by term.[70]

The femur length is a linear measurement of the ossified shaft (diaphysis) of the femur (Fig. 5-6). The slight medial curvature of the bone is disregarded, and the epiphyseal cartilage is not included in the measurement.[73] The femur length is an indicator of growth and can be used to establish gestational age. The femur length is particularly helpful in the third trimester, in which accuracy is similar to the BPD (Table 5-5), and femur length is especially helpful in cases in which the BPD is considered unreliable.[70,74] The proportionality of the femur length to the BPD should also be evaluated and can aid in the detection of a significant skeletal dysplasia.[18,75] Fetuses with these anomalies tend to have femurs that are persistently shortened and are more than 4 mm shorter than the lower limit for the BPD (±2 SD).[76]

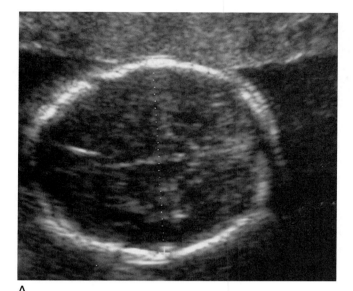

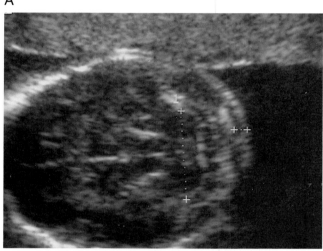

Figure 5–5. A, Transthalamic view of the fetal head, demonstrating the biparietal measurement with the hypoechoic thalami and cavum septi pellucidi visualized during a 20-week anatomic survey. **B,** Transcerebellar view of the fetal head, demonstrating the dumbbell-shaped cerebellum measuring 20.5 mm and the nuchal thickness measuring 3 mm.

The fetal abdomen is measured at the level of the liver, with the umbilical portion of the left portal vein imaged entirely within the liver and equidistant from the abdominal side walls. The stomach is included in this image. The abdominal circumference can be generated in the same way as a head circumference: from either a map reader or a formula for the circumference of a circle (Fig. 5-7).[77] Abdominal measurements are not as accurate as the BPD in establishing gestational age. Instead, the ratio of the head circumference to abdominal circumference (Table 5-6)[77] can be useful in evaluating growth disturbances. Normally, the head is larger than the body in the second and early third trimesters; after 32 weeks, this relationship reverses.[18]

During follow-up sonographic examinations, the gestational age established by the earliest sonographic examination that usually correlates with the last menstrual period (LMP) is considered the baseline. On any subsequent study, interval growth is determined by evaluating the number of weeks elapsed in comparison with the gestational age established by the first study.[8] Interval fetal growth can assist in the determination of fetal macrosomia or intrauterine growth restriction (IUGR). The BPD is the most studied parameter for evaluating longitudinal interval growth.[78]

Estimation of fetal weight can also be a part of fetal growth assessment. Tables that incorporate combinations of head, body, and femur size are available.[79,80] The utility of fetal weight, however, is limited. Fetal weight by itself has a sizable variation (±10%) and does not reflect asymmetric growth. However, if the gestational age has been clearly established (usually by an earlier ultrasound study), the calculated weight can be compared with the expected weight (Table 5-7).[81] If the gestational age is not definitely known, the value of the calculated weight is limited.

Twin Growth

The gestational age of a twin pregnancy is based on the initial sonographic examination, either an average of the two or the age of the larger twin (if there is no discordance in growth). The following is known about twin gestations: (1) the same measurement tables used in the evaluation of singleton pregnancies can be used for twin gestations; (2) normal twin growth parallels singleton growth until at least 30 weeks; and (3) growth decreases later in pregnancy but does not fall below the lower 10th percentile of normal singleton pregnancies.[82]

Twin discordance can be analyzed by comparison of the BPDs, abdominal circumferences, or fetal weights.[83-86] An abdominal circumference difference of at least 20 mm appears to be a more reliable predictor of discordance than a BPD difference of 5 mm. A difference of at least 20% in the estimated fetal weights similarly appears to be a direct way of assessing prenatal discordance. Any of these discrepancies is more likely to be of clinical significance when accompanied by discrepant amniotic sac fluid volumes.

It is important to realize that fetuses tend to crowd each other as they grow, often distorting the head and body measurements.[87] Fetal weight, which reflects composite fetal measurements, can therefore also vary widely. When head and body measurements are discrepant, the fetal femurs should be compared. The femur lengths cannot be distorted by crowding and, if still within 5 mm of each other, most likely reflect normal twin growth.[88]

SECOND- AND THIRD-TRIMESTER FETAL ANATOMY

The anatomy of the fetus should be evaluated systematically to ensure a complete survey of the major fetal organs and structures. The position of the fetus must be assessed with precision for a successful evaluation of the anatomy. The initial evaluation is performed in the transaxial plane, because better images are generally obtained.

Table 5–3. Composite Biparietal Diameters

Biparietal Diameter (mm)	Gestational Age (Weeks)		Biparietal Diameter (mm)	Gestational Age (Weeks)	
	Mean*	Range (90% Variation)†		Mean*	Range (90% Variation)†
20	12.0	12.0	60	23.8	22.3-25.5
21	12.0	12.0	61	24.2	22.6-25.8
22	12.7	12.2-13.2	62	24.6	23.1-26.1
23	13.0	12.4-13.6	63	24.9	23.4-26.4
24	13.2	12.6-13.8	64	25.3	23.8-26.8
25	13.5	12.9-14.1	65	25.6	24.1-27.1
26	13.7	13.1-14.3	66	26.0	24.5-27.5
27	14.0	13.4-14.6	67	26.4	25.0-27.8
28	14.3	13.6-15.0	68	26.7	25.3-28.1
29	14.5	13.9-15.2	69	27.1	25.8-28.4
30	14.8	14.1-15.5	70	27.5	26.3-28.7
31	15.1	14.3-15.9	71	27.9	26.7-29.1
32	15.3	14.5-16.1	72	28.3	27.2-29.4
33	15.6	14.7-16.5	73	28.7	27.6-29.8
34	15.9	15.0-16.8	74	29.1	28.1-30.1
35	16.2	15.2-17.2	75	29.5	28.5-30.5
36	16.4	15.4-17.4	76	30.0	29.0-31.0
37	16.7	15.6-17.8	77	30.3	29.2-31.4
38	17.0	15.9-18.1	78	30.8	29.6-32.0
39	17.3	16.1-18.5	79	31.1	29.9-32.5
40	17.6	16.4-18.8	80	31.6	30.2-33.0
41	17.9	16.5-19.3	81	32.1	30.7-33.5
42	18.1	16.6-19.8	82	32.6	31.2-34.0
43	18.4	16.8-20.2	83	33.0	31.5-34.5
44	18.8	16.9-20.7	84	33.4	31.9-35.1
45	19.1	17.0-21.2	85	34.0	32.3-35.7
46	19.4	17.4-21.4	86	34.3	32.8-36.2
47	19.7	17.8-21.6	87	35.0	33.4-36.6
48	20.0	18.2-21.8	88	35.4	33.9-37.1
49	20.3	18.6-22.0	89	36.1	34.6-37.6
50	20.6	19.0-22.2	90	36.6	35.1-38.1
51	20.9	19.3-22.5	91	37.2	35.9-38.5
52	21.2	19.5-22.9	92	37.8	36.7-38.9
53	21.5	19.8-23.2	93	38.8	37.3-39.3
54	21.9	20.1-23.7	94	39.0	37.9-40.1
55	22.2	20.4-24.0	95	39.7	38.5-40.9
56	22.5	20.7-24.3	96	40.6	39.1-41.5
57	22.8	21.1-24.5	97	41.0	39.9-42.1
58	23.2	21.5-24.9	98	41.8	40.5-43.1
59	23.5	21.9-25.1			

*From weighted least mean square fit equation: $Y + -3.45701 + 0.50157x - 0.00441x^2$.

†For each biparietal diamter, 90% of gestational age data points fell within this range.

From Kurtz AB, Wapner RJ, Kurtz RJ, et al: Analysis of biparietal diameter as an accurate indicator of gestational age. J Clin Ultrasound 8:319, 1980.

Additional views in sagittal, coronal, and oblique planes can be obtained to supplement the evaluation, after the anatomic structures being studied are considered.

Cranial Anatomy

The fetal head is clearly identified from the beginning of the second trimester until term. Both the hyperechoic calvaria and the intracranial anatomy should always be seen. Three axial levels are needed to document the key intracranial structures: transthalamic, transventricular, and transcerebellar. The transthalamic view is the same as that used for the BPD and head circumference (see Fig. 5-5A) measurements. The cavum septi pellucidi is visualized as an anterior midline anechoic structure separating the frontal horns of the lateral ventricles. Posterior to the cavum septi pellucidi, the hypoechoic thalami are separated in the midline by the third ventricle. The presence of the cavum septi pellucidum excludes midline malformations such as all forms of holoprosencephaly and complete agenesis of the corpus callosum.[89]

Table 5–4. Head Circumference Measurements

Head Circumference (mm)	Gestational Age (Weeks)		Head Circumference (mm)	Gestational Age (Weeks)	
	Predicted Mean Values	95% Confidence Limits		Predicted Mean Values	95% Confidence Limits
80	13.4	12.1-14.7	225	24.4	22.1-26.7
85	13.7	12.4-15.0	230	24.9	22.6-27.2
90	14.0	12.7-15.3	235	25.4	23.1-27.7
95	14.3	13.0-15.6	240	25.9	23.6-28.2
100	14.6	13.3-15.9	245	26.4	24.1-28.7
105	15.0	13.7-16.3	250	26.9	24.6-29.2
110	15.3	14.0-16.6	255	27.5	25.2-29.8
115	15.6	14.3-16.9	260	28.0	25.7-30.3
120	15.9	14.6-17.2	265	28.1	25.8-30.4
125	16.3	15.0-17.6	270	29.2	26.9-31.5
130	16.6	15.3-17.9	275	29.8	27.5-32.1
135	17.0	15.7-18.3	280	30.3	27.6-33.0
140	17.3	16.0-18.6	285	31.0	28.3-33.7
145	17.7	16.4-19.0	290	31.6	28.9-34.3
150	18.1	16.5-19.7	295	32.2	29.5-34.8
155	18.4	16.8-20.0	300	32.8	30.1-35.5
160	18.8	17.2-20.4	305	33.5	30.7-36.2
165	19.2	17.6-20.8	310	34.2	31.5-36.9
170	19.6	18.0-21.2	315	34.9	32.2-37.6
175	20.0	18.4-21.6	320	35.5	32.8-38.2
180	20.4	18.8-22.0	325	36.3	32.9-39.7
185	20.8	19.2-22.4	330	37.0	33.6-40.4
190	21.2	19.8-22.8	335	37.7	34.3-41.1
195	21.6	20.0-23.2	340	38.5	35.1-41.9
200	22.1	20.5-23.7	345	39.2	35.8-42.6
205	22.5	20.9-24.1	350	40.0	36.6-43.4
210	23.0	21.4-24.6	355	40.8	37.4-44.2
215	23.4	21.8-25.0	360	41.6	38.2-45.0
220	23.9	22.3-25.5			

From Hadlock FP, Deter RL, Harrist RB, et al: Fetal head circumference: Relation to menstrual age. AJR Am J Roentgenol 138:649,1982.

The transventricular view is at the level above the transthalamic view and identifies the bodies of the lateral ventricles, including the atria. The normal hyperechoic choroid plexus fills more than 60% of the atrium.[90] Because of the normal reverberation artifact on the side closer to the transducer, only the far-sided atrium is usually seen. Because the atria are the most sensitive to the development of hydrocephalus, the atrial measurement allows excellent assessment of the lateral ventricular size.[91] This measurement, obtained with the cursors placed at the junction of the ventricular wall and the ventricular lumen, is easily reproducible and remains constant from 15 to 35 weeks. Early investigators obtained an average measurement of 7.6 ± 0.6 mm, with an upper limit of normal of 10 mm (at 4 SD); others obtained smaller mean diameters but agreed that the upper limit of 10 mm was clinically significant.[92-95] The lateral ventricles do not change in size as the brain grows throughout gestation. The ratio of the lateral ventricular width to the intracranial hemispheric width progressively decreases throughout pregnancy, with the upper limits of normal (±2 SD) measuring 0.74 at 15 weeks, 0.53 at 21 weeks,

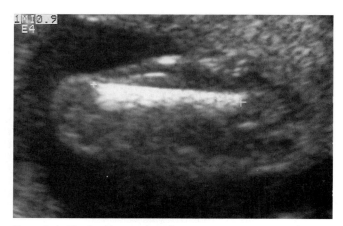

Figure 5–6. The fetal hyperechoic femur measuring 31.8 mm during a 20-week anatomic survey. The femur length is a linear measurement of the ossified shaft (diaphysis) of the femur.

Table 5–5. Femur and Humerus Measurements

Bone Length (mm)	Femur		Humerus	
	Predicted Mean Value	Range, 5th to 95th Percentiles	Predicted Mean Value	Range, 5th to 95th Percentiles
	Gestational Age (Weeks)			
10	12.6	10.4-14.9	12.6	9.9-15.3
11	12.9	10.7-15.1	12.9	10.1-15.6
12	13.3	11.1-15.6	13.1	10.4-15.9
13	13.6	11.4-15.9	13.6	10.9-16.1
14	13.9	11.7-16.1	13.9	11.1-16.6
15	14.1	12.0-16.4	14.1	11.4-16.9
16	14.6	12.4-16.9	14.6	11.9-17.3
17	14.9	12.7-17.1	14.9	12.1-17.6
18	15.1	13.0-17.4	15.1	12.6-18.0
19	15.6	13.4-17.9	15.6	12.9-18.3
20	15.9	13.7-18.1	15.9	13.1-18.7
21	16.3	14.1-18.6	16.3	13.6-19.1
22	16.6	14.4-18.9	16.7	13.9-19.4
23	16.9	14.7-19.1	17.1	14.3-19.9
24	17.3	15.1-19.6	17.4	14.7-20.1
25	17.6	15.4-19.9	17.9	15.1-20.6
26	18.0	15.9-20.1	18.1	15.6-21.0
27	18.3	16.1-20.6	18.6	15.9-21.4
28	18.7	16.6-20.9	19.0	16.3-21.9
29	19.0	16.9-21.1	19.4	16.7-22.1
30	19.4	17.1-21.6	19.9	17.1-22.6
31	19.9	17.6-22.0	20.3	17.6-23.0
32	20.1	17.9-22.3	20.7	18.0-23.6
33	20.6	18.3-22.7	21.1	18.4-23.9
34	20.9	18.7-23.1	21.6	18.9-24.3
35	21.1	19.0-23.4	22.0	19.3-24.9
36	21.6	19.4-23.9	22.6	19.7-25.1
37	22.0	19.9-24.1	22.9	20.1-25.7
38	22.4	20.1-24.6	23.4	20.6-26.1
39	22.7	20.6-24.9	23.9	21.1-26.6
40	23.1	20.9-25.3	24.3	21.6-27.1
41	23.6	21.3-25.7	24.9	22.0-27.6
42	23.9	21.7-26.1	25.3	22.6-28.0
43	24.3	22.1-26.6	25.7	23.0-28.6
44	24.7	22.6-26.9	26.1	23.6-29.0
45	25.0	22.9-27.1	26.7	24.0-29.6
46	25.4	23.1-27.6	27.1	24.6-30.0
47	25.9	23.6-28.0	27.7	25.0-30.6
48	26.1	24.0-28.4	28.1	25.6-31.0
49	26.6	24.4-28.9	28.9	26.0-31.6
50	27.0	24.9-29.1	29.3	26.6-32.0
51	27.4	25.1-29.6	29.9	27.1-32.6
52	27.9	25.6-30.0	30.3	27.6-33.1
53	28.1	26.0-30.4	30.9	28.1-33.6
54	28.6	26.4-30.9	31.4	28.7-34.1
55	29.1	26.9-31.3	32.0	29.1-34.7
56	29.6	27.2-31.7	32.6	29.9-35.3
57	29.9	27.7-32.1	33.1	30.3-35.9
58	30.3	28.1-32.6	33.6	30.9-36.4
59	30.7	28.6-32.9	34.1	31.4-36.9
60	31.1	28.9-33.3	34.9	32.0-37.6
61	31.6	29.4-33.9	35.3	32.6-38.1
62	32.0	29.9-34.1	35.9	33.1-38.7
63	32.4	30.1-34.6	36.6	33.9-39.3
64	32.9	30.7-35.1	37.1	34.4-39.9
65	33.4	31.1-35.6	37.7	35.0-40.6
66	33.7	31.6-35.9	38.3	35.6-41.1
67	34.1	32.0-36.4	38.9	36.1-41.7

From Merz E, Kim-Kern M, Pehl S: Ultrasonic measuration of fetal limb bones in the second and third trimesters. J Clin Ultrasound 15:175, 1987.

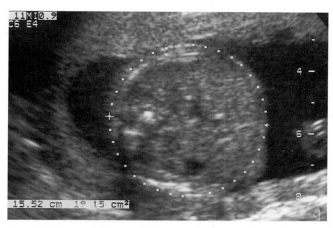

Figure 5–7. Transaxial image of the upper abdomen taken at the area of the liver; the umbilical portion of the left portal vein and the fetal hypoechoic fluid-filled stomach are seen. *Dotted lines* surrounding the outer margins of the abdominal soft tissues are used to calculate the abdominal circumference.

and 0.33 at term.[27,96,97] This ratio has been used by some investigators to evaluate ventriculomegaly but has been found to be inaccurate and has been largely abandoned.[98,99]

The third axial view, the transcerebellar, is obtained by angling the transducer posteriorly from the transthalamic level (see Fig. 5-5B). The posterior fossa, including the cerebellum, cisterna magna, and the posterior nuchal skin, can be imaged in this way. The normal cerebellum

Table 5–6. Head-Abdomen Circumference Ratios

	Ratio of Head Circumference/ Abdominal Circumference	
Gestational Age (Weeks)	Mean	Range, 5th to 95th Percentiles
13-14	1.23	1.14-1.31
15-16	1.22	1.05-1.39
17-18	1.18	1.07-1.29
19-20	1.18	1.09-1.39
21-22	1.15	1.06-1.25
23-24	1.13	1.05-1.21
25-26	1.13	1.04-1.22
27-28	1.13	1.05-1.21
29-30	1.10	0.99-1.21
31-32	1.07	0.96-1.17
33-34	1.04	0.96-1.11
35-36	1.02	0.93-1.11
37-38	0.98	0.92-1.05
39-40	0.97	0.87-1.06
41-42	0.96	0.93-1.00

From Campbell S, Thoms A: Ultrasound measurement of the fetal head to adbomen circumference in the assessment of growth retardation. Br J Obstet Gynaecol 84:165, 1977.

is identified by its hyperechoic vermis in the midline and prominent hypoechoic bilateral hemispheres. The transaxial cerebellar measurement correlates throughout gestation with the BPD and fetal age. The depth of the cisterna magna is measured in the midline from the posterior margin of the cerebellar vermis to the inner surface of the occipital bone. This measurement has a mean of 5 mm and should not exceed 10 mm.[100]

Many major cranial and spinal abnormalities can be detected from the finding of an abnormally large posterior fossa. These anomalies are usually associated with Dandy-Walker malformations and include cisterna magna enlargement and cerebellar hypoplasia.[101] Abnormalities that efface the cisterna magna, particularly the Arnold-Chiari II malformation, can also be detected. This malformation is associated with almost all open spinal meningoceles and myelomeningoceles.[102] In 72% of cases of open neural tube defects, the cerebellum is displaced posteriorly and downward into a characteristic "banana" shape, effacing the cisterna magna.[101] The fetal head may also assume a "lemon" shape, which appears as a biconcavity or scalloping of the frontal bones at the level of the BPD measurement.[96] The mechanism for this "lemon" shape is not well understood and is sometimes seen in normal fetuses or in other anomalies of the fetal head. Both the "banana" and "lemon" signs are best seen before 24 weeks in 98% of cases. After 24 weeks, both these signs are less frequently identified.[101,103]

The posterior fossa view is also helpful in excluding occipital encephaloceles and cystic hygromas. Nuchal skin thickness can also be evaluated in the second trimester. The normal thickness should not exceed 6 mm between 15 and 20 weeks' gestational age. Increased skin thickness is highly suggestive of chromosomal abnormalities, especially trisomy 21.[73,104,105]

The standard cranial imaging planes are usually obtained by the routine transabdominal study. In situations in which the fetal head is deep in the maternal pelvis, however, these imaging planes can be difficult to obtain, and transvaginal scanning may be useful.[106,107]

Spinal Anatomy

Each vertebral level develops from three ossification centers: The single anterior center forms the vertebral body, and the two posterior centers form the neural arches.[108] Careful analysis of all three centers at each vertebral level is necessary to detect spina bifida and vertebral segmentation anomalies. Assessment of the integrity of the overlying posterior soft tissues is also important, inasmuch as they are never normal in an open meningocele or myelomeningocele.

Visualization of the spine in the transaxial plane at each vertebral level is the best projection for evaluating the relationship of the three ossification centers and the overlying soft tissues (Fig. 5-8). If suboptimal, these views can be supplemented with midline sagittal and coronal images. The sagittal view evaluates the anterior center and overlying soft tissues, and the coronal image identifies both posterior centers.[27] The parasagittal view shows the normal curvature of the spine and its tapering toward the sacrum by identifying the anterior center and one of

Table 5–7. Predicted Fetal Weight Percentiles throughout Pregnancy

Gestational Age (Weeks since Last Menstruation)	Smoothed Percentiles				
	10	25	50	75	90
8	—	—	6.1	—	—
9	—	—	7.3	—	—
10	—	—	8.1	—	—
11	—	—	11.9	—	—
12	—	11.1	21.1	34.1	—
13	—	22.5	35.3	55.4	—
14	—	34.5	51.4	76.8	—
15	—	51.0	76.7	108	—
16	—	79.8	117	151	—
17	—	125	166	212	—
18	—	172	220	298	—
19	—	217	283	394	—
20	—	255	325	460	—
21	280	330	410	570	860
22	320	410	480	630	920
23	370	460	550	690	990
24	420	530	640	780	1080
25	490	630	740	890	1180
26	570	730	860	1020	1320
27	660	840	990	1160	1470
28	770	980	1150	1350	1660
29	890	1100	1310	1530	1890
30	1030	1260	1460	1710	2100
31	1180	1410	1630	1880	2290
32	1310	1570	1810	2090	2500
33	1480	1720	2010	2280	2690
34	1670	1910	2220	2510	2880
35	1870	2130	2430	2730	3090
36	2190	2470	2650	2950	3290
37	2310	2580	2870	3160	3470
38	2510	2770	3030	3320	3610
39	2680	2910	3170	3470	3750
40	2750	3010	3280	3590	3870
41	2800	3070	3360	3680	3980
42	2830	3110	3410	3740	4060
43	2840	3110	3420	3780	4100
44	2790	3050	3390	3770	4110

From Brenner WE, Edelman D, Hendricks CH: A standard of fetal growth for the United States of America. Am J Obstet Gynecol 126:555, 1976.

the posterior centers. On occasion, transvaginal scanning may be helpful for examining portions of the spine closest to the cervix.[109]

Most spinal defects occur in the lumbar and sacral regions. By 16 weeks, the spine, although clearly identified, is fully ossified only to the L5 level. Spinal ossification continues in a cephalocaudal direction from L5 to S5, with each additional vertebral level ossifying every 2 to 3 weeks.[110] Therefore, sacral abnormalities may not be appreciated at 16 to 20 weeks, and correlation with the previously discussed intracranial abnormalities associated with the Arnold-Chiari II malformation could be of diagnostic value.

Face and Neck

The basic facial structure is complete by 10 weeks, and the face can be visualized properly as early as 16 weeks. The fetal face is scanned in three planes: transaxial, coronal, and sagittal. The transaxial plane should demonstrate the orbits. Standard graphs for ocular biometry are available, and orbital measurements can be compared.[111] Various coronal planes should demonstrate the anterior cranial fossa, the bony orbits and forehead, the upper lip, and the nostrils. The sagittal, or profile, view gives a global view of the face and the forehead, and the nasal bone and jaw can be visualized. In scans of the fetal face, the orbits

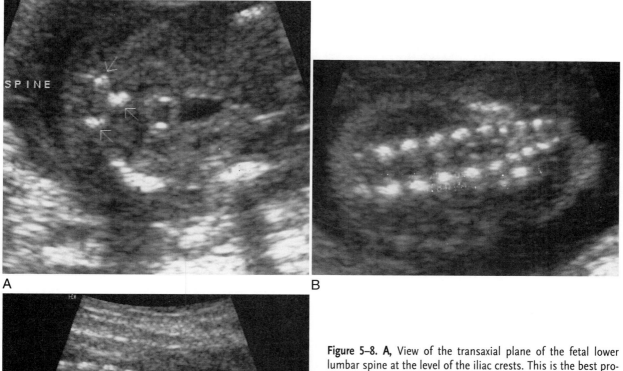

A   B

C

Figure 5–8. A, View of the transaxial plane of the fetal lower lumbar spine at the level of the iliac crests. This is the best projection for evaluating the relationship of the three ossification centers *(arrows)* and the overlying soft tissues. **B,** View of the normal 20-week lower lumbosacral spine, showing the alignment of the vertebral ossification centers. **C,** Normal midline sagittal view of the lumbosacral spine. The *arrow* points to the overlying posterior normal soft tissue. In between, a line of hyperechoic structures represents some of the posterior elements, partially identified in this view.

should be of equal size and without hypertelorism or hypotelorism.[111a] The anechoic lenses should be visualized to determine whether congenital cataracts are present. Both lips should be visualized in both coronal and transaxial planes to look for cleft lip with or without cleft palate, the most common congenital facial malformation (Fig. 5-9).[112,113] The mandible should be seen in profile view. Although, at times, cleft lip and micrognathia may be apparent, they may be difficult to diagnose.[90,114] Cleft palate may go unrecognized if it is not associated with cleft lip.

The neck is usually examined when the head and spine are evaluated. Most neck abnormalities are cystic or solid masses. Posterior masses may be cystic hygromas[115-117] or occipital encephaloceles; anterior masses are usually teratomas.

Cardiac and Chest Anatomy

The obstetric guidelines recommend a four-chamber view of the heart.[8] This can be obtained in 95% of fetuses from 18 weeks to term in a transaxial view of the chest immediately cephalad to the liver (the plane of section for

the abdominal measurements) and above the level of the diaphragm.[118] The four-chamber view should show the right and left ventricles, the interventricular septum, the right and left atria, the interatrial septum and foramen ovale, and the atrioventricular valves. Six anatomic points should be analyzed in this view: cardiac position; cardiac size in relation to the thorax; cardiac atrial and ventricular sizes; appearance of the atrial and ventricular septa; position of the atrioventricular valves; and structure of the myocardium, endocardium, and pericardium.[119]

To determine cardiac position, the position of the fetus must first be identified. Orientation is obtained by using the fetal lie and the position of the fetal spine to establish the right and left sides of the fetus. The heart is expected to be positioned primarily within the left hemithorax, with the cardiac apex pointed at a 45-degree angle toward the left anterior chest wall and with the right ventricular chamber closest to the chest wall.[120] The stomach should be on the left side, concordant with the cardiac apex, and the surrounding lungs should have homogeneous midrange echogenicity.[121]

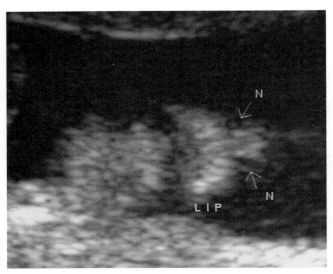

Figure 5–9. Sonographic evaluation of the fetal facial anatomy demonstrating the complete upper lip with the nares *(arrows)*.

Deviation of the heart from its normal position suggests one of the following: the presence of a noncardiac thoracic lesion, a chest wall abnormality, or a situs abnormality. Noncardiac thoracic lesions displace the heart within the thoracic cavity and change the normal surrounding pulmonary echogenicity. These processes include pleural effusions, foregut malformations, abnormalities of pulmonary development (cystic adenomatoid malformation), diaphragmatic hernias, and rare intrathoracic tumors.[121] A chest wall defect is present when the heart is detected outside of the normal thoracic cavity. This anomaly can occur in ectopia cordis or as part of the pentalogy of Cantrell; the former is usually fatal, and the latter includes additional cardiac anomalies. Situs abnormalities may be the result of specific syndromes such as asplenia (bilateral right-sidedness) or polysplenia (bilateral left-sidedness); both are frequently associated with complex congenital heart disease.

The outer diameter of the heart and the fetal thorax increase in size from 16 to 40 weeks.[122-124] The transverse diameter of the heart is measured at the level of the atrioventricular valves in end diastole, whereas the thoracic circumference is measured at the level of the four-chamber view. The ratio of the heart diameter to the thoracic circumference normally remains unchanged at 0.14 throughout the second and third trimesters.[125] The ratio of the thoracic circumference to other biometric parameters (abdominal circumference, head circumference, biparietal diameter, and femur length) also remains constant from 16 to 40 weeks.[122,124-126] Because these chest ratios are independent of gestational age, they may be predictive of chest narrowing with pulmonary hypoplasia, a frequent cause of death in certain skeletal dysplasias and severe early oligohydramnios.

In the four-chamber view, the two ventricles are approximately equal in size throughout the second and third trimesters (Fig. 5-10).[123] The more common cardiac abnormality associated with discrepancy in ventricular

size is hypoplasia of the right or left ventricle.[119,127] The four-chamber view can also detect atrial, atrioventricular, or ventricular septal defects. In the normal fetus, the foramen ovale, a natural atrial septal defect, is patent. Its flap can be identified opening into the left atrium, the most posteriorly situated cardiac chamber. Small septal defects of all types are frequently not appreciated, even with careful scanning, and color-flow Doppler imaging may help in the detection of these smaller defects. Because the leaflets of the tricuspid valve normally insert slightly lower in the ventricular septum and lateral wall than do the mitral valve leaflets, abnormal valve position and appearance are readily detected. This can be seen in Ebstein anomaly with resultant enlargement of the right atrium and in endocardial cushion defects.[118]

Abnormalities of the myocardium and endocardium are rare but have been detected in certain cardiomyopathies such as endocardial fibroelastosis.[128] In rare cases, masses such as rhabdomyomas can arise from the myocardium and be visualized within a ventricle or atrium. A pericardial effusion can develop in a congenital heart disorder or in systemic disorders that result in fetal hydrops.[129]

The four-chamber view detects only 63% of cardiac anomalies.[130] Subtle intracardiac abnormalities and anomalies involving the great vessels are not appreciated. For a more complete analysis, additional left and right outflow tract views have been suggested; they have an increased diagnostic accuracy of 83%.[131-133] The outflow tract views assess the continuity of the aorta with the ventricular septum and the criss-crossing of the aorta and pulmonary artery in their initial course. These views are typically obtained by angling the transducer toward the fetal head from a four-chamber view when the interventricular

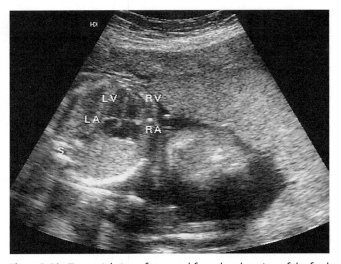

Figure 5–10. Transaxial view of a normal four-chamber view of the fetal heart at approximately 20 weeks. The right atrium (RA) and the right ventricle (RV) are identified with the right ventricular chamber closest to the anterior chest wall. On the left side of the heart, the left atrium (LA) and the left ventricle (LV) are identified closest to the fetal spine (S). The normal foramen ovale, the intact interventricular septum, and the mitral valve are seen.

septum is tangential to the ultrasound beam. When the interventricular septum is perpendicular to the ultrasound beam, these views are obtained by rotating the transducer from the four-chamber view until the aortic outflow tract is observed leaving the left ventricle (the right pulmonary artery is perpendicular to the aorta). Then the transducer is angled until the main pulmonary artery is identified perpendicular to the ascending aorta.

Abdominal and Pelvic Anatomy

The stomach appears as an anechoic structure in the left upper quadrant on the standard transaxial view of the upper abdomen. This is the same view that is used for abdominal measurements. The stomach can be identified after 11 weeks, when the fetus is capable of swallowing sufficient amounts of amniotic fluid.[134] By 14 weeks, the stomach should normally be identified within the time period of a routine examination (approximately 20 minutes). Stomach filling and emptying are variable; therefore, in a small percentage of normal fetuses, the stomach is not visualized. These fetuses require a follow-up study several hours to days later, if scanned between 14 and 19 weeks.[135] By 19 weeks, however, nonvisualization of the stomach or visualization of a very small stomach (less than 1 cm) that does not change size on two scans performed 30 to 60 minutes apart has been associated with an abnormal outcome in almost all cases.[82,135,136] The dynamic structure of the fetal stomach and the intraobserver variability have made it difficult to obtain objective measurements of the fetal stomach size.[137]

Disorders that decrease or prevent fetal swallowing of amniotic fluid cause the nonvisualization of the stomach. These disorders include esophageal atresia (with or without tracheoesophageal fistula), diaphragmatic hernia, facial cleft, significant central nervous system disorders, and severe oligohydramnios from nongastrointestinal causes.[138] Concomitant polyhydramnios can be the result of decreased fetal swallowing, and the likelihood that a nonvisualized stomach represents a structural abnormality (such as esophageal atresia) increases with the severity of polyhydramnios.[138] In contrast, a persistently prominent stomach and duodenum with polyhydramnios strongly suggests an obstruction at the level of the duodenum. Duodenal atresia, associated in some cases with trisomy 21, is the cause in approximately 40% of cases.

The kidneys are routinely imaged in the transaxial plane on either side of the spine, immediately caudad to the liver and spleen. The kidneys can first be visualized at 12 to 14 weeks as bilateral hypoechoic paravertebral structures, but structures within the kidneys cannot be identified until after 16 weeks.[139] As gestation progresses, the renal sinus and the perinephric fat defining the renal margin become more hyperechoic, allowing better visualization of the renal parenchyma.[140] After 30 weeks' gestation, detailed renal anatomy, including the fetal lobulations and medullary pyramids, can often be identified (Fig. 5-11).[141]

The normally hyperechoic central renal collecting system may dilate and be visualized as an anechoic structure situated medial to the kidney. Dilation of this central renal collecting system is termed **pyelectasis.**

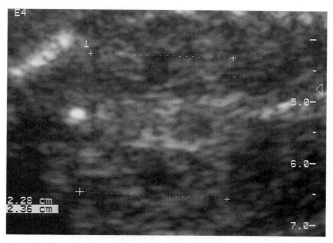

Figure 5–11. Longitudinal view of normal fetal kidneys at approximately 20 weeks. The hyperechoic rim surrounding the kidneys is the normal perinephric fat, which becomes more prominent in the third trimester. The central collecting system of both kidneys is a hypoechoic region and is seen on either side of the spine.

The renal pelvis should be measured in its anteroposterior diameter. In the third trimester, pyelectasis of 5 to 10 mm is often caused by normal bladder reflux and does not represent an obstructive uropathy unless additional calyectasis is identified. When the measurement is greater than 7 mm, a follow-up examination is suggested, frequently postnatally. A measurement of greater than 10 mm indicates urinary obstruction.[142] Mild pyelectasis, less than 5 mm, is generally not considered significant. A measurement of 4 mm or greater before 20 weeks may represent early hydronephrosis and may be a subtle sonographic marker in the detection of fetal aneuploidy, specifically trisomy 21.[143]

A linear relationship exists between renal size and gestational age. Tables are available for renal length, width, and anteroposterior dimension in the second and third trimesters. There are relatively few instances, however, when exact renal measurements are needed. Instead, a ratio of the renal to abdominal circumference at the same level usually suffices, with the ratio remaining constant at 0.27 to 0.30 throughout the second and third trimesters.[144] A bilateral increase in this ratio can diagnose nephromegaly, such as that seen in infantile polycystic kidney disease.

The fetal urinary bladder may be visualized late in the first trimester, shortly after the commencement of fetal urine production, and should be routinely identified by 16 weeks (Fig. 5-12).[141] The normal bladder is a midline, thin-walled, round or ovoid, anechoic structure in the fetal pelvis. In contrast to the stomach, filling and emptying of the urinary bladder are more predictable, occurring in cycles lasting 50 to 155 minutes.[145] If the bladder is not initially seen, sequential scans every 10 to 15 minutes up to 90 minutes always identify a normal bladder. The bladder size and structure should be assessed and changes documented when urinary tract disease is suspected. In posterior urethral valves, for example, the bladder and proximal urethra usually dilate, do not change in caliber, and the thin bladder wall thickens.[145]

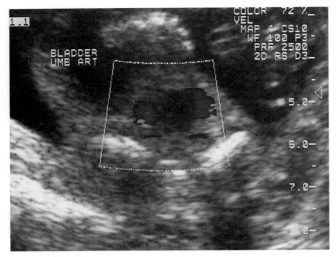

Figure 5–12. Normal urinary bladder is seen as the central hypoechoic area with umbilical artery blood flow seen on both sides. The iliac wings appear as hyperechoic structures posterolateral to the bladder.

Whenever the urinary tract is assessed, amniotic fluid volume should be evaluated. Before 16 weeks' gestation, the kidneys contribute little to amniotic fluid volume. Their role becomes more important during the second half of gestation, when fetal urination produces most of the amniotic fluid.[146] Significant urinary tract impairment involving both kidneys, both ureters, or the bladder is almost always associated with oligohydramnios and may be seen as early as 16 weeks. Most renal, ureteral, and bladder abnormalities are diagnosed after 16 weeks, secondary either to abnormal urine production or an obstructive process.[139] If a unilateral renal process occurs, most commonly either a multicystic dysplastic kidney or a ureteropelvic junction obstruction, amniotic fluid is normal.

Anterior abdominal wall defects can be excluded or detected by an examination of the entire abdominal wall, including identification of the normal umbilical cord insertion (Fig. 5-13). The transaxial plane is the best for demonstrating the anterior abdominal wall. Two defects are typically sought: omphalocele and gastroschisis. Omphalocele is a midline defect that results in herniation of abdominal contents into the base of the umbilical cord. The appearance of omphaloceles varies according to their contents, which can include liver, bowel, mesentery, ascites, and Wharton jelly.[147,148] It is important to realize that normal physiologic herniation of the midgut into the umbilical cord occurs between the 8th and 12th weeks.[149] In up to 20% of normal pregnancies, bowel may still be found outside the abdomen at 12 weeks.[12] Gastroschisis usually occurs to the right of the umbilical cord insertion and typically contains only eviscerated bowel.[150] It is important to remember that the actual umbilical cord insertion is normal in gastroschisis. Atypical abdominal wall defects can also occur in limb–body wall complex, ectopia cordis, cloacal exstrophy, and urachal cyst.[150]

SUMMARY

The routine evaluation of the gravid uterus should have a unified approach for the examination. The American Institute of Ultrasound in Medicine guidelines for the sonographic examination is one proposal for standardization of sonography during pregnancy. Better equipment with improved resolution permits continued identification of additional fetal anatomic structures. The addition of three-dimensional ultrasonography currently provides no additional benefit over two-dimensional imaging; however, it adds new perspectives for evaluation and possible use. As more subtle fetal abnormalities are routinely visualized, it is expected that further updates of the routine obstetric guidelines will occur. It is also anticipated that the role of ultrasonography will expand in the evaluation of fetal well-being and in risk assessment for the inheritance of genetic syndromes.

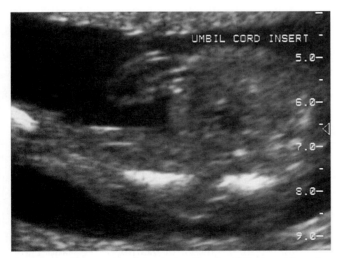

Figure 5–13. The anterior abdominal wall and umbilical cord insertion seen in a transaxial view.

REFERENCES

1. WFUMB Symposium on Safety of Ultrasound in Medicine: Conclusions and recommendations on thermal and non-thermal mechanisms for biological effects of ultrasound. Kloster-Banz, Germany. 14-19 April, 1996. World Federation for Ultrasound in Medicine and Biology. Ultrasound Med Biol 24(Suppl 1):i, S1, 1998.
2. Hershkovitz R, Sheiner E, Mazor M: Ultrasound in obstetrics: A review of safety. Eur J Obstet Gynecol Reprod Biol 101:15, 2002.
3. American College of Obstetrics and Gynecology Committee Opinion: New Ultrasound Output Display Standard, No. 180. Washington, DC, American College of Obstetrics and Gynecology, November 1996.
4. Reece EA, Assimakopoulos E, Zheng X, et al: The safety of obstetric ultrasonography: Concern for the fetus. Obstet Gynecol 76:139, 1990.
5. Stark CR, Orleans M, Haverkamp AD, Murphy J: Short and long term risks after exposure to diagnostic ultrasound in utero. Obstet Gynecol 63:194, 1984.
6. Zisken MC: Intrauterine effects of ultrasound: Human epidemiology. Teratology 59:252, 1999.
7. Salvesen KA: Ultrasound and left-handedness: A sinister association. Ultrasound Obstet Gynecol 19:217, 2002.

8. American Institute of Ultrasound in Medicine: Guidelines for performance of the antepartum obstetrical ultrasound examination. J Ultrasound Med 15:185,1996.

9. Nyberg DA, Laing FC, Filly RA: Threatened abortion: Sonographic distinction of normal and abnormal gestational sacs. Radiology 158:397, 1986.

10. Moore KL: The beginning of development, the first week. In Moore KL (ed): The Developing Human: Clinically Oriented Embryology, 3rd ed. Philadelphia, WB Saunders, 1982, pp 14-39.

11. Levi CS, Lyons EA, Lindsay DJ: Early diagnosis of non-viable pregnancy with endovaginal US. Radiology 167:383, 1988.

12. Green JJ, Hobbins JC: Abdominal ultrasound examination of the first trimester fetus. Am J Obstet Gynecol 159:165, 1988.

13. Levi CS, Lyons EA, Lindsay DJ: Ultrasound in the first trimester of pregnancy. Radiol Clin North Am 28:19, 1990.

14. Yeh H, Rabinowitz JG: Amniotic sac development: Ultrasound features of early pregnancy—the double bleb sign. Radiology 166:97, 1988.

15. Kaufman AJ, Fleischer AC, Thieme GA, et al: Separated chorioamnion and elevated chorion: Sonographic features and clinical significance. J Ultrasound Med 4:119, 1985.

16. Pennell RG, Needleman L, Pajak T, et al: Prospective comparison of vaginal and abdominal sonography in normal early pregnancy. J Ultrasound Med 10:63, 1991.

17. Robinson HP, Fleming JE: A critical evaluation of sonar "crown-rump length" measurements. Br J Obstet Gynecol 82:702, 1975.

18. Blum L, Kurtz AB: Gestational age: What to measure and when. Semin Roentgenol 25:299, 1990.

19. Coulam CB, Britten S, Soenksen DM: Early (34-56 days from last menstrual period) ultrasonographic measurements in normal pregnancies. Hum Reprod 11:1771, 1996.

20. Stefos TI, Lolis DE, Sotiradis AJ, Ziakas GV: Embryonic heart rate in early pregnancy. J Clin Ultrasound 26:33, 1998.

21. Liao AW, Snijders R, Geerts L, Nicolaides KH: Fetal heart rate in chromosomally abnormal fetuses. Ultrasound Obstet Gynecol 16:610, 2000.

22. Van Lith JM, Vissar GH, Mantingh A, Beekhuis JR: Fetal heart rate in early pregnancy and chromosomal disorders. Br J Obstet Gynaecol 99:741, 1992.

23. Mahony BS, Filly RA, Callen PW: Amnionicity and chorionicity in twin pregnancies using ultrasound. Radiology 155:205, 1985.

24. Barss VA, Benacerraf BR, Frigoletto FD Jr: Ultrasonographic determination of chorion type in twin gestation. Obstet Gynecol 66:779, 1985.

25. Hertzberg BS, Kurtz AB, Choi HY, et al: Significance of membrane thickness in the sonographic evaluation of twin gestations. AJR Am J Roentgenol 148:151, 1987.

26. Filly RA: The first trimester. In Callen PW (ed): Ultrasonography in Obstetrics and Gynecology, 2nd ed. Philadelphia, WB Saunders, 1988, pp 19-46.

27. Kurtz AB: The basic ultrasound examination of the uncomplicated pregnancy. Radiol Clin North Am 28:1, 1990.

28. Pennes DR, Bowerman RA, Silver TM: Echogenic adnexal masses associated with first trimester pregnancy: Sonographic appearance and clinical significance. J Clin Ultrasound 13:391, 1985.

29. Willson JR: Genitourinary tract disorders during pregnancy. In Willson JR, Carrington ER (eds): Obstetrics and Gynecology, 9th ed. St. Louis, Mosby–Year Book, 1991, pp 300-312.

30. Snijders RJM, Noble P, Sebire N, Nicolaides KH: UK multicentre project on assessment of risk of trisomy 21 by maternal age and fetal nuchal-translucency thickness at 10-14 weeks gestation. Lancet 351:343, 1998.

31. Nicholaides KH: Increased fetal nuchal translucency at 11-14 weeks. Prenat Diagn 22:308, 2002.

32. De Biasio P, Siccardi M, Volpe G, et al: First-trimester screening for Down's syndrome using nuchal translucency measurement with free β-hCG and PAPP-A between 10-13 weeks of pregnancy—the combined test. Prenat Diagn 19:360, 1999.

33. Zosmer N, Souter VL, Chan CSY, et al: Early diagnosis of major cardiac defects in chromosomally normal fetuses with increased nuchal translucency. Br J Obstet Gynaecol 106:829, 1999.

34. Bilardo CM, Muller MA, Pajkrt E: Outcome of fetuses with increased nuchal translucency. Curr Opin Obstet Gynecol 13:169, 2001.

35. Cicero S, Curcio P, Papageorghiou A, Nicholaides K: Absence of nasal bone in fetuses with trisomy 21 at 11-14 weeks of gestation: An observational study. Lancet 358:1665, 2001.

36. Southall DP, Richards J, Hardwick RA, et al: Prospective study of fetal heart rate and rhythm patterns. Arch Dis Child 55:506, 1980.

37. Allan LD, Anderson RH, Sullivan ID, et al: Evaluation of fetal arrhythmias by echocardiography. Br Heart J 50:240, 1983.

38. Silverman NH, Enderlein MA, Stanger P, et al: Recognition of fetal arrhythmias by echocardiography. J Clin Ultrasound 13:255, 1985.

39. Willson JR: Determination of position and lie in obstetrics and gynecology. In Willson JR, Carrington ER (eds): Obstetrics and Gynecology, 9th ed. St. Louis, Mosby–Year Book, 1991, pp 350-357.

40. Hashimoto BE, Kramer DJ, Brennan L: Amniotic fluid volume: Fluid dynamics and measurement technique. Semin Ultrasound CT MR 14:40, 1993.

41. Lind T, Kendall A, Hytten FE: The role of the fetus in the formation of amniotic fluid. J Obstet Gynecol Br Commonw 79:289, 1972.

42. Nazarian LN, Kurtz AB: Routine ultrasound surveillance of the pregnant uterus. Semin Ultrasound CT MR 14:3, 1993.

43. Goldstein RB, Filly RA: Sonographic estimation of amniotic fluid volume: Subjective assessment versus pocket measurements. J Ultrasound Med 7:363, 1988.

44. Philipson EH, Sokol RJ, Williams T: Oligohydramnios: Clinical associations and predictive value for intrauterine growth retardation. Am J Obstet Gynecol 146:271, 1983.

45. Hill LM: Abnormalities of amniotic fluid. In Nyberg DA, Mahony BS, Pretorius DH (eds): Diagnostic Ultrasound of Fetal Anomalies: Text and Atlas. St. Louis, Mosby–Year Book, 1990, pp 38-66.

46. Schiff E, Ben-Baruch G, Kushner O, et al: Standardized measurement of amniotic fluid volume by correlation of sonography with dye dilution technique. Obstet Gynecol 76:44, 1990.

47. Hoddick WK, Mahony BS, Callen PW, et al: Placental thickness. J Ultrasound Med 4:479, 1985.

48. Spirt BA, Cohen WN, Weinstein HM: The incidence of placental calcification in normal pregnancies. Radiology 142:707, 1982.

49. Spirt BA, Gordon LP: Practical aspects of placental evaluation. Semin Roentgenol 26:32, 1991.

50. Tindall VR, Scott JS: Placental calcification. A study of 3025 singleton and multiple pregnancies. J Obstet Gynecol Br Commonw 72:356, 1965.

51. Grannum PA, Berkowitz RL, Hobbins JC: The ultrasonic changes in the maturing placenta and their relation to fetal pulmonic maturity. Am J Obstet Gynecol 133:915, 1979.

52. Fox H: Pathology of the placenta. Clin Obstet Gynecol 13:501, 1986.

53. Spirt BA, Gordon LP: The placenta as an indicator of fetal maturity: Fact and fancy. Semin Ultrasound 5:290, 1984.

54. Spirt BA, Kagan EH, Rozanski RM: Sonolucent areas in the placenta: Sonographic and pathologic correlation. AJR Am J Roentgenol 131:961, 1978.

55. Harris RD, Simpson WA, Pet LR, et al: Placental hypoechoic/anechoic areas and infarction: A sonographic-pathologic correlation. Radiology 176:75, 1990.

56. Hoogland HJ, deHaan J, Vooys GP: Ultrasonographic diagnosis of intervillous thrombosis related to Rh isoimmunization. Gynecol Obstet Invest 10:237, 1979.

57. Spirt BA, Gordan LP, Kagan EH: Intervillous thrombosis: Sonographic and pathologic correlation. Radiology 146:197, 1983.

58. Mintz MC, Kurtz AB, Arenson R, et al: Abruptio placenta: Apparent thickening of the placenta caused by hyperechoic retroplacental clot. J Ultrasound Med 5:411, 1986.

59. Townsend RR, Laing FC, Jeffrey RB: Placental abruption associated with cocaine abuse. AJR Am J Roentgenol 150:1339, 1988.

60. de Mendonca LK: Sonographic diagnosis of placenta accreta: Presentation of six cases. J Ultrasound Med 7:211, 1988.

61. Finberg HJ, Williams JW: Placenta accreta: Prospective sonographic diagnosis in patients with placenta previa and prior cesarean section. J Ultrasound Med 11:333, 1992.

62. Pasto ME, Kurtz AB, Rifkin MD, et al: Ultrasonographic findings in placenta increta. J Ultrasound Med 2:155, 1983.

63. Bowie JD, Andreotti RF, Rosenberg ER: Sonographic appearance of the uterine cervix in pregnancy: The vertical cervix. AJR Am J Roentgenol 140:737, 1983.

64. Mahony BS, Nyberg DA, Luthy DA, et al: Translabial ultrasound of the third-trimester uterine cervix: Correlation with digital examination. J Ultrasound Med 9:717, 1990.

65. Feingold M, Brook I, Zakut H: Detection of cervical incompetence by ultrasound. Acta Obstet Gynecol Scand 63:407, 1984.

66. Michaels WH, Montgomery C, Karo J, et al: Ultrasound differentiation of the competent from the incompetent cervix. Prevention of preterm delivery. Am J Obstet Gynecol 154:537, 1986.

67. Kurtz AB, Wapner RJ, Kurtz RJ, et al: Analysis of biparietal diameter as an accurate indicator of gestational age. J Clin Ultrasound 8:319, 1980.

68. Doubilet PM, Greenes RA: Improved prediction of gestational age from fetal head measurements. AJR Am J Roentgenol 142:797, 1984.

69. Hadlock FP, Deter RL, Harrist RB, et al: Fetal head circumference: Relation to menstrual age. AJR Am J Roentgenol 138:649, 1982.

70. Benson CB, Doubilet PM: Sonographic prediction of gestational age: Accuracy of second- and third-trimester fetal measurements. AJR Am J Roentgenol 157:1275, 1991.

71. Kopta MM, May RR, Crane JP: A comparison of the reliability of the estimated date of confinement predicted by crown-rump length and biparietal diameter. Am J Obstet Gynecol 145:526, 1983.

72. Smazyal SF, Weisman LE, Hoppler KD, et al: Comparative analysis of ultrasonographic methods of gestational age assessment. J Ultrasound Med 2:147, 1983.

73. Benacerraf BR, Laboda LA, Frigoletto FD Jr: Thickened nuchal fold in fetuses not at risk for aneuploidy. Radiology 184:239, 1992.

74. Jeanty P, Rodesch F, Delbeke D, et al: Estimation of gestational age from measurements of fetal long bones. J Ultrasound Med 3:75, 1984.

75. Merz E, Kim-Kern M, Pehl S: Ultrasonic mensuration of fetal limb bones in the second and third trimesters. J Clin Ultrasound 15:175, 1987.

76. Kurtz AB, Needleman L, Wapner RJ, et al: Usefulness of a short femur in the in utero detection of skeletal dysplasias. Radiology 177:197, 1990.

77. Campbell S, Thoms A: Ultrasound measurement of the fetal head to abdominal circumference ratio in the assessment of growth retardation. Br J Obstet Gynaecol 84:165, 1977.

78. Levi S, Smets P: Intra-uterine fetal growth studied by ultrasonic biparietal measurements: The percentiles of biparietal distribution. Acta Obstet Gynecol Scand 52:193, 1973.

79. Hadlock FP, Harrist RB, Carpenter RJ, et al: Sonographic estimation of fetal weight: The value of femur length in addition to head and abdomen measurements. Radiology 150:535, 1984.

80. Shepard MJ, Richard VA, Berkowitz RL, et al: An evaluation of two equations for predicting fetal weight by ultrasound. Am J Obstet Gynecol 142:47, 1982.

81. Brenner WE, Edelman DA, Hendricks CH: A standard of fetal growth for the United States of America. Am J Obstet Gynecol 126:555, 1976.

82. McKenna K, Goldstein R, Stringer M: Small-absent fetal stomach: Prognostic significance. Radiology 197:729, 1995.

83. Babson SG, Kangas J, Young N, et al: Growth and development of twins of dissimilar size at birth. Pediatrics 33:327, 1964.

84. Brown CE, Guzick DS, Leveno KJ, et al: Prediction of discordant twins using ultrasound measurement of biparietal diameter and abdominal perimeter. Obstet Gynecol 70:677, 1987.

85. Erkkola R, Ala-Mello S, Pirroinen O, et al: Growth discordancy in twin pregnancies: A risk factor not detected by measurements of biparietal diameter. Obstet Gynecol 66:203, 1985.

86. Storlazzi E, Vintzileos AM, Campbell WA, et al: Ultrasonic diagnosis of discordant fetal growth in twin gestations. Obstet Gynecol 69:363, 1987.

87. Shah YG, Graham D, Stinson SK, et al: Biparietal diameter growth in uncomplicated twin gestation. Am J Perinatol 4:229, 1987.

88. Grumbach K, Coleman BG, Arger PH, et al: Twin and singleton growth patterns compared using ultrasound. Radiology 158:237, 1986.

89. Filly RA, Cardoza JD, Goldstein RB, et al: Detection of fetal central nervous system anomalies: A practical level of effort for a routine sonogram. Radiology 172:403, 1989.

90. Pilu G, Romero R, Reece EA, et al: The prenatal diagnosis of Robin anomalad. Am J Obstet Gynecol 154:630, 1986.

91. McGahan JP, Phillips HE: Ultrasonic evaluation of the size of the trigone of the fetal ventricle. J Ultrasound Med 2:315, 1983.

92. Siedler DE, Filly RA: Relative growth of the higher fetal brain structures. J Ultrasound Med 6:573, 1987.

93. Cardoza JD, Goldstein RB, Filly RA: Exclusion of fetal ventriculomegaly with a single measurement: The width of the lateral ventricular atrium. Radiology 169:711, 1988.

94. Alagappan R, Browning PD, Laorr A, et al: Distal lateral ventricular atrium: Reevaluation of normal range. Radiology 193:405,1994.

95. Farrell TA, Hertzberg BS, Kliewer MA: Fetal lateral ventricles: Reassessment of normal values for atrial diameter at US. Radiology 193:409,1994.

96. Johnson ML, Dunne MC, Mack LA, et al: Evaluation of fetal intracranial anatomy by static and real-time ultrasound. J Clin Ultrasound 8:311, 1980.

97. Pretorius DH, Drose JA, Manco-Johnson ML: Fetal lateral ventricular ratio determination during the second trimester. J Ultrasound Med 5:121, 1986.

98. Bowerman RA, DiPietro MA: Erroneous sonographic identification of fetal lateral ventricles: Relationship to the echogenic periventricular "blush." AJNR Am J Neuroradiol 8:661,1987.

99. Hertzberg, Bowie JD, Burger PC, et al: The three lines: Origin of sonographic landmarks in the fetal head. AJR Am J Roentgenol 149:1009, 1987.

100. Mahony BS, Callen PW, Filly RA, et al: The fetal cisterna magna. Radiology 153:773, 1984.

101. Van den Hof MC, Nicolaides KH, Campbell J, et al: Evaluation of the lemon and banana signs in one hundred thirty fetuses with open spina bifida. Am J Obstet Gynecol 162:322, 1990.

102. Goldstein RB, Podrasky AE, Filly RA, et al: Effacement of the fetal cisterna magna in association with myelomeningocele. Radiology 172:409, 1989.

103. Campbell J, Gilbert WM, Nicolaides KH, et al: Ultrasound screening for spina bifida: Cranial and cerebellar signs in a high-risk population. Obstet Gynecol 70:247, 1987.

104. Benacerraf BR, Frigoletto FD Jr: Soft tissue nuchal fold in the second trimester fetus: Standards for normal measurements compared with those in Down syndrome. Am J Obstet Gynecol 157:1146, 1987.

105. Toj A, Simpson GF, Filly RA: Ultrasonically evident fetal nuchal skin thickening: Is it specific for Down syndrome? Am J Obstet Gynecol 156:150, 1987.

106. Benacerraf BR, Estroff JA: Transvaginal sonographic imaging of the low fetal head in the second trimester. J Ultrasound Med 8:325, 1989.

107. Monteagudo A, Reuss ML, Timor-Trisch IE: Imaging the fetal brain in the second and third trimester using transvaginal sonography. Obstet Gynecol 77:27,1991.

108. Moore KL: The nervous system. In Moore KL (ed): The Developing Human: Clinically Oriented Embryology, 3rd ed. Philadelphia, WB Saunders, 1982, pp 375-412.

109. Baxi L, Warren W, Collins MH, et al: Early detection of caudal regression syndrome with transvaginal scanning. Obstet Gynecol 75:486, 1990.

110. Budorick NE, Pretorius DH, Grafe MR, et al: Ossification of the fetal spine. Radiology 181:561, 1991.

111. Mayden KL, Tortora M, Berkowitz RL, et al: Orbital diameters: A new parameter for prenatal diagnosis and dating. Am J Obstet Gynecol 144:289, 1982.

111a. Trout T, Budorick NE, Pretorius DH, et al: Significance of orbital measurements in the fetus. J Ultrasound Med 13: 937, 1994.

112. Saltzman DH, Benacerraf BR, Frigoletto FD: Diagnosis and management of fetal facial clefts. Am J Obstet Gynecol 155:377, 1986.

113. Seeds JW, Cefalo RC: Technique of early sonographic diagnosis of bilateral cleft lip and palate. Obstet Gynecol 62:2S, 1983.

114. Pilu G, Reece EA, Romero R, et al: Prenatal diagnosis of craniofacial malformations with ultrasonography. Am J Obstet Gynecol 155:45, 1986.

115. Frigoletto FD, Birnholz JC, Driscoll SG, et al: Ultrasound diagnosis of cystic hygroma. Am J Obstet Gynecol 136:962,1980.

116. Garden AS, Benzie RJ, Miskin, et al: Fetal cystic hygroma colli: Antenatal diagnosis, significance, and management. Am J Obstet Gynecol 154:221,1986.

117. Pijpers L, Reuss A, Stewart PA, et al: Fetal cystic hygroma: Prenatal diagnosis and management. Obstet Gynecol 72:223, 1988.

118. Copel JA, Pilu G, Green J, et al: Fetal echocardiographic screening for congenital heart disease: The importance of the four-chamber view. Am J Obstet Gynecol 157:648, 1987.

119. McGahan JP: Sonography of the fetal heart: Findings on the four-chamber view. AJR Am J Roentgenol 156:547, 1991.

120. Comstock CH: Normal fetal heart axis and position. Obstet Gynecol 70:255, 1987.

121. Hilpert PL, Pretorius DH: The thorax. In Nyberg DA, Mahony BS, Pretorius DH (eds): Diagnostic Ultrasound of Fetal Anomalies: Text and Atlas. St. Louis, Mosby–Year Book, 1990, pp 262-299.

122. Chitkara U, Rosenberg J, Chervenak FA, et al: Prenatal sonographic assessment of the fetal thorax: Normal values. Am J Obstet Gynecol 156:1069, 1987.

123. DeVore GR, Siassi B, Platt LD: Fetal echocardiography. IV. M-mode assessment of ventricular size and contractility during the second and third trimesters of pregnancy in the normal fetus. Am J Obstet Gynecol 150:981, 1984.

124. Fong K, Ohlsson A, Zalev A: Fetal thoracic circumference: A perspective cross-sectional study with real-time ultrasound. Am J Obstet Gynecol 158:1154, 1988.

125. DeVore GR, Horenstein J, Platt LD: Fetal echocardiography. VI. Assessment of cardiothoracic disproportion: A new technique for the diagnosis of thoracic hypoplasia. Am J Obstet Gynecol 155:1066, 1986.

126. Callan NA, Colmorgen GH, Weiner S: Lung hypoplasia and prolonged preterm ruptured membranes: A case report with implications for possible prenatal ultrasonic diagnosis. Am J Obstet Gynecol 151:756, 1985.

127. Yagel S, Mandelberg A, Hurwitz A, et al: Prenatal diagnosis of hypoplastic left ventricle. Am J Perinatol 3:6, 1986.

128. Achiron R, Malinger G, Zaidel L, et al: Prenatal sonographic diagnosis of endocardial fibroelastosis elastosis secondary to aortic stenosis. Prenat Diagn 8:73, 1988.

129. Nyberg DA, Emerson DS: Cardiac malformations. In Nyberg DA, Mahony BS, Pretorius DH (eds): Diagnostic Ultrasound of Fetal Anomalies: Text and Atlas. St. Louis, Mosby–Year Book, 1990, pp 300-341.

130. Bromley B, Estroff JA, Sanders SP, et al: Fetal echocardiography: Accuracy and limitations in a population at high and low risk for heart defects. Am J Obstet Gynecol 166:1473, 1992.

131. Achiron R, Glaser J, Gelernter I, et al: Extended fetal echocardiographic examination for detecting cardiac malformations in low risk pregnancies. BMJ 304:671,1992.

132. DeVore GR: The aortic and pulmonary outflow tract screening examination in the human fetus. J Ultrasound Med 11:345, 1992.

133. Kirk JS, Riggs TW, Comstock CH, et al: Prenatal screening for cardiac anomalies: The value of routine addition of the aortic root to the four-chamber view. Obstet Gynecol 84:427,1994.

134. Pritchard JA: Fetal swallowing and amniotic fluid volume. Obstet Gynecol 28:606, 1966.

135. Pretorius DH, Gosink BB, Clautice-Engle T, et al: Sonographic evaluation of the fetal stomach: Significance of non-visualization. AJR Am J Roentgenol 151:987, 1988.

136. Millener PB, Anderson NG, Chisholm RJ: Prognostic significance of nonvisualization of the fetal stomach by sonography. AJR Am J Roentgenol 160:827,1993.

137. Zimmer E, Chao CR, Abramovich G, et al: Fetal stomach measurements: Not reproducible by the same observer. J Ultrasound Med 11:663,1992.

138. Nyberg DA: Intra-abdominal abnormalities. In Nyberg DA, Mahony BS, Pretorius DH (eds): Diagnostic Ultrasound of Fetal Anomalies: Text and Atlas. St. Louis, Mosby–Year Book, 1990, pp 342-394.

139. Lawson TL, Foley WD, Berland LL, et al: Ultrasonic evaluation of fetal kidneys. Radiology 138:153, 1981.

140. Bowie JD, Rosenberg ER, Andreotti RF, et al: The changing sonographic appearance of fetal kidneys during pregnancy. J Ultrasound Med 2:505, 1983.

141. Patten RM, Mack LA, Wang KY, et al: The fetal genitourinary tract. Radiol Clin North Am 28:115, 1990.

142. Arger PH, Coleman BG, Mintz MC, et al: Routine fetal genitourinary tract screening. Radiology 156:485, 1985.

143. Benacerraf BR, Mandell J, Estroff JA, et al: Fetal pyelectasis: A possible association with Down syndrome. Obstet Gynecol 76:58, 1990.

144. Grannum PA, Bracken M, Silverman R, et al: Assessment of fetal kidney size in normal gestation by comparison of ratio of kidney circumference to abdominal circumference. Am J Obstet Gynecol 136:249, 1980.

145. Campbell S, Wladimiroff JW, Dewhurst CJ: The antenatal measurement of fetal urine production. Br J Obstet Gynecol 80:680, 1973.

146. Abramovich DR, Garden A, Jandial L, et al: Fetal swallowing and voiding in relation to hydramnios. Obstet Gynecol 54:15, 1979.

147. Nyberg DA, Fitzsimmons J, Mack LA, et al: Chromosomal abnormalities in fetuses with omphalocele: Significance of omphalocele contents. J Ultrasound Med 8:299, 1989.

148. Schaffer RM, Barone C, Friedman AP: The ultrasonographic spectrum of fetal omphalocele. J Ultrasound Med 2:219, 1983.

149. Schmidt W, Yarkoni S, Crelin ES, et al: Sonographic visualization of physiologic anterior abdominal wall hernia in the first trimester. Obstet Gynecol 69:911, 1987.

150. Nyberg DA, Mack LA: Abdominal wall defects. In Nyberg DA, Mahony BS, Pretorius DH (eds): Diagnostic Ultrasound of Fetal Anomalies: Text and Atlas. St. Louis, Mosby–Year Book, 1990, pp 395-432.

CHAPTER 6

Amniocentesis

*Patrice M. L. Trauffer, Ronald J. Wapner,
and Anthony Johnson*

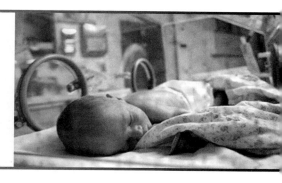

A mniocentesis has been utilized since 1881 to treat obstetric conditions such as hydramnios,[1] but only since 1956 has the procedure been performed to diagnose and evaluate fetal status. Testing during the late 1950s and early 1960s involved aspiration of amniotic fluid to evaluate the impact of maternal Rh sensitization on the fetus,[2] to determine fetal sex by analysis of the Barr body[3-7] and to diagnose rare fetal endocrine and biochemical disorders.[8,9] After the discovery in 1966 by Steele and Breg of the ability to culture and karyotype amniocytes,[10] however, the utilization of amniocentesis rapidly increased. The diagnostic scope of the procedure has continued to expand, and the technique has become accepted by patients as a "safe" form of invasive prenatal diagnosis. As such, it has become the standard to which the safety and accuracy of other invasive prenatal diagnostic procedures are currently compared.

COMPOSITION OF AMNIOTIC FLUID

In the first trimester, amniotic fluid electrolyte composition and osmolality resemble those of a dialysate of maternal and fetal serum and are theorized to be derived from three sources: (1) secretion from the amniotic epithelium; (2) filtration from maternal vessels underlying the decidua and chorion; and (3) fetal vessels along the chorionic plate. Before 15 weeks' gestation, fetal urination does not contribute greatly to the amniotic fluid volume, but it subsequently becomes the largest component, leading to a slight decrease in osmolality.[11] The volume of amniotic fluid varies by gestational age (Fig. 6-1), from 190 mL at 15 to 16 weeks' gestation to a mean peak of 900 mL at 32 to 34 weeks, after which there is a slight decrement until term.[12]

Amniotic fluid changes in content as pregnancy progresses, acquiring proteins and becoming more particulate. Cells within the amniotic fluid emanate either from the fetus (fetal skin, hair, vernix caseosa, gastrointestinal tract, genitourinary system, respiratory tract) or from the extraembryonic membranes.[13] Although the amniotic fluid cell concentration increases with gestational age, only a small portion of these sloughed cells are viable and therefore useful for karyotype analysis. Even these viable cells must be cultured for 4 to 7 days to obtain sufficient mitosis for complete evaluation.[14] However, protein, hormone, enzyme, and DNA analysis can frequently be performed on either the uncultured cells or the cell-free fluid.

INDICATIONS FOR AMNIOCENTESIS

Evaluation of the Fetal Karyotype

Advanced Maternal Age

The most frequent indication for fetal karyotype analysis is advanced maternal age. Although the risk of maternal meiotic nondisjunction leading to fetal aneuploidy increases continuously with maternal age (Table 6-1),[15,16] amniocentesis is routinely offered only to women who will be 35 years old or older at the time of delivery. The choice of 35 as the standard age for offering prenatal diagnosis is somewhat arbitrary but is thought to represent a reasonable balance between the risk of fetal aneuploidy and the hazards of an invasive diagnostic procedure. Trisomy 21 is the most frequent age-related chromosomal abnormality; however, other fetal aneuploidies, both autosomal and sex chromosome, also increase with maternal age (see Table 6-1).[15,16]

The probability of detecting an aneuploid fetus varies with the gestational age at evaluation (see Table 6-1).[15,16] For example, in mothers 35 years of age, there is a 1 per 250 risk of diagnosing a trisomy 21 fetus at a second-trimester amniocentesis but only a 1 per 350 probability of delivering a liveborn child with Down syndrome; this difference is accounted for by the 30% second- and third-trimester loss rate of fetuses with Down syndrome.[17,18]

The paradigm of restricting amniocentesis to the 7.5% of childbearing women 35 years of age or older allows detection of only 20% to 30% of fetuses with Down syndrome. Because the majority of such infants are born to younger women, an efficient and safe technique for screening these pregnancies has been sought.

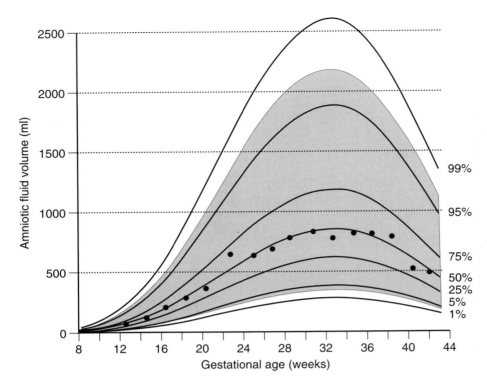

Figure 6–1. Nomogram showing amniotic fluid volumes as a function of gestational age on a linear scale. *Dots* are means for each 2-week interval. Percentiles are calculated from polynomial regression equation and standard deviation of residuals. *Shaded area* covers 95% confidence interval. *(From Brace RA, Wolf EJ: Normal amniotic fluid volume changes throughout pregnancy. Am J Obstet Gynecol 161:382, 1989.)*

Abnormal Maternal Serum Screening for Fetal Aneuploidy

Women carrying a fetus with Down syndrome have a unique pattern of serum biochemical analytes in the second trimester that can be utilized to calculate a more specific risk of Down syndrome than can age alone. The maternal serum pattern associated with trisomy 21 demonstrates a decreased α-fetoprotein level (mean, 0.75 multiple of the median [MOM]),[19] an increased human chorionic gonadotrophin level[20] (mean, 2.0 MOMs), and a decreased unconjugated serum estriol (mean, 0.73 MOMs).[21]

Table 6–1. Crude Maternal Age–Specific Rates (%) of Chromosome Abnormalities

Maternal Age (Years)	From Liveborn Studies		From Amniocentesis*		From Chorionic Villus Sampling†	
	47, +21	All Chromosome Abnormalities	47, +21	All Chromosome Abnormalities	47, +21	All Chromosome Abnormalities
33	0.16	0.29	0.24	0.48	—	—
34	0.20	0.36	0.30	0.66	—	—
35	0.26	0.49	0.40	0.76	0.42	0.77
36	0.33	0.60	0.52	0.95	0.57	1.0
37	0.44	0.77	0.67	1.20	0.75	1.4
38	0.57	0.97	0.87	1.54	1.0	1.8
39	0.73	1.23	1.12	1.89	1.34	2.4
40	0.94	1.59	1.45	2.50	1.79	3.2
41	1.23	2.00	1.89	3.23	2.4	4.2
42	1.56	2.56	2.44	4.00	3.2	5.6
43	2.00	3.33	3.23	5.26	4.2	7.4
44	2.63	4.17	4.00	6.67	5.6	9.8
45	3.33	5.26	5.26	8.33	7.5	12.4

Note: Estimated liveborn statistics.

*Data compiled from 20,000 genetic amniocenteses.

†Data from 3848 chorionic villus sampling studies.

From Hook EB, Cross PK, Jackson L, et al: Maternal age-specific rates of 47, +21 and other cytogenetic abnormalities diagnosed in the first trimester of pregnancy in chorionic villus biopsy specimens: Comparison with rates expected from observations at amniocentesis. Am J Hum Genet 42:797, 1988.

With a combination of these analyte values obtained between 15 and 20 weeks' gestation, in combination with maternal age, pregnant women younger than 35 can be offered a more precise evaluation of their risk of having a child with trisomy 21. If all women younger than 35 years with an analyte-determined risk of trisomy 21 of 1 per 250 or greater are tested, 60% of Down syndrome pregnancies will be identified.[22] Through this approach, amniocentesis would be offered to approximately 5% of the pregnant population younger than 35 years.

Inhibin A, a substance produced by the placenta, has been added as a fourth analyte for these measurements. Modeling of the so-called "quad screen," which includes incorporating inhibin A with α-fetoprotein, human chorionic gonadotropin, and μE3, suggests a detection rate of 70% to 75%, with a 5% false-positive rate.[23]

Screening for Down syndrome is possible during the first trimester with the biochemical analytes pregnancy-associated plasma protein-A (PAPP-A) and free β–human chorionic gonadotropin, in combination with ultrasound measurement of the fetal nuchal translucency. This approach detects approximately 80% of trisomy 21 pregnancies with a 5% false-positive rate.

Another approach to Down syndrome screening is to measure the fetal nuchal translucency and PAPP-A in the first trimester and and wait until the second trimester to measure human chorionic gonadotropin, α-fetoprotein, unconjugated estriol, and inhibin A.[24] This "integrated" or combined screening approach may identify up to 85% of trisomy 21 pregnancies, with a 1.2% false-positive rate. Further evaluation of the integrated test is still required before it can be recommended for use.

At present, invasive testing is offered to all women aged 35 years or older. However, the validity of testing on the basis of maternal age alone has been questioned (e.g., in women aged 35 years or older). New screening tests have altered the situation, and biochemical screening can identify 89% of Down syndrome pregnancies.[25] This detection rate is accomplished if invasive testing is offered when the analyte risk of trisomy 21 is 1 per 250 or higher. With this approach, amniocentesis would be required in only 25% of mothers, but 11% of Down syndrome pregnancies currently detected would be missed. For women whose screen results are negative, the risk of losing a normal pregnancy secondary to amniocentesis is almost threefold higher than the probability of discovering a fetus with Down syndrome. Although more data is required before maternal age alone can be eliminated as an indication for amniocentesis, some women older than 35 are beginning to use serum screening to better evaluate their risk before deciding on amniocentesis.

Previous Child with a Chromosomal Abnormality

The previous birth of a child with a chromosomal abnormality may indicate an increased risk of the same or another abnormality occurring in a subsequent pregnancy.[26,27] The probability of recurrence depends on both the chromosome abnormality involved and the age of the mother at the birth of the affected child. Although certain abnormalities, such as monosomy X, triploidy, and a de novo translocation, are not associated with an increased risk of recurrence, the birth of a child with almost any other autosomal trisomy does indicate an increased risk of recurrence.

The birth of a child with trisomy 21 to a woman younger than 30 years increases the risk of a future child with aneuploidy to approximately 1% to 2%.[26,27] However, if a woman is older than 30 at the birth of a trisomic child, the recurrence risk is not increased beyond that of her age at the next pregnancy. Fewer data are available for determining the recurrence risks for the other common trisomies, such as trisomy 18 and trisomy 13. Those risks appear to be less than that for trisomy 21, however, but are still sufficient to mandate the offer of prenatal testing.

Parental Chromosome Abnormality

For pregnancies in which a parent carries a balanced chromosomal translocation, the parents are routinely offered amniocentesis. Although the rearrangement does not usually cause a phenotypic effect in the carriers, the risk of producing offspring with an imbalance may be as high as 10% to 15%.[28-30] The exact risk to a carrier parent of delivering a viable child with an unbalanced rearrangement is dependent on the specific chromosomes involved, the parent who carries the abnormal chromosome, the type of rearrangement, the specific chromosome breakpoints, and the method of ascertainment of the at-risk family.

Table 6-2 demonstrates the risk of producing offspring with unbalanced translocations for the more common robertsonian translocations, in which two acrocentric chromosomes fuse together at their centromeres, thus reducing the chromosome number in the carrier parent to 45. For the most common 14/21 translocation carried by the mother, the risk is of such magnitude (10% to 15%) that prenatal testing is strongly advised. If the translocation is carried by the father, the risk remains 2% to 4%. For other, less frequent robertsonian translocations, such as those involving chromosomes 13 and 14, the risk of producing living offspring with unbalanced translocations may be low enough that after counseling, the parents may wish to avoid invasive testing. With a 21q/21q translocation, only monosomy 21 (resulting in miscarriage) or trisomy 21 (Down syndrome) can occur; therefore, testing would be superfluous.

Table 6–2. Approximate Risk of Viable Offspring with an Unbalanced Robertsonian Translocation from a Parent with a Balanced Translocation

Parental Translocation	Risk if Maternal Carrier	Risk if Paternal Carrier
13q/14q	<1%	<1%
13q/13q	100%	100%
14q/21q	10%-15%	2%-3%
21q/22q	6%-8%	2%-3%
21q/21q	100%	100%

When one parent carries a balanced reciprocal translocation in which segments of nonhomologous chromosomes are exchanged, predicting the risk of producing a viable fetus with an unbalanced translocation requires considerable cytogenetic evaluation. Ideally, the cytogenetic laboratory can determine the most likely unbalanced gametes, and the potential viability of these can be predicted by review of the literature or catalogs of chromosome rearrangements.[31] When this level of assessment is not feasible, certain general guidelines are helpful. In contrast to robertsonian translocations, the sex of the carrier parent plays only a minor role. The most important predictor of viable offspring with an unbalanced translocation is the mode of ascertainment of the carrier couple. If the couple is ascertained because of the birth of an abnormal liveborn child with an unbalanced translocation, the recurrence risk is as high as 20% to 25%.[28] When the family is ascertained because of recurrent spontaneous abortions, the empirical risk of producing subsequent liveborn children with an unbalanced translocation is less than 5%. Some reciprocal translocation breakpoints are common enough to prompt even more specific counseling. For example, the common 11q/22q translocation, when carried by the mother, carries a 2% to 3% risk of viable offspring.[32]

Fetal Structural Abnormalities Identified on Ultrasound Study

Approximately 10% to 15% of fetuses with ultrasonographically detectable structural abnormalities have a chromosome defect as the cause.[33] Isolated defects have a much lower likelihood (2%) of a chromosomal etiology than do multisystem defects (30%); the frequency of aneuploidy increases with the number of organ systems involved.[33] Table 6-3 lists the risks of fetal chromosomal abnormalities with specific structural defects investigated by amniocentesis. When a fetal abnormality known to be associated with aneuploidy is discovered, karyotyping is indicated because the prognosis, subsequent obstetric management, and neonatal outcome are strongly determined by the result. The diagnostic approach chosen is determined by the gestational age and clinical circumstance. Although cordocentesis allows for a more rapid result, if at least 5 to 7 days are available, amniocentesis is preferred because of the lower risk to the fetus. More rapid processing of amniotic fluid by newer techniques such as fluorescent in situ hybridization (FISH) (see later section on laboratory analysis) may make amniocentesis available even when time is short.

Abnormalities of fetal growth or amniotic fluid volume, unexplained by maternal or obstetric factors, may indicate a chromosomal abnormality and represent another indication for prenatal diagnosis.[33,34] However, severe oligohydramnios may preclude fluid retrieval, and in these instances, placental biopsy or fetal blood sampling may be the more appropriate approach to fetal karyotyping.

Identification of Fetal Single-Gene Disorders

Prenatal diagnosis is available for many mendelian disorders through either molecular techniques or biochemical analysis. In the past, the majority of pregnancies at risk were identified by the previous birth of an affected child. More recently, the identification of a specific genetic error has led to carrier screening and the detection of at-risk families before the birth of an affected child. The availability of both carrier screening and prenatal diagnosis is changing rapidly, and many disorders previously not diagnosable in utero can now be detected by either direct gene analysis or linkage studies. Table 6-4[35-49] lists some common mendelian disorders for which population screening or prenatal diagnosis is available. For less common disorders identified in a specific family, consultation with a genetic center is suggested.

Identification of Fetal Neural Tube Defects

Neural tube defects, which have a prevalence of 1 to 2 per 1000 live births, and ventral wall defects, which occur in 1 per 2000 live births, can be diagnosed by measurement of the amniotic fluid α-fetoprotein level.[50] α-Fetoprotein is a glycoprotein that is produced in the yolk sac and fetal liver, is excreted into fetal serum, and, by 16 weeks' gestation, enters the amniotic fluid by fetal urination. As opposed to maternal serum α-fetoprotein levels, which increase continuously during the second trimester, amniotic fluid α-fetoprotein levels peak at about 12 to 13 weeks' gestation and then decrease as gestation advances. Conditions associated with exposed fetal tissue and with leakage of fetal serum into the amniotic fluid increase the concentration of the protein in both amniotic fluid and maternal blood, inasmuch as the fetal serum level of α-fetoprotein is more than 100 times higher than the amniotic fluid α-fetoprotein level and more than 1000-fold higher than the maternal serum α-fetoprotein level.[51]

Because α-fetoprotein levels vary with gestational age, clinicians must use normative data in which the measured value is compared with the median value for gestational age. Values are reported as MOMs. When a deviation representing 2.0 to 2.5 MOMs is found after the affirmation of correct dating, concern for an anatomic defect is raised. The abnormality may be confirmed and further characterized by evaluation of acetylcholinesterase, an enzyme that is neuronal specific and not routinely present in amniotic fluid. If acetylcholinesterase is present, the risk of an open neural tube defect is more than 97%, and targeted ultrasonography should be utilized to identify the lesion.[52] If acetylcholinesterase is absent, the elevated level of amniotic fluid α-fetoprotein may represent a false-positive finding or contamination with a small amount of fetal blood, or it may be associated with other nonneural anatomic defects. In these cases, a detailed, targeted ultrasound study may help define the nature of the elevation.

As ultrasound imaging and maternal serum α-fetoprotein screening have improved, the use of amniotic fluid α-fetoprotein levels as the primary modality for identifying fetal neural tube defects has diminished. Maternal serum screening identifies 95% of anencephalic fetuses and more than 85% of fetuses with open neural tube defects.[53] Targeted ultrasonography can be used to evaluate cases of elevated levels of maternal

Table 6–3. Incidences of Fetal Chromosome Abnormalities Associated with Various Ultrasonographically Detectable Fetal Malformations

	% with Chromosome Abnormalities		
Malformation	**Isolated Defect Present**	**Multiple Defects* Present**	**Comments**
Central Nervous System			
Strawberry-shaped head	—	80%	Almost exclusively trisomy 18
Ventriculomegaly	5%	30%	Trisomy 18, triploidy, trisomy 21 most common In general, aneuploidy more frequent in mild cases
Holoprosencephaly	0%	30%-50%	Trisomy 13 most frequent
Choroid plexus cyst	2%-3%	50%	Trisomy 18; rarely, trisomy 21
Posterior fossa cyst		50%	Trisomies 18 and 13 most common
Cardiovascular			
Structural cardiac defect	Rare	65%-70%	Trisomies 13, 18, and 21 and 45, XO most common
Lymphatic			
Nuchal edema	40%-60%		Trisomy 21 most likely; also, trisomies 13 and 18
First trimester			
Second trimester	25%		Trisomy 21
Cystic hygroma: second trimester		75%	45XO, especially with hydrops
Skeletal			
Abnormal extremities	Rare	40%	Includes subtle defects of distal extremities
Pulmonary			
Diaphragmatic hernia	Rare	20%-40%	Trisomy 18 most common
Gastrointestinal			
Omphalocele	2%-3%	50%	Trisomy 18 most common; also, trisomy 13
Duodenal atresia	20%	40%-50%	Trisomy 21: not seen on ultrasound study before 20 weeks' gestation
Esophageal atresia	—	80%	Trisomy 18
Genitourinary			
Structural renal defect	2%-3%	25%	
Other			
Nonimmune hydrops	5%-10%	20%	Trisomy 21 most common
Face			
Cleft lip and or palate	Rare	50%	Trisomies 13 and 18
Growth			
Intrauterine growth restriction	2%-3%	30%	Triploidy and trisomy 18 most common, especially when oligohydramnios or polyhydramnios is present

*Additional defects may be subtle and not always identified by ultrasound study.

Modified from Nicolaides K, Snijders RJ, Gosden CM, et al: Ultrasonographically detectable markers of fetal chromosomal abnormalities. Lancet 340:704, 1992.

serum α-fetoprotein and detects all cases of anencephaly and more than 90% of cases of spina bifida.[54] Therefore, a couple with a 2% to 3% risk of a child with a neural tube defect because of the birth of a previously affected infant may elect maternal serum α-fetoprotein screening and targeted ultrasound visualization of the fetal neural axis rather than amniocentesis. Similarly, in a woman with a persistently elevated maternal serum α-fetoprotein level of 2.5 MOMs or higher, the fetus has approximately a 5% to 10% risk of a fetal neural tube defect.[55]

Amniocentesis and measurement of amniotic fluid α-fetoprotein had previously been the definitive diagnostic test. Currently, many couples choose ultrasound imaging and undergo amniocentesis only when scanning cannot adequately visualize the fetal spine. Such patients must be made aware, however, that even experienced clinicians occasionally miss neural tube defects. Despite the lack of complete sensitivity, this approach is suggested for well-informed patients who wish to avoid the potential hazards of amniocentesis.

Table 6–4. Some Common Mendelian Disorders that Can Be Diagnosed In Utero by Amniocentesis

Disorder	Technique for Prenatal Diagnosis with Amniotic Fluid or Chromosome Villi	Population/Carrier Screening Available	Screening Techniques for Carriers	Reference
Autosomal Recessive				
Cystic fibrosis	Molecular identification of mutation or linkage if mutation not known	Yes: population screening not currently recommended Screen family members of affected individuals	Identification of mutation: approximately 90% of carriers identifiable (81% of carrier couples)	36,37
Thalassemia*	Molecular identification of mutation or linkage if mutation not known	Yes : Mediterranean β-thalassemia: Mediterranean, Middle East, Southeast Asia, India, Pakistan; black people α-thalassemia: Southeast Asia	Red blood cell indices: low MCV; Hb A$_2$ level elevated	38
Tay-Sachs disease* (GM$_2$ gangliosidase type 1)	Measurement of hexosaminidase A level	Yes: all Jewish couples should be screened	Reduction of enzyme level in serum; leukocyle enzyme level should be measured if woman is pregnant or taking oral contraceptives	39,40,41
Canavan disease*	Molecular identification of mutation	Yes: all Jewish couples should be screened	Moderate detection of mutation	42
Sickle cell disease*	Molecular identification of the mutation	Yes: all black couples and Hispanic couples should be screened	Hemoglobin electrophoresis is preferred; sickle cell preparation or solubility tests acceptable	43,44
X-Linked				
Duchenne muscular dystrophy	Molecular: deletion found in 60% Linkage if no deletion or mutation identified	Only potential carriers in at-risk families should be screened	Molecular	45,46
Hemophilia A	Specific mutation in some families	Only at-risk family members should be screened	Mutation detection	47
Fragile X syndrome	Identification of DNA expansion within FMR-1 gene	Not routinely recommended	Molecular identification of premutation	48,49

*American College of Obstetrics and Gynecologists currently recommends carrier screening of at-risk couples.[50]

Hb, hemoglobin; MCV, mean corpuscular volume.

THE TECHNIQUE OF AMNIOCENTESIS

Genetic Amniocentesis Performed after 15 Weeks' Gestation

Sampling Technique

Amniocentesis for genetic evaluation has routinely been performed between 15 and 18 weeks' gestation. At this stage, fluid levels (150 to 250 mL) are sufficient so that the fetus can be safely avoided, the uterus is an easily accessible abdominal organ so that the maternal bowel can be avoided, and sufficient viable cells are present so that results will be available in time to allow for the option of pregnancy termination if results are abnormal.

Before the actual amniocentesis, the couple must be extensively counseled, and the genetic risks as well as the risks of the procedure should be discussed in detail. The counseling session should explore the couple's expectations from the procedure and make certain that the limitations of testing are understood. Because more than 70% of pedigree analysis reveals information requiring further comment or counseling, a thorough family history, extended to at least third-degree relatives, is obtained. Likewise, exposure to environmental agents should be reviewed and discussed. Finally, the couple is made aware of the time interval required for laboratory analysis, which varies depending on the specific indication.

A detailed ultrasound evaluation of the pregnancy is performed to confirm appropriate gestational age, ensure viability of the fetus, determine placental location, establish fetal number, and rule out major fetal structural abnormalities or coexisting maternal uterine or pelvic disease. Specifically, measurements of the biparietal diameter, head circumference, abdominal circumference, and femur length should be obtained. If the fetal biometry suggests that the gestation is less than 15 weeks, the patient should be rescheduled. Ultrasound confirmation of the appropriate gestational age is especially important when the amniocentesis is performed as a result of abnormal maternal serum screening results, because an error of 10 days to 2 weeks may alter the interpretation of the analyte-determined risks. The preamniocentesis ultrasound study is intended only to gather limited information related to the pending procedure and is not a detailed evaluation to identify all birth defects.

Once the initial ultrasound study is complete, the gel is cleaned from the maternal abdomen and the skin prepared with an appropriate antiseptic solution. Under real-time ultrasonic guidance, the technician chooses a needle path that avoids penetrating maternal bowel, preferably avoids piercing the placenta, and enters an adequate pocket of amniotic fluid that does not contain fetal parts on umbilical cord. The actual needle insertion should be performed with continuous ultrasonic monitoring of the needle tip, which lowers the incidence of bloody and dry taps and decreases the need for multiple insertions.[56] Furthermore, continuous monitoring reduces the possibility of inadvertent fetal injury, inasmuch as an acute change in fetal position necessitates adjustments of the needle path, before puncturing the amnion in 10% of monitored procedures.[57] This finding is not surprising, considering that the fetus moves more than 200 times every 30 minutes. We have found that a mechanical biopsy guide with a computer generated needle course is helpful in visualizing the anticipated needle path and in maintaining the proper angle and point of entry; however, its use is not essential. Covering the scan head with a sterile glove or, alternatively, scanning from a position lateral to the needle entry site also allows continuous visualization of the needle entry.

After the sampling route is chosen, the needle is inserted with a continuous, controlled thrust into the pocket of amniotic fluid. The stylet is removed, and the initial few drops of fluid are discarded to minimize the risk of maternal cell contamination. Once a free flow of clear fluid is accomplished, a 10- to 30-mL syringe is applied to the needle hub, and 20 to 30 mL of amniotic fluid is aspirated and sent to the laboratory for processing. Attempting to aspirate fluid with the needle adjacent to the fetal membranes may occlude the tip and prevent sampling. Simply rotating the needle 90 to 180 degrees or advancing it until it pierces the wrapping amnion is usually sufficient to initiate flow. If redirection or rotation is not successful in achieving a free flow of clear fluid, the needle should be removed and another insertion site chosen. Another cause of failed sampling is the occurrence of localized uterine contractions,[58] which frequently occur at the needle insertion site. The contraction may obliterate the amniotic fluid space beneath the needle or actually alter the needle path. Ultrasonic guidance allows identification of these contractions and redirection or reinsertion of the needle tip.

On occasion, bloody fluid or even pure blood is retrieved if the needle tip has not completely traversed the uterine wall and placenta. If this occurs, the tip is adjusted until clear fluid is obtained. Although blood-stained amniotic fluid occurs in fewer than 5% of amniocentesis procedures performed with ultrasonic guidance, microscopic evidence of erythrocytes can be found in most specimens. Fortunately, small amounts of blood usually do not adversely affect amniotic cell growth.

In certain cases, transplacental amniocentesis may be unavoidable. Whether this is associated with an increased risk of pregnancy loss continues to be debated.[59-61] In more than half of the amniocentesis procedures in which the placenta is traversed, removal of the needle is followed by an ultrasonically visible intraamniotic hemorrhage.[62] Although the bleeding is usually of short duration, clots and intraamniotic strands, similar in appearance to bands, may be seen.[62] These findings usually resolve in 3 to 10 weeks and do not appear to predispose the fetus to structural anomalies or to significantly increase the pregnancy loss rate. It is prudent to avoid placental perforation; however, if a placenta-free window cannot be found, choosing a sampling site through the lateral, thinnest portion of the placenta avoids inadvertent puncture of the large surface vessels coursing near the cord insertion. Before insertion, color Doppler ultrasound imaging of the proposed insertion site helps identify large vessels. The risks involved in transplacental amniocentesis are not thought to be great enough to preclude the procedure.

There has been a consistent trend over the years to use smaller needles for aspiration. Use of 20- to 22-gauge needles not only is less painful but also has been reported to result in fewer complications than does the 19-gauge and larger needles used previously.[63,64] The possibility that even smaller needles, such as 23- to 25-gauge, may be safer, especially when traversing an anterior placenta, has been suggested. However, any benefit that these small-caliber needles may offer is negated by the increased procedure time required for fluid drainage. At present, we recommend a 20- or 22-gauge spinal needle for genetic amniocentesis.

Techniques to increase the concentration of viable cells in amniotic fluid samples have been sought. Having the patient move about to agitate the fluid and disperse the cells has not been shown to be effective.[65] More recently, it has been demonstrated that additional viable cells can be retrieved by modifying the aspiration technique.[66,67] One approach is to use an exchange apparatus that filters the cells from the fluid and then injects the cell-free fluid back into the amniotic cavity. This allows a larger number of cells to be obtained from each sample and only a small amount of amniotic fluid to be removed.

Complications and Risks of Second-Trimester Amniocentesis

The most frequent complications of amniocentesis, such as vaginal bleeding, rupture of the membranes, chorioamnionitis, and pregnancy loss, also occur in unsampled pregnancies. Therefore, in order to determine the additional risk burden from the procedure, it is necessary to compare studies of amniocentesis with unsampled control populations. Surprisingly, for a commonly performed procedure that has been clinically utilized since the early 1970s, there is a relative paucity of contemporary studies.

Pregnancy loss. The crucial concern for patients undergoing prenatal testing is the risk that the procedure may lead to the loss of a desired pregnancy. A review of contemporary studies performed since 1990 reveal a postprocedure miscarriage rate until 28 weeks' gestation of 1.0% to 2.2%. Although the total postprocedure miscarriage rate is helpful information for patients, it does not represent the rate of procedure-induced miscarriage, because background losses are included.

The prospective, randomized, controlled trial performed by Tabor and associates gives the best analysis of the **procedure-induced** risks of genetic amniocentesis.[68] Study participants were between the ages of 25 and 34 and had no genetic indication for invasive testing but were willing to be randomly assigned to undergo either amniocentesis or no procedure. Amniocentesis was performed by a small number of experienced operators who used standard accepted techniques, including ultrasonic guidance. The group undergoing amniocentesis had an overall loss rate to 28 weeks of 1.7%, in comparison with the control group rate of 0.7% ($p < .01$) (relative risk, 2.3). The authors went on to comment that this 1% difference (95% confidence interval, 0.3% to 1.5%) in fetal loss may represent an underestimate, because the identification and elective termination of karyotypically abnormal fetuses from the amniocentesis group reduced the spontaneous loss rate.

A number of cohort studies have been performed since this report. Most continue to reveal a total postprocedure loss rate of about 1% to 1.5% and an estimated procedure-induced loss rate of about 0.5%.[69-72] Currently, the standard recommendation is that patients be informed that the risk of pregnancy loss from an amniocentesis performed at 15 to 20 weeks' gestation may be as high as 1.0%. However, most centers continue to counsel that the procedure-induced loss rate is more likely to be 0.5%.

Postprocedure vaginal bleeding. Vaginal bleeding after amniocentesis occurs infrequently, usually after difficult procedures, and may be associated with an increased risk of subsequent miscarriage. Bleeding within 6 weeks of the procedure occurs in 0.4% to 2.6% of cases.[63,68,73] In the Medical Research Council report, bleeding did occur more often in sampled patients (1.4%) than in controls (0.4%), and spontaneous miscarriage occurred in 21% of the patients who bled and in none of the control group.[73] A direct correlation between the incidence of bleeding and the number of required needle insertions has also been described.[63]

Amniotic fluid leakage. Leakage of amniotic fluid after a second-trimester diagnostic amniocentesis occurs in 0.8% to 2% of sampled pregnancies; this rate may be up to 1% higher than that seen in unsampled pregnancies.[68,73] In most cases the fluid leakage is self-limited, lasting 1 to 3 days and associated with excellent pregnancy outcome.[74-76] Crandall and colleagues described five cases of amniotic fluid leakage occurring within 2 days of the procedure; all lasted less than 24 hours and ended with normal pregnancy outcome.[74] Gold and associates provided additional evidence that the prognosis for ruptured membranes after amniocentesis is inherently better than that after spontaneous rupture. They treated seven cases of gross rupture of membranes occurring within 24 hours of amniocentesis with hospitalization and strict bed rest until leakage subsided. All leakages ceased within 3 days and amniotic fluid volumes were normal by 7 days. Six of the seven women delivered healthy full-term neonates; in the seventh, an intrauterine demise occurred at 25 weeks.[75]

Infection. Postamniocentesis chorioamnionitis is rare and occurs in 0.5 to 1.5 cases per 1000 procedures performed.[63,77] Infection most often results from the accidental introduction of either skin or bowel flora into the amnionic sac. However, ascending infection is also feasible, especially if chronic amniotic fluid leakage occurs.

The initial signs of a second-trimester intrauterine infection can be quite subtle, and the patient may initially present with only a low-grade fever and flu-like symptoms; however, if ignored, they can rapidly progress to severe chorioamnionitis and maternal sepsis. Uterine tenderness may not be present initially, and a high index of suspicion is necessary to make an early diagnosis. Therefore, in any patient who has recently undergone amniocentesis and presents with fever and no other obvious source, a repeat amniocentesis for Gram stain and culture is indicated. If organisms are present, the prognosis is uniformly dismal, and delay in emptying the uterus does not seem justified.

Rh isoimmunization. A fetal-to-maternal hemorrhage of at least 0.1 mL follows 2% to 3% of second-trimester amniocentesis procedures.[78] This hemorrhage leads to Rh isoimmunization in 2.1% to 5.4% of at-risk pregnancies.[79,80] The Medical Research Council report included 133 Rh D–negative amniocentesis patients who gave birth to Rh-positive babies.[73] Anti-Rho(D) prophylaxis had been given to 59, none of whom was sensitized, whereas in the group not receiving prophylaxis, 5.2% developed antibodies. Dubin and Staisch similarly suggested a 5% risk of new or increased sensitization after genetic amniocentesis.[81] Alternatively, some groups have found no increase in the incidence of sensitization and remain unconvinced that Rho(D) immune globulin prophylaxis is necessary.[68,79] Although this debate persists, it is clear that potential iatrogenic sensitization can be prevented and Rho (D) immune globulin should be given to all Rh D–negative nonsensitized women undergoing amniocentesis. A dose of 100 µg is adequate and is less expensive than the standard 300-µg dose.[82]

Risk of fetal abnormalities. Accidental fetal puncture during amniocentesis usually has no deleterious effects but, on occasion, may result in a minor skin injury with subsequent congenital dimpling. There have, however, been reports of serious fetal damage attributed to amniocentesis needlesticks and include death secondary to exsanguination, cardiac tamponade, severe brain injury, globe injuries with subsequent ocular dysfunction, peritoneal-parietal fistulas, traumatic arteriovenous fistulas, and gangrene of the arm secondary to vascular disruption.[83-88] Fortunately, the use of continuous ultrasound monitoring makes such occurrences infrequent.

The possibility that other congenital anomalies may be increased by amniocentesis continues to be evaluated.

Several reports, including animal studies, have suggested a higher incidence of neonatal respiratory difficulties in sampled pregnancies. Tabor and associates, in a prospective randomized comparison, demonstrated a significant increase in the incidence of both neonatal respiratory distress syndrome and congenital pneumonia in infants whose mothers underwent amniocentesis.[68] The relative risks were 2.1 and 2.5, respectively. Using a primate model, Hislop and colleagues demonstrated altered alveolar number and size, as well as reduction in respiratory airways, when amniocentesis was performed at a comparable gestational age.[89] Other studies, both controlled[73] and uncontrolled,[90-94] have also demonstrated pulmonary alterations in sampled pregnancies, whereas similar studies have failed to confirm these findings.[63,74,95]

Although the debate about neonatal effects remains, a report of the long-term sequelae of genetic amniocentesis may allay some fears. Finegan and associates reported a longitudinal investigation comparing development, behavior, and physical status of 4-year-old children whose mothers had either chosen or declined amniocentesis.[96] The only difference in the two groups was a higher incidence of bilateral middle-ear impedance abnormalities and recurrent ear infections in children exposed to amniocentesis. The authors hypothesized that the reduction in intraamniotic fluid volume led to pressure changes within the ear that disturb normal development.

Perinatal Complications

Perinatal complications have not consistently been found to be increased in patients undergoing amniocentesis. No difference in the incidence of preeclampsia, abruptio placentae, placenta previa, or dysfunctional labor have been demonstrated.[63,68,74] Although Lowe and coworkers did report a higher rate of cesarean section in patients undergoing amniocentesis (17.9%, in comparison with 12.4%),[63] it is unlikely that the second-trimester procedure was causally related. Similarly, findings in the Medical Research Council study that demonstrated a significant increase in placenta previa and abruptio placentae are thought to be more a result of chance than a direct response to the procedure.[73]

Discolored amniotic fluid. Dark or discolored amniotic fluid found at the time of a second-trimester amniocentesis is usually secondary to intraamniotic blood products and is usually not associated with culture failure, but some studies have predicted poor perinatal outcome. In a study performed before the use of ultrasonography, Golbus and associates found that when the amniotic fluid was greenish-brown, a missed abortion was present in 30% of these cases; however, the remaining patients with discolored fluid and a normal karyotype had uncomplicated pregnancies.[97] Hanson and colleagues found red or greenish-brown fluid in 4.6% of amniotic fluid samples from viable pregnancies; 15% of those pregnancies subsequently ended with a fetal or neonatal death.[98] Similarly, Tabor and associates reported a nearly 10-fold relative risk of spontaneous abortion if discolored fluid was withdrawn at amniocentesis.[68] In contrast to these reports, Allen found green or meconium-stained fluid in 1.6% of his cases,[99] with a fetal mortality rate of only 5%.

In practice, although the pregnancy loss rate is most probably increased when dark fluid is obtained, especially when it is brown or dark red, patients can be reassured that once the karyotype is found to be normal, there is no association with fetal abnormalities and that the majority of such pregnancies have excellent outcomes.

Amniocentesis Performed before 14 Weeks' Gestation

One of the major disadvantages of amniocentesis has been that results may be unavailable until 18 to 20 weeks' gestation. The couple receiving abnormal results is then faced with a decision about pregnancy termination after fetal movement has been perceived and the pregnancy is visibly apparent. Not only is pregnancy termination clinically more dangerous at this gestational age, but the psychologic effect is significant. Reports from the mid-1970s suggested that amniocentesis before 15 weeks had an unacceptable procedure and culture failure rate[65,97]; however, the development of high-resolution ultrasonography and direct needle guidance makes the amniotic sac technically accessible as early as 7 weeks' gestation.[99] Simultaneously, the development of improved tissue culture methods has led to improved laboratory success rates and requirements of less fluid and fewer cells for cytogenetic analysis. These technical advances led to attempts at performing amniocentesis earlier in gestation.[100-109]

Sampling Technique

Reports on "early" amniocentesis demonstrate that amniotic fluid can be successfully aspirated and cell cultures established at a rate comparable to that of later procedures.[100-109] However, data on the safety and complications have proved worrisome.

Most studies of early amniocentesis have evaluated procedures performed in the 11th and 12th weeks and have compared these procedures with either those performed after 15 weeks or with chorionic villus sampling. These studies have revealed that amniocentesis before the 13th week is associated with an increased risk of sampling failure and unsuccessful culture.[110,111] Of more concern has been the consistent association of amniocentesis with an increased risk of leakage of amniotic fluid, miscarriage, and talipes equinovarus (clubfoot)[110-112] as defined risks from the largest controlled trials. The risk of talipes is quite dramatic. Whereas it occurs in approximately 1 to 3 births per 1000 in the general population, it is seen in about 1.5% to 1.9% of births after early amniocentesis. When early amniocentesis is followed by leakage of amniotic fluid, clubfoot subsequently occurs in 15% of the neonates.[110] Even without vaginal leakage of fluid, the risk of talipes equinovarus is still increased 10-fold.

Review of the pregnancy anatomy before 14 weeks' gestation gives some understanding about the cause of the problem. The amnionic and chorionic membranes have not fused, and the relatively fragile amnionic membrane is more susceptible to injury that leads to leakage of fluid. The subsequent oligohydramnios may alter the pressure surrounding the fetus, leading to compression or altered fetal movement. There is further evidence that membrane injury plays a role: In pregnancies sampled by transplacental needle passage through an area in which the amnion is adherent, there is a markedly reduced risk of leakage and clubfoot.[113] Although this mechanism seems reasonable, other alternatives have also been described.[114] The current information suggests that amniocentesis should not be performed in the 11th and 12th weeks, especially because chorionic villus sampling is available at this gestational age and has a superior safety profile. Preliminary data suggest that the increased risks of early amniocentesis continue through the 14th week, when the membranes fuse.[113]

SUCCESS AND ACCURACY OF LABORATORY ANALYSIS

After a technically successful amniotic fluid aspiration, the retrieved cells are concentrated by centrifugation and put into tissue culture for a minimum of 5 to 7 days.[115] Final results are usually available within 10 days to 3 weeks. The details of cell culture and analysis are beyond the scope of this chapter and are considered in detail elsewhere.[115,116] From a clinical standpoint, however, it is important to realize that even under ideal laboratory conditions, amniocentesis occasionally fails to yield a result or, worse, may result in a diagnostic error.

Tissue culture failure occurs infrequently (0.2% to 0.6% of cases)[68,97] and results from a paucity of viable cells in the sample, from failure of the cells to grow under laboratory conditions, or because of contamination of the growing culture with infectious organisms. Culture failures are minimized by aspirating a sufficient volume of fluid (20 to 30 mL) and by performing sampling in the middle of the second trimester.[68,97] Although the actual concentration of cells from fluid retrieved earlier than 15 weeks is less than in later gestation,[102] the percentage of viable cells is actually increased. Therefore, culture time for procedures performed between 11 and 14 weeks' gestation is approximately 7 to 12 days, with a total turnaround time similar to that for later amniocentesis.[117,118] However, amniocentesis before 11 weeks' gestation may require slightly longer culture time and still occasionally results in culture failure.[104,105,107,109,117]

Significant diagnostic and clinical errors after amniocentesis are exceedingly rare. In addition to clerical problems from sample handling and mislabeling, however, other errors may occur from either maternal cell contamination or misinterpretation of mosaic results. Pooled data from various U.S. and European centers have shown that although some maternal cells are found in 0.1% to 0.2% of cases,[119] the risk of a major diagnostic error is extremely rare and can be further reduced by discarding the first few milliliters of amniotic fluid during retrieval.

The finding in an amniotic fluid culture of two or more cell lines with different chromosome constitutions is called **mosaicism** and requires careful clinical interpretation. Although the abnormal cell line may represent a significant fetal chromosomal abnormality, it most frequently is a finding secondary to in vitro tissue culture artifacts or to a chromosomal error existing in the extraembryonic membrane but not in the fetus. In the majority of cases, the clinical significance is determined by the specific chromosome abnormality or the distribution of the abnormal cells in culture. To assist in the interpretation of mosaicism, the amniotic fluid cells are cultured on multiple coverslips or in more than one culture vessel. If the aberrant cell line is restricted to a single flask or coverslip, this is considered to be an in vitro clonal event that has no clinical significance for the fetus. Alternatively, when the aberrant cell line is found in multiple culture vessels or colonies, the possibility that the fetus may also carry the abnormal cell line is appreciably increased. Such a finding is present in 0.1% to 0.2% of amniotic fluid samples analyzed[120,121] and requires further analysis for definitive determination of its clinical significance. If mosaicism is found and the abnormal karyotype has previously been reported in dysmorphic liveborn infants, it is necessary to sample additional fetal cell lines such as blood or skin to evaluate the implications. However, in only 60% to 70% of these cases is the abnormal cell line confirmed in the fetus.[120,122]

Molecular cytogenetics may make the culture period obsolete in selected situations. With chromosome-specific probes and FISH, it is now possible to detect certain numeric aberrations in interphase, nondividing cells.[123] Because the viable cells found in amniotic fluid are nucleated, this process eliminates the need for cell cultivation and makes more cells available for screening than does classic cytogenetic analysis. Routinely used probes allow the diagnosis of only the common autosomal trisomies (13, 18, and 21) and sex chromosome aneuploidy and does not identify aberrations involving other chromosomes; therefore, the routine use of FISH is not recommended. This approach is useful when a rapid diagnosis is required and there is a strong clinical suspicion of a common autosomal trisomy.

Amniocentesis in Twins

Amniocentesis is frequently performed for genetic indications on twin gestations because the incidence of twinning, especially dichorionic twinning, increases with advancing maternal age. Because each fetus in a dizygotic gestation carries an independent genetic risk, the probability that one fetus is affected is almost twice the risk for a singleton (see Chapter 17). For example, a 35-year-old woman with a singleton gestation has a 1 per 356 risk of delivering a liveborn child with Down syndrome, whereas a 33-year-old woman with a twin gestation has approximately the same risk (1 per 355). Alternatively, the probability that both fetuses are affected is exceedingly unlikely unless the pregnancy is monozygotic.

Twin Sampling Procedure

The initial step in successfully performing amniocentesis on a twin gestation is a detailed ultrasound study to determine gestational age, fetal positions, location and number of placentas, and characteristics of the separating membrane. In the first trimester, a thin dividing membrane almost certainly confirms a monochorionic gestation[124]; by 16 weeks' gestation, however, this is less certain. Likewise, in the second trimester, the two placentas of a dichorionic gestation may fuse and appear as a single placenta.[124] Therefore, to ensure that accurate genetic information is obtained for each fetus, sampling of each sac is suggested even when the ultrasound study may suggest a monochorionic gestation. This approach also ensures that in the rare cases of monochorionic heterokaryotic twinning, in which one fetus may have a 46,XY karyotype and the other a 45,XO karyotype, a correct diagnosis will be made.

Continuous ultrasound guidance of twin amniocentesis is mandatory. In the most frequently used technique, a 20- or 22-gauge needle is inserted into one sac and 20 to 30 mL of fluid is retrieved. Before the needle is removed, 3 to 5 mL of an inert dye is injected. The presence of microscopic air bubbles mixed with the dye permits visualization of the dye dispersion throughout the amniotic sac. The needle is then removed, and a new needle is inserted into the sac of the coexisting fetus. Clear fluid, without dye, shows that each fetus has been sampled individually. The retrieval of dye-stained fluid strongly suggests that the initial sac was resampled, but in very rare cases this may occur because of a monoamniotic gestation. As ultrasound guidance has improved, some operators have discontinued using dye when a dividing membrane is easily visualized. For experienced operators, this is acceptable, but for those performing only occasional amniocentesis in twin pregnancies, we suggest that this additional step be taken, because inadvertent reinsertion into the initial sac can occur. Either Evans blue or indigo carmine are acceptable dyes. Methylene blue dye, however, has been associated with the occurrence of fetal bowel atresia[125,126] and hemolytic anemia and should *never* be used.

Other techniques for sampling twin gestations have also been described. In one approach, air mixed with indigo carmine dye is injected into the initial sac. The subsequent bubbles are quite easily visualized as they rapidly disperse throughout the sac, enabling the technician to insert the second needle into the opposite, bubble-free sac.[127] This technique is also useful in confirming a monochorionic gestation. An alternative approach has been described in which a single needle is used to sample one sac and is then redirected through the membrane and into the coexisting amnion.[128] Visualizing the perforation of the dividing membrane should confirm that the second sac has been sampled. Although this technique has its advocates, the use of a single needle for sampling both sacs may make laboratory interpretation of abnormalities or mosaicism difficult. Also, the rent in the membrane may become enlarged as the pregnancy progresses, allowing the cord or fetal parts to become entangled or entrapped in the amnion.[129] Finally, another technique has been described in which the first sampling needle is left in place while another amniocentesis is performed with a second needle on the coexisting sac. Visualization of both needles simultaneously provides proof of individual sampling.[130]

It is imperative that the locations of the fetuses, amniotic sacs, and placentas be diagrammed at the time of sampling so that in cases of discordant results, identification of the affected fetus can be accomplished at the time of selective termination (see Chapter 17). Likewise, when samples are submitted to the laboratory, careful labeling of each sample is necessary to ensure its correct association with fetal position.

Complications of Amniocentesis on Twins

Pregnancy loss after genetic amniocentesis on twins occurs more frequently than with singleton gestations (Table 6-5).[131-134] Although a proportion of the additional losses may be attributable to the inherent risks of a twin gestation and unrelated to the procedure, the patient should be counseled that the risk may be two to three times higher than for that of a singleton.

Third-Trimester Amniocentesis

Indications

Amniocentesis was initially described as a third-trimester technique and continues to be useful in the evaluation of many perinatal diagnostic situations. Although a detailed discussion of each is beyond the scope of this chapter,

Table 6–5. Contemporary Studies of Amniocentesis in Twin Gestations

Study Focus	Amniocentesis			
	Wapner et al[131] (1993)	Pijpers et al[132] (1988)	Anderson et al[133] (1991)	Pruggmayer et al[134]
Pregnancies sampled	72	83	339	98
Fetuses sampled	144	160	687	196
Elective abortion				
Pregnancy	1	1	3	0
Singleton	0	0	7	0
Lost to follow-up	1	0	12	0
Delivery cohort				
Pregnancies	70	82	332	98
Fetuses	140	164	666	196
Pregnancy loss at < 28 weeks	2 (2.9%)	4 (4.9%)	12 (3.6%)	8 (8.2%)
Total fetal loss	13 (9.3%)	8 (4.9%)	31 (4.7%)	21 (10.7%)

Table 6–6. Indications for Late Second- and Early Third-Trimester Amniocentesis

Indication for Amniocentesis	Test Performed

Determine fetal lung maturity	Evaluation of AF phospholipids
	  Lecithin:sphingomyelin (L:S) ratio
	  Phosphatidylglycerol

Evaluation of erythroblastosis fetalis
  Evaluate fetal hemolysis
  Determination of fetal blood type
	
	Optical density of amniotic fluid at 450 nm
	Molecular evaluation of the gene for the D antigen

Preterm labor Evaluate for possible chorioamnionitis	 Culture of AF Gram stain of AF Glucose level in AF Interleukin-6 level in AF
Fetal structural abnormality on ultrasound study	Karyotype

Evaluation for fetal infection	Polymerase chain reaction (PCR) for
	  Cytomegalovirus
	  Toxoplasmosis

Evaluation of at-risk couple for fetal PLA 1 status secondary to alloimmune thrombocytopenia	Molecular determination of fetal PCA status

AF, amniotic fluid; PCA, post conceptional age.

Table 6-6 lists the common indications, most of which are discussed in other areas of this book. The most frequent indications are discussed as follows.

Fetal karyotyping. Fetal karyotyping, the major indication at earlier gestational ages, can still be achieved through third-trimester amniocentesis when fetal structural abnormalities are identified by ultrasonography. However, because of the more advanced gestational age, amniocentesis frequently is supplanted by procedures such as fetal blood sampling that yield a result more rapidly. In addition, although third-trimester amniocentesis may harvest a larger volume of cells, these specimens are more difficult to culture because the cells may have decreased replicating capacity and there may be contamination with vernix caseosa or fetal hair. Tissue culture delay is thus longer in this group, although methods to enhance growth and achieve a result are available, and in almost all cases a result is obtained.[135] FISH, described earlier, has been used to obtain rapid identification of the common trisomies (i.e., 13, 18, and 21). Although false-positive FISH results are unlikely, uninformative results do occur. At present, it is recommended that no irreversible clinical decisions be made on the basis of FISH results alone.

Evaluation of preterm labor and chorioamnionitis. Chorioamnionitis, frequently subtle and with minimal clinical symptoms, has been implicated as an cause of preterm labor. Because no medical therapy is currently accepted uniformly for treatment of preterm labor secondary to chorioamnionitis, its presence dictates delivery and contraindicates tocolysis, regardless of gestational age, in order to minimize the fetal and maternal risks. The diagnosis is initially based on clinical symptoms and confirmed by amniotic fluid culture.[136,137] Other amniotic fluid parameters such as abnormal Gram stain,[138] low glucose level,[139-142] elevated white blood cell count,[143] or abnormal leukocyte esterase level[144,145] are also suggestive.

Amniocentesis, therefore, plays a central role in the management of intractable premature labor. In some centers, tocolytic therapy is withheld until after amniocentesis is performed. This serves two purposes: One is to rule out an infectious cause of the premature labor, and the other is to evaluate fetal lung maturity. Appropriate management is then instituted on the basis of these results.

Evaluation of fetal lung maturity. Fetal lung maturity may be determined either directly by determination of amniotic fluid phospholipid levels or indirectly by evaluating amniotic fluid surface tension properties. This investigation is prompted by the onset of premature labor, when early delivery may be indicated because of maternal or fetal disease, or when gestational dating criteria are ambiguous and delivery by induction or cesarean section is elected in the absence of established American College of Obstetricians and Gynecologists criteria.[146] Various tests are employed to detect the presence and amount of specific lecithin or surfactants that predict fetal lung maturity. These include phosphatidylcholine, phosphatidylinositol, and phosphatidylglycerol. Two parameters commonly evaluated in tests of fetal lung maturity are the ratio of lecithin to sphingomyelin and the presence of phosphatidylglycerol. In nondiabetic patients, a ratio of more than 2:1 is associated with a low risk of neonatal respiratory distress syndrome.[147] In all patients, the presence of phosphatidylglycerol is more predictive of fetal lung maturity.[148]

Evaluation of blood group sensitization. Amniocentesis in the third trimester initially came to the fore of obstetric practice in the management of Rh isoimmunization.[2] The hemolysis of fetal red blood cells as a result of fetal antigen and maternal antibody interaction causes elevated levels of bilirubin to be produced. The bilirubin pigment is subsequently eliminated in fetal urine, and its concentration in amniotic fluid is therefore increased. By spectrophotometric analysis of the deviation of the absorbance of the amniotic fluid sample from the standard curve at wavelength 450 (ΔOD 450), the degree of hemolysis can be quantified. Liley developed a curve of normal and abnormal absorbance (ΔOD 450) throughout gestation for management of sensitized pregnancies. Patients can thus be managed with serial amniocentesis to evaluate the degree of fetal hemolysis throughout their pregnancy. The gene for the D antigen has been located and cloned, allowing determination of fetal blood type by evaluation of the amniotic fluid, rather than requiring fetal blood.[149] In cases in which the father is heterozygous at the D locus, a single amniocentesis can determine the fetal blood type; if it is Rh-negative, serial studies are not required.

In 2000, Mari and associates reported a noninvasive approach to the surveillance of red cell alloimmunization. Using Doppler ultrasonography, they measured the peak velocity of systolic blood flow in fetal middle cervical artery. They demonstrated that moderate or severe anemia could be detected by an increase in the velocity of flow.[150] Other studies have since confirmed this, and this approach is rapidly replacing amniocentesis as the primary surveillance tool.

Complications of Third-Trimester Amniocentesis

Complications of amniocentesis in the third trimester are similar to those found at earlier gestational ages and include fetal injury, rupture of membranes, abruptio placentae, introduction of infection, and induction of premature labor.[151] Umbilical cord injury with hemorrhage or thrombosis is more frequent with third-trimester amniocentesis, especially when the amniotic fluid volume is low. Therefore, care must be taken to identify any part of the cord within the anticipated sampling site. If bloody fluid is aspirated, postamniocentesis fetal monitoring is strongly suggested.

Whereas complications of midtrimester amniocentesis either are self-limiting or result in the loss of the pregnancy, in the third trimester they may precipitate the delivery of a premature infant with the attendant neonatal concerns. Thus, the risks and their incidence, approximately 1%, remain the same, but their long-term consequences may be more severe. In third-trimester amniocentesis, attempts to mitigate these risks are similar to those outlined in the previous discussion of midtrimester amniocentesis.

SUMMARY

Amniocentesis is one of the most important and frequently used invasive prenatal diagnostic modalities offered to women throughout pregnancy. In the midtrimester, the primary indication is for evaluation of genetic disorders, predominantly chromosomal abnormalities, as indicated by maternal age, serum screening, or ultrasonographically identified fetal anomalies. Its role in diagnosing single-gene disorders either through DNA molecular analysis or fetal chemistry profiles will continue to expand with progress in the understanding of the underling genetic defect in these conditions. It remains the only way to directly assess α-fetoprotein in pregnancies at risk for open neural tube defects and ventricle wall

defects. At later gestational ages, amniocentesis is employed to document fetal lung maturity, rule out chorioamnionitis, diagnose congenital infection, and monitor fetal hemolysis, in addition to its role in genetic evaluations.

The complication rate associated with amniocentesis is approximately 1% and includes the risk of fetal injury, infection, and pregnancy interruption. These risks are minimized by the use of continuous ultrasound guidance and by operator experience.

REFERENCES

1. Lambl D: Ein seltener Fall von Hydramnios. Zentralbl Gynaekol 5:329, 1881.
2. Bevis DCA: The antenatal prediction of haemolytic disease of the newborn. Lancet 1:395, 1952.
3. Fuchs F, Riis P: Antenatal sex determinants. Nature 177:330, 1956.
4. James F: Sexing foetuses by examination of amniotic fluid. Lancet 1:202, 1956.
5. Makowski EL, Prem KA, Kaiser IH: Detection of sex of fetuses by the incidence of sex chromatin body in nuclei of cells in amniotic fluid. Science 123:542, 1956.
6. Serr DM, Sachs L, Danon M: Diagnosis of sex before birth using cells from the amniotic fluid. Bull Res Counc Isr 58:137, 1955.
7. Shettles LB: Nuclear morphology of cells in human amniotic fluid in relation to sex of infant. Am J Obstet Gynecol 71:834, 1956.
8. Nadler HL: Antenatal detection of hereditary disorders. Pediatrics 42:912, 1968.
9. Jeffcoate TNA, Fliegner JR, Russell SH, et al: Diagnosis of adrenogenital syndrome before birth. Lancet 2:553, 1965.
10. Steele MW, Breg WR Jr: Chromosome analysis of human amniotic fluid cells. Lancet 1:383, 1966.
11. Seeds AE: Current concepts of amniotic fluid dynamics. Am J Obstet Gynecol 138:575, 1980.
12. Brace RA, Wolf EJ: Normal amniotic fluid volume changes throughout pregnancy. Am J Obstet Gynecol 161:382, 1989.
13. Van Leeven L, Jacoby H, Charles D: Exfoliative cytology of amnionic fluid. Acta Cytol 9:442, 1965.
14. Peakman DC, Moreton MF, Corn BJ, et al: Chromosomal mosaicism in amniotic fluid cell culture. Am J Hum Genet 31:149, 1979.
15. Hook EB, Cross PK, Jackson L, et al: Maternal age-specific rates of 47,+21 and other cytogenetic abnormalities diagnosed in the first trimester of pregnancy in chorionic villus biopsy specimens: Comparison with rates expected from observations at amniocentesis. Am J Hum Genet 42:797, 1988.
16. Ferguson-Smith MA, Yates JRW: Maternal age specific rates for chromosome aberrations and factors influencing them: Reports of a collaborative European study on 52,965 amniocenteses. Prenat Diagn 4:5, 1984.
17. Hook EB: Spontaneous deaths of fetuses with chromosomal abnormalities diagnosed prenatally. N Engl J Med 299:1036, 1978.
18. Hook EB: Chromosome abnormalities and spontaneous fetal death following amniocentesis: Further data and associations with maternal age. Am J Hum Genet 35:110, 1983.
19. Cuckle HS, Wald NT Lindenbaum RH: Maternal serum alpha fetoprotein measurement: A screening test for Down syndrome. Lancet 1:926, 1984.

20. Wald NJ, Cuckle HS, Densem JW, et al: Maternal serum screening for Down syndrome in early pregnancy. BMJ 297:883, 1988.
21. Wald NJ, Cuckle H, Densem J, et al: Maternal serum unconjugated estriol as an antenatal screening test for Down syndrome. Br J Obstet Gynaecol 95:334, 1988.
22. Haddow JE, Palomaki GE: Prenatal screening for Down syndrome. In Simpson JL (ed): Essentials of Prenatal Diagnosis. New York, Churchill Livingstone, 1993, pp 44-51.
23. Wald NJ, Huttly WJ, Hackshaw AK: Antenatal screening for Down's syndrome with the quadruple test [Comment]. Lancet 361:835, 2002.
24. Wald NJ, Watt HC, Hackshaw AK: Integrated screening for Down's syndrome based on tests performed during the first and second trimesters. N Engl J Med 341:461, 1999.
25. Haddow JE, Palomaki GE, Knight G, et al: Reducing the need for amniocentesis in women 35 years of age or older with serum markers for screening. New Engl J Med 330:114, 1994.
26. Stene J, Stene E, Mikkelsen M: Risk for chromosome abnormality at amniocentesis following a child with a non-inherited chromosome aberration. Prenat Diagn (Special Issue) 4:81, 1984.
27. Mikkelsen M, Stene J: Previous child with Down syndrome and other chromosome aberration: Group report. In Murken JD, Stenzel-Rutkowske S, Schwinger E (eds): Proceedings on the 3rd European Conference on Prenatal Diagnosis of Genetic Disorders. Stuttgart, Enke, 1979, p 22.
28. Daniel A, Hook EB, Wulf G: Risks of unbalanced progeny at amniocentesis to carrier of chromosome rearrangements: Data from United States and Canadian laboratories. Am J Med Genet 33:14, 1989.
29. Milunsky A: Prenatal diagnosis of chromosome disorders. In Milunsky A (ed): Genetic disorders of the fetus. New York, Plenum Press, 1979, p 108.
30. Boue A, Gallano P: A collaborative study of the segregation of inherited chromosome structural rearrangements in 1356 prenatal diagnoses. Prenat Diagn (Special Issue) 4:45, 1984.
31. Borgaurkos DS: Chromosomal Variations in Man: A Catalog of Chromosomal Variants and Anomalies, 7th ed. New York, Alan R. Liss, 1994.
32. Fraccaro M, Lindstein J, Ford CE, et al: The 11q 22q translocations: A European collaborative analysis of 43 cases. Hum Genet 56:21, 1980.
33. Nicolaides K, Snijders RJ, Gosden CM, et al: Ultrasonographically detectable markers of fetal chromosomal abnormalities. Lancet 340:704, 1992.
34. Gagnon S, Fraser W, Fouquette B, et al: Nature and frequency of chromosomal abnormalities in pregnancies with abnormal ultrasound findings: An analysis of 117 cases with review of the literature. Prenat Diagn 12:9, 1992.
35. Lemna WK, Feldman GL, Kerem B, et al: Mutation analysis for heterozygote detection and the prenatal diagnosis of cystic fibrosis. N Engl J Med 322:291, 1990.
36. Shoshani T, Augarten A, Gazit E, et al: Association of a nonsense mutation (W1232X), the most common mutation in the Ashkenazi Jewish cystic fibrosis patients in Israel, with presentation of severe disease. Am J Hum Genet 50:222, 1992.
37. Kazazian HH Jr: The thalassemia syndromes: Molecular basis and prenatal diagnosis in 1990. Semin Hematol 27:209, 1990.
38. Schneck L, Valenti C, Amsterdam D, et al: Prenatal diagnosis of Tay-Sachs disease. Lancet 1:582, 1970.
39. Navon R, Padeh B: Prenatal diagnosis of Tay-Sachs genotypes. BMJ 4:17, 1971.
40. Pergament E: Prenatal Tay-Sachs diagnosis by chorionic villi sampling [letter]. Lancet 2:286, 1983.
41. American Academy of Pediatrics and American College of Obstetricians and Gynecologists (AAP/ACOG): Position Statement on Screening for Canavan Disease. Washington, DC, AAP/ACOG, 1998.
42. Driscoll MC, Lerner N, Anyane-Yeboa K, et al: Prenatal diagnosis of sickle hemoglobinopathies: The experience of the Columbia University Comprehensive Center for sickle cell disease. Am J Hum Genet 40:548, 1987.
43. Chang JC, Kan YW: A sensitive new prenatal test for sickle-cell anemia. N Engl J Med 307:30, 1982.
44. Ward PA, Hejtmancik JF, Witkowski JA, et al: Prenatal diagnosis of Duchenne muscular dystrophy: Prospective linkage analysis and retrospective dystrophin cDNA analysis. Am J Hum Genet 44:270, 1989.
45. Bakker E, Bonten EJ, Veenema H, et al: Prenatal diagnosis of Duchenne muscular dystrophy: a three-year experience in a rapidly evolving field. J Inherit Metabolic Dis 12:174, 1989.
46. Kasazian HH Jr: The molecular basis of hemophilia A and the present status of carrier and antenatal diagnosis of the disease. Thromb Haemost 70:60, 1993.
47. Yamauchi M, Nagata S, Seki N, et al: Prenatal diagnosis of the fragile X syndrome by direct detection of the dynamic mutation due to an unstable DNA sequence. Clin Genet 44:169, 1993.
48. Murphy PD, Wilmot PL, Shapiro LR: Prenatal diagnosis of fragile X syndrome: Results from parallel molecular and cytogenetic studies. Am J Med Genet 43:181, 1992.
49. American College of Obstetricians and Gynecologists: Antenatal Diagnosis of Genetic Disorders. Technical Bulletin 108. Washington, DC, American College of Obstetricians and Gynecologists, 1986.
50. Adams MJ, Windham GC, James LM, et al: Clinical interpretation of maternal serum alpha-fetoprotein concentrations. Am J Obstet Gynecol 148:241, 1984.
51. Milunsky A: Prenatal diagnosis of neural tube defects. In Milunsky A (ed): Genetic Disorders and the Fetus. New York, Plenum Press, 1979, pp 383-385.
52. Wald NJ, Cuckle HS, Nanchahal K: Amniotic fluid acetylcholinesterase measurements in the prenatal diagnosis of open neural tube defects. Second report of the collaborative acetycholinesterase study. Prenat Diagn 9:813, 1989.
53. State of California, Department of Health Services, Genetics Disease Branch: AFP Screening. Sacramento, CA, California Department of Health, 1991.
54. Nadel AS, Green JK, Holmes LB, et al: Absence of need for amniocentesis in patients with elevated levels of maternal serum alpha-fetoprotein and normal ultrasonographic examinations. New Engl J Med 323:557, 1991.
55. Crandall BF, Robinson L, Grau P: Risks associated with an elevated MSAFP level. Am J Obstet Gynecol 165:581, 1991.
56. Romero R, Jeanty P, Reece EA, et al: Sonographically monitored amniocentesis to decrease intraoperative complications. Obstet Gynecol 65:426, 1985.
57. Lenke RR, Cyr DR, Mack LA: Midtrimester genetic amniocentesis with simultaneous ultrasound guidance. J Clin Ultrasound 13:371, 1985.
58. Finberg HJ, Frigoletto FD: Sonographic demonstration of uterine contraction during amniocentesis. Am J Obstet Gynecol 139:740, 1981.
59. Tabor A, Philip J, Bang J: Safety of amniocentesis. Prenat Diagn 8:167, 1988.
60. Crane JP, Kopta MM: Genetic amniocentesis: Impact of placental position upon the risk of pregnancy loss. Am J Obstet Gynecol 150:813, 1984.

61. Marthin T, Liedgren S, Hammer M: Transplacental needle passage and other risk-factors associated with second trimester amniocentesis [Abstract]. Acta Obstet Gynecol Scand 76(8):728, 1997.

62. Chinn DH, Towers CV, Beeman RG, Miller EI: Sonographically demonstrated intra-amniotic hemorrhage following transplacental genetic amniocentesis. Frequency, sonographic appearance, and clinical significance. J Ultrasound Med 9:495, 1990.

63. Lowe CU, Alexander D, Bryla D, Siegel D: NICHD Amniocentesis Registry. The Safety and Accuracy of Mid-trimester Amniocentesis. U.S. Department of Health, Education, and Welfare publication NIH 78-190. Washington, DC, National Institutes of Health, 1976.

64. Simpson NE, Dallaire L, Miller JR, et al: Prenatal diagnosis of genetic disease in Canada: Report of a collaborative study. Can Med Assoc J 115:739, 1976.

65. Carlan SJ, Papenhausen P, O'Brien WF, et al: Effect of maternal-fetal movement on concentration of cells obtained at genetic amniocentesis. Am J Obstet Gynecol 163:490, 1990.

66. Sundberg K, Smidt-Jensen S, Philip J: Amniocentesis with increased cell yield, obtained by filtration and reinjection of the amniotic fluid. Ultrasound Obstet Gynecol 1:91, 1991.

67. Kennerknecht I, Kramer S, Grab D, Terinde R: Evaluation of amniotic fluid cell filtration: An experimental approach to early amniocentesis. Prenat Diag 13:247, 1993.

68. Tabor A, Philip J, Madsen M, et al: Randomized controlled trial of genetic amniocentesis in 4606 low-risk women. Lancet 1:1287, 1986.

69. Muller F, Thibaud D, Poloce F, et al: Risk of amniocentesis in women screened positive for Down syndrome with second trimester maternal serum markers. Prenat Diagn 22:1036, 2002.

70. Blackwell SC, Abundis MG, Nehra PC: Five-year experience with midtrimester amniocentesis performed by a single group of obstetricians-gynecologists at a community hospital [Abstract]. Am J Obstet Gynecol 186:1130, 2002.

71. Antsaklis A, Papantoniou N, Xygakis A, et al: Genetic amniocentesis in women 20-34 years old: Associated risks [Comment]. Prenat Diag 20:1018, 2000.

72. Reid KP, Gurrin LC, Dickinson JE, et al: Pregnancy loss rates following second trimester genetic amniocentesis. Aust N Z J Obstet Gynecol 39:281, 1999.

73. Medical Research Council Working Party of Amniocentesis: An assessment of the hazards of amniocentesis. Br J Obstet Gynaecol 85(2):1, 1978.

74. Crandall BF, Howard J, Lebherz TB, et al: Follow-up of 2000 second-trimester amnioceteses. Obstet Gynecol 56:625, 1980.

75. Gold RB, Goyert GL, Schwartz DB, et al: Conservative management of second-trimester post-amniocentesis fluid leakage. Obstet Gynecol 74:745, 1989.

76. Borgida AF, Mills AA, Feldman DM, et al: Outcome of pregnancies complicated by ruptured membranes after genetic amniocentesis [Abstract]. Am J Obstet Gynecol 183:937, 2000.

77. Porreco RP, Young PE, Resnik R, et al: Reproductive outcome following amniocentesis for genetic indications. Am J Obstet Gynecol 43:653, 1982.

78. Bowman JM, Pollock JM: Transplacental fetal hemorrhage after amniocentesis. Obstet Gynecol 66:749, 1985.

79. Golbus MS, Stephens JD, Cann HM, et al: Rh isoimmunization following genetic amniocentesis. Prenat Diagn 2:149, 1982.

80. Hill LM, Platt LD, Kellogg B: Rhesus sensitization after genetic amniocentesis. Obstet Gynecol 56:459, 1980.

81. Dubin CF, Staisch KJ: Amniocentesis and fetal-maternal blood transfusion: A review of the literature. Obstet Gynecol Surv 37:272, 1982.

82. Brandenburg H, Jahoda MG, Pijpers L, Wladimiroff JW: Rhesus sensitization after mid-trimester genetic amniocentesis. Am J Genet 32:225, 1989.

83. Manganiello PD, Byrd JR, Tho PT, McDonough PG: A report of the safety and accuracy of mid-trimester amniocentesis at the Medical College of Georgia: Eight and one half years experience. Am J Obstet Gynecol 134:911, 1979.

84. Chong KF, Levitt GA, Lawson J, et al: Subarachnoid cyst with hydrocephalus: A complication of mid-trimester amniocentesis. Prenat Diagn 9:677, 1989.

85. Merlin S, Beyth Y: Unilocular congenital blindness as a complication of mid-trimester amniocentesis. Am J Opthalmol 89:299, 1980.

86. Rickwood AMK: A case of ileal atresia and ileocutaneous fistula caused by amniocentesis. J Pediatr 91:312, 1977.

87. Lamb MP: Gangrene of a fetal limb due to amniocentesis. Br J Obstet Gynaecol 82:829, 1975.

88. Squier M, Chamberlain P, Zaiwalla Z, et al: Five cases of brain injury following amniocentesis in mid-term pregnancy. Dev Med Child Neurol 42:554, 2000.

89. Hislop A, Fairweather DV, Blackwell RJ, Howard S: The effect of amniocentesis and drainage of amniotic fluid on lung development in *Macaca fascicularis*. Br J Obstet Gynaecol 91:835, 1984.

90. Cruikshank DP, Varner MW, Cruikshank JE: Mid-trimester amniocentesis. Am J Obstet Gynecol 146:204, 1983.

91. Sant-Cassia LJ, MacPherson MBA, Tyack AJ: Mid-trimester amniocentesis: Is it safe? A single centre controlled prospective study of 517 consecutive amniocentesis. Br J Obstet Gynaecol 91:736, 1984.

92. Vyas H, Milner AD, Hopkin IE: Amniocentesis and fetal lung development. Arch Dis Child 57:627, 1982.

93. Milner AD, Hoskyns EW, Hopkin IE: The effects of mid-trimester amniocentesis on lung function in the neonatal period. Eur J Pediatr 151:458, 1992.

94. Thompson PJ, Greenough A: Lung volume measured by functional residual capacity in infants following first trimester amniocentesis or chorion villus sampling. Br J Obstet Gynaecol 99:479, 1992.

95. Hunter AGW: Neonatal lung function following mid-trimester amniocentesis. Prenat Diagn 7:433, 1987.

96. Finegan JAK, Quarrington BJ, Hughes HE, et al: Child outcome following mid-trimester amniocentesis: Development, behavior, and physical status at age 4 years. Br J Obstet Gynaecol 97:32, 1990.

97. Golbus MS, Loughman WD, Epstein CJ, et al: Prenatal genetic diagnosis in 3000 amnioceteses. N Engl J Med 300:157, 1979.

98. Hanson FW, Tennant FR, Zorn EM, Samuels S: Analysis of 2136 genetic amnioceteses: Experience of a single physician. Am J Obstet Gynecol 152:436, 1985.

99. Allen R: The significance of meconium in midtrimester genetic amniocentesis. Am J Obstet Gynecol 152:413, 1985.

100. Jorgensen FS, Bang J, Lind AM, et al: Genetic amniocentesis at 7-14 weeks of gestation. Prenat Diagn 12:227, 1992.

101. Assel BG, Lewis SM, Dickerman LH, et al: Single-operator comparison of early and mid–second trimester amniocentesis. Obstet Gynecol 79:940, 1992.

102. Hanson FW, Happ RL, Tennant FR, et al: Ultrasonography-guided early amniocentesis in singleton pregnancies. Am J Obstet Gynecol 162:1376, 1990.

103. Thayer B, Braddock B, Spitzer K, et al: Clinical and laboratory experience with early amniocentesis. Birth Defects 26:58, 1990.

104. Penso CA, Sandstrom MM, Garber MF, et al: Early amnio-centesis: Report of 407 cases with neonatal follow-up. Obstet Gynecol 76:1032, 1990.

105. Nevin J, Nevin NC, Dornan JC, et al: Early amniocentesis: Experience of 222 consecutive patients, 1987-1988. Prenat Diagn 10:79, 1990.

106. Elejalde RE, Elejalde MM, Acuna JM, et al: Prospective study of amniocentesis performed between weeks 9 and 16 of gestation. Am J Med Genet 35:188, 1990.

107. Hackett GA, Smith JH, Rebello MT, et al: Early amniocentesis at 11-14 weeks gestation for the diagnosis of fetal chromosomal abnormality—a clinical evaluation. Prenat Diagn 11:311, 1991.

108. Stripparo L, Buscaglia M, Longatti L, et al: Genetic amniocentesis: 505 cases performed before the sixteenth week of gestation. Prenat Diagn 10:359, 1990.

109. Hanson FW, Smith JH, Rebello MT, et al: Early amniocentesis: outcome, risks, and technical problems at ≤12.8 weeks. Am J Obstet Gynecol 166:1707, 1992.

110. Randomized trial to assess safety and fetal outcome of early and midtrimester amniocentesis. The Canadian Early and Mid-trimester Amniocentesis Trial (CEMAT) Group [Comment]. Lancet 351:9110, 1998.

111. Sundberg K, Bang J, Smidt-Jensen S, et al: Randomised study of risk of fetal loss related to early amniocentesis versus chorionic villus sampling [Comment]. Lancet 350:697, 1997.

112. Nicolaides K, Brizot MdeL, Patel F, Snijders R: Comparison of chorionic villus sampling and amniocentesis for fetal karyotyping at 10-13 weeks' gestation. Lancet 344:435, 1994.

113. Johnson JM, Wilson RD, Singer J, et al: Technical factors in early amniocentesis predict adverse outcome. Results of the Candian Early (EA) versus Mid-trimester (MA) Amniocentesis Trial. Prenat Diagn 19:732, 1999.

114. Farrell SA, Summers AM, Dallaire L, et al: Club foot, an adverse outcome of early amniocentesis: Disruption or deformation? CEMAT. Canadian Early and Mid-Trimester Amniocentesis Trial. J Med Genet 36:843, 1999.

115. Hoehn H: Amniotic fluid cell culture. In Milunsky A (ed): Genetic Disorders and the Fetus, 2nd ed. New York, Plenum Press, 1986, pp 99-114.

116. Martin AO: Characteristics of amniotic fluid cells in vitro and attempts to improve culture techniques. Clin Obstet Gynecol 7:143, 1980.

117. Byrne D, Azar G, Nicolaides K: Why cell culture is successful after early amniocentesis. Fetal Diagn Ther 6:84, 1991.

118. Kerber S, Held KR: Early genetic amniocentesis—4 years' experience. Prenat Diagn 13:21, 1993.

119. Gosden C: Prenatal karyotyping: Amniotic fluid cells or chorion villus samples? In Liu DTY, Symonds EM, Golbus MS (eds): Chorion Villus Sampling. Chicago, Year Book Medical, 1987.

120. Hsu LYF, Perlis TE: United States survey on chromosome mosaicism and pseudomosaicism in prenatal diagnosis. Prenat Diagn 4:97, 1984.

121. Bui TH, Iselius L, Linsten J: European collaborative study on prenatal diagnosis: Mosaicism, pseudomosaicism and single abnormal cells in amniotic fluid cell cultures. Prenat Diagn 4:145, 1984.

122. Worton RG, Stern R: A Canadian collaborative study of mosaicism in amniotic fluid cell cultures. Prenat Diagn 4:131, 1984.

123. Klinger K, Landes G, Shook D, et al: Rapid detection of chromosome aneuploidies in uncultured amniocytes by using fluorescence in situ hybridization (FISH). Am J Hum Genet 51:55, 1992.

124. Kurtz AB, Wapner RJ, Mata J, et al: Twin pregnancies: The accuracy of first trimester abdominal US in predicting chorionicity and amnionicity. Radiology 185:759, 1992.

125. van der Pol JG, Wolf H, Boer K, et al: Jejunal atresia related to the use of methylene blue in genetic amniocentesis in twins. Br J Obstet Gynaecol 99:141, 1992.

126. Nicolini U, Monni G: Intestinal obstruction in babies exposed in utero to methylene blue. Lancet 336:1258, 1990.

127. Tabsch K: Genetic amniocentesis in multiple gestation: A new technique to diagnose monoamniotic twins. Obstet Gynecol 75:296, 1990.

128. Jeanty P, Shah D, Roussis P: Single needle insertion in twin amniocentesis. J Ultrasound Med 9:511, 1990.

129. Megory E, Weiner E, Shalev E, Ohel G: Pseudomonoamniotic twins with cord entanglement following genetic funipuncture. Obstet Gynecol 78:915, 1991.

130. Bahado-Singh R, Schmitt R, Hobbins JC: New technique for genetic amniocentesis in twins. Obstet Gynecol 79:304, 1992.

131. Wapner RJ, Johnson A, Davis G, et al: Prenatal diagnosis in twin gestations: A prospective comparison between second trimester amniocentesis and first trimester chorionic villus sampling. Obstet Gynecol 82:49, 1993.

132. Pijpers L, Jahoda MGJ, Vosters RPL, et al: Genetic amniocentesis in twin diagnosis. Br J Obstet Gynaecol 95:323, 1988.

133. Anderson RL, Goldberg JD, Golbus MS: Prenatal diagnosis in multiple gestation: 20 years' experience with amniocentesis. Prenat Diagn 11:263, 1991.

134. Pruggmayer M, Baumann P, Schutte H, et al: Incidence of abortion after genetic amniocentesis in twin pregnancies. Prenat Diagn 11:637, 1991.

135. Evans MI, Bhatia RK, Bottoms SF, et al: Effects of karyotype, gestational age and medium on the duration of amniotic fluid cell culturing. J Reprod Med 33:765, 1988.

136. Romero R, Sirtori M, Oyarzun E, et al: Infection and labor. V. Prevalence, microbiology, and clinical significance of intraamniotic infection in women with preterm labor and intact membranes. Am J Obstet Gynecol 161:817, 1989.

137. Skoll MA, Moretti ML, Sibai BM: The incidence of positive amniotic fluid cultures in patients with preterm labor with intact membranes. Am J Obstet Gynecol 161:813, 1989.

138. Romero R, Emamian M, Quintero R, et al: The value and limitations of the Gram stain examination in the diagnosis of intraamniotic infection. Am J Obstet Gynecol 159:114, 1988.

139. Romero R, Jimenez C, Lohda A, et al: Amniotic fluid glucose concentration: A rapid and simple method for the detection of intraamniotic infection in preterm labor. Am J Obstet Gynecol 163:968, 1990.

140. Kirshon B, Rosenfeld B, Mari G, et al: Amniotic fluid glucose and intraamniotic infection. Am J Obstet Gynecol 164:818, 1991.

141. Kiltz RJ, Burke MS, Porreco RP: Amniotic fluid glucose concentration as a marker for intra-amniotic infection. Obstet Gynecol 78:619, 1991.

142. Gauthier DW, Meyer WJ, Beiniarz A: Correlation of amniotic fluid glucose concentration and intraamniotic infection in patients with preterm labor or premature rupture of membranes. Am J Obstet Gynecol 165:1105, 1991.

143. Romero R, Quintero R, Nores J, et al: Amniotic fluid white blood cell count: A rapid and simple test to diagnose microbial invasion of the amniotic cavity and predict preterm delivery. Am J Obstet Gynecol 165:821, 1991.

144. Gauthier DW, Meyer WJ: Comparison of Gram stain, leukocyte esterase activity, and amniotic fluid glucose concentration in predicting amniotic fluid culture results in preterm premature rupture of membranes. Am J Obstet Gynecol 167:1092, 1992.

145. Egley CC, Katz VL, Herbert WNP: Leukocyte esterase: A simple bedside test for the detection of bacterial colonization of amniotic fluid. Am J Obstet Gynecol 159:120, 1988.

146. American College of Obstetricians and Gynecologists: Fetal maturity assessment prior to elective repeat cesarean delivery. ACOG Committee Opinion: Committee on Obstetrics: Maternal and Fetal Medicine. Number 98—September 1991. Int J Gynaecol Obstet 38:327, 1992.

147. Gluck L, Kulovich MV, Borer RC, et al: Diagnosis of the respiratory distress syndrome by amniocentesis. Am J Obstet Gynecol 109:440, 1971.

148. Whittle MJ, Wilson AI, Whitfield CR, et al: Amniotic fluid phosphatidyl glycerol and the lecithin/sphingomyelin ratio in the assessment of fetal lung maturity. Br J Obstet Gynaecol 89:727, 1982.

149. Fisk N, Bennett P, Warwick M, et al: Clinical utility of fetal Rh D typing in alloimmunized pregnancies by means of polymerase chain reaction on amniocytes or chorionic villi. Am J Obstet Gynecol 171:50, 1994.

150. Mari G, Deter RL, Rahman F, et al: Non-invasive diagnosis by Doppler ultrasonography of fetal anemia due to maternal red cell immunization. N Engl J Med 342:9, 2000.

151. Gordon MC, Narula K, O'Shaughnessy R, Barth WH Jr: Complications of third-trimester amniocentesis using continuous ultrasound guidance. Obstet Gynecol 99:25509, 2002.

CHAPTER 7

Chorionic Villus Sampling

Ronald J. Wapner

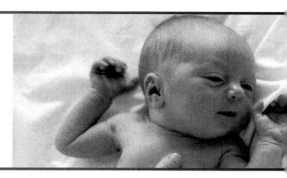

The ability to diagnose fetal disorders by cytogenetic, molecular, and biochemical analysis is one of the most rapidly growing clinical applications of the "new genetics." Since 1980, techniques for first-trimester sampling of chorionic villi have enabled clinicians to make genetic diagnoses in early pregnancy, allowing patients earlier reassurance in most cases or the option of a safer and less psychologically stressful pregnancy termination if the fetus is found to be abnormal. Earlier diagnosis allows couples unwilling to consider second-trimester termination the option of testing. The transition at many centers to first-trimester aneuploid screening through biochemical analyses and nuchal translucency measurement has further enhanced the need for a first-trimester diagnostic procedure.[1]

CHORIONIC VILLUS SAMPLING PROCEDURE: RELATED ANATOMY AND HISTOLOGY

Because anatomic relationships change rapidly with advancing gestational age, the performance of chorionic villus sampling (CVS) requires practical knowledge of developmental embryology. Figure 7-1 illustrates the anatomic arrangements at 9 to 12 weeks from the last menstrual period, which is when CVS is customarily performed. At this time, the gestational sac has not yet filled the entire uterine cavity, and the fetus, surrounded by a relatively small amount of amniotic fluid, is enclosed within the amniotic membrane. The villi over most of the chorionic membrane have degenerated, forming the chorion laeve; those remaining are embedded into the decidua basalis, forming the chorion frondosum, which will ultimately become the placenta. The individual chorionic villi float freely within the blood of the intervillous space and are only loosely attached to the underlying decidua basalis. The extraembryonic coelom, which contains a tenacious mucoid-like substance, is readily evident and separates the thin, wispy, freely mobile amnion from the thick leathery chorion laeve.

As the pregnancy progresses, the gestational sac expands to fill the entire intrauterine cavity and the extraembryonic coelom disappears as the amnion and chorion fuse. The chorion frondosum becomes anchored more deeply into the uterine wall, and the individual villi interdigitate as the placenta takes on the appearance of a single organ.

The chorion frondosum containing the mitotically active villus cells is the targeted preferred biopsy site. The individual villi have a distinctive branched appearance with an outer single cell layer, the syncytiotrophoblast, bordering the proliferative cytotrophoblast. The surface of the villi is punctuated by small buds consisting of an outer syncytial covering surrounding mitotically active cytotrophoblastic cells (Fig. 7-2). In the center of the villus is the mesenchymal core through which fetal capillaries carrying fetal blood cells course (see Fig. 7-2). The cytotrophoblastic buds are the tissue source for the direct preparation of karyotypes, whereas the embryologically distinct mesenchymal core serves as the source of cells for tissue culture.[2]

CHORIONIC VILLUS SAMPLING TECHNIQUES (Fig. 7-3)

As with all prenatal diagnostic procedures, extensive counseling is provided before CVS. The risks, benefits, idiosyncrasies, and limitations of testing must be thoroughly discussed, and other available approaches such as second-trimester amniocentesis must be honestly compared.

Ultrasound evaluation of the pregnancy should be performed before the initial counseling session, because up to 10% of patients may have nonviable pregnancies. In addition to confirmation of viability, measurements of the fetal crown-to-rump length and gestational sac size should be compared with expected values. If the fetal measurement is more than 1 week smaller than predicted by menstrual dates, delaying the procedure until appropriate growth of the crown-to-rump length is demonstrated should be considered, because such early discrepancies may be predictive of an impending miscarriage. The initial scan also

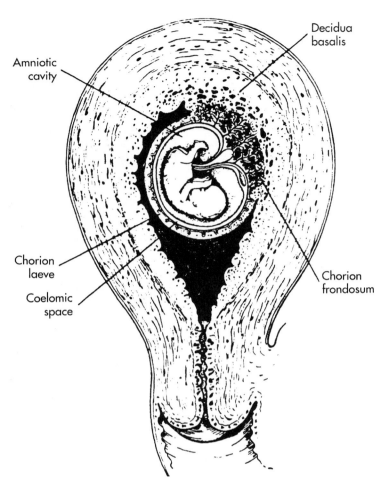

Amniotic
cavity

Decidua
basalis

Chorion
laeve

Coelomic
space

Chorion
frondosum

Figure 7–1. Diagrammatic representation of a 9-week gestation, demonstrating the relationships of the chorionic membranes, amniotic membranes, and extraembryonic coelom. Note that the gestational sac does not fill the entire uterine cavity. *(From Jackson L: First-trimester diagnosis of fetal genetic disorders. Hosp Pract 20[3]:39, 1985.)*

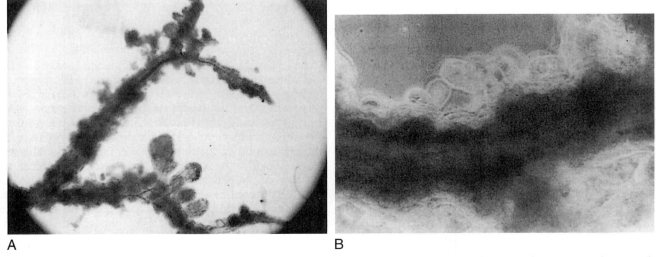

A

B

Figure 7–2. A, Low magnification of a chorionic villus demonstrating the typical branched appearance. Buds are noted. Veins are easily seen within the mesenchymal core. **B,** Higher magnification of a chorionic villus, demonstrating the multiple buds with their syncytiotrophoblastic shell and inner cytotrophoblast.

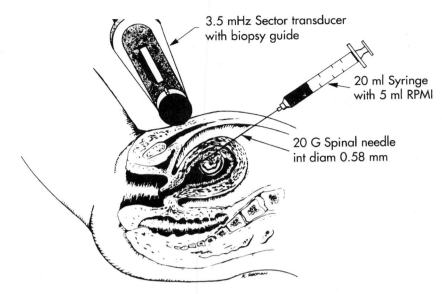

Transabdominal chorionic villus sampling

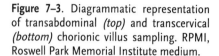

Figure 7–3. Diagrammatic representation of transabdominal *(top)* and transcervical *(bottom)* chorionic villus sampling. RPMI, Roswell Park Memorial Institute medium.

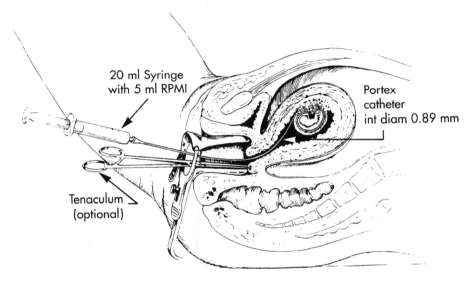

identifies multiple gestations, uterine fibroids, and adnexal disease.

The CVS procedure is scheduled after 70 days' gestation to avoid karyotypically normal and abnormal spontaneous losses that occur most frequently before this time. In addition, as described later in this chapter, sampling before 9 weeks may increase the risk of fetal abnormalities.

On the day of the procedure, ultrasound scanning reconfirms fetal viability and reestablishes the location of the chorion frondosum, which is recognized by its characteristic homogeneous, hyperechoic appearance (Fig. 7-4). The relative relationship of the uterus and cervix is observed, and a sampling approach that allows catheter or needle placement parallel to the chorionic membrane is chosen. Uterine contractions that prevent appropriate placement of the instrument may be present. The clinician should wait 10 to 20 minutes until they dissipate.

Williams and colleagues suggested the use of β-mimetics to eliminate these contractions, although the safety and efficacy of doing this have not been confirmed.[3]

Once the catheter path and uterine position are satisfactory, the patient is placed in the lithotomy position; the vulva, vagina, and cervix are aseptically prepared with povidone-iodine solution; and a speculum is inserted. Transcervical CVS entails the use of a 1.5- to 1.8-mm-diameter polyethylene catheter with a malleable stainless steel stylet that is bent into a slight curve and passed through the cervix until a loss of resistance is detected at the internal os. At this point, the operator waits until the tip of the catheter is visualized by ultrasonography and then directs the catheter into the substance of the chorion frondosum. In order to ensure that sufficient villi are retrieved, the catheter is passed almost to the distal end of the chorion frondosum (see Fig. 7-4). The catheter must

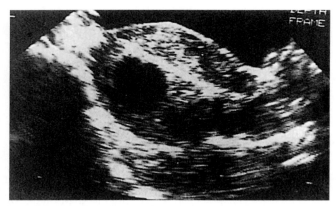

Figure 7–4. Ultrasound image demonstrating proper placement of the chorionic villus sampling catheter within the chorion frondosum.

be inserted slowly, without excessive force, along the unresisting tissue plane provided by the freely floating villi. Proceeding against resistance may disrupt the underlying decidual vessels or cause injury to the chorionic membrane. After catheter location is appropriate, the metal stylet is gently pulled from the catheter and replaced with a 20-mL syringe containing 5 mL of nutrient medium with added heparin. Approximately 15 to 20 mL of negative pressure is applied as the catheter and attached syringe are slowly withdrawn. After successful aspiration, villi can be identified floating within the syringe as white, fluffy, branched structures. If material retrieved is inadequate, as many as two more passes, each with a fresh catheter, may be attempted, although the risk of adverse outcome appears to be proportional to the number of insertions required.[4,5] Whereas one or two insertions are associated with a reasonable pregnancy loss rate, three insertions may lead to fetal loss in excess of 10%.[4] Fortunately, once the technique is mastered, sufficient tissue is retrieved with one or two insertions in more than 97% of patients.

The patient is discharged; no recovery period is required. She is told to contact the sampling center if heavy bleeding, fever, or unusual vaginal discharge develops. Mild to moderate vaginal bleeding or spotting is not uncommon after transcervical CVS and may last for as long as 2 weeks. An ultrasound scan and maternal serum α-fetoprotein measurement should be obtained in the second trimester to provide information about fetal anatomy similar to that obtained with an amniocentesis.

Two techniques for transabdominal CVS have been described. With the "two-needle" technique, a large, 16- to 18-gauge trocar is inserted into the myometrium, and a thinner (19- or 20-gauge) and longer sampling needle is passed through the trocar into the chorion frondosum.[6] The stylet of the sampling needle is replaced with a syringe, and moderate suction is applied. The needle is then passed two to four times through the body of the chorion frondosum in order to aspirate villi. The two-needle technique is theoretically less traumatic than a single-needle approach and has the advantage of allowing the operator to obtain additional villi by reinserting the sampling needle without requiring a second skin puncture.

The "single-needle" approach is quicker, less uncomfortable, able to retrieve adequate tissue with minimal insertions, and appears to be the technique that has gained widest acceptance.[7] For this approach, a 19- or 20-gauge spinal needle is inserted under ultrasonographic guidance into the chorion frondosum parallel to the chorionic plate. In most cases, a relatively empty bladder is preferred so that the uterus is closer to the maternal abdominal wall, minimizing the possibility of inadvertent bowel injury. The tip is initially inserted into the myometrium just above the anticipated sampling site and then slowly advanced through as much of the chorion frondosum as possible. It should be emphasized that the needle should be parallel to the chorionic membrane to ensure the largest sample and to avoid inadvertent puncture of the membrane. Once the needle is in place, the stylet is removed, and a syringe is attached. While continuous negative pressure is applied, the tip of the biopsy needle is passed through the entire length of the chorion frondosum three to four times. The relatively smaller internal diameter of the 20-gauge spinal needle in comparison with that of the transcervical catheter (0.58 mm versus 0.89 mm) accounts for the repetitive passages required in transabdominal sampling. If the sample is inadequate, a new needle is reinserted, and the procedure is repeated. After transabdominal CVS, instructions and recovery are similar to those for transcervical sampling.

Either a transcervical or transabdominal approach can be utilized to retrieve chorionic villi. Each approach has certain advantages (Table 7-1), and most patients can undergo sampling safely and simply by either route.

Table 7–1. Comparison of Transcervical and Transabdominal Chorionic Villus Sampling Procedures

Parameter	Transcervical	Transabdominal
Relative contraindications	Cervical polyps	Interceding bowel
	Retroverted uterus with posterior placenta	Laboratory need for large sample
	Active cervical or vaginal herpes	
Ease of learning	Experience required	Adaptation of amniocentesis technique
Sample size	Large sample; includes whole villi	Smaller: many small pieces
Patient discomfort	Minimal to absent	Moderate
Placental location	Better for posterior placenta	Better for fundal placenta

However, because about 2% to 3% of villi are inaccessible by one route or the other, operators should be capable of performing either technique in order to ensure successful sampling of all patients. Although it may be tempting for an operator already experienced in amniocentesis to learn only transabdominal CVS, mastering the transcervical approach improves sampling efficacy and maximizes safety. If no contraindications are present, the choice of procedure should be based on uterine and placental position. For instance, a retroverted uterus with a posterior placenta renders a transcervical approach technically demanding, whereas a posterior placenta with interceding bowel precludes transabdominal sampling. The sample size from either approach is usually adequate, but the larger bore of the transcervical catheter consistently leads to larger samples, making laboratory preparation easier, especially when samples need to be split for distribution to two or more specialty laboratories.[8,9] Transcervical CVS is a relatively painless procedure. Transabdominal sampling usually entails some patient discomfort, although the pain is well tolerated even when local anesthesia is not used.

Sampling Twin Gestations

CVS can be performed both successfully and safely in twin gestations.[10-12] There are, however, a number of potential pitfalls that are not present when a singleton is sampled. For example, when performing an amniocentesis on twins, dye can be instilled into the first sac to confirm that independent compartments have been entered. No such marker is available for CVS. Therefore, the operator must use meticulous ultrasonographic guidance to be certain that each individual placental site is identified and individually sampled. To avoid potential errors, one should attempt to sample near the cord insertion sites regardless of whether monochorionic or dichorionic placentation is suggested on the ultrasonogram. Samples from each fetus are routinely taken, except for cases in which a membrane is not demonstrated and individual cord insertion sites are not visible. In my experience, utilization of this sampling technique consistently provides correct information about the karyotypes of each pregnancy. However, incorrect sampling can occur, and the patient should be made aware of this possibility. If the operator is not certain that both fetuses have been sampled, amniocentesis should be offered. With experience, this should occur very rarely.

Prospective comparisons between CVS and amniocentesis in twin gestations have confirmed that the procedures are equally safe.[10] Miscarriage of the entire pregnancy after a twin CVS occurs in approximately 2% to 3% of cases,[10,11] which is similar to that reported for amniocentesis (see Chapter 6).

Contamination of one twin's sample with villi from the coexisting fetus can result in significant confusion and potential error. Clinically, this is rarely a problem when karyotyping alone is to be performed, inasmuch as the presence of an abnormal cell line will be identified even if some of these villi are contaminated by the other sample. However, this can lead to seriously inaccurate results when biochemical enzyme analysis on molecular testing is performed. Contamination is best avoided by choosing sampling routes that do not pass through both placental sites. Combinations of abdominal and cervical sampling make this possible. For biochemical or DNA testing, analysis of individual villi rather than their combination into one sample will diminish the possibility of an error.

Discordant results and subsequent requests for selective pregnancy termination are inevitable when high-order gestations are sampled, because 1% to 2% of pregnancies in patients of advanced maternal age have at least one fetus with a karyotype abnormality. Because of this potential, an accurate and detailed diagram of fetal and placental position should be drawn at the time of sampling so that an aneuploid fetus can be identified 1 to 2 weeks later. Even when this is done accurately, there are cases in which subsequent identification of the affected fetus may be inconclusive at the time of reduction. When this problem occurs, a repeat CVS should be performed immediately before the reduction and a 1- to 3-hour direct chromosome preparation used to confirm the karyotype.

Because twins present unique difficulties in prenatal diagnostics, it is suggested that only very experienced operators sample these gestations. Multiple pregnancies of higher order, such as triplets and quadruplets, have been successfully sampled.[13]

SAFETY OF CHORIONIC VILLUS SAMPLING

CVS has been used as a clinical tool since 1980, and more than 400,000 procedures have been evaluated.[14] There have been a number of large prospective comparisons of CVS to second-trimester amniocentesis,[5,15,16] which have demonstrated a comparable pregnancy loss rate and minimal complications. However, sporadic reports have questioned whether under certain circumstances, such as sampling before 9 weeks' gestation, there may be an increased risk of fetal malformation after CVS.[17,18]

Pregnancy Loss

Determining the rate of procedure-induced pregnancy losses for any prenatal diagnostic procedure is complicated by the background miscarriage rates. In 2% to 5% of unsampled pregnancies, fetuses alive at 7 to 12 weeks' gestation are either dead when rescanned between 8 and 20 weeks' gestation or are spontaneously aborted before 28 weeks.[19-22] This background loss rate increases with maternal age and is highest precisely in the age range in which women are most likely to present for prenatal diagnosis.[19,20,23] Because of these data, in studies comparing CVS to second-trimester amniocentesis, patients must be enrolled before the gestational age at which CVS is performed, and then the *total* loss rates are compared. All losses must be included, whether from a spontaneous miscarriage or an induced termination for abnormal results, thereby eliminating any bias that may occur when procedures performed at different gestational ages are compared. This approach also takes into account karyotypically abnormal embryos that are spontaneously aborted before amniocentesis or are electively terminated after CVS.

The best evaluation of the relative safety of CVS in comparison with amniocentesis was in two North American collaborative reports. In early 1989, the Canadian Collaborative CVS–Amniocentesis Clinical Trial Group published a prospective randomized trial comparing CVS with second-trimester amniocentesis.[15] During the study period, patients across Canada were able to undergo only CVS in conjunction with the randomized protocol. There were 7.6% fetal losses (spontaneous abortions, induced abortions, and late losses) in the patients undergoing CVS and 7.0% in those undergoing amniocentesis. Thus, in desired pregnancies, an excess loss rate of 0.6% for CVS over amniocentesis was obtained; this difference was not statistically significant.

Two months after the publication of the Canadian experience, the first American collaborative report appeared. This was a prospective, although nonrandomized, trial of more than 2200 women who chose either transcervical CVS or second-trimester amniocentesis.[5] Patients in both groups were recruited in the first trimester of pregnancy. As in the Canadian study, advanced maternal age was the primary indication for prenatal testing. When the loss rates were adjusted for slight group differences in maternal and gestational ages, an excess pregnancy loss rate of 0.8% referable to CVS over amniocentesis was calculated, which again was not significant.

The United States study investigated numerous predictors of fetal loss. The rates of loss were lowest in cases in which relatively large amounts of tissue were obtained, demonstrating that easy procedures are also the safest. The need for repetitive catheter insertions was significantly associated with pregnancy loss. Among the seven participating centers, the proportion of cases in which more than one insertion was needed varied from 7% to 45%; the centers requiring the fewest insertions had the lowest loss rates. Cases necessitating three or more catheter insertions had a 10.8% spontaneous abortion rate, in comparison with 2.9% of cases necessitating only one pass.

Although the North American trials revealed no statistical difference in pregnancy loss between CVS and amniocentesis, a prospective, randomized, collaborative comparison of more than 3200 pregnancies, sponsored by the European Medical Research Council Working Party on the Evaluation of CVS, demonstrated a 4.6% greater pregnancy loss rate after CVS (95% confidence interval = 1.6% to 7.5%).[24] This difference reflected more spontaneous deaths before 28 weeks' gestation (2.9%), more terminations of pregnancy for chromosomal anomalies (1.0%), and more neonatal deaths (0.3%). Procedures in this study were performed via both the transcervical and transabdominal routes.

The factors contributing to the discrepancies between the results of the European and North American studies remain uncertain. It is probable that operator experience accounted for a large part of this difference. Whereas the United States trial consisted of 7 centers and the Canadian trial 11 centers, the European trial included 31. There were, on average, 325 cases per center in the United States study, 106 in the Canadian study, and only 52 in the European trial. Although no significant change in pregnancy loss rate was demonstrated during the course of the European trial, it appears that the learning curve for both transcervical and transabdominal CVS may exceed 400 or more procedures.[25,26] Operators who have performed less than 100 procedures may have two to three times the postprocedure loss rate of operators who have performed more than 1000 procedures.[26]

Multiple reports from individual centers have confirmed, and even improved upon, the results of these collaborative trials.[27-31] After adjustments for background loss, these studies suggested that in experienced centers, only minimal increases in pregnancy losses are attributable to CVS. For patient counseling, defining the risk of procedure-induced miscarriage as about 0.5% seems appropriate.

Randomized trials have compared the transcervical and transabdominal approaches.[8,9,26,32-34] With more than 1000 patients randomly assigned to each technique, our center has demonstrated comparable loss rates with each approach.[8,26] In addition, equivalent numbers of patients required only one attempt to retrieve tissue (87%) or had unsuccessful procedures (<1%). The United States collaborative CVS project performed a randomized prospective study comparing transcervical and transabdominal CVS and found no difference in the total postprocedure pregnancy loss rates between the two approaches (transcervical, 2.5%; transabdominal, 2.3%).[9] The overall CVS loss rate in this study (2.5%) was 0.8% lower than that in the initial United States study comparing CVS with second-trimester amniocentesis. Because 0.8% was the quantitative difference in loss rates between amniocentesis and CVS in the original study, this suggests that when centers become equivalently experienced, amniocentesis and CVS have the same risk of pregnancy loss. Smidt-Jensen and associates confirmed this in a prospective randomized study in which they found no difference in pregnancy loss between transabdominal CVS and second-trimester amniocentesis.[33]

In conclusion, when the gestational age at sampling is taken into consideration, fetal loss rates for CVS and second-trimester amniocentesis are similar, when equivalent expertise with either approach exists. Integration of both procedures into a center's program offers the most complete, most practical, and safest approach to prenatal diagnosis.[35]

Risk of Fetal Abnormalities after Chorionic Villus Sampling

Although initial reports demonstrated no risk of structural abnormalities after CVS, further experience suggested that CVS was associated with the occurrence of specific fetal malformations when performed at less than 9 weeks' gestation. The first suggestion of this was reported by Firth and colleagues.[17] In their series of 539 CVS-exposed pregnancies, they identified five infants with severe limb abnormalities, all of whom came from a cohort of 289 pregnancies sampled at 66 days' gestation or less. Four of these infants had the unusual and rare oromandibular-limb hypogenesis syndrome, and the fifth had a terminal transverse limb reduction defect. Oromandibular-limb hypogenesis syndrome occurred with a birth prevalence of 1 per 175,000 live births,[36] and limb reduction defects occurred in 1 per 1690 births.[37] In this initial report, all of the limb abnormalities followed transabdominal sampling performed between 55 and 66 days' gestation.

After this initial report, others added supporting cases to this list. Utilizing the Italian multicenter birth defects registry, Mastroiacovo and coworkers reported (in a case-control study) an odds ratio of 11.3 (95% confidence interval = 5.6 to 2.13) for transverse limb abnormalities after first-trimester CVS.[38] It was demonstrated that pregnancies sampled before 70 days, when stratified by gestational age at sampling, had a 20% increased risk of transverse limb reduction defects, whereas those sampled later showed no such increased risk. Since that time, there have been additional reports of transverse limb defects after very early CVS. Most notably, Brambati and associates, an extremely experienced group with no increased risk of limb defects in patients sampled after the 9th week, found a 1.6% incidence of severe limb reduction defects in patients undergoing CVS at 6 and 7 weeks.[39] An informal collaboration of the Fetoscopy Working Group further supported the association of early sampling and limb defects.[40] The data were voluntarily submitted without formal review but revealed an increased incidence of transverse limb defects of 27 per 10,000 when sampling was performed at less than 9.5 weeks. The incidence of 4.7 per 10,000 for procedures performed after 9.5 weeks was consistent with that in the general population.[36] This rate decreased to 0.1% for sampling at 8 to 9 weeks. These observations, although not conclusive, strongly suggest that CVS performed before 9 weeks' gestation significantly increases the risk of severe limb defects.

Most centers have not seen abnormalities when CVS is performed after the 10th week of gestation. Utilizing the extensive experience of the eight centers participating in the United States collaborative evaluation of CVS, Mahoney reported no cases of oromandibular-limb hypogenesis syndrome and no overall increase in the incidence of limb defects.[41] CVS centers in Philadelphia and Milan that have performed a total of 10,000 CVS procedures were unable to confirm the association when CVS was performed beyond the 10th week of gestation.[42] Alternatively, Burton and colleagues reported a cluster of more minor limb reduction defects occurring after procedures at their center.[18] Of 260 procedures, there were four babies with limb reduction defects. All were transverse distal defects involving hypoplasia or absence of fingers and toes. Sampling had been performed at 9.5, 10, 10.5, and 11.5 weeks. In contrast to other clusters, three of the four abnormalities followed transcervical sampling. Although this center's report remained a unique cluster in that the patients were of more advanced gestational age, it raised the question of potential operator-specific contributing factors, because this center's spontaneous miscarriage rate after transcervical sampling was 10.9%. Froster and Jackson reviewed outcomes from almost 200,000 CVS procedures and found no evidence of an increased risk of any type of limb reduction defect when CVS was performed after 9 weeks' gestation.[43]

Mechanisms by which CVS before 9 weeks could lead to fetal malformations continue to be disputed.

Placental thrombosis with subsequent fetal embolization has been suggested but is unlikely because fetal clotting factors appear to be insufficient at this early gestational age. Inadvertent entry into the extraembryonic coelom with resulting amniotic bands has also been suggested but also appears unlikely because actual bands have not been observed in any of the cases. In addition, many of the infants with oromandibular-limb hypogenesis syndrome had other anomalies that could not be accounted for by fetal entanglement or compression. A vascular mechanism appears to be the most plausible.[36] According to this hypothesis, CVS causes direct placental injury or alters the uterine arterial flow, which results in underperfusion of the fetal peripheral circulation. After the initial insult, there may be subsequent rupture of the thin-walled vessels of the distal embryonic circulation, leading to tissue hypoxia, necrosis, and eventually resorption of preexisting structures.[44] A similar mechanism leading to limb defects has been demonstrated in animal models after uterine vascular clamping, maternal cocaine exposure, or even simple uterine palpation.[45,46]

A variation of this hypothesis implicates fetal hemorrhage rather than vasospasm as the etiology of fetal hypoperfusion. Because the fetal and maternal circulations are contiguous, a significant fetal hemorrhage results in a fetal-to-maternal hemorrhage detectable as an increase in the maternal serum α-fetoprotein level. Smidt-Jensen and associates found that fetal loss occurred more frequently among women whose serum α-fetoprotein increased substantially after transabdominal CVS.[47] This suggested that severe fetal hemorrhage may result in fetal loss, whereas lesser degrees may allow the pregnancy to continue, but could result in transient episodes of fetal hypoperfusion.

Quintero and associates have added additional information about the possible etiologic mechanism.[48] Utilizing embryoscopic visualization of the first-trimester embryo, they demonstrated fetal facial, head, and thoracic ecchymotic lesions after traumatically induced detachment of the placenta with subchorionic hematoma formation. No changes in fetal heart rate were seen. Although these lesions consistently appeared after trauma to the placental site, they were produced by the passage of a standard CVS catheter.

Any theory of CVS-induced limb defects must account for the effect of varying fetal sensitivity and should demonstrate a correlation between the severity of the defects and the gestational age at sampling. Firth and colleagues[44] presented evidence that suggested that sampling before 9 weeks' gestation induces severe fetal limb defects, whereas these were not increased after later CVS. Alternatively, Froster and Jackson reviewed the severity of the post-CVS limb defects reported to the World Health Organization registry and found no correlation.[43]

It has been questioned whether CVS after 10 weeks causes more subtle defects such as shortening of the distal phalanx or nail hypoplasia.[49,50] There are few data to substantiate this finding. On the contrary, most experienced centers performing CVS after 10 weeks have not documented an increase in limb defects.[51] These results have led to speculation that the few reported clusters are either statistical flukes or related to center-specific practices.

At present, sampling before 10 weeks' gestation should not be routinely performed. CVS after 10 weeks, performed by experienced clinicians, has minimal to no risk of fetal abnormalities and should continue to be routinely offered.

COMPLICATIONS OF CHORIONIC VILLUS SAMPLING

Bleeding

Vaginal bleeding is uncommon after transabdominal CVS but is seen in 7% to 10% of patients sampled transcervically.[5,24] The bleeding is self-limited, and the pregnancy outcome is excellent. In more than 23,000 CVS procedures performed in our center, clinicians have never needed to terminate a pregnancy or admit a patient for excessive postprocedure bleeding. However, a small subchorionic hematoma may be visualized immediately after sampling in up to 4% of transcervical samples.[52] The hematoma disappears within a few weeks and is only rarely associated with adverse outcome.

Bleeding and hematoma formation result from accidental entry of the instrument into the vascular decidua basalis underlying the chorion frondosum. In these cases, a gritty feeling indicates penetration into the decidual layer. Careful attention to the feel of the catheter and avoiding unnecessary manipulation can prevent most of these hemorrhagic episodes and minimize this complication. With experience, the frequency of post-CVS bleeding is less than 1%.

Infection

Since the initial development of transcervical CVS, there has been concern that transvaginal passage of an instrument could introduce vaginal flora into the uterus. This possibility was confirmed by cultures that isolated bacteria from up to 30% of catheters.[53-58] No association between specific bacteria and adverse pregnancy outcome has been demonstrated.[56] However, Becker and colleagues suggested that in pregnancies in which more than one microorganism was cultured from the cervix, the risk of abortion after transcervical CVS was almost nine times greater than in cases in which no pathogens could be found.[59] Because no specific organism was associated with complications or miscarriage, with the exception of *Neisseria gonorrhoeae*, no other routine preprocedure culture was recommended.

The incidence of post-CVS chorioamnionitis is low.[5,15,54,60] In a study of more than 2000 transcervical CVS procedures, infection was suspected as a possible cause of pregnancy loss in only 0.3% of cases.[5] Infection after transabdominal CVS can occur and, in some cases, is secondary to bowel flora introduced by inadvertent puncture by the sampling needle. In our series of over 23,000 patients, in which prophylactic antibodies were not used, we have not observed any cases of chorioamnionitis requiring uterine evacuation. Our incidence of periabortion chorioamnionitis was 0.08% for both

transcervical and transabdominal sampling, which is about the same as seen in series of spontaneous abortions that have not been sampled.[19,20]

Early in the development of transcervical CVS, two life-threatening pelvic infections were reported.[61,62] Each patient presented with a mild prodrome of maternal myalgias and low-grade fever without localized adnexal or uterine tenderness; this course was similar to the chorioamnionitis seen with intrauterine device retention. Both occurred early in the respective centers' experience and, in both, a single catheter was used for repeat insertions. Since these reports, the practice of using a new sterile catheter for each insertion has been universally adopted, and there have been no additional reports of serious infectious complications.

Rupture of Membranes

Acute rupture of the membranes, documented either by obvious gross fluid leakage or a decrease in measurable amniotic fluid on ultrasonography, is a very rare complication of CVS.[5,24] In our experience, acute rupture of the membranes has not occurred. Attempts to intentionally rupture membranes with a transcervical catheter have confirmed that the chorion can withstand significant punishment without perforation.

Rupture of the membranes days to weeks after the procedure is acknowledged as a possible post-CVS complication. This can result either from injury to the chorion layer, allowing exposure of the amnion to subsequent damage, or from infection. One group reported a 0.3% incidence of delayed rupture of the membranes after CVS,[60] a rate confirmed by Brambati and Varotto.[54]

Unexplained midtrimester oligohydramnios after CVS has been suggested to result from delayed chorioamnion rupture and slow leakage of amniotic fluid. Cheng and coworkers demonstrated an increased incidence of midtrimester oligohydramnios after transcervical CVS that was associated with immediate postprocedure bleeding and an elevated second-trimester maternal serum α-fetoprotein level.[63] Operator experience markedly reduces the risk of this complication, which is probably initiated by the formation of a subchorionic hematoma. The hematoma serves as a nidus for a smoldering infection or irritation of the membranes from the breakdown products from the clot.

Elevated Maternal Serum α-Fetoprotein Levels and Rh Sensitization

An acute rise in maternal serum α-fetoprotein level after CVS has been consistently reported; it implies a detectable degree of fetal maternal bleeding.[64-66] The elevation is transient, occurs more frequently after transabdominal CVS, and appears to be correlated with the quantity of tissue aspirated.[66] Some studies have also demonstrated a correlation between the level of elevation and the incidence of pregnancy loss.[47] Levels drop to normal range by 16 to 18 weeks, thus allowing serum screening for neural tube defects to proceed according to usual prenatal protocols.

In Rh-negative women, this otherwise negligible bleeding accrues special importance, because Rh-positive cells in volumes as low as 0.1 mL can cause Rh sensitization.[67] Because even a single pass of a catheter or needle produces detectable rises in maternal serum α-fetoprotein, all Rh-negative, nonsensitized women undergoing CVS should receive Rho(D) immune globulin.

CVS-induced maternal fetal transfusion can worsen already existing sensitization. Therefore, sampling already sensitized patients is contraindicated.[68] The only exception to this statement would be situations of red blood cell antigen incompatibility in which the CVS is specifically performed to evaluate the fetal blood type. The risk that the procedure may present to the antigen-positive pregnancy must be specifically addressed before sampling, and alternative strategies must be outlined.

Perinatal Complications

There have been no increases in preterm labor, premature rupture of the membranes, numbers of infants small for dates, maternal morbidity, or other obstetric complications in sampled patients.[69] Although the Canadian collaborative study showed an increased perinatal mortality in infants of CVS-sampled patients, with the greatest incidence after 28 weeks, no obvious recurrent event was identified to account for this.[15] To date, no other studies have demonstrated a similar increase in perinatal loss.

Long-Term Infant Development

Long-term infant follow-up has been performed by Chinese investigators who have evaluated 53 children from their initial placental biopsy experience of the 1970s. All were reported in good health, with normal development and school performance.[70]

LABORATORY ASPECTS OF CHORIONIC VILLUS SAMPLING

Immediate Tissue Preparation

The average sample from a CVS aspiration contains 15 to 30 mg (wet weight) of villus material. Transabdominal samples are usually slightly smaller than those retrieved by transcervical sampling but are still quite adequate for routine procedures. The presence of adequate villus tissue can usually be immediately confirmed after aspiration by visual inspection, but a dissecting microscope is occasionally required (see Fig. 7-2A). The villi have a distinct branched fluffy appearance with a central core containing easily visible capillaries. Their appearance is distinctively different from decidual tissue, which has a structureless, sheet-like, membranous appearance.

Isolation of appropriate tissue by the laboratory is done under the dissecting microscope. Meticulous care must be taken to eliminate contaminating decidua, which may be adherent to the villi but is easily teased away. The retrieved sample should be of sufficient size that atypical villi can be discarded. Once clean and free of decidua, the villi are ready for further preparation and analysis.

Cytogenetic Procedures

Villi may be processed for cytogenetic analysis in two separate ways: (1) the "direct method" initially described by Simoni and associates[71] and later modified by others,[72,73] and (2) long-term tissue culture.[74] The direct method can yield karyotypes within 2 to 3 hours, but most laboratories use an overnight incubation and thus report results within 3 to 4 days of the procedure. When tissue culture is used, results should be available in 6 to 8 days. It is recommended that both the direct and culture methods be used with all samples. The direct method provides a rapid result and minimizes decidual contamination. Tissue culture is subject to potential contamination from maternal cells but is better able to evaluate discrepancies between the cytotrophoblast and the actual fetal state.

Biochemical and DNA Procedures

Most biochemical diagnoses can be made with amniotic fluid; cultured amniocytes can also be made from chorionic villi. In many cases, the results are available more rapidly and more efficiently by using villi because sufficient enzyme or DNA is present to allow direct analysis rather than tissue culture. For example, the analysis for Tay-Sachs disease can be performed in less than 30 minutes with fresh villi.[75]

A discussion of individual biochemical diagnoses is beyond the scope of this chapter. Furthermore, it is impractical because techniques are changing rapidly. Because of the rarity of most biochemical disorders, specific diagnoses are usually performed by only a few laboratories. Before performing a CVS, the center analyzing the tissue should be contacted and the details of testing discussed.

DNA may similarly be prepared from villi by standard methods. Approximately 2 to 5 mg of wet tissue are obtained from each average-sized villus, and about 5 μg of DNA may be obtained per milligram of tissue weight. These amounts provide generous samples for standard analysis.

ACCURACY OF CHORIONIC VILLUS SAMPLING CYTOGENETIC RESULTS

A major concern with all prenatal diagnostic procedures is the possibility of discordance between the prenatal cytogenetic diagnosis and the actual fetal karyotype. With CVS, these discrepancies can occur as a result of either maternal tissue contamination or true biologic differences between the extraembryonic tissue and the fetus. Fortunately, genetic evaluation of chorionic villi provides a high degree of diagnostic success and accuracy, particularly in regard to the diagnosis of common trisomies.[76,77] The United States collaborative study revealed a 99.7% rate of successful cytogenetically diagnosis.[77] However, 1.1% of the patients required a second diagnostic test such as amniocentesis or fetal blood analysis to further interpret the results. In most cases, the subsequent study was needed to delineate the clinical significance of mosaic or other ambiguous results (76%), and laboratory failure (20.9%) and maternal cell contamination (MCC) (3.1%) also necessitated follow-up testing. In addition, both false-positive and false-negative results occurred in the early experience with CVS. However, as operators and laboratories have acquired additional experience and expertise in working with villus tissue, clinical interpretation has improved so that errors and the need for follow-up testing has dramatically decreased.

Maternal Cell Contamination

During the initial development of CVS, there was concern that contamination of samples with significant amounts of maternal decidual tissue would lead to diagnostic errors. Small sample size frequently made appropriate tissue selection difficult. As samplers became more adept at removing appropriate quantities of tissue, and as laboratory personnel learned to separate villi from decidua accurately, this problem disappeared. Choosing only whole, clearly typical villous material and discarding any atypical fragments, small pieces, or fragments with adherent decidua will avoid confusion. To allow this capability, sufficient villus material must be available. Therefore, if the initial aspiration is insufficient, a second pass should be performed rather than risking inaccurate results. When proper care is taken and good cooperation and communication exist between the sampler and the laboratory staff, even small amounts of contaminating maternal tissue can be avoided.[78]

Direct preparations of chorionic villi are generally thought to exclude MCC,[71,79] although the chromosomes tend to be of a suboptimal quality in comparison with those in long-term culture. Comparison of direct and long-term culture processing shows a rate of MCC in long-term culture varying from 1.8% to 4%.[78,79] In most cases, the contaminating cells were easily identified as maternal and did not lead to clinical error.

MCC can lead to incorrect sex determination[80,81] and potentially to false-negative diagnosis, although there are no published reports of the latter involving cytogenetic abnormalities. There are, however, reports of false-negative diagnoses of biochemical disorders as a result of MCC, although the frequency is quite low.[82] Interestingly, for reasons still uncertain, MCC occurs more frequently in specimens retrieved by the transcervical route.[79]

Confined Placental Mosaicism

True discrepancies between the karyotype of the villus tissue and the actual fetal karyotype can occur, leading to either false-positive or false-negative clinical results. Although initially there was concern that this problem might invalidate CVS as a prenatal diagnostic tool, subsequent investigations have not only led to a clearer understanding of the clinical interpretation of villus tissue results but also revealed new information about the cause of pregnancy loss, possible causes of intrauterine growth retardation, and the biologic mechanisms for uniparental disomy (UPD).

These discrepancies are now known to occur because the chorionic villi consist of a combination of extra-embryonic tissue sources that became separate and distinct from those of the embryo in early development. Specifically, at approximately the 32- to 64-cell stage, only three or four cells are chosen to become compartmentalized into the inner cell mass to form the embryo, mesenchymal core of the chorionic villi, amnion, yolk sac, and chorion, whereas the remainder become precursors of the extraembryonic tissues.[83]

Mosaicism, the presence in one individual of two cell lines with different chromosome complements, can occur through two possible mechanisms.[84] A meiotic error in the gamete can lead to the formation of a trisomic conceptus which subsequently loses one of the extra chromosomes during mitosis and is "rescued" by reduction to disomy. This alteration results in a mosaic morula in which the percentage of normal cells is dependent on the cell division at which rescue occurred. More abnormal cells are present when correction is delayed to the second or a subsequent cell division. Because the majority of cells in the morula proceed to the trophoblast cell lineage (processed by the direct preparation), it is highly probable that the lineage will continue to contain a significant number of trisomic cells. Alternatively, because only a small number of cells are incorporated into the inner cell mass, involvement of the extraembryonic mesoderm (evaluated by tissue culture) and/or the fetus depends on the chance distribution of the aneuploid progenitor cells. Noninvolvement of the fetal cell lineage results in confined placental mosaicism (CPM), in which the trophoblast and perhaps the extraembryonic mesoderm have aneuploid cells but the fetus is euploid.

Mitotic errors can also produce mosaicism, in which the distribution and percentage of aneuploid cells in the morula or blastocyst depend on the timing of nondisjunction. If mitotic errors occur early in the development of the morula, they may segregate to the inner cell mass and have the same potential to produce an affected fetus or CPM as do meiotic errors. Mitotic errors, occurring after primary cell differentiation or compartmentalization has been completed, lead to cytogenetic abnormalities in only one lineage.

CPM resulting from meiotic rescue can also lead to UPD with the clinical potential of altered fetal growth or development. In this phenomenon, in which the original trisomic embryo is rescued by the loss of one chromosome, the embryo may be left with two chromosomes from the same parent. Because in the trisomic embryo two of the chromosomes come from one parent and one from the other, there is a theoretical one in three chance that the two remaining chromosomes come from the same parent, leading to UPD. UPD may have clinical consequences if the chromosomes involved carry imprinted genes in which expression only occurs in one sex or if the two remaining chromosomes have a mutant recessive gene that becomes homozygous due to UPD. For example, Prader-Willi syndrome results from maternal UPD for chromosome 15 in approximately 15% of cases. In rare cases, CPM for trisomy 15 has been the initial clue that UPD is present and has resulted in an affected child.[85,86] Because of this finding, all cases in which CVS reveals trisomy 15 (either complete or mosaic) should be evaluated for UPD if the amniotic fluid is euploid. Chromosome 16 also appears to be imprinted, and CPM has been reported to lead to severe intrauterine growth restriction, but it can also be compatible with live birth and subsequent normal development, demonstrating that certain genes may function predominantly in the fetal/placental unit.[87,88]

There has been increasing evidence that CPM (unassociated with UPD) can alter placental function and lead to fetal growth failure or perinatal death.[84,89-94] Initial evidence for this development was demonstrated by researchers in Canada, who showed that two of nine fetuses with unexplained intrauterine growth restriction demonstrated placental mosaicism.[89] In more than 4300 CVS samples from our center, mosaicism confined to the placenta was seen in 25 (0.6%). Although the overall fetal loss rate was 2.3%, the rate was 16.7% among the patients with placental mosaicism and rose to 24% when mosaicism was confined exclusively to the cytotrophoblast.[90] From the cases within the United States Collaborative Study, the finding of increased fetal loss with placental mosaicism was confirmed.[91] With few exceptions, most other studies have also confirmed the clinical impact of CPM on placental function. The exact mechanism by which abnormal cells within the placenta alter fetal growth or lead to fetal death is unknown. However, the effect may be limited to specific chromosomes.

The various mechanisms leading to mosaicism, as well as the timing of events, can lead to difficulty in clinical interpretation. With the few exceptions described previously, if the mosaic results are confined to the placenta, fetal development is likely to be normal, whereas mosaic cell lines within the fetus can have significant phenotypic consequences. Therefore, mosaic CVS results necessitate diligent follow-up with amniocentesis or fetal sampling to determine their clinical significance.

Mosaicism occurs after about 1% of all CVS procedures[76,79,95] but is confirmed in the fetus in only 10% to 40% of those cases. This is in contrast to amniocentesis, in which mosaicism is observed in 0.1% to 0.3% of cultures and is confirmed in the fetus in approximately 70% of those cases.[96-98] The probability that the aneuploid cells found at CVS involve the fetus appears to be related to the tissue source in which the aneuploid cells were detected and the specific chromosome involved.[86] Mesenchymal core culture results are more likely to reflect a true fetal mosaicism than is direct preparation.

In one review, Phillips and coworkers demonstrated that autosomal mosaicism involving common trisomies (i.e., 21, 18, and 13) was confirmed in the fetus in 19% of cases, whereas uncommon trisomies involved the fetus in only 3%.[99] When sex chromosome mosaicism was found in the placenta in CVS, the abnormal cell line was confirmed in the fetus in 16% of cases. When a nonfamilial marker chromosome was involved, it was confirmed in the fetus in more than one fourth of cases, whereas mosaic polyploidy was confirmed in only 1 of 28 cases. Chromosomal structural abnormalities were confirmed in 8.6% of cases.

Frequently, when placental mosaicism is discovered, amniocentesis is performed to elucidate the extent of fetal involvement. When mosaicism is limited to the direct preparation only, amniocentesis findings appear to correlate perfectly with fetal genotype.[99] However, when a mosaicism is observed in tissue culture, both false-positive and false-negative amniocentesis results can occur. In these cases, amniocentesis predicts the true fetal karyotype in approximately 94% of cases. Most important

is that these discrepancies may involve the common autosomal trisomies. There have been three cases reported of mosaic trisomy 21 on villus culture, a normal amniotic fluid analysis, and a fetus or newborn with mosaic aneuploidy.[86]

Currently, the following clinical recommendations may be utilized to assist in evaluation of CVS mosaicism. Analysis of CVS samples should, if possible, include both direct preparation and tissue culture. Although the direct preparation is less likely to be representative of the fetus, its use will minimize the likelihood of MCC, and if culture fails, a nonmosaic, normal, direct preparation result can be considered conclusive, although rare cases of false-negative findings of trisomy 21 and 18 have been reported.[100-104] If mosaicism is found on either culture or direct preparation, follow-up testing should be offered. Under no circumstances should a decision to terminate a pregnancy be based entirely on a mosaic CVS result. For CVS findings of mosaicism involving sex chromosome abnormalities, polyploidy, marker chromosomes, structural rearrangements, and uncommon trisomies, the patient can be reassured if amniocentesis results are euploid and detailed ultrasonographic examination is normal. However, no guarantees should be made, and in certain cases, testing for UPD are indicated. If common trisomies 21, 18, and 13 are involved, amniocentesis should be offered, but the patient must be advised of the possibilities of a false-negative result. Follow-up may include detailed ultrasonography, fetal blood sampling, or fetal skin biopsy. At present, the predictive accuracy of these additional tests is uncertain. Finally, preprocedure counseling should always include a discussion of the possibility and implications of mosaic CVS results.

ACCEPTANCE OF CHORIONIC VILLUS SAMPLING

The ability to establish prenatal diagnosis in the first trimester has rapidly gained approval for a number of reasons. Most important is the advantage of added privacy inherent in an earlier procedure. This approach not only provides earlier reassurance when results are normal but also allows an easier and more private pregnancy termination when necessary.

As transabdominal CVS became available, reports appeared that patients preferred that approach to the transcervical technique for factors of comfort, embarrassment, speed, and discomfort. These findings are in contrast to experience at our center, where patients find the transcervical route to be less uncomfortable.

Psychologic studies of women undergoing prenatal diagnosis have found that first-trimester procedures lowered maternal anxiety levels earlier and more consistently than did traditional midtrimester amniocentesis. Measurable and significant decreases in anxiety scores were seen after normal results were available. CVS results, not surprisingly, produced lower scores earlier than did amniocentesis.[105,106] In addition, women undergoing CVS reported greater attachment to the pregnancy during the second trimester than did women undergoing amniocentesis.[107] These authors concluded that the perceived benefits afforded by CVS confirmed earlier reports demonstrating a patient preference for CVS.[108]

Most recently, Down syndrome screening has become possible in the first trimester.[1] The biochemical analyte, pregnancy-associated plasma protein A, is reduced, and levels of the free β subunit of human chorionic gonadotropin are elevated in women carrying fetuses with trisomy 21. In addition, such fetuses are found to have an increase in the amount of fluid behind the neck (the nuchal translucency) when measured between 11 and 14 weeks' gestation. Through the use of a combination of these two biochemical analyses and the ultrasound measurement of the nuchal translucency, first-trimester Down syndrome screening has a detection rate of between 80% and 85% and a 5% false-positive rate at a cutoff of 1:270. This performance is better than standard second-trimester multiple marker screening. As the timing of screening moves from the second to the first trimester, CVS will become the preferred prenatal diagnostic procedure, inasmuch as amniocentesis should not routinely be performed before 15 weeks' gestation.

This increased acceptance of prenatal diagnosis earlier in pregnancy, coupled with the burgeoning ability to manipulate genetic material to give up its information antenatally, has led researchers to realize that as earlier procedures become available, they quickly become the preferred procedure.[109] Twenty years ago, the possibility of diagnosing fetal disorders by sampling the developing placenta was practically unimaginable. Today, because it has proved possible, the next steps are already being performed. Evaluation of fetal cells in maternal blood and gene therapy are modalities under current investigation. In vitro fertilization technology has now made preimplantation genetic diagnosis a reality. One or two blastomeres are sampled from the developing zygote, and the single cells can be analyzed for either cytogenetics or mendelian disorders.[110] By 2015, CVS may exist only as the standard against which to measure the safety and accuracy of the newest technologies.

REFERENCES

1. Wapner RJ, Thom E, Simpson JL, et al: First trimester screening for trisomies 21 and 18. N Engl J Med 349:1405, 2003.
2. Watanabe M, Ito T, Yamatoto M, et al: Origin of mitotic cells of the chorionic villi in direct chromosome analyses. Hum Genet 44:191, 1978.
3. Williams J, Wang B, Rubin C, et al: Evaluation of terbutaline sulfate as a first trimester tocolytic agent in patients undergoing transcervical chorionic villus sampling [abstract 1252]. Am J Hum Genet 49:230, 1991.
4. Jackson LG, Wapner RJ: Risks of chorionic villus sampling. Clin Obstet Gynecol 1:513, 1987.
5. Rhoads GG, Jackson LG, Schlesselman SE, et al: The safety and efficacy of chorionic villus sampling for early prenatal diagnosis of cytogenetic abnormalities. N Engl J Med 320:609, 1989.
6. Smidt-Jensen S, Hahnemann N: Transabdominal chorionic villus sampling for fetal genetic diagnosis. Technical and obstetric evaluation of 100 cases. Prenat Diagn 8:7, 1988.
7. Brambati B, Oldrini A, Lanzani A: Transabdominal chorionic villus sampling: A freehand ultrasound-guided technique. Am J Obstet Gynecol 157:134, 1987.
8. Wapner RJ, Davis GH, Johnson A., et al: A prospective comparison between transcervical and transabdominal chorionic villus sampling [abstract]. Presented at the Society of Perinatal Obstetricians Meeting, 1990, Houston, Texas.
9. Jackson LG, Zachary JM, Fowler SE, et al: A randomized comparison of transcervical and transabdominal chorionic-villus sampling. The U.S. National Institute of Child Health and Human Development Chorionic-Villus Sampling and Amniocentesis Study Group. N Engl J Med 327:594, 1992.
10. Wapner RJ, Johnson A, Davis G, et al: Prenatal diagnosis in twin gestations: A prospective comparison between second trimester amniocentesis and first trimester chorionic villus sampling. Obstet Gynecol 82:49, 1993.
11. Pergament E, Schulman JD, Copeland K, et al: The risk and efficacy of chorionic villus sampling in multiple gestations. Prenat Diagn 12:377, 1992.
12. Brambati B, Tului L, Lanzani A, et al: First trimester genetic diagnosis in multiple pregnancy: Principles and potential pitfalls. Prenat Diagn 11:767, 1991.
13. Eddleman KA, Stone JL, Lynch L, Berkowitz RL: Chorionic villus sampling before multifetal pregnancy reduction [comment]. Am J Obstet Gynecol 183:1078, 2000.
14. Jackson LG: CVS Latest News, vol 32, August 1994.
15. Multicentre randomized clinical trial of chorion villus sampling and amniocentesis. First report. Canadian Collaborative CVS–Amniocentesis Clinical Trial Group. Lancet 1:1, 1989.
16. Kuliev A, Jackson L, Froster U, et al: Chorionic villus sampling safety. Report of World Health Organization/EURO meeting in association with the Seventh International Conference on Early Prenatal Diagnosis of Genetic Diseases. Am J Obstet Gynecol 174(3):8, 1994;
17. Firth HV, Boyd PA, Chamberlain P, et al: Severe limb abnormalities after chorion villus sampling at 56-66 days' gestation. Lancet 337:726, 1991.
18. Burton BK, Schulz CJ, Burd LI: Limb anomalies associated with chorionic villus sampling. Obstet Gynecol 79:726, 1992.
19. Wilson RD, Kendrick V, Witmann BK: Risks of spontaneous abortion in ultrasonographically normal pregnancies. Lancet 2:920, 1984.
20. Gilmore DH, McNay MB: Spontaneous fetal loss rate in early pregnancy. Lancet 1:107, 1985.
21. Casner KA, Christopher CR, Dysert GA: Spontaneous fetal loss after demonstration of a live fetus in the first trimester. Obstet Gynecol 70:827, 1987.
22. Simpson JL, Bombard AT: Chromosomal abnormalities in spontaneous abortion, frequency, pathology, and genetic counseling. In Edmonds K, Bennet MJ (eds): Spontaneous Abortion. London, Blackwell, 1987, p 51.
23. Warburton D, Stein Z, Kline J, et al: Chromosome abnormalities in spontaneous abortion: Data from the New York City Study. In Porter IH, Hook EB (eds): Human Embryonic and Fetal Death. New York, Academic Press, 1980, p 261.
24. Medical Research Council European trial of chorionic villus sampling. MRC working party on the evaluation of chorion villus sampling. Lancet 337:1491, 1991.
25. Saura R, Gauthier B, Taine L, et al: Operator experiences and fetal loss rate in transabdominal CVS. Prenat Diagn 14:70, 1994.
26. Wapner RJ, Barr MA, Heeger S, et al: Chorionic villus sampling: A 10 year, over 13,000 consecutive case experience [abstract]. Presented at the American College of Medical Genetics First Annual Meeting, March 1994, Orlando, Fla.

27. Young SR, Shipley CF, Wade RV, et al: Single-center comparison of results of 1000 prenatal diagnoses with chorionic villus sampling and 1000 diagnoses with amniocentesis. Am J Obstet Gynecol 165:255, 1991.

28. Green JE, Dorfman A, Jones SL, et al: Chorionic villus sampling: Experience with an initial 940 cases. Obstet Gynecol 71:208, 1988.

29. Clark BA, Bissonnette JM, Olson SB, et al: Pregnancy loss in a small chorionic villus sampling series. Am J Obstet Gynecol 161:301, 1989.

30. Gustavii B, Claesson V, Kristoffersson U, et al: Risk of miscarriage after chorionic biopsy is probably not higher than after amniocentesis. Lakartidningen 86:4221, 1989.

31. Jahoda MGJ, Pijpers L, Reuss A, et al: Evaluation of transcervical chorionic villus sampling with a completed follow-up of 1550 consecutive pregnancies. Prenat Diagn 9:621, 1989.

32. Brambati B, Lanzani A, Tului L: Transabdominal and transcervical chorionic villus sampling: Efficacy and risk evaluation of 2411 cases. Am J Hum Genet 35:160, 1990.

33. Smidt-Jensen S, Permin M, Philip J: Sampling success and risk by transabdominal chorionic villus sampling, transcervical chorionic villus sampling, and amniocentesis: A randomized study. Ultrasound Obstet Gynecol 1:86, 1991.

34. Brambati B, Terzian E, Tognoni G: Randomized clinical trial of transabdominal versus transcervical chorionic villus sampling methods. Prenat Diagn 11:285, 1991.

35. Copeland KL, Carpenter RJ, Fenolio KR, et al: Integration of the transabdominal technique into an ongoing chorionic villus sampling program. Am J Obstet Gynecol 161:1289, 1989.

36. Hoyme F, Jones KL, Van Allen MI, et al: Vascular pathogenesis of transverse limb reduction defects. J Pediatr 101:839, 1982.

37. Foster-Iskenius U, Baird P: Limb reduction defects in over 1,000,000 consecutive livebirths. Teratology 39:127, 1989.

38. Mastroiacovo P, Botto LD, Cavalcanti DP: Limb anomalies following chorionic villus sampling: A registry based case control study. Am J Med Genet 44:856, 1992.

39. Brambati B, Simoni G, Traui M: Genetic diagnosis by chorionic villus sampling before 8 gestational weeks: Efficiency, reliability, and risks on 317 completed pregnancies. Prenat Diagn 12:784, 1992.

40. XIII Annual Meeting of the Fetoscopy Working Group, September 1991, Hong Kong.

41. Mahoney MJ: Limb abnormalities and chorionic villus sampling. Lancet 337:1422, 1991.

42. Jackson LG, Wapner RJ, Brambati B: Limb abnormalities and chorionic villus sampling. Lancet 337:1422, 1991.

43. Froster UG, Jackson L: Limb defects and chorionic villus sampling: Results from an international registry 1992-94. Lancet 347:489, 1996.

44. Firth HV, Boyd PA, Chamberlain PF, et al: Analysis of limb reduction defects in babies exposed to chorionic villus sampling. Lancet 343:1069, 1994.

45. Brent RL: Relationship between uterine vascular clamping, vascular disruption syndrome and cocaine teratology. Teratology 41:757, 1990.

46. Webster W, Brown-Woodman T: Cocaine as a cause of congenital malformations of vascular origin: Experimental evidence in the rat. Teratology 41:689, 1990.

47. Smidt-Jensen S, Philip J, Zachary J, et al: Implications of maternal serum alpha-fetoprotein elevation caused by transabdominal and transcervical CVS. Prenat Diagn 14:35, 1994.

48. Quintero R, Romero R, Mahoney M, et al: Fetal haemorrhagic lesions after chorionic villus sampling. Lancet 339:193, 1992.

49. Burton BK, Schulz CJ, Burd LI: Spectrum of limb disruption defects associated with chorionic villus sampling. Pediatrics 91:989, 1993.

50. Olney RS, Khoury MJ, Alo CJ, et al: Increased risk for transverse digital deficiency after chorionic villus sampling: Results of the United States Multistate Case-Control Study, 1988-1992. Teratology 51:20, 1995.

51. Jackson L, Wapner R, Barr-Jackson M: Chorionic villus sampling (CVS) is not associated with an increased incidence of limb reduction defects [abstract]. Presented at the 43rd Meeting of the American Society of Human Genetics, October 1993, New Orleans.

52. Brambati B, Oldrini A, Ferrazzi E, et al: Chorionic villus sampling: An analysis of the obstetric experience of 1000 cases. Prenat Diagn 7:157, 1987.

53. Scialli AR, Neugebauer DL, Fabro SE: Microbiology of the endocervix in patients undergoing chorionic villus sampling. In Fraccaro M, Simoni G, Brambati B (eds): First Trimester Fetal Diagnosis. Berlin, Springer, 1985, pp 69-73.

54. Brambati B, Varotto F. Infection and chorionic villus sampling. Lancet 2:609, 1985.

55. Garden AS, Reid G, Benzie RJ. Chorionic villus sampling. Lancet 1:1270, 1985.

56. McFadyen IR, Taylor-Robinson D, Furr PM, Boustouller YL: Infection and chorionic villus sampling. Lancet 2:610, 1985.

57. Wass D, Bennett MJ: Infection and chorionic villus sampling. Lancet 2:338, 1985.

58. Brambati B, Matarrelli M, Varotto F: Septic complications after chorionic villus sampling. Lancet 1:1212, 1987.

59. Becker R, Mende B, Rodloff AC, et al: Bacteriologic findings before and in transcervical chorionic villi biopsy and their clinical relevance. Geburtshilfe Frauenheilkd 51:704, 1991.

60. Hogge WA, Schonberg SA, Golbus MS: Chorionic villus sampling: Experience of the first 1000 cases. Am J Obstet Gynecol 154:1249, 1986.

61. Barela A, Kleinman GE, Golditch IM, et al: Septic shock with renal failure after chorionic villus sampling. Am J Obstet Gynecol 154:1100, 1986.

62. Blakemore KJ, Mahoney MJ, Hobbins JC: Infection and chorionic villus sampling. Lancet 2:339, 1985.

63. Cheng EY, Luth DA, Hickok D, et al: Transcervical chorionic villus sampling and midtrimester oligohydramnios. Am J Obstet Gynecol 165:1063, 1991.

64. Blakemore KJ, Baumgarten A, Schoenfeld-Dimaio M, et al: Rise in maternal serum alpha-fetoprotein concentration after chorionic villus sampling. Lancet 2:339, 1985.

65. Brambati B, Guercilena S, Bonacchi I, et al: Feto-maternal transfusion after chorionic villus sampling: Clinical implications. Hum Reprod 1:37, 1986.

66. Shulman LP, Meyers CM, Simpson JL, et al: Fetomaternal transfusion depends on amount of chorionic villi aspirated but not on method of chorionic villus sampling. Am J Obstet Gynecol 162:1185, 1990.

67. Zipursky A, Israels LG: The pathogenesis and prevention of Rh immunization. Can Med Assoc J 97:1245, 1967.

68. Moise KJ, Carpenter RJ: Increased severity of fetal hemolytic disease with known rhesus alloimmunization after first trimester transcervical chorionic villus biopsy. Fetal Diagn Ther 5:76, 1990.

69. Williams J 3rd, Medearis AL, Bear MD, Kaback MM: Chorionic villus sampling is associated with normal fetal growth. Am J Obstet Gynecol 157:708, 1987.

70. Angue H, Bingru Z, Hong W: Long-term follow-up results after aspiration of chorionic villi during early pregnancy. In Fraccaro M, Simoni G, Brambati B (eds): First Trimester Fetal Diagnosis. New York, Springer, 1985, p 1.

71. Simoni G, Brambati B, Danesino C, et al: Efficient direct chromosome analyses and enzyme determinations from chorionic villi samples in the first trimester of pregnancy. Hum Genet 63:349, 1983.

72. Handling chorionic villi for direct chromosome studies. Lancet 2:1491, 1983.

73. Bhatia B, Koppitch FC, Sokol RJ, Evans MI: Improving the yield of direct chorionic villus slide preparations. Am J Obstet Gyn 54:408, 1986.

74. Chang HC, Jones OW, Masui H: Human amniotic fluid cells grown in a hormone-supplemented medium: Suitability for prenatal diagnosis. Proc Natl Acad Sci USA 79:4795, 1982.

75. Grebner EE, Jackson LG: Prenatal diagnosis for Tay-Sachs disease using chorionic villus sampling. Prenat Diagn 5:313, 1985.

76. Mikkelsen M, Ayme S: Chromosomal findings in chorionic villi. In Vogel F, Sperling K (eds): Human Genetics. Heidelberg, Springer-Verlag, 1987, p 597.

77. Ledbetter DH, Martin AO, Verlinsky Y, et al: Cytogenetic results of chorionic villus sampling: High success rate and diagnostic accuracy in the United States collaborative study. Am J Obstet Gynecol 162:495, 1990.

78. Elles RG, Williamson R, Niazi D, et al: Absence of maternal contamination of chorionic villi used for fetal gene analysis. N Engl J Med 308:1433, 1983.

79. Ledbetter DH, Zachary JM, Simpson JL, et al: Cytogenetic results from the U.S. collaborative study on CVS. Prenat Diagn 12:317, 1992.

80. Williams J, Medearis AL, Chu WH, et al: Maternal cell contamination in cultured chorionic villi: Comparison of chromosome Q-polymorphisms derived from villi, fetal skin, and maternal lymphocytes. Prenat Diagn 7:315, 1987.

81. Hogge WA, Schonberg SA, Golbus MS: Prenatal diagnosis by chorionic villus sampling: Lessons of the first 600 cases. Prenat Diagn 5:393, 1985.

82. Desnick RJ, Schuette JL, Golbus MS, et al: First trimester biochemical and molecular diagnoses using chorionic villi: High accuracy in the U.S. collaborative study. Prenat Diagn 12:357, 1991.

83. Markert C, Petters R: Manufactured hexaparental mice show that adults are derived from three embryonic cells. Science 202:56, 1978.

84. Wolstenholme J: Confined placental mosaicism for trisomies 2, 3, 7, 8, 9, 16, and 22: Their incidence, likely origins, and mechanisms for cell lineage compartmentalization. Prenat Diag 16:511, 1996.

85. Cassidy SB, Lai LW, Erickson RP, et al: Trisomy 15 with loss of the paternal 15 as a cause of Prader-Willi syndrome due to maternal disomy. Am J Hum Genet 51:701, 1992.

86. Purvis-Smith SG, Saville T, Manass S, et al: Uniparental disomy 15 resulting from "correction" of an initial trisomy 15. Am J Hum Genet 50:1348, 1992.

87. Kalousek DK, Langlois S, Barrett I, et al: Uniparental disomy for chromosome 16 in humans. Am J Hum Genet 52:8, 1993.

88. Post JG, Nijhuis JG: Trisomy 16 confined to the placenta. Prenat Diagn 12:1001, 1992.

89. Kalousek DK, Dill FJ, Pantzar T, et al: Confined chorionic mosaicism in prenatal diagnosis. Hum Genet 77:163, 1987.

90. Johnson A, Wapner RJ, Davis GH, Jackson LG: Mosaicism in chorionic villus sampling: An association with poor perinatal outcome. Obstet Gynecol 75:573, 1990.

91. Wapner RJ, Simpson MS, Golbus MS, et al: Chorionic mosaicism: Association with fetal loss but not with adverse perinatal outcome. Prenat Diagn 12:347, 1992.

92. Goldberg JD, Porter AE, Golbus MS: Current assessment of fetal losses as a direct consequence of chorionic villus sampling. Am J Med Genet 35:174, 1990.

93. Kalousek DK, Howard-Pebbles PN, Olson SB, et al: Confirmation of CVS mosaicism in term placentae and high frequency of intrauterine growth retardation association with confined placental mosaicism. Prenat Diagn 11:743, 1991.

94. Worton RG, Stern R: A Canadian collaborative study of mosaicism in amniotic fluid cell cultures. Prenat Diagn 4:131, 1984.

95. Vejerslev LO, Mikkelsen M: The European collaborative study on mosaicism in chorionic villus sampling: Data from 1986-1987. Prenat Diagn 9:575, 1989.

96. Bui TH, Iselius L, Linsten J: European collaborative study on prenatal diagnosis: Mosaicism, pseudomosaicism and single abnormal cells in amniotic fluid cell cultures. Prenat Diagn 4:145, 1984.

97. Hsu LYF, Perlis TE: United States survey on chromosome mosaicism and pseudomosaicism in prenatal diagnosis. Prenat Diagn 4:97, 1984.

98. Breed ASPM, Mantingh A, Vosters R, et al: Follow-up and pregnancy outcome after a diagnosis of mosaicism in CVS. Prenat Diagn 11:577, 1991.

99. Phillips OP, Tharapel AT, Lerner JL, et al: Risk of fetal mosaicism when placental mosaicism is diagnosed by chorionic villus sampling. Am J Obstet Gynecol 174:850, 1996.

100. Bartels I, Hansmann I, Holland U, et al: Down syndrome at birth not detected by first trimester chorionic villus sampling. Am J Med Genet 34:606, 1989.

101. Lilford RJ, Caine A, Linton G, et al: Short-term culture and false-negative results for Down's syndrome on chorionic villus sampling. Lancet 337:861, 1991.

102. Miny P, Basaran S, Holzgreve W, et al: False-negative cytogenetic result in direct preparations after CVS. Prenat Diagn 8:633, 1988.

103. Simoni G, Fraccaro M, Gimelli G, et al: False-positive and false-negative findings on chorionic villus sampling. Prenat Diagn 7:671, 1987.

104. False-negative finding on chorionic villus sampling. Lancet 2:391, 1986.

105. Robinson GE, Garner DM, Olmsted MP, et al: Anxiety reduction after chorionic villus sampling and genetic amniocentesis. Am J Obstet Gynecol 159:953, 1988.

106. Sjogren B, Uddenberg N: Prenatal diagnosis and psychological distress: Amniocentesis or chorionic villus biopsy? Prenat Diagn 9:477, 1989.

107. Spencer JW, Cox DN: A comparison of chorionic villus sampling and amniocentesis: Acceptability of procedure and maternal attachment to pregnancy. Obstet Gynecol 72:714, 1988.

108. McGovern MM, Goldberg JD, Resnick RJ: Acceptability of chorionic villi sampling for prenatal diagnosis. Am J Obstet Gynecol 155:25, 1996.

109. Evans MI, Drugan A, Koppitch FC, et al: Genetic diagnosis in the first trimester: The norm for the 1990s. Am J Obstet Gynecol 160:1332. 1989.

110. Harper J, Pergament E, Delhanty J: Recent advances in molecular and molecular cytogenetic techniques have enabled the diagnosis of some inherited diseases from a single cell [comment]. Review. Prenat Diagn 18:1343, 1998.

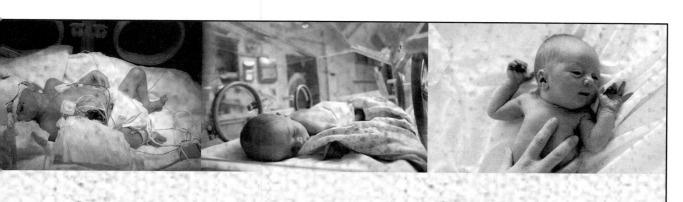

Assessing Fetal Well-Being

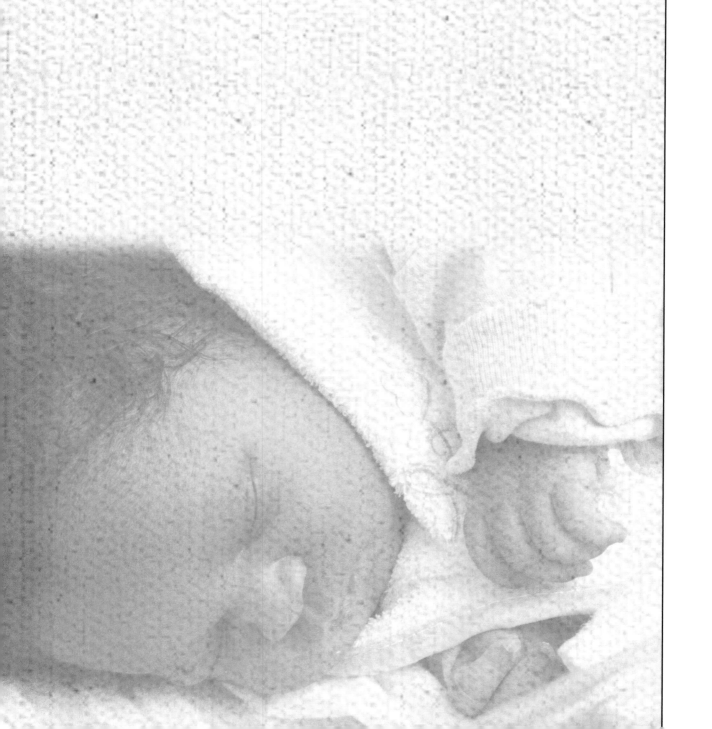

CHAPTER 8

Identification and Management of the Fetus at Risk for Acidosis

Reinaldo Figueroa, Antoun Al Khabbaz, and J. Gerald Quirk

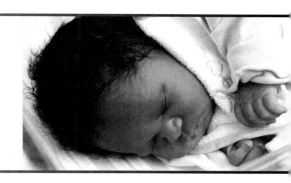

This chapter addresses important clinical issues that regularly concern the obstetrician and pediatrician in the evaluation and care of newborns. An overview of fetal evaluation is essential for a better understanding of common approaches to the clinical care of high-risk and low-risk pregnancies, clinical end points, and known limitations of the available testing modalities. When the fetus is evaluated, most reassuring test results are highly predictive of an apparently normal outcome, but only for limited end points. A normal fetal heart rate (FHR) pattern predicts the birth of an infant with a 5-minute Apgar score of 7 or greater with an accuracy of 99%. In contrast, nonreassuring tests have high false-positive values (>50%) for later morbidity. Similarly, most tests are not adequately sensitive when central nervous system (CNS) dysfunction is used as an end point. Considerable emphasis is directed toward selection of precise clinical terminology.

PERINATAL HYPOXIA-ACIDOSIS AS A CAUSE OF MORBIDITY AND MORTALITY

Occasionally the prospective management of a newborn may be complicated by signs and symptoms suggesting "significant" perinatal hypoxia (more specifically, preexisting intrapartum fetal hypoxia-acidosis). Perinatal hypoxia, when of a significant degree and duration, may result in severe metabolic acidosis, which may contribute to newborn morbidity and mortality. If the hypoxia is severe and persistent, it also may contribute to long-term neurologic deficits.

DEFINITION OF TERMS

Perinatal

The term **perinatal** commonly is misused to include only labor-related events. The term is a broad, inclusive one, however, and includes the periods before (prenatal), during (intrapartum), and after the time of birth (neonatal)

of fetal-neonatal growth and development. It is recommended that the more specific mutually exclusive terms—**prenatal (antenatal), intrapartum,** and **neonatal**—be used to avoid miscommunication.

Asphyxia

Asphyxia is the consequence of persistent hypoxemia of a degree that results in anaerobic metabolism at the tissue level and metabolic acidemia. Hypercarbia also is present in some cases.

Significant

We use the term **significant** as a descriptor when referring to an indicator that reliably can predict clinically relevant end points, such as the degree and duration of hypoxemia-associated acidemia. When present, hypoxia-related acidosis can reliably predict later morbidity, including hypoxic-ischemic encephalopathy and cerebral palsy.

The descriptor *significant* is used with the understanding that reliable predictors for key end points have not been identified yet. There is neither a consensus regarding thresholds nor set criteria that can reliably predict (high positive predictive value) severe fetal metabolic acidemia or a permanent impact on fetal-neonatal organ systems, especially the CNS. This limitation applies to more recently used predictors, such as nonreassuring FHR monitor patterns. Although cord blood gases are not a predictor, no threshold has been determined that reliably predicts biologic injury, and it has been suggested that severe metabolic or mixed metabolic acidosis is required.

ASPHYXIA VERSUS BIRTH ASPHYXIA

The terms *asphyxia* and *birth asphyxia* have been used extensively in the medical literature. In most instances, the usage of the terms has been unsubstantiated by objective evidence or an indication of degree and characteristics. Only more recently have some studies included cord blood gases as an objective end point to assess the presence, degree, and nature (metabolic versus respiratory) of the acidosis.[1] In metabolic terms, asphyxia is not an absolute term. It is a relative term that requires qualification because there is no consensus on its definition or a specific threshold set. To use the term in an unqualified manner has the effect of communicating an impression that all degrees of asphyxia are of equal clinical significance. It is important to define the effects of hypoxia in terms of pH, Pco_2, base deficit, and blood and CNS lactate levels.

Historically, when clinicians have written or spoken of "asphyxia," they often were communicating incorrectly. On the one hand, some referred primarily to severe fetal metabolic acidemia. On the other hand, others (pediatric neurologists, in particular) frequently were speaking of the *result* or impact of a process thought to be secondary to hypoxemia or ischemia. This concept seems to be illustrated by a statement made by Freeman and Nelson[2]: "When describing the situation in the human, we will use the term asphyxia because we do *not* know whether the insult was hypoxic, ischemic, or, more probably, a combination."

Qualifying the term as severe in other than biochemical terms further clouds the issue. Use of the term *severe asphyxia* would imply to clinicians other than neurologists a degree of hypoxemia-acidemia. It seems that neurologists are referring, however, to degrees of effect, without specifying the measurable degree of cause, whether it be hypoxia, hypercapnia, or mechanical (baroreceptor induced). Seldom is there mention of an objective determination (via blood gases) of the degree of hypoxia-acidosis.

Asphyxia is not a prerequisite for the appearance of FHR alterations or low Apgar scores. The following quotation from two prominent investigators, Freeman and Nelson, appears immediately after the previous quotation without qualification regarding pH or oxygen values:

> Less severe degrees of asphyxia in the human fetus are common and may produce signs such as alterations of fetal heart rate and even low Apgar scores. These degrees of asphyxia do not appear to produce permanent neurologic deficits in otherwise normal full-term infants. Even in the presence of more *prolonged or severe asphyxia, manifest in the newborn period as encephalopathy,* most of the primate newborns and most human infants recover with little or no neurologic deficit.[2]

Definition of Birth Asphyxia

A consensus definition with common meaning to all care providers is highly desirable. To avoid confusion, it may be desirable that the term *asphyxia* be dropped and replaced with a more untarnished designation requiring qualification. Should the term *birth asphyxia* continue to be required, it should be used only when certain criteria are met.

Because the term *asphyxia* historically has been used in a different manner by obstetricians, pediatricians, pediatric neurologists, and epidemiologists, we have chosen to use the term *metabolic acidemia-acidosis* throughout this chapter. **Metabolic acidemia-acidosis** describes the clinically relevant biochemical effects of fetal hypoxemia and emphasizes that fetal-newborn acidosis can be described

and quantitated better in terms of pH, Pco_2, base deficit, and lactate level.[3,4]

Until more recently, there were no consensus criteria for the clinical diagnosis of birth asphyxia. Consensus criteria have been established incorporating input from the American Academy of Pediatrics Committee on the Fetus and Newborn and the American College of Obstetricians and Gynecologists (ACOG) Committee on Obstetric Practice.[3,4] It is recommended that the term *birth asphyxia* be reserved for the clinical situation of damaging acidemia, hypoxia, and metabolic acidosis. In addition, a sentinel event capable of interrupting the oxygen supply to the fetus or neonate should be recognized. The ACOG supports the concept that a neonate who has had hypoxia proximate to delivery that is severe enough to result in hypoxic encephalopathy would show other evidence of hypoxic damage, including *all* of the following[3]:

- Profound metabolic or mixed acidemia (pH < 7.00) on an umbilical cord arterial blood sample
- Persistent Apgar scores of 0 to 3 for longer than 5 minutes
- Evidence of neonatal neurologic sequelae (e.g., seizures, coma, hypotonia)
- Multisystem organ failure involving one or more of the following: cardiovascular, gastrointestinal, hematologic, pulmonary, or renal system dysfunction

These are reasonable criteria in that it is likely that a fetus subjected to significant "hypoxemia-acidosis" of a duration and degree severe enough to result in CNS injury would have coexistent multiorgan system injury because the brain and heart are protected by fetal adaptive mechanisms at the expense of less vital tissue and organs.

In 1999, the Perinatal Society of Australia and New Zealand published an international consensus statement on cerebral palsy.[5,6] The essential criteria for defining an acute intrapartum hypoxic event sufficient to cause permanent neurologic impairment were the following:

- Evidence of metabolic acidosis in intrapartum fetal umbilical arterial cord or early neonatal blood samples (pH < 7.00 and base deficit ≥ 12 mmol/L)
- Early onset of severe or moderate neonatal encephalopathy in infants of 34 weeks' gestation or greater
- Cerebral palsy of the spastic quadriparetic or dyskinetic type

Other criteria that together suggest intrapartum timing but by themselves are nonspecific include the following:

- A sentinel (signal) hypoxic event occurring immediately before or during labor
- A sudden, rapid, and sustained deterioration of the FHR pattern usually after the hypoxic sentinel event, when the pattern was previously normal
- Apgar scores of 0 to 6 for longer than 5 minutes
- Early evidence of multisystem involvement
- Early imaging evidence of acute cerebral abnormality

The ACOG and the American Academy of Pediatrics have modified and updated the International Cerebral Palsy Task Force Consensus Statement.[7] It is their belief that the use of these criteria would help to evaluate the probable pathology that caused the cerebral palsy during labor.

Threshold criteria in metabolic terms predictive of *birth asphyxia* are highly desirable. It is likely that the biologic threshold is an umbilical artery pH less than 7.00 and the acidosis is predominantly metabolic in nature. The exact lower limit of the pH (how much lower than 7.00) has not been determined. Eventually, other indicators of end-organ (especially CNS) cellular or tissue damage should be sought, including leakage of specific enzymes or ultrasound evidence of cerebral ischemia.[8]

Hypoxic-ischemic encephalopathy is a subtype of neonatal encephalopathy for which the etiology is considered to be limitation of oxygen and blood flow near the time of birth. The term *hypoxic-ischemic encephalopathy* is appropriate when specifically describing the CNS findings associated with documented severe metabolic acidosis. Although we can measure the severity of the metabolic acidemia, there are no objective means to measure the degree of ischemia in terms of blood flow at the tissue level. We are limited to measuring the effect.

FETAL ASSESSMENT: CLINICAL VALUE AND LIMITATIONS

Early Prenatal Assessment

When a high-risk fetus is studied before labor begins, the determinations are largely nonspecific with the exception of genetic studies and targeted ultrasound studies. This is particularly true when using CNS dysfunction as an end point.

First 20 Weeks

The fetus is relatively inaccessible during the first two trimesters of pregnancy. In early pregnancy, the fetus (according to maternal risk factors) is subject to genetic studies (chorionic villus sampling or genetic amniocentesis) and an ultrasound examination, performed to assess gestational age. Structural abnormalities can be detected, but only in unusual circumstances. In some high-risk situations (e.g., pregestational diabetes mellitus), ultrasound may be indicated to screen for the presence of major congenital anomalies at 18 to 20 weeks of gestation. Detection generally is limited, however, to the most obvious abnormalities in a fetus weighing less than 500 g. Hydrocephalus, holoprosencephaly, anencephaly, and congenital absence of the corpus callosum are common structural problems of the CNS that can be detected. More subtle developmental problems of the CNS are not assessable. In later pregnancy, it may be possible to detect CNS infarction that can occur with maternal cocaine abuse.

Weeks 21 to 30

Few, if any, additional fetal assessments are performed before 28 to 30 weeks of gestation, unless the pregnancy is at high risk for uteroplacental insufficiency (UPI). Risk for UPI may suggest a need for a follow-up scan as part of serial ultrasound determinations for growth. Umbilical artery Doppler velocimetry may be performed, and an elevated systolic-to-diastolic ratio may indicate a fetus that is at risk for uteroplacental insufficiency. The clinical value of these determinations has not been shown for conditions other than intrauterine growth restriction. Doppler velocimetry has not been shown to be valuable as a screening test for detecting fetal compromise in the general obstetric population. Presently, Doppler insonation of other major fetal vessels (e.g., middle cerebral artery) is considered investigational.[9]

Third-Trimester Fetal Evaluation

Biophysical testing of the fetus is done frequently in the last trimester in patients at risk for UPI and with regard to limited end points. Testing frequency varies from one to three times per week depending on the risk factor identified. Table 8-1 summarizes possible nonreassuring findings that may be elicited during prenatal evaluation or labor management. Currently, it is not possible to identify reliably dysfunction of the fetal brain.

Ultrasound

Serial ultrasound examinations may be indicated in the third trimester in patients at risk for UPI to assess fetal growth. If there is delayed growth, ultrasound examination may determine if it is symmetric or asymmetric (head growth dimensions are spared and abdominal circumference—liver, subcutaneous fat—progressively deviates below predicted growth percentiles). Asymmetric growth restriction is associated more commonly with UPI, whereas symmetric growth restriction is associated more commonly with congenital infections, karyotypic abnormalities, and environmental agents, such as external radiation. These generalizations regarding fetal

---

Table 8–1. Possible Nonreassuring Perinatal Indicators

Prenatal Indicators
Nonreactive nonstress test
Positive contraction stress test
Abnormal biophysical profile (score $\leq$6)
Oligohydramnios
Sonographic suggestion of intrauterine growth restriction
Advanced placental maturation on ultrasound

Intrapartum Indicators
Nonreassuring FHR pattern (*repetitive* late or significant
  variable decelerations, prolonged severe decelerations,
  sinusoidal pattern, check mark pattern)[118]
Fetal capillary blood pH suggesting metabolic acidemia

Specific Newborn Observations
Umbilical venous/arterial metabolic acidemia

Nonspecific Newborn Observations
Low Apgar score in term newborn
Need for assisted ventilation
Meconium aspiration syndrome
Persistent fetal circulation in the newborn
Neonatal seizures

FHR, fetal heart rate.

growth may not hold true in circumstances in which there is early or midtrimester onset of preeclampsia. In such cases, growth restriction may be symmetric rather than asymmetric, as classically expected. Occasionally, a third-trimester scan performed for a discrepancy in size and dates serendipitously may uncover an unsuspected periventricular hemorrhage[10-12] or intrauterine seizure activity[13] that otherwise might be attributed to intrapartum or neonatal causes.

Nonstress Test

The nonstress test (NST) is an antenatal test based on the response of the FHR to fetal movement. Although it is a relatively sensitive screening test to identify a fetus at risk, its most important purpose is to provide reassurance that a pregnancy at risk does not require prenatal intervention. Approximately 90% of test results are reassuring. To keep the limitations of the NST in perspective, when compared with traditional adult medical testing procedures, the NST is unsophisticated and represents only a small sample of the total potential observation time in the third trimester. In most cases, these tests are performed once weekly and seldom more than twice weekly.

Reactive nonstress test. The end point of the NST is to observe accelerations of the FHR that peak at 15 beats/min above the baseline and last at least 15 seconds on two occasions within a 20-minute interval. A reactive test result is highly predictive for a normal outcome (high negative predictive value) indicating appropriate fetal cardiovascular adaptations to labor and morbidity independent of gestational age. Survival of the fetus for 1 week or more occurs in greater than 99% of the reactive tests (false-negative rate < 1%).

Nonreactive nonstress test. An NST is nonreactive when there are no FHR accelerations or fetal movements during the testing period. Poor fetal outcome is encountered in 20% of nonreactive NSTs; this test has a high false-positive rate of approximately 80% to 90%, depending on the characteristics of the population tested.

If the NST is nonreactive (and because of the high false-positive rate), additional testing should be performed using the biophysical profile (BPP), contraction stress test (CST), or oxytocin challenge test (OCT). In most cases, reassuring findings on the BPP (score ≥ 8) or CST (normal baseline FHR and absence of late decelerations) provide reassurance that the preceding nonreactive NST was a false-positive test.

Biophysical Profile

The BPP first was reported as an antenatal testing method in 1980. This profile uses a scoring system based on the results of an NST and a real-time ultrasound assessment of fetal breathing movements, fetal tone, fetal gross body movement, and amniotic fluid volume. The profile provides for a maximal score of 10. Each of the five elements is assigned a value of 2 (normal) or 0 (abnormal), with no intermediate values. Since the profile originally was developed, investigators have determined that if the sonographically determined end points are present, it is not necessary to perform the NST portion of the BPP, and the accuracy of the test is not altered.[14] The BPP is discussed in greater detail in Chapter 9.

Contraction Stress Test

The CST uses spontaneously occurring contractions or contractions induced by oxytocin (OCT) or breast stimulation. Three uterine contractions in a 10-minute period are necessary to complete the test. The CST is designed to detect UPI before irreversible fetal damage occurs. The test is contraindicated in patients with a placenta previa, previous classical cesarean delivery, or risk of preterm delivery.

Negative contraction stress test. A negative (reassuring) CST has a normal baseline FHR with no late decelerations. Fetal survival for 1 week is 99% when the CST is negative.

Positive contraction stress test. A CST is positive when there are repetitive or persistent late decelerations. Poor fetal outcome has been observed in approximately 50% of cases when the CST is positive.

Suspicious contraction stress test. If there are intermittent late decelerations, variable decelerations, or an abnormal baseline FHR, the CST is considered suspicious.

Unsatisfactory contraction stress test. A CST in which the recording is of poor quality or there are fewer than three contractions in 10 minutes is considered an unsatisfactory test.

Screening for Oligohydramnios

The presence of oligohydramnios (abnormally low volume of amniotic fluid) increases the risk of adverse fetal outcome because of the preexisting UPI or from compression of the umbilical cord against the uterine wall or other fetal parts. Because fetal urine is the primary source of amniotic fluid in the third trimester, the progressive reduction in amniotic fluid in many cases is thought to reflect a decrease in fetal urine production as a result of UPI. In a growth-restricted fetus, there is shunting of blood away from organs less crucial in fetal life, with preservation of blood flow to the three vital organs (heart, brain, adrenals).

Oligohydramnios may be suspected clinically on the basis of diminished growth of the uterine fundus. Most commonly, oligohydramnios is detected during sonographic evaluation of amniotic fluid volume. Variable decelerations seen on the NST in the latent phase or early in the active phase of labor, at a time when they are not seen commonly, are other possible indications that oligohydramnios is present. Traditionally, oligohydramnios has been diagnosed sonographically by subjective observation or by measuring the depth of the maximal vertical pocket of amniotic fluid. Alternatively, oligohydramnios may be diagnosed when the amniotic fluid index, a summation of the vertical pockets on a four-quadrant assessment of the uterine cavity, is less than expected values.

Despite their clinical utility in providing a source of reassurance in the management of a high-risk fetus, currently available antenatal fetal testing is *not* sensitive or predictive when using prenatal or intrapartum CNS abnormality as an end point. Except in extreme cases, antenatal tests can be reassuring even in the presence of significant CNS anomalies. In rare and extreme cases with obvious antepartum FHR findings that no one would question (e.g., prolonged deceleration to <60 to 70 beats/min for ≥15 minutes), it occasionally is possible to estimate the degree of acidemia arising from prenatal hypoxemic events. In most cases, however, it is not possible to determine reliably the integrity of the fetal CNS before or during labor. As a consequence, the determination of a labor-specific, cause-and-effect conclusion is usually difficult to make with any level of confidence.

Clinical Evolution of Uteroplacental Insufficiency

Prenatal Detection

If significant risk factors for UPI are identified, UPI may be confirmed by the presence of repetitive late decelerations detected during an NST, spontaneous CST (positive CST), or in response to oxytocin-induced contractions on an OCT (positive OCT). Alternatively, the presence of UPI may be suggested by diminution of fetal growth or detection of oligohydramnios. Common clinical examples in which such antenatal testing would be indicated include patients with significant maternal medical problems or fetal risk factors for UPI, intrauterine growth restriction, or post-term pregnancy (postmaturity syndrome).

Prenatal Evolution

Although not specific for UPI, the early evolution of clinical UPI may be suggested by a nonreactive NST. In most cases, additional testing reveals a reassuring CST (negative CST) or BPP (score > 6). If progression of UPI continues, some cases develop a nonreassuring CST (suspicious or positive CST) or BPP (score < 6). At some point, if UPI does not progress rapidly, the fetus may attempt to compensate for the relative hypoxemia to protect the heart, brain, and adrenals by diverting blood flow from less vital tissues (e.g., subcutaneous tissue, muscle, kidneys, and intestines), resulting in asymmetric growth. Compensatory reduction in renal blood flow may result in progressive diminution of fetal urine and amniotic fluid. Oligohydramnios, which may be detected by sonographic evaluation, eventually develops. Fetal demise may occur as a result of progressive UPI or secondary to oligohydramnios-induced umbilical cord compression.

Intrapartum or Postnatal Detection

Risk factors for UPI or fetal growth restriction are detected prospectively in only half of cases. The process may go undetected until the onset of labor or after birth, when obvious intrauterine growth restriction is noticed.

Repetitive late decelerations, with or without reduction of baseline variability, may be detected for the first time during labor as the frequency and intensity of the contractions increase, and the recovery time between contractions decreases. In other situations, repetitive variable decelerations may reflect cord compression from oligohydramnios or entanglement with the fetal body (e.g., nuchal cord). Subcutaneous tissue and muscle wasting or the classic postmaturity syndrome may be noted at birth.

Assessment of Fetus in Labor and at Birth

In most pregnancies, the first meaningful evaluation of fetal function begins after hospital admission for management of labor and delivery. In low-risk patients, prenatal evaluation is limited primarily to the mother, and the fetus is evaluated indirectly, unless risk factors for UPI are identified. Risk factors are detected in only 50% of cases in which it later is determined that the fetus is growth restricted. During active labor, the fetus is screened for periodic hypoxic stresses associated with uterine contractions. Virtually all pregnancies are subject to and most compensate for such hypoxic stresses. The clinical objective is to discriminate between repetitive hypoxic stresses, with minimal metabolic and pathophysiologic consequences, and clinically significant hypoxic stresses resulting in significant metabolic and pathophysiologic alterations. To accomplish this goal, the FHR, an end product of cardiovascular reflexes, is subjected to increased scrutiny during much of the labor process with continuous electronic fetal monitoring (EFM). Although continuous EFM is the standard, intermittent auscultation may be used in some low-risk pregnancies.

Prospectively, the primary clinical problem for the obstetrician is to screen for progressive ongoing fetal acidemia, which has a significant impact on newborn morbidity. EFM screening for clinically significant hypoxemic stress is used routinely during the intrapartum period. EFM ordinarily is not sufficiently predictive of the degree and type (metabolic versus respiratory) of fetal acidemia for it to serve as a reliable measure of the intensity of the cumulative metabolic effect of the hypoxic-acidosis stress.

EFM is, at best, a sensitive screening test for fetal cardiovascular adaptation to labor-related stresses. EFM generates a continuous record of FHR responses to fetal cardiovascular adaptation reflexes involving the brainstem, baroreceptors, chemoreceptors, sympathetic and parasympathetic systems, and, to a lesser degree, higher cortical centers. Table 8-1 summarizes the possible nonreassuring observations that may be detected during prenatal testing, intrapartum or in the newborn.

Although some estimate of the intensity and duration of repetitive hypoxic stresses is possible with EFM, an objective measure of the degree or intensity and characteristics (metabolic versus respiratory) of the resultant acidemia is not possible unless fetal capillary (scalp) blood gases are collected. Scalp blood gas tests are performed only rarely, however, even in university centers. When done, they are performed most commonly not to confirm significant acidemia, but to gain reassurance (scalp pH ≥ 7.25) that the decelerations that are detected are not associated with significant fetal acidemia. If reassurance is achieved, labor can be allowed to continue.

Amniotic fluid is known to have a role as a physical buffer against potential umbilical cord occlusion. The detection of variable decelerations during antenatal

(NST or CST) testing or in early labor, before descent of the presenting part and before a time in which one commonly would observe cord compression patterns, often raises the index of suspicion for fetal oligohydramnios. In other cases, oligohydramnios may be detected when little fluid is released at the time the amniotic sac is ruptured during labor.

ELECTRONIC FETAL HEART RATE MONITORING

Some knowledge of the basic principles of continuous FHR monitoring, including definitions, physiology, and clinical correlations, is mandatory if nonobstetric caregivers are to abstract selectively and review critically available clinical obstetric information (including EFM data). This section provides such a database. FHR physiology and unusual FHR patterns are not discussed in detail. Key definitions, some broad generalizations regarding FHR baseline and periodic changes, and some relatively common clinical correlations are provided. Considerable focus is placed on the importance of adhering to established criteria for pattern recognition, especially with regard to late decelerations. FHR baseline variability is recommended as a means to evaluate the fetal response to, and the cardiovascular impact from, the stress responsible for the pattern detected. Management is discussed to understand better the strategies and limitations of FHR-based labor management.

Baseline Versus Periodic or Episodic Changes

A relative change in baseline rate should be differentiated from a *periodic change* (i.e., acceleration or deceleration). In most cases, periodic changes (accelerations or decelerations) are associated with uterine contractions or fetal movement and do not reflect a true baseline change. The baseline rate is recognized between uterine contractions. The key differences are (1) the duration of the change and (2) the existence of a threshold heart rate. To establish a new baseline (i.e., to change from 140 to 150 beats/min), the change in baseline must persist for at least 10 minutes. Some researchers require a change of longer than 15 minutes.[15] For the purposes of this discussion, periodic FHR changes whose duration is less than 10 to 15 minutes are designated as either a *deceleration* or an *acceleration* depending on the direction of the periodic change.

Baseline Fetal Heart Rate

Baseline FHR is considered normal in the range of 120 to 160 beats/min. Persistence of the FHR outside these limits is defined as follows.

Bradycardia

Bradycardia[16] (or sinus bradycardia) is a persistent baseline FHR change to less than 120 beats/min for 10 minutes or longer.

Tachycardia

Tachycardia[16] is a persistent baseline FHR change greater than 160 beats/min for 10 minutes or longer.

Deceleration Versus Bradycardia

A decrease in FHR potentially could be designated as a deceleration or bradycardia. A deceleration is a short-term (10- to 15-minute), periodic slowing of the FHR below the baseline, whereas a bradycardia must persist for at least 10 to 15 minutes and be below the baseline of 120 beats/min. A deceleration simply may be a decrease of 10 to 20 beats/min below the baseline and stay within the normal baseline range of 120 to 160 beats/min. Within this framework, it is not appropriate to qualify a bradycardia as prolonged, but it is possible to indicate that a deceleration (≤10 to 15 minutes) is prolonged.

Baseline Variability

Variability is the fluctuation of the baseline FHR observed between sequential periodic changes. It is subclassified into short-term (beat-to-beat) and long-term variability.

Beat-to-beat variability is the relatively nonuniform, sawtooth appearance characteristic of the FHR baseline. Short-term variability, or beat-to-beat variability, reflects differences in sequential R-R wave intervals of the fetal electrocardiogram (ECG). If sequential R-R intervals are equal, the baseline is flat (no short-term variability). Normal beat-to-beat variability is generally 2 to 3 beats/min as one evaluates the magnitude of the fluctuation of successive heart rate points. It is considered diminished when the beat-to-beat differences are, on average, 1 beat/min or less. Decreased beat-to-beat variability, in the absence of drugs or other factors known to depress variability, generally is considered the most significant indication of disturbed fetal cardiovascular homeostasis in response to cord compression or UPI.

Long-term variability is reflected by cyclic fluctuations in the FHR baseline that occur at three to five cycles per minute. Long-term variability amplitude is determined by measurement of the oscillations from peak to nadir. In the normal term fetus, the amplitude is usually in the range of 5 to 20 beats/min. Long-term variability is considered reduced when less than 5 beats/min. Generally the magnitude of long-term variability parallels that of short-term variability, with two relatively infrequent exceptions. The first, the *sinusoidal* pattern, is a baseline pattern in which the long-term oscillations are maintained, but there are no superimposed short-term fluctuations. This pattern is observed most commonly with fetal hydrops associated with Rh isoimmunization. At the other extreme, long-term variability may be diminished but short-term variability maintained.

Generalizations About Baseline Variability

Changes in baseline variability are thought to be secondary to an alteration in CNS control, especially the autonomic nervous system. This concept is supported by observations that drugs that depress autonomic reflexes also tend to decrease FHR variability. Maturation of the fetal CNS also is a determinant; variability increases and becomes more cyclic and predictable with advancing gestational age, particularly in the third trimester. Baseline FHR variability may be affected by fetal breathing, body or extremity movements, and state of wakefulness.

The normal fetus has cyclic behavioral states of reduced activity and greater activity. These states usually are defined by the presence or absence of rapid eye movements, physical activity (movement of the trunk and extremities and fetal breathing movements), and FHR variability and presence of accelerations. Cycles of low FHR reactivity correlate with fetal electroencephalogram signs of deep sleep. Fetal electroencephalogram determinations during periods of low reactivity are suggestive of non–rapid eye movement sleep.[17] During the third trimester, term fetuses are normally quiet approximately one third of the time. Quiet periods typically last 20 to 30 minutes, but occasionally last beyond 40 minutes in the third trimester. In general, the fetal reactivity is greatest late at night.[18] As a result of these cycles, fetal reactivity (variability and accelerations) is not always expected to be present. Proper interpretation of any test of fetal well-being that depends on assessment of the FHR as an end point (NST, CST, BPP, EFM) requires an understanding of the impact of the fetal behavioral state. If variability is diminished, the fetal sleep state should be considered as a possibility, and the period of observation should be extended to 30 to 40 minutes. Alternatively the fetus can be stimulated by mechanical or acoustic means.

Decelerations

A deceleration is a periodic slowing of the heart rate of less than 10 minutes' duration. Decelerations most commonly are associated with uterine contractions. Occasionally, they may be associated with fetal movement, particularly if there is coexistent oligohydramnios or cord around the neck.

The FHR is primarily under the control of the fetal autonomic nervous system. Changes detected on continuous EFM may reflect fetal responses to baroreceptor stimulation, or they may reflect hypoxemia arising from umbilical cord compression (variable decelerations) or UPI (late decelerations). In the early stage of hypoxemia, whether from UPI or cord compression, the observed patterns are likely to be reflexive in origin. If hypoxemia is persistent and results in metabolic acidemia, however, some portion of the decelerations is likely to be the result of myocardial depression from myocardial hypoxia. This finding is consistent with animal models wherein the myocardium, similar to the brain, is protected until compensatory mechanisms have been used and presumably are near exhaustion.

It is useful to classify decelerations into three different patterns according to the alterations in FHR that are associated with uterine contractions. Early and late decelerations have a uniform shape and fairly consistent magnitude. Variable decelerations do not have a uniform or predictable relationship in terms of onset, depth, and duration with uterine contractions.

Early Decelerations

Early decelerations are smooth and rounded and mirror the shape of the associated contraction. The deceleration begins early with the uterine contraction, the nadir is coincident with the peak of the contraction, and the return to baseline occurs before the end of the contraction. They generally are thought to be reflexive (vagal) in origin, arising in response to compression of the fetal head.[19] Early decelerations generally are thought to have no major clinical significance other than the need to distinguish them from late or variable decelerations. They do not pose a threat of hypoxia to the fetus.[20] As a result, they are of little consequence to subsequent newborn outcome and are not associated with fetal hypoxemia, fetal acidemia, or low Apgar scores.

Late Decelerations

Late decelerations, in contrast to early decelerations, generally begin shortly after the peak of the contraction and have a relatively constant lag time or delay (approximately 30 seconds) between the onset, peak, and completion of the contraction and the onset, nadir, and return to baseline of the deceleration. In contrast to variable decelerations, repetitive late decelerations are symmetric and uniform in shape, reflect to some extent the magnitude of the associated contraction, and reappear with most significant contractions.[21-23]

Each labor-related uterine contraction induces a periodic, relative decrease in fetal PO_2 and elevation of PCO_2.[24] In a fetus with marginal fetal-placental-maternal exchange, the added stress of repetitive contractions may act in a cumulative manner. If the contractions are persistent and of sufficient magnitude, late decelerations may become manifest.[25-29] The physiology of late decelerations is similar to that of variable decelerations; some late decelerations may have reflexive and hypoxic components.[30,31] In the early phase of progressive fetal hypoxemia, late decelerations are primarily the product of a vagally mediated CNS reflex (in response to fetal hypoxemia).[30] The physiology of late decelerations also is affected by the presence or absence of FHR variability.

Variable Decelerations

Variable decelerations, as the term implies, vary in their appearance and temporal relationship with associated uterine contractions. There is usually an abrupt decrease in FHR from baseline, and there is no relationship between the onset, depth, and duration of the decelerations and the uterine contractions. The pathophysiology of variable decelerations is complex.[22,32-35] The actual mechanism of the deceleration is likely to be a product of baroreceptor and chemoreceptor responses.[34] Variable decelerations arise as a baroreceptor response to the hypertension induced by umbilical artery compression and the chemoreceptor response to fetal hypoxemia. Hypercarbia also may play a role.

The initial component of the slowing of the FHR reflects fetal umbilical artery compression, which induces an increase in fetal blood pressure. Baroreceptors in the aortic arch and carotid bodies are stimulated and respond to the relative increase in blood pressure with a brain stem–mediated reflex, which culminates in a slowing of the FHR. A second delayed component may occur if the variable deceleration is of sufficient magnitude and duration. Because this component is not obliterated by maternal atropine, it is thought to be the result of hypoxemia-induced myocardial depression, and it may share a similar origin with persistent late decelerations.[32]

Accelerations

Accelerations are periodic short-term (<10 minutes) increases in FHR above the baseline. Their appearance often can be correlated with fetal movements or uterine contractions. Accelerations more than 15 beats/min (usually >15 seconds) above the baseline provide reassurance regarding fetal cardiovascular status.[20,36,37] These accelerations correlate well with fetal cardiovascular integrity, particularly when associated with fetal movements. The presence of these accelerations generally is described as *fetal reactivity.*

ELECTRONIC FETAL MONITORING: CLINICAL INTERPRETATION AND MANAGEMENT

Clinical Utility of Secondary Changes in Baseline Fetal Heart Rate

The clinician should avoid the temptation to rely simply on the magnitude of a sequence of decelerations as the sole or even primary clinical FHR parameter to predict the presence and degree of fetal acidemia. First, the decelerations must be repetitive, of a significant magnitude, and nonremediable to pose a potential risk. Even then, if there is sufficient time between repetitive decelerations, the fetus may be able to compensate. The development of progressive changes in baseline FHR, particularly loss of variability and, to a lesser extent, tachycardia, should be evaluated in light of the impact of other factors known to affect baseline variability and rate. The absence of progressive changes suggests that the fetus is compensating.

Baseline Variability: Clinical Correlation

Trends in baseline variability have greater significance than does a change in baseline rate, even if the change eventually is designated as a bradycardia or tachycardia. Baseline variability is accepted widely as the most important FHR parameter for the assessment of fetal cardiovascular status. Trends in baseline variability, in the absence of other known modifiers, may reflect the impact of the stress imposed by cord compression (variable decelerations) or UPI (late decelerations) on the fetus. The clinical impact of repetitive decelerations is assessed largely based on trends in variability.

Normal Variability

Normal baseline variability[38-41] implies a compensated fetal cardiovascular homeostatic system under the control of a functioning autonomic nervous system and, to a lesser extent, higher centers. Coexistence with accelerations provides further evidence of a reassuring fetal status. Normal variability is highly predictive of a nonacidemic fetus.

Decreased or Absent Fetal Heart Rate Variability

Absent or decreased FHR variability has a low positive predictive value for subsequent newborn morbidity because it may be caused by other nonasphyxial causes. Any condition that depresses the autonomic nervous system may reduce variability (Table 8-2).

Table 8–2. Potential Causes of Diminished Variability

Fetal sleep state
Maternal drugs/medications
Hypoxemia/acidemia
Congenital anomalies (anencephaly)
Fetal (supraventricular) tachycardia
Congenital heart disease/heart block
Extreme prematurity
Preexisting neurologic abnormality

Data from Suidan JS, Young BK: Acidosis in the vigorous newborn. Obstet Gynecol 65:361, 1985. [119]

EFM is a sensitive screening device for fetal periodic hypoxemia. In most cases, the fetus subjected to any degree of hypoxemia shows either periodic decelerations (variable or late) or a prolonged deceleration. In most instances, the stress responsible for the hypoxemia generates FHR decelerations before causing a loss of variability.[41,42] If progressive loss of variability follows repetitive late or variable decelerations, there is an increased risk for fetal acidemia and low Apgar scores.

Baseline Variability—Trends in Labor

On admission, the fetus most often shows normal baseline variability. In the absence of repetitive decelerations or medications known to have a significant cardiovascular impact on the fetus, normal variability persists throughout most of labor with the exception of the quiet sleep state. Less frequently, a fetus may show normal variability on admission, followed by progressive loss of variability. If obvious, relatively common causes known to decrease variability, such as narcotics, maternal fever–induced fetal tachycardia, or fetal sleep state, are not operative, the explanation may be provided by coexistent repetitive late or significant variable decelerations. If diminished or absent variability coexists with repetitive late decelerations or significant variable decelerations, the origin of the change in variability is more likely fetal hypoxemia. Generally, significant fetal hypoxemia is not likely in cases showing loss of variability, unless there are coexisting repetitive periodic decelerations.[43]

In some cases, absence of variability with no associated decelerations may be noted on admission. Particularly problematic is a fetus that initially has a normal FHR and absent (flat) baseline variability, with no significant repetitive decelerations or ultrasound findings to provide insight into the pathogenesis of the absent variability. This unexplainable loss of variability can be observed in association with a subsequent vigorous and healthy neonate. These observations are likely to be the product of an in utero event that preceded the period of observation for an unknown time.[43] Such an initial presentation may be associated with preexisting CNS pathology (anencephaly), a developmental CNS defect, or cardiac anomalies.[43]

In other patients who initially have diminished variability, there may be occasional decelerations, but of a magnitude and frequency that ordinarily would not be thought likely to result in loss of variability. Oligohydramnios may be detected on ultrasound or strongly suspected because little fluid is released at the time of membrane rupture. In these situations, the cause of the FHR alteration may be preexisting UPI with or without a previous sublethal cord accident from oligohydramnios. It may be determined later that the fetus has growth restriction or preexisting CNS injury or developmental abnormality.

The sinusoidal baseline pattern is an uncommon form of variability detected in the fetus and neonate. It has been associated with severe fetal anemia and hypoxemia-acidemia and increased perinatal morbidity and mortality. The precise pathophysiology of the sinusoidal FHR pattern is not known.[44] This pattern originally was described as an accompaniment of fetal anemia from Rh isoimmunization.[45-47] It subsequently has been associated with fetal anemia for other reasons and hypoxemia. It is hypothesized that the pattern is due to an alteration of CNS control of the heart, perhaps secondary to preexisting dysfunction in CNS control of the heart or from central or peripheral ischemia. An inverse relationship between sinusoidal amplitude and fetal pH has been shown.[44-47]

If the FHR is observed for the first time immediately preceding in utero death, it may show only a flat baseline with no associated decelerations.[46] There is little in the way of further diagnostic testing to determine the cause. A flat baseline not associated with recurrent decelerations is seen more commonly with normal pH values, however.

Baseline Rate: Clinical Correlations

Baseline rate is the least predictive of the parameters (rate, decelerations, variability) for fetal outcome. Most fetal bradycardias and tachycardias unaccompanied by persistent significant decelerations are not associated with fetal acidemia. The baseline FHR tends to remain relatively constant in the active phase of labor, unless there is an intervening major stress, such as repetitive decelerations or administration of a drug. The isolated observation of tachycardia or bradycardia in the presence of normal variability is generally predictive of a favorable fetal outcome with regard to scalp capillary or cord blood gases.

Bradycardia (100 to 119 beats/min)

Despite the designation *bradycardia*, FHR in the range of 100 to 119 beats/min, especially when accompanied by FHR accelerations and normal variability, is reassuring.[48-51] The reassuring nature of this observation is confirmed by studies that have shown normal fetal scalp blood pH, continuous fetal tissue pH, or umbilical arterial pH at delivery.[52,53]

Marked Bradycardia (<100 beats/min)

A baseline FHR less than 100 beats/min frequently is termed *marked* (sinus) bradycardia. This is a more appropriate term than *severe* bradycardia because favorable clinical outcomes commonly are observed in the presence of bradycardia less than 100 beats/min. The term *severe* has a negative lay connotation. The outcome generally is similar to the outcome observed in association with

bradycardia in the range of 100 to 119 beats/min. One can anticipate that a bradycardia in the range of 80 to 99 beats/min that is associated with normal variability and accelerations generally would result in a favorable outcome.

Tachycardia

The origin of fetal tachycardia is complex. In some instances, tachycardia represents an increase in sympathetic tone, whereas in others it represents a reduction in parasympathetic tone. In either instance, tachycardia may be associated with loss of baseline variability. Unless associated with repetitive decelerations, the tachycardic fetus is likely to be nonacidemic. Maternal fever, amnionitis, and β-mimetic administration are common causes.

Wandering or Unstable Baseline

A wandering baseline is a variant that fluctuates or undulates in an almost unpredictable manner. The undulation may occur before the onset of contractions and may be associated with decelerations. Although there is a strong link between an unstable or wandering baseline and a subsequent unfavorable outcome, the actual mechanism responsible for the pattern has not been established. It is hypothesized that it may reflect an alteration in CNS regulation of the fetal heart. Its presence may indicate the late stage of a fetal response to a stress of considerable intensity and duration. The baseline rate can be observed within the normal and upper limits of the normal range. Variability, although generally absent, occasionally may appear in the initial phase of the evolution of this pattern. If present, decelerations tend to be mild. In its end phase, a wandering baseline generally is characterized by absence of short-term variability and a slow, roller coaster–like downward progression. In such instances, it may be difficult to establish a baseline rate except in hindsight.

Late Decelerations: Clinical Correlations

Late decelerations classically are thought to be a manifestation of clinical or subclinical UPI, which is a clinical syndrome associated with progressive decrease in intervillous space blood flow. Late decelerations detected for the first time in labor may reflect UPI arising before the onset of labor. In the absence of such decelerations, most labor-related late decelerations are a consequence of identifiable and frequently remediable causes (Table 8-3), such as postural hypotension, a recently administered epidural anesthetic, or perhaps oxytocin-induced uterine tachysystole. Notable clinical problems associated with UPI include preeclampsia, insulin-dependent diabetes mellitus, intrauterine growth restriction, and the classic post-term/postmature fetus.[54-56]

Clinical Subclassification of Late Decelerations

Late decelerations[30,57,58] may be classified into two clinical categories with regard to prognosis: decelerations with associated normal baseline variability (reflex late decelerations) and decelerations with diminished or absent variability (nonreflex late decelerations). Physiologically, late decelerations associated with normal beat-to-beat

Table 8–3. Common Clinical Correlations with Late Decelerations

Acute Decrease in Uteroplacental Blood Flow
Maternal hypotension
Epidural/spinal anesthesia
Supine hypotension

Uterine Hyperactivity/Hypertonus
Spontaneous
Oxytocin/prostaglandins
Abruption

Maternal Medical Problems
Pregnancy-induced hypertension
Chronic hypertension
Diabetes mellitus, especially type 1
Sickle cell disease
Collagen vascular disease

Fetal Risk Factors
Intrauterine growth restriction
Postmaturity syndrome

variability are thought to be a vagally mediated chemoreceptor response to hypoxemia.[59-61] Late decelerations of any type may be associated with relative fetal hypoxemia, but the presence of baseline variability and reflex activity within the late decelerations may indicate recent onset of UPI. This finding often is a useful prognostic indicator that anticipates that late decelerations are not likely to be associated with significant fetal metabolic acidemia. These decelerations are more likely to respond to traditional obstetric therapeutic interventions, such as maternal hydration, positional change to improve uterine blood flow, maternal hyperoxia, and reduction of oxytocin administration. Some fetuses that show late decelerations with normal variability can continue to show accelerations in response to fetal movement. Clinically, this category of late decelerations may represent a compensated state.

Repetitive late decelerations with absent or decreased variability (in the absence of another obvious cause, such as narcotic administration) are more likely to be produced by myocardial depression, as opposed to being chemoreceptor reflex mediated.[62] They are less likely to respond to obstetric therapeutic measures and are associated more commonly with some degree of fetal metabolic acidemia.

Narcotics and other drugs are known to depress baseline variability.[63] If narcotics are administered for labor analgesia, the detection of late decelerations with loss of variability may have less significance relative to cardiovascular compromise or risk for significant fetal acidemia. In these cases, therapeutic measures can be instituted and attempts made to gain reassurance while preparing to intervene if therapy is unsuccessful or further testing is nonreassuring. The obstetrician may institute fetal auditory stimulations to elicit return of variability or accelerations. Alternatively, fetal capillary blood sampling can be performed to gain reassurance regarding the fetal biochemical status.

Late decelerations, particularly decelerations in association with normal variability, may be graded as mild, moderate, or severe according to their magnitude below the baseline. These grades have been correlated with scalp blood pH values, with the presence or absence of variability as codeterminant.[41] Some clinicians have designated all late decelerations as "ominous." This type of simplistic terminology and conclusion is best suited for a lay audience and does not consider the many variables that must be integrated to arrive at a final clinical judgment. Use of such terminology with patients and families is not sensitive, particularly when one correlates the presence of late decelerations with subsequent outcome. In the absence of an acute, nonremediable problem, such as an abruption, recently instituted oxytocin, regional anesthesia, or spontaneous uterine tachysystole, late decelerations are thought to reflect the unmasking of preexisting UPI by uterine contractions. This statement does not mean that therapeutic measures would be unsuccessful.

As an isolated observation, late decelerations that are recurrent and nonremediable are of concern, but even then, only an occasional case can be considered *potentially* ominous. Rather, the evolution of secondary changes, such as loss of variability, tachycardia, or only a relative increase in FHR baseline, which develop in association with the recurrent late decelerations, is of greater clinical significance. Development of these secondary changes may reflect progression to fetal acidemia in response to the hypoxemic stress of repetitive contractions. In the case of placental abruption, the nonremediable nature of the condition, rather than the presence of late decelerations per se, may force the obstetrician to intervene if spontaneous delivery is not imminent.

Clinical Management of Late Decelerations

Clinical management in large part depends on the time and circumstances under which the late decelerations are detected. UPI is generally a chronic clinical state that may become manifest for the first time during CST or later during labor. Subclinical UPI may predate the onset of late decelerations elicited on a CST or OCT by days or weeks. The presence or absence of variability provides some prognostic indication regarding the presence of acidosis and the likelihood of a favorable response to therapeutic intervention. Nonetheless, intrauterine resuscitation in the form of lateral positioning of the mother, intravenous fluid administration, and oxygen inhalation generally is initiated in most cases in an attempt to improve fetal status before delivery.

The presence of repetitive late decelerations on a CST or OCT indicates that intervention is required. If variability is present with the late decelerations, vaginal delivery often can be accomplished after implementation of therapeutic measures. If there is decreased or absent variability, the likelihood of cesarean delivery increases. In many situations, there is no urgency to proceed directly to cesarean section, but intrauterine resuscitative measures need to be instituted in preparation for delivery.

A similar thought process is appropriate if late decelerations are detected during labor. Intrauterine resuscitative measures should be attempted, unless there is evidence of rapid, progressive deterioration. In these litigious times, there is often a knee-jerk response to rush the patient quickly to cesarean section. Intrauterine resuscitative measures can be instituted, however, while preparations are made for cesarean section, should therapeutic efforts be unsuccessful. If the magnitude and frequency of the late decelerations diminish with therapy, the urgency to proceed directly to delivery is diminished. Delivery is required expeditiously for fetal indications only when late decelerations are determined to be persistent and nonremediable.

Variable Decelerations: Clinical Correlations

In contrast to late decelerations, repetitive variable decelerations commonly show dramatic departures below the baseline and often persist for 60 or more seconds.[20] Attempts have been made to categorize the severity of variable decelerations by two methods. In one, the number of beats per minute below the baseline characterizes the decelerations; in the other, they are classified according to the nadir of the deceleration. By either method, the duration of the deceleration, particularly when the nadir of the deceleration is less than 70 beats/ min, is a more critical determinant of fetal metabolic alterations.

The grading of the deceleration is not recommended as the sole determinant of clinical management. Grading the magnitude (depth and duration) of variable decelerations is useful, however, as a communication tool and for clinical correlations with fetal or immediate newborn blood gas status. The most commonly applied system was presented by Kubli and colleagues.[20]

Mild Variable Decelerations

Mild variable decelerations are decelerations of less than 30 seconds in duration regardless of the level, or decelerations to 70 to 80 beats/min regardless of the duration.

Moderate Variable Decelerations

Moderate variable decelerations are decelerations with a nadir of less than 70 beats/min for 30 to 60 seconds or a nadir of 70 to 80 beats/min regardless of duration.[20] Mild and moderate variable decelerations are thought to be the product of some degree of short-term (partial) umbilical cord occlusion. In general, these decelerations are not thought to reflect the degree and duration of cord compression required to produce metabolic acidemia. If repetitive mild or moderate variable decelerations are associated with normal variability, the pattern generates no greater clinical concern than a normal tracing showing normal baseline variability, accelerations, and no decelerations.[64]

Severe Variable Decelerations

Severe variable decelerations are repetitive decelerations with a nadir of less than 70 beats/min for at least 60 seconds.[20] The adjective *severe* may be an inappropriate term because it might suggest to some an extreme fetal problem, as opposed to a simple description of the relative magnitude of a deceleration.

The magnitude of a deceleration is not the only determinant of the impact of periodic cord compression.

Adequate recovery time (intercontraction interval) between repetitive variable decelerations is an important determinant of fetal adaptation to the periodic cord compression reflected by the deceleration. An adequate intercontraction interval allows time for the fetus to increase fetal oxygen saturation and reduce PCO_2 to predeceleration levels. If the intercontraction interval is adequate for fetal compensation, and tolerance of the stress is supported by the absence of progressive loss of FHR variability, the term fetus often can tolerate such a pattern for extended periods. The necessity for therapeutic intervention for recurrent variable decelerations is determined by the clinician's experience, the presence of existing or progressive secondary baseline changes, and the fetal response to therapeutic measures. When significant decelerations persist despite therapeutic measures, the management primarily depends on the observed trends in baseline variability and, to a lesser extent, FHR rate.[65] These trends may depend on the recovery (intercontraction interval) time.

When there is significant partial or total cord occlusion, the primary biochemical process during the deceleration/contraction is a progressive increase in PCO_2 and decrease in PO_2. Metabolic acidemia is not thought to be an issue in most instances until occlusion is nearly complete for 60 or more seconds with repetitive contractions. When variable decelerations are prolonged and severe, the clinician can infer that near-total or total cord occlusion is likely during the deceleration.

After release of the cord, usually at the conclusion of the contraction, the biochemical process is reversed. Ordinarily, if there is sufficient recovery time, there is a rapid return to prior pH values in the intercontraction interval because the primary biochemical effect is a periodic deceleration or contraction-limited accumulation of carbon dioxide (respiratory acidemia). In a term fetus, significant metabolic acidemia does not become a threat until the variable decelerations are severe, prolonged, and persistent (less likely when associated with sufficient recovery time between contractions). If severe variable decelerations persist, it becomes more likely that the late component originally described by Barcroft[32] will be activated. Clinically, it is believed that this late component may be reflected by progressive loss of baseline variability.

Clinical Management of Variable Decelerations

Clinical evaluation of the degree of impact of repetitive variable decelerations is a primary issue in the management of labor because 50% of labors have repetitive variable decelerations of some degree. Because the severity of the deceleration cannot be used as the sole predictor of the degree and type of fetal acidemia, other parameters should be evaluated. If repetitive decelerations are persistent, not responsive to therapeutic efforts, and significant (other than an anticipated physiologic response), the FHR baseline may show many secondary changes. The baseline variability may diminish progressively. Although of lesser significance, there also may be either a relative increase in baseline FHR or a progression to tachycardia in the absence of other known causes.

A fetus previously noted to have normal variability, who shows progressive loss of variability in response to

Table 8–4. Evaluation of Variable Decelerations

Reassurance in Presence of Variable Decelerations

Normal or no progressive loss of baseline variability
Rapid return to baseline
Deceleration duration 30-45 sec
Adequate intercontraction/interdeceleration
  recovery time
Normal baseline rate

Nonreassuring Findings in Presence of Variable Decelerations

Progressive loss/absence of variability
Deceleration duration ≥60 sec to 70-80 beats/min
Prolonged return to baseline, especially if
  <70-80 beats/min
Uterine tachysystole (prolonged)/inadequate
  recovery time
Overshoot (especially in preterm fetus)
Nonresponsive to position change or amnioinfusion

repetitive variable decelerations (independent of drugs, sleep state, or amnionitis), is at increased risk for fetal acidemia and low Apgar scores.[66] If variable decelerations persist and have a significant impact on the fetus, the decelerations often show a progressive smoothing, becoming rounded or blunted. The progression through this sequence may be particularly rapid in an extremely immature fetus. If there is absence of variability with repetitive variable decelerations, 67% and 22% of fetuses have an Apgar score less than 7 at 1 and 5 minutes. Table 8-4 summarizes reassuring and nonreassuring observations used to evaluate the impact of the periodic cord compression that induces the variable decelerations in the fetus.

Overshoot is a descriptive term for a smooth acceleration following a prolonged variable deceleration.[65,67] Some newborns later determined to have cerebral palsy are noted, in hindsight, to have shown variable decelerations with so-called overshoot and absent baseline variability.[61] This pattern is observed more frequently in a preterm fetus.

Terminal or Agonal Pattern

Under normal circumstances, variable decelerations reflect an intact compensatory reflex response. With fetal deterioration, however, the decelerations become progressively rounded and blunted, until a smooth, undulating baseline replaces previously noted angular decelerations.[61]

Prolonged Decelerations

Prolonged decelerations are decelerations from a normal FHR to values usually less than 80 beats/min for more than 60 to 120 seconds; beyond 10 minutes, the pattern would be considered as bradycardia. Prolonged decelerations to less than 70 to 80 beats/min are observed in association with persistent cord compression, placental abruption, maternal cocaine abuse, persistent uterine tachysystole, eclampsia, maternal hypotension, and

maternal regional anesthesia. When regional anesthesia or other agents have a causal role in prolonged decelerations, uterine tachysystole with or without hypertonus is a common accompaniment.

Although an uninformed observer may conclude that immediate delivery is the preferable management option when a prolonged deceleration is detected, this is not necessarily so. If the deceleration returns to baseline, a similar deceleration does not recur immediately, and there is adequate recovery time between contractions, the fetus often can recover in utero (intrauterine resuscitation). With time, the variability and the baseline FHR may return to preexisting normal levels, showing the beneficial impact of intrauterine resuscitation.

Rarely, particularly when associated with absence of beat-to-beat variability and a "wandering" baseline, a prolonged deceleration may be associated with a *moribund fetus*. If the patient initially has this pattern, it frequently is not possible to determine its cause. The cause may have been progressive deterioration of a fetus with persistent repetitive late decelerations (UPI or abruption) or recurrent variable decelerations (cord compression) before application of the monitor.

Balancing the Clinical Needs of the Mother and Fetus

Prospective reliable identification of the fetus with intrapartum acidemia is necessary to determine the most appropriate obstetric intervention and to predict which newborn would benefit from early intensive neonatal support. A balance needs to be maintained to avoid overdiagnosis; this minimizes maternal morbidity from operative intervention that does not provide measurable benefit to the fetus. Objective EFM consensus criteria that are highly predictive for the presence of clinically significant acidosis are not available. Although EFM does have a high sensitivity for adverse outcome, it is at the cost of low positive predictive values. As a result, there is considerable variation in obstetric practice with regard to management of EFM patterns. With the current focus on outcome analysis and cost containment, the clinician is faced with the difficulty of balancing the findings of a test that is highly sensitive but has a low predictive value.

The presence of a nonreassuring finding does not require interruption of pregnancy. Nonreassuring findings are prioritized, balanced against existing reassuring observations, and considered in a framework that considers the gestational age, possible response to therapy, and maternal morbidity should intervention occur. These counterbalancing factors are integrated according to the judgment and experience of the obstetrician. If nonreassuring findings are detected antenatally, the obstetrician may insert gestational age and likelihood of successful induction of labor into the clinical decision tree when comparing the benefits of intervention versus nonintervention. Interruption of pregnancy is considered more strongly when there is a failure to respond to prenatal therapeutic measures and when the nonreassuring findings fulfill problem-specific and gestational age–specific criteria for intervention.

The decision process is easier during labor. If therapeutic measures, such as intrapartum oxygen administration, volume expansion, or position change, do not provide acceptable modification of the nonreassuring FHR findings, *and* the combination of findings reaches a critical threshold, intervention via vacuum extraction, forceps, or cesarean section may be considered. The speed with which intervention occurs is modified by the severity and trend of the FHR observation. Stanley[68] suggested the following: "It is likely that only a few children with spastic CP [cerebral palsy] are injured during the labor and delivery (intrapartum) birthing process. Therefore, efforts to further reduce 'birth asphyxia' may have little impact on CP rates."

Much of the preceding discussion relates to the cost-benefit considerations of prospective management. The same limitations become evident, however, when retrospective analysis of clinical information is required in an attempt to assign a cause to newborn morbidity. There are problems in establishing the cause and timing of the origin of the fetal CNS dysfunction. We have little means to evaluate the integrity of the developing CNS at any time, especially in the prenatal period and only indirectly after the onset of labor. The available technologies are not specific, particularly for higher CNS centers. As a result, even if the clinical course is consistent (as opposed to diagnostic) with metabolic acidemia, a firm objective basis to determine reliably when (prenatal versus intrapartum) the dysfunction arose in the perinatal period is lacking. Ultimately, continuous EFM and cord blood gas values, perhaps complemented by sonographic determination of fetal growth and amniotic fluid volume, may help sort out the contribution of prenatal versus intrapartum hypoxemia.

CLINICAL EFFICACY OF CONTINUOUS ELECTRONIC FETAL MONITORING

EFM was introduced on a relatively widespread basis in the mid-1970s after publication of retrospective reports that indicated a correlation between FHR patterns and other indicators of fetal hypoxia (intrapartum fetal death, Apgar scores, and fetal scalp blood pH).[69] These reports suggested that EFM use resulted in a better outcome than was associated with periodic auscultation. There were fewer intrapartum deaths and better outcomes among high-risk fetuses undergoing EFM. It was even suggested that there was better outcome among electronically monitored high-risk fetuses than among low-risk fetuses who were monitored by auscultation. Based on these early retrospective studies, a seemingly reasonable hypothesis developed. The hypothesis was that fetal hypoxemia could be detected early in its course, allowing the obstetrician an earlier opportunity to provide appropriate intervention, reducing the potential long-term impact of ongoing intrauterine hypoxemia during labor. At that time, little was known regarding the prelabor contribution to overall long-term morbidity.

EFM was applied clinically without proof of its value and without considering its implications and associated risk.[70,71] Now its effectiveness is in question. Although careful surveillance of the FHR by continuous EFM does offer a theoretical opportunity to detect nonreassuring

FHR parameters more reliably and an opportunity to modify labor-related periodic hypoxia, there has been a failure to reduce dramatically significant acidosis-related morbidity.[72]

Randomized Electronic Fetal Monitoring Clinical Trials

Later prospective studies designed to assess the efficacy of EFM have been less optimistic, suggesting not only no benefit to routine application of EFM, but also an associated increase in the indication and use of obstetric interventions, including requirement for scalp blood gas sampling, use of forceps, or cesarean section for fetal indications.[72-76]

Haverkamp and colleagues[73,77,78] reported the first prospective randomized trial of intrapartum EFM. The study involved 695 high-risk obstetric patients at term who were assigned randomly to one of three monitoring groups: (1) auscultation (at 15-minute intervals in the first stage of labor and 5-minute intervals in the second stage) alone; (2) EFM alone; or (3) EFM with the option to scalp sample. This study could not determine a benefit for EFM with regard to outcome measures such as neonatal death, Apgar scores, cord blood gases, intensive care nursery admission, or seizures. More disturbingly, the cesarean delivery rate for all indications, including the cesarean delivery rate for fetal distress, was increased in the EFM group.

In the group's second article, Haverkamp and colleagues[77] were able to show the benefit of supplementation of EFM with scalp blood gases as a means to reduce much of the excess rate of cesarean sections in the EFM group. The reduction in need for cesarean section for fetal indication was justified by the presence of a reassuring scalp blood pH that was collected after the detection of nonreassuring FHR observations. This approach indirectly emphasized the high false-positive rate for acidosis when a nonreassuring FHR is the sole indication for cesarean section.

MacDonald and coworkers[76] conducted a prospective study at the National Maternity Hospital in Dublin and the National Perinatal Epidemiology Unit in Oxford, involving 12,964 women and designed to assess the relative value of continuous EFM versus intermittent auscultation. There was an option to perform scalp blood pH analysis in both groups. Because EFM is a continuous screening device that provides greater opportunity to detect changes in the FHR, more than three times (173 versus 49) as many fetal scalp blood pH determinations were performed for nonreassuring FHR observations in the EFM group than in the intermittent auscultation group. Fetal acidemia, using a threshold of less than 7.20 for scalp blood pH, was detected more often in the EFM group (29) than in the intermittent auscultation group (16). Patients in the EFM group were slightly more likely (2.4% versus 2.1%) to undergo cesarean section. There was an increased overall incidence of forceps delivery (8.2% versus 6.3%) and an increased use of forceps in response to nonreassuring FHR observations (2.9% versus 1.2%) in the EFM group. At birth, the incidence of newborns with an umbilical venous pH threshold less than 7.10 was slightly lower (1% versus 2.1%) in the EFM group. The intrapartum death rate was similar for the two groups.

In a prospective nonrandomized study involving approximately 35,000 pregnancies at Parkland Hospital in Dallas, Leveno and associates[74] reported that nonreassuring FHR patterns were detected more frequently in the time frames when universal EFM was used than in the population managed in the time frames when EFM was selected only if high-risk factors were identified. There was also a higher total cesarean rate (11% versus 10.2%) and a small but significant increase (2.6% versus 2.1%) in the number of cesarean sections performed for fetal distress in the population receiving universal EFM.

When only low-risk patients were evaluated, nonreassuring FHR observations also were detected more often (7.6% versus 2.7%), and the cesarean section rate for fetal distress was higher (0.9% versus 0.4%; $P < .01$) in the universal EFM group. Overall, there were no differences in the relative incidence of stillbirths, low Apgar scores, need for assisted ventilation, need for intensive care admissions, or neonatal seizures between the two groups.

Despite inability to determine benefit in predominantly term labors, there was hope that EFM would prove to be beneficial in monitoring a preterm fetus during labor. In 1987, Luthy and associates[75] reported a study of 246 newborns weighing between 700 and 1750 g. Similar to the previous studies involving term fetuses, this study also failed to show a difference in immediate outcome between the newborns monitored electronically and newborns monitored with auscultation.

Impact of Electronic Fetal Monitoring on Long-Term Outcome

EFM has not decreased perinatal mortality.[15] Although some authors have reported that EFM may reduce the incidence of short-term neurologic morbidity, including neonatal seizures,[76] there is little to support the conclusion that there is a beneficial long-term effect in either term or preterm gestations.[76,78] Lumley,[79] in an epidemiologic analysis of prospective randomized studies comparing the course of labor and delivery and outcome in monitored and unmonitored populations, was unable to show a benefit to EFM using neonatal morbidity and development in the first year of life as outcome measures.

Despite all of the advances that have occurred in prenatal and newborn medicine in the last 25 years since completion of the National Collaborative Perinatal Project (NCPP), there has been little or no change in the frequency of cerebral palsy.[68,80-82] The nature of the clinical practice of obstetrics during the 1990s compared with the 1960s, when the NCPP was conducted, should have reduced the consequences of trauma and acidosis-asphyxia because it is likely that modern obstetrics is attended by less trauma and more appropriate and common intervention in labor. Obstetric practice was dramatically different, particularly with regard to frequency of use of oxytocin, high oxytocin dosages used, and limited ability to assess uterine activity except by medical student or nurse palpation. EFM was not available. Forceps (including mid forceps) were used liberally, some at higher stations than would be used today. At delivery, there were no neonatologists. The failure to modify the rate of cerebral palsy is not surprising in view of the findings of the three largest prospective trials addressing the long-term benefits of EFM in term and preterm labor.

In the third article of the Haverkamp series, Langendoerfer and associates[78] evaluated the offspring of the three groups and found no difference in mortality or morbidity, including low Apgar scores, cord arterial pH less than 7.21, seizures, or need for intensive care admissions. Neurologic assessment of the newborn by 72 hours (Brazelton examination) and again at 9 months (the Bayley mental and motor scale scores and the Milani-Comparetti Development Test) did not support the original assumption that obstetric intervention for nonreassuring FHR patterns might improve either the immediate outcome as measured by Apgar score and cord pH or the eventual neurologic outcome. Most disturbingly, despite no obvious benefit in short-term or intermediate-term outcome, there was an increased requirement for cesarean section for fetal distress in the EFM group (6.9% in the EFM versus 0.4% in the auscultated group).[78]

In MacDonald's study,[76] although neurologic abnormalities (seizures, tone and reflex abnormalities, and abnormal neurologic signs) in survivors persisting beyond 1 week were noted to be more frequent in the intermittent auscultation group, later follow-up at 1 year of age showed no difference in the two groups. Shy and colleagues[83] reported the neurologic outcome at 18 months of the preterm newborns from Luthy's 1987 randomized control trial.[75] No benefit was found in the EFM group.

ADJUNCTS TO EXTERNAL FETAL MONITORING

The FHR abnormalities identified on EFM are often nonspecific. Fetal scalp pH determination remains a valid method of intrapartum evaluation. This method is technically cumbersome, however, and often difficult or impossible to perform in situations in which the cervix is minimally dilated or the fetal station is high. Many large centers have eliminated fetal scalp blood sampling and rely on other adjunct methods for evaluation of fetal well-being without increasing adverse perinatal outcomes.[84] These methods include fetal scalp stimulation, fetal vibroacoustic stimulation, and fetal pulse oximetry.

Fetal Scalp Stimulation

The ability of a fetus to respond to scalp stimulation with an acceleration of the heart rate indicates an intact autonomic nervous system. This response often is blunted in the context of acidemia. The FHR acceleration (elevation above the baseline of 15 beats/min for at least 15 seconds) has long been considered to be a reliable sign of fetal well-being.

In 1982, Clark and coworkers[85] analyzed 200 FHR tracings of fetuses that had undergone scalp blood sampling. They found that all fetuses who responded with accelerations had a pH greater than 7.21. After this observation, these investigators conducted a prospective study in which 100 fetuses with heart rate tracings suggestive of acidosis were subjected to scalp stimulation.[86] Each fetus was stimulated for 15 seconds by gentle digital pressure on the scalp followed by a 15-second application of an Allis clamp to the scalp. Scalp blood pH was obtained; 51 fetuses responded with accelerations and all had a scalp pH greater than 7.19. Among fetuses that had a negative (no acceleration) scalp stimulation test, 30 had a pH greater than 7.19, whereas 19 had a pH less than 7.19. The test offered had high sensitivity and negative predictive value but had low specificity.

Elimian and colleagues[87] conducted a similar study on 108 fetuses with nonreassuring FHR tracings. Digital stimulation was performed for 15 seconds, 1 to 2 minutes before pH sampling; 58 fetuses responded with an acceleration of 10 beats/min for at least 10 seconds. All fetuses had a pH greater than 7.20. This approach resulted in a decrease in the need for scalp sampling by 54%. The test still proved to be nonspecific, however. Response of the fetus to scalp stimulation by acceleration has proved to be an excellent predictor of well-being but a less important predictor of fetal compromise.

Fetal Vibroacoustic Stimulation

Vibroacoustic stimulation first was introduced by Sontag and Wallace in 1936.[88] It was studied later during antepartum fetal testing (NST, CST, and BPP)[89-91] and during the intrapartum period.[92] The technique involves placement of an electronic device (an artificial larynx) on the maternal abdomen. The device generates a vibroacoustic stimulus. A reactive response, usually associated with fetal movement, is defined by a FHR acceleration of 15 beats/min sustained over 15 seconds.

Smith and associates[92] subjected 64 patients with nonreassuring FHR tracings to vibroacoustic stimulation for a duration of 3 seconds, followed by fetal scalp sampling. Thirty fetuses were reactive, and all had a pH greater than 7.25. Of the 34 fetuses that did not respond to vibroacoustic stimulation, approximately half were acidotic. The test was only 50% accurate in identifying the acidotic fetus.

Edersheim and colleagues[93] found no incidence of acidosis in the face of a reactive response to vibroacoustic stimulation. They also found that vibroacoustic stimulation was more likely to elicit an acceleration in nonacidotic fetuses than fetal scalp puncture.

Ingemarsson and Arulkumaran[94] recruited 51 women with suspicious FHR tracings for vibroacoustic stimulation. Two of 29 fetuses with reactive responses to vibroacoustic stimulation were acidotic (pH < 7.20). The two acidotic fetuses had the less worrisome respiratory acidosis. In their series, Irion and colleagues[95] found that seven fetuses with pH less than 7.20 had a normal FHR response to acoustic stimulation. The investigators suggested that the stimulus might have been too strong to differentiate the healthy from the nonhealthy fetus.

Accelerations induced by fetal vibroacoustic stimulation seem to be highly indicative of the absence of acidosis. There is roughly a 50% chance of fetal acidosis, however, in the absence of a response to stimulation. Fetal scalp pH determination might be helpful in the latter situation, when technically feasible.

Fetal Pulse Oximetry

Electronic FHR monitoring lacks specificity for detecting fetal compromise. Ominous signs on FHR monitoring indirectly predict fetal hypoxia and acidosis. Pulse oximetry allows for oxygen saturation monitoring. It has improved medical care markedly in many fields, including anesthesiology, critical care, and newborn intensive care.[96]

Peat and colleagues[97] were the first to report the use of pulse oximetry for intrapartum monitoring of fetuses. Adult oximeters were modified for fetal use, and since then, the oximeter has undergone many modifications. The prototype fetal pulse oximeter (Nellcor N-400; Tyco Healthcare Group LP, Nellcor Puritan-Bennett Division, Pleasanton, Calif) has been approved by the U.S. Food and Drug Administration for use as an adjunct to FHR monitoring in labor situations in which there is a nonreassuring FHR tracing. Requirements for use include a singleton fetus at term (>36 weeks' gestation), ruptured membranes, and cervical dilation of more than 2 cm. It should not be used in cases of suspected or documented placenta previa or in obstetric instances requiring immediate delivery. The sensor is placed transvaginally through the dilated cervix to fit between the uterine wall and the soft tissue of the fetal cheek. Many animal and human studies were designed to determine a "critical" arterial oxygen saturation that correlated with fetal acidosis.[98-100] These studies suggest that a decline of saturation to less than 30% is associated significantly with acidosis.

Goffinet and coworkers[101] conducted a prospective multicenter observational study using the Nellcor N-400 fetal oximeter. They found that oxygen saturation values were obtained in 95% of cases with a mean reliable signal time of 64.7% ± 32%. No serious adverse effects were reported in the study population. The investigators found a significant association between low fetal oxygen saturation (<30%) and poor neonatal condition. Carbonne and associates[102] found that intrapartum fetal pulse oximetry can be compared favorably with that of fetal blood analysis using a fetal oxygen saturation of 30% and arterial cord pH of 7.15 as thresholds for abnormal neonatal outcome.

Garite and colleagues,[103] in a multicenter controlled trial, tested the hypothesis of reduction of cesarean delivery rate due to "fetal distress" by the adjunct use of the fetal pulse oximeter in the face of nonreassuring FHR tracing during labor. These investigators reported a reduction of more than 50% in the group of patients in which fetal pulse oximetry and EFM were used compared with the control group in which only EFM was used (4.5% versus 10.2%; P = .007). They found no net difference, however, in the overall cesarean delivery rates in the two groups (29% versus 26%; P = .49). There was a higher rate of cesarean delivery due to dystocia in the study group. The authors postulated that nonreassuring FHR tracings could be indicators for the risk of dystocia. In the study, the median reliable signal time of the pulse oximeter was 67%. The frequencies of various adverse maternal events were similar in the two groups.

The Committee on Obstetric Practice of the ACOG issued an opinion on the use of fetal pulse oximetry as an adjunct to FHR monitoring in labor.[104] The committee did not endorse the adoption of this technology in clinical practice because of concerns about escalation of medical care costs without necessarily improving clinical outcome. The committee recommended further prospective randomized clinical trials to evaluate the use of this new technology.

Fetal Scalp Blood pH

Fetal scalp pH determination first was introduced by Saling in 1962.[105] It later was studied to improve the predictive value of EFM in the face of nonreassuring tracings. Prerequisites for scalp pH determination include ruptured membranes, an engaged fetal head, and a dilated cervix (usually >2 to 3 cm). An amnioscope is inserted through the dilated cervix and applied firmly to the fetal scalp. The scalp is cleaned carefully, and then a thin layer of silicon gel is applied. The scalp is punctured, and approximately 40 mL of fetal blood is collected in a preheparinized glass capillary tube. The sample is transferred to a blood gas analyzer for prompt measurement.[106] A scalp pH greater than 7.25 is usually reassuring. A pH between 7.20 and 7.25 is considered "preacidotic" and necessitates a repeat determination of scalp pH in 20 to 30 minutes. A pH value less than 7.20 is considered acidotic and usually warrants obstetric intervention.

There are several practical problems with fetal scalp pH determination,[107] including technical difficulty in performing the procedure, time delay in obtaining results, unavailability of technical personnel, and insufficient physician training. Also, acidosis usually is intermittent, which necessitates repetitive sampling. The need for fetal scalp pH sampling has been reduced dramatically by the use of other noninvasive tests, such as fetal scalp stimulation or vibroacoustic stimulation.

The ACOG considers assessment of scalp blood pH, if available, to be occasionally helpful.[16] The ACOG acknowledges, however, that it is used uncommonly in current obstetric management.

In a tertiary care center, Hendrix and colleagues[108] performed a retrospective medical record review of 134 patients who underwent cesarean section for nonreassuring FHR tracings. Among patients who had a cervix dilated to more than 3 cm, only 15% underwent scalp pH determination. In a retrospective study, Goodwin and coworkers[84] found that despite the virtual elimination of fetal scalp pH determination in their large teaching service, there was no increase in the cesarean rate for fetal distress and no apparent increase in "perinatal asphyxia."

Continuous measurement of fetal scalp tissue pH using calibrated electrodes[109] and, more recently, a fiberoptic probe with a pH dye indicator,[110] was meant to replace intermittent scalp pH evaluation. Theoretically, it allows monitoring the trend of tissue pH over time. It is not currently used in clinical practice, however, due to technical problems and difficulties associated with continuous measurements.[111]

Fetal Scalp Blood Lactate Concentration

The fetus normally generates its metabolic needs from glucose and glycogen in the presence of oxygen (aerobic metabolism). When hypoxic, the fetus switches to a less efficient anaerobic metabolism to preserve cardiac and brain function in particular. This less efficient metabolism leads to accumulation of lactate and pyruvate and development of lactic acidosis. From a physiologic point of view, lactate can be considered as a direct marker of anaerobic metabolism.[107]

After fetal scalp sampling by the standard technique (described earlier), lactate concentration currently can be measured by an enzymatic reaction (lactate oxidation) with a single-use electrochemical strip. Only 5 µL of blood is needed, and results can be obtained within 60 seconds.

Smith and associates[112] found that infants who had 1-minute Apgar scores less than or equal to 6 had significantly higher lactate levels and lower pH levels than infants who had Apgar scores greater than 7. Westgren and coworkers[113] prospectively randomized 341 patients with nonreassuring FHR tracings into either fetal scalp pH determination or fetal scalp lactate analysis. The investigators were less successful in obtaining a reliable result in the pH group. The patients in the lactate group had fewer scalp incisions per blood sampling attempt, and the result was obtained sooner in the lactate group (2 minutes) compared with the pH group (<4 minutes). There was no difference in the predictive value for perinatal outcome.

More recently, Kruger and colleagues,[114] in a retrospective study, compared the predictive value of fetal scalp blood lactate concentration and pH as markers of "neurologic disability." A total of 326 patients underwent scalp pH and lactate concentration determination. In cases of ominous FHR tracings, lactate was found to be more specific and sensitive than the pH in relation to 5-minute Apgar scores less than 4 and to the development of moderate-to-severe hypoxic-ischemic encephalopathy. They suggested a lactate concentration of 4.8 mmol/L as a suitable cutoff for the prediction of fetal asphyxia. This concentration corresponded to a pH of 7.21 (10th percentile for lactate concentration and 90th percentile for pH level in their study group). Scalp lactate analysis is an attractive alternative for intrapartum fetal monitoring. Further studies are required, however, for standardization of this test.

Recent Developments

New strategies are being developed and implemented with the hope of improving obstetric outcomes. The availability of continuous information of the fetal response to the stress of labor might be a useful tool in modern obstetrics. Presently, there are two such strategies that can be used in addition to the electronic recording of the fetal heart: pulse oximetry and the ST waveform analysis of the fetal ECG.[115-117] Pulse oximetry was discussed earlier in this chapter. It records the level of hypoxemia (oxygenation) in relation to FHR responses during labor.

The second strategy, which is the ST waveform analysis of the fetal ECG, provides information regarding the response of the fetal heart as it is affected by the stress of labor.[116] The fetal ECG may be obtained during labor using the scalp electrode that is used for continuous monitoring of the FHR. The repolarization of the myocardial cells in preparation for the next cardiac contraction is reflected in the ST segment and T wave. Because there is energy consumption during repolarization, when the amount of oxygen supplied to the myocardial cells is insufficient, a negative energy balance occurs, and the myocardial cells produce energy by anaerobic metabolism. The result is an increase in the height of the T wave. This increase can be quantified as the T/QRS ratio, or the ratio between T and QRS amplitude. This process of anaerobic metabolism produces lactate and potassium ions. The potassium ions affect myocardial cell membrane potential and cause an increase of the ST waveform. The fetal response to hypoxia ultimately can lead to an increase in T-wave amplitude and an increase in the T/QRS ratio. The surge of stress hormones during labor can affect ST waveform changes.[116]

A fetus that is unable to respond (growth-restricted fetus) or has not had time to respond (acute abruption) to a hypoxic stress can show ST depression with negative T waves (myocardial hypoxic stress) ultimately leading to a decrease in myocardial activity and cardiac failure.[116] This is called a *biphasic ST event* and presumably is due to an imbalance between the endocardium and the epicardium of the ventricles and the mechanical performance of the myocardium. The perfusion pressure of the endocardium is always lower, but the mechanical stress is always larger; when the myocardium is activated, any decrease in performance causes a biphasic ST.

Factors such as prematurity, infection, fetal tachycardia, myocardial dystrophy, cardiac malformations, long-term stress, and acute hypoxic phase can cause alterations in the balance and performance of the myocardium, and a biphasic ST pattern may be expected.[116] A fetus displaying biphasic ST events is not in a situation of immediate hypoxia and metabolic acidosis, but the fetus can be affected as labor progresses. A fetus that no longer can compensate reacts with biphasic events, and this finding may be a useful marker for the development of severe fetal decompensation.[116]

Two randomized clinical trials, the Plymouth randomized trial[117] and the Swedish multicenter randomized controlled trial,[115] have studied the EFM and ST waveform analysis with standard monitoring. The Plymouth randomized controlled trial studied 2400 high-risk, term deliveries.[117] The investigators found a 46% reduction in operative deliveries for fetal distress in the arm using the ST waveform analysis. They noted that all neonates with ST changes had a pH less than 7.15 and a normal outcome. Although there were no differences in neonatal outcome measures, there were fewer low 5-minute Apgar scores and less metabolic acidosis in the EFM and ST waveform analysis group. There also was a significant reduction in fetal blood sample tests performed. The Swedish multicenter randomized controlled trial studied 4966 women at term.[115] The trial showed a 61% reduction in the number of neonates with metabolic acidosis (pH < 7.05 and base deficit > 12 nmol/L), and there were 28% fewer operative interventions for fetal distress in the EFM and ST waveform analysis arm compared with the EFM arm.[115,116] When the multiple European centers testing the technology validate the findings of the initial studies and it becomes readily available, obstetricians should be trained properly in the use of this new technology so that it becomes a useful tool in their armamentarium.

REFERENCES

1. Ruth VJ, Raivio KO: Perinatal brain damage: Predictive value of metabolic acidosis and the Apgar score. BMJ 297:294, 1988.
2. Freeman JM, Nelson KB: Intrapartum asphyxia and cerebral palsy. Pediatrics 82:240, 1988.
3. American Academy of Pediatrics and American College of Obstetricians and Gynecologists: Guidelines for Perinatal Care, 5th ed. Washington, DC, AAP/ACOG, 2002.
4. American College of Obstetricians and Gynecologists Committee on Obstetric Practice: Inappropriate Use of the Terms Fetal Distress and Birth Asphyxia (Committee Opinion No. 197). American College of Obstetricians and Gynecologists, Washington, DC, February 1998.
5. Freeman RK: Problems with intrapartum fetal heart rate monitoring interpretation and patient management. Obstet Gynecol 100:813, 2002.
6. MacLennan A: A template for defining a causal relationship between acute intrapartum events and cerebral palsy—an international consensus statement. BMJ 319:1054, 1999.
7. American Academy of Pediatrics and American College of Obstetricians and Gynecologists: Neonatal Encephalopathy and Cerebral Palsy: Defining the Pathogenesis and Pathophysiology. Washington, DC, AAP/ACOG, 2003.
8. Graham M, Levene MI, Trounce JQ, et al: Prediction of cerebral palsy in very low birthweight infants: Prospective ultrasound study. Lancet 2:593, 1987.
9. American College of Obstetricians and Gynecologists Committee on Practice Bulletins: Antepartum Fetal Surveillance (Practice Bulletin No. 9). American College of Obstetricians and Gynecologists, Washington, DC, October 1999.
10. Gunn TR, Mok PM, Becroft DM: Subdural hemorrhage in utero. Pediatrics 76:605, 1985.
11. Jackson JC, Blumhagen JD: Congenital hydrocephalus due to prenatal intracranial hemorrhage. Pediatrics 72:344, 1983.
12. Stoddard RA, Clark SL, Minton SD: In utero ischemic injury: Sonographic diagnosis and medicolegal implications. Am J Obstet Gynecol 159:23, 1988.
13. Landy HJ, Khoury AN, Heyl PS: Antenatal ultrasonographic diagnosis of fetal seizure activity. Am J Obstet Gynecol 161:308, 1989.
14. Manning FA, Platt LO, Sipos L: Antepartum fetal evaluation: Development of a fetal biophysical profile. Am J Obstet Gynecol 136:787, 1980.
15. Chalmers I: Randomized control trials of intrapartum monitoring. In Thalhammer O, Baumgarten KV, Polaka A (eds): Perinatal Medicine. Stuttgart, George Thieme, 1979, pp 260-265.
16. American College of Obstetricians and Gynecologists Committee on Technical Bulletins: Fetal Heart Rate Patterns: Monitoring, Interpretation, and Management (Technical Bulletin No. 207). American College of Obstetricians and Gynecologists, Washington, DC, July 1995.
17. Patrick J, Campbell K, Carmichael L, et al: Patterns of gross fetal body movements over 24-hour observation intervals during the last 10 weeks of pregnancy. Am J Obstet Gynecol 142:363, 1982.
18. Patrick J, Campbell K, Carmichael L, et al: Influence of maternal heart rate and gross fetal body movements on the daily pattern of fetal heart rate near term. Am J Obstet Gynecol 144:533, 1982.
19. Paul WM, Quilligan EJ, MacLachlan T: Cardiovascular phenomenon associated with fetal head compression. Am J Obstet Gynecol 90:824, 1964.

20. Kubli FH, Hon EH, Khazin AF, et al: Observations on heart rate and pH in the human fetus during labor. Am J Obstet Gynecol 104:1190, 1969.

21. Caldeyro-Barcia R, Casacuberta C, Bustos R, et al: Correlation of intrapartum change in fetal heart rate with fetal blood oxygen and acid-base state. In Adamsons K (ed): Diagnosis and Treatment of Fetal Disorders. New York, Springer-Verlag, 1968, pp 205-225.

22. Freeman RK, Garite TJ, Nageotte MP: Fetal Heart Rate Monitoring. Baltimore, Williams & Wilkins, 1991.

23. Hon EH: Observations on "pathologic" fetal bradycardia. Am J Obstet Gynecol 77:1084, 1959.

24. Adamsons K, Myers RE: Late decelerations and brain tolerance of the fetal monkey to intrapartum asphyxia. Am J Obstet Gynecol 128:893, 1977.

25. Aarnoudse JG, Huisjes HJ, Gordon H, et al: Fetal subcutaneous scalp Po$_2$ and abnormal heart rate during labor. Am J Obstet Gynecol 153:565, 1985.

26. Caldeyro-Barcia R, Pose SV, Poseiro JJ, et al: Effects of several factors on fetal Po$_2$ recorded continuously in the fetal monkey. In Fluck L (ed): Intrauterine Asphyxia and the Developing Fetal Brain. Chicago, Year Book Medical Publishers, 1977, pp 237-248.

27. Huch A, Huch R, Schneider H, et al: Continuous transcutaneous monitoring of fetal oxygen tension during labour. Br J Obstet Gynaecol 84:4, 1971.

28. James LS, Morishima HO, Daniel SS, et al: Mechanism of late deceleration of the fetal heart rate. Am J Obstet Gynecol 113:578, 1972.

29. Mendez-Bauer C, Arnt IC, Gulin L, et al: Relationship between blood pH and heart rate in the human fetus during labor. Am J Obstet Gynecol 97:530, 1967.

30. Martin CB Jr, de Haan J, van der Wildt B, et al: Mechanisms of late deceleration in the fetal heart rate: A study with autonomic blocking agents in fetal lambs. Eur J Obstet Gynaecol Reprod Biol 9:361, 1979.

31. Myers RE, Mueller-Huebach E, Adamsons K: Predictability of the state of fetal oxygenation from a quantitative analysis of the components of late decelerations. Am J Obstet Gynecol 115:1083, 1973.

32. Barcroft J: Researches on Perinatal Life. Oxford, Blackwell Scientific, 1946, p 124.

33. Gimovsky ML, Caritis SN: Diagnosis and management of hypoxic fetal heart rate patterns. Clin Perinatol 9:313, 1982.

34. Itskovitz J, LaGamma EF, Rudolph AM: Heart rate and blood pressure responses to umbilical cord compression in fetal lambs with special reference to the mechanism of variable deceleration. Am J Obstet Gynecol 147:451, 1983.

35. Kunzel W, Mann LI, Bhakthavathsalan A, et al: Metabolic fetal brain function and cardiovascular observations following total cord occlusion. In Longo L, Reneau D (eds): Fetal and Newborn Cardiovascular Physiology. New York, Garland, 1978, p 301.

36. Krebs HB, Petres RE, Dunn LJ, et al: Intrapartum fetal heart rate monitoring: VI. Prognostic significance of accelerations. Am J Obstet Gynecol 142:297, 1982.

37. Lee CY, DiLoreto PC, Logrand B: Fetal activity acceleration determination for the evaluation of fetal reserve. Obstet Gynecol 48:19, 1976.

38. Braly P, Freeman RK: The significance of fetal heart rate reactivity with a positive oxytocin challenge test. Obstet Gynecol 50:689, 1977.

39. Krebs HB, Petres RE, Dunn LJ: II. Multifactorial analysis of intrapartum fetal heart tracings. Am J Obstet Gynecol 133:773, 1979.

40. O'Gureck JE, Roux JF, Neuman MR: Neonatal depression and fetal heart rate patterns during labor. Obstet Gynecol 40:347, 1972.

41. Paul RH, Suidan AK, Yeh SY, et al: Clinical fetal monitoring: VII. The evaluation and significance of intrapartum baseline FHR variability. Am J Obstet Gynecol 123:206, 1975.

42. Bowes WA, Gabbe SG, Bowes C: Fetal heart rate monitoring in premature infants weighing 1500 grams or less. Am J Obstet Gynecol 137:791, 1980.

43. Garite JT, Linzey EM, Freeman RK, et al: Fetal heart rate patterns and fetal distress in fetuses with congenital anomalies. Obstet Gynecol 53:716, 1979.

44. Young BK, Katz M, Wilson SJ: Sinusoidal fetal heart rate: I. Clinical significance. Am J Obstet Gynecol 136:587, 1980.

45. Baskett TM, Koh KS: Sinusoidal fetal heart pattern: A sign of fetal hypoxia. Obstet Gynecol 44:379, 1974.

46. Cetrulo CL, Schifrin BS: Fetal heart rate patterns preceding death in utero. Obstet Gynecol 48:521, 1976.

47. Richter R, Hohl M, Hammacher K, et al: Significance of oscillation frequency in intrapartum fetal monitoring. Obstet Gynecol 50:694, 1977.

48. Garite JT, Freeman RK: Bradycardias with normal variability usually benign. Contemp Obstet Gynecol 19:29, 1982.

49. Gaziano EP, Freeman DW, Bendel RP: FHR variability and other heart rate observations during second stage labor. Obstet Gynecol 56:42, 1980.

50. Gilstrap LC III, Hauth JC, Toussaint S: Second stage fetal heart rate abnormalities and neonatal acidosis. Obstet Gynecol 62:209, 1984.

51. Low JA, Cox MJ, Karchmar EJ, et al: The prediction of intrapartum fetal metabolic acidosis by fetal heart rate monitoring. Am J Obstet Gynecol 139:299, 1981.

52. Young BK, Katz M, Klein SA, et al: Fetal blood and tissue pH with moderate bradycardia. Am J Obstet Gynecol 135:45, 1979.

53. Young BK, Katz M, Klein SA: The relationship of heart rate patterns and tissue pH in the human fetus. Am J Obstet Gynecol 134:685, 1979.

54. Bekedam DJ, Visser GHA: Effects of hypoxemic events on breathing, body movements, and heart rate variation: A study in growth-retarded human fetuses. Am J Obstet Gynecol 155:52, 1985.

55. Cibils LA: Clinical significance of fetal heart rate patterns during labor: II. Late decelerations. Am J Obstet Gynecol 123:473, 1975.

56. Low JA, Pancham SR, Worthington D: Fetal heart deceleration patterns in relation to asphyxia and weight-gestational age percentile of the fetus. Obstet Gynecol 47:14, 1976.

57. Harris JL, Krueger TR, Parer JT: Mechanisms of late decelerations of the fetal heart rate during hypoxia. Am J Obstet Gynecol 144:491, 1982.

58. Ingemarsson E, Ingemarsson I, Westgren M: Combined decelerations—clinical significance and relation to uterine activity. Obstet Gynecol 58:35, 1981.

59. Hutson JM, Mueller-Heubach E: Diagnosis and management of intrapartum reflex fetal heart rate changes. Clin Perinatol 9:325, 1982.

60. Murata Y, Martin CB Jr, Ikenoue T, et al: Fetal heart rate accelerations and late decelerations during the course of intrauterine death in chronically catheterized rhesus monkeys. Am J Obstet Gynecol 144:218, 1982.

61. Parer JT: Handbook of Fetal Heart Rate Monitoring, 2nd ed. Philadelphia, WB Saunders, 1997.

62. Itskovitz J, Goetzman BW, Rudolph AM: The mechanism of late deceleration of the heart rate and its relationship to oxygenation in normoxemic and chronically hypoxemic fetal lambs. Am J Obstet Gynecol 142:66, 1982.

63. Morishima HO, Daniel SS, Richards RT, et al: The effect of increased maternal PaO$_2$ upon the fetus during labor. Am J Obstet Gynecol 123:257, 1975.

64. Gaziano EP: A study of variable decelerations in association with other heart rate patterns during monitored labor. Am J Obstet Gynecol 135:360, 1979.

65. Goodlin RC: Inappropriate fetal bradycardia. Obstet Gynecol 40:117, 1976.

66. Krebs HB, Petres RE, Dunn LJ: Intrapartum fetal heart rate monitoring: VIII. Atypical variable decelerations. Am J Obstet Gynecol 145:297, 1983.

67. Goodlin RC, Lowe EW: A functional umbilical cord occlusion heart rate pattern: The significance of overshoot. Obstet Gynecol 42:22, 1974.

68. Stanley FJ: The changing face of cerebral palsy? Dev Med Child Neurol 29:263, 1987.

69. Paul RH, Hon EH: Clinical fetal monitoring: V. Effect on perinatal outcome. Am J Obstet Gynecol 118:529, 1974.

70. Banta HD, Thacker SB: Costs and Benefits of Electronic Fetal Monitoring: A Review of the Literature (PHS Publication No. 79-3245). Washington, DC, Department of Health, Education, and Welfare, April 1979.

71. Banta HD, Thacker SB: Assessing the costs and benefits of electronic fetal monitoring. Obstet Gynecol Surv 34:627, 1979.

72. Shiono PH, Fielden JG, McNellis D, et al: Recent trends of cesarean birth and trial of labor rates in the United States. JAMA 257:494, 1987.

73. Haverkamp AD, Thompson HE, McFee JG, et al: The evaluation of continuous fetal heart rate monitoring in high-risk pregnancy. Am J Obstet Gynecol 125:310, 1976.

74. Leveno KJ, Cunningham FG, Nelson S, et al: A prospective comparison of selective and universal electronic fetal monitoring in 34,995 pregnancies. N Engl J Med 315:615, 1986.

75. Luthy DA, Shy KK, van Belle G, et al: A randomized trial of electronic fetal monitoring in preterm labor. Obstet Gynecol 69:687, 1987.

76. MacDonald D, Grant A, Sheridan-Pereira M, et al: The Dublin randomized controlled trial of intrapartum fetal heart rate monitoring. Am J Obstet Gynecol 152:524, 1985.

77. Haverkamp AD, Orleans M, Langendoerfer S, et al: A controlled trial of the differential effects of intrapartum fetal monitoring. Am J Obstet Gynecol 134:399, 1979.

78. Langendoerfer S, Haverkamp AD, Murphy J, et al: Pediatric follow-up of a randomized controlled trial of intrapartum fetal monitoring techniques. Pediatrics 97:103, 1980.

79. Lumley J: Does continuous intrapartum fetal monitoring predict long-term neurological disorders? Paediatr Perinat Epidemiol 2:299, 1988.

80. Blair E, Stanley FJ: Intrapartum asphyxia: A rare cause of cerebral palsy. J Pediatr 112:515, 1988.

81. Hagberg B, Hagberg G, Olow I: The changing panorama of cerebral palsy in Sweden: IV. Epidemiologic trends 1959-1978. Acta Paediatr Scand 73:433, 1984.

82. Paneth N, Kiely J: The frequency of cerebral palsy: A review of population studies in industrial nations since 1950. In Stanley F, Alberman E (eds): The Epidemiology of the Cerebral Palsies. Philadelphia, JB Lippincott, 1984, pp 46-56.

83. Shy KK, Luthy DA, Bennett FC, et al: Effects of electronic fetal-heart-rate monitoring, as compared with periodic auscultation, on the neurologic development of premature infants. N Engl J Med 322:588, 1990.

84. Goodwin TM, Milner-Masterson L, Paul RH: Elimination of fetal scalp blood sampling on a large clinical service. Obstet Gynecol 83:971, 1994.

85. Clark SL, Gimovsky ML, Miller FC: Fetal heart rate response to scalp blood sampling. Am J Obstet Gynecol 144:706, 1982.

86. Clark SL, Gimovsky ML, Miller FC: The scalp stimulation test: A clinical alternative to fetal scalp blood sampling. Am J Obstet Gynecol 148:274, 1984.

87. Elimian A, Figueroa R, Tejani N: Intrapartum assessment of fetal well being: A comparison of scalp stimulation with scalp blood pH sampling. Obstet Gynecol 89:373, 1997.

88. Sontag LW, Wallace RE: Changes in the rate of human fetal heart rate response to vibratory stimuli. Am J Dis Child 51:383, 1936.

89. Inglis SR, Druzin ML, Wagner WE: The use of vibro-acoustic stimulation during the abnormal or equivocal biophysical profile. Obstet Gynecol 82:371, 1993.

90. Read JA, Miller FC: Fetal heart rate acceleration in response to acoustic stimulation as a measure of fetal well-being. Am J Obstet Gynecol 129:512, 1977.

91. Smith CV, Phelan JP, Broussard PM, et al: Fetal acoustic stimulation testing: III. Predictive value of a reactive test. J Reprod Med 33:217, 1988.

92. Smith CV, Nguyen HN, Phelan JP, et al: Intrapartum assessment of fetal well being: A comparison of fetal acoustic stimulation with acid-base determinations. Am J Obstet Gynecol 155:726, 1986.

93. Edersheim TG, Hutson JM, Druzin ML, et al: Fetal heart rate response to vibratory acoustic stimulation predicts fetal pH in labor. Am J Obstet Gynecol 157:1557, 1987.

94. Ingemarsson I, Arulkumaran S: Reactive fetal heart rate response to vibroacoustic stimulation in fetuses with low scalp blood pH. Br J Obstet Gynaecol 96:562, 1989.

95. Irion O, Stuckelberger P, Moutquin JM, et al: Is intra-partum vibratory acoustic stimulation a valid alternative to fetal scalp pH determination? Br J Obstet Gynaecol 103:642, 1996.

96. Dildy GA, Clark SL, Loucks CA: Intrapartum fetal pulse oximetry: Past, present and future. Am J Obstet Gynecol 175:1, 1996.

97. Peat S, Booker M, Lanigan C, et al: Continuous intrapartum measurement of fetal oxygen saturation. Lancet 2:213, 1988.

98. Dildy GA, Thorp GA, Yeast JD, et al: The relationship between oxygen saturation and pH in umbilical blood: Implications for intrapartum fetal oxygen saturation monitoring. Am J Obstet Gynecol 175:682, 1996.

99. Kuhnert M, Seelbach-Gobel B, Butterwegge M: Predictive agreement between the fetal arterial oxygen saturation and fetal scalp pH: Results of the German multicenter study. Am J Obstet Gynecol 178:330, 1998.

100. Nijland R, Jongsma HW, Nijhuis JG, et al: Arterial oxygen saturation in relation to metabolic acidosis in fetal lambs. I. Methodological evaluation. Am J Obstet Gynecol 172:810, 1995.

101. Goffinet F, Langer B, Carbonne B, et al: Multicenter study on the clinical value of fetal pulse oximetry. Am J Obstet Gynecol 177:1238, 1997.

102. Carbonne B, Langer B, Goffinet F, et al: Multicenter study on the clinical value of fetal pulse oximetry. II. Compared predictive values of pulse oximetry and fetal blood analysis. Am J Obstet Gynecol 177:593, 1997.

103. Garite TJ, Dildy GA, McNamara H, et al: A multicenter controlled trial of fetal pulse oximetry in the intrapartum management of nonreassuring fetal heart rate patterns. Am J Obstet Gynecol 183:1049, 2000.

104. American College of Obstetricians and Gynecologists Committee on Obstetric Practice: Fetal Pulse Oximetry (Committee Opinion No. 258). American College of Obstetricians and Gynecologists, Washington, DC, September 2001.

105. Saling E: A new method for examination of the child during labor: Introduction, technique, and principles. Arch Gynecol 197:108, 1962.

106. Greene KR: Scalp blood gas analysis. Obstet Gynecol Clin North Am 26:641, 1999.

107. Clark SL, Paul RH: Intrapartum fetal surveillance: The role of fetal scalp blood sampling. Am J Obstet Gyncol 153:717, 1985.

108. Hendrix NW, Chauhan SP, Scardo JA, et al: Managing nonreassuring fetal heart rate patterns before cesarean delivery: Compliance with ACOG recommendations. J Reprod Med 45:995, 2000.

109. Wood C, Anderson I, Reddy S, et al: Continuous measurement of tissue pH in the human fetal scalp. Br J Obstet Gynaecol 85:668, 1978.

110. Chatterjee MS, Hochberg HM: Continuous intrapartum measurement of tissue pH of the human fetus using newly developed techniques. J Perinat Med 19:92, 1991.

111. McNamara HM, Dildy GA 3rd: Continuous intrapartum pH, pO2, pCO2, and SpO2 monitoring. Obstet Gynecol Clin North Am 26:671, 1999.

112. Smith NC, Soutter WP, Sharp F, et al: Fetal scalp blood lactate as an indicator of intrapartum hypoxia. Br J Obstet Gynaecol 90:821, 1983.

113. Westgren M, Kruger K, Ek S, et al: Lactate compared with pH analysis at fetal scalp blood sampling: A prospective randomized study. Br J Obstet Gynaecol 105:29, 1998.

114. Kruger K, Hallberg B, Blennow M, et al: Predictive value of fetal scalp blood lactate concentration and pH as markers of neurologic disability. Am J Obstet Gynecol 181:1072, 1999.

115. Amer-Wahlin I, Hellsten C, Noren H, et al: Cardiotocography only versus cardiotocography plus ST analysis of fetal electrocardiogram for intrapartum fetal monitoring: A Swedish randomised controlled trial. Lancet 358:534, 2001.

116. Rosen KG: Intrapartum fetal monitoring and the fetal ECG—time for a change. Arch Perinat Med 7:7, 2001.

117. Westgate J, Harris M, Curnow JS, et al: Plymouth randomised trial of cardiotocogram only versus ST waveform plus cardiotocogram for intrapartum monitoring: 2,400 cases. Am J Obstet Gynecol 169:1151, 1993.

118. Cruikshank DP: An unusual fetal heart rate pattern. Am J Obstet Gynecol 130:101, 1978.

119. Suidan JS, Young BK: Acidosis in the vigorous newborn. Obstet Gynecol 65:361, 1985.

CHAPTER 9

The Fetal Biophysical Profile

Andrew Elimian

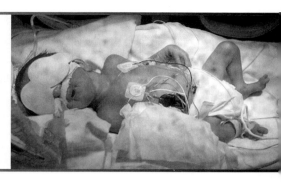

The fetal biophysical profile (BPP) is a technique of fetal risk surveillance based on the combined appraisal of acute and chronic markers of fetal well-being. It is more or less comparable to the Apgar scores used to assess well-being in newborns. It was introduced by Manning and colleagues[1] in 1980 with prevention of fetal death and improvement in perinatal outcome as primary goals. Use of the BPP also has reduced unnecessary intervention in complicated and less complicated pregnancies. In contrast to tests using a single biophysical parameter, such as the nonstress test (NST) and the contraction stress test (CST), the fetal BPP has much lower false-positive and false-negative rates. Although various modifications of the fetal BPP have been attempted, the original technique still is most widely used. This chapter focuses on the physiologic basis, methodology, and clinical applications of the fetal BPP. In addition, the correlation between the biophysical variables and fetal acid-base status, perinatal morbidity and mortality, and long-term neurologic compromise is reviewed. Finally, the use of the BPP in selected clinical circumstances is described.

FETAL ADAPTATION TO ASPHYXIA

Animal and human studies have shown a profound impact on central nervous system (CNS)–regulated fetal biophysical activities, including limbs and breathing movements, in the presence of asphyxia.[2-4] Hypoxemia-induced CNS cellular dysfunction is postulated to be responsible for these changes in biophysical activities. The presumption is that normal biophysical activity implies a functional CNS or, at least, a nonhypoxemic CNS. The chemoreceptors in the fetal aortic and carotid bodies also respond to hypoxemia and partake in the fetal adaptation to asphyxia. Fetal adaptation to asphyxia can be divided into an acute and a chronic response phase mediated by the CNS and the aortic chemoreceptors (Fig. 9-1).

Acute Response

The fetal CNS responds acutely to asphyxia by inhibiting movement-associated fetal heart acceleration, breathing movements, gross body movements, postural tone, and flexor tone. This protective adaptation usually occurs within minutes of an asphyxial insult and yields about a 20% reduction in oxygen[5] requirement and a 30% increase in fetal venous P_{O_2} when fully operational.[6] The dynamic biophysical activities measured during the BPP are controlled by neural activities from different sites in the fetal brain. These sites become functional at different stages of development.[7] The more primitive sites that appear earlier in fetal life require less oxygen for activity and require profound or prolonged hypoxia to become abnormal. The later developing sites require higher levels of oxygen for proper functioning and become abnormal earlier in the progression of hypoxia. Fetal movement and tone, the two earliest fetal biophysical activities, are controlled by cortical centers and appear at 8 and 9 weeks of gestation.[7] These are the last to disappear. Regular fetal breathing is observed after 21 weeks of gestation and is controlled by centers on the ventral surface of the fourth ventricle.[7] Fetal heart reactivity is controlled by the posterior hypothalamus and medulla and functions at the end of the second or beginning of the third trimester. Fetal heart rate (FHR) and fetal breathing are the first parameters to be affected by hypoxia. This serial response allows not only for detection of asphyxia, but also for assessment of its severity and estimation of the risk of demise.

The thresholds of hypoxemia for the acute CNS centers are not fixed. Given sufficient time, they are capable of being reset to lower P_{O_2} values. The mechanism of this resetting is not completely understood. It could be secondary to increased extraction of oxygen from maternal blood, increase in the fetal hemoglobin concentration, and a favorable shift in the oxyhemoglobin dissociation curve. The fetus that already has adapted to chronic

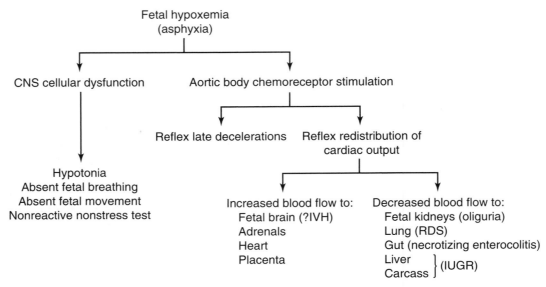

Figure 9–1. Schematic illustration of the fetal biophysical effects of hypoxemia on the fetus. The conditions in parentheses refer to neonatal seque-lae of fetal asphyxia. CNS, central nervous system; IUGR, intrauterine growth restriction; IVH, intraventricular hemorrhage; RDS, respiratory distress syndrome. *(From Manning FA: Fetal assessment by evaluation of biophysical variables—fetal biophysical profile score. In Creasy RK, Resnick R [eds]: Maternal-Fetal Medicine: Principles and Practice, 4th ed. Philadelphia, WB Saunders, 1999, p 320.)*

hypoxemia has variable and significant reduction in reserve and may not be able to compensate for an additional insult. This phenomenon of adaptation in the presence of a reduced or absent reserve might be responsible for the increased sensitivity of the fetal BPP as more abnormal variables are added. Some cases of fetal death have followed a normal test, and an increased risk of perinatal mortality and morbidity can occur when there are oligohydramnios and normal dynamic variables.

Chronic Response

Chronic response is a reflex phenomenon mediated by chemoreceptors in the fetal aortic arch and carotid bodies. In the fetal lamb, hypoxemia results in a significant redistribution of cardiac output. The altered cardiac output leads to an increase in blood flow to the vital organs of the brain, heart, adrenals, and placenta and decreased blood flow to the other organs, including the lungs and kidneys.[8,9] This redistribution ultimately results in decreased amniotic fluid production and oligohydramnios. The concept of asphyxia-induced reflex redistribution may explain the findings of growth restriction and respiratory distress syndrome in a mature neonate, the severity of pulmonary disease in a preterm neonate, and necrotizing enterocolitis and neonatal renal failure. In addition, some adult conditions, such as hypertension, might have their origin in this adaptive reflex according to Barker and colleagues.[10]

The chronic response to asphyxia differs from the acute response in that oligohydramnios and growth restriction develop over days and weeks, rather than minutes. The response is usually progressive and not reversible, and the magnitude usually reflects the severity of the insult. Because of these differences in response

time and manifestations, the combination of acute dynamic variables in association with a marker of chronic status forms the basis of the fetal BPP and affords a much better overall assessment of fetal status and prognosis.

METHODOLOGY

The fetal BPP scoring is based on the evaluation of five discrete biophysical measurements: the NST, fetal breathing movements (FBM), gross body movements, fetal tone, and amniotic fluid volume (Table 9-1). The FHR response to movement is measured by the NST, whereas the other four variables are assessed simultaneously by real-time ultrasonography. The fetal BPP is performed by identifying the largest vertical pocket of amniotic fluid and observing three discrete variables on sonography over 30 minutes. It is best to scan the fetus in a longitudinal plane that shows the face, limbs, and thorax while observing for fetal body movement, breathing movement, and tone. A minimum of 30 minutes of observation is required before absence of a specific variable can be considered abnormal. The five measures are coded as normal, with a score of 2 points, or abnormal, with a score of 0, as seen in Table 9-1.

CRITERIA FOR SCORING

Nonstress Test

A normal score of 2 is assigned when there are two or more episodes of FHR acceleration of at least 15 beats/min for at least 15 seconds associated with fetal movement in 30 minutes. A score of 0 is assigned when there are fewer than two episodes of acceleration of FHR or acceleration of less than 15 beats/min in 30 minutes.

Table 9–1. Biophysical Profile Scoring: Technique and Interpretation

Biophysical Variable	Normal Score (Score = 2)	Abnormal Score (Score = 0)
FBM	At least one episode of FBM of at least 30 sec duration in 30 min observation	Absent FBM or no episode of >30 sec in 30 min
Gross body movement	At least three discrete body/limb movements in 30 min (episodes of active continuous movement considered as single movement)	Two or fewer episodes of body/limb movements in 30 min
Fetal tone	At least one episode of active extension with return of flexion of fetal limb(s) or trunk Opening and closing of hand considered normal tone	Either slow extension with return to partial flexion or movement of limb in full extension Absent fetal movement
FHR	At least two episodes of FHR acceleration of > 15 beats/min and of at least 15 sec duration associated with fetal movement in 30 min	Less than two episodes of acceleration of FHR or acceleration of <15 beats/min in 30 min
Quantitative amniotic fluid volume	At least one pocket of amniotic fluid that measures at least 2 cm in two perpendicular planes	Either no amniotic fluid pockets or a pocket <2 cm in two perpendicular planes

FBM, fetal breathing movements; FHR, fetal heart rate.

From Manning FA: Dynamic ultrasound-based fetal assessment: The fetal biophysical profile score. Clin Obstet Gynecol 38:35,1995. Used with permission of Lippincott-Raven, Philadelphia.

Fetal Breathing Movements

FBM are observable inward movements of the fetal thorax accompanied by descent of the diaphragm, followed by a return to the original position. To avoid mistaking external chest movements for breathing, it is important to observe the thoracic and the abdominal components of fetal breathing. A normal score of 2 is assigned for at least one or more episodes of FBM lasting at least 30 seconds during the 30-minute observation. Episodes of fetal "hiccups" and sighs are counted as evidence of normal FBM. Absence of FBM or an episode of FBM lasting less than 30 seconds is given a score of 0.

Fetal Gross Body Movements

Fetal gross body movements are a single activity or a cluster of activities that involve the limbs or body or both. Isolated movements of hands and arms are considered normal. Episodes of continuous movements involving different parts of the body are considered as single movements. The finding of at least three discrete body and limb movements in 30 minutes, taking care to consider episodes of continuous movement as a single movement, receives a normal score of 2. Two or fewer episodes of gross body movements in the same period are assigned a score of 0.

Fetal Tone

At least one episode of active extension, with return of flexion of fetal limbs or trunk, receives a normal score of 2. Opening and closing of the fetal hand with finger and thumb extension with return to closed fist position usually is considered normal tone. Fetal tone still is considered normal if the hand remains in a closed fist position during the entire 30-minute observation period even in the absence of hand movement. Slow extension with return to partial flexion or movement of the limbs in

full extension or absence of fetal movement is considered abnormal and given a score of 0.

Amniotic Fluid Volume

A normal score of 2 is given when the amniotic fluid measures at least 2 cm in two perpendicular planes, whereas absence of amniotic fluid pockets or a pocket of less than 2 cm in two perpendicular planes is considered abnormal and scored as 0.

INITIATION OF TESTING

The time to initiate testing in pregnancy requires balancing several considerations, including the chances for neonatal survival, severity of maternal disease, risk of fetal death, and potential for complications resulting from false-positive results. Large clinical studies and theoretical models have suggested that initiation of testing at 32 to 34 weeks of gestation is appropriate for most high-risk circumstances.[11-13] In pregnancies with multiple or significantly increased risks for demise, however, it is not unusual to start testing at 26 to 28 weeks of gestation. Testing should not be initiated until active intervention for fetal compromise is possible. Active intervention usually is carried out at a gestational age when extrauterine survival is possible. As the threshold for viability declines, it is plausible that the timing for initiating testing also will decline. The fetal BPP is capable of predicting fetal acidemia in fetuses less than 24 weeks of gestation. As perinatal survival improves further, BPP in the extremely immature fetus may become more common. Each center probably should determine its threshold for viability, but it currently seems to be between 23 and 24 weeks of gestation.

Testing is not indicated in a mature fetus with a good prospect for successful induction or for whom vaginal delivery is contraindicated. These factors negate the primary goal of fetal BPP testing, which is to prevent perinatal death and serious morbidity, because these risks are small in mature fetuses. The fetal BPP might be used, however, to decrease the maternal morbidity associated with failed induction and cesarean section in a patient with an unfavorable cervix.

FREQUENCY OF TESTING

BBP testing once weekly[14] usually is enough for most clinical scenarios except for pregnancies more than 294 days or pregnancies in insulin-dependent diabetics. The clinical circumstance should dictate the frequency of testing rather than a fixed protocol. Increasing the frequency of testing to twice weekly or more usually is appropriate for rapidly developing maternal or fetal conditions, such as chronic abruption, preeclampsia, severe growth restriction, oligohydramnios, and absent or reversed end-diastolic velocities in the umbilical artery. In extremely unstable situations, such as severe alloimmune anemia, it is common to perform testing twice daily until stability is ensured. A decrease in the frequency of testing is appropriate in the setting of stabilizing fetal growth restriction (in which the fetus was tested more frequently at the initiation of testing) and in the case of a woman with perceived decreased fetal movement after several normal tests. Any significant deterioration in the status of the mother or acute decrease in fetal movement requires fetal reevaluation regardless of the time interval from the last test.

ACCURACY OF TESTING

A normal fetal BPP usually is highly reassuring, with a low stillbirth rate of 0.8 per 1000 within 1 week of a normal test result for the traditional BPP[15] and the modified BPP.[13] The negative predictive value for the traditional BPP and the modified BPP is 99.9%. The low false-negative rate depends on the appropriate and timely response to any change in maternal and fetal status and must include retesting or delivery as indicated. The BPP and other forms of antenatal testing cannot predict stillbirths resulting from acute change in maternal or fetal status, such as an acute placental abruption or umbilical cord accidents.

INDICATIONS FOR FETAL BIOPHYSICAL PROFILE

The BPP generally is indicated in pregnancies in which there is an increased risk of fetal demise; maternal conditions and pregnancy-related conditions are included among the indications. Examples of maternal conditions in which the BPP is indicated include antiphospholipid syndrome, hyperthyroidism, hemoglobinopathies (hemoglobin SS, SC, or S-thalassemia), cyanotic heart disease, systemic lupus erythematosus, chronic renal disease, type 1 diabetes mellitus, and hypertensive disorders. Examples of pregnancy-related conditions that require a BPP include pregnancy-induced hypertension, polyhydramnios, oligohydramnios, decreased fetal movement,

intrauterine growth restriction, post-term gestation, isoimmunization, previous unexplained fetal demise, and multiple gestation, especially when there is discrepancy in growth.

CLINICAL MANAGEMENT

An abnormal test result should be considered in the context of the overall clinical picture, keeping in mind the possibility of a false-positive result. Certain maternal conditions, such as diabetic ketoacidosis and pneumonia, can result in an abnormal test, which generally improves as the maternal condition improves. In these circumstances, the fetus could be retested after maternal stabilization. Table 9-2 summarizes the interpretation, risk of perinatal mortality within 1 week in the absence of intervention, and clinical management based on the BPP score. Generally, scores of 10/10, 8/10 with normal fluid, and 8/8 without NST are reliable evidence of a noncompromised fetus that is unlikely to die within 7 days of the test. One usually can defer or avoid intervention for fetal indications. Delivery need not be deferred, however, despite a normal score in certain clinical circumstances, such as postdate with favorable cervix, unstable placenta previa, and worsening preeclampsia. A score of 8/10 with decreased amniotic fluid usually implies a need for delivery if the gestation is 37 weeks or more. At less than 37 weeks, the pregnancy could be followed by more frequent testing (twice or more weekly) until 37 weeks or whenever the BPP becomes abnormal. A score of 6/10 at term and post-term should have a cervical evaluation soon followed by delivery. When the patient is at less than 37 weeks of gestation, the BPP should be repeated the same day or early the next morning. The appropriate management for a fetal BPP of 4/10 or lower is delivery, provided that the pregnancy is of an age at which neonatal survival is possible.

MODIFICATION OF FETAL BIOPHYSICAL PROFILE

Biophysical Profile without Nonstress Test

Five variables constitute the fetal BPP according to the original description, with a maximal normal score of 10/10. This full test requires ultrasound evaluation of breathing, movement, tone, and amniotic fluid volume and recording the FHR trace with an external Doppler monitor. This two-phase testing is time-consuming, costly, and inconvenient. The accuracy of the four ultrasound parameters has been reported to be equivalent to that of the five parameters of the BPP.[16] In addition, the probability of finding a nonreactive NST after a score of 8/8 with the ultrasound parameters is exceedingly small. When one of the four ultrasound parameters is abnormal, however, the chance of an abnormal NST increases significantly and warrants an NST if the test accuracy is to be maintained. Using the protocol that does not include the NST automatically does not compromise the accuracy of the BPP, and generally the test takes less time (usually an average of 8 minutes) and effort.

Table 9–2. Interpretation of Fetal Biophysical Profile Score Results and Recommended Clinical Management

Test Score Result	Interpretation	PNM within 1 Week without Intervention	Management
10 of 10 8 of 10 (normal fluid) 8 of 8 (nonstress test not done)	Risk of fetal asphyxia extremely rare	1/1000	Intervention only for obstetric and maternal factors No indication for intervention for fetal disease
8 of 10 (abnormal fluid)	Probable chronic fetal compromise	89/1000	Determine that there are functioning renal tissue and intact membranes If so, deliver for fetal indications
6 of 10 (normal fluid)	Equivocal test, possible fetal asphyxia	Variable	If the fetus is mature, deliver If the fetus is immature, repeat test within 24 hr If <6/10, deliver
6 of 10 (abnormal fluid)	Probable fetal asphyxia	89/1000	Deliver for fetal indications
4 of 10	High probability of fetal asphyxia	91/1000	Deliver for fetal indications
2 of 10	Fetal asphyxia almost certain	125/1000	Deliver for fetal indications
0 of 10	Fetal asphyxia certain	600/1000	Deliver for fetal indications

PNM, perinatal mortality.

From Manning FA: Dynamic ultrasound-based fetal assessment: The fetal biophysical profile score. Clin Obstet Gynecol 38:37, 1995. Used with permission of Lippincott-Raven, Philadelphia.

Replacement of Largest Vertical Pocket Method with Amniotic Fluid Index

Currently a vertical pocket of 2 cm in two perpendicular planes or more is assigned a score of 2, whereas the absence of a vertical pocket of less than 2 cm is assigned a 0. Studies comparing the use of maximal vertical pocket and the amniotic fluid index (AFI) have yielded similar accuracy in estimating absolute volume and predicting adverse outcome.[17] It seems reasonable to assume that the AFI could be substituted for maximal vertical pocket without any effect on the accuracy of the BPP, although this has not been tested formally in a large obstetric population.

Nonstress Test and Amniotic Fluid Index

A modified BPP consisting of the NST and the AFI has been described and seems to be as accurate as a negative CST.[18] The NST is an immediate indicator of fetal acid-base status, whereas the AFI reflects long-term placental function. The modified BPP is considered normal if the NST is reactive and the AFI is more than 5 and abnormal if either the NST is nonreactive or the AFI is 5 or less. Because the CST is time-consuming and requires stimulation, the modified BPP remains appealing in place of the CST. Its advantage over the traditional BPP is controversial, however. Because the AFI requires the use of ultrasound, it seems logical to collect all four measurements and obviate the need for a formal NST. The data support clinical management based on a BPP score of 8 without the NST. There is no evidence, however, that the selected parameters of the modified BPP are more powerful than the omitted variables. The role of this modification in place of the traditional BPP, or the BPP without the NST, remains to be established. Proponents of this modified BPP point to the added advantage of being able to perceive decelerations during the NST portion of the test, a finding that may be missed when one does the BPP without the NST component.

Placental Grading with Biophysical Profile

Vintzileos and colleagues[19] added placental grading to the lists of variables and expanded the binary score of 0 or 2 to a range of scores of 0, 1, and 2 by taking into account intermediate results (Table 9-3). The possible combinations of variables are considerably higher than those of the traditional BPP. The advantages of this modification over the traditional BPP have not been established. The relationship between placental calcifications and immediate and long-term fetal well-being has not been shown clearly. In general, this modification has not gained general acceptance in clinical practice.

Total Activity Score

Extending the period of ultrasound examination of the fetus to 60 minutes and determining the proportion of this time expended by the fetus for gross body movement and FBM has been shown to be less sensitive in determining acidosis and requires more testing time.[20] Consequently, this modification is the least known and least used.

BIOPHYSICAL PROFILE AND UMBILICAL ACID-BASE VALUES

The technique of cordocentesis has allowed assessment of the fetal umbilical vein pH and its relationship to the BPP. Studies have shown a significant direct correlation between the fetal BPP and umbilical vein pH (Fig. 9-2). Figure 9-3 depicts the probability of fetal acidosis (defined

Table 9–3. Criteria for Scoring Biophysical Parameters*

Nonstress Test
Score 2 (NST 2): ≥ 5 fetal heart rate accelerations of at least 15 beats/min in amplitude and at
  least 15 sec duration associated with fetal movements in a 20-min period
Soce 1 (NST 1): 2-4 accelerations of at least 15 beats/min in amplitude and at least 15 sec duration
  associated with fetal movements in a 20-min period
Score 0 (NST 0): ≤ 1 accelerations in a 20-min period

Fetal Movements
Score 2 (FM 2): At least 3 gross (trunk and limbs) episodes of fetal movements within 30 min.
  Simultaneous limb and trunk movements count as a single movement
Score 1 (FM 1): 1-2 fetal movements within 30 min
Score 0 (FM 0): Absence of fetal movements within 30 min

Fetal Breathing Movements
Score 2 (FBM 2): At least 1 episode of fetal breathing of at least 60 sec duration within a 30-min
  observation period
Score 1 (FBM 1): At least 1 episode of fetal breathing lasting 30-60 sec within 30 min
Score 0 (FBM 0): Absence of fetal breathing or breathing lasting < 30 sec within 30 min

Fetal Tone
Score 2 (FT 2): At least 1 episode of extension of extremities with return to position of flexion
  and 1 episode of extension of spine wiht return to position of flexion
Score 1 (FT 1): At least 1 episode of extension of extremities with return to position of flexion, or
  1 episode of extension of spine with return to flexion
Score 0 (FT 0): Extremities in extension. Fetal movements not followed by return to flexion.
  Open hand

Amniotic Fluid Volume
Score 2 (AF 2): Fluid evident throughout the uterine cavity. A pocket that measures ≥2 cm in
  vertical diameter
Score 1 (AF 1): A pocket that measures < 2 cm but > 1 cm in vertical diameter
Score 0 (AF 0): Crowding of fetal small parts. Largest pocket < 1 cm in vertical diameter

Placental Grading
Score 2 (PL 2): Placental grading 0, 1, or 2
Score 1 (PL 1): Placental posterior difficult to evaluate
Score 0 (PL 0): Placental grading 3

AF, amniotic fluid; FBM, fetal breathing movements; FM, fetal movements; FT, fetal tone; NST, nonstress test; PL, placental grading.

*Maximal score 12; minimal score 0.

From Vintzileos AM, Campbell WA, Ingardia CJ, et al: The fetal biophysical profile and its predictive value. Obstet Gynecol 62:271, 1983.
Reprinted with permission from the American College of Obstetricians and Gynecologists.

as umbilical venous pH ≤ 7.20) as a function of BPP score. The risk of significant metabolic acidemia was approximately 10% for a BPP of 4/10, 20% for a BPP of 2/10, and 100% for a BPP of 0/10. Figure 9-4 shows the relationship between umbilical artery pH at delivery and absence of biophysical activities. The pH was lower when there was absent fetal movement or tone than when FHR reactivity or breathing was absent.

BIOPHYSICAL PROFILE AND PERINATAL MORBIDITY

Various perinatal outcomes either alone or in combination constitute perinatal morbidity. Manning[21] found an inverse linear relationship between the last BPP and fetal distress in labor, 5-minute Apgar score less than 7, operative delivery for fetal distress, birth weight less than the third percentile, and admission to neonatal intensive care

unit, either singly or as a composite morbidity (Fig. 9-5). This relationship probably reflects the role of asphyxia-induced adaptation as a cause or manifestation of most of these morbidities. There was no relationship between the last BPP and the presence or absence of meconium and major congenital anomaly.

BIOPHYSICAL PROFILE AND PERINATAL MORTALITY

The initial prospective blinded study by Manning and coworkers[1] showed a clear relationship between the last score and perinatal mortality. This study showed a range of perinatal mortality from 0% (when all variables were normal) to 60% (when all parameters were abnormal) with intermediate scores yielding intermediate perinatal mortality rates. Since then, many investigators have assessed the clinical usefulness of the BPP in the prevention of

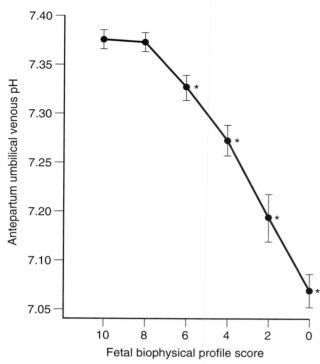

Figure 9–2. Mean umbilical vein pH ($\pm$2 SD) values in fetal blood obtained by cordocentesis, observed for each possible fetal biophysical profile (BPP) score. The mean pH did not vary between scores of 10/10 and 8/10 and was always normal. A progressive and highly significant direct linear relationship was observed between abnormal BPP scores (BPP $\leq$ 6/10) and umbilical vein pH ($R^2 = 0.912$; $P < .01$). *Asterisks* denote a significantly lower mean pH compared with the value recorded for the immediately higher BPP score (student *t*-test; $P < .01$). *(From Manning FA, Snijders R, Harman CR, et al: Fetal biophysical profile scoring: VI. Correlation with antepartum umbilical venous fetal pH. Am J Obstet Gynecol 169:755, 1993.)*

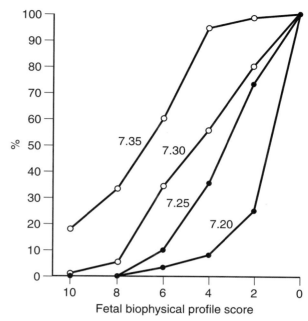

Figure 9–3. Probability (percentage of total observations per category) of antepartum fetal umbilical venous pH declining below an arbitrary value for each biophysical profile score category. The shape of the distribution line varies by select pH cutoff value and conforms to an inverse exponential relationship at a pH of 7.25 and less. *(From Manning FA, Snijders R, Harman CR, et al: Fetal biophysical profile scoring: VI. Correlation with antepartum umbilical venous fetal pH. Am J Obstet Gynecol 169:755, 1993.)*

perinatal death (Table 9-4). Although there has been variation in the reported accuracy, large studies have shown a corrected perinatal mortality of 1.86 to 416 per 1000. Also the corrected perinatal mortality has been shown to be reduced significantly for a tested population compared with an untested population. The more abnormal the BPP scores, the higher the risk of perinatal death. The risk of fetal death with a normal score has been reported to be about 1 in 1000.

BIOPHYSICAL PROFILE AND CEREBRAL PALSY

Perinatal asphyxia in the antepartum, intrapartum, or neonatal period is an acknowledged cause of cerebral palsy. Because the BPP can predict fetal asphyxia, it is plausible that a direct correlation might exist between the last BPP score and the risk of cerebral palsy. A report on a tested population of high-risk fetuses revealed a significant exponential relationship, with a cerebral palsy rate of 0.4 per 1000 when the last BPP score was normal and a rate of 355 per 1000 with a score of 0/10 (Fig. 9-6).[22]

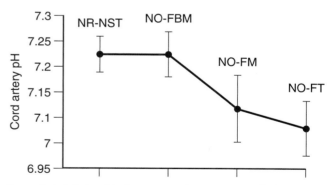

Figure 9–4. Relationship between cord artery pH and absent fetal biophysical activities. The pH tends to be lower in the absence of movements, tone, or both compared with nonreactive nonstress testing, absence of breathing, or both. Results are expressed in means $\pm$ 95% error bars. NO-FBM, absent fetal breathing; NO-FM, absent fetal movements; NO-FT, absent fetal tone; NR-NST, nonreactive nonstress test. *(From Vintzileos AM, Fleming AD, Scorza WE, et al: Relationship between fetal biophysical activities and umbilical cord blood gas values. Am J Obstet Gynecol 165:707, 1991.)*

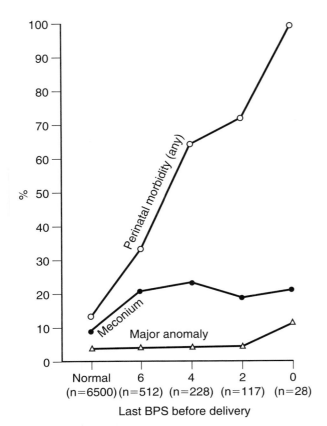

Figure 9–5. Relationship between perinatal mortality, either total or corrected for major anomaly, and the last biophysical profile scoring (BPS) result. This relationship is exponential, yielding a highly significant inverse correlation. *(From Manning FA, Harman CR, Morrison I, et al: Fetal assessment based on fetal biophysical profile scoring: VI. An analysis of perinatal morbidity and mortality. Am J Obstet Gynecol 162:703, 1990.)*

It seems the rate of cerebral palsy in a tested population is significantly less than in a predominately low-risk, untested population, probably due to earlier intervention in deteriorating cases.[22] In essence, the fetal BPP might be a measure available to health care providers to prevent cerebral palsy.

BIOPHYSICAL PROFILE IN SPECIFIC CONDITIONS

Different disease entities have varied presentation, rate of progression, and severity and have different effects on the fetal BPP. Sudden onset and rapid progression may be expected to cause abnormality in some or all of the acute variables, but not in the normal amniotic fluid, whereas indolent diseases may affect the amniotic fluid volume with more or less normal acute variables. Consequently, the BPP may be adaptable to specific disease entities or conditions in terms of initiation, frequency, and interpretation of the testing.

Postdate Fetus

The post-term infant is at increased risk of dysmaturity leading to increased morbidity and mortality.[23,24] As a result, some form of antenatal surveillance is indicated when a pregnancy passes 294 days. One technique is the performance of the BPP twice weekly. Management of the postdate fetus in the presence of a favorable cervix usually involves medical or surgical induction of labor. Cesarean section is done when vaginal delivery is contraindicated by obstetric, maternal, or fetal conditions. It generally is acceptable to undertake cervical ripening followed by induction in a postdate pregnancy with unfavorable cervix. Although it is not known whether antenatal testing of pregnant women between 40 and 42 weeks improves perinatal outcomes, most obstetricians initiate twice-weekly BPP at 41 weeks of gestation.

Diabetes in Pregnancy

Uncontrolled diabetes in pregnancy is associated with increased perinatal mortality and morbidity.[25] In this circumstance, frequent testing is recommended. For well-controlled pregestation diabetes or insulin-requiring gestational diabetes, once- or twice-weekly testing is usually sufficient, starting at about 32 to 34 weeks of gestation. Diabetes associated with other medical conditions, such as hypertension, may warrant early initiation of testing at 28 weeks of gestation. In well-controlled gestational diabetes, the BPP need not be initiated until term.[26] Some obstetricians advocate initial testing at about 36 weeks of gestation in this group, however.

Growth-Restricted Fetus

Perinatal morbidity and mortality are increased significantly in the presence of intrauterine growth restriction.[27] Fetal testing with the BPP plays a significant role in the management of a growth-restricted fetus and may help to select the critical point at which the risk of intrauterine existence outweighs the risk of delivery and neonatal life. The presumed cause of the growth restriction also may determine the need for and the frequency of testing. Doppler velocimetry usually is added because it has been shown to reduce intervention and improve fetal outcome in pregnancies with intrauterine growth restriction.[28] Testing is not useful and not indicated if a major anomaly or chromosomal abnormality is not compatible with extrauterine life. Severity also may affect the frequency of testing. No form of antenatal testing predicts neonatal course in the presence of growth restriction. Antenatal testing seems to help determine the optimal time for delivery.

Multiple Gestation

Multifetal gestation is associated with increased perinatal morbidity and mortality.[29] The role of the BPP in a symmetrically grown twin pregnancy is not well established. The obstetric complications of multiple gestations usually call for some form of testing, however. In triplet or higher order multiple gestations, the BPP is preferable because of difficulty with other forms of testing and their reliability. In the presence of growth restriction in one of the twins at or greater than 34 weeks of gestation, twice-weekly testing

Table 9–4. Relationship of Biophysical Score to Perinatal Death

| Author | No. Patients | No. Tests | Gross Perinatal Mortality (per 1000) | | Corrected Perinatal Mortality (per 1000) | | False-Negative Rate (per 1000) | | False-Positive Rate (%) |
			No.	Rate	No.	Rate	No.	Rate	
Manning	12,620	26,257	93	7.4	24	1.9	8	0.6	—
Baskett	4184	9624	35	8.6	13	3.1*	4	1.0	71.8
Platt	286	1112	4	14.0	2	7.0	2	7.0	71.4
Shime	274	274		0.0		0.0	0		100.0
Schiffrin	240	240	7	44.3	2	12.7	1	6.3	41.6
Vintzileos	342	342	5	33.3	4	26.4		0	60.0
Golde	459	459	2	18.7		0		0	75.0
Manning	19,221	42,286	143	7.95	28	1.95	13	0.676	—
Total	23,780	54,337	206	8	59	2.27	19	0.77	42.6-100

*Lethal anomalies excluded.

From Manning FA: Fetal Medicine: Principles and Practice. Norwalk, Conn, Appleton & Lange, 1995, p 297.

is indicated until delivery for abnormal testing or oligohydramnios at or greater than 37 weeks of gestation. Between 28 and 34 weeks of gestation, frequent testing is indicated because one does not want to compromise the non–growth-restricted twin. At less than 28 weeks of gestation, hopeful expectation with more frequent testing is indicated. In twin-twin gestation, every other day or daily testing may be indicated depending on severity until deterioration of one or both twins. In monoamniotic twins, the safety of the BPP is not established, and delivery usually is undertaken at or greater than 34 weeks of gestation or when lung maturity is shown. A normal BPP in a triplet pregnancy could predict a normal fetus, but an equivocal or abnormal test has limited value in the prediction of fetal compromise. The need for routine use and

benefit of any form of antenatal testing in an uncomplicated multifetal gestation has not been shown. The BPP is known, however, to be as reliable in multifetal gestation as in singleton pregnancies.[30]

Preterm Premature Rupture of Membranes

The BPP is used in the presence of premature rupture of membranes to detect compromise and to predict intra-amniotic infection. Several studies have found that a BPP of 6 or less within 24 hours of delivery correlates with positive amniotic fluid cultures and perinatal infection.[31] Deterioration of score or persistent absence of breathing may be an indication for delivery. Frequency of testing is controversial, with daily testing advocated by some and testing every 48 hours advocated by others. No specific

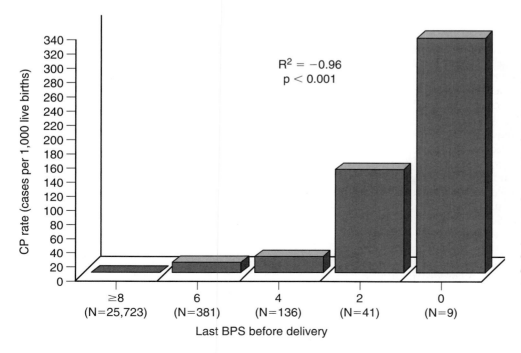

$R^2 = -0.96$
$p < 0.001$

CP rate (cases per 1,000 live births)

Last BPS before delivery

≥8 (N=25,723)   6 (N=381)   4 (N=136)   2 (N=41)   0 (N=9)

Figure 9–6. Relationship between the last biophysical profile score (BPS) and cerebral palsy (CP) at age 5 years. In these 26,288 referred high-risk fetuses subjected to serial biophysical profile testing, an inverse exponential and highly significant relationship between biophysical profile and CP was observed. *(From Manning FA, Bondaji N, Harman CR, et al: Fetal assessment by fetal biophysical profile score: VI. The incidence of cerebral palsy among tested and non-tested perinates. Am J Obstet Gynecol 178:696, 1998.)*

form or frequency of fetal testing has been shown to improve perinatal outcome, however.

Previous Stillbirth

The rate of recurrence and the relationship to the gestational age of the prior stillborn is not known. It has become common practice to initiate weekly testing 2 to 3 weeks before the gestational age of the prior stillborn.[32] More frequent testing may be indicated in extremely anxious patients. Induction usually is undertaken in the presence of minimal deviation or at term (i.e., ≥37 weeks of gestation).

Decreased Fetal Movement

Decreased fetal movement is a common complaint of pregnancy that often needs assessment with the BPP. Decreased fetal movement, with abnormality of one or more of the other parameters of the BPP, is usually an indication for delivery. Immediate delivery is indicated when decreased fetal movement is associated with absence of other parameters of the BPP.

Anomalous Fetus

In the anomalous fetus, absence of the acute variables is difficult to interpret. A change of pattern from normal to abnormal is probably more useful.[32] In these circumstances, one would treat the situation as one would a nonanomalous fetus.

Hypertensive Disease

Chronic hypertension in pregnancy is associated with adverse outcomes, including growth restriction, fetal demise, placental abruption,[33] and a twofold to fourfold increased risk of perinatal mortality.[34,35] Nevertheless, no consensus exists regarding the most appropriate antenatal testing modality or the timing and interval of such testing. The role of BPP in otherwise chronic hypertension in pregnancy is controversial. Frequent testing is indicated in the presence of growth restriction and in superimposed preeclampsia.[36] The frequency depends on the severity of the circumstances and ranges from twice-weekly to daily testing, starting at a gestational age at which extrauterine life is likely (≥26 weeks).

Abnormal Doppler

The perinatal mortality is high in the circumstance of absence or reversed end-diastolic flow often seen in cases of growth restriction. The presence of absent or reversed end-diastolic volume does not mandate delivery, however, unless at term.[37] Between 34 and 37 weeks of gestation, frequent testing with BPP and Doppler is indicated until an abnormal result, mature amniocentesis, or 37 weeks of gestation. At less than 34 weeks of gestation, frequent testing is indicated until deterioration in status.

Systemic Lupus Erythematosus

Pregnant women with autoimmune disorders, including systemic lupus erythematosus, are at increased risk for fetal death,[38] particularly if they have hypertension, renal disease, or antiphospholipid antibodies. Antenatal testing usually is instituted early in pregnancy. Once-a-week

BPP testing usually is begun at 26 to 28 weeks of gestation. Deterioration in clinical status may warrant more frequent testing (every other day or in some circumstances daily). Antenatal testing may be initiated as early as when extrauterine life is possible (23 weeks in women with prior midtrimester fetal death or high titers of antiphospholipid antibodies). Testing in this group of patients with the BPP may be supplemented with umbilical Doppler velocimetry, although the usefulness of this practice has not been established.

REFERENCES

1. Manning FA, Platt LD, Sipos L: Antepartum fetal evaluation: Development of a fetal biophysical profile. Am J Obstet Gynecol 136:787, 1980.
2. Natale R, Clewlow F, Dawes GS: Measurement of fetal forelimb movement in the lamb in utero. Am J Obstet Gynecol 140:545, 1981.
3. Boddy K, Dawes GS, Fisher R, et al: Fetal respiratory movements, electrocortical and cardiovascular responses to hypoxemia and hypercapnia in sheep. J Physiol 243:599, 1974.
4. Martin CB, Murata Y, Petrie RH, et al: Respiratory movements in fetal rhesus monkeys. Am J Obstet Gynecol 119:939, 1974.
5. Rurak DW, Gruber NC: Effect of neuromuscular blockade on oxygen consumption and blood gases. Am J Obstet Gynecol 145:258, 1983.
6. Harman CR, Menticoglou S, Manning FA, et al: Fetal oxygen uptake: A test of placental reserve [abstract]. Proc Soc Obstet Gynecol, Ottawa, 1993.
7. Vintzileos AM, Knuppel RA: Multiple parameter biophysical testing in the prediction of fetal acid-base status. Clin Perinatol 21:823, 1994.
8. Dawes GS, Duncan SLB, Lewis BV, et al: Cyanide stimulation of the systemic arterial chemoreceptors in fetal fetal lambs. J Physiol 201:17, 1969.
9. Cohn HE, Sacks ET, Heyman MA, et al: Cardiovascular responses to hypoxemia and acidemia in fetal lambs. Am J Obstet Gynecol 120:817, 1974.
10. Barker DJP, Osmond C, Golding J, et al: Growth in utero, blood pressure in childhood and adult life and mortality for cardiovascular diseases. BMJ 298:564, 1989.
11. Lagrew DC, Pircon RA, Towers CV, et al: Antepartum fetal surveillance in patients with diabetes: When to start? Am J Obstet Gynecol 168:1820, 1993.
12. Pircon RA, Lagrew DC, Towers CV, et al: Antepartum testing in the hypertensive patient: When to begin. Am J Obstet Gynecol 164:1563, 1991.
13. Rouse DJ, Owen J, Goldenberg RL, Cliver SP: Determinants of the optimal time in gestation to initiate antenatal fetal testing: A decision-analytic approach. Am J Obstet Gynecol 173:1357, 1995.
14. Miller DA, Rabello YA, Paul RH: The modified biophysical profile: Antepartum testing in the 1990s. Am J Obstet Gynecol 174:812, 1996.
15. Manning FA, Morrison I, Harman CR, et al: Fetal assessment based on fetal biophysical profile scoring: Experience in 19,221 referred high-risk pregnancies: II. An analysis of false-negative fetal deaths. Am J Obstet Gynecol 157:880, 1987.
16. Manning FA, Morrison I, Lange IR, et al: Fetal biophysical profile scoring: Selective use of the nonstress test. Am J Obstet Gynecol 156:709, 1987.

17. Moore TR: Superiority of the four-quadrant sum over the deepest-pocket technique in ultrasonographic identification of abnormal amniotic fluid volume. Am J Obstet Gynecol 163:762, 1990.
18. Nageotte MP, Towers CV, Asrat T, et al: The value of a negative antepartum test: Contraction stress test and modified biophysical profile. Obstet Gynecol 84:231, 1994.
19. Vintzileos AM, Campbell WA, Ingardia CJ, et al: The fetal biophysical profile and its predictive value. Obstet Gynecol 62:271, 1983.
20. Ribbert LS, Nicolaides KH, Visser GH: Prediction of fetal acidemia in intrauterine growth retardation: Comparison of quantified fetal activity with the fetal biophysical profile score. Br J Obstet Gynaecol 100:653, 1993.
21. Manning FA: Fetal assessment based on fetal biophysical profile scoring: IV. Positive predictive accuracy of the abnormal test. Am J Obstet Gynecol 162:703, 1990.
22. Manning FA, Bondaji N, Harman CR, et al: Fetal assessment by fetal biophysical profile: VI. The incidence of cerebral palsy among tested and untested perinates. Am J Obstet Gynecol 178:696, 1998.
23. Beischer NA, Brown JB, Smith MA, et al: Studies in prolonged pregnancies: I. The incidence of prolonged pregnancies. Am J Obstet Gynecol 162:698, 1969.
24. American College of Obstetricians and Gynecologists: Ultrasonography in pregnancy (ACOG Technical Bulletin 187). Washington, DC, ACOG, 1993.
25. Moore TR: Diabetes in pregnancy. In Creasy RK, Resnik R: Maternal-Fetal Medicine: Principles and Practice, 4th ed. Philadelphia, WB Saunders, 1999, pp 964-995.
26. American College of Obstetricians and Gynecologists: Gestational Diabetes (ACOG Practice Bulletin 30). Washington, DC, ACOG, 2001.
27. McIntire DD, Bloom SL, Casey BM, Leveno KJ: Birth weight in relation to morbidity and mortality among newborn infants. N Engl J Med 340:1234, 1999.
28. Alfirevic Z, Neilson JP: Doppler ultrasonography in high-risk pregnancies: Systematic review with meta-analysis. Am J Obstet Gynecol 172:1379, 1995.
29. American College of Obstetricians and Gynecologists: Special Problems of Multiple Gestation (ACOG Educational Bulletin 253). Washington, DC, ACOG, 1998.
30. Newman RB, Ellings JM: Antepartum management of the multiple gestation: The case for specialized care. Semin Perinatol 19:387, 1995.
31. Hanley ML, Vintzileos AM: Biophysical testing in premature rupture of the membranes. Semin Perinatol 20:418, 1996.
32. Manning FA: Fetal Medicine: Principles and Practice. Norwalk, Conn, Appleton & Lange, 1995, p 297.
33. Ferrer RL, Sibai BM, Mulrow CD, et al: Management of mild chronic hypertension during pregnancy: A review. Obstet Gynecol 96:849, 2000.
34. Rey E, Couturier A: The prognosis of pregnancy in women with chronic hypertension. Am J Obstet Gynecol 171:410, 1994.
35. Jain L: Effect of pregnancy-induced and chronic hypertension on pregnancy outcome. J Perinatol 17:425, 1997.
36. Report of the National High Blood Pressure Education Program Working Group on High Blood Pressure in Pregnancy. Am J Obstet Gynecol 183:S1, 2000.
37. American College of Obstetricians and Gynecologists. Utility of antepartum umbilical artery Doppler velocimetry in intrauterine growth restriction (ACOG Committee Opinion 188). Washington, DC, ACOG, 1997.
38. Lima F, Buchanan NM, Khamashta MA, et al: Obstetric outcome in systemic lupus erythematosus. Semin Arthritis Rheum 25:184, 1995.

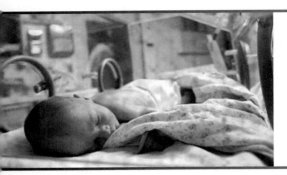

CHAPTER 10

Amniotic Fluid Markers of Fetal Lung Maturity

Cara A. Geary and Jeffrey A. Whitsett

Advances in physiology were translated into improved clinical care in the 1960s and 1970s, enabling the survival of preterm infants with severe respiratory distress syndrome (RDS) for the first time in history. Avery and Meade demonstrated that the lack of pulmonary surfactant was associated with RDS in preterm infants.[1] Thereafter, elucidation of the chemical composition and function of pulmonary surfactant provided a number of useful markers to estimate the risk of RDS after preterm birth. Synthesis of many components of the surfactant system increase with advancing gestational age. Surfactant is secreted by respiratory epithelial cells lining the fetal lung into lung liquid that flows into the amniotic fluid (AF). On the basis of this physiology, various biochemical and biophysical assays were developed to assess fetal lung maturity (FLM) with regard to the presence, quantity, and function of surfactant components in AF, whether obtained by amniocentesis, after rupture of fetal-maternal membranes, or after delivery. Before the development of exogenous surfactant replacement therapy, pulmonary maturity tests were widely used because of the great risk of morbidity and mortality associated with RDS. The effectiveness of surfactant replacement therapy enhanced the survival of preterm infants of increasingly lower gestational ages. Perinatal survival and morbidity are now more strongly influenced by the lack of maturation in other organs, rather than being determined primarily by the developmental status of the surfactant system of the lung. Although these circumstances have altered the patterns of clinical use, FLM testing remains useful in reducing morbidity during the management of preterm delivery.

PULMONARY MATURITY

The lung buds form by weeks 5 to 6 of gestation in the human fetus. Bronchial tubules invade the splanchnic mesenchyme and undergo stereotypic branching to form the major airways. During the canalicular period of lung morphogenesis (between weeks 18 and 24), peripheral saccules dilate, respiratory epithelial cells in the lung periphery become increasingly cuboidal rather than columnar, and biosynthesis of surfactant lipids and proteins begins to increase in pre–type II cells and in type II cells. During the saccular phase, between 24 and 36 weeks' gestation, peripheral airways continue to proliferate and subdivide, and surfactant lipid and protein production increase. Biochemical markers of the surfactant system, including phospholipids and proteins, increase as the type II epithelial cells proliferate and differentiate. Thereafter, the process of alveolarization dominates lung morphogenesis, a process that continues until late childhood. The peripheral saccules septate, forming the alveoli that are lined by cuboidal type II and squamous type I epithelial cells. The alveoli are highly vascularized to facilitate gas exchange. Thus, lung maturation includes a complex process of proliferation, commitment, and differentiation of numerous cell types that are derived from epithelial, stromal, and vascular compartments of the developing lung. In general, AF tests for FLM assess the presence or function of components of pulmonary surfactant and do not address the many other cellular, biochemical, and physiologic processes involved in the maturation of lung function, the latter being increasingly important for survival of infants of extremely young gestational age.

SURFACTANT COMPOSITION

The biochemical composition of mammalian surfactants has been extensively studied in numerous species, including humans (Fig. 10-1). Surfactant composition, whether isolated from AF, lung lavage, or tissue homogenates, is highly conserved in all mammals, consisting of approximately 85% to 90% lipid, 5% to 10% protein, and lesser amounts of carbohydrate. The lipid components consist primarily of phosphatidylcholine, also termed *lecithin*, and neutral lipids (cholesterol, cholesterol esters, triglycerides, and sphingomyelin). The phosphatidylcholine component of pulmonary surfactants is enriched in

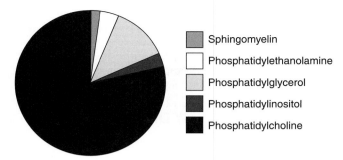

Sphingomyelin
Phosphatidylethanolamine
Phosphatidylglycerol
Phosphatidylinositol
Phosphatidylcholine

Figure 10–1. Lipid composition of surfactant.

dipalmitoylphosphatidylcholine as disaturated phosphatidylcholine (DSPC).[2,3] Phosphatidylcholine, DSPC, and dipalmitoylphosphatidylcholine are used as markers of surfactant sufficiency.

MATURATION OF THE SURFACTANT SYSTEM

Pulmonary surfactant is synthesized primarily by type II epithelial cells lining acinar, saccular, and alveolar regions of the lung. Surfactant phospholipids are synthesized by type II epithelial cells and are transported to and stored in lamellar bodies with the hydrophobic surfactant proteins (SP-B and SP-C) before being secreted into the airspace. After secretion, lamellar bodies unravel to form tubular myelin and monolayered and multilayered phospholipid sheets that lower surface tension at the air-liquid interface. Synthesis of the surfactant phospholipids by type II epithelial cells increases with advancing gestation in all mammals and is enhanced by exposure of the fetus to glucocorticoids. In animal studies, a number of agents (cyclic adenosine monophosphate, β-adrenergic agents, epithelial growth factor, fibroblast growth factors, interleukin-1β, glucocorticoids, thyroid hormones, and estrogen) enhance surfactant synthesis, whereas others (androgens, transforming growth factor-β, insulin) inhibit it. Of these, only glucocorticoids are used clinically to enhance lung function by treatment of the fetus before birth. During labor and delivery, secretion of the surfactant stored in lamellar bodies increases dramatically, expanding the extracellular pool of surfactant that is required for lung function after birth.

AMNIOTIC FLUID PHYSIOLOGY

Composition

AF is composed mainly of water (98% to 99%), electrolytes, and protein secreted by the kidneys and lungs or shed from the skin. Many of the constituents of AF change with gestational age. During midpregnancy, AF contains increasing quantities of creatinine and urea, which probably reflects the maturation of the kidneys. In late pregnancy, AF contains desquamated fetal cells, hair, vernix caseosa, and components secreted from the developing respiratory epithelium, including surfactant lipids and proteins.[4,5]

Volume and Regulation

The volume of AF is tightly regulated, increasing rapidly during the first trimester. In the second trimester, between 22 and 30 weeks' gestation, AF fluid volume stabilizes with an average volume of 750 to 800 mL. AF volume diminishes gradually in the last trimester, decreasing more rapidly after the 39th week.[4,5] During the first trimester, AF is derived primarily from transudation across both fetal and maternal tissues. In the second trimester, the kidneys are the major source of AF. At 20 weeks' gestation, the kidneys produce approximately 120 mL/day or 5 mL/hour of urine. Near term, this rate increases to 800 to 1200 mL/day or 50 mL/hour. The developing fetal lung produces 300 to 400 mL of fluid per day. Approximately 50% of secreted fetal lung fluid is swallowed, and 50% contributes to the AF pool (150 to 200 mL/day). Secretion of lung fluid is influenced by the larynx. Fluid secretion occurs when the larynx opens during fetal breathing movements. The larynx is usually closed, preventing AF from reentering the lungs. Reentry of fluid into the lungs is also minimized by the positive pressure gradient from the lungs to the larynx that maintains the secretion of fetal lung fluid.

AF removal occurs predominantly by fetal swallowing, which begins at 8 to 10 weeks and increases with gestational age. The average swallowed volume is 565 mL/day at term (5% to 10% of the fetal body weight). AF removal can also occur via other routes. Intramembranous transport represents the major alternative pathway for AF clearance, accounting for 200 to 500 mL/day at term. A small volume of AF (10 mL/day) is also removed by a transmembranous route. AF volume increases rapidly after esophageal ligation but returns to normal 2 to 3 weeks later.[4]

FETAL LUNG FLUID PHYSIOLOGY

The lungs begin producing fluid in the canalicular stage of development. The airway epithelia produce approximately 400 mL/day (4.5 mL/kg/hour), and the volume of fluid in the lungs near term is 25 to 40 mL/kg. The net efflux of fluid into the lumen is dependent on active chloride secretion by the epithelia. A tight epithelial layer selectively transports water and electrolytes but generally excludes macromolecules. Thus, little protein efflux occurs across the respiratory epithelia. Fetal lung fluid flows toward and then across the larynx as it opens with fetal breathing movements. The pressure gradient across the larynx is approximately 2 mm Hg, and this resistance to outflow creates pressure within the fetal lung that is important for fetal lung growth. Secreted lung fluid either is swallowed or mixes with the AF.[4] Lung liquid production decreases in the days just before delivery to about 65% of the maximal fetal lung fluid volume. During labor and delivery, fluid secretion ceases and fluid reabsorption begins, clearing approximately 30% of the remaining fetal lung fluid volume. Labor stimulates the release of catecholamines that change the epithelia from net fluid secretion to net fluid reabsorption. Glucocorticoids and catecholamines increase the expression of the sodium channel on the apical membranes of the epithelia, facilitating passive entry of sodium, which is subsequently transported across the basolateral membranes by sodium/potassium–adenosine triphosphatase (Na/K-ATPase).[2] Changes in apical membrane permeability to sodium and an increased expression of Na/K-ATPase cause the epithelia to reabsorb luminal fluid, a process that is maintained throughout adult life. The decrease in fluid production and the onset of lung liquid reabsorption before delivery leave only 35% of the original fetal lung fluid volume to be cleared from the lungs after birth. Most lung fluid is absorbed into the interstitium and moves into the vascular system. Approximately 20% of lung liquid is cleared by the lymphatic vessels. Lung fluid volume after transition is approximately 0.3 mL/kg. Clearance of fetal lung fluid increases with advancing gestational age and is stimulated by a number of endocrine pathways. For example, activity of catecholamine-sensitive clearance pathways is deficient in the preterm lung. In experimental animals, lung fluid clearance can be enhanced by pretreatment of the fetus with corticosteroids or triiodothyroxine.

Failure to clear lung liquid is associated with respiratory distress at birth and probably contributes to the pathogenesis of both RDS and transient tachypnea of the newborn. The process of labor plays an important role in liquid clearance. Delivery by cesarean section without labor bypasses endogenous fluid clearance pathways and is associated with an increased incidence of transient tachypnea of the newborn [5] and RDS.[5-8] Decreased sodium reabsorption was observed in babies delivered by cesarean section without prior labor, in comparison with those delivered by cesarean section with prior labor or delivered vaginally.[6] Decreased sodium reabsorption was also found in preterm neonates with RDS, in comparison with preterm neonates without RDS.[7] In the absence of labor, an additional 25 mL/kg of lung fluid must be reabsorbed after birth.[5]

FETAL LUNG MATURATION TESTING

Management of high-risk pregnancies is often complicated by the presence of risks to both fetus and mother. Preterm delivery places the infant at risk for respiratory disorders and morbidity associated with prematurity. However, delaying delivery may be associated with maternal morbidity from infection, preeclampsia, or other medical problems. Therefore, numerous physiologic, imaging, and biochemical tests have been developed to assess the well-being of both mother and fetus. Of these, AF testing for FLM has been highly useful for assessing the risk of RDS in the fetus. Because RDS is the major neonatal morbid condition associated with third-trimester delivery, FLM tests are most useful in decision making after 28 weeks' gestation. Delivery in the second trimester (at <28 weeks) is often associated with multiple morbid conditions that are not dependent on FLM, including intraventricular hemorrhage, necrotizing enterocolitis, retinopathy of prematurity, and neurodevelopmental abnormalities. In the second trimester, abnormalities in respiratory drive, thoracic cage stability, and the pharyngeal musculature contribute to respiratory insufficiency, placing the neonate at risk for requiring mechanical ventilation and the

subsequent risk of chronic lung disease.[5] Thus, FLM tests are rarely useful in balancing risk-versus-benefit decisions regarding the timing of delivery during the second trimester. In these early gestations, the frequency of morbidity and risk of death are significant enough to warrant continuation of the pregnancy when possible.

RISK OF RESPIRATORY DISTRESS SYNDROME

The surfactant pool size (lung content of phosphatidylcholine) in preterm infants is approximately 2 to 10 mg/kg, much lower than the estimated 100 mg/kg at term. The reduced surfactant pool size and the remarkable clinical response to exogenous surfactant indicate that surfactant deficiency plays an important role in the pathogenesis of RDS in preterm infants.[5] Surfactant pools increase with advancing gestational age, correlating with the decreased risk for RDS (Fig. 10-2).

BASICS OF FETAL LUNG MATURITY TESTS

Most current FLM tests measure one or more components or the function of pulmonary surfactant. The compositions of pulmonary surfactant isolated from the lungs, AF, or bronchoalveolar lavage are similar (see Fig. 10-1). In most FLM tests, a cutoff point that is useful in differentiating "mature" from "immature" determinations is identified. This cutoff point for a "mature" finding is usually set so that the incidence of RDS is 2% or less when mature (false-negative rate).[9] Standard statistical nomenclature for describing results of FLM tests can be confusing because FLM assays generally test for the absence rather than the presence of disease. Thus, sensitivity is the incidence of positive test results that is associated with disease (Table 10-1). Table 10-2 defines the standard

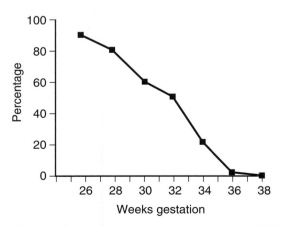

Figure 10–2. Incidence of respiratory distress syndrome (RDS) at various times during gestation without maternal corticosteroid administration. *(Adapted from Haas M, Rice WR: Respiratory distress syndrome for the practicing pediatrician. Pediatr Ann 24:572, 1995.)*

Table 10–1. Standard 2×2 Biostatistics Box Adapted for Fetal Lung Maturity (FLM) Testing

	RDS Present	RDS Absent
FLM test: immature	a: True positive	c: False positive
FLM test: mature	b: False negative	d: True negative

RDS, respiratory distress syndrome.

biostatistical terms as they relate to FLM tests in the literature, although the literature has variable definitions.

Although FLM testing is reliable for predicting the absence of RDS, a major drawback is the inability to predict the presence of RDS. Approximately 50% of infants with "immature" FLM result do not acquire RDS. When the incidence of RDS is low (i.e., at >37 weeks' gestation), FLM testing may not be clinically useful, especially if there are clinical indicators for delivery. However, if elective cesarean delivery after 37 weeks is being considered, FLM testing may be useful because of the increased risk of RDS in infants not undergoing labor (Table 10-3).[10]

AVAILABLE TESTS FOR FETAL LUNG MATURITY

FLM tests in clinical use assess one or more components of the pulmonary surfactant system. Many of the FLM tests, including the lecithin-to-sphingomyelin (L:S) ratio, phosphatidylglycerol, and saturated phosphatidylcholine assays, quantify individual phospholipids present in AF specimens. In contrast, other assays measure characteristics of the various surfactant components to assess

Table 10–2. Standard Biostatistical Terms Applied to Fetal Lung Maturity Testing

Term	Definition
Sensitivity	Percentage of RDS cases correctly identified as immature (sensitivity = a/[a+b])
Specificity	Percentage of cases without RDS correctly identified as mature (specificity = d/[d+c])
Positive predictive value (PPV)	Percentage of infants with an immature result who develop RDS (PPV = a/[a+c])
Negative predictive value (NPV)	Percentage of infants with a mature result who do not develop RDS (NPV = d/[b+d])
Receiver operator curves (ROC)	Plot of sensitivity versus 1-specificity that yields useful information for determining "cutoff" points

RDS, respiratory distress syndrome. For a, b, c, and d, see Table 10-1.

Table 10–3. Characteristics of an Ideal Fetal Lung Maturity Marker

Accessible: amniocentesis or vaginal fluid (after PROM)
Rapid laboratory testing
Reliable in contaminated fluids: meconium, blood, bilirubin
Reliable in complicated pregnancies: DM, PHI, PROM
Accurate predictor of the absence of RDS (high specificity and NPV)
Accurate predictor of the presence of RDS (high sensitivity and PPV)

DM, diabetes mellitus; NPV, negative predictive value; PHI, pregnancy-induced hypertension; PPV, positive predictive value; PROM, premature ruputure of membranes; RDS, respiratory distress syndrome.

surfactant function. For example, microviscosimetry and TDx-FLM tests measure the amount of fluorescent dye incorporated into the lipids in the AF. The lamellar body count (LBC) quantitates the number of lamellar bodies, the active component of pulmonary surfactant, per volume of AF. The optical density FLM test and visual inspection of AF samples have been used to assess fetal lung maturation, because the turbidity of AF is correlated with the concentration of surfactant in AF.

Surfactant spreads rapidly at an air-liquid interface, reduces surface tension, and maintains a stable phospholipid film. Therefore, a number of tests, including the shake test, the foam stability index (FSI), and the tap test were developed to estimate the function of surfactant in AF (Table 10-4).

Lecithin-to-Sphingomyelin Ratio

The L:S ratio was introduced by Roux and colleagues in 1972.[11] Phosphatidylcholine (lecithin) is the most abundant phospholipid in pulmonary surfactant. AF phosphatidylcholine content increases gradually until approximately the 34th week of gestation, and then its concentration increases more rapidly. In the L:S ratio, the content of lecithin is provided as a ratio with sphingomyelin, a nonspecific lipid present in AF. AF sphingomyelin falls, whereas phosphatidylcholine generally increases after 32 weeks' gestation. Surfactant in AF is precipitated with cold acetone, and both lecithin and sphingomyelin levels are determined after chromatography. In a normal pregnancy, the L:S ratio is less than 0.5 at 20 weeks of gestational age and increases gradually to 1.0 at about 32 weeks. The incidence of RDS is low (<2%) at any gestational age if the L:S ratio is higher than 2. An L:S ratio of 2.0 or higher is usually achieved by 35 weeks of gestational age in a normal fetus. The RDS risk is relatively low at intermediate L:S values (1.5 to 2.0), and the incidence of RDS is high with L:S ratios of less than 1.0.[5] Approximately 55% of neonates with an L:S ratio of less than 2.0 do not develop RDS.[12] Technical limitations of L:S ratio calculation include the expense of equipment, the technical expertise required, the long assay time, and

Table 10–4. Tests of Fetal Lung Maturation

Quantification of surfactant components
  Lecithin-to-sphingomyelin (L:S) ratio
  Phosphatidylglycerol
  Saturated phosphatidylcholine
  Lung profile
  Microviscometer assay of phospholipids
  Surfactant-to-albumin polarization
  Lamellar body count
Tests of amniotic fluid turbidity
  Optical density
  Visual inspection
Tests of surfactant function
  Foam stability index
  Shake test
  Tap test

the lack of 24-hour availability in many hospitals. AF specimens require immediate cooling and centrifugation. If not assayed immediately, samples must be frozen to minimize enzymatic breakdown of lecithin. In addition, the L:S ratio is not valid for AF samples contaminated with blood and meconium.[5,13] Although the L:S ratio has been considered the "gold standard" to which all other FLM tests are compared, newer FLM tests are proving superior to the L:S ratio in their accuracy, precision, and predictive values. A College of American Pathologists Survey found L:S determinations to have an unacceptable level of variation in the range of most clinical concern (Fig. 10-3).[14]

Phosphatidylglycerol

AF phosphatidylglycerol has been widely used to assess the risk of RDS. Although phosphatidylglycerol is not required for surfactant function, it is made almost exclusively by type II pneumocytes, and its presence in AF is strongly associated with pulmonary maturity. AF concentrations

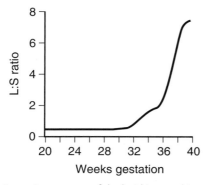

Figure 10–3. Approximate curve of the lecithin-to-sphingomyelin (L:S) ratio during gestation. *(Adapted from Jobe A: Evaluation of fetal lung maturation. In Creasy RK, Resnik R [eds]: Maternal-Fetal Medicine, 4th ed. Philadelphia, WB Saunders, 1999, pp. 402-422.)*

of phosphatidylglycerol change dramatically with increasing gestational age. Phosphatidylglycerol is almost undetectable until about 35 weeks' gestation, and then it increases dramatically and remains elevated for the remainder of gestation. Studies comparing phosphatidylglycerol and L:S ratio found that false-positive and false-negative rates are lower for phosphatidylglycerol than for the L:S ratio. Phosphatidylglycerol was initially assayed by thin-layer chromatography, a method similar to that for L:S measurements. Phosphatidylglycerol is now commonly assayed by a rapid, less expensive slide agglutination test (Amniostat-FLM).[13,15] The Amniostat assay detects phosphatidylglycerol in approximately 90% of samples in which thin-layer chromatography yielded positive results. The phosphatidylglycerol assay is not altered by AF contaminants and can be used on free-flowing vaginal pool samples in patients with premature rupture of membranes (PROM).[14,16] A unique disadvantage to the phosphatidylglycerol test is the interference caused by specimens contaminated with certain bacteria that contain phosphatidylglycerol within their cell membrane.[14,17]

Disaturated Phosphatidylcholine

Approximately 50% of the phosphatidylcholine in pulmonary surfactant is saturated, a characteristic that enhances the stability of the surfactant film. Disaturated phosphatidylcholine (DSPC) in AF is generally measured by thin-layer chromatography and is a better predictor of lung maturity than is the L:S ratio.[18] DSPC was correctly predictive of RDS in 82% of cases, in comparison with the L:S prediction rate of 56%, and had a false-mature rate of only 1.1% (versus 4.7% for the L:S). Unlike the L:S ratio, DSPC measurement is accurate in the presence of blood, meconium, and gestational diabetes. Unfortunately, as with the L:S, measuring DSPC requires expensive equipment, long assay times, and specifically trained personnel and is therefore not widely used.[13,18]

Lung Profile

The lung profile quantifies multiple phospholipid components (saturated phosphatidylcholine, phosphatidylglycerol, and phosphatidylinositol) present in surfactant. Because each phospholipid has its own characteristic developmental profile, this assay provides information on various constituents contributing to surfactant function and may improve prediction of RDS. Unfortunately, the test has many of the same disadvantages of that of the L:S measurement and is not widely used.[5,13]

Microviscosimeter Assay of Phospholipids

In the microviscosimeter assay, a fluorescent, lipid-soluble dye partitions into lipids within the AF sample. When the dye incorporates into phospholipid membranes, including surfactant, its fluorescence is quenched. The amount of dye unincorporated into lipid is estimated by measuring the fluorescence. The more fluorescence there is, the less the dye partitioned into the phospholipids, which indicates immaturity. An FLM analyzer (FELMA) machine is used for this test. Although faster, easier, and at least as reliable as the L:S ratio, the test is limited by interference by AF contaminants and the high cost of the FELMA.[13,19-21]

TDx-Fluorescent Polarization

The TDx-FLM assay involves the use of a lipid-soluble, fluorescent dye whose emission depends on whether the dye is incorporated into phospholipids or is associated with albumin. The TDx analyzer is an automated fluorescent polarimeter that measures the fluorescence present in a 1-mL sample of AF after normalization to the concentration of albumin in the sample. A value of 50 to 70 mg of surfactant per gram of albumin is usually used to define maturity. The TDx assay is rapid, readily standardized among laboratories, produces few false-mature results, and therefore widely used.[12-14,22-24]

Lamellar Body Count

The LBC measures the numbers of lamellar bodies present in AF. Lamellar bodies are small, concentrically layered organelles containing surfactant lipids and protein that are produced by the type II pneumocytes and secreted into the fetal lung fluid (or alveolar air space after delivery). In normal gestations, the numbers of lamellar bodies in AF increase linearly until 36 weeks and then increase exponentially until term.[25] Lamellar bodies are approximately the same size as platelets and are measured in a standard electronic cell counter.

A meta-analysis found the LBC to perform better than the L:S ratio.[26] Meconium has a small effect on the LBC. The LBC can be adjusted for contaminating blood. In the first 20 minutes after collection, the cell counter enumerates both platelets and lamellar bodies, artificially increasingly the LBC (<5% increase). Over the next few hours, coagulation of blood in the sample traps lamellar bodies and decreases the LBC. This effect is significant only if the AF hematocrit exceeds 1%. Although not ideal, the test can be used for assessment of FLM in vaginal pool samples if the AF is actively flowing and does not contain abundant mucus. Mucus interferes with the cell counter and artificially increases the LBC.[27] The LBC is rapid, inexpensive, and widely available. Because lamellar bodies pellet after centrifugation, a consensus report recommended that AF samples not be centrifuged before the LBC.[28] Unlike other FLM tests, the LBC provides an immature cutoff point (<15,000 lamellar bodies/μL for noncentrifuged samples), below which the risk of RDS is quite high (~46%) in comparison with the 12.5% incidence of RDS in the transitional range (15,000 to 50,000 lamellar bodies/μL). Comparison of LBC with L:S or phosphatidylglycerol assays revealed that 19.4% of the samples were "mature" in the "immature" group and 63% were "mature" in the "transitional" group.[27,28] When the LBC was used as a screening test in which only "transitional" results were further evaluated with a second FLM test, the need for validation of 76% of samples was eliminated.[29]

Optical Density

Optical density of AF at 650 nm may be predictive of pulmonary maturity, performing as well as the L:S ratio.[30-32]

The mature cutoff for this optical density is 0.15. The test is not compromised by the presence of blood, but it is influenced by the presence of meconium. Centrifugation dramatically alters optical density results, because any centrifugation removes surfactant components.[14] The optical density measurement is rapid, and equipment is readily available in most laboratories.

Visual Inspection

Immature lungs can be predicted with surprising accuracy by visual inspection of the AF. Surfactant in AF causes the fluid to become turbid. When untrained observers evaluated samples against known controls or evaluated whether newspaper print could be read through the AF sample, the results were comparable to those for L:S and phosphatidylglycerol measurement.[13,33,34] This test is compromised by the presence of blood or meconium in the AF. Because of its lack of objectivity, clinicians are unlikely to base clinical decisions on this test.

Shake Test

The shake test and the foam stability index (FSI) are based on the principle that surfactant in AF forms a stable foam layer when shaken. These assays assess the stability of foam in the presence of increasing concentrations of an antifoaming agent, ethanol. AF is diluted to 47.5% ethanol and shaken, and the presence of foam at the surface of the liquid is assessed. Foam indicates maturity. The diagnostic utility of the shake test was comparable with that of the L:S ratio. A more recent study found that the shake test was less predictive than phosphatidylglycerol measurement.[35] Unfortunately, AF contaminants interfere with the shake test. In addition, an "immature" result is associated with a poor positive predictive value (overestimation of the risk of developing RDS), and it should be followed by another FLM test.[13,36]

Foam Stability Index

The FSI is a modification of the shake test and involves adding increasing concentrations of ethanol to the AF.[37,38] Of 134 infants in whom the ethanol concentration forming a stable foam layer was greater than 47%, 133 did not have RDS.[38] Although the FSI is rapid and widely available, AF contaminants increase the index, and the FSI should not be used in the presence of blood or meconium. Because the commercial test (Lumadex) is no longer available, variability in this test is a concern. Also, because ethanol is hygroscopic and the concentration intervals in the test are small (1% increments), the FSI is subject to error.[14]

Tap Test

The tap test involves mixing 1 mL of AF, 1 drop of 6 N hydrochloric acid, and 1.5 mL of diethyl ether. After tapping the sample four times, the presence of bubbles in the ether layer at 2, 5, and 10 minutes is assessed. In the presence of surfactant, bubbles disappear. The test has a negative predictive value of higher than 94% and a positive predictive value of approximately 50%. Like most

FLM tests, contaminants in the AF interfere with the test, and it is not widely used.[13,38]

Comparison of Fetal Lung Maturity Tests

Table 10-5 is a comparison of the five most commonly used and most thoroughly investigated FLM tests. Table 10-6 lists clinical considerations involved with these tests.

Cost-Effectiveness of Fetal Lung Maturity Testing

Cost analysis of FLM testing in a tertiary care setting revealed that FLM testing for preterm labor was worthwhile only for fetuses at moderate risk for developing RDS.[40] When the risk of RDS was higher than 17% (at <34 weeks), it was most cost-effective to administer corticosteroids and delay labor. When the risk of RDS was moderate (at 34 to 36 weeks), it was most cost-effective to perform FLM testing and then make management decisions on the basis of the FLM result. When the risk of RDS was less than 2% (at >36 weeks), neither tocolysis nor FLM testing was cost-effective (but this finding did not apply to elective deliveries).

Diagnostic Pathways

Many institutions have adopted a clinical pathway approach for FLM testing.[12,22,25,26,28] In general, testing is initiated with one or more screening tests and ends with a phospholipid assay. Initial screening tests are rapid, inexpensive, and produce few false-mature results, but they produce high false-immature rates. If the test result indicates immaturity, a second FLM test—often another rapid, inexpensive test—is performed. If the results again indicate immaturity, a final FLM test is performed. A "mature" result on any test is considered to represent lung maturation. When LBC is used as a screening test, only transitional results are followed by additional testing. Figure 10-4 shows a potential diagnostic pathway.

FETAL LUNG MATURITY TESTING IN SPECIFIC CLINICAL SETTINGS

Certain maternal and fetal conditions may influence the timing and effect of fetal lung maturation. Although stress is commonly considered to induce lung maturation, studies evaluating the effect of various conditions on FLM tests have yielded conflicting findings. For example, pregnancy-induced hypertension and PROM have long been considered to enhance lung maturation. However, studies suggest that neither condition affects lung maturation.[41-43] The influence of several maternal conditions on fetal lung maturation is less ambiguous. Substance abuse and multiple gestations appear to accelerate fetal lung maturation, whereas poorly controlled diabetes delays fetal lung maturation. Most other maternal and fetal conditions necessitate further study to determine their true effect on lung maturation.

Maternal Hypertension

Hypertension complicates 7% to 10% of all pregnancies. Increased risk of intrauterine growth restriction and stillbirth associated with maternal hypertension makes early delivery desirable in certain situations. Both

chronic hypertension and pregnancy-induced hypertension may be associated with accelerated fetal lung maturation; however, findings of clinical studies have been conflicting.[42,43]

Gestational Diabetes

A delay in maturity indicated by FLM tests was associated with pregnancies complicated by poorly controlled diabetes mellitus.[13] Timing of maturity as indicated by FLM tests in well-controlled diabetes mellitus were similar to those in uncomplicated pregnancies.[18,44,45] Phosphatidylglycerol may be the preferred FLM test for poorly controlled diabetes mellitus.[14]

Intrauterine Growth Restriction

Intrauterine growth restriction (IUGR) is a common complication in pregnancies and has many causes, some intrinsic to the fetus (e.g, chromosomal abnormalities) and some secondary to maternal conditions (placental insufficiency, collagen vascular diseases, hypertension). Fetal lung maturation may be accelerated in some cases of IUGR, depending on the cause of the IUGR. Unfortunately, studies to date have been inconclusive in this regard.[43,46]

Multiple Gestation

Multiple gestations are at increased risk for premature delivery. Although constituting only 1% to 2% of all pregnancies, they account for approximately 10% of patients admitted to neonatal intensive care units. After 31 weeks, FLM tests indicate maturity 2 to 3 weeks earlier in twins than in singletons.[13,47] The high concordance in FLM tests in twins older than 32 weeks suggests that only one sac requires sampling. Before 32 weeks, discordance is greater; therefore, both sacs should be sampled.[48]

Prolonged Premature Rupture of Membranes

PROM occurs in approximately 10% of all pregnancies. Balancing the risks of infection and pulmonary hypoplasia against those of prematurity to determine the optimal time for delivery is difficult. PROM may be associated with accelerated fetal lung maturation,[41,49-51] but FLM testing is difficult and of questionable utility after rupture of membranes.[52] Amniocentesis after PROM is often technically challenging. Vaginal pool samples of AF are not as reliable as those obtained by amniocentesis. Free-flowing fluid that is relatively clear of bacteria can be used for phosphatidylglycerol assays, TDx-FLM, or LBC. The presence of bacteria in the sample may result in a false-positive phosphatidylglycerol result, inasmuch as some bacteria (*Gardnerella vaginalis*, *Listeria* species, *Escherichia coli*) contain phosphatidylglycerol.[9,17,53] In addition, the maturation of surfactant components induced by PROM may not appear in AF in a timely manner.

Substance Abuse

Both maternal smoking and cocaine abuse have been found to accelerate fetal lung maturation. Both are associated with a decreased incidence of RDS and an increased mature FLM rate at younger gestational ages.[54]

Table 10-5. Comparison of the Five Most Common Fetal Lung Maturation Tests

Test	Lecithin-Sphingomyelin	PG	TDx-FLM Assay	Foam Stability Index	Lamellar Body Count
Assay	Thin-layer chromatography: ratio of saturated phosphatidylcholine to sphingomyelin	Slide agglutination assay for PG (Amniostat)	Differential polarization of chromophore between surfactant and albumin	Functional assay of surfactant's ability to create foam with increasing EtOH	Electronic cell counter based on similar size of lamellar bodies to that of platelets
Date assay introduced	1972	1983	1992	1978	1989
Mature value	>2.0	Present	>70 mg/g albumin	>48%	>50,000
Transitional value	1.5-2.0	Trace	50-70 mg/g albumin	47%	15,000-50,000
Immature value	<1.5	Absent	<50 mg/g albumin	<47%	<15,000
					Mature Immature
Sensitivity	64%-92%	81%-100%	93%-100%	87%-100%	89% 62%
Specificity	74%-100%	43%-100%	88%	97%	64% 90%
PPV	32%-43%	15%-73%	20%-47%	35%	25% 96%
NPV	97%	95%-100%	96%-100%	100%	98% 95%
Equipment	TLC equipment	Spectrophotometer	Fluorimeter	Reagents	Cell counter
Availability	Not readily available, may need to be sent to reference laboratory for analysis	Available	Available	Available	Available in almost every laboratory
Test time	Slow (3-5 hr)	Rapid (25 min)	Rapid (<1 hr)	Rapid (30 min)	Rapid (<20 min)
Technical expertise	High	Moderate	Moderate	Moderate	Minimal
AF volume			1 mL		200 µL
Interlaboratory precision	Poor	Good	Good	Good	Good
Direct laboratory cost	$30	$40	$40	$50	$4
Meconium staining	↓ Ratio	Unaffected	Interferes with test	↑ False mature	↑ Count by ≤5000
Blood staining	↓ Ratio	Unaffected	Interferes with test	↑ False mature	Biphasic interference (modest; see text)
Bacterial contamination	—	Some bacteria are PG positive	Interferes with test	↑ False mature	↑ False immature
Vaginal pool sample	Mucus ↑ false immature	Often adequate (bacteria can interfere)	Interferes with test	↑ False mature	Interference if mucus present
Poorly controlled DM	↑ False mature	Unaffected	Interferes with test	—	Unknown
Comments	"Gold standard" to which all other tests have been compared to date	Good choice for contaminated amniotic fluid, poorly controlled DM, or low-risk population	Good choice for high-risk populations	Lumadex kit no longer available (↑ variability with hand-mixed reagents)	See ref. 27
References	5, 12-14, 25-28	5, 9, 12-14, 16, 25, 28, 35, 46	12-14, 24, 47	9, 12-14	12-14, 25-29

AF, amniotic fluid; DM, diabetes mellitus; EtOH, ethanol; FLM, fetal lung maturity; PG, phosphatidylglycerol; PPV, positive predictive value; TLC, total lung capacity.

Table 10–6. Clinical Considerations with Fetal Lung Maturity (FLM) Testing

Gestational age–associated morbid conditions of prematurity
Fetal condition in utero
Maternal condition warranting preterm delivery
Effect of test result on management decisions
Effect of amniotic fluid contaminants on FLM test
    Blood, meconium, bacteria, vaginal debris
Maternal conditions affecting lung development
    Diabetes, pregnancy-induced hypertension, prolonged premature rupture of membranes, placental insufficiency multiples, substance abuse
Effect of corticosteroids on utility of FLM test results

Corticosteroids

Corticosteroids decrease the risk of RDS and decrease the severity of RDS in infants who develop the disease.[5,55] Lung function generally improves within 48 hours after prenatal glucocorticoid therapy. However, results of DSPC, L:S, and phosphatidylglycerol analysis do not change after corticosteroid treatment.[56] This disparity is probably caused by the influence of corticosteroids on various aspects of lung morphogenesis, differentiation, and function, in addition to enhancing synthesis of surfactant. One study found that the use of corticosteroids did not affect the negative predictive value of the L:S, phosphatidylglycerol, or LBC tests.[28]

Abnormal Amniotic Fluid Volume

With the exception of L:S, which corrects for AF volume, polyhydramnios would be expected to dilute surfactant components and result in falsely low FLM test results. Likewise, false-maturity findings would be expected in the presence of oligohydramnios. However, only acute (<1 week) changes in AF were associated with falsely low FLM test results. Chronic oligohydramnios or polyhydramnios did not influence FLM tests.[57]

SUMMARY

A number of useful tests have been developed for the assessment of the risk of RDS after preterm birth. Diligent standardization and judicious clinical use of these assays can serve to optimize the timing of delivery, in an attempt to minimize unnecessary risk to the fetus for RDS. Unnecessary preterm delivery continues to be a significant cause of morbidity and even mortality for preterm infants. AF testing for pulmonary maturity should therefore be carefully applied to the decision-making algorithms with regard to the timing of preterm birth.

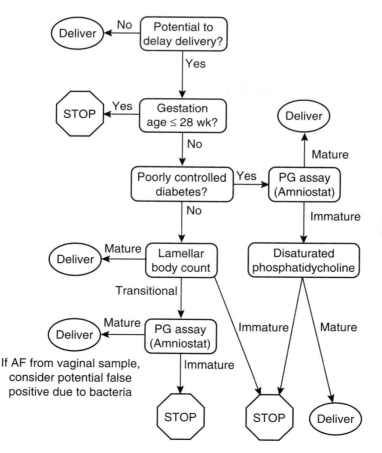

Figure 10–4. Potential pathway for utilizing fetal lung maturity testing. AF, amniotic fluid; PG, phosphatidylglycerol.

If AF from vaginal sample, consider potential false positive due to bacteria

REFERENCES

1. Avery ME, Mead J: Surface properties in relation to atelectasis and hyaline membrane disease. Am J Dis Child 97:517, 1959.
2. Whitsett JA: Composition of pulmonary surfactant lipids and proteins. In Polin RA, Fox WW (eds): Fetal and Neonatal Physiology, 2nd ed. Philadelphia, WB Saunders, 2004, pp 1005-1013.
3. Harwood JL: Lung surfactant. Prog Lipid Res 26:211, 1987.
4. Brace RA, Resnik R: Dynamics and disorders of amniotic fluid. In Creasy RK, Resnik R (eds): Maternal-Fetal Medicine, 4th ed. Philadelphia, WB Saunders, 1999, pp 404-422.
5. Jobe A: Evaluation of fetal lung maturation. In Creasy RK, Resnik R (eds): Maternal-Fetal Medicine, 4th ed. Philadelphia, WB Saunders, 1999, pp 404-422.
6. Gowen CW Jr, Lawson EE, Gingras J, et al: Electrical potential difference and ion transport across nasal epithelium of term neonates: Correlation with mode of delivery, transient tachypnea of the newborn, and respiratory rate. J Pediatr 113:121, 1988.
7. Barker PM, Gowen CW, Lawson EE, Knowles MR: Decreased sodium ion absorption across nasal epithelium of very premature infants with respiratory distress syndrome (see comments). J Pediatr 130:373, 1997.
8. Haas M, Rice WR: Respiratory distress syndrome for the practicing pediatrician. Pediatr Ann 24:572, 1995.
9. Spinnato JA 2nd: Maturity testing with preterm premature rupture of the membranes. Clin Perinatol 28:819, 2001.
10. Wax JR, Herson V, Carignan E, et al: Contribution of elective delivery to severe respiratory distress at term. Am J Perinatol 19:81, 2002.
11. Roux JF, Nakamura J, Brown E, et al: The lecithin-sphingomyelin ratio of amniotic fluid: An index of fetal lung maturity? Pediatrics 49:464, 1972.
12. Ravel R: Tests in obstetrics: Fetal maturity tests. In: Clinical Laboratory Medicine, 6th ed. St. Louis, Mosby–Year Book, 1995, pp 549-550.
13. Field NT, Gilbert WM: Current status of amniotic fluid tests of fetal maturity. Clin Obstet Gynecol 40:366, 1997.
14. Dubin SB: Assessment of fetal lung maturity. Practice parameter. Am J Clin Pathol 110:723, 1998.
15. Garite TJ, Yabusaki KK, Moberg LJ, et al: A new rapid slide agglutination test for amniotic fluid phosphatidylglycerol: Laboratory and clinical correlation. Am J Obstet Gynecol 147:681, 1983.
16. Benoit J, Merrill S, Rundell C, Meeker CI: Amniostat-FLM: An initial clinical trial with both vaginal pool and amniocentesis samples. Am J Obstet Gynecol 154:65, 1986.
17. Beazley D, Lewis R: The evaluation of infection and pulmonary maturity in women with premature rupture of the membranes. Semin Perinatol 20:409, 1996.
18. Delgado JC, Greene MF, Winkelman JW, Tanasijevic MJ: Comparison of disaturated phosphatidylcholine and fetal lung maturity surfactant/albumin ratio in diabetic and nondiabetic pregnancies. Am J Clin Pathol 113:233, 2000.
19. Gonen R, Tal J, Oettinger M, et al: Assessment of fetal lung maturity by a microviscosimeter. Obstet Gynecol 51:422, 1978.
20. Golde SH, Vogt JF, Gabbe SG, Cabal LA: Evaluation of the FELMA microviscosimeter in predicting fetal lung maturity. Obstet Gynecol 54:639, 1979.
21. Blumenfeld TA, Cheskin HS, Shinitzky M: Microviscosity of amniotic fluid phospholipids, and its importance in determining fetal lung maturity. Clin Chem 25:64, 1979.
22. Bonebrake RG, Towers CV, Rumney PJ, Reimbold P: Is fluorescence polarization reliable and cost efficient in a fetal lung maturity cascade? Am J Obstet Gynecol 177:835, 1997.
23. Elrad H, Beydoun SN, Hagen JH, et al: Fetal pulmonary maturity as determined by fluorescent polarization of amniotic fluid. Am J Obstet Gynecol 132:681, 1978.
24. Fantz CR, Powell C, Karon B, et al: Assessment of the diagnostic accuracy of the TDx-FLM II to predict fetal lung maturity. Clin Chem 48:761, 2002.
25. Beinlich A, Fischass C, Kaufmann M, et al: Lamellar body counts in amniotic fluid for prediction of fetal lung maturity. Arch Gynecol Obstet 262:173, 1999.
26. Wijnberger LD, Huisjes AJ, Voorbij HA, et al: The accuracy of lamellar body count and lecithin/sphingomyelin ratio in the prediction of neonatal respiratory distress syndrome: A meta-analysis. BJOG 108:583, 2001.
27. Neerhof MG, Dohnal JC, Ashwood ER, et al: Lamellar body counts: A consensus on protocol. Obstet Gynecol 97:318, 2001.
28. Neerhof MG, Haney EI, Silver RK, et al: Lamellar body counts compared with traditional phospholipid analysis as an assay for evaluating fetal lung maturity. Obstet Gynecol 97:305, 2001.
29. Lewis PS, Lauria MR, Dzieczkowski J, et al: Amniotic fluid lamellar body count: Cost-effective screening for fetal lung maturity. Obstet Gynecol 93:387, 1999.
30. Sbarra AJ, Selvaraj RJ, Cetrulo CL, et al: Positive correlation of optical density at 650 nm with lecithin/sphingomyelin ratios in amniotic fluid. Am J Obstet Gynecol 130:788, 1978.
31. Cetrulo CL, Sbarra AJ, Selvaraj RJ, et al: Amniotic fluid optical density and neonatal respiratory outcome. Obstet Gynecol 55:262, 1980.
32. Bustos R, Estol P, Fasanello A, et al: Optical density at 650 nm in amniotic fluid, L/S ratio and foam test as indicators of fetal lung maturity. J Perinat Med 8:278, 1980.
33. Sbarra AJ, Chaudhury A, Cetrulo CL, et al: A rapid visual test for predicting fetal lung maturity. Am J Obstet Gynecol 165:1351, 1991.
34. Strong TH Jr, Hayes AS, Sawyer AT, et al: Amniotic fluid turbidity: A useful adjunct for assessing fetal pulmonary maturity status. Int J Gynaecol Obstet 38:97, 1992.
35. Kucuk M: Tap test, shake test and phosphatidylglycerol in the assessment of fetal pulmonary maturity. Int J Gynaecol Obstet 60:9, 1998.
36. Rodriguez-Macias KA: A comparison of three tests for determining fetal pulmonary maturity. Int J Gynaecol Obstet 51:39, 1995.
37. Sher G, Statland BE, Knutzen VK: Diagnostic reliability of the lecithin/sphingomyelin ratio assay and quantitative foam stability index test: Results of a comparative study. J Reprod Med 27:51, 1982.
38. Sher G, Statland BE, Freer DE, Kraybill EN: Assessing fetal lung maturation by the foam stability index test. Obstet Gynecol 52:673, 1978.
39. Socol ML, Sing E, Depp OR: The tap test: A rapid indicator of fetal pulmonary maturity. Am J Obstet Gynecol 148:445, 1984.
40. Myers ER, Alvarez JG, Richardson DK, Ludmir J: Cost-effectiveness of fetal lung maturity testing in preterm labor. Obstet Gynecol 90:824, 1997.
41. Hallak M, Bottoms SF: Accelerated pulmonary maturation from preterm premature rupture of membranes: A myth. Am J Obstet Gynecol 169:1045, 1993.
42. Ferroni KM, Gross TL, Sokol RJ, Chik L: What affects fetal pulmonary maturation during diabetic pregnancy? Am J Obstet Gynecol 150:270, 1984.
43. Barkai G, Mashiach S, Lanzer D, et al: Determination of fetal lung maturity from amniotic fluid microviscosity in high-risk pregnancy. Obstet Gynecol 59:615, 1982.

44. Kjos SL, Walther FJ, Montoro M, et al: Prevalence and etiology of respiratory distress in infants of diabetic mothers: Predictive value of fetal lung maturation tests. Am J Obstet Gynecol 163:898, 1990.

45. Piper JM, Langer O: Does maternal diabetes delay fetal pulmonary maturity? Am J Obstet Gynecol 168:783, 1993.

46. Gross TL, Sokol RJ, Wilson MV, et al: Amniotic fluid phosphatidylglycerol: A potentially useful predictor of intrauterine growth retardation. Am J Obstet Gynecol 140:277, 1981.

47. McElrath TF, Norwitz ER, Robinson JN, et al: Differences in TDx fetal lung maturity assay values between twin and singleton gestations. Am J Obstet Gynecol 182:1110, 2000.

48. Whitworth NS, Magann EF, Morrison JC: Evaluation of fetal lung maturity in diamniotic twins. Am J Obstet Gynecol 180:1438, 1999.

49. Kulovich MV, Hallman MB, Gluck L: The lung profile. I. Normal pregnancy. Am J Obstet Gynecol 135:57, 1979.

50. Richardson CJ, Pomerance JJ, Cunningham MD, Gluck L: Acceleration of fetal lung maturation following prolonged rupture of the membranes. Am J Obstet Gynecol 118:1115, 1974.

51. Namavar Jahromi B, Ardekany MS, Poorarian S: Relationship between duration of preterm premature rupture of membranes and pulmonary maturation. Int J Gynaecol Obstet 68:119, 2000.

52. Refuerzo JS, Blackwell SC, Wolfe HM, et al: Relationship between fetal pulmonary maturity assessment and neonatal outcome in premature rupture of the membranes at 32-34 weeks' gestation. Am J Perinatol 18:451, 2001.

53. Edwards RK, Duff P, Ross KC: Amniotic fluid indices of fetal pulmonary maturity with preterm premature rupture of membranes. Obstet Gynecol 96:102, 2000.

54. Hanlon-Lundberg KM, Williams M, Rhim T, et al: Accelerated fetal lung maturity profiles and maternal cocaine exposure. Obstet Gynecol 87:128, 1996.

55. Lyons CA, Garite TJ: Corticosteroids and fetal pulmonary maturity. Clin Obstet Gynecol 45:35, 2002.

56. Farrell PM, Engle MJ, Zachman RD, et al: Amniotic fluid phospholipids after maternal administration of dexamethasone. Am J Obstet Gynecol 145:484, 1983.

57. Nelson GH, Nelson SJ: Theoretical effects of amniotic fluid volume changes on surfactant concentration measurements. Am J Obstet Gynecol 152:870, 1985.

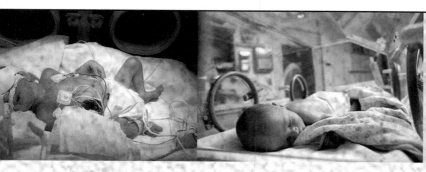
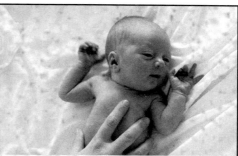

Fetal Intervention

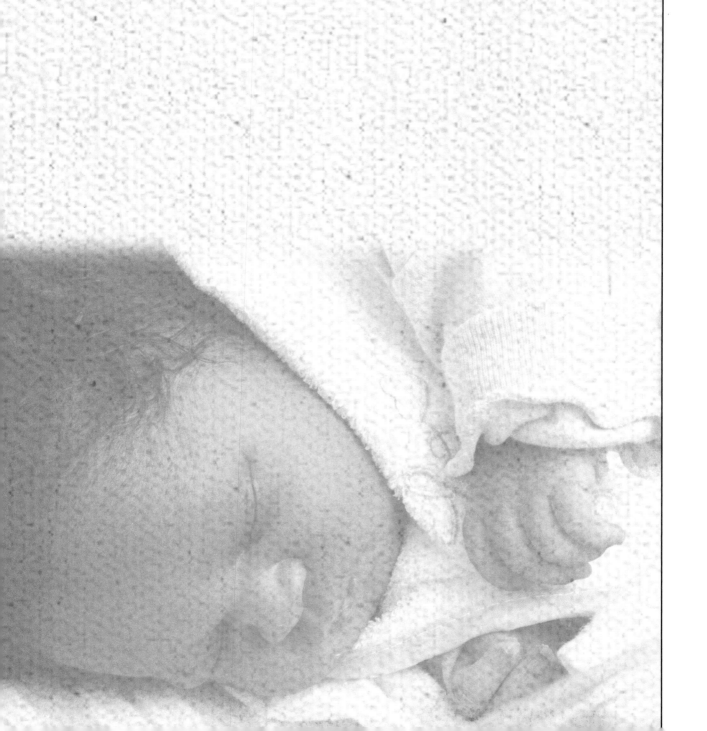

CHAPTER 11

Intrauterine Growth Restriction

Muhammad Subhani

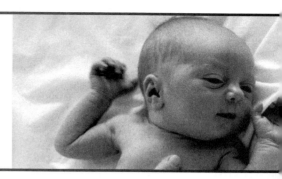

Intrauterine growth restriction (IUGR) is a pathophysiologic process characterized by the failure of a pregnancy to achieve its intrinsic growth potential. **Intrauterine growth restriction** is the preferred term rather than **intrauterine growth retardation,** to avoid a negative connotation similar to mental retardation.

Since 1919,[1] it has been known that infants with birth weight less than 2500 g (low birth weight) are vulnerable to various complications. The misconception of prematurity as a causative factor in all low-birth-weight infants was dismissed after the introduction of growth curves in 1963 by Lubchenco[2] for infants between the gestational ages of 26 and 42 weeks. Newborn infants since that time have been classified into one of three categories: appropriate for gestational age (AGA), or infants whose growth is between the 10th and 90th percentiles; large for gestational age (LGA), or infants whose growth is above the 90th percentile; and small for gestational age (SGA), or infants whose growth is below the 10th percentile (Fig. 11-1). The terms *IUGR* and *SGA* traditionally have been used synonymously, although there are some differences, as noted subsequently. This classification unambiguously separated AGA infants from SGA and LGA infants; the latter subgroups are susceptible to complications specific to each of the categories.

The determination of adequate intrauterine growth of any infant on initial examination after birth customarily is made by plotting the values of birth weight, length, and head circumference on one of several available normative graphs. Although etiologic factors may be similar for SGA and IUGR in some instances, they are separate entities. This differentiation has practical application because the diagnosis of SGA does not point toward any specific pathology. Approximately 70% of infants identified as SGA on the basis of being in less than the 10th percentile of birth weight simply represent the extreme of the spectrum of neonatal size[3]; they have no significant pathologic abnormality. Only the affected remaining infants justifiably can be labeled as IUGR; these infants are at risk for associated complications. The absence of clinical (Fig. 11-2) and laboratory evidence for IUGR in an infant who otherwise is classified as SGA indicates the attainment of the infant's predetermined potential for intrauterine growth without any restrictions. The diagnosis of IUGR implies a pathologic process necessitating further etiologic evaluation and intervention, if applicable. The diagnosis of SGA does not proclaim IUGR automatically, and the similarities do not justify the erroneous use of these two terms as synonyms. Cassidy[4] and Wilcox[5] have addressed this important issue.

INCIDENCE

The significant disproportion between the incidence of growth restriction and complications arising from this diagnosis necessitates an accurate estimation of its incidence. A true determination is difficult, not only in different regions of the world, but also in the United States. The reason for this difficulty is that demographic data frequently are collected only as low birth weight, which includes AGA infants as well. In addition, race, gender, and definition criteria have made it difficult to have a uniform identification of this entity. Where some information does exist, however, significant differences in the incidence of IUGR can be seen between developed and underdeveloped nations (i.e., 4% to 8% versus 6% to 30).[6-10]

MORTALITY AND MORBIDITY

The perinatal morbidity and mortality for IUGR infants are estimated at approximately 20%, which is disproportionately high for a 3% to 10% incidence of IUGR births in the United States.[11-14] In the developing world, the range is even wider, with figures of 3% to 30% and an even higher rate of complications.[15,16] In general, premature IUGR infants have a higher mortality rate, but it also is high in mature infants with IUGR.[17] Some causes of IUGR lead to preterm deliveries. In this subset of infants, increased mortality is seen after birth from prematurity-related complications (e.g., respiratory distress syndrome,

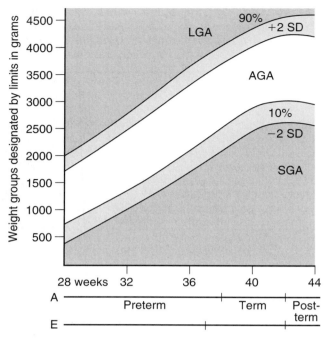

Figure 11–1. Diagram comparing suggested standards of birth weight for gestational age. The darker gray areas include weights above and below 2 SDs from the mean; the lighter gray areas include the additional ranges beyond the 10th and 90th percentiles (10%, 90%) for a middle-class population in Portland, Oregon. At the bottom, the ranges for preterm, term, and post-term birth are those suggested by the American Academy of Pediatrics (A) and the Second European Congress of Perinatal Medicine (E). Use of the term *prematurity* to indicate a birth weight less than 2501 g or in any other sense should be avoided because of past misuse. *(Modified from Elliot K, Knight J [eds]: Pathology of the deprived fetus and its supply line. In Size at Birth. Ciba Foundation Symposium [New Ser] 27:3-19.)*

sepsis, intraventricular hemorrhage, and asphyxia). Intrauterine demise surpasses the above-mentioned premature mortality, occurring most commonly between 38 and 42 weeks of gestation, a time when the complications of prematurity no longer can be considered contributing

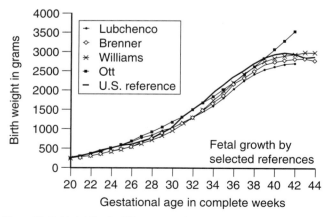

Figure 11–2. Variability in different growth curves. *(From Alexander GR, Himes JH, Kaufman RB, et al: A United States national reference for fetal growth. Obstet Gynecol 87:163, 1996.)*

factors. Sciscione and associates,[18] after adjusting the birth weight standards of maternal and infant characteristics, found a better correlation of predictable mortality in SGA infants. Acceleration of maturity in response to the stress of IUGR as a protective effect for the infant remains a disputed issue, owing to conflicting results by various studies.

LIMITATIONS OF GROWTH CHARTS

The introduction of growth curves by Lubchenco and colleagues[2,19,20] was followed by the appearance of charts by Usher and McLean,[21] Babson and Benda,[22] and Gruenwald.[23] Lubchenco's data were questioned because they were derived at high altitude in Denver, Colorado, and might not be universally applicable to all populations. Although these growth charts differ by less than 10% for a given percentile at a given gestational age, an infant plotted on the 5th percentile on one chart may belong to the 10th percentile on another growth curve chart. Ethnic and racial differences, in addition to various other factors, are responsible for these variances. An ideal growth curve not only would take these into consideration, but also eliminate all possible etiologic factors for IUGR (e.g., pregnancies affected by maternal smoking or pregnancy-induced hypertension). All these commonly used growth charts are incapable of fulfilling these criteria and consequently remain susceptible to biases.

It is imperative to determine an accurate gestational age so that the values of growth parameters can be plotted appropriately. Inadvertent biases by physicians can occur at several points. Except in pregnancies that are the consequence of in vitro fertilization or pregnancies followed from early gestation, there always remains a possibility of discrepancy between the gestational age approximated by the date of last menstrual period versus an examination (prenatal maternal physical examination, ultrasound, or both). Among birth weight, length, and head circumference, the latter two are observer dependent. They also are subject to large variations from medical conditions that potentially could alter them just before delivery (e.g., excessive molding and extreme breech presentations). Although refinements have been made, the standard neonatal examinations (Ballard,[24,25] Dubowitz,[26] and Lubchenco[19,20] examinations) based on the physical and neurologic characteristics for the assessment of gestational age also are viewer dependent. Any or all of these factors may lead to a diagnosis of IUGR, when it actually does not exist.

Far less variability is noted for the growth charts available from antenatal ultrasound measurements. The foremost difference between these and the postnatal growth charts is that these correspond to serial measurements from the same infant over time, whereas the postnatal growth charts use a single value near the time of delivery. Riddle and colleagues[27] showed that current growth charts are inadequate to estimate birth weight before 30 weeks of gestation.

DEFINITION

No single optimal definition exists to describe IUGR, partially due to the fact that the prenatal diagnostic criteria differ from the postnatal criteria. The use of birth weight as a measure to grade the adequacy of intrauterine growth retrospectively is a crude method at best to define IUGR. Most clinicians agree, however, that an infant is IUGR if the birth weight is below the 10th percentile for a given gestational age. This definition routinely is considered synonymous with SGA.[6,28-40] Some define IUGR, however, only if the infant's birth weight is below the third percentile[41-44] or when the infant's birth weight is 2 SD below the mean for a given gestational age. As previously noted, there also are several standard growth charts that represent different populations. An infant determined to have IUGR on one growth chart may not show the same findings on another chart.

DIAGNOSIS

As a result of improved prenatal care in modern obstetrics, especially the use of ultrasound technology, the diagnosis of IUGR has been made prenatally with increasing accuracy. The biggest impact of this early diagnosis is in cases incompatible with life (e.g., trisomy 18). This approach assists parents in making decisions about termination of pregnancy and concurrently avoiding unnecessary maternal interventions in hopeless situations. Timing and mode of delivery and selection of appropriate diagnostic modalities for further evaluation after birth also are guided by the initial findings.

Antenatal Diagnosis

Appropriate antenatal monitoring, where available, now can diagnose most cases before birth. Depending on the etiology, however, not all infants may show signs of IUGR until late in pregnancy. Development of placental insufficiency not severe enough to warrant close follow-up in a pregnancy that otherwise had shown appropriate growth until 34 weeks of gestation may culminate in an infant born at full term with manifestations of IUGR.

Before the era of ultrasound, estimation of the gestational age was made by calculating the expected date of confinement from the date of the last menstrual period, with supporting evidence from maternal weight gain and fundal height. Irregular menstrual cycles and inaccurate date information from the mother often made the last menstrual period method unreliable, however, and the maternal weight gain and fundal height lack specificity. Biochemical diagnostic modalities used in the past for detection of IUGR, such as maternal serum and urine estriol,[45,46] human placental lactogen,[47] amniotic fluid 3-methylhistidine-to-creatinine molar ratio,[48] serum cystine aminopeptidase (oxytocinase),[49] Schwangerschaft protein,[46,50] glucose tolerance testing,[51] and foam stability index[52] have been rendered obsolete due to the ease of use, safety, and accuracy of ultrasound.

Ultrasound has emerged as the gold standard not only for the initial estimation of the gestational age, but also for serial growth monitoring. The most preferable time for the first sonogram in any confirmed pregnancy is between 16 and 20 weeks of gestation, a time when most accurate verification of last menstrual period is possible with simultaneous identification of major malformations. Depending on the initial findings, the obstetrician can

determine the need for repeat ultrasound examination. In most cases, the recommended follow-up timing is between 3 and 4 weeks. In all but unusual cases, this date can be ascertained only after serial measurements. In severe cases, even an isolated value is considered sufficient, however. Certain risk factors have an established relationship to IUGR, and their presence in any pregnancy warrants screening and follow-up.

The diagnosis of IUGR by prenatal ultrasound rests on the abnormal findings of either fetal weight or measurements of biparietal diameter (BPD), head circumference (HC), fetal weight, femur length (FL), and abdominal circumference (AC). Curves now are available for antenatal growth by ultrasound at different gestational ages. Use of multiple measurements versus a single parameter increases the overall accuracy of the results. BPD alone cannot be considered an accurate indicator of IUGR because it may be affected by asymmetry and can be altered by the shape of the head (e.g., dolichocephaly). AC signifies the nutritional status of the abdominal viscera and is altered with wasting. Estimation of fetal weight requires simultaneous use of more than one measurement to achieve optimal accuracy.

Various ratios have been generated by combining these individual measurements, which are more reliable predictors of IUGR. The HC/AC ratio detects IUGR when wasting of abdominal viscera is seen without reduction in HC (i.e., asymmetric, or head-sparing, type). The two most commonly used ratios are the HC/AC ratio and FL/AC ratio. The latter is performed only if there is a problem in obtaining the former due to fetal positioning. The values and interpretation of the HC/AC ratio and FL/AC ratio are presented in Tables 11-1 and 11-2. The use of intrauterine prenatal ponderal indices has been described by using the fetal body length, FL, and the fetal weight, but these indices carry a higher risk of error due to cubing of the fetal body length.

In addition to the above-mentioned individual measurements and ratios, ultrasound has been used for Doppler flow studies, placental grading, and amniotic fluid volume. Doppler flow studies specifically encompass two

Table 11–1. Head Circumference-to-Abdominal Circumference Ratio

Normal Values	
<32 wk gestation	>1
32-34 wk gestation	Approximately 1
>34 wk gestation	<1
Asymmetric IUGR	
(Head remains larger than body, i.e., AC)	Increased ratio
Symmetric IUGR	
HC and AC are reduced	Normal ratio

AC, abdominal circumference, HC, head circumference, IUGR, intrauterine growth restriction.

Table 11–2. Femur Length-to-Arm Circumference Ratio

Normal values: 21–37 wk gestation	22
IUGR	>23.5

IUGR, intrauterine growth restriction.

significant advantages. First, abnormalities are detectable early in gestation when other diagnostic modalities, such as the biophysical profile, are not valid. Second, Doppler flow studies are a great tool to determine the urgency of delivery time. Among many vessels, umbilical artery waveform has been used with the greatest success and most consistent results. Values of blood flow in systolic and diastolic phases are available. In the presence of IUGR, resistance may be detected during diastole, which could increase to the point that the diastolic flow is reversed. This change leads to a decreased systolic-to-diastolic ratio. Kingdom and associates[53] described the correlation between abnormal artery velocimetry, placental pathology, and IUGR. If normal values of systolic-to-diastolic ratio usually indicate fetal well-being, the absence or reversal of end-diastolic flow is associated with increases in perinatal morbidity and mortality and long-term poor neurologic outcome (see Table 11-6).[54]

Cerebral vascular dilation on ultrasound also may be noted in cases of IUGR, a compensatory mechanism for preserving blood flow, brain growth, and function. Splunder and coworkers[55] showed that redistribution of blood flow occurs in favor of the fetal brain, despite the change from a low uteroplacental vascular resistance to a high vascular resistance. Flow velocity waveforms at cardiac and venous levels change independently from arterial downstream impedance, suggesting the role of other factors, such as a time delay between change in umbilical flow and change in umbilical downstream impedance. Loy and associates[56] did not find any significant difference between normal infants and infants with IUGR for the vascular resistance response after vibroacoustic stimulation, suggesting preservation of vascular resistance regulation. The study results reaffirmed the previously noted finding, however, that the ratio of cerebral to umbilical resistance may be a more accurate test than the cerebral or umbilical artery alone to discriminate between a normal infant and an infant with IUGR.

The frequent finding of oligohydramnios with IUGR has been studied by Manning and colleagues[55] and Moore and Cayle.[56] A value of maximal vertical pocket of amniotic fluid (also called the *amniotic fluid index*) of less than 75 mm, depending on gestational age, and an amniotic fluid index of less than 50 mm, independent of gestational age, have been described in association with IUGR. Finally, a normal placenta shows signs of "aging" with increasing thickness due to calcium deposition. An increased thickness with estimated fetal weight of less than 2700 g after 36 weeks of gestation suggests IUGR.

Ultrasound also can help to distinguish a SGA infant from an infant with IUGR, using the above-mentioned fetal growth parameters, amniotic fluid volume, placental grading, and Doppler study of the umbilical arteries.[53] SGA infants, similar to normal fetuses, show an increase in umbilical blood flow accompanied by an increase in end-diastolic velocity in the Doppler waveform.[59,60] Infants with IUGR have an abnormally low umbilical arterial flow, manifested by absent or reverse end-diastolic flow. This change is the end result of placental villus dysfunction.[61,62] Todros and associates[63] showed that compared with absent or reverse end-diastolic flow, the placentas from growth-restricted fetuses with positive end-diastolic flow showed a normal pattern of stem artery development, accompanied by increased capillary angiogenesis and terminal villus development, suggesting an adaptive pathway for the placenta in the face of uteroplacental ischemia. Gardeil and colleagues[64] detected IUGR prenatally in 76% of infants whose birth weight was less than the 10th percentile at 38 weeks of gestation by using a cutoff point of 5 mm of subcutaneous fetal abdominal fat. Abnormal results also were associated with low ponderal index results. This simple and fast technique does not have significant value if used alone, but it could be used as a screening test to enhance existing sonographic measurements.

Postnatal Diagnosis

IUGR can appear as a total surprise after birth in cases of poor or no prenatal care or after its development in late gestation. An infant whose growth parameters fall into the AGA category still can be diagnosed with relative IUGR. Infants born at 37 to 38 weeks of gestation with a birth weight of 2900 g, whose parents previously had infants born at the same gestational age with birth weights of 3200 to 3700 g, have relative IUGR. These infants, although they fit into the AGA group for weight, still exhibit restriction of intrauterine growth by failing to achieve an average weight according to race and gender already set by two previous siblings. The pediatrician or any other caregiver is responsible for diagnosing IUGR as soon as possible after birth so that the specific complications can be anticipated and managed appropriately.

The postnatal diagnosis of IUGR consists of plotting birth weight, length, and head circumference on one of the several available growth charts, after gestational age has been established accurately. A final diagnosis cannot be made, however, without ascertaining certain clinical features (Box 11-1). The introduction of a modified scoring system for gestational age by Ballard and colleagues[25] for extremely premature infants has addressed this important issue with some accuracy. Other practical limitations of growth charts were described earlier, however. Infants classified as IUGR according to the gestational age–specific weight, height, and HC who fail to show the clinical features of IUGR should be diagnosed SGA rather than IUGR.

CLINICAL FEATURES

Some or all of the features listed in Box 11-1 are present to various extents in IUGR infants.

Box 11–1	Clinical Features of Intrauterine Growth Restriction

Relatively large head compared with whole body

Shrunken abdomen with "scaphoid" appearance (must be distinguished from diaphragmatic hernia)

Loose skin, sometimes dry, peeling with the appearance of "hanging," occasionally meconium stained

Long fingernails, especially in term and post-term infants with severe intrauterine growth restriction, occasionally meconium stained

Face with shrunken appearance or wizened

Widened or overriding cranial sutures, anterior fontanelle larger than usual

Thin umbilical cord, sometimes meconium stained

TYPES

Two types of IUGR traditionally have been described—symmetric (or non–head sparing) and asymmetric (or head sparing)—although overlap does exist (Table 11-3). A simple approach to comprehend these two types lies in the appreciation of the fact that the process of intrauterine growth comprises three continuous stages of hyperplasia, hyperplasia and hypertrophy, and hypertrophy (Table 11-4). The timing and the extent of the restriction in growth lead to one of these types. Two varieties of growth restriction in reference to the growth curves obtained for the BPD have been described. In the *late flattening (asymmetric)* type, BPD remained normal until flattening was noted in late gestation (HC = height × weight). The *low profile (symmetric)* type showed abnormally low BPD from the beginning of gestation. BPD is proportionally decreased compared with the weight and length in the latter type.

The ponderal index, a measurement of soft tissue and muscle mass, commonly is used to differentiate between these two varieties because it is unaffected by race, gender, or menstrual age. Judicious use of this index can identify infants who are nutritionally deprived with poor subcutaneous tissue.

$$\text{Ponderal index} = \text{body weight (g)} \times [100/\text{crown-heel length (cm)}]$$
$$\text{Normal} = 2.32 - 2.85\ (2.32 = \text{thin AGA},$$
$$2.85 = \text{obese AGA})$$

Also, measurement of the severity of asymmetric IUGR infants can be assessed because the closer the ponderal index is to 2.32, the less the sparing of the head. A normal birth weight may be found in an infant who still may have an abnormal ponderal index. In the combined type of IUGR, infants may have skeletal shortening.

ETIOLOGY

Categorization of numerous causes for IUGR into a few groups is difficult. For convenience, the causes can be divided broadly into fetal, maternal, and placental factors (Table 11-5). Penrose and Penrose[65] and Polani[66] estimated that approximately 40% of the total birth weight variation is due to maternal and fetal genetic factors (approximately half in each), and the rest is due to fetal environment.

Fetal Factors

Epidemiologic Variables

In any population, 20% of birth weight variability can be attributed to fetal genotype, as noted by the studies of

Table 11-3. Symmetric and Asymmetric Intrauterine Growth Restriction

	Symmetric	Asymmetric
Etiology	Usually intrinsic to the infant	Usually extrinsic to the infant
Affected gestation	Quite early, in first trimester	Most in third trimester, some in late second trimester onward
Body affected	Yes	Yes
Bone growth affected	Yes	No
Biparietal diameter	Low profile type	Low flattening type
Brain affected	Yes, symmetrically to body size	No (known as "brain sparing")
Ponderal index	Normal	Low
Genetic disorders	Yes	No
Risk for hypoglycemia	Low	High
Risk for perinatal asphyxia	Low	High
Blood flow in internal carotid artery	Normal	Redistribution
Maternal and fetal arterial waveform velocity	Normal	Decreased
Glycogen and fat content	Relative	Decreased
Fetal distress	No	Yes
Examples	Chromosomal disorders, genetic disorders, infectious (e.g., TORCH)	Chronic fetal distress, preeclampsia, chronic hypertension

TORCH, toxoplasmosis, rubella, cytomegalovirus, herpes simplex.

Table 11–4. Stages of Intrauterine Growth

	Hyperplasia	Hyperplasia and Hyperptrophy	Hypertrophy
Period of gestation	4-20 wk	20-28 wk	28-40 wk
Process	Active mitosis	Active mitosis, but decreasing	Slow mitosis
DNA activity	Same as protein content	Slower than protein	Protein well in excess of DNA
Others	—	—	Rapid increase of fat, muscle, and connective tissue
Result of insult	Decrease in cell number and size (symmetric type)	Decrease in cell number and size (symmetric type)	Normal cell number, but restriction of cell size (asymmetric type)

monozygotic and dizygotic twins. Girls are diagnosed more often with IUGR[67,68] than boys (15.4% versus 8.5%), being 5% (150 g) lighter and 1.2% (0.9 cm) shorter.[21,69] This gender-specific difference is not apparent, however, before 28 weeks of gestation.[2]

Genetic and Chromosomal Abnormalities

Altogether, genetic and chromosomal causes account for approximately 5% to 20% cases of IUGR, and most of them lead to the symmetric type of IUGR. Autosomal chromosomal disorders come to attention more often because all except some cases of X or Y chromosome disorders culminate in early abortions. Among the most notable are trisomy disorders (e.g., trisomies 21, 18, and 13). Trisomy 21 does not show extreme IUGR, however, and usually arises late in gestation. The other two trisomies show significant IUGR from early gestation. Minor deletion and translocation disorders also are associated with IUGR. With an increase in the number of congenital defects, the frequency of IUGR also is increased.[70] Abnormalities of fetal development and somatic growth may have a common etiology, or growth failure may

Table 11–5. Causes of Intrauterine Growth Restriction

Fetal Causes	Maternal Causes	Placental Causes
Genetic	Undernutrition	Uteroplacental vascular
Mucolipidoses	Smoking	insufficiency
Seckel syndrome	Alcohol	Essential hypertension
Cornelia de Lange syndrome	Drugs	Preeclampsia
Syndrome of hypoplastic anemia	Narcotics (heroin, cocaine,	Placental abruption
with triphalangeal thumbs	morphine, marijuana)	Diabetes mellitus
CHARGE complex	Steroids	Renal disease
Pena-Shokeir phenotype	Anticonvulsants (barbiturates,	Collagen disorders
(pseudotrisomy 18)	phenytoin, trimethadione)	Cyanotic heart disease
Chromosomal	Warfarin	
Trisomies 8,13, 18, and 21	Thalidomide	
4p syndrome	Antineoplastic agents	
5p syndrome	Isotretinoin	
13q, 18p, 18q syndromes	Lithium	
Triploidy	Chronic maternal illness	
XO	Socioeconomic status	
XXY, XXXY, XXXXY	Multiple gestation	
XXXXX		
Infectious		
TORCH		
Toxoplasmosis		
Malaria		
Syphilis		
Varicella		
Changas disease		
Inborn errors of metabolism		

make the fetus more susceptible to malformation or vice versa.[71]

Neonatal Infections

Fetal infections are responsible for 5% to 10% of cases of IUGR. Although the placenta acts as a first-line defense against organisms, some still can reach the infant. The results are most devastating when infections occur in the first trimester. Etiologically, viruses are the most frequent offenders. Although all viruses encompassing TORCHES (toxoplasmosis, rubella, cytomegalovirus, herpes, syphilis) have been implicated, direct evidence suggesting definite involvement for IUGR is available only for cytomegalovirus and rubella.[72,73] Inhibition of cell division and cell death lead to a reduction in cell number. Pathologically, cytolysis dominates the picture in both viruses. In addition, cytomegalovirus infection is characterized by obliterative angiopathy, whereas rubella shows an invasive propensity for endothelial cells.[74] The evidence for herpesvirus and human immunodeficiency virus is unclear. Among bacteria, syphilis has been implicated in IUGR. Protozoan infections caused by *Toxoplasma gondii*, *Plasmodium*, and *Trypanosoma cruzi* also can result in IUGR.

Maternal Factors

Epidemiologic Factors

Considerable differences in mean birth weight attributable to ethnicity and race have been well described[15,75] (e.g., the average birth weight in New Guinea is 2400 g versus 3800 g in the West Indies). Significant diversity is discernible even among different European nationalities.[67] The maternal height and weight also are linked to the size of the fetus,[76-80] and considerable differences of 750 g have been noted.[68] The effect of altitude is evident from underestimation of the 10th percentile of birth weights after 32 weeks of gestation and the mean birth weight after 35 weeks of gestation in the well-known Lubchenco growth charts, which were based on a Denver, Colorado, population, almost 5,000 to 10,000 feet above sea level.[2,21,23,30]

Growth retardation is diagnosed more commonly in first-born infants, typically being smaller than subsequent siblings,[68,81] with elimination of this effect by the third pregnancy.[82] This finding is in contrast to adolescent mothers, whose later born infants weigh less than the previously born sibling. The most probable explanation is the nutritional requirement by the growing adolescent mother herself, which may affect the fetus. Independent of socioeconomic factors, black[83,84] and Chinese[85,86] infants have lower mean birth weights and higher rates of low birth weight than white infants.

Multiple Gestations

McKeown and Record[87] described the decrease in mean birth weight with increasing number, noticeable after 30 weeks of gestation[23] and in multiple gestations.[87] Twin gestations contribute to 3% or less of cases of IUGR because the incidence of multiple gestations is less than 1%. Finding appropriate catch-up growth in mildly growth-restricted twins at 1 year reaffirms the inability of the internal maternal milieu to provide appropriate nutrition to the fetus, rather than fetal inability for full expression of the growth potential.

Hypoxia

Hypoxia and ischemia, localized or generalized, can engender IUGR. This effect can be seen in maternal cyanotic heart disease, pulmonary diseases, and hemoglobinopathies. Similarly, hypoxia noted in nonindigenous women moving to altitudes higher than 10,000 feet have resulted in clinically significant reduction in birth weight, with associated placental hypertrophy as a compensatory mechanism.[88,89]

Smoking, Alcohol, and Drugs

It is estimated that approximately 10% of pregnant women regularly abuse drugs, and mothers frequently abuse more than one drug. It is difficult to estimate the relative share and the exact mechanism for IUGR with any specific drug. Nonetheless, alcohol, cigarette smoking, and cocaine have been studied extensively. Cigarette smoking occurs in 25% of pregnancies in the United States, with an increased risk of IUGR 2.4 times higher than the nonsmoking population. An average reduction in birth weight of 170 g and 300 g have been reported with cigarette smoking of 10 and 15 cigarettes per day respectively. In the United States, 65% of fetuses are exposed to alcohol during pregnancy, with abuse occurring in approximately 11%. Fetal alcohol syndrome with poor postnatal growth indicates the effect of alcohol on the reduction of the number of fetal cells in early pregnancy. Cocaine has been implicated in uterine vasospasm and reduced fetal blood flow. The variables of poor socioeconomic status and poor or no prenatal care also are present in most cases and are considered significant contributors to poor growth in utero.

Hypertensive and Autoimmune Disorders

Vascular disorders encompassing autoimmune disease, associated with lupus eythematosus, chronic hypertension, pregnancy-induced hypertension, preeclampsia and eclampsia, and insulin-dependent diabetes mellitus, are well established as causes of IUGR. Associated abnormalities depend on the cause: vascular insufficiency in advanced diabetes mellitus, attenuated trophoblastic invasion in pregnancy-induced hypertension, and decreased uteroplacental flow. Disorders of hypertension are of special importance because of their relative frequency. Preeclampsia is seen in 6% to 8% of all pregnancies with significantly high maternal and fetal mortality rates of 0.5% to 17% and 8% to 17%. Fetal growth is not jeopardized if chronic hypertension is well controlled. Pregnancy-induced hypertension, even before it becomes clinically significant, potentially can affect fetal growth, which can be appreciated by reduced uterine blood flow with Doppler studies. The effect of maternal hyperglycemia in moderate diabetes mellitus without major vascular involvement results in an increased birth weight—an effect offset by the vascular pathology seen in severe diabetes mellitus, which results in IUGR.

Inadequate Maternal Nutrition

Adverse environmental conditions associated with poor socioeconomic status usually lead to poor prepregnancy maternal nutrition, bad nutritional habits, late or no prenatal care, and drug abuse. All are known etiologic factors for IUGR. Augmentation in birth weight is possible with improvement of the environmental status and nutrition, as noticed in Japanese infants born to mothers with better nutrition and living conditions after the war.

The first-trimester fetal nutritional requirements, which are insignificant in amount because the fetus is quite small, almost always are fulfilled by maternal nutrition reserves. Exceptions occur in cases of severe preconceptional maternal malnutrition and prolongation of this status. A 400- to 600-g difference in birth weight was observed in the Leningrad famine with poor maternal intake. The results of the Holland famine have shown that the most noticeable reduction in birth weight occurred when fetuses were deprived of adequate nutrition in the third trimester, the trimester of maximal fetal growth. Prepregnancy weight and weight gain during pregnancy are important determining factors. These factors remain independent of each other. Prepregnancy body mass index has been used by many clinicians to reduce the risk of IUGR by determining the target weight gain during pregnancy, excluding obese mothers.

Caloric amount, rather than protein provision, is thought to be more important for intrauterine growth.[90] Increased fetal adiposity without increase in length, HC, or muscle mass is noted with increased caloric intake. Contrary to expectation, delayed fetal growth has been reported with increased protein intake.[91] Although improper nutrition does not play a significant role in the United States, reduction in low birth weight rate from 28% to 5% was noted in Gambia when mothers had positive caloric balance.[92] Decreased serum levels of zinc[93-95] and folate[96] have been associated with IUGR in some studies.

The "selfish mother hypothesis" is the opposite of one of the adaptations seen in a normal pregnancy. Normally, insulin resistance occurs in the late trimester to satisfy the increased fetal growth by facilitating the decreased use of maternal substrate uptake and their divergence to the fetus. This alteration from the norm leads to deposition of glycogen and fat in the fetus. Placental somatomammotropin, a lipolytic hormone, rapidly mobilizes free fatty acids and ketone bodies to serve as alternate substrate during fasting periods. Obese mothers and some mothers with insulin resistance exhibit the selfish mother hypothesis, with fasting hypoglycemia and flattened glucose clearance. The end result is the use of the ingested calories or their deposition into maternal tissues, rather their transfer to the fetus, leading to IUGR.[97,98]

Placental Factors

Placental growth and maturity herald fetal growth except in late gestation, when simultaneous decline in placental growth is observed with equivalently attenuated fetal weight gain, suggesting placental function decline.[99] A correlation exists between the birth weight and placental weight and villous surface area. In all but a few cases, a small placenta is considered synonymous with IUGR. The abnormality may be noted in weight only or may be found with associated vascular abnormalities. Not all placentas of affected infants show gross or histologic abnormalities, however.

The supply of the nutrients, oxygen, and hormones through the "placental bridge" can be influenced significantly by various physical and anatomic abnormalities. A common pathology in early gestation leading to IUGR is the attenuation of cytotrophoblast invasion or its abnormal differentiation, both of which lead to decreased uteroplacental blood flow. Uteroplacental flow-velocity waveform studies in hypertensive mothers have been used to diagnose abnormal waveforms, denoting abnormally increased resistance to blood flow. As noted by Easterling and associates,[100] high-resistance hypertension is much more likely to produce low birth weight compared with low-resistance hypertension. An adversely affected syncytiotrophoblast in late pregnancy can cause decreased production of human placental lactogen, leading to poor fetal growth as a result of failure of stimulation of insulin-like growth factor and lack of availability of nutrient substrates.

COMPLICATIONS

Neonatal Complications

Perinatal Asphyxia

Infants with IUGR remain at high risk for one or all of the neonatal asphyxial syndromes during labor. They are incapable of sustaining brief periods of hypoxia associated with labor contractions, which otherwise are well tolerated by unaffected infants, because their internal milieu already is compromised by chronic intrauterine hypoxia. If recognized early enough, the infant might be delivered before a precarious situation develops. Severe cases or poor recognition of IUGR may result in fetal demise, and autopsy readily shows the involved pathology. Low and associates[101] showed that approximately 50% of IUGR infants show signs of acidosis at the time of delivery. Involvement of an expert team capable of handling these difficult cases cannot be overemphasized.

Hypothermia

Although the IUGR infant may be hyperthermic in utero owing to placental insufficiency, the infant remains at risk of hypothermia after birth. These infants have low reserves of brown fat, although they show normal responses to cold by increased muscular activity and catecholamine (norepinephrine) release. These responses may be abolished by central nervous system depression, however, frequently present in these infants. Further attenuation of heat production occurs if hypoxia and hypoglycemia are concomitantly present. These infants also possess an increased surface area-to-body mass ratio. Collectively, these factors lead to significant decreases in temperature after birth.[102]

Polycythemia and Hyperviscosity

Goldberg and colleagues[103] and Humbert and associates[104] reported that a central hematocrit value of greater than 60% is found in about 50% term SGA infants, and approximately 17% have hematocrit values greater than 65% compared with 5% in AGA term infants. Various explanations for this finding include an increase in erythropoietin levels[105-107] and maternal-fetal transfusion, secondary to chronic hypoxia. Even when true polycythemia is not present, these infants have hematocrit levels higher than normal.[107] The end result is the increased propensity for sludging of red blood cells in the microvasculature and decreased perfusion. This process can affect any body tissue, but necrotizing enterocolitis,[108] presumably due to associated mesenteric blood flow changes, can be particularly devastating in this condition.

Miscellaneous Complications

Abnormalities have been detected in the polymorphonuclear and the lymphocyte cell lines. These abnormalities may persist into childhood, rendering theses children more susceptible to infections. Quantitative and qualitative functions are depressed in the lymphocytes. Placental insufficiency, leading to poor transfer of antibody, is presumed to be responsible for the abnormally low levels of IgG.[109] The augmented levels of IgM, if present, suggest fetal infection, being produced by the fetus itself instead of being transported across the placenta. Reduction in thymic tissue is noted in 50% of infants, and peripheral T lymphocytes are reduced.[110] Chandra[111] and Pittard and coworkers[112] described the impaired cutaneous hypersensitivity and phytohemagglutinin responses, which are qualitative abnormalities of T lymphocytes. Attenuated chemotaxis and bactericidal activity have been shown by Prokopowicz and associates.[113]

Long-Term Complications

Growth Potential

A generalized observation for infants with IUGR regarding postnatal growth is that they tend to be slimmer and shorter than other infants, and their growth pattern correlates with the birth weight and length.[114-118] Previous studies have shown that term infants with asymmetric IUGR do show catch-up growth,[119-121] but some of these infants were diagnosed with IUGR on the basis of low ponderal index despite normal birth weight. Some authors have shown

that height and weight of asymmetrically growth-restricted infants remained low in midchildhood.[122] It is difficult to interpret these results when all of them do not follow the same defining criteria. Strauss and Dietz,[123] after evaluating 55,760 infants at gestational age more than 37 weeks enrolled in the National Collaborative Perinatal Project, showed that height and weight of infants born with IUGR at 7 years of age remained 0.5 SD less than infants born without IUGR. These investigators concluded that long-term growth deficits associated with IUGR are largely independent of prenatal or postnatal environmental factors. They were unable to document any difference in body proportionality between infants with IUGR who approached their sibling's growth and infants who did not. In addition, it was shown previously that body proportionality may not always be a reliable predictor of future growth potential.[124,125]

Neurologic Complications

Identifying IUGR as an isolated cause for neurodevelopmental problems is arduous because it is almost impossible to separate infants with IUGR from the diagnoses, which themselves can lead to neurologic problems. Some studies have shown minimal difference in IQ changes after exclusion of infections and anomalies as etiologies.[126-128] Most other studies without the removal of these confounding variables showed problems in school performance and behavior, however.[127,129-137] Prognosis is especially poor if IUGR is associated with prematurity.[128,138-140] Poor developmental outcome[124,133,141-143] has been associated with IUGR that involves poor head growth (symmetric type). HC remains a strong predictor of subsequent neurologic development. Impairments of verbal outcome,[142] visual recognition memory,[141] and general neurodevelopmental outcome[143] have been found to be altered at 7 years. Cognitive disabilities (e.g., problematic recognition memory) are seen more frequently than motor disabilities.[141] In 1997, Goldenburg and associates[144] showed a difference in IQ of an average of 3.3% less in infants with IUGR at 5 years of age compared with AGA infants, becoming more pronounced with 6.6% lower scores on standard intelligence tests in cases of combined IUGR and prematurity. Strauss and Dietz,[123]

Table 11–6. Fetal, Neonatal/Infancy, and Adult Disorders That Might Result from Fetal Programming as a Consequence of Fetal Undernutrition at Different States of Gestation

	First Trimester	Second Trimester	Third Trimester
Consequences	Low growth trajectory	Disturbed fetal-placental relationships	Brain growth sustained, but not body
Fetal adaptation	Down-regulation of fetal growth	Insulin resistance	Growth factor(s) resistance/deficiency
Anthropometry	Symmetric	Mixed	Asymmetric
Infant growth	Reduced infant growth	Reduced infant growth	Catch-up growth possible
Adult life	Increased BP	Increased BP, NIDDM. ischemic heart disease	Increased BP, NIDDM, hypercholesterolemia, ischemic heart disease

BP, blood pressure: NIDDM, non–insulin-dependent diabetes mellitus.

From Barker D: Mothers, Babies, and Diseases Later in Life. London, BMJ Books, 1994.

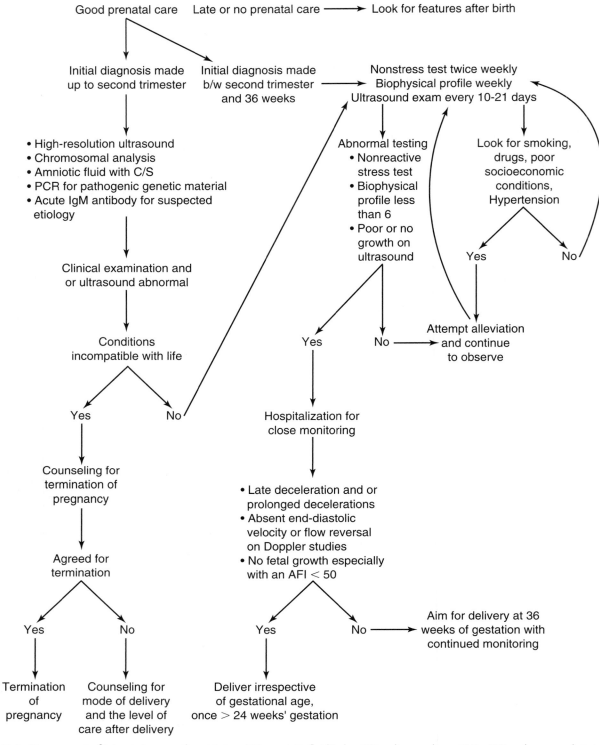

Figure 11–3. Management of intrauterine growth restriction. AFI, amniotic fluid index; C/S, culture and sensitivity; PCR, polymerase chain reaction.

after eradicating the confounding variables of genetic and environmental factors, concluded that IQ and Bender-Gestalt scores were significantly lower in infants with IUGR compared with IQ in infants born without IUGR. There were no significant differences in IQ or Bender-Gestalt scores between siblings born with and without IUGR. IUGR had little impact on intelligence and motor development except when associated with large deficits in HC. The tests used in this study lacked sufficient specificity and sensitivity, however, to identify subtle effects, such as spatial working memory, recognition memory, or memory strategy, which may be important in school performance even when no significant deficiency in IQ exists. The question of normality of neurodevelopment in the presence of head sparing remains unanswered. Until more conclusive study results are available, it would be judicious to follow these infants closely.

Complications Later in Life

Miscellaneous complications noted later in life,[145-151] with poorly defined mechanisms, are summarized in Table 11-6.

MANAGEMENT

A simple management scheme is not possible to define, owing to the many etiologies associated with IUGR. The specific management is focused toward eradication or alleviation of the cause in each case. When diagnosed, depending on the etiology, gestational age, and status of the fetus, the crucial decision of allowing the pregnancy to proceed versus delivering the infant has been facilitated greatly with the sophisticated technology of ultrasound and improved obstetric care. Close surveillance is required with the ultimate goal of delivering an infant as close to term gestation as possible except in conditions incompatible with life, in which case termination of pregnancy is considered. In general, cases of asymmetric IUGR are more amenable to favorable response and good prognosis with intervention than the symmetric type. The asymmetric type, occurring later in gestation, usually does not involve chromosomal, genetic, or infectious causes (common causes of symmetric type), for which little management could be offered, despite early diagnosis.

Infants with IUGR preferably should be delivered in centers where a team of obstetricians, neonatologists, and nursing staff is familiar with the management of these high-risk infants. An overview of the management scheme is presented in an algorithm in Figure 11-3.

REFERENCES

1. Yloppo A: Das Wachstum der Fruhgeborenen von des Geburt biszum Schulater. Z Kinderhielkd 24:111, 1919.
2. Lubchenco LO, Hausman C, Dressler M, et al: Intrauterine growth as estimated from liveborn birth-weight data at 24 to 42 weeks gestation. Pediatrics 32:793, 1963.
3. Ott WJ: The diagnosis of altered fetal growth. Obstet Gynecol Clin North Am 15:237, 1988.
4. Cassidy G: The small-for-date infant. In Avery GB (ed): Neonatology: Pathophysiology and Management of the Newborn. Philadelphia, JB Lippincott, 1981, p 263.
5. Wilcox AJ: Intrauterine growth retardation: Beyond birth weight criteria. Early Hum Dev 8:189, 1983.
6. Galbraith RS, Karchman EJ, Piercy WN, et al: The clinical prediction of intrauterine growth retardation. Am J Obstet Gynecol 133:281, 1979.
7. Gruenwald P: Chronic fetal distress and fetal insufficiency. Biol Neonate 5:215, 1963.
8. Scott KE, Usher R: Fetal malnutrition: Its incidence, causes and effects. Am J Obstet Gynecol 94:951, 1966.
9. Lugo G, Cassady G: Intrauterine growth retardation: Clinicopathological findings in 233 consecutive infants. Am J Obstet Gynecol 109:615, 1971.
10. Kramer M: Determinants of low birth weights: Methodological assessment and meta-analysis. Bull World Health Organ 65:663, 1987.
11. Erhardt CL, Joshi GB, Nelson FG, et al: Influence of weight and gestation on perinatal and neonatal mortality by ethnic group. Am J Public Health 54:1841, 1964.
12. Manra LR: Intrapartum fetal morbidity and mortality in intrauterine growth retarded infants. J Am Osteopath Assoc 80:101, 1980.
13. Morrison I, Olsen J: Weight-specific still births and associated causes of death: An analysis of 765 stillbirths. Am J Obstet Gynecol 152:975, 1985.
14. Piper JM, Xenakis EM-J: Do growth-retarded premature infants have different rates of perinatal morbidity and mortality than appropriately grown premature infants? Obstet Gynecol 87:169, 1996.
15. Meredith HV: Body weight at birth of viable human infants: A worldwide comparative treatise. Hum Biol 42:217, 1970.
16. Villar J, Belzian JM: The relative contribution of prematurity and fetal growth retardation in low birth weight in developing and developed societies. Am J Obstet Gynecol 143:793, 1982.
17. Mellin GW: Fetal life tables: A means of establishing perinatal rates of risk. JAMA 180:91, 1962.
18. Sciscione AC, Gorman R, Callan NA, et al: Adjustment of birth weight standards for maternal and infant characteristics improves the prediction of outcome in the small-for-gestational age infant. Am J Obstet Gynecol 175:544, 1996.
19. Lubchenco LO, et al: Clinical estimation of gestational age. In Kempe CH (ed): Current Pediatrics Diagnosis and Treatment. Los Altos, CA, Lange, 1974.
20. Lubchenco LO, et al: The High Risk Infant. Philadelphia, WB Saunders, 1976, pp 65-68.
21. Usher RH, McLean F: Intrauterine growth of live born Caucasian infants at sea level: Standards obtained from measurements in 7 dimensions of infants born between 25 and 44 weeks. J Pediatr 74:901, 1969.
22. Babson SG, Benda GI: Growth curves for the clinical assessment of infants of varying gestational age. J Pediatr 89:814, 1976.
23. Gruenwald P: Growth of human fetus: I. Normal growth and its variation. Am J Obstet Gynecol 94:112, 1966.
24. Ballard JL, Novak KK, Driver M: A simplified score for assessment of fetal maturation of early newborn infants. J Pediatr 95:769, 1979.
25. Ballard JL, Khoury JC, Wedig K, et al. New Ballard score, expanded to include extremely premature infants. J Pediatr 119:417, 1991.
26. Dubowitz LM, Dubowitz V, Goldberg C: Clinical assessment of gestational age in the newborn infant. J Pediatr 77:1, 1970.
27. Riddle W, et al: Interpolation of growth curves. Poster No. 1825, Poster presentation at the Society of Pediatric Research, Boston, April 30, 2001.

28. Arias F: The diagnosis and management of intrauterine growth retardation. Obstet Gynecol 49:293, 1977.

29. Battaglia FC: Intrauterine growth retardation. Am J Obstet Gynecol 106:1103, 1970.

30. Battaglia FC, Lubchenco LO: A practical classification of newborn infants by weight and gestational age. J Pediatr 71:159, 1967.

31. Belizan J, Villar JC, Nardin JC, et al: Diagnosis of intrauterine growth retardation by a simple clinical method: Measurement of uterine height. Am J Obstet Gynecol 131:643, 1978.

32. Casalino M: Intrauterine growth retardation: A neonatologist approach. J Reprod Med 14:248, 1975.

33. Croall J, Sheriff S, Matthew J: Non-pregnant plasma volume and fetal growth retardation. Br J Obstet Gynaecol 85:90, 1978.

34. Hill DE: Physical growth and development after intrauterine growth retardation. J Reprod Med 21:343, 1978.

35. Hobbins JC, Berkowitz RL, Grannum PAT: Ultrasonography and the diagnosis of IUGR. Clin Obstet Gynecol 20:957, 1977.

36. Koops BL: Neurologic sequelae in infants with intrauterine growth retardation. Am J Obstet Gynecol 106:1103, 1970.

37. Little D, Campbell S: Ultrasound evaluation of intrauterine growth retardation. Radiol Clin North Am 20:335, 1982.

38. Redmond GP: Effect of drugs on intrauterine growth. Clin Perinatol 6:5, 1979.

39. Walther FJ, Ramackers LHJ: Development aspects of subacute fetal distress—behavior problems and dysfunction. Early Hum Dev 6:1, 1982.

40. Chandra RK: Fetal malnutrition and postnatal immunocompetence. Am J Dis Child 129:450, 1975.

41. Daikoku NH, Johnson JW, Graf C, et al: Patterns of intrauterine growth retardation. Obstet Gynecol 54:211, 1979.

42. Daikoku NH, Tyson JE, Graf C, et al: The relative significance of human placental lactogen in the diagnosis retarded fetal growth. Am J Obstet Gynecol 135:516, 1979.

43. Jones RAK, Robertson NRC: Problems of the small-for-dates baby. Clin Obstet Gynecol 11:499, 1984.

44. Starfield B, Shapiro S, McCormick M, et al: Mortality and morbidity in infants with intrauterine growth retardation. J Pediatr 101:978, 1982.

45. Beischer NA, Brown JB: Current status of estrogen assays in obstetrics and gynecology: II. Estrogen assays in late pregnancy. Obstet Gynecol 27:303, 1972.

46. Klopper A: The diagnosis of growth retardation by biochemical methods. Clin Obstet Gynecol 11:437, 1984.

47. Spellacy WN, Buhi WC: Human placental lactogen and intrauterine growth retardation. Obstet Gynecol 97:446, 1976.

48. Midonik M, Lavin JP, Gimmon Z, et al: The use of amniotic fluid 3-methyl histidine to creatinine molar ratio for the diagnosis of intrauterine growth retardation. Obstet Gynecol 60:288, 1982.

49. Lin CC, Moawad AH, River P, et al: Amniotic C-peptide as an index for intrauterine fetal growth. Am J Obstet Gynecol 139:390, 1981.

50. Gordon YB, Grudzinskas JG, Jeffrey D, et al: Concentration of pregnancy-specific beta$_1$-glycoprotein in maternal blood in normal pregnancy and intrauterine growth retardation. Lancet 1:331, 1977.

51. Khouzami UA, Ginsburg DS, Daikoku NH, et al: The glucose tolerance test as a means of identifying intrauterine growth retardation. Am J Obstet Gynecol 139:423, 1981.

52. Sher G, Statland BE, Knutzen VR: Evaluation of small third trimester fetuses using foam stability index. Obstet Gynecol 58:314, 1981.

53. Kingdom JCP, Burrell SJ, et al: Pathology and clinical implications of abnormal umbilical artery Doppler waveforms. Ultrasound Obstet Gynecol 9:271, 1997.

54. Valacamonico A, Danti L, Frusca T, et al: Absent end-diastolic velocity in umbilical artery: Risk of neonatal morbidity and brain damage. Am J Obstet Gynecol 170:796, 1994.

55. Splunder P, et al: Fetal atrioventricular, venous, and arterial flow velocity waveforms in the small for gestational age fetus. Pediatr Res 42:765, 1997.

56. Loy GL, Lin CC, Chien EK, et al: Cerebral and umbilical vascular resistance response to vibroacoustic stimulation in growth restricted fetuses. Obstet Gynecol 90:947, 1997.

57. Manning FA, Hill LM, Platt LD: Qualitative amniotic fluid volume determination by ultrasound: Antepartum detection of intrauterine growth retardation. Am J Obstet Gynecol 139:254, 1981.

58. Moore TR, Cayle JE: The amniotic fluid index in normal human pregnancy. Am J Obstet Gynecol 162:1168, 1990.

59. Hendricks S, Sorensen TK, Wang KY, et al: Doppler umbilical artery waveform indices—normal values from fourteen to forty-two weeks. Am J Obstet Gynecol 161:761, 1989.

60. Burke G, Stuart B, Crowley P, et al: Is intrauterine growth retardation with normal umbilical artery blood flow a benign condition? BMJ 300:1044, 1990.

61. Macara L, Kingdom JC, Kaufmann P, et al: Structural analysis of placental terminal villi from growth-restricted pregnancies with abnormal umbilical artery Doppler waveforms. Placenta 17:37, 1996.

62. Krebs C, Macara LM, Leiser R, et al: Intrauterine growth restriction with absent end-diastolic flow velocity in the umbilical artery is associated with maldevelopment of the placental terminal villus tree. Am J Obstet Gynecol 75:1534, 1996.

63. Todros T, Sciarrone A, Piccoli E, et al: Umbilical Doppler waveforms and placental villous angiogenesis in pregnancies complicated by fetal growth restriction. Obstet Gynecol 93:499, 1999.

64. Gardeil F, Greene R, Stuart B, et al: Subcutaneous fat in the fetal abdomen as a predictor of growth restriction. Obstet Gynecol 94:209, 1999.

65. Penrose LS, Penrose LS (eds): Recent Advances in Human Genetics. London, Churchill Livingstone, 1961.

66. Polani PE: Chromosomal and other genetic influences on birth weight variation. In Elliot K, Knight J (eds): Size at Birth. Amesterdam, Associated Scientific Publishers, 1974.

67. Keirse MJ: Epidemiology and aetiology of the growth retarded baby. Clin Obstet Gynecol 11:415, 1984.

68. Thompson FM, Billewics WC, Hytten FE: The assessment of fetal growth. J Obstet Gynaecol Br Commonw 75:903, 1968.

69. Fisher DA: Intrauterine growth retardation: Endocrine receptor aspect. Semin Perinatol 8:37, 1984.

70. Khoury MJ, Erikson JD, Cordero JF, et al: Congenital malformations and intrauterine growth retardation: A population study. Pediatrics 82:83, 1998.

71. Spiers P: Does growth retardation predispose the fetus to congenital malformation? Lancet 1:312, 1982.

72. Berge P, Stagno S, Federer W, et al: Impact of asymptomatic congenital cytomegalovirus infection size at birth and gestational duration. Pediatr Infect Dis 9:170, 1990.

73. Vorherr H: Factors influencing fetal growth. Am J Obstet Gynecol 142:577, 1982.

74. Nimrod CA: The biology of normal growth and deviant fetal growth. In Reece EA, Hobbins JC, Mahoney MJ, Petrie RH (eds): Medicine of the Fetus and Mother. Philadelphia, JB Lippincott, 1992.

75. Aubry RH, Beydun S, Cabalum MT, et al: Fetal growth retardation. In Bolognese RJ, Schawrtz RH (eds): Perinatal Medicine. Baltimore, Williams & Wilkins, 1977, p 175.

76. Casalino M: Intrauterine growth retardation—a neonatologist's approach. J Reprod Med 14:248, 1975.

77. Metcof J: Maternal nutrition and fetal development. Early Hum Dev 4:99, 1980.

78. Morton NE: The inheritance of human birth weight. Ann Hum Genet 20:125, 1955.

79. Polani PE: Chromosomal and other genetic influences on birth weight variations in size at birth. Ciba Foundation Symposium 27. Amsterdam, Excerpta Medica, 1974, pp 127-160.

80. Walton A, Hammond J: The maternal effects on growth and confirmation in Shire horse–Shetland pony crosses. Proc R Soc G Brit 125:311, 1938.

81. Smith DW: Clinical Approach to Deformation Problems: Recognizable Patterns of Human Deformation. Philadelphia, WB Saunders, 1981, p 101.

82. Camilleri AP, Cremona V: The effect of parity on birth weight. J Obstet Gynaecol Br Commonw 77:145-147, 1970.

83. David R: Race, birth weight, and mortality rate. J Pediatr 116:19, 1990.

84. Kleinman JC, Kessel SS: Racial differences in low birth weight: Trends and risk factors. N Engl J Med 317:749, 1987.

85. Cheng MCE, Chew PCT, Ratnam SS: Birthweight distribution of Singapore Chinese, Malay and Indian infants from 34 weeks to 42 weeks gestation. J Obstet Gynaecol Br Commonw 79:149, 1972.

86. Yip R, Li Z, Wan-Hwa C: Race and birth weight: The Chinese example. Pediatrics 87:688, 1991.

87. McKeown R, Record RG: Observation of fetal growth in multiple pregnancy in man. J Endocrinol 8:386, 1952.

88. Yip R: Altitude and birth weight. J Pediatr 111:869, 1987.

89. Lichty JA, Ting RY, Bruns PD, et al: Studies of babies born at high altitude. Am J Dis Child 93:666, 1957.

90. Stein Z, Susser M, Rush D: Prenatal nutrition and birth weight: Experiments and quasi-experiments in the past decade. J Reprod Med 21:287, 1987.

91. Rush D, Stein Z, Susser M: A randomized controlled trial of prenatal nutritional supplementation in New York City. Pediatrics 68:783, 1980.

92. Prentice AM, Whitehead RG, Watkinson M, et al: Prenatal dietary supplementation of African women and birth weight. Lancet 1:489, 1983.

93. Meadows NJ, Ruse W, Smith MF, et al: Zinc and small babies. Lancet 2:1135, 1981.

94. Wells JL, James DK, Luzton R, et al: Maternal leukocyte zinc deficiency at start of third trimester as a predictor of fetal growth retardation. BMJ 294:1054, 1987.

95. Neggers YH, Cutter JR, Alvarez JO, et al: The relationship between maternal serum zinc levels during pregnancy and birthweight. Early Hum Dev 25:75, 1991.

96. Goldenberg RL, Tamura T, Cliver SP, et al: Serum folate and fetal growth retardation: A matter of compliance? Obstet Gynecol 79:71, 1992.

97. Abell DA, Beischer NA: The relationship between maternal glucose tolerance and fetal size at birth. Aust N Z J Obstet Gynaecol 16:1, 1976.

98. Langer O, Damus K, Maiman M, et al: A link between relative hypoglycemia-hypoinsulinemia during oral glucose tolerance tests and intrauterine growth retardation. Am J Obstet Gynecol 155:711, 1986.

99. Molteni RA, Stys SJ, Battaglia FC: Relationship of fetal and placental weight in human beings: Fetal/placental weight ratios at various gestational ages and birth weight distributions. Reprod Med 152:975, 1978.

100. Easterling TR, Benedetti TJ, Carlson, KC, et al: The effect of maternal hemodynamics on fetal growth in hypertensive pregnancies. Am J Obstet Gynecol 165:902, 1991.

101. Low JA, Boston RW: Fetal asphyxia during the antepartum period in intrauterine growth retarded infants. Am J Obstet Gynecol 113:351, 1972.

102. Sinclai J: Heat production and thermoregulation in the small for date infant. Pediatr Clin North Am 17:147, 1970.

103. Wirth FH, Goldberg KE: Neonatal hyperviscosity, incidence and effect of partial plasma exchange transfusion [abstract]. Pediatr Res 19:372, 1975.

104. Humbert JR, Abelson JH: Polycythemia in small for gestational age infants. J Pediatr 75:812, 1969.

105. Meberg A: Hematologic syndrome of growth-retarded infants. Am J Dis Child 143:1260, 1947.

106. Cassady G: Body composition in intrauterine growth retardation. Pediatr Clin North Am 17:79, 1970.

107. Snijders RJM, Abbas A, Melby O, et al: Fetal plasma erythropoietin concentration in severe growth retardation. Am J Obstet Gynecol 168:615, 1993.

108. Hackett GA, Canpbell S, Gamsu H, et al: Doppler studies in the growth retarded fetus and prediction of neonatal necrotizing enterocolitis, haemorrhage and neonatal morbidity. BMJ 294:13, 1987.

109. Ferguson S: Prolonged impairment of cellular immunity in children with intrauterine growth retardation. J Pediatr 93:52, 1978.

110. Chandra RK, Matsumura T: Ontogenic development of the immune system and effects of fetal growth retardation. J Perinat Med 7:279, 1979.

111. Chandra RK: Immunocompetence in low birth weight infants after intrauterine malnutrition. J Perinat Med 7:279, 1979.

112. Pittard WB 3rd, Miller K, Sorenson RU, et al: Normal lymphocyte response to mitogen in term and premature neonates following normal and abnormal intrauterine growth. Clin Immunol Immunopathol 30:178, 1984.

113. Prokopowicz J, Ziobro J, Iwaszko-Krawczuk W: Bactericidal capacity of plasma and granulocytes in small-for-dates newborns. Acta Paediatr Acad Sci Hung 16:267, 1975.

114. Binkin NJ, Yip R, Fleshood L, Trowbridge FL et al: Birth weight and childhood growth. Pediatrics 82:828, 1988.

115. Fitzhardinge PN, Inwood S: Long-term growth in small-for-age date children. Acta Pediatr Scand (Suppl) 27:349, 1989.

116. Walther FJ: Growth and development of term disproportionate small-for-age gestational age infants at the age of 7 years. Hum Dev 18:1, 1988.

117. Tenovuo A, Piekkala P, Kero P: Growth of 519 small for gestational age infants during the first two years of life. Acta Pediatr Scand 76:636, 1987.

118. Piekkala P, Kero P, Sillanpaa M, et al: The somatic growth of a regional birth cohort of 351 preterm infants durimg the first two years of life. J Perinat Med 17:41, 1989.

119. Davies DP, Platts P, Pritchard JM, et al: Nutritional status of light-for-dates infants at birth and its influence on early postnatal growth. Arch Dis Child 54:703-706, 1979.

120. Holmes GI, Miller HC, Hassanein K, et al: Postnatal somatic growth in infants with atypical fetal growth patterns. Am J Dis Child 131:1078, 1977.

121. Villar J, Smeriglio V, Martorell R, et al: Heterogeneous growth and mental development of intrauterine growth-retarded infants during the first 3 years of life. Pediatrics 74:783, 1984.

122. Walther FJ, Ramaekers LHJ: Growth in early childhood of newborns affected by disproportionate intrauterine growth retardation. Acta Pediatr Scand 71:651, 1982.

123. Strauss R, Dietz W, et al: Growth and development of term children born with low birth weight: Effects of genetic and environmental factors. J Pediatr 133:67, 1998.

124. Harvey D, Prince J, Bunton J, et al: Abilities of children who were small-for-gestational-age-babies. Pediatrics 69:296, 1982.

125. Villar J, Belzian JM: Heterogenous postnatal growth patterns of intrauterine growth retarded infants (IUGR). Am J Clin Nutr 35:860, 1982.

126. Berg AT: Childhood neurology morbidity and its association with gestational age, intrauterine growth retardation and antenatal stress. Pediatr Perinat Epidemiol 2:229, 1988.

127. Matilainen R, Heinonen K, Siren-Tiusanen H: Effect of intrauterine growth retardation (IUGR) on the psychological performance of preterm at preschool age. J Child Psychol Psychiatry 29:601, 1988.

128. Pena IC, Teberg AJ, Finello KM: The premature small for gestational age during the first year of life: Comparison by birth weight and gestational age. J Pediatr 113:1066, 1988.

129. Holst K, Anderson E, Philip J, et al: Antenatal and perinatal conditions correlated to handicap among 4-year-old children. Am J Perinatol 6:258, 1989.

130. Schauseil-Zipf U, Hamm W, Stenzel B, et al: Severe intrauterine growth retardation, obstetrical management and follow up studies in children between 1970 and 1985. J Obstet Gynaecol Reprod Biol 30:1, 1989.

131. Touwen BC, Hadders-Algra M, Huisjes HJ: Hypotonia at six years in prematurely small-for-gestational age children. Early Hum Dev 17:79, 1988.

132. Matilainen R, Heinonen K, Siren-Tiusanen H, et al: Neurodevelopmental screening of growth-retarded-prematurely born children before school. Eur J Pediatr 146:453, 1987.

133. Low JA, Galbraith RS, Muir D, et al: Intrauterine growth retardation: A study of long-term morbidity. Am J Obstet Gynecol 142:670, 1982.

134. Hill R, Verniaud WM, Deter RL, et al: The effect of intrauterine malnutrition on the term infant: A 14-year progressive study. Acta Paediatr Scand 73:482, 1984.

135. Ounsted MK, Moar VA, Scott A: Children of deviant birth weight at the age of seven years: Health, handicap, size, and developmental staus. Early Hum Dev 9:323, 1984.

136. Villar J, de Onis M, Kestler E, et al: The differential neonatal morbidity of the intrauterine growth retardation syndrome. Am J Obstet Gynecol 163:151, 1990.

137. Vohr BR, Oh W, Rosenfield AG, et al: The preterm small for gestational age infant: A two-year follow up study. Am J Obstet Gynecol 133:425, 1979.

138. Babson SG, Henderson NB: Fetal undergrowth: Relation of head growth to later intellectual performance. Pediatrics 53:890, 1974.

139. Robertson CM, Etches PC, Kyle JM: Eight-year school performance and growth of preterm, small for gestational age infants: A comparative study with subjects matched for birth weight or for gestational age. J Pediatr 116:19, 1990.

140. Ruys-Dudok van Heel I, de Leeuw R: Clinical outcome of small for gestational age preterm infants. J Perinat Med 17:77, 1989.

141. Rutstein RP, Wesson MD, Gotlieb S, Biasini FJ: Clinical comparison of the visual parameters in infants with intrauterine growth retardation vs. infants with normal birth weight. Am J Optom Physiol Opt 63:697, 1986.

142. Pollitt E, Gorman KS: Nutritional deficiencies as developmental risk factors. In Nelson CA (ed): Infants and Children at Risk: Integrating Biological, Psychological and Social Risk Factors. Minnesota Symposia on Child Psychology. Hillsdale, NJ, Lawrence Erlbaum Associates, 1994, pp 121-144.

143. Berg AT: Indices of fetal growth retardation, perinatal hypoxia and childhood neurological morbidity. Early Hum Dev 19:271, 1989.

144. Goldenburg RL, DuBard MB, Cliver SP, et al: Pregnancy outcome and intelligence at age five years. Am J Obstet Gynecol 175:1511, 1996.

145. Smart J: Undernutrition, learning and memory: Review of experimental studies. In Taylor TG, Jenkins NK (eds): Proceedings of XII International Congress of Nutrition. London, Edward Arnold, 1981, p 221.

146. Barker DJP: Fetal and infant origins of adult disease. BMJ 310:111, 1993.

147. Snoeck A, Remacle C, Reusens B, et al: Effects of a low protein diet during pregnancy on the fetal rat endocrine pancreas. Biol Neonate 57:107, 1990.

148. Dahri S, Snoeck A, Reusens B, et al: Islet function in offspring of mothers on a low protein diet during pregnancy. Diabetes 40:115, 1991.

149. Cherif H, Reusens B, Dahri S, et al: Effect of an isocaloric low protein diet during gestation on rat on an in vitro insulin secretion by islets of the offspring. Diabetologia A80:37, 1994.

150. Rasschaert J, Reusens B, Dahri S, et al: Impaired activity of rat pancreatic islet mitochondrial glycerophosphate dehydrogenase in protein malnutrition. Endocrinology 136:2631, 1995.

151. Hay WW Jr, Catz CS, Grave GD, Yaffe SJ: Workshop summary: Fetal growth—its regulation and disorders. Pediatrics 99:585, 1997.

CHAPTER 12

Hydrops Fetalis

David M. Coulter

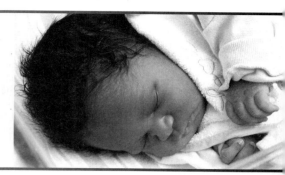

For the obstetrician and perinatologist, hydrops fetalis represents a diagnostic challenge and raises significant questions about fetal management and delivery. For the neonatologist, hydrops may also present a diagnostic dilemma and presents the prospect of a difficult delivery room resuscitation, as well as challenging and complicated management issues in the neonatal intensive care unit. This chapter addresses the extensive differential diagnosis of hydrops, its pathophysiologic mechanisms, the prognosis of hydrops, and management of the fetus and neonate with hydrops.

Fetal hydrops was first described in 1609[1] and for the next three centuries was considered a single pathologic entity. Ballantyne's pathology text, published in 1892, raised the possibility that hydrops represented a final common pathway for a number of different pathologic processes.[2] Diamond and colleagues first recognized hydrops as the consequence of severe erythroblastosis fetalis.[3] In 1943, Potter distinguished immune hydrops attributable to erythroblastosis fetalis from nonimmune hydrops, the hydrops associated with other entities.[4] Although this distinction made sense in an era in which the overwhelming majority of cases of hydrops were attributable to erythroblastosis, it is less useful now, when hemolytic disease causes relatively few cases.

DEFINITION

Hydrops fetalis, or fetal anasarca, results from the abnormal accumulation of interstitial fluid in the fetus. Its clinical spectrum ranges from small pleural effusions or ascites and minimal tissue edema to massive pleural effusions and ascites with severe edema that stiffens the extremities, obliterates facial features, and makes neonatal resuscitation impossible. There are no clear, consensus-reached criteria for ultrasound diagnosis of fetal hydrops. However, a reasonable and practical set of criteria is the presence of excess fluid in at least one potential space (pericardial or pleural fluid, or ascites) together with skin edema (>5 mm thick) or fluid in two potential spaces.[5,6]

In hydropic pregnancies, the placenta is large and edematous with swollen villi and immature-appearing fetal vessels. Sonographically, in hydrops caused by anemia, hydrops may first appear as a pericardial effusion and then progress to pleural effusions, ascites, and finally generalized edema. If the anemia is treated effectively, these changes resolve in reverse order of appearance.[7]

DIFFERENTIAL DIAGNOSIS

A broad spectrum of clinical entities is associated, presumably causally, with hydrops fetalis.[8,9] Table 12-1 lists most reported conditions.[10-25] However, some of these associations are based only on single case reports, and it should be emphasized that association does not establish causation.

Five disease processes cause 63% of all cases of hydrops: cardiovascular processes, chromosomal disorders, thoracic processes, twinning, and anemia.[8]

PATHOPHYSIOLOGY

Hydrops fetalis results from an imbalance in the movement of fluid between the vascular and extravascular spaces that results in the excessive accumulation of interstitial fluid in the fetus. Thus, the pathophysiologic process of hydrops is determined by the factors that mediate this fluid movement. Potential mechanisms include

1. Increased capillary permeability
2. Decreased plasma colloid osmotic pressure
3. Decreased lymph flow
4. Increased capillary hydrostatic pressure
5. Impaired placental clearance of excess fetal fluid

Available data implicate the first four but provide no information regarding the fifth.

Acute vascular volume expansion in the fetal sheep, a stress that should increase capillary hydrostatic pressure, is partially compensated by increased fluid flow across

Table 12–1.   Clinical Conditions Associated with Hydrops Fetalis

Maternal conditions	Diabetes
	Anemia
	Hypoproteinemia
	Thyrotoxicosis[10]
Anemia	
Hemolytic	Alloimmune
	α-Thalassemia
	Red blood cell enzyme deficiencies
Other	Fetal-maternal hemorrhage
	Twin-twin transfusion (donor)
Cardiac	Arrhythmias: supraventricular tachycardia, atrial flutter, heart block
	Structural anomalies (mainly associated with atrioventricular regurgitation): ASD, VSD, hypoplastic left heart, subaortic obstruction, aortic stenosis,[11] pulmonary valve insufficiency, Ebstein anomaly
	Cardiomyopathy
	Myocarditis
	Premature closure of foramen ovale
	Premature closure of ductus arteriosus (maternal treatment with nonsteroidal anti-inflammatory drugs)
	Myocardial tumor: teratoma, tuberous sclerosis with cardiac rhabdomyoma
	Intrapericardial teratoma
	Endocardial fibroelastosis
Infections	Viruses: cytomegalovirus, coxsackievirus, rubella, herpes simplex, human herpesvirus 6,[12] varicella, respiratory syncytial virus, parvovirus B19, adenovirus[13]
	Toxoplasmosis
	Bacterial (syphilis, *Listeria* species)
	Chagas disease
	Leptospirosis
Placental and umbilical cord abnormalities	Chorioangioma (placenta, chorionic vessels, or umbilical vessels)
	True knot of umbilical cord
	Torsion of umbilical cord
	Angiomyxoma of umbilical cord
	Aneurysm of umbilical artery
	Hemorrhagic endovasculitis of placenta
	Chorionic vein thrombosis
	Placental and umbilical vein thrombosis
Fetal vascular abnormalities	Arteriovenous malformations
	Hemangioma of liver
	Angio-osteohypertrophy (Klippel-Trenauney-Weber syndrome)
	Generalized arterial calcification
	Hemangioendothelioma
Vascular accidents	Inferior vena cava thrombosis
	Twin-twin transfusion (recipient)
	Maternal-fetal hemorrhage
Lymphatic abnormalities	Pulmonary lymphangiectasia
	Cystic hygroma
	Turner syndrome
	Noonan syndrome
	Multiple pterygium syndrome
Brain lesions	Absence of corpus callosum
	Encephalocele
	Intracranial hemorrhage
	Holoprosencephaly
Intrathoracic space-occupying lesions	Diaphragmatic hernia
	Adenomatoid malformation of lung
	Bronchogenic cyst
	Mediastinal teratoma
	Extralobar pulmonary sequestration
	Chylothorax
Gastrointestinal	Bowel obstruction: atresias, imperforate anus, volvulus
	Meconium peritonitis

Table 12–1. Clinical Conditions Associated with Hydrops Fetalis—cont'd

Renal and urinary	Congenital nephrosis (Finnish type)
	Obstructive uropathy
	Renal vein thrombosis
Neoplasms	Neuroblastoma
	Choriocarcinoma
	Sacrococcygeal teratoma
	Hepatoblastoma
	Wilms tumor[14]
Storage diseases	Glycogen storage diseases
	Lysosomal storage disorders[15]
	Mucopolysaccharidosis types IVA, VII
	Gaucher disease type 2
	Sialidosis
	GM_1 gangliosidosis
	Galactosialidosis
	Niemann-Pick disease type C
	Disseminated lipogranulomatosis (Farber disease)
	Infantile free sialic acid storage disease
	Mucolipidosis type II (type I cell disease)
	Hemochromatosis[16]
	Other
Chromosomal abnormalities	Trisomy 10, 13, 15, 16, 18, 21 mosaicism[17]
	Triploidy
	Tetraploidy
	XO
	5Q+[18]
	11p+
	12p tetrasomy (Pallister-Killian syndrome)[19]
	13q–
	17q–
	18q+
Skeletal dysplasias	Osteogenesis imperfectra
	Osteopetrosis
	Restrictive thoracic osteodystrophies
	Short-limbed dwarfism syndromes
	Greenberg dysplasia[20,21]
Neuromuscular disorders	Myotonic dystrophy
	Myopathies
Other	Bowel obstruction with perforation and meconium peritonitis
	Obstructive uropathy
	Congenital nephrosis
	Infant of a diabetic mother
	Neu-Laxova syndrome
	Congenital erythropoietic porphyria[22]
	Fryns syndrome[23]
	Cardiofaciocutaneous syndrome[24]
	Cumming syndrome[25]
	Idiopathic

ASD, atrial septal defect; VSD, ventricular septal defect.

the placenta from the fetal to the maternal vascular compartment.[26] However, after volume loading, a greater portion of the infused fluid enters the interstitial space in the fetus than in the adult animal,[27] an indication that there are fetal mechanisms that permit greater movement of fluid into the interstitium and then restrict its reuptake into the circulation.

Brace summarized factors that promote increased formation of extracellular fluid in the fetus.[28] First, substantially more fluid is filtered across fetal capillaries than across adult capillaries. Second, fetal capillaries are more permeable to proteins than are the capillaries of adult animals, leading to lower ratios between vascular and extravascular colloid oncotic pressures and thereby impairing reuptake of the excess filtered fluid into the vascular space. Third, the interstitial space of the fetus is more compliant than that of the adult; therefore, a larger amount of fluid can move into the interstitium without increasing hydrostatic pressure, a driving force for reuptake of fluid by capillaries. Thus, any stimulus that leads to increased formation of interstitial fluid in the adult has an exaggerated effect in the fetus.

Besides reuptake into capillaries, the only other avenue of egress for fluid in the fetal interstitium is via the lymphatic vessels. The increased rate of formation of interstitial fluid in the normal sheep fetus is therefore compensated by markedly increased thoracic duct lymph flow.[29] Ligation of the thoracic duct in fetal sheep caused hydrops in one of 11 animals, but excision of thoracic lymphatic vessels consistently produced hydrops.[30] There are physiologic limitations to lymphatic drainage in the fetus. Thoracic duct flow is much more sensitive to venous pressure in fetuses than it is in older animals, and flow decreases markedly with small increases in outflow pressure (Fig. 12-1).[31,32] As a result, any process that increases central venous pressure (CVP) or intrathoracic pressure in the fetus can be expected to decrease lymphatic drainage, expand the interstitial fluid compartment, and lead eventually to hydrops.

Data from animal experiments, as well as observations in human fetuses with hydrops, underscore the central role of elevated CVP in the genesis of hydrops. In the fetal sheep, inflation of a balloon in the right hemithorax increased CVP and consistently produced hydrops that resolved when the balloons were deflated.[33] Two animal models, electronically driven tachycardia[34-36] and rapidly induced anemia,[37] both in fetal sheep, illustrated the development of hydrops as venous pressure rose and

lymphatic flow fell. In fetal sheep maintained anemic (at a hematocrit of 12%) by daily partial exchange transfusions, hydrops developed in only the six animals whose CVP became elevated. Regardless of cause, most hydropic human fetuses have elevated CVP.[38] In fetuses with immune hydrops, elevated CVP was present before intrauterine transfusion and decreased to normal levels after intrauterine transfusion and resolution of hydrops.[39]

In theory, reduced plasma colloid oncotic pressure could contribute to development of hydrops, but animal data and human experience do not substantiate this possibility. A 41% reduction in total serum protein in fetal lambs produced a corresponding decrease in colloid oncotic pressure but failed to produce hydrops.[40] In the animal models of hydrops caused by tachycardia or anemia, development of hydrops was not related to changes in colloid oncotic pressure.[35,37] Many infants who are born hydropic have normal levels of serum proteins. Infants with congenital analbuminemia have decreased colloid oncotic pressure but are not born with significant edema or hydrops.[41,42]

Polyhydramnios is often a presenting sign of hydrops. Increased amniotic fluid volume could be attributed to fetal diuresis, increased fluid transport across the fetal surface of the placenta, or decreased clearance of amniotic fluid. The main source of amniotic fluid is fetal urine output. Levels of digoxin-like immunoreactive substance, a promoter of natriuresis, and of atrial natriuretic peptide are elevated in hydropic fetuses.[43] In the tachycardic fetal sheep, atrial natriuretic peptide levels increase with the development of hydrops and decrease as hydrops resolves.[44] It appears that fetal diuresis in response to expansion of fetal intravascular fluid is the cause of the polyhydramnios associated with hydrops. The roles of fluid transport across the fetal side of the placenta and altered clearance of amniotic fluid remain unexplored.

MATERNAL DIAGNOSTIC ASSESSMENT

Typically, hydrops is diagnosed during routine obstetric ultrasound examination or during ultrasound assessments indicated for evaluating polyhydramnios, pregnancy-induced hypertension, multiple gestation, or fetal arrhythmia. Referral to a perinatal center for further assessment and management is indicated. The diagnostic workup begins with careful documentation of the medical and family history and a thorough ultrasound examination, including fetal echocardiography. The goals of this evaluation are to define the extent of the hydrops and to provide an anatomic diagnosis, if possible. Other diagnostic testing is based on the early presentation and initial diagnostic testing. It may include maternal blood testing (for hemolytic disease, fetomaternal hemorrhage, hemoglobinopathies, or fetal infection), fetal electrocardiography to evaluate arrhythmia, amniocentesis (to assess possible fetal infection or chromosomal abnormalities), fetal thoracentesis (to assess possible chylothorax), and cordocentesis (to diagnose chromosomal anomalies, hemoglobinopathies, anemia, or infection, as well as to assess fetal acid-base status). Table 12-2 lists specific testing that may be useful to evaluate hydrops.

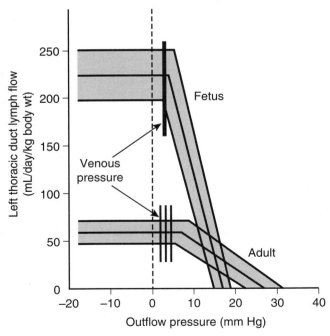

Figure 12–1. The relationship between left thoracic duct lymph flow and outflow pressure in chronically catheterized fetal and adult sheep. *Stippled area* is mean ± 2 × standard error of the mean. *(From Brace RA: Fluid distribution in the fetus and neonate. In Polin RA, Fox WW [eds]: Fetal and Neonatal Physiology, 3rd ed. Philadelphia, WB Saunders, 2004, pp 1341-1350.)*

Table 12–2. Evaluation of Fetal Hydrops

History

Age, parity, gestation
Pregnancy history
  Miscarriages, fetal demise
  Previous infants with isoimmune hemolytic disease
  Previous infants with jaundice
Medical and obstetric history
  Use of illicit drugs
  Receipt of blood products
  Transplant recipient
  Risk factors for sexually transmitted diseases
Family history
  Hereditary or metabolic diseases
  Asian or Mediterranean ancestry (risk of α-thalassemia)
Recent infections and contacts
  Occupational exposure to infants or young children
  Pet cat in household
Medications
Reason for referral

Maternal Laboratory Studies

Complete blood cell count
Blood type and indirect Coombs antibody screen
Hemoglobin electrophoresis
Kleihauer-Betke test
Infection screening: coxsackievirus, cytomegalovirus,
  rubella, parvovirus, *Toxoplasma* species, syphilis, group B
  Streptococcus, Listeria monocytogenes
Autoantibody screen: anti-Ro and anti-La
Triple screen
Oral glucose tolerance test

Amniotic Fluid Testing

Karyotype
Culture or PCR for TORCH, parvovirus

α-Fetoprotein
Restriction endonucleases (thalassemias)
Define fetal lung maturity

Fetal Studies

Detailed ultrasound study
  For anatomic abnormalities
  To evaluate extent edema and effusions
  To rule out multiple gestation
  Amniotic fluid index
  Placental morphology and thickness
  Doppler flow studies
    Umbilical artery
    Middle cerebral artery
    Tricuspid ejection velocity
Echocardiography
  Anatomy
  Arrhythmia
Fetal blood testing
  Karyotype
  Complete blood count
  Blood type and Coombs test
  Hemoglobin electrophoresis
  Blood chemistry profiles, albumin and gas
    measurements
  Metabolic testing: Tay-Sachs disease, Gaucher disease,
    gangliosidosis
  Total immunoglobulin M
  G6PD in male fetuses
  Culture or PCR for TORCH, parvovirus
Fetal fluid testing (if aspirated for therapeutic reasons)
  Culture or PCR for TORCH, parvovirus
  Biochemistry: protein
  Cell count

G6PD, glucose-6-phosphate dehydrogenase; PCR, polymerase chain reaction; TORCH, toxoplasmosis, other infections, rubella, cytomegalovirus, and herpes simplex.
Modified from Swain S, Cameron AD, McNay MB, et al: Prenatal diagnosis and management of nonimmune hydrops fetalis. Aust N Z J Obstet Gynecol 39:285, 1999.

Pregnancy Complications

A woman carrying an affected fetus may have polyhydramnios. Reduction amniocentesis decreases discomfort and respiratory distress and may prevent or treat associated preterm labor. A syndrome that resembles preeclampsia (mirror syndrome) can occur and may be the presenting sign of a hydropic pregnancy. Other complications include preterm labor, malpresentation, antepartum or postpartum hemorrhage, retained placenta, and difficulties with vaginal delivery.[1]

PROGNOSIS

The prognosis of hydrops fetalis diagnosed in utero remains quite bleak. It depends in part on gestational age at diagnosis, probably because more severe fetal abnormalities tend to produce hydrops earlier in gestation.[45] This observation is also explained by the technical difficulties of effective interventional fetal therapy very early

in gestation. The prognosis also depends on fetal condition at the time of diagnosis; more severely affected fetuses are more likely to die. Beyond these issues, the prognosis depends almost entirely on the underlying diagnosis and the degree of prematurity at delivery. Mortality rates of infants in whom hydrops was diagnosed in utero ranged from 50% to 98% in older reported series[46] and from 51% to 87% in recent reports.[47,48] This variability probably reflects both the diagnostic composition of the reported group and evolving standards of care. An undefined portion of this mortality is attributable to pregnancy terminations, 65% in one reported series.[49]

Spontaneous resolution can occur. Some causes of hydrops are amenable to intrauterine therapy. Hemolytic anemias and the anemia caused by parvovirus[50,51] can be effectively treated by intrauterine transfusions, with resolution of the hydrops and a probability of delivering a healthy infant near term. Similarly, cardiac tachyarrhythmias in the absence of structural heart disease usually respond well to intrauterine therapy and carry a good prognosis.

Other authors have reported very high neonatal mortality rates among infants with idiopathic nonimmune hydrops. However, I have observed that virtually all "idiopathic" cases referred to our tertiary care center are caused by chylothorax. This problem was not recognized as a cause of hydrops in many older reports. It can be palliated in utero by thoracoamniotic shunting.[52,53] Excess mortality has been described among infants who have pleural effusions and is probably attributable in part to secondary pulmonary hypoplasia. Survival improved dramatically in infants who had been treated with pleural-amniotic shunting. In our experience, most such infants who are admitted to a tertiary center survive. It is thus possible that the prognosis for that portion of idiopathic hydrops attributable to pleural effusions, diagnosed antenatally and effectively palliated, may be better than previously reported. Further improvement in postnatal survival of infants with chylothorax may come with more effective medical management. Octreotide may produce prompt resolution of ongoing pleural effusions.[54]

It can be extremely difficult to resuscitate and care for hydropic infants, and these problems are compounded when the infant is born prematurely. It is hoped that advances in neonatal therapy will improve the outlook for infants born with hydrops. However, one report indicated that newer treatment modalities such as surfactant replacement, antenatal steroids, and high-frequency ventilation have not had much of an effect on the survival of these patients.[47]

Hydrops per se has no effect on long-term outcome. Infants who received intrauterine transfusions for hemolytic disease had normal long-term outcomes,[55] as did a group of infants who had nonimmune hydrops.[56] Hydrops does pose significant risks of morbidity and mortality in the neonatal period. Severe and refractory neonatal hypoglycemia, a frequent neonatal complication of hydrops, can have adverse effects on the central nervous system.

FETAL MANAGEMENT

Potentially treatable causes of hydrops include tachyarrhythmias (administration of digoxin or other drugs to the mother, direct intravascular drug treatment of the fetus), heart failure (digoxin), fetal anemia (intrauterine intravascular transfusion), twin-twin transfusion syndrome (ablation of placental vascular anastomoses), cystic hygroma (from sclerotherapy), and pleural effusions (thoracic-amniotic shunting). Tachyarrhythmias and anemia are most amenable to fetal therapy. Fetal surgery has been reported to be successful for some lesions (cystic adenomatoid malformations of the lung, sacrococcygeal teratoma) but remains experimental.[57] Amniocentesis may be indicated for hydrops associated with severe polyhydramnios. Pregnancy termination, even in the third trimester, can be an acceptable option when hydrops is caused by lethal conditions.[58]

Phibbs[59] suggested a prognosis-based management strategy after completion of diagnostic studies:

1. *The underlying condition is lethal.* Fetal therapy is not necessary. Cesarean section is not indicated for fetal distress but may be required for maternal indications. Termination of the pregnancy is an option for the parents.
2. *The long-term prognosis is very poor.* Termination of pregnancy is an option before 24 gestational weeks. Parents should be counseled against cesarean section for fetal distress.
3. *The condition can be treated in utero and prognosis is acceptable.* Therapy should be recommended and continued until the fetus is sufficiently mature in order to optimize chances of survival and minimize serious complications of prematurity. If earlier delivery is required for fetal indications, glucocorticoids should be administered to promote fetal maturation, and delivery should take place in a center where neonatal intensive care is immediately available.
4. *Treatment is possible only after delivery, and prognosis is acceptable.* Delivery should take place in a center with immediate availability of neonatal intensive care, when risk from fetal condition exceeds risks associated with prematurity.
5. *No diagnosis can be made.* Delivery should take place in a center with immediate availability of neonatal intensive care. Because of the poor prognosis in idiopathic cases, termination before 24 gestational weeks is an option for the parents.

DELIVERY AND NEONATAL MANAGEMENT

Planning for the delivery of a hydropic fetus requires close collaboration between the perinatologist and the neonatologist. If massive pleural effusions are present, it is my experience and that of others[60] that resuscitation can be greatly aided by prenatal thoracentesis. Cesarean section delivery has been recommended because of the known risk of soft tissue dystocia.[61] Hydropic fetuses should be delivered in centers with full neonatal intensive care capabilities, including high-frequency ventilation, as well as pediatric surgery facilities if the fetus has a defined surgical condition. A neonatologist should be available at the delivery to deal with anticipated complications, potentially including an extremely difficult neonatal resuscitation.

The following equipment should be immediately available in the resuscitation area:

1. Cardiorespiratory monitor
2. Pulse oximeter
3. Endotracheal intubation supplies (laryngeal edema may require use of a smaller than expected endotracheal tube)
4. Equipment for emergency thoracentesis and paracentesis: plastic intravenous catheters over needles of at least 18-gauge size (smaller catheters are not rigid enough and tend to kink), stopcocks, extension tubing, and 30- to 50-mL syringes; the use of steel "butterfly" needles is discouraged because of the potential risk of

lacerating lungs or abdominal structures as fluid is aspirated
5. Equipment for tube thoracostomy
6. Equipment for umbilical arterial and venous cannulation, including pressure transducers connected, calibrated, and ready for use
7. Supplies for exchange transfusion
8. Specimen tubes for diagnostic testing

Prenatal ultrasound assessment of the fetus aids in preparation for resuscitation. The presence of massive ascites or pleural effusions necessitates preparation for immediate thoracentesis and/or paracentesis. As noted previously, if these fluid accumulations can be drained before delivery, resuscitation is made much easier. If severe anemia is anticipated, unmatched type O, Rh-negative, packed red blood cells should be immediately available.

Respiratory depression is common in hydropic neonates. Most require endotracheal intubation during neonatal resuscitation. Failure to achieve adequate lung expansion after endotracheal intubation necessitates emergency drainage of thoracic and abdominal fluid accumulations. Most delivery room mortality occurs because of failure to establish adequate gas exchange. Ascitic fluid can be drained rapidly until ventilation delivers adequate tidal volumes. In one series, the mean volume of ascitic fluid removed was 72 mL, and the largest volume was 435 mL. Thoracic fluid volume averaged 58 mL, with a maximum of 130 mL.[46] Pleural and peritoneal catheters should be taped in place so that further aspiration of fluid can be performed as needed. Chylothorax often continues to produce massive volumes of fluid, and prolonged use of thoracostomy tubes is necessary to prevent embarrassment of pulmonary function. In such cases, vigilance for infection is imperative.

Initial laboratory assessments should include immediate hematocrit and blood gas measurements. Pleural and ascitic fluid should be sent for cell counts and other testing as indicated. The remainder of the laboratory assessment should be governed by the suspected diagnosis or the differential diagnosis and modified by results of antenatal testing. Potentially useful tests are listed in Table 12-2. As with fetal assessments, testing can be focused on the basis of initial clinical and laboratory information.

Anemia is treated with partial exchange transfusion with packed red blood cells; the goal is a hematocrit over 35%. The typical infant with immune hydrops and severe anemia has a normal circulating blood volume[62,63]; therefore, exchange should be isovolemic. The vascular volume status in cases of nonimmune hydrops has not been studied, but it may depend on the cause of the hydrops. Measured volume in one case of hydrops caused by supraventricular tachycardia was either normal or slightly increased, depending on the estimated baseline weight.[64] In the presence of signs of hypovolemia, packed red blood cells can serve for volume expansion.

Although the primary process of hydrops is fluid retention, epiphenomena contribute to the complications seen in neonates. Hypoglycemia occurs frequently and can begin as early as 1 minute after birth; therefore, it

necessitates immediate attention and close monitoring. Hyperinsulinemia is attributed to islet cell hyperplasia that occurs for unclear reasons in nonimmune hydrops.[65] In immune hydrops, data suggest that hemoglobinemia causes inactivation of insulin[66] with resultant islet cell hyperplasia. Pulmonary hypoplasia may complicate management of infants who have long-standing compromise of pulmonary expansion or limited fetal breathing movements (massive pleural effusions or ascites, abdominal or thoracic space-occupying lesions). The neonatal course of such infants can further be compromised by pulmonary hypertension.

If not recognized in utero, supraventricular tachycardia may pose a difficult diagnostic dilemma. Affected infants can be born with severe hydrops and a normal heart rate. The tachycardia may not recur for a prolonged time— 3 weeks in one case treated in my institution.

Subsequent management depends on the underlying disease process. Fluid overload responds to diuretics, and these agents also help improve pulmonary function. Hydropic infants can lose 30% or more of their birth weight as they diurese. To aid in managing fluid therapy, it may be convenient to estimate the infant's dry weight. The head is usually grossly swollen, and occipitofrontal head circumferences are thus unreliable. However, length is little affected by hydrops; therefore, the infant's length can be applied to standard intrauterine growth curves to estimate the dry weight (same percentile weight for the measured length at the estimated gestational age (e.g., a 33-week hydropic infant with birth weight of 2680 g and length of 41.5 cm is in the 25th percentile; the estimated dry weight, the 25th percentile weight at 33 weeks, is 1750 g).

To provide adequate information for genetic counseling for future pregnancies, infants who die from hydrops must undergo thorough investigation if the cause of the hydrops is unknown. Karyotyping is essential, because hydrops can thoroughly mask dysmorphic features. Other laboratory studies should include assessment for infectious causes and hemoglobin electrophoresis. An autopsy is ideal, but in the presence of parental resistance, postmortem magnetic resonance imaging studies can establish important anatomic diagnoses. Pathologic examination of the placenta can also provide essential information.

REFERENCES

1. Forouzan I: Hydrops fetalis: Recent advances. Obstet Gynecol Surv 52:130, 1997.
2. Ballantyne JW: The Diseases and Deformities of the Fetus. Edinburgh, Oliver and Boyd, 1892.
3. Diamond LK, Blackfan KD, Baty JM: Erythroblastosis fetalis and its association with universal edema of the fetus, icterus gravis neonatorum and anemia of the newborn. J Pediatr 12:269, 1932.
4. Potter EL: Universal edema of the fetus unassociated with erythroblastosis. Am J Obstet Gynecol 46:130, 1943.
5. Mahoney BS, Callen PW, Chinn DH, Golbus MS: Severe nonimmune hydrops fetalis: Sonographic evaluation. Radiology 151:757, 1984.

6. Romero R, Pilu G, Jeanty P, et al: Nonimmune hydrops fetalis. In Prenatal Diagnosis of Congenital Anomalies. Norwalk, Conn, Appleton & Lange, 1988, pp 414-426.

7. DeVore G: Personal communication, June 1988.

8. Machin GA: Hydrops revisited: Literature review of 1,414 cases published in the 1980's. Am J Med Genet 34:366, 1989.

9. Jones DC: Nonimmune fetal hydrops: Diagnosis and fetal management. Semin Perinatol 19:447, 1995.

10. Stulberg RA, Davies GA: Maternal thyrotoxicosis and fetal nonimmune hydrops. Obstet Gynecol 95:1036, 2000.

11. Schmider SA, Henerich W, Dahnert I, Dudenhausen JW: Prenatal therapy of non-immunologic hydrops caused by severe aortic stenosis. Ultrasound Obstet Gynecol 16:275, 2000.

12. Ashshi AM, Cooper RJ, Klapper PE, et al: Detection of human herpes virus 6 DNA in fetal hydrops. Lancet 355:1519, 2000.

13. Towbin JA, Griffin LD, Martin AB, et al: Intrauterine viral myocarditis presenting as nonimmune hydrops fetalis: Diagnosis by polymerase chain reaction. Pediatr Infect Dis J 13:144, 1994.

14. Vadeyar S, Ramsay M, James D, O'Neill D: Prenatal diagnosis of congenital Wilms' tumor (nephroblastoma) presenting as fetal hydrops. Ultrasound Obstet Gynecol 16:80, 2000.

15. Stone DL, Sidransky E: Hydrops fetalis: Lysosomal storage disorders in extremis. Adv Pediatr 46:409, 1999.

16. Kassem E, Dolfin, T, Litmanowitz, I, et al: Familial perinatal hemochromatosis: A disease that causes recurrent non-immune hydrops. J Perinat Med 27:122, 1999.

17. Knoblauch H, Sommer D, Zimmer C, et al: Fetal trisomy 10 mosaicism: Ultrasound, cytogenetic, and morphologic findings in early pregnancy. Prenat Diagn 19:330, 1999.

18. Witters I, Van Buggenout G, Moerman P, Fryns JP: Prenatal diagnosis of de novo distal 5q duplication associated with hygroma colli, fetal oedema and complex cardiopathy. Prenat Diagn 18:1304, 1998.

19. Langford K, Hodgson S, Seller M, Maxwell D: Pallister-Killian syndrome presenting through nuchal translucency screening for trisomy 21. Prenat Diagn 20:670, 2000.

20. Madazli R, Askoy F, Ocak V, Atasu T: Detailed ultrasonographic findings in Greenberg dysplasia. Prenat Diagn 21:65, 2001.

21. Horn LC, Faber R, Meiner A, et al: Greenberg dysplasia: First reported case with additional non-skeletal malformations and without consanguinity. Prenat Diagn 20:1008, 2000.

22. Daikha-Dahmane F, Dommergues M, Narcy M, et al: Congenital erythropoietic porphyria: Prenatal diagnosis and autopsy findings in two sibling fetuses. Pediatr Dev Pathol 4:180, 2001.

23. Ramsing M, Gillesses-Kaesbach G, Holzgreve W, et al: Variability in the phenotypic expression of Fryns' syndrome: A report of two sibships. Am J Med Genet 95:415, 2000.

24. Grebe TA, Clericuzio C: Neurologic and gastrointestinal dysfunction in cardio-facio-cutaneous syndrome: Identification of a severe phenotype. Am J Med Genet 95:144, 2000.

25. Perez del Rio MJ, Fernandez-Toral J, Madrigal, B, et al: Two new cases of Cumming syndrome confirming autosomal recessive inheritance. Am J Med Genet 82:340, 1999.

26. Brace RA, Moore TR: Transplacental, amniotic, urinary and fetal fluid dynamics during very-large-volume fetal intravenous infusions. Am J Obstet Gynecol 164:907, 1991.

27. Brace RA: Fetal blood volume responses to intravenous saline solution and dextran. Am J Obstet Gynecol 147:777, 1983.

28. Brace RA: Fluid distribution in the fetus and neonate. In Polin RA, Fox WW, Abman SH (eds): Fetal and Neonatal Physiology, 3rd ed. Philadelphia, WB Saunders, 2004, pp 1341-1350.

29. Brace RA: Thoracic duct lymph flow and its measurement in the chronically catheterized sheep fetus. Am J Physiol 256:H16, 1989.

30. Andrus RL, Brace RA: The development of hydrops fetalis in the ovine fetus after lymphatic ligation or excision. Am J Obstet Gynecol 102:1331, 1990.

31. Brace RA, Valenzuela GJ: Effects of outflow pressure and vascular volume loading on thoracic duct lymph flow in adult sheep. Am J Physiol 258:R240, 1990.

32. Brace RA: Effects of outflow pressure on fetal lymph flow. Am J Obstet Gynecol 160:494, 1989.

33. Rice HE, Estes JM, Hedrick MH, et al: Congenital cystic adenomatoid malformation: A sheep model of fetal hydrops. J Pediatr Surg 29:692, 1994.

34. Nimrod C, Davies D, Harder J, et al: Ultrasound evaluation of tachycardia-induced hydrops in the fetal lamb. Am J Obstet Gynecol 157:655, 1987.

35. Gest AL, Hansen TL, Moise AA, et al: Atrial tachycardia causes hydrops in fetal lambs. Am J Physiol 258:H1159, 1990.

36. Gest AL, Martin GC, Moise AA, et al: Reversal of blood flow with atrial tachycardia and hydrops in fetal sheep. Pediatr Res 28:223, 1990.

37. Blair DK, VanderStraten MC, Gest AL, et al: Hydrops in fetal sheep from rapid induction of anemia. Pediatr Res 35:560, 1994.

38. Weiner CP: Umbilical pressure measurement in evaluating nonimmune hydrops fetalis. Am J Obstet Gynecol 168:817, 1993.

39. Weiner CP, Pelzer GD, Heilskov J: The effect of intravascular transfusion on umbilical venous pressure in anemic fetuses with and without hydrops. Am J Obstet Gynecol 161:1498, 1989.

40. Moise KR Jr, Carpenter RJ, Hesketh DE: Do abnormal Starling forces cause fetal hydrops in red blood cell alloimmunization? Am J Obstet Gynecol 167:907, 1992.

41. Barnes SE, Bryan EM, Harris DA, et al: Oedema in the newborn. Mol Aspects Med 1:187, 1976.

42. Cormode EJ, Lyster DM, Israels S: Analbuminemia in a neonate. J Pediatr 86:862, 1975.

43. Weiner CP, Robillard JE: Atrial natriuretic factor, digoxin-like immunoreactive substance, norepinephrine, epinephrine and plasma renin activity in human fetuses and their alterations by fetal disease. Am J Obstet Gynecol 159:1353, 1988.

44. Nimrod C, Harder J, Davies D, et al: Atrial natriuretic peptide production in association with nonimmune fetal hydrops. Am J Obstet Gynecol 159:625, 1988.

45. Santolaya J, Alley D, Jaffe R, et al: Antenatal classification of hydrops fetalis. Obstet Gynecol 79:256, 1992.

46. Carlton DP, McGillivray BC, Schreiber MD: Nonimmune hydrops fetalis: A multidisciplinary approach. Clin Perinatol 16:839, 1989.

47. Wy CA, Sajous CH, Loberiza F, Weiss MG: Outcome of infants with a diagnosis of hydrops fetalis in the 1990s. Am J Perinatol 16:561, 1999.

48. Swain S, Cameron AD, McNay MB, Howatson AG: Prenatal diagnosis and management of nonimmune hydrops fetalis. Aust N Z J Obstet Gynecol 39:285, 1999.

49. Heironen S, Markku R, Kirkinen P: Etiology and outcome of second trimester non-immunological fetal hydrops. Acta Obstet Gynecol Scand 79:15, 2000.

50. Rodis JF, Borgida AF, Wilson M, et al: Management of parvovirus infection in pregnancy and outcomes of hydrops; A survey of members of the Society of Perinatal Obstetricians. Am J Obstet Gynecol 179:985, 1998.

51. Odibo AO, Campbell WA, Feldman D, et al: Resolution of human parvovirus B19–associated nonimmune hydrops after intrauterine transfusion. J Ultrasound Med 17:547, 1998.

52. Aubard Y, Derouineau I, Aubard V, et al: Primary fetal hydrothorax: A literature review and proposed antenatal clinical strategy. Fetal Diagn Ther 13;325, 1998.

53. Aguirre OA, Finley BE, Ridgway LE 3rd, et al: Resolution of unilateral fetal hydrothorax with associated non-immune hydrops after intrauterine thoracentesis. Ultrasound Obstet Gynecol 5:346, 1995.

54. Coulter DM: Successful treatment with octreotide of spontaneous chylothorax in a premature infant. J Perinatol 24:194, 2004.

55. Hudon L, Moise KJ Jr, Hegemeier SE, et al: Long-term neurodevelopmental outcome after intrauterine transfusion for the treatment of fetal hemolytic disease. Am J Obstet Gynecol 179:858, 1998.

56. Haverkamp F, Noeker M, Gerresheim G, Fahnenstich H: Good prognosis for psychomotor development in survivors with nonimmune hydrops fetalis. BJOG 107:282, 2000.

57. Bullard KM, Harrison MR: Before the horse is out of the barn: Fetal surgery for hydrops. Semin Perinatol 19:462, 1995.

58. Chervenak F, Farley M, Walters L, et al: When is termination of pregnancy during the third trimester morally justifiable? N Engl J Med 310:501, 1984.

59. Phibbs R: Hydrops fetalis. In Spitzer AR (ed): Intensive Care of the Fetus and Neonate. St. Louis, CV Mosby, 1996, pp 149-156.

60. Takeuchi K, Moriyama T, Oomori S, et al: Management of acute chylothorax with hydrops fetalis diagnosed in the third trimester of pregnancy. Fetal Diagn Ther 14:264, 1999.

61. Bianchi DW, Crombleholme TM, D'Alton ME: Fetology. New York, McGraw-Hill, 2000, pp 959-965.

62. Phibbs RH, Johnson P, Tooley WH, et al: Cardiorespiratory status of erythroblastotic infants, II: Blood volume, hematocrit, and serum albumin concentration in relation to hydrops fetalis. Pediatrics 53:13, 1974.

63. Nicolaides KH, Clewell WH, Rodeck CH: Measurement of human fetoplacental blood volume in erythroblastosis fetalis. Am J Obstet Gynecol 157:50, 1987.

64. Cowan RH, Waldo AL, Harris HB: Neonatal paroxysmal supraventricular tachycardia with hydrops. Pediatrics 55:428, 1975.

65. Mostoufe-Zahah M, Weiss LM, Driscoll SG: Nonimmune hydrops fetalis: A challenge in perinatal pathology. Hum Pathol 16:785, 1985.

66. Brown G, Brown R, Hey E: Fetal hyperinsulinism in rhesus immunization. Am J Obstet Gynecol 131:682, 1978.

CHAPTER 13

The Fetus with a Treatable Endocrine and Metabolic Disorder

Guy Rosner, Shai Ben Shahar, Yuval Yaron, and Mark I. Evans

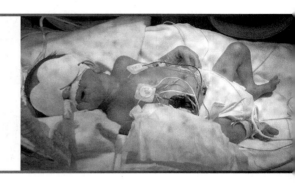

The Human Genome Project has provided mapping of many disease-associated genes and enabled better approaches to diagnosis and primary prevention. Some metabolic and endocrine disorders, such as congenital adrenal hyperplasia (CAH) and cardiac arrhythmias also may be amenable to pharmacologic interventions, however.[1,2] This chapter focuses on fetal endocrine and metabolic diseases in which pharmacologic therapy during pregnancy may ameliorate or even prevent the disease state. The use of folic acid supplementation for the prevention of neural tube defects (NTDs) is discussed separately at the end of the chapter.

ENDOCRINE DISORDERS

Adrenal Disorders: Congenital Adrenal Hyperplasia

Treatment of CAH during fetal life is a well-described and excellent example of the pharmacologic prevention of a birth defect. CAH consists of a group of metabolic disorders, all of which are characterized by an enzymatic defect in the steroidogenetic pathway. As a result of the enzyme defect, and to maintain cortisol production, there is a compensatory increase in adrenocorticotropic hormone secretion, which leads to overproduction of the steroid precursors in the adrenal cortex—the adrenal hyperplasia.

All forms of CAH are inherited in an autosomal recessive manner. The phenotype of each form is determined by the severity of the cortisol deficiency and the nature of the steroid precursors that accumulate proximal to the enzymatic block. The most common abnormality, responsible for greater than 90% of patients with CAH, is caused by a deficiency of the 21-hydroxylase (21-OH) enzyme. Other, less common causes for CAH include deficiencies in 11β-hydroxylase, 17α-hydroxylase, and 3β-hydroxysteroid-dehydrogenase. Diminished 21-OH activity results in accumulation of 17-hydroxyprogesterone (17-OHP) as a result of its decreased conversion to 11-deoxycorticosterone. The excess 17-OHP is converted via androstenedione to androgens, the levels of which increase by several hundred–fold (Fig. 13-1). The excess androgens cause virilization of the undifferentiated female external genitalia. The degree of virilization may vary from mild clitoral hypertrophy to complete formation of a phallus and scrotum. In contrast, genital development in male fetuses usually is normal. The excess androgens cause postnatal virilization in both genders and may manifest in precocious puberty.

The "classic" form of CAH involves a severe enzyme deficiency or even a complete block of enzymatic activity, which is associated in two thirds to three fourths of patients with salt loss that may be life-threatening. The classic form is easy to recognize in newborn girls but may be overlooked in boys, who may present at a later stage with severe dehydration or death. The estimated incidence of classic CAH is 1:5000 to 1:60,000, depending on the ethnic background. The "nonclassic" attenuated form of 21-OH deficiency results in partial blockade of the enzymatic activity and usually is clinically apparent as simple virilization in women only later in life. It is estimated to occur in approximately 3.5% of Ashkenazi Jews and approximately 2% of Hispanics.[3] The gene for 21-OH is in close linkage to the HLA major histocompatibility complex on the short arm of chromosome 6.[4] The gene for 21-OH (CYP21B) has been mapped, allowing direct mutation analysis in informative families.[5]

Historically, in the late 1970s and early 1980s, the diagnosis of CAH was made on amniocentesis by the finding of elevated levels of 17-OHP in the supernatant. With the development of chorionic villus sampling in the latter part of the 1980s, linkage-based molecular diagnosis in the first trimester became available. Since discovery and mapping of the gene, direct DNA mutation analysis has become the routine approach.

The fetal adrenal gland can be suppressed pharmacologically by maternal replacement doses of dexamethasone.[6] The suppression can prevent masculinization of affected female fetuses in couples who are carriers of classic CAH (fetuses at risk for nonclassic CAH do not

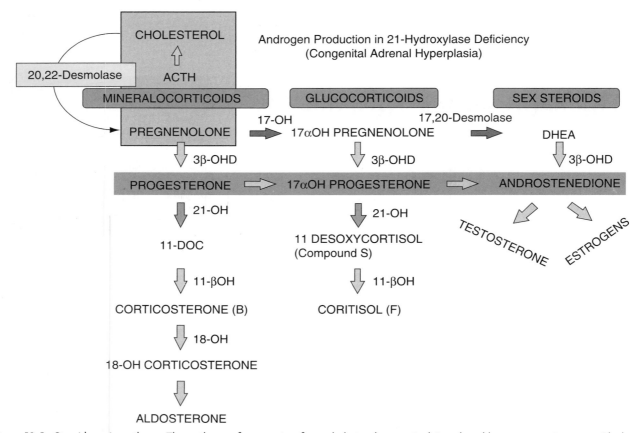

Figure 13–1. Steroidogenic pathway. The pathway of conversion from cholesterol to cortisol is vulnerable to enzymatic errors. Blockage at 21-hydroxylase leads to overproduction of 17-hydroxyprogesterone, which ultimately leads to excess androgens that produce masculinization of the external genitalia. ACTH, adrenocorticotropic hormone.

require any prenatal treatment). In the first attempt to prevent female genital birth defects in 1982, Evans and colleagues[6] administered dexamethasone to a carrier mother beginning at 10 weeks of gestation. Serial maternal estriol and cortisol levels indicated that adrenal gland suppression had been achieved. The female fetus was born at 39 weeks of gestation with normal external genitalia. Forrest and David[7] employed a similar protocol beginning at 9 weeks of gestation to treat several fetuses at risk for CAH. Female fetuses subsequently confirmed to be affected with severe CAH were spared masculinization of the external genitalia. Several hundred pregnant women and their fetuses since have been treated, with prevention of masculinization in more than 85% of affected female fetuses.[8]

Because the differentiation of the external genitalia begins at about 7 weeks of gestation, diagnosis by amniocentesis or chorionic villus sampling comes far too late to prevent masculinization. For carrier parents at risk of having an affected fetus, pharmacologic therapy has to be initiated before diagnosis. This approach suggests that therapy must be administered to all patients at risk, despite the fact that the chance of an affected female fetus for carrier parents is only 1 in 8 (i.e., 1/4 affected × 1/2 female). Direct DNA diagnosis or linkage studies may be performed by chorionic villus sampling in the first trimester. As a result, for seven out of eight patients, therapy can be discontinued as soon as the diagnosis of male sex is made or if CAH is ruled out. If the fetus is found to be an affected female, however, therapy is continued throughout gestation. Stress-dose corticosteroids should be given to the mother during labor and gradually tapered postpartum. If the fetus is a male or is unaffected, therapy can be discontinued at the time of diagnosis. No consistent untoward effects on fetuses have been reported, but long-term safety studies have not been published yet. Greater weight gain, edema, and striae were noticed in treated mothers, but no increased risk of hypertension or gestational diabetes was noted.[8]

Inclusion criteria of the European Society for Pediatric Endocrinology and Wilkins Pediatric Endocrine Society[9] for prenatal treatment of CAH include (1) a previously affected sibling or first-degree relative with known mutation causing classic CAH proven by DNA analysis, (2) reasonable expectation that the father is the same as the proband's, (3) availability of rapid and quality genetic analysis, (4) therapy started less than 9 weeks after the last menstrual period, (5) lack of intent for therapeutic abortion, and (6) reasonable expectation of the patient's compliance. The treatment requires a professional team that includes an expert in high-risk obstetrics, a pediatric endocrinologist, a genetic counselor, and availability of a molecular genetic laboratory.

Thyroid Disorders

Hypothyroidism

Congenital hypothyroidism affects about 1:3000 to 1:4000 infants.[10] About 85% of cases are the result of thyroid dysgenesis, a heterogeneous group of developmental defects characterized by an inadequate amount of thyroid tissue. Congenital hypothyroidism is associated only rarely with errors of thyroid hormone synthesis, thyroid-stimulating hormone (TSH) insensitivity, or absence of the pituitary gland. Fetal hypothyroidism may not manifest in a goiter before birth because maternal thyroid hormones may cross the placenta. Congenital hypothyroidism presenting with a goiter can be found in only about 10% to 15% of cases, with an estimated prevalence of 1:30,000 to 1:50,000 live births.[11]

Fetal goiterous hypothyroidism is caused in most instances by maternal exposure to thyrostatic agents used to treat maternal hyperthyroidism.[12] These drugs include propylthiouracil (PTU), the inadvertent use of radioactive iodine in pregnant women, or iodide exposure. Maternal ingestion of amiodarone or lithium also may cause hypothyroidism in the fetus. Finally, fetal hypothyroidism may result from transplacental passage of maternal blocking antibodies (known as *TBIAb* or *TBII*) or rarely may be due to defects in fetal thyroid hormone biosynthesis.[10]

Fetal goiterous hypothyroidism may lead to severe fetal and neonatal consequences. An enlarged goiter may cause esophageal obstruction and subsequent polyhydramnios, which may result in preterm delivery or premature rupture of membranes. Rarely a goiter may lead to high-output heart failure due to high vascular flow in the goiter.[13] A large fetal goiter can cause extension of the fetal neck, leading to dystocia. The effects of fetal hypothyroidism itself may be devastating. Without treatment, postnatal growth delay and severe mental retardation may ensue. Even with immediate diagnosis and treatment at birth, long-term follow-up of children with congenital hypothyroidism has shown that they have lower scores on perceptual-motor, visual-spatial, and language tests.[14]

In suspicious cases, an extensive maternal and family history should be obtained. In patients with a positive history, maternal thyroid hormone levels and blocking immunoglobulin levels should be measured. In addition, all women with a history of any thyroid disease (hypothyroidism and hyperthyroidism) are advised to have monthly fetal ultrasound scans to screen for fetal goiter, polyhydramnios, or fetal tachycardia.[14]

Occasionally, fetal goiterous hypothyroidism may be identified by a routine ultrasound study, often performed because of increased uterine size from polyhydramnios caused by esophageal obstruction and impaired swallowing. Sometimes a fetal goiter may be discovered incidentally on a routine scan. Before the advent of cordocentesis, amniotic fluid levels of TSH and free thyroxine (T_4) were used as potential indicators of fetal

thyroid function. These proved to be inconsistent, however.[15] With cordocentesis, fetal thyroid status can be evaluated directly and accurately; fetal response to therapy can be measured reliably using available appropriate nomograms for fetal serum levels of free T_4, total T_4, free triiodothyronine (T_3), total T_3, and TSH.[16,17] In utero treatment initially was suggested by Van Herle and colleagues[18] using intramuscular injection of levothyroxine sodium. Subsequent studies have indicated, however, that intra-amniotic administration of T_4 may be superior and can lead to resolution of the polyhydramnios as well. The dose of the injected drug may be refined using the fetal thyroid profile in the amniotic fluid and the thyroid size.[19] The doses commonly used for treatment range from 200 to 500 mg by intra-amniotic administration every week.[23] With this regimen, fetal goiters have been shown to regress, hyperextension of the fetal head has been shown to resolve, and fetal and newborn TSH levels have normalized.[19]

Hyperthyroidism

Neonatal hyperthyroidism is rare, with an incidence of 1:4000 to 1:40,000 live births.[11] Fetal thyrotoxic goiter usually is secondary to maternal autoimmune disease, principally Graves disease or Hashimoto thyroiditis. Twelve percent of infants of mothers with a known history of Graves disease are affected with neonatal thyrotoxicosis, which may occur even if the mother is euthyroid.[20] Similar to hypothyroidism, inherent to the underlying mechanism is the transplacental passage of maternal IgG antibodies. In this case, the antibodies, known as *TSAb* or *TSI*, are directed predominantly against the TSH receptor.

Usually the investigation of fetal hyperthyroidism begins only after the discovery of fetal goiter. Often the goiter is diagnosed on ultrasound in patients referred for elevated thyroid-stimulating antibodies. In some cases, fetal goiters are realized serendipitously on routine ultrasonography. Other goiters may be discovered in patients referred for scan because of polyhydramnios. In addition to the risks related to the goiter itself, untreated fetal hyperthyroidism may be associated with a mortality rate of 12% to 25% because of high-output cardiac failure.[21] When a fetal goiter is identified, biochemical evaluation is indicated. Historically, amniotic fluid levels of TSH and free T_4 were used as potential indicators of fetal thyroid function. These measurements proved inconsistent, however, in that amniotic fluid levels of these hormones do not always correlate with serum levels. Some controversy still exists regarding their use, although they may be beneficial in centers that do not have available cordocentesis.[22] As previously stated, cordocentesis allows reliable assessment of fetal thyroid status and TSH,[23,24] and treatment can be planned accordingly.

When the diagnosis of fetal hyperthyroidism is confirmed, fetal treatment should be initiated. Authors have attempted to treat fetal hyperthyroidism with maternally administered antithyroid drugs. Porreco and Bloch[25] reported maternal treatment of fetal thyrotoxicosis with PTU, which resulted in a good outcome.[25] The initial dose used was 100 mg orally three times a day, which was decreased later to 50 mg orally three times a day. Wenstrom and associates[21] described a favorable outcome using maternal methimazole to treat fetal hyperthyroidism in a patient who could not tolerate PTU failure. Hatjis[26] also treated fetal goiterous hyperthyroidism with a maternal dose of 300 mg of PTU. This patient required supplemental levothyroxine (Synthroid), however, to remain euthyroid. There was good fetal outcome in this case as well.

INBORN ERRORS OF METABOLISM

Methylmalonic Acidemia

The methylmalonic acidemias (MMAs) are a group of enzyme-deficiency diseases inherited in an autosomal recessive manner that result from one of several genetically distinct causes. Some cases are caused by mutations in the gene encoding methylmalonyl–coenzyme A mutase, whereas others are due to a defect that reduces the biosynthesis of adenosylcobalamin from vitamin B_{12}. The disease is characterized by a broad clinical spectrum ranging from a benign condition to fatal neonatal disease. In the severe form, MMA is characterized by severe metabolic acidosis, developmental delay, and biochemical abnormalities that include methylmalonic aciduria, long-chain ketonuria, and intermittent hyperglycinemia. Patients with defects in adenosylcobalamin biosynthesis may respond to administration of large doses of vitamin B_{12}, which may enhance the amount of active holoenzyme (mutase apoenzyme plus adenosylcobalamin). A proposed mechanism for the neurologic abnormalities observed in MMA was suggested by a group of Brazilian investigators[27] who administered methylmalonic acid to rats during the first month of life. Significant diminutions of myelin content and of ganglioside N-acetylneuraminic acid were noted in the cerebrum.

Ampola and colleagues[28] were the first to attempt prenatal diagnosis and treatment of a vitamin B_{12}–responsive variant of MMA. These authors followed the pregnancy of a patient who previously had lost an infant to severe acidosis and dehydration at age 3 months. The diagnosis of MMA was made posthumously by chemical analysis of blood and urine. In the subsequent pregnancy, amniocentesis at 19 weeks revealed elevated methylmalonic acid in the amniotic fluid. Cultured amniocytes also showed defective propionate oxidation and undetectable levels of adenosylcobalamin. When adenosylcobalamin was added, normal succinate oxidation and methylmalonyl–coenzyme A mutase activity were noted. These studies established that the fetus also had MMA apparently from deficient synthesis of adenosylcobalamin. It already had been known that fetal MMA is associated with increased methylmalonic acid excretion in the maternal urine.

Ampola and colleagues[28] documented increased methylmalonic acid in maternal urine at 23 and 25 weeks of gestation. Late in the pregnancy, cyanocobalamin (10 mg/day) was administered orally to the mother in divided doses. The treatment altered the maternal serum vitamin B_{12} level only marginally. There was a slight reduction, however, of maternal urinary methylmalonic acid excretion that remained severalfold above normal. At approximately 34 weeks of gestation, 5 mg/day of cyanocobalamin was administered intramuscularly. The maternal serum B_{12} level rose gradually to more than six times above normal and was accompanied by a progressive decrease in urinary methylmalonic acid excretion. Maternal urinary methylmalonate was only slightly above the normal range when delivery occurred at 41 weeks. Amniotic fluid methylmalonic acid concentrations were three times the normal mean at 19 menstrual weeks and four times the normal mean at term, despite prenatal treatment. Postnatally the diagnosis of MMA was confirmed. The infant had no acute neonatal complications and had an extremely high serum vitamin B_{12} level. Long-term postnatal management involved protein restriction, although no continuous vitamin B_{12} treatment was required. In this instance, prenatal treatment improved the fetal and, secondarily, the maternal biochemistry. Whether there was any significant clinical benefit to the fetus with in utero treatment cannot be assessed adequately. It seems likely that reducing the fetal burden of methylmalonic acid should have some beneficial effect on fetal development and could reduce the risks in the neonatal period.

Andersson and coworkers[29] followed a cohort of eight children with MMA for 5.7 years. Congenital malformations were described, reinforcing the deleterious effects of prenatally abnormal cyanocobalamin metabolism. Growth was improved significantly in most cases after initiation of therapy postnatally, and microcephaly resolved in one case. Developmental delay of variable severity always was present, however, regardless of treatment onset. These data suggest that prenatal therapy of MMA may be effective and may ameliorate some of the prenatal effects. Evans and colleagues[30] documented the changing dosage requirements necessary over the course of pregnancy to maintain adequate levels of vitamin B_{12}. They sequentially followed maternal plasma and urine levels in a prenatal treated pregnancy.[30] Data such as these suggest that modulation of maternal-fetal pharmacologic interchange of therapeutic drugs would be difficult to control with precision.

Multiple Carboxylase Deficiency

Biotin-responsive multiple carboxylase deficiency is an inborn error of metabolism caused by diminished activity of the mitochondrial biotin-dependent enzymes (pyruvate carboxylase, propionyl–coenzyme A carboxylase, and α-methylcrotonyl–coenzyme A carboxylase). The condition may arise from mutations in the holocarboxylase synthetase gene mapped to chromosome 21q22.1 or the biotinidase gene localized to chromosome 3p25.[31-35] Affected patients present as newborns or in early childhood with dermatitis, severe metabolic acidosis, and a characteristic pattern of organic acid excretion. It has been shown that metabolism in patients or in their cultured cells can be restored toward normal levels by biotin supplementation. Prenatal diagnosis can be made by demonstration of elevated levels of typical organic acids (3-hydroxyisovalerate, methylcitrate) in the amniotic fluid or in the chorionic villi. The existence of a mild form of holocarboxylase synthetase deficiency can complicate prenatal diagnosis, however, because organic acid levels in amniotic fluid might be normal.[36] Prenatal diagnosis must be performed by enzyme assay in cultured fetal cells in biotin-restricted medium.

Roth and colleagues[37] treated a fetus without prenatal diagnosis in a case in which two previous siblings had died of multiple carboxylase deficiency. The first sibling had died within 3 days of birth, and in the second sibling, the diagnosis of biotin-responsive carboxylase deficiency was made posthumously. Because the mother was first seen at 34 weeks of gestation, prenatal diagnosis was not attempted. Because of severe neonatal manifestations in previous offspring and because of the probable harmlessness of biotin, oral administration was begun at a dose of 10 mg/day. There were no apparent untoward effects, and maternal urinary biotin excretion increased by a factor of approximately 100 during biotin administration. Nonidentical twins subsequently were delivered at term. Cord blood and urinary organic acid profiles were normal, and cord blood biotin concentrations were four to seven times greater than normal. The neonatal course for both twins was unremarkable. Subsequent study of the cultured fibroblasts of both twins indicated that the cells of twin B (but not of twin A) had virtually complete deficiency of all three carboxylase activities. Genetic complementation studies confirmed that despite the normal clinical presentation during the newborn period, twin B was homozygous for the disease mutation.

Packman and colleagues[38] also have reported the prenatal diagnosis and treatment of biotin-responsive multiple carboxylase deficiency for a mother who previously had given birth to a boy with the neonatal-onset form of this disease. In the subsequent pregnancy, maternal urine organic acid profiles were normal. Carboxylase activities were assayed in cultured amniotic fluid cells obtained by amniocentesis at 17 menstrual weeks. In biotin-restricted medium, the amniotic cells showed the characteristic severe reduction in carboxylase activities. Since these initial reports of prenatal administration of biotin to fetuses affected with this disorder, other cases have been published,[36,39] providing further compelling evidence that biotin administration antenatally is taken up effectively by the fetus and prevents functional deficiency of the carboxylases in an affected newborn. No toxicity from treatment was observed. Because experience with this treatment is confined to a few cases, however, it is reasonable to carry out prenatal diagnosis and only then to initiate treatment with biotin in any affected fetus.

Smith-Lemli-Opitz Syndrome

Smith-Lemli-Opitz syndrome (SLOS) is a dysmorphologic syndrome that first was reported in 1964.[40] Features include characteristic facies; growth restriction; mental retardation; and anomalies of the heart, kidneys, central nervous system, and limbs. Cleft palate, postaxial polydactyly, syndactyly of the toes, and cataracts are seen often in affected patients. The Y-shaped syndactyly of the second and third toes is specific for this disorder and is seen in greater than 90% of affected patients. Affected patients typically present with a narrow forehead, ptosis, anteverted nares, low-set ears, and micrognathia.

Boys may present with ambiguous genitalia. In contrast with CAH, patients with SLOS are deficient in cholesterol and lack steroid precursors. This abnormality leads to lack of androgens, which results in undermasculinization of the male genitalia. Patients with the severe form of the syndrome present not only with these dysmorphologic findings, but also with a high rate of neonatal mortality.[41] The incidence of SLOS is estimated to be 1:20,000 to 1:40,000 live births,[42] and it seems to be most common in whites of Northern European origin, with an estimated carrier frequency of 1:70.[43] In 1993, the cause of SLOS was discovered to be an inborn error of cholesterol biosynthesis due to a deficiency of the enzyme dehydrocholesterol-Δ^7 reductase.[42,44-46] The gene for 7-dehydrocholesterol-Δ^7 reductase has been localized to chromosome 11q12-13.[46]

As a result of this enzymatic defect, there is a characteristic biochemical pattern of reduced cholesterol levels and elevated 7-dehydrocholesterol (DHC) and 8-DHC levels in all body fluids and tissues, including red blood cells, fibroblasts, amniotic fluid, and chorionic villi. The values observed in affected patients may be extremely variable. The diagnosis is made primarily by the presence of the cholesterol precursor, 7-DHC, and not by the deficiency of cholesterol. The level of 7-DHC in affected patients is 100 to 1000 times normal. Unaffected individuals have levels of 7-DHC and 8-DHC of less than 1 mg/dL, whereas patients with SLOS have levels of 7 to 20 mg/dL or greater. Clinical manifestations correlate with cholesterol levels. Severely affected patients have low levels (usually <10 to 15 mg/dL), whereas patients with more mild manifestations may present with levels of 40 to 70 mg/dL. Prenatal diagnosis of SLOS has been available since 1994 by either amniocentesis or chorionic villus sampling.[47-49]

Since the identification of the cholesterol metabolic defect in SLOS, a treatment protocol has been attempted providing exogenous cholesterol. This form of therapy now has been provided to many patients with SLOS for the past several years in many centers in the United States and internationally,[50-52] with the goal of raising cholesterol levels and decreasing the precursors 7-DHC and 8-DHC. It has been shown that dietary cholesterol supplementation can restore a normal growth pattern in children and adolescents with SLOS, alleviate behavioral abnormalities, and improve general health.[50-53]

Fetal therapy strategies theoretically may include providing cholesterol to the mother or to the fetus. The former approach is not possible, however, because cholesterol does not cross the placenta well during the second trimester, and there is no evidence that it crosses the placenta in the third trimester. Cholesterol is available only in a crystalline form that cannot be given intravenously or intramuscularly. It is impractical to inject cholesterol into the amniotic fluid because it would precipitate. Cholesterol can be given to the fetus, however, by giving fresh frozen plasma in the form of low-density lipoprotein cholesterol. A group at Tufts University has attempted treatment antenatally in several affected fetuses. In cases in which treatment was started late in pregnancy, the results were inconclusive. Although few descriptions of fetal therapy for SLOS exist, the latest report of antenatal treatment comes from the same group of investigators.[54] Therapy was begun at 34 weeks of gestation and resulted in increased fetal cholesterol levels and red blood cell mean corpuscular volume, with subtle improvement in fetal growth as assessed by consequent fetal weight plots. No significant changes in 7-DHC and 8-DHC levels were observed, however, emphasizing further the inconclusiveness of that treatment. Nevertheless, the main point of these studies was that the provision of cholesterol to the fetus as early as possible would result in the greatest clinical benefit because significant development of the central nervous system and myelination occurs before birth.

Galactosemia

Galactosemia is an inborn error of metabolism caused by diminished activity of the enzyme galactose-1-phosphate uridyltransferase (GALT). It is inherited as an autosomal recessive trait and results in cataracts, growth deficiency, and ovarian failure. Clinical symptoms appear in the neonatal period and can be ameliorated by elimination of galactose from the diet. Cellular damage from galactosemia is thought to be mediated by accumulation of galactose-1-phosphate intracellularly and galactitol in the lens. The *GALT* gene, localized to chromosome 9p13, is the only known gene to be associated with galactosemia. Several disease-causing mutations commonly are encountered in classic galactosemia, with the most frequently observed being the Q188R classic mutation. Mutational analysis is available for the six classic galactosemia alleles (Q188R, S135L, K285N, L195P, Y209C, F171S) and for the N314D Duarte variant mutation.[55] In cases in which disease-causing mutations are not identified (10% to 29% of cases of classic galactosemia), GALT sequence analysis may be performed to detect private mutations. Galactosemia can be diagnosed prenatally by study of cultured amniocytes and chorionic villi.

There are suggestions that the early postnatal treatment of galactosemic individuals with a low-galactose diet may not be sufficient to ensure normal development. Some authors have speculated that prenatal damage to galactosemic fetuses could contribute to subsequent abnormal neurologic development and to lens cataract formation. It has been recognized that female galactosemics, even when treated from birth with galactose deprivation, have a high frequency of primary or secondary amenorrhea because of ovarian failure. This problem occurs because oocytes already have been damaged irreversibly long before birth. There also may be some subtle abnormalities of male gonadal function.

Exposure to a high-galactose diet has been considered to represent an animal model for human galactosemia. Chen and colleagues[56] observed a reduction in the oocyte content of rat ovaries after prenatal exposure to a 50% galactose diet. No analogous alterations in the testes were observed in prenatally treated males. Experiments in rats suggest that toxicity to the female gonads from galactose or its metabolites is most obvious during the premeiotic stages of ovarian development. Impaired germ cell migration leading to the development of gonads with deficient initial pools of germ cells was proposed as the causal link between galactosemia and premature ovarian failure.[57]

These observations in animals and humans have led to speculation that galactose restriction during pregnancy may be desirable if the fetus is affected with galactosemia. In the human female, ovarian meiosis begins at 12 weeks and is complete by 28 menstrual weeks. Ovarian damage and perhaps neurologic or lens abnormalities might occur before the usual time when prenatal diagnosis by amniocentesis can be accomplished. Anticipatory treatment in pregnancies at risk for a galactosemic fetus might be initiated best early in gestation or even preconceptionally.

Despite these experiments and speculations, we are unaware of studies that adequately assess the impact of prenatal administration of a low-galactose diet to galactosemic infants. Such data, especially prospectively controlled, would be difficult to obtain. Nevertheless, prenatal galactose restriction is probably desirable in galactosemia and should be harmless. There is little reason to suppose that galactose restriction would have adverse consequences because galactosemic fetuses and normal fetuses are capable of some endogenous galactose synthesis.

MULTIFACTORIAL DISORDERS

Neural Tube Defects

NTDs are malformations secondary to abnormal neural tube closure between 3 and 4 weeks of gestation. The cause is complex and imperfectly understood with genetic and environmental factors involved. Animal studies suggest that NTDs can arise from a variety of vitamin or mineral deficiencies. Historical data in humans suggest increased NTD frequencies in subjects with poor dietary histories or with intestinal bypasses. Biochemical evidence of suboptimal nutrition is present in some women bearing infants with NTDs. Analysis of recurrence patterns within families and of twin-twin concordance data provides evidence of a genetic influence in nonsyndromal cases, although factors such as socioeconomic status, geographic area, occupational exposure, and maternal use of antiepileptic drugs also are associated with variations in the incidence of NTDs.[58] In 1980, Smithells and colleagues[59,60] suggested that vitamin supplementation containing 0.36 mg of folate could reduce the frequency of NTD recurrence by sevenfold in women with one or more prior affected children. For almost a decade, there was a great deal of controversy regarding the benefit of folate supplementation for the prevention of NTDs.[61-64]

In 1991, a randomized, double-blinded trial designed by the MRC Vitamin Study Research Group showed that preconceptional folate reduces the risk of recurrence in high-risk patients.[65] Subsequently, it was shown that preparations containing folate and other vitamins also reduce the occurrence of first-time NTDs.[66] In response to these findings, guidelines were issued calling for consumption of 4 mg/day of folic acid by women with a prior child affected with an NTD for at least 1 month before conception through the first 3 months of pregnancy.

In addition, 0.4 mg/day of folic acid is recommended to all women planning a pregnancy to be taken before conception occurs. The data on NTD recurrence prevention now are well established, and prevention became routine for high-risk cases. As of January 1998, the U.S. Food and Drug Administration mandated that breads and grains be supplemented with folic acid. The impact of food fortification with folic acid on NTDs during the years 1990 through 1999 was evaluated by assessing birth certificate reports before and after mandatory fortification.[67] It was found that the birth prevalence of NTDs decreased by 19%. The continuing decline in NTD rates is due to the introduction and increased use of prenatal diagnosis in addition to the population-wide increases in blood folate levels since food fortification was mandated.[68] Evans and associates[69] showed a nearly 30% decrease in high maternal serum α-fetoprotein values in the United States, when values from 2000 are compared with 1997 values, before the introduction of general folic acid supplementation.

Folate plays a central part in embryonic and fetal development because of its role in nucleic acid synthesis, which is mandatory for the widespread cell division during embryogenesis. Folate deficiency can occur because of low dietary folate intake or because of increased metabolic requirements, as seen in genetic alterations, such as polymorphism of the thermolabile enzyme methyltetrahydrofolate reductase (MTHFR). A metabolic effect of folate deficiency is homocysteine elevation in blood. As mentioned, the thermolabile variant of MTHFR, 677TT, is a known risk factor for NTD. Evidence regarding a second polymorphism in the same gene, 1298AC, does not support its role in NTD, however.[70] Additionally, numerous studies analyzing MTHFR variants have resulted in positive associations with increased NTD risk only in certain populations, suggesting that these variants are not large contributors to the cause of NTD.[71] It seems inadvisable to have parents prospectively tested for MTHFR variants. Reinforcement to the assumption that additional candidate genes other than MTHFR may be responsible for an increased risk to NTDs comes from the NTD collaborative group of Duke University.[72] A total of 175 American white NTD patients and their families were examined for the thermolabile variant of MTHFR. Although a significant association was found comparing patients and controls, no such association was found in patients' parents.

Two other key enzymes in the metabolic pathway of homocysteine are methionine synthase (MTR) and methionine synthase reductase (MTRR). MTR polymorphism and a specific (A66G) MTRR polymorphism have been found to be associated with an increased risk for NTD. The NTD risk was not influenced by maternal preconception folic acid intake at doses of 0.4 mg/day. Because of limited sample size, however, further studies are needed to draw meaningful inferences.[73] Other candidate genes suggested as risk factors for NTD (mainly spina bifida) are polymorphisms in the mitochondrial membrane transporter gene *UCP2*.[74] Despite previous studies suggesting that zinc deficiency may play a role in the cause of NTDs,[75,76] further studies found this observation to be inconclusive.[77,78] Methionine deficiency might be involved in NTD because a 30% to 55% reduction in the risk of having an NTD-associated pregnancy was reported when methionine intake was greater than the lowest quartile of intake; there was a further reduction in risk with greater methionine intake.[79]

Preconception folic acid intake as a sole vitamin or as multivitamin supplementation reduces the risk of recurrent and first-time NTDs. Additionally, folic acid and multivitamin supplementation reduces the occurrence of some other congenital anomalies seen in the urinary tract and cardiovascular systems and anomalies involving the limbs and face (orofacial clefting).

PHARMACOLOGIC AND NUTRITIONAL APPROACHES

It might be appropriate to consider suppressing excessive cholesterol production prenatally in severe hypercholesterolemia when a safe and effective agent for accomplishing this becomes available (although there is no clear evidence for hypercholesterolemic prenatal damage). If cysteamine or related agents were to prove to be an effective treatment for lethal variants of cystinosis, prenatal therapy might be considered because excessive and possibly harmful cystine accumulation is evident even in cystinotic fetuses. Cysteamine levels have been detected in chorionic villi, and significant elevations at 10 weeks of gestation have been hypothesized. Inhibitors of γ-glutamyl transpeptidase, if safe, would elevate intracellular glutathione levels and inhibit oxoproline production in glutathione synthase deficiency, averting the characteristic neonatal acidosis.

In theory, it would be desirable to minimize copper accumulation in Wilson disease at an early point in gestation. If and when reliable prenatal diagnosis of Wilson disease is possible, cautious administration of penicillamine prenatally might be considered. This would be a double-edged sword, however, because the teratogenic potential of penicillamine would demand careful evaluation. Batshaw and colleagues[80] treated certain urea cycle defects by administering arginine and benzoate. Because hyperammonemia in some of these entities develops acutely after birth, it might be desirable to consider pretreating the fetus with these compounds just before or during labor to minimize postnatal hyperammonemia. Conversely, it may be desirable to consider drug avoidance as an approach to fetal treatment. Fetuses with glucose-6-phosphate dehydrogenase deficiency are sensitive to a variety of drugs that induce hemolysis. It probably would be appropriate to avoid administering these agents to women carrying or known to be at risk for carrying fetuses deficient in glucose-6-phosphate dehydrogenase.

Umbilical cord catheterization under ultrasound guidance may lead to the development of other types of fetal treatment.[81] Systems such as gene replacement are being developed for certain lysosomal storage disorders. Progress is being made in postnatal experimental models on administration of thymic cells for certain immune deficiency states, bone marrow transplantation for a variety of genetic disorders, and gene transfer. The development of better and earlier techniques for prenatal treatment will be complex, especially with regard to gene transfer; progress will be made, however, and access to the fetal vasculature may be required for these methods to have a chance for success.

Bone marrow transplantation or thymic cell infusion is a specialized example of organ transplantation. In the future, fetal organ transplantation may become possible and may open many prospects for surgical treatment of certain biochemical genetic disorders.

One also can speculate about the therapeutic possibilities involving compounds administered directly into the amniotic fluid or into the fetal intestinal tract. It might be possible to administer thyroid hormone in this fashion or to prevent meconium ileus in cystic fibrosis by instilling not yet determined enzymes into the fetal intestinal tract.

Although a multitude of metabolic disorders exist, prenatal treatment for most has never been attempted or considered. The discovery of new disease-associated genes and prenatal carrier testing may allow preconceptional carrier detection in the future, without the tragedy of first having an affected child. This detection may provide targeted therapy in families who choose to continue the pregnancy and offer the prospect of improved outcome by ameliorating at least some of the prenatal deleterious effects of the metabolic disease.

REFERENCES

1. Evans MI, Pinsky WW, Johnson MP, Schulman JD: Medical fetal therapy. In Evans MI (ed): Reproductive Risks and Prenatal Diagnosis. Norwalk, CT, Appleton & Lange, 1992, p 236.
2. Johnson MP, Evans MI, Quintero RA, Flake AW: In utero therapy of the fetus. In Gleisher N, Buttino L Jr, Elkayam U, et al (eds): Principles and Practice of Medical Therapy in Pregnancy, 3rd ed. Norwalk, CT, Appleton & Lange, 1998.
3. Speiser PW, Dupont B, Rubinstein P, et al: High frequency of nonclassical steroid 21-hydroxylase deficiency. Am J Hum Genet 37:650, 1985.
4. Dupont B, Oberfield SE, Smithwick EM, et al: Close genetic linkage between HLA and congenital adrenal hyperplasia (21-hydroxylase deficiency). Lancet 2:1309, 1977.
5. White PC, Grossberger D, Onufer BJ, et al: Two genes encoding steroid 21-hydroxylase are located near the genes encoding the fourth component of complement in man. Proc Natl Acad Sci U S A 82:1089, 1985.
6. Evans MI, Chrousos GP, Mann DL, et al: Pharmacologic suppression of the fetal adrenal gland in utero: Attempted prevention of abnormal external genital masculinization in suspected congenital adrenal hyperplasia. JAMA 253:1015, 1985.
7. Forrest M, David M: Prenatal treatment of congenital adrenal hyperplasia due to 21-hydroxylase deficiency [abstract y11]. Presented at Seventh International Congress of Endocrinology, Quebec, Canada, 1984.
8. New MI, Carlson A, Obeid J, et al: Prenatal diagnosis for congenital adrenal hyperplasia in 532 pregnancies. Clin Endocrinol Metab 86:5651, 2001.
9. Clayton PE, Miller WL, Oberfield SE, et al, ESPE/LWPES CAH Working Group: Consensus statement on 21-hydroxylase deficiency from the European Society for Paediatric Endocrinology and the Lawson Wilkins Pediatric Endocrine Society. Horm Res 58:188, 2002.
10. Fisher DA, Klein AH: Thyroid development and disorders of thyroid function in the newborn. N Engl J Med 304:702, 1981.
11. Fisher DA: Neonatal thyroid disease of women with autoimmune thyroid disease. Thyroid Today 9:1, 1986.
12. Volumenie JL, Polak M, Guibourdenche J, et al: Management of fetal thyroid goitres: A report of 11 cases in a single perinatal unit. Prenat Diagn 20:799, 2000.
13. Morine M, Takeda T, Minekawa R, et al: Antenatal diagnosis and treatment of a case of fetal goitrous hypothyroidism associated with high-output cardiac failure. Ultrasound Obstet Gynecol 19:506, 2002.
14. Rovet J, Ehrlich R, Sorbara D: Intellectual outcome in children with fetal hypothyroidism. J Pediatr 110:700, 1987.
15. Sack J, Fisher DA, Hobel CJ, Lam R: Thyroxine in human amniotic fluid. J Pediatr 87:364, 1975.
16. Thorpe-Beeston JG, Nicolaides KH, McGregor AM: Fetal thyroid function. Thyroid 2:207, 1992.
17. Ballabio M, Nicolini U, Jowett T, et al: Maturation of thyroid function in normal human fetuses. Clin Endocrinol 31:565, 1989.
18. Van Herle AJ, Young RT, Fisher DA, et al: Intra-uterine treatment of a hypothyroid fetus. J Clin Endocrinol Metab 40:474, 1973.
19. Gruner C, Kollert A, Wildt L, et al: Intrauterine treatment of fetal goitrous hypothyroidism controlled by determination of thyroid-stimulating hormone in fetal serum: A case report and review of the literature. Fetal Diagn Ther 16:47, 2001.
20. Bruinse HW, Vermeulen-Meiners C, Wit JM: Fetal treatment for thyrotoxicosis in nonthyrotoxic pregnant women. Fetal Ther 3:152, 1988.
21. Wenstrom KD, Weiner CP, Williamson RA, Grant SS: Prenatal diagnosis of fetal hyperthyroidism using funipuncture. Obstet Gynecol 76:513, 1990.
22. Sack J, Fisher DA, Hobel CJ, Lam R: Thyroxine in human amniotic fluid. J Pediatr 87:364, 1975.
23. Thorpe-Beeston JG, Nicolaides KH, McGregor AM: Fetal thyroid function. Thyroid 2:207, 1992.
24. Ballabio M, Nicolini U, Jowett T, et al: Maturation of thyroid function in normal human fetuses. Clin Endocrinol 31:565, 1989.
25. Porreco RP, Bloch CA: Fetal blood sampling in the management of intrauterine thyrotoxicosis. Obstet Gynecol 76:509, 1990.
26. Hatjis CG: Diagnosis and successful treatment of fetal goitrous hyperthyroidism caused by maternal Graves' disease. Obstet Gynecol 81(5 Pt 2):837, 1993.
27. Brusque A, Rotta L, Pettenuzzo LF, et al: Chronic postnatal administration of methylmalonic acid provokes a decrease of myelin content and ganglioside N-acetylneuraminic acid concentration in cerebrum of young rats. Braz J Med Biol Res 34:227, 2001.
28. Ampola MG, Mahoney MI, Nakamura E, et al: Prenatal therapy of a patient with vitamin B responsive methylmalonic acidemia. N Engl J Med 293:313, 1975.
29. Andersson HC, Marble M, Shapira E: Long term outcome in treated combined methylmalonic acidemia and homocysteinemia. Genet Med 1:146, 1999.
30. Evans MI, Duquette DA, Rinaldo P, et al: Modulation of B12 dosage and response in fetal treatment of methylmalonic aciduria (MMA): Titration of treatment dose to serum and urine MMA. Fetal Diagn Ther 12:21, 1997.
31. Leon Del Rio A, Leclerc D, Gravel RA: Isolation of a cDNA encoding human holocarboxylase synthetase by functional complementation of a biotinauxotroph of E. coli. Proc Natl Acad Sci U S A 92:4626, 1995.

32. Suzuki Y, Akoi Y, Ishida Y, et al: Isolation and characterization of mutations in the holocarboxylase synthetase cDNA. Nat Genet 8:122, 1994.

33. Akoi Y, Suzuki Y, Sakamoto O, et al: Molecular analysis of holocarboxylase synthetase deficiency: A missense mutation and a single base deletion are predominant in Japanese patients. Biochim Biophys Acta 1272:168, 1995.

34. Dupuis L, Leon-Del-Rio A, Leclerc D, et al: Clustering of mutations in the biotin-binding region of holocarboxylase synthetase in biotin responsive multiple carboxylase deficiency. Hum Mol Genet 5:1011, 1996.

35. Popmponio RJ, Hymes J, Reynolds TR, et al: Mutation in the human biotinidase gene that cause profound biothinidase deficiency in symptomatic children: Molecular, biochemical, and clinical analysis. Pediatr Res 42:840, 1997.

36. Suormala T, Fowler B, Jakobs C, et al: Late onset holocarboxylase synthetase deficiency: Pre- and post-natal diagnosis and evaluation of effectiveness of antenatal biotin therapy. Eur J Pediatr 157:570, 1998.

37. Roth KS, Yang W, Allen L, et al: Prenatal administration of biotin: Biotin responsive multiple carboxylase deficiency. Pediatr Res 16:126, 1982.

38. Packman S, Cowan MJ, Golbus MS, et al: Prenatal treatment of biotin responsive multiple carboxylase deficiency. Lancet 1:1435, 1982.

39. Thuy LP, Jurecki E, Nemzer L, et al: Prenatal diagnosis of holocarboxylase synthetase deficiency by assay of the enzyme in chorionic villus material followed by prenatal treatment. Clin Chim Acta 284:59, 1999.

40. Smith DW, Lemli L, Opitz JM: A newly recognized syndrome of multiple congenital anomalies. J Pediatr 64:210, 1964.

41. Curry CJR, Carey JC, Holland JS: Smith-Lemli-Opitz syndrome—type II: Multiple congenital anomalies with male pseudohermaphroditism and frequent early lethality. Am J Med Genet 26:45, 1987.

42. Opitz JM: RSH-SLO ("Smith-Lemli-Opitz") syndrome: Historical, genetic, and development considerations. Am J Med Genet 50:344, 1994.

43. Kelley RI: A new face for an old syndrome. Am J Med Genet 65:251, 1997.

44. Kelley RI: Diagnosis of Smith-Lemli-Opitz syndrome by gas chromatography/mass spectrometry of 7-dehydrocholesterol in plasma, amniotic fluid and cultured skin fibroblasts. Clin Chim Acta 236:45, 1995.

45. Tint GS, Irons M, Elias E, et al: Defective cholesterol biosynthesis associated with the Smith-Lemli-Opitz syndrome. N Engl J Med 330:107, 1994.

46. Waterham HR, Wijburg FA, Hennekam RCM, et al: Smith-Lemli-Opitz is caused by mutations in the 7-dehydrocholesterol reductase gene. Am J Hum Genet 63:329, 1998.

47. Johnson JA, Aughton DJ, Comstock CH, et al: Prenatal diagnosis of Smith-Lemli-Opitz syndrome, type II. Am J Med Genet 49:240, 1994.

48. Hobbins JC, Jones OW, Gottesfeld MD, Persutte W: Transvaginal ultrasonography and transabdominal embryoscopy in the first-trimester diagnosis of Smith-Lemli-Opitz syndrome, type II. Am J Obstet Gynecol 171:546, 1994.

49. Sharp P, Haan E, Fletcher JM, et al: First trimester diagnosis of Smith-Lemli-Opitz syndrome. Prenat Diagn 17:355, 1997.

50. Irons M, Elias E, Tint GS, et al: Abnormal cholesterol metabolism in the Smith-Lemli-Opitz syndrome: Report of clinical and biochemical findings in 4 patients and treatment in 1 patient. Am J Med Genet 50:347, 1994.

51. Irons M, Elias ER, Abuelo D, et al: Treatment of Smith-Lemli-Opitz syndrome: Results of a multicenter trial. Am J Med Genet 68:311, 1997.

52. Elias ER, Irons MB, Hurley AD, et al: Clinical effects of cholesterol supplementation in six patients with the Smith-Lemli-Opitz syndrome (SLOS). Am J Med Genet 68:305, 1997.

53. Nowaczyk MJM, Whelan DT, Heshka TW, Hill R: Smith-Lemli-Opitz syndrome: A treatable inherited error of metabolism causing mental retardation. Can Med Assoc J 161:165, 1999.

54. Irons MR, Nores J, Stewart TL, et al: Antenatal therapy of Smith-Lemli-Opitz syndrome. Fetal Diagn Ther 14:133, 1999.

55. Elsas LJ: Prenatal diagnosis of galactose-1-phosphate uridyltransferase (GALT) deficient galactosemia. Prenat Diagn 21:302, 2001.

56. Chen YT, Mattis'on DR, Feigenbaum L, et al: Reduction in oocyte number following prenatal exposure to a high galactose diet. Science 314:1145, 1981.

57. Bandyopadhyay S, Chakrabarti J, Banerjee S, et al: Prenatal exposure to high galactose adversely affects initial gonadal pool of germ cells in rats. Hum Reprod 18:276, 2003.

58. Frey L, Hauser WA: Epidemiology of neural tube defects. Epilepsia 44(suppl 3):4, 2003.

59. Smithells RW, Sheppard S, Schorah CJ, et al: Possible prevention of neural tube defects by preconceptual vitamin supplementation. Lancet 1:399, 1980.

60. Smithells RW, Nevin NC, Seller MJ, et al: Further experience of vitamin supplementation for prevention of neural tube defect recurrences. Lancet 1:1027, 1983.

61. Younis JS, Granat M: Insufficient transplacental digoxin transfer in severe hydrops fetalis. Am J Obstet Gynecol 157:1268, 1987.

62. Mills JL, Rhoads GG, Simpson JL, et al: The absence of a relation between the periconceptional use of vitamins and neural-tube defects. N Engl J Med 321:430, 1989.

63. Mulinare J, Cordero JF, Erickson JD, Berry RJ: Periconceptional use of multivitamins and the occurrence of neural tube defects. JAMA 260:3141, 1988.

64. Schulman JD: Treatment of the embryo and the fetus in the first trimester: Current status and future prospects. Am J Med Genet 35:197, 1990.

65. MRC Vitamin Study Research Group: Prevention of neural tube defects: Results of the MRC vitamin study. Lancet 338:132, 1991.

66. Czeizel AE, Dudas I: Prevention of the first occurrence of neural-tube defects by preconceptional vitamin supplementation. N Engl J Med 327:1832, 1992.

67. Honein MA, Paulozzi LJ, Mathews TJ, et al: Impact of folic acid fortification of the US food supply on the occurrence of neural tube defects. JAMA 285:2981, 2001.

68. Olney RS, Mulinare J: Trends in neural tube defect prevalence, folic acid fortification, and vitamin supplement use. Semin Perinatol 26:277, 2002.

69. Evans MI, Llurba E, Landsberger EJ, et al: Impact of folic acid supplementation in the United States: Markedly diminished high maternal serum AFPs. Obstet Gynecol 103:474, 2004.

70. Parle-McDermott A, Mills JL, Kirke PN, et al: Analysis of MTHFR 1298AC and 677 CT polymorphisms as risk factor neural tube defects. J Hum Genet 48:190, 2003.

71. Finnell RH, Shaw GM, Lammer EJ, Volcik KA: Does prenatal screening for 5,10-methylenetetrahydrofolate reductase (MTHFR) mutations in high-risk neural tube defect pregnancies make sense? Genet Test 6:47, 2002.

72. Rampersaud E, Melvin EC, Siegel D, et al: Updated investigations of the role of methylenetetrahydrofolate reductase in human neural tube defects. Clin Genet 63:210, 2003.

73. Zhu H, Wicker NJ, Shaw GM, et al: Homocysteine remethylation enzyme polymorphisms and increased risks for neural tube defects. Mol Genet Metab 78:216, 2003.

74. Volocik KA, Shaw GM, Zhu H, et al: Risk factors for neural tube defects: Associations between uncoupling protein 2 polymorphisms and spina bifida. Birth Defects Res Part A Clin Mol Teratol 67:158, 2003.

75. Sever LE: Zinc deficiency in man. Lancet 1:887, 1973.

76. McMichael AJ, Dreosti IE, Gibson GT: A prospective study of serial maternal serum zinc levels and pregnancy outcome. Early Hum Dev 7:59, 1982.

77. Stoll C, Dott B, Alembik Y, Koehl C: Maternal trace elements, vitamin B_{12}, vitamin A, folic acid, and fetal malformations. Rep Toxicol 13:53, 1999.

78. Hambidge M, Hackshaw A, Wald N: Neural tube defects and serum zinc. Br J Obstet Gynaecol 100:746, 1993.

79. Shoob HD, Sargent RG, Thompson SJ, et al: Dietary methionine is involved in the etiology of neural defect-affected pregnancies in humans. J Nutr 131:2653, 2001.

80. Batshaw M, Brusilow S, Waber L, et al: Treatment of inborn errors of urea synthesis: Activation of alternative pathways of waste nitrogen synthesis and excretion. N Engl J Med 306:1387, 1982.

81. Nicolaides KH, Thorpe-Beeston JG, Noble P: Cordocentesis. In Eden RD, Boehm H (eds): Assessment and Care of the Fetus: Physiological, Clinical and Medico Legal Principles. Norwalk, CT, Appleton & Lange, 1990, p 291.

CHAPTER 14

Stem Cells and Gene Therapy

Laura S. Haneline and Mervin C. Yoder

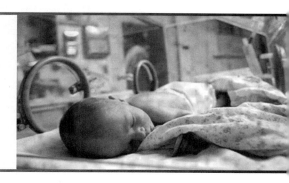

Modern medicine has affected all aspects of life, but probably no two topics have been so widely discussed in the recent popular press as stem cells and gene therapy. The field of stem cell biology is currently highly controversial. Although the potential applications of these cells for use in the treatment of human diseases are theoretically enormous, a clear understanding is needed of the biology of these cells and the complexities involved in differentiating stem cells into mature cells. A fair appraisal of the current state of the use of stem cells in the treatment of human diseases compared with the widely publicized therapeutic claims could be summarized as an "overselling" of the benefits of stem cells. A similar phenomenon occurred in gene therapy. Introducing genes into cells to treat inherited disorders, cure cancer, and diminish the impact of degenerative diseases in affected patients was highly touted, and great expectations arose, but the reality of gene therapy to treat human disorders subsequently became more circumspect. As stated by Verma, "The reality is that the timeline of promises kept is unpredictable, but the reaction to unfulfilled expectations is predictable."[1] Similarly, President George W. Bush stated, "...while we're all hopeful about the potential of this research, no one can be certain that the science will live up to the hope it has generated."[2]

This chapter introduces the reader to stem cell biology and gene therapy. First, several terms that partition stem cell biology into embryonic and adult categories are defined. A brief overview of stem cell isolation and characterization and methods for differentiating stem cells into mature cells follows. The stem cell overview concludes with a comparison of the biologic properties of embryonic and adult stem cells and some illustrations of the current uses of stem cells in treatments for human disorders. An introduction to gene therapy includes overviews of the major viral vectors for gene therapy. The principles of vector development for each virus, examples of the use of the vector in preclinical animal models of disease, and illustrations of the use of these systems for treatment of human clinical disorders comprise the gene therapy review.

STEM CELLS

Definitions

The human body is composed of approximately 200 kinds of cells. At birth and throughout life, all of the cells of the body share a common ancestry, having been derived from a single fertilized egg. The fertilized egg, or zygote, is referred to as a **totipotent cell** because it has the potential to form all of the cells necessary to form an entire embryo during development in utero. In essence, the zygote is the "mother" of all stem cells.

Stem cells are cells residing in embryonic, fetal, or adult tissues that have the capacity for prolonged self-renewal (cell division giving rise to at least one daughter cell possessing all of the potential of the parental cell) and the ability to give rise to mature cells that make up the tissues and organs of the body. **Pluripotent** stem cells possess the capacity to give rise to cells developing from all three embryonic germ layers—ectoderm, endoderm, and mesoderm. **Unipotent** or **bipotent** stem cells give rise to cells from one or two of the germ layers.

Embryonic stem (ES) cells are derived from cells of the inner cell mass of the mammalian blastocyst (Fig. 14-1) on culture of the cells in vitro under specific conditions. ES cells are pluripotent and show unlimited self-renewal potential in vitro. Murine ES cells retain the potential to form a complete embryo when reinjected into the inner cell mass of a recipient blastocyst and transferred into the womb of a pseudopregnant mouse. Murine and human ES cells form teratomas (benign tumors composed of multiple differentiated cell lineages) on transplantation into immunodeficient mice.[3]

Embryonic germ (EG) cells are derived from the developing gonads of fetal mammals.[4-6] The germ cells present in the developing gonads become EG cells on in vitro culture. Human EG cells, including individual clonal lines, display pluripotent differentiation potential in vitro.[7]

Adult stem cells are self-renewing cells residing in numerous tissues throughout the body (embryo, fetus, infant, or adult) that give rise to cells that mature into all of

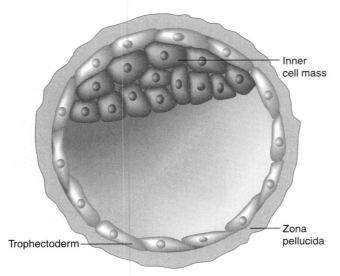

Figure 14–1. Human preimplantation blastocyst. Embryonic stem cells are derived in vitro from cells isolated from the inner cell mass.

the specialized cells that compose a specific tissue or organ. Adult stem cells have been identified in the bone marrow, blood, brain, skeletal muscle, gastrointestinal tract, pancreas, dental pulp, skin, liver, cornea, and retina.[8] Evidence suggests that some adult stem cells may be pluripotent.[9,10] Adult stem cells are rare cells that have not yet been shown to self-renew in an unlimited fashion in vitro. Adult stem cells also have been called *somatic stem cells* to clarify that they are not germ cells (sperm or oocyte). The term *postnatal stem cells* also has been used to delineate adult stem cells present in animals after birth from the stem cells present during embryonic and fetal development.

Adult stem cells generally give rise to cells specific for the tissue within which they reside; however, more recent studies have provided evidence that some adult stem cells are capable of being "reprogrammed" to differentiate into mature cells of another tissue (Fig. 14-2). Adult stem

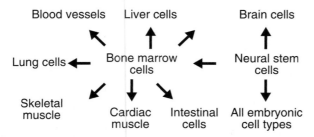

Figure 14–2. Diverse differentiation potential of stem cells isolated from the bone marrow and brain. Bone marrow cells not only produce blood cells, but also can be induced to differentiate into a variety of other cells comprising other tissues after transplantation. Neural stem cells are capable of differentiating into cells derived from all three embryonic germ layers (ectoderm, mesoderm, and endoderm), including bone marrow cells.

cells that can be reprogrammed display a characteristic called **plasticity**.[11] Adult stem cell plasticity is a poorly understood process that is difficult to prove experimentally. Rigorous criteria have been proposed to limit the use of this term to conditions in which a clone of cells derived from one tissue has been shown to give rise to functional cells of another tissue in vivo on transplantation.[12] **Clonality** refers to an entire group of cells being derived from a single cell. Few studies characterizing adult stem cells have been conducted at the clonal level.

Isolation and Characterization

The isolation and characterization of all ES, EG, and adult stem cells cannot be covered in this overview. The isolation and general description of murine and human ES and hematopoietic stem cells (HSC) are discussed. Interested readers are referred to several excellent publications discussing the isolation of murine and human EG cells and adult neural, hepatic, skeletal muscle, gastrointestinal tract, and skin stem cells.[13-19]

Murine Embryonic Stem Cells

Murine ES cells were isolated in 1981 by two groups of investigators who reported that cells from the inner cell mass of the murine blastocyst could be maintained in vitro in a pluripotent state under defined conditions.[20,21] Growth of the cells from the inner cell mass required a coculture system using pre-established murine embryonic fibroblast feeder monolayers. Subsequent studies indicated that murine ES cells required leukemia inhibitory factor (LIF) to be present in the culture medium to maintain high proliferative potential and to prevent loss of pluripotency and induction of cellular differentiation.[22] ES cells can be maintained indefinitely without chromosomal aberrations under these culture conditions and contribute to the formation of extraembryonic, fetal, and germ cell lineages on reintroduction into donor blastocysts and transfer into the fallopian tubes of pseudopregnant mice.[23]

Murine ES cells grow in tight compact colonies on mouse feeder layers or on nonadhesive culture dishes in the presence of LIF. The ES cells express several cell surface markers, including stage-specific antigen 1 (SSEA-1) and alkaline phosphatase. The nuclear transcription factor, Oct-4, is highly expressed, and this factor serves as a marker of the self-renewal potential of the ES cells. Murine ES cells form teratomas on injection into recipient mice.[24]

The ability to culture pluripotent cells in vitro has permitted novel insights and greater accessibility into gene expression and cellular differentiation pathways than previously available when attempting to study the murine postimplantation embryo in situ. Removal of LIF from the culture medium initiates murine ES cell differentiation. Plating LIF-deprived ES cells on nonadhesive culture plates or semisolid medium (methylcellulose) or placing ES cells into suspended drops of culture medium induces the cells to form spherical structures called *embryoid bodies* (EB).[25] Within the EB, cells derived from the embryonic germ layers develop with similar relationships to those of the developing embryo: embryonic endoderm on the exterior of the EB and mesoderm and ectoderm on the interior surrounding a fluid-filled cavity (yolk sac–like).

Disaggregation of the EB and replating the differentiating ES cells on various culture substrates, varying culture media with added growth factors or morphogens, or implantation subcutaneously into immunocompromised mice results in differentiation of the ES cells into multiple mature cell types, including neurons, pancreatic cells, blood cells, endothelial cells, cardiomyocytes, skeletal muscle cells, adipocytes, and numerous other cells.[26] By extrapolation, the ability of murine ES cells to proliferate extensively in vitro and to be differentiated into specific cell types underlies the current enthusiasm for studying human ES cells as a future means to create mature cells that can replace aged or damaged cells in human patients.

Murine ES cells can be genetically manipulated during in vitro culture. One of the most powerful approaches to understanding gene function is via mutational analysis. By altering the gene sequence and observing a change in a biologic activity of the animal, one may infer a role for the normal gene product in that particular biologic process.[27,28] A variety of genetic mutations in murine ES cells have been created using insertional mutagenic strategies, ES cell reintroduction into blastocysts to generate germline chimeras, and breeding analysis to identify recessive lethal mutations.[29] An alternative approach is to disrupt a normal gene through generation of a site-specific targeted mutation via homologous recombination of the cloned DNA sequences and the corresponding genomic locus in the ES cells. By selecting in vitro for the ES cells in which the cloned DNA sequence has been incorporated into the genome and transfer of the mutation into the germline (via ES cell injection into donor blastocysts and chimeric mouse generation), one is able to analyze the biologic consequence of disrupting a particular gene or a portion of that gene. This strategy is commonly referred to as generating a mouse *knockout*.[30]

Murine ES cells are pluripotent cells that serve as a novel reagent to study normal murine development, molecular pathways of cellular differentiation, genetic control of embryogenesis, and gene function during development. The culture conditions required to maintain ES cell pluripotency have proved invaluable to the derivation of human ES cells. Murine ES cells will continue to serve as a model system for analysis of gene function in the age of human gene discovery.

Human Embryonic Stem Cells

The isolation, characterization, and methods of derivation of human ES cells were first reported in 1998.[3] Cleavage-stage human embryos created via in vitro fertilization for clinical purposes were donated for research purposes by the donor families after informed consent and institutional review board approval of the study. From the 36 donor embryos, 20 were grown successfully to the blastocyst stage (day 5 postfertilization), immunosurgery was performed to remove the trophoblast cells, and inner cell mass cells were plated on murine fibroblast feeder cell layers (similar to derivation of murine ES cells). Five ES cell lines from five separate embryos were derived. These five ES cell lines continuously proliferated for

6 months and have been successfully cryopreserved. The karyotype of the ES cells was normal with three lines being female and two male. Removing the ES cells from the murine feeder layers resulted in differentiation of the cells. If the ES cells were allowed to overgrow and "pile up" on the feeder layers, however, the ES cells also underwent differentiation. Human LIF addition to the human ES cells plated in the absence of mouse feeder layers failed to maintain ES cell pluripotency and growth. Although mouse feeder layers are sufficient to maintain human and murine ES cell self-renewal, LIF alone is sufficient to maintain murine, but not human, ES cells in the absence of feeder layers.

The morphology of human ES cells is similar to murine ES cells. Both show a high nuclear-to-cytoplasmic ratio with prominent nucleoli. Human ES cells form colonies in vitro that are not as compact as murine ES cells but are similar to rhesus monkey ES cells.[31] Human ES cells express the cell surface markers SSEA-3 and alkaline phosphatase. Oct-4 expression is high, consistent with the self-renewal potential of these cells. Similar to murine ES cells, human ES cells express high levels of telomerase, an enzyme that lengthens telomeres. Telomere length maintenance is a property of self-renewing cells and some cancer cells.

The most favored test of human ES cell pluripotency is injection of the cells into immunocompromised mice and observing for the formation of human teratomas. All five of the original ES cell lines produced teratomas on intramuscular injection into mice. Analysis of the tissue in the teratomas showed that derivatives of all three embryonic germ layers were present.[3] Two cloned human ES cell lines have been derived from one of the original ES cell lines. The cloned human ES cells formed teratomas in vivo similar to the original ES cell population.[32,33] This result confirms that the progeny of a single human ES cell retain pluripotency despite the fact that these cells have been passaged extensively in vitro.

Advances in the in vitro differentiation of human ES cells into specific lineages have been reported.[32] Addition of retinoic acid and nerve growth factor to cultured human ES cells was reported to enhance neuronal cell differentiation significantly.[34] The differentiated cells showed extensive outgrowth of neuronal processes and expression of neuron-specific molecules. Co-culture of human ES cells with murine bone marrow or yolk sac cell lines induced hematopoietic differentiation in vitro.[35] The ES cell–derived hematopoietic cells expressed known human hematopoietic cell surface antigens and transcription factors. When plated in colony-forming cell assay cultures containing hematopoietic growth factors, numerous hematopoietic progenitor populations were identified. Hematopoietic cell maturation appeared to be normal. Finally, plating of human ES cells in conditions that promote EB formation resulted in spontaneous contractions occurring in 8.1% of the EB.[36] Cells from the areas of spontaneous contractions expressed cardiac-specific proteins and mRNA for cardiac-specific transcription factors and displayed morphologic evidence of sarcomeric organization and intercalated disk formation connecting adjacent cells. In addition, the ES cell–derived cells exhibited cardiomyocyte-like calcium ion transients that were synchronous with the recorded contractions and responded to positive and negative chronotropic agents. These data suggest that human ES cells can be differentiated into neurons, hematopoietic cells, and cardiomyocytes in vitro. At present, it is unknown if these cells would function in vivo, a crucial experimental hurdle for which new transplantation models may be required.

The current controversy regarding the use of human ES cells involves numerous arguments beyond the scope of this review.[37-41] For some individuals, use of human embryos for any research purposes is unethical. Others distinguish between (1) embryos created by in vitro fertilization and donated for research from (2) embryos created using donor oocytes specifically for research and (3) embryos made for research by transfer of somatic cell nuclei to donor enucleated oocytes (nuclear transfer or nuclear cloning).[42] Therapeutic cloning involves transfer of the nucleus from the somatic cells of a donor into an enucleated donor oocyte for the purpose of making medically useful cells and tissues via blastocyst generation, inner cell mass harvest, and generation of ES cells.[43] Using the nucleus of a somatic cell from a patient with a particular organ failure theoretically would permit generation of immunologically compatible cells (from the ES cells generated) that could be used to repair the damaged organ. This nuclear transfer technology differs from that used to help infertile couples.[44] In 2001, President George W. Bush announced that National Institutes of Health funds could be used to support research on the more than 60 human ES cell lines that already existed worldwide.[2] National debate continues regarding ethical questions surrounding the use of human embryos for research, research on human ES cells, and human nuclear cloning experiments.

Adult Stem Cells

Mouse hematopoietic stem cells. Hematopoiesis is the process of blood cell production. Although red blood cells were first observed microscopically in the late 1600s, tools to isolate and characterize HSC and their progeny have become available only since the mid-20th century.[45] In the mid-1940s, exposure to ionizing radiation was found to cause life-threatening lowering of all circulating blood cell concentrations (pancytopenia). Animals could be protected from the hematologic effects of radiation by cells residing in the spleen and bone marrow.[46-48] In 1961, in vivo transplantation techniques were reported that permitted analysis of HSC clonality, extensive self-renewal capacity, and multipotentiality.[49] Techniques were developed in the mid-1960s to permit the culture of mouse bone marrow cells in vitro, and the identification of a hierarchy of hematopoietic progenitor cells with different capacities to give rise to certain kinds of blood cells was reported.[50-52] Methods to highly purify HSC from mouse bone marrow have become available only since the 1980s.[53-56] The most recent advances have permitted isolation of a nearly pure population of mouse HSC.[9,57]

The primary site of hematopoiesis changes during murine development. Blood cells first emerge in the extraembryonic yolk sac.[58] On the 10th day of gestation (mouse pregnancy is completed in 20 days), blood cells colonize the developing liver, and this organ becomes the major site of hematopoiesis by the 12th day of gestation. Four days before birth, blood cells colonize the developing bone marrow and spleen, and after delivery, these sites become the lifelong source of hematopoietic cells for the animal.[59] HSC emerge in embryonic life in a pattern similar to the appearance of the mature blood cells, although distinct developmental differences in HSC homing and engraftment are apparent.[60,61]

Murine HSC are defined as self-renewing cells with the potential to repopulate all hematopoietic lineages of mature cells on transplantation into a recipient animal.[62] Murine HSC are heterogeneous, with some cells showing the capacity to repopulate all lineages for a short time (<4 months), whereas other cells repopulate the recipient animal long term (>4 months).[62] The long-term repopulating cells isolated from mouse bone marrow are generally present in a quiescent state; however, a natural slow turnover (self-renewal divisions) of these cells can be detected.[63,64] Murine HSC are rare cells with an approximate frequency of 1/100,000 marrow cells.[65] Culture of isolated murine HSC ex vivo generally is associated with loss of repopulating ability, but several advances have permitted some HSC maintenance for a short period in vitro.[66-68]

Although bone marrow HSC are recognized as the source of all circulating blood cells, studies have suggested that the differentiation potential of HSC may not be restricted to blood cell lineages alone. HSC have been shown to give rise to hepatocytes on injection into recipient animals with inherited or induced hepatic injury.[69,70] Analysis of the mechanisms involved suggests that fusion of the bone marrow–derived cells with hepatocytes is the most likely method of marrow-derived cell contribution to the liver repopulation that occurs in injury models of liver regeneration.[71] HSC that repopulate the marrow of lethally irradiated hosts also ameliorate the myocardial injury caused by coronary artery ligation in instrumented mice.[72] A single HSC may give rise to hematopoietic cells and epithelial cells in multiple organs in recipient mice.[9] These results suggest that HSC, one example of adult stem cells, may show greater differentiation potential than previously realized. Whether adult stem cells circulate and regularly participate in tissue homeostasis or become engaged in multilineage differentiation only under circumstances of significant tissue injury or disease remains to be determined.

The relatively slow proliferation, lack of significant self-renewal divisions in vitro, and rarity of HSC highlight the current known properties of all adult stem cells and are among the major apparent differences between adult stem cells and ES cells. These differences have led some to predict that ES cells may serve better as a source of differentiated cells for cell-based therapies in human patients. A preliminary report indicates, however, that a rare murine bone marrow cell displays properties similar to ES cells.[73] This adult progenitor cell has been passaged for more than 120 population doublings with no shortening of telomere length (cells express telomerase), and high levels of Oct-4 are expressed. Clonal cell lines have been established that display pluripotent differentiation capacity. If substantiated by further study in the mouse and if present in the human, these results would show that certain adult stem cells display properties almost equivalent to those of ES cells.

Human hematopoietic stem cells. Using experimental methods extrapolated from the murine model, HSC have been isolated from human subjects. Human HSC are present in fetal liver, umbilical cord blood, and bone marrow and can be mobilized into the peripheral blood for collection by apheresis.[74-76] As with the murine system, human hematopoiesis seems to be composed of a hierarchy of cells with progressive levels of lineage commitment and cellular differentiation as evidenced by the results of a variety of in vitro and in vivo assays.[56] In vitro colony-forming cell assays are used to define lineage-committed or multipotential hematopoietic progenitors. Long-term, culture-initiating cell assays detect the presence of hematopoietic cells that give rise to hematopoietic progenitor cells in vitro and correlate in frequency with transplantable HSC. Limitations in the ability of these in vitro assays to predict stem cell function precisely has led to development of murine assays of human HSC function. Human bone, fetal liver, or thymus tissue can be engrafted into tissues of immunodeficient mice, and transplanted human HSC engraft in these explanted human tissues in vivo.[77] Alternatively, certain strains of immunodeficient mice accept human HSC transplants, and most, although not all, lineages of human cells are produced in the recipient mice.[78]

Using all the aforementioned assays, investigators have been able to isolate and characterize the human HSC. Human cells with repopulating activity express the cell surface antigens CD34 and CD90, but not the antigens found on the surface of mature blood cells.[79] Human HSC can be enriched from donor tissue using cell surface expression of the CD34 antigen, and the number of CD34+ cells transplanted per kilogram of patient weight correlates with successful engraftment.[80] Only 1% to 2% of marrow cells express the CD34 antigen. As with murine HSC, human HSC generally lose repopulating ability on isolation and in vitro culture, and attempts at expanding HSC in vitro for transplantation purposes have not been successful.[81,82] One more recent advance has been the use of chemotherapeutic agents or hematopoietic growth factors to mobilize CD34-expressing HSC from the marrow into the peripheral blood of patients.[83] Large numbers of mobilized HSC and progenitor cells can be collected by apheresis and further enriched for cells expressing CD34. This procedure is gaining acceptance as a standard method for isolating sufficient numbers of HSC for human transplantation. Methods are available to isolate HSC from human tissues throughout the stages of human development. An encouraging report suggests that human HSC may expand ex vivo when cultured in hypoxic conditions and maintain in vivo repopulating ability (tested in immunodeficient mice).[84] If reproduced by studies conducted in large animals or in human clinical trials, this method of expanding stem cells may prove to be clinically relevant in enhancing stem cell engraftment.

In 1959, Thomas and colleagues[85] reported that treatment of leukemia patients with supralethal doses of irradiation and transplantation with donor bone marrow cells from their identical twin resulted in prompt hematopoietic recovery. Although the patients later died as a result of leukemia, these patients were the first to receive a marrow transplant successfully as therapy. The strategy of using myeloablative doses of chemotherapy and radiation was to overcome the host's immune response to allow the transplanted bone marrow cells to engraft and to eradicate the underlying hematologic malignancy. This has been a successful strategy, and many patients have benefited, although the chemotherapy and irradiation are associated with significant toxicities that limit this treatment to more healthy patients. A more recent experimental approach is to prepare patients with reduced or no pretransplant conditioning and to administer immunosuppressive medications post-transplantation.[86] This new approach of nonmyeloablative stem cell transplantation may become an optimal method for replacement of host hematopoietic cells with donor HSC and serve as a platform for cellular or gene therapies or both.

GENE THERAPY

Transfer of genes into cells in vivo to correct an existing genetic defect has been a target since the 1980s.[87] A variety of transfer vectors have been developed; these generally can be divided into viral and nonviral vectors. For the purposes of this review, an overview is provided of the most commonly used viral vectors for gene therapy. The field of nonviral vectors has been reviewed elsewhere.[88,89] The principle of gene therapy is simple. Insert a gene into a patient to express an essential gene product that functions normally to replace the gene product that is defective and causing disease. A successful gene therapy strategy would address several issues, including (1) delivery of a gene that encodes for a gene product that reverses the pathophysiologic progression of the patient's disease, (2) use of a transfer vector that causes the gene to be expressed by the appropriate cells within the body, and (3) provision of a vector delivery system for introducing the gene into the body.[88] Although gene therapy has been shown to be an efficacious therapy, there have been numerous pitfalls and side effects that have slowed the promise of this potentially revolutionary treatment paradigm.[90]

An overview of each of the major vector systems is presented. Where indicated, comments on the use of the vector in human gene therapy are made.

Retrovirus Vectors

Retroviruses were among the first viral vectors developed to introduce recombinant DNA into target cells for gene therapy.[91,92] Significant advances in understanding of retroviral biology have occurred since the original descriptions of retrovirus-mediated gene transfer into murine hematopoietic stem and progenitor cells in 1984 and 1985.[93-96] This knowledge has resulted in improved vector design and transduction protocols to enhance gene transfer efficiency in human cells. Information acquired from the study of retroviruses has provided insights into the design of newer viral vectors (i.e., lentivirus) and a novel strategy to follow the fate and proliferation patterns of individual stem cells to understand basic stem cell biology better.

Recombinant retroviral vectors used for gene delivery were based on the Moloney murine leukemia virus (MMLV) and were modified from wild-type MMLV to eliminate possible replication-competent retrovirus production from target cells, in addition to including therapeutic genes (Fig. 14-3).[91,92] The primary modifications were to delete genes necessary for viral particle packaging (*gag, pol,* and *env*) and to replace them with therapeutic genes. The recombinant retroviral vector still encodes long terminal repeats that contain promoter, enhancer, and DNA integration elements and a ψ sequence necessary for recognition of retroviral RNA, as opposed to other cellular RNAs, to be packaged into a viral particle. Recombinant retroviral vectors (constructed as plasmid DNA) are transfected into packaging cells to engineer a stable, high-titer retrovirus packaging cell line.

Packaging cell lines are typically immortalized fibroblasts that have had crucial components of virion assembly (*gag, pol,* and *env* genes) introduced into their genome.

Because these three genes do not contain a ψ sequence, however, they are not packaged in the virion, making the retrovirus incapable of replication when integrated into the target cell's genome. *Gag* encodes virion core structural proteins. *Pol* encodes a reverse transcriptase necessary for RNA transcription into DNA before integration can occur. *Env* encodes virion envelope glycoproteins that are recognized by specific receptors on target cells and are required for virion entry into the cell. The *env* gene was separated from *gag* and *pol* genes to reduce further the probability of replication-competent retrovirus production through homologous recombination.[97,98]

Retroviral vectors exhibit many qualities desired from an ideal viral vector. Development of a stable, moderately high-titer packaging cell line allows for the relative ease of reproducible retrovirus production, which can be prepared in quantities large enough to be clinically useful. Retroviral integration into the host cell's genome should permit stable, long-term expression of a therapeutic protein in the transduced cell and in the progeny of that cell. In addition, efficient transduction of many cell types that are actively dividing at the time of infection can be achieved with retroviruses.

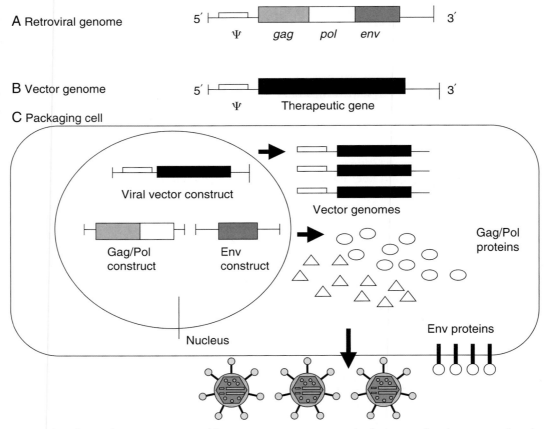

Figure 14–3. Retrovirus-based gene therapy vectors. **A,** Wild-type retrovirus genome encodes for *gag, pol,* and *env* genes. A packaging sequence or ψ allows retroviral RNA to be recognized and packaged into virion particles. **B,** Retroviral vectors used for gene delivery replace *gag, pol,* and *env* genes with a therapeutic gene of interest. **C,** Packaging cells are genetically engineered to contain a Gag/Pol construct and an Env construct to decrease the likelihood of replication-competent retrovirus generation. The viral vector construct is transfected into packaging cells. Viral vector RNA is recognized and packaged with Gag and Pol proteins into a virion particle that is coated with Env proteins. Virions are released into the supernatant overlaying the packaging cells.

Although retroviral vectors have many of the attributes of an ideal gene delivery vehicle, significant problems limit extensive use of these vectors for all potential clinical applications. To obtain lifelong expression of recombinant proteins, stem cells have been targeted so that repeated treatments would not be required, decreasing the risk of an immunologic response. Because of the relative ease of harvesting HSC, the hematopoietic system has been used as a model system to study extensively methods that enhance transduction efficiency and result in sustained recombinant protein expression. The lessons learned from the hematopoietic system are likely to have an impact on the ability to treat multiple inherited and acquired disorders using other target cell populations. Major limitations for using retrovirus-mediated gene transfer as a viable therapy continue to be low transduction efficiency and sustained recombinant protein expression. A review of strategies to overcome both of these problems follows.

Successful transduction of a target cell by a retrovirus involves three crucial steps, as illustrated in Figure 14-4: binding to a specific receptor, reverse transcription, and integration. Deficiencies in two of these processes (receptor binding and integration) pose significant obstacles in achieving high levels of HSC transduction. One approach to enhance the efficiency of retrovirus binding and entry into stem cells has been to substitute alternative envelope glycoprotein genes (*env*) in packaging cells to target virion binding to different receptors.[99] This modification, referred to as *retroviral pseudotype*, alters the range of cells targeted due to specific receptor expression patterns. Table 14-1 summarizes retroviral envelope pseudotypes and the receptors targeted. Ecotropic and amphotropic pseudotyping were among the first described and have been studied extensively.[98] More recent studies suggest, however, that newer alternative envelope glycoproteins are capable of transducing a higher proportion of human stem cells compared with the earlier envelope pseudotypes.[100-107] Currently, several investigators are attempting to optimize gene transfer efficiency by modifying the retroviral envelope, making this an exciting area of investigation to follow in the near future.

An additional hindrance to efficient transduction is that limited numbers of retroviral receptors are expressed

Table 14–1. Retroviral Envelope Pseudotypes

Retroviral Envelope Pseudotype	Receptor Name
Ecotropic	m-CAT
Amphotropic	Pit-2
Gibbon ape leukemia virus (GALV)	Pit-1
Vesicular stomatitis virus (VSV-G)	Unknown
Retrovirus (10A1)	Pit-1 and Pit-2
Feline leukemia virus group B (FeLV-B)	Pit-1
Feline leukemia virus group C (FeLV-C)	FLVCR
Simian type D retrovirus RD 114	RDR

on human HSC.[99] The observation that transduction efficiency could be enhanced by coculturing stem cells on either packaging cells or a stromal layer[108] led to the novel approach of increasing gene transfer efficiency by colocalizing the HSC and virion using fibronectin, an important extracellular matrix protein.[109-111] Fibronectin contains binding sites for cell adhesion molecules (VLA-4 and VLA-5), which mediate HSC binding, and a heparin binding site, which aids virion binding through surface glycoproteins (Fig. 14-5). Studies using recombinant fibronectin fragments containing these sites revealed that colocalization of stem cell and virion significantly enhances gene transfer efficiency.[110,112] This observation was instrumental in assessing the potential therapeutic benefit of retrovirus-mediated gene transfer because coculturing techniques could not be used clinically owing to multiple safety concerns and technical difficulties in maintaining large-scale cocultures.

Optimizing retrovirus integration in HSC is a particularly challenging issue due to two facts that seem to be mutually exclusive: active cell division is mandatory for integration to occur, yet a defining property of HSC is their relative quiescence. To circumvent this problem, strategies have been evaluated that induce cycling in these cells to increase transduction efficiency, including cytokine/growth factor stimulation or treatment with cyclin-dependent kinase inhibitors.[78] Initiation of stem cell cycling may induce differentiation instead of stem cell replication or self-renewal, making these methods less than optimal given the current understanding of stem cell biology. In addition, this approach does not work for nondividing tissues (i.e., brain, heart, lung, pancreas), which makes the inability of retroviruses to infect nondividing cells a major drawback restricting clinical utility.

Successful transduction is the first step toward gene therapy; however, it may not be the most difficult barrier to treating human disease. In addition to the obstacles discussed earlier that hinder transduction efficiency, investigators have encountered problems with the level of sustained recombinant protein expression. Normal endogenous protein expression is tightly regulated in all cells, and the regulation of specific proteins differs between cell types. Thus, it is not difficult to imagine how either low or high levels of a particular protein could be

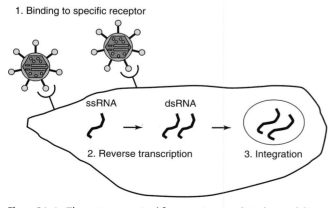

Figure 14–4. Three steps required for retrovirus-mediated gene delivery into target cells.

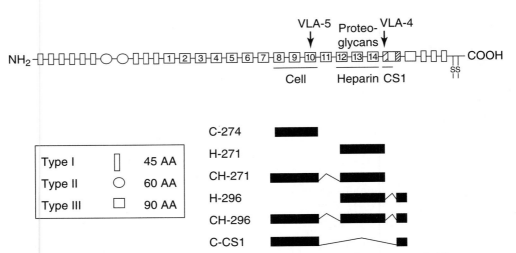

Figure 14–5. Fibronectin structure of A chain. Schematic of fibronectin illustrates types I through III amino acid (AA) repeat sequences and various binding domains. Below the fibronectin molecule are schematics of recombinant fibronectin fragments that have been used to evaluate functional binding domains for retrovirus-mediated gene transduction. The cell domain binds VLA-5, the heparin domain mediates adhesion through surface proteoglycans, and the CS1 domain binds VLA-4. VLA-4 and VLA-5 are adhesion molecules expressed on the surface of multiple cell types.

detrimental or limit the functional capabilities of a protein. The ability of a cell to up-regulate or down-regulate expression may be crucial for specific protein function.

Controlling recombinant protein expression may be more complex than initially anticipated. Recombinant protein expression is affected by promoter and enhancer elements in the long terminal repeat sequences of the retroviral vector and by the number and site of integrations in the target cell. Additional unknown factors probably have a role as well. Several investigators have described a phenomenon termed *transcriptional silencing,* in which transcription of retroviral sequences ceases, extinguishing a cell's ability to produce the desired protein.[113] To address some of these issues regarding levels of protein expression, many investigators are exploring the possibility of tightly regulating expression of retroviral encoded genes using self-inactivating vectors.[114-116] In these vectors, retroviral promoter and enhancer sequences are replaced with either tissue-specific endogenous promoters or regulatable promoters so that expression can be turned on and off. Regulating when and in what tissues a protein is expressed may reduce unwanted side effects, improve protein function, and enhance clinical efficacy. Further studies evaluating the optimal promoter or enhancer sequences (or both) to target specific cell populations are currently under way.

Additional risks are (1) the potential for an immunologic response against either retroviral proteins or the expressed therapeutic protein and (2) disruption of a normal gene sequence/function by insertion of retroviral DNA (insertional mutagenesis). Currently, no cases have been reported that describe an immunologic response against retroviral proteins. Although this is reassuring, it does not exclude the possibility that an immunologic response may occur in individual patients or with expression of specific proteins, an important safety consideration when designing gene therapy clinical trials. Two cases of insertional mutagenesis

with subsequent progression to leukemia have now been reported, however.[117,118]

Early optimism for treating children with X-linked severe combined immunodeficiency disorder (SCID) was dampened by complications involving insertional mutagenesis. Initially, three young children (ages 1 to 11 months) with X-linked SCID were treated successfully in Paris, France.[119] These children had a mutation in the γ chain (γc) subunit of multiple cytokine receptors resulting in an early block in T-cell and natural killer cell differentiation. Bone marrow cells were harvested from these patients, transduced with a retrovirus containing the normal γc gene, and infused back into the patients. Ten months after transplantation, all three patients had normal lymphocyte functions and seemed to be cured clinically. Eleven patients were enrolled in the French gene therapy trial for the treatment of SCID, which promised to be a cure for this lethal disorder. Two children have now developed a T-cell leukemia, due at least in part to disruption of a known tumor suppressor gene involved in T-cell leukemias (LMO-2).[117] Numerous national and international committees have discussed the risks and benefits of continuing gene therapy trials,[118,120] an ethical dilemma that continues to trouble clinicians trying to develop lifesaving therapies without creating life-threatening problems. More recent reviews highlight relevant considerations for the continuation of gene therapy clinical trials.[121,122]

In addition to the potential direct clinical applications of retroviruses, they can be used to follow the fate and proliferation patterns of individual stem cells to understand basic stem cell biology better. This experimental method has been used to document HSC migration from fetal liver to bone marrow and to show that individual HSC proliferation and differentiation patterns fluctuate over time.[123,124] When a retrovirus infects a stem cell, random retroviral integration results in a unique genetic "mark" of the stem cell and all its differentiated progeny, which allows for the detection of changes in clonal expansion or proliferative fates of an individual stem cell. Using molecular biology techniques, such as Southern blotting or inverse polymerase chain reaction, unique integration patterns can be detected to examine the behavior of individual stem cells. Conceptually, this is a powerful tool in understanding stem cell biology. With the rapidly growing area of adult stem cell plasticity research and the realization of potential clinical applications, it is apparent that techniques such as retroviral genetic marking are necessary to prove whether a single adult stem cell is pluripotential and can be reprogrammed into different cellular fates, depending on the environmental stimuli encountered.

Adeno-Associated Virus Vectors

Adeno-associated viruses (AAVs) are single-stranded DNA viruses that are members of the Parvoviridae family. These 20- to 30-nm, nonenveloped viruses are among the smallest viruses known to exist. AAVs constitute the *Dependovirus* genus and are called such because of the requirement for a helper virus to enable a productive viral infection. These viruses have a broad host range and cause no disease in human subjects.[125]

Under nonpermissive conditions, a cellular AAV infection is followed by integration of the virus into the host genome. In human subjects, wild-type AAVs integrate site specifically into the q arm of chromosome 19. When integrated, the virus remains dormant until the cell is subsequently infected with a helper virus, such as adenovirus or herpesvirus. The presence of the helper virus (permissive conditions) rescues the integrated AAV genome from the host chromosome and leads to the production of a lytic cycle.[125] This natural predilection to integrate site specifically is one major attribute of AAVs that has led to the development of these viruses as vectors for gene transfer.[126] The genomes of multiple AAV serotypes have been isolated and sequenced.[127] Distinctive features include a standard genomic composition of 4680 nucleotides that includes two large open reading frames for several structural (capsid) proteins and some nonstructural, regulatory (rep) proteins. A unique aspect of the AAV genomic

sequence is the presence of 145-nucleotide palindromic, inverted terminal repeats (Fig. 14-6). When the DNA is folded on itself to maximize potential base pairing, the overall palindrome forms a T-shaped structure. These terminal repeats are required for the replication and packaging of the AAV genome.

Use of AAV serotype 2 (AAV2) as a viral transduction vector was first reported in 1984.[128] The AAV2 capsid proteins were deleted, and the bacterial neomycin resistance gene was inserted. This recombinant plasmid was transfected into human cells that previously had been infected with adenovirus to supply the helper virus function. To supply the missing capsid proteins, it was necessary to cotransfect a second plasmid containing the missing structural proteins but no other elements that would permit AAV2 packaging. This double transfection into helper virus–infected cells permitted harvesting of recombinant AAV2 virions at nearly 1 million infectious particles per milliliter of cell culture supernatant. In subsequent years, it has become known that the inverted terminal repeats are the only *cis*-acting elements (DNA sequence contiguous to the inserted gene of interest) required for the development of recombinant AAV vectors. Additional improvements included construction of a plasmid containing all of the adenoviral gene elements that were sufficient to serve as helper elements to provide permissive conditions for recombinant AAV2 virion production in human cells in vitro and to produce AAV2 without adenoviral contamination.[129]

The specific steps required for successful infection of cells with recombinant AAV2 have been only recently identified. Given the broad host range of wild-type AAV infectivity, many scientists were surprised to learn in 1998 that AAV2 infection requires target cell expression of heparan sulfate proteoglycan (HSPG).[130] Subsequent studies showed that HSPG and fibroblast growth factor receptor 1 are required for AAV2 binding and internalization into target cells.[131] AAV2 also may bind to certain cell surface adhesion molecules that promote AAV2 binding and cellular entry.[132] On internalization, the AAV2 must traffic to the cell nucleus, a process influenced by certain intracellular signaling pathways. Finally, the most

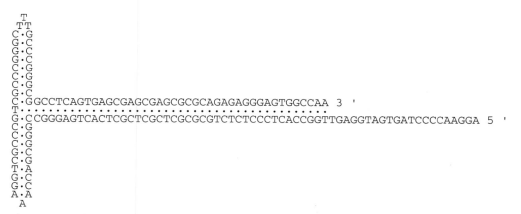

Figure 14–6. The adeno-associated virus (AAV) inverted terminal repeats are 145 nucleotides in length. The palindromic sequence allows the DNA to fold to form a stable hairpin T structure.

significant rate-limiting step in the efficiency of AAV2 vector transduction may be in the synthesis of the complementary strand to the single AAV2 virion DNA in the infected cell nucleus.[133] Expression from recombinant AAV2 in cells in vivo and in vitro correlates with the formation of duplex DNA. Advances in understanding these basic aspects of AAV2 biology have permitted improved vector design, higher titers of recombinant virions produced, and improved efficiency of AAV2 transduction in vitro and in vivo.[134]

AAVs display many properties that are advantageous to use as gene transfer vectors. AAVs are nonpathogenic in humans, although nearly 90% of adult subjects are seropositive. AAVs infect dividing and nondividing cells, integrate into the host chromosome, and show long-term expression in vivo, and there is low probability of vector rescue because all viral coding sequences have been deleted from current AAV vectors. Recombinant AAV vectors can be produced in high titer and are resistant to heat and chemical solvents.[126] A limitation of AAVs is that the gene of interest to be inserted into the recombinant AAV backbone can be no longer than 4.5 to 5 kb. Larger DNA inserts would not be packaged because the normal AAV genome is restricted to 4.68 kb, and the structural proteins cannot enclose a larger DNA component. Several more recent advances may overcome this limitation by relying on the known property that AAVs form concatamers (either integrated into the host genome or as episomal templates into the cytoplasm) after cell infection.[135,136]

The most widely studied and used AAV for gene transfer is AAV2. This serotype may be more limited for human use than some of the other serotypes because nearly 90% of individuals may have circulating neutralizing antibodies to the AAV2 virions. Comparison of several AAV serotypes reveals some similarities and differences with regard to immune recognition in human subjects. Types 1, 2, and 3 are highly homologous with respect to viral capsid amino acid composition and binding to HSPG. Although neutralizing antibody to all three of these serotypes has been documented, AAV1 has never been isolated from a clinical sample. Types 4 and 5 are distinctly different, and antibodies raised to these virions do not cross-react with each other or any of the other serotypes. Varying the capsid structure of recombinant AAVs results in differential tissue tropism when injected intravenously into experimental mice. This variation in tissue infectivity may be another potential advantage when the specific cell surface receptors for each serotype are known, and the regulation of cellular expression of these receptors is determined.[134]

Use of recombinant AAVs for efficient gene transfer into the central nervous system, muscle, lung, gut, liver, blood, and eye in several mammalian systems has provided sufficient preclinical data to initiate human clinical trials.[127] Treatment of mice and hemophilic dogs with a single intramuscular injection of AAV-encoding blood coagulation factor IX resulted in sustained (1 and 2.5 years) expression of the factor at levels sufficient to correct the hemophilic phenotype. Based on these and other preclinical safety data, a recombinant AAV encoding the human factor IX coding sequence was constructed and tested in a phase I human clinical trial.[137] Adult patients with factor IX deficiency receiving replacement therapy were given a single intramuscular injection in a dose-escalation design. Data from the first three patients (lowest dose) indicate that the AAV provirus is present in the skeletal muscle site and factor IX is expressed. Factor IX was present in the serum above the preinjection baseline level in one of the three subjects. No toxicities were observed in these first three patient volunteers; however, one ongoing concern is whether the vector may infect the germ cells of the patients and potentially be transmittable in reproductively active subjects. These preliminary data suggest that AAV-mediated gene therapy for hemophilia B is safe and has the potential to be efficacious in affected patients; however, testing at higher doses is required to confirm this speculation.[137]

Adenovirus Vectors

Adenoviruses are large viruses with a complex icosahedral capsid giving the virus a distinctive morphology.[138] The virus genome is arranged as a linear sequence of double-stranded DNA ending in inverted terminal repeats (similar to the AAVs). The 36 kb of DNA encode for more than 50 polypeptides. Adenoviruses have a broad host range and infect dividing and nondividing cells, including even highly differentiated cells, such as skeletal muscle, lung, brain, and heart. Because wild-type adenoviruses deliver their genome to the nucleus and can replicate with high efficiency, these viruses have long been considered prime candidates as gene transfer vectors.[139]

More than 50 different human adenoviral serotypes have been identified.[138] Serotypes 1, 2, 4, 5, and 7 are common causes of disease in patients. Adenoviral infections present in human subjects as a "common cold" or as an influenza-like illness with acute pharyngitis, conjunctivitis, or pneumonia. Most adults have been exposed to multiple adenoviral serotypes as children, and more than 90% express neutralizing antibodies to adenoviruses. Current adenoviral vectors are derived from adenovirus serotypes 2 and 5.

The natural infectious cycle of adenoviruses can be divided into two phases. The early phase is characterized by entry of the virus into the cell, passage of the adenoviral genome into the host nucleus, and selective transcription and translation of viral genes. This early phase modulates the host cellular biochemistry and physiology to facilitate viral gene transcription and translation of proteins necessary for the encapsidation of the replicated viral genome into mature virions in the late phase of the infectious cycle. The entire adenoviral life cycle can be accomplished in permissive cells in 10 to 14 hours, and one infected cell can produce 10,000 virions.

Four primary sets of gene products are important in promoting the early adenoviral gene transcription phase.[138] The E1, E2, and E4 gene products play important roles in initiation of viral gene transcription, modulation of the host cell metabolism to facilitate viral replication, and replication of the entire adenoviral genome. The E3 genes seem dispensable for the viral life cycle but play an important role in attempting to subvert host defense immune mechanisms that normally eradicate virally infected cells. These four sets of genes have been the prime targets to remove to create recombinant adenoviral vectors for gene transfer.

In the first generation of adenoviral vectors, the E1 region alone or the E1 and E3 regions were removed to create room for insertion of a therapeutic gene and to prevent initiation of viral gene transcription.[139] An example of a typical vector is depicted in Figure 14-7, in which a plasmid containing the gene of interest has been inserted into the former E1 gene position of a serotype 5 adenoviral genome. The inserted plasmid contains the left adenoviral inverted terminal repeat, an encapsidation signal, and the promoters and enhancers to drive expression of the gene of interest. A simian virus 40 (SV40) polyadenylation signal also has been inserted to promote mature mRNA transcripts of the gene of interest. The recombinant adenoviral plasmids are transfected into 293 human epithelial cells (embryonic kidney) that are known to express the E1 adenoviral proteins constitutively. The 293 cells provide the "missing" E1 adenoviral proteins that have been deleted from the recombinant adenoviral plasmid and together provide all the necessary proteins for replication of the recombinant adenoviral genome (containing the gene of interest) and sustain mature virion production.

Even in the absence of the E1 gene products, some transcription of the adenoviral genes in the recombinant adenoviral plasmid was found to occur when the vectors were injected in vivo. These proteins caused typical responses in the host cells that activated an immune response, including T cell–mediated destruction of the transduced cells.[140] The immune response rapidly diminished expression of the gene of interest in the host.[141] Newer vectors have been created in which the E2 or E4 genes or both or nearly all of the viral genes (gutless vectors) have been removed.[142] This last group of vectors contains only the inverted terminal repeats and packaging sequence in addition to the gene of interest. Helper virus and the recombinant gutless vectors are propagated in appropriate host cells, and the recombinant virions are

purified to remove the helper virus. Although these viruses have decreased toxicity in animals, infusion of an E1/E4–deleted recombinant adenovirus into the hepatic artery of a human patient with partial ornithine transcarbamylase deficiency resulted in the first reported fatality from gene therapy.[91]

Adenoviral vectors have been administered to experimental animals to transduce liver, skeletal muscle, heart, brain, lung, pancreas, and a variety of tumors.[138,143] The first human clinical trials using recombinant adenoviruses involved delivering the cystic fibrosis gene to the respiratory epithelium of affected adult volunteers.[144] These early trials were unable to show clinical efficacy.[145] Adenoviral vectors continue to be attractive candidate vectors for treatment of cancer.[146] A variety of replication-selective adenoviral vectors have been created as oncolytic agents.[147]

Lentivirus Vectors

Lentiviruses are a distinct family of retroviruses that possess many of the positive features of other retroviral vectors, including stable genomic integration and lack of immunogenicity. The major advantage of lentiviral vectors is the unique ability to infect nondividing cells,[148,149] including quiescent stem cells and terminally differentiated cells (i.e., neurons, cardiomyocytes, hepatocytes). This characteristic of lentiviruses broadens their potential clinical applications, making them a particularly attractive viral vector system. Previous information acquired from studying retroviruses is being used to optimize the development of lentiviral vectors, advancing understanding of lentiviral biology at an astonishing pace. Current knowledge, which is truly in its infancy, suggests that lentiviral vectors are more complex than other retroviral vectors. This section provides only basic information. For more inquisitive readers, reviews by Lever[150] and Trono[151] are recommended additional resources along with independent literature reviews to obtain the most up-to-date information.

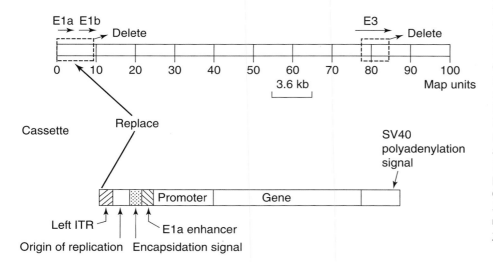

Adenovirus type 5

Figure 14–7. Diagram of a prototypical first-generation recombinant replication-defective adenovirus vector. The E1 and E3 regions of the type 5 adenoviral genomic DNA are deleted. An expression cassette containing essential *cis*-acting viral elements at the left end (inverted terminal repeat [ITR]), a promoter, and the gene of interest plus polyadenylation signals is inserted in the former E1 position. The recombinant adenovirus genome is packaged in an embryonic human kidney cell line (293 cells) that provides adenovirus E1 gene products *trans* to the recombinant E1-deficient genome. *(Modified from Brody SL, Crystal RG: Adenovirus-mediated in vivo gene transfer. Ann N Y Acad Sci 716:90-101, 1994.)*

The initial lentiviral vectors for gene transfer were described in 1990 and were based on human immunodeficiency virus (HIV-1).[152] The HIV genome encodes some of the same components as other retroviruses *(gag, pol,* and *env)*. The additional complexity of the HIV genome is illustrated, however, by the existence of many accessory genes *(tat, nef, rev, vpr, vpu,* and *vif)*, as shown in Figure 14-8.[92] Much of the HIV genome has been deleted from current lentiviral vectors with the intention of eliminating replication-competent lentivirus production to decrease the risk of HIV infection and acquired immunodeficiency syndrome (AIDS), without diminishing gene transfer capabilities.[153] Although these manipulations seem to reduce the potential for replication-competent lentivirus production, the concentration of viral particles produced or lentivirus titer is significantly lower, making the application of these viruses in gene transfer protocols more challenging.

Besides deleting HIV accessory genes, additional modifications have been necessary to transduce a wide variety of cell types and to increase the ease of high-titer lentivirus production. One crucial manipulation was to change the envelope protein because HIV normally targets a specific T-lymphocyte subset (CD4 cells). Currently the envelope pseudotype used most frequently is the vesicular stomatitis

virus G protein (VSV-G), which allows for a broader spectrum of cells to be infected by lentiviruses.[154] Several cell types have been targeted successfully with VSV-G pseudotyped lentiviruses, including retinal cells, pancreatic islet cells, HSC, hepatocytes, neurons, muscle, respiratory epithelium, and cells of the inner ear.[151,154-158] In addition, VSV-G pseudotyping facilitates the enhancement of lentivirus titer using centrifugation methods,[100] which overcomes the obstacles encountered after deletion of other HIV genes.

To improve the reproducibility and ease of lentivirus production, it was necessary to develop a stable lentiviral packaging cell line. Initial attempts to create a lentiviral packaging cell line proved to be difficult due to the cytopathic effects of lentiviruses on packaging cells themselves. To avoid these toxic effects, a cell line was developed that contained a tetracycline-inducible expression system, which results in reasonable lentivirus titers that can be concentrated using centrifugation methods.[159,160]

Other promising lentiviral vector alterations include the addition of sequences that facilitate initiation of reverse transcription, nuclear transport, or efficiency of translation.[161-163] In addition, to increase further the safety of these vectors, self-inactivating lentiviral vectors have been developed.[164] Because of the theoretical risk of developing

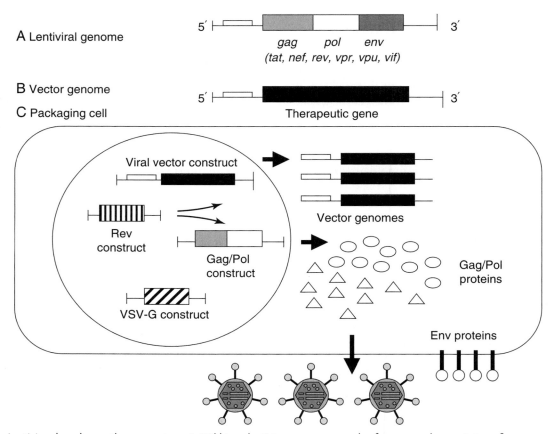

Figure 14–8. Lentivirus-based gene therapy vectors. **A,** Wild-type lentivirus genome encodes for *gag, pol, env, tat, nef, rev, vpr, vpu,* and *vif* genes. A packaging sequence or ψ allows lentiviral RNA to be recognized and packaged into virion particles. **B,** Lentiviral vectors used for gene delivery replace lentiviral genes with a therapeutic gene of interest. **C,** Packaging cells are cotransfected with a Rev construct, Gag/Pol construct, VSV-G construct, and viral vector construct, and the lentiviral virion production is similar to other retroviruses.

AIDS with HIV-based constructs, vectors are being developed that are based on lentiviruses that do not cause human disease, including simian, equine, feline, and sheep viruses.[158,165-171] Presently, there is no evidence of recombinant HIV production from target cells transduced with the current HIV-based vectors. In addition, there is no evidence at this point that vectors based on non-HIV lentiviruses offer any additional benefits to the originally described HIV vectors.

Although the potential benefits of lentiviral vectors seem extraordinary, the theoretical risks may prohibit or significantly limit their use on human patients. No clinical trials are currently under way; however, many investigators are exploring this possibility. Although considerable progress already has been made in understanding lentivirus biology, the evaluation of these vectors remains in beginning stages. With the potential impact on treating human disease, lentiviral research will be an exciting area to follow over the next several years. As previously learned from experience with retroviral vectors, however, the reality of using gene therapy as a routine treatment for inherited or acquired disorders is unpredictable, given the likelihood of encountering unknown future obstacles.

Herpes Simplex Virus Vectors

Herpes simplex virus (HSV) is a neurotropic, enveloped, double-stranded DNA virus. The HSV genome is composed of 152 kb of DNA and encodes for 84 gene products. As with the other viral vectors, the gene products of the HSV genome have been categorized as essential or nonessential (for purposes of deletion and insertion of genes of interest) based on whether expression is required for viral replication in permissive cells.[172]

Some unique aspects of the HSV-1 life cycle make this virus an attractive vector candidate. After a primary infection with the virus, viral particles may enter sensory neurons, innervating the area of infection. The viral genome is carried to the neuronal body, where the DNA enters the nucleus. Two pathways may be taken. If the lytic pathway is chosen, the virus undergoes viral replication, viral packaging, and cell lysis with release of mature infectious virions. Alternatively the viral DNA may enter a latent phase, in which the HSV genome exists in an episomal state for up to the life of the individual. This ability of the virus to exist in a latent state in neurons may be useful for therapeutic transgene expression in neurons.[173]

Because wild-type HSV infection and replication in a cell generally result in cell lysis, vector construction requires that the genes involved in HSC replication be inactivated. A series of immediate-early genes are essential for initiating viral gene transcription. Disrupting one or more of these immediate-early genes formed the basis of the earliest HSV vectors. Deletion of these genes alone was insufficient, however, to prevent cytotoxicity, and many other HSV genes have been targeted for deletion to improve utility of HSV vectors.[173]

HSV vectors have been used to transduce neurons in vivo in many experimental animal models of human neurologic disorders. These vectors have been used successfully to express neurotropic factors in neurons in models of neuropathic diseases.[174] HSV vectors have

Table 14–2. Advantages and Disadvantages of Simian Virus 40 Viral Vectors

Advantages
Wide diversity of cells infected
Infects quiescent and dividing cells
Integrates into host cell genome
Deleting *Tag* makes replication incompetent
Packaging cell lines available
No associated human disease

Disadvantages
Potential reacquisition of *Tag* from packaging cells
Virus titering time-consuming
Small genome size of simian virus 40 constructs may limit the size of therapeutic genes

been used to express analgesic molecules intrasynaptically and avoid systemic side effects of some medications.[175] Neuroprotection of the central nervous system also has been shown via HSV-mediated transient expression of certain gene products.[176] Many studies have produced HSV vectors for delivery of antitumor genes to malignant cells.[177-179] Further modifications of HSV vectors may permit use of these neurotropic vectors in human clinical trials.

Simian Virus 40 Vectors

To conclude this review of viral vectors for gene transfer, SV40 vectors are briefly discussed. SV40 is a double-stranded circular DNA papovavirus that was engineered into a unique gene delivery system in 1996.[180] To decrease the risk of replication-competent SV40 production, the large T antigen gene *(Tag)* was deleted from SV40 constructs and replaced with a cloning site for introducing therapeutic genes easily. Packaging cells then provide *Tag* for virion production. The advantages and disadvantages of SV40 viral vectors are outlined in Table 14-2.[180] Probably the major advantage of SV40 viral vectors is the ability to transduce nondividing cells. Most work to date has focused on transduction of hepatocytes, hematopoietic progenitor cells, and T lymphocytes.[181-184] Currently, no clinical trials are being conducted. Scientists are actively investigating the potential of using SV40 vectors, however, as a novel treatment strategy for HIV-infected individuals.[185,186]

REFERENCES

1. Verma I: Are the benefits of stem cells being oversold? Mol Ther 4:161, 2001.
2. Vogel G: Bush squeezes between the lines on stem cells. Science 293:1242-1245, 2001.
3. Thomson JA, Itskovitz-Eldor J, Shapiro SS, et al: Embryonic stem cell lines derived from human blastocysts. Science 282:1145, 1998.
4. Shamblott M, Axelman J, Wang S, et al: Derivation of pluripotent stem cells from cultured human primordial germ cells. Proc Natl Acad Sci U S A 95:13726, 1998.

5. Matsui Y, Zsebo K, Hogan B: Derivation of pluripotential embryonic stem cells from murine primordial germ cells in culture. Cell 70:841, 1992.

6. Labosky P, Barlow D, Hogan B: Embryonic germ cell lines and their derivation from mouse primordial germ cells. Germline Dev 182:157, 1994.

7. Shamblott M, Axelman J, Littlefield J, et al: Human embryonic germ cell derivatives express a broad range of developmentally distinct markers and proliferate extensively in vitro. Proc Natl Acad Sci U S A 98:113, 2001.

8. Slack J: Skinny dipping for stem cells. Nat Cell Biol 3:E205-E206, 2001.

9. Krause DS, Theise N, Collecter M, et al: Multi-organ, multilineage engraftment by a single bone marrow-derived stem cell. Cell 105:369, 2001.

10. Clarke D, Johansson CB, Wilbertz J, et al: Generalized potential of adult neural stem cells. Science 288:1660, 2000.

11. Orkin S: Stem cell alchemy. Nat Med 6:1212, 2000.

12. Anderson D, Gage F, Weissman I: Can stem cells cross lineage boundaries? Nat Med 7:393, 2001.

13. Layer P, Rothermel A, Willbold E: From stem cells toward neural layers: A lesson from re-aggregated embryonic retinal cells. Neuroreport 12:A39, 2001.

14. Vessey C, de la Hall P: Hepatic stem cells: A review. Pathology 33:130, 2001.

15. Fuchs E, Segre J: Stem cells: A new lease on life. Cell 100:143, 2000.

16. Lagasse E, Shirzura J, Uchida N, et al: Toward regenerative medicine. Immunity 14:425, 2001.

17. Oshima H, Rochat A, Kedzia C, et al: Morphogenesis and renewal of hair follicles from adult multipotent stem cells. Cell 104:233, 2001.

18. Uchida N, Buck D, He D, et al: Direct isolation of human central nervous system stem cells. Proc Natl Acad Sci U S A 97:14720, 2000.

19. Toma J, Akhavan M, Fernanades K, et al: Isolation of multipotent adult stem cells from the dermis of mammalian skin. Nat Cell Biol 3:778, 2001.

20. Martin G: Isolation of a pluripotent cell line from early mouse embryos cultured in medium conditioned by teratocarcinoma stem cells. Proc Natl Acad Sci U S A 78:7634, 1981.

21. Evans M, Kaufman M: Establishment in culture of pluripotential cells from mouse embryos. Nature 292:145, 1981.

22. Nichols J, Evans E, Smith A: Establishment of germ-line-competent embryonic stem (ES) cells using differentiation inhibiting activity. Development 110:1341, 1990.

23. Beddington R, Robertson E: An assessment of the developmental potential of embryonic stem cells in the midgestation embryo. Development 105:733, 1989.

24. Kirschstein R: Stem Cells: Scientific Progress and Future Research Directions, Washington, DC, National Institutes of Health, 2001, p 5.

25. O'Shea K: Embryonic stem cell models of development. Anat Rec 257:32, 1999.

26. Weiss M, Orkin S: In vitro differentiation of murine embryonic stem cells. J Clin Invest 97:591, 1996.

27. Beddington R: Mouse mutagenesis: From gene to phenotype and back again. Curr Biol 8:R840, 1998.

28. Mills A, Bradley A: From mouse to man: Generating megabase chromosome rearrangements. Trends Genet 17:331, 2001.

29. Robertson E: Using embryonic stem cells to introduce mutations into the mouse germ line. Biol Reprod 44:238, 1991.

30. Capecchi M: The new mouse genetics: Altering the genome by gene targeting. Trends Genet 5:70, 1989.

31. Thomson J, Kalishman J, Golos T, et al: Isolation of a primate embryonic stem cell line. Proc Natl Acad Sci U S A 92:7844, 1995.

32. Odorico J, Kaufman D, Thomson J: Multilineage differentiation of human embryonic stem cell lines. Stem Cells 19:193, 2001.

33. Amit M, Carpenter M, Inokuma M, et al: Clonally derived human embryonic stem cell lines maintain pluripotency and proliferative potential for prolonged periods of culture. Dev Biol 227:271, 2000.

34. Schuldinger M, Eiges R, Eden A, et al: Induced neuronal differentiation of human embryonic stem cells. Brain Res 913:201, 2001.

35. Kaufman D, Hanson E, Lewis R, et al: Hematopoietic colony-forming cells derived from human embryonic stem cells. Proc Natl Acad Sci U S A 98:10716, 2001.

36. Kehat I, Kenyagin-Karsenti D, Snir M, et al: Human embryonic stem cells can differentiate into myocytes with structural and functional properties of cardiomyocytes. J Clin Invest 108:407, 2001.

37. Guenin L: Morals and primordials. Science 292:1659, 2001.

38. Juengst E, Fossel M: The ethics of embryonic stem cells—now and forever, cells without end. JAMA 284:3180, 2000.

39. Robertson J: Human embryonic stem cell research: Ethical and legal issues. Nat Rev Genet 2:74, 2001.

40. Winston R: Embryonic stem cell research: The case for. Nat Med 7:396, 2001.

41. Antoniou M: Embryonic stem cell research: The case against. Nat Med 7:397, 2001.

42. McLaren A: Important differences between sources of embryonic stem cells. Nature 408:513, 2000.

43. Lanza R, Caplan A, Silver L, et al: The ethical validity of using nuclear transfer in human transplantation. JAMA 284:3175, 2000.

44. Kubiak J, Johnson M: Human infertility, reproductive cloning and nuclear transfer: A confusion of meanings. BioEssays 23:359, 2001.

45. Wintrobe M: Milestones on the path of progress. In Wintrobe M (ed): Blood, Pure and Eloquent. New York, McGraw-Hill, 1980, pp 1-31.

46. Jacobson L, Marks E, Gaston E, et al: Role of the spleen in radiation injury. Proc Soc Exp Biol Med 70:7440, 1949.

47. Ford C, Hamerton J, Barnes W, et al: Cytological identification of radiation-chimaeras. Nature 177:452, 1956.

48. Lorenz E, Uphoff D, Reid T, et al: Modification of irradiation injury in mice and guinea pigs by bone marrow injections. J Natl Cancer Inst 12:197, 1951.

49. Till J, McCulloch E: A direct measurement of the radiation sensitivity of normal mouse bone marrow cells. Radiat Res 14:213, 1961.

50. Pluznik D, Sachs L: The cloning of normal "mast" cells in tissue culture. J Cell Comp Physiol 66:319, 1965.

51. Bradley T, Metcalf D: The growth of mouse bone marrow cells in vitro. Aust J Exp Biol Med Sci 44:287, 1966.

52. Axelrad A, McLeod D, Shreeve M, et al (eds): Properties of Cells That Produce Erythrocytic Colonies In Vitro, vol 74. In Robinson W (series ed): Hemopoiesis in Culture. Washington, DC, National Institutes of Health, 1974, p 205.

53. Visser JWN, Bauman JGJ, Mulder AH, et al: Isolation of murine pluripotent hemopoietic stem cells. J Exp Med 59:1576, 1984.

54. Visser J, VanBekkum D: Purification of pluripotent hemopoietic stem cells: Past and present. Exp Hematol 18:248, 1990.

55. Spangrude G, Heimfeld S, Weissman I: Purification and characterization of mouse hematopoietic stem cells. Science 241:58, 1988.

56. Spangrude GJ, Cooper DD: Paradigm shifts in stem-cell biology. Semin Hematol 37:3, 2000.

57. Osawa M, Hanada K, Hamada H, et al: Long-term lympho-hematopoietic reconstitution by a single CD34-low/negative hematopoietic stem cell. Science 273:242, 1996.

58. Palis J, Yoder M: Yolk sac hematopoiesis—the first blood cells of mouse and man. Exp Hematol 29:927, 2001.

59. Yoder MC: Embryonic hematopoiesis. In Christensen RD (ed): Hematologic Problems of the Neonate. Philadelphia, WB Saunders, 2000, pp 3-19.

60. Yoder M: Introduction: Spatial origin of murine hematopoietic stem cells. Blood 98:3, 2001.

61. Yoder M, Palis J: Ventral (yolk sac) hematopoiesis in the mouse. In Zon L (ed): Hematopoiesis. London, Oxford University Press, 2001, pp 180-191.

62. Orlic D, Bodine D: What defines a pluripotent hematopoietic stem cell (PHSC): Will the real PHSC please stand up! Blood 84:3991, 1994.

63. Weissman I: Stem cells: Units of development, units of regeneration, and units in evolution. Cell 100:157, 2000.

64. Bradford G, Williams B, Rossi R, et al: Quiescence, cycling, and turnover in the primitive hematopoietic stem cell compartment. Exp Hematol 25:445, 1997.

65. Zhong R, Astle C, Harrison D: Distinct developmental patterns of short-term and long-term functioning lymphoid and myeloid precursors defined by competitive limiting dilution analysis in vivo. J Immunol 157:138, 1996.

66. Purton LE, Bernstein ID, Collins SJ: All-trans retinoic acid enhances the long-term repopulating activity of cultured hematopoietic stem cells. Blood 95:470, 2000.

67. Fraser C, Szilvassy S, Eaves C, et al: Proliferation of totipotent hematopoietic stem cells in vitro with retention of long-term competitive in vivo reconstituting ability. Proc Natl Acad Sci U S A 89:1968, 1992.

68. Miller C, Eaves C: Expansion in vitro of adult murine hematopoietic stem cells with transplantable lympho-myeloid reconstituting ability. Proc Natl Acad Sci U S A 94:13648, 1997.

69. Lagasse E, Connors H, Al-Dhalimy M, et al: Purified hematopoietic stem cells can differentiate into hepatocytes in vivo. Nat Med 6:1229, 2000.

70. Theise N, Badve S, Saxena R, et al: Derivation of hepatocytes from bone marrow cells in mice after radiation-induced myeloablation. Hepatology 31:235, 2000.

71. Wang X, Willenbring H, Akkarl Y, et al: Cell fusion is the principal source of bone-marrow-derived hepatocytes. Nature 422:897, 2003.

72. Jackson K, Mijka S, Wang H, et al: Regeneration of ischemic cardiac muscle and vascular endothelium by adult stem cells. J Clin Invest 107:1395, 2001.

73. Jiang Y, Jahagirdar B, Reinhardt R, et al: Pluripotency of mesenchymal stem cells derived from adult marrow. Nature 418:41, 2002.

74. Huang S, Law P, Young D, et al: Candidate hematopoietic stem cells from fetal tissues, umbilical cord blood vs. adult bone marrow and mobilized peripheral blood. Exp Hematol 26:1162, 1998.

75. Broxmeyer H, Hangoc G, Cooper S, et al: Growth characteristics and expansion of human umbilical cord blood and estimation of its potential for transplantation in adults. Proc Natl Acad Sci U S A 89:4109, 1992.

76. Cairo M, Wagner J: Placental and/or umbilical cord blood: An alternative source of hematopoietic stem cells for transplantation. Blood 90:4665, 1997.

77. Namikawa R, Weilbaecher K, Kaneshima H, et al: Long-term human hematopoiesis in the SCID-hu mouse. J Exp Med 172:1055, 1990.

78. Dao MA, Taylor N, Nolta JA: Reduction in levels of the cyclin-dependent kinase inhibitor p27(kip-1) coupled with transforming growth factor beta neutralization induces cell-cycle entry and increases retroviral transduction of primitive human hematopoietic cells. Proc Natl Acad Sci U S A 95:13006, 1998.

79. Baum C, Weissman I, Tsukamoto A, et al: Isolation of a candidate human hematopoietic stem-cell population. Proc Natl Acad Sci U S A 89:2804, 1992.

80. Gratama JW, Keeney M, Sutherland DR, et al: The real CD34+ events: Simplicity versus accuracy and flexibility [letter; comment]. Exp Hematol 27:975, 1999.

81. Srour EF, Abonour R, Cornetta K, et al: Ex vivo expansion of hematopoietic stem and progenitor cells: Are we there yet? J Hematother 8:93, 1999.

82. Verfaillie C: Can human hematopoietic stem cells be cultured ex vivo. Stem Cells 12:466, 1995.

83. Siena S, Bregni M, Brando B, et al: Circulation of CD34+ hematopoietic stem cells in the peripheral blood of high-dose cyclophosphamide-treated patients: Enhancement by intravenous recombinant human granulocyte-macrophage colony-stimulating factor. Blood 74:1905, 1989.

84. Danet G, Pan Y, Luongo J, et al: Expansion of human SCID-repopulating cells under hypoxic conditions. J Clin Invest 112:126, 2003.

85. Thomas E, Storb R, Clift R, et al: Bone-marrow transplantation. N Engl J Med 292:832, 1975.

86. Slavin S: New strategies for bone marrow transplantation. Curr Opin Immunol 12:542, 2000.

87. Anderson W, Fletcher J: Gene therapy in human beings: When is it ethical to begin? N Engl J Med 303:1293, 1980.

88. Ledley F: Nonviral gene therapy: The promise of genes as pharmaceutical products. Hum Gene Ther 6:1129, 1995.

89. Nishikawa M, Huang L: Nonviral vectors in the new millennium: Delivery barriers in gene transfer. Hum Gene Ther 12:861, 2001.

90. Leiden J: Gene therapy—promise, pitfalls, and prognosis. N Engl J Med 333:871, 1995.

91. Somia N, Verma IM: Gene therapy: Trials and tribulations. Nat Rev Genet 1:91, 2000.

92. Verma IM: From reverse transcriptase to gene therapy: A marvelous journey. Harvey Lect 95:43, 1999.

93. Williams D, Lemischka I, Nathan D, et al: Introduction of new genetic material into pluripotent haematopoietic stem cells of the mouse. Nature 310:476, 1984.

94. Miller AD, Eckner RJ, Jolly DJ, et al: Expression of a retrovirus encoding human HPRT in mice. Science 225:630, 1984.

95. Dick JE, Magli MC, Huszar D, et al: Introduction of a selectable gene into primitive stem cells capable of long-term reconstitution of the hemopoietic system of W/Wv mice. Cell 42:71, 1985.

96. Keller G, Paige C, Gilboa E, et al: Expression of a foreign gene in myeloid and lymphoid cells derived from multipotent haematopoietic precursors. Nature 318:149, 1985.

97. Markowitz D, Goff S, Bank A: A safe packaging line for gene transfer: Separating viral genes on two different plasmids. J Virol 62:1120, 1988.

98. Danos O, Mulligan RC: Safe and efficient generation of recombinant retroviruses with amphotropic and ecotropic host ranges. Proc Natl Acad Sci U S A 85:6460, 1988.

99. Barrette S, Orlic D: Alternative viral envelopes for oncoretroviruses to increase gene transfer into hematopoietic stem cells. Curr Opin Mol Ther 2:507, 2000.

100. Burns JC, Friedmann T, Driever W, et al: Vesicular stomatitis virus G glycoprotein pseudotyped retroviral vectors: Concentration to very high titer and efficient gene transfer into mammalian and nonmammalian cells. Proc Natl Acad Sci U S A 90:8033, 1993.

101. Kelly PF, Vandergriff J, Nathwani A, et al: Highly efficient gene transfer into cord blood nonobese diabetic/severe combined immunodeficiency repopulating cells by oncoretroviral vector particles pseudotyped with the feline endogenous retrovirus (RD114) envelope protein. Blood 96:1206, 2000.

102. Kelly PF, Carrington J, Nathwani A, et al: RD114-pseudotyped oncoretroviral vectors: Biological and physical properties. Ann N Y Acad Sci 938:262, 2001.

103. Quigley JG, Burns CC, Anderson MM, et al: Cloning of the cellular receptor for feline leukemia virus subgroup C (FeLV-C), a retrovirus that induces red cell aplasia. Blood 95:1093, 2000.

104. Kiem HP, Heyward S, Winkler A, et al: Gene transfer into marrow repopulating cells: Comparison between amphotropic and gibbon ape leukemia virus pseudotyped retroviral vectors in a competitive repopulation assay in baboons. Blood 90:4638, 1997.

105. Sugai J, Eiden M, Anderson MM, et al: Identification of envelope determinants of feline leukemia virus subgroup B that permit infection and gene transfer to cells expressing human Pit1 or Pit2. J Virol 75:6841, 2001.

106. Barrette S, Douglas J, Orlic D, et al: Superior transduction of mouse hematopoietic stem cells with 10A1 and VSV-G pseudotyped retrovirus vectors. Mol Ther 1:330, 2000.

107. Gatlin J, Melkus MW, Padgett A, et al: Engraftment of NOD/SCID mice with human CD34(+) cells transduced by concentrated oncoretroviral vector particles pseudotyped with the feline endogenous retrovirus (RD114) envelope protein. J Virol 75:9995, 2001.

108. Moore KA, Deisseroth AB, Reading CL, et al: Stromal support enhances cell-free retroviral vector transduction of human bone marrow long-term culture-initiating cells. Blood 79:1393, 1992.

109. Moritz T, Dutt P, Xiao X, et al: Fibronectin improves transduction of reconstituting hematopoietic stem cells by retroviral vectors: Evidence of direct viral binding to chymotryptic carboxy-terminal fragments. Blood 88:855, 1996.

110. Hanenberg H, Xiao XL, Dilloo D, et al: Colocalization of retrovirus and target cells on specific fibronectin fragments increases genetic transduction of mammalian cells. Nat Med 2:876, 1996.

111. Pollok KE, Williams DA: Facilitation of retrovirus-mediated gene transfer into hematopoietic stem and progenitor cells and peripheral blood T-lymphocytes utilizing recombinant fibronectin fragments. Curr Opin Mol Ther 1:595, 1999.

112. Kimizuka F, Taguchi Y, Ohdate Y, et al: Production and characterization of functional domains of human fibronectin expressed in Escherichia coli. J Biochem (Tokyo) 110:284, 1991.

113. Palmer TD, Rosman GJ, Osborne WR, et al: Genetically modified skin fibroblasts persist long after transplantation but gradually inactivate introduced genes. Proc Natl Acad Sci U S A 88:1330, 1991.

114. Hofmann A, Nolan GP, Blau HM: Rapid retroviral delivery of tetracycline-inducible genes in a single autoregulatory cassette. Proc Natl Acad Sci U S A 93:5185, 1996.

115. Yu SF, von Ruden T, Kantoff PW, et al: Self-inactivating retroviral vectors designed for transfer of whole genes into mammalian cells. Proc Natl Acad Sci U S A 83:3194, 1986.

116. Hwang JJ, Li L, Anderson WF: A conditional self-inactivating retrovirus vector that uses a tetracycline-responsive expression system. J Virol 71:7128, 1997.

117. Check E: A tragic setback. Nature 420:116, 2002.

118. European Society of Gene Therapy: French gene therapy group reports on the adverse event in a clinical trial of gene therapy for X-linked severe combined immune deficiency (X-SCID). Position statement from the European Society of Gene Therapy. J Gene Med 5:82, 2003.

119. Cavazzana-Calvo M, Hacein-Bey S, de Saint Basile G, et al: Gene therapy of human severe combined immunodeficiency (SCID)-X1 disease. Science 288:669, 2000.

120. Marshall E: Gene therapy: What to do when clear success comes with an unclear risk? Science 298:510, 2002.

121. Kohn DB, Sadelain M, Glorioso JC: Occurrence of leukaemia following gene therapy of X-linked SCID. Nat Rev Cancer 3:477, 2003.

122. Baum C, Dullmann J, Li Z, et al: Side effects of retroviral gene transfer into hematopoietic stem cells. Blood 101:2099, 2003.

123. Jordan CT, Lemischka IR: Clonal and systemic analysis of long-term hematopoiesis in the mouse. Genes Dev 4:220, 1990.

124. Clapp DW, Freie B, Lee W-H, et al: Molecular evidence that in situ-transduced fetal liver hematopoietic stem/progenitor cells give rise to medullary hematopoiesis in adult rats. Blood 86:2113, 1995.

125. Berns K, Linden R: The cryptic life style of adeno-associated virus. BioEssays 17:237, 1995.

126. Muzyczka N: Use of adeno-associated virus as a general transduction vector for mammalian cells. Curr Top Microbiol Immunol 158:97, 1992.

127. Samulski J, Sally M, Muzyczka N: Adeno-associated viral vectors. In Friedman T (ed): The Development of Human Gene Therapy. Cold Spring Harbor, NY, Cold Spring Harbor Laboratory Press, 1999.

128. Hermonat P, Muzyczka N: Use of adeno-associated virus as a mammalian DNA cloning vector: Transduction of neomycin resistance into mammalian tissue culture cells. Proc Natl Acad Sci U S A 81:6466, 1984.

129. Ferrari F, Xiao X, McCarty D, et al: New developments in the generation of Ad-free, high-titer rAAV gene therapy vectors. Nat Med 3:1295, 1997.

130. Summerford C, Samulski R: Membrane-associated heparan sulfate proteoglycan is a receptor for adeno-associated virus type 2 virions. J Virol 72:1, 1998.

131. Qing K, Mah C, Hansen J, et al: Human fibroblast growth factor receptor 1 is a co-receptor for infection by adeno-associated virus 2. Nat Med 5:71, 1999.

132. Summerford C, Bartlett JS, Samulski J: aVb5 integrin: A co-receptor for adeno-associated virus 2 infection. Nat Med 5:78, 1999.

133. McCarty D, Monahan P, Samulski J: Self-complementary recombinant adeno-associated virus (scAAV) vectors promote efficient transduction independently of DNA synthesis. Gene Ther 8:1248, 2001.

134. Rabinowitz JE, Samulski J: Building a better vector: The manipulation of AAV virions. Virology 278:301, 2000.

135. Yan Z-J, Zhang Y, Duan D, et al: Trans-splicing vectors expand the utility of adeno-associated virus for gene therapy. Proc Natl Acad Sci U S A 97:6716, 2000.

136. Sun L, Li J, Xiao X: Overcoming adeno-associated virus vector size limitation through viral DNA heterodimerization. Nat Med 6:599, 2000.

137. Kay M, Manno C, Ragni M, et al: Evidence for gene transfer and expression of factor IX in haemophilia B patients treated with an AAV vector. Nat Genet 24:257, 2000.

138. Russell W: Update on adenovirus and its vectors. J Gen Virol 81:2573, 2000.

139. Berkner K: Expression of heterologous sequences in adenoviral vectors. Curr Top Microbiol Immunol 158:39, 1992.

140. Yang Y, Li Q, Ertl H, et al: Cellular and humoral immune responses to viral antigens create barriers to lung-directed gene therapy with recombinant adenoviruses. J Virol 69:2004, 1995.

141. Yang Y, Wilson J: Clearance of adenovirus-infected hepatocytes by class-I restricted CD4+ CTLs in vivo. J Immunol 155:2564, 1995.

142. Hitt M, Addison C, Graham F: Human adenovirus vectors for gene transfer into mammalian cells. Adv Pharm 40:137, 1997.

143. Bramson J, Graham F, Gauldie J: The use of adenoviral vectors for gene therapy and gene transfer in vivo. Curr Opin Biotechnol 6:590, 1995.

144. Brody S, Crystal R: Adenovirus-mediated in vivo gene transfer. Ann N Y Acad Sci 716:90, 1994.

145. Alton E, Kitson C: Gene therapy for cystic fibrosis. Expert Opin Investig Drugs 9:1523, 2000.

146. Roth J, Cristiano R: Gene therapy for cancer: What have we done and where are we going? J Natl Cancer Inst 89:21, 1997.

147. Heise C, Kirn D: Replication-selective adenoviruses as oncolytic agents. J Clin Invest 105:847, 2000.

148. Lewis P, Hensel M, Emerman M: Human immunodeficiency virus infection of cells arrested in the cell cycle. EMBO J 11:3053, 1992.

149. Bukrinsky MI, Haggerty S, Dempsey MP, et al: A nuclear localization signal within HIV-1 matrix protein that governs infection of non-dividing cells. Nature 365:666, 1993.

150. Lever AM: Lentiviral vectors: Progress and potential. Curr Opin Mol Ther 2:488, 2000.

151. Trono D: Lentiviral vectors: Turning a deadly foe into a therapeutic agent. Gene Ther 7:20, 2000.

152. Page KA, Landau NR, Littman DR: Construction and use of a human immunodeficiency virus vector for analysis of virus infectivity. J Virol 64:5270, 1990.

153. Zufferey R, Nagy D, Mandel RJ, et al: Multiply attenuated lentiviral vector achieves efficient gene delivery in vivo. Nat Biotechnol 15:871, 1997.

154. Naldini L, Blomer U, Gallay P, et al: In vivo gene delivery and stable transduction of nondividing cells by a lentiviral vector. Science 272:263, 1996.

155. An DS, Kung SK, Bonifacino A, et al: Lentivirus vector-mediated hematopoietic stem cell gene transfer of common gamma-chain cytokine receptor in rhesus macaques. J Virol 75:3547, 2001.

156. Akkina R, Walton R, Chen M, et al: High-efficiency gene transfer into CD34+ cells with a human immunodeficiency virus type 1-based retroviral vector pseudotyped with vesicular stomatitis virus envelope glycoprotein G. J Virol 70:2581, 1996.

157. Kafri T, Blomer U, Peterson DA, et al: Sustained expression of genes delivered directly into liver and muscle by lentiviral vectors. Nat Genet 17:314, 1997.

158. Wang G, Slepushkin V, Zabner J, et al: Feline immunodeficiency virus vectors persistently transduce nondividing airway epithelia and correct the cystic fibrosis defect. J Clin Invest 104:R55, 1999.

159. Kafri T, van Praag H, Ouyang L, et al: A packaging cell line for lentivirus vectors. J Virol 73:576, 1999.

160. Xu K, Ma H, McCown TJ, et al: Generation of a stable cell line producing high-titer self-inactivating lentiviral vectors. Mol Ther 3:97, 2001.

161. Follenzi A, Ailles LE, Bakovic S, et al: Gene transfer by lentiviral vectors is limited by nuclear translocation and rescued by HIV-1 pol sequences. Nat Genet 25:217, 2000.

162. Zennou V, Petit C, Guetard D, et al: HIV-1 genome nuclear import is mediated by a central DNA flap. Cell 101:173, 2000.

163. Zufferey R, Donello JE, Trono D, et al: Woodchuck hepatitis virus posttranscriptional regulatory element enhances expression of transgenes delivered by retroviral vectors. J Virol 73:2886, 1999.

164. Miyoshi H, Blomer U, Takahashi M, et al: Development of a self-inactivating lentivirus vector. J Virol 72:8150, 1998.

165. Johnston JC, Gasmi M, Lim LE, et al: Minimum requirements for efficient transduction of dividing and nondividing cells by feline immunodeficiency virus vectors. J Virol 73:4991, 1999.

166. Schnell T, Foley P, Wirth M, et al: Development of a self-inactivating, minimal lentivirus vector based on simian immunodeficiency virus. Hum Gene Ther 11:439, 2000.

167. Poeschla EM, Wong-Staal F, Looney DJ: Efficient transduction of nondividing human cells by feline immunodeficiency virus lentiviral vectors. Nat Med 4:354, 1998.

168. Mitrophanous K, Yoon S, Rohll J, et al: Stable gene transfer to the nervous system using a non-primate lentiviral vector. Gene Ther 6:1808, 1999.

169. Olsen JC: Gene transfer vectors derived from equine infectious anemia virus. Gene Ther 5:1481, 1998.

170. Pandya S, Boris-Lawrie K, Leung NJ, et al: Development of an Rev-independent, minimal simian immunodeficiency virus-derived vector system. Hum Gene Ther 12:847, 2001.

171. Berkowitz RD, Ilves H, Plavec I, et al: Gene transfer systems derived from Visna virus: Analysis of virus production and infectivity. Virology 279:116, 2001.

172. Krisky D, Marconi P, Oligino T, et al: Development of herpes simplex virus replication-defective multigene vectors for combination gene therapy applications. Gene Ther 5:1517, 1998.

173. Burton E, Wechuck J, Wendell S, et al: Multiple applications for replication-defective herpes simplex virus vectors. Stem Cells 19:358, 2001.

174. Goins W, Yoshimura N, Phelan M, et al: Herpes simplex virus mediated nerve growth factor expression in bladder and afferent neurons: Potential treatment for diabetic bladder dysfunction. J Urol 165:1748, 2001.

175. Goss J, Mata M, Goins W, et al: Antinociceptive effect of a genomic herpes simplex virus-based vector expressing human proenkephalin in rat dorsal root ganglion. Gene Ther 8:551, 2001.

176. Yamada M, Natsume A, Mata M, et al: Herpes simplex virus vector-mediated expression of Bcl-2 protects spinal motor neurons from degeneration following root avulsion. Exp Neurol 168:225, 2001.

177. Marconi P, Tamura M, Moriuchi S, et al: Connexin 43-enhanced suicide gene therapy using herpesviral vectors. Mol Ther 1:71, 2000.

178. Rubzam L, Boucher P, Murphy P, et al: Cytotoxicity and accumulation of ganciclovir triphosphate in bystander cells cocultured with herpes simplex virus type 1 thymidine kinase-expressing human glioblastoma cells. Cancer Res 59:669, 1999.

179. Hamel W, Magnelli L, Chiarugi V, et al: Herpes simplex virus thymidine kinase/ganciclovir-mediated apoptotic death of bystander cells. Cancer Res 56:2697, 1996.

180. Strayer DS: SV40 as an effective gene transfer vector in vivo. J Biol Chem 271:24741, 1996.

181. Strayer DS: Effective gene transfer using viral vectors based on SV40. Methods Mol Biol 133:61, 2000.

182. Sauter BV, Parashar B, Chowdhury NR, et al: A replication-deficient rSV40 mediates liver-directed gene transfer and a long-term amelioration of jaundice in Gunn rats. Gastroenterology 119:1348, 2000.

183. Strayer DS, Zern MA: Gene delivery to the liver using simian virus 40-derived vectors. Semin Liver Dis 19:71, 1999.

184. BouHamdan M, Duan LX, Pomerantz RJ, et al: Inhibition of HIV-1 by an anti-integrase single-chain variable fragment (SFv): Delivery by SV40 provides durable protection against HIV-1 and does not require selection. Gene Ther 6:660, 1999.

185. Jayan GC, Cordelier P, Patel C, et al: SV40-derived vectors provide effective transgene expression and inhibition of HIV-1 using constitutive, conditional, and pol III promoters. Gene Ther 8:1033, 2001.

186. BouHamdan M, Strayer DS, Wei D, et al: Inhibition of HIV-1 infection by down-regulation of the CXCR4 co-receptor using an intracellular single chain variable fragment against CXCR4. Gene Ther 8:408, 2001.

CHAPTER 15

Pharmacology in the Fetus and Newborn

Sylvain Chemtob and Jacob V. Aranda

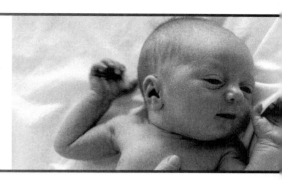

THE FETUS AND THE NEWBORN: THE ULTIMATE THERAPEUTIC ORPHANS

Neonatal Drug Use and Exposure

Advances in neonatal care have led to the increased survival and improved outcome of newborns, especially infants with low birth weight or who are extremely premature. At least 85% of children who are born weighing less than 1000 g survive.[1-3] A 50% survival rate is now reported among those born at 23 to 24 weeks of gestation. The improved survival rate and outcome result from improvements in care, the use of potent pharmacologic agents (e.g., steroids, diuretics, inotropic agents), and new molecular entity agents (e.g., pulmonary surfactant, nitric oxide). Multiple therapeutic agents are often administered simultaneously to the critically ill infant, each drug having the potential to interact with each other. Extensive pharmacoepidemiologic studies in neonatal intensive care units have shown that at least 150 agents are used during the neonatal period. Each infant in a newborn intensive care unit receives an average of 5.6 drugs, and at least 15% of infants in the neonatal intensive care unit receive 10 or more drugs, with some exposed to as many as 34 agents.[4-6] Except for a few antimicrobial agents, surfactant, recombinant erythropoietin, and other drugs (e.g., caffeine, citrate), none of the medications used in infants is approved for use in newborns, and even less so in the premature newborns and those with extremely low birth weight. Much like older children, newborns can be considered "therapeutic orphans." Studies on drugs for diseases unique to newborns (respiratory distress syndrome, necrotizing enterocolitis, retinopathy of prematurity) are needed in order to allow proper labeling of these drugs for affected infants.

EFFECT OF FETAL/NEONATAL MATURITY ON DRUG DOSE AND RESPONSE

Among the newborn population, substantial differences in drug metabolism, disposition, and plasma clearance exist mainly as a function of fetal maturity at birth and the added effect of advancing postnatal age. Premature neonates born at 22 to 23 weeks' gestation (just over 50% of the normal gestation period) are now considered viable. Their extreme immaturity is not limited to the lungs; it affects all organs, including the brain, kidneys, gastrointestinal system, and hepatic system. In the immature neonate, these organs exhibit substantial functional deficiency in comparison with those in the full-term newborn. Renal function such as glomerular filtration rate is very low at birth and is directly related to gestational age.[7,8] This immaturity affects clinical practice, as illustrated for gentamicin (given to almost all infants with respiratory distress and suspected infection), for which the dose interval of the same amount of drug (milligrams per kilogram of body weight) varies from every 36 hours in infants younger than 26 weeks' gestation to every 12 hours in full-term newborns.

Data on pharmacokinetics, metabolism, and disposition of drugs in the neonate[9,10] allow for certain generalizations. The rates of drug biotransformation and overall elimination are extremely variable among infants, generally slow, and directly related to fetal maturity or gestational and postconception age. This phenomenon is further complicated by the substrate dependency of the maturational changes in drug metabolism and elimination and their marked vulnerability to pathophysiologic states such as perinatal asphyxia. Moreover, unlike adults, newborns may activate alternative biotransformation in accord with enzyme availability, such as the methylation of theophylline to caffeine.[11] Thus, extrapolation of clinical pharmacology data from adults, young infants, and older children to the newborn cannot be justified and may often result in therapeutic tragedies. Numerous well-known therapeutic disasters in the past (e.g., chloramphenicol gray baby syndrome, kernicterus caused by sulfa drugs, cystic brain lesions caused by hexachlorophene [pHisoHex], hepatorenal failure and death caused by vitamin E formulations) resulted from lack of knowledge or appreciation of the unique functional status of the newborn. Reports of cardiac arrhythmia and prolonged QT intervals with cisapride[12] illustrate the ongoing problem of therapeutic misadventures in neonatology; this prokinetic agent was extensively used in newborns and young infants with gastroesophageal reflux and apnea despite an absence of data about its efficacy, kinetics, or safety. Again, dosage and therapeutic regimens were largely derived from adult data. These concepts are elaborated in this chapter.

BASIC PRINCIPLES

As noted, newborns, especially those born prematurely, are exposed to a large number of different drugs. The response of the newborn to various agents is often different from that observed in the adult, not only because of age-dependent differences in the pharmacodynamics but also because of pharmacokinetics.

The major need in neonatal pharmacologic therapy is the formulation of a distinct and rational therapeutic plan in which the ultimate individualization of drug dosage is based on careful assessment of the patient. In order to apply a sound approach in pharmacologic therapeutics for the newborn, knowledge of fundamental principles of pharmacology is essential for optimizing drug treatment and minimizing adverse effects in the newborn. An understanding of the essentials of pharmacokinetics enables the clinician to improve individualization of drug therapy, as well as to enhance the clinician's assessment of new agents or new applications of established drugs. This chapter reviews basic principles in pharmacology as they pertain to pharmacokinetics and pharmacodynamics, as well as basic changes during development that affect pharmacokinetics and dynamics in the newborn.

Drug Absorption

The majority of drugs administered to the premature newborn are injected via the intravenous route and therefore are not affected by factors that govern systemic absorption. However, certain agents are administered intramuscularly (e.g., vitamin K), via an enteral route (e.g., thiazides, caffeine), or percutaneously (e.g., topical antiseptics, analgesics, theophylline). Regardless of the route of administration, drugs must cross cell membranes in order to reach their sites of action. Therefore, the mechanisms by which drugs cross membranes and the physicochemical properties of molecules and membranes are important to consider in drug transfer. Several properties of the drug molecule influence the mechanism by which a drug traverses the cell membrane. The factors involved in these transfers include lipid solubility, degree of ionization (pK_a), molecular weight (usually <600 D), and protein binding. In addition, the type of transfer process affects transport of the molecules of interest.

Transport Mechanisms

Passive diffusion. Passive diffusion is the major transmembrane process for many small drugs.[13] According to Fick's first law of diffusion, drug molecules diffuse from a region of high drug concentration to a region of low drug concentration. As mentioned, several factors affect the rate of diffusion. Among these, the ionization state of the molecule is affected by the pH on both sides of the membrane, according to the Henderson-Hasselbalch equation ($pH = pK_a + log [base/acid]$). Thus, for instance, acidic compounds, such as salicylic acid, are less ionized when the environmental pH is low, facilitating its diffusion.

Active transport. Active transport is a carrier-mediated transmembrane process that plays an important role in the renal and biliary secretion of many drugs and metabolites. Active transport is characterized by a transfer of molecules against a concentration gradient. Thus, energy must be consumed to achieve this process; this system is saturable. An example of this transport system is the organic acid secretory pathway in the renal tubule, which allows secretion of furosemide, ethacrynic acid, and indomethacin.[14]

Facilitated diffusion. Facilitated diffusion is also a carrier-mediated transport system; in contrast to active transport, this type of transport moves along a concentration gradient. This system, which does not require energy input, is also saturable and selective for the drug. Transporters involved in facilitated diffusion are the organic cation transporters, the organic anion transporters, and the oligopeptide transporters, including PepT1 (which incorporates numerous drugs within cells)[15-17]; drugs transported by these transporters include corticosterone, ethacrynic acid, and captopril, respectively. These transporters are present not only in the intestine but also in the liver, brain, and kidneys, affecting drug elimination and distribution.[18]

Pinocytosis. Pinocytosis, the process of engulfing large molecules, is the proposed absorption system[19] for oral polio vaccine and immunoglobulins, as well as possibly oligonucleotides, in the intestines of neonates.

Pore transport. Pore transport applies to very small molecules (e.g., urea, water); proteins responsible for transport of water and urea have been characterized and are classified as aquaporins and urea transporters, respectively.[20,21]

Membrane Transporters

Transporters are membrane-integrated proteins that facilitate movement of nutrients such as amino acids, dipeptides and tripeptides, sugars, nucleosides, vitamins, and bile acids into cells. In the intestine, it has become increasingly clear that several of these transporters play a significant role in drug absorption. Cellular import of numerous nutrients and drugs depends on transporters that are classified as primary, secondary, and tertiary. Primary transporters—specifically, the adenosine triphosphate (ATP)–binding cassette transporters such as multidrug resistance (MDR) protein and breast cancer resistance protein—utilize energy from ATP as their driving force; secondary and tertiary transporters utilize voltage and ion gradients generated by primary transporters/exchangers.[18] Sodium and protons are frequently cotransported with the compound of interest. Because the activity of a given transporter is a function of the electrochemical gradient driving force, the efficiency of the transport is influenced by the activity of the Na^+/H^+-antiporter and of the Na^+/HCO_3^- symporter.

A number of membrane transporters play key roles in drug import and distribution; in this role, they also enhance clearance of drugs from the fetus, as has been demonstrated for the ATP-dependent breast cancer resistance protein. These membrane transporters include the H^+/dipeptide symporters, facilitative glucose transporter-related proteins, Na^+/glucose and Na^+/nucleoside cotransporters, amino acid transporters, Na^+/neurotransmitter symporters, and the organic cation and anion transporters.[15-17,22] The H^+/dipeptide symporters carry cephalosporins and angiotensin-converting enzyme inhibitors; the organic cation transporters carry antihistaminics, β blockers, cimetidine, and metformin; and the organic anion transporters carry aspirin, indomethacin, and methotrexate. These ports of entry, along with their structural polymorphisms, influence pharmacokinetics.[18]

Kinetics of Absorption

Most pharmacokinetic models assume a first-order absorption, which takes into account a first-order rate of change in the amount of drug absorbed and a first-order rate of drug elimination. This can be described in the following one-compartment model equation:

$$\partial D_B/\partial t = FK_aD_{si} - K_{el}D_B$$

where $\partial D_B/\partial t$ is the rate of change of drug in the body (D_B); F is the fraction absorbed (see later section on bioavailability); K_a and K_{el} are the absorption and elimination constants, respectively; and D_{si} is the drug at the site of absorption. Although many drugs follow multiple-compartment kinetics, the K_a may still be calculated from a one-compartment model.[23] The importance of the K_a lies in the design of a multiple-dosage regimen. Knowledge of the K_a and K_{el} allows for the prediction of the peak and trough steady-state plasma drug concentrations ($C_{ss\,max}$ and $C_{ss\,min}$) after multiple dosing concentrations[24] (see later section on clinical pharmacokinetics):

$$C_{ss\,max} = (FD_{si}/V_d)/(1 - e^{-K_{el}\tau})$$

$$C_{ss\,min} = C_{ss\,max} \bullet e^{-K_{el}\tau}$$

where τ is the dosing interval and V_d is the volume of distribution. These equations show that these concentrations depend on the absorption rate, the volume of distribution, and K_{el} (and consequently on clearance; see later section on clinical pharmacokinetics), and the dosing interval.

Factors that Affect Drug Absorption

The systemic absorption of a drug from its site of administration depends on the factors just discussed, which constitute the **physicochemical properties** of the agent and of the membrane. In addition, other factors have a major contribution to absorption; these include the **disintegration, dissolution**, and **solubility** of the compound; the **blood flow** to the site of absorption; the **surface area** of absorption; **transit time** of the drug, as in the case of gastrointestinal tract administration; the **export of drugs** by P-glycoproteins in enterocytes, the activity of which can be altered through genetic polymorphisms; and in situ **metabolism of the agent**,[25] including a first-pass effect. A first-pass effect is defined as the process of rapidly taking up and metabolizing an agent into inactive compounds by the liver, immediately after enteric absorption

and before it reaches the systemic circulation, as is the case with morphine, isoproterenol, propranolol, and hydralazine. Each of the factors affecting absorption taken separately or combined may have profound effects on the efficacy and toxicity of a drug.

When absorption of drugs through the gastrointestinal tract of the newborn is evaluated, the developmental stages of this organ must be taken into account. The few studies of enteral drug absorption have revealed full maturation by approximately 4 months after birth.[26] Interestingly, intestinal length, in relation to other anthropometric measurements, and villous formation are not underdeveloped in the young infant[27] and are thus not limiting factors for absorption.

On the other hand, **gastric acid secretion** is low in very young preterm infants, in comparison with adults,[28] and could potentially reduce absorption of weak acids and bases if given enterally. In contrast, lipid-soluble drugs, such as methylxanthines, are more easily absorbed by newborns than by older children.[29] Newborns also exhibit low bile salt secretory ability.[30] This deficiency may also reduce absorption of lipid-soluble vitamins, such as vitamins D and E.[31,32] Adequate absorption of vitamin E has been observed in premature infants,[33] however, possibly as a result of lower intake of iron.[34]

Another important difference for drug absorption between neonates and adults is the type and degree of **bacterial colonization** of the gut. The development of the intestinal flora has been shown to affect the absorption of vitamin K.[35] Thus, maturation of the gastrointestinal tract may explain some of the characteristics of intestinal absorption of drugs in the growing child.

Enzymatic development of the gastrointestinal tract may also alter drug absorption. The elevated activity of β-glucuronidase in the newborn may deconjugate glucuronide-conjugate drugs[36] and enhance reabsorption of the agent into the systemic circulation; this effect may prolong the pharmacologic activity of certain agents, such as indomethacin.[37] The presence of ATP-dependent P-glycoproteins in the intestinal epithelium apical brush border, as well as the canalicular face of hepatocytes, facilitates drug export and reduce bioavailability.[38] Decreased expression of P-glycoproteins of variable polymorphisms influences drug absorption in the developing child.[18,39] The same applies to intestinal drug-metabolizing enzymes, particularly CYP1A1, whose activity appears to increase as the person ages,[40] whereas glutathione S-transferase activity decreases with age.[41]

In addition to the gastrointestinal changes that occur with development, drug absorption is also altered by disease conditions of the infant. Diseases of genetic (e.g., cystic fibrosis), microbial, or circulatory origin (e.g., necrotizing enterocolitis) may alter the intestinal mucosa and limit absorptive surface.

Bioavailability

Bioavailability is the fraction of the administered dose that reaches the systemic circulation. Calculating bioavailability does not take into consideration the rate at which the drug is absorbed. The absolute availability of a drug may be measured by comparing the respective area under the plasma concentration curves (AUC) after oral (PO) and intravenous (IV) administration. This measurement may be performed as long as V_d and K_{el} are independent of the route of administration:

$$\text{Absolute availability} = (AUC_{PO}/dose_{PO})/(AUC_{IV}/dose_{IV})$$

Bioavailability is relevant when we take into account the percentage of *active* drug reaching the central compartment. As previously described, multiple factors alter the absorption of drugs. Thus, the bioavailability of an agent is influenced by the same factors.

Distribution

The **disposition** of a drug is its passage in the body from absorption to excretion. After absorption, a drug is distributed to various body compartments. This distribution determines its efficacy, as well as its toxicity. The distribution of drugs is influenced by several factors, including the size of the body water and lipid compartments, regional hemodynamics, and the degree of binding of drugs to plasma and tissue proteins. The initial phase of distribution reflects regional blood flow. Organs supplied with high perfusion, such as the brain, heart, and kidneys, are the first to be exposed to the drug. A second phase of distribution involves a large fraction of the body mass, which includes the muscle and adipose tissue. In addition to regional circulation, factors determining diffusion of drugs to the tissues also play an important role in the distribution. These consist of the same factors that influence the passage of drugs across membranes, as discussed previously, and those that contribute to the degree of protein binding. Accordingly, the apparent V_d of xenobiotics (as well as of endogenous agents) is composed of the various distribution compartments and is expressed by the following equation:

$$V_d = \text{(total drug in the body)/(concentration of drug in plasma)}$$

If equilibration of the drug is assumed to be instant after administration, V_d can be determined by extrapolating the drug concentration at time 0 (C_0) and dividing the dose of drug administered by the concentration of drug at time 0 (C_0). However, this equation can be applied only to a single-compartment model. V_d may be calculated more accurately with the following equation, which is independent of the model used:

$$V_d = \text{dose}/K_{el}[AUC]_0^\infty$$

Physiologic and Pathologic Factors Affecting Distribution of Drugs

Body water. The factors that influence the distribution of drugs in the body are subject to developmental changes. The amount and distribution of total body water undergoes marked changes in the perinatal period.[42] Total body water and extracellular fluid volume decrease with increasing gestational age. After birth, total body water decreases, and the volume of intracellular fluid increases in relation to that of the extracellular fluid. In the full-term newborn, the degree of insensible water is linked to the metabolic rate of the infant, as is the case in the older child.[43] In the preterm newborn, there is no fixed relationship between metabolic rate and insensible

water loss. In the infant with very low birth weight, evaporative heat loss is substantially greater than that produced by basal metabolic rate.[33,44] This loss results from the immaturity of the cornified layer of the skin and the larger ratio of body surface area to body mass in the young infant.[42] For the same reason, topical absorption of drugs in young infants exceeds that of adults.[45]

Many disorders of the newborn can also affect total body water and, thus, the distribution of drugs. Renal and hepatic dysfunctions may have important consequences on both elimination and distribution of xenobiotics. In addition, excess body fluid volume secondary to the syndrome of inappropriate secretion of antidiuretic hormone, resulting from pulmonary or central nervous system disorders, also influences the distribution of drugs. Certain drugs can also modify total body water. For instance, frequent administration of diuretics reduces body water[46,47] and the drugs' apparent volume of distribution.[48] Thus, the neonatal changes in total body water volume and the ratio of extracellular to intracellular fluid volume may have profound effects on drug distribution.

Lipid mass. The degree and disposition of the lipid mass in the body also affect drug distribution. The adipose tissue mass changes markedly during development, increasing from 1% to 15% of total body mass between 28 and 40 weeks of gestation[49] and continuing to rise to 25% of body mass by 1 year of age.

Another system that contains a high proportion of lipids is the central nervous system. Normally, the maximal increment in weight of the human brain occurs in the few weeks before term. In contrast, extensive myelination occurs postnatally.[50] The distribution of drugs to the central nervous system is unique in that entry of drugs into this system is restricted. Endothelial cells of brain capillaries, in contrast to those in other areas, form a blood-brain barrier that limits the penetration of hydrophilic substances into the brain. Consequently, ionized molecules, such as quaternary amines (e.g., neostigmine), have limited access to the central nervous system. In contrast, lipid-soluble compounds, such as chloramphenicol and phenobarbital, traverse the blood-brain barrier.

Transporters. As indicated previously, transporters are key determinants in the pharmacokinetic characteristics of drugs. A number of transporters have been cloned and are expressed in various tissues, including the epithelium of intestines and kidneys; in hepatocytes; and in brain endothelial cells. The developmental profile infers increased expression with age for a number of major transporters.[39,51,52] Polymorphisms of P-glycoproteins, organic anion transporters, and cation transporters have been described. A number of single-nucleotide polymorphisms have revealed loss of function.[18] Altogether, these developmental and genetic changes affect the volume of distribution of numerous drugs.

Systemic and regional hemodynamics. A major determinant of drug distribution is the combination of cardiac output and blood flow to various organs. Marked changes in the neonatal circulation take place in the perinatal period.[53-55] Important changes in regional blood flow may occur as a result of a patent ductus arteriosus,[56] sudden changes in blood gases secondary to pulmonary disorders, and a narrow range of organ blood flow autoregulation[57-59] in the stressed preterm infant. Persistence of a patent ductus arteriosus is also associated with retention of fluid and the development of congestive heart failure, which aggravates the increase in body water.[60] A similar situation can also be observed with noncyanotic congenital heart malformations. The variations in blood flow and total body fluid that result from these disorders and those secondary to developmental changes may alter the rate of drug distribution.

Protein binding. The degree of drug binding to plasma proteins has several consequences resulting from its effect on the distribution of a pharmacologic agent.[61] The degree of binding is inversely related to V_d as it maintains the drug in the vascular space. This adherence affects the renal and plasma clearance, the half-life, and the efficacy of the agent at its site of action.

Several factors modify the binding of drugs to plasma proteins: the amount of plasma-binding proteins, the number of binding sites, the affinity of the drug for the protein, and factors that alter drug-protein binding, such as blood pH, levels of free fatty acids, bilirubin concentration, presence of other drugs, and disease states (e.g., renal failure, liver failure).

Albumin binds principally to acidic drugs, whereas basic agents are bound to lipoproteins, β globulins, and α_1-acid glycoproteins.[62] Albumin contains a few high-affinity and several low-affinity binding sites.[63] In the preterm newborn, both albumin and α_1-acid glycoprotein concentrations and binding affinities are deficient, resulting in an increased fraction of free drug[64,65] and less drug in the vascular compartment.[66] Numerous conditions may further reduce the binding of drugs to proteins. Among the most described are changes in pH. Decreases in pH enhance the dissociation of weak acids from their albumin-binding sites. Thus, the commonly observed acidosis in premature infants may significantly change the binding of drugs to plasma proteins. The elevated plasma free fatty acid content of the newborn may also alter drug binding to plasma proteins.[67,68] However, this effect may not be as important as previously described.[69] The presence of maternal drugs that have crossed the placenta or other agents concomitantly administered to the infant may also compete for the same plasma protein-binding sites of drugs given to the newborn. Finally, the presence of fetal albumin may also affect drug binding.[64]

The potential interference of endogenous compounds, particularly unconjugated bilirubin in the newborn, on drug-protein binding has been addressed.[70] A displacement of bilirubin from its albumin-binding site may result in free circulating unconjugated bilirubin, which can penetrate the brain and predispose the newborn to kernicterus. However, it has been demonstrated that bilirubin is tightly bound to albumin and may itself displace drugs from their protein-binding sites.[70] In addition, free bilirubin is only sparingly lipophilic. Thus,

these factors can only partially contribute to the development of bilirubin-induced encephalopathy. Nonetheless, a few drugs can alter the binding affinity of albumin for bilirubin, as is the case with certain nonsteroidal anti-inflammatory agents (phenylbutazone and ibuprofen), and sulfonamides.[70,71]

The volume of distribution of certain compounds is also affected by their binding to proteins outside the vascular space. For instance, digoxin exhibits a higher degree of binding to myocardial and skeletal proteins in the newborn than in the adult.[72,73] This increased binding results in an augmented apparent V_d of digoxin.

Thus, multiple factors influence the distribution of drugs in the body.[74] These factors are themselves affected by development, genetics, and diseases of the newborn infant. Major changes in the distribution of fluids and fat and their proportion in relation to body mass occur at the end of gestation and during the neonatal period. Perinatal and neonatal alterations in cardiac output and regional blood flow, secondary to physiologic and pathophysiologic changes, also take place. For several drugs, the degree of drug binding to plasma proteins also varies between the newborn and adult. Furthermore, changes in the expression of transporters occur with development. Appropriate considerations of these various factors in the neonatal period enables adjustment of drug dosage in the newborn.[18]

Drug Elimination

The relatively high lipophilicity of many drugs does not allow their elimination to occur readily. After filtration through the glomerulus or passage into the bile, these agents are rapidly absorbed by the renal tubule or gastrointestinal mucosa, respectively. Consequently, the elimination of most drugs from the body involves the process of biotransformation, followed by excretion. In this section, we review the different biotransformation processes that take place in the body and the mechanisms of renal drug excretion, with particular reference to developmental aspects.

Drug Biotransformation

Drug biotransformation converts drug molecules into more polar derivatives. As drug molecules become less lipid soluble, they diffuse less readily across cell membranes. Consequently, these converted molecules do not reach their sites of action and are also not reabsorbed by the renal tubule. Thus biotransformation of drugs not only facilitates their excretion from the body but also may diminish their pharmacologic activity.

The metabolism of drugs does not always produce inactive compounds. Initial biotransformation of certain agents results in the formation of active metabolites. For instance, codeine is demethylated to morphine, diazepam is dealkylated to nordiazepam and subsequently hydroxylated to oxazepam, acetylsalicylic acid is hydrolyzed to salicylic acid, and theophylline is methylated to caffeine. Furthermore, as discussed subsequently, oxidation of certain aromatic compounds produces highly reactive electrophiles. Therefore, biotransformation can produce relatively innocuous metabolites or highly toxic compounds.

The mechanisms affecting the biotransformation of drugs are usually the same as those that metabolize endogenous products (e.g., hormones). Most biotransformation takes place in the liver, but some may occur at other sites, such as the kidneys, intestinal mucosa, and lungs. Biotransformation reactions can be divided into two phases: phase I, the **nonsynthetic reactions**, and phase II, **synthetic or conjugation reactions**. The great majority of phase I reactions (oxidation, reduction, and hydrolysis) are catalyzed by microsomal enzymes; other than glucuronidation, phase II reactions are extramicrosomal (Table 15-1).

Phase I Reactions (Nonsynthetic Reactions)

The enzymes involved in phase I reactions, notably the mixed-function oxidases or monooxygenases, are localized in the smooth endoplasmic reticulum. They consist of three principal components: an electron transporter, reduced nicotine adenine dinucleotide phosphate (NADPH)–cytochrome P-450 reductase (a flavoprotein), and one of the many cytochrome P-450 isozymes (designated CYP along with a number that refers to the gene family and subfamily to which they belong), which are oxidase hemoproteins.[75,76] The reaction requires both NADPH and molecular oxygen, which results in the oxidation of compounds by one atom of oxygen (thus, the name *monooxygenase*) and formation of water after reduction of the second oxygen atom.

The reactions catalyzed by the microsomal monooxygenases include aromatic ring and aliphatic side chain hydroxylation, *N*- and *O*-dealkylation, deamination, sulfoxidation, *N*-oxidation, *N*-hydroxylation, nitroreduction, and azoreduction. Epoxides are also formed by monooxygenases, converting aromatic moieties of agents to arene and alkene oxides. These electrophilic compounds can react avidly with proteins and nucleic acids, exerting potential mutagenic and carcinogenic effects.[77]

Several drugs can inhibit cytochrome P-450 enzyme activity. For example, cimetidine, spironolactone, and propylthiouracil inhibit cytochrome P-450 activity, slowing elimination. Other drugs can induce specific cytochrome P-450 isozymes, such as phenobarbital (CYP3A), rifampin (CYP1A, CYP2C), and 3-methylcholanthrene (CYP1A).

Of the nearly 1000 known cytochrome P-450s, only about 50 are functionally active in humans; these are divided into 17 families and a number of subfamilies.

Table 15–1. Biotransformation Reactions

Reaction	Examples of Drug Substrates
Phase I (Nonsynthetic Reactions)	
Oxidation	
Aromatic ring hydroxylation	Phenytoin, phenobarbital
Aliphatic hydroxylation	Ibuprofen
N-hydroxylation	Acetaminophen
N-, *O*-, *S*-dealkylation	Morphine, codeine
Deamination	Diazepam
Sulfoxidation, *N*-oxidation	Cimetidine
Reduction	
Azoreduction	Chloramphenicol
Nitroreduction	Ethanol
Alcohol dehydrogenase	
Hydrolysis	
Ester hydrolysis	Acetylsalicylic acid
Amide hydrolysis	Indomethacin
Phase I (Enzymes)	
CYP1A1/2	Caffeine, theophylline
CYP2C	Warfarin, ibuprofen, phenytoin, omeprazole, diazepam
CYP2D6	Codeine, imipramine, propranolol, timolol, tamoxifen
CYP2E1	Acetaminophen, caffeine, tamoxifen
CYP3A	Erythromycin, midazolam, 6β-hydroxycortisol
Phase II (Synthetic [Conjugation] Reactions)	
Glucuronide conjugation	Morphine, acetaminophen
Glycine conjugation	Salicylic acid
Sulfate conjugation	Acetaminophen, α-methyldopa
Glutathione conjugation	Ethacrynic acid
Methylation	Dopamine, epinephrine
Acetylation	Sulfonamides, clonazepam

Adapted from Correia MA, Castagnoli N: Pharmacokinetics II: Drug biotransformation. In Katzung BG (ed): Basic and Clinical Pharmacology. Norwalk, Conn, Appleton & Lange, 1986, pp 35-43.

The majority of all drug metabolism is catalyzed by CYP1, CYP2, and CYP3 families; the other families catalyze the synthesis and degradation of steroids, fatty acids, vitamins, and other endogenous compounds. Although individual CYP isoforms tend to have substrate specificities, overlap is common. CYP3A4 and CYP3A5 are similar isoforms, which together are involved in metabolism of approximately 50% of drugs. CYP2C and CYP2D6 also catalyze the metabolism of many drugs. CYP1A1/2, CYP2A6, CYP2B1, and CYP2E1 are involved to a lesser degree in drug metabolism but are rather implicated in activation of procarcinogenic agents, including aromatic amines and aromatic hydrocarbons.

The cytochrome P-450–dependent monooxygenase system develops in fetal life, but, in general, its activity in the fetus and newborn remains considerably lower than that found in adult liver.[78,79] The diminished enzyme activity may be clinically important because drugs that are oxygenated slowly by these enzymes (e.g., phenobarbital and phenytoin) can exhibit a prolonged half-life in the young infant[80]; this change is especially the case for CYP2A, CYP2B6, CYP2C, and CYP3A4/5 (Table 15-2). CYP1A2 exhibits the most delayed expression and begins to appear at 1 to 3 months of postnatal age[81]; CYP2C and CYP3A4/5 appear during the first postnatal week,[82,83] soon followed by CYP2D6.[84] Accordingly, there are significant differences in the developmental expression of the three important gene families implicated in xenobiotic metabolism. Drugs converted by CYP2D6 and CYP3A7, such as carbamazepine, dextromethorphan, and tricyclic antidepressants, are eliminated in the newborn nearly as rapidly as in the adult,[79] whereas those metabolized primarily by CYP1A2, such as caffeine and theophylline, exhibit a prolonged half-life in the neonate (see Table 15-1).[85] Of interest, CYP2E1 is induced and metabolized by ethanol in the fetus and has been proposed to be implicated in the development of fetal alcohol syndrome.[86]

A few of the oxidative and reductive reactions are produced by enzymes (not cytochrome P-450) present in the mitochondria and cytosol of the liver and other tissues. These enzymes include those involved in oxidation of alcohols and aldehydes; alcohol and aldehyde dehydrogenases; and enzymes that partake in the metabolism of catecholamines, tyrosine hydroxylase, and monoamine oxidase. Although the activity of some of these enzymes can be detected early in gestation, their full activity is reached only in early childhood,[87] but ontogenic differences are observed. For example, class I alcohol dehydrogenase, the major ethanol-metabolizing enzyme, but not class III alcohol dehydrogenase appears well expressed in the fetal liver.[88]

Phase II Reactions (Synthetic Reactions)

Phase II reactions consist of conjugations, whereby molecules naturally present in the body are combined with the drug or other molecules. The drug may have first undergone a phase I reaction, or the original drug may be directly conjugated. Conjugation converts drugs into more polar compounds, which are pharmacologically less active and are more readily excreted. Although it was previously thought that conjugation reactions represented true inactivation and detoxification reactions, it is currently known that certain conjugation reactions may lead to the formation of hepatotoxic compounds (e.g., N-acetylation of isoniazid).

Glucuronidation.
Formation of glucuronide is the principal conjugation reaction. Natural substrates of this pathway include bilirubin and thyroxine. Many drugs containing hydroxyl, amino, carboxyl, thiol, and phenolic groups also utilize the same pathway. Examples of these drugs include morphine, acetaminophen, phenytoin, sulfonamides, chloramphenicol, salicylic acid, and indomethacin.

The conjugation of a compound with glucuronic acid results in the production of a strongly acidic substance that is more water soluble at physiologic pH than is the parent compound. This process reduces its transfer across membranes and, consequently, facilitates its dissociation with its receptive site, as well as enhances its elimination in urine and bile. The fate of glucuronidated drugs in urine or bile depends on their molecular size. Compounds with relatively low molecular weights are almost completely excreted in urine, whereas those with high molecular weights (>500 D) are eliminated almost entirely in bile.

Glucuronides are eliminated by the kidneys, primarily by glomerular filtration. Biliary excretion of drugs conjugated to glucuronic acid occurs by simple diffusion or by active secretion. Once in the intestine, these drugs may be reabsorbed after being hydrolyzed by glucuronidase; the activity of the latter is increased in the fetus and newborn.[36]

Drugs or conditions that inhibit glucuronidation prolong the pharmacologic activity of these agents. This inhibition may occur at the level of glucuronic acid

| Table 15–2. | Ontogeny of Human Phase I and Phase II Metabolizing Enzymes |

Enzyme	Fetus	Newborn	Infant	Adult
Phase I				
CYP1A1	+	–	–	–
CYP1A2	–	–	+	+
CYP2C	–	+	+	+
CYP2D6	+/–	+	+	+
CYP2E1	+/–	+	+	+
CYP3A7	+	+	–	–
CYP3A4/5	–	+	+	+
Phase II				
UGT1A1	–	+	+	+
UGT1A3	+/–	+/–	+	+
UGT2B7	+/–	+/–	+	+
GSTA	+/–	+/–	+	+
SULT1A1	+/–	+/–	+	+
SULT1A3	+	+	+	+/–

MGT, UDP-glucuronosyltransferase; GST, glutathione S-transferase; SULT, sulfotransferase.

Adapted from Hines and McCarver[79] and from McCarver and Hines.[115]

synthesis (e.g., by certain steroid hormones) or at the level of the uridine diphosphate–glucuronyl transferase activity itself. In the human fetus and newborn, glucuronidation reactions are slow but mature rapidly postnatally (see Table 15-2).[89] This maturation is clearly illustrated with the metabolism of bilirubin. Reduced activity of the 2B isoform in early life is responsible for the gray baby syndrome secondary to chloramphenicol administration.

Other synthetic conjugation reactions. Other conjugation reactions include those with glycine, sulfates, glutathione, methyl, and acetyl groups. The activity of these various transferases is also generally lower in the fetus and newborn than in the adult (see Table 15-2).[90]

Factors Affecting Biotransformation

Development and biotransformation. Several factors may alter the rate, extent, and type of biotransformation reactions. As pointed out previously, there are marked changes in biotransformation during development. The cytochrome P-450–dependent monooxygenase system develops in fetal life, but in general its activity in the fetus and newborn remains considerably lower than that found in adult liver.[91] Consequently, certain drugs such as phenytoin and phenobarbital are oxidized slowly in the young infant by these enzymes, which prolongs their half-life.[92] In addition, the ontogeny of metabolizing enzymes in tissues other than the liver is particularly

Table 15–3. Comparative Plasma Half-Lives of Miscellaneous Drugs in Newborns and Adults

	Plasma Half-Life (hr)	
	Newborn	**Adult**
Analgesics-Antipyretics		
Acetaminophen	3.5	2.2
Phenylbutazone	21-34	12-30
Indomethacin	7.5-51.0	6
Meperidine	22	3.5
Anesthetics		
Bupivacaine	25	1.3
Mepivacaine	8.7	3.2
Anticonvulsants		
Phenytoin	21	11-29
Carbamazepine	8-28	21-36
Phenobarbital	82-199	24-140
Diazepam	25-100	15-25
Other Drugs		
Caffeine	100	6
Theophylline	30	6
Furosemide	7.7-19.9	0.5
Chloramphenicol	14-24	2.5
Salicylates	4.5-11.5	2.7
Digoxin	52	31-40

Data from Aranda et al,[116] Morselli et al,[37] and Morselli.[117]

relevant for CYP1A1, CYP3A4, CYP3A5, and uridine diphosphate–glucuronyl transferases.

Table 15-3 presents the approximate prolongation of the plasma half-lives of certain drugs in the newborn in relation to adults. Many drugs such as indomethacin, caffeine, and theophylline are eliminated much more slowly in the neonate. Interestingly, despite the close structural resemblance of drugs such as caffeine and theophylline, their elimination rates may vary significantly. Thus, application of dose rates for theophylline to caffeine in the treatment of neonatal apnea would lead to marked accumulation of caffeine in the blood. Other drugs, such as carbamazepine, are eliminated as readily in the infant as in the adult.

For a number of drugs administered to the neonate, the rate of elimination increases rapidly during the first postnatal week, as observed for phenytoin and phenobarbital. Nonetheless, large interindividual variability in plasma half-lives is detected in the neonate, but the half-life shortens with maturation. This finding means that some neonates receiving a standard recommended dose may exhibit subtherapeutic drug concentrations in the plasma, whereas in others the upper limit of the presumed therapeutic range may be exceeded. In neonates given phenobarbital for seizures, repeated doses of 5 mg/kg/day can yield mean plasma concentrations of about 40 mg/L during the first week, whereas a lower dosage (2.5 to 5 mg/kg/day) can yield plasma concentrations below 15 mg/L by the second and third weeks. This warrants monitoring of plasma concentrations. Adjustment of dosage on the basis of plasma concentrations of the drug and accounting for a rapid postnatal increase in drug clearance may result in maintenance of plasma concentrations of phenobarbital within the suggested therapeutic range (15 to 25 mg/L). In contrast, caffeine clearance exhibits negligible maturational changes in the neonatal period. Adult rates of elimination are achieved at about 3 to 4 months and may be exceeded thereafter.

The need to eliminate xenobiotic compounds from the body in the presence of decreased oxidative and conjugative pathways in the fetus and neonate may lead to activation and/or use of available biotransformation pathways. For example, premature neonates given theophylline may produce caffeine via methylation pathways, which are active as early as the first trimester, as shown in human hepatic organ culture studies. Because minimum oxidative function is present at this stage of gestation, the relative increase in activity of the methylase pathway leads to the production of caffeine as one of the major metabolites of theophylline in the human fetus and newborn. Both caffeine and theophylline exhibit similar pharmacologic activity but variable specific potency. Therefore, interpretation of clinical effect must account for both methylxanthines.

Environment and biotransformation. Environmental influences can also affect drug metabolism by inducing or inhibiting metabolic activities. For instance, calcium channel blockers, antifungal agents, and macrolide antibiotics are potent inhibitors of CYP3A enzymes, quinidine inhibits CYP2D6, and other compounds such as cimetidine, amiodarone, and fluoxetine reduce activity of many cytochrome P-450 enzymes. A number of agents, including anticonvulsants and aromatic hydrocarbons, can, on the other hand, stimulate induction of certain cytochrome P-450 subfamilies and isoforms.

Genetics and biotransformation. Genetic influences on metabolic enzyme activity is the rule rather than the exception; however, the interplay between genetics and ontogeny on drug metabolism remains largely unknown. A gene of one member of the cytochrome P-450 enzyme system, CYP2D6, has been extensively studied and found to exhibit approximately 70 single-nucleotide polymorphisms, many of which lead to diminished enzyme activity. These polymorphisms may significantly affect drugs metabolized by CYP2D6, such as β blockers, codeine, dextromethorphan, and nortriptyline. Similar observations have been made for CYP2C9 and CYP2C19, which metabolize phenytoin and omeprazole, respectively.[93] In the case of CYP3A enzymes, no significant functional polymorphisms have been yet identified; hence, factors regulating gene expression are more important to explain the interindividual variability (>10-fold). Genetic polymorphism is also clinically observed for phase II enzymes. *N*-acetylation of isoniazid stands out as one of the most remarkable ones, whereby polymorphism of *N*-acetyltransferase-2 gene leads to two populations of acetylators: fast and slow.[93] Hence, environment and genetics exert major influences on biotransformation, which in turn contributes significantly to explain interpersonal differences; these factors play a lesser role on renal excretion of drugs.

Other factors and biotransformation. Other factors that affect biotransformation include blood flow to the liver, gender of the patient, and disease states. Blood flow may be the limiting factor controlling drug elimination of certain drugs (e.g., morphine, meperidine, propranolol, and verapamil). These drugs, often termed **flow-limited** drugs, are so readily metabolized by the liver that hepatic clearance is essentially equal to liver blood flow. In contrast, the biotransformation of **capacity-limited** drugs (e.g., phenytoin, theophylline, diazepam, and chloramphenicol) is determined by the liver's metabolizing capacity rather than by hepatic blood flow.[94] The effect of gender in the newborn remains unclear but is probably not as important as in the adult.

Overall available data allow the following generalizations regarding drug metabolism in the fetus and newborn:

1. The rates of drug biotransformation and overall elimination are slow.
2. The rate of drug elimination from the body exhibits marked variability among patients.
3. The maturational changes in drug metabolism and disposition as a function of postnatal age are extremely variable and depend on the substrate or drug being used, although they progress relatively rapidly over the first postnatal month.
4. Neonatal drug biotransformation and elimination are vulnerable to pathophysiologic states.
5. Neonates may exhibit activation of alternate biotransformation pathways.

Renal Excretion of Drugs

The renal excretion of drugs and their metabolites occurs through three major processes: glomerular filtration, active tubular secretion, and passive tubular reabsorption. The ultimate elimination rate of a drug, after its entry into the tubule, depends on its lipophilicity and ionization state (environmental pH dependent). This process is similar to that which applies for absorption and distribution.

Glomerular filtration of drugs. The amount of drug filtered through the glomerulus depends on a molecular size smaller than that of albumin (69,000 D) and its plasma protein binding. Almost all non–protein-bound drugs are filtered. Glomerular filtration rate increases during fetal developmental but remains low in the newborn, in contrast to that of the adult.[95,96] Certain conditions of the newborn, such as asphyxia, severe respiratory insufficiency, and patent ductus arteriosus, are associated with a decrease in glomerular filtration rate. Certain agents (e.g., indomethacin, tolazoline) may impede their own excretion by reducing glomerular filtration rate.[97,98]

Active tubular transport of drugs. A number of transport systems found in the proximal tubule are involved in the energy-dependent secretion of organic compounds (endogenous or exogenous).[99] One such system transports organic anions, including drug conjugates with glucuronic acid, glycine, and sulfates; drugs that use this excretory system include penicillins, furosemide, and chlorothiazide. The other transport system secretes organic cations, such as histamine and choline. Multidrug resistance proteins 1, 3, 5, and 6 are localized at the basolateral membrane, whereas isoforms 2 and 4 are found at the brush-border membrane of tubular epithelium. These transporters generally operate as efflux pumps. A counteracting mechanism involves the peptide transporters PEPT1 and, especially, PEPT2, which are present at the apex of the proximal tubular epithelium; these transporters operate as influx pumps. All transporters described are energy dependent. In the case of organic cation, organic anion, and peptide transporters, cellular import requires an electrochemical gradient, especially of Na⁺, which is largely maintained by the Na^+/K^+-ATPase pump, whereas multidrug resistance proteins are directly ATP dependent.[100] Membrane transporters, mainly located in the distal tubule, operate to reabsorb drugs from the tubular lumen back into circulation; this reabsorption occurs mostly by nonionic diffusion.

Tubular secretion of organic anions and cations is also lower in newborns than it is in adults. This developmental characteristic explains the prolonged half-life of certain agents that use this system of elimination in the newborn, as is the case with furosemide, penicillins, and glucuronidated drugs.

Passive tubular reabsorption of drugs. This form of renal excretion of drugs is regulated by three factors: the concentration gradient across the tubular membrane, the ionization state of the compound in the tubular fluid (which depends on the drug's pK_a and the tubular fluid pH), and the lipid solubility of the drug. These characteristics of the agent can be used to enhance their renal excretion. For instance, alkalinization of the urine can increase by up to sixfold the elimination of salicylic acid.

Developmental aspects of renal drug excretion. The kidneys are the most important organs for drug elimination in the newborn. The most frequently used drugs in neonates, such as antimicrobial agents, are excreted via this route. Renal elimination of these drugs reflects and depends on neonatal renal function, characterized by low glomerular filtration rate, low effective renal blood flow, and low tubular function, in comparison with those in the adult. Neonatal glomerular filtration rate is about 30% of the adult value and is greatly influenced by gestational age at birth. The most rapid changes occur during the first week of life, and these events are reflected by the plasma disappearance rates of aminoglycosides, which are eliminated mainly by glomerular filtration. These changes have been considered in the dosage regimen recommended for these drugs and other antibiotics.

Effective renal blood flow may influence the rate at which drugs are presented to and eliminated by the kidneys. Effective renal blood flow, as measured by para-aminohippuric acid (PAH) clearance, is substantially lower in infants than in adults, even when PAH extraction values are correlated (i.e., PAH extraction is 60% in infants, in comparison with >92% in adults). Available data suggest that effective renal blood flow is low during the first 2 days of life (34 to 99 mL/min/1.73 m²), which increases to 54 to 166 mL/min/1.73 m² by 14 to 21 days and further increases to adult values of about 600 mL/min/1.73 m² by age 1 to 2 years.

Although pharmacokinetic behavior of drugs eliminated via the neonatal kidneys does not exhibit the variability observed with those that undergo hepatic biotransformation, a relative unevenness is observed, as seen for many antimicrobials such as ampicillin. As is the case with biotransformation, this interindividual variability in renal elimination at birth does narrow with advancing age. Accordingly, plasma half-life of drugs eliminated by kidneys also shortens progressively after birth, achieving adult rates within the first postnatal month. In the clinical setting, these developmental changes require adjustment of maintenance dosages. The drug-dependent variability in the elimination process may reflect in part the major renal mechanisms of drug excretion: that drugs that undergo elimination mainly via glomerular filtration (e.g., aminoglycosides) are excreted more rapidly than those requiring primarily tubular excretion (e.g., penicillins). These differences may reflect neonatal glomerular preponderance.

Effects of Disease on Drug Disposition

Most pharmacokinetic parameters have been determined for healthy or moderately ill individuals. Unfortunately, in neonatology, as in other intensive care settings, drugs are often used on very sick patients in which pharmacokinetics are affected. Disease states (e.g., congestive heart failure, liver disease) are conditions well recognized to affect drug elimination. The same applies to pathologic insults (e.g., hypoxia, asphyxia); for instance, neonates with seizures who experience perinatal asphyxia may have higher steady-state plasma concentrations of phenobarbital than do those without asphyxia. Consequently, adjustment in drug dosage is critical to avoid toxicity. For this purpose, understanding the pathophysiology of a specific clinical condition and its pharmacologic consequences is of utmost importance for appropriate drug therapy. This section addresses the issue of diseases that can influence drug disposition in the newborn.

Cardiovascular disease. Cardiac output is a major determinant of drug elimination. Heart failure produces a decrease in cardiac output that alters the regional distribution of blood flow, with preferential circulation to the brain, heart, and kidneys. Under these circumstances, the liver often suffers from hypoxia from pulmonary edema, decreased hepatic blood flow, and increased portal venous pressure.[101,102] These consequences on hepatic tissue decrease the liver clearance of many drugs.

Congestive heart failure is also associated with a reduction in renal blood flow and glomerular filtration rate.[103] This compromise in renal function contributes to a decrease in drug elimination. In newborns with congestive heart failure, elevated plasma levels of digoxin have been observed.

Renal disease. The kidneys are a major source of drug elimination. Hence, alterations in function significantly influence the pharmacokinetics of numerous drugs that depend to a large extent (>90% of the total clearance) on this form of elimination.[99] Several factors affect the clearance of drugs from the kidneys during renal insufficiency. As glomerular filtration rate falls, there is a decrease in drugs eliminated principally via this route, such as digoxin, aminoglycosides, and cephalosporins. Reduction in tubular function plays a significant role for agents that utilize this route of elimination, such as penicillins and furosemide. In addition, changes in plasma and urine pH alter the excretion of ionized drugs. Uremia is also associated with alterations in cardiac output, liver function, and blood-brain barrier permeability, which further contribute to the changes in drug disposition.[104]

The relevance of drug accumulation lies in the pharmacologic activity and/or toxicity of the unexcreted products. Nomograms can assist in modifying drug dosage in renal failure; these should be adjusted to age.

Liver disease. Because the liver is a major site of drug disposition, hepatic failure alters drug excretion[105] by affecting plasma protein binding, liver circulation, and intrinsic biotransformation. The excessive variability in liver dysfunction makes it difficult to formulate specific dosage recommendations. Marked changes in pharmacokinetics, like those seen with renal insufficiency, have not been observed in severe liver failure.[106] Nonetheless, dosages of drugs eliminated mainly by hepatic biotransformation should generally be reduced in patients with severe liver disease.

Clinical Pharmacokinetics

The fundamental assumption of clinical pharmacokinetics is that a relationship exists between the concentration of a drug at its site of action and its serum or plasma level. The concentration of drug in the blood enables the clinician to monitor the dose-response relationship by extrapolation and to predict its kinetics. Consequently, drug levels in blood enable appropriate individual dosing adjustments.

The distribution of drugs in the body is governed by multiple factors. Pharmacokinetic principles can be understood only with regard to the distribution of drugs in the various compartments. A compartment is not necessarily a defined physiologic or anatomic site but is considered one or many tissues that are similar in affinity for a drug. The factors that determine the movement of a drug in and out of compartments are those that affect distribution. Therefore, the lipophilicity, ionization state, transporters, and protein binding of a drug, as well as regional blood flow, regulate the extent and rate of passage of an agent into and out of a compartment.

Distribution

The simplest model is the single-compartment model. In this model, it is assumed that after administration of a drug, immediate equilibration of its concentration is achieved in all major tissues. First-order kinetics apply to this model; therefore, the rate of change in the amount of drug in the body is a constant fraction of the amount of drug present at the time. Thus, the higher the dose, the greater the elimination rate from the compartment. In a multicompartment model analysis, it is assumed that all rate processes for the passage of drug from one compartment to another exhibit first-order kinetics. Therefore, the plasma level–time curve for a drug that seems to exhibit a multicompartment model of distribution is described by the summation of the several first-order rate processes.

The rate of disappearance of a drug concentration according to first-order kinetics can be expressed as

$$\partial C/\partial t = -kC$$

where C is the concentration of the drug and k the first-order elimination rate constant, expressed in units of $time^{-1}$ (e.g., $hours^{-1}$). Integration of this equation yields the drug concentration at a time t:

$$\log C = -kt/2.3 + \log C_0, \text{ or } C = C_0 e^{-kt}$$

where C_0 is the concentration at time 0. Thus, the slope of the log of the concentration-time curve is $-k/2.3$.

Drug half-life and loading dose. From the preceding equation ($\log C = -kt/2.3 + \log C_0$), we can obtain the **first-order half-life:**

$$t_{1/2} = 0.693/k$$

The time required for the concentration to decrease by one half is a constant determined by k and is independent of the initial drug concentration. Thus, the time it takes to achieve a steady-state plasma concentration, or the time it takes to eliminate the near totality of the drug, is equal to five half-lives. In order to expedite achievement of average steady-state plasma concentrations ($C_{ss\ av}$), a loading dose (D_L) can be given:

$$D_L = C_{ss\ av} \bullet V_d$$

Maintenance dose. The dose necessary to maintain the steady-state concentration (the maintenance dose, D_{ss}) can be calculated from the following equation:

$$D_{ss} = (0.693 \bullet C_{ss\ av} \bullet V_d \bullet \tau)/t_{1/2}$$

where τ is the dosing interval. Thus D_{ss} is also equal to the rate of drug elimination during τ.

Optimal dosing schedule. By setting the maximum and minimum effective steady-state concentrations for a multiple dosing regimen, it is possible to determine the **optimal dosing schedule** once the $t_{1/2}$ is known. With the same equation to calculate the concentration at a time t, $\log C = -kt/2.3 + \log C_0$, and by substituting C for $C_{ss\ min}$ and C_0 for $C_{ss\ max}$, an optimal dosing interval, τ, can be determined:

$$\tau = \log(C_{ss\ max}/C_{ss\ min}) \bullet 3.3 \bullet t_{1/2}$$

Drug clearance. Drug clearance can be defined as the plasma volume in the vascular compartment that is cleared of the drug as a function of time. Clearance (Cl) is defined as excretion rate per plasma concentration. Clearance can be expressed by the following equation:

$$Cl = D_0/[AUC]_0^t$$

By rearranging the equation according to the equation expressing V_d (see distribution shown previously),

$$Cl = V_d \bullet k$$

Zero-Order Kinetics

When elimination processes become saturated, disposition of certain drugs occurs via zero-order kinetics. In contrast to a first-order process, in which the fraction of drug eliminated is constant, in a zero-order process the elimination rate is constant per se; that is, the drug is eliminated at a constant rate. Consequently, the zero-order $t_{1/2}$ is not constant but is proportional to the initial amount or concentration of the drug:

$$t_{1/2} = 0.5C_0/k_0$$

where k_0 is the zero-order rate constant. Many drugs exhibit zero-order kinetics with elevated concentrations; as the drug concentrations decline, first-order kinetics prevail. Examples of drugs that exhibit saturation kinetics include salicylates, phenylbutazone, phenytoin, diazepam, and chloramphenicol.

Drug Monitoring in the Clinical Setting

In the clinical setting, therapeutic drug monitoring of a number of agents such as anticonvulsants (phenytoin, phenobarbital, carbamazepine), antimicrobials (gentamicin, tobramycin, chloramphenicol), cardiac glycosides (digoxin), and methylxanthines (caffeine, theophylline) is often useful in individualizing drug therapy. Rapid microassay techniques such as enzyme multiplied immunoassay technique and high-pressure liquid chromatography require small volumes of blood samples and are well suited for neonates. Therapeutic drug monitoring to verify appropriateness of the drug dosing is useful for adjusting the dosage and preventing undesired therapeutic effects as a result of developmental and pathophysiologic changes. Because most drugs used in neonates exhibit first-order kinetics, change in dosage is proportional to the change in plasma drug concentration at steady state. Thus, a plasma phenobarbital concentration of 10 mg/L at a dosage of 5 mg/kg/day would be expected to increase by 100% to 20 mg/L if the dosage were doubled to 10 mg/kg/day; conversely, a plasma phenobarbital concentration of 10 mg/L would be halved if the phenobarbital dose were reduced by half. These predictions are expected to occur at steady state, at which the fraction of the drug dose eliminated from the body is usually held constant.

GENERAL PRINCIPLES OF PHARMACODYNAMICS: DRUG-RECEPTOR INTERACTION

Pharmacodynamics is defined as the biochemical and physiologic effects of drugs. This aspect of pharmacology is the raison d'être of pharmacotherapeutics.

Sites of Drug Action (Concept of Receptors)

Drugs may act outside the cell, at the cell membrane, or inside the cell. The effect of certain drugs action may or may not be mediated by interaction with receptor sites. For instance, there are drugs that act on *extracellular* products of cells. For instance, chelating agents, such as dimercaprol and penicillamine, bind circulating metals. The action of these agents can be considered truly extracellular.

However, most drugs bind to specific *receptor* sites. This renders specificity to drug *action* and refers not only to distribution but also to the specificity of the drug action. Receptors consist of macromolecules that recognize and bind specific ligands and translate this binding into propagation of an intracellular message, either directly (e.g., nicotinic receptor: ion transport) and/or by virtue of a second messenger (e.g., protein kinase C, angiotensin II). The receptive site of drugs can also be the active site of enzymes with which the drug binds and competes with the natural substrate or a complementary strand of nucleic acid.[107] The concept of receptors suggests the existence of functional domains on the receptor molecule, a ligand-binding domain and an effector domain. Such conceptualization of the receptor is consistent with the mode of action of agonists and antagonists. The concept of drug-receptor interaction is now generalized and applies to most drugs utilized, including inhaled anesthetics.[108]

The actions of drugs on receptors is dependent on receptor density, receptor confirmation and activity, and effector signaling pathways. These factors are all subject to genetic, developmental, and pathologic influences.[93,109-111] Genetic variations in drug targets have been clearly described to exert profound effects on drug efficacy. Well-characterized examples apply to gene variants of β_2 adrenoceptors, 5-lipoxygenase, and angiotensin-converting enzyme, which affects response of agonists and antagonists for asthma and hypertension.[112] Along these lines, age-dependent differences in the interaction of a drug with its specific receptor have also been demonstrated (e.g., warfarin and cyclosporine).[113,114] Thus a complex interplay among ontogeny, genetics, and disease condition affects pharmacodynamics in young children.

COLLABORATIVE TRIALS FOR NEONATAL DRUG USE

In view of the particular limitations of the premature and full-term newborns to handle drugs, along with their distinctive and unusual dosage requirements, there are increasing endeavors by neonatologists to conduct appropriate drug studies in the newborn. Studies that have been especially successful were sponsored and initiated by pharmaceutical industries. Examples of these studies include those for Exosurf, Curosurf, and Survanta, involving at least 35 controlled trials, recombinant erythropoietin with more than 15 studies, and investigator-initiated collaborative trials, as was the case for nitric oxide in neonatal pulmonary hypertension, indomethacin in ductus arteriosus closure, and antenatal phenobarbital or indomethacin for the prevention of intraventricular hemorrhage. These studies revealed that multicenter collaborative trials provide particularly meaningful data for drug evaluation in large populations of sick newborns, especially those of very low birth weight (<1000 g).

REFERENCES

1. Allen MC, Donohue PK, Dusman AE: The limit of viability—neonatal outcome of infants born at 22 to 25 weeks' gestation. N Engl J Med 329:1597, 1993.
2. Hack M, Fanaroff AA: Outcomes of extremely-low-birth-weight infants between 1982 and 1988. N Engl J Med 321:1642, 1989.
3. Robertson PA, Sniderman SH, Laros RK Jr, et al: Neonatal morbidity according to gestational age and birth weight from five tertiary care centers in the United States, 1983 through 1986. Am J Obstet Gynecol 166:1629, 1992.
4. Aranda JV, Cohen S, Neims AH: Drug utilization in a newborn intensive care unit. J Pediatr 89:315, 1976.
5. Aranda JV, Collinge JM, Clarkson S: Epidemiologic aspects of drug utilization in a newborn intensive care unit. Semin Perinatol 6:148, 1982.
6. Aranda JV, Portuguez-Malavasi A, Collinge JM, et al: Epidemiology of adverse drug reactions in the newborn. Dev Pharmacol Ther 5:173, 1982.
7. Guignard JP, Dubourg L, Gouyon JB: Diuretics in the neonatal period. Rev Med Suisse Romande 115:583, 1995.
8. van den Anker JN: Pharmacokinetics and renal function in preterm infants. Acta Paediatr 85:1393, 1996.
9. Gilman JT, Gal P: Pharmacokinetic and pharmacodynamic data collection in children and neonates. A quiet frontier. Clin Pharmacokinet 23:1, 1992.
10. Rane A, Wilson JT: Clinical pharmacokinetics in infants and children. Clin Pharmacokinet 1:2, 1976.

11. Bory C, Baltassat P, Porthault M, et al: Metabolism of theophylline to caffeine in premature newborn infants. J Pediatr 94:988, 1979.
12. Farrington E: Cardiac toxicity with cisapride. Pediatr Nurs 22:256, 1996.
13. Schanker LS: Passage of drugs across body membranes. Pharmacol Rev 14:501, 1962.
14. Quamme GA: Loop diuretics. In Dirks JH, Sutton RAL (eds): Diuretics: Physiology, Pharmacology and Clinical Use. Philadelphia, WB Saunders, 1986, pp 86-116.
15. Burckhardt G, Wolff NA: Structure of renal organic anion and cation transporters. Am J Physiol 278:F853, 2000.
16. Lee VH, Sporty JL, Fandy TE: Pharmacogenomics of drug transporters: The next drug delivery challenge. Adv Drug Deliv Rev 50:S33, 2001.
17. Zhang L, Brett CM, Giacomini KM: Role of organic cation transporters in drug absorption and elimination. Annu Rev Pharmacol Toxicol 38:431, 1998.
18. Mizuno N, Niwa T, Yotsumoto Y, et al: Impact of drug transporter studies on drug discovery and development. Pharmacol Rev 55:425, 2003.
19. Bode F, Baumann K, Kinne R: Analysis of the pinocytic process in rat. Biochim Biophys Acta 433:294, 1976.
20. Matsuzaki T, Tajika Y, Tserentsoodol N, et al: Aquaporins: A water channel family. Anat Sci Int 77:85, 2002.
21. Sands JM: Mammalian urea transporters. Annu Rev Physiol 65:543, 2003.
20. Sadee W, Drubbisch V, Amidon GL: Biology of membrane transporter proteins. Pharm Res 12:1823, 1995.
23. Shargell L, Yu ABC: Applied Biopharmaceutics and Pharmacokinetics. New York, Appleton-Century-Crofts, 1980, pp 68-84.
24. Winter ME: Basic Clinical Pharmacokinetics. San Francisco, Applied Therapeutics, 1980, pp 46-48.
25. Hall SD, Thummel KE, Watkins PB, et al: Molecular and physical mechanisms of first-pass extraction. Drug Metab Dispos 27:161,1999.
26. Heimann G: Enteral absorption and bioavailability in children in relation to age. Eur J Clin Pharmacol 18:43, 1980.
27. Weaver LT, Austin S, Cole TJ: Small intestinal length: A factor essential for gut adaptation. Gut 32:1321, 1991.
28. Euler AR, Byrne WJ, Meis PJ, et al: Basal pentagastrin-stimulated acid secretion in newborn human infants. Pediatr Res 13:36, 1979.
29. Neese AL, Soyka LF: Development of a radioimunoassay for theophylline: Application to studies in premature infants. Clin Pharmacol Ther 21:633, 1977.
30. Watkins JB, Szczepanik P, Gould JB, et al: Bile salt metabolism in the human premature infant: Preliminary observations of pool size and synthesis rate following prenatal administration of dexamethasone and phenobarbital. Gastroenterology 69:706, 1975.
31. Hillman LS, Martin LA, Haddad JG: Absorption and maintenance dosage of 25-hydroxycholecalciferol (25-HCC) in premature infants. Pediatr Res 13:400, 1979.
32. Melhorn DK, Gross S: Vitamin E-dependent anemia in the premature infant. II. Relationships between gestational age and absorption of vitamin E. J Pediatr 79:581, 1971.
33. Bell EF, Brown EJ, Milner R, et al: Vitamin E absorption in small premature infants. Pediatrics 63:830, 1979.
34. Graeber JE, Williams ML, Oski FA: The use of intramuscular vitamin E in the premature infant: Optimum dose and iron interaction. J Pediatr 90:282, 1977.
35. Gustaffson BE, Daft FS, McDaniel EG, et al: Effects of vitamin K–active compounds and intestinal microorganisms in vitamin K–deficient germ-free rats. J Nutr 78:461, 1962.
36. Yaffe SJ, Stern L: Clinical implications of perinatal pharmacology. In Mirkin BL (ed): Perinatal Pharmacology and Therapeutics. New York, Academic Press, 1976, pp 355-428.
37. Morselli PL, Franco-Morselli R, Bossi L: Clinical pharmacokinetics in newborns and infants: Age-related differences and therapeutic implications. Clin Pharmacokinet 5:485, 1980.
38. Matheny CJ, Lamb MW, Brouwer KR, et al: Pharmacokinetic and pharmacodynamic implications of P-glycoprotein modulation. Pharmacotherapy 21:778, 2001.
39. Tsai CE, Daood MJ, Lane RH, et al: P-glycoprotein expression in mouse brain increases with maturation. Biol Neonate 81:58, 2002.
40. Stahlberg MR, Hietanen E, Maki M: Mucosal biotransformation rates in the small intestine of children. Gut 29:1058, 1998.
41. Gibbs JP, Liacouras CA, Baldassano RN, et al: Up-regulation of glutathione S-transferase activity in enterocytes of young children. Drug Metab Dispos 27:1466, 1999.
42. Costarino A, Baumgart S: Modern fluid and electrolyte management of the critically ill premature infant. Pediatr Clin North Am 33:153, 1986.
43. Winters RW: Maintenance fluid therapy. In Winters RW (ed): The Body Fluids in Pediatrics. Boston, Little, Brown, 1973, pp 113-133.
44. Williams PR, Oh W: Effects of radiant warmer on insensible water loss in newborn infants. Am J Dis Child 128:511, 1974.
45. West DP, Worobec S, Solomon LM: Pharmacology and toxicology of infant skin. J Invest Dermatol 76:147, 1981.
46. Chemtob S, Doray JL, Laudignon N, et al: Alternating sequential dosing with furosemide and ethacrynic acid in drug tolerance in the newborn. Am J Dis Child 143:850, 1989.
47. Segar J, Robillard JE, Johnson K, et al: Addition of metolazone to overcome tolerance to furosemide in infants with bronchopulmonary dysplasia. J Pediatr 120:966, 1992.
48. Chemtob S, Papageorgiou A, du Souich P, et al: Cumulative increase in serum furosemide concentration following repeated doses in the newborn. Am J Perinatol 4:203, 1987.
49. Widdowson EM: Growth and composition of the fetus and newborn. In Assali NS (ed): Biology of Gestation, vol 2. New York, Academic Press, 1968, pp 1-49.
50. Davison N, Dobbing J: Myelination as a vulnerable period in brain development. Br Med Bull 22:40, 1966.
51. Dutt A, Priebe TS, Teeter LD, et al: Postnatal development of organic cation transport and mdr gene expression in mouse kidney. J Pharmacol Exp Ther 261:1222, 1992.
52. Li N, Hartley DP, Cherrington NJ, et al: Tissue expression, ontogeny, and inducibility of rat organic anion transporting polypeptide 4. J Pharmacol Exp Ther 301:551, 2002.
53. Iwamoto HS, Teitel D, Rudolph AM: Effects of birth-related events on blood flow distribution. Pediatr Res 22:634, 1987.
54. Klopfenstein HS, Rudolph AM: Postnatal changes in the circulation, and the responses to volume loading in sheep. Circ Res 42:839, 1978.
55. Teitel DF, Iwamato HS, Rudolph AM: Effects of birth-related events on central blood flow patterns. Pediatr Res 22:557, 1987.
56. Gersony WM: Patent ductus arteriosus in the neonate. Pediatr Clin North Am 33:545, 1986.
57. Chemtob S, Beharry K, Rex J, et al: Changes in cerebrovascular prostaglandins and thromboxane as a function of systemic blood pressure: Relationship to cerebral blood flow autoregulation of the newborn. Circ Res 67:674, 1990.
58. Hernandez MJ, Brennan RW, Bowman GS: Autoregulation of cerebral blood flow in the newborn dog. Brain Res 184:199, 1980.

59. Papile LA, Rudolph AM, Heymann MA: Autoregulation of cerebral blood flow in the preterm fetal lamb. Pediatr Res 19:159, 1985.

60. Guignard JP, Gouyon JB: Body fluid homeostasis in the newborn infant with congestive heart failure: Effects of diuretics. Clin Perinatol 15:447, 1988.

61. Krasner J, Yaffe SJ: Drug-protein binding in the neonate. In Morselli PL, Garattini S, Sereni F (eds): Basic and Therapeutic Aspects of Perinatal Pharmacology. New York, Raven Press, 1975, pp 357-366.

62. Dayton PG, Israili ZH, Perel JM: Influence of binding on drug metabolism and distribution. Ann N Y Acad Sci 226:172, 1973.

63. Vallner JJ: Binding of drugs by albumin and plasma protein. J Pharm Sci 66:447, 1977.

64. Ehrnebo M, Agurell S, Jalling B, et al: Age differences in drug binding by plasma proteins: Studies on human foetuses, neonates and adults. Eur J Clin Pharmacol 3:189, 1971.

65. Piafsky KM, Mpamugo L: Dependence of neonatal drug binding on α_1-acid glycoprotein concentration. Clin Pharmacol Ther 29:272, 1981.

66. Boreus LO: Principles of Pediatric Pharmacology (Monographs in Clinical Pharmacology, vol 6). New York, Churchill Livingstone, 1982.

67. Friedman Z, Danon A, Lamberth EL Jr, et al: Cord blood fatty acid composition in infants and in their mothers during the third trimester. J Pediatr 92:461, 1978.

68. Thiessen H, Jacobsen J, Brodersen R: Displacement of albumin-bound bilirubin by fatty acids. Acta Pediatr 61:285, 1972.

69. Fredholm BB, Rane A, Persson B: Diphenylhydantoin binding to proteins in plasma and its dependence on free fatty acid and bilirubin concentration in dogs and newborn infants. Pediatr Res 9:26, 1975.

70. Brodersen R, Friis-Hansen B, Stern L: Drug-induced displacement of bilirubin from albumin in the newborn. Dev Pharmacol Ther 6:217, 1983.

71. Cooper-Peel C, Brodersen R, Robertson A: Does ibuprofen affect bilirubin-albumin binding in newborn infant serum? Pharmacol Toxicol 79:297, 1996.

72. Andersson KE, Bertler A, Wettrell G: Post-mortem distribution and tissue concentration of digoxin in infants and adults. Acta Paediatr 64:497, 1975.

73. Lang D, Hofstetter R, von Bernuth G: Postmortem tissue and plasma concentrations of digoxin in newborns and infants. Eur J Pediatr 128:151, 1978.

74. Aranda JV: Factors associated with adverse drug reactions in the newborn. Pediatr Pharmacol 3:245, 1983.

75. Beaune PH, Kremers PG, Kaminsky LS, et al: Comparison of monooxygenase activities and cytochrome P-450 isozyme concentrations in human liver microsomes. Drug Metab Dispos Biol Fate Chem 14:437, 1986.

76. Coon MJ, Inouye: Biochemical properties of cytochrome P-450 in relation to steroid oxygenation. Ann N Y Acad Sci 458:216, 1985.

77. Rane A, Gustafsson JA: Formation of a 16,17-trans-glycolic metabolite from a 16-dihydro-androgen in human fetal liver microsomes. Clin Pharmacol Ther 14:833, 1973.

78. de Wildt SN, Kearns GL, Leeder JS, et al: Cytochrome P450 3A: Ontogeny and drug disposition. Clin Pharmacokinet 37:485, 1999.

79. Hines RN, McCarver DG: The ontogeny of human drug-metabolizing enzymes: Phase I oxidative enzymes. J Pharmacol Exp Ther 300:355, 2002.

80. Battino D, Estienne M, Avanzini G: Clinical pharmacokinetics of antiepileptic drugs in paediatric patients. Part II. Phenytoin, carbamazepine, sulthiame, lamotrigine, vigabatrin, oxcarbazepine and felbamate. Clin Pharmacokinet 29:341, 1995.

81. Sonnier M, Cresteil T: Delayed ontogenesis of CYP1A2 in the human liver. Eur J Biochem 251:893, 1998.

82. Kinirons MT, O'Shea D, Kim RB, et al: Failure of erythromycin breath test to correlate with midazolam clearance as a probe of cytochrome P4503A. Clin Pharmacol Ther 66:224, 1999.

83. Lacroix D, Sonnier M, Moncion A, et al: Expression of CYP3A in the human liver—evidence that the shift between CYP3A7 and CYP3A4 occurs immediately after birth. Eur J Biochem 247:625, 1997.

84. Treluyer JM, Jacqz-Aigrain E, Alvarez F, et al: Expression of CYP2D6 in developing human liver. Eur J Biochem 202:583, 1991.

85. Aranda JV, Collinge JM, Zinman R, et al: Maturation of caffeine elimination in infancy. Arch Dis Child 54:946, 1979.

86. Lieber CS: Cytochrome P-4502E1: Its physiological and pathological role. Physiol Rev 77:517, 1997.

87. Smith M, Hopkinson DA, Harris H: Developmental changes and polymorphism in human alcohol dehydrogenase. Ann Hum Genet 34:251, 1971.

88. Giacoia GP, Catz CS: Drugs and pollutants in breast milk. Clin Perinatol 6:181, 1979.

89. Mahu JL, Preaux AM, Mavier P, et al: Characterization of microsomal bilirubin and p-nitrophenol uridine diphosphate glucuronosyltransferase activities in human liver: A comparison with rat liver. Enzyme 26:93, 1981.

90. Radde IC: Drug metabolism. In MacLeod SM, Radde IC (eds): Textbook of Pediatric Clinical Pharmacology. Littleton, Mass, PSG Publishing, 1985, pp 56-71.

91. Aranda JV, MacLeod SM, Renton KW, et al: Hepatic microsomal drug oxidation and electron transport in newborn infants. J Pediatr 85:534, 1974.

92. Neims AH, Warner M, Loughnan PM, et al: Developmental aspects of the hepatic cytochrome P450 monooxygenase system. Annu Rev Pharmacol Toxicol 16:427, 1976.

93. Weinshilboum R: Inheritance and drug response. N Engl J Med 348:529, 2003.

94. Wilkinson GR, Shand DG: Commentary: A physiological approach to hepatic drug clearance. Clin Pharmacol Ther 18:377, 1975.

95. Leake RD, Trygstad CW, Oh W: Inulin clearance in the newborn infant: Relationship to gestational and postnatal age. Pediatr Res 10:759, 1976.

96. Robillard JE, Kulvinskas C, Sessions C, et al: Maturational changes in the fetal glomerular filtration rate. Am J Obstet Gynecol 122:601, 1975.

97. Catterton Z, Sellers B Jr, Gray B: Inulin clearance in the premature infant receiving indomethacin. J Pediatr 96:737, 1980.

98. Ward RM: Pharmacology of tolazoline. Clin Perinatol 11:703, 1984.

99. Welling PG, Craig WA: Pharmacokinetics in disease states modifying renal function. In Benet LZ (ed): The Effect of Disease States on Drug Pharmacokinetics. Washington, DC, American Pharmaceutical Association, 1976, pp 155-167.

100. Russel FG, Masereeuw R, van Aubel RA: Molecular aspects of renal anionic drug transport. Annu Rev Physiol 64:563, 2002.

101. Tokola O, Pelkonen O, K Adarki NT, et al: Hepatic drug-oxidizing enzyme systems and urinary D-glucaric acid excretion in patients with congestive heart failure. Br J Clin Pharmacol 2:429, 1975.

102. Vesell ES: Disease as one of many variables affecting drug disposition and response: Alterations of drug disposition in liver disease. Drug Metab Rev 8:265, 1978.

103. Feld LG, Springate JE, Fildes RD: Acute renal failure. I. Pathophysiology and diagnosis. J Pediatr 109:401, 1986.

104. Fabre J, Balant L: Renal failure, drug pharmacokinetics and drug action. Clin Pharmacokinet 1:99, 1976.

105. Roberts R, Branch R, Desmond P, et al: The influence of liver diseases on drug disposition. Baillieres Clin Gastroenterol 8:105, 1979.

106. Wilkinson GR: Influences of liver disease on pharmacokinetics. In Evans WE, Schentag JJ, Jusko WJ (eds): Applied Pharmacokinetics: Principles of Therapeutic Drug Monitoring. San Francisco, Applied Therapeutics, 1980, pp 57-75.

107. Cohen JS, Hogan ME: The new generic medicines. Sci Am 271:76, 1994.

108. Campagna JA, Miller KW, Forman SA: Mechanisms of actions of inhaled anesthetics. N Engl J Med 348:2110, 2003.

109. Kearns GL, Abdel-Rahman SM, Alander SW, et al: Developmental pharmacology—drug disposition, action, and therapy in infants and children. N Engl J Med 349:1157, 2003.

110. Kobayashi H, Cazzaniga A, Spano P, Trabucchi M: Ontogenesis of α- and β-receptors located on cerebral microvessels. Brain Res 242:358, 1982.

111. Li DY, Chatterjee T, Fernandez H, et al: Fewer PGE_2 and $PGF_{2\alpha}$ receptors in brain synaptosomes of newborn than of adult pigs. J Pharmacol Exp Ther 267:1292, 1993.

112. Evans WE, McLeod HL: Pharmacogenomics—drug disposition, drug targets, and side effects. N Engl J Med 348:538, 2003.

113. Marshall JD, Kearns GL: Developmental pharmacodynamics of cyclosporine. Clin Pharmacol Ther 66:66, 1999.

114. Takahashi H, Ishikawa S, Nomoto S, et al: Developmental changes in pharmacokinetics and pharmacodynamics of warfarin enantiomers in Japanese children. Clin Pharmacol Ther 68:541, 2000.

115. McCarver DG, Hines RN: The ontogeny of human drug-metabolizing enzymes: Phase II conjugation enzymes and regulatory mechanisms. J Pharmacol Exp Ther 300:361, 2002.

116. Aranda JV, Turmen T, Cote-Boileau T: Drug monitoring in the perinatal patient: Uses and abuses. Ther Drug Monit 2:39, 1980.

117. Morselli PL: Clinical pharmacokinetics in neonates. Clin Pharmacokinet 1:8198, 1976.

CHAPTER 16

Surgery for Fetal Malformations

Hanmin Lee and Michael R. Harrison

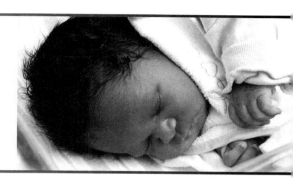

Advances in radiology and sampling techniques have given clinicians a window into the womb with which to make diagnoses of fetal abnormalities. Early in utero diagnosis affords families further time to make informed decisions regarding the pregnancy. Most prenatally diagnosed anomalies are best treated by standard postnatal care because the remainder of the gestation would not adversely affect the developing fetus. Some are best treated by early delivery, if the condition poses an imminent threat to the fetus and the fetus is of viable gestational age. A small subset of fetuses with anomalies that cause progressive injury may respond favorably to fetal intervention. The pathophysiology of these anomalies has been delineated over the course of 20 years by serial in utero and postnatal monitoring. Advances in ultrasonography, computed tomography, and magnetic resonance imaging (MRI) have increased the sensitivity and specificity of detecting fetal anomalies. Over this same period, techniques for open hysterotomy and minimal access hysteroscopy for purposes of in utero intervention have been established, first in animal models and subsequently in humans. With regard to all fetal interventions, maternal safety is paramount. This chapter presents an overview of fetal surgery and then reviews specific diseases amenable to fetal surgery and the techniques used to treat these anomalies.

GENERAL PRINCIPLES

The treatment of a fetus with an anomaly that is potentially correctable in utero is complicated by the potential for harm to the mother. Perhaps the only parallel in medicine in which a person undergoes a significant operative intervention for the benefit of another without direct health benefits to himself or herself is that of living, related transplantation of the kidney or liver. Transplantation of these organs has now extended to living, nonrelated transplantation. In living donor organ transplantation, the donor undergoes a major surgical procedure (i.e., nephrectomy or partial hepatectomy) for the potential benefit of another with no direct health benefit to himself or herself. In fetal surgery, the mother undergoes a major surgical procedure for the potential benefit of the fetus without any direct health benefit to herself.

The most important consideration in fetal surgery is the safety of the mother. Extensive research has been conducted to determine if fetal surgery can be performed safely with respect to the mother. The initial investigation began with thousands of fetal surgical interventions in small and large animal models, including primates.[1-8] This investigation resulted in the refinement of surgical, obstetric, and anesthetic techniques with the conclusion that fetal surgery could be performed safely in humans. In addition, fetal surgery should be considered only if the in utero anomaly has been shown by experimental animal models and clinical observation in humans to have severe irreversible consequences, and experimental animal data show that fetal surgery could be beneficial.

The first open fetal surgical procedure was performed in the 1980s at the University of California San Francisco (UCSF).[9] The initial review of maternal outcome after open fetal surgery showed no mortality and no detectable adverse effect on future fertility. The main complication was preterm labor; gestational age at delivery ranged from 25 to 35 weeks. In more than 150 subsequent cases at UCSF, we have had no maternal mortality after fetal surgery and no known adverse effects on fertility. Several significant morbidities exist for women undergoing fetal surgery, however. Bleeding and infection are potential complications of any surgery and may occur in fetal surgery as well. Midgestation hysterotomy is not performed in the lower uterine section, and all future deliveries should be by cesarean section because of the risk of uterine rupture with vaginal delivery. Fetal surgery does not seem to have an adverse effect on future fertility.[10,11] A review of the first 50 fetal surgical cases performed at UCSF revealed no infections, but 6 patients required blood transfusions. Perhaps the most significant morbidity arises from preterm labor. Four patients developed pulmonary edema while receiving high-dose tocolytic medications.

The pulmonary edema resolved with cessation of tocolytics in all four cases.

Families are counseled extensively regarding potential risks and benefits. Families who are candidates for fetal intervention at the Fetal Treatment Program at UCSF routinely meet with fetal treatment coordinators, perinatologists, geneticists, neonatologists, anesthesiologists, obstetric nursing staff, social workers, radiologists, and pediatric general surgeons. In addition, pediatric subspecialists are available for consultation when appropriate, such as neurosurgeons for in utero myelomeningocele (MMC) repair. Appropriate available treatment options, potentially including termination, early delivery, or fetoscopic or open fetal intervention, are discussed, as is continued observation. The decision is often a difficult one for a family to make for a variety of logistical, financial, religious, and ethical reasons as well as concern for the safety of the mother and fetus. Meeting with specialists from different fields, sometimes over several days, gives a family different viewpoints and the time to make a well-informed decision. At UCSF, all cases with the potential to undergo fetal intervention are discussed extensively with the multidisciplinary team at a weekly fetal treatment meeting. Pertinent diagnostic studies are reviewed, and a consensus is reached for further workup, treatment, or both.

TRAVERSING THE UTERUS

Surgery for malformations detected in utero can be categorized technically into three general categories: (1) ultrasonographically guided percutaneous intervention, (2) fetoendoscopically guided (Fetendo) intervention, and (3) directly visualized intervention via hysterotomy. In all three instances, two factors are of utmost importance: the position of the placenta and the position of the fetus. These must be accurately identified by ultrasonography. The presence of a skilled sonographer is particularly crucial in minimal access cases because the sonographer serves as the only real-time intrauterine "visualization" in some procedures and augments the use of fetoscopy in others.

For all fetal surgical procedures, the mother is placed in either a supine or lithotomy position. The left side of the table should be tilted downward to minimize pressure by the gravid uterus on the inferior vena cava. Anesthesia ranges from local and sedation for some minimally invasive procedures to general and epidural for open fetal procedures.

Ultrasonographically guided percutaneous procedures are performed for a variety of fetal anomalies. Beyond simple needle drainage procedures, the most common types of procedures are shunts from a fetal cavity to the amniotic sac. These procedures are performed with real-time continuous ultrasound guidance. We also have used percutaneous radiofrequency ablation for the treatment of a variety of fetal anomalies. The catheters and radiofrequency devices have an outer diameter of 2 to 2.5 mm, and the procedures can be performed percutaneously with low risk for uterine rupture and bleeding. There has been no evidence that uterine closure is necessary in these cases.

With regard to Fetendo procedures, the initial port site is identified by ultrasonography and is chosen based on a placenta-free area of the uterus that would allow optimal visualization of intrauterine structures. Fetoscopic procedures can be performed either percutaneously or via a limited maternal laparotomy incision. In contrast to other endoscopic surgical procedures, carbon dioxide is generally not used to create a space because it has been reported to cause fetal acidosis. Most clinicians have used warmed isotonic crystalloid solutions or amniotic fluid to create a clear visual field and space for intervention. These fluids can be pumped in through a side port on the trocar for the fetoscope. For fetoscopy, 1- to 5-mm endoscopes are generally used; the smaller scopes in this range may be placed entirely percutaneously with minimal risk for uterine rupture. We generally prefer minilaparotomy and uterine closure when using 5-mm or larger trocars. Fetal interventions can be performed through a working port on the trocar for the fetoscope or via accessory ports placed with ultrasonographic and fetoscopic guidance.[12,13]

In performing open fetal surgery, a low transverse abdominal incision is made. The rectus muscle and fascia are divided either transversely or vertically in the midline, depending on the degree of exposure necessary. A large abdominal ring retractor is placed for exposure and to prevent lateral compression of the uterine vessels. The placenta should be avoided in all instances of open fetal procedures and is marked with ultrasound guidance. If an open hysterotomy is used, specially designed uterine staplers and back-biting uterine clamps are essential in controlling myometrial bleeding. The fetus is monitored with pulse oximetry on an exposed limb. Exposure of the fetus is minimized to the appropriate body part. The fetus is bathed in warm saline. After repair of the defect, the fetus is returned to the uterus and the uterine defect is closed with continuous sutures and fibrin glue. The amniotic cavity is filled with warm normal saline such that low-normal levels of fluid exist. The skin is closed with subcuticular sutures and a clear dressing so that postoperative monitoring, including ultrasonography, may be performed. Monitoring for uterine irritability and adequate tocolysis are particularly important in open fetal procedures.[14]

Potential complications may result from any procedure that violates the uterine integrity. Bleeding may result from any surgical intervention and in fetal surgery may arise from the abdominal wall, the uterine wall, or the placenta. The inferior epigastric vessels should be avoided in percutaneous or minilaparotomy procedures or ligated and divided in open hysterotomy procedures. The lateral aspects of the uterus should be avoided because the uterine vessels arise laterally. The placenta should be avoided in all cases involving a maternal hysterotomy and, if possible, in percutaneous procedures.

Membrane rupture remains one of the greatest obstacles to successful fetal surgery and may occur whether a minimally invasive approach or open technique is used. Contributing causes include inadequate membrane closure, chorioamnionitis, membrane separation, and uterine contractions. Meticulous sterile technique, careful membrane and uterine closure, and adequate tocolysis are important considerations in minimizing the risk of membrane rupture. In addition, further research is necessary in determining the physical and biochemical properties of the membranes that make them susceptible to rupture. Tocolytic agents used perioperatively include halogenated inhalational agents, magnesium sulfate, β-sympathomimetics, indomethacin, and nitroglycerin.[15-17]

ANOMALIES AMENABLE TO FETAL SURGERY

Congenital Hydronephrosis

Optimal clinical management of fetal obstructive uropathy requires a thorough understanding of its pathophysiology and natural history in the developing fetus. Unrelieved obstruction of the urinary tract causes progressive damage to the developing kidney, resulting in dysplastic renal morphogenesis. Decreased fetal urine production causes oligohydramnios, resulting in potentially fatal pulmonary hypoplasia. Numerous experimental models in animals have shown that in utero decompression of bilateral fetal hydronephrosis can ameliorate pulmonary hypoplasia and preserve renal function, depending on the timing of therapy and the duration of the obstruction.[18-22]

The challenge in managing fetuses with bilateral hydronephrosis lies in the selection of a fetus with a dilated urinary tract for whom fetal intervention is appropriate (i.e., a fetus with obstruction severe enough to compromise renal and pulmonary function at birth, but not so severe that the damage is irreversible). Appropriate selection of fetuses for prenatal intervention can now be performed based on an improved understanding of the natural history and pathophysiology of the disease and qualitative and quantitative tests of renal function. Fetal urologic evaluation begins with ultrasonography. The findings of uniformly fatal lesions, such as bilateral renal agenesis, severe renal hypoplasia, or bilateral multicystic dysplasia, preclude further evaluation or treatment.

When sonography shows bilateral hydronephrosis, the initial assessment of fetal renal function is the determination of the quantity of amniotic fluid. Because most amniotic fluid in middle and late pregnancy is a product of fetal urination, a normal amount of amniotic fluid usually implies the presence of at least one functioning kidney. Decreasing amniotic fluid volume on serial ultrasound examinations in the setting of bilateral hydronephrosis may indicate deteriorating renal function. Amniotic fluid status is predictive only in the extremes,[23] however (i.e., normal volume late in gestation suggests adequate function, whereas severe oligohydramnios early in gestation suggests poor function). Sonographic examination of the urinary bladder and kidneys is an unreliable indicator of fetal renal function. Although the urine-filled bladder can be visualized easily by ultrasonography at 15 weeks of gestation, urine reaccumulation after bladder aspiration or furosemide stimulation can be deceiving. Similarly, sonographic appearance of the kidneys lacks the sensitivity and specificity to predict renal function.[24] In a series of 49 cases correlating renal ultrasound appearance with histopathology, the presence of cortical cysts or increased echogenicity was highly predictive of renal dysplasia; the absence of these findings does not preclude renal dysplasia, however.

Ultrasonography can accurately show the gross anatomy of a dilated urinary tract and provide some qualitative information about renal function. Ultrasonography cannot accurately determine the degree of renal dysfunction or dysplasia, however, and sonography is of limited prognostic value in many cases. Analysis of fetal urine provides a more direct and quantitative method to evaluate fetal renal function. The composition of fetal urine, a hypotonic ultrafiltrate of fetal serum, remains constant throughout gestation until just before term. The total urine output is a combination of glomerular filtration, tubular reabsorption, and secretion. Changes in fetal urine electrolyte composition or volume may reflect changes in renal function. Previously, we reviewed the management of 40 fetuses with bilateral hydronephrosis and oligohydramnios to determine the prognostic value of fetal urine composition in predicting normal renal and pulmonary function at birth.[23]

The prognostic criteria of urine composition (sodium < 100 mEq/L, chloride < 90 mEq/L, osmolarity < 210 mOsm) and normal-appearing fetal kidneys on ultrasonography have proved to predict reliably neonatal and long-term outcome after in utero urinary tract decompression. More recently reported methods using proton nuclear magnetic resonance spectroscopy of fetal urine and measurements of calcium and β2-microglobulin levels in fetal urine may improve further prenatal selection for fetal intervention.[25] To achieve accurate measurements of renal function, the bladder should be aspirated three times. The first tap measures urine that has been in the bladder for a variable length of time. The second tap measures urine in the collecting systems, and the third tap measures fresh urine and best reflects renal function.

Initial evaluation should include ultrasonography to confirm the diagnosis, delineate the anatomy of the obstruction, define the status of the amniotic fluid, and exclude associated life-threatening anomalies. If no associated anomalies are detected, and the amniotic fluid volume is normal, the pregnancy should be followed by serial ultrasonography. If the amniotic fluid volume remains adequate, the mother should receive routine obstetric care and the fetus can be evaluated and treated postnatally. If the fetus presents with oligohydramnios or develops decreasing amniotic fluid volume, a prognostic evaluation should be done, including (1) assessment of amniotic fluid volume; (2) sonographic visualization of the renal parenchyma; and (3) fetal bladder aspiration to determine urine sodium, chloride, and osmolarity.

The indications for prenatal intervention are narrow. Prenatal intervention should be reserved for fetuses with adequate renal function for postnatal survival and pulmonary immaturity precluding early delivery. Methods of urinary tract decompression include vesicoamniotic shunt placement and open fetal surgery. Fetal surgery is appropriate only for select fetuses diagnosed in the late first and early second trimesters, with associated oligohydramnios, favorable urine electrolytes, and normal renal parenchyma on ultrasonography.

Of the more than 300 cases of fetal hydronephrosis that have been referred to the Fetal Treatment Center at UCSF, only 8 patients have met the indications for open fetal surgery.[3] Fetal hydronephrosis was the first anomaly for which fetal surgery was performed. The first open case for hydronephrosis was performed in 1981, and the patient received bilateral ureterostomies.[9] The next seven patients had bladder marsupialization at 18 to 24 weeks of gestation.

Six of the eight pregnancies were delivered by cesarean section at 32 to 36 weeks of gestation. Because of our inability to predict irreversible fetal renal failure early in our experience, a seventh fetus never drained urine well, and this fetus was removed at reexploration. An eighth fetus, although adequately decompressed, died 2 weeks after the procedure from pulmonary immaturity and hypoplasia—the mother discontinued her tocolytic therapy, resulting in premature delivery.

Four of the six fetuses delivered had return of normal amniotic fluid dynamics, and all four had adequate pulmonary function at birth. Two other neonates died at birth secondary to pulmonary hypoplasia. Of the surviving four infants, one had normal renal function but died of unrelated causes at 9 months of age, one has grown and developed normally but developed chronic renal insufficiency at 3 years and received a successful kidney transplant, and the last two children have normal renal function at ages 3 and 5 years.

Increasingly, congenital hydronephrosis has been treated with catheter decompression, either by ultrasound guidance or by fetoscopic guidance. Several groups around the world have performed vesicoamniotic shunting with varying success.[26,27] Although vesicoamniotic shunting probably does not relieve urinary obstruction as reliably as open fetal surgery due to catheter malfunction and obstruction, the procedure is less problematic for the mother than open fetal surgery.

In a few highly selected cases, open decompression of the obstructed urinary tract can restore amniotic fluid dynamics and prevent the development of fatal pulmonary hypoplasia. In the future, fetoscopic surgery may provide a less invasive approach to decompress the fetal bladder. The effect of fetal urinary tract decompression on long-term renal function remains unknown, however, and is the subject of ongoing studies.

Congenital Diaphragmatic Hernia

Despite advances in postnatal methods of respiratory support, survival for infants born with congenital diaphragmatic hernia (CDH) remains only 60% to 70%.[28] Additionally, survival for all fetuses diagnosed with CDH may be only 20% to 27%, owing to in utero demise or death of infants with unrecognized CDH.[29] Of the surviving children, many have long-term ventilatory and supplemental oxygen requirements secondary to pulmonary parenchymal and vascular hypoplasia and developmental delays and feeding difficulties. Most theories regarding the cause of CDH support the presence of a simple defect in the diaphragm embryologically, leading to pulmonary hypoplasia from compression of the developing lung. We have theorized that in utero intervention may allow increased antenatal lung growth and increased pulmonary function and survival postnatally. In a fetal lamb model, we showed that compression of the lungs during the last trimester, either with an intrathoracic balloon or by creation of a diaphragmatic hernia, results in fatal pulmonary hypoplasia. Removal of the compressing lesion allows the lung to grow and develop sufficiently to permit survival at birth.[30]

The first attempts at fetal surgery for CDH were centered around in utero diaphragmatic hernia repair. The results proved that fetal surgery for CDH was feasible but did not show an overall survival benefit.[31] The subset of fetuses with severe lung hypoplasia has exceedingly high postnatal mortality, however, and these fetuses are identifiable prenatally by ultrasonography and MRI. The factors associated with poor outcome that can be assessed prenatally by ultrasonography are (1) the presence of liver herniation into the chest and (2) a low lung-to-head ratio (LHR). In one study from our institution, survival was 100% in fetuses with CDH without liver herniation and 56% in fetuses with CDH with liver herniation into the chest. The LHR is calculated as the area of the contralateral lung at the level of the cardiac atria divided by the head circumference. This LHR value has been shown to correlate in a statistically significant fashion with survival: 100% survival with an LHR greater than 1.35, 61% survival with an LHR between 0.6 and 1.35, and 0% survival with an LHR less than 0.6.[32] Ultrasonography also is crucial in identifying other anomalies associated with CDH. The most common secondary anomalies are cardiac anomalies, and the survival of patients with a CDH and an intracardiac anomaly is dismal.[33] Other common sites for anomalies include urinary, central nervous system, musculoskeletal, genital, and gastrointestinal. Chromosomal abnormalities have been found in 3.6% to 9% of cases, particularly trisomies 18 and 21.[34,35] Volumetric analysis of lung size in fetuses with CDH with MRI techniques is a promising new method of evaluating relative lung volume.[36]

We have found over the course of 10 years that we can identify fetuses with CDH with expected poor outcome. During the same period, extensive animal studies and observation in fetuses born with congenital high airway obstruction have proved that lung growth may be driven by tracheal obstruction or occlusion, leading to pressurized fluid accumulating in the airway.[37,38] This realization led to the study of lung distention by tracheal occlusion or by partial or complete liquid ventilation as a method of achieving lung growth postnatally.[39,40] Our group focused on in utero tracheal occlusion as a method of augmenting lung growth in fetuses with CDH.[41,42] Our preliminary study examined the effect of extrinsic tracheal occlusion by the placement of an obstructing clip in utero using both open and Fetendo techniques. We found in a few patients that survival was increased in the Fetendo group but not the open group compared with the control group, which consisted of patients undergoing standard postnatal care. This study led to the current National Institutes of Health (NIH)–funded trial comparing in utero tracheal occlusion with standard postnatal care using minimal access techniques. The method of tracheal occlusion has evolved to that of internal tracheal occlusion employing a detachable balloon device using Fetendo techniques (Fig. 16-1).

Congenital Cystic Adenomatoid Malformation of the Lung and Sacrococcygeal Teratoma

Most solid tumors diagnosed in utero are benign in nature, and many regress. Some solid tumors grow so large, however, that they obstruct central venous return by mass effect or cause high-output cardiac failure. In the most severe cases, this condition results in hydrops fetalis as exhibited by skin and scalp edema; fluid in the pleural, pericardial, and peritoneal cavities; and placentomegaly. The natural history of hydrops is fetal demise in most instances. The tumors that most commonly result in hydrops in utero are congenital cystic adenomatoid malformation of the lung (CCAM) and sacrococcygeal teratoma (SCT). The experience with fetal surgery for these lesions is reviewed.

CCAM is a cystic pulmonary lesion with a broad spectrum of initial presentation. It is characterized by overgrowth of respiratory bronchioles with the formation of cysts of various sizes. Classification of CCAM has centered around the sizes of the cysts.[43,44] Children and infants diagnosed with CCAM with a paucity of symptoms undergo elective resection. A fetus diagnosed with a CCAM should undergo serial surveillance studies. A small subset of fetuses with large lesions develops nonimmune hydrops fetalis. The natural history of most of these fetuses is that of rapidly progressive deterioration and in utero demise.

If the fetus is of a viable gestational age in the presence of hydrops, early delivery should be considered. In instances in which one dominant macrocystic lesion is present in a previable fetus, thoracoamniotic shunt may reverse the hydrops fetalis. Needle drainage has not proved to be an effective option because rapid reaccumulation of fluid occurs. Fetal thoracotomy with resection is an option in a previable fetus without the presence of a dominant cyst. The fetal thoracic space is exposed through a fifth intercostal space thoracotomy after maternal hysterotomy. The lobe containing the CCAM is easily identified and is brought out through the wound. The pulmonary hilar structures are mass ligated using an endoloop or a vascular endostapling device. The thoracotomy is closed in layers.[43,45]

The experience with CCAM at UCSF and the Children's Hospital of Philadelphia was reviewed. A total of 134 women pregnant with fetuses with CCAM were diagnosed in utero. Of this group, 120 elected to continue their pregnancies. A total of 79 fetuses had no evidence of hydrops. Of these, 76 were followed expectantly, and all survived. Three fetuses without evidence of hydrops with large dominant cysts underwent thoracoamniotic shunt placement, and all three survived. Twenty-five hydropic fetuses were followed with no intervention. All mothers delivered prematurely, and all fetuses died perinatally. Sixteen fetuses with hydrops underwent intervention: 13 had open fetal surgery, and 3 had thoracoamniotic shunt placement. In the group that had shunt placement, 2 of 3 survived, and 8 of 13 survived in the open fetal surgery group.

SCT is a rare tumor that is being diagnosed with increasing frequency in utero, allowing for the observation of the prenatal natural history of the disease and appropriate perinatal management. As with CCAM, fetuses with SCT are susceptible to in utero demise. SCT tumors can grow to a tremendous size in relation to the fetus, resulting in a vascular shunt and, in the extreme form, high output failure and nonimmune hydrops. Additionally, some tumors bleed either within the tumor or externally and may cause fetal anemia and hypovolemia. Other potential problems with a fetus with a large SCT are dystocia and preterm labor from increased fetal size.

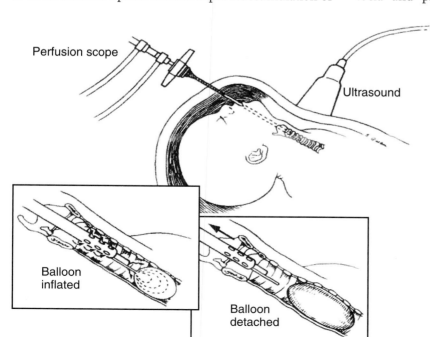

Perfusion scope

Ultrasound

Balloon inflated

Balloon detached

Figure 16–1. Using sonographic and endoscopic guidance, the fetal trachea is cannulated with the telescope. After inflation, the balloon is detached proximal to the carina *(inset)*.

Delivery can be particularly difficult when the diagnosis has not been made prenatally. Traumatic delivery may result in hemorrhage or tumor rupture. Most clinicians favor cesarean delivery for fetuses with large SCTs. Prenatal diagnosis and careful obstetric planning are crucial in the appropriate management of a fetus with an SCT.

The experience with prenatally diagnosed SCT was reviewed at UCSF. Of the 17 fetuses, 12 developed hydrops, whereas 5 did not. All five of the nonhydropic fetuses delivered near term and survived. Of the 12 hydropic fetuses, 7 underwent fetal intervention with 3 survivors. Five hydropic fetuses were followed without fetal intervention, and none of this group survived.[46] Hydrops in fetuses with SCTs has been shown in other groups to correlate with an exceedingly high rate of fetal demise.[47-49] The most common method of fetal intervention is hysterotomy with resection of the tumor. A predominantly cystic lesion may be amenable to percutaneous drainage or placement of a shunt. Effectively debulking the tumor with percutaneous coagulation, such as with radiofrequency ablation to decrease the vascular shunt, is a minimally invasive alternative to open resection that warrants further investigation.

Twin Anomalies

Complications of monochorionic twin pregnancies are relatively common, occurring in 10% to 15% of twin pregnancies.[50] The most common anomaly is twin-twin transfusion syndrome (TTTS), a condition in which intertwin vasculatures communicate via placental vessels. As a result of these vascular connections, transfusions occur between the twins via arterioarterial, arteriovenous, and venovenous anastomoses. These vascular connections are often multiple, and flow may occur in both directions. Complications arise when there is net flow of blood from one twin (donor) to the other (recipient). As a result of the transfusion, both twins may experience hemodynamic compromise. The donor twin has diminished cardiac output and may sustain low-flow injuries, particularly to the brain and the kidneys. Conversely, the recipient twin has increased cardiac output and may sustain high-output cardiac failure. Clinically, TTTS is manifested by size discordance. Progressive disease is evidenced by oligohydramnios in the donor twin and polyhydramnios in the recipient twin. Advanced disease is evidenced by the absence of urine in the bladder of the donor twin and hydrops fetalis in one or both twins. Mortality of TTTS diagnosed in the second trimester is greater than 80% and may occur in the donor twin, the recipient twin, or both twins.[51] Additionally, when one monozygotic twin dies in utero, significant risks exist in the other twin, including ischemic brain or renal injury or death.[52,53] Long-term outcome of surviving twins has not been rigorously studied.

Because of the high morbidity and mortality with TTTS, clinicians have attempted a variety of treatments aimed at achieving improved outcome in one or both twins. The most commonly used treatment is high-volume amnioreduction of the fluid of the polyhydramniotic sac. Because polyhydramnios may incite labor, the initial aim of amnioreduction was to reduce uterine volume to decrease preterm labor and increase gestation. Additionally, amnioreduction may have some unknown benefit in treating TTTS. High-volume amnioreduction resulted in survival of 58% of twins from the International Amnioreduction Registry.[51] Septostomy, or creation of a hole in the intertwin membrane, has been used by some to equilibrate pressures in the donor and recipient amniotic sacs.[54]

Several groups have used fetoscopic guidance to laser-ablate intertwin vascular connections. This procedure can be done nonselectively, by ablating all inter-twin connections, or selectively, by ablating only arteriovenous connections with flow in the causative direction. Fetoscopic laser ablation can be performed either percutaneously using 1- to 3-mm endoscopes or by maternal laparotomy with 4- to 5-mm endoscopes. A maternal laparotomy is favored with use of the larger scopes to close the large uterine defect created by placement of these devices. All scopes are placed through ports that have side channels for irrigation and placement of the laser. Survival for TTTS using laser ablation of vascular connections has been 50% to 67%.[55-59] Several multi-institutional trials are currently under way to compare the efficacy of large-volume amnioreduction and laser ablation in the treatment of TTTS.

Twin-reverse arterial perfusion sequence occurs in 1% of monozygotic twins and 3% of triplets. This condition occurs in multiple gestations in which one fetus is acardiac and usually acephalic with the presence of intertwin arterioarterial and venovenous connections in the presence of a monozygotic placenta. Flow to the acardiac, acephalic twin is achieved retrograde from the normal, or pump, twin. The pump twin is at high risk to develop high-output cardiac failure with 50% to 75% mortality without treatment. Most recent therapies have been aimed at dividing the vascular connections between the pump twin and the acardiac twin by stopping blood flow through the umbilical cord of the acardiac twin. This therapy has been performed in a variety of methods, including umbilical cord ligation with fetoscopic guidance or percutaneous injection of thrombogenic coils or fibrin glues.[60,61] We have employed percutaneous, ultrasonographically guided ablation of the umbilical cord of the acardiac twin using radiofrequency coagulation. We have had greater than 90% survival using this technique without evidence of neurologic injury to the pump twin.

Myelomeningocele

MMC is a relatively common birth defect that is associated with significant neurologic deficits. Neurologic sequelae include loss of hind-limb function, loss of bowel and bladder function, and hydrocephalus and the development of hindbrain herniation (Chiari II malformation). The degree of neurologic injury depends on a variety of factors, predominantly the extent and location of the open neural tube defect, with more cephalad and larger lesions generally leading to more extensive debilitation. Current therapy consists of postnatal closure of the open neural tube defect and extensive rehabilitation. Most of the neurologic deficits are relatively fixed by birth, however, and are not reversible. With advances in fetal diagnosis and

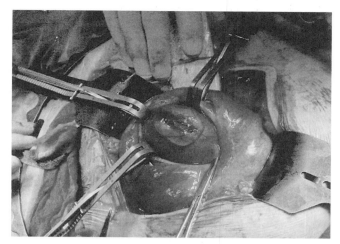

Figure 16–2. Myelomeningocele defect in a fetus before repair.

therapy, researchers hypothesized that prenatal intervention for MMC might prevent or lessen some of the neurologic sequelae of the disease. Fetal models of MMC were created and repaired in rats, lambs, and monkeys.[5,6,8,62-64] The data from these experiments showed that animals undergoing correction of the MMC defect had improved neurologic function, including hind-limb movement, compared with control animals who did not undergo repair.[5,7]

These data led to pilot trials of in utero MMC repair in humans. MMC is the first nonlethal anomaly for which fetal surgery has been undertaken. Repair has been approached via open hysterotomy and fetoscopic techniques and with primary repair and skin allografts.[65-67] Several groups including ours have reported successful technical repair, primarily with open fetal surgery.[67,68] Figure 16-2 shows an MMC defect in a fetus before repair. In utero repair has not shown improvement of hind-limb function or improved bowel or bladder function compared with historical controls. There has been some evidence, however, that hindbrain herniation and hydrocephalus may be lessened by in utero repair compared with historical controls of postnatal repair. Based on these results and the animal studies, the NIH has currently funded a prospective, multi-institutional, randomized trial to investigate the effectiveness of in utero MMC repair.

FUTURE OF FETAL SURGERY

Fetal surgery is a rapidly evolving multidisciplinary field. Until fairly recently, only fetal malformations that were likely to result in in utero or postnatal demise were considered for fetal surgery due to the inherent risks to the mother. MMC was the first nonlethal anomaly treated by fetal surgery. As minimal access techniques improve and are applied to fetal surgery, resulting in decreasing morbidity to the mother, indications for in utero intervention will continue to broaden. Future procedures will rarely require a maternal hysterotomy. In utero gene therapy for metabolic deficiencies and tissue engineering

for organ and tissue deficits will become a reality. As the field of fetal surgery expands, practitioners must remain dedicated to rigorous scientific quality assurance. In utero procedures performed in humans should be grounded in basic science research and animal models that show the likelihood of benefit for the fetus.

SUMMARY

Fetal surgery is a promising novel therapy for a variety of prenatally diagnosed conditions. Fetal intervention for anomalies that have a high mortality have shown improved survival compared with historical controls. Currently, NIH-funded trials comparing fetal surgery with standard therapy are either under way or soon to be started for CDH, TTTS, and MMC. As the field of fetal surgery grows, maternal safety must continue to be the first priority.

REFERENCES

1. Adzick NS, Harrison MR, Glick PL, et al: Fetal surgery in the primate: III. Maternal outcome after fetal surgery. J Pediatr Surg 21:477, 1986.
2. Adzick NS, Harrison MR: Fetal surgical therapy. Lancet 343:897, 1994.
3. Harrison MR, Adzick NS: The fetus as a patient: Surgical considerations. Ann Surg 213:279, 1991.
4. Rice HE, Estes JM, Hedrick MH, et al: Congenital cystic adenomatoid malformation: A sheep model of fetal hydrops. J Pediatr Surg 29:692, 1994.
5. Meuli M, Meuli-Simmen C, Hutchins GM, et al: In utero surgery rescues neurological function at birth in sheep with spina bifida. Nat Med 1:342, 1995.
6. Meuli M, Meuli-Simmen C, Yingling CD, et al: Creation of myelomeningocele in utero: A model of functional damage from spinal cord exposure in fetal sheep. J Pediatr Surg 30:1028, 1995.
7. Meuli M, Meuli-Simmen C, Yingling CD, et al: In utero repair of experimental myelomeningocele saves neurological function at birth. J Pediatr Surg 31:397, 1996.
8. Michejda M: Intrauterine treatment of spina bifida: Primate model. Z Kinderchir 39:259, 1984.
9. Harrison MR, Golbus MS, Filly RA, et al: Fetal surgery for congenital hydronephrosis. N Engl J Med 306:591, 1982.
10. Farrell JA, Albanese CT, Jennings RW, et al: Maternal fertility is not affected by fetal surgery. Fetal Diagn Ther 14:190, 1999.
11. Longaker MT, Golbus MS, Filly RA, et al: Maternal outcome after open fetal surgery: A review of the first 17 human cases. JAMA 265:737, 1991.
12. VanderWall KJ, Meuli M, Szabo Z, et al: Percutaneous access to the uterus for fetal surgery. J Laparoendosc Surg 6(Suppl 1):S65, 1996.
13. VanderWall KJ, Bruch SW, Meuli M, et al: Fetal endoscopic ('Fetendo') tracheal clip. J Pediatr Surg 31:1101, 1996.
14. Harrison MR, Adzick NS: Fetal surgical techniques. Semin Pediatr Surg 2:136, 1993.
15. Cauldwell CB, Rosen MA, Jennings R: Anesthesia and monitoring for fetal intervention. In Harrison MR, Evans MI, Adzick NS, Holzgreve W (eds): The Unborn Patient. Philadelphia, WB Saunders, 2001, p 149.
16. Rosen MA: Anesthesia for procedures involving the fetus. Semin Perinatol 15:410, 1991.

17. Rosen MA: Anesthesia for fetal procedures and surgery. Yonsei Med J 42:669, 2001.

18. Glick PL, Harrison MR, Halks-Miller M, et al: Correction of congenital hydrocephalus in utero: II. Efficacy of in utero shunting. J Pediatr Surg 19:870, 1984.

19. Glick PL, Harrison MR, Golbus MS, et al: Management of the fetus with congenital hydronephrosis: II. Prognostic criteria and selection for treatment. J Pediatr Surg 20:376, 1985.

20. Glick PL, Harrison MR, Adzick NS, et al: Correction of congenital hydronephrosis in utero: IV. In utero decompression prevents renal dysplasia. J Pediatr Surg 19:649, 1984.

21. Glick PL, Harrison MR, Noall RA, et al: Correction of congenital hydronephrosis in utero: III. Early mid-trimester ureteral obstruction produces renal dysplasia. J Pediatr Surg 18:681, 1983.

22. Harrison MR, Golbus MS, Filly RA, et al: Fetal hydronephrosis: Selection and surgical repair. J Pediatr Surg 22:556, 1987.

23. Crombleholme TM, Harrison MR, Golbus MS, et al: Fetal intervention in obstructive uropathy: Prognostic indicators and efficacy of intervention. Am J Obstet Gynecol 162:1239, 1990.

24. Mahony BS, Filly RA, Callen PW, et al: Fetal renal dysplasia: Sonographic evaluation. Radiology 152:143, 1984.

25. Lipitz S, Ryan G, Samuell C, et al: Fetal urine analysis for the assessment of renal function in obstructive uropathy. Am J Obstet Gynecol 168(1 Pt 1):174, 1993.

26. Freedman AL, Johnson MP, Smith CA, et al: Long-term outcome in children after antenatal intervention for obstructive uropathies. Lancet 354:374, 1999.

27. Coplen DE: Prenatal intervention for hydronephrosis. J Urol 157:2270, 1997.

28. Clark RH, Hardin WD Jr, Hirschl RB, et al: Current surgical management of congenital diaphragmatic hernia: A report from the Congenital Diaphragmatic Hernia Study Group. J Pediatr Surg 33:1004, 1998.

29. Harrison MR, Bjordal RI, Langmark F, et al: Congenital diaphragmatic hernia: The hidden mortality. J Pediatr Surg 13:227, 1978.

30. Adzick NS, Outwater KM, Harrison MR, et al: Correction of congenital diaphragmatic hernia in utero: IV. An early gestational fetal lamb model for pulmonary vascular morphometric analysis. J Pediatr Surg 20:673, 1985.

31. Harrison MR, Adzick NS, Flake AW, et al: Correction of congenital diaphragmatic hernia in utero: VI. Hard-earned lessons. J Pediatr Surg 28:1411, 1993.

32. Metkus AP, Filly RA, Stringer MD, et al: Sonographic predictors of survival in fetal diaphragmatic hernia. J Pediatr Surg 31:148, 1996.

33. Sharland GK, Lockhart SM, Heward AJ, et al: Prognosis in fetal diaphragmatic hernia. Am J Obstet Gynecol 166(1 Pt 1):9, 1992.

34. Bollmann R, Kalache K, Mau H, et al: Associated malformations and chromosomal defects in congenital diaphragmatic hernia. Fetal Diagn Ther 10:52, 1995.

35. Dillon E, Renwick M, Wright C: Congenital diaphragmatic herniation: Antenatal detection and outcome. Br J Radiol 73:360, 2000.

36. Coakley FV, Lopoo JB, Lu Y, et al: Normal and hypoplastic fetal lungs: Volumetric assessment with prenatal single-shot rapid acquisition with relaxation enhancement MR imaging. Radiology 216:107, 2000.

37. DiFiore JW, Fauza DO, Slavin R, et al: Experimental fetal tracheal ligation and congenital diaphragmatic hernia: A pulmonary vascular morphometric analysis. J Pediatr Surg 30:917, 1995.

38. DiFiore JW, Fauza DO, Slavin R, et al: Experimental fetal tracheal ligation reverses the structural and physiological effects of pulmonary hypoplasia in congenital diaphragmatic hernia. J Pediatr Surg 29:248, 1994.

39. Wilson JM, DiFiore JW, Peters CA: Experimental fetal tracheal ligation prevents the pulmonary hypoplasia associated with fetal nephrectomy: Possible application for congenital diaphragmatic hernia. J Pediatr Surg 28:1433, 1993.

40. Nobuhara KK, Fauza DO, DiFiore JW, et al: Continuous intrapulmonary distension with perfluorocarbon accelerates neonatal (but not adult) lung growth. J Pediatr Surg 33:292, 1998.

41. Hedrick MH, Ferro MM, Filly RA, et al: Congenital high airway obstruction syndrome (CHAOS): A potential for perinatal intervention. J Pediatr Surg 29:271, 1994.

42. Hedrick MH, Estes JM, Sullivan KM, et al: Plug the lung until it grows (PLUG): A new method to treat congenital diaphragmatic hernia in utero. J Pediatr Surg 29:612, 1994.

43. Adzick NS, Harrison MR, Flake AW, et al: Fetal surgery for cystic adenomatoid malformation of the lung. J Pediatr Surg 28:806, 1993.

44. Adzick NS, Harrison MR, Glick PL, et al: Fetal cystic adenomatoid malformation: Prenatal diagnosis and natural history. J Pediatr Surg 20:483, 1985.

45. Adzick NS, Harrison MR, Crombleholme TM, et al: Fetal lung lesions: Management and outcome. Am J Obstet Gynecol 179:884, 1998.

46. Westerburg B, Feldstein VA, Sandberg PL, et al: Sonographic prognostic factors in fetuses with sacrococcygeal teratoma. J Pediatr Surg 35:322, 2000.

47. Flake AW, Harrison MR, Adzick NS, et al: Fetal sacrococcygeal teratoma. J Pediatr Surg 21:563, 1986.

48. Flake AW: Fetal sacrococcygeal teratoma. Semin Pediatr Surg 2:113, 1993.

49. Bond SJ, Harrison MR, Schmidt KG, et al: Death due to high-output cardiac failure in fetal sacrococcygeal teratoma. J Pediatr Surg 25:1287, 1990.

50. Sebire NJ, Snijders RJ, Hughes K, et al: The hidden mortality of monochorionic twin pregnancies. Br J Obstet Gynaecol 104:1203, 1997.

51. Fisk N: The fetus with twin-twin transfusion syndrome. In Harrison MR, Evans MI, Adzick NS, Hozgreve W (eds): The Unborn Patient. Philadelphia, WB Saunders, 2001, p 341.

52. Fusi L, Gordon H: Twin pregnancy complicated by single intrauterine death: Problems and outcome with conservative management. Br J Obstet Gynaecol 97:511, 1990.

53. Fusi L, McParland P, Fisk N, et al: Acute twin-twin transfusion: A possible mechanism for brain-damaged survivors after intrauterine death of a monochorionic twin. Obstet Gynecol 78(3 Pt 2):517, 1991.

54. Saade GR, Belfort MA, Berry DL, et al: Amniotic septostomy for the treatment of twin oligohydramnios-polyhydramnios sequence. Fetal Diagn Ther 13:86, 1998.

55. Quintero RA, Comas C, Bornick PW, et al: Selective versus non-selective laser photocoagulation of placental vessels in twin-to-twin transfusion syndrome. Ultrasound Obstet Gynecol 16:230, 2000.

56. Quintero RA, Bornick PW, Allen MH, et al: Selective laser photocoagulation of communicating vessels in severe twin-twin transfusion syndrome in women with an anterior placenta. Obstet Gynecol 97:477, 2001.

57. Ville Y, Hecher K, Gagnon A, et al: Endoscopic laser coagulation in the management of severe twin-to-twin transfusion syndrome. Br J Obstet Gynaecol 105:446, 1998.

58. Feldstein VA, Machin GA, Albanese CT, et al: Twin-twin transfusion syndrome: The 'Select' procedure. Fetal Diagn Ther 15:257, 2000.

59. Deprest JA, Van Schoubroeck D, Evrard VA, et al: Fetoscopic Nd:YAG laser coagulation for twin-twin transfusion syndrome in cases of anterior placenta. J Am Assoc Gynecol Laparosc 3(4 Suppl):S9, 1996.

60. Deprest JA, Van Ballaer PP, Evrard VA, et al: Experience with fetoscopic cord ligation. Eur J Obstet Gynecol Reprod Biol 81:157, 1998.

61. Quintero RA, Reich H, Puder KS, et al: Brief report: Umbilical-cord ligation of an acardiac twin by fetoscopy at 19 weeks of gestation. N Engl J Med 330:469, 1994.

62. Meuli-Simmen C, Meuli M, Hutchins GM, et al: The fetal spinal cord does not regenerate after in utero transection in a large mammalian model. Neurosurgery 39:555, 1996.

63. Heffez DS, Aryanpur J, Hutchins GM, et al: The paralysis associated with myelomeningocele: Clinical and experimental data implicating a preventable spinal cord injury. Neurosurgery 26:987, 1990.

64. Heffez DS, Aryanpur J, Rotellini NA, et al: Intrauterine repair of experimental surgically created dysraphism. Neurosurgery 32:1005, 1993.

65. Bruner JP, Tulipan NE, Richards WO: Endoscopic coverage of fetal open myelomeningocele in utero. Am J Obstet Gynecol 176(1 Pt 1):256, 1997.

66. Bruner JP, Tulipan NB, Richards WO, et al: In utero repair of myelomeningocele: A comparison of endoscopy and hysterotomy. Fetal Diagn Ther 15:83, 2000.

67. Bruner JP, Tulipan N, Paschall RL, et al: Fetal surgery for myelomeningocele and the incidence of shunt-dependent hydrocephalus. JAMA 282:1819, 1999.

68. Adzick NS, Sutton LN, Crombleholme TM, et al: Successful fetal surgery for spina bifida. Lancet 352:1675, 1998.

CHAPTER 17

Multifetal Pregnancy Reduction and Selective Termination

Richard L. Fischer and Ronald J. Wapner

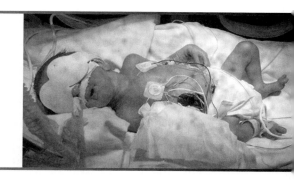

Although they provide significant benefits to most couples, the development of more sophisticated and complex reproductive technologies also may lead to complex clinical situations. The accidental production of **high-order multiple gestations** of three or more fetuses has resulted primarily from either the aggressive use of ovulation-inducing agents or the use of in vitro fertilization techniques. The identification in early pregnancy of a multiple gestation in which only one fetus was genetically or anatomically abnormal only became possible as ultrasound visualization improved and intrauterine diagnostic procedures became standard. Before 1980, the options available to these couples, many of whom had long-standing infertility, were limited: either terminate the entire pregnancy, or continue a pregnancy with the potential of either an extreme preterm delivery or the birth of a handicapped infant.

With the development of high-resolution ultrasonography and continuing experience with ultrasonically guided procedures, the option of intrauterine termination of one or more fetuses from a multiple gestation has emerged as a therapeutic option. Cases in which an *abnormal* fetus is specifically targeted for termination is called **selective termination** or **selective reduction**. In contrast, when a high-order multiple gestation is reduced to improve perinatal outcome, the term **multifetal pregnancy reduction (MFPR)** has been coined.[1] This chapter reviews the indications, techniques, and potential complications of these two procedures and addresses some of the controversies surrounding their usage.

MULTIFETAL PREGNANCY REDUCTION

The spontaneous occurrence of a multiple gestation is relatively uncommon. With the increasing use of assisted reproductive techniques, however, the incidence has increased markedly.[2] Presently, most high-order multiple gestations are a result of reproductive technology.[3,4] It is estimated that the rate of twins is 5% to 10% with use of clomiphene citrate (Clomid; Serophene) and 10% to 40%

with use of human menopausal gonadotropin (Pergonal).[5,6] Three or even more fetuses occur in 2% to 3% of human menopausal gonadotropin inductions, resulting in a condition some have referred to as **high-order** or **grand multiple gestations**. In vitro fertilization and gamete or zygote intrafallopian transfer result in high-order multiple gestations approximately 4% of the time.[7]

Multifetal pregnancies present an increased risk of maternal and perinatal complications. Maternal anemia, deep venous thrombosis, gestational diabetes, postpartum hemorrhage, and preeclampsia occur more frequently with multiple gestations. The high risk of preterm labor and the need for tocolytic agents expose the mother to additional potential complications, the most severe of which occur more frequently with multiple gestations (e.g., pulmonary edema). In addition to the medical hazards, there are social and financial considerations for parents of multiple gestations, which may be compounded further if one or more children are handicapped as a result of extreme prematurity.

Fetal risks are related predominantly to prematurity but include growth restriction and an increased risk of congenital anomalies. The perinatal morbidity and mortality resulting from pregnancies containing three or more fetuses are difficult to determine accurately because reported series are small and subject to reporting bias (Table 17-1).[8-19] There is, however, unanimous consensus that gestational age at delivery is inversely proportional to the number of fetuses. The average gestational age at delivery is 35.5 weeks for twins, 33.5 weeks for triplets, and 31.5 weeks for quadruplets, despite advances in tocolytic therapy and home uterine activity monitoring. Owing to the inability to prevent preterm delivery in such high-order multiple gestations, techniques were developed to improve outcome by reducing the number of viable fetuses.

Techniques

Transabdominal Approach

The most commonly used technique for MFPR is transabdominal injection of **potassium chloride (KCl)** into the

Table 17-1. Pregnancy Outcome of Published Series of Multiple Gestations

Study	No. Fetuses	No. Cases	<28 wk No.	(%)	28-31 wk No.	(%)	32-36 wk No.	(%)	≥37 wk No.	(%)	Uncorrected PNM (per 1000)	Dates
Keith, 1980[8*‡]	Twins	588	24	4	31	5	140	24	372	63	72	1971-1975
Medearis, 1979[9†]	Twins	2831	105	4	145	5	800	28	1781	63	116	1972-1976
Australia IVF, 1988[10]	Twins	169	8	5	10	6	63	38	86	52	N/A	1979-1988
Savona-Ventura & Grech, 1988[11*]	Twins	190	7	4	11	6	44	23	128	67	98	1983-1985
Itzkowic, 1979[12]	Triplets	59	6	10	9	15	29	49	15	25	232	1946-1976
Holcberg, 1982[13]	Triplets	31	5	16	6	19	16	52	4	13	312	1960-1979
Australia IVF, 1988[10]	Triplets	32	1	3	11	36	18	58	1	3	N/A	1979-1985
Newman, 1989[14*]	Triplets	198	10	5	36	18	127	64	24	12	66	1985-1988
Vervliet, 1989[15]	Triplets	15	1	17	3	20	10	67	1	7	N/A	1985-1988
Lipitz, 1989[16§]	Triplets	78	8	10	12	16	46	60	11	14	93	1975-1988
Lipitz, 1990[17]	Quadruplets	8	2	25	0	0	6	75	0	0	313	1975-1989
Gonen, 1990[18]	Quadruplets	5	0	0	5	100	0	0	0	0	100	1978-1988
Vervliet, 1989[15]	Quadruplets	6	2	33	1	17	3	50	0	0	N/A	1985-1988
Collins & Bleyl, 1990[19]	Quadruplets	71	9	13	25	35	34	48	3	4	147	1980-1989
Lipitz, 1990[17]	Quintuplets	2	0	0	2	100	0	0	0	0	0	1975-1989
Gonen, 1990[18]	Quintuplets	1	0	0	1	100	0	0	0	0	0	1978-1988
Lipitz, 1990[17]	Sextuplets	1	0	0	1	100	0	0	0	0	167	1975-1989

Note: Includes series providing gestational age at delivery.

*Data modified to fit gestational age grouping.

†Gestational age at delivery for "uncomplicated" twin pregnancies only. PNM refers to all 3594 twin pregnancies from 1972-1976.

‡Gestational age at delivery not stated in 21 twin pregnancies.

§One patient who delivered two infants at 27 weeks and one at 38 weeks excluded.

PNM, perinatal mortality.

From Fischer RL, Wapner RJ: Surgical therapy. In Barnea ER, Hustin J, Jauniaux E (eds): The First Twelve Weeks of Gestation. New York, Springer Verlag, 1992.

fetal thoracic cavity. The most fundal fetuses are technically most accessible, whereas the fetus overlying the cervical os usually is avoided to prevent delayed rupture of a necrotic sac and subsequent ascending infection. A 22-gauge spinal needle is directed into the fetal pericardial area, and 0.2- to 0.4-mL increments of a 2-mEq/mL KCl solution are injected until cardiac asystole occurs. Direct injection into the fetal heart is not required. The quantity of KCl required usually ranges from 0.4 to 9 mEq. Near-immediate resumption of cardiac activity may occur occasionally, so leaving the needle in place for 1 to 3 minutes after obtaining initial asystole is advised.[20-22] After death is confirmed, the needle is withdrawn from the fetus, and 5 to 10 mL of amniotic fluid is removed, which decreases the volume of fluid to be resorbed and seems to minimize postprocedure vaginal fluid leakage.[22,23]

Delayed resumption of fetal cardiac activity may occur in approximately 1% to 3% of MFPR cases and mandates repeat ultrasound examination 30 minutes after the procedure. Reinjection of KCl can occur at a time when identification of the initially injected fetus is certain. Reinitiation of cardiac activity beyond this time has not been reported.

The timing of transabdominal MFPR may range from 9 to 13 weeks of gestation, with most centers performing the procedure between weeks 10 and 11.[3] Because the phenomenon of a "vanishing" coexisting fetus may occur 21.2% of the time after fetal heart activity has been documented,[24] delaying the procedure until at least 9 to 10 weeks allows for spontaneous reduction in fetal number, which avoids unnecessary procedures and minimizes postprocedure loss of the remaining embryos. There is little benefit and potential harm in delaying MFPR beyond the end of the first trimester because a higher loss rate and earlier gestational age at delivery occurs when the procedure is performed after 13 weeks of gestation.[3,4] Table 17-2 lists the characteristics of series reporting at least 20 cases of transabdominal MFPR.[3,20,22,25-29]

Transvaginal Approach

For transvaginal MFPR, a 16- or 18-gauge long needle is guided by transvaginal ultrasonography through the vaginal fornix and uterine wall into a gestational sac. A smaller gauge needle is inserted through the larger one, directed into the fetal thorax and used for the KCl injection. A single-needle technique, without the outer guide

Table 17–2. Transabdominal Multifetal Pregnancy Reduction*

Author	Year	No. Patients	Gestational age (wk) (mean or range)	Loss rate (%) (<24 wk)	Comments
Evans[25]	1990	20	9-12	22.7	
Donner[26]	1990	23	9-13	13.0	
Wapner[22]	1990	38	9-13	2.6	
Dommergues[27]	1991	35	8-14	23.0	Used mechanical trauma, injection of air, saline, or KCl
Tabsh[28]	1993	131	11-13	4.9	
Boulot[29]	1993	35	9.7 ± 1.4	11.4	Used KCl or NSS
Berkowitz[20]	1993	200	10-13	9.5	
Evans[3]	1993	463	10.8 ± 2.0	16.2	May include data from Evans, Berkowitz, Wapner, Dommergues, Boulot

*From series reporting 20 cases or more. Unless otherwise stated, multifetal pregnancy reduction performed by intrathoracic KCl injection.

KCl, potassium chloride, NSS, normal saline solution.

needle, is preferred by others and seems to be equally efficacious.[30,31] Although the transabdominal MFPR approach seeks to avoid the sac overlying the internal os for fear of increased loss rates, Timor-Tritsch and colleagues[30] observed comparable transvaginal loss rates when the lower embryo was terminated.

Although most transvaginal procedures are performed at a gestational age similar to the transabdominal technique, the superior resolution of first-trimester vaginal sonography has led to attempts at earlier procedures in which puncture and aspiration of the gestational sac or embryo are performed at 5 to 8 weeks of gestation.[32-35] A 25- to 30-cm long, 18-gauge needle is directed transvaginally into the uterus, and the needle is positioned close to or within the embryo. Sudden, rapid suction with a 20-mL syringe results in partial or complete aspiration of the embryo.[7,34] The theoretical advantage of these earlier procedures is that no toxic substances are injected, and there is less necrotic tissue to be resorbed. This earlier approach does not allow, however, for the occurrence of spontaneous loss of one or more of the fetuses and does not allow for prereduction ultrasound detection of fetal anomalies.[30,31] In one series of transvaginal reductions, 13.4% of pregnancies had a death of one fetus

before the MFPR procedure. Additionally, two pregnancies that underwent early MFPR subsequently were discovered to have fetal anomalies that might have been detectable by endovaginal ultrasonography if MFPR had been delayed until 9.5 weeks.[30] Proponents of the earlier performance of transvaginal MFPR, however, point out the inherent difficulty of assessing anatomy at 10 weeks, not just on one fetus, but on four or five.[34] Table 17-3 lists series of at least 10 cases of transvaginal MFPR that have been published.[7,30,31,34,35]

Associated Risks

Pregnancy Loss

Loss rates after MFPR vary significantly from center to center and range from 0% to 40% (see Tables 17-2 and 17-3). The presence of relatively small numbers from some centers and the incorporation by pioneering centers of their early losses resulting from inexperience make a determination of the true loss rate difficult to estimate. Evans and associates[3] attempted a more accurate approximation by using a multicenter compilation of consecutive and completed pregnancies after transabdominal MFPR. A total of 463 procedures were recorded, including 18 sets

Table 17–3. Transvaginal Multifetal Pregnancy Reduction

Author	Year	No. Patients	Gestational age (wk) (mean or range)	Loss rate (%) (<24 wk)	Comments
Shalev[35]	1989	10	8-11	10.0	
Yovel[31]	1992	20	11-12	0.0	Mechanical trauma and NSS
Vauthier-Brouzes[7]	1992	22	5.3	0.0	Fetal puncture and aspiration
Itskovitz-Eldor[34]	1992	19	7-8	0.0	Embryo/sac aspiration
Timor-Tritsch[30]	1993	134	Not stated	12.6	Last 85 MFPR performed at or after 9.5 wk

*From series reporting 10 cases or more. Unless otherwise stated, MFPR performed by intrathoracic potassium chloride injection.

MFPR, multifetal pregnancy reduction, NSS, normal saline solution.

of twins, 175 sets of triplets, 193 sets of quadruplets, 52 sets of quintuplets, 14 sets of sextuplets, 7 sets of heptuplets, 3 sets of octuplets, and 1 set of nontuplets. All of the procedures were performed successfully with one needle insertion per embryo. Fifty-seven pregnancies were reduced to singletons, 380 to twins, and 26 to triplets. The total pregnancy loss rate was 16.2%, with cumulative loss rates of 3%, 3.9%, and 4.6% at 1, 2, and 4 weeks post-MFPR. Higher loss rates were observed with larger starting and finishing numbers of fetuses. The loss rate for pregnancies reduced to twins was 6.7% when starting with triplets, 15.3% when starting with quadruplets, and 29.5% when starting with quintuplets.

The results of the multicenter study most likely represent maximal loss rates because each center's outcome improved as experience was gained. In our experience at Jefferson Medical College, postprocedure pregnancy loss to 28 weeks of gestation was 3.4% in more than 300 procedures. This is the total loss rate and not the rate of procedure-induced losses. Because twin gestations are known to have an increased risk of fetal loss, a substantial percentage of the postprocedure losses may be accounted for by background losses. In our own experience, the perinatal loss rate for pregnancies reduced to twins was similar to that of unreduced twins.[36]

The gestational age at delivery is related primarily to the number of fetuses remaining post-MFPR and is consistent with gestational ages expected in unreduced pregnancies; in the multicenter study, singletons delivered at 37.1 weeks, twins at 35.6 weeks, and triplets at 33.3 weeks. In 35 pregnancies undergoing MFPR, an additional fetus was lost after the procedure, and this postprocedure pregnancy loss was associated with an increased risk of preterm delivery.[3] The gestational age at delivery for pregnancies losing at least one fetus was 29.7 weeks compared with 33.1 weeks when no additional fetuses died.

Presently, most reported outcome experience is with transabdominal MFPR, with only a few studies adequately comparing the transabdominal and transvaginal approaches. Shalev and coworkers[35] observed a loss rate of 10% with transvaginal KCl injection compared with 40% with the transabdominal route. This difference was attributed to avoidance of multiple uterine punctures when the double-needle, transvaginal approach was used. Yovel and colleagues[31] also compared the two approaches, using intrathoracic mechanical disruption coupled with saline injection. A loss rate of 10% was observed with the transabdominal route performed at 11 to 12 weeks compared with 0% loss rate in the transvaginal group performed at 8 to 10 weeks. The authors concluded that the two methods were of comparable safety. As experience is gained with endovaginal ultrasonography, the transvaginal technique may increase in popularity.

Infection

Serious maternal infection, usually chorioamnionitis, has occurred after MFPR and can develop from either an ascending transcervical organism or contamination from inadvertent puncture of the maternal bowel. These situations occur infrequently, with most series of transabdominal procedures having an infection rate of less than 1%.

In our own experience of more than 300 transabdominal cases, we have observed only two infections. Timor-Tritsch and colleagues[30] observed three infections in their series of 134 transvaginal MFPR procedures. Two responded to oral antibiotics, whereas one required intravenous antibiotics and uterine evacuation.

The initial presentation of an intrauterine infection can be minor and misleading, often beginning with a low-grade fever and influenza-like symptoms. This condition has been known to progress insidiously, and septic shock has occurred when unattended. Because uterine tenderness and purulent vaginal discharge may be late-presenting symptoms, a high clinical index of suspicion is required to diagnose the early manifestations. Intravenous antibiotic therapy and uterine evacuation are required for severe infections. Although successful use of antibiotics without termination of the pregnancy has been reported for mild infections,[30] the extent of infection and details of the cases are not described.

There is a lack of agreement regarding the routine use of prophylactic antibiotics, regardless of the route of MFPR. Some centers routinely use them,[20,28,29,31] whereas others do not.[22,27,30] No comparative studies have shown improvement in pregnancy outcome when prophylactic antibiotics are used.

Risk to Surviving Fetuses

Thrombotic complications in surviving fetuses whose co-twins have died spontaneously have been reported; they include multicystic encephalomalacia, hydranencephaly, renal cortical necrosis, and small bowel atresia.[37] Sudden death of the co-twin also has been reported. These complications have occurred almost exclusively in monochorionic gestations, of which greater than 85% contain vascular anastomoses within the placenta.[38] Two mechanisms of fetal injury have been hypothesized. In one theory, thromboplastin from the necrotic conception crosses to the living fetus, causing disseminated intravascular coagulation and subsequent fetal hemorrhage or infarction. Alternatively, a sudden hemodynamic shift across the anastomotic placental vessels may result in hypovolemia, hypotension, and local ischemia.

Congenital abnormalities similar to those seen with the spontaneous demise of a co-twin have been reported after MFPR, but a causal relationship seems dubious, especially when the remaining fetuses are dichorionic. Boulot and associates[39] described two separate cases of "anencephaly-like malformations" in remaining fetuses after first-trimester MFPR by transabdominal intrathoracic hypertonic saline injection. The chorionicity was not reported. In both cases, supposedly "normal" embryos had been observed by transvaginal ultrasonography before MFPR. Encephaloceles also have been discovered in remaining fetuses in other studies of MFPR.[28,30] Although the cause of these anomalous fetuses might be attributable to the procedure or to the prolonged retention of a dead uterine cohabitant, they most likely represent previously unrecognized abnormalities. Because most reports of post-MFPR follow-up, including the multicenter study, have not observed an increase in fetal anomalies, the risk of injury to the remaining fetus is seen almost exclusively in monochorionic gestations. We presently recommend that when a monochorionic twin gestation is observed within a high-order multiple gestation, either both fetuses should be terminated or the twin gestation should be left undisturbed. Because a monochorionic gestation may have significantly increased perinatal risks, intentionally leaving this situation may be unwise, if it can be avoided.

Because high-order multiple gestations have an increased risk of fetal structural abnormalities, many of which would not be identified on first-trimester ultrasonography, fetal anatomy should be assessed in the surviving fetus at 18 to 20 weeks of gestation after first-trimester MFPR of any chorionicity. The parents should be made aware before MFPR of the possibility of a previously unrecognized anomaly in one of the surviving infants.

Only limited information is available on the physical and mental development of surviving co-sibs. All studies to date have failed to show any difference in gestational age at delivery, birth weight, and incidence of infants small for gestational age, however, when pregnancies reduced to twins have been compared with spontaneous twins.[36,40] In the only study of long-term follow-up of MFPR, Brandes and colleagues[41] assessed seven children (one triplet and two twin sets) at 1 year of age and beyond and compared them with an appropriately matched control group. No differences were observed in either physical or mental development. Although these results are encouraging, further studies are needed to confirm these findings.

Maternal Coagulopathy

Maternal disseminated intravascular coagulation is a well-known complication of prolonged retention of a dead fetus and is thought to be due to release of thromboplastin from the degenerating fetus into the maternal circulation. Although theoretically possible, no cases of post-MFPR disseminated intravascular coagulation have been reported. Postprocedure monitoring of maternal coagulation status is not recommended.

Rh Sensitization

Regardless of the technique used for MFPR, there is the potential for transfer of fetal red blood cells into the maternal circulation. Rh immune globulin should be administered after MFPR to all Rh-negative women.

Neural Tube Screening after Multifetal Pregnancy Reduction

Maternal serum α-fetoprotein (AFP) is used as a second-trimester screen for fetal neural tube defects and more recently for Down syndrome. After MFPR, however, the release of AFP from the deceased fetuses causes elevated maternal AFP levels, and use of this serum marker for diagnostic purposes is unreliable. Grau and associates[42] evaluated 22 women who had maternal serum AFP screening after MFPR to twins, and all but one had levels greater than 4.5 multiples of the median (MOM), the cutoff used for twins. The average elevated maternal serum AFP level was 9.4 MOM, with a range of 5 to 19 MOM. Post-MFPR amniocentesis was subsequently performed, with 24.5% having amniotic fluid AFP levels greater than 2 MOM. One was positive for acetylcholinesterase.

Despite these elevated amniotic fluid AFP levels, no liveborn infant was found to have a neural tube defect. From this experience, we recommend that maternal serum AFP screening *not* be performed after first-trimester MFPR, and if amniocentesis is performed post-MFPR, the amniotic fluid AFP levels must be interpreted with caution. In lieu of AFP screening, all remaining fetuses should be evaluated by ultrasonography in the second trimester.

Cytogenetic Testing and Multifetal Pregnancy Reduction

Many women undergoing assisted reproductive technology are of advanced maternal age when a successful pregnancy is achieved. Prenatal cytogenetic diagnosis of these pregnancies can be performed either by **chorionic villus sampling (CVS)** before MFPR or by a subsequent second-trimester amniocentesis. Although many centers have opted for amniocentesis, others have shown that CVS before the reduction can be performed safely and accurately. With this approach, a karyotypically abnormal embryo can be identified and intentionally terminated in the first trimester. This approach avoids the need for a riskier second-trimester selective termination. Although CVS in experienced centers can karyotype all membranes of a multiple gestation reliably,[43] the procedure can be complex, and the potential exists for cross-contamination of chorionic villi leading to inaccurate results or inadequate sampling of individual sacs. In our center, we routinely perform CVS on the three or four lowest sacs 5 to 7 days before the planned reduction. If an abnormal karyotype is identified, the affected fetus can be intentionally terminated at the time of the MFPR. We have found fetal location to remain stable over this brief period. A meticulous map of fetal position must be drawn at the time of CVS to ensure later fetal identification.

REMAINING CONTROVERSIES INVOLVING MULTIFETAL PREGNANCY REDUCTION

How Many Fetuses Warrant Multifetal Pregnancy Reduction?

Controversy exists over the number of fetuses for which MFPR should be offered. Many centers do not reduce twins to a singleton because they believe that the favorable outcome of most twin gestations makes this an elective procedure.[25] Others have honored such requests, albeit reluctantly, on the grounds of the legal right of a woman's choice to abortion and the purported intent of the mother to terminate the entire gestation should MFPR not be performed.[22,30]

In light of advances in neonatal care, some investigators have questioned the need for MFPR on triplets.[44,45] Porreco and coworkers[46] compared 13 pregnancies in which triplets were reduced to twins with a control group of 11 triplet gestations that either declined or were not offered MFPR during the same time period. Although the numbers in each group were small, there were no significant differences in maternal complications, such as preterm labor, preterm premature rupture of membranes, placental abruption, and pregnancy-induced hypertension. Additionally, other parameters of perinatal outcome, such as gestational age at delivery, birth weight, neonatal hospital days, and neonatal complications, were similar. Higher rates of medical intervention, such as tocolysis and prolonged hospitalization, were noted, however, for the nonreduced triplet pregnancies.

Other reports have not been so optimistic, with maintained triplets having worse perinatal outcomes than triplets reduced to twins or spontaneous twins. Melgar and colleagues[45] compared five pregnancies reduced from triplets to twins with 20 sets of nonreduced triplets and showed a significant improvement in the mean gestational age at delivery, from 34.8 weeks in the twin group to 33.1 weeks in the pregnancies maintained as triplets. Additionally, the average length of stay in the neonatal intensive care unit was 8 days in the twins group compared with 20.7 days for the nonreduced triplets. Two reports have shown further the potential hazard of triplet gestations.[36,47] In their comparison of maintained triplets with triplets reduced to twins, Macones and colleagues[36] showed a significant difference in the perinatal outcome. The maintained triplets had an average gestational age at delivery that was 4 weeks less, the birth weight was decreased by more than 1 pound, and the perinatal mortality rate was increased fivefold. More recently, Yaron and associates[47] looked at the reduction of triplets to twins and compared the data of unreduced triplets with two large populations of twins. These data show substantial improvement of reduced twins compared with triplet pregnancies. Data from collaborative series suggest that pregnancy outcomes for gestations reduced from quadruplets or triplets to twins do at least as well as gestations starting as twins, supporting some cautious aggressiveness in infertility situations to secure optimal outcomes (Table 17-4).

Although the controversy over the optimal starting and ending number of fetuses continues, we believe that all patients with triplets or more should be told of the availability of the procedure. Patients with quadruplets or more can be counseled that there is a consensus that reduction improves perinatal outcome. Couples with triplet gestations must understand that although the overall perinatal mortality with triplets has improved and may approach that of twins,[48] the gestational age at delivery and birth weight still remain less than their twin counterparts.[49] At present, the issue of when MFPR should be offered remains a personal decision between the well-informed patient and her physician.

How Many Fetuses Should Remain?

Because reduction to a singleton would leave no allowance for a subsequent spontaneous loss of the remaining fetus and because the perinatal outcome for twins is acceptable, most centers reduce to a twin gestation unless otherwise requested by the patient.[25,35,50] Leaving this margin to allow for spontaneous losses seems warranted because in the multicenter study,[3] 35 of 463 pregnancies (7.6%) reduced to twins were complicated by the subsequent death of one fetus with successful continuation of the pregnancy. Dommergues and coworkers[27] questioned the need, however, for maintaining an "extra" fetus because spontaneous loss occurred only once in 58 MFPR procedures, and the perinatal outcome was optimal when the pregnancy was reduced to a singleton. Similarly, in 26 cases of MFPR to a single fetus reported by Salat-Baroux and colleagues,[51] there was only one pregnancy loss, which occurred early in their experience and was most likely procedure related.

At present, most operators continue to leave twins remaining, believing that the excellent perinatal outcome of most twin gestations makes reduction to a singleton primarily a social or financial decision. Reduction to a single fetus is suggested routinely, however, when there

Table 17-4. Reduced versus Unreduced Triplets Comparison

Years		MFPR Cases				
			Deliveries (wk)			
	Losses < 24 wk	24-28	29-32	33-36	>37	
1980s	6.7%	6.1%	9.1%	36.9%	47.9%	
1990-1994	5.7%	5.2%	9.9%	39.2%	45.2%	
1995-1998	4.5%	3.2%	6.9%	28.3%	55.1%	
1998-2002 (mean GA 35.5, PMR 10.0/1000) 1998-2002	5.1%	4.6%	10.8%	41.8%	37.6%	
1998-2002 (3 → 1) (mean GA 39.5, PMR 0/1000)	8.0%	4.0%	12.0%	4.0%	72.0%	

Nonreduced Triplets	Losses < 24 wk	Mean GA	PMR
1998 (Leondires)	9.9%	33.3	55/1000
1999 (Angel)	8.0%	32.3	29/1000
1999 (Lipitz)	25.0%	33.5	109/1000
2002 (Francois)	8.3%	31.0	57.6/1000

GA, gestational age; MFPR, multifetal pregnancy reduction; PMR, perinatal mortality rate.

From Evans MI, Krivchenia EL, Gelber SE, Wapner RJ: Selective reduction. Clin Perinatol 30:103, 2003.

are significant medical situations that would put a twin gestation at increased risk. Uterine malformations, history of prior preterm delivery, diethylstilbestrol exposure, and the presence of monochorionic twins in a triplet pregnancy justify serious consideration of reduction to a singleton.[20,28]

Ethical, Legal, and Religious Considerations Involving Multifetal Pregnancy Reduction

Rarely has there been more intense ethical debate in perinatal medicine than in the area of MFPR.[52-55] To some, MFPR represents a significant scientific breakthrough that allows patients with little hope for a normal pregnancy outcome to deliver healthy infants. To others, especially those who oppose elective abortion, it represents an abuse of medical technology with unwarranted destruction of healthy fetuses. Although a full discussion of these issues is beyond the scope of this chapter, many excellent publications are available.

All sides seems to agree that the ideal solution to the medical, ethical, and legal dilemma would be to limit the number and extent of grand multiple gestations, reducing the number of MFPR procedures that need to be performed.[56] For women undergoing ovulation induction, close surveillance of estradiol levels and follicle number and growth can reduce the need for MFPR. Should hyperstimulation occur, the excess follicles can be aspirated before ovulation, leaving two to three follicles. This approach has been termed *selective follicular reduction* by one author.[57] Additionally, limitation of the number of preembryos and oocytes transferred in in vitro fertilization and gamete intrafallopian transfer would reduce the incidence of such high-order multiple gestations. Toward that end, the Voluntary Licensing Authority in England has placed a limit on embryos and oocytes transferred to three, with four allowable under "exceptional" clinical conditions.[58] It is hoped that these measures will modify the role of MFPR to that of an interim procedure until adequate prevention of grand multiple gestation can be achieved.[53]

Discussion

Because of the relative infancy of MFPR, there are few studies to evaluate the long-term effects on the surviving fetuses and the mother. Developmental studies on the infants and psychological profiles on women who have terminated wanted fetuses are necessary to determine the appropriateness of continuing MFPR. At present, it would seem reasonable, however, for individuals experienced in ultrasonically guided procedures to continue to offer MFPR to women with high-order multiple gestations in an attempt to reduce perinatal morbidity and mortality. As with any surgical procedure, the risks and benefits of MFPR and alternative therapies should be discussed thoroughly with the patient. The collaborative loss rate numbers (i.e., 4.5% for triplets, 8% for quadruplets, 11% for quintuplets, and 15% for sextuplets or more) seem reasonable to present to families considering the procedure. Ethical and emotional issues should be explored and discussed openly before, during, and after MFPR has been performed.[59]

SELECTIVE TERMINATION

First-trimester or second-trimester prenatal diagnostic testing leads to the discovery of fetuses with genetic or anatomic abnormalities sufficiently early in gestation to allow the option of pregnancy termination. The likelihood of diagnosing an abnormality is increased in multiple gestations, which not only have an increased risk of a fetal structural defect,[60] but also have an increased probability of a karyotypic abnormality (Box 17-1). A woman with a twin gestation undergoing genetic testing for advanced maternal age has a 67% higher risk of carrying at least one chromosomally abnormal fetus than a woman of the same age carrying a singleton.[61] If the twins are a result of ovulation induction, in vitro fertilization, or gamete intrafallopian transfer, in which dizygotic pregnancies are more likely, her risk of a fetus with a chromosomal abnormality is twofold higher than for a singleton pregnancy.

In the past, when an abnormal fetus was identified in a multiple gestation, options only included terminating the entire pregnancy or continuing with a known anomalous fetus. More recently, selective termination of the affected fetus, while leaving the normal sib or sibs undisturbed, has developed as an alternative.

Technique

Selective termination has been attempted since 1978 by many techniques, including fetal cardiac puncture, exsanguination, air embolization, and surgical removal of the abnormal embryo (see Table 17-4). Presently, intracardiac KCl is the least invasive approach, is not hampered by air distortion of the ultrasound image, and has the lowest loss rate. As a result, it has become the procedure of choice for most operators.

In the second trimester, selective termination is performed by ultrasonically guided injection of KCl (2 mEq/mL) into the fetal cardiac region. To cause fetal

---

Box **17–1**	Genetic Risks for Twin Pregnancy: Chromosomal Abnormalities[48]

Assumptions:
1. X = age-related risk of newborn with chromosomal abnormality for a singleton pregnancy
2. $1/3$ of twins are monozygotic (MZ), $2/3$ are dizygotic (DZ)

Risk of both fetuses affected:
$$1/3 \text{ MZ} \cdot X + 2/3 \text{ DZ} (X \cdot X) = 1/3 X + 2/3 X^2 \approx 1/3 X$$
$$(2/3 X^2 \text{ is negligible and can be excluded})$$

Risk of only one fetus affected:
$$1/3 \text{ MZ} \cdot 0 + 2/3 \text{ DZ}[X(1 - X) + (1 - X)X] =$$
$$2/3 (X - X^2 + X - X^2) = 2/3 (2X - 2X^2) =$$
$$4/3 X (2X^2 \text{ is negligible})$$

Risk of at least one fetus affected:
$$1/3 X + 4/3 X = 5/3 X$$

For almost certain dizygotic twins (IVF, ovulation induction),
$$MZ = 0 \text{ and } DZ = 1, \text{ so}$$

Risk of both fetuses affected: X^2
Only one affected: $2X - 2X^2 \approx 2X$
At least one affected: $X^2 + 2X - 2X^2 \approx 2X$

death, 2 to 10 mEq of KCl usually is required, in contrast to 1 to 3 mEq of KCl employed with first-trimester procedures. Additionally, because the fetal thorax is larger in the second trimester, the KCl must be injected either directly into the heart or into the pericardiac region. As with MFPR, prophylactic antibiotics are used by some authors, depending on the difficulty of the procedure and preference of the operator.

Selective termination requires precise identification of the affected fetus. This approach is facilitated if the abnormal fetus has an anatomic marker identifiable by ultrasonography, such as fetal gender or the presence of a specific anomaly. If no such marker exists, the detailed diagram of fetal and placental orientation drawn at the time of initial CVS or amniocentesis must be relied on. Although reversal of positions has been reported,[62] it is only rarely observed. In our experience, specifically detailing fetal and placental position at the time of sampling allows almost certain identification of the affected fetus 3 weeks later. In some cases, residual dye injected at the time of the original amniocentesis may be observed at the time of selective termination, further confirming fetal identification. In cases in which there are no ultrasonic markers, no residual dye, inaccurate drawings, a significant time lag from the original diagnostic procedure, or any question as to the location of the affected fetus, however, repeat cytogenetic or biochemical analysis should be performed before termination. Fetal blood sampling, direct analysis of chorionic villi retrieved by placental biopsy, or fluorescent in situ hybridization of amniocytes can facilitate this procedure. Additionally, at the time of selective reduction, a sample of fetal tissue (usually amniotic fluid) must be analyzed to confirm termination of the correct fetus.

Safety of Selective Termination

The pregnancy loss rate associated with selective termination is difficult to assess accurately because most publications have been case reports, subject to reporting bias. Additionally, the operators whose experience is outlined in Table 17-4 used a variety of techniques before intracardiac KCl became the primary modality. Of the eight pregnancy losses reported before the multicenter study, three occurred with air embolism,[63] and five occurred in monochorionic gestations[22,64] (see the following section on selective termination in monochorionic gestations). Of the combined 22 cases of dichorionic twins selectively terminated by intracardiac KCl, all co-twins survived, with a mean gestational age at delivery of 36.7 weeks (range 31 to 40 weeks).

Because of the relative paucity of large numbers of selective terminations, Evans and colleagues[4] combined the experience of nine centers in four countries to determine risk more accurately. A total of 183 cases were compiled, which were performed by intracardiac or intraumbilical KCl, fetal exsanguination, or air embolization. There were 169 sets of twins, 11 sets of triplets, and 3 sets of quadruplets. Indications included chromosomal abnormalities (52.5%), structural anomalies (41.5%), and mendelian disorders (6%). As with MFPR, there was a 100% technical success of selective termination. The total pregnancy loss rate (before 24 weeks) was 12.6%. Loss rates were directly proportional to the gestational age at which selective reduction was performed, with a 5.4%

loss rate if performed at or before 16 weeks compared with 14.4% if performed on or after 17 weeks. Additionally, the likelihood of preterm delivery also was directly proportional to gestational age at selective termination. The mode of selective termination also influenced the loss rate, with a rate of 8.3% for KCl injection versus 41.7% for air embolization.

No evidence of maternal disseminated intravascular coagulation has been observed after selective termination, despite the relatively advanced gestational ages of some procedures. It is suggested that coagulation profiles need not be followed after selective termination.

Selective Termination in Monochorionic Gestations

The monochorionic gestation discordant for a genetic or anatomic abnormality represents an unusual variation and a dilemma for the physician. Although monochorionic placentation occurs exclusively in monozygotic gestations, cytogenetic discordancy can occur as a result of postzygotic nondisjunction in one of the fetuses, resulting in one normal and one mosaic fetus. This condition is called **heterokaryotic twinning**. If this nondisjunction involves the Y chromosome, discordancy for gender may occur.[65] Structural anomalies also can occur in only one twin of a monozygotic pair as a result of unique environmental events, such as vascular disruptions, viral infections, amnion rupture with amniotic band syndrome, or deformation syndromes.

The selective termination of one fetus of a monochorionic pair is fraught with risk for the intended survivor. Golbus and coworkers[64] reported five cases of monochorionic gestations selectively terminated by various methods, including cardiac tamponade, air embolization, intracardiac KCl, and hysterotomy. Four of the five co-twins died within 4 to 12 hours, with the only survivor occurring after hysterotomy and extraction of the abnormal fetus. Similarly, in our own experience, all selective terminations of monochorionic gestations have resulted in fetal death of the planned survivor.

The pathogenesis of the demise presumably is related to the anastomotic connections within the placenta, which are almost always present in monochorionic gestations. Death may occur by two possible mechanisms—transfer of the feticidal agent or thromboplastin or, more likely, sudden hemodynamic shifts.

Present experience suggests that should one fetus of a monochorionic pair have to be terminated, it should be performed either by hysterotomy or possibly umbilical cord ligation. Both of these approaches are significantly more invasive than the techniques used for selective termination of dichorionic twins and present a major risk to the remaining fetus and the mother. In most cases, continuation of the pregnancy must be given serious consideration despite the fetal abnormality. Couples for whom this approach is not acceptable should be referred to centers experienced in these more invasive procedures.

First-Trimester Selective Termination

With the increased use of CVS and the demonstration that the procedure can be undertaken safely and accurately in twin gestations,[43,66] cytogenetically discordant pregnancies are being identified earlier with selective termination in the first trimester.[22,67,68] The procedure is accomplished by intrathoracic KCl injection in a manner identical to that for MFPR. Because there are unlikely to be ultrasound markers to identify the affected fetus, however, the importance of detailed mapping of fetal and placental position at the time of initial testing is mandatory. Although our experience has shown consistently that the fetal position remains unchanged, we continue to confirm the abnormal diagnosis before reduction by repeating the CVS on the affected fetus on the same day as the planned termination. Two-hour rapid karyotyping of the chorionic villi is used. Additionally, 5 to 10 mL of amniotic fluid is retrieved during the termination procedure and submitted for further confirmation of the diagnosis.

Selective Termination for Twin-Twin Transfusion Syndrome

A serious complication of monochorionic gestations is that of the twin-twin transfusion syndrome, in which a hemodynamic imbalance exists in the intraplacental vascular anastomoses between the two fetuses, leading to chronic shunting of blood from the donor twin to the recipient twin. The recipient twin usually becomes plethoric, with increased size and polyhydramnios. The donor twin, in contrast, becomes growth restricted and, owing to the lack of renal perfusion, develops oligohydramnios. The thin amniotic membrane surrounding the donor twin may closely envelop the fetus, leading to constricted movement and the typical "stuck twin" appearance. Perinatal mortality is extremely high with this syndrome, especially when the diagnosis is made in the second trimester. Many therapies have been advocated, such as aggressive amniocentesis[69] and laser ablation of anastomotic blood vessels on the fetal surface of the chorion.[70] Because most of the anastomoses occur deep within the cotyledons, however, laser ablation therapy has limited utility.

With the increasing use of selective termination, investigators have sought to apply it to this unique condition. Wittmann and associates[71] were the first to report selective termination of a donor twin at 25 weeks of gestation. The fetus, which measured only 19 weeks in size by ultrasonic biometry, was terminated by bolus injection of 5 mL of saline into the pericardiac space. After selective termination, the amniotic fluid volume around the remaining fetus normalized, and the patient ultimately was delivered at 37 weeks of gestation of a viable infant who remained well throughout the observation period of 1 year. The same authors subsequently reported two unsuccessful attempts.[72] In one case, the remaining fetus died in utero, whereas in the second the infant died in the neonatal period. We are aware of other unsuccessful attempts at selective termination for twin-twin transfusion and recommend against its use until the pathophysiology of the condition is more clearly understood and better techniques are developed to evaluate the anastomosis.

Selective Termination for Lethal Anomalies

Information is limited regarding the best approach for a multiple gestation containing a fetus with a lethal anomaly. It may be argued that this circumstance should not justify an invasive procedure because the outcome for the anomalous infant would not ultimately be altered, and the procedure may add additional risks to the remaining normal infant. The risks imposed on the remaining fetus and the mother by not performing a selective termination also must be considered, however. When the fetal abnormality is known to present an increased risk of extreme preterm delivery (e.g., polyhydramnios from anencephaly), selective termination may be justified from a risk-versus-benefit viewpoint. The mother's emotional well-being must be considered because without selective termination, she would be forced to carry a fetus that is destined to die. The parents of these complex pregnancies must be intimately involved in all decision making.

Legal Issues Involving Selective Termination

The legal issues surrounding selective termination are similar to those for abortion of a singleton. Strictly interpreted, selective termination is not an abortion, however, because the latter term implies the evacuation of the uterus. Previous laws, which do not address the issue of in utero termination of affected fetuses, may not rigidly apply. It is believed by most to represent a variation of abortion, however, and to date no laws have been enacted that would proscribe its performance. A survey by Evans and associates[73] of maternal-fetal medicine specialists, geneticists, clergy, and ethicists indicated that most respondents accepted selective termination for fetal anomalies, with the acceptance rate increasing with the severity of the anomaly and the decreasing gestational age at termination.

Discussion

As is the case with MFPR, selective termination requires continued evaluation of its safety and long-term effects on the surviving fetus or fetuses. The mere presence of a coexisting abnormal fetus does not make selective termination mandatory. If the fetal anomaly is lethal and not known to be associated with factors that would cause significant perinatal complications, the relative risk of selective termination must be weighed against the medical and emotional risks of expectant management. At present, parents of genetically or anatomically discordant twins who opt for selective termination should be referred to centers with experience in these procedures.

SUGGESTED READINGS

Aberg A: Cardiac puncture of fetus with Hurler's disease avoiding abortion of unaffected co-twin. Lancet 2:990, 1978.

Antsaklis A, Politis J, Karagiannopoulos C, et al: Selective survival of only the healthy fetus following prenatal diagnosis of thalassemia major in binovular twin gestation. Prenat Diagn 4:289, 1984.

Beck L, Terinde R, Rohrborn G, et al: Twin pregnancy, abortion of one fetus with Down's syndrome by sectio parva, the other delivered mature and healthy. Eur J Obstet Gynecol Reprod Biol 12:267, 1980.

Blaskiewicz R: Transabdominal multifetal pregnancy reduction: Report of 40 cases [letter]. Obstet Gynecol 76:735, 1990.

Boulot P, Hedon B, Pelliccia G, et al: Obstetrical results after embryonic reductions performed on 34 multiple pregnancies. Hum Reprod 5:1009, 1990.

Caspi E, Ronen J, Schreyer P, et al: The outcome of pregnancy after gonadotropin therapy. Br J Obstet Gynaecol 83:967, 1976.

Fischer RL: Quadruplet pregnancy: Contemporary management and outcome [letter]. Obstet Gynecol 81:476, 1993.

Gemmette EV: Selective pregnancy reduction: Medical attitudes, legal implications, and a viable alternative. J Health Polit Policy Law 16:383, 1991.

Grazi RV, Wolowelsky JB: Multifetal pregnancy reduction and disposal of untransplanted embryos in contemporary Jewish law and ethics. Am J Obstet Gynecol 165:1268, 1991.

Hobbins JC: Selective reduction—a perinatal necessity? N Engl J Med 318:1062, 1988.

Howie PW: Selective reduction in multiple pregnancy. BMJ 297:433, 1988.

Kerenyi KD, Citkara U: Selective birth in twin pregnancy with discordancy for Down's syndrome. N Engl J Med 304:1525, 1981.

Persson PH, Grennert L: Towards a normalization of the outcome of twin pregnancy. Acta Genet Med Gemellol 28:341, 1979.

Petres R, Redwine F: Selective birth in twin pregnancy [letter]. N Engl J Med 305:1218, 1981.

Pijpers L, Jahoda MG, Reuss A, et al: Selective birth in a dizygotic twin pregnancy with discordancy for Down's syndrome. Fetal Ther 4:58, 1989.

Redwine FO, Hays PM: Selective birth. Semin Perinatol 10:73, 1986.

Rodeck CH: Fetoscopy in the management of twin pregnancies discordant for a severe abnormality. Acta Genet Med Gemellol 33:57, 1984.

Rosner F: Pregnancy reduction in Jewish law [letter]. Am J Obstet Gynecol 168:278, 1993.

Walters WA: Selective termination in multiple pregnancy [editorial]. Med J Aust 152:451, 1990.

Wass D, Bennett M, Garrett W, et al: Selective termination in the first trimester [letter]. Aust N Z J Obstet Gynaecol 27:171, 1987.

REFERENCES

1. Berkowitz RL, Lynch L: Selective reduction: An unfortunate misnomer. Obstet Gynecol 75:873, 1990.
2. Grutzner-Konnocke H, Grutzner P, Grutzner U, et al: Higher order multiple births: Natural wonder or failure of therapy? Acta Genet Med Gemellol 39:491, 1990.
3. Evans MI, Dommergues M, Wapner RJ, et al: Efficacy of transabdominal multifetal pregnancy reduction: Collaborative experience among the world's largest centers. Obstet Gynecol 82:61, 1993.
4. Evans MI, Goldberg JD, Dommergues M, et al: Efficacy of second-trimester selective termination for fetal abnormalities: international collaborative experience among the world's largest centers. Am J Obstet Gynecol 171:90, 1993.
5. ACOG Technical Bulletin 120: Medical Induction of Ovulation. Washington, DC, American College of Obstetricians and Gynecologists, 1988.
6. Schenker JG, Yarkoni S, Granat M: Multiple pregnancies following induction of ovulation. Fertil Steril 35:105, 1981.
7. Vauthier-Brouzes D, Lefebvre G: Selective reduction in multifetal pregnancies: Technical and psychological aspects. Fertil Steril 57:1012, 1992.
8. Keith L, Ellis R, Berger GS, et al: The Northwestern University multihospital twin study: I. A description of 588 twin pregnancies and associated pregnancy loss, 1971 to 1975. Am J Obstet Gynecol 138:78, 1980.
9. Medearis AL, Jonas HS, Stockbauer JW, et al: Perinatal deaths in twin pregnancy. Am J Obstet Gynecol 134:413, 1979.
10. Australia IVF Collaborative Group: In-vitro fertilization pregnancies in Australia and New Zealand. Med J Aust 148:429, 1988.
11. Savona-Ventura C, Grech ES: Multiple pregnancy in the Maltese population. Int J Gynaecol Obstet 26:41, 1988.
12. Itzkowic D: A survey of 49 triplet pregnancies. Br J Obstet Gynaecol 86:23, 1979.
13. Holcberg G, Biale Y, Lewenthal H, et al: Outcome of pregnancy in 31 triplet gestations. Obstet Gynecol 59:472, 1982.
14. Newman R, Hamer C, Miller M: Outpatient triplet management: A contemporary review. Am J Obstet Gynecol 161:547, 1989.
15. Vervliet J: Management and outcome of 21 triplet and quadruplet pregnancies. Eur J Obstet Gynecol Reprod Biol 33:61, 1989.
16. Lipitz S, Reichman B, Paret G, et al: The improving outcome of triplet pregnancies. Am J Obstet Gynecol 161:1279, 1989.
17. Lipitz S, Frenkel Y, Watts C, et al: High-order multifetal gestation—management and outcome. Obstet Gynecol 76:215, 1990.
18. Gonen R, Heyman E, Asztalos EV, et al: The outcome of triplet, quadruplet, and quintuplet pregnancies managed in a perinatal unit: Obstetric, neonatal, and follow-up data. Am J Obstet Gynecol 162:454, 1990.
19. Collins M, Bleyl J: Seventy-one quadruplet pregnancies: Management and outcome. Am J Obstet Gynecol 162:1384, 1990.
20. Berkowitz RL, Lynch L, Lapinski R, et al: First-trimester transabdominal multifetal pregnancy reduction: A report of two hundred completed cases. Am J Obstet Gynecol 169:17, 1993.
21. Lynch L, Berkowitz RL, Chitkara U, et al: First-trimester transabdominal multifetal pregnancy reduction: A report of 85 cases. Obstet Gynecol 75:735, 1990.
22. Wapner RJ, Davis GH, Johnson A, et al: Selective reduction of multifetal pregnancies. Lancet 335:90, 1990.
23. Still K, Kolatat T, Corbett T, et al: Early third trimester selective feticide of a compromising twin. Fetal Ther 4:837, 1989.
24. Landy HJ, Weiner S, Corson SL, et al: The "vanishing twin": Ultrasonographic assessment of fetal disappearance in the first trimester. Am J Obstet Gynecol 155:14, 1986.
25. Evans MI, May M, Drugan A, et al: Selective termination: Clinical experience and residual risks. Am J Obstet Gynecol 162:1568, 1990.
26. Donner C, McGinnis JA, Simon P, et al: Multifetal pregnancy reduction: A Belgian experience. Eur J Obstet Gynecol Reprod Biol 38:183, 1990.
27. Dommergues M, Nisand I, Mandelbrot L, et al: Embryo reduction in multifetal pregnancies after infertility therapy: Obstetrical risks and perinatal benefits are related to operative strategy. Fertil Steril 55:805, 1991.
28. Tabsh K: A report of 131 cases of multifetal pregnancy reduction. Obstet Gynecol 82:57, 1993.
29. Boulot P, Hedon B, Pelliccia G, et al: Multifetal pregnancy reduction: A consecutive series of 61 cases. Br J Obstet Gynaecol 100:63, 1993.
30. Timor-Tritsch IE, Peisner DB, Monteagudo A, et al: Multifetal pregnancy reduction by transvaginal puncture: Evaluation of the technique used in 134 cases. Am J Obstet Gynecol 168:799, 1993.
31. Yovel I, Yaron Y, Amit A, et al: Embryo reduction in multifetal pregnancies using saline injection: Comparison between the transvaginal and transabdominal approach. Hum Reprod 7:1173, 1992.
32. Birnholz JC, Dmowski WP, Binor Z, et al: Selective continuation in gonadotropin-induced multiple pregnancy. Fertil Steril 5:873, 1987.

33. Itskovitz J, Boldes R, Thaler I, et al: Transvaginal ultrasonography-guided aspiration of gestational sacs for selective abortion in multiple pregnancy. Am J Obstet Gynecol 160:215, 1989.

34. Itskovitz-Eldor J, Drugan A, Levron J, et al: Transvaginal embryo aspiration—a safe method for selective reduction in multiple pregnancies. Fertil Steril 58:351, 1992.

35. Shalev J, Frenkel Y, Goldenberg M, et al: Selective reduction in multiple gestations: Pregnancy outcome after transvaginal and transabdominal needle-guided procedures. Fertil Steril 52:416, 1989.

36. Macones GA, Schemmer G, Pritts E, et al: Multifetal reduction of triplets to twins improves perinatal outcome. Am J Obstet Gynecol 169:982, 1993.

37. Hoyme HE, Higginbottom MC, Jones KL: Vascular etiology of disruptive structural defects in monozygotic twins. Pediatrics 67:288, 1981.

38. Benirschke K: Twin placenta in perinatal mortality. N Y State J Med 61:1499, 1961.

39. Boulot P, Hedon B, Deschamps F, et al: Anencephaly-like malformation in surviving twin after embryonic reduction. Lancet 335:1155, 1990.

40. Donner C, de Maertelaer V, Rodesch F: Multifetal pregnancy reduction: Comparison of obstetrical results with spontaneous twin gestations. Eur J Obstet Gynecol Reprod Biol 44:181, 1992.

41. Brandes JM, Scher A, Itzkovits J, et al: Growth and development of children conceived by in vitro fertilization. Pediatrics 90:424, 1992.

42. Grau P, Robinson L, Tabsh K, et al: Elevated maternal serum alpha-fetoprotein and amniotic fluid alpha-fetoprotein after multifetal pregnancy reduction. Obstet Gynecol 76:1042, 1990.

43. Wapner RJ, Johnson A, Davis G, et al: Prenatal diagnosis in twin gestations: A comparison between second-trimester amniocentesis and first-trimester chorionic villus sampling. Obstet Gynecol 82:49, 1993.

44. Lorenz J, Terry J: Selective reduction of multifetal pregnancies [letter]. N Engl J Med 319:949, 1988.

45. Melgar CA, Rosenfeld DL, Rawlinson K, et al: Perinatal outcome after multifetal reduction to twins compared with nonreduced multiple gestations. Obstet Gynecol 78:763, 1991.

46. Porreco RP, Burke MS, Hendrix ML: Multifetal reduction of triplets and pregnancy outcome. Obstet Gynecol 78(part 1): 335, 1991.

47. Yaron Y, Bryant-Greenwood PK, Dave N, et al: Multifetal pregnancy reduction (MFPR) of triplets to twins: Comparisons with non-reduced triplets and twins. Am J Obstet Gynecol 180:1268, 1999.

48. Sassoon DA, Castro LC, Davis JL, et al: Perinatal outcome in triplet versus twin gestations. Obstet Gynecol 75: 817, 1990.

49. Weissman A, Jakobi P: Triplet pregnancies—are we really doing better [letter]? Am J Obstet Gynecol 163:1716, 1990.

50. Dumez Y, Oury JF: Method for first trimester selective abortion in multiple pregnancy. Contr Gynecol Obstet 15:50, 1986.

51. Salat-Baroux J, Aknin J, Antoine JM, et al: The management of multiple pregnancies after induction for superovulation. Hum Reprod 3:399, 1988.

52. Diamond E: Selective reduction of multifetal pregnancies [letter]. N Engl J Med 319:950, 1988.

53. Evans MI, Fletcher JC, Zador IE, et al: Selective first-trimester termination in octuplet and quadruplet pregnancies: Clinical and ethical issues. Obstet Gynecol 71:289, 1988.

54. Weiner J: Selective first-trimester termination in octuplet and quadruplet pregnancies: Clinical and ethical issues [letter]. Obstet Gynecol 72:821, 1988.

55. Zaner R, Boehm F, Hill G: Selective termination in multiple pregnancies: Ethical considerations. Fertil Steril 54:203, 1990.

56. Selective fetal reduction [editorial]. Lancet 2:773, 1988.

57. MacDonald RR: Selective reduction in multifetal pregnancy [editorial]. Eur J Obstet Gynecol Reprod Biol 38:181, 1991.

58. Brahams D: Assisted reproduction and selective reduction of pregnancy. Lancet 2:1409, 1987.

59. ACOG Committee Opinion 94: Multifetal Pregnancy Reduction and Selective Fetal Termination. Washington, DC, American College of Obstetricians and Gynecologists, 1991.

60. Luke B, Keith LG: Monozygotic twinning as a congenital defect and congenital defects in monozygotic twins. Fetal Diagn Ther 5:61, 1990.

61. Hunter AGW, Cox DM: Counseling problems when twins are discovered at genetic amniocentesis. Clin Genet 16:34, 1979.

62. Benke PJ: Twins discordant for Down's syndrome. Clin Genet 21:104, 1982.

63. Chitkara U, Berkowitz RL, Wilkins IA, et al: Selective second-trimester termination of the anomalous fetus in twin pregnancies. Obstet Gynecol 73:690, 1989.

64. Golbus MS, Cunningham N, Goldberg JD, et al: Selective termination of multiple gestations. Am J Med Genet 31:339, 1988.

65. Schmidt R, Sobel EH, Nitowsky HM, et al: Monozygotic twins discordant for sex. J Med Genet 13:64, 1976.

66. Pergament E, Schulman JD, Copeland K, et al: The risk and efficacy of chorionic villus sampling in multiple gestations. Prenat Diagn 12:377, 1992.

67. Brambati B, Formigli L, Tului L: Selective reduction of quadruplet pregnancy at risk of β-thalassasemia. Lancet 336:1325, 1990.

68. Mulcahy M, Roberman B, Reid S: Chorion biopsy, cytogenetic diagnosis and selective termination in a twin pregnancy at risk of haemophilia [letter]. Lancet 2:866, 1984.

69. Elliot JP, Urig MA, Clewell WH: Aggressive therapeutic amniocentesis for treatment of twin-twin transfusion syndrome. Obstet Gynecol 77:537, 1991.

70. De Lia JE, Cruikshank DP, Keye WR: Fetoscopic neodymium:YAG laser occlusion of placental vessels in severe twin-twin transfusion syndrome. Obstet Gynecol 75:1046, 1990.

71. Wittmann BK, Farquharson DF, Thomas WD, et al: The role of feticide in the management of severe twin transfusion syndrome. Am J Obstet Gynecol 155:1023, 1986.

72. Baldwin VJ, Wittmann BK: Pathology of intragestational intervention in twin-to-twin transfusion syndrome. Pediatr Pathol 10:79, 1990.

73. Evans MI, Drugan A, Bottoms SF, et al: Attitudes on the ethics of abortion, sex selection, and selective pregnancy termination among health care professionals, ethicists, and clergy likely to encounter such situations. Am J Obstet Gynecol 164:1092, 1991.

CHAPTER 18

Diagnosis and Treatment of Preterm Labor

Curtis L. Lowery and E. Albert Reece

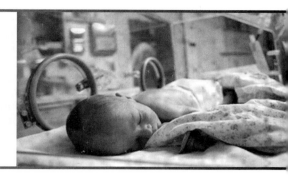

The 1996 U.S. vital statistics report indicated that the rate of preterm birth rose from 9.4% to 11% between 1981 and 1996, a net increase of 17%. From 1995 to 1996 alone, the rate of twin pregnancies increased by 4%, and that of triplet or higher gestations, by 19%.[1] Since 1980, the rate of twin births has increased more than a third, and the rate of triplet or higher order gestations has quadrupled. Advances in assisted reproductive technology have allowed older infertile couples to reproduce, which has led to an explosion in the numbers of multiple-fetus pregnancies.[2] This population of older women has a high rate of preterm birth not only because of the higher incidence of multiple gestation but also because of age-related medical problems that lead to more preterm deliveries.

Preterm labor, defined as labor occurring before 37 weeks' gestation, almost certainly represents a multifactorial, clinical syndrome in which multiple diverse conditions (e.g., fever, convulsions, hypertension) follow a common pathway, resulting in premature delivery. It is the leading cause of premature birth, which represents only 7% to 10% of all births but accounts for more than 85% of perinatal complications and deaths.[3] At times, preterm birth may be of benefit to the mother, the fetus, or both, if the result is decreased mortality or morbidity (e.g., placental abruptions, severe preeclampsia, in utero infections).

CONDITIONS ASSOCIATED WITH PREMATURITY

Berkowitz and Papiernik provided a complete review of demographic factors associated with preterm birth.[4] Although most studies have shown a strong association between socioeconomic status and preterm birth, socioeconomic status is more probably a marker for types of behavior that predispose the patient to preterm birth than a direct cause of preterm delivery. The inconsistencies in the correlation of socioeconomic status and other indirect factors such as limited health care access and risk behavior may explain the variations in the magnitude of the effects of socioeconomic status on preterm birth rates. There is a stronger correlation between socioeconomic status and preterm birth in whites than in African Americans.[5] This phenomenon is demonstrated by the fact that the relative risk of African Americans, whose overall risk for preterm delivery is 2.0 to 2.5 times greater than that in white patients, rises in the youngest gestational age range to 3.5.[6,7] This risk has been shown to correlate across socioeconomic status, and, at present, there is no explanation for this increased incidence of preterm birth in the African American population. Although much less studied, other ethnic groups do not seem to show as great a disparity from the white population as does the African American population.[8]

Other social factors have been shown to affect the incidence of preterm birth. For example, Berkowitz and Papiernik reported that the incidence of preterm birth is higher among unmarried mothers even when corrected for socioeconomic factors. They also described a significant association between preterm birth and low prepregnancy maternal weight. Closer inspection of the latter finding revealed that, rather than a continuous diminution in risk with increasing prepregnancy weight across all groups of patients, the greatest risk for preterm birth is seen in white patients in the lowest socioeconomic level.[9-11] One of the greatest risk factors associated with preterm delivery is the history of a previous preterm birth. Again, according to Berkowitz and Papiernik, a history of a single preterm birth results in a relative risk of 3.0, which increases with each subsequent preterm birth.[4]

The relationship between spontaneous abortion and preterm birth is not as well established. Some studies have demonstrated a stronger association between multiple spontaneous abortions when the abortions occurred in the second trimester rather than the first. Multiple gestation is strongly predictive for preterm delivery; most studies have shown that 25% to 50% of multiple gestations are delivered before term. In addition, there is an observed J-shaped curve that demonstrates an increased risk for patients younger than 20 and older than 35 years of age, which remains valid today.[1-3]

Adverse lifestyle practices have often been linked with an increased risk of preterm delivery. There is much evidence of a correlation between cocaine exposure and preterm delivery. Although adequate prenatal care seems to reduce the effect in these patients, their risk remains elevated.[12] In interpreting this information, it is important to remember that content variables play a major role in studies conducted with drug-abusing populations. In order to identify drug-abusing patients, researchers and clinicians have relied heavily on self-reporting and anonymous drug screens, techniques that are inherently flawed. Blood and urine screening have short windows of laboratory detection, and self-reporting is subject to patient reliability.[13] These problems may have resulted in a selection bias that identifies heavy drug users more frequently than those who use drugs only intermittently or occasionally during pregnancy. Most drug abusers use multiple illicit drugs, as well as tobacco and alcohol, and it is therefore difficult to separate the effects of these other substances from that of the cocaine. Cigarette smoking has been strongly associated with low birth weight, but only a moderate association with prematurity has been shown.[14] In general, smoking tends to create a selection bias for race and socioeconomic status, and it is impossible to adequately separate these confounding variables in the retrospective studies.[15-18] In a review article published in 2002, Leviton and Cowan looked at caffeine consumption and pregnancy outcome and noted mixed findings in the literature. The authors observed that an "association between caffeine consumption and spontaneous abortion may well reflect the Stein-Susser epiphenomenon (women with prominent nausea tend to reduce caffeine consumption and nausea appears to be a marker of good implantation), perhaps reflecting a favorable balance of hormones produced by a healthy placenta."[19] People who use caffeine heavily also tended to smoke more frequently and may underreport their cigarette use. In this case, caffeine use may be a marker for other social problems, including smoking.

The effect of stress on pregnancy outcome has also been the focus of much investigation. The interpretation of these studies is hampered by methodologic concerns, including variations in the definitions of stress, restriction of studies to special populations, small sample size, and poorly defined measurements of stress. Stress in pregnancy may express itself in different ways, such as depression and decreased appetite. A number of reports have described the adverse impact of poor weight gain during pregnancy on preterm delivery. The important question is whether the decreased weight gain is a marker for other complex social problems during pregnancy or a causative factor that results directly in preterm delivery.[20-22] Adequate social support, however, has not resulted in the reduction of preterm delivery.[23-25] In the one report that found a reduction of prematurity in populations given sufficient social support, there was no decrease in prematurity rates in the lowest socioeconomic class or among women who lived alone.[26] Overall life stress is probably not associated with a significantly

increased risk of preterm delivery.[27,28] However, a high-risk pregnancy may itself create, and expose the mother to, high levels of psychologic stress.[29]

Reviews of the literature regarding sexual intercourse and orgasm during pregnancy show no clear consensus.[30-34] There is some evidence that women in a stable monogamous relationship may safely continue to have intercourse during pregnancy; other reports indicate that women who remain sexually active because of abusive relationships or prostitution are more likely to deliver prematurely. These two examples demonstrate the dramatically different results in studies that evaluate sexual intercourse and pregnancy outcome. Sexual intercourse should not be actively discouraged in obstetric patients who are not at risk for premature delivery.

The relationship of the frequency of cervical examinations and the risk for preterm labor was studied in a randomized controlled trial performed in seven European countries. Two policies were compared: the attempt to perform a cervical examination at every prenatal visit (2803 women) and the avoidance of cervical examination if possible (2799).[35] The median number of cervical examinations was 6 in the experimental group and 1 in the controls. There were 6.7% preterm (at <37 weeks) deliveries in the experimental group and 6.4% in the control group (risk ratio = 1.05; 95% confidence interval [CI] = 0.85 to 1.29, nonsignificant). The low birth weight rate was 6.6% in the experimental group and 7.7% in the controls (nonsignificant). Premature rupture of membranes (PROM) was not seen significantly more frequently in the experimental group (27.1% vs. 26.5%). In this large controlled trial, there was no benefit or added risk from routine cervical examinations during the pregnancy. On the basis of the literature noted here, however, routine digital examinations of the cervix cannot be recommended. This statement does not preclude examination of patients with a history of incompetent cervix or patients with a cervical cerclage in place. Likewise, patients who complain of painful uterine contractions should undergo digital cervical examination.

DIAGNOSIS OF PRETERM LABOR

Despite the millions of dollars annually spent in the United States on biomedical research and clinical testing, the precise physiologic processes that lead to full-term births remain mysterious, and the physiology of preterm labor is even more poorly understood. Preterm labor is a clinical diagnosis made by the documentation of cervical changes with or without the presence of documented uterine contractions. It is commonly believed that tocolytic therapy is less effective with advanced cervical dilation, but it is also known that at least 25% to 75% of patients with regular preterm uterine contractions deliver at term without tocolytic therapy.[36,37] On the one hand, aggressive and early treatment of preterm labor with tocolytic agents may be more effective at reducing preterm delivery. This approach, however, results in the unnecessary exposure of many pregnant women and fetuses to the adverse side effects of tocolytic agents. Clinicians currently lack tools capable of differentiating

Table 18–1. Relative Risk of Premature Delivery, Based on Cervical Length at 24 and 28 Weeks' Gestation

Cervical Length	Relative Risk	95% Confidence Interval
24 Weeks		
40 mm, ≤75th percentile	1.98	1.20-3.27
35 mm, ≤50th percentile	2.35	1.42-3.89
30 mm, ≤25th percentile	3.79	2.32-6.19
26 mm, ≤10th percentile	6.19	3.84-9.97
22 mm, ≤5th percentile	9.49	5.95-15.15
13 mm, ≤1st percentile	13.99	7.89-24.78
28 Weeks		
40 mm, ≤75th percentile	2.80	1.41-5.56
35 mm, ≤50th percentile	3.52	1.79-6.92
30 mm, ≤25th percentile	5.39	2.82-10.28
26 mm, ≤10th percentile	9.57	5.24-17.48
22 mm, ≤5th percentile	13.88	7.68-25.10

$P < .001$ for values at or below the 50th percentile, and $P = .003$ for values at or below the 75th percentile.

true preterm labor from false preterm labor and therefore often administer treatment to patients who are not in true preterm labor. Risk factors associated with preterm labor are numerous and varied (see Fig. 18-1). Although tests exist to detect factors associated with preterm labor, they are inherently unreliable, predicting no more than 50% of cases of preterm deliveries.[38] Other studies have shown that dilation of the cervix may be a normal anatomic variation, particularly in multiparous patients, and that there is no significant increase risk of preterm delivery.[39-41] This practice leads to unnecessary hospitalization and the exposure of mothers and fetuses to potentially harmful pharmacologic side effects. A secondary effect is the increase in health care costs.

Preterm labor is almost certainly a multifactorial disease process whose common pathway includes uterine contractions, cervical changes, and/or PROM. The implementation of tocolytic treatment has focused on the gestational age range between 24 and 34 weeks, during which it is believed that reduction in the incidence of preterm birth has the greatest effect on neonatal morbidity and mortality.[42] The incidence of preterm birth increases with increasing gestational age, and there is a simultaneous change in the inciting mechanisms of preterm labor as pregnancy progresses. Between 24 and 29 weeks, infection of the maternal-fetal compartments is the most common cause of preterm labor.[43] After 29 weeks, most preterm labor is either idiopathic or iatrogenic (delivery is indicated to reduce either maternal or fetal jeopardy). The majority of clinical trials of tocolytic efficacy, however, have dealt with the onset of labor during this period because of the larger incidence of preterm labor and births at this time during gestation. Thus, the literature largely reflects studies of premature labor between 29 and 34 weeks, which is most commonly idiopathic preterm labor.

Preterm labor is clearly multifactorial in origin; however, for the sake of discussion, it is possible to classify this disease into two pathways: the intrinsic (or idiopathic) and the extrinsic. The intrinsic classification should be used when it is not possible to identify causative factors before, during, or after the preterm birth. It is possible that many intrinsic premature births may, in fact, be the result of external disease factors that clinicians do not yet have the clinical sophistication to identify and diagnose. It is known, for example, that erroneous external signals (e.g., hormonal, neural) may reach the uterus and initiate preterm labor.[44] In most instances, these changes lead to either a decrease in uterine resistance to contractility, an increase in contractile stimulation, or both. The uterus is simply responding to these signals by preparing for delivery, albeit prematurely. The internal control signals reach the uterus and initiate and increase uterine activity. These contractions initiate cervical changes and result in active labor (Fig. 18-1).

The extrinsic pathway is characterized by events associated with overt and clinically detectable events within the gravid uterus itself. This pathway is exemplified by premature separation of the placenta, chorioamnionitis, and overdistention of uterine size or shape. These pathologic conditions are often detectable before the onset of contractions within the uterus. Treatment of many of the conditions in the extrinsic pathway may be relatively contraindicated, and the likelihood of a significant reduction in preterm birth within this group is limited at best.

TESTS FOR THE DIAGNOSIS OF PRETERM LABOR

Digital Cervical Examinations

Painless dilation of the cervix may represent cervical incompetence, preterm labor, or, more commonly, normal anatomic changes of pregnancy. The use of cervical dilation as a predictor of preterm birth has been studied by many groups.[45-49] The cervical examinations were performed as early as 20 to 24 weeks and were performed at selected times throughout the pregnancy. The positive predictive value of cervical dilation has ranged between 6% and 28%, and these changes present a twofold to fourfold increase in preterm delivery when cervical dilation is noted. There is variation in findings by clinical examiners, and the reproducibility of the digital cervical examination has therefore been poor. Because there must be significant dilation in the cervix before the clinicians can confirm these changes, there is less chance that tocolytic therapy will actively prevent premature delivery.

Sonographic Cervical Examination

One theory as to why digital cervical examinations lack positive predictive value for the diagnosis of preterm labor is that there is great individual variability in the digital cervical examination between clinicians. There is consistency between examiners when the cervix is dilated more than 3 cm but almost no consistency in measurements less than 3 cm or in assessment of cervical effacement.[50] For cervical examinations to be useful as predictors

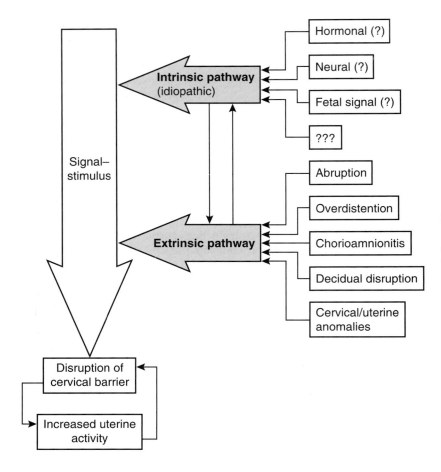

Figure 18–1. The two pathways of preterm labor. *(From Abrahams C, Katz M: A perspective on the diagnosis of preterm labor. J Perinat Neonat Nurs 16[1]:1-11, 2002.)*

of preterm labor, a more consistent method of cervical measurements must be developed. Zador and colleagues first reported on the use of ultrasonography to assess cervical length in 1976.[51] In this study of active labor, spring-loaded clips containing a piezoelectric crystal were replaced on the internal and external os of the cervix, and ultrasonography was used to measure the distance between the clips in order to assess shortening of the cervix. The first study to determine normal cervical length was performed by Zemlyn in 1981.[52] Although this study was designed to be an evaluation of the use of ultrasonography to predict placenta previa, it was noted that the average cervix measured between 2.5 and 3.0 cm. There has been debate as to whether transabdominal or transvaginal ultrasonography provides the best measurements of cervical length. One of the first investigators to compare transabdominal ultrasonography with transvaginal ultrasonography of the cervix was Andersen in 1991.[53] In the discussion of this article, Andersen advocated the sole use of transvaginal evaluation of the cervix because the proximity of the optimal focal length allowed close inspection of the cervical canal. The transvaginal ultrasound examination eliminated the bladder as a confounding variable and made evaluation of cervical length possible in almost all patients.

Unfortunately, the majority of articles that have attempted to assess cervical length measurements in the prediction of preterm labor have been limited by low patient numbers, bias in patient selection, and absence of statistical significance. The Maternal-Fetal Medicine National Institutes of Health Network in 1996 (Preterm Prediction Trial) conducted a study in which a large number of patients were included to overcome many of these criticisms.[54] In this study, the researchers evaluated the cervical length of 2915 women at 24 weeks of pregnancy and then 2531 of the same women at 28 weeks. These women were not at risk for preterm delivery and were selected from the routine obstetric populations at 10 university centers. The mean cervical length at 24 weeks' gestation was 34.0 ± 7.8 mm for nulliparous women and 36.1 ± 8.4 mm in parous women. The mean cervical length at 28 weeks of pregnancy was 32.6 ± 8.1 mm for nulliparous women and 34.5 ± 8.7 mm for parous women. Women with values at or below a particular percentile for cervical length at 24 weeks were compared with those who had cervical length values above the 75th percentile (see Table 18-1).

Table 18-1 shows that there is a significant relationship between a decrease in the cervical length below the 75th percentile and an increasing relative risk of preterm labor

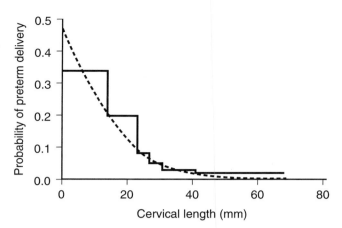

Figure 18–2. Estimated probability of spontaneous preterm delivery before 35 weeks' gestation from the logistic regression analysis *(dashed line)* and the observed frequency of spontaneous preterm delivery *(solid line)* according to the cervical length measured by transvaginal ultrasonography at 24 weeks' gestation. *(From Iams JD, Goldenberg RL, Meis PJ, et al: The length of the cervix and the risk of spontaneous premature delivery. National Institute of Child Health and Human Development Maternal-Fetal Medicine Unit Network. N Engl J Med 334:569, 1996. By permission of Massachusetts Medical Society.)*

and delivery. In Figure 18-2, it is evident that there is a flattening of the risk for preterm delivery at 30 mm. Before this measurement, there is a steep upward trend in the risk for delivery as the cervical measurement decreases.

Figure 18-2 shows the results of transvaginal ultrasound measurements at 24 weeks and the probability of preterm

delivery before 35 weeks, in which the estimated probability of preterm delivery from the logistic regression analysis was used. At approximately 30 mm, there is a flattening of the curve, and women with a cervical length of 30 mm had a 6.19 relative risk for preterm delivery, in comparison with women with a cervical length of 40 mm (75th percentile).

In Figure 18-3, the relative risk of preterm delivery in comparison to the cervical length measurements is plotted in millimeters. It is clear from this figure that as cervical length decreases, the relative risk of preterm birth increases significantly. It is interesting to note that there was no value of cervical length for which there was no risk of premature delivery or below which the probability of preterm birth is 100%. The logistic regression analysis indicated that for each increase of 1 mm in cervical length, the odds ratio for preterm delivery was 0.91 (95% CI = 0.89 to 0.93). A change in cervical length between the 24- and 28-week visits had a small but significant association with the risk of preterm delivery that was independent of the initial cervical length. Among the 56.3% of subjects whose cervix decreased in length between 24 and 28 weeks, the rate of preterm delivery was 4.2%, in comparison with 2.1% among those whose cervix did not decrease in length (relative risk = 2.03; 95% CI = 1.28 to 3.22). This study confirms the work of others that decreased cervical length measurements made by transvaginal ultrasonography are correlated with an increased probability of preterm birth.[53,55]

In addition to cervical length and measurements, the presence or absence of funneling was also evaluated in the preterm prediction trial. In that study, there were 185 subjects at 24 weeks (6.3%) and 232 subjects at 28 weeks (9.2%) whose cervix had a funnel at the internal cervical

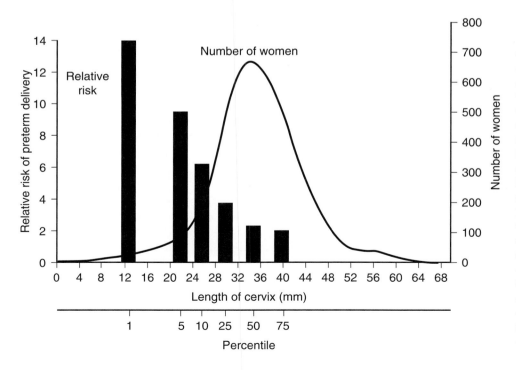

Figure 18–3. Distribution of patients *(solid line)* among percentiles for cervical length by transvaginal ultrasonography at 24 weeks' gestation and the relative risk *(bars)* for spontaneous preterm delivery before 35 weeks' gestation according to percentiles for cervical length. The risks among women with values at or below the 1st, 5th, 10th, 25th, 50th, and 75th percentiles for cervical length are compared with the risk among women with values above the 75th percentile. *(From Iams JD, Goldenberg RL, Meis PJ, et al: The length of the cervix and the risk of spontaneous premature delivery. National Institute of Child Health and Human Development Maternal Fetal-Medicine Unit Network. N Engl J Med 334(9):569, 1996. By permission of Massachusetts Medical Society.)*

os on ultrasound examination, a finding reported to indicate an increased risk of premature delivery.[56] Although funneling in this study was also associated with increased risk of preterm delivery—at 24 weeks, the relative risk was 5.02 (95% CI = 3.53 to 7.15) and at 28 weeks, the relative risk was 4.78 (95% CI = 3.18 to 7.19)—there was great variation in the incidence of reporting of funneling across the 10 centers. This led the investigators to believe that there was inconsistency in the definition of funneling between centers and raised the question of the clinical usefulness of this measurement.

BIOCHEMICAL MARKERS

Fetal Fibronectin Testing

Fetal fibronectin collected from vaginal swabs has been used as a screening test for preterm delivery. Elevated levels of fetal fibronectin may reflect the separation of the fetal membranes from maternal deciduas.[57] In a low-risk population screen between 22 and 24 weeks, a positive fetal fibronectin test result had a 13% predictive value for spontaneous preterm delivery before 28 weeks and a 36% prediction for delivery before 37 weeks.[58] In 1998, Iams and associates combined the use of fetal fibronectin, cervical length, and obstetric history to determine the risk for preterm delivery (Table 18-2).[59] Of importance is that patients with a positive fetal fibronectin result, a history of preterm birth, and a cervical length of less than 25 mm had only a 64% chance of premature delivery. This test may be most useful in limiting unnecessary hospitalizations. A negative fetal fibronectin result is highly predictive that preterm delivery will not occur within 7 days of testing,[60-63] but a positive fetal fibronectin result does not appear to be highly predictive of preterm birth (see Table 18-2).

Salivary Estriol Testing

Serum estrogen levels have been shown to increase before parturition in both animal and human studies.[64,65] Saliva has been shown to be an easily collectible source for measurement of hormones in pregnancy, and these salivary hormone values closely reflect serum levels. Darne and colleagues at the University College Hospital in London first documented an increase in salivary estriol in samples collected from pregnant women longitudinally during pregnancy.[66] Because pregnant women often have ptyalism, it is easy to collect a 1-mL specimen of saliva. Ninety percent of the estriol in saliva is unconjugated, and intraindividual and intersample variations are quite small.[67] The samples are stable at room temperature and can be collected and mailed to reference laboratories without fear of degradation of the sample. Administration of glucocorticoids has been shown to reduce salary estriol to levels 23% lower than pretreatment values for at least 1 week after administration.[68]

McGregor and associates first studied salivary estriol testing longitudinally on 241 women without symptoms and risk of preterm labor.[69] Weekly salivary estriol analyses were performed from 22 weeks until delivery. The authors noted a surge in serum estriol levels approximately 3 weeks before delivery in both full-term and preterm patients. Overall, this level yielded a sensitivity of 71% and a specificity of 77% in predicting preterm labor. In the low-risk group, according to the Creasy score, serial salivary estriol testing was found to have a sensitivity of 92%, a specificity of 74%, a false-positive rate of 26%, and a negative predictive value of 95% for premature labor (Fig. 18-4).

In a larger, more definitive follow-up study, McGregor and associates[70] performed a triple-blind multicenter trial to examine the performance of weekly (from 22 weeks onward) salivary estriol measurements in asymptomatic women with singleton pregnancies judged to be at low risk or high risk (by the Creasy score). The outcome assessed was onset of labor followed by preterm delivery. A single positive salivary estriol test result, defined as 2.1 ng/dL or higher, followed 1 week later by a confirmatory positive test result, yielded a sensitivity of 40%, a specificity of 93%, a positive predictive value of 19%, and a negative predictive value of 97% (Table 18-3).

Table 18–2. Fetal Fibronectin and Risk for Preterm Birth

| | History of Delivery (%) | | | |
Cervical Length	At 18-26 Weeks	At 27-31 Weeks	At 32-36 Weeks	At ≥37 Weeks
Fetal fibronectin negative				
≤25 mm	25	25	25	6
26-35 mm	14	14	13	3
>35 mm	7	7	7	1
Fetal fibronectin positive				
≤25 mm	64	64	63	25
26-35 mm	46	45	45	14
>35 mm	28	28	27	7

This table incorporates information from the most recent previous pregnancy, fetal fibronectin status, and cervical length at 24 weeks' gestation to predict the risk for preterm birth before 35 weeks' gestation in the current pregnancy. Risk for preterm birth is given as a percentage.

Adapted from Iams JD, Goldenberg RL, Mercer BM, et al: The Preterm Prediction Study: Recurrence risk of spontaneous preterm birth. Am J Obstet Gynecol 178:1035, 1998.

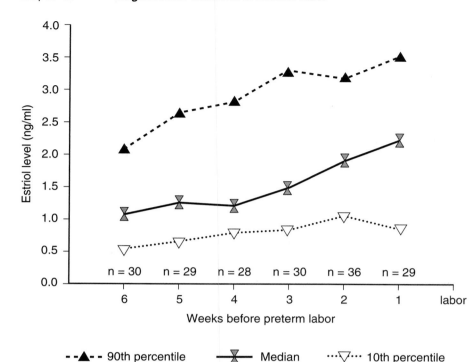

Figure 18–4. Highest weekly saliva estriol levels in women with a single fetus and preterm labor, independent of delivery. *(From McGregor JA, Jackson M, Lachelin GCL, et al: Salivary estriol as risk assessment for preterm labor: A prospective trial. Am J Obstet Gynecol 173:1337, 1995.)*

In another study by Robertson and coworkers, the use of salivary estriol as a predictor of preterm birth was tested on 145 women presenting with signs and symptoms of preterm labor.[71] When a threshold of 2.1 ng/dL was used, the following was observed: a positive predictive value of 57% and a negative predictive value of 88% for delivery in less than 7 days, and a positive predictive value of 64% and a negative predictive value of 85% for delivery in less than 14 days. A prospective pilot analysis of serial salivary estriol used in 53 twin pregnancies yielded the same receiver-operator curve analytic threshold level as did singleton pregnancies (2.1 ng/dL).[72]

As with fetal fibronectin, the clinical usefulness of salivary estriol appears to be its negative predictive value. Through the use of salivary estriol testing, patients' fears may be alleviated and prolonged hospital stays avoided. For women with a positive test result, more intense surveillance and implementation of treatment modalities are merited. Currently, there is a 24-hour turnaround time for the salivary estriol assay, and the lack of rapid testing has limited the widespread application of this modality. Because fetal fibronectin testing is now available at the bedside, this biochemical assay has gained greater clinical acceptance.

Table 18–3. Test Characteristics of Salivary Estriol for Prediction of Preterm Birth

Clinical Presentation and No. of Patients	Delivery Interval (days)	Sensitivity (%)	Specificity (%)	Positive Predictive Value (%)	Negative Predictive Value (%)
Women with symptoms*					
145	<7	33[†]	95[†]	57	88
145	≤14	31[†]	96[†]	64	85
Women without symptoms‡					
At low risk: 508	<36	42	93	14	98
At high risk: 218	<36	39	90	26	94
All: 726	<36	40	93	19	97

*Adapted from Heine RP, McGregor JA, Goodwin TM, et al: Serum salivary estriol to detect an increased risk of preterm birth. Obstet Gynecol 96:490, 2000.
†Calculation from published data.
‡Adapted from McGregor JA, Jackson M, Lachelin GCL, et al: Salivary estriol as risk assessment for preterm labor: A prospective trial. Am J Obstet Gynecol 173:1337, 1995. Reported values are for the predictive accuracy of a single salivary estriol ≥ 2.1 ng/mL, followed by a confirmatory retest.

From Mozurkewich E, Hayashi R: Biochemical markers of preterm birth. Postgrad Obstet Gynecol 20:4, 2000.

Other Biochemical Markers of Preterm Labor

Several biochemical markers have been associated with preterm delivery, including activin, inhibin, follistatin,[73,74] fibronectin,[57,58,75] collagenase,[76] and tissue inhibitors of metalloproteinases.[77] To date, only fibronectin has been used in a screening test for preterm delivery.

ELECTROMECHANICAL DETECTION OF UTERINE ACTIVITY

Ambulatory Uterine Monitoring

It has been known that uterine activity occurs sporadically throughout pregnancy and increases in the third trimester.[78] Although both full-term and preterm patients may exhibit an increase in the frequency of uterine activity, fewer than 25% of patients delivering prematurely exhibit an increase in contractions before delivery.[79] The uterine activity patterns of normal full-term labors span a broad range of frequencies, and arbitrary cutoff points do not appear to provide sufficient discrimination to prevent overdiagnosis of preterm labor.[57,80]

Most home uterine activity monitoring (HUAM) devices have been shown to be sensitive in the detection of uterine contraction frequency[81,82] but have failed to quantify the duration or amplitude of the contractions.[83] Quantification of contraction duration or frequency may be necessary to adequately predict the onset of labor. In a study by Paul and Smeltzer, monitoring with a guard ring–type surface transducer was compared directly with intrauterine pressure monitoring.[81] They found that the occurrences of uterine activity and quiescence were accurately noted by the guard ring device, but the intensity of uterine contractions was usually underestimated. It is not obvious that HUAM devices can quantify uterine activity to the level necessary to predict the onset of preterm labor.

From the start of the HUAM trials, there has been a question whether uterine activity monitoring or the frequent daily interactions with patient were most effective in reducing the incidence of preterm birth. In a large clinical trial by Dyson and associates, this question appeared to have been answered.[84] In this trial, the investigators found that the timing of delivery was unaffected by either the use of HUAM or by daily nursing contact, in comparison with maternal uterine self-palpation and weekly nursing contact. As might be anticipated, the patients receiving daily nursing contact or HUAM had a higher incidence of emergency room visits and subsequent admission and use of tocolytic agents. Unfortunately, the incidence of preterm births was not reduced as a result of these more intense interventions.

There have been six published meta-analyses of the major HUAM trials (Table 18-4).[85-90]

The designs of many of these trials varied according to the minimum number of HUAM transmissions daily, the timing of transmissions, the ability of patients to transmit more often, and the level of feedback provided by monitoring nurses. It is not clear that the individual studies before Dyson and associates' study[84] and the Collaborative Home Uterine Monitoring Study[90] had significant power to establish the value of HUAM for the prevention of preterm birth. These two large studies together contained more than twice as many enrollees as have the other studies to date. Because of the selection criteria that included hypothesis-driven design, precision in allocation, and tracking with intent to treat, both of these two studies are of the highest quality. The primary end point of most of these studies is to detect a difference in cervical dilation and diagnosis of preterm labor. This outcome would be meaningless if infant survival were not improved. As a general rule, the lack of preestablished uniform definitions of preterm labor or threshold for referral to hospitals produces heterogeneity in diagnosis and treatment protocols, which virtually ensure great diversity in the study populations. It appears that these inconsistencies make the blending of the different study populations a questionable exercise at best (Table 18-5).

The critical question regarding the use of HUAM is whether the earlier diagnosis of preterm labor can lead to reduction in the incidence of preterm birth. The information in Table 18-5, as well as the cumulative meta-analyses of the high-quality studies, lead us to believe that the early diagnosis does not in fact lead to reduction in preterm birth. This failure may be the result of many factors; however, the most obvious must be the lack of demonstrated efficacy of tocolytic agents.[91] Although early studies have demonstrated a beneficial effect of HUAM, more recent, well-controlled trials have not identified any clinical benefit. It is possible that HUAM devices may offer limited benefit to select segments of the population who reside a great distance from their caregivers or

Table 18–4. Critical Analyses of Home Uterine Activity Monitoring

Report	Number of Studies	Earlier Detection of Preterm Labor	Lower Rate of Preterm Birth
Sachs et al (1991)[87]	7	Yes	Not consistent
Grimes and Schultz (1992)[86]	5	NA	No
McLean et al (1993)[89]	5	Yes	Yes
USPSTF (1993)[88]	7	Yes	Not consistent
Keirse (1995)[223]	5	Yes	Yes
Colton et al (1995)[85]	6	Yes	Yes

NA, not available; USPSTF, U.S. Preventive Services Task Force.

Table 18–5. Summary of Selected Prospective Trials of Home Uterine Activity Monitoring

Trial	Gestation Age (wk) at PTL (Monitor/Control)	Rate of PTL (%) (Monitor/Control)	PTB*
Katz et al (1983)[225]	28/31	51/45	.29
Iams et al (1988/90)[79]	—	36/34	.92
Morrison (1990)[†]	28/29	71/67	.32
Hill (1990)[‡]	—	43/36	.76
Dyson (1991)[§]	29/29	34/34	1.18
			.77[‖]
Mou (1991)[¶]	33/33	25/24	.59
Wapner (1995)**	33/33	24/22	—
CHUMS (1995)[90]	32/32	24/24	1.06
			.94[‖]
Dyson et al (1998)[84]	31/31	22/27	1.0/1.0

*Odds ratios for PTBs at <37 weeks.

†Morrison JC, Pittman KP, Martin RW, McLaughlin BN: Cost/health effectiveness of home uterine activity monitoring in a Medicaid population. Obstet Gynecol 76(1 Suppl):76S-81S. 1990.

‡Hill WC, Fleming AD, Martin RW, et al: Home uterine activity monitoring is associated with a reduction in preterm birth. Obstet Gynecol 76(1 Suppl)L\:13S-18S, 1990.

§Dyson DC, Crites Y, Ray D: Home monitoring of uterine activity. N Engl J Med 326:1223, 1992.

‖Odds ratios for PTBs at <37 weeks in twins only.

¶Mou SM, Sunderji SG, Gall S, et al. Multicenter randomized clinical trial of home uterine activity monitoring for detection of preterm labor. Am J Obstet Gynecol 165(Pt 1):858-66, 1991.

**Wapner RJ, Cotton DB, Artal R, et al: A randomized multicenter trial assessing a home uterine activity monitoring device used in the absence of daily nursing contact. Am J Obstet Gynecol 172:1026-34, 1995.

CHUMS, collaborative home uterine monitoring study group; PTB, preterm birth; PTL, preterm labor.

possibly in pregnancies with high-order multiple gestations. It is doubtful that this clinical device should be applied routinely for at-risk populations.

Electromyographic Signals

Proper diagnosis of labor is one of the major challenges faced by obstetricians. There are no accurate or completely objective methods to predict the onset of labor, differentiate true and false labor both for full-term and preterm patients, and determine whether false labor will progress to true labor within a certain time. At present, the progress of labor is monitored by recording the changes in the cervical state and by measuring the rate, duration, and amplitude of uterine contraction with the tocodynamometer or the intrauterine pressure catheter. Because of the poor predictive power of the tocodynamometer and the invasive nature of the intrauterine pressure catheter, neither technique has been beneficial in the prediction of preterm labor or the diagnosis of true labor at term. Unwanted hospital stays and treatment could be avoided if physicians were able to differentiate more objectively between true labor and false labor.

In order to understand the mechanism of labor, many studies have been conducted to record the electrical activity of the uterus in humans and animals with both internal electrodes and abdominal surface electrodes.[78,92-98] The electrical activity of the uterine contraction results from the generation and transmission of action potentials in the myometrial cells of the uterine muscle. The electrical activity arising from these cells excites the neighboring cells because they are coupled by electronic synapses called *gap junctions*. Garfield and colleagues and others have shown that the gap junctions are sparse throughout pregnancy but increase during labor in various species.[99-104] It was also observed that these gap junctions disappeared within 24 hours of delivery. The increase in the gap junction number and their electrical transmission provides better coupling between the cells and results in synchronization and coordination of the contractile events in the uterus. These studies show that the propagation of the electrical activity over the entire uterus from the increase in gap junction area at term is related to successful progress of labor and delivery of the fetus.[105] Buhimschi and colleagues performed simultaneous recording of electromyographic (EMG) activity directly from the uterus and abdominal surface of rats.[97] They proved that the EMG activity recorded from the rat's abdominal surface mirrors the activity generated in the uterus. In a further human study in which electrodes were placed on the maternal abdomen, they showed that it is possible to use surface EMG activity to follow the evolution of uterine contractility during pregnancy.[106] Using fast Fourier transform spectral analysis, it was observed that the uterine EMG bursts in patients during active labor peaked at a frequency of 0.71 ± 0.05 Hz, whereas in nonlaboring full-term patients, the peak was around 0.48 ± 0.03 Hz. Also, the peak amplitude values were lower for patients not in labor than for patients in active labor. Some of the earlier studies[78,98] actually reported the existence of two types of frequencies relating to bursts of EMG activity: the slow wave (<0.1 Hz), lasting a few seconds with an amplitude of about 5 mV, and a superimposed fast wave (0.3 to 2.0 Hz) with an amplitude of 50 μV. These observations indicate that frequency content and the amplitude of an EMG burst could be a valuable parameter to track the changes in uterine activity during pregnancy and through labor.

Although widely studied for decades, uterine EMG signals have yet to be used routinely in clinics for assessing or identifying uterine contractions. In order to develop this technique as a clinical tool for better diagnosis of labor, clinicians must first extract and display the information contained in the EMG burst activity. The key parameters that need to be extracted to characterize an EMG burst are time, frequency, and amplitude. Except for one study on rats,[6] most studies in the past have used the standard fast Fourier transform to analyze the frequency information contained in the uterine EMG signals. Although this is a very effective technique for extracting the frequency content of the signal, it is obtained at the cost of losing time information contained in the original signal. In other words, fast Fourier transform analysis reveals the spectral content of the signal without any information on when it occurs. For EMG monitoring to become a widely useful clinical tool the effectiveness for diagnosis of preterm labor or labor at term must be demonstrated. Although it has been widely demonstrated that EMG signals in patients before labor differ from those in patients in labor, a transition state has not yet been well described or clinically demonstrated. In addition, no instruments capable of displaying this information in a meaningful fashion for clinicians are commercially available.

Magnetomyography: Measurement of Magnetic Activity

All electrophysiologic phenomena are characterized by the flow of ion currents within the body. These currents are, of course, detectable by measuring potentials inside or on the surface of the body. According to the physics of electromagnetism, the flow of current will also result in a magnetic field. Consequently, common clinical electrophysiologic measurements such as the electrocardiogram, electroencephalogram, and electromyogram have magnetic homologues: the magnetocardiogram, the magnetoencephalogram, and the magnetomyogram, respectively.[1,107] Eswaran and coworkers[108] showed that it is possible to noninvasively record the magnetic field corresponding to uterine electrophysiologic activity. The advantage of performing these magnetic field recordings is that they are much less dependent on tissue conductivity, and the signals are detectable outside the boundary of the skin without the need for electrical contact with the body. Unlike electrical recordings, the magnetic recordings are independent of any kind of reference, thus ensuring that each sensor mainly records localized activity. These magnetomyographic recordings were performed with a 151-channel magnetic field sensor array called SARA (SQUID [superconducting quantum interference device] Array for Reproductive Assessment). SARA (Fig. 18-5) is a passive device that records tiny magnetic field fluctuations generated by flow of current in the human body.

With the SARA instrument, it has been demonstrated that it is possible to determine the regions of localized activation (Fig. 18-6), propagation velocity, and direction and the spread of uterine electrophysiologic activity as a function of distance. Currently, SARA is a research tool and, with further development, could potentially be a clinical tool for predicting the onset of full-term labor and the presence of preterm labor.

INFECTIONS AND PREMATURE DELIVERY

Preterm labor and PROM account for 80% of all preterm births. The remaining 20% are medically indicated deliveries for maternal or fetal reasons.[109] The possible association between preterm birth and an infectious process was defined as early as 1940.[110] There is increasing evidence that urinary tract infections, intrauterine infections, and bacterial vaginosis are associated with an increase risk of spontaneous preterm delivery.[111-115] Infants born prematurely as a result of a maternal infectious process may have infection themselves, in addition to the complications of prematurity.[116,117] The proposed mechanism of infection leading to preterm birth is the ascension of

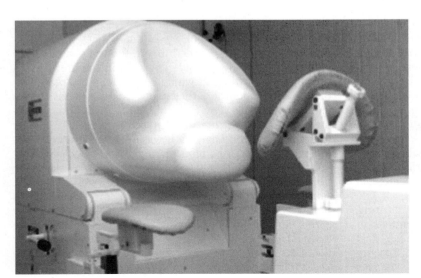

Figure 18–5. A view of the 151-channel SARA (SQUID [superconducting quantum interference device] Array for Reproductive Assessment) system with sensor array built to match the shape of a gravid abdomen.

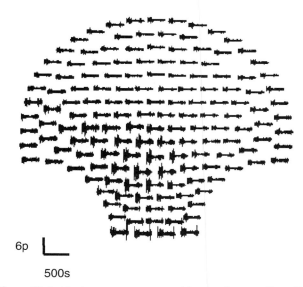

6p

500s

Figure 18–6. Uterine magnetomyographic signals recordings from 151 channels with strong uterine activity seen in the lower left side of the abdomen.

microorganisms from the cervix or vagina into the uterine cavity and the subsequent infection of the fetal membranes and decidua. Once the organisms gain access to the uterine cavity, they invade the amniotic sac and release lipopolysaccharides and other toxins that recruit monocytes and mononuclear phagocytes. Cytokines are released by the monocytes and motor code phagocytes and lead to the release of prostaglandins, which results in the subsequent preterm labor.[118,119]

Periodontal Disease and Preterm Labor

In 1996, Offenbacher and colleagues at the University of North Carolina reported a case-control study of 124 pregnant mothers that demonstrated a 7.5- to 7.9-fold increased risk for premature birth in mothers with severe periodontal disease.[120] It is theorized that the periodontal infections serve as reservoirs of gram-negative organisms, lipopolysaccharides, and inflammatory mediators that include prostaglandin E_2 and tissue necrosis factor, which may trigger a hormonal cascade that leads to preterm labor or PROM. In 1994, Collins and associates performed experiments with pregnant hamsters that demonstrated this reservoir model.[121] In a follow-up case control study by Offenbacher and colleagues, a dose-response relationship between maternal gingival circular fluid prostaglandin E_2 and decreasing birth weight was demonstrated.[122] More recently, a randomized controlled trial was performed on 400 women in Santiago, Chile, by Lopez and coworkers.[123] In this study, pregnant women with periodontal disease were randomly assigned to either a group receiving dental treatment before 28 weeks ($n = 200$) or a control group that received dental treatment only after delivery ($n = 200$). The primary end point was birth before 37 weeks or at a birth weight of less than 2500 g. The incidence of prematurity/low birth weight (PLBW) was 1.84% (3 of 163) in the treatment group and

10.11% (19 of 188), in the control group (odds ratio = 5.49; 95% CI = 1.65 to 18.22; $P = .001$). Multivariate logistic regression analysis showed that periodontal disease was the strongest factor related to PLBW (odds ratio = 4.70; 95% CI = 1.29 to 17.13). Other factors significantly associated with such deliveries were previous PLBW (odds ratio = 3.98; 95% CI = 1.11 to 14.21), fewer than six prenatal visits (odds ratio = 3.70; 95% CI = 1.46 to 9.38), and low maternal weight gain (odds ratio = 3.42; 95% CI = 1.16 to 10.03). The conclusion of this study was that periodontal disease significantly increases the risk of preterm birth and that treatment during pregnancy reduces the association with preterm birth.

In another study of periodontal disease and preterm labor, 69 mothers were selected: 13 were periodontally healthy, and 56 had varying stages of periodontal disease.[124] They and their newborns formed the study population. Presence and severity of periodontal disease were clinically determined with the Russell periodontal index. The nutritional evaluation of the newborns was determined by the Lubchenco modified growth pattern. A decrease in the average neonatal weight and gestational age was observed as the mother's level of periodontal disease increased. Correlation analysis demonstrated a highly significant clinical relationship between more severe periodontal disease and lower birth weight ($r = -0.49$; $P < .01$). A highly significant relationship was also clinically demonstrated between increasing periodontal disease severity and decreasing gestational age of the newborns ($r = -0.59$; $P < .01$). There were significant differences in the weight and gestational age of the newborns of mothers with periodontal disease. This study, along with the previously described studies, points out the probable association of periodontal disease, preterm labor, and low birth weight in infants.

Antibiotics and Preterm Labor Prevention

Many studies have attempted to evaluate the potential link between intrauterine infections and preterm labor. Evidence shows that cytokine release and the subsequent production of prostaglandins may lead to preterm contractions, weakening of the chorionic and amniotic membranes, and cervical softening and dilation. Once initiated, this cascade is difficult to stop. This association between preterm labor and infections has led to the theory that antibiotic therapy may be useful in the prevention of preterm birth.

Preterm birth may be prevented before the onset of labor by the prophylactic use of antibiotics to reduce the incidence of vaginal and cervical bacterial colonization. Bacterial vaginosis (*Gardnerella vaginalis*) and associated vaginal bacteria (e.g., *Mycoplasma hominis, Ureaplasma urealyticum*) have been correlated with preterm labor, preterm birth, chorioamnionitis, and low birth weight.[115] Identification of bacterial vaginosis as an isolated risk factor has created much controversy. The timing of treatment, the appropriate antibiotic selection, and whether treatment actually reduces prematurity and the rate of neonatal complications are the subjects of much debate. Gravett and coworkers[125] theorized in 1986 that vaginal bacterial could ascend through the cervix and infect the decidua, which would then lead to preterm labor and PROM. Bacterial vaginosis was found in vaginal fluid of 43% of their study population, and bacteria were cultured from amniotic fluid in 24% of amniocentesis specimens. They found that in women with preterm labor, bacterial vaginosis colonization of amniotic fluid was associated with a significantly shorter latency period, decreased success rate of parenteral tocolysis, and a significantly increased rate of intrapartum chorioamnionitis. Morales and associates[126] evaluated 80 patients with a history of spontaneous preterm birth or prolonged PROM in a previous pregnancy for the presence of bacterial vaginosis between 13 and 20 weeks' gestation. The women were randomly assigned to receive oral metronidazole (250 mg orally three times daily for 7 days) or placebo. This study concluded that after patients at risk were identified, oral antibiotics were significantly beneficial in reducing preterm labor, preterm birth, prolonged PROM, and low birth weight (<2500 g).

McGregor and associates[127] in 1994 and Joesoef and colleagues[128] in 1995 failed to demonstrate a reduction in perinatal morbidity by treatment of vaginosis with the use of clindamycin vaginal cream. These groups concluded that upper genitourinary tract infection must have occurred early in the process and that the use of systemic antibiotics would be necessary to produce a clinical effect. Hauth and coworkers performed a randomized, controlled study to evaluate the use of systemic antibiotics in the reduction of preterm birth.[129] Metronidazole and erythromycin were used in the treatment group ($n = 433$), and the control group ($n = 191$) was given a placebo. Overall, the investigators found a reduction in the incidence of preterm delivery from 36% to 26% with antibiotic treatment ($P = .01$). The correlation between treatment and a reduced incidence of preterm labor and delivery was significant only in the women with a positive bacterial vaginosis screen result at study entry. Of these 258 women, the preterm delivery rate was reduced from 49% to 31% with antibiotic treatment.

Prophylactic antibiotic therapy has not always been shown to be effective for reducing preterm birth in the asymptomatic patient. In a double-blind, placebo-controlled, randomized trial designed to evaluate the efficacy of metronidazole versus placebo treatment in asymptomatic patients infected with *Trichomonas* species, Carey and Klebanoff demonstrated an increased rate of preterm delivery in the antibiotic treatment group.[130] The investigators recommended that the asymptomatic patient infected with *Trichomonas* species not be treated with antibiotics. In a clinical trial by the National Institute of Child Health and Human Development Network of Maternal-Fetal Medicine Units, 1953 women who had no symptoms but had positive findings of bacterial vaginosis, were randomly assigned to receive 2 g of oral metronidazole or placebo.[131] All subjects were between 16 and 24 weeks pregnant. Diagnostic studies were repeated between 24 and 30 weeks, and a second treatment was administered, again double-blind. Preterm delivery occurred in 12.2% of the metronidazole recipients and in 12.5% of the placebo recipients (relative risk = 1.0; 95% CI = 0.8 to 1.2). Treatment did not prevent preterm

deliveries that resulted from spontaneous labor (5.1% in the metronidazole recipients vs. 5.7% in the placebo recipients) or spontaneous rupture of the membranes (4.2% vs. 3.7%), nor did it prevent delivery before 32 weeks (2.3% vs. 2.7%). Treatment with metronidazole did not reduce the occurrence of preterm labor, intraamniotic or postpartum infections, neonatal sepsis, or admission of the infant to the neonatal intensive care unit.

Antibiotic Treatment of Women in Preterm Labor

In 1991, using, a placebo-controlled trial with intravenous clindamycin, McGregor and associates[132] were unable to demonstrate that antibiotic therapy was effective in the treatment of preterm labor. This study did demonstrate pregnancy prolongation in women who had bacterial vaginosis. Stratification by gestation age showed that the largest interval to delivery occurred in those less than 33 weeks' gestation (40 days vs. 28 days; $P < .05$). In a three-arm study by Morales and associates,[133] ampicillin (500 mg orally every 6 hours), erythromycin (500 mg orally every 6 hours), or placebo was administered to individuals with a diagnosis of preterm labor (>1 cm at presentation). The antibiotics were administered for 10 days, regardless of culture results. This study was able to demonstrate a significant lengthening of the latency period in women administered either antibiotic regimen in relation to placebo (31.7 ± 23.2 days and 28.5 ± 19 days vs. 16.6 ± 17.7 days; $P < .01$ and $P < .05$, respectively). There was no demonstrated decrease in neonatal or maternal morbidity.

Newton and colleagues performed two studies of antibiotic treatment and prevention of preterm delivery in 1989[134] and 1991.[135] In the first study, the patients were randomly assigned to receive either (1) ampicillin, 2 g intravenously every 6 hours, followed by erythromycin, 333 mg orally every 8 hours for 1 week, or (2) a matching placebo. In a second study, either ampicillin with sulbactam (1 g every 6 hours for 3 days) or a matching placebo was administered. Magnesium sulfate, ritodrine, indomethacin, or a combination of these was used concomitantly to enhance pregnancy prolongation. No benefit was demonstrated with the use of antibiotics in the prevention of preterm delivery in either study.

A randomized, multicenter trial of antibiotic therapy for 275 patients in preterm labor, funded by the National Institute of Child Health and Human Development, was reported in 1993 by Romero and associates.[136] These patients received either intravenous ampicillin and erythromycin, followed by oral amoxicillin/erythromycin base, or a matching placebo regimen. This study also failed to demonstrate improvement in the latency period for preterm labor and delivery, and it did not demonstrate substantial decreases in maternal or neonatal morbidity rates in patients with antibiotic therapy.

Cox and coworkers investigated the use of antibiotics in patients not receiving tocolytic medications.[137] In a double-blind, placebo-controlled trial, patients were randomly assigned to receive ampicillin (2 g) and sulbactam (1 g), intravenously every 6 hours in eight doses), followed by amoxicillin–clavulanic acid (250 mg orally every 8 hours for 5 days), or placebo medications at the same time intervals as those receiving treatment. Seventy-eight participants between 24 and 34 weeks pregnant in preterm labor were involved in this study. As in other studies, there was no significant prolongation in the pregnancy, reduction in neonatal or maternal morbidity, or improvement in neonatal survival in the antibiotic-treated group.

McCaul and colleagues[138] performed a trial of antibiotic therapy for women with either preterm labor or prolonged PROM. One-hundred-eighty-seven patients were randomly assigned to receive ampicillin or placebo. Prolongation of the latency period was demonstrated only for the women with prolonged PROM (17.8 ± 27.0 days versus 8.1 ± 11.2 days; $P = .04$).

Svare and associates[139] published results of a trial in 1997 in which they examined ampicillin and metronidazole treatment in idiopathic preterm labor. In this multicenter, double-blind, placebo-controlled study, patients were randomly assigned to receive parenteral antibiotics (ampicillin, 2 g intravenously every 6 hours for 24 hours, and metronidazole, 500 mg intravenously every 8 hours for 24 hours), followed by oral antibiotics for 1 week (pivampicillin, 500 mg orally every 8 hours, and metronidazole, 400 mg orally every 8 hours) or a placebo regimen. With 112 participants, they were able to demonstrate a significant prolongation of pregnancy (47.5 days versus 27 days; $P < .05$), a decreased incidence of preterm birth (42% versus 65%; $P < .05$), and a lower rate of neonatal intensive care unit admissions (40% versus 63%; $P < .05$). They could not demonstrate improvement in maternal or neonatal infectious morbidity.

There have been many results from the use of antibiotic treatment of preterm labor. Although some studies have demonstrated the ability of antibiotics to prolong the pregnancy, no study has demonstrated a significant reduction in maternal or neonatal morbidity. There is great concern that the widespread use of antibiotics will produce an increase in the incidence of bacterial resistance, ultimately leading to even more devastating infections. In addition, there have been limited studies of antibiotic transfer into the fetal compartment, particularly the fetal brain. There is some concern that partial treatment of in utero infections could result in the prolongation of pregnancy but also in the continued exposure of the fetus to infection. At present, without further evidence that the antibiotic treatment significantly improves morbidity for the fetus or mother, antibiotic treatment in pregnancy for the treatment of preterm labor should be used with extreme reservation.

REGULATION OF UTERINE CONTRACTIONS

Parturition has been studied for many decades in animals, nonhuman primates, and humans, but despite this work, the mechanisms controlling uterine contractions in the human are not well understood. The exogenous hormones oxytocin and progesterone are known to be uterotonic agents; however, these hormones are unlikely to play the major role in the initiation of parturition. There are two differing hypotheses that provide a framework for understanding the initiation of labor.[140] The first major hypothesis is that the uterus is, by nature, quiescent and remains so until activated by external forces (perhaps oxytocin and prostaglandin $F_{2\alpha}$ and/or unknown factors from mother or fetus). Under this hypothesis, labor must be initiated. The second major hypothesis is that the uterus is by nature active and labor must be suppressed. Under this theory, to initiate labor, the suppression must be removed in order for the uterus to begin to contract. Nitric oxide has been shown to suppress uterine activity in vitro.[141-143]

The most commonly accepted mechanism for the initiation of a smooth muscle contraction involves an increase in intracellular calcium. The two major determinants of myometrial contractility are the intracellular calcium concentration and the activity of the calcium-dependent enzyme myosin light-chain kinase (MLCK).[144] The intracellular calcium either may be released from the endoplasmic reticulum or may enter the cell from external sources. The intracellular calcium ion (Ca^{2+}) concentration increases in response to agonist stimulation.[140] The resting intracellular concentration of calcium is between 50 to 150 nM, but during a contraction, there is a thousandfold increase in the concentration. The intracellular calcium binds with the protein calmodulin, and the complex binds to and thus activates MLCK. MLCK transfers the terminal phosphate from adenosine triphosphate (ATP) to the contractile protein myosin (Figs. 18-7 and 18-8).

Calcium binds with the protein calmodulin, and the complex binds to and thus activates MLCK, which transfers the terminal phosphate from ATP to one of two myosin light chains. The MLCK phosphorylation can be reversed by the action of a myosin light-chain phosphatase. The phosphorylation of myosin light chains increases the conformational association of actin and myosin, which results in hydrolysis of ATP by the myosin head region of the protein. The conformational changes that occur in a sequential manner as ATP is first hydrolyzed, followed by adenosine diphosphate and phosphate leaving their binding sites, result in movement of myosin on the actin filament. Many thousands of these events occur in unison, resulting in force generation by the tissue.

Stimulation of the β_2 receptor by a β_2-sympathomimetic agonist (ritodrine) activates adenylyl cyclase, resulting in accumulation of cyclic adenosine monophosphate (cAMP) and subsequent activation of cAMP-dependent protein kinase (cAMP-PK), which consists of two regulatory subunits bound to two catalytic subunits (Fig. 18-9). The binding of cAMP to the regulatory subunits causes the dissociation of the catalytic subunits, which are then capable of phosphorylating MLCK along with other cellular substrates. Once phosphorylated, MLCK is not able to interact with calcium-calmodulin and is incapable of phosphorylating the myosin light chains. This in turn results in the absence of myosin-actin interaction and subsequent relaxation of the smooth muscle. Actions of cyclic nucleotides such as cAMP can also lead

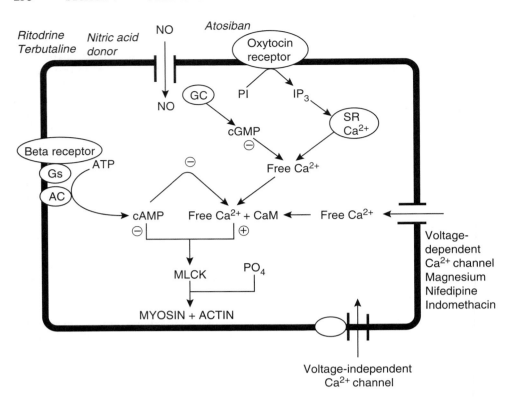

Figure 18–7. Mechanisms of myometrial contractility. See text for details. AC, adenylylate cyclase; ATP, adenosine triphosphate; Ca^{2+}, calcium ion; CaM, calmodulin; cAMP, cyclic adenosine monophosphate; cGMP, cyclic guanosine monophosphate; GC, guanylate cyclase; Gs, guanylyl nucleotide regulatory protein; IP_3, inositol triphosphate; MLCK, myosin light-chain kinase; NO, nitric oxide; PI, phosphatidylinositol; PO_4, phosphate.

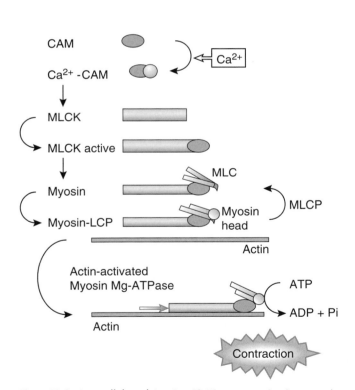

Figure 18–8. Intracellular calcium ion (Ca^{2+}) concentration increases in response to agonist stimulation. ADP, adenosine diphosphate; ATPase, adenosine triphosphatase; CAM, calmodulin; LCP, light-chain phosphate; Mg, magnesium; MLC, myosin light chain; MLCP, myosin light-chain phosphate; MLCK, myosin light-chain kinase; Pi, phosphatidylinositol.

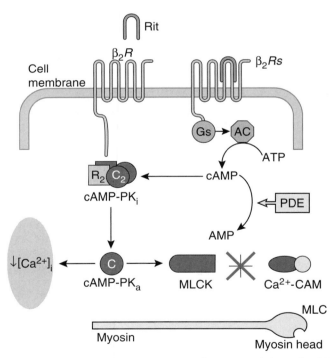

Figure 18–9. The β_2-adrenergic receptor (β_2R) is coupled to adenylyl cyclase (AC) by a trimeric stimulatory guanosine triphosphate-binding protein (Gs). AMP, adenosine monophosphate; ATP, adenosine triphosphate; C_2, catalytic subunit; $[Ca^{2+}]_i$, intracellular calcium ion; CAM, calmodulin; cAMP, cyclic adenosine monophosphate; MLC, myosin light chain; MLCK, myosin light-chain kinase; PDE, phosphodiesterase; PK_a, protein kinase a; PK_i, protein kinase i; R_2, regulatory subunit; Rit, ritodrine.

to decreased concentrations of intracellular Ca^{2+} that favor relaxation by lowering the activation state of MLCK.

The conformational change induced by the phosphorylation of the protein myosin increases the association with the protein actin. This new confirmation, together with the corresponding activation of the myosin Mg^+-ATPase and the hydrolysis of ATP, develops the mechanical force that serves as the energy required to generate force and cause the actin and myosin complex to move in relation to one another, which, in turn, results in cell shortening.[145] At a tissue level, the activated myosin protein slides along the actin and results in a significant shortening of the uterine cell. As all the smooth muscle cells shorten together, the uterine contraction is generated. The presence of a phosphatase (myosin light-chain phosphatase), potentially regulated by increased levels of cyclic nucleotides such as cAMP and cyclic guanosine monophosphate and by noncyclic nucleotide-dependent phosphorylation, causes removal of the phosphate from the myosin light chain, allowing the cell to relax. Further control of the uterine contraction is accomplished through the proteins calponin and caldesmon. These proteins normally inhibit the interaction between actin and myosin, but when phosphorylated, this inhibition is lost.[146] This system, referred to as *thin-filament regulation*, allows differing amounts of tension for one concentration of Ca^{2+} and may play a role in the maintenance of uterine quiescence during pregnancy. It may also be part of the mechanism of labor.[147]

It has been proposed that parturition be divided into four hypothetical phases: phase 0 (quiescent), phase 1 (activation), phase 2 (stimulation), and phase 3 (involution) (Fig. 18-10).[148,149] Phase 0 accounts for 95% of pregnancy. During this phase, uterine activity is suppressed through inhibitors, including progesterone, prostacyclin, relaxin, nitric oxide, parathyroid hormone–related peptide, corticotropin-releasing hormone, human placental lactogen, and calcitonin gene–related peptide.[38] Phase 1 accounts for about 5% of pregnancy, and during this phase, levels of uterotonic inhibitors decrease, whereas estrogens and contraction-associated proteins increase. Inhibition and control of important factors, including gap junction proteins (particularly connexin 43) and myometrial oxytocin receptors, are important; prostaglandin receptors (especially prostaglandin F receptors), calcium channels, and some sodium channels[150] are all increased. The maturation of the fetal hypothalamic-pituitary-adrenal system results in an increase in fetal and placental corticotropin-releasing hormones, which results in increased secretion of estrogens. These changes result in a significant alteration in the hormonal milieu of the pregnancy, and there is a marked increase in myometrial excitability. There is also an increase in responsiveness to uterotonic agents and, finally, in electrical coupling. This preparatory or activation phase requires coordination between the uterus, cervix and fetal membranes and involves the endocrine, immune, and neural control systems.[151,152]

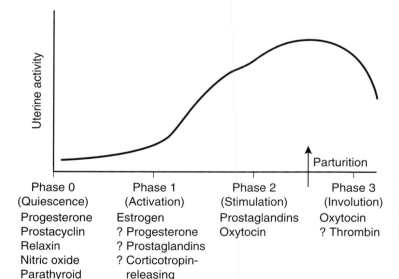

Figure 18–10. Regulation of uterine activity during pregnancy and labor. The regulation of uterine activity during pregnancy and labor can be divided into four distinct physiologic phases—quiescence, activation, stimulation, and involution—that are or may be influenced by a number of stimulatory and inhibitory factors. Question marks indicate a possible influence. (*Adapted from Challis JR, Lye SJ, Gibb W: Prostaglandins and parturition. Ann N Y Acad Sci 828:254, 1997.*)

MECHANISMS OF PRETERM LABOR

Lockwood and Kuczynski proposed a conceptual model of preterm labor in which there are four pathways: (1) maternal and fetal stress (activation of the maternal and fetal hypothalamic-pituitary-adrenal axis); (2) inflammatory pathway (decidual, chorioamnionic, or systemic tissue infections); (3) decidual hemorrhage; and (4) pathologic uterine distention.[153] Stress to the mother or fetus may activate the maternal fetal hypothalamic-pituitary-adrenal axis and result in preterm labor.[154,155]

Inflammation activates the cytokine system, leading to an increase in inflammatory factors and release of uterotonic substances.[156-159] Gomez and associates suggested that both preterm labor and PROM may be adaptive mechanisms that occur when the fetus is exposed to a hostile intrauterine environment such as infection.[158] If the infection results in production of uterotonic agents, preterm labor occurs, but if the response to the infection is the production of proteases, PROM may result. Placental hemorrhage activates a proteolytic cascade that can produce uterotonic agents and proteases. Overdistention of the uterus (polyhydramnios, multiple gestation, or overexpansion of the uterine cavity as a result of uterine anomalies) produces gap junctions, increases oxytocin receptors, produces prostaglandin synthesis, and activates cytokines.

PRETERM LABOR SUPPRESSION

Since 1960, a host of tocolytic therapies have become available for the treatment of preterm labor. All these therapies have been used despite the lack of a clear understanding of the causes of preterm labor or the long-term effects of the therapeutic interventions. To date, no therapy has demonstrated a reduction in perinatal mortality. There are still several fundamental questions that should be answered about tocolytic therapy:

1. Can preterm labor be accurately diagnosed?
2. Does treatment of preterm labor prolong pregnancy, reduce the incidence of preterm delivery, and increase actual birth weight?
3. Does treatment of preterm labor reduce perinatal morbidity and mortality?
4. What are the side effects for the mother and fetus, and does the benefit of treatment exceed the risk of exposure to the side effects of these powerful drugs?
5. How should new modalities such as prenatal steroids and surfactant therapy (which have improved neonatal survival) be used to modify preterm labor treatment strategies?

Although it is difficult to make the diagnosis of preterm labor, 50% of patients in controlled trials, treated with placebo therapy, go on to deliver at term. Generally accepted criteria for the diagnosis of preterm labor are (1) regular uterine contractions associated with cervical changes; (2) regular contractions and cervical dilation of at least 2 cm or effacement of 80% or more; or (3) regular contractions and effacement with ruptured membranes. Knowledge of biochemical markers such as fetal fibronectin and salivary estriol has enabled clinicians to withhold therapy for patients who lack these markers and can be used to limit the number of patients exposed to unnecessary treatment. To date, these tests have lacked positive predictive powers. Again, clinicians are often placed in the difficult position of balancing risk versus benefits of treatment with a test that has a high false-positive rate. It is possible that these biochemical tests may be combined with other, newer testing modalities such as cervical sonography and transabdominal electrophysiologic monitoring of the uterus to improve positive predictive values. Through this cross correlation of different testing modalities, it may be possible to improve the positive predictive value of the diagnosis of preterm labor and reduce unnecessary tocolytic therapy.

Answering the second question is more difficult. Large preterm labor prevention studies have shown that prolongation of gestation can be safely accomplished for only 24 to 48 hours. Prolongation of labor beyond this period has not been readily demonstrated, and there is dispute regarding the true efficacy of tocolysis. There is no evidence that tocolytic therapy has resulted in an increase in gestational age at delivery or improvements in birth weights of infants of patients receiving this therapy. Also, there is little proof that these therapies are effective in significantly prolonging the pregnancy beyond this short window of suppression. Likewise, there is no information to support the belief that tocolytic therapy has had a major effect on improving neonatal morbidity and mortality.

Most tocolytic agents produce side effects that can be potentially dangerous in the mother and, to a certain extent, the fetus. Therefore, the issue of benefit versus risk should always be weighed when the use of tocolytic agents is considered. Patient care must be individualized, and consultation with neonatology colleagues must be sought. Gestational age or estimated fetal weight can be used as a guide to decide whether to institute tocolytic therapy. In most major perinatal centers, nondiabetic patients 34 to 35 weeks pregnant or in whom estimated fetal weights exceed 2500 g are not empirically treated with tocolytic agents to prolong gestation, inasmuch as the perinatal survival rate at that gestational age is virtually 100%.

In view of these statements and findings, it seems that the focus should be on improving the diagnosis of preterm labor and limiting the unnecessary exposure of patients to the potential toxic side effects of these agents. Aggressive treatment of premature infants has resulted in improvement in neonatal survival of infants of gestational ages exceeding 28 weeks. The improvements in survival of these older infants should allow clinicians to focus on treatment of preterm labor in pregnancies in which the fetus is not as close to term. It is in this group of infants that tocolytic therapy may have better benefit-to-risk ratios.

Before initiation of tocolytic therapy, the following prerequisites should be met:

1. A diagnosis of preterm labor.
2. A gestational age of more than 23 weeks but less than 34 weeks.

3. An absence of medical and obstetric contraindications to labor suppression.

Absolute contraindications to labor suppression are as follows:

1. Intrauterine fetal demise.
2. Fetal anomalies incompatible with survival.
3. Fetal distress.
4. Severe intrauterine growth restriction.
5. Intrauterine infection.
6. Severe maternal hemorrhage.
7. Eclampsia or severe preeclampsia.

Relative contraindications to labor suppression are as follows:

1. Mild chronic hypertension.
2. Mild abruptio placentae.
3. Stable placenta previa.
4. Maternal cardiac disease.
5. Hyperthyroidism.
6. Uncontrolled diabetes mellitus.
7. Fetal distress.
8. Fetal anomaly.
9. Mild growth retardation.
10. Cervix more than 5 cm dilated.

As noted, the false-positive diagnosis of preterm labor is common, and as many as 50% to 70% of patients with the clinical diagnosis of preterm labor are delivered at term.[160] It is also important to note that at least 18% of women seen for evaluation of preterm labor who are discharged without treatment later return to deliver prematurely.[161] Many of the signs and symptoms of preterm labor are very nonspecific. Patients may report symptoms of pubic pressure, increased vaginal discharge, backache, and mild cramping. Because tocolytic therapy poses significant risk to the mother and fetus, it is important to use more objective criteria to make the diagnosis of preterm labor. Reasonable criteria for the diagnosis of preterm labor include documented uterine contractions (four in 20 minutes for 1 to 2 hours), intact membranes with documented cervical change, cervical effacement of 80%, or cervical dilation of more than 2 cm.[162]

Goals of Preterm Labor Suppression

Methods designed to identify women at risk for preterm labor and to intervene with preventive measures have largely been unsuccessful. The success of screening programs that use risk scoring indices, HUAM, ultrasound evaluation of cervical length, serial digital cervical examinations, fetal fibronectin testing, and salivary estriol testing depends on effective therapies to prevent preterm delivery once the diagnosis has been made. Without effective clinical treatment measures, even the screening programs that are highly successful in identifying women at risk for preterm birth do not successfully reduce the preterm delivery rate. Morbidity rates decrease with each week of increasing gestational age, but severe mortality remains significantly elevated in the infants born before 28 weeks' gestation.[163] Although rates of patent ductus arteriosus, intraventricular hemorrhage,

and necrotizing enterocolitis significantly decline after 32 weeks' gestational age, respiratory distress syndrome continues to occur up until 36 weeks.[164]

It is clear that parturition begins long before the clinically detectable signs and symptoms of labor. The process of labor is heralded by the appearance of myometrial gap junctions, enhanced myometrial contractility, changes in cervical collagens and matrix, and the appearance of oxytocin receptors. With the introduction of antenatal glucocorticoid therapy, the introduction of surfactant therapy to reduce neonatal respiratory distress syndrome, and significant improvements in neonatal intensive care nursery survival statistics, the traditional clinical goals of preterm labor suppression have been significantly altered. In view of the neonatal benefit from antenatal administration of corticosteroids, a main goal of tocolytic therapy is to prolong delivery for 24 to 48 hours.[165] Most tocolytic agents have been able to accomplish this short-term goal. A second but equally important short-term goal of suppression therapy is to prevent delivery long enough to allow transfer of the mother to the tertiary care facility, where a higher level of neonatal care is available. The acute management of the extremely premature infant is crucial to preventing long-term morbidity and mortality. Infants born in facilities lacking capabilities for immediate resuscitation of severely premature infants do not fare as well as those born in tertiary care centers.

Mechanisms of Preterm Labor Suppression

Bed Rest and Hydration

There is no evidence to support the use of bed rest in the treatment of preterm labor.[157,166] The use of bed rest in the treatment of twin pregnancies has been more extensively studied than that for the singleton pregnancy. These studies showed no reduction in the incidence of preterm labor; in fact, one study showed a higher incidence of preterm birth in the women routinely assigned to bed rest.[167] Although seemingly benign at first, strict bed rest poses a risk of maternal thromboembolism. In a study by Kovacevich and colleagues on patients with PROM, there were 15.6 cases of thromboembolism per 1000 women assigned to bed rest, in comparison to 0.8 cases per 1000 women not assigned to bed rest.[168] In another study, Danilenko-Dixon and associates did not demonstrate an increase in incidence of thromboembolism in patients confined to bed rest.[169] Women assigned to bed rest should be observed closely for signs and symptoms of deep vein thrombosis. Symptoms of deep vein thrombosis include muscle pain, calf tenderness, swelling, positive Hollman sign, or dilated superficial veins. It is also important to remember that prolonged bed rest poses significant psychosocial and financial problems to women and their families. Women subjected to prolonged hospital stays and confined to strict bed rest may demonstrate anxiety, depression, hostility, and emotional and intellectual lability. Bed rest should be considered a therapeutic modality and should be subjected to the same rigorous clinical evaluations as any other therapeutic intervention. This modality is not without cost to the women themselves, their families, and the health care delivery system as a whole, and it may pose some direct medical risk to the mothers from the hazards of thromboembolism.

A decrease in intravascular volume has been associated with an increase in the frequency of uterine contractions. Although it has become standard therapy to treat preterm contractions with hydration, there is no objective evidence that this therapy can decrease the incidence of preterm delivery.[170] Because many of these patients need tocolytic therapy with further hydration, there is a risk that the extra fluid given during hydration will increase the risks of intravascular fluid overload and of the subsequent development of pulmonary edema. Hydration therapy should be limited to 500 mL or less.

Gap Junctions

The development of gap junctions is one of the principal changes that occur in association with labor at term and during preterm labor.[171] Progesterone is one of the most powerful inhibitors of gap junction formation, and it is through the inhibition of the gap junction formation that progesterone maintains myometrial suppression.

The various classes of tocolytic agents act directly on the myocyte by reducing intracellular calcium, activating cAMP, inhibiting production of prostaglandins, or blocking the oxytocin receptor. The ultimate result is to prevent myosin-actin interaction rendering the myometrium unresponsive to stimulation. Pharmacologic suppression of preterm labor has taken advantage of several potential intervention points in the contractions cascade. One obvious point for therapeutic intervention is the phosphoregulation/dephosphoregulation of the myosin light chain.[172,173]

Unfortunately, many of the potential intervention sites of the contraction cascade are not specific for uterine smooth muscle and have equal effects on vascular and gastrointestinal smooth muscle. Reduction of intracellular calcium has been shown to reduce smooth muscle activity. Intracellular calcium may be reduced either (1) by increasing the efflux of Ca^{2+} from the cell and/or increasing the uptake of Ca^{2+} into internal stores or (2) by blocking Ca^{2+} uptake into the cell or preventing its release from the internal stores. Nifedipine has been shown to block calcium entry through voltage-sensitive channels. The difficulty with such therapies has been that nifedipine-sensitive Ca^{2+} channels are present on many cell types, not just myometrium, and pharmacologic effects are not limited to contraction suppression.

Myometrial cells have both α_1- and β_2-adrenergic receptors on their external surface. Stimulation of the β_2-adrenergic receptor activates adenylyl cyclase, and this results in the accumulation of cAMP and subsequent activation of cAMP-dependent protein kinase, which, along with specific phosphatase regulation, is capable of phosphorylating MLCK at its site of interaction with calmodulin.

Despite the introduction of several new classes of tocolytic agents since the mid-1990s, the incidence of preterm birth has remained unchanged. Therapeutic agents currently used for treatment of premature labor include β-mimetic agonists (e.g., ritodrine, terbutaline, fenoterol), magnesium sulfate, calcium channel blockers (nifedipine, nicardipine), prostaglandin synthetase inhibitors (indomethacin and related drugs), and oxytocin antagonists. However, the only approved drug for the treatment of preterm labor is ritodrine hydrochloride (Yutopar), which was approved by the U.S. Food and Drug Administration (FDA) in 1980.[174]

Preterm birth results from spontaneous labor (50% of preterm births) or spontaneous preterm rupture of membranes (25% of preterm births) or is caused intentionally for fetal-maternal benefit (25% of preterm births); in this last case, the delivery is classified as indicated.[109] A higher proportion of preterm births follows PROM in the African American population than in the general population. African Americans have a twofold increased risk of premature birth and a threefold increased risk of very early preterm birth. This disparity in the overall preterm birth rates, particularly in very premature infants, is responsible for the twofold difference in infant mortality seen between African Americans and whites in the United States.[175-177] In general, the risk of prematurity for most Hispanic and Asian women is approximately equal to that of the white population. Within each of these ethnic groups, high income and post–high school education are usually associated with lower preterm birth rates (Fig. 18-11).[178]

β-ADRENERGIC AGENTS

β Adrenergic agents (also referred to as β mimetics or β sympathomimetics) are derivatives of epinephrine and norepinephrine. β_1-Adrenergic receptors predominate in the heart, the small intestine, and adipose tissue. β_2-Adrenergic receptors are found in the smooth muscle of the uterus, blood vessels, diaphragm, and bronchioles. Ritodrine, terbutaline, salbutamol, fenoterol, and hexoprenaline are all more selective for the β_2-adrenergic receptor.[179] These agents inhibit uterine activity through activation of the β_2 receptor, but all have varying effects on the β_1 receptor as well. Also, the β_2-receptor effects are not limited to the uterus, and there are physiologic effects caused by the activation of this receptor in other tissues. Ritodrine hydrochloride is the most commonly prescribed β-adrenergic agent in the United States, and it remains the only FDA-approved tocolytic drug.[180]

Efficacy

Since 1970, there have been many randomized placebo-controlled studies of ritodrine. In the first prospective double-blind, placebo-controlled trial of ritodrine in 1971, delivery was delayed 7 days in 80% of the ritodrine recipients and in 48% of the placebo recipients. However, the protocol was criticized because the placebo group was secondarily treated with oral ritodrine after 48 hours of intravenous infusion of placebo solution.[181] In the phase III clinical trial for the FDA, Merkatz and coworkers reported a multicenter series of randomized, prospective, double-blind, controlled trials of 313 singleton pregnancies with intact membranes. Ritodrine was found to be superior in attaining more than 36 weeks of gestation (52% of women taking ritodrine versus 38% of controls; $P < .05$)

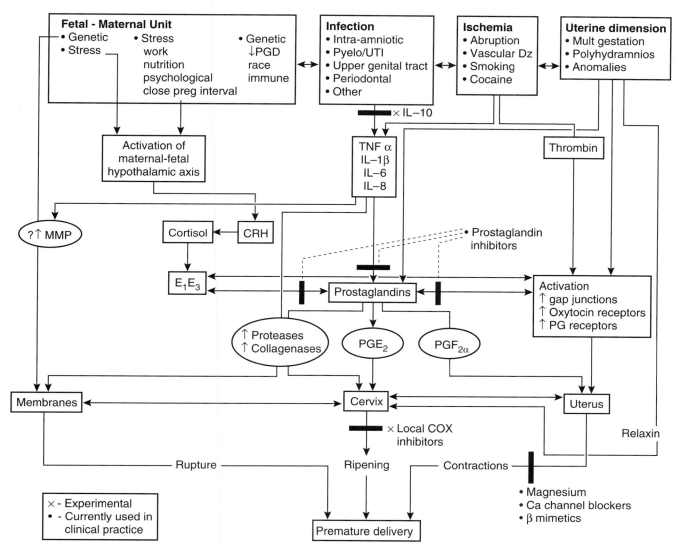

Figure 18-11. Etiologic pathways leading to preterm birth. COX, cyclooxygenase; CRH, corticotropin-releasing hormone; Dz, disease; E_1, estrone; E_3, estriol; IL-1β, interleukin-1β; IL-6, interleukin-6; IL-8, interleukin-8; IL-10, interleukin 10; MMP, metalloproteinases; Mult, multiple; PG, prostaglandin; PGD, prostaglandin dehydrogenase; PGE_2, prostaglandin E_2; $PGF_{2\alpha}$, prostaglandin $F_{2\alpha}$; preg, pregnancy; Pyelo, pyelonephritis; TNF-α, tumor necrosis factor α; UTI, urinary tract infection. *(Adapted by Rodts-Palenik S, from Norwitz ER, Robinson JN: A systematic approach to the management of preterm labor. Semin Perinatol 25:223, 2001; American College of Obstetricians and Gynecologists: Preterm labor and delivery. In Obstetrics: An Update in Obstetrics and Gynecology, 2nd ed. Washington DC, American College of Obstetricians and Gynecologists, 1999; Goldenberg RL, Hauth JC, Andrew WW: Intrauterine infection and preterm delivery. N Engl J Med 342:1500, 2000; Romero R, Tinnakorn C, Gomez R, et al: Does the human fetus rupture the membranes in preterm PROM? Am J Obstet Gynecol 185:S71, 2002; and Weiss G: Endocrinology of parturition. J Clin Endocrinol Metab 85:4421, 2000.)*

and in mean pregnancy days gained (32.6% of ritodrine recipients versus 21.3% of controls, $P < .001$).[182] In a meta-analysis of the literature performed by King and colleagues,[36] ritodrine was effective in prolonging delivery by 48 hours (odds ratio = 0.59; CI = 0.42 to 0.83). A more marked effect is seen at 24 hours with an odds ratio of 0.29 (CI = 0.21 to 0.41). This meta-analysis even supported a decrease in preterm deliveries with an odds ratio of 0.71 (CI = 0.53 to 0.96). This review by King and colleagues of randomized, controlled trials of β-adrenergic

agents not only confirmed short-term delay in delivery but also suggested that treatment may reduce the frequency of preterm birth and low birth weight.

A decrease in perinatal mortality has not been clearly shown with ritodrine or any other tocolytic agent. It has been argued that no study has had a sample size sufficient for evaluating this outcome, particularly because perinatal mortality is so low in recruited preterm subjects, who are commonly between 32 and 34 weeks pregnant. Merkatz and coworkers showed decreased neonatal death (5% versus 13%; $P < .05$) and neonatal respiratory distress syndrome (11% versus 20%; $P = .05$) in patients treated with ritodrine in comparison with controls.[182] The Canadian Preterm Labor Investigators Group showed mortality rates in ritodrine and placebo cohorts similar to those found by Merkatz and coworkers with a comparable cause of death distribution. Similar data with regard to morbidity caused by respiratory distress, patent ductus arteriosus, intraventricular hemorrhage, infection, seizures, hypotension, and hypoglycemia were also reported.[91]

Mechanism of Action

The β agonist binds to its membrane receptor, and this complex acts through the guanylyl nucleotide regulatory protein to activate adenylyl cyclase. The resultant increase in cytoplasmic cAMP decreases intracellular free calcium and directly inhibits MLCK. Decreased activity of MLCK decreases phosphorylation of myosin and results in decreased myocyte contractility (see Fig. 18-11). Continued exposure of the β-adrenergic receptor to the β agonist leads to a decrease in organ response, termed *tachyphylaxis*. This change may be secondary to the desensitization and down-regulation of membrane receptors.[183,184] The rapidity and magnitude of these receptor changes and reduced response may be dose related.

Maternal cardiovascular side effects seen with β-adrenergic agents include hypotension, tachycardia, and cardiac arrhythmias. Tachycardia is the most common side effect and is observed in the majority of affected patients. Widening of pulse pressure with diastolic hypotension is also common. Severe systolic hypotension is infrequent, however. Although cardiac arrhythmias are frequently observed, ischemic electrocardiographic changes and angina pectoris are relatively rare.[185] Electrocardiographic changes suggestive of ischemia, such as ST depression, T-wave flattening or inversion, and prolonged QT interval, have been noted. Maternal ST depression has been commonly noted but is probably not reflective of myocardial ischemia.[186] It is controversial as to whether β agonists may be safely continued in the asymptomatic pregnant woman who shows minor electrocardiographic changes. There have been reports of maternal deaths from myocardial infarction during β-adrenergic treatment for preterm labor.

The incidence of pulmonary edema during β-adrenergic treatment for preterm labor has been reported at 5%. The cause of the development of pulmonary edema during β-adrenergic treatment is unknown. Conditions that put the patient at risk for the development of pulmonary edema during tocolytic therapy include overhydration, prolonged treatment (>24 hours), tachycardia, elevated cardiac output, excessive volume expansion, decreased plasma oncotic pressure, and increased vascular permeability secondary to infection. Cardiogenic dysfunction does not appear to be necessary for the development of this problem during therapy.[187,188]

Metabolic effects of β-adrenergic receptor agonists include alterations in glucose, insulin, potassium, and lactic acid levels.[189-191] Parenteral administration of β agonists results in an acute rise in plasma glucose concentrations.

This increase appears to be mediated by direct β-adrenergic stimulation of the maternal pancreas to secrete glucagon, which in turn results in gluconeogenesis and glycogenolysis. The serum potassium decreases during the first few hours of parenteral infusion but then normalizes to preinfusion levels with prolonged therapy. Replacement is rarely needed. It is recommended that glucose and serum potassium levels be monitored during infusion.

Fetal Side Effects

Placental transfer occurs rapidly with maternal ritodrine infusion, and fetal effects that resemble those in the mother are seen. Fetal heart rates increase after ritodrine infusion,[179,180,192] but these increases tend to be milder than those seen in the mother. Fetal cardiac dysrhythmias also occur, but they are rare.[179] Higher serum concentrations of erythropoietin have been found in newborns exposed to ritodrine in utero. This finding suggests that β-adrenergic exposure subjects the fetus to hypoxia, which results in blood cell expansion as a compensatory mechanism. Much less common fetal cardiac effects include fetal heart failure, fetal myocardial ischemia, hydrops fetalis, and ventricular septal hypertrophy. The increase in energy expenditure with β-adrenergic agents could potentially increase fetal oxygen requirements.[193] β-Adrenergic agents therefore should not be administered in the setting of fetal compromise. Metabolic effects include fetal hyperglycemia and hyperinsulinemia.[194] After delivery, the neonate is at risk for hypoglycemia, ileus, hypotension, and hyperbilirubinemia. The incidence of neonatal effects can be reduced when the interval from medication administration to delivery is longer than 24 hours. Administration of certain β-adrenergic agonists has been related to increased neonatal intraventricular hemorrhage in comparison with magnesium sulfate and no treatment.[195]

Pharmacology of β-Adrenergic Agents

Ritodrine

Ritodrine hydrochloride can be administered by the oral, intramuscular, or intravenous route. This agent is metabolized by the liver to sulfate and glucuronide forms and, to a large extent, is excreted in the free or conjugated form by the kidneys.[196,197] Hepatic metabolism varies from individual to individual and causes differences in ritodrine clearance among individuals. Therefore, the dosage in each patient must be individually tailored, according to desired clinical effects versus side effects. After intravenous administration, ritodrine rapidly leaves the intravascular space and binds to extravascular tissues, a reversible process. This pool contributes to the slow elimination rate of the drug, which occurs after the first rapid decrease in contractions.[196] When a ritodrine infusion is stopped, the plasma concentration rapidly falls until extravascular ritodrine returns to the circulation and is cleared. The elimination half-life is 150 minutes. The ritodrine concentration at a steady state increases by 28 ng/mL for each 50-g/minute increase in the infusion rate. A steady state is reached after four to five half-lives, and for ritodrine this is about 10 hours. The ritodrine concentration rises rapidly after intramuscular injection, and peak concentration is achieved in 30 minutes. After a 10-mg intramuscular injection, a peak plasma concentration of 53 ng/mL is reached.

We recommend that for intravenous administration, the infusion begin at 50 µg/minute and increase every 20 minutes until uterine quiescence is achieved, unacceptable side effects occur, or a maximum infusion rate of 350 µg/min is reached. Once labor is inhibited, the labor-inhibiting infusion rate is maintained for 60 minutes and then decreased by 50 µg/minute every 30 minutes until the lowest effective rate is achieved (but not less than 50 µg/minute). The lowest effective infusion rate is then arbitrarily maintained for 12 hours.[196] If labor recurs within this 12-hour period, then the protocol should be reinitiated. Side effects that warrant lowering or discontinuation of the medication include tachycardia of more than 130 beats per minute, hypotension with diastolic blood pressure less than 140 mm Hg, chest pain, or shortness of breath.

The effectiveness of ritodrine after repeated intramuscular injections is comparable with that after continuous intravenous infusions. When ritodrine is given orally (maximum recommended daily dose is 120 mg), it achieves a steady-state concentration of 7 ng/mL. This level is one fourth of the lowest blood level associated with that recommended for intravenous infusion.

Terbutaline

Although terbutaline is not approved by the FDA for the treatment of preterm labor, it is currently used widely, and much data about its usage have accumulated. Terbutaline can be given via the oral, subcutaneous, or intravenous route. The half-life after intravenous injection is 3.7 hours. When a single 0.25-mg intravenous injection is given, a peak plasma concentration of 15 ng/mL is reached. Therapeutic levels are between 5 and 15 ng/mL. After that peak, the plasma level is quickly reduced to less than 2 ng/mL in 2 hours. An oral 5-mg dose of terbutaline results in a peak concentration at 4 hours of 5 µg/mL. Because of pharmacokinetic properties, oral terbutaline is superior to oral ritodrine in achieving an adequate plasma level.

Infusions of terbutaline can be started at 5 to 10 µg/minute and increased 5 to 10 µg/minute every 20 to 30 minutes to a maximum rate of 25 µg/minute. Maintaining this therapy for 12 hours is recommended after labor is successfully inhibited. Similar precautions regarding side effects, as described for ritodrine treatment, should be used for terbutaline. As noted in the introduction, the use of maintenance therapy after initial treatment has not been shown to be of any clinical benefit and should probably be abandoned. Subcutaneous terbutaline in a dose of 0.25 to 0.5 mg can be given in boluses for acute suppression of contractions in preterm labor. Initially, the drug can be given every 20 minutes for a maximum of two to three doses and then repeated every 3 to 4 hours. In an effort to overcome the down-regulation effects of β receptors, continuous infusions of terbutaline have been introduced. Portable subcutaneous infusion

pumps can be used to administer very low doses of terbutaline (0.3 to 0.5 mg/hour) with additional intermittent boluses of 0.25 mg at times of peak uterine activity.

Terbutaline administration via a subcutaneous pump has been described as an acceptable method for maintenance therapy because of the ability to administer lower dosages by this route. A lower dosage of terbutaline is thought to reduce the incidence of desensitization of β-adrenergic receptors and reduce the incidence of side effects. Desensitization results in less effectiveness of the medication over time. Bader and Braden and associates collected data on more than 8000 women during a 6-year period. They reported an incidence of pulmonary edema and other adverse cardiac events that were no higher than what has been observed with administration of oral terbutaline.[198,199] Guinn and colleagues also did not find any major complications among women receiving subcutaneous terbutaline pump therapy.[200] Unfortunately, the efficacy of subcutaneous terbutaline pump therapy is no better than that of oral therapy in prolonging pregnancy.[201] In comparison with placebo, subcutaneous terbutaline pump therapy did not prolong pregnancy, increase gestational age at delivery, reduce the rate of premature deliveries, or prevent recurrent preterm labor.

Contraindications

β Agonists should be avoided or used with extreme caution in women with cardiac disease, untreated hyperthyroidism, and uncontrolled diabetes mellitus. Women with controlled diabetes may require serial evaluations of glucose, potassium, and urine ketones. Parenteral insulin infusion may be warranted.

MAGNESIUM SULFATE

Efficacy

In a retrospective review by Elliott, magnesium sulfate was shown to be effective in delaying delivery of patients in preterm labor.[202] Magnesium sulfate prevented delivery within 24 hours in 78% (214), within 48 hours in 76% (208), within 72 hours in 70% (191), and to more than 7 days in 51% (140) of 274 patients with intact membranes. Like other tocolytic agents, magnesium sulfate was less effective with cervical dilation. Magnesium sulfate prevented delivery for at least 48 hours in 87% (150) of 173 patients with cervical dilation of less than 2 cm, in 62% (53) of 85 patients with cervical dilation of 3 to 5 cm, and in 31% (5) of 16 patients with cervical dilation of more than 6 cm.

Hollander and associates compared magnesium sulfate to ritodrine and found equal efficacy between the drugs.[203] A randomized, controlled trial conducted by Cox and coworkers showed no benefit in labor suppression when magnesium sulfate was compared with no treatment.[204] The work of Cox and coworkers has been criticized for its magnesium sulfate dosing protocol. They gave a 4-g bolus, followed by an infusion of only 2 g/hour, with an increase to 3 g/hour if contractions persisted. Lifson and colleagues reported that 90% of patients with cervical change treated with a magnesium sulfate intravenous bolus of 4 g, followed by an infusion rate of 4 g/hour or more, remained undelivered at 3 days; this finding was similar to the previously reported efficacy.[205]

In a study published in 1997, Macones and coauthors undertook an objective evaluation of all randomized controlled trials in which magnesium sulfate was used as tocolytic therapy.[206] Twelve trials were identified for evaluation, but four studies were eliminated because they failed to compare magnesium sulfate with any other treatment. Thus, a total of eight randomized trials comparing magnesium sulfate with placebo or β agonists for tocolysis were identified and subjected to independent review by two or more reviewers. The following outcomes were evaluated: (1) delivery delay of more than 48 hours, (2) delivery delay of more than 1 week, (3) frequency of delivery after 37 weeks, (4) frequency of major adverse drug events (pulmonary edema, myocardial ischemia, serious cardiac arrhythmia), (5) frequency of medication discontinuation because of side effects, and (6) mean latency period (interval from random assignment until delivery). There were no significant differences in tocolytic effects between magnesium sulfate and either ritodrine or placebo.

The authors noted that there were surprisingly few trials comparing magnesium sulfate to placebo but that magnesium sulfate was no better in prolonging gestation than was placebo. The small number of patients included in these clinical trials made the studies subject to possible type II error (beta errors). The authors also noted that "in order to detect a relative risk of 1.5 for delivery after 37 weeks for those treated with magnesium sulfate compared with placebo (assuming α = 0.05, β = 0.20, control rate = 0.25), approximately 231 patients would be required in each group, in contrast with the total of 191 treated or untreated patients enrolled in the available trials."[206] It is interesting to note that magnesium sulfate performed as well as the β-adrenergic agents despite having performed no better than the placebo in the placebo trials. The β agonists were associated with a higher incidence of treatment discontinuations or interruptions by maternal factors than were the magnesium sulfate. The authors questioned whether magnesium sulfate performed as well as the β-adrenergic agents or whether each agent failed to adequately suppress labor (Table 18-6).

Mechanism of Action

In the smooth muscles, increased extracellular magnesium competes with calcium at both voltage-dependent and voltage-independent sites. Excess magnesium depresses the peripheral neuromuscular system by its action (reduction) on the amplitude of the motor endplate potential, reduction of the motor endplate sensitivity, and inhibition of acetylcholine release. In addition, high magnesium concentrations increase the activity of the magnesium/calcium ATPase and thereby increase calcium extrusion from the smooth muscle cell. Magnesium thus decreases the amount of calcium available for light-chain phosphorylation and the contractile cascade.[207-209] Magnesium may also directly compete with intracellular calcium by decreasing the calcium-calmodulin binding affinity to MLCK, thereby inhibiting myometrial contractility.

Pharmacology and Dosage

Magnesium sulfate is believed to inhibit uterine activity when serum magnesium levels are between 5 and 8 mg/dL. Magnesium levels do not guide management decisions independently. Adjustment is typically based on uterine activity and maternal side effects. Higher serum magnesium levels are associated with maternal toxicity. Respiratory depression may occur with serum magnesium levels between 13 and 15 mg/dL or higher. Loss of patellar reflexes usually precedes respiratory depression and is associated with serum magnesium levels between 8.4 and 12 mg/dL. Frequent assessment of deep tendon reflexes is warranted in order to evaluate potential toxicity. Impaired renal function and decreased urine output promote magnesium retention and may potentiate magnesium toxicity. Intake and output levels are routinely measured, and the physician is notified of decreased urine output.

Normal serum magnesium concentrations in pregnant women are 1.8 ± 0.6 mg/dL. Spontaneous myometrial contractions are inhibited in vitro with concentrations of 9.6 to 12 mg/dL. Although the serum concentrations necessary to inhibit preterm labor are unclear, in human clinical trials, concentrations of 5 to 7.5 mg/dL appear to be effective. According to one study, there was no relationship between magnesium serum levels and tocolysis.[209a] Plasma concentration is determined by the infusion rate and glomerular filtration rate.

Commonly used intravenous dosages, such as a bolus of 4 g followed by a 1-, 2-, or 3-g continuous infusion per hour, result in serum concentrations of 4.0, 5.1, and 6.4 mg/dL, respectively. In contrast, 1 g of magnesium sulfate given orally increases the serum concentration by as much as 1.2 mg/dL. The recommended dosage for preterm labor inhibition is a bolus of 4 to 6 g of magnesium sulfate given over approximately 15 to 20 minutes, followed by a maintenance dose of 2 g/hour. This dose can be increased up to 4 g/hour with caution.[203,209a] Calcium and magnesium compete for a common reabsorptive site in the loop of Henle.[209b] Consequently, ionized serum calcium concentration decreases by 25% and parathyroid hormone concentration increases by 32%, preventing further calcium loss.[209c] Seventy-five percent of the magnesium sulfate is excreted during the infusion, and 90% by 24 hours after the infusion. Extreme caution should be exercised when there is evidence of renal compromise,[209b] because the excretion of magnesium sulfate is primarily via the kidneys. Magnesium sulfate takes 40 hours to be excreted by the full-term neonate, whereas preterm newborns and asphyxiated infants maintain magnesium levels for longer periods.[209d,209e,214]

Maternal Side Effects

Magnesium sulfate is usually well tolerated by patients receiving this drug for tocolysis.[180,192] Flushing, nausea and vomiting, sensation of warmth, lethargy, and dry mouth occur in 45% of women receiving magnesium sulfate infusion. Other side effects include headache and general muscle weakness.[179,194] Magnesium sulfate promotes smooth muscle relaxation. Therefore, transient

Table 18–6. Comparisons of Tocolytic Therapies with Magnesium Sulfate

Author	Description of Patient Selection	Description of Therapeutic Regimens	Blinded Randomization	Blinded Observers	Comparability of Groups Assessed	Intention to Treat
Miller et al	Yes	Yes	Yes	Unknown	Yes	Yes
Cotton et al	Yes	Yes	Unknown	Unknown	Yes	Yes
Tchillinguirian et al	Yes	Yes	Unknown	Unknown	Yes	Yes
Beall et al	Yes	Yes	Unknown	No	Yes	Unknown
Hollander et al	Yes	Yes	Unknown	No	Yes	Yes
Wilkins et al	Yes	Yes	Yes	No	Yes	Yes
Cox et al	Yes	Yes	Yes	Unknown	Yes	Yes
Chau et al	Yes	Yes	No	Unknown	Yes	Yes

Author	Preterm Labor Definition	MgSO$_4$ Loading Dose (g)	Maximum Maintenance Dosage (g/hr)	Placebo	Other Active Agents	Oral Therapy
Miller et al	Regular contractions	4	2	No	IV terbutaline	Yes
Cotton et al	Cervical change, or >2 cm, or >80% or SROM and 3 contractions in 10 min	4	2	Yes	IV terbutaline	No
Tchillinguirian et al	One premature labor unit	4	2	No	Ritodrine	Yes
Beall et al	Cervical change or contractions every 10 min	4	3.5	No	IV ritodrine, terbutaline	Yes
Hollander et al	Cervical change or >2 cm or >80% and 3 contractions in 10 min	4	Based on Mg levels	No	Ritodrine	Yes
Wilkins et al	Cervical change or ≥2 cm or ≥50% and contractions every 5 min	4	Based on Mg levels	No	Ritodrine	Yes
Cox et al	>1 cm, <5 cm and regular contractions	4	3	Yes	None	No
Chau et al	Cervical change or >2 cm or >80% and 3 contractions every 10 minutes	4	4	No	Subcutaneous terbutaline	Yes

IV, intravenous; SROM, spontaneous rupture of membranes.

From Macones GA, Sehdev HM, Berlin M, et al: Evidence for magnesium sulfate as a tocolytic agent. Obstet Gynecol Surv 52:652, 1997.

hypotension[210] from peripheral vasodilation can be anticipated, especially during the loading dose. Pulmonary edema may occur in association with magnesium sulfate but is almost always caused by fluid overload, and limiting the fluid intake to less than 2500 mL/day can decrease the risk of this occurrence.[180,211,212] Magnesium sulfate promotes calcium excretion in the kidney and may result in hypocalcemia.[179,180] Treatment for hypocalcemia is almost never necessary, but reductions in bone density have been reported during prolonged treatments.

The magnesium ion competes with calcium. With increasing concentrations of magnesium, all muscles of the body can be affected. Loss of patellar reflexes can be observed with magnesium concentrations of 8.4 to 12 mg/dL, respiratory depression begins with levels of 13 to 15 mg/dL, and asystole can occur with levels of 30 mg/dL. Blurred vision and diplopia occur in about 70% of patients.

Ischemia, maternal hypotension, and pulmonary edema have been reported,[202] although at much lower levels than with ritodrine. The incidence of pulmonary edema is less than 1%.[202] Serum calcium decreases and urinary excretion of calcium increases with magnesium sulfate treatment. The antidote for magnesium toxicity is the slow intravenous administration of 1 g of calcium gluconate.

Fetal Side Effects

Magnesium sulfate crosses the placenta and reaches the fetal compartment, where it is maintained at a steady state. Neonates, especially preterm and asphyxiated infants, excrete magnesium sulfate slowly.[213] It has been reported that with mean umbilical cord magnesium concentrations of 3.6 mg/dL, there is no significant alteration in neurologic state or Apgar scores of newborns at delivery. Nevertheless, when umbilical magnesium levels are higher (between 4 and 11 mg/dL), it is common to observe decreased muscle tone and drowsiness. Magnesium sulfate has been associated with decreased fetal breathing movement,[179,180] blunted response to vibroacoustic stimulation, and nonreactive results on nonstress testing.[179,210] Fetal heart rate variability may be decreased secondary to the central nervous system depressant effects of magnesium.[180]

With prolonged treatment or high maternal magnesium levels (6 to 8 mg/dL), it is common to observe a decrease in fetal heart rate variability and a decrease in the biophysical profile score (mainly as a result of decreased breathing). Maternal treatment lasting more than 1 week results in half of the fetuses showing evidence of long bone demineralization. In fact, a case of congenital rickets has been reported after maternal magnesium therapy.[214] Magnesium sulfate may interfere with fetal bone development, and radiographic bone abnormalities have been documented. Neonatal side effects include hypocalcemia,[179] hypotonia, drowsiness, and respiratory depression.[192] Potentiation of its anticalcium effects with concurrent usage of nifedipine (calcium channel blocker) has been reported and can be dangerous. It appears that the sublingual administration of nifedipine is the offending route of administration for this side effect, on the basis of its rapid action.

Some epidemiologic data have suggested a possible fetal neuroprotective effect and decreased incidence of cerebral palsy with antenatal magnesium sulfate exposure.[215,216] A concern has been raised for increasing rates of perinatal mortality associated with high doses of magnesium sulfate, but this concern has not been supported.[216,217] Currently, there is an ongoing study by the Maternal-Fetal Medicine Network to further evaluate fetal and neonatal effects of magnesium sulfate. The current concerns regarding potential safety of magnesium sulfate, coupled with the lack of evidence that this drug is effective at prolonging the pregnancy even 24 to 48 hours, warrant reevaluation of the use of this drug for tocolytic therapy.[218]

Contraindications

Because of the risk of cardiorespiratory depression, magnesium sulfate infusion should be avoided in patients with myasthenia gravis, heart block, and myocardial damage. Patients with renal insufficiency should be monitored closely for evidence of toxicity.

PROSTAGLANDIN SYNTHETASE INHIBITORS

Prostaglandins stimulate myometrial gap junction formation and raise intracellular calcium levels by increasing calcium flux across the cell membrane. They stimulate calcium release from the sarcoplasmic reticulum and are intimately involved in parturition. Prostaglandins are formed by the conversion of arachidonic acid by the cyclooxygenase enzyme. Prostaglandin synthetase inhibitors block the production of arachidonic acid by interfering with the cyclooxygenase enzyme. Although prostaglandin synthetase inhibitors have few maternal side effects and are effective tocolytic agents, identified harmful fetal effects include decreased fetal urine production and constriction of the ductus arteriosus. These problems have limited the widespread use of these drugs as primary tocolytic agents.

Efficacy

The use of indomethacin as a tocolytic agent has been studied since the mid-1970s. Like most other tocolytic agents, indomethacin has not been rigorously evaluated in multiple randomized, controlled trials. Two early reports comparing indomethacin with placebo in a double-blind, prospective manner showed statistically higher rates of labor inhibition in the indomethacin-treated patients than in patients treated with placebo.[219,220] There have been only three reports that compared indomethacin and placebo in a randomized, controlled manner.[221,222] In 1995, Keirse published a meta-analysis in the Cochrane Pregnancy and Childhood Database.[223] The meta-analysis of the studies indicate that indomethacin was more effective than placebo in delaying delivery for 48 hours, delaying delivery for 7 to 10 days, prolonging the pregnancy beyond 37 weeks, and decreasing the incidence of low birth weight in infants. There was no difference in rates of fetal death, neonatal deaths, and respiratory distress syndrome between the treatment and placebo recipients. Spearing performed a small trial of 42 patients in which indomethacin was given in addition to ethanol and compared to ethanol administration alone. This study did not show a significant benefit from the addition of indomethacin (odds ratio = 0.33; 95% CI = 0.06 to 1.73).[224] Katz and colleagues assigned, in an alternating manner, 120 women at less than 35 weeks' gestation with preterm labor to one of two treatment groups: intravenous ritodrine only or ritodrine and indomethacin.[225] Again, the differences between these two groups were not statistically significant. Gamissans and associates performed two double-blind trials.[226,227] In both trials, women were treated with ritodrine and randomly assigned to receive either indomethacin or placebo. Among those who received indomethacin plus ritodrine, there was a decrease in delivery within 7 days and a decrease of delivery before 37 weeks, in comparison with the placebo recipients.

Several studies have compared indomethacin as a first-line agent alone to an alternative tocolytic drug. These studies are difficult to interpret because the effects of the secondary drugs are always suspect and indomethacin's absolute tocolytic effect in comparison with no treatment cannot be evaluated. Morales and associates[228,229] compared indomethacin with intravenous magnesium sulfate or ritodrine. The results show that indomethacin and a comparable tocolytic agent are equally effective in delaying delivery for 48 hours (approximately 85% to 90% in each group). Similarly, Kurki and associates performed a randomized, double-blind comparison between indomethacin and nylidrin (a β-sympathomimetic agent) in the treatment of preterm labor.[230] In this study, indomethacin was significantly more effective than nylidrin in delaying delivery for 48 hours and beyond 37 weeks. In addition, patients treated with indomethacin experienced fewer adverse drug effects.

Subclinical infection has been implicated as an etiologic factor in preterm delivery. Newton and colleagues[135] therefore performed a randomized, double-blind clinical trial in which they compared a combination therapy of magnesium sulfate, indomethacin, and ampicillin-sulbactam with single-agent tocolysis with magnesium sulfate. The investigators reported no difference between the two regimens with regard to delivery delay, incidence of preterm delivery, and neonatal outcome.

Some researchers have compared indomethacin with another nonsteroidal anti-inflammatory agent. For example, Carlan and coauthors reported that indomethacin and sulindac were equally successful in delaying delivery for 48 hours and for 7 days.[231] Sulindac appeared to decrease the amniotic fluid volume less than indomethacin when used for the acute treatment of preterm labor. Other investigators[232,233] compared indomethacin with an oral β-sympathomimetic tocolytic drug (after short-term parenteral therapy) for efficacy and safety as a prolonged tocolytic therapy. In comparison with the β-sympathomimetic drug, indomethacin was equally effective as a tocolytic but more commonly resulted in oligohydramnios and vasospasm of the ductus arteriosus.

At least three randomized placebo-controlled trials and four non–placebo-controlled trials supported indomethacin as effective in delaying delivery for at least 48 hours, for 7 to 10 days, and beyond 37 weeks. It is important to remember that these conclusions are derived from a review of a heterogenous collection of studies. Also, these studies had small numbers of subjects, and it is impossible to make statements regarding neonatal safety. Finally, the majority of the studies were performed before the use of antenatal corticosteroids and the use of surfactant in newborns, and it is impossible to determine the impact of these therapeutic modalities on neonatal outcomes.

Mechanism of Action

Prostaglandins increase uterine contractility by enhancing the production of myometrial gap junctions and by stimulating calcium release from the sarcoplasmic reticulum.[234] Prostaglandin synthetase inhibitors inactivate cyclooxygenase, the enzyme that regulates the production of the first prostaglandin intermediate, from arachidonic acid. By inhibiting prostaglandin production, prostaglandin synthetase inhibitors inhibit myometrial contractility by blocking gap junction formation and preventing prostaglandin-mediated increases in intracellular calcium.[144]

Maternal Side Effects

Indomethacin is the most studied prostaglandin synthetase inhibitor used for tocolysis. Indomethacin interferes with conversion of thromboxane to prostacyclin. There is concern that this could lead to a predisposition to hemorrhage because thromboxane is involved in platelet aggregation.[234] This effect might be compounded by the suppression of uterine activity, inasmuch as these contractions are necessary to control hemorrhage in the postpartum period. Lunt and colleagues showed that even though indomethacin prolonged bleeding time, there was no prolongation in prothrombin time or active partial thromboplastin time.[235] Also, this group did not identify any evidence of postpartum hemorrhage in any of their patients, but they did suggest that hemorrhage was still a theoretical risk. Indomethacin can interfere with the gastrointestinal mucosal barrier and may exacerbate peptic ulcer disease. Indomethacin should not be used in patients with a history of this condition.[235] Gastrointestinal irritation in women with outcome peak ulcer disease is demonstrated by excessive nausea and heartburn.[180]

Fetal Side Effects

Indomethacin readily crosses the placenta and has a direct effect on fetal prostaglandin synthesis.[232] Indomethacin has been associated with oligohydramnios in the fetus, most likely as a result of effects on fetal renal blood flow. The angiotensin-aldosterone system is affected by prostaglandin production, and it is through this mechanism these drugs may have their effects. Fortunately, effects of indomethacin on fetal urine production have been reversible, and the oligohydramnios usually corrects with discontinuation of the medications.[232,235]

Constriction of the ductus arteriosus has also been associated with indomethacin use.[236] Constriction of the ductus arteriosus is more likely to occur with fetal exposure after 31 to 32 weeks, but complete closure could result in intrauterine fetal demise. Although no fetal deaths associated with indomethacin exposure have actually been documented, ductal vasospasm, when seen in fetuses, occurred with exposures beyond 48 hours.[237,238] Like renal blood flow, ductal constriction has been shown to diminish on discontinuation of the indomethacin.[232,237] Exposures longer than 48 hours have also been associated with the development of pulmonary hypertension and an increasing incidence of necrotizing enterocolitis in premature infants born after exposure.[233] A higher incidence of neonatal intraventricular hemorrhage among infants with extremely low birth weight has been reported,[239] and prolonged exposure (up to 5 weeks) has been associated with fetal anuria, renal microcystic lesions, and neonatal death.[192] However, other studies reveal no significant increase in necrotizing enterocolitis and intraventricular hemorrhage with indomethacin tocolysis,[221,240,241] which suggests that the differing effects are more likely due to the reasons for tocolysis as opposed to the drug itself.

Ultrasonography should be performed weekly to evaluate the amniotic fluid volume in patients taking indomethacin. The harmful fetal effects from indomethacin exposure, particularly when used longer than 48 hours, should make the clinician wary of using this drug as a first-line tocolytic agent.

Pharmacology

Indomethacin, the prototype of prostaglandin synthase inhibitors, is rapidly absorbed after both oral and rectal administration. Indomethacin freely crosses the placenta with comparable maternal and fetal concentrations, and peak plasma concentrations are reached in 1 to 2 hours. Indomethacin is metabolized by the liver and excreted by the kidney. Maternal serum half-life is 5.8 hours, with a range of 2.5 to 11.2 hours. In contrast, the fetus excretes indomethacin relatively slowly (half-life, 14.7 hours), ranging from hours to days.[242] Indomethacin can be administered orally or rectally with a 50- to 100-mg loading dose, followed by 25 mg every 4 to 6 hours.[222,243] Indomethacin is metabolized extensively by the liver, and 10% is excreted unchanged in the urine. Frequent evaluations of the amniotic fluid index and fetal cardiac function may be warranted if indomethacin is continued longer than 48 hours.

Contraindications

Maternal contraindications to the usage of indomethacin include a maternal history of gastrointestinal ulcer or hemorrhage, renal disease, bleeding disorders, and hypersensitivity. Fetal contraindications include oligohydramnios, gestational age of more than 34 weeks, and fetal cardiac disease.

CALCIUM CHANNEL BLOCKERS

Nifedipine, a prototype of calcium channel blockers, seems to be an effective tocolytic agent. The calcium channel antagonists are organized into three classes on the basis of their chemical structure. Nifedipine and nicardipine, two agents of the dihydropyridine class of calcium channel blockers, are the preferred agents for tocolysis because they more selectively inhibit uterine contractions with minimal effects on the maternal cardiovascular system.[244] Verapamil, but not nifedipine, impairs atrioventricular conduction and can cause cardiac dysfunction. The use of verapamil for treating preterm labor was first reported in 1972. Effectiveness of treatment could not be shown because dosage was limited after cardiovascular side effects.

Efficacy

There have been no randomized placebo-controlled trials to evaluate the efficacy of nifedipine, or any of the calcium channel blockers, for the treatment of preterm labor. There have been several small studies comparing nifedipine with other tocolytic agents. Most of the existing tocolytic trials of nifedipine have been small heterogenous studies in which this drug was compared with ritodrine in the treatment of preterm labor.[245-253] Despite the small number of existing trials, the calcium channel blockers may be effective tocolytic agents and, at the same time, may have fewer maternal and fetal side effects.[254]

In a study by Read and Welby, nifedipine was compared to ritodrine in 40 patients in a randomized fashion. Unfortunately, the control group with no treatment was not randomized and was cared for by another physician. Of the three groups, 13 of 20 failed therapy in the no treatment control group, 11 failed treatment in the ritodrine group, and only 5 patients failed treatment in

the nifedipine group.[251] Nifedipine was significantly better than both the placebo and ritodrine groups. In 1997, Papatsonis and associates conducted a multicenter study of 185 women treated for preterm labor between 20 and 33 weeks of gestation and demonstrated superior efficacy of nifedipine over ritodrine in delaying delivery at 24 hours, at 48 hours, and at 1 and 2 weeks.[255] Two meta-analyses also demonstrated nifedipine to be more effective than the β agonists in delaying preterm birth and improving neonatal outcome.[256,257] Moreover, only a handful of investigators evaluated the use of calcium channel blockers for the treatment of preterm labor in multiple gestations.[245,248,250] In a review of the management of preterm labor in multiple gestations, the use of calcium channel blockers was advocated over β-adrenergic agents because of the benefits of maternal safety, in view of the expanded maternal intravascular volume.[258]

Nifedipine has been studied more than the other calcium channel blockers for the treatment of preterm labor. At present, there have been no large prospective, randomized, controlled trials in which nifedipine has been compared with placebo. Most studies have been small trials in which nifedipine was compared with other tocolytic agents, most often ritodrine. These trials have shown either equal tocolytic effects or superior labor prolongation with fewer side effects in comparison with ritodrine. Because the studies have had relatively small numbers of subjects, maternal and fetal side effects cannot yet be adequately assessed; however, as yet, untoward events have not been identified.

Mechanism of Action

Calcium channel blockers (e.g., nicardipine) inhibit uterine contractions by reducing intracellular calcium through a blockade of the voltage-dependent calcium channels and by blocking release of calcium from the sarcoplasmic reticulum. Therefore, less intracellular calcium is available for the phosphorylation of light-chain kinase and the contractile cascade. Nifedipine and nicardipine are potent inhibitors of uterine muscle contractions in vitro.

It has been demonstrated that there is an endogenous inhibitor of uterine activity that is present in the chorion, decidua, and placenta of nonlaboring patients at term.[259-261] Levels of this endogenous calcium channel blocker diminish toward term and may play a role in maintaining uterine quiescence before the onset of labor.[259]

Maternal Side Effects

Calcium channel blockers can cause vasodilation, decreased peripheral vascular resistance, tachycardia, nausea, headache, and hypertension.[252] The most common side effects are flushing (96%), and headache (38%).[247] This vasodilation is less severe than that seen with ritodrine and is more easily tolerated by the mother.[262] The maternal side effects associated with nifedipine are consistently milder and more tolerable than those associated with either the β-adrenergic tocolytics or magnesium sulfate, which accounts for its lower incidence of discontinuation by patients.[246,248,256,257,263,264] A modest decrease in diastolic blood pressure occurs approximately

10 minutes after the initial sublingual dose, or 20 minutes after the second oral dose, and is generally transient and not clinically significant.[262] This decrease is often accompanied by a clinically insignificant, mild, unsustained increase in the maternal heart rate. Both ritodrine and nifedipine produce hyperglycemia, but the increase in serum glucose produced by nifedipine (consistently less than 120 mg/dL) is less significant than that induced by ritodrine.

There have been two reports of serious maternal complications during the use of nifedipine treatment of preterm labor.[265,266] In one study, a patient receiving nifedipine was said to have experienced a myocardial infarction, and in a second study, hepatic toxicity was reported. In the report of hepatotoxicity, the patient had twins, received terbutaline, intravenous magnesium, subcutaneous terbutaline, indomethacin, subcutaneous terbutaline pump infusion, and finally nifedipine tocolysis. The liver enzyme levels became elevated, and nifedipine was discontinued. From the study, it is unclear which treatments might have resulted in hepatic toxicity.

Nifedipine must not be used in conjunction with magnesium sulfate. There have been several case reports in which nifedipine was used in conjunction with magnesium sulfate, and there was evidence that the patients developed neuromuscular blockade.[267,268] This blockade occurred even when levels of magnesium sulfate were subtherapeutic, but it was reversible with calcium gluconate.

Fetal Side Effects

Original animal data demonstrated a decrease in fetal arterial partial pressure of oxygen and in pH when nifedipine or nicardipine was infused in monkeys or sheep.[269-271] Nevertheless, these effects have not been substantiated in published human studies. Neonates whose mothers were treated with nifedipine had similar morbid conditions as those whose mothers were treated with β adrenergics. In addition, Doppler flow studies did not reveal evidence of umbilical circulatory compromise in the infants with nifedipine-treated mothers. Doppler studies of the middle cerebral, renal, and umbilical arteries as well as the ductus arteriosus, aortic, and pulmonary valves of human fetuses have failed to show changes during nifedipine administration.[272] In addition, Apgar scores and cord pHs of neonates exposed to antepartum nifedipine are not significantly different from those of control neonates receiving other tocolytic agents or no agent.[246,249,255,263,273,274] In the only multicenter, prospective, randomized, controlled trial of the use of nifedipine, Papatsonis and associates, in fact, showed that there was a lower incidence of respiratory distress syndrome, intraventricular hemorrhage, jaundice, and admission to the neonatal intensive care unit among neonates exposed to nifedipine than among those exposed to intravenous ritodrine.[255] This finding was thought to result from improved efficacy of preterm labor treatment in the nifedipine group and from a direct effect on pulmonary blood flow and fetal blood pressure. Similarly, a meta-analysis of 679 patients who received either nifedipine or β-adrenergic tocolysis confirmed less respiratory distress syndrome and fewer neonatal intensive care unit admissions in the nifedipine recipients.[257]

Pharmacology and Dosage

Oral administration of nifedipine results in peak levels within 30 to 60 minutes, in contrast to the sublingual route, which peaks within minutes.[275] Nifedipine is partially bound in the circulation with a bioavailability of 65%. Nifedipine is metabolized by the liver, and 70% to 80% of its metabolites are excreted by the kidneys; the remaining 20% to 30% are excreted in the feces. The half-life of nifedipine is 2 hours.

When utilized as a tocolytic agent, both sublingual and oral administrations result in pharmacokinetics similar to those in nonpregnant volunteers. Regardless of the mode of administration, significant variability occurs between patients in the plasma concentration and the half-life of this drug. This variability is attributed to differences in first-pass metabolism and gastric absorption of the drug. On average, the maternal half-life of the drug is approximately 1.5 hours, whereas the half-life in the neonate is much longer, approximately 26.5 hours. This difference is attributable to the immaturity of the fetal and neonatal liver. As opposed to sublingual loading, no cumulative increase in maximum maternal plasma concentration of nifedipine occurs with oral administration of 20 mg every 6 hours. Subsequently, prolonged dosing can be given for tocolysis without concern for cumulative effects.

The usual recommended dosage is 10 mg sublingually (by breaking the capsule), which can be repeated once or twice in 20-minute intervals if contractions continue.[252] These sublingual doses are followed by oral doses of 10 to 20 mg every 4 to 6 hours up to a maximum dosage of 120 mg/day. One investigator noted better tocolytic efficacy with slightly higher dosages up to 160 mg/day.[255] Because of risk of neuromuscular blockade, nifedipine or other calcium channel blockers should not be used in conjunction with magnesium sulfate.

Contraindications to Calcium Channel Blockers

Known hypersensitivity and heart block are maternal contraindications to the use of calcium channel blockers for almost any indication. Significant maternal hypotension is a contraindication to calcium channel blocker tocolysis, and concomitant use with magnesium sulfate should be avoided because of reports of neuromuscular blockade.

OXYTOCIN ANTAGONISTS

A newer class of medications, oxytocin antagonists, with atosiban as the prototype, is being studied in humans.[276] Atosiban suppresses uterine contractions in women with threatened preterm labor. Goodwin and colleagues reported at the Society of Gynecologic Investigation in 1996 that atosiban resulted in cessation of contractions or significant reduction in frequency in 83% of patients with established preterm labor without significant side effects.[277] If these studies are confirmed, oxytocin antagonists should be a very desirable and clinically useful group of tocolytic agents.

Efficacy

In a randomized, double-blind, placebo-controlled trial, there was a significantly greater decrease in mean contraction frequency in patients receiving a 2-hour infusion of atosiban (55.3 ± 36.3) than in those treated with bed rest and hydration (26.7 ± 40.4) for threatened preterm labor, defined as more than four contractions per hour without evidence of cervical change.[277]

In a nonrandomized, open-label trial for patients in preterm labor, 70.5% (43) of 61 patients receiving atosiban for up to 12 hours remained undelivered after 48 hours. Cessation of uterine contractions was found in 62.3% of patients, with the mean time to cessation being 4.6 ± 3.2 hours. The rate of successful tocolysis was related to the degree of initial cervical dilation. Atosiban, however, has been withdrawn from the FDA application process, reportedly because of disappointing results of a placebo-controlled, randomized, clinical trial.[179]

Mechanism of Action

Atosiban is a selective oxytocin-vasopressin receptor antagonist capable of inhibiting oxytocin-induced myometrial contractions. The mechanism appears to be competitive inhibition of oxytocin receptors in the myometrium and decidua. Oxytocin stimulates contractions by stimulating the conversion of phosphatidylinositol to inositol triphosphate. This binds to a protein in the sarcoplasmic reticulum, leading to calcium release into the cytoplasm. Thus, oxytocin antagonists result in a decrease in intracellular free calcium that results in decreased myometrial contractility.[144]

Maternal Side Effects

Because oxytocin receptors are found mostly in the reproductive tract, atosiban has the advantage of being highly organ-specific; therefore, there are only local side effects from the use of this drug. In placebo-controlled trials, there were no differences in side effects between atosiban and the placebo, except for local tissue reaction at the slight of the drug injection.[278]

Fetal Side Effects

In a study by Romero and associates, there was a higher death rate in fetuses less than 28 weeks in the atosiban treatment group.[278] Atosiban crosses the placenta with a mean maternal-fetal ratio of 12. Although the adverse effects caused by atosiban cannot be excluded, it should be noted that these fetal-infant deaths were associated with infection and extreme prematurity. Despite randomization, most of the preterm infants (less than 28 weeks) were assigned to the atosiban group.

Pharmacology

Atosiban is a nonapeptide that has been approved for use in Europe. Atosiban has not been approved by the FDA and is currently not available for use in the United States. In Europe, this agent is administered intravenously for acute tocolysis, and initial and terminal half-lives are 13 and 102 minutes, respectively. The regimen used in the largest randomized studies begins with an intravenous bolus of 6.75 mg, followed immediately by a 300-µg/minute intravenous infusion for 3 hours, and then 100 µg/minute for up to 45 hours.

Contraindications

There are no absolute maternal contraindications described. Because of the study that showed a higher death rate in fetuses younger than 28 weeks, it has been suggested that the use of atosiban be limited to older fetuses.

NITRIC OXIDE DONORS

Efficacy

Nitroglycerin is a potent smooth muscle relaxant that has been used to relax the uterus for obstetric procedures. It has been used for removal of retained placenta, correction of uterine inversion, facilitation of fetal extraction during cesarean delivery, and intrapartum version of second twins. Cessation of uterine contractions have been reported with nitroglycerin administration in sheep and rhesus monkeys.[279,280] Observational studies with trinitrate patches reported potential for nitroglycerin as a tocolytic agent but were limited by the nature of the studies. El-Sayed and coworkers compared intravenous nitroglycerin with magnesium sulfate for treatment of preterm labor in a randomized study. The patients treated with intravenous nitroglycerin had more frequent tocolytic failures and higher incidence of discontinuation as a result of hypotension, which caused the study to be discontinued midway.[281] The use of high-dose intravenous nitroglycerin as a tocolytic agent is not supported at this time. Future research with different delivery methods or dosages may yield different results.

Mechanism of Action

Nitroglycerin is frequently used in pregnancy for rapid uterine relaxation during breech extraction, uterine inversion, retained placenta, and version. Nitric oxide donors, like nitroglycerin, activate the cyclic guanosine monophosphate pathway involved in smooth muscle relaxation. The activation of cyclic guanosine monophosphate results in decreased intracellular free calcium that leads to decreased activation of MLCK and decreased myometrial contractility.

Maternal Side Effects

The primary side effect is maternal hypotension, related to smooth muscle relaxation of blood vessels. Symptoms include headache, light-headedness, nausea, and vomiting. Preexisting maternal hypotension is suggested as an exclusion criterion in studies.

Fetal Side Effects

There are no clear data indicating that nitric oxide donor therapy adversely affects the infant. There are no significant differences in neonatal hemodynamics, Apgar scores, or umbilical cord gases in cases of nitroglycerin exposure at elective cesarean delivery in comparison with controls.[282]

Pharmacology

Nitric oxide donors have been administered intravenously and by transdermal patch. The dosages and routes of administration have varied in studies but are primarily titrated to cessation of contractions while maintaining adequate blood pressure. The transdermal regimen used in the largest multicenter study was an initial 10-mg transdermal glyceryl trinitrate patch applied to the skin of the abdomen. If, after 1 hour, there was no reduction in contraction frequency or strength, an additional patch was applied. No more than two patches were administered simultaneously, and these were left in place for 24 hours, after which they were removed and the patient was reassessed.[283]

Contraindications

Because nitric oxide donors cause maternal vasodilation and cause dramatic affects on maternal blood pressure, they should not be used when there is significant maternal hypotension or when there is evidence of fetal distress. Likewise, these agents should not be used when there is evidence of maternal hemorrhage, except as treatment for retained placenta and acute hemorrhage.

COMBINATION TOCOLYTIC THERAPY

There have been a limited number of studies that attempted to assess the efficacy of combined labor-inhibiting agents. Before consideration of the initiation of a second tocolytic drug, the patient's medical status should be reassessed. Intraamniotic infection and abruption should be aggressively ruled out before a second-line tocolytic medication is added. Amniocentesis should be used liberally to evaluate the amniotic fluid for the presence of infection and blood, as well as to assess the status of fetal pulmonary maturation. Two randomized controlled trials have addressed combination versus single-agent therapy with ritodrine and magnesium sulfate. Whereas one study by Hatjis and associates showed benefit from the combined therapy,[284] other studies have not demonstrated an improvement in contraction suppression.[285] Maternal side effects were found to be significantly increased when combined agents are used. In another study, neuromuscular blockade was reported when magnesium sulfate and nifedipine were used in combination.[268] Myocardial infarction has been reported when nifedipine was administered after ritodrine tocolysis in a previously healthy young patient. In view of the limited data and concerns over patient safety, combined tocolytic therapy should not be used routinely.

MAINTENANCE THERAPY AFTER ACUTE TOCOLYSIS

Extended Parenteral Tocolytic Therapy

Women with preterm contractions may often have repeated visits to the labor and delivery department and/or may remain for extended periods within the hospital with frequent episodes of uterine activity. These women may require extended parenteral tocolytic therapy. Women with these problems include those with high-order multiple pregnancies, those with advanced cervical dilation, and those for whom compliance is an issue.[211,286]

Kosasa and coworkers studied 1000 consecutive women in preterm labor or with ruptured membranes treated as inpatients with a combination of intravenous terbutaline (maximum 80-μg/minute infusion) and magnesium sulfate to achieve a serum level of 6.5 to 7.5 mg/dL (6.5 g/hour maximum dose).[212] This long-term tocolytic therapy extended gestation by 61 ± 23.6 days in 751 women with intact membranes and by 20.5 ± 17.4 days in 24 parturients with ruptured membranes. Nausea was the most commonly observed side effect (25%), but vomiting occurred only rarely. Dudley and colleagues also administered extended parenteral therapy with magnesium sulfate to 111 patients. Sixty patients were treated for 48 to 72 hours, but 29 received the drug for 3 to 10 days; 22 additional patients were treated longer than 10 days.[287] Prolonged hospitalization is expensive, separates the patient from the family, interferes with adequate rest, and increases maternal stress. Before subjecting mothers to this aggressive therapy, clinicians should strongly consider the potential benefits and risks from such therapy, and this intervention should probably be reserved for patients not close to term.

A less costly method of treating these special patients involves the outpatient use of a programmable pump that administers basal and bolus doses of β-agonist drugs such as terbutaline. This technique takes advantage of the concept that intermittent terbutaline dosing in small amounts along with low-level basal administration avoids tachyphylaxis.[288] For example, typical oral dosages of terbutaline range from 30 to 40 mg/day, whereas subcutaneous terbutaline infusion dosages average 2 to 4 mg/day. A substantial decrease in the dosage of drug necessary to achieve uterine quiescence, decreased variance in intestinal absorption, improved patient compliance, avoidance of multiple daily drug doses, and lack of need for self-medication at night enhance the utility of this therapeutic approach.

Twenty-two scientific studies using this technique in almost 5000 subjects have been published as of this writing in peer-reviewed literature. Twenty trials involving more than 4800 patients reported enhanced pregnancy prolongation of 3.7 to 8.4 weeks, a mean gestational age at delivery of 35.8 weeks, fewer recurrent episodes of preterm labor, and fewer early deliveries, particularly before 34 weeks, in comparison with control patients receiving standard oral therapy or taking no tocolytics. The two trials reporting no benefit enrolled 42 and 52 patients with preterm labor within the same institution and randomly assigned them to receive oral terbutaline, subcutaneous terbutaline infusion, or subcutaneous saline infusion.[200,289] In the 20 investigations in which efficacy was found, patients were discharged with daily skilled nursing contact, home uterine contraction monitoring for 2 hours/day, and 24-hour availability of emergency contact for monitoring transmission to adjust subcutaneous terbutaline therapy.

As with many drugs administered parenterally, safety has also been an important issue. Because of the low dosage, the incidence of side effects with subcutaneous terbutaline infusion is quite low. Perry and associates found that only 47 of 8709 patients (0.54%) had pulmonary problems while receiving subcutaneous terbutaline.[290] Of these, only 5 women with complications were being treated with only terbutaline therapy in the home, whereas the other 42 received several concomitant tocolytic agents or large amounts of intravenous fluids or had severe pregnancy-induced hypertension and/or multiple gestations (all in the hospital). When such complications do develop, they usually occur in association with factors other than drug therapy.

In summary, prolonged tocolytic therapy may be of benefit in treatment of patients with refractory premature labor. Traditional methods of inpatient treatment protocols of these patients have relied on prolonged stays in labor and delivery units with repeated sessions of intravenous administration of tocolytic agents. This approach is expensive and stressful to patients and should be reserved for women for which there is a clear benefit for prolonging the pregnancy. Subcutaneous outpatient terbutaline therapy has been studied. Although enabling the patient to leave the hospital and live with her family appears to be a reasonable approach, these studies have failed to show a significant prolongation of the pregnancy or a reduction in newborn morbidity and mortality. As with all forms of tocolytic therapy, there is limited evidence that this therapeutic modality changes neonatal outcome.

Oral Maintenance Therapy

Once a patient has been successfully treated for preterm labor, either she may remain on suppressive therapy, usually with oral agents, or she may be re-treated as necessary should preterm contractions resume. To study this approach, patients have been discharged with a variety of oral agents. Although there is a scientific rationale for this approach, a meta-analysis failed to show benefit. Sanchez-Ramos and colleagues evaluated 12 randomized, clinical trials of maintenance tocolysis involving 1590 patients (855 treated and 735 receiving placebo/no treatment).[291] The predominant tocolytic class was β agonists with seven trials of oral or subcutaneous terbutaline, three trials of oral ritodrine, one trial with oral sulindac, and one trial with subcutaneous atosiban. This meta-analysis showed that maintenance tocolytic therapy was not associated with a significant reduction in the rates of recurrent preterm labor or preterm delivery, with pooled odds ratios of 0.95 (95% CI = 0.77 to 1.17) and 0.81 (95% CI = 0.64 to 1.28), respectively. Maintenance therapy was not associated with an increase in mean gestational age at delivery, but more days were gained, with a pooled difference in mean interval from randomization to delivery between treatment and comparison of 4.34 days (95% CI = 3.10 to 5.75). A slight reduction in the incidence of recurrent preterm labor was seen in patients who received the same agent for acute and maintenance tocolysis (odds ratio = 0.59; 95% CI = 0.41 to 0.85). The study included neonatal outcomes, such as birth weight, incidence of

respiratory distress syndrome, and perinatal mortality; there was no benefit from the use of maintenance tocolytic therapy with regard to these outcomes. It was the recommendation of this group that oral tocolytic therapy not be utilized for maintenance treatment.

In a randomized, controlled trial, Carr and associates found that maintenance therapy with oral nifedipine after magnesium sulfate tocolysis did not significantly prolong pregnancy. Gestational age at delivery was 35.4 ± 3.2 weeks versus 35.3 ± 3.2 weeks in the nifedipine recipients and no-treatment recipients, respectively. The number of days gained in utero was 37 ± 23.9 versus 32.8 ± 20.4 for nifedipine and no-treatment recipients, respectively.[292] There are no data in the literature to support the use of oral tocolytic agents as maintenance therapy after successful parenteral treatment.

TOCOLYTIC THERAPY IN MULTIPLE GESTATIONS

The increasing numbers of multiple gestations place these pregnancies at greater risk for tocolytic complications than singleton pregnancies. Affected patients are more likely to have vascular and cardiovascular effects as a result of these therapies. Multiple gestations also require higher infusion rates and more frequent incremental increases in the doses of intravenous agents because of an increased glomerular filtration rate and higher levels of hepatic metabolism associated with the multiple gestation. Higher serum levels of magnesium sulfate are required for tocolysis of preterm labor in the multiple pregnancy (7.0 to 7.5 mg/dL).[293] Unfortunately, an increased risk of adverse effects associated with these tocolytics is often a byproduct of higher dosages. The side effects are less tolerable in the pregnant patient already under stress from the physiologic discomforts inherent in multiple gestations, and in some cases, these complications can be life-threatening.

Although the efficacy of ritodrine is equivalent in singleton and multiple gestations, the complication rate is unquestionably higher in multiple gestations. A 34.4% incidence of cardiovascular complications was observed in women with multiple gestations treated with ritodrine, in comparison with a 4.0% incidence of cardiovascular complications in women with singleton pregnancies.[294] The inherent ability of the β agonists to expand plasma volume is compounded if they are delivered in saline-containing solutions.[179] Isotonic saline administration should be avoided in the preterm labor treatment of women with multiple gestations. The use of dextrose in water as the drug delivery vehicle tends to reduce the incidence of pulmonary edema in the treatment of these patients.

Because the diastolic blood pressure is lower in women with multiple gestations than that in women with single gestations, effects on the cardiovascular system may be more profound in this group of women. β-Adrenergic agents have multiple effects on the heart, including tachycardia, rhythm disturbances, subendocardial ischemia, and cardiac failure. An increase in the systolic blood pressure, coupled with a decrease in the diastolic blood pressure, is commonly observed during tocolysis with β-adrenergic agents, especially terbutaline. Such changes generally occur with no significant change in the mean blood pressure and usually are of minimal, if any, clinical consequence in singleton pregnancy. Because the diastolic blood pressure in women with multiple gestations is lower than that of women with singleton pregnancies, this group of patients is predisposed to developing profound reductions in blood pressure during β-adrenergic tocolysis. These hazards are of considerable concern, and β-adrenergic agents should be used with caution in the treatment of preterm labor in women with multiple gestations.

Indomethacin has been used in multiple gestations not only as a tocolytic but also as a valuable intervention to treat symptomatic polyhydramnios. When the use of this agent is considered, it is important to remember that the effects of indomethacin on amniotic fluid vary between pregnancies and in individual fetuses.[295,296] For any given fetus, the incidence of oligohydramnios increases with increasing dose of the drug, but the effect of indomethacin on an individual fetus cannot be predicted. Ultrasonography should be used to assess the amniotic fluid volume of each fetus, and indomethacin should be discontinued should any fetus develop oligohydramnios.

Table 18–7. Comparisons of Tocolytic Agents

Adverse Effect	Ritodrine/ Terbutaline	Magnesium Sulfate	Calcium Channel Blocker	Indomethacin
Maternal				
Tachycardia	•		•	
Systolic hypotension	•			
Cardiac arrhythmias	•			
Angina pectoris	•			
Pulmonary edema	•	•		
Hyperglycemia	•			
Other	•			
Anxiety	•			
Shortness of breath	•			
Tremors	•			
Nausea	•	•	•	•
Headache	•	•	•	
Hypoglycemia	•			
Hyperinsulinemia	•			
Decreased patellar reflexes		•		
Respiratory depression		•		
Asystole		•		
Flushing		•		
Nystagmus		•		
Dizziness		•		
Fetal and Neonatal				
Lethargy		•		
Blurred vision and diplopia		•		
Ischemia		•		
Hypertension		•	•	
Decreased muscle tone and drowsiness		•		
Fetal heart rate variability		•		
Long bone demineralization		•		
Vasodilation			•	
Decreased peripheral vascular resistance			•	
Hepatotoxicity			•	
Decreased arterial P_{O_2} and pH (animal studies only)			•	
Vomiting				•
Drug rash				•
Fetal ductus constriction				•
Decreased fetal urine output				•
Increased neonatal morbidity				•
Necrotizing enterocolitis				•
Intracranial hemorrhage				•
Patent ductus arteriosis				•

P_{O_2}, partial pressure of oxygen.

Indomethacin may be particularly damaging to the fetal kidney, because of the reduction in dilatory effects that the prostaglandins have on renal blood flow.[297] Fetuses with compromised circulation, such as those affected by twin-twin transfusion syndrome, may have elevated circulating levels of angiotensin II that enhance the vasoconstrictive actions of prostaglandin inhibition. The use of indomethacin in such compromised fetuses is probably contraindicated (Table 18-7).

REFERENCES

1. Ventura SJ, Martin JA, Curtin SC, Mathews TJ: Report of final natality statistics, 1996. Mon Vital Stat Rep 46(11 Suppl):2, 13, 1998.
2. Newman RB, Luke B: Multifetal Pregnancy: A Handbook for the Care of the Pregnant Patient. Philadelphia, Lippincott Williams & Wilkins, 2000.
3. Rush RW, Keirse MJNC, Howat P, et al: Contribution of preterm delivery to perinatal mortality. BMJ 2:965, 1976.
4. Berkowitz GS, Papernik E: Epidemiology of preterm birth. Epidemiol Rev 15:414, 1993.
5. Kleinman JC, Kessel SS: Racial differences in low birthweight: Trends and risk factors. N Engl J Med 317:749, 1987.
6. Blackmore CA, Savitz DA, Edwards LJ, et al: Racial differences in the patterns of preterm delivery in Central North Carolina. Pediatr Perinat Epidemiol 9:281, 1995.
7. National Center for Health Statistics: Vital Statistics of the United States 1988, vol 1. Natality. Hyattsville, Md, National Center for Health Statistics, 1988.
8. Shiono PH, Klebanoff MA: Ethnic differences in preterm and very preterm delivery. Am J Public Health 76:1317, 1986.
9. Kramer MS, Coates AL, Michoud M-C, et al: Maternal anthropometry and idiopathic preterm labor. Obstet Gynecol 86:744, 1995.
10. Lang JM, Lieberman E, Cohen A: A comparison of risk factors for preterm labor and term small-for-gestational-age birth. Epidemiology 7:369, 1996.
11. Siega-Riz, Adair LS, Hobeal CJ: Maternal underweight status and inadequate rate of weight gain during the third trimester pregnancy increases the risk of preterm delivery. J Nutr 126:146, 1996.
12. McGregor SM, Keith LG, Bachichi JA, et al: Cocaine abuse during pregnancy: Correlation between prenatal care and perinatal outcome. Obstet Gynecol 74:882, 989.
13. Klein J, Ng SKC, Schittini M, et al: Cocaine use during pregnancy: Since the detection by hair assay. Am J Public Health 87:352, 1997.
14. Institute of Medicine, Committee to Study the Prevention of Low Birthweight: Preventing Low Birthweight. Washington, DC, National Academy Press, 1985.
15. Lazvaroni F, Bonassi S, Magani M, et al: Moderate drinking and outcome of pregnancy. Eur J Epidemiol 9:599, 1993.
16. MacDonald LD, Peacock JL, Anderson HR: Marital status: Associations with social and economic circumstances, psychological state and outcomes of pregnancy. J Public Health 14:26, 1992.
17. Verkerk PH, van Noord-Zaabstri BM, Florey C, et al: The effect of moderate maternal alcohol consumption on birthweight and gestational age in low risk population. Early Hum Dev 32:121, 1993.
18. Borges G, Lopez-Cervantes M, Medina-Mori ME, et al: Alcohol consumption, low birth weights and preterm delivery in the National Addiction Survey (Mexico). Int J Addict 28:355, 1993.
19. Leviton A, Cowan L: A review of the literature relating caffeine consumption by women to their risk of reproductive hazards. Food Chem Toxicol 40:1271, 2002.
20. Preentzen BH, Johnson JWC, Simpson S: Nutrition and hydration: Relationship to preterm myometrial contractility. Obstet Gynecol 70:887, 1987.
21. Virji SK, Cottington E: Risk factors associated with preterm deliveries among racial groups in the national sample of unmarried mothers. Am J Perinatol 8:347, 1991.
22. Krimer MS, McLeaen FH, Eason BL, et al: Maternal nutrition and spontaneous preterm birth. Am J Epidemiol 136:574, 1992.
23. Hebegaard M, Henriksen TB, Echer NJ, et al: Do stressful life events effects duration of gestation and risk of preterm delivery? Epidemiology 7:339, 1996.
24. Norbeck JS, Tilden VP: Life stress, social support, and emotional disequilibrium in complications of pregnancy: A prospective, multivariate study. J Health Soc Behav 24:30, 1983.
25. Pagel MD, Smilkstein G, Regen H, Montano D: Psychosocial influences all newborn outcomes: A controlled prospective study. Soc Sci Med 30:597, 1990.
26. Bryce RL, Stanley FJ, Garner JB: Randomized, controlled trial of antenatal social support to prevent preterm birth. Br J Obstet Gynaecol 98:1001, 1991.
27. Honnor MJ, Zubrick SR, Spanley FJ: The role of life advanced in different categories of preterm birth in a group of women with previous poor pregnancy outcome. Eur J Epidemiol 10:181, 1994.
28. Lobel M, Dunkel-Schetter C, Scrimshaw SC: Prenatal maternal stress and prematurity: A prospective study of socioeconomically disadvantaged women. Health Psychol 11:32, 1992.
29. Hebegaard M, Henriksen TB, Echer NJ, et al: Do stressful life events affect duration of gestation and risk of preterm delivery? Epidemiology 7:339, 1996.
30. Solberg BA, Butler J, Wagner NN: Sexual behavior in pregnancy. N Engl J Med 288:1098, 1973.
31. Rayburn WF, Wilson EA: Coital activity and premature delivery. Am J Obstet Gynecol 137:972, 1980.
32. Mills JL, Harlap S, Harley EE: Should coitus late in pregnancy be discouraged? Lancet 2:136, 1981.
33. Ekwo EE, Gosselink CA, Woolson R, et al: Coitus late in pregnancy: Risk of preterm rupture of amniotic sac membranes. Am J Obstet Gynecol 168:22, 1993.
34. Read JS, Klebanoff MA: Sexual intercourse during pregnancy and preterm delivery: Effects of vaginal microorganisms. The Vaginal Infections and Prematurity Study Group. Am J Obstet Gynecol 168:514, 1993.
35. Buekens P, Alexander S, Boutsen M, et al: Randomised controlled trial of routine cervical examinations in pregnancy. European Community Collaborative Study Group on Prenatal Screening. Lancet 344:841, 1994.
36. King JF, Grant A, Keirse MJNC, Chalmers I: Beta mimetics in preterm labour: An overview of randomized controlled trials. Br J Obstet Gynaecol 95:211, 1988.
37. Marshall CL, Hayashi RH: Obstetrics management of the very low birth weight fetus. Clin Perinatol 13:251, 1986.
38. Norwitz ER, Robinson JN, Challis JRG: The control of labor. N Engl J Med 341:660, 1999.
39. Parikh MN, Mehta AC: Internal cervical os during the second half of pregnancy. J Obstet Gynaecol Br Commonw 68:818, 1961.

40. Schaffner F, Schanzer SN: Cervical dilation in the early third trimester. Obstet Gynecol 27:130, 1966.

41. Floyd WS: Cervical dilatation in the mid-trimester of pregnancy. Obstet Gynecol 18:380, 1961.

42. Creasy RK, Merkatz IR: Prevention of preterm birth: Clinical opinion. Obstet Gynecol 76(Suppl):2, 1990.

43. Hauth JC, Andrews WW, Goldenberg RL: Infection-related risk factors predictive of spontaneous preterm labor and birth. Prenat Neonat Med 3:86, 1998.

44. Lockwood CJ, Dudenhausen JW: New approaches to the prediction of preterm delivery. J Perinatol Med 21:441, 1993.

45. Mercer BM, Goldenberg RL, Das A, et al: The Preterm Prediction Study: A clinical risk assessment system. Am J Obstet Gynecol 174:1885, 1996.

46. Papiernik E, Bouyer J, Collin D, et al: Precocious cervical ripening and preterm labor. Obstet Gynecol 67:238, 1986.

47. Wood C, Bannerman RHO, Booth RT, Pinkerton JHM: The prediction of premature labor by observation of the cervix and external tocography. Am J Obstet Gynecol 91:396, 1965.

48. Leveno KJ, Cox K, Roark ML: Cervical dilation and prematurity revisited. Obstet Gynecol 68:434, 1986.

49. Stubbs TM, Van Dorsten P, Miller MC: The preterm cervix and preterm labour: Relative risks, predictive values, and change over time. Am J Obstet Gynecology 155:829, 1986.

50. Holcomb WL, Smeltzer JS: Cervical effacement: Variation in belief among clinicians. Obstet Gynecol 78:43, 1991.

51. Zador I, Neuman MR, Wolfson RN: Continuous monitoring of the cervical dilatation during labor by ultrasound transit time measurement. Med Biol Eng Comput 14:229, 1976.

52. Zemlyn S: The length of the uterine cervix and its significance. J Clin Ultrasound 9:267, 1981.

53. Andersen HF: Transvaginal and transabdominal ultrasonography of the uterine cervix during pregnancy. J Clin Ultrasound 19:77, 1991.

54. Iams JD, Goldenberg RL, Meis PJ, et al: The length of the cervix and the risk of spontaneous premature delivery. N Engl J Med 334:567, 1996.

55. Andersen HF, Nugent CE, Wanty SD, Hayashi RH: Prediction of risk for preterm delivery by ultrasonographic measurement of cervical length. Am J Obstet Gynecol 163:859, 1990.

56. Okitsu O, Mimura T, Nakayama T, Aono T: Early prediction of preterm delivery by transvaginal ultrasonography. Ultrasound Obstet Gynaecol 2:402, 1992.

57. Lockwood CJ, Senyei AE, Dische MR, et al: Fetal fibronectin in cervical and vaginal secretions as a predictor of preterm delivery. N Engl J Med 325:669, 1991.

58. Goldenberg RL, Mercer BM, Meis PJ, et al: The Preterm Prediction Study: Fetal fibronectin testing and spontaneous preterm birth. Obstet Gynecol 87:643, 1996.

59. Iams JD, Goldenberg RL, Mercer BM, et al: The Preterm Prediction Study: Recurrence risk of spontaneous preterm birth. Am J Obstet Gynecol 178:1035, 1998.

60. Lopez RL, Francis JA, Garite TJ, Dubyak JM: Fetal fibronectin detection as a predictor of preterm birth in actual clinical practice. Am J Obstet Gynecol 182:1103, 2000.

61. Peaceman AM, Andrews WW, Thorp JM, et al: Fetal fibronectin as a predictor of preterm birth in patients with symptoms: A multicenter trial. Am J Obstet Gynecol 177:13, 1997.

62. Joffe GM, Jacques D, Bemis-Heys R, et al: Impact of the fetal fibronectin assay on admissions for preterm labor. Am J Obstet Gynecol 180:581, 1999.

63. Nageotte MP, Casal D, Senyei AE: Fetal fibronectin in patients at increased risk for premature birth. Am J Obstet Gynecol 170:20, 1994.

64. Tulchinsky D, Hobel CJ, Yeager E, Marshall JR: Plasma estrone, estradiol, estriol, progesterone, and 17-hydroxy-progesterone in human pregnancy. I. Normal Pregnancy. Am J Obstet Gynecol 112:1095, 1972.

65. Liggens GC: Initiation of labor. Biol Neonate 55:366, 1989.

66. Darne J, McGarrigle HHG, Lachlin GCL: Increased saliva oestriol to progesterone ratio before idiopathic preterm delivery: A possible predictor for preterm labor? BMJ 294:270, 1987.

67. Voss HF: Saliva as a fluid for measurement of estriol levels. Am J Obstet Gynecol 180:S226, 1999.

68. Hendershott CM, Dullien V, Goodwin TM: Serial beta-methasone administration: Effect on maternal salivary estriol levels. Am J Obstet Gynecol 180:S219, 1999.

69. McGregor JA, Jackson M, Lachelin GCL, et al: Salivary estriol as risk assessment for preterm labor: A prospective trial. Am J Obstet Gynecol 173:1337, 1995.

70. McGregor JA, Heine RP, Artal R, et al: Results of a prospective blinded, multicenter trial of salivary estriol for risk of preterm labor and delivery [abstract]. Am J Obstet Gynecol 178:S18, 1998.

71. Robertson PA, McGregor JA, Varner M, et al: The role of salivary estriol in predicting symptomatic patients [abstract]. Presented at the 68th Annual Clinical Meeting of the American College of Obstetricians and Gynecologists, April 1998, Atlanta.

72. Heine RP, McGregor JA, Goodwin TM, et al: Serial salivary estriol to detect an increased risk of preterm birth. Obstet Gynecol 96:490, 2000.

73. Petraglia F: Inhibin, activin and follistatin in the human placenta: A new family of regulatory proteins. Placenta 18:3, 1997.

74. Petraglia F, De Vita D, Gallinelli A, et al: Abnormal concentration of maternal serum activin-A in gestational diseases. J Clin Endocrinol Metab 80:558, 1995.

75. Iams JD, Casal D, McGregor JA, et al: Fetal fibronectin improves the accuracy of diagnosis of preterm labor. Am J Obstet Gynecol 173:141, 1995.

76. Rajabi M, Dean DD, Woessner JF Jr: High levels of serum collagenase in premature labor: A potential biochemical marker. Obstet Gynecol 69:179, 1987.

77. Clark IM, Morrison JJ, Hackett GA, et al: Tissue inhibitor of metalloproteinases: Serum levels during pregnancy and labor, term and preterm. Obstet Gynecol 83:532, 1994.

78. Zahn V: Uterine contractions during pregnancy. J Perinat Med 12:107, 1984.

79. Iams JD, Johnson FF, Hamer C: Uterine activity and symptoms as predictors of preterm labor. Obstet Gynecol 76(Suppl):42, 1990.

80. Newman RB, Gill PJ, Campion S, et al: The influence of fetal number on antepartum uterine activity. Obstet Gynecol 73:695, 1989.

81. Paul MJ, Smeltzer JS: Relationship of measured external tocodynometry with measured internal uterine activity. Am J Perinatol 8:417, 1991.

82. Hess LW, McCaul JF, Perry KG, et al: Correlation of uterine activity using the Term Guard monitor versus standard external tocodynamometry compared with the intrauterine pressure catheter. Obstet Gynecol 76(Suppl):52, 1990.

83. Scheerer LJ, Campion S, Katz M: Ambulatory tocodynamometry data interpretation: Evaluating variability and reliability. Obstet Gynecol 76(Suppl):67, 1990.

84. Dyson DC, Danbe KH, Bamber JA, et al: Monitoring women at risk for preterm labor. N Engl J Med 338:15, 1998.

85. Colton T, Kayne HL, Zhang Y, et al: A meta-analysis of home uterine activity monitoring. Am J Obstet Gynecol 173:1499, 1995.

86. Grimes DA, Schultz KF: Randomized controlled trials of home uterine activity monitoring: A review and critique. Obstet Gynecol 79:137, 1992.

87. Sachs BP, Hellerstein S, Freeman RK, et al: Sounding board. Home uterine activity monitoring: Does it prevent prematurity? N Engl J Med 325:1374, 1991.

88. U.S. Preventive Services Task Force: Home uterine activity monitoring for preterm labor. JAMA 270:371, 1993.

89. Mclean M, Walters WAW, Smith R: Prediction and early diagnosis of preterm labor: A critical review. Obstet Gynecol Surv 48:209, 1993.

90. A multicenter randomized controlled trial of home uterine monitoring: Active versus sham device. The Collaborative Home Uterine Monitoring Study (CHUMS) Group. Am J Obstet Gynecol 173:1120, 1995.

91. The Canadian Preterm Labor Investigators Group: Treatment of preterm labor with the beta-adrenergic agonist ritodrine. N Engl J Med 327:308, 1992.

92. Devedeux D, Marque C, Mansour S, et al: Uterine electromyography—a critical review. Am J Obstet Gynecol 169:1636, 1993.

93. Garfield RE, Chwalisz K, Shi L, et al: Instrumentation for the diagnosis of term and preterm labour. J Perinat Med 26:413, 1998.

94. Kuriyama H, Caspo AI: A study of parturient uterus with the microelectrode technique. Endocrinology 68:1010, 1961.

95. Steer CM: The electrical activity of the human uterus in normal and abnormal labor. Am J Obstet Gynecol 68:867, 1954.

96. Mansour S, Duchene J, Germain G, Marque C: Uterine EMG: Experimental and mathematical determination of relationship between internal and external recordings. IEEE EMBS 3:485, 1991.

97. Buhimschi C, Boyle MB, Saade GR, Garfield RE: Uterine activity during pregnancy and labor assessed by simultaneous recordings from the myometrium and abdominal surface in the rat. Am J Obstet Gynecol 178:811, 1998.

98. Wolfs G, van Leeuwen M, Rottinghuis H, Boeles JT: An electromyographic study of the human uterus during labor. Obstet Gynecol 37:241, 1971.

99. Garfield RE, Blennerhasset MG, Miller SM: Control of myometrial contractility: Role and regulation of gap junctions. In Clarke JR (ed): Oxford Review of Reproductive Biology, vol 10. Oxford, England, Oxford University Press, 1988, pp 436-490.

100. Miyoshi H, Boyle MB, MacKay LB, Garfield RE: Gap junction currents in cultured muscle cells from human myometrium. Am J Obstet Gynecol 178:588, 1998.

101. Miller SM, Garfield RE, Daniel EE: Improved propagation in myometrium associated with gap junctions during parturition. Am J Physiol 256:C130, 1989.

102. Garfield RE, Hayashi RH: Appearance of gap junctions in the myometrium of women during labor. Am J Obstet Gynecol 140:254, 1981.

103. Garfield RE, Sims S, Kannan MS, Daniel EE: Possible role of gap junctions in activation of myometrium during parturition. Am J Physiol 235:C168, 1978.

104. Garfield RE, Sims S, Daniel EE: Gap junctions: Their presence and necessity in myometrium during parturition. Science 198:958, 1977.

105. Garfield RE, Saade G, Buhimschi C, et al: Control and assessment of uterus and cervix during pregnancy and labour. Hum Reprod Update 4:673, 1998.

106. Buhimschi C, Boyle MB, Garfield RE: Electrical activity of the human uterus during pregnancy as recorded from abdominal surface. Obstet Gynecol 90:102, 1997.

107. Williamson SJ, Romani GL, Kaufman L: Biomagnetism: An Interdisciplinary Approach. New York, Plenum Press, 1983.

108. Eswaran H, Preissl H, Wilson JD, et al: First magnetomyographic recordings of uterine activity with spatial-temporal resolution using a 151-channel sensor array. Am J Obstet Gynecol 187:145, 2002.

109. Tucker JM, Goldenberg RL, Davis RO, et al: Etiologies of preterm birth in an indigent population: Is prevention a logical expectation? Obstet Gynecol 77:343, 1991.

110. Zahl PA, Bjerknes C: Induction of decidua-placental hemorrhage in mice by the endotoxins of certain gram-negative bacteria. Proc Soc Exp Biol Med 54:329, 1943.

111. Kass EH: Pyelonephritis and bacteriuria. A major problem in preventive medicine. Ann Intern Med 56:46, 1962.

112. Romero R, Oyarzun E, Mazor M, et al: Meta-analysis of the relationship between asymptomatic bacteriuria and preterm delivery/low birth weight. Obstet Gynecol 73:576, 1989.

113. Andrews WW, Hauth JC, Goldenberg RL, et al: Amniotic fluid interleukin-6: Correlation with upper genital tract microbial colonization and gestational age in women delivered after spontaneous labor versus indicated delivery. Am J Obstet Gynecol 173:606, 1995.

114. Goldenberg RL, Andrews WW, Yuan AC, et al: Sexually transmitted diseases and adverse outcomes of pregnancy. Clin Perinatol 24:23, 1997.

115. Hillier SL, Nugent RP, Eschenbach DA, et al: Association between bacterial vaginosis and preterm delivery of a low-birth-weight infant. N Engl J Med 333:1737, 1995.

116. Yoon BH, Romero R, Kim CJ, et al: High expression of tumor necrosis factor-alpha and interleukin-6 in periventricular leukomalacia. Am J Obstet Gynecol 177:406, 1997.

117. Alexander JM, Gilstrap LC, Cox SM, et al: Clinical chorioamnionitis and the prognosis for very low birth weight infants. Obstet Gynecol 91:725, 1998.

118. Genazzani AR, Petraglia F, Volpe A, et al (eds): Advances in Gynecological Endocrinology, vol I. Carnforth, England, Parthenon, 1988, p 487.

119. Romero R, Mazor M, Wu YK, et al: Infection in the pathogenesis of preterm labor. Semin Perinatol 12:262, 1988.

120. Offenbacher S, Katz V, Ferpik G, et al: Periodontal infections as a possible risk factor for preterm low birth weight. J Periodontol 67:1103, 1996.

121. Collins JG, Windley HW III, Larnolb RR, et al: Effects of a *Porphyromonas gingivalis* infection on inflammatory mediator response and pregnant outcome in the hamster. Infect Immun 62:4356, 1994.

122. Offenbacher S, Jared HL, O'Reilly PG, et al: Potential pathogenic mechanisms of periodontitis associated pregnancy complications. Ann Periodontol 3:233, 1998.

123. Lopez NJ, Smith PC, Gutierrez J: Periodontal therapy may reduce the risk of preterm low birth weight in women with periodontal disease: A randomized controlled trial. J Periodontol 73:911, 2002.

124. Romero BC, Chiquito CS, Elejalde LE, Bernardoni CB: Relationship between periodontal disease in pregnant women and the nutritional condition of their newborns. J Periodontol 73:1177, 2002.

125. Gravett MG, Eshenbach DA, Holmes KK: Preterm labor associated with subclinical amniotic fluid infection and with bacterial vaginosis. Obstet Gynecol 67:229, 1986.

126. Morales WJ, Schorr S, Albritton J: Effect of metronidazole in patients with preterm birth in preceding pregnancy and bacterial vaginosis. A placebo-controlled, double-blind study. Am J Obstet Gynecol 171:345, 1994.

127. McGregor JA, French JI, Jones W, et al: Bacterial vaginosis is associated with prematurity and vaginal fluid mucinase and sialidase: Results of a controlled trial of topical clindamycin cream. Am J Obstet Gynecol 170:1048, 1994.

128. Joesoef MR, Hillier SL, Wiknjosastro G, et al: Intravaginal clindamycin treatment for bacterial vaginosis: Effects on preterm delivery and low birth weight. Am J Obstet Gynecol 173:1527, 1995.

129. Hauth JC, Goldenberg RL, Andrews WW, et al: Reduced incidence of preterm delivery with metronidazole and erythromycin in women with bacterial vaginosis. N Engl J Med 333:1732, 1995.

130. Carey JC, Klebanoff M: Metronidazole treatment increased the risk of preterm birth in asymptomatic women with *Trichomonas*. Am J Obstet Gynecol 182:S13, 2000.

131. Carey JC, Klebanoff MA, Hauth JC, et al: Metronidazole to prevent preterm delivery in pregnant women with asymptomatic bacterial vaginosis. National Institute of Child Health and Human Development Network of Maternal-Fetal Medicine Units. N Engl J Med 342:534, 2000.

132. McGregor JA, French JI, Seo K: Adjunctive clindamycin therapy for preterm labor: Results of a double-blind, placebo-controlled trial. Am J Obstet Gynecol 165(4 Pt 1): 867, 1991.

133. Morales WJ, Angel JD, O'Brian WF, et al: A randomized study of antibiotic therapy in idiopathic preterm labor. Obstet Gynecol 72:829, 1988.

134. Newton ER, Dinsmoor MJ, Gibbs RS: A randomized, blinded, placebo-controlled trial of antibiotics in idiopathic preterm labor. Obstet Gynecol 74:562, 1989.

135. Newton ER, Shields L, Ridgway LE III, et al: Combination antibiotics and indomethacin in idiopathic preterm labor: A randomized, double-blind clinical trial. Am J Obstet Gynecol 165:1753, 1991.

136. Romero R, Sibai BM, Caritis S, et al: Antibiotic treatment of preterm labor with intact membranes: A multicenter, randomized, double-blinded, placebo-controlled trial. Am J Obstet Gynecol 169:764, 1993.

137. Cox SM, Bohman VR, Sherman L, et al: Randomized investigation of antimicrobials for the prevention of preterm birth. Am J Obstet Gynecol 174:206, 1996.

138. McCaul JF, Perry KG, Moore JL, et al: Adjunctive antibiotic treatment of women with preterm rupture of membranes or preterm labor. Int J Gynecol Obstet 38:19, 1992.

139. Svare J, Langhoff-Roos J, Andersen LF, et al: Ampicillin-metronidazole treatment in idiopathic preterm labour: A randomized controlled multicentre trial. Br J Obstet Gynaecol 104:892, 1997.

140. Buxton IL, Crow W, Mathew SO: Regulation of uterine contraction: Mechanisms in preterm labor. AACN Clin Issues 11:271, 2000.

141. Maher JE, Cliver SP, Goldenberg RL, et al: The effect of corticosteroid therapy in the very premature infant. March of Dimes Multicenter Study Group. Am J Obstet Gynecol 170:869, 1994.

142. Bradley KK, Buxton ILO, Barber JE, et al: Nitric oxide relaxes human myometrium by a cGMP-independent mechanism. Am J Physiol 44:C1668, 1998.

143. Kuenzli KA, Bradley ME, Buxton ILO: Cyclic GMP–independent effects of nitric oxide on guinea-pig uterine contractions. Br J Pharmacol 119:737, 1996.

144. Jeyabalan A, Caritis SN: Pharmacologic inhibition of preterm labor. Clin Obstet Gynecol 45:99, 2002.

145. Wray S: Uterine contraction and physiological mechanisms of modulation. Am J Physiol 33:C1, 1993.

146. Bolton TB, Prestwich SA, Zholos AV, Gordienko DV: Excitation-contraction coupling in gastrointestinal and other smooth muscles. Annu Rev Physiol 61:85, 1999.

147. Riemer RK, Heymann MA: Regulation of uterine smooth muscle function during gestation. Pediatr Res 44:615, 1998.

148. Challis JRG, Gibb W: Control of parturition. Prenat Neonat Med 1:283, 1996.

149. Cunningham FG, MacDonald PC, Gant NF, et al: Williams Obstetrics, 19th ed. Norwalk, Conn, Appleton & Lange, 1993, pp 298-299.

150. Lye SJ: Myometrial physiology and parturition. In Rodeck CH, Whittle MJ (eds): Fetal Medicine: Basic Science and Clinical Practice. London, Churchill-Livingstone, 1997.

151. Chwalisz K, Garfield RE: Regulation of the uterus and the cervix during pregnancy and in labor: Role of progesterone and nitric oxide. Ann N Y Acad Sci 828:238, 1997.

152. Chwalisz K, Garfield RE: Role of nitric oxide in the uterus and cervix: Implications for the management of labor. J Perinat Med 26:448, 1998.

153. Lockwood CJ, Kuczynski E: Markers of risk for preterm delivery. J Perinat Med 27:5, 1999.

154. Castracane VD: Endocrinology of preterm labor. Clin Obstet Gynecol 31:533, 2000.

155. Lockwood CJ: Stress-associated preterm delivery: The role of corticotropin-releasing hormone. Am J Obstet Gynecol, 180:S264, 1999.

156. Dudley DJ: Immunoendocrinology of preterm labor: The link between corticotropin-releasing hormone and inflammation. Am J. Obstet Gynecol, 180:S251, 1999.

157. Goldenberg RL, Hauth JC, Andrews WW: Intrauterine infection and preterm labor. N Engl J Med, 342:1500, 2000.

158. Gomez R, Romero R, Edwin SS, David C: Pathogenesis of preterm labor and premature rupture of membranes associated with intraamnionic infection. Infect Dis Clin North Am 11:135, 1997.

159. Saji F, Samejima Y, Kamiura S, et al: Cytokine production in chorioamnionitis. J Reprod Immunol 47:85, 2000.

160. Caritis S, Darby M, Chan L: Pharmacologic treatment of preterm labor. Clin Obstet Gynecol 31:635, 1988.

161. Pircon RA, Strassner HT, Kirz DS, et al: Controlled trial of hydration and bed rest alone in the evaluation of preterm uterine contractions. Am J Obstet Gynecol 161:775, 1989.

162. Gonik B, Creasy RK: Preterm labor—its diagnosis and management. Am J Obstet Gynecol 154:3, 1986.

163. Lefebvre F, Glorieux J, St-Laurent-Gagnon T: Neonatal survival and disability rate at age 18 months for infants born between 23 and 28 weeks of gestation. Am J Obstet Gynecol 174:833, 1996.

164. Robertson PA, Sniderman SH, Laros RK Jr, et al: Neonatal morbidity according to gestational age and birth weight from five tertiary care centers in the United States, 1983 through 1986. Am J Obstet Gynecol 166:1629, 1992.

165. Ventura SJ, Martin JA, Curtin SC, et al: Births: Final data for 1999. Natl Vital Stat Rep 49:1, 2001.

166. Maloni JA, Breninski-Tonmasi JE, Johnson LA: Antepartum bed rest: Effect upon the family. J Obstet Gynecol Neonat Nurs 30:165, 2001.

167. Saunders MC, Dick JS, Brown IM, et al: The effects of hospital admission for bed rest on the duration of twin pregnancy: A randomised trial. Lancet 2:793, 1985.

168. Kovacevich GJ, Gaich SA, Lavin JP, et al: The prevalence of thromboembolic events among women with extended bedrest prescribed as part of the treatment for premature labor or preterm premature rupture of membranes. Am J Obstet Gynecol 182:1089, 2000.

169. Danilenko-Dixon DR, Heit JA, Silverstein MC, et al: Risk factors for deep vein thrombosis and pulmonary embolism during pregnancy or postpartum: A population-based, case-control study. Am J Obstet Gynecol 184:104, 2001.

170. Flynn K: Preterm labor and premature rupture of membranes. In Mandeville LK, Troiano NH (eds): High Risk and Critical Care Intrapartum Nursing, 2nd ed. Philadelphia, Lippincott Williams & Wilkins, 1999.

171. Lye SJ: The initiation and inhibition of labour: Toward a molecular understanding. Semin Reprod Endocrinol 12:284, 1994.

172. Haway DR, DePaoli-Roach AA: Dephosphorylation of myosin by the catalytic subunit of a type-2 phosphatase produces relaxation of chemically skinned uterine smooth muscle. J Biol Chem 260:9965, 1985.

173. Word RA: Myosin phosphorylation and the control of myometrial contraction/relaxation. Semin Perinatol 19:3, 1995.

174. Barden TP, Peter JB, Merkatz IR: Ritodrine hydrochloride: A beta-mimetic agent for use in preterm labor. Obstet Gynecol 56:1, 1980.

175. Gardner MO, Goldenberg RL: The influence of race and previous pregnancy outcome on outcomes in current pregnancy. Semin Perinatol 19:191, 1995.

176. Goepfert AR, Goldenberg RL: Prediction of prematurity. Curr Opin Obstet Gynecol 8:417, 1996.

177. Shiono PH, Klebanof MA, Graubard BI, et al: Birthweight among women of different ethnic groups. JAMA 255:48, 1986.

178. Creasy RK, Gummer BA, Liggins GC: System for predicting spontaneous preterm birth. Obstet Gynecol 55:692, 1980.

179. Hearne AE, Nagey DA: Therapeutic agents in preterm labor: Tocolytic agents. Clin Obstet Gynecol 43:787, 2000.

180. Hill WH: Risks and complications of tocolysis. Clin Obstet Gynecol 38:725, 1995.

181. Wesselius-deCasparis A, Thiery M, Sian A, et al: Results of double-blind, multicentre study with ritodrine in premature labor. BMJ 3:141, 1971.

182. Merkatz IR, Peter JB, Barden TP: Ritodrine hydrochloride: A betamimetic agent for use in preterm labor II. Evidence of efficacy. Obstet Gynecol 56:7, 1980.

183. Harden T: Agonist-induced desensitization of the beta-adrenergic receptor–linked adenylate cyclase. Pharmacol Rev 35:5, 1983.

184. Caritis SN, Chiao JP, Moore JJ, et al: Myometrial desensitization after ritodrine infusion. Am J Physiol 253:E410, 1987.

185. Benedetti T: Maternal complications of parenteral beta sympathomimetic therapy for preterm labor. Am J Obstet Gynecol 145:1, 1983.

186. Hendricks S, Keroes J, Katz M: Electrocardiographic changes associated with ritodrine-induced maternal tachycardia and hypokalemia. Am J Obstet Gynecol 154:921, 1986.

187. Caritis S, Toig G, Heddinger L, et al: A double-blind study comparing ritodrine and terbutaline in the treatment of preterm labor. Am J Obstet Gynecol 150:7, 1984.

188. Ingemarrson I, Bentsson B: A five-year experience with terbutaline for preterm labor: Low rate of severe side effects. Obstet Gynecol 66:176, 1985.

189. Young DC, Toofanian A, Leveno KJ: Potassium and glucose concentrations without treatment during ritodrine tocolysis. Am J Obstet Gynecol 145:105, 1983.

190. Lunell NO, Joelsson I, Larsson A, et al: The immediate effect of a beta-adrenergic agonist (salbutamol) on carbohydrate and lipid metabolism during the third trimester of pregnancy. Acta Obstet Gynecol Scand 56:475, 1977.

191. Spellacy WN, Cruz AC, Buhi WC, et al: The acute effects of ritodrine infusion on maternal metabolism: Measurements of levels of glucose, insulin, glucagon, triglycerides, cholesterol, placental lactogen, and chorionic gonadotropin. Am J Obstet Gynecol 131:637, 1978.

192. Iams JD: Preterm birth. In Gabbe SG, Niebyl JR, Simpson JL (eds): Obstetrics: Normal and Problem Pregnancies, 4th ed. New York, Churchill Livingstone, 2002, pp 755-826.

193. Smigaj D, Roman-Drago NM, Amini SB, et al: The effect of oral terbutaline on maternal glucose metabolism and energy expenditure in pregnancy. Am J Obstet Gynecol 178:1041, 1998.

194. Creasy RK: Preterm birth prevention: Where are we? Am J Obstet Gynecol 168:1223, 1993.

195. Groome LJ, Goldenberg RL, Cliver SP, et al: Neonatal periventricular-intraventricular hemorrhage after maternal beta-sympathomimetic tocolysis. The March of Dimes Multicenter Study Group. Am J Obstet Gynecol 167:873, 1992.

196. Caritis SN, Venkataramanan R, Darby MJ, et al: Pharmacokinetics of ritodrine administered intravenously. Recommendations for changes in the current regimen. Am J Obstet Gynecol 162:429, 1990.

197. Caritis SN, Lin LS, Toig G, et al: Pharmacodynamics of ritodrine in pregnant women during preterm labor. Am J Obstet Gynecol 147:752, 1983.

198. Bader AM, Boudier E, Martinez C, et al: Etiology and prevention of pulmonary complications following beta-mimetic mediated tocolysis. Eur J Obstet Gynecol 80:133, 1998.

199. Braden GL, Von Oeyen PT, Germain J, et al: Ritodrine- and terbutaline-induced hypokalemia in pre-term labor: Mechanisms and consequences. Kidney Int 51:1867, 1997.

200. Guinn DA, Goepfert AR, Owen J, et al: Terbutaline pump maintenance therapy for prevention of preterm delivery: A double-blind trial. Am J Obstet Gynecol 179:874, 1998.

201. Parilla BV, Dooley SL, Minogue JP, Socol ML: The efficacy of oral terbutaline after intravenous tocolysis. Am J Obstet Gynecol 169:965, 1993.

202. Elliott JP: Magnesium sulfate as a tocolytic agent. Am J Obstet Gynecol 147:277, 1983.

203. Hollander DI, Nagey DA, Pupkin MJ: Magnesium sulfate and ritodrine hydrochloride: A randomized comparison. Am J Obstet Gynecol 156:631, 1987.

204. Cox SM, Sherman ML, Leveno KJ: Randomized investigation of magnesium sulfate for prevention of preterm birth. Am J Obstet Gynecol 163:767, 1990.

205. Lifson MS, Nagey DA, Coulson CC, et al: Efficacy of magnesium sulfate in the treatment of preterm labor: Predictors of failure. J Matern Fetal Invest 1:197, 1991.

206. Macones GA, Sehdev HM, Berlin M, et al: Evidence for magnesium sulfate as a tocolytic agent. Obstet Gynecol Surv 52:652, 1997.

207. Ohki S, Ikura M, Zhang M: Identification of magnesium binding sites and the role of magnesium on target recognition by calmodulin. Biochemistry 36:4309, 1997.

208. Sanborn BM: Ion channels and the control of myometrial electrical activity. Semin Perinatol 19:31, 1995.

209. Monga M, Creasy RK: Pharmacologic management of preterm labor. Semin Perinatol 19:84, 1995.

209a. Madden C, Owen J, Hauth C: Magnesium tocolysis: Serum levels versus success. Am J Obstet Gynecol 162:1177, 1990.

209b. Cruikshank DP, Pitkin RM, Donnelly E, et al: Urinary magnesium, calcium, and phosphate excretion during magnesium sulphate infusion. Obstet Gynecol 58:430, 1981.

209c. Cruikshank DP, Pitkin RM, Reynolds WA, et al: Effects of magnesium sulphate treatment on perinatal calcium metabolism. I. Maternal and fetal responses. Am J Obstet Gynecol 134:243, 1979.

209d. Smith LG Jr, Burns PA, Schanler RJ: Calcium homeostasis in pregnant women receiving long-term magnesium sulphate therapy for preterm labor. Am J Obstet Gynecol 167:45, 1992.

209e. Holcomb WS Jr, Shackelford GD, Petrie RH: Magnesium tocolysis and neonatal bone abnormalities: A controlled study. Obstet Gynecol 78:611, 1991.

210. Higby K, Xenakis EMJ, Pauerstein CJ: Do tocolytics stop preterm labor? A critical and comprehensive review of efficacy and safety. Am J Obstet Gynecol 168:1247, 1993.

211. Creasy RK, Iams JD: Preterm labor and delivery. In Creasy RK, Resnik R (eds): Maternal-Fetal Medicine, 4th ed. Philadelphia, WB Saunders, 1999.

212. Kosasa T, Busse R, Wahl N, et al: Long-term tocolysis with combined intravenous terbutaline and magnesium sulfate: A 10-year study of 1,000 patients. Obstet Gynecol 84:369, 1994.

213. Yeast JD, Halberstadt C, Meyer BA, et al: The risk of pulmonary edema and colloid osmotic pressure changes during magnesium sulfate infusion. Am J Obstet Gynecol 169:1566, 1993.

214. Green KW, Key TC, Coen R, et al: The effects of maternally administered magnesium sulfate on the neonate. Am J Obstet Gynecol 146:29, 1983.

215. Nelson KB, Grether JK: Can magnesium sulfate reduce the risk of cerebral palsy in very low birthweight infants? Pediatrics 95:263, 1995.

216. Schendel DE, Berg CJ, Yeargin-Allsop M: Prenatal magnesium sulfate exposure and the risk for cerebral palsy or mental retardation among very low birth-weight children aged 3 to 5 years. JAMA 276:1805, 1996.

217. Mittendorf R, Covert R, Boman J: Is tocolytic magnesium sulphate associated with increased total pediatric mortality? Lancet 350:1517, 1997.

218. Scudiero R, Khoshnood B, Pryde PG, et al: Perinatal death and tocolytic magnesium sulfate. Obstet Gynecol 96:178, 2000.

219. Zuckerman H, Reiss U, Rubinstein I: Inhibition of human premature labor by indomethacin. Obstet Gynecol 44:787, 1974.

220. Zuckerman H, Shalev E, Gilad G, et al: Further study of the inhibition of premature labor by indomethacin. Part I. J Perinat Med 12:19, 1984.

221. Panter K, Hannah M, Amankwa K, et al: The effect of indomethacin tocolysis in preterm labour on perinatal outcome: A randomized placebo-controlled trial. BJOG 106:467, 1999.

222. Niebyl JR, Blake DA, White RD, et al: The inhibition of premature labor with indomethacin. Am J Obstet Gynecol 136:1014, 1980.

223. Keirse MJNC: Indomethacin tocolysis in preterm labour. In Enkin M, Keirse MJNC, Renfrew MJ, Neilson J (eds): Pregnancy and Childbirth Module. Cochrane Database of Systematic Reviews. London, BMJ Publishing, 1995.

224. Spearing G: Alcohol, indomethacin and salbutamol. A comparative trial of their use in preterm labor. Obstet Gynecol 53:171, 1979.

225. Katz Z, Lancet M, Yemini M, et al: Treatment of premature labor contractions with combined ritodrine and indomethacin. Int J Gynaecol Obstet 21:337, 1983.

226. Gamissans O, Canas E, Cararach V, et al: A study of indomethacin combined with ritodrine in threatened preterm labour. Eur J Obstet Gynecol Reprod Biol 8:123, 1978.

227. Gamissans O, Balasch J: Prostaglandin synthetase inhibitors in the treatment of preterm labor. In Fuchs F, Stubblefield P (eds): Preterm Birth: Causes, Prevention and Management. New York, Macmillan, 1984.

228. Morales W, Smith S, Angel J, et al: Efficacy and safety of indomethacin versus ritodrine in the management of preterm labor: A randomized study. Obstet Gynecol 74:567, 1989.

229. Morales W, Madhav H: Efficacy of indomethacin compared with magnesium sulfate in the management of preterm labor: A randomized study. Am J Obstet Gynecol 169:97, 1993.

230. Kurki T, Eronen M, Lumme R, Ylikorkala O: A randomized double-dummy comparison between indomethacin and nylidrin in threatened preterm labor. Obstet Gynecol 78:1093, 1991.

231. Carlan S, O'Brien W, O'Leary T, Mastrogiannis D: Randomized comparative trial of indomethacin and sulindac for the treatment of refractory preterm labor. Obstet Gynecol 79:223, 1992.

232. Bivins H, Newman R, Fyfe D, et al: Randomized trial of oral indomethacin and terbutaline sulfate for the long-term suppression of preterm labor. Am J Obstet Gynecol 169:1065, 1993.

233. Besinger R, Niebyl J, Keyes W, Johnson T: Randomized comparative trial of indomethacin and ritodrine for the long-term treatment of preterm labor. Am J Obstet Gynecol 164:981, 1991.

234. Macones GA, Marder SJ, Clothier B, Stamilio DM: The controversy surrounding indomethacin for tocolysis. Am J Obstet Gynecol 184:264, 2001.

235. Lunt CC, Satin AJ, Barth WH, Hankins GDV: The effect of indomethacin tocolysis on maternal coagulation status. Obstet Gynecol 84:820, 1994.

236. Rasanen J, Jouppila P: Fetal cardiac function and ductus arteriosus during indomethacin and sulindac therapy for threatened preterm labor: A randomized study. Am J Obstet Gynecol 173:20, 1995.

237. Vermillion ST, Scardo JA, Lashus AG, Wiles HB: The effect of indomethacin tocolysis on fetal ductus arteriosus constriction with advancing gestational age. Am J Obstet Gynecol 177:256, 1997.

238. Vermillion ST, Newman RP: Recent indomethacin tocolysis is not associated with neonatal complications in preterm infants. Am J Obstet Gynecol 181(5 Pt 1):1083, 1999.

239. Iannucci TA, Bensinger RE, Fisher SG, et al: Effect of dual tocolysis on the incidence of severe intraventricular hemorrhage among extremely low birth weight infants. Am J Obstet Gynecol 175:1043, 1996.

240. Gardner M, Owen J, Skelly S, et al: Preterm delivery after indomethacin: A risk factor for neonatal complications? J Reprod Med 41:903, 1996.

241. Vermillion S, Newman R: Recent indomethacin tocolysis is not associated with neonatal complications in preterm infants. Am J Obstet Gynecol 181:1083, 1999.

242. Bhat R, Vidyasager D, Vadapalli MO, et al: Disposition of indomethacin in preterm infants. J Pediatr 95:313, 1979.

243. Zuckerman H, Shalev E, Gilad G, et al: Further study of the inhibition of premature labor by indomethacin. Part II double-blind study. J Perinat Med 12:25, 1984.

244. Granger S, Hollingsworth M, Weston A: A comparison of several calcium antagonists on uterine, vascular, and cardiac muscles from the rat. Br J Pharmacol 85:255,1985.

245. Kupferminc M, Lessing JB, Yaron Y, et al: Nifedipine versus ritodrine for suppression of preterm labor. Br J Obstet Gynaecol 100:1090, 1993.

246. Van Dijk KG, Dekker G, van Geijn HP: Ritodrine and nifedipine as tocolytic agents: A preliminary comparison. J Perinat Med 23:409, 1995.

247. Garcia-Velasco JA, Gonzalez Gonzalez A: A prospective, randomized trial of nifedipine vs. ritodrine in threatened preterm labor. Int J Gynaecol Obstet 61:239, 1998.

248. Koks CA, Brolmann HA, de Kleine MJ, et al: A randomized comparison of nifedipine and ritodrine for suppression of preterm labor. Eur J Obstet Gynecol Reprod Biol 77:171, 1998.

249. Meyer W, Randall H, Graves W: Nifedipine versus ritodrine for suppressing preterm labor. J Reprod Med 35:649, 1990.

250. Janky E, Leng JJ, Cormier PH, et al: A randomized study of the treatment of threatened premature labor. Nifedipine versus ritodrine. J Gynecol Biol Reprod 19:478, 1990.

251. Read M, Welby D: The use of a calcium channel antagonist (nifedipine) to suppress preterm labor. Br J Obstet Gynaecol 93:933, 1986.

252. Ferguson JE, Dyson D, Schutz T, et al: A comparison of tocolysis with nifedipine or ritodrine: Analysis of efficacy and maternal, fetal, and neonatal outcome. Am J Obstet Gynecol 163:105, 1990.

253. Bracero L, Leikin E, Kirshenbaum N, et al: Comparison of nifedipine and ritodrine for the treatment of preterm labor. Am J Perinatol 8:365, 1991.

254. Rodts-Palenik S, Morrison JC: Tocolysis: An update for the practitioner. Obstet Gynecol Surv 57(5, Suppl 2):S9, 2002.

255. Papatsonis DN, VanGeijn HP, Ader HJ, et al: Nifedipine and ritodrine in the management of preterm labor. A randomized multicenter trial. Obstet Gynecol 90:230, 1997.

256. Oei SG, Mol BW, de Kleine MJ, et al: Nifedipine versus ritodrine for suppression of preterm labor: A meta-analysis. Acta Obstet Gynecol Scand 78:783, 1999.

257. Tsatsaris V, Papasotsonis D, Goffinet F, et al: Tocolysis with nifedipine or beta-adrenergic agonists: A meta-analysis. Obstet Gynecol 97:840, 2001.

258. Vayssiere C: [Special management for threatened preterm delivery in multiple pregnancies]. J Gynecol Obstet Biol Reprod (Paris) 31(7 Suppl):5S114, 2002.

259. Emery SP, Idriss E, Richmonds C, et al: Human fetal membranes release a Ca^{++} channel inhibitor. Am J Obstet Gynecol 179:989, 1998.

260. Collins PL, Moore JJ, Idriss E, Kulp TM: Human fetal membranes inhibit calcium L-channel activated uterine contractions. Am J Obstet Gynecol 175:1173, 1996.

261. Carroll E, Gianipoulos J, Collins P: Abnormality of calcium channel inhibitor released from fetal membranes in preterm labor. Am J Obstet Gynecol 184:356, 2001.

262. Ferguson JE, Dyson DC, Holbrook RH, et al: Cardiovascular and metabolic effects associated with nifedipine and ritodrine tocolysis. Am J Obstet Gynecol 161:788, 1989.

263. Glock JL, Morales WJ: Efficacy and safety of nifedipine versus magnesium sulfate in the management of preterm labor: A randomized study. Am J Obstet Gynecol 169:960, 1993.

264. Murray C, Haverkamp A, Orleans M, et al: Nifedipine for treatment of preterm labor: A historic prospective study. Am J Obstet Gynecol 167:52, 1992.

265. Sawaya GF, Robertson PA: Hepatotoxicity with the administration of nifedipine for the treatment of preterm labor. Am J Obstet Gynecol 167:512, 1992.

266. Oei SG, Oei SK, Brolmann HA: Myocardial infarction during nifedipine therapy for preterm labor. N Engl J Med 340:154, 1999.

267. Ben-Ami M, Gilady Y, Shalev E: The combination of magnesium sulphate and nifedipine: A cause of neuromuscular blockade. Br J Obstet Gynaecol 101:262, 1994.

268. Snyder S, Cardwell M: Neuromuscular blockade with magnesium sulfate and nifedipine. Am J Obstet Gynecol 161:35, 1989.

269. Ducsay CA, Thompson JS, Wu AT, et al: Effects of calcium entry blocker (nicardipine) tocolysis in rhesus macaques: Fetal plasma concentrations and cardiorespiratory changes. Am J Obstet Gynecol 157:1482, 1987.

270. Parisi V, Salinas J, Stockmar E: Fetal vascular responses to maternal nicardipine administration in the hypertensive ewe. Am J Obstet Gynecol 161:1035, 1989.

271. Harake B, Gilbert RD, Ashwal S, et al: Nifedipine. Effects on fetal and maternal hemodynamics in pregnant sheep. Am J Obstet Gynecol 157:1482, 1987.

272. Mari G, Kirshon B, Moise K, et al: Doppler assessment of the fetal and uteroplacental circulation during nifedipine therapy for preterm labor. Am J Obstet Gynecol 161:1514, 1989.

273. Papatsonis D, Kok J, van Geijn H, et al: Neonatal effects of nifedipine and ritodrine for preterm labor. Obstet Gynecol 95:477, 2000.

274. Ray D, Dyson D, Crites YM: Nifedipine tocolysis and neonatal acid-base status at delivery. Am J Obstet Gynecol 170:387, 1994.

275. Ferguson JE, Schutz T, Perske R, et al: Nifedipine pharmacokinetics during preterm labor tocolysis. Am J Obstet Gynecol 161:1485, 1989.

276. Andersen LF, Lyndrup J, Akerlund M, et al: Oxytocin receptor blockade: A new principle in the treatment of preterm labor? Am J Perinatal 6:196, 1989.

277. Goodwin TM, Valenzuela G, Silver H, et al: Treatment of preterm labor with the oxytocin antagonist atosiban. Am J Perinatol 13:143, 1996.

278. Romero R, Sibai BM, Sanchez-Ramos L, et al: An oxytocin receptor antagonist (atosiban) in the treatment of preterm labor: A randomized, double-blind, placebo-controlled trial with tocolytic rescue. Am J Obstet Gynecol 182:1173, 2000.

279. Jennings RW, MacGillivray TE, Harrison MR: Nitric oxide inhibits preterm labor in rhesus monkey. J Matern Fetal Med 2:170, 1993.

280. Heymann MA, Bootstaylor B, Roman C, et al: Glyceryl trinitrate stops active labor in sheep. In Moncada S, Feelisch M, Busse R, et al (eds): The Biology of Nitric Oxide. London, Portland, 1994, pp 201-203.

281. El-Sayed YY, Riley ET, Holbrook RH, et al: Randomized comparison of intravenous nitroglycerin and magnesium sulfate for treatment of preterm labor. Obstet Gynecol 93:79, 1999.

282. David M, Halle H, Lichtenegger W, et al: Nitroglycerin to facilitate fetal extraction during cesarean delivery. Obstet Gynecol 91:119, 1998.

283. Lees CC, Lojacono A, Thompson C, et al: Glyceryl trinitrate and ritodrine in tocolysis: An international multicenter randomized study. Obstet Gynecol 94:403, 1999.

284. Hatjis C, Swain M, Nelson L, et al: Efficacy of combined administration of magnesium sulfate and ritodrine in the treatment of preterm labor. Obstet Gynecol 69:317, 1987.

285. Ferguson J, Hensleigh P, Kredenster D: Adjunctive use of magnesium sulfate with ritodrine for preterm labor tocolysis. Am J Obstet Gynecol 148:166, 1984.

286. Wilkins IA, Goldberg JD, Phillips RN, et al: Long-term use of magnesium sulfate as a tocolytic agent. Obstet Gynecol 67:38S, 1986.

287. Dudley D, Gagnon D, Varner M: Long-term tocolysis with intravenous magnesium sulfate. Obstet Gynecol 73:373, 1989.

288. Lam F, Elliott J, Jones JS, et al: Clinical issues surrounding the use of terbutaline sulfate for preterm labor. Obstet Gynecol Surv 53:S85, 1998.

289. Wenstrom KD, Weiner CP, Merrill D, et al: A placebo-controlled randomized trial of the terbutaline pump for - prevention of preterm delivery. Am J Perinatol 14:87, 1997.

290. Perry KG Jr, Morrison JC, Rust OA, et al: Incidence of adverse cardiopulmonary effects with low-dose continuous terbutaline infusion. Am J Obstet Gynecol 173:1273, 1995.

291. Sanchez-Ramos L, Kaunitz AM, Gaudier FL, et al: Efficacy of maintenance therapy after acute tocolysis: A meta-analysis. Am J Obstet Gynecol 181:484, 1999.

292. Carr DB, Clark AL, Kernek K, et al: Maintenance oral nifedipine for preterm labor: A randomized clinical trial. Am J Obstet Gynecol 181:822, 1999.

293. Elliott JP, Radin TG: Serum magnesium levels during magnesium sulfate tocolysis in high-order multiple gestations. J Reprod Med 40:450, 1995.

294. Gabriel R, Harika G, Saniez D, et al: Prolonged intravenous ritodrine therapy: A comparison between multiple and singleton pregnancies. Eur J Obstet Gynecol Reprod Biol 57:65, 1994.

295. Hill L, Lazebnik N, Many A: Effect of indomethacin on individual amniotic fluid indices in multiple gestations. J Ultrasound Med 15:395, 1996.

296. Deeny M, Haxton M: Indomethacin use to control polyhydramnios complicating triplet pregnancy. Br J Obstet Gynaecol 100:281, 1993.

297. Sideris EB, Yokochi K, Van Helder T: Effects of indomethacin and prostaglandins E_2, I_2, and D_2 on the fetal circulation. Adv Prostaglandin Thromboxane Leukot Res 12:477, 1983.

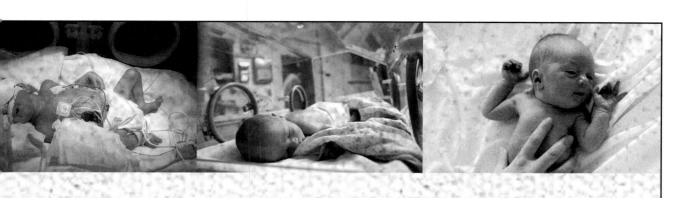

Maternal Factors Influencing Neonatal Outcome

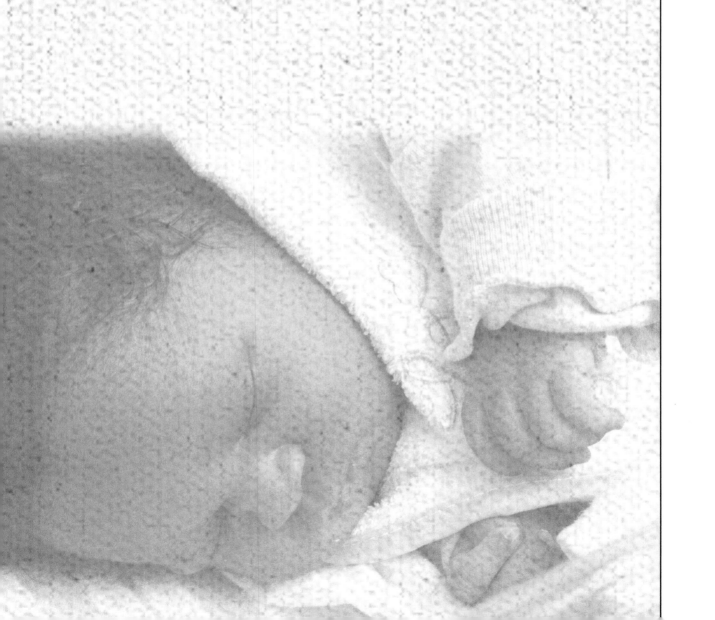

CHAPTER 19

Maternal Illness and the Effects on the Fetus

M. Shannon Burke and Tara Becker

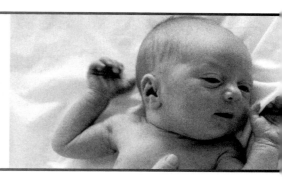

A ny medical or surgical condition can occur during pregnancy. Many of these conditions can be grouped together to understand the approach to their diagnosis, management, and treatment. Pregnancy complicating these illnesses may change one's approach to a certain extent, but in general, pregnant patients should be managed similarly to nonpregnant women. A few diseases are specific to pregnancy, and occasionally pregnancy uncovers a previously existing medical illness.

General guidelines include the attempt to control the signs of the medical illness effectively before a pregnancy occurs if possible. With chronic illnesses, adequate control should be sustained for 6 months before pursuing pregnancy. If medication changes need to be made for better control or because there are drugs with fewer problems during pregnancy, these changes should be made and the patient should be stabilized. Medications should be reviewed[1] for the possible effects on the fetus, and if there is a common problem with that drug, other alternatives should be explored. The U.S. Food and Drug Administration has approved a rating system for medications during pregnancy based on the information that is available from animal studies and reports of medication use during pregnancy and lactation (Table 19-1).[2]

In counseling patients, physicians must explain that drugs are not evaluated specifically for their effects on the developing fetus or their use in pregnancy.[3,4] Medications that are needed to control a patient's medical condition should not be discontinued without an alternative medication or a plan for observing the patient specifically for a change in the symptoms. The patient and her family should be counseled about the effects of her disease and the medications on the pregnancy with the best information possible. The patient should understand her options and be made aware of the potential problems.

When evaluating the use of medications in pregnancy, three areas should be considered: (1) possible effects on the development of the fetus before 12 weeks of gestation, when a medication may be teratogenic; (2) medications that may alter the normal fetal physiology, resulting in poor fetal growth or organ function; and (3) pharmacologic or dosing changes that may be peculiar to pregnancy or cause accumulation on the fetal side of the maternal-fetal circulation.[5]

PHYSIOLOGY

Chronic illness in the mother potentially can affect the infant before birth. Most often the effect is placental insufficiency, which results in deficient growth of the infant. Placental trophoblastic development begins immediately after implantation with invasion of the maternal blood by uteroplacental spiral arteries. Placental angiogenesis continues until 24 weeks. Failure of this development leads to microscopic structural abnormalities that represent the changes that contribute to placental ischemia.[6] This process also may lead to decreased amniotic fluid and nonreassuring fetal status.

During pregnancy, there is an increase in maternal blood volume that is necessary to provide appropriate blood flow for the mother and to supply the growing uterus and fetus with adequate nutrition. Any maternal disease state that causes vascular depletion or vasoconstriction has an impact on the increase in maternal blood volume and uterine blood flow. When there is diminished uterine flow, the placental growth is not stimulated, and there is poor placental invasion into the uterine muscle. This deficiency results in a small, inefficient placenta that is less capable of pulling oxygen from the maternal blood and removing waste from the fetal compartment. The chronic low oxygen environment leads to decreased fetal growth and ultimately to decreased fetal urine output, causing oligohydramnios or decreased amniotic fluid volume. The fetus must be evaluated throughout the pregnancy as a part of the profile of the maternal illness.[7-11]

Table 19–1. Definitions of Medication Risk Factors by the U.S. Food and Drug Administration

Category	Definition of Risk Factor	Examples of Medication
A	Controlled studies in women fail to show a risk to the fetus in the first trimester (and there is no evidence of risk in later trimesters) and the possibility of harm appears remote.	Prenatal vitamins Thyroid medication Magnesium sulfate
B	Either animal reproduction studies have not shown a fetal risk but there are no controlled studies in pregnant women, or animal reproduction studies have shown an adverse effect that was not confirmed in controlled studies in the first trimester (and there is no evidence of risk in later trimesters).	Aspartame Dexchlorpheniramine Penicillin Cephalosporins Metronidazole Bacitracin Ethambutol
C	Either studies in animals have revealed adverse effects on the fetus (teratogenic, embryocidal, or other) and there are no controlled studies in women, or animal studies are not available. Drugs should be given only if the potential benefit justifies the potential risk to the fetus.	Aspirin Isoniazid Hydralazine Labetalol Betamethasone Dexamethasone Prochlorperazine (Compazine)
D	There is positive evidence of human fetal risk, but the benefits for use in pregnant women may be acceptable despite the risk.	Phenytoin Valproic acid Lithium
X	Studies in animals or humans have shown fetal abnormalities and/or there is evidence of fetal risk based on human experience, and the risk of the use of the drug in pregnant women clearly outweighs any possible benefit. The drug is contraindicated in women who are or may become pregnant.	Isotretinoin (Acutane) Diethylstilbestrol (DES) Methotrexate Aminopterin Thalidomide Ergotamine Radioactive markers

Modified from Risk factor definitions for medications. Fed Reg 45:37434, 1980.

FREQUENCY OF CONCURRENT MEDICAL PROBLEMS

The medical illnesses most frequently encountered[12] during the childbearing years include hypertension, asthma, diabetes, epilepsy, cardiac disease, thromboembolic disorders, and thyroid disorders. Less frequently, but still of concern, are immunologic and rheumatologic diseases, hemoglobinopathies, gastrointestinal disorders, and neurologic disorders. In this chapter, many of these conditions are outlined with respect to the potential effects on the pregnancy. More extensive discussions of hypertension, preeclampsia, diabetes, infections, antenatal fetal assessment, and pharmacology of the fetus and newborn are found in other chapters of this book.

Medical illnesses of the mother may be assessed for the severity of effect on the pregnancy by the relationship to fetal outcome. Fetal death before delivery is a finite end point that can give an indication of risk by medical problem (Table 19-2).[13]

HYPERTENSION

Hypertension occurs in about 6% to 8% of all pregnancies in the United States.[14-16] Hypertensive disorders during pregnancy are the second leading cause of maternal mortality, causing 15% of deaths. Many of these patients

Table 19–2. Maternal Medical Disease and Rate of Stillbirth Infants

Medical Condition	Stillbirths per 1000 Live Births
All pregnancies	6-7
Diabetes, gestational	5-15
Diabetes, type 1	6-10
Diabetes, type 2	35
Chronic hypertension	5-25
Superimposed preeclampsia	52
Mild preeclampsia	9
Severe preeclampsia	21
Eclampsia	18-48
HELLP syndrome	51
Hyperthyroidism, stable	0-36
Thyrotoxicosis, uncontrolled	100-156
Hypothyroidism, subclinical	0-15
Hypothyroidism, overt	15-125
Obesity > 150 lb	15-20
Systemic lupus erythematosus (SLE)	40-150
SLE with anticardiolipin	800
Renal insufficiency, mild	15
Renal insufficiency, moderate	32-200
Cholestasis of pregnancy	12-30

HELLP, hemolysis, elevated liver enzymes, and low platelet count.

Modified from Simpson L: Maternal medical disease: Risk of antepartum fetal death. Semin Perinatal 26:42, 2002.

have no prior history. Chronic hypertension is diagnosed if it is detected before the 20th week of pregnancy. Hypertension is defined as greater than 140 mm Hg systolic blood pressure or 90 mm Hg diastolic blood pressure. Severe hypertension is diagnosed with a systolic blood pressure of 160 mm Hg or a diastolic blood pressure of 110 mm Hg.[17] The risk in the pregnancy is greatest in women with a history of long-standing chronic hypertension, women with renal or vascular disease, women who are older than 40 years old, and women with either gestational or preexisting diabetes. When hypertension is identified, the perinatal mortality is tripled, and the frequency of placental abruption is doubled.[18]

Medications

Treatment regimens have not been studied in a randomized fashion, although some medications have been used for many years because hypertension is a common problem during pregnancy (Table 19-3). Methyldopa has the longest history of use in pregnancy.[19-21] It has been preferred because animal models have shown that an increase in uterine blood flow occurs with methyldopa. There are limits to increasing doses because it may have a sedative effect and cause headache. Labetalol has come into greater use because it can be given twice a day and has fewer side effects at higher doses.[22,23] Side effects are unusual but may include dizziness and nausea. Labetalol is a combined α and β blocker and should be avoided in anyone with severe asthma. Hydralazine has been popular as an oral medication in the past, but it is not used as frequently with the availability of newer medications.[24,25] Hydralazine in intravenous doses is still the most frequent medication for severe, unresponsive hypertension. Nifedipine[26,27] also has gained in popularity and may be given as a once-daily dose with the slow-release product. Side effects are usually mild and include headache and dyspepsia.[28]

β-Blockers, such as propranolol and atenolol, are avoided during pregnancy because they have been associated with fetal growth restriction and hypoglycemia in the neonate.[29-31] Angiotensin-converting enzyme inhibitors cannot be used during pregnancy.[32,33] They have been found to result in renal failure in the fetus when used after the second trimester. Intrauterine exposure results in oligohydramnios and potentially pulmonary hypoplasia from the lack of amniotic fluid. The decreased urine output may continue into the neonatal period.[34]

Antepartum Management

During the antepartum period, maternal renal function and other possible underlying disorders should be evaluated. Management of underlying disease and blood pressure control with medication are the most important goals. Patients with hypertension during pregnancy should come for more frequent prenatal visits to assess their response to medications, to check for urine protein, and to evaluate fetal growth.[35] Antenatal surveillance with nonstress testing and assessment of amniotic fluid should begin at 34 weeks in a well-controlled patient with no other underlying disease. Surveillance should begin earlier if diabetes, renal disease, or vascular disease is associated with hypertension. Preeclampsia occurs more frequently in women with preexisting hypertension and is distinct from chronic hypertension. Fetal growth by ultrasound should be assessed on a regular schedule throughout the pregnancy. If fetal growth retardation or decreased amniotic fluid is detected, Doppler flow evaluations may be useful in determining the severity of placental insufficiency. Consideration should be given to delivery by term rather than continuing antenatal surveillance.[36,37]

MATERNAL CARDIAC DISEASE

Clinical Diagnosis

Hemodynamic changes of pregnancy include a 30% to 50% increase in cardiac output. Cardiac output reaches a maximum by the 24th week of pregnancy.[38] The increase is maintained until the third trimester, when there is a slight decrease. Total blood volume increases by approximately 25% by the second trimester.[11] In a normal pregnancy, women may complain of dyspnea, orthopnea, dizziness, fatigue, edema, and weight gain. Many pregnant women normally have a systolic flow murmur during pregnancy due to the increased cardiac output and blood volume. The severity of these symptoms may suggest maternal cardiac disease, such as a severe dyspnea with reduced activity levels, syncope, or cardiac dysrhythmias. Symptoms not present in normal pregnancy include hemoptysis, chest pain, cyanosis, clubbing, or diastolic murmurs. Diastolic murmurs and harsh or loud systolic murmurs are not commonly associated with normal pregnancy.[39]

Table 19-3. Hypertensive Medications

Medication	Brand Name	Starting Oral Dose	Maximal Dose
Methyldopa	Aldomet	250 mg bid	3000 mg/day
Labetalol	Normodyne	100 mg bid	2400 mg/day
Nifedipine	Procardia	10 mg tid	180 mg/day
Nifedipine	Procardia XL	30 mg/day	120 mg/day
Hydralazine	Apresoline	10-25 mg qid	100 mg/day

Functional Classification of Heart Disease

Because pregnancy is associated with increased cardiac output and decreased vascular resistance that results in an increased stroke volume, pregnancy must be considered the ultimate stress test in a heart that has marginal function. Congenital heart disease in women has replaced rheumatic heart disease as the major cause of maternal cardiac abnormalities.[40] It has been reported that 0.8% of pregnancies are complicated by maternal congenital heart disease.[41] When a woman with congenital heart disease becomes pregnant, it is important to counsel her that 3.5% to 14% of maternal heart lesions may be seen in offspring. The recurrence rate varies with the family history and the cardiac lesion, but it seems that there is a 2.23 times greater overall risk of a congenital lesion in the infant.[42,43]

Of obstetric patients with heart disease, 80% have lesions that do not interfere with their activity and are considered New York Heart Association class I or class II. Most patients who decompensate and require additional care are class I and class II simply because most cardiac patients are class I and class II. Cardiac evaluation should be considered in any woman contemplating pregnancy if she has a history of a heart murmur; episodes of syncope, chest pain, exercise intolerance, or cyanosis; a family history of left-sided heart problems, such as aortic stenosis; or a history of rheumatic fever.[44]

Many patients with congenital heart disease have had complete repairs of lesions with no residual hemodynamic effects. Cardiac lesions, with or without repairs, that continue to be associated with maternal cyanosis and elevated maternal hematocrit are particularly associated with worse maternal outcomes, fewer live-born infants, and poor fetal growth. The worst fetal outcomes are associated with a maternal hematocrit greater than 50% secondary to cyanosis.[43,45] Cardiac lesions associated with pulmonary hypertension have a maternal mortality rate of up to 50%, and these lesions are associated with a particularly poor outcome in pregnancy.[8]

The key determinant of maternal outcome is the actual cardiac lesion. Clarifying the anatomic and physiologic problems is crucial in predicting the course of the pregnancy. Obtaining old medical records, a current echocardiographic evaluation, and cardiac consultation are essential to management of any patient with a significant history of a cardiac lesion. Clark[46] developed a staging of cardiac lesions based on expected maternal mortality (Table 19-4).

Cardiac Dysrhythmias

Bradyarrhythmias do not occur frequently during pregnancy but should be evaluated for their impact on maternal hemodynamics. Occasionally, placement of a pacemaker becomes necessary. Cardioversion has been used during pregnancy without apparent harm to the fetus.[47,48] Tachyarrhythmias are more common during pregnancy and usually require only decreased activity and elimination of any stimulants, such as caffeine and nicotine. Treatment with antiarrhythmic drugs may be used if necessary.

Peripartum Cardiomyopathy

Cardiomyopathy occurs most frequently in women with preexisting hypertension.[49] It is a dilated form of left ventricular heart failure in women with no previously known heart disease. The echocardiogram shows poor contractility and dilation of the left ventricle and atrium.[50] The condition generally occurs late in the pregnancy or after delivery.[51] Therapy includes diuretics, sodium

Table 19-4. Maternal Mortality Related to Cardiac Diagnosis

Group 1 (mortality < 1%)	Atrial septal defect, uncomplicated
	Ventricular septal defect, uncomplicated
	Patent ductus arteriosus, uncomplicated
	Pulmonary or tricuspid insufficiency
	Corrected tetralogy of Fallot
	Porcine valve replacement
	Mitral stenosis — NYHA classes I and II
Group 2 (mortality 5-15%)	Mitral stenosis with atrial fibrillation
	Mitral stenosis — NYHA classes III and IV
	Aortic stenosis
	Coarcation of the aorta, uncomplicated
	Uncorrected tetralogy of Fallot
	Post myocardial infarction
	Marfan syndrome with an aortic root < 4 cm
	Prosthetic valve replacement
Group 3 (mortality 25-50%)	Any lesion associated with pulmonary hypertension
	Coarctation of the aorta, complicated
	Marfan syndrome with an aortic root > 4 cm
	Peripartum cardiomyopathy

NYHA, New York Heart Association.

Modified from Clark S: Cardiac desease in pregnancy. Crit Care Clin 7:777, 1991.

restriction, digoxin, and limitation of physical activity. Treatment also may include afterload reduction with hydralazine, or prazosin (Minipress).[52] Captopril (Capoten) should not be used in pregnant patients. Anticoagulants are used if there is an arrhythmia or significant enlargement of the atria. A good prognosis depends on the absence of cardiomegaly 6 months after the diagnosis. The recurrence risk in subsequent pregnancies is extremely high.[53]

General Management Principles

The initial approach to cardiac disease in pregnancy is to make an accurate diagnosis of the specific cardiac disorder. Electrocardiographic and echocardiographic data are particularly useful to assist in management of the pregnancy. Cardiac catheterization generally is not necessary for diagnosis but may be required to exclude pulmonary hypertension. The symptoms of cardiac disease are related to physical exertion, which may require bed rest, and to cardiac overload, which may be prevented with dietary salt restriction. Antibiotic prophylaxis for bacterial endocarditis is recommended for most cardiac conditions. Patients with pulmonary hypertension, cardiomyopathy, or Marfan syndrome with a dilated aortic root should discuss prevention or termination of pregnancy. Having a relationship with a cardiologist is important for the patient throughout her life and is helpful during pregnancy if there are problems.[54]

Management during Labor and Delivery

Pulmonary edema and arrhythmias are the most frequent problems seen in women with cardiac disease during labor and delivery. Careful monitoring of the maternal vital signs and central hemodynamic monitoring by Swan-Ganz catheter may be necessary with significant cardiac disease. Fetal heart tones should be assessed continuously. Careful fluid management in patients with mitral stenosis and aortic stenosis is important.

Anticoagulants should be discontinued before labor begins; this often suggests the need for a planned induction after anticoagulants are discontinued and for appropriate personnel to be available for the delivery. Fetal complications often are related to premature delivery or poor fetal growth because of decompensation. Acute maternal decompensation may cause fetal bradycardia.

Patients with cardiac disease can deliver vaginally without additional complications, although an extremely prolonged second stage with excessive effort is best avoided for maternal benefit. A patient with pulmonary hypertension who continues her pregnancy may require cesarean section with epidural anesthesia and intensive monitoring.[8,39]

Fetal Echocardiography with Maternal Cardiac Disease

Recurrence risks are such with most cardiac lesions that when either parent or siblings have a cardiac defect, fetal echocardiography should be done at 20 to 22 weeks of gestation to assess the fetal cardiac structure. Fetal echocardiography detects approximately 80% of fetal cardiac abnormalities, but detection rates depend on the anomaly.[55-57]

MATERNAL RENAL DISORDERS

Pregnancy is associated with anatomic changes of the urinary tract marked by dilation of the ureters and collecting system. The dilation is greater in the right renal pelvis than on the left because of pressure on the ureter from dextrorotation of the uterus. Progesterone causes decreased tone in the collecting system, contributing to this dilation. Early in pregnancy, renal blood flow and glomerular filtration rate are increased by approximately 50% to 80%.

Urinary Tract Infection

Asymptomatic bacteriuria[58] occurs more commonly during pregnancy and should be screened during the first prenatal visit. Bacteriuria may lead to pyelonephritis three to four times more often in pregnancy because of the dilation of the ureters and poor emptying of the bladder. Urinary infections should be treated with antibiotics with follow-up cultures and antibiotic suppression if there are recurrent urinary tract infections. Pyelonephritis during pregnancy may be associated more frequently with bacteremia, pneumonia, pulmonary edema, and septic shock because of the relative immunosuppression of pregnancy.[59] Maternal tachycardia and markedly elevated temperatures (103° F [39° C]) are associated with an increase in respiratory complications.[60] Initial outpatient treatment is effective in uncomplicated pyelonephritis.[61] Patients should be watched carefully and should be hospitalized for intravenous antibiotics if they are not responding to outpatient measures. Occasionally a fever persists despite antibiotic therapy, and a renal ultrasound for possible obstructive uropathy should be considered.[62]

Acute Renal Failure

Acute renal failure in pregnancy may be due to hypovolemia from antepartum hemorrhage, sepsis, dehydration, preeclampsia, or placental abruption. Volume expansion with careful monitoring reverses the concentrated urine and oliguria in most cases. If extreme hypovolemia occurs for a prolonged period, acute tubular necrosis may occur with any of the above-mentioned conditions. Acute tubular necrosis usually is associated with cortical necrosis and disseminated intravascular coagulation. The condition is most often characterized by severe oliguria, which resolves in less than 6 weeks. Renal dialysis and careful management of fluids and electrolyte status are necessary. Treatment of the inciting cause of acute tubular necrosis is the primary objective in supportive medical therapy.[63]

Chronic Renal Failure

Mild renal insufficiency may be associated with increased proteinuria during pregnancy, which should return to baseline in the postpartum period. Blood pressure may be increased for the first time during pregnancy. Pregnancy outcome is usually good.[64] Renal insufficiency with a serum creatinine greater than 1.4 mg/dL has been shown to progress to end-stage renal disease in about 30% of pregnancies. To achieve a good outcome, control of hypertension is essential in all patients with moderate renal insufficiency. Perinatal outcome has improved since the 1990s, perhaps due to improved treatment for hypertension.[65]

There is a marked increase in preeclampsia (60%), preterm delivery (55% to 60%), fetal growth restriction (31% to 37%), and perinatal mortality (7% to 16%).[66]

For the best prognosis, chronic renal failure should be in remission.[65,67,68] Hypertension and serum creatinine greater than 1.5 mg/dL are general predictors of a poor overall prognosis.[69] Steroids and cytotoxic agents can be used in pregnancy if necessary. Patients with renal homografts have a high rate of preeclampsia, premature delivery, and intrauterine growth restriction. Patients who are taking immunosuppressive drugs because of a renal transplant have completed normal pregnancies. There is little evidence to show an increase in congenital malformations.[70]

Polycystic kidney disease is the third most common cause of renal failure in the general population. It is a dominantly inherited disease, which is associated with asymptomatic hypertension, flank pain, hematuria, and large flank masses. This disease usually presents in the third or fourth decade of life and has a 30% association with intracranial berry aneurysms.[71]

MATERNAL PULMONARY DISORDERS

Pregnant patients experience a feeling of breathlessness even at rest. There is no increase in respiratory rate or vital capacity in pregnancy, although oxygen consumption, tidal volume, and minute ventilation increase. Despite the increase in minute ventilation, it represents only a small proportion of the mother's capacity to increase minute ventilation; patients are less disabled during pregnancy by respiratory problems than they are by cardiac diseases.[72]

Bronchial Asthma

Asthma is a common medical illness in women of childbearing age, affecting about 1% of pregnant patients. Asthma has a variable effect in pregnancy, with 35% to 42% of patients deteriorating, 18% to 28% experiencing improvement, and 33% to 40% remaining the same during pregnancy.[73] Bronchospasm and increased airway secretions characterize asthma. There may be an allergic component associated with adult asthma. Patients with an asthma attack usually present with shortness of breath, wheezing, and coughing. Asthma is most serious for patients who are delivered by cesarean section, for adolescents, and for African Americans.

Medications used before pregnancy are generally appropriate for continued use. The use of a short-acting, symptom-relieving medication such as an inhaler and a long-term medication to decrease the underlying inflammation is recommended. β-Sympathomimetic agents, such as terbutaline, can be administered orally or by inhalation. Cromolyn, inhaled or administered orally, can be used for its anti-inflammatory activity to inhibit the antigen-induced sensitivity of the pulmonary tissue.[74] Inhaled or systemic corticosteroids may be necessary to control asthma, but the doses should be kept to a minimum because of an association with premature rupture of membranes and early delivery.[75] Oral theophylline medications have been used extensively in the past and

still may be used if there is poor control with other medications. Achieving and maintaining adequate theophylline levels during pregnancy requires monitoring plasma drug levels because pregnancy increases protein binding and liver metabolism, which results in decreased medication levels. The newer leukotriene receptor antagonists seem to be useful in treating asthma, but little information is available regarding the effects on the fetus.[76] The pulmonary status usually can be evaluated serially by simple peak flow measurements done in the clinic or by the patient at home.

Treatment of acute attacks requires rapid evaluation of the severity. In extremely severe attacks, mechanical ventilation is occasionally required. Inhaled nebulized short-acting β-sympathomimetic agents are the first-line treatment. Oxygen should be administered to maintain a Po_2 greater than 85 mm Hg to ensure fetal oxygenation. Intravenous hydration, aminophylline, and subcutaneous terbutaline may be given as necessary. Subcutaneous epinephrine should be avoided. Evidence of infection as the inciting cause should be investigated with a chest x-ray, sputum Gram stain, cultures, and a complete blood count. In patients who have been previously steroid dependent, intravenous steroid therapy should be administered for 24 hours, followed by a weaning regimen to oral prednisone.[77]

Prostaglandin $F_{2\alpha}$ (Hemabate) is a strong bronchoconstrictor and should be avoided if uterine atony occurs. Narcotics may cause respiratory depression and should be used with caution.

Fetal outcome is related to the frequency and extent of respiratory compromise during the pregnancy. Fetal growth restriction and oligohydramnios potentially result from severe asthma. Antenatal surveillance should include serial ultrasound for documentation of fetal growth and a biophysical profile for evaluation of amniotic fluid and fetal well-being. Doppler flow assessment of the umbilical and uterine vessels may be helpful if there is evidence of fetal compromise.[78]

Cystic Fibrosis

The incidence of cystic fibrosis is approximately 1 in 2000 live births, making it one of the most common genetic disorders. Survival to the childbearing years has improved dramatically as a result of improved pulmonary therapy and the use of antibiotics. Cystic fibrosis affects multiple organ systems with an underlying defect, resulting in increased pulmonary secretions, diabetes from decreased pancreatic enzymes, infertility, and hepatic cirrhosis. The best outcomes are achieved when the maternal pulmonary status is maximized before pregnancy. Possible predictors of poor pregnancy outcome are the presence of cor pulmonale, emphysema, recurrent pulmonary infections, chronic hypoxia with an arterial Po_2 of less than 60 mm Hg, and a vital capacity of less than 50%. Aggressive management of infection and pulmonary function is essential. The forced expiratory volume and forced vital capacity can be used to monitor pulmonary status and should be assessed monthly during pregnancy.[79]

Prenatal diagnosis is much more accessible now than it was in the past. Current recommendations include carrier screening of all pregnant couples. Because this is an autosomal recessive disease, family members of a cystic fibrosis patient should be offered carrier testing.[80]

Pulmonary Embolism

Pulmonary embolism occurs in approximately 1 to 2 per 1000 pregnancies and, if left untreated, is associated with a high mortality.[81] The top three causes of maternal mortality in all countries include pulmonary embolism.[82] Mortality decreases to less than 1% with appropriate and rapid anticoagulation treatment. Patients with pulmonary embolism may present with chest pain, dyspnea, hemoptysis, or symptoms of a deep venous thrombosis in the lower extremities. On arterial blood gas analysis, there is usually a respiratory alkalosis and hypoxemia with a decreased P_{CO_2}. Occasionally, Doppler flow studies of the extremities are positive for a deep venous thrombosis, and treatment can begin based on that information. A ventilation-perfusion scan or spiral computed tomography can be done during pregnancy to confirm the diagnosis.[83]

Management of pulmonary embolism should include maximal improvement of oxygen levels to maintain the maternal P_{O_2} at greater than 85 mm Hg whenever possible to ensure adequate fetal oxygenation. Anticoagulation with heparin should be accomplished intravenously and continued for several days. Full anticoagulation for 3 months should be continued after a significant venous thromboembolism during pregnancy. Subcutaneous heparin should be given in doses adequate to double the partial thromboplastin time. Warfarin should not be used during pregnancy because of a documented teratogenic syndrome associated with first-trimester use and because of neonatal bleeding if used at the end of pregnancy.[84] Low-molecular-weight heparin has been used during pregnancy with some success, and currently there are no documented fetal problems with its use.[85] The primary advantage of low-molecular-weight heparin is once-daily dosing. This advantage is lost when used in pregnancy because it is necessary to administer it every 12 hours to maintain a therapeutic anti–factor Xa level, especially during the third trimester.[86,87]

Because the increased coagulation state of pregnancy does not diminish until 6 weeks postpartum, anticoagulation should be continued until that time. Warfarin can be given for anticoagulation after delivery, even if the patient is breast-feeding.

Pulmonary embolism or venous thrombosis may be associated with an increased thrombotic tendency from several hematologic deficiencies that have been identified previously.[88,89] Hypercoagulation conditions and the suggested testing are delineated in Table 19-5. Disorders may be recognized because of a history of venous thromboembolism, early severe preeclampsia, fetal growth restriction, placental abruption, early recurrent miscarriage, or intrauterine fetal death.[90] Patients who are identified with an underlying coagulation disorder should be referred to their family health care provider postpartum for consideration of possible anticoagulation throughout their life. Many of these disorders are genetic, and other relatives should be offered evaluation for the disorder.

MATERNAL ENDOCRINE DISORDERS

Thyroid Disorders

Thyroid disorders in pregnancy can be understood only by taking into consideration the normal changes of pregnancy. There is an increased amount of estrogen during normal pregnancy that results in increased serum thyroid-binding globulin, increased measurement of total thyroxine (T_4), and decreased resin triiodothyronine uptake. Free T_4, free T_4 index, and thyroid-stimulating hormone (TSH) are not changed during pregnancy, so they are the best indicators for diagnostic purposes. In the management of thyroid disorders in pregnancy, it is useful to remember that TSH and thyroid replacement medication do not cross the placenta well. Iodine, antithyroid medications, and thyroid immunoglobulin antibodies cross the placenta and stimulate the fetal thyroid.[91]

Table 19–5. Hypercoagulation Conditions

Condition	Population Frequency	Inheritance	Effect of Heparin on Testing	Testing During Pregnancy
Factor V Leiden mutation	5-9%	AD	None	DNA evaluation, not protein C resistance in pregnancy
Prothrombin mutation	2-4%	AD	None	DNA evaluation
Hyperhomocystinemia (correlated to MTHFR mutation)	1-11%	AR	None	Fasting homocystine levels cause thrombosis, NTD, coronary disease
Protein C deficiency	0.2-0.5%	AD	Decreases	Functional activity
Protein S deficiency	0.08%	AD	Decreases	Functional activity antigen, total and free
Antithrombin III deficiency	0.02-0.2%	AD, point mutation	Decreases	Most coagulopathic deficiency
Anticardiolipin syndrome	<1%	Acquired	None	Anticardiolipin IgG antibodies, activated PTT

AD, autosomal dominant; AR, autosomal recessive; MTHFR, methylenetetrahydrofolate reductase; NTD, neural tube defect; PTT, partial thromboplastin time.

Modified from Lockwood C: Inherited thrombophilias in pregnancy patients: Detection and treatment paradigm. Obstet Gynecol 99:333, 2002.

Hyperthyroidism

Hyperthyroidism occurs in approximately 1 in 1000 of all pregnancies. The most common cause of hyperthyroidism is chronic autoimmune hyperthyroidism, also called *Graves disease*. Patients may present with heat intolerance, weight loss or failure to gain weight in pregnancy, an increased appetite, weakness or tremor, and/or exophthalmosis. The patient may have an enlarged, soft thyroid gland and may have an increased resting pulse rate. Diagnosis can be made on the basis of an increased free T_4 index or an elevated free T_4. Although women may not be severely symptomatic with hyperthyroidism during pregnancy, it should be treated because of the possible poor perinatal outcome. Hyperthyroidism of the mother may lead to fetal growth restriction and oligohydramnios.[92]

Ultrasound evaluation of the pregnancy should be obtained because the presenting symptoms of hydatidiform mole may be hyperthyroidism. Serial ultrasound studies should be obtained throughout the pregnancy to assess fetal growth and well-being. Fetal heart rate assessment should be performed at every prenatal visit.

Management of Graves disease during pregnancy generally means a choice between surgical or medical intervention. Ablation with radioactive iodine (^{131}I) is contraindicated during pregnancy because the fetal thyroid actively absorbs ^{131}I.[93]

Therapy with propylthiouracil (PTU) should be initiated as soon as possible. When thyroid function tests indicate control has been obtained, the dosage of PTU should be reduced to the minimum needed to maintain control. The ideal level of PTU is less than 100 mg/day by the last 3 months of pregnancy so that there would be a minimal effect on the neonate. Methimazole generally is not recommended because of a reported, although controversial, association with cutis aplasia in the fetus. Methimazole also has been reported to be associated with choanal atresia.[94]

If surgical management is necessary for maternal control, medications should be used to normalize the laboratory parameters before surgery. To avoid miscarriage, the second trimester of pregnancy is considered the preferred time for surgical intervention. Postoperatively, thyroid replacement therapy is needed to maintain thyroid function tests in the euthyroid range for a normal pregnancy.

Patients with autoimmune thyroid disease have thyroid-stimulating immunoglobulins or long-acting thyroid stimulators that are present even after the mother has received surgical or ^{131}I therapy for her disease. This antibody is capable of crossing the placenta and may cause significant fetal hyperthyroidism despite the euthyroid condition in the mother.[95] The fetus may become markedly hyperthyroid in such a circumstance and have severe intrauterine growth restriction, oligohydramnios, and tachycardia. Under some circumstances, it may be useful to evaluate the fetal status with percutaneous umbilical blood sampling.[96] A fetal goiter may be noted on ultrasound assessment. In the worst situations, the fetus can have an actual thyrotoxicosis, also known as a *thyroid storm*. Fetal thyrotoxicosis may occur in only 1% of women with hyperthyroidism, but the fetal mortality may be 30%.[41] In these cases, to control the fetal response, the mother may have to be treated with competing thyroid replacement and PTU.[97,98]

Women who present with an acute thyroid storm have symptoms of dehydration, high fever, and tachycardia. The diagnosis of acute hyperthyroidism may be confused with preeclampsia in pregnancy. Patients are at particular risk during pregnancy and must be treated urgently with intravenous β blockers such as propranolol and PTU in an intensive care setting until they are stabilized.

Hypothyroidism

Hypothyroidism is uncommon in pregnancy because most patients are infertile if there is clinically significant disease. Hypothyroidism may result from a primary disorder or secondarily from previous ablation with ^{131}I or surgery. Patients present most often with cold intolerance, excessive weight gain, constipation, dry skin, and fatigue. Levels of T_4 and resin triiodothyronine uptake are low for normal pregnancy, and TSH levels are markedly elevated. Treatment for hypothyroidism should be aggressive during pregnancy because of poor perinatal outcome and decreased neonatal mental development.[99] Hypothyroidism should be treated with thyroid replacement medications, such as L-thyroxine. The dosage should be adjusted to maintain free T_4 and TSH levels within the midnormal range for pregnancy, and levels should be assessed on a regular schedule throughout the pregnancy. Medication adjustments are required in 75% of women who are on thyroid replacement therapy during pregnancy. There is an increased rate of fetal growth restriction and preeclampsia in women with thyroid disease in pregnancy.

Hyperprolactinemia

Hyperprolactinemia generally causes amenorrhea, oligomenorrhea, short luteal phase, or galactorrhea. Patients receiving therapy for hyperprolactinemia with bromocriptine or cabergoline should have the drug discontinued when pregnancy occurs. Before the pregnancy, the patient should have an appropriate workup with cranial computed tomography (CT) looking for a pituitary tumor. Microadenomas enlarge during pregnancy less than 2% of the time and are generally symptomatic only 1.6% of the time. Women with macroadenomas before pregnancy have asymptomatic enlargement of their tumor 15% of the time, and 8.9% have symptomatic tumor enlargement during pregnancy. In women with symptomatic macroadenomas that have not responded to medical therapy and who desire pregnancy, limited transsphenoidal decompression followed by a dopamine agonist may be considered. Symptoms of tumor enlargement include visual defects and headaches.[100] Prolactin levels during pregnancy are not indicators of current tumor status because they are normally elevated during pregnancy. There do not seem to be any other complications with hyperprolactinemia in pregnancy, and these women can breast-feed successfully when no tumor-related symptoms are present.

MATERNAL GASTROINTESTINAL DISEASES

Anatomic changes occur in the gastrointestinal tract in all pregnancies due to the increasing volume of the uterus. Most pregnant patients experience appetite changes, nausea and vomiting, constipation, heartburn, and hemorrhoids. Gastrointestinal disorders do not increase during pregnancy, but the diagnosis may be difficult because of the changes during pregnancy.

Hyperemesis Gravidarum

Nausea and vomiting are common in pregnancy. Nausea occurs in 60% and vomiting occurs in 70% of all pregnant women.[101] The rapid elevation of human chorionic gonadotropin may be the cause of nausea and vomiting. In most patients, nausea and vomiting resolve during the second trimester, and less than 1% require medical intervention.[102] Patients who require some therapy may respond to vitamin B_6 and doxylamine.[103] Patients who do not respond to simple therapy may present with dehydration and ketonuria and may have fluid and electrolyte imbalances. These patients must be admitted to the hospital for intravenous hydration and correction of electrolytes. Initially, patients should refrain from oral intake until their vomiting has been controlled. When they are able to begin oral intake, it should be done slowly with liquids first, and then with dry carbohydrate foods.[104] No antiemetic medications have been thoroughly studied for pregnancy. Promethazine (Phenergan), prochlorperazine (Compazine), ondansetron (Zofran), and metoclopramide (Reglan) all have been used to keep the patient hydrated and eating reasonably well.[105] Thyroid function should be evaluated to detect possible hyperthyroidism.[106] Patients also should be evaluated with ultrasonography because hydatidiform mole and multiple gestations may present as severe hyperemesis.

Biliary Disease

Asymptomatic biliary stones can be seen in 3.5% of women undergoing a routine ultrasonography for obstetric reasons.[107] Symptomatic cholecystitis requiring the removal of the gallbladder during pregnancy occurs in 1 in 1000 to 3000 pregnant women. Symptoms include tenderness over the right upper quadrant, low-grade fever, and jaundice.[108] On laboratory evaluation, these patients may have hyperbilirubinemia, increased hepatic enzymes, and at times an elevated white blood cell count. Alkaline phosphatase is elevated three- to fourfold during normal pregnancy. Medical treatment should be initiated with hospitalization, gastrointestinal rest with nasogastric suctioning, intravenous hydration, and antibiotics. Cholecystectomy becomes necessary only in patients with markedly symptomatic stones or frequent attacks of cholecystitis or biliary colic. Surgical treatment usually is not necessary because the acute infection resolves, but definitive treatment in patients who do not respond to medical therapy should not be delayed. Increased maternal and fetal mortality rates are associated with untreated cholecystitis and with subsequent pancreatitis.[109,110] Laparoscopic intervention has become widely accepted for surgery during pregnancy.[111] It is crucial in patients presenting with symptoms of biliary disease to obtain laboratory evaluation to rule out preeclampsia with the HELLP variant (hemolysis, elevated liver profile, and low platelets), which presents as epigastric or right upper quadrant pain.

Pancreatitis

Pancreatitis is a rare diagnosis in pregnancy, occurring in 1 in 1000 to 10,000 pregnancies. It must be recognized and treated because of the increase in maternal and perinatal mortality associated with the diagnosis.[112] Acute pancreatitis usually presents as a rapid onset of severe midepigastric pain that may radiate through to the back. Nausea and vomiting, fever, tachycardia, and possibly hypotension may be present. The patient may have an ileus and abdominal tenderness; ascites and pleural effusions occasionally are seen. A gallbladder ultrasonogram for biliary stones should be obtained. On laboratory evaluation, the patient may have an elevated white blood cell count, hemoconcentration, increased liver enzymes, and increased serum bilirubin levels. Serum amylase levels may be elevated 12 to 24 hours after the acute onset of the illness.[113] Treatment includes intravenous hydration with correction of any electrolyte abnormality. Patients must receive nasogastric suction, antibiotic therapy, and analgesia. Pancreatitis in pregnancy is associated most often with predisposing factors, such as biliary tract disease, trauma, or alcoholism.[114]

Inflammatory Bowel Disease

Inflammatory bowel disease includes ulcerative colitis or Crohn disease (regional enteritis). These conditions are generally chronic and indolent. Both of these diseases are subject to remissions and exacerbations that do not seem to be increased during pregnancy.[115] Both conditions present as urgency of defecation, crampy lower abdominal pain, and watery diarrhea. Patients may have blood or mucus in their stools, and they may have weight loss. Medications indicated for the treatment of ulcerative colitis and Crohn disease include sulfasalazine and corticosteroids, which seem to have acceptable risks during pregnancy. Mercaptopurine and azathioprine should be used with caution. Methotrexate is contraindicated in pregnancy.[116] Control of the chronic illness before pregnancy is the most important issue.[117] If chronic inflammatory bowel disease is present, it is preferable that the disease be in remission for at least 6 months before pregnancy. Evaluation of possible malnutrition should be done with particular concern regarding folic acid and vitamin B_{12} deficiencies. There have been reports of increased miscarriage rates and preterm deliveries in patients who have active disease during pregnancy.[118] Development of toxic megacolon is associated with a particularly poor outcome and should be treated immediately.

Intrahepatic Cholestasis

Intrahepatic cholestasis is a condition unique to pregnancy, usually in the third trimester. Patients present with severe generalized pruritus. Laboratory tests may show a cholestatic elevation of bile acid and alkaline phosphatase levels and mild elevations of transaminase levels. The level of elevation of bile acids has not been correlated with fetal outcome. The baseline value of alkaline phosphatase is often elevated in normal pregnancy. Hyperbilirubinemia may be seen but is usually less than 5 mg/dL. Coagulation abnormalities generally are not seen in this condition.[119] Patients often experience a recurrence in subsequent pregnancies or with the use of oral contraceptives. Some reports show increased risk of perinatal mortality or fetal distress associated with this illness, and antenatal surveillance has been recommended.[120,121] The premature delivery rate was increased to 41% in one study.[122]

Treatment is directed at reduction of the pruritus with oral or topical antihistamines, phenobarbital, or cholestyramine. Most of these treatments have not been successful. A new medication, ursodeoxycholic acid, has been reported in the literature to reduce pruritus and decrease fetal risk. There are limited reports on the use of ursodeoxycholic acid in pregnancy, and it is generally not being used at this time.[123,124] Amniocentesis for fetal lung maturity and consideration of early labor induction may be indicated if the pruritus is severe. The pruritus begins to fade soon after delivery. If the prothrombin time is elevated, patients should be treated with vitamin K for maternal benefit.

MATERNAL IMMUNOLOGIC DISORDERS

Autoimmune disorders, also known as *collagen vascular disease* or *connective tissue disease,* are acquired conditions that affect multiple organs and are predominantly found during the childbearing years.

Systemic Lupus Erythematosus

Systemic lupus erythematosus (SLE) is a rare disease occurring in approximately 1 in 5000 pregnancies. Women are affected 10 times more often than men. SLE is a pathologic hyperactivity of B lymphocytes with production of autoantibodies. Most patients present with arthritis, skin rashes, and hematologic abnormalities. Occasionally, patients also have cardiovascular or renal complications or both. All of the specific criteria of the American Rheumatology Association are rarely seen in young women with SLE. Diagnosis is made primarily on the finding of positive antinuclear antibodies in serum from women with these symptoms.[125] Nonsteroidal antiinflammatory drugs (NSAIDs) and prednisone are the mainstays of therapy in patients with active lupus. NSAIDs cannot be used on a regular basis during pregnancy because they result in decreased amniotic fluid. Frequently, antimalarial drugs are used to treat lupus patients. These drugs have not been studied for use during pregnancy, but case reports suggest there are no fetal complications from using them throughout pregnancy.[126,127] Occasionally, immunosuppressive or cytotoxic drugs are required for control of symptoms. The most common drug is azathioprine or cyclophosphamide. In contrast to other autoimmune diseases, SLE is not likely to improve with pregnancy. About 30% of women with SLE remain stable during pregnancy. Patients who are in a clinical remission 6 months before pregnancy are most likely to remain in remission during the pregnancy. Patients with

SLE are more likely to develop preeclampsia and thrombocytopenia during pregnancy. Premature delivery (18%) and fetal growth restriction (25%) are the most common complications of pregnancy in women with SLE.[128,129]

All complications, including pregnancy loss, are increased in women with SLE who have antiphospholipid antibodies, lupus anticoagulant, or β₂-glycoprotein antibodies present.[130] These patients are prone to thrombosis, intrauterine growth restriction, severe early-onset preeclampsia, premature delivery, and recurrent pregnancy loss. Lupus anticoagulant originally was identified in patients with lupus, but it often occurs in patients without any other symptoms of SLE. Interventions discussed in the section on thrombotic conditions must be considered for this subgroup of patients.[131]

Women with positive anti-SS-A/Ro or anti-SS-B/La antibodies[132] are specifically at risk for developing intrauterine fetal complete heart block and neonatal lupus. The estimated frequency of this occurring is 0.5% to 2% of infants. The chance of a second affected child is increased to 10% to 20%.[133] Complete heart block appears in the fetus at about 20 weeks of gestation (range, 16 to 30 weeks) and usually is represented by a constant fetal heart rate of less than 70 beats/min. Fetal mortality with complete heart block is 20% or greater. The fetus requires careful monitoring for heart failure during the pregnancy, and most infants need cardiac pacing during the first year of life.[134,135] In the future, additional markers may be identified that allow clinicians to isolate which infants may be at greatest risk for heart block.[136,137] Currently, there are no known therapies to avoid the development of complete heart block when antibodies are present.

Patients with nephritis associated with SLE (15% to 20%) also have the best prognosis if the following conditions are present: (1) the patient has been in remission for more than 6 months, (2) serum creatinine level is less than 1.5 mg/dL, (3) proteinuria is less than 3 g/day, and (4) patient is not hypertensive. Patients with lupus nephritis are particularly vulnerable to complications of pregnancy, including increased miscarriage rate (15%), premature delivery (30% to 40%), intrauterine growth restriction (20% to 30%), and preeclampsia (30%).[138,139] Lupus flare may occur any time during the pregnancy or postpartum and may present with a variety of signs and symptoms.[140]

Rheumatoid Arthritis

Rheumatoid arthritis complicates pregnancy in 1 in 1000 to 2000 cases. It is the most common systemic rheumatic disease and occurs in young women three times as often as in young men. Patients usually present with pain and swelling in one or more joints, usually in the upper extremities. Most patients have a positive serum rheumatoid factor. Pregnancy causes a remission in most patients, but these patients may experience an exacerbation within 6 months postpartum.[141] The mainstays of therapy for rheumatoid arthritis are aspirin, NSAIDs, and corticosteroids. Large doses of salicylates or NSAIDs are contraindicated in pregnancy because of complications with fetal oliguria and ultimately decreased amniotic fluid.[142,143] Penicillamine and methotrexate have been used for treatment of rheumatoid arthritis, but these agents are considered teratogenic and should be avoided during pregnancy. Antimalarials may be used in pregnancy if needed for control of symptoms. Azathioprine has been used safely during pregnancy. Therapy with gold salts has been shown to have long-term effectiveness but should be avoided in pregnancy if possible.[144,145] Most patients remain stable or possibly improve during their pregnancy and do not require more than small doses of NSAIDs during the pregnancy.

NEUROLOGIC DISORDERS

Seizures

Epilepsy presents in 0.3% to 0.6% of pregnant women, with approximately 70% having grand mal seizures. Most patients present with a previously diagnosed seizure disorder and have undergone active treatment with antiepileptic drugs. Several studies have shown that seizure activity remains constant in approximately 50% of patients, increases in approximately 40%, and decreases in 10%.

Choosing a single, effective medication that prevents seizures during pregnancy and that has the least association with fetal developmental problems is the challenge in managing epilepsy.[146] Most medications available for seizure control are considered category D2 except for newer medications with which there is less experience. Women with seizures should be counseled about the effects of medications and that the value of the medication for preventing seizures is greater than the potential effect of the medication on the fetus. Using the medication that is most directed to the type of seizure the patient has and trying to use only one drug are the most important goals (Table 19-6).[147] Drug levels must be monitored during pregnancy because levels may drop secondary to an increase in liver metabolism, renal excretion, and volume of distribution that happens naturally in pregnancy. It is crucial to avoid seizures during pregnancy and to maintain therapeutic levels of antiepileptic drugs. Preventing seizures is important because of the decreased oxygenation to the fetus that occurs during a seizure.[147] Medication levels should be assessed on a regular schedule throughout pregnancy. If an attempt is made to withdraw antiepileptic medications, this should occur 1 year before a planned pregnancy, and the patient should be completely stable before conception.

Phenytoin is still the most commonly used medication for generalized seizure disorders. There seems to be a phenytoin syndrome of congenital malformations, including cleft lip and palate, midline cardiac defects, facial anomalies, microcephaly, intrauterine growth restriction, and mental retardation.[148] The conclusion that phenytoin may cause these congenital malformations is confused by information that women with epilepsy have an increased congenital malformation rate over the general population, even when they are not on antiepileptic medication.

Phenobarbital is another drug frequently used for generalized seizures, but it is rarely effective as a single agent. Phenobarbital may affect fetal brain growth and should be avoided if possible.

Carbamazepine and valproic acid are used frequently for generalized seizure disorders and are associated with an increased incidence of 1% to 2% for neural tube defects in the fetus.[149,150] Trimethadione is used for petit mal seizures and has been associated with a 50% rate of the phenytoin syndrome.[151] It is believed that all antiepileptic medications have some teratogenic potential. The second-generation antiepileptics, such as lamotrigine and gabapentin, may have advantages over the older drugs, but few registry data are available at this time for the potential fetal teratogenic effects. Valproic acid, carbamazepine, and trimethadione especially should be avoided during the first trimester of pregnancy. Changing or discontinuing drugs should be done carefully during pregnancy if the patient is well controlled on her current medications.[152]

Folic acid in the maternal diet before pregnancy and during the first trimester has been shown to decrease the frequency of neural tube defects in the

Table 19–6. Antiepileptic Medications

Medication	Risk*	Enzyme Inducing	Coverage
Valproic acid	D	N	Broad spectrum
Phenytoin	D	Y	General
Phenobarbital	D	Y	General
Carbamazepine	D	Y	Partial
Ethosuximide	C	Y	Absence
Lamotrigine	C	N	Broad spectrum
Oxcarbazepine	C	Y	Partial
Gabapentin	C	N	Partial
Levetiracetam	C	N	Broad spectrum
Topiramate	C	Y	Broad spectrum
Zonisamide	C	N	Broad spectrum
Trimethadione	D	Y	Petit mal

*See Table 19–1 for definitions of risk factors C and D.

Modified from Delgado-Escueta A, Janz D: Consensus guidelines: Preconceptional counseling, management and care of the women with leprosy. Neurology 42:149, 1992 (ref. 146)

general population. This benefit has not been shown with valproic acid, but increased folate is still recommended.[153]

Prenatal diagnosis should be offered, including a maternal serum α-fetoprotein determination at 15 to 21 weeks of gestation. A targeted fetal ultrasound study to evaluate the fetal central nervous system, face, lip, and heart should be done at midtrimester, usually between 18 and 22 weeks of gestation. Targeted fetal echocardiography also should be considered. Serial ultrasound studies to document fetal head growth may be useful.

Enzyme-inducing seizure medications have been said to increase neonatal bleeding episodes because of a decrease in vitamin K. The only prospective evaluation of neonatal complications to date does not support an increase in neonatal bleeding.[154] There is no evidence that treating the mother with vitamin K before delivery is useful in preventing fetal bleeding problems because it cannot be shown to cross the placental barrier.[155,156] A consensus recommends giving vitamin K, 10 mg/day, for the last month of pregnancy despite a lack of evidence to support the practice.[157] Newer antiepileptic agents have the advantage of not causing as much enzyme induction and may cause fewer problems with vitamin K depletion.[158] Newer medications that are not enzyme inducing are more compatible with oral contraceptive pills because they do not decrease the contraceptive effects of the hormones.[149]

Patients who present with their first seizure in pregnancy should be completely evaluated by a neurologist with a CT scan, electroencephalogram, and lumbar puncture, as necessary. New-onset seizures occasionally occur during pregnancy and may recur only during pregnancy; this occurs in less than 25% of patients with seizures. New-onset seizures are most often related to trauma, tumors, drug toxicity, or alcohol withdrawal. Occasionally, metabolic abnormalities may lead to convulsions in pregnancy and should be investigated.[157]

Cerebrovascular Accidents

The risk of stroke in a pregnant patient is 13 times the risk in a nonpregnant patient of the same age. Subarachnoid hemorrhage is five times higher in pregnancy.[159] Ischemic and hemorrhagic cerebrovascular accidents occur more frequently in African American women, women who smoke cigarettes, and women with diabetes.[160]

Ruptured aneurysms and arteriovenous malformations are the most common causes of subarachnoid hemorrhage. Patients present with severe headache, loss of consciousness, nuchal rigidity, and lateralizing signs. Seizures may be the presenting sign. When these complications occur in pregnancy, they generally occur after 28 weeks of gestation. Patients with this presentation need an appropriate neurologic workup with cranial CT scanning or other necessary imaging studies and lumbar puncture.[161]

Pregnant patients may present with intracerebral hemorrhage, arterial occlusive disease, or cerebral venous thrombosis similar to nonpregnant patients. There may be a small increase in the risk of arterial occlusive disease during pregnancy. Cerebral venous thrombosis and intracerebral hemorrhage are associated with the onset of preeclampsia in pregnancy. These patients also may present with headache, changes in consciousness, and seizures. Patients must have an appropriate workup with the help of a neurologist and should be treated appropriately with supportive care, antiepileptics, anticoagulation, and control of hypertension when necessary. Patients with cerebrovascular accidents during pregnancy should be delivered by cesarean section only for obstetric indications.[162]

Ischemic strokes have a low risk of recurrence in subsequent pregnancies in young women. The highest risk time period for ischemic stroke seems to be during the postpartum period rather than during the pregnancy.[163] Rates of stroke are increased in pregnancy when associated with cigarette smoking, preeclampsia, multiple gestation, antiphospholipid syndrome, and operative delivery.[164]

Migraine Headache

Headache is one of the most common reasons for outpatient visits, affecting 20% of all women. A survey of experts in headache management showed that the triptan medications are far superior to other treatments for migraine headaches. Sumatriptan is a category C medication. The Glaxo-Wellcome Registry included 312 registrants through 1999 with no increase in birth defects noted. In some patients, tricyclic antidepressants and selective serotonin reuptake inhibitors also have been used for headache management. Ergotamines should be avoided during pregnancy because they have been shown to decrease uterine blood flow.[165] Migraine headaches may improve, decrease, or occur for the first time during pregnancy. Neurodiagnostic testing, in consultation with a neurologist, should proceed as needed to determine any organic basis for the headache.[166]

Spinal Cord Lesions

Spinal cord lesions at T5 or higher are associated with a serious peripartum complication called *autonomic hyperreflexia*. Piloerection may be the only symptom, but serious hypertensive crises and cerebrovascular accidents can occur. Prophylaxis against this reaction can be accomplished with epidural anesthesia early in labor. Surveillance during the pregnancy for urinary tract infection, anemia, preterm labor, normal bowel function, and prevention of skin ulcers is crucial. Perception of uterine activity is absent for women with high lesions, and monitoring for cervical change is helpful.[167,168]

MATERNAL HEMATOLOGIC DISORDERS

Anemia refers to a lowered level of hemoglobin resulting in decreased oxygen-carrying capacity. Nutritional deficiencies leading to anemia are a major health risk worldwide, even in developed countries with availability of high-quality, fortified diets.[169] An implied benefit to identification and treatment of anemia is derived from epidemiologic studies, but there are no randomized trials showing clinically relevant outcomes correlated with hematocrit levels.[170] The current targets were established based on the maximal hemoglobin levels that can be obtained with iron supplementation and appropriate nutrition. Developing functional goals related to maternal and infant outcomes would improve the focus of programs to address mild to moderate anemia.[171] Severe anemia is associated with a 3.5 times greater risk of maternal mortality, but anemia may represent a marker for other problems leading to mortality.[172,173]

Any discussion of hematologic changes in pregnancy must take into account the physiologic changes of pregnancy. A physiologic anemia of pregnancy results in an average hematocrit of 33.5% (range, 31% to 36%) in the second trimester. This change seems to occur because of a physiologic dilution caused by an increase in plasma volume that occurs before a commensurate increase in red blood cells.[17] Other hematologic changes include the total neutrophil count that increases during pregnancy so that the total white blood count ranges from 9,000 to 15,000. In general, the platelet count, prothrombin time, and partial thromboplastin time do not change during pregnancy. Measurable fibrinogen is increased in pregnancy, with the normal range up to 600 mg/dL.

Microcytic or Normocytic Anemias

Iron deficiency anemia causes 75% of anemia in pregnancy.[174] There is an increased need for iron during pregnancy, and some women are unable to take iron orally because of gastrointestinal intolerance.[175,176] Usually a mild normocytic, normochromic anemia is seen on the peripheral blood smear. Serum iron levels may decrease to less than 60 mg/dL, and transferrin saturation may be less than 15%. Generally, 60 mg of elemental iron per day (300 mg of ferrous sulfate or gluconate) is advised beginning early in pregnancy. If iron deficiency anemia develops, three times the prophylactic dose of iron should be given along with a prenatal vitamin tablet. Rarely is parenteral iron therapy required for iron deficiency anemia that has not responded to oral therapy or in patients who cannot tolerate orally administered iron.[177]

Macrocytic Anemias

Nutritional deficiencies of folic acid are responsible for a megaloblastic anemia of pregnancy with macrocytic cells on the peripheral smear. Serious anemia due to folic acid deficiency is unusual in the United States and generally responds quickly to oral folic acid supplementation of 1 mg/day. Serum folic acid levels also may be decreased by exposure to phenytoin, barbiturates, and large amounts of alcohol. Vitamin B_{12} deficiency producing pernicious anemia is rare in young women on a regular diet.[178]

Sickle Cell Anemia

Sickle cell anemia is caused by the inheritance of an autosomal recessive gene for an amino acid in the β chain of hemoglobin that results in production of abnormal hemoglobin. Heterozygous sickle cell trait is found in the United States in approximately 8.5% of African Americans, and it is seen in whites and Asians. Hemoglobin S is the most common hemoglobin disorder in the United States. Sickle cell carriers do not show the manifestations of the disease but may have mild anemia; they are more prone to urinary tract infections and should be screened on a regular basis for asymptomatic bacteriuria.[179] Appropriate genetic counseling is important, and

the patient's partner should be screened for sickle cell trait. Prenatal testing of amniotic fluid is available for sickle cell.[180] If an infant is born to parents who are both carriers of sickle cell trait, the nursery should be alerted because the infant has a 25% chance of being affected by sickle cell disease. Many states now mandate sickle cell screening of all neonates.

Most patients with homozygous sickle cell disease have had repeated sickle cell crises throughout life, which are characterized by limb and abdominal pain. Diagnosis is best made by hemoglobin electrophoresis to determine if the patient has homozygous sickle cell disease or hemoglobin SC disease. Patients with SC disease have less severe anemia and fewer crises during pregnancy. If a crisis does occur with SC disease, it can be as severe as SS disease. Patients should be observed carefully throughout the pregnancy to ensure that hematocrit levels remain greater than 30%. Folic acid supplementation of 1 mg/day should be given. Maintaining good maternal hydration and avoiding infections sometimes can prevent a crisis.

Sickle crises should be managed with exchange transfusion, analgesia, oxygen therapy, intravenous hydration, and treatment of any infections. Antepartum testing should be initiated about 32 weeks of gestation. Infants of pregnancies complicated by sickle cell disease are frequently delivered before 37 weeks, have growth restriction, and have increased postpartum infections. Overall, maternal and neonatal outcomes can be good with careful management.[181] Prophylactic transfusion results in significant decreases of pain crises and severe anemia, but also results in patients receiving more frequent transfusions than patients treated based solely on hemoglobin values. No significant differences were seen in other maternal or neonatal outcomes with prophylactic versus treatment regimens.[182]

Thalassemia

Thalassemia is classified by the type of hemoglobin chain that is inadequately produced. This may be the α or β hemoglobin. Heterozygous β-thalassemia trait (also called *thalassemia minor*) patients have a mild hypochromic microcytic anemia resembling iron deficiency anemia. The diagnosis may be made from a low mean corpuscular volume less than 80 mm^3 on a routine complete blood count.[183] The hemoglobin electrophoresis has a high hemoglobin A_2 level (>3.5%) and may have a high fetal hemoglobin. No treatment is necessary for these patients, but the father should be screened, and genetic counseling should be offered.

β-Thalassemia major occurs with homozygous β-chain abnormalities resulting in a severe blood disorder. Patients have severe anemia and may die from heart failure. Early and intensive blood transfusion protocols are necessary to keep the hemoglobin level higher than 10 g/dL. Prenatal diagnosis is available with polymerase chain reaction and high-throughput DNA sequencing.[184] The α-thalassemias occur in four different states, depending on the number of α genes that have been deleted or have mutated. Bart hemoglobin results from the homozygous form in which no α hemoglobin can be produced, and it is incompatible with life. Hemoglobin H disease is missing three α chains, and these patients have a severe hypochromic, microcytic anemia with poikilocytosis. α-Thalassemia minor has two deleted genes and presents with a mild anemia.[185] The mean corpuscular volume is less than 80 mm³ in α-thalassemia also, but electrophoresis is normal. Molecular genetic testing is required to make the diagnosis. If both partners are diagnosed as carriers, genetic counseling and testing should be offered.[180]

Platelet Disorders

Normal platelet count in pregnancy may decrease to 100,000/μL and be completely normal. After excluding an intercurrent disease, such as leukemia, lymphoma, metastatic neoplasia, or megaloblastic anemia, and potential drug exposures, significant thrombocytopenia is usually considered to be immune thrombocytopenia. Patients should be screened for lupus erythematosus with an antinuclear antibody profile.

If the mother has preexisting immune thrombocytopenia and shows a circulating IgG antibody against platelets, the antibody is able to cross the placenta and may cause neonatal thrombocytopenia. In this circumstance, neonatal evaluation before delivery may be indicated, although the necessity is questioned because the potential risk of neonatal bleeding is low. If there is a maternal antibody present, it may be appropriate to evaluate the level of fetal platelets by percutaneous umbilical blood sampling before labor.[186] Fetal scalp sampling during labor also has been proposed, but it is not as reliable as percutaneous umbilical blood sampling for predicting fetal platelet count. These pregnancies most often deliver at term. It is believed that the infants may be at increased risk of intracranial hemorrhage due to thrombocytopenia if the platelet count is less than 50,000/μL at the time of birth. If the fetal platelet count is less than 50,000/μL, the current recommendation is to deliver the infant by cesarean section.[187]

The rate of positive platelet antibodies is high in women with benign gestational thrombocytopenia, preeclampsia, and immune thrombocytopenia. It is hoped that newer glycoprotein-specific assays will be of greater assistance in distinguishing situations in which the neonate may be at risk of having thrombocytopenia from passage of maternal antibodies.[188]

When the diagnosis of immune thrombocytopenia is made, patients are initially treated with oral prednisone, 5 to 40 mg/day, until a platelet count greater than 100,000/μL is achieved. If steroids do not cause an improvement in platelet count, a splenectomy may be necessary, although this is best avoided during pregnancy. Occasionally, immunosuppression with azathioprine has been used with immune thrombocytopenia. This is probably an acceptable therapy after the first trimester. Intravenous gamma globulin therapy to improve platelet count before delivery also has been given, although the improvement lasts only a few days.

SUMMARY

Any proposed medical or surgical therapy should consider the coexisting pregnancy, but the care of the pregnant woman should not be less because she is pregnant. The fetus has the greatest chance for a healthy survival if the mother is healthy. Most therapies, medications, and interventions are not studied specifically on pregnant patients because of ethical concerns. Evaluation of some of the possible effects can be made based on the understanding of basic physiology and the pharmacokinetics of the medications involved in treatment.

Assessment of the fetus is essential during any pregnancy that may be affected by maternal illness. A variety of tests are available for evaluation of the fetus, and these tests are especially valuable when the test is reassuring. It has become clear that evaluation of amniotic fluid volume by ultrasound is important in a fetus that may be affected by a maternal condition that causes decreased uterine blood flow, placental insufficiency, or fetal heart failure.[189,190] A greater focus on drug registries for pregnancies exposed to medications and increased attempts to obtain evidence-based data may help the movement toward more focused care of the pregnant woman and her child.

REFERENCES

1. Briggs G, Freeman R, Yaffe S: Drugs in Pregnancy and Lactation. Baltimore, Williams & Wilkins, 2001.
2. Risk factor definitions for medications. Fed Reg 45:37434, 1980.
3. Lo W, Friedman J: Teratogenicity of recently introduced medications in human pregnancy. Obstet Gynecol 100:465, 2002.
4. Rubin P: Drug treatment during pregnancy. BMJ 317:1503, 1998.
5. Hansen W, Yankowitz J: Pharmacologic therapy for medical disorders during pregnancy. Clin Obstet Gynecol 45:136, 2002.
6. Kingdom J: Oxygen and placental vascular development. Adv Exp Med Biol 474:259, 1999.
7. Burton G: Nutrition of the human fetus during the first trimester—a review. Placenta 22(A):S70, 2001.
8. Clark S, Cotton D, Hankins G, et al: Critical Care Obstetrics. Boston, Blackwell Scientific, 1991.
9. Cunningham F, Gant N, Leveno K, et al: Maternal adaptation to pregnancy. In: Williams Obstetrics, 21st ed. New York, Appleton & Lange, 2001, pp 167-200.
10. Frederiksen M: Physiologic changes in pregnancy and their effect on drug disposition. Semin Perinatol 25:120, 2001.
11. Hytten, Paintin D: Increase in plasma volume during normal pregnancy. J Obstet Gynaecol Br Commonw 70:402, 1963.
12. Mason E, Montello-Rosene K, Powrie R: Medical problems during pregnancy. Med Clin North Am 82:246, 1998.
13. Simpson L: Maternal medical disease: Risk of antepartum fetal death. Semin Perinatol 26:42, 2002.
14. Report of National High Blood Pressure Education Program Working Group on high blood pressure in pregnancy. Am J Obstet Gynecol 183:S1, 2000.
15. American Academy of Pediatrics: Transfer of drugs and other chemicals into human milk. AAP Committee on Drugs. Pediatrics 108:776, 2001.
16. Sibai B: Chronic hypertension in pregnancy. Obstet Gynecol 100:369, 2002.
17. Anderson A, Lichorad A: Hypertensive disorders, diabetes mellitus, and anemia: Three common medical complications of pregnancy. Primary Care Clin Office Pract 27:185, 2000.

18. Smulian J, Ananth C, Vintzileos A, et al: Fetal deaths in the United States: Influence of high-risk conditions and implications for management. Obstet Gynecol 100:1183, 2002.

19. Montan S, Anandakumar C, Arulkumaran S, et al: Effects of methyldopa on uteroplacental and fetal hemodynamics in pregnancy-induced hypertension. Am J Obstet Gynecol 168:152, 1993.

20. Rosenthal T, Oparil S: The effect of antihypertensive drugs on the fetus. J Hum Hypertens 16:293, 2002.

21. Sibai B: Treatment of hypertension in pregnant women. N Engl J Med 335:257, 1996.

22. El-Qarmalawi A, Morsy A, Al-Fadly A, et al: Labetalol vs. methyldopa in the treatment of pregnancy-induced hypertension. Int J Gynaecol Obstet 49:125, 1995.

23. Mahmoud T, Bjornsson S, Calder A: Labetalol therapy in pregnancy induced hypertension: The effects on fetoplacental circulation and fetal outcome. Eur J Obstet Gynecol Reprod Biol 50:109, 1993.

24. Fairlie F, Walker J: Maternal and fetal haemodynamics in hypertensive pregnancies during maternal treatment with intravenous hydralazine or labetalol. Br J Obstet Gynaecol 98:1186, 1991.

25. Powers D, Papadakos P, Wallin J: Parenteral hydralazine revisited. J Emerg Med 16:191, 1998.

26. Aali B, Nejad S: Nifedipine or hydralazine as a first-line agent to control hypertension in severe preeclampsia. Acta Obstet Gynecol Scand 81:25, 2002.

27. Papatsonis D, Lok C, Bos J, et al: Calcium channel blockers in the management of preterm labor and hypertension in pregnancy. Eur J Obstet Gynecol Reprod Biol 45:122, 2001.

28. Magee L, Schick B, Donnenfeld A, et al: The safety of calcium channel blockers in human pregnancy: A prospective, multicenter cohort study. Am J Obstet Gynecol 174:823, 1996.

29. Butters L, Kennedy S, Rubin P: Atenolol in essential hypertension during pregnancy. BMJ 301:587, 1990.

30. Lydakis C, Lip G, Beevers M, et al: Atenolol and fetal growth in pregnancies complicated by hypertension. Am J Hypertens 12:541, 1999.

31. Magee LA, Duley L: Oral beta-blockers for mild to moderate hypertension during pregnancy. Cochrane Database Syst Rev (B):CD002863, 2003.

32. Chisholm C, Chescheir N, Kennedy M: Reversible oligohydramnios in a pregnancy with angiotensin-converting enzyme inhibitor exposure. Am J Perinatol 14:511, 1997.

33. Shotan A, Widerhorn J, Hurst A, et al: Risks of angiotensin-converting enzyme inhibition during pregnancy: Experimental and clinical evidence, potential mechanisms, and recommendations for use. Am J Med 96:451, 1994.

34. Hanssens M, Keirse M, Vankelecom F: Fetal and neonatal effects of treatment with angiotensin-converting enzyme inhibitors in pregnancy. Obstet Gynecol 78:128, 1991.

35. ACOG Committee on Practice Bulletins: ACOG Practice Bulletin. Chronic hypertension in pregnancy. Obstet Gynecol 98(Suppl):177, 2001.

36. ACOG Practice Bulletin 9: Antepartum Fetal Surveillance. Washington, DC, American College of Obstetricians and Gynecologists, 1999.

37. Magann E: Antenatal testing among 1001 patients at high risk: The role of ultrasonographic estimate of amniotic fluid volume. Am J Obstet Gynecol 180:1330, 1999.

38. Brown M, Gallery E: Volume homeostasis in normal pregnancy and pre-eclampsia: Physiology and clinical implications. Baillieres Clin Obstet Gynecol 8:287, 1994.

39. Elkayam U: Pregnancy and cardiovascular disease. In Braunwald E, Zipes DP, Libby P (eds): A Textbook of Cardiovascular Medicine, 6th ed. Philadelphia, WB Saunders, 2001, pp 2172-2178.

40. Lim S: Rheumatic heart diseases in pregnancy. Ann Acad Med Singapore 31:340, 2002.

41. Shillingford A, Weiner S: Maternal issues affecting the fetus. Clin Perinatol 28:31-70, 2001.

42. Boughman J, Berg K, Astemborski J, et al: Familial risks of congenital heart defect assessed in a population-based epidemiologic study. Am J Med Genet 26:839, 1987.

43. Whittemore R, Hobbins J, Engle M: Pregnancy and its outcome in women with and without surgical treatment of congenital heart disease. Am J Cardiol 50:641, 1982.

44. Colman J, Sermer M, Seaward P, et al: Congenital heart disease in pregnancy. Cardiol Rev 8:166, 2000.

45. Patton D, Lee W, Cotton D: Cyanotic maternal heart disease in pregnancy. Obstet Gynecol Surv 45:756, 1990.

46. Clark S: Cardiac disease in pregnancy. Crit Care Clin 7:777, 1991.

47. Chow T, Galvin J, McGovern B: Antiarrhythmic drug therapy in pregnancy and lactation. Am J Cardiol 82:581, 1998.

48. Page R: Treatment of arrhythmias during pregnancy. Am Heart J 130:871, 1995.

49. Ford R, Barton J, O'Brien J, et al: Demographics, management, and outcome of peripartum cardiomyopathy in a community hospital. Am J Obstet Gynecol 182:1036, 2000.

50. Heider A, Kuller J, Strauss R, et al: Peripartum cardiomyopathy: A review of the literature. Obstet Gynecol Surv 54:526, 1999.

51. Bernstein P, Magriples U: Cardiomyopathy in pregnancy: A retrospective study. Am J Perinatol 18:163, 2001.

52. Lage S, Kopel L, Medeiros C, et al: Angiotensin II contributes to arterial compliance in congestive heart failure. Am J Physiol Heart Circ Physiol 283:1424, 2002.

53. Pearson G, Veille J, Rahimtoola S, et al: Peripartum cardiomyopathy. National Heart, Lung, and Blood Institute and Office of Rare Diseases (National Institutes of Health). JAMA 283:1183, 2000.

54. Gei A, Hankins G: Cardiac disease and pregnancy. Obstet Gynecol Clin North Am 28:465, 2001.

55. Ferencz C, Boughman J, Neill C, et al: Congenital cardiovascular malformations: Questions on inheritance. Baltimore-Washington Infant Study Group. J Am Coll Cardiol 14:756, 1989.

56. McCurdy C, Reed K: Basic technique of fetal echocardiography. Semin Ultrasound CT MRI 14:267, 1993.

57. Rossiter J, Callan N: Prenatal diagnosis of congenital heart disease. Obstet Gynecol Clin North Am 20:485, 1993.

58. Connolly A, Thorp J: Urinary tract infections in pregnancy. Urol Clin North Am 26:778, 1999.

59. Cunningham F, Lucas M, Hankins G: Pulmonary injury complicating antepartum pyelonephritis. Am J Obstet Gynecol 156:797, 1987.

60. Towers C, Kaminsakas C, Garite T, et al: Pulmonary injury associated with antepartum pyelonephritis: Can patients at risk be identified? Am J Obstet Gynecol 164:974, 1991.

61. Wing D, Hendershott C, Debuque L, et al: Outpatient treatment of acute pyelonephritis in pregnancy after 24 weeks. Obstet Gynecol 94:683, 1999.

62. Bjerklund-Johansen T: Diagnosis and imaging in urinary tract infection. Curr Opin Urol 12:39, 2002.

63. Jones D, Hayslett J: Outcome of pregnancy in women with moderate or severe renal insufficiency. N Engl J Med 335:226, 1996.

64. Katz A, Hayslett J, Singson E, et al: Pregnancy in women with kidney disease. Kidney Int 18:192, 1980.

65. Jungers P, Chauveau D, Choukroun G, et al: Pregnancy in women with impaired renal function. Clin Nephrol 47:281, 1997.

66. Hou S: Pregnancy in women with chronic renal disease. N Engl J Med 312:836, 1985.

67. Cunningham F, Cox S, Harstad T, et al: Chronic renal disease and pregnancy outcome. Am J Obstet Gynecol 163:453, 1990.

68. Dunne F, Chowdhury T, Harland A, et al: Pregnancy outcome in women with insulin-dependent diabetes mellitus complicated by nephropathy. Q JM 92:451, 1999.

69. Bar J: Prediction of pregnancy outcome in subgroups of women with renal disease. Clin Nephrol 53:437, 2000.

70. Lessan-Pezeshki M: Pregnancy after renal transplantation: Points to consider. Nephrol Dial Transplant 17:703, 2002.

71. Wilson P, Guay-Woodford L: Pathophysiology and clinical management of polycystic kidney disease in women. Semin Nephrol 19:123, 1999.

72. Ie S, Rubio E, Alper B, Szerlip HM: Respiratory complications of pregnancy. Obstet Gynecol Surv 57:39, 2002.

73. Nelson-Piercy C: Asthma in pregnancy. Thorax 56:325, 2001.

74. Shatz M: Asthma and pregnancy. Lancet 353:1202, 1999.

75. Park-Wyllie L, Mazzotta P, Pastuszak A, et al: Birth defects after maternal exposure to corticosteroids: Prospective cohort study and meta-analysis of epidemiological studies. Teratology 62:385, 2000.

76. Shatz M, Zeiger R, Harden K, et al: The safety of asthma and allergy medications during pregnancy. J Allergy Clin Immunol 100:301, 1997.

77. Bubak M, Li J: Asthma in adolescents and adults. In Rakel RE (ed): Conn's Current Therapy, 54th ed. Philadelphia, WB Saunders, 2002, pp 777-779.

78. Vergani P, Roncaglia N, Andreotti C, et al: Prognostic value of uterine artery Doppler velocimetry in growth-restricted fetuses delivered near term. Am J Obstet Gynecol 187:932, 2002.

79. Olson G: Cystic fibrosis in pregnancy. Semin Perinatol 21:307, 1997.

80. Henneman L, Poppelaars F, tenKate L: Evaluation of cystic fibrosis carrier screening programs according to genetic screening criteria. Genet Med 4:241, 2002.

81. Dizon-Townson D: Pregnancy related venous thromboembolism. Clin Obstet Gynecol 45:363, 2002.

82. Greer I: Thrombosis in pregnancy: Maternal and fetal issues. Lancet 353:1258, 1999.

83. Nilsson T, Olausson A, Johnsson H, et al: Negative spiral CT in acute pulmonary embolism. Acta Radiol 43:486, 2002.

84. Hall J, Pauli R, Wilson K: Maternal and fetal sequelae of anti-coagulation during pregnancy. Am J Med 68:122, 1980.

85. Pettila V, Kaaja R, Leinonen P: Thromboprophylaxis with low molecular weight heparin (dalteparin) in pregnancy. Thromb Res 96:275, 1999.

86. Bonnar J, Green R, Norris L: Inherited thrombophilia and pregnancy: The obstetric perspective. Semin Thromb Hemost 24:49, 1998.

87. Ensom M, Stephenson M: Low-molecular-weight heparins in pregnancy. Pharmacotherapy 19:1013, 1999.

88. Lockwood C: Inherited thrombophilias in pregnancy patients: Detection and treatment paradigm. Obstet Gynecol 99:333, 2002.

89. McColl M, Walker I, Greer I: The role of inherited thrombophilia in venous thromboembolism associated with pregnancy. Br J Obstet Gynaecol 106:756, 1999.

90. Kupferminc M, Eldor A, Steinman N, et al: Increased frequency of genetic thrombophilia in women with complications of pregnancy. N Engl J Med 340:9, 1999.

91. American College of Obstetricians and Gynecologists: ACOG Practice Bulletin. Clinical management guidelines for obstetrician-gynecologists. Number 37, August 2002. Thyroid disease in pregnancy. Obstet Gynecol 100:387, 2002.

92. Matsuura N, Harada S, Ohyama Y, et al: The mechanisms of transient hypothyroxinemia in infants born to mothers with Graves' disease. Pediatr Res 42:214, 1997.

93. Lazarus J: Epidemiology and prevention of thyroid disease in pregnancy. Thyroid 12:861, 2002.

94. Greenberg F: Choanal atresia and athelia: Methimazole teratogenicity or a new syndrome? Am J Med Genet 28:931, 1987.

95. Laurberg P, Nygaard B, Glinoer D, et al: Guidelines for TSH-receptor antibody measurements in pregnancy. Eur J Endocrinol 139:584, 1998.

96. Weiner C: Fetal blood sampling and fetal thrombocytopenia. Fetal Diagn Ther 10:173, 1995.

97. Wallace C, Couch R, Ginsberg J: Fetal thyrotoxicosis: A case report and recommendations for prediction, diagnosis and treatment. Thyroid 5:125, 1995.

98. Weetman A: Graves' disease. N Engl J Med 343:1236, 2000.

99. Smallridge R, Ladenson P: Hypothyroidism in pregnancy: Consequences to neonatal health. J Clin Endocrinol Metab 86:2349, 2001.

100. Molitch M: Pituitary diseases in pregnancy. Semin Perinatol 22:457, 1998.

101. Hod M, Orvieto R, Kaplan B, et al: Hyperemesis gravidarum: A review. J Reprod Med 39:605, 1994.

102. Nelson-Piercy C: Hyperemesis gravidarum. Curr Obstet Gynaecol 7:98, 1997.

103. Pastuszak A: Doxylamine/pyridoxine for nausea and vomiting of pregnancy. Can Pharm J 128:39, 1995.

104. ManStuijvenberg M, Schabort I, Labadarios D, et al: The nutritional status and treatment of patients with hyperemesis gravidarum. Am J Obstet Gynecol 172:1585, 1995.

105. Jewell D, Young G: Interventions for nausea and vomiting in early pregnancy. Cochrane Database Syst Rev (2): CD000145, 2000.

106. Goodwin T, Montero M, Mestman J: Transient hyperthyroidism and hyperemesis gravidarum: Clinical aspects. Am J Obstet Gynecol 167:648, 1992.

107. Sama C, Labate A, Taroni F, et al: Epidemiology and natural history of gallstone disease. Semin Liver Dis 10:149, 1990.

108. Graham G, Baxi L, Tharakan T: Laparoscopic cholecystectomy during pregnancy: A case series and review of the literature. Obstet Gynecol Surv 53:566, 1998.

109. Dixon N, Faddis D, Silberman H: Aggressive management of cholecystitis during pregnancy. Am J Surg 154:292, 1987.

110. Lee S, Bradley J, Mele M, et al: Cholelithiasis in pregnancy: Surgical versus medical management. Obstet Gynecol 95:S70, 2000.

111. Cosenza C, Saffari B, Jabbour N, et al: Surgical management of biliary gallstone disease during pregnancy. Am J Surg 178:545, 1999.

112. Mayer I, Hussain H: Abdominal pain during pregnancy. Gastroenterol Clin North Am 27:1, 1998.

113. Strickland D, Hauth J, Widsh J, et al: Amylase and isoamylase activities in serum of pregnant women. Obstet Gynecol 63:389, 1984.

114. United Kingdom guidelines for the management of acute pancreatitis. British Society of Gastroenterology. Gut 42 (Suppl 2):S1, 1998.

115. Baiocco P, Korelitz B: The influence of inflammatory bowel disease and its treatment on pregnancy and fetal outcome. J Clin Gastroenterol 6:211, 1984.

116. Rajapakse R, Korelitz B: Inflammatory bowel disease during pregnancy. Curr Treat Options Gastroenterol 4:245, 2001.

117. Korelitz B: Inflammatory bowel disease and pregnancy. Gastroenterol Clin North Am 27:213, 1998.

118. Willoughby C: Fertility, pregnancy and inflammatory bowel disease. In Allan R, Keighley M, Hawkins C, et al (eds): Inflammatory Bowel Disease. New York, Churchill-Livingstone, 1990, pp 547-558.

119. Mullally B, Hansen W: Intrahepatic cholestasis of pregnancy: Review of the literature. Obstet Gynecol Surv 57:47, 2001.

120. Davies M, daSilva R, Jones S, et al: Fetal mortality associated with cholestasis of pregnancy and the potential benefit of therapy with ursodeoxycholic acid. Gut 37:580, 1995.

121. Rioseco A, Ivankovic M, Manzur A, et al: Intrahepatic cholestasis of pregnancy: A retrospective case control of perinatal outcome. Am J Obstet Gynecol 170:890, 1994.

122. Bacq Y, Sapey T, Brechot M, et al: Intrahepatic cholestasis of pregnancy: A French prospective study. Hepatology 26:358, 1997.

123. Brites D, Rodrigues C, Oliveira N, et al: Correction of maternal serum bile acid profile during ursodeoxycholic acid therapy in cholestasis of pregnancy. J Hepatol 28:91, 1998.

124. Mazella G, Nicola R, Francesco A, et al: Ursodeoxycholic acid administration in patients with cholestasis of pregnancy: Effects on primary bile acids in babies and mothers. Hepatology 33:504, 2001.

125. Cortes-Hernandez J, Ordi-Ros J, Paredes F, et al: Clinical predictors of fetal and maternal outcome in systemic lupus erythematosus: A prospective study of 103 pregnancies. Rheumatology 41:643, 2002.

126. Al-Herz A, Schulzer M, Esdaile J: Survey of antimalarial use in lupus pregnancy and lactation. J Rheumatol 29:700, 2002.

127. Borden M, Parke A: Antimalarial drugs in systemic lupus erythematosus: Use in pregnancy. Drug Saf 24:1055, 2001.

128. Kari J: Pregnancy outcome in connective tissue disease. Saudi Med J 22:590, 2001.

129. Yasmeen S, Wilkins E, Field N, et al: Pregnancy outcomes in women with systemic lupus erythematosus. J Matern Fetal Med 10:91, 2001.

130. Chi H: Recent advances in the diagnosis of antiphospholipid syndrome. Int J Hematol 76(Suppl 2):47, 2002.

131. Kiss E, Bhattoa H, Bettembuk P, et al: Pregnancy in women with systemic lupus erythematosus. Eur J Obstet Gynecol Reprod Biol 101:129, 2002.

132. Buyon J, Winchester R, Slade S, et al: Identification of mothers at risk for congenital heart block and other neonatal lupus syndromes in their children: Comparison of enzyme-linked immunoabsorbent assay and immunoblot for measurement of anti-SS-A/Ro and anti-SS-B/La antibodies. Arthritis Rheum 36:1263, 1993.

133. Brucato A, Doria A, Frassi M, et al: Pregnancy outcome in 100 women with autoimmune diseases and anti-Ro/SSA antibodies: A prospective controlled study. Lupus 11:716, 2002.

134. Friedman D, Rupel A, Glickstein J, et al: Congenital heart block in neonatal lupus: The pediatric cardiologist's perspective. Indian J Pediatr 69:517, 2002.

135. Julkunen H, Kaaja R, Wallgren E, et al: Isolated congenital heart block: Fetal and infant outcome and familial incidence of heart block. Obstet Gynecol 82:11, 1993.

136. Julkunen H, Kaaja R, Siren M, et al: Immune-mediated congenital heart block (CHB): Identifying and counseling patients at risk for having children with CHB. Semin Arthritis Rheum 28:97, 1998.

137. Salomonsson S: A serologic marker for fetal risk of congenital heart block. Arthritis Rheum 46:1233, 2002.

138. Julkunen H: Pregnancy and lupus nephritis. Scand J Urol Nephrol 35:319, 2001.

139. Moroni G, Quaglini S, Banfi G, et al: Pregnancy in lupus nephritis. Am J Kidney Dis 40:713, 2002.

140. Kochenour N, Branch D, Rote N, et al: A new postpartum syndrome associated with antiphospholipid antibodies. Obstet Gynecol 69:460, 1987.

141. Wilder R: Neuroendocrine-immune system interactions and autoimmunity. Annu Rev Immunol 13:307, 1995.

142. Moise K: Indomethacin therapy in the treatment of symptomatic polyhydramnios. Clin Obstet Gynecol 34:310, 1991.

143. Nelson J, Hughes K, Smith A, et al: Maternal-fetal disparity in HLA class II alloantigens and the pregnancy-induced amelioration of rheumatoid arthritis. N Engl J Med 329:466, 1993.

144. Brooks P: Clinical management of rheumatoid arthritis. Lancet 341:286, 1993.

145. Kallen B: Drug treatment of rheumatic diseases during pregnancy: The teratogenicity of antirheumatic drugs—what is the evidence? Scand J Rheumatol 27:119, 1998.

146. Crawford P: Best practice guidelines for the management of women with epilepsy. Seizure 8:201, 1999.

147. Delgado-Escueta A, Janz D: Consensus guidelines: Preconceptional counseling, management and care of the pregnant woman with epilepsy. Neurology 42:149, 1992.

148. Hanson J, Smith D: The fetal hydantoin syndrome. J Pediatr 87:285, 1975.

149. Morrell M: The new antiepileptic drugs and women: Efficacy, reproductive health, pregnancy and fetal outcome. Epilepsia 37:34, 1996.

150. Rosa F: Spina bifida in infants of women treated with carbamazepine during pregnancy. N Engl J Med 324:674, 1991.

151. Goldman A, Yaffe S: Fetal trimethadione syndrome. Teratology 17:103, 1978.

152. Holmes L, Harvey E, Coull B, et al: The teratogenicity of anticonvulsant drugs. N Engl J Med 344:1132, 2001.

153. Hansen D, Grafton T, Dial S, et al: Effect of supplemental folic acid on valproic acid-induced embryotoxicity and tissue zinc levels in vivo. Teratology 52:277, 1995.

154. Kaaja E, Kaaja R, Matila R, et al: Enzyme-inducing antiepileptic drugs in pregnancy and the risk of bleeding in the neonate. Neurology 58:549, 2002.

155. Pschirrer E, Monga M: Seizure disorders in pregnancy. Obstet Gynecol Clin 28:601, 2001.

156. Thorp J, Gaston L, Caspers D, et al: Current concepts and controversies in the use of vitamin K. Drugs 49:376, 1995.

157. Zahn C, Morrell M, Collins S, et al: Consensus statements: Medical management of epilepsy. Neurology 51:949, 1998.

158. Kwan P, Brodie M: Effectiveness of first antiepileptic drug. Epilepsia 42:1255, 2001.

159. Fox M, Harms R, Davis D: Selected neurologic complications of pregnancy. Mayo Clin Proc 65:1595, 1990.

160. Jaigobin C, Silver F: Stroke and pregnancy. Stroke 31:2948, 2000.

161. Pettitti D, Sidney S, Quesenberry C, et al: Incidence of stroke and myocardial infarction in women of reproductive age. Stroke 28:280, 1997.

162. Mas J, Lamy C: Stroke in pregnancy and the puerperium. J Neurol 245:305, 1998.

163. Lamy C: Ischemic stroke in young women: Risk of recurrence during subsequent pregnancies. Neurology 55:269, 2000.

164. Ros H, Lichtenstein P, Bellocco R, et al: Pulmonary embolism and stroke in relation to pregnancy: How can high-risk women be identified? Am J Obstet Gynecol 186:198, 2002.

165. Evans R, Lipton R: Topics in migraine management: A survey of headache specialists highlights some controversies. Neurol Clin 19:1, 2001.

166. Silberstein S: Migraine and pregnancy. Neurol Clin 15:209, 1997.

167. Sasa H, Komatsu Y, Kobayashi M: Labor and delivery of patients with spinal cord injury. Int J Gynecol Obstet 63:189, 1998.

168. Wanner M, Rageth C, Zach G: Pregnancy and autonomic hyperreflexia in patients with spinal cord lesions. Paraplegia 25:482, 1987.

169. Baker W: Iron deficiency in pregnancy, obstetrics and gynecology. Hematol Oncol Clin North Am 14:1061, 2000.

170. Cuervo L, Mahomed K: Treatments for iron deficiency anemia in pregnancy. Cochrane Database Syst Rev (2): CD003094, 2001.

171. Beaton G: Iron needs during pregnancy: Do we need to rethink our targets? Am J Clin Nutr 72:265, 2000.

172. Brabin B, Hakimi M, Pelletier D: An analysis of anemia and pregnancy-related maternal mortality. J Nutr 131: 604S, 2001.

173. Haram K, Nilsen S, Ulvik R: Iron supplementation in pregnancy: Evidence and controversies. Acta Obstet Gynecol Scand 80:683, 2001.

174. Progress in chronic disease prevention. Anemia during pregnancy in low-income women—United States, 1987. MMWR Morb Mortal Wkly Rep 39:73, 1990.

175. CDC criteria for anemia in children and childbearing-aged women. MMWR Morb Mortal Wkly Rep 38:400, 1989.

176. Sifakis S, Pharmakides G: Anemia in pregnancy. Ann N Y Acad Sci 900:125, 2000.

177. Bayoumeu F, Subiran-Buisset C, Baka N, et al: Iron therapy in iron deficiency anemia in pregnancy: Intravenous route versus oral route. Am J Obstet Gynecol 186:518, 2002.

178. Frenkel E: Clinical and laboratory features and sequelae of deficiency of folic acid (folate) and vitamin B_{12} (cobalamin) in pregnancy and gynecology. Hematol Oncol Clin North Am 14:1079, 2000.

179. Baill I, Witter F: Sickle cell trait and its association with birthweight and urinary tract infections in pregnancy. Int J Gynaecol Obstet 33:19, 1990.

180. American College of Obstetrics Gynecology: Genetic testing for hemoglobinopathies. ACOG Committee Opinion No. 238. Obstet Gynecol 96:1, 2000.

181. Sun P, Wilburn W, Raynor B, et al: Sickle cell disease in pregnancy: Twenty years of experience in Grady Memorial Hospital. Am J Obstet Gynecol 184:1127, 2001.

182. Koshy M, Burd L, Wallace D, et al: Prophylactic red-cell transfusions in pregnant patients with sickle cell disease. N Engl J Med 319:1447, 1989.

183. Kazazian H, Boehm C: Molecular basis and prenatal diagnosis of beta-thalassemia. Blood 72:1107, 1988.

184. Chern S, Chen C: Molecular prenatal diagnosis of thalassemia in Taiwan. Int J Gynaecol Obstet 69:103, 2000.

185. Cao A, Rosatelli M, Monni G, et al: Screening for thalassemia: A model of success. Obstet Gynecol Clin North Am 29:305, 2002.

186. Samuels P, Bussel J, Braitman L, et al: Estimation of the risk of thrombocytopenia in the offspring of pregnant women with presumed immune thrombocytopenic purpura. N Engl J Med 323:229, 1990.

187. Johnson J, Samuels P: Review of autoimmune thrombocytopenia: Pathogenesis, diagnosis, and management in pregnancy. Clin Obstet Gynecol 42:317, 1999.

188. Lescale K, Edelman K, Cines D, et al: Antiplatelet antibody testing in thrombocytopenic pregnant women. Am J Obstet Gynecol 174:1014, 1996.

189. Nageotte M, Towers C, Asrat T, et al: The value of a negative antepartum test: Contraction stress test and modified biophysical profile. Obstet Gynecol 84:231, 1994.

190. Vintzileos A: Antenatal assessment for the detection of fetal asphyxia. Ann N Y Acad Sci 900:137, 2000.

CHAPTER 20

Diabetes During Pregnancy

David J. Garry

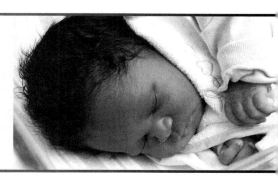

Diabetes mellitus complicates 3% to 10% of pregnancies. During the 20th century, perinatal morbidity and mortality rates declined from 50% to the current rates of 2% to 5%.[1,2] This dramatic improvement resulted from the introduction of insulin, aggressive management practices in diabetic control, and modern surveillance techniques. This chapter reviews diabetes mellitus in pregnancy with a discussion of potential complications and more recent approaches in management.

PATHOPHYSIOLOGY

Pregnancy has been considered to be an "insulinogenic" and a "diabetogenic" state. Hyperplasia of pancreatic β cells, secondary to estrogen and progesterone elevations, results in increased insulin production.[3,4] Human chorionic somatomammotropin, formerly called *human placental lactogen*, is a single-chain polypeptide (191 amino acids) produced by the syncytiotrophoblast of the placenta that acts as an insulin antagonist. Levels of placental steroids and peptides increase as pregnancy progresses. This linear rise in human chorionic somatomammotropin, estrogens, and progesterone with elevated levels of cortisol and prolactin results in increased glucose production, decreased glucose tolerance, and insulin resistance.[5] These adaptive changes act in concert to facilitate placental glucose transport, promoting fetal anabolism, and allow for diversion of glucose from maternal skeletal muscle to adipose tissue for enhancement of maternal anabolism.[6,7]

DIABETES CLASSIFICATION

The American Diabetes Association has classified diabetes mellitus into several categories (Table 20-1).[8] Women with type 1 diabetes are typically diagnosed in childhood and rarely diagnosed during pregnancy. Type 2, or insulin-resistant diabetes, is difficult to diagnose during pregnancy and can be confused with severe gestational diabetes mellitus (GDM). A definitive diagnosis of type 2 diabetes mellitus requires glucose tolerance testing after

the pregnancy. In the 1940s, White[9] proposed an alternative classification system that stratified the disease by onset, duration, and end-organ complications of diabetes. *Class A* refers to GDM; *classes B, C*, and *D* include pregestational diabetes of varying durations; and *classes F, R*, and *H* refer to diabetes with overt end-organ disease.[9] The White classification system fails to differentiate diabetes by pathophysiology, however, and should no longer be used.

GESTATIONAL DIABETES MELLITUS

Screening for GDM is recommended at 24 to 28 weeks of gestation for all pregnant women in a two-step approach. First, a 50-g oral glucose challenge test is administered. Women with a serum value greater than 140 mg/dL (>7.8 mmol/L) after 1 hour must take the second-step, 3-hour, 100-g oral glucose tolerance test (GTT). The diagnosis of GDM is made when two or more GTT values are abnormal: fasting level equal to or greater than 95 mg/dL (≥5.3 mmol/L), 1-hour level equal to or greater than 180 mg/dL (≥10 mmol/L), 2-hour level equal to or greater than 155 mg/dL (≥8.6 mmol/L), or 3-hour level equal to or greater than 140 mg/dL (≥7.8 mmol/L). This two-step approach identifies approximately 80% of women with GDM.[10] Using a glucose challenge test cutoff value of greater than 130 mg/dL (>7.2 mmol/L) increases the sensitivity to 90% but results in more women undergoing a GTT. Alternative diagnostic cutoff values have been proposed. These values affect the sensitivity and specificity of testing, but no data from clinical trials have determined which values are associated with better outcome. Women with a history of GDM (recurrence rate is 35% to 50%), a strong family history of diabetes mellitus, a history of a prior unexplained stillbirth, a prior macrosomic newborn, a history of a major fetal anomaly not associated with a syndrome, or an obese maternal body habitus may benefit from screening in the first or second trimester. Women who screen negative in the first or second trimester should be retested in the third trimester.

Table 20–1. Classification of Diabetes Mellitus

Category	Description
I	Type 1 diabetes mellitus (β-cell destruction/insulin deficiency)
	Immune mediated
	Idiopathic
II	Type 2 diabetes mellitus (insulin resistance/deficiency)
III	Other specific types
	Genetic defect β-cell function
	Genetic defect insulin action
	Diseases of the pancreas
	Endocrinopathies
	Drug/chemical induced
	Infection mediated
	Other immune mediated
	Other genetic syndromes
IV	Gestational diabetes mellitus

Adapted from Expert committee on the diagnosis and classification of diabetes mellitus. Diabetes Care 24:S5, 2001.

When the diagnosis of GDM is established, management includes nutritional therapy, exercise, and insulin if necessary to achieve glucose control. Dietary modifications are the first step, using an approximate 30- to 35-kcal/kg diet based on prepregnancy body weight for nonobese women. Moderate caloric restrictions for obese (body mass index > 30) women may improve pregnancy outcome.[67] Exercise in women diagnosed with GDM reduces the need for insulin and improves pregnancy outcome.[70] Targeted self-monitoring values for optimal control are fasting whole-blood glucose values less than or equal to 95 mg/dL (≤5.3 mmol/L) and 2-hour postprandial whole-blood glucose values less than or equal to 120 mg/dL (≤6.7 mmol/L). For patient convenience, 1-hour postprandial glucose values of less than 140 mg/dL (<7.8 mmol/L) may be used. When target values are repetitively exceeded, insulin therapy is initiated for glycemic control.

Historically, oral agents for management of diabetes have been contraindicated in pregnancy because of concerns of possible teratogenicity and potential fetal hyperinsulinemia. More recently, oral glyburide, a second-generation sulfonylurea, has been shown to have similar effects on glucose control and pregnancy outcome compared with insulin therapy, with no report of adverse fetal outcome.[11] In addition, metformin, an oral antihyperglycemic agent not related to sulfonylureas, has been used in women with polycystic ovarian syndrome and infertility to facilitate ovulation and improved pregnancy rates.[68] Metformin therapy throughout pregnancy in women with polycystic ovarian syndrome has been shown to reduce first-trimester losses without apparent teratogenicity.[69]

The greatest risk associated with GDM is fetal macrosomia and associated complications, including birth trauma, hyperbilirubinemia, polycythemia, hypocalcemia, respiratory distress, and need for cesarean delivery. Another concern is the clear association between development of preeclampsia (sixfold increase) and pregnancy-induced hypertension (fivefold increase) and GDM.[72] The development of these maternal and fetal morbidities is related to the degree of glycemic control obtained during the gestation. The lifetime risk for developing type 2 diabetes mellitus for women diagnosed with GDM varies from 19% to 87%, and current recommendations include postpartum evaluation of glucose impairment with either a fasting plasma glucose or a 2-hour, 75-g oral GTT.[71]

FETAL MALFORMATIONS

The risk of a major birth defect in the general population is 1% to 2%, whereas the risk in a woman with overt diabetes is increased fourfold to eightfold. The most common malformations include neural tube defects, cardiac defects, and renal anomalies.[12] There is no increase in fetal anomalies in children of diabetic fathers or in women with GDM. This suggests that glycemic control, with avoidance of excessive hyperglycemia and hypoglycemia during embryogenesis, is an important factor in the development of these birth defects.[13,14] The frequency of fetal anomalies as related to glycemic control correlates linearly with maternal glycohemoglobin (hemoglobin A_{1c} [HbA_{1c}]). Risks for fetal malformation with HbA_{1c} less than 7% approaches the general population risks of 1% to 2%. When HbA_{1c} values are 7.2% to 9.1%, there is a fetal malformation rate of 14%. An HbA_{1c} of 9.2% to 11.1% denotes a 23% malformation rate, and an HbA_{1c} greater than 11.2% is associated with a malformation rate equal to or greater than 25%.[15,16]

Optimizing glycemic control before conception has the potential for improving the outcome for the pregnancy. In addition, hypervitamin therapy has shown a potential for decreasing the malformation rate. Folate supplementation has reduced neural tube defects and cardiac defect risks.[17,18] Counseling should incorporate vitamin usage into nutritional therapy.

FETAL GROWTH

Acceleration of fetal growth secondary to excessive glucose load has resulted in a 20% to 33% incidence of macrosomia in diabetic patients. **Macrosomia** is defined as birth weight greater than 90% for gestational age or greater than 4000 g.[44] The fetus of a diabetic gestation deposits weight primarily in the trunk and abdominal areas with normal growth of the head and extremities.[19,20] This central deposition of fat, differing from the nondiabetic fetus, may result in increased morbidity during vaginal delivery. Delivery of the fetal head followed by entrapment of the larger trunk can result in shoulder dystocia. The general incidence of shoulder dystocia has been reported to be 3% or less in infants weighing more than 4000 g; however, the incidence of shoulder dystocia in the diabetic population approaches 31%.[21] Other neonatal morbidities in these macrosomic diabetic newborns include severe hypoglycemia, neonatal jaundice, hyperbilirubinemia, polycythemia, hypocalcemia, neonatal acidosis, and brachial plexus injury.[22-24]

Severe type 1 or 2 diabetes mellitus with associated significant vasculopathy commonly results in severely decreased uteroplacental perfusion and intrauterine growth restriction of the fetus. The cause of intrauterine growth restriction also can originate from fetal structural anomalies and other maternal disorders. Serial clinical and sonographic evaluation of fetal growth has become a mainstay in management.

PREMATURITY

Iatrogenic and idiopathic preterm deliveries are a problem for diabetic pregnancies.[25] Iatrogenic preterm delivery often is related to preeclampsia and hypertensive disorders, which complicate 10% of GDM pregnancies and 8% to 16% of types 1 and 2 diabetic gestations.[26] Historically, overt diabetic gestations were delivered early for prevention of intrauterine fetal death, but this practice resulted in other newborn complications associated with prematurity, including neonatal death. The timing of the delivery is a controversial point in management of the diabetic pregnancy. Glycemic control, fetal status, and other maternal complications necessitate individualization in the decision-making process.

Spontaneous preterm delivery rates for pregestational diabetic pregnancies range from 12% to 17% and are considerably greater than control populations (7% to 10%).[73-75] Management of premature labor with β-adrenergic tocolytic agents and glucocorticoid administration for enhancement of fetal lung maturity has been associated with worsening of maternal glucose control. The incidence of GDM is increased in women with premature labor when β-adrenergic agents and corticosteroids are used for treatment.[27] β-Adrenergic agents affect maternal glucose metabolism through decreased peripheral insulin sensitivity and increased endogenous glucose production.[28] β-Adrenergics such as ritodrine and terbutaline are often avoided in diabetic patients; magnesium sulfate and nifedipine are better options for tocolysis. After steroid administration, glycemic control may require temporary insulin therapy for women with GDM and adjusted dosing for types 1 and 2 pregnant diabetics.

STILLBIRTH

Unexplained stillbirths have declined from 30% to 2% to 4% over the past 50 years.[47] The incidence of intrauterine fetal demise in types 1 and 2 diabetic gestations still remains higher, however, than in the general population. The precise mechanism of intrauterine fetal death in pregnancies of diabetic women is unknown. When adequate maternal glycemic control is maintained, stillbirth is rare. Several factors may relate to the increased risk of sudden fetal death. Uteroplacental blood flow in diabetic gestations is diminished compared with that of a normal gestation. This impairment in blood flow correlates with the degree of glycemic control.[48] In sheep, sustained hyperglycemia with hyperinsulinemia resulted in decreased fetal oxygenation, hypoxemia, and fetal death.[49] Extramedullary hematopoiesis, which has been recognized in stillborn fetuses of diabetic women, suggests chronic intrauterine hypoxia as a cause of these losses. Polycythemia, which occurs more frequently in newborns

of diabetic women, is also related to chronic intrauterine hypoxemia secondary to abnormalities in maternal glycemic control.[50,51] Elevated erythropoietin levels have been obtained in umbilical cord blood of diabetic infants.[52] Fetal oxygenation worsens with poor glycemic control, shifting the maternal oxyhemoglobin dissociation curve to the left and resulting in increasing hemoglobin affinity with reduced red blood cell oxygen delivery at the tissue level.[53]

MATERNAL MANAGEMENT

The management of glycemic control revolves around nutritional modification, exercise, and insulin therapy. Care should begin before conception with optimization of glycemic control, updated vaccinations, vitamin therapy, and well-designed support systems. Most diabetic women do not present until after conception has occurred. Nutritional approaches vary, and a single uniform diet for all patients is unrealistic. A general approach is a 30- to 35-kcal/kg diet based on ideal body weight with distribution of caloric content as follows: 10% to 20% protein, less than 10% saturated fats, and 60% to 70% from monounsaturated fats and carbohydrates.[38] An association between lowered IQ and altered behavioral and intellectual development in offspring with maternal ketonemia has led to efforts to avoid accelerated starvation secondary to severe caloric restriction.[45] First-trimester dietary modifications often are required due to persistent nausea and vomiting. Finally, the addition of fiber supplementation has been shown to improve glucose control during pregnancy.[39]

Women with diabetes who lead an active life should be encouraged to continue a reduced program of exercise during pregnancy.[40] Women who do not routinely exercise can initiate limited programs, such as walking, to improve glycemic control and overall outcome of the gestation. Decreased placental blood flow, lasting 30 minutes after cessation of exercise in diabetic pregnant women, suggests caution or avoidance of exercise routines in the third trimester.[54] Other obstetric complications also may necessitate restrictions on or elimination of exercise.

Insulin is the mainstay in the management of types 1 and 2 diabetes mellitus. The goal of insulin therapy is glycemic control with maintenance of fasting finger-stick glucose values less than 95 mg/dL (<5.3 mmol/L) and a 2-hour postprandial value less than 120 mg/dL (<6.7 mmol/L). Finger-stick glucose values should be monitored several times daily (fasting and postprandial), and insulin dosages should be adjusted periodically. Episodes of hyperglycemia and hypoglycemia should be avoided, and a glucagon kit should be prescribed for emergency self-treatment of hypoglycemia.[41] Most women can be maintained on a combination of intermediate-acting and short-acting insulins. During an uncomplicated pregnancy, there is a normal increase in insulin level secondary to the relative insulin resistance that occurs from elevated human chorionic somatomammotropin and other pregnancy-related hormonal responses. The insulin requirement for type 1 diabetics decreases minimally in the first trimester and subsequently increases, whereas type 2 diabetics show a sharp initial increase in requirement and a continued demand for the remainder of the gestation.[55] A reasonable initial insulin dose is 0.7 U/kg of ideal body weight in the first trimester, 0.8 U/kg in the second trimester, and 1 U/kg in the third trimester. For multiple-dose therapy, two thirds of the total calculated dose is administered in the morning (before breakfast), and one third is administered in the evening. The morning dose is divided into intermediate-acting insulin (two thirds of the total) and short-acting insulin (one third of the total) 15 to 30 minutes before breakfast. The evening dose is divided into short-acting insulin (half of the total) given 15 to 30 minutes before dinner and intermediate-acting insulin (half of the total) at bedtime. Several alternative insulin protocols are available with the goal of glycemic control.

Other considerations in glycemic control include the dawn phenomenon and Somogyi phenomenon. The dawn phenomenon, secondary to nocturnal growth hormone secretion, involves an initial decrease in insulin requirements followed by early morning (5:00 to 8:00 AM) increases in plasma glucose and insulin requirements.[56] The Somogyi phenomenon or effect is a paradoxic situation of insulin-induced posthypoglycemic hyperglycemia.[57]

Subcutaneous insulin pump therapy has shown some advantages, with improvement in managing nausea and vomiting of pregnancy, reductions in hyperglycemic and hypoglycemic events, and improved management in the postpartum period when insulin requirements fluctuate.[42] Insulin pump therapy during pregnancy, whether initiated or continued, is associated with similar glycemic control, perinatal outcome, and cost factors when compared with a multiple-dose insulin protocol.[58] The type of insulin used in the continuous subcutaneous insulin infusion device has been regular (short-acting) insulin or insulin lispro (ultra-short-acting). The object of pump therapy is to mimic the action of normal pancreatic β cells. The pump delivers a basal rate and bolus doses. Insulin doses are based on blood glucose test results. Continuous subcutaneous insulin infusion use requires an optimal patient who is comfortable with mechanical devices, self-motivated, lacks skin hypersensitivity to tape, monitors blood glucose regularly, and understands her disease process.[76]

The occurrence of diabetic ketoacidosis (DKA) in pregnancy ranges from 1% to 3% with rare maternal mortality (<1%).[59,60] The most common causes of DKA are infectious (30%), noncompliance (20%), new-onset disease (25%), and idiopathic (25%).[61] There is no consensus regarding the precise definition of DKA. Lack of effective insulin, hyperglycemia, and ketonemia all are components of DKA. The fetus is in significant jeopardy in the setting of DKA, reflected in a fetal loss rate of 9%.[62] The mainstay of treatment in DKA is fluid and electrolyte replacement with insulin therapy (Table 20-2).

Vascular complications, including nephropathy, retinopathy, neuropathy, and coronary artery disease, should be considered when drafting a management plan. A baseline 24-hour urine specimen, frequent urinalysis with culture, ophthalmologic evaluation, and electrocardiogram provide evidence of end-organ status during the gestation. The effect of pregnancy on the diabetic kidney is related to the degree of compromise before the gestation. If the prepregnancy creatine clearance is less than 80 mL/min or proteinuria is greater than 2 g/24 hours, there is an average 50% postpregnancy loss in renal function and an overall increased perinatal loss rate.[63] Proliferative diabetic retinopathy, a serious cause of maternal blindness, is exacerbated by the pregnant state. In women with minimal or no retinopathy, there is a 10% risk of progression of eye disease and a 30% risk of progression for women having mild to severe preexisting retinal disease.[64] Ophthalmologic evaluation and laser photocoagulation therapy are safe to perform during pregnancy.[43]

FETAL SURVEILLANCE

Because of the increased risk of perinatal mortality and morbidity in the fetus and newborn of diabetic women, the role of fetal surveillance encompasses (1) identification of congenital malformations, (2) evaluation of the fetal size, and (3) reassurance of fetal well-being. Biochemical and sonographic modalities are employed in the first and second trimesters to identify fetuses with congenital malformations. Nuchal translucency at 11 to 14 weeks, coupled with free human chorionic gonadotropin-β and pregnancy-associated plasma protein A, allows early identification of potential aneuploidy, congenital cardiac defects, and other genetic syndromes.[30,31] Traditional biochemical screening at 15 to 20 weeks with maternal serum α-fetoprotein, human chorionic gonadotropin, and estriol allows for detection of 90% of neural tube defects and identifies 60% of fetal aneuploidy. Most importantly, a second-trimester detailed sonographic evaluation of fetal anatomy can detect many of the fetal malformations associated with diabetes. With baseline congenital cardiac disease occurring in 2% to 4% of types 1 and 2 diabetics, fetal echocardiography has become a major component of fetal evaluation at 20 to 22 weeks of gestation.

The association of diabetes and fetal growth abnormalities has led to the incorporation of serial sonography into the management plans. The identification of intrauterine growth restriction associated with diabetes strengthens the need for fetal testing of well-being. Conversely the sonographic diagnosis of a macrosomic infant, with an estimated fetal weight greater than 90% for gestational age, also may alter management. An abdominal circumference greater than 75% for gestational age when measured at 29 to 33 weeks allows identification of women with GDM who might benefit from insulin therapy.[32] In addition, the sonographic diagnosis of an estimated fetal weight equal to or greater than 4250 to 4500 g at term can alter delivery mode. Women with macrosomic fetuses should be offered elective cesarean section to decrease the incidence of birth trauma.[33,34,83]

Fetal surveillance for well-being is recommended in diabetic pregnancies. There is a lack of a general consensus, however, on exact gestational age for the start of testing, frequency of testing, or which antepartum test should be performed. In well-controlled GDM gestations, antepartum fetal testing is initiated at 40 weeks.[35,65] For type 1 diabetes, type 2 diabetes, and uncontrolled GDM, assessment of fetal well-being usually is initiated at 32 to 34 weeks

Table 20-2. Management of Diabetic Ketoacidosis

Initial management	Identify underlying/precipitating cause
	If infectious, begin antimicrobial therapy
	Measure blood glucose, electrolytes, and serum ketones
	Assess magnitude of dehydration, hyperosmolarity, and acidosis
Fluid management	Calculate degree of dehydration
	Deficit = (serum sodium/140)(ideal body weight in kg)(0.6)
	Correct for glucose [true serum sodium = (glucose/3)/18]
	Replace fluid deficit
	Restore circulatory function with normal saline solution and maintain
	at 500-1000 mL/hr for the first hr; 250-500 mL/hr for the second through eighth hr;
	adjust rate for next 12-24 hr
Insulin management	Continuous IV insulin infusion of 5-10 U/hr
	Follow glucose hourly, and adjust insulin to decrease glucose 60-90 mg/dL/hr
	Continue IV insulin until ketoacidosis has cleared, then switch to subcutaneous insulin
Electrolyte management	Initiate potassium supplementation at 10-30 mmol/hr in IV fluids (if serum potassium
	< 5 mmol/L with good renal output)
	Follow electrolytes hourly, and maintain potassium with additions to IV fluids
Other issues	Low-dose heparin for prevention of thromboembolic disease
	Phosphate replacement
	Bicarbonate for impending cardiovascular collapse
	Follow neurologic symptoms
	Treatment of cerebral edema is IV mannitol, 1 g/kg body weight

of gestation. Concomitant maternal or fetal conditions affecting these gestations dictate the appropriate gestational age for initiation of antepartum testing.[35-37] The nonstress test, biophysical profile, umbilical artery Doppler, and contraction stress test constitute the current armamentarium of antepartum tests for fetal well-being. Most protocols for type 1 diabetes, type 2 diabetes, and uncontrolled GDM use twice-weekly fetal testing. The intervention for abnormal antepartum testing approximates 5% of pregnancies complicated by diabetes, and the frequency of intrauterine death with testing is 3 per 1000 pregnancies.[35]

DELIVERY

The delivery of the newborn in diabetic gestations consists of two main considerations: timing and mode. Improvements in management and surveillance have diminished the necessity for early delivery. Several factors influence the timing and mode of delivery, including glycemic control, prior obstetric history, concomitant maternal disease, presence of a fetal anomaly, fetal size, fetal well-being, and status of the maternal cervix.

In the United States, elective delivery occurs in approximately 10% to 20% of diabetic gestations.[66] In insulin-dependent diabetics, induction of labor may be planned at 38 weeks or later. If the cervix is unfavorable and glucose is well controlled with no evidence of fetal macrosomia, however, expectant management until 40 weeks with fetal surveillance is practical.[77] Delivery without documented fetal lung maturity is recommended when there is compromise to the life of the mother or significant risk of compromise of the fetus. These scenarios are related primarily to coexisting maternal hypertensive diseases, preeclampsia, or eclampsia. Delivery is recommended when fetal lung maturity is documented

and there is poor glycemic control, a stable intrauterine growth-restricted fetus, equivocal antepartum testing, suspected fetal macrosomia, or worsening chronic hypertension. Poor glycemic control has been related to delayed fetal lung maturation and subsequent neonatal respiratory distress syndrome.[78] A lecithin-to-sphingomyelin ratio greater than 2 in conjunction with the presence of phosphatidylglycerol equal to or greater than 2% to 5% phospholipids are the traditional amniotic fluid markers of fetal lung maturation. The TDx-FLM (Abbott Diagnostics, Abbott Park, IL), a rapid test of fetal lung maturity, can be considered mature at 55 mg/g for nondiabetic gestations and mature at 70 mg/g for diabetic gestations.[79] Each institution needs to review the neonatal outcomes of diabetic gestations (type 1 diabetes, type 2 diabetes, and GDM) as related to the amniotic fluid fetal lung maturity marker or combination of markers.

A common neonatal morbidity with diabetic gestations is neonatal hypoglycemia secondary to fetal hyperinsulinemia. Use of glucose-containing intravenous solutions during labor, subsequent maternal hyperglycemia, and fetal hyperinsulinemia have been described in normal and diabetic gestations.[80,81] Precise maternal glycemic control during labor is needed. On the morning of labor induction or cesarean section, breakfast and normal insulin dosage should be withheld, and a 5% dextrose in saline solution intravenous infusion should be started. Maternal glucose values are monitored every 1 to 2 hours and maintained between 70 and 120 mg/dL. If glucose values exceed 120 mg/dL, insulin is added for continuous infusion. A pediatrician or clinician skilled in newborn resuscitation should be present for delivery. After delivery, the insulin requirements of type 1, type 2, and uncontrolled GDM diabetics are suppressed, making continued monitoring of glycemic control required. Breast-feeding for diabetic mothers is encouraged, although maintaining good diabetic control requires greater effort and flexibility because of the increased metabolic demands.[82]

There is considerable controversy regarding the mode of delivery in diabetic gestations. Cesarean section should be reserved for situations in which risks of delayed delivery would further compromise mother or fetus, sonographic estimated fetal weight is equal to or greater than 4250 to 4500 g, there is a refusal of trial of labor with a previous cesarean delivery, and other obstetric indications exist that preclude vaginal delivery.

REFERENCES

1. Peel J: A historical review of diabetes and pregnancy. J Obstet Gynaecol Br Commonw 79:385, 1972.
2. Lassman-Vague V, Thiers D: Maternal and fetal prognosis during pregnancy of diabetic women. Diabetes Metab 16:149, 1990.
3. Kalkhoff RK: Metabolic effects of progesterone. Am J Obstet Gynecol 142:735, 1982.
4. Costini NV, Kalhott RK: Relative effects of pregnancy, estradiol and progesterone on the plasma insulin and pancreatic islet insulin secretion. J Clin Invest 50:992, 1971.
5. Hollingsworth DR: Alterations of maternal metabolism in normal and diabetic pregnancies: Differences in insulin dependent, non-insulin dependent and gestational diabetes. Am J Obstet Gynecol 146:417, 1983.
6. Leturque A, Ferre P, Burnol AF, et al: Glucose utilization rates and insulin sensitivity in vivo in tissues of virgin and pregnant rats. Diabetes 135:172, 1986.
7. Freinkel N: The Banting Lecture 1980. Of pregnancy and progeny. Diabetes 29:1023, 1980.
8. Expert committee on the diagnosis and classification of diabetes mellitus. Diabetes Care 24:S5, 2001.
9. White P: Pregnancy complicating diabetes. Am J Med 7:609, 1949.
10. Expert committee on the diagnosis and classification of diabetes mellitus. Diabetes Care 23:S4, 2000.
11. Langer O, Conway DL, Berkus MD, et al: A comparison of glyburide and insulin in women with gestational diabetes mellitus. N Engl J Med 343:1134, 2000.
12. Cousins L: The California Diabetes and Pregnancy Programme: A state-wide collaborative programme for the pre-conception and prenatal care of diabetic women. Ballieres Clin Obstet Gynaecol 5:443, 1991.
13. Sadler TW, Hunter ES 3rd, Wynn RE, et al: Evidence for multifactorial origin of diabetes induced embryopathies. Diabetes 38:70, 1989.
14. Sadler TW, Hunter ES 3rd, Balkan W, et al: Effects of maternal diabetes on embryogenesis. Am J Perinatol 5:319, 1988.
15. Lucus MJ, Leveno KJ, Williams ML, et al: Early pregnancy glycosylated hemoglobin, severity of diabetes, and fetal malformation. Am J Obstet Gynecol 161:426, 1989.
16. Greene MF: Spontaneous abortions and major malformations in women with diabetes mellitus. Semin Reprod Endocrinol 17:127, 1999.
17. Czeizel AE: Prevention of congenital abnormalities by periconceptional multivitamin supplementation. BMJ 306:1645, 1993.
18. Botto LD, Mulinare J, Erickson JD: Occurrence of congenital heart defects in relation to maternal mulitivitamin use. Am J Epidemiol 151:878, 2000.
19. Reece EA, Winn HN, Smikle C, et al: Sonographic assessment of growth of the fetal head in diabetic pregnancies compared with normal gestations. Am J Perinatol 7:18, 1990.
20. Landon MB, Mintz MC, Gabbe SG: Sonographic evaluation of fetal abdominal growth: Predictor of the large-for-gestational-age infant in pregnancies complicated by diabetes mellitus. Am J Obstet Gynecol 160:115, 1989.
21. Acker DB, Sachs BP, Friedman EA: Risk factors for shoulder dystocia. Obstet Gynecol 66:762, 1985.
22. Mimouni F, Miodovnik M, Rosenn B, et al: Birth trauma in insulin-dependent diabetic pregnancies. Am J Perinatol 9:205, 1992.
23. Ballard JL, Rosenn B, Khoury JC, et al: Diabetic fetal macrosomia: Significance of disproportionate growth. J Pediatr 122:115, 1993.
24. Hunter DJ, Burrows RF, Mohide PT, et al: Influence of maternal insulin-dependent diabetes mellitus on neonatal morbidity. Can Med Assoc J 149:47, 1993.
25. Scholl TO, Sowers M, Chen X, et al: Maternal glucose concentration influences fetal growth, gestation, and pregnancy complications. Am J Epidemiol 154:514, 2001.
26. Cousins L: Pregnancy complications among diabetic women: Review 1965-1985. Obstet Gynecol Surv 42:140, 1987.
27. Fisher JE, Smith RS, Lagrandeur R, et al: Gestational diabetes mellitus in women receiving beta-adrenergics and corticosteroids for threatened preterm delivery. Obstet Gynecol 90:880, 1997.
28. Smigaj D, Roman-Drago NM, Amini SB, et al: The effect of oral terbutaline on maternal glucose metabolism and energy expenditure in pregnancy. Am J Obstet Gynecol 178:1041, 1998.
29. Cundy T, Gamble G, Townend K, et al: Perinatal mortality in Type 2 diabetes mellitus. Diabet Med 17:33, 2000.
30. Michailidis GD, Economides DL: Nuchal translucency measurement and pregnancy outcome in karyotypically normal fetuses. Ultrasound Obstet Gynecol 17:102, 2001.
31. Nicolaides KH, Heath V, Liao AW: The 11-14 week scan. Baillieres Best Pract Res Clin Obstet Gynaecol 14:581, 2000.
32. Buchanan TA, Kjos SL, Montoro MN, et al: Use of fetal ultrasound to select metabolic therapy for pregnancies complicated by gestational diabetes. Diabetes Care 17:275, 1994.
33. Rossavik IK, Joslin GL: Macrosomatia and ultrasonography: What is the problem? South Med J 86:1129, 1993.
34. Landon MB, Gabbe SG: Antepartum fetal surveillance in gestational diabetes mellitus. Diabetes 34(Suppl):50, 1985.
35. Landon MB, Gabbe SG: Fetal surveillance and timing of delivery in pregnancy complicated by diabetes mellitus. Obstet Gynecol Clin North Am 23:109, 1996.
36. Lagrew DC, Pircon RA, Towers CV, et al: Antepartum fetal surveillance in patients with diabetes: When to start? Am J Obstet Gynecol 168:1820, 1993.
37. Landon MB, Gabbe SG: Fetal surveillance in the pregnancy complicated by diabetes mellitus. Clin Obstet Gynecol 34:535, 1991.
38. Nutritional recommendations and principles for people with diabetes mellitus. Diabetes Care 24:S45, 2001.
39. Gabbe SG, Cohen AW, Herman GO, et al: Effect of dietary fiber on the oral glucose tolerance test in pregnancy. Am J Obstet Gynecol 143:514, 1982.
40. ACOG Practice Bulletin 30: Gestational Diabetes. Washington, DC, American College of Obstetricians and Gynecologists, September 2001.
41. Rayburn W, Piehl E, Sanfield J, et al: Reversing severe hypoglycemia during pregnancy with glucagon therapy. Am J Perinatol 4:259, 1987.
42. Lenhard MJ, Reeves GD: Continuous subcutaneous insulin infusion: A comprehensive review of insulin pump therapy. Arch Intern Med 161:2293, 2001.

43. Klein BEK, Moss SE, Klein R: Effect of pregnancy on progression of diabetic retinopathy. Diabetes Care 13:34, 1990.

44. ACOG Practice Bulletin 22: Fetal Macrosomia. Washington, DC, American College of Obstetrics and Gynecology, November 2000.

45. Rizzo T, Metzger BE, Burns WJ, et al: Correlations between antepartum maternal metabolism and intelligence of offspring. N Engl J Med 325:911, 1991.

46. Green DW, Khoury J, Mimouni F: Neonatal hematocrit and maternal glycemic control in insulin-dependent diabetes. J Pediatr 120:302, 1992.

47. Essex NL, Pyke DA: Management of maternal diabetes in pregnancy. In Sutherland HW, Stowers JM (eds): Carbohydrate Metabolism in Pregnancy and the Newborn. Berlin, Springer, 1979, pp 357-368.

48. Nylund L, Lunell NO, Lewander R, et al: Uteroplacental blood flow in diabetic pregnancy: Measurements with indium 113m and a computer-linked gamma camera. Am J Obstet Gynecol 144:298, 1982.

49. Phillips AF, Dublin JW, Matty PJ, et al: Arterial hypoxemia and hyperinsulinemia in the chronically hyperglycemic fetal lamb. Pediatr Res 16:653, 1982.

50. Mimouni F, Miodovnik M, Siddiqi TA, et al: Neonatal polycythemia in infants of insulin-dependent diabetic mothers. Obstet Gynecol 68:370, 1986.

51. Green DW, Khoury J, Mimouni F: Neonatal hematocrit and maternal glycemic control in insulin-dependent diabetes. J Pediatr 120:302, 1992.

52. Widness JA, Susa JB, Garcia JF, et al: Increased erythropoietin in infants born to diabetic mothers and in hyperinsulinaemic rhesus fetuses. J Clin Invest 67:637, 1981.

53. Landon MB, Gabbe SG: Fetal surveillance and timing of delivery in pregnancy complicated by diabetes mellitus. Obstet Gynecol Clin North Am 23:109, 1996.

54. Rauramo I, Forss M: Effect of exercise on placental blood flow in pregnancies complicated by hypertension, diabetes or intrahepatic cholestasis. Acta Obstet Gynecol Scand 67:15, 1988.

55. Langer O, Anyaegbunam A, Brustman L, et al: Pregestational diabetes: Insulin requirements throughout pregnancy. Am J Obstet Gynecol 159:616, 1988.

56. Koivisto VA, Yki-Jarvinen H, Helve E, et al: Pathogenesis and prevention of the dawn phenomenon in diabetic patients treated with CSII. Diabetes 35:78, 1986.

57. Campbell IW: The Somogyi phenomenon: A short review. Acta Diabetol Lat 13:68, 1976.

58. Gabbe SG, Holing E, Temple P, et al: Benefits, risks, costs and patient satisfaction associated with insulin pump therapy for pregnancy complicated by type I diabetes mellitus. Am J Obstet Gynecol 182:1283, 2000.

59. Kilvert JA, Nicholson HO, Wright AD: Ketoacidosis in diabetic pregnancy. Diabet Med 10:278, 1993.

60. Ramin KD: Diabetic ketoacidosis in pregnancy. Obstet Gynecol Clin North Am 26:481, 1999.

61. Lebovitz HE: Diabetic ketoacidosis. Lancet 345:767, 1995.

62. Cullen MT, Reece EA, Homko CJ, et al: The changing presentations of diabetic ketoacidosis during pregnancy. Am J Perinatol 13:449, 1996.

63. Biesenbach G, Stoger H, Zazgornik J: Influence of pregnancy on progression of diabetic nephropathy and subsequent requirement of renal replacement therapy in female type I diabetic patients with impaired renal function. Nephrol Dial Transplant 7:105, 1992.

64. Chew EY, Mills JL, Metzger BE, et al: Metabolic control and progression of retinopathy. The Diabetes in Early Pregnancy Study. National Institute of Child Health and Human Development Diabetes in Early Pregnancy Study. Diabetes Care 18:631, 1995.

65. Kjos SL, Leung A, Henry OA, et al: Antepartum surveillance in diabetic pregnancies: Predictors of fetal distress in labor. Am J Obstet Gynecol 173:1532, 1995.

66. Landon MB, Gabbe SG, Sachs L: Management of diabetes mellitus and pregnancy: A survey of obstetricians and maternal-fetal specialists. Obstet Gynecol 75:635, 1990.

67. Dornhorst A, Nicholls JS, Probst F, et al: Calorie restriction for treatment of gestational diabetes. Diabetes 40(Suppl 2): 161, 1991.

68. Batukan C, Baysal B: Metformin improves ovulation and pregnancy rates in patients with polycystic ovary syndrome. Arch Gynecol Obstet 265:124, 2001.

69. Glueck CJ, Phillips H, Cameron D, et al: Continuing metformin throughout pregnancy in women with polycystic ovary syndrome appears to safely reduce first-trimester spontaneous abortion: A pilot study. Fertil Steril 75:46, 2001.

70. Jovanovic-Peterson L, Durak EP, Peterson CM: Randomized trial of diet versus diet plus cardiovascular conditioning on glucose levels in gestational diabetes. Am J Obstet Gynecol 161:415, 1989.

71. O'Sullivan JB: Diabetes mellitus after GDM. Diabetes 29(Suppl 2):131, 1991.

72. Joffe GM, Esterlitz JR, Levine RJ, et al: The relationship between abnormal glucose tolerance and hypertensive disorders of pregnancy in healthy nulliparous women. Calcium for Preeclampsia Prevention (CPEP) Study Group. Am J Obstet Gynecol 179:1032, 1998.

73. Greene MF, Hare JW, Krache M, et al: Prematurity among insulin-requiring diabetic gravid women. Am J Obstet Gynecol 161:106, 1989.

74. Hanson U, Persson B: Outcome of pregnancies complicated by type 1 insulin-dependent diabetes in Sweden: Acute pregnancy complications, neonatal mortality and morbidity. Am J Perinatol 10:330, 1993.

75. Sibai BM, Caritis SN, Hauth JC, et al: Preterm delivery in women with pregestational diabetes mellitus or chronic hypertension relative to women with uncomplicated pregnancies. Am J Obstet Gynecol 183:1520, 2000.

76. Saudek CD: Novel forms of insulin delivery. Endocrinol Metab Clin North Am 26:599, 1997.

77. Kjos SL, Henry OA, Montoro M, et al: Insulin-requiring diabetes in pregnancy: A randomized trial of active induction of labor and expectant management. Am J Obstet Gynecol 169:611, 1993.

78. Piper JM, Xenakis EM, Langer O: Delayed appearance of pulmonary maturation markers is associated with poor glucose control in diabetic pregnancies. J Matern Fetal Med 7:148, 1998.

79. Del Valle GO, Adair CD, Ramos EE, et al: Interpretation of the TDx-FLM fluorescence polarization assay in pregnancies complicated by diabetes mellitus. Am J Perinatol 14:241, 1997.

80. Soler NG, Soler SM, Malins JM: Neonatal morbidity among infants of diabetic mothers. Diabetes Care 1:340, 1978.

81. Grylack LJ, Chu SS, Scanlon JW: Use of intravenous fluids before cesarean section: Effects on perinatal glucose, insulin, and sodium homeostasis. Obstet Gynecol 63:654, 1984.

82. Gagne MP, Leff EW, Jefferis SC: The breast-feeding experience of women with type I diabetes. Health Care Women Int 13:249, 1992.

83. Conway DL, Langer O: Elective delivery of infants with macrosomia in diabetic women: Reduced shoulder dystocia versus increased cesarean deliveries. Am J Obstet Gynecol 178:922, 1998.

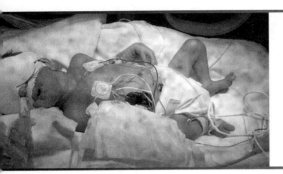

Hypertensive Disorders in Pregnancy

Michael D. Hnat and Baha M. Sibai

Hypertensive disorders are the most common medical complications of pregnancy, with a reported incidence ranging between 5% and 10%,[1] and they account for a major cause of maternal and perinatal mortality and morbidity worldwide.[2] The three most common forms of hypertension in pregnancy are chronic essential hypertension, acute gestational hypertension, and preeclampsia. Chronic hypertension constitutes 30% of the cases, and the other types are responsible for the remaining 70%.[3]

CLASSIFICATIONS AND DEFINITIONS

According to the Working Group Report on Hypertension in Pregnancy, hypertension can be classified into four categories: (1) chronic hypertension, (2) preeclampsia-eclampsia, (3) preeclampsia superimposed upon chronic hypertension, and (4) gestational hypertension.[4]

The diagnosis of chronic hypertension in pregnancy is usually based on the presence of one or more of the following: (1) a history of hypertension before pregnancy, (2) persistent elevations of the blood pressure above 140/90 mm Hg before week 20 of gestation, or (3) hypertension that persists beyond day 42 after delivery.[4] Preeclampsia is a form of hypertension that is unique to human pregnancy and usually occurs after 20 weeks of pregnancy, except in pregnancies involving hydatidiform moles or hydrops. The hallmark of preeclampsia is hypertension with proteinuria (0.3 g or more in a 24-hour specimen). The disease is further subdivided into mild or severe according to the severity of the hypertension or end-organ involvement. Eclampsia is the occurrence of seizures not attributable to other causes. The diagnosis of superimposed preeclampsia is generally based on the exacerbation of hypertension with the development of new-onset proteinuria. In pregnancies complicated by chronic hypertension, with the appearance of new-onset proteinuria, the development of symptoms is more important for confirming the diagnosis than is the level of blood pressure. As a result, Sibai recommended that the diagnosis of superimposed preeclampsia be made on the basis of exacerbated hypertension plus the development of substantial proteinuria (at least 0.5 g/24 hours) or symptoms during the second half of the pregnancy. In women receiving antihypertensive drugs, this diagnosis should be made solely on the basis of new-onset proteinuria, clinical symptoms, or thrombocytopenia.[5] On occasion, it is difficult to make the diagnosis because of the physiologic drop in blood pressure (sometimes to normotensive levels) during the midtrimester in patients with chronic hypertension.[3,6] This decrease is particularly important in patients who first receive prenatal care in the second or third trimester. Of importance is that in some women, the elevation of blood pressure at less than 20 weeks of pregnancy may be caused by preeclampsia.[7]

Chronic Hypertension

The reported incidence of chronic hypertension in pregnancy ranges from 1% to 3%. Ninety percent of the patients suffer from essential hypertension, whereas 10% have secondary hypertension.[7] Hypertension in pregnancy can be classified into mild to moderate (between 140 to 159 mm Hg systolic pressure and/or between 90 to 109 mm Hg diastolic pressure) and severe (>160 mm Hg systolic pressure and/or >110 mm Hg diastolic pressure). Alternatively, chronic hypertensive patients can be divided into low-risk and high-risk groups (Box 21-1).[7]

Pregnancies complicated by chronic hypertension are reportedly associated with an increased incidence of perinatal and maternal complications such as superimposed preeclampsia, abruptio placentae, fetal growth restriction, preterm birth, and perinatal mortality. The reported incidence of superimposed preeclampsia has ranged from 4.7% to 52%, depending on the population studied, the severity of hypertension at the onset of pregnancy, and the diagnostic criteria used. The incidence of superimposed preeclampsia is high among patients in the high-risk group (25% to 52%).[5] The reported incidence of abruptio placentae has ranged from 0.45% to 10%; the incidence is lowest among women with mild uncomplicated

<table>
<tr><td>**Box 21–1**</td><td>**High-Risk Characteristics**</td></tr>
</table>

Maternal age older than 40 years
Duration of hypertension more than 15 years
Blood pressure ≥ 160/100 mm Hg early in pregnancy
Diabetes (classes B to F)
Renal disease (all causes)
Cardiomyopathy
Connective tissue disease
Coarctation of the aorta
Presence of lupus anticoagulant
Previous pregnancy with perinatal loss
Previous abruptio placentae
Previous stroke

hypertension and highest in pregnancies complicated by severe superimposed preeclampsia.[5,8,9] Superimposed preeclampsia and abruptio placentae are responsible for most cases of intrauterine growth restriction (IUGR), preterm delivery, and perinatal deaths. In general, perinatal morbidity and mortality are not increased in uncomplicated mild chronic hypertension, although they are markedly increased in patients with severe disease, in those with renal disease, and in cases complicated by superimposed preeclampsia.[3,9-11]

Mild Chronic Hypertension

Mild chronic hypertension represents 95% of cases of chronic hypertension in pregnancy. One of the earliest and largest studies dealing with hypertension in pregnancy was by Dunlop, who described pregnancy outcome in 1226 women with mild to moderate essential hypertension who were treated and delivered during the decade from 1955 to 1964. The use of antihypertensive drugs was not mentioned in this report. His findings revealed that patients with mild chronic hypertension had a pregnancy outcome that was superior to that of the general obstetric population. The worst perinatal outcome occurred in the group that developed superimposed preeclampsia.[8]

Chesley reported a perinatal mortality of 3.2% in 593 pregnancies with uncomplicated chronic hypertension managed between 1972 and 1974. During the same

period, the perinatal loss in the general obstetric population was 4.2%. Antihypertensive drugs were not used unless the diastolic pressure was 110 mm Hg or more. The diagnosis of superimposed preeclampsia was made in 5.7% of the patients, and the perinatal mortality rate among these patients was 21.4%. Pregnancies with uncomplicated mild chronic hypertension had a perinatal outcome similar to that of normal pregnancies, whereas the development of superimposed preeclampsia was associated with poor perinatal outcome.[6]

Sibai and colleagues studied pregnancy outcome in 211 women with mild chronic hypertension. All hypertensive medications were discontinued at the time of the first prenatal visit and restarted only if blood pressure exceeded 160/110 mm Hg. Ten percent developed superimposed preeclampsia, 1.4% developed abruptio placentae, and 12% delivered at less than 37 weeks of pregnancy. The perinatal mortality rate was 28.1 per 1000, and 7.9% of the babies had IUGR. Overall, most of the poor perinatal outcomes occurred in patients with superimposed preeclampsia. For patients without this complication, the perinatal outcome was superior to that of the general obstetric patients (Table 21-1).[3] Mabie and associates studied 169 pregnancies in 156 women with chronic hypertension. Antihypertensive medications were given if the diastolic blood pressure exceeded 90 mm Hg. Overall, the perinatal mortality rate was 28.4 per 1000. Superimposed preeclampsia developed in 34.3% of the patients, 1.8% had abruptio placentae, and 14.8% had IUGR.[12]

There are numerous clinical reports (retrospective and prospective) describing pregnancy outcome in treated women with chronic hypertension. The findings of these studies have been conflicting because of the difference in the definition, management, and populations studied. Five prospective controlled trials compared methyldopa with either a placebo regimen or no treatment (Table 21-2).[7] In two independently controlled trials, antihypertensive medications were associated with an improved perinatal outcome. In both these studies, the incidence of superimposed preeclampsia was unaffected by the use of the drugs.[13-15] On the other hand, Arias and Zamora were unable to demonstrate any clear fetal benefit from antihypertensive therapy in pregnant patients with mild chronic hypertension. It is interesting that, in

Table 21–1. Pregnancy Outcome in 211 Women with Mild Chronic Hypertension

	With Preeclampsia (N = 21)	Without Preeclampsia (N = 190)
Mean gestational age (wk)	35.8	39.3
<37 weeks	15 (71.4%)	11 (5.8%)
Mean birth weight (g)	2345	3210
SGA	7 (33.3%)	10 (5.3%)
Perinatal deaths	5 (23.8%)	1 (0.5%)
Abruptio placentae	2 (9.5%)	1 (0.5%)

SGA, small for gestational age.

Adapted from Sibai BM, Abdella TN, Anderson GD: Pregnancy outcome in 211 patients with mild chronic hypertension. Obstet Gynecol 61:571, 1983.

Table 21–2. Pregnancy Outcome in Randomized Controlled Trials of Chronic Hypertension

Author(s)	Gestation at Entry (wk)*	Gestation at Delivery (wk)*	Birth Weight (g)	IUGR (%)	Preeclampsia (%)
Leather et al.[13]					
Control (N = 24)	<28	36.5	2520		?
Treated (N + 23)		38.0	2840	NA	?
Redman et al.[14,15]					
Control (N = 107)	20.6 ± 0.5	38.1 ± 0.2	3130 ± 49		4.7
Treated (N = 101)	21.9 ± 0.5	38.1 ± 0.2	3090 ± 60	NA	6.7
Arias and Zamora[16]					
Control (N = 29)	16.4 ± 1.1	38.3 ± 0.4	3011 ± 103	14.2	10.3
Treated (N = 29)	14.7 ± 1.0	38.1 ± 0.5	2926 ± 131	14.2	3.4
Weitz et al.					
Placebo (N = 12)	<34	37.6 ± 0.5	2820	25	33.3
Treated (N = 13)		39.0 ± 0.4	3140	0	38.4
Sibai et al.[10]					
Control (N = 90)	11.3 ± 0.2	39.0 ± 0.2	3123 ± 69	8.9	15.6
Treated (N = 173)	11.2 ± 0.2	38.7± 0.2	3060 ± 72	7.5	17.3

*Data expressed as mean ± standard error of the mean (SEM) when SEM is available.

IUGR, intrauterine growth retardation; Preeclampsia, increased blood pressure plus proteinuria; NA, not available.

spite of the lack of improvement in perinatal outcome, the incidence of pregnancy-aggravated hypertension was significantly reduced in their treated group.[16]

Sibai and colleagues conducted a randomized clinical trial in which they compared the use of no therapy with the use of either methyldopa or labetalol in the management of 263 women with mild chronic hypertension in pregnancy. In the untreated group, antihypertensives were used only if systolic blood pressure exceeded 160 mm Hg or if diastolic blood pressure exceeded 110 mm Hg. There was no difference regarding the incidence of superimposed preeclampsia, abruptio placentae, cesarean delivery, or neonatal outcome (Table 21-3).[10]

Blake and MacDonald treated hypertensive patients with atenolol, methyldopa, and bendrofluazide. Their intention was to reduce the blood pressure as closely as possible to the average normal level for the particular stage of pregnancy. The control patients were given only methyldopa or no treatment. Blake and MacDonald found that intensive treatment of hypertension in pregnancy might prevent the maternal manifestations of preeclampsia, specifically proteinuria. However, such treatment was found to decrease the mean birth weight and to increase the numbers of infants with low birth weight. These adverse effects were of such concern that the ethical committee recommended that the study be concluded early.[17]

Three prospective controlled trials compared methyldopa with a β-blocker for mild hypertension in pregnancy. Gallery and associates found greater plasma volume expansion, larger neonatal birth weights, and no perinatal deaths among oxprenolol-treated patients.[18] In contrast, Fidler and coworkers found no difference in pregnancy outcome and neonatal birth weight. They also found that the oxprenolol-treated group had a higher incidence of abnormal fetal heart rate tracings during labor.[19] Plouin and colleagues found no difference in the neonatal heart

Table 21–3. Pregnancy Outcome in 26 Women with Mild Hypertension According to Treatment

	No Treatment (N = 90 [%])	Treatment (N = 173 [%])
Superimposed preeclampsia	14 (15.6)	30 (17.3)
Abruptio placentae	2 (2.2)	3 (1.7)
Perinatal deaths	1 (1.1)	2 (1.1)
Preterm (<37 weeks)	9 (10)	21 (12.1)
Small for gestational age	8 (8.9)	13 (7.5)

Adapted from Sibai BM, Mabie WC, Shamsa F, et al: A comparison of no medications versus methyldopa or labetalol in chronic hypertension during pregnancy. Am J Obstet Gynecol 162:960, 1990.

rate, blood pressure, or respiratory rate between the methyldopa-treated and the labetalol-treated groups. They concluded that labetalol is as safe as methyldopa for the fetus and newborn.[20]

Severe Chronic Hypertension

There are few reports describing pregnancy outcome in women with severe hypertension. Most of these studies were conducted before 1950 and did not mention the use of antihypertensive drugs. As a result, the reported maternal and perinatal outcomes were invariably poor. Increase in perinatal morbidity was related mainly to the increased incidence of superimposed preeclampsia (25% to 30%) or abruptio placentae (5% to 10%).[21,22]

In 1966, Kincaid-Smith and associates reported a perinatal loss of 9.3% among 32 severely hypertensive women treated with methyldopa. The findings of their study suggested a potential improvement in perinatal outcome. The incidence of superimposed preeclampsia, however, remained high (38%).[23]

Sibai and Anderson reported pregnancy outcome in 44 women with severe hypertension who started prenatal care in the first trimester. Hypertension was first treated with intravenous hydralazine, and all patients subsequently received oral methyldopa and hydralazine. Fifty-two percent developed superimposed preeclampsia, and 2.3% had abruptio placentae. The perinatal mortality rate was 25%. All perinatal deaths and most of the poor outcomes were related to delivery of a premature neonate and to superimposed preeclampsia.[9] It is important to note that good perinatal outcome in such pregnancies is possible in the absence of superimposed preeclampsia, although it is not possible to predict who will develop superimposed preeclampsia.[7]

Effects of Antihypertensive Medications on the Fetus and Neonate

β-blockers are thought to increase uterine muscle tone; cause IUGR; block the tachycardic response to hypoxia; and result in neonatal respiratory depression, bradycardia, and hypoglycemia.[24] In experimental animal studies, acute administration of β blockers reduced uteroplacental circulation in rats[25] and caused reduction in fetal tolerance to hypoxia when given to acutely hypoxic sheep.[26,27] In humans, several studies have addressed this issue: Plouin and colleagues reported that pindolol does not compromise the uteroplacental blood flow and does not affect fetal heart rate.[28] Moreover, pindolol had no significant metabolic effect on the mother and fetus[29] and has been used in pregnancy without teratogenic or other side effects.[19,30,31] Bott-Kanner and associates studied the effects of early antihypertensive treatment with pindolol. Although they found no adverse effects on either mother or fetus, no beneficial effects were demonstrated.[32] Pickles and colleagues showed no adverse effects on fetal growth with labetalol treatment.[33] Fabrigues and associates studied the neonatal outcome of patients treated with atenolol and showed no significant adverse effects on the fetus.[34]

Chronic use of atenolol during pregnancy has been consistently associated with reduced fetal weights as well as placental function.[8,35-37] Montan and coworkers performed Doppler flow ultrasonographic studies on 14 women with pregnancy-associated hypertension before and during the first and third days of treatment with atenolol. They found that the baseline blood flow characteristics were normal in the fetus and in the maternal arcuate artery, in comparison with fetuses in uncomplicated pregnancies of corresponding gestational ages. Volumetric blood flow remained unchanged in the fetal descending aorta and in the umbilical vein during atenolol treatment, whereas pulsatility index increased in the fetal descending aorta and in the arcuate artery. These findings suggested that the peripheral vascular resistance, in both the maternal and fetal sides of the placenta, increased during short-term antihypertensive treatment with atenolol.[38] Montan and coworkers later compared atenolol with pindolol and found significant effects on uteroplacental and fetal hemodynamics—although in the normal range—with the use of atenolol but not with pindolol. This study raised concerns about further deterioration in hemodynamics in a compromised fetus. They also found significantly lower placental weights in the atenolol-treated group.[37] In 1990, Butters and colleagues compared atenolol with placebo. The infants of the two groups had similar gestational age at delivery, but those whose mothers were treated with atenolol had significantly lower birth weights and lower placental weights than did those whose mothers took the placebo.[35] Thus, the use of atenolol for treatment of chronic hypertension in pregnant women should be avoided.

Another drug commonly used in pregnancy is methyldopa, and its long-term safety for the mother and the fetus has been adequately assessed. Methyldopa was thought to decrease the head circumference if used between 16 to 20 weeks of pregnancy. The reduction in head circumference was not related to either the amount of methyldopa used or to the duration of its use.[39] Leather and associates[13] and Redman and colleagues[15] reported no increase in perinatal deaths among patients treated with methyldopa. Redman and colleagues also found that methyldopa had no significant effect on fetal weight, placental weight, or maturity of the newborn.[15] Furthermore, long-term follow-up until the children were 7 years of age revealed no residual neurologic deficits.[40]

The use of calcium channel blockers in the pregnant animal model was reportedly associated with a decrease in placental blood flow and development of fetal hypoxemia and acidosis.[41-44] Parisi and coworkers studied the effects of maternal nicardipine therapy on fetal placental blood flow and cardiorespiratory status in the hypertensive pregnant ewe. After maternal infusion of angiotensin II, nicardipine was infused, and fetal and maternal blood flow were measured. Nicardipine reversed maternal hypertension; however, it decreased placental blood flow and increased vascular resistance. Parisi and coworkers noted the deaths of 5 of 15 fetuses 65 minutes after nicardipine infusion.[42,43] Ducsay and colleagues administered nicardipine to rhesus monkeys having spontaneous contractions and noted the development of fetal acidosis and hypoxemia.[41] Ahokas and associates used a different calcium channel blocker, nifedipine, and found that blood flow was not significantly altered in the spontaneously hypertensive rat.[45] Cameron and coworkers studied the effects of nicardipine when used for the acute reduction of blood pressure in patients with preeclampsia. There was no significant difference in either the pulsatility index or resistance index of the uteroplacental or umbilical vessels within 60 minutes of a single oral dose of nicardipine.[46] Lindow and associates, using the radioisotope method, determined an index of uteroplacental blood flow. There was no significant change in the blood flow index after a single sublingual dose of nifedipine, despite a significant fall in blood pressure.[47] Hanretty and colleagues were unable to demonstrate a change in Doppler waveforms within 8 hours of a single 20-mg oral dose of nifedipine in nine pregnant women with proteinuria and hypertension.[48] Mari and coworkers performed Doppler studies of the uteroplacental and fetal circulations in patients with preterm labor who were treated with nifedipine for tocolysis. No significant difference was found in flow velocity waveforms 5 hours after the initial dose.[49] Moretti and associates examined the effects of long-term oral nifedipine therapy in patients with preeclampsia well before delivery. Baseline Doppler studies were performed immediately before treatment, repeated after steady state was reached (48 hours), and then performed at 3-day intervals until delivery. Long-term use of nifedipine was associated with significant decrease in maternal blood pressure but had no significant effect on the resistance indices in any of the vessels studied or on cord blood gases.[50]

The use of diuretics in mild, long-term hypertension is highly controversial. Sibai and colleagues reported that patients with long-term hypertension who were treated with diuretics had a marked reduction in plasma volume in comparison with a well-matched group of patients not treated with similar medications. Such patients demonstrated a rebound expansion in plasma volume when diuretics were discontinued.[51] In another study, Sibai and colleagues showed that diuretics prevent normal plasma volume expansion in hypertensive pregnancies without influencing perinatal outcome.[52]

Angiotensin-converting enzyme (ACE) inhibitors, such as captopril, enalapril, and lisinopril, are becoming widely used as first-line therapy for chronic hypertension in the nonpregnant state. In the experimental animal mode, captopril causes abortion and fetal death, apparently by reducing the uteroplacental perfusion. In human pregnancy, ACE inhibitors have been associated with several fetal and neonatal complications, which include neonatal hypotension, fetal growth restriction, oligohydramnios, neonatal anuria, renal failure, and neonatal death.[53-56] Thus, the use of ACE inhibitors should be avoided in pregnancy, along with the use of angiotensin receptor blockers.

From the preceding discussion, it can be concluded that antihypertensive medications are not without side effects and should not be used unless benefits from such treatment are well documented.

Recommended Management of Patients with Chronic Hypertension

Management of the patient with chronic hypertension should begin before pregnancy. The patient is encouraged to have her blood pressure checked several times before pregnancy and to establish the cause of the hypertension and the severity of her hypertension in the nonpregnant state. The patient is then advised to seek prenatal care once pregnancy is confirmed. Early prenatal care ensures accurate determination of gestational age and the severity of the woman's hypertension in the first trimester. For patients in whom hypertension is seen for the first time during pregnancy, the first step in management should include evaluation of the hypertension. Attention should be paid to the following: the duration of hypertension; use of antihypertensive medications; history of cardiac or renal disease, diabetes, or thyroid disease; and the outcome of previous pregnancies (superimposed preeclampsia, abruptio placentae, perinatal outcome, congestive heart failure).

On the basis of the initial assessment findings, the patient is classified as having low-risk or high-risk chronic hypertension. In pregnancies in patients considered to be at high risk, maternal and perinatal complications are increased.[9,25,57-61] As a result, these patients should be managed in consultation with a maternal-fetal specialist. In addition, patients with chronic renal disease—particularly those with primary glomerular diseases and significant renal function impairment (serum creatinine level > 2.5 mg/dL)—should be managed in consultation with a nephrologist.

Antihypertensive medications must be used in all women with severe hypertension. In addition, there are short-term maternal benefits with treatment of mild hypertension and target organ damage, such as diabetes mellitus, renal disease, and cardiac dysfunction.[26,62] Antihypertensive drugs such as atenolol and ACE inhibitors should be discontinued if possible in patients because of the potential adverse maternal and fetal side effects[52,56,63] and should be replaced with nifedipine, labetalol, or methyldopa as needed. If maternal blood pressure is not well controlled with maximum doses of methyldopa (4 g/day), then a second drug such as labetalol or nifedipine may be added.[21,64] In some of these patients, blood pressure may be difficult to manage, which mandates the use of multiple oral drugs, as well as intravenous therapy.[9]

During the course of pregnancy, the patient is to be observed carefully for the development of superimposed preeclampsia. The timing of prenatal visits is then adjusted on the basis of maternal and fetal conditions. Fetal evaluation includes serial ultrasonography for fetal growth, antepartum fetal testing with the use of the nonstress test, and/or the biophysical profile. In women with high-risk chronic hypertension, fetal testing may need to be started at 28 weeks and then repeated weekly or more often, depending on fetal condition (superimposed preeclampsia, suspected fetal growth restriction). The biophysical profile needs to be determined only when the nonstress test result is nonreactive.

The pregnancy may then be continued to term or until onset of superimposed preeclampsia or development of fetal growth restriction or fetal distress. The development of superimposed preeclampsia is an indication for hospitalization. Subsequent management depends on the severity of the preeclampsia and fetal gestational age. The development of superimposed preeclampsia is an indication for delivery in all patients in whom the fetus's gestational age is beyond 34 weeks. If superimposed preeclampsia develops before this time, the pregnancy may be monitored expectantly with close evaluation of maternal and fetal well-being.[65]

In general, most patients with mild chronic hypertension (low-risk group) have pregnancy outcomes similar to those of the general obstetric population. These patients have a good perinatal outcome regardless of whether they use antihypertensive medication.[3,66] Thus, all antihypertensive medications may be discontinued in patients receiving such therapy at the time of first prenatal visits. Prior observations have revealed that approximately 50% of pregnant patients with mild chronic hypertension demonstrate a significant reduction in their blood pressure to normotensive levels during the second trimester; only 4% of those patients subsequently require antihypertensive therapy for exacerbation of hypertension to severe levels. An additional third of the patients have no change in blood pressure in the second trimester; 16% of those patients subsequently require antihypertensive therapy. The remaining 17% demonstrate an increase in blood pressure during the second trimester, and 32% of those patients subsequently develop severe hypertension in the third trimester.[1] Thus, the blood pressure change in the second trimester may be used as a prognostic indicator for the future development of exacerbation in hypertension. In addition, Chesley and Annitto showed that women with chronic hypertension had greater decreases in their blood pressure during pregnancy than do normotensive patients.[21] The development of exacerbated hypertension alone is not an indication for delivery. These patients may be safely treated with methyldopa as needed. Subsequent management is then similar to that in the high-risk group.

If the patient is well motivated, she can be instructed in self-determination of blood pressure, as recommended by Zuspan and Rayburn.[67] This approach avoids the phenomenon of "white coat hypertension" that is associated with a visit to a physician's office and thus precludes the unnecessary initiation or increase in the dosage of antihypertensive drugs. At present, it is recommended that patient-recorded measurements of blood pressure be used to supplement those recorded in the doctor's office.[67]

Early onset of prenatal care and close antepartum and intrapartum assessments of fetal well-being are responsible for the improved perinatal outcome in pregnancies complicated by mild chronic hypertension.[3,10] Fetal evaluation includes serial ultrasonography for fetal growth and antepartum fetal testing, as described previously. The nonstress test is usually started at 34 weeks and repeated weekly. These pregnancies should be continued until onset of labor or term. The development of superimposed preeclampsia or severe IUGR is an indication for hospitalization and for close evaluation of maternal and fetal well-being. Subsequent management depends on fetal gestational age and results of antepartum fetal testing.

Preeclampsia

Preeclampsia occurs in 2% to 6% of pregnancies, according to the diagnostic criteria used and the population studied. It is principally a disease of nulliparous women, with an incidence ranging from 3% to 7% of nulliparous women,[66,68-70] in comparison with 0.8% to 5% of multiparous women.[71,72] In addition, preeclampsia is significantly increased in multifetal pregnancies, in women with previous preeclampsia, and in patients with certain medical disorders (Box 21-2). The cause of preeclampsia is unknown. Some of the theories that are associated with its origin include vascular endothelial damage, abnormal trophoblast invasion, coagulation abnormalities, immunologic events, genetic predisposition, and dietary deficiencies or excesses. Over the years, more than 100 clinical, biophysical, and biochemical tests have been recommended to identify patients at risk for preeclampsia. However, none of these has proved to be a sufficient or reliable screening test for preeclampsia.[73-75] The same remains true for the prevention of preeclampsia. Various methods for preventing or reducing the incidence of preeclampsia have been reported in the literature (Box 21-3). Again, these methods have not been shown to reduce the rate of preeclampsia, except possibly vitamins C and E.

Preeclampsia is a clinical syndrome that embraces a wide spectrum of signs and symptoms. Although hypertension is the traditional hallmark of the disease, preeclampsia can manifest in the form of either a capillary leak (edema, proteinuria) or a spectrum of abnormal hemostasis with multiple organ dysfunction, which results in clinical manifestations without the presence of hypertension. The diagnosis of preeclampsia is based on blood pressure criteria, as well as proteinuria, and is defined primarily as gestational hypertension plus proteinuria. Edema is no longer considered part of the diagnosis of preeclampsia,[76-78] because it is a common finding in normal pregnancy and because approximately one third of preeclamptic women never demonstrate the presence of edema.[79]

Box 21–2	**Risk Factors for Preeclampsia**

Nulliparity
Family history of preeclampsia
Obesity
Multifetal gestation
Preeclampsia in previous pregnancy
Poor outcome in previous pregnancy
   Intrauterine growth restriction
   Abruptio placentae
   Fetal death
Preexisting medical conditions
   Chronic hypertension
   Renal disease
   Diabetes mellitus
Thrombophilias
   Antiphospholipid antibody syndrome
   Protein C, protein S, or antithrombin deficiency
   Factor V Leiden

Box 21-3   Prior Methods Used to Prevent Preeclampsia

Antihypertensive drugs
Antithrombotic agents
Calcium
Dipyridamole
Fish oil and evening primrose oil
Heparin
High-protein and low-salt diet
Low-dose aspirin
Magnesium
Nutritional supplementation (protein)
Vitamins C and E
Zinc

The diagnosis of preeclampsia requires the presence of hypertension with proteinuria. Proteinuria is defined as a concentration of 0.1 g or more of protein per liter of urine in at least two random urine specimens collected 4 hours or more apart or 0.3 g or more in a 24-hour collection. The definitive test for the diagnosis of proteinuria should be quantitative measurement of total protein excretion over a 24-hour period. The concentration of urinary protein is highly variable and is influenced by several factors.[80,81] Studies have demonstrated the poor correlation of proteinuria found on urinary dipstick tests with the total concentration in 24 hours.[39,82-84] Preeclampsia should be considered in the absence of proteinuria when gestational hypertension is present with association of signs or symptoms suggestive of significant end-organ involvement (cerebral symptoms, epigastric or right upper quadrant pain plus nausea or vomiting, fetal growth restriction, or abnormal laboratory test results such as thrombocytopenia and abnormal liver enzyme levels).[69,85]

The diagnosis of preeclampsia and the severity of the disease process are generally based on maternal blood pressure measurements. In mild preeclampsia, the diastolic blood pressure should range from 90 to less than 110 mm Hg, and the systolic pressure, from 140 to less than 160 mm Hg, on two occasions at least 4 to 6 hours apart. Criteria for severe preeclampsia are listed in Box 21-4. In addition, eclampsia is the occurrence of seizures not attributable to other causes.

Box 21-4   Criteria for Diagnosing Severe Preeclampsia

Blood pressure ≥ 160 mm Hg or diastolic
   pressure ≥ 110 mm Hg, recorded on at least two
   occasions, 6 hours apart with patient on bed rest
Proteinuria (≥5 g in 24 hours)
Oliguria (≤400 mL in 24 hours)
Abnormal liver function
Persistent cerebral or visual disturbances
Persistent epigastric pain
Pulmonary edema or cyanosis
Persistent thrombocytopenia
Evidence of HELLP (hemolysis, elevated liver enzymes,
   low platelets) syndrome

A rise in blood pressure (by 30 mm Hg systolic and 15 mm Hg diastolic) has been used in the past as a criterion for the diagnosis of preeclampsia. Because a gradual increase in blood pressure from second to third trimester is seen in most normotensive pregnancies, this definition is usually unreliable. When using this particular definition, Villar and Sibai showed a low sensitivity and positive predictive value in 700 primigravidae for the prediction of preeclampsia.[86] Two other studies reported similar pregnancy outcomes among women who remained normotensive and those who demonstrated a 15-mm Hg rise in diastolic blood pressure.[13,87,88] It must be emphasized that the presence of symptoms suggesting end-organ involvement is more important than the absolute blood pressure reading in establishing the diagnosis of preeclampsia. After all, there is more to preeclampsia than the presence of hypertension.[89]

Laboratory abnormalities are nonspecific in preeclampsia; however, they reflect the derangements of the multiple organ system involved. The most common hematologic abnormality in women with preeclampsia is thrombocytopenia. The serum uric acid is frequently elevated (>6 mg/dL). The serum creatinine level is rarely elevated if the diagnosis is made early in the course of the disease. Thrombocytopenia can be part of the syndrome of hemolysis, elevated liver enzymes, and low platelets (HELLP syndrome). Liver dysfunction in the absence of the HELLP syndrome results in mild elevation of serum transaminase levels and possibly an increase in indirect bilirubin level. Routine evaluation of other coagulation factors is recommended only when the platelet counts are less than $100,000/mm^3$ or when abruptio placentae is suspected.

Mild Preeclampsia

Patients with mild preeclampsia should be evaluated at the time of diagnosis for maternal and fetal conditions. Patients with mild preeclampsia are at slightly increased risk for development of abruptio placentae and convulsions, particularly in cases occurring long before term.[73,90] Therefore, women with mild disease who have favorable cervical conditions at or near term should undergo induction of labor.

When mild preeclampsia is diagnosed before the 37th week of pregnancy, the optimal management is controversial. There are considerable differences in opinion regarding the need for hospitalization, recommended maternal activity and diet, and the use of antihypertensive drugs, sedatives, and anticonvulsant prophylaxis.[5,91,92]

Traditionally, management of patients with mild preeclampsia consisted of bed rest in the hospital for the duration of the pregnancy. This approach was thought to enhance fetal survival and diminish the frequency of progression to severe disease.[70,93] Several studies have challenged the benefits of prolonged antepartum hospitalization.[31,44,94,95] Two studies of outcome in women with mild hypertension at less than 37 weeks of pregnancy without proteinuria, who were randomly prescribed either rest in the hospital or normal activity at home, concluded that management at home was safe and cost effective.[94,95] Two other studies reported that management could be done safely and efficiently in day care units, in comparison with the hospital.[31,44]

Gilstrap and colleagues studied 545 women with mild preeclampsia at 25 to 38 weeks of pregnancy who remained in the hospital until delivery. During hospitalization, the patients were given a regular diet, with no limits on activity. Salt restriction and antihypertensive drugs were not used. The duration of pregnancy prolongation was 2 to 120 days (average, 24 days). Eighty-one percent of the patients became normotensive within 5 days, 13% continued to have intermittent hypertension, and 6% had a poor response.[90]

Sibai reported on 186 women with mild preeclampsia hospitalized at 26 to 35 weeks. They were given a regular diet, no salt restriction, and no limit on activity. As part of a randomized clinical trial, 100 patients received labetalol. The duration of pregnancy prolongation was 4 to 80 days (average, 21 days).[1] Similarly, Mathews studied pregnancy outcome in 135 women with mild preeclampsia long before term who were randomly prescribed either bed rest in the hospital or normal activity at home. There was no difference in maternal or perinatal outcome between these two groups.[95]

Feeney conducted a prospective study that included 465 women. These patients were managed at home and were visited by midwives two to three times per week for measurement of abdominal size, blood pressure, and urine protein, and evaluation of fetal movement charts. The outcome was compared with that of 438 patients managed in the traditional way. Feeney concluded that home management was safe and cost effective.[96] From these studies, it appears that early and prolonged hospitalization for these patients enhances fetal survival and diminishes the frequency of progression to severe diseases. In many such instances, this treatment arrests the clinical course of the disease or improves it long enough to enable the fetus to achieve maturity without jeopardizing maternal safety. This treatment is also cost effective, in view of the cost of prolonged intensive care required by a premature infant.

Several clinical reports (controlled and uncontrolled) have described the use of various antihypertensive drugs to prolong gestation and improve perinatal outcome in women with mild preeclampsia long before term. Most studies compared β-blocker treatment with placebo and had controversial results with regard to neonatal morbidity.[24,28,97,98] Furthermore, the sample size was not adequate in any of these studies for evaluating perinatal mortality. None of these studies showed a better perinatal outcome in comparison with studies that included hospitalization only for management of mild preeclampsia.[5] The only possible benefit of such treatment is the lower incidence of progression to severe hypertension.

In a prospective, randomized trial comparing no pharmacologic treatment with nifedipine therapy in the management of mild preeclampsia long before term, Sibai and colleagues found that nifedipine was effective in reducing maternal blood pressure, both systolic and diastolic. However, this reduction in blood pressure was not associated with a reduction in antepartum hospital days in the nifedipine recipients. Of more importance, there was no difference in gestational age at delivery between the groups.[99]

Management. Our management plan for patients with mild preeclampsia is summarized in Figure 21-1. Patients with mild preeclampsia require maternal and fetal evaluation at the time of diagnosis. Diuretics and antihypertensive drugs are not prescribed, and sedatives are not used. Initially, fetal evaluation should include serial ultrasonography for evaluation of fetal growth and antenatal testing.

Maternal evaluation includes daily maternal weighing and frequent blood pressure monitoring while the patient is awake. All patients should be educated about reporting symptoms of impending eclampsia (headache, visual disturbances, or epigastric pain). Laboratory evaluation should include measurement of urine protein, hematocrit, and platelet count, and liver function tests every 3 to 4 days. This evaluation is extremely important, because patients may develop thrombocytopenia and elevations in liver enzyme levels with minimal blood pressure elevations.

If the patient's blood pressure improves or remains stable in the absence of either significant proteinuria (<1000 mg/24 hours) or maternal symptoms (headache, visual disturbances, or epigastric pain), outpatient observation may be considered on a selective basis. This form of management is appropriate in reliable patients during the early stages of the disease, when there is no evidence of fetal jeopardy (i.e., abnormal testing or abnormal fetal growth).[100] A typical regimen for such patients consists of modified rest at home, home blood pressure monitoring as needed, and daily urine protein dipstick testing. The patient should also be instructed to count fetal movements and should be warned about symptoms of impending eclampsia. Hospitalization is indicated when maternal condition worsens (i.e., acute hypertension or substantial proteinuria develops) for prompt evaluation of maternal and fetal status. Delivery is indicated after 37 weeks of gestation as soon as the cervix is in a favorable condition or at 40 completed weeks.[5]

Severe Preeclampsia

Pregnancies complicated by severe preeclampsia are associated with increased rates of maternal and perinatal morbidity and mortality. The perinatal survival rate is poor if the disease develops before 23 weeks; however, it improves when the disease occurs at or after 25 weeks.[101] Severe preeclampsia was once thought to have beneficial effects on the preterm fetus as a result of intrauterine stress that accelerated neonatal lung maturity and neurologic development. However, Schiff and colleagues reported no significant difference in the incidence of immature lung maturity tests between women with preeclampsia and matched controls.[102] Surprisingly, the rate of respiratory distress syndrome was greater among the women with preeclampsia than among the controls, but the difference was not significant. In addition, fetal neurologic and physical development, as defined by the Ballard score, were not found to be accelerated at the time of delivery in infants born to women with preeclampsia.[103]

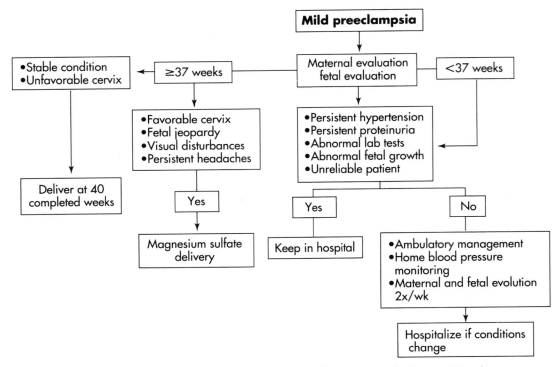

Figure 21–1. Recommended management of mild preeclampsia at the University of Tennessee Medical Center, Memphis.

Other studies have indicated that neonatal complications in preterm infants of preeclamptic mothers are related to prematurity rather than preeclampsia. Benedetti and colleagues reported that the rate of neonatal survival among infants of severe preeclamptic gestations with birth weights between 600 and 1400 g was no different than the rate for infants of nonpreeclamptic gestations with similar birth weights.[104] Friedman and coworkers showed in a matched cohort study that there were no significant differences between premature neonates born to women with preeclampsia at 24 to 35 weeks and those born to normotensive women with preterm labor with regard to neonatal death, respiratory distress syndrome, severe intraventricular hemorrhage, necrotizing enterocolitis, and sepsis.[105]

A few reports have discussed laboratory abnormalities in neonates of severe preeclamptic patients. Monroe and associates in 1979 reported that 57% of neutrophil counts of infants born to hypertensive women fell below the normal reference range.[106] Brazy and coworkers in 1982 reported that thrombocytopenia occurred in 47% of infants born to preeclamptic mothers, but only a small number of these infants develop overt hemolysis. Those authors suggested that a statistical correlation between maternal platelet count and disseminated intravascular coagulation occurred in infants of mothers who had a platelet count below 50,000/mm³. Those authors also found significantly higher incidences of growth restriction, microcephaly, thrombocytopenia, leukopenia, neutropenia, low Apgar scores, patent ductus arteriosus, hypotonia, gastrointestinal hypomotility, and delayed adaptation in premature infants born to severely preeclamptic mothers.[83]

Koenig and Christensen in 1989 reported that 49% of newborns of hypertensive mothers have neutropenia, which is transient (1 to 60 hours) in 83% of those infants and prolonged (3 to 30 days) in 17%. This disorder was more prevalent among preterm and growth-restricted newborns and among newborns whose mothers had severe hypertension or hypertension and HELLP syndrome. Nosocomial infections occurred during the first 2½ weeks of life in 23% of the newborns with neutropenia but in only 3% of those without this disorder. Koenig and Christensen suggested that neutropenia was the result of diminished neutrophil production.[107]

Sibai and colleagues reported on 303 pregnancies complicated by severe preeclampsia. There were 28 stillbirths and 15 neonatal deaths; thus, the corrected perinatal mortality rate was 135 per 1000. The rate of perinatal survival was zero when preeclampsia developed before 28 weeks but rose to 100% when disease developed after 36 weeks of gestation. The rate of perinatal mortality among the infants of the women with chronic hypertension was 32%, as opposed to 7.7% among those of the women without chronic hypertension. Thirty-six percent of the stillbirths were associated with abruptio placentae. There was a 20% incidence of IUGR; the incidence of growth restriction was higher in the group with chronic hypertension, especially if the preeclampsia developed before 28 weeks. The severity and incidence of neonatal complications were also closely linked to gestational age at delivery.[108] Szymonowicz and Yu compared the immediate neonatal and long-term performance of 35 very low birth weight (VLBW) infants born to mothers with severe preeclampsia to 35 infants born to normotensive mothers and matched for gestation, sex, and survival. All the VLBW survivors had a clinical, neurologic, and psychologic assessment at 2 years of age. The infants of preeclamptic mothers had a higher incidence of hematologic abnormalities in the neonatal period. The systolic blood pressure on admission was lower in the babies of the preeclamptic group, who also required a higher volume of blood or colloid in the first 24 hours after birth to maintain normal blood pressure. There were no significant differences between the two groups in other neonatal complications. There was no significant difference in height and head circumference at the 2-year assessment; however, weight remained significantly lower in the preeclampsia group. The mean psychomotor development index on the Bayley Scales of Infant Development was similar in the two groups. Survivors in the preeclamptic group, however, had a significantly lower mean developmental index.[109]

Ounsted and coworkers collected data on growth and development at the age of 7.5 years for 56 children whose mothers had had hypertension with superimposed preeclampsia. They compared these data with the results from 76 children whose mothers had had only hypertension. No difference was found between the two groups in weight and head circumference (all the mean values were above the median for age). The frequencies of impairment of sight, hearing, or other handicaps did not differ in the two groups. The two groups had similar scores for different intellectual abilities. For perceptual matching, children who had been small for gestational age at birth had lower scores than the others.[91] Zeben-van der Aa and associates studied the long-term outcome at 2 years of age of 300 living infants born at less than 32 weeks of gestation to mothers with hypertensive disorders of pregnancy and compared it to that of infants born to normotensive women of a similar gestational age. They concluded that such infants born alive have better survival chances without an increase in handicap risk, irrespective of their intrauterine growth.[110]

Management. There is universal agreement that all severely preeclamptic patients should be delivered if the disease develops after 34 weeks or if there is evidence of the following before 35 weeks: rupture of membranes, severe growth restriction, or maternal or fetal distress. Appropriate management consists of parenteral magnesium sulfate ($MgSO_4$) to prevent convulsions and control of maternal blood pressure within a safe range, followed by induction of labor to achieve delivery. If delivery of a preterm infant is anticipated at a level I or level II hospital, the mother should be transferred to a tertiary care center with adequate neonatal intensive care facilities.[5]

There has been disagreement concerning the management of patients at or before 34 weeks. Some institutions consider delivery as the definitive therapy for all cases, regardless of gestational age; others recommend prolongation of pregnancy in all severely preeclamptic gestations until the development of fetal lung maturity, the development of fetal or maternal distress, or achievement of a gestational age of 36 weeks. Some of the measures used in these cases have included one or more of the following: antihypertensive agents, diuretics, sedatives,

chronic parenteral $MgSO_4$, plasma volume expanders, and antithrombotic agents.[5] One of the earliest studies dealing with conservative management was that by Nochimson and Petrie. They delayed delivery of patients with severe hypertension at 27 to 33 weeks for 48 hours to permit steroid acceleration of fetal lung maturity.[111] Rick and colleagues also delayed delivery 48 to 72 hours when the lecithin-to-sphingomyelin ratio revealed immature fetal lungs.[112]

Martin and Tupper described the results of conservative management in 55 women with severe preeclampsia before 36 weeks. The patients were treated with bed rest, oral phenobarbital, diuretics, and antihypertensive agents. Parenteral $MgSO_4$ was used if maternal hyperreflexia was present or if maternal blood pressure exceeded 170/110 mm Hg. Martin and Tupper could prolong these pregnancies for an average of 19.2 days. Such pregnancies resulted in three stillbirths and two neonatal deaths, which represented a perinatal mortality rate of 8.9%. In addition, 56.6% of the neonates were severely growth restricted and 9% were asphyxiated.[113]

Odendaal and coworkers reported on 129 patients with severe preeclampsia before 34 weeks who were treated with bed rest, $MgSO_4$, and various antihypertensive drugs. The pregnancies were prolonged for an average of 11 days with a perinatal mortality rate of 32%. Abruptio placentae was the cause of 36% of intrauterine deaths.[114]

In a prospective randomized study, Odendaal and coworkers described the outcome of 58 women with severe preeclampsia at 28 to 34 weeks. These patients were treated with $MgSO_4$, hydralazine, and corticosteroids for fetal lung maturity. All received intensive maternal and fetal evaluation in a high-risk obstetric ward. Twenty patients were delivered within 48 hours of hospitalization for maternal and/or fetal reasons, and the other 38 were randomly assigned to receive either aggressive or expectant management. Aggressively managed patients were given steroids and delivered within 72 hours. Patients assigned to expectant management were treated with prazosin to maintain blood pressure between 140/90 and 150/100 mm Hg. In addition, they received frequent evaluations of maternal and fetal well-being. These patients were delivered at 34 weeks or earlier in the presence of fetal or maternal distress. The total average days of pregnancy prolongation in the conservatively managed group was 9 days, and the average days of pregnancy prolongation after randomization was 7.1 days (range, 2 to 18). The authors found fewer neonatal complications and a lower number of days spent in the neonatal intensive care unit for the women receiving expectant management.[114]

In another prospective randomized study, expectant management was compared with aggressive treatment of severe preeclampsia at 28 to 32 weeks' gestation and demonstrated a reduction in neonatal complications and neonatal stay in the newborn intensive care unit without a significant increase in maternal morbidity.[115] Patients were carefully selected before random assignment to expectant or aggressive management. Exclusion criteria included maternal medical disease (renal diseases, diabetes, collagen vascular disease), multifetal gestation, bleeding, eclampsia, HELLP syndrome, and severe IUGR.

For the women receiving expectant management, the average pregnancy prolongation was 15.4 ± 6.6 days and was not affected by the amount of proteinuria at randomization. Maternal indications for delivery were thrombocytopenia, uncontrolled severe hypertension, headache or blurred vision, epigastric pain, severe ascites, and maternal demand. Other indications included fetal compromise, achievement of 34 weeks' gestation, preterm labor, or rupture of membranes and vaginal bleeding. There were no cases of fetal or neonatal deaths, eclampsia, pulmonary edema, renal failure, or disseminated coagulopathy in either group.[115]

Fenakel conducted a clinical trial on 51 patients with severe preeclampsia between 26 and 36 weeks. These patients were randomized to either nifedipine or hydralazine. They found better blood pressure control, a lower incidence of fetal distress, and a better perinatal outcome in the group managed by nifedipine.[116]

Severe preeclampsia in the second trimester is an obstetric dilemma. Aggressive management with immediate delivery results in extremely high rates of perinatal morbidity and mortality, but attempts at prolonging pregnancy might result in fetal demise or asphyxia in utero and may expose the mother to severe morbidity and even mortality.[117] Pattinson and associates studied 34 patients with severe preeclampsia before 28 weeks who were managed conservatively with bed rest, antihypertensive drugs, and frequent fetal and maternal evaluation. All 11 pregnancies less than 24 weeks ended with perinatal deaths. The 34 fetuses with a gestational age between 24 and 27 weeks had a 38% survival rate.[118]

Sibai and colleagues studied 109 patients with severe preeclampsia at 19 to 27 weeks. Twenty-five patients diagnosed with preeclampsia were seen at 24 weeks or less, and pregnancy termination was recommended. Ten patients accepted termination, but 15 refused and were managed expectantly for an average of 19.4 days. These 15 pregnancies resulted in 11 fetal deaths and 3 neonatal deaths, an overall perinatal survival of 6.7%. In addition, three had HELLP, two developed abruptio placentae, and one had eclampsia. The authors concluded that expectant management is not justified in women with severe preeclampsia at less than or equal to 24 weeks. Eighty-four patients were between 24 and 27 weeks; 30 patients underwent immediate delivery because of their own or the attending physician's desire, whereas 54 were managed expectantly with antihypertensive medications and daily evaluation of fetal and maternal conditions. For the women receiving expectant management, the rate of perinatal survival was significantly higher and the rates of acute and long-term neonatal morbidity were lower. In addition, maternal complications were infrequent in both groups. Sibai and colleagues concluded that expectant management for women with severe preeclampsia at more than 24 weeks is possible but should be done selectively only in a tertiary care center with adequate intensive care facilities (Table 21-4).[66]

The majority of the studies mentioned have shown only that expectant management is possible and beneficial in a select group of patients with severe preeclampsia; they excluded patients with severe IUGR and HELLP syndrome. The presence of IUGR appears to be detrimental rather than protective for neonatal survival in severe preeclampsia and limits expectant management.[69,119] In a retrospective study, Witlin and others reported that the rate of IUGR increased with an increase in gestational age and latency period during expectant management in a series of 195 neonates born of women with severe preeclampsia.[120] In multivariate analysis ($P = .038$; odds ratio = 13.2; 95% confidence interval = 1.16 to 151.8) and univariate analysis ($P = .001$; odds ratio = 5.88; 95% confidence interval = 1.81 to 192), IUGR decreased survival. Because prolongation of an adverse intrauterine environment may worsen rather than improve fetal outcome, patients with fetuses who have severe IUGR or oligohydramnios and patients with nonreassuring antenatal testing should not receive expectant management.

Chammas and colleagues recommended delivery of a neonate with IUGR 48 hours after the first dose of betamethasone.[69] In this retrospective study, patients with severe preeclampsia at less than 34 weeks were managed expectantly at Chammas and colleagues' institution. On admission, fetal weights estimated by ultrasound in 19% and 11% of the fetuses were below the 5th percentile and between the 5th and 10th percentiles, respectively. The mean gestational age on admission was 31.1 ± 1.9 weeks

Table 21-4. Pregnancy Outcome in Women with Severe Preeclampsia at 25 to 27 Weeks of Pregnancy

	Expectant Management (N = 54)	Aggressive Management (N = 30)	P
Delivery gestational age (wk)	28.0 ± 1.2	26.3 ± 0.8	<0.0001
Birth weight (g)	880 ± 212	709 ± 159	<0.0001
Perinatal death (%)	13 (24)	20 (67)	<0.0005
Days in NICU (mean ± SD)	70 ± 32	115 ± 94	<0.02
Small for gestational age (%)	26 (48)	10 (33)	NS
Intraventricular hemorrhage (%)	22 (41)	22 (71)	<0.007

NICU, neonatal intensive care unit; NS, nonsignificant; SD, standard deviation.

From Sibai BM, Akl S, Fairlie F, Moretti M: A randomized protocol for managing severe preeclampsia in the second trimester. Am J Obstet Gynecol 163:733, 1990.

for women whose fetuses were suspected of having IUGR and 29.3 ± 2.8 weeks (P = .034) for those without IUGR. The mean latency interval was 3.1 ± 2.1 days for neonates with IUGR, which was significantly shorter than the latency for neonates with no IUGR (6.6 ± 6.1 days). The rates for maternal and fetal indications were similar in both groups. There were no differences in Apgar scores, cord pH, and length of stay in the neonatal intensive care unit between the groups. There were two neonatal deaths caused by prematurity, but none occurred in the infants with IUGR. Because the mean latency period for neonates with IUGR was only 3.1 ± 2.1 days, Chammas and colleagues concluded that neonates with IUGR did not benefit from a delay in delivery for 1 to 2 days after steroids took effect.[69]

Our management plan for patients with severe preeclampsia is as follows. Patients with early severe preeclampsia are admitted initially to the labor and delivery area for continuous evaluation of maternal and fetal conditions for at least 24 hours. During observation, they receive a continuous infusion of MgSO$_4$ to prevent convulsions, as well as bolus doses of hydralazine (5 to 10 mg), 10 mg of oral nifedipine, or 20 mg of intravenous labetalol as needed to keep diastolic blood pressure below 110 mm Hg. Maternal evaluation includes continuous monitoring of blood pressure, heart rate, cerebral status, and the presence of epigastric pain. Laboratory evaluation includes but is not limited to a complete blood cell count with platelet counts and renal-hepatic profiles. Fetal evaluation includes a biophysical profile and an ultrasonographic assessment of fetal growth.

For patients developing severe preeclampsia long before term, Figure 21-2 shows the recommended management plan. Patients with persistent severe hypertension (despite the use of antihypertensive medications) or other signs of maternal or fetal deterioration are delivered within 24 hours, regardless of the fetus's gestational age or lung maturity. In addition, fetuses at gestational ages of more than 34 weeks are usually delivered within 24 hours. Fetuses at gestational ages between 32 and 34 weeks are delivered if there is evidence of fetal lung maturity or after steroid administration. Women between 24 and 32 weeks receive individualized management based on their clinical response during the observation period. All these women receive steroids for fetal lung maturity. Some demonstrate marked diuresis and improvement in blood pressure during the observation period. If maternal and fetal evaluations reveal normal findings during the observation period, MgSO$_4$ is discontinued, and the patients are monitored in the high-risk ward. They receive antihypertensive medications to keep the diastolic blood pressure between 90 to 100 mm Hg with daily evaluation of maternal and fetal well-being. Nifedipine, 10 mg, may be administered every 6 hours and increased to every 4 hours for a maximum of 20 mg every 4 hours. If this dosage is not adequate, oral labetalol, 200 mg, can be given every 8 hours and increased to a maximum of 600 mg every 6 hours. In general, most of these patients will require delivery within 2 weeks. However, some patients might continue the pregnancy for several weeks. The course of pregnancy in such patients is unpredictable; therefore, management should be performed only in a tertiary care center.[5,117]

A trial of labor should be attempted, and a cesarean section is reserved for the usual obstetric indications. Severe preeclampsia is not an indication for cesarean sections. In patients with unfavorable cervical conditions and whose fetuses have a gestational age of less than 30 weeks, it is appropriate to consider an elective cesarean section. Epidural anesthesia is the anesthetic of choice in women with preeclampsia. Conduction anesthesia is contraindicated for reasons such as an infection at the puncture site or a coagulopathy.

HELLP Syndrome

In 1989, Weinstein coined the expression "HELLP syndrome" for a unique variant of preeclampsia.[121] Hemolysis, defined as the presence of microangiopathic hemolytic anemia, is the hallmark of the HELLP syndrome. The reported incidence of this syndrome in preeclampsia has ranged from 2% to 12%.[122] The HELLP syndrome may develop before or after delivery. In the postpartum period, the time of onset of the manifestations may range from a few hours to 7 days; the majority of cases develop within 48 hours after delivery.

Various criteria are used to diagnose HELLP syndrome. A platelet count of less than 100,000/mm^3 has been the most consistent finding among various criteria to diagnose HELLP syndrome. Martin and associates devised the following classification based on platelet count nadir. Class 1 HELLP syndrome was defined as a platelet nadir below 50,000/mm^3, class 2 as a platelet nadir between 50,000 and 100,000/mm^3, and class 3 as a platelet nadir between 100,000 and 150,000/mm^3.[123] Sibai recommended uniform and standardized laboratory values be used to diagnose this syndrome (Box 21-5).[122]

Patients with HEELP syndrome may have a variety of unusual signs and symptoms. A majority of the patients present long before term, complaining of epigastric or right upper quadrant pain (65%); some have nausea or vomiting (50%); and others have nonspecific viral syndrome–like symptoms. Ninety percent of patients give a history of malaise for the previous few days. Hypertension and proteinuria may be absent or slight. Severe hypertension is not a constant or even a frequent finding in HELLP syndrome. Various medical and surgical disorders may be confused with HELLP syndrome. Appendicitis, gallbladder disease, gastroenteritis, hyperemesis gravidarum, peptic ulcer, and viral hepatitis are some examples.

Management of preeclamptic patients presenting with the HELLP syndrome is controversial.[121] Several therapeutic modalities are described in the literature and are similar to those used in the management of severe preeclampsia long before term (see Fig. 21-2). Investigators from the Netherlands reported that expectant management is possible in women with HELLP syndrome before 34 weeks.[124,125] Using plasma volume expansion, Visser and Wallenburg were able to prolong pregnancy a median of 10 days (range, 0 to 62). Overall, the rate of perinatal mortality was 14.1%, and no maternal complications occurred.[124]

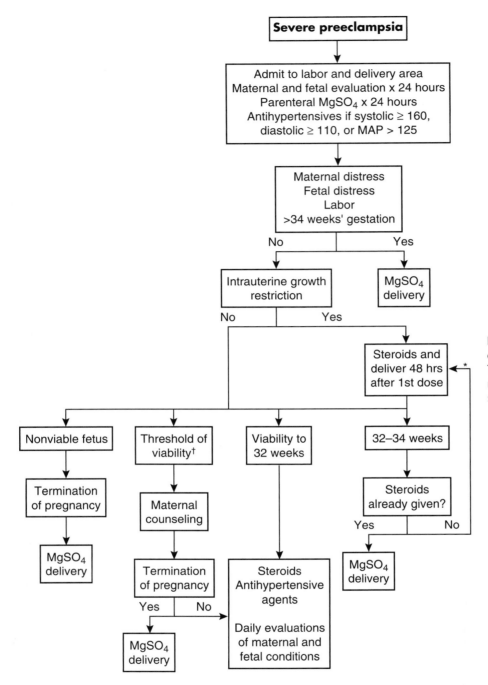

Figure 21–2. Recommended management of severe preeclampsia at the University of Tennessee Medical Center, Memphis. MAP, mean arterial pressure; MgSO₄, magnesium sulfate.

†Threshold of viability is dependent upon tertiary care center, and is usually around 23–24 weeks' gestation.
*Alternate treatment may include amniocentesis for fetal lung maternity.

Poor maternal and perinatal outcomes have been associated with pregnancies complicated by preeclampsia and the HELLP syndrome. The reported rate of perinatal mortality has ranged from 7.7% to 60%, and the rate of maternal mortality from 0% to 24%. Most of these patients require transfusions of blood and blood products and are at increased risk for the development of acute renal failure, pulmonary edema, ascites, pleural effusions, abruptio placentae, and hepatic rupture.[126-130] Abramovici and colleagues showed neonatal morbidity and mortality were related to gestational age rather than to the presence or absence of the HELLP syndrome in severe preeclampsia.[131]

Eclampsia

Eclampsia is defined as the occurrence of convulsions or coma unrelated to other cerebral conditions with signs

Box 21–5	Criteria for the Diagnosis of HELLP Syndrome

Hemolysis

Abnormal peripheral blood smear
Increased bilirubin level (>1.2 mg/dL)
Increased lactic dehydrogenase level (>600 IU/L)

Elevated Liver Enzymes

Increased aspartate aminotransaminase level (≥72 IU/L)
Increased lactic dehydrogenase level (>600 IU/L)

Thrombocytopenia

Platelet count < 100,00/mm³

and symptoms of preeclampsia. Convulsions may occur before, during, or after delivery. Half of all cases of eclampsia usually occur before the onset of labor; the other 50% are equally divided between the intrapartum and postpartum periods. Eclampsia that occurs before the 20th week or more than 48 hours after delivery is rare and has been termed **atypical eclampsia**. The pathophysiologic events leading to convulsions remain unknown. The incidence of eclampsia ranges from 1 per 147 to 1 per 3448 pregnancies[131,132] and is as high as 3.6% in twin pregnancies. The rate of maternal mortality is reported to vary between 0% and 13%, and that of perinatal mortality, between 10% and 28%. Abruptio placentae, IUGR, prematurity, and hypoxic episodes during the convulsions are frequently implicated as the causes of perinatal mortality.[20,80,120,134-136] Infants with low birth weight (premature and/or IUGR) and those with whom abruptio placentae occurred are also highly susceptible to intrapartum hypoxia and trauma and present numerous neonatal problems. Moreover, these infants are at increased risk for delayed physical growth and neurologic development.[86,137]

Sibai and colleagues reported the immediate outcomes and long-term follow-up outcomes of the surviving infants of 109 eclamptic mothers. The total perinatal mortality rate was 10.7%, and the neonatal mortality rate was 4%. This study revealed an increased incidence of prematurity, IUGR, fetal asphyxia, acidosis, and abruptio placentae in eclampsia occurring before delivery. These same factors may be responsible for most of the early neonatal complications encountered in infants of eclamptic mothers. Fifty-six percent of deliveries were premature, and abruptio placentae complicated 22.5% of the pregnancies. Thirty percent of the premature infants were growth restricted[86]; that number is similar to those reported by Lopez-Llera and associates (27%)[138] and Brazy and coworkers (29%).[83] It is important to note that IUGR was present in only the premature infants. Moreover, IUGR was symmetric (affecting weight, length, and head circumference) in all growth-restricted infants before 32 weeks of gestation. Except for the higher hematocrit values in infants of eclamptic mothers, the incidence of abnormal hematologic laboratory findings was comparable with that in the premature control group. There was no difference in regard to thrombocytopenia, leukopenia, or disseminated intravascular coagulation.[36]

Moreover, there was no correlation between the presence and severity of thrombocytopenia in eclamptic mothers and their infants.[139] Most of the hematologic findings seen in infants born to eclamptic mothers are probably secondary to sepsis, hypoxia, or acidosis, which may suppress the bone marrow production or increase peripheral sequestration. The long-term follow-up data, up to 4 years of age, seem favorable in the absence of complications such as IUGR, prematurity, and abruptio placentae. Somatic growth for weight and height in infants of eclamptic mothers is similar to that seen in premature and/or IUGR controls. In fact, the somatic growth for weight and height was normal on follow-up in most infants who were neurologically normal.[86]

In 1990, Sibai reported the perinatal outcome of 254 pregnancies complicated by eclampsia. The total perinatal mortality rate was 11.8%, and most deaths were secondary to extreme prematurity, IUGR, congenital infections, congenital anomalies, and abruptio placentae. In fact, abruptio placentae was responsible for 68% of the perinatal deaths.[140] The outcome of 28 premature infants and 14 full-term infants of eclamptic mothers for up to 50 months was reported.[140] Of the 12 infants who were small for gestational age by weight at birth, 8 showed catch-up growth at an average of 20.6 months (range, 2 to 48 months). In all, only two of the infants remained growth restricted by weight, height, and head circumference; both were mentally retarded. A total of three infants had major neurologic deficits resulting in cerebral palsy and mental retardation on follow-up evaluation. General health continued to be a problem for the premature infants during the first year of life. Several were hospitalized several times for either pulmonary or neurologic complications.

Delivery of the fetus and placenta is the definitive treatment of eclampsia. Once convulsions and severe hypertension are well controlled and the patient has been stabilized, preparation for delivery should be initiated. Severe fetal bradycardia and late decelerations are frequently seen during and immediately after eclamptic convulsions that may be secondary to maternal hypoxia and acidosis. Management of such patients should aim to correct maternal hypoxia and acidosis, which is commonly followed by a gradual recovery of the fetal heart rate pattern.[141,142] All patients should have continuous fetal observation. Intravenous oxytocin may be used to induce labor. Women with unfavorable cervical conditions and at 30 weeks or less are then delivered electively by cesarean section. $MgSO_4$ is the drug of choice for prevention and treatment of eclampsia. Five randomized studies compared the use of $MgSO_4$ with other anticonvulsants,[30,105,143,144] the largest being that of the Eclampsia Trial Collaborative Group.[145] $MgSO_4$ proved superior in preventing seizures. A loading dose of 6 g of $MgSO_4$ should be given over a 15- to 20-minute period, followed by 2 g/hour to maintain adequate serum levels. Approximately 10% to 15% of women have a second convulsion after receiving the intravenous loading dose. An additional 2-g bolus can be given intravenously over 3 to 5 minutes. No more than 8 g of $MgSO_4$ should be given over a short period of time to control convulsions.[135]

SUMMARY

Hypertensive disorders are the most common complications of pregnancy and certainly contribute to maternal and neonatal morbidity and mortality. The ultimate goals of therapy must always be safety of the mother first and then the delivery of a live, mature newborn who will not require intensive and prolonged neonatal care. Definitive therapy in the form of delivery is the desired goal because it is the only cure for preeclampsia. In some cases, however, such an approach is not in the best interest of the fetus. As a result, the decision between immediate delivery and expectant management depends on one or more of the following: maternal and fetal status at the time of initial evaluation, fetal gestational age, presence of labor, and the wishes of the mother. This management scheme presented is only a guideline and should be combined with clinical judgment, which plays a considerable role in the management of these patients.

Acknowledgment

Special thanks are given to Ihab M. Usta for her contributions to this chapter. Dr. Usta was the author of this chapter in the first edition.

REFERENCES

1. Sibai BM: Preeclampsia-eclampsia. Curr Prob Obstet Gynecol Fertil 13:1, 1990.
2. Sibai BM: Drug therapy: Treatment of hypertension in pregnant women. N Engl J Med 335:257, 1996.
3. Sibai BM, Abdella TN, Anderson GD: Pregnancy outcome in 211 patients with mild chronic hypertension. Obstet Gynecol 61:571, 1983.
4. Report of the National High Blood Pressure Education Program Working Group on High Blood Pressure in Pregnancy. Am J Obstet Gynecol 183:S22, 2000.
5. Sibai BM: Diagnosis and management of chronic hypertension in pregnancy. Obstet Gynecol 78:451, 1991.
6. Chesley LC: Hypertension and renal disease. In: Hypertensive Disorders in Pregnancy, 2nd ed. New York, Appleton-Century-Crofts, 1978, pp 478-485.
7. Sibai BM: Chronic hypertension in pregnancy. Clin Perinatol 18:833, 1991.
8. Dunlop JCH: Chronic hypertension and perinatal mortality. Proc R Soc Med 59:838, 1966.
9. Sibai BM, Anderson GD: Pregnancy outcome of intensive therapy in severe hypertension in first trimester. Obstet Gynecol 67:517, 1986.
10. Sibai BM, Mabie WC, Shamsa F, et al: A comparison of no medications versus methyldopa or labetalol in chronic hypertension during pregnancy. Am J Obstet Gynecol 162:960, 1990.
11. Sibai BM, Villar MA, Mabie WC: Acute renal failure in hypertensive disorders of pregnancy: Pregnancy outcome and remote prognosis in thirty-one consecutive cases. Am J Obstet Gynecol 162:777, 1990.
12. Mabie WC, Gonzalez AR, Sibai BM, et al: A comparative trial of labetalol and hydralazine in the acute management of severe hypertension complicating pregnancy. Obstet Gynecol 70:328, 1987.
13. Leather HM, Humphreys DM, Baker PB, et al: A controlled trial of hypotensive agents in hypertension in pregnancy. Lancet 1:488, 1968.
14. Redman CWE, Beilin LJ, Bonnar J, et al: Fetal outcome in trial of antihypertensive treatment in pregnancy. Lancet 2:753, 1976.
15. Redman CWG, Beilin LJ, Bonnar J: Treatment of hypertension in pregnancy with methyldopa: Blood pressure control and side effects. Br J Obstet Gynaecol 84:419, 1977.
16. Arias F, Zamora J: Antihypertensive treatment and pregnancy outcome in patients with mild chronic hypertension. Obstet Gynecol 53:489, 1979.
17. Blake S, MacDonald D. The prevention of the maternal manifestations of preeclampsia by intensive antihypertensive treatment. Br J Obstet Gynaecol 98:244, 1991.
18. Gallery EDM, Saunders DM, Hyom N, et al: Randomized comparison of methyldopa and oxprenolol for treatment of hypertension in pregnancy. BMJ 1:1591, 1979.
19. Fidler J, Smith V, Fayers P, et al: Randomized controlled comparative study of methyldopa and oxprenolol in treatment of hypertension in pregnancy. BMJ 286:1927, 1983.
20. Plouin PF, Breart G, Millard F, et al: Comparison of antihypertensive efficacy and perinatal safety of labetalol and methyldopa in the treatment of hypertension in pregnancy: A randomized controlled trial. Br J Obstet Gynaecol 95:868, 1988.
21. Chesley LC, Annitto JE: Pregnancy in the patient with hypertensive disease. Am J Obstet Gynecol 53:372, 1947.
22. Landesman R, Holze E, Scherr L: Fetal mortality in essential hypertension. Obstet Gynecol 6:354, 1955.
23. Kincaid-Smith P, Bullen M, Mills J: Prolonged use of methyldopa in severe hypertension in pregnancy. BMJ 1:274, 1966.
24. Rubin PC: Beta-blockers in pregnancy. N Engl J Med 305:1323, 1981.
25. Hou SH, Grossman SD, Madias NE: Pregnancy in women with renal disease and moderate renal insufficiency. Am J Med 78:185, 1985.
26. Hokegard KH, Karlsson K, Kjellmer I, et al: Effect of nifedipine on Doppler flow velocity waveforms in severe preeclampsia. BMJ 299:1205, 1989.
27. Kjellmer I, Dagbjartsson A, Hrbek A, et al: Maternal beta-adrenoreceptor blockade reduces fetal tolerance to asphyxia. Acta Obstet Gynecol Scand Suppl 118:75, 1984.
28. Plouin PF, Breart G, Llado J, et al: A randomized comparison of early with consecutive use of antihypertensive drugs in management of pregnancy-induced hypertension. Br J Obstet Gynaecol 97:134, 1990.
29. Friedman EA, Neff RK: Hypertension-hypotension in pregnancy. JAMA 239:2249, 1978.
30. Dommissse J: Phenytoin sodium and magnesium sulphate in the management of eclampsia. Br J Obstet Gynaecol 94:104, 1990.
31. Soothill PW, Ajayi R, Campbell S, et al: Effects of a fetal surveillance unit on admission of antenatal patients to hospital. BMJ 303:269, 1991.
32. Bott-Kanner G, Hirsch M, Friedman S, et al: Antihypertensive therapy in the management of hypertension in pregnancy: A clinical double-blind study of pindolol. Clin Exp Hypertens 11:207, 1992.
33. Pickles CJ, Symonds EM, Broughton PF: The fetal outcome in a randomized double-blind controlled trial of labetalol versus placebo in pregnancy-induced hypertension. Br J Obstet Gynaecol 96:38, 1989.
34. Fabrigues G, Alvarez L, Varas Juri P, et al: Effectiveness of atenolol in the treatment of hypertension during pregnancy. Hypertension 19(Suppl II):129, 1992.
35. Butters L, Kennedy S, Rubin P: Atenolol in essential hypertension during pregnancy. BMJ 301:587, 1990.

36. Lip GYH, Beevers M, Churchill D, et al: Effect of atenolol on birth weight. Am J Cardiol 79:1436, 1997.
37. Montan S, Ingermarsson I, Marshal K, et al: Randomized controlled trial of atenolol and pindolol in human pregnancy: Effects on fetal hemodynamics. BMJ 304:946, 1992.
38. Montan S, Liedholm H, Lingman G, et al: Fetal and uteroplacental hemodynamics during short-term atenolol treatment of hypertension pregnancy. Br J Obstet Gynaecol 94:312, 1987.
39. Meyer NL, Mercer BM, Friedman SA, Sibai BM: Urinary dipstick protein: A poor predictor of absent or severe proteinuria. Am J Obstet Gynecol 170:137, 1994.
40. Redman CW: Treatment of hypertension in pregnancy. Kidney Int 18:267, 1980.
41. Ducsay CA, Thompson JS, Wu AT, et al: The effects of calcium entry blocker (nicardipine) tocolysis in rhesus macaques: Fetal plasma concentrations and cardiorespiratory changes. Am J Obstet Gynecol 157:1482, 1987.
42. Parisi VM, Salinas JM, Stockmar EJ: Fetal vascular responses to maternal nicardipine administration in the hypertensive ewe. Am J Obstet Gynecol 161:1035, 1989.
43. Parisi VM, Salinas JM, Stockmar EJ: Placental vascular responses to nicardipine in the hypertensive ewe. Am J Obstet Gynecol 161:1039, 1989.
44. Tsujiei M, Furuhashi N, Kimura H, et al: Effects of nifedipine on placental blood flow, placental weight and fetal weight in normotensive and spontaneously hypertensive rats. Gynecol Obstet Invest 34:193, 1992.
45. Ahokas RA, Sibai BM, Mabie WC, et al: Nifedipine does not adversely affect uteroplacental blood flow in the hypertensive term-pregnant rat. Am J Obstet Gynecol 159:440, 1988.
46. Cameron AD, Walker JJ, Mathara AM, et al: The effect of antihypertensive therapy on the Doppler waveform in the maternal and fetal vascular system. In Abstracts of the Second International Doppler Society Meeting, Paris, 7th Meeting, 1989.
47. Lindow SW, Davies N, Davey DA, et al: The effect of sublingual nifedipine on uteroplacental blood flow in hypertensive pregnancy. Br J Obstet Gynaecol 95:1276, 1988.
48. Hanretty KP, Whittle JM, Howie CA, et al: Effect of nifedipine on Doppler flow velocity waveforms in severe preeclampsia. BMJ 299:1205, 1989.
49. Mari G, Kirshon B, Moise K, et al: Doppler assessment of the fetal and uteroplacental circulation during nifedipine therapy for preterm labor. Am J Obstet Gynecol 161:1514, 1989.
50. Moretti MM, Fairlie FM, Akl S, et al: The effect of nifedipine therapy on fetal and placental Doppler waveforms in preeclampsia remote from term. Am J Obstet Gynecol 163:1844, 1990.
51. Sibai BM, Abdella TN, Anderson GD, et al: Plasma volume findings in pregnancy women with mild hypertension: Therapeutic considerations. Am J Obstet Gynecol 145:539, 1983.
52. Sibai BM, Grossman RA, Grossman HG: Effects of diuretics on plasma volume in pregnancies with long term hypertension. Am J Obstet Gynecol 150:831, 1984.
53. Hanssens M, Keirse MJNC, Vandelecom F, Van Assche FA: Fetal and neonatal effects of treatment with angiotensin-converting enzyme inhibitors in pregnancy. Obstet Gynecol 171:128, 1991.
54. Kreft-Jais C, Plouin PF, Tchobroutsky C, Boutroy MJ: Angiotensin-converting enzyme inhibitors during pregnancy: A survey of 22 patients given captopril and 9 given enalapril. Br J Obstet Gynaecol 95:420, 1988.
55. Lumbers ER, Burrell JH, Menzies RI, et al: The effects of converting enzyme inhibitor (captopril) and angiotensin II on fetal renal functions. Br J Pharmacol 110:821, 1993.
56. Rosa FW, Bosco LA, Graham CF, et al: Neonatal anuria with maternal angiotensin converting enzyme inhibitor. Obstet Gynecol 74:371, 1989.
57. Abe S, Amagasaki Y, Konishi K, et al: The influence of antecedent renal disease on pregnancy. Am J Obstet Gynecol 153:508, 1985.
58. Branch DW, Andres R, Digre KB, et al: The association of antiphospholipid antibodies with severe preeclampsia. Obstet Gynecol 73:541, 1989.
59. Cunningham FG, Cox SM, Harstad TW, et al: Chronic renal disease and pregnancy outcome. Am J Obstet Gynecol 163:453, 1990.
60. Mabie WC, Pernoll MK, Biswas MK: Chronic hypertension in pregnancy. Obstet Gynecol 67:197, 1986.
61. Scott JR, Rote NS, Branch DW: Immunologic aspects of recurrent abortion and fetal death. Obstet Gynecol 70:645, 1987.
62. Mabie WC, Ratts TE, Ramanathan Kb, et al: Circulatory congestion in obese hypertensive women: A subset of pulmonary edema in pregnancy. Obstet Gynecol 72:553, 1988.
63. Schoenfeld A, Segal J Friedman S, et al: Adverse reactions to antihypertensive drugs in pregnancy. Obstet Gynecol Surv 41:67, 1986.
64. Greer W, Walker JJ, Bjornsson S, et al: Second line therapy with nifedipine combined with atenolol in the management of severe preeclampsia. Clin Exp Hypertens B 8:277, 1989.
65. Sibai BM, Akl S, Fairlie F, Moretti M: A randomized protocol for managing severe preeclampsia in the second trimester. Am J Obstet Gynecol 163:733, 1990.
66. Sibai BM, Hauth J, Caritis S, et al: Hypertensive disorders in twin versus singleton pregnancies. Am J Obstet Gynecol 182:938, 2000.
67. Zuspan FP, Rayburn WF: Blood pressure self-monitoring during pregnancy: Practical considerations. Am J Obstet Gynecol 164:2, 1991.
68. Chammas MF, Nguyen TM, Li MA, et al: Expectant management of severe preterm preeclampsia: Is intrauterine growth restriction an indication for immediate delivery? Am J Obstet Gynecol 183:853, 2000.
69. Hauth JC, Ewell MG, Levine RJ, et al: Pregnancy outcomes in healthy nulliparas who developed hypertension. Calcium for Preeclampsia Prevention Study Group. Obstet Gynecol 95:24, 2000.
70. Knuist M, Bonsel GJ, Zondervan HA, Treffers PE: Intensification of fetal and maternal surveillance in pregnant women with hypertensive disorders. Int J Gynecol Obstet 61:127, 1998.
71. Campbell DM, MacGillivray I: Preeclampsia in twin pregnancies: Incidence and outcome. Hypertens Pregnancy 18:197, 1999.
72. Long PA, Abell DA, Beischer NA: Parity and preeclampsia. Aust N Z J Obstet Gynaecol 19:203, 1979.
73. Dekker GA, Sibai BM: Early detection of preeclampsia. Am J Obstet Gynecol 165:160, 1991.
74. Friedman SA, Lindheimer MD: Prediction and differential diagnosis. In Lindheimer MD, Roberts JM, Cunningham GF (eds): Chesley's Hypertensive Disorders in Pregnancy. Stamford, CT, Appleton & Lange, 1999, p 201.
75. Myatt L, Miodovnik M: Prediction of preeclampsia. Semin Perinatol 23:45, 1999.
76. ACOG Technical Bulletin 29: Chronic hypertension in pregnancy. Washington, DC, American College of Obstetricians and Gynecologists, July 2001.
77. Brown MA, Hague WM, Higgins J, et al: The detection, investigation, and management of hypertension in pregnancy. Full consensus statement of recommendations from the Council of the Australian Society for the Study of Hypertension in Pregnancy. Aust N Z J Obstet Gynaecol 40:139, 2000.

78. Helewa ME, Burrows RF, Smith J, et al: Report of the Canadian Hypertension Society Consensus Conference: 1. Definitions, evaluation and classification of hypertensive disorders in pregnancy. Can Med Assoc J 157:715, 1997.

79. Mattar F, Sibai BM: Eclampsia. VIII. Risk factors for maternal morbidity. Am J Obstet Gynecol 182:307, 2000.

80. Barton JR, Witlin AG, Sibai BM: Management of mild preeclampsia. Clin Obstet Gynecol 42:455, 1999.

81. Halligan AWF, Bell SC, Taylor DJ: Dipstick proteinuria: Caveat emptor. Br J Obstet Gynaecol 106:1113, 1999.

82. Brazy JE, Grimn JK, Little VA: Neonatal manifestations of severe maternal hypertension occurring before the thirty-sixth week of pregnancy. J Pediatr 100:165, 1982.

83. Kuo VS, Kuomantakis G, Gallery FDM: Proteinuria and its assessment in normal and hypertensive pregnancy. Am J Obstet Gynecol 167:723, 1992.

84. Saudan P, Burrows RF, Smith J, et al: Does gestational hypertension become pre-eclampsia? Br J Obstet Gynaecol 105:1177, 1988.

85. Sibai BM, Anderson GD, Abdella TN, et al: Eclampsia. II. Neonatal outcome, growth, and development. Am J Obstet Gynecol 146:307, 1983.

86. Villar MA, Sibai BM: Clinical significance of elevated mean arterial blood in second trimester and threshold increase in systolic or diastolic pressure during third trimester. Am J Obstet Gynecol 60:419, 1989.

87. Levine RJ, Ewell MG, Hauth JC, et al: Should the definition of preeclampsia include a rise in diastolic blood pressure of ≥15 mm Hg to a level <90 mm Hg in association with proteinuria? Am J Obstet Gynecol 183:787, 2000.

88. North RA, Taylor RS, Schellenberg J-C: Evaluation of a definition of pre-eclampsia. Br J Obstet Gynaecol 106:767, 1999.

89. Roberts JM, Redman CWE: Pre-eclampsia is more than pregnancy-induced hypertension. Lancet 341:1447, 1993.

90. Gilstrap LC, Cunningham GF, Whalley PJ: Management of pregnancy-induced hypertension in the nulliparous patient remote from term. Semin Perinatol 2:73, 1978.

91. Ounsted M, Cockburn J, Moar VA, et al: Maternal hypertension with superimposed preeclampsia: Effects on child development at 7½ years. Br J Obstet Gynaecol 90:644, 1983.

92. Witlin AG, Sibai BM: Hypertension. Clin Obstet Gynecol 41:533, 1998.

93. Lydakis C, Lip Gy, Beevers M, Beevers DG: Atenolol and fetal growth in pregnancies complicated by hypertension. Am J Hypertens 12:541, 1999.

94. Constantine G, Beevers DG, Reynolds AL, et al: Nifedipine as a second line antihypertensive drug in pregnancy. Br J Obstet Gynaecol 94:1136, 1987.

95. Mathews DD: A randomized controlled trial of bed rest and sedation or normal activity and non-sedation in the management of non-albuminuric hypertension in late pregnancy. Br J Obstet Gynaecol 84:108, 1977.

96. Feeney JG: Hypertension in pregnancy managed by community midwives. BMJ 288:1046, 1984.

97. Sibai BM, Gonzalez AR, Mabie WC, et al: A comparison of labetalol plus hospitalization versus hospitalization alone in the management of preeclampsia remote from term. Obstet Gynecol 70:323, 1987.

98. Wichman K, Ryden E, Kalbery BE: A placebo controlled trial of metoprolol in the treatment of hypertension in pregnancy. Scand J Clin Lab Invest 44:90, 1984.

99. Sibai BM, Anderson GD, McCubbin JH: Eclampsia. II. Clinical significance of laboratory findings. Obstet Gynecol 59:153, 1982.

100. Barton JR, Stanziano GI, Sibai BM: Monitored outpatient management of mild gestational hypertension remote from term. Am J Obstet Gynecol 170:1765, 1994.

101. Sibai BM, Taslimi M, Abdella TN, et al: Maternal perinatal outcome of conservative management of severe preeclampsia in mid-trimester. Am J Obstet Gynecol 152:32, 1987.

102. Schiff E, Friedman SA, Mercer BM, Sibai BM: Fetal lung maturity is not accelerated in preeclamptic pregnancies. Am J Obstet Gynecol 169:1096, 1993.

103. Chari RS, Friedman SA, Schiff E, et al: Is fetal neurologic and physical development accelerated in preeclampsia? Am J Obstet Gynecol 174:829, 1996.

104. Benedetti TJ, Benedetti JF, Stenchever MA: Severe preeclampsia: Maternal and fetal outcome. Clin Exp Hypertens 243:401, 1982.

105. Friedman SA, Schiff E, Koa L, Sibai BM: Neonatal outcome after preterm delivery for preeclampsia. Am J Obstet Gynecol 172:1785, 1995.

106. Monroe BL, Weinberg AG, Rosenfield CR, et al: The neonatal blood count in health and disease. I. Reference values for neutrophilic cells. J Pediatr 95:89, 1979.

107. Koenig JM, Christensen RD: Incidence, neutrophil kinetics, and natural history of neonatal neutropenia associated with maternal hypertension. N Engl J Med 321:557, 1989.

108. Sibai BM, Spinnato JA, Watson DL, et al: Pregnancy outcome in 303 cases with severe preeclampsia. Obstet Gynecol 64:319, 1984.

109. Szymonowicz W, Yu VYH: Severe pre-eclampsia and infants of very low birth weight. Arch Dis Child 62:712, 1987.

110. Zeben-van der Aa DM, Verwey RA, Verloove-Vanhorick SP, et al: Maternal hypertension and very pre-term infants' mortality and handicaps. Eur J Obstet Gynecol Reprod Biol 39:87, 1991.

111. Nochimson DJ, Petrie RH: Glucocorticoid therapy for induction of pulmonary maturity in severely hypertensive gravid women. Am J Obstet Gynecol 133:449, 1979.

112. Rick PS, Elliot JP, Freeman RK: Use of corticosteroids in pregnancy-induced hypertension. Obstet Gynecol 55:206, 1980.

113. Martin TN, Tupper WRC: The management of severe toxemia in patients less than 36 weeks gestation. Obstet Gynecol 54:602, 1975.

114. Odendaal HJ, Pattinson RC, Bam R, et al: Aggressive or expectant management for patients with severe preeclampsia between 28-34 weeks' gestation: A randomized controlled trial. Obstet Gynecol 76:1070, 1990.

115. Sibai BM, Mercer BM, Schiff E, Friedman SA: Aggressive versus expectant management of severe preeclampsia at 28 to 32 weeks' gestation: A randomized controlled trial. Am J Obstet Gynecol 171:818, 1994.

116. Fenakel K, Fenakel E, Apppleman Z, et al: Nifedipine in the treatment of severe preeclampsia. Obstet Gynecol 77:331, 1991.

117. Sibai BM: Management of preeclampsia. Clin Perinatol 18:793, 1991.

118. Pattinson RC, Odendaal HJ, Du Toit R: Conservative management of severe proteinuria hypertension before 28 weeks' gestation. S Afr Med J 73:516, 1988.

119. Wightman H, Hibbard BM, Rosen M: Perinatal mortality and morbidity associated with eclampsia. BMJ 2:235, 1978.

120. Witlin AG, Saade GR, Mattar F, Sibai BM. Predictors of neonatal outcome in women with severe preeclampsia or eclampsia between 24 and 33 weeks' gestation. Am J Obstet Gynecol 182:607, 2000.

121. Weinstein L: Syndrome of hemolysis, elevated liver enzymes, and low platelet count: A severe consequence of hypertension in pregnancy. Am J Obstet Gynecol 142:159, 1982.

122. Sibai BM: The HELLP syndrome (hemolysis, elevated liver enzymes, and low platelets): Much ado about nothing? Am J Obstet Gynecol 162:311, 1990.

123. Martin JN Jr, Files JC, Black PG, et al: Plasma exchange for preeclampsia. I. Postpartum use of persistently severe preeclampsia-eclampsia with HELLP syndrome. Am J Obstet Gynecol 162:126, 1990.

124. Van Pampus MG, Wolf H, Westerberg SM, et al: Maternal and perinatal outcome after expectant management of the HELLP syndrome compared with preeclampsia without HELLP syndrome. Eur J Obstet Gynecol Reprod Biol 76:31, 1998.

125. Visser W, Wallenburg HC: Temporising management of severe pre-eclampsia with and without the HELLP syndrome. Br J Obstet Gynaecol 102:111, 1995.

126. Abroug F, Boujdaria R, Nouira S, et al: HELLP syndrome: Incidence and maternal-fetal outcome—a prospective study. Intensive Care Med 18:274, 1992.

127. Audibert F, Friedman SA, Frangieh AU, Sibai BM: Clinical utility of strict diagnostic criteria for the HELLP (hemolysis, elevated liver enzymes, and low platelets) syndrome. Am J Obstet Gynecol 175:460, 1996.

128. Sibai BM, Ramadan MK: Acute renal failure in pregnancies complicated by hemolysis, elevated liver enzymes, and low platelets. Am J Obstet Gynecol 168:1682, 1993.

129. Tompkins MJ, Thiagarajah S: HELLP syndrome: The benefit of corticosteroids. Am J Obstet Gynecol 181:304, 1999.

130. Tuffnell DJ, Lilford RJ, Buchan PC, et al: Randomized controlled trial of day care for hypertension in pregnancy. Lancet 339:224, 1992.

131. Abramovici D, Friedman SA, Mercer BM, et al: Neonatal outcome in severe preeclampsia at 24 to 36 weeks' gestation: Does the HELLP (hemolysis, elevated liver enzymes, and low platelet count) syndrome matter? Am J Obstet Gynecol 180:221, 1999.

132. Ferraz EM, Sherline DM: Convulsive toxemia of pregnancy (eclampsia). South Med J 69:2, 1976.

133. Moar VA, Jefferies MA, Mutch LMM, et al: Neonatal head circumference and the treatment of maternal hypertension. Br J Obstet Gynaecol 85:933, 1978.

134. Lopez-Llera M: Main clinical types and subtypes of eclampsia. Am J Obstet Gynecol 166:4, 1992.

135. Poprapakkhan S: An epidemiologic study of eclampsia. Obstet Gynecol 54:26, 1979.

136. Zuspan FP: Problems encountered in the treatment of pregnancy induced hypertension. Am J Obstet Gynecol 131:591, 1978.

137. Sibai BM, McCubbin JH, Anderson GD, et al: Eclampsia. I. Observations of 67 recent cases. Obstet Gynecol 58:609, 1981.

138. Lopez-Llera M, Hernandez Horta JL, Huttick F: Retarded fetal growth in eclampsia. J Reprod Med 9:229, 1972.

139. Sibai BM, Anderson GD: Hypertension. In Gabbe SE, Niebyl JR, Simpson JL (eds): Obstetrics: Normal and Problem Pregnancy, 2nd ed. New York, Churchill Livingston, 1991, pp 993-1055.

140. Sibai BM: Eclampsia. VI. Maternal-perinatal outcome in 254 consecutive cases. Am J Obstet Gynecol 163:1049, 1990.

141. Boehm FH, Growdon JH: The effect of eclamptic convulsions on the fetal heart rate. Am J Obstet Gynecol 120:851, 1974.

142. Paul RH, Kee SK, Berstein SG: Changes in fetal heart rate: Uterine contraction patterns associated with eclampsia. Am J Obstet Gynecol 130:165, 1978.

143. Bhalla AK, Dhall GI, Dhall K: A safer and more effective treatment regimen for eclampsia. Aust N Z J Obstet Gynecol 34:144, 1994.

144. Crowther C: Magnesium sulphate versus diazepam in the management of eclampsia: A randomized controlled trial. Br J Obstet Gynaecol 97:110, 1990.

145. The Eclampsia Trial Collaborative Group: Which anticonvulsant for women with eclampsia? Evidence from the Collaborative Eclampsia Trial. Lancet 345:1455, 1995.

SUGGESTED READINGS

Banias BB, Devoe LD, Nolan TE: Severe preeclampsia in preterm pregnancy between 26 and 32 weeks' gestation. Am J Perinatol 9:357, 1992.

Barton JR, Bergauer NK, Jacques DL, et al: Does advanced maternal age affect pregnancy outcome in women with mid hypertension remote from term? Am J Obstet Gynecol 176:1236, 1997.

Bell SC, Halligan AWF, Martin J, et al: The role of observer error in antenatal dipstick proteinuria analysis. Br J Obstet Gynaecol 106:1177, 1999.

Beurel JN Jr: Eclampsia in lowland gorilla. Am J Obstet Gynecol 141:345, 1981.

Blickstein I, Ben-Hur H, Borenstein R: Perinatal outcome of twin pregnancies complicated with preeclampsia. Am J Perinatol 9:258, 1992.

Brown MA, Buddle ML: Inadequacy of dipstick proteinuria in hypertensive pregnancy. Aust N Z J Obstet Gynaecol 35:366, 1995.

Crawther CA, Boumeester AM, Ashwist HM: Does admission to hospital for bed rest prevent disease progression or improve fetal outcome in pregnancy complicated by non-proteinuric hypertension? Br J Obstet Gynaecol 99:13, 1992.

Dekker GA, Sibai BM: Pathogenesis and etiology of preeclampsia. Am J Obstet Gynecol 179:1359, 1998.

Dubois D, Petitcolas J, Temperville B, et al: Treatment of hypertension in pregnancy with beta-adrenoreceptor antagonists. Br J Clinic Pharmacol 13(Suppl):375, 1982.

Friedman SA, Schiff E, Kao L, Sibai BM: Phenytoin versus magnesium sulfate in patients with eclampsia: Preliminary results from a randomized trial [abstract 452]. Poster presented at 15th Annual Meeting of the Society of Perinatal Obstetricians, Atlanta, GA, January 23-28, 1995. Am J Obstet Gynecol 172:384, 1995.

Karlsson K, Lundgren Y, Ljungblad U: The acute effects of a nonselective beta adrenergic blocking agent in hypertensive rats. Acta Obstet Gynecol Scand Suppl 118:81, 1984.

Lindheimer MD, Katz AI: Sodium and diuretics in pregnancy. N Engl J Med 288:891, 1973.

Lunell NO, Nylund L, Lewander R, Sarby B: Uteroplacental blood flow in pre-eclampsia measurements with indium-113m and a computer-linked gamma camera. Clin Exp Hypertens B 1:105, 1982.

Magee LA, Ornstein MP, von Dadelzsen P: Management of hypertension in pregnancy. BMJ 318:1332, 1999.

Moller B, Lindmark G: Eclampsia in Sweden, 1976-1980. Acta Obstet Gynaecol Scand 65:307, 1986.

Pritchard JA, Cunningham FG, Pritchard SA: The Parkland Memorial Hospital protocol for treatment of eclampsia: Evaluation of 245 cases. Am J Obstet Gynecol 148:951, 1984.

Pritchard JA, Pritchard SA: Standardized treatment of 154 consecutive cases of eclampsia. Am J Obstet Gynecol 123:543, 1975.

Saudan PJ, Brown MA, Farrell T, Shaw L: Improved methods in assessing proteinuria in hypertensive pregnancy. Br J Obstet Gynaecol 104:1159, 1997.

Sibai BM: Management and counseling of patients with preeclampsia remote from term. Clin Obstet Gynecol 35:426, 1992.

Sibai BM, Barton JR, Akl S, et al: A randomized prospective comparison of nifedipine and bed rest versus bed rest alone in the management of preeclampsia remote from term. Am J Obstet Gynecol 167:879, 1992.

Sibai BM, Caritis SN, Thom E, et al: Prevention of preeclampsia with low-dosage aspirin in healthy nulliparous pregnant women. N Engl J Med 329:1213, 1993.

Sibai BM, Schneider JM, Morrison JC, et al: The late postpartum eclampsia controversy. Obstet Gynecol 55:74, 1980.

Suckerman-Voldman E: Pindolol therapy in pregnant hypertensive patients. Br J Clin Pharmacol 13:379S, 1982.

Weitz C, Khouzami V, Maxwell K, Johnson JW: Treatment of hypertension in pregnancy with methyldopa: Randomized double blind study. Int J Gynaecol Obstet 25:35, 1987.

Woods JB, Blake PG, Perry KG, et al: Ascites: A portent of cardiopulmonary complications in the preeclamptic patient with the syndrome of hemolysis, elevated liver enzymes, and low platelets. Obstet Gynecol 80:87, 1992.

CHAPTER 22

Oligohydramnios and Polyhydramnios

Jeffrey P. Phelan

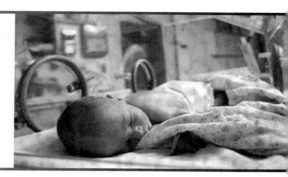

A mniotic fluid and its significance have mystified clinicians for centuries. In early times, scientists believed that amniotic fluid nourished the fetus.[1] As this belief was chiseled away, amniotic fluid dynamics has been found to be a major factor in maintaining or determining fetal integrity. A normal or above-normal amniotic fluid volume allows regular fetal movement, protects the fetus from cord compression during contractions and fetal movement, and helps maintain a stable thermal environment.

Because amniotic fluid plays such an important role in the developing fetus, disorders in amniotic fluid volume, such as oligohydramnios and polyhydramnios, and their clinical significance in antenatal and intrapartum fetal care are the focus of this chapter.

AMNIOTIC FLUID VOLUME CHANGES

In addition to changes in the amniotic fluid content, the amniotic fluid volume expands dramatically during pregnancy. The amniotic fluid volume increases progressively until the early third trimester. From that point until term, the amniotic fluid volume remains relatively constant. It is estimated that during the period from 37 weeks to 41 weeks, the amniotic fluid volume declines about 10%. After the estimated date of delivery, there is an estimated 33% decline in amniotic fluid volume during each week.[2-5]

In the first half of pregnancy, amniotic fluid volume increases in relation to fetal weight and the permeability of the fetal skin.[6] This change is reflected in the composition of the amniotic fluid, and it mirrors, to some extent, extracellular fluid and fetal urinary output.

In the latter half of pregnancy, the regulation of amniotic fluid volume involves the complex interaction of fetal swallowing, tracheal fluid production, and urination. Although the role of fetal swallowing in controlling amniotic fluid volume has not been adequately defined, fetal swallowing is known to play a dominant role when the amniotic fluid volume is normal. With advancing gestational age, fetal pulmonary or tracheal fluid secretions increase and probably play an important role in the pathogenesis of polyhydramnios.[6]

Finally, the latter half of pregnancy should be characterized as the renal phase of amniotic fluid volume production. Fetal renal function becomes maximal near term.[7] Beyond week 42 of gestation, fetal urine production declines and provides a reasonable explanation for the higher rates of oligohydramnios observed in these postdate pregnancies.[2,3,8,9] Thus, oligohydramnios is related to inadequate renal perfusion[10] and serves as a sign of intrafetal shunting.[11]

AMNIOTIC FLUID VOLUME ASSESSMENT: THE AMNIOTIC FLUID INDEX

Methods to assess the amniotic fluid volume include invasive techniques (such as dye dilution, which requires amniocentesis)[2,3,12] and noninvasive techniques (ultrasonography).[13-17] With the introduction of ultrasonography, invasive techniques were reserved for research purposes to quantify the amniotic fluid volume. Similarly, single-pocket techniques[13,14,16] have been supplanted by the more descriptive amniotic fluid index first described by Phelan and colleagues[17] in 1987.

Currently, the amniotic fluid index is the primary method of assessing the amniotic fluid volume in the United States and the world. This assessment[17] requires the use of the umbilicus and linea nigra as reference points. The umbilicus is used to delineate the upper and lower halves of the uterus. The linea nigra is then used to delineate the right and left halves of the uterus. The transducer is placed on the maternal abdomen along the longitudinal axis of the mother and perpendicular to the floor. The vertical diameter of the largest pocket in each quadrant is measured. The measurements obtained from each quadrant are summed. If the umbilical cord or a fetal limb is in the center of the pocket with fluid above and below these parts, the pocket is measured from top to bottom and through the cord or extremity. If, however, there is no amniotic fluid below the part, the measurement is extended to the uppermost portion of the part. The sum of all four quadrants' measurements represents the amniotic fluid index in centimeters for that patient.

In low-risk pregnancies, the mean amniotic fluid index is 16.2 ± 5.3 cm.[18] Phelan and Martin established definitions for oligohydramnios and polyhydramnios.[19] According to these authors, oligohydramnios is defined as an amniotic fluid index of less than 5.1 cm,[17] and polyhydramnios is considered to be present whenever the amniotic fluid index is higher than 25.0 cm.[18,19]

A comparison of all the known techniques to measure the amniotic fluid volume demonstrated that the amniotic fluid index was the superior technique.[20,21] For example, Moore[20] and Rutherford and associates[21] were able to show comparable to superior results with the amniotic fluid index over the single-pocket techniques,[13,14,16] which were not affected by fetal movement[22] or by interobserver or intraobserver differences.[23,24]

In summary, the amniotic fluid index is simple, easy to perform, and reproducible, and it provides a description, although linear, of the amniotic fluid volume. Thus, the amniotic fluid index provides a semiquantitative measurement of the amniotic fluid volume,[25,26] and 1 cm of amniotic fluid index appears to correspond to about 50 mL of amniotic fluid.[27] In addition to being able to more easily identify amniotic fluid volume disorders, the amniotic fluid index is correlated with changes in the amniotic fluid volume during pregnancy.[18] These findings suggest that it is clinically useful for monitoring the amniotic fluid volume in patients with premature rupture of the membranes[28] or in amniotic fluid volume reduction therapy.[29]

AMNIOTIC FLUID VOLUME DISORDERS

Polyhydramnios

Polyhydramnios represents the pathologic accumulation of amniotic fluid and is associated with high rates of perinatal morbidity and mortality. Polyhydramnios is defined as an amniotic fluid volume in excess of 2000 mL or an amniotic fluid index of more than 25.0 cm.[18,30] Under these circumstances, the incidence of polyhydramnios in the general population ranges from 0.2% to 1.6%.[31-35] However, this incidence is considerably lower in a nonreferral population.[31]

The more severe the polyhydramnios, the more likely there is to be a clinical reason for the excess fluid.[33] For example, Hill and coworkers[33] were able to identify a cause in 17% of patients with mild polyhydramnios. Among patients with severe polyhydramnios, an explanation for the higher volume of fluid was found in 91%.[33] When a basis for the polyhydramnios can be found, the diagnosis usually belongs, but is not limited, to the following categories[19]: fetal malformations, genetic disorders, diabetes mellitus, Rh sensitization, and congenital infections.[36]

In the patient with suspected polyhydramnios, the first step should be a referral to a maternal-fetal medicine specialist skilled in the art of ultrasonography and genetic evaluations. In that visit, the polyhydramnios

Table 22–1. Fetal Malformations That Have Been Associated with Polyhydramnios

Central nervous system
  Anencephaly
  Hydrocephaly
  Encephalocele
Gastrointestinal
  Gastroschisis
  Omphalocele
  Tracheoesophageal fistula
Respiratory tract
  Pulmonary hypoplasia
  Chylothorax

From Phelan JP, Martin GI: Polyhydramnios: Fetal and neonatal implications. Clin Perinatol 16:987, 1989.

must be confirmed. Once it is confirmed, a targeted ultrasound evaluation of the more commonly identified fetal malformations is obstetrically necessary (Table 22-1).

In general, polyhydramnios is most often associated with some impairment of fetal swallowing. This finding is especially true in fetuses with trisomies 13 and 18. In the case of central nervous system abnormalities, the pathophysiologic mechanism may also be related to the transudation of fluid across the fetal meninges or the lack of antidiuretic hormone with resultant polyuria.[37]

In contrast, gastrointestinal tract abnormalities are not related to the fetal inability to swallow; instead, they usually result from an obstructive process, such as duodenal atresia. The closer the obstruction is to the oropharynx, the greater is the likelihood of a pathologic accumulation of amniotic fluid. In the case of an omphalocele or a gastroschisis, the polyhydramnios is believed to be caused by the transudation of fluid from the lesion into the amniotic fluid.

Amniotic fluid also plays a direct role in pulmonary development and contributes, in part, to lung growth. In the fetal lungs, the flow of tracheal fluid is bidirectional, with a net outward flow of fetal lung fluid. If there is an interruption of this exchange process across the surface area of the lungs, as in cases of bilateral pulmonary hypoplasia, polyhydramnios may occur.[38]

In addition to fetal structural malformations, chromosomal and genetic abnormalities are also increased in patients with polyhydramnios. In fact, the incidence of chromosomal abnormalities may approach 35%.[39] The most common chromosomal abnormalities involve trisomies 13, 18, and 21. Neuromuscular disorders that affect fetal swallowing may also result in polyhydramnios.

In the absence of an apparent sonographic abnormality, the clinical evaluation should also include, but not be limited to, screening tests for toxoplasmosis, cytomegalovirus, diabetes mellitus, and Rh sensitization. If results of these evaluations are negative, amniotic fluid volume reduction with prostaglandin synthetase inhibitors such as indomethacin appears to be a reasonable therapeutic option.[29,40-43]

Amniotic Fluid Volume Reduction

Therapeutic reduction of the amniotic fluid volume may be obstetrically necessary to benefit or maintain the pregnancy, because uncorrected severe polyhydramnios can be associated with a number of obstetric complications (Table 22-2).

To reduce the amniotic fluid volume and thus the risks associated with severe polyhydramnios, amniocentesis or prostaglandin inhibitors have been advocated. The use of frequent, often daily amniocentesis to reduce the amniotic fluid volume is fraught with tremendous difficulty and may be associated with higher risks of maternal or fetal infection, as well as rupture of membranes. Moreover, the amniotic fluid volume turns over every 2 to 3 hours.[12] Thus, any effort to reduce the amniotic fluid volume with amniocentesis often requires the permanent placement of an intrauterine catheter to enable gradual amniotic fluid drainage and to avoid repeated amniocentesis. Either approach is associated with considerable discomfort for the patient and exposes her and her fetus to a significant risk of infection and decompression-related complications, such as abruption.[19]

As an alternative, prostaglandin synthetase inhibitors have been advocated as a noninvasive technique to reduce the amniotic fluid volume.[28,39-42] Indomethacin at a dose of 25 mg orally every 6 hours appears to produce fetal antidiuresis, mediated by a decrease in free water clearance.[43] The reduction in free water clearance appears to result from increased plasma arginine vasopressin.[43] These reductions in amniotic fluid volume do not appear to occur with the use of β-mimetics, magnesium sulfate, or aspirin therapy.[41,44]

While patients are receiving indomethacin therapy for the treatment of premature labor or to reduce the amniotic fluid volume, the amniotic fluid volume should be monitored frequently with the amniotic fluid index. The amniotic fluid index appears to be ideally designed to assist in the clinical management of these patients. For example, amniotic fluid index changes can be monitored and recorded. This evaluation enables the clinician to effectively monitor the effect, if any, of indomethacin therapy on the amniotic fluid volume. If the amniotic fluid volume returns to normal, the indomethacin can be discontinued. In the typical case, the amniotic fluid volume rises steadily. Future therapy is dictated by the patient's gestational age and the subsequent volume of amniotic fluid.

Table 22-3. Fetal and Placental Conditions That May Be Associated with Oligohydramnios

Urinary tract malformations
Chronic abruption
Ruptured membranes
Intrauterine growth restriction
Postdate pregnancy

From Phelan JP: Amniotic fluid assessment and significance of contaminants. In Reece EA, Hobbins JC, Mahoney MJ, Petrie RH (eds): Medicine of the Fetus and Mother. Philadelphia, Lippincott-Raven, 1992, pp 777-788.

Oligohydramnios

Oligohydramnios is defined as an amniotic fluid volume of less than 400 mL or an amniotic fluid index of less than 5.1 cm.[2,3,17,18,24-26,30] Multiple causes (Table 22-3) and consequences (Table 22-4) of this condition have been identified. In patients with oligohydramnios, the clinical focus depends primarily on the trimester of pregnancy and the cause, if known, for the oligohydramnios. For example, the finding of second-trimester oligohydramnios should alert the clinician to the possibility of a urinary tract malformation in the fetus or preterm premature rupture of the membranes.[6] In contrast, third-trimester oligohydramnios is a sign of possible ruptured membranes, intrauterine growth impairment, or intrafetal shunting.[10,11] The rate of oligohydramnios is highest in postdate pregnancies.[45]

Second-trimester oligohydramnios is associated with a poor prognosis for the fetus. In circumstances of preterm premature rupture of the membranes long before term, a more favorable prognosis is encountered.[46,47] In contrast, fetus-induced oligohydramnios carries the least favorable prognosis. In a study of 34 pregnancies with oligohydramnios and without premature rupture of the membranes, 9 fetuses (26%) had congenital malformations, 11 fetuses (32%) died in utero, and 6 fetuses (18%) had an entirely normal outcome.[48] Although the finding of second-trimester oligohydramnios is not necessarily hopeless, the likelihood that the neonate will be viable and normal is markedly reduced.

Prolonged exposure to oligohydramnios, however, can also lead to deformation syndromes, such as cranial, facial, or skeletal abnormalities, or to bilateral pulmonary

Table 22-2. Clinical Conditions That Can Be Associated with Severe Polyhydramnios

Premature labor
Placental abruption
Puerperal hemorrhage
Perinatal mortality
Maternal respiratory difficulties

From Phelan JP: Amniotic fluid assessment and significance of contaminants. In Reece EA, Hobbins JC, Mahoney MJ, Petrie RH (eds): Medicine of the Fetus and Mother. Philadelphia, Lippincott-Raven, 1992, pp 777-788.

Table 22-4. Potential Consequences of Oligohydramnios

Fetal deformation
Umbilical cord compression
Meconium passage
Fetal demise
Belated pulmonary hypoplasia
Intrauterine infection

From Phelan JP: Amniotic fluid assessment and significance of contaminants. In Reece EA, Hobbins JC, Mahoney MJ, Petrie RH (eds): Medicine of the Fetus and Mother. Philadelphia, Lippincott-Raven, 1992, pp 777-788.

hypoplasia. Of patients with oligohydramnios, 10% to 15% develop a deformation syndrome,[49,50] and 17% exhibit pulmonary hypoplasia.[51,52] In patients with oligohydramnios unrelated to premature rupture of the membranes, urinary tract malformations are most commonly seen. In addition to a targeted ultrasound evaluation, the furosemide test,[6] amnioinfusion,[53] or subtotal immersion[54] may be necessary to increase the amniotic fluid volume or to confirm a renal abnormality. As part of the evaluation, if technically feasible, amniocentesis to determine the fetal karyotype may be helpful in the subsequent management of these pregnancies. Often, however, a percutaneous umbilical blood sample or a placental biopsy may be necessary to obtain a chromosomal sample.

Third-trimester oligohydramnios should alert the clinician to these aforementioned possibilities but should also give rise to the clinical suspicion of intrauterine growth restriction, a postdate pregnancy, or premature rupture of the membranes. The finding of oligohydramnios in the third trimester is associated with increased incidence of cord compression, variable fetal heart rate decelerations, meconium-stained amniotic fluid, fetal heart rate nonreactivity, and adverse perinatal outcome. Unlike oligohydramnios caused by premature rupture of the membranes,[52] this kind of oligohydramnios is related to intrafetal shunting[10,11] and is associated with a less favorable fetal outcome.

As shown by Rutherford and associates[21] and by Jeng and colleagues,[25] there is an inverse relationship between amniotic fluid volume and pregnancy outcome. The lower the amniotic fluid volume, the higher are the percentages of fetal heart rate abnormalities (such as decelerations and nonreactivity), meconium-stained amniotic fluid, and perinatal morbidity and mortality. Thus, in the case of third-trimester oligohydramnios, ultrasound evaluation often requires fetal heart rate monitoring to determine fetal condition. Regardless of the nonstress test results, third-trimester oligohydramnios that is unrelated to premature rupture of the membranes should alert the clinician to the potential for fetal compromise. When oligohydramnios is identified in the full-term or post-term patient, delivery should be considered. Although induction of labor is considered acceptable, the clinician should consider offering the patient a cesarean delivery.

Patients with third-trimester oligohydramnios are also potential candidates for amnioinfusion. Amnioinfusion, however, should be limited to appropriately grown singleton pregnancies in a vertex presentation with a reactive fetal heart rate pattern and a normal baseline rate before the infusion.[55] This recommendation is made because of the known inverse relationship between the amniotic fluid index and the incidence of fetal heart rate abnormalities and adverse pregnancy outcome.[21]

As mentioned, fetus-induced oligohydramnios is a sign of intrafetal shunting.[10,11] This statement indicates that fetuses with this form of oligohydramnios have an increased susceptibility to cord compression and a prolonged fetal heart rate deceleration. If the prolonged fetal heart rate deceleration does not respond to remedial measures and terbutaline, the end result could be fetal brain injury. Theoretically, the basis for amnioinfusion is that the lower the amniotic fluid volume, the higher is the likelihood that umbilical cord compression will produce fetal heart rate decelerations. With restoration of the amniotic fluid volume by saline amnioinfusion, the cesarean delivery rate can be reduced 90% in these patients.[56-60] At the same time, saline amnioinfusion can improve the outcome in patients with thick meconium,[59,61] and, theoretically, reduce the incidence of meconium aspiration syndrome.

In a group of patients with oligohydramnios, Strong and associates infused saline during the intrapartum period and were able to significantly lower rates of meconium passage, severe variable decelerations, end-stage bradycardia, and operative deliveries for fetal distress.[60] Moreover, as demonstrated by Nageotte and colleagues[57] and Strong and associates,[60] higher umbilical arterial blood pH values were also observed in the infusion recipients.

Saline amnioinfusion is useful for the correction of repetitive variable decelerations or prolonged fetal heart rate decelerations and also for the restoration of an inadequate amniotic fluid volume.[60,62] If amnioinfusion is implemented to expand the fluid volume, repeated infusions may be necessary to maintain the patient's volume during labor. Therefore, ultrasound assessment of the amniotic fluid volume during labor may be necessary to ensure that the patient has evidence of a normal amniotic fluid volume. As a rule, an amniotic fluid index of 1 cm is equivalent to approximately 50 mL of amniotic fluid. In the Strong and associates' series,[60] the amniotic fluid index was kept above 8 cm. At this level, a significantly lower risk of intrapartum fetal distress was observed.

REFERENCES

1. Denman T: An Introduction to the Practice of Midwifery. London, Bliss & White, 1815.
2. Beischer NA, Brown JB, Townsend L: Studies in prolonged pregnancy. III. Amniocentesis in prolonged pregnancy. Am J Obstet Gynecol 193:496, 1969.
3. Gadd RL: The volume of the liquor amnii in normal and abnormal pregnancies. J Obstet Gynecol Br Commonw 73:11, 1966.
4. Queenan JT: Amniocentesis. In Queenan JT (ed): Management of High Risk Pregnancy. Oradell, NJ, Medical Economics Books, 1985, p 201.
5. Queenan JT, Thompson W, Whitfield CR, et al: Amniotic fluid volumes in normal pregnancies. Am J Obstet Gynecol 114:34, 1972.
6. King JC: Oligohydramnios. In Charles D, Glover DD (eds): Current Therapy in Obstetrics. Philadelphia, BC Decker, 1988, p 46.
7. Kurjak A, Kirkinen P, Latin V, et al: Ultrasonic assessment of fetal kidney function in normal and complicated pregnancies. Am J Obstet Gynecol 141:266, 1981.
8. Eden RD, Gergely RZ, Schifrin BS, et al: Comparison of antepartum testing schemes for the management of the post date pregnancy. Am J Obstet Gynecol 144:683, 1982.
9. Phelan JP, Platt LD, Yeh SY, et al: The role of ultrasound assessment of amniotic fluid volumes in the management of the post date pregnancy. Am J Obstet Gynecol 151:304, 1985.
10. Oz AU, Holub B, Medilcioglu I, et al: Renal artery Doppler investigation of the etiology of oligohydramnios in postterm pregnancy. Obstet Gynecol 100:715, 2002.

11. Phelan JP, Kim JO: Fetal heart rate observations in the brain-damaged infant. Semin Perinatol 24:221, 2000.

12. Vosburgh GH, Flexner LB, Cowie DB, et al: The rate of renewal in woman of the water and sodium of the amniotic fluid as determined by tracer techniques. Am J Obstet Gynecol 56:1156, 1948.

13. Chamberlain PF, Manning FA, Morrison I, et al: Ultrasound evaluation of amniotic fluid volume. I. The relationship of marginal and decreased amniotic fluid volumes to perinatal outcome. Am J Obstet Gynecol 150:245, 1984.

14. Crowley P, O'Herlihy C, Boylan P: The value of ultrasound measurement of amniotic fluid volume on the management of prolonged pregnancies. Br J Obstet Gynecol 91:444, 1984.

15. Gohari P, Berkowitz RL, Hobbins JC, et al: Prediction of IUGR by total intrauterine volume. Am J Obstet Gynecol 127:255, 1977.

16. Manning FA, Hill LM, Platt LD: Qualitative amniotic fluid volume determination by ultrasound: Antepartum detection of intrauterine growth retardation. Am J Obstet Gynecol 139:254, 1981.

17. Phelan JP, Smith CV, Broussard P, et al: Amniotic fluid volume assessment with the four-quadrant technique at 36-42 weeks' gestation. J Reprod Med 32:540, 1987.

18. Phelan JP, Ahn MO, Smith CV, et al: Amniotic fluid index measurements during pregnancy. J Reprod Med 32:627, 1987.

19. Phelan JP, Martin GI: Polyhydramnios: Fetal and neonatal implications. Clin Perinatol 16:987, 1989.

20. Moore TR: Superiority of the four-quadrant sum over the single-deepest-pocket technique in ultrasonographic identification of abnormal amniotic fluid volumes. Am J Obstet Gynecol 163:762, 1990.

21. Rutherford SE, Phelan JP, Smith CV, et al: The four quadrant assessment of amniotic fluid volume: An adjunct to antepartum fetal heart rate testing. Obstet Gynecol 70:533, 1987.

22. Wax JR, Costigan K, Callan NA, et al: Effect of fetal movement on the amniotic fluid index. Am J Obstet Gynecol 168:188, 1993.

23. Bruner JP, Reed GW, Sarno AP, et al: Intraobserver and interobserver variability of the amniotic fluid index. Am J Obstet Gynecol 168:1309, 1993.

24. Rutherford SE, Phelan JP, Smith CV, et al: The four quadrant assessment of amniotic fluid volume: Interobserver and intraobserver variation. J Reprod Med 32:597, 1987.

25. Jeng CJ, Jou TJ, Wang KG, et al: Amniotic fluid index measurement with the four-quadrant technique during pregnancy. J Reprod Med 35:674, 1990.

26. Moore TR, Cayle JE: The amniotic fluid index in normal human pregnancy. Am J Obstet Gynecol 162:1168, 1990.

27. Strong T, Hetzler G, Paul RH: Amniotic fluid volume increase after amnioinfusion of a fixed volume. Am J Obstet Gynecol 162:746, 1990.

28. Smith CV, Greenspoon J, Phelan JP, et al: The clinical utility of the nonstress test in the conservative management of patients with preterm spontaneous premature rupture of the membranes. J Reprod Med 32:1, 1987.

29. Cabrol D, Landesman R, Muller J, et al: Treatment of polyhydramnios with prostaglandin synthetase inhibitor (indomethacin). Am J Obstet Gynecol 157:422, 1987.

30. Pritchard JA, MacDonald PC: Diseases and abnormalities of the placenta and fetal membranes. In: Williams' Obstetrics, 15th ed. New York, Appleton-Century-Crofts, 1976, p 476.

31. Alexander EX, Spintz HB, Clark RA: Sonography of polyhydramnios. AJR Am J Roentgenol 138:343, 1982.

32. Barry AP: Hydramnios: A survey of 100 cases. Br J Med Sci 61:257, 1953.

33. Hill L, Breckle R, Thomas ML, et al: Polyhydramnios: Ultrasonically detected prevalence and neonatal outcome. Obstet Gynecol 69:21, 1987.

34. Hobbins JC, Grannum PA, Berkowitz RL, et al: Ultrasound in the diagnosis of congenital anomalies. Am J Obstet Gynecol 134:331, 1979.

35. Karmer E: Hydramnios, oligohydramnios and fetal malformations. Clin Obstet Gynecol 9:508, 1966.

36. Ledger WJ: Maternal infection with adverse fetal and newborn outcomes. In Ledger WJ (ed): Infection in the Female. Philadelphia, Lea & Febiger, 1986, p 197.

37. Wallenburg HC, Wladimiroff JW: The amniotic fluid: Polyhydramnios and oligohydramnios. J Perinat Med 5:233, 1977.

38. Mendelsohn G, Hutchins GM: Primary pulmonary hypoplasia. Am J Dis Child 131:1220, 1977.

39. Platt LD, Devore GR, Lopez E, et al: Role of amniocentesis in ultrasound-detected fetal malformations. Obstet Gynecol 68:153, 1986.

40. Goldenberg RL, Davis RO, Baker RC: Indomethacin induced oligohydramnios. Am J Obstet Gynecol 160:1196, 1989.

41. Hickok DE, Hollenbach KA, Reilly SF, et al: The association between decreased amniotic fluid volume and treatment with nonsteroidal anti-inflammatory agents for preterm labor. Am J Obstet Gynecol 160:1525, 1989.

42. Kirshon B, Mari G, Moise KJ Jr: Indomethacin therapy in the treatment of symptomatic polyhydramnios. Obstet Gynecol 75:202, 1990.

43. Walker MPR, Moore TR, Cheung CY, et al: Indomethacin-induced urinary flow rate reduction in the ovine fetus with reduced free water clearance and elevated plasma arginine vasopressin levels. Am J Obstet Gynecol 167:1723, 1992.

44. Maher JE, Owen J, Hauth J, et al: The effect of low-dose aspirin on fetal urine output and amniotic fluid volume. Am J Obstet Gynecol 169:885, 1993.

45. Phelan JP: The postdate pregnancy: An overview. Clin Obstet Gynecol 32:221, 1989.

46. Garite TJ: Premature rupture of the membranes: The enigma of the obstetrician. Am J Obstet Gynecol 151:1001, 1985.

47. Wilson JC, Levy DL, Wilds PL: Premature rupture of membranes prior to term: Consequences of nonintervention. Obstet Gynecol 60:601, 1982.

48. Mercer LJ, Brown LG: Fetal outcome with oligohydramnios in the second trimester. Obstet Gynecol 67:840, 1986.

49. King JC, Mitzner W, Butterfield AB, et al: Effect of induced oligohydramnios on fetal lung development. Am J Obstet Gynecol 154:823, 1986.

50. Nimrod C, Varela-Bittings F, Machin G, et al: The effect of very prolonged membrane rupture on fetal development. Am J Obstet Gynecol 148:540, 1984.

51. Nimrod C, Davies D, Iwanicki S, et al: Ultrasound prediction of pulmonary hypoplasia. Obstet Gynecol 68:495, 1986.

52. Perlman M, Williams J, Hirsch M: Neonatal pulmonary hypoplasia after prolonged leakage of amniotic fluid. Arch Dis Child 51:349, 1976.

53. Quetel TA, Mejides AA, Salman FA, et al: Amnioinfusion: An aid in the ultrasonographic evaluation of severe oligohydramnios in pregnancy. Am J Obstet Gynecol 167:333, 1992.

54. Strong TH: Reversal of oligohydramnios with subtotal immersion: A report of five cases. Am J Obstet Gynecol 169:1595, 1993.

55. Pitt C, Sanchez-Ramos L, Kaunitz AM, et al: Prophylactic amnioinfusion for intrapartum oligohydramnios: A meta-analysis of randomized control trials. Obstet Gynecol 96:861, 2000.

56. Miyazaki FS, Taylor NA: Saline amnioinfusion for relief of variable or prolonged decelerations: A preliminary report. Am J Obstet Gynecol 146:670, 1983.

57. Nageotte MP, Freeman RK, Garite TJ, et al: Prophylactic intrapartum amnioinfusion in patients with preterm premature rupture of the membranes. Am J Obstet Gynecol 153:557, 1985.

58. Ogita S, Imanaka M, Matsumoto M, et al: Transcervical amnioinfusion of antibiotics: A basic study for managing premature rupture of membranes. Am J Obstet Gynecol 158:23, 1988.

59. Sadovsky Y, Amon E, Bade ME, et al: Prophylactic amnioinfusion during labor complicated by meconium: A preliminary report. Am J Obstet Gynecol 161:613, 1989.

60. Strong TH, Hetzler G, Sarno AP, et al: Prophylactic intrapartum amnioinfusion: A randomized clinical trial. Am J Obstet Gynecol 162:1370, 1990.

61. Macri CJ, Schrimmer DB, Leung A, et al: Prophylactic amnioinfusion improves outcome of pregnancy complicated by thick meconium and oligohydramnios. Am J Obstet Gynecol 167:117, 1992.

62. Sarno AP, Ahn MO, Phelan JP: Intrapartum amniotic fluid volume at term: Association of ruptured membranes, oligohydramnios and increased fetal risk. J Reprod Med 35:719, 1990.

CHAPTER 23

Substance Use During Pregnancy

Hallam Hurt

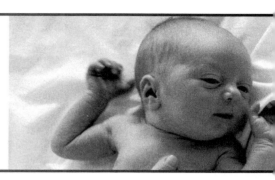

Substance use during pregnancy is not a new phenomenon, but the increase in cocaine use by pregnant women that began in the late 1980s has intensified national interest in maternal substance use and its effect on the fetus and newborn. This chapter describes a general approach to the substance-using woman and her infant and specific approaches for management of newborns exposed in utero to cocaine, narcotics, alcohol, marijuana, cigarettes, and amphetamines.

GENERAL APPROACH TO MOTHER

Care of a pregnant substance user involves much more than attention to the particular substances being used. Evaluation of the woman's general health and lifestyle is crucial to improving the outcome of the pregnancy (Table 23-1). Many substance users have erratic, late, or no prenatal care, and interventions may be delayed until late in pregnancy or may not occur until the time of delivery. When a pregnant substance user comes in contact with the health care system, an immediate, urgent attempt must be made to investigate medical, economic, and social factors influencing the mother and her pregnancy (Table 23-2). Before addressing particular concerns related to use of specific substances, several issues common to substance-using women are discussed.

Detection and Documentation of Substance Use

Screening for substance use in pregnant women is controversial, raising medical, legal, and social concerns. Identification of the substance user can facilitate, however, obtaining appropriate care for her. Knowledge of certain substances to which the fetus has been exposed is helpful in anticipatory care of the newborn. Guidelines concerning screening vary. The efficacy and use of specific screening procedures should be discussed among responsible individuals within institutions, and protocols should be designed according to these discussions and according to federal guidelines. An honest discussion with the mother held in a nonthreatening environment often results in the mother being forthcoming regarding substance use. Information gathered by this approach is far preferable to confrontations. Screening without consent carries legal ramifications.

Detection of substance use by pregnant women can be done by interview, urine testing, and, more recently, hair analysis. Interview and urine screen are the more common methods. Urine screens are noninvasive, and the sample is easily collected. Drawbacks in general are that only recent substance use is detected, and false-negative results may be high. Hair analysis is invasive but allows an accurate screen and an assessment of the chronicity of substance usage. The hair nearest the scalp reflects the most recent use, whereas hair most distant from the scalp reflects usage earlier in pregnancy.[1,2]

A newborn's in utero exposure to drugs is most commonly documented through a positive maternal history or urine screen and a urine screen of the infant. If infant urine is being used, it must be collected as soon as possible after delivery because a delay allows metabolism and excretion of the substance to occur before collection. Another method of screening infants is analysis of meconium. Ostrea and colleagues[2,3] showed a high sensitivity and specificity of meconium analysis for presence of cocaine, morphine, and marijuana. In addition, meconium analysis may give some evidence of chronicity of use. Ostrea and colleagues[4] suggested that substances found in meconium passed in the first 10 hours after delivery corresponded to substance use in the first 20 weeks of gestation, substances in meconium passed in the next 11 to 20 hours corresponded to substance use between 21 and 30 weeks of gestation, and substances in meconium passed later corresponded to substance use after 30 weeks of gestation.

General Health

Frequently, substance users show a general inattention to their own health and to the health of their fetus. Poor nutrition, coupled with erratic or poor prenatal care, is often seen. Whenever the pregnant substance user enters the health care system, the personnel involved in her care

Table 23–1. General Approach to Mother*

General health	Perform careful physical examination
	Provide nutritional counseling
Pregnancy	Establish gestational age of fetus
	Evaluate fetal size and growth
	Evaluate fetal well-being
	Schedule prenatal appointments
Substance use	Obtain careful history
	Consider obtaining toxicology screen; discuss with mother[†]
	Counsel about potential effects of substances on fetus
	Refer to drug treatment program
Infections	Assess for gonococcus, chlamydia, bacterial vaginosis, group B streptococcus, hepatitis, herpes
	Obtain serology for syphilis
	Place tuberculin skin test
	Counsel regarding testing for human immunodeficiency virus status
Social	Obtain social service consultation

*A nonjudgmental attitude facilitates data collection and encourages patient compliance.

[†]As per institutional, state, or national guidelines.

should obtain a detailed history and attempt to establish gestational age and well-being of the fetus. Substance users, often fearful of legal ramifications of substance use, are best dealt with in a nonjudgmental manner. The first visit is a time to establish rapport. This approach, coupled with encouragement, increases the likelihood of the substance user meeting future prenatal appointments and seeking drug treatment.

Polysubstance Use

Most pregnant women who use one substance use others. A careful history of substance use (amount and frequency) per trimester should be obtained. Consideration should be given to screening the urine; if screening is performed, it should be discussed first with the mother.

Infections

The lifestyle of many substance users involves multiple sexual partners, prostitution as a means to obtain drugs, and sharing of materials necessary for intravenous drug use. The likelihood of sexually transmitted diseases in a pregnant substance user is high. At prenatal visits or at delivery if this is the first encounter with medical care, the woman (with appropriate counseling and consent) should be evaluated for infections, including chlamydia, bacterial vaginosis, group B streptococcus, gonorrhea, syphilis, hepatitis, herpes, tuberculosis, and human immunodeficiency virus (HIV).

Socioeconomic Status

Substance use knows no social barriers. In the inner city, however, substance use is concentrated in the lower socioeconomic classes. The pregnant substance user presenting for health care, regardless of socioeconomic status, should be seen by a social worker who can interview her to establish the circumstances of her current living conditions, assess her immediate needs, and begin planning for needs of the infant after delivery. Referrals for counseling should be made. Although an affluent substance user would not require financial assistance, other support measures and referrals to substance use programs should be made.

GENERAL APPROACH TO INFANT

An infant born to a substance user requires a careful general evaluation (Table 23-3) and particular attention to adverse effects known to be secondary to the specific substances to which he or she was exposed. The general approach includes the following guidelines.

Resuscitation and Stabilization

Because drug users frequently have had no or poor prenatal care, often little is known about the pregnancy at the time of the mother's admission to the labor and delivery suite. The pediatric team should be prepared to resuscitate the infant. Infants exposed to certain substances, in

Table 23–2. When First Presentation of Substance User to Health Care System Is during Labor

The following must be accomplished quickly:
  Alert pediatric team
  Obtain history for estimated gestational age, intercurrent illness
  Obtain prenatal laboratory tests, especially maternal blood type and hepatitis status
  Assess for rupture of membranes, meconium-stained fluid; consider use of antibiotics if membranes are ruptured
  Assess for presence of sexually transmitted diseases
  Obtain ultrasound for estimated fetal weight and gestational age

Table 23–3. General Approach to Infant

Birth	Resuscitate as needed
	Admit to general nursery unless otherwise indicated by gestational age, clinical condition, or history of maternal narcotic use
	Document maternal substance use patterns and prenatal care
	Consider obtaining urine/meconium for toxicology*
	Counsel mother regarding breast-feeding
Physical examination	Assess for presence of malformations
	Obtain specific diagnostic evaluations, such as cranial and renal ultrasounds, based on clinical indications only†
Gestational age and size	Perform careful evaluation for gestational age
	Plot growth parameters on standard growth chart
	Anticipate problems related to gestational age, size
	If growth retardation or microcephaly present, evaluate for etiology, including screening for congenital infection
Infections	
Acute bacterial	If premature or prolonged rupture of membranes, foul-smelling amniotic fluid, elevated maternal temperature: obtain CBC w/differential, blood culture, lumbar puncture, initiate antibiotics
Sexually transmitted/other diseases	Screen mother/infant (chlamydia, herpes, gonococcus, syphilis, hepatitis, human immunodeficiency virus, tuberculosis); initiate therapy per results
	Administer hepatitis vaccine if mother's hepatitis status is unknown
Social	Obtain social service consultation
	Initiate careful discharge planning, including appointments for follow-up of medical and neurodevelopmental status

*As indicated per institutional, state, or national guidelines.

†Subject to change pending evaluation of new data regarding consequences of gestational drug exposure.

particular, cocaine, are more likely to be compromised at birth from conditions such as asphyxia due to abruptio placentae. Overall, the frequency of prematurity and growth restriction is increased in infants born to substance users. The presence or absence of these conditions dictates specifics of care necessary at delivery and on admission to the nursery.

Gestational Age and Size

The estimated gestational age of the fetus of a substance user is often unknown. If possible, an ultrasound examination before delivery can give the pediatric team an estimated gestational age and fetal weight. After delivery and stabilization of the infant, a careful physical examination should be performed to detect malformations and to establish gestational age. All growth measurements should be plotted on standard growth charts, with attention to whether the infant is small for gestational age because numerous illicit substances can cause growth restriction. If growth restriction is present, other etiologies, such as congenital infections and chromosomal abnormalities, should be considered; growth restriction secondary to substance use is a diagnosis of exclusion. The incidence of prematurity is increased in women using a variety of substances. If preterm delivery occurs, problems associated with prematurity should be anticipated.

Bacterial Infections and Sexually Transmitted Diseases

Substance-using women may present for delivery with a history of ruptured membranes for several days.

Acute bacterial infection in the infant should be anticipated. If the obstetrician has initiated antibiotics in the mother, the pediatrician should consider treating the infant. If the obstetrician has not treated the mother with prolonged rupture of membranes, careful evaluation of the infant, including complete blood count, differential count, and blood culture, should be obtained. The decision to initiate antibiotics then is based on clinical judgment and laboratory results.

The incidence of sexually transmitted diseases is increased in substance users, with some reports showing 50% of cocaine users to have a documented infection during pregnancy. The evaluation of the infant for infectious diseases can be combined with the obstetrician's evaluation of the mother. If the obstetrician is obtaining studies to determine the presence of HIV in the mother, the pediatrician may wait for these results before initiating studies in the infant. Data concerning maternal exposure to infections with chlamydia, hepatitis, herpes, gonorrhea, syphilis, HIV, and tuberculosis are crucial to providing optimal care to the infant.

SPECIFIC SUBSTANCES

Cocaine

Cocaine, an alkaloidal agent derived from the plant *Erythroxylon coca,* is sold illegally in the United States for recreational use. Its use by pregnant women has increased dramatically in recent years. Modes of cocaine use are several, with the more frequent being intranasal or smoking. "Crack" cocaine, which is smoked, is the form most often used by inner city populations. Cocaine is a central nervous system (CNS) stimulant that alters mood and causes physiologic effects, such as tachycardia, hyperthermia, and hypertension. It blocks the reuptake of catecholamines at nerve terminals, increasing their concentrations in the peripheral nervous system and CNS.[5] Identification of the cocaine user is usually through interview and urine screens; hair analysis also has been used.[1]

The effects of cocaine in pregnancy have been studied by many investigators. Studies by Moore and associates[6] and Woods and colleagues[7] using pregnant ewes showed a dose-dependent decrease in uterine blood flow shortly after the ewes were injected with cocaine. The maternal systolic blood pressure increased within 1 minute and returned to baseline in approximately 10 minutes. The fetal blood pressure increased as well, lagging behind the maternal changes by several minutes. Of additional concern, these changes were accompanied by decreases in fetal oxygenation.

Decrease in uterine blood flow and the accompanying fetal hypoxemia are widely regarded as the cause of growth restriction in infants born to mothers using cocaine. Some investigators suggest, however, that the growth restriction in cocaine-exposed fetuses is more likely mulifactorial because cocaine-using mothers often use other substances known to reduce fetal weight, such as marijuana, alcohol, and tobacco. The women themselves may be poorly nourished.[8] Additional effects of cocaine on pregnancy include an increase in the incidence of preterm births and a possible increase in the incidence of abruptio placentae.[9]

Numerous effects of maternal cocaine use on the fetus and newborn have been suggested. Animal studies by some investigators showed an increase in congenital malformations in fetuses exposed to cocaine, whereas other studies did not show an increase.[10,11] Other literature supports the suggestion that cocaine is a teratogen and describes fetal vascular disruption in animals exposed to cocaine in utero.[12] This defect is believed to be secondary to an interruption of blood flow, which results in disruption of a previously normally formed part of the body. Although Hoyme and coworkers[13] reported findings in human infants consistent with this mechanism, a more recent study did not identify an increased number or consistent pattern of abnormalities.[14]

CNS bleeding and structural abnormalities were reported in one study in which mothers used cocaine and methamphetamine.[15] Several subsequent studies showed no increase in CNS hemorrhages.[16,17] Perinatal cerebral infarction secondary to maternal cocaine use also has been reported.[18] In addition to these reports of CNS structural abnormalities, some investigators have documented abnormal electroencephalogram tracings in infants exposed to cocaine in utero.[19]

A possible increase in genitourinary malformations in infants exposed to cocaine in utero is controversial. Early reports and one large retrospective study[20] suggested an increase, whereas more recent reports showed no increased risk.[21,22]

Two reports suggested an increased incidence of necrotizing enterocolitis in infants exposed to cocaine in utero.[23,24] The postulated mechanism was a decrease in intestinal blood flow experienced by the infant in utero.

Respiratory pattern abnormalities and an increase in sudden infant death syndrome (SIDS) are reported in infants exposed to cocaine in utero. The etiology of the increase in SIDS, as with other sequelae associated with cocaine exposure, may be multifactorial. Home monitoring is not recommended.[25]

The neurodevelopmental outcome of infants exposed to cocaine is a point of much interest and some controversy.[26] The potential for adverse outcome is suggested from animal studies and some human studies. Reports suggest that learning difficulties, abnormal play behavior, and potential effects on language skills occur with increased frequency in cocaine-exposed infants.[27,28] Other investigators have not reported these findings.[29,30] Because of the high likelihood of maternal polysubstance use and the influence of factors such as low socioeconomic status, any studies suggesting adverse long-term outcome in cocaine-exposed infants must carefully control for these confounding factors. In a cohort of inner city children followed since birth (half with cocaine exposure and half controls), there was no difference in developmental or intelligence quotient found; however, both groups performed below test norms.[31,32] Although there are conflicting reports regarding effect of gestational cocaine exposure on "macro" outcomes such as IQ, there are increasing concerns for more subtle adverse effects of gestational exposure. Mayes[33] suggested an emerging "cocaine baby syndrome," which includes abnormal arousal and attentional processing. Currently this is an active area of investigation by many researchers.

Management

A cocaine-using woman should be counseled about potential effects of cocaine use on her pregnancy, including risks for abruptio placentae, fetal growth restriction, preterm delivery, congenital malformations, and possible long-term adverse neurodevelopmental effects on the infant. She should be counseled to stop drug use and enter a drug treatment program. Because of the high likelihood of polysubstance use, sexually transmitted diseases, and chaotic social living conditions in cocaine-using women, additional medical investigations and social service intervention are crucial to ensure an improved outcome of pregnancy for the mother and the infant.

The newborn of a cocaine-using woman should have a careful physical examination and gestational age assessment at the time of delivery. If there are no perinatal conditions that demand special attention, infants exposed to cocaine in utero do not require admission to a newborn intensive care unit.

At this time, there are no recommendations that infants exposed to cocaine in utero have cranial or renal ultrasound examinations unless dictated by abnormal clinical condition, and there are no recommendations that cocaine-exposed infants be discharged on home monitors. Infants of cocaine users should be observed carefully, however, for feeding intolerance and be evaluated for exposure to sexually transmitted diseases. Their home environment should be assessed by social services before discharge from the hospital, with the discharge being delayed until an adequate caregiving situation is established. It is crucial that careful follow-up plans be established so that these infants can be evaluated for possible adverse neurodevelopmental outcome.

Cocaine-using mothers should not breast-feed their infants. Cocaine is found in breast milk, and cocaine intoxication has been described in infants breast-fed by their mothers.[34]

Narcotics

Opium, derived from the poppy *Papaver somniferum,* has been used for centuries as an analgesic. Among its derivatives are meperidine, heroin, methadone, and codeine. Specific opiate receptors have been located in the brain, but the exact mechanism by which these substances produce their effects is not known. Narcotics can be used by numerous routes: oral, intranasal, pulmonary (smoking), intramuscular, and intravenous. The effects of narcotic addiction on pregnancy are numerous and include virtually all the problems described in Table 23-1 and medical problems associated with intravenous substance use, such as cellulitis, thrombophlebitis, endocarditis, hepatitis, and presence of HIV. Identification of opiate use in a pregnant woman is primarily by interview or screen.

Because withdrawal of opiates in a pregnant woman can be associated with significant fetal distress and even death, detoxification of women during pregnancy is rarely attempted; rather, methadone maintenance programs are encouraged. Methadone can be taken orally, it is long acting, and its administration decreases the use of street drugs and the risks attendant to their use. Establishing a methadone dosing and maintenance program frequently requires admission of the pregnant addict to a substance abuse unit. Because withdrawal causes adverse effects in the fetus, narcotic antagonists (naloxone) should not be used in pregnant addicts unless absolutely necessary for the mother's health.[35]

Effects of heroin on the fetus and the newborn include growth restriction, prematurity, fetal distress, perinatal asphyxia, increased incidence of meconium-stained amniotic fluid, and withdrawal symptoms. A lower incidence of jaundice and respiratory distress syndrome has been reported.[36]

Withdrawal occurs in approximately 85% of infants born to narcotic-addicted mothers.[36] All narcotic-exposed infants should be monitored carefully, which may include admission to a newborn intensive care unit or special care nursery. As noted with heroin-addicted mothers, heroin-exposed infants with perinatal problems should not receive narcotic antagonists because their administration may precipitate seizures. The onset of withdrawal symptoms in a neonate occurs any time from the first 48 hours postdelivery to approximately 2 weeks postdelivery. The timing is related to the mother's daily dose and length of her addiction; in general, withdrawal seems more severe in infants whose mothers have used large amounts of the substance for an extended period.[37] Withdrawal from methadone has been reported to occur later than withdrawal from heroin. The classic signs of neonatal abstinence are listed in Table 23-4.

These signs have been codified into a neonatal abstinence scoring system that allows management and treatment of the infant according to individual scores (Fig. 23-1). Pharmacologic interventions described by Finnegan[37] are initiated when the total abstinence score is 8 or higher for three consecutive scorings or when the average of any three consecutive scorings is 8 or higher. Before pharmacotherapy is initiated, neonatal conditions that could cause similar signs, such as hypocalcemia, hypoglycemia, hypomagnesemia, hypothermia, and sepsis, should be considered and eliminated as causative factors. The pharmacotherapeutic agents most useful in neonatal abstinence syndrome are paregoric and phenobarbital. For precise directions for scoring, daily management of the infant, and use of pharmacotherapeutic drugs, the reader is referred to a review article.[37]

Management

A narcotic-using woman should be informed of the potential adverse effect on the fetus and counseled to cease use of these agents. Pregnant addicts should be entered in a methadone maintenance program. The newborn of an addict should be admitted to a neonatal intensive care unit or a nursery where careful observation and monitoring can be performed. The infant should receive a careful physical examination, gestational age and size for gestational age should be determined, and the infant should be monitored for withdrawal.

Additional diagnostics for opiate-exposed neonates, beyond those dictated by size, gestational age, and obvious

Table 23–4. Signs of Neonatal Abstinence

Central nervous system
  Excessive or continuous high-pitched crying
  Sleeplessness
  Hyperactivity
  Tremors
  Hypertonia
  Myoclonic jerks
  Seizures
Gastrointestinal
  Excessive sucking
  Poor feeding
  Regurgitation or vomiting
  Loose or watery stools
Other
  Sweating
  Fever
  Yawning
  Sneezing
  Mottling
  Nasal stuffiness
  Nasal flaring
  Tachypnea
  Excoriation (secondary to excessive movement)

Neonatal Abstinence Scoring System

System	Signs and Symptoms	Score	AM	PM	Comments
Central nervous system disturbances	Excessive high-pitched (or other) cry	2			Daily weight
	Continuous high-pitched (or other) cry	3			
	Sleeps < 1 hour after feeding	3			
	Sleeps < 2 hours after feeding	2			
	Sleeps < 3 hours after feeding	1			
	Hyperactive Moro reflex	2			
	Markedly hyperactive Moro reflex	3			
	Mild tremors disturbed	1			
	Moderate-severe tremors disturbed	2			
	Mild tremors undisturbed	3			
	Moderate-severe tremors undisturbed	4			
	Increased muscle tone	2			
	Excoriation (specific area)	1			
	Myoclonic jerks	3			
	Generalized convulsions	5			
Metabolic/vasomotor/respiratory disturbances	Sweating	1			
	Fever < 101° F (99-100.8° F/37.2-38.2° C)	1			
	Fever > 101° F (38.4° C and higher)	2			
	Frequent yawning (> 3-4 times/interval)	1			
	Mottling	1			
	Nasal stuffiness	1			
	Sneezing (> 3-4 times/interval)	1			
	Nasal flaring	2			
	Respiratory rate > 60/min	1			
	Respiratory rate > 60/min with retractions	2			
Gastrointestinal disturbances	Excessive sucking	1			
	Poor feeding	2			
	Regurgitation	2			
	Projectile vomiting	3			
	Loose stools	2			
	Watery stools	3			
	TOTAL SCORE				
	INITIALS OF SCORER				

Figure 23–1. Neonatal abstinence scoring system. *(From Finnegan LP: Neonatal abstinence syndrome: Assessment and pharmacotherapy. In Rubaltelli FF, Granati B [eds]: Neonatal Therapy: An Update. Amsterdam, Elsevier Science, 1986. Copyright F. Rubaltelli.)*

problems at delivery, are not indicated. SIDS is reported to be increased in infants of opiate addicts[38]; however, home monitoring is not routinely recommended. Long-term behavior problems in children exposed to narcotics in utero have been suggested. The true source of these problems is difficult to define because narcotic-exposed newborns also may experience a long period of withdrawal, which could affect behavior. If these infants are placed with the addicted mother or in a less than optimal socioeconomic situation, these factors themselves could affect outcome.[35] Regardless of the cause of adverse neurodevelopmental or behavioral outcomes, infants exposed to narcotics in utero should be followed carefully so that interventions, if indicated, can be instituted.

Heroin crosses into breast milk. The American Academy of Pediatrics (AAP) considers heroin use a contraindication for breast-feeding.[39]

Alcohol

Alcohol use among women is common, with an estimated 8% to 11% of women of childbearing age classified as either problem drinkers or alcoholics. Alcohol crosses the placenta freely. Although it acts primarily as a CNS depressant in adults, it is believed to be a teratogen in the fetus. Suggested mechanisms for this effect include increased cellular peroxidase activity; decreased DNA synthesis; and impaired cellular growth, differentiation, and migration. Interference in amino acid transport across the placenta may account for the adverse effect on fetal growth.[40]

Identification of alcohol use in pregnancy usually occurs through patient interview; the identification of use and documentation of the amount of alcohol consumed can be difficult because of patient denial. It is particularly important to determine the degree of maternal alcohol consumption because heavy use is associated with a spectrum of fetal effects called the **fetal alcohol syndrome (FAS)**.

Moderate alcohol use in pregnancy is associated with an increased risk for spontaneous abortions. Low birth weight is more frequent in infants born to women who consume alcohol, even in the absence of full-blown FAS. Some reports show an increase in abruptio placentae in pregnancies of women who consume alcohol.[40]

The effects of alcohol on the fetus range from prenatal growth reduction to FAS. The diagnosis of FAS, proposed by the Fetal Alcohol Study Group of the Research Society on Alcoholism, is made when at least one abnormality from each category shown in Table 23-5 is present.[40] In addition to items listed in the table, infants may show other stigmata of dysmorphogenesis, including joint anomalies, small distal phalanges, small fifth fingernails, heart murmur, ventricular septal defect, atrial septal defect, ptosis, cleft lip or palate, micrognathia, mottling, webbed neck, cervical vertebral anomalies, rib anomalies, and hypoplastic labia majora.[41]

The incidence of FAS varies with the ethnic population and the geographic area under consideration. Overall in the United States, FAS rates are estimated to range from 1 case per 300 to 1 or 2 cases per 1000 live births. FAS is now thought to be a leading cause of mental retardation in the United States. FAS reportedly occurs only in infants born to frankly alcoholic mothers whose intake is 8 to 10 drinks or more per day. Although the American Council on Science and Health recommends that pregnant women limit alcohol consumption to no more than two drinks daily (1 oz or 30 mL of absolute alcohol), most health care professionals recommend total abstinence from alcohol as the best course for pregnant women.[36,42]

Management

Pregnant women who admit to alcohol use should be informed of possible fetal effects. Some experts recommend termination of pregnancy in women with heavy use in the first trimester. Women should be counseled to cease alcohol use or, at minimum, to limit consumption to no more than two drinks daily.

Table 23-5. Criteria for the Diagnosis of Fetal Alcohol Syndrome According to the Fetal Alcohol Study Group*

Prenatal and/or postnatal growth retardation; failure to thrive (weight, length, and/or head circumference < 10th percentile)

Central nervous system involvement includes signs of neurologic abnormalities (irritability in infancy and hyperactivity during childhood), developmental delay, hypotonia, or intellectual impairment (mild to moderate mental retardation)

Characteristic facial dysmorphology (at least two of three)
Microcephaly (head circumference < 3rd percentile)
Microphthalmia and/or short palpebral fissures
Poorly developed philtrum
Thin upper lip (vermilion border)
Flattening or absence of the maxilla

*One abnormality from each group must be present.

Modified from Pietrantoni M, Knuppel RA: Alcohol use in pregnancy. Clin Perinatol 81:93, 1991.

Care of the infant born to an alcohol-using mother includes (1) evaluation for acute intoxication—infants born to intoxicated women may smell of alcohol and have cord blood alcohol levels indicating they are legally drunk; (2) observation for withdrawal[43]; and (3) evaluation for evidence of FAS—infants exposed to alcohol in utero should have a careful evaluation for stigmata of FAS. In some cases, evaluation by a geneticist may be helpful.

Infants with prenatal alcohol exposure are at high risk for adverse neurodevelopmental outcome. There should be careful discharge planning with attention to scheduling follow-up visits.

Alcohol crosses into breast milk. The AAP considers maternal alcohol use usually compatible with breast-feeding,[39] although some literature[44] suggests that infants chronically exposed may have lower scores on the Psychomotor Development Index of the Bayley Scales of Infant Development.

Marijuana

Marijuana, derived from *Cannabis sativa,* is the most commonly used illicit drug among women of childbearing age with estimates of use among pregnant women ranging from 3% to 16%.[45] It is smoked for its hallucinogenic properties. The major psychoactive ingredient is Δ-9-tetrahydrocannabinol (THC). Metabolites of THC can be detected in the urine 1 to 2 weeks after last use.[46] Identification of marijuana use is through interview and urine screen.

The effect of maternal marijuana use on the fetus and newborn is best described as controversial. There are conflicting reports on the effect of marijuana on intrauterine growth, incidence of prematurity, malformations, and long-term developmental and neurobehavioral outcome. Studies that show an effect on growth in general do not show dramatic effects. Although malformations have been reported,[47,48] no consistent pattern has been documented, and in many cases pregnancy was complicated by polysubstance use. Although some studies show no differences on scores of the Bayley Scales of Infant Development or on the scores of the Wechsler Preschool and Primary Scales of Intelligence,[49] others suggest long-term effects on neurocognitive function, with deficits in vigilance and increased impulsive and hyperactive behaviors.[50]

The conflicting reports surrounding effects of marijuana on pregnancy and the newborn may arise from confounding from effects of other substances the pregnant woman may be using. Further investigations are needed to define specific effects of marijuana more fully.

Management

Management of the pregnant marijuana user should concentrate on defining use, if any, of other substances; counseling to stop use of marijuana; and attention to lifestyle needs. Management of the newborn should involve a careful physical examination and assessment of growth and size for gestational age. No further diagnostics are necessary unless dictated by individual infant condition.

THC is excreted in breast milk. The AAP considers use of marijuana during breast-feeding to be contraindicated.[39]

Cigarettes

Cigarette smoking is common among women, with some estimates of use among pregnant women of 25%. Identification of cigarette use in pregnancy is through interview. In cigarette-smoking women there is an increased risk of fetal growth restriction. The mechanism for growth restriction is uncertain but may include fetal hypoxia from carbon monoxide production or from nicotine-induced vasospasm. An average growth reduction of approximately 200 g can be anticipated in term infants whose mothers smoke one pack of cigarettes per day.[51] Additional concerns in infants born to cigarette smokers include increased risk for SIDS,[52] increased blood pressure,[53] effects on early infant lung function,[54] and vascular retinal abnormalities[55] in infants born to cigarette smokers.

Management

Management of pregnant smokers should include counseling to stop or decrease smoking during pregnancy. Attention should be given to defining any other substance use. A newborn exposed to cigarette use in utero should have a careful physical examination. Growth parameters should be plotted on standard charts, and size for gestational age should be assessed. Any infant with significant growth restriction also should be evaluated for causes other than maternal cigarette use, including evaluations for congenital infection, chromosomal abnormalities, and syndromes with prenatal growth deficiency. There are numerous reports of increased risk of SIDS in infants of mothers who smoked during pregnancy; however, currently there is no recommendation that these infants be discharged on home monitors. The AAP considers nicotine use to be contraindicated during breast-feeding.[39]

Amphetamines

Amphetamines are sympathomimetic drugs that act as CNS stimulants. Their mechanism of action seems to be through release of neurotransmitters from presynaptic neurons. Routes of use include oral, nasal, and intravenous administration. Women, including pregnant women, may take amphetamines for appetite suppression and illicitly for stimulant effects.[36] Identification of amphetamine use is through interview and urine screen.

Amphetamine addiction in pregnancy is associated with shortened gestation and growth restriction.[56] As with other illicit substances, however, it is difficult to separate the effect of amphetamine use alone from the frequently coexisting polysubstance use and attendant lifestyle factors. Infant amphetamine withdrawal, described by several investigators, consists of shrill cry, irritability, jerking, sneezing, diaphoresis, and drowsiness.[57,58] Amphetamine use seems to carry little risk of teratogenicity, although some concern exists for an increase in cardiac defects in a fetus exposed to amphetamines.[59] One report of infants exposed to methamphetamine and cocaine in utero showed an increased risk of cranial abnormalities detected by ultrasound.[15] The mechanism of cerebral injury is believed to be secondary to vasoconstriction.

Management

Pregnant women using amphetamines should be counseled to stop use and to enroll in a substance use treatment program. The newborn should receive a careful physical examination with particular attention to the cardiovascular system and CNS. Assessment for gestational age and size for gestational age should be carried out. Monitoring for withdrawal should be instituted. To date, there is no clear indication for further diagnostics unless indicated by individual infant condition.

Amphetamines are found in breast milk. The AAP recommends that amphetamine-using mothers not breast-feed their infants.[39]

Ecstasy

Methylenedioxymethamphetamine (Ecstasy) use has increased, particularly in young women of childbearing age. Ecstasy has hallucinogenic properties; the mechanism of action is similar to that of amphetamines. Identification of use is through history.

Despite the increase in ecstasy use, there are few data regarding effects on human pregnancy. One prospective follow-up of 136 infants with gestational exposure suggested, however, a significantly increased risk of congenital defects, with a predominance of cardiovascular (26 per 1000 live births [3 to 90]) and musculoskeletal anomalies (38 per 1000 live births [8 to 109]). Birth weights were in the expected range for term infants.[60]

Management

Management of pregnant ecstasy users should include counseling to cease use. Use of other substances should be defined, with appropriate counseling given. Management of the newborn should involve a careful physical examination, with attention to the cardiovascular and musculoskeletal systems. No further diagnostics are necessary unless dictated by an individual infant's condition.

REFERENCES

1. Graham K, Koren G, Klein J, et al: Determination of gestational cocaine exposure by hair analysis. JAMA 262:3328, 1989.
2. Ostrea EM Jr, Welch RA: Detection of prenatal drug exposure in the pregnant woman and her newborn infant. Clin Perinatol 18:629, 1991.
3. Ostrea EM Jr, Matias O, Keane C, et al: Spectrum of gestational exposure to illicit drugs and other xenobiotic agents in newborn infants by meconium analysis. J Pediatr 133:513, 1998.
4. Ostrea EM Jr, Brady M, Gause S, et al: Drug screening of newborns by meconium analysis: A large-scale, prospective, epidemiologic study. Pediatrics 89:107, 1992.
5. Farrar HC, Kearns GL: Cocaine: Clinical pharmacology and toxicology. J Pediatr 115:665, 1989.
6. Moore TR, Sorg J, Miller L, et al: Hemodynamic effects of intravenous cocaine on the pregnant ewe and fetus. Am J Obstet Gynecol 155:883, 1986.
7. Woods JR, Plessinger MA, Clark K: Effect of cocaine on uterine blood flow and fetal oxygenation. JAMA 257:957, 1987.
8. Zuckerman B, Frank DA, Hingson R, et al: Effects of maternal marijuana and cocaine use on fetal growth. N Engl J Med 320:762, 1989.
9. MacGregor SN, Keith LG, Chasnoff IJ: Cocaine use during pregnancy: Adverse perinatal outcome. Am J Obstet Gynecol 157:686, 1987.
10. Fantel AG, Macphail BJ: The teratogenicity of cocaine. Teratology 26:17, 1982.
11. Mahalik MP, Gautieri RF, Mann DE Jr: Teratogenic potential of cocaine hydrochloride in CF-1 mice. J Pharm Sci 190:703, 1990.
12. Webster WS, Brown-Woodman PD: Cocaine as a cause of congenital malformations of vascular origin: Experimental evidence in the rat. Teratology 41:689, 1990.
13. Hoyme HE, Jones KL, Dixon SD, et al: Prenatal cocaine exposure and fetal vascular disruption. Pediatrics 85:743, 1990.
14. Behnke M, Eyler FD, Garvan CW, et al: The search for congenital malformations in newborns with fetal cocaine exposure. Pediatrics 107:E74, 2001.
15. Dixon SD, Bejar R: Echoencephalographic findings in neonates associated with maternal cocaine and methamphetamine use: Incidence and clinical correlates. J Pediatr 115:770, 1989.
16. Dusick AM, Covert RF, Schreiber MD, et al: Risk of intracranial hemorrhage and other adverse outcomes after cocaine exposure in a cohort of 323 very low birth weight infants. J Pediatr 122:438, 1993.
17. Frank DA, McCarten K, Cabral H, et al: Cranial ultrasounds in term newborns: Failure to replicate excess abnormalities in cocaine exposed. Pediatr Res 31:247A, 1992.
18. Chasnoff IJ, Bussey ME, Savich R, et al: Perinatal cerebral infarction and maternal cocaine use. J Pediatr 108:456, 1986.
19. Legido A, Clancy RR, Spitzer AR, et al: Electroencephalographic and behavioral-state studies in infants of cocaine-addicted mothers. Am J Dis Child 146:748, 1992.
20. Chavez GF, Mulinare J, Cordero JF: Maternal cocaine use during early pregnancy as a risk factor for congenital urogenital anomalies. JAMA 262:795, 1989.
21. Rajegowda BK, Lala R, Nagaraj A, et al: Results of renal ultrasound in babies born to cocaine (CO) abusing mothers. Pediatr Res 31:407A, 1992.
22. Rosenstein BJ, Wheeler JS, Heid PL: Congenital renal abnormalities in infants with in utero cocaine exposure. J Urol 144:110, 1990.
23. Porat R, Brodsky N: Cocaine: A risk factor for necrotizing enterocolitis. J Perinatol 11:30, 1991.
24. Telsey AM, Merrit TA, Dixon SD: Cocaine exposure in a term neonate: Necrotizing enterocolitis as a complication. Clin Pediatr 27:547, 1988.
25. Bauchner H, Zuckerman B: Cocaine, sudden infant death syndrome, and home monitoring [editorial]. J Pediatr 117:904, 1990.
26. Frank DA, Augustyn M, Knight WG, et al: Growth, development, and behavior in early childhood following prenatal cocaine exposure: A systematic review. JAMA 285:1613, 2001.
27. Rodning C, Beckwith L, Howard J: Prenatal exposure to drugs: Behavioral distortions reflecting CNS impairment? Neurotoxicology 10:629, 1989.
28. Singer LT, Arendt R, Minnes S, et al: Developing language skills of cocaine-exposed infants. Pediatrics 107:1057, 2001.
29. Hurt H, Brodsky NL, Betancourt L, et al: Play behavior in toddlers with in utero cocaine exposure: A prospective, masked, controlled study. J Dev Behav Pediatr 17:373, 1996.
30. Hurt H, Brodsky NL, Betancourt L, et al: Cocaine-exposed children: Follow-up through 30 months. J Dev Behav Pediatr 16:29, 1995.
31. Hurt H, Malmud E, Betancourt LM, et al: A prospective comparison of developmental outcome of children with in utero cocaine exposure and controls using the Battelle Developmental Inventory. J Dev Behav Pediatr 22:27, 2001.
32. Hurt H, Malmud EK, Betancourt LM, et al: Inner-city children perform poorly on intelligence testing regardless of in utero cocaine exposure. Arch Pediatr Adolesc Med 151:1237, 1997.
33. Mayes LC: Developing brain and in utero cocaine exposure: Effects on neural ontogeny. Dev Psychopathol 11:685, 1999.
34. Chasnoff IJ, Lewis DE, Squires L: Cocaine intoxication in a breast-fed infant. Pediatrics 80:836, 1987.
35. Hoegerman G, Schnoll S: Narcotic use in pregnancy. Clin Perinatol 18:51, 1991.
36. Briggs GG, Freeman RK, Yaffe SJ: Drugs in Pregnancy and Lactation: A Reference Guide to Fetal and Neonatal Risk, 4th ed. Baltimore, Williams & Wilkins, 1994.
37. Finnegan LP: Neonatal abstinence syndrome. In Nelson NM (ed): Current Therapy in Neonatal-Perinatal Medicine. Philadelphia, BC Decker, 1990.
38. Finnegan L: In-utero opiate dependence and sudden infant death syndrome. Clin Perinatol 6:163, 1979.
39. American Academy of Pediatrics Committee on Drugs: Transfer of drugs and other chemicals into human milk. Pediatrics 93:137, 1994.
40. Pietrantoni M, Knuppel RA: Alcohol use in pregnancy. Clin Perinatol 18:93, 1991.
41. Jones KL: Fetal alcohol effects. In: Smith's Recognizable Patterns of Human Malformation, 4th ed. Philadelphia, WB Saunders, 1988, pp 491-494.
42. Council on Scientific Affairs, AMA: Fetal effects of maternal alcohol use. JAMA 249:2517, 1983.
43. Coles CD, Smith IE, Fernhoff PM, et al: Neonatal ethanol withdrawal: Characteristics in clinically normal, nondysmorphic neonates. J Pediatr 105:445, 1984.

44. Little RE, Anderson KW, Ervin CH, et al: Maternal alcohol use during breast-feeding and infant mental and motor development at one year. N Engl J Med 321:425, 1989.

45. National Institute on Drug Abuse: National Household Survey on Drug Abuse: Main Findings 1985. Rockville, MD, National Institute on Drug Abuse, 1998.

46. Gold MS: Marijuana. New York, Plenum, 1989.

47. Hingson R, Alpert JJ, Dooling N, et al: Effects of maternal drinking and marijuana use on fetal growth and development. Pediatrics 70:539, 1982.

48. Qazi QH, Mariano E, Milman DH, et al: Abnormalities in offspring associated with prenatal marijuana exposure. Dev Pharmacol Ther 8:141, 1985.

49. Fried PA, Watkinson B: 12- and 24-month neurobehavioral follow-up of children prenatally exposed to marijuana, cigarettes and alcohol. Neurotoxicol Teratol 10:305, 1988.

50. Fried PA, Watkinso B, Gray R; Differential effects on cognitive functioning in 9- to 12-year olds prenatally exposed to cigarettes and marijuana. Neurotoxicol Teratol 20:293, 1998.

51. Martinez A, Partridge JC, Bean X, et al: Perinatal substance abuse. In Taeusch HW, Ballard RA (eds): Avery's Diseases of the Newborn, 7th ed. Philadelphia, WB Saunders, 1998, pp 103-118.

52. Hoffman HJ, Hillman LS: Epidemiology of the sudden infant death syndrome: Maternal, maternal, neonatal and postnatal risk factors. Clin Perinatol 19:717, 1992.

53. Beratis NG, Panagoulias D, Varvarigou A: Increased blood pressure in neonates and infants whose mothers smoked during pregnancy. J Pediatr 128:806, 1996.

54. Hanrahan JP, Tager IB, Segal MR, et al: The effect of maternal smoking during pregnancy on early infant lung function. Am Rev Respir Dis 145:1129, 1992.

55. Beratis NG, Varvarigou A, Katsibris J, et al: Vascular retinal abnormalities in neonates of mothers who smoked during pregnancy. J Pediatr 136:760, 2000.

56. Little BB, Snell LM, Gilstrap LC 3rd: Methamphetamine abuse during pregnancy: Outcome and fetal effects. Obstet Gynecol 72:541, 1988.

57. Eriksson M, Larsson G, Winbladh B, et al: The influence of amphetamine addiction on pregnancy and the newborn infant. Acta Paediatr Scand 67:95, 1978.

58. Ramer CM: The case history of an infant born to an amphetamine-addicted mother. Clin Pediatr 13:596, 1974.

59. Nora JJ, Vargo TA, Nora AH, et al: Dexamphetamine: A possible environmental trigger in cardiovascular malformations. Lancet 1:1290, 1970.

60. McElhatton PR, Bateman DN, Evans C, et al: Congenital anomalies after prenatal ecstasy exposure. Lancet 354:1441, 1999.

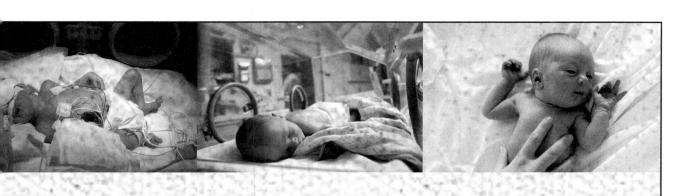

Management Considerations
in the High-Risk Pregnancy

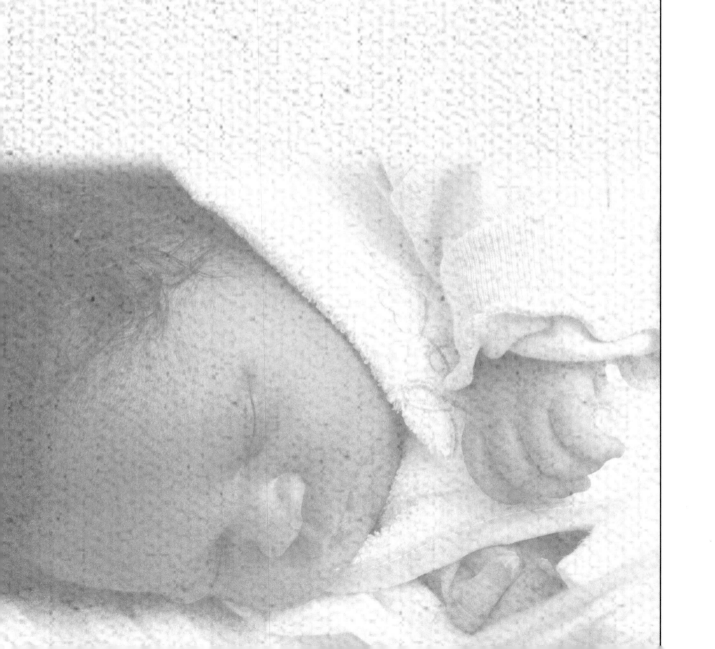

CHAPTER 24

Preterm Labor

Reinaldo Figueroa and Paul L. Ogburn, Jr.

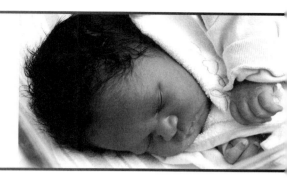

Preterm labor and the resulting preterm birth are major unsolved problems in obstetric care. Although advances in obstetrics and neonatology have resulted in significant improvements in perinatal outcomes, preterm delivery still is associated with more perinatal morbidity and mortality than any other obstetric condition except for birth defects.[1] In developed countries, approximately 5% to 10% of all pregnancies result in preterm delivery; most of these are a result of preterm labor.[2,3]

Preterm delivery, or delivery occurring before the completion of 37 weeks of gestation, can be spontaneous or indicated. Spontaneous preterm delivery includes preterm labor; preterm rupture of membranes; and related conditions, such as cervical incompetence or amnionitis.[4] Spontaneous deliveries account for approximately 70% to 80% of all preterm deliveries.[5-7] Indicated deliveries account for 20% to 30% of preterm deliveries and include medical or obstetric conditions that increase the risk for a maternal or fetal adverse outcome.[8-10] Conditions such as preeclampsia, intrauterine growth restriction, placental abruption, placenta previa, and fetal demise are responsible for most indicated preterm deliveries. These topics are discussed elsewhere in this book.

In the 1980s and 1990s, the use of assisted reproductive technologies, such as in vitro fertilization and gamete intrafallopian transfer, and ovulation induction to achieve successful pregnancies revolutionized the field of infertility. In singleton gestations conceived after in vitro fertilization, however, the risks of preterm delivery and neonates with low birth weight are reported to be increased compared with pregnancies conceived spontaneously.[11,12] The incidence of multiple gestations has increased as these assisted reproductive technologies have improved and become more widely available.[13] In the United States, twin live births accounted for 28.1 per 1000 live births in 1997, an increase from 18.9 per 1000 live births in 1980.[14] The rate of triplet and higher order multiple births in the United States was 193.5 per 100,000 live births in 1998, a fivefold increase from 37 per 100,000 live births in 1980.[14]

In the United States, the preterm delivery rate has increased steadily from 9.4% in 1981 to 11.8% in 1999.[1] Preterm delivery is associated with 70% of neonatal and infant deaths.[15] The total expenditure for maternal hospitalization due to preterm labor with or without delivery has been estimated to be greater than $820 million.[16] Annual health care costs from premature births are estimated to be billions of dollars for neonatal intensive care alone.[17] Since the 1990s, there has been an increase in the survival of extremely premature infants. Survival rates for neonates at 22 weeks are 0 to 21%; at 23 weeks, 5% to 46%; at 24 weeks, 40% to 59%; at 25 weeks, 60% to 82%; and at 26 weeks, 75% to 93%.[18] Of survivors, 20% to 25% have at least one major disability; 50% of disabled infants have more than one major disability.[18] Half of all extremely premature infants have one or more subtle neurodevelopmental disabilities in the school and teenage years.[18] Preterm labor has significant consequences for public health in the United States. The risk factors for preterm labor are presented in Table 24-1.

MECHANISMS OF PRETERM LABOR

Risk Factors

Epidemiologic factors that have been associated with preterm delivery include nonwhite race, maternal age younger than 17 years or older than 35 years, low socioeconomic status, and low prepregnancy weight.[19-23] Smoking increases the risk of preterm delivery and low birth weight, and it may increase the risk for spontaneous abortion.[24-26] Cocaine use has been associated with preterm delivery.[27-29]

A history of preterm delivery is a significant risk factor for future preterm delivery (Table 24-2).[20,30,31] This risk is particularly significant if the preterm birth occurred in the second trimester. The risk of delivering prematurely in a subsequent pregnancy is increased sixfold to eightfold whether the patient had rupture of membranes or not.[32] Vaginal bleeding in more than one trimester has been associated with an increase in preterm delivery.[33]

Table 24–1. Risk Factors for Preterm Labor

Factor	Preterm Labor Rate (%)
Multiple gestations	51
Dilated cervix at 32 wk	43
Abdominal surgery during pregnancy	41
Effaced cervix at 32 wk	33
Uterine anomaly	33
Exposure to diethylstilbestrol	33
Prior preterm delivery	31
Irritable uterus	29
Hydramnios	26
Prior preterm labor	25
History of cone biopsy	22
Bleeding after 12 wk	21
Two or more second-trimester abortions	20
Febrile illness	17

Adapted from Iams JD, Johnson FF, Creasy RK: Prevention of preterm birth. Clin Obstet Gynecol 31:599, 1988.

Uterine anomalies also have been associated with preterm delivery (Table 24-3).[34-36] Women with myomas have an increased risk of preterm delivery, especially if the myomas are large.[37,38] Cervical conization has been associated with an increased risk of preterm delivery.[39,40] A study showed that induced abortions may be associated with preterm delivery in subsequent pregnancies.[41]

As mentioned earlier, multiple gestations have resulted in an increase in the incidence of preterm births. Multiple gestations account for 13% of all preterm births. It is possible that the use of assisted reproductive technologies adds to the prematurity risk of multiple gestations, although the reports are inconsistent.[42,43]

Occupational exertion among pregnant women has been implicated in the increasing rate of preterm delivery.[44,45] Although an earlier study showed that there was an increase in infants with low birth weight and not in preterm delivery among working women,[46] a more recent study has shown an increase in spontaneous preterm birth associated with long periods of standing (>40 hr/wk).[47]

Intrauterine infection has been associated with preterm labor and preterm delivery, particularly among the subset of women who have progressive labor that is ultimately refractory to tocolysis.[48-51] Such intrauterine infection may be present even in the absence of clinical maternal infection and has been diagnosed via positive culture of amniocentesis-derived amniotic fluid in patients with intact membrane and idiopathic preterm labor.[51-55] Elevated levels of amniotic fluid cytokines, particularly interleukin-6, tumor necrosis factor, and interleukin-1, have been associated with intrauterine infection and preterm delivery.[53,56-58]

Iams and colleagues[59] reported their experience in frequency of preterm labor based on associated pregnancy complications (see Table 24-1). Although there are historical risk factors that can alert clinicians to the potential risk of preterm birth, it may be that the best predictors of low risk for preterm birth in a current pregnancy are ultrasound showing a cervical length greater than 25 mm without funneling seen at the internal os and the absence of fetal fibronectin detected in the upper vagina.[60]

Biochemical Mechanisms

Many different factors are believed to trigger preterm labor.[61-65] Possible mechanisms for preterm labor include (1) inflammatory responses associated with infection,[66,67] fevers, flares of systemic lupus erythematosus, and inflammatory bowel disease; (2) tissue ischemia or acidosis associated with placental insufficiency, placental abruption, fetal growth restriction, and diabetic ketoacidosis; (3) uterine stretching or irritation associated with multiple gestations, polyhydramnios, degenerating myomas, abdominal surgery, uterine anomalies, and incompetent cervix; (4) hormonal changes associated with stress,[68] prolonged standing, and other conditions; and (5) idiopathic causes (may include racial variation and familial increased incidence of preterm labor).

Term and preterm labor may share a common final pathway composed of uterine contractility, cervical dilation, and activation of the membranes.[69] Romero and

Table 24–2. Preterm Birth and Postobstetric Outcome*

No. of Mothers	First Birth	Second Birth	Subsequent Preterm Birth %	Relative Risk
25,817	Not preterm		4.4	1.0
1860	Preterm		17.2	3.9
24,689	Not preterm	Not preterm	2.6	0.6
1540	Preterm	Not preterm	5.7	1.3
1128	Not preterm	Preterm	11.1	2.5
320	Preterm	Preterm	28.4	6.5

*Based on 27,677 mothers with their first three singleton births, Norway, 1967 to 1976.

Adapted from Bakketeig LS, Hoffman HJ: Epidemiology of preterm births. In Elder MG, Hendricks CH (eds): Preterm Labor. London, Butterworths, 1981.

Table 24-3. Uterine Anomalies and Pregnancy Outcome

Uterine Anomaly	No. of Patients	Pregnancies	No. of Abortions (%)	No. of Preterm Labor (%*)	Fetal Survival Rate (%)
Unicornuate	10	15	7 (47)	3 (38)	40
Didelphic	13	25	8 (32)	6 (35)	64
Bicornuate	62	144	40 (28)	28 (27)	64
Septate	41	81	21 (26)	7 (12)	77

*Calculated as percentage of pregnancies >20 weeks' gestation.

Adapted from Heinonen PK, Saarikoski S, Pystynen P: Reproductive performance of women with uterine anomalies. Acta Obstet Gynecol Scand 61:157, 1982.

colleagues[69] described what they called the **preterm labor syndrome,** suggesting that preterm labor is a pathologic condition resulting from multiple etiologies. Term labor results from multifactorial physiologic events eventually activating the components of the final common pathway. Preterm labor results from pathologic processes that activate some of the components of the term labor pathway. Term labor and preterm labor are associated with an increase in uterine contractility. There is an increase in myometrial gap junction formation and up-regulation of myometrial oxytocin receptors. The cervix, composed primarily of connective tissue, undergoes changes in preparation for parturition in normal labor and preterm labor. The biochemical events associated with cervical ripening are a decrease in total collagen content, an increase in collagen solubility, and an increase in collagenolytic activity. Another similarity between term labor and preterm labor is activation of the decidua and membranes, which occurs through a series of biochemical and anatomic events. The membranes separate from the decidua, allowing for rupture of membranes and postpartum expulsion of the placenta. Degradation of the extracellular matrix (fibronectin) and the enzymatic activity of the matrix metalloproteinases have been implicated in decidual and membrane activation.[70] These changes seen in human labor at term occur gradually over days to weeks. When the uterus and the cervix are prepared, endocrine or paracrine factors from the fetoplacental unit switch the irregular uterine contractions to a pattern of regular contractions.[71] This switch in uterine contractility may be coordinated by the fetus through different mechanisms, including the influence of the fetus on placental steroid hormone production, mechanical distention of the uterus, secretion of neurohypophyseal hormones, and stimulation of prostaglandin synthesis.[64,65]

Many different pathologic conditions have been associated with preterm delivery. Approximately 25% of preterm labors are believed to result from intraamniotic infection.[67,72,73] In this hostile environment to the fetus, the fetoplacental unit is believed to trigger labor prematurely. Elevated levels of lipoxygenase and cyclooxygenase pathway products can be shown in many women with infection.[74,75] Increased concentrations of cytokines in the amniotic fluid of these women have been found.[53,56-58]

Some women who deliver prematurely have been found to have lesions in the maternal and fetal vasculature.[76]

These lesions have been identified as failure of physiologic transformation of the spiral arteries, atherosis, maternal or fetal arterial thrombosis, and a decrease in the number of arterioles in the villi.[69] Preterm labor could result from uteroplacental ischemia caused by maternal vascular lesions, whereas fetal compromise from fetal lesions could lead to preterm labor.[69]

Uterine overdistention could result in preterm labor. Women with multiple gestations, polyhydramnios, or müllerian duct abnormalities are at increased risk of preterm delivery. It is suspected that uterine overdistention may activate a pressor-sensitive system causing labor.[69] Stretching of the chorioamniotic membranes can induce production of cytokines by the membranes initiating parturition. Other authors have shown that women with multiple gestations or polyhydramnios have enhanced amniotic expression and activity of cyclooxygenase-2.[77] The expression of cyclooxygenase-2 mediates labor in humans.[78,79]

Cervical disease as a result of a congenital disorder, surgical trauma, or traumatic damage to the structural integrity of the cervix can lead to preterm delivery. Cervical incompetence is seen now as part of a continuum with preterm labor and could be responsible for some cases of preterm delivery.[62]

Abnormal allograft reaction and allergic phenomena have been proposed as potential mechanisms of preterm labor.[69] Low endogenous calcium inhibitor activity in fetal membranes has been suggested as a possible cause of idiopathic preterm labor.[80] Another possible cause of idiopathic preterm labor is deficiency of the enzyme 15-hydroxyprostaglandin dehydrogenase, the enzyme responsible for degrading the primary prostaglandins.[81] Present in the chorion and decidua, deficiency of this enzyme may impair the ability of the fetal membranes to metabolize the primary prostaglandins, allowing prostaglandin E_2 to initiate contractions. A physiologic mechanism for preterm labor secondary to placental abruption has been proposed when thrombin was found to be a powerful uterotonic agent.[82,83]

The production of adrenal and hypothalamic stress hormones can be increased by maternal and fetal stress. The increase in these hormones can enhance the expression of corticotropin-releasing hormone in the placenta, decidua, and amniochorion.[68] Corticotropin-releasing hormone increases prostaglandin production from the decidua and amniochorion, causing uterine contractility. Corticotropin-releasing hormone also could be increased as a result of uteroplacental vascular ischemia and fetal hypoxemia caused by decidual hemorrhage.

ASSESSMENT OF RISK FACTORS FOR PRETERM LABOR

Much research has been done in an attempt to allow for the early diagnosis of preterm labor and to predict women at highest risk for developing preterm labor. More intensive preterm labor surveillance programs could be instituted for pregnancies found to be at increased risk. In predicting whether a woman is at risk of preterm delivery, there is the hope an intervention would be available to diagnose preterm labor earlier, to improve the effectiveness of treatment (delaying delivery), and to improve the neonatal outcome. An important intervention is the opportunity to administer maternal corticosteroid therapy as recommended by the National Institutes of Health because it is strongly associated with decreased morbidity and mortality.[84-86] Tocolytic therapy can be given to the mother to prolong pregnancy so that corticosteroids can be administered.

Risk Scoring Systems

Risk scoring systems based on history and epidemiologic data have been designed to determine the risk of preterm delivery.[87-92] These systems were intended as screening profiles, to stratify women within the general population into high-risk and low-risk groups for preterm delivery so that high-risk patients could be followed in a more intensive manner during their pregnancies.

In general, risk scoring systems have been unable to identify reliably women who will give birth preterm. Because approximately 50% of preterm deliveries occur in a first pregnancy,[93] this single limitation of risk factor scoring systems renders them particularly ineffective. The low sensitivity of the systems used in these studies shows that 70% of women who ultimately deliver before term may not be categorized.[88,89,91,92,94] The low positive predictive values imply that three quarters of women categorized "high risk" eventually have term deliveries and not only are categorized incorrectly, but also are subjected unnecessarily to potentially costly intervention programs (Table 24-4).

Bacterial Vaginosis

Bacterial vaginosis is a common alteration of the normal vaginal flora in which the normal lactobacilli-predominant flora is replaced by *Gardnerella vaginalis*, *Mobiluncus* species, anaerobes, and mycoplasmas.[95] It has been found in 10% to 20% of pregnant women[96] and more frequently in African American women than in white women.[97] Although the major symptom of bacterial vaginosis is malodorous vaginal discharge, 50% of women with bacterial vaginosis do not have symptoms.[98]

The presence of bacterial vaginosis has been associated with spontaneous preterm delivery, midtrimester loss, premature rupture of membranes, chorioamnionitis, and amniotic fluid colonization.[99-103] Bacterial vaginosis has been associated with histologic chorioamnionitis and postpartum endometritis.[53,103,104]

Varying results have been obtained from many trials of screening and treatment for bacterial vaginosis in pregnant women to reduce the incidence of preterm delivery.[105-110] Initial studies in which women at risk for delivering prematurely were screened for bacterial vaginosis and treated with antibiotics (metronidazole/erythromycin or metronidazole alone) showed that there was a reduction in the risk of preterm birth and infectious morbidity, suggesting treatment was beneficial.[106,110] More recently, other randomized studies using vaginal clindamycin cream or 2-g doses of metronidazole have not confirmed these findings.[105,107] Five trials that included women in a general obstetric population and women without risk factors for preterm birth were reviewed in a meta-analysis.[111] The difference in the rate of preterm birth between the treated and placebo groups was not statistically significant. Antibiotic therapy in the form of amoxicillin, clindamycin, and metronidazole was effective at eradicating bacterial vaginosis. When the subgroup of women with a previous preterm birth was studied, a significant reduction in the risk of preterm birth was seen in the antibiotic group.[111]

In the most recent and largest double-blinded, randomized controlled trial, no benefit was seen of treating women with asymptomatic bacterial vaginosis with two 2-g doses of metronidazole at 16 to 24 weeks of gestation and a repeat dose at 24 to 30 weeks.[105] There was no reduction in the rates of preterm birth or other adverse neonatal outcomes. Treating women did not reduce the occurrence of preterm labor, intraamniotic or postpartum infections,

Table 24–4. Risk Scoring Systems for Predicting Preterm Delivery

Study	Incidence of PTL/PTD (%)	Population	Sensitivity (%)	Specificity (%)	PPV (%)	NPV (%)
Herron et al, 1982[88]	PTL 4.7	1150, middle-class urban	55.6	84.7	17.0	97.5
Main et al, 1987[89]	PTD 14.8	391, inner city	25.9	79.9	18.3	86.1
Mueller-Heubach and Guzick, 1989[91]	PTD 8	4591, inner city	39.4	84.3	21.9	92.6
Owen et al, 1990[92]	PTD 8.5	7478, inner city	30.0	86.8	21.1	91.3

NPV, negative; PPV, positive predictive value; PTD, preterm delivery; PTL, preterm labor.

neonatal sepsis, or admissions to the neonatal intensive care unit.

Currently the U.S. Preventive Services Task Force recommends that low-risk women should not be screened for bacterial vaginosis because there is good evidence that screening and treatment of bacterial vaginosis in asymptomatic women does not improve outcomes such as preterm labor and preterm delivery.[112] There is insufficient evidence to recommend screening and treating high-risk women for bacterial vaginosis because good-quality studies have had conflicting results.[112] The conflicting results of these studies could be related to the timing of administration of antibiotics and the route and dosage of antibiotics. Because of the association of bacterial vaginosis with endometritis and first-trimester loss, it has been suggested that the risk of preterm labor may be reduced if the woman is treated in the first trimester or before conception.[113-116]

Fetal Fibronectin

Fetal fibronectin is a glycoprotein found in plasma and in the extracellular matrix. It is produced by a variety of cell types, including the fetal membranes, and it functions as an adhesion binder of the placenta and membranes to the decidua.[117] It is normally present in cervical and vaginal secretions until 16 to 20 weeks of gestation.[118] It also can be detected in cervicovaginal secretions in term pregnancies with intact membranes, suggesting its appearance may be related to the birth process.

Many trials have shown an association with the presence of fetal fibronectin between 20 and 34 weeks of gestation and preterm birth.[119-123] In addition, the risk of preterm birth when the test result is negative is low.[118,120,121] It is believed that fetal fibronectin is a marker for the disruption of the chorioamnion and underlying decidua due to inflammation or infection.[118] A positive fetal fibronectin test in the midtrimester has been associated with subsequently diagnosed chorioamnionitis.[124]

A meta-analysis by Leitich and colleagues[125] concluded that the presence of fetal fibronectin in vaginal or cervical secretions is a moderate predictor of preterm birth. It has a sensitivity of 61% and a specificity of 83% when the outcome studied is delivery at less than 34 weeks of gestation.[19] When the relationships between fetal fibronectin, a short cervix, presence of bacterial vaginosis, and traditional risk factors for spontaneous preterm birth were analyzed, it was found that the most significant association with preterm birth were a positive fetal fibronectin test, a cervical length less than 25 mm, and a history of preterm birth.[60]

The usefulness of the fetal fibronectin test seems to be its negative predictive value because it helps in reducing unnecessary interventions in symptomatic women. The negative predictive value of the fetal fibronectin in symptomatic women ranges from 69% to 92% before 37 weeks of gestation. A woman with a negative test result has a greater than 95% chance of not delivering within the next 14 days.[19,84,122,126]

No effective intervention is available to reduce the preterm birth risk of a woman with a positive fetal fibronectin test. Routine screening of low-risk, asymptomatic women is not yet recommended because the incidence of preterm birth in this population is low.[125] Screening high-risk, asymptomatic women may be helpful in identifying a subgroup of women who are not likely to deliver prematurely.[127]

Recommendations for the use of this test in specific high-risk groups are that the sampling be performed no earlier than 24 weeks and 0 days of gestation and no later than 34 weeks and 6 days of gestation in a woman with an intact amniotic membrane and cervical dilation of less than 3 cm.[19,123] The specimen collection should be done before a digital examination and before the use of lubricants to prevent false-positive and false-negative results.[127] Blood, amniotic fluid, recent intercourse, and a recent digital examination may give a false-positive result; lubricants may give a false-negative result.[127] The results must be available from a laboratory within 24 hours to allow for clinical decision making.[19]

Salivary Estriol

Some preterm births are preceded by activation of the fetal hypothalamic-pituitary-adrenal axis. Dehydroepiandrosterone (DHEAS) is produced by the fetal adrenal gland, converted to 16α-OH-DHEAS in the fetal liver, and then converted to estriol by the placenta. This process results in increased placental estrogen synthesis. Levels of estriol rise throughout pregnancy with an accelerated increase 5 weeks before term birth.

Studies have shown that maternal levels of serum estriol and salivary estriol increase before the onset of spontaneous term and preterm labor.[128] A surge of estriol precedes spontaneous labor by 2 to 3 weeks, with elevations occurring earlier in gestations that deliver preterm. Maternal salivary estriol levels show diurnal variation, with a surge beginning at 10 PM and peaking between 2 AM and 4 AM.[129] Estriol levels may be suppressed by betamethasone administration.[130]

Salivary estriol has been found to be more predictive of preterm labor than traditional risk assessment.[131,132] In studies evaluating the usefulness of salivary estriol in predicting the onset of preterm labor, the salivary estriol test had a positive predictive value ranging from 7% to 25% in low-risk women and from 25% to 48% in high-risk women. In addition, the salivary estriol test had a high negative predictive value ranging from 95% to 98% in low-risk women and from 89% to 94% in high-risk women.[131,132] The salivary estriol test has a high false-positive rate when delivery before 37 weeks of gestation is used as the outcome measure.[131] Gingivitis, bleeding gums, and smoking affect the accuracy of the test. The high percentage of false-positive results limits the usefulness of the test because it could add significantly to the cost of prenatal care, particularly if used in a low-risk population.[19]

Cervical Ultrasonography

Transvaginal ultrasonography has been shown to be more accurate than transabdominal ultrasonography or digital examination in assessing the length of the cervix.[133,134] In 1996, Iams and colleagues[135] showed an association between cervical length and preterm delivery in a prospective blinded trial. The normal distribution of cervical length in pregnancy after 22 weeks of gestation was established, and women with progressively shorter cervices experienced increased rates of preterm delivery.[135] The association of cervical shortening with preterm delivery has been confirmed by other studies.[136-139] The performance of the test has varied widely. Leitich and colleagues[140] performed a systematic review of 35 studies using cervical length to predict preterm delivery. The test was found to have sensitivities of 68% to 100% and specificities of 44% to 79%.[140] Guzman and Ananth[141] reviewed seven major studies in low-risk and high-risk populations. The sensitivity and positive predictive values for delivery before 32 and 35 weeks of gestation were studied. For deliveries before 32 weeks of gestation, the sensitivities were 1% to 82% and the positive predictive values were 11% to 52%.[141] Higher sensitivities for the test were obtained in high-risk patients, especially women with a history of mid-trimester loss.[141]

The use of cervical length measurement by transvaginal ultrasonography combined with other methods of screening has been documented.[142] A short cervix (defined as <25 mm), particularly if associated with a positive fetal fibronectin result, was found to be a strong predictor of preterm birth.[142] The sequential use of cervical length and fetal fibronectin have been employed to stratify risk groups and discern the etiology of preterm birth.[60] The presence of either a cervix less than 25 mm in length at less than 35 weeks of gestation or a positive fetal fibronectin result was strongly associated with preterm birth, especially in women with a history of preterm birth.[60]

Cervical sonography may play a role in high-risk populations, such as women with a history of preterm delivery, rupture of membranes, cervical surgery, or diethylstilbestrol exposure.[143] In low-risk populations, the role of cervical length measurement is not as clear because most cases of spontaneous preterm labor occur in women with no known risk factors. At present, cervical length measurement has limited clinical applicability because the precise gestational age for examination, the cutoff cervical length, the need for repeat examinations, and the frequency of these examinations have not been defined.[143] It has not been established that detection of a short cervix improves pregnancy outcome, so the routine use of cervical length measurement is not recommended.[84]

Home Uterine Activity Monitoring

Home uterine activity monitoring (HUAM) has been proposed as a method for predicting preterm birth in high-risk women. Some investigators believed that early detection of uterine contractions would lead to earlier diagnosis of preterm labor. Early treatment with tocolytic agents then could be accomplished successfully.

Some women who subsequently deliver preterm show an increase in uterine activity earlier in pregnancy than women who give birth at term.[144] Because uterine contractions may not be recognized by the patient,[145,146] emphasis was placed on patient education to recognize uterine activity. Many patients could not recognize uterine contractions by self-palpation.[147]

In HUAM, electronic recordings of uterine contractions are transmitted to a health care practitioner on a daily basis. The transmissions are interpreted, and the patient is given advice. Many randomized controlled trials examining the efficacy of HUAM have published results.[148-154] These studies are difficult to compare because they vary in design, inclusion criteria, and measurements of end points and outcomes.[19] Limitations such as a small sample size preclude reaching meaningful conclusions.

Initial studies, criticized for their flawed design, used the rate of preterm delivery as their end point.[19,155,156] It was concluded that high-risk women using HUAM had earlier preterm labor detected with less cervical dilation and lower preterm birth rates. Variations in study design included minimal number of transmissions daily, the timing of transmissions, the ability of patients to transmit more often, and the level of feedback provided by monitoring nurses.[157] It has been suggested that the results of other studies should be dismissed because of the many errors and biases.[19,158] The largest study showed no improvement in rate of preterm delivery at less than 35 weeks of gestation and in neonatal outcome.[148]

In 1993, the U.S. Preventive Services Task Force performed an independent review and concluded they had insufficient evidence to recommend for or against HUAM in high-risk pregnancies.[159] The role for HUAM in preventing preterm birth has not been shown. HUAM is not recommended currently as a screening tool in asymptomatic low-risk women.[19,160,161]

MEASURES TO PREVENT PRETERM DELIVERIES

Once premature labor has started, several interventions have been used to stop it. Initially, bed rest and hydration are instituted to improve circulation and treat dehydration. When the decision to start tocolytic therapy has been made, different pharmacologic agents may be used: β-sympathomimetics, magnesium sulfate, and calcium channel blockers decrease myometrial intracellular calcium availability; prostaglandin synthetase inhibitors (indomethacin) decrease the conversion of arachidonic acid to prostaglandins. In addition, underlying infections are treated with antibiotics to decrease infection as a source of tissue necrosis and cytokine release.

Bed Rest

In the management of preterm labor, bed rest often is recommended because of the belief that rest may decrease uterine activity. Bed rest has been shown to improve uteroplacental blood flow, leading to a slight increase in birth weight. Goldenberg and colleagues[162] were unable to show a decrease in the incidence of preterm delivery.

Bed rest may be deleterious to the mother. The deleterious consequences of bed rest may include thromboembolic disease, muscle atrophy, bone demineralization, impaired glucose tolerance, heartburn, constipation, and the potential for a longer postpartum recovery period.[163,164] There is little evidence for the benefit of bed rest in preventing preterm delivery, although the information available does not rule out a benefit.

Hydration

Hydration is another common recommendation for the treatment of preterm labor. Intravenous hydration with 500 to 1000 mL of a crystalloid solution is used initially to treat preterm labor and may be helpful in some instances because it decreases uterine contractility.[165,166] It has been postulated that the circulating levels of antidiuretic hormone are affected by volume expansion. Indirectly, the circulating levels of oxytocin are affected, decreasing uterine contractility.[167] Hydration has not been shown to be significantly effective in stopping early preterm labor.[165,166,168] Because patients in preterm labor additionally receive tocolytic agents, fluid overload and pulmonary edema may occur if hydration is not monitored carefully.[169] Helfgott and colleagues[168] found that bed rest with hydration and sedation and bed rest with hydration alone were of no more benefit than simple bed rest for patients with preterm uterine contractions and intact membranes.

Antibiotics

Infections of the lower genital tract have been associated with preterm delivery.[170-175] Colonization of the lower genital tract may serve as a marker of upper genital tract infection or may lead to direct migration of organisms to the decidua, fetal membranes, and amniotic fluid.

During prenatal care, women should be screened for gonorrhea and chlamydia and treated, if positive, to prevent spread to sexual partners and the newborn. In addition, treatment may improve the pregnancy outcome as shown in nonrandomized trials.[171,176] Screening and treatment for asymptomatic bacteriuria has been standard practice to prevent pyelonephritis. An association between asymptomatic bacteriuria and preterm delivery has been shown.[170,177] Trichomoniasis should be treated in pregnancy because some studies have shown adverse pregnancy outcomes in women with this condition.[171,174,175,178] There are no randomized studies to support its treatment to prevent preterm birth. Bacterial vaginosis has been associated with preterm delivery and infants with low birth weight.[100-103,108] Routine screening of women at high risk for preterm delivery is controversial. The U.S. Preventive Services Task Force concluded that the evidence was insufficient to recommend for or against routinely screening high-risk pregnant women for bacterial vaginosis.[112] Asymptomatic women at low risk of preterm delivery should not be screened for bacterial vaginosis based on evidence from the literature.[112] Genital tract colonization of mycoplasmas has not been associated with preterm delivery; treatment for the purpose of decreasing the risk of preterm delivery is not indicated. Finally, genital colonization of group B streptococcus should not be treated during the antepartum period because it has not been shown to be effective in preventing preterm delivery or decreasing the risk of early neonatal sepsis.[179] Routine use of antibiotics for pregnancy prolongation in preterm labor with intact membranes is not indicated because published studies have not shown a benefit

consistently.[172,180,181] In addition, the rates of chorioamnionitis, endometritis, maternal infection, neonatal pneumonia or sepsis, necrotizing enterocolitis, and neonatal death did not decrease by the use of antibiotics. In patients in preterm labor with intact membranes, antibiotics should be given as prophylaxis to prevent neonatal sepsis by group B streptococcus.[179] In patients with premature rupture of membranes, antibiotics may be given in addition to prevent group B streptococcal sepsis, to prolong pregnancy, and to decrease complications.[172]

Cervical Cerclage

Cervical cerclage has been used to improve the outcome of women with previous preterm births. The results of these studies have been inconsistent.[182-184] Other studies assessing the value of cervical ultrasonography to guide who would receive the cerclage have been carried out.[185] Some investigators have evaluated conservative management as an alternative to cerclage placement in women with second-trimester sonographic evidence of cervical dilation.[183,185] No differences in outcome were seen. It seems that transvaginal sonographic examination of the cervix followed with cerclage placement, when indicated, is a safe alternative to elective cerclage.[143]

TOCOLYSIS

The evaluation of studies attempting to use a variety of pharmacologic agents to inhibit preterm labor is made difficult by a lack of uniformity in defining the condition being treated. When contractions alone are used as the single diagnostic variable, the error in diagnosing preterm labor is 40% to 70%.[186] In many randomized controlled trials of tocolytic therapy, 30% to 90% of patients receiving placebo have had delivery delayed for 48 hours, with 30% to 40% ultimately reaching term.[187,188] A wide variety of treatment protocols have been used. Finally, only 10% to 20% of women at risk for preterm delivery are candidates for tocolytic use.[189]

Preterm labor is diagnosed between 20 and 37 weeks of gestation with documented uterine contractions, with intact membranes; documented cervical change or cervical dilation of at least 2 cm; or at least 80% effacement on presentation.[190] The diagnosis also is made in the presence of uterine contractions and spontaneous rupture of membranes (Table 24-5).

In a preterm woman presenting with concerns of contractions or labor, external fetal heart rate monitoring and uterine contraction monitoring are instituted. A thorough history is obtained, focusing specifically on duration of symptoms, possibility of membrane rupture, and prior obstetric history. The mother's vital signs are recorded, looking specifically for maternal fever or tachycardia. The uterine fundus is palpated to discern fetal presentation and to detect the presence of uterine tenderness, which would suggest clinical chorioamnionitis. The woman also is evaluated for pyelonephritis or suprapubic tenderness suggesting cystitis, both of which are associated with preterm labor.

A sterile speculum examination is performed before digital examination of the cervix in all cases of possible

Table 24–5. Criteria for Diagnosis of Preterm Labor

Gestation 20-37 wk
  and
Documented uterine contractions (4 in 20 min, 8 in 60 min)
  and
Ruptured membranes *or* Intact membranes
          and
        Documented cervical change
          or
        Cervical effacement of 80%
          or
        Cervical dilation of 2 cm

preterm labor. If preterm rupture of the membranes is diagnosed either by grossly evident pooling of fluid in the vaginal vault or by microscopically apparent ferning in secretions obtained via swab from the vaginal vault, digital examination is deferred. In the absence of premature rupture of membranes and persistence of contractions, preterm labor is diagnosed either via initial cervical evaluation or by serial examinations over 6 to 12 hours, preferably by a single examiner. Laboratory studies should include a urine specimen for microscopic evaluation along with cultures from the genital area for gonorrhea and chlamydia (cervix) and group B streptococcus (rectum and vaginal introitus). If preterm labor is diagnosed, antibiotic chemoprophylaxis for group B streptococcus is administered intrapartum to prevent vertical transmission and early-onset neonatal sepsis.[179,191] In addition, a course of corticosteroid therapy is initiated for acceleration of fetal lung maturity.[86,192]

The routine use of amniocentesis to guide management of preterm labor is controversial. Amniocentesis may be done to search for intrauterine infection in the presence of maternal fever, without an obvious localizing source and preterm labor, or in the absence of fever, in women refractory to first-line tocolytic therapy. Amniocentesis also may be used when the gestational age is in question or when growth restriction is suspected.

Tocolytic therapy is considered only when preterm labor is diagnosed. Because tocolytic therapy may result in untoward maternal and fetal effects, use of tocolytics should be limited to women in true preterm labor at high risk for spontaneous birth. The risks and benefits of tocolytic therapy must be considered, balancing the negligible improvements in perinatal morbidity and mortality in the face of pulmonary maturity at 34 weeks or more against the side effects of tocolytic agents.[193-195]

Evaluation of a patient for contraindications to the use of tocolytics in general or to the use of specific tocolytic agents is undertaken next. Contraindications include fetal death, fetal distress when immediate delivery would improve the fetal outcome, and severe fetal malformation. If maternal infection is present, appropriate antibiotic therapy should be initiated. The patient should be evaluated for metabolic abnormalities that might contribute to uterine activity or that might be associated with significant maternal morbidity or mortality if inappropriate

tocolytic therapy is initiated. Examples of maternal conditions that might be affected adversely by inappropriate tocolytic therapy include thyroid storm; diabetes mellitus, especially ketoacidosis; maternal cardiac disease; and placental abruption (Table 24-6). At hospitals without appropriate neonatal resources, identifying women at risk allows for appropriate maternal transport to a tertiary care center. Conversely, identifying women at low risk for preterm delivery would avert the use of unnecessary interventions.

Tocolytics should be used to delay delivery with the hope of improving neonatal outcomes. It has been recognized that tocolytic agents stop contractions and do not treat the condition causing preterm labor. To prevent preterm delivery, the condition initiating the preterm labor must be treated. Specific benefits that may be achieved by delaying the delivery are improving neonatal outcome by the administration of corticosteroid therapy, transferring the mother to a tertiary care facility, and allowing time for other treatments to work (i.e., antibiotics if chorioamnionitis is suspected).[196]

To justify the use of aggressive tocolysis to prolong pregnancy and improve neonatal outcome, the following factors need to be taken into consideration: (1) the likelihood of neonatal survival and morbidity at the initiation of therapy, (2) the likely prolongation of pregnancy from the time of diagnosing preterm labor, and (3) improvement in neonatal outcome at the time delivery is either imminent or permitted. As improvements in neonatal care have made quality survival possible at earlier gestational ages, attention has centered on prolonging preterm gestation at the earlier limits of viability. A multicenter study of more than 20,000 accurately dated pregnancies showed that after 34 weeks the incidences of high-grade intraventricular hemorrhage, necrotizing enterocolitis, and sepsis are virtually 0, whereas morbidity related to

Table 24–6. Contraindications to Tocolytic Therapy for Preterm Labor

Absolute Contraindications
Severe pregnancy-induced hypertension
Severe abruptio placentae
Severe bleeding from any cause
Chorioamnionitis
Fetal death
Fetal anomaly incompatible with life
Severe fetal growth restriction

Relative Contraindications
Mild chronic hypertension
Mild abruptio placentae
Stable placenta previa
Maternal cardiac disease
Hyperthyroidism
Uncontrolled diabetes mellitus
Fetal distress
Fetal anomaly
Mild fetal growth restriction
Cervix > 5 cm dilated

respiratory distress syndrome decreases to less than 15%.[195] There seems to be significant neonatal benefit in prolonging pregnancy by 1 week in the period from 24 to 26 weeks.[197-199] Even smaller delays in delivery in this period can improve survival significantly.[200] In addition, because infants with very low birth weight born in tertiary care centers seem to do better overall than infants transported to a tertiary neonatal center,[201,202] it can be argued that even short-term tocolytic success that allows maternal transport to an appropriate center for delivery is warranted by improved neonatal outcome.

Lastly, before consideration of individual tocolytic agents, neonatal outcome statistics need to be viewed carefully. Most of these tocolytic trials were conducted before the era of postnatal administration of surfactant. Although maternally administered corticosteroids have shown consistent benefit in reducing the incidence of respiratory distress syndrome in gestations greater than 28 weeks,[203] they have not shown comparable benefit in gestations of 24 to 28 weeks.[204] There is evidence, however, to support a synergistic effect of antenatal corticosteroids and postnatal surfactant before the 28-week period.[205-207]

Information from the Neonatal Research Network of the National Institute of Child Health and Human Development shows that the neonatal survival rate increases from 0% at 21 weeks of gestation to 75% at 25 weeks of gestation (Table 24-7).[197,198] In addition, neonatal survival increases from 11% at 401 to 500 g birth weight to 75% at 701 to 800 g birth weight (Table 24-8).[197,198] Neonatal morbidity in the form of intraventricular hemorrhage, periventricular leukomalacia, chronic lung disease, necrotizing enterocolitis, nosocomial infections, and retinopathy of prematurity contributes to the significant number of extremely premature neonates with disabilities in mental and psychomotor development,

Table 24-7. Newborn Deaths by Gestational Age

Completed Weeks of Gestation	No. of Deaths	Percentage of Deaths
21	12	100
22	56	79
23	216	70
24	301	50
25	379	25
26	436	20
27	519	10
28	569	8
29	535	5
30	472	3
31	362	5
32	225	7
33	185	5
>34	156	5

Adapted from Lemons JA, Bauer CR, Oh W, et al: Very low birth weight outcomes of the National Institute of Child Health and Human development Neonatal Research Network, January 1995 through December 1996. Pediatrics 107:E1, 2001.

Table 24-8. Newborn Deaths by Birth Weight

Birth Weight (g)	No. of Deaths	Percentage of Deaths
401-500	195	89
501-600	317	71
601-700	449	38
701-800	439	25
801-900	419	12
901-1000	462	10
1001-1100	398	8
1101-1200	430	5
1201-1300	465	5
1301-1400	488	3
1401-1500	571	3

Adapted from Lemons JA, Bauer CR, Oh W, et al: Very low birth weight outcomes of the National Institute of Child Health and Human development Neonatal Research Network, January 1995 through December 1996. Pediatrics 107:E1, 2001.

neuromotor function, or sensory and communication function.[198] The most commonly used tocolytic agents are magnesium sulfate, β-adrenergic agonists, prostaglandin synthetase inhibitors, and calcium channel blockers.

Magnesium Sulfate

Magnesium is the most commonly used parenteral tocolytic agent in the United States. Magnesium inhibits myometrial activity in vitro and in vivo, presumably depressing myometrial contractility by altering calcium uptake, binding, and distribution in smooth muscle cells. Many actions of magnesium sulfate have been proposed, but the precise mechanism of action is unknown.[208] Therapy is administered via continuous infusion at 2 to 4 g/hr, usually after a 4- to 6-g loading bolus has been infused over 15 to 30 minutes. Serum concentrations of 5 to 8 mg/dL seem to be necessary to reduce uterine activity.[209]

Flushing, dizziness, and nausea are commonly observed with magnesium therapy, usually during infusion of the loading dose. Blurred vision also frequently is reported and is an effect of the drug on the small extraocular muscles. The loss of deep tendon reflexes can be seen at magnesium levels of 7 to 10 mEq/L, whereas respiratory depression may occur at levels of 10 to 12 mEq/L. Pulmonary edema has been reported with magnesium sulfate therapy.[210] In contrast to the β-agonists, magnesium sulfate does not produce a profound tachycardia and may be used more safely in preterm labor complicated by hypertension, diabetes, most heart diseases, and maternal bleeding. Absolute contraindications include myasthenia gravis and heart block. Concurrent use of magnesium sulfate and calcium channel blockers can result in profound hypotension.

Reports of fetal effects of maternal magnesium therapy are conflicting. The passage of magnesium through the placenta may result in loss of fetal heart reactivity or decrease in fetal breathing movements.[211] Transient respiratory and motor depression have been reported with blood magnesium levels of 4 to 11 mEq/L.[209,212] Demineralization of bone has been described with prolonged use of magnesium.[213] Antenatal exposure to magnesium sulfate may be associated with a decreased incidence of cerebral palsy, suggesting a fetal neuroprotective effect.[214,215]

β-Adrenergic Agonists

Ritodrine is the only agent approved by the U.S. Food and Drug Administration to treat preterm labor. Ritodrine is a nonselective β agonist; administration stimulates β_2-adrenergic receptors found in smooth muscle of the uterus and β_1-adrenergic receptors in the heart and small intestine, resulting in undesired side effects.[216] β_2-Adrenergic stimulation of smooth muscle receptors leads to activation of adenylate cyclase, which increases intracellular concentrations of cyclic adenosine monophosphate (AMP), decreasing levels of calcium available to the myosin-actin contractile unit. Continued exposure to β-adrenergic agonists leads to a reduced effectiveness, a phenomenon called *tachyphylaxis*.[217] In vitro studies performed using strips of continuously perfused human myometrium suggest that this effect is secondary to down-regulation of β receptors.[218]

Ritodrine and terbutaline have been the two most commonly used β agonists. Ritodrine is no longer available because the manufacturer withdrew it from the market. Terbutaline is available for use by intravenous, subcutaneous, and oral routes. The subcutaneous route of terbutaline may be used for acute tocolysis, but it does not allow immediate discontinuation if side effects occur.[219] Also, subcutaneous terbutaline needs to be dosed too frequently to be acceptable to patients for maintenance therapy. The continuous subcutaneous administration of terbutaline in low dosages using an infusion pump also has been reported. It has been hypothesized that terbutaline pump therapy avoids the down-regulation of the myometrial β receptors, which otherwise would lead to decreasing effectiveness.[220] Continuous oral maintenance with terbutaline has not been shown to be effective in preventing preterm birth.

Maternal cardiovascular side effects are the ones most commonly encountered during β-adrenergic therapy. Serious complications, such as cardiac arrhythmias, hypotension, myocardial ischemia, and pulmonary edema, have been reported in 1% to 5% of cases.[217] Tachycardia alone, necessitating discontinuation of therapy, occurs in 10% of patients.[221,222] Pulmonary edema is the most commonly seen serious side effect and is a result of combined aggressive intravenous hydration, increased cardiac output, and β-adrenergic stimulation of the renin-aldosterone system and decrease in colloid osmotic pressure. Pulmonary edema may be avoided by limiting fluid intake, dose, and duration of β-sympathomimetic therapy.[223,224] In addition, cyclic AMP production alters maternal carbohydrate metabolism, resulting in potentially serious hyperglycemia. It has been seen during oral maintenance therapy with terbutaline (although not with ritodrine).[225] Because of its significant potential for side effects, β-agonist tocolysis is contraindicated in women with uncontrolled insulin-dependent diabetes mellitus, underlying cardiac disease, and untreated hyperthyroidism.

β-Agonists readily cross the placenta, and fetal tachycardia may be apparent on external fetal heart rate monitoring. Data from controlled clinical trials show no difference in neonatal morbidity or mortality between mothers treated with β-adrenergic agents and mothers treated with placebo. The β-sympathomimetics may produce hyperinsulinemia and neonatal hypoglycemia. Studies of children examined 6 years after exposure found no significant difference in neurologic testing, growth patterns, or overall behavior.[226]

Prostaglandin Synthetase Inhibitors (Indomethacin)

Zuckerman and colleagues[227] were the first to report the use of the prostaglandin synthetase inhibitor indomethacin to treat preterm labor successfully in 80% of 50 patients treated for 24 hours. A subsequent randomized, double-blind, placebo-controlled study yielded similar results in a smaller study population; patients also were treated for a 24-hour period.[228] Prostaglandin synthetase inhibitors may exert an effect on transmembrane calcium flux.[229,230] They are reversible competitive inhibitors of cyclooxygenase; they reduce the levels of prostaglandins and diminish myometrial contractility. Short-term therapy with indomethacin may be as effective as ritodrine and seems to have fewer side effects.[231] The dose used is 50 to 100 mg initially, followed by 25 mg every 4 to 6 hours. Because of the potential risk of fetal death with closure of the ductus arteriosus during long-term use, indomethacin therapy usually is limited to 48 hours.[186]

Maternal side effects attributable to the prostaglandin synthetase inhibitors are minimal and usually are related to gastrointestinal irritation (nausea, dyspepsia, vomiting). They are contraindicated in patients with known gastric ulcers. The prostaglandin synthetase inhibitors also are contraindicated in women with bleeding disorders because they can increase bleeding time by reducing levels of thromboxane synthesis in platelets, which inhibits normal platelet aggregation. Other contraindications are hepatic dysfunction, renal dysfunction, and asthma in aspirin-sensitive patients.[217]

In direct contrast to the intravenous agents, use of the prostaglandin synthetase inhibitors has raised concern over fetal side effects.[232-236] The sensitivity of the fetal ductus arteriosus to constrictive effects of indomethacin has been shown beginning at 27 weeks and reaching a maximum by 30 weeks of gestation, with more than half of exposed fetuses exhibiting some degree of ductal constriction by 32 weeks.[237] It has been found that short-term indomethacin treatment up to 34 weeks is not associated with premature closure of the ductus or persistent fetal circulation.[233,238,239] Other side effects have included transient renal insufficiency, inhibition of newborn hemostasis, and necrotizing enterocolitis.[240-245] Necrotizing enterocolitis may be related to a loss in the bowel's ability to autoregulate oxygen consumption, leading to intestinal ischemia. Even more controversial is the relationship between indomethacin and intraventricular hemorrhage. Although some studies suggest a decreased incidence of intraventricular hemorrhage when indomethacin has been administered neonatally,[246] presumably through an inhibition of free radical production by the cerebral microcirculation,[247] other reports have not supported this association. Some studies have found an increased incidence of intraventricular hemorrhage in newborns exposed in utero to indomethacin,[248-250] whereas others have not.[250] These fetal side effects make indomethacin a potentially dangerous tocolytic agent for long-term administration.[251-258]

In situations when indomethacin is used for less than 72 hours, no special surveillance is recommended. With longer use, surveillance consisting of weekly evaluation of blood flow through the ductus arteriosus should be instituted at 27 weeks, with therapy being stopped in any case by 32 weeks.[259] Reports of prostaglandin synthetase inhibitor–related oligohydramnios also make weekly ultrasound evaluation of amniotic fluid volume a necessity in all pregnancies undergoing long-term treatment.[260]

Calcium Channel Blockers

Calcium channel blockers have been shown to inhibit uterine activity induced by oxytocin, prostaglandins, and ergonovine maleate.[261,262] They also have suppressed spontaneous and methergine-induced uterine activity in vivo and in the postpartum period.[263] They seem to block the voltage-dependent calcium channels in myometrial cells.[264] They may increase calcium efflux from the cell by inhibiting the release of intracellular calcium from sarcolemmal stores.[217]

Nifedipine has been the drug most commonly tested. It compared favorably with ritodrine in efficacy in arresting preterm labor in published randomized trials.[265-269] Nifedipine is administered orally. A dose of 10 mg orally every 20 minutes for four doses followed by 20 mg orally every 4 to 8 hours has been recommended.[270] Maternal side effects, such as tachycardia, palpitations, headaches, and cutaneous flushing, are well tolerated.

The main concern with regard to fetal safety when calcium channel blockers are used as tocolytics is the potential to affect uterine blood flow and fetal oxygenation. The generalized vasodilation seen during use of these agents has been shown to lower the systemic blood pressure and uterine blood flow in unanesthetized animals.[271] Short-term nifedipine therapy seems not to affect fetal cardiac function or peripheral vascular function.[272] Acid-base studies of umbilical cord blood have not revealed fetal hypoxia or acidosis.[273-275]

Other Agents

Because the available tocolytic agents have been unable to decrease the preterm delivery rate and its neonatal consequences, investigators have studied or are in the process of investigating other pharmacologic agents, such as oxytocin receptor antagonists (atosiban), nitric oxide donors (nitroglycerin), and cyclooxygenase-2 inhibitors.[276-278] The use of these agents as tocolytics should be considered investigational at this time, and they should be used only in centers where appropriate research and patient safeguards are in place.

Classic treatment of preterm labor has included bed rest, hydration, hospitalization, and offering emotional support and comfort (using sedation, analgesics, or both). Although not usually considered "tocolytic therapy," these forms of treatment may be the effective part of any treatment for preterm labor. We also have noticed that treatment with blood transfusions has stopped contractions of preterm labor in triplet pregnancies complicated by significant anemia.

Multiple Agents or Serial Agent Tocolysis

Sometimes patients in true preterm labor do not respond to the use of a single tocolytic agent. In these circumstances, one should suspect that a subclinical infection or placental abruption might be responsible for the preterm labor. These conditions are associated with significant maternal and fetal morbidity and should be ruled out before multiple agents are used.

The mechanism of action of each agent needs to be considered when considering multiple-agent therapy. It has been suggested that dual-agent therapy might be more efficacious because it combines different physiologic mechanisms. There is an increase in side effects reported when more than one tocolytic agent is used.

Nifedipine should not be used in conjunction with magnesium because they act as neuromuscular depressants in their dual actions as calcium antagonists.[279] The combination of magnesium sulfate and β-sympathomimetics has been proposed by some, presumably because the efficacy of the tocolytic therapy is improved, while the dose of β-sympathomimetics is decreased.[280-282] The long-term combination therapy of magnesium sulfate and β-sympathomimetics has a much higher risk of pulmonary edema, however.[193,265,282,283]

In patients not responding to magnesium sulfate, adding indomethacin if the gestation is less than 32 weeks for a period of 48 hours may be beneficial.[284] The use of indomethacin and magnesium sulfate may be the safest combination available.[196] Indomethacin decreases maternal renal function and specifically decreases magnesium ion excretion. Patients receiving this form of dual-agent tocolysis are at heightened risk for magnesium toxicity. The combination of indomethacin and nifedipine may be tried. The combination of β-sympathomimetics and nifedipine may produce maternal diastolic hypotension and cardiovascular problems and should be employed carefully.[285] β-Sympathomimetics and indomethacin also have been tried.[286,287] The use of combination tocolytic therapy is not generally recommended and should be reserved for use in unique clinical situations and at centers where close monitoring of experimental treatments can be maintained.

Maintenance Tocolytic Therapy

The benefit of long-term maintenance tocolytic therapy has not been shown. Most reports studying oral tocolytics have involved small numbers of patients. Because of the small sample size of these studies, two meta-analyses were carried out to evaluate the efficacy of these drugs. The findings of these meta-analyses did not support the long-term use of maintenance oral β-agonist tocolytics after the treatment of an acute episode of preterm labor.[288,289]

In some situations, patients remain hospitalized and receive parenteral tocolytic therapy for a prolonged period. Prolonged hospitalization is associated with increases in maternal stress, inadequate rest, maternal complications, and increased costs. Some clinicians may justify this approach if there is an improvement in neonatal outcome. The outpatient use of a programmable pump that administers basal and bolus doses of terbutaline is a less costly method.[220] In general, an improvement in outcome has not been shown with the long-term use of tocolytic therapy.

Although controversy remains about the effectiveness of tocolytic therapy per se, the following actions are generally accepted interventions to either decrease preterm births or improve perinatal outcomes for premature infants: (1) decrease the incidence of illicit drug use and cigarette smoking in pregnancy, (2) decrease iatrogenic multiple gestations by improved treatment of infertility, (3) transfer the mother to the tertiary hospital before birth of the premature infant, and (4) administer corticosteroids to the mother 48 hours before birth.

RISKS OF SUCCESSFUL TOCOLYSIS

There is a growing body of evidence associating complications of pregnancy, such as intrauterine infection, growth restriction, and placental abruption, with preterm delivery.[23] Fetal infection has been recognized as an etiologic factor of cerebral palsy. More premature neonates have been found to be smaller for gestational age than term neonates. If a suboptimal or hostile environment is associated with preterm delivery, successful tocolysis might place the fetus at risk for further growth impairment or death. Perhaps these patients should undergo serial ultrasound evaluations for growth and biophysical well-being.

REFERENCES

1. Ventura SJ, Martin JA, Curtin SC, et al: Births: Final data for 1999. Nat Vital Stat Rep 49:1, 2001.
2. Burke C, Morrison JJ: Perinatal factors and preterm delivery in an Irish obstetric population. J Perinat Med 28:49, 2000.
3. Creasy RK: Preterm birth prevention: Where are we? Am J Obstet Gynecol 168:1223, 1993.
4. Creasy RK, Iams JD: Preterm labor and delivery. In Creasy RK, Resnik R (eds): Maternal-Fetal Medicine: Principles and Practice, 4th ed. Philadelphia, WB Saunders, 1999, pp 494-520.
5. Ianucci TA, Tomich PG, Gianopoulos JG: Etiology and outcome of extremely low-birth weight infants. Am J Obstet Gynecol 174:1896, 1996.
6. Main DM, Gabbe SG, Richardson D, et al: Can preterm deliveries be prevented? Am J Obstet Gynecol 151:892, 1985.
7. Meis PJ, Ernest JM, Moore ML, et al: Regional program for prevention of premature birth in northwestern North Carolina. Am J Obstet Gynecol 157:550, 1987.
8. Goldenberg RL, Rouse DJ: Prevention of premature birth. N Engl J Med 339:313, 1998.
9. Meis PJ, Goldenberg RL, Mercer BM, et al: The preterm prediction study: Risk factors for indicated preterm births. Am J Obstet Gynecol 178:562, 1998.
10. Savitz DA, Blackmore CA, Thorp JM: Epidemiologic characteristics of preterm delivery: Etiologic heterogeneity. Am J Obstet Gynecol 164:467, 1991.
11. Tanbo T, Dale PO, Lunde O, et al: Obstetric outcome in singleton pregnancies after assisted reproduction. Obstet Gynecol 86:188, 1995.
12. Verlaenen H, Cammu H, Derde MP, et al: Singleton pregnancy after in vitro fertilization: Expectations and outcome. Obstet Gynecol 86:906, 1995.
13. Kiely JL: What is the population based risk of preterm birth among twins and other multiples? Clin Obstet Gynecol 41:3, 1998.
14. Ventura SJ, Martin JA, Curtin SC, et al: Births: Final data for 1998. Nat Vital Stat Rep 48:1, 2000.
15. Copper RL, Goldenberg RL, Creasy RK, et al: A multicenter study of preterm birth weight and gestational age-specific neonatal mortality. Am J Obstet Gynecol 168:78, 1993.
16. Nicholson WK, Frick KD, Powe NR: Economic burden of hospitalizations for preterm labor in the United States. Obstet Gynecol 96:95, 2000.
17. Skolnick AA, Mark D: AMA's Science Reporters Conference focuses on contraception and prevention of premature births. JAMA 276:1538, 1996.
18. Lorenz JM: The outcome of extreme prematurity. Semin Perinatol 25:348, 2001.
19. American College of Obstetricians and Gynecologists: ACOG Practice Bulletin. Assessment of risk factors for preterm birth. Clinical management guidelines for obstetricians-gynecologists. Obstet Gynecol 98:709, 2001.
20. Bakketeig LS, Hoffman HJ: Epidemiology of preterm birth: Results from a longitudinal study of births in Norway. In Elder MG, Hendricks CH (eds): Preterm Labor. London, Butterworths, 1981.
21. Lumley J: The epidemiology of preterm birth. Baillieres Clin Obstet Gynaecol 7:477, 1993.
22. Robinson JN, Regan JA, Norwitz ER: The epidemiology of preterm labor. Semin Perinatol 25:204, 2001.
23. Wen SW, Goldenberg RL, Cutter GR, et al: Intrauterine growth retardation and preterm delivery: Perinatal risk factors in an indigent population. Am J Obstet Gynecol 162:213, 1990.
24. Cnattingius S, Forman MR, Berendes HW, et al: Effect of age, parity and smoking on pregnancy outcome: A population based study. Am J Obstet Gynecol 168:16, 1993.
25. Cnattingius S, Granath F, Petersson G, et al: The influence of gestational age and smoking habits on the risk of subsequent preterm deliveries. N Engl J Med 341:943, 1999.
26. Walsh RA: Effects of maternal smoking on adverse pregnancy outcomes: Examination of the criteria of causation. Hum Biol 66:1059, 1994.
27. Chasnoff I, Griffeth D, MacGregor S, et al: Temporal patterns of cocaine use in pregnancy. JAMA 261:1714, 1989.
28. Cherukuri R, Minkoff H, Hansen RL, et al: A cohort study of alkaloidal cocaine ("crack") in pregnancy. Obstet Gynecol 72:147, 1988.
29. Spence MR, Williams R, DiGegorio GJ, et al: The relationship between recent cocaine use and pregnancy outcome. Obstet Gynecol 78:326, 1991.
30. Adams MM, Elam-Evans LD, Wilson HG, et al: Rates and factors associated with recurrence of preterm delivery. JAMA 283:1591, 2000.
31. Mercer BM, Goldenberg RL, Moawad AH, et al: The preterm prediction study: Effect of gestational age and cause of preterm birth on subsequent outcome. Am J Obstet Gynecol 181:1216, 1999.
32. Ekwo EE, Gosselink CA, Moawad A: Unfavorable outcome in penultimate pregnancy and premature rupture of membranes in successive pregnancy. Obstet Gynecol 80:166, 1992.

33. Strobino B, Pantel-Silverman J: Gestational vaginal bleeding and pregnancy outcome. Am J Epidemiol 129:806, 1989.

34. Cooney MJ, Benson CB, Doubilet PM: Outcome of pregnancies in women with uterine duplication anomalies. J Clin Ultrasound 26:3, 1998.

35. Heinonen PK: Unicornuate uterus and rudimentary horn. Fertil Steril 68:224, 1997.

36. Heinonen PK, Saarikoski S, Pystynen P: Reproductive performance of women with uterine anomalies. Acta Obstet Gynecol Scand 61:157, 1982.

37. Davis JL, Ray-Mazumder S, Hobel CJ, et al: Uterine leiomyomas in pregnancy: A prospective study. Obstet Gynecol 75:41, 1990.

38. Rice JP, Kay HH, Mahoney BS: The clinical significance of uterine leiomyomas in pregnancy. Am J Obstet Gynecol 160:1212, 1989.

39. Kristensen J, Langhoff-Roos J, Wittrup M, et al: Cervical conization and preterm delivery/low birth weight: A systematic review of the literature. Acta Obstet Gynecol Scand 72:640, 1993.

40. Raio L, Ghezzzi F, DiNaro E, et al: Duration of pregnancy after carbon dioxide laser conization of the cervix: Influence of cone height. Obstet Gynecol 90:978, 1997.

41. Zhou W, Sorensen HT, Olsen J: Induced abortion and subsequent pregnancy duration. Obstet Gynecol 94:948, 1999.

42. Minakami H, Sayama M, Honma Y, et al: Lower risks of adverse outcome in twins conceived by artificial reproductive techniques compared with spontaneously conceived twins. Hum Reprod 13:2005, 1998.

43. Moise J, Laor A, Amon Y, et al: The outcome of twin pregnancies after IVF. Hum Reprod 13:1702, 1998.

44. Hoffman HJ, Bakketeig LG: Risk factors associated with the occurrence of preterm birth. Clin Obstet Gynecol 27:539, 1984.

45. Papiernik E: Proposals for a programmed prevention policy of preterm birth. Clin Obstet Gynecol 27:614, 1984.

46. Grunebaum A, Minkoff H, Blake D: Pregnancy among obstetricians: A comparison of births before, during, and after residency. Am J Obstet Gynecol 157:79, 1987.

47. Luke B, Mamelle N, Keith L, et al: The association between occupational factors and preterm birth: A United States nurses' study. Am J Obstet Gynecol 173:849, 1995.

48. Duff P, Kopelman JN: Subclinical intra-amniotic infection in asymptomatic patients with refractory preterm labor. Obstet Gynecol 69:756, 1987.

49. Dunlow S, Duff P: Microbiology of the lower genital tract and amniotic fluid in asymptomatic preterm patients with intact membranes and moderate to advanced degrees of cervical effacement and dilatation. Am J Perinatol 7:235, 1990.

50. Hameed C, Tejani N, Verma UL, et al: Silent chorioamnionitis as a cause of preterm labor refractory to tocolytic therapy. Am J Obstet Gynecol 149:726, 1984.

51. Watts DH, Krohn MA, Hillier SL, et al: The association of occult amniotic fluid infection with gestational age and neonatal outcome among women in preterm labor. Obstet Gynecol 79:351, 1992.

52. Bobitt JR, Ledger WJ: Unrecognized amnionitis and prematurity: A preliminary report. J Reprod Med 19:8, 1977.

53. Hillier SL, Witkin SS, Krohn MA, et al: The relationship of amniotic fluid cytokines and preterm delivery, amniotic fluid infection, histologic chorioamnionitis, and chorioamnion infection. Obstet Gynecol 81:941, 1993.

54. Romero R, Sirtori M, Oyarzun E, et al: Infection and labor: V. Prevalence, microbiology, and clinical significance of intraamniotic infection in women with preterm labor and intact membranes. Am J Obstet Gynecol 161:817, 1989.

55. Skoll MA, Moretti ML, Sibai BM: The incidence of positive amniotic fluid cultures in patients in preterm labor with intact membranes. Am J Obstet Gynecol 161:813, 1989.

56. Romero R, Avila C, Santhanam U, et al: Amniotic fluid interleukin-6 in preterm labor. J Clin Invest 85:1392, 1990.

57. Romero R, Brody DT, Oyarzun E, et al: Infection and labor: III. Interleukin-1: A signal for the onset of parturition. Am J Obstet Gynecol 160:1117, 1989.

58. Romero R, Manogue KR, Mitchell MD, et al: Infection and labor: IV. Cachectin-tumor necrosis factor in the amniotic fluid of women with intraamniotic infection and preterm labor. Am J Obstet Gynecol 161:336, 1989.

59. Iams JD, Johnson FF, Creasy RK: Prevention of preterm birth. Clin Obstet Gynecol 31:599, 1988.

60. Goldenberg RL, Iams JD, Das A, et al: The preterm prediction study: Sequential cervical length and fetal fibronectin testing for the prediction of spontaneous preterm birth. Am J Obstet Gynecol 182:636, 2000.

61. Goldenberg RL, Iams JD, Mercer BM, et al: The preterm prediction study: The value of new vs. standard risk factors in predicting early and all spontaneous preterm births. Am J Public Health 88:233, 1998.

62. Iams JD: Preterm birth. In Gabbe SG, Niebyl JR, Simpson JL (eds): Obstetrics: Normal and Problem Pregnancies, 4th ed. New York, Churchill Livingstone, 2002.

63. Lettieri L, Vintzileos AM, Rodis JF, et al: Does "idiopathic" preterm labor resulting in preterm birth exist? Am J Obstet Gynecol 168:1480, 1993.

64. Norwitz ER, Robinson JN: A systematic approach to the management of preterm labor. Semin Perinatol 25:223, 2001.

65. Norwitz ER, Robinson JN, Challis JR: The control of labor. N Engl J Med 341:660, 1999.

66. Goldenberg RL, Hauth JC, Andrews WW: Intrauterine infection and preterm delivery. N Engl J Med 342:1500, 2000.

67. Romero R, Avila C, Brekus CA, et al: The role of systemic and intrauterine infection in pre-term parturition. Ann N Y Acad Sci 662:355, 1991.

68. Lockwood CJ: Stress-associated preterm delivery: The role of corticotropin-releasing hormone. Am J Obstet Gynecol 180: S264, 1999.

69. Romero R, Gomez R, Mazor M, et al: The preterm labor syndrome. In Elder MG, Romero R, Lamont RF (eds): Preterm Labor. New York, Churchill Livingstone, 1997.

70. Maymon E, Romero R, Pacora P, et al: Evidence for the participation of interstitial collagenase (matrix metalloproteinase 1) in preterm premature rupture of membranes. Am J Obstet Gynecol 183:914, 2000.

71. Challis JRG, Matthews SG, Gibb W, et al: Endocrine and paracrine regulation of birth at term and preterm. Endocr Rev 21:514, 2000.

72. Dudley DJ: Pre-term labor: An intra-uterine inflammatory response syndrome? J Reprod Immunol 36:93, 1997.

73. Tucker JM, Goldenberg RL, Davis RO, et al: Etiologies of preterm birth in an indigent population: Is prevention a logical expectation? Obstet Gynecol 77:343, 1991.

74. Romero R, Emamian M, Wan M, et al: Prostaglandin concentrations in amniotic fluid of women with intraamniotic infection and preterm labor. Am J Obstet Gynecol 157:1461, 1987.

75. Romero R, Munoz H, Gomez R, et al: Increase in prostaglandin bioavailability precedes the onset of human parturition. Prostaglandins Leukot Essent Fatty Acids 54:187, 1996.

76. Arias F, Rodriguez L, Rayne SC, et al: Maternal placental vasculopathy and infection: Two distinct subgroups among

patients with preterm labor and preterm ruptured membranes. Am J Obstet Gynecol 160:585, 1993.

77. Leguizamon G, Smith J, Younis H, et al: Enhancement of amniotic cyclooxygenase type 2 activity in women with preterm delivery associated with twins or polyhydramnios. Am J Obstet Gynecol 184:117, 2001.

78. Sawdy RJ, Slater DM, Dennes WJ, et al: The roles of the cyclo-oxygenases types one and two in prostaglandin synthesis in human fetal membranes at term. Placenta 21:54, 2000.

79. Slater D, Dennes W, Sawdy R, et al: Expression of cyclo-oxygenase types-1 and -2 in human fetal membranes throughout pregnancy. J Mol Endocrinol 22:125, 1999.

80. Caroll EM, Gianopoulos JG, Collins PL: Abnormality of calcium channel inhibitor release from fetal membranes in preterm labor. Am J Obstet Gynecol 184:356, 2001.

81. Challis JRG, Gibb W: Control of parturition. Prenat Neonat Med 1:283, 1996.

82. Elovitz MA, Ascher-Landsberg J, Saunders T, et al: The mechanisms underlying the stimulatory effects of thrombin on myometrial smooth muscle. Am J Obstet Gynecol 183:674, 2000.

83. Elovitz MA, Saunders T, Ascher-Landsberg J, et al: Effects of thrombin on myometrial contractions in vitro and in vivo. Am J Obstet Gynecol 183:799, 2000.

84. Agency for Healthcare Research and Quality: Management of Preterm Labor. Evidence Report/Technology Assessment No. 18. Rockville, MD, Agency for Healthcare Research and Quality, 2000.

85. Murphy K, Aghajafari F, Hannah M: Antenatal corticosteroids for preterm birth. Semin Perinatol 25:341, 2001.

86. National Institutes of Child Health and Development: Effect of corticosteroids for fetal maturation on perinatal outcomes. NIH Consensus Statement 12:1, 1994.

87. Creasy RK: Lifestyle influences on prematurity. J Dev Physiol 15:15, 1991.

88. Herron MA, Katz M, Creasy RK: Evaluation of a preterm birth prevention program: Preliminary report. Obstet Gynecol 59:452, 1982.

89. Main DM, Richardson D, Gabbe SG, et al: Prospective evaluation of risk scoring system for predicting preterm delivery in black inner city women. Obstet Gynecol 69:61, 1987.

90. Mercer BM, Goldenberg RL, Das A, et al: The preterm prediction study: A clinical risk assessment system. Am J Obstet Gynecol 174:1885, 1996.

91. Mueller-Heubach E, Guzich DS: Evaluation of risk scoring in a preterm birth prevention study of indigent patients. Obstet Gynecol 160:829, 1989.

92. Owen J, Goldenberg RL, Davis RO, et al: Evaluation of a risk scoring system as a predictor of preterm birth in an indigent population. Am J Obstet Gynecol 163:873, 1990.

93. Hewitt BG, Newnham JP: A review of the obstetric and medical complications leading to the delivery of infants of very low birthweight. Med J Aust 149:234, 1988.

94. Creasy RK, Gummer BA, Liggins GC: System for predicting spontaneous preterm birth. Obstet Gynecol 55:692, 1980.

95. Spiegel CA, Amsel R, Eschenbach DA, et al: Anaerobic bacteria in nonspecific vaginitis. N Engl J Med 303:601, 1980.

96. Martius J, Roos T: The role of urogenital tract infections in the etiology of preterm births: A review. Arch Gynecol Obstet 258:1, 1996.

97. Royce RA, Jackson TP, Thorp JM Jr, et al: Race/ethnicity, vaginal flora patterns, and pH during pregnancy. Sex Transm Dis 26:96, 1999.

98. Eschenbach DA: History and review of bacterial vaginosis. Am J Obstet Gynecol 169:441, 1993.

99. Hay PE, Lamont RF, Taylor-Robinson D, et al: Abnormal bacterial colonization of the genital tract and subsequent preterm delivery and late miscarriage. BMJ 308:295, 1994.

100. Hillier SL, Nugent RP, Eschenbach DA, et al: Association between bacterial vaginosis and preterm delivery of a low-birth-weight-infant. N Engl J Med 333:1737, 1995.

101. Llahi-Camp JM, Rai R, Ison C, et al: Association of bacterial vaginosis with a history of second trimester miscarriage. Hum Reprod 11:1575, 1996.

102. Meis PJ, Goldenberg RL, Mercer B, et al: The preterm prediction study: Significance of vaginal infections. Am J Obstet Gynecol 173:1231, 1995.

103. Silver HM, Sperling RS, St Gibbs RS: Evidence relating bacterial vaginosis to intraamniotic infection. Am J Obstet Gynecol 161:808, 1989.

104. Martius J, Eschenbach DA: The role of bacterial vaginosis as a cause of amniotic fluid infection, chorioamnionitis and prematurity—a review. Arch Gynecol Obstet 247:1, 1990.

105. Carey JC, Klebanoff MA, Hauth JC, et al: Metronidazole to prevent preterm delivery in pregnant women with asymptomatic bacterial vaginosis. N Engl J Med 342:534, 2000.

106. Hauth JC, Goldenberg RL, Andrews WW, et al: Reduced incidence of preterm delivery with metronidazole and erythromycin in women with bacterial vaginosis. N Engl J Med 333:1732, 1995.

107. Joesoef MR, Hillier SL, Wiknjosastro G, et al: Intravaginal clindamycin treatment for bacterial vaginosis: Effects on preterm delivery and low birth weight. Am J Obstet Gynecol 173:1527, 1995.

108. Kekki M, Kurki T, Pelkonen J, et al: Vaginal clindamycin in preventing preterm birth and peripartal infections in asymptomatic women with bacterial vaginosis: A randomized, controlled trial. Obstet Gynecol 97:643, 2001.

109. Kurkinen R, Vuopala S, Koskela M, et al: A randomised controlled trial of vaginal clindamycin for early pregnancy bacterial vaginosis. Br J Obstet Gynaecol 107:1427, 2000.

110. Morales WJ, Schorr S, Albritton J: Effect of metronidazole in patients with preterm birth in preceding pregnancy and bacterial vaginosis: A placebo-controlled, double-blind study. Am J Obstet Gynecol 171:345, 1994.

111. Brocklehurst P, Hannah M, McDonald H: Interventions for treating bacterial vaginosis in pregnancy. Cochrane Review. In: The Cochrane Library, Issue 2, 2001.

112. Guise JM, Mahon SM, Aickin M, et al: Screening for Bacterial Vaginosis in Pregnancy: Systematic Evidence Review. (AHRQ/Publication No. AHRQ01-S001). Rockville, MD, Agency for Healthcare Research and Quality, 2001.

113. Korn AP, Bolan G, Padian N, et al: Plasma cell endometritis in women with symptomatic bacterial vaginosis. Obstet Gynecol 85:387, 1995.

114. Kurki T, Sivonen A, Renkonen OV, et al: Bacterial vaginosis in early pregnancy and pregnancy outcome. Obstet Gynecol 80:173, 1992.

115. Ralph SG, Rutherford AJ, Wilson JD: Influence of bacterial vaginosis on conception and miscarriage in the first trimester: Cohort study. BMJ 319:220, 1999.

116. Ugwumadu AHN: Bacterial vaginosis in pregnancy. Curr Opin Obstet Gynecol 14:115, 2002.

117. Feinberg RF, Kliman HJ, Lockwood CJ: Is oncofetal fibronectin a trophoblast glue for implantation? Am J Pathol 138:537, 1991.

118. Lockwood CJ, Senyei AE, Dische MR, et al: Fetal fibronectin in cervical and vaginal secretions as predictor of preterm delivery. N Engl J Med 325:669, 1991.

119. Goldenberg RL, Mercer BM, Iams JD, et al: The preterm prediction study: Patterns of cervicovaginal fetal fibronectin as predictors of spontaneous preterm delivery. Am J Obstet Gynecol 177:8, 1997.

120. Iams JD, Casal D, McGregor JA, et al: Fetal fibronectin improves the accuracy of diagnosis of preterm labor. Am J Obstet Gynecol 173:141, 1995.

121. Lockwood CJ, Wein R, Lapinski R, et al: The presence of cervical and vaginal fetal fibronectin predicts preterm delivery in an inner-city obstetric population. Am J Obstet Gynecol 169:798, 1993.

122. Malak TM, Sizmur F, Bell SC, et al: Fetal fibronectin in cervicovaginal secretions as a predictor of preterm birth. Br J Obstet Gynaecol 103:648, 1996.

123. Peaceman AM, Andrews WW, Thorp JM, et al: Fetal fibronectin as a predictor of preterm birth in patients with symptoms: A multicenter trial. Am J Obstet Gynecol 177:13, 1997.

124. Goldenberg RL, Thom E, Moawad AH, et al: The preterm prediction study: Fetal fibronectin, bacterial vaginosis, and peripartum infection. Obstet Gynecol 87:656, 1996.

125. Leitich H, Egarter C, Kaider A, et al: Cervicovaginal fetal fibronectin as a marker for preterm delivery: A meta-analysis. Am J Obstet Gynecol 180:1169, 1999.

126. Inglis SR, Jeremias J, Kuno K, et al: Detection of tumor necrosis factor-alpha, interleukin-6, and fetal fibronectin in the lower genital tract during pregnancy: Relation to outcome. Am J Obstet Gynecol 171:5, 1994.

127. Andersen HF: Use of fetal fibronectin in women at risk for preterm delivery. Clin Obstet Gynecol 43:746, 2000.

128. Goodwin TM: A role for estriol in human labor, term and preterm. Am J Obstet Gynecol 180:S208, 1999.

129. McGregor JA, Hastings C, Roberts T, et al: Diurnal variation in salivary estriol level during pregnancy: A pilot study. Am J Obstet Gynecol 180:S223, 1999.

130. Hendershott CM, Dullien V, Goodwin TM: Serial betamethasone administration: Effect on maternal salivary estriol levels. Am J Obstet Gynecol 180:S219, 1999.

131. Heine RP, McGregor JA, Dullien VK: Accuracy of salivary estriol testing compared to traditional risk factor assessment in predicting preterm birth. Am J Obstet Gynecol 180:S214, 1999.

132. McGregor JA, Jackson GM, Lachelin GC, et al: Salivary estriol as risk assessment for preterm labor: A prospective trial. Am J Obstet Gynecol 173:1337, 1995.

133. Colombo DF, Iams JD: Cervical length and preterm labor. Clin Obstet Gynecol 43:735, 2000.

134. Sonek JD, Iams JD, Blumenfeld M, et al: Measurement of cervical length in pregnancy: Comparison between vaginal ultrasonography and digital examination. Obstet Gynecol 76:172, 1990.

135. Iams JD, Goldenberg RL, Meis PJ, et al: The length of the cervix and the risk of spontaneous premature delivery. N Engl J Med 334:567, 1996.

136. Berghella V, Tolosa JE, Kuhlman K, et al: Cervical ultrasonography compared with manual examination as a predictor of preterm delivery. Am J Obstet Gynecol 177: 723, 1997.

137. Crane JM, Van den Hof M, Armson BA, et al: Transvaginal ultrasound in the prediction of preterm delivery: Singleton and twin gestations. Obstet Gynecol 90:357, 1997.

138. Hassan SS, Romero R, Berry SM, et al: Patients with an ultrasonographic cervical length < or = 15 mm have nearly a 50% risk of early spontaneous preterm delivery. Am J Obstet Gynecol 182:1458, 2000.

139. Watson WJ, Stevens D, Welter S, et al: Observations on the sonographic measurement of cervical length and the risk of preterm birth. J Matern Fetal Med 8:17, 1999.

140. Leitich H, Brunbauer M, Kaider A, et al: Cervical length and dilatation of the internal cervical os detected by vaginal ultrasonography as markers for preterm delivery: A systematic review. Am J Obstet Gynecol 181:1465, 1999.

141. Guzman ER, Ananth CV: Cervical length and spontaneous prematurity: Laying the foundation for future interventional randomized trials for the short cervix. Ultrasound Obstet Gynecol 18:195, 2001.

142. Iams JD, Goldenberg RL, Mercer BM, et al: The preterm prediction study: Recurrence risk of spontaneous preterm birth. Am J Obstet Gynecol 178:1035, 1998.

143. Welsh A, Nicolaides K: Cervical screening for preterm delivery. Curr Opin Obstet Gynecol 14:195, 2002.

144. Nageotte MP, Dorchester W, Porto M, et al: Quantitation of uterine activity preceding preterm, term and postterm labor. Am J Obstet Gynecol 158:1254, 1988.

145. Katz M, Newman RB, Gill PJ: Assessment of uterine activity in ambulatory patients at high risk of preterm delivery. Am J Obstet Gynecol 154:44, 1986.

146. Newman RB, Gill PJ, Wittreich P, et al: Maternal perception of prelabor uterine activity. Obstet Gynecol 68:765, 1986.

147. Brustman L, Langer O, Anyaegbunam A: Education does not improve patient perception of preterm contractions. Obstet Gynecol 76:97, 1990.

148. Dyson DC, Crites YM, Ray DA, et al: Prevention of preterm birth in high-risk patients: The role of education and provider contact versus home uterine monitoring. Am J Obstet Gynecol 164:756, 1991.

149. Dyson DC, Danbe KH, Bamber JA, et al: Monitoring women at risk for preterm labor. N Engl J Med 338:15, 1998.

150. Hill WC, Fleming AD, Martin RW, et al: Home uterine activity monitoring is associated with a reduction in preterm birth. Obstet Gynecol 76:13S, 1990.

151. Iams JD, Johnson FF, O'Shaugnessy RW, et al: A prospective random trial of home uterine activity monitoring in pregnancies at increased risk of preterm labor. Am J Obstet Gynecol 157:638, 1987.

152. Morrison JC, Martin JM, Martin RW, et al: Prevention of preterm birth by ambulatory assessment of uterine activity: A randomized study. Am J Obstet Gynecol 156:536, 1987.

153. Wapner RJ, Cotton DB, Artal R, et al: A randomized multicenter trial assessing a home uterine activity monitoring device used in the absence of daily nursing contact. Am J Obstet Gynecol 172:1026, 1995.

154. Watson DL, Welch RA, Mariona FG, et al: Management of preterm labor patients at home: Does daily uterine activity monitoring and nursing support make a difference? Obstet Gynecol 76:32S, 1990.

155. Grimes DA, Schulz KF: Randomized controlled trials of home uterine activity monitoring: A review and critique. Obstet Gynecol 79:137, 1992.

156. Sachs BP, Hellerstein S, Freeman R, et al: Home monitoring of uterine activity: Does it prevent prematurity? N Engl J Med 325:1374, 1991.

157. Devoe LD, Ware DJ: Home uterine activity monitoring: A critical review. Clin Obstet Gynecol 43:778, 2000.

158. Keirse MJ, Van Hoven M: Reanalysis of a multireported trial on home uterine activity monitoring. Birth 20:117, 1993.

159. United States Preventive Services Task Force: Home uterine activity monitoring for preterm labor. JAMA 270:371, 1993.

160. Colton T, Kayne HL, Zhang Y, et al: A metaanalysis of home uterine activity monitoring. Am J Obstet Gynecol 173:1499, 1995.

161. Collaborative Home Uterine Monitoring Study Group (CHUMS): A multicenter randomized controlled trial of home uterine monitoring: Active versus sham device. Am J Obstet Gynecol 173:1120, 1995.

162. Goldenberg RL, Cliver SP, Bronstein J, et al: Bed rest in pregnancy. Obstet Gynecol 84:131, 1994.

163. Kovacevich GJ, Gaich SA, Lavin JP, et al: The prevalence of thromboembolic events among women with extended bed rest prescribed as part of the treatment for premature labor of preterm premature rupture of membranes. Am J Obstet Gynecol 182:1089, 2000.

164. Maloni JA, Chance B, Zhang C, et al: Physical and psychosocial side effects of antepartum hospital bed rest. Nurs Res 42:197, 1993.

165. Pircon RA, Strassner HT, Kirz DS, et al: Controlled trial of hydration and bed rest versus bed rest alone in the evaluation of preterm uterine contractions. Am J Obstet Gynecol 161:775, 1989.

166. Valenzuela G, Cline S, Hayashi RH: Follow-up of hydration and sedation in the pretherapy of premature labor. Am J Obstet Gynecol 147:396, 1983.

167. Cobo E, Cifuentes R, de Villamizar M: Inhibition of menstrual uterine motility during water diuresis. Am J Obstet Gynecol 132:313, 1978.

168. Helfgott AW, Willis DC, Blanco JD: Is hydration and sedation beneficial in the treatment of threatened preterm labor? A preliminary report. J Matern Fetal Med 3:37, 1994.

169. Guinn DA, Goepfert AR, Owen J, et al: Management options in women with preterm uterine contractions: A randomized clinical trial. Am J Obstet Gynecol 177:814, 1997.

170. Gibbs RS, Romero R, Hillier SL: A review of premature birth and subclinical infection. Am J Obstet Gynecol 166:1515, 1992.

171. Hardy PH, Nell EE, Spence MR, et al: Prevalence of six sexually transmitted diseases among pregnant intercity adolescents and pregnancy outcome. Lancet 2:333, 1984.

172. Locksmith G, Duff P: Infection, antibiotics, and preterm delivery. Semin Perinatol 25:295, 2001.

173. McGregor JA, French JI, Parker R, et al: Prevention of premature birth by screening and treatment for common genital tract infections: Results of a prospective controlled evaluation. Am J Obstet Gynecol 173:157, 1995.

174. Minkoff H, Grunebaum AN, Schwarz RH, et al: Risk factors for prematurity and premature rupture of membranes: A prospective study of the vaginal flora in pregnancy. Am J Obstet Gynecol 150:965, 1984.

175. Read JS, Klebanoff MA: Sexual intercourse during pregnancy and preterm delivery: Effects of vaginal microorganisms. Am J Obstet Gynecol 168:514, 1993.

176. Sarell PM, Pruett KA: Symptomatic gonorrhea during pregnancy. Obstet Gynecol 32:670, 1968.

177. Romero R, Oyarzun E, Mazor M, et al: Meta-analysis of the relationship between asymptomatic bacteriuria and preterm delivery/low birth weight. Obstet Gynecol 73:576, 1989.

178. Mason PR, Brown IM: Trichomonas in pregnancy. Lancet 2:1025, 1980.

179. American College of Obstetricians and Gynecologists: Prevention of early-onset group B streptococcal disease in newborns. ACOG Committee Opinion: No. 279, December 2002. Obstet Gynecol 100:1405, 2002.

180. Kenyon SL, Taylor DJ, Tarnow-Mordi W: Broad-spectrum antibiotics for spontaneous preterm labour: The ORACLE II randomised trial. Lancet 357:989, 2001.

181. Romero R, Sibai B, Caritis S, et al: Antibiotic treatment of preterm labor with intact membranes: A multicenter, randomized, double-blinded, placebo-controlled trial. Am J Obstet Gynecol 169:764, 1993.

182. Althuisius SM, Dekker GA, van Geijn HP, et al: Cervical Incompetence Prevention Randomized Cerclage Trial (CIPRACT): Study design and preliminary results. Am J Obstet Gynecol 183:823, 2000.

183. Hassan SS, Romero R, Maymon E, et al: Does cervical cerclage prevent preterm delivery in patients with a short cervix? Am J Obstet Gynecol 184:1325, 2001.

184. Novy MJ, Gupta A, Wothe DD, et al: Cervical cerclage in the second trimester of pregnancy: A historical cohort study. Am J Obstet Gynecol 184:1447, 2001.

185. Rust OA, Atlas RO, Jones KJ, et al: A randomized trial of cerclage versus no cerclage among patients with ultrasonographically detected second-trimester preterm dilatation of the internal os. Am J Obstet Gynecol 183:830, 2000.

186. Caritis SN, Darby MJ, Chan L: Pharmacologic treatment of preterm labor. Clin Obstet Gynecol 31:635, 1988.

187. Keirse MJNC, Grant A, King JF: Preterm labour. In Chalmers I, Enkin M, Keirse MJNC (eds): Effective Care in Pregnancy and Childbirth. New York, Oxford University Press, 1989.

188. King JF, Grant A, Keirse MJNC, et al: Beta-mimetics in preterm labour: An overview of the randomized controlled trials. Br J Obstet Gynaecol 95:211, 1988.

189. Zlatnick FJ: The applicability of labour inhibitors to the problem of prematurity. Am J Obstet Gynecol 113:704, 1972.

190. Gonik B, Creasy RK: Preterm labor—its diagnosis and management. Am J Obstet Gynecol 154:3, 1986.

191. Boyer KM, Gotoff SP: Prevention of early-onset neonatal group B streptococcal disease with selective intrapartum chemoprophylaxis. N Engl J Med 314:1665, 1986.

192. ACOG Technical Bulletin 206: Premature Labor. Washington, DC, American College of Obstetricians and Gynecologists, September 1995.

193. Higby K, Xenakis EMJ, Pauerstein CJ: Do tocolytic agents stop preterm labor? A critical and comprehensive review of efficacy and safety. Am J Obstet Gynecol 168:1247, 1993.

194. Richter R: Evaluation of success in treatment of threatening preterm labor by betamimetic drugs. Am J Obstet Gynecol 127:482, 1977.

195. Robertson PA, Sniderman SH, Laros RK, et al: Neonatal morbidity according to gestational age and birth weight from five tertiary centers in the United States, 1983 through 1986. Am J Obstet Gynecol 166:1629, 1992.

196. Katz VL, Farmer RM: Controversies in tocolytic therapy. Clin Obstet Gynecol 42:802, 1999.

197. American College of Obstetricians and Gynecologists: ACOG Practice Bulletin: Clinical Management Guidelines for Obstetrician-Gynecologists: No. 38, September 2002. Perinatal care at the threshold of viability. Obstet Gynecol 100:617, 2002.

198. Lemons JA, Bauer CR, Oh W, et al: Very low birth weight outcomes of the National Institute of Child Health and Human Development Neonatal Research Network, January 1995 through December 1996. Pediatrics 107:E1, 2001.

199. Silver RK, MacGregor SN, Farrell EE, et al: Perinatal factors influencing survival at twenty-four weeks' gestation. Am J Obstet Gynecol 168:1724, 1993.

200. Goldenberg RL, Nelson KG, Davis RO, et al: Delay in delivery: Influence of gestational age and the duration of delay on perinatal outcome. Obstet Gynecol 64:480, 1984.

201. Kitchen W, Ford GW, Doyle LW, et al: Outcome of extremely low birth-weight infants in relation to the hospital of birth. Aust N Z J Obstet Gynaecol 24:1, 1984.

202. Nwaesei CG, Young DC, Byrne JM, et al: Preterm birth at 23 to 26 weeks' gestation: Is active obstetric management justified? Am J Obstet Gynecol 157:890, 1987.

203. Crowley P, Chalmers I, Keirse MJNC: The effects of corticosteroid administration before preterm delivery: An overview of the evidence from controlled trials. Br J Obstet Gynaecol 97:11, 1990.

204. Garite TJ, Keegan KA, Freeman RK, et al: A randomized trial of ritodrine tocolysis versus expectant management in patients with premature rupture of membranes at 25 to 30 weeks of gestation. Am J Obstet Gynecol 157:388, 1987.

205. Davey AM, Sherer DM, Abramowicz JS, et al: Does antenatal maternal betamethasone administration reduce neonatal morbidity following immediate surfactant therapy at delivery [abstract]? Am J Obstet Gynecol 166:276, 1992.

206. Jobe AH, Mitchell BR, Gunkel JH: Beneficial effects of the combined use of prenatal corticosteroids and postnatal surfactant on preterm infants. Am J Obstet Gynecol 168:508, 1993.

207. Kwong MS, Egan EA, Notter RA: Synergistic responses of antenatal betamethasone and tracheal instillation of calf lung surfactant extract at birth [abstract]. Pediatr Res 21:458, 1986.

208. Ramsey PS, Rouse DJ: Magnesium sulfate as a tocolytic agent. Semin Perinatol 25:236, 2001.

209. Petrie RH: Tocolysis using magnesium sulfate. Semin Perinatol 5:266, 1981.

210. Elliot JP, O'Keeffe DF, Greenberg P, et al: Pulmonary edema associated with magnesium sulfate and betamethasone administration. Am J Obstet Gynecol 134:717, 1979.

211. Peaceman AM, Meyer BA, Thorp JA, et al: The effect of magnesium sulfate tocolysis on the fetal biophysical profile. Am J Obstet Gynecol 161:771, 1989.

212. Savory J, Monif G: Serum calcium levels in cord sera of the progeny treated with magnesium sulfate for toxemia of pregnancy. Am J Obstet Gynecol 110:556, 1971.

213. Holcomb WL, Shackelford GD, Petrie RH: Magnesium tocolysis and neonatal bone abnormalities: A controlled study. Obstet Gynecol 78:611, 1991.

214. Nelson KB, Grether JK: Can magnesium sulfate reduce the risk of cerebral palsy in very low birthweight infants? Pediatrics 95:263, 1995.

215. Schendel DE, Berg CJ, Yeargin-Allsop M: Prenatal magnesium sulfate exposure and the risk for cerebral palsy or mental retardation among very low-birth-weight children aged 3 to 5 years. JAMA 276:1805, 1996.

216. Caritis SN, Lin LS, Toig G, et al: Pharmacodynamics of ritodrine in pregnant women during preterm labor. Am J Obstet Gynecol 147:752, 1983.

217. Jeyabalan A, Caritis SN: Pharmacologic inhibition of preterm labor. Clin Obstet Gynecol 45:99, 2002.

218. Ke R, Vohra M, Casper R: Prolonged inhibition of human myometrial contractility by intermittent isoproterenol. Am J Obstet Gynecol 149:841, 1984.

219. Stubblefield PG, Heyl PS: Treatment of premature labor with subcutaneous terbutaline. Obstet Gynecol 59:457, 1982.

220. Lam F, Gill P, Smith M, et al: Use of the subcutaneous terbutaline pump for long-term tocolysis. Obstet Gynecol 72:810, 1988.

221. Merkatz IR, Peter JB, Borden TP: Ritodrine hydrochloride: A beta-mimetic agent for use in preterm labor: II. Evidence of efficacy. Obstet Gynecol 56:7, 1980.

222. Robertson PA, Herron M, Katz M, et al: Maternal morbidity associated with isoxsuprine and terbutaline tocolysis. Eur J Obstet Gynecol Reprod Biol 11:317, 1981.

223. Caritis S, Toig G, Heddinger L, et al: A double-blind study comparing ritodrine and terbutaline in the treatment of preterm labor. Am J Obstet Gynecol 150:7, 1984.

224. Ingemarrson I, Bentsson B: A five-year experience with terbutaline for preterm labor: Low rate of severe side effects. Obstet Gynecol 66:176, 1985.

225. Main EK, Main DM, Gabbe SG: Chronic oral terbutaline therapy is associated with maternal glucose intolerance. Am J Obstet Gynecol 157:644, 1987.

226. Hadders-Algra, Touwen BCL, Huisjes HJ: Long-term follow-up of children prenatally exposed to ritodrine. Br J Obstet Gynaecol 93:156, 1986.

227. Zuckerman H, Reiss U, Rubinstein I: Inhibition of human premature labor by indomethacin. Obstet Gynecol 44:787, 1974.

228. Niebyl JR, Blake DA, White RD, et al: The inhibition of premature labor with indomethacin. Am J Obstet Gynecol 136:1014, 1980.

229. McCoshen JA, Hoffman DR, Kredentser JV, et al: The role of fetal membranes in regulating production, transport, and metabolism of prostaglandin E_2 during labor. Am J Obstet Gynecol 163:1632, 1990.

230. Vermillion ST, Landen CN: Prostaglandin inhibitors as tocolytic agents. Semin Perinatol 25:256, 2001.

231. Besinger RE, Niebyl JR, Keyes WG: Randomized comparative trial of indomethacin and ritodrine for the long-term treatment of preterm labor. Am J Obstet Gynecol 164:981, 1991.

232. Csaba IF, Sulyok E, Ertl T: Clinical note: Relationship of maternal treatment with indomethacin to persistence of fetal circulation syndrome. J Pediatr 92:484, 1978.

233. Dudley DK, Hardie MJ: Fetal and neonatal effects of indomethacin used as a tocolytic agent. Am J Obstet Gynecol 151:181, 1985.

234. Goudie BM, Dossetor JB: Effect on the fetus of indomethacin given to suppress labor. Lancet 1:1187, 1989.

235. Manchester D, Margolis HS, Sheldon RE: Possible association between maternal indomethacin therapy and primary pulmonary hypertension of the newborn. Am J Obstet Gynecol 126:467, 1976.

236. Morales WJ, Smith SG, Angel JL, et al: Efficacy and safety of indomethacin in the treatment of preterm labor: A randomized study. Obstet Gynecol 74:567, 1989.

237. Moise KJ: The effect of advancing gestational age on the frequency of fetal ductal constriction secondary to maternal indomethacin use. Am J Obstet Gynecol 168:1350, 1993.

238. Niebyl JR, Witter FR: Neonatal outcome after indomethacin treatment of preterm labor. Am J Obstet Gynecol 155:747, 1986.

239. Zuckerman H, Shalev E, Gilad G, et al: Further study of the inhibition of premature labor by indomethacin: Part I. Clinical experience. J Perinat Med 12:19, 1984.

240. Betkurur MV, Yeh TF, Miller K, et al: Indomethacin and its effect on renal function and urinary kallikrein excretion in premature infants with patent ductus arteriosus. Pediatrics 68:99, 1981.

241. Cifuentes RF, Olley PM, Balfe JW, et al: Indomethacin and renal function in premature infants with persistent patent ductus arteriosus. J Pediatr 95:583, 1979.

242. Friedman ZI, Whitman V, Maisels MJ, et al: Indomethacin disposition and indomethacin induced platelet dysfunction in premature infants. J Clin Pharmacol 18:272, 1978.

243. Kirshon B, Moise KJ, Wasserstrum N, et al: Influence of short-term indomethacin therapy on fetal urinary output. Obstet Gynecol 72:51, 1988.

244. Major CA, Lewis DF, Harding JA, et al: Tocolysis with indomethacin increases the incidence of necrotizing enterocolitis in the low birth weight neonate. Am J Obstet Gynecol 170:102, 1994.

245. Vanhaesebrouck P, Thiery M, Leroy LG, et al: Oligohydramnios, renal insufficiency, and ileal perforation in preterm infants after intrauterine exposure to indomethacin. J Pediatr 113:738, 1988.

246. Bandstra ES, Montalvo BM, Goldberg RN, et al: Prophylactic indomethacin for prevention of intraventricular hemorrhage in premature infants. Pediatrics 82:533, 1988.

247. Pickard JD, Tampura I, Stewart M, et al: Prostacyclin, indomethacin, and the cerebral circulation. Brain Res 197:425, 1980.

248. Baerts W, Fetter WF, Hop WJ, et al: Cerebral lesions in preterm infants after tocolytic indomethacin. Dev Med Child Neurol 32:910, 1990.

249. Ianucci TA, Besinger RE, Fisher SG, et al: Effect of dual tocolysis on the incidence of severe intraventricular hemorrhage among extremely low-birth weight infants. Am J Obstet Gynecol 175:1043, 1996.

250. Suarez RD, Grobman WA, Parilla BV: Indomethacin tocolysis and intraventricular hemorrhage. Obstet Gynecol 97:921, 2001.

251. Eronen M, Pesonen E, Kurki T, et al: Increased incidence of bronchopulmonary dysplasia after antenatal administration of indomethacin to prevent preterm labor. J Pediatr 124:782, 1994.

252. Gardner M, Owen J, Skelly S, et al: Preterm delivery after indomethacin: A risk factor for neonatal complications? J Reprod Med 41:903, 1996.

253. Gerson A, Abbasi S, Johnson A, et al: Safety and efficacy of long-term tocolysis with indomethacin. Am J Perinatol 7:71, 1990.

254. Macones GA, Marder SJ, Clothier B, et al: The controversy surrounding indomethacin for tocolysis. Am J Obstet Gynecol 184:264, 2001.

255. Norton M, Merrill J, Cooper B, et al: Neonatal complications after the administration of indomethacin for preterm labor. N Engl J Med 25:1603, 1993.

256. Panter K, Hannah M, Amankwa K, et al: The effect of indomethacin tocolysis in preterm labor on perinatal outcome: A randomized placebo-controlled trial. Br J Obstet Gynaecol 106:467, 1999.

257. Souter D, Harding J, McCowan L, et al: Antenatal indomethacin—adverse fetal effects confirmed. Aust N Z J Obstet Gynaecol 38:11, 1998.

258. Vermillion S, Newman R: Recent indomethacin tocolysis is not associated with neonatal complications in preterm infants. Am J Obstet Gynecol 181:1083, 1999.

259. Tulzer G, Gudmundsson S, Tews G, et al: Incidence of indomethacin-induced human fetal ductal constriction. J Matern Fetal Invest 1:267, 1992.

260. Carlan SJ, O'Brien WF, O'Leary TD, et al: Randomized comparative trial of indomethacin and sulindac for the treatment of refractory preterm labor. Obstet Gynecol 79:223, 1992.

261. Ulmsten U, Andersson KE, Wingerup L: Treatment of premature labor with the calcium antagonist nifedipine. Arch Gynecol 229:1, 1980.

262. Veille JC, Bissonnette JM, Hohimer AR: The effect of a calcium channel blocker (nifedipine) on uterine blood flow in the pregnant goat. Am J Obstet Gynecol 154:1160, 1986.

263. Forman A, Gandrup P, Andersson KE, et al: Effects of nifedipine on spontaneous and methylergometrine-induced activity post partum. Am J Obstet Gynecol 144:442, 1982.

264. Carsten ME, Miller JD: A new look at uterine musculature contraction. Am J Obstet Gynecol 157:1303, 1987.

265. Ferguson JE, Dyson DC, Holbrook RH, et al: Cardiovascular and metabolic effects associated with nifedipine and ritodrine tocolysis. Am J Obstet Gynecol 161:788, 1989.

266. Janky E, Leng JJ, Cormier PH, et al: A randomized study of the treatment of threatened premature labor: Nifedipine versus ritodrine. J Gynecol Obstet Biol Reprod 19:478, 1990.

267. Meyer WR, Randall HW, Graves WL: Nifedipine versus ritodrine for suppressing preterm labor. J Reprod Med 35:649, 1990.

268. Read MD, Wellby DE: The use of a calcium antagonist (nifedipine) to suppress preterm labour. Br J Obstet Gynaecol 93:933, 1986.

269. Tsatsaris V, Papatsonis D, Goffinet F, et al: Tocolysis with nifedipine or beta-adrenergic agonists: A meta-analysis. Obstet Gynecol 97:840, 2001.

270. Papatsonis DN, Van Geijn HP, Ader HJ, et al: Nifedipine and ritodrine in the management of preterm labor: A randomized multicenter trial. Obstet Gynecol 90:230, 1997.

271. Lirette M, Holbrook H, Katz M: Cardiovascular and uterine blood flow changes during nicardipine HCl tocolysis in the rabbit. Obstet Gynecol 69:79, 1987.

272. Mari G, Kirshon B, Moise KJ, et al: Doppler assessment of the fetal and uteroplacental circulation during nifedipine therapy for preterm labor. Am J Obstet Gynecol 161:1514, 1989.

273. Ferguson JE, Dyson DC, Schutz T, et al: A comparison of tocolysis with nifedipine or ritodrine: Analysis of efficacy and maternal, fetal, and neonatal outcome. Am J Obstet Gynecol 163:105, 1990.

274. Papatsonis DN, Kok JH, Van Geijn HP, et al: Neonatal effect of nifedipine and ritodrine for preterm labor. Obstet Gynecol 95:477, 2000.

275. Ray D, Dyson D, Crites Y: Nifedipine tocolysis and neonatal acid-base status at delivery. Am J Obstet Gynecol 12:113, 1994.

276. Bukowski R, Saade GR: New developments in the management of preterm labor. Semin Perinatol 25:272, 2001.

277. Romero R, Sibai BM, Sanchez-Ramos L, et al: An oxytocin receptor antagonist (atosiban) in the treatment of preterm labor: A randomized, double-blind, placebo-controlled trial with tocolytic rescue. Am J Obstet Gynecol 182:1173, 2000.

278. Worldwide Atosiban versus Beta-agonists Study Group: Effectiveness and safety of the oxytocin antagonist atosiban versus beta-adrenergic agonists in the treatment of preterm labour. Br J Obstet Gynaecol 108:133, 2001.

279. Snyder SW, Cardwell MS: Neuromuscular blockade with magnesium and nifedipine. Am J Obstet Gynecol 61:35, 1989.

280. Ferguson JE, Hensleigh PA, Kredenster D: Adjunctive use of magnesium sulfate with ritodrine for preterm labor tocolysis. Am J Obstet Gynecol 148:166, 1984.

281. Hatjis C, Swain M, Nelson L, et al: Efficacy of combined administration of magnesium sulfate and ritodrine in the treatment of preterm labor. Obstet Gynecol 69:317, 1987.

282. Kosasa TS, Busse R, Wahl N, et al: Long-term tocolysis with combined intravenous terbutaline and magnesium sulfate: A 10-year study of 1,000 patients. Obstet Gynecol 84:369, 1994.

283. Ogburn PL, Hansen CA, Williams PP, et al: Magnesium sulfate and β-mimetic dual-agent tocolysis in preterm labor after single agent failure. J Reprod Med 3:583, 1985.
284. Lewis DF, Grimshaw A, Brooks G, et al: A comparison of magnesium sulfate and indomethacin to magnesium sulfate only for tocolysis in preterm labor with advanced cervical dilation. South Med J 88:737, 1995.
285. Oei SG, Oei SK, Brolmann HAM: Myocardial infarction during nifedipine therapy for preterm labor. N Engl J Med 339:154, 1999.
286. Gamissans O, Canas E, Cararach V, et al: A study of indomethacin combined with ritodrine in threatened preterm labour. Eur J Obstet Gynecol Reprod Biol 8:123, 1978.

287. Katz Z, Lancet M, Yemini M, et al: Treatment of premature labor contractions with combined ritodrine and indomethacin. Int J Gynaecol Obstet 21:337, 1983.
288. Macones GA, Berlin M, Berlin JA: Efficacy of oral beta-agonist maintenance therapy in preterm labor: A meta-analysis. Obstet Gynecol 85:313, 1995.
289. Sanchez-Ramos L, Kaunitz AM, Gaudier FL, et al: Efficacy of maintenance therapy after acute tocolysis: A meta-analysis. Am J Obstet Gynecol 181:484, 1994.

CHAPTER 25

Premature Rupture of Membranes: Diagnosis and Management

Linda Chan, Meena Khandelwal, and John S. Hammes*

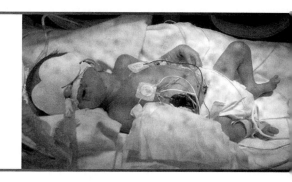

Premature rupture of membranes (PROM) refers to rupture of the amniotic membranes before the onset of labor; it occurs in 8% to 10% of term pregnancies. **Preterm PROM (PPROM)** is rupture of membranes before 37 weeks of gestation. The incidence of PROM in the National Institute of Child Health and Human Development (NICHD) preterm prediction study was 4.5%, and PROM accounted for 32.6% of all preterm births.[1] PPROM complicates 1.7% of all pregnancies but contributes to 20% of all perinatal deaths.[2] In women with PROM at term, most (70%) begin labor within 24 hours, and nearly all (95%) begin labor by 72 hours.[3] In women with preterm PROM, a meta-analysis of 13 randomized trials reported that 75% delivered within 1 week of diagnosis.[4] In PPROM, the latency period to delivery is inversely proportional to the gestational age.[5] In patients with midtrimester PROM, the mean latency period may range from 10.6 to 21.5 days.[6]

Maternal and fetal complications from PROM include intrauterine infection, placental abruption, breech presentation, prolapsed umbilical cord, fetal heart rate (FHR) abnormalities, fetal distress, and prolonged hospital stay. Neonatal morbidity and mortality are predominantly due to infection and complications of prematurity. Morbidities of prematurity include respiratory distress syndrome (RDS), intraventricular hemorrhage (IVH), necrotizing enterocolitis (NEC), patent ductus arteriosus, retinopathy of prematurity, and chronic lung disease. In cases of extreme prematurity, attempts at prolonging gestation are worthwhile, given that the chance of fetal survival increases for each day the fetus stays in the uterus. In PPROM occurring at gestational ages less than 23 weeks, the fetus is at high risk for structural and developmental abnormalities. Complications of prolonged PPROM and oligohydramnios

include pulmonary hypoplasia and oligohydramnios sequence. Oligohydramnios sequence consists of Potter facies, which is characterized by abnormal flattened facial appearance with low-set compressed ears, and deformities of the extremities including flexion contractures.[7]

Several small studies have observed spontaneous cessation of fluid leakage in 2.6% to 11% of patients with PPROM.[8] Most women who have PPROM are unlikely, however, to carry their pregnancy to full term. Multiple risk factors are associated with PROM (Table 25-1).[1,9]

PPROM may be iatrogenic, occurring in 1.2% of genetic amniocenteses, 3% to 5% of diagnostic fetoscopies, and approximately 10% of operative fetoscopies.[10] Borgida and associates[11] retrospectively reviewed patients with PPROM secondary to genetic amniocentesis. They found that these

Table 25–1. Risk Factors for Premature Rupture of Membranes

Low socioeconomic status
Sexually transmissible infections
Preterm labor in index pregnancy
Vaginal bleeding
Cervical colonization
Cigarette smoking during pregnancy
Uterine distention
  Polyhydramnios
  Multiple gestation
Cevical incompetence
α-1-Antitrypsin deficiency
Bacterial vaginosis
Combination risk factors
  Previous preterm birth from PPROM
  Short cervix
  Positive fetal fibronectin
Idiopathic

PPROM, preterm premature rupture of membranes.
Adapted from references 1 and 9.

*Views expressed in this chapter are those of the authors and do not reflect the official policy of the Department of the Navy, the Department of Defense, or the United States government.

patients had significantly longer latency periods (124 versus 28 days) and delivered at more advanced ages (34.2 versus 21.6 weeks) than women with spontaneous PPROM.[11] Although membranes may seal spontaneously in iatrogenic PPROM, patients remain at risk for pregnancy loss.[10]

ETIOLOGY

The etiology of PROM is an area of active investigation. Evidence suggests that PROM results from a complex interplay of factors. These factors are biomolecular (i.e., impaired enzyme regulation, breakdown of collagen) and mechanical (i.e., distention of the uterus from the developing fetus, gravitational forces), which act to disrupt the normal structural arrangement of the chorioamniotic membranes. Figure 25-1 illustrates the predominant pathophysiologic mechanisms leading to PROM.

Defects in Collagen

The amniochorion is a two-layered membrane consisting largely of cells embedded in collagenous and noncollagenous matrix. Placental collagenase and amniotic fluid trypsin increase during pregnancy, probably as a result of decreased regulatory inhibition. If this inhibition is disordered, an exaggerated response and disruption in the collagen matrix occurs, leading to PROM. Congenital defects in collagen production, such as Ehlers-Danlos syndrome and α_1-antitrypsin deficiency, are risk factors for PROM. This fact supports a role for defects in collagen production in the pathophysiology of PROM.[12]

Nutritional deficiencies and smoking also may lead to defective collagen synthesis via reduced availability of ascorbic acid and copper.[3,13]

Matrix Metalloproteinases

Collagenases, which are normally present in the amniotic fluid, also play a role in PROM. These enzymes normally assist in the remodeling of collagen in the cervix and in a process known as *cervical ripening*. Accumulating evidence suggests that the activity of various collagenases, also called *matrix metalloproteinases (MMPs)*, is deranged in PROM. Studies have shown increased MMP-2 and MMP-9 (also known as *gelatinase B*) concentrations in the amniotic fluid of women with PPROM.[14] Two other collagenases, MMP-8 and MMP-13, have the ability to cleave collagen types I, II, and III, which lend the amnion its tensile strength. MMP-8 was found to be dramatically increased in the amniotic fluid of patients with infection, probably via elaboration by activated neutrophils.[15] Amniotic MMPs, of which there are more than 20 reported to date, are a subject of current investigation; however, their clinical utility and application in management of PROM still await future clinical trials.

Infection and Inflammation

Infectious agents and host inflammatory response have been investigated extensively in the etiology of PROM. In cases of PROM occurring before term, approximately one third of patients show microbial invasion of the amniotic cavity. Anaerobic bacteria isolated from the amniotic fluid

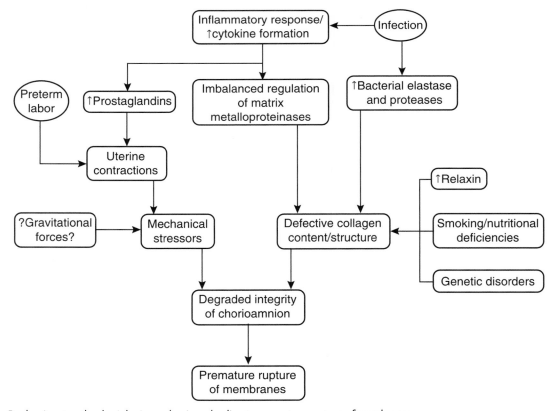

Figure 25–1. Predominant pathophysiologic mechanisms leading to premature rupture of membranes.

of women with PROM produce elastase. This enzyme may damage the connective tissue of the chorioamnion and contribute to PROM.[16]

In addition to an increase in some MMPs and elastase, infection may result in inflammation. Inflammatory cells, such as monocytes, neutrophils, and macrophages, may elaborate reactive oxygen species, which are capable of damaging collagen and amniotic epithelium.[13] Evaluation of the amniotic fluid of women with positive microbial growth has shown significantly elevated markers of inflammation (i.e., interleukin-6, interleukin-1β, tumor necrosis factor, and leukocytes) compared with fluid from patients with negative cultures.[17] Many interleukins, including interleukin-1β and interleukin-6, may lead to increased prostaglandin elaboration, hastening the onset of labor. Release of cytokines (tumor necrosis factor and interleukins) in clinical or subclinical chorioamnionitis is implicated in the increased incidence of cerebral palsy, periventricular leukomalacia, and IVH with PPROM.[18-20]

Hormones

Stress, hypoxia, and infection may lead to activation of the fetal hypothalamic-pituitary-adrenal axis, leading to an increase in corticotropin-releasing hormone, corticotropin, and cortisol. These changes may stimulate prostaglandin E_2, which is associated with PROM.[3,21] Another area of investigation includes relaxin, a peptide hormone that facilitates parturition by causing relaxation of the symphysis pubis. It is up-regulated in PROM. The exact nature of the role of relaxin in PROM requires further elucidation.[22]

Uterine Activities

As gestation progresses, several significant events that may predispose to PROM take place. Uterine activity increases, and the uterus is distended by the developing pregnancy. These mechanical stresses result in downward pressure on the chorioamnion and lead to a loss of intrinsic elasticity. Concurrently, as the pregnancy progresses, the phospholipids between the chorion and the amnion decline, which also may predispose the membranes to rupture by shear forces.[12] Factors that also contribute to augmented uterine contractility include preterm labor and increased prostaglandin release from several sources, as outlined previously.[3]

Occupational Fatigue

Physical stress contributes to PROM. Among nulliparous women, the risk of PPROM increases in proportion to increased occupational fatigue. In one study, sources of occupational fatigue included upright posture, working with industrial machines, physical exertion, repetitive or boring work, and work in a cold, wet, or noisy area. Women not working outside the home had the lowest incidence of PPROM. Women working with four or more of these sources of occupational fatigue had the highest incidence of PROM.[23]

CLINICAL PRESENTATION

Early diagnosis of PROM in pregnancy is important to optimize early intervention and to improve neonatal outcome. Presenting symptoms of PROM range from asymptomatic to fever, abdominal pain, and cramps in the setting of labor and ascending infection of the genital tract. The differential diagnosis of PROM includes urinary leakage, cervicitis, excessive vaginal discharge, and pooling of semen. The NICHD Maternal-Fetal Medicine Units Network found that a combination of short cervical length, previous preterm birth caused by PROM, and positive fetal fibronectin screening test was highly associated with preterm delivery by PROM in the current pregnancy.[1]

DIAGNOSIS

The diagnosis of PROM is based primarily on history and physical examination. Cervical inspection with a sterile speculum is recommended for the assessment of cervical dilation and the presence of amniotic fluid in the posterior fornix of the vagina. Clear fluid accumulation in the posterior vaginal fornix supports and clear fluid emanating from the cervical canal confirms the diagnosis of PROM. Sterile swabs should be used to obtain endocervical cultures for *Chlamydia trachomatis* and *Neisseria gonorrhoeae*. Distal vaginal and rectal cultures should be taken to rule out group B streptococcus (GBS) colonization of the genital tract.

Digital cervical examination in women with preterm PROM shortens the latency period and should be avoided unless labor is imminent. Even one or two digital cervical examinations have been shown to shorten rupture-to-delivery interval by 2 days.[24] Imseis and colleagues[25] showed that digital examination introduces vaginal flora into the cervical canal. In 80% of their patients, there was a heavier growth or a greater number of different organisms after a digital cervical examination was performed.[25] Cervical evaluation by sterile speculum examination correlates reasonably well with digital examination and is usually sufficient for the obstetrical management of PROM.[26]

Laboratory Tests

Several simple tests may help to confirm the diagnosis of PROM. The pH of vaginal secretions is usually 4.5 to 6.0, whereas the pH of amniotic fluid is normally greater than 7.1. Nitrazine paper, a pH indicator, turns blue at a pH of 6 to 6.5 or higher. A blue-colored nitrazine test from a swab of the vaginal fluid supports the diagnosis of PROM. Blood, bacterial vaginosis, and semen also may change the color of the nitrazine paper, giving a false-positive test. Alternatively a false-negative test may occur if there is insufficient amniotic fluid in the vagina at the time of sampling. Another confirmatory diagnostic test for PROM is the ferning test. Amniotic fluid has increased sodium chloride content, and when it dries, a fernlike pattern of crystals, or arborization, appears. The ferning test is performed by placing a sample of vaginal fluid on a microscope slide and allowing it to air dry. Viewed under a light microscope, ferning confirms the presence of amniotic fluid.[9]

Ultrasound Evaluation

Transabdominal ultrasonography is important in the setting of PROM. It is used to confirm fetal presentation, assess gestational age, estimate fetal weight, and rule out major fetal malformations. Ultrasound also may be used to confirm the diagnosis of ruptured fetal membranes by the evaluation of the status of amniotic fluid volume. Visualization of oligohydramnios in the absence of fetal urinary tract malformations or fetal growth restriction suggests that the diagnosis of ruptured membranes is highly likely. In the setting of oligohydramnios, however, sonographic survey of fetal anomalies may be hampered by lack of contrast owing to inadequate amniotic fluid volume. Performance of weekly transvaginal ultrasound examinations to assess cervical length has been evaluated and was found not to confer an increase in infectious complications in women with PPROM.[27] Further clinical trials are needed, however, to evaluate whether endovaginal ultrasound and cervical length improve the management or outcome in pregnancies complicated by PPROM. At this time, the routine use of endovaginal ultrasound for assessment of cervical length in women with PPROM is not recommended.

Amniocentesis

Ultrasound-guided transabdominal amniocentesis, with instillation of indigo carmine dye (1 mL in 9 mL of sterile normal saline) may be useful in cases in which the diagnosis of PROM is equivocal. If blue fluid emanates from the vagina within 30 minutes of instillation, the test confirms PROM.[9]

Amniocentesis also may be useful in assessing for infection and determining fetal lung maturity status. Studies of amniocentesis in PPROM suggest that fluid is obtained successfully in at least 72% of attempts in studies performed before 1996. The success rate of amniocentesis in oligohydramnios has improved with advances in high-resolution ultrasound capability, although it is dependent on the experience of the operator. Known complications of amniocentesis include bleeding and injury to the fetus; however, they are rare, with one retrospective review finding no significant complications in 91 cases.[28] Although this procedure is relatively safe and technically feasible, its overall utility in PROM remains disputed. Whether the routine use of amniocentesis in PROM improves clinical outcome warrants additional prospective controlled studies.

Assessment of Fetal Lung Maturity

Amniotic fluid may be collected from the vaginal pool or via amniocentesis for the assessment of fetal pulmonary maturity. The maturity status of the fetal lung is an important factor in determining the timing for delivery and the need for antenatal corticosteroids of a near-term fetus.

Many tests are available to evaluate pulmonary fetal maturity. A complete discussion of them is beyond the scope of this chapter. The generally accepted standard is the amniotic lecithin-to-sphingomyelin ratio. Fetal lungs are considered to be mature when this ratio is greater than or equal to 2. The presence of phosphatidylglycerol in amniotic fluid also suggests a mature fetal lung profile. Another test, FLM II assay (Fetal Lung Maturity II, Abbott Laboratories, Abbott Park, IL), uses fluorescence to quantitate the ratio between surfactant and albumin in amniotic fluid. A mature fetal pulmonary profile is defined as a surfactant/albumin value of 55 mg/g or greater. A borderline test is defined as values between 40 mg/g and 54 mg/g, and a result of less than 40 mg/g is considered immature. A retrospective study by Edwards and colleagues[29] evaluated the use of this test in preterm PROM. They found that when this test result showed mature lungs, the negative predictive value was 97.6%.[29]

DIAGNOSIS OF CHORIOAMNIONITIS

Chorioamnionitis is an important source of maternal and neonatal morbidity and mortality that is associated with PROM. Women with chorioamnionitis may present with temperature greater than 38° C (>100.4° F), leukocytosis, maternal or fetal tachycardia (or both), uterine tenderness, or labor. Normal amniotic fluid is amber or yellow in color and is clear in appearance. Amniotic fluid that is cloudy or meconium stained, is foul smelling, or has a glucose concentration less than 20 mg/dL suggests intrauterine infection. Gram stain of the amniotic fluid may be useful in looking for the presence of leukocytes and bacteria. This test has a sensitivity of 23% to 60%. A negative Gram stain has a negative predictive value of 70% to 80%.[30,31] Growth of organisms on culture of amniotic fluid confirms intrauterine infection. Amniotic fluid cytokines may be elevated in chorioamnionitis. Interleukin-6 or interleukin-1β concentration in amniotic fluid shows diagnostic promise, but its use currently is limited to research settings.[31]

GROUP B STREPTOCOCCUS PROPHYLAXIS

GBS genital colonization affects 10% to 30% of pregnant women and is an important source of neonatal morbidity and mortality from early-onset disease. Early-onset GBS disease usually presents as sepsis, pneumonia, or meningitis with case-fatality rates of 5% to 20%. Risk factors for early-onset GBS disease include a prior infant with invasive GBS disease, GBS bacteriuria in the current pregnancy, a history of preterm delivery at less than 37 weeks, ruptured membranes greater than 18 hours, and fever greater than 38° C. The incidence of GBS disease also is higher among infants born to African-American women, to Hispanic women, and to women younger than 20 years of age. Intrapartum administration of antibiotics to a pregnant woman has been shown to reduce early-onset neonatal GBS disease. Intrapartum chemoprophylaxis should be initiated with intravenous penicillin G. Penicillin G is preferred over ampicillin because the former has a narrower spectrum and may be less likely to result in selection of antibiotic-resistant organisms. Clindamycin or erythromycin may be used if β-lactam allergy is present.[32]

The Committee on Obstetric Practice from the American College of Obstetricians and Gynecologists supports the Centers for Disease Control and Prevention recommendations that obstetric providers adopt a culture-based strategy for the prevention of early-onset GBS disease in newborns. All pregnant women should have vaginal and rectal GBS screening cultures obtained at 35 to 37 weeks of gestation, except if they had GBS bacteriuria during the current pregnancy or had a previous infant with invasive

GBS disease. Indications for intrapartum antibiotic prophylaxis under a universal prenatal screening strategy are (1) previous infant with invasive GBS disease, (2) positive bacteriuria during current pregnancy, (3) positive GBS screening culture during current pregnancy, and (4) unknown GBS status with presence of any one of the following intrapartum risk factors: delivery at less than 37 weeks of gestation, ruptured membranes greater than 18 hours, or fever greater than 38° C. Intrapartum antibiotic prophylaxis is not indicated in (1) previous pregnancy with a positive GBS screening culture, (2) planned cesarean section delivery in the absence of labor or ruptured membranes regardless of maternal GBS culture status, and (3) negative vaginal and rectal GBS screening culture in late gestation during the current pregnancy, regardless of intrapartum risk factors. If chorioamnionitis is suspected, however, broad-spectrum antibiotic therapy that includes an agent known to be active against GBS should replace GBS prophylaxis.[32]

ANTIBIOTICS

As previously noted, infection plays an important role as a cause or consequence of PPROM. Many clinical trials of antimicrobial therapy with PPROM have been conducted in the hopes of decreasing associated maternal and neonatal morbidity and mortality. Almost all of these trials showed success of antimicrobial therapy in prolonging latency-to-delivery interval. The two largest meta-analyses support a role for antibiotics in decreasing the frequency of postpartum endometritis.[4,33] With the exception of the NICHD and ORACLE 1 studies, most of the trials lacked adequate power to assess neonatal outcomes. Table 25-2 highlights results of several studies of antibiotics and neonatal outcomes in PPROM.[4,33-39]

The ORACLE 1[39] study was a large prospective trial of women with PPROM randomized to (1) erythromycin, (2) amoxicillin/clavulanic acid (Augmentin), (3) both, or (4) placebo for 10 days. This study enrolled 4826 women with PPROM at less than 37 weeks of gestation, of which approximately 50% of cases were at less than 32 weeks of gestation. GBS colonization status was not known. In a subanalysis, the investigators found that treatment of singleton pregnancy with erythromycin resulted in reduced neonatal death, chronic lung disease, or major sonographic cerebral abnormality before discharge compared with the other three treatment arms. Any use of Augmentin resulted in a significant increase in NEC (1.8%) compared with either erythromycin or placebo (0.7%) (P = .0005). It was unclear why erythromycin was superior to the combination of erythromycin and Augmentin.[39] It has been speculated that β-lactams, by destroying bacteria, may release endotoxins and prostaglandins, which may worsen outcomes compared with the suppressive effect of macrolide antibiotics.[33] A limitation of this study is that use of antenatal corticosteroids and tocolytics was not controlled.

The other large prospective trial was completed by collaborators for the NICHD Maternal-Fetal Medicine Units Network. These investigators also examined the effect of antibiotics on perinatal outcome in PPROM.

Patients with PPROM between 24 and 32 weeks of gestation were randomized to antibiotics (intravenous ampicillin and erythromycin for 48 hours followed by oral amoxicillin and erythromycin for 5 days) versus placebo. Women were not permitted corticosteroids after enrollment. Among mothers receiving antibiotics, latency and birth weight were increased. Similarly, infants born to mothers treated with antibiotics had less RDS and were less likely to have more than one of the component outcomes of fetal/infant death, severe IVH, grade 2 or 3 NEC, or sepsis within 72 hours of birth. The incidence of NEC in the antibiotic group was 2.3% compared with 5.8% in the control group (P = .03). The antibiotic group had a lower incidence of clinical amnionitis than the placebo group, although postpartum endometritis was similar regardless of whether antibiotics were used. Also the incidence of composite fetal-infant morbidity was less among women not colonized with GBS.[38] It was unclear what the effect of withholding corticosteroids was in this setting. A meta-analysis by Leitich and colleagues[37] could not show an additive effect in smaller trials using corticosteroids and antibiotics concomitantly; they showed that glucocorticoids diminished the effect of antibiotic treatment.

Three observational studies cited prolonged PPROM, chorioamnionitis, and maternal infection as major obstetric risk factors for cerebral palsy and other neurodevelopmental impairment.[18-20] The ORACLE 1 investigators found fewer major cerebral abnormalities on cranial ultrasound in infants whose mothers were given erythromycin.[39] This finding suggests that childhood disability may be related more to infection rather than to duration of PPROM.

TOCOLYTICS

Tocolytics are medications that cause uterine smooth muscle relaxation and are given to women at risk for preterm delivery. Common agents used include magnesium sulfate, terbutaline, indomethacin, and nifedipine. The tocolytic agent of choice in the setting of PPROM is intravenous magnesium sulfate. It lacks the tachycardic effect of nifedipine and terbutaline and does not mask fever as may indomethacin. Magnesium sulfate is associated with decreased risk for cerebral palsy.[40] Numerous trials advocate short-term (24 to 48 hours) use of parenteral tocolytics to prolong the pregnancy for administration of corticosteroids and antibiotics.[41-47] Prolonged tocolysis does not improve neonatal outcome, however, and may increase maternal infections.[47]

CORTICOSTEROIDS

The National Institutes of Health (NIH) Consensus Development Panel concluded that antenatal corticosteroid treatment decreased the frequency of neonatal RDS, IVH, and neonatal death and that administration of corticosteroids is advocated in pregnancies at risk for preterm birth. Data suggest that glucocorticoids in the setting of PPROM also reduce the risk of NEC.[48] The NIH consensus statement recommended that all fetuses between 24 and 34 weeks of gestation at risk for preterm

Table 25-2. Antibiotic Therapy and Neonatal Outcomes in Preterm Premature Rupture of Membranes

Author Year (No. Studies)	No. Patients	Antibiotics Used	NEC	RDS	Pneumonia or Oxygen Required	Sepsis or +BC	IVH or Abnormal US	BPD or Chronic Lung Disease	Neonatal Mortality	Comments
Meta-analyses and Clinical Reviews										
Ohlsson, 1989[34] (2 studies)	407	Tetracycline, cephalexin	—	—	—	↔	—	—	↔	—
Arheart, Mercer,[4] 1995 (13 studies)	1594	Various	↔	↔	→	→	→	—	↔	Variable use of steroids and tocolytics
Ananth et al, 1996[35] (9 studies)	957	Various	↔	↔	—	↔	—	—	→	Variable use of steroids and tocolytics
Egarter et al, 1996[36] (7 studies)	657	Ampicillin, penicillin, mezlocillin, erythromycin	↔	↔	—	→	→	—	↔	Glucocorticoids and tocolytics not used
Leitich et al, 1998[37] (5 studies)	509	Various	↔	↔	—	↔	↔	—	↔	Glucocorticoids used
Kenyon and Boulvain,[33] 1999/2001 (12 studies)	1685	Various	↔	↔	→	→	↔	—	↔	Variable use of steroids and tocolytics
Large Prospective Randomized Studies										
Mercer et al, 1997[38]	614	Ampicillin, erythromycin, amoxicillin*	→	→	(GBS-negative patients only)	↔	↔	→	↔	No glucocorticoids or tocolytics; PDA↓; ↑gastrointestinal symptoms in treatment group
Kenyon et al (ORACLE 1),[39] 2001	4826	Erythromycin, amoxicillin clavulanate (Augmentin)†	↑ with Augmentin ↔ with erythromycin	↔	→	→	↔	↔	↔	Glucocorticoids used

*Intravenous ampicillin and erythromycin for 48 hours followed by amoxicillin and erythromycin for 5 days.

†Four study arms: erythromycin, or Augmentin, or erythromycin + Augmentin, or placebo for 10 days.

Frequency: ↑ = increase; ↓ = decrease; ↔ = no change; — = data not available.

+BC, positive blood cultures; BPD, bronchopulmonary dysplasia; GBS, group B streptococcus; IVH, intraventricular hemorrhage; NEC, necrotizing enterocolitis; RDS, respiratory distress syndrome; US, ultrasound.

delivery be considered candidates for antenatal treatment with corticosteroids. In the presence of PPROM, antenatal corticosteroids are recommended for women at less than 30 to 32 weeks of gestation in the absence of chorioamnionitis. Treatment consists of two 12-mg doses of betamethasone, given intramuscularly 24 hours apart, or four 6-mg doses of dexamethasone, given intramuscularly 12 hours apart. The benefits of antenatal corticosteroids are additive to the benefits derived from surfactant therapy. Whether this therapy increases either neonatal or maternal infection is unclear. The risk of death from prematurity is greater, however, than the danger from infection.[49] Crowley[50] reviewed 18 trials and confirmed that antenatal corticosteroids are effective in preventing neonatal mortality (odds ratio 0.60, 95% confidence interval 0.48 to 0.75), RDS (odds ratio 0.53, 95% confidence interval 0.44 to 0.63), and IVH. In the same review, there was no reduction in the risk for NEC or chronic lung disease. No adverse outcome of prophylactic corticosteroids for the treatment of preterm birth has been identified.[50]

Optimal benefit of antenatal corticosteroids begins 24 hours after initiation of therapy and lasts 7 days. Treatment with corticosteroids for less than 24 hours still is associated with substantial reductions in neonatal mortality, RDS, and IVH, however, and corticosteroids should be given unless imminent delivery is anticipated. Data are insufficient to establish the clinical effect of corticosteroids beyond 7 days of treatment. There is inadequate evidence to argue for or against the use of corticosteroids at gestational age of greater than 34 weeks at delivery. The use of corticosteroids in mothers expected to deliver after 34 weeks is not recommended, unless there is evidence of pulmonary immaturity.[49]

Given that the clinical effect of corticosteroids is not known beyond 7 days, many clinicians have repeated weekly courses of corticosteroids in women who remain undelivered, but who are at continued risk of preterm birth. An increasing body of retrospective and post hoc data raises the concern, however, of adverse maternal and neonatal effects from repeated courses of antenatal corticosteroids. Maternal adverse effects include an increase in chorioamnionitis and gestational diabetes. Neonates may have lower rates of RDS and oxygen use but may encounter reduced birth and brain weight, impaired neonatal immune and adrenal function, and increased risk of sepsis and death.[50,51] An NIH consensus panel concluded that as a result of inconsistency of studies, it is impossible to make an unequivocal statement regarding repeated courses of steroids. The panel recommended use of repeat courses only for patients enrolled in randomized, controlled trials.[52]

MANAGEMENT

Maternal-Fetal Surveillance

When PROM is diagnosed, the woman should be observed initially for any signs and symptoms of infection, vaginal bleeding, and onset of labor. The fetus should be assessed for signs of well-being and be monitored for any signs of umbilical cord compression or distress. Cardiotocography, real-time ultrasonography, and maternal perception of fetal movement are techniques used to monitor fetal well-being. Hypoxemia and acidemia affect FHR pattern, fetal movement, and tone. In response to hypoxemia, a decrease in renal blood flow secondary to redistribution of fetal blood flow may lead to oligohydramnios.

A nonstress test (NST) is a tracing of the FHR pattern. Its use assumes that normal fetuses have acceleration of the heart rate of at least 15 beats above baseline that lasts for at least 15 seconds. A normal or reactive NST is when there are two or more FHR accelerations in 20 minutes with or without discernible fetal movement. A nonreactive NST occurs when FHR accelerations do not meet the above-mentioned criteria in 40 minutes. A nonreactive NST is common in preterm infants. It is observed in 50% of infants from 24 to 28 weeks of gestation and in 15% of infants from 28 to 32 weeks of gestation. A previously reactive NST that becomes nonreactive is worrisome for poor fetal oxygenation status and may require further evaluation with a biophysical profile (BPP). Other nonreassuring findings on NSTs include repetitive or prolonged variable FHR decelerations.[53]

The BPP consists of five components: NST, fetal movement, fetal tone, fetal respiration, and amniotic fluid volume. The last four components are measured by ultrasonography. A fetus is considered healthy when the NST is reactive and fetal movement, tone, and respiration are present with a normal amniotic fluid volume (single vertical pocket of at least 2 cm). Each of the five components of the BPP is given a score of either 0 (abnormal) or 2 (normal). The scores are summed to yield a composite BPP score. A composite BPP score of 8 or 10 is considered normal, a score of 6 is equivocal, and a score of 4 is considered abnormal. A modified BPP consists of only two components: NST and amniotic fluid index (the summation of umbilical cord free vertical pockets of amniotic fluid in the four quadrants of the gravid uterus). The modified BPP is considered normal if the NST is reactive and the amniotic fluid index is greater than 5.[53]

Nonreactive NSTs and BPP scores of 6 or less have been associated with perinatal infection. A randomized trial comparing these two modalities in women with PPROM revealed that both are relatively insensitive (39.1% and 25%) at detecting infectious complications.[54] Most authorities recommend some sort of daily fetal assessment after PPROM. Although BPP or NST is commonly performed, evidence that these tests directly improve perinatal outcome in this setting is lacking.[9]

Indications for Delivery

In the setting of PROM, the presence of chorioamnionitis or signs of nonreassuring maternal or fetal status are indications for prompt delivery of the infant. An infected premature newborn fares poorly compared with a noninfected premature infant, and an infected mother can be overwhelmed by sepsis. In the absence of clinical chorioamnionitis, the obstetric management of PROM varies and depends largely on gestational age at presentation. Management schema is different at term (>37 weeks' completed gestation), at preterm (<30 to 32 weeks' gestation), and at close to term (32 to 36 6/7 weeks' gestation).

The mode of delivery depends on fetal presentation and presence of fetal or obstetric indications for cesarean section. Early involvement of the neonatologist is warranted for all women with preterm PROM. Wherever possible, women with PPROM should be delivered in a hospital with personnel skilled in the intensive care of the fetus and neonate and with proper equipment for resuscitation and management of preterm infants.

Term Premature Rupture of Membranes

The overwhelming risk of PROM at or beyond 37 weeks of gestation is infection. Labor and delivery usually follow PROM at term. In one trial, half of women with PROM at term who were managed expectantly delivered within 5 hours, and 95% delivered within 28 hours.[9]

Management of women who present at term with ruptured membranes and an unfavorable cervix is controversial. Induction of a woman with term PROM and an unfavorable cervix may result in a higher rate of cesarean birth. Delayed induction may lessen the need for cesarean section but may increase the infectious risk to mother and fetus. A meta-analysis evaluated this issue in detail. In this meta-analysis, three different management schemas were evaluated: immediate oxytocin induction, conservative management (delayed oxytocin induction), and cervical ripening (prostaglandin preparation followed by oxytocin induction). Studies included in this meta-analysis defined early intervention groups as induction from immediately after to within 12 hours of membrane rupture. The delayed induction group was defined as induction between 24 and 96 hours after membrane rupture. In the cervical ripening agent group, oxytocin was begun after varying lengths of time in the absence of labor. Delayed induction resulted in more maternal infections than immediate induction with oxytocin or prostaglandins followed by oxytocin. Serious neonatal infections, defined as culture-proven neonatal septicemia, meningitis, or pneumonia, and cesarean deliveries were not significantly different among the three management schema.[55]

In a prospective study of low-risk patients, Shalev and coworkers[56] found no difference between induction at 12 hours after rupture of membranes and induction after 72 hours of expectant management with respect to infectious complications and pregnancy outcome. These authors also pointed out, however, that conservative management is associated with an increased cost of prolonged hospitalization.[56]

Women should be informed of the benefits and risks of different options of immediate induction versus delayed induction with PROM at term. According to the American College of Obstetricians and Gynecologists, women with term PROM may be induced at the time of presentation or be observed for 24 to 72 hours for the onset of spontaneous labor.[9] In a study of 5041 women with term PROM, however, it seemed that women preferred induction of labor to expectant management.[57] In term PROM, clinical chorioamnionitis and maternal colonization with GBS are the most important predictors of subsequent neonatal infection.[58]

Preterm Premature Rupture of Membranes

The obstetric management of pregnancies with PROM varies and depends on gestational age at presentation. At less than 32 weeks of gestation, expectant management is warranted in an effort to minimize the risks of prematurity, in the absence of contraindications for continued pregnancy. GBS genital colonization status needs to be determined and followed by a protocol for intrapartum prophylaxis as appropriate. Antibiotics have been shown to prolong latency-to-delivery interval and improve perinatal outcome in PPROM and should be included in the management of PPROM.[9,38] Erythromycin alone[39] or the combination of erythromycin with ampicillin or amoxicillin seems to be safe in PPROM.[38] In view of the findings of the ORACLE 1 study, amoxicillin/clavulanic acid (Augmentin), previously widely used in PPROM, cannot be routinely recommended due to an increased risk of NEC.[39] Antenatal corticosteroids have been shown to decrease neonatal RDS, IVH, and neonatal death. In the absence of clinical chorioamnionitis, the administration of corticosteroid is recommended in pregnancies with PPROM at less than 32 weeks of gestation.[49]

At gestational ages between 32 and 37 weeks, the decision for immediate delivery versus expectant management depends on whether the fetus is closer to 32 weeks or closer to 37 weeks of gestation. Balancing the hazards of ascending infection and cord prolapse against prematurity-related risk is a complicated process about which there is little consensus. Several studies supported immediate delivery rather than expectant management in PPROM occurring after 32 to 34 weeks of gestation,[59-62] whereas another concluded that expectant management is safe between 34 and 37 weeks.[63]

A prospective study by Mercer and colleagues[59] examined this issue among women presenting at 32 to 37 weeks of gestation. Patients were randomized to immediate induction versus expectant management, and no prophylactic antibiotics were administered. Maternal and infant hospitalization was prolonged in the expectantly managed group. Chorioamnionitis and fetal heart rate abnormalities also were significantly increased. Although confirmed culture-proven rates of sepsis were not different, rates of suspected sepsis and antibiotic use were greater among neonates in the expectant management group. Rates of NEC, RDS, IVH, and pneumonia were not different in either group.[59] Similarly a randomized prospective study of women with PROM at 34 to 37 weeks of gestation concluded that immediate induction was warranted, owing to decreased neonatal infectious morbidity in these patients.[61]

In contrast, another study that retrospectively compared patients delivering between 34 and 37 weeks of gestation did not find significant differences in neonatal and maternal morbidity and mortality between patients with PROM and patients without PROM. This study did show, however, that neonatal intensive care unit (NICU) length of stay differed by gestational age and concluded that unless another indication for delivery (e.g., chorioamnionitis or fetal distress) is present, expectant management is a safe and reasonable course of action.[63]

In PPROM between 32 and 37 weeks of gestation, the option of immediate delivery versus expectant management is contingent on the gestational age–related neonatal survival and morbidity statistics, which may vary among different geographic locations and patient populations. Neonatal complications with potential long-term consequences, such as grade 3 or 4 IVH and NEC, are rare after 34 weeks of gestation. The contemporary mortality rate for infants delivered after 32 weeks' gestation is less than 2% with an incidence of RDS of 22% at 32 weeks,[62] whereas the incidence of RDS is decreased to 5% at 34 to 37 weeks of gestation.[61] The preponderance of reports supports active management toward delivery in women with PPROM after 34 weeks of gestation with[59] or without documented fetal lung maturity status, even at gestational ages as early as 30 to 34 weeks.[64] If fetal lungs are documented to be immature, the fetus still may benefit from a course of antenatal corticosteroids and a 24- to 48-hour delay in delivery after initiation of treatment for the medication to take effect.[9]

If expectant management is considered, one must keep in mind that the mean latency-to-delivery interval at gestational ages between 32 and 37 weeks is brief (range 22 to 119 hours).[59,61] In a study of PPROM between 32 and 36 weeks, only 10% of the cohort had latencies of 48 hours, and only 2.5% had latencies of 7 days.[62] Additional benefits in reducing morbidity related to prematurity may be limited due to the short latency-to-delivery interval.

Induction of Labor

Women with PROM at or near term may be induced with the goal of achieving vaginal delivery in the absence of indications for a cesarean section. Indications for induction of labor are not absolute; rather they should consider gestational age, status of mother and fetus, fetal presentation, and cervical condition. If the patient's cervix is favorable for induction, labor may be induced with oxytocin infusion. If the cervix is not ripe for induction, cervical ripening may be initiated with prostaglandin E_2 preparations (dinoprostone) or the synthetic prostaglandin E_1 analogue, misoprostol (Cytotec). Monitoring FHR and uterine contractions is recommended as for any high-risk pregnancy.

Uterine hyperstimulation (single contractions lasting >2 minutes or contraction frequency >5 in 10 minutes) is a potential complication of pharmacologic induction and may lead to fetal distress if it is persistent. Intravaginal prostaglandin E_2 for induction of labor in women with PROM seems to be safe and effective. One dose of intravaginal misoprostol induced labor in 86% of patients at term. The use of intravaginal misoprostol for induction of labor has been studied extensively and found to be safe and effective. Its use may reduce the need for oxytocin as well. Smaller doses of misoprostol (25 µg) may be less likely to result in uterine hyperstimulation.[65]

It is important that misoprostol not be used in women with prior cesarean section or major uterine surgery due to the risk of uterine rupture.[66] A Cochrane Review of randomized trials revealed that induction of labor with prostaglandins at 34 or more weeks of gestation decreased the risk of chorioamnionitis and admission to NICUs, with no increased risk of cesarean section.[60]

Cerclage and Preterm Premature Rupture of Membranes

Repetitive second-trimester spontaneous abortions in some women may be attributed to cervical incompetence and present with silent dilation of the cervix without uterine contractions. Cerclage, the placement of a circumferential suture in the cervical stroma, is the treatment for cervical incompetence in an attempt to prolong the pregnancy. The most common complication after cerclage placement is PPROM, affecting 22% to 24% of elective procedures with undilated cervix and 20% to 72% of emergent (salvage) cerclages.[67-69] Cervical dilation at the time of cerclage placement correlates with the incidence of PPROM and may explain the variability in the emergent cerclage group.[68] After PPROM, imminent delivery ensues in 22% to 29% of women due to active labor, fetal compromise, or chorioamnionitis.[70-72] Maternal and neonatal outcome in women with cervical cerclage is not affected as long as the cerclage is removed on admission to the hospital.[70,73] The optimal timing of cerclage removal after PPROM is controversial, however. The risks of premature delivery must be balanced with the risks of neonatal and maternal sepsis. Other maternal complications of retained cerclage may include vaginal bleeding, cervical laceration, and amputation.

Delaying cerclage removal prolonged pregnancy 8.5 days versus 2.5 days in patients whose cerclage was removed immediately, but also resulted in higher rates of neonatal sepsis.[74] In another study, neonatal mortality was reported as 70% in patients with retained cerclage versus 10% with immediate cerclage removal.[75] These studies were conducted before routine use of antibiotics or steroids.

A retrospective review assessed outcomes with delayed cerclage removal in the setting of PPROM with the use of antibiotics and antenatal steroids in most patients. Patients whose cerclage removal was delayed had a latency period of 10.1 days compared with 5 days in patients whose removal was immediate.[72] Rates of neonatal and maternal infection did not differ significantly; neonatal outcomes, such as mortality, RDS, birth weight, and duration of NICU stay, likewise did not differ significantly.[71,72]

The few studies that evaluated the impact of delaying cerclage removal after PPROM all were limited by their retrospective nature, small sample size, and possible selection bias.[71,72,75] Given that major complications from prematurity are low after 32 weeks of gestation, we recommend removal of the cerclage in patients presenting with PPROM after 32 weeks.[49] In gestational ages less than 32 weeks, antenatal corticosteroids are indicated as per NIH guideline, and the optimal time for cerclage removal should be individualized, taking into account the risks of prematurity versus the risks of infection. With the use of antibiotics with or without tocolytics, the mean latency-to-delivery interval was 119 hours in the immediate cerclage removal group versus 244 hours in the delayed cerclage removal group. It seemed that an attempt to prolong pregnancy with cerclage in situ after PPROM is safe for at least 48 hours with the use of antibiotics.[72]

Hospitalization versus Home Care

Women with PROM at term are probably best served by hospitalization. Hannah and colleagues[76] analyzed data from the International Term PROM study and found that nulliparas managed at home had an increased risk of requiring antibiotics before delivery and that neonates born of mothers managed at home had a twofold increased risk of infection compared with neonates born of mothers managed in the hospital.

In women with PPROM, management usually requires hospitalization with bed rest and pelvic rest. One small, randomized trial carefully selected women with PPROM to home management or hospitalization after an initial 72 hours of inpatient observation. No difference in maternal or neonatal outcome in this highly selected group was apparent, and antenatal costs were reduced by 50% in the home management group. Small savings in the antepartum period could be easily superseded, however, by even a few extra days of NICU hospitalization for the neonate.[77]

EXPERIMENTAL MANAGEMENT TECHNIQUES

Amnioinfusion

PPROM with oligohydramnios is associated with a higher risk of umbilical cord compression, chorioamnionitis, neonatal sepsis, shorter latency period, pulmonary hypoplasia, and neonatal mortality. Amnioinfusion is the instillation of normal saline or lactated Ringer's solution via transabdominal or transcervical routes to restore amniotic fluid volume. This is done to mitigate against the above-mentioned complications from oligohydramnios.

A case series evaluated serial transabdominal amnioinfusions in 49 women with PPROM at less than 26 weeks of gestation. Neonatal survival was 92% for the 13 patients who did not have oligohydramnios. The remaining 36 women with persistent oligohydramnios with an amniotic fluid pocket of less than 2 cm underwent serial amnioinfusion. Eleven (30%) of these women responded with their amniotic fluid pocket restored to greater than 2 cm for 48 hours. Patients with persistent oligohydramnios were found to have shorter latencies, higher rates of pulmonary hypoplasia, worse neurologic outcomes, and lower neonatal survival compared with patients without oligohydramnios. All of the 20 women with amniotic fluid greater than 2 cm either spontaneously or after amnioinfusion had good long-term neurologic outcomes, and only one newborn had pulmonary hypoplasia.[78] Another study of transabdominal amnioinfusion in pregnancies with PPROM at 25 to 32 weeks of gestation reported an increase in latency-to-delivery interval and improved neonatal outcome with amnioinfusion.[79]

In a randomized study of amnioinfusion in 66 patients with PPROM, no significant differences in the end points of Apgar scores, infectious morbidity, or neonatal death were seen between control and amnioinfusion groups. There are currently inadequate data to guide clinical practice regarding the use of amnioinfusion in the setting of PPROM, although it may prove useful in selected cases.[80]

Amniosealants

Attempts have been made to reseal the break or site of rupture in the amniotic membranes that leads to amniorrhexis. Resealing was first suggested by Genz in 1979,[81] but not until more recently has it gained renewed interest. Materials used include transvaginal fibrin sealants,[81-83] blood patch,[84] transabdominal amniopatch[10] (combination of autologous or allogeneic platelets and cryoprecipitate), and gelatin sponge.[85] All reports to date on the use of amniosealants for the treatment of PPROM consist of case reports and case series. Neonatal survival ranged from 3 of 7 (43%) using an amniopatch at 15 to 22 weeks of gestation[10] to 7 of 13 (54%) using fibrin sealants at less than 24 weeks of gestation.[86] A case series of 47 patients reported 80% neonatal survival with fibrin sealants versus 43% survival in the control group.[87] Some authors advocate cerclage placement in combination with amniosealant,[81,87] and other authors promote the addition of amnioinfusion.[85] All of the aforementioned techniques remain experimental.

Prevention of Premature Rupture of Membranes

Preventing PROM is a worthwhile goal. In view of the putative pathophysiologic role of infection in PROM, antibiotic therapy has been evaluated extensively as a means of prevention. A randomized trial of metronidazole in women with bacterial vaginosis failed to prevent PROM or premature delivery.[88]

There has been considerable interest in the development of general and specific inhibitors of MMPs for the treatment of periodontal disease and arthritis and for the prevention of tumor metastasis. These agents include tetracycline-type antibiotics; synthetic MMP inhibitors, such as batimastat (which selectively chelates the zinc atom at the active site of the enzymes), and the native tissue inhibitors of metalloproteinases, TIMP-1 and TIMP-2. The ability of these substances to prevent or retard changes in the extracellular matrix of fetal membranes before PPROM occurs has yet to be evaluated.[3] Laboratory and theoretical evidence supports a role for vitamin C and vitamin E supplementation in reducing the risk for PPROM; however, neither has been studied in a controlled fashion.[13]

REFERENCES

1. Mercer BM, Goldenberg RL, Meis PJ, et al, for the NICHD Maternal-Fetal Medicine Units Network: The preterm prediction study: Prediction of preterm premature rupture of membranes through clinical findings and ancillary testing. Am J Obstet Gynecol 183:738, 2000.
2. Cunningham FG, Gant NF, Leveno KJ, et al: Preterm birth. In: Williams Obstetrics. New York, McGraw Hill, 2001, p 689.
3. Parry S, Strauss JF: Mechanisms of disease: Premature rupture of the fetal membranes. N Engl J Med 338:663, 1998.
4. Mercer BM, Arheart KL: Antimicrobial therapy in expectant management of preterm premature rupture. Lancet 346:1271, 1995.
5. Carroll SG, Blott M, Nicolaides KH: Preterm prelabor amniorrhexis: Outcome of live births. Obstet Gynecol 86:18, 1995.

6. Schucker JL, Mercer BM: Midtrimester premature rupture of the membranes. Semin Perinatol 20:389, 1996.

7. Richards DS: Complications of prolonged PROM and oligohydramnios. Clin Obstet Gynecol 41:817, 1998.

8. Mercer BM: Management of preterm rupture of the membranes. Clin Obstet Gynecol 41:872, 1998.

9. American College of Obstetricians and Gynecologists: Premature Rupture of Membranes. Clinical Management Guidelines for Obstetrician-Gynecologists Number 1. Washington, DC, ACOG, 1998.

10. Quintero RA, Morales WJ, Allen M, et al: Treatment of iatrogenic previable premature rupture of membranes with intra-amniotic injection of platelets and cryoprecipitate (amniopatch): Preliminary experience. Am J Obstet Gynecol 181:744, 1999.

11. Borgida AF, Mills AA, Feldman DM, et al: Outcome of pregnancies complicated by ruptured membranes after genetic amniocentesis. Am J Obstet Gynecol 183:937, 2000.

12. Polzin WJ, Brady K: The etiology of premature rupture of the membranes. Clin Obstet Gynecol 41:810, 1998.

13. Woods J, Plessinger M, Miller R: Vitamins C and E: Missing links in preventing preterm premature rupture of membranes. Am J Obstet Gynecol 185:5, 2001.

14. Fortunato SJ, Menon R: Distinct molecular events suggest different pathways for preterm labor and premature rupture of membranes. Am J Obstet Gynecol 184:1399, 2001.

15. Maymon E, Romero R, Pacora P, et al: Evidence for the participation of interstitial collagenase (matrix metalloproteinase 1) in preterm premature rupture of membranes. Am J Obstet Gynecol 183:913, 2000.

16. Mikamo H, Kawazoe K, Yasumasa S, et al: Elastase activity of anaerobes isolated from amniotic fluid with preterm premature rupture of membranes. Am J Obstet Gynecol 180:378, 1999.

17. Yoon BH, Romero R, Park JS, et al: Microbial invasion of the amniotic cavity with *Ureaplasma urealyticum* is associated with a robust host response in fetal, amniotic, and maternal compartments. Am J Obstet Gynecol 184:1399, 1998.

18. Verma U, Tejani N, Klein S, et al: Obstetric antecedents of intraventricular hemorrhage and periventricular leukomalacia in the low-birth-weight neonate. Am J Obstet Gynecol 176:275, 1997.

19. Murphy DJ, Sellers S, MacKenzie IZ, et al: Case-control study of antenatal and intrapartum risk factors for cerebral palsy in very preterm singleton babies. Lancet 346:1449, 1995.

20. Spinillo A, Capuzzo E, Stronati M, et al: Effect of preterm premature rupture of membranes on neurodevelopmental outcome: Follow up at two years of age. Br J Obstet Gynaecol 102:882, 1995.

21. Vermeulen GM: Spontaneous preterm birth: Prevention, management and outcome. Eur J Obstet Gynecol Reprod Biol 92:1, 2000.

22. Bryant-Greenwood GD, Miller LK: Human fetal membranes: Their preterm premature rupture. Biol Reprod 63:1575, 2000.

23. Newman RB, Goldenberg RL, Moawad AH, et al: Occupational fatigue and preterm premature rupture of membranes. Am J Obstet Gynecol 184:438, 2001.

24. Alexander JM, Mercer BM, Miodovnik M, et al, for the NICHD Maternal-Fetal Unit Network: The impact of digital cervical examinations on expectantly managed preterm ruptured membranes. Am J Obstet Gynecol 183:1003, 2000.

25. Imseis HM, Trout WC, Gabbe SG: The microbiologic effect of digital cervical examination. Am J Obstet Gynecol 180:578, 1999.

26. Munson LA, Graham A, Koos BJ, et al: Is there a need for digital examination in patients with spontaneous rupture of the membranes? Am J Obstet Gynecol 153:562, 1985.

27. Carlan SJ, Richmond LB, O'Brien JM: Randomized trial of endovaginal ultrasound in preterm premature rupture of membranes. Obstet Gynecol 89:458, 1997.

28. Blackwell SC, Berry SM: Role of amniocentesis for the diagnosis of subclinical intra-amniotic infection in preterm rupture of the membranes. Curr Opin Obstet Gynecol 101:541, 1999.

29. Edwards RK, Duff P, Ross KC: Amniotic fluid indices of fetal pulmonary maturity with preterm premature rupture of membranes. Obstet Gynecol 96:102, 2000.

30. Coultrip LL, Grossman JH: Evaluation of rapid diagnostic tests in the detection of microbial invasion of the amniotic cavity. Am J Obstet Gynecol 167:1231, 1992.

31. Greig PC: The diagnosis of intrauterine infection in women with preterm premature rupture of the membranes (PPROM). Clin Obstet Gynecol 41:849, 1998.

32. American College of Obstetricians and Gynecologists: Prevention of Early-Onset Group B Streptococcal Disease in Newborns. ACOG Committee Opinion 279. Washington, DC, ACOG, 2002.

33. Kenyon S, Boulvain M: Antibiotics for preterm premature rupture of the membranes (Cochrane review). In: The Cochrane Library, Issue 1. Oxford, Update Software, 2001.

34. Ohlsson A: Treatments of preterm premature rupture of the membranes: A meta-analysis. Am J Obstet Gynecol 160:890, 1989.

35. Ananth CV, Guise JM, Thorp JM: Utility of antibiotic therapy in preterm premature rupture of membranes: A meta-analysis. Obstet Gynecol Surv 51:324, 1996.

36. Egarter C, Leitich H, Karas H, et al: Antibiotic treatment in preterm premature rupture of membranes and neonatal morbidity: A meta-analysis. Am J Obstet Gynecol 174:589, 1996.

37. Leitich H, Egarter C, Reisenberger K, et al: Concomitant use of glucocorticoids: A comparison of two metaanalyses on antibiotic treatment in preterm premature rupture of membranes. Am J Obstet Gynecol 178:899, 1998.

38. Mercer BM, Miodovnik M, Thurnau GR, et al, for the NICHD Maternal-Fetal Medicine Units Network: Antibiotic therapy for reduction of infant morbidity after preterm premature rupture of the membranes. JAMA 278:989, 1997.

39. Kenyon SL, Taylor DJ, Tarnow-Mordi P, for the ORACLE Collaborative Group: Broad-spectrum antibiotics for preterm premature rupture of the membranes: The ORACLE 1 randomised trial. Lancet 357:979, 2001.

40. Matsuda Y, Kouno S, Hiroyama Y, et al: Intrauterine infection, magnesium sulfate exposure and cerebral palsy in infants born between 26 and 30 weeks of gestation. Eur J Obstet Gynecol Reprod Biol 91:159, 2000.

41. Christensen KK, Ingemarsson I, Leideman T, et al: Effect of ritodrine on labor after premature rupture of the membranes. Obstet Gynecol 55:187, 1980.

42. Levy DL, Warsof SL: Oral ritodrine and preterm premature rupture of membranes. Obstet Gynecol 66:621, 1985.

43. Dunlop PDM, Crowley PA, Lamont RF, et al: Preterm ruptured membranes, no contractions. J Obstet Gynecol 7:92, 1986.

44. Garite TJ, Keegan KA, Freeman RK, et al: A randomized trial of ritodrine tocolysis versus expectant management in patients with premature rupture of membranes at 25 to 30 weeks of gestation. Am J Obstet Gynecol 157:388, 1987.

45. Weiner CP, Renk K, Klugman M: The therapeutic efficacy and cost-effectiveness of aggressive tocolysis for premature labor associated with premature rupture of the membranes. Am J Obstet Gynecol 159:216, 1988.

46. Matsuda Y, Ikenoue T, Hokanishi H: Premature rupture of the membranes—aggressive versus conservative approach: Effect

of tocolytic and antibiotic therapy. Gynecol Obstet Invest 36:102, 1993.

47. Decavalas G, Mastrogiannis D, Papadopoulos V, et al: Short-term versus long-term prophylactic tocolysis in patients with preterm premature rupture of membranes. Eur J Obstet Gynecol Reprod Biol 59:143, 1995.

48. Harding JE, Pang JM, Knight DB, et al: Do antenatal corticosteroids help in the setting of preterm rupture of membranes? Am J Obstet Gynecol 184:131, 2001.

49. Effect of corticosteroids for fetal maturation on perinatal outcomes, February-March 2, 1994. Am J Obstet Gynecol 173:246, 1995.

50. Crowley P: Prophylactic corticosteroids for preterm birth (Cochrane review). In: The Cochrane Library, Issue 2. Oxford, Update Software, 2000.

51. Walfisch A, Hallak M, Mazor M: Multiple courses of antenatal steroids: risks and benefits. Obstet Gynecol 98:491, 2001.

52. National Institutes of Health: Report of the Consensus Development Conference on Antenatal Corticosteroids Revisited: Repeat Courses. Bethesda, MD, National Institute of Child Health and Human Development, 2000, 17:1-10.

53. American College of Obstetricians and Gynecologists: Antepartum Fetal Surveillance. Clinical Management Guidelines for Obstetrician-Gynecologists Number 9. Washington, DC, ACOG, 1999.

54. Lewis DF, Adair CD, Weeks JW, et al: A randomized trial of daily nonstress testing versus biophysical profile in the management of preterm premature rupture of membranes. Am J Obstet Gynecol 181:1495, 1999.

55. Mozurkewich EL, Wolf FM: Premature rupture of membranes at term: A meta-analysis of three management schemes. Obstet Gynecol 89:1035, 1997.

56. Shalev E, Peleg D, Eliyahu S: Comparison of 12- and 72-hour expectant management of premature rupture of membranes in term pregnancies. Obstet Gynecol 85:766, 1995.

57. Hannah ME, Ohlsson A, Farine D, et al: Induction of labor compared with expectant management of prelabor rupture of the membranes at term. N Engl J Med 334:1005, 1996.

58. Seaward PG, Hannah ME, Myhr TL, et al: International multicenter term PROM study: Evaluation of predictors of neonatal infection in infants born to patients with premature rupture of membranes at term. Am J Obstet Gynecol 179:635, 1998.

59. Mercer BM, Crocker LG, Boe NM, et al: Induction versus expectant management in premature rupture of the membranes with mature amniotic fluid at 32 to 36 weeks: A randomized trial. Am J Obstet Gynecol 169:775, 1993.

60. Tan BP, Hannah ME: Prostaglandins for prelabour rupture of membranes at or near term (Cochrane review). In: The Cochrane Library, Issue 3.Oxford, Update Software, 2001.

61. Naef RW, Albert JR, Ross EL, et al: Premature rupture of membranes at 34 to 37 weeks' gestation: Aggressive versus conservative management. Am J Obstet Gynecol 178:126, 1998.

62. Neerhof MG, Cravello C, Haney EI, et al: Timing of labor induction after premature rupture of membranes between 32 and 36 weeks' gestation. Am J Obstet Gynecol 180:349, 1999.

63. Steinfeld JD, Lenkoski C, Lerer T, et al: Neonatal morbidity at 34-37 weeks: The role of ruptured membranes. Obstet Gynecol 94:120, 1999.

64. Cox SM, Leveno KJ: Intentional delivery versus expectant management with preterm ruptured membranes at 30-34 weeks' gestation. Obstet Gynecol 86:875, 1995.

65. American College of Obstetricians and Gynecologists: Induction of Labor. Clinical Management Guidelines for Obstetrician-Gynecologists Number 10. Washington, DC, ACOG, 1999.

66. American College of Obstetricians and Gynecologists: Response to Searle's Drug Warning on Misoprostol. ACOG Committee Opinion 248.Washington, DC, ACOG, 1999.

67. Charles D, Edwards WB: Infectious complications of cervical cerclage. Am J Obstet Gynecol 141:1065, 1981.

68. Treadwell MC, Bronsteen RA, Bottoms SF: Prognostic factors and complication rates for cervical cerclage: A review of 482 cases. Am J Obstet Gynecol 165:555, 1991.

69. Harger JH: Comparison of success and morbidity in cervical cerclage procedures. Obstet Gynecol 56:543, 1990.

70. Yeast JD, Garite TR: The role of cervical cerclage in the management of preterm premature rupture of the membranes. Am J Obstet Gynecol 158:106, 1988.

71. McElrath TF, Norwitz ER, Lieberman ES, et al: Management of cervical cerclage and preterm premature rupture of membranes: Should the stitch be removed? Am J Obstet Gynecol 183:840, 2000.

72. Jenkins TM, Berghella V, Shlossman PA, et al: Timing of cerclage removal after preterm premature rupture of membranes: Maternal and neonatal outcomes. Am J Obstet Gynecol 183:847, 2000.

73. Blickstein J, Katz Z, Lancet M, et al: The outcome of pregnancies complicated by preterm premature rupture of membranes with and without cerclage. Int J Obstet Gynecol 28:237, 1989.

74. Kuhn RJP, Pepperell RJ: Cervical ligation: A review of 242 pregnancies. Aust N Z J Obstet Gynaecol 17:79, 1977.

75. Ludmir J, Bader T, Chen L, et al: Poor perinatal outcome associated with retained cerclage in patients with premature rupture of membranes. Obstet Gynecol 84:823, 1994.

76. Hannah ME, Hodnett ED, Willan A, et al: Induction of labor compared with expectant management for prelabor rupture of the membranes at term. Obstet Gynecol 96:533, 2000.

77. Carlan SJ, O'Brien WF, Parsons MT, et al: Preterm premature rupture of membranes: A randomized study of home versus hospital management. Obstet Gynecol 81:61, 1993.

78. Locatelli A, Vergani P, Di Pirro G, et al: Role of amnioinfusion in the management of premature rupture of the membranes at <26 weeks' gestation. Am J Obstet Gynecol 183:878, 2000.

79. Garzetti GG, Ciavattini A, De Cristofaro F, et al: Prophylactic transabdominal amnioinfusion in oligohydramnios in preterm premature rupture of membranes: Increase of amniotic fluid index during latency period. Gynecol Obstet Invest 44:249, 1997.

80. Hofmeyr GJ: Amnioinfusion for preterm rupture of membranes (Cochrane review). In: The Cochrane Library, Issue 2.Oxford, Update Software, 2001.

81. Genz HJ: [Treatment of premature rupture of membranes by means of fibrin adhesion.] Med Welt 30:1557, 1979.

82. Uchida K, Terada S, Hamasaki H: Intracervical fibrin instillation as an adjuvant to treatment for second trimester rupture of membranes. Arch Gynecol Obstet 255:95, 1994.

83. Sciscione AC, Manley JS, Pollock M, et al: Intracervical fibrin sealants: A potential treatment for early preterm premature rupture of membranes. Am J Obstet Gynecol 184:368, 2001.

84. Sener T, Ozalps S, Hassa H, et al: Maternal blood clot patch therapy: A model for postamniocentesis amniorrhea. Am J Obstet Gynecol 177:1535, 1997.

85. O'Brien JM, Mercer BM, Barton JR, et al: An in vitro model and case report that used gelatin sponge to restore amniotic fluid volume after spontaneous premature rupture of the membranes. Am J Obstet Gynecol 185:1094, 2001.

86. Catalano A, Zardini E: La rottura intempestiva delle membrane: Evoluzione spontanea dell'evento e suo approccio terapeutico mediante una colla di fibrina umana. Min Ginecol 46:675, 1994.

87. Baumgarten K, Moser S: The technique of fibrin adhesion for premature rupture of membranes during pregnancy. J Perinat Med 14:43, 1986.

88. Carey JC, Klebanoff MA, Hauth JC, et al, for the NICHD Maternal-Fetal Unit Network: Prevent preterm delivery in pregnant women with asymptomatic bacterial vaginosis. N Engl J Med 342:534, 2000.

CHAPTER 26

Maternal Fever and Chorioamnionitis

Stephen J. Smith and Stuart Weiner

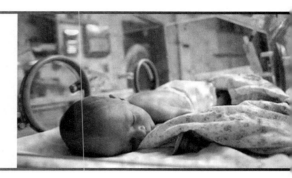

Although maternal fever has profound physiologic and teratogenic effects in animals, the impact on the human fetus is unclear. There is a close tie between maternal and fetal body temperature because of the mechanisms of fetal thermoregulation. It does seem likely, therefore, that in certain situations, maternal fever may have a significant effect on the development and physiology of the human fetus. Fever may also be a symptom of chorioamnionitis. Although maternal complications from chorioamnionitis have significantly decreased since the 1950s, this entity continues to be a major etiologic factor in neonatal morbidity and mortality.

MATERNAL FEVER

Physiology and Purpose

The causes and physiologic mechanisms of fever do not differ between nonpregnant and pregnant women. A febrile reaction may be caused by allergic reactions, malignancy, autoimmune disorders, and infection. Exogenous pyrogens are the initial mediators for fever.[1] These substances, usually microbial endotoxins or exotoxins, induce the production of endogenous pyrogens, including interleukin,[1] tumor necrosis factor, and interferons, by host cells.[2,3] Endogenous pyrogens then act on the anterior hypothalamus to cause local production of prostaglandins, which, in turn, elevate the thermal set point. Under central nervous system modulation, heat production is increased by changes in metabolic rate and muscle contraction (e.g., shivering). Heat loss is minimized by cutaneous vasoconstriction.

Fever is generally self-limited. Centrally acting substances, including vasopressin and α-melanotropin, may suppress temperature elevation at the level of the hypothalamus.[4,5] Evaporation of sweat and vasodilatation are common mechanisms of heat loss that lower temperature.

Experimental evidence suggests that the purpose of fever is to create an environment in which host defenses are more active and bacteria are more susceptible to these defenses. It has been shown in vitro that some pathogens are inhibited by or, at least, more susceptible to, antibiotics at temperatures in the febrile range.[6] At similar temperature ranges, neutrophil, T cell, and monocyte function are enhanced in vitro.[7,8] These effects, however, may be reversed at extremely high temperatures (>42° C).[8]

The Fetus and Maternal Fever

Fetal Thermoregulation

In order to understand the effect of maternal temperature change on the fetus, the thermoregulatory mechanisms in the fetus must be discussed. The fetus is highly active metabolically and therefore produces substantial quantities of heat. This heat accumulates until a fetal-maternal temperature gradient is established. In the human, a 0.5° C gradient is necessary to ensure a steady state of heat transfer from fetus to mother. The two mechanisms of heat elimination are (1) conduction of heat through fetal skin, amniotic fluid, and uterine wall and (2) convective heat exchange between the fetal and maternal circulations in the placenta. The latter mechanism is thought to be primary.[9] Because these mechanisms are based on a heat gradient from fetus to mother, there is a tight linkage between fetal and maternal temperature. As maternal temperature varies, fetal temperature closely follows.

Effect on the Uteroplacental Unit

In instrumented animal models, maternal hyperthermia and the associated hypoventilation result in decreased uterine and umbilical artery blood flow.[10,11] These changes are associated with fetal acidosis and hypoxia. Also, because placental heat exchange is the primary mode of heat dissipation in these fetal animals, decreased placental flow decreases fetal heat exchange, resulting in a worsening of the metabolic status.[10]

There are few data describing the fetal metabolic, respiratory, and cardiovascular responses to maternal fever in humans. It seems probable that fetal hypothermia in the human results in an increased metabolic rate and oxygen requirement. Maternal fever occurring in association with another stress, such as labor or placental insufficiency, may therefore put the fetus at risk for distress. For example, at the height of maternal fever during labor, the fetus is more likely to show a worrisome heart rate pattern, as manifested by tachycardia, decreased variability, and late decelerations. Resolution of the fever by administration of pyrolytics (such as acetaminophen) to the mother is associated with resolution of the abnormal heart rate pattern.[12]

Teratogenic Effect

Hyperthermia has been shown to cause abortion and fetal malformations in experimental animals. The type of defect is determined by the embryonic stage at the time of exposure. The incidence and severity of malformation are determined by the degree of hyperthermia. It appears that the minimum temperature elevation necessary to cause defects is 2.0° to 2.5° C above the normal body temperature for that species (the threshold elevation). This degree of temperature elevation must persist for approximately 1 hour (the threshold duration).[13] Central nervous system abnormalities, such as neural tube defects, microphthalmia, cranial nerve defects, and behavior abnormalities, are the most common types of malformations seen in association with experimentally induced hyperthermia.[14]

The teratogenic effect of maternal fever on the human fetus is unclear. The primary concern is the effect of maternal fever on the embryo during neural tube closure on days 21 to 28 after conception. Numerous case reports and older epidemiologic studies have linked maternal hyperthermia to neural tube defects in the fetus.[15] These studies, however, are plagued by small numbers and retrospective design. The most informative investigation of this issue was an epidemiologic study by Milunsky and coworkers.[16] From a cohort of 23,491 women undergoing maternal serum α-fetoprotein value testing or amniocentesis, 5566 women were identified with first-trimester heat exposure (from a hot tub, a sauna, fever, and/or an electric blanket). The adjusted relative risks were 2.8 for hot tub use (95% confidence interval [CI] = 1.2 to 6.5), 1.8 for sauna (95% CI = 0.4 to 7.8), 1.8 for fever (95% CI = 0.8 to 4.1), and 1.2 for electric blanket (95% CI = 0.5 to 2.6). These statistics suggest a possible association between first-trimester heat exposure and neural tube defects but are far from conclusive.

In summary, absolute proof of a causal connection between maternal fever and malformations in the human fetus is not established. However, animal data and retrospective and epidemiologic studies in humans have raised concerns. How, then, should the pregnant women with fever be managed? A reasonable approach is the recommendation of maternal serum α-fetoprotein testing and targeted ultrasound examination for the patient who reports a high fever (>102° F [39° C] of >24 hours' duration) in the early first trimester. For low fevers of short duration, reassurance is offered.

CHORIOAMNIONITIS

Definition of Terms

Many terms have been used to describe the condition of infection of the uterus and its contents during pregnancy. Among these are chorioamnionitis, intraamniotic infection (IAI), amnionitis, and intrauterine infection. In this chapter, IAI is defined as the presence of bacteria in the amniotic fluid. IAI may be clinically evident or subclinical. In prospective studies, Gibbs and associates' criteria for clinical IAI were maternal temperature greater than 100° F [38° C], along with two or more of the following characteristics: maternal or fetal tachycardia, foul odor of the amniotic fluid, or maternal leukocytosis. All patients had ruptured membranes.[17,18] Subclinical IAI is the absence of overt clinical signs in the presence of a positive amniotic fluid culture.

Epidemiology

Incidence

The traditionally quoted incidence of IAI is 1% to 2%. In three retrospective studies, Gibbs and associates reported the incidence at 0.8%, 0.9%, and 1.3%.[19-21] However, two other prospective studies show a significantly increased incidence. Soper and colleagues reported an incidence of 10.5% in a predominantly indigent black population,[22] and Newton and associates reported an incidence of 4.3% in a primarily Mexican-American population.[23] Possible explanations for this difference are (1) underestimation of the true incidence in retrospective studies; (2) a difference in patient population; (3) longer duration of ruptured membranes, inasmuch as the majority of patients with ruptured membranes are managed expectantly; and (4) a difference in the criteria for diagnosis.

Risk Factors

Risk factors for the development of clinical IAI in laboring patients include low parity, duration of internal monitoring, duration of ruptured membranes, number of vaginal examinations, and duration of labor.[22,23] The nulliparous patient with a long labor, multiple vaginal examinations, and prolonged internal monitoring and membrane rupture is at high risk for IAI.

Association with Preterm Labor and Preterm Premature Rupture of Membranes

The frequency of IAI in patients in preterm labor with intact membranes ranges from 0% to 61%. Most of these cases of IAI are subclinical, except for the symptom of preterm labor. Advanced cervical dilation and poor response to tocolytic agents are factors associated with IAI in this setting.[24] The prevalence of positive amniotic fluid culture in patients with preterm premature rupture of membranes (PROM) is 30%.[25] In addition, subclinical IAI is present in up to 75% of patients with preterm PROM in active labor.[26] Despite the obvious association between preterm labor and preterm PROM and subclinical IAI, a definite cause-and-effect relationship is difficult to establish, although causation in both directions is a clinically accepted axiom.

Pathogenesis

Bacteria may gain access to the intrauterine environment by four possible pathways: (1) ascending from the lower genital tract, (2) hematogenous spread, (3) retrograde movement from the peritoneal cavity through the fallopian tubes, and (4) introduction during invasive procedures.

Ascending Route

Ascending spread of microorganisms is believed to be the most common pathway of IAI. Three pieces of evidence support this concept of pathogenesis. First, in twin gestations with bacteria present in at least one sac (as determined by amniocentesis), the presenting sac is involved in virtually all instances.[27] Furthermore, the second sac is not involved unless the presenting sac is. When the same microorganism is present in both sacs, there is a larger inoculum size in the presenting sac.[27] Second, the microorganisms in the lower genital tract are similar to those causing IAI.[28-31] Third, the inflammatory response is generally more intense at the site of the membrane rupture.[32]

Two theories explaining the mechanism of ascending infection have been offered. The first is that ascending bacteria may diffusely colonize the decidua, chorion, and amnion, gaining access to the amniotic fluid at a relatively late stage. The second possibility is that after ascending through the cervix, bacteria immediately traverse the chorioamnion, thus colonizing the amniotic fluid early in the infection process. Romero and associates' description of the histologic patterns of the chorion-decidua interface and amnion in patients with subclinical IAI and intact membranes seems to support a contribution from both theories.[33] Two distinct histologic patterns were described. The first, a marginating pattern, consisted of neutrophils piled up diffusely along the interface between the chorion/amnion and the decidua, which was suggestive of the presence of chemotactic stimuli within the amniotic fluid. This pattern was significantly associated with a positive amniotic fluid culture and suggested that bacteria traversed the membranes early in the infection process. The resulting immunologic reaction was directed toward the bacteria within the amniotic fluid. The second pattern, a nonmarginating pattern, was characterized by locally destructive, necrotizing inflammation within the chorion-decidua interface in response to foci of bacteria. The prevalence of positive amniotic fluid cultures in this group was low. This pattern suggests that infection was confined to the chorion/amnion and decidua.[33]

Hematogenous Route

Maternal bloodborne microorganisms may gain access to the intraamniotic cavity transplacentally. *Listeria monocytogenes,* a small gram-positive bacillus present in milk and soft cheeses, most frequently causes perinatal infection by this mechanism.[34,35]

Retrograde Route

Retrograde seeding of the intraamniotic cavity during peritonitis has been described. This is an extremely rare event.

Procedure-Related Introduction

Bacteria may gain inadvertent entry into the amniotic fluid during invasive procedures. The incidence of IAI after second-trimester amniocentesis is about 1 per 1000.[36]

Infectious complications after cordocentesis occur in approximately 0.5% of cases.[37]

The overall rate of IAI after cervical cerclage may be as high as 7%.[38] This incidence is markedly increased, possibly up to 40%, when emergency salvage cerclage is used in the 19- to 24-week gestation complicated by cervical dilation and exposure of the bulging membranes to vaginal flora.[39] In most cases of salvage cerclage, colonization of the amniotic fluid can be demonstrated with amniocentesis before placement of the cerclage. Romero and associates noted positive amniotic fluid cultures in 51% of 14- to 24-week gestations complicated by cervical dilation of more than 2 cm.[40]

Immunologic Properties of Amniotic Fluid and Cervix

Numerous reports have described the antibacterial activity of amniotic fluid. Various substances, including B-lysin,[41] lysozyme,[42] immunoglobulins,[43] and low-molecular-weight peptide-zinc complex[43-47] have been proposed as the cause of this antibacterial property. The clinical significance of these inhibitory properties and their effects on IAI are unknown. Interestingly, Blanco and coworkers noted that the amniotic fluid in patients with IAI was significantly less likely to be inhibitory to *Escherichia coli.*[48] Whether a decrease in these amniotic fluid immunologic properties predisposes a patient to IAI is unknown.

The cervix also contributes to the host defense against IAI. Cervical mucus provides a physical and chemical barrier to microbial invasion. In vitro, cervical mucus has a strong inhibitory effect on bacteria, comparable with that of ampicillin.[49]

Microbiology

The microorganisms causing IAI are the same as those seen in the majority of gynecologic infections: a polymicrobial milieu consisting of the endogenous flora of the bowel and vagina. In a study of 52 patients with IAI, Gibbs and associates showed an average of 2.2 isolates per specimen of amniotic fluid, with aerobic and anaerobic pathogens occurring in equal frequency.[18] Table 26-1 describes the organisms and their distribution in 404 patients with IAI.[50] The mostly commonly isolated organisms in this series were gram-negative anaerobes, group B streptococci, *Gardnerella vaginalis,* and the genital *Mycoplasma* species. Rare causes of IAI include *L. monocytogenes, Haemophilus influenzae,* and *Candida albicans.* Candidal IAI is reported almost exclusively in association with a retained intrauterine device or cerclage.[51,52]

The qualitative bacteriologic processes of amniotic fluid in cases of IAI involving full-term versus preterm gestations differ. Hillier, in culturing the chorioamnion in placentas above and below 34 weeks of gestation, found that group B streptococci, fusobacterium, and peptostreptococcus were significantly related to preterm delivery.[53] Sperling and colleagues stratified for birth weight (<2500 g or >2500 g) in 404 cases of IAI and found a significant increase in the presence of gram-negative anaerobes in the group with low birth weight.[50] This study suggests that preterm labor and delivery may result from subclinical IAI caused by gram-negative anaerobes.

Table 26–1. Organisms Isolated in Amniotic Fluid in 404 Cases of Intraamniotic Infection

Organism	No. of Infants (%)
Group B streptococci	59 (14.6)
Escherichia coli	33 (8.2)
Enterococci	22 (5.4)
Gardnerella vaginalis	99 (24.5)
Peptostreptococcus species	38 (9.4)
Bacteroides bivius	119 (29.5)
Bacteroides fragilis	14 (3.5)
Fusobacterium species	22 (5.4)
Any gram-negative anaerobe	115 (38.4)
Mycoplasma hominis	123 (30.4)
Ureaplasma urealyticum	190 (47.0)

From Sperling RS, Newton E, Gibbs RS: Intraamniotic infection in low-birthweight infants. J Infect Dis 157:113, 1988.

Diagnosis

Although diagnosis of clinical IAI is often straightforward, subclinical IAI remains a difficult diagnostic dilemma. Because of its association with preterm labor and PROM, early and accurate diagnosis of subclinical IAI is desirable. The major goal of early diagnosis is delivery before the onset of fetal infection.

Physical Examination

Classically, the diagnosis of chorioamnionitis is a clinical one. The clinical diagnosis of IAI is based on the presence of maternal fever and tachycardia, fetal tachycardia, uterine contractions and tenderness, and a foul odor of the amniotic fluid. The relative frequencies of these symptoms in cases of IAI are shown in Table 26-2. Unfortunately, when cases of subclinical IAI are included, physical examination is an insensitive indicator of IAI in general.

Maternal Laboratory Parameters

Both maternal leukocytosis and elevated C-reactive protein levels have been used for the diagnosis. Neither is predictive of IAI. As seen in Table 26-2, maternal leukocytosis occurs with highly variable frequency in clinical IAI.

C-reactive protein has been shown to have poor positive and negative predictive values.[54,55]

Amniocentesis

Direct examination of amniotic fluid through amniocentesis is often necessary to aid in the diagnosis of subclinical IAI. Although culture of amniotic fluid offers the most accurate results, this information is usually unavailable for 48 to 72 hours. Therefore, several other techniques have been devised for rapid diagnosis. These include Gram stain, white blood cell (WBC) count, glucose concentration measurement, limulus amebocyte lysate assay, gas-liquid chromatography of bacterial products, measurement of leukocyte esterase activity, and lactate dehydrogenase (LDH) measurement.

Culture. Amniotic fluid culture is the best available clinical method for accurate diagnosis of IAI. Fluid should be cultured for aerobic and anaerobic bacteria, along with *Mycoplasma hominis* and *Ureaplasma urealyticum*. However, because results are delayed 2 to 3 days, it is usually impractical to base management decisions on culture results alone.

Gram stain. The Gram stain for detection of bacteria in amniotic fluid is an inexpensive and widely available test for rapid diagnosis of IAI. According to a compilation of various reports, the sensitivity and specificity of the Gram stain are approximately 57% and 97%, respectively (Table 26-3).[56-63,65,66] The sensitivity of the test is directly proportional to inoculum size. In the presence of more than 10^5 colony-forming units/mL, the sensitivity approaches 80%.[49] *Mycoplasma* and *Ureaplasma* organisms are not detectable by Gram stain and therefore are a cause of false-negative results. The Gram stain should be interpreted by experienced personnel to significantly improve accuracy.[64] Centrifugation of the amniotic fluid specimen apparently does not improve sensitivity or specificity.[62]

Leukocytes in amniotic fluid. Garite and Freeman initially found no correlation between the presence of leukocytes in amniotic fluid and culture results.[57] Romero and associates, however, showed a strong association between more than 30 WBCs per high-power field and a

Table 26–2. Findings in Clinical Intraamniotic Infection

Finding	Gibbs et al.[18] N = 52	Ferguson et al.[19] N = 107	Hauth et al.[21] N = 103
Temperature > 100° F (%)	100*	48	99.2
Maternal tachycardia (%)	83	NA	19.4
Leukocytosis (%)	69	17	NA
Fetal tachycardia (%)	60	39	82.0
Uterine tenderness (%)	17	52	16.5
Foul odor (%)	8	45	8.7

*Criteria for diagnosis included temperature > 100° F. NA, not addressed in study.

Table 26–3. Sensitivity and Specificity of Gram Stain in Diagnosing Intraamniotic Infection

Study	Sensitivity	Specificity
Elimian et al.[56]	75.0% (9/12)	100.0% (92/92)
Garite and Freeman[57]	70.0% (14/20)	97.0% (64/66)
Garry et al.[58]	75.0% (12/16)	99.1.% (114/115)
Grecci et al.[59]	44.4% (4/9)	94.7% (89/94)
Hussey et al.[60]	45.0% (9/20)	97.0% (129/133)
Romero et al.[61]	79.1% (19/24)	99.6% (239/240)
Romero et al.[62]	44.8% (13/29)	97.6% (83/85)
Romero et al.[63]	60.8% (14/23)	90.5% (38/42)
Skoll et al.[65]	28.6% (2/7)	95.8% (115/120)
Vintzileos et al.[66]	60.0% (9/15)	81.4% (35/43)
Total	57.1% (105/175)	96.9% (998/1030)

positive amniotic fluid culture.[62] Examination for WBCs at the time of Gram stain may be helpful. The identification of abundant WBCs (>30 per high-power field) in association with bacteria reduces the likelihood of a false-positive result. Abundant WBCs in the absence of bacteria suggests that a *Mycoplasma* organism is causing IAI.

Amniotic fluid glucose concentration. Measurement of the amniotic fluid glucose concentration is also a rapid, inexpensive, and widely available test. The sensitivity, specificity, and positive and negative predictive values of multiple studies are reviewed in Table 26-4.[56-58,64,67-70] Comparison of these studies is difficult because of the different glucose levels used as cutoff points. In general, low amniotic fluid glucose concentration is specific for IAI. The lack of sensitivity limits the clinical usefulness of this measurement. It should be used in combination with other rapid tests, such as the Gram stain.

Limulus amebocyte lysate assay. This assay detects the lipopolysaccharide of the cell wall in gram-negative bacteria. In detection of IAI, its sensitivity is 69% and its specificity is 95.2%.[62]

Gas-liquid chromatography. Short-chain organic acids are byproducts of bacterial metabolism and their detection by gas-liquid chromatographic analysis has been proposed for the diagnosis of IAI. This method has limited clinical usefulness. Its sensitivity and specificity in subclinical IAI are poor, and it requires a laboratory procedure with limited availability.[71]

Leukocyte esterase test. This simple test detects the presence of WBCs in amniotic fluid. The sensitivity and specificity range from 80% to 91% and 81% to 95%, respectively.[60,72]

Lactate dehydrogenase. Garry and coworkers, using an LDH value of more than 419 U/L, showed a sensitivity, specificity, positive predictive value, and negative predictive value of 75%, 90%, 50%, and 96%, respectively, in predicting a positive amniotic fluid culture in 131 women presenting with preterm labor.[58] Elimian and colleagues noted a sensitivity, specificity, positive predictive value, and negative predictive value of 83%, 92%, 59%, and 98%, respectively, when they used an LDH maximum of 400 U/L.[56] LDH measurement is another rapid, readily

Table 26–4. Amniotic Fluid Glucose Concentration in the Prediction of Intraamniotic Infection

Study	Sensitivity	Specificity	Positive Predictive Value	Negative Predictive Value
Elimian et al.[56] (<14 mg/dL)	83.3%	89.1%	50.0%	97.6%
Garry et al.[58] (<17 mg/dL)	81.2%	93.0%	61.9%	97.3%
Gauthier et al.[67] (<16 mg/dL)	79.1%	94.2%	86.9%	90.2%
Grecci et al.[59] (<20 mg/dL)	44.4%	88.9%	26.7%	94.3%
Greig et al.[68] (<11 mg/dL)	54.5%	100%	100%	80.0%
Kirshon et al.[69] (<10 mg/dL)	75.0%	100%	100%	90.0%
Klitz et al.[70] (<5 mg/dL)	64.3%	98.6%	90.0%	93.4%
Romero et al.[64] (<14 mg/dL)	86.9%	91.7%	62.5%	97.8%

available test to assist in the diagnosis of IAI. In comparison with other rapid tests, LDH has similar diagnostic accuracy in predicting a positive amniotic fluid culture, although it has not been as extensively evaluated as the Gram stain or glucose concentration measurement.

Summary. There are significant limitations in accurately diagnosing subclinical IAI with the tests just described. Amniotic fluid cultures are limited by inavailability of results in a timely manner and by the inability to isolate an infectious agent because of low levels of inoculum, previous antibiotic treatment, or the presence of a microorganism that cannot be cultured. Although each rapid test has respectable specificity, there is a significant risk for a false-negative result. In other words, a negative test result cannot be used to exclude the diagnosis of IAI, but a positive result is a very specific diagnostic marker for IAI. A currently reasonable approach to the diagnosis of subclinical IAI is the use of a combination of rapid tests, such as Gram stain, glucose measurement, and leukocyte esterase determination, to guide clinical management.

Future tests. Our understanding of the maternal and fetal response to IAI is in its infancy. Of prime interest currently is the infection-induced stimulation of maternal and fetal immune cells to produce cytokines in the presence of bacterial invasion of the amniotic cavity. It is thought that cytokine production then leads to synthesis and release of prostaglandins, which stimulate cervical ripening and uterine contractions. This cascade is a proposed explanation for preterm labor in association with IAI. In the setting of IAI, preterm delivery is associated with elevated levels of several cytokines, including interleukin-1, interleukin-6 (IL-6), interleukin-8 (IL-8), interleukin-16, interleukin-18, and tumor necrosis factor α.[73-77]

The detection of these cytokines in amniotic fluid may prove a useful rapid marker for the diagnosis of subclinical IAI. It appears that IL-6 is the cytokine most closely associated with IAI, histologic chorioamnionitis, and the presence of bacteria in the chorioamnion.[74] An elevated IL-6 concentration in amniotic fluid has a sensitivity ranging from 80.9% to 83.3% and a specificity ranging from 69.2% to 75% in predicting a positive amniotic fluid culture.[59,77] IL-6 concentration was a better predictor of IAI than Gram stain, glucose measurement, and WBC count in patients with preterm PROM in at least one study.[77]

Cytokines have been isolated in cervical and vaginal secretions. Elevated cervical and vaginal fluid concentrations of IL-6 and IL-8 have been associated with IAI.[78,79] Although these studies are preliminary, this concept may prove to be a noninvasive method to aid in the diagnosis.

Another emerging technology is the use of polymerase chain reaction (PCR) to detect intraamniotic bacteria. Preliminary studies suggest that PCR gene amplification of bacterial 16S recombinant DNA gene in amniotic fluid has a greater sensitivity than culture in detecting IAI.[80,81] General clinical use of PCR is currently limited by labor intensiveness, its high cost, the extreme measures

needed to prevent contamination, and its inability to identify the specific microorganism causing infection. In research studies, PCR seems to be replacing culture as the gold standard for the diagnosis of IAI.

Fetal Surveillance Techniques

The biophysical profile (BPP), nonstress test (NST), and Doppler velocimetry of the umbilical artery have been proposed as aids in the diagnosis of subclinical IAI with varying success. Virtually all studies addressing these techniques have been performed in the setting of preterm PROM.

Vintzileos and associates used daily modified BPPs in patients with preterm PROM as an early predictor of IAI. A BPP score of less than 8 within 24 hours of delivery had a sensitivity, specificity, and positive and negative predictive values of 80%, 97.6%, 92.3%, and 93.2%, respectively, in detecting amnionitis, possible neonatal sepsis, and confirmed neonatal sepsis.[66] In addition, the presence of fetal breathing was extremely reliable in excluding infection (negative predictive value = 95.3%).[82] Other authors have not confirmed the usefulness of the BPP or its components in predicting subclinical IAI. Del Valle and colleagues found no difference in the BPP scores in cases of confirmed amnionitis or neonatal sepsis versus those without.[83] Likewise, Miller and coworkers found no difference in BPP scores between patients with and without clinical IAI.[84] Neither set of authors showed a significant difference between patients with and without infection when analyzing the individual components of the BPP. Also, in contrast to Vintzileos and associates, Gonen and colleagues showed that the NST was not useful for predicting congenital sepsis, inasmuch as 11 of 13 fetuses with congenital sepsis had reactive NSTs within 24 hours of birth.[85]

Lewis and associates performed the only prospective randomized trial comparing a daily BPP with a daily NST in the prediction of infection in the setting of preterm PROM.[86] The sensitivity, the specificity, and the positive and negative predictive values of each test are presented in Table 26-5. Both tests are similar in their effectiveness, demonstrating poor sensitivity and acceptable specificity. Of significance in today's health care environment was the reduced daily cost of the NST in comparison with the BPP ($1731 versus $2917; $P < .001$).

In general, the NST and BPP are not sensitive indicators of IAI, but they appear to be the best form of fetal surveillance available at this time. The question remains as to how the BPP and NST fit into the scheme of diagnostic tests for subclinical IAI. Roussis and coworkers showed that deterioration in the BPP or NST over time was highly suggestive of infection[87]; specifically, an initially reactive NST that became nonreactive in association with absence of fetal breathing was suggestive of infection (66%). The use of either a daily NST or a daily BPP is acceptable in the evaluation of a patient at high risk for development of IAI, such as in the case of preterm PROM. Emphasis should be placed on the deterioration of BPP score or NST as being suggestive of infection.

Umbilical artery velocimetry currently has no role as a predictor of IAI. Neither Carroll and associates[88] nor

Table 26-5. Clinical Utility of the NST and BPP in Predicting Intraamniotic Infection

Test	Sensitivity	Specificity	Positive Predictive Value	Negative Predictive Value
Daily NST	39.1%	84.6%	52.9%	75.9%
Daily BPP	25.0%	92.9%	66.7%	68.4%

BPP, biophysical profile; NST, nonstress test.

From Lewis DF, Adair CD, Weeks JW, et al: A randomized clinical trial of daily nonstress testing versus biophysical profile in the management of preterm premature rupture of membranes. Am J Obstet Gynecol 181:1495, 1999.

Leo and colleagues[89] reported a significant difference in umbilical artery Doppler indices in patients with and without IAI in PROM. A rising trend of the systolic-to-diastolic ratio of the umbilical artery within the normal range has been reported in cases of subclinical IAI in PROM.[90] However, it currently has no clinical utility in assessing the fetus at risk for infection.

Management

When IAI is diagnosed, delivery should be expedited. Isolated case reports describe the use of intensive antimicrobial therapy rather than delivery when IAI is documented in the previable fetus, with resultant eradication of bacterial colonization of the amniotic fluid.[91,92] This investigational management approach seems appropriate only in rare circumstances and only at tertiary perinatal centers.

Route of Delivery

Vaginal delivery is preferred in cases of IAI; cesarean section is reserved for the usual obstetric indications. This statement is based on three important considerations. First, neonatal morbidity and mortality rates are unchanged, regardless of the interval from diagnosis of IAI to delivery.[20,21,56] However, the literature does not address the effect of a diagnosis to delivery interval of more than 12 hours on maternal and neonatal complications. Therefore, a delay in delivery much beyond 12 hours should be avoided. Second, during labor in the presence of IAI, there is no increase in the incidence of birth asphyxia in the absence of other signs of other fetal jeopardy, such as ominous fetal heart rate patterns.[93] Third, maternal morbidity rates increase significantly with the use of cesarean section.[94] When abdominal delivery is necessary, a transperitoneal low transverse incision is most commonly used today. There is no apparent advantage to the extraperitoneal approach with modern antibiotics.

Course of Labor

Labor is more often dysfunctional when clinical IAI is present. Soper and colleagues found significant increases in cesarean rate (58.1% versus 5.9%; $P < .0001$), use of oxytocin (79.1% versus 33.4%; $P < .0001$), and length of both the latent ($P = .0001$), and active ($P = .009$) phases of labor in cases of IAI versus controls.[22] It is difficult to determine whether IAI is a cause or an effect of dysfunctional labor, because there is evidence to support both mechanisms. In vitro experiments show that bacterial isolates decrease the motility of myometrial strips.[95] Work done by Silver and associates also suggested a causal relationship between high-virulence bacteria in amniotic fluid and protracted labor.[96] Patients with IAI caused by high-virulence organisms have a significantly lower cervical dilation rate, a higher maximum rate of oxytocin use, and a higher rate of cesarean section for dystocia. Satin and colleagues investigated whether clinical IAI had an inhibitory or stimulatory effect on labor and drew a different conclusion. They examined three groups of patients: those with clinical IAI diagnosed before oxytocin use, those in whom IAI was diagnosed after oxytocin use, and a control group. Clinical IAI diagnosed before oxytocin infusion was associated with shorter intervals between oxytocin initiation and delivery (4.3 vesus 5.6 hours; $P = .04$) and had no effect on the cesarean section rate, in comparison to controls. In contrast, IAI diagnosed late in labor was associated with a longer interval between oxytocin initiation and delivery (12.6 versus 7.9 hours; $P < .0001$) and an increased rate of cesarean section for dystocia (40% versus 10%; $P < .0001$).[97] These data suggest that IAI diagnosed before labor may have a stimulatory effect on uterine activity, whereas IAI diagnosed after initiation of oxytocin may be a marker of dystocia rather than a cause of dysfunctional labor.

There are no clear guidelines for selection of anesthetic techniques during labor complicated by IAI. The incidence of bacteremia in clinical IAI is approximately 8%.[94,98] Therefore, there is a theoretical risk of seeding the epidural space in the bacteremic patient by using regional anesthesia. Unfortunately, maternal characteristics, including mean temperature and leukocyte counts, are not helpful for predicting bacteremia.[98] No prospective studies have examined the potential complications of regional anesthesia in patients with IAI. In two retrospective studies, a total of 784 patients with either clinical or histologic chorioamnionitis received regional anesthesia.[98,99] None, including 16 patients with bacteremia, had infectious complications related to the anesthesia. However, the number of bacteremic patients in these studies was too low for drawing firm conclusions. Therefore, regional anesthesia may be used with caution when bacteremia is suspected.

The obstetrician should be alerted to the possibility of postpartum hemorrhage after labor complicated by IAI, usually caused by atony of the infected uterus. Affected patients are at increased risk for severe postpartum hemorrhage, which is more often refractory to oxytoxics.[100]

Use of Antibiotics

For several years, controversy existed with regard to when antibiotics should be administered for IAI: during labor or after cord clamping, so as to not affect culturing or treatment of the neonate. In the late 1980s, three studies—one retrospective, one nonrandomized, and one prospective and randomized—established as standard the administration of intrapartum antibiotics as soon as the diagnosis of IAI is made. Gilstrap and coworkers, in a retrospective study of treatment during and after labor, found no difference in maternal complication rate.[101] A significant difference was found in the frequency of positive blood cultures for group B streptococci in neonates younger than 35 gestational weeks with regard to whether the mothers were given antibiotics during versus after labor (0 of 133 versus 8 of 14; $P < .05$). Sperling and colleagues, in a nonrandomized study, also found no difference in maternal outcome with regard to timing of antibiotic administration. However, a significant decrease was found in the incidence of neonatal sepsis between the women treated during labor (2.8%) and those treated after labor (19.6%; $P < .001$).[102] The best designed study was the prospective randomized trial by Gibbs and associates, who administered ampicillin and gentamicin, with clindamycin added in the case of cesarean section. Significant differences between women receiving intrapartum treatment and those receiving postdelivery treatment were noted in the incidence of neonatal sepsis (0% versus 21%; $P = .03$); duration of neonatal hospital stay (3.8 versus 5.7 days; $P = .02$); and the maternal postpartum hospital stay, mean febrile days, and mean postpartum temperature ($P = .05$).[17] These data argue strongly in favor of intrapartum antibiotic treatment for IAI. The neonatal management is modified accordingly.

The standard antibiotics used for IAI are ampicillin and gentamicin. These have been extensively evaluated in many studies. Because of the failure rate of ampicillin and gentamicin in cases of IAI in which infants were delivered by cesarean section, the postoperative addition of an antibiotic with effective anaerobic coverage, such as clindamycin, has been advocated.[94] The newer broad-spectrum penicillins and cephalosporins achieve therapeutic levels in cord blood and placental tissue and are probably just as effective as the traditional ampicillin

and gentamicin.[103] However, these antibiotics have not been extensively evaluated in prospective randomized trials.

The maternal postpartum treatment of IAI is controversial. Some physicians elect to continue antibiotics empirically until the woman is afebrile and asymptomatic, whereas others discontinue antibiotics after delivery. Two trials examined this question. Barry and colleagues, investigating women with chorioamnionitis who delivered vaginally, administered postpartum antibiotics to one group and placebo to another group. There were no cases of endometritis in the placebo recipients.[104] Turnquest and associates investigated the same question in women with intrapartum chorioamnionitis who delivered by cesarean section. There was no significant difference in the rate of endometritis between the postpartum gentamicin/clindamycin recipients and the placebo recipients (14.8% versus 21.8%; $P = .32$).[105] An obvious deficiency of these studies was the small sample sizes and therefore the inability to exclude a type II error. Larger randomized, prospective trials are necessary to clarify this issue.

Neonatal Outcome

It was traditionally thought that IAI was primarily an infection of the mother, involving the placenta, amniotic fluid, and the chorioamnion. It was believed that the fetus was infected infrequently. New developments suggest that the fetus is indeed infected more frequently, develops an inflammatory response, and may be at high risk for long-term neurologic morbidity.

Short Term

Among neonates who are premature and have low birth weight, there appears to be an increase in mortality and immediate morbidity as a result of exposure to IAI. Both Garite and Freeman[57] and Morales,[106] in looking at gestations less than 34 weeks with preterm PROM, found significant increases in perinatal death, respiratory distress syndrome, and neonatal infection in the infants with IAI in comparison with control groups (Table 26-6). Sperling and colleagues showed the greater predisposition of the infants with low birth weight to the effects of IAI. After stratifying for birth weight in a group of patients with clinical IAI, a significant difference was seen in early sepsis (16.2% versus 4.1%; $P = .005$) and death from sepsis (10.8% versus 0%; $P < .001$) between infants weighing less than and more than 2500 g, respectively.[50]

Alexander performed a cohort analysis of all singleton live-born infants weighing 500 to 1500 g delivered at his

Table 26-6. Short-Term Perinatal Outcome

	Garite and Freeman[57]			Morales[106]		
	IAI	Control	p	IAI	Control	p
Perinatal death	13%	3%	<.05	25%	6%	<.01
Respiratory distress syndrome	34%	16%	<.01	62%	35%	<.01
Neonatal infection	17%	7%	<.05	28%	11%	<.01

IAI, intraamniotic infection.

institution between 1988 to 1996. Ninety-five of 1367 infants with very low birth weight (7%) were born to mothers with clinical chorioamnionitis. Neonatal sepsis, respiratory distress syndrome, seizure in the first 24 hours of life, IVH (grade 3 or 4), and periventricular leukomalacia were significantly increased with chorioamnionitis.[107]

It appears that the term neonate tolerates IAI better than the preterm infant. Information addressing mortality and immediate morbidity in the term infant, however, is sparse. Alexander and associates performed a retrospective cohort study of all live-born full-term infants weighing more than 2500 g born in their institution between 1988 and 1997. Of 101,170 full-term infants, 5144 were exposed to clinical chorioamnionitis. Chorioamnionitis was significantly associated with the need for delivery room resuscitation and with neonatal pneumonia and sepsis.[108] Despite the possible increase in sepsis and pneumonia in the full-term neonate, IAI appears to have minimal effect on mortality.[20,108,109]

Long Term

Since the early 1990s, IAI has been implicated as a potential cause of cerebral palsy. Several studies show a significant association between clinical and histologic chorioamnionitis and cerebral palsy in preterm infants.[110-113] In addition, clinical and histologic chorioamnionitis is associated with cystic periventricular leukomalacia, a lesion in the white matter of the brain that is predictive of cerebral palsy in preterm neonates.[114-118] Wu and Colford performed a meta-analysis of studies that addressed the association between (1) clinical and histologic chorioamnionitis and (2) cerebral palsy or cystic periventricular leukomalacia. In preterm infants, clinical chorioamnionitis was significantly associated with both cerebral palsy (relative risk = 1.9; 95% CI = 1.4 to 2.5) and periventricular leukomalacia (relative risk = 3.0; 95% CI = 2.2 to 4.0). Histologic chorioamnionitis was significantly associated with periventricular leukomalacia (relative risk = 2.1; 95% CI = 1.5 to 2.9).[119]

There is some information linking IAI and cerebral palsy in full-term infants. In a population-based case-control study, Grether and Nelson found a significant association between clinical chorioamnionitis and unexplained cerebral palsy (odds ratio = 9.3; 95% CI = 2.7 to 31.0).[121] Histologic evidence of placental infection was also associated with cerebral palsy.

Three theories have been postulated to explain the mechanism of brain injury in the fetus exposed to IAI. Grether and Nelson suggested that maternal mediators of infection, such as cytokines, nitric oxide, or free radicals may cross the placenta and the blood-brain barrier of the fetus, inducing injury.[120] Other investigators suggested that brain injury results from direct invasion of fetal brain tissue by bacteria. A third and quite probable mechanism is that the fetal inflammatory response to infection produces brain tissue damage. Evidence is emerging to support this mechanism. First, the fetus is known to produce inflammatory cytokines, including interleukin-1β, IL-6, and tumor necrosis factor α. Second, elevation of interleukin-1β and IL-6 levels in the amniotic fluid is associated with the development of cerebral palsy and periventricular leukomalacia.[121] Third, IL-6 and tumor

necrosis factor α have been identified at autopsy in the periventricular area in the majority of neonates with periventricular leukomalacia.[122]

Maternal Outcome

Maternal mortality from IAI has become increasingly rare. Gibbs and Locke reported 10 deaths from clinical IAI among 501 maternal deaths from 1969 to 1973.[123] However, in a compilation of major studies encompassing 1974 to 1991, there were no maternal deaths in 1421 cases of IAI.[17,20,21,50,57,97,101,124] Maternal morbidity most commonly includes fever and endometritis; septic shock and septic pelvic thrombophlebitis are rarer. Rates of morbidity after cesarean section are significantly increased over those after vaginal delivery.[20,21]

SUMMARY

Maternal fever and chorioamnionitis present challenging diagnostic and management dilemmas, especially in the preterm pregnancy. Despite imprecise tools for definitive diagnosis of IAI, perinatologists, in consultation with neonatal colleagues, must balance the fetal/neonatal risks of infection against the maternal and neonatal morbidity associated with delivery. Until the advent of artificial surfactant therapy, the morbidity expected from hyaline membrane disease after an elective preterm delivery often led to a decision to observe until IAI was certain. With the dramatic improvement in therapy for neonatal respiratory distress syndrome since the early 1990s, however, a move toward earlier delivery, when IAI is only suspected, may often be warranted to minimize neonatal infectious comorbidity. As the maternal and fetal immune response to IAI is further elucidated and diagnostic tests are refined, it is probable that interventions, such as preterm delivery, antibiotics, and even anticytokine therapy, will be more selectively and effectively administered to the woman with IAI in order to optimize maternal and neonatal outcome.

REFERENCES

1. Dinarello CA, Cannon JG, Wolff SM: New concepts on the pathogenesis of fever. Rev Infect Dis 10:168, 1988.
2. Endres S, VanderMeer JWM, Dinarello CA: Interleukin-1 in the pathogenesis of fever. Eur J Clin Invest 17:469, 1987.
3. Nakamura H, Seto Y, Motoyoshi S, et al: Recombinant human tumor necrosis factors causes long-lasting and prostaglandin-mediated fever, with little tolerance, in rabbits. J Pharmacol Exp Ther 245:336, 1988.
4. Naylor AM, Cooper KE, Veale WL: Vasopressin and fever: Evidence supporting the existence of an antipyretic system in the brain. Can J Physiol Pharmacol 65:1333, 1987.
5. Veale WL, Kasting NW, Cooper KE: Arginine vasopressin and endogenous antipyresis: Evidence and significance. Fetal Proc 40:2750, 1981.
6. Mackowiak PA: Direct effects of hyperthermia on pathogenic microorganisms: Teleologic implications with regard to fever. Rev Infect Dis 3:508, 1981.
7. Jampel HD, Duff GW, Gershon RK, et al: Fever and immunoregulation. III. Fever augments the primary in vitro humoral immune response. J Exp Med 157:1229, 1983.

8. Van Oss CJ, Absolom DR, Moore LL, et al: Effect of temperature on the chemotaxis, phagocytic engulfment, digestion and O_2 consumption of human polymorphonuclear leukocytes. J Reticuloendothel Soc 27:561, 1980.

9. Rudelstorfer R, Tabsh K, Khoury A, et al: Heat flux and oxygen consumption of the pregnancy uterus. Am J Obstet Gynecol 154:462, 1986.

10. Morishima HO, Glaser B, Niemann WH, James LS: Increased uterine activity and fetal deterioration during maternal hyperthermia. Am J Obstet Gynecol 121:531, 1975.

11. Oakes GK, Walker AM, Ehrenkranz RA, et al: Uteroplacental blood flow during hyperthermia with and without respiratory alkalosis. J Appl Physiol 41:197, 1976.

12. Kirshon B, Moise KJ, Wasserstrum N: Effect of acetaminophen on fetal acid-base balance in chorioamnionitis. J Reprod Med 34:955, 1989.

13. Graham JM, Edwards MJ, Edwards MJ: Teratogen update: Gestational effects of maternal hyperthermia due to febrile illness and resultant patterns of defects in humans. Teratology 58:209, 1998.

14. Edwards MJ, Shiota K, Smith MS, Walsh DA: Hyperthermia and birth defects. Reprod Toxicology 9:411, 1995.

15. Warkany J: Teratogen update: Hyperthermia. Teratology 33:365, 1986.

16. Milunsky A, Ulcickas M, Rothman KJ, et al: Maternal heat exposure and neural tube defects. JAMA 268:882, 1992.

17. Gibbs RS, Dinsmoor MJ, Newton ER, Ramamurthy RS: A randomized trial of intrapartum versus immediate postpartum treatment of women with intra-amniotic infection. Obstet Gynecol 72:823, 1988.

18. Gibbs RS, Blanco JD, St. Clair PJ, Castaneda YS: Quantitative bacteriology of amniotic fluid from women with clinical intraamniotic infection at term. J Infect Dis 145:1, 1982.

19. Ferguson MG, Rhodes PG, Morrison JC, Puckett CM: Clinical amniotic fluid infection and its effect on the neonate. Am J Obstet Gynecol 151:1058, 1985.

20. Gibbs RS, Castillo MS. Rodgers PJ: Management of acute chorioamnionitis. Am J Obstet Gynecol 136:709, 1980.

21. Hauth JC, Gilstrap LC 3rd, Hankins GD, Connor KD: Term maternal and neonatal complications of acute chorioamnionitis. Obstet Gynecol 66:59, 1985.

22. Soper DE, Mayhall CG, Dalton HP: Risk factors for intraamniotic infection: A prospective epidemiologic study. Am J Obstet Gynecol 161:562, 1989.

23. Newton ER, Prihoda TJ, Gibbs RS: Logistic regression analysis of risk factors for intraamniotic infection. Obstet Gynecol 73:571, 1989.

24. Armer TI, Duff P: Intraamniotic infection in patients with intact membranes and preterm labor. Obstet Gynecol Surv 46:589, 1991.

25. Romero R, Ghidini A, Mazor M, Behnke E: Microbial invasion of the amniotic cavity in premature rupture of membranes. Clin Obstet Gynecol 34:769, 1991.

26. Romero R, Quintero R, Oyarzun E, et al: Intraamniotic infection and the onset of labor in preterm premature rupture of the membranes. Am J Obstet Gynecol 159:661, 1988.

27. Romero R, Shamma F, Avila C, et al: Infection and labor. VI. Prevalence, microbiology, and clinical significance of intraamniotic infection in twin gestations with preterm labor. Am J Obstet Gynecol 163:757, 1990.

28. Jeppson KG, Reimer LG: *Eikenella corrodens* chorioamnionitis. Obstet Gynecol 78:503, 1991.

29. Rusin P, Adam RD, Peterson EA, et al: *Haemophilus influenzae:* An important cause of maternal and neonatal infections. Obstet Gynecol 77:92, 1991.

30. Silver HM, Sperling RS, St. Clair PJ, Gibbs RS: Evidence relating bacterial vaginosis to intraamniotic infection. Am J Obstet Gynecol 161:808, 1989.

31. Wong GP, Cimolai N, Dimmick JE, Martin TR: *Pasteurella multocida* chorioamnionitis from vaginal transmission. Acta Obstet Gynecol Scand 71:384, 1992.

32. Benirschke K, Driscoll SG: The Pathology of the Human Placenta. Berlin, Springer-Verlag, 1967.

33. Romero R, Salafia CM, Athanassiadis AP, et al: The relationship between acute inflammatory lesions of the preterm placenta and amniotic fluid microbiology. Am J Obstet Gynecol 166:1382, 1992.

34. Khong TY, Frappell JM, Steel HM, et al: Perinatal listeriosis. A report of six cases. Br J Obstet Gynaecol 93:1083, 1986.

35. Romero R, Winn HN, Wan M, Hobbins JC: *Listeria monocytogenes* chorioamnionitis and preterm labor. Am J Perinatol 5:286, 1988.

36. Turnbull AC, MacKenzie IZ: Second trimester amniocentesis and termination of pregnancy. BMJ 39:315, 1983.

37. Ludomirski A, Winer S, Craparo FJ, Bolognese RJ: Fetal cordocentesis at Pennsylvania Hospital: Experience with 400 procedures. Paper presented at the Annual Meeting of the American College of Obstetricians and Gynecologists, May 24, 1989, Atlanta.

38. Aarnoudge JO, Huisjes HI: Complications of cervical cerclage. Acta Obstet Gynecol Scand 58:255, 1979.

39. Charles D, Edwards WR: Infectious complications of cervical cerclage. Am J Obstet Gynecol 141:1065, 1981.

40. Romero R, Gonzalez R, Sepulveda W, et al: Infection and labor. VIII. Microbial invasion of the amniotic cavity in patients with suspected cervical incompetence: Prevalence and clinical significance. Am J Obstet Gynecol 167:1086, 1992.

41. Ford LC, DeLonge RJ, Lebherz TB: Identification of bactericidal factor (B-lysin) in amniotic fluid at 40 weeks gestation. Am J Obstet Gynecol 127:788, 1977.

42. Cherry SH, Filler M, Harvey H: Lysozyme content of amniotic fluid. Am J Obstet Gynecol 116:639, 1973.

43. Larsen B, Snyder IS, Galask RP: Bacterial growth inhibition by amniotic fluid. I. In vitro evidence for bacterial growth-inhibiting activity. Am J Obstet Gynecol 119:492, 1974.

44. Larsen B, Snyder IS, Galask RP: Bacterial growth inhibition by amniotic fluid. II. Reversal of amniotic fluid bacterial growth inhibition by addition of a chemically defined medium. Am J Obstet Gynecol 119:497, 1974.

45. Schlievert P, Larsen B, Johnson W, Galask RP: Bacterial growth inhibition by amniotic fluid. III. Demonstration of the variability of bacterial growth inhibition by amniotic fluid with a new plate-count technique. Am J Obstet Gynecol 122:809, 1975.

46. Schlievert P, Larsen B, Johnson W, Galask RP: Bacterial growth inhibition by amniotic fluid. IV. Studies on the nature of bacterial inhibition with the use of plate-count determinations. Am J Obstet Gynecol 122:814, 1975.

47. Schlievert P, Johnson W, Galask, RP: Bacterial growth inhibition by amniotic fluid. VI. Evidence for a zinc-peptide antibacterial system. Am J Obstet Gynecol 125:906, 1976.

48. Blanco JD, Gibbs RS, Krebs LF, Castaneda YS: The association between the absence of amniotic fluid bacterial inhibitory activity and intra-amniotic infection. Am J Obstet Gynecol 143:749, 1982.

49. Romero R, Gomez R, Araneda H, et al: Cervical mucus inhibits microbial growth: A host defense mechanism to prevent ascending infection in pregnant and non-pregnant women. Paper presented at the Annual Meeting of the Society of Perinatal Obstetricians, February 8-11, 1993, San Francisco.

50. Sperling RS, Newton E, Gibbs RS: Intraamniotic infection in low-birthweight infants. J Infect Dis 157:113, 1988.

51. Mazor M, Chaim W, Sepulveda W, Glezerman M: Prevalence and clinical significance of fungal invasion of the amniotic cavity in preterm labor and preterm PROM. Paper presented at the Annual Meeting of the Society of Perinatal Obstetricians, February 8-11, 1993, San Francisco.

52. Smith CV, Horenstein J, Platt LD: Intraamniotic infection with *Candida albicans* associated with a retained intra-uterine contraceptive device: A case report. Am J Obstet Gynecol 159:123, 1988.

53. Hillier SL, Witkin SS, Krohn MA, et al: The relationship of amniotic fluid cytokines and preterm delivery, amniotic fluid infection, histologic chorioamnionitis, and chorioamnion infection. Obstet Gynecol 81:941, 1993.

54. Ernest JM, Swain M, Block SM, et al: C-reactive protein: A limited test for managing patients with preterm labor or preterm rupture of membranes? Am J Obstet Gynecol 156:449, 1987.

55. Cammu H, Goossens A, Derde MP, et al: C-reactive protein in preterm labour: Association with outcome of tocolysis and placental histology. Br J Obstet Gynaecol 96:314, 1989.

56. Elimian A, Figueroa R, Canterino J, et al: Amniotic fluid complement C3 as a marker of intra-amniotic infection. Obstet Gynecol 92:72, 1998.

57. Garite TJ, Freeman RK: Chorioamnionitis in the preterm gestation. Obstet Gynecol 59:539, 1982.

58. Garry D, Figueroa R, Aguero-Rosenfeld M, et al: A comparison of rapid amniotic fluid markers in the prediction of microbial invasion of the uterine cavity and preterm delivery. Am J Obstet Gynecol 175:1336, 1996.

59. Grecci LS, Gilson GJ, Nevils B, et al: Is amniotic fluid analysis the key to preterm labor? A model using interleukin-6 for predicting rapid delivery. Am J Obstet Gynecol 179:172, 1998.

60. Hussey MJ, Levy ES, Pombar X, et al: Evaluating rapid diagnostic tests of intra-amniotic infection: Gram stain, amniotic fluid glucose level and amniotic fluid to serum glucose level ratio. Am J Obstet Gynecol 179:650, 1998.

61. Romero R, Sirtori M, Oyarzun E, et al: Infection and labor. V. Prevalence, microbiology, and clinical significance of intraamniotic infection in women with preterm labor and intact membranes. Am J Obstet Gynecol 161:817, 1989.

62. Romero R, Emamian M, Quintero R, et al: The value and limitations of the Gram stain examinations in the diagnosis of intraamniotic infection. Am J Obstet Gynecol 159:114, 1988.

63. Romero R, Kadar N, Hobbins JC, Duff GW: Infection and labor: The detection of endotoxin in amniotic fluid. Am J Obstet Gynecol 157:815, 1987.

64. Romero R, Jimenez C, Lohda AK, et al: Amniotic fluid glucose concentration: A rapid and simple method for detection of intraamniotic infection in preterm labor. Am J Obstet Gynecol 163:968, 1990.

65. Skoll MA, Morett ML, Sibai BM: The incidence of positive amniotic fluid cultures in patients in preterm labor with intact membranes. Am J Obstet Gynecol 161:813, 1969.

66. Vintzileos AM, Campbell WA, Nochimson DJ, et al: Fetal biophysical profile versus amniocentesis in predicting infection in preterm premature rupture of the membranes. Obstet Gynecol 68:488, 1986.

67. Gauthier DW, Meyer WJ, Bieniarz A: Correlation of amniotic fluid glucose concentration and intraamniotic infection in patients with preterm labor or premature rupture of membranes. Am J Obstet Gynecol 165:1105, 1991.

68. Greig PC, Ernest JM, Teot L: Low amniotic fluid glucose levels are a specific but not a sensitive marker for subclinical intrauterine infections in patients in preterm labor with intact membranes. Am J Obstet Gynecol 171:365, 1994.

69. Kirshon B, Rosenfeld B, Mari G, Belfort M: Amniotic fluid glucose and intraamniotic infection. Am J Obstet Gynecol 164:818, 1991.

70. Klitz RJ, Burke MS, Porreco RP: Amniotic fluid glucose as a marker for intraamniotic infection. Obstet Gynecol 78:619, 1991.

71. Romero R, Scharf K, Mazor M, et al: The clinical value of gas-liquid chromatography in the detection of intra-amniotic microbial invasion. Obstet Gynecol 72:44, 1988.

72. Hoskins IA, Johnson T, Winkel CA: Leukocyte esterase activity in human amniotic fluid for the rapid detection of chorioamnionitis. Am J Obstet Gynecol 157:730, 1987.

73. Athayde N, Romero R, Maymon E, et al: Interleukin-16 in pregnancy, parturition, rupture of fetal membranes, and microbial invasion of the amniotic cavity. Am J Obstet Gynecol 182:135, 2000.

74. Pacora P, Romero R, Maymon E, et al: Participation of the novel cytokine interleukin 18 in the host response to intra-amniotic infection. Am J Obstet Gynecol 183:1138, 2000.

75. Romero R, Avila C, Santhanam U, Sehgal PB: Amniotic fluid interleukin 6 in preterm labor. Association with infection. J Clin Invest 85:1392, 1990.

76. Yoon BH, Romero R, Park JS, et al: Microbial invasion of the amniotic cavity with *Ureaplasma urealyticum* is associated with a robust response in fetal, amniotic and maternal compartments. Am J Obstet Gynecol 179:1254, 1998.

77. Romero R, Yoon BH, Mazor M, et al: A comparative study of the diagnostic performances of amniotic fluid glucose, white blood cell count, interleukin-6, and Gram stain in the detection of microbial invasion in the patients with preterm premature rupture of membranes. Am J Obstet Gynecol 69:839, 1993.

78. Hitti J, Hillier SL, Agnew KJ, et al: Vaginal indicators of amniotic fluid infection in preterm labor. Obstet Gynecol 97:211, 2001.

79. Jun JK, Yoon BH, Romero R, et al: Interleukin-6 determinations in cervical fluid have diagnostic and prognostic value in preterm premature rupture of membranes. Am J Obstet Gynecol 183:868, 2000.

80. Hitti J, Riley DE, Krohn MA, et al: Broad-spectrum bacterial rDNA polymerase chain reaction assay for detecting amniotic fluid infection among women in premature labor. Clin Infect Dis 24:1228, 1997.

81. Markenson GR, Martin RK, Tillotson-Criss M, et al: The use of polymerase chain reaction to detect bacteria in amniotic fluid in pregnancies complicated by preterm labor. Am J Obstet Gynecol 177:1471, 1997.

82. Vintzileos AM, Campbell WA, Nochimson DJ: Fetal breathing as a predictor of infection in premature rupture of the membranes. Obstet Gynecol 67:813, 1986.

83. Del Valle GO, Joffe GM, Izquierdo LA, et al: The biophysical profile and the nonstress test: Poor predictors of chorioamnionitis and fetal infection in prolonged preterm premature rupture of membranes. Obstet Gynecol 80:106, 1992.

84. Miller JM Jr, Kho MS, Brown HL, Gabert HA: Clinical chorioamnionitis is not predicted by an ultrasonic biophysical profile in patients with premature rupture of membranes. Obstet Gynecol 76:1051, 1990.

85. Gonen R, Ohlsson A, Farine D, Milligan JE: Can the nonstress test predict congenital sepsis? Am J Perinat 8:91, 1991.

86. Lewis DF, Adair CD, Weeks JW, et al: A randomized clinical trial of daily nonstress testing versus biophysical profile in the management of preterm premature rupture of membranes. Am J Obstet Gynecol 181:1495, 1999.

87. Roussis P, Rosemond RL, Glass C, Boehm FH: Preterm premature rupture of membranes: Detection of infection. Am J Obstet Gynecol 165:1099, 1991.

88. Carroll SG, Papaioannou S, Nicolaides KH: Doppler studies of the placental and fetal circulation in pregnancies with preterm prelabor amniorrhexis. Ultrasound Obstet Gynecol 5:184, 1995.

89. Leo MV, Skurnick JH, Ganesh VV, et al: Clinical chorioamnionitis is not predicted by umbilical artery Doppler velocimetry in patients with premature rupture of membranes. Obstet Gynecol 79:916, 1992.

90. Fleming AD, Salafia CM, Vintzileos AM, et al: The relationships among umbilical artery velocimetry, fetal biophysical profile, and placental inflammation in preterm premature rupture of the membranes. Obstet Gynecol 164:38, 1991.

91. Cruikshank DP, Warenski IC: First-trimester maternal *Listeria monocytogenes* sepsis and chorioamnionitis with normal neonatal outcome. Obstet Gynecol 73:469, 1989.

92. Romero R, Scioscia AL, Edberg SC, Hobbins JC: Use of parenteral antibiotic therapy to eradicate bacterial colonization of amniotic fluid in premature rupture of the membranes. Obstet Gynecol 67:15S, 1986.

93. Maberry MC, Ramin SM, Gilstrap LC 3rd, et al: Intrapartum asphyxia in pregnancies complicated by intra-amniotic infection. Obstet Gynecol 76:351, 1990.

94. Gibbs RS, Duff P: Progress in the pathogenesis and management of clinical intraamniotic infection. Am J Obstet Gynecol 164:1317, 1991.

95. Leck BF, McDonald D, Vaughan J: The spontaneous motility of human myometrial strips in vitro and its modification by some bacterial extracts. J Physiol 324:42P, 1981.

96. Silver RK, Gibbs RS, Castiulo M: Effect of amniotic fluid bacteria on the course of labor in nulliparous women at term. Obstet Gynecol 68:587, 1986.

97. Satin AJ, Maberry MC, Leveno KJ, et al: Chorioamnionitis: A harbinger of dystocia. Obstet Gynecol 79:913, 1992.

98. Bader AM, Gilbertson L, Kirz L, Datta S: Regional anesthesia in women with chorioamnionitis. Reg Anesth 17:84, 1992.

99. Goodman EJ, DeHorta E, Taguiam JM: Safety of spinal and epidural anesthesia in parturients with chorioamnionitis. Reg Anesth 21:436, 1996.

100. Hayashi RH, Castillo MS, Noah ML: Management of severe postpartum hemorrhage with a prostaglandin $F_{2-alpha}$ analogue. Obstet Gynecol 63:806, 1984.

101. Gilstrap LC 3rd, Leveno KJ, Cox SM, et al: Intrapartum treatment of acute chorioamnionitis: Impact on neonatal sepsis. Am J Obstet Gynecol 159:579, 1988.

102. Sperling RS, Ramamurthy RS, Gibbs RS: A comparison of intrapartum versus immediate postpartum treatment of intra-amniotic infection. Obstet Gynecol 70:861, 1987.

103. Maberry MC, Trimmer KJ, Bawdon RE, et al: Antibiotic concentration in maternal blood, cord blood and placental tissue in women with chorioamnionitis. Gynecol Obstet Invest 33:185, 1992.

104. Barry C, Hansen KA, McCaul JF: Abbreviated antibiotic therapy for clinical chorioamnionitis: A randomized trial. J Matern Fetal Med 3:216, 1994.

105. Turnquest MA, How HY, Cook CR, et al: Chorioamnionitis: Is continuation of antibiotic therapy necessary after cesarean section? Am J Obstet Gynecol 1798:1261, 1998.

106. Morales WJ: The effect of chorioamnionitis on the developmental outcome of preterm infants at one year. Obstet Gynecol 70:183, 1987.

107. Alexander JM, Gilstrap LC, Cox SM, et al: Clinical chorioamnionitis and the prognosis for very low birth weight infants. Obstet Gynecol 91:725, 1998.

108. Alexander JM, McIntire DM, Leveno KJ: Chorioamnionitis and the prognosis for term infants. Obstet Gynecol 94:274, 1999.

109. Yoder PR, Gibbs RS, Blanco JD, et al: A prospective controlled study of maternal and perinatal outcome after intra-amniotic infection at term. Am J Obstet Gynecol 145:695, 1983.

110. Allan WC, Vohr B, Makuch RW, et al: Antecedents of cerebral palsy in a multicenter trial of indomethacin for intraventricular hemorrhage. Arch Pediatr Adolesc Med 151:580, 1997.

111. Cooke RW: Cerebral palsy in very low birthweight infants. Arch Dis Child 65:201, 1990.

112. Jacobson B, Hagberg G, Hagberg B, et al: Cerebral palsy in preterm infants: A population based analysis of antenatal risk factors. Am J Obstet Gynecol 182(Suppl):S29, 2000.

113. Nelson KB, Ellebery JH: Predictors of low and very low birthweight and the relation of these to cerebral palsy. JAMA 254:1473, 1985.

114. Baud O, Foix-L'Helias L, Kaminski M, et al: Antenatal glucocorticoid treatment and cystic periventricular leukomalacia in very premature infants. N Engl J Med 341:1190, 1999.

115. Leviton A, Paneth N, Reuss ML, et al: Maternal infection, fetal inflammatory response and brain damage in very low birth weight infants. Developmental Epidemiology Network Investigators. Pediatr Res 46:566, 1999.

116. Perlman JM, Risser R, Broyles RS: Bilateral cystic periventricular leukomalacia in the premature infant: Associated risk factors. Pediatrics 97:822, 1996.

117. Roland EH, Magee JF, Rodriguez E, et al: Placental abnormalities: Insights into pathogenesis of cystic periventricular leukomalacia. Am Neurol 40:3213, 1996.

118. Zupan V, Gonzalez P, Lacaze-Masmonteil T, et al: Periventricular leukomalacia: Risk factors revisited. Dev Med Child Neurol 38:1061, 1996.

119. Wu YW, Colford JM: Chorioamnionitis as a risk factor for cerebral palsy: A meta-analysis. JAMA 284:1417, 2000.

120. Grether JK, Nelson KB: Maternal infection and cerebral palsy in infants of normal birth weight. JAMA 278:207, 1997.

121. Yoon BH, Jun JK, Romero R, et al: Amniotic fluid inflammatory cytokines (interleukin-6, interleukin-1 beta, and tumor necrosis factor-alpha), neonatal brain white matter lesion and cerebral palsy. Am J Obstet Gynecol 177:19, 1997.

122. Yoon BH, Romero R, Kim CJ, et al: High expression of tumor necrosis factor-alpha and interleukin-6 in periventricular leukomalacia. Am J Obstet Gynecol 177:406, 1997.

123. Gibbs CE, Locke WE: Maternal deaths in Texas 1969-1973. A report of 501 consecutive maternal deaths from the Texas Medical Association's Committee on Maternal Heath. Am J Obstet Gynecol 126:687, 1976.

124. Duff P, Sanders, R, Gibbs RS: The course of labor in term patients with chorioamnionitis. Am J Obstet Gynecol 147:391, 1983.

CHAPTER 27

Meconium and the Compromised Fetus and Neonate

Mamta Fuloria and Thomas E. Wiswell

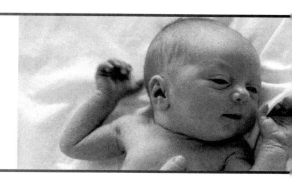

The term **meconium** is derived from the Greek word *meconium-arion*, which means "opium-like." Aristotle likely coined this term for two reasons: (1) he believed that meconium induced fetal sleep, and (2) initially, processed poppy seeds are a black, tarry slurry resembling meconium. It is probable that he recognized the association between the presence of meconium in the amniotic fluid and the occurrence of neonatal depression and fetal deaths.

Meconium-stained amniotic fluid (MSAF) is present in approximately 13% of all deliveries,[1,2] with the incidence increasing with advancing gestational age in all ethnic groups. There is a 1.5-fold increased risk of MSAF in African American women compared with white women.[3]

Regardless of the reason for meconium passage, its presence may be associated with adverse fetal and neonatal outcomes, including death, acute respiratory complications, and long-term pulmonary and neurologic abnormalities. Historically, **meconium aspiration syndrome (MAS)** developed in 5% to 12% of infants born through MSAF.[1,2] More recent evidence suggests, however, that in developed nations, a smaller proportion of meconium-stained infants develop the disorder (1.6% to 3.6%).[4,5] The proportion apparently has declined since 1990.[4] Although many changes in obstetric practice have occurred in recent years (e.g., amnioinfusion), the major reason for the reduction in MAS seems to be the decline in births at gestational ages beyond 41 weeks. Of infants with MAS, 30% to 50% require mechanical ventilation.[1,2,6,7] One third of infants with MAS have accompanying persistent pulmonary hypertension of the newborn (PPHN).[8] The mortality associated with MAS is 4% to 19%.[6,7,9] Much of this mortality is attributable to PPHN. Long-term pulmonary sequelae associated with MAS include abnormal pulmonary function tests (e.g., increased functional residual capacity) and airway hyperreactivity during infancy[10] and later childhood.[11,12] Yuksel and colleagues[10] showed that infants who required a higher degree of respiratory support in the neonatal period, particularly for long periods, subsequently had more symptoms and were more likely to require bronchodilator therapy.

Infants born through moderately thick or thick-consistency MSAF have a sevenfold increased risk of developing early-onset neonatal seizures and a fivefold increased likelihood of hypotonia compared with infants born through thin meconium-stained or clear amniotic fluid.[13] It is presumed that these findings are secondary to in utero, intrapartum, or postnatal hypoxic-ischemic events. Some investigators have observed an increased likelihood of cerebral palsy in surviving infants with a low Apgar score who were born through MSAF.[14]

PATHOPHYSIOLOGY OF MECONIUM PASSAGE

Meconium is composed primarily of water (72% to 80%); other components include gastrointestinal secretions, bile, bile acids, pancreatic secretions, mucus, vernix caseosa, lanugo, blood, cellular debris, and swallowed amniotic fluid.[1,15] Meconium is found in the gastrointestinal tract at 10 to 16 weeks of gestation. Typically, at birth, 60 to 200 g of meconium may be present in the intestinal tract of a term infant.

In utero passage of meconium is rare before 37 weeks of gestation.[16] MSAF is noted, however, in one third to one half of pregnancies lasting beyond 42 weeks of gestation.[17,18] The lack of strong peristalsis, a tonically constricted anal sphincter, and the presence of a terminal cap of viscous meconium inhibit in utero passage of meconium. The levels of motilin, a promotility hormone, have been shown to be higher in term and post-term infants compared with preterm infants,[19] a finding that supports the hypothesis that maturation of the gastrointestinal tract plays an important role in the physiologic passage of meconium. Rubin and coworkers[20] showed that interfacial tension of meconium is strongly associated with the gestational age of infants, with meconium passed by preterm infants having higher interfacial tension compared with meconium passed by term infants. The gestational age–dependent differences in adhesiveness of meconium, which may be related to surfactant in swallowed amniotic fluid, may be responsible in part for preterm neonates not being as likely to pass meconium *in utero* compared with term neonates.

In most instances, *in utero* passage of meconium is likely a physiologic maturational event. This event also is associated, however, with antepartum or intrapartum fetal hypoxia, acidemia, or both.[18,21] Alexander and associates[3] observed a twofold increase in the incidence of MSAF if fetal stress was present. Fetal hypoxia may result in increased intestinal peristalsis and relaxation of the anal sphincter, with resultant passage of meconium. A fetus in distress potentially could gasp and aspirate meconium, a phenomenon more likely to occur in term and post-term compared with preterm infants. In addition, oligohydramnios may result in compression of the fetal head or the umbilical cord, leading to a vagal response that stimulates meconium passage.

PATHOPHYSIOLOGY OF MECONIUM ASPIRATION SYNDROME

Regardless of the reason for the *in utero* passage of meconium, respiratory symptoms can be secondary to aspiration of meconium prenatally or at the time of delivery. Many of the associated respiratory symptoms of MAS are due to altered pulmonary vascular structure,[22] reactivity related to perinatal hypoxia, or directly to the meconium itself.

An ominous heart rate tracing and evidence of severe fetal asphyxia, including low umbilical artery pH and Apgar scores, are predictive of a prolonged need for mechanical ventilation in infants with MAS.[23] In a large multicenter clinical trial,[24] we showed a direct relationship between the thickness of meconium and severity of respiratory disease. Additionally, we observed that neonates born through thick-consistency MSAF were significantly more likely to develop MAS compared with infants born through thin-consistency (odds ratio 9.85, confidence interval 4.39, 22.08) or moderately thick–consistency MSAF (odds ratio 3.93, confidence interval 1.88, 6.65). The latter findings previously had been anecdotally reported.[25]

Figure 27-1 shows the pathophysiology of the development of MAS. Aspiration of meconium can cause either partial or total mechanical obstruction of the airways. Partial obstruction of airways may result in a "ball-valve effect," with gas trapping and the potential for development of air leaks. Complete airway obstruction leads to alveolar collapse and development of ventilation-perfusion mismatch. In an adult rabbit model of MAS, Tyler and colleagues[26] noted early onset of airway obstruction with alveolar collapse, ventilation-perfusion mismatch, and increased functional residual capacity. Studies in animal models[27] with MAS and in neonates with mild MAS[28] (neonates who did not require mechanical ventilation) have shown lower dynamic and specific lung compliance during the illness.

The presence of meconium in the airways can induce an inflammatory response with resultant chemical pneumonitis, protein leak, and surfactant inactivation secondary to the protein leak. In a retrospective review of autopsied cases with histologic evidence of meconium exposure,[29] 67% of all cases with pulmonary inflammation were observed to be secondary to meconium aspiration. In a rabbit model of MAS, the later stages of the disease are characterized by microvascular endothelial cell damage with development of an intrapulmonary shunt, alveolar collapse, and cellular necrosis, consistent with chemical pneumonitis.[26] *In vitro* studies have shown alveolar macrophage and cord blood neutrophil dysfunction, as evidenced by increased superoxide anion[30] and thromboxane[31] production from alveolar macrophages, increased neutrophil chemotaxis,[32] and inhibition of neutrophil oxidative burst and phagocytosis.[33]

With a pulsating bubble surfactometer or a Wilhelmy balance, meconium has been shown to inhibit pulmonary surfactant function directly in a dose-dependent manner.[34-36] Bae and colleagues[37] showed that meconium alters the ultrastructure of surfactant, with the normal loosely stacked layers being replaced by spherical lamellar and folded linear structures. This alteration in surfactant structure was associated with a significant increase in surface tension of the mixture. At low concentrations of meconium, Higgins and coworkers[38] showed absence of toxicity to rat alveolar type II pneumocytes. At higher concentrations of meconium (>1%), they showed dose-dependent cytotoxicity that was inhibited in the presence of heat-treated meconium, suggesting that a protein moiety may be partly responsible for this action. Antunes and colleagues[39] showed decreased production of surfactant protein B (SP-B) in the presence of high concentrations of meconium. In a rat model of MAS, decreased levels of SP-A and SP-B have been shown in bronchoalveolar lavage fluid, suggesting either a decreased production or increased degradation of surfactant proteins in the presence of meconium.[40]

In addition to these effects, PPHN may develop secondary to acidosis, hypoxemia, or hypercapnia associated with *in utero* or postnatal meconium aspiration. Additionally, fetal stress associated with acute or chronic in utero hypoxia can result in remodeling or altered reactivity of the pulmonary vasculature, with subsequent development of PPHN.

CLINICAL FEATURES

The clinical presentation of infants born through MSAF may depend on the degree of *in utero* or postnatal hypoxia and the consistency of aspirated meconium. Infants born through thick-consistency meconium and infants who are depressed at birth are more likely to develop respiratory complications.[1,2,5,24,25] Infants born through thin-consistency meconium and infants who are "apparently vigorous" at birth are at lower risk for respiratory complications. We have defined "apparent vigor" immediately after birth[24] as the initial presence of a heart rate greater than 100 beats/min in an infant who also shows reasonable respiratory effort and good tone. In a large multicenter clinical trial,[24] 3% of vigorous infants born through any consistency of MSAF developed MAS. Only 1% of vigorous infants born through thin-consistency MSAF developed MAS compared with 7% of vigorous infants

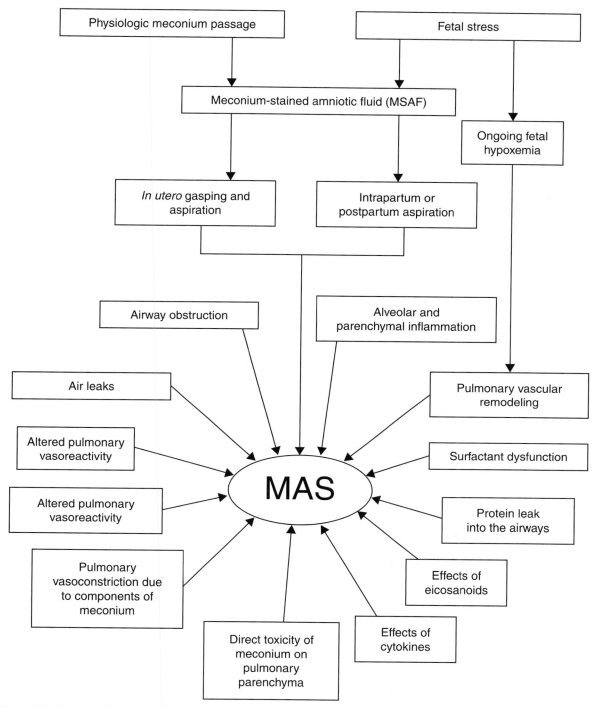

Figure 27–1. The complex pathophysiology of meconium passage and the development of meconium aspiration syndrome (MAS).

born through thick-consistency MSAF. Additionally, we found the incidence of any respiratory complication (including MAS, transient tachypnea of the newborn, pneumothorax, sepsis/pneumonia, PPHN, and pulmonary edema) to be significantly higher in infants born through thick-consistency compared with thin-consistency MSAF (15% versus 2%).[24] In the same investigation, approximately half of the infants with MAS needed

respiratory support with either mechanical ventilation or continuous positive airway pressure. The need for increasing levels of respiratory support also was directly related to the consistency of MSAF.

Infants with MAS are often post term and may exhibit signs of respiratory distress or neurologic depression or both at birth. These infants may develop pulmonary hypertension, with significant hypoxemia, hypercapnia,

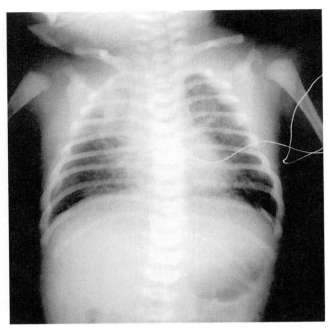

Figure 27–2. The "classic" radiographic findings of MAS: patchy perihilar infiltrates. Multiple other radiographic findings can be seen in affected infants.

Table 27-1. Investigations of Patients with Meconium Aspiration Syndrome

Routine Investigations
Complete and differential blood count
Blood cultures
Chest radiography
Arterial blood gases

Other Investigations as Indicated
Echocardiography, if severe hypoxemia is present, to evaluate for
    Pulmonary hypertension
    Cardiac contractility
    Ventricular filling
    Structural cardiac anomalies
Evaluation for perinatal asphyxia, if suspected
    Placenta, membranes, and umbilical cord examination by a pathologist
    Urine output and monitoring of serial BUN and creatinine
    Serial complete blood counts for platelet count, total lymphocyte count, nucleated red blood cell count
    Monitoring for hypoglycemia and hypocalcemia
    Close monitoring of neurologic status (e.g., tone, state of consciousness, presence of seizures)
    Serial liver function tests, particularly AST, ALT, and GGT
    Consider neuroimaging if abnormal neurologic findings are present
Serum electrolytes

ALT, alanine aminotransferase; AST, aspartate aminotransferase; BUN, blood urea nitrogen; GGT, γ-glutamyltransferase.

acidosis, and right-to-left shunting of blood at the ductus arteriosus or the foramen ovale or both. Typical findings on chest radiography include diffuse patchy infiltrates (Fig. 27-2), areas of consolidation, and hyperinflation. Other radiographic findings include the presence of a pneumothorax and cardiomegaly if significant antenatal or perinatal hypoxia was present.

EVALUATION OF INFANTS WITH MECONIUM ASPIRATION SYNDROME

Table 27-1 presents recommendations for evaluation of infants with suspected MAS. Routinely, a complete blood count with differential, one or more blood cultures, a chest radiograph, and arterial blood gases are obtained as needed. Other investigations may be warranted in infants with MAS. Because PPHN frequently accompanies MAS, if significant hypoxemia is present in infants with MAS, echocardiography should be performed. With echocardiography, one may assess the presence of right-to-left shunting at the ductus arteriosus and the foramen ovale; this technique also is helpful in evaluating cardiac contractility, ventricular filling, and presence of structural congenital heart lesions.

Frequently the presence of MSAF and MAS is associated with perinatal asphyxia. The term *perinatal asphyxia* is often used with imprecision. In the *Guidelines for Perinatal Care*[41] of the American Academy of Pediatrics and the American College of Obstetricians and Gynecologists, it is recommended that the term *asphyxia* be reserved to describe a neonate with all of the following conditions: (1) profound metabolic or mixed acidemia (pH < 7.00) on an umbilical cord artery blood sample, if obtained;

(2) Apgar score 0 to 3 for longer than 5 minutes; (3) neonatal neurologic manifestations, such as seizures, coma, or hypotonia; and (4) multisystem organ dysfunction (e.g., cardiovascular, liver, renal). If perinatal asphyxia is suspected, we recommend multiple studies, including (1) examination of the placenta, amnion and chorion, and umbilical cord by a pathologist; (2) urine output and serial blood urea nitrogen and creatinine measurements; (3) serial complete blood counts, particularly platelet count, absolute lymphocyte count, and nucleated red blood cell count; (4) serial blood glucose and calcium levels; (5) close monitoring of neurologic status (e.g., tone, state of consciousness), with electroencephalography as indicated; and (6) neuroimaging, if abnormal neurologic findings are present.

MONITORING OF INFANTS WITH MECONIUM ASPIRATION SYNDROME

To manage infants with MAS appropriately, many factors need to be monitored closely. Heart rate, respiratory rate, and blood pressure can be evaluated continuously on the current generation of monitors typically found in newborn intensive care units. Acid-base status, oxygenation, and ventilation can be assessed with arterial blood gases. In the sickest infants, blood gases can be obtained via an umbilical arterial catheter or a peripheral arterial line. In less ill patients or infants in whom arterial access cannot be obtained, some clinicians opt to monitor oxygen saturation continuously with pulse oximetry and to obtain capillary blood gases to assess pH and trends in partial pressure of carbon dioxide (PCO_2) levels. Others monitor PCO_2 status with end-tidal PCO_2 monitors. Intermittent arterial "sticks" may be performed to verify an infant's status.

PREVENTION OF MECONIUM ASPIRATION SYNDROME

Prenatal Strategies

Amnioinfusion

Since the initial description of amnioinfusion for the relief of repetitive intrapartum variable decelerations in the 1980s, substantial interest has been generated in the use of amnioinfusion for the prevention of neonatal morbidity associated with MSAF. It has been postulated that increasing amniotic fluid volume would dilute meconium, with a possible decrease in the toxic effects secondary to various meconium components. In the presence of oligohydramnios, amnioinfusion may relieve cord compression, potentially decreasing fetal hypoxia and acidosis, further meconium passage, fetal gasping, and *in utero* aspiration of meconium. A meta-analysis[42] of randomized clinical trials assessing the efficacy of amnioinfusion for the management of moderate-consistency or thick-consistency meconium staining of the amniotic fluid during labor showed a reduction in the incidence of the diagnosis of MAS. Others[43] have reported no beneficial effects of the procedure. Amnioinfusion has been associated with an increase in the incidence of uterine tetany, more instrumented and operative deliveries, more fetal heart rate abnormalities, and higher incidences of maternal endometritis and neonatal sepsis. Based on the existing data, we do not believe there is conclusive evidence that amnioinfusion prevents MAS. Larger, randomized clinical trials are needed to assess the effect of amnioinfusion on neonatal morbidity and mortality related to MSAF and possible maternal complications with greater certainty.

Intrapartum Strategies

Cesarean Section

It has been speculated that removing the meconium-stained fetus from the uterus before the stresses of vaginal delivery would decrease the likelihood of aspirating meconium. Most anecdotal reports indicate an increased incidence of MAS among infants born operatively. Meydanli and colleagues[44] performed a randomized, controlled trial in 70 singleton pregnancies complicated by thick-consistency MSAF. The mothers were randomized to either elective cesarean section or to vaginal delivery. The incidence of MAS was significantly greater among infants delivered via cesarean section.

Maternal Sedation or Paralysis

The use of sedatives and paralytics in the mother has been proposed as a potential therapy to prevent MAS. It has been suggested that after crossing the placenta, these agents sedate or paralyze the fetus, preventing gasping and subsequent meconium aspiration. There are no data to indicate, however, that this strategy is beneficial in the prevention of MAS. Because use of sedation and paralysis carries potential risks for the mother and the child, this strategy should not be used to prevent MAS.

Oropharyngeal Suctioning

Carson and colleagues[45] described a decrease in the incidence of MAS in a cohort of infants after oropharyngeal suctioning at the perineum compared with historical controls. Although this difference was not significant, they advocated this therapy in all infants born through MSAF. There was widespread acceptance of this strategy. Falciglia and coworkers[46,47] were unable, however, to show the strategy's efficacy in either an observational[46] or historical controlled[47] study.

Vain and associates[5] reported findings from a large randomized, controlled trial designed to assess potential benefits of oropharyngeal and nasopharyngeal suctioning of meconium-stained neonates before delivery of their shoulders. More than 2500 infants in the trial were randomized to receive suctioning or expectant management. The investigators were unable to show any advantages of intrapartum suctioning in preventing MAS, need for mechanical ventilation, or death from the disorder.

Cricoid Pressure, Epiglottal Blockage, and Thorax Compression

Several unproven therapies[48] have been suggested as being beneficial in preventing MAS, including use of cricoid pressure, epiglottal blockage, and compression of the thorax. Cricoid pressure involves applying pressure to the airway to prevent meconium from descending into the lungs. With epiglottal blockage, one or more fingers are placed down an infant's airway to apply pressure on the epiglottis and block the airway. Both of these maneuvers have the potential to traumatize the airway and induce a vagal response. Compression of the thorax involves encircling a neonate's chest with the hands and applying pressure to prevent the newborn from inhaling deeply and aspirating more meconium. This, too, is a potentially dangerous practice with the possibility of trauma and aspiration secondary to chest recoil when the encircling hands are removed. Because of the potential for harm with absolutely no evidence of benefit, none of these maneuvers should be used.

Postnatal Strategies

Tracheal Suctioning

Until more recently, considerable controversy has existed regarding the initial delivery room resuscitation of a neonate born through MSAF. In a retrospective study, Ting and Brady[9] showed a 70% decreased risk of developing MAS in infants who received endotracheal suctioning soon after birth. Prospective studies evaluating the effectiveness of immediate tracheal suctioning for the prevention of MAS have shown variable results, with some showing a decreased likelihood of respiratory complications after tracheal suctioning[49,50] and others showing either no difference[51] or even an increased risk.[52,53] Based on the available data in 1992, the American Academy of Pediatrics and American Heart Association recommended intrapartum oropharyngeal suctioning at the perineum and tracheal suctioning of depressed infants and infants born through thick, particulate meconium.[54] In a large (>2000 neonates), prospective, randomized, multicenter controlled clinical trial, we[24] were unable to show any difference in the incidence of MAS and other respiratory complications in apparently vigorous neonates who were randomized to intubation and tracheal suctioning compared with expectant management. Additionally, we observed an increased likelihood of all respiratory complications in infants born through moderately thick–consistency (6.3%) and thick-consistency (15.4%) MSAF compared to infants born through thin-consistency MSAF (2.3%). Similarly the incidence of MAS was 0.8% with thin-consistency MSAF compared with 7.2% with thick-consistency MSAF. The incidence of complications secondary to tracheal suctioning was low, with all complications being mild and transient.[24] Based on the findings of this study, the *Neonatal Resuscitation Textbook*[55] of the American Academy of Pediatrics and American Heart Association recommends tracheal suctioning only in infants born through MSAF who are not vigorous at birth, have respiratory distress, or both.

Chest Physiotherapy

In any infant, the objectives of chest physiotherapy are to prevent accumulation of debris and to improve mobilization of airway secretions, with consequent improvement in gas exchange. It stands to reason that chest physiotherapy would perform a similar function in neonates who have aspirated meconium. Data to support this practice are lacking, however. Numerous complications, including pneumothoraces, hypoxemia, arrhythmias, and tissue damage, have been reported with this procedure; its routine use in infants who have aspirated meconium is not justified.

MANAGEMENT OF INFANTS WITH MECONIUM ASPIRATION SYNDROME

Conventional Management

Because the alleviation of hypoxemia can decrease mortality and morbidity, it is crucial that critically ill infants be identified rapidly and treatment instituted as soon as possible. Management of infants with MAS is mainly supportive. Placement of central arterial and venous catheters (umbilical arterial and venous catheters) is important to monitor blood gases and blood pressure and to provide access for medications and nutrition. Close attention should be paid to fluid intake, and urine output and serum electrolytes should be monitored.

Because it can be difficult to differentiate between MAS and pneumonia/sepsis, these infants should be treated with antibiotics for at least 48 to 72 hours pending blood culture results. Ampicillin and gentamicin are usually used because they cover the most commonly encountered gram-positive and gram-negative organisms

causing neonatal sepsis during the immediate newborn period.

Depending on the severity of respiratory distress, respiratory support should be provided. Conventional support ranges from supplemental oxygen via an oxyhood or nasal cannula, to nasal continuous positive airway pressure, to mechanical ventilation using standard time-cycled, pressure-limited infant ventilators. Because of the high risk of air leak, some clinicians prefer administering oxygen to a fraction of inspired oxygen of 1.00 before using positive pressure. Although some clinicians are proponents of early use of nasal continuous positive airway pressure, others believe it should be avoided because of the risk of air leak. There have been no studies to delineate advantages of any particular mode of conventional ventilation (e.g., intermittent mandatory ventilation versus assist-control ventilation). From the late 1970s through the late 1980s, the management of PPHN was often with hyperventilation.[56] Because PPHN is associated frequently with MAS, many neonatologists routinely hyperventilate infants with the latter disorder, despite the lack of supportive evidence. The goal of this approach is to achieve hyperoxia (PaO_2 levels typically > 120 to 150 mm Hg) and alkalosis (pH > 7.50). Sometimes, extraordinarily low $PaCO_2$ values (10 to 15 mm Hg) are seen with hyperventilation. Conversely, some clinicians advocate the concept of "gentle" ventilation, in which pH levels of 7.15 to 7.20 are accepted, as are PaO_2 levels of 35 to 40 mm Hg and $PaCO_2$ levels of 70 mm Hg or greater. There are no randomized, controlled trials that have supported any particular approach versus another one, and there are no data to support acceptance of extreme values of pH, PaO_2 or $PaCO_2$. We believe it is reasonable to try to achieve the following: (1) pH 7.25 to 7.45, (2) PaO_2 60 to 80 mm Hg, and (3) $PaCO_2$ 35 to 55 mm Hg. We recognize, however, that it may be difficult to achieve blood gas values in these ranges, particularly during the most severe course of the disorder. Other "conventional" therapies for MAS include routine use of sedation (e.g., fentanyl), paralysis (e.g., with pancuronium), alkalosis (infusions with bicarbonate), and therapy with pressors (dopamine and dobutamine). There are virtually no data to support *routine* use of any of the latter therapies. We do support their use when clinically indicated.

Beyond Conventional Management

High-frequency ventilation has been used in neonates since the early 1980s. HFV is often used as a "rescue" mode of ventilation in neonates with MAS who are failing conventional management, and some clinicians advocate high-frequency ventilation use as the initial method of ventilation in infants with MAS. There are no randomized, controlled trials, however, to support high-frequency ventilation use as either a primary or a rescue mode of ventilation for MAS. The sole randomized, controlled trial related to this disorder was in term infants with respiratory failure who were thought to be candidates for extracorporeal membrane oxygenation (ECMO).[57] Many of the included infants had MAS. In that particular trial, however, the infants randomized to high-frequency oscillatory ventilation did no better than infants treated conventionally.

Infants with PPHN are often severely hypoxemic and hemodynamically unstable. The use of inhaled nitric oxide (iNO), a selective pulmonary vasodilator, may help improve oxygenation in some instances. The U.S. Food and Drug Administration approved the use of iNO in term infants with hypoxic respiratory failure associated with clinical or echocardiographic evidence of pulmonary hypertension. iNO is not approved as a primary therapy for MAS; infants must have evidence of PPHN. The use of iNO does not decrease mortality or duration of hospitalization, and it does not improve neurologic outcome. Additionally, of the several large trials assessing iNO use in infants with PPHN, only one showed that infants with MAS would benefit (less need for ECMO).[58] It is believed that iNO decreases extrapulmonary right-to-left shunting and ventilation-perfusion mismatch by causing pulmonary vasodilation in well-aerated lung fields. In a randomized clinical trial, Kinsella and colleagues[59] showed that high-frequency oscillatory ventilation (for alveolar recruitment and maintenance of optimal lung volume) combined with iNO therapy was more efficacious than either therapy alone in improving oxygenation in infants with MAS.

Several investigators have shown that meconium inhibits surfactant function in a dose-dependent manner.[34-36] In vitro, this inhibition can be overcome with high concentrations of surfactant. The major effects of meconium seem to be (1) a physical effect on the phospholipid monolayer, (2) alteration of surfactant morphology, and (3) cellular effects on the type II pneumocytes. Bae and colleagues[37] showed that a meconium-to-surfactant ratio exceeding 2.0 was associated with a significant increase in the minimal surface tension of Surfacten (the Japanese equivalent of beractant [Survanta]). This increase in surface tension corresponded to ultrastructural changes in the surfactant, with the normal, loosely stacked layers being replaced by spherical lamellar and folded linear structures. Higgins and associates[38] showed toxicity to rat cultured alveolar type II cells with high concentrations of meconium. In a rat model of MAS, decreased levels of SP-A and SP-B were observed in bronchoalveolar lavage fluid.[40] Considering these data, it seems logical to theorize that surfactant replacement therapy in infants with MAS would improve the pulmonary outcomes.

Small retrospective studies have shown variable responses to surfactant therapy.[60-63] Some trials indicated improved oxygenation, whereas others had inconsistent results. This variability in response to exogenous surfactant could be secondary to the method of delivery, timing of administration, amount delivered, distribution of the substance, or specific preparation used. In a small, prospective, randomized, controlled trial, Findlay and colleagues[64] used Survanta at a dose of 6 mL/kg (1.5 times the standard dose used for respiratory distress syndrome) infused over 20 minutes. Compared with control infants, infants receiving surfactant infusions had a shorter hospital course, fewer air leaks, and a lesser requirement for ECMO. The investigators did not observe any improvement in the respiratory status of the study infants, however, until the second dose of surfactant, a finding suggestive of inadequate initial dosing with surfactant in these infants. In a larger randomized, controlled trial,

Lotze and coworkers[65] randomized 328 term-gestation infants with respiratory failure (approximately half of whom had MAS) to either bolus therapy with Survanta at standard doses or conventional management. The infants treated with surfactant had a lesser requirement for ECMO. All other end points were equivalent between groups.

Because it is impossible to know the exact amount of meconium aspirated by a particular infant and its effect on surfactant function, it would not be feasible to estimate a "correct" dose of surfactant for each affected infant without performing bronchoalveolar lavage and estimating surfactant function in the lavage fluid. Surfactant boluses are more likely to reach areas with better aeration compared with areas that are collapsed or contain debris, resulting in further ventilation-perfusion mismatch. A reasonable alternative to administration of bolus exogenous surfactant to these infants would be lavage of the airways with dilute surfactant. Lavage of airways with surfactant also may help remove residual meconium and inflammatory mediators, with subsequent decrease in pulmonary symptoms secondary to airway obstruction and inflammation. In animal models with MAS, surfactant lavage (compared with no lavage or saline lavage) has been shown to result in improved gas exchange and increased meconium recovery.[66,67] In adult rabbits and rhesus monkeys with experimental MAS,[68] bronchoalveolar lavage with dilute lucinactant (Surfaxin) resulted in a rapid and sustained improvement in oxygenation compared with no treatment, saline lavage, or bolus Surfaxin administration. Surfaxin is a synthetic surfactant containing a protein mimic of surfactant protein B. We performed a pilot clinical trial in infants with MAS using bronchoalveolar lavage with dilute Surfaxin.[69] We found this therapy to be safe and to show apparent efficacy. There was a more rapid and sustained improvement in oxygenation and a decreased duration of mechanical ventilation. Currently, a large, multicenter, randomized, controlled trial is being conducted to elucidate further the safety and efficacy of surfactant lavage using Surfaxin compared with standard care for the treatment of infants with moderate to severe MAS. Until completion of this or other randomized clinical trials, bronchoalveolar lavage with surfactant for the treatment of MAS should be considered an experimental therapy.

More research is needed to establish the exact role of surfactant in the management of infants with MAS, including the optimal doses, timing of administration, type of surfactant used, and mode of delivery (bolus, continuous infusion, or lavage). The Food and Drug Administration has yet to approve any surfactant for either bolus or lavage treatment of MAS.

Aspiration of meconium has been shown to be associated with inflammatory changes in the lungs. These changes include an increase in the absolute neutrophil count and chemotactic activity,[70] increased production of superoxide anion[30] and mediators such as thromboxane[31] by alveolar macrophages, and decreased neutrophil oxidative burst and phagocytosis.[33] Because glucocorticoids have potent anti-inflammatory properties, it is conceivable that they could ameliorate, in part, the inflammation associated with aspiration of meconium and possibly improve oxygenation. Davey and colleagues[70] have shown decreased alveolar white blood cells in tracheal aspirate from infants with MAS who were treated early with dexamethasone. In a small, randomized, clinical trial, Wu and colleagues[71] showed improved oxygenation and ventilation indices and decreased duration of mechanical ventilation in infants with MAS who were treated early with dexamethasone. In the treatment and the control groups, the patients were not very sick (<50% required mechanical ventilation), however. Although the results of this trial are promising, the role of steroids, including patient selection, dosage, type of steroid used, and appropriate timing of administration, needs to be investigated further.

Foust and colleagues[72] showed that meconium-stained lambs with respiratory distress can be treated successfully with partial or total liquid ventilation with rapid improvement in oxygenation and dynamic lung compliance and decrease in lung barotrauma. The unique ability of perflubron to dissolve large quantities of oxygen and carbon dioxide at atmospheric pressure can be useful in ventilating neonates with MAS, providing the much needed time for the lungs to recuperate from the meconium aspiration. In contrast to its effect on surfactant activity, meconium does not seem to alter the surface tension of perflubron in vitro. The high density and low surface tension of perflubron, along with its ability to decrease the interfacial tension of meconium-saline suspensions, may help clear meconium from the airways of neonates with MAS. The reduction in interfacial tension also may result in improved lung compliance. Further research is needed to delineate the role of liquid ventilation in the management of neonates with MAS.

Severely hypoxemic infants, or infants not responding to any of the aforementioned therapies, may benefit from ECMO.[73] Neonates with MAS constitute approximately one third of all infants who are managed with ECMO. ECMO is described in more detail elsewhere in this book.

SUMMARY

The occurrence of MSAF is a relatively common problem. MAS is a complex disorder, with symptoms ranging from mild respiratory distress to PPHN and death in some infants. The importance of this clinical syndrome lies in the significant morbidity and mortality attributable to it. The limited understanding of the pathophysiology of MAS has hampered the development of newer and better treatment options for these infants. Currently, the management of MSAF and of infants who develop MAS is mainly supportive. The use of exogenous surfactant has been shown to improve oxygenation in infants with MAS; however, the type of surfactant, optimal dose, timing, and route of administration need further investigation. The role of other therapies, including amnioinfusion for the prevention of MAS, surfactant lung lavage, use of steroids, and liquid ventilation, needs further evaluation. It is hoped that ongoing and future research will lead to improved clinical management of affected neonates.

REFERENCES

1. Wiswell TE, Bent RC: Meconium staining and the meconium aspiration syndrome. Pediatr Clin North Am 40:955, 1993.
2. Cleary GM, Wiswell TE: Meconium-stained amniotic fluid and the meconium aspiration syndrome: An update. Pediatr Clin North Am 45:511, 1998.
3. Alexander GR, Hulsey TC, Robillard P-Y, et al: Determinants of meconium-stained amniotic fluid in term pregnancies. J Perinatol 14:259, 1994.
4. Yoder BA, Kirsch EA, Barth WH, et al: Changing obstetric practices associated with decreasing incidence of meconium aspiration syndrome. Obstet Gynecol 99:731, 2002.
5. Vain N, Szyld E, Prudent L, et al: Oro- and nasopharyngeal suction of meconium-stained neonates before delivery of their shoulders does not prevent meconium aspiration syndrome: Results of the international, multicenter, randomized, controlled trial (RCT) [abstract 2206]. Pediatr Res 51:379A, 2002.
6. Wiswell TE, Tuggle JM, Turner BS: Meconium aspiration syndrome: Have we made a difference? Pediatrics 85:715, 1990.
7. Coltart TM, Byrne DL, Bates SA: Meconium aspiration syndrome: A 6-year retrospective study. Br J Obstet Gynaecol 96:411, 1989.
8. Fleischer A, Anyaegbunam A, Guidette D, et al: A persistent clinical problem: Profile of the term infant with significant respiratory complications. Obstet Gynecol 79:185, 1992.
9. Ting P, Brady JP: Tracheal suction in meconium aspiration. Am J Obstet Gynecol 122:767, 1975.
10. Yuksel B, Greenough A, Gamsu HR: Neonatal meconium aspiration syndrome and respiratory morbidity during infancy. Pediatr Pulmonol 16:358, 1993.
11. Macfarlane PI, Heaf DP: Pulmonary function in children after neonatal meconium aspiration syndrome. Arch Dis Child 63:368, 1988.
12. Swaminathan S, Quinn J, Stabile MW, et al: Long-term pulmonary sequelae of meconium aspiration syndrome. J Pediatr 114:356, 1989.
13. Berkus MD, Langer O, Samueloff A, et al: Meconium-stained amniotic fluid: Increased risk for adverse neonatal outcomes. Obstet Gynecol 84:115, 1994.
14. Nelson KB, Ellenberg JH: Obstetric complications as risk factors for cerebral palsy or seizure disorder. JAMA 251:1843, 1984.
15. Holtzman RB, Banzhaf WC, Silver RK, et al: Perinatal management of meconium staining of the amniotic fluid. Clin Perinatol 16:825, 1989.
16. Matthews TG, Warshaw JB: Relevance of the gestational age distribution of meconium passage in utero. Pediatrics 64:30, 1979.
17. Usher RH, Boyd ME, McLean FH, et al: Assessment of fetal risk in postdate pregnancies. Am J Obstet Gynecol 158:259, 1988.
18. Miller FC, Read JA: Intrapartum assessment of the postdate fetus. Am J Obstet Gynecol 141:516, 1981.
19. Lucas A, Adrian TE, Christofides N, et al: Plasma motilin, gastrin, and enteroglucagon and feeding in the human newborn. Arch Dis Child 55:673, 1980.
20. Rubin BK, Tomkiewicz RP, Patrinos ME, et al: The surface and transport properties of meconium and reconstituted meconium solutions. Pediatr Res 40:834, 1996.
21. Nathan L, Leveno KJ, Carmody TJ, et al: Meconium: A 1990s perspective on an old obstetric hazard. Obstet Gynecol 83:329, 1994.

22. Murphy JD, Vawter GF, Reid LM: Pulmonary vascular disease in fatal meconium aspiration. J Pediatr 104:758, 1984.

23. Hernandez C, Little BB, Dax JS, et al: Prediction of the severity of meconium aspiration syndrome. Am J Obstet Gynecol 169:61, 1993.

24. Wiswell TE, Gannon CM, Jacob J, et al: Delivery room management of the apparently vigorous meconium-stained neonate: Results of the multicenter, international collaborative trial. Pediatrics 105:1, 2000.

25. Rossi EM, Philipson EH, Williams TG, et al: Meconium aspiration syndrome: Intrapartum and neonatal attributes. Am J Obstet Gynecol 161:1106, 1989.

26. Tyler DC, Murphy J, Cheney FW: Mechanical and chemical damage to lung tissue caused by meconium aspiration. Pediatrics 62:454, 1978.

27. Tran N, Lowe C, Sivieri EM, et al: Sequential effects of acute meconium aspiration on pulmonary function. Pediatr Res 14:34, 1980.

28. Yeh TF, Lilien LD, Barathi A, Pildes RS: Lung volume, dynamic lung compliance, and blood gases during the first 3 days of postnatal life in infants with meconium aspiration syndrome. Crit Care Med 10:588, 1982.

29. Burgess AM, Hutchins GM: Inflammation of the lungs, umbilical cord and placenta associated with meconium passage in utero. Pathol Res Pract 192:1121, 1996.

30. Kojima T, Hattori K, Fujiwara T, et al: Meconium-induced lung injury mediated by activation of alveolar macrophages. Life Sci 54:1559, 1994.

31. Khan AM, Shabarek FM, Colasurdo GN, et al: Meconium stimulates production of thromboxanes from human epithelial cell A549. Pediatr Res 43:288A, 1998.

32. de Beaufort AJ, Pelikan DMV, Elferink JGR, et al: Pneumonitis following meconium aspiration: Neutrophil chemotaxis induced by interleukin-8 present in meconium. Pediatr Res 43:171A, 1998.

33. Clark P, Duff P: Inhibition of neutrophil oxidative burst and phagocytosis by meconium. Am J Obstet Gynecol 173:1301, 1995.

34. Moses D, Holm BA, Spitale P, et al: Inhibition of pulmonary surfactant function by meconium. Am J Obstet Gynecol 164:477, 1991.

35. Clark DA, Nieman GF, Thompson JE, et al: Surfactant displacement by meconium free fatty acids: An alternative explanation for atelectasis in meconium aspiration syndrome. J Pediatr 110:765, 1987.

36. Sun B, Curstedt T, Robertson B: Surfactant inhibition in experimental meconium aspiration. Acta Paediatr 82:182, 1993.

37. Bae C-W, Takahashi A, Chida S, et al: Morphology and function of pulmonary surfactant inhibited by meconium. Pediatr Res 44:187, 1998.

38. Higgins ST, Wu A-M, Sen N, et al: Meconium increases surfactant secretion in isolated rat alveolar type II cell. Pediatr Res 39:443, 1996.

39. Antunes MJ, Friedman M, Greenspan JS, et al: Meconium decreases surfactant protein B levels in rat fetal lung explants. Pediatr Res 41:137A, 1997.

40. Cleary GM, Antunes MJ, Ciesielka DA, et al: Exudative lung injury is associated with decreased levels of surfactant proteins in a rat model of meconium aspiration. Pediatrics 100:998, 1997.

41. American Academy of Pediatrics and the American College of Obstetricians and Gynecologists: Guidelines for Perinatal Care. Elk Grove Village, IL, American Academy of Pediatrics, 2002, pp 196-197.

42. Pierce J, Gaudier FL, Sanchez-Ramos L: Intrapartum amnioinfusion for meconium-stained fluid: Meta-analysis of prospective clinical trials. Obstet Gynecol 95:1051, 2000.

43. Spong CY: Amnioinfusion: Indications and controversies. Contemp Obstet Gynecol 42:138, 1997.

44. Meydanli MM, Dilbaz B, Caliskan E, et al: Risk factors for meconium aspiration syndrome in infants born through thick meconium. Int J Gynecol Obstet 72:9, 2001.

45. Carson B, Losey RW, Bowes WA Jr, et al: Combined obstetric and pediatric approach to prevent meconium aspiration syndrome. Am J Obstet Gynecol 126:712, 1976.

46. Falciglia HS: Failure to prevent meconium aspiration syndrome. Obstet Gynecol 71:349, 1988.

47. Falciglia HS, Henderschott C, Potter P, et al: Does DeLee suction at the perineum prevent meconium aspiration syndrome? Am J Obstet Gynecol 167:1243, 1992.

48. Wiswell TE: Handling the meconium-stained infant. Semin Neonatol 6:225, 2001.

49. Gregory GA, Gooding CA, Phibbs RH, et al: Meconium aspiration in infants: A prospective study. J Pediatr 85:848, 1974.

50. Suresh GK, Sarkar S: Delivery room management of infants born through thin meconium stained liquor. Indian Pediatr 31:1177, 1994.

51. Daga SR, Dave K, Mehta V, et al: Tracheal suction in meconium stained infants: A randomized controlled study. J Trop Pediatr 40:198, 1994.

52. Yoder BA: Meconium-stained amniotic fluid and respiratory complications: Impact of selective tracheal suction. Obstet Gynecol 83:77, 1994.

53. Linder N, Aranda JV, Tsur M, et al: Need for endotracheal intubation and suction in meconium-stained neonates. J Pediatr 112:613, 1998.

54. Committee on Neonatal Ventilation/Meconium/Chest Compressions: Guidelines proposed at the 1992 National Conference on Cardiopulmonary Resuscitation and Emergency Cardiac Care, Dallas, 1992. JAMA 268:2276, 1992.

55. Kattwinkel J, Niermeyer S, Denson SE, et al: Neonatal Resuscitation Textbook, 4th ed. Elk Grove Village, IL, American Academy of Pediatrics, 2000.

56. Walsh MC, Stork EK: Persistent pulmonary hypertension of the newborn: Rational therapy based on pathophysiology. Clin Perinatol 28:609, 2001.

57. Clark RH, Yoder BA, Sell MS: Prospective, randomized comparison of high-frequency oscillation and conventional ventilation in candidates for extracorporeal membrane oxygenation. J Pediatr 124:447, 1994.

58. Clark RH, Kueser TJ, Walker MW, et al: Low-dose nitric oxide therapy for persistent pulmonary hypertension of the newborn. Clinical Inhaled Nitric Oxide Research Group. N Engl J Med 342:469, 2000.

59. Kinsella JP, Troug WE, Walsh WF, et al: Randomized, multicenter trial of inhaled nitric oxide and high-frequency oscillatory ventilation in severe, persistent pulmonary hypertension of the newborn. J Pediatr 131:55, 1997.

60. Khammash H, Perlman M, Wojtulewicz J, et al: Surfactant therapy in full-term neonates with severe respiratory failure. Pediatrics 92:135, 1993.

61. Halliday HL, Speer CP, Robertson B, and Collaborative Surfactant Study Group: Treatment of severe meconium aspiration syndrome with porcine surfactant. Eur J Pediatr 155:1047, 1996.

62. Auten RL, Notter RH, Kendig JW, et al: Surfactant treatment of full-term newborns with respiratory failure. Pediatrics 87:101, 1991.

63. Blanke JG, Jorch G: Surfactant therapy in severe neonatal respiratory failure—multicenter study: II. Surfactant therapy in 10 newborn infants with meconium aspiration syndrome. Klin Padiatr 205:75, 1993.

64. Findlay RD, Taeusch HW, Walther FJ: Surfactant replacement therapy for meconium aspiration syndrome. Pediatrics 97:48, 1996.

65. Lotze A, Mitchell BR, Bulas DI, et al: Multicenter study of surfactant (beractant) use in the treatment of term infants with severe respiratory failure. J Pediatr 132:40, 1998.

66. Paranka MS, Walsh WF, Stancombe BB: Surfactant lavage in a piglet model of meconium aspiration syndrome. Pediatr Res 31:625, 1992.

67. Ohama Y, Itakura Y, Koyama N, et al: Effect of surfactant lavage in a rabbit model of meconium aspiration syndrome. Acta Paediatr Jap 36:236, 1994.

68. Cochrane CG, Revak SD, Merritt TA, et al: The efficacy and safety of KL4-surfactant in preterm infants with respiratory distress syndrome. Am J Respir Crit Care Med 153:404, 1996.

69. Wiswell TE, Knight GR, Finer NN, et al: A multicenter, randomized, controlled trial comparing the safety and effectiveness of Surfaxin (lucinactant) to standard care for treatment of the meconium aspiration syndrome (MAS). Pediatrics 109:1081, 2002.

70. Davey AM, Becker JD, Davis JM: Meconium aspiration syndrome: Physiological and inflammatory changes in a newborn piglet model. Pediatr Pulmonol 16:101, 1993.

71. Wu JM, Yeh TF, Wang JY, et al: The role of pulmonary inflammation in the development of pulmonary hypertension in newborn with meconium aspiration syndrome (MAS). Pediatr Pulmonol 18(Suppl):205, 1999.

72. Foust R III, Tran NN, Cox C, et al: Liquid assisted ventilation: An alternative ventilatory strategy for acute meconium aspiration injury. Pediatr Pulmonol 21:316, 1996.

73. Kim ES, Stolar CJ: ECMO in the newborn. Am J Perinatol 17:345, 2000.

CHAPTER 28

Third-Trimester Hemorrhage

Dawnette Lewis, Richard E. Broth, and Ronald Bolognese

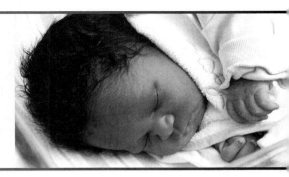

Third-trimester obstetric blood loss is associated with significant risks for poor perinatal outcome and increased maternal morbidity and mortality. The most common causes of third-trimester bleeding are placenta previa, abruptio placentae, and, less commonly, vasa previa, which can potentially result in fetal exsanguination secondary to vessel rupture. These three entities present difficult diagnostic and management challenges to the clinician. Other clinical situations that create additional risk factors for bleeding include placenta accreta, increta, and percreta. Although improved antenatal and neonatal management have resulted in decreases in morbidity and mortality, the serious clinical problems inherent as a result of third-trimester hemorrhage necessitate correct diagnosis and management for optimizing maternal and perinatal outcome.

PLACENTA PREVIA

Historically, placenta previa was diagnosed clinically by digital examination under "double setup" conditions. Transabdominal ultrasonography enabled clinicians to visualize a low-lying placenta. With the evolution of transvaginal ultrasound technology, however, clinicians are better able to describe the location of the placenta in relation to the cervix. The type of placenta previa is defined by its proximity to the internal cervical os. A placental edge more than 2 cm from the internal cervical os is considered normal placentation, an edge within 2 cm is considered marginal, and anything overlying the internal os is considered a complete placenta previa (Figs. 28-1 and 28-2).

Incidence and Etiology

The incidence of placenta previa is quoted as approximately 3% to 5% in the midtrimester and falls to almost 0.3% to 0.7% among full-term pregnancies.[1,2] Risk factors associated with placenta previa include history of cesarean delivery, advanced maternal age, multiparity, history of placenta previa, spontaneous and induced abortions, cigarette smoking, cocaine use, African and Asian ethnicity, and multiple gestation.[2-18] It is postulated that damage to the endometrium and myometrium can predispose to a low implantation of the placenta and may increase the risk of placenta previa. Despite this theory, the cause of placenta previa remains obscure. Abnormally low placental implantation increases the likelihood of fetal malpresentation, and an increased congenital malformation rate is also associated with placenta previa.[1,19]

Interestingly, independent studies have demonstrated that women with placenta previa have a lower risk of hypertensive complications of pregnancy than do normal controls. The researchers theorized that because of altered placental perfusion, maternal blood flow is improved at the placental site in women with placenta previa, which would provide better blood flow and prevent hypoxia to the trophoblasts in comparison with the normally implanted placenta.[20-22]

Maternal Morbidity and Mortality

Significant morbidity is associated with maternal blood loss resulting from placenta previa. In comparison with pregnancies with normal placentation, the combination of antepartum and intrapartum blood loss is greater and could increase the need for maternal transfusion. Maternal morbidity in patients with diagnosed placenta previa is related to antepartum hemorrhage, the possibility of coexistent placental abruption, and mode of delivery, inasmuch as most patients with placenta previa undergo cesarean delivery. It has been reported that the total estimated blood loss and the need for blood transfusions are increased with complete placenta previa in comparison with a marginal placenta previa.[23] Iyasu and coworkers in a 9-year epidemiologic study of placenta previa in the United States, found that women with placenta previa were 14 times more likely to have a related abruption than were controls.[1] There is also the additional maternal risk related to cesarean delivery, which includes maternal infection, hemorrhage, thromboembolism, and potential injury to adjacent intraabdominal organs.

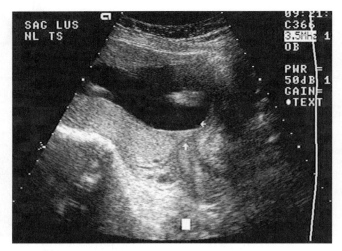

Figure 28–1. Complete posterior placenta previa, sagittal view.

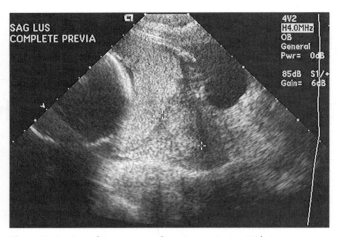

Figure 28–2. Complete anterior placenta previa, sagittal view.

Women with previous uterine incision from a prior cesarean section or other uterine procedures and who have an additional diagnosis of placenta previa are at particularly increased risk for placenta accreta, increta, and percreta. Taylor and associates, in a population-based, case-control study, evaluated the relationship between induced/spontaneous abortions and placenta previa, which showed an increased incidence of placenta previa in women with more than one induced or spontaneous abortion (Table 28-1).[6]

Neonatal Morbidity and Mortality

Preterm labor, preterm delivery, low birth weight, stillbirth, neonatal deaths, and perinatal deaths are associated with pregnancies complicated by placenta previa. Despite the aggressive use of tocolytic agents and maternal transfusion to prolong pregnancy, McShane and colleagues found that two thirds of patients were delivered before 36 weeks' gestation as a complication of placenta previa and found a 22% incidence of respiratory distress syndrome related to prematurity.[19] An association between intrauterine growth restriction has been reported in several studies but disputed by others.[24,25] It has also been suggested that a relationship exists between antepartum and intrapartum blood loss and neonatal anemia.[19,26]

Diagnosis

A diagnosis of placental previa is usually made with the presence of "painless vaginal bleeding" in the third trimester of pregnancy. Approximately 20% of cases of placental previa are associated with abdominal pain, because preterm labor or placental abruption may further complicate the clinical picture.

The diagnostic modality in pregnancy when placenta previa is suspected is transvaginal ultrasonography; transabdominal ultrasonography can be associated with both false-positive and false-negative diagnoses.[27] Since its introduction in 1988 to detect placenta previa, transvaginal ultrasonography has proved to be a more sensitive and specific study for diagnosis than transabdominal ultrasonography.[28-30] Farine and associates

Table 28–1. Odds Ratios for Placenta Previa According to Abortion History among Women with Two or More Prior Pregnancies

Abortion History	Cases (*N* = 317)	Controls (*N* = 864)	Odds Ratio	95% Confidence Interval
No. of induced abortions				
0	201 (63%)	613 (71%)	1.00	—
1	69 (22%)	150 (17%)	1.41	1.01-1.99
≥2	47 (15%)	101 (12%)	1.34	0.89-2.02
No. of spontaneous abortions				
0	165 (52%)	528 (61%)	1.00	—
1	84 (27%)	220 (25%)	1.27	0.92-1.76
≥2	68 (21%)	116 (13%)	1.64	1.11-2.44

From Taylor VM, Kramer MD, Vaughan TL, et al: Placenta previa in relation to induced and spontaneous abortion: A population-based study. Obstet Gynecol 82:88, 1993.

mentioned several advantages of transvaginal versus abdominal ultrasonography, including better visualization of the cervical internal os and its relationship to placental location, which results in improved diagnostic accuracy with posterior previas.[28] The sensitivity and negative predictive value of transvaginal sonography is reported to be as high as 100%, and specificity was calculated to be as high as 98.8% in another review.[29,31] Translabial ultrasonography yields similar results as transvaginal ultrasonography.[32,33]

Numerous questions regarding the safety of transvaginal ultrasonography were initially raised, but multiple studies have demonstrated its safety in women with placenta previa. There appears to be no increase in vaginal bleeding after this procedure.[28,30,31] Timor-Tritsch and Yunis demonstrated the safety of transvaginal ultrasonography by describing the angle of the transvaginal probe in relation to the external cervical os.[30] With transvaginal imaging, the image of the vagina and cervix are at a 40- to 49-degree angle to each other, which makes it impossible to enter the external cervical os with a vaginal probe.[28,30,32]

Magnetic resonance imaging (MRI) is a newer technology advocated by several authors for evaluation of suspected cases of placenta previa. The stated benefits of MRI include multiplanar imaging capabilities, potentially better tissue differentiation, and the ability to differentiate blood from other fluids.[34,35]

Management

Obstetric management of the patient with third-trimester hemorrhage is dictated by the severity of the blood loss and the gestational age of the fetus. Initial evaluation should be done in the hospital. Immediate intravenous access should be obtained, and the patient's blood should be typed and crossmatched for packed red blood cells, should a transfusion be necessary. As with all emergencies, the pregnant woman should be stabilized before any attempt to save the fetus is made. Once the mother is stabilized, the fetus may need to be delivered if fetal compromise is present.

If both mother and fetus are clinically stable, then conservative management may be applicable if the fetus is premature. Consideration should be given to administering betamethasone for fetal lung maturity if the fetus is between 24 and 34 weeks of gestational age. One course of corticosteroids is recommended by the National Institutes of Health since the benefits of repeated courses of betamethasone are unknown. This government office is currently conducting a randomized controlled trial of single versus repeated courses of betamethasone.[36] A type and crossmatch of the pregnant patient should be maintained with the goal of keeping the hematocrit level at 30% or higher. Iron supplementation is also given to anemic patients. Erythropoietin can also be used to increase red blood cell mass in anemic patients.[37-40] There are instances in which the blood from the bleeding placenta previa can cause preterm labor or preterm contractions. Towers and coworkers reported the use of tocolytic agents as safe in the management of third-trimester bleeding.[41] Their retrospective study concluded that tocolytic use did not appear to increase rates of maternal

or neonatal morbidity and mortality.[41] If coexistent placental abruption is suspected, laboratory evaluation for maternal disseminated intravascular coagulation should be performed. In addition, a Kleihauer-Betke test should be conducted to assess potential fetal-to-maternal hemorrhage. The Rh-negative mother with bleeding should also receive Rh immune globulin to prevent Rh sensitization. Arias reported that cervical cerclage in patients with placenta previa improved outcomes,[42] but the efficacy of this treatment has not been corroborated. Cobo and associates replicated Arias's study and found that cervical cerclage did not provide any additional benefit in improving outcomes of pregnancies complicated by placenta previa.[43]

Once the pregnant patient with placenta previa is stabilized in hospital, consideration may be given to outpatient management. Several investigators have compared conservative and expectant management of patients with placenta previa.[3,23,44-46] D'Angelo and Irwin expectantly managed 38 patients with third-trimester placenta previa on either an inpatient or outpatient basis. Their results suggested improved outcomes in the inpatient group, with lower rates of neonatal morbidity and larger neonates who delivered at more advanced gestational ages in comparison with those managed as outpatients. In addition, total hospital costs for mother and neonate were 67% higher in the outpatient-managed patients.[44] Wing and colleagues, in a subsequent randomized, controlled trial of inpatient versus outpatient expectant management of placenta previa, showed no difference in neonatal morbidity between the two groups and reported no neonatal deaths. Cost analysis based on maternal hospital days demonstrated a net savings of $15,080 per patient if women were managed as outpatients.[46]

If outpatient management is utilized as a treatment option, the patient is placed on strict bed rest, except for bathroom privileges, and pelvic rest for the remainder of the pregnancy, because strenuous activity might stimulate vaginal bleeding and precipitate hemorrhage. Extreme caution is used with outpatient management because repeat bleeding episodes are unpredictable and often asymptomatic, and extensive hemorrhage may occur. The patient should have immediate access to a telephone and live within 10 to 15 minutes' driving distance from the hospital. We recommend in-hospital bed rest for the rest of the pregnancy after a third episode of vaginal bleeding.

Ultrasonography may be used to monitor fetal growth in patients with placenta previa because of the possibility of intrauterine growth restriction.[24,25]

Cesarean delivery is the accepted method of delivery in all cases of placenta previa. An amniocentesis for fetal lung maturity should be considered at 36 weeks' gestation. If there is accurate dating of the pregnancy by a first-trimester ultrasonogram, amniocentesis may be deferred and a planned elective delivery scheduled at 37 weeks' gestation. At all times, the clinician must weigh the risk of possible life-threatening maternal hemorrhage with prematurity. Because of the likelihood of excessive bleeding during surgery, at least 2 units of blood should be available for possible transfusion. Finally, in patients suspected of having abnormal implantation of the placenta, such as placenta accreta, increta, and percreta, precautions are taken in the event of massive intraoperative blood loss resulting from the adherent placenta.

PLACENTA ACCRETA, INCRETA, AND PERCRETA

Incidence and Etiology

Adherent placenta approaching or invading through myometrial tissue represents the pathologic finding of placenta accreta, increta, and percreta. The overall incidence is 1 per 7000, but it has been reported to vary from 1 per 540 to 1 per 70,000.[47] The placenta is normally separated from the myometrium by the decidua basalis and the fibrinoid layer of Nitabuch. Clinically, because the normal cleavage plane between placenta and decidua is absent, these abnormalities cause failure of normal placental separation after delivery, which often results in massive hemorrhage. Abnormal formation of the decidua basalis frequently results from uterine scarring after previous cesarean section or another procedure, such as dilatation and curettage.

Clark and colleagues documented the association between placenta previa, previous cesarean delivery, and abnormal placental implantation (Table 28-2).[48] They reported that the risk of placenta previa ranges from 1% without a history of uterine surgery and increases to 10% with four or more previous cesarean sections. They also found that when placenta previa was associated with previous cesarean section, the risk of placenta accreta increased dramatically. The risk of placenta accreta was 24% with one previous cesarean delivery and increased to 67% after four or more prior cesarean deliveries.[48] Other studies have also reported on the association between placenta accreta and placenta previa inpatients with a history of uterine scars.[17,21,49]

Several authors have described an association between unexplained elevations of maternal serum α-fetoprotein and subsequent placenta accreta/increta. This association may be the result of abnormal placentation or abnormal placental function.[50,51]

Ophir and coworkers described one case of placenta increta and one case of placenta percreta, both associated with elevated maternal serum creatinine kinase concentration.

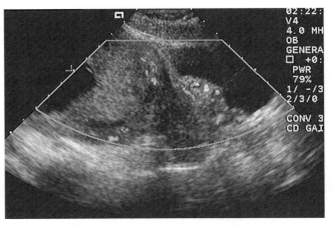

Figure 28-3. Placenta previa with placenta accreta, shown by power Doppler imaging. Note proximity to the bladder.

The authors hypothesized that because placental villi invade the myometrium, this can cause muscle damage and that creatinine kinase can be used as a possible marker of placenta accreta/increta/percreta.[52]

Diagnosis

Ultrasonography is an important tool for delineating placental location and implantation. Certain ultrasound criteria have been used to diagnose placenta accreta, increta, and percreta: thinning or loss of the normal hypoechoic zone beneath the placenta, the presence of intraplacental lacunae or lakes, thinning or disruption of the normally hyperechoic uterine serosa-bladder interface, and visualization of focal exophytic masses, with the latter two findings raising the possibility of placenta percreta.[53-56] Because of the clinical association of an anterior placenta previa in a patient with previous cesarean section, the obstetrician should suspect the possibility of placenta accreta (Figs. 28-3 and 28-4).

MRI may be useful in the diagnosis of placenta percreta, as described by Thorp and associates in a patient

Table 28-2. Placenta Previa with Prior Uterine Incision(s): Effect on Incidence of Placenta Accreta

No. of Prior Cesarean Sections	Placenta Previa (N = 286)	Placenta Previa/ Accreta (N = 29)	Percentage
0	238	12	5
1	25	6	24
2	15	7	47
3	5	2	40
4	3	2	67

From Clark, SL, Koonings PP, Phelan JP: Placenta previa/accreta and prior cesarean section. Obstet Gynecol 66:89, 1985.

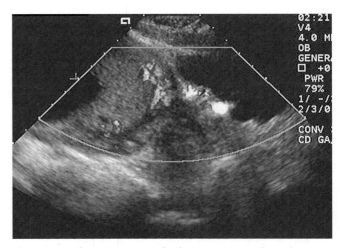

Figure 28-4. Placenta previa with placenta accreta, shown by power Doppler imaging. Note proximity to the bladder.

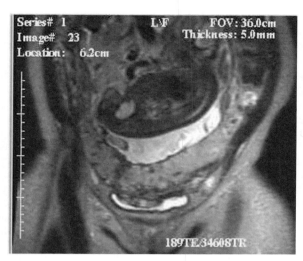

Figure 28–5. Magnetic resonance image of placenta previa/accreta.

with placental invasion through the uterine serosa and into the bladder base (Figs. 28-5 and 28-6).[57]

Clinically, suspicion of abnormal placental adherence is raised if, during the third stage of labor, the placenta fails to separate from the uterine wall in its usual way or, on attempt to manually remove the placenta, a normal cleavage plane cannot be identified. In these cases, attempts to remove the placenta may result in massive maternal hemorrhage.

Management and Outcome

The risk of maternal death from massive blood loss is increased in patients with placenta accreta, increta, and percreta, which highlights the importance of proper surgical preparation.[47,49,58] Clark and colleagues[59] and Stanco and associates[60] noted that 30% and 50%, respectively, of emergency peripartum hysterectomies in their series were performed for placenta accreta or percreta. In general, hysterectomy is the procedure of choice in patients with placenta accreta to avoid complications from severe hemorrhage. In Breen and coworkers' series of 40 patients with placenta accreta, increta, or percreta, 38 underwent

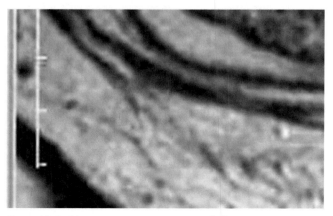

Figure 28–6. Magnetic resonance image of placenta previa/accreta with suspected placenta percreta.

hysterectomy, and other series noted a similarly increased need for removal of the uterus.[47] Conservative therapy, such as uterine packing of the lower uterine segment and the use of methotrexate, may help avoid hysterectomy but is reserved for the rare hemodynamically stable patient who wants to preserve future fertility.[61-64]

Maternal blood loss may be quite large in patients with placenta accreta. Read and colleagues noted an estimated delivery and immediate postpartum blood loss of 3800 mL in all patients and almost 5000 mL if the pregnancy was associated with placenta previa.[49] The mean number of red blood cell transfusions was 7.9; almost 20% of these patients developed coagulation abnormalities.[23,49] Similar findings, with the additional morbid conditions of hypotensive shock and enterotomy, were reported by Miller and associates.[17]

The obstetrician, gynecologic oncologist, and urologist should take a multidisciplinary approach in the management of these complicated patients. At least 4 units of crossmatched red blood cells should be available at the time of surgery, in addition to other blood components such as fresh-frozen plasma and platelets.

ABRUPTIO PLACENTAE

Abruptio placentae, or placental abruption, is defined as the separation of a normally implanted placenta from the uterine wall before the birth of a fetus after 20 weeks' gestation.[65,66] It is associated with significant rates of maternal and fetal morbidity and mortality. The causes are numerous, and although the diagnosis is a clinical one, it is important to attempt to elicit the cause. Abruption is a well-known cause of third-trimester bleeding, and the diagnosis and management can be a challenge for the obstetrician.

The incidence of abruption has been quoted at 11.5 per 1000 deliveries[67] or approximately 1 per 120 deliveries[68-70]; 1% to 2% of those threaten the life of the fetus.[67,70,71] Abruption accounts for approximately 6% to 12% of maternal mortality[70,72] and 20% to 40% of perinatal mortality, mostly from issues related to prematurity.[67] Forty percent occur after 37 weeks and are managed by delivery.[69,70,73,74] Of these, almost 90% of affected fetuses are small for gestational age, which is suggestive of a chronically abnormal maternal-fetal interface. Of affected fetuses that are less than 37 weeks of gestational age, almost one third deliver within 7 days.[75,76]

There are many conditions and causes that contribute to abruption. These include advanced maternal age, multiparity, tobacco use, cocaine use, trauma, membrane rupture, hypertension (chronic and gestational), diabetes, renal disease, chorioamnionitis, multiple gestation, history of abruption, thrombophilia, short umbilical cord, and dietary deficiencies. No common denominator has been identified as the cause, but a few scenarios have been suggested. These can be divided into those originating from an arterial source and those from a venous source. Arterial bleeding contributing to abruption seems to be related to spiral arteriole disease stemming from such processes as hypertension, trauma, and uterine decompression and from effects of cocaine use and smoking.

This is the more severe form, in which severe abruption can cause acute fetal compromise, necessitating delivery.[73] Venous bleeding occurs at the outermost portions of the intervillous space with an obscure bleeding site. With increasing pressure, there may be rupture of some venous channels, causing a hematoma that is usually self-limited and usually does not cause a disruption of the uteroplacental function. Most of these cases are transient, but if the bleeding continues, there is further separation of the placenta and a resultant decrease in maternal-fetal oxygen exchange through the placenta.[77] The condition in which the bleeding progresses into or through the myometrium is a Couvelaire uterus. Only 25% of placental abruptions can be diagnosed by ultrasonography.[75]

Women who have a history of placental abruption have a recurrence risk of 5.5% to 16%,[78] whereas those with an obstetric history complicated by two prior abruptions have a significant risk, as high as 25%.[79] In general, abruptions that occur in a subsequent pregnancy tend to be more severe and occur earlier in gestation.

Hypertensive Disease

Pritchard and associates in 1970 showed an association between abruption and hypertension.[71] Since then, this phenomenon has been studied in more detail. Severe preeclampsia is most closely associated with abruption (risk ratio = 38.8), followed by chronic hypertension with superimposed preeclampsia and chronic hypertension. There is no association with mild preeclampsia.[80] Of the patients who have eclampsia complicated by abruption, more than half have had no prenatal care.[69] Many authors have correlated the degree of hypertension with perinatal mortality,[81,82] but others have shown no association.[75,83,84] There is no correlation of severity with systolic, diastolic, or mean arterial pressures; quantitative proteinuria; epigastric pain; vaginal bleeding; gestational age at delivery; or laboratory values.[69]

Preterm Premature Rupture of Membranes

Acute and chronic abruption have been linked to preterm premature rupture of membranes (PPROM), although the exact mechanism is unknown. One explanation is abrupt uterine compression from the loss of fluid, which triggers placental separation. The other theory is that the abruption is caused by a subacute infection, which is evident from pathologic specimens but not from clinical findings.[73,85,86] The incidence of abruption in PPROM has been shown to be as high as 7%, especially with severe oligohydramnios,[87] and the mean gestational age at delivery in these patients is 28 weeks.[73]

Illicit Drug Use

Since the early 1980s, cocaine use has become more prevalent, increasingly among pregnant women.[88] It is derived from the leaves of the *Erythroxylon coca* plant and causes such effects as vasoconstriction, tachycardia, and transient hypertension by increasing central nervous system stimulation. It does so by blocking dopamine and norepinephrine reuptake at the presynaptic adrenergic nerve endings.[89] This stimulation, in turn, causes a sympathetic response that can lead to the events that are ultimately responsible for placental abruption. The incidence of placental abruption among substance abusers is 13% to 17%; for cocaine users, it is approximately 13.4%, as opposed to approximately 1% in controls.[90] The premise that the vasoconstriction properties can cause umbilical artery vasoconstriction led to the idea of testing fetal blood flow with Doppler ultrasonography for abnormalities in patients who use cocaine, to predict pregnancy complications. Hoskins and colleagues discovered that in all cases that resulted in abruption, systolic/diastolic ratios were abnormally elevated, and they hypothesized that this was secondary to placental vascular dysfunction, whereby the vasospasm resulted in a separation between the placenta and uterus.[90] They also observed that there was an association between (1) abnormal Doppler signals and (2) intrauterine growth restriction and smallness for gestational age. Tobacco smoking is known to be associated with abruptio placentae. Smoking reduces the risk of preeclampsia; however, when both occur in concert, there is an increased risk of abruption.

Maternal Trauma

Trauma has been shown to affect 1 in 12 pregnancies in some manner.[91] The most common cause of blunt abdominal trauma is motor vehicle accidents, followed by falls and domestic abuse/assaults.[74] Although most cases tend to have favorable outcomes, many considerations are involved, including gestational age at the time of injury, extent of injury, and mechanism of injury. Pregnancies complicated by domestic violence have an increased incidence of PROM, preterm labor, and abruption. Studies show that more than 50% of fetal losses after abdominal trauma were the result of placental abruption.[92] The mechanism seems to be a shearing effect at the interface between the elastic myometrium and the inelastic placenta. This shearing effect is independent of placental location.[91] Women should be encouraged to be cautious to avoid abdominal trauma and to properly fasten their seatbelts with both the lap belt and shoulder harness while riding in an automobile, because this has been shown to have a positive effect on outcome severity.[93]

Other Factors

Several other situations have been correlated with placental abruption. Multiparous women have a higher incidence than do nulliparous women,[80] and the risk increases further with grand multiparity (five to eight previous live births) and great-grand multiparity (more than eight previous live births).[94] Twin gestation increases the risk for abruption twofold over that of a singleton pregnancy.[95] Women who have undergone a prior cesarean delivery have a 30% increase in the incidence of placental abruption in comparison with those who have had a prior vaginal delivery.[96]

Abruption can also be seen in patients who have a heritable thrombophilia. These patients have a statistically increased prevalence of mutations in the genes encoding for factor V Leiden, prothrombin, methylenetetrahydrofolate reductase, and homocysteine.[70] In one study, of 29 patients in whom placental abruption was diagnosed, 8 (27.6%) were found to have the factor V Leiden mutation (3 homozygotes and 5 heterozygotes), in comparison with 1 (3.4%) of 29 controls.

Maternal Morbidity

Maternal morbidity (Table 28-3) and mortality as a consequence of abruption is directly related to the amount of hemorrhage leading to hypovolemia, shock, and coagulopathy. Blood loss in excess of 1500 mL has been reported.[82] Many coexisting conditions have been associated with abruption, as noted in Table 28-3, with stillbirth being 11 times more common and coagulopathies more than 50 times more common in this subset of patients than in controls. Almost 40% of patients require blood or blood products for replacement and correction of their coagulopathy, which thus confers transfusion risks on the patient as well.[97] In addition to the aforementioned risks, more than 50% of the fetuses show signs of distress with a significant abruption. They require delivery by cesarean section, which increases maternal morbidity and mortality.[67,83]

Perinatal Morbidity and Mortality

Abruption carries a mortality rate of 20% to 40%; fetal demises account for 25% of the perinatal deaths.[67] Because more than half of abruptions occur before 37 weeks and 70% before 36 weeks, the morbidity and mortality are heavily associated with gestational age at delivery. In pregnancies complicated with preterm PROM, the mean gestational age at delivery is 28 weeks, and many of these neonates suffer long-term sequelae of their prematurity. Some of the affected fetuses have further complications from their chronic vascular issues, leading to decreased weight and growth.

Diagnosis

The diagnosis of placental abruption is mainly a clinical one. In severe cases, there is no time to rely on any other diagnostic studies that may useful in less acute situations.

Usually the constellation of vaginal bleeding, abdominal pain, and a tender, "rock-hard" abdomen are enough to make the diagnosis, but not all need be present for the diagnosis. In fact, many cases of abruption are concealed, as explained earlier, and vaginal bleeding is not present. Tocometry may reveal uterine tetany, hyperstimulation, or just irregular contractions. After 20 weeks' gestation, fetal cardiac monitoring can be performed by either external Doppler evaluation or ultrasonography to assess the fetal heart rate. In cases of more than 20% abruption, fetal heart rate abnormalities are seen, and there is a significant increase in perinatal death.[98] As already noted, ultrasonography detects only between 25% and 36% of abruptions,[99] and, therefore, the absence of findings does not rule out placental abruption. Blood may be seen in retroplacental, submembranous, or subchorionic locations. Laboratory values that may be helpful include elevated coagulation values, decreased platelet counts, decreased levels of antithrombin III and fibrinogen, and a positive result of a Kleihauer-Betke test for fetomaternal hemorrhage.

Management

Management of these patients can be complicated and is dictated by the severity of the abruption and the gestational age at which this occurs. As noted with placenta previa, patients with severe hemorrhage need to be stabilized in a hospital environment and given intravenous fluids and blood products as needed, with full fetal and maternal uterine monitoring. If both the mother and fetus are stable, conservative management may be employed. In two studies of patients with fewer than one contraction every 10 minutes over a 4-hour period, none had evidence of placental abruption[92,100]; such patients may even be discharged home after 4 to 6 hours of observation. Of those with uterine contractions of greater frequency, approximately 20% have evidence of abruption and need to be managed closely. Controlled and appropriate use of

Table 28–3. Estimated Rate of Selected Obstetric Conditions per 1000 Deliveries and Corresponding Rate Ratios among Women with and without Abruptio Placentae

Coexisting Condition	Rate		Rate Ratio	95% CI
	With Abruptio Placentae	No Abruptio Placentae		
Preterm premature rupture of membranes	58.6	32.1	1.8	1.3-2.6
Preterm labor	335.4	43.5	7.5	6.8-8.3
Chorioamnionitis	15.2	6.1	2.5	1.6-3.9
Coagulopathies	25.2	0.5	54.1	32.8-89.4
Preeclampsia/eclampsia	52.8	27.8	1.9	1.5-2.4
Chronic hypertension	7.3	3.3	2.2	1.1-2.3
Gestational hypertension	9.4	5.8	1.6	0.8-3.3
Twins	23.5	8.5	2.8	1.8-4.2
Stillbirth	70.8	12.5	11.1	8.9-13.8
Cesarean delivery	528.0	203.4	2.6	2.4-2.8

CI, confidence interval.

From Saftlas AF, Olson DR, Atrash HK, et al: National trends in the incidence of abrutio placentae, 1979-1987. Obstet Gynecol 78:1081, 1991.

tocolytic agents does not appear to increase rates of morbidity or mortality in these situations. In one study, 73% of patients with suspected abruption whose fetuses were at a gestational age of less than 36 weeks were treated with magnesium sulfate tocolysis without ill effect.[41] If the conservative approach is taken and the patient remains pregnant, appropriate antepartum monitoring and sonography should be implemented, and corticosteroids should be given to the newborn for lung maturity. As with placenta previa, all women with an Rh-negative blood type without sensitization should receive Rh immune globulin (RhoGAM). In cases of abruption after 36 weeks, or with severe cases, delivery is indicated. Most situations necessitate cesarean delivery for fetal or maternal indications, but vaginal delivery is not contraindicated.

VASA PREVIA

Vasa previa is a much less common cause of third-trimester hemorrhage. Vasa previa is the condition in which vessels run through the membranes below the presenting part and run over or close to the internal cervical os, unsupported by placenta or cord. Since 1831, about 250 cases have been reported in the literature.

The estimated incidence of vasa previa is 1 per 2500 deliveries. Risk factors for vasa previa include in vitro fertilization, multiple gestation, placenta previa, and bilobed and succenturiate-lobed placenta. This diagnosis carries a high fetal mortality of up to 50%; the risk to the mother is low because the bleeding is entirely fetal. Bleeding may result from torn umbilical vessels both before and after rupture of the membranes.[101-103]

Diagnosis

Before ultrasound technology, the diagnosis was usually made at the time of delivery. There are many case reports or case series in the literature in regard to antenatally diagnosed vasa previa.[103-110]

Fung and Lau reported three cases of antenatally diagnosed vasa previa and provide a good review of the literature since 1980, which differentiates neonatal outcome based on antepartum versus intrapartum diagnosis of vasa previa (Table 28-4).[105,106]

These data emphasize the importance of using transvaginal ultrasonography to confirm the diagnosis of suspected vasa previa.

If vasa previa is clinically suspected as a possible cause of third trimester bleeding, the Apt, Ogita, and Loendersloot tests can be performed to differentiate

Table 28–4. Fetal Outcome According to the Time of Diagnosis of Vasa Previa

Time of Diagnosis of Vasa Previa	No. of Fetuses	No. of Fetuses with Anemia or Requiring Transfusion	No. of Stillbirths and Neonatal Deaths	No. of Fetuses with Unknown Outcome
Antenatal	22	1	0	0
No history of vaginal bleeding	16	0	0	0
History of antepartum bleeding	6	1	0	0
Intrapartum or postpartum	31	13	7	0
No intrapartum bleeding, no history of vaginal bleeding	6	0	1	0
Hemorrhage (vasa previa not diagnosed antenatally) Intrapartum bleeding	5	1	4	0
Spontaneous	12	8	1	0
After manipulation (digital examination, AROM, or FSE)	8	4	1	0
Total	53	14	7	0

AROM, artificial rupture of membranes; FSE, fetal scalp electrode.

From Fung TY, Lau TK: Poor perinatal outcome associated with vasa previa: Is it preventable? A report of three cases and review of the literature. Ultrasound Obstet Gynecol 12:430, 1998.

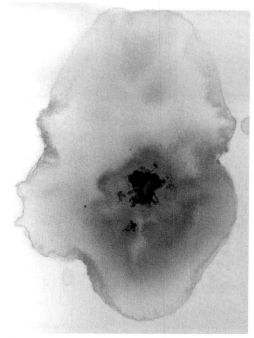

A

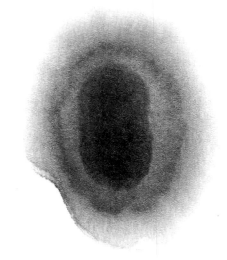

B

Figure 28-7. Apt test showing maternal blood **(A)** and fetal blood **(B)**.

between fetal and maternal hemoglobin. After addition of an alkaline solution (sodium hydroxide or potassium hydroxide) to the sample of blood, fetal hemoglobin resists oxidation and remains pinkish-red, whereas maternal hemoglobin changes to a dark brown color (Fig. 28-7). Since bleeding from a vasa previa is usually accompanied by fetal compromise and delivery is expedited, there is rarely time to perform these tests.

REFERENCES

1. Iyasu S, Saftlas AK, Rowley DL, et al: The epidemiology of placenta previa in the United States, 1979 through 1987. Am J Obstet Gynecol 168:1424, 1993.
2. Rzios N, Doran TA, Miskin M, et al: Natural history of placenta previa ascertained by diagnostic ultrasound. A J Obstet Gynecol 133:287, 1979.
3. Brenner WE, Edelman DA, Hendricks CH: Characteristics of patients with placenta previa and results of "expectant management." Am J Obstet Gynecol 132:180, 1978.
4. Higgins SD, Garite TL: Late abruptio placentae in trauma patients: Implications for monitoring. Obstet Gynecol 63:10, 1984.
5. Strong TH, Brar HS: Placenta previa in twin gestations. J Reprod Med 34:415, 1989.
6. Taylor VM, Kramer MD, Vaughan TL, et al: Placenta previa in relation to induced and spontaneous abortion: A population-based study. Obstet Gynecol 82:88, 1993.
7. Zhang J, Savitz DA: Maternal age and placenta previa: A population-based, case-control study. Am J Obstet Gynecol 168:641, 1993.
8. Handler AS, Mason ED, Rosenberg DL, et al: The relationship between exposure during pregnancy to cigarette smoking and cocaine use and placenta previa. Am J Obstet Gynecol 170:884, 1994.
9. Taylor VM, Kramer MD, Vaughan TL, et al: Placenta previa and prior cesarean delivery: How strong is the association? Obstet Gynecol 84:55, 1994.
10. Thomas AG, Alvarez M, Friedman F Jr, et al: The effect of placenta previa on blood loss in second-trimester pregnancy termination. Obstet Gynecol 84:58, 1994.
11. Hershkowitz R, Fraser D, Mazor M, et al: One or multiple previous cesarean sections are associated with similar increased frequency of placenta previa. Eur J Obstet Gynecol 62:185, 1995.
12. Monica G, Lilja C: Placental previa, maternal smoking and recurrence risk. Acta Obstet Gynecol Scand 74:341, 1995.
13. Ananth CV, Wilcox AJ, Savitz DA, et al: Effect of maternal age and parity on the risk of uteroplacental bleeding disorders in pregnancy. Obstet Gynecol 88:511, 1996.
14. Andres RL: The association of cigarette smoking with placenta previa and abruptio placentae. Sem Perinatol 20:154, 1996.
15. Chelmow D, Andrew DE, Baker ER: Maternal cigarette smoking and placenta previa. Obstet Gynecol 87:703, 1996.
16. Hemminiki E, Merilainen J: Long-term effects of cesarean sections: Ectopic pregnancies and placental problems. Am J Obstet Gynecol 174:1569, 1996.
17. Miller DA, Chollet JA, Goodwin TM: Clinical risk factors for placenta previa–placenta accreta. AM J Obstet Gynecol 177:210, 1997.
18. Frederiksen MC, Glassenberg R, Sitka CS: Placenta previa: A 22-year analysis. Am J Obstet Gynecol 180:1432, 1999.
19. McShane PM, Heyl PS, Epstein MF: Maternal and perinatal morbidity resulting from placenta previa. Obstet Gynecol 65:176, 1985.
20. Leiberman JR, Fraser D, Kasis A, et al: Reduced frequency of hypertensive disorders in placenta previa. Obstet Gynecol 77:83, 1991.
21. Ananth CV, Smullian JC, Vintzileos AM: The association of placenta previa with history of cesarean delivery and abortion: A metaanalysis. Am J Obstet Gynecol 177:1071, 1997.
22. Cnattinguis S, Mills JL, Yuen J, et al: The paradoxical effect of smoking in preeclamptic pregnancies: Smoking reduces the incidence but increases the rates of perinatal mortality,

abruptio placentae, and intrauterine growth restriction. Am J Obstet Gynecol 177:156, 1997.

23. Cotton DB, Read JA, Paul RH, et al: The conservative aggressive management of placenta previa. Am J Obstet Gynecol 137:687, 1980.

24. Comeau J, Shaw L, Campbell C, et al: Early placenta previa and delivery outcome. Obstet Gynecol 61:577, 1983.

25. Wolf EJ, Mallozzi A, Rodis JF, et al: Placenta previa is not an independent risk factor for a small for gestational age infant. Obstet Gynecol 77:707, 1991.

26. Newton ER, Barss V, Cetrulo CL: The epidemiology and clinical history of asymptomatic midtrimester placenta previa. Am J Obstet Gynecol 148:743, 1984.

27. Laing FC: Placenta previa: Avoiding false-negative diagnosis. J Clin Ultrasound 9:109, 1981.

28. Farine D, Fox HE, Jacobson S, et al: Vaginal ultrasound for diagnosis of placenta previa. Am J Obstet Gynecol 159:566, 1988.

29. Farine D, Peisner DB, Timor-Tritsch IE: Placenta previa—is the traditional diagnostic approach satisfactory? J Clin Ultrasound 18:328, 1990.

30. Timor-Tritsch IE, Yunis RA: Confirming the safety of transvaginal sonography in patients suspected of placenta previa. Obstet Gynecol 81:742, 1993.

31. Leerentveld RA, Gilberts E, Arnold M, et al: Accuracy and safety of transvaginal sonographic placental location. Obstet Gynecol 76:759, 1990.

32. Dawson WB, Dumas MD, Romano WM, et al: Translabial ultrasonography and placenta previa: Does measurement of the os-placenta distance predict outcome? J Ultrasound Med 15:441, 1996.

33. Timor-Tritsch IE, Monteagudo A: Diagnosis of placenta previa by transvaginal sonography. Ann Med 25:279, 1993.

34. Kay HH, Spritzer CE: Preliminary experience with magnetic resonance imaging in patients with third-trimester bleeding. Obstet Gynecol 78:424, 1991.

35. Powell MC, Buckley J, Price H, et al: Magnetic resonance imaging and placenta previa. Am J Obstet Gynecol 154:565, 1986.

36. National Institutes of Health: Antenatal corticosteroids revisited: Repeat courses. NIH Consensus Statement. 17:1, 2000.

37. Goldberg M: Erythropoiesis, erythropoietin, and iron metabolism in elective surgery: Preoperative strategies for avoiding allogeneic blood exposure. Am J Surg 70:37s, 1995.

38. Scott L, Ramin SM, Hanson J, et al: Erythropoietin use in pregnancy: Two cases and a review of the literature. Obstet Gynecol 1:22, 1995.

39. Harris S, Payne G, Putman J: Erythropoietin treatment of erythropoietin-deficient anemia without renal disease during pregnancy. Obstet Gynecol 87:812, 1996.

40. Braga J, Marques R, Branco A, et al: Maternal and perinatal implications of the use of human recombinant erythropoietin. Acta Obstet Gynecol Scand 75:449, 1996.

41. Towers CV, Pircon RA, Heppard M: Is tocolysis safe in the management of third-trimester bleeding? Am J Obstet Gynecol 180:1572, 1999.

42. Arias F: Cervical cerclage for temporary treatment of patients with placenta previa. Obstet Gynecol 71:545, 1988.

43. Cobo E, Conde-Agudelo A, Delgado J, et al: Cervical cerclage: An alternative for the management of placenta previa. Am J Obstet Gynecol 179:122, 1998.

44. D'Angelo LJ, Irwin LF: Conservative management of placenta previa: A cost-benefit analysis. Am J Obstet Gynecol 149:320, 1984.

45. Silver R, Depp R, Sabbagha RE, et al: Placenta previa: Aggressive expectant management. Am J Obstet Gynecol 150:15, 1984.

46. Wing DA, Paul RH, Millar LK: Management of symptomatic placenta previa: A randomized, controlled trial of inpatient versus outpatient expectant management.. Am J Obstet Gynecol 175:806, 1996.

47. Breen JL, Neubecker R, Gregori CA, et al: Placenta accreta, increta, and percreta. A survey of 40 cases. Obstet Gynecol 49:43, 1977.

48. Clark SL, Koonings PP, Phelan JP: Placenta previa/accreta and prior cesarean section. Obstet Gynecol 66:89, 1985.

49. Read JA, Cotton DB, Miller FC: Placenta accreta: Changing clinical aspects and outcome. Obstet Gynecol 56:31, 1980.

50. McCool RA, Bombard AT, Bartholomew DA, Calhoun BC: Unexplained positive/elevated maternal serum alpha-fetoprotein associated with placenta increta. J Reprod Med 37:826, 1992.

51. Zelop C, Nadel A, Frigoletto FD, et al: Placenta accreta/percreta/increta: A cause of elevated maternal serum alpha-fetoprotein. Obstet Gynecol 80:693, 1992.

52. Ophir E, Tendler R, Odeh M, et al: Creatine kinase as a biochemical marker in diagnosis of placenta increta and percreta. Am J Obstet Gynecol 180:1039, 1999.

53. Finberg HJ, Williams JW: Placenta accreta: Prospective sonographic diagnosis in patients with placenta previa and prior cesarean section. J Ultrasound Med 11:333, 1992.

54. Guy GP, Peisner DB, Timor-Tritsch IE: Ultrasonographic evaluation of uteroplacental blood flow patterns of abnormally located and adherent placentas. Am J Obstet Gynecol 163:723, 1990.

55. Pasto ME, Kurtz AB, Rifkin MD, et al: Ultrasonographic findings in placenta increta. J Ultrasound Med 2:155, 1983.

56. Tabsh KM, Brinkman CR, King W: Ultrasound diagnosis of placenta increta. J Clin Ultrasound 10:288, 1982.

57. Thorp JM, Cooncell RB, Sandridge DA, et al: Antepartum diagnosis of placenta previa percreta by magnetic resonance imaging. Obstet Gynecol 80:506, 1992.

58. Fox H: Placenta accreta, 1945-1969. Obstet Gynecol Surv 27:475, 1972.

59. Clark SL, Yeh SY, Phelan JP, et al: Emergency hysterectomy for obstetric hemorrhage. Obstet Gynecol 64:376, 1984.

60. Stanco LM, Schrimmer DB, Paul RH, et al: Emergency peripartum hysterectomy and associated risk factors. Am J Obstet Gynecol 168:879, 1993.

61. Cox SM, Carpenter RJ, Cotton DB: Placenta percreta: Ultrasound diagnosis and conservative surgical management. Obstet Gynecol 71:454, 1988.

62. Druzin ML: Packing of lower uterine segment for control of postcesarean bleeding in instances of placenta previa. Surg Gynecol Obstet 169:543, 1989.

63. Matthews NM, McGowan LM, Patten P: Placenta previa accreta with delayed hysterectomy. Aust N Z Obstet Gynaecol 36:476, 1996.

64. Silver LE, Hobel CJ, Lagasse L, et al: Placenta previa percreta with bladder involvement: New considerations and review of the literature. Ultrasound Obstet Gynecol 9:131, 1997.

65. Creasy RK, Resnik R: Maternal Fetal Medicine, 4th ed. Philadelphia, WB Saunders, 1999, p 621.

66. Alexander JD, Schneider FD: Vaginal bleeding associated with pregnancy. Primary Care 27:137, 2000.

67. Saftlas AF, Olson DR, Atrash HK, et al: National trends in the incidence of abruptio placentae, 1979-1987. Obstet Gynecol 78:1081, 1991.

68. Knab DR: Abruptio placentae: An assessment of the time and method of delivery. Obstet Gynecol 52:625, 1978.

69. Witlin AG, Saade GR, Mattar F, et al: Risk factors from abruptio placentae and eclampsia: Analysis of 445 consecutively managed women with severe preeclampsia and eclampsia. Am J Obstet Gynecol 180:1322, 1999.

70. Ananth CV, Wilcox AJ: Placental abruption and perinatal mortality in the United States. Am J Epidemiol 153:332, 2001.

71. Pritchard JA, Mason R, Corley M, et al: Genesis of severe abruption. Am J Obstet Gynecol 108:22, 1970.

72. Atrash HK, Koonin LM, Lawson HW, et al: Maternal mortality in the United States, 1979-1986. Obstet Gynecol 76:1055, 1990.

73. Elliot JP, Gilpin B, Strong TH, et al: Chronic abruption-oligohydramnios sequence. J Reproductive Med 43:418, 1998.

74. Pak LL, Reece EA, Chan L: Is adverse pregnancy outcome predictable after blunt abdominal trauma? Am J Obstet Gynecol 179:1140, 1998.

75. Sholl JS: Abruptio placentae: Clinical management in non-acute cases. Am J Obstet Gynecol 156:40, 1987.

76. Bond AL, Edersheim TG, Curry L, et al: Expectant management of abruptio placentae before 35 weeks gestation. Am J Perinatol 6:121, 1989.

77. Harris BA Jr, Gore H, Flowers CE Jr: Peripheral placental separation: A possible relationship to premature labor. Obstet Gynecol 66:774, 1985.

78. Pritchard JA, Bekken AL: Clinical and laboratory studies on severe abruptio placentae. Am J Obstet Gynecol 97:681, 1967.

79. Hibbard BM, Jeffcoate TN: Abruptio placentae. Obstet Gynecol 27:155, 1966.

80. Ananth CV, Savitz DA, Bowes WA, et al: Influence of hypertensive disorders and cigarette smoking on placental abruption and uterine bleeding during pregnancy. Br J Obstet Gynaecol 104:572, 1997.

81. Abdella TN, Sibai BM, Hays JM, et al: Relationship of hypertensive disease to abruptio placentae. Obstett Gynecol 63:365, 1984.

82. Golditch IM, Boyce NE: Management of abruptio placentae. JAMA 212:288, 1970.

83. Eriksen G, Wohlert M, Ersbak V, et al: Placental abruption. A case control investigation. Br J Obstet Gynaecol 98:448, 1991.

84. Paterson MEL: The aetiology and outcome of abruptio placentae. Acta Obstet Gynecol Scand 58:31, 1979.

85. Darby MJ, Caritis SN, Shen-Schwartz S: Placental abruption in the preterm gestation: An association with chorioamnionitis. Obstet Gynecol 74:88, 1989.

86. Taefi P, Kaiser TF, Sheffer JB, et al: Placenta percreta with bladder invasion and massive hemorrhage. Report of a case. Obstet Gynecol 36:686, 1970.

87. Vintzileos AM, Campbell WA, Nochimson DJ, et al: Preterm premature rupture of the membranes: A risk factor for development of abruptio placentae. Am J Obstet Gynecol 156:1235, 1987.

88. Slutsker L: Risks associated with cocaine use during pregnancy. Obstet Gynecol 79:778, 1992.

89. Acker D, Sachs BP, Tracey KJ, et al: Abruptio placentae associated with cocaine use. Am J Obstet Gynecol 146:220, 1983.

90. Hoskins IA, Friedman DA, Frieden FJ, et al: Relationship between antepartum cocaine abuse, abnormal umbilical artery Doppler velocimetry, and placental abruption. Obstet Gynecol 78:279, 1991.

91. Pearlman MD, Tintinalli JE, Lorenz RP: Blunt abdominal trauma during pregnancy. N Engl J Med 323:1609, 1990.

92. Pearlman MD, Tintinalli JE, Lorenz RP: A prospective controlled study of outcome after trauma during pregnancy. Am J Obstet Gynecol 162:665, 1990.

93. Pearlman MD, Klinich KD, Schneider LW, et al: A comprehensive program to improve safety for pregnant women and fetuses in motor vehicle crashes: A preliminary report. Am J Obstet Gynecol 182:1554, 2000.

94. Babinszki A, Kerenyi T, Torok O, et al: Perinatal outcome in grand and great-grand multiparity: Effects of parity on obstetric risk factors. Am J Obstet Gynecol 181:669, 1999.

95. Ananth CV, Smullian JC, Demissie K, et al: Placental abruption among singleton and twin births in the United States: Risk factor profiles. Am J Epidemiol 153:771, 2001.

96. Lydon-Rochelle M, Holt VL, Easterling TR: First birth cesarean and placental abruption or previa at second birth. Obstet Gynecol 97:765, 2001.

97. Hurd WW, Miodovnik M, Hertzberg V, et al: Selective management of abruptio placentae: A prospective study. Obstet Gynecol 61:467, 1983.

98. Nyberg DA, Mack LA, Benedetti TJ, et al: Placental abruption and hemorrhage: Correlation of sonographic with fetal outcome. Radiology 164:357, 1987.

99. Signore C, Sood A, Richards D: Second-trimester vaginal bleeding: Correlation of ultrasonographic findings with perinatal outcome. Am J Obstet Gynecol 178:336, 1998.

100. Dahmus MA, Sibai BM: Blunt abdominal trauma: Are there predictive factors for abruptio placentae or maternal fetal distress? Am J Obstet Gynecol 169:1054, 1993.

101. Pent D: Vasa previa. Am J Obstet Gynecol 134:151, 1979.

102. Dougall A, Baird CH: Vasa previa—report of three cases and review of literature. Br J Obstet Gynaecol 94:712, 1987.

103. Oyelese KO, Turner M, Lees C, et al: Vasa previa: An avoidable obstetric tragedy. Obstet Gynecol Surv 54:138, 1999.

104. Lee W, Lee VL, Kirk JS, et al: Vasa previa: Prenatal diagnosis, natural evolution, and clinical outcome. Obstet Gynecol 95:572, 2000.

105. Oyelese KO, Schwarzler P, Coates S, et al: A strategy for reducing the mortality rate from vasa previa using transvaginal sonography with color Doppler. Ultrasound Obstet Gynecol 12:434, 1998.

106. Fung TY, Lau TK: Poor perinatal outcome associated with vasa previa: Is it preventable? A report of three cases and review of the literature. Ultrsound Obstet Gynecol 12:430, 1998.

107. Hertzberg BS, Kliewer MA: Vasa previa: Prenatal diagnosis by transperineal sonography with Doppler evaluation. J Clin Ultrasound 26:405, 1998.

108. Sauerbrei EE, Davies GL: Diagnosis of vasa previa with endovaginal color Doppler and power Doppler sonography: Report of two cases. J Ultrasound Med 17:393, 1998.

109. Nomiyama M, Tyota Y, Kawano H: Antenatal diagnosis of velamentous umbilical cord insertion and vasa previa with color Doppler imaging. Ultrasound Obstet Gynecol 12:426, 1998.

110. Chasnoff I, Burns WJ, Schnoll SH, et al: Cocaine use in pregnancy. N Engl J Med 313:666, 1985.

CHAPTER 29

Management of Multiple Gestations

Daniel W. Skupski and Frank A. Chervenak

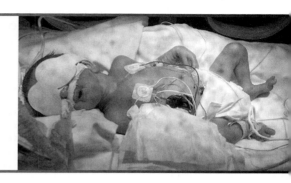

The incidence of twins worldwide is about 1 per 80 pregnancies (1.25%).[1] The frequency of monozygotic twins is constant throughout the world, regardless of maternal age, parity, or race, all three of which have the most influence on the rate of dizygotic twinning. The incidence of monozygotic twinning is between 3.5 and 4 per 1000 births.[2] The frequencies of triplets and other higher order gestations that occur naturally can be estimated through the Hellin hypothesis.[1] According to this calculation, if the incidence of naturally occurring twins in a given population is n, the incidence of triplets will be 1 per n^2, the incidence of quadruplets will be 1 per n^3, and so on. In the United States, where $n = 85$, the incidence of naturally occurring triplets would be 1 per 7,225, that of quadruplets would be 1 per 614,125, and so on.

Assisted reproductive technologies in the United States have led to an increase in the incidence of multiple-gestation pregnancies.[3] Among patients treated with clomiphene citrate, the twinning rate is between 6.8% and 17%.[4] Treatment with gonadotropins may result in a rate between 18% and 53.5%.[4] After in vitro fertilization, the incidence of twins depends on the number of embryos transferred into the uterus and on the maternal age. The rate of multiple gestations ranges from 10.8% to 45.7%.[3] Younger maternal age and an increased number of embryos transferred lead to higher rates of multiple gestations.[3]

Multiple gestations contribute significantly to perinatal mortality. Twins account for approximately 12.6% of the perinatal mortality, although they account for only about 2.5% of the population.[5] The overall rate of perinatal mortality for twins in developed countries is approximately 50 per 1000 births.[5,6] The perinatal mortality rate for triplets is even higher, about 119 per 1000 births.[7] The majority of perinatal morbidity in multiple gestations results from preterm delivery and intrauterine growth restriction (IUGR).[8-12] The average length of gestation decreases inversely with the number of fetuses present (Table 29-1).[8] Some authors have presented mortality data showing that multiple-gestation neonates are "healthier"

for each birth weight or gestational age.[13] This is apparently an effect of the concrete measurement scale used. When these data are adjusted to a relative scale (e.g., z scores), the effect showing that multiple gestations are less likely to die is eliminated.[14] Thus, the clinical impression that multiple-gestation neonates are more likely to die is borne out in the statistical analysis of data from large birth registries.[14]

DIAGNOSIS OF MULTIPLE GESTATION

The most useful clinical tool for the diagnosis of multiple gestation is the measurement of a fundal height or a uterine size larger than expected for date. The widespread availability of diagnostic ultrasonography and maternal serum screening has led to early diagnosis of multiple gestation. The diagnosis is almost always made before delivery.[15] The largest randomized controlled trial of diagnostic ultrasonography, the Routine Antenatal Diagnostic Imaging with Ultrasound Study (RADIUS), demonstrated the early diagnosis of twins in all cases in which ultrasonography was performed.[16] Maternal serum α-fetoprotein elevation, which occurs in 20% to 30% of

Table 29–1. Average Length of Pregnancy Relative to the Number of Fetuses*

Number of Fetuses	Number of Pregnancies	Days of Completed Gestation
1	82	271
2	21	246
3	5	234
4	3	205

*In pregnancies beyond 20 weeks with accurate dates.

Adapted from Caspi E, Ronen J, Schreyer P, et al: The outcome of pregnancy after gonadotropin therapy. Br J Obstet Gynaecol 83:967, 1976.

patients with twin gestations, can also be a clue toward the diagnosis. If this elevation is greater than four multiples of the median and twins are seen, further evaluation is indicated.[17] If the extreme elevation remains unexplained after follow-up ultrasonography and amniocentesis, the twins still need to be watched closely, because a poor perinatal outcome has been associated with this population of twins.[17]

The diagnostic method of choice is clearly ultrasonography.[18] In the first trimester, multiple sacs can be seen with transabdominal ultrasonography at 6 weeks, embryos within the sacs can be seen at 7 weeks, and fetal hearts can be identified between 7 and 8 weeks.[19] All these landmarks are seen approximately 1 to 2 weeks earlier with the transvaginal approach.[20] It is prudent to reserve the diagnosis of multiple gestation until two or more fetal poles with two or more fetal hearts are seen, because of the high frequency of the "vanishing twin" in scans taken during early pregnancy.[21]

Zygosity and Chorionicity

The two basic types of twin gestations are monozygous and dizygous. **Monozygous** refers to progeny resulting from the fertilization of one ovum by one sperm. **Dizygotic** gestations result from the fertilization of two separate ova by two separate sperm, which allows for genotypic dissimilarity. Multiple gestations of higher order can be composed of any combination of monozygotic, dizygotic, or multizygotic gestations. In describing multiple gestations, the terms "identical" and "fraternal" should be avoided, because they refer only to phenotypic likeness, although in general "identical" implies monozygosity and "fraternal" is meant to describe dizygosity. In spontaneous conceptions, approximately 30% of multiple gestations are monozygous and 70% are dizygous.[22] The increase in multiple dizygotic gestations as a result of assisted reproductive technologies has led to a decrease in the percentage of monozygous

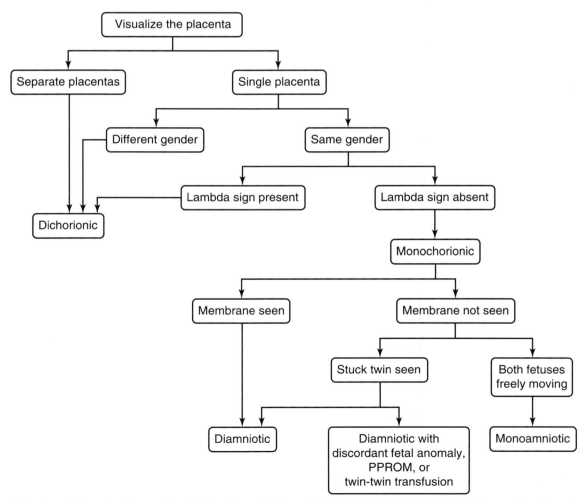

Figure 29–1. Second-trimester ultrasound evaluation of amnionicity and chorionicity. PPROM, preterm premature rupture of membranes.

Table 29–2. Antenatal Diagnostic Tests in Multiple Gestations

Test	Reason	Gestational Age
Transvaginal ultrasonography	To determine chorionicity and accurate dating	6-10 weeks
Transvaginal ultrasonography	To determine amnionicity	10-14 weeks
MSAFP*	To screen for neural tube defects	15-17 weeks
Transabdominal and transvaginal ultrasonography	To screen for fetal anomalies and cervical length	About 20 weeks
Transabdominal ultrasonography	To screen for IUGR	About every 4 weeks after 20 weeks
NST and AFI or BPP	To screen for FHR abnormalities/acidemia	Weekly after 26-28 weeks†

*Often omitted if amniocentesis is planned because amniotic fluid α-fetoprotein is routinely performed and is more precise than MSAFP.

†More frequently if clinical conditions are suggestive of a higher risk.

AFI, amniotic fluid index; BPP, biophysical profile; FHR, fetal heart rate; IUGR, intrauterine growth restriction; MSAFP, maternal serum α-fetoprotein; NST, nonstress test.

fetuses (i.e., <30%). Nevertheless, the rate of monozygous multiple gestations has been found to be two to three times higher in iatrogenic pregnancies than in spontaneous conceptions.[23,24]

There are three types of twin placentas: monoamniotic-monochorionic, diamniotic-monochorionic, and diamniotic-dichorionic. All dizygous twins have dichorionic (and therefore diamniotic) placentas, but monozygous gestation can result in any of the three configurations.[25] Examination of the placenta after birth aids in determination of zygosity. Differing gender establishes twins as dizygous for approximately 35% of twin gestations. Careful study of the placenta leads to the proper diagnosis in an additional 20%. Most of the remaining 45% of same-gender dichorionic twins are dizygotic. Other methods to determine zygosity after birth in these cases are blood grouping and molecular genetic techniques. Molecular genetic techniques can also be used in the antenatal period.[26]

Ultrasonography is instrumental in diagnosing chorionicity and amnionicity (Fig. 29-1). The perinatal mortality rate is lowest in dichorionic twins, about 9%. Thus, a systematic approach to the diagnosis of chorionicity is helpful.[18,19] Multiple gestations should be scanned routinely at several times during the pregnancy, as shown in Table 29-2. Chorionicity is best determined between 6 and 12 weeks of gestation.[18] During the first trimester of a dichorionic pregnancy, trophoblastic tissue from the chorion laeve has not degenerated; this leaves a greater distance between the sacs within the uterus than is seen with monochorionicity (Fig. 29-2).[18]

In the second or third trimesters, gender and number of placental masses are determined first. Discordant gender indicates that the pregnancy is dizygotic and, therefore, that the placenta is dichorionic. Likewise, if two separate placental disks are seen, the gestation is dichorionic. Difficulty in determining chorionicity can arise if fetal position prevents gender determination or if an

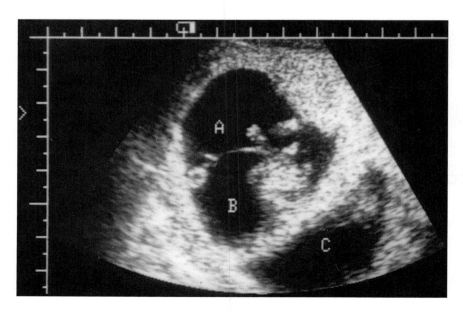

Figure 29–2. Ultrasound image of dichorionic, triamniotic triplets in the first trimester. The thin membrane between triplets A and B indicates monochorionicity. The thick membrane between triplets B and C indicates dichorionicity. Note the ease in determining chorionicity.

accessory lobe of the placenta exists; attention is then turned to the dividing membrane. If evaluation of gender and number of placentas identifies twins of the same gender and a shared placenta, attention is also turned to the dividing membrane.

Four methods of determining chorionicity have been described. The first method, indicating dichorionicity, is the presence of two completely separate placentas.[27] The second method has been described as the "twin peak" or lambda sign.[28] This sign is the appearance of a triangular projection of chorionic tissue protruding toward the amniotic cavity from the placenta at the interface between the dividing membrane and the placental chorionic surface in pregnancies with a single placental zone. A "twin peak" indicates dichorionicity. The third method determines membrane thickness; this method correctly identifies chorionicity in 80% to 90% of patients.[29] A monochorionic membrane should be thin and hairlike. A dichorionic membrane is thick and more easily visualized. The fourth method involves actual counting of the layers in a dividing membrane. When this is possible, the correct diagnosis can be made in almost all cases, but it is not always possible.[30] Monochorionic membranes should have only two layers; dichorionic membranes should consist of three or four visible layers. The first two methods are the easiest and most technically feasible to use; determining membrane thickness and counting membrane layers provide no greater accuracy than determination of the "twin peak" sign.[31]

Visualization of the membrane may be difficult with oligohydramnios involving one twin. In this case, the membrane may be completely apposed to the body of the fetus, which no longer has any fluid around it. If this is so, however, this fetus is trapped against the uterine wall. Therefore, even if the mother moves or a significant amount of time has elapsed, this "stuck twin" does not move. This sign aids in differentiating this situation from a monoamniotic pregnancy.[19]

A monoamniotic sac is one without a visible separating membrane. This finding should be confirmed on multiple examinations before a definitive diagnosis is made. Monoamniotic twins are rare, occurring in only 1% of twin gestations.[32] Antenatal diagnosis is important because of a mortality rate of 50% to 60% associated with monoamniotic twins.[32] Amnionicity is best determined between 10 and 14 weeks of gestation.[18] Very early in the first trimester (i.e., 6 to 10 weeks) the amnion may be difficult or impossible to visualize; a definitive diagnosis should be delayed until approximately 10 weeks of gestation.[18]

ABNORMALITIES OF MULTIPLE GESTATION

Fetal Anomalies

The incidence of fetal anomalies in multiple gestations is 1.5 to 3 times higher than that of singleton gestations.[33,34] This increase arises from the higher percentage of structural defects found in monozygotic twin gestation. In higher order multiple gestations, there is an even greater chance that one fetus will have an anomaly.

Management of any of the anomalies that can be seen among twins, and management of any karyotypic abnormality that is found, depends on the severity of the anomaly, as well as on the gestational age at which it is diagnosed. The patient, in conjunction with her partner, must make the final decision about management. One option is selective termination of one fetus.

Schinzel and colleagues described three helpful categories in which to organize the anomalies encountered in multifetal pregnancies, described as follows.[35]

Anomalies of Twinning

The event of monozygous twinning itself is thought to be "teratogenic" by some authors. Some anomalies are thought to be a consequence of the "teratogenic" event. Midline defects such as neural tube defects, anencephaly, sirenomelia, holoprosencephaly, and exstrophy of the cloaca, as well as conjoined twins (described later), are examples.[36] Nance proposed that this group of defects involving midline structures must be in some way linked to the twinning process.[37]

Vascular Connections

Other anomalies to consider are those resulting from vascular interchange between the fetuses. In monochorionic (and thus always monozygous) gestations, there are vascular connections between the twins (within the placenta) in 100% of the cases.[25] When one twin dies, hemorrhage from the living twin into the dead twin's dilated vascular space can result in microcephaly, hydranencephaly, a porencephalic cyst, intestinal atresia, aplasia cutis, limb amputation, or death of the second twin.[38]

Compression Deformities

It is thought that minor foot deformities (clubfoot), skull asymmetry, and congenital dislocation of the hip seen in multiple gestations (particularly in higher order multifetal pregnancies) are caused by intrauterine crowding.[35,39]

Monoamniotic Gestations

Monoamniotic pregnancies are associated with an extremely high rate of perinatal mortality. These pregnancies require intensive fetal surveillance and were traditionally delivered by cesarean section at 36 weeks of gestation. The extremely high rates of mortality, caused in part by cord entanglement even before 36 weeks of gestation, has led many centers to opt for elective cesarean delivery at 32 weeks of gestation.[40,41]

Conjoined Twins

Conjoined twins deserve special mention because they are specific to multiple gestations. The incidence ranges from 1 per 50,000 to 1 per 100,000 births, or approximately 1 per 600 twin births.[42,43] The cause of the conjoining is thought to be incomplete division of the monozygotic embryo at the time of cleavage of the embryonic disk. This development may occur through one of two mechanisms. The classic model suggests that conjoined twins occur due to a very late split in the embryonic process. The hatching model hypothesizes that the inner cell mass splits during the process of embryo extrusion from the zona pellucida, but the split is incomplete and conjoined twins result.[44,45] Most commonly, such twins are joined at the chest (thoracopagus).[42] Conjoined twins have been detected by ultrasonography in the first trimester.[45] Conjoined twins are stillborn in 40% of births, and, in many instances, the remaining newborns are severely premature.[46] If the fetuses are dead or have little chance of surviving and are small enough to be delivered vaginally, this route would be preferable. If conjoined twins have a possibility of survival, delivery should be by cesarean section, with appropriate neonatal support. For some patients, even when their fetuses are dead, abdominal delivery is necessary to avoid maternal trauma. The degree of fusion of the twins and the number, type, and extent of fusion of shared organs help determine the appropriateness of surgical separation.

The advances of three-dimensional ultrasonography and power Doppler imaging show promise in allowing careful mapping of the extent of organ sharing before birth.[47] This allows the surgical team to prepare in advance of the time of birth, as well as more informed counseling for the parents.

Monochorionic Gestations

Monochorionic gestations have higher rates of fetal growth restriction, morbidity, and mortality than do dichorionic gestations.[48] In addition, twin-twin transfusion is a dreaded complication of monochorionic gestations; there have been only two reports of this syndrome occurring in dichorionic gestations in which, unlike most cases, vascular connections were present.[49,50] A large proportion of these complications probably arises from placental variables, including patterns of vascular connections and unequal sharing of placental mass.[48] The presence of blood flow redistribution (brain sparing) is indicative of impending or actual fetal growth restriction and can be detected by Doppler ultrasound studies.[51] Fetoscopic laser occlusion of chorioangiopagus vessels (to be described) has been performed in the setting of growth restriction of one fetus, but it is uncertain whether any form of treatment or intervention is beneficial in this situation.[52]

Twin-Twin Transfusion Syndrome

The abnormality of vascular connections between placentas has been reported to complicate nearly 100% of monochorionic placentas studied.[53] When arterial-venous connections are uncompensated and unidirectional blood flow results, the abnormality of twin-twin transfusion syndrome can occur.[1] In its most severe form, the donor fetus is growth restricted or possibly hydropic as a result of high-output cardiac failure, with anemia, hypotension, and oligohydramnios. The recipient of the transfusion is more active, has increased amniotic fluid as a result of increased urination, and has congestive heart failure as a result of circulatory overload. The recipient twin also has hypervolemia, hypertension, plethora, and thromboses of peripheral vessels (Fig. 29-3). The sonographic findings are varied, but objective sonographic diagnostic criteria for the antenatal period have been published (Table 29-3).[54] The degree of morbidity from the syndrome may depend not only on the caliber of the vessels involved but also

---

Table 29–3. Ultrasound Criteria for the Antenatal Diagnosis of Twin-Twin Transfusion Syndrome

Second-Trimester Diagnostic Criteria

Monochorionic gestation
  Same gender
  Single placental mass
  Thin dividing membrane
  Lack of lambda or twin peak sign
Abnormal amniotic fluid volume*
  One twin with oligohydramnios, deepest vertical
    pocket ≤ 2.0 cm
  Other twin with polyhydramnios, deepest vertical
    pocket ≥ 8.0 cm
Persistent fetal bladder findings*
  Small or no bladder visualized in twin with
    oligohydramnios
  Large bladder visualized in twin with polyhydramnios

Helpful Diagnostic Clues

Estimated fetal weight discordance (≥20% of larger
  twin's estimated weight)
Appearance of a "stuck" twin*
Hydrops fetalis (presence of one or more of the
  following in either twin)
  Skin edema (≥5-mm thickness)
  Pericardial effusion
  Pleural effusion
  Ascites
Doppler studies
  Absent diastolic flow in umbilical artery (donor)
  Umbilical venous pulsations
  Abnormal ratio of umbilical artery pulsatility index
    to middle cerebral artery pulsatility index

*Serial scanning may be necessary.

---

on the gestational age of the pregnancy and the presence or absence of any compensatory connections (arterioarterial or venovenous). The perinatal mortality rate is 80% to 100% without treatment and 40% to 50% with treatment.[55-58]

Several methods of treatment for twin-twin transfusion syndrome have been reported (Table 29-4).[55,59-61] The introduction of each new therapy has led to increasing rates of survival of fetuses and neonates with twin-twin transfusion syndrome (Table 29-5).[55-58,60-73] This probably results from a combined effect of better experience with the procedures and improvements in neonatal care.[74] As Table 29-5 shows, survival rates with the therapies listed do not differ significantly. Selective termination by umbilical cord ligation or cautery is too recent for comparison.[59,75] The current overall survival rate is approximately 60% with any therapy.[76] Several authors have examined the rate of affected pregnancies with at least one survivor, demonstrating a 70% to 75% rate for serial amnioreduction and fetoscopic laser occlusion of chorioangiopagus vessels.[60,73]

An important finding is that approximately 10% of survivors have long-term neurologic damage.[77] This should be included in the counseling of patients at the

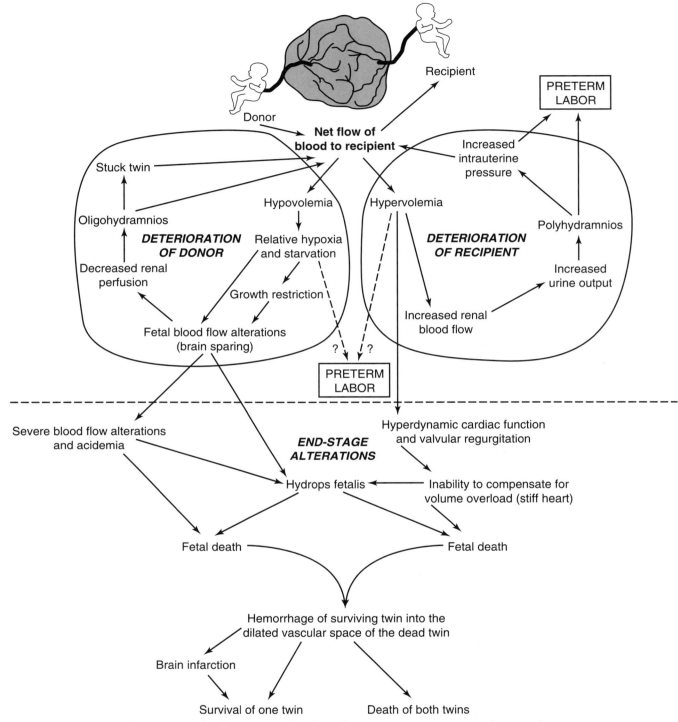

Figure 29–3. Fetal and intrauterine physiologic changes in severe twin-twin transfusion syndrome.

time of diagnosis.[78] There is an increased chance that classical cesarean delivery will be necessary, which leads to a higher risk of adverse outcomes in future pregnancies. For many of the aforementioned reasons, termination of pregnancy should be discussed as an option for management of the pregnancy when twin-twin transfusion syndrome is diagnosed early in the second trimester.

Single Fetal Death in Utero

A single fetal death, which complicates 0.5% to 6.8% of multiple gestations, can be diagnosed by ultrasonography.[79,80]

Table 29-4. Management Options in Severe Twin-Twin Transfusion Syndrome

Noninvasive
  Bed rest
  Maternal digoxin to treat fetal heart failure
  Ultrasound and Doppler assessment for optimal
    timing of delivery
  Tocolysis for preterm labor

Invasive
  Amniodrainage or amnioreduction
  Septostomy of the intertwin membrane
  FLOC—fetoscopic laser ablation of chorioangiopagus
    vessels
  Selective termination
    Hysterotomy
    Intracardiac injection of cardiotoxic substances
    Umbilical cord injection of caustic substances
    Umbilical cord ligature—ultrasonographically
      guided endoscopic approach
    Umbilical cord bipolar coagulation—
      ultrasonographically guided

Abortion

The risk of major morbidity or death for the surviving twin has been reported to be as high as 46%; the highest risk is in monochorionic twin pairs.[81] The prognosis depends on the cause of the initial demise, as well as the type of placentation—and therefore the presence or absence of shared circulation—and the estimated gestational age at delivery. The management of multiple gestations with a single fetal death includes delivery after 34 weeks of gestation after documentation of lung maturity in the surviving fetus or fetuses. Before 34 weeks, expectant management with close surveillance seems prudent.[80] Both serial ultrasonography and twice-weekly fetal heart rate testing in the form of the nonstress test (NST) are recommended. Delivery may become necessary before 34 weeks or at documentation of fetal lung maturity if stress in utero of the surviving fetus or fetuses becomes apparent. The mode of delivery is usually determined by other obstetric indications but may be affected by the position of the dead fetus. Careful evaluation of fetal remains and the placentas can aid in establishing a cause of death, which may be important for the management of subsequent pregnancies.[82]

Preterm Labor and Preterm Delivery

Preterm delivery remains the leading cause of morbidity and mortality in multiple gestation. The incidence of preterm delivery among twins is between 20% and 50%[83,84] and is even higher for triplets (75%) and higher

Table 29-5. Survival Rates in Case Series of Twin-Twin Transfusion Syndrome

Author	Year	Treatment	Survival Rate (%)
Bebbington[62]	1989	None	47
Bebbington[62]	1989	Amnioreduction*	0
Mahoney[56]	1990	None	20
Mahoney[56]	1990	Amnioreduction	69
Urig[57]	1990	None	0
Urig[57]	1990	Amnioreduction	39
Gonsoulin[63]	1990	Amnioreduction	21
Elliott[64]	1991	Amnioreduction	79
Saunders[65]	1992	Amnioreduction	37
Pinette[66]	1993	None	75
Pinette[66]	1993	Amnioreduction	83
Fries[67]	1993	Amnioreduction	50
Reisner[68]	1993	None	40
Reisner[68]	1993	Amnioreduction	74
Ville[58]	1995	FLOC	52
DeLia[55]	1995	FLOC	53
Ville[69]	1996	Amnioreduction	50
Dennis[70]	1997	None	50
Dennis[70]	1997	Amnioreduction	82
Saade[61]	1998	Septostomy	83
Ville[71]	1998	FLOC	55
Zikulnig[72]	1999	FLOC	64
Hecher[73]	1999	FLOC	61
Mari[60]	2001	Amnioreduction	60

*Amnioreduction used only for maternal respiratory compromise.

FLOC, fetoscopic laser occlusion of chorioangiopagus vessels.

Table 29–6. Risk Factors in Multiple Gestation

Higher order multiple gestations
Fetal anomaly
Monozygosity/monochorionicity
Monoamnionicity
Twin-twin transfusion syndrome
Single fetal death
Polyhydramnios
Growth discordancy/intrauterine growth restriction of
   one or more fetuses
MSAFP > 4 multiples of the median
Antepartum bleeding
Pregnancy-induced hypertension/preeclampsia
Preterm labor
Preterm premature rupture of membranes
Detection of multiple fetuses late in pregnancy

MSAFP, maternal serum α-fetoprotein (level).

order multiple gestations.[85] The average number of completed weeks of gestation at delivery is inversely related to the number of fetuses (see Table 29-1).[8] Theories about the underlying causes for these complications include increased uterine tone from distention, increased intraamniotic pressure, increased readiness of the myometrium, and uteroplacental insufficiency.[86] Overall, little progress has been made in this particular area of management of multiple gestations. Patient education, early referral to a specialist, and antepartum care in a special clinic are all measures aimed at earlier identification of the problem of premature labor.[87] Risk assessment, combined with serial cervical examinations, may also help identify patients at highest risk for premature birth (Table 29-6).

Home uterine activity monitoring was previously thought to lead to earlier identification of premature uterine activity and allow treatment to prevent preterm delivery. Randomized controlled clinical trials have shown, however, that home uterine activity monitoring does not lead to decreased rates of preterm delivery.[88-90] However, careful surveillance in form of daily patient contact may be of value.

Advances have been made in the prediction of preterm birth in multiple gestations through transvaginal ultrasound evaluation of the cervix with or without other serum markers.[91-94] However, the prevention of preterm birth remains an elusive goal.

MANAGEMENT OF PRETERM LABOR

Multifetal Pregnancy Reduction

Higher order multiple fetuses are frequently delivered prematurely.[95] Antepartum management of these pregnancies should employ all available noninvasive measures to prolong gestation.[95] Bed rest and tocolytic agents should also be used liberally.[95] Multifetal pregnancy reduction of one or more embryos in the first trimester is an invasive modality that has been shown to be of benefit

in reducing the complications of severe prematurity for these fetuses.[96,97] The procedure has a complication rate or pregnancy loss rate of 6% to 10%, which decreases with more operator experience.[98,99] We currently offer multifetal pregnancy reduction to all multiple-gestation patients in the first trimester who conceived by assisted reproductive technology and who carry pregnancies of three or more fetuses.

Cerclage

Prophylactic cerclage for multiple gestations does not yet have a proven benefit and is not without significant risks.[100,101] In our opinion, a cerclage should be placed only when cervical incompetence is present. Transvaginal ultrasonography has been evaluated as a screening tool. Cervical cerclage has shown mixed results on prolongation of pregnancy or prevention of preterm birth when a short cervix (<25 mm) or dilation of the internal cervical os is seen on transvaginal ultrasonograms in a singleton pregnancy.[102,103] When the length of the cervix is extremely short (i.e., <15 mm for singleton gestations) in the early part or middle of the second trimester, the role of cerclage is controversial.[104,105]Thus, there may be a role for routine transvaginal ultrasonography in the assessment of cervical length in multiple gestations. However, the length of the cervix at which cerclage should be placed in multiple gestations is uncertain, because the normal amount of cervical shortening that occurs with advanced gestation happens to a greater degree in multiples compared with singletons.[100]

There is great difficulty in making clinical decisions in this area for several reasons. First, on the basis of transvaginal ultrasound screening for cervical length, there are no clearly established indications for placement of cerclage. Second, the distinction between preterm labor and a relative weakness of the cervix is difficult. Last, cerclage removal should be performed in the setting of intractable preterm labor, but this is a difficult clinical decision in many cases. Further study in this area is needed.

Bed Rest

The value of bed rest in prevention of prematurity remains controversial. Much of the confusion in the literature results from a lack of unanimity among protocols and a predominance of retrospective data. The Cochrane Review of evidence-based medicine contains a meta-analysis that included six trials (>600 women and >1400 fetuses) showing no benefit of hospitalization with bed rest for preventing preterm delivery in multiple gestations.[106] Hospitalized bed rest is disruptive and costly and cannot be recommended on the basis of the available evidence. However, certain complications, such as premature cervical dilation, recurrent uterine contractions, and suspected IUGR, may warrant prolonged hospitalization for rest and closer observation.

This review does not answer the question of whether any type of bed rest is beneficial. It has been found that up to 81% of perinatal mortality in twins occurs before the 29th week of gestation.[15] Therapeutic bed rest to prevent premature birth would be needed before this period. The common practice in multiple gestations is to recommend some limitations of activity (e.g., avoidance of exercise, heavy lifting, and/or sexual activity) during or after the second trimester. It is uncertain whether controlled trials will ever be performed to answer this question.

Tocolysis

Tocolysis has been regarded both as a prophylactic and as a therapeutic means of managing prematurity. The current consensus does not support the routine use of prophylactic tocolytic agents.[107] However, intravenous tocolytic agents for the treatment of preterm labor in multiple gestations continue to be widely used, on the basis of their efficacy in several trials.[108,109] Intravenous tocolysis appears to allow pregnancies to be prolonged 2 to 7 days. This effect is highly desirable because the time allows maternally administered corticosteroids to enhance fetal lung maturation.[108] Because of the increased maternal blood volume and cardiac output of a multiple pregnancy, however, the margin of safety with the use of tocolytic agents is narrow.[110] Careful fluid management and monitoring of cardiovascular status are critical in the prevention of pulmonary edema and other maternal complications.[111]

Steroid Administration

The use of steroids for treating known or suspected pulmonary immaturity has been shown to be efficacious in certain patients carrying singleton pregnancies.[112] Their use in multifetal pregnancies, however, has long been controversial. A collaborative study did not demonstrate a benefit from dexamethasone for twins or triplets, and the authors postulated that the dynamics and concentrations of the steroid might be altered when multiple fetuses are present.[112] Nevertheless, the National Institutes of Health published a statement firmly recommending that antenatal corticosteroids for fetal lung maturation be used in all multiple gestations that undergo preterm labor.[113] A follow-up statement has firmly recommended against multiple courses of maternal steroids for repetitive episodes of preterm labor, because of the adverse fetal effects of increased neonatal sepsis and increased fetal growth restriction; more is not necessarily better.[114]

Intrauterine Growth Restriction

The use of ultrasound imaging is central to the diagnosis of the problems that twins face in utero. There is a difference between normal fetal growth in twins and that in singletons.[115,116] IUGR occurs in only 5% to 7% of singleton pregnancies, but it may complicate as many as 47% of multiple gestations.[117] Indeed, objective evidence of IUGR after delivery (neonatal body water turnover) has been found in up to 70% of twin neonates.[118] Because growth is a dynamic process, serial scanning during pregnancy is necessary.

Fetal assessment by ultrasonography is currently recommended every 4 weeks, beginning at 26 weeks, and as frequently as every 2 weeks if IUGR is suspected. This minimizes the risks of IUGR, which include fetal demise, deranged electrolyte physiologic processes, and long-term neurologic damage. The relative uteroplacental

insufficiency that underlies IUGR in twin gestations is believed to become significant at the onset of the third trimester. Multiple gestations of higher order may be at risk even sooner. IUGR can be predicted from an estimated fetal weight that is calculated through multiple parameters.[119,120] The four underlying causes of weight discordance are twin-twin transfusion syndrome, IUGR of one twin, hydrops of one twin, and macrosomia of one twin. When IUGR affects one or more fetuses, management is similar to that of IUGR in a singleton. Bed rest and expectant management with close fetal surveillance are indicated. Doppler blood flow studies are important for determining the severity of IUGR and can help in a decision for iatrogenic preterm delivery.[120] If 37 weeks of gestation is reached or if amniocentesis shows the presence of fetal lung maturation, delivery should be carried out. Before 37 weeks of gestation, the risks of prematurity must be weighed against the risks of continued stress in utero, and frequent fetal assessment in mandatory. Before documented maturity of all fetuses, delivery becomes mandatory only when fetal assessment shows evidence of fetal acidemia. Fetal acidemia can be detected by electronic fetal heart rate monitoring or by the fetal biophysical profile (BPP). In contrast, for severely premature fetuses, allowing one fetus to die in utero in order to avoid severe prematurity for both should be considered, although this should not be contemplated for monochorionic twins because of the high rate of death or brain damage in the surviving twin.[81]

Acute and Chronic Polyhydramnios

"Acute" polyhydramnios, in which a large amount of amniotic fluid accumulates rapidly, is a phenomenon that complicates 5% to 8% of multiple gestations.[86] Chronic polyhydramnios, in which the increased fluid is present for a longer duration during the pregnancy (i.e., during the second and third trimesters) is more likely to be associated with an anomaly of the fetus.[121] An acute increase in fluid is associated with an extremely high rate of fetal mortality from severe prematurity if it occurs in the second trimester. Frequent amniocentesis to reduce fluid volume and delay delivery is an option.[122] The risks with frequent amniocentesis include abruption, infection, and premature labor.[85] We believe amniocentesis should be considered for premature labor with acute polyhydramnios and that amniocentesis should be performed to relieve maternal respiratory embarrassment.

Pregnancy-Induced Hypertension/Preeclampsia

Antepartum management of multiple fetuses includes the treatment of the many maternal complications of these pregnancies. Pregnancy-induced hypertension, preeclampsia, or both are seen in as many as 37% of multiple gestations, and the incidence increases with each increase in the number of fetuses.[111,123] The cause is thought to be related to a relative decrease or limitation of uteroplacental blood flow when more than one placenta is present.[124,125] Not only are the rates of pregnancy-induced hypertension and preeclampsia higher than those in singleton pregnancies, but also the onset is often earlier and the severity is greater. The risks from this disease to mother and fetus, as well as the diagnosis and management of hypertension in pregnancy, are similar in singleton and twin gestations.

Hemorrhage

Antepartum and postpartum hemorrhage are more common with multiple fetuses, leading to an increased need for surgical intervention and an increased risk of blood loss.[126,127] Abruptio placentae is primarily responsible for the increase in antepartum hemorrhage.[127] Prompt evaluation of any antepartum vaginal bleeding is necessary. Routine use of uterotonic agents in the immediate postpartum period can decrease the incidence and severity of postpartum hemorrhage.

FETAL ASSESSMENT

There is a wide range of practices across the country for the antenatal assessment of fetal well-being in multiple gestations. There are few or no evidence-based data to demonstrate the optimal scheme. We believe that antenatal fetal assessment of multiple gestations is important because of the high perinatal mortality rate (>9%). Because these tests are potentially lifesaving, we begin performing these tests at 26 to 28 weeks of gestation.

There are two methods for antenatal assessment: ultrasound monitoring and fetal heart rate monitoring. Ultrasonography is used for assessment of fetal growth, the BPP, and estimation of amniotic fluid volume. Fetal heart rate monitoring can be performed as a NST or a contraction stress test (CST).

The diagnostic tests that are commonly employed for multiple gestations are summarized in Table 29-2.

Ultrasonography

Ultrasonography is used to monitor growth, monitor amniotic fluid volume, describe placentation, and diagnose fetal death, all of which are relatively long-term markers of fetal status in utero. Ultrasonography is also used to guide invasive procedures. Fetal growth should be assessed routinely in multiple gestations about every 4 weeks, as described in the section on IUGR. Assessment of amniotic fluid volume is generally performed once or twice weekly during the third trimester as an adjunct to the NST.

Amniotic Fluid Volume Assessment

Ultrasound evaluation of amniotic fluid is important in evaluating multiple gestations. Increased or decreased fluid may be the first sign of a new problem, such as IUGR, discordance from a transfusion syndrome, or hydrops. Altered fluid volume signals the need for closer surveillance with the other modes of fetal surveillance. Third-trimester assessment of amniotic fluid volume, when performed in combination with the NST (see the following section), should be performed at least weekly. The use of a deepest vertical pocket measurement or the four-quadrant amniotic fluid index has been validated for use in twin gestations.[129]

Nonstress Testing and Contraction Stress Testing

The primary method of choice for antenatal fetal assessment is the NST, an acute measure of fetal well-being,

combined with the ultrasound assessment of amniotic fluid volume, a chronic measure of fetal well-being.[130] There are no contraindications to the NST, and it can be performed simultaneously (and thus efficiently) on multiple fetuses.[131] The NST is generally performed weekly or twice weekly, and amniotic fluid volume is assessed weekly. The NST is reliable and has high predictive value when the results are normal.[132] When the results are abnormal, there is a much lower positive predictive value, and another test such as vibroacoustic stimulation is generally used to differentiate a fetal sleep state from the presence of fetal acidemia.[133]

The CST is rarely used in a multiple gestation, because the CST requires that uterine contractions be induced. Because of the propensity for preterm labor, multiple gestation is considered a contraindication to the CST. If a CST occurs because of spontaneous uterine contractions, it can be interpreted as if a formal CST had been performed.

Biophysical Profile

The fetal BPP is a reliable method of fetal surveillance and can be used as a means of follow-up of a nonreactive NST result.[134] Of importance is that the BPP includes both acute and chronic measures of fetal well-being. It is, of course, more time consuming for a multiple gestation, but there are no contraindications to this procedure. Its sensitivity and specificity have been found to be as high for twins as for singletons.[134] The BPP has been used as the primary method of fetal surveillance in higher order multiple gestations, because of the technical difficulty in obtaining adequate fetal heart rate monitoring when the NST is performed.[135]

Doppler Velocimetry

Doppler velocimetry is an acceptable method of evaluating placental impedance in singleton pregnancies, as discussed in the section on IUGR. For twins, ultrasound findings in combination with Doppler velocimetry in multiple fetal vessels are helpful in the diagnosis of IUGR and twin-twin transfusion syndrome.[72,136]

Invasive Procedures

When indicated, invasive testing can be performed safely for diagnosis of chromosomal anomalies and infectious diseases affecting the fetus and for the treatment of fetal alloimmunization in multiple gestations. The options are chorionic villus sampling, amniocentesis, and cordocentesis or percutaneous umbilical blood sampling.

Although chorionic villus sampling is technically challenging and requires experienced operators, it has been shown to be as safe as amniocentesis for the diagnosis of chromosomal anomalies in multiple gestations.[137] There is a small rate of twin-twin villus contamination (3 per 161) that may preclude correct detection of abnormal results or of gender.[137] Amniocentesis as a follow-up test may be necessary in a small percentage of cases.

Amniocentesis has been extensively studied in multiple gestations. There appears to be a slightly higher pregnancy loss rate with traditional amniocentesis in multiple gestations than in singleton pregnancies.[138] Modern techniques include ultrasound guidance, avoidance of the placenta if possible, a separate needle insertion for each fetus, avoidance of dye injection, and avoidance of puncture of the intertwin membrane. Placental traversing of the needle is associated with a slightly higher rate of pregnancy loss.[139] Injection with methylene blue dye is associated with the development of intestinal atresia in as high as 19% (17 per 89) of cases and with a higher rate of fetal death.[128,140] There is a suggestion that the risk of intestinal atresia may still be present with indigo carmine dye, which has been used almost exclusively since about 1990.[141] Our practice is to use dye injection if an ultrasonogram shows that one of the sacs is difficult to access. Puncture of the intertwin membrane is associated with the development of a pseudomonoamniotic twin gestation and possible fetal demise from cord entanglement.[142]

Cordocentesis or percutaneous umbilical blood sampling can be performed in a twin gestation for appropriate indications.[143,144] The exact risks of the procedure, however, are not well defined in multiple gestations.

INTRAPARTUM MANAGEMENT

Labor

The patient with a multiple gestation is known to have a greater level of uterine activity throughout gestation, including the latent phase of labor.[145] For both multiparas and nulliparas, the latent phase of labor is shorter, because such patients usually present with more advanced cervical changes.[146] The overall duration of labor is not significantly different in comparison with singletons because the active phase is longer.[147,148] Uterine overdistention and malpresentation cause a lack of regular frequent uterine contractions, or dysfunctional labor, and this is the main cause of the prolongation of the active phase of labor.[146-149] Oxytocin augmentation is indicated in multiple gestations when prolongation or arrest of the active phase of labor is diagnosed. Because an overdistended uterus is at higher risk for rupture, it is optimal to use an intrauterine pressure catheter to guide the infusion of oxytocin.

With the availability of intrapartum ultrasonography and continuous fetal heart rate monitoring, the time interval between the delivery of twins is not a critical factor in obtaining a successful outcome.[150,151] Fetal status can be monitored throughout labor and delivery by electronic fetal heart rate monitoring. The characteristics of fetal heart rate patterns that may signal hypoxia or, more important, acidemia, are the same as those in singleton gestations: namely, lack of beat-to-beat variability, abnormal baseline fetal heart rate, presence of decelerations, lack of return to the previous baseline after decelerations, and lack of spontaneous or induced accelerations.[133]

Antepartum care of twins or higher order multiple gestations should be carried out by experts familiar with their special needs. These pregnancies should be delivered only in centers with capabilities for real-time ultrasonography, electronic fetal heart rate monitoring, and immediate cesarean delivery when necessary.

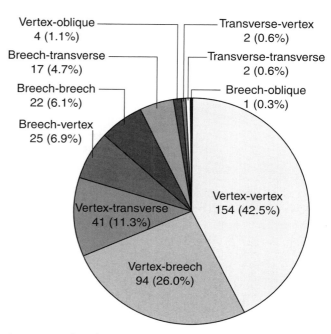

Figure 29–4. The relative occurrence rates of the possible combinations of twin presentations in 362 patients. *(From Chervenak FA, Johnson RE, Youch S, et al: Intrapartum management of twin gestation. Obstet Gynecol 65:119, 1985.)*

Mode of Delivery

The intrapartum management of twins begins with a consideration of the relative presentations of twin A and twin B (Fig. 29-4). The possible combinations are varied, but three broad categories provide a working classification: vertex-vertex (vertext twin A, vertex twin B), vertex-nonvertex (vertex twin A, nonvertex twin B), and nonvertex twin A (Fig. 29-5). Our management plan, based on this classification, is illustrated in Figure 29-6.

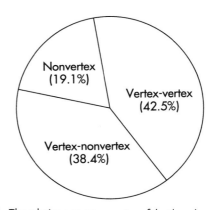

Figure 29–5. The relative occurrence rates of the three broad categories of twin presentations: vertex-vertex, vertex-nonvertex, and nonvertex twin A. *(From Adams D, Chervenak F: Multifetal pregnancies: Epidemiology, clinical characteristics, and management. In Reece E, Hobbins J, Mahoney M, Petrie R [eds]: Medicine of the Fetus and Mother. Philadelphia, JB Lippincott, 1992, p 267.)*

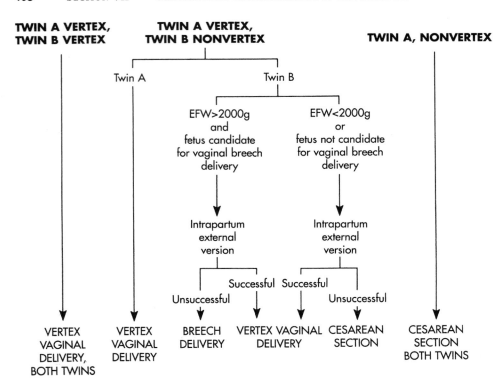

Figure 29–6. Outline of proposed intrapartum management of twin gestation. EFW, estimated fetal weight. *(From Chervenak FA, Johnson RE, Youch S, et al: Intrapartum management of twin gestation. Obstet Gynecol 65:119, 1985.)*

Nonvertex Twin A

Vaginal delivery has not been documented to be safe in any study of twins when twin A is nonvertex. In addition, a large randomized controlled trial has demonstrated that even in experienced obstetricians' hands, singleton breech vaginal deliveries were fraught with significantly more neonatal death and permanent injury than when cesarean delivery was planned.[152] It is reasonable to expect that the breech-presenting first twin has the same risks. For these reasons, we recommend cesarean section for this subgroup. However, Blickstein and associates supported vaginal delivery of the breech-presenting first twin when the estimated fetal weight is more than 2000 g.[153]

Twin A Vertex, Twin B Vertex

There is widespread agreement that vaginal delivery of vertex-vertex twins is appropriate.[150,154,155] After delivery of twin A, the status of twin B should be assessed with ultrasonography and fetal heart rate monitoring. The vertex of twin B should be brought into the pelvis by further labor, whereupon amniotomy should be performed and vaginal delivery accomplished with continued fetal heart rate monitoring. Uterine activity can be augmented with oxytocin when uterine contractions are infrequent. If at any point close monitoring reveals fetal heart rate deterioration, we do not recommend the additional insult of an internal podalic version or difficult forceps delivery. Instead, cesarean delivery should be performed immediately. In addition, cesarean delivery may become indicated for failure of descent.

One area of controversy involves the fetuses of very low birth weight presenting as vertex, including those weighing less than 1500 g.[154] We believe that vaginal delivery is appropriate for these fetuses in the absence of convincing clinical data that cesarean section is beneficial.[150,155]

Twin A Vertex, Twin B Nonvertex

Cesarean delivery of all vertex-breech and vertex-transverse twin presentations is an option that is currently accepted.[155] This approach is recommended by some authors because of the possibility of birth trauma and birth asphyxia to the vaginally delivered nonvertex twin.[154-156] To avoid routine cesarean section in this setting, two other options exist. There appears to be no difference in neonatal outcomes between planned cesarean delivery and planned vaginal delivery for this subgroup of patients.[157]

Successful external version of the second twin has been reported by several investigators.[150,154,156,158] The size of both fetuses should be assessed sonographically. If twin B is much larger (i.e., >500-g difference), then version and attempted vaginal delivery are best avoided. If external version is chosen, epidural anesthesia to provide abdominal wall relaxation is optimal, and this can be provided early in the course of labor and reinforced as needed and immediately before delivery. Ultrasonographic guidance, along with continuous heart rate surveillance, facilitates the procedure. With this management scheme, version has been found to be a safe and effective procedure to accomplish vaginal vertex delivery.[159]

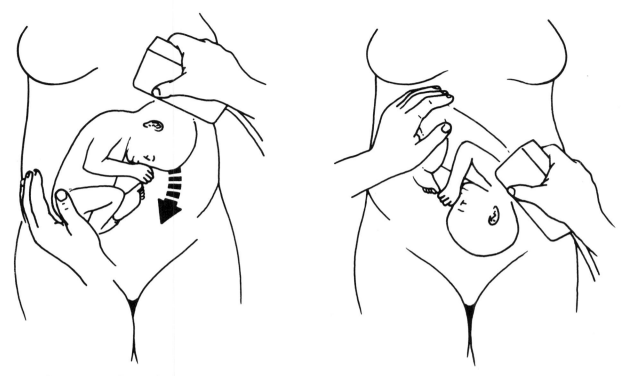

Figure 29–7. The maneuver of external version. *(From Chervenak FA, Johnson RE, Berkowitz RL, et al: Intrapartum external version of the second twin. Obstet Gynecol 62:160, 1983.)*

The maneuver is shown in Figure 29-7. Gentle pressure with the transducer or with the clinician's hands is used to guide the vertex toward the pelvis. The shortest arc between the vertex and the pelvic inlet should be followed first. The version can be accomplished as either a forward or a backward roll, but in all patients, undue force must be avoided; a gentle approach may avoid complications such as direct fetal trauma, ruptured uterus, and abruptio placentae. When the vertex is brought to the pelvic inlet, the membranes are ruptured and delivery is accomplished, with oxytocin augmentation as needed. If the version is unsuccessful, vaginal breech or cesarean delivery should be carried out. If the fetal heart rate deteriorates, cesarean delivery should be performed immediately.

Vaginal breech delivery of the second twin is a second option for avoiding routine abdominal delivery of vertex-nonvertex twins.[150,160-164] This approach depends on the estimated fetal weights according to ultrasonograms. For twins estimated to weigh more than 2000 g on ultrasonograms, several studies have not found an excessive risk of birth trauma when these second twins are delivered vaginally as breech.[150,160,162,163] Neonatal mortality continues to result primarily from breech delivery of premature infants. For breech delivery to be considered, the standard criteria for singleton pregnancy should be met: an adequate maternal pelvis, a flexed fetal head, and an estimated fetal weight of 2000 to 3500 g.[165]

Twins presenting as breech and estimated to weigh less than 2000 g potentially have very low birth weight. For these fetuses, there is a lack of data demonstrating the safety of vaginal breech delivery.[150,166] At this time, we agree with other authors that these infants—whether singleton or multiple gestation—should be delivered by cesarean section through an adequate uterine incision.[150,166]

There are several exceptions to the foregoing management plans, including elective cesarean delivery after documentation of fetal lung maturity, monoamniotic twins, conjoined twins, and other congenital anomalies. Monoamniotic twins are optimally delivered by cesarean section at 32 to 36 weeks of gestation.[40,41,46] In most instances of conjoined twins, abdominal delivery is indicated as described earlier.[167] Many of the other congenital anomalies seen more frequently among twins can also necessitate cesarean delivery. If one or both of a pair have severe IUGR, the stress of labor and vaginal delivery may be contraindicated.

Triplets and Higher Order Multiple Gestations

Modern management of higher order multiple gestations includes some or all of the following: multifetal pregnancy reduction, bed rest at 16 weeks of gestation until delivery, home uterine activity monitoring, frequent use of intravenous tocolysis, or terbutaline pump tocolysis for preterm labor and cesarean delivery.[168]

To avoid birth trauma, our approach to triplets and higher order multiple gestations is cesarean delivery. However, some authors advocate vaginal delivery by an experienced operator, even when there may be three or more fetuses; a clear improvement in outcome resulting from abdominal delivery has not been proved.[169-176]

REFERENCES

1. Benirschke K, Kim CK: Multiple pregnancy (first of two parts). N Engl J Med 288:1276, 1973.
2. Bulmer MG: The familial incidence of twinning. Ann Hum Genet 24:1, 1960.
3. Schieve LA, Peterson HB, Meikle SF, et al: Live-birth rates and multiple-birth risk using in vitro fertilization. JAMA 282:1832, 1999.
4. Schenker JG, Yarkoni S, Granat M: Multiple pregnancies following induction of ovulation. Fertil Steril 35:105, 1981.
5. Powers WF, Kiely L: The risks confronting twins: A national perspective. Am J Obstet Gynecol 170:456, 1994.
6. Howarth GR, Pattinson RC, De Jong G: Total perinatal-related wastage in twin pregnancies. S Afr Med J 80:31, 1991.
7. Berkowitz R, Lynch L, Stone J, Alvarez M: The current status of multifetal pregnancy reduction. Am J Obstet Gynecol 174:1265, 1996.
8. Caspi E, Ronen J, Schreyer P, Goldberg MD: The outcome of pregnancy after gonadotropin therapy. Br J Obstet Gynaecol 83:967, 1976.
9. Crosignani PG, Rubin BL: Multiple gestation pregnancy—the ESHRE Capri Workshop Group. Hum Reprod 15:1856, 2000.
10. Derom R, Vlietinck R, Derom C, et al: Perinatal mortality in the East Flanders Prospective Twin Survey. Eur J Obstet Gynaecol Reprod Biol 41:25, 1991.
11. Keith L, Ellis R, Berger GS, et al: The Northwestern University multihospital twin study. Am J Obstet Gynecol 138:781, 1980.
12. Senat MV, Ancel PY, Bouvier-Colle MH, Bréart G: How does multiple pregnancy affect maternal mortality and morbidity? Clin Obstet Gynecol 1:79, 1998.
13. Cheung YB, Yip P, Karlberg J: Mortality of twins and singletons by gestational age: A varying-coefficient approach. Am J Epidemiol 152:1107, 2000.
14. Lie RT: Invited commentary: Intersecting perinatal mortality curves by gestational age—are appearances deceiving? Am J Epidemiol 152:1117, 2000.
15. Chervenak FA, Youcha S, Johnson RE, et al: Antenatal diagnosis and perinatal outcome in a series of 385 consecutive twin pregnancies. J Reprod Med 29:727, 1984.
16. Ewigman BG, Crane JP, Frigoletto FD, et al: Effect of prenatal ultrasound screening on perinatal outcome. N Engl J Med 329:821, 1993.
17. Redford DHA, Whitfield CR: Maternal serum alpha fetoprotein in twin pregnancies uncomplicated by neural tube defect. Am J Obstet Gynecol 152:550, 1985.
18. Chasen ST, Skupski DW: Early recognition of iatrogenic multiple pregnancy. In Blikstein I, Keith LG (eds): Iatrogenic Multiple Pregnancy. Carnforth, United Kingdom, Parthenon Publishing, 2000, pp 97-116.
19. Chitkara U, Berkowitz RL: Assessment of multiple pregnancy. In Chervenak FA, Isaacson G, Campbell S (eds): Textbook of Obstetric and Gynecologic Ultrasound. Boston, Little, Brown, 1993, pp 413-420.
20. Timor-Tritsch IE: Sonoembryology. In Timor-Tritsch IE, Rottem S (eds): Transvaginal Sonography, 2nd ed. New York, Elsevier, 1991, pp 225-298.
21. Landy HJ, Keith L, Keith D: The vanishing twin. Acta Genet Med Gemellol (Roma) 31:179, 1982.
22. Benirschke K: Accurate recording of twin placentation. A plea to the obstetrician. Obstet Gynecol 18:334, 1961.
23. Sherer DM, Bombard AT, Kellner LH, Divon MY: Noninvasive first-trimester screening for fetal aneuploidy. Obstet Gynecol Surv 52:123, 1997.
24. Snijders RJM, Johnson S, Sebire NJ, et al: First-trimester ultrasound screening for chromosomal defects. Ultrasound Obstet Gynecol 7:216, 1996.
25. Benirschke K, Kaufmann P: Pathology of the Human Placenta, 4th ed. New York, Springer, 2000, pp 804-826.
26. Kovacs B, Shabahrami B, Platt LD: Molecular genetic prenatal determination of twin zygosity. Obstet Gynecol 72:954, 1988.
27. Mahoney BS, Filly RA, Callen PW: Amnionicity and chorionicity in twin pregnancies: Prediction using ultrasound. Radiology 155:205, 1985.
28. Finberg HJ: The "twin peak" sign: Reliable evidence of dichorionic twinning. J Ultrasound Med 1992. 11:571-7.
29. Townsend RR, Simpson GF, Filly RA: Membrane thickness in the ultrasound prediction of chorionicity of twin gestations. J Ultrasound Med 7:327, 1985.
30. Vayssiere CF, Heim N, Camus EP, et al: Determination of chorionicity in twin gestations by high-frequency abdominal ultrasonography: Counting the layers of the dividing membrane. Am J Obstet Gynecol 175:1529, 1996.
31. Sepulveda W, Sebire NJ, Hughes K, et al: The lambda sign at 10-14 weeks of gestation as a predictor of chorionicity in twin pregnancies. Ultrasound Obstet Gynecol 7:421, 1996.
32. Udom-Rice I, Skupski DW, Chervenak FA: Intrapartum management of multiple gestation. Semin Perinatol 19:424, 1995.
33. Hendricks CH: Twinning in relation to birth weight, mortality, and congenital anomalies. Obstet Gynecol 27:47, 1966.
34. MacGillivray I: Epidemiology of twin pregnancy. Semin Perinatol 10:4, 1986.
35. Schinzel AA, Smith DW, Miller JR: Monozygotic twins and structural defects. J Pediatr 95:921, 1979.
36. Windham GC, Bjerkedal T, Sever LE: The association of twinning and neural tube defects: Studies in Los Angeles, California and Norway. Acta Genet Med Gemellol (Roma) 31:165, 1982.
37. Nance WE: Malformations unique to the twinning process. Prog Clin Biol Res 69:123, 1981.
38. Fusi L, McParland P, Fisk N, et al: Acute twin-twin transfusion: A possible mechanism for brain-damaged survivors after intrauterine death of a monochorionic twin. Obstet Gynecol 78:517, 1991.
39. Little J, Bryan E: Congenital anomalies in twins Semin Perinatol 10:50, 1986.
40. Beasley E, Megerian G, Gerson A, Roberts NS: Monoamniotic twins: Case series and proposal for antenatal management. Obstet Gynecol 93:130, 1999.
41. Peek MJ, McCarthy A, Kyle P, et al: Medical amnioreduction with sulindac to reduce cord complications in monoamniotic twins. Am J Obstet Gynecol 176:334, 1997.
42. Mariona FG: Anomalies specific to multiple gestations. In Chervenak FA, Isaacson G, Campbell S (eds): Textbook of Obstetric and Gynecologic Ultrasound. Boston, Little, Brown, 1993, pp 1051-1062.
43. Vaughn TC, Powell LC: The obstetrical management of conjoined twins. Obstet Gynecol (Suppl) 53:67, 1979.
44. Sills ES, Tucker MJ, Palermo GD: Assisted reproductive technologies and monozygous twins: Implications for future study and clinical practice. Twin Res 3:217, 2000.
45. Skupski D, Streltzoff J, Hutson JM, et al: Early diagnosis of conjoined twins in a triplet pregnancy following in vitro fertilization and assisted hatching. J Ultrasound Med 14:611, 1995.
46. Sutter J, Arab H, Manning FA: Monoamniotic twins: Antenatal diagnosis and management. Am J Obstet Gynecol 155:836, 1986.

47. Bega G, Wapner R, Lev-Toaff A, Kuhlman K: Diagnosis of conjoined twins at 10 weeks using three-dimensional ultrasound: A case report. Ultrasound Obstet Gynecol 16:388, 2000.

48. Gaziano EP, De Lia JE, Kuhlmann RS: Diamniotic monochorionic twin gestations: An overview. J Matern Fetal Med 9:89, 2000.

49. Lage JM, Vanmarter LJ, Mikhail E: Vascular anastomoses in fused, dichorionic twin placentas resulting in twin transfusion syndrome. Placenta 10:55, 1989.

50. Molnar-Nadasdy G, Altshuler G: Perinatal pathology casebook. A case of twin transfusion syndrome with dichorionic placentas. J Perinatol 16:507, 1996.

51. Gaziano E, Gaziano C, Brandt D: Doppler velocimetry determined redistribution of fetal blood flow: Correlation with growth restriction in diamniotic monochorionic and dizygotic twins. Am J Obstet Gynecol 178:1359, 1998.

52. Quintero RA, Bornick PW, Morales WJ, Allen MH: Selective photocoagulation of communicating vessels in the treatment of monochorionic twins with selective growth retardation. Am J Obstet Gynecol 185:689, 2001.

53. Robertson EG, Neer KJ: Placental injection studies in twin gestation. Am J Obstet Gynecol 147:170, 1983.

54. Skupski DW: Current perspectives on twin-to-twin transfusion syndrome. In Chervenak FA, Kurjak A (eds): Fetal Medicine: The Clinical Care of the Fetus as a Patient. Carnforth, United Kingdom, Parthenon Publishing, 1999, pp 205-210.

55. De Lia J, Kuhlmann RS, Harstad TW, Cruikshank DP: Fetoscopic laser ablation of placental vessels in severe previable twin-twin transfusion syndrome. Am J Obstet Gynecol 172:1202, 1995.

56. Mahoney BS, Petty CN, Nyberg DA, et al: The "stuck twin" phenomenon: Ultrasonographic findings, pregnancy outcome, and management with serial amniocenteses. Am J Obstet Gynecol 163:1513, 1990.

57. Urig MA, Clewell WH, Elliott JP: Twin-twin transfusion syndrome. Am J Obstet Gynecol 163:1522, 1990.

58. Ville Y, Hyett J, Hecher K, Nicolaides K: Preliminary experience with endoscopic laser surgery for severe twin-twin transfusion syndrome. N Engl J Med 332:224, 1995.

59. Deprest JA, Audibert F, Van Schoubroeck D, et al: Bipolar coagulation of the umbilical cord in complicated monochorionic twin pregnancy. Am J Obstet Gynecol 182:340, 2000.

60. Mari G, Roberts A, Detti L, et al: Perinatal morbidity and mortality rates in severe twin-twin transfusion syndrome: Results of the International Amnioreduction Registry. Am J Obstet Gynecol 185:708, 2001.

61. Saade GR, Belfort MA, Berry DL, et al: Amniotic septostomy for the treatment of twin oligohydramnios-polyhydramnios sequence. Fetal Diagn Ther 13:86, 1998.

62. Bebbington MW, Wittman BK: Fetal transfusion syndrome: Antenatal factors predicting outcome. Am J Obstet Gynecol 160:913, 1989.

63. Gonsoulin W, Moise KJ Jr, Kirshon B, et al: Outcome of twin-twin transfusion diagnosed before 28 weeks of gestation. Obstet Gynecol 75:214, 1990.

64. Elliot JP, Urig MA, Clewell WH: Aggressive therapeutic amniocentesis for treatment of twin-twin transfusion syndrome. Obstet Gynecol 77:537, 1991.

65. Saunders NJ, Snijders RJ, Nicolaides KH: Therapeutic amniocentesis in twin-twin transfusion syndrome appearing in the second trimester of pregnancy. Am J Obstet Gynecol 166:820, 1992.

66. Pinette MG, Yuqun P, Pinette SG, Stubblefield PG: Treatment of twin-twin transfusion syndrome. Obstet Gynecol 82:841, 1993

67. Fries MH, Goldstein RB, Kilpatrick SJ, et al: The role of velamentous cord insertion in the etiology of twin-twin transfusion syndrome. Obstet Gynecol 81:569, 1993.

68. Reisner DP, Mahoney BS, Petty CN, et al: Stuck twin syndrome: Outcome in thirty-seven consecutive cases. Am J Obstet Gynecol 169:991, 1993.

69. Ville Y, Sideris I, Nicolaides KH: Amniotic fluid pressure in twin-to-twin transfusion syndrome: An objective prognostic factor. Fetal Diagn Ther 11:176, 1996.

70. Dennis LG, Winkler CL: Twin-to-twin transfusion syndrome: Aggressive therapeutic amniocentesis. Am J Obstet Gynecol 177:342, 1997.

71. Ville Y, Hecher K, Gagnon A, et al: Endoscopic laser coagulation in the management of severe twin-twin transfusion syndrome. Br J Obstet Gynaecol 105:446, 1998.

72. Zikulnig L, Hecher K, Bregenzer T, et al: Prognostic factors in severe twin-twin transfusion syndrome treated by endoscopic laser surgery. Ultrasound Obstet Gynecol 14:380, 1999.

73. Hecher K, Plath H, Bregenzer T, et al: Endoscopic laser surgery versus serial amniocenteses in the treatment of severe twin-twin transfusion syndrome. Am J Obstet Gynecol 180:717, 1999.

74. Skupski DW: Changes in survival of preterm singletons versus twins delivered after twin-twin transfusion syndrome over the calendar years 1970-1994. Fetal Diagn Ther 13:334, 1998.

75. Nicolini U, Poblete A, Boschetto C, et al: Complicated monochorionic twin pregnancies: Experience with bipolar cord coagulation. Am J Obstet Gynecol 185:703, 2001.

76. Skupski DW: Twin-to-twin transfusion syndrome: An update. Croat Med J 41:228, 2000.

77. Mari G, Detti L, Oz U, Abuhamad AZ: Long-term outcome in twin-twin transfusion syndrome treated with serial aggressive amnioreduction. Am J Obstet Gynecol 183:211, 2000.

78. Skupski DW, Chervenak FA: Twin-twin transfusion syndrome: An evolving challenge. Ultrasound Review Obstet Gynecol 1:28, 2001.

79. Dudley DK, D'Alton ME: Single fetal death in twin gestations. Semin Perinatol 10:65, 1986.

80. Hanna JH, Hill JM: Single intrauterine fetal demise in multiple gestation. Obstet Gynecol 63:126, 1984.

81. Nicolini U, Poblete A: Single intrauterine death in monochorionic twin pregnancies. Ultrasound Obstet Gynecol 14:297, 1999.

82. Magee JF: Investigation of stillbirth. Pediatr Dev Pathol 4:1, 2001.

83. Syrop CH, Varner MW: Triplet gestation: Maternal and neonatal implications. Acta Genet Med Gemellol (Roma) 34:81, 1985.

84. Watson P, Campbell DM: Preterm deliveries in twin pregnancies in Oxford. Acta Genet Med Gemellol (Roma) 35:193, 1986.

85. Newton ER: Antepartum care in multiple gestation. Semin Perinatol 10:19, 1986.

86. Skupski D, Chervenak F: Management of multiple gestation pregnancies. In Spitzer AR (ed): Intensive Care of the Fetus and the Neonate. St. Louis, Mosby–Year Book, 1996, pp 315-325.

87. ACOG Practice Bulletin 31: Assessment of Risk Factors for Preterm Birth. Washington, DC, American College of Obstetricians and Gynecologists, January 2001.

88. Devoe LD, Ware DJ: Home uterine activity monitoring: A critical review. Clin Obstet Gynecol 43:778, 2000.

89. Iams JD, Johnson FF, O'Shaughnessy RW, West LC: A prospective random trial of home uterine activity monitoring in pregnancies at increased risk of preterm labor. Am J Obstet Gynecol 157:638, 1987.

90. Mou SM, Sunderji SG, Gall S, et al: Multicenter randomized clinical trial of home uterine activity monitoring for detection of preterm labor. Am J Obstet Gynecol 165:858, 1991.

91. Goldenberg RL, Iams JD, Das A, et al: The preterm prediction study: Sequential cervical length and fetal fibronectin testing for the prediction of spontaneous preterm birth. National Institute of Child Health and Human Development Maternal-Fetal Medicine Units Network. Am J Obstet Gynecol 182:636, 2000.

92. Guzman ER, Walters C, O'Reilly-Green C, et al: Use of cervical ultrasonography in prediction of spontaneous preterm birth in twin gestations. Am J Obstet Gynecol 183:1103, 2000.

93. Skentou C, Souka AP, To MS, et al: Prediction of preterm delivery in twins by cervical assessment at 23 weeks. Ultrasound Obstet Gynecol 17:7, 2001.

94. Yang JH, Kuhlman K, Daly S, Berghella V: Prediction of preterm birth by second trimester cervical sonography in twin pregnancies. Ultrasound Obstet Gynecol 15:288, 2000.

95. ACOG Educational Bulletin 253: Special Problems of Multiple Gestation. Washington, DC, American College of Obstetricians and Gynecologists, November 1998.

96. Berkowitz RL, Lynch L, Chitkara U, et al: Selective reduction of multifetal pregnancies in the first trimester. N Engl J Med 318:1043, 1988.

97. Lynch L, Berkowitz RL, Chitkara U, Alvarez M: First trimester transabdominal multifetal pregnancy reduction: A report of 85 cases. Obstet Gynecol 75:735, 1990.

98. Evans MI, Dommergues M, Wapner RJ, et al: International collaborative experience of 1789 patients having multifetal pregnancy reduction: A plateauing of risks and outcomes. J Soc Gynecol Invest 3:23, 1996.

99. Evans MI, Berkowitz RL, Wapner RJ, et al: Improvement in outcomes of multifetal pregnancy reduction with increased experience. Am J Obstet Gynecol 184:97, 2001.

100. Elimian A, Figueroa R, Nigam S, et al: Perinatal outcome of triplet gestation: Does prophylactic cerclage make a difference? J Matern Fetal Med 8:119, 1999.

101. Parilla BV, Haney EI, MacGregor SN: Cervical incompetence in multiple gestations. Obstet Gynecol 97:S29, 2001.

102. Final report of the Medical Research Council/Royal College of Obstetricians and Gynaecologists multicentre randomised trial of cervical cerclage. MRC/RCOG Working Party on Cervical Cerclage. Br J Obstet Gynaecol 100:516, 1993.

103. Rust OA, Atlas RO, Jones KJ, et al: A randomized trial of cerclage versus no cerclage among patients with ultrasonographically detected second-trimester preterm dilation of the internal os. Am J Obstet Gynecol 183:830, 2000.

104. Hassan SS, Romero R, Maymon E, et al: Does cervical cerclage prevent preterm delivery in patients with a short cervix? Am J Obstet Gynecol 184:1325, 2001.

105. Heath VC, Souka AP, Erasmus I, et al: Cervical length at 23 weeks of gestation: The value of Shirodkar suture for the short cervix. Ultrasound Obstet Gynecol 12:318, 1998.

106. Crowther CA: Hospitalisation and bed rest for multiple pregnancy. Cochrane Database Syst (1):CD000110, 2001.

107. Skaerris J, Aberg A: Prevention of prematurity in twin pregnancy by orally administered terbutaline. Acta Obstet Gynecol Scand (Suppl) 108:39, 1982.

108. Canadian Preterm Labor Investigators Group: Treatment of preterm labor with the beta-adrenergic agonist ritodrine. N Engl J Med 327:308, 1992.

109. O'Connor MC, Murphy H, Dalrymple IJ: Double blind trial of ritodrine and placebo in twin pregnancy. Br J Obstet Gynaecol 86:706, 1979.

110. Hankins GDV: Complications of beta-sympathomimetic tocolytic agents. In Clark SL, Cotton DB, Hankins GDV, Phelan JP (eds): Critical Care Obstetrics, 2nd ed. Cambridge, Mass, Blackwell Scientific, 1991, pp 223-250.

111. Skupski D, Chervenak F: Maternal complications of multiple gestation. In Gall S (ed): Multiple Pregnancy and Delivery. St. Louis, Mosby–Year Book, 1996, pp 199-222.

112. Collaborative Group on Antenatal Steroid Therapy: Effects of antenatal dexamethasone administration on the prevention of respiratory distress syndrome. Am J Obstet Gynecol 141:276, 1981.

113. Effect of antenatal steroids for fetal maturation on perinatal outcomes. NIH Consens Statement 12(2):1, 1994.

114. Antenatal corticosteroids revisited: Repeat courses. NIH Consens Statement 17(2):1, 2000.

115. Chervenak FA, Skupski DW, Romero R, et al: How accurate is fetal biometry in the assessment of fetal age? Am J Obstet Gynecol 178:678, 1997.

116. Socol ML, Tamura RK, Sabbagha RE, et al: Diminished biparietal diameter and abdominal circumference growth in twins. Obstet Gynecol 64:235, 1984.

117. Chitkara U, Berkowitz GS, Levine R, et al: Twin pregnancy: Routine use of ultrasound examinations in the prenatal diagnosis of intrauterine growth retardation and discordant growth. Am J Perinatol 2:49, 1985.

118. MacLennan AH, Millington G, Grieve A, et al: Neonatal body water turnover: A putative index of perinatal morbidity. Am J Obstet Gynecol 139:948, 1981.

119. Estorlazzi AM, Vintzileos A, Campbell WA, et al: Ultrasonic diagnosis of discordant fetal growth in twin gestations. Obstet Gynecol 69:363, 1987.

120. Ott WJ: Sonographic diagnosis of intrauterine growth restriction. Clin Obstet Gynecol 40:787, 1997.

121. Jones KL: Dysmorphology: An approach to a child with structural defects. Curr Prob Pediatr 8:3, 1978.

122. Elliott JP, Sawyer AT, Radin TG, Strong RE: Large-volume therapeutic amniocentesis in the treatment of hydramnios. Obstet Gynecol 84:1025, 1994.

123. McMullen PF, Norman RJ, Marivate M: Pregnancy induced hypertension in twin pregnancy. Br J Obstet Gynaecol 91:240, 1984.

124. Skupski D, Nelson S, Kowalik A, et al: Multiple gestations from in vitro fertilization: Successful implantation alone is not associated with subsequent preeclampsia. Am J Obstet Gynecol 175:1029, 1996.

125. Skupski D: Multiple gestations from in vitro fertilization: Successful implantation alone is not associated with subsequent preeclampsia [reply to letter]. Am J Obstet Gynecol 177:492, 1997.

126. Kovacs BW, Kirschbaum TH, Paul RH: Twin gestations. I. Antenatal care and complications. Obstet Gynecol 74:313, 1989.

127. Spellacy WN, Handler A, Ferre CD: A case-control study of 1253 twin pregnancies from a 1982-1987 perinatal database. Obstet Gynecol 75:168, 1990.

128. van der Pol JG, Wolf H, Boer K, et al: Jejunal atresia related to the use of methylene blue in genetic amniocentesis in twins. Br J Obstet Gynaecol 99:141, 1992.

129. Chau AC, Kjos SL, Kovacs BW: Ultrasonographic measurement of amniotic fluid volume in normal diamniotic twin pregnancies. Am J Obstet Gynecol 174:1003, 1996.

130. Blake GD, Knuppel RA, Ingardia CJ, et al: Evaluation of non-stress fetal heart rate testing in multiple pregnancy. Obstet Gynecol 63:528, 1984.

131. Devoe LD, Azor H: Simultaneous nonstress fetal heart rate testing in twin pregnancy. Obstet Gynecol 58:450, 1981.

132. Lenstrup C: Predictive value of antepartum nonstress testing in multiple pregnancies. Acta Obstet Gynecol Scand 63:597, 1984.

133. Skupski DW: What is fetal distress? In Chervenak FA, Kurjak A (eds): New Perspectives on the Fetus as Patient. Carnforth, United Kingdom, Parthenon Publishing, 1996, pp 455-470.

134. Lodeiro JG, Vintzileos AM, Feinstein SJ, et al: Fetal biophysical profile in twin gestations. Obstet Gynecol 67:824, 1986.

135. Elliott JP, Finberg HJ: Biophysical profile testing as an indicator of fetal well-being in high-order multiple gestations. Am J Obstet Gynecol 172:508, 1995.

136. Joern H, Rath W: Correlation of Doppler velocimetry findings in twin pregnancies including course of pregnancy and fetal outcome. Fetal Diagn Ther 15:160, 2000.

137. Wapner RJ, Johnson A, Davis G, et al: Prenatal diagnosis in twin gestations: A comparison between second-trimester amniocentesis and first-trimester chorionic villus sampling. Obstet Gynecol 82:49, 1993.

138. Pruggmayer M, Baumann P, Schutte H, et al: Incidence of abortion after genetic amniocentesis in twin pregnancies. Prenat Diagn 11:637, 1991.

139. Tabor A, Philip J, Madsen M, et al: Randomised controlled trial of genetic amniocentesis in 4606 low-risk women. Lancet 1:1287, 1986.

140. Kidd SA, Lancaster PA, Anderson JC, et al: Fetal death after exposure to methylene blue dye during mid-trimester amniocentesis in twin pregnancy. Prenat Diagn 16:39, 1996.

141. Gluer S: Intestinal atresia following intraamniotic use of dyes. Eur J Pediatr Surg 5:240, 1995.

142. Megory E, Weiner E, Shalev E, Ohel G: Pseudomonoamniotic twins with cord entanglement following genetic funipuncture. Obstet Gynecol 78:915, 1991.

143. Moise KJ, Cotton DB: Discordant fetal platelet counts in a twin gestation complicated by idiopathic thrombocytopenic purpura. Am J Obstet Gynecol 156:1141, 1987.

144. Shah DM, Jeanty P, Dev VG, et al: Diagnosis of trisomy 18 in monozygotic twins by cordocentesis. Am J Obstet Gynecol 160:214, 1989.

145. Newman RB, Gill PJ, Katz M: Uterine activity during pregnancy in ambulatory patients: Comparison of singleton and twin gestations. Am J Obstet Gynecol 154:530, 1986.

146. Friedman EA, Sachtleben MR: The effect of uterine overdistension on labor. I. Multiple pregnancy. Obstet Gynecol 23:164, 1964.

147. Bender S: Twin pregnancy: A review of 472 cases. J Obstet Gynaecol Br Emp 59:510, 1952.

148. Garrett WJ, Phil D: Uterine overdistension and the duration of labour. Med J Aust 47:376, 1960.

149. MacGillivray I: Labour in multiple pregnancies. In MacGillivray I, Nylander PPS, Corney G (eds): Human Multiple Reproduction. Philadelphia, WB Saunders, 1975, pp 147-159.

150. Chervenak FA, Johnson RE, Youcha S, et al: Intrapartum management of twin gestation. Obstet Gynecol 65:119, 1985.

151. Rayburn WF, Lavin JP, Miodovnik M, Varner MW: Multiple gestations: Time interval between delivery of the first and second twins. Obstet Gynecol 63:502, 1984.

152. Hannah ME, Hannah WJ, Hewson SA, et al: Planned caesarean section versus planned vaginal birth for breech presentation at term: A randomised multicentre trial. Term Breech Trial Collaborative Group. Lancet 356:1375, 2000.

153. Blickstein I, Goldman RD, Kupferminc M: Delivery of breech first twins: A multicenter retrospective study. Obstet Gynecol 95:37, 2000.

154. Barrett JM, Staggs SM, Van Hooydonk JE, et al: The effect of type of delivery upon neonatal outcome in premature twins. Am J Obstet Gynecol 143:360, 1982.

155. Cetrulo C: The controversy of mode of delivery in twins: The intrapartum management of twin gestation. Semin Perinatol 10:39, 1986.

156. Kelsick F, Minkoff H: Management of the breech second twin. Am J Obstet Gynecol 144:783, 1982.

157. Rabinovici J, Barkai G, Reichman B, et al: Randomized management of the second nonvertex twin: Vaginal delivery or cesarean section. Am J Obstet Gynecol 156:52, 1987.

158. Ranney B: The gentle art of external cephalic version. Am J Obstet Gynecol 116:239, 1973.

159. Chervenak FA, Johnson RE, Berkowitz RL, et al: Intrapartum external version of the second twin. Obstet Gynecol 62:160, 1983.

160. Acker D, Leiberman M, Holbrook H, et al: Delivery of the second twin. Obstet Gynecol 59:710, 1982.

161. Chauhan SP, Roberts WE, McLaren RA, et al: Delivery of the nonvertex second twin: Breech extraction versus external cephalic version. Am J Obstet Gynecol 173:1015, 1995.

162. Chervenak FA, Johnson RE, Berkowitz RL, et al: Is routine cesarean section necessary for vertex-breech and vertex-transverse twin gestation? Am J Obstet Gynecol 148:1, 1984.

163. Collea JV, Chein C, Quilligan EJ: The randomized management of term frank breech presentation: A study of 208 cases. Am J Obstet Gynecol 137:235, 1980.

164. Greig PC, Veille JC, Morgan T, Henderson L: The effect of presentation and mode of delivery on neonatal outcome in the second twin. Am J Obstet Gynecol 167:901, 1992.

165. Collea JV, Rabin SC, Weghorst GR, Quilligan EJ: The randomized management of term frank breech presentation: Vaginal delivery versus cesarean section. Am J Obstet Gynecol 131:186, 1978.

166. Kauppila O, Groncoos M, Aro P, et al: Management of low birth weight breech delivery: Should cesarean section be routine? Obstet Gynecol 57:289, 1981.

167. Filler RM: Conjoined twins and their separation. Semin Perinatol 10:82, 1986.

168. Elliott JP, Radin TG: Quadruplet pregnancy: Contemporary management and outcome. Obstet Gynecol 80:421, 1992.

169. Alamia V, Royek AB, Jackle RK, Meyer BA: Preliminary experience with a prospective protocol for planned vaginal delivery of triplet gestations. Am J Obstet Gynecol 179:1133, 1998.

170. Byrne BM, Rasmussen MJ, Stronge JM: A review of triplet pregnancy. Ir Med J 86:55, 1993.

171. Dommergues M, Mahieu-Caputo D, Mandelbrot L, et al: Delivery of uncomplicated triplet pregnancies: Is the vaginal route safer? A case-control study. Obstet Gynecol 172:513, 1995.

172. Gonen R, Heyman E, Asztalos EV, et al: The outcome of triplet, quadruplet, and quintuplet pregnancies managed in a perinatal unit: Obstetric, neonatal, and follow-up data. Am J Obstet Gynecol 162:454, 1990.

173. Kaufman GE, Malone FD, Harvey-Wilkes KB, et al: Neonatal morbidity and mortality associated with triplet pregnancy. Obstet Gynecol 91:342, 1998.

174. Keith LG, Ameli S, Keith DM: The Northwestern University triplet study. I: Overview of the international literature. Acta Genet Med Gemellol (Roma) 37:55, 1988.

175. Loucopoulos A, Jewelewicz R: Management of multifetal pregnancies: Sixteen years' experience at the Sloane Hospital for Women. Am J Obstet Gynecol 143:902, 1982.

176. Ron-El R, Caspi E, Schreyer P, et al: Triplet and quadruplet pregnancies and management. Obstet Gynecol 57:458, 1981.

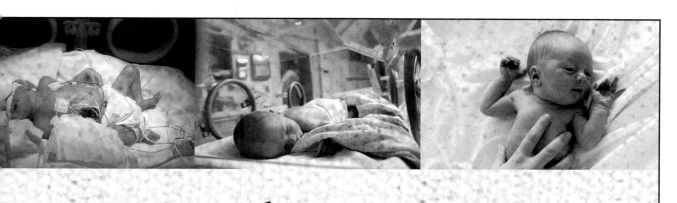

Neonatal Resuscitation

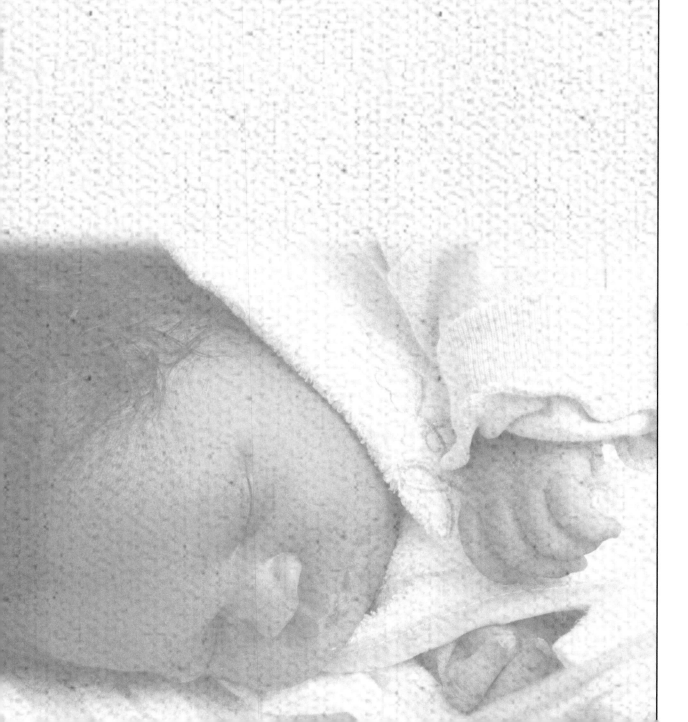

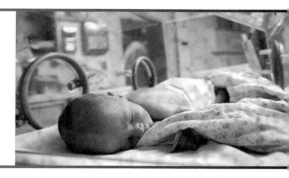

CHAPTER 30

Delivery Room Resuscitation

Steven M. Donn and Roger G. Faix

The first minutes after birth may pose severe biologic challenges to the newborn that can radically influence the remainder of the infant's life. Although numerous maternal, placental, and fetal conditions may, at times, induce fetal compromise and interfere with the physiologic transition to extrauterine existence, difficulties also occasionally occur after an unremarkable pregnancy, labor, and delivery. Timely intervention by skilled clinicians may facilitate survival and prevention or amelioration of organ injury.

NORMAL FETAL PHYSIOLOGY

Intrauterine fetal health depends on perfusion of the uteroplacental unit and umbilical cord, as well as the oxygen and nutrient content of both maternal and fetal blood. Delivery of oxygen and nutrients to the fetus takes place across the placenta, as does the removal of carbon dioxide and other metabolic waste products. Breathing movements are frequently seen in the healthy fetus, although the fetal lungs play a minimal role in the intrauterine sustenance of the fetus. Because fluid fills the lungs and envelops the infant, no significant fetal pulmonary gas exchange can take place.

The normal fetal circulatory pattern is very different from that required after birth, but it is quite satisfactory for survival in the womb (Fig. 30-1).[1,2] The blood with the highest oxygen content in the fetus is found in the umbilical vein as it exits the placenta, the organ of gas exchange. Although the partial pressure of oxygen (pO_2) in this site is typically only 35 to 40 mm Hg or less under normal circumstances, the high affinity of fetal hemoglobin for oxygen may result in up to 80% saturation, a level that is adequate to fulfill the metabolic needs of the fetal tissues under normal circumstances. This relatively well-oxygenated blood courses through the ductus venosus into the inferior vena cava and is delivered to the right atrium. Blood flow is then split into two streams by the crista dividens. Approximately 60% of the blood is shunted directly across the patent foramen ovale into the left atrium; from there it crosses the mitral valve into the left ventricle and is pumped into the ascending aorta, perfusing the coronary and carotid arteries. This particular arrangement ensures that two of the most vital organs, the myocardium and brain, receive blood with a relatively high oxygen content, suitable for the metabolic needs of these organs.

The remaining 40% of the inferior vena caval blood is delivered to the right atrium and is mixed with deoxygenated blood from the superior vena cava, crosses the tricuspid valve into the right ventricle, and then travels to the pulmonary artery. Once in the pulmonary artery, most of the blood bypasses the lungs by crossing the patent ductus arteriosus into the descending aorta. This preferential course reflects the relatively low fetal vascular resistance in the systemic circuit and high resistance in the pulmonary pathway. The high capacitance and low impedance properties of the placenta are major factors in the decreased resistance of the systemic circuit. The low ambient oxygen content in the perivascular and endothelial tissue of the pulmonary vessels results in hypoxic vasoconstriction. Local elaboration of vasodilating endogenous prostanoids and adenosine has been implicated in maintaining patency of the ductus arteriosus.[3,4] As a consequence of high pulmonary vascular resistance, only about 10% of the blood that reaches the pulmonary artery actually flows through the intrapulmonary vessels. Because there is a relatively small amount of blood flowing through the lungs, there is a correspondingly small amount of blood returning from the lungs via the pulmonary veins into the left atrium. Decreased pulmonary venous return results in atrial pressure that is lower in the left atrium than the right. The functional sequela is that the one-way flap valve of the foramen ovale is maintained in the open position, thus permitting shunting of blood directly from the right atrium to the left.

Pulmonary blood flow is quite low in the fetus but does not impair fetal well-being, because the placenta performs the gas exchange function. Fetal pulmonary blood flow is sufficient if it fulfills the nutritive requirements of the

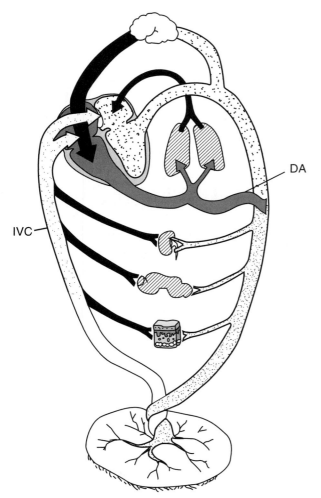

Figure 30–1. Circulation in the normal fetus. (Oxygen content corre-lates inversely with density of *stippling;* magnitude of blood flow is approximated by size of depicted vessel.) Freshly oxygenated blood leaves placenta by umbilical vein and courses through ductus venosus into the inferior vena cava (IVC), joining blood from the viscera. More than half the IVC flow crosses the foramen ovale to the left atrium, where it mixes with the small pulmonary venous return. This relatively well-oxygenated blood is delivered to the ascending aorta and thence to the myocardium and brain. The remaining IVC flow mixes with superior vena cava blood and reaches the right ventricle. Because of high pulmonary vascular resistance, most blood reaching the pulmonary artery flows preferentially across the ductus arteriosus (DA) and into the descending aorta. *(From Phibbs RH: Delivery room management of the newborn. In Avery GB [ed]: Neonatology: Pathophysiology and Management of the Newborn, 3rd ed. Philadelphia, JB Lippincott, 1987, p 213.)*

lungs for adequate growth so that the gas exchange function can be assumed after birth.

TRANSITIONAL PHYSIOLOGY

Successful extrauterine transition requires adequate neu-rologic drive for respiratory effort, mobilization of alveolar fluid to permit entry and egress of respiratory gases, and

a change in circulatory pattern to increase pulmonary blood flow for gas exchange. The placenta is cut off from the infant's circulation at birth by clamping and transect-ing the umbilical cord. This alteration causes a sharp increase in systemic vascular resistance. As the infant takes his or her first vigorous breaths and generates appropriately high transpulmonary pressures, alveolar fluid is hydrostatically driven across the alveolar epithe-lium into the interstitium and then taken up by the pul-monary circulation and lymphatic vessels.[5] An additional factor that contributes to the resorption of alveolar fluid is the role of labor and its associated hormonal changes, which up-regulate alveolar epithelial pumps that convert the fluid flux in the lungs from net secretion to net absorption. At the same time, gaseous inflation mechan-ically stretches intraparenchymal structures and facili-tates pulmonary vasodilation. As atmospheric oxygen enters the alveoli and increases the pH and PO_2 of blood and, subsequently, the pulmonary perivascular and endothelial tissues, the pulmonary vasomotor tone further decreases, and the ductus arteriosus may begin to con-strict. Local perturbations in prostanoid, adenosine, nitric oxide, and other endothelium-associated pathways have all been hypothesized to play a role in these vascular changes.[6-10] The combination of increased systemic and decreased pulmonary vascular resistance results in enhanced pulmonary blood flow by reducing the right-to-left shunt across the ductus arteriosus into the descend-ing aorta. The sharp rise in pulmonary blood flow is followed by an increase in pulmonary venous return with an attendant elevation of left atrial pressure. The rise in pressure causes the flap of the foramen ovale to close, thereby removing another avenue of pulmonary bypass (Fig. 30-2).

Some infants do not undergo a smooth transition to extrauterine life. Lack of robust, regular spontaneous res-piratory effort at birth interferes with mobilization of alveolar fluid, inflation of alveoli for gas exchange, and reduction of pulmonary vascular resistance. The absence of respiratory effort may result from a variety of processes, some of which are relatively benign and readily reversible (such as transplacental delivery of maternal anesthetic agents), and others that may be more malignant and refractory (such as severe protracted hypoxic-ischemic insults). If adequate lung expansion is not attained and sustained, hypoxia and acidosis rapidly progress. In preterm infants, this may adversely affect an already mar-ginal surfactant balance and interfere with alveolar recruitment and ventilation-perfusion matching. In full-term or post-term infants, the large number of muscular-ized or partially muscularized arteries in the pulmonary circulation may respond with persistence or even exacer-bation of vasoconstriction. The increase in pulmonary vascular resistance may exceed the rise in systemic resist-ance generated by the cutting off of the placenta from the circulation. As a circulatory consequence of this change, blood reaching the pulmonary artery may follow the path of least resistance, crossing the ductus arteriosus and delivering deoxygenated blood into the descending aorta rather than to the lungs. The reduced pulmonary blood flow yields decreased pulmonary venous return. Left atrial

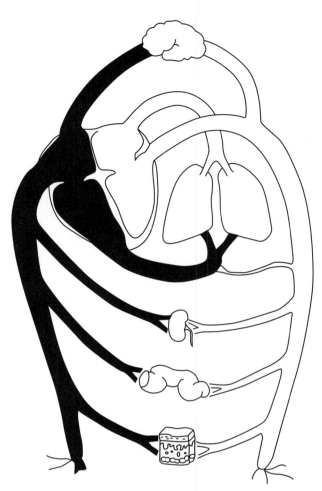

Figure 30–2. Circulation in the normal newborn. After expansion of the lungs and clamping of the umbilical cord, pulmonary blood flow increases, left atrial and systemic arterial pressures rise, and pulmonary artery and right-sided heart pressures fall. The foramen ovale closes when atrial pressure on the left side is greater than that on the right side. Both inferior and superior vena caval blood then flow to the right ventricle and are pumped to the pulmonary artery. The rise in systemic arterial pressure and the drop in pulmonary artery pressure then favor left-to-right flow through the ductus arteriosus, which eventually constricts and closes. *(From Phibbs RH: Delivery room management of the newborn. In Avery GB [ed]: Neonatology: Pathophysiology and Management of the Newborn, 3rd ed. Philadelphia, JB Lippincott, 1987, p 214.)*

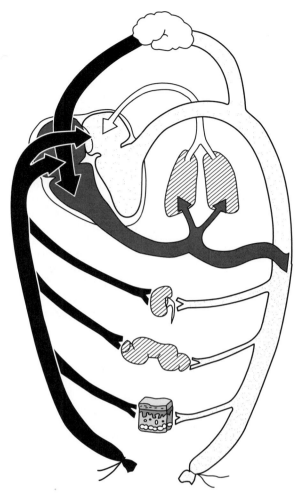

Figure 30–3. Neonatal circulation after perinatal asphyxia and incomplete lung expansion. Because of high pulmonary vascular resistance, pulmonary blood flow is low, and right-to-left flow across the ductus to the descending aorta is significant. Because pulmonary venous return is low, left atrial pressure is lower than that in the right atrium, with resultant patency of the foramen ovale and mixture of right and left atrial blood. As a result, blood with suboptimal oxygen content reaches the ascending aorta for myocardial and brain perfusion, and blood with even lower oxygen content supplies the postductal descending aorta and associated organs. *(From Phibbs RH: Delivery room management of the newborn. In Avery GB [ed]: Neonatology: Pathophysiology and Management of the Newborn, 3rd ed. Philadelphia, JB Lippincott, 1987, p 214.)*

pressure is lower than right atrial pressure, with attendant right-to-left shunting across the foramen ovale and an additional decrement in pulmonary blood flow (Fig. 30-3). If this circulatory pattern persists, progressive hypoxemia and acidosis may develop with increased potential for organ injury and mortality.

PHYSIOLOGY OF RESUSCITATION

In most infants who require resuscitation, properly performed positive-pressure ventilation with 100% oxygen is sufficient to revive the infant. This maneuver mobilizes alveolar fluid, facilitates alveolar recruitment, induces reduction of pulmonary vascular resistance, and supports good pulmonary gas exchange with an improved systemic circulation and acid-base status. In the context of prolonged hypoxic-ischemic insults, anomalies of the cardiopulmonary system, or superimposed pathologic processes (such as sepsis, acute hemorrhage, or pneumothorax), normal blood flow and adequate gas exchange may not occur. Even positive-pressure ventilation may fail because of impaired myocardial function, deficient oxygen-carrying capacity, hypoplastic vital organs, or abnormal vascular tone or integrity. Additional interventions are necessary for infants who do not respond to positive-pressure ventilation.

Effective resuscitation requires timely communication, skilled personnel, and proper equipment. It is useful to prospectively identify factors predictive of an increased likelihood that the infant will need neonatal resuscitation or specialized neonatal care (Box 30-1). Knowledge of specific problems may influence decisions regarding maternal transfer, intrapartum management, and the postnatal resuscitation of the infant. The presence of risk conditions must be communicated to clinicians who are responsible for the delivery room management and postnatal care of the infant. Many infants who require resuscitation, however, have no risk factors identified before delivery. Accordingly, appropriate equipment and trained personnel must be present at all deliveries. Unavailability of needed staff and equipment after a compromised infant has been delivered increases the likelihood of organ injury and makes resuscitation much more difficult.[11,12]

INTRAUTERINE FETAL RESUSCITATION

If the mother undergoes a severe, life-threatening insult such as vehicular trauma, thromboembolic catastrophe, amniotic fluid embolus, or acute exacerbation of an underlying disease that necessitates her own resuscitation, uteroplacental perfusion and the fetus may be severely compromised as well. Depending on gestational age, the severity of maternal compromise, and the probability of maternal recovery, the fetus may benefit most from aggressive maternal resuscitation or rapid evacuation from the critically hostile intrauterine environment.[13] Special considerations for pregnancy have been incorporated into the guidelines of the American Heart Association for cardiopulmonary resuscitation and emergency cardiovascular care.[14] Most of the recommended maneuvers have potential benefit for the fetus as well as for the mother.

In many circumstances, maternal compromise is absent, noncontributory, or rapidly reversible, and effective resuscitation can be accomplished in utero. Intrauterine resuscitation is generally aimed at rapidly stabilizing the fetus so that either the pregnancy can be continued or a controlled, safe delivery can be performed under nonemergency circumstances. If the fetus fails to respond rapidly, or if clinical findings strongly suggest the presence of a condition for which intrauterine resuscitation is unlikely to be effective, careful consideration of emergency delivery is indicated.

A single case report described the use of transabdominal intrauterine chest compressions under sonographic guidance in the successful resuscitation and long-term survival of a 29-week fetus who sustained acute bradycardia and subsequent asystole during an intrauterine packed red blood cell transfusion.[15] Although cordocentesis has been used increasingly for fetal diagnosis and therapy, it is not typically used for acute administration of resuscitative medications because it can be time consuming and involves significant inherent risks. In most circumstances, it is probably better to rapidly initiate other

---

Box 30–1   Partial List of Risk Factors Associated with an Increased Need for Neonatal Resuscitation

Antepartum (Maternal)

Diabetes mellitus
Hypertension
Substance abuse
Vascular disease
Vasoactive medications
Smoking
Poor maternal weight gain
Myasthenia gravis
Sexually transmitted disease
Prior fetal/neonatal death
No prenatal care
Chronic disease
Anemia
Hemorrhage
Maternal age <16 or >35 years
Polyhydramnios/oligohydramnios
Decreased fetal movement
Placental anomaly
Uterine or cervical anomaly

Intrapartum

Multiple gestation
Nonvertex presentation
Postdatism
Macrosomia/microsomia
Maternal hypotension
Abruptio placentae or placenta previa
Umbilical cord accidents
Maternal infection
Operative delivery (with use of forceps, vacuum, or cesarean section)
General anesthesia
Spinal anesthesia
Maternal sedation
Polyhydramnios/oligohydramnios
Fetal anomaly
Prematurity
Prolonged labor
Meconium-stained amniotic fluid
Abnormal fetal heart rate pattern
Prolonged second stage of labor

Postpartum (Neonatal)

Apnea
Bradycardia
Respiratory distress
Hypoperfusion
Anemia/pallor
Congenital anomaly
Infection
Prematurity
Birth trauma

Adapted from Faix RG: Neonatal resuscitation. In Donn SM, Faix RG (eds): Neonatal Emergencies. Mt Kisco, NY, Futura, 1991, p 19.

interventions or delivery. If the fetus is previable and the need for resuscitation arises during an invasive intrauterine procedure, the access offered by cordocentesis may enable more aggressive intervention than might otherwise be possible. Cordocentesis in a previable fetus with hydrops was reported to result in fetal cardiac arrest; only transiently successful resuscitation was conducted with intracardiac epinephrine and fetal transfusion.[16] The long-term outcome and advisability of aggressive resuscitation under such circumstances remains unclear.

Maternal repositioning may alleviate fetal compromise from vascular compression.[17,18] If the mother is supine, the gravid uterus may impinge on the maternal aorta or inferior vena cava with resultant uteroplacental hypoperfusion. Assumption of the left lateral decubitus position reduces such extrinsic compression of maternal great vessels. Umbilical cord compression is often suggested by variable fetal heart rate decelerations. Impingement may occur between two fetal structures, the fetus and the uterine wall or other pelvic structures, or by elongation of the cord during fetal descent. If the fetal membranes have already ruptured, cord prolapse should be excluded. If prolapse is found, the mother should be placed in the Trendelenburg position and the presenting part manually elevated to minimize cord compression, while preparation for emergency abdominal delivery is initiated. Successful decompression of the cord, elevation of fetal structures, and reduction of uterine contractions have also been achieved by rapid retrograde distention of the maternal urinary bladder.[19] In the absence of prolapse, several nonsupine positions may be used to reduce umbilical compromise. Resolution of the characteristic variable decelerations usually indicates success (see Box 30-1).

Supplemental maternal oxygen increases maternal pO_2 much more dramatically than fetal pO_2. Because of the high oxygen affinity of fetal hemoglobin and the steep slope of the fetal hemoglobin-oxygen dissociation curve at the low intrauterine pO_2 found in normal and mild to moderately hypoxic intrauterine circumstances, maternal oxygen administration can produce a modest but potentially critical improvement in fetal oxygen saturation and oxygen content.[20,21] One study demonstrated a mean increase in fetal arteriolar oxygen saturation of 11% within 5 to 10 minutes after maternal administration of 100% oxygen.[20] Although the resultant fetal arterial oxygen content may be much lower than that seen in normal extrauterine circumstances, the improvement may be sufficient to ensure adequate oxygen delivery to vital organs and hence prevent or minimize hypoxic-ischemic injury.

Tetanic uterine contractions may interfere with utero-placental perfusion in the otherwise healthy fetus. This abnormality is most readily detected in women with ruptured membranes who have monitoring of intrauterine pressure and fetal heart rate. If these contractions are associated with the pharmacologic use of oxytocin, the short half-life of the medication usually allows rapid resolution after cessation of the continuous oxytocin infusion. If tetany is spontaneous or refractory to cessation of oxytocin administration, and if placental abruption can be ruled out, judicious administration of tocolytic agents

may be beneficial.[22-25] In the growth-restricted or chronically underperfused fetus, the already tenuous uteroplacental circulation may be seriously compromised by normal uterine contractions, and tocolytic therapy may also be considered in the presence of fetal distress.[26,27] The clinician should be aware, however, that reported improvements in fetal heart tracings have not always been accompanied by corresponding statistically significant improvements in cord blood pH, lactate, or clinically important measures of well-being.[28,29] Well-designed, adequately powered studies are too few to conclude that tocolytic agents are indicated for suspected intrapartum fetal distress.[28] Deliberations should include potential benefits and adverse effects of tocolytic agents on both the mother and infant.

Amnioinfusion, the intrauterine instillation of warmed saline solution, has been successfully used for reduction of presumed umbilical cord compression that is refractory to maternal repositioning.[30,31] In the presence of meconium-stained amniotic fluid, this technique appears to reduce the incidence and severity of neonatal meconium aspiration syndrome.[32-34] Improved fetal and maternal outcomes with intrapartum oligohydramnios, premature rupture of membranes at less than 26 weeks' gestation, and chorioamnionitis have also been noted.[35-37] Not surprisingly, multiple adverse effects have also been observed, including (but not limited to) the introduction of infection, excessive uterine distention, migration of fluid to other body cavities, and placental abruption. There is at least one report of amnioinfusion-induced malpresentation with fetal demise.[38] If amnioinfusion is used, care should be taken to avoid dystocia and compression of the umbilical cord and placenta, which may arise from iatrogenic polyhydramnios and intrauterine hypertension.[39] Careful consideration of benefits and potential complications is warranted.

The implementation of such maneuvers depends on the timely detection of potentially reversible life-threatening fetal compromise by judicious obstetric surveillance with sonography, fetal heart rate monitoring, biochemical testing, pulse oximetry,[40] and other techniques.[41] At least one retrospective report from a single institution, however, documented that the recommendations of the American College of Obstetricians and Gynecologists for further assessment and management of nonreassuring intrapartum fetal heart rate patterns were used in fewer than 50% of appropriate cases.[42] Conventional methods for intrauterine resuscitation include maternal positioning, administration of supplemental maternal oxygen, alteration of the position of the fetus or cord, amnioinfusion, and tocolysis.

NEONATAL RESUSCITATION

As the intrauterine environment is made as hospitable as possible and steps are undertaken to facilitate or forestall delivery, preparation for the postnatal resuscitation and stabilization should proceed concurrently. At least two staff members who are skilled and experienced in neonatal resuscitation should be present at all deliveries,[11] although some authors recommend that at least three such staff members be available.[43,44] It is more critical that qualified resuscitation staff members possess the necessary skills and experience than specific professional titles. If there are no identified high-risk factors, it is acceptable for the resuscitation team to include the health care professional performing the delivery.[11] If high-risk factors are present, the resuscitation team should be responsible only for the infant. Separate resuscitation teams should be provided for each infant in the event of a multiple birth. Resuscitation equipment (Box 30-2) should be present in the delivery area and ready for immediate use.[45] The resuscitation team should review the equipment, ensure that it is functional, and activate the radiant warmer, oxygen, and suction well before the infant is delivered.

The age-old mnemonic of the "ABCs" of resuscitation is still valid today and continues to form the basis of neonatal resuscitation. Most difficulties resulting in maladaptation are respiratory in nature; thus, great attention must be given to pulmonary resuscitation. On occasion, prolonged asphyxia also leads to myocardial depression, necessitating additional resuscitative measures.

Box 30–2	Basic Equipment for Neonatal Resuscitation

Gloves and gowns
Radiant warmer
Prewarmed blankets
Stethoscope
Suction bulb
Regulatable suction source
Suction catheters: 5.0-, 8.0-, 10.0-French
Suction traps
Reservoir for meconium suctioning from endotracheal tube
Oxygen source with flowmeter
Infant resuscitation bag with manometer (must have 100% O$_2$ adaptor if self-inflating model is used)
Face masks: newborn and premature sizes
One or more laryngoscopes with functioning batteries
Laryngoscope blades: straight, sizes 0 and 1, with functioning light bulbs
Endotracheal tubes: uncuffed, sizes 2.5, 3.0, 3.5, and 4.0 mm
Endotracheal tube stylets (if desired)
Umbilical catheters: 3.5-, 5.0-, and 8.0-French
Feeding tube: 5.0- and 8.0-French
Sterile umbilical vessel catheterization tray
Syringes: 1, 3, 5, 10, 20 mL
Three-way stopcock
Needles (including butterfly type)
Cardiorespiratory monitor with electrocardiographic display
Fluid for parenteral administration: dextrose, normal saline
Medication, including the following:
  Epinephrine, 1:10,000
  4.2% sodium bicarbonate
  Naloxone hydrochloride
  Volume expander (e.g., normal saline, Ringer's lactate)

Adapted from Faix RG: Neonatal resuscitation. In Donn SM, Faix RG (eds): Neonatal Emergencies. Mt Kisco, NY, Futura, 1991, p 20.

Airway

The unique features that distinguish the airway of the newborn include its small caliber, the deficiency of cartilaginous support, and the viscous fluids (such as mucus or meconium) with which it is usually filled at the time of birth. These features must be considered when resuscitation is begun.

According to Poiseuille's law, the flow through a tube is proportional to the fourth power of the radius of the tube.[46] Thus, the relatively small size of the newborn's trachea can severely limit gas flow.[47] This limitation can be compounded by viscous fluids or particulate material within the airways, as well as a tendency for the smaller airways to collapse at end expiration. Early measures in resuscitation are thus directed at clearing the airway of secretions and maximizing the cross-sectional area of the trachea. The infant should be placed in an appropriate position; first the mouth and then the nose should be suctioned until clear. Ideally, the infant should be in a supine position, and the head and neck should be placed in the neutral position during the initial stabilization. This can be facilitated by placing a rolled towel beneath the infant's shoulder blades. The warming bed should also be flat, or the infant's trachea may not be optimally patent. Controversy still exists as to the best approach to airway management in the presence of meconium-stained amniotic fluid. It seems clear that "obstetric" suctioning of the upper airway while the infant's head is on the perineum is prudent and carries minimal risk,[48] but it is not universally accepted that every meconium-stained infant requires endotracheal suctioning. Infants who have respiratory depression at birth and who require positive-pressure ventilation should certainly have tracheal secretions suctioned before the application of positive-pressure ventilation. Failure to do so may not only hinder gas exchange but may also drive particulate matter deeper into the tracheobronchial tree, where it may cause greater harm.[49] On the other hand, active, vigorous infants who are meconium-stained may not derive much benefit from tracheal suctioning and may even react adversely.[50-53] The approach of performing direct laryngoscopy and suctioning the trachea only if meconium is seen at the vocal cords does not seem justified, because 15% to 20% of infants who have aspirated meconium have "clean" vocal cords.[54]

Endotracheal intubation may be necessary to secure the airway, particularly if secretions are copious. The proper size tube is one that fits snugly but not tightly. A small oral air leak around the tube is permissible if adequate chest excursions occur during inspiration. Table 30-1 lists suggested guidelines for initial endotracheal tube size (internal diameter) and depth of insertion (measured at the lip for orotracheal tubes) on the basis of birth weight. Placement should be confirmed, first clinically by assessing equality of breath sounds and chest excursions and, later, radiographically. Optimal placement occurs when the endotracheal tube tip is midway between the vocal cords and the carina.

Breathing

Pulmonary resuscitation also involves the facilitation of transition from a fluid-filled lung to an air-filled lung.[2]

Table 30-1. Recommended Endotracheal Tube Sizes and Depths of Insertion at Lip

Birth Weight (g)	Size (mm)	Depth (Cm)
<1000	2.5	7
1000-2000	3.0	8
2001-3000	3.5	9
3001-4000	4.0	10

Depending on several factors, including morphologic and biologic maturity, the opening pressure required for the initial expansion of the lungs may be considerable. Pressures of greater than 30 cm H_2O in the full-term infant and pressures up to 50 cm H_2O in the preterm infant are occasionally necessary.[55] Thus, it is not surprising that some infants are unable to inflate their lungs, especially if concomitant disease is present. If the airway is patent, positive-pressure ventilation may be applied by a bag-and-mask technique, with either an anesthesia-type or a self-inflating bag and an appropriate-sized mask that covers the infant's nose and mouth (but not the eyes) and makes a good seal. Positive-pressure ventilation should then be delivered at a rate of 40 to 60 breaths per minute, sufficient to result in a rise of the chest wall and adequate breath sounds on auscultation. The use of a pressure manometer may be helpful in guiding inflation pressures and in establishing initial ventilator settings if mechanical ventilation becomes necessary. Positive-pressure ventilation should generally continue until the infant is exhibiting sufficient spontaneous effort and maintaining a normal heart rate. The infant should be weaned gradually and not abruptly. If it appears that bag-and-mask support will be more than a temporary measure, endotracheal intubation is recommended.

There has been an interest in the use of room air, rather than increased oxygen concentrations, to resuscitate respiration-depressed newborns. The underlying rationale for this is the decreased potential for generating numerous reactive free radicals, such as peroxynitrite, and the depletion of antioxidants, leading to lipid peroxidation and possible damage to protein and DNA.[56] Preliminary clinical trials, performed primarily in underdeveloped settings, have thus far not demonstrated a disadvantage to resuscitation using room air compared with 100% oxygen.[57,58] Markers of oxidative stress have also been shown to be decreased when room air is used.[59] Although this is an intriguing premise, it must at present be considered investigational until further clinical trials prove long-term safety and efficacy.

Circulation

Major circulatory considerations concern facilitation of the fetal-to-neonatal transition, maintenance of cardiac output, and establishment of adequate tissue perfusion. Augmentation of myocardial performance by appropriate oxygenation, attention to acid-base balance, and provision of an adequate blood volume are also crucial at this time.

If proper pulmonary resuscitation fails to bring about the anticipated cardiac response—a sustained heart rate of more than 100 beats per minute—within 20 to 30 seconds, additional measures should be instituted. If the heart rate is less than 60, external cardiac massage should be started by initiating chest compressions and ventilation at a combined rate of 120 beats per minute, consisting of 90 compressions and 30 breaths. The infant should be reassessed for spontaneous cardiac activity after 20 to 30 seconds of combined positive-pressure ventilation and chest compressions. If the heart rate is still less than 60 beats per minute, the use of epinephrine is indicated. A 1:10,000 dilution is given in a dose of 0.1 to 0.3 mL/kg and may be administered through an endotracheal tube, intravenously, or, in rare instances, by intracardiac injection (Table 30-2). Some authorities recommend increasing subsequent doses if the initial response is not optimal. The higher end of the dose range is suggested if the endotracheal route is used, although this method should be used only if no alternative access is available. It may be repeated at 5-minute intervals.

Circulatory concerns also need to address vascular access, because other pharmacologic agents or blood volume expanders may be required. Umbilical venous catheterization is usually the most readily and easily accessible conduit for this purpose.[60] It also enables sampling of venous blood for analysis of acid-base balance, blood gases, and other laboratory values (Box 30-3).

Drugs

A limited number of resuscitative drugs are used in the delivery room setting. Clinicians involved in neonatal resuscitation must be thoroughly familiar with the indications, precautions, and complications associated with each of these agents. These are summarized in Table 30-2, along with the dosages, concentrations, and routes of delivery for the most commonly administered agents.

Environment

Thermoregulation is a critical event in transition. Hypothermia may result in multiple untoward effects (especially an increase in oxygen consumption and basal metabolic rate, and a leftward shift of the oxygen-hemoglobin dissociation curve) that may potentially impair transition and be deleterious to the infant's well-being.[61] Most hypothermia is avoidable with some forethought. The resuscitation area to which the newborn is brought should be preheated with a radiant warmer. The infant should be dried rapidly after birth to minimize evaporative heat loss. Drying may be deferred if the infant is respiration-depressed and born amid meconium, because drying may trigger respiratory gasping that may produce or exacerbate meconium aspiration before tracheal suction can be performed. All wet towels should be promptly removed from contact with the infant. Personnel must be aware that they may block the radiant heat from reaching the infant if they lean over the baby on the resuscitation table. Inspired respiratory gases should be adequately warmed and humidified, and intravenous fluids should be warmed to body temperature before administration. Avoidance of drafts and convective heat loss is another important consideration.

Table 30–2. Drugs Commonly Used for Neonatal Resuscitation

Agent	Indications	Concentration	Dose	Route	Precautions	Complications
Dextrose	Hypoglycemia	10%	2 mL/kg	IV	Maintain euglycemia	Hyperglycemia Hyperosmolality
Epinephrine	Bradycardia	1:10,000	0.1–0.3 mL/kg	ET IV IC	Avoid administration through arterial catheter	Hyperglycemia Tachycardia Increased oxygen consumption
Sodium bicarbonate	Metabolic acidosis	0.5 mEq/mL (4.2%)	1–2 mEq/kg	IV	Ensure adequate ventilation	Hypercarbia Hypernatremia Hyperosmolality Hypokalemia
THAM (trishydroxymethyl aminomethane)	Acidosis	0.3 M	4–8 mL/kg	IV	—	Hypoglycemia Respiratory depression Vascular sclerosis
Naloxone	Narcotic-induced respiratory depression	0.4 or 1.0 mg/mL	0.1 mg/kg	IV IM SC ET	Maternal history of opiate or narcotic abuse	May initiate acute withdrawal syndrome in infant of addicted mother
Volume expanders (administer over 15-30 minutes) Blood Colloid Crystalloid	 Hypovolemia Hypovolemia Hypovolemia	 — — —	 10–20 mL/kg 10–20 mL/kg 10–20 mL/kg	 IV IV IV	 — — —	 — — —

ET, endotracheal tube; IC, intracardiac; IM, intramuscular; IV, intravenously; SC, subcutaneous.

Box 30–3 Outline of Initial Conduct of Neonatal Resuscitation

Thermoregulation

Radiant warmer
Dry infant, remove wet towels; if infant is depressed and amniotic fluid was meconium-stained, defer this step until after
  tracheal suction

Ensure Airway Patency

Proper placement of head and neck in neutral position
Suction mouth, then nose
If amniotic fluid was meconium-stained:
  Obstetrician should suction nose, oropharynx, and hypopharynx after delivery of head
  Consider tracheal intubation and suctioning with an adaptor and regulated suction (maximum −80 to −100 mm Hg) if the
    infant has respiratory depression
  After tracheal toilet, aspirate gastric contents at or beyond 5 minutes of life

Gentle but Firm Stimulation: Slap Soles, Rub Back for a Few Seconds

Assess Concurrently

Is the infant making adequate respiratory effort?
  If no, initiate positive-pressure ventilation (PPV) with >80% oxygen; assess efficacy by breath sounds, chest excursions
Is the heart rate >100/minute?
  If no, initiate PPV with >80% oxygen
Is central cyanosis present?
  If no, observe
  If yes, and adequate respiratory effort, and heart rate >100, administer free-flow oxygen ≥80%; initiate PPV with >80% oxygen
    if no response in 20 sec.

If PPV Is Necessary, Reassess after 20 Seconds while Delivering ≥80% Oxygen Free-Flow

If spontaneous respiratory effort and heart rate >100, observe for cyanosis and attempt to wean free-flow oxygen
If no spontaneous respiratory effort or heart rate <100, resume PPV
  If heart rate <60, institute cardiac massage; assess efficacy by umbilical or brachial pulses
  If heart rate >60, PPV alone; consider naloxone if maternal opiate use within 4 hours of delivery

If Continued PPV with or without Cardiac Massage Necessary, Reassess after 20 to 30 Seconds

If spontaneous respiratory effort and heart rate >100, observe for cyanosis and attempt to wean free-flow oxygen
If no spontaneous respiratory effort or heart rate <100, resume PPV
  If heart rate <60 and not rising, also resume cardiac massage and prepare to administer epinephrine
  If heart rate >60, PPV alone

**Serial Reassessment Every 20 to 30 Seconds during PPV with or without Cardiac Massage as Needed; Epinephrine May
Be Repeated Every 5 Minutes**

Place Orogastric Tube after 2 Minutes; Aspirate Stomach and Place Tube To "Chimney"

Establish Vascular Access

Obtain blood gas, hematocrit, other necessary laboratory tests
Initiate glucose infusion

If Blood Gas Reveals Severe Metabolic Acidosis, Sodium Bicarbonate or THAM May Be Used to Treat

**If Infant Fails to Respond Appropriately, Consider Pneumothorax, Hypovolemia, Congenital Anomaly, or Other Confounders
Listed in Box 30-1**

Document Events and Times

Call for Additional Help as Needed

THAM, trishydroxymethyl aminomethane.

Adapted from Faix RG: Neonatal resuscitation. In Donn SM and Faix RG, editors: Neonatal Emergencies, Futura, Mount Kisco, NY,
1991, p. 22, with permission.

DELIVERY ROOM RESUSCITATION OF THE NEWBORN

Although the basic tenets of neonatal resuscitation have been reflected in clinical practice for decades, it took a considerable time to develop a consistent approach. Members of the American Heart Association and the American Academy of Pediatrics created and implemented a standardized approach to neonatal resuscitation that includes a certification program for health care providers. First introduced in 1986, the Neonatal Resuscitation Program has become widely accepted as a standard for delivery room cardiopulmonary resuscitation and emergency cardiac care. Readers are referred to the *Instructor's Manual for Neonatal Resuscitation*[12] in its entirety. Box 30-3 represents a condensed outline of neonatal resuscitation based on the guidelines recommended by the American Heart Association/American Academy of Pediatrics Neonatal Resuscitation Steering Committee in 2003.[45]

SPECIAL RESUSCITATION PROCEDURES

A thorough knowledge of mechanical procedures is required of individuals responsible for neonatal resuscitation. Those procedures include endotracheal intubation, external cardiac massage (Box 30-4), umbilical vein catheterization, pneumothorax evacuation by needle thoracentesis, and intracardiac injection (Box 30-5).[62] It is essential that a health care facility providing delivery services have a requisite number of individuals trained and experienced in resuscitation procedures to ensure an appropriate response to problems whenever they arise.

Box 30–4 Technique of External Cardiac Massage

Equipment

Flat, Hard Surface

Preparation

Provide firm surface under infant; hands of the resuscitator may be a good alternative to ensure a firm surface
Place hands around infant with fingertips beneath the thoracic spine
Place overlapping thumbs over lower third of sternum
Alternative approach is to place fingertips over lower third of sternum (avoid xiphoid) perpendicular to plane of chest with other hand under back

Procedure

Depress thumbs (or fingertips) sufficiently to depress sternum one-third the anteroposterior diameter of the chest
Release pressure without breaking contact
Interpose chest compressions with positive-pressure ventilation at 3:1 ratio (three compressions, one ventilation every 2 seconds)
Have assistant assess efficacy by palpating umbilical or brachial pulses
Continue at rate of 120 compressions/min

Box 30–5 Technique of Intracardiac Injection

Equipment

Syringe (3-5 mL)
Needle (22 g, 1-1½ inch)
Iodine solution
Epinephrine 1:10,000, 1.0 mL

Preparation

Patient in supine position
Determine anatomic location of heart: may be altered, e.g., by presence of tension pneumothorax
Prepare site with iodine solution

Procedure

Needle may be inserted in subxiphoid location and directed toward left shoulder, or inserted perpendicular to chest wall in left fourth intercostal space between midclavicular line and left sternal border
Apply slight negative pressure to syringe as needle is advanced; blood return signals entry into heart
Inject drug
Remove needle
Continue chest compressions to allow distribution of drug

THE PROBLEMATIC RESUSCITATION

The failure of an infant to respond to resuscitation may be the result of numerous factors. Some of these may be procedurally related, including improper performance of resuscitation, or a result of mechanical problems with equipment or endotracheal tube difficulties. Other factors to consider include pathologic problems that must be alleviated (such as hypovolemia or pneumothorax), effects of maternal anesthesia or analgesia, anomalous conditions, or the sequelae of traumatic birth injuries (Box 30-6).[45] Attention must be paid to both mechanical and pathophysiologic factors.

WHEN TO STOP RESUSCITATION

Among the most difficult issues is when to terminate resuscitative efforts in an infant who is not responding to an appropriately performed resuscitation, especially in view of the long-term neurologic condition as the most important outcome measure. The decision is often clouded by a lack of understanding of the event or events that led to neonatal depression and the need for resuscitation. However, there is some evidence that newborns may tolerate a significantly prolonged resuscitation, with a relatively low incidence of neurologic deficit in survivors. Table 30-3 demonstrates the effect of the prolongation of a low Apgar score (0 to 3) on the development of cerebral palsy. Even if the score is depressed for 15 minutes, nearly two of every three survivors fail to develop cerebral palsy.[63] It seems prudent that, rather than developing an arbitrary set of circumstances for terminating a resuscitation, each case should be determined on its own merits and the ultimate determination made by the most experienced physician involved in the procedure.

Box 30–6	Common Problems Interfering with Effective Resuscitation

Improper performance
Head and neck position
Airway patency
Mask size and application
Adequacy of bag compression
Sternal placement of fingers
Firm surface under infant
Adequacy of sternal compression
Mechanical difficulties:
    Oxygen not turned on
    Airway connectors loose or unconnected
    Oxygen tubing misrouted or unconnected
Endotracheal tube problems:
    Right main bronchus
    Esophagus
    Occlusion
    Leak
Hypovolemia
Pneumothorax or other intrathoracic air leak
Maternal medication (opiate, anesthetic)
Congenital anomaly of cardiopulmonary system or airway
Birth trauma
Inappropriate route of medication
Do not give sodium bicarbonate endotracheally
Do not give epinephrine subcutaneously or
    intramuscularly

Adapted from Faix RG: Neonatal resuscitation. In Donn SM, Faix RG (eds): Neonatal Emergencies. Mt Kisco, NY, Futura, 1991, p 28.

DOCUMENTATION

Although the most significant aspects of resuscitation involve patient management issues, it is crucial that a complete and accurate record be made of what transpires during the process. A recorder who is assigned to keep meticulous track of events and times is invaluable. This is especially true in the delivery room, in which, in the context of today's medicolegal environment, documentation

Table 30–3. Relationship of Depressed Apgar Scores (≤3) to Survival and Chronic Neurologic Disability in Infants Weighing More than 2500 g at Birth

Duration (Minutes)	Death in First Year (%)	Cerebral Palsy (%)
1	5.6	1.5
5	15.5	4.7
10	34.4	16.7
15	52.5	36.0
20	59.0	57.1

Adapted from Nelson KB, Ellenberg JH: Apgar scores as predictors of chronic neurologic disability. Pediatrics 68:36, 1981. Copyright American Academy of Pediatrics.

may be a key element in refuting subsequent allegations of medical negligence.[64]

Many institutions have simplified the approach to documentation by using preprinted forms for all cardiopulmonary arrests/resuscitations. These generic forms can be applied to the delivery room setting, provided that the appropriate dose, concentration, and volume of drug are recorded, with additional notation of narrative material as needed. Great care should be taken to record exact times and sequences of events. If, under hectic circumstances, recording is done on scrap paper (such as a paper towel), it should be transcribed into the medical record along with an appropriate explanation. Clinicians must remember that in later years, when events and outcomes may be called into question, the only documentation of the event may be what appears in the medical record.

REFERENCES

1. Dawes GS: Fetal and Neonatal Physiology. Chicago, Year Book Medical, 1968, pp 29-40.
2. Nelson NM: Respiration and circulation before birth. In Smith CA, Nelson NM (eds): The Physiology of the Newborn Infant. Springfield, Ill, Charles C Thomas, 1976, pp 15-117.
3. Clyman RI: Ductus arteriosus: Current theories of prenatal and postnatal regulation. Semin Perinatol 11:64, 1987.
4. Mentzer RM Jr, Ely SW, Lasley RD, et al: Hormonal role of adenosine in maintaining patency of ductus arteriosus in fetal lamb. Ann Surg 202:223, 1985.
5. Bland RD, Hansen TN, Haberkern CM: Lung fluid balance in 5 lambs before and after birth. J Appl Physiol 102:992, 1982.
6. Abman SH, Chatfield BA, Hall SL, et al: Role of EDRF during transition of pulmonary circulation at birth. Am J Physiol 259:H1921, 1990.
7. Frantz E, Soifer SJ, Clyman RI, et al: Bradykinin produces pulmonary vasodilation in fetal lambs: Role of prostaglandin production. J Appl Physiol 67:1512, 1989.
8. Konduri GG, Theodorou AA, Mukhopadhay A, et al: Adenosine triphosphate and adenosine increase the pulmonary blood flow to postnatal levels in fetal lambs. Pediatr Res 31:451, 1992.
9. Leffler CW, Hessler JR, Green RS: The onset of breathing at birth stimulates pulmonary vascular prostacyclin synthesis. Pediatr Res 18:938, 1984.
10. Soifer SJ, Morin FC III, Kaslow DC, et al: The developmental effects of prostaglandin D_2 on the pulmonary and systemic circulations in newborn lambs. J Dev Physiol 5:237, 1983.
11. Bloom RS, Cropley C: Textbook of Neonatal Resuscitation. Dallas, American Heart Association and American Academy of Pediatrics, 1987.
12. Instructor's Manual for Neonatal Resuscitation, 4th ed. Elk Grove Village, American Heart Association/American Academy of Pediatrics, 2003.
13. Dildy GA, Clark SL: Cardiac arrest during pregnancy. Obstet Gynecol Clin North Am 22:303, 1995.
14. American Heart Association: Cardiopulmonary resuscitation and emergency cardiovascular care. Part 8: Advanced challenges in resuscitation. Section 3: Special challenges in ECC. Cardiac arrest associated with pregnancy. Circulation 102(Suppl 1):I229, 2000.
15. Nicolaides KH, Rodeck CH: In utero resuscitation after cardiac arrest in a fetus. BMJ 288:900, 1984.

16. Elliott JP, Foley MR, Finberg HJ: In utero fetal cardiac resuscitation: A case report. Fetal Diagn Ther 9:226, 1994.

17. Bieniarz J, Branda LA, Maqueda E, et al: Aortocaval compression by the uterus in late pregnancy. III. Unreliability of the sphygmomanometric method in estimating uterine artery pressure. Am J Obstet Gynecol 102:1106, 1968.

18. Lin C-C: Intrauterine fetal resuscitation. In Lin C-C, Verp MS, Sabbagha RE (eds): High-Risk Fetus: Pathophysiology, Diagnosis, and Management. New York, Springer-Verlag, 1993, pp 667-668.

19. Runnebaum IB, Katz M: Intrauterine resuscitation by rapid urinary bladder instillation in a case of an excessively long umbilical cord. Eur J Obstet Gynecol Reprod Biol 84:101, 1999.

20. McNamara H, Johnson N, Lilford R: The effect on fetal arteriolar oxygen saturation resulting from giving oxygen to the mother measured by pulse oximetry. Br J Obstet Gynaecol 100:446, 1993.

21. Meschia G: Placental respiratory gas exchange and fetal oxygenation. In Creasy R, Resnik R (eds): Maternal-Fetal Medicine: Principles and Practice, 2nd ed. Philadelphia, WB Saunders, 1989, p 303-313.

22. Lipshitz J, Klose CW: Use of tocolytic drugs to reverse oxytocin-induced uterine hypertonus and fetal distress. Obstet Gynecol 66:16S, 1985.

23. Tejani NA, Verma UL, Chatterjee S, et al: Terbutaline in the management of acute intrapartum fetal acidosis. J Reprod Med 28:857, 1983.

24. Valenzuela GJ, Foster TC: Use of magnesium sulfate to treat hyperstimulation in term labor. Obstet Gynecol 75:762, 1990.

25. Vigil-DeGracia P, Simiti E, Lora Y: Intrapartum fetal distress and magnesium sulfate. Int J Gynaecol Obstet 68:3, 2000.

26. Cabero L, Vaz-Romero M, Cerquiera MJ: Conservative treatment of intrapartum fetal acidosis with a beta-mimetic agent. Eur J Obstet Gynecol Reprod Biol 28:185, 1988.

27. Lipshitz J: Use of a b2-sympathomimetic drug as a temporizing measure in the treatment of acute fetal distress. Am J Obstet Gynecol 129:31, 1977.

28. Kulier R, Gulmezoglu AM, Hofmeyr GJ, et al: Beta-mimetics in fetal distress: Randomized, controlled trial. J Perinatal Med 25:97, 1997.

29. Nordstrom L, Chua S, Persson B, et al: Intrapartum tocolysis has no effect on fetal lactate concentration. Eur J Obstet Gynecol Reprod Biol 89:165, 2000.

30. Miyazaki FS, Nevarez F: Saline amnioinfusion for relief of repetitive variable decelerations: A prospective randomized study. Am J Obstet Gynecol 153:301, 1985.

31. Miyazaki FS, Taylor NA: Saline amnioinfusion for relief of variable or prolonged decelerations. A preliminary report. Am J Obstet Gynecol 146:670, 1983.

32. Pierce J, Gaudier FL, Sanchez-Ramos L: Intrapartum amnioinfusion for meconium-stained fluid: Meta-analysis of prospective clinical trials. Obstet Gynecol 95:1051, 2000.

33. Sadovsky Y, Amon E, Bade ME, et al: Prophylactic amnioinfusion during labor complicated by meconium: A preliminary report. Am J Obstet Gynecol 161:613, 1989.

34. Wenstrom KD, Parsons MT: The prevention of meconium aspiration in labor using amnioinfusion. Obstet Gynecol 73:647, 1989.

35. Locatelli A, Vergani P, DiPirro G, et al: Role of amnioinfusion in the management of premature rupture of the membranes at <26 weeks' gestation. Am J Obstet Gynecol 183: 878, 2000.

36. Parilla BV, McDermott DM: Prophylactic amnioinfusion in pregnancies complicated by chorioamnionitis: A prospective, randomized trial. Am J Perinatol 15:649, 1998.

37. Pitt C, Sanchez-Ramos L, Kaunitz AM, et al: Prophylactic amnioinfusion for intrapartum oligohydramnios: A meta-analysis of randomized controlled trials. Obstet Gynecol 96:861, 2000.

38. Washburne JF, Chauhan SP, Magann EF, et al: Amnioinfusion-induced malpresentation. J Miss State Med Assoc 39:240, 1998.

39. Tabor BL, Maier JA: Polyhydramnios and elevated intrauterine pressure during amnioinfusion. Am J Obstet Gynecol 156:130, 1987.

40. Garite TJ, Dildy GA, McNamara H, et al: A multicenter controlled trial of fetal pulse oximetry in the intrapartum management of nonreassuring fetal heart rate patterns. Am J Obstet Gynecol 183:1049, 2000.

41. Lindsay MK: Intrauterine resuscitation of the compromised fetus. Clin Perinatol 26:569, 1999.

42. Hendrix NW, Chauhan SP, Scardo JA, et al: Managing nonreassuring fetal heart rate patterns before cesarean delivery. Compliance with ACOG recommendations. J Reprod Med 45:995, 2000.

43. Jacobs MM, Phibbs RH: Prevention, recognition, and treatment of perinatal asphyxia. Clin Perinatol 16:785, 1989.

44. Moore JJ, Andrews L, Henderson C, et al: Neonatal resuscitation in community hospitals: A regional-based, team-oriented training program coordinated by the tertiary center. Am J Obstet Gynecol 161:849, 1989.

45. Faix RG: Neonatal resuscitation. In Donn SM, Faix RG (eds): Neonatal Emergencies. Mt. Kisco, NY, Futura, 1991, pp 15-30.

46. Comroe JH: Physiology of Respiration. Chicago, Year Book Medical, 1965, pp 114-116.

47. Oca MJ, Becker MA, Dechert RE, Donn SM: Relationship of neonatal endotracheal tube size and airway resistance. Respir Care 47:994, 2002.

48. Carson BS, Losey RW, Bowes WA, et al: Combined obstetric and pediatric approach to prevent meconium aspiration syndrome. Am J Obstet Gynecol 126:712, 1976.

49. Barks JDE: Meconium aspiration and other neonatal aspiration syndromes. In Donn SM, Faix RG (eds): Neonatal Emergencies. Mt. Kisco, NY, Futura, 1991, pp 169-177.

50. Halliday H: Endotracheal intubation at birth for preventing morbidity and mortality in vigorous, meconium-stained infants born at term. Cochrane Database Syst Rev (1):CD000500, 2001.

51. Linder N, Aranda JV, Tsur M, et al: Need for endotracheal intubation and suction in meconium-stained neonates. J Pediatr 112:613, 1988.

52. Liu WF, Harrington T: The need for delivery room intubation of thin meconium in the low-risk newborn: A clinical trial. Am J Perinatol 15:675, 1998.

53. Wiswell TE, Gannon CM, Jacob J, et al: Delivery room management of the apparently vigorous meconium-stained neonate: Results of the multi-center, international collaborative trial. Pediatrics 105:1, 2000.

54. Gregory GA, Gooding CA, Phibbs RH, et al: Meconium aspiration in infants—a prospective study. J Pediatr 85:848, 1974.

55. Vyas H, Milner A, Hopkins I, et al: Physiologic responses to prolonged and slow rise inflation in the resuscitation of the complicated newborn infant. J Pediatr 99:635, 1981.

56. Saugstad OD: Resuscitation of newborn infants with room air or oxygen. Semin Neonatol 6:233, 2001.

57. Saugstad OD, Rootwelt T, Aalen O: Resuscitation of asphyxiated newborn infants with room air or oxygen: An international controlled trial. The Resair 2 study. Pediatrics 102:e1, 1998.

58. Vento M, Asensi M, Sastre J, et al: Six years of experience with the use of room air for the resuscitation of asphyxiated newly born term infants. Biol Neonate 79:261, 2001.

59. Vento M, Asensi M, Sastre J, et al: Resuscitation with room air instead of 100% oxygen prevents oxidative stress in moderately asphyxiated term neonates. Pediatrics 107:642, 2001.

60. Feick HJ, Donn SM: Vascular access and blood sampling. In Donn SM, Faix RG (eds): Neonatal Emergencies. Mt. Kisco, NY, Futura, 1991, pp 31-50.

61. Marks KH: Thermal and caloric balance. In Nelson NM (ed): Current Therapy in Neonatal-Perinatal Medicine, 2nd ed. Philadelphia, BC Decker, 1990, pp 366-369.

62. Donn SM (ed): The Michigan Manual: A Guide to Neonatal Intensive Care, 2nd ed. Armonk, NY, Futura, 1997, pp 10-17.

63. Nelson KB, Ellenberg JH: Apgar scores as predictors of chronic neurologic disability. Pediatrics 68:36, 1981.

64. Donn SM, Goldman EB: Documentation. In Donn SM (ed): The Michigan Manual: A Guide to Neonatal Intensive Care, 2nd ed. Armonk, NY, Futura, 1997, pp 423-425.

CHAPTER 31

Examination of the Critically Ill Neonate

Thomas E. Wiswell and Alan R. Spitzer

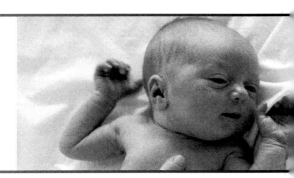

Since the early 1960s, remarkable advances have occurred in the care of newborn infants. Mortality rates are strikingly lower, and care is provided for babies whose birth weights and gestational ages, as well as congenital malformations, were previously incompatible with survival. In many nurseries, babies weighing less than 500 g at birth and as young as 23 weeks' postmenstrual age are now capable of survival, although intact neurologic survival is still relatively uncommon. Above 600 g, however, survival rates increase dramatically, and neurodevelopmental outcome improves substantially as well. Many factors have contributed to improved outcome (Table 31-1). These factors include improved management of the high-risk pregnancy, earlier recognition of life-threatening illnesses (such as necrotizing enterocolitis), regionalized care both for mothers at tertiary centers before delivery and for neonates after birth, the ability to effectively treat newborns with specifically designed ventilators, improved surgical techniques, new methods of prenatal diagnosis, acceleration of lung maturation (steroids), tocolysis, surfactant, total parenteral nutrition, thermoregulation, extracorporeal membrane oxygenation, and neonatal transport systems.

The perinatal period (from the onset of labor to 7 days of age), however, remains the most critical period of life: The risk of dying is higher during this interval than at any other time during a person's life. Even in 2002, 0.7% or more of all liveborn infants died during the first year of life, approximately 27,000 annually in the United States. Seven percent to 10% of newborns are born after a preterm gestation (as many as 16% of black infants), and they are at greater risk for death or disability. Six percent of all newborns require some degree of resuscitation immediately after birth. Two percent to 5% of all neonates require intensive care. Although many of these children are born prematurely, full-term infants are affected as well. The numbers of infants with extremely low birth weight (ELBW) who survive are increasing, although many of these children have sequelae, such as bronchopulmonary dysplasia and retinopathy of prematurity.

To optimize care for the fetus and newborn and achieve intact outcome, we need to determine which infants are critically ill or at risk for subsequent problems. Skilled initial examination of these individuals, as well as sequential follow-up evaluation, adds important information that allows recognition of disease states and enables optimal therapy.

FETAL ASSESSMENT AND DELIVERY ROOM EXAMINATION

Many determinants have been associated with adverse outcomes of the fetus. A partial list of these factors is presented in Table 31-2 (Most of these problems are discussed elsewhere in this book, and the reader is referred to those chapters.) If any of these variables has been identified, the mother and developing fetus should be assessed more frequently. If any of these risk factors has been noted during the pregnancy, a pediatrician or another person skilled in neonatal resuscitation should be present at delivery. However, approximately 40% of neonates who require resuscitation in the delivery room have *not* been previously identified as being at "high risk." The physical findings detected during the first minutes of a newborn's life may therefore dictate whether that child lives and whether the infant will have neurologic sequelae. At times, fetal disorders may have been diagnosed during gestation and a decision is made not to intervene if the child requires resuscitation (for example, anencephaly or trisomy 13). Not so clear-cut, however, is the case of the infant with ELBW (especially <600 g or <24 weeks' gestation). Fetal estimates of weight and gestational age are often inaccurate, and the child may be more mature than previously thought. An accurate scale must be available so that a child's birth weight can be assessed rapidly. Some physicians do not resuscitate if one of the following situations occurs:

1. The neonate's gestational age is less than 24 weeks.
2. Birth weight is within a certain level (400 to 600 g).

Table 31–1. Some of the Factors Contributing to Improved Neonatal Outcome: 1964 to 2003

Improved prenatal and perinatal obstetric management
Enhanced prenatal assessment techniques
Fetal ultrasonography
Prenatal genetic and metabolic diagnosis
Prenatal assessment of lung maturity
Fetal interventional strategies and techniques
Tocolysis
Antepartum referrals to tertiary centers
Tertiary care centers for neonates
Early recognition of illness risk and severity
Neonatal transport
The Neonatal Resuscitation Program
Improved thermal stability
Improved methods of mechanical ventilation
Hastening of lung maturation with steroids
Better surgical techniques for the neonate
Total parenteral nutrition
Surfactant therapy
Collaborative multicenter trials

Table 31–2. Risk Factors for Adverse Fetal or Neonatal Outcome

Antepartum
Congenital infection
Minimal, late, or no prenatal care
Placenta previa
Maternal substance abuse
Fetal malformations
Multiple gestation
Increased or decreased amniotic fluid volume
Blood group incompatability
Increased (>35 years) or decreased (16 years) maternal age
Maternal diabetes
Maternal medications (such as anticonvulsants, lithium)
Maternal connective tissue disorders (such as systemic lupus erythematosus)
Intrauterine growth restriction
Largeness for gestational age
Prematurity (≤37 weeks)
Postmaturity (≥42 weeks)
Other chronic maternal problems
  Thyroid
  Cardiovascular
  Metabolic or other endocrinologic
  Renal
  Neuromuscular
History of genetically inherited diseases (such as cystic fibrosis, neural tube defects)
Decreased fetal activity
History of sexually transmitted diseases (including HIV)
Previous child with congenital malformations
Previous stillbirths
Maternal hypertension (chronic or pregnancy induced)
Immature fetal lungs
Isoimmune thrombocytopenia
Third-trimester bleeding
Uterine structural anomalies
Previous child with chromosomal abnormality
Prenatal diagnosis (in current pregnancy) of chromosomal abnormality
Severe anemia
Nutritional disorders (malnutrition, anorexia, hyperemesis)

Intrapartum
Chorioamnionitis
Maternal urinary tract infection
Abnormal fetal presentation (breech or transverse lie)
Fetal heart rate abnormalities
Meconium-stained amniotic fluid
Maternal drug abuse
Premature rupture of membranes
Prolonged rupture of membranes
Cesarean section delivery
Instrument-assisted delivery (forceps or vaccum)
Abruption of the placenta

HIV, human immunodeficiency virus.

3. The infant with obvious ELBW is in "dire straits" (low heart rate with no respiratory effort).
4. The neonate with ELBW is severely bruised.
5. The child cannot be readily intubated with 2.5-mm inner diameter endotracheal tube.

In cases in which the fetus has ELBW or has a suspected lethal malformation, the parents should be counseled before delivery about their desires regarding resuscitative efforts. If there is any doubt regarding viability in a particular neonate, resuscitative efforts should be instituted. There are no laws mandating that these efforts be continued if the child's status changes at a later point.

How does a clinician assess a neonate during the immediate postpartum period? The most common way is to use the Apgar scoring system (Table 31-3). This score is a critical, systematic, and continuous method of assessing a neonate's condition, resuscitation requirements, and response to resuscitative efforts. The value of the Apgar score has been repeatedly validated. Although other scoring systems, such as the Score for Neonatal Acute Physiology, have been introduced to try to improve upon the predictive value of the Apgar score, the Apgar score is the one that is applied for most births throughout the United States and conveys a significant amount of information to the caregivers of any child. The five components of the Apgar system are heart rate, respiratory effort, color, tone, and reflex irritability (response to noxious stimuli). A score of 0 to 2 is given for each of these variables at 1 and 5 minutes. If the 5-minute Apgar score is less than 7, additional scores are commonly obtained at 5-minute intervals until the infant is 20 minutes of age or until there are two successive scores of 7 or higher. There should be no delay in resuscitative efforts (that is, until the 1-minute Apgar score is assigned) for the child who obviously needs resuscitation. Intervention should begin immediately in

Table 31-3. The Apgar Scoring System

Component	Score		
	0	1	2
Heart rate	Absent	<100/min	>100/min
Respirations	Limp	Slow, irregular	Good, crying
Muscle tone	Limp	Some flexion	Active motion
Reflex irritability (insertion of catheter into nostrils)	No response	Grimace	Cough or sneeze
Color	Blue or pale	Body pink, hands and feet blue	Completely pink

A score of 0 to 2 is assigned for each component at 1 and 5 minutes. If the 5-minute score is less than 7, additional scores should be performed every 5 to 20 minutes until scores are 7 or higher.

such cases. The standard of the American Academy of Pediatrics, the American College of Obstetricians and Gynecologists (ACOG), and the American Heart Association is that someone skilled in neonatal resuscitation should be present in the delivery room whenever a baby is born. An excellent source for training is the Neonatal Resuscitation Program course developed jointly by the American Academy of Pediatrics and American Heart Association (see Chapter 30).

A health care provider in the delivery room should perform a brief physical examination of the child. A more detailed evaluation takes place later. The most severely ill neonates usually manifest their problems immediately after birth. They often need resuscitation and stabilization in the delivery room, followed by intensive care. If a hospital is unable to care for critically ill neonates, arrangements should be made for transfer to a tertiary care center as soon as possible. Ninety percent of the hospitals in the United States in which babies are delivered do not have level II or III nurseries. Many infants who are thought initially to be "well" and are placed in the "well-baby" nursery subsequently manifest symptoms of underlying malformations or illnesses. Examples of such children include those with sepsis or congenital heart disease. The symptoms of such infants are often first noted by nursing personnel, as the initial well-baby physical examination may not take place until the child is 6 to 24 hours old. In some cases, critical illness may not yet be apparent even at this time. Mothers or nurses may be the first to note cyanosis, apnea, or feeding difficulties, because they spend substantially more time with the child than does an examining physician. The observations of nonphysicians should never be discounted, although some parents are easily alarmed by benign findings or conditions. Their concerns should never be ignored, however, because adverse sequelae might be prevented.

POSTDELIVERY EXAMINATION

One of the most important aspects of the physical examination is assessment of the child's gestational age. Dubowitz and colleagues first described an easy-to-perform method in 1970.[1] This was modified into an even simpler

assessment by Ballard in 1979,[2] with a more recent modification in 1991 (which includes the very premature infant) (Fig. 31-1).[3] These systems use aspects of physical and neuromuscular maturity to determine the gestational age.

Whether in the delivery room or in the nursery, the health care provider needs to recognize whether the child's symptoms represent a life-threatening condition. If so, these findings need to be addressed before a detailed examination is performed. If the child is stable, however, a more extensive physical examination of the newborn can be performed. Several in-depth guides for physical examination of the well neonate are listed in the suggested readings for this chapter.

This chapter describes the key components of the physical examination of a critically ill neonate. In this circumstance, the initial assessment is commonly made simultaneously with procedures or with the institution of therapy. Important initial information that is crucial in this situation includes physical measurements of the child (weight, length, head circumference, and abdominal circumference) and vital signs (heart rate, respiratory rate, and blood pressure). Oxygen saturation is increasingly included as part of the assessment of vital signs.

At the time of the examination, the seriously ill baby is often wearing clothing and diapers or is covered with drapes. Because every area of the child must be evaluated, these coverings must be removed during the course of the assessment. The critically ill neonate is apt to be connected to a vast array of sophisticated monitoring equipment (e.g., cardiorespiratory monitors, oxygen saturation monitors) and a mechanical ventilator and may have several arterial and venous catheters in place. The inexperienced health care provider may focus excessively on this equipment or laboratory evaluations, rather than on the baby. In this age of technologic wizardry, too little credence and importance are given to the basic skills of physical examination. Both subtle and gross abnormalities that reflect major illness may not be elicited with exclusive reliance on technology but, however, may be found with this "hands-on" evaluation.

In initiating the physical examination, the examiner should have warmed hands and equipment during the evaluation. Adequate hand washing is absolutely essential

Neuromuscular Maturity

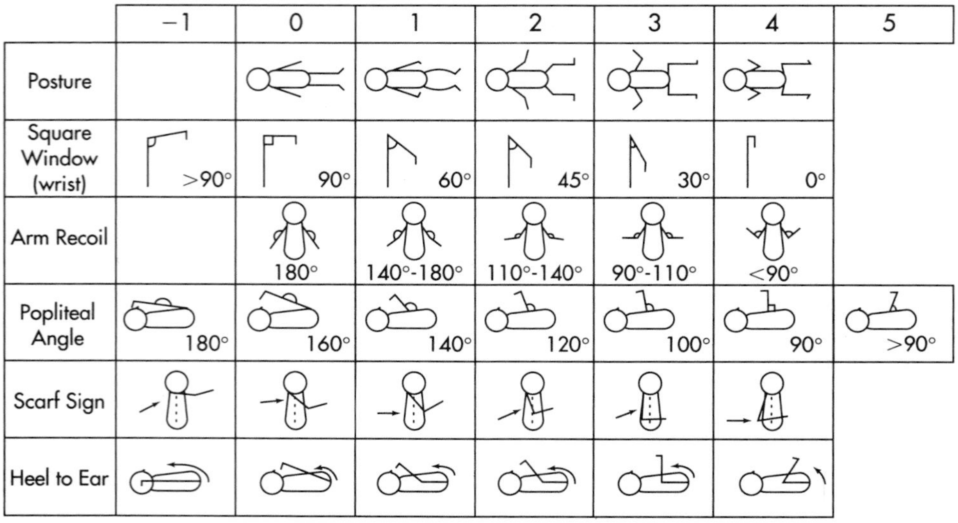

	−1	0	1	2	3	4	5
Posture							
Square Window (wrist)	>90°	90°	60°	45°	30°	0°	
Arm Recoil		180°	140°–180°	110°–140°	90°–110°	<90°	
Popliteal Angle	180°	160°	140°	120°	100°	90°	>90°
Scarf Sign							
Heel to Ear							

Physical Maturity

								Maturity Rating	
Skin	sticky friable transparent	gelatinous red, translucent	smooth pink, visible veins	superficial peeling and/or rash. few veins	cracking pale areas rare veins	parchment deep cracking no vessels	leathery cracked wrinkled	**score**	**weeks**
Lanugo	none	sparse	abundant	thinning	bald areas	mostly bald		−10	20
								−5	22
Plantar Surface	heel-toe 40–50 mm: −1 < 40 mm: −2	> 50 mm no crease	faint red marks	anterior transverse crease only	creases ant. 2/3	creases over entire sole		0	24
								5	26
Breast	imperceptible	barely perceptible	flat areola no bud	stippled areola 1–2 mm bud	raised areola 3–4 mm bud	full areola 5–10 mm bud		10	28
								15	30
								20	32
Eye/Ear	lids fused loosely: −1 tightly: −2	lids open pinna flat stays folded	sl. curved pinna; soft; slow recoil	well-curved pinna; soft but ready recoil	formed and firm instant recoil	thick cartilage ear stiff		25	34
								30	36
Genitals male	scrotum flat, smooth	scrotum empty faint rugae	testes in upper canal rare rugae	testes descending few rugae	testes down good rugae	testes pendulous deep rugae		35	38
								40	40
Genitals female	clitoris prominent labia flat	prominent clitoris small labia minora	prominent clitoris enlarging minora	majora and minora equally prominent	majora large minora small	majora cover clitoris and minora		45	42
								50	44

Figure 31–1. Ballard Modification of Dubowitz Examination for gestational age assessment.

before and immediately after touching the infant. Nothing prevents nosocomial infections better than good hand washing. Nosocomial infections occur in a sizable proportion (if not the majority) of sick infants who require prolonged hospitalization. Furthermore, all examining equipment (e.g., stethoscope, otoscope) should be carefully cleaned between uses (a minimum of wiping off with alcohol should be performed).

Sequence of Examination

What is the best sequence of examination? Procedures that cause the baby the least stress should be performed first. The evaluation should be gentle, unrushed, and minimally disturbing to the infant. Nothing in the examination is more important than observation. The examiner can often assess even subtle abnormalities by simply inspecting the child for a few moments. To elicit nuances of some disorders, nothing is more valuable to the examiner than repeated practice. The experiences gleaned from examining scores of healthy, as well as sick, infants help the examiner more readily detect deviations.

During the initial inspection of the infant, several aspects of the examination should be assessed: (1) overall size and contour (including the head, trunk, abdomen, and extremities); (2) color; (3) respiratory pattern and presence of distress; (4) posture and tone; (5) state of alertness; (6) gross anatomic malformations or injuries; and (7) presence of spontaneous or rhythmic movements.

A general rule is that any child with one anatomic malformation is more likely to have additional anomalies.

After observation of the child, the examiner should auscultate the heart, lungs, and abdomen, because it is necessary that the child remain quiet and nonagitated. If the child remains quiet, palpation of the abdomen can then be performed. A gentle touch, even with deep palpation, often leads to a successful examination. The specific items assessed in examination of the heart, lungs, and abdomen are described later.

We next attempt to examine the child's eyes. The slope of the eyes and the intrapupillary distance should be assessed (wide-spaced eyes versus narrow-spaced eyes). Using one hand, we try gently to separate the upper and lower eyelids. The color of the sclera should be assessed, as should the presence of any iris or eyelid abnormalities (such as colobomata). With the ophthalmoscope, we try to tangentially examine the eye for corneal and lens opacities. The presence and extent of lens vessels can be used to estimate the gestational age of a premature infant. At this time, the pupillary response to light is checked. Visualization of the fundus is performed to ascertain whether there is a normal pink retina ("red reflex") and a clear visual tract.

We then proceed to examine the child from head to toe, and we closely inspect and palpate each area. If the child is clinically stable, a "full" assessment is performed. We first examine the child's head, looking for molding, a caput succedaneum (edema of the scalp caused by pressure), or a cephalohematoma (caused by subperiosteal hemorrhage). The size and contours of the head (the presence of obvious megalencephaly, hydrocephaly, or microcephaly) should be noted, as should the occipital-frontal circumference. The sutures and the fontanels are palpated. Are the sutures mobile, separated, contiguous, overlapping, or physically fused? Are both the anterior and posterior fontanels open and soft, or are they tense and bulging? The anterior fontanel is usually several times larger than the posterior and is more easily found, even with overriding sutures. Is there a third fontanel (often present with chromosomal disorders)? Because of molding, the examiner may have to wait 1 or 2 days before being able to adequately evaluate the fontanels and sutures.

Visible Skull Defects

Visible skull defects need close consideration. A defect in the skin (cutis aplasia) may be associated with trisomy 13, and an indentation or dimple may indicate a depressed skull fracture. Aberrant bulging of tissue (not always cystic in nature), regardless of the location on the skull, may be characteristic of an encephalocele. Encephaloceles, although most commonly found in the occipital area, may be located elsewhere on the head (parietally, intranasally). The skull bones themselves should also be palpated. A "ping-pong ball" response (craniotabes) is often associated with metabolic bone disorders. Unusual whorls or hair patterns may be the only visible manifestation of certain underlying brain malformations. Is the amount of hair excessive? Does the hair extend excessively down the forehead or down the nape of the neck? If there is a suspicion of hydrocephalus or hydranencephaly, the clinician should transilluminate the skull. Finally, in an infant with either unexplained congestive heart failure or numerous hemangiomas, auscultation of the anterior fontanel may reveal a bruit, which may be a manifestation of aberrant intracranial vascular shunting of blood.

The ears should be externally inspected for location (e.g., whether they are low set), position, and rotation. The placement of the ears is typically defined by drawing an imaginary line from the outer canthus of the eye to the occiput. The pinna of the ear should lie above that line in normal circumstances. Are the pinnae underdeveloped or otherwise malformed? Are preauricular skin tags present? Are the ear canals patent? Can the tympanic membranes, which are often obscured by vernix, be visualized? All these factors may give clues to certain malformation syndromes.

Patency of the nostrils can be assessed by either auscultation of air flow at each orifice or by the passage of a soft catheter. Is there nasal flaring? Is the philtrum of the upper lip normal? Are the lips and palate intact, or has clefting occurred during gestation? Soft palate clefts are often small and not easily detected. Are there any intraoral cysts or other masses? Is the tongue excessively large? Are the mandible and maxilla of normal size and configuration? Are the mouth and other facial movements symmetric when the child is crying?

On inspection and palpation of the neck, are there any obvious fissures, cysts, or masses? If so, their location should be further assessed. Are these lesions in the midline, or is their origin in the lateral regions of the neck? In addition, neck mobility should be evaluated. Excessive posterior nuchal skin (webbing) should also be noted.

On examination of the chest, unusual protrusion or an inward configuration of the sternum should be noted. An unusually small or bell-shaped thorax may be seen with pulmonary hypoplasia. An increased anterior-posterior chest diameter is common with the air trapping of meconium aspiration syndrome. Intercostal retractions always mean either volume loss from the lungs or inspiratory obstruction, and more detailed evaluation, especially by chest radiograph, is necessary. Is the chest symmetric? Are supernumerary nipples present? Is breast tissue hypertrophy (normal-from maternal hormones) or a breast abscess present? Is there a discharge from the nipple area ("witches' milk," pus, blood, or mucus)? Are the breath sounds equal and symmetric? Are there bowel sounds in the chest? Are rhonchi, rales, grunting, or stridor audible on auscultation? The examiner should consider transilluminating the chest if a pneumothorax, pneumomediastinum, or pneumopericardium is suspected (distant or absent breath sounds, distant cardiac sounds). The examiner should also palpate the clavicles, because fractures may be associated with crepitus over the affected area.

Examination of the Heart

Examination of the heart is an essential part of the assessment. Persistent global cyanosis (nonperipheral or noncircumoral) may indicate structural cardiac malformations. The point of maximum impulse should be observed or palpated. An abnormal "heave" of the chest may be indicative of aberrant ventricular enlargement. Pulses should be palpated in all four extremities. Weak or absent pulses, as well as the presence of bounding pulses, are abnormal findings. Weakness of all pulses may indicate diminished cardiac output, peripheral vasoconstriction, or hypoplastic left heart syndrome. "Bounding" pulses, in which an abnormally vigorous pulse is felt, are commonly found after several days of life in premature infants with a patent ductus arteriosus. In affected infants, pulses are often palpated in the palms of the hands. If lower extremity pulses are diminished, four-extremity blood pressures should be obtained. Grossly disparate blood pressures between the upper and lower extremities may be indicative of an aortic coarctation. For any noninvasive blood pressure measurement, use of appropriate cuff sizes is of paramount importance.

Palpation and auscultation of the heart may reveal a shift in cardiac position from the normal expected area. The examiner must consider abnormal cardiac location caused by displacement (such as pneumothorax or diaphragmatic hernia) or dextrocardia.

The normal neonatal heart rate ranges from 120 to 160 beats per minute. Agitation or medications (theophylline, pancuronium) may increase the rate. Persistent heart rates of less than 90 beats per minute are abnormal in a neonate, even during relaxed, deep sleep. Heart rates below 80 usually indicate conduction disturbances of the heart. Regularity of the heart rate should be noted.

Auscultation may be difficult because of the rapidity of the heart rate and the presence of other distracting sounds (particularly mechanical ventilation). Distraction because of the former may be overcome with concentration and experience; the latter may be dealt with by briefly disconnecting the child from the ventilator. Murmurs are uncommonly associated with structural cardiac anomalies. In fewer than 5% to 10% of times that neonatal murmurs are heard, a malformation is present. Furthermore, with the many structural cardiac malformations, murmurs are sometimes not heard. The most commonly auscultated murmurs are flow murmurs that represent transition from the fetal circulation (perinatal adaptations). The murmur of tricuspid regurgitation is common in asphyxiated neonates and in those with persistent pulmonary hypertension. The murmur of a patent ductus arteriosus is often heard among premature infants, particularly as they are recovering from respiratory distress syndrome. A persistent murmur in a healthy, full-term neonate should be further evaluated, as should any murmur in a critically ill baby. This evaluation should minimally consist of palpation of pulses and blood pressure measurements in all four extremities, liver palpation, chest radiograph, electrocardiogram, and echocardiogram. An arterial blood gas measurement should be considered, particularly if cyanosis is present.

Examination of the Abdomen

The abdomen of the newborn is usually rounded in appearance, is soft to palpation, and moves synchronously with spontaneous or mechanical breaths. A scaphoid appearance at birth is often seen in infants with a congenital diaphragmatic hernia. Serial observations of the abdomen and abdominal circumference measurements are important if intraabdominal pathologic processes are suspected. Inspection of the abdomen is useful in the presence of obstruction, ileus, peritonitis, or necrotizing enterocolitis. The examiner may easily note abdominal wall erythema, visible bowel loops, distended vessels, or overall distention. Bowel sounds should be auscultated before palpation. Bowel obstruction may be associated with high-pitched, normal, or decreased bowel sounds. The examiner must perform palpation with warmed hands while the child is as relaxed as possible. It is performed gently and systematically, because all four quadrants are evaluated. Palpation of the liver, spleen, bladder, and kidneys should be attempted. The liver is normally palpable 0.5 to 2 cm below the costal margin. The spleen is either not palpable or is palpable only 0.5 to 1 cm below the costal margin. The most common abnormal palpable masses are of renal origin (hydronephrosis and multicystic kidney). Diastasis recti is a common benign finding and is detectable as a longitudinal gap in the musculature of the midline of the abdomen. Is periumbilical erythema present? Is the umbilicus meconium stained, withered, or dystrophic? Can three umbilical vessels (two arteries and one vein) be identified? Is drainage from the cord present? Is an umbilical hernia present? If so, is it reducible?

The back of the neonate should be examined for the presence of unusual tissue (such as tufts of hair), masses, other dermatologic findings (such as hemangiomas), or a pilonidal dimple or sinus. Many of these findings are associated with spina bifida occulta. The examiner should note any obvious deformities of the spine (dysraphism, masses).

In infant boys, the prepuce normally covers the entire glans of the penis. Thus, a physiologic (nonobstructive) phimosis is present. The shaft of the penis should be inspected for the presence of epispadias or hypospadias. The testes should be identified and palpated. Are they present in the scrotum or the canal, or are they not palpable? Hydroceles are commonly observed in neonates. They are typically unilateral and result in increased scrotal size with a tight, cystic appearance. In infant girls, the clitoris should be inspected for abnormal size. The labia, particularly the labia minora, are relatively large in neonates, especially among premature infants. Mucoid or bloody vaginal discharges during the first week of life are common (a benign response to the withdrawal of maternal hormones), as are mucoid tags on the wall of the vagina. Reference values are available for penile and clitoral size for various gestational ages. Inguinal hernias are common among premature infants. It is important to note whether the hernias are easily reducible.

The anus and rectum should be checked carefully for patency, position, and size. Blood is often found in the stool of critically ill neonates. Although it may be an insignificant finding in many instances, it may also herald the development of necrotizing enterocolitis. The anus should be checked carefully for the presence of fissures, which may be the source of the blood.

The extremities should be examined for the presence of structural malformation (clubfoot, polydactyly). Range of motion should be assessed. Are movements and sensation normal? Are the extremities of equal size bilaterally? Are the nails normal? Aberrant dermatoglyphics are common among children with chromosomal disorders, particularly trisomies 13, 18, and 21. The hips need to be evaluated for possible dislocation with the Barlow and Ortolani maneuvers. Part of the Dubowitz examination is assessment of the popliteal angle. In premature infants with intracranial hemorrhages, this maneuver often reveals decreased extension. Fixed contractures of the joints (arthrogryposis) may be found in children with abnormalities of the central nervous system, peripheral nerves, or skeletal muscles. Acutely or chronically ill newborns may develop deep-seeded infections of the joints, bones, or soft tissue. Catheter sites, whether they are infiltrated or not, need to be frequently examined for infection, edema, or ischemia.

Neurologic Examination

The essentials of the neurologic examination can be accomplished while the other portions of the physical examination (the neurologic examination is described in greater detail in Chapter 52) are performed. Observation is critical. Does the infant make normal, responsive, symmetric movements? Are the posture and tone normal? Tone depends on gestational age, as well as illness. Is the response to stimuli normal? Several basic reflexes should be assessed: the Moro, plantar, palmar, sucking, rooting, stepping, tonic neck, crossed extension, and deep tendon reflexes. Is there excessive head lag? Is the child hyperirritable or inconsolable? What is the level of consciousness—that is, is the child alert, lethargic, or comatose? Does the child have normal sleep states?

Throughout the examination, the child is assessed for dermatologic findings. There are many common variants in newborns (capillary hemangiomas, icterus, Mongolian spots, and so on). All of the dermatologic findings, normal and otherwise, should be recorded. Both capillary and strawberry hemangiomas seem to be more common in premature neonates, for reasons that are unclear.

SPECIAL CONSIDERATIONS

The Premature Infant

The number of premature infants who survive has increased dramatically since the early 1970s. The threshold of viability (in terms of gestational age and birth weight) continues to progress downward, although there does appear to be a limit at 23 weeks' postmenstrual age. Clinicians need to be cognizant of the strikingly different appearance of premature babies in comparison with full-term infants, differences that are proportional to the degree of prematurity. For example, an 800-g child at 25 weeks of gestational age is noticeably different in appearance from a 1400-g premature infant at 30 weeks of gestational age, who in turn looks very different from a 3200-g, full-term, healthy neonate.

Effect of Prematurity or Illness on the Examination

The premature infant may not tolerate aspects of the physical examination as well as a full-term child. Furthermore, any critically ill child, regardless of gestational age, may respond adversely to the examination. Those with persistent pulmonary hypertension should be minimally disturbed, because irritation in such a child as a response to stimuli can predispose to worsening of the right-to-left shunting. Similarly, a septic, hypotensive child can have detrimental reactions to stimuli, as can an irritable child with chronic lung disease.

Neonates may react with oxygen desaturation, bronchospasm, bradycardia, tachycardia, or alterations (increases or decreases) in blood pressures. If any of these reactions occur, particularly if they are sustained, the examination should be interrupted and deferred for the time being. The clinician should resume the examination only when it is clear that the child's values have returned to baseline. If it takes more than a minute to do so, the degree of illness is likely to be very serious. Clinical judgment is essential in the decision to discontinue various aspects of the examination. Because each child's tolerance and response are different, there is no blanket recommendation regarding curtailing the examination of all neonates of a certain gestational age or with a particular diagnosis. The examiner has to weigh the value of the information that can be gleaned against the adverse effect on the child. Because the heart rate, respiratory rate, blood pressure, and oxygen saturation are monitored in virtually all critically ill neonates, an unpropitious response to aspects of the evaluation is usually immediately evident.

Ill children are often connected to an array of life-sustaining systems, including indwelling catheters, ventilators, and monitors. Many essential functions are performed with these devices (such as dopamine infusion to maintain blood pressure support or connection to a ventilator to avoid hypoxemia and hypercarbia). The examiner must take care not to disrupt the functions these devices provide (e.g., accidentally dislodging an endotracheal tube or a chest tube).

Technologic advances may hamper the examiner, and a child in an incubator is more difficult to access than one on a radiant warmer. In an infant being treated with high-frequency ventilation, the heart and lungs may not be auscultated easily unless the devices are transiently disconnected. Newer technologies, such as liquid ventilation or inhalational nitric oxide, may preclude an adequate examination, because their interruption could adversely affect the baby.

Influence of Medications

Numerous medications may influence the findings on a child's examination. Maternally administered narcotics or general anesthesia can lead to hypotonia and an inadequate respiratory effort in an infant. The use of magnesium for maternal hypertension or preeclampsia may also depress the child's values and make the examination difficult. Drugs given to the baby, such as fentanyl or pancuronium, may affect the examination dramatically (e.g., changes in tone, respirations, responsivity, heart rate, and blood pressure). The examiner needs to know whether such medications are influencing the examination of an individual newborn.

ADJUNCTIVE ASSESSMENT

There are a number of ways to increase the amount of information concerning a particular child. Some of these ways involve invasive technologies; others do not.

Additional data can be obtained with the use of ultrasound assessment, electroencephalography, electrocardiography, roentgenograms (with or without contrast material), computed tomography, magnetic resonance imaging, pulmonary function testing, angiography, bronchoscopy, nuclear scans, mass spectroscopy, and positron emission tomography. However, many of these techniques are not portable and can be performed only in specialized locations because of the size, type, or weight of the equipment. These locations can be a great distance from the nursery: for example, on a different floor of the hospital or in another facility. Transport of the critically ill neonate has its own inherent risks. Once again, the clinician must balance the information that can be gained versus the risks to the child.

REFERENCES

1. Dubowitz L, Dubowitz V, Goldberg C: Clinical assessment of gestational age in the newborn infant. J Pediatr 77:1, 1970.
2. Ballard JL, Novak KK, Driver M: A simplified score for assessment of fetal maturity of newly born infants. J Pediatr 95:769, 1979.
3. Ballard JL, Khoury JC, Wedig K, et al: New Ballard score, expanded to include extremely premature infants. J Pediatr 119:417, 1991.

SUGGESTED READINGS

Algranati PS: The Pediatric Patient: An Approach to History and Physical Examination. Baltimore, Williams & Wilkins, 1992.

Neonatal Resuscitation Manual. Elk Grove Village, Ill, American Heart Association and the American Academy of Pediatrics, 2003.

Athreya BH, Silverman BK, Spitzer AR: Pediatric Physical Diagnosis. Norwalk, Conn, Appleton-Century-Crofts, 1985.

Arias E, MacDorman MF, Strobino DM, Guyer B: Annual summary of vital statistics—2002. Pediatrics 112:1215, 2003.

Beachy P, Deacon J (eds): Core curriculum for neonatal intensive care nursing. Philadelphia, WB Saunders, 1993.

Behrman RE, Kliegman RM, Jenson HB: Nelson Textbook of Pediatrics, 17th ed. Philadelphia, WB Saunders, 2003.

Buyse ML (ed): Birth Defects Encyclopedia. Dover, Mass, Center for Birth Defects Information Services, 1990.

Cloherty JP, Stark AR (eds): Manual of Neonatal Care, 5th ed. Boston, Little, Brown, 2004.

Creasy RK, Resnik R (eds): Maternal-Fetal Medicine: Principles and Practice, 5th ed. Philadelphia, WB Saunders, 2003.

Davis DJ: How aggressive should delivery room cardiopulmonary resuscitation be for extremely low birth weight neonates? Pediatrics 92:447, 1993.

Fanaroff AA, Martin RJ (eds): Neonatal-Perinatal Medicine, 6th ed. St. Louis, Mosby–Year Book, 2002.

Freeman RK, Poland RL, Hauth JC, et al (eds): Guidelines for Perinatal Care, 5th ed. Elk Grove Village, Ill, American Academy of Pediatrics and American College of Obstetricians and Gynecologists, 2003.

Hittner HM, Hirsch NJ, Rudolph AJ: Assessment of gestational age by examination of the anterior vascular capsule of the lens. J Pediatr 1:455, 1977.

Hoekelman RA, Friedman SB, Nelson NM, et al (eds): Primary pediatric care, 2nd ed. St. Louis, Mosby–Year Book, 1992.

Jones KL: Recognizable Patterns of Human Malformation, 5th ed. Philadelphia, WB Saunders, 1997.

Klaus MH, Fanaroff AA: Care of the high-risk neonate, 5th ed. Philadelphia, WB Saunders, 2002.

Long WA: Fetal and Neonatal Cardiology. Philadelphia, WB Saunders, 1990.

Manning FA: Fetal monitoring. Clin Perinatol 16:583, 1989.

McMillan JA, DeAngelis CD, Feigin RD, et al (eds): Oski's Pediatrics, 3rd ed. Baltimore, Williams & Wilkins, 1999.

Moss GD, Cartlidge PHT, Speidel BD, et al: Routine examination in the neonatal period. BMJ 302:878, 1991.

Seidel HM, Rosenstein BJ, Pathak A: Primary Care of the Newborn. St. Louis, Mosby–Year Book, 1993.

Taeusch HW, Ballard RA, Avery ME (eds): Schaeffer and Avery's Diseases of the Newborn, 7th ed. Philadelphia, WB Saunders, 1998.

Volpe JJ: Neurology of the Newborn, 4th ed. Philadelphia, WB Saunders, 2001.

Willett MJ, Patterson M, Steinbock B: Manual of Neonatal Intensive Care Nursing. Boston, Little, Brown, 1986.

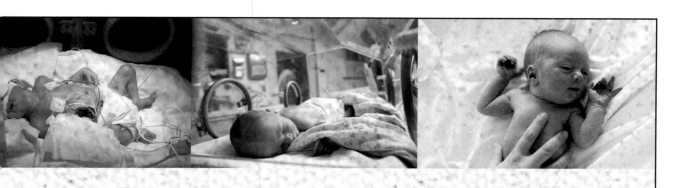

Intensive Care of Neonates:
General Considerations

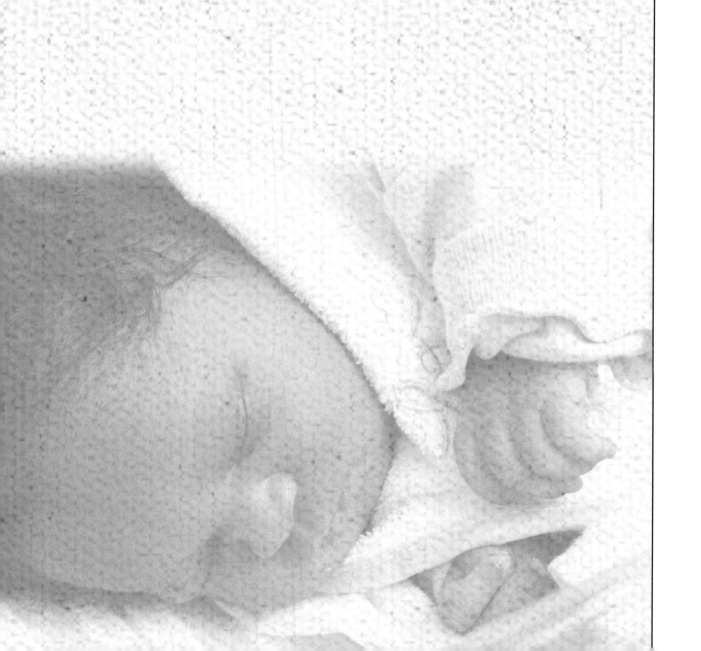

CHAPTER 32

Radiology in the Intensive Care Nursery

George W. Gross

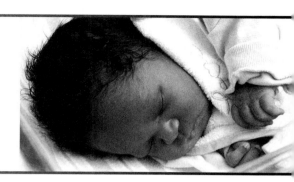

I maging of newborns requires modifications to the techniques applied to children and adolescents. If the newborn is in the intensive care nursery (ICN), particular care must be devoted to maintaining the patient's fragile clinical state. Because it usually is too hazardous to move a premature or critically ill newborn to the radiology department, portable imaging studies are often essential. Portable studies are usually of lesser overall diagnostic quality than nonportable studies performed in the radiology department using standard imaging equipment. Examinations such as the barium swallow and barium enema, which require fluoroscopic imaging, may be precluded because of the inability to transport the patient. Portable ultrasound equipment may not have all the imaging and recording features that are available on nonportable units.

IMAGING TECHNIQUES

Portable Radiography

Portable radiographic units are of the capacitor-discharge or battery-operated types with variable kilovoltage (kVp) and milliamperage (mA) selections.[1] Any mobile unit used in neonatal radiography must be small enough to fit between the Isolette and any overhead heating or monitoring equipment (Fig. 32-1).[1] To overcome patient motion, an output of at least 100 mA is necessary to permit sufficiently short exposure times.[1] Standard portable neonatal chest radiography uses a 40-inch distance and an average technique of 50 to 60 kVp at 0.8 to 1.2 mA.[1]

Nongrid cassettes with 400-speed, rare-earth, film-screen combinations should be used to minimize patient dose.[1] Exposure doses are in the range of 5 mrad for a portable anteroposterior chest radiograph to 8 mrad for a portable anteroposterior abdominal radiograph.[1] Nursing and other personnel in the ICN receive negligible radiation exposure and need not leave the room or wear a protective apron as long as they are at least 1 foot from the primary, vertically oriented x-ray beam.[1]

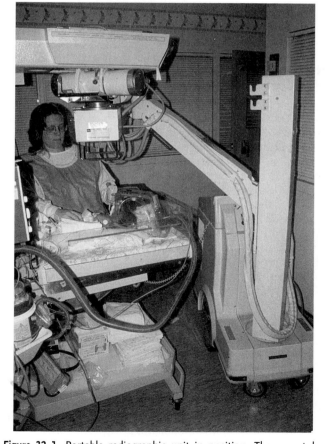

Figure 32-1. Portable radiographic unit in position. The x-ray tube and housing are positioned over the patient and beneath the overhead heating unit. A cassette holding the radiographic film to be exposed is placed beneath the mattress or padding under the patient. A lead apron typically is worn by the technologist because of proximity to the patient.

Special Projections

Conventional portable chest and abdominal radiography in the ICN involves an anteroposterior view as the minimal study and does not require repositioning of the neonate from the customary supine position. Lateral views of the chest and abdomen can be "cross-table," using a horizontally oriented x-ray beam and requiring no patient repositioning. Recumbent, nonsupine lateral views of the chest, with the patient turned up onto one side, tend to yield images of better diagnostic value. Routine use of a portable lateral view of the chest in ICN patients is *not* warranted.[2] Decubitus views of the abdomen, particularly the left decubitus position (left side down), are most helpful in excluding free intraperitoneal air, which tends to migrate to the space between the right lateral abdominal wall and liver. Neonatal magnification radiography has been advocated as a means of improving anatomic definition and reducing patient radiation exposure, but it has not achieved general acceptance.[3-5]

Fluoroscopy

Fluoroscopy, or dynamic radiography, of the newborn's gastrointestinal tract or airway may be clinically important, but it requires patient transport to the radiology department and is often precluded by the patient's critical clinical status.[1] Intubation or other life-support apparatus complicates, but does not preclude, the use of fluoroscopy.

Nonportable and Portable Contrast Studies of the Gastrointestinal Tract

Contrast examination of the gastrointestinal tract in neonates and infants should be performed, if possible, in the radiology fluoroscopic suite, permitting optimal anatomic definition and functional evaluation and control over ingested or infused contrast material. For routine intestinal examinations, barium sulfate is the contrast agent of choice.[1,6]

If contrast examination of the intestinal tract is to be performed and there is concern for bowel perforation, water-soluble contrast agents should be substituted for barium.[1] Hyperosmolar agents, such as diatrizoate (Hypaque or Renografin), draw fluid into the bowel lumen and can produce dehydration and electrolyte imbalance.[1,7] Newer, nonionic iso-osmolar water-soluble agents, such as iopamidol (Isovue), are expensive but safer, cause negligible fluid shift, are not absorbed from the bowel, and provide good opacification over a prolonged period.[1]

If fluoroscopic examination is precluded by the patient's critical clinical status and patient management requires assessment of the status of the intestinal tract (intestinal perforation, bowel obstruction, necrotizing enterocolitis [NEC]), portable contrast examination of the gastrointestinal tract in the ICN is possible.[8] After positioning of an end-hole-only catheter in the stomach and confirmation of satisfactory position of the catheter by an abdominal radiograph, 5 to 10 mL of nonionic, water-soluble iodinated contrast material (e.g., Isovue) is injected into the stomach with the patient turned up onto the right side to promote passage into the bowel. Delayed abdominal radiographs at periodic intervals (based on rate of progression of contrast material) are obtained, until contrast material has reached the colon or rectum. Additional contrast material in 5-mL increments can be injected as required. Bowel perforation appears as contrast material diffusing into the peritoneal cavity (either localized or generalized) or as excretion of contrast material by the kidneys. Obstruction appears as dilated loops of bowel and lack of proper progression of contrast material down the intestinal tract.

Ultrasonography

Because of its portability and ability to differentiate between solid tissue and simple and complex fluid collections, ultrasonography has important imaging applications in the ICN (Fig. 32-2). The most important application of sonography in the ICN at present is in the

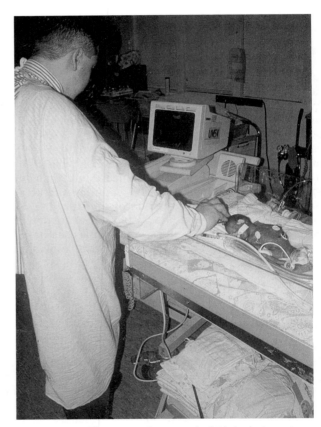

Figure 32–2. Portable sonographic unit at bedside in the intensive care nursery. If the patient is in an Isolette, the sonographic transducer, held by the technologist, reaches the patient through an opening in the Isolette, to minimize disturbance of the patient's environment. The sonographic transducer is positioned for neonatal cranial sonography via the anterior fontanelle. Sonographic contact gel is applied to the transducer head to optimize ultrasound beam transmission. Behind the control panel is the monitor for image viewing. The desired images are "frozen," then either photographed on radiographic film or transferred to an ultrasound picture archiving and communication system for later viewing. Most newer portable ultrasound units have videotaping or "clip store" viewing capabilities or both for real-time imaging review and color Doppler and power Doppler imaging capabilities.

imaging of the neonatal brain. Identification and characterization of pleural and peritoneal fluid collections and assessment of the status of the heart (echocardiography), solid organs, and vessels of the abdomen and retroperitoneum are other important applications.[9,10] Extracardiac thoracic sonography can differentiate drainable pleural fluid collections from pleural thickening, accurately characterize chest and mediastinal masses, guide aspiration and drainage procedures, and allow rapid diagnosis of causes of unilateral opaque hemithorax.[9] Pulsed Doppler and color-Doppler sonography are adjunct sonographic imaging modalities to evaluate blood vessel patency and vascular flow patterns.[11]

Computed Tomography

Computed tomography (CT) lacks portability and has limited use in a critically ill ICN patient. Imaging of the brain as a follow-up to cranial sonography is the primary neonatal application of CT at present. CT is the most sensitive imaging modality for identifying calcification.[12] Direct coronal CT scanning of the neonatal chest is feasible but not applicable to an intubated premature infant.[13]

Magnetic Resonance Imaging

Similar to CT, magnetic resonance imaging (MRI) lacks portability and has had little use in the ICN population to date. Imaging of the brain has been the primary use of MRI in neonates. MRI presents additional problems with patient monitoring and sedation, which are often essential in a neonate.

Nuclear Medicine Procedures

Many nuclear medicine procedures have applicability to pediatric patients.[1] Renal scintigraphy and radionuclide bone scanning are the primary applications of nuclear medicine in neonates. Image recording is typically via a gamma camera; some models have portable capability. Technetium-99m is the most widely used radioisotope because it has a short half-life and low patient-absorbed radiation doses.[1]

Angiography and Interventional Procedures

Angiography in ICN patients may be accomplished via iodinated contrast injection through indwelling vascular catheters (e.g., an umbilical arterial line), but it has had limited application in the ICN population. Interventional procedures, such as drainage of fluid collections, typically are guided by ultrasonography because of its portable capability. Tracheobronchography in neonates and infants on mechanical ventilation can be accomplished using nonionic water-soluble contrast media.[14]

Digital Imaging

Instead of recording the radiographic image directly on film, as occurs with conventional radiography, digital imaging employs either a photostimulable phosphor system (**computed radiography**) or a series of detectors (**digital radiography**) to record quantitatively transmitted x-rays in an area of specific size, called a **pixel**.[7,15] High-quality chest and abdominal radiographs are obtainable using a digital system.[15-17] The potential advantages of digital radiography are a decrease in radiation dose, an increase in image quality, improved diagnostic information from image manipulation, and the potential for transferring images electronically to a picture archiving and communication system or to remote sites (e.g., the ICN).[7,15,17]

RADIATION SAFETY AND PROTECTION

The portable radiographic unit used in the ICN must meet radiation protection standards as determined by the National Council on Radiation Protection. The x-ray tube is shielded, and the emitted x-ray beam is confined to the minimal area required for appropriate imaging, via collimation. Gonadal shielding is used unless the shielding would obscure areas of important imaging evaluation. The typical vertical beam radiography used in the ICN requires nursing and other personnel to be only 1 foot away from the primary x-ray beam. It does not require any lead shielding.[1]

The whole-body radiation dose for a two-view (anteroposterior and lateral) portable chest examination of a neonate varies with exposure factors, but it is generally in the range of 25 to 60 microsieverts (μSv), with a mean of 40 μSv.[18] One year of exposure to natural background radiation is 3 millisieverts (μSv), which is 75 times the dose from one portable chest examination.[18] Patient dosage reduction can be achieved through a combination of x-ray beam hardening via filtration, decreased x-ray attenuation by the cassette, and faster film-screen combinations.[19,20] Low-dose neonatal chest radiographic systems can have reduced image sharpness, however.[19,20]

MISCELLANEOUS PRECAUTIONS AND TECHNICAL CONSIDERATIONS

Protection of the neonate from infection should include clean but nonsterile gowning and handwashing by the technologist.[1,21] The importance of handwashing cannot be overemphasized, especially in a unit in which multiple films must be obtained at one time. In addition, cassettes used for examination of infectious infants should be cleaned with an antiseptic before being used on another patient.[21] Additional cleanliness of cassettes is achieved by wrapping in a disposable plastic bag or sterile sheet.[1]

Maintenance of patient body temperature in the Isolette is essential. The opening in the main door of the Isolette should be kept closed and should be opened as infrequently and briefly as possible.[21] Care must be taken not to disrupt any of the life-support lines and catheters, and the assistance of the nursing personnel in patient positioning and restraint should be encouraged.[1,21]

CATHETERS, TUBES, AND MONITORS EMPLOYED IN NEONATAL CARE

External monitors are usually at least partially opaque and recognizable on standard radiographic projections. Internally positioned catheters and tubes vary considerably

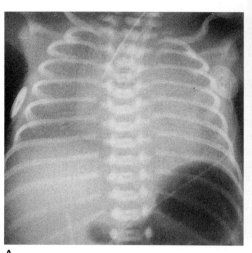

A

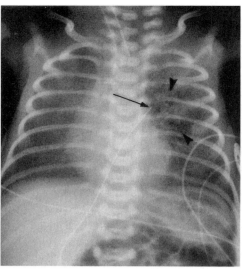

B

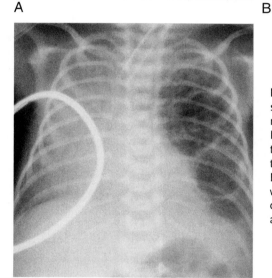

C

Figure 32–3. A, Portable anteroposterior chest radiograph in a premature newborn with severe respiratory distress syndrome and on mechanical ventilation shows diffuse pulmonary granularity consistent with the clinical diagnosis of respiratory distress syndrome. No complication of ventilatory assistance is present. **B,** Two days later, central lucency in the left lung *(arrowheads)* has developed, suggesting interstitial pulmonary air. Note the tip of the umbilical venous catheter in a left upper lobe pulmonary vein *(arrow)*. Endotracheal tube position is good. **C,** By 13 days of age, overexpansion of the left lung with coarse cystic change reflecting much worse pulmonary interstitial emphysema has developed. Relative increase in density of the right lung may reflect in part compressive atelectasis. No pneumothorax occurred in this neonate.

in their radiopacity (or "whiteness") on the radiograph, and many can be difficult to identify and localize with accuracy.

The tip of the endotracheal tube should project about halfway between the medial ends of the clavicles and carina to be in optimal position (Figs. 32-3B, 32-4A, 32-5, and 32-6). If positioned too low, the endotracheal tube tip projects at the carina or may enter the right main bronchus as a result of its closer orientation to the alignment of the trachea (Figs. 32-7B, 32-8, and 32-9). Location of the tip of the endotracheal tube above the thoracic inlet is considered too high (Figs. 32-10 and 32-11). Inadvertent intubation of the esophagus is uncommon (Figs. 32-12 and 32-13). If assisted ventilation beyond 2 to 3 months is necessary, a tracheostomy tube is usually substituted for the endotracheal tube. The preferred tracheostomy tube tip position is about 1 to 1.5 cm above the carina (Fig. 32-14).

The umbilical venous line tip should be near the junction of the right atrium and the inferior vena cava, and the umbilical arterial line tip should project between the third and fifth lumbar vertebrae to be positioned below the major tributaries of the abdominal aorta (Fig. 32-15; see Fig. 32-6). Some neonatologists prefer a "high" umbilical arterial line, in which case the catheter tip should project between the seventh and ninth thoracic vertebral bodies (Fig. 32-16; see also Fig. 32-9). Umbilical venous and arterial catheter malposition is common (Figs. 32-16 through 32-23; see also Fig. 32-3). Precise determination of umbilical venous catheter position is frequently impossible (see Fig. 32-19). Central venous catheter tip position in the superior vena cava or right atrium is preferred (Fig. 32-24).[22] Associated right atrial thrombus formation can be monitored using echocardiography.[22]

Frequently malpositioned, the nasogastric tube tip should be in the proximal portion of the stomach, where

Text continues on p 452.

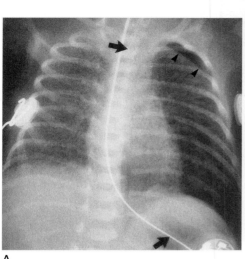

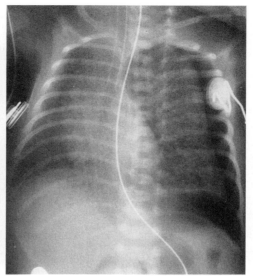

A

B

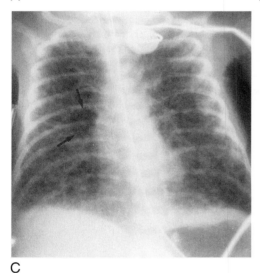

C

Figure 32–4. A, Portable anteroposterior chest radiograph in a 2-day-old premature infant with respiratory distress syndrome shows diffuse increase in pulmonary density compatible with respiratory distress syndrome and accompanied by diffuse interstitial pulmonary emphysema. In addition, there is a left pneumothorax *(arrowheads)*. The pneumothorax tends to collect anterior to the lung in these supine neonates in the intensive care nursery and is usually larger than suggested by the typical anteroposterior supine chest radiograph. The endotracheal and nasogastric tubes *(arrows)* are in good position. **B,** Repeat chest radiograph same day as in **A** after sudden clinical deterioration shows increase in size of the left pneumothorax, now with a tension component. Note the fine cystic changes within the lungs, best seen on the left, reflecting pulmonary interstitial emphysema. **C,** Four days later, there is marked hyperinflation of both lungs with a coarse appearance to the lung parenchyma, reflecting worsening pulmonary interstitial emphysema. Overlying the right hilum is a larger, focal pulmonary cyst *(arrows)*. The left pneumothorax had been aspirated and did not recur.

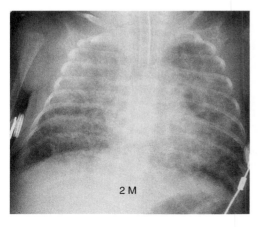

Figure 32–5. A 2-month-old premature infant with respiratory distress syndrome on mechanical ventilation with high ventilatory pressure settings since birth. There are coarse cystic changes throughout both lungs, reflecting severe bronchopulmonary dysplasia. The endotracheal tube is in good position.

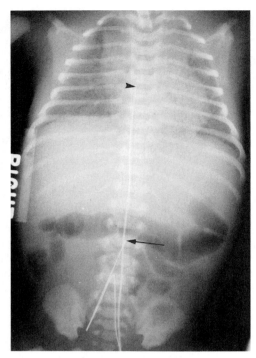

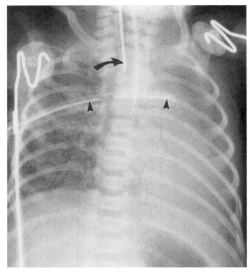

Figure 32–6. A premature newborn with respiratory distress. Diffuse pulmonary granularity with air bronchograms is suggestive of respiratory distress syndrome but in this patient reflected β-streptococcal pneumonia, which can have a radiographic appearance identical to respiratory distress syndrome. Premature rupture of the maternal membranes had occurred. The tip of the umbilical venous catheter *(arrowhead)* is high in the right atrium, higher in position than generally preferred. At L3, the umbilical arterial catheter tip *(arrow)* is in good position of a "low" umbilical artery catheter.

Figure 32–8. A premature infant with respiratory distress syndrome on mechanical ventilatory assistance. The tip of the endotracheal tube is at the carina, too low in location. The end of the nasoenteric tube *(arrow)* is in the upper thoracic esophagus, much too high. The single right pleural chest tube *(arrowheads)* placed for control of a prior pneumothorax extends well across the midline and may have penetrated into the left lung. There is a relative increase in density in the left lower lung zone that suggests partial left lower lobe atelectasis.

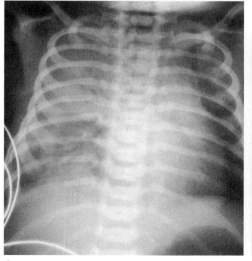

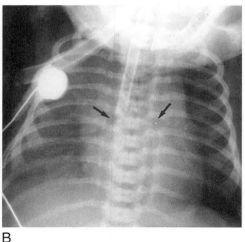

A   B

Figure 32–7. A newborn with postnatal respiratory distress caused by aspiration pneumonia. **A,** The initial postnatal radiograph shows patchy increase in density primarily of the right lung. **B,** Repeat chest radiograph later in the day and after intubation shows improvement in lung aeration and decrease in density but with the tip of the endotracheal tube at the orifice of the right main bronchus, too low in position. Note the right and left main bronchi *(arrows)*. Although the carina often is not well seen on the anteroposterior chest radiograph, its approximate location can be determined by identifying the main bronchi and tracing them in a medial and cephalad direction to their approximate junction point.

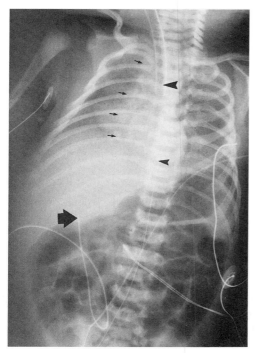

Figure 32–9. A newborn with respiratory distress syndrome. The tip of the endotracheal tube *(large arrowhead)* is at the carina, too low in position. The tip of the umbilical arterial line *(small arrowhead)* overlies T8, satisfactory for a "high" umbilical arterial line but too high for the preferred "low" umbilical arterial line, where the tip should be between L3 and L5. The tip of the umbilical venous line *(large arrow)* projects at the inferior edge of the liver, too low in position but with precise location indeterminate. The patient is rotated to the right, as indicated by the anterior ends of the right ribs projecting much further laterally than do the anterior ends of the left ribs. A vertical line of round opacities projecting over the thorax to the right of midline *(small arrows)* reflects the sternal ossification centers and should not be mistaken for pathology. Normally, on a nonrotated anteroposterior chest radiograph, the sternal ossification centers overlie the spine and are obscured. The intestinal gas pattern is normal, and there is no indication of hepatosplenomegaly.

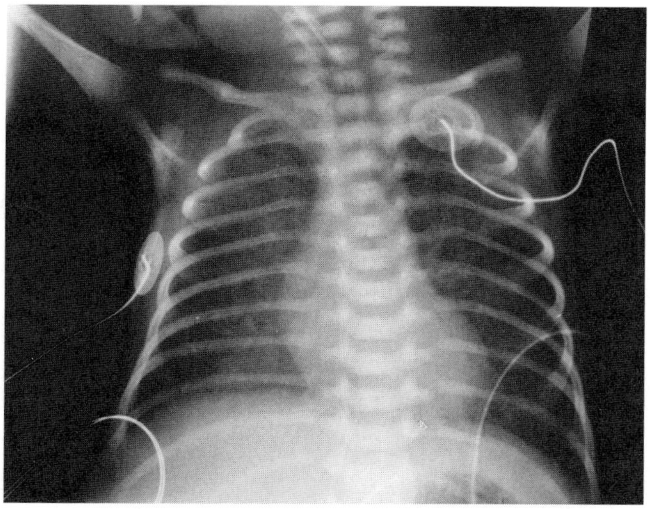

Figure 32–11. The endotracheal tube projects approximately 1 cm above the thoracic inlet (as indicated by the medial ends of the clavicles) and is too high in position. The radiograph is overpenetrated (too dark), which tends to underestimate the severity of pulmonary disease. Underpenetration of the radiograph has the opposite effect.

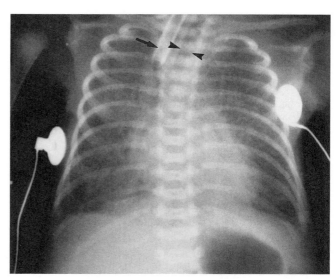

Figure 32–12. The endotracheal tube is malpositioned in the esophagus. The endotracheal tube *(arrow)* is adjacent to but separate from the trachea *(arrowheads)*.

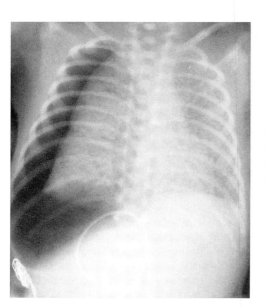

Figure 32–10. A premature newborn with respiratory distress syndrome and on mechanical ventilatory assistance. In addition to diffuse pulmonary granularity reflecting the atelectasis of respiratory distress syndrome, there is mottled pulmonary lucency suggesting pulmonary interstitial emphysema. Additionally a right tension pneumothorax with depression of the right diaphragm and mild mediastinal shift to the left are present.

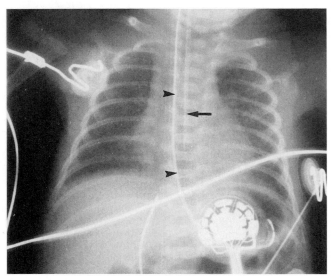

Figure 32–13. The precise location of the endotracheal tube *(arrow)* is indeterminate, but the fact that it extends well below the carina indicates that it cannot be situated in the trachea. Because it precisely parallels the nasogastric catheter *(arrowheads)*, the endotracheal tube was believed to be in the esophagus.

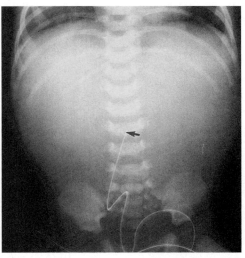

Figure 32–15. Portable anteroposterior supine abdominal radiograph shows complete absence of intestinal gas, which usually reflects absence of swallowing of air caused by paralysis with Pavulon in a patient on assisted mechanical ventilation or with severe central nervous system depression due to perinatal asphyxia. The tip of the umbilical arterial line overlies L3 *(arrow)*. Preferred umbilical arterial line tip position is between L3 and L5, below the major abdominal organ tributaries of the aorta.

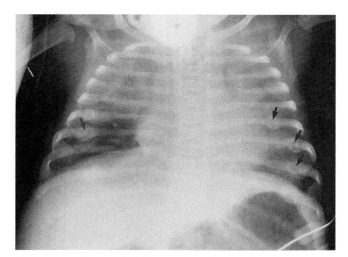

Figure 32–14. A 4-month-old premature infant with bronchopulmonary dysplasia and with a tracheostomy tube for long-term assisted ventilation. The tracheostomy tube is in good position. Diffuse increase in lung density reflects bronchopulmonary dysplasia. There are healing fractures of several ribs bilaterally *(arrows)* resulting from chest physical therapy. Undermineralized ribs in chronically ill neonates are prone to fracturing when subjected to even the relatively mild stress of chest physical therapy to maintain airway patency and help drain secretions.

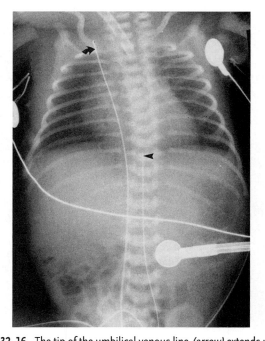

Figure 32–16. The tip of the umbilical venous line *(arrow)* extends up the superior vena cava, ending approximately in the internal jugular vein, much too high in position. The tip of the umbilical arterial line *(arrowhead)* overlies the ninth thoracic vertebral body. This umbilical arterial line position would be satisfactory for a "high" line, but most neonatologists prefer the umbilical arterial line to end in the region of L3 and L4.

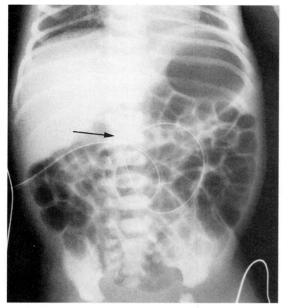

Figure 32–17. Anteroposterior abdominal radiograph obtained to evaluate position of an umbilical venous line. The tip *(arrow)* of the umbilical venous line projects below the edge of the liver, indicating that it is in the umbilical vein, too low in position. The abdomen is normal in appearance, with widely distributed air in nondilated loops of bowel, no suggestion of abdominal mass or fluid collection, and normal liver and spleen size.

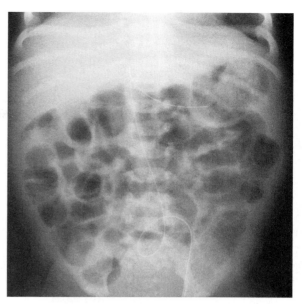

Figure 32–18. The umbilical venous catheter extends to the liver, then deviates sharply to the left upper quadrant, within the splenic vein.

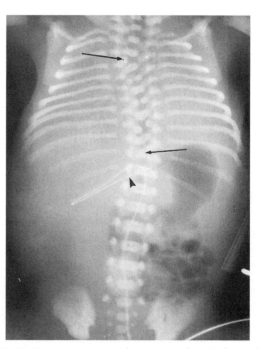

Figure 32–20. A premature (27 weeks gestational age) infant with postnatal respiratory distress. There is near-complete opacification of the lungs with associated air bronchograms, which reflects respiratory distress syndrome (hyaline membrane disease). The umbilical venous catheter *(arrowhead)* is doubled back on itself in the right portal vein. There is incomplete extension of ingested air into the intestinal tract, with bowel gas limited to the stomach, duodenum, and jejunum, with no gas in the right side of the abdomen. This radiograph was obtained within a few hours of birth, so the distribution of intestinal gas can be considered normal. A right-sided abdominal mass must be considered, however, if this gas pattern persists after 24 to 48 hours of life. Note the extensive dysraphism of the thoracic spinal segment *(arrows)*, which would raise the possibility of other associated anomalies as part of the VATER (vertebral defects, imperforate anus, tracheoesophageal fistula, and radial and renal dysplasia) association.

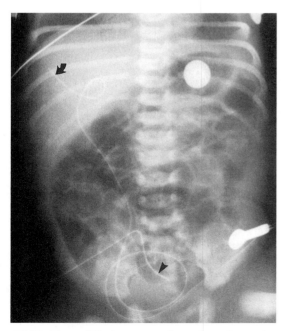

Figure 32–19. The umbilical venous catheter *(arrow)* extends to the right upper quadrant, with a configuration highly atypical for being in the right portal vein. An intraperitoneal location to the umbilical venous catheter is a realistic concern (see Fig. 32-21). The umbilical arterial catheter *(arrowhead)* extends only to the midpelvis region and is probably near the junction of the umbilical and hypogastric arteries.

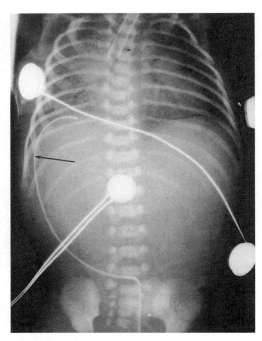

Figure 32–21. The umbilical venous catheter *(arrow)* has a configuration incompatible with an intravenous location. The catheter had perforated the umbilical vein and extended into the peritoneal cavity, causing a hemoperitoneum.

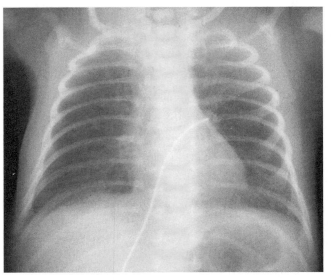

Figure 32–23. The tip of this malpositioned umbilical venous line has traversed the right atrium, foramen ovale, and left atrium and has come to reside in a left upper lobe pulmonary vein. Umbilical venous catheters that have been advanced too far frequently end up in a similar location. The preferred location of the tip of the umbilical venous catheter is at the inferior vena cava–right atrial junction or low in the right atrium.

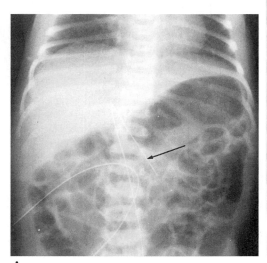

A

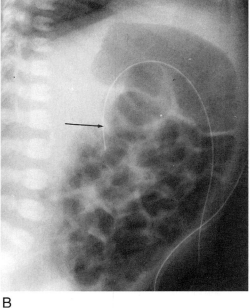

B

Figure 32–22. Anteroposterior **(A)** and lateral **(B)** views show the umbilical venous catheter *(arrow)* extending to the margin of the liver. It then abruptly turns caudally, appearing to lie in the superior mesenteric vein.

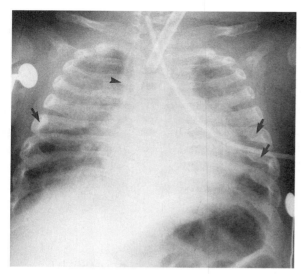

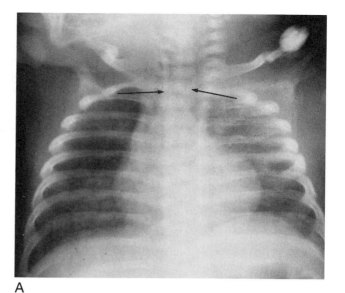

A

Figure 32–24. A 6-month-old premature infant with bronchopulmonary dysplasia and requiring continuing mechanical ventilatory assistance via endotracheal tube. Note the deformity of multiple ribs bilaterally *(arrows)*, reflecting healed fractures secondary to chest physical therapy. The tip of the central venous line *(arrowhead)* is in the superior vena cava, in satisfactory position. The endotracheal tube also is in good position.

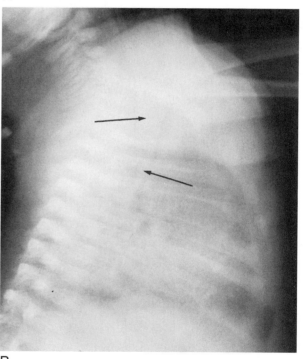

B

Figure 32–26. **A** and **B,** Passage of a nasogastric tube in a 7-week-old infant with bronchopulmonary dysplasia was followed by coughing and increased respiratory distress. The faintly opaque tube *(arrows)* can be seen to double back on itself in the esophagus at the level of the thoracic inlet, then extend into the trachea. Malposition of nasogastric tubes usually involves insufficient advancement of the tubes, such that their tip is usually in the distal esophagus.

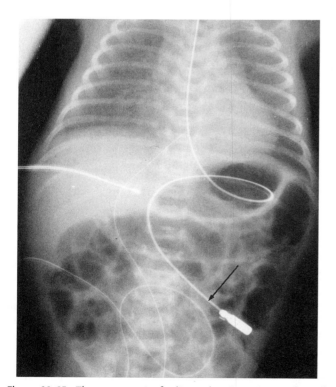

Figure 32–25. The nasoenteric feeding tube *(arrow)* extends well beyond the stomach into the proximal jejunum, in satisfactory position. The umbilical arterial catheter tip is satisfactorily positioned low in the right atrium.

secretions tend to pool with the patient in the supine position (Figs. 32-25 and 32-26; see also Figs. 32-4A and 32-8). If a suction catheter with more widely spaced side holes is employed, the most proximal side hole should be in the distal esophagus. Pleural chest tubes must have all end and side holes within the pleural space (Fig. 32-27B and C). If placed for drainage of a pneumothorax, the pleural chest tube should be directed anteriorly to where pleural air tends to collect with the neonate in the supine position and posteriorly when drainage of pleural fluid

collections is the objective. Disruption or breaking of a life-support tube or catheter is an infrequent complication (Fig. 32-28).

THORAX

Normal Appearances

Fetal lung fluid is almost completely cleared and replaced with air by the initial few breaths after birth.[23]

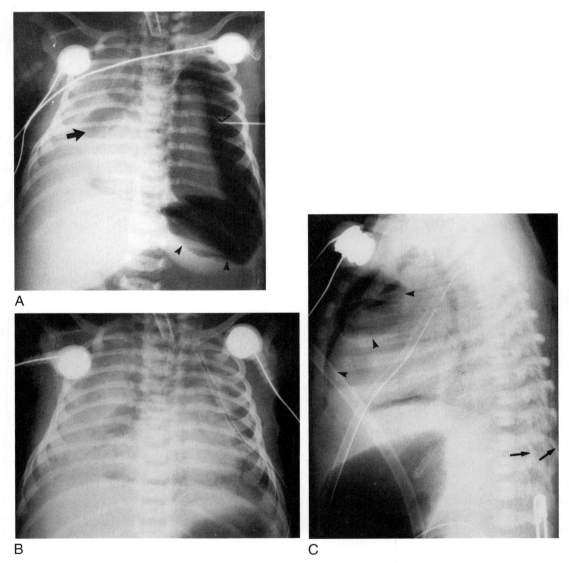

Figure 32–27. A newborn with respiratory distress syndrome and on mechanical ventilation. Complete collapse of both lungs **(A)** is associated with a left tension pneumothorax, mediastinal shift to the right, and central parenchymal cyst in the right lung *(arrow)*. Aspiration of air from the left pleural space was not successful in controlling the tension pneumothorax. Note the needle in the left pleural space *(open arrow)* and the pronounced depression of the left diaphragm *(arrowheads)* caused by the tension pneumothorax. Anteroposterior supine **(B)** and cross-table lateral **(C)** views taken the same day after placement of a left pleural chest tube show satisfactory control of the left pneumothorax and improved aeration of the right lung primarily. The parenchymal cyst overlying the right hilum persists. The lateral view shows the residual pleural air *(arrowheads)* better, located anteriorly because of the patient's supine position, than does the anteroposterior view. Pleural chest tube position appears entirely satisfactory based on the anteroposterior view alone, whereas the lateral projection shows the tip of the chest tube to be relatively posterior. Anterior chest tube position is preferred for drainage of pneumothoraces; posterior position is preferred for drainage of pleural fluid collections. Patient rotation as present on the lateral projection can be estimated by the degree of separation of the sets of posterior ribs *(arrows)*.

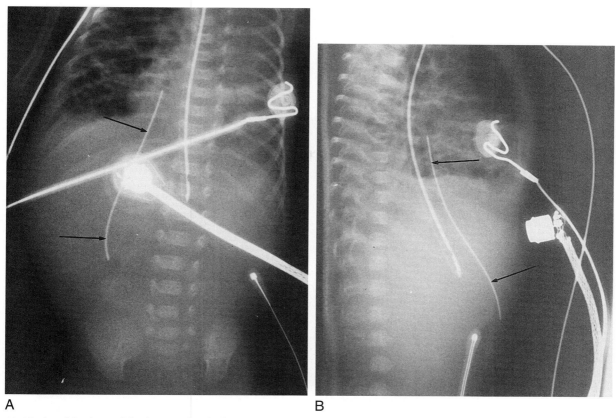

A   B

Figure 32–28. A and **B,** This umbilical venous line broke; the residual segment *(arrows)* extends through the liver into the right atrium. The nasogastric tube is well positioned in the stomach. There is severe, unilateral (right-sided) pulmonary interstitial emphysema.

The expanded lungs of the newborn, on the anteroposterior radiograph, have a relatively uniform lucency with only mild increase in density in the hilar regions.[23] Aerated lung is seen extending to the inner margins of the ribs. The cardiothymic contour to the mediastinum is highly variable, but a generous amount of mediastinal soft tissue is normally present.[23,24] Normal thymus frequently is misinterpreted as upper lobe consolidation or a mediastinal mass (Fig. 32-29). The mediastinal and diaphragmatic margins should be sharply defined.[25] A properly exposed chest radiograph shows rib and vertebral structures. The liver and stomach should be definable in the right and left upper abdominal quadrants (Fig. 32-30).

On the lateral view, the heart and thymus project in the low anterior and high anterior thorax.[23] Air should be evident in the trachea and is frequently evident in the esophagus.[23] Smooth doming of the diaphragms should be present.[23]

Normal Variations

A chest radiograph exposed during relative expiration shows a variable and occasionally striking degree of generalized opacity throughout the lungs that can simulate pathology. The midportion of the diaphragms should be at the level of the ninth posterior or sixth anterior ribs if the radiograph is obtained during reasonable inspiration.[1]

Deviation of the incident x-ray beam from a true anteroposterior orientation can significantly affect the appearance of normal thoracic structures. The more apical lordotic (i.e., oriented from low anterior to high posterior) the projection, the higher the anterior ends of the ribs project relative to the posterior ribs and spine and the lower the lung volumes (Figs. 32-31, 32-32A, and 32-33). Patient rotation to one side or the other results in an asymmetrical projection of ribs relative to the lungs, with anterior rib ends on the side of rotation projecting further lateral than present on the opposite side (Figs. 32-34 and 32-35; see also Figs. 32-3, 32-9, and 32-32B).[24]

Interlobar fissures, usually the minor fissure on the right, are often seen on the chest radiograph and should be considered a normal finding, especially if they are thin and sharply defined. Pleural fluid can accumulate in fissures, however, and accentuate their appearance.[23]

Normally the trachea in a neonate straightens and increases slightly in diameter during inspiration and narrows and buckles to the side opposite the aortic arch (usually to the right) during expiration.[23,24] A buckled appearance to the trachea on the anteroposterior and lateral chest radiograph may be a common normal variation (Fig. 32-36).[23,24] If the trachea is deviated from midline in a smooth manner, increased concern for intrathoracic pathology is warranted. Anterior indentation of the

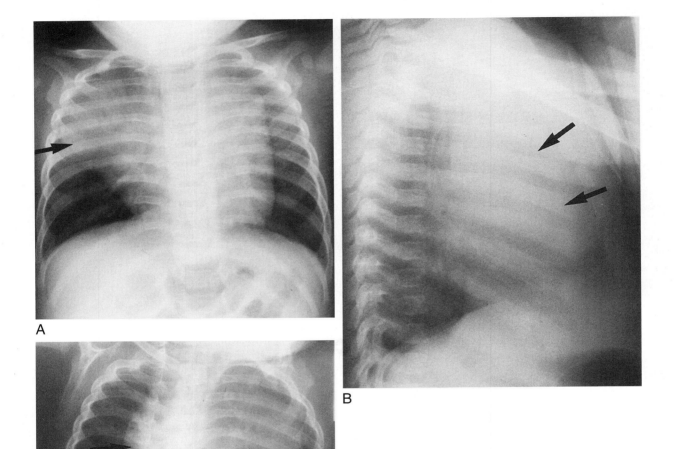

A

B

C

Figure 32–29. There is atypical-appearing soft tissue density overlying the right upper lobe on the frontal view **(A)** and in the upper retrosternal region on the lateral view **(B)** *(arrows)*. Is this a normal thymus with an atypical radiographic appearance, or is there a thymic or other mediastinal mass? Chest fluoroscopy with spot radiography and with the patient rotated slightly to the left **(C)** shows a common configuration to a normal but prominent right thymic lobe *(arrow)*. No further imaging or evaluation was required.

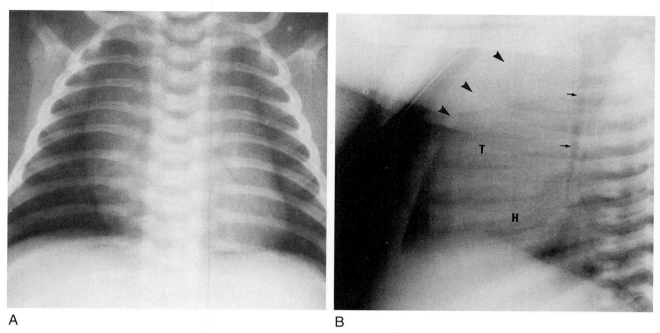

A   B

Figure 32–30. A, Portable anteroposterior chest radiograph shows a normal cardiothymic silhouette, clear and normally aerated lungs, normal pulmonary blood flow, and normal regional skeletal structures. **B,** Corresponding lateral view shows a normal thymus *(T)* and heart *(H)*. The trachea *(arrows)* and spine are normal. Note the sternal ossification centers *(arrowheads)*.

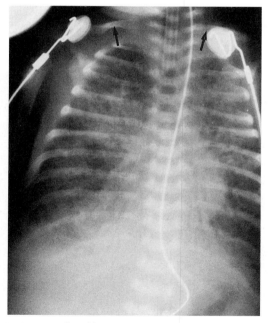

Figure 32–31. A 10-day-old premature neonate with severe respiratory distress caused by *Pseudomonas* pneumonia. The lungs show diffuse, inhomogeneous increase in opacity and severe hyperinflation. The projection is apical lordotic, as indicated by the clavicles *(arrows)* projecting above the first ribs and the anterior ends of most of the ribs projecting higher than the posterior rib segments. The endotracheal and nasogastric tubes are in good position.

trachea, as seen on the lateral chest radiograph, is attributed to normal encroachment by the innominate artery and is rarely, if ever, of any clinical significance.[23]

Skin redundancy, combined with the recumbent patient position during radiography, often results in a sharply marginated change in density overlying the lung field that can simulate a pneumothorax, but which represents a skin-fold artifact only (Fig. 32-37).[23,24] Orientation of the line of density change significantly different from the inner thoracic margin, extension of the line beyond the thorax, and presence of lung parenchymal density in the more lucent region lateral to the line all suggest a skin-fold artifact.[23]

On a rotated anteroposterior chest radiograph, the sternal ossification centers can project as a vertically oriented row of opaque densities (see Fig. 32-9). Apparatus related to mechanical ventilatory assistance and maintaining stable patient environment can produce a variety of density artifacts on the chest radiograph (Figs. 32-38 and 32-39; see also Fig. 32-35). Neurologically impaired newborns may have a bell-shaped thoracic configuration on the anteroposterior chest radiograph (Fig. 32-40).

Cardiac Disorders, Including Congenital Cardiac Disease

In-depth discussion of congenital and acquired cardiac disease in the newborn is beyond the scope of this chapter. Cardiac disease in neonates and infants is usually congenital and impossible to evaluate thoroughly by chest radiography alone. Echocardiography with pulsed and

Text continues on p 459.

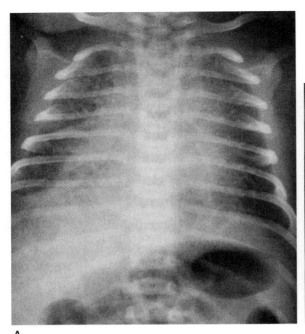

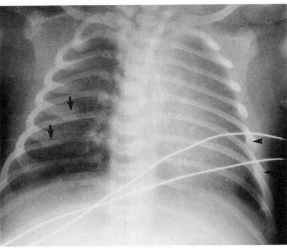

A

B

Figure 32–32. Postnatal respiratory distress in a near-term newborn delivered by cesarean section. **A,** Initial chest radiograph taken within hours of birth shows a sharp, diffuse, and bilateral increase in interstitial pulmonary density with obscuration of the cardiac borders and probably a small right pleural effusion. The position of the clavicles well above the first ribs indicates this to be an apical lordotic projection. **B,** Repeat chest radiograph the following day shows pronounced clearing of the pulmonary density and a near-normal appearance to the lungs. This rapid improvement in interstitial pulmonary density strongly suggests retained fetal lung fluid or transient tachypnea of the newborn as the underlying abnormality. If this pattern of density persists beyond 48 hours of life, transient tachypnea of the newborn ceases to be a reasonable diagnostic consideration, and neonatal pneumonia or aspiration is more likely. Note the degree of rotation of the patient to the left, as indicated by the anterior ends of the right ribs *(arrows)* projecting over the right lung field compared with the anterior ends of the left ribs *(arrowheads)* projecting further laterally.

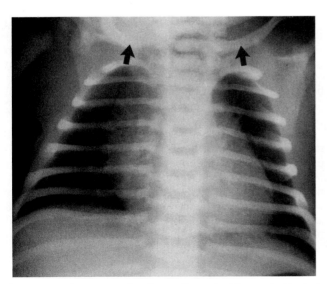

Figure 32–33. Anteroposterior chest radiograph with an apical lordotic orientation results in the clavicles *(arrows)* projecting above the first ribs and the anterior ends of the upper ribs projecting higher than the posterior portion. Portable chest radiography in the intensive care nursery results frequently in apical lordotic frontal views, which tend to underestimate lung volume. The cardiothymic silhouette and lungs are normal, with no demonstrated intrathoracic abnormality.

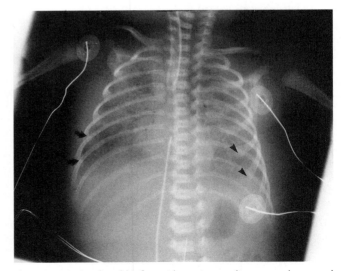

Figure 32–34. A 4-day-old infant with respiratory distress syndrome and on assisted ventilation. Uneven distribution of surfactant administered via the endotracheal tube has resulted in asymmetric and heterogeneous lung opacification. The patient is rotated to the right, as indicated by the projection of the anterior ends of the right ribs *(arrows)* further lateral than are the anterior ends of the left ribs *(arrowheads)*. Projection of mediastinal structures in the thorax can be significantly affected by patient rotation, which should be assessed on all films.

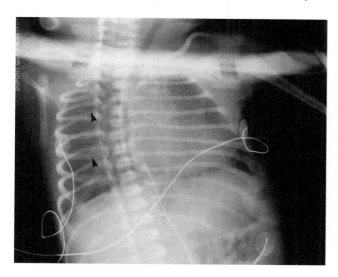

Figure 32–35. There is pronounced rotation of the patient to the left for this anteroposterior portable chest radiograph, as indicated by the left ribs projecting in greater profile and the anterior ends of the right ribs *(arrowheads)* projected over the medial portion of the right hemithorax, close to the spine. Note the density artifact at the upper margin of the thorax produced by the overlying Oxyhood.

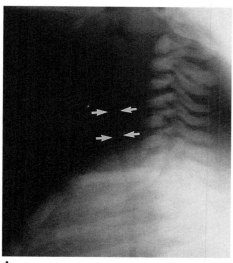

A

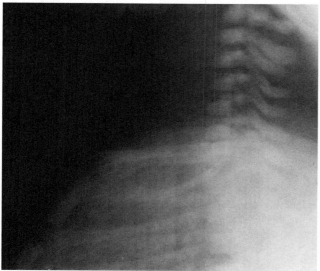

B

Figure 32–36. Lateral views of the upper airway in a neonate. During inspiration **(A)**, the trachea tends to have a straight alignment *(arrows)*, but to buckle anteriorly **(B)** and on the anteroposterior view (not shown) to the side opposite the aortic arch during expiration. This represents normal physiologic variation in tracheal configuration.

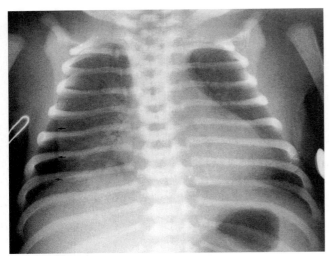

Figure 32–37. A sharply marginated, slightly curved change in density is present in the right lower lung zone *(arrows)*. The presence of parenchymal lung density lateral to this density change and its oblique orientation relative to the inner thoracic margin suggest correctly that a skin fold rather than a pneumothorax accounts for this density change.

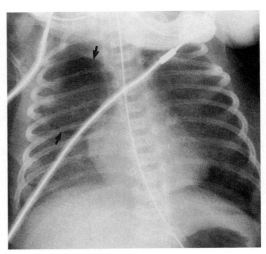

Figure 32–39. The round area of lucency *(arrows)* overlying the right upper lung field is caused by a hole in the top of the Isolette being interposed between the x-ray tube and the patient, decreasing the x-ray beam attenuation and increasing the film exposure (making it "darker") at the hole site. The perfectly round margins of the lucency suggest that it is not part of the patient but rather reflects a man-made structure.

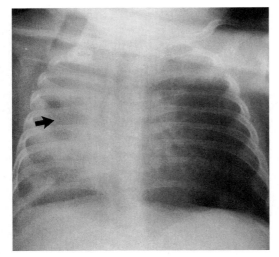

Figure 32–38. Opacification and volume loss of the right lung are accompanied by a large right lung cyst *(arrow)*, reflecting staphylococcal pneumonia with pneumatocele formation. The transversely oriented density overlying the upper thorax reflects the edge of an Oxyhood.

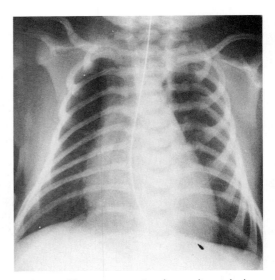

Figure 32–40. Portable anteroposterior chest radiograph shows a relatively narrower upper thoracic cage compared with the lower portion, termed the *bell-shaped thorax* and often a reflection of an underlying neurologic abnormality. This infant had myotonic dystrophy.

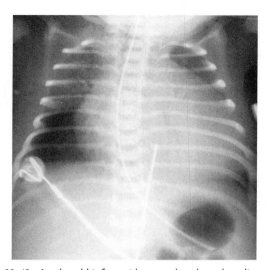

Figure 32–41. A 1-day-old infant with a greatly enlarged cardiac silhouette caused by cardiomyopathy on the basis of severe birth asphyxia. Reliable assessment of cardiac size is frequently difficult on the usual portable anteroposterior chest radiograph taken in the intensive care nursery because of variations in respiration, phase of cardiac cycle, and radiographic magnification.

color Doppler imaging forms the basis of the evaluation of cardiac disease in the newborn.

The chest radiograph can provide important supplemental information in the evaluation of the newborn's cardiovascular system. A general assessment of cardiac size and pulmonary blood flow can be obtained (Fig. 32-41).[23,26] Heart size can be estimated, with a cardiothoracic ratio, on the portable supine anteroposterior chest radiograph, with greater than 60% suggesting cardiac enlargement or pericardial effusion (Fig. 32-42). The normal-sized heart appears as an oval or egg-shaped soft tissue structure, elevated posteriorly, on the lateral chest radiograph. As the heart enlarges, the cardiac configuration becomes progressively rounder. Pulmonary blood flow is grossly evaluated as normal, increased, decreased, or bizarre, as seen with collateral circulation to the lungs.[23] Pulmonary blood flow often appears decreased and heart size appears normal for several days after birth, even in the presence of congenital cardiac disease, because of persistence of high pulmonary vascular resistance.[23] Laterality of the aortic arch, pattern of abdominal situs, and any associated rib or thoracic spinal anomaly usually can be determined from the chest radiograph (Fig. 32-43).

Patients suspected of having heterotaxia syndrome and derangement of solitus asymmetry initially should have plain films of the chest and abdomen to determine cardiac and gastric positions and to assess pulmonary vascularity.[27] Because plain films alone are inaccurate in determining visceroatrial situs in 30% of cases, supplemental

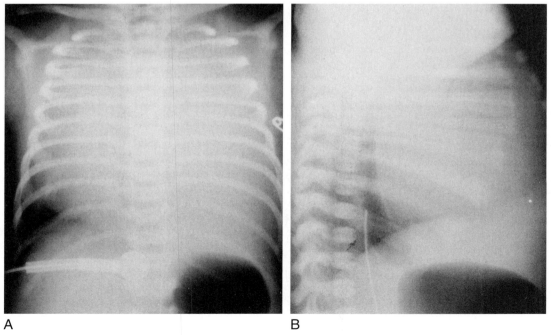

A   B

Figure 32–42. Anteroposterior **(A)** and lateral **(B)** views in a newborn with respiratory distress. The cardiothymic silhouette extends the entire width of the thoracic cage on the anteroposterior view, much more than would normally occur. The anteroposterior cardiac dimension on the lateral view is excessively large, confirming enlargement of the heart rather than a prominent but otherwise normal thymus. Echocardiography showed a large pericardial effusion. Differentiation of cardiac enlargement/dilation from pericardial fluid collections is not reliable on the neonatal chest radiograph.

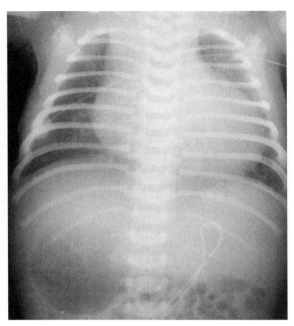

Figure 32–43. A cyanotic newborn with complex congenital cardiac disease. In addition to enlargement of the cardiac silhouette, there is at least mild vascular congestion. The cardiac apex is on the left. Abdominal situs inversus is indicated by the stomach being in the right upper quadrant, the liver in the left. When the cardiac apex and stomach are on opposite sides, as in this patient, there almost always is complex congenital cardiac disease.

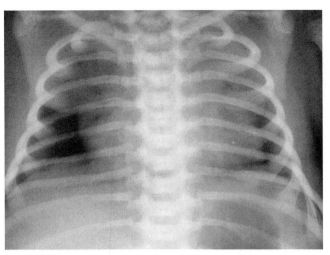

Figure 32–44. A newborn with mild respiratory distress, not requiring assisted ventilation. Oligohydramnios had been present in utero. Radiographically the lungs are clear, but overall lung volumes appear decreased, suggesting pulmonary hypoplasia. The upper thoracic soft tissue density is produced by a normal thymus. The diagnosis of pulmonary hypoplasia by chest radiography is difficult, in part because of the variation in lung volumes normally seen.

imaging with sonography, selective radionuclide spleen scanning, or MRI should be performed.[27]

Pulmonary Disorders Causing Neonatal Respiratory Distress

Developmental Anomalies

Pulmonary hypoplasia. Reflecting decreased lung size caused by reduction in functioning pulmonary units, pulmonary hypoplasia can vary considerably in severity and clinical significance.[10,23,28] More severe degrees of pulmonary hypoplasia can present in full-term infants as severe respiratory distress that may progress rapidly from severe hypoxemia to death.[10] Tachypnea, cyanosis, and difficulty in achieving adequate ventilation are common clinical signs.[10]

With bilateral pulmonary hypoplasia, the lungs radiographically may appear clear but unusually small, and the diagnosis frequently is suggested only with serial radiographs (Fig. 32-44).[10,23] Complications, such as pneumomediastinum, pneumothorax, and pneumoperitoneum, occur with increased frequency.[23] Unilateral pulmonary hypoplasia appears radiographically as a small, hyperlucent lung with decreased pulmonary blood flow and a shift of the mediastinum to the affected side.[10,23,28,29] Accurate quantitation of hypoplasia is impossible by chest radiography.

Congenital diaphragmatic hernia. Left sided in 65% to 80% of cases, congenital diaphragmatic hernia (CDH) involves the intrathoracic extension of a variable amount of intra-abdominal structures (bowel, stomach, spleen, liver) through a posterior diaphragmatic defect at the pleuroperitoneal canal.[1,10,23,28-31] Bilateral pulmonary hypoplasia, more severe on the side of herniation, is invariably present.[10,23,29-32] A rare anterior CDH has associated anterior abdominal wall and sternal defects, including omphalocele.[33]

Chest radiograph findings consist of air-containing or fluid-containing bowel on the side of herniation, contralateral displacement of the heart and other mediastinal structures, compression of the contralateral lung, and reduced size of the abdomen with decreased or absent air-containing intra-abdominal bowel (Fig. 32-45).[1,10,23,28,29,34] There is little or no visible aerated lung on the side of the herniation.[10,23,29,32]

Smaller right-sided diaphragmatic defects may be occluded by the liver and may not involve intrathoracic herniation of abdominal contents.[10,23,28] With large right-sided diaphragmatic defects, the liver may herniate into the chest and produce a large thoracic soft tissue mass with absence of an intra-abdominal liver shadow.[10,23,29] Increasingly, CDH is diagnosed by antenatal sonography, with the demonstration of fluid-filled bowel at the level of the heart on transverse sonographic images of the fetal thorax.

After surgical repair of a CDH, the volume of the hypoplastic lungs is usually shown.[29] As a result of the low, fixed position of the repaired diaphragm and reduced volume of the ipsilateral hypoplastic lung, a large "ex vacuo" pleural air collection, easily mistaken for a tension pneumothorax, is typically present.[29] Computer-assisted analysis of the lung area on the anteroposterior chest radiograph may help predict outcome in CDH infants postoperatively but not preoperatively.[35] Because of hypoxemia and pulmonary hypertension, newborns with

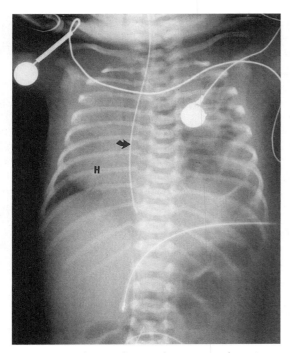

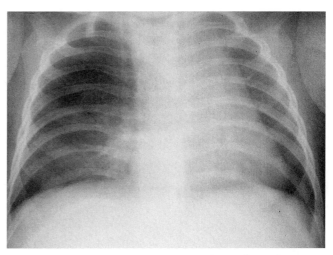

Figure 32–46. A 3-day-old neonate had this chest radiograph to evaluate tachypnea. There is relative hyperlucency and hyperinflation of the upper portion of the right lung in conjunction with partial compressive atelectasis of the right lower lobe. Congenital lobar emphysema involving the right upper lobe was found at surgery.

Figure 32–45. A newborn with immediate postnatal respiratory distress. Anteroposterior view of the chest and upper abdomen shows a bubbly, cystic appearance to the left hemithorax reflecting intrathoracic bowel. The heart *(H)* is displaced to the right. The position of the nasogastric tube *(arrow)* indicates rightward shift of the esophagus as well. Note the continuity of bowel extending from the left upper quadrant into the left hemithorax. The abdomen frequently has a scaphoid appearance because of the absence of intra-abdominal bowel.

a CDH may be managed with extracorporeal membrane oxygenation (ECMO), either before or after surgical repair.[32]

Congenital lobar emphysema. Usually the result of partial obstruction of a lobar bronchus, congenital lobar emphysema is characterized by marked overinflation of a single lobe of the lung.[1,10,23,28,29,34,36] The pattern of involvement is left upper lobe (50%), right middle lobe (30%), and right upper lobe (20%); involvement of lower lobes or multiple lobes is rare.[1,10,23,28,29]

Gradually progressing respiratory distress, almost always starting before 6 months of age and manifest at birth in one third of cases, is the most common clinical presentation.[10,29,36] Choking or feeding difficulties, vomiting, cyanosis, or signs of respiratory infection also can occur.[10] Associated anomalies occur in 14% to 50% of cases and usually involve the cardiovascular system (especially ventricular septal defect or patent ductus arteriosus).[10,36]

Radiographically the involved lobe initially may appear opaque because of distention with fluid and accompanied by contralateral mediastinal shift. As the fluid clears and is replaced by air over a 1-day to 2-week period, the radiographic appearance may change to a reticular pattern, then to the characteristic hyperlucent appearance (Fig. 32-46).[1,10,23,29,32,34] Compression of adjacent lung and contralateral mediastinal shift also is present.[10,23,29,32] In questionable cases, a ventilation-perfusion lung scan may be of diagnostic help; the scan shows decreased perfusion and absence of ventilation of the involved lobe.[10,36] CT of the thorax can confirm the diagnosis by showing stretched, attenuated vessels within the hyperlucent lobe.[29,36]

Congenital cystic adenomatoid malformation. A hamartomatous lesion of the lung that is characterized by an overgrowth of terminal bronchioles, congenital cystic adenomatoid malformation (CCAM) occurs in three relatively distinct patterns: type I, larger, variable-sized cysts with normal adjacent lung; type II, multiple small cysts and little pulmonary mass effect; and type III, dilated bronchial-like structures and a solid space-occupying intrathoracic mass.[10,28-30,37-39] Type I accounts for 70% of CCAM; type II, for 20%; and type III, for 10%.[10,29,38,39]

Most cases present during the neonatal period with respiratory distress.[23,28,38,39] The radiographic appearance of CCAM is variable. It may appear initially as a solid intrapulmonary mass (Fig. 32-47).[10,23,32,37-39] With clearing of the fluid, multiple small bubbly lucencies may be present.[10,23,32,34,37-39] With type I CCAM, the larger cysts may progressively enlarge and can mimic intrathoracic bowel seen with CDH.[10,29,34,38] Type II lesions may appear as heterogeneous areas of uniform small cysts.[38] Type III lesions are usually large and homogeneous and more suggestive of parenchymal consolidation or mass than a cystic lesion.[37,38] CT can provide excellent supplemental information on lesion anatomy that correlates well with pathologic evaluation of CCAM.[40]

Primary Pulmonary Disease

Transient tachypnea of the newborn. Also referred to as **wet lung disease, transient respiratory distress of the newborn,** or **neonatal retained fluid syndrome,** transient tachypnea of the newborn reflects self-limited, transient, postnatal respiratory distress lasting less than 48 hours,

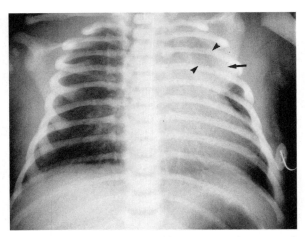

Figure 32–47. A newborn with mild respiratory distress and on mechanical ventilation. Antenatal sonography had suggested a left-sided chest mass. Anteroposterior chest radiograph shows an increase in soft tissue density occupying the upper third of the left hemithorax *(arrow)* with suggestion of a central area of lucency *(arrowheads)*. A congenital cystic adenomatoid malformation was found at surgery.

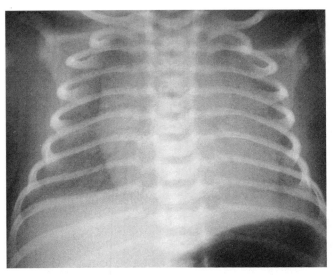

Figure 32–48. Respiratory distress syndrome in a near-term neonate is indicated by diffuse pulmonary granularity accompanied by air bronchograms. Lung volumes are normal to low-normal, which is typical for patients with respiratory distress syndrome and not on mechanical ventilatory assistance. When on a ventilator, lung volumes frequently increase significantly in response to high-pressure settings.

usually in a term newborn and more commonly occurring in neonates delivered by cesarean section.[1,10,23,41]

The typical radiographic appearance is of increased, delicate interstitial markings bilaterally, often more pronounced on the right in conjunction with small pleural effusions and mild prominence to the cardiothymic silhouette (see Fig. 32-32).[1,10,23,41] The lungs tend to be mildly overinflated.[10,41] Mild alveolar opacification may be present on radiographs obtained early in the postnatal course.[1,10,23] The diagnosis is usually confirmed when follow-up radiographs show resolution of these changes within 24 to 48 hours, in conjunction with improvement in clinical status.[1,10,23,41]

Respiratory distress syndrome. Reflecting pulmonary immaturity and a deficiency of pulmonary surfactant, respiratory distress syndrome (RDS), also commonly referred to as **hyaline membrane disease**, occurs predominantly in premature infants.[1,10,23,32,42] RDS presents as respiratory distress within 8 hours of birth, with tachypnea, grunting, retractions, and cyanosis of varying severity.[10,23,42]

The radiographic appearance of RDS is typically a diffuse increase in granular opacity throughout both lungs, accompanied by air bronchograms (Fig. 32-48; see also Figs. 32-3A, 32-10, and 32-20).[10,23,32,42] Lung volume is reduced before intubation but is more variable and may be increased when the neonate receives assisted ventilation (Fig. 32-49).[10,23] The increase in pulmonary opacity generally correlates with the severity of respiratory distress.[10] By the onset of clinical respiratory distress, the chest radiograph is usually abnormal.[10] A normal chest radiograph in a newborn with respiratory distress after 8 hours of life basically excludes RDS as the underlying cause.[1,10]

The radiographic appearance of RDS has been divided arbitrarily into four levels based on severity of disease.[10] Grade I RDS reflects the earliest stage, with alveolar atelectasis involving primarily the more dependent or

posterior portions of the lungs. Radiographically a mild, fine reticulogranular appearance to the lungs is present, and air bronchograms are limited. Grade II RDS involves extension of the atelectasis to the more anterior or nondependent portions of the lungs, with increase in overall pulmonary granularity, less sharply defined cardiac margins, and more prominent air bronchograms. Grade III RDS involves further increase in pulmonary opacification,

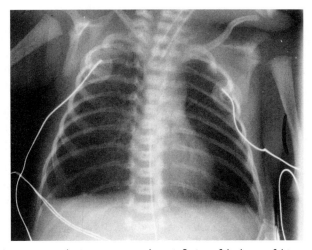

Figure 32–49. There is pronounced overinflation of the lungs of this newborn with respiratory distress syndrome and on high-pressure mechanical ventilation. The highest portion of each diaphragm should project approximately at the level of the posterior portion of the ninth rib or the anterior end of the sixth rib. In this neonate, they project considerably lower. In general, the more overinflated the lungs are, the more lucent and less opaque they appear for a given degree of intrinsic disease.

obscuration of the cardiac and diaphragmatic margins, and increased air bronchograms. With severe RDS (grade IV), the lungs are opaque, and the cardiomediastinal margins are completely obscured.

With improvement in the underlying atelectasis of RDS, the lungs become progressively better aerated, often in a patchy, irregular pattern.[10,42] Intratracheal instillation of surfactant can result in rapid clinical improvement and a more rapid rate of radiographic clearing of the lungs.[32,42-47] The pattern of radiographic clearing of RDS pulmonary density after surfactant instillation is variable.[42,43,48] Use of bovine surfactant extract resulted in a decreased incidence of pneumothorax and pulmonary interstitial emphysema and an increase in asymmetrical pulmonary densities in one study.[49] Recurrent lung opacity after an initial positive response to surfactant therapy can reflect such factors as edema from barotraumas, shunting from a patent ductus arteriosus, neurogenic edema from intracranial hemorrhage, and pneumonia.[50] Recurrent lung opacities also may be a predictor of chronic lung disease in a premature infant.[50]

Physiologic closure of the ductus arteriosus usually occurs in the first 4 days of life in healthy term and most premature infants of 30 weeks of gestational age or greater, including infants with uncomplicated RDS.[1,51] A hemodynamically significant left-to-right shunt via a patent ductus arteriosus often develops 5 to 7 days postnatally in infants with RDS.[1,10,23] The radiographic findings of patent ductus arteriosus superimposed on RDS consist of cardiomegaly, pulmonary vascular congestion, and pulmonary edema.[23] The chest radiograph typically shows an interval increase in heart size and diffuse pulmonary density only (Fig. 32-50).[1,23] Atelectasis, pneumonia, and pulmonary hemorrhage all are frequent coexisting conditions in premature newborns with RDS and may alter the appearance of the lungs from the typical granularity of RDS in variable ways.[42] A chest radiographic scoring system based on multiple factors has been proposed as a means to quantitate the severity of neonatal respiratory distress and to predict chronic respiratory problems.[52]

Complications of mechanical ventilation. The positive-pressure ventilation and oxygen therapy required to manage a neonate with RDS and other pulmonary disorders adequately can result in "air block" complications.[10,23,32,42] With rupture of terminal bronchioles and alveoli, intrapulmonary air may leak into the pulmonary interstitium, with subsequent dissection along the interlobular septa and their lymphatics.[1,10,23,32,42] Pulmonary interstitial emphysema may be segmental, lobar, diffuse, or bilateral and contributes to further loss of lung compliance and impairment of ventilation and gas exchange.[10,23,32] Radiographically, pulmonary interstitial emphysema appears as variable microcystic or linear lucencies localized or diffusely distributed in the lung parenchyma, with an increase in lung volumes and pseudoclearing of the pulmonary granularity of RDS (Figs. 32-51 through 32-54; see also Figs. 32-3B, 32-4A and C, and 32-10).[1,10,23,30] Three types of interstitial air bubbles have been described: type I, seen in the early phase of RDS and representing overdistended terminal bronchioles and

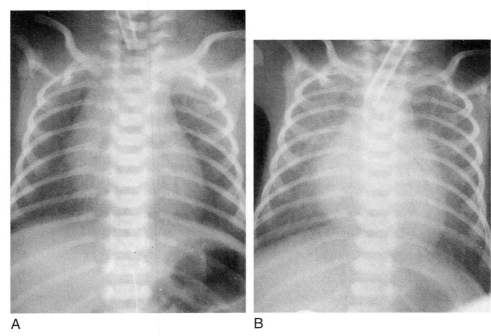

A   B

Figure 32–50. A 4-day-old infant with respiratory distress syndrome and mild pulmonary opacification **(A)**. Two days later, in conjunction with increasing distress, bounding pulses, and audible murmur, chest radiograph **(B)** shows an increase in cardiac size and generalized pulmonary density, findings suggesting a left-to-right shunt via a patent ductus arteriosus. Echocardiography was confirmatory. The ductus closed with indomethacin administration.

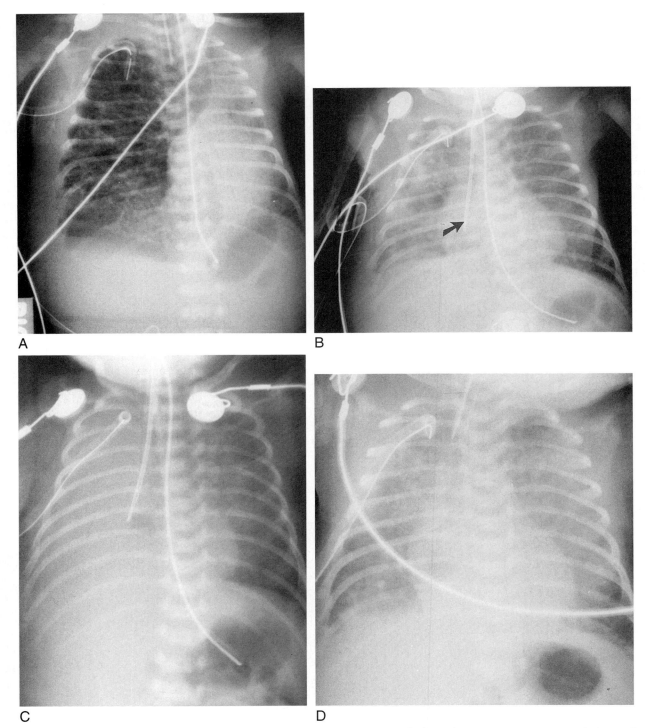

Figure 32–51. A, A premature neonate with severe respiratory distress syndrome, requiring high ventilatory pressure settings. Marked overinflation and irregular cystic changes of the right lung reflect severe pulmonary interstitial emphysema. An accompanying right pneumothorax is incompletely controlled by a single pleural chest tube. **B,** One day later, selective catheterization and occlusion of the right main bronchus was performed to control the pulmonary interstitial emphysema. The catheter *(arrow)* is positioned satisfactorily in the right main bronchus, but the inflated balloon is radiolucent and not visible on the radiograph. Significant improvement in the hyperinflation and interstitial air involving the right lung is already apparent. **C,** By the following day, the right lung is collapsed with complete resolution of the pulmonary interstitial emphysema. The right pneumothorax does not persist. **D,** After deflation of the balloon and removal of the catheter, the right lung is similar in appearance to the left. The pulmonary interstitial emphysema and pneumothorax remain resolved.

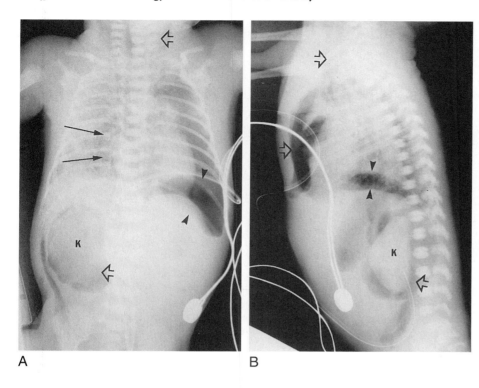

A   B

Figure 32–52. A premature newborn with severe respiratory distress syndrome on assisted ventilation. Anteroposterior **(A)** and lateral **(B)** views of the chest and abdomen show predominantly right-sided pulmonary interstitial emphysema *(arrows)*, a left pneumothorax *(arrowheads)*, and a pneumomediastinum with air tracking up into the neck and down into the retroperitoneum *(open arrows)*, surrounding the right kidney *(K)*.

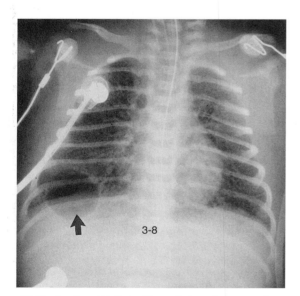

Figure 32–53. A 3-day-old infant with respiratory distress syndrome and on mechanical ventilation. In addition to generalized pulmonary interstitial emphysema bilaterally, a large parenchymal cyst *(arrow)* developed at the right lung base. Spontaneous rupture of these cysts can result in the sudden development of a pneumothorax.

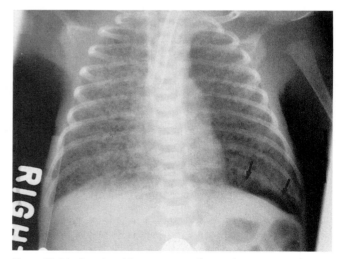

Figure 32–54. A 6-day-old premature infant with respiratory distress syndrome and on mechanical ventilation developed diffuse microcystic pulmonary changes reflecting pulmonary interstitial emphysema and accompanied by a small, partially subpulmonic left pneumothorax *(arrows)*.

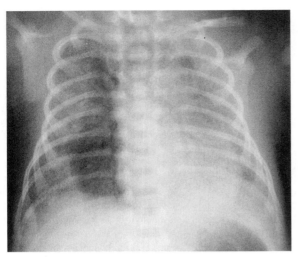

Figure 32–55. Relative lucency of the medial half of the right lung field compared with the lateral portion is an abnormal appearance and suggests a pneumothorax with the pleural air localizing medially and anteriorly. Generalized pulmonary granularity with air bronchograms reflects respiratory distress syndrome. The pattern of density of the lungs on an anteroposterior supine chest film should not show an increase in lucency progressing from the lateral lung margin to the mediastinum; if present, pneumothorax or pneumomediastinum must be considered.

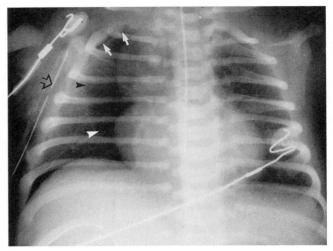

Figure 32–56. Signs of a right-sided pneumothorax in a newborn with mild respiratory distress syndrome are definition of a free pleural edge laterally *(white arrows)*, increased lucency over the medial portion of the right lung *(arrowhead)*, and unusually sharp definition of the right mediastinal border compared with the left side. A single right-sided chest tube in the lateral chest wall soft tissues is malpositioned *(open arrow)*.

alveolar ducts; type II, representing pulmonary interstitial emphysema related to positive-pressure assisted ventilation; and type III, representing distended alveolar groups in a damaged lung of chronic bronchopulmonary dysplasia (BPD).[53] A larger, localized cystic air collection within the pulmonary interstitium, usually right-sided, may be present occasionally (see Fig. 32-53).[1,54] Air subsequently can dissect centrally to the mediastinum, resulting in a pneumomediastinum or, rarely, a pneumopericardium.[42] It also may rupture into the pleural space, resulting in a pneumothorax (Fig. 32-55; see also Fig. 32-10).[1,10,23,32,42] Intravascular extension of air resulting in air embolism occurs rarely and is almost invariably fatal.[42] Pulmonary interstitial emphysema is considered a finding with potentially ominous clinical consequences and is typically treated with high-frequency ventilation, selective bronchial occlusion, or placement of the neonate in a lateral decubitus position (see Fig. 32-51).[54-58]

Pneumothorax is suggested by separation of the visceral pleural surface and lung from the inner thoracic margin with no lung parenchymal density within the area of hyperlucency, relative lucency of the hemithorax medially, and overall hyperlucency of a hemithorax when pleural air is localized anterior to the lung (Fig. 32-56; see also Figs. 32-4A, 32-51A, 32-54, and 32-55).[1,10,23] Trapping of air in the pleural space can result in a tension pneumothorax, which is suggested by partial collapse of the lung, depression of the ipsilateral diaphragm, and contralateral mediastinal shift (see Figs. 32-4B and 32-52).[1,10,23] In neonates with unilateral or bilateral anterior tension pneumothorax, compression of the thymus can result in

an upper mediastinal pseudomass on the anteroposterior chest radiograph.[59] Although infrequently obtained, the cross-table lateral chest radiograph can permit optimal evaluation of the relative position of the lung, intrapleural air, and tip of any pleural chest tube in a supine neonate with a pneumothorax compared with the supine anteroposterior chest view alone or in combination with a vertical-beam lateral view.[23]

Pneumothoraces judged to be clinically significant typically are treated with a pleural chest tube, which is opaque and readily definable on the chest radiograph (see Fig. 32-51A). Most chest tubes have one end hole and one side hole within 2 cm of the tube tip. Both holes must be within the pleural space. The portable anteroposterior view with the patient supine does not allow determination of relative position of the chest tube in the anteroposterior plane and cannot define a possible mismatch between anteriorly collected pleural air and a posteriorly positioned chest tube (see Fig. 32-27B). A lateral projection may be necessary to make this determination (see Fig. 32-27C). Lateral migration of pleural chest tubes occurs frequently in ICN patients (Fig. 32-57; see also Fig. 32-56).

A chest tube inserted for treatment of a pneumothorax may inadvertently perforate the lung.[60] This complication is suggested by the occurrence of persistent or repeated pneumothoraces despite the presence of a pleural chest tube and development of atelectasis or infiltrate near the end of the chest tube (see Fig. 32-8).[60]

A pneumomediastinum is suggested on the anteroposterior radiograph by central thoracic lucency extending to both sides of midline, isolation of the thymic lobes, and dissection of air as streaky lucencies into the neck and supraclavicular regions (Fig. 32-58; see also Fig. 32-52).[10,23,42]

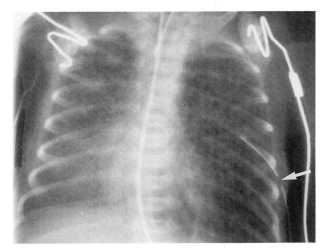

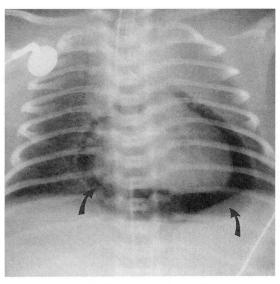

Figure 32–57. A left pleural chest tube placed for treatment of a pneumothorax has migrated laterally, with its side hole *(arrow)* outside of the left pleural space. There is sharp hyperinflation of the left lung, partly caused by pulmonary interstitial emphysema.

Figure 32–59. A 2-day-old infant with respiratory distress syndrome, on assisted ventilatory support. Anteroposterior chest radiograph after sudden clinical deterioration shows the heart to be silhouetted by a zone of lucency reflecting a pneumopericardium *(arrows)*. In contrast to pneumomediastinum, a pneumopericardium has air extending around the heart, including the inferior margin, but not into the upper mediastinum and lower neck region.

Retrocardiac mediastinal air does not elevate the thymic lobes.[61] Pneumopericardium, which usually occurs with high-pressure mechanical ventilation but has been described in high-frequency ventilation, is suggested by low central thoracic lucency that extends beneath the cardiac shadow but does not extend into the upper thorax (Fig. 32-59).[1,10,23,62]

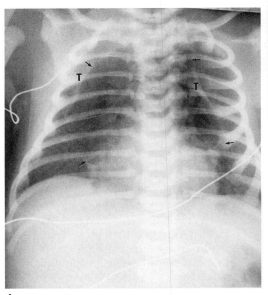

A

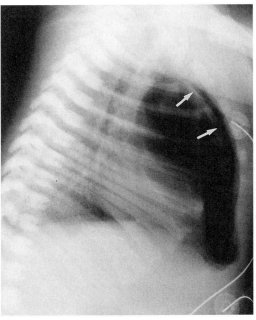

B

Figure 32–58. A, A large pneumomediastinum *(arrows)* is present in a newborn with respiratory distress caused by meconium aspiration. The right and left lobes of the thymus *(T)* are silhouetted medially and laterally by air in the mediastinum and lungs. **B,** Lateral view shows mediastinal air anteriorly with isolation of the thymus *(arrows)*. Pneumomediastinum is usually not of significant clinical concern and rarely requires any specific intervention.

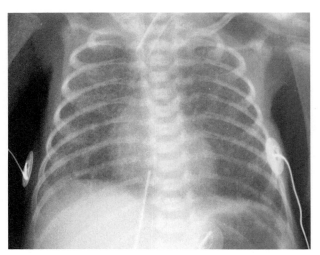

Figure 32–60. The mild, diffuse, hazy-to-granular increase in pulmonary density in a 2-week-old premature infant maintained on high ventilatory pressure settings since birth most likely reflects chronic lung disease (bronchopulmonary dysplasia). Endotracheal tube and umbilical venous line positions are satisfactory.

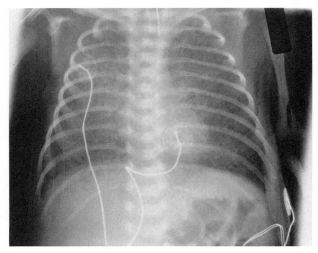

Figure 32–61. Maintained on high-pressure mechanical ventilation since birth, a 21-day-old premature infant has developed a diffusely hazy to mildly coarse pattern of increased lung density bilaterally that most likely reflects chronic lung disease (bronchopulmonary dysplasia). Lung volumes are moderately increased, likely because of high-pressure settings. Heart size is normal, decreasing the probability of congestive heart failure accounting for or contributing to the pulmonary density. At this age, respiratory distress syndrome should have resolved or progressed on to bronchopulmonary dysplasia.

Bronchopulmonary dysplasia (chronic lung disease). BPD, occasionally referred to as *chronic lung disease,* is a form of chronic lung injury resulting from artificial ventilation and supplemental oxygen therapy applied to newborns with respiratory failure of several possible etiologies, usually RDS.[10,23,32,42,63,64] Evidence suggests that increased ventilatory volume plays a greater role in the development of BPD than does increased ventilatory pressure.[65] The incidence of BPD is higher in infants who develop pulmonary interstitial emphysema.[64]

The original description of BPD involved four radiographic stages.[1,10,42,64] Initially, in stage I, diffuse pulmonary granularity and air bronchograms characteristic of RDS are seen on the chest radiograph.[42] In stage II, from 4 to 10 days of age, the lungs show increased consolidation and a coarse reticulonodular pattern of density.[42] During stage III, from 10 to 20 days, cystic areas of variable size develop and are accompanied by hyperinflation of the lungs.[42] In stage IV, beginning at 20 to 30 days of age, a radiographic picture of generalized emphysema with strandlike pulmonary densities or areas of atelectasis is present. Cardiomegaly caused by cor pulmonale may be present. These classic stages of progression of BPD are seen infrequently today because of changes in the therapy of RDS and other causes of neonatal respiratory distress.[1]

Most cases of BPD at present show diffuse parenchymal granularity initially (Fig. 32-60), gradually evolving into a diffuse, hazy appearance to the lungs (type 1 BPD) or bilateral pulmonary hyperinflation with coarse interstitial densities (type 2 BPD) (Fig. 32-61; see also Figs. 32-3C, 32-5, 32-14, and 32-24).[10,66,67] RDS complicated by pulmonary interstitial emphysema or pneumothorax is more likely to evolve into type 2 BPD.[67] The histologic changes of BPD are interstitial edema initially, followed by interstitial fibrosis, smooth muscle hypertrophy of bronchial walls, and thickened vascular walls.[32,66] Patients who have

BPD and who have had surgical closure of a patent ductus arteriosus may develop asymmetrical postoperative changes of BPD, typically worse on the right.[68]

Infants who survive BPD usually show a gradual improvement in hyperinflation and pulmonary densities, with a normal chest radiograph appearance by 3 or 4 years of age.[1] Chest CT provides excellent delineation of the pulmonary sequelae of BPD, which include multifocal areas of hyperinflation, linear opacities, and absence of bronchiectasis.[69]

Chest physical therapy is used to maintain airway patency and assist in clearing of secretions. When chest physical therapy is combined with the typically undermineralized bones of ICN patients, however, rib fractures often result in neonates with BPD (see Figs. 32-14 and 32-24).

Immature lung syndrome. Immature lung syndrome, similar to RDS, occurs in smaller premature newborns (usually <1500 g birth weight).[1,10,70] In contrast to RDS, immature lung syndrome usually involves the onset of respiratory distress only after 1 week, tends to run a more chronic course, and is less likely to evolve into severe BPD.[1,10] This entity is thought to be due to decreased alveolarization from nutritional and growth failure, common in these extremely-low-birth-weight infants.

Initial chest radiographs may show mild hypoaeration but are otherwise normal.[1,10] Ill-defined fluffy densities in the perihilar regions with few, if any, associated air bronchograms may be the only radiographic abnormalities.[1,10] The radiographic changes may remain stable for 1 to 2 months or gradually clear.[10] The development of

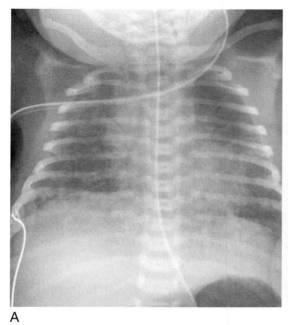

A

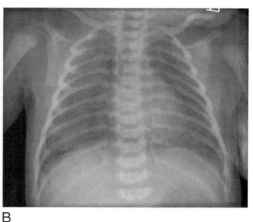

B

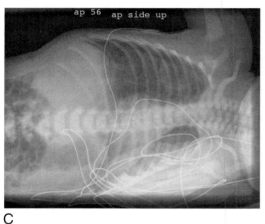

C

Figure 32–62. Portable anteroposterior chest radiograph **(A)** in a 42-week gestational age newborn with meconium below the vocal cords. There is diffuse, coarse accentuation of lung markings bilaterally, accompanied by relative hyperinflation of the lungs, which is consistent with meconium aspiration syndrome. Anteroposterior supine **(B)** and left decubitus **(C)** views in another newborn with moderately severe meconium aspiration show coarse accentuation of lung marking bilaterally. In addition, there is increased lucency at the medial and inferior margins of the right lung that is highly suspicious for an associated pneumothorax. The left decubitus view **(C)** confirms the pneumothorax, with pleural air localizing between the right lateral chest wall and the right lung.

air-block complications and BPD is less common than with RDS.[10]

Meconium aspiration syndrome. Variable in its severity and occurring in 1 to 3 per 1000 live births, meconium aspiration syndrome is usually most severe in a postmature newborn of 42 or greater weeks of gestational age.[10,23,71] Coarse, irregular peribronchial interstitial densities, accompanied by generalized pulmonary hyperinflation that may be severe, constitute the typical radiographic changes (Fig. 32-62).[1,10,23,71] Segmental or lobar areas of atelectasis are also common.[10,23,71] One third of newborns with meconium aspiration syndrome require mechanical ventilation.[72] Pneumothorax and other forms of air block occur frequently in association with more severe degrees of meconium aspiration syndrome (see Fig. 32-62B and C).[1,10,23] Radiographic clearing may require several days or weeks.[1,10,23] The radiographic findings are not specific and may be produced by neonatal pneumonia or pulmonary hemorrhage.[10] A history of meconium staining or meconium below the vocal cords is required for diagnosis.[10]

Neonatal pneumonia. Pneumonia in neonates and infants may be acquired antenatally, caused by transplacental transmission of infectious organisms (usually viral), or caused by aspiration of infected amniotic fluid, usually in association with prolonged rupture of maternal membranes.[1,10,23,32,73] Alternatively, neonatal pneumonia may be acquired perinatally or postnatally.[1,10,23,32,73] Neonatal pneumonias are more often bacterial than viral.[1,10,23,73,74] Group B streptococcal sepsis is one of the most common causes of neonatal pneumonia and sepsis.[72,75] Fungal agents, which may be endemic to certain geographic areas, infrequently can produce pulmonary infection in compromised neonates.[76] *Chlamydia trachomatis* and *Ureaplasma urealyticum* are two other agents thought to cause neonatal pneumonia frequently.[72] The clinical signs and physical presentation of neonatal pneumonia are extremely variable and nonspecific.[1,10,23]

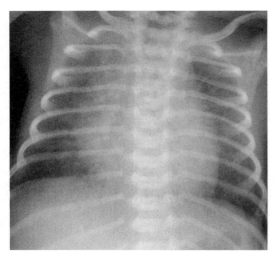

Figure 32–63. A newborn with mild respiratory distress. Delivery was associated with prolonged rupture of membranes. Anteroposterior chest radiograph shows a mild, diffuse increase in pulmonary interstitial markings, which is most suggestive of transient tachypnea of the newborn but which in this patient represented neonatal pneumonia. The radiographic appearance of both can be virtually identical.

The chest radiograph findings in neonatal pneumonia also are variable and nonspecific (Fig. 32-63; see also Figs. 32-7A and 32-31).[1,10,23,77] Four patterns of pulmonary density change seen in neonatal pneumonia are coarse, stringy densities widely distributed throughout the lungs; focal or lobar consolidation; diffuse pulmonary granularity suggestive of RDS; and scattered patchy densities in one or both lungs.[10,23,77]

Although usually not organism specific, certain radiographic findings may suggest the infectious agent.[10] A moderate or large pleural effusion suggests staphylcoccal infection, and cavitation in an area of previous consolidation suggests *Staphylococcus* or *Klebsiella* infection

(see Fig. 32-38).[1,10,30] Diffuse pulmonary granularity with air bronchograms caused by pneumonia is likely to be caused by group B streptococcus (see Fig. 32-6).[1,10,23] Pneumonia superimposed on chronic lung disease in a premature neonate is suggested by clinical deterioration associated with progressive coarse, diffuse consolidation of the lungs on the chest radiograph.[32]

Atelectasis. Most normal newborns achieve complete aeration of the lungs with the initial few breaths.[23] Very immature or neurologically impaired newborns may show homogeneously opaque and small lungs caused by incomplete expansion.[23]

Segmental, lobar, or total collapse of a lung is relatively common and usually reflects mechanical obstruction of a bronchus, which may be extrinsic (mass or vascular structure) or intrinsic (mucous or meconium plug, malpositioned endotracheal tube) (Figs. 32-64 and 32-65; see also Fig. 32-8).[23,78] Right upper lobe atelectasis is common and has a characteristic appearance, with upward displacement and bowing of the minor fissure.[78] Atelectasis in a neonate is frequently superimposed on a preexisting pulmonary process (see Figs. 32-3C and 32-8). The use of DNase to treat atelectasis caused by airway blockage from excessive mucus has been reported.[79]

Hyperinflation of a lung or segment. Hyperinflation of a lung or segment results in an area of hyperlucency with diminished vascular density. In addition to congenital lobar emphysema, hyperinflation can result from bronchial compression by mass or vessel, malpositioned endotracheal tube, or mucous plugging of a bronchus.[78]

Persistent fetal circulation syndrome. If, after birth, the high fetal pulmonary vascular resistance does not decrease as expected and pulmonary artery pressure exceeds systemic pressure, right-to-left shunting through the foramen ovale and patent ductus arteriosus occurs.[10,23] **Persistent fetal circulation syndrome** and

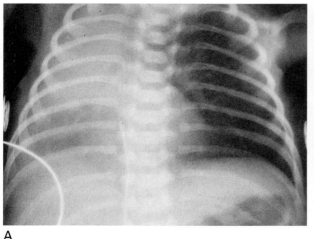

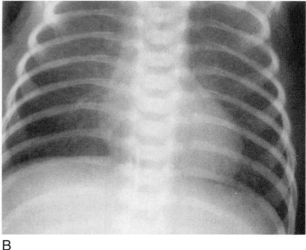

A   B

Figure 32–64. A, Generalized atelectasis of the right lung with shift of mediastinal structures to the right is present on this morning film. **B,** Repeat chest radiograph that evening shows complete resolution of the right-sided atelectasis with return of normal aeration. Rapid development and resolution of pulmonary densities strongly suggest atelectasis as the underlying abnormality.

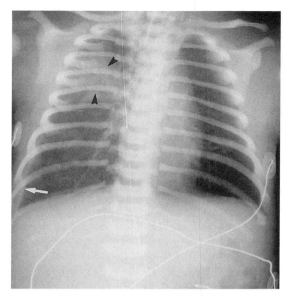

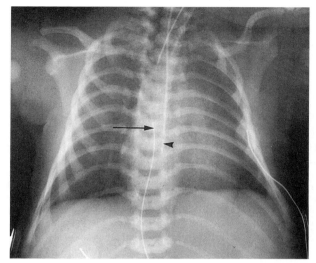

Figure 32–65. In addition to marked hyperinflation of the lungs and partial right upper lobe atelectasis *(arrowheads)*, there is widening of right lower lateral pleural space caused by pleural fluid *(arrow)*. Although usually reflecting an effusion, this finding is nonspecific and could reflect hemothorax, chylothorax, or even pyothorax. Because the intensive care nursery patient typically is in the supine position, pleural fluid collections tend to localize posteriorly and are seen "en face" on the typical anteroposterior portable radiograph. As a result, pleural fluid may present as a generalized increase in density of the hemithorax with little or no widening of the pleural space laterally. Alternatively, pleural fluid may appear as a soft tissue "cap" over the apex of the aerated lung.

Figure 32–66. Portable anteroposterior chest radiograph in a newborn with respiratory distress and mild cyanosis, requiring assisted ventilation and intubation. Heart size is normal, and both lungs are clear, probably even hyperlucent with decreased pulmonary vascular density. These findings in a newborn with respiratory distress suggest primary pulmonary hypertension of the newborn or persistent fetal circulation, involving right-to-left shunting at the foramen ovale or ductus arteriosus. Endotracheal tube position is satisfactory. The tip of the umbilical venous line *(arrow)* is probably in the lower superior vena cava, higher than preferred. The nasogastric tube *(arrowhead)* ends in the distal esophagus and should be advanced.

persistent pulmonary hypertension of the newborn are the terms applied to this situation.[10,23] The presumed etiology is hypoxia that results in pulmonary arteriolar vasoconstriction and elevation of pulmonary arterial pressure.[10,23] Inhaled nitric oxide is widely used to improve oxygenation in persistent pulmonary hypertension of the newborn in newborns.[80] Persistent pulmonary hypertension is a common indication for ECMO rescue therapy when intensive standard medical management fails.[81]

In the primary form, without associated cardiac or pulmonary disease, the lungs appear clear, the pulmonary vascular density is normal or decreased, and the heart is mildly enlarged (Fig. 32-66).[10,23] In the secondary form, in which the pulmonary hypertension is associated with pulmonary disease such as meconium aspiration syndrome or neonatal pneumonia, the radiographic appearances reflect the primary pulmonary disease process.[10,23]

Pulmonary hemorrhage. Minimal pulmonary hemorrhage is usually clinically inapparent and causes no specific chest radiograph findings.[10,23] Massive pulmonary hemorrhage, relatively uncommon and usually occurring in association with other neonatal pulmonary and nonpulmonary disorders, appears radiographically as fluffy, predominantly alveolar opacities of the lungs (Fig. 32-67).[10,23,56,82-85] The changes are usually bilateral but may be asymmetrical.[10] Massive pulmonary hemorrhage causes airless, opaque lungs, often with associated pleural effusions.[10] When

pulmonary hemorrhage occurs in conjunction with other primary pulmonary or cardiac disease, the radiographic findings may be primarily those of the concurrent pulmonary process.[10,23]

Aspiration pneumonitis. Vomiting and swallowing dysfunction are the usual causes of aspiration and subsequent pneumonitis.[10] Associated abnormalities include esophageal atresia, pharyngeal incoordination, vascular ring, gastroesophageal reflux, high intestinal obstruction, and significant central nervous system pathology.[10]

In most cases of aspiration pneumonitis in newborns, patchy densities are seen in the right upper lobe and perihilar regions because of their dependent position in the typically supine newborn (Fig. 32-68).[10] Aspiration caused by high intestinal obstruction has associated gastric and proximal small bowel distention radiographically.[10] Massive aspiration may present with bilateral fluffy infiltrates.[10] With chronic aspiration, resultant fibrosis appears as chronic coarse opacities in the lung fields on the chest radiograph.[10]

Infant of a diabetic mother. Initially the chest radiographic findings mimic transient tachypnea of the newborn, with accentuated interstitial markings and cardiomegaly[10] or regional distribution of granular densities.[86] Mild hyperaeration of the lungs is usually present.[10,86] Compared with uncomplicated transient tachypnea of the newborn, clearing of the pulmonary density and resolution of the cardiac enlargement are usually slower in an

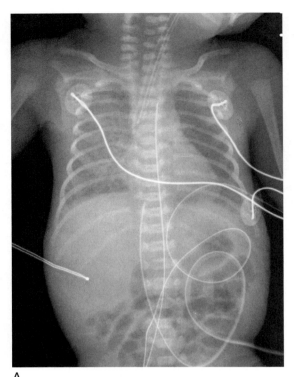

A

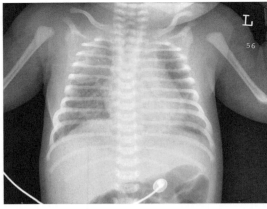

Figure 32–68. A newborn with aspiration pneumonitis in the early post-natal period. There is a bilateral patchy, nonhomogeneous (greater in the right upper and left lower lobes) increase in pulmonary density. The pulmonary infiltrates cleared with antibiotic therapy and assisted ventilation.

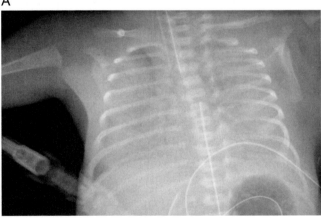

B

Figure 32–67. A 3-day-old premature newborn with respiratory distress syndrome. **A,** Portable anteroposterior chest radiograph shows asymmetrical lung opacification (greater on the right) due to uneven distribution of surfactant. The endotracheal tube is low in position. **B,** Portable anteroposterior chest radiograph the following day shows a severe, diffuse, bilateral increase in pulmonary opacification, which was accompanied by blood emanating from the endotracheal tube. Subsequent chest radiographs showed progressive resolution of the acute pulmonary hemorrhage in a heterogeneous pattern.

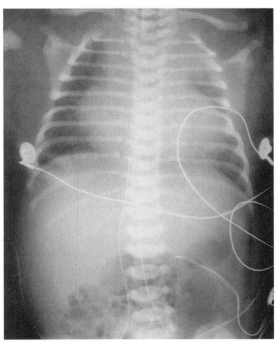

Figure 32–69. An infant of a diabetic mother shows cardiomegaly, mild vascular congestion of the lungs, and increased prominence to the liver, suggesting hepatomegaly. Mild generalized thickening of soft tissues is also present.

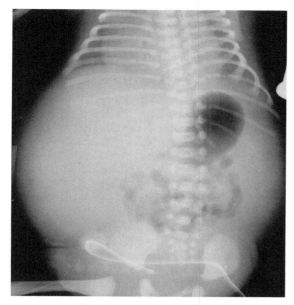

Figure 32–70. A newborn with immune hydrops fetalis and with a distended abdomen caused by massive ascites. Anteroposterior abdominal radiograph shows bulging of both flanks, a generalized increase in soft tissue density in the abdomen, and centralization of bowel containing air, which tends to shift toward the midline in the most anterior, nondependent portion of the abdomen. There also is a mild degree of generalized soft tissue edema.

infant of a diabetic mother.[10] Most patients have a radiographically normal heart size within 1 week.[10]

The chest radiograph findings may suggest congestive heart failure or neonatal hydrops fetalis and may be indistinguishable from the findings of congenital heart disease (Fig. 32-69).[10] An infant of a diabetic mother is suggested by prominent subcutaneous fat and large body size for gestational age.[10,23]

Erythroblastosis fetalis. Erythroblastosis fetalis is a hemolytic disorder of the fetus and newborn that is caused by incompatibility between fetal or newborn red blood cells and maternal antibodies.[10] The severity of the hemolytic disease is reflected in the radiographic findings (Figs. 32-70 and 32-71).[10] Generalized anasarca produces a large-for-gestational-age infant.[10] In addition to hydrops, cardiomegaly, attributed to anemia and high-output failure, is present.[10] Pericardial effusions and hypoaeration of the lungs (caused by diaphragmatic elevation by abdominal organomegaly or ascites) can accentuate the enlargement of the cardiac silhouette.[10] Prominence of the pulmonary vasculature, pulmonary edema, and pleural effusions also may be present.[10] Marked hepatosplenomegaly caused by extramedullary hematopoiesis and cardiac failure is common.[10] Resolution of these radiographic changes in neonates who survive is usually gradual.[10]

Pleural Fluid Collections

Widening of the pleural space (unilateral or bilateral) by soft tissue density material (fluid) in a neonate most commonly reflects a chylothorax, although pleural effusion, empyema, and hemorrhage can produce a similar radiographic appearance (see Fig. 32-65).[1,10,29,30] There may be an associated lung parenchymal abnormality, such as neoplasm, sequestration, or infectious process.[10,87] Because the ICN patient is usually positioned supine, pleural fluid tends to collect posteriorly, in the dependent portion of the pleural space. As a result, on the usual anteroposterior supine portable chest radiograph, pleural fluid may appear only

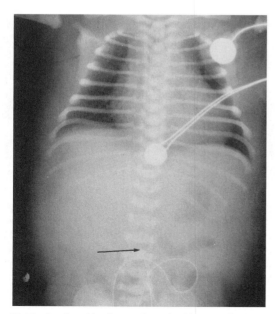

Figure 32–71. A 1-day-old infant with erythroblastosis fetalis and generalized edema accompanied by cardiomegaly and ascites. Note the generalized increase in soft tissue thickness throughout the thorax and abdomen. The tip of the umbilical arterial catheter *(arrow)* overlies the L3-4 disk space, in good position.

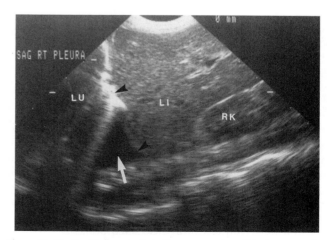

Figure 32–72. Sagittally oriented ultrasonography of the lower portion of the right thorax shows anechoic (echo-free) fluid *(arrow)* in the lower right pleural space, reflecting pleural effusion. LI, liver; LU, lung; RK, right kidney. *Arrowheads* indicate diaphragm.

as a generalized increase in density of the hemithorax. Sonography assists in identifying and further characterizing pleural fluid collections (Fig. 32-72).

Mediastinal and Pulmonary Masses

Mediastinal masses in neonates and infants are uncommon; 60% are neurogenic in origin and located in the posterior mediastinum.[23] Teratomas and dermoids are anterior mediastinal in location and constitute 12% to 20% of masses.[23] Bronchogenic or duplication cysts typically are located in the middle mediastinum and may contain an air-fluid level.[30,37] There are miscellaneous rare mediastinal tumors and cysts.[88]

All mediastinal masses have predominantly soft tissue density on plain radiographs.[23] Teratomas and dermoids may contain calcification and fat density areas, and neuroblastomas may contain irregular or granular calcifications.[23] Anterior mediastinal masses frequently displace or narrow the trachea, middle mediastinal masses indent the esophagus, and posterior mediastinal masses may have associated spine erosion or deformity.[23,37] Ultrasonography, CT, MRI, and barium swallow studies are supplemental imaging procedures used in the evaluation of mediastinal masses.[23,37] An atypical configuration of the normal thymus can simulate an upper mediastinal mass on the chest radiograph, but it should not produce deviation or deformity of the trachea.[89] Thoracic sonography shows the normal thymus and allows exclusion of a true mediastinal mass.[89,90]

Pulmonary sequestration is a rare congenital anomaly involving nonfunctioning pulmonary tissue with no normal connection with the bronchial tree or pulmonary arteries and with systemic arterial supply.[1,10,23,91] Radiographic presentation may be as a homogeneous soft tissue mass, a large cyst containing air or fluid, or a combination of both, usually in the left lower hemithorax.[10,23,37,92] Demonstration of the systemic arterial supply to the sequestration can be by angiography, MRI, or, more recently, duplex or color Doppler sonography.[10,37,91] Spontaneous resolution of the masslike density has been reported.[93]

Primary pulmonary tumors are rare in neonates and infants, the most frequently reported being pulmonary blastoma, which has malignant and metastatic potential.[23,94] Pulmonary hemangioma can cause respiratory distress in the neonate.[95] Pulmonary varix and arteriovenous malformations may appear as a nodular shadow with associated feeding vessels.[23]

Extracorporeal Membrane Oxygenation

ECMO is a form of cardiopulmonary bypass used to treat term or near-term newborns with severe but reversible cardiac or pulmonary failure who have failed maximal ventilatory and medical support.[32,65,71,96] To optimize success rate and minimize duration of required ECMO support, the infant's lung disease should be fully reversible within 10 to 14 days.[32,96] Most ECMO candidates have an underlying pulmonary disease with associated pulmonary hypertension, resulting in right-to-left shunting.[71,96] Meconium aspiration syndrome, sepsis, neonatal pneumonia, CDH, and severe hyaline membrane disease are the most common pulmonary processes leading to ECMO.[32,71,96]

The ECMO apparatus includes a membrane oxygenator, a heating unit, and a roller occlusion pump.[71,96] In veno-arterial ECMO, carotid arterial and jugular venous cannulas are placed on the right side of the neck at initiation of ECMO bypass.[96] Desaturated blood is removed via the jugular venous cannula, oxygenated in the external circuit, then returned to the patient via the carotid arterial cannula.[96] The right internal jugular vein is ligated. The right common carotid artery was formerly ligated but now is usually surgically reconstructed.[96] In veno-venous ECMO, a single double-lumen venous catheter is inserted into the right internal jugular vein with its tip in the right atrium.[71] Requiring relative hemodynamic stability and good cardiac function, veno-venous ECMO avoids the need for surgical disruption of the right common carotid artery and is increasingly replacing veno-arterial ECMO whenever feasible.[71]

Patients are anticoagulated with heparin throughout their course of ECMO and are at increased risk for hemorrhagic complications, most frequently involving the central nervous system.[32,96] Repaired CDH patients on ECMO have a high incidence of thoracic hemorrhagic complications as well.[96,97]

The chest radiograph before ECMO reflects the nature and severity of the underlying disease process causing respiratory failure.[96] The findings can range from

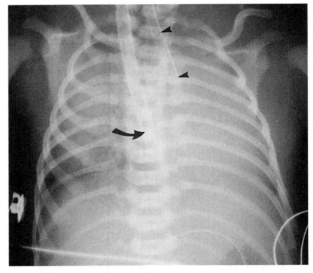

Figure 32–73. A term neonate with severe respiratory failure caused by meconium aspiration, incompletely responsive to maximal conventional medical support. With a predicted mortality of greater than 80%, the patient was placed on extracorporeal membrane oxygenation (ECMO). Desaturated blood is removed from the patient via the jugular venous cannula *(arrow)*, with the preferred tip location in the right atrium. After oxygenation in an external membrane oxygenator, blood is returned to the patient via a carotid arterial cannula *(arrowheads)*, whose preferred tip position is in the aortic arch. Both cannulas appear to be in good location and were functioning well. Patients are maintained on low ventilatory pressure settings throughout ECMO and remain intubated. Complete or near-complete opacification of the lungs occurs during ECMO in most patients, reflecting a combination of alveolar edema and atelectasis.

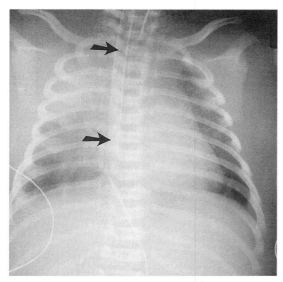

Figure 32–74. A term newborn with severe respiratory failure caused by neonatal pneumonia. The infant was placed on extracorporeal membrane oxygenation. A double-lumen veno-venous cannula *(arrows)* is in good position, with its tip in the right atrium. The single-cannula venovenous system requires better cardiac function but obviates the need to ligate or reconstruct surgically the right common carotid artery.

hyperlucent lungs in primary pulmonary hypertension of the newborn to diffuse pulmonary parenchymal infiltrates with or without hyperinflation.[96] Air-block complications of mechanical ventilation, such as pulmonary interstitial emphysema and pneumothorax, are common.[96] Heart size can range from normal to greatly enlarged, depending on degree of cardiac dysfunction.

After placement of the patient on ECMO, the chest radiograph shows the opaque ECMO cannula (veno-venous ECMO) or cannulas (veno-arterial ECMO) extending intrathoracically from the right side of the neck (Figs. 32-73 and 32-74).[71,96] The jugular venous (dual-cannula system) and veno-venous (single-cannula system) cannulas extend down along the right mediastinal margin, traversing the superior vena cava and ending in the right atrium, the preferred tip location.[96] The shorter carotid arterial cannula of the veno-arterial system extends obliquely to overlie the left upper mediastinal region, with the preferred cannula tip site being the aortic arch.[96] Because the patient is on low-pressure mechanical ventilation throughout ECMO, an endotracheal tube is in place.[96] Various other support lines and catheters, such as pleural chest tubes and umbilical arterial and venous catheters, may be present.[96]

Most neonates show progressive opacification of the lung fields during ECMO, reflecting a combination of alveolar edema and atelectasis.[71,96] Both lungs become completely opaque and airless during ECMO in most patients.[71,96] The opacification resolves as pulmonary function and compliance improve and the underlying disease process resolves.[96] Pleural effusions are common during ECMO and may be masked by the generalized pulmonary opacification, in which case thoracic sonography may be used to identify pleural fluid collections.[96]

With termination of ECMO, pulmonary opacity of varying severity, occasionally worse than on the pre-ECMO chest radiographs, may persist for days or weeks despite the clinical improvement.[96] A variety of radiographically definable thoracic complications may occur during ECMO, including ECMO cannula malposition and migration, chest tube migration, pneumothoraces, pulmonary and pleural hemorrhages, and atelectasis.[97]

ABDOMEN

Normal Appearances and Common Variations

Interpretation of plain films of the abdomen in neonates and infants is difficult, in part because of the quantity of bowel and soft tissue structures present. The right upper quadrant of the abdomen should normally be homogeneous soft tissue density, reflecting the liver primarily (see Fig. 32-17). The inferior hepatic margin should run obliquely in the right upper quadrant, from lower laterally to higher medially. No calcification or air should be included within the margins of the liver. A smaller area of soft tissue density, representing the spleen, may be present in the extreme left upper quadrant of the abdomen (see Fig. 32-17). As delineated by air, the stomach should be in the left upper quadrant, medial to the splenic shadow (see Fig. 32-17). The remainder of the abdomen is usually a mixture of soft tissue and air density, depending on the quantity of intestinal gas present (see Fig. 32-17). Because of the relative lack of fat in the neonate, the kidneys, psoas muscles, and other retroperitoneal structures are typically not delineated on conventional radiographs, although a thin, sharply marginated lucent stripe representing properitoneal fat is often seen along the lateral abdominal wall on the anteroposterior supine radiograph.

As the newborn swallows, air enters the intestinal tract, with progressive replacement of intraluminal fluid (see Fig. 32-20). Air is usually noted within the stomach within 10 to 15 minutes of birth, within the proximal small bowel by 30 to 60 minutes, throughout the small bowel by 6 hours, and throughout the colon by 12 to 24 hours.[23] Differentiation of loops of small bowel from colon on conventional radiographs is usually not possible in neonates and infants. The overall quantity of bowel gas normally tends to be greater in neonates and infants than in older children and adults.

Fluid-filled segments of bowel can appear as soft tissue "masses" on the anteroposterior supine radiograph; fluid accumulating in the fundus of the stomach is the most frequent cause of this pseudomass appearance.[23] Umbilical hernias and stumps can project as round or oval soft tissue masses.[23] Their margins are unusually sharply defined, however, because of surrounding air.[23] Likewise, intact meningoceles and myelomeningoceles can produce a soft tissue mass appearance overlying the abdomen, but they are accompanied by dysraphic changes of the adjacent lumbar spine.[23] Distention of the urinary bladder can produce a lower abdominal and pelvic "mass" effect (Fig. 32-75A).

A generalized increase in intestinal gas can occur in infants with respiratory distress caused by excessive

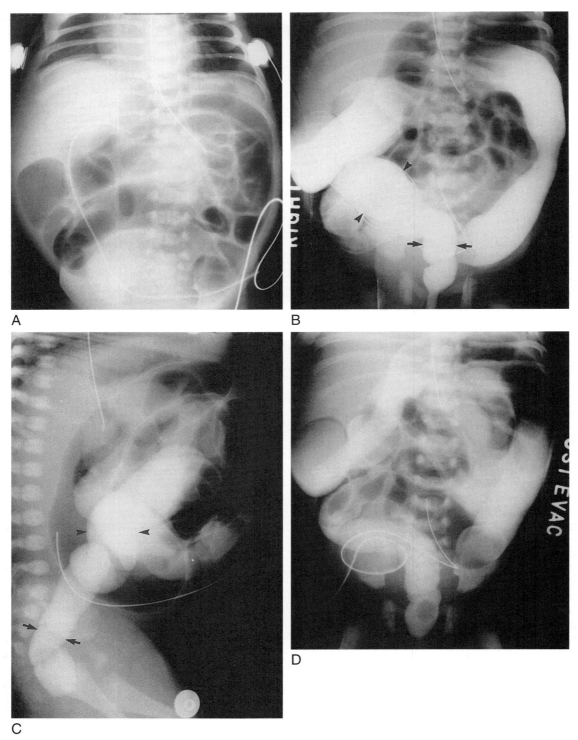

Figure 32–75. A 3-day-old infant with progressive abdominal distention and failure to pass meconium. Anteroposterior abdominal radiograph **(A)** shows moderate gaseous distention of multiple loops of bowel. Soft tissue fullness in the pelvis and lower abdomen reflected a distended urinary bladder, although a soft tissue mass also would be a consideration, especially in a female neonate. It is frequently impossible to differentiate dilated colon from small bowel in the newborn, based on the abdominal radiograph. Because of the presence of dilated bowel, the next indicated imaging procedure would be a barium enema. Anteroposterior **(B)** and lateral **(C)** views show relative narrowing and lack of distensibility of the rectum *(arrows)* compared with the sigmoid colon *(arrowheads)*. This change in colon caliber and configuration is called the *transition zone* and is highly suggestive of Hirschsprung's disease. The aganglionic rectum is narrower than the normally innervated sigmoid colon, with the transition zone representing the segment of change from abnormal (rectum) to normal (sigmoid) innervation. Postevacuation radiograph **(D)** indicates no apparent colonic emptying, an abnormal finding that further suggests the diagnosis of Hirschsprung's disease. Rectal biopsy was confirmatory.

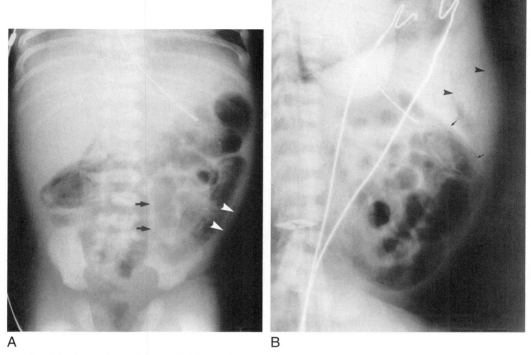

A   B

Figure 32–76. An 11-day-old infant with rapid onset of abdominal tenderness and distention accompanied by blood-tinged stool after start of oral feeding. **A,** Anteroposterior abdominal radiograph shows multiple, mildly distended loops of bowel with a mild increase in soft tissue spacing *(arrows)* between intraluminal air that suggests bowel wall thickening or intraperitoneal fluid. Intramural bowel air *(arrowheads)* on the left reflects pneumatosis intestinalis and confirms the clinical suspicion of necrotizing enterocolitis. **B,** In addition to showing distended bowel and pneumatosis intestinalis *(arrows)*, the cross-table lateral view shows extensive portal venous air *(arrowheads)*. Should intestinal perforation with a relatively small amount of intraperitoneal air occur as a complication of necrotizing enterocolitis, the cross-table lateral view of the abdomen would be at a disadvantage in showing the free air because of the location of intraluminal air in the region where free intraperitoneal air would collect.

swallowing of air. With passage of time and meconium, this appearance typically resolves. Benign gaseous distention of the bowel is common in premature infants treated with nasal continuous positive airway pressure.[98] An airless appearance to the abdomen is seen occasionally in neonates and infants, usually in conjunction with intubation and after administration of neuromuscular paralyzing agents (see Fig. 32-15). Other causes include excessive vomiting and prolonged nasogastric suction.

Necrotizing Enterocolitis

The role of radiology in the management of NEC is to assist in making the correct diagnosis, monitor the progression of the disease, and identify any complications.[23] The initial plain film finding in NEC is usually bowel dilation caused by ileus.[1,23,99] Although there is no pattern of bowel distention that is specific for NEC, disproportionate dilation of bowel in the right lower quadrant, especially if the pattern of dilation persists over 1 day or more, is suggestive of NEC.[1,99] More generalized bowel distention also can be an early sign of NEC, however.[23] If, in addition, there is an increase in soft tissue separation between individual intraluminal bowel gas collections, inflammatory bowel wall thickening, or intraperitoneal

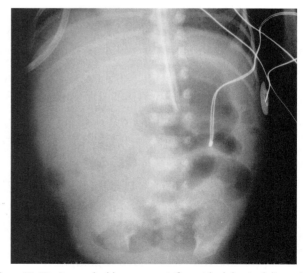

Figure 32–77. A 4-week-old premature infant with abdominal distention and tenderness. Dilated loops of bowel are present in the left abdomen, and there is increased soft tissue density with a few small collections of bowel gas in the right abdomen. No actual intramural bowel air is definable. The increased soft tissue and dilated loops of bowel, in the appropriate clinical setting, suggest necrotizing enterocolitis. Necrotic bowel due to necrotizing enterocolitis was present at surgery and resected.

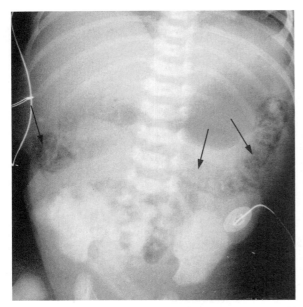

Figure 32–78. A 3-day-old infant with abdominal tenderness and blood in stool after beginning feeding. There is extensive pneumatosis intestinalis *(arrows)* of a predominantly cystic or submucosal nature involving the transverse colon, as a reflection of necrotizing enterocolitis.

fluid interspersed among bowel, NEC is considerably more likely (Figs. 32-76 and 32-77).[23,99]

Air within the bowel wall, or pneumatosis cystoides intestinalis, is the radiographic sign most pathognomonic for NEC in premature neonates (Fig. 32-78; see also Fig. 32-76).[1,23,99,100] This intramural air can occur in differing patterns, depending on location of the air.[1,23] Submucosal air usually has a bubbly or microcystic appearance; subserosal air typically is more linear or curvilinear in appearance.[1,23,99] The cystic pattern can be difficult to distinguish from intraluminal air mixed with stool or meconium with a high degree of confidence.[1,23,99]

Extension of intramural air into the intestinal venous system can result in a branching pattern of lucency within the central portion of the liver, reflecting portal venous air (see Fig. 32-76).[99] Improvement in therapy has made this finding, which is uncommon, a much less ominous reflection of NEC than was formerly the case. Sonography of the abdomen can show portal venous gas and bowel wall thickening in infants with NEC before the appearance of signs of NEC on plain abdominal radiographs.[22,23,99,100]

Perforation of diseased bowel usually results in intraperitoneal extension of bowel air.[23] The resultant pneumoperitoneum may present as an area of relative lucency overlying the right upper quadrant, primarily on the anteroposterior supine radiograph (Figs. 32-79A, 32-80, and 32-81). The falciform ligament can be outlined on both sides by free intraperitoneal air (see Figs. 32-79A, 32-80, and 32-81). Definition of the mucosal and the serosal surfaces of loops of bowel indicates bowel perforation and free intraperitoneal air (see Fig. 32-79A). If the amount of intraperitoneal air is limited, the left decubitus

anteroposterior radiograph of the abdomen may be essential in detection of the free air, which collects between the liver and lateral abdominal wall (see Fig. 32-79C).

In addition to bowel perforation with free intraperitoneal air shown on abdominal radiographs, there are other radiographic changes that may make surgical intervention appropriate or necessary in neonates with NEC.[23,102,103] In some cases of perforation, no free air is detected, usually in cases in which little or no bowel gas was present before perforation.[23] Additionally, in the presence of peritonitis, perforation may be accompanied by an increase in abdominal girth and overall radiographic density because of accumulation of intraperitoneal fluid.[23] Occasionally, bowel perforation with NEC is accompanied by a sudden decrease in amount of intestinal gas but without development of free intraperitoneal air.[23] Focally dilated loops of bowel that persist without change from radiograph to radiograph suggest ischemic, necrotic bowel, necessitating surgical intervention.[23]

Occasionally, neither the clinical nor the plain radiographic appearance in an infant allows the diagnosis of NEC to be made or excluded with confidence. In such cases, portable examination of the intestinal tract using nonionic (low osmolality), water-soluble contrast material may identify signs of NEC or exclude the diagnosis.[8]

When NEC is diagnosed and appropriate treatment is instituted, serial abdominal radiographs (typically, anteroposterior supine and left decubitus views) are indicated to follow progression or regression of radiographic findings and to look for complications, such as bowel necrosis and perforation.[1] The appropriate interval between radiographic examinations is variable and should be determined by the level of suspicion of NEC and the severity of clinical findings.[1] In general, abdominal radiographs should be obtained every 6 to 12 hours during the active phase of NEC, unless there is a sudden change in clinical status that suggests an acute-onset complication.[1]

Neonates successfully treated for NEC are at risk for development of post-NEC strictures.[23,99] Development of abdominal distention accompanied by new bowel dilation on abdominal radiographs suggests post-NEC stricture formation.[23,99] Contrast examination of the intestinal tract is indicated to evaluate for focal, persistent bowel narrowing.[23] A much less common complication of NEC is the formation of an enteric fistula, which requires contrast examination of the intestinal tract for diagnosis.[104]

Neonatal Intestinal Obstruction

Intestinal Atresias

Esophageal atresia and tracheoesophageal fistula.
Esophageal atresia and tracheoesophageal fistula consist of three types of abnormality, which have differing radiographic findings: esophageal atresia without tracheoesophageal fistula, esophageal atresia with tracheoesophageal fistula, and tracheoesophageal fistula with intact esophagus.[1,23,99,105] In cases of esophageal atresia without or with fistula, a distended, partially air-filled proximal esophageal segment is usually seen on chest radiographs (Figs. 32-82A and 32-83A).[23,29] On the lateral projection, the trachea is usually anteriorly displaced and narrowed, on a

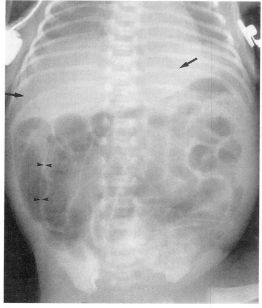

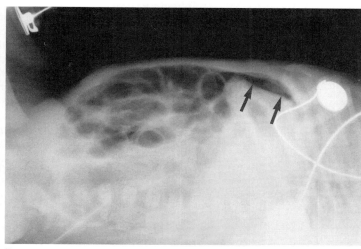

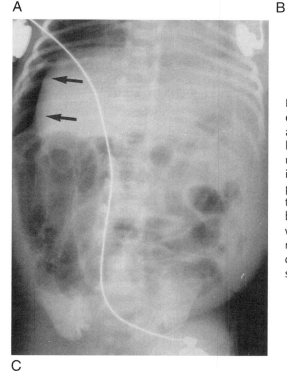

A

B

C

Figure 32–79. A 9-day-old infant with intestinal perforation caused by necrotizing enterocolitis. **A,** There are two radiographic signs of free intraperitoneal air on the anteroposterior supine film; a zone of relatively greater lucency *(arrows)* overlying the liver with greater opacity on either side; and sharp definition of both sides of individual loops of bowel *(arrowheads)*, rather than just the inner margin, caused by adjacent intraperitoneal air. Mild bowel distention is also present, but there is no definable pneumatosis intestinalis. **B,** The free intraperitoneal air *(arrows)* as seen on the cross-table lateral view is not easily distinguished from the much more copious intraluminal bowel gas, although differentiation can be made. **C,** The left decubitus anteroposterior view shows better the free intraperitoneal air *(arrows)*, which has collected high in the right upper quadrant between the liver and lateral abdominal wall. In general, the left decubitus view of the abdomen is superior to the cross-table lateral view in identifying smaller amounts of free intraperitoneal air.

developmental basis (see Figs. 32-82B and 32-83B).[23] An enteric catheter ends or loops back on itself at the site of atresia (see Figs. 32-82C and D and 32-83A and B).[1,29,99] If no fistula is present between the tracheobronchial tree and distal esophageal segment, the abdomen is airless because of the absence of intestinal gas.[1,23,29,97] If a distal fistula is present, air-containing bowel is seen on abdominal radiographs (see Fig. 32-82).[1,23,29,99] Esophageal atresia with obstruction of a distal tracheoesophageal fistula, resulting in a gasless abdomen, has been reported.[106]

In cases of H-type tracheoesophageal fistula with intact esophagus, clinical presentation is usually in infancy or early childhood, and the most likely radiographic presentation is of pulmonary infiltrates caused by aspiration pneumonia.[23,29,99]

Should confirmation of esophageal atresia beyond plain radiographs be required, distention of the blind-ending esophageal pouch with air injected through an enteric tube, with simultaneous radiography, should suffice.[1] Injection of contrast material into the proximal

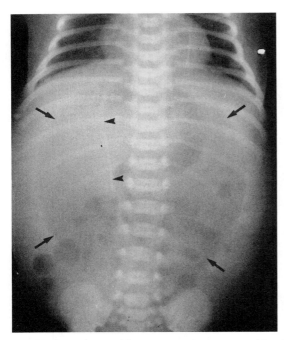

Figure 32–80. A newborn with pneumoperitoneum resulting from spontaneous perforation of the terminal ileum, cause indeterminate. There is a large central lucency *(arrows)* in the abdomen reflecting the free air collecting in the most anterior, nondependent portion of the abdomen. Air outlines both sides of the falciform ligament *(arrowheads)* in the right upper quadrant. Such large amounts of free intraperitoneal air are readily identified on the anteroposterior supine radiograph, and a supplementary left decubitus view is not necessary for diagnosis.

esophageal pouch is potentially dangerous because of possible aspiration and should be avoided.[1,23] Radiologic demonstration of an H-type fistula requires slow injection of contrast material via an end-hole esophageal catheter being gradually withdrawn toward the hypopharynx.[29] Prone positioning of the infant with horizontal-beam lateral fluoroscopy optimizes definition of an H-type fistula.[29]

Ventilation of newborns with tracheoesophageal fistula and RDS may be compromised by tracheal gas flow diversion through the fistula.[107] Placement of a gastrostomy tube for gastric decompression, surgical ligation of the fistula, occlusion of the fistula via a balloon catheter, and use of high-frequency jet ventilation are potentially effective therapeutic measures.[107] Esophageal atresia and tracheoesophageal fistula is a component of the VATER or VACTERL association of anomalies that may include vertebral, anorectal, cardiac, tracheoesophageal, renal, and radial ray limb abnormalities.[29]

Duodenal atresia. Associated with Down syndrome, duodenal atresia typically presents radiographically as air distention of the stomach and proximal duodenum above the usual site of atresia at or below the ampulla of Vater.[1,23,99] This "double-bubble" sign is seen with duodenal atresia and annular pancreas (Fig. 32-84).[1,23,99] The plain film appearance is characteristic, and further imaging before surgical correction is not necessary.[1,23] In the rare anomaly wherein a double limb of the pancreatic ductal system is present, with one limb originating above and the other below the site of atresia, bowel gas may pass beyond the site of duodenal atresia into small bowel and colon.[1,23] Duodenal atresia appears on antenatal sonograms as a similar, double-bubble, fluid-filled structure in the upper abdomen of the fetus.[23]

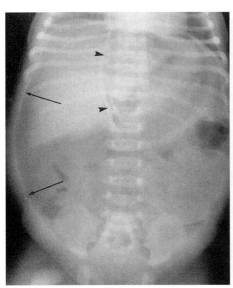

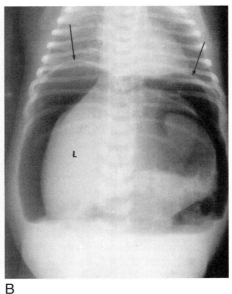

A

B

Figure 32–81. A newborn developed a massive pneumoperitoneum caused by spontaneous perforation of the stomach. **A,** Anteroposterior supine view shows relative lucency throughout the abdomen, with a clear difference in density between the abdominal cavity and lateral abdominal wall *(arrows)*. The falciform ligament is outlined by free air *(arrowheads)*. **B,** Upright view better illustrates the amount of free air. Note the thin hemidiaphragms *(arrows)* separating the thoracic and abdominal cavities. L, liver.

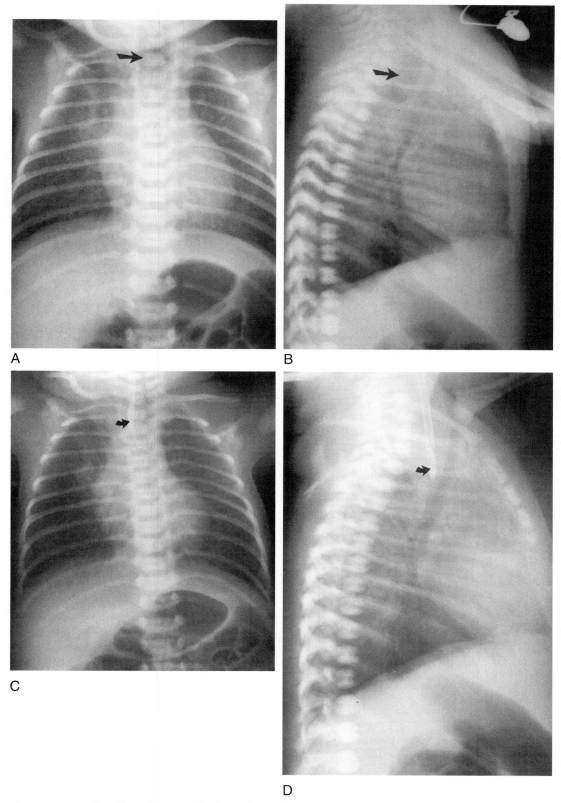

Figure 32–82. Anteroposterior **(A)** and lateral **(B)** portable chest radiographs show increased lucency at the base of the neck *(arrows)* with mild anterior bowing of the trachea as seen on the lateral view, reflecting esophageal atresia. Air in the intestinal tract indicates the presence of a fistula between the tracheobronchial tree and the distal esophageal segment. This was a type C esophageal atresia, with a distal fistula, by far the most common form of esophageal atresia. Anteroposterior **(C)** and lateral **(D)** views after attempted passage of a nasogastric catheter show the catheter tip *(arrow)* to end near the blind-ending proximal esophageal pouch.

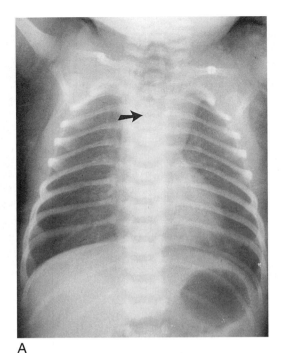

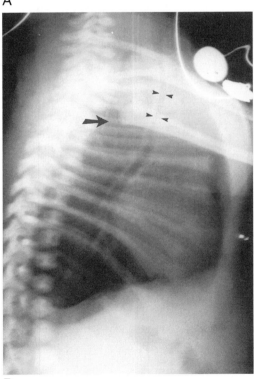

Figure 32–83. Anteroposterior **(A)** and lateral **(B)** views show distention of a blind-ending proximal esophageal pouch *(arrows)* associated with type C esophageal atresia with a fistula between the tracheobronchial tree and the distal esophageal segment. This fistula is implied by the presence of air in the intra-abdominal intestinal segment. There is associated narrowing of the adjacent trachea *(arrowheads)*, a commonly associated finding. An enteric tube is curled in the proximal esophageal pouch.

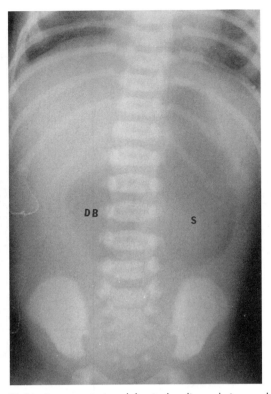

Figure 32–84. Anteroposterior abdominal radiograph in a 2-day-old infant shows a gasless abdomen except for air within the stomach *(S)* and distended duodenal bulb *(DB)*. This pattern of air distribution in a newborn usually reflects duodenal atresia, although an annular pancreas can cause a similar appearance. Antenatal sonography identifies fluid rather than air distention of the stomach and first duodenal segment. Down syndrome is of clinical concern with the imaging findings of duodenal atresia.

Jejunal and ileal atresia. The radiographic appearance of small bowel atresia depends on the site of obstruction (Figs. 32-85 and 32-86; see also Figs. 32-21 and 32-22). Dilated intestine is present in all cases.[1,23] If the site of atresia is high in the jejunum, only a few loops of bowel can be seen.[1,23] The further distal the site of obstruction, the greater the number of dilated loops of bowel and air-fluid levels that are present.[1,23]

Obstruction judged to be high in the jejunum is a surgical management problem, and no further imaging is usually necessary.[23] More distal small bowel obstruction usually requires a contrast study of the colon to exclude malrotation and volvulus as the cause. With distal small bowel atresia, a microcolon of greatly reduced caliber is present.[23] Irregular or linear intramural calcifications also may be present in infants with small bowel atresia.[23]

Other intestinal atresias. Pyloric atresia and other forms of congenital gastric outlet obstruction occur rarely.[23,108,109] The stomach is distended, and little or no small bowel and colonic air is present on abdominal radiographs.[23,108,109] The upper gastrointestinal series shows complete or near-complete obstruction at the antropyloric region.[108,109]

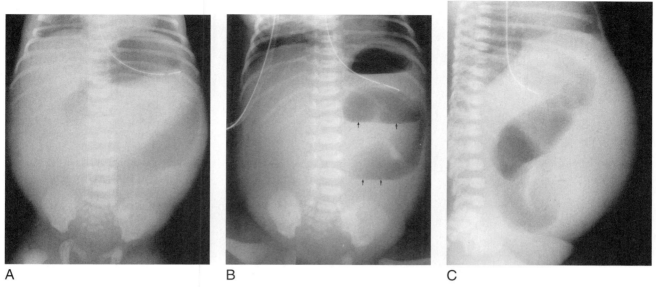

A   B   C

Figure 32–85. Anteroposterior supine **(A)** and upright **(B)** and lateral recumbent **(C)** views show abdominal distention with increased soft tissue density suggesting intra-abdominal fluid and distention of several loops of bowel with fluid and air. Air-fluid levels are present on the upright film *(arrows)*. This pattern of bowel distention suggests proximal small bowel obstruction. Atresia of the proximal jejunum accompanied by ascites was identified at surgery.

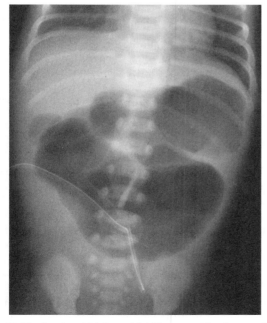

Figure 32–86. A 2-day-old infant with bilious vomiting but no abdominal distention. Intestinal malrotation with volvulus was suspected clinically. Anteroposterior abdominal radiograph shows gaseous distention of proximal bowel, greater in length than can be accounted for by stomach and duodenum alone. There is no demonstrable distal bowel gas and no suggestion of intra-abdominal fluid. Proximal jejunal atresia was present at surgery.

Colonic atresia can be of four types: type I, or membranous atresia; type II, with the atresia consisting of a thin fibrous band; type III, or complete atresia with no connecting band; and type IV, or multiple atresias.[1,23,99] The colon proximal to the site of atresia appears greatly dilated on plain radiographs and contains a mixture of meconium and air.[23,99] Barium enema shows variable shortening of the colon, depending on the site of atresia, and a microcolon caliber.[23,99] The proximal colon beyond the site of atresia may appear hook shaped or dilated (the "windsock" sign).[23] Multiple atresias represent 6% to 29% of all atresias, most of which are jejunal and ileal in location.[110]

Malrotation and Ladd's bands or volvulus. The developing intestinal tract in the fetus is located outside the abdomen during part of intrauterine life but returns to the abdomen for completion of 270 degrees of rotation.[1,23,99] Normal bowel fixation results in the mesenteric root extending from the left upper to right lower retroperitoneum (representing the ligament of Treitz and ileocecal junction).[1,23,99] The normally long mesenteric root prevents midgut torsion or volvulus.[1]

In malrotation, the ligament of Treitz is positioned caudally and to the right, and the ileocecal junction tends to be high and to the left.[23] The resultant short mesenteric root can be associated with formation of intraperitoneal bands (Ladd's bands) or torsion of the bowel (volvulus).[1,23,99] Ladd's bands typically obstruct the third or fourth portions of the duodenum and produce a radiographic appearance of high bowel obstruction.[1,23,99] Volvulus initially involves mechanical obstruction of the bowel lumen but can progress to vascular compromise, bowel ischemia, and possible necrosis with subsequent perforation.[23,99]

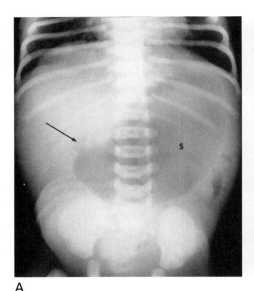

A

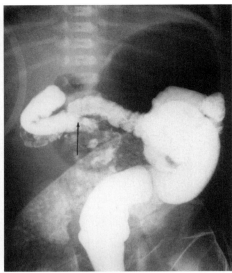

B

Figure 32–87. A newborn with bilious vomiting. **A,** Anteroposterior abdominal radiograph shows gaseous distention of the stomach *(S)* and limited air in nondilated duodenum *(arrow)*. **B,** To evaluate for malrotation and possible volvulus, barium enema was performed, which showed an abnormally high cecum *(arrow)* as an indication of malrotation. Because of the high degree of clinical concern for associated volvulus, emergency laparotomy was performed, which identified malrotation and high duodenal obstruction caused by Ladd's bands. Volvulus was not present, however.

Clinically, infants with malrotation and obstructing Ladd's bands or volvulus have bilious vomiting.[1,23,99,102] If volvulus is suspected clinically, emergency radiographic evaluation with plain radiographs and a contrast study of the intestinal tract are indicated.[1,23]

Plain abdominal radiographs in malrotation with obstructing Ladd's bands usually show high intestinal obstruction, with distention of the stomach and duodenum and with limited bowel gas distally (Fig. 32-87A).[1,23] Abdominal films are not reliable in excluding an associated volvulus, with the findings varying from normal to small bowel obstruction.[1,23,100]

Contrast examination of the intestinal tract from above shows the distal duodenal obstruction in cases of obstructing Ladd bands and low and rightward malposition of the ligament of Treitz in malrotation without obstructing bands.[1,23,99] If volvulus is present, a corkscrew appearance to the proximal small bowel may be seen if obstruction is partial or intermittent or a beaked appearance to the end of bowel if obstruction is complete.[1,23,99] If a contrast enema is performed, the cecum is abnormally high and leftward in location, but the actual point of obstruction is not visualized (Fig. 32-87B).[1,23] Abdominal sonography has identified midgut volvulus.[111]

Gastric volvulus is a rare surgical emergency in infancy and childhood.[112] The volvulus can be either organoaxial (around a line joining the esophageal hiatus and pylorus [two thirds of cases]) or mesentericoaxial (around a line joining the greater and lesser curves).[112] Most cases are secondary to deficient fixation of the stomach.[112] Abdominal radiographs in mesentericoaxial volvulus show the stomach to be spherical on supine films, and two fluid levels are present on the erect film—one in the fundus and one in the antrum (higher).[112] Barium studies show the obstruction and an upside-down configuration to the stomach.[112] More difficult to diagnose on plain films and barium studies,

organoaxial volvulus involves a horizontal lie to the stomach and a single fluid level.[112]

Hirschsprung's disease. Hirschsprung's disease, or aganglionosis, involves a variable length of colon, beginning at the anorectal junction and proceeding proximally in a continuous pattern of involvement.[1,23,99] Most cases are limited to the distal colonic segment (the rectum and distal rectosigmoid regions).[1,23,99] Total colonic aganglionosis is rare, and skip areas of involvement are believed not to exist.[1,23,99]

Although usually presenting in childhood with abnormal patterns of stooling and fecal soiling, Hirschsprung's disease may produce intestinal obstruction with vomiting, failure to pass meconium within 24 hours, or diarrhea in the neonatal period.[1,23,99] If Hirschsprung's disease is suspected clinically, contrast examination of the colon is indicated.[23,99,113]

Plain abdominal films usually show distended, partially air-filled small bowel, often with limited or no air in the rectum (see Fig. 32-75).[1,23] This pattern is nonspecific, however, and can be produced by other colon obstructions, such as meconium plug syndrome and neonatal small left colon syndrome.[23]

The most common finding on barium enema examination is a "transition zone" in the rectosigmoid region, with maximal rectal diameter being less than that of more proximal colon (see Fig. 32-75B and C).[1,23] The ratio of maximal rectal diameter to that of colonic diameter is termed the **rectosigmoid index.** The rectosigmoid index is greater than 1 in normal patients and less than 1 in patients with Hirschsprung's disease.[1,23] Less frequently seen is an irregular or spiculated appearance to the sigmoid colon, thought to reflect spasm.[23,99] Delayed 24- or 48-hour abdominal radiographs usually show prolonged retention of barium in the colon.[1,23] Of neonates with Hirschsprung's disease, 25% show a normal colonic configuration, and a normal barium enema in the neonatal

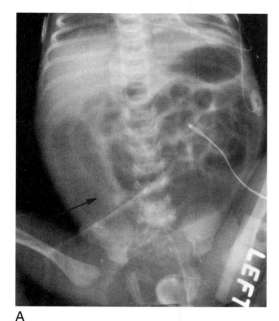

A

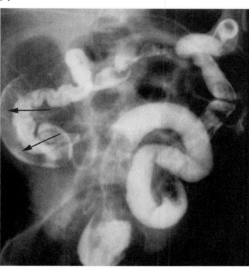

B

Figure 32–88. A 1-day-old premature newborn with progressive abdominal distention and failure to pass meconium. **A,** Anteroposterior supine abdominal radiograph shows multiple dilated, air-filled loops of bowel in the right and lower portions of the abdomen. A cluster of tiny lucencies *(arrow)* in the right lower quadrant is compatible with the "soap-bubble" appearance of meconium plugging the terminal ileum. There is no air in the rectum, and the abdomen is otherwise normal. **B,** Contrast enema shows a small-caliber colon (microcolon) and plugging of the terminal ileum by meconium, as outlined by contrast material *(arrows)*. All of the distended bowel is shown to be small bowel. This appearance is characteristic of meconium ileus.

period does not fully exclude the diagnosis.[23,113] In this case, if clinical suspicion of Hirschsprung's disease is high in the presence of a normal barium enema, rectal biopsy should be performed anyway. No bowel preparation before the barium enema is necessary.[99]

Meconium ileus. Typically associated with cystic fibrosis, meconium ileus reflects impaction of thick, tenacious meconium in the distal small bowel, with resultant obstruction at the distal ileal level.[1,23,99,114] Ileal atresia or stenosis, ileal perforation, meconium peritonitis, and volvulus without or with pseudocyst formation are common complications of the meconium impaction.[1,23,99,114]

Plain abdominal radiographs usually show numerous air-filled loops of small bowel, suggesting low small bowel obstruction (Fig. 32-88A).[1,23,99,114] Air-fluid levels may be absent or limited because of the thickness of the meconium.[1,23,99] A mixture of meconium and air can produce a "soap-bubble" appearance to bowel in the right lower quadrant of the abdomen.[1,23,99]

If meconium ileus is suspected clinically, a contrast enema is indicated for diagnosis and possible therapy (Fig. 32-88B).[1,23,99] Although barium is satisfactory for diagnostic purposes, the iodine-containing, water-soluble contrast agent diatrizoate (Gastrografin) is generally preferred.[1,23,114] Gastrografin, being hypertonic, draws fluid into the bowel lumen and enhances the possibility of loosening the impacted meconium to permit spontaneous passage without the need for surgical intervention.[1,23,114] Gastrografin contains polysorbate 80 (Tween 80), a surface tension–reducing and emulsifying agent that assists in meconium passage as well.[23] Care must be taken to maintain satisfactory fluid and electrolyte balance, however.[23,99,114]

Meconium plug syndrome. Delayed passage of meconium can occur with a normally innervated but functionally immature colon.[1,23,99] Characteristically, meconium fills the left side of the colon and causes partial bowel obstruction that can vary in severity.[23] Diminished or absent passage of meconium is associated with abdominal distention in the newborn.[1,23] Plain abdominal films show numerous air-filled, dilated loops of bowel with a paucity of air-fluid levels and absence of rectal air (Fig. 32-89A).[1,23,99] Barium enema examination is required for diagnosis.[1,23,99] Barium characteristically flows around extensive intraluminal rectal and left-sided colonic meconium (Fig. 32-89B).[1,23,99] Colonic caliber is normal or slightly increased. With subsequent evacuation of barium and meconium, the bowel dilation and abdominal distention resolve.[1,23] Meconium plug syndrome infrequently may have coexisting Hirschsprung's disease.[1,23]

Neonatal small left colon syndrome. Considered to reflect functional immaturity of the colon, the neonatal small left colon syndrome is characterized by abdominal distention in the newborn accompanied by dilated loops of bowel on abdominal radiographs.[1,23,99] Barium enema examination shows relative narrowing of the left colon to about the splenic flexure, where there is a "transition zone" to a larger caliber colon more proximally, simulating Hirschsprung's disease.[1,99] Rectal biopsy shows normal ganglionic innervation of the colon, however.

Annular pancreas. Reflecting an anomalous band of pancreatic tissue that encircles the second portion of the duodenum, annular pancreas usually is associated with duodenal stenosis or atresia but can be an isolated

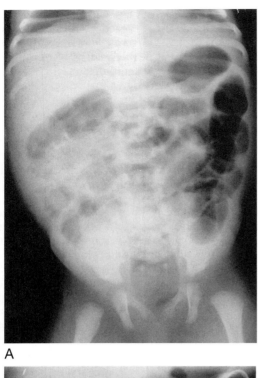

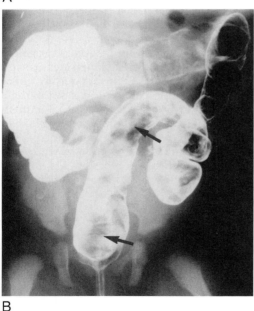

Figure 32–89. A 2-day-old infant with mild abdominal distention and failure to pass meconium. **A,** Anteroposterior abdominal radiograph shows mild distention of bowel but is otherwise unremarkable. Air is present in the rectum. **B,** Barium enema was performed to evaluate for possible obstruction. Copious meconium was identified in the rectum and left colon *(arrows)*, suggesting the diagnosis of meconium plug syndrome. The barium enema was diagnostic and therapeutic, with the meconium being promptly expelled and the intestinal distention resolved. The patient did not have Hirschsprung's disease, which occurs in approximately 10% of newborns with meconium plug syndrome.

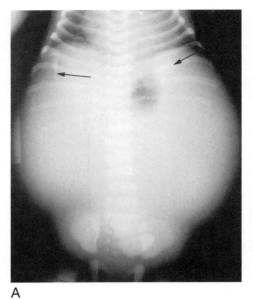

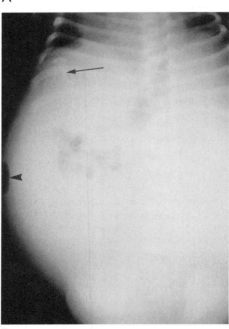

Figure 32–90. A 1-day-old infant with massively distended abdomen and ballotable intra-abdominal fluid. Anteroposterior supine **(A)** and left decubitus **(B)** radiographs show severe abdominal distention with bulging flanks and diffusely increased soft tissue density. Intestinal gas is limited to the stomach and proximal small bowel, which are not dilated. Intra-abdominal calcification is present in both upper quadrants *(arrows)*, reflecting meconium peritonitis. The decubitus view shows a small amount of free air rising to the nondependent portion of the abdomen *(arrowhead)*. Ultrasonography confirmed massive intra-abdominal fluid. Meconium peritonitis with intestinal perforation and pseudocyst formation was present at surgery.

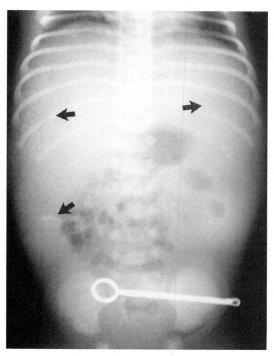

Figure 32–91. A newborn with mild abdominal distention. Anteroposterior abdominal radiograph shows multiple, widely scattered intraabdominal calcifications *(arrows)*, reflecting meconium peritonitis caused by intestinal perforation in utero. There is no bowel dilation to indicate associated intestinal obstruction caused by atresia resulting from the intestinal perforation and meconium extrusion.

abnormality.[99] When forming a complete ring, annular pancreas results in duodenal obstruction that is often complete and that mimics duodenal atresia.[99] The double-bubble sign is often present on plain abdominal radiographs.[99]

Intestinal Perforation

Intestinal perforation in utero can result in intraperitoneal extrusion of meconium and meconium peritonitis, which may calcify and appear as irregular opaque densities on the abdominal radiograph (Figs. 32-90 and 32-91).[99] Intestinal atresia and abdominal pseudocyst formation are additional possible complications (see Fig. 32-90).[99]

Box 32–1	Etiology of Neonatal Intestinal Perforation

Necrotizing enterocolitis
Idiopathic gastric perforation
Associated with distal intestinal obstruction
  Imperforate anus
  Hirschsprung's disease
  Immature colon syndrome
  Meconium ileus

Modified from Kirks DR (ed): Practical Pediatric Imaging: Diagnostic Radiology of Infants and Children, 2nd ed. Boston, Little, Brown, 1991.

Intestinal perforation in the neonatal period can reflect a variety of causes (Box 32-1) and occur from stomach to colon.[97,115,116] The radiographic diagnosis of intestinal perforation depends on demonstration of free intraperitoneal air in most cases (see Figs. 32-80, 32-81, and 32-90). A relative increase in lucency in the upper central abdominal region on the usual anteroposterior supine abdominal radiograph and delineation of the falciform ligament by free air are the primary radiographic signs of perforation (see Figs. 32-80 and 32-81). The left decubitus anteroposterior abdominal radiograph is the best single film for showing small amounts of free air in the neonate. The cross-table lateral film of the abdomen has the advantage of not requiring repositioning of the patient, but smaller amounts of free intraperitoneal air may be masked by normal intraluminal gas in the nondependent, anterior portion of the abdomen. Upright films are seldom obtained on newborns and young infants, especially if their clinical condition is precarious (see Fig. 32-81).

If bowel perforation occurs in conjunction with little or no bowel gas, diagnosis may not be possible by plain radiographs. Intraperitoneal fluid has the same overall density as intraluminal fluid and regional soft tissues (see Fig. 32-90). If bowel perforation is strongly suspected and no free intraperitoneal air is shown on plain radiographs, a contrast study of the upper intestinal tract using nonionic water-soluble contrast material is indicated.[117] Good bowel opacification is preserved without dilution, absorption of the contrast agent from the bowel lumen is minimal in the absence of intrinsic bowel disease, and extravasation of contrast material into the peritoneal cavity may be shown.[117]

Spontaneous intestinal perforation in very-low-birthweight neonates without NEC can be suspected when there is bluish discoloration of the abdomen. It may be associated with coagulase-negative staphylococcal infection and may not have free intraperitoneal air on abdominal radiographs.[118]

Intestinal (Paralytic) Ileus

Intestinal or paralytic ileus reflects distention of bowel caused by decreased bowel peristalsis rather than mechanical obstruction. Although the extent of bowel distention can vary with ileus, a more generalized bowel distention pattern, especially if air is definable in the rectum, is most suggestive of ileus (Fig. 32-92). Air-fluid levels tend to be prominent and widespread.[23] In contrast to mechanical obstruction, small-to-large bowel proportions remain the same, with relatively greater large bowel diameter compared with small bowel diameter.[23]

Omphalocele and Gastroschisis

Omphalocele is a deficiency of the ventral abdominal wall at the umbilicus, with resultant herniation of viscera into the base of the umbilical cord.[1,119] The contents are covered by a thin membrane consisting of peritoneum and amnion.[1,119] The umbilical cord inserts at the apex of the omphalocele.[1] The size and contents of an omphalocele are variable. More than two thirds of patients with omphalocele have associated anomalies, most commonly involving the gastrointestinal tract.[1] Malrotation is always present.[1]

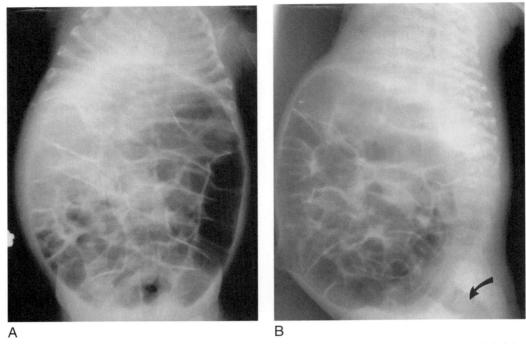

A

B

Figure 32–92. A 4-month-old ventilated ex-premature infant with severe bronchopulmonary dysplasia who developed marked abdominal distention. Anteroposterior supine **(A)** and lateral recumbent **(B)** radiographs show moderate-to-marked gaseous distention of virtually the entire small bowel and colon. Air in the rectum *(arrow)* would reasonably exclude bowel obstruction as the cause of the intestinal distention. This degree of generalized, rather than localized, bowel distention suggests ileus as the cause. Necrotizing enterocolitis would not give such diffuse bowel distention. Sepsis was the presumed cause of this infant's intestinal distention.

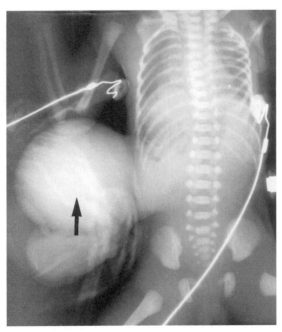

Figure 32–93. A newborn with midline anterior abdominal wall defect, well encapsulated, reflecting an omphalocele *(arrow)*. Associated intestinal malrotation is almost always present.

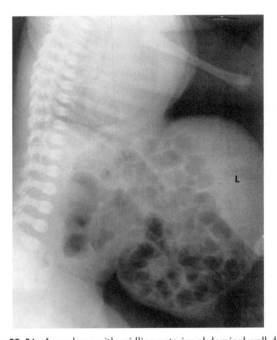

Figure 32–94. A newborn with midline anterior abdominal wall defect and a huge encapsulated omphalocele containing liver (L) and bowel. Omphaloceles and gastroschises are frequently identified on antenatal sonography. Postnatal imaging of the abdomen and associated defect is seldom required, although imaging of other organ systems to assess for possible associated anomalies is often necessary.

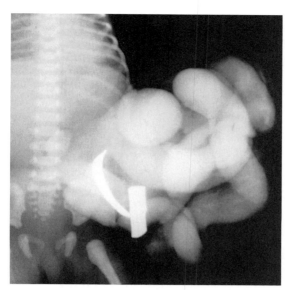

Figure 32–95. A newborn with a paramedian anterior abdominal wall defect, from which project multiple loops of fluid-filled bowel without a confining membrane. These findings are characteristic of gastroschisis, which has a lower incidence of associated anomalies than does omphalocele.

The diagnosis of omphalocele is made clinically. Abdominal radiographs show a sharply marginated, midline, anterior abdominal wall mass that contains bowel and possibly solid organs (Figs. 32-93 and 32-94).[1] Although no further imaging of the omphalocele itself is indicated, evaluation of the cardiovascular, urinary, and intestinal structures by echocardiography, renal sonography, and contrast studies of the intestinal tract may be necessary for assessment of extent of associated anomalies.

Gastroschisis is a defect of the ventral abdominal wall lateral to the midline, with a normally positioned umbilicus and no membrane or sac covering the herniated bowel.[1,23,119,120] Associated anomalies are less common and severe with gastroschisis compared with omphalocele.[1] Malrotation is always present, and intestinal atresia may be associated.[1,120] Abdominal radiographs in patients with gastroschisis show extra-abdominal viscera without a smooth and sharply marginated covering membrane (Fig. 32-95).[1]

Biliary Atresia and Neonatal Hepatitis

Biliary atresia is the most common congenital abnormality of the biliary system. It usually presents with prolonged jaundice, may have associated congenital anomalies, and involves the inability to excrete bile with resultant conjugated hyperbilirubinemia.[1,99]

Idiopathic neonatal hepatitis is the most common primary liver disorder in early infancy. It accounts for 35% to 45% of cases of neonatal cholestasis and is usually evident in the first week of life.[99] Although the etiology of biliary atresia and neonatal jaundice is unknown, viral infection is implicated.[23] Early surgical intervention is essential for the optimal treatment of biliary atresia but has little or no benefit for neonatal hepatitis.[23]

Box 32–2 | **Etiology of Abdominal Masses in the Newborn**

Urinary Tract

Hydronephrosis
Multicystic dysplastic kidney
Mesoblastic nephroma
Wilm's tumor
Infantile polycystic kidney disease
Renal vein thrombosis

Genital

Hydrometrocolpos (female)
Ovarian cysts (female)
Teratoma

Adrenal/Retroperitoneal

Adrenal hemorrhage
Neuroblastoma

Gastrointestinal/Abdomen

Complicated volvulus
Complicated meconium ileus
Pseudocyst proximal to atresia
Intestinal duplication
Mesenteric/omental cyst
Hepatoblastoma
Hemangioma/hemangioendothelioma (liver)
Hamartoma (liver)
Choledochal cyst

Modified from Hartman GE, Shochat SJ: Abdominal mass lesions in the newborn: Diagnosis and treatment. Clin Perinatol 16:123, 1989; and Kirks DR (ed): Practical Pediatric Imaging: Diagnostic Radiology of Infants and Children, 2nd ed. Boston, Little, Brown, 1991.

Imaging of and differentiation between biliary atresia and neonatal hepatitis consists of abdominal sonography and hepatobiliary scanning.[1] Abdominal radiography is of little or no value in the evaluation of neonatal jaundice. Sonography is used primarily to exclude other causes of neonatal obstructive jaundice, such as choledochal cyst, inspissated bile syndrome, or obstructing mass.[99] The gallbladder is normal in neonatal hepatitis, usually but not always small or absent with biliary atresia.[99]

Hepatobiliary scintigraphy is the best noninvasive method of differentiating neonatal hepatitis from biliary atresia.[99] With the former, hepatic uptake of isotope varies from normal to poor, and isotope excretion into the bowel is present.[1] With the latter, hepatic uptake of isotope is normal, but there is no passage of isotope into bowel.[1]

Neonatal Abdominal Masses

Abdominal masses in the newborn period are relatively common and have multiple possible etiologies (Box 32-2).[23,121,122] More than 50% originate in the genitourinary tract.[23,122] In any neonate with a suspected abdominal mass, initial imaging should consist of plain abdominal radiographs to search for calcifications or fatty density that might assist in characterizing the lesion and

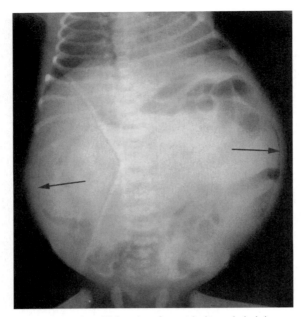

Figure 32–96. A 2-day-old female infant with distended abdomen and firm abdominal mass encompassing most of the abdomen on physical examination. Anteroposterior supine abdominal radiograph shows an increase in soft tissue density in the central portion of the abdomen with displacement of air-filled bowel toward the periphery. The mass has compressed several segments of bowel in the abdominal flanks *(arrows)*. A mesenteric hemangioma was found at surgery.

Box 32–3	Etiology of Neonatal Ascites

Genitourinary

Posterior urethral valves
Congenital nephrosis

Gastrointestinal

Meconium peritonitis caused by intestinal perforation
Fetal appendicitis with rupture
Perforation of Meckel's diverticulum
Imperforate anus

Hepatobiliary

Hepatitis, cytomegalovirus, other infections
Biliary atresia
Metabolic disorders (glycogen storage disease, galactosemia)
Spontaneous common bile duct perforation

Cardiac

Rh disease
Severe anemia secondary to thalassemia, hemorrhage
Major congenital cardiac disease
Arrhythmia (e.g., supraventricular tachycardia)
Arteriovenous malformation

Miscellaneous

Chylous ascites
Congenital lymphatic obstruction
Traumatic disruption of the thoracic duct
Congenital infection (syphilis, cytomegalovirus, toxoplasmosis)

Modified from Avery ME, First LR (eds): Pediatric Medicine. Baltimore, Williams & Wilkins, 1989.

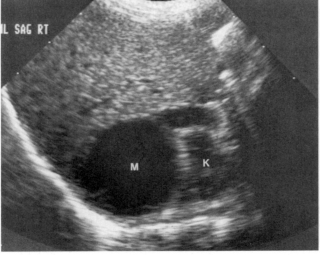
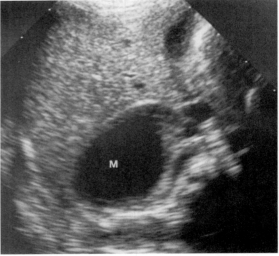

A   B

Figure 32–97. Sagittal **(A)** and transverse **(B)** sonograms of the right upper abdomen in a newborn with jaundice and a palpable mass. There is a largely anechoic mass (M) in the right upper retroperitoneum, adjacent to the upper pole of the right kidney (K), which is characteristic in appearance for an adrenal hemorrhage. Subsequent sonography showed progressive decrease in size of the hemorrhage.

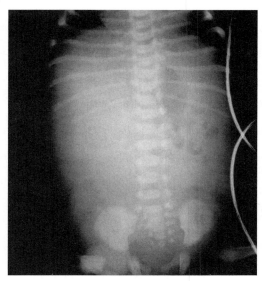

Figure 32–98. A newborn male infant with moderate abdominal distention. Portable anteroposterior abdominal radiograph shows a diffuse increase in soft tissue density throughout most of the abdomen except for the left upper quadrant, where limited intestinal gas in nondistended loops of bowel is present. The radiographic findings are nonspecific and could reflect intraperitoneal fluid (e.g., ascites), an abdominal or retroperitoneal mass, or fluid-filled loops of bowel (in view of the early postnatal state). Ultrasonography is the next appropriate imaging procedure for evaluation of the abdomen under these circumstances (see Fig. 32-100).

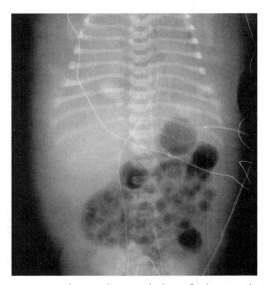

Figure 32–99. A newborn with severe hydrops fetalis secondary to Rh incompatibility. Anteroposterior radiograph of the chest and abdomen shows several changes secondary to the hydrops, including generalized body anasarca, bilateral large pleural effusions, and massive ascites, which have caused shift of air-filled loops of bowel to the central, nondependent portion of the abdomen.

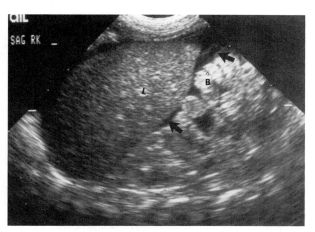

Figure 32–100. Sagittally oriented ultrasonography of the right upper quadrant shows several small areas of anechoic (echo-free) fluid *(arrows)* representing ascites, which was widespread in the abdomen. Fluid-filled bowel represented most of the non–air-containing portions of the abdomen. Abdominal sonography is the preferred imaging modality for identifying and localizing ascites and other abdominal fluid collections in young children. B, bowel; L, liver.

to be certain that dilated bowel is not being misinterpreted clinically as a mass lesion.[23,122] Radiographically an abdominal mass appears as an area of increased soft tissue density within the abdomen, often displacing air-filled loops of bowel (Fig. 32-96).

Sonography of the abdomen and pelvis would be the next imaging study in any neonate with an abdominal mass.[23,122] In almost all cases, sonography shows the organ of origin and internal structure (solid versus cystic versus mixed solid and cystic) of the mass (Fig. 32-97).[121,122] Additional imaging would depend on sonographic findings but might not be necessary before surgery.[23,122]

Intraperitoneal Fluid

Intraperitoneal fluid in neonates and infants can have multiple causes or associated abnormalities (Box 32-3). Whether representing ascites, blood, or more complex collections, intraperitoneal fluid appears on the abdominal radiograph as an increase in soft tissue density between individual loops of air-containing bowel (Fig. 32-98). With larger amounts of fluid, air-containing bowel tends to move anteriorly and medially in the supine neonate, appearing on the anteroposterior radiograph as centralized bowel gas with increased soft tissue in the abdominal flanks (Fig. 32-99). Sonography is excellent at identifying free intraperitoneal fluid and showing its internal characteristics (Fig. 32-100).

References

1. Kirks DR (ed): Practical Pediatric Imaging: Diagnostic Radiology of Infants and Children, 2nd ed. Boston, Little, Brown, 1991.
2. Franken EA Jr, Yu P, Smith WL, et al: Initial chest radiography in the neonatal intensive care unit: Value of the lateral view. AJR Am J Roentgenol 133:43, 1979.

3. Brasch RC: Portable infant elevator for neonatal magnification radiography. AJR Am J Roentgenol 132:1016, 1979.
4. Brasch RC, Gould RG: Direct magnification radiography of the newborn infant. Radiology 142:649, 1982.
5. Nikesch W, Kuntzler CM, Cushing FR: Neonatal magnification radiography using standard-focus X-ray tubes. AJR Am J Roentgenol 141:665, 1983.
6. Cohen M, Towbin R, Baker S, et al: Comparison of Iohexol with barium in gastrointestinal studies of infants and children. AJR Am J Roentgenol 156:345, 1991.
7. Cohen MD, Katz BP, Kalasinski LA, et al: Digital imaging with a photostimulable phosphor in the chest of newborns. Radiology 181:829, 1991.
8. Keller MS, Chawla HS: Neonatal metrizamide gastrointestinal series in suspected necrotizing enterocolitis. Am J Dis Child 139:713, 1985.
9. Glasier CM, Leithiser RE Jr, Williamson SL, et al: Extracardiac chest ultrasonography in infants and children: radiographic and clinical implications. J Pediatr 114:540, 1981.
10. Sty JR, Wells RG, Starshak RJ, et al: Diagnostic Imaging of Infants and Children, vol. III. Gaithersburg, MD, Aspen, 1992.
11. Shiraishi H, Yanagisawa M: Bidirectional flow through the ductus arteriosus in normal newborns: Evaluation by Doppler color flow imaging. Pediatr Cardiol 12:201, 1991.
12. Bisceglia M, Donaldson JS: Calcification of the ligamentum arteriosum in children: A normal finding on CT. AJR Am J Roentgenol 156:351, 1991.
13. Rencken IO, Sola A, Gould R, et al: Direct coronal CT scanning of the neonatal chest. Pediatr Radiol 29:451, 1999.
14. Riebel T, Wartner R: Use of non-ionic contrast media for tracheobronchography in neonates and young infants. Eur J Radiol 11:120, 1990.
15. Cohen MD, Long B, Cory DA, et al: Digital imaging of the newborn chest. Clin Radiol 40:365, 1989.
16. Gross GW, Ehrlich SM, Wang Y: Diagnostic quality of portable abdominal radiographs in neonates with necrotizing enterocolitis: Digitized vs nondigitized images. AJR Am J Roentgenol 154:779, 1990.
17. Nakano Y, Odagiri K: Use of computed radiography in respiratory distress syndrome in the neonatal nursery. Pediatr Radiol 19:167, 1989.
18. Arroe M: The risk of x-ray examinations of the lungs in neonates. Acta Pediatr Scand 80:489, 1991.
19. Burton EM, Kirks DR, Strife JL, et al: Evaluation of a low-dose neonatal chest radiographic system. AJR Am J Roentgenol 151:999, 1988.
20. Roehrig H, Krupinski EA, Hulett R: Reduction of patient exposure in pediatric radiology. Acad Radiol 4:547, 1997.
21. Wilmot DM, Sharko GA (eds): Pediatric Imaging for the Technologist. New York, Springer-Verlag, 1987.
22. Marsh D, Wilkerson SA, Cook LN, et al: Right atrial thrombus formation screening using two-dimensional echocardiograms in neonates with central venous catheters. Pediatrics 81:284, 1988.
23. Swischuk LE (ed): Imaging of the Newborn, Infant, and Young Child, 3rd ed. Baltimore, Williams & Wilkins, 1989.
24. Ryan S, Folan-Curran J: Embryology and anatomy of the neonatal chest. In Donoghue V (ed): Radiological Imaging of the Neonatal Chest. Berlin, Springer-Verlag, 2002, pp 1-8.
25. Oh KS, Newman B, Bender TM, et al: Radiologic evaluation of the diaphragm. Radiol Clin North Am 26:355, 1988.
26. Smevik B, Stake G: Congenital heart and great vessel disease. In Donoghue V (ed): Radiological Imaging of the Neonatal Chest. Berlin, Springer-Verlag, 2002, pp 111-170.
27. Hernanz-Schulman M, Genieser NB, Friedman D, et al: Current evaluation of the patient with abnormal viscero-atrial situs. AJR Am J Roentgenol 154:797, 1990.
28. Newman B, Oh KS: Abnormal pulmonary aeration in infants and children. Radiol Clin North Am 26:323, 1988.
29. Ryan S: Postnatal imaging of chest malformations. In Donoghue V (ed): Radiological Imaging of the Neonatal Chest. Berlin, Springer-Verlag, 2002, pp 93-109.
30. Alford BA, McIlhenny J, Jones JE, et al: Asymmetric radiographic findings in the pediatric chest: Approach to early diagnosis. Radiographics 13:77, 1993.
31. Cullen ML, Klein MD, Philippart AL: Congenital diaphragmatic hernia. Surg Clin North Am 65:1115, 1985.
32. Wood BP: The newborn chest. Radiol Clin North Am 31:667, 1993.
33. Milne LW, Morosin AM, Campbell JR, et al: Pars sternalis diaphragmatic hernia with omphalocele: A report of two cases. J Pediatr Surg 25:726, 1990.
34. Donnelly LF, Frush DP: Localized radiolucent chest lesions in neonates: Causes and differentiation. AJR Am J Roentgenol 172:1651-1658, 1999.
35. Dimitriou G, Greenough A, Davenport M, et al: Prediction of outcome by computer-assisted analysis of lung area on the chest radiograph of infants with congenital diaphragmatic hernia. J Pediatr Surg 35:489, 2000.
36. Stigers KB, Woodring JH, Kanga JF: The clinical and imaging spectrum of findings in patients with congenital lobar emphysema. Pediatr Pulmonol 14:160, 1992.
37. Haddon MJ, Bowen AD: Bronchopulmonary and neurenteric forms of foregut anomalies: Imaging for diagnosis and management. Radiol Clin North Am 29:2414, 1991.
38. Rosado-de-Christenson ML, Stocker JT: Congenital cystic adenomatoid malformation. Radiographics 11:865, 1991.
39. Sittig SE, Asay GF: Congenital cystic adenomatoid malformation in the newborn: Two case studies and review of the literature. Respir Care 45:1188, 2000.
40. Kim WS, Lee KS, Kim IO, et al: Congenital cystic adenomatoid malformation of the lung: CT-pathologic correlation. AJR Am J Roentgenol 168:47, 1997.
41. Donoghue V: Transient tachynea of the newborn. In Donoghue V (ed): Radiological Imaging of the Neonatal Chest. Berlin, Springer-Verlag, 2002, pp 45-47.
42. Donoghue V: Hyaline membrane disease and complications of its treatment. In Donoghue V (ed): Radiological Imaging of the Neonatal Chest. Berlin, Springer-Verlag, 2002, pp 1-8.
43. Clarke EA, Siegle RL, Gong AK: Findings on chest radiographs after prophylactic pulmonary surfactant treatment of premature infants. AJR Am J Roentgenol 153:799, 1989.
44. Edwards DK, Hilton SVW, Merritt TA, et al: Respiratory distress syndrome treated with human surfactant: Radiographic findings. Radiology 157:329, 1985.
45. Gortner L: Natural surfactant for neonatal respiratory distress syndrome in very premature infants: A 1992 update. J Perinat Med 20:409, 1992.
46. Levine D, Edwards DKE III, Merritt TA: Synthetic vs human surfactants in the treatment of respiratory distress syndrome: Radiographic findings. AJR Am J Roentgenol 157:371, 1991.
47. Wood BP, Sinkin RA, Kendig JW, et al: Exogenous lung surfactant: Effect on radiographic appearance in premature infants. Radiology 165:11, 1987.
48. Slama M, Andre C, Huon C, et al: Radiological analysis of hyaline membrane disease after exogenous surfactant treatment. Pediatr Radiol 29:56, 1999.
49. Soll RF, Horbar JD, Griscom NT, et al: Radiographic findings associated with surfactant treatment. Am J Perinatol 8:114, 1991.

50. Odita JC: The significance of recurrent lung opacities in neonates on surfactant treatment for respiratory distress syndrome. Pediatr Radiol 31:87, 2001.
51. Reller MD, Colasurdo MA, Rice MJ, et al: The timing of spontaneous closure of the ductus arteriosus in infants with respiratory distress syndrome. Am J Cardiol 66:75, 1990.
52. Yuksel B, Greenough A, Karani J, et al: Chest radiographic scoring system for use in pre-term infants. Br J Radiol 64:1015, 1991.
53. Swischuk LE: Bubbles in hyaline membrane disease: Differentiation of three types. Radiology 122:417, 1977.
54. Williams DW, Merten DF, Effmann EL, et al: Ventilator-induced pulmonary pseudocysts in preterm neonates. AJR Am J Roentgenol 150:885, 1988.
55. Bancalari E, Goldberg RN: High-frequency ventilation in the neonate. Clin Perinatol 14:581, 1987.
56. Bandari V, Gagnon C, Rosenkrantz T, et al: Pulmonary hemorrhage in neonates of early and late gestation. J Perinat Med 27:369, 1999.
57. Chua RNS, Yoder MC: Management of unilateral pulmonary cystic emphysema with selective bronchial intubation and high frequency jet ventilation in two infants. Pediatr Pulmonol 9:122, 1990.
58. Schwartz AN, Graham CB: Neonatal tension pulmonary interstitial emphysema in bronchopulmonary dysplasia: Treatment with lateral decubitus positioning. Radiology 161:351, 1986.
59. O'Keeffe FN, Swischuk LE, Stansberry SD: Mediastinal pseudomass caused by compression of the thymus in neonates with anterior pneumothorax. AJR Am J Roentgenol 156:145, 1991.
60. Strife JL, Smith P, Dunbar JS, et al: Chest tube perforation of the lung in premature infants: Radiographic recognition. AJR Am J Roentgenol 141:73, 1983.
61. Rosenfeld DL, Cordell CE, Jadeja N: Retrocardiac pneumomediastinum: Radiographic findings and clinical implications. Pediatrics 85:92, 1990.
62. Neal RC, Beck DE, Smith VC, et al: Neonatal pneumopericardium with high-frequency ventilation. Ann Thorac Surg 47:274, 1989.
63. Lanning P, Tammela O, Koivisto M: Radiological incidence and course of bronchopulmonary dysplasia in 100 consecutive low-birth-weight neonates. Acta Radiol 36:353, 1995.
64. Northway WH Jr: Bronchopulmonary dysplasia: Then and now. Arch Dis Child 83:1070, 1990.
65. Twomey A: Update on clinical management of neonatal chest conditions. In Donoghue V (ed): Radiological Imaging of the Neonatal Chest. Berlin, Springer-Verlag, 2002, pp 9-32.
66. Hoffer FA, Ablow RC: The cross-table lateral view in neonatal pneumothorax. AJR Am J Roentgenol 142:1283, 1984.
67. Hyde I, English RE, Williams JD: The changing pattern of chronic lung disease of prematurity. Arch Dis Child 64:448, 1989.
68. Steinberg JDJ, Oetomo SB, Martijn A: Asymmetrical pulmonary changes in premature infants with surgical closure of a persistent ductus arteriosus. Br J Radiol 63:22, 1990.
69. Oppenheim C, Mamou-Mani T, Sayegh N, et al: Bronchopulmonary dysplasia: Value of CT in identifying pulmonary sequelae. AJR Am J Roentgenol 163:169, 1994.
70. Edwards DK, Jacob J, Gluck L: The immature lung: Radiographic appearance, course, and complications. AJR Am J Roentgenol 135:659, 1980.
71. Owens CM: Meconium aspiration. In Donoghue V (ed): Radiological Imaging of the Neonatal Chest. Berlin, Springer-Verlag, 2002, pp 49-61.
72. Manson D: Diagnostic imaging of neonatal pneumonia. In Donoghue V (ed): Radiological Imaging of the Neonatal Chest. Berlin, Springer-Verlag, 2002, pp 63-73.
73. Wiswell TE, Tuggle JM, Turner BS: Meconium aspiration syndrome: Have we made a difference? Pediatrics 85:715, 1990.
74. Levy I, Rubin LG: *Legionella* pneumonia in neonates: A literature review. J Perinatol 18:287, 1998.
75. Kalliola S, Vuopio-Varkila J, Takala AK, et al: Neonatal group B streptococcal disease in Finland: A ten-year nationwide study. Pediatr Infect Dis J 18:806, 1999.
76. Child DD, Newell JD, Bjelland JC, et al: Radiographic findings of pulmonary coccidioidomycosis in neonates and infants. AJR Am J Roentgenol 145:261, 1985.
77. Haney PJ, Bohlman M, Sun CC: Radiographic findings in neonatal pneumonia. AJR Am J Roentgenol 143:23, 1984.
78. Markowitz RI, Fahey JT, Hellenbrand WE, et al: Bronchial compression by a patent ductus arteriosus associated with pulmonary atresia. AJR Am J Roentgenol 144:535, 1985.
79. El Hassan NO, Chess PR, Huysman MW, et al: Rescue use of DNase in critical lung atelectasis and mucus retention in premature neonates. Pediatrics 108:468, 2001.
80. Kinsella JP, Abman SH: Inhaled nitric oxide and high frequency oscillatory ventilation in persistent pulmonary hypertension of the newborn. Eur J Pediatr 157(suppl 1):S28, 1998.
81. Perez-Benavides F, Boynton BR, Desai NS, et al: Persistent pulmonary hypertension of the newborn infant: Comparison of conventional versus extracorporeal membrane oxygenation in neonates fulfilling Bartlett's criteria. J Perinatol 13:181, 1993.
82. Berger TM, Allred EN, Van Marter LJ: Antecedents of clinically significant pulmonary hemorrhage among newborn infants. J Perinatol 20:295, 2000.
83. Kluckow M, Evans N: Ductal shunting, high pulmonary blood flow, and pulmonary hemorrhage. J Pediatr 137:68, 2000.
84. Lin TW, Su BH, Lin HC, et al: Risk factors of pulmonary hemorrhage in very-low-birth-weight infants: A two-year retrospective study. Acta Paediatr Taiwan 41:255, 2000.
85. Tomaszewska M, Stork E, Minich NM, et al: Pulmonary hemorrhage: Clinical course and outcomes among very-low-birth-weight infants. Arch Pediatr Adolesc Med 153:715, 1999.
86. Duara S, Spackman TJ, Boutwell WC, et al: A newly recognized profile in neonatal lung disease with maternal diabetes. AJR Am J Roentgenol 144:529, 1985.
87. Vade A, Kramer L: Extralobar pulmonary sequestration presenting as intractable pleural effusion. Pediatr Radiol 19:333, 1989.
88. Gupta R, Carachi R: Pseudopericardial cyst in a neonate—a case report and review of the literature. Z Kinderchir 44:162, 1989.
89. Han BK, Babcock DS, Oestreich AE: Normal thymus in infancy: Sonographic characteristics. Radiology 170:471, 1989.
90. Lemaitre L, Marconi V, Avni R, et al: The sonographic evaluation of normal thymus in infants and children. Eur J Radiol 7:130, 1987.
91. Smart LM, Hendry GMA: Imaging of neonatal pulmonary sequestration including Doppler ultrasound. Br J Radiol 64:324, 1991.
92. Rosado-de-Christenson ML, Fraizer AA, Stocker JT, et al: Extralobar sequestration: Radiologic-pathologic correlation. Radiographics 13:425, 1993.
93. Sintzoff SA, Avni EF, Rocmans P Jr, et al: Pulmonary sequestration-like anomaly presenting as a spontaneously resolving mass. Pediatr Radiol 21:143, 1991.

94. Jetley NK, Bhatagar V, Krishna A, et al: Pulmonary blastoma in a neonate. J Pediatr Surg 23:1009, 1988.

95. Sennhauser FH, Stokes KB, Campbell NT, et al: Pulmonary haemangioma: A cause of neonatal respiratory distress. Pediatr Surg Int 4:127, 1989.

96. Gross GW: The chest radiograph in the neonate on ECMO. Radiol Rep 2:291, 1990.

97. Gross GW, Cullen J, Kornhauser MS, et al: Thoracic complications of extracorporeal membrane oxygenation: findings on chest radiographs and sonograms. AJR Am J Roentgenol 158:353, 1992.

98. Jaile JC, Levin T, Wung JT, et al: Benign gaseous distension of the bowel in premature infants treated with nasal continuous airway pressure: a study of contributing factors. AJR Am J Roentgenol 158:125, 1992.

99. Sty JR, Wells RG, Starshak RJ, et al: Diagnostic Imaging of Infants and Children, vol. I. Gaithersburg, MD, Aspen, 1992.

100. Boulton JE, Ein SH, Reilly BJ, et al: Necrotizing enterocolitis and volvulus in the premature neonate. J Pediatr Surg 24:901, 1989.

101. Merritt CRB, Goldsmith JP, Sharp MJ: Sonographic detection of portal venous gas in infants with necrotizing enterocolitis. AJR Am J Roentgenol 143:1059, 1984.

102. Ghory MJ, Sheldon CA: Newborn surgical emergencies of the gastrointestinal tract. Surg Clin North Am 65:1083, 1985.

103. Ross MN, Wayne ER, Janik JS, et al: A standard of comparison for acute surgical necrotizing enterocolitis. J Pediatr Surg 24:998, 1989.

104. Levin TL, Brill PW, Winchester P: Enteric fistula formation secondary to necrotizing enterocolitis. Pediatr Radiol 21:309, 1991.

105. Martin LW, Alexander F: Esophageal atresia. Surg Clin North Am 65:1099, 1985.

106. Goh DW, Brereton RJ, Spitz L: Esophageal atresia with obstructed tracheoesophageal fistula and gasless abdomen. J Pediatr Surg 26:160, 1991.

107. Donn SM, Zak LK, Bozyniski EA, et al: Use of high-frequency jet ventilation in the management of congenital tracheoesophageal fistula associated with respiratory distress syndrome. J Pediatr Surg 25:1219, 1990.

108. Moore CCM: Congenital gastric outlet obstruction. J Pediatr Surg 24:1241, 1989.

109. Muller M, Morger R, Engert J: Pyloric atresia: Report of four cases and review of the literature. Pediatr Surg Int 5:276, 1990.

110. Chittmittrapap S: Pyloric atresia associated with ileal and rectal atresia. Pediatr Surg Int 3:426, 1988.

111. Leonidas JC, Magid N, Soberman N, et al: Midgut volvulus in infants: Diagnosis with US. Radiology 179:491, 1991.

112. Cameron AEP, Howard ER: Gastric volvulus in childhood. J Pediatr Surg 22:944, 1987.

113. Martin LW, Torres AM: Hirschsprung's disease. Surg Clin North Am 65:1171, 1985.

114. Rescorla F, Grosfeld JL, West KJ, et al: Changing patterns of treatment and survival in neonates with meconium ileus. Arch Surg 124:837, 1989.

115. Tan CEL, Kiely EM, Brereton RJ, et al: Neonatal gastrointestinal perforation. J Pediatr Surg 24:888, 1989.

116. Weinberg G, Kleinhaus S, Boley SJ: Idiopathic intestinal perforations in the newborn: An increasingly common entity. J Pediatr Surg 24:1007, 1989.

117. Clarke EA, Dutton NE: Use of Iohexol in the early determination of gastrointestinal perforation. J Pediatr Surg 23:1027, 1988.

118. Meyer CL, Payne NR, Roback SA: Spontaneous isolated intestinal perforations in neonates with birth weights under 1000 grams not associated with necrotizing enterocolitis. J Pediatr Surg 26:714, 1991.

119. Martin LW, Torres AM: Omphalocele and gastroschisis. Surg Clin North Am 65:1235, 1985.

120. Shah R, Woolley MM: Gastroschisis and intestinal atresia. J Pediatr Surg 26:788, 1991.

121. Hartman GE, Shochat SJ: Abdominal mass lesions in the newborn: Diagnosis and treatment. Clin Perinatol 16:123, 1989.

122. Merten DF, Kirks DR: Diagnostic imaging of pediatric abdominal masses. Pediatr Clin North Am 32:1397, 1985.

CHAPTER 33

Fetal and Neonatal Thermal Regulation

Sudhish Chandra and Stephen Baumgart

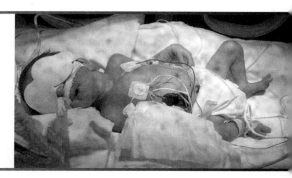

Ecology. The scientific study of living things in relation to their environment. Note that ecology is not synonymous with the environment.

Webster's Abridged Dictionary

BRIEF HISTORY OF INCUBATION[1]

In Ancient Egypt, incubation was a practice of animal husbandry to increase agrarian productivity and was handed down from father to son.[2] As chick embryos grew with gestation, their metabolic rate increased such that incubation required less and less exogenous heat during progression through 21 days of gestation. This gradual decrease in heat applied has been termed **graded incubation**.

The obstetrician Tarnier (an enthusiast of aviaries) first applied this principle of graded incubation systematically to human premature infants in Paris in 1830, using a covered incubator chamber that he called a *couveuse*. Tarnier's students, Budin and Auvard, modified his couveuse by adding a thermometer and regulatory alarms to alert the infant's attendant to deviations from prescribed environmental temperature.[3] Over the next 60 years in Tarnier's and Budin's clinic, refinements of incubation techniques resulted in an increased survival rate from 38% to 66% of premature infants weighing less than 2000 g at birth.[4]

In the United States, modification and commercial manufacture of Budin's incubator was pursued in Chicago and Boston, resulting in the Rotch Incubator, which was displayed at the Chicago's Columbian Exposition in 1893.[3,5-7] During the first half of the 20th century, various means for temperature regulation of incubator environments were explored. In 1933, Blackfan and Yaglou[8] reported better rectal temperature maintenance when humid saturation was applied to the air within the incubator chamber. Their recommended incubator air temperature was nearly 25°C, with 88% relative humidity.[8] This increased humidity subsequently was associated with bacterial infections, however.

By 1940, in the United States, Chappel, working at Pennsylvania Hospital and Thomas Jefferson Medical College Hospital in Philadelphia, in an effort to avoid bacterial infection associated with the use of saturated humid environments, added the principle of air isolation to incubator technology.[9] Chappel's incubators were vented outside the hospital to avoid contamination of other infants. In 1958, Silverman and colleagues[10] suggested using higher air temperatures instead of humidity to avoid this complication. Incubator temperatures in Silverman's dry incubators ranged from 29° C to 31° C.[10] These authors exhibited significantly improved survival rates using these higher temperatures.

Cross and Hill[11-13] proposed the concept of a **thermal neutral temperature range** for nurturing ovine and human neonates in artificially incubated environments. The thermal neutral temperature for premature newborns is analogous to the adult **thermal comfort zone**, in which adults (at rest in a single layer of clothing) remain comfortable without physiologic thermal adaptive response (either shivering or sweating). By 1962, Bruck[14,15] had shown **minimal observed metabolic rate (MOMR)** of oxygen consumption as an indication of thermal neutrality in newborns nurtured within specific and narrow ranges of environmental temperature in incubators. By 1969, Hey and Katz[16-18] had extensively described thermal neutral environments for premature infants and developed the Hey and Katz nomograms for incubator temperature regulation consistent with the ancient Egyptians' graded incubation concept. Nevertheless, achieving thermal neutral conditions in modern neonatal intensive care units outside of laboratory controlled conditions remains an elusive goal.

PHYSICAL AVENUES OF HEAT TRANSFER[19]

Shown in Table 33-1, the four avenues for infant heat exchange within the nursery environment are summarized by earth, air, fire, and water. *Earth* represents conduction, which is the transfer of heat from solid object to solid object through surface-to-surface contact. *Air* represents

Table 33–1. Four Avenues of Physical Heat Transfer

Earth	=	Conduction
Air	=	Convection
		Natural
		Forced
Fire	=	Radiation
Water	=	Evaporation (or condensation)

convection, which may occur through two mechanisms, natural and forced. *Fire* represents heat exchange through radiation (direct heat transfer by infrared electromagnetic waves). *Water* represents the loss of latent heat through evaporation or the deposition of heat from water condensation. Analyzing each of these mechanisms separately is necessary to understand completely each infant's unique thermal equilibrium. Probably no two infants achieve the same equilibrium despite the fact that they may be nurtured in similar incubator devices and under similar physical conditions.

Conduction

Conductive heat loss to cooler surfaces in contact with an infant's skin depends on the conductivity of the surface material and its temperature. Usually, infants are nursed on insulating mattresses and blankets that minimize conductive heat loss to nearly zero. Intuitively, care must be exercised to maintain dry layers of insulation in contact with an infant's skin to maintain optimal external insulation, especially in preterm infants with little insulating subcutaneous fat.

Convection

Convective heat transfer in general comprises movement of heat through a fluid medium, either a liquid (e.g., blood flow; see physiology section later) or a gas (e.g., environmental air). Two mechanisms determine convective heat transfer from infants into the environmental air.

Natural Convection

Natural convection results simply from the gradient of temperature between the infant's skin surface and the surrounding still air.[20,21] In general, this temperature gradient is approximately 10° C (25° C air to 35° C skin). Natural convection forms geometric **convection cells** over the curved surfaces of the infant lying supine within an incubator or on an open cot. These convection cells form as warm air naturally rises from the skin, conveying heat and body moisture away from the surface of the infant. As warm air rises, it subsequently cools and falls back toward the infant, forming a convection cell. Several cells may form over the curvature of the infant's body. Surface area, posture, and body geometry play an important role in the rate of convective heat loss from the skin. An infant flexed in the fetal position leaves less surface area exposed to the airborne environment and experiences less convective heat loss.[22] An infant extended flaccidly is able to dissipate more heat. Posture may be the first clue to the thermal comfort or discomfort of a newborn.

Forced Air Convection

The second form of convection is the result of **forced convective** air movement. In forced convection, exogenously applied energy moves an air mass past the infant's skin at a longitudinal rate. The rate of forced convective heat loss is exponentially proportional to the rate of air movement.[21] The effect of forced convection in disrupting the microenvironment of warm, humid air layered near an infant's skin usually is not appreciated in the nursery, where drafts, air turbulence, and consequently exacerbated heat loss may occur. Within convection-warmed incubators (warmed air is forced into the incubator by a fan), manufacturers strive to render the air near the infant as still as possible to prevent forced convective heat loss. Estimates of natural and forced air convective heat loss from premature neonates nursed within standard incubators indicate their success because natural convection is the only major loss likely to occur.[23] Care must be exercised, however, not to disrupt air flow inside incubators with padding, toys, or respiratory equipment that delivers oxygen flow.

Radiation

Radiant heat transfer is probably the least intuitive aspect of heat loss or heat gain in newborn incubation. Radiant heat transfer occurs as the result of infrared electromagnetic transmission of energy from one warm body to another cooler one. Bodies of different temperatures determine the direction and magnitude of heat transfer, with the warm body irradiating to the cooler one *down* the temperature gradient. A radiant heat transfer constant (Stefan-Boltzman constant), the physical emissivity properties of the infant's skin and plastic walls (ε_{skin}, ε_{walls}), the infant's exposed body surface area and posture, and the temperature gradient determine the rate of infrared radiant heat loss or gain.[19] Characteristically, in a standard single-walled incubator, heat transfers from the infant's skin, which is warmer, to the surrounding cooler walls of the plastic incubator's interior. The incubator plastic then reradiates heat to the cooler nursery walls and windows. The plastic incubator's walls are opaque to the transmission of infrared energy and absorb nearly all of the infant's irradiated heat. The temperature of the walls of the incubator are determined not only by the incubator's internal air, which is artificially warmed, but also by the external air of the surrounding nursery, which is generally about 10°C cooler than the infant's incubator. An infant's posture also may affect radiant heat loss by increasing or reducing the exposed radiating surface area. Nonevaporative heat loss (**operant temperature**) is approximately determined 60% by average wall temperature and 40% by air temperature inside the incubator.

Evaporation

For several reasons, a premature newborn in particular may lose large amounts of water through evaporation from the surface of the skin.[20,22,24-31] The infant's first encounter with evaporative heat loss occurs in the delivery room, where the infant is sheathed with amniotic fluid and exposed to the cool, dry air of the delivery suite. Premature infants in particular may be subject to particularly excessive

Table 33–2. Body Surface Area–to–Body Mass Ratio Comparison in Adults and Low-Birth-Weight Neonates

	Body Mass (kg)	BSA (m²)	Mass/BSA (cm²/kg)
Adult	70.0	1.73	250
LBW premature	1.5	0.13	670
Very LBW	0.5	0.07	1400

BSA, body surface area; LBW, low birth weight.

Adapted from Costarino AT, Baumgart S: Water metabolism in the neonate. In Cowett KM (ed): Principles of Perinatal-Neonatal Metabolism. New York, Springer-Verlag, 1991, pp 623-649.

evaporative heat loss by virtue of a thin epidermal layer lacking keratinized epithelium, which serves as a vapor barrier for older infants and adults to prevent excessive evaporative losses. Excessive heat loss is exacerbated by a thin dermis and lack of subcutaneous fascia, which provide insulation for infants at term.

Additionally, premature neonates may lose excessive amounts of water and heat due to an increased body surface area-to-body mass ratio, as shown in Table 33-2.[32] In Table 33-2, a 70-kg adult having 1.73 m² body surface area manifests a 250 cm²/kg ratio, whereas a 1.5-kg premature infant (despite having a much smaller surface area) has an almost threefold increase in surface area-to-body

mass ratio. In particular, an extremely-low-birth-weight premature infant (≤500 g at birth) may have a body surface area exposed per kilogram of body mass greater than six times an adult. Simple geometry dictates that insensible water loss evaporating from the skin of a very-low-birth-weight premature infant conveys heat away from the body at a rate at least six times that of an adult. Finally, the mass of a very-low-birth-weight infant comprises 80% to 90% water, which is exposed to the external environment through a nonkeratinized, extremely thin epidermal barrier.[33]

Hammarlund and Sedin[27] summarized in a series of elegant studies the rate of transepidermal water (and evaporative heat) loss in premature newborns nurtured in incubators throughout the first month of life at different gestational ages (Fig. 33-1). Figure 33-1 shows that an infant 26 weeks' or less gestation may, in the first 48 hours of life, lose 60 g of water/m²/hr, or greater than 180 mL/kg/day. Approximately 0.6 kcal/mL is lost through latent heat of evaporation. Consequently an extremely-low-birth-weight premature infant may lose greater than 100 kcal/kg/day simply through evaporation from the skin.

PHYSIOLOGY OF THERMAL RESPONSE

Fetal Thermoregulation

The human fetus (similar to all mammals) generates heat through several energy-dependent, exothermic metabolic processes. Estimates from calorimetric studies in fetal sheep and indirect calorimetry performed in human

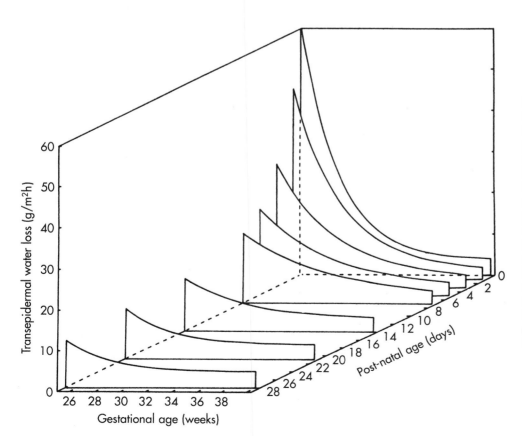

Figure 33–1. Insensible water evaporation from the skin of premature infants of varied gestational and postnatal ages. There is an exponential increase in the rate of cooling through evaporation in younger, less mature subjects. This difference may be due to body surface geometry, lack of keratin in the cornified epithelium of the epidermis, and a large proportion of body mass composed of water in these infants. See text for a detailed discussion of these factors. *(From Sedin G, Hammarlund K, Nilsson GE, et al: Measurements of transepidermal water loss in newborn infants. Clin Perinatol 12:79, 1985.)*

newborns shortly after birth suggest that the rate of heat production ranges from 33 to 47 kcal/kg/min (2.3 to 3.3 W/kg) in these mammals.[34,35] Although some of this heat production may be dissipated from the fetal skin through the amniotic fluid and into the uterine wall, it is estimated that less than 20% of the maternal-fetal temperature gradient composes fetal-uterine heat transfer. Probably of greater importance in the fetal elimination of intrinsic metabolic heat production is placental blood flow. Specifically, the investigations of fetal-maternal temperature gradients have shown that a minimal gradient of 0.45° C to 0.5° C is a sufficient arterial-venous difference across the umbilical circulation to eliminate entirely the metabolic rate of heat produced during fetal life.[36-38]

The mother also constitutes a massive heat reservoir. When elevated maternal temperature degrades the fetal capacity to eliminate metabolic heat produced, fetal fever may ensue, resulting in the van't Hoff effect, whereby fatal hyperthermia may occur. For these reasons, pregnant women should avoid hyperthermic states through fever control during acute illnesses or by avoiding extremes of environmental temperature (e.g., prolonged hot baths).

Transition from the Uterine Environment: Physiology of Cold Stress Response

Fetal mechanisms for cold stress response are not particularly active prenatally. These mechanisms are mitigated by the sympathetic nervous system and brown fat and are discussed in more detail subsequently.[39-41] Immediately upon birth, however, the fetal reliance on the maternal heat reservoir and on placental blood flow ceases. Characteristically the infant is born wet into a cold and hostile environment.

Inevitably, rapid environmental cooling ensues, with body temperatures dropping at a rate of 0.2° C/min to 1° C/min, depending on the maturity of the infant and the environmental factors encountered. Shivering (characteristic of nonmammalian species at birth and requiring vast amounts of adenosine triphosphate as an immediate skeletal muscle energy source) is not active in the human newborn thermal response. A human neonate's primary response when acutely exposed to a cold environment comprises increased infant voluntary muscular activity, vasoconstriction, and **nonshivering thermogenesis**.[39] Infants are able to maintain an increased metabolic rate of heat production under delivery room conditions only for minutes to at most a few hours using these mechanisms. Thereafter, energy stores become depleted, and hypothermia ensues rapidly.

As shown in Figure 33-2, an epinephrine-mediated thermal response occurs acutely on parturition.[42] This surge occurs through the sympathetic nervous system and through neurohumoral secretion via the para-aortic sympathetic nodes and the fetal adrenal glands. Pursued to an extreme, norepinephrine-mediated peripheral vasoconstriction and pulmonary vasoconstriction occur with subsequent deterioration of oxygenation and circulation. Tissue hypoxia with accumulation of lactic acidosis results from anaerobic metabolism and may precipitate the ultimate demise of the unaided neonate. Tissue hypoxia lowers metabolic rate and blunts thermal response, accelerating the development of acute hypothermia.

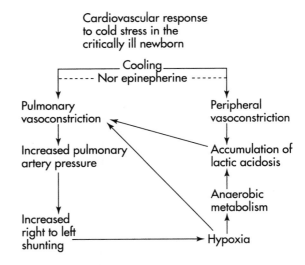

Figure 33–2. Schematic representation of norepinephrine-mediated responses to cold stress at birth in neonates. Cold stress increases metabolic rate and brown fat oxidation, which may be mediated by norepinephrine as well. See text for details. *(From Baumgart S: Incubation of the human newborn infant. In Pommerance J, Richardson CJ [eds]: Issues in Clinical Neonatology. Norwalk, CT, Appleton & Lange, 1992, pp 139-150.)*

Afferents

Homeothermic response to a cold environment begins with the sensation of temperature. Traditional physiology identifies two temperature-sensitive sites—the hypothalamus and the skin. Sensation of cold by neonatal skin triggers a cold-adaptive response long before core sensors in the hypothalamus (which are blunted) come into play. Some investigators conjecture that neonatal cold reception resides primarily in the skin, whereas warm reception resides in the hypothalamus. Both sensors are probably integrated, however, because cold sensory response is inhibited by core sensor hyperthermia and vice versa. Peripheral skin cold sensation is teleologically important because early detection of heat loss from the skin aids in the infant's timely response for maintaining core temperature.

Central Regulation

Integration of multiple skin temperature inputs probably occurs in the hypothalamus. No single control temperature seems to exist, however. Under different environmental conditions, temperature of the skin may fluctuate 8° to 10° C, and temperature of the hypothalamus may vary by 0.5° C. Diurnal temperature fluctuations; variations with general sympathetic tone; and blunted regulation with asphyxia, hypoxemia, and central nervous system malformations also exist. Premature infants may regulate core temperature near 37.5° C, whereas term infants may respond to maintain a core temperature of 36.5° C. Because important thermoregulatory processes are triggered by 0.5° C, deviation at any temperature-sensitive site is important.

Efferents

The effector limb of the neonatal thermal response is mediated primarily by the sympathetic nervous system, although infant behavior also may be involved. The earliest maturing response is vasoconstriction in deep dermal arterioles, resulting in reduced flow of warm blood from the infant's core into the exposed periphery of the skin's circulation. Additionally, reduction of skin blood flow effectively places a layer of insulating fat between the core and the exposed skin in a term infant. Reduced subcutaneous fat content in low-birth-weight infants diminishes this effective insulating property. Vasoconstriction nevertheless remains a premature newborn's first line of defense, and the response is present even in the most immature infants.[19]

Brown fat constitutes a second sympathetic effector organ that provides a metabolic source of nonshivering thermogenesis.[39] Brown fat is located in axillary, mediastinal, paraspinal, perinephric, and other regions of the newborn. Adipocyte membranes show numerous norepinephrine/epinephrine receptor sites for sympathetically enervated and humoral stimulation. With cold stress, these receptors stimulate production of cyclic adenosine monophosphate, inducing lipoprotein lipase activity. Thyroid hormone is permissive to this effect, and a thyroid surge in neonates also characterizes cold stimulation from birth.[43-45] Electron microscopy shows an abundance of mitochondria to hydrolyze and re-esterify triglycerides and to oxidize free fatty acids.[46] In a term infant, these reactions are exothermic and may increase metabolic rate by twofold or more. The brown appearance of brown fat is produced by proliferative blood vessels, which conduct the produced heat into the central venous circulation. Preterm infants have little or no brown fat, however, and may not be capable of any more than a 25% increase in metabolic rate despite the most severe cold stress.[47]

Finally, evidence suggests that control of voluntary muscle tone, posture, and increased motor activity with agitation may serve to augment heat production in skeletal muscle via glycogenolysis and glucose oxidation. Most of these substrates are deposited in accelerated fashion over the last trimester of gestation. A premature human infant remains particularly vulnerable to cold stress. Clinical observations of infant posture, behavior, and skin perfusion and measurements of the skin-to-core temperature gradient ultimately may provide the most useful guidelines for assessing infant comfort during incubation.

Intervention in Early Cold Stress

Intervention in cold stress in the immediate newborn period includes the following actions: (1) Drying infants in the delivery room interrupts the process of evaporative heat loss, (2) bundling (swaddling) infants to prevent exposure to cool air interrupts convective heat loss and provides insulation to retain heat generated metabolically, and (3) placing the newborn in the mother's arms (in particular, into her axillary fold) engenders conductive heat transfer from the mother to the infant and reduces cold stress. Alternatively, after an infant is dried and placed onto dry batting, a variety of warming devices may be used.

A convectively warmed incubator enclosure with air temperatures ranging from 35°C to 37°C or alternatively a radiant warmer bed platform may be provided, and a variety of swaddling heat shields have been advocated to prevent excessive cold exposure in premature infants.[20,48-50]

When outside the delivery room environment, infants generally are placed in either an incubator or a bassinet, and temperature is monitored closely and maintained through the first 2 to 3 hours of transitional care, either by warming the air within the incubator or by careful monitoring of the bundled, cot-nursed infant. Premature infants or infants who are small for gestation nevertheless may experience the consequences of a cool environment, wherein core temperature is maintained normal at the expense of metabolically generated heat.[10]

ECOLOGY OF HUMAN INCUBATION

General Metabolic Heat Balance Equation

The general metabolic heat balance equation is expressed as follows:

$$\dot{Q}_{metabolic} + \dot{Q}_{stored} = \dot{Q}_{conduction} + \dot{Q}_{convection} + \dot{Q}_{radiation} + \dot{Q}_{evaporation}$$

where $\dot{Q}$ is the rate of heat change (gain or loss), either through heat storage (resulting in an increase in body temperature) or produced through metabolism (left side of the equation, often expressed in kcal/kg/hr, kJ/kg/day, W/m²), and is balanced exactly by the sum of the rates of heat losses (right side of this equation).[51] For homeothermy to occur, $\dot{Q}_{stored}$ should equal zero (neither heat gain nor heat loss sufficient to alter body temperature). If increases in heat loss to the environment occur, the physiologic responses enumerated previously are stimulated, resulting in an increase in metabolic rate of substrate consumption and a commensurate increase in $\dot{Q}_{metabolic}$. Correction of body temperature occurs, but at the expense of energy. As with all mammals, even the smallest premature infant surviving where metabolic rate measurements can be made shows this homeothermic tendency.

Glass and coworkers[52] investigated the deleterious effects in premature infants nurtured in dry, ambient air environments of either 35°C or 36.5°C in the first few days of life. Significant differences in weight gain were shown, with warmer infants achieving better growth. Rectal temperatures assessed in both groups of infants were considered normal, and the authors concluded that thermogenic response in the slightly cooler infants was sufficient to consume calories, which otherwise might have been used for growth. These authors subsequently noted that graded temperature regulation within incubators (to promote a thermal neutral environment) was essential not only to the survival of preterm infants, but also to reduce their morbidity and achieve optimal growth after premature birth.

Thermal Neutral Concept[11-18,53]

The **thermal neutral environment** is shown conceptually in Figure 33-3.[42] Environmental temperature is plotted against the infant's metabolic rate of heat production (indicated in the figure indirectly by rate of oxygen

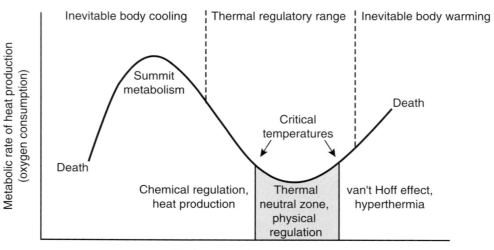

Figure 33–3. Conceptual representation of the thermal neutral temperature range for newborns. Environmental temperature is indicated on the horizontal axis, and metabolic rate response to environmental temperature variation is indicated on the vertical axis as rate of oxygen consumption. The shaded region depicts the upper and lower limits of nonmetabolic thermal regulatory response (e.g., vasoconstriction), termed **critical temperatures**. Beyond the critical temperature range, metabolic rate increases with either cold stress *(left)* or the van't Hoff effect with inevitable body core warming *(right)*. When cold stress exceeds the body's compensatory capacity for increased heat production, inevitable core temperature cooling occurs with eventual death of the organism. See text for details. *(From Baumgart S: Incubation of the human newborn infant. In Pommerance J, Richardson CJ [eds]: Issues in Clinical Neonatology. Norwalk, CT, Appleton & Lange, 1992, pp 139-150.)*

consumption). The premise underlying Figure 33-3 is that although newborns (particularly premature infants) cannot shiver, they respond to environmental cooling by increasing the metabolic rate of heat production. The shaded region of this graph is designated the **thermal neutral temperature zone**. Within this narrow range of environmental temperatures (bordered by a low **critical temperature** on the left and a high critical temperature on the right), the infant may control body temperature near normal using mechanisms of physical regulation alone (e.g., vasoconstriction), without necessitating an increase in metabolic rate. Below the critical temperature of the thermal neutral zone, the infant's metabolic rate increases in a dramatic thermoregulatory response.

Body temperature may be maintained outside the thermal neutral zone by an increased metabolic rate of heat production. Infants near term may increase metabolic rate by 200% to 300% in an effort to maintain a constant core body temperature. Because core temperature is maintained at the expense of metabolic energy expenditure, simply monitoring core body temperature (rectal or axillary) is insufficient to detect whether an infant is within the thermal neutral zone of environmental temperature. When environmental temperature has decreased past a maximal or summit metabolism, inevitable body cooling occurs, resulting in deep hypothermia. If pursued to an extreme, the infant may die as a result of hypothermic exposure.

In contrast, an inappropriately high environmental temperature results in inevitable body heating (see Fig. 33-3). Beyond the infant's ability to dissipate body heat, the

van't Hoff effect ensues with inevitable body warming. Metabolic rate proceeds at an accelerated rate, resulting in excess heat production without sufficient heat elimination. Ultimately, body temperature increases to where infants experience seizures and die. Thermoregulation for neonates is a fairly complex process with maintenance of physical and physiologic parameters required to maintain a noncompromised, homeothermic state characteristic of mammalian physiology.

CONVENTIONAL CONVECTION-WARMED INCUBATORS

Convection Warming: Air versus Skin Temperature Servocontrol

Characteristically the modern incubator incorporates a transparent, plastic hood positioned over the infant with various access ports. Hand holes provide access with least interruption of air warming; in addition, a larger door may be opened, permitting access to the infant for handling and procedures. Underneath the bed surface on which the infant lies is a tungsten electric warming element. Air is forced over the warming element by a fan incorporated into the heating device. Air circulates within the incubator hood, usually in a drumlike fashion, attempting to maintain still air at the center of the incubator near the infant's skin. Temperature may be regulated electronically at the incubator's control panel to determine thermostatically the air temperature within the hood (to provide the optimal thermal neutral environment), or alternatively the infant's skin temperature may be controlled thermostatically to maintain a constant skin temperature, usually measured over the infant's abdomen (see later).[16,54] Regulation of each of these temperatures is described briefly.

Air Temperature Control

Figure 33-4 shows the Hey and Katz air temperature nomogram for premature neonatal incubation in a single-wall device, comparing infants weighing 1 kg at birth with infants weighing 2 kg at birth and defining thermal neutral incubator operating temperatures recommended (vertical axis in °F or °C).[16-18] The horizontal axis represents the infant's postnatal age in days to approximately 1 month. The principle of graded incubation is shown in this nomogram. The authors hastened to add in a caption to this figure, however, that nursery air temperatures less than 27° C or relative humidity less than 50% renders this nomogram inaccurate unless significant upward adjustment of the incubator's **operant temperature** (a weighted mean of measured wall and air temperatures) is made.

Skin Surface Control

As a result of the difficulties in determining the exact thermal neutral environment by defining all of the infant and environmental parameters described earlier (including air temperature, air velocity, relative humidity, mean inner wall temperature, infant skin temperature, surface area,

and positional geometry for all nursery environments), Silverman and colleagues[54] reasoned that any set of environmental conditions that guaranteed a **normothermic** skin surface temperature would be sufficient to attenuate thermoregulatory response, mediated in humans predominantly by skin temperature sensation. These authors defined a skin temperature set point between 36.2° C and 36.5° C over the anterior abdominal wall for thermostatic control of incubator air temperature warming to guarantee a MOMR of oxygen consumption and a thermal neutral environment. Servocontolled skin temperature has now become the standard of care for regulating incubator heating in many nurseries in North America and Europe.

Evaporation and Humidification in Incubators

Convection-warmed incubators are extremely complex environments. One example of this complexity is shown in Figure 33-5, adapted from a study of partitional calorimetry performed by Okken and colleagues.[55] Two specially constructed incubators were compared. The first partition (left) describes a natural (still air) convection-warmed incubator, wherein air rose passively from heating elements located underneath the infant's mattress to warm the interior of the incubator hood. The second partition represents a standard fan-forced convection incubator as described previously. As seen in Figure 33-5, nonevaporative heat loss (the sum of convection, radiation, and conduction) was 60% compared with 47% in the forced convection–warmed

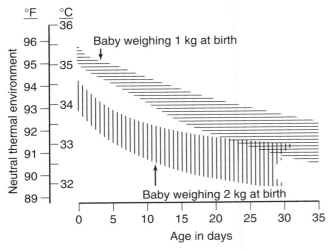

Figure 33–4. Hey and Katz's nomogram for determining incubator interior air temperature by assessing infant body weight (and gestation) and postnatal age. The principle of graded incubation is shown by the lower air temperature required to nurture older, more mature subjects. The authors add in a footnote that nursery air temperature outside the single-walled, convection-warmed incubator chamber should approximate 25°C. Room temperatures less than this value may lower incubator wall temperature significantly, increase radiant heat loss from the infant's skin to the interior wall of the incubator chamber, and result in infant cooling. Hey and Katz recommend adjusting incubator operative temperature by 1°C, for deviation of the nursery's ambient air temperature from 27°C. *(From Hey EN, Katz G: The optimum thermal environment for naked babies. Arch Dis Child 45:328, 1970.)*

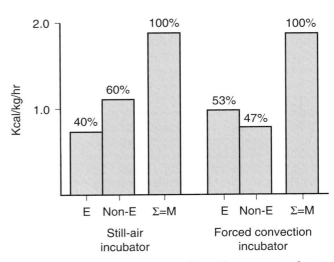

Figure 33–5. Partitional calorimetry performed for premature infants in two different types of convection-warmed incubators, natural and forced air. The rate of evaporative (E) heat loss is greater proportionally for infants nurtured in a conventional forced air–warmed environment than the rate of nonevaporative (non-E) heat loss from convection, conduction, and radiation. Heat balance is regulated by metabolic rate (M) and nonmetabolic mechanisms for thermal conservation (e.g., vasoconstriction). *(Adapted from Okken A, Blijham C, Franz W, et al: Effects of forced convection of heated air on insensible water loss and heat loss in preterm infants in incubators. J Pediatr 101:108, 1982.)*

incubator. Evaporative heat loss was 13% higher, however, in the forced convection–warmed environment. These authors attributed the increased evaporative heat loss in a forced convection–warmed incubator to disturbance of the layer of humid, moist air near the infant's skin. The relationship between convection and evaporation is shown by this elegant experiment.

Artificial humidification within the incubator hood has been used commonly (in Europe) to reduce excessive evaporative heat loss and to prevent dehydration. Humidification inside incubator hoods usually is accomplished by passive evaporation of water from a reservoir pan incorporated near the heating element and in the air pathway underneath the incubator mattress.[56] Other attempts at humidification of incubators in the past employed nebulized mist in an effort to supersaturate the infant's environment.[57,58] This technique resulted in the proliferation of *Pseudomonas* infections from 1950 to 1970 and was resoundingly rejected in a series of case studies.[57-60]

Running incubator hoods dry results in relative humidity levels less than 10% to 15% when nursery air is warmed and recirculated within the infant's chamber, promoting excessive insensible water (and heat) loss.[56] The incubator compensates for this excessive heat loss by increasing ambient air temperature within the incubator hood to maintain the infant's body temperature. A vicious cycle is established wherein excessive evaporation results in increased incubator operating temperature, which results in excessive evaporative loss. In response to these concerns, the American Academy of Pediatrics in their incubator recommendations suggested that an intermediate humidification level of 40% to 50% be employed using water in the vapor form (rather than nebulized particulate water, which may foster bacterial growth).[61]

An investigation of incubator humidification was conducted by Harpin and Rutter.[56] In a retrospectively controlled series of infants, 33 infants were nurtured in humidified incubators saturated between 80% and 90% relative humidity. Infants were less than 30 weeks of gestation and less than 2 weeks of age. Two infants acquired *Pseudomonas* sepsis, and one died. A group of 29 infants of similar gestation and maturity was nurtured in the dry incubation group; one acquired *Pseudomonas* sepsis and died. None of these infants died as a result of infection during the course of the study in the first few weeks of life. The authors recommended that humidification be used routinely only in the first 2 to 4 weeks of life and only with intermittent periods of dry incubator operation for at least 12 hours to prevent colonization of the incubator. Although this practice has not found general favor in the United States, humidification early in life may be prudent for incubation of a very-low-birth-weight infant in whom heat and water losses are excessive and perhaps pathologic. Modern incubators now may incorporate temperature and humidity control devices to prevent condensation at relative humidity levels greater than 80% and, it is hoped, diminish the risk of infection.

Radiant Heat Transfer in Incubators and Double Walls

An example of the importance of radiant heat transfer is shown in Figure 33-6,[23] which compares two incubators

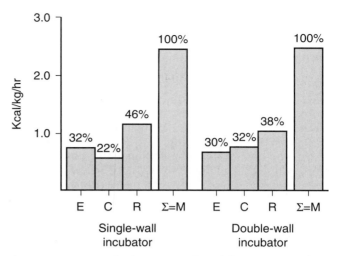

Figure 33–6. Partitional calorimetry performed for premature infants nursed in two different types of convection-warmed incubators, single walled and double walled. Radiant (R) heat loss by infants nurtured within a double-walled chamber is significantly reduced. The incubator's (skin) servocontrolled air temperature is compensatorily less to maintain homeothermy. In contrast, a higher air temperature is required to nurture infants in a single-walled chamber because infant radiant heat loss to the cooler single wall is higher. Convective (C) and evaporative (E) heat losses and metabolic rate (M) of heat produced by the infant, which balances the sum of heat losses, also are shown. *(Adapted from Bell EF, Rios GR: A double-walled incubator alters the partition of body heat loss of premature infants. Pediatr Res 17:135, 1983.)*

of different design. On the left, partitional calorimetry is shown for a standard, single-walled incubator; on the right, a double-walled incubator is depicted. The double-walled incubator (Air Shields, C100 Isolette) comprises a plastic chamber similar to the single-walled incubator with an additional inner wall suspended several centimeters separate from the outer wall of the incubator. Warmed air is circulated by forced convection between these two incubator walls, warming the outer and the inner surfaces of the inner wall and the inner surface of the outer wall of the incubator. The result is homogeneously elevated inner wall plastic temperature about 10° C warmer than the single-walled device. The infant's skin radiates to the infrared-opaque inner wall instead of to the colder outer wall of the incubator, down a much-reduced temperature gradient.

Figure 33-6 shows that radiant heat loss to the walls of the incubator (directly exposed to the infant's skin) is significantly reduced in the double-walled incubator. Paradoxically, convective heat loss is higher in the double-walled incubator because a lower air temperature is required to warm the infant when radiant heat loss is conserved. In the single-walled incubator, convective heat transfer is less the result of the higher incubator air temperature required to balance increased radiant heat loss. Because vapor pressure was constant in these studies regardless of incubator air temperature, evaporative heat loss was almost the same in both incubator devices.

The benefit derived from the double-walled incubator was a more homogeneous partition comparing evaporation, convection, and radiation in the double-walled device with the single-walled device. The interplay of environmental variables is seen to be important in determining the net heat balance for infants nurtured in these devices.

Incubator Homeothermy

All of the aforementioned incubator studies showing a thermal neutral environment under a variety of controlled conditions and governing incubator air temperature, incubator air humidity, wall temperature, and nursery environmental temperature were performed at steady-state conditions. Measurements of infant metabolic rate similarly were performed when the infant was at rest, postprandial, and, in general, naked and supine. As stated earlier, steady-state conditions may not be the reality for a premature neonate nurtured within an incubator hood governed by a thermostatically regulated servocontrol system and subjected to the many variations in the modern neonatal intensive care environment. Hand ports and doors may be open and closed several times a day to perform nursing procedures; minor surgical procedures; and x-ray, ultrasound, and echocardiographic examinations. The incubator ports may be opened more than once an hour in some nursery situations.

Figure 33-7 shows the characteristics of two incubators and their thermostatic regulatory mechanisms for controlling air temperature at a constant level near thermal neutral temperature for premature newborns when the major access panel is opened and closed.[62] Some of these devices are able to respond in such a way as to maintain or slightly overshoot the thermal neutral temperature. Any enclosed device when opened for a significant amount of time cannot interrupt the entry of cool surrounding nursery air.

When the doors of these incubators subsequently are closed, incubator temperatures may rebound. Overdamping of the servocontrol system in some instances may result in overshoot and undershoot of mid-hood incubator air temperature (as shown in Fig. 33-7) for 1 hour after the door has been closed. Conceivably, these temperature fluctuations over or under thermal neutral temperature may become part of an infant's routine experience during intensive care. When using incubators for nurturing premature infants, it is recommended that these devices be interrupted as little as possible. Such a *laissez-faire* approach may be impractical, however, for acute management of a critically ill newborn.

Prematurity and Conventional Incubation

In a classic study of partitional calorimetry, Wheldon and Rutter[21] described the complete thermal balance of a series of infants nurtured in a partially humidified, single-walled, forced convection–warmed incubator. As shown in Figure 33-8 at the top, a group of infants with a mean weight of 1.58 kg showed nearly similar radiant, convective, and evaporative heat losses, which when summed approximately balanced the infant's metabolic rate. When the same incubator device controlled body temperature

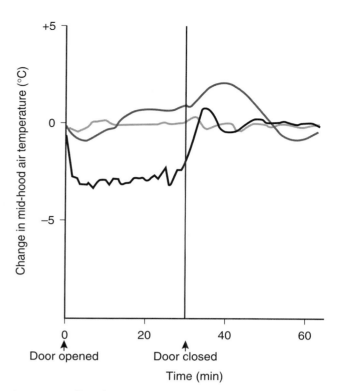

Figure 33–7. Effect of opening and closing the incubator front panel on interior air temperature servocontrolled to maintain a steady-state air temperature near a thermal neutral condition for premature neonates. Three different commonly used devices of different manufacture are represented to show different control responses to perturbation of the steady state. Overshoot and undershoot of temperature homeostasis is shown commonly. These air temperature variations may persist past 1 hour after returning the incubator panel to a closed position. *(From Bell EF, Rios GR: Performance characteristics of two double-walled infant incubators. Crit Care Med 11:663, 1983.)*

for a 1.08-kg infant (Fig. 33-8B), the incubator behaved differently. Radiant heat loss by comparison was low, whereas convective heat loss became negative. In other words, convection became a heat gain because the incubator's air temperature was greater than the infant's skin temperature.

As a result of warming, vapor pressure decreased, and evaporative heat loss became high. Evaporative heat loss alone was greater in the 1.08-kg infant than the sum of radiant, conductive, and convective losses and was greater than the infant's metabolism. This striking change in incubator temperature homeostasis was brought about by the small size of the infant, which resulted in relatively large evaporative and radiant heat loss components, necessitating a compensatory increase in incubator heat produced by forced convection. Most incubators in the United States incorporate temperature safety features that do not permit air temperature greater than body temperature for longer than 0.5 hour. Many incubator designs may not warm adequately a very-low-birth-weight infant (less than 1 kg), particularly early in life when evaporative losses are extremely high.[25,29] This tendency may

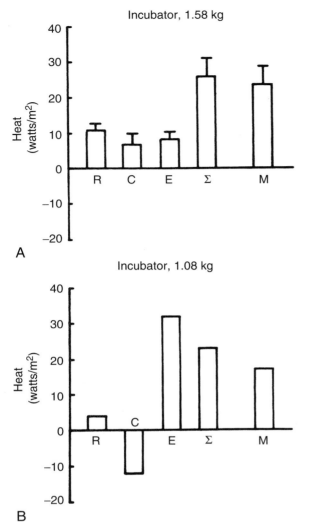

Figure 33–8. Partitional calorimetry for two premature infant populations nurtured in standard fashion within a single-walled, convection-warmed incubator. The larger infants **(A)** experience moderate convective (C), radiant (R), and evaporative (E) heat losses, which are balanced exactly by metabolic rate (M) of heat production. In contrast, the very-low-birth-weight infant depicted in **B** experiences significantly larger evaporative (E) heat loss, such that the (skin temperature) servocontrolled incubator compensates by increasing air temperature *greater than* skin temperature, promoting convective (C) heat *gain*, which is indicated as a *negative heat loss* in this graph. Similarly, warming of the incubator's walls by the superheated air renders radiant (R) heat loss negligible. This infant's environment is thermally unstable, with body temperature balanced between large convective heat gain and evaporative heat loss. The infant's metabolic rate (M) is small in magnitude in comparison and may not be sufficient to regulate the infant's body temperature at steady state. *(Adapted from Wheldon AE, Rutter N: The heat balance of small babies nursed in incubators and under radiant warmers. Early Hum Dev 6:131, 1982.)*

be countered by either humidifying the incubator or defeating the temperature-limiting safety feature, permitting incubator air temperature to be greater than body temperature. Neither of these strategies has achieved popularity among incubator design engineers because of the liabilities involved with either infection with excess humidification or hyperthermia with excess warming capability (see earlier discussion of humidification).

OPEN RADIANT WARMER BED

The radiant warmer bed comprises an open bed platform topped with a foam mattress and usually covered with cotton blankets on which a critically ill newborn infant lies without a plastic enclosure. Suspended from a pylon approximately 80 to 90 cm above this platform is a radiant heat source composed of an electrically heated metal alloy wire coiled within a quartz tube. A thermostatic skin servocontrol mechanism regulates electrical power to the alloy wire, generating radiant heat in the middle portion of the infrared spectrum. The wavelengths emitted range from 1000 to 3000 nm. The surrounding quartz envelope absorbs this infrared energy and re-emits electromagnetic radiation in longer wavelengths (>3000 nm). At full power, the sum of infrared irradiance is less than 100 mW/cm^2 of surface area irradiated on the bed platform below. The heat delivered in the near-infrared spectrum (<1000 nm) is less than 10 mW/cm^2 of surface area irradiated. Although controversial, these levels of radiant exposure in the infrared spectrum are believed to be biologically safe for the developing skin and eyes in a premature newborn.[63]

Additionally, a series of polished aluminum baffles distributes energy emitted by the radiant heating element evenly over the surface of the bed platform. Figure 33-9 shows a typical mapping of a radiant warmer bed surface while receiving radiant heat at half-power.[22] Generally, within the operating range for premature newborns weighing 1 to 1.5 kg, the radiant power density delivered is shown by the highlighted area in the center of this diagram (14.8 to 17.4 mW/cm^2), well below the 50 to 60 mW/cm^2 believed to be potentially deleterious.[63] The head, foot, and sides of the radiant warmer bed platform receive less radiant power and less warming than is delivered to the center of the bed platform. Optimally, infants are positioned in the center of this area.

The infant's posture and position under the radiant warming element may affect the effective radiative surface exposed. The infant's curved body surfaces affect direct versus indirect radiant heat transfer. The infant not only faces the warmer directly above (where radiant heat density is greatest), but also to the sides, where the radiant heater's power density drops to zero. Laterally the infant is irradiating heat away from the body to the much cooler walls of the nursery. Radiant delivery is complex, comprising radiant heat delivery, which is absorbed by the infant, and radiant heat losses to the sides.[64]

Partitional Calorimetry under Radiant Warmers

Figure 33-10 shows complete partitional calorimetry performed under radiant warmers in a series of premature infants.[64] Radiant heat losses under a radiant warmer and

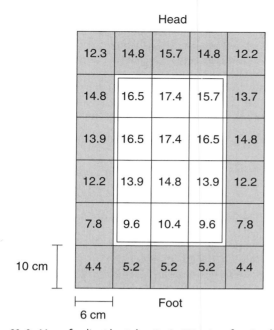

Figure 33–9. Map of radiant heat density (mW/cm² surface irradiated) delivered to bed surface under usual operating conditions for a radiant warmer. The central portion of the bed maintains nearly uniform distribution for infants nurtured near the mattress' center region. Radiant power density diminishes laterally at the bed's margins. *(From Baumgart S, Engle WD, Fox WW, Polin RA: Radiant warmer power and body size as determinants of insensible water loss in the critically ill neonate. Pediatr Res 15:1495, 1981.)*

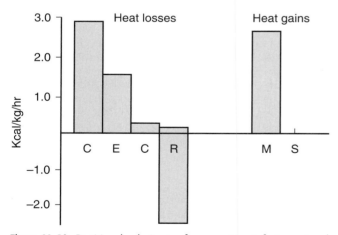

Figure 33–10. Partitional calorimetry for premature infants nurtured naked and supine on a radiant warmer bed servocontrolled to maintain abdominal skin temperature between 36.5°C and 37.2°C. Dynamic equilibrium is achieved when radiant heat delivered from the warmer balances large convective, evaporative, and radiant heat losses. Metabolic rate of heat production is relatively small compared with the magnitude of physical heat exchange with the surrounding environment. *(Adapted from Baumgart S: Radiant heat loss versus radiant heat gain in premature neonates under radiant heaters. Biol Neonate 57:10, 1990.)*

heat gains are shown. The effects of evaporation, convection, and conduction and of infant metabolic heat production also are depicted. Heat loss is composed of 64% convection to the surrounding cool air of the nursery's environment (air temperature 25° C). Most convective heat loss occurs through natural convection, whereas a minor component of heat loss is through forced convective air movement from doors opening and closing within the nursery, nursery personnel bustling near the bedside, and the cycling of heating and cooling vents supplying the nursery's ambient air temperature control.

Turbulent convective air movements also contribute to evaporative heat loss, which constitutes 30% of total heat loss in Figure 33-10. This situation is analogous to the observation of Okken and coworkers[55] (see Fig. 33-5) wherein convection of forced air contributed to disruption of a thin microenvironment of humidified, warm air layered near the infant's skin, potentiating evaporative loss. Under a radiant warmer, owing to indirect heating of the bed's surface, conductive heat loss in this diagram is less than 4%, and radiant heat losses from the infant's sides toward the nursery's walls constitutes less than 2% of total heat loss.

Thermal equilibrium is maintained under a radiant warmer by a striking replacement of heat losses (through convection, evaporation, conduction, and radiation), by radiant heat gain directly from the warming element. Almost 58% of heat replacement is derived from the servocontrolled radiant warmer element. Metabolic heat production constitutes only 42% of the thermal balance and is overpowered by radiant heat replacement.

Convective heat loss is the single largest component of heat loss for infants nurtured under radiant warmers, followed by evaporation. Heat loss is replaced in a nonhomogeneous fashion by the radiant warming element located above the infant. Radiant temperature may be lower at the sides of the infant, and uneven heating and cooling effects (a balance between convective turbulence, evaporation, and overhead radiant warming) may be felt at the infant's skin.

Radiant Warmers versus Incubators[65]

Insensible Water Loss

When open radiant warmer beds were first introduced into neonatal intensive care units in the early 1970s, several authors published results suggesting an increased insensible water loss (and evaporative heat loss) for critically ill premature infants nurtured under these conditions.[32] Several of these studies failed to control for ambient vapor pressure (a function of air temperature and relative humidity), however, for infants nurtured within closed incubator environments versus under open radiant warmers. Two studies on insensible water loss incurred within incubators and under radiant warmers are summarized in Figure 33-11.[42] The dotted line in Figure 33-11 represents insensible water loss for infants ranging in weight from 1 to 2 kg.[31] Insensible water loss for infants weighing less than 1 kg was extrapolated linearly. Infants in this study were nurtured in incubators with moderate humidification. In an analogous study,

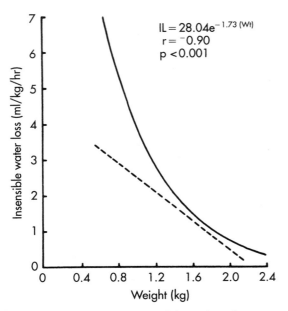

$IL = 28.04e^{-1.73 \,(Wt)}$
$r = ^{-}0.90$
$p < 0.001$

Figure 33–11. Evaporative water (and heat) loss for premature neonates of comparable birth weight range determined for infants nurtured under radiant warmers *(solid line)* and within single-wall, convection-warmed incubators *(not humidified)* set to maintain thermal neutral conditions *(broken line)*. Water and heat loss is comparable for infants in the low-birth-weight range greater than 1.1 kg. Data for very-low-birth-weight infants less than 0.8 kg are lacking, however, for infants nurtured in incubators. Linear extrapolation of water loss data may underestimate evaporative rates in these tiny infants. *(From Baumgart S: Incubation of the human newborn infant. In Pommerance J, Richardson CJ [eds]: Issues in Clinical Neonatology. Norwalk, CT, Appleton & Lange, 1992, pp 139-150.)*

infants ranging in weight from 0.67 to 2.2 kg who were nurtured under radiant warmers were measured to determine their insensible water loss.[25] A geometric rise in insensible water loss occurred with infants with less than 1 kg birth weight. At birth weights greater than 1 kg, insensible water losses between incubator-nurtured and radiant warmer–nurtured infants were roughly equivalent. The divergence occurs probably more as a function of body geometry as infants become smaller, manifesting a geometrically larger surface area.

Similar rates of water loss were reported by Sedin and associates[29] measuring transcutaneous evaporation using another technique and cited in Figure 33-1. Together, these studies suggest that insensible water loss is less a function of the heat source used, but rather reflects infant geometry, skin maturity, and ambient vapor pressure. Use of water-saturated environments within incubators may all but eliminate insensible water loss and evaporative heat loss.[56]

Metabolic Rate

Because of the relatively large fluctuations in convective evaporative and radiant heat transfer for infants nursed under radiant warmers, several authors have criticized these devices as ineffective in producing a thermal neutral environment. In 1984, Le Blanc[66] summarized several studies in a single meta-analysis comparing radiant warmer technology with convectively heated incubators for infants nurtured alternatively in each of these environments. The thermal neutral environment was defined for each warming device as the MOMR of oxygen consumption (mL/kg/min), when skin temperature was servocontrolled between 36° C and 36.5° C and thermal equilibrium had been achieved at steady-state conditions (without any interruption of the incubator) for several hours. Eleven of 16 infants showed slightly higher rates of oxygen consumption when nursed at similar temperatures under radiant warmers. Mean results showed oxygen consumption of 6.84 ± 0.37 SEM versus 7.45 ± 0.44 mL/kg/min, an increase of 8.8% in metabolic rate under radiant warmers.

Variations in Assessment of Infant Metabolic Rate

Assessment of infant metabolic rate in the intensive care nursery, particularly for critically ill neonates, may not approximate the steady-state conditions of LeBlanc[66] when the assumptions of MOMR are observed. The accepted method for assessing metabolic rate (the most popular one used in critically ill newborn infants) is indirect calorimetry. Metabolic gas exchange is measured as the difference between inspired and expired concentrations of oxygen and carbon dioxide. Airflow into or out of the infant's environment is assessed to determine volume of gas exchange.

Typically, oxygen consumption ranges from 5 to 10 mL/kg/min, and carbon dioxide production ranges from 3.5 to 10 mL/kg/min, rendering a respiratory quotient (carbon dioxide production divided by oxygen consumption) that ranges from 0.7 to 1. As shown in Table 33-3,[67] the exothermic caloric value of oxygen consumption and carbon dioxide production is approximately 5 kcal/L of oxygen consumed for carbohydrate metabolism, with a respiratory quotient of 1.

Infants nurtured in various incubation environments are evaluated for oxygen consumption and carbon dioxide production in which standard calorimetry technique dictates that MOMR of oxygen consumption be used to compare environmental conditions. The assumptions involved in the calculation of MOMR are (1) that the infant is at rest and asleep, (2) that the infant is postprandial at least 2 to 3 hours, and (3) that the infant resides at thermal neutral temperature conditions.

Table 33–3. Caloric Value of Oxygen Consumed and Carbon Dioxide Produced by Oxidation of Carbohydrate, Fat, and Protein

Substrate	Oxygen (kcal/L)	Carbon Dioxide (kcal/L)	Respiratory Quotient
Carbohydrate	5.05	5.05	1.00
Fat	4.69	6.63	0.71
Protein	4.49	5.60	0.80

After Karlberg P: Determination of standard energy metabolism (basal metabolism) in normal infants. Acta Paediatr Scand 41 (suppl):89, 1952.

Table 33–4. Typical Oxygen Consumption Values (mL/kg/min) During Early Neonatal Development at Resting Thermoneutral Conditions

	Birth	3-5 Days	1-2 Weeks
Term	4.5	6.0	7.0
Premature	4.5-5.5	—	8.0-9.0
Small for gestational age	>5.5	>6.5	>8.0-9.0

Approximated from Hull D, Small, ORC: Heat production in the newborn. In Sinclair JC (ed): Temperature Regulation and Energy Metabolism in the Newborn. New York, Grune & Stratton, 1978; pp 129-156.

Typical oxygen consumption values shortly after birth, at 3 days of age, and at 1 to 2 weeks of age are shown in Table 33-4.[47] Typically, premature infants show slightly higher oxygen consumption values than term infants, and small-for-gestational-age infants manifest oxygen consumption values slightly higher than these. The minimal requirement for oxygen consumption in these studies shows a metabolic rate of caloric expenditure of roughly 65 to 75 kcal/kg/day. Additionally, beyond this amount, 9 to 10 kcal/kg/day may be required for growth. Intensive care conditions provided for critically ill neonates rarely approximate the conditions, however, of a growing premature infant at rest and at steady state.

Major factors affecting the rate of oxygen consumption include temperature, whereby summit metabolism may reach 200% to 300% of MOMR. An infant's activity (particularly when cold stressed) additionally may increase oxygen consumption 100% to 200%, as the infant cries and moves. Finally, feeding, even with intravenous nutrition, triggers specific dynamic action (the heat of digestion) and increases metabolic rate by about 25%.

Figure 33-12 shows results of oxygen consumption measurements from studies conducted in our intensive care nursery in a 1.2-kg infant nurtured naked and supine under a radiant warmer while intubated endotracheally and receiving ventilatory support.[68] During this 90-minute period, oxygen consumption may be seen to fluctuate

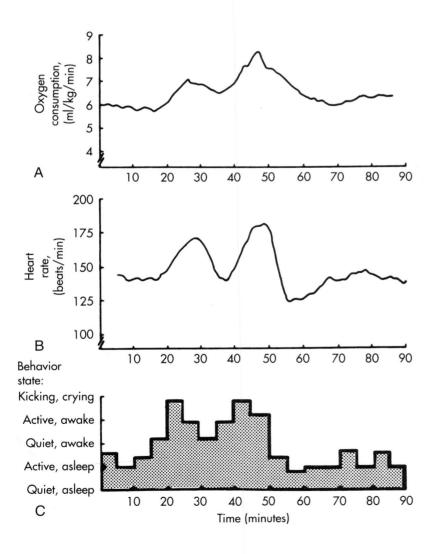

Figure 33–12. **A-C,** Example of non–steady-state variation in metabolic rate of oxygen consumption in a 1.2-kg infant nurtured under a skin temperature servocontrolled (35.5°C) radiant warmer **(A)**. Infant agitation is represented by an increased behavior score shown in the histogram **(C)**. Heart rate parallels oxygen consumption and behavior **(B)**. *(From Baumgart S: Partitioning of heat losses and gains in premature newborn infants under radiant warmers. Pediatrics 75:89, 1985.)*

between 6 mL/kg/min and 9 mL/kg/min and is paralleled closely by the infant's heart rate in beats per minute (to deliver oxygen to the tissues). Finally, the infant's behavior is noted in the bottom graph and roughly parallels the previous two graphs.

These observations of infant behavior affecting metabolism are typical of many premature infants, even when critically ill and receiving mechanical ventilation. Criteria of determining MOMR would suggest that oxygen consumption for this subject is 6 mL/kg/min. The integrated sum of behavior over the entire 90 minutes of the study period would reflect a higher rate of metabolism than this, however. Such observations have led Schulze and associates[69] to speculate that thermal neutral environments should be evaluated over periods considerably longer than 10 to 30 minutes of MOMR at steady state.

Thermal Neutral Temperature under Radiant Warmers

Figure 33-13 shows the metabolic rate of oxygen consumption (in mL/kg/min) on the vertical axis over three 90-minute study periods for the same infant in Figure 33-12 at three different radiant warmer servocontrol skin temperatures: 35.5° C, 36.5° C, and 37.5° C.[70] At the cooler temperature, 35.5° C, MOMR is equal to approximately 6 mL/kg/min. At 36.5° C, MOMR is equal to about 4.3 mL/kg/min, which is significantly lower. At 37.5° C, metabolic rate is significantly lower still at about 4 mL/kg/min. From these studies over longer durations of time, it seems clear that infant behavior may constitute a significant part of the metabolic rate determination and that behavioral peaks may affect significantly the definition of a thermal neutral zone. This result was corroborated by Bruck and Parmelee[14] in the early 1960s for larger infants nurtured inside convection-warmed incubators.

In Figure 33-14, 18 premature infants nurtured under radiant warmers showed a thermal neutral environmental temperature (approximately 36.2° C to 36.5° C servocontrolled anterior abdominal wall skin temperature), wherein all infant behavior was incorporated.[70] As shown in this graph, metabolic rate approximated 7.2 mL/kg/min at the warmer's 36.5° C skin temperature set point. Increasing anterior abdominal skin temperature beyond this point by 1° C resulted in no significant further reduction in metabolic rate.

As shown in Figure 33-15, the gradient between peripheral skin temperatures (measured on the heel), core temperature (measured rectally), and mean skin temperature (sampled at the heel, abdomen, and cheek) widened with decreasing anterior abdominal wall skin servocontrol temperature.[70] In particular, when servocontrolled to 37.5° C, these infants rapidly approached mean skin temperatures nearly equal to servocontrolled skin temperature. The gradient for heat loss (through convection) narrowed sufficiently for many of these infants to manifest fever (38.2° C to 38.5° C). We recommend avoiding skin control temperatures greater than 36.7° C to 37° C for infants in the weight range studied (0.87 to 1.60 kg).

A moderate skin temperature between 36.5° C and 37.2° C corresponds to the thermal neutral zone for premature infants under a radiant warmer. Beyond this level, there is risk for hyperthermia. The thermal neutral environment under a radiant warmer does not constitute a homeothermic steady state. Nevertheless the radiant warmer environment seems necessary to deliver heat continuously to critically ill infants requiring intensive care intervention. The uninterrupted steady-state studies performed in premature growing infants do not apply to critically ill infants. Care for critically ill infants within

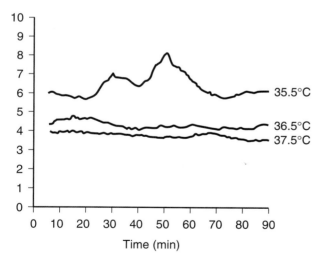

Figure 33–13. Same 1.2-kg infant as in Figure 33-12, nurtured under a radiant warmer servocontrolled to maintain abdominal skin temperature variously at 35.5° C, 36.5° C, and 37.5° C. Infant agitation and minimal observed oxygen consumption at steady state diminish significantly with higher skin temperature maintenance. *(From Malin S, Baumgart S: Optimal thermal management for low birth weight infants nursed under high-power radiant warmers. Pediatrics 79:47, 1987.)*

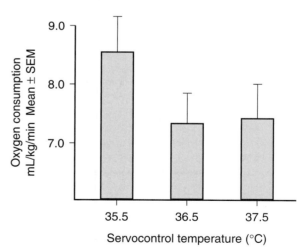

Figure 33–14. Summary of thermal neutral temperature conditions shown for 18 premature neonates (0.9 to 1.8 kg) nurtured under radiant warmers with skin temperature servocontrolled. The lowest thermally neutral temperature limit for the servocontrol set point was between 36.2° C and 36.7° C (median 36.5° C). *(From Malin S, Baumgart S: Optimal thermal management for low birth weight infants nursed under high-power radiant warmers. Pediatrics 79:47, 1987.)*

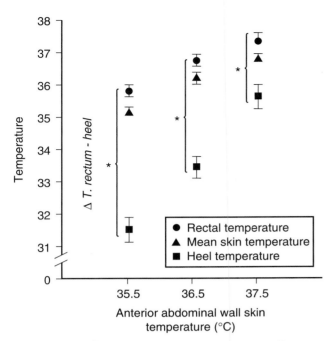

Figure 33–15. Heel temperature, core temperature, mean skin temperature, and servocontrolled abdominal skin temperature for the 18 infants shown in Figure 33-13. The gradient between peripheral and core temperature maintenance increases with cold stress and diminishes with high temperature maintenance to a point at which the heat loss gradient to the environment reverses. Inadvertent radiant heat warming of the infant's core may result with the latter condition and resulted in significant hyperthermia in almost half of the study subjects. The lowest safe and thermally neutral abdominal skin temperature for servocontrol in these studies was determined to be between 36.5° C and 37.0° C. Frequent monitoring of core temperatures to ensure less than 37.2° C to 37.5° C core temperature maintenance is required for infants nurtured in this fashion. *(From Malin S, Baumgart S: Optimal thermal management for low birth weight infants nursed under high-power radiant warmers. Pediatrics 79:47, 1987.)*

incubator environments results in frequent interruption of the incubator's function and similar inhomogeneous thermal control. A best compromise depends on individual clinical practice. Some clinical adaptations evaluated for use with radiant warmers are discussed in the next section.

SPECIAL INCUBATION STRATEGIES

A variety of different shielding techniques have been proposed for use in infants nurtured under radiant warmers or in incubators in an attempt to render their environments more uniformly homeothermic. A brief summary of some of these strategies follows.

Rigid Plastic Body Hoods as Heat Shields

Several authors have proposed a 1- to 3-mm thickness of plastic used as a miniature incubator hood and placed over infants on open radiant warmer beds. Yeh and coworkers[71] reported that insensible water loss was significantly less for infants nurtured using such a device (2.35 mL/kg/hr versus 1.70 mL/kg/hr evaporative loss). Bell and colleagues,[72] attempting to replicate this study, failed to show a significant difference in water loss using a rigid plastic body hood under radiant warmers (3.40 mL/kg/hr versus 3.37 mL/kg/hr). The configuration of the plastic hoods used in each of these studies was different, in some cases permitting free air exchange at the open ends of the hood. The interposition of radiant energy opaque plastic between the infant and the radiant warming element may have interfered with the delivery of radiant heat to the infant's skin. In a study in our nursery,[73] 85% of radiant warmer power was interrupted and absorbed by the plastic heat shield. Typically the plastic heated to 42° C. In response, the radiant warmer's servocontrolled heater output increased commensurately to maintain abdominal skin temperature at 36.5° C. Insensible water loss was unaffected by use of this rigid plastic body hood. Use of plastic hoods with a respiratory humidifier (a technique never validated) encourages "rain-out" condensation and bacterial colonization with water-borne pathogens. Disruption of the radiant warmer's servocontrol mechanism by the interposition of an opaque, plastic heat sink between the infant and the warmer seems to be a futile strategy.

Hybrid Incubator/Radiant Warmer Design

A more promising new development in commercial convection-warmed incubator and radiant warming technology is a hybrid design, combining these two separate warming modes into one device. In the incubator mode, movable plastic walls enclose the tiny premature infant, providing servocontrolled air warming, and the overhead radiant warmer is turned off. In the radiant warmer mode, the plastic walls are retracted to the sides, and the radiant warmer rapidly fires up to maintain servocontrolled skin temperature during procedures. The infant is not moved during the transition, and no plastic barrier is interposed between the infant and the radiant heater when on. The servocontrol algorithms and the integrity of the plastic enclosure in incubator mode are critical to the performance of such devices; the utility of these products is not yet proved.

Occlusive Plastic Blankets or Bags

In contrast to a rigid plastic body hood (and less cumbersome than the hybrid design), we have advocated the use of a flexible plastic blanket made of plastic wrap.[20,74] This device is thin enough to permit free radiant heat exchange between the infant and the warmer.[73] The flexible plastic blanket conforms closely to the infant's body and reduces the effect of convection in disrupting the microenvironment of warm, humid air near the infant's skin, successfully reducing insensible water loss.[20] As a result of the reduction in convective and evaporative heat losses under radiant warmers, the servocontrolled radiant heat required to maintain thermal equilibrium is reduced by 30%.[74] Insensible water loss commensurately is diminished from approximately 2 mL/kg/hr to 1.2 mL/kg/hr. Oxygen consumption is reduced from approximately 9 mL/kg/min to 8 mL/kg/min. The net effect of plastic wrap blanket heat shielding under radiant warmers is to render the environment more homeothermic, with lower power required to achieve thermal equilibrium from the radiant warmer and the infant's own rate of metabolic heat production.

Vohra and colleagues[75] evaluated a polyethylene plastic bag to promote temperature maintenance during resuscitation performed at delivery (under radiant warmers) and during the transport of infants to the neonatal intensive care unit. A significantly higher admission rectal temperature and subsequent improved survival were reported for infants less than 28 weeks of gestation. A larger, randomized trial of this technique may be warranted.

Adverse effects with plastic blankets or bags have been cited. In particular, for very-low-birth-weight premature infants less than 0.80 kg, the immature skin may stick to the plastic causing maceration, and in cases in which skin temperature servocontrol fails, life-threatening hyperthermia may result. When using these devices, nursing care requires avoiding direct skin contact with the plastic and vigilant infant temperature assessment independent of the servocontroller. Nevertheless, to date, plastic blankets are the most effective technique for rendering infants under radiant warmers more consistently thermally neutral.

Semiocclusive Artificial Skin

A new and exciting strategy for reduction in insensible water loss in extremely-low-birth-weight premature infants nurtured under radiant heaters (and within dry incubators) is covering the exposed surfaces of immature skin with semiocclusive polyurethane dressings (Tegederm, 3M, St. Paul, MN; and Opsite, Smith and Nephew, Largo, FL).[76] In early studies using this technique covering the chest and abdomen of premature infants, we evaluated transcutaneous evaporation directly using an evaporimeter. Compared with adjacent skin sites that were not dressed with the artificial polyurethane skin, insensible water loss from days 1 to 4 of life was reduced by 30% to 50%. On careful removal of the artificial polyurethane dressing, skin moisture barrier development was commensurate with development over the adjacent naked skin sites tested.

A report by Porat and Brodsky[77] cited preliminary results of applying an adherent polyurethane layer over the entire torso and extremities of extremely-low-birth-weight infants less than 800 g. Improved fluid and electrolyte balance, a reduced incidence of patent ductus arteriosus and intraventricular hemorrhage, and improved survival were shown with use of this form of plastic shielding. These results are preliminary, and further studies are required before routine application of artificial polyurethane skin dressings adherent to premature neonates can be advocated.

Petroleum Emollients[78-80]

Another occlusive dressing for the skin of low-birth-weight preterm infants during the first week of life is the application of Aquaphor. Although early results were encouraging for preserving skin integrity and perhaps controlling excessive dehydration in incubators,[79] the findings of a multicenter randomized trial are still wanting.[78] Some anecdotal reports suggest that bacterial infections may be more common with use of this technique.[80]

Until the results of the multicenter trial are conclusive, clinicians should exercise critical judgment before adopting this practice.

SPECIAL CLINICAL SCENARIOS

Kangaroo Care[81]

Kangaroo care refers to warming by skin-to-skin contact with the mother or father whereby premature infants are held naked between the axillary folds or the breasts mimicking a kangaroo's pouch. First implemented in Bogotá, Colombia, this method was popularized for nonintubated premature infants in Scandinavian and European countries in the 1980s. Kangaroo care has been shown to promote a thermal neutral metabolic response and temperature stability in stable growing premature infants. Early studies suggested a significant reduction in early mortality and morbidity, enhanced mother-infant attachment, increased infant alertness, more stable sleep patterns, better weight gain, and earlier hospital discharge. During kangaroo care, infants with bronchopulmonary dysplasia have better oxygenation, and other infants show less periodic breathing and reduced apnea. In the modern nursery, kangaroo care may be initiated even during mechanical ventilation in stable infants. The infant should be covered with a blanket to avoid outward convective and evaporative heat losses, and sessions (initially limited to 0.5 to 1 hour) can be increased successively up to 4 hours. To our knowledge, no adverse reports have been published, and its use in many nurseries is increasing.

Extremely-Low-Birth-Weight Infants

Temperature maintenance of an extremely premature infant (<750 g) should be part of resuscitation from the time of delivery. Despite radiant warming in the delivery room and convective incubation during transport, these infants nevertheless become hypothermic. They are born wet and prone to excessive transepidermal evaporative and convective heat losses. Suboptimal radiant heating, blowing noncontrolled warm, humidified air under plastic blankets (probably not as effective as the still air envelope conserved by the blanket), and the pressure for performing procedures with surgical drapes blocking radiant heat delivery may worsen heat loss.

Quickly drying the infant, properly placing the infant directly under the radiant heater at birth, and covering the infant's head are small but important steps of temperature resuscitation. Other techniques might be considered from birth, such as use of the plastic bag described by Vohra and coworkers[75] and a plastic wrap or blanket or polyurethane drape during umbilical catheterization. Finally, these infants should be rewarmed adequately under a radiant warmer before transferring to an incubator because early transfer may prolong thermal recovery in these hypoxic infants, who are incapable of generating enough metabolic heat. The use of incandescent light bulbs as an uncontrolled heat source for supplemental radiant heat delivery in incubators not only is inefficient, but also interferes with incubator function and can produce dangerous burns due to uneven heat distribution.

There are no data describing the best rate of rewarming hypothermic infants. A closely monitored rate of temperature increase of about 1° C to 2° C/hr seems reasonable but may not be achievable, especially in incubators delivering air temperatures less than 37° C. Alternatively a radiant warmer skin servocontrol temperature can be set 1° C higher than the infant's temperature and gradually increased until a normal core temperature is achieved. Hybrid incubators also can be used as radiant warmer beds and may be helpful in such rewarming scenarios.

Neonatal Fever—A Problem of Temperature Elevation[82-84]

Craig[82] defined neonatal **pyrexia** as a rectal (core body) temperature greater than 37.4° C; however, other investigators accept normal temperatures up to 37.8° C.[10] Of all newborns admitted to the regular newborn nursery, 1% to 2.5% develop fever judged by rectal or axillary temperatures, depending on the limits chosen. Sepsis is uncommon but is the most dreaded cause of fever in the newborn period. In reality, fever is an inconsistent and infrequent sign of sepsis (<10% of febrile neonates have culture-proven sepsis), and temperature elevation may be seen with several other clinical entities.

Mechanisms Producing Neonatal Fever

Mechanisms producing neonatal fever are incompletely understood. Fever most commonly results from disturbances in the complex interactions between central heat conservation and heat dissipation mechanisms at the hypothalamic level, caused by various immunogenic pyrogens (commonly prostaglandin E_2). Newborn infants of different animal species react in peculiar ways to different known pyrogens; human newborns may have severe documented bacterial infections without increased body temperature or even manifest hypothermia.

In addition, exposure to excess heat or insulation (excessive swaddling) can increase core temperature of newborns quickly due to their poor heat dissipation mechanisms (absence of sweating). This overheating commonly occurs when term infants are nursed in uncontrolled incubators or under radiant warmers. Temperature elevation also may occur with increased infant metabolic rate, as seen with skeletal muscle rigidity and status epilepticus. Another cause of temperature elevation is observed occasionally in well, breast-feeding newborns on the third to fourth day of life and is believed to result from dehydration secondary to insufficient milk production. Finally, there are more recent reports of an increased incidence of neonatal fever in infants of mothers receiving epidural analgesia. The mechanisms for temperature elevation in these latter two cases (see later) are unknown.

Determining the Cause of Fever

Sepsis is an uncommon but probably the most treatable life-threatening cause of high fever (especially temperature >38° C to 39° C). Paradoxically, septic neonates more frequently present with hypothermia. Most neonatal febrile episodes are noted on the first day of life (54% in one series); however, any fever occurring on the third day of life and fever greater than 39° C have been correlated with a significantly higher chance of bacterial disease and some viral diseases, particularly herpes simplex encephalitis.

Hyperthermia resulting from overheating has been reported in term or preterm infants as a complication of improper use of shielding devices or from excessive environment heating in equatorial and tropical countries. Dehydration fever is infrequently recognized in the newborn period, usually occurring in healthy breast-fed term infants on the third or fourth day of life. Temperature may range from 37.8° C to 40° C. Rehydration leads to resolution of fever and is key to the diagnosis of this entity.

In two more recent reports, fever was much more common in neonates born to mothers receiving epidural analgesia during labor compared with infants born to mothers without epidurals (7.5% versus 2.5%; 14.5% versus 1%).[83,84] With increasing use of epidural analgesia during labor, the recognition of epidural neonatal fever is an important consideration in evaluation of a febrile neonate.

Unusual and uncommon causes of neonatal fever include neonatal typhoid fever, congenital malaria (Third World countries), and hepatitis B vaccination. In addition, temperature elevations may be seen with central nervous system malformations, subarachnoid or other intracranial hemorrhages, and on rare occasions neonatal spinal neurenteric cyst (especially in the presence of prolonged fever of >3 weeks with myelopathy).

Management

The clinical problem is that fever may be the only indication for severe bacterial disease. The relevant perinatal history should be evaluated for risk factors mitigating a laboratory evaluation or presumptive treatment for infection. Signs suggesting sepsis (diminished activity, irritability, seizures) should be assessed. All neonates with fever should be evaluated for hydration, weight loss, and foci of infection (cellulitis, septic arthritis or osteomyelitis, omphalitis, or presence of colonized foreign bodies, as a central venous line). Febrile neonates without a clinical history or signs of infection present a challenge, and data are insufficient in the literature about appropriate management. An infant's environment should be examined for overheating, and in breast-feeding infants with fever at 3 to 4 days and excessive weight loss, dehydration fever should be considered and treated to establish this diagnosis. Mothers receiving epidural analgesia often manifest shivering with their temperature increase, and they experience a rapid defervescence after discontinuation of the epidural infusion. Recognition of this pattern may avoid unnecessary sepsis evaluations in neonates with fever in the first day of life.

SUMMARY

Since the principle of *graded incubation* was first applied to premature human neonates, survival has been enhanced. The complexity of neonatal care has exploded in recent years to include many techniques and manipulations of these fragile patients. Care must be taken to provide an uninterrupted source of infant warming adequate not only to maintain body temperature, but also to reduce thermal stress and the metabolic demand associated with it. As clinicians strive to nurture smaller infants, they must be aware that the problem of heat loss and cold stress increases geometrically as body size diminishes. In the hectic intensive care nursery environment, frequently temperature regulation is either forgotten or delegated to machinery ill-equipped to respond to thermal fluctuations in a timely manner. Incubators are probably best for the nurturance of premature, growing infants who require little manipulation or intervention. Radiant warmers may be required for the delivery of intensive care with uninterrupted heat delivery. As much as possible, shielding infants from the harsh extrauterine environment is desirable. Finally, preservation of the delicate microenvironment of warm, humid air that resides near an infant's skin within 1 to 2 mm is vital for maintaining homeothermy.

REFERENCES

1. Cone TE: History of the Care and Feedings of the Premature Infant. Boston, Little, Brown, 1985.
2. Cadman WH: The Artificial Incubating Establishments of the Egyptians. Report of the 1913 Meeting of the British Association for the Advancement of Science, London, 1914.
3. Marx S: Incubation and incubators. Am Med Surg Bull 9:311, 1896.
4. Berthod P: La Couveuse et le Gavage a la Maternite de Paris (thesis). Paris, G. Rougier, 1887.
5. Mauriceau F: Traite des Maladies des Femmes Grosses et Accouchees. Paris, Chez l'Auteur, 1669, p 100.
6. Rotch TM: Description of a new incubator. Arch Pediatr 10:661, 1893.
7. Southwick GR: The care of weak, or prematurely born infants. N Engl Med Gaz 25:310, 1890.
8. Blackfan KD, Yaglou CP: The premature infant: A study of effects of atmospheric conditions on growth and on development. Am J Dis Child 46:1175, 1933.
9. Bolt RA: The mortalities of infancy. In Abt I-A (ed): Pediatrics, vol. 2. Philadelphia, WB Saunders, 1923.
10. Silverman WA, Fertig JW, Berger AP: The influence of the thermal environment upon the survival of the newly born premature infant. Pediatrics 22:876, 1958.
11. Cross KW, Dawes GS, Mott JC: Anoxia, oxygen consumption and cardiac output in newborn lambs and adult sheep. J Physiol 146:316, 1959.
12. Hill JR, Rahimtulla KA: Heat balance and the metabolic rate of newborn babies in relation to environmental temperature, and the effect of age and of weight on basal metabolic rate. J Physiol 180:239, 1965.
13. Hill JR: The oxygen consumption of newborn and adult mammals: Its dependence on the oxygen tension in the inspired air and on the environmental temperature. J Physiol 149:346, 1959.
14. Bruck K, Parmelee AH, Bruck M: Neutral temperature range and range of "thermal comfort" in premature infants. Biol Neonate 4:32, 1962.
15. Bruck K: Temperature regulation in the newborn infant. Biol Neonate 3:65, 1961.
16. Hey EN, Katz G: The optimum thermal environment for naked babies. Arch Dis Child 45:328, 1970.
17. Hey EN: The relation between environmental temperature and oxygen consumption in the new-born baby. J Physiol 200:589, 1969.
18. Hey EN: Thermal neutrality. Br Med Bull 31:69, 1975.
19. Sinclair JC: Metabolic rate and temperature control. In Smith CA, Nelson NM (eds): The Physiology of the Newborn Infant. Springfield, IL, Charles C Thomas, 1976, pp 354-415.
20. Baumgart S, Engle WD, Fox WW, et al: Effect of heat shielding on convective and evaporative heat losses and on radiant heat transfer in the premature infant. J Pediatr 99:948, 1981.
21. Wheldon AE, Rutter N: The heat balance of small babies nursed in incubators and under radiant warmers. Early Hum Dev 6:131, 1982.
22. Baumgart S, Engle WD, Fox WW, Polin RA: Radiant warmer power and body size as determinants of insensible water loss in the critically ill neonate. Pediatr Res 15:1495, 1981.
23. Bell EF, Rios GR: A double-walled incubator alters the partition of body heat loss of premature infants. Pediatr Res 17:135, 1983.
24. Baumgart S, Engle WD, Fox WW, Polin RA: Radiant energy monitoring as a measurement of insensible water loss in critically ill neonates under radiant warmers. Pediatr Res 14:590A, 1980.
25. Baumgart S, Langman CB, Sosulski R, et al: Fluid, electrolyte and glucose maintenance in the very low birth weight infant. Clin Pediatr 21:199, 1982.
26. Bell EF, Neidich GA, Cashore WJ, et al: Combined effect of radiant warmer and phototherapy on insensible water loss in low-birth weight infants. J Pediatr 94:810, 1979.
27. Hammarlund K, Sedin G: Transepidermal water loss in newborn infants: VIII. Relation to gestational age and postnatal age in appropriate and small for gestational age infants. Acta Paediatr Scand 72:721, 1983.
28. Hey EN, Katz G: Evaporative water loss in the newborn baby. J Physiol (Lond) 200:605, 1969.
29. Sedin G, Hammarlund K, Nilsson GE, et al: Measurements of transepidermal water loss in newborn infants. Clin Perinatol 12:79, 1985.
30. Williams PR, Oh W: Effects of radiant warmer on insensible water loss in newborn infants. Am J Dis Child 128:511, 1974.
31. Wu PYK, Hodgman JE: Insensible water loss in preterm infants: Changes with postnatal development and non-ionizing radiant energy. Pediatrics 54:704, 1974.
32. Costarino AT, Baumgart S: Water metabolism in the neonate. In Cowett RM (ed): Principles of perinatal-neonatal metabolism. New York, Springer-Verlag, 1991, pp 623-649.
33. Costarino AT, Baumgart S: Modern fluid and electrolyte management of the critically ill premature infant. Pediatr Clin North Am 33:153, 1986.
34. Power GG, Kawamura T, Dale PS, et al: Temperature responses following ventilation of the fetal sheep in utero. J Dev Physiol 8:477, 1986.
35. Ryser G, Jequier E: Study by direct calorimetry of thermal balance on the first day of life. Eur J Clin Invest 2:176, 1972.
36. Morishima HO, Yeh MN, Niemann WH, et al: Temperature gradient between fetus and mother as an index for assessing intrauterine fetal condition. Am J Obstet Gynecol 129:443, 1977.
37. Power GG, Schroder H, Gilbert RD: Measurement of fetal heat production using differential calorimetry. J Appl Physiol 57:917, 1984.
38. Schroder H, Gilbert RD, Power GG: Computer model of fetal-maternal heat exchange in sheep. J Appl Physiol 65:460, 1988.
39. Alexander G, Williams D: Shivering and non-shivering thermogenesis during summit metabolism in young lambs. J Physiol (Lond) 198:251, 1968.
40. Hodgkin DD, Gilbert RD, Power GG: In vivo brown fat response to hypothermia and norepinephrine in the ovine fetus. J Dev Physiol 10:383, 1988.

41. Schroder H, Huneke B, Klug A, et al: Fetal sheep temperatures in utero during cooling and application of triiodothyronine, norepinephrine, propranolol and suxamethonium. Pflugers Arch 410:376, 1987.

42. Baumgart S: Incubation of the human newborn infant. In Pommerance J, Richardson CJ (eds): Issues in Clinical Neonatology. Norwalk, CT, Appleton & Lange, 1992, pp 139-150.

43. Bray GA, Goodman HM: Studies on the early effects of thyroid hormones. Endocrinology 76:323, 1965.

44. Klein AH, Reviczky A, Padbury JF: Thyroid hormones augment catecholamine-stimulated brown adipose tissue thermogenesis in the ovine fetus. Endocrinology 114:1065, 1984.

45. Swanson HE: Interrelations between thyroxin and adrenalin in the regulation of oxygen consumption in the albino rat. Endocrinology 59:217, 1956.

46. Silva JE, Larsen PR: Adrenergic activation of triiodothyronine production in brown adipose tissue. Nature 305:712, 1983.

47. Hull D, Smales ORC: Heat production in the newborn. In Sinclair JC (ed): Temperature Regulation and Energy Metabolism in the Newborn. New York, Grune & Stratton, 1978, pp 129-156.

48. Baum JD, Scopes JW: The silver swaddler. Lancet 1:672, 1968.

49. Besch NJ, Perlstein PH, Edwards NK, et al: The transparent baby bag. N Engl J Med 284:121, 1971.

50. Dahm LS, James LS: Newborn temperature: Heat loss in the delivery room. Pediatrics 49:504, 1972.

51. Hardy JD, Gagge AP, Rapp GM: Proposed standard system of symbols for thermal physiology. J Appl Physiol 27:439, 1969.

52. Glass L, Silverman WA, Sinclair JC: Effect of the thermal environment on cold resistance and growth of small infants after the first week of life. Pediatrics 41:1033, 1968.

53. Bruck K: Heat production and temperature regulation. In Stave U (ed): Perinatal Physiology. New York, Plenum, 1978, pp 455-498.

54. Silverman WA, Sinclair JC, Agate FJ Jr: The oxygen cost of minor changes in heat balance of small newborn infants. Acta Pediatr Scand 55:294, 1966.

55. Okken A, Blijham C, Franz W, et al: Effects of forced convection of heated air on insensible water loss and heat loss in preterm infants in incubators. J Pediatr 101:108, 1982.

56. Harpin VA, Rutter N: Humidification of incubators. Arch Dis Child 60:219, 1985.

57. Moffet HL, Allan D, Williams T: Survival and dissemination of bacteria in nebulizers and incubators. Am J Dis Child 114:13, 1967.

58. Moffet HL, Allan D: Colonization of infants exposed to bacterially contaminated mists. Am J Dis Child 114:21, 1967.

59. Brown DG, Baublis J: Reservoirs of *pseudomonas* in an intensive care unit for newborn infants: mechanism of control. J Pediatr 90:453, 1977.

60. Hoffman MA, Finberg L: *Pseudomonas* infections in infants associated with high humidity environments. J Pediatr 46:626, 1955.

61. American Academy of Pediatrics and American College of Obstetricians and Gynecologists: Guidelines for Perinatal Care, 2nd ed. Elk Grove Village, IL, AAP/ACOG, 1988, p 278.

62. Bell EF, Rios GR: Performance characteristics of two double-walled infant incubators. Crit Care Med 11:663, 1983.

63. Baumgart S, Knauth A, Casey FX, et al: Infrared eye injury not due to radiant warmer use in premature neonates. Am J Dis Child 147:565, 1993.

64. Baumgart S: Radiant heat loss versus radiant heat gain in premature neonates under radiant heaters. Biol Neonate 57:10, 1990.

65. Meyer MP, Payton MJ, Salmon A, et al: Clinical comparison of radiant warmer and incubator care for preterm infants from birth to 1800 grams. Pediatrics 108:395, 2001.

66. LeBlanc MH: Relative efficacy of radiant and convective heat in incubators in producing thermoneutrality for the premature. Pediatr Res 18:425, 1984.

67. Karlberg P: Determination of standard energy metabolism (basal metabolism) in normal infants. Acta Paediatr Scand 41(Suppl):89, 1952.

68. Baumgart S: Partitioning of heat losses and gains in premature newborn infants under radiant warmers. Pediatrics 75:89, 1985.

69. Schulze K, Kairan R, Stefanski M, et al: Spontaneous variability in minute ventilation, oxygen consumption and heart rate of low birth weight infants. Pediatr Res 15:1111, 1981.

70. Malin S, Baumgart S: Optimal thermal management for low birth weight infants nursed under high-power radiant warmers. Pediatrics 79:47, 1987.

71. Yeh TF, Amma P, Lillian LD, et al: Reduction of insensible water loss in premature infants under the radiant warmer. J Pediatr 94:651, 1979.

72. Bell EF, Weinstein MR, Oh W: Heat balance in premature infants: Comparative effects of convectively heated incubator and radiant warmer, with and without plastic heat shield. J Pediatr 96:460, 1980.

73. Baumgart S, Fox WW, Polin RA: Physiologic implications of two different heat shields for infants under radiant warmers. J Pediatr 100:787, 1982.

74. Baumgart S: Reduction of oxygen consumption, insensible water loss and radiant heat demand using a plastic blanket for low birth weight infants under radiant warmers. Pediatrics 74:1022, 1984.

75. Vohra S, Frent G, Campbell V, et al: Effect of polyethylene occlusive skin wrapping on heat loss in very low birth weight infants at delivery: A randomized trial. J Pediatr 134:547, 1999.

76. Knauth A, Gordin M, McNelis W, et al: A semipermeable polyurethane membrane as an artificial skin in premature neonates. Pediatrics 83:945, 1989.

77. Porat R, Brodsky N: Effect of Tegederm use on outcome of extremely low birth weight (ELBW) infants, Pediatr Res 33:231(A), 1993.

78. Edwards WH, Conner JM, Soll RF, for the Vermont Oxford Network: The effect of Aquaphor original emollient ointment on nosocomial sepsis rates and skin integrity in infants of birth weight 501-1000 grams. Pediatr Res 49:388A, 2001.

79. Nopper AJ, Horii KA, Sookdeo-Drost S, et al: Topical ointment therapy benefits premature infants. J Pediatr 128:660-669, 1996.

80. Oski K, Pappagallo M, Lerer T, Hussain N: Does use of Aquaphor (Aq) in extremely low birth weight infants (ELBW) increase the risk for nosocomial sepsis? Pediatr Res 49:227A, 2001.

81. Anderson GC: Current knowledge about skin-to-skin (kangaroo care) for preterm infants. J Perinatol 11:216, 1991.

82. Craig WS: The early detection of pyrexia in the newborn. Arch Dis Child 41:448, 1963.

83. Lieberman E, Lan JM, Frigoletto F Jr, et al: Epidural analgesia, intrapartum fever, and neonatal sepsis evaluation. Pediatrics 99:415, 1997.

84. Pleasure JR, Stahl GE: Do epidural anesthesia-related maternal fevers alter neonatal care? Pediatr Res 27:221A, 1990.

CHAPTER 34

Neonatal Nurse Practitioners in the Neonatal Intensive Care Unit

Patricia C. Mele and Claudia C. Herbert

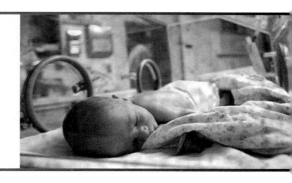

The role of the neonatal nurse practitioner (NNP) has been defined by the National Association of Neonatal Nurses (NANN): "a registered nurse with clinical expertise in neonatal nursing who has received formal education with supervised clinical experience in the management of sick newborns and their families."[1] This definition is also accepted by the Committee on the Fetus and Newborn of the American Academy of Pediatrics.[2] The NNP manages a caseload of patients with collaboration, consultation, and general supervision from a neonatologist.[1] NNPs are licensed to care for patients from birth at any gestational age until 2 years of age. Because the NNP is an advanced practice nurse, the role of the NNP may also extend into research, consultation, administration, education, and community service.[1]

HISTORY AND EVOLUTION OF THE NEONATAL NURSE PRACTITIONER ROLE

Historically, the role of the NNP has been somewhat ambiguous. The1960s was a period of numerous societal and health care delivery changes. Women assumed more active positions on issues related to their professional life, their reproductive life, and their own health care. Women prevailed in the field of nursing and other professions that were previously more male oriented. The feminist movement identified with and supported the enhancement of the nursing profession. The role of the nurse practitioner evolved during this era; the first nurse practitioner program began at the University of Colorado in 1965.[2] Factors leading to further development of the practitioner's role were the increasing technology and complexity of neonatal care, physician shortages, and nurses' desire for autonomy and increased responsibility in medical practice.[3] Also during this decade, neonatology became recognized as a subspecialty within pediatrics. Insurance companies began paying for neonatal care, and the crucial role of the family in the nurturance of infants

born prematurely was acknowledged. Delivery of care and the development of new treatments for high-risk neonates progressed at a rapid rate. The federal government recognized the need for higher levels of skill and knowledge to care for this population of children.[2]

In the 1970s, the first sub-board examinations of the American Board of Pediatrics in neonatal-perinatal medicine were held, and the first federal grants were provided to further the development of education programs for the health care providers for these children.[2] The evolution and expansion of the NNP's role was further expedited by supply and demand; the population of sicker and smaller newborns was growing, and there was a shortage of medical staff to care for them adequately. Pediatricians had had little exposure to neonatology practices during their residency training in the period before 1970, and there was a shortage of trained neonatologists graduating from a limited number of specialty fellowships during the 1970s. The American Board of Pediatrics and the Liaison Committee on Medical Education ruled that in a 3-year pediatric residency, no resident should receive more than 6 months in a subspecialty area.[2] As the resident training programs decreased their enrollments and restricted work hours, critical care coverage was disproportionately reduced even further.

Development and nationwide implementation of regionalized neonatal intensive care during the 1970s and 1980s further intensified the conflict between neonatal intensive care unit (NICU) staffing and the role of residents during their training. With a growing emphasis on primary care during their training, pediatric residents were less well equipped to provide highly technologic neonatal care. The Committee on the Fetus and Newborn of the American Academy of Pediatrics published a statement in 1982 on neonatal nurse clinicians (now called NNPs) that strongly supported their role as members of the health care team.[4]

The utilization of NNPs as specialized care providers in the NICU became cost imperative in tertiary hospital settings.[5] Pediatricians were unwilling or unable to function as neonatologists. Nurses were required to expand their roles in the NICU through advanced practice. Safety, effectiveness, and efficiency of NNPs in the delivery of primary care are now well established. In summary, the increased survival rates of infants with extremely low birth weights, the shortages of physicians trained in neonatal intensive care, and the nursing profession's emphasis on the development of advanced practice nursing roles have provided the opportunity to introduce NNPs into tertiary care neonatal settings.[6]

The NNP has blended nursing and medicine into a unique profession that delivers high-quality, consistent, holistic care to critically ill neonatal infants and to their families. Health care is more consistent, and families are comforted by the presence of familiar faces. The NNP also becomes a true advocate for care as the roles of the neonatology attending physician, fellow, and pediatric resident all tend to be more fragmented, inasmuch as they rotate through the NICU usually on a monthly basis. This tiny patient population has dictated the evolution of a combined nursing-medicine specialty in health care: the NNP in the NICU.

EDUCATION AND CERTIFICATION

Originally, NNPs in the NICU were trained in hands-on techniques by physicians and without formal graduate education in nursing: "Because most of the established nursing education community at that time viewed nurse practitioner preparation as medical education, the early NNP programs were hospital based, continuing education programs, which awarded a certificate to its graduates (hence the name *certificate programs*). Over time, the role was seen as an expanded nursing role, and the preparation of NNPs moved into the mainstream of graduate education."[7] Creating new programs, based on nursing, with an emphasis on graduate education was an important development in the evolution of the NNP role. University-based NNP graduate programs provided advanced practice nursing with education, knowledge, and skills shared by advanced practice nurses in other specialties. "Common educational preparation will assure the credibility of NNPs within the nursing profession, in the eyes of non-nursing health care professionals, and ultimately, in the eyes of the public."[5]

In view of the widely recognized need for consistency in education and the development of clinical competence, NNP programs gradually instituted graduate preparation programs. In 1987, there were 29 NNP programs. Eighteen of these programs were continuing education or certification programs consisting of 9 months of full-time study: 3 months of didactic teaching and 6 months of internship experience. Eleven other programs were graduate university-based programs, usually 24 months in length, depending on part-time versus full-time study requirements.[1,2]

In 1989, the NANN developed a specialized task force to review inconsistencies in NNP education nationally. In 1994, NANN published the *Program Guidelines for Neonatal Nurse Practitioner Education Preparation* (NANN, Educational Task Force).[8] By the year 2000, the National Certification Corporation for the Obstetric, Gynecologic, and Neonatal Nursing Specialties began to enforce minimal education requirements for graduates to be considered eligible for taking the National Certification Examination. These requirements included graduation from a postbaccalaureate educational program that prepares nurse practitioners, and either a graduate degree in the specialty or a post-masters' certificate in the specialty was awarded. The program curriculum had to reflect the content of the NNP examination. Today, there are approximately 35 NNP programs in the United States. The original program guidelines for NNP educational preparation are being revised to reflect current NNP practices. These documents describe outcome competencies for professional nurse practice that each program graduate must meet to function as an advanced practice nurse at the novice level in a NICU. These competencies have been established in accordance with the scope of practice of NNPs in a manner consistent with public health and safety.[9] NANN currently recommends that "...the NNP should complete a formal program of graduate nursing education that includes health policy, research, theory development, and leadership. Graduate education should surround a focus of advanced neonatal concepts and practice. Placing educational programs for the NNP in this environment prepares the nurse for a variety of advanced practice roles and increases the potential for professional growth and improved practice outcomes."[1,5]

With these changes in educational requirements, a pathway to ensure the continuing practice of certificate-prepared NNPs was considered. "Grandfathering" steps were discussed, but a national agreement regarding recertification was not established. There are several variations of the grandfathering process that are independently configured from state to state. Master's degree completion programs offer additional graduate-level study to UU NNPs in flexible curricula that emphasize theory and practice in primary care of the neonate at high risk. The largest program of this kind in the United States exists at the State University of New York at Stony Brook School of Nursing and is offered via computer-mediated didactic instruction and community-based clinical instruction.

Much uncertainty in education, certification, and recertification for the NNPs in the NICU remains, however. Some units include pediatric, perinatal, and family nurses. There exists ethical controversy as to the adequacy of didactic and clinical preparation from these other disciplines in nursing in comparison with that of more formalized NNP education. Again, the NANN task force is reviewing all of these areas to standardize the education and ensure competency of the persons practicing and providing the NNP education.

THE ROLE OF THE NEONATAL NURSE PRACTITIONER

The nurse practitioner's role was limited initially to caring for well newborns in level 1 neonatal nurseries and step-down care units. Today, the NNP practices routinely in tertiary and quaternary units caring for the most acutely ill patients. The NNP brings specialized knowledge and clinical expertise to treating patients in the NICU, in the delivery room, on transport, in follow-up high-risk developmental clinics, and in community hospitals. As the NNPs' expertise has continued to infiltrate the NICU, it has also become important for their participation in other leadership activities. The NNP should be actively involved in developing new approaches to neonatal care. This concept requires the NNPs' participation in research and education.

An advanced practice nurse may be a clinical nurse specialist or a nurse practitioner. The role of the clinical nurse specialist centers on improving patient outcomes through education and leadership. The NNP provides primary care to a caseload of patients in collaboration with a neonatologist.[5] In the NICU, the NNP monitors patients from admission to discharge. The average patient load in the NICU is 6 to 10 patients per practitioner. The NNPs know their patients and families personally and provide continuity of daily care. Management involves (but is not limited to) delivery room resuscitations; physical examinations and assessments; admission and discharge responsibilities; daily nutritional assessments; ordering and prescribing ventilation, medications, parenteral fluid administration, nutrition, and immunizations; and ordering and interpreting radiologic studies, laboratory studies, and other diagnostic tests. Technical procedures include endotracheal intubations, arterial and venous umbilical catheter placements, percutaneous central line placements, arterial and venous punctures and/or cannulations, lumbar punctures, suprapubic bladder aspirations, thoracotomy and chest tube insertions, ventricular taps, synovial taps, pericardiac needle aspirations, circumcisions, and minor suturing. Often, as the most experienced person, the NNP leads resuscitations. An integral aspect of the NNP role is the provision of emotional support and information to families regarding the diagnosis, care, treatment, and outcomes of their infants.

The daily routines and responsibilities of the NNP involve the collaboration of multiple members of the patient care team. Patient and family care is determined and provided through a multidisciplinary approach. The situations of the babies and families are discussed with the attending neonatologists, neonatal fellows, residents, staff nurses, social workers, clinical nurse specialists, respiratory therapists, obstetricians, radiologists, and various consultants. A daily management plan is agreed upon in collaboration with the team. In critical care, there are clinical situations that require immediate decisions and interventions that the NNP performs independently. Discharge planning, parent teaching, and communication with private medical care providers after discharge is a crucial element of meeting these babies' and families' needs.

Attending and participating in conferences and hospital committees further broadens the scope of NNP practice, allowing for ongoing education and updating standards of practice to enhance patient care. These groups and activities include the discharge planning committee, quality assurance committee, transport committee, pharmacy committee, pediatric conferences, perinatal conferences, and regular continuing education.

In these capacities, the role of the NNP extends beyond the NICU. Care is also provided to neonates in affiliated community hospital delivery rooms and nurseries. NNPs act as consultants and have also begun to fill various community roles to support the care of fragile newborns after hospital discharge.[10]

Many NNPs hold joint appointments in schools of nursing and medicine as clinical instructors. The NNP formally plays a role as a preceptor to NNP students. Clinical training and education is provided to pediatric residents, neonatal fellows, and the NICU and community hospital nursing staff through hands on-teaching, as well as formal lectures.

Organizationally, NNP administration in hospitals is conducted under the aegis of the Department of Nursing, the Department of Medicine, or both. This organizational structure often causes a great deal of confusion. Controversies arise with schedules, payroll, evaluation, and reporting mechanisms. The NNPs participate in both departments. This may lead to problems with job satisfaction, longevity, and burnout, and should be carefully addressed to minimize conflict.

COST AND EFFECTIVENESS

Legislative and economic cost-containment reforms are dramatically altering the health care environment and patient care delivery systems. Many organizations have been forced to redesign services to decrease costs of delivering care, while continuing to provide quality services and maintain or improve patient outcomes. Many tertiary care facilities have responded to the declining postgraduate medical funding by supplementing medical house staff with nurse practitioners. This change is most common in pediatrics in the neonatal intensive care arena.[11]

Current information indicates that advanced practice nurses are cost effective and provide quality care. Factors assessed include increased client satisfaction, reduced malpractice coverage requirements, early discharge, and patient outcomes comparable with or better than those of house staff physician colleagues. Early studies showed the clinical nurse specialist to be instrumental in the early discharge of infants with low birth weights, which resulted in decreased cost.[12] A more recent study of care provided in a tertiary setting showed that the NNP-managed group of preterm infants had decreased length of stay and that costs were decreased, in comparison with the house staff–managed patients and costs. Although most advanced practice nurses are employed in outpatient settings, NNPs and clinical nurse specialists have successfully practiced in NICUs since 1980.[5]

Several studies have compared infants cared for by NNPs with those cared for by residents. The results supported the use of NNPs as an alternative to pediatric residents in delivering care to critically ill neonates.[6,13-16] Moreover, other published reviews have indicated that the level of care provided by NNPs is equivalent or superior to those of other models of care.[17] Research demonstrates that care delivered by NNPs is comparable to that of physicians in terms of knowledge base, problem solving, and communication and in the outcomes of morbidity, mortality, process of care, number of hospital days, parental satisfaction, and types of infants cared for.[18]

A detailed retrospective study compared the cost and quality outcomes of two matched groups of infants in a NICU. One group was cared for by NNPs, and the other group, by the traditional house staff team model. The infant groups were matched by place of birth, gestational age, birth weight, sex, race, and Apgar scores at birth. Quality of care was determined by examining specific outcomes that related to care rendered. Outcomes included length of hospital stay, days spent receiving oxygen, days spent receiving mechanical ventilation, morbidity, and mortality. Costs included charges accrued by the infants for pharmaceuticals, laboratory evaluations, radiologic studies performed, respiratory therapy and supplies, and the total hospital and NICU charges. The infants cared for by the NNPs in collaboration with attending neonatologists received care equal to that of the house staff–managed group at lower cost and with greater continuity and consistency. Cost effectiveness of the NNP group was documented as $18,240 less per infant than that of infants managed by the medical house staff. The differences seen were attributed to the NNPs' unique blend of knowledge, communication skills, and continuous presence, in addition to early identification of service coordination needs.[11]

Although clinical nurse specialist/NNPs are paid higher salaries than resident house staff, the differences are not enough to make a substantial effect on overall costs. Although salaries are a significant portion of the overall costs for delivering care to NICU infants, savings in overhead and materials more than compensate to pay for using the NNP model of NICU care delivery.[6]

SUMMARY

The NNP brings together an exceptional culmination of experiences. Blending nursing experiences with advanced medical knowledge enables the NNP to provide extraordinary care focused on this special population of infants and families. Advanced practice nurses as a group must continue to improve cost-effective, quality care delivery to their patients and families. During the current era of health care cutbacks, the role of the nurse practitioner continues to infiltrate the health arena and is increasingly accepted by the community. The NNP model should continue to become more familiar to patients, families, and other clinical specialties outside the NICU academic setting.

REFERENCES

1. National Association of Neonatal Nurses: NANN Standards of Education and Practice for Neonatal Nurse Practitioner Programs. Glenview, Ill, 2002, pp 1-19.
2. Fara A, Bieda A, Shiao S: The history of the neonatal nurse practitioner in the United States. Neonatal Netw 15:11-19, 1996.
3. Clancy G, Maguire D: Advanced practice nursing in the neonatal intensive care unit. Crit Care Nurs Clin North Am 7:71, 1995.
4. Little G, Buss-Frank M: Transition from housestaff in the neonatal intensive care unit: A time to review, revise and reconfirm. Am J Perinatol 13:127, 1996.
5. National Association of Neonatal Nurses: Position statement on graduate education for entry into neonatal nurse practitioner practice. Neonatal Netw 14:52-54, 1995.
6. Mitchell-DiCenso A, Guyatt G, Marrin M: A controlled trial of nurse practitioners in neonatal intensive care. Pediatrics 98:1143, 1996.
7. Strodtbeck F, Trotter C, Lott J: Coping with transition: Neonatal nurse practitioner education for the 21st century. J Pediatr Nurs 13:272, 1998.
8. National Association of Neonatal Nurses, Educational Task Force: Program Guidelines for Neonatal Nurse Practitioner Education Preparation. Glenview, Ill, 1994.
9. Cavaliere T, Sansoucie D: The use of family nurse practitioners and pediatric nurse practitioners as providers of neonatal intensive care: Safe practice or risky business? Newborn Infant Rev 1:142, 2001.
10. Ruth-Sanchez V, Lee K, Basque E: A descriptive study of current neonatal nurse practitioner practice. Neonatal Netw 15:23, 1996.
11. Bissinger R, Allred C, Arford P: A cost effective analysis of neonatal nurse practitioners. Nurs Econ 15:92-99, 1997.
12. National Association of Neonatal Nurses: Position statement for advanced nursing practice. Neonatal Netw 14:59-60, 1995.
13. Carzoli R, Martinez-Cruz M, Cuevas L: Comparison of neonatal nurse practitioners, physician assistants, and residents in the neonatal intensive care unit. Arch Pediatr Adolesc Med 148:1271, 1994.
14. Martin R, Fenton L, Leonardson G, Reid TJ: Consistency of care in an intensive care nursery staffed by nurse clinicians. Am J Dis Child 139:169, 1985.
15. Schulman M, Lucchese K, Sullivan A: Transition from housestaff to nonphysicians as neonatal intensive care providers: Cost, impact on revenue, and quality of care. Am J Perinatol 12:442, 1995.
16. Schultz J, Liptak G, Fioravanti J: Nurse practitioners' effectiveness in NICU. Nurs Manage 25:50, 1994.
17. Buus-Frank M, Conner-Bronson J, Mullaney D: Evaluation of the neonatal nurse practitioner role: The next frontier. Neonatal Netw 15:31-40, 1996.
18. Beal J, Steven K, Quin M: Neonatal nurse practitioner role satisfaction. J Perinat Neonatal Nurs 11:65, 1997.

SUGGESTED READINGS

Beal J: A nurse practitioner model of practice. MCN Am J Matern Child Nursing 25:18, 2000.
Beal J, Tiani T, Sara T: The role of the neonatal nurse practitioner in the post NICU follow-up. J Perinat Neonatal Nurs 13:78, 1999.
Britton J: Neonatal nurse practitioner and physician use on a newborn resuscitation team in a community hospital. J Pediatr Health Care 11:61, 1997.
Brown S, Grimes D: A meta-analysis of nurse practitioners and nurse midwives in primary care. Nurs Res 44:332, 1995.
Casselden D: The role of the neonatal nurse practitioner. Nurs Times 91:42, 1995.
Collins C, Butler F, Guildner S: Models for community-based long term care for the elderly in a changing health system. Nurs Outlook 45:59, 1997.
Crawly J: Oxford health services NPs direct reimbursement care providers. Clinician News 1:1, 1997.

Dillon A, George S: Advanced neonatal nurse practitioners in the United Kingdom: Where are they and what do they do? J Adv Nurs 25:257, 1997.

Fagin C: Cost effectiveness. Nursing's value proves itself. Am J Nurs 90:16, 1990.

Feldman M, Ventura M, Crosby F: Studies of nurse practitioner effectiveness. Nurs Res 36:303, 1987.

Hall M, Smith S, Jackson J, et al: Neonatal nurse practitioners—a view from perfidious Albion? Arch Dis Child 67:458, 1992.

Hunsberger M, Mitchell A, Blatz S, et al: Definition of an advanced nursing practice role in the NICU: The clinical nurse specialist/neonatal practitioner. Clin Nurse Spec 6:91, 1992.

Karlowicz M, McMurray J: Comparison of neonatal nurse practitioners' care and residents' care of extremely low-birth-weight infants. Arch Pediatr Adolesc Med 154:1123, 2000.

Lowes R: The new generation of providers: What do PA, NP, and CNM spell? Med Econ 6:156, 2000.

Maguire D: Multidisciplinary collaboration in neonatal intensive care. Nurs Adm Q 18:18-22, 1994.

McCourt M, Griffin C: Comprehensive primary care follow-up for premature infants. J Pediatr Health Care 14:270, 2000.

Mitchell A, Watts J, Whyte R: Evolution of graduating neonatal nurse practitioners. Pediatrics 88:789, 1991.

Nagle C, Perlmutter D: The evolution of the nurse practitioner role in the neonatal intensive care unit. Am J Perinatol 17:225, 2000.

Ruth-Sanchez V: Facilitators of and constraints to neonatal nurse practitioner practice: Comparing nursing and medical models. J Am Acad Nurse Pract 8:175, 1996.

Smith A: Will cutting back on MD residents help or hurt PAs, NPs, and hospitals? Clin News 1, 1997.

Trotter C, Danaher R: Neonatal nurse practitioners: A descriptive evaluation of an advanced practice role. Neonatal Netw 13:39, 1994.

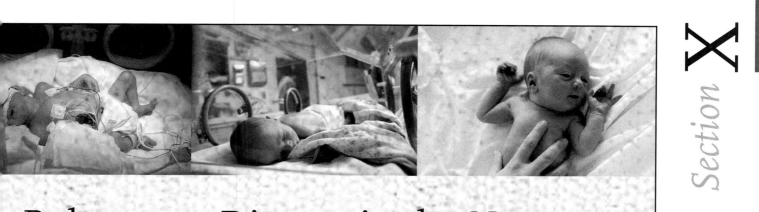

Pulmonary Disease in the Neonate

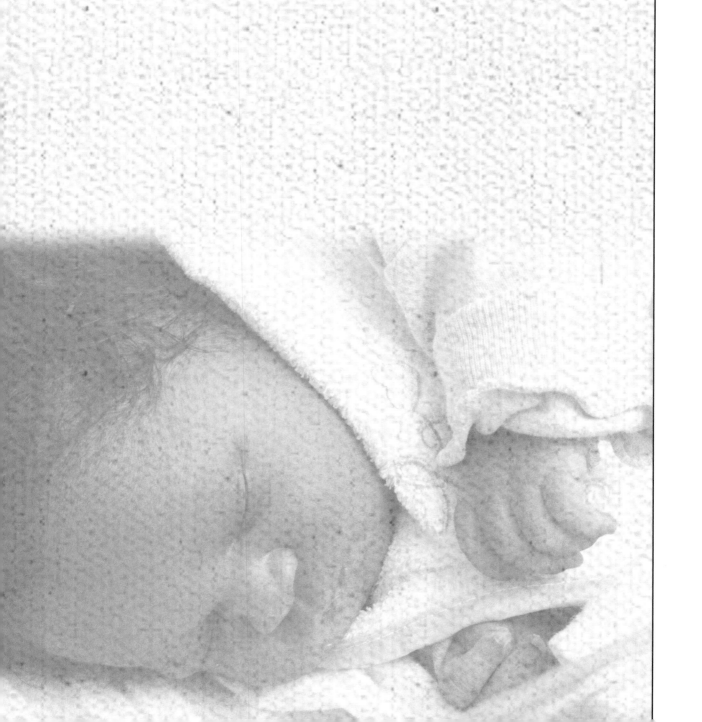

Blood Gas Interpretation

Michael S. Kornhauser

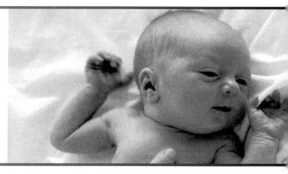

A thorough understanding of blood gases is essential to proper evaluation and management of neonates in the intensive care unit setting. **Blood gases** provide information on oxygenation, carbon dioxide (CO_2) homeostasis, and acid-base balance and are the most important tool used in evaluating the adequacy of pulmonary function. Blood gases also guide oxygen (O_2) and ventilatory therapy in newborns with respiratory failure and are a useful diagnostic tool in patients with disorders involving the cardiac, renal, or central nervous system.[1] Abnormal blood gas values can occur with dysfunction in each of these organ systems, and subsequent improvements in blood gases often signify an improvement of the underlying disorder.

The proper interpretation of blood gases is important in neonatal medicine and is one cornerstone on which good patient care is based. The intricacies of blood gases must be understood by the practitioner. This chapter gives a broad overview concerning the methodology and interpretation of blood gases, with particular reference to physiologic principles and to points of clinical importance in the newborn period.

BLOOD GAS MEASUREMENTS

Definitions and Normal Values

Fundamental to all blood gas reports are the values for pH, Po_2, and Pco_2. These values are measured directly by **blood gas analyzers**. **pH** is a value without units and is equal to the negative log of the hydrogen ion (H^+) concentration in the blood ($pH = -\log [H^+]$). The derivation of pH is discussed later in the section on acid-base disturbances. Po_2 refers to the partial pressure of dissolved O_2, and Pco_2 refers to the partial pressure of dissolved CO_2 in the blood. Pao_2 and $Paco_2$ refer to the partial pressures of the O_2 and CO_2 in arterial blood. The partial pressure of O_2 or CO_2 can be thought of as the force exerted by O_2 or CO_2 molecules that drives them to leave the bloodstream. Partial pressure is measured in millimeters of mercury (mm Hg) or torr units, with 1 torr equaling 1 mm Hg.

Other values included in the blood gas report are calculated values, including bicarbonate (sometimes called *actual bicarbonate,* or [HCO_3^-]), standard bicarbonate, and base excess. These values are reported in milliequivalents per liter (mEq/L). The method of their calculation is discussed in the section on acid-base disturbances.

The **saturation of hemoglobin (Hb) (So_2)** in blood gas reports refers to the percentage of Hb-carrying O_2. **Sao_2** refers to the Hb saturation of arterial blood. Hb saturation may be measured directly in vitro with oximetry, or it can be calculated using the **oxyhemoglobin dissociation curve**, which relates So_2 to Po_2. The accuracy of both of these methods can be influenced by the types of Hb present, including fetal Hb.[2] The accuracy of calculated So_2 is affected by other factors in addition to the amount of fetal Hb present that influence the position of the oxyhemoglobin dissociation curve.

The normal blood gas values for newborns undergo marked changes with age, and these values are different from those of older children and adults. The changes in normal values reflect the cardiopulmonary adjustments that occur as the newborn adapts from intrauterine to extrauterine life. Representative normal values for the first 7 days of life are shown in Table 35-1.[3]

Blood Gas Electrodes

Blood gas analyzers use electrodes to measure changes in voltage and current that occur when reference electrolyte solutions are exposed to O_2, CO_2, and H^+ from sampled blood. These values then are related to the Po_2, Pco_2, and pH of the sample.

The electrode that measures Po_2 is known as the **Clark electrode.**[4] In this system, O_2 from the sampled blood is allowed to diffuse into an electrolyte solution via an O_2-permeable membrane. A platinum cathode and a silver/silver chloride anode are placed into the electrolyte solution, and a constant voltage is applied across them. This process causes O_2 and water to react at the cathode, consuming electrons. Simultaneously, silver and chloride react at the anode and release electrons into solution. The net result

Table 35–1.   Values for pH, P_{CO_2}, P_{O_2}, and Standard Bicarbonate in Cord Blood and in Arterial Blood at Different Ages during the Neonatal Period

		UV	UA	5-10 min	20 min	30 min	60 min	5 hr	24 hr	2 days	3 days	4 days	5 days	6 days	7 days
pH	n	45	27	44	28	62	43	36	72	53	49	38	40	35	42
	Mean	7.32	7.242	7.207	7.263	7.297	7.332	7.339	7.369	7.365	7.364	7.37	7.371	7.369	7.371
	SD	0.055	0.059	0.051	0.04	0.044	0.031	0.028	0.032	0.028	0.027	0.027	0.031	0.023	0.026
	Range	7.178 7.414	7.111 7.375	7.091 7.302	7.18 7.33	7.206 7.38	7.261 7.394	7.256 7.389	7.29 7.448	7.314 7.438	7.304 7.419	7.32 7.44	7.296 7.43	7.321 7.423	7.32 7.431
P_{CO_2} mm Hg	n	44	27	43	28	62	43	36	71	53	49	39	40	35	42
	Mean	37.8	49.1	46.1	40.1	37.7	36.1	35.2	33.4	33.1	33.1	34.3	34.8	34.8	35.9
	SD	5.6	5.8	7	6	5.7	4.2	3.6	3.1	3.3	3.4	3.8	3.5	3.6	3.1
	Range	26 52	35 60	35 65	31 58	28 54	28 45	29 45	27 40	26 43	26 40	27 43	28 41	28 42	30 42
St. bic mEq/L	n	44	27	42	28	61	42	36	71	53	49	38	40	35	42
	Mean	20	18.7	16.7	17.5	18.2	19.2	19.4	20.2	19.8	19.7	20.4	20.6	20.6	21.8
	SD	1.4	1.8	1.6	1.3	1.5	1.2	1.2	1.3	1.4	1.4	1.7	1.7	1.9	1.3
	Range	15.5 22.5	14 21	12.5 20.5	14 20	15 21	16 21.5	16 22	18 23.5	16.5 24.5	16 23.5	17.5 25	17.5 24.5	17 24.5	18.5 26
P_{O_2} mm Hg	n	45	29	42	24	54	31	30	62	47	42	33	32	30	38
	Mean	27.4	15.9	49.6	50.7	54.1	63.3	73.7	72.7	73.8	75.6	73.3	72.1	69.8	73.1
	SD	5.7	3.8	9.9	11.3	11.5	11.3	12	9.5	7.7	11.5	9.3	10.5	9.5	9.7
	Range	15 40	7 23	33 75	31 85	31 85	38 83	55 106	54 95	62 91	56 102	60 93	56 102	55 96	57 94

Results are reported as mean and standard deviation.

St. bic, standard bicarbonate; UA, umbilical artery; UV, umbilical vein.

Adapted from Koch G, Wendel H: Adjustment of arterial blood gases and acid-base balance in the normal newborn infant during the first week of life. Biol Neonate 12:136, 1968. With permission from S Karger, Basel AG, Switzerland.

is a flow of electrons from the anode to replace electrons consumed in the reduction of O_2 at the cathode. The amount of electrical current generated by this process is directly proportional to the amount of O_2 dissolved in the electrolyte solution. Because the Po_2 of the blood sample determines the amount of O_2 dissolved in solution, measurement of the electrical current allows calculation of the Po_2.

H^+ concentration and pH are determined using the **Sanz electrode.**[5,6] In this system, a reference solution with a known pH and the sampled blood with an unknown pH are separated by a pH-sensitive glass electrode. H^+ can diffuse into the glass in proportion to the H^+ concentration within each solution.[7] This process causes a loss of H^+ from each solution and generates a voltage potential between solutions. The voltage changes generated in this process (between measuring and reference electrodes), together with the known pH of the reference solution, can be used to solve for the pH of the sampled blood.

Pco_2 is measured using a modified version of the pH electrode. In this system, a reference solution with known pH and a bicarbonate solution are separated by pH-sensitive glass. CO_2 from the sampled blood diffuses through a CO_2-permeable membrane into the bicarbonate solution. The reaction between CO_2 and bicarbonate generates H^+ in amounts proportional to the amount of dissolved CO_2 in solution. This process causes a change in the pH of the bicarbonate solution and a voltage change between the bicarbonate solution and the reference solution. The change in voltage is proportional to the amount of CO_2 dissolved in solution and is proportional to the Pco_2. The electrode that measures Pco_2 is known as the **Severinghaus electrode.**[8]

The pH electrode provides the most precise measurement, with electrode accuracy equal to ±0.01 unit.[9] The Pco_2 electrode is accurate to $\pm2\%$. The Po_2 electrode is the least precise electrode, with accuracy equal to $\pm3\%$.[9] If the Po_2 is greater than 100 mm Hg, the accuracy of the measurement is $\pm10\%$.

Blood Gas Sampling Sites

Arterial blood gases provide the most accurate assessment of O_2 and CO_2 homeostasis and acid-base balance. Arterial blood gases are the same regardless of the site from which they are drawn except in cases of right-to-left ductal shunting and in certain congenital heart defects. If arterial catheters are in place, the blood gas is easily obtained, and the results reflect steady-state conditions (the effects of crying and patient agitation are avoided). Arterial blood gases are the gold standard against which other methods of blood gas assessment are compared.

The measurement of arterial blood gases requires either peripheral arterial puncture or catheterization of an umbilical or peripheral artery. Although these procedures commonly are performed in neonatal intensive care units, they can be technically difficult and time-consuming. Additionally, arterial blood gas sampling has certain risks, such as infection,[10,11] thrombosis,[12] excessive bleeding,[13] embolism,[14] and nerve damage.[15] Blood gas sampling from other sites is sometimes preferable.

The most useful alternative site for blood gas analysis is from a capillary sample. "Arterialized" capillary blood can be obtained by puncturing an area, usually the heel, which previously has been warmed with compresses or in a warm water bath. Heating the skin increases blood flow through the capillary bed, so values for capillary pH and Pco_2 usually correlate closely with values from arterial specimens.[16] Capillary pH generally shows a closer correlation to arterial values than does capillary Pco_2.[17] Poor tissue perfusion (from shock, hypotension, or peripheral vasoconstriction) or inadequate warming of the heel leads to a significantly lower pH and higher Pco_2 in capillary specimens compared with arterial values.[16,18] Capillary Po_2 does not correlate well with arterial Po_2, especially for arterial Po_2 values greater than about 60 mm Hg.[19,20] Capillary blood specimens cannot exclude hyperoxemia, an important issue particularly for preterm newborns.[21] At arterial Po_2 levels less than 60 mm Hg, properly collected capillary Po_2 yields values that are about 10 mm Hg less than values from arterial samples.[22] Potential complications from capillary blood gas sampling are less severe than complications from arterial sampling but can include cellulitis, abscess formation, and osteomyelitis.[23]

Venous blood is another potential specimen for blood gas sampling. Mixed venous blood (from the pulmonary artery or right heart) can give a gross idea of arterial pH and Pco_2.[24,25] Compared with arterial values, the pH is about 0.04 units lower and Pco_2 is about 8 mm Hg higher in mixed venous samples.[25] Mixed venous Po_2 is not useful in assessing Pao_2, but it can be useful (together with mixed venous O_2 saturation [Svo_2]) in the assessment of tissue oxygenation. If venous blood is sampled peripherally, values for pH and Pco_2 may vary significantly from those of arterial blood, depending on tissue perfusion and metabolic rate distal to the site of venipuncture. Peripheral venous blood gas samples are of limited value.

Factors Affecting Accuracy of Measurements

Several factors may lead to errors in blood gas measurements.[26-28] A common problem is air bubbles that come in contact with the blood sample after blood gas collection. When this occurs, the partial pressures of O_2 and CO_2 within the blood equilibrate with the partial pressures of O_2 and CO_2 within the air bubble(s). Because room air has a Po_2 of about 150 mm Hg and a Pco_2 of essentially zero, air bubbles cause the Po_2 and Pco_2 of the blood sample to move toward these levels. The effect on the Po_2 measurement is the most pronounced, with Po_2 levels increasing or decreasing from the true value toward 150 mm Hg.[29] Pco_2 levels tend to decrease and pH tends to increase, but these changes are not as large as the changes occurring with Po_2. The duration of contact between air bubbles and the blood sample is a more important factor in measurement error than the size of the bubbles.[29] Air bubbles should be removed from the blood gas sample as soon as possible.

Delay in processing the blood gas is another common cause of error. Cellular metabolism continues after the blood sample has been taken, leading to continued O_2

Table 35–2. Effects of Metabolism on Blood Gases at 37° C

Measurement	Direction	Magnitude/hr
pH	Decrease	0.05
$Paco_2$	Increase	5 mm Hg
Pao_2	Decrease	150 mm Hg*
		200 mm Hg†

*Initial Po_2 > 250 mm Hg.

†Initial Po_2 < 150 mm Hg.

From Malley WJ: Clinical Blood Gases: Applications and Noninvasive Alternatives. Philadelphia, WB Saunders, 1990.

consumption and CO_2 production within the sample.[30] The effects of metabolism at body temperature on pH, Po_2, and Pco_2 are shown in Table 35-2.[7] The magnitude of change in Po_2 is related to the initial Po_2 level, with higher Po_2 levels decreasing at a faster rate. If there is a significant delay from the time the sample is drawn until it is analyzed, there can be significant alterations in blood gas values. To lessen this problem, blood gas samples can be placed in an iced water bath; this slows metabolism by a factor of 10 and stabilizes pH, Po_2, and Pco_2 values until the specimen is analyzed.[30]

Other factors can affect blood gas results. Inadvertent mixture of venous or capillary blood during an arterial puncture lowers Po_2 and, to a lesser extent, increases Pco_2 and decreases pH. This effect depends on the volume of blood that contaminates the arterial specimen. Patient agitation also can introduce inaccuracy, with crying and hyperventilation decreasing Pco_2. Excessive heparinization of blood gas syringes used to be a common cause of error, but this problem has largely been eliminated since the advent of preheparinized syringes. The major effect of excessive heparin is the reduction of Pco_2, with minimal effects on Po_2 and pH.[7,31]

ASSESSMENT OF OXYGENATION

Oxygen Transport

O_2 diffuses from the alveoli into the pulmonary capillaries and is transported to the tissues in a dissolved state within the plasma and in combination with Hb. Both forms of O_2 transport depend on the Pao_2.

The amount (or volume) of O_2 transported dissolved in plasma is relatively small and depends on the solubility of O_2 in plasma. At body temperature, the solubility coefficient for O_2 is 0.003 mL O_2/100 mL of blood/mm Hg Po_2.[7] The relationship between dissolved O_2 content and Po_2 is linear, with the amount of O_2 dissolved in plasma progressively increasing as the Po_2 increases.

Most O_2 carried within the blood is transported in combination with Hb. Hb exists either in an oxygenated (saturated) state or in a deoxygenated (desaturated) state. When combined with O_2, Hb carries approximately 1.34 mL O_2/g Hb (some suggest that this figure is actually 1.39 mL O_2/g Hb).[32] The relationship between Hb saturation

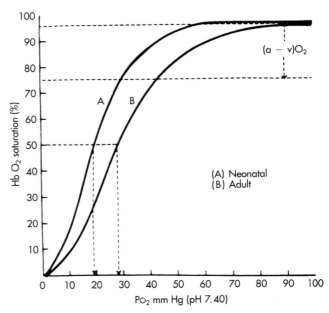

Figure 35–1. Oxyhemoglobin dissociation curves of blood from term infants at birth and from adults. *(From Delivoria-Papadopoulos M, DiGiacomo JE: Oxygen transport and delivery. In Polin RA, Fox WW [eds]: Fetal And Neonatal Physiology. Philadelphia, WB Saunders, 1992, p 807.)*

and Po_2 is shown in Figure 35-1, which compares the oxyhemoglobin dissociation curve for newborns and adults.[33] The vertical axis in Figure 35-1 also can be plotted as the amount of O_2 carried in combination with Hb because this value is directly related to So_2. In contrast to the linear relationship between Po_2 and the amount of O_2 dissolved in plasma, the relationship between Po_2 and the amount of O_2 combined with Hb is sigmoidal. Figure 35-1 also shows the Po_2 at which Hb is 50% saturated. This is known as the P_{50} of Hb, a value that is higher in adults than in newborns. The difference between arterial and venous Hb saturation also is shown in Figure 35-1.

The O_2 content of blood is equal to the amount of O_2 dissolved in plasma plus the amount of O_2 carried by Hb. The arterial blood O_2 content can be calculated as follows for a Pao_2 of 100 mm Hg, assuming 16 g Hb/100 mL blood with Sao_2 = 99%:

O_2 dissolved in plasma = (0.003 mL O_2/100 mL blood/ mm Hg) × (100 mm Hg) = *0.3 mL O_2/100 mL blood*

O_2 carried by Hb = 16 g Hb/100 mL × 1.34 mL O_2/g Hb × 0.99 = *21.2 mL O_2/100 mL blood*

Total arterial O_2 content = *0.3 mL O_2/100 mL + 21.2 mL O_2/100 mL* = 21.5 mL O_2/100 mL blood (or 21.5 vol%)

In this example, Hb carries about 70 times more O_2 than is carried dissolved in plasma. The total O_2 content of blood is primarily dependent on So_2 and Hb concentration, with changes in either of these values causing proportional changes in blood O_2 content. Po_2 also is related to blood O_2 content, but more indirectly, through its sigmoidal relationship with So_2. Changes in Po_2 do not cause proportional changes in blood O_2 content; rather, there are varying effects, depending on the portion of the oxyhemoglobin dissociation curve that is involved.

To illustrate further the importance of the O_2-carrying capacity of Hb, consider a hypothetical situation in which plasma without red blood cells passes through the lungs. If pulmonary function is normal, the PaO_2 and the amount of O_2 carried dissolved in arterial blood are normal. Without Hb to combine with O_2, however, the total O_2 content of the arterial blood is low. Using the preceding calculation, the O_2 content in this hypothetical case would be 0.3 mL/100 mL blood.

Tissue O_2 **delivery** is another important factor in assessing O_2 transport. The amount of O_2 delivered per unit time to the tissues is equal to the cardiac output times the total arterial O_2 content.[7] Tissue O_2 delivery depends on four main factors: pulmonary function, cardiac filling and function, Hb level, and Hb saturation (as determined by the PO_2 and the oxyhemoglobin dissociation curve). O_2 delivery is higher in newborns compared with adults.[34]

Tissues O_2 **consumption** also is important for assessing oxygenation and can be calculated using the Fick equation[7]:

$$O_2 \text{ consumption} = \text{cardiac output} \times$$
$$(\text{arterial } O_2 \text{ content} - \text{mixed venous } O_2 \text{ content})$$

This equation describes the amount of O_2 extracted per unit time at the capillary level and taken up by the tissues. Mixed venous blood O_2 content can be calculated in the same way as arterial O_2 content, when SvO_2 and mixed venous PO_2 have been determined. If cardiac output is known, tissue O_2 consumption can be calculated. O_2 consumption also is elevated in newborns compared with adults.[34]

The actual driving force for diffusion of O_2 into the cell is determined by the PO_2 gradient between the capillary and the cell.[33] Cellular PO_2 is maintained within a narrow range, so capillary PO_2 is the primary factor that determines the rate of O_2 diffusion into the cell.[33] The PO_2 of mixed venous blood (PvO_2) sometimes is used to represent the average end-capillary O_2 tension, which promotes O_2 diffusion.[7] If the PvO_2 decreases, the O_2 pressure gradient between the capillary and cell is decreased, limiting the rate of O_2 diffusion into the cell. This change can lead to tissue hypoxia.[33]

Role of Hemoglobin

There are several important implications to the sigmoidal relationship between PO_2 and SO_2. The shape of the curve allows a large increase in blood O_2 content as venous blood passes through the lungs. This is shown schematically in Figure 35-2.[35] In this example, Hb is 75% saturated at a venous PO_2 of 40 mm Hg, which is a point along the steep part of the Hb dissociation curve. As the PO_2 increases to an arterial level of 70 mm Hg, there is a large increase in SO_2 and a large increase in blood O_2 content. As PaO_2 increases further, there is only a small additional increase in SaO_2 because the PaO_2 is now on the flat upper part of the oxyhemoglobin dissociation curve. *Total* blood O_2 content does not increase dramatically at this point. The amount of *dissolved* O_2 progressively increases, but this increase is a relatively insignificant part of total arterial blood O_2 content (in the physiologic range of PaO_2).

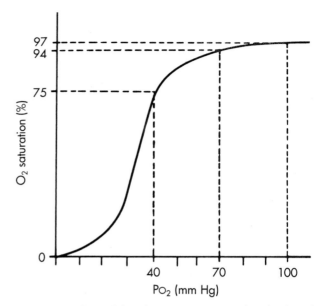

Figure 35–2. Oxyhemoglobin dissociation curve. Selected values for PO_2 and the corresponding percent oxygen saturation are shown. (*Adapted from Burgess WR, Chernick V: Respiratory Therapy in Newborn Infants and Children, 2nd ed. New York, Thieme, 1986, p 44. Copyright Thieme Medical Publishers Inc., 1986.*)

The upper portion of the oxyhemoglobin dissociation curve is not without benefit, however. It offers a protective effect by minimizing changes in arterial blood O_2 content with variations in PaO_2; relatively large decreases from normal PaO_2 levels are necessary before SaO_2 and O_2 content are significantly affected.

At the tissue level, the curve operates in reverse. PO_2 decreases from arterial levels (along the flat upper part of the curve) to venous levels (along the steep middle part of the curve). This allows for large decreases in SO_2 and release of relatively large amounts of O_2 to the tissues. As mentioned, capillary PO_2 determines the rate of O_2 diffusion into the cell.

The shape of the oxyhemoglobin dissociation curve determines how best to assess arterial oxygenation. On the flat upper part of the dissociation curve, where there is little change in SaO_2 for large changes in PaO_2, PaO_2 is a better indicator of arterial O_2 status. On the steep part of the dissociation curve, where there are large changes in SaO_2 for small changes in PaO_2, SaO_2 is a better indicator of arterial oxygenation.[36]

Shifting of the Oxyhemoglobin Dissociation Curve

The position of the oxyhemoglobin dissociation curve is not static; it can shift to the left or to the right in response to various conditions. Factors that cause a shift in the curve are shown in Figure 35-3.[37] These variables include changes in pH, PCO_2, temperature, and levels of 2,3-diphosphoglycerate (2,3-DPG). 2,3-DPG is an organophosphate that is synthesized within red blood cells as a by-product of the glycolytic pathway.[38-40] 2,3-DPG binds to Hb, which affects Hb and O_2 interactions.[41-43]

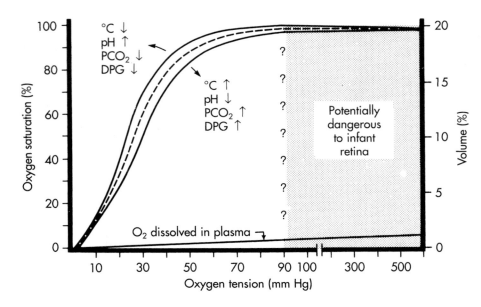

Figure 35–3. Factors that shift the oxyhemoglobin dissociation curve. *(Adapted from Klaus MH, Fanaroff AA: Care of the High Risk Neonate. Philadelphia, WB Saunders, 1986, p 173.)*

A decrease in pH or an increase in P_{CO_2}, temperature, or 2,3-DPG level shifts the oxyhemoglobin dissociation curve to the right. This shift decreases the affinity of Hb for O_2, resulting in a lower S_{O_2} for any given P_{O_2} and a higher value for P_{50}. Hb readily releases O_2 to the tissues with rightward shifting of the curve, but O_2 binding to Hb becomes more difficult, with complete saturation of Hb requiring higher O_2 tensions.[44]

The curve shifts to the left with an increase in pH or a decrease in P_{CO_2}, temperature, or 2,3-DPG level. A leftward shift increases the affinity of Hb for O_2, resulting in a higher S_{O_2} for any given P_{O_2} and a lower value for P_{50}. This shift reduces the ability of Hb to release O_2, but makes it easier for Hb to combine with O_2 at lower O_2 tensions.

The ability of the curve to shift left or right is used to physiologic advantage to facilitate O_2 loading and unloading at the pulmonary and tissue levels. As red blood cells pass through the lung to combine with O_2, CO_2 is released,

and P_{CO_2} decreases. This decrease in P_{CO_2} causes the oxyhemoglobin dissociation curve to shift to the left, which promotes O_2 uptake by Hb. This effect maximizes Sa_{O_2} and arterial blood O_2 content at any given level of Pa_{O_2}. The phenomenon of increased Hb affinity for O_2, when it is not in combination with CO_2, is called the **Bohr effect**.[32]

At the tissue level, cellular metabolism increases local temperature, P_{CO_2}, and H^+ concentration. These factors cause the oxyhemoglobin dissociation curve to shift to the right and promote O_2 release from Hb. This effect is shown in Figure 35-4.[7] In this example, the amounts of O_2 released from Hb are shown for an arterial P_{O_2} of 100 mm Hg and a venous P_{O_2} of 40 mm Hg. Curve C, which is shifted to the right, allows the greatest decrease in O_2 content between arterial and venous blood, maximizing O_2 release from Hb to the tissues. For comparison, curve B is shown, which is shifted to the left; it minimizes the amount of O_2 released by Hb.

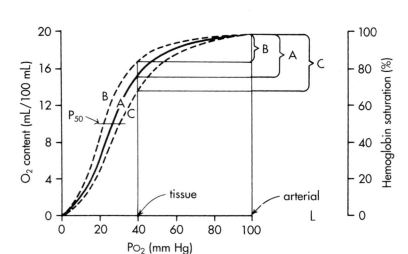

Figure 35–4. Effects of shifts of the oxyhemoglobin dissociation curve on tissue oxygen delivery. A shift to the right *(curve C)* increases oxygen release, and a shift to the left *(curve B)* decreases oxygen release. $P_{50} = P_{O_2}$ at 50% hemoglobin saturation with oxygen. *(Adapted from Malley WJ: Clinical Blood Gases: Applications and Noninvasive Alternatives. Philadelphia, WB Saunders, 1990, p 93.)*

Pathologic shifting of the oxyhemoglobin dissociation curve can occur and may adversely affect the normal binding of O_2 with Hb. The curve may shift excessively to the left in cases of severe alkalosis/hypocarbia (sometimes iatrogenically induced in the treatment of neonatal pulmonary hypertension) or with certain abnormal forms of Hb.[45] As noted, SaO_2 and arterial blood O_2 content are enhanced when the oxyhemoglobin dissociation curve shifts to the left. This effect is evident only at SaO_2 levels less than 100%, however. When Hb is 100% saturated with O_2, additional leftward shifting of the oxyhemoglobin dissociation curve provides no further benefit in increasing arterial blood O_2 content. Additional leftward shifting of the curve increasingly "tightens" the binding of O_2 to Hb, however. This effect means that PvO_2 must decrease to less than normal levels for O_2 to be released from Hb to the tissues. A low value for PvO_2 can impair the rate of diffusion of O_2 into the cells, possibly resulting in tissue hypoxia.

If the curve shifts excessively to the right, Hb releases more O_2 at given PaO_2 and PvO_2 levels, and O_2 unloading to the tissues increases. This effect may be outweighed by an inadequate SaO_2, however, and inadequate arterial blood O_2 content (if PaO_2 is in the physiologic range). When there is excessive rightward shifting of the oxyhemoglobin dissociation curve, tissue hypoxia can result.

Fetal Hemoglobin

Fetal Hb (Hb F) constitutes approximately 75% to 85% of a full-term newborn's Hb.[46] Hb F differs from adult Hb (Hb A) in that Hb F has two γ chains in place of the two β chains of Hb A.[45] Hb F and Hb A also differ with respect to the position of the oxyhemoglobin dissociation curve, which is shifted to the left for Hb F. A newborn has lower levels of 2,3-DPG than those found in later life, which partly accounts for this leftward shift.[32,47] Also, 2,3-DPG affects the O_2 affinity of Hb F only about 40% as much as it affects that of Hb A, a factor that likewise leads to leftward shifting of the curve.[34] Premature newborns exhibit a further shift to the left of the oxyhemoglobin dissociation curve because of even higher levels of Hb F and lower levels of 2,3-DPG than the levels found in full-term newborns.[33]

The position of the oxyhemoglobin dissociation curve for Hb F maximizes arterial O_2 content and tissue O_2 release at the arterial and venous O_2 tensions that exist in utero.[48] After birth, the O_2 affinity of Hb quickly decreases, and the dissociation curve shifts to the right.[49] This process teleologically makes sense because the postpartum neonate is exposed to higher O_2 tensions than in utero; an increased affinity of Hb for O_2 is not advantageous because PaO_2 levels increase postnatally. The progressive rightward shift of the oxyhemoglobin dissociation curve in newborns is illustrated in Figure 35-5.[49] An increase in 2,3-DPG levels and a decrease in the percentage of Hb F jointly account for this phenomenon.[50]

Figure 35-6 shows the relationship between advancing newborn age and O_2 unloading from Hb.[51] The amount of O_2 released to the tissues is shown in the hatched areas, and in this example is equal to the difference between arterial and venous O_2 content as O_2 tensions decline

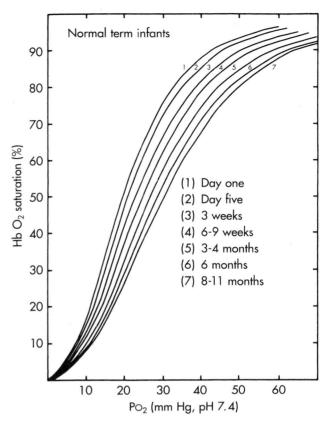

Figure 35–5. Oxyhemoglobin dissociation curve of term infants at different postnatal ages. *(Adapted from Delivoria-Papadopoulos M, Roncevic NP, Oski FA: Postnatal changes in oxygen transport of term, premature, and sick infants: The role of red cell 2,3-diphosphoglycerate and adult hemoglobin. Pediatr Res 5:235, 1971.)*

from a point of 95% SaO_2 to a venous PO_2 of 40 mm Hg. Figure 35-6 shows that tissue O_2 release increases with age. This increase compensates for the reduction in arterial O_2-carrying capacity that occurs in progressively older infants as Hb concentration decreases. Although the affinity of Hb for O_2 decreases, Hb still is able to remain almost fully saturated with O_2, as a result of the higher PaO_2 levels of older infants. SaO_2 is maintained on the flat upper part of the oxyhemoglobin dissociation curve.

Hypoxemia and Hypoxia

Hypoxemia is defined as a PaO_2 value that is below normal. Box 35-1 lists possible causes for a low PaO_2.[22] **Hypoxia** is defined as inadequate O_2 delivery and release to the tissues, at a level below tissue metabolic needs. Although hypoxemia and hypoxia are closely related, these terms cannot be used interchangeably. Hypoxemia, particularly if severe, often causes hypoxia. If the cardiac output or Hb concentration increases, however, or if metabolic rate decreases, tissue oxygenation can be maintained at adequate levels, even with slightly to moderately low PaO_2 values. Hypoxemia can occur without coexistent hypoxia.

Similarly, hypoxia can be present without hypoxemia. In conditions that decrease cardiac output or in cases of moderate to severe anemia, tissue O_2 delivery may be

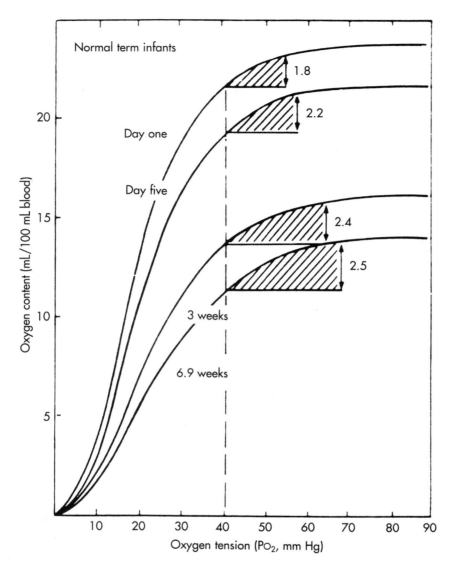

Figure 35–6. Changing relationship between oxygen unloading from hemoglobin and advancing age. Although total oxygen-carrying capacity decreases because of decreasing hemoglobin levels, the amount of oxygen unloaded to the tissues increases. *(From Delivoria-Papadopoulos M, Roncevic NP, Oski FA: Postnatal changes in oxygen transport of term, premature, and sick infants: The role of red cell 2,3-diphosphoglycerate and adult hemoglobin. Pediatr Res 5:235, 1971.)*

inadequate despite a normal PaO$_2$. This situation also can occur when the metabolic rate is elevated (e.g., during fever or excessive activity from seizures) because tissue O$_2$ demands may be higher than the amount of O$_2$ that can be delivered per unit time. Tissue hypoxia at normal PaO$_2$ levels also can occur when the oxyhemoglobin dissociation curve shifts markedly to the left because Hb tends to "hold onto" O$_2$ and not release it to the tissues.[45] Failure of O$_2$ use at the cellular level, as occurs in cyanide poisoning, also can cause hypoxia without concomitant hypoxemia.

Hypoxia is of more clinical importance than hypoxemia. The assessment of hypoxia can be difficult, however. Although hypoxemia is assessed easily by measuring PaO$_2$, there is no direct test for hypoxia. Rather, different laboratory and clinical indices are used in conjunction to evaluate for the presence of hypoxia. Measurement of PaO$_2$ and SaO$_2$ is the obvious first step in assessing the adequacy of tissue oxygenation. Tissue hypoxia is likely with moderately to severely decreased PaO$_2$ and SaO$_2$

levels, particularly if there is simultaneous metabolic acidosis (caused by lactic acid). SaO$_2$ is more closely related to arterial blood O$_2$ content than PaO$_2$, so it is a better indicator of hypoxia. An SaO$_2$ greater than 90% generally is considered acceptable for adults[7,52]; this value may be lower in neonates. The toxicity of O$_2$, particularly to preterm newborns, has been shown in multiple studies, and the optimal SaO$_2$ in these patients is not precisely known.[53,54]

Recommended SaO$_2$ values differ depending on the underlying disease process and degree of maturity.[55] One caveat to interpreting SaO$_2$ is that when the oxyhemoglobin dissociation curve shifts to the left, SaO$_2$ is higher for any given value of PaO$_2$. Although the SaO$_2$ may seem adequate, the increase in Hb's affinity for O$_2$ may prevent adequate O$_2$ release to the tissues.

Lactic acid (normal range 0.26 to 2.2 mmol/L) accumulates during tissue hypoxia as cells switch from aerobic to anaerobic metabolism.[56] Metabolic acidosis from increased blood lactic acid levels often is an indicator of hypoxia. Lactic acid may accumulate in conditions other

Box 35–1 | Causes for a Low P_{O_2} and a High P_{CO_2}

Hypoventilation

Inadequate respiratory effort
  Central nervous system depression
    Asphyxia
    Trauma
    Intracranial hemorrhage
    Maternal drugs
    Central nervous system immaturity
    Apnea of prematurity
    Neuromuscular disease
    Myasthenia gravis
    Phrenic nerve palsy
    Myopathies
  Mechanical ventilator settings
    Rate or pressure or both too low
Upper airway not patent
  Choanal atresia
  Laryngeal web
  Mucus, blood, or meconium blocking upper airway
  Mucus, blood, or meconium blocking
    endotracheal tube
  Displaced or kinked endotracheal tube
  External compression of airway
Decreased lung tissue
  Pulmonary hypoplasia
    Thoracic dystrophy
    Diaphragmatic hernia
    Potter syndrome
Decreased lung compliance
  Atelectasis
    Respiratory distress syndrome
  Pneumothorax

Abnormal pulmonary interstitium
  Interstitial edema
  Interstitial emphysema
  Interstitial fibrosis
  End-tidal pressure too high

Abnormal Ventilation-Perfusion Ratio

Obstruction of small airways
  Meconium aspiration
  Atelectasis
    Respiratory distress syndrome
    Pneumothorax
  Alveolar exudate
    Pneumonia
  Alveolar fluid
    Transient tachypnea
    Congenital heart disease
    Fluid overload

Increased Extrapulmonary Right-to-Left Shunt

Pulmonary vasoconstriction
  Respiratory distress syndrome
  Low pH
  Severe infection
  Idiopathic persistent pulmonary hypertension
Pulmonary hypoplasia with decreased pulmonary
    vasculature
  Thoracic dystrophy
  Diaphragmatic hernia
  Potter syndrome
  Cyanotic heart disease

From Phillips BL, McQuitty J, Durand DJ: Blood gases: Technical aspects and interpretation. In Goldsmith JP, Karotkin EH, Barker S (eds): Assisted Ventilation of the Neonate, 2nd ed. Philadelphia, WB Saunders, 1988, p 227.

than hypoxia, however. In adults, liver disease and certain drugs and toxins can elevate blood lactic acid levels.[7,57,58] Also, elevations in blood pyruvate cause lactic acid levels to increase. Lactic acidosis is not a specific marker for hypoxia.[59] Additionally, some studies have shown a poor correlation between decreased tissue O_2 delivery and increased lactic acid levels, suggesting that lactic acidosis is not a sensitive marker for hypoxia.[60] This lack of sensitivity may be due in part to the nonlinear rise in lactic acid levels that occur during progressive hypoxia.[61] Also, because lactic acid is normally metabolized by the liver, elevated levels can be temporary.[59] In certain instances, until blood flow is restored to areas of low perfusion, lactic acid levels may not be elevated in the central bloodstream.[56] The absence of lactic acidosis does not imply the absence of hypoxia.

The measurement of mixed venous P_{O_2} and S_{VO_2} is another method used to assess for hypoxia. In adults, normal P_{VO_2} is about 40 mm Hg (range 35 to 45 mm Hg),[7,62] and normal S_{VO_2} is about 75% (range 68% to 77%).[63] The value of these mixed venous O_2 indices is that they reflect the equilibrium between O_2 delivery to the tissues and tissue O_2 consumption. If O_2 consumption remains constant, conditions that decrease O_2 delivery to the tissues (either decreased arterial O_2 content or decreased cardiac output) cause the P_{VO_2} and S_{VO_2} to decrease; these decreases are evident from an examination of the Fick equation. Low P_{VO_2} and S_{VO_2} values are believed to indicate tissue hypoxia. Although some authors believe that P_{VO_2} and S_{VO_2} are the best overall indicators of tissue hypoxia,[64] others have shown a poor correlation between these indices and other indicators of tissue hypoxia.[65] There is also some debate as to which of these two indices is superior in assessing tissue oxygenation.[62,66] If the oxyhemoglobin dissociation curve shifts markedly to the left, S_{VO_2} may be a less useful value because venous blood is more saturated at any given P_{VO_2}.[62] In conditions causing cellular metabolic dysfunction with inability to use O_2 (e.g., cyanide poisoning), venous O_2 indices are high despite tissue hypoxia. More recently, some authors have advocated the technique of partial venous occlusion to measure fractional O_2 extraction and S_{VO_2}.[56] This technique holds promise as a noninvasive method to assess for hypoxia and has been shown to be useful in differentiating between symptomatic and asymptomatic anemia.[67]

Other biochemical markers have been used on a research basis to assess for tissue hypoxia, although these are not part of the standard blood gas report. One of the most studied of these markers is hypoxanthine. Hypoxanthine is a breakdown product of adenosine triphosphate. Under aerobic conditions, hypoxanthine is metabolized to inosine monophosphate and uric acid. Under conditions of tissue hypoxia, the metabolic pathways of hypoxanthine are blocked, and hypoxanthine levels increase.[68] Animal studies have shown linear increases in plasma hypoxanthine levels during prolonged hypoxemia.[68] Increases in hypoxanthine levels in these studies have correlated well with increased blood lactic acid levels. Studies on human newborns have shown increased hypoxanthine levels in neonates with birth asphyxia.[69] Hypoxanthine seems to be a better marker for the potential complications of birth asphyxia than lactic acid in these studies.[69] More recent studies have shown that hypoxanthine is elevated in preterm newborns who develop periventricular leukomalacia, which occurs secondary to hypoxia-ischemia, and in infants who die of sudden infant death syndrome.[70,71] Some investigators have suggested that hypoxanthine should be the gold standard in assessing for tissue hypoxia.[72] At this point, however, hypoxanthine assays remain primarily a research tool and are not routinely available. Other biochemical markers that also hold promise in the evaluation of hypoxia include plasma vasopressin and erythropoietin levels. Vasopressin levels are elevated in the cerebrospinal fluid of newborns with birth asphyxia, and the severity of asphyxia correlates with the degree of elevation of vasopressin.[73] Erythropoietin levels are elevated in states of chronic in utero hypoxia.[74]

There is presently no one practical laboratory test that is sensitive and specific in assessing hypoxia in all situations. The physical examination is a valuable adjunct, in that hypoxia may affect vital signs, perfusion, and other physiologic functions. The adequacy of tissue oxygenation probably is best diagnosed by using simultaneous clinical and laboratory observations.

ASSESSMENT OF CARBON DIOXIDE HOMEOSTASIS

CO_2 is the principal waste product in aerobic metabolism and is removed from the bloodstream via the lungs.[75] The amount of CO_2 entering the blood depends on the metabolic rate and on the respiratory quotient of the substrate being metabolized. The **respiratory quotient** refers to the ratio of CO_2 production to O_2 consumption. The respiratory quotient is 1 for carbohydrates, 0.8 for protein, and 0.7 for fat.[76]

CO_2 readily diffuses from the bloodstream into the alveoli so that CO_2 tensions within the blood and alveolar air can be assumed to be equal.[77] As such, $Paco_2$ directly reflects the adequacy of alveolar ventilation with respect to CO_2 production and with respect to metabolic rate.[77]

Carbon Dioxide Transport

CO_2 transport is more complicated than O_2 transport. CO_2 is transported in the plasma in three ways: as dissolved CO_2, as bicarbonate ions ($[HCO_3^-]$), and in combination with plasma proteins.[78] Additionally, CO_2 is carried in the red blood cell, primarily in combination with Hb.[78] Figure 35-7 schematically shows mechanisms for CO_2 transport.[35]

About 5% to 10% of CO_2 is carried dissolved in plasma.[79] The dissolved CO_2 exerts a pressure that is measured as Pco_2. A small portion of dissolved CO_2 (approximately 0.1%) combines with water to form carbonic acid (H_2CO_3). This process, known as the **hydrolysis reaction**, moves forward slowly in plasma because of the absence of enzymatic catalysis.[77] CO_2 also combines with proteins in the plasma to form carbamino compounds; this accounts for approximately 2% of CO_2 transport.[35]

About 90% to 95% of CO_2 enters the red blood cell.[77] Most intracellular CO_2 combines with water to form

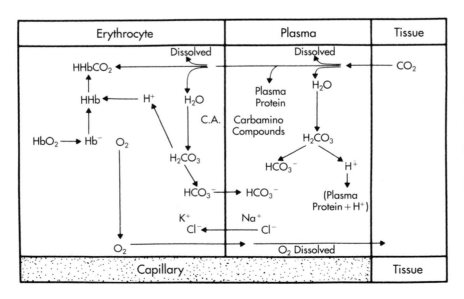

Figure 35–7. Mechanisms for carbon dioxide transport in tissue. C.A., carbonic anhydrase. *(Adapted from Burgess WR, Chernick V: Respiratory Therapy in Newborn Infants and Children, 2nd ed. New York, Thieme, 1986, p 48. Copyright Thieme Medical Publishers, Inc., 1986.)*

H_2CO_3 in the hydrolysis reaction. H_2CO_3 then dissociates almost completely to form H^+ and HCO_3^-. Red blood cells contain high quantities of carbonic anhydrase; this enzyme promotes the hydrolysis reaction to move forward within the red blood cell. The carbonic anhydrase activity of term newborns is lower than that of adults and is lower still in preterm newborns; this factor does not seem to limit CO_2 transport in the neonatal period, however.[80,81]

HCO_3^- generated in the hydrolysis reaction diffuse into the plasma, moving down concentration gradients. Meanwhile, H^+ combines with Hb, which acts as a buffer. To maintain electrical neutrality, chloride ions (Cl^-) move into the red blood cell as HCO_3^- moves out, a phenomenon known as the **chloride shift**.[35] The conversion of CO_2 to HCO_3^- within the red blood cell accounts for 80% to 85% of total CO_2 transport within the blood.

CO_2 also is carried in combination with Hb in the red blood cell, accounting for approximately 10% of total CO_2 transport.[7] The affinity of Hb for CO_2 is greater when Hb is desaturated. This phenomenon is known as the **Haldane effect** and is an important factor at the tissue level, promoting CO_2 uptake by Hb as O_2 is released.[82]

At the level of the lung, the process just described is reversed. This reversal is shown in Figure 35-8.[35] HCO_3^- diffuses down concentration gradients into the red blood cell and together with H^+ released from Hb reform CO_2. CO_2 leaves the red blood cell and together with the CO_2 in the plasma is excreted via the lung. The affinity of Hb for O_2 increases as CO_2 is released from Hb.

The CO_2 content of blood is higher than the O_2 content at similar CO_2 or O_2 tensions. This difference is shown in Figure 35-9.[83] The solubility of CO_2 in blood is higher than that of O_2 (0.07 mL CO_2/100 mL/mm Hg P_{CO_2} versus 0.003 mL O_2/100 mL/mm Hg P_{O_2}), which partially accounts for the higher CO_2 content.[7] The relationship between P_{CO_2} and CO_2 content is essentially linear, which is in contrast to the sigmoidal relationship between P_{O_2} and O_2 content.

ASSESSMENT OF ACID-BASE BALANCE

An **acid** is a substance that releases H^+ into solution. A **base** is a substance that removes H^+ from solution. The acidity or alkalinity of a solution, or the equilibrium between acids and bases, is assessed by the measurement of pH. As mentioned, *pH* refers to the negative log of the H^+ concentration (pH = $-\log$ [H^+]). Because H^+ is present at low concentrations in the blood, pH is the preferable term to use when assessing H^+ content.

H^+ concentration must be kept in a narrow range to maintain normal cellular function. The lungs, kidneys, and blood buffers are involved jointly in maintaining normal [H^+] and pH. The lungs and kidneys control pH by adjusting the amount of acids and bases in the blood. The lungs adjust H_2CO_3 levels through the excretion of CO_2, and the kidneys adjust bicarbonate levels and excrete fixed acids (sulfuric, phosphoric, hydrochloric, and organic acids) produced during metabolism. The role of the kidneys is discussed later in the section on acid-base disturbances. Blood buffers act by preventing large swings in pH during acute changes in acid-base balance.

Carbonic Acid Chemistry

H_2CO_3 is the major acid excreted by the body.[84] An understanding of H_2CO_3 chemistry is important to the understanding of acid-base balance. As mentioned, CO_2 produced from tissue metabolism can combine with water in the plasma as follows:

$$CO_2 \text{ (dissolved)} + H_2O \leftrightarrow H_2CO_3 \leftrightarrow H^+ + HCO_3^-$$

This reaction is shifted far to the left because most CO_2 remains in the dissolved state within the plasma. Nevertheless, small amounts of H_2CO_3 are formed, and H_2CO_3 dissociates to form H^+ and HCO_3^-. There is a direct relationship between the concentrations of dissolved CO_2 and H_2CO_3 in the plasma; changes in [dissolved CO_2] are followed by changes in the same direction in [H_2CO_3].

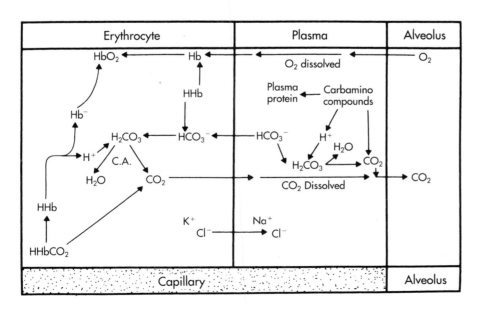

Figure 35–8. Mechanisms for carbon dioxide transport in the lung. C.A., carbonic anhydrase. (*Adapted from Burgess WR, Chernick V: Respiratory Therapy in Newborn Infants and Children, 2nd ed. New York, Thieme, 1986, p 49. Copyright Thieme Medical Publishers, 1986.*)

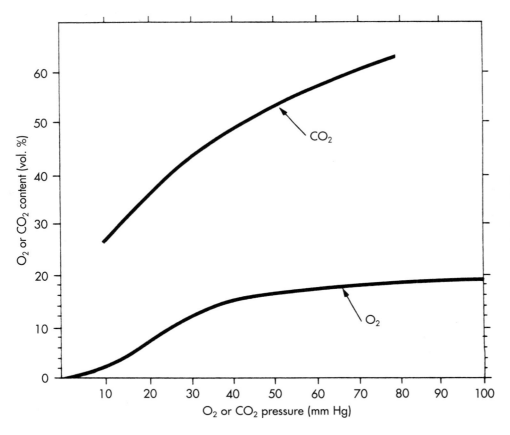

Figure 35–9. Carbon dioxide and oxygen dissociation curves of blood. *(From Comroe JH: The Transport of Oxygen by Blood in the Physiology of Respiration. Chicago, Year Book Medical Publishers, 1965, p 165.)*

The Henderson-Hasselbalch equation can be derived from the dissociation reaction of H_2CO_3 and can be used to quantitate acid-base balance. Its derivation is as follows:

$$K = [H^+][HCO_3^-]/[H_2CO_3]$$

where K = dissociation constant for H_2CO_3. Converting to the log form:

$$\log K = \log ([H^+][HCO_3^-]/[H_2CO_3])$$

or

$$\log K = \log [H^+] + \log ([HCO_3^-]/[H_2CO_3])$$

Converting to pH:

$$-\log [H^+] = -\log K + \log ([HCO_3^-]/[H_2CO_3])$$

or

$$pH = pK_a + \log ([HCO_3^-]/[H_2CO_3])$$

Because H_2CO_3 concentration is directly proportional to the amount of dissolved CO_2 in the plasma, the expression can be modified as follows:

$$pH = pK_a + \log ([HCO_3^-]/[\text{dissolved } CO_2])$$

The amount of dissolved CO_2 depends on the P_{CO_2} and the solubility of CO_2 in the plasma. The solubility of CO_2 may be reported in units of mEq/L (as opposed to mL CO_2/100 mL blood) and is equal to 0.03 mEq/L/mm Hg P_{CO_2}.[46] Also, pK_a is equal to 6.1. The equation may be modified as follows:

$$pH = 6.1 + \log ([HCO_3^-]/[0.03 \times P_{CO_2}])$$

This equation represents the final form of the Henderson-Hasselbalch equation, describing the relationship of pH to plasma bicarbonate concentration and to P_{CO_2}. Because pK_a is a constant, it is the ratio of $[HCO_3^-]$ to P_{CO_2} that determines pH. The kidneys regulate $[HCO_3^-]$, and the lungs control P_{CO_2}, so the Henderson-Hasselbalch equation also may be expressed as pH = kidneys/lungs.[7]

Blood Buffers

Blood buffers refer to systems that attempt to minimize changes in pH despite acute changes in acid or base concentrations. Buffers act by converting strong acids to weak acids (which produce fewer H^+) and by converting strong bases to weak bases (which combine with fewer H^+). In this way, changes in $[H^+]$ are minimized. Buffering reactions occur quickly after sudden changes in acid-base balance.

The most important buffering system is the bicarbonate buffer system. An example of how this system works in buffering an acid is as follows:

Hydrochloric acid (a strong acid) + $NaHCO_3$ (sodium bicarbonate) → H_2CO_3 (a weak acid) + NaCl

Because H_2CO_3 is a weak acid, it dissociates to a lesser extent than hydrochloric acid, producing fewer H^+ ions and minimizing changes in pH. The bicarbonate buffer system is referred to as an **open buffer system**, meaning that the body can remove products of buffering reactions.[46] In the previous example, as H_2CO_3 levels increase during buffering, H_2CO_3 continuously forms CO_2

through the hydrolysis reaction; CO_2 is excreted via the lungs. This process prevents the buildup of buffering products and allows bicarbonate buffering reactions to proceed.

Other buffer systems in the body are closed systems, meaning that as the products of buffering accumulate, they cannot be excreted. This process tends to limit continued buffering reactions in these systems. Plasma proteins, organic and inorganic phosphates, and Hb all provide buffering reactions as closed systems.[7]

Acid-Base Disturbances

The four basic disturbances in acid-base balance are respiratory acidosis, respiratory alkalosis, metabolic acidosis, and metabolic alkalosis. Each of these disturbances is subject to compensatory mechanisms to bring pH back into the normal range. pH is usually not completely "normalized," however. In adults, maximal compensatory mechanisms in severe acid-base disorders usually bring pH back to about 50% of normal.[7]

Table 35-3 shows a method of basic acid-base blood gas classifications.[79] Disorders are grouped as either primarily respiratory in nature (an increase or decrease in P_{CO_2}), or primarily metabolic in nature (an increase or decrease in $[HCO_3^-]$ and base excess). Respiratory and metabolic acid-base disorders are classified further as uncompensated, partly compensated, or completely compensated. Primary respiratory acid-base disorders are compensated by metabolic adjustments, and vice versa. This compensatory effect is evident from the Henderson-Hasselbalch equation, which shows that a relatively constant ratio of $[HCO_3^-]$ to P_{CO_2} is necessary to maintain pH in the normal range. By examining the pH, P_{CO_2} and $[HCO_3^-]$ (or base excess), a specific acid-base disturbance can be properly assigned to one of the classifications in Table 35-3. One problem that may arise is the determination of which abnormality is the primary acid-base problem and which is the compensatory mechanism. If a particular patient has a normal pH, but the P_{CO_2} and $[HCO_3^-]$ are elevated, the blood gas disturbance may represent either a compensated respiratory acidosis or a compensated metabolic alkalosis. Usually the clinical course of the patient and prior experience clarify compensatory mechanisms from the primary acid-base disorder.

As noted, the indices indicating metabolic acid-base balance are calculated values. These indices most commonly include actual bicarbonate ($[HCO_3^-]$), standard bicarbonate, and base excess. $[HCO_3^-]$ is determined using the Henderson-Hasselbalch equation, when pH and P_{CO_2} have been measured. $[HCO_3^-]$ also can be derived from the total CO_2, which is a value routinely reported with serum electrolyte measurements. Total CO_2 is a measure of the total amount of CO_2 transported within the plasma. As mentioned, most CO_2 (80% to 85%) is transported as bicarbonate. The total CO_2 in serum electrolyte reports approximates the value for $[HCO_3^-]$ obtained in blood gas measurements and can be used to verify the accuracy of the blood gas report.

$[HCO_3^-]$ is not an absolute indicator of metabolic acid-base status because alterations in *respiratory* acid-base balance (i.e., changes in P_{CO_2}) also have a small effect on $[HCO_3^-]$.[35] This effect is evident from examining the hydrolysis reaction, which shows that as P_{CO_2} and [dissolved CO_2] vary, so does $[HCO_3^-]$. The ratio between changes in P_{CO_2} to changes in $[HCO_3^-]$ is about 10:1 when P_{CO_2} increases greater than 40 mm Hg and is about 5:1 when P_{CO_2} decreases less than this value.[85] There needs to be significant hypercarbia or hypocarbia for $[HCO_3^-]$ to be affected substantially by changes in P_{CO_2}.

The measurement of standard bicarbonate is designed to obviate the effect of P_{CO_2} on $[HCO_3^-]$ and is included in the typical blood gas report. In this in vitro test, blood is equilibrated to a P_{CO_2} of 40 mm Hg at 37° C, and the $[HCO_3^-]$ is determined. This method theoretically provides a more accurate index of metabolic acid-base balance than does $[HCO_3^-]$. Standard bicarbonate reflects in vitro conditions, however, and the results can differ from the "true" value for standard bicarbonate if the measurement could be performed in vivo.[35] Under most circumstances, standard bicarbonate and $[HCO_3^-]$ values are similar, unless there is significant hypercarbia or hypocarbia.

Base excess is another metabolic acid-base index.[86] Base excess is equal to the observed blood buffer base minus the normal blood buffer base. It is a reflection of the effect of all blood buffers, not just bicarbonate. Under conditions of metabolic acidosis, buffering capacity is consumed, and the base excess is negative; this condition also is referred to as a **base deficit**. Base excess is calculated from a Siggaard-Anderson nomogram, which relates P_{CO_2}, pH, Hb concentration, and base excess. This nomogram was developed from data obtained in vitro.[35] As such, and similar to standard bicarbonate, the determination of base excess may not exactly reflect the "true" base excess in vivo.

Primary Respiratory Disorders and Compensatory Mechanisms

Respiratory acidosis is the most important disorder in this group because of its frequency and potentially life-threatening nature. Uncompensated, or acute, respiratory

Table 35-3. Blood Gas Classifications

Classification	pH	Pa_{CO_2}	$[HCO_3^-]$	BE
Respiratory disorder				
Uncompensated acidosis	↓	↑	N	N
Partly compensated acidosis	↓	↑	↑	↑
Compensated acidosis	N	↑	↑	↑
Uncompensated alkalosis	↑	↓	N	N
Partly compensated alkalosis	↑	↓	↓	↓
Compensated alkalosis	N	↓	↓	↓
Metabolic disorder				
Uncompensated acidosis	↓	N	↓	↓
Partly compensated acidosis	↓	↓	↓	↓
Compensated acidosis	N	↓	↓	↓
Uncompensated alkalosis	↑	N	↑	↑
Partly compensated alkalosis	↑	↑	↑	↑
Compensated alkalosis	N	↑	↑	↑

Arrows, elevated or depressed values; BE, base excess; HCO_3^-, bicarbonate; N, normal.

From Chatburn RL, Carlo WA: Assessment of neonatal gas exchange. In Carlo WA, Chatburn RL (eds): Neonatal Respiratory Care, 2nd ed. Chicago, Year Book Medical Publishers, 1988.

acidosis is due to alveolar hypoventilation and is heralded by an increase in P_{CO_2} with a decrease in pH. For every increase in P_{CO_2} of 10 mm Hg, the pH decreases by about 0.07 unit.[87] Causes of hypoventilation are listed in Box 35-1. [HCO_3^-] and base excess are normal in acute respiratory acidosis because there is no time for renal compensation.

In adults, renal compensatory mechanisms usually begin about 12 to 24 hours after the onset of respiratory acidosis, with complete compensation taking 3 to 5 days to occur.[88] The timing of renal compensation has not been as well studied in neonates. The kidneys compensate by excreting more H^+ and by increasing bicarbonate reabsorption. Most of these processes take place in the proximal tubule. The mechanisms involved are complex but can be summarized as follows (Fig. 35-10).[76] Plasma CO_2 diffuses into the renal tubular cells, and under the influence of carbonic anhydrase, breaks down to form HCO_3^- and H^+. H^+ is then secreted into the glomerular filtrate in exchange for sodium. Sodium is actively transported back into the blood, accompanied by HCO_3^-. In the glomerular filtrate, secreted H^+ and filtered bicarbonate form H_2CO_3 under the influence of brush border carbonic anhydrase. H_2CO_3 subsequently dissociates to CO_2 and water. CO_2 is reabsorbed into the tubular cell to enter the hydrolysis reaction, and water is excreted. Phosphate and ammonia in the glomerular filtrate also can combine with secreted H^+, allowing further excretion of hydrogen and reabsorption of bicarbonate. Some free H^+ also is found in the urine. As blood P_{CO_2} increases, the reactions in the tubular cells are driven forward, with further bicarbonate reabsorption and hydrogen secretion.

The ability of the neonatal kidney to compensate for respiratory acidosis depends on gestational and chronologic age. Full-term and preterm newborns have a decreased renal threshold for bicarbonate compared with older children. The renal bicarbonate threshold is defined as the plasma [HCO_3^-] at which bicarbonate is no longer completely reabsorbed in the renal tubule; this threshold value is lower in preterm than in full-term newborns.[88] Studies indicate that urine acidification also is reduced in newborns, particularly in preterm newborns.[88] Urine acidification and bicarbonate reabsorptive mechanisms seem to increase over the first few weeks of postnatal life.

Uncompensated (or acute) **respiratory alkalosis** is the other primary respiratory disorder in this category and is due to alveolar hyperventilation. Arterial hypoxemia can cause hyperventilation through stimulation of the peripheral chemoreceptors.[36,89] Painful stimuli and conditions causing abnormal stimulation of the central nervous system (infection, fever) are other causes of hyperventilation.[36] Renal compensation in acute respiratory alkalosis occurs within 1 to 2 days in adults and is the opposite of that found in respiratory acidosis: bicarbonate is excreted, and hydrogen ions are conserved.

Primary Metabolic Disorders and Compensatory Mechanisms

Metabolic acidosis is due to an increase in the body's fixed acid concentration or a decrease in normal blood base.[90] In uncompensated metabolic acidosis, there is a decrease in pH, with a decrease in [HCO_3^-] and an increase in base deficit (more negative base excess). The most common cause for metabolic acidosis in a neonatal intensive care unit probably is lactic acidosis from tissue hypoxia.[87] Other causes for metabolic acidosis in neonates include sepsis, inborn errors of metabolism, renal failure, total parenteral nutrition, and bicarbonate loss, either from diarrhea or from immature renal bicarbonate reabsorptive mechanisms. The anion gap ([Na^+] − [Cl^-] − [HCO_3^-]) is normal (12 to 14 mEq/L) when metabolic acidosis is secondary to loss of bicarbonate and is increased when metabolic acidosis is secondary to an increase in fixed acid concentration (most commonly lactic acid).

In an otherwise normal patient, metabolic acidosis without respiratory compensation is unusual. A decrease in pH almost immediately stimulates hyperventilation, with ensuing hypocarbia and a shift in pH toward normal.[35] Adequate respiratory compensation for metabolic

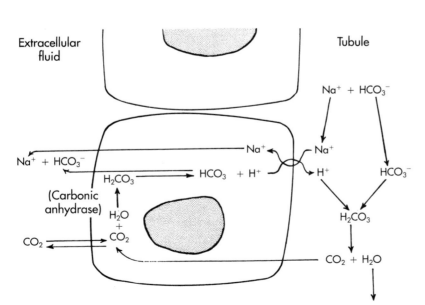

Figure 35–10. Mechanisms of renal compensation for primary respiratory acid-base disorders. *(Adapted from Guyton AC: Textbook of Medical Physiology, 4th ed. Philadelphia, WB Saunders, 1971.)*

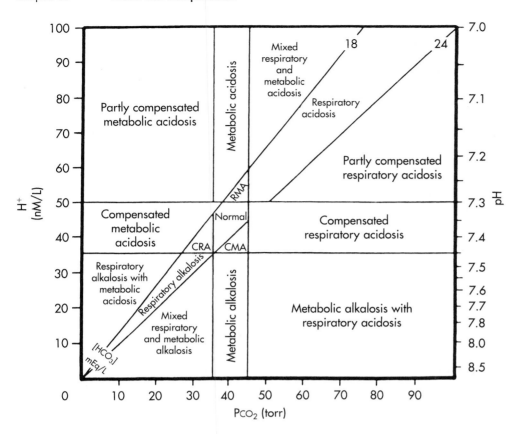

Figure 35–11. A neonatal acid-base map. CMA, compensated metabolic alkalosis; CRA, compensated respiratory alkalosis; RMA, mixed respiratory and metabolic acidosis. *(From Chatburn RL, Carlo WA: Assessment of neonatal gas exchange. In Carlo WA, Chatburn RL [eds]: Neonatal Respiratory Care, 2nd ed. Chicago, Year Book Medical Publishers, 1988, p 58.)*

acidosis may not occur, however, in the presence of pulmonary or central nervous system disease.[79]

Metabolic alkalosis is caused by either a loss of fixed acid or a gain of blood base. Gastric fluid loss, as with vomiting or continuous gastric suction, leads to a loss of hydrochloric acid and metabolic alkalosis. Hypokalemia, hypochloremia, diuretic therapy, excessive bicarbonate administration, and adrenal hypersecretion are other causes of metabolic alkalosis.[87] Compensation in metabolic alkalosis is achieved through hypoventilation and hypercarbia. In adults, this compensatory mechanism is more incomplete because hypercarbia (and possibly concurrent hypoxia) ultimately stimulate ventilatory efforts.[7]

Acid-Base Map

The classification of acid-base disorders shown in Table 35-3 identifies basic disorders and their compensatory mechanisms, but it may not be helpful in properly identifying mixed acid-base disturbances. Mixed disturbances are common and can occur in a variety of scenarios. Severe respiratory distress syndrome can cause a mixed respiratory and metabolic acidosis, owing to coexisting hypercarbia and lactic acidosis from hypoxia. Fulminating neonatal sepsis also is a common cause for a mixed respiratory and metabolic acidosis. In pulmonary hypertension,

hyperventilation and bicarbonate administration sometimes are used together therapeutically; this leads to a mixed respiratory and metabolic alkalosis.

Some mixed acid-base disturbances initially may appear as compensated simple acid-base problems. An example of this complexity can occur during the treatment of chronic lung disease with diuretics. The P_{CO_2} and $[HCO_3^-]$ generally are elevated in this situation, appearing as a metabolic alkalosis compensating for a respiratory acidosis. If the pH is **overcompensated** (pH > 7.45), however, the metabolic alkalosis would not just be a compensatory mechanism, but would represent an additional primary metabolic disorder induced by the use of diuretics.

To help in the assessment of simple and mixed acid-base disorders, a neonatal *acid-base map* based on the Henderson-Hasselbach equation has been developed and is shown in Figure 35-11.[79] Normal values in this system are pH = 7.30 to 7.45, P_{CO_2} = 35 to 45 mm Hg, and $[HCO_3^-]$ = 18 to 24 mEq/L. By plotting the pH, P_{CO_2}, and $[HCO_3^-]$ on the map, simple and mixed acid-base disturbances can be classified properly.

REFERENCES

1. Burton GG, Hodgkin JE: Respiratory Care: A Guide to Clinical Practice, 2nd ed. Philadelphia, JB Lippincott, 1984.

2. Kafer ER: Blood gases. In Long WA (ed): Fetal and Neonatal Cardiology. Philadelphia, WB Saunders, 1990, pp 277-300.

3. Koch G, Wendel H: Adjustment of arterial blood gases and acid-base balance in the normal newborn infant during the first week of life. Biol Neonate 12:136, 1968.

4. Clark LC Jr: Monitor and control of blood and tissue oxygen tensions. Trans Am Soc Artif Intern Organs 2:41, 1956.

5. National Committee for Clinical Laboratory Standards: Tentative Standard for Definitions of Quantities and Conventions Related to Blood pH and Gas Analysis. NCCLS Publication C12-T. Villanova, PA, NCCLS, 1982.

6. Sanz MC: Ultramicro methods and standardization of equipment. Clin Chem 3:406, 1957.

7. Malley WJ: Clinical Blood Gases: Applications and Noninvasive Alternatives. Philadelphia, WB Saunders, 1990.

8. Severinghaus JW, Bradley AF: Electrodes for blood P_{O_2}, and P_{CO_2} determinations. J Appl Physiol 13:515, 1958.

9. Winckers EK, Teunissen AJ, Van den Camp RA, et al: A comparative study of the electrode systems of three pH and blood gas apparatus. J Clin Chem Clin Biochem 16:175, 1978.

10. Adam RD, Edwards LD, Becker CC, et al: Semiquantitative cultures and routine tip cultures on umbilical catheters. J Pediatr 100:123, 1982.

11. Casalino MD, Lipsitz PJ: Contamination of umbilical catheters. J Pediatr 78:1077, 1971.

12. Goetzmann BW, Stadalnik RC, Bogren HG, et al: Thrombotic complications of umbilical artery catheters: A clinical and radiographic study. Pediatrics 56:374, 1975.

13. Miller D, Kirkpatrick BV, Kodroff M, et al: Pelvic exsanguination following umbilical artery catheterization in neonates. J Pediatr Surg 14:264, 1979.

14. O'Neill JA, Neblett WW Jr, Born ML: Management of major thromboembolic complications of umbilical artery catheters. J Pediatr Surg 16:972, 1981.

15. Pape KE, Armstrong DL, Fitzhardinge PM: Peripheral median nerve damage secondary to brachial arterial blood gas sampling. J Pediatr 93:852, 1978.

16. Gandy G, Grann L, Cunningham N, et al: The validity of pH and P_{CO_2} measurement in capillary samples of sick and healthy newborn infants. Pediatrics 34:192, 1964.

17. Courtney SE, Kaye RW, Breakie LA, et al: Capillary blood gases in the neonate: A reassessment and review of the literature. Am J Dis Child 144:168, 1990.

18. Brouillette RT, Waxman DH: Evaluation of the newborn's blood gas status. Clin Chem 43:215, 1997.

19. Duc CV, Comarasamy N: Digital arterial oxygen tension as a guide to oxygen therapy in the newborn. Biol Neonate 24:134, 1974.

20. Koch G, Wendel H: Comparison of pH, carbon dioxide tension, standard bicarbonate, and oxygen tension in capillary blood and in arterial blood during the neonatal period. Acta Paediatr Scand 56:10, 1967.

21. McLain BI, Evans J, Dear PR: Comparison of capillary and arterial blood gas measurements in neonates. Arch Dis Child 63:743, 1988.

22. Phillips BL, McQuitty J, Durand DJ: Blood gases: Technical aspects and interpretation. In Goldsmith JP, Karotkin EH, Barker S (eds): Assisted Ventilation of the Neonate, 2nd ed. Philadelphia, WB Saunders, 1988, pp 213-232.

23. Short BL, Avery GA: Capillary-blood sampling. In Fletcher MA, MacDonald MG, Avery GB (eds): Atlas of Procedures in Neonatology. Philadelphia, JB Lippincott, 1983, pp 97-100.

24. Gambino SR, Thiede WH: Comparisons of pH in human arterial, venous and capillary blood. Am J Clin Pathol 32:298, 1959.

25. Phillips B, Peretz DI: A comparison of central venous and arterial blood gas values in the critically ill. Ann Intern Med 70:745, 1969.

26. Elser RC: Quality control of blood gas analysis: A review. Respir Care 31:807, 1986.

27. Fan LE, Dellinger KT, Mills AL, et al: Potential errors in neonatal blood gas measurements. J Pediatr 97:650, 1980.

28. Mellor LD, Innanen VT: A source of error in determination of blood gases. Clin Chem 29(Pt 1):395, 1983.

29. Biswas CK, Ramos JM, Agroyannis B, et al: Blood gas analysis: Effect of air bubbles in syringe and delay in estimation. BMJ 284:923, 1982.

30. Adams AP, Hahn CEW: Principles and Practice of Blood Gas Analysis. London, Franklin Scientific Products, 1979.

31. Hutchison AS, Ralson SH, Dryburgh FJ, et al: Too much heparin: Possible source of error in blood gas analysis. BMJ 287:1131, 1983.

32. Comroe JH: Physiology of Respiration, 2nd ed. Chicago, Year Book Medical Publishers, 1974.

33. Delivoria-Papadopoulos M, DiGiacomo JE: Oxygen transport and delivery. In Polin RA, Fox WW (eds): Fetal and Neonatal Physiology. Philadelphia, WB Saunders, 1992, pp 801-813.

34. Kafer ER: Neonatal gas exchange and oxygen transport. In Long WA (ed): Fetal and Neonatal Cardiology. Philadelphia, WB Saunders, 1990, pp 97-117.

35. Burgess WR, Chernick V: Respiratory Therapy in Newborn Infants and Children, 2nd ed. New York, Thieme, 1986.

36. Czervinske MP: Arterial blood gas analysis and other cardiopulmonary monitoring. In Koff PB, Eitzman DV, Neu J (eds): Neonatal and Pediatric Respiratory Care. St. Louis, Mosby, 1988, pp 260-281.

37. Klaus MH, Fanaroff AA: Care of the High Risk Neonate. Philadelphia, WB Saunders, 1986.

38. Chanutin A, Curnish RR: Effect of organic phosphates on the oxygen equilibrium of human erythrocytes. Arch Biochem Biophys 121:96, 1967.

39. Oski FA: Red cell metabolism in the newborn infant: V. Glycolytic intermediates and glycolytic enzymes. Pediatrics 44:84, 1969.

40. Rapoport S, Guest GM: Distribution of acid-soluble phosphorus in the blood cells of various vertebrates. J Biol Chem 138:269, 1941.

41. Benesch R, Benesch RE: The effect of organic phosphates from the human erythrocyte on the allosteric properties of hemoglobin. Biochem Biophys Res Commun 26:162, 1967.

42. Chauntin A, Curnish RR: Effect of organic and inorganic phosphates on the oxygen equilibrium of human erythrocytes. Arch Biochem Biophys 121:96, 1967.

43. Oski FA, Gottlieb AJ, Miller WW, et al: The effects of deoxygenation of adult and fetal hemoglobin on the synthesis of red cell 2,3-diphosphoglycerate and its in vivo consequences. J Clin Invest 49:400, 1970.

44. Bellingham AJ, Detter JC, Lenfant C, et al: Regulatory mechanism of haemoglobin oxygen affinity in acidosis and alkalosis. J Clin Invest 50:700, 1971.

45. Oski FA, Nathan DG: Hematology of Infancy and Childhood. Philadelphia, WB Saunders, 1993.

46. Kirschbaum TH: Fetal hemoglobin composition as a parameter of the oxyhemoglobin dissociation curve of fetal blood. Am J Obstet Gynecol 84:477, 1962.

47. Oski FA, Delivoria-Papadopoulos M: The red cell 2,3-diphosphoglycerate and tissue oxygen release. J Pediatr 77:941, 1970.

48. Smith CA, Nelson NM: The Physiology of the Newborn Infant, 4th ed. Springfield, Ill, Charles C Thomas, 1976.

49. Delivoria-Papadopoulos M, Roncevic NP, Oski FA: Postnatal changes in oxygen transport of term, premature, and sick infants: The role of red cell 2,3-diphosphoglycerate and adult hemoglobin. Pediatr Res 5:235, 1971.

50. Delivoria-Papadopoulos M, Morrow G, Oski FA, et al: Exchange transfusion in the newborn infant with fresh and "old" blood: The role of storage of 2,3-diphosphoglycerate, hemoglobin-oxygen affinity, and oxygen release. J Pediatr 6:898, 1971.

51. Roberton NRC, Rennie JM: Textbook of Neonatology, 3rd ed. Edinburgh, Churchill Livingstone, 1999.

52. Mertzlufft F: Normal and therapeutic threshold values for arterial O_2 saturation. In Zander R, Mertzlufft F (eds): The Oxygen Status of Arterial Blood. Basel, Karger, 1991, pp 228-232.

53. Saugstad OD: Is oxygen more toxic than currently believed? Pediatrics 108:1203, 2001.

54. Tin W, Milligan WA, Pennefather P, et al: Pulse oximetry, severe retinopathy, and outcome at one year in babies less than 28 weeks gestation. Arch Dis Child Fetal Neonatal Educ 184:F106, 2001.

55. Poets CF: When do infants need additional inspired oxygen? A review of the current literature. Pediatr Pulmonol 26:424, 1998.

56. Wardle SP, Weindling AM: Peripheral oxygenation in preterm infants. Clin Perinatol 26:947, 1999.

57. Heinig RE, Clarke EF, Waterhouse C: Lactic acidosis and liver disease. Arch Intern Med 13:1229, 1979.

58. Tietz NW: Fundamentals of Clinical Chemistry, 3rd ed. Philadelphia, WB Saunders, 1987, p 659.

59. Dantzker DR, Gutierrez G: The assessment of tissue oxygenation. Respir Care 30:456, 1985.

60. Astiz ME, Rackow EC, Kaufman B, et al: Relationship of oxygen delivery and mixed venous oxygenation to lactic acidosis in patients with sepsis and acute myocardial infarction. Crit Care Med 16:655, 1988.

61. Heironomus TW, Bageant RA: Mechanical Artificial Ventilation, 3rd ed. Springfield, Ill, Charles C Thomas, 1977.

62. Snyder JV: Assessment of systemic oxygen transport. In Snyder JV, Pinsky MR (eds): Oxygen Transport in the Critically Ill. Chicago, Year Book Medical Publishers, 1987, pp 179-198..

63. Nelson LD: Mixed venous oximetry. In Snyder JV, Pinsky MR (eds): Oxygen Transport in the Critically Ill. Chicago, Year Book Medical Publishers, 1987, pp 235-248.

64. Demers RR, Irwin RS, Braman SS: Criteria for optimum PEEP. Respir Care 22:596, 1977.

65. Noble WH, Kay JC: Effect of continuous positive-pressure ventilation and oxygenation after pulmonary microemboli in dogs. Crit Care Med 13:412, 1985.

66. Brandt L: The significance of the mixed venous O_2 status as a complement to the arterial O_2 status. In Zander R, Mertzlufft F (eds): The Oxygen Status of Arterial Blood. Basel, Karger, 1991, pp 238-263.

67. Wardle SP, Weindling AM: Peripheral fractional oxygen extraction and other measures of tissue oxygenation to guide blood transfusions in preterm newborns. Semin Perinatol 25:60, 2001.

68. Saugstad OD: Hypoxanthine as an indicator of hypoxia: Its role in health and disease through free radical production. Pediatr Res 23:143, 1988.

69. Thiringer K: Cord plasma hypoxanthine as a measure of foetal hypoxia. Acta Paediatr Scand 72:231, 1983.

70. Russell GA, Jeffers G, Cooke RW: Plasma hypoxanthine: A marker for hypoxic-ischaemic induced periventricular leucomalacia? Arch Dis Child 67(4 Spec No):388, 1992.

71. Rognum TO, Saugstad OD: Hypoxanthine levels in vitreous humor: Evidence of hypoxia in most infants who died of sudden infant death syndrome. Pediatrics 87:306, 1991.

72. Pietz J, Guttenberg N, Gluck L: Hypoxanthine: New standard for asphyxia. Pediatr Res 21:373A, 1987.

73. Bartrons J, Figueras J, Jimenez R, et al: Vasopressin in cerebrospinal fluid of newborns with hypoxic-ischemic encephalopathy: Preliminary report. J Perinat Med 21:399, 1993.

74. Varvarigou A, Beratis NG, Makri M, et al: Increased levels and positive correlation between erythropoietin and hemoglobin concentrations in newborn children of mothers who are smokers. J Pediatr 124:480, 1994.

75. West JB: Ventilation Blood Flow and Gas Exchange, 3rd ed. London, Blackwell Scientific, 1977.

76. Guyton AC: Textbook of Medical Physiology, 4th ed. Philadelphia, WB Saunders, 1971.

77. Shapiro BA, Peruzzi WT, Kowzelowski-Templin R: Clinical Application of Blood Gases, 5th ed. St. Louis, Mosby-Year Book, 1994.

78. Roughton FJW: Transport of oxygen and carbon dioxide. In Fenn WO, Rahn H (eds): Handbook of Physiology. Washington, DC, American Physiological Society, 1964, pp 767-826.

79. Chatburn RL, Carlo WA: Assessment of neonatal gas exchange. In Carlo WA, Chatburn RL (eds): Neonatal Respiratory Care, 2nd ed. Chicago, Year Book Medical Publishers, 1988, pp 40-60.

80. Kleinman LI, Petering HG, Sutherland JM: Blood carbonic anhydrase activity and zinc concentration in infants with respiratory-distress syndrome. N Engl J Med 277:1157, 1967.

81. Stave U: Perinatal Physiology. New York, Plenum, 1978.

82. Christiansen J, Douglas CG, Haldane JS: The absorption and dissociation of carbon dioxide by human blood. J Physiol (Lond) 48:244, 1914.

83. Comroe JH, Forster RE, Dubois AB, et al: The Lung: Clinical Physiology and Pulmonary Function Tests. Chicago, Year Book Medical Publishers, 1962.

84. Masoro EJ, Seigel PD: Acid-Base Regulation: Its Physiology, Pathophysiology and Interpretation of Blood-Gas Analysis, 2nd ed. Philadelphia, WB Saunders, 1977.

85. Narins RG, Emmett M: Simple and mixed acid-base disorders: A practical approach. Medicine (Baltimore) 59:161, 1980.

86. Collier CR, Hackney JD, Mohler JG, et al: Use of extracellular base excess in diagnosis of acid-base disorders: A conceptual approach. Chest 61:65, 1972.

87. Keener PA: Disorders of acid-base balance. In Schreiner RL, Kisling JA (eds): Practical Neonatal Respiratory Care. New York, Raven Press, 1982.

88. Brewer ED: Urinary acidification. In Polin RA, Fox WW (eds): Fetal and Neonatal Physiology. Philadelphia, WB Saunders, 1992, pp 1258-1260.

89. Flenley DC: Oxygen transport in chronic ventilatory failure. In Payne JP, Hill DW (eds): Oxygen Measurements in Biology and Medicine. Boston, Butterworth, 1975.

90. Van Slyke DD: Studies of acidosis. J Biol Chem 48:153, 1921.

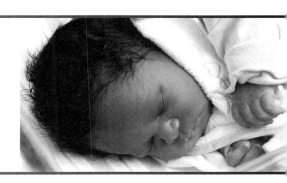

CHAPTER 36

Apnea of Prematurity and Apparent Life-Threatening Events

Joseph D. DeCristofaro

pnea of prematurity (AOP) is one of the most common diagnoses made in the neonatal intensive care unit (NICU). It occurs in more than 85% of infants born at less than 34 weeks of gestational age,[1] and its incidence varies inversely with gestational age. Nearly 100% of infants born before 26 weeks of gestation experience an apneic episode during their NICU hospital stay.

Apnea is the cessation of breathing. In the preterm infant, AOP has been defined in many ways, and there is no general consensus regarding the definition of pathologic apnea. Apnea has been considered significant if it lasts for a prolonged period of time; this is an important distinction, because short pauses in breathing occur in all individuals. In research and clinical studies, apnea has been defined as cessation of breathing longer than 10 seconds,[2,3] 15 seconds,[4,5] 20 seconds,[6] or 30 seconds,[7] depending on the author. The most consistent definition for pathologic apnea is a respiratory pause of 15 seconds' duration, associated with a heart rate drop and/or a color change. Pathologic apnea was defined at the National Institute of Child Health and Human Development consensus conference of 1986 as pauses of 20 seconds' duration or longer or as pauses of less than 20 seconds but associated with bradycardia or cyanosis.[8] This definition has remained in the medical literature for many years. This definition of pathologic apnea was chosen somewhat arbitrarily, however, and it has not been specifically associated with either a poor outcome or pathologic processes. Indeed, many infants have apneic pauses that persist beyond 20 seconds, which go undetected and self-correct with no caregiver intervention.[9] To date, not a single pathologic apnea has been linked with any dysfunctional outcome in an infant. It has never been conclusively demonstrated that a single apneic pause, if undetected, may result in sudden infant death syndrome (SIDS).

TYPES OF APNEA

Apnea has been classified into three types (Fig. 36-1): central, obstructive, and mixed. **Central apnea** is a pause in breathing with the absence of respiratory effort or diaphragmatic activity. During periods of **obstructive apnea**, airflow is absent, but respiratory muscle contractions continue, indicating an ongoing effort to breathe. **Mixed apnea** is a combination of these two, most often a central apnea of at least 3 seconds followed by an obstructive component. The proportion with which these three types of apneas occur varies in the literature.[1,10,11] Indeed, the percentage of apnea types also seems to change over the first few days of life.[1] Certainly, central and mixed apneas occur with the greatest frequency. The most recent literature suggests that mixed apnea is the most common, because many of the central apneas, when carefully studied, are found to have some obstructive component. For example, infants who have a central apnea of 15 seconds' duration but who demonstrate obstruction within the first few recovery breaths are exhibiting mixed apneas in the strictest sense of the term. This is often difficult to document, and documentation depends on the method used for detection.

Many methods for detection of apnea exist. Different methods used to detect respiration significantly alter the reporting of type of apneas. Initially, the two-channel pneumocardiogram was used to detect apnea. This technique involves the use of chest wall electrodes that measure the change in transthoracic impedance as the chest wall moves and also record the trend of the heart rate. However, this method fails to pick up obstructive apneas when used alone, inasmuch as continued respiratory effort is seen in the thoracic impedance channel, even when airflow is obstructed. In order to define obstructive apnea with greater confidence, multichannel recording must be performed, involving the addition of a channel in which airflow can be assessed simultaneously with thoracic impedance. When there is evidence of continued breathing effort but absent airflow, obstruction may be present (see Fig. 36-1). It is especially important to note that clinical apnea may not be appropriately detected by simple observation alone. Several studies in the literature[11-15] have described series of infants with

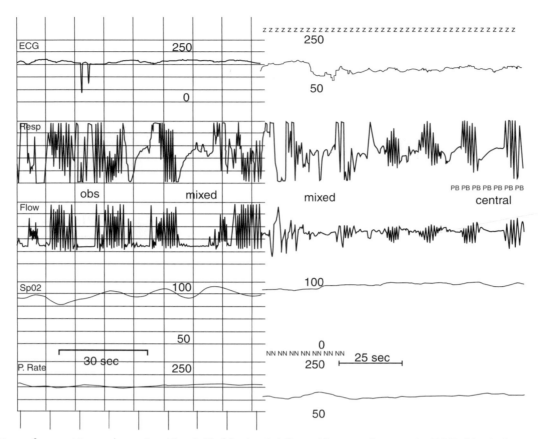

Figure 36–1. Types of apnea: (1) central, seen in 40% to 60% of the time in infants with apnea of prematurity (AOP); (2) mixed, seen in 40% to 70% of the time in infants with AOP; and (3) obstructive (obs), seen rarely (10%) in infants with AOP. These two tracings demonstrate two methods of detecting airflow. The grid on the left shows airflow as detected by end-tidal carbon dioxide, and the tracings on the right show airflow as detected by thermistor probe. The absence of airflow, as shown by a flat line in the middle channel, depicts apnea. Absence of chest wall movement on the respiratory channel, along with the absence of flow in the middle channel, is best seen on the tracing on the right, an example of periodic breathing. ECG, electrocardiogram; Resp, respirations; SpO_2, oxygen saturation; P. Rate, pulse rate.

very frequent and occasionally prolonged apnea episodes that were not detected clinically by the nursing or medical staffs caring for these infants. In some cases, apnea-related events resulted in prolonged hospitalization or readmission to the hospital for apparent life-threatening events (ALTEs). Unless some type of multichannel recording is performed in an infant, it is not certain that a child has no apnea.

Newer technologic methods attempt to detect both central and obstructive apneas noninvasively. For example, Weese-Mayer and colleagues described their experience with the Collaborative Home Infant Monitoring Evaluation (CHIME) monitor, a respiratory inductance plethysmographic method for detection of central and obstructive apneas.[16] With the inductance method, movements in the chest wall and abdomen are recorded and added together to help detect an obstructive event. During obstructive apnea, these movements of the chest and abdomen occur in opposite directions, blunting the cumulative waveform. In this study, the inductance plethysmography method was combined with either a nasal end-tidal carbon dioxide or a thermistor probe to

detect airflow. Weese-Mayer and colleagues studied 422 infants, with a cumulative total of 233 episodes of apnea longer than 16 seconds. There was complete agreement among the three methods in only 87 (37%) of these events. The CHIME monitor detected 55% of the obstructed events that were detected by the end-tidal carbon dioxide method. The thermistor probe detected fewer events than did the end-tidal carbon dioxide method. Thus, end-tidal carbon dioxide and thermistor probe with impedance appear to detect more apneas than does the inductance plethysmography method. These data indicate why the percentage of central, obstructive, and mixed apneas may differ from one author to another and why results often depend on the methodology used for detection.

The duration of apnea has been linked with the degree of change in the heart rate and oxygen saturation. Upton and associates reported a positive correlation between oxygen desaturations and the duration of an apnea and more severe saturation when bradycardia accompanied the event.[3] Ramanathan and coworkers found a strong correlation between the duration of apnea and the degree of oxygen desaturation.[9] Similarly, Carbone and colleagues found that the longest apneas in preterm infants resulted in the greatest changes in heart rate and oxygen saturation.[17] However, there was a poor correlation between the fall in heart rate and the degree of desaturation.

CAUSES OF APNEA

AOP is often considered a diagnosis of exclusion because there are many other possible causes of apnea. Because AOP is so common, however, especially in the most premature infants, it should be anticipated. Other common causes of apnea in infants include bacterial and viral infections such as sepsis, pneumonia, and meningitis. Viral infections, especially respiratory syncytial virus, have been associated with the new onset of apnea in the presence of an increased nasal discharge and cough (Fig. 36-2). Metabolic disorders have been linked to apnea and include medium chain acyl–coenzyme A dehydrogenase deficiency, biotinidase deficiency, and hypophosphatasia. Central nervous system disorders[18] (Fig. 36-3) may also manifest as apnea in the newborn and must be considered in the differential diagnosis (Table 36-1). Infants with apnea require prompt attention and need a workup for their apnea, and a detailed differential

diagnosis should be considered (Table 36-2, Fig. 36-4; see also Table 36-1 and Figs. 36-2 and 36-3).

AOP has many proposed causes.[10] These include immaturity of the respiratory region of the brain, depression of central inspiratory activity, upper airway obstruction and flaccidity, decreased ventilatory response to carbon dioxide, instability of the compliant chest wall, and hypoxic depression. Many of these mechanisms are likely to be acting in concert in the preterm infant with AOP.

A peculiar breathing pattern found in almost all infants, including full-term infants, is periodic breathing. This respiratory pattern is characterized by a repetition of three apneic pauses of 3 to 19 seconds' duration, interrupted by spurts of breathing for less than 20 seconds. The frequency of periodic breathing tends to increase with decreasing gestational age. Preterm infants can spend a significant amount of time in periodic breathing, with more than 40% of their total sleep time demonstrating this pattern. Although it is often considered to be a benign disorder, infants with periodic breathing can have associated drops in heart rate and oxygen saturation.[19] These heart decelerations are usually not low enough to produce bradycardia; otherwise, they would be classified as pathologic apnea. In some cases, however, periodic breathing may be associated with repetitive oxygen desaturation, even while the heart rate is maintained at a

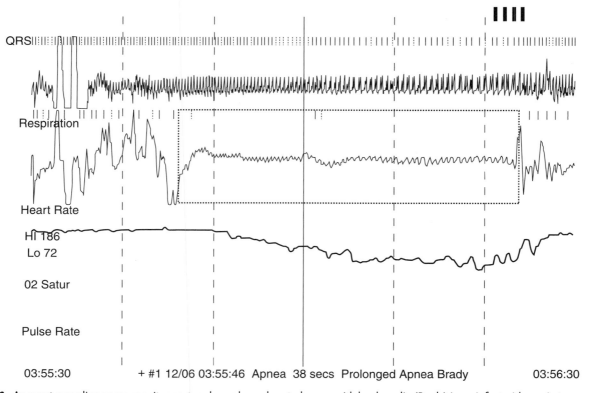

Figure 36–2. An event-recording apnea monitor captured a prolonged central apnea with bradycardia (Brady) in an infant with respiratory syncytial virus. Each vertical line represents a 10-second interval. The four *thick bars* at the top right of this tracing represent the four beeps of the apnea monitor alarm. This was a self-corrected event. The monitor failed to sound an alarm for apnea that was set for 20 seconds because it detected the heart pulsations as chest wall movement on the respiratory channel, or cardiovascular artifact. The monitor did sound an alarm for bradycardia. O_2 Satur, oxygen saturation.

ECG-QRS

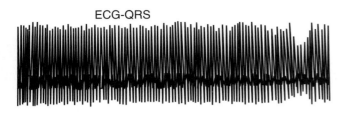

HR Trend BPM

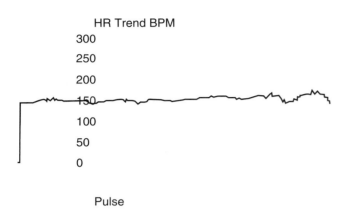

Pulse

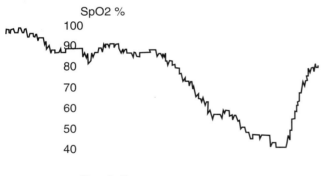

SpO2 %

Respiration

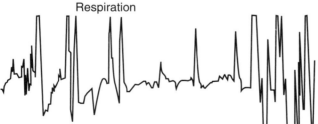

Figure 36–3. Tracings of an infant with known apnea secondary to a myelomeningocele and Arnold-Chiari II malformation. He had new-onset prolonged apneas, with stridor and cyanosis and a ventriculoperitoneal shunt malfunction. BPM, beats per minute; ECG, electrocardiogram; HR, heart rate; SpO_2, oxygen saturation.

Table 36–1.   Central Nervous System Lesions at Birth Manifesting with Apnea

Trauma
Infratentorial bleeding
Spinal cord injury
Perinatal asphyxia

Congenital Brain Disorder
Familial multisystem atrophy
Degenerative infantile thalamic degeneration
Infantile neuroaxonal dystrophy
Pena-Shokeir syndrome type I
Werdnig-Hoffman disease

Brain Tumors
Glioma
Teratoma

Brain Malformations
Arnold-Chiari malformation
Achondroplasia
Osteogenesis imperfecta
Dandy-Walker malformation
Joubert syndrome
Miller-Dieker syndrome
Congenital central hypoventilation syndrome
Familial lissencephaly
Möbius syndrome

Modified from Brazy JE, Kinney HC, Oakes WJ: Central nervous system structural lesions causing apnea at birth. J Pediatr 111:163, 1987.

consistent level. The physiologic consequences of periodic breathing with oxygen desaturation are not known.

In preterm infants, periodic breathing may be induced by hypoxemia[20] and reduced by supplemental oxygen administration. In fact, supplemental oxygen administration in preterm infants can alter not only the respiratory pattern but also the overall sleep architecture in the short term.[21] Methylxanthine therapy can also decrease or eliminate periodic breathing. Kelly and Shannon found an increased rate of periodic breathing in infants with ALTE.[22] In addition, an association between excessive (>5%) periodic breathing in full-term infants and subsequent sudden infant death has been described. This report raised concern over an identifiable risk for the development of SIDS, but this association has not been corroborated in subsequent studies.

AOP often manifests within the first 24 hours after birth in preterm infants without respiratory distress. In babies with respiratory distress, the onset of AOP usually begins as the respiratory distress syndrome is resolving, generally toward the end of the first week after birth.[23] The use of prenatal steroids has resulted in a decreased incidence of respiratory distress syndrome, but this has not affected the frequency of AOP.[24] Infants born as part of a multiple-gestation pregnancy have the same incidence of AOP as gestational age–matched singletons.[24]

Table 36–2. Causes of Apnea in the Infant

Central nervous system	Intracranial bleeding
	Seizure
	Structural malformations (see Table 36-1)
Gastrointestinal	Feeding bradycardias
	GERD
	Necrotizing enterocolitis
Genetic	X-linked Leigh syndrome
Hormonal	Hypothyroidism
Infection	Sepsis
	Meningitis
	Pneumonia
	Viral syndrome
	RSV
Medication	Narcotics
	PGE_1
	Amikacin
Metabolic	Hyponatremia
	Hypermagnesemia
	Hypoglycemia
	Urea cycle defects
	Biotinidase deficiency
	Other inborn errors of metabolism
Oxygenation problems	Hypoxemia
Syndromes	Stuve-Wiedemann syndrome
	Arthrogryposis
	Cornelia de Lange syndrome
	Pierre Robin syndrome
Thermal stress	Hyperthermia

GERD, gastroesophageal reflux disease; PGE_1, prostaglandin E_1; RSV, respiratory syncytial virus.

The developmental outcome in infants with apnea is generally favorable. Koons and associates found no difference in infant development when applying Bayley Scales of Infant Development scores in infants with persistent apnea versus those without apnea.[25] They also found no difference in the incidence of cerebral palsy, speech delay, or retinopathy of prematurity between the two groups. Similarly, Nelson and coworkers found no difference in development between infants treated with theophylline for AOP and those without apnea.[26] Cheung and colleagues more recently reported outcomes in 164 infants with persistent apnea beyond 35 weeks' postmenstrual age (PMA) versus those in whom the apnea had resolved.[27] They performed 24-hour four-channel pneumography on this group of infants and monitored them to a median of 24 months. They reported a worse outcome in the infants who had frequent apneic episodes and in those with lower oxygen desaturation associated with the apnea, especially in infants with grades III and IV intraventricular hemorrhage. These findings suggest that AOP should not necessarily be considered "normal" and necessitates aggressive evaluation and management.

Apnea in infants may be of clinical concern when the episodes occur with sufficient frequency that they result in significant bradycardia or desaturation. The definition of significant bradycardia depends on the age of the infant and also varies among authors. Equally hard to define is a "significant" desaturation. Physiologically, heart rate decelerations in full-term infants have been shown to result in decreased brain blood flow velocities on Doppler imaging when the heart rate fell to 80 beats per minute.[28] Other methods including nuclear magnetic

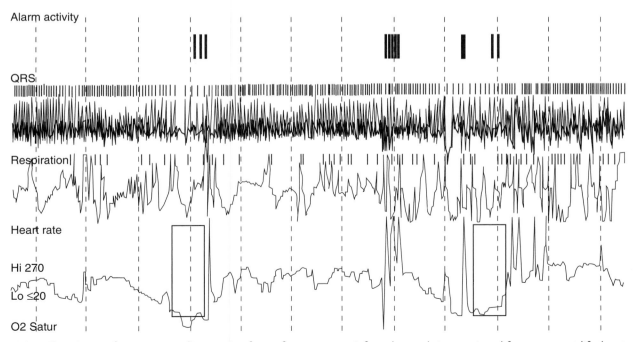

Figure 36–4. The printout of an event-recording monitor from a former preterm infant who was being monitored for an apparent life-threatening event that occurred 1 month earlier. Her prior printouts were normal, without true apnea or bradycardia events. She had been well until shortly before this recording, when she started having new-onset monitor alarms associated with coughing fits and cyanosis. Her nasopharyngeal swab for pertussis culture was positive. O_2 Satur, oxygen saturation.

resonance–spectroscopy have shown that decreased brain oxygenation can occur with apnea and bradycardia with accompanying oxygen desaturation, although apparently not with a desaturation alone.[29] Pratesi and Donzelli reported similar findings in 5 preterm infants.[30] Other investigators have described periods of cerebral deoxygenation in the presence of apnea, with a strong correlation between apnea duration and brain deoxygenation.[31]

The technique of near infrared spectroscopy may be a more important indicator of potential harm than peripheral oxygen saturation monitoring, because the same apnea that results in brain deoxygenation may have no effect on peripheral oxygen saturation.[30,32] Watkin and associates found that only the larger changes in cerebral deoxygenation had an associated drop in peripheral oxygen saturation.[33] As noted earlier in this chapter, even relatively brief periodic breathing can result in recurrent periodic cerebral deoxygenation,[34] a problem that appears to be worse in the supine position.[35] These results call into question the optimal sleep position for the preterm infant with excessive periodic breathing. Together, the data suggest that apnea, even in the absence of bradycardia or desaturation, may be physiologically important. Whether this portends any long-term developmental disadvantage is unknown.

MEDICAL TREATMENT OF APNEA OF PREMATURITY

Treatment for AOP should be considered when the apnea results in recurrent bradycardia or desaturation, even when the infant spontaneously terminates the episodes. Treatment should also be considered for some infants with increased periodic breathing or prolonged central apneas even in the absence of desaturations or bradycardia. Treatment of AOP should begin with the most benign of treatments. The treatment choices include supplemental oxygen, continuous positive airway pressure (CPAP), and medications. Infants in whom these interventions fail require intubation and mechanical ventilation. Severe, intractable apnea remains the only absolute indication for mechanical ventilation during the neonatal period.

Hypoxemia has been shown to increase the amount of apnea and periodic breathing in preterm infants, and oxygen supplementation can decrease these events in some infants. However, supplemental oxygen treatment has not been shown to consistently reduce the frequency of significant apnea in preterm infants. Although some studies have indicated that apnea frequency declines, other studies have not been as conclusive in this regard. Supplemental oxygen, however, does reduce the amount of desaturation associated with AOP and remains an important adjunct to care. Conversely, hyperoxia may also be detrimental to the preterm infant. It alters sleep architecture[21] and may contribute to the pathogenesis of bronchopulmonary dysplasia and retinopathy of prematurity. The use of unrestricted supplemental oxygen treatment is not advisable, and children who receive oxygen for the treatment of apnea with desaturation should be monitored carefully for potential complications of therapy.

CPAP has been shown to decrease the amount of mixed and obstructive apneas.[36] CPAP appears to treat apnea by splinting the airway and improving alveolar ventilation and oxygenation. Many different devices exist for the administration of CPAP. The advantage of one type of appliance over another for the treatment of AOP has not been reported. Another treatment for AOP with positive pressure is nasal intermittent positive-pressure ventilation (NIPPV). This technique, first reported in 1989, was initially found to have no advantage over CPAP.[37] In a more recent randomized trial, however, NIPPV was shown to be more effective than CPAP in decreasing apnea in symptomatic preterm infants.[38] The authors studied 34 infants in whom treatment with oxygen and aminophylline failed. They found both CPAP and NIPPV efficacious in decreasing apneas. Bubble CPAP may provide similar fluctuations in airway pressure to simulate NIPPV plus conventional CPAP. The use of NIPPV for AOP may help prevent more invasive interventions but needs further study to confirm these short-term effects and long-term efficacy and to determine the rate of possible complications.[39]

Many medications have been used to treat AOP. These include methylxanthines, doxapram, and other supplements (Table 36-3). Kuzemko and Paala first reported using aminophylline to treat preterm infants with apnea in 1973 through rectal suppositories.[40] Aminophylline and theophylline use proliferated during the 1980s but has largely been replaced by caffeine as the medication of choice.[41] Caffeine has many advantages over aminophylline: Caffeine is rapidly absorbed when administered orally; it may be administered once daily and has a wide therapeutic window of efficacy. Many physiologic and pharmacologic effects of caffeine have been reported (Table 36-4).[42,43] Toxic effects of caffeine have typically been reported only at levels above 50 mg/dL,[44] unlike theophylline, which has a much narrower therapeutic window. Ergenekon and colleagues,[45] however, reported a very large overdose of caffeine citrate in which an infant received an oral dose of 600 mg/kg of caffeine citrate, or 300 mg/kg of caffeine base. The infant was symptomatic for 96 hours with tachycardia, agitation, irritability, tachypnea, diuresis, electrolyte disturbance, hyperglycemia, and metabolic acidosis. The infant did not have seizures.

The short-term use of methylxanthines for the treatment of apnea in preterm infants was reviewed by Henderson-Smart and Steer.[46] This review supported the short-term use of methylxanthines to reduce the number of apneic attacks in preterm infants. Methylxanthines act in several ways. They block adenosine receptors in the central nervous system and are phosphodiesterase inhibitors, increasing second messenger cyclic adenosine monophosphate. The therapeutic range for methylxanthine dosing treatments is shown in Table 36-3. Caffeine dosing protocols vary to some extent. Bolus dosing ranges from 10 mg/kg to as high as 50 mg/kg of caffeine base.[41] Caffeine has a half-life of about 100 hours[47,48] that decreases over time as the infant matures. The rate of caffeine metabolism is increased after 60 days of life and tends to be higher in infant girls than infant boys.[49]

Table 36-3. Pharmacotherapy for the Treatment of Apnea

| | Methylxanthines | |
	Theophylline	Caffeine
Chemical structure	1,3-dimethylxanthine	1,3,7-Trimethylxanthine
Half-life	30 hr (15-50) in preterm newborns 20 hr in older preterm infants 6.7 hr by 6 mo	100 hr in preterm newborns 40 hr by 4 mo (46 wk PMA) Less in girls
Clearance	20-25 mL/kg/hr in preterm newborns 40 mL/kg/hr older preterm infants	9 mL/kg/hr in preterm infants >100 mL/kg/hr by 6 mo
Apparent volume of distribution	0.7 L/kg (0.3-1.1) in preterm newborns Less in the older infant	0.8-0.9 L/kg in infants Same volume of distribution as adult
Absorption	100% when given PO in chidren Less in the preterm infant Erratic when given per rectum	100% in infants and adults when given orally

Metabolism	In preterm infant, liver cytochrome p450
	  is major site of metabolism. Up to 50%
	  of drug, however, is excreted unchanged
	  by the kidney
	Liver oxidation, demethylation, and
	  methylation (to caffeine)
		Up to 86% of drug is excreted unchanged
		  by the kidney in preterm infants
		Liver is the major site of metabolism in adults
		
		Liver demethylation

Loading dose	5-6 mg/kg	20-50 mg/kg (citrate)
Maintenance dosage	2 mg/kg every 8-12 hr	5-6 mg/kg/day (citrate)
Serum levels	Trough level, 5-15 mg/dL	Trough level, 8-25 mg/dL
Metabolism affected by	Smoking: increases excretion Phenobarbital: increases clearance Phenytoin: increases clearance Rifampin: increases clearance Erythromycin: decreases clearance Cimetidine: decreases clearance	Cholestasis: delays clearance

Less efficacious treatments: doxapram, primidone, atropine, naloxone, almitrine, and L-carnitine.

PMA, postmenstrual age; PO, per os (orally).

Table 36-4. Effects of Caffeine

Physiologic Effects

Increased frequency of breathing
Decreased carbon dioxide levels
Decreased apnea frequency
Increased minute ventilation
Increased ventilatory response to hypercarbia
Decreased hypoxemia and hypoxic episodes
Increased central inspiratory drive
Increased diaphragmatic excursion
Increased transmission of neuronal impulses

Pharmacologic Effects

Tachycardia
Increased oxygen consumption
Increased metabolic rate
Poor weight gain[42]
Decreased cerebal blood flow velocity and intestinal
  blood flow velocity with high bolus dose (50 mg/kg of
  caffeine citrate)[43]
Diuresis
Agitation and jitteriness
Glucose intolerance
Lower seizure threshold
Decreased lower esophageal sphincter tone

The blood levels for caffeine need to be checked less frequently than those for theophylline, perhaps once weekly or every other week, with a therapeutic range of 8 to 30 mg/dL. In rare cases, in some infants who rapidly metabolize caffeine, dosing may need to be increased to twice or three times per day.

Doxapram is a centrally acting drug, stimulating the medullary neurons as well as the chemoreceptors. It has been used extensively in adults and is commercially available as an intravenous preparation with benzyl alcohol added as the preservative. The presence of benzyl alcohol makes it difficult to use in the growing preterm infant. The loading dose of doxapram is 3 mg/kg, and the maintenance drip consists of 0.5 to 2.5 mg/kg/hour, titrated to effect. The efficacy of doxapram is improved when it is used in conjunction with methylxanthines. However, its use in preterm infants should be avoided because of the known toxicity of benzyl alcohol and other adverse effects shown in more recent studies. Maillard and associates[50] reported a prolongation in the corrected QT interval in infants being treated with doxapram without reported ventricular arrhythmias. Of even greater concern is the dose-related effect on developmental outcome. Sreenan and coworkers reported a greater developmental delay in infants weighing less than 1250 g who were treated with doxapram, an effect associated with the total dose given the duration of treatment.[51] This suggests that an alternative treatment for these infants should be strongly considered before doxapram is administered. Other supplements have been examined for treating AOP. Carnitine, for example, has been reported to have no significant effect on AOP.[52,53]

Infants in whom all these interventions fail need to be intubated and placed on mechanical ventilation. In the more immature infants who are already intubated, apnea may manifest with desaturation and a slowing heart rate. Dimaguila and associates described preterm infants who presented with apneas while being ventilated with a low-pressure strategy (Fig. 36-5).[54] The hypoxemia started with body movements and a heart rate acceleration and was followed by a drop in spontaneous tidal volume and ventilator-delivered tidal volume. The heart rate decreased as the hypoxemia continued. These events were more common in the supine position. These and other data suggest that the optimal sleep position in preterm infants recovering from respiratory distress syndrome may be prone. In the asymptomatic preterm baby, the prone sleep position also results in decreased awakenings and less heart rate variability, with no difference in sleep states or total sleep, in comparison with the supine position.[55] Although the prone position in infants with resolving respiratory disease appears to be beneficial, the risk of SIDS, as with full-term infants, does appear to be higher in this position than in the supine position. Therefore, unless there are specific contraindications to supine sleep, the supine position should be recommended at the time of discharge. If the infant has been sleeping prone because of earlier difficulties with oxygenation, the nursing staff should gradually adjust sleep position by putting the child in a supine position at least several days before discharge.

The resolution of apnea in the preterm infant is a major concern when discharge is considered. Indeed, several studies have shown that infants thought to be ready for discharge were still having significant numbers of desaturations.[19,56] Nursing documentation is notoriously inaccurate in detecting significant apneic events in preterm infants.[12,57,58] In some centers, this has resulted in the testing of an infant's breathing pattern before discharge, even in asymptomatic preterm infants. Testing helps determine the maturity of cardiorespiratory pattern and the frequency of pathologic apneas and is often performed with event recording[59] or continuous multichannel recording. Differences in determining physiologic maturation may account for differences in interhospital discharge timing.[60]

APPARENT LIFE-THREATENING EVENTS

ALTE was defined at a consensus conference held by the National Institute of Child Health and Human Development in 1986 as an episode that is frightening to the observer and characterized by some combination of apnea, color change, marked change in muscle tone, choking, or gagging.[8] The definition is rather subjective; the interpretation of the event is left to the eyes of the beholder. The frequency of ALTE is quoted as occurring in approximately 2% to 3% of the general population, although the exact incidence is not well established. The cause of an ALTE, in most cases, remains idiopathic. When investigations are pursued to determine a possible cause, the most consistent associated finding is gastroesophageal reflux (GER), because reflux is so common in young infants.[6] Whether the reflux is causal or even associated with ALTE in these events is controversial. Other causes of ALTE (Table 36-5) include metabolic, infectious, seizure, and child abuse or Munchausen syndrome by proxy. Munchausen syndrome is thought to play a role in as many as 5% of infants in whom SIDS had been erroneously diagnosed.

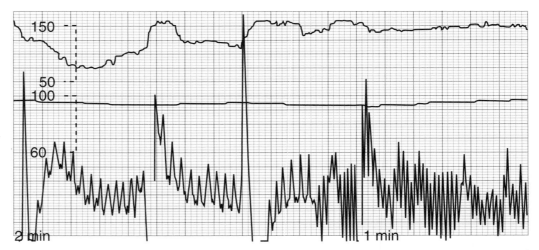

Figure 36-5. Oxypneumogram showing heart rate trend (top tracing), oxygen saturation (middle tracing), and impedance (bottom tracing). These are the tracings of an infant 25 weeks of gestational age on a ventilator with assist-control, with a backup rate of 60 breaths per minute. At the start of the tracing, the infant became apneic. The ventilated breaths are shown as the constant rhythmic movements of the same intensity. This infant was receiving supplemental oxygen that prevented hypoxemia, but the ventilated breaths alone could not prevent the bradycardia to 75 beats per minute.

Table 36–5. Differential Diagnosis of Apparent Life-Threatening Events

Idiopathic
Gastroesophageal reflux disease (GERD)
Seizure disorder
Munchausen syndrome by proxy (MSBP)
Metabolic disorder
    Hypoglycemia
    Hyponatremia
    Hypothyroidism
    MCAD deficiency
    Biotinidase deficiency
Infection
    Viral syndrome
    Bacterial infection
Cardiac
    Congenital heart disease or heart failure
    Cardiac arrhythmia: prolonged QTc
Airway abnormalities
    Bronchomalacia
    Choanal stenosis
    Micrognathia with Pierre Robin syndrome
    Piriform aperture stenosis

MCAD, medium-chain acyl–coenzyme A dehydrogenase; QTc, corrected QT interval.

Infants who have suffered an ALTE are not a homogeneous group. When these infants have been studied with polysomnography, various findings have been reported, including prolonged sleep apnea, excessive periodic breathing, decreased ventilatory response to carbon dioxide, decreased ventilatory response to hypoxia, increased numbers of mixed and obstructive apneic episodes, and altered heart rate variability.[61-66] These mixed findings, full of inconsistencies, lend further support to the notion that the diagnosis of ALTE represents a wastebasket for multiple causes.

Although no consistent polysomnographic findings have been reported in infants with ALTE in the short term, there may be a sleep disorder that becomes more apparent over time. Guilleminault and associates reported their 10-year experience with a complete database of 346 infants in whom ALTE was diagnosed, who were studied with polysomnography, and who underwent follow-up studies.[67] They found that more than half of their patients had an obstructive breathing disorder that became more apparent over time. Two thirds of this group also had a mild facial dysmorphism that was more clearly identifiable by 6 months of age. Thus, a subgroup of patients who suffer an ALTE appear to eventually manifest associated anatomic problems that may account for the disordered breathing of obstructive sleep apnea. A strong family history of sleep-disordered breathing was found for about half of the infants in whom obstructive sleep apnea was diagnosed.[68] Thus, there is an association between ALTE in infancy and later obstructive sleep apnea. A positive family history of obstructive sleep apnea may be a clue to help identify infants who are at risk for developing this problem.

Infants who have been vigorously resuscitated from an ALTE should be admitted to the hospital for evaluation. The usual workup for ALTE may include cardiorespiratory monitoring, serum electrolyte measurements, a blood culture, and perhaps chest radiography and electrocardiography or electroencephalography with cerebral imaging. Depending on the history elicited, a pH probe and or barium swallow study may be helpful. The admission in uncomplicated cases may last 72 hours, but in some cases the workup can be completed in a shorter time.[69] Covert surveillance has also become part of the workup on occasion, especially in cases in which the ALTE is recurrent.[70] These recordings help confirm the diagnosis of Munchausen syndrome by proxy.

Newer technologic methods incorporating videotaping with event recording were reported by Brouillette and coworkers.[71] These authors utilized audiovisual equipment to videotape the infant being monitored by an event-recording apnea monitor to evaluate sleep position and movements in the infant during events. They recorded 65 true events in 13 infants; of these, 20 events (30%) resolved at the same time that the monitor alarm went on. Thus, apnea monitors may provide more than an alert to the caregivers: It may also serve as an "alert" for the infant by providing auditory stimulation to arouse from the event.

Normative data for the natural occurrence of mixed and obstructive apneas in full-term infants 2 to 28 weeks of age have been reported. Kato demonstrated that mixed and obstructive apneas are rarely seen in overnight polysomnographic studies (>1000 infants).[72] When seen, they occurred most commonly in infants at 2 to 7 weeks of age, are of short duration, and rarely occur after 7 weeks.

Treatment of ALTE is largely directed toward identifying a possible precipitating cause. In idiopathic ALTE, caffeine therapy has been used when apneas have been documented, although apnea is not consistently detected. One group successfully used acetazolamide for idiopathic ALTE, 7 mg/kg/day divided three times daily for 6 weeks.[73] This drug alters the pH in the cerebrospinal fluid and, presumably, the brain, thereby increasing the respiratory drive. Interestingly, this treatment also resulted in an improvement in baseline oxygen saturation. Additional trials are necessary to corroborate these findings and to investigate possible side effects.

APNEA AND GASTROESOPHAGEAL REFLUX DISEASE

Controversy shrouds the issue of GER and apnea. Although both are common in preterm infants, a cause-and-effect relationship has been difficult to prove. Infants with awake apneas have been described to have GER-related apnea events,[74] but they represent a very tiny portion of the overall ALTE or apnea population of patients. Thach and Menon reported a mechanism for apnea during reflux in a series of studies.[75,76] In these studies, instillation of a liquid into the oropharynx resulted in respiratory pauses and airway closure, followed by swallowing. This mechanism has also been postulated to occur in respiratory syncytial virus–associated apneas (see Fig. 36-2).

A myriad of studies investigating the association between apnea and GER has yielded equivocal results. Certainly, if such a temporal association exists, it is not a predominant cause of apnea and not a consistent finding. Treatment of AOP with antireflux medications has no consistent effect on improving apneas.[77] An example of a GER-related apnea is shown in Figure 36-6.

Variation in the identification of reflux accounts for some of the inconsistency. Although the pH probe has

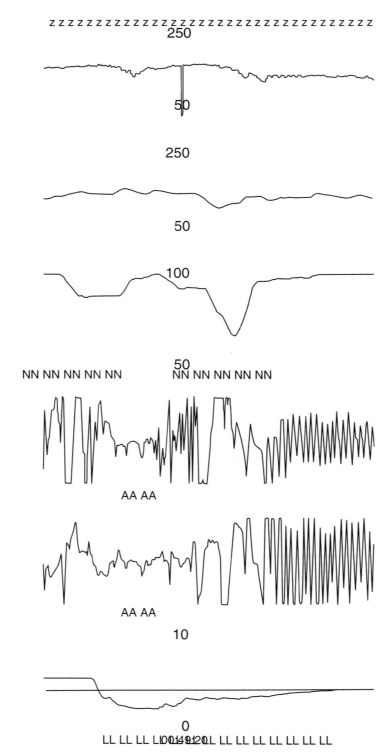

Figure 36–6. Multichannel recording showing the tracing of the esophageal pH probe channel at the bottom. The top tracing shows the heart rate trend from electrocardiography; the next tracing shows the heart rate pulse from the pulse oximeter; the third tracing shows the oxygen saturation; the fourth tracing is from the thermistor probe; and the fifth tracing shows chest wall impedance. A line is drawn across the pH probe channel at value of 4, the level considered to be significant acidosis. The infant had an oxygen desaturation associated with the onset of gastroesophageal reflux disease.

long been regarded as the "gold standard" for identification of GER, it is not an infallible method. This technique cannot detect the level to which reflux rises in the esophagus, for example, or whether the reflux is resulting in aspiration. The identification of postcibal reflux can be difficult to detect, especially when the infant is drinking a nonacidic (infant formula) liquid during the study. Glucose water and apple juice have an acidic pH and have been used in older infants during pH probe studies to help in the detection of postcibal events.

Thus, the use of a single pH probe to identify esophageal acid reflux in infants fed milk formula may result in missing postcibal episodes of reflux. Peter and colleagues,[78] moreover, reported the use of a new multiple intraluminal impedance technique to allow for detection of minuscule amounts of fluid moving in the esophagus. Although the 19 infants in their investigation were studied for only 6 hours each, more than 500 reflux episodes were detected, with 2000 apneas (median of 9-second duration) and 188 desaturations to less than 80%. Nevertheless, no temporal association was found between fluid reflux and apnea, bradycardia (heart rate <100), or desaturation. Only in 9 cases of the 188 desaturations did reflux precede the event. Apneas, bradycardias, or desaturations were as likely to occur during reflux as during no reflux episodes. Although this method may accurately detect minuscule volumes of fluid fluxes in the esophagus, their physiologic significance has yet to be reported. This study clearly demonstrated that reflux is more common and frequent than previously thought.

APPARENT LIFE-THREATENING EVENTS AND GASTROESOPHAGEAL REFLUX DISEASE

Infants commonly have episodes of spitting up after a feeding or before the next feeding without any physiologic or pathologic significance. Clinically significant reflux is that which results in recurrent aspiration pneumonia, failure to thrive, or recurrent ALTE. Infants with ALTE have more irregular breathing and obstructive apneas than do control infants.[79,80] Sheikh and associates[81] found that two thirds of their infants with ALTE had GER disease, documented either by pH probe or by barium swallow study. However, a temporal relationship between ALTE and GER has been difficult to document in many cases.[82]

APNEA MONITORS

Apnea monitors were first introduced in the 1970s after the studies of Steinschneider suggested a relationship between apnea and SIDS.[83] The family on which many of these studies was based, however, was later found to have asphyxiated their children, undermining much of the apnea hypothesis. The apnea theory of SIDS, however, placed apnea monitors at the forefront of preventative care. Apnea programs began to proliferate in the 1980s. However, although for many infants the apnea monitor alarms go on, most of these alarms are false.[84]

Nevertheless, monitors do provide some reassurance and empowerment for the caregivers, so that they can intervene when the monitor detects and sounds the alarm for serious events. Moreover, there are anecdotal reports of infants who experience a cyanotic episode that was detected by apnea monitoring, alerting the caregiver to initiate resuscitative efforts, thereby "saving" the infant. These episodes are tantamount to an ALTE. Without the warnings of an apnea monitor alarm, parents and physicians often question what might have happened to the infant had there been no monitor in place. In addition, there are numerous reports of infants who have had apnea monitors prescribed but who died while not on the monitor, which also reinforces the notion of the protective effect of these monitors.

Although monitors now capture and record events thought to be dangerous or pathologic, studies suggest that these severe events occur in normal full-term newborns.[9] Extreme events, defined as apneic episodes exceeding 30 seconds or accompanied by 10 seconds of bradycardia (heart rate < 60 beats per minute in infants younger than 44 weeks' PMA; heart rate < 50 beats per minute in infants 44 weeks' PMA or older), occurring after hospital discharge were seen even in full-term infants. However, these extreme events were found 18 times more frequently in symptomatic preterm infants and 10 times more frequently in asymptomatic preterm babies than in healthy full-term infants. Extreme events tended to recur in infants within 6 weeks of the prior event and were rare after 43 weeks' PMA. Thus, even "normal" full-term infants experience extreme events that are self-resolving (monitor alarm was off), which raises the significance of these episodes. It is conceivable that under certain circumstances, these events might become more serious if, for some reason, the child were not able to self-resuscitate.

In infants who have died while being monitored with event-recording apnea monitors, bradyarrhythmias have been the most common abnormal waveforms recorded, not central apnea. These findings suggest that severe hypoxemia was already present at the start of the recorded event.[85,86] Many infants in these studies were found to be gasping, a physiologic response to profound hypoxemia.

To determine how often full-term infants have hypoxemia, Hunt and coworkers described longitudinal data on oxygen saturations in full-term healthy newborns during the first 6 months of life.[87] They found that acute desaturation of less than 90% occurred in more than half of normal full-term infants. When hypoxemia was found, it often occurred more than once, and lasted more than 5 seconds. None of the infants in this study received any kind of intervention. In preterm infants, normative oximetry data were reported by Poets and associates.[14] Among preterm infants with a history of ALTE, oxygenation was found to be abnormal in more than 50%, and clinically undetected baseline hypoxemia was present in more than 20%.

The use of apnea monitors varies considerably from region to region. Although one hospital may monitor many of its infants after discharge, others, virtually next door, may not. This variation confirms that there is no real standard of care for apnea monitors.[88] Indeed, researchers from Pediatrix, a large national association of neonatologists with geographically diverse NICUs, have shown that the discharging physician's preference was the most dependent variable related to an infant's discharge with an apnea monitor.[89] Contrary to what would be expected, they also found that discharge with an apnea monitor was not associated with a shorter length of hospital stay. In fact, other studies have linked apnea monitor discharge with a higher rate of rehospitalization,[59,90] perhaps because of the need to reevaluate the reasons for apnea monitor alarms.

Indications for apnea monitoring after discharge therefore vary greatly among physicians. Searching for a margin of safety for discharge,[91] or the "safe" time interval between the last noted clinical event and the time of discharge, is arbitrary at best. Difficulties lie in the definition of "significant event" and the method of detecting such events (nursing documentation versus cardiorespiratory monitoring surveillance). Nevertheless, there are clinical indicators that are used to determine readiness for discharge home from the NICU. These include the ability of the infant to feed and grow, to maintain body temperature in an open crib, and to have cardiorespiratory stability. In NICUs with apnea programs, infants with unresolved AOP or infants who have suffered a significant ALTE are often discharged with an apnea monitor.

Unresolved AOP can be defined as the persistence of apneic events for which some kind of intervention is required before discharge. Use of methylxanthines is not necessarily an indication for home monitoring. Infants with controlled apnea, specifically those with no nursing intervention within a week and a normal event recording, may be safely discharged on methylxanthine therapy without a monitor.[59] Using this approach, we have identified a population at high risk who are monitored and a group at lower risk whose AOP is well controlled with medication. It must be remembered, however, that an occasional infant may have increasing apnea as the methylxanthine level decreases, and a home monitor can alert caregivers to that possibility.

Infants with an ALTE are often prescribed a home monitor, especially children who needed resuscitation to resolve their event. Other infants for whom home apnea monitoring should be considered are those with severe bradycardia with feedings, those with bronchopulmonary dysplasia who are receiving supplemental oxygen, those with tracheostomy, and those with orofacial malformations that result in recurring obstructive apneas (e.g., Pierre Robin syndrome)[92] and siblings of a SIDS victim whose parents desire monitoring.

The prescription of apnea monitors simply requires a prescription from a physician and a letter describing medical necessity with the diagnosis that justifies its use. Clearly, the difficulty lies not with the prescribing of the monitor but in the follow-up of the patient until the monitor can be safely discontinued. Caregivers need to learn how to respond to the monitor alarms, when to notify the apnea program about a problem, when to call the respiratory company (which rented the monitor to them) for an equipment problem, and when to call the infant's primary care provider. Parents must be trained in infant cardiopulmonary resuscitation and must be instructed not to intervene immediately for every monitor alarm. Hence, before prescribing an apnea monitor for an infant, the physician must consider whether it is really necessary for the patient and whether the parents can handle both the equipment and any potential interventions that may be necessary.

Indications for discontinuation of home apnea monitoring depend largely on the initial indication for monitoring. Infants who are monitored for unresolved AOP should be monitored until the AOP has resolved. This generally occurs within a few weeks after 40 weeks' PMA. Some infants, however, may manifest apnea well beyond their original due date. Some of the most prematurely born infants may take a longer time to resolve their apnea.[93] Thus, a "normal" monitor download after stopping methylxanthines is often a prerequisite for discontinuation. In general, most preterm infants discharged with an apnea monitor are younger than 36 weeks' PMA and are off their monitor by 42 weeks' PMA.[24,59,94]

For infants who are monitored for idiopathic ALTE, monitoring is generally continued for some event-free interval. Many programs use a 2-month event-free interval as one criterion for discontinuation of the monitor. A shorter period of time is reasonable, in view of data from the CHIME study,[9] showing that extreme events (see previous description) tend to not recur after 6 weeks. Monitoring of infants with ALTE in which the cause of the event was identified may not be necessary. However, when they are monitored, a similar event-free interval may be used as a criterion for discontinuation.

Siblings of infants who have died of SIDS are sometimes monitored in an attempt to prevent death in the sibling. This is based on the assumption that monitors can prevent SIDS and that such siblings are at greater risk for an adverse outcome. However, monitors have not been shown to prevent SIDS, and such siblings may not be at greater risk for SIDS.[92] Data from several studies are equivocal about this point. Nevertheless, when these siblings are placed on apnea monitors, indications used for discontinuation include the anniversary date of death or age of the SIDS victim or 6 months of age in the sibling, whichever is earlier.

REFERENCES

1. Barrington K, Finer N: The natural history of the appearance of apnea of prematurity. Pediatr Res 29:372, 1991.
2. Jones RA: Apnea of immaturity. 1. A controlled trial of theophylline and face mask continuous positive airway pressure. Arch Dis Child 57:761, 1982.
3. Upton CJ, Milner AD, Stokes GM: Apnea, bradycardia, and oxygen saturation in preterm infants. Arch Dis Child 66:381, 1991.
4. Hiatt IM, Hegyi T, Indyk L, et al: Continuous monitoring of PO_2 during apnea of prematurity. J Pediatr 98:288, 1981.
5. Boros SJ, Reynolds JW: Prolonged apnea of prematurity: Treatment with continuous airway distending pressure delivered by nasopharyngeal tube. Clin Pediatr 15:123, 1976.

6. Gerhardt T, Bancalari E: Apnea of prematurity: I. Lung function and regulation of breathing. Pediatrics 74:58, 1984.

7. Lagercrantz H, Broberger U, Milerad J, von Euler C: Ventilatory studies in two older infants with prolonged apnea. Acta Paediatr Scand 69:545, 1980.

8. Little GA, Ballard RA, Brooks JG, et al: National Institutes of Health Consensus Development Conference on Infantile Apnea and Home Monitoring, Sept 29 to Oct 1, 1986. Pediatrics 79:292, 1987.

9. Ramanathan R, Corwin MJ, Hunt CE, et al: Cardiorespiratory events recorded on home monitors: Comparison of healthy infants with those at increased risk of SIDS. JAMA 285:2199, 2001.

10. Ruggins NR: Pathophysiology of apnea in preterm infants. Arch Dis Child 66:70, 1991.

11. Spitzer AR, Fox WW: Infant apnea. Pediatr Clin N Am 33:561, 1986.

12. Southall DP, Levitt GA, Richards JM, et al: Undetected episodes of prolonged apnea and severe bradycardia in preterm infants. Pediatrics 72:541, 1983.

13. Samuels MP, Poets CF, Stebbens VA, et al: Oxygen saturation and breathing patterns in preterm infants with cyanotic episodes. Acta Paediatr 81:875, 1992.

14. Poets CF, Samuels MP, Southall DP: Epidemiology and pathophysiology of apnea of prematurity. Biol Neonate 65:211, 1994.

15. Barrington KJ, Finer N, Li D: Predischarge respiratory recordings in very low birth weight newborn infants. J Pediatr 129:934, 1996.

16. Weese-Mayer DE, Corwin MJ, Peucker MR, et al: Comparison of apnea identified by respiratory inductance plethysmography with that detected by end-tidal CO_2 or thermistor. Am J Respir Crit Care Med 162:471, 2000.

17. Carbone T, Marrero LC, Weiss J, et al: Heart rate and oxygen saturation correlates of infant apnea. J Perinatol 19:44, 1999.

18. Brazy JE, Kinney HC, Oakes WJ: Central nervous system structural lesions causing apnea at birth. J Pediatr 111:163, 1987.

19. Poets CF, Stebbens VA, Alexander JR, et al: Oxygenation and breathing patterns in infancy. 2: Preterm infants at discharge from special care. Arch Dis Child 66:574, 1991.

20. Parkins KJ, Poets CF, O'Brien LM, et al: Effect of exposure to 15% oxygen on breathing pattern and oxygen saturation in infants: An interventional study. BMJ 316:887, 1998.

21. Simakajornboun N, Beckerman RC, Mack C, et al: Effect of supplemental oxygen on sleep architecture and cardiorespiratory events in preterm infants. Pediatrics 110:884, 2002.

22. Kelly DH, Shannon DC: Periodic breathing in infants with near-miss sudden infant death syndrome. Pediatrics 63:355, 1979.

23. Carlo WA, Martin RJ, Versteegh FG, et al: Effect of respiratory distress syndrome on chest wall movements and respiratory pauses in preterm infants. Am Rev Respir Dis 126:103, 1982.

24. DeCristofaro JD, Biswas S, Nitu M, Katz S: Apnea of prematurity, length of stay, and NICU admission in 31-34 weeks gestational age multiple births. Pediatr Res 44:994A, 1998.

25. Koons AH, Mojica N, Jadeja N, et al: Neurodevelopmental outcome of infants with apnea of infancy. Am J Perinatol 10:208, 1993.

26. Nelson RM, Resnick MB, Holstrum WJ, Eitzman DV: Developmental outcome of premature infants treated with theophylline. Dev Pharmacol Ther 1:274, 1980.

27. Cheung PY, Barrington KJ, Finer NN, Robertson CM: Early childhood neurodevelopment in very low birth weight infants with predischarge apnea. Pediatr Pulmonol 27:14, 1999.

28. Perlman JM, Volpe JJ: Episodes of apnea and bradycardia in the preterm newborn: Impact on cerebral circulation. Pediatrics 76:333, 1985.

29. Livera LN, Spencer SA, Thorniley MS, et al: Effects of hypoxaemia and bradycardia on neonatal cerebral haemodynamics. Arch Dis Child 66:376, 1991.

30. Pratesi S, Donzelli G: Evaluation of cerebral oxygenation in newborns with prematurity apnea: New frequency domain NIR oximeter. Acta Biomedica Ateneo Parmense 71(Suppl 1): 609, 2000.

31. Urlesberger B, Kaspirek A, Pichler G, Muller W: Apnoea of prematurity and changes in cerebral oxygenation and cerebral blood volume. Neuropediatrics 30:29, 1999.

32. Jenni OG, Wolf M, Hengartner M, et al: Impact of central, obstructive and mixed apnea on cerebral hemodynamics in preterm infants. Biol Neonate 70:91, 1996.

33. Watkin SL, Spencer SA, Dimmock PW, et al: A comparison of pulse oximetry and near infrared spectroscopy (NIRS) in the detection of hypoxaemia occurring with pauses in nasal airflow in neonates. J Clin Monit Comp 15:441, 1999.

34. Urlesberger B, Pichler G, Gradnitzer E, et al: Changes in cerebral blood volume and cerebral oxygenation during periodic breathing in term infants. Neuropediatrics 31:75, 2000.

35. Pichler G, Schomlzer G, Muller W, Urlesberger B: Body position–dependent changes in cerebral hemodynamics during apnea in preterm infants. Brain Devel 23:395, 2001.

36. Miller MJ, Carlo WA, Martin RJ: Continuous positive airway pressure selectively reduces obstructive apnea in preterm infants. J Pediatr 106:91, 1985.

37. Ryan CA, Finer NN, Peters KL: Intermittent positive pressure ventilation offers no advantage over nasal continuous positive airway pressure in apnea of prematurity. Am J Dis Child 143:1196, 1989.

38. Lin C-H, Wang S-T, Lin Y-J, Yeh T-F: Efficacy of nasal intermittent positive pressure ventilation in treating apnea of prematurity. Pediatr Pulmonol 26:349, 1998.

39. Lemyre B, Davis PG, DePaoli AG: Nasal intermittent positive pressure ventilation (NIPPV) versus nasal continuous positive airway pressure (NCPAP) for apnea of prematurity. Cochrane Database Syst Rev (1):CD002272, 2002.

40. Kuzemko JA, Paala J: Apnoeic attacks in the newborn treated with aminophylline. Arch Dis Child 48:404, 1973.

41. Scanlon JEM, Chin KC, Morgan MEI, et al: Caffeine or theophylline for neonatal apnea? Arch Dis Child 67:425, 1992.

42. Bauer J, Maier K, Linderkamp O, Hentschel R: Effect of caffeine on oxygen consumption and metabolic rate in very low birth weight infants with idiopathic apnea. Pediatrics 107:660, 2001.

43. Hoecker C, Nelle M, Poeschl J, et al: Caffeine impairs cerebral and intestinal blood flow velocity in preterm infants. Pediatrics 109:784, 2002.

44. Davis JM, Metrakos K, Aranda JV: Apnea and seizures. Arch Dis Child 61:791, 1986.

45. Ergenekon E, Dalgi N, Assot E, et al: Caffeine intoxication in a preterm neonate. Paediatr Anaesth 11:737, 2001.

46. Henderson-Smart DJ, Steer P: Methylxanthine treatment for apnea in preterm infants. Cochrane Database Syst Rev (3):CD000140, 2001.

47. Aranda JV, Gorman W, Bergsteinsson H, Gunn T: Efficacy of caffeine in the treatment of apnea in the low-birth-weight infant. J Pediatr 90:467, 1977.

48. LeGuennec J-C, Brillon B, Pare C: Maturational changes of caffeine concentration and disposition in infancy during maintenance therapy for apnea of prematurity: Influence of gestational age, hepatic disease, and breast-feeding. Pediatrics 76:834, 1985.

49. Al-Alaiyan S, al-Rawithi S, Rains D, et al: Caffeine metabolism in preterm infants. J Clin Pharmacol 41:620, 2001.

50. Maillard C, Boutroy MJ, Fresson J, et al: QT interval lengthening in preterm infants treated with doxapram. Clin Pharmacol Therap 70:540, 2001.

51. Sreenan C, Etches PC, Demianczuk N, Robertson CM: Isolated mental developmental delay in very low birth weight infants: Association with prolonged doxapram therapy for apnea. J Pediatr 139:832, 2001.

52. O'Donnel J, Finer NN, Rich W, et al: Role of L-carnitine in apnea of prematurity: A randomized controlled trial. Pediatrics 109:622, 2002.

53. Whitfield J, Smith T, Sollohub H, et al: Clinical effects of L-carnitine supplement on apnea and growth in very low birth weight infants. Pediatrics 111:477, 2003.

54. Dimaguila MAVT, Di Fiore JM, Martin RJ, Miller MJ: Characteristics of hypoxemic episodes in very low birth weight infants on ventilatory support. J Pediatr 130:577, 1997.

55. Goto K, Mirmiran M, Adams MM, et al: More awakenings and heart rate variability during supine sleep in preterm infants. Pediatrics 103:603, 1999.

56. Razi NM, DeLauter M, Pandit PB: Periodic breathing and oxygen saturation in preterm infants at discharge. J Perinatol 22:442, 2002.

57. Graff M, Soriano C, Rovell K, et al: Undetected apnea and bradycardia in infants. Pediatr Pulmonol 11:195, 1991.

58. Spear ML, Stefano H, Spitzer AR: Prolonged apnea and oxyhemoglobin desaturation in asymptomatic preterm infants. Pediatr Pulmonol 13:151, 1992.

59. Subhani M, Katz S, DeCristofaro JD: Prediction of post-discharge complications by predischarge event recordings in infants with apnea of prematurity. J Perinatol 20:92, 2000.

60. Eichenwald EC, Blackwell M, Lloyd JS, et al: Inter-neonatal intensive care unit variation in discharge timing: Influence of apnea and feeding management. Pediatrics 108:928, 2001.

61. Edner A, Katz-Salamon M, Lagerkrantz H, et al: Heart rate variability in infants with apparent life-threatening events. Acta Pediatr 89:1326, 2000.

62. Hunt CE: Apnea and SIDS. In Kliegman RM, Nieder ML, Super DM (eds): Practical Strategies in Pediatric Diagnosis and Therapy. Philadelphia, WB Saunders, 1996, pp 135-147.

63. Leistner HL, Haddad GG, Epstein RA, et al: Heart rate and heart rate variability during sleep in aborted SIDS. J Pediatr 97:51, 1980.

64. Pincus SM, Cummins TR, Haddad GG: Heart rate control in normal and aborted-SIDS infants. Am J Physiol 264:R638, 1993.

65. Poets CF, Samuels MP, Noyes JP, et al: Home event recordings of oxygenation, breathing movements and heart rate and rhythm in infants with recurrent life-threatening event. Pediatrics 123:693, 1993.

66. Ruggins NR, Milner AD: Site of upper airway obstruction in infants following an apparent life-threatening event. Pediatrics 91:595, 1993.

67. Guilleminault C, Pelayo R, Leger D, Philip P: Apparent life-threatening events, facial dysmorphia and sleep-disordered breathing. Eur J Pediatr 159:444, 2000.

68. Guilleminault C, Pelayo R, Leger D, et al: Sleep-disordered breathing and upper-airway anomalies in first-degree relatives of ALTE children. Pediatr Res 50:14, 2001.

69. Tal Y, Tirosh E, Even L, Jaffe M: A comparison of the yield of a 24 h versus 72 h hospital evaluation in infants with apparent life-threatening events. Eur J Pediatr 158:954, 1999.

70. Byard RW, Burnell RH: Covert video surveillance in Munchausen syndrome by proxy. Ethical compromise or essential technique? Med J Aust 160:352, 1994.

71. Brouillette RT, Tsirigotis D, Leimanis A, et al: Computerised audiovisual event recording for infant apnoea and brady-cardia. Med Biol Eng Comp 38:477, 2000.

72. Kato I, Franco P, Groswasses J, et al: Frequency of obstructive and mixed sleep apneas in 1,023 infants. Sleep 23:487, 2000.

73. Philippi H, Bieber I, Reitter B: Acetazolamide treatment for infantile central apnea. J Clin Neurol 16:600, 2001.

74. Spitzer AR, Boyde JT, Tuchman DN: Awake apnea-relationship to gastroesophageal reflux. J Pediatr 104:200, 1984.

75. Thach BT, Menon A: Pulmonary protective mechanisms in human infants. Am Rev Respir Dis 131:S55, 1985.

76. Thach BT: Reflux associated apnea in infants: Evidence for a laryngeal chemoreflex. Am J Med 103:120S, 1997.

77. Kimball AL, Carlton DP: Gastroesophageal reflux medications in the treatment of apnea in premature infants. J Pediatr 138:355, 2001.

78. Peter CF, Sprodowski N, Bohnhorst B, et al: Gastroesophageal reflux and apnea of prematurity: No temporal relationship. Pediatrics 109:8, 2002.

79. Guilleminault C, Ariagno R, Korobkin R, et al: Mixed and obstructive sleep apnea and near-miss for SIDS: 2. Comparisons of near-miss and normal infants by age. Pediatrics 64:882, 1979.

80. Kahn A, Blum D, Waterschoot P, et al: Effects of obstructive sleep apneas and transcutaneous oxygen pressure in control infants, siblings of sudden infant death syndrome victims, and near miss infants: Comparison with the effects of central apneas. Pediatrics 70:852, 1982.

81. Sheikh S, Stephen T, Fraser A, Eid N: Apparent life-threatening episodes in infants. Clin Pulmonol Med 7:81, 2000.

82. Arad-Cohen N, Cohen A, Tirosh E: The relationship between gastroesophageal reflux and apnea in infants. J Pediatr 137:321, 2000.

83. Steinschneider A: Prolonged apnea and the sudden infant death syndrome: Clinical and laboratory observations. Pediatrics 50:646, 1972.

84. Weese-Mayer DE, Silvestri JM: Documented monitoring: An alarming turn of events. Clin Perinatol 19:891, 1992.

85. Poets CF, Meny RG, Chobanian MR, Bonofiglo RE: Gasping and other cardiorespiratory patterns during sudden infant deaths. Pediatr Res 45:350, 1999.

86. Meny RG, Carroll JL, Carbone MT, Kelly DH: Cardio-respiratory recordings from infants dying suddenly and unexpectedly at home. Pediatrics 93:44, 1994.

87. Hunt CE, Corwin MJ, Lister G, et al: Longitudinal assessment of hemoglobin oxygen saturation in healthy infants during the first 6 months of age. J Pediatr 135:580, 1999.

88. Meadows W, Mendez D, Lantos J, et al: What is the legal "standard of medical care" when there is no standard medical care? A survey of the use of home apnea monitoring by neonatology fellowship training programs in the United States. Pediatrics 89:1083, 1992.

89. Perfect Sychowski S, Dodd E, Thomas P, et al: Home apnea monitor use in preterm infants discharged from newborn intensive care units. J Pediatr 139:245, 2001.

90. Malloy MH, Graumbard B: Access to home apnea monitoring and its impact on rehospitalization among very low birth weight infants. Arch Pediatr Adolesc Med 149:326, 1995.

91. Darnall RA, Kattwinkel J, Nattie C, Robinson M: Margin of safety for discharge after apnea in preterm infants. Pediatrics 100:795, 1997.

92. Committee on Fetus and Newborn, American Academy of Pediatrics: Apnea, sudden infant death syndrome, and home monitoring. Pediatr 111:914, 2003.

93. Eichenwald EC, Aina A, Stark AR: Apnea frequently persists beyond term gestation in infants delivered at 24 to 28 weeks. Pediatrics 100:354, 1997.

94. Nwokolo N, Nitu M, Katz S, DeCristofaro JD: Resolution of apnea of prematurity in 24-28 week gestational age infants is no different from preterms 31-34 weeks gestational age. Pediatr Res 45:1480A, 1999.

CHAPTER 37

Sudden Infant Death Syndrome

Carl E. Hunt

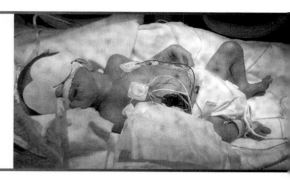

Sudden infant death syndrome (SIDS) is defined as the death of an infant that is sudden, unexpected by history, and unexplained by a thorough postmortem examination, which includes a complete autopsy, investigation of the scene of death, and review of the medical history.[1] An autopsy is essential in all sudden and unexpected infant deaths because the history and investigation of the scene do not exclude all known causes of sudden infant death, including unsuspected congenital abnormalities and fatal child abuse.

Comprising over 8% of all infant mortality in the United States, SIDS was the third leading cause of infant mortality in 2001, ranked below congenital anomalies (20%) and disorders relating to short gestation/low birth weight (16%). About 2230 infants died of SIDS in the United States in 2001, a rate of 0.55 per 1000 live births, and preliminary data suggest a lower rate for 2002.[2]

SIDS is the most common cause of postneonatal infant mortality in developed countries, generally accounting for 40% to 50% of infant deaths between 1 month and 1 year of age and about 20% of all deaths in infants discharged from a neonatal intensive care unit (NICU). Among full-term infants, SIDS is rare before 1 month of age; the incidence peaks at 2 to 4 months of age, and 95% of all cases have occurred by 6 months of age. In preterm infants, SIDS occurs at a younger postconceptional age but older postnatal age than in full-term infants.[3]

PATHOLOGY

There is no autopsy finding pathognomonic of SIDS, and no finding is required for the diagnosis. There are, however, some common findings.[4] Petechial hemorrhages are found in more than 90% of cases and may be more extensive than in other causes of infant mortality. Pulmonary edema is often present and may be substantial.

Autopsy studies demonstrate structural evidence (tissue markers) indicative of preexisting, chronic low-grade asphyxia in nearly two thirds of SIDS victims.[5] These tissue markers include persistence of adrenal brown fat, hepatic erythropoiesis, brain stem gliosis, and other structural abnormalities. In addition to astrogliosis, the brain stem abnormalities include persistent dendritic spines and hypomyelination.[6] The primary areas of persisting brain stem dendritic spines are in the magnocellular nucleus of the reticular formation and dorsal and solitary nuclei of the vagal nerve. Significant increases in the number of reactive astrocytes in the medulla have also been observed in SIDS victims; these increases are not confined to areas related to respiratory neuroregulation.[7] Substance P, a neuropeptide transmitter found in selected sensory neurons of the central nervous system, is present in increased amounts in the pons of SIDS victims.[8] Quantitative three-dimensional anatomic studies indicate that a small subset of SIDS victims has hypoplasia of the arcuate nucleus; this region is a site of cardiorespiratory control in the ventral medulla and is integrated with other regions that regulate arousal, autonomic function, and chemosensory function.[9] Neurotransmitter studies have also identified receptor abnormalities in the arcuate nucleus in some SIDS victims, including significant decreases in binding to kainate receptors, muscarinic cholinergic receptors, and serotonergic receptors.[10] There is a positive correlation between decreased density of muscarinic cholinergic and kainate receptors. The neurotransmitter deficits in the arcuate nucleus in SIDS victims thus involve more than one receptor type relevant to autonomic control overall and especially to cardiorespiratory control, including arousal responsiveness. Finally, tyrosine hydroxylase immunoreactivity in two brain stem areas, vagal nuclei and the reticularis superficialis ventrolateralis, suggests that adrenaline and noradrenalin neurons are altered in SIDS victims.[11,12]

Other postmortem observations are also consistent with preexisting, low-grade, chronic asphyxia. SIDS infants as a group have both prenatal and postnatal growth restriction and elevated blood cortisol levels.[5,13] Vascular endothelial growth factor, which is up-regulated by hypoxia, is elevated in the cerebrospinal fluid of SIDS victims in comparison with controls, which confirms that SIDS is preceded by hypoxia and suggests that it is prolonged hypoxia.[14] The elevated levels of hypoxanthine in vitreous humor observed in SIDS victims further indicate a relatively long period of tissue hypoxia preceding death.[15] Because adenosine, a precursor of hypoxanthine, is a respiratory inhibitor, these observations thus indicate a potentially important interaction between asphyxia and hypoventilation; in response to asphyxia from any cause, the secondary acceleration of adenosine monophosphate catabolism and adenosine accumulation creates a vicious cycle, leading to progressive hypoventilation.

RISK FACTORS FOR SIDS

Genetic Risk Factors

Sequencing the approximately 30,000 genes in the human genome is resulting in fundamental changes in the way physicians think about the role of specific gene products in facilitating adverse pathophysiologic responses that result in SIDS.[16] To the extent that impaired neural control of breathing is relevant to SIDS, data linking specific genotypes to brain stem regulation of breathing control are rapidly accumulating. Adaptation to an environmental risk such as hypoxia, for example, involves complex regulation of gene expression in precise brain stem sites, and normal postnatal cardiorespiratory control depends on genes that control prenatal development.

Neural control of breathing and sleep are closely integrated, and abnormalities in regulation of sleep and circadian rhythmicity can thus result in impairments in cardiorespiratory integration and arousal responsiveness from sleep.[17] Circadian rhythmicity has been extensively studied in animals, and homologous counterparts of essential circadian clock genes isolated in *Drosophila* species have been identified in mammals.[16] Because the sleep-wake cycle is under control of the circadian clock, these circadian master genes, as well other sleep-related genes, probably influence sleep regulation.

Targeted gene inactivation studies in animals have identified several genes involved with prenatal brain stem development of respiratory control, including arousal responsiveness.[16] During embryogenesis, for example, the survival of specific cellular populations that constitute the respiratory neuronal network is regulated by neurotrophins, a multigene family of growth factors and receptors. Brain-derived neurotrophic factor is required for development of normal breathing behavior in mice; newborn mice lacking this factor exhibit ventilatory depression in association with apparent loss of peripheral chemoafferent input.[17] Ventilation is depressed, and hypoxic ventilatory drive is deficient or absent.

Krox-20, a homeobox gene important for hindbrain morphogenesis, also appears to be required for normal development of the respiratory central pattern generator.[18] Animals with *Krox-20*–null mutations exhibit an abnormally slow respiratory rhythm and increased incidence of respiratory pauses, and this respiratory depression can be further modulated by endogenous enkephalins. Inactivation of *Krox-20* may result in absence of a rhythm-promoting reticular neuronal group localized in the caudal pons and could thus be a cause of life-threatening apnea.[16]

Brain stem muscarinic cholinergic pathways are important in ventilatory responsiveness to CO_2.[16] The muscarinic system develops from the neural crest, and the *ret* protooncogene is important for this development. *Ret* knockout mice have a depressed ventilatory response to hypercarbia, which implicates absence of the *ret* gene as a cause of impaired hypercarbic responsiveness and hence potentially relevant to SIDS. Diminished ventilatory responsiveness to hypercarbia has also been demonstrated in male newborn mice heterozygous for *Mash-1*.[19] There is a molecular link between *ret* and *Mash-1,* and the latter is expressed in embryonic neurons before the former in vagal neural crest derivatives and in brain stem locus coeruleus neurons, an area involved with arousal responsiveness. *Mash-1* may thus be involved in respiratory control development through mechanisms linked to the X chromosome. Abnormality of this gene is one possible genetic basis for the increased frequency of SIDS among boys and for the impaired arousal responsiveness thought to be critically important in the pathophysiologic process of SIDS.[16,20]

Serotonin exerts potent excitatory effects on respiratory control in the brain. Many genes are involved in the control of serotonin synthesis, storage, membrane uptake, and metabolism of serotonin. The transporter gene is located on chromosome 17, and variations in the promoter region of the serotonin transporter gene appear to have a role in serotonin membrane uptake and regulation. Several transporter polymorphisms have been described, including one in the promoter region; the long ("L") allele increases effectiveness of the promoter and hence would lead to reduced serotonin concentrations at nerve endings in comparison to the short ("S") allele. The "L/L" genotype is associated with increased serotonin transporters on neuroimaging and increased postmortem binding. Studies in white, African American, and Japanese infants indicate that SIDS victims are more likely than controls to have the "L" allele.[21]

Environmental Risk Factors

A number of environmental risk factors have been associated with SIDS.[20] Some of these risk factors may directly increase risk for SIDS, whereas others may be surrogates for more fundamental underlying disorders. The modifiable environmental risk factors (e.g., sleep position) have been the focus of targeted risk-reduction campaigns that have resulted in substantial reductions in the prevalence of SIDS.

Nonmodifiable Environmental Risk Factors

Lower socioeconomic status is associated with higher risk for SIDS.[20] Rates of SIDS are two to three times higher among Native American and African American infants than among white, Hispanic, and Asian/Pacific Islander infants. Although one explanation for these higher rates may be a higher concentration of socioeconomic risk factors, further study is needed to better understand the causes of racial disparity in SIDS in order to intervene appropriately. Boys are 30% to 50% more likely to be affected than girls, although this male predominance has not been found among native populations in the United States, Australia, or New Zealand (e.g., Native American, Eskimo, aborigine, Maori). There is also a seasonal pattern for SIDS: Cases occur two to three times more commonly in cold seasons than in the warmer months.

Modifiable Environmental Risk Factors

All of these risk factors are at least potentially modifiable.[20] Some (e.g., sleep position) have been amenable to postnatal intervention, but many require a change in behavior before or during pregnancy (e.g., cigarette smoke exposure). Some, such as prematurity, are still at best only partially modifiable. SIDS victims are more commonly of higher birth order, independent of maternal age, and the condition is associated with a short interpregnancy interval. The incidence of SIDS is higher among infants with low birth weight, preterm infants, and those with intrauterine growth restriction. Mothers of SIDS victims generally receive less prenatal care and initiate care later in pregnancy; a two to three times higher risk is associated with late or no prenatal care. An increased SIDS risk is associated with numerous obstetric factors, which suggests that the in utero environment of future SIDS victims is suboptimal. Relative growth failure is evident postnatally and prenatally. The number of postnatal routine care visits and of immunizations is significantly less for SIDS victims than for normal infants, which suggests that postnatal care is also suboptimal. SIDS is associated with reported illness in the last 2 weeks of life and an increased frequency of doctor's office visits in the last week, especially for gastrointestinal illness and/or appearing droopy or listless. Future SIDS victims have also been observed to have repeated fatigue during feedings and profuse sweating during sleep. The fatigue is unexplained except insofar as it may be secondary to an intercurrent acute illness. The sweating may be explained by intercurrent febrile illness, by thermal stress related to prone sleep position, or by overbundling, but it could also be indicative of an autonomic deficit.[16,20]

Sleeping position. The declines in SIDS rates of 50% or more occurring in numerous countries since 1992 can be attributed largely to reductions from placing babies prone for sleep. A meta-analysis of 17 case-control studies published before 1993 revealed a combined odds ratio of 2.8 (95% confidence interval [CI] = 2.1 to 3.6) for SIDS in infants sleeping in the prone position.[20] Studies published since 1992 have confirmed this strong association between prone sleeping and SIDS. These dramatic decreases in SIDS rates have generally not been associated with significant decreases in other risk behaviors. The 40% reduction in SIDS rates in the United States during the period 1992 to 1998 as prone prevalence decreased by approximately 50%, however, was also associated with a 25% decrease in maternal reporting of smoking during pregnancy.

As prone sleeping rates have declined after SIDS risk reduction campaigns, side sleeping has emerged as an independent risk factor for SIDS, with a relative risk of 2.0 in comparison with supine sleeping. As a result, the

American Academy of Pediatrics has recommended since 1996 that supine sleeping be the preferred sleeping position for all infants.[22]

In addition to prone and side sleeping, unsafe sleeping practices also include soft sleep surfaces and soft bedding.[20] Soft bedding, covers over the head, and sleeping under a comforter (duvet) have also emerged as more significant risk factors as prone prevalence has decreased. Bed sharing has been implicated as another risk factor for SIDS risk, but studies have not classified risk for SIDS according to reason for bed sharing and have only partially adjusted for other pertinent risk factors.

Attention has also focused on the potential role of unaccustomed prone sleeping (infants usually placed nonprone but placed prone for the last sleep) and secondary prone sleeping (infants placed nonprone for sleep but found prone).[20] Both secondary prone sleeping and unaccustomed prone sleeping have been associated with significantly higher risk for SIDS than has usually sleeping prone, especially for infants usually sleeping supine.[23] About 20% of all SIDS deaths in the United States occur in child care settings,[24] and these deaths have been associated at least in part with secondary or unaccustomed prone sleeping.

When the recommendation for nonprone sleeping was originally released, there was concern that supine sleeping could be associated with an increase in adverse consequences such as aspiration, vomiting, and trouble sleeping. Subsequent studies, however, have not identified any adverse consequences of supine sleeping in comparison with prone sleeping.[25] No symptom or illness was increased among nonprone sleepers during the first 6 months, and some illnesses were actually less common, especially ear infections. Aspiration has not been observed to occur more frequently in infants sleeping supine, and aspiration deaths have not increased in the United Kingdom despite prone prevalence rates as low as 2%. In addition, infants sleeping supine do not appear to be at increased risk for episodes of apnea or cyanosis.

Preterm infants were initially excluded from "back-to-sleep" campaigns. This exclusion was based on data at younger postnatal ages indicating that ventilation was optimal when the infant slept prone, especially when still symptomatic from hyaline membrane disease. Studies have since confirmed, however, that both preterm and full-term infants are at greater risk for SIDS when sleeping prone or on the side.[20] The odds ratios for SIDS at birth weights of less than 2500 g are 83 and 36.6 for prone and side sleeping, respectively, and the odds ratios at less than 37 weeks' gestational age are 48.8 and 40.5, respectively. When preterm infants are sufficiently mature and healthy to be discharged home without supplemental oxygen, there is no clinically significant impairment in respiratory status when they are sleeping supine in comparison with prone. The American Academy of Pediatrics has therefore recommended since 2000 that all infants sleep supine at home, regardless of gestational age at birth,[22] but adherence to this recommendation remains limited. Infants weighing less than 1500 g at birth are more likely to be placed to sleep in the prone position at home than are infants with a birth weight of 1500 to 2499 g (26% versus 14%) even though risk for SIDS is higher at birth weights of less than 1500 g than at more than 1500 g.[26] Strategies are needed to reassure health care providers that the supine position for sleeping is as safe and effective in preterm as in full-term infants and that they should model safe sleeping practices in the NICU as the discharge planning process begins.

Smoking. Maternal smoking during pregnancy has consistently been associated with increased risk of SIDS.[20] The relative risk is in the range of 4.7 and represents one of the most significant modifiable risk factors after declines in prone sleeping. There appears to be a small independent effect of paternal smoking during pregnancy, but studies examining the influence of other household members have been inconsistent. Infants dying from SIDS tend to have higher concentrations of nicotine in their lungs than do control infants, regardless of reported smoking exposure.[27] Elimination of prenatal exposure to cigarette smoke could theoretically reduce the risk of SIDS approximately 30% to 40%.[28] It is difficult to assess the independent effect of postnatal exposure to cigarette smoke because smoking exposure during and after pregnancy are highly correlated, but studies do suggest that eliminating postnatal exposure to environmental cigarette smoke might further reduce risk for SIDS. In some studies of bed sharing as a risk factor for SIDS, this association has been linked with postnatal maternal smoking.

There are several potential mechanisms to explain why cigarette smoke exposure is a risk factor for SIDS. Maternal smoking can potentiate hyperplasia of pulmonary neuroendocrine cells, and dysfunction of these cells may contribute to the pathophysiologic process of SIDS.[16] Both animal and clinical studies indicate decreased ventilatory and arousal responsiveness to hypoxia after fetal exposure to nicotine.[29] The age-specific attenuation of hypoxic defenses after nicotine exposure is suggestive of impaired brain catecholamine metabolism. In vitro studies suggest that smoking increases risk for SIDS through greater susceptibility to viral and bacterial infections and enhanced bacterial binding after passive coating of mucosal surfaces with smoke components.[30]

Exposure to drugs or alcohol. Most studies, after adjusting for cigarette smoke exposure, have not identified an association between SIDS and maternal alcohol use during or after pregnancy.[20] One study among Northern Plains Indians, however, identified an increased frequency of binge drinking during pregnancy of 73% in mothers of SIDS victims, in comparison with 45% in control mothers.[31]

Maternal drug use during pregnancy is a risk factor for SIDS, with a twofold increased risk of SIDS observed in the National Institute of Child Health and Human Development's Cooperative Epidemiological Study after adjusting for birth weight, race, and age.[32] Another study identified a sevenfold-increased risk for SIDS among infants of substance-abusing mothers in comparison with drug-free mothers.[33] Relative risks vary from 3.1 (95% CI = 0.43 to 21.74) for phencyclidine and 6.9 (95% CI = 4.04 to 11.68) for cocaine to 15.1 (95% CI = 6.30 to 36.20) for opiates. The variable and sometimes conflicting

results appear related (1) at least in part to failure to control for confounding variables and (2) sometimes to inadequate sample size.

Overheating. The association between overheating and SIDS has led to the hypothesis that hyperthermia may be an important link in the causal pathway.[20] Various indicators of overheating have been identified, including increased ambient temperature, high body temperature, sweating, and excessive clothing or bedding. Interactions between overheating and prone sleep position have also been identified; higher ambient temperature and excess thermal insulation have been associated with increased risk of SIDS in infants sleeping prone.

Infections. No clear association has been identified between SIDS and specific viral or bacterial pathogens.[20] It has been suggested that upper respiratory infections or other minor illnesses in conjunction with other factors, such as prone sleeping, may play a role in the pathogenesis of SIDS. Deficient inflammatory responsiveness to infection has also been hypothesized to be a mechanism for SIDS.[16,30,34] Partial deletions in the C4 gene may contribute to this apparent link between upper respiratory infection and SIDS. Mast cell degranulation has been reported in SIDS victims; this is consistent with an anaphylactic reaction to a bacterial toxin, and some family members of SIDS victims also have mast cell hyperrelease and degranulation, which suggests that there is a genetic component to risk for an anaphylactic reaction.[35]

Gene-Environment Interactions

The abundant associations between environmental factors and SIDS do not preclude important polygenic risks for SIDS in which genes interact in different environments to increase or decrease risk for SIDS.[16] There are many examples of interactions between genetic susceptibility and environmental factors to result in clinical disease. Asthma, for example, shows polygenic inheritance and genetic heterogeneity.[36] Multiple independent segregating genes are required for phenotypic expression, and different combinations of gene variants can contribute to the phenotype in different families.

In regard to SIDS, there appears to be an interaction between prone/side sleep position and impaired cardiorespiratory control, especially impaired ventilatory and arousal responsiveness.[16,20] Face-down or nearly face-down sleeping does occasionally occur in prone-sleeping infants and can result in episodes of airway obstruction and asphyxia in healthy full-term infants.[37] All these healthy infants aroused before the face-down or face-nearly-down position became life-threatening, but infants with insufficient arousal responsiveness to asphyxia would be at risk for fatal asphyxia. Sleeping on a very soft surface would further increase the risk of life-threatening asphyxia in the face-down or nearly face-down sleeping positions. Both hypercarbia and hypoxemia have been documented in clinical and experimental studies as consequences of rebreathing or upper airway obstruction in association with prone sleeping.

Some investigators attribute the risk of prone sleeping to thermal stress, hypothesizing that (face-down) prone sleeping causes a clinically significant degree of thermal stress.[16] Any thermal stress could further compromise infants with deficient cardiorespiratory control. There thus may be links between modifiable risk factors such as soft bedding, prone sleep position, and thermal stress and links between genetic risk factors such as cardiorespiratory control deficits (ventilatory and arousal abnormalities) and temperature/metabolic regulation deficits.

The increased risk for SIDS associated with fetal and postnatal exposure to cigarette smoke also appears to depend at least in part on genetic risk factors.[16] Both lambs and human infants demonstrate impaired ventilatory and arousal responsiveness to hypoxia associated with fetal exposure, and postnatal nicotine exposure in piglets may interfere with normal autoresuscitation after apnea.[29] In addition, fetal rat exposure to maternal smoking reduces protein kinase C within the dorsocaudal brain stem, which would impair ventilatory and arousal responsiveness to hypoxia.[16]

INFANT GROUPS AT INCREASED RISK FOR SIDS

Unexplained Apparent Life-Threatening Events

An apparent life-threatening event (ALTE) is defined as a sudden, unexpected change in an infant that is frightening to the caregiver but does not lead to death or persistent collapse.[38] Most affected patients are younger than 12 months and generally younger than 6 months of age. Episodes are characterized by some combination of apnea, color change, change in muscle tone, choking, and gagging. About 40% to 50% of ALTEs cannot be explained by the history and clinical evaluation and are therefore classified as idiopathic. The percentage of idiopathic cases is probably higher when symptoms are sleep related. Incidence rates for an ALTE vary from 0.5 to 10.0 per 1000 live births; this 20-fold difference is probably related to different case definitions and methods of ascertainment. Most studies of ALTEs do not include information about birth weight and gestational age, but the incidence in preterm infants has been estimated to be in the range of 8% to 10%.[39] In the Collaborative Home Infant Monitoring Evaluation (CHIME), 30% of 152 infants with an idiopathic ALTE were 37 weeks of gestational age or younger at birth.[40] Preterm infants thus are at increased risk for an idiopathic ALTE, but it is unknown to what extent this might be related to a prior history of apnea of prematurity or to persisting symptoms of apnea of prematurity.

Infants with an idiopathic ALTE are at increased risk for SIDS, but there is no consensus as to the magnitude of this risk or the extent to which prematurity or apnea of prematurity might be a related factor. A history of an earlier idiopathic ALTE has been reported in 5% to 9% of SIDS victims.[20,38,40] The risk of SIDS appears to increase with two or more idiopathic events, but no definitive incidence rates are available. In the CHIME study, the relative risk of having at least one extreme event was increased in preterm infants with a history of an idiopathic ALTE but only until about 43 weeks' postconception age.[40]

Infants experiencing an idiopathic ALTE are candidates for home memory monitoring. In such patients, memory monitors can be useful in determining risk for, and timely identification of, recurrent life-threatening episodes and are perhaps useful in reducing the risk for neurodevelopmental sequelae from subsequent events.[41] There are no data to indicate, however, that the risk for SIDS can be reduced by using a home monitor.[22]

Subsequent Siblings of a SIDS Victim

The extent to which the risk for SIDS may be increased in subsequent siblings has been controversial.[16] One contributor to this controversy has been the uncertainty about the frequency with which intentional suffocation is misclassified as SIDS. Clarification of the role of intentional suffocation as a cause of sudden unexpected death in infancy has been impaired by the lack of objective criteria for diagnosis. On the basis of cases in which a few families had multiple sudden, unexpected infant/child fatalities and the parents later confessed to or were convicted of homicide, however, some health professionals have stated that only homicide runs in families and all second cases of SIDS in a family should be investigated for possible homicide. Such opinions notwithstanding, a familial metabolic disorder should be considered in families with multiple unexplained infant deaths, especially when the history is atypical for SIDS. In addition, there are also substantial data indicating that the next-born siblings of first-born infants dying of any cause are at significantly increased risk for infant death from the same cause, including SIDS.[16] The relative risk is 9.1 for concordance of cause of recurrent death versus 1.6 for a discordant cause of death, and the relative risk for recurrence of each cause of infant death is similar for SIDS (95% CI = 5.4 to 5.8) and for each of the other causes (range = 4.6 to 12.5). The relative risk for recurrent postperinatal infant mortality from the same general cause was significantly increased in the next-born and all subsequent siblings in another study, and the relative risk was 7.2 (95% CI = 3.0 to 17.3) for recurrence of a non-SIDS cause of death, in comparison with 5.4 for recurrence of SIDS.[16]

In a case-control study of all sudden unexpected infant deaths among 473,000 live births, families in whom the deaths were explained by the postmortem evaluation had a significantly increased likelihood of having had a previous infant death, in comparison with controls (odds ratio = 5.96; 95% CI = 1.29 to 27.63).[16] SIDS infants were similarly more likely than controls to have had a previous sibling death (odds ratio = 3.82; 95% CI = 1.58 to 9.22) and to have had a previous stillbirth (odds ratio = 2.82; 95% CI = 1.16 to 6.85).

The risk for recurrent infant mortality in subsequent siblings from the same cause as the index sibling thus appears to be increased to a similar degree for both explained causes and for SIDS. These increased risks in families with SIDS victims are consistent with genetic risk factors interacting with environmental risk factors, including genetic factors such as brain stem abnormalities in autonomic control.

Prematurity

Numerous studies have identified low birth weight as a risk factor for SIDS.[3,16,20,42] There is an inverse relationship between risk for SIDS and birth weight/gestational age (Table 37-1). The lesser risk of SIDS with birth weight of less than 1000 g versus 1000 g or more probably reflects greater reluctance to identify SIDS as the cause of death at birth weights lower than 1000 g. SIDS, however, should be the correct diagnosis whenever the death is sudden, unexpected, and unexplained by the postmortem examination. The environmental risk factors associated with SIDS in preterm infants are not substantially different from those observed in full-term infants, including the increased risk associated with nonsupine sleep positions.[3,42] However, the postnatal age of preterm

Table 37–1. Epidemiologic Factors Associated with Increased Risk for Sudden Infant Death Syndrome in Preterm Infants

Factor	Adjusted Odds Ratio
Birth Weight (grams)	
500-999	3.1*
1000-1499	3.8*
1500-2499	2.5*
>2499	1.0
Gestational Age (weeks)	
17-28	2.9*
29-32	2.8*
33-36	1.8*
>36	1.0
Race	
Nonblack	1.0
Black	1.7*
Gender	
Male	1.5*
Female	1.0
Maternal Age (years)	
<18	1.7*
18-35	1.0
>35	0.5*
Maternal Education (years)	
<12	1.7*
≥12	1.0
Pregnancies	
1	0.6*
2-3	1.0
>3	1.1*
Maternal Smoking	
No	1.0
Yes	2.8*

*Statistically significant difference in comparison with reference group.

Adapted from Malloy M, Freeman DH: Birth weight– and gestational age–specific sudden infant death syndrome mortality: United States, 1991 versus 1995. Pediatrics 105:1227, 2000.

Table 37–2. Postconceptional and Postnatal Ages of Sudden Infant Death Syndrome Victims

Gestational Age	Postconceptional Age	Postnatal Age
24-28	44*	18†
29-32	45*	16†
33-36	47*	11
>36	50	11

All ages are in weeks.

*p < .05 in comparison to >36 weeks, gestational age.

†p < .05 in comparison to the two older groups.

Adapted from Malloy MH, Hoffman HJ: Prematurity, sudden infant death syndrome, and age of death. Pediatrics 96:464, 1995.

infants dying of SIDS is about 5 to 7 weeks older than that of full-term infants, and the postconceptional age is 4 to 6 weeks younger than that of full-term infants (Table 37-2).

Early reports suggested a relationship between bronchopulmonary dysplasia and risk for SIDS.[20] However, there was no control group matched for gestational age and birth weight. A prospective control study identified comparable incidences of ALTEs in infants with bronchopulmonary dysplasia (8.9%) and in matched control preterm infants (10.5%), but the study was too small to yield any data regarding relative risk for SIDS with respect to bronchopulmonary dysplasia.[43]

Prospective identification of future SIDS victims has been an even greater challenge in preterm infants than in full-term infants because of the greater variability in the results of physiologic assessments due to variable postconceptional and postnatal age. It has been difficult to determine the extent to which cardiorespiratory patterns in preterm infants outside the normal range for full-term infants are "normal" for that postconceptional age or whether they represent a risk for clinically significant events at home or for SIDS.[20,44] Sleep laboratory recordings at 36 to 44 weeks postconceptional age in 92% of preterm infants born at 25 to 36 weeks' gestation with clinical and/or hospital monitor-detected cyanosis, apnea, or bradycardia yielded values that exceeded the range established for full-term infants.[45] The findings included apnea longer than 20 seconds, periodic breathing for more than 15% of sleep time, episodes of heart rate less than 80 beats per minute (bpm), feeding hypoxia, and hypercarbia. Although all these infants were discharged on a home monitor without memory, only 16% had apparent serious events that received parental intervention, and there was no correlation between parental reports of clinically significant events and the predischarge recording. In preterm infants weighing less than 1500 g at birth and having no clinical cardiorespiratory symptoms at the time of NICU discharge, cardiorespiratory pattern values were above the 95th percentile for healthy full-term infants for apnea density in 18%, for periodic breathing in 15%, and for longest apnea in 17%.[44] These values above the 95th percentile were associated with a younger postconceptional age than were all the values of the preterm infants below the 95th percentile (36 versus 37.5 weeks, respectively). The CHIME study documented a higher relative risk for at least one extreme event at home only in premature infants, in comparison with healthy full-term infants, and only to about 43 weeks of postconceptional age.[40] The CHIME study provides no insights, however, about the extent to which risk for SIDS might be related to frequency or severity of extreme events. Hence, even though 18.5% of SIDS victims are premature[26] and the risk of SIDS progressively increases as birth weight decreases, preterm infants destined to die of SIDS still cannot be accurately identified prospectively.

Physiologic Studies in Groups at Increased Risk for SIDS

A brain stem abnormality related to neuroregulation of cardiorespiratory control and other autonomic functions is consistent with the autopsy findings in SIDS victims and with the clinical findings in physiologic studies performed in infants at increased risk for SIDS, a few of whom later died of SIDS.[20] The observed abnormalities include differences related to respiratory pattern, chemoreceptor sensitivity, control of heart and respiratory rate or variability, cardiorespiratory interaction, and hypoxic arousal responsiveness.

Respiratory Pattern

The respiratory pattern abnormalities have included prolonged apnea, excess brief apneic episodes, and periodic breathing. Dynamic respiratory patterning in infants subsequently dying of SIDS has indicated restricted breath-to-breath respiratory rate variability at slow respiratory rates, caused by absence of normally present influences affecting breathing.

Chemoreceptor Sensitivity

Some infants at increased risk for SIDS have diminished ventilatory responsiveness to hypercarbia and/or to hypoxia. Such assessments, however, are too costly and time consuming for routine clinical use, and the extent of individual overlap between normal and at-risk infants precludes accurate identification of infants who will die of SIDS. Chemoreceptor sensitivity studies have generally not been performed in preterm infants and would be even less useful than in full-term infants because of potential confounding by persisting lung disease and/or incomplete brain stem maturation.

Arousal Responses

Absence of arousal responsiveness renders infants incapable of responding effectively to sleep-related asphyxia from any cause. Infants at increased risk for SIDS who have diminished ventilatory responsiveness to hypercarbia and/or hypoxia generally have a concomitant abnormality in hypercarbic and/or hypoxic arousal responsiveness. A deficit in arousal responsiveness may be a necessary prerequisite for SIDS but may be insufficient to cause SIDS in the absence of other genetic or environmental risk factors. Victims of SIDS may also have deficient autoresuscitation (gasping) as a component of the asphyxic arousal response deficit.[46] A failure of

autoresuscitation in victims of SIDS would be the final and most devastating physiologic failure.

Hypoxic and hypercapnic arousal responses have been performed in some preterm infants approaching 40 weeks of postconceptional age. However, because of the confounding effects of variable neurophysiologic and respiratory maturation, it has not been possible to establish normative values. In full-term infants with idiopathic apparent life-threatening events, however, the occurrence and severity of recurrent symptoms have been correlated with arousal responsiveness.[20]

A relationship exists between arousal and postnatal age in full-term infants but has not been systematically assessed in preterm infants. Most full-term infants younger than 9 weeks arouse in response to mild hypoxia, but only 10% to 15% of normal infants older than 9 weeks do so.[47] These data thus suggest that as full-term infants mature, their ability to arouse in response to mild-moderate hypoxic stimuli diminishes as they reach the age range of greatest risk for SIDS.

Current methods for assessing arousal responsiveness in infants are cumbersome and time consuming. Furthermore, the overlap in individual values between healthy full-term controls and infants in groups at increased risk for SIDS precludes any prospective identification of infants destined to die of SIDS.

Temperature Regulation

Increased body or environmental temperature or both are associated with SIDS.[20] There are complex interactions between temperature regulation and cardiorespiratory control. The increased sleep-related sweating that does occur in some infants who have had an idiopathic ALTE may be caused by alveolar hypoventilation and secondary asphyxia or by autonomic dysfunction as part of a more generalized deficiency in brain stem function, or it may be an indication of overheating.

Cardiac Control

The ability to shorten QT interval as heart rate increases is impaired in some SIDS infants, which suggests that such infants may be predisposed to ventricular arrhythmia.[20] Infants later dying of SIDS have higher heart rates in all sleep-waking states and diminished heart rate variability during wakefulness. Infants with SIDS also have significantly lower heart rate variation at the respiratory frequency across all sleep-waking cycles. Even in early infancy, therefore, future SIDS victims differ in the extent to which cardiac and respiratory activities are coupled. Although heart rate variability has been studied in preterm infants, only full-term infants have been included in the studies that have a control group.

Part of the decrease in heart rate variability and increase in heart rate observed in infants who later die of SIDS may be related to decreased vagal tone. This could be related to vagal neuropathy, to brain stem damage in areas responsible for parasympathetic cardiac control, or to other factors. Furthermore, because the greatest reduction in all types of heart rate variability occurs while the infant is awake, these reductions may be related to the reduced motility retrospectively reported in SIDS victims and also observed in infants at increased risk for SIDS.[48] In a comparison of heart rate power spectra before and after obstructive apneic episodes in infants, future SIDS victims did not have the decreases in power ratios of low frequency to high frequency observed in control infants. Some future SIDS victims thus have different autonomic responsiveness to obstructive apnea, which perhaps indicates impaired autonomic nervous system control (dysautonomia) that could be associated with higher vulnerability to external or endogenous stress factors and could result in reduced electrical stability of the heart, leading to ventricular fibrillation.[49]

The CHIME Study

The CHIME study was performed with a specially designed memory monitor in which respiratory inductance plethysmography was used for breath detection; thus, the monitor detected obstructed breaths as well as central apneic episodes.[40] Healthy full-term infants, premature infants, subsequent siblings of SIDS victims, and infants with a prior idiopathic ALTE were monitored during the first 6 months after birth. The events stored for analysis included events exceeding conventional alarm thresholds (apnea lasting 20 seconds or longer, or heart rate of less than 60 to 80 bpm for 5 seconds or longer, depending on postconceptional age) and extreme events (apnea lasting 30 seconds or longer, or heart rate of less than 50 to 60 bpm for 5 seconds or longer, depending on postconceptional age).

Conventional events were common in all groups, and at least one occurred in 41% of infants in the CHIME study. Extreme events occurred in 10% of all the infants. In total, 653 extreme events were observed during 718,358 hours of monitoring. Of those conventional events with apnea lasting 20 seconds or longer, 50% included three or more obstructed breaths. Among extreme events with apnea lasting 30 seconds or longer, 70% included three or more obstructed breaths. In general, the degree of hypoxemia increased with increasing duration of apnea or bradycardia, and 25% of extreme events were associated with a decrease in O_2 saturation of 10% or more.

Extreme events occurred at a higher frequency only in premature infants in comparison with healthy full-term infants and were most frequent in preterm infants 34 weeks of gestational age or younger and weighing less than 1750 g at birth. Among these preterm infants, the relative risk of at least one extreme event was 18.0 in those who had persisting symptoms related to apnea of prematurity at the time of NICU discharge and was 10.1 in those who had no symptoms related to apnea of prematurity for at least 5 days before NICU discharge. In these two groups, the risk of at least one extreme event remained higher than that in the healthy full-term infants until approximately 43 weeks of postconceptional age. Of all infants with at least one extreme event, 52% experienced a second extreme event. Among those with at least two extreme events, 57% experienced a third. Among those with at least three extreme events, 80% experienced a fourth.

The CHIME study was not designed to determine whether using a home monitor reduces risk for SIDS or whether infants experiencing extreme events are more likely to die of SIDS. The CHIME data do define for the first time the risk of occurrence and the timing of extreme cardiorespiratory events according to postconceptional age during early postnatal development. Also of importance is that these data document a high frequency of obstructed breaths during events. Because all home monitors currently prescribed involve the use of transthoracic impedance for breath detection and thus cannot detect obstructed breaths, the CHIME data should be important in designing the next generation of home monitors and in determining whether an infant is likely to be at risk for a potentially life-threatening event.

Terminal Recordings in SIDS Victims

Home cardiorespiratory monitors with memory capability have recorded some terminal events in SIDS victims.[50] In most instances, there has been sudden and rapid progression of severe bradycardia, too soon to be explained by progressive desaturation from prolonged central apnea. These observations are consistent with an abnormality in autonomic control of heart rate variability or with hypoxemia secondary to obstructive apnea as the precipitating mechanism for the severe bradycardia.

In all these terminal recordings, breathing was detected by transthoracic impedance, which cannot detect obstructed breaths, and most monitors did not include recordings of O_2 saturation. Therefore, it is not possible to reach any conclusions regarding whether the first component of the terminal event is apnea, bradycardia, or desaturation unrelated to apnea or bradycardia.

Prospective Screening

The prospective studies performed in full-term and preterm infants in the sleep laboratory or at home have focused primarily on respiratory pattern, cardiac abnormalities, or both. Neither has demonstrated sufficient sensitivity and specificity to be clinically useful as a screening test, even when obstructive apnea can be identified.[20] The relationship between prolonged apnea of prematurity or delayed maturation of cardiorespiratory pattern and risk of SIDS also remains unclear. It is not known whether increased risk for a cardiorespiratory event in preterm infants in comparison with full-term infants has any clinical significance; nor is it known whether infants with a history of apnea of prematurity are at greater risk for SIDS than are gestational age–matched preterm infants without such a history. The CHIME study does provide new insights about the risk for conventional and extreme events according to postconceptional and postnatal age but no insights regarding prospective identification of future SIDS victims.[40]

Home memory monitors can record respiratory pattern, heart rate and electrocardiographic variables, and oxygenation.[40,51] The CHIME study suggests that the next generation of home memory monitors may need to be able to detect obstructed breaths as well as central apnea in order to yield any progress in identification of future SIDS victims. In the interim, however, it is not possible for home memory monitoring to identify any specific cardiorespiratory pattern or other abnormality that has sufficient sensitivity and specificity to have predictive value for SIDS.

REDUCING RISK FOR SIDS

The international back-to-sleep campaigns have significantly reduced environmental risks for SIDS and have been associated with reductions in SIDS rates of 50% or more beginning in the late 1980s. Despite the successes with risk reduction, however, there is no intervention that can be guaranteed to prevent SIDS in individual infants. Home electronic surveillance for apnea and bradycardia has been utilized since the early 1980s, but no suitably designed prospective studies have been performed, and hence no data exist to support a role for home cardiorespiratory monitors in preventing SIDS.[52]

Limited data are available from the National Maternal and Infant Health Survey regarding extent of home monitor use in preterm and full-term SIDS victims and live controls.[53] The prevalence estimates for monitor use for birth weights of 500 to 1499 g, 1500 to 2499 g, and 2500 g or more were 20%, 3%, and 1% in African Americans, as opposed to 44%, 9%, and 1% for other infants. In no instance was there a significant difference in prevalence of home monitor use in SIDS versus case controls, and in African American infants weighing 500 to 1499 g at birth, the adjusted odds ratio for SIDS was significantly higher (3.9) with a home monitor. This higher odds ratio probably reflects a higher risk for SIDS in the infants monitored in this retrospective nonrandomized observational study.

Preventing extreme events such as those observed in the CHIME study may be necessary if home monitors are to have any potential for reducing risk for SIDS.[40] Even if prolonged apnea, including obstructed breaths, is not a primary autonomic abnormality contributing to risk for SIDS, home monitoring could still be potentially helpful if apnea of any type causing bradycardia or hypoxemia as part of the terminal event could be detected reliably and sufficiently early to enable intervention before the onset of life-threatening hypoxemia. However, this hypothesis remains untested, and neither home electronic surveillance with current technology nor any other intervention can be recommended as a strategy to prevent SIDS. Despite absence of any proven prospective intervention to prevent SIDS, dramatic decreases in population-based risk can be achieved by eliminating modifiable risk factors associated with SIDS.

Another limitation in determining the efficacy of home monitoring as an intervention has been inconsistent or low compliance with the prescribed regimen. Anecdotal postmortem interviews with parents of SIDS victims dying with a monitor in the home have suggested that 50% or more of such families were not utilizing the home monitor at the time death occurred.[20] Of alarms set off by monitors with standard transthoracic impedance methods for breath detection, fewer than 10% are related to physiologic events.[54] Initial parental difficulties with frequent monitor alarms unassociated with clinical significance may thus easily lead to parental frustration and noncompliance. The best predictor of monitor use in the first 5 weeks of use of the CHIME home monitor was the extent of successful use during the first week.

SUMMARY

Significant advances have been achieved in regard to the pathophysiologic processes of SIDS, potentially important genetic and environmental risk factors, and gene-environment interactions. Significant reductions in overall SIDS mortality have occurred in association with marked reductions in prone and side sleeping, the environmental risk factors for which modification has been most successful to date. In individual infants, however, there is no accurate method for prospectively identifying infants destined to die of SIDS or, if identified, an effective intervention.

REFERENCES

1. Willinger M, James LS, Catz C, et al: Defining the sudden infant death syndrome (SIDS): deliberations of an expert panel convened by the National Institute of Child Health and Human Development. Pediatr Pathol 11:677, 1991.
2. Arias E, Mac Dorman MF, Strobino DM, Guyer B: Annual summary of vital statistics: 2002. Pediatrics 112:1215, 2003.
3. Martin JA, Ventura SJ, MacDorman MF, Strobino DM: Annual summary of vital statistics—1998. Pediatrics 104:1229, 1999.
4. Malloy MH, Hoffman HJ: Prematurity, sudden infant death syndrome, and age of death. Pediatr 96:464, 1995.
5. Valdes-Dapena M: The sudden infant death syndrome: Pathologic findings. Clin Perinatol 19:701, 1992.
6. Naeye RL: Sudden infant death syndrome, is the confusion ending? Mod Pathol 1:169, 1988.
7. Quattrochi JJ, McBride PT, Yates AJ: Brainstem immaturity in sudden infant death syndrome: A quantitative rapid Golgi study of dendritic spines in 95 infants. Brain Res 325:39, 1985.
8. Kinney HC, Burger PC, Harrell FE Jr, Hudson RP Jr: "Reactive gliosis" in the medulla oblongata of victims of the sudden infant death syndrome. Pediatrics 72:181, 1983.
9. Obonai T, Takashima S, Becker LE, et al: Relationship of substance P and gliosis in medulla oblongata in neonatal sudden infant death syndrome. Pediatr Neurol 15:189, 1996.
10. Filiano JJ, Kinney HC: Arcuate nucleus hypoplasia in the sudden infant death syndrome. J Neuropathol Exp Neurol 51:394, 1992.
11. Kinney HC, Panigrahy A, Filiano JJ, et al: Brainstem serotonergic receptor binding in the sudden infant death syndrome. J Neuropathol Exp Neurol 59:377, 2000.
12. Hasan SU, Simakajornboon N, MacKinnon Y, Gozal D: Antenatal cigarette smoke exposure induces selective changes in expression of protein kinase C (PKC) isoforms within the dorsocaudal brainstem of the neonatal rat. Pediatr Res 47(Part 2):360A, 2000.
12. Obonai T, Yasuhara M, Nakamura T, Takashima S: Catecholamine neuron alteration in the brainstem of sudden infant death syndrome victims. Pediatrics 101:285, 1998.
13. Naeye RL, Fisher R, Rubin HR, et al: Selected hormone levels in victims of the sudden infant death syndrome. Pediatrics 65:1134, 1980.

14. Jones KL, Krous HF, Nadeau J, et al: Vascular endothelial growth factor in the cerebrospinal fluid of infants who died of sudden infant death syndrome: Evidence for antecedent hypoxia. Pediatrics 111:358, 2003.

15. Rognum TO, Saugstad OD: Hypoxanthine levels in vitreous humor: Postmortem evidence of hypoxia. Pediatrics 87:306, 1991.

16. Hunt CE: Sudden infant death syndrome and other causes of infant mortality. Am J Respir Crit Care Med 164:346, 2001.

17. Katz DM, Balkowiec A: New insights into the ontogeny of breathing from genetically engineered mice. Curr Opin Pulm Med 3:433, 1997.

18. Fortin G, Dominguez del Toro E, Abadie V, et al: Genetic and developmental models for the neural control of breathing in vertebrates. Respir Physiol 122:247, 2000.

19. Dauger S, Renolleau S, Vardon G, et al: Ventilatory responses to hypercapnia and hypoxia in *Mash*-1 heterozygous newborn and adult mice. Pediatr Res 46:5354, 1999.

20. Hunt CE, Hauck FR: Sudden infant syndrome. In Behrman RE, Kliegman RM, Jenson HB (eds): Nelson Textbook of Pediatrics, 17th ed. Philadelphia, Elsevier Science, 2004, pp 1380-1385.

21. Weese-Mayer DE, Berry-Kravis EM, Maher BS, et al: Sudden infant death syndrome: Association with a promoter polymorphism of the serotonin transporter gene. Am J Med Genet 117A:268, 2003.

22. American Academy of Pediatrics Task Force on Infant Sleep Position and Sudden Infant Death Syndrome: Changing concepts of sudden infant death syndrome: Implications for infant sleep environment and sleep position. Pediatrics 105:650, 2000.

23. Cote A, Gerez T, Brouillette RT, Laplante S: Circumstances leading to a change to prone sleeping in sudden infant death syndrome victims. Pediatrics 106:E86, 2000.

24. Moon RY, Patel KM, Shaefer SJ: Sudden infant death syndrome in child care settings. Pediatrics 106:295, 2000.

25. Hunt CE, Lesko SM, Vezina RM, et al: Infant sleep position and associated health outcomes. Arch Pediatr Adolesc Med 157:469, 2003.

26. Vernacchio L, Corwin MJ, Lesko SM, et al: Sleep position of low birth weight infants. Pediatrics 111:633, 2003.

27. McMartin KI, Platt MS, Hackman R, et al: Lung tissue concentrations of nicotine in sudden infant death syndrome (SIDS). J Pediatr 140:205, 2002.

28. Wisborg K, Kesmodel U, Henriksen TB, et al: A prospective study of smoking during pregnancy and SIDS. Arch Dis Child 83:203, 2000.

29. Froen JF, Akre H, Stray-Pedersen B, Saugstad OD: Adverse effects of nicotine and interleukin-1B on autoresuscitation after apnea in piglets: Implications for sudden infant death syndrome. Pediatrics 105:E52, 2000.

30. Gordon AE, El Ahmer OR, Chan R, et al: Why is smoking a risk factor for sudden infant death syndrome? Child Care Health Dev 28(Suppl 1):23, 2002.

31. Iyasu S, Randall LL, Welty TK, et al: Risk factors for sudden infant death syndrome among Northern Plains Indians. JAMA 288:2717, 2002.

32. Hoffman HJ, Hillman LS: Epidemiology of the sudden infant death syndrome: Maternal, neonatal, and postneonatal risk factors. Clin Perinatol 19:717, 1992.

33. Ward SLD, Bautista D, Chan L, et al: Sudden infant death syndrome in infants of substance-abusing mothers. J Pediatr 117:876, 1990.

34. Blackwell CC, Weir DM, Busuttil A: Infection, inflammation and sleep: More pieces to the puzzle of sudden infant death syndrome (SIDS). APMIS 107:455, 1999.

35. Gold Y, Goldberg A, Sivan Y: Hyper-releasability of mast cells in family members of infants with sudden infant death syndrome and apparent life-threatening events. J Pediatr 136:460, 2000.

36. Sanford AJ, Pare PD: The genetics of asthma. Am J Respir Crit Care Med 161:S202, 2000.

37. Waters KA, Gonzalez AJC, Morielli A, Brouillette RT: Face-straight-down and face-near-straight-down positions in healthy, prone-sleeping infants. J Pediatr 128:616, 1996.

38. Samuels MP: Apparent life-threatening events: Pathogenesis and management. In Lenfant CL (ed): Sleep and Breathing in Children. New York, Marcel Dekker, 2000, pp 423-441.

39. Barrington KJ, Finer N, Li D: Predischarge respiratory recordings in very low birth weight newborn infants. J Pediatr 129:934, 1996.

40. Ramanathan R, Corwin MJ, Hunt CE, et al: Cardiorespiratory events recorded on home monitors. Comparison of healthy infants with those at increased risk for SIDS. JAMA 285:2199, 2001.

41. Hunt CE, Baird T, Tinsley L, et al: Cardiorespiratory events detected by home memory monitoring during early infancy and neurodevelopmental outcome at one year of age. J Pediatr, in press.

42. Malloy M, Freeman DH: Birth weight– and gestational age–specific sudden infant death syndrome mortality: United States, 1991 versus 1995. Pediatrics 105:1227, 2000.

43. Gray PH, Rogers Y: Are infants with bronchopulmonary dysplasia at risk for sudden infant death syndrome? Pediatrics 93:774, 1994.

44. Hageman JR, Holmes D, Suchy S, Hunt CE: Respiratory pattern at hospital discharge in asymptomatic preterm infants. Pediatr Pulmonol 4:78, 1988.

45. Rosen CL, Glaze DG, Frost JD: Home monitor follow-up of persistent apnea and bradycardia in preterm infants. Am J Dis Child 140:547, 1986.

46. Poets CF, Meny RG, Chobanian MR, Bonofiglo RE: Gasping and other cardiorespiratory patterns during sudden infant deaths. Pediatr Res 45:350, 1999.

47. Davidson-Ward SL, Bautista DB, Keens TG: Hypoxic arousal responses in normal infants. Pediatrics 89:860, 1992.

48. Einspieler C, Widder J, Holzer-Sutter A, Kenner T: The predictive value of behavioural risk factors for sudden infant death. Early Hum Dev 18:101, 1998.

49. Franco P, Szliwowski H, Dramaix M, Kahn A: Decreased autonomic responses to obstructive sleep events in future victims of sudden infant death syndrome. Pediatr Res 46:33, 1999.

50. Meny RG, Carroll JL, Carbone MT, Kelly DH: Cardiorespiratory recordings from infants dying suddenly and unexpectedly at home. Pediatrics 93:44, 1994.

51. Hunt CE, Hufford DR, Bourguignon C, Oess MA: Home documented monitoring of cardiorespiratory pattern and O_2 saturation in healthy infants. Pediatr Res 39:216, 1996.

52. Committee on Fetus and Newborn, American Academy of Pediatrics: Apnea, sudden infant death syndrome, and home monitoring. Pediatrics 111:914, 2003.

53. Malloy MH, Hoffman HJ: Home apnea monitoring and sudden infant death syndrome. Prev Med 25:645, 1996.

54. Silvestri J, Hufford DR, Durham JD, et al: Assessment of compliance with home cardiorespiratory monitoring in infants at risk of sudden infant death syndrome. J Pediatr 127:384, 1995.

CHAPTER 38

Differential Diagnosis of Neonatal Respiratory Disorders

Kolawole O. Solarin, Alan Zubrow, and Maria Delivoria-Papadopoulos

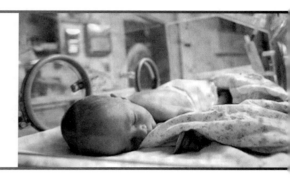

One of the major causes of perinatal morbidity and mortality is the inability of the newborn infant to transition successfully to air breathing at the time of delivery. **Pulmonary gas exchange** in the newborn results from the interaction of physiologic, biochemical, and morphologic factors that may come into play anytime from conception through the postpartum period and thereafter. These factors are influenced by abnormalities of growth and differentiation of the developing lung, lung immaturity secondary to preterm delivery, and complications occurring during the perinatal period. The overall effect is the birth of an infant who presents with **respiratory distress** at birth or shortly thereafter. Some of the disorders causing respiratory problems in the newborn are life-threatening, and misunderstanding of the pathophysiology may lead to incorrect therapeutic choices, delays in treatment, adverse side effects, and a worse prognosis. Because most of the disease processes are not characterized by one crucial symptom, the correct diagnosis is made by a combination of clues. This chapter discusses the initial assessment, interpretation of symptoms and signs, and pathophysiology of most of the respiratory disorders that present around the time of delivery. These disorders can be congenital, can be secondary to prematurity, or can result from perinatal complications (e.g., sepsis or birth asphyxia). More detailed information on investigations and management of these disorders are discussed in other relevant chapters of this book.

INTERPRETING SYMPTOMS AND SIGNS OF RESPIRATORY DISTRESS IN THE NEWBORN

The medical history, clinical symptoms and signs, especially those affecting the respiratory tract, biochemical data, and results of the imaging studies provide crucial information. Together with an understanding of the underlying pathophysiology, a diagnosis can be reached, and a treatment plan can be determined.

Nasal Flaring

Although nasal flaring can be seen in normal infants during feeding and possibly when stooling, it is usually a sign of respiratory distress in newborns. Nasal flaring is in an attempt to decrease airway resistance and consequently work of breathing because newborns are obligatory nasal breathers. It is often described as mild, moderate, or severe and can be used as a quick estimate of improvement or worsening of respiratory problems in the delivery room. Absence of nasal flaring has been reported, however, in a newborn with bilateral choanal stenosis, presenting with respiratory distress.[1]

Grunting

Grunting is an attempt to maintain or increase the functional residual capacity during expiration by closing the vocal cords. The grunting sound is heard as air is forced through the partially closed cords. It can be continuous or intermittent depending on the etiology and severity of the respiratory disorder. Grunting also can be used clinically to assess worsening or improvement of respiratory status. Most newborns with moderate or severe respiratory distress syndrome, atelectasis, and lung collapse tend to grunt.[2]

Abnormal Respiratory Rate

The respiratory rate is one of the frequently monitored vital signs in the intensive care nursery. It is a function of alveolar ventilation and reflects the work of breathing. The respiratory rate can increase or decrease and may be associated with other symptoms and signs of respiratory distress. **Tachypnea** due to the stress of labor and delivery and the events associated with the transition from fetal to neonatal life tends to resolve shortly after birth. Disorders of the lung parenchyma, including pneumonia, atelectasis, and respiratory distress syndrome, often lead to an increase in respiratory rate. Decreased respiratory rate with a longer inspiratory time can be seen in disorders in which there is obstruction in the airway, such as a laryngeal subglottic web. Abnormalities in the respiratory rate also occur as a result of skeletal and neuromuscular disorders, intrauterine exposure to certain drugs (e.g., opiates), and abnormalities of acid-base homeostasis.

Retractions of the Chest Wall

Retractions can be subcostal, intercostal, substernal, or a combination of all three. They tend to be seen frequently because the chest of the newborn, especially the preterm neonate, is very compliant. Retractions occur in situations when the lungs are stiff, when there is obstruction of the airway, or when there are morphologic anomalies of the thoracic wall. In disorders in which the lungs are stiff, such as respiratory distress syndrome and pneumonia, excess negative intrapleural pressure is generated to overcome poor lung compliance in the presence of a compliant chest wall. This pressure change is accompanied by the use of accessory muscles for respiration and subsequently retractions with each contraction of the diaphragm. Significant obstruction in the airway also tends to lead to use of the accessory muscles because of increased airway resistance. In some cases, all types of retractions may be seen occurring at the same time.

Cyanosis

Newborns with respiratory disease can present with central cyanosis. It may be due to hypoventilation, ventilation-perfusion inequality, diffusion abnormalities, or cardiac disease (due to right-to-left shunting). Ventilation-perfusion inequality can occur with various lesions in the lung, including atelectasis, pneumonia, and meconium aspiration. The response to oxygen supplementation helps to differentiate a true pulmonary disease from a cyanotic heart defect or persistent pulmonary hypertension. Exposure to higher concentrations of supplemental oxygen usually results in improvement in PaO_2 in pulmonary disease but does not lead to any significant increase in cyanotic cardiac disease. Persistent pulmonary hypertension may or may not respond to supplemental oxygen. Cardiac causes of cyanosis always should be considered when there is cyanosis and no respiratory symptoms, especially if there is a cardiac murmur. Peripheral cyanosis is fairly common in newborns, and in most cases, it is not clinically significant.

Apnea

Apnea is the total absence of gas exchange and can occur in the newborn period. It is considered significant if it persists for more than 20 seconds or is accompanied by other clinical signs, including bradycardia, cyanosis, and oxygen desaturation. Apnea that occurs immediately after delivery or in the postnatal period can result from perinatal asphyxia, infection, intracranial hemorrhage, hypothermia, obstruction of the airway, seizures, or other central nervous system lesions. **Apnea of prematurity** that occurs in preterm infants is rarely seen in full-term infants or in the first 24 to 48 hours after birth. Apnea of prematurity should be differentiated from periodic breathing, which is usually a cluster of apneic episodes

lasting for less than 15 seconds with no associated cardiovascular symptoms and signs. It is considered normal in preterm patients, but may have significant physiologic implications in a small subgroup of premature neonates.

Oxygen Saturation and Blood Gas Analysis

Assessment of oxygen saturation, PaO_2, PCO_2, and pH is crucial in the evaluation and management of respiratory distress, especially in infants who require oxygen and ventilatory support. These blood gas values can be monitored easily. Most newborns in respiratory distress often require frequent blood gas analysis from an indwelling arterial catheter, most commonly placed in the umbilical artery.

Oxygen readily combines with hemoglobin in a reversible reaction to form oxyhemoglobin.[3] The amount of oxygen combined with hemoglobin depends on the PaO_2, making this determination important in the assessment of respiratory status and oxygenation. A small amount of oxygen is carried that is dissolved in blood. The relationship between oxygen saturation and PaO_2 is explained by the **oxygen dissociation curve** (Fig. 38-1). The amount of oxygen combined with hemoglobin increases steadily until the partial pressure is about 50 mm Hg. After this, the curve tapers and becomes flatter.[4-6] At a partial pressure of approximately 90 mm Hg, the blood is about 100% saturated. From Figure 38-1, it is impossible to estimate correctly the PaO_2 by the oxygen saturation when it is higher than 95%. The oxygen dissociation curve is shifted to the right by increases in hydrogen ion concentration, temperature, PCO_2, and the concentration of 2,3-diphosphoglycerate.[7-10]

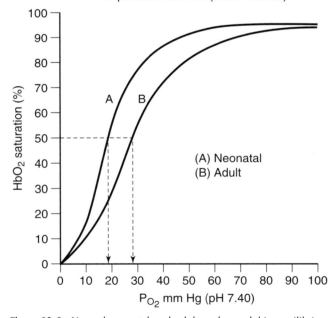

Figure 38–1. Normal neonatal and adult oxyhemoglobin equilibrium curves (mean value).

Measured arterial blood Pao_2 is influenced by factors including the ability of the lung to exchange oxygen adequately at the alveolar level, the capability of the blood to carry oxygen, ventilation, the presence of ventilation-perfusion mismatch, and shunting of blood from right to left, depending on the disease process. In hypoxemia, lactic acid accumulates in the tissues because aerobic oxidation ceases and is replaced by anaerobic respiration. Release of lactic acid into the blood leads to metabolic acidosis by disrupting the acid-base balance in the blood. The aforementioned factors also influence the Pco_2.[11] Because about 60% of carbon dioxide is dissolved in blood, leading to the formation of bicarbonate, changes in Pco_2 can affect the acid-base balance. Changes in Pco_2 may lead to respiratory acidosis or respiratory alkalosis depending on whether it is increased or decreased. These changes also can be reflected as base deficit or excess on blood gas analysis.[10] The relationship between pH, Pco_2, and bicarbonate is explained by the **Henderson-Hasselbalch equation**:

$$pH = pK_a + \log (HCO_3^-/0.03\ Pco_2)$$

where pK_a is the dissociation constant of carbon dioxide, $0.03\ Pco_2$ is the concentration of dissolved carbon dioxide, and HCO_3^- is the concentration of bicarbonate. As the value of $0.03\ Pco_2$ changes secondary to retention or excessive loss of carbon dioxide, the pH decreases or increases. In cases of respiratory failure, the blood gas analysis typically shows significant evidence of metabolic acidosis, hypercapnia, and hypoxemia.

Chest Radiograph and Other Imaging Studies

The chest radiograph is crucial for diagnostic and management purposes in infants with respiratory distress. Disease processes that cause respiratory distress can be observed within the lung parenchyma or outside the lungs but within the chest or airway. Specific findings on the chest radiograph are discussed subsequently with the associated lesions. More conclusive imaging studies may be suggested by findings on the initial chest radiograph.

RESPIRATORY DISTRESS CAUSED BY CONGENITAL MORPHOLOGIC DISORDERS OF THE LUNG AND AIRWAY

Most major developmental disorders of the lung tend to arise at the early stages of organogenesis. During the embryonic period (0 to 7 weeks), the respiratory diverticulum and primary bronchopulmonary divisions are formed.[12,13] The epithelium of the lung at this stage is columnar. The next 8 to 9 weeks of development is the pseudoglandular stage (8 to 16 weeks). This stage involves the formation of all of the conducting airways down to the terminal bronchioles along with the appearance of cuboidal epithelial cells in addition to the columnar cells. Major developmental anomalies that occur during this period include tracheoesophageal fistula, pulmonary agenesis, congenital pulmonary cysts, bronchial anomalies, and choanal atresia.

Tracheoesophageal Fistula

Tracheoesophageal fistula is a relatively common problem in the newborn. The incidence is reported to be about 1 in 4000 to 5000 live births. The lesion is thought to occur by 4 weeks of gestation. The trachea arises from a diverticulum on the ventral surface of the embryonic foregut. The most common anatomic type (85%) is the distal tracheoesophageal fistula with a blind upper esophageal pouch and a lower esophageal segment connected to the trachea.[14,15] Infants with this type of tracheoesophageal fistula typically present in respiratory distress with coughing spells and choking as a result of oral secretions that may be excessive. These infants can become cyanotic. When esophageal atresia is present, it is usually impossible to pass a nasogastric suction catheter beyond 8 to 10 cm. A chest radiograph often reveals the catheter coiled in the esophagus, which in most cases ends up as a pouch.

Congenital Pulmonary Cysts

Congenital pulmonary cysts are relatively uncommon. These lesions are thought to result from a separation of a portion of the developing lung parenchyma that subsequently forms cystic lesions. Some cysts may communicate with the bronchial branches of the trachea. They can be intrapulmonary or extrapulmonary depending on their relationship to the trachea or major bronchi. A large extrapulmonary cyst can cause compression of the airway, and the infant presents in severe respiratory distress with inspiratory stridor and wheezing.[16,17] Chest radiographs typically show hyperinflation of one lung if there is bronchial obstruction. Death resulting from airway obstruction by a large extrapulmonary cyst has been reported.

The most common congenital pulmonary cyst is **congenital cystic adenomatoid malformation (CCAM)**. CCAM is intrapulmonary and characterized by persistence of undifferentiated airway epithelium.[16] The proximal columnar cells lining the early airway epithelium do not transition to more flattened cells of the distal airways. There also is associated overgrowth of mesenchymal tissue, forming solid or cystic lesions depending on whether there is communication with the airway. The cysts can be single or multiple, small (<1 mm) or large (>2 mm). Multiple small cysts have been associated with other fetal anomalies and a poor prognosis. Severe respiratory problems may occur at birth if there is associated pulmonary hypoplasia, hydrops, or mediastinal shift.[16-18] A case of spontaneous pneumothorax resulting from CCAM has been reported.[19] Reports suggest that bronchogenic cysts, CCAM, and pulmonary sequestration may have a common embrologic link.[20,21]

The coexistence of CCAM with recombinant chromosome 18 (partial deletion of 18p and partial duplication of 18p) also has been reported. It is suggested that fetal and parental karyotyping be considered in cases of CCAM.[22] Lesions that may resemble congenital pulmonary cysts on chest radiographs include lobar emphysema, pneumothorax, bronchogenic cyst, congenital diaphragmatic hernia (CDH), and pulmonary sequestration.

Congenital Lobar Emphysema

Congenital lobar emphysema occurs in 1 in 6000 newborns and is more common in boys. In this lesion, the affected lobe is uniformly distended; usually the upper and middle lobes are affected. Reports have suggested there is a deficiency of cartilage in these patients, which may be inherited.[23] About 10% to 15% of these patients have associated cardiac lesions. Affected newborns may present with severe respiratory symptoms soon after birth, subcostal and intercostal retractions, tachypnea, and cyanosis.[24,25] Chest radiographs show a hyperinflated area of the lung with possible compression of adjacent lung tissue. The hyperinflated area usually is not well demarcated and can be confused with a pneumothorax.

Eventration of the Diaphragm

Newborns with the congenital (nonparalytic) variety of **eventration of the diaphragm** may present with respiratory distress because of poor lung reserve or paradoxical movement of the diaphragm. It is more common on the left side. The affected area of the diaphragm is usually less muscular and may not be thicker than a thin membrane. The affected part of the diaphragm tends to be abnormally high on the chest radiograph. It is usually an incidental finding, and most affected patients are asymptomatic. A suspected eventration of the diaphragm must be differentiated from CDH. Magnetic resonance imaging and ultrasonography can be used to differentiate the two lesions prenatally.[26]

Lobar Sequestration

In **lobar sequestration**, an area of lung parenchyma does not communicate normally with the airways, pulmonary artery, and sometimes pulmonary vein. The sequestrated lung tends to receive its arterial blood supply from vessels arising from the aorta, whereas the veins may drain to different areas, including the pulmonary veins, azygos veins, and hemiazygos veins. There are two types of sequestration: the extralobar type, in which the cyst is separated from the normal lung, and the intralobar type, in which the cyst is part of the normal lung. Most intralobar sequestrations are located in the left lower lobe, whereas extralobar sequestrations generally are located in the posterior mediastinum. It is speculated that lobar sequestration develops from a second tracheobronchial bud from the primitive foregut that occurs around 4 weeks of gestation. Aberrant expression of the homeobox gene *Hoxb-5* has been implicated in the development of bronchopulmonary sequestration. This homeobox gene is necessary for normal branching of the airways during development.[27]

Extralobar lesions generally do not cause any symptoms. Although most intralobar lesions tend to present after the neonatal period, lesions that have been reported in the neonate cause respiratory distress by compressing normal lung. Intralobar sequestration usually presents as a cystic lesion on the chest radiograph. Pulmonary sequestration has been reported, however, which presents as a suprarenal lesion in a neonate.[28]

Congenital Diaphragmatic Hernia

CDH develops because of persistence of the pleuroperitoneal canal in the posterolateral portion of the diaphragm. Normally the closure of the pleuroperitoneal canal occurs around 8 weeks of gestation. A diaphragmatic hernia tends to occur if this defect persists after the return of the midgut back to the abdominal cavity.[29] This alteration allows for herniation of abdominal contents through the defect. The size of the herniated portion can vary from very small to large enough to contain most of the gut, spleen, or liver. Pulmonary complications that occur as a result of the hernia are probably independent of its size and depend more on the period in which the hernia develops during lung development.[30] Associated deficiency of surfactant is believed to contribute to the severity of the respiratory problems in affected newborns.[31] There can be bilateral lung hypoplasia, which tends to be more severe on the side of the hernia. Lung weight, lung volume, and airway generations can be decreased.[32] Pulmonary arterioles can be muscular, predisposing some of the affected newborns to pulmonary hypertension. The defect is more common on the left side in greater than 85% of affected infants.

The incidence of CDH is 1 in 3000 to 4000 live births. Chromosomal defects, including trisomies 18 and 21 and Fryns syndrome, a rare autosomal recessive disorder, have been associated with occurrence of CDH.[33] Anomalies of other organs, including the brain, the heart, and the limbs, have been reported in about 30% to 40% of patients with CDH. Bilateral hernias are rare and usually fatal. The diagnosis of CDH can be made during pregnancy by fetal ultrasound. Postnatally, symptoms and time of presentation vary inversely with the severity of the lung hypoplasia. Typically, infants present immediately after delivery with severe respiratory distress that usually requires intubation in the delivery room. Infants are often cyanotic, and the abdomen may be scaphoid because of herniation of the abdominal contents into the thoracic cavity. A radiograph of the chest and abdomen is usually diagnostic. There are loops of bowel in the affected hemithorax, a shift of the mediastinum away from the hemithorax with the herniation, and a gasless abdomen. The clinical presentation of patients with this condition represents the summation of the extent of the herniation of abdominal contents into the abdomen, pulmonary hypoplasia, and cardiac compromise. This condition must be differentiated from CCAM and other cystic lesions of the lung.

Pulmonary Hypoplasia

Hypoplastic lung can occur in association with various conditions, including oligohydramnios, bilateral dysplastic kidneys, severe posterior urethral valves, and CDH. The number of airway generations and alveoli are less than normal, resulting in respiratory distress in affected newborns.[34] This change is due to arrest of lung development and differentiation, and in the case of oligohydramnios, there is compression of the thorax and lung due to lack of fluid. Oligohydramnios may be caused by a chronic leak of amniotic fluid from premature rupture of membranes or occur as a result of renal agenesis leading to a lack of production of amniotic fluid. In oligohydramnios caused by a chronic leak of amniotic fluid, the severity of lung disease and respiratory distress depends on the timing of the leak and extent. In some cases, the pulmonary hypoplasia is so severe that it is not compatible with postnatal life. Most infants with renal agenesis tend to have lethal pulmonary hypoplasia.

Choanal Atresia

Newborns with **choanal atresia** can present with respiratory distress and cyanosis immediately after birth, especially if the disorder is bilateral. This distress occurs because infants are obligate nasal breathers until they are about 4 to 6 weeks old. Most infants with this disorder (80% to 90%) have unilateral lesions, however. The incidence is 1 in 5000, and it is twice as common in girls. Isolated choanal atresia has been reported in siblings.[35]

Choanal atresia is believed to occur because the buconasal membrane fails to rupture. Normal rupture occurs around 7 weeks of gestation. About 90% of the atresias are bony, whereas the remaining 10% are membranous.[36] About one third to half of affected infants have associated anomalies, including the **CHARGE** (*c*oloboma of the eyes, *h*eart defects, renal *a*nomaly, *r*etardation of growth and mental development, *e*ar anomalies with hearing loss) association.[37,38] Typically, newborns with bilateral choanal atresia present at birth with respiratory distress and cyanosis that resolves with crying; these infants are pinker when they cry compared with when they are not crying. The diagnosis is suspected further in the delivery room if a 6-Fr to 8-Fr catheter cannot be passed into the nasopharynx. The diagnosis can be confirmed with a computed tomography scan. An artificial airway should be provided in the delivery room, and the infant should be evaluated thoroughly for other associated lesions.

RESPIRATORY DISTRESS CAUSED BY ABNORMALITIES OF PULMONARY SURFACTANT

The later stages of lung development begin with the canaliculi stage (16 to 25 weeks). The lung is regarded as potentially viable for gas exchange by the end of this stage. Significant developments during this period include lung epithelial cell differentiation, pulmonary acinar formation, and surfactant production. In the saccular stage (25 to 38 weeks) of lung development, the acinar tubules dilate and become much thinner.[13] There also is a reduction in the amount of interstitial tissue. The final branching of the airway generations from 18 to 23 occurs in this stage. The last stage of lung development is the alveolar stage, which extends from term to 2 to 8 years.

The main neonatal respiratory disorder related to these later stages of lung development is the **respiratory distress syndrome**, owing to premature delivery and inadequate pulmonary surfactant. In addition to the relative deficiency of surfactant, the premature lung is structurally underdeveloped for postnatal life. More recent publications have described a variety of lung disorders resulting from abnormalities in the protein component of surfactant in which affected patients present with severe respiratory distress in the newborn period. These disorders, which can be lethal, have been described only in newborns born at term.[39]

Pulmonary Surfactant

Pulmonary surfactant is a surface-active complex mixture of phospholipids and specific proteins that are synthesized and secreted into the alveolar space by the type II cells of the lung. The phospholipid component helps to reduce surface tension at the alveolar surface. The protein part plays a major role in the adsorption and spreading of surfactant phospholipids at the air-liquid interface and possibly in host defense functions.[40,41] By weight, surfactant contains 80% phospholipids, 10% other lipids, and 10% proteins.[42] Phosphatidylcholine constitutes about 70% to 80% of the phospholipid component of surfactant by dry weight. Saturated phosphatidylcholine (dipalmitoylphosphatidylcholine), which is more than 50% of the phosphatidylcholine component, is the main surface-active constituent of surfactant. Surfactant also contains 5% to 10% phosphatidylethanolamine, phosphatidylserine, sphingomyelin, phosphatidylinositol, and phosphatidylglycerol.[43] The presence of phosphatidylglycerol in amniotic fluid and the ratio of phosphatidylcholine to sphingomyelin are used as markers to determine lung maturity.[44] As the premature lung matures, the level of phosphatidylinositol decreases as phosphatidylglycerol appears. Likewise, the sphingomyelin content in amniotic fluid tends to decreases as term approaches, whereas the phosphatidylcholine level increases.

There are two groups of surfactant proteins: the hydrophilic surfactant proteins A and D (SP-A and SP-D) and the hydrophobic surfactant proteins B and C (SP-B and SP-C). SP-A and SP-D do not seem to have a primary role in the biophysical functions of surfactant.[45] They belong to a family of C-type lectins known to be involved with host defense against viral and bacterial pathogens.[46] SP-B and SP-C are known to enhance the surface tension–lowering properties of surfactant and facilitate its adsorption and spread.[47]

Synthesis of the phospholipid and protein components of surfactant takes place in the type II cells and is developmentally regulated. Synthesis of phosphotidylcholine involves the reaction of cytidine diphosphocholine and deacylated phosphatidic acid. The rate-regulatory enzyme in phosphatidylcholine synthesis is choline-phosphate cytidyltransferase. Its activity is known to increase as gestation progresses and can be stimulated by glucocorticoids.[41]

SP-B and SP-C initially are synthesized as larger polypeptides but post-translationally processed to smaller proteins.[48] The gene for SP-B is located on chromosome 2. The SP-B gene contains 11 exons. SP-B proprotein contains 381 amino acids, whereas the mature protein is a 79-amino acid polypeptide. Mature peptide corresponds to codon 201 through 279 of the SP-B mRNA.[47] The important role of mature SP-B in surfactant function is shown by the fact that infants born with hereditary SP-B deficiency have severe respiratory distress syndrome and die despite adequate medical intervention.[49] In addition to its action of helping the spread and biophysical action of the phospholipid content of surfactant in the air-liquid interface of the lung, SP-B is important for the formation of lamellar bodies. These are storage organelles for surfactant in the type II cell before the surfactant is released into the airspace. Infants with hereditary SP-B deficiency lack lamellar bodies.[39]

The mature SP-C protein consists of 33 to 35 amino acids. It is processed by cleavage of a 191- to 197-amino acid primary translation product. The gene for SP-C is located on chromosome 8.[48] The role of SP-C in enhancing the surface tension–lowering action and spread of surfactant in the air-liquid interface is well shown. Most exogenous surfactant preparations used to treat respiratory disease of the newborn now contain SP-B and SP-C in addition to the phospholipid component. The surfactant phospholipid components, SP-B, SP-C, and possibly SP-A are stored in lamellar bodies before being secreted out of the type II cells to form tubular myelin.

Respiratory Distress Syndrome

Respiratory distress syndrome is the most common respiratory disorder observed in premature infants and is caused by a relative or total lack of surfactant.[50] It is a leading cause of morbidity and mortality in the neonatal period. Apart from a premature delivery, other risk factors for surfactant deficiency include maternal diabetes mellitus and perinatal asphyxia. The incidence of respiratory distress syndrome increases with decreasing gestational age. It is more common in boys. Respiratory distress syndrome is mainly due to deficiency of surfactant, but the etiology can be multifactorial. Deficiency of pulmonary surfactant leads to decreased functional residual capacity, atelectasis, and ventilation-perfusion mismatch. Arterial blood gas analysis often reveals a low Po_2, an increased Pco_2, and a metabolic acidosis. Affected infants usually develop respiratory distress at the time of birth or shortly thereafter. They present with nasal flaring, tachypnea, retractions, grunting, cyanosis, and a requirement for supplemental oxygen. Rales and poor air entry into both lung fields may be appreciated on auscultation. The infant may be pale with poor perfusion of the extremities. Severely affected infants often require intubation in the delivery room and exogenous surfactant administration. Typical findings on the chest radiograph include diffuse reticulogranular pattern, air bronchograms, and atelectasis. The heart size is usually normal, unless there are other problems, such as a patent ductus arteriosus causing congestive cardiac failure or another cardiac lesion, especially if the mother had diabetes during the pregnancy. These radiographic findings also are observed in infants with infections due to bacterial organisms (especially group B streptococcus), and empirical treatment should be started as soon as possible. Total and differential white blood cell counts are usually within the normal range in respiratory distress syndrome.

Hereditary Surfactant Protein-B Deficiency

Reports have described term infants presenting with respiratory distress that is progressive and is usually lethal.[49,51,52] The symptoms, signs, and radiologic findings are identical to findings observed in infants with respiratory distress syndrome associated with prematurity. These symptoms and signs do not resolve, however, with the administration of exogenous surfactant. This disease, termed **hereditary SP-B deficiency**, is due to mutations in the *SP-B* gene leading to a total or partial deficiency of the SP-B protein. The incidence is unknown, but the disease has been found predominantly in infants born to parents of northern European descent. About 15 mutations have been identified, but the most common, termed *121 ins 2*, accounts for about 70% of reported cases. The 121 ins 2 is due to a frame-shift mutation that disrupts codon 121 of the SP-B mRNA, resulting in premature termination of translation and consequently lack of SP-B. Infants homozygous for the 121 ins 2 mutation lack SP-B.[53,54] The only available treatment option for infants with total lack of SP-B is lung transplantation.[49] Carriers for the deficiency do not seem to have the disease. Although hereditary SP-B deficiency has been described only in term infants, there is no reason not to expect its occurrence in preterm infants.

Transient Tachypnea of the Newborn

Transient tachypnea of the newborn is a self-limited condition commonly seen in term and preterm infants. Affected infants usually present at birth or shortly thereafter with tachypnea, retractions, respiratory distress, and grunting, and they may require supplemental oxygen. The symptoms, which are usually mild, may persist for hours to a few days. Respiratory failure due to transient tachypnea of the newborn is rare. Infants with transient tachypnea of the newborn are otherwise well. The hallmark suggesting the diagnosis is evidence of interstitial fluid and prominent interlobar fissures on the chest radiograph. Other common findings on the chest radiograph include increased hilar markings and mild cardiomegaly. Known risk factors include asphyxia, maternal sedation, delivery by cesarean section, and prematurity. It is believed that transient tachypnea of the newborn results from delayed clearance of fetal lung fluid, which leads to poor lung compliance and subsequent respiratory distress. The fetal lung is filled with fluid from about 16 weeks of gestation until term, and this fluid has to be cleared after birth for adequate pulmonary gas exchange to occur. Production of this fluid normally tends to decrease a few days before delivery, and some of the fluid is cleared during labor and delivery. The remaining fluid is normally absorbed into the pulmonary vessels and lymphatics within a few hours after birth. An initial mild deficiency of surfactant also has been implicated as a cause of transient tachypnea of the newborn.

RESPIRATORY DISTRESS CAUSED BY INFECTION

Neonatal Pneumonia

Neonatal pneumonia can be due to bacterial, viral, or other infectious agents acquired transplacentally, perinatally, or postnatally. When there is a suspicion of a bacterial infection, antibiotics should be started as soon as possible.

The history, physical examination, and maternal evaluation for risk factors determine the early empirical treatment in asymptomatic newborns. The newborn's presentation depends on the causative organism. For most viral pathogens, infection is acquired transplacentally, and the severity depends on when the fetus was infected in utero. Respiratory symptoms and signs can vary from mild to severe, and in some cases, respiratory failure is present at the time of birth. Respiratory distress may be accompanied by other signs, including exanthems, low birth weight, microcephaly, petechiae, purpura, hepatosplenomegaly, thrombocytopenia, and jaundice, which may further suggest a viral etiology. Varicella pneumonia often is associated with significant mortality. Chest radiographs in newborns with viral pneumonia tend to be nonspecific.

Newborns with bacterial pneumonia can deteriorate rapidly with evidence of shock, meningitis, and respiratory failure. Initial laboratory screens for sepsis may reveal neutropenia or leukocytosis, bandemia, thrombocytopenia, and a high C-reactive protein level. Chest radiographs of infants with neonatal pneumonia, especially group B streptococci, are sometimes indistiguishable from those with respiratory distress syndrome due to surfactant deficiency.

Other agents causing pneumonia in newborns include *Candida albicans,*[55] *Chlamydia trachomatis,* and *Ureaplasma urealyticum.*[56] In congenital candidiasis, respiratory symptoms may be associated with erythematous maculopapular lesions on the trunk and extremities.[55]

RESPIRATORY DISTRESS CAUSED BY ASPIRATION OF MECONIUM

Meconium Aspiration Syndrome

Meconium in the airway and airspaces of the lungs of a newborn causes respiratory distress due to blockage of the airway, inactivation of surfactant, direct damage to lung parenchyma, initiation of events leading to pulmonary hypertension, atelectasis, and ventilation-perfusion mismatch.[57] Affected infants can present with mild-to-moderate respiratory distress, but rapid progression to respiratory failure with cyanosis and pulmonary hypertension is common.[58,59] The passage of meconium before delivery is associated with fetal asphyxia, and it usually is seen in post-term infants. Most infants with meconium-stained amniotic fluid are asymptomatic and have no meconium below the cords on intubation. Typically, infants with **meconium aspiration syndrome** have meconium-stained amniotic fluid, and some have meconium below the cords on intubation.[60] A chest radiograph may show generalized coarse infiltrates in both lung fields and hyperaeration. These infants are specifically prone to air leaks, especially pneumothoraces.[57] The amount of meconium sunctioned on intubation and the extent of aspiration seen on chest radiographs may not correlate with clinical presentation or severity of the disease. Some infants with no meconium below the cords have been found to have extensive meconium aspiration on chest radiograph and severe respiratory distress, clinically suggesting that meconium was aspirated before delivery.

Persistent Pulmonary Hypertension

Respiratory distress due to **persistent pulmonary hypertension** can be lethal in the newborn period. In persistent pulmonary hypertension, the fetal circulatory pattern, in which there is high pulmonary vascular resistance and minimal blood flow to the lung, is maintained after birth. This pattern results in hypoxemia because most of the blood getting to the right side of the heart is shunted through the patent ductus arteriosus to the systemic circulation. This pattern of flow progressively can result in respiratory failure with cyanosis and significant metabolic acidosis. Evidence suggests surfactant deficiency is present in persistent pulmonary hypertension.[61] Affected infants tend to have minimal increases in P_{O_2} after exposure to supplemental oxygen if persistent pulmonary hypertension is severe. These infants often show evidence of shunting on pulse oximetry monitoring using preductal and postductal probes. Infants usually are born at term and may have only mild parenchymal disease on chest radiographs. Shunting of blood from the right side to the left side of the heart due to a cardiac lesion must be excluded by echocardiography and Doppler. Other disorders associated with development of persistent pulmonary hypertension in the newborn are listed in Box 38-1.

RESPIRATORY DISTRESS CAUSED BY AIR LEAKS

Pneumothorax and Pulmonary Interstitial Emphysema

Pneumothorax and pulmonary interstitial emphysema are the most frequent of all the air-leak syndromes seen in the newborn period. Other forms of air leaks, including pneumomediastinum and pneumopericardium, are less commonly seen. Risk factors include use of mechanical ventilation and continuous positive-pressure ventilation in a newborn with primary lung parenchymal disease.

Clinically significant **pneumothorax** usually causes sudden worsening of respiratory status that does not resolve until the air is evacuated. Other signs and symptoms include tachypnea, retractions, grunting, cyanosis, poor perfusion of the extremities, and decreased air entry to the affected part of the lung on auscultation. If there is associated shift of the heart to the opposite side, there is

---

Box 38–1 | **Diseases Associated with Persistent Pulmonary Hypertension**

Respiratory distress syndrome
Sepsis
Perinatal hypoxia
Congenital diaphragmatic hernia
Pulmonary hypoplasia
Polycythemia
Pneumonia
Meconium aspiration syndrome
Postmaturity
Idiopathic causes

Box 38–2	Other Causes of Respiratory Distress in the Newborn

Ascites
Massive hepatosplenomegaly
Anemia
Hydrops
Polycythemia
Rickets
Neonatal hyperthyroidism
Hypophosphatasia
Thanatophoric dwarfism
Jeune asphyxiating thoracic dystrophy
Kyphosis
Scoliosis
Intracranial hemorrhage
Interventricular hemorrhage
Tetralogy of Fallot
Vascular ring
Pericardial cyst
Pericardial teratoma
Posterior urethral valves
Goiter
Thyroglossal duct cyst
Cystic hygroma
Neonatal vallecular cyst
Anterior neck cysts arising from the III and IV
   pharyngeal pouches
Macroglossa
Duchenne muscular dystrophy
Myotonic dystrophy
Werdnig-Hoffmann spinal muscular dystrophy
Hypoglycemia
Metabolic acidosis
Tumor
Hemangioma
Neuroblastoma
Arteriovenous malformation
Schwannoma
Teratoma

decreased air entry to both sides of the lung even with unilateral pneumothorax. Pneumothorax can be diagnosed quickly at the bedside by transilluminating the chest wall. Findings on chest radiographs include air in the pleural space, displacement of the mediastinum to the contralateral side, displacement of the diaphragm downward, and collapse of the ipsilateral lung.

Pulmonary interstitial emphysema tends to occur more frequently in preterm infants who are mechanically ventilated. Air tracks into the perivascular and peribronchial tissues with rupture of alveoli, leading to further worsening of the respiratory status. It may be unilateral or bilateral and can progress to pneumothorax or pneumomediastinum. The risk of bronchopulmonary dysplasia is higher in these patients. Chest radiographs show air in interstitial spaces of the lung.

OTHER DISORDERS

Many other disorders that present in the neonatal period may have associated respiratory distress (Box 38-2). Discussion of these disorders is beyond the scope of this chapter. The reader should consult other chapters in this book for detailed information.

REFERENCES

1. Dave A: Absent nasal flaring in newborn with bilateral respiratory distress. Pediatrics 109:989, 2002.
2. Yao AC, Lind J, Vuorenkoski V: Expiratory grunting in the normal late clamped neonate. Pediatrics 48:865, 1971.
3. Astrup P: Red cell pH and oxygen affinity of hemoglobin. N Engl J Med 283:202, 1970.
4. Beresch R, Beresch RE: The effect of organic phosphates from the human erythrocyte on the allosteric properties of hemoglobin. Biochem Biophys Res Communications 26:162, 1967.
5. Chanutin A, Curnish R: Effect of organic and inorganic phosphates on the oxygen equilibrium of human erythrocytes. Arch Biochem Biophys 121:96, 1967.
6. Sacks LM, Delivoria-Papadopoulos M: Hemoglobin-oxygen interactions. Semin Perinatol 8:168, 1984.
7. Delivoria-Papadopoulos M, Roncervis NP, Oski FA, et al: Postnatal change in oxygen transport in term, premature and sick infants: The role of the red cell 2,3-diphosphoglycerate and adult hemoglobin. Pediatr Res 5:235, 1971.
8. Oski FA, Delivoria-Papadopoulos M: The shift to the left. Pediatrics 48:853, 1971.
9. Oski FA, Gottlieb AJ, Delivoria-Papadopoulos M, et al: Red cell 2,3-diphosphoglycerate levels in subjects with chronic hypoxia. N Engl J Med 280:1165, 1969.
10. West JB: Respiratory Physiology: The Essentials, 7th ed. Philadelphia, Lippincott Williams & Wilkins, 2004, pp 84-88.
11. Laffey JG, Kavanagh BP: Medical progress: Hypocapnia. N Engl J Med 347:43, 2002.
12. Burri PW: Development and growth of the human lung. In: Handbook of Physiology: The Respiratory System. Bethesda, MD, American Physiological Society, 1985.
13. Inselman LS, Mellins RB: Growth and development of the lung. J Pediatr 98:1, 1981.
14. Foglia RP: Esophageal disease in the pediatric age group. Surg Clin North Am 4:785, 1994.
15. Holder TM, Cloud DT, et al: Esophageal atresia and tracheoesophageal fistula: A survey of its members by the Surgical Section of the American Academy of Pediatrics. Pediatrics 34:542, 1964.
16. Heydanus R, Stewart PA, Wladimiroff JW, Los FJ: Prenatal diagnosis of congenital cystic adenomatoid malformation: A report of seven cases. Prenat Diagn 13:65, 1993.
17. Al-Bassam, Al-Rabeeah, Al-Nassar S, et al: Congenital cystic disease of the lung in infants and children. Eur J Pediatr Surg 9:364, 1999.
18. Sittig SE, Asay GF: Cystic adenomatoid malformation in the newborn: Two case studies and review of the literature. Respir Care 45:1188, 2000.
19. Gardikis S, Didilis V, Polychrodinis A, et al: Spontaneous pneumothorax resulting from congenital cystic adenomatous malformation in a preterm infant: Case report and literature review. Eur J Plast Surg 12:195, 2002.
20. Bratu I, Flageole H, Chen MF, et al: The multiple facets of pulmonary sequestration. J Pediatr Surg 36:784, 2001.
21. MacKenzie TC, Guttenberg ME, Nisenbaum HL, et al: A fetal lesion consisting of bronchogenic cyst, bronchopulmonary sequestration, and congenital cystic adenomatoid malformation: the missing link? Fetal Diag Ther 16:193, 2001.
22. Roberts D, Sweeney E, Walkinshaw S: Congenital cystic adenomatoid malformation of the lung coexisting with

recombinant chromosome 18: A case report. Fetal Diag Ther 16:65, 2001.

23. Roberts PA, Holland AJ, Halliday RJ, et al: Congenital lobar emphysema: Like father, like son. J Pediatr Surg 37:799, 2002.

24. Al-Salem AH: Congenital lobar emphysema. Saudi Med J 23:335, 2002.

25. Olutoye OO, Coleman BG, Adzick NS: Prenatal diagnosis and management of congenital lobar emphysema. J Pediatr Surg 35:792, 2000.

26. Tsukahara Y, Ohno T, Itakura A, et al: Prenatal diagnosis of congenital diaphragmatic eventration by magnetic resonance imaging. Am J Perinatol 18:241, 2001.

27. Volpe MV, Archavachotokul K, Bhan I, et al: Association of bronchopulmonary sequestration with expression of the homeobox protein Hoxb-5.J Pediatr Surg 35:1817, 2000.

28. Chan YF, Oldfield R, Vogel S, et al: Pulmonary sequestration presenting as a prenatally detected suprarenal lesion in a neonate. J Pediatr Surg 35:1367, 2000.

29. Golombek SG: The history of congenital diaphragmatic hernia from 1850 to the present. J Perinatol 22:242, 2002.

30. Jesudason EC: Challenging embryological theories on congenital diaphragmatic hernia: Future therapedic implications for pediatric surgery. Ann R Coll Surg Engl 84:252, 2002.

31. Glick PL, Stannard VA, Leach CL, et al: Pathophysiology of congenital diaphragmatic hernia: II. The fetal lamb CDH model is surfactant deficient. J Pediatr Surg 27:382, 1992.

32. Kitagawa M: Lung hypoplasia in congenital diaphragmatic hernia: A quantitative study of airway, artery, and alveolar development. Br J Surg 58:342, 1971.

33. Fryns JP: A new lethal syndrome with cloudy cornea, diaphragmatic defects and distal limb deformities. Hum Genet 50:65, 1979.

34. Ratan SK, Grover SB: Lung agenesis in a neonate presenting with contralateral mediastinal shift. Am J Perinatol 18:441, 2001.

35. Brenner KE, Oca MJ, Donn SM: Congenital choanal atresia in siblings. J Perinatol 20:443, 2000.

36. Koga K, Kawashiro N, Araki A, et al: Radiographic diagnosis of congenital bony nasal stenosis. Int J Pediatr Otorhinolaryngol 59:29, 2001.

37. Hall BD: Choanal atresia and associated multiple anomalies. J Pediatr 95:395, 1979.

38. Keller JL, Kacker A: Choanal atresia, CHARGE association, and congenital nasal stenosis. Otolaryngol Clin North Am 33:1343, 2000.

39. Beers MF, Hamvas A, Moxley MA, et al: Pulmonary surfactant metabolism in infants lacking surfactant protein B. Am J Respir Cell Mol Biol 22:380, 2000.

40. Kallapur S, Ikegami M: The surfactants. Am J Perinatol 17:335, 2000.

41. Rooney SA, Young SL, Mendeloon CR: Molecular and cellular processing of lung surfactant. FASEB J 8:957, 1994.

42. Jobe AH, Ikegami M: Biology of surfactant. Clin Perinatol 28:655, 2001.

43. van Golde LM: The pulmonary surfactant system: Biochemical aspects and functional significance. Physiol Rev 68:374, 1988.

44. Gluck L, Kulovich MV, Boser RC Jr, Keidel WN: The interpretation and significance of the lecithin/sphingomyelin ratio in amniotic fluid. Am J Obstet Gynecol 120:142, 1974.

45. Weaver TE: Synthesis processing and secretion of surfactant proteins B and C. Biochim Biophys Acta 1408:173, 1998.

46. Wright L: Immunomodulatory functions of surfactant. Physiol Rev 77:931, 1977.

47. Hawgood S, Benson BJ, Schilling J, et al: Nucleotide and amino acid sequences of pulmonary surfactant protein SP 18 and evidence of cooperation between SP18 and SP 28-36 in surfactant lipid absorption. Proc Natl Acad Sci U S A 8:75, 1989.

48. Beers MF: Molecullar processing and cellular metabolism of surfactant protein C. In Rooney SA (ed): Lung Surfactant: Cellular and Molecular Processing. Austin, TX: RG Landes, 1998, pp 93-124.

49. Thompson MW: Surfactant protein B deficiency: Insights into surfactant function through clinical surfactant protein deficiency. Am J Med Sci 321:26, 2001.

50. Avery ME, Mead J: Surface properties in relation to atelectasis and hyaline membrane disease. J Dis Child 97:517, 1959.

51. Acharyya S, Acharyya K: Surfactant protein B: A rare lethal condition in newborn. Indian Pediatr 38:1039, 2001.

52. Ballard PL, Nogee LM, Beers MF, et al: Partial deficiency of surfactant protein B in an infant with chronic lung disease. Pediatrics 96:1046, 1995.

53. Nogee LM, Wert SE, Profitt SA, et al: A mutation in the surfactant protein B gene responsible for fatal neonatal respiratory disease in multiple kindreds. J Clin Invest 93: 1860, 1994.

54. Nogee LM, Wert SE, Proffit SA, et al: Allelic heterogeneity in hereditary surfactant protein B deficiency. Am J Respir Crit Care Med 161:973, 2000.

55. Macphail GL, Taylor GD, Bucanan-Chell M, et al: Epidemiology, treatment and outcome of candidemia: A five-year review at three Canadian hospitals. Mycoses 45:141, 2002.

56. Viscardi RM, Manimtim WM, Sunn CC, et al: Lung pathology in premature infants with *Ureaplasma urealyticum* infection. Pediatr Dev Pathol 5:141, 2002.

57. Wiswell TE: Handling the meconium stained infant. Semin Neonatol 6:225, 2001.

58. Davis PJ, Shekerdemian LS: Meconium aspiration syndrome and extracorporeal membrane oxygenation. Arch Dis Child Fetal Neonat Ed 84:F1, 2001.

59. Theophilopolos D, Plaza M, Gilbert-Barness E, et al: Clinico-pathology conference: Infant with meconium-stained amniotic fliud, poor Apgar scores, hypoxia, and respiratory problems. Pediatr Pathol Mol Med 20:209, 2001.

60. Mangararo R, Mami C, Palmara A, et al: Incidence of meconium aspiration syndrome in term meconium stained babies managed at birth with selective tracheal intubation. J Perinat Med 29:465, 2001.

61. Hallman M, Kankaanpaa K: Evidence of surfactant deficiency in persistence of the fetal circulation. Eur J Pediatr 134:129, 1980.

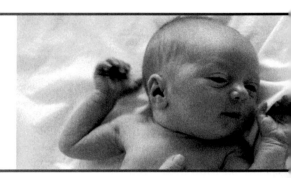

CHAPTER 39

Nitric Oxide and Alternative Pulmonary Vasodilators

Nicolas F. M. Porta and Robin H. Steinhorn

The discovery of endothelium-derived nitric oxide (NO) as a major regulator of vascular tone, as well as subsequent intense research efforts directed toward understanding its role in clinical medicine, has dramatically changed the practice of neonatology. In less than a decade, the use of inhaled NO (iNO) as a selective pulmonary vasodilator progressed from experimental therapy to standard of care for infants with persistent pulmonary hypertension of the newborn (PPHN). Because iNO is now a widely available therapy approved by the U.S. Food and Drug Administration for full-term infants with hypoxic respiratory failure, understanding the indications, outcomes, and limitations of this therapy is increasingly important.

NITRIC OXIDE

NO is an inorganic, gaseous free radical that was discovered in the late 1980s to be the main constituent of the endothelium-derived relaxing factor.[1] After 1990, NO replaced prostacyclin as the agent most extensively studied in the perinatal pulmonary circulation, and the investigators who first described NO–cyclic guanosine monophosphate (cGMP) signaling were awarded the Nobel Prize in Medicine in 1998.

Endogenously, NO is produced from the terminal nitrogen of L-arginine by nitric oxide synthase (NOS) (Fig. 39-1). There are three known isoforms of NOS. Neuronal NOS (nNOS or NOS I) and endothelial NOS (eNOS or NOS III) are low-output, constitutively expressed isoforms whose activity is regulated by calcium and calmodulin. Inducible NOS (iNOS or NOS II) is a high-output NOS whose expression is induced by cytokines and other agents and whose activity is largely or completely independent of calcium. All three isoforms are present and developmentally regulated in the fetal lung,[2-4] and physiologic studies indicate that all three are potential sources of NO leading to vascular smooth muscle relaxation in the perinatal pulmonary circulation.[5-7]

The best described action of NO is its activation of soluble guanylate cyclase, a heterodimer with α and β subunits. After activation, soluble guanylate cyclase converts guanosine triphosphate to the second messenger cGMP.[8,9] Through activation of specific kinases, cGMP decreases free cytosolic calcium concentration, which results in smooth muscle cell relaxation.

Cyclic nucleotide phosphodiesterases (PDE) constitute the only known pathway for the hydrolysis of cGMP and control the intensity and duration of its signal transduction.[10,11] Eleven families of PDE isoenzymes have been identified, and at least four PDE isoenzymes have been identified in human pulmonary artery.[12] Type 5 (PDE5), a cGMP-binding, cGMP-specific isoform, is found in especially high concentrations in the lung.[11,13,14]

The Role of Nitric Oxide Signaling in the Perinatal Lung

Understanding the physiology of the normal pulmonary vascular transition that occurs at birth, as well as the pathophysiologic mechanisms underlying PPHN, is important for optimal use of iNO and other pulmonary vasodilators.

In fetal life, high pulmonary vascular resistance is maintained by hypoxia. The initial dramatic pulmonary vasodilatation and decrease in pulmonary vascular resistance normally seen after birth are stimulated by the combination of rhythmic ventilation of the lung and increase in alveolar oxygen tension.[15] Each of these stimuli by itself decreases pulmonary vascular resistance and increases pulmonary blood flow, but the largest effects are seen when the two events occur simultaneously.[16]

Pulmonary endothelial cells play a central role in the pulmonary vascular transition through the production and release of numerous mediators that act on the smooth muscle cells. The main endothelial products currently believed to be responsible for the pulmonary vasodilatation at transition include arachidonic acid metabolites and NO. Prostacyclin is the arachidonic acid metabolite most studied in the transition of the pulmonary circulation at birth.

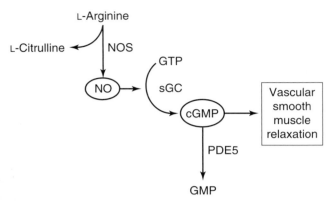

Figure 39–1. Nitric oxide signaling pathway in regulation of vascular tone. Nitric oxide (NO) is synthesized by nitric oxide synthase (NOS) from the terminal nitrogen group of L-arginine. NO stimulates soluble guanylate cyclase (sGC), which converts guanosine triphosphate (GTP) to cyclic guanosine monophosphate (cGMP). cGMP indirectly decreases free cytosolic calcium, which results in smooth muscle relaxation, which in turn leads to vascular dilation. Type 5 phosphodiesterase (PDE5) hydrolyzes cGMP, thus regulating the intensity and duration of its vascular effects. GMP, guanosine monophosphate.

Prostacyclin may be important in pulmonary vasodilatation after rhythmic distention of the lung, but it does not appear to play an important role in the pulmonary vascular response to oxygenation in the fetus.[17] Despite a large body of research, the importance of prostacyclin in the transition at birth remains unclear. In contrast, the production of NO has been shown to be fundamental to the pulmonary vascular response to oxygen in the fetus and at birth.[5,18] Furthermore, acute or chronic inhibition of NOS in fetal lambs produces pulmonary hypertension after delivery, which indicates its importance in the normal pulmonary vascular transition.[19]

The expression of the key enzymes responsible for production and response to NO (e.g., NOS, soluble guanylate cyclase, PDE5) follows distinct developmental time lines, with peak expression occurring during the perinatal period.[2,20-22] It is interesting to speculate that this developmental pattern primes the newborn to respond particularly well to endogenous and exogenous NO.

Abnormalities of Transition: Persistent Pulmonary Hypertension of the Newborn

PPHN is failure of the normal circulatory transition that follows birth and complicates approximately 2 per 1000 live births.[23] PPHN causes substantial morbidity and mortality in otherwise normal full-term infants. With inadequate pulmonary perfusion, neonates develop refractory hypoxemia, respiratory distress, and acidosis. Appropriate and timely interventions are essential to prevent progression to circulatory failure and death.

Clinically, PPHN is most often recognized in full-term or near-term neonates, but it can occur in premature neonates as well. PPHN is often associated with perinatal distress and typically manifests as respiratory distress and cyanosis within 6 hours of birth. Laboratory findings

may include low glucose, hypocalcemia, polycythemia, or thrombocytopenia. Radiographic findings are variable, depending on the primary disease associated with PPHN. Classically, the chest radiograph in idiopathic PPHN is clear with decreased vascular markings. In general, the degree of hypoxemia is more marked than the severity of radiographic lung disease.

It is important to realize that not all full-term infants who are hypoxemic have PPHN. PPHN is characterized by extrapulmonary shunt, in which high pulmonary artery pressure at systemic levels leads to right-to-left shunting of blood flow across the ductus arteriosus or foramen ovale. In many infants with parenchymal lung disease, hypoxemia results from intrapulmonary shunt or ventilation-perfusion mismatch and may not be associated with the shunting of blood flow across the patent ductus arteriosus and patent foramen ovale. Pulmonary vascular resistance may be elevated in hypoxemic newborns without PPHN, but without extrapulmonary shunting, it does not contribute significantly to hypoxemia. Therefore, echocardiography is an essential tool for determining the specific cause of hypoxemia.

Respiratory failure and hypoxemia in the full-term newborn result from a heterogeneous group of disorders, and the therapeutic approach and response often depend on the underlying disease. PPHN often results when structurally normal pulmonary vessels constrict in response to alveolar hypoxia caused by hypoventilation or by parenchymal disorders such as hyaline membrane disease or meconium aspiration syndrome (MAS). However, PPHN can also occur idiopathically in the absence of underlying parenchymal disease. In these cases, the syndrome is the result of an abnormally remodeled vasculature that develops in utero in response to prolonged fetal stress, hypoxia, and/or pulmonary hypertension. Excessive and peripheral muscularization of pulmonary arterioles can be seen in these cases. Finally, PPHN is commonly associated with lung hypoplasia, as seen in congenital diaphragmatic hernia. These underlying causes of PPHN are structurally quite different, and functional differences in response to vasodilators such as iNO are commonly observed. Knowledge of biologic alterations seen with PPHN is instrumental in expanding available therapeutic options.

Alterations of Endogenous Nitric Oxide Production in PPHN

As noted previously, inhibition of NOS in lambs produces pulmonary circulatory changes consistent with PPHN after delivery.[19,24] These lambs have hypoxemia as a result of shunting of deoxygenated blood across the foramen ovale, which suggests that inhibition or decreased activity of NOS could cause acute PPHN in some human infants. However, persistent pulmonary hypertension develops in these lambs without associated pulmonary vascular remodeling. Therefore, reduction of endogenous NO production alone is probably not sufficient to produce the full physiologic and anatomic picture of PPHN.

Mice with targeted disruption of eNOS offer an important experimental approach to the study of PPHN, although measurements of pulmonary hemodynamics are currently not feasible in newborn mice. Disruption of eNOS expression has not been reported to increase perinatal mortality. However, adult eNOS −/− mice respond to mild hypoxia with exaggerated pulmonary hypertension and an increase in muscularization in peripheral arterioles.[25,26] It is possible that decreased NOS expression in human infants produces similar exaggerated responses to hypoxia.

The animal model that most closely approximates human PPHN involves fetal occlusion of the ductus arteriosus in sheep, which leads to anatomic and physiologic alterations in the newborn lambs that are similar to clinical PPHN.[27,28] These lambs have decreased expression and activity of eNOS and soluble guanylate cyclase in their lung parenchyma and pulmonary arteries.[29-32] The net effect of these alterations leads to decreased NO-cGMP signaling. These studies demonstrate that alterations of the fetal circulation associated with transient increased pulmonary blood flow and shear stress can disrupt normal NO signaling and produce pulmonary hypertension after birth.

It is difficult to measure endogenous NO production in the newborn, and direct assay of NO production by pulmonary cells versus other cell types is not yet possible. Therefore, the few studies in human infants all have been based on more global measures of NO production. Urinary nitrites and nitrates are lower in infants with PPHN than in healthy full-term infants.[33] Plasma cGMP concentrations are also low in infants with PPHN and increase rapidly in response to iNO.[34] Expression of eNOS was found to be absent in umbilical vein endothelial cells cultured from four of six meconium-stained infants who subsequently developed PPHN.[35] Together, these studies provide indirect evidence for a deficiency of endogenous NO production in infants with PPHN. However, it is difficult to be certain whether the absence of eNOS produces PPHN or whether the vascular changes of PPHN result in decreased expression of eNOS.

Clinical Evidence of Efficacy of Inhaled Nitric Oxide

Before the availability of iNO, specific pulmonary vasodilatation was not clinically possible, and infants with PPHN received supportive care with aggressive ventilator management, in whom alkalosis was often induced with hyperventilation and/or infusion of alkali.[23] The most severely affected infants were treated with prolonged cardiopulmonary bypass with extracorporeal membrane oxygenation (ECMO) with its associated cost, morbidity, and mortality.

Some key features of NO make it a perfect candidate for a selective pulmonary vasodilator. It has a rapid and potent vasodilator effect. Because it is a small gas molecule, NO can be delivered through a ventilator directly to airspaces approximating the pulmonary vascular bed. Once in the blood stream, NO binds avidly to hemoglobin, which further limits its ability to exert systemic vasodilator effects. In a variety of animal models of pulmonary hypertension, iNO was shown to produce selective pulmonary vasodilatation after brief exposures. In the early 1990s, the first report in humans showed that brief exposures to iNO decreased pulmonary vascular resistance in adults with pulmonary hypertension.[36] Soon afterward, two

separate reports described dramatic improvements in oxygenation in severely hypoxic infants with PPHN.[37,38] This was followed by an animal study that showed that 24-hour periods of NO inhalation improved survival and did not produce lung injury in newborn lambs with PPHN after ductal ligation.[39]

The early animal studies and human case reports rapidly led investigators to develop multicenter randomized, placebo-controlled, blinded trials to test the effectiveness of iNO in full-term and near-term infants with PPHN.[40-44] These trials demonstrated that iNO significantly decreased the need for ECMO in newborns with PPHN.

Several of the randomized trials had sufficient numbers of patients to assess response as a function of the underlying lung disease, and these studies showed that the response to iNO is dependent on the underlying cause of PPHN. The most consistent finding was that iNO does not reduce the need for ECMO in infants with unrepaired congenital diaphragmatic hernia.[44,45] The infants with congenital diaphragmatic hernia enrolled in these two studies had relatively severe illness at the time of enrollment, as measured by oxygenation index. Although it is possible that iNO may be beneficial if delivered before onset of severe respiratory failure, this has not yet been demonstrated.

In the Neonatal Inhaled Nitric Oxide Study Group (NINOS) trial,[45] infants with hypoxemia associated with parenchymal lung disease caused by respiratory distress syndrome (RDS) and MAS were less likely to respond to iNO than were those with a predominance of vascular disease (Fig. 39-2). However, in the subsequent Clinical Inhaled Nitric Oxide Research Group Initiative (CINRGI) trial, in which lung expansion was first optimized with high-frequency ventilation and surfactant, infants with RDS and MAS responded well, as evidenced by a decreased need for ECMO (Fig. 39-3).[44]

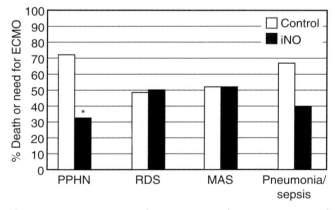

Figure 39–2. Outcome according to primary diagnosis in Neonatal Inhaled Nitric Oxide Study (NINOS). Data are expressed as percentages of infants who died or required extracorporeal membrane oxygenation (ECMO) according to primary diagnosis. Inhaled nitric oxide (iNO) decreased death or need for ECMO only among infants with idiopathic persistent pulmonary hypertension of the newborn (PPHN) in this trial, and it had no significant effect on infants with respiratory distress syndrome (RDS) or meconium aspiration syndrome (MAS). Asterisk indicates significant difference between the iNO recipients and controls (P < .05). (Data from reference 45.)

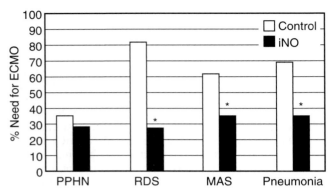

Figure 39–3. Outcome according to primary diagnosis in the Clinical Inhaled Nitric Oxide Research Group Initiative (CINRGI) trial. Data are expressed as percentages of infants requiring extracorporeal membrane oxygenation (ECMO) according to primary diagnosis. Inhaled nitric oxide (iNO) decreases the need for ECMO in infants with idiopathic persistent pulmonary hypertension of the newborn (PPHN) caused by parenchymal lung diseases. *Asterisks* indicate significant difference between iNO recipients and controls (P < .05). MAS, meconium aspiration syndrome; RDS, respiratory distress syndrome. *(Data from reference 44.)*

Meta-analysis has reinforced the finding that iNO reduces the need for ECMO in infants with hypoxic respiratory failure (Fig. 39-4).[46,47] Although iNO decreases the need for ECMO, it does not appear to reduce mortality rate or length of hospitalization. Although iNO has not been shown to significantly reduce morbid conditions such as chronic lung disease, follow-up studies of infants indicate that it does not increase abnormalities of lung function in the first year of life.[48] In addition, follow-up studies to 18 to 24 months of infants enrolled in the NINOS trial showed that iNO does not significantly increase the incidence of adverse neurodevelopmental sequalae.[49]

Finally, the use of iNO in premature infants younger than 34 weeks of gestational age has been reported.[50] Although adverse effects have not yet been found, the use of iNO in premature infants remains investigational, and multicenter trials nearing completion will determine whether there is a benefit.

Initiation of Inhaled Nitric Oxide

Current recommendations for the use of iNO are based on the results of the large, randomized, placebo-controlled clinical trials noted previously, which showed decreased need for ECMO in full-term or near-term infants (older than 34 weeks' gestation) with hypoxemic

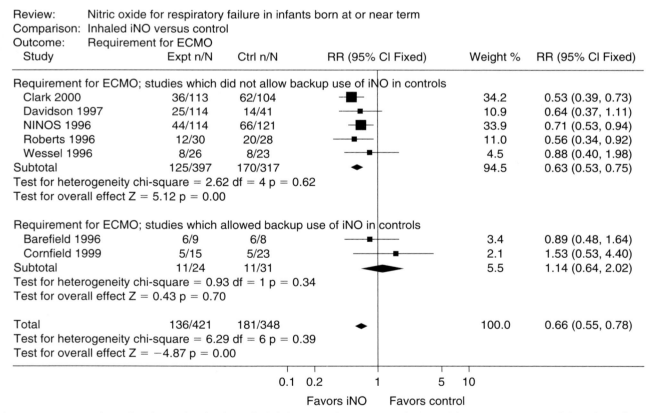

Study	Expt n/N	Ctrl n/N	RR (95% CI Fixed)	Weight %	RR (95% CI Fixed)
Review:	Nitric oxide for respiratory failure in infants born at or near term				
Comparison:	Inhaled iNO versus control				
Outcome:	Requirement for ECMO				
Requirement for ECMO; studies which did not allow backup use of iNO in controls					
Clark 2000	36/113	62/104		34.2	0.53 (0.39, 0.73)
Davidson 1997	25/114	14/41		10.9	0.64 (0.37, 1.11)
NINOS 1996	44/114	66/121		33.9	0.71 (0.53, 0.94)
Roberts 1996	12/30	20/28		11.0	0.56 (0.34, 0.92)
Wessel 1996	8/26	8/23		4.5	0.88 (0.40, 1.98)
Subtotal	125/397	170/317		94.5	0.63 (0.53, 0.75)
Test for heterogeneity chi-square = 2.62 df = 4 p = 0.62					
Test for overall effect Z = 5.12 p = 0.00					
Requirement for ECMO; studies which allowed backup use of iNO in controls					
Barefield 1996	6/9	6/8		3.4	0.89 (0.48, 1.64)
Cornfield 1999	5/15	5/23		2.1	1.53 (0.53, 4.40)
Subtotal	11/24	11/31		5.5	1.14 (0.64, 2.02)
Test for heterogeneity chi-square = 0.93 df = 1 p = 0.34					
Test for overall effect Z = 0.43 p = 0.70					
Total	136/421	181/348		100.0	0.66 (0.55, 0.78)
Test for heterogeneity chi-square = 6.29 df = 6 p = 0.39					
Test for overall effect Z = −4.87 p = 0.00					

0.1   0.2   1   5   10

Favors iNO   Favors control

Figure 39–4. Meta-analysis of randomized trials of use of inhaled nitric oxide (iNO) in newborns with hypoxemic respiratory failure shows that iNO decreases requirement for extracorporeal membrane oxygenation (ECMO). CI, confidence interval; Ctrl n/N, numbers of control subjects; Expt n/N, experimental numbers of subjects; RR, relative risk. *(From Barrington KJ, Finer NN: Nitric oxide for respiratory failure in infants born at or near term. Cochrane Database Syst Rev [4]:CD000509, 2001, with permission. Copyright Cochrane Library.)*

respiratory failure.[41,44] Although infants were eligible for enrollment in these trials with an oxygenation index exceeding 25, the mean oxygenation index of the patients enrolled in both trials was nearly 40. There are currently no studies that indicate that iNO benefits infants with less severe respiratory failure, such as those with an oxygenation index of less than 25. Although experimental data indicate that prolonged inhalation of low doses of iNO may be beneficial in animal models of pulmonary hypertension,[51] there is not sufficient evidence that this approach benefits human infants who have pulmonary hypertension beyond the first week or two of life.

An initial echocardiographic evaluation establishes the presence of pulmonary hypertension. In addition, it allows the clinician to rule out structural congenital heart disease as a cause of hypoxemia and to diagnose congenital heart lesions for which iNO treatment would be contraindicated. The use of iNO is contraindicated in congenital heart disease that is dependent on right-to-left shunting across the ductus arteriosus. This would include critical aortic stenosis, interrupted aortic arch, and hypoplastic left heart syndrome. Decreasing pulmonary vascular resistance with iNO in these conditions could lead to systemic hypoperfusion. In addition, iNO may worsen pulmonary edema in infants with obstructed total anomalous pulmonary venous return caused by the fixed venous obstruction. The use of iNO should be reserved for postoperative care in these patients after the obstruction has been surgically corrected.

When there is a poor response to iNO, the clinician should carefully consider whether ventricular function is adequate. For instance, left ventricular dysfunction is often associated with high left atrial and pulmonary venous pressures; iNO alone may not produce a sustained improvement in oxygenation if pulmonary venous hypertension and pulmonary edema are present.

Dose

Early studies in animals and infants used iNO doses as high as 80 to 100 parts per million (ppm). However, large clinical trials have not produced evidence that inhalation of these high doses produces better outcomes than lower doses (20 ppm). For instance, infants enrolled in the NINOS trial had iNO initiated at 20 ppm, but the dose could be increased to 80 ppm if there was no response.[41] Of the 112 infants, 55 (49%) failed to respond to 20 ppm iNO with an increase in arterial O_2 pressure of more than 20 mm Hg; of these, only 12 (22%) responded with an increase in arterial O_2 pressure of more than 10 mm Hg when the dose was increased. In a second trial, infants were randomly assigned to receive iNO at 5, 20, or 80 ppm or placebo.[42] No dose-dependent differences were observed, as measured by sustained improvement in oxygenation in response to 5, 20, and 80 ppm iNO.

Although no dose-dependent difference in oxygenation has been demonstrated, seven neonates with persistent pulmonary hypertension had pulmonary arterial pressure directly measured during inhalation of NO.[52] The iNO produced peak improvement in oxygenation at 5 ppm, but peak improvement in the ratio of pulmonary to systemic arterial pressure did not occur until a NO dose of 20 ppm.

These data suggest that oxygenation does not always reflect an optimal decrease in pulmonary vascular resistance and that 20 ppm may be the most appropriate initial dose for the treatment of PPHN.

Some studies have examined the clinical effects of starting therapy with lower doses. One group of investigators randomly assigned infants with PPHN to receive an initial iNO dose of 2 or 20 ppm[53] and found that infants who received 2 ppm did not have any improvement in oxygenation. Furthermore, these infants had no improvement in oxygenation even after iNO was increased to 20 ppm. This observation is significant because it implies that administration of a subtherapeutic dose of iNO may adversely affect the clinical response to a therapeutic dose of iNO. However, another study enrolled infants with an oxygenation index of less than 25 and showed that iNO at 1 to 2 ppm was as effective as higher concentrations. Those authors also noted that low doses did not attenuate responses to higher doses of iNO.[54] Although these results need to be confirmed, this study suggests that attempts to start at lower doses of iNO may be safe and effective in infants with moderate respiratory disease.

Ventilator Strategies

As noted, severe parenchymal lung disease may be associated with poor responsiveness to iNO in newborns with PPHN. In the initial NINOS trial, iNO did not reduce need for ECMO in infants with RDS and MAS.[41] In subsequent trials in which lung expansion was first optimized with surfactant and/or high-frequency ventilation, infants with RDS and MAS had significant reductions in ECMO use if assigned to receive iNO.[44] An additional randomized multicenter trial demonstrated that for infants with PPHN associated with severe parenchymal disease, response rates for high-frequency oscillatory ventilation (HFOV) and iNO together were better than HFOV alone or iNO with conventional ventilation.[43] These results have led to the recommendation that lung inflation should be optimized with HFOV before use of iNO.

Parenchymal lung disease of full-term and near-term infants is often associated with surfactant deficiency and/or inactivation. Surfactant dysfunction has been demonstrated in MAS, with a concentration-dependent inhibition of pulmonary surfactant activity occurring at meconium concentrations much lower than those required for inhibition by plasma protein and blood cell components.[55] Single-center trials have shown that surfactant improves oxygenation in infants with MAS,[56] and a large multicenter trial demonstrated that surfactant treatment decreased the need for ECMO, regardless of center-to-center variability in ventilator management strategy.[57] The reduction in need for ECMO was most apparent in infants with primary diagnoses of MAS or sepsis. Thus, surfactant may be an important tool in optimizing lung inflation before or during the use of iNO in infants with parenchymal lung disease.

Although inadequate lung inflation may lead to poor responsiveness to iNO, it is important to use powerful strategies such as HFOV with care. Overexpansion of the lung beyond 9 or 10 ribs may paradoxically worsen pulmonary hypertension because overdistended alveoli may compress capillaries and small arterioles. Optimal, not maximal, expansion should be the goal.

Toxicity of Inhaled Nitric Oxide

It is important to monitor for potential toxic effects associated with the use of iNO.[58] The reaction of NO with oxygen produces NO_2, which is highly toxic to pulmonary epithelial cells. Current delivery devices measure NO_2 continuously at the bedside with electrochemical cells. NO binding to hemoglobin produces methemoglobin. Activity of methemoglobin reductase is often reduced in the neonatal period, and high levels of methemoglobin could aggravate hypoxia. Methemoglobin levels should be measured several times during the first 24 hours of therapy and then at 24-hour intervals. Fortunately, NO_2 levels higher than 5 ppm and methemoglobin levels higher than 5% have generally been reported only in infants receiving high doses of iNO (80 ppm).[42]

An additional concern is that NO increases platelet cGMP, which inhibits platelet aggregation and could increase bleeding complications. Although iNO increases bleeding time in healthy adults,[59] bleeding complications, including intracranial hemorrhage, have not been increased in infants treated with iNO. However, if unexpected bleeding occurs in the clinical setting, discontinuation of iNO should be considered.

Extremely hypoxic infants who are candidates for iNO therapy are typically treated with high fractions of inspired oxygen, which leads to oxidative stress in the lung. Increased production of peroxynitrite through reaction of NO with superoxide ion produced in inflamed lungs can lead to further oxidative damage to all pulmonary cells and nitration of proteins. Damaged cells and inactivated proteins and enzymes can lead to further hypoxia and failed vasodilatation. Continued requirement for aggressive respiratory support can lead to chronic lung injury, which can eventually become irreversible.

Weaning and Rebound Pulmonary Hypertension

Once a pulmonary vascular response to 20 ppm is established and stable, efforts to wean from both iNO and fraction of inspired O_2 should be made, knowing that the combination of these two gases can generate several toxic products. In general, we recommend that weaning begin within 24 hours of initiation of iNO. During weaning from iNO, the goal should be adequate oxygenation rather than hyperoxia. Once oxygenation is established, iNO can frequently be easily decreased to low doses of 5 ppm within 24 hours. Subsequently, most infants tolerate continued weaning from iNO over several days until 1 to 2 ppm is reached. Recommendations for weaning from iNO are varied, and various large trials have used different protocols effectively.

A frequent and dramatic problem with iNO therapy is the development of rebound pulmonary hypertension.[60] This is the clinical finding that acute withdrawal of iNO can be associated with a dramatic worsening of hypoxia. This phenomenon occurs even in patients who had no initial improvement with initiation of iNO.[61] Various

mechanisms have been proposed for this phenomenon. The simplest explanation is that the rebound reflects worsening of the underlying condition or ongoing need for iNO despite clinical improvement. However, in vitro studies and clinical experience indicate that rebound pulmonary hypertension results from more complex cellular mechanisms. First, exogenous NO does not appear to inhibit NOS expression,[62] but it does inhibit NOS activity and endogenous production of NO.[63] Purified NOS becomes nitrated when exposed to NO donors, and NOS activity is inhibited by exposure to peroxynitrite. Second, iNO can lead to increased production of competing vasoconstrictors, such as endothelin.[64] Endothelin is a vasoactive peptide with powerful vasoconstrictive properties. During iNO therapy, although pulmonary vasodilatation is promoted, endothelin accumulates. When iNO is interrupted, endothelin action becomes unopposed, which leads to net vasoconstriction.

Although weaning is usually well tolerated, stopping iNO can be more problematic. This is particularly true if the patient has been exposed to higher doses for several days, and weaning and discontinuation should be done cautiously in order to avoid rebound pulmonary hypertension. We recommend stepwise weaning to 1 ppm and then discontinuation of iNO from that dose. Mild hypoxemia necessitating a transient increase in inspired oxygen is still sometimes seen. This is often tolerated, although some infants respond only to reinstitution of iNO. Subsequent attempts at withdrawing iNO are often successful with slow but deliberate final weaning. The iNO delivery device allows weaning to 0.5 ppm before final discontinuation.

Use of Nitric Oxide in the Non-ECMO Center

Because of the relative ease of delivery of iNO, this therapy is already used at many centers that do not provide ECMO. Although iNO produces a marked improvement in oxygenation in many infants with PPHN, this improvement is not always sustained. The ideal clinical use of iNO should never cause delay in transfer to an ECMO center.

Withdrawal of iNO during transport to an ECMO center should be expected to produce rebound pulmonary hypertension and acute deterioration. Therefore, continuing iNO during transport is essential. When there is a lack of improvement or deterioration despite iNO treatment in institutions that cannot offer more advanced rescue therapy, provisions must be in place to accomplish transport to the ECMO center without interruption of iNO treatment. If a center does not provide ECMO, it should work in collaboration with an ECMO center to prospectively establish appropriate iNO failure criteria and mechanisms for the timely transfer of infants to the collaborating ECMO center.[65] A hospital that does not provide ECMO is responsible for the guarantee of uninterrupted iNO delivery during transport to an ECMO center before initiating therapy.[65]

Finally, because the use of iNO has not been demonstrated to reduce need for ECMO in infants with congenital diaphragmatic hernia, we recommend that iNO be used in these infants in non-ECMO centers only for acute stabilization, if necessary, followed by immediate transfer to a center that can provide ECMO.

Enhancement of Inhaled Nitric Oxide Effect

As with the preclinical testing for iNO use in PPHN, the understanding of the cellular mechanisms that impair the clinical response to iNO has been gained largely from the study of animal models. Many investigators have studied experimental lambs with persistent pulmonary hypertension after antenatal ligation of the ductus arteriosus because of the vascular alterations in the multiple enzymes that are responsible for NO-cGMP signaling. Other investigators have examined cultured vascular smooth muscle cells and found that NO donor compounds and cytokines decrease soluble guanylate cyclase expression. These studies indicate that other important environment stimuli potentially modulate responsiveness to NO.[66,67]

Because the response to iNO is believed to be mediated primarily by activation of soluble guanylate cyclase and activation of cGMP-dependent protein kinase, enhancement of cGMP accumulation by other mechanisms is being investigated in the treatment of PPHN. Inhibition of cGMP-metabolizing PDE5 activity may increase cGMP concentrations and increase the efficacy of iNO. Dipyridamole, which has been used for many years to inhibit platelet aggregation, inhibits cGMP metabolism. Although there have been anecdotal reports of its use in human infants,[68,69] dipyridamole may be associated with systemic hypotension in the neonatal period[70] and must be used with caution in this age group. More potent and specific experimental inhibitors of PDE5 have been tested with encouraging results, which indicates the feasibility of this therapeutic strategy.

Sildenafil is a potent and highly specific PDE5 inhibitor approved by the U.S. Food and Drug Administration for the treatment of male erectile dysfunction. In experimental lambs with pulmonary hypertension induced by a thromboxane analogue, both enteric and aerosolized sildenafil dilated the pulmonary vasculature and augmented the pulmonary vascular response to iNO.[71,72] Intravenous sildenafil was found to be a selective pulmonary vasodilator with efficacy equivalent to iNO in a piglet model of meconium aspiration.[73] Reports of the use of enteric sildenafil in adults and pediatric patients with pulmonary hypertension are appearing.[74] Sildenafil may attenuate rebound pulmonary hypertension after withdrawal of iNO in this population.[75] Studies to date have been limited in newborns, because sildenafil is available only in enteric forms. However an intravenous preparation is now under investigation in adults and newborns with pulmonary hypertension.

New studies indicate that scavengers of reactive oxygen species, such as superoxide dismutase, may augment responsiveness to iNO. Because iNO is usually delivered with high concentrations of oxygen, there is a concern about enhanced production of free radicals such as superoxide. Superoxide combines rapidly with NO to form peroxynitrite, a potent oxidant. Superoxide dismutase scavenges and converts superoxide radical to hydrogen peroxide, which is subsequently converted to water by the enzyme catalase. In lambs with pulmonary hypertension, a single dose of intratracheal recombinant human superoxide dismutase dilated the pulmonary circulation and enhanced the pulmonary vascular effects of iNO.[76] This therapeutic approach may have multiple beneficial effects: scavenging superoxide may make iNO more available to stimulate vasodilatation and may also reduce oxidative stress and limit lung injury. Human trials are expected to begin soon.

ALTERNATIVE PULMONARY VASODILATORS

Although iNO is often effective and sufficient for reversing PPHN, alternative therapies may be useful when response to NO is not adequate or sustained. The best-known alternative agent is probably tolazoline, which is a potent endothelium-independent vasodilator. Unfortunately, the efficacy of tolazoline was limited by systemic hypotension, and it is no longer manufactured in the United States.

Like cGMP, cyclic adenosine monophosphate (cAMP) also stimulates vasodilatation, and therapies aimed at increasing cAMP levels have been used for pulmonary hypertension. Using milrinone to inhibit PDE3, a phosphodiesterase that metabolizes cAMP, is one potential approach. Milrinone has been shown to decrease pulmonary artery pressure and resistance and to act additively with iNO in animal studies.[77] Systemic hypotension may limit the usefulness of milrinone.

Prostacyclin stimulates membrane-bound adenylate cyclase, thus increasing cAMP levels. In addition, prostacyclin inhibits pulmonary artery smooth muscle cell proliferation in vitro.[78] Although the use of systemic infusions of prostacyclin has been limited by the development of systemic hypotension,[79] inhaled prostacyclin has been shown to have vasodilator effects limited to the pulmonary circulation.[80] Reports of its use in children have been positive, but reports of inhaled prostacyclin use in infants with pulmonary hypertension have been rare to date.[81,82] The actions of inhaled prostacyclin and iNO appear to be additive in humans[83] and even synergistic in animal studies.[84] Rebound pulmonary hypertension after withdrawal of iNO has been mitigated by intravenous prostacyclin in children with pulmonary hypertension after congenital heart disease.[85] We used inhaled prostacyclin to treat four infants with severe PPHN who were unresponsive to iNO, and we observed rapid improvements in oxygenation in all four infants.[86]

Many other vasodilators have been investigated, and some may be useful as adjuvant therapies in the management of infants with severe PPHN who do not adequately respond to iNO.[87] Magnesium sulfate has vasodilator effects through antagonism of calcium entry into vascular smooth muscle cells. Improved oxygenation after intravenous magnesium sulfate infusion in infants with PPHN has been reported, but the potential for systemic vasodilatation and hypotension will probably limit clinical use. Adenosine and adenosine triphosphate cause NO-dependent pulmonary vasodilatation in fetal lambs,[88] and pilot studies indicate a potential benefit in infants.[89] Moya and colleagues suggested that treatment with a unique gas, O-nitrosoethanol, may increase the endogenous pool of S-nitrosothiols in the airway and circulation, thereby providing a new treatment strategy for PPHN.[90] They found that O-nitrosoethanol produced sustained improvements in postductal arterial oxygenation and systemic hemodynamics in seven neonates.[91]

SUMMARY

The use of iNO has significantly decreased the need for ECMO in full-term infants with hypoxic respiratory failure. Awareness of the scientific basis for, and human experience with, the use of iNO is imperative in order to use this powerful therapy in the most safe and effective manner. Meanwhile, ongoing investigation of the causes of respiratory failure is essential for bringing additional effective therapies to the bedside. The ultimate goal is not only to further decrease the need for ECMO but also to decrease rates of mortality and morbidity and to improve the overall outcome for this high-risk population of infants.

REFERENCES

1. Ignarro LJ, Buga GM, Wood KS, et al: Endothelium-derived relaxing factor produced and released from artery and vein is nitric oxide. Proc Natl Acad Sci U S A 84:9265, 1987.
2. North AJ, Star RA, Brannon TS, et al: Nitric oxide synthase type I and type III gene expression are developmentally regulated in rat lung. Am J Physiol Lung Cell Mol Physiol 266:L635, 1994.
3. Loesch A, Burnstock G: Ultrastructural localization of nitric oxide synthase and endothelin in rat pulmonary artery and vein during postnatal development and aging. Cell Tissue Res 283:355, 1996.
4. Xue C, Reynolds PR, Johns RA: Developmental expression of NOS isoforms in fetal rat lung: Implications for transitional circulation and pulmonary angiogenesis. Am J Physiol Lung Cell Mol Physiol 270:L88, 1996.
5. Tiktinsky MH, Morin FC III: Increasing oxygen tension dilates fetal pulmonary circulation via endothelium-derived relaxing factor. Am J Physiol Heart Circ Physiol 265:H376, 1993.
6. Rairigh RL, Storme L, Parker TA, et al: Role of neuronal nitric oxide synthase in regulation of vascular and ductus arteriosus tone in the ovine fetus. Am J Physiol Lung Cell Mol Physiol 278:L105, 2000.
7. Rairigh RL, Parker T, Ivy DD, et al: Role of inducible nitric oxide synthase in the pulmonary vascular response to birth-related stimuli in the ovine fetus. Circ Res 88:721, 2001.
8. Ignarro LJ, Harbison RG, Wood KS, Kadowitz PJ: Activation of purified soluble guanylate cyclase by endothelium-derived relaxing factor from intrapulmonary artery and vein: Stimulation by acetylcholine, bradykinin and arachidonic acid. J Pharmacol Exp Ther 237:893, 1986.
9. Murad F: Cyclic guanosine monophosphate as a mediator of vasodilatation. J Clin Invest 78:1, 1986.
10. Schmidt HHHW, Lohmann SM, Walter U: The nitric oxide and cGMP signal transduction system: Regulation and mechanism of action. Biochim Biophys Acta 1178:153, 1993.
11. Thompson WJ: Cyclic nucleotide phosphodiesterases: Pharmacology, biochemistry and function. Pharmacol Ther 51:13, 1991.
12. Rabe KF, Tenor H, Dent G, et al: Identification of PDE isozymes in human pulmonary artery and effect of selective PDE inhibitors. Am J Physiol Lung Cell Mol Physiol 266:L536, 1994.
13. Saeki T, Saito I: Isolation of cyclic nucleotide phosphodiesterase isozymes from pig aorta. Biochem Pharmacol 46:833, 1993.
14. Thomas MK, Francis SH, Corbine JD: Characterization of a purified bovine lung cGMP-binding cGMP phosphodiesterase. J Biol Chem 265:14964, 1990.
15. Fineman JR, Soifer SJ, Heymann MA: Regulation of pulmonary vascular tone in the perinatal period. Annu Rev Physiol 57:115, 1995.
16. Teitel DF, Iwamoto HS, Rudolph AM: Changes in the pulmonary circulation during birth-related events. Pediatr Res 27:372, 1990.
17. Morin FC III, Egan EA, Norfleet WT: Indomethacin does not diminish the pulmonary vascular response of the fetus to increased oxygen tension. Pediatr Res 24:696, 1988.
18. Cornfield DN, Reeve HL, Talorova S, et al: Oxygen causes fetal pulmonary vasodilatation through activation of a calcium-dependent potassium channel. Proc Natl Acad Sci U S A 93:8089, 1996.
19. Fineman JR, Wong J, Morin FC III, et al: Chronic nitric oxide inhibition in utero produces persistent pulmonary hypertension in newborn lambs. J Clin Invest 93:2675, 1994.
20. Bloch KD, Filippov G, Sanchez LS, et al: Pulmonary soluble guanylate cyclase, a nitric oxide receptor, is increased during the perinatal period. Am J Physiol Lung Cell Mol Physiol 272:L400, 1997.
21. Hanson KA, Burns F, Rybalkin SD, et al: Developmental changes in lung cGMP phosphodiesterase-5 activity, protein, and message. Am J Respir Crit Care Med 158:279, 1998.
22. Sanchez LS, Del La Monte SM, Filippov G, et al: Cyclic-GMP–binding, cyclic-GMP–specific phosphodiesterase gene expression is regulated during rat pulmonary development. Pediatr Res 43:163, 1998.
23. Walsh-Sukys MC, Tyson JE, Wright LL, et al: Persistent pulmonary hypertension of the newborn in the era before nitric oxide: Practice variation and outcomes. Pediatr 105:14, 2000.
24. Abman SH, Chatfield BA, Hall SL, McMurtry IF: Role of endothelium-derived relaxing factor during transition of pulmonary circulation at birth. Am J Physiol Heart Circ Physiol 259:H1921, 1990.
25. Fagan KA, Fouty BW, Tyler RC, et al: The pulmonary circulation of homozygous or heterozygous eNos-null mice is hyperresponsive to mild hypoxia. J Clin Invest 103:291, 1999.
26. Steudel W, Scherrer-Crosbie M, Bloch KD, et al: Sustained pulmonary hypertension and right ventricular hypertrophy after chronic hypoxia in mice with congenital deficiency of nitric oxide synthase 3. J Clin Invest 101:2468, 1998.
27. Morin FC III: Ligating the ductus arteriosus before birth causes persistent pulmonary hypertension in the newborn lamb. Pediatr Res 25:245, 1989.
28. Abman SH, Accurso FJ: Acute effects of partial compression of ductus arteriosus on fetal pulmonary circulation. Am J Physiol Heart Circ Physiol 26:H626, 1989.
29. Black SM, Fineman JR, Steinhorn RH, et al: Altered molecular expression of nitric oxide synthase in a lamb model of increased pulmonary blood flow. Am J Physiol Heart Circ Physiol 275:H1643, 1998.

30. Shaul PW, Yuhanna IS, German Z, et al: Pulmonary endothelial NO synthase gene expression is decreased in fetal lambs with pulmonary hypertension. Am J Physiol Lung Cell Mol Physiol 272:L1005, 1997.

31. Steinhorn RH, Millard SL, Morin FC III: Persistent pulmonary hypertension of the newborn: Role of nitric oxide and endothelin in pathophysiology and treatment. Clin Perinatol 22:405, 1995.

32. Tzao C, Nickerson PA, Russell JA, et al: Pulmonary hypertension alters soluble guanylate cyclase activity and expression in pulmonary arteries isolated from fetal lambs. Pediatr Pulmonol 31:97, 2001.

33. Dollberg S, Warner BW, Myatt L: Urinary nitrite and nitrate concentrations in patients with idiopathic persistent pulmonary hypertension of the newborn and effect of extracorporeal membrane oxygenation. Pediatr Res 37:31, 1995.

34. Christou H, Adatia I, Van Marter LJ, et al: Effect of inhaled nitric oxide on endothelin-1 and cyclic guanosine 5′−monophosphate plasma concentrations in newborn infants with persistent pulmonary hypertension. J Pediatr 130:603, 1997.

35. Villaneuva ME, Zaher FM, Svinarich DM, Konduri GG: Decreased gene expression of endothelial nitric oxide synthase in newborns with persistent pulmonary hypertension. Pediatr Res 44:338, 1998.

36. Pepke-Zaba J, Higenbottam TW, Dinh-Xuan AT, et al: Inhaled nitric oxide as a cause of selective pulmonary vasodilatation in pulmonary hypertension. Lancet 338:1173, 1991.

37. Kinsella JP, Shaffer E, Neish SR, Abman SH: Low-dose inhalational nitric oxide in persistent pulmonary hypertension of the newborn. Lancet 340:819, 1992.

38. Roberts JD, Polaner DM, Lang P, Zapol WM: Inhaled nitric oxide in persistent pulmonary hypertension of the newborn. Lancet 340:818, 1992.

39. Zayek M, Wild LM, Roberts JD, Morin FC III: Effect of nitric oxide on survival and lung injury in newborn lambs with persistent pulmonary hypertension. J Pediatr 123:947, 1993.

40. Roberts JD, Fineman J, Morin FC III, et al: Inhaled nitric oxide gas improves oxygenation in PPHN. N Engl J Med 336:605, 1997.

41. Neonatal Inhaled Nitric Oxide Study Group: Inhaled nitric oxide in full-term and nearly full-term infants with hypoxic respiratory failure. N Engl J Med 336:597, 1997.

42. Davidson D, Barefield ES, Kattwinkel J, et al: Inhaled nitric oxide for the early treatment of persistent pulmonary hypertension of the term newborn: A randomized, double-masked, placebo-controlled, dose-response, multicenter study. Pediatrics 101:325, 1998.

43. Kinsella JP, Truog WE, Walsh WF, et al: Randomized, multicenter trial of inhaled nitric oxide and high-frequency oscillatory ventilation in severe, persistent pulmonary hypertension of the newborn. J Pediatr 131:55, 1997.

44. Clark RH, Kueser TJ, Walker MW, et al: Low dose nitric oxide therapy for persistent pulmonary hypertension of the newborn. N Engl J Med 342:469, 2000.

45. Neonatal Inhaled Nitric Oxide Study Group: Inhaled nitric oxide and hypoxic respiratory failure in infants with congenital diaphragmatic hernia. Pediatrics 99:838, 1997.

46. Finer NN, Barrington KJ: Nitric oxide therapy for the newborn infant. Semin Perinatol 24:59, 2000.

47. Barrington KJ, Finer NN: Nitric oxide for respiratory failure in infants born at or near term. Cochrane Database Syst Rev (4):CD000509, 2001.

48. Dobyns EL, Griebel J, Kinsella JP, et al: Infant lung function after inhaled nitric oxide therapy for persistent pulmonary hypertension of the newborn. Pediatr Pulmonol 28:24, 1999.

49. Neonatal Inhaled Nitric Oxide Study Group: Inhaled nitric oxide in term and near-term infants: Neurodevelopmental follow-up of the Neonatal Inhaled Nitric Oxide Study Group (NINOS). J Pediatr 136:611, 2000.

50. Kinsella JP, Walsh WF, Bose CL, et al: Inhaled nitric oxide in premature neonates with severe hypoxaemic respiratory failure: A randomised controlled trial. Lancet 354:1061, 1999.

51. Roberts JD, Roberts CT, Jones RC, et al: Continuous nitric oxide inhalation reduces pulmonary arterial structural changes, right ventricular hypertrophy, and growth retardation in the hypoxic newborn rat. Circ Res 76:215, 1995.

52. Tworetzky W, Bristow J, Moore P, et al: Inhaled nitric oxide in neonates with persistent pulmonary hypertension. Lancet 357:118, 2001.

53. Cornfield DN, Maynard RC, deRegnier RO, et al: Randomized, controlled trial of low-dose inhaled nitric oxide in the treatment of term and near-term infants with respiratory failure and pulmonary hypertension. Pediatrics 104:1089, 1999.

54. Finer NN, Sun JW, Rich W, et al: Randomized, prospective study of low-dose versus high-dose inhaled nitric oxide in the neonate with hypoxic respiratory failure. Pediatrics 108:949, 2001.

55. Moses D, Holm BA, Spitale P, et al: Inhibition of pulmonary surfactant function by meconium. Am J Obstet Gynecol 164:477, 1991.

56. Findlay RD, Taeusch W, Walther FJ: Surfactant replacement therapy for meconium aspiration syndrome. Pediatrics 97:48, 1996.

57. Lotze A, Mitchell BR, Bulas DI, et al: Multicenter study of surfactant (beractant) use in the treatment of term infants with severe respiratory failure. Survanta in Term Infants Study Group. J Pediatr 132:40, 1998.

58. Weinberger B, Laskin DL, Heck DE, Laskin JD: The toxicology of inhaled nitric oxide. Toxicol Sci 59:5, 2001.

59. Hogman M, Frostell C, Arnberg H, Hedenstierna G: Bleeding time prolongation and NO inhalation. Lancet 341:1664, 1993.

60. Miller OI, Tang SF, Keech A, Celermajer DS: Rebound pulmonary hypertension on withdrawal from inhaled nitric oxide. Lancet 346:51, 1995.

61. Davidson D, Barefield ES, Kattwinkel J, et al: Safety of withdrawing inhaled nitric oxide therapy in persistent pulmonary hypertension of the newborn. Pediatrics 104:231, 1999.

62. Yuhanna IS, MacRitchie AN, Lantin-Hermosos RL, et al: Nitric oxide (NO) upregulates NO synthase expression in fetal intrapulmonary artery endothelial cells. Am J Respir Cell Mol Biol 21:629, 1999.

63. Black SM, Heidersbach RS, McMullan DM, et al: Inhaled nitric oxide inhibits NOS activity in lambs: Potential mechanism for rebound pulmonary hypertension. Am J Physiol Heart Circ Physiol 277:H1849, 1999.

64. McMullan DM, Bekker JM, Johengen MJ, et al: Inhaled nitric oxide–induced rebound pulmonary hypertension: Role for endothelin-1. Am J Physiol Heart Circ Physiol 280:H777, 2001.

65. American Academy of Pediatrics Committee on the Fetus and Newborn: Use of inhaled nitric oxide. Pediatrics 106:344, 2000.

66. Filippov G, Bloch DB, Bloch KD: Nitric oxide decreases stability of mRNAs encoding soluble guanylate cyclase subunits in rat pulmonary artery smooth muscle cells. J Clin Invest 100:942, 1997.

67. Takata M, Filippov G, Liu H, et al: Cytokines decrease sGC in pulmonary artery smooth muscle cells via NO-dependent

and NO-independent mechanisms. Am J Physiol Lung Cell Mol Physiol 280:L272, 2001.

68. Kinsella JP, Torielli F, Ziegler JW, et al: Dipyridamole augmentation of response to nitric oxide. Lancet 346:647, 1995.

69. Thebaud B, Saizou C, Farnoux C, et al: Dypiridamole, a cGMP phosphodiesterase inhibitor, transiently improves the response to inhaled nitric oxide in two newborns with congenital diaphragmatic hernia. Intensive Care Med 25:300, 1999.

70. Dukarm RC, Morin FC III, Russell JA, Steinhorn RH: Pulmonary and systemic effects of the phosphodiesterase inhibitor dipyridamole in newborn lambs with persistent pulmonary hypertension. Pediatr Res 44:831, 1998.

71. Weimann J, Ullrich R, Hromi J, et al: Sildenafil is a pulmonary vasodilator in awake lambs with acute pulmonary hypertension. Anesthesiology 92:1702, 2000.

72. Ichinose F, Erana-Garcia J, Hromi J, et al: Nebulized sildenafil is a selective pulmonary vasodilator in lambs with acute pulmonary hypertension. Crit Care Med 29:1000, 2001.

73. Shekerdemian LS, Ravn HB, Penny DJ: Intravenous sildenafil lowers pulmonary vascular resistance in a model of neonatal pulmonary hypertension. Am J Respir Crit Care Med 165:1098, 2002.

74. Bigatello LM, Hess D, Dennehy KC, et al: Sildenafil can increase the response to inhaled nitric oxide. Anesthesiology 92:1827, 2000.

75. Atz AM, Wessel DL: Sildenafil ameliorates effects of inhaled nitric oxide withdrawal. Anesthesiology 91:307, 1999.

76. Steinhorn RH, Albert G, Swartz DD, et al: Recombinant human superoxide dismutase enhances the effect of inhaled nitric oxide in persistent pulmonary hypertension. Am Rev Respir Crit Care Med 164:834, 2001.

77. Deb B, Bradford K, Pearl RG: Additive effects of inhaled nitric oxide and intravenous milrinone in experimental pulmonary hypertension. Crit Care Med 28:795, 2000.

78. Wharton J, Davie N, Upton PD, et al: Prostacyclin analogues differentially inhibit growth of distal and proximal human pulmonary artery smooth muscle cells. Circulation 102:3130, 2000.

79. Rubin LJ, Groves BM, Reeves JT, et al: Prostacyclin-induced acute pulmonary vasodilatation in primary pulmonary hypertension. Circulation 66:334, 1982.

80. Zobel G, Dacar D, Rodl S, Friehs I: Inhaled nitric oxide versus inhaled prostacyclin and intravenous versus inhaled prostacyclin in acute respiratory failure with pulmonary hypertension in piglets. Pediatr Res 38:198, 1995.

81. Santak B, Schreiber M, Kuen P, et al: Prostacyclin aerosol in an infant with pulmonary hypertension. Eur J Pediatr 154:233, 1995.

82. Soditt V, Aring C, Groneck P: Improvement of oxygenation induced by aerosolized prostacyclin in a preterm infant with persistent pulmonary hypertension of the newborn. Intensive Care Med 23:1275, 1997.

83. Rocca GD, Coccia C, Pompei L, et al: Hemodynamic and oxygenation changes of combined therapy with inhaled nitric oxide and inhaled aerosolized prostacyclin. J Cardiothorac Vasc Anesth 15:224, 2001.

84. Hill LL, Pearl RG: Combined inhaled nitric oxide and inhaled prostacyclin during experimental chronic pulmonary hypertension. J Appl Physiol 86:1160, 1999.

85. Hermon M, Golej J, Burda G, et al: Intravenous prostacyclin mitigates inhaled nitric oxide rebound effect: A case control study. Artif Organs 23:975, 1999.

86. Kelly LK, Porta NF, Goodman DM, et al: Inhaled prostacyclin for term infants with persistent pulmonary hypertension refractory to inhaled nitric oxide. J Pediatr 141:830, 2002.

87. Weinberger B, Weiss K, Heck DE, et al: Pharmacologic therapy of persistent pulmonary hypertension of the newborn. Pharmacol Ther 89:67, 2001.

88. Konduri GG, Mital S: Adenosine and ATP cause nitric oxide–dependent pulmonary vasodilatation in fetal lambs. Biol Neonate 78:220, 2000.

89. Konduri GG, Garcia DC, Kazzi NJ, Shankaran S: Adenosine infusion improves oxygenation in term infants with respiratory failure. Pediatrics 97:295, 1996.

90. Moya MP, Gow AJ, McMahon TJ, et al: S-nitrosothiol repletion by an inhaled gas regulates pulmonary function. Proc Natl Acad Sci U S A 98:5792, 2001.

91. Moya MP, Gow AJ, Califf RM, et al: Inhaled ethyl nitrite gas for persistent pulmonary hypertension of the newborn. Lancet 360:141, 2002.

CHAPTER 40

Pulmonary Function Testing in the Sick Newborn

Vinod K. Bhutani and Emidio M. Sivieri

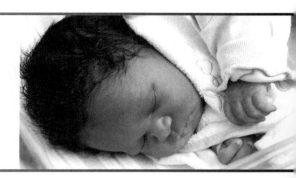

Neonatal pulmonary functions are altered in any newborn with respiratory disease and manifestations of disordered gas exchange, pulmonary mechanics, respiratory energetics, or cyclical and breathing patterns. Knowledge of pulmonary physiology is the basis of the understanding of these disorders, objective measurement (by practical and user-friendly technology), and bedside application for improved outcome. This chapter describes clinical applications of these neonatal pulmonary functions. Details on techniques to measure pulmonary functions are described in articles listed in the Suggested Readings. Clinicians who care for newborns with respiratory illnesses are encouraged to review this literature and to seek innovative strategies to apply the principles of neonatal pulmonary physiology and to enhance the care of a sick newborn.

BASIS FOR CLINICAL APPLICATIONS

To define better physiologic goals of respiratory support and to achieve a "normalized" gas exchange with appropriate ventilation-perfusion matching necessitate an understanding of the physiology of respiratory failure. Correction of neonatal respiratory failure with the least respiratory intervention or barotrauma has to be achieved to provide optimal oxygenation and carbon dioxide (CO_2) elimination. The definition of "optimal" or **normalized gas exchange** for a neonate has been a subject of extensive debate. Normal gas exchange values usually are based on population studies (Table 40-1). Each neonate has a specific and narrow range of oxygen tensions, CO_2 levels, and pH range, however, beyond which respiratory responses are initiated to correct the perturbation. Encompassing this narrow range, there is a reasonably wide margin of "safety" or insufficiency beyond which hypoxic collapse or CO_2 narcosis occurs (Fig. 40-1). These ranges allow a clinician to select, at his or her discretion, the optimal levels of gas exchange based on disease state,

physiologic considerations, and technical limitations. The clinical goals are to maintain individualized ranges of optimal oxygenation, optimal CO_2 clearance, and synchronous ventilatory support and to do so with least level of barotrauma.

PHYSIOLOGIC BACKGROUND FOR NEONATAL PULMONARY FUNCTIONS

Pulmonary mechanics are best understood by viewing the respiratory system in a simplistic format of a linear respiratory model. By making the fewest assumptions, the driving pressure required to move gas in and out of the lungs and maintain ventilation is the sum of the pressure required to overcome elastic, resistive, and inertial respiratory loads (Table 40-2). During spontaneous breathing and conventional ventilation, inertial forces are usually negligible. In these conditions, driving pressure is correlated to ventilation and $PaCO_2$ as a function of elastic and resistive loads.

Physiologic feedback mechanisms that control the level of ventilation are well known and studied; these include mechanisms that stimulate the peripheral and central chemoreceptors and mechanisms that influence stretch receptors. Interactions of these dual feedback systems are essential to appropriate and precise ventilatory responses (Fig. 40-2). When a clinician assumes respiratory support of an individual infant, a fundamental understanding of interactions of oxygenation, CO_2 elimination, acid-base status, and pulmonary graphics (which provide an insight of pulmonary mechanics) enhances bedside decision making. Neonatal respiratory dysfunction is secondary to decreased lung compliance, increased airway compliance, increased thoracic compliance, or decreased respiratory muscle strength, which either individually or in combination predisposes to respiratory failure as evidenced by hypoxemia or hypercapnia or both.

Table 40–1. Optimal and Normalized Gas Exchange Ranges

Normal values for population group
Normal values for an individual
Physician discretion for a desired range based on
  Disease state
  Equipment capability
  Physiologic consideration
Technical limitations

Table 40–2. Pulmonary Mechanics Equations

Equation 1	Driving pressure = volume/compliance + resistance × flow + inertial resistance × flow
Equation 2	Driving pressure = volume/compliance + resistance × flow
Equation 3	$cm\ H_2O = (mL \div mL/cm\ H_2O) + (cm\ H_2O/mL/sec \times mL/sec)$
Equation 4	Driving pressure = elastic load (tidal volume ÷ compliance) + resistive load (pulmonary resistance × airflow)

CLINICAL ASSESSMENT OF NEONATAL PULMONARY FUNCTIONS

Bedside evaluation of history, clinical assessment, blood gas and acid-base profiles, and the interaction of the infant to any supportive respiratory devices enhances the bedside application of pulmonary physiologic principles, especially for a neonate with respiratory distress. The noninvasive assessment of the three respiratory signals provides objective, valuable online data that may be used in an adjunctive manner to monitor, interpret, and define the severity of dysfunction. These data do not provide a clinical diagnosis but can be useful in the following ways: (1) evaluation of alteration or limitation in inspiratory/expiratory airflow; (2) evaluation of driving pressure, work, and the effort to maintain minute ventilation; (3) evaluation and calculation of the elastic and resistive components of pulmonary dysfunction; (4) calculation of the inspiratory, expiratory, and total lung time constants; (5) evaluation of the interaction between spontaneous breathing and conventional mechanical ventilation,

including continuous positive airway pressure; (6) evaluation of the degree of response to a therapeutic intervention (e.g., changes in ventilator settings, medications, or posture); and (7) evaluation of the evolution and resolution of the respiratory disease.

Driving pressure is the pressure gradient required to achieve tidal volume. During spontaneous breathing, it is the net change in intrapleural pressure, and the physiologic value in a healthy term neonate ranges from 4 to 5 cm H_2O. During positive-pressure ventilation, the net driving pressure is the gradient between the peak inflating pressure and the **positive end-expiratory pressure (PEEP)**. At any given point in the respiratory cycle, the driving pressure is the sum of elastic and resistive pressures (Fig. 40-3). Clinical conditions associated with altered loads and the therapies used to reduce these loads are listed in Table 40-3.

Elastic pressure is the pressure required to inflate the lung. It is measured from a point of "no airflow" at

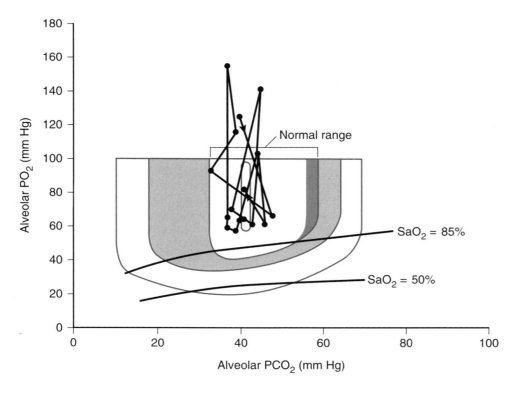

Figure 40–1. Assessment of normal gas exchange.

CONTROL OF NEONATAL VENTILATION
CONCEPTS FOR SIMULATED TRAINING

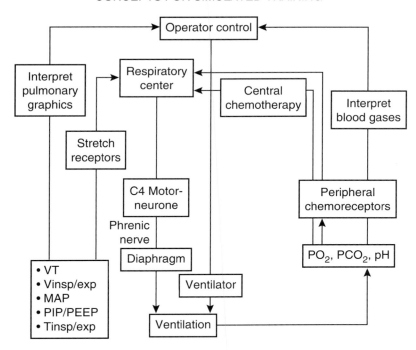

Figure 40–2. Control of neonatal ventilation: theoretical concepts of interaction pulmonary mechanics.

the start of lung expansion to point of "no airflow" at the end of lung expansion. In relationship to tidal volume, it is a measure of lung compliance. When measured during spontaneous breathing (e.g., from end expiration to end inspiration), elastic pressure represents the dynamic change and is used to quantitate dynamic compliance. Under experimental conditions, when pressures have been allowed to equilibrate for some time, the net change in pressure is a more precise measure of elasticity and quantifies the static compliance.

Resistive pressure is the pressure required beyond the elastic pressure to overcome the viscoelastic properties of the lung (as attributed by the airways and to the airflow) and represents the deviation from the linear direction of the elastic pressure. There are inspiratory and expiratory components to resistive pressure (see Fig. 40-3). Values reach a peak at maximal (inspiratory/expiratory) airflow and are measured at midrespiratory cycles—midinspiration and midexpiration.

Pulmonary graphic assessment of the **pressure-volume loops** uniquely describes the inspiratory and

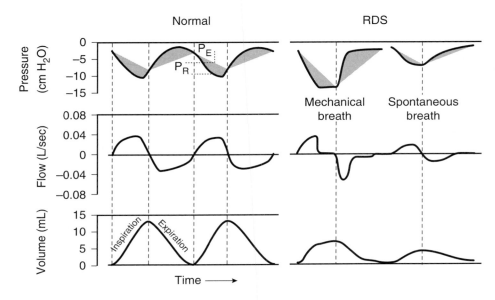

Figure 40–3. Scalar pressure, flow, and volume relationship. Resistive and elastic pressures (P_R and P_E) are shaded in the driving pressure tracing. RDS, respiratory distress syndrome.

Table 40–3. Clinical Conditions Associated with Altered Loads

Diseases with High Elastic Load	Reduction of Elastic Load	Diseases with Resistive Loads	Reduction of Resistive Load
Respiratory distress syndrome	Surfactant replacement	Early meconium aspiration syndrome	Differentiate resistive load from that due to bronchomalacia
Congenital pneumonia	Positive end-expiratory pressure	Airway obstructive disease	or bronchospasm
Meconium aspiration syndrome (late)	Prenatal glucocorticoid therapy	Reactive airway disease	Judicious use of positive end-expiratory pressure: "splint airways"
Pulmonary edema	Systemic steroid therapy	Obstructive tracheal lesions	Bronchodilator therapy: decrease tone
Immature lung	Superoxide-dismutase therapy	Bronchopulmonary dysplasia	Inhaled or systemic steroid therapy
Decreased lung volume: pulmonary hypoplasia, congenital diaphragmatic hernia, end-stage bronchopulmonary dysplasia	Partial liquid ventilation \ Total liquid ventilation	Congenital anomalies	Minimize airway mucosal or structural barotrauma

expiratory phases of tidal breathing. A two-dimensional relationship of tidal volume and driving pressure describes the loop. The slope represents the elastic properties of the breath, whereas the deviations of the loop represent the resistive components. Inspiratory and expiratory components help differentiate the location of the resistive load to the respective phases of a respiratory cycle. The loop, or hysteresis, also assesses work of breathing and the energy expenditure for each breath. It represents the sum of energy lost to both resistive elastic loads. Loss due to elastic load may be considered as a "potential loss." A product of tidal volume and driving pressure, the values may be calculated as joules, calories, or oxygen expenditure.

SPECIFIC CLINICAL APPLICATIONS TO IMPROVE RESPIRATORY MANAGEMENT

Clinical directions to the neonatal respiratory team that supervises the technologies of respiratory support (respiratory therapists, nurses, physicians) include the delivery of oxygen and ventilatory support: use of mean airway pressure (conventional or high-frequency ventilation), end-distending pressure (continuously or with cyclic ventilatory support), airflow, and the ratio of ventilatory cycling (inspiratory/expiratory ratio and rates). Of these variables, several need to be optimized for individual magnitude and the interdependence of each other. Some of the strategies that we have used are discussed subsequently.

Optimizing Peak Inflating Pressure

If an infant is being managed on pressure-limited ventilatory support, visualizing the concomitant tidal volume may corroborate the selection of a chosen peak inflating pressure. A suggested goal would be to ventilate initially at the low "normal" value of tidal volume (e.g., 5 to 6 mL/kg). This strategy provides for a more objective approach than choosing the peak inflating pressure on the basis of auscultation for adequate breath sounds during manual ventilation. Similarly the tidal volume actually delivered to a neonate can be measured when setting the volume support during volume-controlled ventilation.

Optimizing Peak End-Expiratory Pressure

It is feasible to define an optimal end-distending pressure using pulmonary graphics; however, the process is complex and at present not user-friendly. Using a combination of the effects of driving pressure on tidal volume and visual changes in pressure-volume relationships, one can ascertain whether incremental changes in PEEP lead to pulmonary overdistention or underdistention or are moving to a linear component of the pressure-volume relationship (see example in Fig. 40-4). Because the clinical goal is to ventilate at the linear portion of the pressure-volume loop, bedside incremental changes in PEEP should be done only by experienced clinicians who can assess accurately the changes in measured data and calculate the impact of PEEP manipulation.

Optimizing Circuit Airflow

Usually the circuit airflow of the ventilator has not been an active decision of the clinician and has been based on manufacturer's guidelines. Excessive circuit airflow can lead to overdistention (Fig. 40-5) and inadvertent excessive PEEP. Both of these effects lead to hypoventilation and subsequent hypercapnia. The pulmonary graphic manifestations would be lower tidal volumes, wider pulmonary hysteresis, pressure overdistention, and perhaps turbulence in the airflow signal. These would be corrected immediately by a bedside maneuver to reduce the

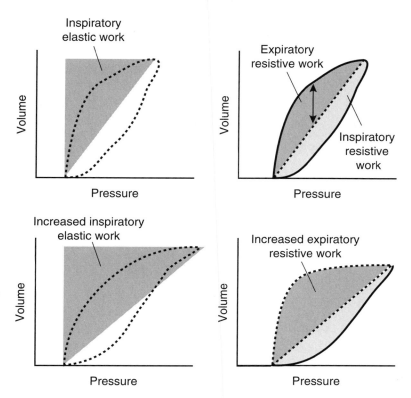

Figure 40–4. Pressure-volume relationships with delineation of elastic and resistive pressure loads.

circuit airflow. Another option to set the circuit airflow is to base the setting on an eightfold level of the desired minute ventilation (tidal volume and respiratory frequency). Circuit airflow is set, at the operator's discretion, to flow from inspiratory to expiratory circuits. The magnitude depends on the patient's minute ventilation. Excessive circuit airflow can lead to turbulence and may impede expiratory flow from the patient, whereas low circuit airflow may limit inspiratory airflow rate and lead to hypoventilation.

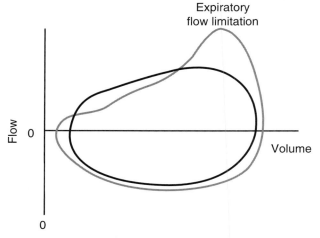

Figure 40–5. Respiratory flow-volume relationships.

Optimizing Inspiratory Time

Inspiratory time (and the expiratory time) may be increased or decreased by the physician as a response to change in the mean airway pressure and oxygenation. These decisions usually are made on clinical decisions and based on the physiologic understanding of respiratory time constants (product of compliance and resistance). In addition to the impact on oxygenation, the concomitant and often indirect beneficial or deleterious effects of the new inspiratory time can be assessed on the pulmonary graphics. These include the effects on tidal volume, inspiratory and expiratory hysteresis, pressure-volume relationship (e.g., overdistention from excessive mean airway pressure), and flow-volume relationships (e.g., expiratory flow limitation from excessive and inadvertent PEEP) as sequelae of shortened expiratory time.

Optimizing Synchrony and Rate of Ventilatory Support

Real-time evaluation of synchronous ventilation on the graphic displays is helpful for nurses, respiratory therapists, and physicians to assess nonventilatory means to correct asynchronous ventilation. The clinical value of the visual display allows for early response to a neonate's discomfort. Infants who continue to "fight" the ventilator and are not amenable to bedside comforting and nursing measures may show their response to ventilatory technologies based on synchronized ventilation.

Optimizing Tidal Volume

The tidal volume is evident with the placement of the pneumotachometer, and the digital readout provides the variability that is evident between spontaneous, mechanical, and augmented breaths. The optimal peak inflating pressure can be ascertained by adjusting to appropriate tidal volume (providing a more objective assessment to auscultation). In a clinical condition, when the infant is breathing synchronously or when spontaneous breathing has been diminished or abolished, the steady measures of tidal volume provide clinically useful information. First, when the tidal volume value is 5 to 8 mL/kg and there are no signs of pressure-volume overdistention, the clinician may ascertain that ventilation is at optimal **functional residual capacity (FRC)**. Incremental changes (by 1 cm H_2O) in PEEP and peak inflating pressure (such that the driving pressure is unchanged) should not result in an appreciable change in tidal volume. The rationale for this observation is that if the infant is being ventilated at optimal FRC (at the linear component of the respiratory pressure-volume curve), slight movements along the curve should maintain the tidal volume. Second, if the tidal volume is less than 5 mL/kg, either the infant is being ventilated at a low lung volume (an increase in peak inflating pressure would improve the tidal volume), or the infant is being ventilated at high lung volume (a decrease in peak inflating pressure would improve the tidal volume). Low values may lead to hypoventilation, and high values (>8.5 mL/kg) may lead to tidal volume overdistention. Lastly, if the tidal volume is greater than 8 mL/kg, pressure-volume and flow-volume curves should be evaluated for pulmonary overdistention and increased resistive work of breathing. Inspiratory and expiratory values should be similar. Any limitations are best assessed by tidal flow-volume loops: a two-dimensional relationship of tidal volume to inspiratory and expiratory airflow. This loop relationship describes the manner of flow, its peak, its acceleration and deceleration slopes, and the presence of any limitations and is useful in differentiating any obstructive airflow lesions.

Optimizing Inspired Oxygen

The process of plotting serial arterial blood gases on the P_{O_2}-P_{CO_2} nomogram (Fig. 40-6) provides the clinician a perspective on the extent of the variation induced either by disease or by the operator. Operator-driven swings in oxygenation may be minimized by prospective decisions (e.g., use of the alveolar gas equation; Table 40-4) or by invoking changes in a cautious and incremental manner. Strategies to achieve optimal oxygen exchange are (1) increase of alveolar oxygen tension by increasing the inspired oxygen (Table 40-5), (2) increase of the surface area of lungs during expiration (use of PEEP or surfactant to distend or recruit alveolar surface area), and (3) increase of surface area of lungs during inspiration by applying a higher mean airway pressure (by inflating pressure, increasing inspiratory time, or prolonging inspiration).

Optimizing Carbon Dioxide Exchange

The relationship between alveolar ventilation and arterial CO_2 tension is incredibly linear and may be used as an advantage in defining desired goals for "permissive" hypercapnia. Selection of a P_{CO_2} value of 50 mm Hg in lieu of the "normal" value of 40 mm Hg is a choice of defining a 25% deviation; this may indicate hypoventilation by 25%. This decision could be an elective clinical maneuver, but the clinician needs to ensure that the decision is not a passive one such that atelectatic lungs are being ventilated. The plotting of serial blood gases on

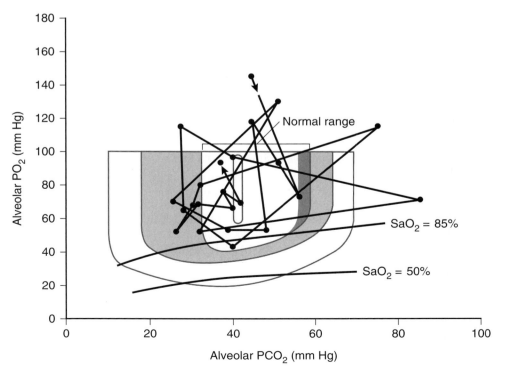

Figure 40–6. Oxygen–carbon dioxide variation in a sick newborn.

Table 40–4. Alveolar Gas Equation

Relationship of inspired oxygen (F_{IO_2}) and arterial
   oxygen tension (Pa_{O_2})
$PA_{CO_2} = P_{ICO_2} - (PA_{CO_2}/R) + PA_{CO_2} \times F_{IO_2} \times (I - R)/R$
$PA_{CO_2} = (F_{ICO_2})(PB - 47) - (PA_{CO_2}/R) + PA_{CO_2} \times F_{ICO_2}$
   $\times (I - R)/R$

Table 40–5. Strategies to Achieve Optimal Oxygen Exchange

Goals	Strategies (may use algebraic equations)
Oxygenation	Increase alveolar oxygen tension
	Alveolar gas equation
	Rule of "seven"
	Adjust for change in altitude
	Adjust for change in Pa_{CO_2}
	Adjust for respiratory quotient
	Adjust for change in temperature
CO_2 elimination	Alveolar ventilation inversely correlated to Pa_{CO_2}
	Alveolar ventilation is (Vt – Vd) × rate
	Provided dead space is constant: proportional changes in Vt or rate lead to proportional changes in alveolar ventilation and Pa_{CO_2}

a P_{O_2}-P_{CO_2} nomogram (see Fig. 40-6) provides the clinician with a direct visual impact of the recent gas exchange history so that prospective decisions are made consciously and conscientiously.

The sum of tidal volume of all breaths delivered during a minute period is the minute ventilation. A product of tidal volume and breathing frequency or sum of alveolar ventilation and dead space ventilation also represents the minute ventilation. Minute ventilation (minus dead space) is inversely correlated to arterial CO_2. Increase in tidal volume or increase of respiratory rates decreases the minute ventilation, but it is the alveolar ventilation that is directly and inversely to PA_{CO_2} and Pa_{CO_2}. The interaction of tidal volume to alveolar ventilation needs a frequent assessment of dead space to ensure a constant relationship.

MINIMIZING THE LEVEL OF INTERVENTION OR BAROTRAUMA

The key to successful ventilation is to deliver the least level of ventilatory support to allow breathing to remain at the infant's FRC. Lung volume at which respiratory cycles occur during spontaneous breathing is the FRC (i.e., volume of air present in the lung that is in communication with the airways at the end of a tidal expiration). Optimal FRC value is at about 40% of total lung capacity—30 to 35 mL/kg—and represents the most linear component of the static pressure-volume relationship of the lung. FRC primarily increases with body length (Fig. 40-7). As shown

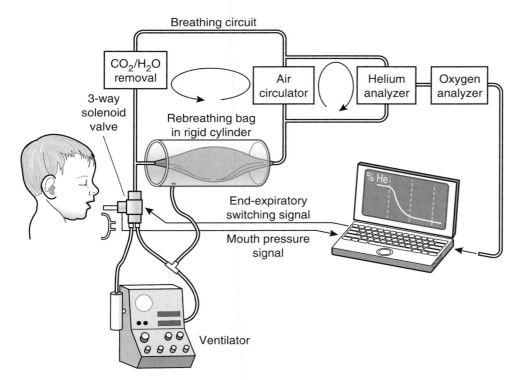

Figure 40–7. Measurement of functional residual capacity (FRC) by helium dilution technique.

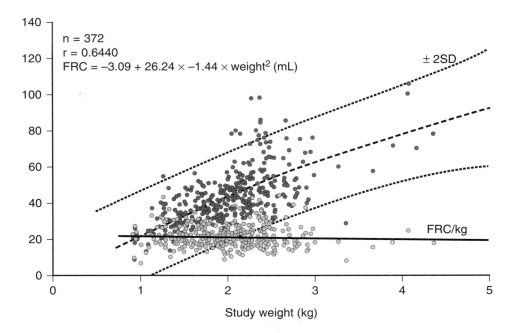

Figure 40–8. Functional residual capacity (FRC) measurements in healthy term and preterm newborns as a function of body weight.

in Figure 40-6, ventilating at high or low FRC requires higher inflating pressures compared with ventilation at the most linear component of the respiratory pressure-volume loop. At this lung volume, the change in tidal volume requires the least inflating pressure. The challenge for a neonatologist managing a sick newborn is that the FRC of an infant with respiratory disease is altered: FRC is low in the presence of elastic lung disease and high in the presence of resistive disease. FRC is often unpredictable in infants with evolving bronchopulmonary dysplasia, who have a varying combination of elastic and resistive lung disease. Resistive loads caused by mechanical ventilation or induced barotrauma augment the fluctuations in FRC.

Actual measurements of FRC in "healthy" preterm neonates, infants who had respiratory distress syndrome, and infants with bronchopulmonary dysplasia are limited (Fig. 40-8). User-friendly and accurate technologies to measure FRC in sick and preterm neonates are currently unavailable. Major limitations have been the bedside ability to measure with reasonable accuracy of ±1 mL (±10% of FRC values observed in infants with respiratory distress syndrome). Indirect estimates of FRC (other than chest radiographs) rely on interpretation of pulmonary graphics (identification of tidal pressure-volume overdistention) and measures of tidal volume with incremental changes of driving pressure.

FRC adjustments may be made by incremental changes to end-distending pressure or by achieving adequate lung inflation through inspiratory time and adequate lung deflation by manipulating expiratory time. Bedside evidence of respiratory barotrauma can be due to driving pressure–induced overdistention (high tidal volume), volume-induced overdistention (high FRC due to excessive airflow or inadvertent PEEP), measurements of large tidal volume (>8.5 mL/kg), or actual evidence of high or low FRC.

USE OF TIME CONSTANTS TO DEFINE OPTIMAL FUNCTIONAL RESIDUAL CAPACITY

Surface area of the lung during expiration, to define optimal FRC, can be influenced by time determinants for inspiration or expiration. Adequate exhalation is as important as achieving optimal inflation. The adequacy of respiratory airflow is affected by resistive and elastic properties of the lung: Resistive properties slow the equilibration time, and elastic properties hasten the equilibration time. The product of resistance and compliance is termed the **time constant** and represents the time required to achieve approximately 63% equilibration of pressure and volume change (based on natural log function) (Table 40-6); fivefold time constant is the amount of time to allow for 99% equilibration of each cycle. Examples of increased

Table 40–6. Time Constant Equations

Equation 1	Time constant (τ) = (compliance) × (resistance)
Equation 2	$\tau = C \times R$
Equation 3	sec = (mL/cm H_2O) × (cm H_2O/mL/sec)
Equation 4	Time constant is the time that allows for 63% equilibration change of tidal volume or driving pressure during either inspiration or expiration
Equation 5	Fivefold time constant is the time that allows for 99% equilibration change. This time duration is equivalent to the minimal inspiratory or expiratory time during a respiratory cycle

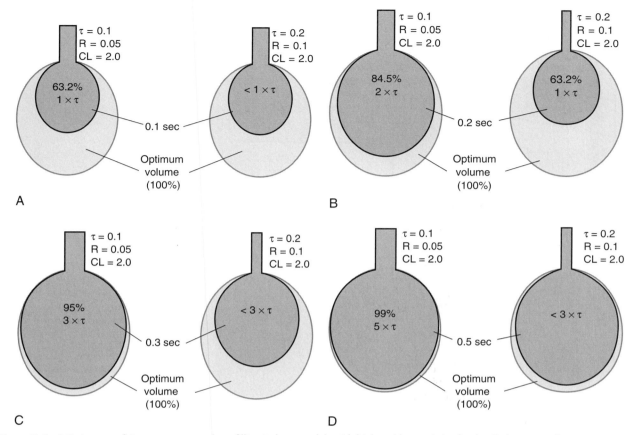

Figure 40–9. A-D, Impact of time constants on lung filling in lung models with high and low resistive loads. CL, lung compliance.

resistive and elastic loads on inspiratory time are illustrated in Figure 40-9.

INTERDEPENDENCE OF RESPIRATORY SUPPORT

The relationships between mean airway pressure and oxygenation and between alveolar ventilation and CO_2 elimination have been discussed earlier. During ventilation, attainment of optimal and normalized gas exchange is inextricably linked and intertwined with neonatal pulmonary mechanics and their interdependent interactions to ventilatory support parameters. Several of these effects are predictable and have been modeled on simplified linear models. These allow for a calculated and practical model such that adaptive technologies may be applied. Adaptive modeling of neonatal oxygen control already has been feasible with spontaneous breathing and is being studied during mechanical ventilation. Predictive modeling of CO_2 control is far more complex and may be accomplished by pseudoadaptive and bedside calculation strategies. Availability of smart, online, and interactive software and processing technologies has the potential to use bedside pulmonary mechanics to modulate neonatal gas exchange during mechanical ventilation.

SUMMARY

Clinical pulmonary functions currently available are tidal volume, calculation (or estimation) of time constants, pressure-volume relationship, and flow-volume relationship (pulmonary graphics). Interpretation of these data from physiologic perspectives allows for a better understanding of the evolution of pulmonary dysfunction as a sick neonate deals with acute lung disease, then either recovers or progresses to a subacute and even chronic lung disease with eventual recovery. FRC measurements (when available) and their interpretation with pulmonary graphics would enhance the objective assessment of pulmonary functions. The eventual clinical outcome of a sick newborn would be measured not only by the newborn's survival, incidences of bronchopulmonary dysplasia, chronic lung disease, days on oxygen and ventilatory support, and neurologic sequelae, but also by the magnitude of objective recovery from neonatal lung disease (Fig. 40-10). Optimal management of a sick newborn with respiratory disease should be grounded in an understanding of the ongoing pulmonary physiologic derangements, the impact of technologic interventions on these parameters, and a bedside evaluation of these interactions such that ensuing recovery is associated with minimal sequelae.

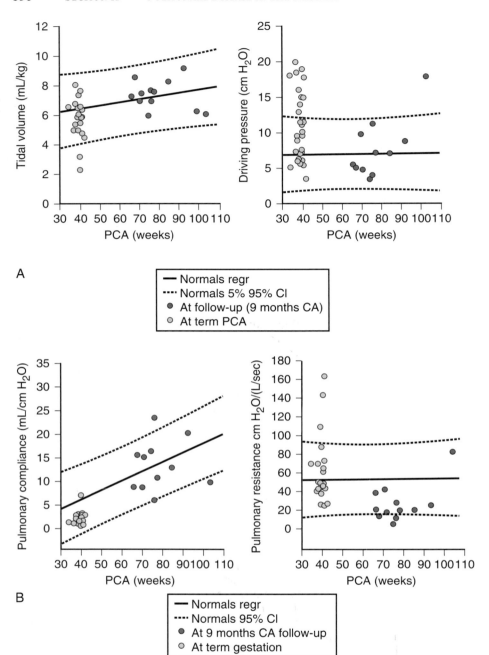

A

Legend:
— Normals regr
---- Normals 5% 95% CI
● At follow-up (9 months CA)
○ At term PCA

B

Legend:
— Normals regr
---- Normals 95% CI
● At 9 months CA follow-up
○ At term gestation

Figure 40–10. Pulmonary follow-up in infants with birth weights less than 750 g. PCA, postconception age.

Suggested Readings

Bhutani VK, Shaffer TH, Vidyasager D (eds): Neonatal Pulmonary Function Testing. Ithaca, NY, Perinatology Press, 1988.

Bhutani VK, Siveri EM, Abbasi S: Evaluation of pulmonary function in the neonate. In Polin RA, Fox WW (eds): Fetal and Neonatal Physiology, 2nd ed. Philadelphia, WB Saunders, 1999, pp 1143-1164.

Comroe JH: Physiology of Respiration, 2nd ed. Chicago, Year Book Medical Publishers, 1974.

Polgar G, Promadhat V: Pulmonary Function Testing in Children. Philadelphia, WB Saunders, 1971.

West JB: Respiratory Physiology: The Essentials. Oxford, Blackwell Scientific Publications, 1974.

CHAPTER 41

Neonatal Bronchoscopy

Neil N. Finer

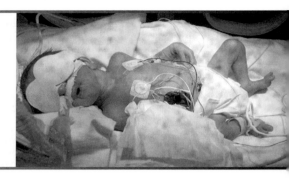

Bronchoscopy, or visualization of the upper and lower airways by use of rigid or flexible instruments, is an integral part of critical care medicine. Because of size limitations, **flexible fiberoptic bronchoscopy** has become an option for pediatric and, more recently, neonatal intensive care only with the development of small-diameter endoscopes. Rigid bronchoscopy has been possible with a 2.5-mm rigid bronchoscope, the most popular being the Storz (Karl Storz GMGH & Co., Tuttlingen, Germany) with the Hopkins telescopic rods. The true external diameter of a 2.5-mm rigid bronchoscope is 4 mm, however, making this scope difficult to use in infants with extremely low birth weight. The Hopkins rod lens provides excellent resolution. Although meant to be inserted through the endoscope, the telescopes occasionally can be used alone for visualization of the airways, and I have found this technique useful occasionally in infant airways.

Flexible fiberoptic bronchoscopes were first introduced in 1969. These first instruments were approximately 6 mm in outside diameter. The first fiberoptic instrument that was useful in neonates was the 3.5-mm BF3C4 Olympus bronchoscope (Olympus Corporation of America, Melville, NY) with a 1.2-mm suction channel. Subsequently, smaller fiberoptic bronchoscopes have been developed and now are available in a 1.8-mm size. The first experience using a pediatric fiberoptic flexible bronchoscope was described by Wood and Sherman.[1] My more recent experience has been principally with the 2.2-mm flexible fiberoptic scopes (BF N20; Olympus America, Melville NY), the smallest flexible bronchoscopes available with flexible tips.[2]

Shortly after the introduction of fiberoptic bronchoscopy into our neonatal intensive care unit, we acquired a camera and a video adapter with a camera controller (MV9370; Circon Video Systems, Santa Barbara, Calif) so that we could record endoscopies. I have always used a split-beam adapter so that the operator can visualize the airway directly because even the best cameras and video systems cause some distortion in color and reduce resolution. Currently, we use an Olympus camera with split-beam adapter (Olympus Model No. OTV-F2; Olympus America, Melville, NY). In addition, we place a small microphone near the infant's mouth to record breathing in nonintubated infants so that we can evaluate the effects of inspiration and expiration. We have found that video recording of bronchoscopy is a valuable adjunct to endoscopy in critically ill neonates and children. Such recording tends to shorten the viewing time when one is attempting to show findings to colleagues, trainees, or parents. In addition, when there has been some diagnostic doubt, often a careful review of the videotape serves to clarify findings. This is especially true in evaluating vocal cord abnormalities. Finally, the availability of videotape allows us to obtain consultation with colleagues without subjecting the infant to repeat endoscopy.

Fiberoptic endoscopy of the neonate can be done either through the endotracheal tube (ETT) or via the natural airway. The available instruments allow visualization through the smallest ETT (2.5 mm) that is used in the intensive care unit (Fig. 41-1). Until more recently, however, these smallest flexible-tip bronchoscopes did not have a suction channel, and the vision may become obscured, although we have found that by gentle flexion and extension of the tip a clear field can be restored. There is now a 2.7-mm fiberoptic endoscope that has a small suction channel; this is useful, but the small size of this channel limits the ability to remove debris and thick

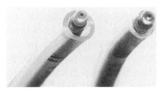

Figure 41–1. An end-on view of the 2.2-mm bronchoscope (BF N20; Olympus America, Melville, NY) inserted through a 2.5-mm endotracheal tube on the right and through a 3.0-mm endotracheal tube on the left. This tube fits snugly through the smaller tube.

viscid secretions.[3] In addition, this endoscope cannot pass through a 2.5-mm ETT. The Visicath fiberoptic endoscopes (Microvasive Inc, Milford, Mass) have suction channels, but these are small, and the endoscope does not have a flexible tip.

For nonintubated neonates, we prefer the transnasal route for visualization of the upper airway, which includes the nasopharynx, posterior oropharynx, larynx, and trachea. With current endoscopes, this examination can be performed in infants with birth weights of 500 g. The transnasal route provides an excellent view of the entire upper airway, including the posterior aspect of the tongue.

Small bronchoscopes without flexible tips also are available (PF185; Olympus America, Melville, NY), including the previously described fiberoptic catheters that may be considered as disposable bronchoscopes (Microvasive Inc., Milford, Mass). Finer and Etches[4] and Shinwell and colleagues[5] have used these devices repeatedly. These devices provide reasonable optics but must be handled with great care because any acute bend can fracture the fiberoptic bundles. The accompanying handheld light source produces less light than dedicated standalone units, but the portability, ease of use, and rapid setup are advantageous for acute situations. I believe, however, that a proper dedicated fiberoptic bronchoscope with light source is preferable.

PREPARATION FOR BRONCHOSCOPY

Methodology

Because of the small size of the ultrathin endoscopes, the brightest light source available is recommended, especially for video endoscopy. We currently use a xenon light source (CLV-10; Olympus America, Melville, NY). For urgent endoscopies, we use a smaller portable light source that can be carried rapidly to any bedside (Olympus Model No. ILK-3; Olympus America, Melville NY). The use of a teaching head may reduce the amount of available light.

The bronchoscope can be introduced into the infant's nares for evaluation of the upper airway, larynx, and trachea in nonintubated infants. Although it may seem that oral insertion of the endoscope provides a more direct route, visualization of the larynx is more difficult by this route because of the anterior position of the neonatal larynx. In addition, fiberoptic bronchoscopic intubation is much more difficult using the oral route. When evaluating spontaneously breathing infants, we use a single nasal prong to provide oxygen during the procedure. In unstable, spontaneously breathing infants, the bronchoscope can be passed through an adapter connected to a mask continuous positive airway pressure setup.[6] For ventilated infants, we use a standard bronchoscopy adapter and apply a fingertip from a sterile glove over the proximal end of the adapter (Fig. 41-2). A small hole is created in the latex to allow the passage of the scope. Using this method, an infant may continue to receive ventilatory support, albeit with markedly increased airway resistance. We always try to keep the procedure as short

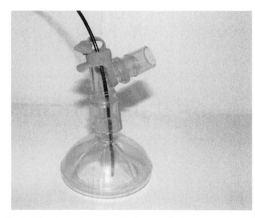

Figure 41–2. The bronchoscope is inserted through a bronchoscope adapter, and then through a face mask. It would be used for an unstable, nonintubated infant who requires continuous positive airway pressure or positive-pressure breaths during the procedure. This adapter can be used for infants receiving mechanical ventilation as well.

as possible, and when determining ETT position or the presence of an ETT plug, the entire procedure should be completed in less than 20 seconds.

Premedication

A great deal has been written about premedication for adult endoscopy, but premedication in neonatal endoscopy often is poorly described or simply not given, with comments to indicate that such sedation was not required. With increasing concern for pain management in neonates and the obvious discomfort associated with transnasal fiberoptic bronchoscopy or a rigid oral endoscopy, safe and effective sedation is required. Following the technique of Wood,[7] we have used 2 mg/kg of meperidine (Demerol) administered intravenously, or 0.1 mg/kg of morphine with topical lidocaine (Xylocaine) to the nares for transnasal endoscopies. It is important to give this premedication at least 5 to 10 minutes before the procedure to obtain adequate sedation. In addition, for intubated infants, we use 4 to 7 mg/kg of 1% lidocaine via the ETT injected through a feeding tube at the tip of the ETT so that it is delivered to the distal trachea, carina, and main stem airways. We also prepare a syringe of naloxone, 0.1 mg/kg, to be administered if the infant shows signs of reduced ventilation or frank apnea. We have found that this premedication is usually well tolerated, but in growing premature infants, especially infants with apnea of prematurity, an occasional infant has increased apnea. In these infants, we prefer to give 1 mg/kg of meperidine or 0.05 mg/kg of morphine followed by supplemental doses if an adequate level of sedation is not obtained. In older infants and children, we have used a combination of demerol plus midazolam, 30 to 100 µg/kg, but we have found that midazolam has not been necessary for most of our neonatal endoscopies. In a highly unstable neonate, such as an infant with persistent fetal circulation with associated severe hypoxemia who shows a poor tolerance to handling, we prefer to use anesthetic doses of fentanyl, 10 μg/kg, before the procedure, usually in combination with a paralytic agent.[8] We have not found premedication with atropine to be necessary. Secretions can be removed with suctioning before the procedure, and a decreasing heart rate is usually an indication that the procedure has been too lengthy, especially if the bronchoscope is below the vocal cords. One approach to provide anesthesia to the airway involves the use of nebulized lidocaine, which may be effective in decreasing airway reactivity.[8]

Monitoring

All infants undergoing endoscopy are monitored continuously for heart rate, pulse oximetry, and blood pressure if an arterial line is in situ. Virtually all endoscopies are performed in the neonatal intensive care unit on an overhead warmer. Supplemental oxygen is administered before the procedure to increase the infant's saturation to a level greater than 95%.

Our preferred endoscope at present is the 2.2-mm fiberoptic scope with a flexible tip (BF N20; Olympus America, Melville NY). All infants experience a small decrease in oxygen saturation while the bronchoscope is in the airway. Our experience has shown an inevitable decrease in oxygen saturation in a significant portion of infants, especially in infants with respiratory distress or infants who were not well sedated before the procedure, Vigneswaran and Whitfield[10] noted a 14.2 mm Hg decrease in transcutaneous PaO$_2$ with fiberoptic bronchoscopy, and more recently, Cohn and associates[11] noted that 31% of such procedures resulted in transient oxygen saturation, and 14% resulted in transient bradycardia. Proper preoxygenation, adequate monitoring, and keeping the procedure to the minimal time required can minimize this complication.

INDICATIONS

The indications for bronchoscopy in the neonate are divided into urgent and elective.

Urgent Indications

The most common urgent indication for endoscopy is suspected airway obstruction in an intubated neonate or in a neonate who has just been extubated. For an intubated neonate, the axiom "when in doubt pull it out" usually applies. In certain circumstances, however, it is preferable to be certain that the ETT needs to be removed. In addition, the airways below the tip of the ETT may be occluded. Removal of the tube in these cases would be counterproductive. Bronchoscopy can confirm the position of an ETT as being either in the trachea or in one of the main stem bronchi. This procedure can be confusing for an inexperienced operator; however, it can be taught easily using an animal model and subsequently performed with a high degree of diagnostic accuracy.[12,13] In my experience, it is common initially for operators to believe that they are visualizing the carina when they are well within the right main stem bronchus and looking at the right middle and lower lobe orifices, and other authors have noted the same difficulty.[14] The diagnosis of

acute obstruction secondary to a plug, foreign material, or a blood clot at the distal end of the ETT is confirmed easily by endoscopy because vision is obscured by the plug at the end of the ETT. For an infant who has an acute deterioration with either a misplaced or obstructed ETT, fiberoptic bronchoscopy can be performed within 60 seconds of the decision that it is required, which is far quicker than it takes to obtain a chest radiograph.

Certain neonates may show evidence of airway obstruction after extubation. This obstruction may be related to a floppy upper airway, severe laryngomalacia secondary to prolapsing epiglottis or arytenoids or both, vocal cord paralysis, laryngeal edema, mucous plugging, or upper airway obstruction from the tongue falling against the posterior pharyngeal wall. In such circumstances, urgent endoscopy can confirm the diagnosis and facilitate further management.

A few infants are born with dysmorphic airways, often associated with a hypoplastic mandible or maxilla. Examples are infants with Pierre Robin syndrome with micrognathia, microglossia, cleft palate, Goldenhar syndrome, and Treacher Collins syndrome, wherein direct visualization of the larynx is often difficult to impossible. In addition, infants with large heads from hydrocephalus and infants with other malformations, such as occipital encephaloceles, may prove difficult to intubate.

Before the development of ultrathin bronchoscopes, many techniques had been described to intubate such infants, including the use of a ureteral catheter fitted with a central guidewire.[15] Others have described the technique of using the bronchoscope to determine visually the course of a guidewire to facilitate intubation over the laryngoscope.[16] Vauthy and Reddy[17] suggested the use of the flexible fiberoptic bronchoscope for establishment of airways in infants and children with airway obstruction. When experience has been gained with the ultrathin bronchoscopes, bronchoscopic transnasal intubation can be accomplished quickly and easily.[18] A bronchoscope is passed through the ETT with the proximal ventilator connector removed. The ETT is wedged on the proximal end of the bronchoscope. The bronchoscopy proceeds as usual, and the infant is administered oxygen. For neonates who require manual ventilation with a bag and mask or who are hypoxic, this technique can be modified so that it is performed through a bag and mask with a bronchoscopic adapter placed at the connection between the mask and the bag (see Fig. 41-2). The operator can perform the endoscopy while the infant is receiving bag-and-mask ventilation. This approach usually results in adequate oxygenation and ventilation and removes the urgency for the procedure. The laryngeal mask airway also may be used to provide intermittent positive-pressure ventilation during the endoscopy and may be useful for difficult fiberoptic intubations.[19-22]

When the bronchoscope is positioned in the lower trachea, the ETT is passed over the instrument, through the nose, and into the trachea, taking care to maintain the position of the scope, with the length of the scope outside the nares being kept as taut as possible to facilitate the passage of the ETT. Final positioning of the ETT is confirmed visually through the bronchoscope. We have never had to perform an urgent tracheostomy or surgically obtain an airway in the neonatal intensive care unit in 20 years, with the single exception of an infant who was born with complete proximal laryngotracheal agenesis. The use of ultrathin bronchoscopes for the establishment of difficult pediatric airways is well described in the anesthesia literature[16,23,24]; I believe these techniques are extremely useful in neonates with dysmorphic or otherwise abnormal upper airways. I have now performed transnasal fiberoptic intubation in 50 neonates with a variety of disorders[18] and have performed this procedure during a transport at a referring hospital for an infant with Treacher Collins syndrome and airway obstruction who could not be intubated using a laryngoscope. The ultrathin bronchoscope and light source are small and easily included with other transport gear.

Infants with severe laryngeal or upper tracheal stenosis after extubation may prove difficult to intubate. Occasionally we have intubated such infants using a rigid Storz-Hopkins telescope (No. 27018B, 3.0 mm, length 19 cm; Karl Storz GMGM & Co., Tuttlinger, Germany). In such circumstances, we have passed a No. 3 or larger ETT over the telescopic rod and intubated the infant under direct vision, passing the telescopic rod gently past the narrowed airway segment. The ETT is passed over the bronchoscope to establish an airway. We have used this technique to intubate an infant who was born with a severe cystic hygroma involving the anterior and lateral neck such that urgent tracheotomy would have proved difficult or impossible because the cystic hygroma protruded approximately 3 inches anterior to the trachea over the entire anterior and lateral aspects of the neck. Using a laryngoscope, it was not possible to visualize the larynx. Blind intubation was unsuccessful, and the larynx could not be visualized with the fiberoptic bronchoscope. After administration of muscle relaxation and bag and mask ventilation to maximize the oxygen saturation, the larynx was identified with the Storz 3.0-mm bronchoscope and Hopkins telescope. Intubation was performed over the Hopkins telescope.

Elective Indications

The determination of the position of the distal tip of the ETT in intubated neonates has been the subject of many studies.[13,25-27] A variety of methods, including palpation,[25,28] ultrasonography,[29] transtracheal illumination,[14] and magnetic detection,[30] have been reported.

Many studies have shown the value of the flexible bronchoscope for determining ETT position in older infants and children. In studies by Dietrich and colleagues,[12,13] the carina was not seen on x-ray in 15 of 24 patients, whereas the carina was seen clearly with a bronchoscope in 22 of 24 patients. These investigators also showed that the time to confirm ETT position was 40 seconds for the endoscope versus 30 minutes for x-ray. Fiberoptic bronchoscopy can be used to confirm the position of the ETT in neonates, and similar to older children, this evaluation correlates well with radiography.[10,27] I believe that fiberoptic bronchoscopy should be considered the gold standard for determination of ETT position because radiographs themselves do not provide

confirmation of ETT position in infants with abnormal tracheas. Bronchoscopy determines the relationship of the ETT to the carina no matter where it is positioned. In addition, bronchoscopy can confirm the movement of the ETT with head flexion and extension[27] and allow appropriate ETT position to allow for such movement.

Previous authors have used the disposable Visicath fiberoptic endoscopes of 1.3- or 2.0-mm size. These endoscopes pass through the smallest ETTs (2.5 mm), and although they increase airway resistance, this effect is minimal in 3.0-mm and larger tubes. One of the channels can be used for the administration of oxygen at low flow to maintain oxygenation. These endoscopes do not have flexible tips and consequently are misdirected easily into the tracheal mucosa and often cannot be positioned without significant alteration of the infant's head position. The advantage of these devices is that they are readily and rapidly available without the need to set up a light source and with the availability of a suction channel. My experience with this suction channel is that it most often does not remove thick secretions. Shinwell[31] reported complete or partial resolution of atelectasis, however, in 10 infants using these endoscopes. In addition, my experience has been similar to that of Dietrich and colleagues[12] in that minimal training is required to teach operators how to recognize adequate ETT position.

The next most common indication for nonurgent endoscopy in neonates is upper airway obstruction, which most commonly presents with stridor. This condition may occur after extubation or after delivery in infants with congenital anomalies. As can be seen from Table 41-1, which represents a 7-year experience with neonatal bronchoscopy, in my experience, the most common abnormality in the upper airway is laryngomalacia secondary to prolapsing arytenoids, posterior prolapse, collapse of the

Table 41–1. Neonatal Fiberoptic Bronchoscopy Findings: A 7-Year Experience

Diagnosis	No.	%
Upper airway (N = 144)		
Laryngomalacia	45	31.3
Subglottic narrowing, edema, web, stenosis	16	11.1
Vocal cord paralysis, unilateral or bilateral	11	7.6
Subglottic narrowing	4	2.7
Lower airway (N = 220*)		
Tracheomalacia	28	12.7
Bronchomalacia	10	4.5
Tracheal/bronchial granulations	42	19
Obstructed/dislodged ETT	18	23.6 via ETT only
Bronchoscopic intubations	40	

*76 via endotracheal tube (ETT); 144 transnasal, in nonintubated infants.

epiglottis, or a combination of these conditions. Other common findings include laryngeal edema, bilateral or unilateral vocal cord paralysis, acquired subglottic stenosis, webs, and subglottic cysts. These findings are consistent with other reported experience.[32] Cohen and associates[33] described their use of 10 years of endoscopy and tracheotomy in the neonate period and reviewed 124 neonates. This study confirmed the frequent occurrence of laryngomalacia followed by subglottic stenosis as a cause for laryngeal lesions. Holinger[32] pointed out that 45% of all patients with an airway anomaly had at least one associated abnormality involving the respiratory tract that may have contributed to the patient's symptoms. Other diagnoses include subglottic hemangiomas. Although the subglottic area can be difficult to visualize, with experience and the use of videobronchoscopy, this area can be well visualized without the need for rigid laryngoscopy.[34] The complete differential diagnosis of stridor in a neonate is large and has been reviewed by Wiatrak and Cotton.[35]

Other nonurgent indications include recurrent atelectasis associated with intubation[31] or after extubation to determine if there are tracheal abnormalities, such as tracheomalacia, tracheobronchomalacia, or other forms of abnormal tracheal anatomy. We have diagnosed an atretic left main stem orifice and small distal left-sided orifices in an infant who presented with an opaque left hemithorax. A subsequent bronchogram confirmed a left-sided hypoplasia, and a subsequent ventilation-perfusion study showed absence of perfusion of this lung.

Unusual Indications

There are many unique clinical situations in which the ultrathin flexible bronchoscope can be invaluable. We have used the endoscope for placement of a Fogarty catheter into a tracheoesophageal fistula to prevent progressive bowel distention and to allow resolution of lung disease before surgical repair. Bloch and Filston[36] described the use of the previously described Visicath endoscope to identify the stomach and to facilitate a gastrostomy in such an infant. A Fogarty balloon catheter was tied to the bronchoscope, which was retracted into the trachea, and then the balloon was inflated to occlude the fistula. We have performed a similar procedure using the 2.2-mm bronchoscope via the ETT. The Fogarty catheter was passed between the tracheal wall and the outer wall of the ETT and guided into position into the fistulous tract by the bronchoscope. The balloon was inflated to allow gastric decompression until the airway disease resolved, at which time complete surgical correction was undertaken. This approach may not always be successful because the use of high ventilatory pressures may force the balloon into the stomach.[37] Bloch and Filston[36] also reported the use of a transtracheal technique for placement of a Fogarty catheter; such a technique is a useful option in infants who may not be ready for complete surgical correction because of significant lung disease or other complications.

Neonates with severe unilateral pulmonary interstitial emphysema or persistent unilateral air leaks also may benefit from intermittent occlusion of the ipsilateral main stem bronchus. We have used the flexible endoscope to position a Fogarty balloon catheter to occlude the ipsilateral main stem bronchus for a short period, which has been associated with a rapid resolution of the interstitial emphysema in selected infants. Occasionally a beneficial result occurs after selective intubation, which can be guided by the flexible endoscope.

More recently, endoscopy skills have been required for the initial stabilization of infants who were diagnosed in utero with congenital airway obstruction, called **congenital high airway obstruction syndrome (CHAOS)**. Findings may include enlarged lungs, inverted diaphragms, a dilated trachea distal to the obstruction, and ascites. There are many reports of the planned **ex utero intrapartum treatment (EXIT)** procedure, which allows bronchoscopic evaluation of the airway and placement of an ETT where possible or a tracheostomy while the infant continues to receive placental support. This procedure has been used at birth for infants who received fetal surgical intervention for congenital diaphragmatic hernia with the placement of a tracheal plug or clip, which is then removed immediately after delivery. Other procedures performed using the EXIT procedure include orotracheal intubation, tracheostomy, tracheostomy with retrograde orotracheal intubation, tracheoplasty, central line placement, and instillation of surfactant.[38,39]

REVIEW OF LITERATURE

Although there are numerous articles reviewing individual institutional experiences with flexible fiberoptic endoscopy in infants and children, most of these articles describe experiences in older infants and children, with few subjects being true neonates. In addition, some of these reports involve the use of nondirectional flexible bronchoscopes, which, in my experience, are less optimal than endoscopes with flexible tips.[1,7,40-43]

Fan and Flynn[44] described the initial neonatal experience using flexible bronchoscopy. These authors consecutively evaluated 41 neonates who had been intubated for respiratory distress and were examined at extubation. Nine developed stridor; one neonate required a tracheostomy. These authors also showed a variety of lesions in these patients, including ulceration, granulation, and evidence of supraglottic or subglottic edema. The authors concluded that there were many minor lesions in asymptomatic infants, results consistent with our observations.[45]

In recent years there have been large series describing rigid and flexible endoscopy in neonates. The largest series using rigid endoscopy is that of Lindahl and colleagues.[46] These authors performed 196 bronchoscopies on 132 neonates with a variety of lesions, including esophageal atresia, gastrointestinal malformation, and diaphragmatic hernia. They used the Storz bronchoscope and Wolf 9.5 and 10 Charrier cystoscopes (Richard Wolf GMBH, Knittlingen, Germany) and a Storz 10 Charrier cystorectoscope. They performed many procedures, including lavage on 67 occasions and dilations for endoscopic abrasions on 32 occasions. They found no complications in 97 diagnostic procedures, but there were 7 complications in 99 therapeutic endoscopies, including

5 pneumothoraces, a right lower lobe bronchial rupture, and a rupture of the pulmonary artery during endobronchial removal of an obstructing granuloma. All patients survived. The most common indication was difficulty with artificial ventilation.

A series of 37 flexible bronchoscopies in 33 infants in the neonatal intensive care unit was performed by de Blic and coworkers[47] using the 2.2-mm flexible ultrathin bronchoscope. Twenty-eight of these procedures were done via the ETT before tracheostomy in nine spontaneously breathing infants. In 21 of these infants, the indication was persistent atelectasis or emphysema, followed by unexplained acute respiratory distress in 10 and stridor in 3. These authors and others have shown that flexible endoscopy can be useful in infants with bronchopulmonary dysplasia. Cohn and associates[11] evaluated 129 endoscopies in 47 children with a history of bronchopulmonary dysplasia. Only 19 of these children were younger than 3 months of age at the time of endoscopy. These authors noted that 30% of the patients had tracheobronchomalacia, a percentage similar to our observations in infants with bronchopulmonary dysplasia. It is important to confirm these diagnoses because wheezing infants may not respond to bronchodilator therapy if they have tracheomalacia.

Table 45-1 depicts our experience using flexible fiberoptic endoscopy over a 7-year period. We now have evaluated more than 250 neonates. In the 7-year experience, 65 of the procedures were performed in intubated neonates and 135 in nonintubated neonates. The diagnoses showed a preponderance of upper airway abnormalities and acute indications for lower airway obstruction. Among these infants, we evaluated a cohort of 55 infants who had been intubated for 1 week or longer to determine whether routine endoscopy was indicated.[45] Although we found many minor abnormalities in these infants, we detected no significant pathology in infants who did not have clinical abnormalities, such as stridor or other forms of respiratory difficulty. As a result of these observations, we do not recommend routine endoscopy for any asymptomatic neonate.

Since the late 1990s, we and others have noted a marked decrease in the airway sequelae of infants with very low birth-weight.[48] This decrease may be due in part to the decreased length of time that such infants are intubated, but it is surprising when one considers the smaller size of the airways in infants with birth weights less than 600 g and the relatively large diameter of the 2.5-mm ETT used in these infants. We have now had four cases of significant subglottic stenosis or granulation tissue during the past 6 years in the neonatal intensive care unit at the University of California, San Diego, an interval during which we treated more than 600 infants of less than 1500-g birth weight who required intubation and mechanical ventilation.[49] This finding may reflect the marked decline in spontaneous unplanned extubations, which decreased from 14% in 1992 to 7% in 2002. Over this same interval, a greater percentage of bronchoscopic evaluations have been for upper airway problems, including the evaluation of stridor in nonventilated infants, the evaluation of choanal patency, and evaluations to determine the presence of significant reflux to the laryngeal airway.

I anticipate that for detailed endoscopic evaluation of airways in infants in whom bronchoscopy does not provide definitive diagnosis, newer techniques, such as virtual bronchoscopy, will be extremely informative.[50,51] Virtual endoscopy provides computer-generated, three-dimensional visualization of a cavity by reconstructing two-dimensional computed tomography or magnetic resonance imaging data. Virtual endoscopy has the added benefit of the ability to assess the transmural extent of disease and view the airway distal to areas of luminal compromise.

SUMMARY

The ultrathin fiberoptic bronchoscope, which can pass easily through even the smallest currently used ETTs, provides a rapid method to diagnose congenital and acquired airway lesions and to assess ETT position and patency. This tool can provide neonatologists with the ability to establish secure endotracheal airways in infants with micrognathia, cleft palate, and other disorders and to diagnose a variety of abnormalities in the upper and lower airway. Neonatal flexible bronchoscopy can be learned by anyone with sufficient interest, can be lifesaving, and should be available for the management of critically ill neonates.

REFERENCES

1. Wood RE, Sherman JA: Pediatric flexible bronchoscopy. Ann Otol Rhinol Laryngol 89:414, 1980.
2. Finer NN, Etches PC: Fiber-optic bronchoscopy in the neonate. Pediatr Pulmonol 7:116, 1989.
3. Hasegawa S, Hitomi S, Murakawa M, Mori K: Development of an ultrathin fiberscope with a built-in channel for bronchoscopy in infants. Chest 110:1543-1546, 1996.
4. Etches PC, Finer NN: Use of an ultrathin fiberoptic catheter for neonatal endotracheal tube problem diagnosis. Crit Care Med 17:202, 1989.
5. Shinwell ES, Higgins RD, Auten RL, et al: Fiberoptic bronchoscopy in the treatment of intubated neonates. Am J Dis Child 143:1064, 1989.
6. Erb T, Hammer J, Rutishauser M, Frei FJ: Fiber-optic bronchoscopy in sedated infants facilitated by an airway endoscopy mask. Paediatr Anaesth 9:47, 1999.
7. Wood RE: Spelunking in the pediatric airways: Explorations with the flexible fiberoptic bronchoscope. Pediatr Clin North Am 31:785, 1984.
8. Yaster M: The dose response of fentanyl in neonatal anesthesia. Anesthesiology 66:433, 1987.
9. Gjonaj ST, Lowenthal DB, Dozor AJ: Nebulized lidocaine administered to infants and children undergoing flexible bronchoscopy. Chest 112:1665, 1997.
10. Vigneswaran R, Whitfield JM: The use of a new ultra-thin fiberoptic bronchoscope to determine endotracheal tube position in the sick newborn infant. Chest 80:174, 1981.
11. Cohn RC, Kercsmar C, Dearborn D: Safety and efficacy of flexible endoscopy in children with bronchopulmonary dysplasia. Am J Dis Child 142:1225, 1988.
12. Dietrich KA, Conrad SA, Romero MD, et al: Accuracy of flexible fiberoptic endoscopy in identifying abnormal endotracheal tube positions. Pediatr Emerg Care 4:257, 1990.

13. Dietrich KA, Strauss RH, Cabalka AK, et al: Use of flexible fiberoptic endoscopy for determination of endotracheal tube position in the pediatric patient. Crit Care Med 16:884, 1988.

14. Stewart RD, LaRosee A, Kaplan RM, et al: Correct positioning of an endotracheal tube using a flexible lighted stylet. Crit Care Med 18:97, 1990.

15. Gouvemeur JM: Using an ureteral catheter as a guide in difficult neonatal fiberoptic intubation. Anesthesiology 66:436, 1987.

16. Howardy-Hansen P, Berthelsen P: Fiber-optic bronchoscopic nasotracheal intubation of a neonate with Pierre Robin syndrome. Anaesthesia 43:121, 1988.

17. Vauthy PA, Reddy R: Acute upper airway obstruction in infants and children: Evaluation by the fiberoptic bronchoscope. Otol Rhinol Laryngol 89:417, 1980.

18. Finer NN, Muzyka D: Flexible endoscopic intubation of the neonate. Pediatr Pulmonol 12:48, 1992.

19. Brimacombe J, Newell S, Swainston R, et al: A potential new technique for awake fiber-optic bronchoscopy—use of the laryngeal mask airway. Med J Aust 156:876, 1992.

20. Dich-Nielsen JO, Nagel P: Flexible fiber-optic bronchoscopy via the laryngeal mask. Acta Anaesth Scand 37:17, 1993.

21. Ellis DS, Potluri PK, O'Flaherty JE, Baum VC: Difficult airway management in the neonate: A simple method of intubating through a laryngeal mask airway. Paediatr Anaesth 9:460, 1999.

22. Wilson IG: The laryngeal airway in paediatric practice [editorial]. Br J Anaesth 70:124, 1993.

23. Biban P, Rugolotto S, Zoppi G, et al: Fiberoptic endotracheal intubation through an ultra-thin bronchoscope with suction channel in a newborn with difficult airway. Anesth Analg 90:1007, 2000.

24. Kleeman PP, Jantzen JPAH, Bonfils P: The ultra-thin bronchoscope in management of the difficult paediatric airway. Can J Anaesth 34:606, 1987.

25. Bednarek FRJ, Kuhns LR: Endotracheal tube placement in infants determined by suprasternal palpation: A new technique. Pediatrics 56:224, 1975.

26. Loew A, Thibeault DW: A new and safe method to control the depth of endotracheal tube intubation in neonates. Pediatrics 54:506, 1974.

27. Rotschild A, Chitayat D, Putennan ML, et al: Optimal positioning of endotracheal tubes for ventilation of preterm infants. Am J Dis Child 145:1007, 1991.

28. Kuhns LR, Poznanski AK: Endotracheal tube position in the infant. Pediatrics 78:991, 1971.

29. Slovis TL, Poland RL: Endotracheal tubes in neonates: Sonographic positioning. Radiology 160:262, 1986.

30. Blayney M, Costello S, Perlman M, et al: A new system for location of endotracheal tube in preterm and term neonates. Pediatrics 87:44, 1991.

31. Shinwell ES: Ultrathin fiber-optic bronchoscopy for airway toilet in neonatal pulmonary atelectasis. Pediatr Pulmonol 13:48, 1992.

32. Holinger LD: Etiology of stridor in the neonate, infant and child. Ann Otol Rhinol Laryngol 89:397, 1980.

33. Cohen SR, Eavey RD, Desmond MS, et al: Endoscopy and tracheotomy in the neonatal period: A 10-year review. Ann Otol Rhinol Laryngol 86:577, 1977.

34. Hawkins DB, Dark RW: Flexible laryngoscopy in neonates, infants, and young children. Ann Otol Rhinol Laryngol 96:81, 1987.

35. Wiatrak BJ, Cotton RT: Diagnosis and treatment of lesions of the upper airway: Part I. The neonate. Semin Respir Med 11:152, 1990.

36. Bloch EC, Filston HC: A thin fiberoptic bronchoscope as an aid to occlusion of the fistula in infants with tracheo-esophageal fistula. Anesth Analg 67:791, 1988.

37. Berry FA: Basic considerations. In Berry FA (ed): Anesthetic Management of Difficult and Routine Pediatric Patients. New York, Churchill Livingstone, 1986.

38. DeCou JM, Jones DC, Jacobs HD, Touloukian RJ: Successful ex utero intrapartum treatment (EXIT) procedure for congenital high airway obstruction syndrome (CHAOS) owing to laryngeal atresia. J Pediatr Surg 33:1563, 1998.

39. Mychaliska GB, Bealer JF, Graf JL, et al: Operating on placental support: The ex utero intrapartum treatment procedure. J Pediatr Surg 32:227-230, 1997.

40. Fan LL, Sparks LM, Fix EJ: Flexible fiberoptic endoscopy for airway problems in a pediatric intensive care unit. Chest 93:556, 1988.

41. Ward RF, Arnold JE, Healy GB: Flexible minibronchoscopy in children. Ann Otol Rhinol Laryngol 96:645, 1987.

42. Wood RE: Clinical applications of ultrathin flexible bronchoscopes. Pediatr Pulmonol 1:244, 1985.

43. Wood RE, Azizkhan RG, Sidman J, et al: Surgical applications of ultrathin flexible bronchoscopes in infants. Ann Otol Rhinol Laryngol 100:116, 1991.

44. Fan LL, Flynn JW: Laryngoscopy in neonates and infants: Experience with the flexible fiberoptic bronchoscope. Laryngoscope 91:451, 1981.

45. Finer NN, Etches PC, Tarn A: Neonatal airway injury after prolonged ventilation. Pediatr Res 33:325A, 1993.

46. Lindahl H, Rintala R, Malinen L, et al: Bronchoscopy during the first month of life. Pediatr Surg 27:548, 1992.

47. de Blic J, Delacourt C, Scheinmann P: Ultrathin flexible bronchoscopy in neonatal intensive care units. Arch Dis Child 66:1383, 1991.

48. daSilva O, Stevens D: Complications of airway management in very-low-birth-weight infants. Biol Neonate 75:40, 1999.

49. Rich W, Finer NW, Vaucher YE: Ten-year trends in neonatal assisted ventilation of very low-birthweight infants. J Perinatol 23:660, 2003.

50. Fried MP, Moharir VM, Shinmoto H, et al: Virtual laryngoscopy. Ann Otol Rhinol Laryngol 108:221, 1999.

51. Hartnick CJ, Emery KH, Chung S, Myer CM: Imaging case study of the month: Pediatric virtual bronchoscopy. Ann Otol Rhinol Laryngol 111:281, 2002.

CHAPTER 42

Oxygen Therapy

Carla M. Weis, Cynthia A. Cox, and William W. Fox

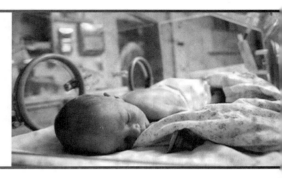

The goal of oxygen (O_2) therapy is to achieve adequate delivery of O_2 to the tissues without creating O_2 toxicity. The optimal use of O_2 in effecting the delicate balance between sufficient O_2 delivery and toxicity has been the subject of many publications. An understanding of the physiology of oxygenation, the various available modes for measuring oxygenation, and the potential toxicity of O_2 is fundamental for the clinician caring for the fetus or neonate.

PHYSIOLOGIC CONSIDERATIONS

Oxygen Transport

The transport of O_2 from the environment to the tissues depends on the orchestration of several interrelated physiologic systems. This process begins in the lung and is affected by the amount of O_2 entering the lung and the adequacy of gas exchange within the lung. When O_2 has reached the blood, the ability of O_2 to bind with hemoglobin (Hb) plays a vital role in O_2 transport. The integrity of the cardiovascular system is responsible for blood flow to the tissues and to the lung and is determined mainly by cardiac output. Malfunction within any of these systems can compromise O_2 delivery. Box 42-1 lists general conditions that can lead to poor tissue oxygenation.

Alveolar-Arterial Oxygen Pressure Difference

Generally the clinician measures the arterial or peripheral **partial pressure of O_2 (Po_2)** in the blood and correlates this result with the **expected arterial O_2 concentration**, knowing the inspired O_2 percentage (and alveolar level). The comparison between alveolar and arterial O_2 levels is termed the **alveolar-arterial O_2 pressure difference ($P[A - a]o_2$)**. The level of $P(A - a)o_2$ correlates with severity of pulmonary illness. Values of $P(A - a)o_2$ have been used to assess degree of illness and to predict subsequent outcome of infants with hyaline membrane disease and of infants with persistent pulmonary hypertension and associated clinical conditions.

To determine the $P(A - a)o_2$, one first must calculate the expected alveolar Po_2 using the following simplified calculation:

$$[Fio_2(P_{atm} - PH_2O)] - Pco_2 = \text{alveolar } Po_2$$

Where Fio_2 is fractional inspired O_2 concentration, P_{atm} is atmospheric pressure, PH_2O is water vapor pressure, and Pco_2 is partial pressure of carbon dioxide (CO_2) in the alveolus, which is approximately equal to the partial pressure of CO_2 in the blood.

With 100% inspired O_2 concentration (at sea level) and Pco_2 40 mm Hg, the expected alveolar Po_2 (expressed as either mm Hg or torr) would be:

$$[1.0(760 \text{ mm Hg} - 47 \text{ mm Hg})] - 40 \text{ mm Hg} = 673 \text{ mm Hg (or torr)}$$

After the alveolar concentration is determined, the arterial Po_2 (Pao_2) is subtracted to calculate the $P(A - a)o_2$. The calculated $P(A - a)o_2$ increases with increasing inspired O_2 concentration. The $P(A - a)o_2$ quantitates ventilation-perfusion ($\dot{V}/Q$) mismatch. In normal adults breathing room air, this value ranges from 10 to 20 mm Hg. Normal neonates have values 40 to 50 mm Hg, and they may remain in the 20 to 40 mm Hg range for days after birth because of the substantial amount of shunting present in the newborn.[1,2] When a normal adult breathes 100% O_2, the Pao_2 is approximately 600 mm Hg compared with approximately 300 mm Hg in a newborn.[3] In a sick neonate on 100% O_2, $P(A - a)o_2$ of greater than 300 mm Hg is considered to be elevated. This difference generally is caused by one of three pulmonary-cardiac interactions:

1. A diffusion block at the alveolar-capillary level
2. A $\dot{V}/Q$ mismatch in the lungs
3. A fixed right-to-left shunt (intracardiac)

Alveolar-capillary block refers to thickening of the distance between alveolus and capillary bed, usually not seen in the newborn. Most diseases of the neonate that present with hypoxemia have right-to-left shunting primarily caused by $\dot{V}/Q$ mismatching or fixed right-to-left (intracardiac) shunting. A $\dot{V}/Q$ mismatch can occur as a result of ventilated areas that are poorly perfused (increasing physiologic dead space) or perfused areas that are poorly ventilated (intrapulmonary shunt). Underventilated alveoli exist whenever inspired air is unable to reach the alveolar-capillary membrane (e.g., pneumonia, atelectasis, pulmonary edema).

To distinguish between hypoxia caused by $\dot{V}/Q$ mismatch and that caused by fixed intracardiac (right-to-left) shunting, the hyperoxia test is performed. For this test, the infant is placed in 100% O_2, and an arterial blood gas is performed after 5 to 10 minutes. A PaO_2 less than 150 mm Hg strongly suggests that there is right-to-left shunting caused by cyanotic congenital heart disease (fixed shunt), although severe pulmonary hypertension with right-to-left shunting via the ductus arteriosus and foramen ovale also may occur in this way. This test can aid in the diagnosis of cyanotic congenital heart disease, and it has been used prognostically.[4-6] In the case of pulmonary disease, the resulting determination of the $P(A - a)O_2$ reflects the severity of disease. The $P(A - a)O_2$ has been used as a predictor of mortality and has become part of the entry criteria for many extracorporeal membrane oxygenation programs. In a retrospective review of 30 infants with persistent pulmonary hypertension of the newborn, Beck and associates[7] determined that a $P(A - a)O_2$ of 610 mm Hg for 8 consecutive hours would predict a mortality of 79%.

In recent years, the oxygenation index (OI) has been found to be a more sensitive prognostic indicator than $P(A - a)O_2$ for neonatal pulmonary disease because the mean airway pressure (MAP) is considered in the calculation.[8] An infant's OI is calculated by the formula: (MAP) · (FIO_2/PaO_2). The OI has been used to quantitate postsurfactant responses and to evaluate infants before extracorporeal membrane oxygenation therapy in many centers.[9-11] Its value for extracorporeal membrane oxygenation lies in statistics that reveal an 80% mortality with an OI greater than 40.[9] An OI of 25 is reported to predict a 50% mortality.[9]

Arterial Partial Pressure of Oxygen and Oxygen Saturation

Until the early 1980s, neonatal O_2 therapy relied on measurement and evaluation of PaO_2. (The Clark electrode for measurement of PO_2 was the earliest method for evaluating arterial blood gases.) Now, because of ease of measurement, clinicians rely more on pulse oximetry for continuous monitoring, while correlating O_2 saturation with PaO_2 intermittently. The danger of relying solely on O_2 saturation is hyperoxia. The risk of O_2 toxicity is correlated with the PaO_2 and not the O_2 saturation. For this reason, clinicians attempt specific control of PaO_2, maintaining

levels less than 80 mm Hg. There are other reasons why PaO_2, rather than O_2 saturation, can be useful. Values of PaO_2 range from 0 to greater than 600 mm Hg, whereas values of O_2 saturation range from 0 to 100%. PaO_2 measurements offer a wider range compared with O_2 saturation, which enables the clinician to evaluate patient status (i.e., an infant with a PaO_2 of 300 mm Hg probably has a better pulmonary status than an infant with a PaO_2 of 100 mm Hg at the same FIO_2). In addition, studies that suggest the determination of pulmonary prognosis can be based on $P(A - a)O_2$[4-6] rely on measurement of PaO_2. Essentially the PaO_2 and the O_2 saturation offer different information, and although they are intimately and directly related to each other, this relationship can vary with changing physiologic states. The clinician caring for neonates must understand the relationship between PaO_2 and O_2 saturation.

Under normal conditions, 97% of O_2 transported from the lungs to the tissue is carried by Hb, and approximately 3% is dissolved in plasma. It is the dissolved component that determines PO_2 in the blood. The PO_2 quantitates the pressure exerted by this gas to diffuse to an area of lower pressure. This pressure is expressed as mm Hg or torr.

O_2 saturation differs from PO_2 in that it represents the percent of Hb that is saturated with O_2. Because the transport of O_2 within the blood is achieved almost entirely by Hb, O_2 saturation can be a measure of the O_2 load in the blood stream, but the amount of Hb must be considered to assess O_2 content.

O_2 content of the blood is the volume of O_2 contained in whole blood (expressed as volume percent). This O_2 load is divided between two compartments: O_2 bound to Hb and O_2 dissolved in plasma, with virtually all of the O_2 load carried by Hb. At a PaO_2 of 100 mm Hg, Hb (at normal levels) carries approximately 100 times more O_2 than does plasma (which carries only 0.3 mL O_2/100 mL). Because Hb plays such an important role in determining O_2 content, conditions of anemia may affect O_2 content and O_2 delivery significantly. The O_2 content of blood primarily depends on the amount of Hb *and* how much of it is saturated. At 100% saturation, each gram of Hb binds a total of 1.34 mL of O_2. As Hb becomes more saturated, its O_2 binding is enhanced (i.e., cooperative binding, or **heme-heme interaction**), and it becomes easier to saturate, until complete saturation is approached; this explains the sigmoidal shape of the oxyhemoglobin equilibrium curve (Hb/O_2 dissociation/saturation curve) (Fig. 42-1). At a PaO_2 of 100 mm Hg, Hb is near complete saturation. Increasing the O_2 beyond this point increases the PaO_2 rapidly, but the increase in the total O_2 content of the blood is negligible. Technically, Hb is not 100% saturated until the PaO_2 reaches 250 mm Hg.[12]

At a PaO_2 less than 100 mm Hg, one must look at the oxyhemoglobin equilibrium curve to determine the exact O_2 saturation of Hb. Each curve is characterized by a P_{50} value. The **P_{50}** is the partial pressure of O_2 at which Hb is 50% saturated. As noted in Figure 42-1, the oxyhemoglobin equilibrium curve depends on Hb type (e.g., fetal versus adult) and varying physiologic conditions. The curve is shifted to the right (meaning lower O_2 saturation at a comparable PO_2) in the face of acidosis or increased

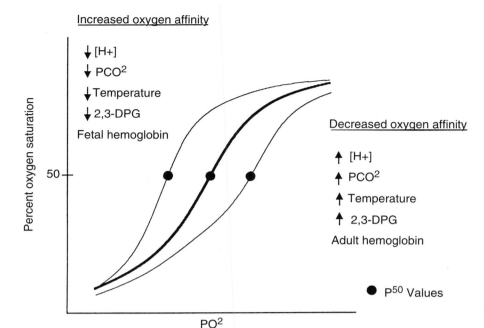

Increased oxygen affinity

$\downarrow$ [H+]

$\downarrow$ PCO^2

$\downarrow$ Temperature

$\downarrow$ 2,3-DPG

Fetal hemoglobin

Percent oxygen saturation

50 —

Decreased oxygen affinity

$\uparrow$ [H+]

$\uparrow$ PCO^2

$\uparrow$ Temperature

$\uparrow$ 2,3-DPG

Adult hemoglobin

● P^{50} Values

PO^2

Figure 42–1. The oxyhemoglobin saturation curves. Factors that shift the curve and increase or decrease oxygen affinity are indicated. 2,3-DPG, 2,3-diphosphoglycerate.

PCO_2 (Bohr effect), increased temperature, or increased concentration of 2,3-diphosphoglycerate, as in adult Hb. Conversely the oxyhemoglobin equilibrium curve is shifted to the left (higher O_2 saturation at a comparable PO_2) in the opposite physiologic conditions: alkalosis, low PCO_2, low temperature, or low levels of 2,3-diphosphoglycerate, as in fetal Hb.[13]

The physiologic effects of shifts in the oxyhemoglobin equilibrium curve are important to understand (Table 42-1). The unloading of O_2 from the blood to the tissue relies on the diffusion gradient between the partial pressure of O_2 in tissue and the partial pressure of O_2 in the blood (determined by the O_2 dissolved in plasma). If the partial pressure

of O_2 in the blood is high, a greater diffusion gradient is set up between blood and tissue, allowing for "easier" O_2 delivery to tissues. With a right-shifted curve (higher P_{50}), O_2 is bound to Hb less tightly and reaches equilibrium (i.e., released from and bound to Hb) at relatively higher partial pressures, enhancing unloading of O_2 to tissues. This situation is physiologically optimal for tissue O_2 uptake, especially during increased tissue metabolism. As the blood reaches the tissue, the by-products of metabolism (i.e., increased temperature, acidosis, and PCO_2 diffusing into the blood) act to increase the P_{50} and shift the curve to the right. Areas where O_2 consumption is highest allow an exaggerated diffusion gradient for O_2 between the blood and tissue, enhancing O_2 delivery.

When the oxyhemoglobin equilibrium curve is left shifted (lower P_{50}), O_2 is bound to Hb more tightly and reaches equilibrium (i.e., released from and bound to Hb) at relatively lower partial pressures, enhancing loading of O_2 to Hb. This situation is physiologically optimal for fetoplacental O_2 exchange and for O_2 exchange within the lung.

For the fetus, who exists in a state of relative hypoxemia, the effect of fetal Hb is that fetal systemic blood contains a higher O_2 saturation and an increased O_2 content at lower PO_2 levels. This allows efficient extraction of O_2 from the placenta. Although O_2 delivery to fetal tissues is not as efficient under these circumstances, it is offset, to some extent, by the greater slope of the left-shifted curve so that a comparable decrease in PO_2 results in a relatively larger decrease in saturation and a relatively enhanced unloading of O_2. Also, teleologically, fetal extraction of O_2 from the placenta is more important for survival than tissue O_2 delivery because without extraction there can be no delivery.

In the lungs, shifting of the oxyhemoglobin equilibrium curve facilitates respiratory gas exchange. As CO_2 is

Table 42–1. Shifts in Oxyhemoglobin Equilibrium Curve

	Left Shift	Right Shift
Causes	Alkalosis	Acidosis
	Decreased CO_2	Increased CO_2
	Decreased temperature	Increased temperature
	Decreased 2,3-DPG	Increased 2,3-DPG
Effects	Increased affinity	Decreased affinity
	Decreased P_{50}	Increased P_{50}
	Unloads at lower PO_2	Unloads at higher PO_2
Importance (advantages)	Blood O_2 uptake	Tissue O_2 uptake
	Fetus	Increased tissue metabloism
	Lungs	

2,3-DPG, 2,3-diphosphoglycerate.

released from red blood cells into the alveoli and the P_{CO_2} in the blood decreases, the curve is shifted to the left. This shift enhances uptake of O_2 from the alveoli into the blood.

There are times when a leftward shift of the oxyhemoglobin equilibrium curve may not be favorable. In a mechanically ventilated neonate who is hyperventilated, either intentionally or unintentionally, the resulting leftward shift of the curve may produce or aggravate hypoxia in the critically ill neonate.[14]

Oxygen Delivery and Consumption

The goal of O_2 therapy is to deliver O_2 successfully to the tissues.[15] Ideally, for a critically ill patient, the goal of therapy should be to match O_2 delivery to O_2 consumption instead of simply trying to achieve "normal" values. O_2 consumption is defined as the quantity of O_2 extracted from the capillary beds as blood passes to the venous side and is influenced by the metabolic needs of the tissues. In well newborns breathing room air, O_2 consumption can be measured by determining the difference between the inspired and expired O_2 concentrations. O_2 consumption measurements in critically ill newborns with varying metabolic needs are difficult to obtain, however. Clinically, there are methods that allow the estimation of O_2 use by the tissues to assess the effectiveness of tissue O_2 delivery. The mixed venous (pulmonary artery) O_2 tension has been called "the most reliable single physiologic indicator of the overall balance between oxygen supply and demand"[16] (see later). This value is the blood O_2 tension that has equilibrated with the tissues. A low or decreasing mixed venous P_{O_2} represents a detrimental imbalance between O_2 consumption and O_2 delivery. Disturbances in this balance can result from one or more of the following:

1. Inadequate O_2, Hb, or cardiac output
2. Increased demand (beyond available compensation)
3. Inadequate perfusion
4. Disruption of cellular O_2 metabolism

Several other measurements also are useful in assessing O_2 delivery (Box 42-2). The **O_2 content** of blood is determined by knowing P_{O_2}, Hb concentration, and percent saturation. **O_2 delivery** is calculated by the product of O_2 content and cardiac output. These concepts are clinically important, and intensivists caring for adults, using Swan-Ganz catheters, routinely measure cardiac output and calculate O_2 delivery in critically ill adults.[16-19] By calculating the O_2 content of arterial and venous blood, an estimate of **O_2 consumption** can be obtained by multiplying the difference between arterial and venous content by the cardiac output. (Some of these measurements are inaccurate in the presence of cardiac shunts, for example, a patent ductus arteriosus.) Because cardiac output measurements are not commonly done in neonatal intensive care units, O_2 consumption can be estimated by using the difference between the arterial O_2 content and the venous O_2 content. This calculation can provide valuable information when trying to match O_2 delivery and O_2 demand. Techniques to evaluate O_2 delivery and O_2 consumption presently are not used widely in neonates but may have value in the future.

Box 42–2 Three Methods Used to Quantitate Oxygen Therapy

1. O_2 Content (Arterial and Venous)

$$O_2 \text{ content (arterial)} \begin{cases} PaO_2 \\ \text{Hemoglobin concentration} \\ \text{Hemoglobin saturation} \\ \text{Mixed venous } P_{O_2} \end{cases} O_2 \text{ content (venous)}$$

$$\begin{aligned} O_2 \text{ content} \\ (mL\ O_2/dL) \end{aligned} = \begin{aligned} &[\text{Hb concentration (g/dL)} \times \\ &1.34\ mL/g \times \text{Hb saturation}] + \\ &[PO_2/100 \times 0.3\ mL/dL] \end{aligned}$$

2. Oxygen Delivery

$$\begin{aligned} O_2 \text{ delivery} \\ (mL\ O_2/min) \end{aligned} = O_2 \text{ content} \times \begin{aligned} \text{Cardiac output} \\ (dL/min) \end{aligned}$$

3. Oxygen Consumption

$$\begin{aligned} O_2 \text{ consumption} \\ (mL\ O_2/min) \end{aligned} = \begin{bmatrix} O_2 \text{ content(arterial)} - O_2 \text{ content} \\ \times \text{ Cardiac Output} \qquad \text{(venous)} \\ (dL/min) \end{bmatrix}$$

O_2 consumption can be increased substantially in intensive care nursery patients for a variety of reasons. Studies performed in adult intensive care units show specific clinical situations in which O_2 consumption is increased. Decreased pulmonary compliance or tachypnea may consume 25% to 40% of O_2 transported in the spontaneously breathing patients.[20] Chest physiotherapy can increase O_2 consumption by 35%.[21] Surgical trauma can be associated with a 10% to 30% increase and severe infections with a 50% increase in O_2 consumption.[22] Although these studies were done on adults, these issues have clinical relevance in a neonatal intensive care setting.

MEASUREMENTS

Pulse Oximetry

Measurement of O_2 saturation by pulse oximetry is now the most widely used noninvasive form of O_2 monitoring. The pulse oximeter consists of a light-emitting and light-sensing cuff that can be placed around a whole extremity to monitor arterial pulsations closely. Light of different wavelengths is transmitted through the blood by a light-emitting element and detected by a sensor. The transmitted light is either red light at a 660-nm wavelength or infrared light at a 940-nm wavelength. At 660 nm, oxyhemoglobin is more transparent than deoxyhemoglobin; however, at 940 nm, the opposite effect occurs. The difference in absorption of light at these two wavelengths, detected by the sensor, allows calculation of an Hb-to-Hb O_2 ratio, or percent saturation of Hb.[23] Other compounds, such as carboxyhemoglobin or methemoglobin, might cause interference if they are not specifically screened,[24,25] but these compounds usually are not present in high enough concentration to cause error in O_2 saturation values.[26]

Commercially available O_2 saturation devices are user friendly in that they do not require frequent rotation of sampling sites, do not burn, have a rapid response, do not require calibration, and display pulse strength (helping to differentiate artifact from true readings). They are, however, subject to movement artifact and require location of an acceptable pulse.

Partial Pressure of Oxygen in Blood

Umbilical Artery Catheters

Sampling from umbilical arterial catheters is the most common way to measure PaO_2 and to monitor the effectiveness of O_2 therapy intermittently in the critically ill neonate. The relatively large umbilical arteries are easier to catheterize than peripheral vessels in delivery room emergencies and in the intensive care nursery, and the procedure can be painless. Also, because the catheters reside in large vessels, they last longer than peripheral catheters.

There has been extensive discussion about high (T6 to T10) or low (L3 to L4) umbilical artery catheter-tip placement.[27-29] It has been suggested that high catheters have potentially more risk of developing thrombosis or releasing emboli to the mesenteric or renal arteries.[30] Complications from low catheters may be more frequent, although milder (vasospasm), and easier to identify.

Vascular spasm is the most common complication of umbilical arterial catheters and encompasses a wide spectrum of presentations. This spasm most often involves blanching of one or both lower extremities. When blanching or cyanosis occurs, catheter placement must be reviewed radiologically, infusion content must be verified, and the opposite extremity should be warmed (including the femoral area). Warming one extremity creates simultaneous vasodilation of the opposite extremity, and heat damage to the underperfused extremity is avoided. The catheter should be removed promptly if vasospasm persists.

Sepsis also is a common complication with *any* type of indwelling catheter left in place for longer than a few days, and umbilical lines are no exception.[31] With regard to umbilical artery catheters, previous recommendations suggesting that they be used for less than 1 week have changed with prolonged intensive care of very-low-birth-weight infants. In these infants, arterial access is so difficult that catheters sometimes may be left in place for 1 month, with careful daily assessment. In all cases, the necessity of arterial blood gas monitoring must be weighed against the risk of infection from umbilical lines.

Peripheral Arterial Lines

In larger infants or in infants in whom umbilical catheterization is unsuccessful, percutaneous peripheral artery catheterization is recommended.[32] Sites commonly used for percutaneous arterial catheterization are the radial and posterior tibial arteries. These catheters are used for blood sampling and blood pressure monitoring. They are not used for fluid and blood infusions or drug administration,[33] in contrast to umbilical artery catheters.

Patency of the catheter is maintained with a heparinized saline infusion. Care of the radial arterial catheter includes restraining the arm and observing any changes in circulation in the extremity. The length of time the catheter remains functional often is related to the meticulous care given to the catheter and the catheter insertion site.

Capillary Blood Gas

Obtaining capillary blood gases has been commonplace in intensive care nurseries since the 1960s, when studies showed a good correlation of pH and PCO_2 between arterial and capillary samples.[34,35] The O_2 tension may not be reliable, especially at higher values of PaO_2.[12] Care must be taken to warm the extremity adequately before sampling to arterialize the capillary blood. Excessive squeezing should be avoided.

Potential sampling sites include the heels and fingers. When using the heel, only the medial and lateral aspects of the plantar surface should be used. As a result of multiple heel punctures, calcified heel nodules may develop and can persist for several months to years. Calcaneal osteochondritis is another potential complication of using the heel for sampling.

Venous Blood Gas

A venous blood gas can give the clinician a general idea about systemic pH and PCO_2. The venous PCO_2 is approximately 5 mm Hg higher than arterial values, and the pH may be slightly lower. Venous samples vary according to the site from which they are obtained.[36] A venous blood gas cannot be used to monitor arterial oxygenation, although a **mixed venous** sample may give information on tissue oxygenation.

Mixed Venous Partial Pressure of Oxygen

Another important way to monitor O_2 therapy is to evaluate mixed venous PO_2.[16,18,37-39] Neonatologists have begun to realize the importance of this measurement since its extensive use in monitoring extracorporeal membrane oxygenation therapy. In neonates, umbilical venous catheter samples can be used to reflect mixed venous PO_2 (if the catheter is in the inferior vena cava). True mixed venous (pulmonary artery) PO_2 is an indicator of tissue oxygenation because this value is the O_2 tension of blood that has equilibrated with the tissues. In many situations, monitoring of mixed venous PO_2 can be useful to evaluate the effectiveness of O_2 delivery.

Changes in tissue oxygenation can be reflected in the mixed venous PO_2. Normal mixed venous PO_2 should be in the range of 40 mm Hg, or 75% mixed venous saturation. This fact shows that approximately 25% of the O_2 bound to Hb is consumed by the tissues. In critically ill neonates, if a decreased mixed venous PO_2 occurs, it indicates that tissue O_2 delivery is insufficient relative to O_2 needs, and tissue hypoxia can result. With a 12 mm Hg decrease in mixed venous PO_2 to 28 mm Hg, the Hb saturation is 50%, representing a doubling of O_2 consumption[16] (i.e., 50% of bound O_2 extracted instead of 25%). In this situation, O_2 delivery needs to be increased. If tissue hypoxia persists or is extreme, severely damaged tissue may decrease its O_2 extraction (a functional systemic shunt), resulting in a rising mixed venous Po_2. This situation also can occur in sepsis or other capillary leak syndromes that lead to increased extracellular fluid. This increase creates a greater diffusion distance and impedes O_2 delivery. In these cases, although an increasing mixed venous Po_2 can be expected, if additional O_2 delivery is inadequate, a normal mixed venous Po_2 may occur and be misleading.

A decreasing value indicates a detrimental imbalance between O_2 delivery and O_2 consumption, and an increasing value should warn of microvascular insufficiency or extreme hypoxia. A stable value can be reassuring and indicate appropriate O_2 delivery.

Oxygen Trend Monitoring

Transcutaneous Po_2 monitoring was introduced in 1974.[40] The technology for this device consists of a platinum cathode and a silver/silver chloride anode that is bathed in an electrolyte solution. Heating of the electrode (to ~44° F) is necessary to produce local vasodilation and increases O_2 delivery to the skin for more accurate measurement. This device is effective for trend monitoring of Po_2, but it must be calibrated and correlated with an arterial blood gas. Accuracy is affected by skin thickness and skin blood flow, and the skin probes are generally less effective in infants older than 1 month of age. Clinical use of transcutaneous Po_2 monitors is complicated by the fact that these electrodes produce local heating and erythema of the skin in small premature infants, and monitoring sites must be rotated every 3 to 4 hours. For the most part, O_2 saturation measurement has eliminated transcutaneous Po_2 monitoring.

OXYGEN TOXICITY

The side effects of inadequate O_2 administration are well known and include acidosis, cell death, and failure of specific organs. The most important sequela of hypoxemia is neurologic damage, but the kidneys, lungs, and gastrointestinal tract also are highly susceptible to low O_2 levels. Administration of excessive levels of O_2 in neonates also has been implicated in organ damage. O_2 radical disease can be implicated in the pathogenesis of most of the complications of prematurity.[41]

Retinopathy of Prematurity

Few subjects have caused more consternation for the clinician than the condition called **retinopathy of prematurity (ROP)**, a vasoproliferative retinal disorder. The medical (and legal) problem with this condition is that early uncontrolled epidemiologic studies suggested that excessive inspired O_2 and increased O_2 tension in the blood were related to retinal damage and, in extreme cases, blindness in neonates.[42,43] For years after these initial studies, great care was exercised to control Po_2 within specific ranges. Review of subsequent literature reveals the following facts:

1. Infants born after 33 to 34 weeks of gestation or weighing greater than 1500 g rarely develop ROP.
2. The incidence of the disease is inversely proportional to gestational age and birth weight, with the most premature infants showing an 80% incidence.
3. Very premature infants can develop the condition when inspired O_2 and blood O_2 tensions are carefully controlled[44,45] and even when in room air.
4. The greater the duration of elevated blood O_2 tension, the greater the risk of ROP.[1]

One theory of pathogenesis of ROP suggests that the initial event is vasoconstriction of immature retinal vessels caused by increased Pao_2. If this vasoconstriction persists, the vessels sclerose or become permanently occluded. When Pao_2 levels are reduced to "normal," there is endothelial proliferation at the margins of vascular occlusion. Extension of this "ridge" of cellular proliferation may cause hemorrhage and retinal detachment. Another theory suggests that ischemia and reperfusion injuries can result in free radical release, damaging cell membranes and creating a vasoproliferative response.[46,47]

For prevention of ROP, several approaches have been suggested. First, one should maintain the lowest inspired O_2 concentrations possible to prevent hypoxemia. Subsequently, it was suggested that higher O_2 saturation levels should be maintained to avoid fluctuating O_2 levels, which may produce alternating spasm and dilation of the retinal vessels. The STOP-ROP Multicenter Study Group reported no benefit to supplemental O_2 (oxygen saturation of 96% to 99%) on prethreshold ROP compared with using goal oxygen saturation values of 89% to 94%, while also finding no additional progression of ROP.[48] Finally, several studies suggest that the antioxidant vitamin E may reduce the incidence and severity of ROP.[46,49,50]

Pulmonary Oxygen Toxicity

The most common chronic pulmonary problem in small premature infants is bronchopulmonary dysplasia, more liberally referred to as **chronic lung disease**. O_2 toxicity in the lungs has been studied carefully in animal models.[51-54] Exposure of monkey lung to 100% O_2 produced a sequence of events. Initially there were few changes, but after 100 hours the lung became more edematous, and the epithelial layer was destroyed. After 1 week of high O_2 exposure, type I cells were replaced by type II cells, and more extensive edema occurred. Some studies have shown the beginning of fibrosis at this stage and loss of ciliary function and proteolytic damage. Others have shown an increase in lung hyaluronan and lung water content.[54]

The most pronounced damage to the lung from O_2 occurs when the lung is immature. A developing lung with immature architecture and less natural defenses that is exposed to positive-pressure ventilation with O_2 exhibits damage most rapidly.

The STOP-ROP Multicenter Study Group reported an increased risk of pneumonia or exacerbation of chronic lung disease or both at 3 months corrected age with supplemental O_2 (Pox 96% to 99%).[48] Van Marter and colleagues[55] showed that infants with chronic lung disease were more likely to have been exposed to higher inspired O_2 concentrations, even though Pox values were not different. They reported that most of the increased risk of chronic lung disease was explained simply by the initiation of mechanical ventilation.

With regard to the development of chronic lung disease, studies suggest that oxidative stress may not be as important as previously suggested.[56,57] For these infants, the fear of O_2 toxicity must be balanced with previous knowledge that higher O_2 saturation values (93% to 95%) are associated with improved weight gain and a reduction in pulmonary artery pressure and airway resistance and less sudden infant death.[56]

Oxygen Free Radicals

In recent years, numerous studies have described the molecular basis for O_2 toxicity.[58-61] Evidence suggests that the univalent reduction of O_2 and formation of toxic free radical compounds may be an important mechanism for O_2 toxicity. These radical species include superoxide anion, singlet O_2, hydrogen peroxide, and hydroxyl radicals. Damage is initiated by lipid peroxidation, inactivating sulfhydryl enzymes, and damaging nucleic acids. The lung is equipped with antioxidant enzymes to protect it from injury by O_2 free radicals.[62-64] Superoxide dismutase catalyzes the conversion of superoxide anion to hydrogen peroxide, whereas catalase and glutathione peroxidase help to convert hydrogen peroxide to water. It seems that the protection from free radical formation is a developmental process that is inadequate at birth in premature infants.[65-67]

CLINICAL MANAGEMENT

In the Delivery Room

Saugstad and coworkers,[68] in the Resair 2 study, and others[69] have shown that most newborns can be resuscitated equally efficiently with room air as with 100% O_2. Animal studies of meconium aspiration also have shown room air and 100% O_2 to be equally efficient for reoxygenation.[70] Other studies have suggested detrimental effects, owing to oxidative stress, when using 100% O_2 for resuscitation in preterm and term newborns.[54,71-73] Although 100% O_2 continues to be standard practice and the recommendation of the American Academy of Pediatrics, more studies are expected and may lead to future clinical trials.

In the Nursery

Guidelines for control of O_2 in neonates are changing. Formerly, most textbooks recommended maintaining PaO_2 between 50 mm Hg and 80 mm Hg. Now there is a trend toward accepting lower PaO_2 values in smaller neonates. In earlier work, Rhodes and colleagues[74] mechanically ventilated 150 small infants (<1500 g) and allowed PaO_2 values as low as 35 mm Hg before inspired O_2 concentrations were increased. Although there were other management criteria (i.e., pH >7.2), the incidence of bronchopulmonary dysplasia was low (in the range of 3%); developmental follow-up was not reported. More recently, Tin and associates[75] retrospectively examined 295 preterm (<28 weeks) infants and found a fourfold increase in ROP requiring cryotherapy if O_2 saturation values were 88% to 98% versus 70% to 90% and other outcome differences and no difference in survival or cerebral palsy. Attempting to keep O_2 saturation at a normal "physiologic" level may do more harm than good in infants of less than 28 weeks of gestation.

In an attempt to prevent bronchopulmonary dysplasia and other potential effects of O_2 toxicity, clinicians are trying to use less exposure to mechanical ventilation and O_2. As clinicians are beginning to accept higher PCO_2 values, so are they accepting lower O_2 saturation values.[75-77] Using available data, neonatologists now are considering goal O_2 saturation ranges for ventilated preterm infants 30 weeks of gestation or less to be approximately 85% to 92% and avoiding an O_2 saturation greater than 94%, while having judicious indications for increasing baseline O_2 levels.

For spontaneously breathing preterm infants, the use of recently described normal reference ranges may be more appropriate.[78] These infants breathing room air exhibit a median O_2 saturation value of 97% and rarely have O_2 saturation values less than 92%, whereas infants on supplemental O_2 rarely have O_2 saturation values less than 90%. Beyond these guidelines, tighter goal ranges for these infants perhaps should be dictated by their degree of, and risk for, ROP and chronic lung disease.

As mentioned earlier, it is accepted that very-low-birth-weight infants (without hypovolemia or anemia) can achieve adequate tissue oxygenation with lower $Hb-O_2$ saturations than previously believed. There is a poor correlation, however, between PaO_2 and O_2 saturation, in part because of the fetal nature of the oxyhemoglobin equilibrium curve. The PaO_2 required to attain 90% saturation (i.e., P_{90}) may be 41 mm Hg[79]; a more mature infant may have higher requirements. In vivo studies of preterm infants indicate that to keep PaO_2 values between 50 and 70 mm Hg, O_2 saturation values of 85% to 94% need to be accepted; however, at 94% saturation, PaO_2 may vary from 63 to 119 mm Hg.[80] Also, an individual patient's O_2 demand, relative to O_2 delivery, may vary considerably over time and always should be considered. An O_2 saturation of 86% has different clinical implications for an infant with a hematocrit of 26% versus 36%. Measuring inferior vena cava PO_2 or central venous saturation to approximate mixed venous PO_2 may prove to be helpful in this regard because these values provide a better measure of the adequacy of tissue delivery compared with arterial tension. Following arterial O_2 content is technically easier (see Box 42-1), only requiring PaO_2, O_2 saturation, and Hb, and should receive more attention than the O_2 saturation alone.

SUMMARY

Many clinical factors, including blood flow, Hb, and PaO_2, contribute to tissue oxygenation and influence O_2 therapy. Optimizing blood pressure and hematocrit can allow a minimal PaO_2 to achieve adequate oxygenation.

It is difficult to define optimal oxygenation for a premature infant or adequate delivery of O_2 to the tissues while avoiding toxicity. Ideally the ability to monitor O_2 delivery and O_2 consumption would allow optimal management of a critically ill neonate. These measurements are not done routinely, however, and direct measurements are often impossible in the nursery at present. The discussion continues over what constitutes adequate PaO_2 or O_2 saturation for neonates, and in practice, this value is variable and dependent on the individual infant's condition.

There does not seem to be much debate that in an extremely preterm infant, a PaO_2 greater than 80 mm Hg can be toxic and that a PaO_2 greater than 40 mm Hg is usually sufficient. It is not nearly this simple, however, to generate O_2 saturation guidelines for preterm infants. Not only is there poor correlation between O_2 saturation and PaO_2, but also, more importantly, the focus needs to be on arterial O_2 content, and there is *no* direct correlation between PaO_2 or O_2 saturation and arterial O_2 content because O_2 content also depends on Hb concentration. In addition, the O_2 content of a preterm infant needs to be considered on an individual basis and at any given point in time. Only then can one intelligently assess the cause-and-effect relationships of O_2 therapy and the associated complications of prematurity.

REFERENCES

1. Kinsey VE, Arnold HJ, Kalina RE: PaO_2 levels and retrolental fibroplasia: A report of the cooperative study. Pediatrics 60:655, 1977.
2. Poets CF: When do infants need additional inspired oxygen? A review of the current literature. Pediatr Pulmonol 26:424, 1998.
3. Martin RJ, Klaus MH, Fanaroff AA: Respiratory problems. In Klaus MH, Fanaroff AA (eds): Care of the High-Risk Neonate. Philadelphia, WB Saunders, 1986.
4. Krummel TM, Greenfield LJ, Kirkpatrick BV: Alveolar-arterial oxygen gradients versus the neonatal pulmonary insufficiency index for prediction of mortality in ECMO candidates. J Pediatr Surg 91:380, 1984.
5. Marsh TD, Wilkerson SA, Cook LN: Extracorporeal membrane oxygenation selection criteria: Partial pressure of arterial oxygen versus alveolar-arterial oxygen gradient. Pediatrics 82:162, 1988.
6. Ormazabal MA, Kirkpatrick BV, Muller DG: Alteration of alveolar-arterial O_2 gradient (A-a)DO_2 in response to tolazoline as a predictor of outcome in neonates with persistent pulmonary hypertension. Pediatr Res 14:607, 1980.
7. Beck R, Anderson KD, Pearson GD: Criteria for extracorporeal membrane oxygenation (ECMO) in a population of infants with persistent pulmonary hypertension of the newborn (PPHN). J Pediatr Surg 21:297, 1986.
8. Hallman M, Merritt A, Jarvenpaa AL: Exogenous human surfactant for treatment of severe respiratory distress syndrome: A randomized prospective clinical trial. J Pediatr 106:963, 1985.
9. Bartlett RH, Gazzaniga A, Toomasian J: Extracorporeal membrane oxygenation (ECMO) in neonatal respiratory failure: 100 cases. Ann Surg 204:236, 1986.
10. Baumgart S, Hirschl RB, Butler SZ, et al: Diagnosis-related criteria in the consideration of extracorporeal membrane oxygenation in neonates previously treated with high-frequency jet ventilation. Pediatrics 89:491, 1992.
11. Ortiz RM, Cilley RE, Bartlett RH: Extracorporeal membrane oxygenation in pediatric respiratory failure. Pediatr Clin North Am 34:39, 1987.
12. Phillips BL, McQuitty J, Durand DJ: Blood gases: Technical aspects and interpretation. In Goldsmith JP, Karotkin EH (eds): Assisted Ventilation of the Neonate. Philadelphia, WB Saunders, 1988.
13. Hay WWJ: Physiology of oxygenation and its relation to pulse oximetry in neonates. J Perinatol 7:309, 1987.
14. Woodson RD: Physiological significance of oxygen dissociation curve shifts. Crit Care Med 7:368, 1979.
15. Finch CA, Lenfant C: Oxygen transport in man. N Engl J Med 286:407, 1972.
16. McGee WT, Veremakis C, Wilson GL: Clinical importance of tissue oxygenation and use of the mixed venous blood gas. Res Med 4:15, 1988.
17. Danek SJ, Lynch JP, Weg JG, et al: The dependence of oxygen delivery in the adult respiratory distress syndrome. Am Rev Respir Dis 122:387, 1980.
18. Gore JM, Sloan K: Use of continuous monitoring of mixed venous saturation in the coronary care unit. Chest 86:757, 1984.
19. Zion MM, Balkin J, Rosenmann D, et al: Use of pulmonary artery catheters in patients with acute myocardial infarction. Chest 98:1331, 1990.
20. Roussos C, Macklen PT: The respiratory muscles. N Engl J Med 307:786, 1982.
21. Weissman C, Kemper M, Damask MC: Effect of routine intensive care interactions on metabolic rate. Chest 86:815, 1984.
22. Kinney JM, Duke JH, Long CL: Tissue fuel and weight loss after injury. J Clin Pathol 23(suppl 4):65, 1970.
23. Wukitsch MW, Peterson MT, Tobler DR: Pulse oximetry: Analysis of theory, technology, and practice. J Clin Monit 4:290, 1988.
24. Barker SJ, Tremper KK: The effect of carbon monoxide inhalation on pulse oximetry and transcutaneous PO_2. Anesthesiology 66:677, 1987.
25. Watcha MF, Connor MT, Hong AV: Pulse oximetry in methemoglobinemia. Am J Dis Child 143:845, 1989.
26. Hay WWJ, Thilo F, Curlander JB: Pulse oximetry in neonatal medicine. Clin Perinatol 18:441, 1991.
27. Harris MS, Little GA: Umbilical artery catheters: High, low, or no. J Pediatr Med 6:15, 1978.
28. Kitterman JA, Phibbs RH, Tooley WH: Catheterization of umbilical vessels in newborn infants. Pediatr Clin North Am 17:895, 1970.
29. Mokrohisky ST, Levine RL, Blumhagen JD: Low positioning of umbilical artery catheters increases associated complications in newborn infants. N Engl J Med 299:561, 1978.
30. Bott WW, Gow R, Whyte H: Complications resulting from use of arterial catheters: Retrograde flow and rapid elevation in blood pressure. Pediatrics 76:250, 1985.
31. Balagtas RC, Bell CE, Edward LD, et al: Risk of local and systemic infections associated with umbilical vein catheterization: A prospective study in 86 newborn patients. Pediatrics 48:359, 1971.
32. MacDonald MG, Eichelberger MR: Peripheral arterial cannulation. In Fletcher MA, MacDonald MG, Avery GB (eds): Atlas of Procedures in Neonatology. Philadelphia, JB Lippincott, 1983.
33. Todres ID, Rogers MC, Shannon DC: Percutaneous catheterization of the radial artery in the critically ill neonate. J Pediatr 87:273, 1975.
34. Bannister A: Comparison of arterial and arterialized capillary blood in infants with respiratory distress. Arch Dis Child 44:726, 1969.
35. Gandy G, Grann L, Cunningham N: The validity of pH and PCO_2 measurements in capillary samples of sick and healthy newborn infants. Pediatrics 34:192, 1964.
36. Shapiro BA, Harrison RA, Walton JR: Clinical Application of Blood Gases. Chicago, Year Book Medical Publishers, 1977.
37. Kandel G, Aberman A: Mixed venous oxygen saturation: Its role in the assessment of the critically ill patient. Arch Intern Med 143:1400, 1983.
38. Kazarian KK, DelGuercio LR: The use of mixed venous blood gas determinations in traumatic shock. Ann Emerg Med 9:179-182, 1980.

39. Lee J, Wright F, Barber R: Central venous oxygen saturation in shock. Anesthesiology 36:472, 1972.

40. Huch R, Lubberg DW, Huch A: Reliability of transcutaneous monitoring of arterial P_{O_2} in newborn infants. Arch Dis Child 49:213, 1974.

41. Saugstad OD: Oxygen radical disease in neonatology. Semin Neonatol 3:229, 1998.

42. Kinsey VE, Jacobus J, Hemphill F: Retrolental fibroplasia: Cooperative study of retrolental fibroplasia and the use of oxygen. AMA Arch Ophthalmol 56:418, 1956.

43. Patz A, Eastham A, Higginbotham DH: Oxygen studies in retrolental fibroplasia in experimental animals. Am J Ophthalmol 36:1511, 1953.

44. Kalina RE: Treatment of retrolental fibroplasia. Surv Ophthalmol 24:229, 1980.

45. Lucey JF, Dangman B: A reexamination of the role of oxygen in retrolental fibroplasia. Pediatrics 73:82, 1984.

46. Johnson L, Quinn GE, Abbasi S, et al: Effect of sustained pharmacologic vitamin E levels on incidence and severity of retinopathy of prematurity: A controlled clinical trial. J Pediatr 114:827, 1989.

47. Penn JS, Tolman BL, Lowery LA: Variable oxygen exposure causes preretinal neovascularization in the newborn rat. Invest Ophthalmol Vis Sci 34:576, 1993.

48. STOP-ROP Multicenter Study Group: Supplemental therapeutic oxygen for prethreshold retinopathy of prematurity (STOP-ROP), a randomized, controlled trial: I. Primary outcomes. Pediatrics 105:295, 2000.

49. Johnson L, Schaffer D, Boggs TR: The premature infant, vitamin E deficiency and retrolental fibroplasia. Am J Clin Nutr 27:1158, 1974.

50. Johnson L, Schaffer D, Quinn GE, et al: Vitamin E supplementation and the retinopathy of prematurity. Ann N Y Acad Sci 393:473, 1982.

51. DeLemos RA, Coalson JJ, Gerstmann DR: Oxygen toxicity in the premature baboon with hyaline membrane disease. Am Rev Respir Dis 136:677, 1988.

52. Kapanci Y, Weibel E, Kaplan H: Pathogenesis and reversibility of the pulmonary lesions of oxygen toxicity in monkeys: II. Ultrastructural and morphometric studies. Lab Invest 20:101, 1969.

53. Kaplan H, Robinson F, Kapanci Y: Pathogenesis and reversibility of the pulmonary lesions of oxygen toxicity in monkeys: I. Clinical and light microscopic studies. Lab Invest 20:94, 1969.

54. Johnsson H, Eriksson L, Jonzon A, et al: Lung hyaluronan and water content in preterm and term rabbit pups exposed to oxygen or air. Pediatr Res 44:716, 1998.

55. Van Marter LJ, Allred EN, Pagano M, et al: Do clinical markers of barotraumas and oxygen toxicity explain interhospital variation in rates of chronic lung disease? Pediatrics 105:1194, 2000.

56. Buss IH, Darlow BA, Winterbourn CC: Elevated lipid carbonyls and lipid peroxidation products correlating with myeloperoxidase in tracheal aspirates from premature infants. Pediatr Res 47:640, 2000.

57. Winterbourn CC, Chan T, Buss IH, et al: Protein carbonyls and lipid peroxidation products as oxidation markers in preterm infant plasma: Associations with chronic lung disease and retinopathy and effects of selenium supplementation. Pediatr Res 48:84, 2000.

58. Freeman BA: Hyperoxia increases radical production in rat lung homogenates. Arch Biochem Biophys 216:477, 1982.

59. Freeman BA, Crapo JD: Hyperoxia causes increased oxygen radical production in rat lungs and lung mitochondria. J Biol Chem 256:10986, 1981.

60. Freeman BA, Crapo JD: Biology of disease: Free radicals and tissue injury. Lab Invest 47:412, 1982.

61. Wispe JR, Roberts RJ: Molecular basis of pulmonary oxygen toxicity. Clin Perinatol 14:651, 1987.

62. Forman HJ, Fisher AB: Antioxidant defenses. In Gilbert DL (ed): Oxygen and Living Processes: An Interdisciplinary Approach. New York, Springer-Verlag, 1981.

63. Frank L: Protection from oxygen toxicity with endotoxin: Role of the endogenous antioxidant enzymes of the lung. J Clin Invest 65:1104, 1980.

64. White CW: Pulmonary oxygen toxicity: Cellular mechanisms of oxidant injury and antioxidant defense. In Bancalari E, Stocker JT (eds): Bronchopulmonary Dysplasia. New York, Hemisphere, 1988.

65. Bonuccelli CM, Permutti S, Sylvester JT: Developmental differences in catalase activity in hypoxia-hyperoxic effects of fluid balance in isolated lamb lungs. Pediatr Res 33:519, 1993.

66. Frank L, Sosenko IRS: Development of lung antioxidant enzyme systems in late gestation: Possible implications for the prematurely born infant. J Pediatr 110:9, 1987.

67. Roberts RJ: Antioxidant systems of the developing lung. In Farrell PM, Taussig LM (eds): Bronchopulmonary Dysplasia and Related Chronic Respiratory Disorders. 90th Ross Conference on Pediatric Research, Ross Labs, Columbus, OH, 1986.

68. Saugstad OD, Rootwelt T, Aalen O: Resuscitation of asphyxiated newborn infants with room air or oxygen: an international controlled trial: The Resair 2 study. Pediatrics 102:e1, 1998.

69. Ramji S, Ahuja S, Thirupuram S, et al: Resuscitation of asphyxic newborn infants with room air or 100% oxygen. Pediatr Res 34:809, 1993.

70. Tollofsrud PA, Solas AB, Saugstad OD: Newborn piglets with meconium aspiration resuscitated with room air or 100% oxygen. Pediatr Res 50:423, 2001.

71. Kutzche S, Ilves P, Kirkeby OJ, Saugstad OD: Hydrogen peroxide production in leukocytes during cerebral hypoxia and reoxygenation with 100% or 21% oxygen in newborn piglets. Pediatr Res 49:834, 2001.

72. Temesvari P, Karg E, Bodi I, et al: Impaired early neurologic outcome in newborn piglets reoxygenated with 100% oxygen compared with room air after pneumothorax-induced asphyxia. Pediatr Res 49:812, 2001.

73. Vento M, Aseni M, Sastre J, et al: Resuscitation with room air instead of 100% oxygen prevents oxidative stress in moderately asphyxiated term neonates. Pediatrics 107:642, 2001.

74. Rhodes PG, Graves GR, Patel DM, et al: Minimizing pneumothorax and bronchopulmonary dysplasia in ventilated infants with hyaline membrane disease. J Pediatr 103:634, 1983.

75. Tin W, Milligan DWA, Pennefather P, Hey E: Pulse oximetry, severe retinopathy, and outcome at one year in babies of less than 28 weeks' gestation. Arch Dis Child Fetal Neonatal Educ 84:F106, 2001.

76. Saugstad OD: Is oxygen more toxic than currently believed? Pediatrics 108:1203, 2001.

77. Saugstad OD: Chronic lung disease: Oxygen dogma revisited. Acta Paediatr 90:113, 2001.

78. Ng A, Subhedar N, Primhak RA, Shaw NJ: Arterial oxygen saturation profiles in healthy preterm infants. Arch Dis Child Fetal Neonatal Educ 79:64, 1998.

79. Emond D, Lachance C, Gagnon J, et al: Arterial partial pressure of oxygen required to achieve 90% saturation of hemoglobin in very low birth weight newborns. Pediatrics 91:602, 1993.

80. Wasunna A, Whitelaw AGL: Pulse oximetry in preterm infants. Arch Dis Child 62:957, 1987.

CHAPTER 43

Continuous Positive Airway Pressure

Carla M. Weis, Cynthia A. Cox, and William W. Fox

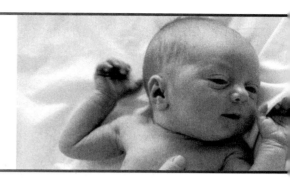

Continuous **positive airway pressure (CPAP)** is defined as the application of positive airway pressure throughout the respiratory cycle. Distending pressure continues to be provided throughout expiration, allowing lung stability. Because this pressure produces lung distention, it also is known as **continuous distending pressure**.[1] This pressure has no distending effect during inspiration, however, because of the much higher inspiratory pressure that supersedes it.

There has been a strong focus more recently on the potential benefits of using nasal CPAP as the initial form of support, including in the delivery room, referred to as **early CPAP,** for respiratory distress syndrome (RDS), instead of endotracheal positive-pressure ventilation.[2-7] This approach can provide the lung stability that is necessary in the face of surfactant deficiency, while avoiding the trauma of positive-pressure ventilation. This chapter addresses this and all other potential uses of CPAP and reviews the pulmonary physiology related to CPAP, which leads to optimal application.

The idea that positive airway pressure applied at end expiration would provide lung stability originated partially from observations by Harrison and colleagues in 1968,[8] who described grunting in neonates as naturally producing end-expiratory pressure. In 1971, Gregory and associates[9] introduced the clinical use of end-distending pressure in neonates. Before the development of CPAP, most ventilation of neonates was performed with a positive-pressure inspiratory phase and a passive expiratory phase, and distending pressure at end expiration was allowed to decline to 0 cm H_2O,[10] allowing unstable alveoli to collapse at end expiration. By applying CPAP, lung stability was conferred.

The term *CPAP,* by convention, usually indicates that the infant is breathing spontaneously, without ventilator assistance. Many different devices or methods have been used to apply CPAP to spontaneously breathing infants.[11] Four of these are listed in Table 43-1 along with advantages and disadvantages of each. The first three (endotracheal CPAP,[9,12,13] nasopharyngeal CPAP,[14,15] and nasal prongs) are the most commonly used and generate continuous *positive* airway pressure. The fourth (negative end-expiratory pressure) uses a negative extrathoracic pressure, also known as **continuous negative pressure**.[16,17] Using this method, an equal or greater effect on functional residual capacity (FRC) and dynamic lung compliance can be achieved,[18] while avoiding invasive techniques (e.g., endotracheal intubation) and perhaps avoiding compromise to venous return. Other methods used in the past to apply continuous distending pressure include a sealed facemask,[19-21] head box,[22,23] and face chamber.[24]

Infants who are intubated and connected to a ventilator circuit have a similar application of positive end-expiratory pressure (PEEP). When CPAP is used in a spontaneously breathing patient or is added to a ventilated infant (PEEP), the airway pressure never reaches 0 cm H_2O, and the lungs are not allowed to collapse. Physiologically, CPAP and PEEP are the same. For the remainder of this chapter, *CPAP* refers to this physiologic effect and is not indicative of a specific delivery mode unless specified.

PHYSIOLOGIC EFFECTS

Beneficial physiologic effects of CPAP are created by an increase in transpulmonary pressure with a resultant increase in FRC, stabilization of an unstable chest wall, and improvement in ventilation-perfusion ($\dot{V}/Q$) ratios.[25-28] These effects result in improved oxygenation and ventilation.[29] The major effect of CPAP is to optimize lung volume, specifically FRC.[30] The selection of an appropriate level of CPAP for an individual infant depends on the physiology, disease condition, and size of the infant. Table 43-2 summarizes the use of high and low levels of CPAP in terms of various neonatal situations, their physiology, and the rationale for their use.

Physiology

Over a range of CPAP levels (from low to high), three main physiologic parameters can be affected: pulmonary

Table 43–1. Continuous Distending Pressure: Modes of Application

Device	Advantages	Disadvantages
Endotracheal CPAP (endotracheal tube in trachea)	Most complete seal Stays in place Optimal transmission of pressure Intubated infant ready for ventilation Suctioning access	Higher airway resistance Pharyngeal groove if long-term orally Tracheal/subglottic stenosis
Nasopharyngeal CPAP (shortened endotracheal tube inserted nasally to posterior pharynx Nasal prongs/nasal mask	Better stability than prongs Allows patients more activity than prongs More optimal delivery pressure than prongs Noninvasive Lightweight	Increases airway resistance Plugging Nasopharyngeal irritation Easily dislodged Requires head stabilization Nasal septal damage with prongs if long-term use Mucous plugging Increases airway resistance
Negative end-expiratory pressure	Noninvasive Venous return not compromised	Hypothermia Large device Aerophagia

CPAP, continous positive airway pressure.

Pulmonary Mechanics

Because CPAP is the major factor that determines lung volume, the clinician always must keep in mind the relationship between pressure and volume (dynamic lung compliance). As Figure 43-1 shows, in region A, the lung volume is low (as in RDS) and lung compliance (pressure/volume slope) is low. As lung volume increases (region B) and an optimal volume is reached, lung compliance increases. Finally, if lung volume is increased even more (region C), the lungs become overdistended (as in meconium aspiration syndrome), and compliance is low. This diagram is the best way to understand the relationship between pressure and volume (dynamic lung compliance), with the idea in mind that lung volume can be controlled by CPAP. In cases A and C, one can attempt to adjust end-distending pressure to bring lung volume back to region B: optimal FRC, which results in optimal compliance and the lowest work of breathing.

Lung volume also is related to airway resistance (Fig. 43-2). Lung volume varies inversely with airway resistance so that with low lung volumes, airway resistance is high.[31] If insufficient CPAP is being used and atelectasis is not resolved, airway resistance and work of breathing are higher. Because an infant supported with a CPAP device is spontaneously breathing, the focus of

Table 43–2. Clinical Conditions and Their Continuous Positive Airway Pressure (CPAP) Requirements

High CPAP		Low CPAP	
Condition	Rationale	Condition	Rationale
High O$_2$ requirement	Alveolar recruitment	Low O$_2$ requirement	Less need for recruiting alveoli
Large infant	Relatively low chest wall compliance	Small infant	Relatively high chest wall compliance
Decreased lung compliance	Effective distention	Increased lung compliance	Achieve same volume with less pressure
Atelectasis	Alveolar recruitment and stabilization	Resolved atelectasis	Less need for recruiting alveoli
Obstructive lung disease	Stabilize obstructed airways	Initiating treatment (early disease)	Requires minimal pressure support
Severe lung disease	Effective distention	Weaning treatment (resolving disease)	Requires minimal pressure support
		Apnea	Stabilizes airway if obstructive

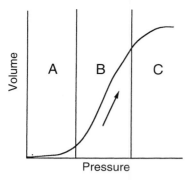

Figure 43–1. Pressure-volume relationship of the lung. The slope represents dynamic lung compliance. *Region A*: low volume, low compliance. *Region B*: optimal lung volume, optimal lung compliance. *Region C*: high volume, low compliance.

treatment is to reduce the infant's workload. Current CPAP devices use an infant flow driver (e.g., Aladdin Infant Flow System, Hamilton Medical, Reno, NV; Hudson Infant Nasal CPAP System, Hudson Respiratory Care, Tenecula, CA), designed to reduce workload. These systems create a Venturi effect in airflow resulting in variable pressures during the respiratory cycle (versus continuous pressure and flow) to minimize expiratory resistance, while maintaining a continuous distending pressure. Compared with constant flow nasal CPAP, these devices can decrease work of breathing,[32] while effecting greater lung recruitment.[33] Essentially, CPAP can improve distribution of ventilation to optimize FRC and optimize lung compliance and airway resistance.

Cardiovascular Stability

CPAP, as a regulator of lung volume, can influence cardiovascular stability. CPAP at high levels may have direct cardiovascular effects that are detrimental. If excessive levels of CPAP are used, the airway pressure is

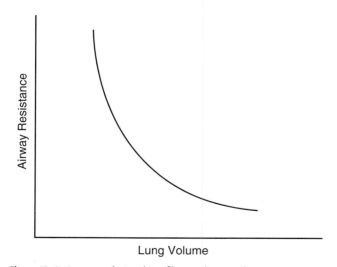

Figure 43–2. Inverse relationship of lung volume and airway resistance; as lung volume is increased, airway resistance decreases.

transmitted to the pleural space, and intrapleural pressure is increased above normal. The right-sided cardiac structures (vena cava and right atrium) are relatively thin walled and compliant. These intrathoracic structures are compressed, and venous return is compromised. The decreased venous return results in diminished cardiac output. Manifestations of this decreased cardiac output include metabolic acidosis, tachycardia, and decreased arterial blood pressure. The level of CPAP that constitutes "excessive" depends on lung compliance. The clinician managing patients on CPAP always must be aware that if lung compliance is low, less intra-airway pressure is transmitted to the pleural space, and less cardiac compromise occurs. All patients receiving CPAP must be maintained in a euvolemic state. Hypovolemia predisposes infants to more circulatory depression if excessive CPAP is used.

Inappropriately high levels of CPAP may be recognized in several ways. First, arterial blood gases may reflect metabolic acidosis caused by excessive CPAP, which impedes venous return to the heart and subsequently reduces cardiac output. This acidosis most frequently occurs in infants in whom CPAP is increased too rapidly or in infants who have rapidly improving lung compliance. Additionally, excessive CPAP may cause pulmonary overdistention, decreased dynamic lung compliance, and increased carbon dioxide retention.[12] A trial of lower CPAP or increased fluids should be considered if metabolic acidosis persists. Metabolic acidosis also may develop if CPAP is too low and hypoxemia exists.

Pulmonary Vascular Resistance

The level of CPAP, whether too high or too low, can significantly affect pulmonary vascular resistance and $\dot{V}/Q$ matching.[34] Overdistention of the lung may cause direct pressure on pulmonary arterioles or capillaries, increasing pulmonary vascular resistance and pulmonary artery pressure.[35] When applying inappropriately low levels of CPAP, atelectasis is not resolved. Atelectasis results in shunting of blood away from collapsed alveoli and regional increases in pulmonary vascular resistance.

Whenever excessive or insufficient levels of CPAP are applied, $\dot{V}/Q$ matching is disturbed. Optimal $\dot{V}/Q$ ratios are not achieved, and partial pressure of oxygen (Po_2) is not be optimized, unless an optimal level of CPAP is used.

Renal Effects

Renal effects of CPAP seem to be directly related to cardiac output. If optimal levels of CPAP are applied, $\dot{V}/Q$ ratios are optimal, and the patient is not hypovolemic, there should be no direct effects on renal function. Renal function may be improved under conditions when Po_2 is optimized. Several studies have suggested that the secretion of aldosterone, antidiuretic hormone, and antinatriuretic factor are affected by the application of CPAP.[36-38] These studies are contradictory, however. It is unlikely that renal blood flow is adversely affected if CPAP is used appropriately. As lung compliance and oxygenation increase, CPAP should be weaned to avoid the transmission of pressure and unfavorable cardiovascular effects.

It has been well established that by day 2 or 3 of life in infants with uncomplicated RDS, a diuretic phase occurs.[39,40] Concomitant with this diuretic phase, lung compliance improves rapidly.[41] In this phase of disease, peak inspiratory pressure and CPAP (or PEEP) levels should be weaned rapidly.

Cerebral Effects

Similar to the pulmonary and renal effects of CPAP, the intracranial effects of CPAP are directly related to the level of positive pressure applied to the airway *and* the lung compliance, affecting blood flow. To influence cerebral perfusion pressure, the airway distending pressure must be excessive enough, relative to lung compliance, to be transmitted to the pleural space and to the superior vena cava.

The association between high-frequency ventilation (HFV) and intraventricular hemorrhage continues to be a topic of study and controversy. Potential causes of intraventricular hemorrhage during HFV include the relatively increased CPAP applied when using this form of ventilation, which can create high intrathoracic pressure leading to cerebral venous congestion and the easily achieved hypocarbia.[42] A review of currently available data suggests that standard application of HFV probably does not increase the risk of intraventricular hemorrhage or periventricular leukomalacia (PVL).[43]

Epidemiologically, CPAP use has been associated with an increased incidence of intracranial bleeding when the head box system is used.[22,23,44] The relationship, if any, between the use of other CPAP application methods and the incidence of intracranial hemorrhage is difficult to determine and remains unclear at this time.

Disease Conditions

Lung Disease

In most cases of neonatal premature lung disease, atelectasis with low lung volume is the major problem, often as a result of surfactant deficiency. Application of CPAP prevents lung collapse at end expiration and increases lung volume until an optimal lung volume is reached (if an optimal level of CPAP is applied). The lung volume changes can be followed by serial chest x-rays of FRC measurements. Lung volume on x-ray is evaluated by counting total ribs from the apex of the lung to the level of the diaphragm. Generally, location of the diaphragm at the level of about seven to eight ribs represents normal lung expansion. The effect of progressively increasing CPAP in a critically ill infant is observed by obtaining serial arterial blood gases or oxygen saturation. As CPAP is increased, Po_2 and oxygen saturation improve until overdistention occurs; oxygenation then decreases.[29] Partial pressure of carbon dioxide (Pco_2) usually increases also, unless lung volume is initially suboptimal. In such cases, Pco_2 may decrease as $\dot{V}/Q$ matching improves.

In other neonatal lung diseases (e.g., aspiration syndromes), in contrast to having collapsed alveoli, there may be primarily airway obstruction and air trapping with overdistention. CPAP can stabilize partially or totally obstructed airways at end expiration, preventing air trapping. In this case, because trapped gas is released, the actual thoracic gas volume may decrease after CPAP is applied. Because aspiration syndromes generally occur in bigger infants with decreased lung compliance, the CPAP levels used are generally higher.[13]

If lung volume is optimally regulated with CPAP, the airway obstruction or alveolar atelectasis improves. It is not clear whether CPAP recruits collapsed alveoli or just maintains alveolar volume after it has been recruited by peak inspiratory pressure.[45] It is clear that a high level of inspiratory pressure is required to reopen a totally collapsed alveolus, but after the air sac is open, pressure levels in the CPAP range can maintain patency.[46]

A major component of the effectiveness afforded by HFV is the idea of optimizing lung inflation and maintaining recruited alveoli with CPAP.[43] With high-frequency oscillatory ventilation, often a "high lung volume strategy" is employed.[43] A relatively high mean airway pressure (MAP) is maintained, while high-frequency and low-volume tidal breaths oscillate above (inspiratory) and below (expiratory) this recruiting lung volume. Even when a "low lung strategy" is used (as for air leaks), the concept of maintaining recruited alveoli still is a mainstay of this form of ventilation. A high-frequency jet ventilator works in tandem with a conventional ventilator to supply the CPAP necessary to maintain alveolar recruitment.

Apnea

Apnea is a common problem encountered in premature infants. **Obstructive apnea** is caused by a collapsible airway, and **central apnea** is caused by altered regulation of the central nervous system. The application of CPAP can stabilize airways, maintain optimal lung volume, or influence pulmonary reflexes, resulting in decreased occurrence of apneic episodes.[47,48] For many infants, the problem results from a combination of obstructive and central apnea, called **mixed apnea**. The effectiveness of CPAP in the treatment of obstructive and mixed apnea has been shown.[49] In either case, low levels of CPAP are appropriate. In some cases of central apnea, CPAP may work only because it stimulates the infant in some way. Other cases of central apnea respond because of lung volume adjustment. Clinically, the ability of CPAP to decrease effectively the frequency of apneic episodes in infants is variable, reflecting the varied causes of neonatal apnea.[50] Despite the many causes of neonatal apnea, optimal lung inflation often can reverse the process.[51,52]

OPTIMAL CONTINUOUS POSITIVE AIRWAY PRESSURE

Optimal CPAP has been defined on the basis of several different parameters.[34,53-55] In clinical usage, the term **optimal CPAP** usually means the level of CPAP that produces the highest Po_2 without secondary complications. One needs to achieve a balance between low levels of CPAP resulting in suboptimal oxygenation and high levels transmitting excessive pressure to the intrapleural space, creating acidosis or carbon dioxide retention. Other definitions of optimal CPAP are based on pulmonary

Table 43–3. Optimal Continuous Positive Airway Pressure: Definition in Different Clinical Conditions

	Physiology	Basis of Definition of Optimal CPAP
Acute RDS (worsening or weaning)	Significant A-a gradient Rapidly changing compliance	PaO_2 Oxygen saturation Oxygen delivery
Small premature infant weaning off CPAP	Small A-a gradient Weak respiratory muscles Increased chest wall compliance	Lung compliance (see Fig. 43-1)
BPD on 60% oxygen	Decreased compliance Increased resistance A-a gradient not labile	Pulmonary mechanics: resistance and compliance
4-day-old with RDS and PDA	Congestive heart failure Pulmonary edema	Balance between cardiac output and pulmonary blood flow

BPD, bronchopulmonary dysplasia, CPAP, continuous positive airway pressure; PDA, patent ductus arteriosus; RDS, respiratory distress syndrome.

function testing and include measurement of dynamic compliance or pulmonary resistance. The definition of optimal CPAP usually varies according to the disease state of the patient and the objective of the clinician (Table 43-3).

Ideally, one can obtain arterial blood gases along with simultaneous measurement of pleural pressure (esophageal catheter), central venous pressure, and pulmonary function studies to determine optimal CPAP. In practice, one usually adjusts CPAP to 1 cm above and 1 cm below current levels and obtains Po_2 or lung compliance values after waiting 10 to 15 minutes. This practice has been called a **CPAP/PEEP grid** and provides the most practical management information. Interpreting this grid depends on one's specific goals in managing a particular patient.

In an acutely ill premature infant with RDS who has a rapidly changing compliance, oxygenation is a major problem. In these infants with high inspired oxygen concentrations, optimal CPAP usually is defined in terms of oxygenation. Similarly, optimal CPAP can be defined in terms of optimal oxygen delivery (cardiac output × arterial oxygen content).

In other patients, such as small infants being weaned from mechanical ventilation, in whom oxygenation is not a major problem, airway resistance, lung compliance, and work of breathing may prevent extubation or further weaning. In this case, the definition of optimal CPAP may be based on measurements of pulmonary mechanics obtained by bedside pulmonary function testing. In addition, for bigger patients with bronchopulmonary dysplasia (BPD), optimal CPAP might be determined by lowest airway resistance. In most patients, a balance between two or three of these factors must be used when evaluating a CPAP/PEEP grid.

CLINICAL USE OF CONTINUOUS POSITIVE AIRWAY PRESSURE

With an understanding of the physiologic effects of CPAP, the application of CPAP is beneficial in many clinical conditions in neonates.

Early Continuous Positive Airway Pressure

Small infants have low ventilatory reserves, tire easily, and precipitously develop respiratory failure. Prevention of atelectasis in small neonates may preserve surfactant production[56] and maintain optimal lung compliance.

As suggested from early studies,[16,57-59] earlier use of nasal CPAP now is being recommended, especially for small premature infants,[60,61] and may decrease the incidence of BPD.[2,4,60,62] In the first minutes after birth, the combination of surfactant deficiency and structural lung immaturity enables the premature lung to sustain much more injury than mature lungs. During this time, even relatively normal tidal volumes can be damaging.[63] Early use of surfactant and early application of CPAP can offer some protection. No randomized trial comparing early CPAP and mechanical ventilation has been published to date, however. A ventilation strategy that includes moderate permissive hypercapnia ($PaCO_2$ 45 to 60 mm Hg) has been suggested to contribute less pulmonary trauma and lead to a decreased incidence of BPD.[64] Permissive hypercapnia still is considered experimental, however, because there are no prospective, controlled trials in neonates, and the potential for adverse effects exists.[42] Early CPAP has been shown to reduce the need for intubation in very-low-birth-weight infants independent of PcO_2 values.[2] Early CPAP and hypercarbia potentially can be ideal partners in the prevention of BPD.

Initiating Continuous Positive Airway Pressure

The initiation of extratracheal CPAP (e.g., nasal prongs) in an infant should be considered when the infant has x-ray signs of atelectasis, has chest wall retractions, requires greater than 50% inspired oxygen, or displays rapidly progressive lung disease. Even infants with low fraction of inspired oxygen requirements may benefit from the use of CPAP application, especially early use.

CPAP levels less than 4 cm H_2O pressure are rarely used with extratracheal CPAP; pressures greater than 6 cm H_2O are more common because pressure is lost through the mouth or is not transmitted effectively. If no improvement occurs, or if the infant exhibits agitation,

Table 43-4. Continuous Positive Airway Pressure (CPAP)

Low (2-3 cm H₂O)		Medium (4-7 cm H₂O)	
Use	Side Effects	Use	Side Effects
Maintenance of lung volume in very-low-birth-weight infants During weaning During hyperventilation for PPHN No role with nasal CPAP	May be too low to maintain adequate lung volume or adequate oxygenation CO₂ retention	Increasing lung volume in surfactant deficiency, such as RDS Stabilizing areas of atelectasis Stabilizing obstructed airways	If lungs have normal C_L: May overdistend May impede venous return Air leak

High (8-10 cm H₂O)		Ultrahigh (11-15 cm H₂O)	
Use	Side Effects	Use	Side Effects
Preventing alveolar collapse with poor C_L and poor lung volume Improving distribution of ventilation	Pulmonary air leak Decreased C_L if overdistended May impede venous return (metabolic acidosis) May increase PVR CO₂ retention	Tracheal or bronchial collapse Markedly decreased C_L or severe obstruction Preventing white-out or reestablishing lung volume during ECMO Only used with ETT CPAP	Same as "High" levels, depending on C_L

C_L, lung compliance; ECMO, extracorporeal membrane oxygenation; ETT, endotracheal tube; PPHN, persistent pulmonary hypertension of the newborn; PVR, pulmonary vascular resistant; RDS, respiratory distress syndrome.

endotracheal CPAP should be considered, with or without mechanical ventilation.

Endotracheal CPAP levels of 4 to 5 cm H₂O pressure generally are used initially, and a Po_2 response should be observed within 15 to 20 minutes. If an increase in Po_2 does not occur, CPAP should be increased in 1-cm increments until "high" levels (based on weight and condition) are achieved. Table 43-4 summarizes the range of levels of CPAP used in most neonates and their uses and side effects.[65] These levels are for endotracheal CPAP in which the pressure is effectively transmitted to the airways. Classically an initial CPAP level in the low-to-moderate range yields a more beneficial effect, in terms of improved oxygenation, for newborns with RDS.[29] (In practice, although levels of CPAP are being increased, inspired oxygen is increased in 10% increments.)

At the high-pressure end of the CPAP spectrum are older infants with BPD and tracheomalacia. In these infants with low lung compliance, hyperactive airways, and collapsible tracheas, the use of 14 or 15 cm H₂O pressure may be necessary for tracheal or airway stability. These levels of CPAP are always applied to infants receiving mechanical ventilation. Similarly high levels of CPAP, with or without background ventilation, have been recommended for neonates on extracorporeal membrane oxygenation.[66] These neonates are generally bigger infants with low lung compliance who benefit from alveolar recruitment. It seems that institution of higher CPAP levels in these patients helps prevent the white-out stage of extracorporeal membrane oxygenation and may permit earlier weaning from the extracorporeal membrane oxygenation circuit.

Weaning Continuous Positive Airway Pressure

When weaning from PEEP/CPAP, a general rule is to decrease CPAP as inspired oxygen requirement decreases. This approach takes into consideration that oxygen requirements in most infants relate inversely to lung compliance. An infant requiring low inspired oxygen has higher lung compliance and needs less CPAP. Evaluation and comparison of chest x-rays for evidence of atelectasis or overinflation also are useful during weaning.

For endotracheal CPAP, infants often are extubated from 3 to 4 cm H₂O; lower levels are rarely used because an extubated infant can generate 2 to 3 cm H₂O with spontaneous breathing. For infants on nasal CPAP, there is dissipation of the applied CPAP across the nasopharyngeal airway (and sometimes through the mouth). These infants generally do not benefit, and could be compromised, with CPAP levels less than 4 or 5 cm H₂O.

References

1. Ahumada CA: Continuous distending pressure. In Goldsmith JP, Karotkin EH (eds): Assisted Ventilation of the Neonate, 2nd ed. Philadelphia, WB Saunders, 1988, pp 128-145.
2. Gitterman MK, Fusch C, Gitterman AR, et al: Early nasal continuous positive airway pressure treatment reduces the need for intubation in very low birth weight infants. Eur J Pediatr 156:384, 1997.
3. Kamper J: Early nasal continuous positive airway pressure and minimal handling in the treatment of very-low-birth-weight infants. Biol Neonate 76(suppl 1):22, 1999.

4. Roberton NR: Early nasal CPAP reduces the need for intubation in VLBW infants. Eur J Pediatr 157:438, 1998.

5. Verder H, Albertsen P, Ebbesen F, et al: Nasal continuous positive airway pressure and early surfactant therapy for respiratory distress syndrome in newborns of less than 30 weeks' gestation. Pediatrics 103:24, 1999.

6. Wung JT: CPAP: Devices, indications and complications/mechanical ventilation of the newborn. 6th Annual Conference Respiratory Care of the Newborn, Columbia Presbyterian Medical Center, New York, 1993.

7. Wung JT: Respiratory management for low-birth-weight infants. Crit Care Med 9(suppl):S364, 1993.

8. Harrison VC, de Heese HV, Klein M: The significance of grunting in hyaline membrane disease. Pediatrics 41:549, 1968.

9. Gregory GA, Kitterman JA, Phibbs RH, et al: Treatment of the idiopathic respiratory distress syndrome with continuous positive airway pressure. N Engl J Med 284:1333, 1971.

10. Fox WW, Berman LS, Dinwiddie R, et al: Tracheal extubation of the neonate at 2-3 cm H_2O continuous positive airway pressure (CPAP). Pediatrics 59:257, 1977.

11. Gregory GA: Devices for applying continuous positive airway pressure. In Thibeault DW, Gregory GA (eds): Neonatal Pulmonary Care. Menlo Park, CA, Addison-Wesley, 1986, pp 307-320.

12. Brady JP, Gregory GA: Assisted ventilation. In Klaus MH, Fanaroff AA (eds): Care of the High-Risk Neonate, 3rd ed. Philadelphia, WB Saunders, 1986, pp 202-219.

13. Fox WW, Berman LS, Downes JJ, et al: The therapeutic application of end expiratory pressure in the meconium aspiration syndrome. Pediatrics 56:214, 1975.

14. Boros SJ, Reynolds JW: Prolonged apnea of prematurity: Therapy with continuous airway distending pressure delivered by nasopharyngeal tube. Clin Pediatr 15:123, 1976.

15. Novogroder M, MacKuanying N, Eidelman A, et al: Nasopharyngeal ventilation in respiratory distress syndrome. J Pediatr 82:1059, 1973.

16. Gerard P, Fox WW, Outerbridge EW, et al: Early versus late introduction of continuous negative pressure in the management of idiopathic respiratory distress syndrome. J Pediatr 87:591, 1975.

17. Outerbridge E, Roloff D, Stern L: Continuous negative pressure in the management of severe respiratory distress syndrome. J Pediatr 81:384, 1972.

18. Shoptaugh M, Cvetnic WG, Hallman M, et al: Pulmonary mechanics generated by positive end-expiratory and continuous negative pressure. J Perinatol 13:341, 1993.

19. Allen L, Blake A, Durbin G, et al: CPAP and mechanical ventilation by face mask in newborn infants. BMJ 4:137, 1975.

20. Allen LP, Reynolds EOR, Rivers RPA, et al: Controlled trial of continuous positive airway pressure given by face mask for hyaline membrane disease. Arch Dis Child 52:373, 1977.

21. Pape KE, Armstrong DL, Fitzhardinge PM: Central nervous system pathology associated with mask ventilation in the very low birth weight infant: A new etiology for intracerebellar hemorrhages. Pediatrics 58:473, 1976.

22. Turner T, Evans J, Brown J: Monoparesis: Complication of CPAP. Arch Dis Child 50:128, 1975.

23. Vert P, Andre M, Sibout M: CPAP and hydrocephalus. Lancet 2:319, 1973.

24. Ahlstr Adom H, Jonson B, Svenningsen NW: Continuous positive airways pressure treatment by a face chamber in idiopathic respiratory distress syndrome. Arch Dis Child 51:13, 1976.

25. Field D, Milner AD, Hopkins IE: Effects of positive end expiratory pressure during ventilation of the preterm infant. Arch Dis Child 60:843, 1985.

26. Gregory GA, Kitterman JA, Phibbs RH, et al: Increase in lung volume and absence of right to left shunt with continuous positive airway pressure in idiopathic respiratory distress. Pediatr Res 6:149, 1972.

27. Haman S, Reynolds EOR: Methods for improving oxygenation in infants mechanically ventilated for severe hyaline membrane disease. Arch Dis Child 48:612, 1973.

28. Saunders RA, Milner AD, Hopkins IE: The effects of CPAP on lung mechanics and lung volumes in the neonate. Biol Neonate 29:178, 1976.

29. Fox WW, Gewitz MH, Berman LS, et al: The PaO_2 response to changes in end expiratory pressure in the newborn respiratory distress syndrome. Crit Care Med 5:226, 1977.

30. Fox WW, Schwartz JG, Shaffer TH: The effects of endotracheal leaks on functional residual capacity determination in the intubated neonate. Pediatr Res 13:60, 1979.

31. Nunn JF: Applied Respiratory Physiology, 3rd ed. Boston, Butterworths, 1987.

32. Pandit PB, Courtney SE, Pyon KH, et al: Work of breathing during constant- and variable-flow nasal continuous positive airway pressure in preterm neonates. Pediatrics 108:682, 2001.

33. Courtney SE, Pyon KH, Saslow JG, et al: Lung recruitment and breathing pattern during variable versus continuous flow nasal continuous positive airway pressure in premature infants: An evaluation of three devices. Pediatrics 107:304, 2001.

34. Suter PM, Fairley HB, Isenberg MD: Optimum and expiratory airway pressure in patients with acute pulmonary failure. N Engl J Med 292:284, 1975.

35. Fox WW, Duara S: Clinical management of persistent pulmonary hypertension of the neonate. J Pediatr 103:505, 1983.

36. Annat G, Viale JP, Xuan BB, et al: Effect of PEEP ventilation on renal function, plasma renin, aldosterone, neurophysins and urinary ADP, and prostaglandins. Anesthesiology 58:136, 1983.

37. Bark H, LeRoith D, Nyska M, et al: Elevation in plasma ADH levels during PEEP ventilation in the dog: Mechanisms involved. Am J Physiol 239:E474, 1980.

38. Hall SV, Johnson EE, Hedley-Whyte J, et al: Renal hemodynamics and function with continuous positive pressure ventilation in dogs. Anesthesiology 41:452, 1974.

39. Langman CB, Engle WD, Baumgart S, et al: The diuretic phase of respiratory distress syndrome and its relationship to oxygenation. J Pediatr 98:562, 1981.

40. Spitzer AR, Fox WW, Delivoria-Papadopoulos M: Maximum diuresis—a factor in predicting recovery from respiratory distress syndrome and the development of bronchopulmonary dysplasia. J Pediatr 98:476, 1981.

41. Heaf DP, Belik J, Spitzer AR, et al: Changes in pulmonary function during the diuretic phase of respiratory distress syndrome. J Pediatr 101:103, 1982.

42. Wiswell TE, Gannon CM, Graziani LJ, Spitzer AR: Hypercapnia during the first 3 days of life increases the risk for the development of severe intracranial hemorrhage in the very low birthweight, conventionally-ventilated premature infant. Pediatr Res 43:203A, 1998.

43. Keszler M, Durand DJ: Neonatal high-frequency ventilation: Past, present, and future. Clin Perinatol 28:579, 2001.

44. Gabriele G, Rosenfeld CR, Fixler DE, et al: Continuous airway pressure breathing with the head box in the newborn lamb: Effects on regional blood flow. Pediatrics 59:858, 1977.

45. Shaffer TH, Delivoria-Papadopoulos M: Alteration in pulmonary function of premature lambs due to PEEP. Respiration 36:183, 1978.

46. Shaffer TH, Koen PA, Moskowitz GD, et al: PEEP: Effects on lung mechanics of premature lambs. Biol Neonate 34:1, 1978.

47. Kattwinkel J, Nearman HS, Fanaroff AA, et al: Apnea of prematurity: Comparative therapeutic effects of cutaneous stimulation and nasal CPAP. J Pediatr 86:588, 1976.

48. Speidel BD, Dunn PM: Use of nasal CPAP to treat severe recurrent apnea in very preterm infants. Lancet 2:658, 1976.

49. Miller MJ, Carlo WA, Martin RJ: Continuous positive airway pressure selectively reduces obstructive apnea in preterm infants. J Pediatr 106:91, 1985.

50. Miller MJ, Martin RJ: Pathophysiology of apnea of prematurity. In Polin RA, Fox WW (eds): Fetal and Neonatal Physiology, vol 1, 3rd ed. Philadelphia, WB Saunders, 1992, pp 905-918.

51. Angell-James JE, Daly MD: The effects of artificial lung inflation on reflexly induced bradycardia associated with apnoea in the dog. J Physiol 274:349, 1978.

52. Halbower AC, Jones MD Jr: Physiologic reflexes and their impact on resuscitation of the newborn. Clin Perinatol 26:621, 1999.

53. Bonta BW, Uauy R, Warshaw JB, et al: Determination of optimal CPAP for the treatment of IRDS by measurements of esophageal pressure. J Pediatr 91:449, 1977.

54. Innes M, Coates AL, Collinge JM, et al: Measurement of pleural pressure in neonates. J Appl Physiol 52:491, 1982.

55. Tauswell AK, Clubb RA, Smith BT, et al: Individualized CDP applied within six hours of delivery in infants with respiratory distress syndrome. Arch Dis Child 55:33, 1980.

56. Lawson EE, Birdwell RL, Huang PS: Augmentation of pulmonary surfactant secretion by lung expansion at birth. Pediatr Res 13:611, 1979.

57. Boros SJ, Reynolds JW: Hyaline membrane disease treated with early nasal end-expiratory pressure: One year's experience. Pediatrics 56:218, 1975.

58. John E, Thomas DB, Burnard ED: Influence of early introduction of CPPB on the course of HMD. Aust Paediatr J 12:276, 1976.

59. Krouskop RW, Brown EG, Sweet AY: The early use of continuous positive airway pressure in the treatment of idiopathic respiratory distress syndrome. J Pediatr 87:263, 1975.

60. Avery ME, Tooley WH, Keller JB, et al: Is chronic lung disease in low birthweight infants preventable? A survey of eight centers. Pediatrics 79:26, 1987.

61. Jones DB, Deveau D: Nasal prong CPAP: A proven method for reducing chronic lung disease. Neonatal Network 10:7, 1991.

62. Horbar JD, McAuliffe TL, Adler SM, et al: Vartiability in 28-day outcomes for very low birth weight infants: An analysis of 11 neonatal intensive care units. Pediatrics 82:554, 1988.

63. Jobe AH, Ikegami M: Mechanisms initiating lung injury in the preterm. Early Hum Dev 53:81, 1998.

64. Ambalavanan N, Carlo WA: Hypocapnia and hypercapnia in respiratory management of newborn infants. Clin Perinatol 28:517, 2001.

65. Spitzer AR, Shaffer TH, Fox WW: Assisted ventilation: Physiologic implications and complications. In Polin RA, Fox WW (eds): Fetal and Neonatal Physiology, vol 1. Philadelphia, WB Saunders, 1992, pp 894-913.

66. Keszler M, Subramanian KNS, Smith YA, et al: Pulmonary management during extracorporeal membrane oxygenation. Crit Care Med 17:495, 1989.

CHAPTER 44

Positive-Pressure Ventilation: The Use of Mechanical Ventilation in the Treatment of Neonatal Lung Disease— General Principles of Care

*Alan R. Spitzer**

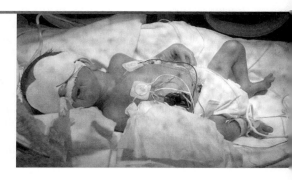

Positive-pressure mechanical ventilation with the use of pressure-limited ventilators remains the most common approach for the treatment of respiratory failure in neonatal intensive care units in the United States. Since the previous edition of this text, mechanical ventilators have changed significantly, although the fundamental physiology of positive-pressure ventilation remains intact. The most dramatic changes, however, have involved the introduction of a variety of novel variations for the delivery of positive-pressure ventilation. Most of these new approaches are designed to reduce either volutrauma or barotrauma to the lung, theoretically diminishing the risk of bronchopulmonary dysplasia (BPD). Although many of these therapies appear promising, none have clearly been shown to either eliminate BPD or reduce hospital length of stay, especially for neonates with extremely low birth weight (≤1000 g). These infants, in particular, have emerged as a primary focus of attention in the neonatal intensive care unit (NICU). Although these infants represent only a small part of admissions to the NICU (5% to 8%), they remain hospitalized for long periods and consume a disproportionate number of hospital days. In addition, they often have the highest rates of mortality and morbidity, both acute and long-term. Because of these issues, positive-pressure ventilation remains a critical focal point of care, not only from a pulmonary perspective but also from a neurodevelopmental viewpoint. At the turn of the millennium, it is no longer sufficient to ensure pulmonary recovery alone. Intact neurologic outcome must also be considered a priority with any approach to care of the neonate with lung disease.

For the larger infant with pulmonary problems, positive-pressure ventilation is also an essential part of care. For these neonates, the use of more advanced forms of ventilatory support, such as synchronized intermittent mandatory ventilation (SIMV),[1] assist/control (A/C) ventilation,[2] high-frequency jet ventilation (HFJV),[3,4] high-frequency oscillatory ventilation (HFOV),[5] inhalational nitric oxide (iNO) therapy,[6] or extracorporeal membrane oxygenation (ECMO),[7] has not altered the central role of positive-pressure conventional mechanical ventilation. The purpose of this chapter, therefore, is to review the uses of pressure-limited, time-cycled, positive-pressure ventilation in the management of neonatal respiratory failure in both premature and full-term neonates.

DESIGN PRINCIPLES

Classification

Positive-pressure mechanical ventilators are referred to by most clinicians as either "volume" or "pressure" types. **Volume-preset** ventilators deliver the same tidal volume of gas with each breath, regardless of the pressure that is needed. **Pressure-preset** ventilators, in contrast, are designed to deliver a volume of gas until a preset limiting pressure designated by the physician is reached. The remainder of volume in the unit is then released into the atmosphere. As a result, the tidal volume that is delivered to the patient by pressure-preset ventilators with each breath may be variable, but the peak pressure delivered to the airway remains constant. The flow generation necessary to drive pressure-preset ventilators may occur in the following ways: constant-flow generator (high-pressure gas source or compressor), non–constant-flow generator (cam-operated piston), or a constant-pressure generator (weighted bellows).

*This chapter represents an adaptation of Chapters 9 and 13 from Goldsmith JP, Karotkin EH: Assisted Ventilation of the Neonate, 4th ed. Philadelphia, WB Saunders, 2003.

Ventilators have been introduced that have the capability of serving as either volume- or pressure-controlled, time-cycled ventilators, depending on the operator's preference (e.g., Bird V.I.P., Bird Products Co., Palm Springs, Calif). These units have significant advantages for some patients and represent an important advance in the technology of ventilator development. In addition, new modifications of ventilator circuits allow a variety of pressure assist modes, designed to reduce the effort required (especially in the infant with extremely low birth weight) to generate, sustain, and terminate a ventilator breath.[8] Termination of inspiration is now recognized to be an important component of ventilator control, because prolongation of inspiration may lead to air trapping, air leak, and chronic lung injury. Furthermore, the use of microprocessors allows ventilators to be modified to perform very small, but theoretically beneficial, modifications to pressure, flow, and volume throughout the ventilatory cycle. Through such mechanisms, approaches such as proportional assist ventilation (PAV) and respiratory muscle unloading (RMU) can be achieved during the ventilatory cycle, a feat that would have been impossible as recently as the late 1990s.[9] With these techniques, pressure at the airway is increased during inspiration in proportion to the inspired tidal volume (with restrictive lung disease) or to flow (with resistive or obstructive airway disease) to diminish the elastic work of breathing. Many of these approaches are described in greater detail both elsewhere in this chapter and in other sections of this book.

Volume versus Pressure Ventilators

For many years, an ongoing debate has persisted in neonatal respiratory care as to the relative merits of volume-controlled versus pressure-controlled mechanical ventilation for the neonate.[10] This debate has been mirrored by the debate of whether it is barotrauma (pressure injury) or volutrauma (volume injury) that primarily damages the lung during mechanical ventilation in the treatment of neonatal respiratory disease.[11,12] As a result, many neonatologists decide to use a ventilator on the basis of their familiarity with individual units (most commonly, the ventilator used in the nursery in which they trained!), personal bias, or anecdotal information. It is apparent that each type of ventilator can provide appropriate support if the clinician understands the basic principles of physiology that support mechanical ventilation.

As mentioned previously, volume-preset ventilators deliver the same tidal volume with each breath. Areas of the lung that are atelectatic from collapsed or obstructed airways require a higher opening pressure, which can often be achieved with a volume-preset ventilator. Most of this volume, however, is preferentially delivered into segments of the lung that remain partially inflated and more compliant. Consequently, the volume-preset ventilator, although delivering a more consistent tidal volume, may overdistend the "healthier" areas of the lung and promote air leaks. Furthermore, these ventilators, although delivering the preset volume, may lose some of that volume around the endotracheal tube because the neonatal endotracheal tube is uncuffed. Current ventilator monitors can actually measure the amount of this volume loss by comparing inspiratory flow and expiratory return through the endotracheal tube adapter. Modifications have allowed some ventilators to adjust for this volume loss. In diseases in which shifting or migratory atelectasis is commonplace (e.g., BPD), with frequent compliance changes, the delivery of a consistent tidal volume may prevent the episodes of oxygen (O_2) desaturation that occur frequently.

With pressure-controlled ventilation, the volume of gas delivered to the terminal air spaces depends on the compliance of the lungs and, to a lesser degree, that of the airway and of the thoracic wall. With a decrease in compliance (increased lung stiffness), the preset pressure is reached more rapidly during gas compression and delivery, and residual volume is released to the atmosphere. As a result, tidal volume decreases, and if ventilation is inadequate, the physician must compensate for this loss of volume by increasing the peak inspiratory pressure (PIP). Nevertheless, because of the types of pulmonary diseases most often encountered in the neonate, pressure-controlled ventilators often offer advantages in management of the critically ill neonate.

Theoretical Advantages of Pressure-Preset Ventilators

There are several major advantages to the use of pressure-preset ventilators. First, these ventilators can use simple flowmeters or pressure meters to monitor ventilator gas delivery. Therefore, the design of these ventilators is much simpler (fewer working parts) and more compact; some models operate by means of a pressure source alone (no electricity needed); and they incur decreased costs. Volume-preset ventilators, in comparison, require a piston or volume meter to regulate breath size, in addition to the pressure metering. Volume-preset ventilators therefore have more working parts and more complex metering requirements, and, in general, they incur higher costs. In the more modern ventilator units with SIMV, A/C capability, pressure assist modes, or both pressure and volume capability, the devices are more complex, and the cost typically exceeds that of the volume-preset ventilator alone. The disadvantages in cost and complexity of such units, however, are compensated for by their enhanced flexibility in clinical use.

Pressure-preset ventilators are, in general, relatively simple to operate. As a result, fellows, house staff, and nurse practitioners, as well as others, can be taught the basic principles of therapy more easily. The pressure delivered to the infant can be immediately read from the meter, and adjustments to therapy can be made once appropriate monitoring has been performed or an arterial blood gas level is obtained. With volume-preset ventilators, either compliance of the ventilator and tubing must be known and calculated to assess volume or a rough guess must be made as to the volume required and delivered to the infant. The calculations involved are often complex and difficult for physicians in training to grasp readily. The differences between pressure-preset and volume-preset monitors have decreased with the addition of the various other modalities used in mechanical ventilation. In general, however, there are fewer preliminary calculations that physicians must make for using pressure ventilators.

PIP is thought to be directly related to the likelihood of development of air leaks and chronic lung disease in the newborn.[13] Judicious use of PIP, with constant monitoring of that factor, may aid in reducing these complications. Again, the theoretical considerations of pressure injury, as opposed to volume injury, enter into the discussion. If the physician firmly believes that volume injury is the primary reason for the development of either air leaks or chronic lung disease in neonates, cautious monitoring of volume delivery to the lung may be preferred. In actual practice, however, it is so difficult to divorce pressure- from volume-related injury that this controversy may be far more theoretical than practical.

Because the same pressure is provided to the infant with each ventilator breath, the physician does not have to constantly review pressure delivery and the risk it poses, even as compliance, waveform, and respiratory rate change during the illness. With volume ventilation, as compliance improves (e.g., during recovery from respiratory distress syndrome [RDS]), volume delivery may rapidly become excessive, and injury may occur. With pressure ventilation, excessive volume is always dumped from the ventilator circuit once the preset pressure is reached. Overdistention of the lung is therefore less likely, although air leaks and BPD can occur with any form of mechanical ventilation.

Lastly, the distinction between pressure- and volume-support ventilation has continued to blur even further with the introduction of volume-guarantee ventilation (Drager Babylog 8000 Ventilator, Telford, Pa), perhaps achieving simultaneously the best of both approaches to neonatal ventilation. With volume guarantee, a targeted mean tidal volume or minute ventilation for an infant can be ensured, while operator control of peak airway pressure is still maintained. A predetermined tidal volume is thereby ensured even when PIP is elevated, which would normally result in tidal volume loss to the atmosphere. In one study, a modest reduction in PIP for infants with very low birth weight was achieved with this form of mechanical ventilation, and gas exchange was well maintained.[14] This form of ventilation will no doubt be evaluated further in the near future.

Basic Ventilator Design

Commonly used infant pressure-preset ventilators operate on similar principles, as illustrated in Figure 44-1. Through some newer technologic advances, such as the dual microprocessor units that open and close a series of solenoid valves in the Infant Star Ventilator (Infrasonics, Inc., San Diego, Calif), this approach is modified to some extent. The underlying concept, however, is the same in that a preset pressure allows a certain volume of gas to be delivered to the patient until the desired pressure is reached. In addition, the provision of additional ventilator capabilities, such as A/C ventilation and SIMV, requires sophisticated microprocessor assistance during mechanical ventilation. The microprocessor must be able to assess ventilator cycle timing, the changeover from inspiration to expiration and from expiration to inspiration, and the relative pressure, flow rate, and tidal volume levels during ventilatory cycling. Without this capability, many

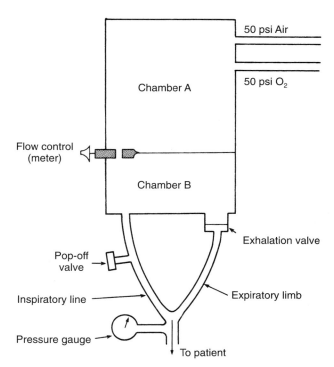

Figure 44–1. Diagram of the basic system utilized in infant positive-pressure ventilators. The pressure source is compressed air, O_2, or both, from a wall source to chamber A. A flowmeter between chambers A and B regulates air flow to chamber B, which operates at a much lower pressure. The pressure gauge and pop-off valve prevent the pressure from exceeding 50 to 70 cm H_2O. The ventilator is cycled by the opening and closing of the expiratory valve, which prevents CO_2 accumulation in the tubing. psi, pounds per square inch.

of the newer ventilatory modalities would not be possible. To assist in this regard, especially if ventilator graphics monitoring is also used, flow sensor capability is also needed. Many ventilators therefore have a low-volume pressure transducer within, or added to, the ventilator circuit (usually at the proximal airway) to measure gas flow into and out of the patient. In their basic design, however, ventilators basically remain pistons that deliver a volume of gas under pressure to the lung.

In the system illustrated in Figure 44-1, a pressure source of either compressed air, O_2, or both from a wall source is introduced into chamber A. The wall pressure is approximately 50 to 150 cm H_2O. This pressure is never applied directly to the infant but acts as a driving force for the ventilator. Mixing of compressed air and O_2 occurs in a blender before the gases reach the chamber; therefore, a known concentration of O_2 is delivered to the infant. A second chamber, chamber B, is added, and a flowmeter or resistor is inserted between the two chambers to regulate the amount of air flow delivered into chamber B, which is smaller in the diagram and operates at a much lower pressure.

From the diagram, it is apparent that if the flow rate between the two chambers is high and if the system were closed, the smaller chamber (B) could eventually reach driving pressure levels. Because chamber B interfaces with the infant, a maximum of 70 cm H_2O should rarely, if ever, be exceeded. For this reason, a pressure gauge and a "pop-off" regulating valve are added to the system to prevent excessive pressures from developing in chamber B (and in the infant's airway).

In addition, an exhalation valve is added to the system. When it is open, a continuous flow occurs through the system, preventing accumulation of excessive CO_2 in the tubing. On closure of this valve, pressure increases in chamber B, the ventilator tubing, and the infant's airway until the preset pressure level is reached. The ventilator is cycled by the opening and closing of the expiratory valve or by the solenoid system in the Infant Star Ventilator. In the Infant Star and the Bird V.I.P. ventilators, there is an additional "demand flow" modification in which the negative pressure created in the circuit during a patient's spontaneous breath is augmented by an additional fast-response demand valve that increases flow through the circuit, easing work of breathing. In the Newport Wave Ventilator (Newport Medical Instruments, Inc., Newport Beach, Calif), there is a separation of the spontaneous flow system from the mechanical breath system called the DuoFlow System. This system acts as a separate-standing continuous positive airway pressure (CPAP) unit during spontaneous respiration in the exhalation phase of respiration.

Lastly, the design of the system is such that the "upstroke" of the ventilator during inhalation can be modified by flow rate between chambers A and B. If flow is high, inspiratory pressure is reached quickly, and the respiratory waveform is "squared" (Fig. 44-2). If flow is reduced, the rate of rise of the inspiratory pressure is lessened, and the waveform appears more sinusoidal. Because sudden distention of the airways is thought by some neonatologists to contribute to tracheobronchomalacia and BPD, most current ventilators produce a more sinusoidal waveform.[15] Ventilator design since the 1990s has incorporated more sinusoidal gas delivery, even though evidence of the effect of waveform on development of chronic respiratory complications is not substantial.

Cycling

In conventional positive-pressure ventilators, the cycling process determines the method by which the inspiratory phase is initiated and terminated. Volume-preset ventilators are cycled when a preset volume is attained. Most standard pressure-preset ventilators are regulated by either an electrical timer (time cycled) or by a pneumatic timer (pressure cycled). The pneumatic-cycled ventilators have a small chamber in which pressure increases to a preset level and subsequently closes the inspiratory valve.

Although these ventilators are called "pressure-preset" ventilators by clinicians who set the machines according to desired inspiratory pressure, they are technically known as **flow generators** because the power source produces such high pressure that even if the infant's lung compliance or airway resistance changes, the inspiratory flow rate is not affected. Examples of the most common time-cycled and pressure-cycled ventilators in current use are listed in Table 44-1. Some ventilators have two or more cycling modes and are called **mixed-cycle** ventilators. These are generally volume-cycled ventilators with an additional time-cycled control. The control capabilities of each ventilator, and the differences between the methods in which pressures and volumes are delivered, sustained, and terminated are important to understand but beyond the scope of this discussion. Clinicians are strongly urged to carefully review the operator's manual for each specific ventilator in order to avoid any error in management.

If the physician operates pressure-preset ventilators at a high respiratory rate, the flow rate must be sufficiently high to deliver a full tidal breath or reach the desired pressure in a brief period of time. In addition, if inspiratory time (T_I) is short, a higher flow rate may be necessary to deliver the required volume and pressure in the limited time period.[16] Consequently, the physician should avoid excessive ventilator rates (>70 breaths per minute) in most infants with neonatal lung diseases. Because of the reduced compliance that is often present in these restrictive lung

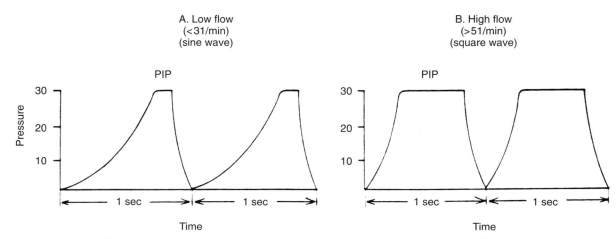

Figure 44–2. Comparison of ventilator waveforms. **A,** Relative sine waveform. **B,** Relative square waveform. PIP, peak inspiratory pressure.

Table 44–1. Commonly Used Neonatal Positive-Pressure Ventilators

Bird V.I.P Infant/Pediatric Ventilator
Bird V.I.P Gold Infant/Pediatric Ventilator
Bear Cub 750psv Infant Ventilator
Infant Star Ventilator
Sechrist IV-200 SAVI Ventilator
Newport Wave Ventilator
Drager Babylog 8000 Plus Infant Care Ventilator
Siemens Servo 300 Ventilator

diseases, the combination of short inspiration and reduced compliance may result in little more than dead space ventilation and gas trapping.

An addition to many neonatal ventilators is the concept of **termination sensitivity**. Termination sensitivity is a ventilator control that the clinician can set to terminate a ventilator breath at a specific percentage of peak flow during inspiration (Fig. 44-3). Termination sensitivity is an effective way to limit prolongation of the inspiratory phase of the ventilatory cycle. If a termination sensitivity of 5% to 10% is set, inspiration ceases when inspiratory flow decreases to 5% to 10% of peak flow. A termination sensitivity of 5% to 10% usually limits inspiration to 0.2 to 0.3 second during neonatal mechanical ventilation. In practice, however, it is often preferable to simply set the T_I that is desired directly on the ventilator and turn off the termination sensitivity control.

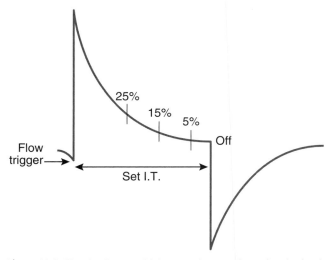

Figure 44–3. Termination sensitivity or expiratory trigger. Inspiration is initiated by a change of flow at the airway. When the lungs have inflated, flow decreases at the proximal airway, resulting in breath termination. The point of termination can be adjusted by the clinician, and represents a percentage of peak inspiratory flow. For example, a 10% termination sensitivity ends the breath when flow is 10% of peak flow. I.T., inspiratory termination. *(From Becker MA, Donn SM: Graphics monitoring. In Sinha SK and Donn SM [eds]: Manual of Respiratory Care. Armonk, NY, Futura, 2000, p 166.)*

PROCEDURE FOR INITIATING MECHANICAL VENTILATION

Mechanical ventilation of the newborn, especially in infants with extremely low birth weight (<1000 g), is associated with numerous complications. Before administering this therapy, all clinical personnel must be thoroughly familiar with the operation of ventilators and the physiologic principles that govern their use. Mechanical ventilation is 5% device-related and 95% physiologic principles in delivering optimal patient care. Unfortunately, too many clinicians become overly concerned with the "hardware" of mechanical ventilation and forget that the "software"—the decisions governing use of the devices—is far more important. With the increasing complexity of modern neonatal mechanical ventilators, however, it is becoming more difficult to avoid becoming enmeshed in hardware issues, even when it is unclear whether the newer modifications provide any substantial clinical benefit. It is therefore essential to have a comprehensive understanding both of the equipment being used and of the controls that that equipment offers in treating the critically ill neonate. The discussion throughout the remainder of this chapter therefore focuses primarily on the physiologic principles of neonatal respiratory care, although some of the newer technologic manipulations that can be achieved with modern neonatal ventilators are also presented.

First Steps

Although the procedures in this section may appear routine and simple, they are crucial because errors made at this point may be life-threatening (e.g., if the gas sources are not connected to the ventilator correctly). In addition, although this discussion focuses primarily on the pulmonary physiology and ventilator management of the infant, physicians should never overlook many of the important peripheral issues for successful respiratory care, such as infection surveillance and control, nutritional support, fluid and electrolyte management, comfort and pain relief of the infant, and emotional support for the family. A discussion with the family early in the child's hospitalization about the benefits and perils of ventilatory assistance can be extremely important in reducing the understandable concern of the family.

When not in use, the ventilator should be carefully cleaned, the circuits sterilized, and the unit stored in a clean, dry area. A plastic cover should be placed over the ventilator. Periodic infection control surveillance and culturing of ventilator equipment are valuable practices. When the ventilator is removed from storage, the following steps should be taken:

1. The electrical connections should be checked. Only grounded (three-pronged) sources should be used. Any unit that undertakes the care of neonates on ventilators must have access to backup generators in case of power failure in the nursery.
2. The O_2 and room air gas sources should be connected to the wall, and the required pressure must be adequate to drive most conventional ventilators (approximately 50 psi). Wall gauges should monitor this pressure.

3. All connections must fit securely, and the correct ventilator tubing and circuitry should be placed for the specific ventilator. The endotracheal tube must fit tightly into the ventilator connector; otherwise, air leaks may result. Circuits should never be jury-rigged if appropriate connectors are unavailable. These kinds of modifications can be lethal to an infant if a circuit comes apart at a critical point in care.

4. Humidification systems must be properly filled and checked. Newer units that utilize hydrophobic humidification techniques, especially those with heated filaments in the tubing, may not show droplet formation, which indicates saturation of the gas. Alternative methods of periodically checking the humidifiers for adequate humidification are therefore essential. Inadequately humidified gas can injure the airway and has been linked to necrotizing tracheobronchitis.[17]

5. Temperature devices should be examined periodically to ensure appropriate and accurate temperature of the gas entering the lungs. Inspired gas should be approximately at body temperature (35° to 36° C [±2° C]). Inadequately warmed gas can produce bronchospasm, especially in the chronically ventilated infant, whereas excessively heated gas can inflame the immature airway.[18]

Ventilator Controls

The ventilator controls that are commonly found on many pressure-controlled ventilators include the following:

1. Fraction of inspired O_2 concentration (FIO_2)
2. PIP
3. Positive end-expiratory pressure (PEEP)
4. Rate
5. Ventilator flow rate
6. T_I (some other ventilators may also have expiratory time [T_E] or inspiratory-to-expiratory [I/E] ratio)
7. Assist sensitivity
8. Termination sensitivity
9. Selection of SIMV/CPAP mode or A/C mode for either volume or pressure ventilation
10. Graphics monitoring
11. Ventilator alarm settings

From these controls, waveform and mean airway pressure (MAP) may be indirectly selected. Newer ventilators also digitally display controls. The external waveform monitor on the Bird V.I.P. has unusually extensive capabilities, including demonstration of flow-volume and pressure-volume loops. In addition, ventilators may have the following additional control capability:

1. Demand flow
2. Exhalation assist
3. Manual breath
4. Pressure support modes
5. High-frequency modes

Although sales representatives often stress the utility of these additional capabilities, the scientific evidence that underscores the value of these modifications is somewhat limited; however, increasing numbers of investigations appear to show some benefit from these modifications.

The use of SIMV and A/C have become widespread and do appear to offer demonstrable advantages in neonatal respiratory care.[19,20]

High-frequency ventilators (see Chapters 45 and 46) have additional controls, such as peak-to-peak pressure, jet valve on-time, amplitude, and sigh frequency and duration. The reader is referred to these chapters for more detailed discussion of these ventilators.

Fraction of Inspired Oxygen

Oxygen is probably the most commonly used drug in neonatal intensive care, but it is rarely thought of as such by physicians. Appropriate use of O_2 is highly therapeutic in most cases of neonatal cardiopulmonary disease. In addition to relieving hypoxemia, oxygen's action as a pulmonary vasodilator in cases of persistent pulmonary hypertension of the newborn (PPHN) may be invaluable.[21] Inadequate O_2 administration with consequent hypoxemia, however, may result in severe neurologic injury. Excessive variation in O_2 administration has been implicated as one of the provocative factors in retinopathy of prematurity[22] (not purely a high level of supplemental oxygen as was previously thought),[23] with subsequent retinal scarring and loss of vision, as well as in BPD,[24] leading to further O_2 or ventilator dependency. Accurate measurement of O_2 administration and arterial O_2 tension (PaO_2) or oxygen saturation is therefore mandatory in any neonate who requires O_2 therapy.

Regulation of ambient O_2 concentration during mechanical ventilation is performed by blenders. Commercial blenders precisely mix O_2 and compressed air into desired concentrations of O_2 as determined by the patient's O_2 requirements. Many ventilators, particularly the newer units, have blenders incorporated into their design. Older ventilators have separate blenders that can be attached to the O_2 inflow source on the ventilator. Blenders are usually easy to operate and work by simply dialing in the desired O_2 concentration. Although blenders are generally very accurate, the clinician must employ an additional device periodically to check that the blender is actually delivering the desired O_2 concentration to the patient. Portable O_2 analyzers or continuous in-line sensing devices may be used to check the inspired O_2 concentration at the connector of the patient to the ventilator.

Administration of poorly humidified oxygen may result in bronchospasm and airway injury in neonates. It is important that oxygen be warmed to 35° or 36° C to reduce the risk of airway problems. When any gases administered to patients are warmed and humidified, excessive humidification may get into the circuit and produce "rain-out," or the formation of droplets that can drip into the airway. A heating wire within the ventilator circuitry can reduce the severity of this problem.

Peak Inspiratory Pressure

With pressure-limited ventilators, PIP is the primary factor used to deliver tidal volume. The difference in pressures between PIP and end-distending pressure (PEEP) is the primary determinant of tidal volume in these machines. In most modern ventilators, PIP can be directly selected by the physician, but the operator should be aware that PIP may change if either flow rate or the I/E ratio is changed. In some older, pressure-cycled ventilators (BABYbird, Palm Springs, Calif), PIP is regulated by a combination of the flow rate, respiratory rate, and I/E ratio.

When starting levels of PIP are selected, several physiologic factors must be considered: the infant's weight, gestational age, and postnatal age; the type and severity of the disease process; and lung compliance, airway resistance, and time constant of the lung. A **time constant**, which is the product of compliance and resistance, is the unit of time necessary for the alveolar pressure to reach 63% of the total change in airway pressure during positive-pressure ventilation. Time constants can be measured during inspiration and expiration. If, for example, inspiration lasts for a period of time equal to one time constant, then 63% of the difference in pressure between airway opening and alveoli equilibrates, and a proportional volume of gas enters the airways of the lung. With additional time during inspiration for further pressure equilibration, an additional 63% of the remaining pressure equilibrates (total = 86% now, or 63% + [63% × the remaining 37%]), and an additional equivalent volume of gas follows. After three to five time constants, little additional pressure change occurs, and gas volume delivery is therefore essentially complete (Fig. 44-4).

With reduced compliance, as seen in RDS, the time constant decreases, so that pressure equilibration occurs during a shortened inspiration and expiration. Inspiration and expiration, with volume movement of gas in and out of the lungs, therefore occur in a shorter time period than is seen in normal lungs. When the time constant of the lung becomes so short during either inspiration or expiration that pressure equilibration cannot occur, then either inadequate delivery of volume during inspiration may result or air trapping and incremental overdistention of the lung during expiration may ensue. This latter phenomenon appears to be very important in

the development of air leak syndromes during neonatal ventilation.[25]

Before attachment of any patient to the ventilator, inspiratory pressure should be carefully checked to be certain that it is neither excessive nor inadequate. The adapter that connects to the endotracheal tube should be occluded, and the pressure gauge on the ventilator should be checked, with adjustments made as necessary. Once the patient is attached to the ventilator, the PIP should be rechecked to be certain it has not changed significantly from what was observed with the adapter occluded. If it has changed more than 2 to 3 cm H_2O, the operator must consider the possibility of air leak or an obstructed endotracheal tube.

Considerable controversy exists regarding the level of PIP that should be used for infants with respiratory disease. It appears that as a basic principle, the lowest PIP that adequately ventilates the patient is usually the most appropriate. Another important consideration in this regard is the overall approach to mechanical ventilation that is used. In general, the use of A/C ventilation results in a need for lower PIP than may be seen with either conventional mechanical ventilation (with pressure that is entirely operator selected) or SIMV. With A/C ventilation, infants usually tend to increase their ventilatory rate somewhat to compensate for the lower PIP selected by the clinician. This strategy is usually effective unless the clinician selects a PIP that is inadequate for providing adequate gas exchange and only dead space ventilation occurs. Simply increasing the PIP slightly may be sufficient to achieve success if the arterial carbon dioxide tension ($Paco_2$) remains excessively elevated (>55 mm Hg). In some clinical circumstances, such as acute RDS, this style of ventilatory support may be beneficial and may reduce exposure to higher PIP. It appears that the incidence of pulmonary complications (air leaks and BPD) may also be reduced with this technique.[26]

In contrast, some neonatologists, fearful of barotrauma at all costs, may persistently utilize an inadequate PIP for excessively long periods. On the basis of the infant's size, some physicians arbitrarily set a certain PIP level above which they do not venture, even when ventilation remains grossly insufficient as seen in arterial blood gases. In contrast to the excellent and well-conceived "gentle ventilation" approach developed by Jen-Tien Wung at the Children's Hospital of New York (formerly Babies Hospital), protracted hypercarbia and respiratory acidosis can result in serious systemic and neurologic injury. A study by Vannucci and colleagues indicated that in an animal model, extreme hypercapnia ($Paco_2$ > 100 mm Hg) may result in cardiac depression and reduced cerebral blood flow, with subsequent hypoxic-ischemic brain injury.[27] The necessity of adequate gas exchange under all circumstances therefore cannot be overemphasized. It does no good to avoid barotrauma while the patient dies or suffers significant injury from insufficient gas exchange that results in long-term morbidity. Appropriate PIP can usually be judged on clinical examination (chest movement and breath sounds) and on the basis of blood gas analysis.

Table 44-2 summarizes advantages and side effects of different pressure ranges. Barotrauma can be reduced

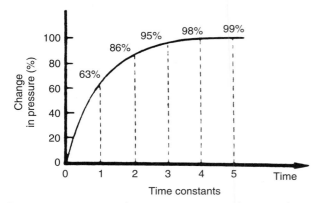

Figure 44–4. Percentage change in pressure in relation to the time (in time constants) allowed for equilibration. As a longer time is allowed for equilibration, a higher percentage change in pressure occurs. The same rule governs the equilibration for step changes in volume. *(From Carlo WA, Martin RJ: Principles of assisted ventilation. Pediatr Clin North Am 33:221, 1986.)*

Table 44–2. Peak Inspiratory Pressure

Low (20 cm H$_2$O)		High (20 cm H$_2$O)	
Advantages	**Adverse Effects**	**Advantages**	**Adverse Effects**
Fewer side effects, especially BPD, PAL Normal lung development may proceed more rapidly	Insufficient ventilation; may not control PaCO$_2$ ↓ Pao$_2$, if too low Generalized atelectasis may occur (may be desirable in some cases of air leaks)	May help reexpand atelectasis ↓ Paco$_2$ ↑ Pao$_2$ Decrease pulmonary vascular resistance	Associated with ↑ PAL, BPD May impede venous return May decrease cardiac output

BPD, bronchopulmonary dysplasia; Paco$_2$, arterial carbon dioxide tension; PAL, pulmonary air leaks; Pao$_2$, arterial oxygen tension.

with the use of lower PIP, and the incidence of air leaks and chronic lung disease may be decreased. There are, however, few data to suggest definite value in extreme pressure reduction with permissive hypercapnia.[28,29] Normal lung development may also be enhanced by lower PIP, although there is evidence that even distribution of gas throughout the lung may be more important than low pressure. High-frequency ventilation (HFV) appears to decrease barotrauma to some extent by providing such gas distribution. Again, the clinician must provide adequate PIP to deliver an appropriate tidal volume (V$_T$) to the patient. Low V$_T$ from low PIP may reduce minute ventilation (V$_E$ = rate × V$_T$), resulting in elevated Paco$_2$ and hypoxemia. Because long-term follow-up on children treated with this approach has not been extensive to date, the degree of morbidity is not known.

High PIP should usually be avoided because of the risk of air leaks, such as pneumothorax, interstitial emphysema, and pneumomediastinum. Furthermore, high intrathoracic pressure, when transmitted to the myocardium, may impede venous return to the heart and decrease cardiac output. There appears to be a neutral range of Paco$_2$. Although a high or low Paco$_2$ by itself may not be harmful, it may be related to alterations in cardiac output that can produce injury to the central nervous system. Certain clinical conditions, however, may warrant the use of high PIP. In patients with markedly decreased compliance or in those in whom lung volume is decreased from atelectasis, a high PIP may be needed to maintain adequate gas exchange or to reexpand collapsed sections of the lung. Also, some physicians treat pulmonary hypertension with high PIP to hyperventilate patients intentionally to a lower Paco$_2$ in an effort to decrease pulmonary artery pressure.[21] As a general rule, however, hyperventilation has been shown to induce a variety of neurologic injuries in infants and is no longer a recommended therapy for PPHN.[30]

Positive End-Expiratory Pressure

Although it has been used since Gregory and colleagues' original work in 1970 to 1971, CPAP has reemerged as a highly effective way to initiate ventilatory assistance in infants with the lowest birth weights, with the least risk of airway and neurologic injury.[31,32] Furthermore, extubation to CPAP after mechanical ventilation appears to decrease the likelihood of reintubation and reduces the frequency of apnea.[33,34] Most infants should receive a trial of CPAP before initiation of mechanical ventilation. There is some information indicating that there are outcome differences in the methods by which CPAP is delivered.[35] In addition, some groups suggest that "bubble" or underwater CPAP may be more effective than ventilator-delivered CPAP. It is difficult to reconcile how relatively small pressure differences could be reflected in an infant's outcome, however, in view of the normal attenuation of pressures down the airway. Further studies should be forthcoming in this regard.

While a neonate is on the ventilator, the use of PEEP or continuous distending pressure has become a standard technique for ventilatory treatment. The approach to treatment is similar to that recommended for CPAP in the spontaneously breathing patient. Selection of the appropriate PEEP depends on the size of the patient, the pathophysiologic features of the disease process, and the goals of treatment. In most clinical situations, there appears to be an "optimal PEEP" below which lung volumes are not well maintained and above which the lungs become overdistended.[36] On most ventilators, PEEP is selected simply by setting the desired pressure. The clinician must be aware, however, that the chosen PEEP may be altered by other ventilator variables. For example, if expiratory time is too short or if airway resistance is increased, a degree of inadvertent PEEP that is additive to the selected level may be generated.[37,38] This inadvertent PEEP in such situations may contribute to gas trapping and increase the potential for air leaks.

The major benefits of PEEP are similar to those seen with CPAP in the spontaneously breathing infant. PEEP stabilizes and recruits lung volume, improves compliance (to a certain point, after which compliance may actually decrease), and improves ventilation-perfusion matching in the lung.

Table 44–3. Continuous Positive Airway Pressure (CPAP) or Positive End-Expiratory Pressure (PEEP)

Low (2–3 cm H_2O)		Medium (4–7 cm H_2O)		High (>8 cm H_2O)	
Advantages	Adverse Effects	Advantages	Adverse Effects	Advantages	Side Effects
Used during late phases of weaning	May be too low to maintain adequate lung volume	Recruits lung volume with surfactant deficiency states (e.g., RDS)	May overdistend lungs with normal compliance	Prevents alveolar collapse in surfactant deficiency states with severely decreased C_L	PAL
Maintenance of lung volume in very premature infants with low FRC	CO_2 retention from V/Q mismatch, inasmuch as alveolar volume is inadequate	Stabilizes lung volume once recruited		Improves distribution of ventilation	Decreases compliance of lung overdistends
Useful in some infants with extremely low birth weight on A/C ventilation		Improves V/Q matching			May impede venous return to the heart May increase PVR CO_2 retention

A/C, assist/control; C_L, lung compliance; FRC, functional residual capacity; PAL, pulmonary air leak; PVR, pulmonary vascular resistance; RDS, respiratory distress syndrome; V/Q, ventilation-perfusion.

Table 44-3 summarizes the effects of CPAP or PEEP at various levels. PEEP less than 2 cm H_2O is not recommended, except in rare instances, because the presence of an endotracheal tube bypasses the normal airway mechanics that typically provide a low level of end-distending pressure during spontaneous breathing.[39] Furthermore, the resistance of the endotracheal tube necessitates a certain PEEP level if the atelectasis that is produced by an inspiratory load in the presence of inadequate PEEP is to be avoided.

Low PEEP levels (2 to 3 cm H_2O) are usually used during weaning phases of ventilatory management, and some infants with extremely low birth weight on A/C support may be adequately treated at these levels. When such levels are provided early in the course of disease in larger infants, however, atelectasis may result with CO_2 retention. In most clinical circumstances, medium levels of PEEP (4 to 7 cm H_2O) are most often appropriate. Such levels allow appropriate maintenance of lung volumes but minimize the potential side effects associated with higher PEEP and pulmonary overdistention. PEEP levels above 8 cm H_2O are rarely used in conventional mechanical ventilation because of the risk of pulmonary air leaks and reduction of cardiac output. With HFJV, however, higher PEEP may sometimes be needed to ensure adequacy and maintenance of lung volume.[3] Severe respiratory failure in larger infants may also necessitate high PEEP levels (8 to 10 cm H_2O and above) for a period, until an alternative therapy (HFJV or ECMO) can be initiated. Extreme vigilance for pneumothoraces, pneumomediastinum,

increased pulmonary vascular resistance, and inadequate cardiac output is essential at any level of CPAP or PEEP, but especially at the higher levels of support.

Rate or Frequency of Ventilation

Respiratory rate is one of the primary determinants of minute ventilation in mechanical ventilation (minute ventilation = respiratory rate × V_T) (Table 44-4). No conclusive studies demonstrate the optimal ventilatory rate for the treatment of neonatal respiratory disease. Some studies have indicated improved oxygenation at higher rates (≥60 breaths per minute).[40] Other studies have historically suggested more success with slower rates (≤40 breaths per minute).[41] As with other previously mentioned ventilator controls, the best rate in a given situation depends on several variables, including size of the infant, type and stage of the disease, presence of complications, and clinical response. Furthermore, the successful introduction of high-frequency ventilators suggests that frequency may be important only in reference to other controls being used at that time. For example, very high rates can be successfully used if PIP (and consequently V_T) and T_I can be reduced simultaneously. Without such a reduction, high frequencies might result in severe complications. In conventional ventilation, especially during A/C ventilation, high frequencies may be spontaneously generated by an infant with PIP kept at a minimum level. Many infants subsequently "autowean" their rate as lung compliance improves. This circumstance, however, is very different from that of the patient

Table 44-4. Neonatal Mechanical Ventilatory Rates

Slow (≤40 bpm)		Medium 40–60 bpm		Rapid (≥60 bpm)	
Advantages	Adverse Effects	Advantages	Adverse Effects	Advantages	Side Effects
↑Pao$_2$ with increased MAP	Must increase PIP to maintain minute ventilation	Mimics normal ventilatory rate	May not provide adequate ventilation in some cases	Higher Pao$_2$ (may be the result of air trapping)	May exceed time constant and produce air trapping
Useful in weaning	↑PIP may cause barotrauma	Effectively treats most neonatal lung diseases	↑PIP may still be needed to maintain minute ventilation	May allow ↓PIP and V$_T$	May cause inadvertent PEEP
Used with square-wave ventilation	Patient may require paralysis	Usually does not exceed time constant of lung, so air trapping is unlikely		Hyperventilation may be useful in PPHN	May result in change in compliance (frequency dependence of compliance)
Needed when I/E ratio is inverted				May reduce atelectasis	Inadequate V$_T$ and minute ventilation if only dead space is ventilated

I/E, inspiratory/expiratory; bpm, breaths per minute; MAP, mean airway pressure; Pao$_2$, arterial oxygen tension; PEEP, positive end-expiratory pressure; PIP, peak inspiratory pressure; PPHN, persistent pulmonary hypertension of the neonate; V$_T$, tidal volume.

intentionally treated with hyperventilation to deliberately lower Paco$_2$.

In most instances, whether the clinician selects a high or low respiratory rate, the goal of therapy is the reduction of barotrauma with an associated decrease in air leaks and chronic lung disease. Again, neurologic effects from whatever ventilatory technique is used must always be taken into consideration. Both high and low ventilatory rates can achieve these objectives if the physician has an overall strategy for ventilator management, such as that outlined later in this chapter. Most complications involving ventilator rates occur because the clinician fails to recognize the effect of rate change on other aspects of ventilatory care. For example, if higher rates are selected, a prolonged T$_I$ and an inadequate T$_E$ may result in decreased compliance and air trapping, if the time constant of the lung does not adequately allow for gas exit. Thus, ventilatory changes cannot be entertained without an evaluation of the overall effects of that decision.

In addition to the considerations already noted, it is essential that the capabilities of the ventilator in use be examined to be certain that what is selected for the patient is actually delivered by the machine. Boros[42] and Simbruner and Gregory[43] showed that there is significant variability among ventilators to deliver pressures and V$_T$, especially at higher frequencies. Some ventilators have exhalation-assist modes to help in alleviating gas trapping

in the tubing at higher rates, but this provision does not ensure consistent V$_T$ delivery.

Physicians who prefer slower rate ventilation often cite the work of Haman and Reynolds[41] and Boros,[42] who demonstrated that lower rates, when delivered with higher MAPs, produced better oxygenation. Again, lower rates can be used successfully, with a minimum of complications, if the clinician is aware of the potential sources of problems for the infants being treated. Slower rate ventilation could not have been developed without modification of ventilator circuitry to provide continuous gas flow, rather than intermittent flow. This modification, introduced by Kirby and associates[44] in the early 1970s, has now been extended in some ventilators to include a separate circuit entirely for spontaneous breathing. Before the introduction of continuous flow, an infant who attempted to breathe against a closed valve would rebreathe exhaled gas, with a potential increase in Paco$_2$. With constant flow in a time-cycled device, the physician could now choose to provide a predetermined amount of mechanical ventilation in combination with spontaneous breathing. This technique is referred to as intermittent mandatory ventilation (IMV) and it has been a useful adjunct to ventilator weaning. With the current ability to synchronize the ventilator to the infant's breathing (as in SIMV), the technique has become increasingly important as a weaning approach. As the pulmonary disease improves, the infant receives fewer machine breaths, and spontaneous breathing is allowed to increase.

Ventilator rate is usually controlled by directly selecting the rate in time-cycled machines, which constitute the majority of neonatal ventilators today. In pressure-cycled machines, the rate is changed by altering T_I, T_E, or the I/E ratio.

Inspiratory-to-Expiratory Ratio

Possible variations in I/E ratios are summarized in Table 44-5. The ability to select an I/E ratio varies from ventilator to ventilator. In some pressure-cycled units, both T_I and T_E can be directly selected to produce the desired I/E ratio. On most units, however, the T_I is selected, and, in combination with the desired frequency, the I/E ratio is then automatically set. In patient-triggered ventilation, however, with the termination sensitivity set at 5% to 10%, the I/E ratio may become variable, inasmuch as the flow characteristics of the inspiratory phase of ventilation alter the duration of inspiration from breath to breath. If a specific I/E ratio is desired, the termination sensitivity must be shut off.

I/E ratio has been considered an important variable in ventilator management strategies, beginning with Reynolds and Tagizadeh's[45] work, which emphasized its role in controlling oxygenation. In their studies, the I/E ratio was reversed (>1:1), with inspiration longer than expiration. More recently, however, the I/E ratio has been regarded as less important than the T_I. There is still a great deal of debate among neonatologists regarding the optimal T_I for neonatal mechanical ventilation. Increasingly, emphasis has been placed on shorter T_I, with the belief that airway and lung injury will be reduced. It is evident, however, that if T_I is reduced too much, opening pressure within the lung is not reached and only dead space

ventilation occurs. As a result, one should try to balance a shorter T_I with adequate gas entry into the lung. In general, we now use a starting T_I of 0.3 to 0.4 second for most neonatal ventilation, shorter than was previously described in the first edition of this book.

Selecting any two of the four variables (T_I, T_E, I/E, and rate) automatically determines the other two. Choosing a T_I of 0.5 second with an I/E of 1:1 automatically provides a T_E of 0.5 second and a rate of 60 breaths per minute. Furthermore, if rate is decreased to 30 breaths per minute and the I/E is left at 1:1, then the T_I increases to 1 second, possibly increasing the risk of airway overdistention and air leak. Consequently, many physicians prefer to set a T_I that they believe is adequate and are not as concerned about the I/E ratio directly. It is my preference, in general, to select a T_I of 0.3 to 0.4 second during the acute phases of most neonatal lung diseases to avoid air trapping. Further recommendations about appropriate I/E ratios, however, depend on the type, severity, and stage of the disease being treated. It is evident, however, that the I/E ratio decreases as ventilatory rates are slowed if the T_I remains constant. This approach provides a higher MAP and better oxygenation during the early phases of disease. As the infant's status improves, the slowing of the ventilator rate extends expiration and automatically decreases I/E and MAP, when it is often appropriate to do so.

An additional caution about prolonged I/E ratios involves cardiac output considerations. Increasing the duration of inspiration enhances the amount of intrathoracic pressure that is transmitted to the heart. Venous return may be compromised, and cardiac output may be decreased. In addition, if an air leak develops, it may further result in impaired venous return. As a result,

Table 44–5. Ratio Control in Neonatal Mechanical Ventilation

Inverse (>1:1)		Normal (1:1 to 1:3)		Prolonged Expiratory (<1:3)	
Advantages	Adverse Effects	Advantages	Adverse Effects	Advantages	Adverse Effects
↑ MAP	May have insufficient emptying time, and air trapping may result	Mimics natural breathing pattern	Insufficient emptying at highest rates	Useful during weaning, when oxygenation is less of a problem	Low T_I may decrease tidal volume
↑ Pao_2 in RDS	May impede venous return to the heart	May give best ratio at higher rates		May be more useful in diseases such as MAS, when air trapping is a part of the disease process	Higher flow rates may have to be used, which may not be optimal for distribution of ventilation
May enhance alveolar recruitment when atelectasis is present	Increases pulmonary vascular resistance and worsens diseases such as PPHN, CHD Worsened PAL				May ventilate more dead space

CHD, congenital heart disease; MAP, mean airway pressures; MAS, meconium aspiration syndrome; PAL; pulmonary air leak; Pao_2, arterial oxygen tension; PPHN, persistent pulmonary hypertension of the neonate; RDS, respiratory distress syndrome; T_I, inspiration time.

Table 44–6. Flow Rates in Neonatal Ventilation

Low Rate (0.5 to 3 L/min)		High Rate (4–10 L/min or more)	
Advantages	Adverse Effects	Advantages	Adverse Effects
Slower inspiratory time, more sine wave	Hypercapnia, if flow rate is not adequate to remove CO_2 from the system	Produces more square wave ventilatory pattern	↑ Barotrauma
Less barotraumas to airways	At high ventilator rate, low flow may not enable the machine to reach PIP	↑ Pao_2	In moderate to severe RDS, may produce more airway injury
	↓ Pao_2 in some cases	Needed to deliver high PIP with rapid ventilator rates	
		Prevents CO_2 retention	

Pao_2, arterial oxygen tension; PIP, peak inspiratory pressure; Pao_2, oxygen tension; RDS, respiratory distress syndrome.

prolonged I/E has been associated with an increased risk of intraventricular hemorrhage. I therefore use reversed I/E only as a last resort to try to improve oxygenation, most often in cases in which another way of increasing oxygenation more effectively cannot be found. Since the introduction and widespread use of high-frequency ventilators, iNO therapy, and ECMO, prolonged I/E has rarely been used in our nurseries.

Flow Rate

Flow rates used for neonatal mechanical ventilation are summarized in Table 44-6. Flow rate is an important determinant of the ability of the ventilator to deliver desired levels of PIP, waveform, I/E ratios, and, in some cases, respiratory rate. A minimum flow at least two times an infant's minute ventilation is usually required (neonatal minute ventilation typically ranges from approximately 0.2 to 1.0 L/min), but the usual operating range during mechanical ventilation is usually 4 to 10 L/min.

When low flow rates are used, the time it takes to reach PIP is longer, and the pressure curve has a lower plateau and appears similar to a sine waveform (see Fig. 44-2). Normal neonatal spontaneous breath patterns are shaped like a sine waveform. Because maldistribution of ventilation occurs in many neonatal respiratory diseases, there may, theoretically, be a reduction of barotrauma with this pattern of waveform. With sine wave ventilation, however, if the flow rate is too low in relation to minute ventilation, dead space ventilation may increase because effective opening pressure for the airways is not reached within an appropriate time. As a result, hypercapnia may result. In addition, if higher ventilator rates are used on sine waveform ventilators, inadequate flows may also result in dead space ventilation because the ventilator does not reach PIP in the allocated time. Opening pressure of the lung is not reached, and gas exchange is reduced.

Higher flow rates are needed if square wave ventilation (see Fig. 44-2) is desired on standard ventilators. Also, at higher rates, a high flow may be necessary to attain a high or adequate PIP (and adequate V_T) because T_I is short. Carbon dioxide rebreathing is also prevented in the

ventilator tubing at higher flow rates. The most common complication of high flow rates is an increased incidence of air leaks because maldistribution of ventilation results in a rapid pressure increase in nonobstructed or nonatelectatic airways and alveoli.

Waveforms

The waveforms commonly used in neonatal ventilation are described and summarized in Table 44-7. Waveforms are typically not selected by the physician in prescribing mechanical ventilation but are often the result of other factors, including ventilator design. Many of the considerations regarding waveform are discussed earlier (see "Flow Rate"). Sine wave breathing approximates normal spontaneous respiration more closely than does a square waveform. The smoother increase in inspiratory pressure may be advantageous for infants with maldistribution of ventilation, which is commonly seen in many neonatal lung diseases.

Square waveform breathing improves oxygenation, when used with slower rates and longer T_I. Square waveform breathing, in general, also provides a higher MAP than does sine waveform breathing if identical PIP is used, because the PIP is reached more rapidly with square waveforms.[42] The longer time at PIP with square waveforms may assist in opening atelectatic areas of the lung in some instances, although overdistention of inflated areas and air leaks may also occur. With square waveforms and reversed I/E ratios, venous return to the heart and cardiac output may decrease.

The use of graphics monitoring is helpful in examining pressure-limited and volume-limited breaths to obtain a better understanding of how these differ. Figure 44-5 shows the differences between the waveforms in these approaches to positive-pressure ventilation.

Mean Airway Pressure

Although no current mechanical ventilator allows the operator to select MAP (the SensorMedics [Conshohocken, Pa] high-frequency oscillator is an exception), this ventilator variable is considered to be important because of its

Table 44–7. Wave Forms in Neonatal Mechanical Ventilation

Sine Wave		Square Wave	
Advantages	Adverse Effects	Advantages	Adverse Effects
Smoother increase of pressure	Lower mean airway pressure	Higher MAP for equivalent PIP	With high flow, the ventilation may be applying higher pressure to normal airways and alveoli
More like normal respiratory pattern		Longer time at PIP may open atelectatic areas of lung and improve distribution of ventilation	Venous return is impeded if longer T_I is used or I/E ratio is reversed

I/E, inspiratory/expiratory; MAP, mean airway pressure; PIP, peak inspiratory pressure; T_I, inspiratory time.

relationship to oxygenation.[46] The clinician typically measures MAP by determining the mean of instantaneous readings of pressure within the airway during a single respiratory cycle. In waveform terminology, the MAP is equal to the area under the pressure curve for a single respiratory cycle divided by the duration of the cycle, or the integral of the pressure during a respiratory cycle. MAP is higher in square waveform ventilation than in sine waveform ventilatory patterns when PIP and duration of PIP are equal. No studies to date have specifically implicated MAP as the primary determinant of air leaks or chronic lung disease. Increases in oxygenation, however, are directly related to increases in MAP. It is nonetheless evident that some changes in MAP, particularly with a short T_I, may not be reflected in increased oxygenation. The ventilator control variables that influence MAP are PIP, PEEP, I/E ratio, and waveform.

Because pulmonary barotrauma may be correlated with high PIP that is unevenly distributed throughout the lung,[47] efforts have been made to ventilate patients with lower PIP and slower ventilatory frequency while MAP is maintained. To accomplish this pattern of ventilator support, T_I must be increased, which also changes the I/E ratio. As MAP increases, alveolar recruitment occurs,

reducing alveolar-arterial O_2 delivery gradient and increasing arterial oxygenation. Techniques to recruit alveolar volume by using sustained inflation and higher MAP during HFOV appear to be effective, although less so during conventional positive-pressure ventilation.[48] The use of high MAP may be required during acute phases of neonatal lung disease, especially RDS, when compliance is low. In less severely affected infants and during recovery, high MAP may interfere with venous return, as seen with elevated PEEP. The clinician must be particularly cautious after surfactant administration in the infant with low birth weight, because compliance and functional residual capacity changes may occur very rapidly.[49] If efforts to reduce PIP and MAP are not made quickly, lung overdistention, with the potential risk for air leaks, may occur. It is also thought that sudden changes in compliance may predispose some infants to pulmonary edema and pulmonary hemorrhage.[50]

An alternative approach to ventilation, first developed by Wung and coworkers at Babies Hospital in New York, downplays the importance of close management of higher PIP and MAP.[51] In that approach, lower PIP and MAP are commonly selected even during acute phases of illness, and arterial blood gas measurements of pH and CO_2 tension that may be outside the normal range are accepted. Wung and coworkers have been very successful with what has often been described as "gentle ventilation," but the clinician should *always* attempt to ventilate infants as "gently" as possible. The goal of any strategy of ventilatory management is to provide adequate gas exchange with the lowest settings possible. Wung and coworkers' approach to ventilation is discussed further later in the section Approaches to Neonatal Ventilation.

THE MANAGEMENT OF RESPIRATORY FAILURE WITH POSITIVE-PRESSURE VENTILATORS

Definition of Respiratory Failure

There currently is no universally accepted definition for respiratory failure in the neonatal period. Because of the complexity of interplay between clinical and laboratory

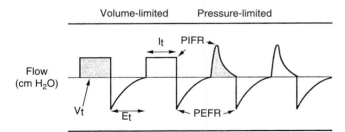

Figure 44–5. Flow waveforms for both volume- and pressure-limited breath types. Inspiratory flow is above baseline, whereas expiratory flow is below. Peak inspiratory flow rate (PIFR) and peak expiratory flow rate (PEFR) are shown. E_t, expiratory time; I_t, inspiratory time; V_t, tidal volume. *(From Nicks JJ: Graphics monitoring. In Sinha SK and Donn SM [eds]: Manual of Neonatal Respiratory Care. Armonk, NY, Futura, 2000, p 65.)*

relationships in determining respiratory failure, management of this problem in the neonate is rarely simple and straightforward. Respiratory failure usually includes two or more criteria from the following clinical and laboratory categories:

Clinical criteria
   Retractions (intercostal, supraclavicular, suprasternal)
   Grunting
   Respiratory rate of more than 60 breaths per minute
   Central cyanosis
   Intractable apnea
   Decreased activity and movement
Laboratory criteria
   $Paco_2$ of more than 60 mm Hg
   Pao_2 of less than 50 mm Hg or O_2 saturation of less than 80%, with an Fio_2 of 1.0
   pH of less than 7.25

The clinical severity of presentation of respiratory failure can be extremely variable in the neonatal period. Some infants exhibit severe distress immediately, whereas others may have marked abnormalities in arterial blood gas levels and yet appear to be far less compromised. Close observation of infants is crucial in this setting. Retractions typically indicate a significant loss of lung volume. The infant then attempts to recruit alveolar volume by increasing respiratory effort, but the excessively compliant neonatal chest wall makes this effort somewhat futile in most cases. Rather than acting as a rigid strut, the neonatal thorax collapses, and the negative intrapleural pressure that is generated fails to reopen alveoli that are atelectatic. Grunting often accompanies retractions, particularly in the neonate with RDS. Grunting is an expiratory effort against a partially closed glottis that elevates the end-expiratory pressure in an attempt to increase residual lung volume and oxygenation. It is also usually indicative of volume loss in the lung. Retractions and grunting should therefore be considered ominous signs of impending respiratory failure during the neonatal period, particularly in the infant who weighs less than 1500 g. Both retractions and grunting are occasionally seen, however, in the neonate with cold stress, in which case these signs should last for no longer than 2 to 4 hours, once the child has been warmed appropriately. The clinician should therefore always maintain appropriate thermal stability for any infant; otherwise, the medical care may become far more complex than is necessary.

If significant grunting and retractions are observed in an infant, early ventilatory assistance should be offered. Infants should be placed on nasal CPAP very quickly in an attempt to halt progressive volume loss in the lung. Nasal CPAP is often initiated in the delivery room, especially in the very smallest infants, as the examiner determines the need for surfactant administration. Occasionally an infant may be briefly intubated to administer surfactant and then returned to CPAP. If such measures are ineffective, however, intubation and mechanical ventilation may be required, because metabolic derangement in these infants may proceed rapidly once the child can no longer support gas exchange. Late institution of mechanical support is often less effective and the

complications and associated morbidity are far greater than those seen with early intervention. Although the larger, more mature infant may have greater reserve and tolerate respiratory insufficiency for a longer period than the premature infant, the physician should keep in mind that recovery from respiratory failure rarely occurs in any infant during the neonatal period without some form of respiratory assistance. An aggressive (but gentle) early approach is often preferable in neonates, regardless of the disease.

Connecting the Patient to the Ventilator

The ventilator should be selected according to the size of the child, the disease to be treated, and the severity of the disease. It is important to try to visualize the potential changes in the disease that may await an infant in the days ahead and to select a ventilator that is capable of meeting the requirements for therapy in that child. Few events are more frustrating than having to change a ventilator in midtreatment because the ventilator in current use does not have a needed capability. Fortunately, most neonatal ventilators introduced since the 1990s have quite exceptional capabilities in comparison with earlier models that were far more limited.

Before a child is treated with a ventilator, the following considerations should be kept in mind:

1. The endotracheal tube should be well secured and appropriately positioned. The tip of the endotracheal tube should be located about 1 to 2 cm above the carina. Breath sounds should be equal after insertion, and a chest radiograph should be obtained before mechanical ventilation is initiated, to ensure correct placement of the tube and to permit the physician to monitor changes in the disease with treatment.
2. Once the patient is connected to the ventilator, the clinical observations and mechanical factors listed in Table 44-8 should be followed. Vascular access is an important part of management and should occur shortly after initiation of ventilatory support, if not before that time. Nursing staff often have a catheter placed peripherally as rapidly as intubation can occur.

Table 44–8. Preliminary Review for Initiating Ventilatory Support

Clinical Signs	Mechanical Factors
Color	Oxygen supply
Respiratory rate	Endotracheal tube placement
Breathing pattern	Ventilator circuit humidification
Retractions and grunting	Humidifier and heater function
Chest and abdominal synchrony	Chest radiograph
Synchrony with the ventilator (consider assist/control or SIMV)	Intravascular access

SIMV, synchronized intermittent mandatory ventilation.

Ventilator Management

Since the previous edition of this book, a number of ventilator variables have been added to some units that increase their capabilities. SIMV and A/C ventilation have become standard approaches; modalities such as proportional assist ventilation and tidal volume–guaranteed ventilation represent some more recent modifications. The benefits of all these newer strategies of treatment are still somewhat uncertain, and their usefulness and effects on long-term outcomes remain to be determined. This section concentrates on the basics of ventilator management that are common to most pressure- and time-cycled machines. It is, however, difficult to describe the use of positive-pressure ventilation without describing an overall management strategy for the particular circumstance of ventilator use. When appropriate, some brief discussion about the various new ventilator capabilities is provided, as well as mention of how these capabilities might affect the patient's management.

Arterial blood gas analysis remains the "gold standard" for the assessment of effective gas exchange (see Chapter 35). It is essential for the clinician to understand which ventilator controls are most likely to correct or change specific blood gas abnormalities. Table 44-9 summarizes these adjustments. In general, it is sound practice to adjust only one ventilator control at a time. Multiple changes made simultaneously are difficult to interpret, and the clinical care of the patient may be made more difficult to assess. The importance of an overall scheme of management for ventilatory care of a neonate cannot be overemphasized. Regardless of the approach to ventilation that is used, the clinician should not simply respond randomly to blood gas measurements; instead, he or she should set specific goals that should be progressively approached throughout care. Furthermore, it is crucial that the physician of record articulate this approach to everyone involved in the care of the infant. There is nothing more frustrating than coming to a child's bedside only to find that the changes made (especially during the night) on the ventilator, although not incorrect on a blood gas–by–blood gas basis, have nevertheless resulted in a child's making little overall progress, inasmuch as the specific goals of treatment were not clear.

The initiation of mechanical ventilation is often unnecessarily complicated. A scheme for the initiation of ventilation is shown in Figure 44-6. If the clinician has a clear understanding of the goals of ventilatory support, steady progress toward those goals should be readily attainable. Once the clinician has decided that intervention is needed, the steps outlined in Table 44-10 should be followed. Adjustment of ventilation after stabilization of the infant is detailed in Figure 44-7. Some additional comments are appropriate in relation to this approach to management.

The use of surfactant has become a standard adjunct to ventilatory management of the neonate. A more detailed discussion of surfactant therapy is presented in Chapter 10. Although optimal surfactant treatment is still not established at present, the practice at most level III neonatal intensive care units has been to use surfactant liberally and early in the infant diagnosed with RDS (caused by surfactant deficiency). Data suggest that early use of surfactant, as soon as the diagnosis of RDS is made, has better results than does later rescue use after the disease is well established.[52] Other neonatal lung diseases may also respond to surfactant administration, because inactivation of surfactant is commonly seen with acidosis or with the presence of meconium in the airway and lungs.[53] The evidence in these diseases, however, is less extensive than what has been published for treatment of RDS. Furthermore, it does appear that there are some differences with regard to surfactant replacement in meconium aspiration syndrome that must be considered when exogenous surfactants are used.

Table 44-9. Mechanical Ventilator Settings Used to Adjust Arterial Blood Gases

$Paco_2$	Pao_2	Respiratory Acidosis (Low pH)	Metabolic Acidosis (Low pH)
Rate and PIP (determine minute ventilation; ↑ rate or ↑ PIP causes ↓ CO_2)	F_{IO_2} ↑ O_2 causes ↑ Pao_2	Same controls as $Paco_2$	Volume expansion or sodium bicarbonate
I/E ratio (determines duration of inspiration and expiration; longer expiration causes ↓ $Paco_2$)	PEEP (↑ PEEP causes ↑ Pao_2)		May correct with improved oxygenation and ventilation, as perfusion improves
PEEP (if too high or too low, may cause ↑ $Paco_2$)	T_I or I/E ratio (↑ T_I causes ↑ Pao_2; ↓ T_I causes ↓ Pao_2 in general) PIP (↑ PIP usually causes ↑ Pao_2; effect is less than others listed)		Caution: high PEEP may result in metabolic acidosis because of impaired venous return

F_{IO_2}, fraction of inspired oxygen; I/E, inspiratory/expiratory; $Paco_2$, arterial carbon dioxide tension; Pao_2, arterial oxygen tension; PEEP, positive end-expiratory pressure; PIP, peak inspiratory pressure; T_I, inspiratory time.

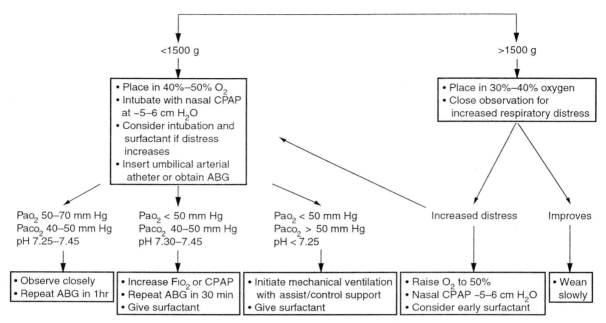

1. Clinical diagnosis of neonatal lung disease
   (tachypnea, cyanosis, retractions, grunting, nasal flaring, apnea,
   decreased activity)
2. Confirmatory studies (CXR, ABG,CBC, etc.)

Figure 44–6. Initial management plan for the neonate with pulmonary disease. ABG, arterial blood gas analysis; CBC, complete blood count; CPAP, continuous positive airway pressure; CXR, chest radiograph; F_{IO_2} = fraction of inspired oxygen; $Paco_2$, arterial carbon dioxide tension; Pao_2, arterial oxygen tension.

Table 44–10. Initiation of Mechanical Ventilation in Neonatal Lung Disease

1. Intubate infant; secure endotracheal tube adequately
2. Place pressure manometer in gas flow line and begin manual ventilation to determine appropriate pressure for ventilation
3. Begin manual inflation with
   F_{IO_2} = 0.5
   Rate at 40–50 bpm
   Initial PIP at 12–15 cm H_2O
   Initial PEEP at 4–5 cm H_2O
   I/E ratio at 1:1 to 1:2
4. Observe infant for
   Cyanosis
   Chest wall excursion
   Capillary perfusion
   Breath sounds
5. If ventilation is inadequate, increase PIP by 1 cm H_2O every few breaths, until air entry seems adequate
6. If oxygenation is poor, and cyanosis remains, increase F_{IO_2} by 5% every minute until cyanosis is abolished
7. Measure ABGs
8. Adjust ventilation as indicated by ABG results (see Fig. 44-8)

ABG, arterial blood gas; bpm, breaths per minute; F_{IO_2}, fraction of inspired oxygen; I/E, inspiratory/expiratory; PEEP, positive end-expiratory pressure; PIP, peak inspiratory pressure.

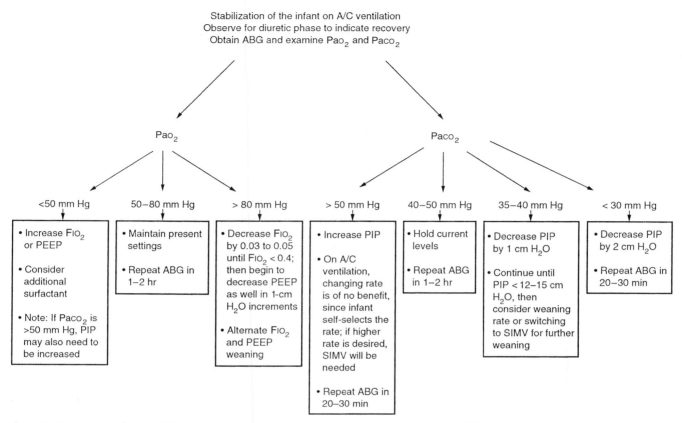

Figure 44-7. An approach to ventilator management after stabilization in neonatal lung disease. ABG, arterial blood gas analysis; A/C, assist/-control; FIO$_2$, fraction of inspired oxygen; PaCO$_2$, arterial carbon dioxide tension; PaO$_2$, arterial oxygen tension; PEEP, positive end-expiratory pressure; PIP, peak inspiratory pressure; SIMV, synchronized intermittent mandatory ventilation.

Peptide-containing surfactants (KL4) appear to be more resistant than the modified natural surfactants currently in use.[54] Several surfactants are now approved by the U.S. Food and Drug Administration for use in the United States. Beractant (Survanta), colfosceril palmitate (Exosurf), calfactant (Infasurf), and poractant alfa (Curosurf) are all available and have their various advocates among neonatologists.

Depending on the specific surfactant used and the infant's response, one to four doses of the drug are given. It is important that the clinician observe the infant closely during the surfactant administration process. Although most infants tolerate the procedure well, some children do experience oxygen desaturation. Other infants may improve rapidly, and overventilation can occur with the possibility of air leaks. The risk of pulmonary hemorrhage is also slightly higher in some infants who are treated with surfactant.[50] Furthermore, excessively low PaCO$_2$ during the first days of life has been associated with an increased risk of cerebral palsy in some children.[55]

The use of pulmonary function testing may also guide ventilator management. The use of pulmonary graphics monitoring, either as an intrinsic part of the ventilator or as an adjunct, has become increasingly widespread. Although not as precise as pulmonary function determined independently of the ventilator, these units are extremely helpful in guiding ventilator management. Tidal volumes, minute ventilation, ventilator leak, chest wall distortion, flow-volume loops, pressure-volume loops, and several other functions can be readily evaluated. Overall lung volumes cannot be determined, however, except through the use of measurements of functional residual capacity by either nitrogen washout or helium dilution. Some interpolation methods that are less difficult to perform, but somewhat less precise, have also been studied.[56] Improved functional residual capacity is probably the most important effect of surfactant administration in many disease conditions. With newer graphics monitors, however, much of the necessary information can be evaluated several times daily in managing neonates on ventilatory support. Pulmonary function testing is described in greater detail in Chapter 40.

The management strategy outlined in Figure 44-7 is applicable to nearly all types of neonatal lung disease. The basic principles that guide this approach are as follows.

First, it is generally accepted that the most damaging aspects of neonatal ventilation, or the leading causes of lung injury, are FIO$_2$ and PIP. Although it is not always possible to limit the use of FIO$_2$ and PIP during the most critical phases of illness, the clinician should try to reduce the levels of these controllable variables as soon as the infant shows signs of improvement. This algorithm for ventilator management is therefore designed to reduce FiO_2 and PIP as primary initiatives and to decrease rate and PEEP later. My practice now is to initiate positive-pressure ventilation in the A/C mode, especially in infants with very low birth weight. Because of its design, A/C weaning occurs primarily by decreasing FiO_2 and PIP, not the rate or PEEP. I have therefore found that the basic principles outlined in the previous edition of this book not only remain applicable but also are actually facilitated by the use of A/C ventilation.

Second, it is preferable to make frequent small changes in ventilator support rather than infrequent larger changes in degree of support. Commonly, ventilator management is approached with no overall plan in mind. In many nurseries, an arterial blood gas level is obtained at a random time, and the neonatologist makes a change on the basis of that single blood gas analysis. Often, the changes may be reasonable, but they can be inappropriate because they do not take place within a defined strategy for weaning. The child ultimately winds up on a level of support that appears odd, but ventilator changes were not necessarily incorrect on a blood gas–by–blood gas basis. The clinician simply did not have a coherent plan for ventilator management. For example, a child may wind up receiving a PIP of 25 cm H_2O and a rate of 5 to 10 breaths per minute as weaning progresses because of low $PaCO_2$ levels. Each decision might have been correct, but the overall "balance" of ventilatory support is not optimal (although occasionally, as in a child with chronic BPD, such support levels may be necessary). It is therefore important to develop a sense for overall balance of ventilator support, such as that listed in Table 44-11. If the ventilator settings vary much from the overall patterns across any row in this table, the physician should consider a ventilator strategy that brings the patient's support back into a more appropriate combination of settings. Table 44-11 assumes an approximate I/E ratio of 1:1 to 1:3 and an initial backup ventilator rate of 40 to 60 breaths per minute. Normal arterial blood gas values for this table are as follows:

$$PaO_2 = 60 \text{ to } 80 \text{ mm Hg}$$

$$PaCO_2 = 40 \text{ to } 50 \text{ mm Hg}$$

$$pH = 7.25 \text{ to } 7.45$$

VENTILATOR WEANING

As previously indicated, my suggested approach to ventilator weaning is indicated in Figure 44-7. Once an infant has remained stable for at least 24 hours, I gradually begin to decrease the two factors that appear to have the greatest toxicity for the lung—O_2 and PIP—while leaving the infant initially on A/C ventilation. The weaning approach is very gradual, and frequent small changes are preferred to infrequent, larger decreases in support. The goal is to allow the infant to assume gradual, progressive responsibility for gas exchange while ventilator support is decreased. As FiO_2 and PIP are decreased, we usually switch an infant back to SIMV when the FiO_2 is below 0.4 and the PIP is approximately 12 cm H_2O. The factor that has made this approach possible was the introduction of IMV, now synchronized to the infant's own breathing as SIMV.

The general approach to SIMV weaning is to decrease the number of ventilator breaths progressively while the infant steadily increases spontaneous respiratory effort. No prospective controlled studies, however, clearly demonstrate the benefit of this approach in the sick neonate. Theoretically, however, this system does afford several advantages:

1. It allows a gradual transition from mechanical ventilation to spontaneous breathing.
2. It eliminates the need for special bedside equipment to provide PEEP during weaning. (Some individuals, however, believe that there is a difference between ventilator-delivered and underwater-delivered or "bubble" CPAP. This issue still needs to be studied. There do appear to be differences among CPAP devices, however, in some cases.[35])
3. It avoids the need for expensive and complicated sigh mechanisms seen in some ventilators.

Table 44–11. Guidelines for Ventilator Care*

Inspired O_2 (%)	PEEP (cm H_2O)	PIP (<1500 g) cm H_2O	PIP (>1500 g) cm H_2O	Rate (bpm)
100%	6–8	25–30	25–30	40–60
90%, 80%	5–7	25–30	25–30	40–60
70%, 60%	5	20–25	22–30	35–50
50%	4	20–25	22–30	30–45
40%	3–4	15–20	18–25	20–35
30%	2–3	10–18	15–22	<30 (wean)

*These values are only guidelines that may not be appropriate in all clinical situations. In general, they should be viewed as the maximum necessary levels of support. At the highest support levels, standard positive-pressure ventilation may no longer be appropriate and alternative (high-frequency ventilation, inhaled nitric oxide, extracorporeal membrane oxygenation) should be considered on an individual basis. The reader should also note that the acceptable levels of PIP have been lowered from prior iterations of this chart, because I no longer believe that infants should receive peak pressures > 30 cm H_2O, except in unique cases.

bpm, breaths per minute; PEEP, positive end-expiratory pressure; PIP, peak inspiratory pressure.

4. It has been shown to increase lung volume in infants.
5. There is a decreased need to use muscle relaxants or sedation to prevent patients from fighting the ventilator during weaning.
6. It may assist in coordinating respiratory muscular efforts during weaning.

In practice, however, simply weaning the ventilator rate, especially in infants with low birth weight, does not work well, and it may expose the infant to excessive PIP during weaning. As a result, the approach, as shown in Figure 44-7, advocates decreasing pressure first to a low level (<15 cm H_2O) before SIMV weaning. In this way, the risk of barotrauma and late air leak development is reduced.

Weaning should usually be initiated as soon as possible after the infant has demonstrated stability for at least 4 to 8 hours and when arterial blood gas values suggest that ventilatory needs are decreasing. Before initiation of weaning, a chest radiograph should be obtained as a baseline against which to compare, if problems arise during the weaning process. Pulmonary function testing or examination of graphics monitoring is also very helpful in gauging the capacity for weaning. Increases in compliance and functional residual capacity typically herald recovery from pulmonary disease in the neonate. It has also been demonstrated that, in infants with RDS, a diuretic phase occurs immediately before the improvement in pulmonary mechanics. Thus, an increase in urine output (>3 mL/kg/hour) may be a helpful observation during treatment.[57]

Studies have suggested that even the smallest infants may be weaned from positive-pressure ventilation to nasal CPAP very effectively.[58] Without nasal CPAP, progressive atelectasis often occurs because the very compliant chest wall does not maintain lung volume well in these infants. Nasal CPAP often helps avoid the need for reintubation. Some work has suggested that nasal SIMV may be even more advantageous, but studies thus far are limited.[53] Once extubation is planned, we usually place an infant on nasal CPAP for a minimum of 2 to 3 days. This therapy is usually well tolerated, but the clinician must be attentive to stomach distention and nasal erosion.

During weaning, it is also important to monitor the infant's complete blood cell count; electrolyte, calcium, glucose, and blood urea nitrogen levels; fluid balance; and urine specific gravity. Metabolic disturbances that manifest as abnormalities in these studies may affect weaning rate and prolong duration of support and length of stay. Appropriate caloric balance is also essential for successful weaning. The infant who is nutritionally depleted does not wean or extubate as well as the child who is in positive caloric balance. Calories may be given enterally or parenterally. Intubation has not been a contraindication to feeding in infants with low birth weight. Feeding should always be stopped, however, at least 4 hours before an extubation attempt, or a nasogastric tube should be inserted and the stomach emptied. After extubation, feeding should be withheld for a minimum of 4 to 6 hours.

Extubation

Some clinicians have difficulty managing the patient at the time of extubation. Although ventilator care is often meticulous and thoughtful, extubation often seems to be chaotic and haphazard. The child who is to be extubated should be prepared for the procedure, as with any medical intervention. Extubation is reasonable when the child is receiving less than 40% O_2 and when the ventilator support has decreased to a rate of 10 breaths per minute and a PIP of 10 to 12 cm H_2O. Since the late 1980s, infants have been have rarely allowed to wean to endotracheal tube CPAP alone; we prefer to extubate from a rate of 5 to 10 breaths per minute. In our experience, the child who is intubated but on CPAP of only 2 to 4 cm H_2O expends increased effort in work of breathing that wastes calories and energy unnecessarily. Our success rate has improved with extubation from low-level ventilatory support.

The decision to extubate should be made well in advance of the procedure. A chest radiograph should be obtained before extubation to be certain that a baseline study is available should problems arise after extubation. Radiographs are repeated at 2 and 24 hours after extubation to evaluate atelectasis. Respiratory therapists are notified, and the equipment that is desired after extubation is immediately available. Infants with very low birth weight are usually extubated to a nasal CPAP of 5 to 6 cm H_2O; the child who weighs more than 1000 g is placed in a humidified oxygen hood or provided O_2 through a nasal cannula at the desired concentration. The child is typically treated at first with an O_2 concentration that is 5% above that received while he or she was still mechanically ventilated, until stable.

The child to be extubated should have all facial tape carefully removed so that skin injury to the face can be avoided. The endotracheal tube is connected to a Mapleson bag, and the child is given a prolonged sigh of 15 to 20 cm H_2O while the endotracheal tube is extracted. This sigh prevents negative pressure from developing in the airway, which occurs on tube removal and may cause atelectasis. The infant is then placed in the desired environment (often with nasal CPAP in the case of the infant with very low birth weight) and watched closely for several minutes. Pulse oximetry at this time is invaluable. Oxygen saturation should be kept at a minimum of 92%. Upon extubation, there should be no significant respiratory distress, or it should last only momentarily. Signs of respiratory difficulty include tachypnea, retractions, pallor, cyanosis, agitation, and lethargy. If distress is significant, it is prudent to replace the endotracheal tube and repeat the trial in 2 days. If a child fails two attempts at extubation, we perform flexible fiberoptic bronchoscopy on the infant to be certain that there are no obstructive lesions in the airway. If the result of this study is negative, we initiate dexamethasone treatment (0.5 mg/kg/day in two divided doses beginning 48 hours before extubation, continuing for 24 hours after extubation, if successful) to reduce any airway edema. In addition, methylxanthines, such as caffeine citrate or theophylline, may decrease resistance and increase respiratory drive, enhancing the likelihood of successful extubation. There are no controlled studies that demonstrate the effectiveness of this approach, but the anecdotal findings are that it appears to benefit some children.

If a child cannot be extubated after several repeated attempts, the diagnosis of laryngotracheomalacia must be considered. Some of these infants may not successfully be extubated, and tracheostomy must be considered. I do *not* perform a tracheostomy, however, until it is certain that a child cannot be extubated and that this fact has been demonstrated at least four times over several weeks. Such cases are exceedingly rare.

Accidental extubation occasionally occurs in all nurseries for a variety of reasons. The tape around the endotracheal may loosen, or the movement of the child may free the tube and dislodge it. If extubation occurs, I carefully assess the infant to determine his or her readiness for extubation at the time of the event. If extubation was thought to be days away and the child appears to be exerting excessive effort, the endotracheal tube is immediately replaced. Allowing the child to become unnecessarily distressed at this point further delays ultimate extubation and should be avoided. If the child appears comfortable, however, we monitor pulse oximetry to be sure that the infant remains well oxygenated, and we obtain a chest radiograph and arterial blood gas levels. If these are acceptable, the child can remain extubated with very careful observation.

COMPLICATIONS OF MECHANICAL VENTILATION

The potential complications of neonatal mechanical ventilation are substantial, and a partial list is presented in Table 44-12. Many of these complications can be avoided or minimized with the approaches to care outlined in this chapter. The most commonly seen clinical circumstance that produces immediate concern involves sudden deterioration of an infant on a ventilator. In such circumstances, the child may appear well one moment but rapidly become cyanotic, with pallor, bradycardia, hypotension, and hypercapnia the next. An approach to this situation is shown in Figure 44-8.

If the physician demonstrates that progression of lung disease is the cause of deterioration, then a more advanced form of therapy, such as HFV or ECMO, must be considered. These treatments appear to be effective for some infants who require rescue therapy for severe cardiopulmonary disease. They are discussed in Chapters 45, 46, and 47.

Protective Lung Strategies for the Fetus and Neonate, and Management of Ventilation in the Delivery Room

Effective pulmonary management of the infant with respiratory failure begins during prenatal care and in the delivery room. There is evidence that many premature infant deliveries are the result of maternal chorioamnionitis, which is often accompanied by elevated cytokine production.[59,60] Because tocolytic therapy is required very frequently in premature labor or with premature rupture of membranes, the premature neonate may be exposed in utero to high levels of cytokines or other vasoactive

Table 44–12. Complications of Mechanical Ventilation

Airway injury
Tracheal inflammation
Tracheobronchomalacia
Subglottic stenosis
Granuloma formation
Palatal grooving
Nasal septal injury
Necrotizing tracheobronchitis

Air leaks
Pulmonary interstitial emphysema
Pneumothorax
Pneumomediastinum
Pneumopericardium
Pneumoperitoneum
Hyperinflation

Endotracheal tube complications
Dislodgment
Obstruction
Accidental extubation
Airway erosion

Cardiovascular complications
Decreased cardiac output
Patent ductus arteriosus
Intraventricular hemorrhage

Chronic lung injury
Bronchopulmonary dysplasia
Acquired lobar emphysema

Miscellaneous
Retinopathy of prematurity
Apnea
Infection
Feeding intolerance
Developmental delay

substances, which may make subsequent resuscitation and ventilatory management more difficult.[61,62] The obstetrician therefore has the complex and unenviable task of attempting to decide whether a fetus will do better outside the uterus than if he or she remains inside. To date, there are few data that can successfully answer this thorny question. Clearly, in the presence of evolving infection and fever, or with worsening preeclampsia, delivery of the fetus is essential. But in the afebrile mother who has repeatedly threatened premature labor, no answers currently exist. Is an infant better with aggressive tocolysis at 25 to 26 weeks, or is the long-term risk actually lower ex utero? What about the infant who is beyond 27 to 28 weeks? Where can the line to deliver be successfully drawn, and what are the resulting pulmonary and neurodevelopmental consequences? It is likely that this research issue will be aggressively pursued in the very near future.

The development of adequate pulmonary blood flow, functional residual capacity, and ventilation-perfusion matching, with uniform distribution of lung surfactant,

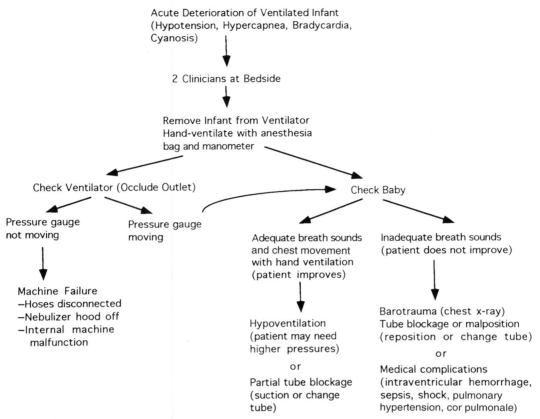

Figure 44–8. Algorithm demonstrating approach to the ventilated infant with sudden, acute deterioration. *(From Gottschalk SK, King B, Schuth CR: Basic concepts in positive pressure ventilation of the newborn. Perinatol Neonatol 4:15, 1980.)*

can be affected by the management in the first few minutes after birth. Animal studies demonstrate that airway and lung parenchymal injury can occur with only a few large breaths at the time of birth.[63-66] This potential injury is exacerbated in the preterm infant, in whom the immature airway structure can be easily disrupted by pressure deformation. The resulting loss in airway integrity can lead to an escalating cycle of airway collapse and distal atelectasis, the need for increased inflation pressures, and further airway injury. Bjorklund and associates demonstrated in an animal model that manual ventilation with only six large tidal breaths after birth can alter lung function.[66] In addition to airway injury, tidal breathing in the delivery room can cause alterations in surfactant function. These changes may result from parenchymal disruption with protein leak and surfactant inactivation.[67,68] Hence, tidal breaths in the delivery room can reduce the efficacy of exogenous surfactant administration, while simultaneously disrupting the integrity of the airway structure and the pulmonary parenchyma. As a result, even in infants shortly after birth, the physician attempting to reduce pulmonary trauma in the neonate may be fighting a losing battle.

The early instillation of exogenous surfactant appears to reduce the lung injury and protein leak associated with preterm delivery.[69] This protection is diminished if this therapy is delayed more than 30 minutes after birth.[70] Although distribution of exogenous surfactant is improved with instillation during the first few minutes after birth, the outcome of infants with very low birth weight is probably improved if instillation is delayed until adequate respiration is established.[71] Our ability to predict infants who will develop respiratory distress syndrome is limited for preterm infants born later in gestation (>32 weeks); therefore, most practices limit the use of prophylactic exogenous surfactant administration to the early-gestation premature infant.

The optimal delivery room management of the preterm neonate would therefore include the gentle establishment of a functional residual capacity and matched pulmonary blood flow, with the even distribution of pulmonary surfactant. These events might be accomplished by the early institution of CPAP or by delivery room initiation of mechanical ventilation with low tidal volumes. The exogenous surfactant can be instilled once the infant is stabilized. Although the institution of mechanical ventilation in the very preterm infant may be necessary, delaying intubation in this population and observing to see whether the infant needs ventilation may not necessarily be detrimental.[72] Newer technology may allow for the early institution of controlled continuous positive airway pressure or HFV soon after birth, necessitating the presence of ventilators in the delivery room. It is becoming increasingly clear, however, that hand ventilation with nonhumidified gas at high inflation pressures in the delivery room is not optimal and may provoke substantial airway injury during neonatal resuscitation. Furthermore, the uncontrolled use of oxygen, a long-term mainstay of resuscitation, has been questioned by studies indicating that room air resuscitation may be advantageous for long-term outcome.[73] To date, no studies have examined room air resuscitation in infants with low birth weight, particularly with regard to pulmonary injury.

Conventional Ventilation

The management of neonatal respiratory failure has changed dramatically since the 1960s. Some of these therapies, such as the use of endogenous surfactant, HFV, and iNO have been shown to diminish mortality or diminish the need for more invasive therapy such as extracorporeal life support.[7,14] Defining specific management strategies to improve outcomes, however, has not been as well documented. It is clear that even slightly different pulmonary approaches, even when utilizing similar medications and ventilators, can result in different outcomes. As a result, the incidence of chronic lung disease varies among different intensive care nurseries.[1,2] Because there are many variables that affect the pulmonary outcome of an infant, determining which factors primarily contribute to these differences is difficult. The multivariate analyses of Van Marter and coworkers,[74] however, suggested that most of the increased risk for chronic lung disease among infants with very low birth weight was explained simply by the decision to initiate mechanical ventilation. Graziani and associates, using regression analysis, also showed that the decision to initiate mechanical ventilation had significant neurologic implications for infants with very low birth weight.[55] Horbar and colleagues also demonstrated that strategies could be effectively changed through a multidisciplinary collaborative quality improvement program, with resultant diminished chronic lung disease.[75]

Optimizing neonatal management includes reducing the ventilator-related lung injury. The specific ventilator variable that induces the greatest injury has remained controversial. As mentioned in the earlier discussion on positive-pressure ventilation outlining the various ventilator approaches, the attempt to completely eliminate lung injury in the neonate has been less than successful. Because it is possible to achieve the same tidal volume, minute ventilation, and gas exchange with different ventilator settings, it is important to try to determine which variable achieves adequate gas exchange with the least potential iatrogenic injury. Animal studies suggest that tidal breathing (volutrauma), as well as ventilating the atelectatic lung (atelectotrauma), cause injury.[76-81] The size of the breath may therefore be more important than the inflating pressure in determining the risk for chronic lung disease. In the atelectatic lung, adequate minute ventilation is achieved by overinflating already expanded lung regions, thereby causing damage to those ventilated

regions. Hence, utilizing an adequate amount of end-expiratory pressure or MAP to optimize alveolar volume recruitment, may diminish lung injury.

Although less information is available on other ventilator controls, for conventional ventilators used to support infants with restrictive lung disease, shorter T_I with more rapid rates and low flow rates (to prevent turbulent gas flow in the airways) appear to be preferable.[82-85] In addition, the use of a disease-specific ventilator approach that changes as the lung mechanics change may be most beneficial. Hence, the concept of patient-triggered ventilation, especially proportional assist ventilation, may prove increasingly useful as experience is gained with that approach.

Advances in technology have allowed the introduction of patient-triggered ventilation and online lung mechanics from conventional ventilators. These advances allow for more accurate monitoring of the infant's status, as well as allowing a wide array of new ventilator modalities such as synchronized, pressure support, proportional assist, and A/C ventilation. In addition, the clinician can utilize the graphics information from several new ventilators to make more rapid changes, thereby reducing injury. These techniques may improve outcomes of infants, although further work on these techniques needs to pursued.[86,87] In addition, new techniques of reducing trauma during conventional ventilation, such as tracheal gas insufflation, continue to be introduced and need more widespread evaluation.[88]

Once an infant is being treated with mechanical ventilation and is stabilized, weaning from the ventilator is always challenging. Mechanical breaths, even at low ventilator settings, can induce lung injury. When the infant finally does begin weaning progressively, the decision to finally remove the mechanical ventilator is also difficult. Both nasal SIMV and variable-flow nasal CPAP may allow small infants to successfully wean off the ventilator more quickly.[35,89]

Approaches to Neonatal Ventilation

The general strategy described in this chapter for mechanical ventilation of the neonate is only one of many approaches to respiratory support of the newborn infant. Numerous other methods that work equally well when used by experienced clinicians have been described in the literature. The number of different strategies has seemingly expanded exponentially, although the evidence supporting one approach over another is very sparse at present. All such techniques, however, are guided by certain basic physiologic principles and consistency of management in an individual nursery. Table 44-13 lists some alternative styles of mechanical ventilation of the newborn and the basic principles on which the techniques are based. These techniques of neonatal ventilation are discussed briefly.

The first systematic approach to mechanical ventilation was devised by Reynolds and Tagizadeh during the early 1970s.[45] This technique, commonly referred to as **slow-rate ventilation**, used a ventilator rate of 20 to 30 breaths per minute and a reversed I/E ratio (2:1 to 4:1) to improve oxygenation. This method did improve oxygenation by

Table 44–13. Historical and New Approaches to Neonatal Mechanical Ventilation

Approach	Rationale	Technique
Slow rate ventilation (Reynolds and Tagizadeh[45])	Improve oxygenation, decrease barotrauma	Rate at 20–30 bpm Increase in MAP with longer T_I, or reversal of I/E ratio
"Gentle ventilation" or permissive hypercapnia (Wung et al[51])	Accept higher $Paco_2$ and lower pH in order to reduce airway and lung injury Focus on adequate oxygenation	Rate of 20–40 bpm, but increase rate preferentially to PIP Keep PIP low, accept $Paco_2$ up to 60 mm Hg, occasionally higher pH can be as low as 7.15–7.20 for brief periods
Rapid rate ventilation (Bland et al[40])	Use rapid rate and hand ventilation to achieve oxygenation at lower PIP Reduce barotrauma, accept some inadvertent PEEP	Rate of 60–80 bpm, higher at times, to maximum of 120–150 bpm Keep low PIP, use shortened T_I
Hyperventilation (Peckham and Fox[21])	Use rapid rate and PIP as necessary to reduce $Paco_2$ to the *highest* level at which oxygenation occurs Reduce right-to-left shunting by decreasing pulmonary artery pressure In general, used to treat PPHN; should be used cautiously in other diseases, because of risk of air leak	Rate of 60–150 bpm Use PIP to reduce $Paco_2$ to 35 mm Hg or less Achieve the *highest* $Paco_2$ that allows oxygenation Periodically challenge infant by decreasing support to see whether PPHN has resolved or transition phase has begun
High-frequency jet ventilation (HFJV) (Spitzer et al[3])	Use rate of 400–500 bpm at reduced pressure in the treatment of severe lung disease or pulmonary air leak Extremely low tidal volume Background sigh used to improve oxygenation	Rate of 400–500 bpm; T_I of 0.02 sec Background sigh rate by conventional ventilator of 5–10 bpm with T_I of 0.5 sec Avoid excessively low $Paco_2$, common in HFJV Maintain alveolar volume with PEEP
High-frequency oscillatory ventilation (HFOV), high-volume strategy (deLemos et al[47])	Use rate of 600–900 bpm with alveolar recruitment technique to increase lung volume Allows use of HFOV with decreased tidal volume and reduces lung injury	Rate of 600–900 bpm Give prolonged inflation periodically with bag and mask or ventilator control to recruit volume in lung Wean by decreasing oscillatory pressure
Patient-triggered ventilation: SIMV and assist/control (Donn and Sinha[8])	Allow patient to trigger and self-regulate (to some extent) level of ventilatory support that is required, thereby reducing barotrauma With SIMV, patient breaths and ventilator breaths are synchronized to avoid "stacking" of pressures and simultaneous patient and ventilator breath With A/C, patient triggers ventilator to deliver all breaths. Both forms have backup rate if patient becomes apneic	SIMV: set ventilator rate at about 40–45 to start; use approach similar to conventional IMV, keeping pressures at a minimum to exchange gas adequately, while reducing barotrauma Assist/control: set PIP and PEEP for adequate gas exchange, allow patient to increase rate of breathing to blow off CO_2 In both cases, give adequate F_{IO_2} to keep Pao_2 at 60–60 mm Hg
Tidal volume–guided ventilation or tidal volume–guaranteed ventilation	Consistent delivery of a uniform minimum tidal volume, while maintaining the ability to set pressure limits	Clinician sets upper limit of pressure and desired V_T; ventilator attempts to deliver guaranteed tidal volume with lowest possible pressure If pressure is inadequate to deliver volume, unit alarms to alert physician to increase pressure limit or lower V_T

Continued

Table 44-13. Historical and New Approaches to Neonatal Mechanical Ventilation—cont'd

Approach	Rationale	Technique
Proportional assist ventilation (PAV) and respiratory muscle unloading (RMU) (*Schulze and Bancalari*[96])	Microprocessor-controlled feedback loop to assist mechanical ventilation Process allows clinician to provide support throughout the ventilatory cycle to ease work of breathing for the infant Ventilator senses flows throughout respiratory cycle	With PAV, desired assist flow above baseline is generated during inspiration to overcome airway and ventilator resistance During RMU, the reverse occurs as circuit pressure falls below baseline and respiratory muscles are unloaded, further easing work of breathing
Tracheal gas insufflation	Provision of fresh gas into the distal tube reduces anatomic dead pace and lowers tidal volume and pressure requirements	Small continuous gas injection into the distal endotracheal tube is given at 0.5 L/min with another form of ventilation simultaneously being used, or with spontaneous breathing on CPAP

bpm, breaths per minute; CPAP, continuous positive airway pressure; FIO_2, fraction of inspired oxygen; I/E, inspiratory to expiratory; IMV, intermittent mandatory ventilation; MAP, mean airway pressure; $Paco_2$, arterial carbon dioxide tension; Pao_2, arterial oxygen tension; PEEP, positive end-expiratory pressure; PIP, peak inspiratory pressure; PPHN, persistent pulmonary hypertension of the newborn; SIMV, synchronized intermittent mandatory ventilation; T_I, inspiratory time; V_T, tidal volume.

increasing MAP, but it also had some associated problems. Air trapping and elevated $Paco_2$ levels were common, and the incidence of intraventricular hemorrhage was much higher than that reported by other investigators. Consequently, this approach soon fell out of favor and, except for rare instances of oxygenation difficulty, is rarely used today.

In the mid-1970s, Bland and coworkers reported on a series of infants treated with more **rapid ventilation**, in whom hand ventilation was often used to improve gas exchange.[40] They used lower pressures but rates of more than 100 breaths per minute in an attempt to decrease the risk of chronic lung disease. This approach was one of the first to emphasize the potential that higher rates and lower pressures might have in reducing lung injury in neonates. The results, although favorable, probably arose from some inadvertent PEEP, and the inconsistency of hand ventilation was unsatisfactory in many nurseries. They did suggest, however, that rapid rates could be successfully used in some infants.

Several years later, Peckham and Fox explored the possibility of using higher rates and pressures to lower the $Paco_2$ and pulmonary vascular resistance intentionally.[21] This **hyperventilation technique** is still used in some nurseries for the treatment of PPHN. Initially, the authors advocated rates as high as 150 breaths per minute, but they subsequently suggested that some of the complications of hyperventilation could be avoided through the use of slower rates (60 breaths per minute) and sufficient PIP to lower the $Paco_2$ to the point at which oxygenation improves. This technique has been criticized as being "overly aggressive" by some clinicians, many of whom fail to understand the goals of therapy. This treatment is

designed to ventilate an infant to the $Paco_2$ level at which adequate oxygenation is first seen (the "critical $Paco_2$"). Many physicians mistakenly believe that simply "cranking up the ventilator" to achieve the lowest $Paco_2$ is the primary goal; this results in needless barotrauma. Of more importance, there is evidence that neurologic injury, especially cerebral palsy and hearing loss, may be more common in infants who are hyperventilated.[30] Because of these risks, I have attempted to use approaches to ventilatory assistance that were less likely to provoke neurologic injury. It cannot be stressed enough that continued use of high pressures for prolonged periods of ventilatory support are associated with pulmonary and central nervous system injury and should be avoided whenever possible. It may be more preferable in many instances for example, to refer an infant for ECMO care—rather than continue high-pressure ventilation.

If it is used at all, hyperventilation should be initiated cautiously in PPHN. Once the rate of 60 breaths per minute is set, the PIP should be increased until the $Paco_2$ begins to fall. At some point, oxygenation suddenly improves. This level is the critical $Paco_2$. The Pao_2 should be kept at approximately 100 to 120 mm Hg to assist in pulmonary vasodilatation. PEEP is usually maintained at 2 to 5 cm H_2O unless the patient also has pneumonitis and volume recruitment within the lung is necessary to sustain oxygenation. Paralysis is sometimes necessary during this phase of illness, although it should be induced judiciously. Paralysis removes the work of breathing contributed by the patient and may result in sudden deterioration of blood gases. If patients appear to be "fighting the ventilator," it is usually the result of hypoxemia or hypercarbia. Improvement in gas exchange through an alternative ventilatory approach often reduces the agitation of the infant, while avoiding paralysis. In addition, external stimulation should be kept to a minimum. Vasopressor agents (dopamine or dobutamine) are often beneficial, and intravenous administration of sodium bicarbonate may help in alkalization. Tolazoline is not generally beneficial, and its use has been abandoned by many clinicians, especially since iNO therapy became available. The adverse effects of systemic vasodilatation and hypotension with tolazoline usually outweigh any pulmonary benefits. The manufacturer has apparently agreed with this concept and has removed it from the market.

Once the infant has been stable for 12 to 24 hours, it is appropriate to challenge the infant by allowing the $Paco_2$ to increase slightly (3 to 5 mm Hg) by decreasing the PIP by 1 to 2 cm H_2O. Excessively large decreases in PIP in the early phases of this disease can often result in sudden, marked deterioration ("flip-flop"), from which recovery is difficult. If oxygenation remains adequate, it is likely that the child has entered the transitional phase of PPHN, and slow, cautious weaning can proceed. Weaning of PIP and Fio_2 should always be in small increments (1 cm H_2O or 2% Fio_2) and infrequent, to avoid flip-flop. The goal should be to have the child receive less than 50% O_2 and a PIP of 25 cm H_2O within 48 hours. Once these levels are reached, management usually poses few difficulties.

The concept of minimizing volutrauma and atelectrauma is best seen in the use of HFV, which often reduces $Paco_2$ with less barotrauma to the airways and lungs. HFV has been well-established as an effective rescue tool for infants requiring high levels of respiratory support in RDS and for infants with pulmonary air leaks.[25,41] My approach since the early 1990s has been to use this ventilatory strategy rather than conventional ventilation with hyperventilation, because of the reduced barotrauma and the improved outcomes. HFV is effective in only 38% of patients with severe PPHN and meconium aspiration, however, which suggests that more than 60% may need either iNO or ECMO.[3] It is possible, however, to learn in 6 hours or less which infant will respond to HFV and which will probably not.[41] It does not appear that conventional ventilation in such circumstances is preferable to HFV or likely to produce better outcomes. The benefit of prophylactic HFV has, however, been demonstrated in several different preterm animal models.[90] Translating this animal work to show effectiveness as a preventive strategy against lung injury in infants, however, has been difficult. This technique has become more complicated by the advances in respiratory therapies that are improving conventional ventilation outcomes. HFV, both HFJV and HFOV, is extremely useful in limiting barotrauma in tiny premature infants. It has been my experience that HFJV is somewhat more useful when air leaks (pneumothorax or pulmonary interstitial emphysema) are present, whereas HFOV may be slightly more advantageous in situations of oxygenation difficulties. Both units are extremely effective, however, when used appropriately. It is, as yet, unclear that HFV is the treatment of choice in early, uncomplicated RDS in infants with extremely low birth weight. Some studies

have suggested a greater likelihood of neurologic injury when HFV is used early in the course of illness, rather than as a rescue therapy for air leak or high levels of conventional ventilator support, although a more recent trial was far more encouraging in this regard.[91,92] At present, it appears that HFV should be used primarily as a rescue modality for complications of more standard positive-pressure ventilation.

The introduction and the U.S. Food and Drug Administration's approval of iNO as an adjunct to therapy in PPHN has been shown to be beneficial in some cases of PPHN (see Chapter 39), but it does not appear to have a significant lung protective role, inasmuch as it is typically used only when there is already some evidence of airway and lung injury.[6] Nitric oxide acts as a direct pulmonary vasodilator when given through a separate circuit to the patient on a ventilator. It appears to work most effectively in PPHN syndromes with little debris in the airway. Meconium aspiration syndrome with PPHN seems to respond more poorly than the "pure" forms of pulmonary hypertension. Approximately 30% to 40% of infants with PPHN respond to this therapy, and ECMO may be avoided in a number of situations. Some studies have also suggested a benefit in oxygenation for the premature infant with RDS, a lung disease that always has some element of increased pulmonary vascular resistance.[93] In premature infants, however, there may be some adverse consequences in terms of cerebral vasodilatation and intracranial hemorrhage, although long-term outcome does not appear to be adversely influenced in any way in the few studies described to date.[94,95] Currently, iNO is not approved for any use in the neonate other than PPHN, and further studies in the premature population are needed before any clear recommendation can be made regarding its use. Arterial oxygenation appears to improve rapidly, even at nitric oxide concentrations as low as 1 to 2 ppm. The treatment currently is very expensive, however, and not approved for the infant with RDS or in any form of prophylactic care. As a result, iNO has little role as a lung protective strategy in infants with very low birth weight. Of perhaps greater concern is the excessively prolonged use of iNO in an attempt to avoid ECMO in the most severely affected larger patients. In these instances, iNO may actually increase exposure to high ventilator pressures, prolong the ultimate length of stay, increase the risk of BPD, and be associated with a higher likelihood of neurologic injury. Infants should respond rapidly to iNO or they should be referred to an experienced ECMO center in order to avoid these injuries.

In contrast to hyperventilation, Wung and coworkers at Babies Hospital in New York introduced the concept of **gentle ventilation** in the mid-1980s.[51] They advocated the use of rates of 20 to 40 breaths per minute and sufficient pressures to allow adequate oxygenation while tolerating a $Paco_2$ that was as high as 60 to 70 mm Hg, rather than injure the lung by using higher pressures. If $Paco_2$ could not be controlled, they recommended the use of more rapid rates (120 to 140 breaths per minute) to try to decrease $Paco_2$. If this attempt failed, they suggested returning to the previous lower rates. The pH in this system was sometimes kept at low levels (to 7.15) for periods of time as long as 24 hours. Weaning was accomplished with reduction in pressures as the infant's status improved. The results appear to be comparable with those from hyperventilation, but with the added benefit of less chronic lung injury in the patient with PPHN. The use of this technique in premature infants with RDS has also been reported, with an incidence of BPD that is very low (approximately 5%).[1] Wung and coworkers suggested that the use of this approach may further decrease the need for ECMO in PPHN. The number of infants actually described in the medical literature managed with this approach to date has been small, however, and follow-up data on the results of this approach are still very limited. In certain nurseries, it does appear that "gentle ventilation" is a valuable tool for some infants with severe respiratory disease. What Wung and coworkers demonstrated, is that the lungs of a critically ill neonate are fragile and need to be treated as such. Furthermore, their approach has shown neonatologists that tolerance of slightly higher CO_2 levels is preferable to continued battering of the lung with high-pressure ventilation.

The concept of "gentile ventilation" illustrates one of the most confusing aspects of managing respiratory distress in the newborn: namely, when, and to what degree, to intervene. The introduction of mechanical ventilation is potentially detrimental, and deciding to place an infant on mechanical ventilator support remains a difficult decision. In addition, determining what measurements (e.g., blood gases, graphics monitoring) should guide ventilator changes remains unclear. Permissive hypercapnia in preterm infants seems safe and may reduce the duration of assisted ventilation.[28] This strategy has particular appeal in that hypocarbia may be related to brain injury.[19,95] Severe hypercarbia may also cause brain injury, however, which strongly suggests that there are excellent physiologic reasons why nature has seen fit to establish eucapnic ventilation as the normal range.[27] When a strategy of permissive hypercapnia is used, it is important to minimize atelectasis, as the recruitment and derecruitment of lung regions are not optimal. In addition, although data look promising when this strategy is implemented, long-term follow-up of infants managed with high CO_2 levels has not been explored.

Patient-triggered ventilation, as previously indicated, has now become a very standard part of the repertoire of neonatologists. In general, patient-triggered ventilation consists of two forms of mechanical ventilation: SIMV and A/C. With SIMV, the ventilator is synchronized to the infant's breathing pattern. If the patient-triggering threshold is met within a specific time window (depending on the preset ventilator rate), a ventilator breath is not delivered and the infant breathes spontaneously. On the other hand, a ventilator breath is delivered if the infant fails to breathe. Examination of the infant's breathing pattern with SIMV therefore reveals both spontaneous breaths and ventilator breaths. The value of this form of support is that pressures within the airway are not stacked, so that airway and lung injury are theoretically reduced, and gas is not inadvertently "dumped" from the ventilator because airway pressures are reached prematurely. Although for many neonatologists SIMV is the

primary mode of ventilator support for neonates, it appears to have greater benefit as a weaning tool or if overdistention is present with A/C, particularly in infants with extremely low birth weight who have either RDS or pulmonary insufficiency of prematurity.

A/C ventilation is also a form of patient-triggered support. With A/C, each infant breath that reaches the trigger threshold initiates a full ventilator breath. If the infant is apneic, or the effort is inadequate to trigger a ventilator breath, the ventilator delivers a preset backup rate to the infant. All breaths in this form of ventilation therefore appear similar and are entirely ventilator derived, and no spontaneous infant breaths ever occur on A/C support (unless the generated pressure is so low that it fails to trigger the ventilator). With A/C, the infant is fully synchronized to the ventilator. With the use of termination sensitivity as an adjunct, T_I is limited to a percentage of maximum flow and air trapping can usually be reduced or eliminated.

A/C is a very effective form of initial treatment for many infants in the early stages of a variety of neonatal lung diseases. It has been my experience that the use of A/C limits pressure exposure for the infant, and I often select a rate with a lower pressure than would usually be set on SIMV. Minute ventilation is higher on A/C than on SIMV.[26] It is more difficult, however, to wean infants from A/C, some overdistention occasionally occurs if there is excessive neural drive to breathe, and prolonged use of A/C may lead to some diaphragmatic muscle atrophy and further weaning difficulty. Consequently, we often move an infant from A/C to SIMV when the infant begins to show signs of recovery from the lung disease. With A/C, physicians must also be cautious of "autocycling" of the ventilator. This problem can occur when there is erroneous triggering of the ventilator from leaks in the system, buildup of humidity in the circuit, or sensing of the cardiac pulsations as breaths. Frequent breaths are delivered unnecessarily to the infant. We have also seen an occasional infant on A/C support who does well while awake, with good gas exchange, but has inadequate blood gases while sleeping or if sedated. In such cases, it would be helpful to have the capability of utilizing two separate ventilator settings, one for waking periods and one during apneic support when slightly more pressure may be necessary for gas exchange. To date, however, no neonatal ventilator has the capability of selecting multiple ventilator settings simultaneously that could be triggered automatically under selected conditions.

An adjunct therapy during patient-triggered ventilation is **pressure support ventilation**, in which spontaneous infant breaths are partially or fully augmented by an inspiratory pressure assist above baseline PEEP. This modification eases the work of breathing by allowing additional pressure delivery to overcome the various sources of resistance encountered by the infant (e.g., endotracheal tube, circuitry, valves). This form of therapy may be used alone or, more commonly, in association with SIMV ventilation. Because it is fully synchronized with the infant's ventilation, it can be used to treat infants who are becoming fatigued from work of breathing, for sedated infants, and for infants in a weaning phase of ventilation who are first beginning to reuse their respiratory musculature. When used in conjunction with SIMV, it is important that the SIMV rate is not set too high; otherwise, the infant has no impetus to breathe, and one of the primary purposes of pressure support is nullified.

Tidal volume–guided ventilation or **volume-guaranteed ventilation** is a new approach to therapy in which the clinician sets a mean tidal volume to be delivered by the ventilator, while still allowing management of ventilator pressures. It is, in essence, a variation of pressure support ventilation, in which volume, not pressure, guides the delivery of an augmented breath. The goal in this form of ventilation is to minimize variation in delivery of tidal volume, thought to be the cause of pulmonary barotrauma in many infants. Volume guarantee is available on the Drager Babylog 8000 ventilator and is used in conjunction with patient-triggered modalities. When the physician sets the upper limit of PIP during patient-triggered support, the ventilator attempts to deliver the set guaranteed tidal volume, using the lowest airway pressure possible. When the expired tidal volume exceeds the upper limit PIP, the ventilator uses a lower PIP on the next breath. If the set tidal volume cannot be delivered within the PIP set by the clinician, an alarm alerts the operator to reset the PIP to a higher level or to adjust the guaranteed tidal volume to a lower level. Although data to date are not substantial, it does appear that volume guarantee can achieve similar levels of gas exchange with slightly lower mean levels of PIP.[14] Further refinement of this patient-triggered approach is likely in the near future. Additional modifications may occur, such as guaranteed minute ventilation, in which a desired minute ventilation is designated, with the ventilator providing a mix of guaranteed tidal volume and frequency to provide the desired minute ventilation.

PAV and RMU require even more sophisticated computer assistance to achieve their effects. These innovative approaches control, through a servo, ventilator pressure throughout inspiration (in the case of PAV) or throughout the entire respiratory cycle (during RMU). With both forms of ventilator support, the infant's respiratory effort is continuously monitored. During inspiration, as with pressure support ventilation, pressure rises above baseline to produce the desired inspiratory resistive unloading, thereby easing work of breathing. During exhalation, circuit pressure falls below baseline end-distending pressure, facilitating elastic and resistive unloading throughout that phase of the respiratory cycle (Figs. 44-9 and 44-10). With this form of support, the resulting airway pressure is a moving variable that changes with the needs of the infant at any point during the respiratory cycle and is a weighted summation of a combination of airflow and tidal volume above the baseline (usually PEEP) level. Although human infant studies with PAV and RMU are somewhat limited at present, work from Schulze and Bancalari and colleagues appear very encouraging.[9,19,96] In a trial that examined the relative effects on infants with low birth weight treated with IMV, A/C, and PAV, PAV appeared to maintain equivalent arterial oxygenation at lower airway and transpulmonary pressures than did the other two modalities. During PAV, the oxygenation index was also reduced by 28%, with no evidence of more frequent apnea or other complications. An intriguing finding was a decrease in both systolic and diastolic beat-to-beat variability with PAV, which suggested that additional overall cardiovascular stability is offered to infants treated with this form of support. Furthermore, a more recent study indicated that there was less thoracoabdominal synchrony during PAV in preterm infants.[97] Currently, few centers use this form of ventilatory support, because it is

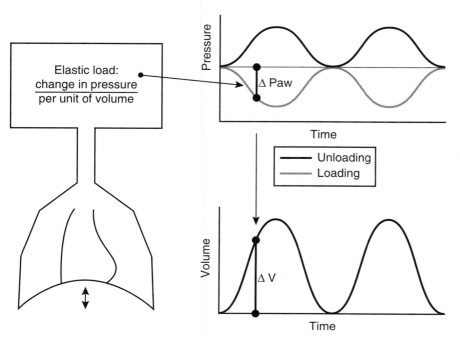

Figure 44–9. Mechanical model of respiratory elastic loading and unloading during the respiratory cycle. Airflow increases during inspiratory to augment the breath and reduce the work of breathing for the infant. Δ Paw, change in peak airway pressure; Δ V, change in volume. *(From Schulze A, Bancalari E: Proportional assist ventilation in infants. Clin Perinatol 28:561, 2001.)*

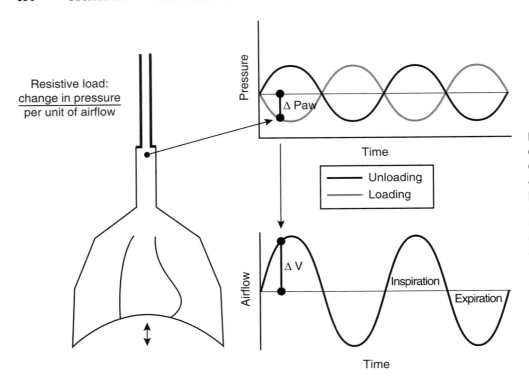

Figure 44–10. Mechanical model of resistive loading and unloading during the respiratory cycle. ΔPaw, change in peak airway pressure; ΔV, change in volume. *(From Schulze A, Bancalari E: Proportional assist ventilation in infants. Clin Perinatol 28:561, 2001.)*

Resistive load:
change in pressure
per unit of airflow

Pressure

ΔPaw

Time

Unloading
Loading

Airflow

ΔV

Inspiration
Expiration

Time

still in early trials, but the concepts appear very promising. Additional larger scale trials will unquestionably be conducted in the very near future.

The added space of the ventilator adaptor and the endotracheal tube add a significant amount of anatomic dead space during mechanical ventilation, particularly to the airway of an infant with an extremely low birth weight (<1000 g). Through a mechanism of tracheal gas insufflation, fresh gas is delivered to the more distal part of the endotracheal tube and aids in washing out CO_2 from the airway. PIP can usually be decreased, as can tidal volume.[33] These factors may reduce barotrauma and volutrauma in these infants, and early trials appear promising.

COMMENTARY

Respiratory insufficiency remains a frequent and challenging complication of birth. Managing the pulmonary status of a sick neonate is a great responsibility. The decision to place an infant on respiratory support and the selection of appropriate ventilator settings should be made with an understanding of the ramifications of those decisions. When many breaths are imposed on an infant each minute, even small deviations from perfection can be significant and potentially catastrophic, in terms of both lung injury and long-term neurologic impairment. There is evidence that despite advances in technology, length of hospital stay for the preterm population has begun to increase, and BPD remains a complication of significance in every nursery.

As is evident from much of this discussion, the technologic innovations in positive-pressure ventilation have been quite substantial and, no doubt, confusing to many

neonatologists. There are likely to be even more in the future, as computer technology becomes even faster in execution speed. Although many of these techniques may offer theoretical benefits to infants, actual demonstration of substantial clinical value has been quite sparse in many cases. Moreover, some approaches are so new that they have been limited to small pilot trials thus far. The clinician should always keep in mind that most infants with lung disease can be very successfully ventilated with standard positive-pressure ventilators without all the investigative modifications or without bells and whistles. In the care of an extremely premature infant whose lungs are never supposed to undergo positive-pressure ventilation (or even air breathing) at such an early stage of development, it may simply not be possible to limit the pulmonary injury that occurs in many infants. In addition, no approach to ventilatory support should ever be used unless the physician is well aware of the potential risks, both acute and long-term, especially with regard to neurologic injury and neurodevelopmental handicap. In my work over many years, the follow-up of our patients has been instrumental in allowing us to work to improve outcomes. Although this information was occasionally disappointing to us at first, the obligation to publish this work and consider alternatives has been important in our own education and, we hope, to other clinicians. We therefore believe that all neonatologists have an obligation to examine their infants carefully and publish their findings, so that others can benefit from their accomplishments as well as from their errors. No approach to respiratory support is complete without such information.

Although studies will ultimately help to frame a preferred sequence of ventilators, modalities, and therapies that provide optimal lung protection for a general population of infants, the care will always need to be individualized. No neonate is supposed to have gas forced into the lungs under positive pressure, and all ventilators therefore represent a paradox: they keep infants alive, but at some cost to the infant. As physicians continue to undertake the care of ever tinier and more fragile infants, as well as larger infants with pulmonary insufficiency, they will continue to have infants who manifest many long-term problems. Ultimately, optimal pulmonary outcomes can be achieved only when it can be guaranteed that neurodevelopmental outcomes will be as good as possible.

REFERENCES

1. Greenough A, Milner AD, Dimitriou G: Synchronized mechanical ventilation for respiratory support in newborn infants. Cochrane Database Syst Rev (1):CD000456, 2001.
2. Abubakar KM, Keszler M: Patient-ventilator interactions in new modes of patient-triggered ventilation. Pediatr Pulmonol 32:71, 2001.
3. Spitzer AR, Butler S, Fox WW: Ventilatory response of combined high frequency jet ventilation and conventional mechanical ventilation for the rescue treatment of severe neonatal lung disease. Pediatr Pulmonol 7:244, 1989.
4. Baumgart S, Hirschl RB, Butler SZ, et al: Diagnosis-related criteria in the consideration of extracorporeal membrane oxygenation in neonates previously treated with high frequency jet ventilation. Pediatrics 89:491, 1992.
5. Bhuta T, Clark RH, Henderson-Smart DJ: Rescue high frequency oscillatory ventilation vs conventional ventilation for infants with severe pulmonary dysfunction born at or near term. Cochrane Database Syst Rev (1):CD002974, 2001.
6. Finer NN, Barrington KJ: Nitric oxide for respiratory failure in infants born at or near term. Cochrane Database Syst Rev (2):CD000399, 2001.
7. Hintz SR, Suttner DM, Sheehan AM, et al: Decreased use of neonatal extracorporeal membrane oxygenation (ECMO): How new treatment modalities have affected ECMO utilization. Pediatrics 106:1339, 2000.
8. Donn SM, Sinha SK: Newer modes of mechanical ventilation for the neonate. Curr Opin Pediatr 13:99, 2001.
9. Schulze A, Gerhardt T, Musante G, et al: Proportional assist ventilation in low birth weight infants with acute respiratory disease: A comparison to assist/control and conventional mechanical ventilation. J Pediatr 135:339, 1999.
10. Sinha SK, Donn SM, Gavey J, McCarty M: Randomised trial of volume controlled versus time cycled, pressure limited ventilation in preterm infants with respiratory distress syndrome. Arch Dis Child Fetal Neonatal Ed 77:F202, 1997.
11. Dreyfuss D, Saumon G: Barotrauma is volutrauma, but which volume is the one responsible? Intensive Care Med 18:139, 1992.
12. Gannon CM, Wiswell TE, Spitzer AR: Volutrauma, $PaCO_2$ levels, and neurodevelopmental sequelae following assisted ventilation. Clin Perinatol 25:159, 1998.
13. Ratner I, Hernandez J, Accurso F: Low peak inspiratory pressures for ventilation of infants with hyaline membrane disease. J Pediatr 100:801, 1982.
14. Cheema IU, Ahluwahia JS: Feasibility of tidal volume-guided ventilation in newborn infants: A randomized, crossover trial using the volume guarantee modality. Pediatrics 107:1323, 2001.
15. Truog WE, Jackson LC: Alternative modes of ventilation in the prevention and treatment of bronchopulmonary dysplasia. Clin Perinatol 19:621, 1992.
16. Boros SJ, Bing BR, Mammel MC, et al: Using conventional ventilators at unconventional rates. Pediatrics 74:487, 1984.
17. Hanson JB, Waldstein G, Hernandez JA, et al: Necrotizing tracheobronchitis: An ischemic lesion. Am J Dis Child 142:1094, 1988.
18. Greenspan JS, DeGuilio PA, Bhutani VK, et al: Airway reactivity as determined by a cold air challenge in infants with bronchopulmonary dysplasia. J Pediatr 114:452, 1988.
19. Schulze A: Enhancement of mechanical ventilation of neonates by computer technology. Semin Perinatol 24:429, 2000.
20. Kapasi M, Fujino Y, Kirmse M, et al: Effort and work of breathing in neonates during assisted patient-triggered ventilation. Pediatr Crit Care Med 2:9, 2001.
21. Peckham GJ, Fox WW: Physiologic factors affecting pulmonary artery pressure in infants with persistent pulmonary hypertension. J Pediatr 93:1005, 1978.
22. Cunningham S, McColm JR, Wade J, et al: A novel model of retinopathy of prematurity simulating preterm oxygen variability in the rat. Invest Ophthalmol Vis Sci 41:4275, 2000.
23. STOP-ROP Study Group: Supplemental Therapeutic Oxygen for Prethreshold Retinopathy Of Prematurity (STOP-ROP), a randomized, controlled trial. I: Primary outcomes. Pediatrics 105:295, 2000.
24. Jobe AH, Ikegami M: Prevention of bronchopulmonary dysplasia. Curr Opin Pediatr 13:124, 2001.
25. Keszler M, Donn SM, Bucciarelli RL, et al: Multicenter controlled trial comparing high-frequency jet ventilation and conventional mechanical ventilation in newborn infants with pulmonary interstitial emphysema. J Pediatr 119:85, 1991.
26. Mrozek JD, Bendel-Stenzel EM, Meyers PA, et al: Randomized controlled trial of volume-targeted synchronized ventilation and conventional intermittent mandatory ventilation following initial exogenous surfactant therapy. Pediatr Pulmonol 29:11, 2000.
27. Vannucci RC, Towfighi J, Brucklacher RM, Vannucci SJ: Effect of extreme hypercapnia on hypoxic-ischemic brain damage in the immature rat. Pediatr Res 49:799, 2001.
28. Mariani G, Cifuentes J, Carlo WA: Randomized trial of permissive hypercapnia in preterm infants. Pediatrics 104:1082, 1999.
29. Woodgate PG, Davies MW: Permissive hypercapnia for the prevention of morbidity and mortality in mechanically ventilated newborn infants. Cochrane Database Syst Rev (2):CD002061, 2001.
30. Graziani LJ, Desai S, Baumgart S, et al: Clinical antecedents of neurologic and audiologic abnormalities in survivors of neonatal ECMO—a group comparison study. J Child Neurol 12:415, 1997.
31. Gregory GA, Kitterman JA, Phibbs RH, et al: Treatment of the idiopathic respiratory-distress syndrome with continuous positive airway pressure. N Engl J Med 284:1333, 1971.
32. De Klerk A, De Klerk R: Nasal continuous positive airway pressure and outcomes of preterm infants. J Paediatr Child Health 37:161, 2001.
33. Lemyre B, Davis PG, De Paoli AG: Nasal intermittent positive pressure ventilation (NIPPV) versus nasal continuous positive airway pressure (NCPAP) for apnea of prematurity. Cochrane Database Syst Rev (3):CD002272, 2000.
34. Davis PG, Henderson-Smart DJ: Nasal continuous positive airways pressure immediately after extubation for preventing morbidity in preterm infants. Cochrane Database Syst Rev (3):CD000143, 2000.

35. Courtney SE, Pyon KH, Saslow JG, et al: Lung recruitment and breathing pattern during variable versus continuous flow nasal continuous positive airway pressure in premature infants: An evaluation of three devices. Pediatrics 107:304, 2001.

36. Bonta BW, Vavy R, Warshaw JB, et al: Determination of optimal continuous airway pressure for the treatment of RDS by measurement of esophageal pressure. J Pediatr 91:449, 1977.

37. Stenson BJ, Glover RM, Wilkie RA, et al: Life-threatening inadvertent positive end-expiratory pressure. Am J Perinatol 12:336, 1995.

38. da Silva WJ, Abbasi S, Pereira G, Bhutani VK: Role of positive end-expiratory pressure changes on functional residual capacity in surfactant treated preterm infants. Pediatr Pulmonol 18:89, 1994.

39. Fox WW, Berman LS, Dinwiddie R, et al: Tracheal extubation of the neonate at 2-3 cm H_2O continuous positive airway pressure. Pediatrics 59:257, 1977.

40. Bland RD, Kim MH, Light MJ, et al: High frequency mechanical ventilation in severe hyaline membrane disease. An alternative treatment? Crit Care Med 8:275, 1980.

41. Haman S, Reynolds EOR: Methods of improving oxygenation in infants mechanically ventilated for severe hyaline membrane disease. Arch Dis Child 48:617, 1973.

42. Boros SJ: Variations in inspiratory-expiratory ratio and air pressure wave form during mechanical ventilation: The significance of mean airway pressure. J Pediatr 94:114, 1979.

43. Simbruner G, Gregory GA: Performance of neonatal ventilators: The effects of changes in resistance and compliance. Crit Care Med 9:509, 1981.

44. Kirby R, Robinson EJ, Schulz J, et al: Continuous flow ventilation as an alternative to assisted or controlled ventilation in infants. Anesth Analg 51:871, 1971.

45. Reynolds EOR, Tagizadeh A: Improved prognosis of infants mechanically ventilated for hyaline membrane disease. Arch Dis Child 49:505, 1974.

46. Boros SJ, Mabaln SV, Ewald R, et al: The effect of independent variations in inspiratory-expiratory ratio and end expiratory pressure during mechanical ventilation in hyaline membrane disease: The significance of mean airway pressure. J Pediatr 91:794, 1977.

47. Meredith KS, deLemos RA, Coalson JJ, et al: Role of lung injury in the pathogenesis of hyaline membrane disease in premature baboons. J Appl Physiol 66:2150, 1989.

48. Bond DM, McAloon J, Froese AB: Sustained inflations improve respiratory compliance during high-frequency oscillatory ventilation but not during large tidal volume positive-pressure ventilation in rabbits. Crit Care Med 22:1269, 1994.

49. Goldsmith LS, Greenspan JS, Rubinstein SD, et al: Immediate improvement in lung volume after exogenous surfactant: Alveolar recruitment versus increased distension. J Pediatr 119:424, 1991.

50. Soll RF: Prophylactic synthetic surfactant for preventing morbidity and mortality in preterm infants. Cochrane Database Syst Rev (2):CD001079, 2000.

51. Wung JT, James LS, Kilchevsky E, James E: Management of infants with severe respiratory failure and persistence of the fetal circulation, without hyperventilation. Pediatrics 76:488, 1985.

52. Yost CC, Soll RF: Early versus delayed selective surfactant treatment for neonatal respiratory distress syndrome. Cochrane Database Syst Rev (2):CD001456, 2000.

53. Wiswell TE: Advances in the treatment of the meconium aspiration syndrome. Acta Paediatr Suppl 90:28, 2001.

54. Herting E, Rauprich P, Stichtenoth G, et al.: Resistance of different surfactant preparations to inactivation by meconium. Pediatr Res 50:44, 2001.

55. Graziani LJ, Spitzer AR, Mitchell DG, et al: Mechanical ventilation in preterm infants: Neurosonographic and developmental studies. Pediatrics 90:515, 1992.

56. Riou Y, Storme L, Leclerc F, et al: Comparison of four methods for measuring elevation of FRC in mechanically ventilated infants. Intensive Care Med 25:1118, 1999.

57. Spitzer AR, Fox WW, Delivoria-Papadopoulos M: Maximal diuresis—a factor in predicting recovery from RDS and the development of bronchopulmonary dysplasia. J Pediatr 98:476, 1981.

58. Higgins RD, Richter SE, Davis JM: Nasal continuous positive airway pressure facilitates extubation of very low birth weight neonates. Pediatrics 88:999, 1991.

59. Vigneswaran R: Infection and preterm birth: Evidence of a common causal relationship with bronchopulmonary dysplasia and cerebral palsy. J Paediatr Child Health 36:293, 2000.

60. Krohn MA, Hitti J: Characteristics of women with clinical intra-amniotic infection who deliver preterm compared with term. Am J Epidemiol 147:111, 1998.

61. Kashlan F, Smulian J, Shen-Schwarz S, et al: Umbilical vein interleukin 6 and tumor necrosis factor alpha plasma concentrations in the very preterm infant. Pediatr Infect Dis J 19:238, 2000.

62. Baud O, Emilie D, Pelletier E, et al: Amniotic fluid concentrations of interleukin-1beta, interleukin-6 and TNF-alpha in chorioamnionitis before 32 weeks of gestation: Histological associations and neonatal outcome. Br J Obstet Gynaecol 106:72, 1999.

63. Panitch HB, Deoras KS, Wolfson MR, Shaffer TH: Functional changes in airway smooth muscle structure-function relationships. Pediatr Res 31:151, 1992.

64. Bhutani VK, Rubenstein D, Shaffer TH: Effect of positive pressure on the mechanical behavior of the developing rabbit trachea. Pediatr. Res 15:829, 1981.

65. Shaffer TH, Bhutani VK, Wolfson MR, Tran NN: In-vivo mechanical properties of the developing airway. Pediatr Res 25:143, 1989.

66. Bjorklund LJ, Ingimarsson J, Curstedt T, et al: Manual ventilation with a few large breaths at birth compromises the therapeutic effect of subsequent surfactant replacement in immature lambs. Pediatr Res 42:348, 1997.

67. Berry D, Jobe A, Ikegami M: Leakage of macromolecules in ventilated and unventilated segments of preterm lamb lungs. J Appl Physiol 70:423, 1991.

68. Nilsson R, Grossmann G, Robertson B: Lung surfactant and the pathogenesis of neonatal bronchiolar lesions induced by artificial ventilation. Pediatr Res 12:249, 1978.

69. Seidner SR, Ikegami M, Yamada T, et al: Decreased surfactant dose-response after delayed administration to preterm rabbits. Am J Respir Crit Care Med 152:113, 1995.

70. Kendig JW, Notter RH, Cox C, et al: A comparison of surfactant as immediate prophylaxis and as rescue therapy in newborns of less than 30 weeks gestation. N Engl J Med 324:865, 1991.

71. Soll RF: Clinical trials of surfactant therapy in the newborn. In Robertson B, Taeusch HW (eds): Surfactant Therapy for Lung Disease. New York, Marcel Dekker, 1995, pp 407-422.

72. Linder W, Vofsbeck S, Hummler H, Pohlandt F: Delivery room management of extremely low birth weight infant: Spontaneous breathing or intubation? Pediatrics 103:961, 1999.

73. Vento M, Asensi M, Sastre J, et al.: Resuscitation with room air instead of 100% oxygen prevents oxidative stress in moderately asphyxiated term neonates. Pediatrics 107:642, 2001.

74. Van Marter LJ, Allred EN, Pagano M, et al: Do clinical markers of barotrauma and oxygen toxicity explain interhospital variation in rates of chronic lung disease? The Neonatology Committee for the Developmental Network. Pediatrics 105:1194, 2000.

75. Horbar JD, Rogowski J, Plsek PE, et al: Collaborative quality improvement for neonatal intensive care. Pediatrics 107:14, 2001.

76. Jobe A, Ikegami M: Mechanisms initiating lung injury in the preterm. Early Hum Dev 53:81, 1998.

77. Dreyfuss D, Saumon G: Role of tidal volume, FRC, and end-inspiratory volume in the development of pulmonary edema following mechanical ventilation. Am Rev Respir Dis 148:1194, 1993.

78. Slutsky AS: Lung injury caused by mechanical ventilation. Chest 116(Suppl):9S, 1999.

79. Muscedere JG, Mullen JB, Gan K, Slutsky AS: Tidal ventilation at low airway pressures can augment lung injury. Am J Respir Crit Care Med 149:1327, 1994.

80. Heicher DA, Kasting DS, Harrod JR: Prospective clinical comparison of two methods for mechanical ventilation of the neonate: Rapid rate and short inspiratory time versus slow rate and long inspiratory time. J Pediatr 98:957, 1981.

81. Clark RH, Slutsky AS, Gerstmann DR: Commentary: Lung protective strategies of ventilation in the neonate: What are they? Pediatrics 105:112, 2000.

82. Oxford Region Controlled Trial of Artificial Ventilation (OCTAVE): Multi-centre randomised controlled trial of high versus low frequency positive pressure ventilation in 346 newborn infants. Arch Dis Child 66:770, 1991.

83. Greenough A, Pool J, Gamsu H: Randomized controlled trial of two methods of weaning from high frequency positive pressure ventilation. Arch Dis Child 64:834, 1989.

84. Spahr RC, Klein AM, Brown DR, et al: Hyaline membrane disease: A controlled study of inspiratory to expiratory ratio in its management by ventilator. Am J Dis Child 134:373, 1980.

85. Bernstein G, Marnnion FL, Heldt GP, et al: Randomized multicenter trial comparing synchronized conventional intermittent mandatory ventilation in neonates. J Pediatr 128:453, 1996.

86. DeBoer RC, Ansari NA, Baumer JH, et al: Mode of ventilation in neonatal RDS: Effect on the stress response. Prenatal Neonatal Med 1:266, 1996.

87. Nicks JJ, Becker MA, Donn SM: Bronchopulmonary dysplasia: Response to pressure support ventilation. J Perinatol 14:495, 1994.

88. Oliver RE, Rozycki HJ, Greenspan JS, et al: Tracheal gas insufflation (TGI) as a lung protective strategy: Physiologic, histologic, and biochemical markers. Pediatr Res 49:272A, 2001.

89. Barrington KJ, Bull D, Finer N: Randomized trial of nasal synchronized intermittent mandatory ventilation compared to continuous positive airway pressure after extubation of very low birth weight infants. Pediatrics 107:638, 2001.

90. deLemos RA, Coalson JJ, Gerstmann DR, et al: Ventilatory management of infant baboons with hyaline membrane disease: The use of high frequency ventilation. Pediatr Res 21:594, 1987.

91. The HIFI Group: A collaborative randomized trial of high frequency oscillatory ventilation versus conventional mechanical ventilation in the treatment of respiratory failure in preterm infants. N Engl J Med 320:88, 1989.

92. Courtney SE, Durand DJ, Asselin JM, The Neonatal Ventilation Study Group: Early high frequency oscillatory ventilation (HFOV) vs synchronized intermittent mandatory ventilation (SIMV) in very low birth weight (VLBW) infants. Pediatr Res 49:387A, 2001.

93. Hoehn T, Krause MF, Buhrer C: Inhaled nitric oxide in premature infants—a meta-analysis. J Perinat Med 28:7, 2000.

94. Bennett AJ, Shaw NJ, Gregg JE, Subhedar NV: Neurodevelopmental outcome in high-risk preterm infants treated with inhaled nitric oxide. Acta Paediatr 90:573, 2001.

95. Wiswell TE, Graziani LJ, Kornhauser MS, et al: Effects of hypocarbia on the development of cystic periventricular leukomalacia in premature infants treated with high-frequency ventilation. Pediatrics 98:918, 1996.

96. Schulze A, Bancalari E: Proportional assist ventilation in infants. Clin Perinatol 28:561, 2001.

97. Musante G, Schulze A, Gerhardt T, et al: Proportional assist ventilation decreases thoracoabdominal asynchrony and chest wall distortion in preterm infants. Pediatr Res 49:175, 2001.

CHAPTER 45

High-Frequency Jet Ventilation

Martin Keszler

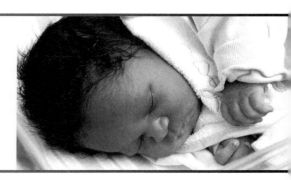

Despite advances in obstetric care and increased use of antenatal steroids and surfactant replacement therapy, treatment of respiratory failure continues to present significant challenges. Although death from respiratory failure is now uncommon, the incidence of chronic lung disease remains unacceptably high.

Because chronic lung disease is one of the leading causes of prolonged hospitalization and significant respiratory and developmental disabilities, many approaches in modern neonatal care have focused on methods that might reduce the incidence of this dreaded complication. **High-frequency ventilation (HFV)** seemed to hold much promise in this area, as a result of its ability to provide excellent gas exchange with lower pressure amplitude. By 2000, **high-frequency jet ventilation (HFJV)** had firmly established itself as an important tool in the therapeutic armamentarium of neonatologists. Despite more than 20 years of laboratory and clinical research and several hundred publications, however, the exact role of HFJV (and other HFV techniques) remains controversial. At one end of the spectrum, a few clinicians use HFJV as a primary mode of ventilation for infants who require ventilatory support, whereas at the other extreme are clinicians who view HFJV strictly as a rescue technique, only to be used when conventional mechanical ventilation (CMV) has failed. Most clinicians seem to possess an intermediate level of enthusiasm, using HFJV as an early rescue mode in infants who are judged to be at high risk of complications with CMV or have developed air leak, even though they are maintaining adequate gas exchange on CMV. This chapter summarizes the state of the art of HFJV based on available literature and my extensive personal experience with this technique dating back to the early 1980s.

BRIEF HISTORY

The development of HFJV traces its earliest origins to the observations of Henderson and colleagues,[1] who first showed that gas exchange could occur at tidal volumes (VT) smaller than anatomic dead space. The true beginnings of HFV date back to Emerson in the United States[2] and Lunkenheimer in Germany,[3] who developed devices and concepts that evolved into modern high-frequency flow interrupters and oscillators. Subsequently, Sanders[4] noted that when oxygen was delivered via the side arm of a bronchoscope in short bursts, rather than continuously, the carbon dioxide (CO_2) accumulation that previously limited bronchoscopy to only a few minutes was markedly reduced. The Sanders jet was the first practical device that used the basic principle of jet ventilation and is the forerunner of modern jet ventilators. Building on these ideas, Klain and Smith[5] introduced jet ventilation into adult critical care in the mid-1970s. Heijman and Sjöstrand in Sweden[6] first introduced concepts of high-frequency positive-pressure ventilation into clinical practice in infants and children at about the same time, and Marchak and associates[7] reported the first use of high-frequency oscillatory ventilation (HFOV) in infants in 1981.

At about the same time, investigators working at the University of Arizona developed a high-frequency jet ventilator based on fluidic technology. Harris and colleagues at Tucson Medical Center applied the first prototype unit clinically in 1979 to a premature infant with intractable respiratory failure (T. Harris, personal communication, 1987).

At the University of Minnesota, Boros and colleagues[8,9] treated a series of 25 infants between 1980 and 1983 with an electronically controlled solenoid valve jet ventilator (IDC VS-600; Instrument Development Corporation, Pittsburgh, Pa). Simultaneously, initially using a prototype fluidic jet ventilator similar to the one used by Harris and later the IDC VS-600, I successfully treated several preterm infants with severe respiratory distress syndrome (RDS) and air leak at Children's Hospital, Akron, Ohio. The jet injector was a right-angle metal cannula within a connector that fit into a standard endotracheal tube adapter.

A randomized clinical trial of HFJV in infants with RDS and pulmonary interstitial emphysema (PIE) was initiated at Children's Hospital in Akron in 1981 but was abandoned quickly after necrotizing tracheobronchitis was noted in an infant who died of nonrespiratory causes. Similar lesions were reported later by Ophoven and coworkers[10] and other investigators, and this led to a temporary dampening of enthusiasm for HFJV.

In time, these lesions were found to be caused by lack of humidification in the early jet devices. It was soon shown that similar lesions could be reproduced in animals using other HFV devices; Wiswell and colleagues[11,12] found that necrotizing tracheobronchitis could result from ischemia of the submucosal layer when high intratracheal pressure was generated, particularly when combined with hypotension.

In the clinical setting, where HFJV was used in extremely ill infants with hemodynamic instability and hypotension requiring high ventilator pressures, it is not surprising that necrotizing tracheobronchitis was observed with some frequency in the early days of HFJV. Kirpalani and associates[13] subsequently showed an identical lesion in infants treated with conventional mechanical ventilation. When it was recognized that necrotizing tracheobronchitis was not an inherent risk of HFJV, the interest in HFJV returned to its former level by the mid-1980s.

Parallel development of a jet ventilator similar to the IDC-600 occurred at Rainbow Babies' and Children's Hospital, Cleveland, Ohio. Different versions of this unit were used for the short-term treatment of 12 premature infants with severe hyaline membrane disease reported in 1984.[14] A specially designed heating and humidification system for the jet gas was developed jointly by investigators in Cleveland and Akron, avoiding further problems with airway damage.[15] A randomized trial comparing effectiveness of short-term (48 hours) use of this jet ventilator with conventional mechanical ventilation in severe hyaline membrane disease, reported in 1987, showed similar gas exchange with lower mean airway pressures and no increase in complications.[16]

These early jet ventilators had many limitations. Accurate measurement of airway pressures or V_T was not feasible because fresh gas was introduced through a jet nozzle into the distal end of the patient circuit at the endotracheal tube adapter, creating a Venturi effect. As a result, negative pressures were produced at the usual site of airway pressure monitoring.

Monitoring of airway pressure required placement of a second cannula beyond the tip of the endotracheal tube, which could not be accomplished safely in infants with small endotracheal tubes. With these early jet ventilators, clinicians were required to manipulate the driving pressure manually until adequate chest rise was seen, and they relied on blood gas monitoring to guide further adjustments.

In response to these challenges, engineers at Bunnell, Incorporated (Salt Lake City, Utah), designed a high-frequency jet ventilator (Bunnell Life Pulse) specifically for infants. The device was modeled in many ways after pressure-limited infant ventilators already in common use, with peak inspiratory pressure (PIP) as the major control variable: PIP is set by the operator, and then held constant by a built-in, microprocessor-based servocontrol mechanism (see Device Description later).

GAS EXCHANGE DURING HIGH-FREQUENCY JET VENTILATION

Despite many years of successful clinical use and a large body of published literature, understanding of the exact mechanisms of gas exchange during HFJV remains incomplete. Traditional respiratory physiology is inadequate to explain gas exchange with V_T at or below the anatomic dead space. Extensive laboratory and clinical evidence shows that HFV devices are efficient at CO_2 removal. Some alternative mechanism must be operative during HFV to facilitate gas exchange.

Several theories have been proposed to explain gas exchange at high frequencies. Most of the proposed mechanisms have in common the concept that gas exchange occurs in part by enhanced molecular diffusion resulting from increased mixing of gases in the airways. The details of these mechanisms, which include bulk flow, pendelluft, Taylor-type dispersion, and radial diffusion, are beyond the scope of this chapter and have been elegantly described in classic articles by Chang[17] and Venegas and Fredberg.[18]

Unique to HFJV is the concept of **spike formation**. Henderson first described this phenomenon in his classic 1915 paper.[1] He showed that a high-velocity impulse of gas penetrates through the dead space gas resident in the upper airway, rather than pushing it ahead of it as occurs with gas flow at low velocities. This spike enhances bulk flow of gas in the upper airway by largely bypassing anatomic dead space and provides more efficient gas mixing in the more distal lung (Fig. 45-1).

Mathematical models predict and empirical observations support the formation of coaxial rotational outflow of gas along the periphery of the airway simultaneously with the movement of gas inward in a spike form down the center of the airway (Fig. 45-2). The position of the endotracheal tube seems to be important in the efficiency of spike formation and gas mixing.[19] Other factors that reduce the effectiveness of spike formation and impair ventilation include the presence of thick secretions and debris in the airways.

As with all forms of mechanical ventilation, the factors affecting oxygenation and ventilation are interrelated, but distinct. In most neonatal lung diseases, the primary problem causing hypoxemia is diffuse atelectasis, which leads to ventilation-perfusion mismatch and intrapulmonary shunt. As mean airway pressure is increased, the degree of atelectasis is reduced, and ventilation-perfusion matching is improved. In general, increasing mean airway pressure with any high-frequency device results in improved oxygenation.

Similar to CMV, mean airway pressure with HFJV is affected by multiple factors, including end-expiratory pressure, PIP, inspiratory time–to–expiratory time ratio (I/E), and the superimposed "conventional" breaths. Because mean airway pressure is not set directly, it is important to be mindful of the variables that affect it to avoid inadvertent changes that may lead to deterioration in oxygenation caused by an unintended fall in mean airway pressure.

The relationship between ventilation (CO_2 removal) and ventilator settings is more complex for HFV than it is

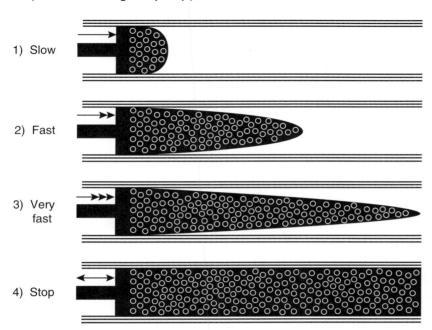

1) Slow

2) Fast

3) Very fast

4) Stop

Figure 45–1. Spike formation at high flow velocities.

for CMV. With CMV, CO_2 removal is proportional to alveolar minute ventilation (i.e., the product of respiratory frequency and V_T [$f \times V_T$]). In HFV, CO_2 removal occurs by a combination of enhanced diffusion and other phenomena that eliminate or reduce effective dead space so that CO_2 removal is roughly proportional to the product of HFV frequency and the *square* of the HFV V_T ($f \times [V_T]^2$). This relationship between CO_2 elimination and the square of V_T seems to apply equally to both forms of HFV and has been validated in numerous animal models.[20-22]

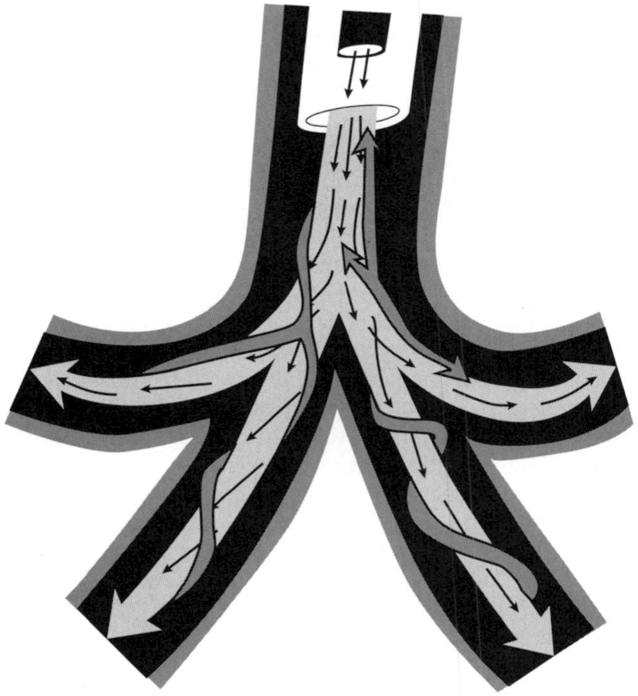

In practical terms, the above-delineated relationship means that small adjustments in HFV pressure amplitude (ΔP) or V_T have a large effect on CO_2 elimination. Consequently, CO_2 elimination is relatively frequency independent and is controlled primarily by adjusting ΔP, accomplished by the independent adjustment of positive end-expiratory pressure (PEEP) and PIP.

An important difference between HFV devices and conventional ventilators is the relationship between the pressure amplitude measured at the endotracheal tube and the pressure amplitude that is delivered to the alveoli. With conventional ventilators operating at relatively low frequencies, gas exchange occurs almost entirely by bulk flow (convection), and the pressure applied at the airway opening is transmitted fully to the alveoli. With HFJV, convection also occurs in the large airways, but it is driven primarily by the kinetic energy of the gas emerging at high velocity from the jet orifice. With the extremely short inspiratory time, pressure transmission to distal areas of the lung is attenuated. Beyond the first few generations of the airways, gas exchange during HFJV occurs predominantly by enhanced diffusion, and the pressure amplitude and volume swings seen in terminal airways and alveoli are substantially less than the amplitude measured in the trachea. This reduction in distal pressure and V_T is common to all forms of HFV, and it is believed to be the mechanism responsible for the reduction of lung injury with HFV.

With each patient and device, it is important to choose a frequency that achieves optimal gas exchange without gas trapping. Excessively high frequencies can cause gas trapping when expiratory time becomes insufficient to achieve complete exhalation. This trapping results in CO_2 retention and impairment of venous return owing to increased intrathoracic pressure. Because of the inherent differences in the way in which gas delivery is accomplished, the

Figure 45–2. Rotational coaxial flow during high-frequency jet ventilation.

optimal frequencies for HFJV are lower than those for HFOV.

The optimal range of HFV frequencies depends on the size of the patient and the patient's intrinsic lung mechanics.[18] In general, the smaller the patient, the higher the optimal frequency, and vice versa. When determining the optimal ventilator frequency, the most important aspect of lung mechanics is the time constant, the product of compliance and resistance: $C_{dyn} \times R_{aw}$. In general, patients with short time constants (low lung compliance and low airway resistance) can be ventilated effectively at higher frequencies than patients with longer time constants (high lung compliance or high airway resistance or both). There is no simple way to calculate ideal frequencies for each of the HFV devices for an individual patient; one must rely on clinical experience and trial and error adjustments.

DEVICE DESCRIPTION

The Bunnell Life Pulse ventilator is the only jet ventilator approved by the Food and Drug Administration available in the United States for the treatment of infants. Servocontrol of PIP is accomplished by the ventilator's microprocessor, which compares the PIP level set by the operator with the actual PIP measured continuously in the distal airway, and the driving or "servo" pressure behind the inspiratory pulses is increased or decreased in proportion to the difference between the set and actual PIP. These moment to moment adjustments in servopressure are accomplished by an array of precision solenoid valves supplying the pressure chamber that pressurizes the circuit.

Actual delivery of the jet pulses is by way of an electromagnetically controlled pinch valve in the "patient box" controlled by the same microprocessor (Fig. 45-3). Moving the pinch valve and pressure transducer into the patient box placed close to the patient is an important advance, resulting in much less dampening of the jet pulse and more accurate pressure monitoring. This allows the Bunnell jet to operate efficiently at much higher frequencies than the early prototype devices. The clinician sets the same variables on the front panel of the Bunnell jet as he or she is accustomed to setting on conventional ventilators—PIP (range 8 to 50 cm H_2O), frequency or rate (range 240 to 660 breaths/min), and jet valve "on time," which is comparable to inspiratory time (range 0.020 to 0.034 seconds).

The humidification system for the Bunnell unit also is feedback controlled for maintaining appropriate temperature, humidity, and water level and preventing excessive condensation. The humidifier cartridge and circuit were designed to withstand the relatively high servopressure and at the same time offer a minimum of compressible volume.

Working with Mallinckrodt, Incorporated (St. Louis), the Bunnell engineers also helped develop the Hi-Lo jet triple-lumen endotracheal tube, which made accurate airway pressure monitoring and feedback control of PIP possible. One lumen carried pressure signals from the distal tip of the endotracheal tube back to the jet's pressure transducer located in the patient box for monitoring and servocontrol purposes. The second lumen carried the jet pulses released through the pinch valve down to its distal opening or jet injector, which was located far enough up in the lumen of the main tube that it did not interfere with pressure measurements. The third and main lumen of the jet tube was connected with the conventional ventilator circuit for delivery of background PEEP and occasional intermittent mandatory ventilation (IMV) breaths or "sighs."

More recently, the inconvenience associated with the need to reintubate patients with the triple-lumen tube has been eliminated with the development of a special endotracheal tube adapter known as the LifePort (Bunnell, Inc., Salt Lake City, Utah). This device incorporates the jet stream delivery and pressure measurement lumens into the walls of the adapter (Fig. 45-4). The accuracy and efficiency of the system have been validated thoroughly, and its availability has greatly improved the ease of use of the jet ventilator.

LABORATORY STUDIES

A wealth of data from animal studies dating back 20 years suggests that in diseases characterized primarily by atelectasis, HFV leads to better lung inflation and less alveolar and airway damage than does conventional tidal ventilation.[23,24] This observation has been shown in preterm animals and in animal models of surfactant deficiency and lung injury induced by saline lavage. There are not as many laboratory studies with HFJV as there are with oscillatory ventilation, but many of the HFOV results probably can be generalized to include all HFV devices, as long as a similar strategy designed to optimize lung volume is used.

Several early HFJV studies focused on showing the effect of jet ventilation on lung parenchyma of healthy and saline-lavaged animals.[25,26] These studies showed a lesser degree of injury in animals ventilated with HFJV. Subsequently a series of studies was performed by several groups of investigators in animal models of meconium aspiration syndrome. The results are contradictory, with some studies showing apparent advantages of HFJV and others showing no differences. These conflicting results are likely due to differences in the ventilatory strategies and the animal models used.

Mammel and coworkers[27] found no advantage of HFJV in a feline model of aspiration using HFJV at a relatively high frequency immediately after instillation of meconium. They noted difficulty with ventilation and oxygenation and documented elevated pulmonary artery pressures and pulmonary vascular resistance in the HFJV group. These findings are consistent with gas trapping due to airway obstruction and inadequate expiratory time.

Trindade and associates[28] also compared IMV with HFJV with a low airway pressure strategy in a meconium aspiration model and showed no differences in gas exchange, lung mechanics, or hemodynamic variables. In contrast, we studied HFJV alone and HFJV combined with low-rate IMV in a canine model of meconium aspiration and found improved ventilation and oxygenation at lower mean and peak airway pressures, particularly in the animals ventilated with HFJV combined with low-rate

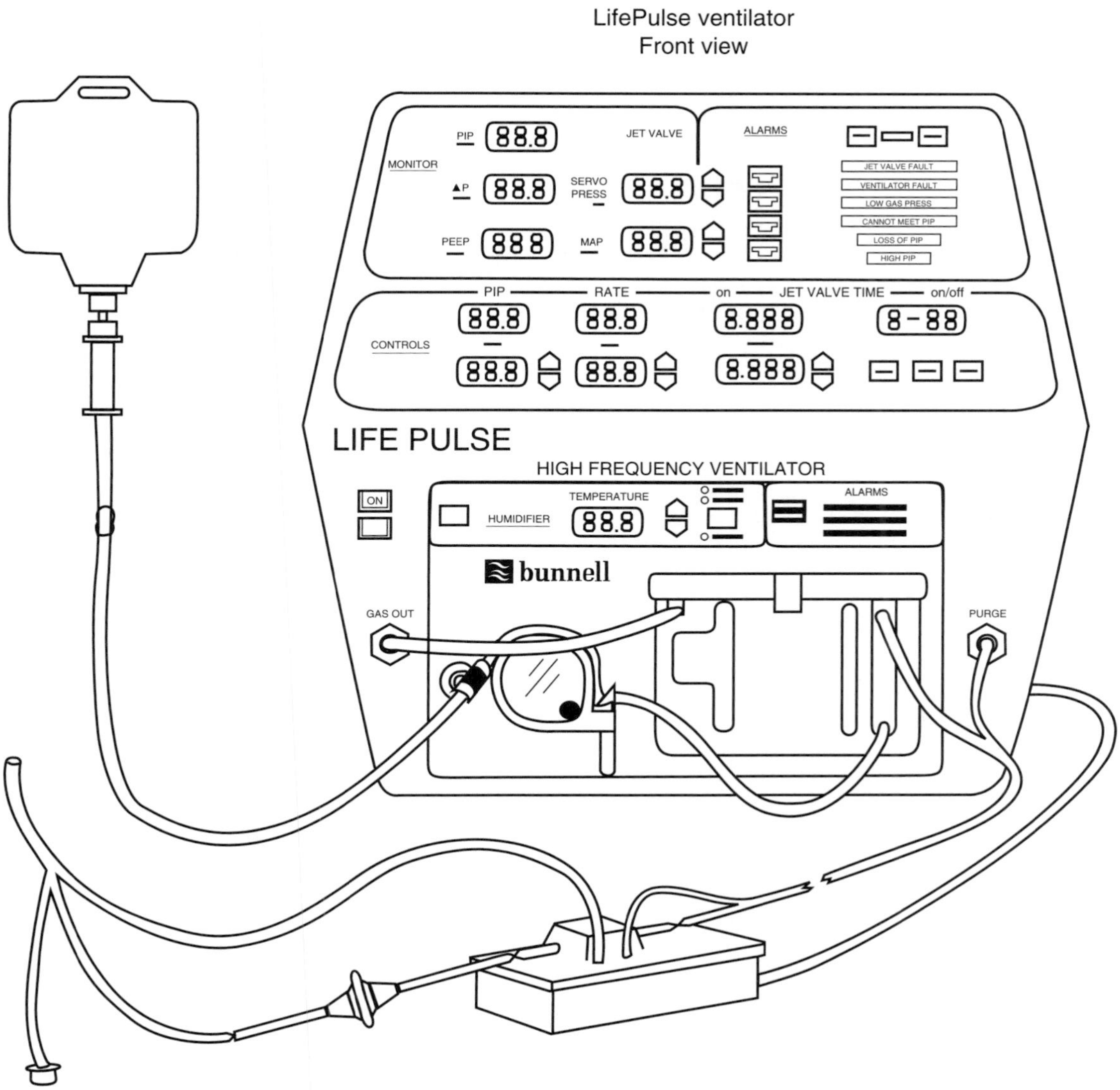

LifePulse ventilator
Front view

Figure 45–3. Bunnell LifePulse jet ventilator and patient box. *(Courtesy of Bunnell, Inc., Salt Lake City, Utah.)*

IMV.[29] There were no adverse hemodynamic effects of HFJV and no elevation of pulmonary vascular resistance.

In contrast to the Mammel and Trindade studies, we used a slightly more dilute mixture of meconium, allowed the animals to stabilize for 30 minutes on CMV, suctioned the trachea before the onset of ventilation, and used a slower HFJV rate (i.e., longer expiratory time). The "combined HFJV" animals had significantly lower histologic lung injury scores compared with the tidal ventilation group.[30] The benefit of superimposed conventional breaths was probably the result of improved alveolar recruitment, made necessary by the fact that the meconium resulted in surfactant inactivation.

Wiswell and colleagues[31] investigated the effects of four different ventilators on gas exchange and lung histology in newborn piglets and reported that animals ventilated with HFJV or with high-frequency flow interrupter (HFFI) had significantly fewer histologic abnormalities than animals ventilated with conventional IMV. More

recently, in an elegant study, Wiswell and colleagues[32] compared the effects of surfactant therapy with HFJV and CMV on ventilator variables, gas exchange, and lung histology in a piglet model of meconium aspiration syndrome. These investigators were unable to show benefit of surfactant therapy or of HFJV compared with CMV.

The hemodynamic effects of HFJV were examined by many authors. Despite some inconsistency in the findings, it generally can be concluded that in animals with some degree of hemodynamic compromise, HFJV results in less circulatory impairment compared with CMV.[33-36]

CLINICAL STUDIES

Rescue Studies

The focus of early work with HFJV was the treatment of air leak. Most of the 25 patients treated by Boros and colleagues[9] in the early 1980s had air leak complicating

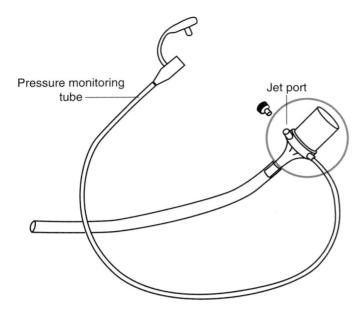

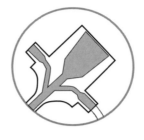

Figure 45–4. The LifePort jet adapter. *(Courtesy of Bunnell, Inc., Salt Lake City, Utah.)*

RDS. In 1984, Harris and Christensen[37] reported promising results in a series of 20 patients with PIE treated with HFJV. Spitzer and coworkers[38] reported in 1989 an impressive 54% survival in what was then by far the largest clinical series of 176 patients, most of whom had severe RDS complicated by air leak. The results in these extremely ill infants were quite encouraging.

The Spitzer study provided the first set of useful guidelines for clinical management and a sound basis for continued investigation of the efficacy and safety of this device. Similar to the previously mentioned studies, the lack of a control population made it difficult to establish unequivocally the beneficial effects of this therapy. Nonetheless, it was a turning point in the history of HFJV and clearly established this technique as an important clinical tool.

Subsequently, Baumgart and associates[39] described a series of potential candidates for extracorporeal membrane oxygenation (ECMO) who were treated with HFJV, also with apparently encouraging results. Infants with homogeneous lung disease (RDS or pneumonia) seemed to respond better than infants with meconium aspiration or lung hypoplasia. Although nearly all infants showed initial improvement in gas exchange, infants who survived continued to improve, whereas nonsurvivors began to deteriorate by 6 hours of therapy.

Based on a series of 28 infants with poor initial response to exogenous surfactant, Davis and colleagues[40] suggested that the combination of HFJV and exogenous surfactant may be more effective than either technique alone. This hypothesis has not been tested in a randomized controlled study, however.

Building on these earlier experiences, the multicenter randomized trial of HFJV by Keszler and associates[41] specifically focused on infants with RDS complicated by PIE. Because this was a rescue study, the age at randomization was nearly 2 days, and all of the infants had severe

lung disease. The major finding was that HFJV led to significantly faster and more frequent resolution of PIE. When rescue crossover of infants who were failing CMV is accounted for, survival was improved with the use of HFJV (65% versus 47%; $P < .05$). Gas exchange also was improved with HFJV, and there was a modest trend toward less chronic lung disease with HFJV (50% versus 67%; $P = .17$).

Several other studies focused on treatment of air leak. Gonzalez and coworkers[42] showed a substantial decrease in leak through chest tubes in a group of infants with bronchopleural fistula when they were switched from CMV to HFJV. Similarly, improved gas exchange and reduced flow through tracheoesophageal fistula was shown by Goldberg and colleagues[43] and by Donn and associates.[44] The advantages of HFJV in these patients may be in the ability to ventilate them with extremely short inspiratory times.

Uncomplicated Respiratory Distress Syndrome

The first randomized controlled trial of HFJV by Carlo and colleagues[45] used a low-pressure strategy and a device that is not commercially available. The study employed a sequential analysis study design with power assumptions based on an 85:15 advantage of one therapy over the other. Consequently, this trial included only 42 patients and did not have the statistical power to show anything but extreme differences in outcome. Although the study showed no benefit in the HFJV-treated patients, its negative conclusion is clearly susceptible to type II statistical error for smaller, yet clinically important differences in outcome.

In a later multicenter randomized clinical trial that included 133 infants who had significant RDS despite surfactant therapy, Keszler and associates[46] found a reduction in chronic lung disease at 36 weeks' corrected age (20% versus 40%; $P < .05$) and less need for home oxygen therapy (6% versus 23%; $P < .01$) in infants treated with HFJV. There was no increase in complications, including intraventricular hemorrhage (IVH) and periventricular leukomalacia (PVL). At the same time, a similar but smaller single-center study by Wiswell and colleagues[47] failed to show any pulmonary benefit.

In the Wiswell study, the mean age at randomization was 7 hours, and the incidence of IVH/PVL was one of the primary outcome variables evaluated. Severe IVH occurred in 22% of the CMV infants and 41% of the HFJV infants; cystic PVL occurred in 6% of CMV infants and 31% of HFJV infants. A radiologist masked to study group and with special expertise in interpretation of neonatal ultrasonograms read all the cerebral ultrasonograms. This study was stopped by its Data Monitoring and Safety Committee because of the high incidence of IVH/PVL in the HFJV patients.[47]

These two studies were done concurrently and under a similar protocol, using the same device, but with one key difference—only the multicenter trial specified an HFJV ventilator strategy aimed at optimizing lung volume. Although exposure to hypocarbia was not found to be an independent predictor of neuroimaging abnormalities in the Wiswell study, a larger sample size might have shown a role for this or other factors. A subsequent publication that included patients from the randomized trial and other patients treated with HFJV at the same institution did show that prolonged exposure to hypocarbia was a predictor for neuroimaging abnormalities in HFJV patients.[48] Earlier published data also from this group described a dramatically increased incidence of PVL and cerebral palsy in conventionally ventilated preterm infants exposed to marked hypocarbia,[49] findings consistent with the results of other studies.[50,51]

In contrast to Wiswell's single-center study, the larger multicenter trial showed no overall increase in IVH or PVL, but did show an interesting difference between two subgroups of HFJV patients. Even though a well-defined optimal volume strategy of HFJV was prescribed, a substantial proportion of the HFJV patients were ventilated using a traditional low-pressure strategy of HFJV, similar to that used in the Wiswell study. Although this protocol deviation detracted from the overall quality of the study, it provided an opportunity to compare the two strategies of HFJV.

This post-hoc analysis must be interpreted with caution, but it showed a much lower incidence of IVH/PVL in the optimal volume subgroup (9% versus 33% in the low-pressure group; CMV = 28%). The low-pressure subgroup of HFJV had significantly lower arterial partial pressure of CO_2 ($PaCO_2$) compared with CMV and the optimal volume HFJV subgroup.[46] These findings are consistent with data obtained using HFOV and suggest that different ventilator strategies may lead to important differences in outcome.

OTHER INDICATIONS FOR HIGH-FREQUENCY JET VENTILATION

Several uncontrolled series of patients suggested effectiveness of HFJV as a rescue treatment in potential candidates for ECMO. Only one randomized controlled study

has been completed—a single-center study of HFJV versus CMV for near-ECMO patients by Engle and coworkers,[52] which was limited by the inclusion of only 24 infants. HFJV improved gas exchange and showed a trend to less frequent need for ECMO. None of the 9 HFJV survivors had chronic lung disease compared with 4 of 10 CMV infants. These differences were not statistically significant, but the study was extremely small and susceptible to type II statistical error.

Intuitively, when abdominal distention, massive edema, or other pathophysiology limits chest wall and diaphragmatic motions, small VT of HFJV would be expected to offer an advantage over large VT breathing. We reported improved ventilation and hemodynamic variables in 20 such patients when switched from CMV to HFJV.[53] The role of HFJV in supporting patients with increased intraabdominal pressure is supported further by an animal study that showed improved gas exchange and better hemodynamics with HFJV in an animal model of increased intraabdominal pressure.[54]

Two clinical trials specifically addressed the hemodynamic effects of HFJV. Meliones and colleagues[55] reported decreased airway pressures, lower pulmonary vascular resistance, and improved cardiac index in term infants with congenital heart disease after a Fontan procedure. Davis and associates[56] showed that the use of HFJV during cardiothoracic surgery in infants undergoing Blalock-Taussig shunts was associated with improved oxygenation at a decreased mean airway pressure. The technical aspects of the surgery seemed to be facilitated by the decreased motion of the intrathoracic structures.

Although, intuitively, HFJV offers an advantage over CMV in infants with pulmonary hypoplasia, such as congenital diaphragmatic hernia, no randomized controlled studies exist to substantiate this impression. Anecdotally, however, most tertiary centers where HFJV is available routinely use this therapy as first-line treatment in infants with pulmonary hypoplasia.

CHOICES OF HIGH-FREQUENCY JET VENTILATION

Clinicians may be faced with the decision as to which type of HFV should be used in a given patient and perhaps which device to purchase for the neonatal intensive care unit. In the absence of any controlled clinical trials directly comparing HFOV with HFJV, these decisions usually are based on personal preference and prior experience. In practical terms, the choice comes down to that between HFJV and HFOV because the Infant Star flow interrupter is no longer in production.

Despite their mechanical and physiologic differences, the HFV devices available in the United States are more similar than dissimilar. Both offer the advantage of using extremely small VT to avoid the larger cyclic volume changes that are required with CMV. Both devices can (and usually should) be used with a strategy aimed at optimizing lung volume.

The outdated concept that HFJV does not achieve good oxygenation stemmed from the emphasis on low airway pressures that became a standard approach to the use of

HFJV. This strategy was appropriate for the treatment of air leak, which was the predominant use of HFJV in the early years but is not an inherent feature of HFJV. The availability of background sighs to provide ongoing volume recruitment may allow the maintenance of similar lung volume with lower mean airway pressure compared with HFOV, but this has not been systematically studied.

In most situations, the user's familiarity with the operation of the particular device and attention to the choice of a ventilatory strategy that is best suited to the patient's pulmonary condition is probably more important than the differences between the devices.

One major difference between the devices is the I/E ratio. There is some evidence that one of the key elements in treating PIE is a short inspiratory time. In this area, the jet ventilator with an approximately 1:6 I/E ratio may have an advantage over the oscillator with a 1:1 or 1:2 ratio. Also, because of the manner in which the inspiratory gas flow travels down the center of the airway at high velocity with little lateral pressure on the airway wall, HFJV seems to be more suitable for ventilation of infants with disruptions of the large airways. It is my impression that in most centers with access to both modalities, HFJV is the preferred device for treatment of air leak.

CLINICAL INDICATIONS FOR HIGH-FREQUENCY JET VENTILATION

There is no uniformity of opinion as to the specific indications for HFV in general, and this controversy is equally true for HFJV. This uncertainty stems in part from the differing results of the published clinical studies and in part from the availability of therapeutic options, such as exogenous surfactant and synchronized, volume-targeted ventilatory modes, which were not available when the early studies of HFJV were conducted. Although there is a wide variation in how published data are interpreted and consequently in how HFJV is used in the United States, several general conclusions can be drawn. These are discussed subsequently and summarized in Table 45-1.

First, HFJV is clearly preferable to CMV (and probably to HFOV) for the treatment of air leak syndromes, such as PIE, bronchopleural fistula, or tracheoesophageal fistula. The data from animal studies, data from numerous case reports, the HFJV data of Gonzalez and colleagues,[42] and data from the PIE controlled trial[41] all support this conclusion. Based on available experience, any patient with air leak should be treated with HFJV until at least 24 hours after the air leak has resolved.

Second, HFJV is indicated in patients with severe uniform lung disease, such as RDS, who require substantial pressures and are at high risk of developing complications of CMV. The data from animal studies support the argument that use of small V_T at high frequencies allows more uniform lung inflation and causes less damage to severely noncompliant lungs than the larger V_T of CMV. As a rough guideline, I believe that most patients with uniform lung disease who require inspiratory pressures greater than 23 to 25 cm H_2O or fraction of inspired oxygen (F_{IO_2}) greater than 0.4 to 0.6 despite appropriate PEEP could benefit from HFV with no evidence of superiority of HFOV or HFJV.

Table 45-1. General Indications for High-Frequency Jet Ventilation

Air leak syndromes (e.g., PIE, BPF, TEF)	HFJV is the preferred ventilator mode.
Severe uniform disease (RDS)	HFJV allows more uniform lung inflation and causes less damage to severely noncompliant lungs. No evidence of HFJV versus HFOV superiority here.
Severe nonuniform disease (e.g., aspiration syndromes)	HFJV is often quite effective and should always be tried before ECMO. (Use lower high-frequency ventilation rate and shorter I/E in these patients, e.g., 300 breaths/min and 1:9.)
Pulmonary hypoplasia (e.g., congenital diaphragmatic hernia)	HFJV and HFOV usually maintain adequate gas exchange using much smaller tidal volumes.
Severe chest wall restriction and/or upward pressure on the diaphragm due to abdominal distention	HFJV is preferred ventilator mode.
Severe respiratory failure and PPHN (ECMO and inhaled INO candidates)	HFJV may help avoid ECMO and improve NO effectiveness.
Preterm infants with RDS	HFJV and HFOV may reduce chronic lung disease; however, hyperventilation must be avoided to prevent neurologic injury.

BPF, bronchopulmonary fistula; ECMO, extracorporeal membrane oxygenation; HFJV, high-frequency jet ventilation; HFOV, high-frequency oscillatory ventilation; I/E, inspiratory-to-expiratory ratio; NO, nitric oxide; PIE, pulmonary interstitial emphysema; PPHN, persistent pulmonary hypertension of the newborn; RDS, respiratory distress syndrome; TEF, tracheoesophageal fistula.

Third, HFJV also may be preferable to CMV for patients with severe nonuniform disease, such as aspiration syndromes. The studies by Wiswell and coworkers[31] using the piglet model of meconium aspiration syndrome and Keszler and colleagues[29] using a canine model suggest that HFJV causes less damage to these lungs than does CMV. Although these conditions have not been as well studied in humans, there is a great deal of anecdotal experience to suggest that at least some infants with severe nonhomogeneous disease do well with HFJV.

Meconium aspiration syndrome is a heterogeneous syndrome, which evolves over time. Airway obstruction usually predominates in the early stages. Although HFJV may facilitate mobilization of secretions, the presence of debris in the airways may interfere with efficient ventilation.

In infants in whom the surfactant inhibitory effect of meconium predominates and in the subsequent inflammatory stages of meconium aspiration syndrome, HFJV is often effective. It is reasonable to offer a trial of HFJV to all patients with severe aspiration syndrome who are at risk of requiring more invasive therapies, such as ECMO. These infants tend to have relatively long time constants, however, and may develop gas trapping on HFJV; these infants may do better on CMV. When HFJV is used in these infants, slower frequencies (as low as 300 breaths/min, where I/E = 1:9, must be employed because of the longer time constants) are used to minimize the chance of gas trapping. Other than the apparent improved clearance of secretions with HFJV, there is little evidence of superiority of either device.

Fourth, HFJV may have a role in patients with pulmonary hypoplasia, such as is seen with diaphragmatic hernia. Although this has not been well studied, there is a good deal of anecdotal evidence for improved gas exchange with both types of HFV in such infants. It is reasonable to assume that the ideal method of ventilating these small lungs is with a high-frequency device that allows one to maintain adequate gas exchange while using extremely small VT.

Fifth, HFJV is a preferred mode of ventilation when severe chest wall restriction or upward pressure on the diaphragm due to abdominal distention interferes with tidal ventilation and causes hemodynamic embarrassment.

Sixth, based on extensive anecdotal experiences from most centers offering ECMO and the clinical trial of Engle and associates,[52] I believe that a trial of HFJV is appropriate in term infants with severe respiratory failure who are potential candidates for ECMO. Patients with significant parenchymal lung disease who require inhaled nitric oxide therapy may benefit from the improved lung aeration afforded by HFV to optimize the delivery of the therapeutic agent at the alveolar level. Both devices seem to be similarly effective in avoiding the need for ECMO, and both devices support the administration of inhaled nitric oxide.

Finally, an argument can be made that HFV, including HFJV, may be the preferred mode of ventilation for all preterm infants with RDS. Extensive animal data and the

clinical trials of Keszler and colleagues,[46] Gerstmann and associates,[58] and the Neonatal Ventilation Study Group[59] support this approach. Many centers have adopted HFV as a primary mode of ventilation. Anecdotally, these clinicians believe that this is an effective approach, which may lead to a decrease in the incidence of chronic lung disease. The enthusiasm for the routine use of HFV as a primary mode of ventilation continues to be tempered, however, by the lingering concerns about the ease with which inadvertent hyperventilation can occur and the possibility of neurologic injury.

VENTILATORY STRATEGIES

The way in which HFJV is used has evolved over time because understanding of the interaction of the ventilator and pulmonary pathophysiology has increased and because the patient population being treated today is different than it was in the 1980s. In the early days of HFJV, the technique was used for rescue of patients failing CMV and was seen primarily as a means of reducing airway pressure and the lung injury associated with overdistention and air leak. With the elegant studies by the groups led by deLemos[60,61] and Froese,[62-64] subsequently confirmed by many controlled clinical trials, we have come to understand that the greatest advantage of HFV is the ability to achieve uniform lung expansion and to support a patient at higher mean airway pressures without excessive tissue stretching.

With the growing understanding that avoiding atelectasis is as important as avoiding overdistention, the general approach to most patients treated with HFOV and HFJV emphasizes lung recruitment and maintenance of the distending airway pressure above the critical closing pressure. This concept has been shown to be equally true for both types of HFV, although it has been adopted more slowly by users of HFJV. HFJV does have the demonstrated ability to support gas exchange at lower airway pressures in patients in whom this strategy is appropriate (i.e., air leak syndrome).

The following guidelines for the use of the Bunnell Life Pulse HFJV are based on my clinical experience and research and on input from dozens of other clinicians who have used HFJV since the 1980s. They represent an approach to maintaining lung volumes within the narrow ideal range between atelectasis and overdistention and to weaning patients actively from mechanical ventilation. The strategies are based on the assumption that blood gases and lung inflation should be kept within certain target ranges and that patients who are stable within these target ranges should be actively weaned, with a goal to extubation as soon as possible.

These guidelines address typical premature infants with predominantly atelectatic lung disease. It is crucial that the clinician carefully assesses the patient's pulmonary pathophysiology and determine which problem (e.g., atelectasis, air leak, airway obstruction, air trapping, decreased pulmonary blood flow) is predominantly responsible for the gas exchange defect. Only then can one design the optimal ventilation strategy that is appropriate for the particular patient at that time. The specific strategies appropriate in different disease processes are summarized in Table 45-2. The evolution of the disease process must be re-evaluated frequently and the ventilatory strategy adjusted accordingly.

Target Ranges for Blood Gas Values

The target range for oxygen is based on postductal pulse oximetry, with the ideal value for most patients being approximately 90% to 95% saturation. Assuming a strategy of modest permissive hypercapnia, the $PaCO_2$ should be approximately 40 to 55 mm Hg in most patients without PIE, gross air leak, hyperinflation, or chronic changes on chest radiographs. Higher $PaCO_2$ values may be tolerated in patients with these complications. In most patients, arterial pH should be at least 7.25, although pH ranging from 7.20 to 7.25 may be acceptable.

Table 45–2. Matching Ventilator Strategy and Disease Process

Disease Process	Pathophysiology	Strategy/Goals	Initial Settings	Weaning
Air leak syndrome (PIE, pneumothorax)	PIE: gas interstitium compressing alveoli, airways and pulmonary venules. Pneumothorax: loss of VT through chest tube	Minimize distending and peak pressure, accept lower PaO_2, higher FIO_2 and $PaCO_2$, target lower lung volume	Drop PIP by 10–20% from value on CV; PEEP 4–6 cm H_2O; avoid background sigh if severe PIE	Lower PIP aggressively. Look for atelectasis and increase PEEP as needed
Severe uniform lung disease (RDS)	Atelectasis, hypoxemia, lungs highly susceptible to volutrauma and oxygen exposure	Recruit lung volume, achieve optimal expansion, avoid overventilation. Use frequent x-ray to guide management	PIP initially same as CV, but must be dropped quickly; once lung volume is recruited, PEEP 6–9 cm H_2O, depending on FIO_2	Wean FIO_2 before MAP. May need to increase PEEP to avoid drop in MAP when PIP is lowered
Nonuniform disease (MAS)	Uneven aeration, risk of gas trapping, surfactant inactivation, inflammation, high risk of air leak. Atelectasis or gas trapping may predominate	Tailor strategy to predominant pathophysiology. Avoid gas trapping, optimize lung volume	Lower frequency (300–360), PIP to achieve minimal acceptable PCO_2. Moderate PEEP 5–8 cm H_2O.	Lower PIP and use PEEP to avoid loss of lung volume
Chest wall restriction (severe NEC, repaired gastroschisis)	Restricted chest and/or diaphragmatic movement, atelectasis, hemodynamic impairment	Recruit lung volume, avoid atelectasis, minimize adverse hemodynamic effects	Adjust PIP to achieve adequate chest wall movement. Sufficient PEEP to maintain FRC (usually 6–8 cm H_2O).	Wean PIP to avoid hypocarbia, maintain MAP with PEEP
Lung hypoplasia (CDH)	Small, atelectasis-prone lungs, susceptible to volutrauma, pulmonary hypertension	Gently recruit lung volume, avoid overexpansion, minimize adverse hemodynamic effects	Set PIP at lowest level to achieve adequate ventilation. Fast rates okay as time constants are short. Sufficient PEEP to maintain FRC (usually 6–8 cm H_2O)	Wean carefully but fast enough to avoid overexpansion and air leak
Obstructive disease (BPD)	Long time constants, risk of gas trapping, nonuniform inflation	Achieve adequate gas exchange with minimal pressures, optimize lung volume, improve uniformity of inflation	Lower frequencies due to long time constants, moderate PEEP to optimize gas distribution and splint airways open	Wean slowly Rapid improvement is not anticipated

BPD, bronchopulmonary dysplasia; CDH, congenital diaphragmatic hernia; CV, conventional ventilation; FRC, functional residual capacity; MAP, mean airway pressure, MAS, meconium aspiration syndrome; NEC, necrotizing enterocolitis; PEEP, positive end-expiratory pressure; PIE, pulmonary interstitial emphysema; PIP, positive inspiratory pressure; VT, tidal volume.

Initial High-Frequency Ventilation Settings

The Bunnell Life Pulse typically is started at a frequency of 7 Hz = 420 breaths/min (higher or lower rate may be appropriate, depending on time constants) and inspiratory time of 0.02 seconds. When switching from CMV, the PEEP is increased to the range of 6 to 8 cm H_2O, depending on the degree of atelectasis and oxygen requirement. Historically, reluctance to use adequate PEEP has hindered the effectiveness of HFJV in RDS. One of the key advantages of HFV is, however, the ability to use higher mean and end-expiratory pressures safely because of the lower ΔP.

Background IMV at a rate of 2 to 5 breaths/min is initiated with an inspiratory time of 0.4 to 0.5 second. The PIP is maintained initially at the original value on the HFJV and CMV to achieve alveolar recruitment. Within a few minutes, however, the improved lung expansion results in better lung compliance, and the PIP must be lowered promptly by 10% to 20% to avoid overventilation. Further weaning of PIP should be guided by adequacy of chest wall movement or transcutaneous Pco_2 monitoring. When HFJV is the initial ventilatory mode, PIP should be started at a value consistent with the patient's disease process and its severity, starting low (16 to 18 cm H_2O) and increasing as needed to achieve a perceptible chest wall movement.

Adjusting High-Frequency Ventilation Settings to Optimize Lung Inflation and Oxygenation

In the early stages of uncomplicated RDS, hypoxemia is the result of ventilation-perfusion mismatch and is readily corrected when optimal lung expansion is reached. In such patients, the adequacy of oxygenation is an excellent guide to the need for mean airway pressure.

When initiating early HFJV, the strategy consists of progressively increasing mean airway pressure by increasing PEEP (and to a lesser degree PIP) until Fio_2 less than or equal to 0.35 is reached. When this is not readily achieved with several mean airway pressure increases of 10% to 20%, further management should be guided by chest radiographs. Excessively high mean airway pressure may lead to overinflation and can cause hypoxemia secondary to increased pulmonary vascular resistance. For this reason, radiographic assessment of lung volume also is essential in patients with more complex pulmonary pathophysiology.

The magnitude of mean airway pressure adjustment should be proportional to the degree of underinflation or overinflation. The usual increment is 10% to 15% of the initial value. Even relatively small changes in mean airway pressure can result in significant changes in lung inflation. When atelectasis occurs because of excessive weaning or suctioning, it becomes necessary to re-expand the lungs by some form of volume recruitment maneuver.

With HFJV, the background IMV rate serves as intermittent sigh breaths, which is usually adequate to recruit lung volume with only a modest increase in the HFJV and background PIP. It is crucial, however, to increase the PEEP sufficiently to maintain this recruitment.

The adequacy of selected PEEP level can be tested by transiently discontinuing the sigh breaths and observing pulse oximetry readings. If PEEP is adequate, oxygen saturation is maintained at the same level. If saturation gradually drifts down over several minutes, the selected PEEP level is insufficient to maintain lung inflation and needs to be increased (Fig. 45-5). Background IMV may facilitate alveolar re-recruitment in such cases, and when lung volume is recruited successfully, IMV peak pressure and rate usually can be lowered again to avoid alveolar overdistention. The HFJV PIP also may need to be lowered at this point to avoid overventilation.

Target Ranges for Lung Inflation

It is difficult to measure lung volumes accurately on HFJV, but they can be approximated from chest radiographs. A radiograph is a two-dimensional representation of a three-dimensional object, but as a first approximation, the position of the hemidiaphragms is a reasonable marker for lung inflation. The evaluation of lung inflation should take into account, however, not only the position of the diaphragms, but also the relative flatness of the diaphragms, whether the heart silhouette is narrow, and the appearance of the lung parenchyma. Optimal lung inflation for most patients is achieved when the top margin of the dome of the right hemidiaphragm is located between the bottom of the eighth rib and midway between the ninth and tenth ribs. For patients with PIE or bronchopleural fistula, the ideal lung inflation is one rib less than for patients without air leak. Overaggressive weaning of pressure aimed at resolving air leak may lead to atelectasis, however, which would require higher PIP to correct.

Adjusting High-Frequency Jet Ventilation Settings Based on Arterial Partial Pressure of Carbon Dioxide

At a given HFJV frequency, $Paco_2$ is primarily determined by pressure amplitude (ΔP). When a frequency appropriate for the infant's size and clinical condition is chosen, changes in frequency should be reserved for situations in which there is reason to believe that the patient's condition has changed in a way that affects the time constants. Frequencies greater than 500 bpm are seldom used. The direction of change is usually to decrease frequency because time constants tend to increase over time.

Adjustment of amplitude (accomplished primarily by adjusting PIP) should be guided by adequacy of chest wall movement or transcutaneous Pco_2 monitoring or both, in addition to blood gases. The magnitude of amplitude changes should be proportional to the desired change in $Paco_2$. The usual range is 5% to 10%. Repeated small adjustments may be preferable to infrequent large changes. When large changes in lung compliance occur because of lung volume recruitment or surfactant administration, however, aggressive lowering of ΔP may be needed to avoid inadvertent hypocarbia. Transcutaneous Pco_2 monitoring is helpful in recognizing and correcting this problem.

PEEP is likely to need to be increased during weaning to avoid an inadvertent decrease in mean airway pressure. This is analogous to decreasing the pressure amplitude on HFOV whereby the positive and negative deflections from mean pressure are decreased. The short HFJV I/E ratio makes PEEP changes have a larger impact, however, on mean pressure than PIP changes (Fig. 45-6). Inspiratory time usually is maintained at the shortest value of 0.02 second.

FINDING OPTIMAL PEEP DURING HFJV

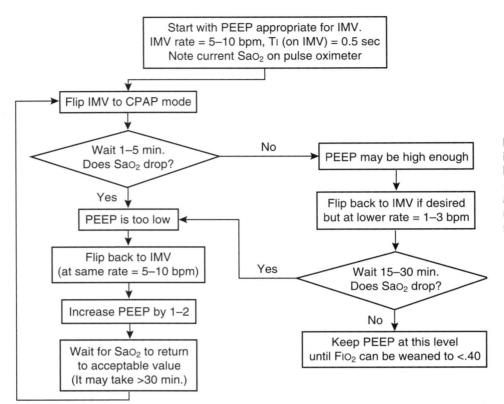

Figure 45–5. Determining optimal positive end-expiratory pressure (PEEP) level on high-frequency jet ventilation (HFJV). CPAP, continuous positive airway pressure; IMV, intermittent mechanical ventilation; Sao_2, oxygen saturation; Tı, inspiration time.

When CO_2 retention is unresponsive to an increase in ΔP, a decrease in frequency should be considered to eliminate the possibility of inadvertent PEEP due to gas trapping. (With inspiratory time held constant, Vт does not change with changes in frequency, so lowering HFJV rate should result in an increase in $Paco_2$. If gas trapping is present, however, lowering frequency lowers the *effective* PEEP, and $Paco_2$ decreases due to the increase in ΔP and consequently Vт.) In most cases, inadvertent PEEP may be detected by an increase in the monitored PEEP on the front panel of the Life Pulse ventilator when no increase in PEEP has been made on the conventional ventilator. Monitored mean airway pressure also increases in such cases.

Weaning High-Frequency Jet Ventilation

One area of HFV management that has not been well studied is the question of when (or whether) patients on HFJV should be weaned to CMV. The only clinical trial that directly addressed this issue was by Clark and colleagues,[65] which showed that infants who were treated with HFOV alone did better than infants who were changed from HFOV to CMV after 72 hours. Although there are some advantages to having a patient on CMV (e.g., Vт can be measured accurately, fewer chest radiographs may be needed, it may be easier for the parents to hold the infant), there are few compelling physiologic reasons to change infants from HFJV to CMV during the acute stage of the disease.

We have managed patients on HFJV successfully for several weeks and routinely extubated patients directly from HFJV. In general, we would suggest continuing HFJV until extubation or for as long as the patient is continuing to improve.

For patients who are no longer improving beyond 2 to 4 weeks of age, a trial of an alternative mode of ventilation is indicated. At this stage of the lung disease, increased airway resistance is likely to have developed, and this factor

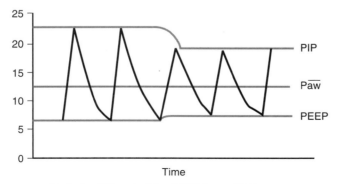

Reducing PIP and raising PEEP keeps P͞aw constant

Figure 45–6. Relationship between positive inspiratory pressure (PIP), positive end-expiratory pressure (PEEP), and mean airway pressure (P͞aw).

may render HFJV less effective. If the decision is made to continue HFJV, lower frequencies may be appropriate in these patients to accommodate the longer time constants. Controlled data regarding the effectiveness of HFJV in infants with chronic lung disease are lacking, although anecdotally, some seem to benefit.[66]

Assuming the goal is to wean the patient actively toward extubation, patients who are stable within the target ranges for lung inflation and blood gases should be weaned on a regular basis. It is important to balance the desire to wean patients with the need to avoid atelectasis when the distending airway pressure declines below the critical closing pressure of the lungs.

FIO_2 should be weaned first in response to good oxygenation. In most cases, mean airway pressure should not be weaned until the FIO_2 is less than 0.4. In general, we have found that with stable patients in the first 1 or 2 weeks of their disease, an attempt should be made to lower mean airway pressure, amplitude, or both at least every 6 to 12 hours. Patients with more chronic disease may not tolerate such an aggressive weaning schedule.

Infants with very low birth weight usually can be extubated as soon as they have been weaned to PIP of about 12 cm H_2O, mean airway pressure of 6 to 8 cm H_2O, and FIO_2 less than or equal to 0.25 to 0.30. Older, larger infants can be extubated from higher settings when they show good, sustained respiratory effort.

Suctioning during High-Frequency Jet Ventilation

Routine suctioning should be avoided in most patients to avoid loss of lung volume that invariably occurs with disconnection from the ventilator. In patients who do have significant secretions or in whom there is clinical suspicion of airway obstruction, suctioning can be accomplished in two ways. In relatively stable patients, the ventilator can be placed in standby mode briefly for the duration of the procedure and restarted as soon as completed. The ventilator takes some time to return to the full level of support. In unstable patients, placing the ventilator in standby mode may not be tolerated well. In such patients, it is preferable to suction with the ventilator running. In this case, suction must be applied throughout the procedure (during insertion of the catheter and its withdrawal) so that excessive pressure does not build up in the airway.

SUMMARY

Laboratory and clinical investigations of HFV have contributed a great deal to understanding of the pathophysiology of respiratory failure and lung injury. HFJV is now generally recognized as an effective rescue therapy in a variety of conditions leading to respiratory failure. The role of HFJV as a primary mode of ventilation remains a subject of ongoing debate, however.

Enthusiasm for HFJV as a primary mode of ventilation continues to be tempered by lingering concerns about the possibility of neurologic injury. At the same time, advances in CMV modes have led to some degree of convergence of HFV and tidal ventilation. This logical result of improved understanding of respiratory pathophysiology makes the benefits of HFV more difficult to discern.

REFERENCES

1. Henderson Y, Chillingworth FD, Whitney JL: The respiratory dead space. Am J Physiol 38:1, 1915.
2. Emerson JH: Apparatus for vibrating portions of a patient's airway. Patent No. 2918197, Washington, DC, U.S. Patent Office, Dec. 29, 1959.
3. Lunkenheimer PP, Rafflenbeul W, Keller H, et al: Application of transtracheal pressure-oscillations as a modification of "diffusion respiration." Br J Anaesth 44:627, 1972.
4. Sanders RD: Two ventilating attachments for bronchoscopes. Delaware Med J 39:170, 1967.
5. Klain M, Smith RB: High-frequency percutaneous transtracheal jet ventilation. Crit Care Med 5:280, 1977.
6. Heijman K, Sjöstrand U: Treatment of the respiratory distress syndrome: A preliminary report. Opusc Med 19:235, 1974.
7. Marchak BE, Thompson WK, Duffy MB, et al: Treatment of RDS by high-frequency oscillatory ventilation: A preliminary report. J Pediatr 99:287, 1981.
8. Pokora T, Bing DX, Mammel MC, et al: Neonatal high-frequency jet ventilation. Pediatrics 72:27, 1983.
9. Boros SJ, Mammel MC, Coleman JM, et al: Neonatal high-frequency jet ventilation: Four years' experience. Pediatrics 75:657, 1985.
10. Ophoven JP, Mammel MC, Gordon MJ, et al: Tracheobronchial histopathology associated with high frequency jet ventilation. Crit Care Med 12:829, 1984.
11. Wiswell TE, Clark RH, Null DM, et al: Tracheal and bronchial injury in high-frequency flow interruption compared with conventional positive-pressure ventilation. J Pediatr 112:249, 1988.
12. Wiswell TE, Bley JA, Turner BS, et al: Different high-frequency ventilator strategies: Effect on the propagation of tracheobronchial histopathologic changes. Pediatrics 85:70, 1990.
13. Kirpalani H, Higa T, Perlman M, et al: Diagnosis and therapy of necrotizing tracheobronchitis in ventilated neonates. Crit Care Med 13:792, 1985.
14. Carlo WA, Chatburn RL, Martin RJ, et al: Decrease in airway pressure during high-frequency jet ventilation in infants with respiratory distress syndrome. J Pediatr 104:101, 1984.
15. Chatburn RL, McClellan LD: A heat and humidification system for high-frequency jet ventilation. Respir Care 27:1386, 1982.
16. Carlo WA, Chatburn RL, Martin RJ: Randomized trial of high-frequency jet ventilation versus conventional ventilation in respiratory distress syndrome. J Pediatr 110:275, 1987.
17. Chang H: Mechanisms of gas transport during ventilation by high-frequency oscillation. J Appl Physiol 56:553, 1984.
18. Venegas JG, Fredberg JJ: Understanding the pressure cost of ventilation: Why does high-frequency ventilation work? Crit Care Med 22:S49, 1994.
19. Mullet WJ: Investigations of Convective Transport during High-Frequency Ventilation in Neonates. Philadelphia, University of Pennsylvania, 1991 [doctoral thesis].
20. Venegas JG, Hales CA, Strieder DJ: A general dimensionless equation of gas transport by high-frequency ventilation. J Appl Physiol 60:1025, 1986.
21. Venegas JG, Custer J, Kamm RD, Hales CA: Relationship for gas transport during high-frequency ventilation in dogs. J Appl Physiol 59:1539, 1985
22. Boynton BR, Hammond MD, Fredberg JJ, et al: Gas exchange in healthy rabbits during high-frequency oscillatory ventilation. J Appl Physiol 66:1343, 1989.
23. deLemos RA, Coalson JJ, Gerstmann DR, et al: Ventilatory management of infant baboons with hyaline membrane disease: The use of high frequency ventilation. Pediatr Res 21:594, 1987.

24. Hamilton PP, Onayemi A, Smyth JA, et al: Comparison of conventional and high frequency ventilation: Oxygenation and lung pathology. J Appl Physiol 55:131, 1983.

25. Keszler M, Klein R, McClellan L, et al: Effects of conventional and high-frequency ventilation on lung parenchyma. Crit Care Med 10:514, 1982.

26. Quan SF, Militzer HW, Calkins JM, et al: Comparison of high-frequency jet ventilation with conventional mechanical ventilation in saline-lavaged rabbits. Crit Care Med 12:759, 1984.

27. Mammel MC, Gordon MJ, Connett JE, Boros SJ: Comparison of high-frequency jet ventilation and conventional mechanical ventilation in a meconium aspiration model. J Pediatr 103:630, 1983.

28. Trindade O, Goldberg RN, Bancalari E, et al: Conventional vs high-frequency jet ventilation in a piglet model of meconium aspiration: Comparison of pulmonary and hemodynamic effects. J Pediatr 107:115, 1985.

29. Keszler M, Molina B, Siva Subramanian KN: Combined high-frequency jet ventilation in a meconium aspiration model. Crit Care Med 14:34, 1986.

30. Keszler M, Klappenbach RS, Reardon E: Lung pathology after high-frequency jet ventilation combined with slow intermittent mandatory ventilation in a canine model of meconium aspiration. Pediatr Pulmonol 4:144, 1988.

31. Wiswell TE, Foster NH, Slayter MV, Hachey WE: Management of a piglet model of the meconium aspiration syndrome with high-frequency or conventional ventilation. Am J Dis Child 146:1287, 1992.

32. Wiswell TE, Peabody SS, Davis JM, et al: Surfactant therapy and high-frequency jet ventilation in the management of a piglet model of the meconium aspiration syndrome. Pediatr Res 36:494, 1994.

33. Otto CW, Quan SF, Conhan TJ, et al: Hemodynamic effects of high-frequency jet ventilation. Anesth Analg 62:298, 1983.

34. Chiaranda M, Rubini A, Fiore G, et al: Hemodynamic effects of continuous positive-pressure ventilation and high-frequency jet ventilation with positive end-expiratory pressure in normal dogs. Crit Care Med 12:750, 1984.

35. Courtney SE, Spohn WA, Weber KR, et al: Cardiopulmonary effects of high frequency positive pressure ventilation vs. jet ventilation in respiratory failure. Am Rev Respir Dis 139:504, 1989.

36. Suguihara C, Bancalari E, Goldberg RN, et al: Hemodynamic and ventilatory effects of high-frequency jet and conventional ventilation in piglets with lung lavage. Biol Neonate 51:241, 1987.

37. Harris TR, Christensen RD: High-frequency jet ventilation treatment of pulmonary interstitial emphysema. Pediatr Res 19:326A, 1984.

38. Spitzer AR, Butler S, Fox WW: Ventilatory response of combined high frequency jet ventilation and conventional mechanical ventilation for the rescue treatment of severe neonatal lung disease. Pediatr Pulmonol 7:244, 1989.

39. Baumgart S, Hirschl RB, Butler SZ, et al: Diagnosis-related criteria in the consideration of extracorporeal membrane oxygenation in neonates previously treated with high frequency jet ventilation. Pediatrics 89:491, 1992.

40. Davis JM, Richter SE, Kendig JW, et al: High-frequency jet ventilation and surfactant treatment of newborns with severe respiratory failure. Pediatr Pulmonol 13:108, 1992.

41. Keszler M, Donn S, Bucciarelli R, et al: Multi-center controlled trial of high-frequency jet ventilation and conventional ventilation in newborn infants with pulmonary interstitial emphysema. J Pediatr 119:85, 1991.

42. Gonzalez F, Harris T, Black P, et al: Decreased gas flow through pneumothoraces in neonates receiving high-frequency jet versus conventional ventilation. J Pediatr 110:464, 1987.

43. Goldberg L, Marmon L, Keszler M: High-frequency jet ventilation decreases flow through tracheo-esophageal fistula. Crit Care Med 20:547, 1992.

44. Donn SM, Zak LK, Bozynski ME, et al: Use of high-frequency jet ventilation in the management of congenital tracheoesophageal fistula associated with respiratory distress syndrome. J Pediatr Surg.25:1219, 1990.

45. Carlo WA, Siner B, Chatburn RL, et al: Early randomized intervention with high-frequency jet ventilation in respiratory distress syndrome. J Pediatr 117:765, 1990.

46. Keszler M, Modanlou HD, Brudno DS, et al: Multi-center controlled clinical trial of high-frequency jet ventilation in preterm infants with uncomplicated respiratory distress syndrome. Pediatrics 100:593, 1997.

47. Wiswell TE, Graziani LJ, Kornhauser MS, et al: High-frequency jet ventilation in the early management of respiratory distress syndrome is associated with a greater risk for adverse outcomes. Pediatrics 98:1035, 1996.

48. Wiswell TE, Graziani LJ, Kornhauser MS, et al: Effects of hypocarbia on the development of cystic periventricular leukomalacia in premature infants treated with HFJV. Pediatrics 98:918, 1996.

49. Graziani LJ, Spitzer AR, Mitchell DG, et al: Mechanical ventilation in preterm infants: Neurosonographic and developmental studies. Pediatrics 90:515, 1992.

50. Calvert SA, Hoskins EM, Fong KW, Forsyth SC: Etiological factors associated with the development of periventricular leukomalacia. Acta Pediatr Scand 76:254, 1987.

51. Fujimoto S, Togari H, Yamaguchi N, et al: Hypocarbia and cystic periventricular leukomalacia in premature infants. Arch Dis Child 71:F107, 1994.

52. Engle WA, Yoder MC, et al: Controlled prospective randomized comparison of HFJV and CV in neonates with respiratory failure and persistent pulmonary hypertension. J Perinatol 17:3, 1997.

53. Keszler M, Jennings LL: High-frequency jet ventilation in infants with decreased chest wall compliance. Pediatr Res 41:257A, 1997.

54. Keszler M, Goldberg LA, Wallace A: High frequency jet ventilation in subjects with low chest wall compliance. Pediatr Res 33:331A, 1993.

55. Meliones JN, Bove EL, Dekeon MK, et al: High-frequency jet ventilation improves cardiac function after the Fontan procedure. Circulation 84(Suppl III):364, 1991.

56. Davis D, Russo P, Greenspan J, et al: High frequency jet ventilation in infants undergoing Blalock-Taussig shunts. Ann Thorac Surg 57:845, 1994.

57. Kinsella JP, Truog WE, Walsh WF, et al: Randomized, multicenter trial of inhaled nitric oxide and high-frequency oscillatory ventilation in severe, persistent pulmonary hypertension of the newborn. J Pediatr 131:55, 1997.

58. Gerstmann DR, Minton SD, Stoddard RA, et al: The Provo multicenter early high-frequency oscillatory ventilation trial: Improved pulmonary and clinical outcome in respiratory distress syndrome. Pediatrics 98:1044, 1996.

59. Courtney SE, Durand DJ, Asselin JM, Hudak ML, Aschner JL, Shoemaker CT. High-frequency oscillatory ventilation versus conventional mechanical ventilation for very-low-birth-weight infants. N Engl J Med 347:643, 2002.

60. deLemos RA, Coalson JJ, Meredith KS, et al: A comparison of ventilation strategies for the use of high-frequency oscillatory ventilation in the treatment of hyaline membrane disease. Acta Anaesthesiol Scand 33:102, 1989.

61. Kinsella JP, Gerstmann DR, Clark RH, et al: High-frequency oscillatory ventilation versus intermittent mandatory ventilation: Early hemodynamic effects in the premature baboon with hyaline membrane disease. Pediatr Res 29:160, 1991.

62. McCulloch PR, Forkert PG, Froese AB: Lung volume maintenance prevents lung injury during high-frequency oscillatory ventilation in surfactant deficient rabbits. Am Rev Respir Dis 137:1185, 1988.

63. Froese AB: Role of lung volume in lung injury: HFO in the atelectasis-prone lung. Acta Anaesthesiol Scand 90:126, 1989.

64. Froese AB, McCulloch PR, Fugiura M, et al: Optimizing alveolar expansion prolongs the effectiveness of exogenous surfactant therapy in the adult rabbit. Am Rev Respir Dis 148:569, 1993.

65. Clark RH, Gerstmann DR, Null DM Jr, deLemos RA: Prospective randomized comparison of high-frequency oscillatory and conventional ventilation in respiratory distress syndrome. Pediatrics 89:5, 1992.

66. Friedlich P, Subramanian N, Sebald M, Noori S, Seri I. Use of high-frequency jet ventilation in neonates with hypoxemia refractory to high-frequency oscillatory ventilation. J Matern Fetal Neonatal Med 13:398, 2003.

CHAPTER 46

High-Frequency Oscillatory Ventilation

C. Michael Cotten and Reese H. Clark

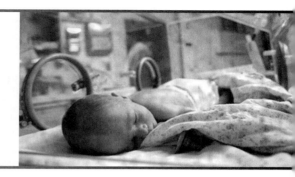

Despite improvements in respiratory care, ventilator-induced lung injury remains an important cause of morbidity and mortality in neonates.[1,2] Experimental evidence has shown that large tidal volumes (VT) of gas damage the developing lung.[3-5] In addition, animal experiments have demonstrated that reinflating atelectatic lungs can cause lung injury. The use of exogenous surfactant[6,7] and gentler strategies of conventional ventilation[8] has reduced, but not eliminated, ventilator-induced lung injury.

The development of high-frequency ventilators has been driven by the hope of finding a method of accomplishing adequate gas exchange in a manner that minimizes lung injury.[9-12] Animal experiments have suggested that when used with a strategy that promoted lung inflation, high-frequency ventilation promotes better gas exchange and reduced lung injury compared with conventional ventilation.[13-17] Clinical research in neonatal intensive care units has been less definitive. Some trials have indicated a reduction in pulmonary morbidity; others have shown no effect or potential harm.[18]

In this chapter, we review the mechanisms of lung injury and discuss how high-frequency ventilation decreases lung injury while permitting adequate gas exchange. We present clinical trials and meta-analyses reviewing use of high-frequency oscillatory ventilation (HFOV) for neonates with various problems and discuss how HFOV interacts with other therapies, particularly surfactant and inhaled nitric oxide. Finally, we discuss the complications thought to be associated with high-frequency ventilation.

MECHANISMS OF LUNG INJURY

Volume-Induced Lung Injury

The use of large VT to accomplish adequate ventilation is a major cause of lung damage **(volutrauma)**.[5,19-22] When VT is limited, the use of high airway pressures alone does not produce as much damage.[5,21-23] Rapid changes in lung volume may be more important than changes in airway

pressure in the propagation of lung injury.[3,24,25] In animals with normal lungs, large VT ventilation damages the pulmonary capillary endothelium, alveolar and airway epithelium, and basement membranes.[3,24,25] This mechanical damage causes fluid, protein, and blood to leak into the airways, alveoli, and lung interstitium, initiating a sequence that can lead to progressive respiratory failure. The mere initiation of ventilation in preterm animal models with respiratory distress syndrome increases expression of inflammatory mediators,[4,26] and this inflammatory response is not limited to the lung. Ventilator-induced lung injury is associated with increases in systemically circulating inflammatory mediators that may cause multisystem injury and multiorgan failure.[27-29]

Lung Injury Associated with Atelectasis

Atelectotrauma refers to the observation that ventilating a collapsed lung causes much more injury than ventilating an optimally inflated lung.[22] Opening and closing of lung units creates surface forces that can denude the surface epithelium. The most severe lung injury seen in animal models of lung disease occurs when atelectotrauma and volutrauma are combined. Use of zero end-expiratory pressure (allowing the lung to collapse) combined with use of large VT creates the greatest degree of lung injury.[26,30] Optimizing functional residual capacity improves ventilation-perfusion matching, decreases intrapulmonary shunt, limits dead space volume (VDS), and allows each VT breath to be distributed more evenly throughout the lung. Optimizing lung inflation and alveolar ventilation (cycling VT from normal functional residual capacity to a peak lung volume lower than total lung capacity) reduces the potential for lung injury.[26,30]

HIGH-FREQUENCY OSCILLATION

History

The ideas behind HFOV extend back to 1915[31,32] with rapid puffs of cigarette smoke displacing gas. In 1959, Emerson[33] built and patented a high-frequency oscillator.[12,34]

In 1972, Lunkenheimer and colleagues[35] reported that paralyzed dogs could be supported for 40 minutes by oscillating gas at V_T less than V_{DS}.

Later in the 1970s, four "physician volunteers" were ventilated successfully with an oscillator for 12 minutes and maintained normal arterial partial pressure of carbon dioxide ($PaCO_2$).[35-37] In the 1980s, 12 patients with a variety of respiratory problems, including an infant with respiratory distress syndrome, were ventilated for 1 hour with high-frequency oscillation.[36,37] These studies suggested that high-frequency oscillation decreases ventilation-perfusion mismatch for patients with shunts and provides adequate gas exchange. The strategy was based on the idea that oscillation would facilitate gas diffusion. Investigators reasoned that facilitated diffusion, rather than convection, would decrease the effect of time constants on gas exchange and would increase the areas within a diseased lung that could participate in gas exchange.[23,35,37-43] To implement the theories, positive end-expiratory pressure was used to regulate mean lung volume, and oscillations (rather than convection) were used to move gas in and out of the lung.[44] Ventilation was controlled by oscillator amplitude, and the provision of adequate bypass flow removed carbon dioxide displaced from the alveoli.[36]

In the 1980s, the focus was on using high-frequency ventilation to accomplish gas exchange using small V_T to avoid barotrauma.[9,45,46] Although ventilation was well maintained, oxygenation was not. Animal experiments showed that to maintain oxygenation in animals with acute lung injury, lung volume needs to be recruited.[13,17,44,47] Clinical trials began in the late 1980s and continue today. There is increasing evidence for the importance of optimizing mean lung volume and avoiding lung overinflation as detailed in the animal work of the 1980s.

Mechanics and Gas Exchange Using High-Frequency Oscillatory Ventilation

In general, a high-frequency oscillator generates pressure oscillation around a set mean airway pressure. Adjusting flow into and out of the patient's ventilator circuit controls mean airway pressure. Exhalation is active because of the biphasic pressure waveform. The clinician can adjust mean airway pressure to affect mean lung volume without changing the pressure oscillation. Pressure amplitude, rather than peak and trough pressures, can be adjusted to alter V_T and ventilation. Changes in pressure amplitude do not alter mean airway pressure or mean lung volume significantly.[18] Many different devices have been used to provide high-frequency oscillation, and studies of these devices show large variations in machine performance and differences in the complexity of operation as neonatal ventilators.[48,49] None of the tested devices has been shown to be equivalent.

There are no clinical comparisons between different types of high-frequency ventilation. Each type has its own potential risks and theoretical benefits. The physician caring for patients treated with a specific type of high-frequency ventilator must know the appropriate use and limitations of the device. Application of any of these ventilators outside of the manufacturers' guidelines must be considered experimental and should be offered only under the direction of carefully designed study protocols.

Oxygenation

Strategies employed to improve oxygenation during high-frequency ventilation are similar to strategies used during conventional ventilation. To optimize oxygen delivery, assisted ventilation should maximize ventilation-perfusion matching without impairing cardiac output. During high-frequency ventilation, lung volume is held relatively constant, and the inflation-deflation cycle is reduced relative to conventional ventilation. Conceptually, high-frequency ventilation allows the use of high end-expiratory pressure that maintains lung volume without requiring the use of high peak inspiratory pressures or large V_T to maintain ventilation.

Effective oxygenation with HFOV depends on optimizing lung volume and maintaining functional residual capacity.[13,14,44,47,50] Animal studies evaluating the use of HFOV for hyaline membrane disease have shown that use of lower mean airway pressures than those used with conventional ventilation is associated with progressive loss of lung volume and severe hypoxia.[13,14,44,47,51] Using mean airway pressures higher than those used with conventional ventilation have maintained lung volume, improved gas exchange, normalized the pattern of lung inflation, and reduced lung injury.[14,17,44,47,52] The strategy of using a higher mean airway pressure has been called a **high lung volume strategy**, but the target is not hyperinflation; instead, it is optimal mean lung volume.[13,53]

Despite careful management, lung units (especially the dependent portion of the lung) can become atelectatic. This change can occur with disconnection from the ventilator for suctioning or with ventilation without end-expiratory pressure, or it can be due to progression of the patient's disease. High-frequency breaths, with inspiratory times measured in milliseconds, are unlikely to overcome the atelectatic lung units' impedance and open atelectatic alveoli. When using a high-frequency oscillator and dealing with atelectasis, some clinicians use sustained (10 to 30 seconds) lung inflation greater than the estimated opening pressure to recruit collapsed alveoli. Clinically, this recruitment is accomplished by increasing the mean airway pressure by 2 to 5 cm H_2O for a brief period until oxygenation improves. The goal of a sustained inflation is to supersede opening pressure of the lung and return to the more stable volume on the exhalation limb of the pressure-volume curve. With devices that allow concurrent use of a conventional ventilator, lung recruitment often is accomplished by providing a large V_T breath (sighs).[54,55] The conventional ventilator intermittently interrupts the high-frequency breaths and delivers a larger V_T breath to recruit collapsed areas of the lung.[54] Sustained inflations can improve oxygenation, but if poorly timed or controlled, they can decrease cardiac output, reduce blood flow to the brain, and increase lung injury.[18,52,56,57]

Defining and measuring optimal lung volume for the prevention of lung injury and maintenance of oxygenation is difficult. Most investigators use the chest radiograph, indirect measures of cardiac output, and arterial-to-alveolar partial pressure of oxygen (PaO_2/PAO_2) ratio to assess lung inflation. At present, the best determinants of low lung volume are a chest radiograph showing atelectasis along with a PaO_2/PAO_2 ratio showing poor oxygenation. Other clues include increased (for less volume) or decreased (for more volume) patient respiratory effort.

When the chest radiograph shows lung hyperinflation and there are clinical signs of decreased cardiac output, lung volume is too high. In older children, mixed venous oxygen content and cardiac output also can be monitored and are helpful in assessing the impact of any type of assisted ventilation on cardiac output. Future development of lung volume assessment, such as respiratory inductive plethysmography, will help clinicians assess better the adequacy of lung volume and make volume recruitment maneuvers safer.[58]

Ventilation

One basic tenet of respiratory physiology is that alveolar ventilation (VA) is the product of breathing rate (f) and VT minus VDS:

$$VA = f \bullet (VT - VDS)$$

This equation predicts that if VT is less than or equal to the VDS, alveolar ventilation should not occur. Animal experiments with high-frequency ventilation have shown that adequate ventilation can be achieved using VT less than the VDS.[12,59-62] During high-frequency ventilation, carbon dioxide output (VCO2) is still related to frequency and VT, but with modifications

$$VCO_2 = f^a \bullet VT^b$$

where a has been estimated to be between 0.75 and 1.24 and b between 1.5 and 2.2, close to 2 with sinusoidal oscillations. Although VT is small, minor changes can elicit large changes in ventilation. The VT delivered to the alveolus depends on the ventilator frequency and the impedance of the respiratory system.[49]

Impedance is the pressure cost to move gas, and it is based on the combination of the inert property of the gas, the airway resistance, and lung compliance. Impedance varies with frequency.[23] If the clinician increases ventilator frequency, impedance increases and VT delivered to the alveolus decreases.[60] Changes in endotracheal tube size, airway resistance, and lung compliance affect impedance and, along with ventilator frequency, can affect $PaCO_2$ more significantly than similar changes occurring during the narrow range of frequencies and the high peak pressures used for conventional ventilation.[63]

Another important difference between high-frequency ventilation and conventional ventilation is the distribution of gas transport. During conventional ventilation, the distribution of gas transport is affected primarily by the lung unit's time constant, the product of airway resistance and lung unit compliance (TC [in seconds] = R [cm H_2O/ L/sec] × C [L/cm H_2O]). In animals with lung disease, each lung unit has different compliance and airway resistance. Alveolar ventilation is greater in lung units with low resistance and higher compliance compared with high airway resistance and low compliance units. The more normal lung units with low resistance and high

compliance are cycled through larger volume changes and as a result may be injured. During high-frequency ventilation, the distribution of gas transport seems to be more uniform, but also is affected by VT, frequency, respiratory system mechanics, and uniformity of the lung disease.

The reasons for the enhanced gas transport with low VT, high-frequency ventilation are unknown, but several theories, based on experimental lung models, attempt to explain the phenomenon. Similar to conventional ventilation, some **convective bulk flow ventilation** occurs in the most proximal airways and alveoli, and molecular diffusion explains gas exchange across alveolar capillary membranes. One potential difference in gas transport is the way alveoli interact during high-frequency ventilation. The difference in time constants among alveoli in a diseased lung is overcome when an inflated alveolus empties into downstream "slower" alveoli.[12] This oscillation of gas between lung units with different time constants is called the **Pendelluft effect**. In addition to Pendelluft, the **velocity profile** of gas delivered at high frequency allows forward flow of fresh gas in the center of the airway, while mixed alveolar gas exits at the periphery; the more rapid the velocity in, the more effective the removal. When delivered at high velocity, there also is enhanced dispersion of gas known as **Taylor dispersion**.[12]

At present, there are no human data comparing the effectiveness of different VT and frequencies in the prevention of lung injury. Future research may define disease-specific frequencies and VT that maximize uniformity of gas transport and minimize the pressure cost of ventilation for each of the high-frequency ventilators.

EFFICACY OF HIGH-FREQUENCY OSCILLATORY VENTILATION

Animal Studies

Prevention of Lung Injury

In a premature baboon model of hyaline membrane disease, HFOV reduces the occurrence of air leak, prevents the evolution of hyaline membrane disease, promotes uniform lung inflation, and improves gas exchange and lung mechanics.[17,47] In rhesus monkeys with hyaline membrane disease, HFOV improves gas exchange and reduces exudative alveolar edema.[15,16] Adult rabbits rendered surfactant deficient by repeated lung lavage also respond to the use of HFOV with improved gas exchange and reduced lung injury.[13,14,64,65] Compared with conventional ventilation, HFOV reduces the amount of inflammatory mediators (thromboxanes and platelet-activating factor) and the number of leukocytes recovered in lung lavage samples from animals with acute lung injury.[66]

HFOV is most effective in the treatment of surfactant-deficient animals when it is applied early and with a strategy designed to recruit and maintain lung inflation. Use of HFOV after 8 hours of conventional ventilation improves gas exchange and lung inflation compared with continued use of conventional ventilation.[67] This relatively late use of HFOV does not reduce acute lung injury, however, as effectively as use immediately after delivery.[67]

Use of High-Frequency Oscillation with Surfactant

Data on the combined use of high-frequency oscillation and exogenous surfactant indicate a synergistic effect in reducing ventilator-induced lung injury. Proteinaceous alveolar edema in monkeys with hyaline membrane disease is reduced by HFOV and exogenous surfactant, but the combination results in the least amount of edema.[16] When compared with administration of surfactant with conventional ventilation, the use of surfactant with HFOV improves gas exchange, improves pulmonary mechanics, and increases the phospholipid quantities recovered from lung lamellar body and lavage fluid in surfactant-depleted adult rabbits.[14,16] In adult rabbits injured with *N*-nitroso-*n*-methylurethane, HFOV reduces the conversion of alveolar surfactant large aggregates into less functional small aggregate forms.[68] Although animal studies show that surfactant and HFOV synergistically reduce lung injury, it is unclear whether the use of HFOV improves the distribution of exogenous surfactant within the lung.[69,70]

Human Studies

Premature Neonates

Clinical trials comparing the use of HFOV and conventional ventilation in neonates with hyaline membrane disease have not been as encouraging as animal data. Most clinical trials have failed to show significant improvements in outcomes. The explanation of these contradictory results most likely is related to the heterogeneity of neonates with hyaline membrane disease, the timing and strategy of high-frequency ventilation employed, the intercenter variability in neonatal management, and improvements in conventional ventilation. Animal studies are designed so that confounding variables can be carefully controlled. In human studies, it is difficult to control all the potential confounding variables. What has become increasingly clear is that the strategy with which HFOV is used is important.[71-74]

Hyaline Membrane Disease

There have been several clinical studies of the use of HFOV in the treatment of premature neonates.[8,46,75-82] A more recent meta-analysis[83] has summarized the accumulated evidence on whether the elective use of HFOV compared with conventional ventilation in preterm infants decreases the incidence of chronic lung disease without adverse effects. This Cochrane analysis included only randomized controlled trials comparing HFOV and conventional ventilation in preterm neonates with respiratory distress syndrome. Eight eligible studies have compared HFOV with conventional ventilation.[8,46,76,77,79-81,84] Meta-analysis has shown no difference in mortality. There is a trend toward decreases in chronic lung disease in survivors. There is also an increase in severe (grades 3 and 4) intraventricular hemorrhage, however, in the HFOV group. Use of HFOV is also associated with a small but significant increase in air leak syndrome. This meta-analysis is dominated by the large HIFI study, which did not specifically use the high-volume strategy, and had major center differences in outcomes.

In the subgroup of two trials[46,77] *not* using a high-volume strategy, including the HIFI trial, HFOV has no effect on the rate of chronic lung disease; however, periventricular leukomalacia is increased (summary relative risk 1.64 [1.02 to 2.64]). In the subgroup of six trials in which a high-volume strategy was used, HFOV results in more favorable pulmonary outcomes.[8,76,79-81,84] Rates of chronic lung disease in survivors at 28 to 30 days and the use of oxygen at 36 to 37 weeks' postmenstrual age or discharge are reduced. The analysis of these six high-volume strategy studies shows no differences in the rates of intraventricular hemorrhage or periventricular leukomalacia.

Subsequent to the Cochrane analysis, a multicenter trial has compared early HFOV with synchronized intermittent mandatory ventilation and V_T monitoring for the treatment of very-low-birth-weight neonates with respiratory distress.[82] Eligible infants weighed between 601 and 1200 g, were less than 4 hours old, had received one dose of surfactant, and required ventilation with a mean airway pressure greater than 6 cm H_2O and fraction of inspired oxygen (F_{IO_2}) greater than 0.25. Ventilator management was governed by protocols designed to optimize lung inflation and blood gases and included weaning and extubation criteria. Of 500 patients enrolled, 245 were randomized to HFOV and 255 were randomized to synchronized intermittent mandatory ventilation. Patients randomized to HFOV are more likely to be alive and off oxygen at 36 weeks' corrected age (56% versus 47%; $P = .036$). Infants randomized to HFOV also are extubated earlier from their primary disease and are less likely to be treated with systemic steroids. HFOV is not associated with increased risk of intracranial hemorrhage, cystic periventricular leukomalacia, or other complications of prematurity.

Only three of the published trials have included neurodevelopmental follow-up, with the meta-analysis showing a modestly increased risk of neurodevelopmental abnormality (summary relative risk 1.26 [1.01 to 1.58]).[46,83,84] The HIFI trial included 386 of 504 survivors (77%) and has shown an increased risk to infants treated with high-frequency ventilation of more often having a Bayley score less than 83 and a neurologic defect.[46] The trial by Ogawa and coworkers,[84] which used a high-volume strategy, has shown no difference with developmental delay at 12 months in 9% of children from each study group.

Lastly, Johnson and colleagues have shown that infants treated with HFOV have similar outcomes to those treated with conventional ventilation. There were no differences in the treatment groups in chronic lung disease, air leak, or brain injury.[85]

In a long-term follow-up study (6 years), Gerstmann and colleagues[86] have reported data on postdelivery neurodevelopmental and pulmonary function. Preterm infants originally randomized to conventional ventilation after surfactant treatment are found to have evidence of obstructive pulmonary disease manifested as increased residual volume and decreased peak expiratory flow. These changes are not found in the children who were randomized to HFOV. The authors speculated that early HFOV, when used with a lung recruitment strategy in combination with surfactant replacement, may ameliorate acute neonatal lung injury, which predisposes some preterm infants to develop chronic lung disease.

The devices used varied from trial to trial, as did the strategies of "conventional support." In the trial published by Moriette and colleagues,[80] the oscillations were generated using a 1:1 inspiratory-to-expiratory time ratio. Other studies have used a 1:2 ratio.[82,86] Although meta-analysis is helpful in providing summary information, it does not replace the need to read closely the details of methods and findings of each specific trial. We believe device type influences performance and outcome.

Pulmonary Interstitial Emphysema

Many of the preliminary evaluations of high-frequency ventilation involved preterm infants with air leak syndromes. Keszler and colleagues[87] have reported the largest series. Their multicenter controlled trial comparing high-frequency jet ventilation ($n = 74$) with conventional ventilation ($n = 70$) has shown that newborn infants with pulmonary interstitial emphysema are more likely to respond to high-frequency jet ventilation than to continued conventional ventilation (61% versus 37%; $P < .01$). In addition, high-frequency jet ventilation improves gas exchange at lower peak and mean airway pressures and is associated with a more rapid resolution of pulmonary interstitial emphysema. When corrected for the crossover design, infants treated with high-frequency jet ventilation have a better survival rate than neonates treated with conventional ventilation (65% versus 47%; $P < .05$). The incidence of chronic lung disease, intraventricular hemorrhage, patent ductus arteriosus, and new air leak is similar for both groups.

Uncontrolled rescue studies evaluating the efficacy of HFOV in neonates with air leak syndromes before the surfactant era have shown similar results and indicate that high-frequency ventilation may be a valuable management tool in the treatment of air leak syndromes.[56,88-90] The reported rates of death (20% to 68%) and chronic lung disease (50% to 100%) are high in all these studies, however. Surfactant therapy has reduced greatly the occurrence of air leak syndrome, and the need for high-frequency ventilation as a rescue tool has been diminished.

Extracorporeal Membrane Oxygenation Candidates

A prospective randomized comparison of HFOV and conventional ventilation has shown that HFOV is a more effective rescue tool than conventional ventilation.[91] Of the patients who do not respond to conventional ventilation, 63% respond to HFOV with improved oxygenation, but only 23% of the HFOV treatment failures respond to conventional ventilation. The two groups do not differ with respect to their need for extracorporeal membrane oxygenation (ECMO), ventilator or hospital days, chronic lung disease, or survival. Only 46% of the patients who meet ECMO criteria require ECMO. Several rescue studies have supported the observation that high-frequency oscillation improves gas exchange in near-term neonates with severe respiratory failure.[92-95]

Using high-frequency oscillation to treat ECMO candidates does not appear to increase morbidity. The incidence

of chronic lung disease and intracranial hemorrhage in ECMO candidates managed successfully with HFOV is lower than in neonates who do not respond to HFOV and require ECMO.[95,96] Neonates who require ECMO are generally sicker, however, and more often have lung hypoplasia syndromes than neonates successfully treated with high-frequency ventilation.

Extracorporeal Membrane Oxygenation Criteria and High-Frequency Ventilation

ECMO is useful in the management of life-threatening respiratory failure.[97] There is debate, however, over what defines life-threatening respiratory failure. The use of high-frequency ventilation in neonates considered candidates for ECMO has complicated this definition further because of the relatively high mean airway pressures used and its significance in calculating oxygenation index (mean airway pressure $\times$ [FIO_2/PaO_2]).[95]

The ability of HFOV to improve gas exchange in ECMO candidates has appeared to be disease specific.[95] HFOV improves gas exchange in 88% of neonates with hyaline membrane disease, 79% with pneumonia, 51% with meconium aspiration, and 22% with congenital diaphragmatic hernia. Failure to show an improvement in the PaO_2/PAO_2 ratio after 6 hours of HFOV is predictive of a need for ECMO.

These reports indicate that some neonates with severe respiratory failure should be offered a trial of HFOV only when ECMO is available. Neonates with an oxygenation index greater than 0.40 and a diagnosis of meconium aspiration or congenital diaphragmatic hernia often do not respond to HFOV.[91,92,95] For most of these patients, ECMO may improve survival, and delayed referral to ECMO centers may increase their risk of morbidity and mortality. Any patient whose oxygenation is poor despite a 4- to 8-hour trial of HFOV should be considered for immediate transfer to an ECMO center. These transfers can be complicated by the unavailability of HFOV transport systems and difficulty in restarting conventional ventilation.

High-Frequency Oscillatory Ventilation and Congenital Diaphragmatic Hernia

Three studies offer promise from the early use of HFOV for patients with congenital diaphragmatic hernia.[98-100] All these studies are observational reports, but all show survival for patients with isolated congenital diaphragmatic hernia of greater than 75%. Miguet and coworkers[100,101] have used HFOV for 18 consecutive patients (14 with isolated congenital diaphragmatic hernia) with an initial mean airway pressure of 15 cm H_2O and amplitude of at least 30 cm H_2O; thus, hyperventilation was avoided and ECMO did not have to be used. Thirteen of the 14 patients with isolated congenital diaphragmatic hernia survived. In the study by Reyes and colleagues,[98] 14 (78%) of 18 patients ventilated with HFOV within the first 3 hours of life survived. Somaschini and associates[99] used HFOV as the primary ventilatory mode to support 28 patients with isolated congenital diaphragmatic hernia, and 25 (89%) survived. Although not definitive, the results of these studies suggest that HFOV may have a role to play in the management of neonates with congenital diaphragmatic hernia.

Use of High-Frequency Oscillation with Inhaled Nitric Oxide

Inhaled nitric oxide improves gas exchange and reduces the use of ECMO in near-term neonates with severe respiratory failure.[102-104] The combined use of HFOV and inhaled nitric oxide seems to be more effective than either therapy alone in the management of neonates with lung disease and pulmonary hypertension.[105] This finding was particularly true for neonates with respiratory distress syndrome or meconium aspiration syndrome.[105] Similar to HFOV alone, the efficacy of HFOV and inhaled nitric oxide in neonates with congenital diaphragmatic hernia has not been shown.[102-104,106] The combined use of HFOV and inhaled nitric oxide requires a careful definition of treatment failure. Delayed transport of critically ill neonates to higher levels of care can have lethal consequences.

COMPLICATIONS

Complications reported to be associated with HFOV include decreased cardiac output, hypotension, intraventricular hemorrhage, periventricular leukomalacia,[107] mucous plugging, and necrotizing tracheobronchitis.[108]

Cardiac Output Effects

The interaction of airway pressure with cardiac output is related to lung compliance and lung volume. The use of high mean airway pressure can cause lung overinflation, reduced venous return, increased pulmonary vascular resistance, reduced left ventricular filling, and reduced cardiac output.[100,101,109-111] In patients with marginal cardiac output, the constant distending airway pressure associated with the use of HFOV can seriously compromise cardiac output. Animal and human studies have shown that when used with a strategy that avoids lung hyperinflation, HFOV does not reduce cardiac output, but with an emphasis on the "open lung" strategies, vigilant assessment of cardiac output is necessary when initiating HFOV and when pressures are increased.[112] The clinician must be wary of the infant recovering from acute lung disease because the same mean airway pressure previously necessary to maintain adequate lung volume can lead rapidly to overdistention and cardiovascular compromise with improving lung compliance.[47]

Intracranial Injury: Intraventricular Hemorrhage and Periventricular Leukomalacia

The causes of intraventricular hemorrhage and periventricular leukomalacia are multifactorial; a cause-and-effect association between HFOV and intracranial hemorrhage is difficult to assess. More recent meta-analyses suggest that the association between high-frequency ventilation and intracranial pathology may be related more to how high-frequency ventilation is used rather than to whether it is used.[71,72] High-frequency ventilation can produce rapid changes in $Paco_2$, which can cause sudden changes in cerebral blood flow and which may lead to neurologic complications.[107,113,114] Safe use of any high-frequency ventilator requires close, careful monitoring of $Paco_2$ and avoidance of hypocarbia.

Tracheal Injury

Tracheal injury is a potential complication of any form of ventilatory support that requires endotracheal intubation. Necrotizing tracheobronchitis is a severe form of tracheal injury that is often life-threatening. Early reports have suggested that high-frequency jet ventilation is associated with a high incidence of necrotizing tracheobronchitis.[115,116] Further studies have suggested that inadequate humidification of the inspired gas, decreased tracheal blood flow, and the use of high airway pressure are more important than the mode of ventilation in the cause of this disease.[108,117] In a study evaluating the efficacy of high-frequency jet ventilation in the treatment of pulmonary interstitial emphysema, the occurrence of airway obstruction in neonates treated with high-frequency jet ventilation is no different than in neonates treated with conventional ventilation.[87] The diagnosis of necrotizing tracheobronchitis should be considered in neonates with severe sudden airway obstruction because early recognition and treatment are lifesaving.

SUMMARY

Despite improvements in respiratory care, ventilator-induced lung injury remains an important cause of morbidity and mortality in neonatal patients who require assisted ventilation. Animal data clearly show that high-frequency ventilation can reduce lung injury successfully in experimental models of acute lung injury. Animal models and human research show that the efficacy of high-frequency ventilation depends on optimizing lung volume and avoiding lung overinflation. When used with a strategy that allows the lung to collapse or is associated with hyperventilation, high-frequency ventilation does not reduce lung injury and is associated with significant brain injury. When used with a strategy that promotes lung recruitment, high-frequency ventilation effectively reduces the occurrence of chronic lung disease and is not associated with significant brain injury. Future development of devices that allow accurate monitoring of lung volume while using HFOV will help optimize achieving the "open lung" strategy.

Similar to every tool used to support critically ill neonates, high-frequency ventilation requires a careful clinician and health care team. As therapies and technology evolve, there remains nothing more important than each member of the health care team spending time at the bedside. Their critical continuous evaluation of an infant's response to therapy is essential to promotion of optimal outcome.

REFERENCES

1. STOP-ROP Study Group: Supplemental Therapeutic Oxygen for Prethreshold Retinopathy Of Prematurity (STOP-ROP), a randomized, controlled trial: I. Primary outcomes. Pediatrics 105:295, 2000.

2. Van Marter LJ, Allred EN, Pagano M, et al: Do clinical markers of barotrauma and oxygen toxicity explain interhospital variation in rates of chronic lung disease? Pediatrics 105:1194, 2000.

3. Parker JC, Hernandez LA, Peevy KJ: Mechanisms of ventilator-induced lung injury. Crit Care Med 21:131, 1993.

4. Jobe AH, Ikegami M: Mechanisms initiating lung injury in the preterm. Early Hum Dev 53:81, 1998.

5. Dreyfuss D, Saumon G: Ventilator-induced lung injury: Lessons from experimental studies. Am J Respir Crit Care Med 157:294, 1998.

6. Jobe AH, Ikegami M: Surfactant and acute lung injury. Proc Assoc Am Physicians 110:489, 1998.

7. Jobe AH, Ikegami M: Surfactant for acute respiratory distress syndrome. Adv Intern Med 42:203, 1997.

8. Gerstmann DR, Minton SD, Stoddard RA, et al: The Provo multicenter early high-frequency oscillatory ventilation trial: Improved pulmonary and clinical outcome in respiratory distress syndrome. Pediatrics 98:1044, 1996.

9. Froese AB, Bryan AC: High frequency ventilation [editorial]. Am Rev Respir Dis 123:249, 1981.

10. Froese AB: High frequency ventilation: current status. Can Anaesth Soc J 31:S9, 1984.

11. Froese AB, Butler PO, Fletcher WA, Byford LJ: High-frequency oscillatory ventilation in premature infants with respiratory failure: A preliminary report. Anesth Analg 66:814, 1987.

12. Froese AB, Bryan AC: High frequency ventilation. Am Rev Respir Dis 135:1363, 1987.

13. Froese AB: Role of lung volume in lung injury: HFO in the atelectasis-prone lung. Acta Anaesthesiol Scand 90:126, 1989.

14. Froese AB, McCulloch PR, Sugiura M, et al: Optimizing alveolar expansion prolongs the effectiveness of exogenous surfactant therapy in the adult rabbit. Am Rev Respir Dis 148:569, 1993.

15. Jackson JC, Truog WE, Standaert TA, et al: Effect of high-frequency ventilation on the development of alveolar edema in premature monkeys at risk for hyaline membrane disease. Am Rev Respir Dis 143:865, 1991.

16. Jackson JC, Truog WE, Standaert TA, et al: Reduction in lung injury after combined surfactant and high-frequency ventilation. Am J Respir Crit Care Med 150:534, 1994.

17. Meredith KS, deLemos RA, Coalson JJ, et al: Role of lung injury in the pathogenesis of hyaline membrane disease in premature baboons. J Appl Physiol 66:2150, 1989.

18. Clark RH: High-frequency ventilation. J Pediatr 124:661, 1994.

19. Ikegami M, Kallapur S, Michna J, Jobe AH: Lung injury and surfactant metabolism after hyperventilation of premature lambs. Pediatr Res 47:398, 2000.

20. Jobe AH, Ikegami M: Lung development and function in preterm infants in the surfactant treatment era. Annu Rev Physiol 62:825, 2000.

21. Dreyfuss D, Martin LL, Saumon G: Hyperinflation-induced lung injury during alveolar flooding in rats: Effect of perfluorocarbon instillation. Am J Respir Crit Care Med 159:1752, 1999.

22. Slutsky AS: Lung injury caused by mechanical ventilation. Chest 116:9S, 1999.

23. Venegas JG, Fredberg JJ: Understanding the pressure cost of ventilation: Why does high-frequency ventilation work? Crit Care Med 22:S49, 1994.

24. Tremblay LN, Slutsky AS: Ventilator-induced injury: From barotrauma to biotrauma. Proc Assoc Am Physicians 110:482, 1998.

25. Hernandez LA, Peevy KJ, Moise AA, Parker JC: Chest wall restriction limits high airway pressure-induced lung injury in young rabbits. J Appl Physiol 66:2364, 1989.

26. Michna J, Jobe AH, Ikegami M: Positive end-expiratory pressure preserves surfactant function in preterm lambs. Am J Respir Crit Care Med 160:634, 1999.

27. Ranieri VM, Suter PM, Tortorella C, et al: Effect of mechanical ventilation on inflammatory mediators in patients with acute respiratory distress syndrome: A randomized controlled trial. JAMA 282:54, 1999.

28. Ranieri VM, Giunta F, Suter PM, Slutsky AS: Mechanical ventilation as a mediator of multisystem organ failure in acute respiratory distress syndrome [letter]. JAMA 284:43, 2000.

29. Acute Respiratory Distress Syndrome Network: Ventilation with lower tidal volumes as compared with traditional tidal volumes for acute lung injury and the acute respiratory distress syndrome. N Engl J Med 342:1301, 2000.

30. Takata M, Abe J, Tanaka H, et al: Intraalveolar expression of tumor necrosis factor-alpha gene during conventional and high-frequency ventilation. Am J Respir Crit Care Med 156:272, 1997.

31. Henderson Y, Chillingworth F, Wilkinson MH: The respiratory dead space. Am J Physiol 18:1, 1915.

32. Bryan AC: The oscillations of HFO. Am J Respir Crit Care Med 163:816, 2001.

33. Emerson JH: Apparatus for vibrating portions of a patient's airway. United States Patent Office 1959; Serial no. 491, 699, patented Dec. 29, 1959.

34. Slutsky AS, Drazen FM, Ingram RHJ, et al: Effective pulmonary ventilation with small-volume oscillations at high frequency. Science 209:609, 1980.

35. Lunkenheimer PP, Frieling G, Whimster WF: High frequency ventilation 20 years of endeavour reviewed: Why an expert meeting now? Acta Anaesthesiol Scand 90:1, 1989.

36. Butler WJ, Bohn DJ, Bryan AC, et al: Ventilation by high-frequency oscillation in humans. Anesth Analg 59:577, 1980.

37. Marchak BE, Thompson WK, Duffty P, et al: Treatment of RDS by high-frequency oscillatory ventilation: A preliminary report. J Pediatr 99:287, 1981.

38. Chan V, Greenough A, Milner AD: The effect of frequency and mean airway pressure on volume delivery during high-frequency oscillation. Pediatr Pulmonol 15:183, 1993.

39. Chan V, Greenough A, Dimitriou G: High frequency oscillation, respiratory activity and changes in blood gases. Early Hum Dev 40:87, 1995.

40. Fredberg JJ: Augmented diffusion in the airways can support pulmonary gas exchange. J Appl Physiol 49:232, 1980.

41. Fredberg JJ, Keefe DH, Glass GM, et al: Alveolar pressure nonhomogeneity during small-amplitude high-frequency oscillation. J Appl Physiol 57:788, 1984.

42. Freitag L, Bremme J, Schroer M: High frequency oscillation for respiratory physiotherapy. Br J Anaesth 63:44S, 1989.

43. Venegas JG, Yamada Y, Custer J, Hales CA: Effects of respiratory variables on regional gas transport during high-frequency ventilation. J Appl Physiol 64:2108, 1988.

44. Kolton M, Cattran CB, Kent G, et al: Oxygenation during high-frequency ventilation compared with conventional mechanical ventilation in two models of lung injury. Anesth Analg 61:323, 1982.

45. Frantz ID, Werthammer J, Stark AR: High-frequency ventilation in premature infants with lung disease: Adequate gas exchange at low tracheal pressure. Pediatrics 71:483, 1983.

46. HIFI Study Group: High-frequency oscillatory ventilation compared with conventional mechanical ventilation in the treatment of respiratory failure in preterm infants. N Engl J Med 320:88, 1989.

47. Kinsella JP, Gerstmann DR, Clark RH, et al: High-frequency oscillatory ventilation versus intermittent mandatory ventilation: Early hemodynamic effects in the premature baboon with hyaline membrane disease. Pediatr Res 29:160, 1991.

48. Fredberg JJ, Glass GM, Boynton BR, Frantz ID: Factors influencing mechanical performance of neonatal high-frequency ventilators. J Appl Physiol 62:2485, 1987.

49. Hatcher D, Watanabe H, Ashbury T, et al: Mechanical performance of clinically available, neonatal, high-frequency, oscillatory-type ventilators. Crit Care Med 26:1081, 1998.

50. Walsh MC, Carlo WA: Determinants of gas flow through a bronchopleural fistula. J Appl Physiol 67:1591, 1989.

51. Ackerman NB Jr, Coalson JJ, Kuehl TJ, et al: Pulmonary interstitial emphysema in the premature baboon with hyaline membrane disease. Crit Care Med 12:512, 1984.

52. Walsh MC, Carlo WA: Sustained inflation during HFOV improves pulmonary mechanics and oxygenation. J Appl Physiol 65:368, 1988.

53. Froese AB: High-frequency oscillatory ventilation for adult respiratory distress syndrome: Let's get it right this time! [editorial; comment]. Crit Care Med 25:906, 1997.

54. Bond DM, Froese AB: Volume recruitment maneuvers are less deleterious than persistent low lung volumes in the atelectasis-prone rabbit lung during high-frequency oscillation. Crit Care Med 21:402, 1993.

55. Bond DM, McAloon J, Froese AB: Sustained inflations improve respiratory compliance during high-frequency oscillatory ventilation but not during large tidal volume positive-pressure ventilation in rabbits. Crit Care Med 22:1269, 1994.

56. Clark RH, Gerstmann DR, Null DM, et al: Pulmonary interstitial emphysema treated by high-frequency oscillatory ventilation. Crit Care Med 14:926, 1986.

57. Walker AM, Brodecky VA, de Preu ND, Ritchie BC: High-frequency oscillatory ventilation compared with conventional mechanical ventilation in newborn lambs: Effects of increasing airway pressure on intracranial pressures. Pediatr Pulmonol 12:11, 1992.

58. Göthberg S, Parker TA, Griebel J, et al: Lung volume recruitment in lambs during high-frequency oscillatory ventilation using respiratory inductive plethysmography. Pediatr Res 49:38, 2001.

59. Chan V, Greenough A: The effect of frequency on carbon dioxide levels during high frequency oscillation. J Perinat Med 22:103, 1994.

60. Fredberg JJ, Allen J, Tsuda A, et al: Mechanics of the respiratory system during high frequency ventilation. Acta Anaesthesiol Scand 90:39, 1989.

61. Fredberg JJ: Pulmonary mechanics during high frequency ventilation. Acta Anaesthesiol Scand 90:170, 1989.

62. Slutsky AS: Nonconventional methods of ventilation. Am Rev Respir Dis 138:175, 1988.

63. Gerstmann DR, Fouke JM, Winter DC, et al: Proximal, tracheal, and alveolar pressures during high-frequency oscillatory ventilation in a normal rabbit model. Pediatr Res 28:367, 1990.

64. Byford LJ, Finkler JH, Froese AB: Lung volume recruitment during high-frequency oscillation in atelectasis-prone rabbits. J Appl Physiol 64:1607, 1988.

65. Hamilton PP, Onayemi A, Smyth JA, et al: Comparison of conventional and high-frequency ventilation: oxygenation and lung pathology. J Appl Physiol 55:131, 1983.

66. Kawano T: High frequency oscillation. Acta Paediatr Jpn 34:631, 1992.

67. deLemos RA, Coalson JJ, deLemos JA, et al: Rescue ventilation with high frequency oscillation in premature baboons with hyaline membrane disease. Pediatr Pulmonol 12:29, 1992.

68. Kerr CL, Veldhuizen RA, Lewis JF: Effects of high-frequency oscillation on endogenous surfactant in an acute lung injury model. Am J Respir Crit Care Med 164:237, 2001.

69. Heldt GP, Merritt TA, Golembeski D, et al: Distribution of surfactant, lung compliance, and aeration of preterm rabbit lungs after surfactant therapy and conventional and high-frequency oscillatory ventilation. Pediatr Res 31:270, 1992.

70. Walther FJ, Kuipers IM, Gidding CE, et al: A comparison of high-frequency oscillation superimposed onto backup mechanical ventilation and conventional mechanical ventilation on the distribution of exogenous surfactant in premature lambs. Pediatr Res 22:725, 1987.

71. Bhuta T, Henderson SD: Elective high-frequency oscillatory ventilation versus conventional ventilation in preterm infants with pulmonary dysfunction: Systematic review and meta-analyses. Pediatrics 100:E6, 1997.

72. Bhuta T, Henderson-Smart DJ: Elective high frequency jet ventilation versus conventional ventilation for respiratory distress syndrome in preterm infants. Cochrane Database Syst Rev CD000328, 2000.

73. Bhuta T, Henderson-Smart DJ: Rescue high frequency oscillatory ventilation versus conventional ventilation for pulmonary dysfunction in preterm infants. Cochrane Database Syst Rev CD000438, 2000.

74. Cools F, Offringa M: Meta-analysis of elective high frequency ventilation in preterm infants with respiratory distress syndrome. Arch Dis Child Fetal Neonatal Educ 80:F15, 1999.

75. Claris O, Salle BL: High frequency oscillatory ventilation and the prevention of chronic lung disease. Pediatr Pulmonol 16(suppl):33, 1997.

76. Clark RH, Gerstmann DR, Null DMJ, deLemos RA: Prospective randomized comparison of high-frequency oscillatory and conventional ventilation in respiratory distress syndrome. Pediatrics 89:5, 1992.

77. Rettwitz-Volk W, Veldman A, Roth B, et al: A prospective, randomized, multicenter trial of high-frequency oscillatory ventilation compared with conventional ventilation in preterm infants with respiratory distress syndrome receiving surfactant. J Pediatr 132:249, 1998.

78. Rimensberger PC, Beghetti M, Hanquinet S, Berner M: First intention high-frequency oscillation with early lung volume optimization improves pulmonary outcome in very low birth weight infants with respiratory distress syndrome. Pediatrics 105:1202, 2000.

79. Thome U, Kössel H, Lipowsky G, et al: Randomized comparison of high-frequency ventilation with high-rate intermittent positive pressure ventilation in preterm infants with respiratory failure. J Pediatr 135:39, 1999.

80. Moriette G, Paris-Llado J, Walti H, et al: Prospective randomized multicenter comparison of high-frequency oscillatory ventilation and conventional ventilation in preterm infants of less than 30 weeks with respiratory distress syndrome. Pediatrics 107:363, 2001.

81. Plavka R, Kopecký P, Sebron V, et al: A prospective randomized comparison of conventional mechanical ventilation and very early high frequency oscillatory ventilation in extremely premature newborns with respiratory distress syndrome. Intensive Care Med 25:68, 1999.

82. Courtney SE, Durand DJ, Asselin JM, et al: Early high frequency oscillatory ventilation vs synchronized intermittent mandatory ventilation for very low birth weight infants. N Engl J Med 347:643, 2002.

83. Henderson-Smart DJ, Bhuta T, Cools F, Offringa M: Elective high frequency oscillatory ventilation versus conventional ventilation for acute pulmonary dysfunction in preterm infants. Cochrane Database Syst Rev CD000104, 2001.

84. Ogawa Y, Miyasaka K, Kawano T, et al: A multicenter randomized trial of high frequency oscillatory ventilation as compared with conventional mechanical ventilation in preterm infants with respiratory failure. Early Hum Dev 32:1, 1993.

85. Johnson AH, Peacock JL, Greenough A, et al: High-frequency oscillatory ventilation for the prevention of chronic lung disease of prematurity. N Engl J Med. 347:633, 2002.

86. Gerstmann DR, Wood K, Miller A, et al: Childhood outcomes following early high-frequency oscillatory ventilation for neonatal respiratory distress syndrome. Pediatrics 108:617, 2001.

87. Keszler M, Donn SM, Bucciarelli RL, et al: Multicenter controlled trial comparing high-frequency jet ventilation and conventional mechanical ventilation in newborn infants with pulmonary interstitial emphysema. J Pediatr 119:85, 1991.

88. Carlo WA, Chatburn RL, Martin RJ, et al: Decrease in airway pressure during high-frequency jet ventilation in infants with respiratory distress syndrome. J Pediatr 104:101, 1984.

89. Carlo WA, Chatburn RL, Martin RJ: Randomized trial of high-frequency jet ventilation versus conventional ventilation in respiratory distress syndrome. J Pediatr 110:275, 1987.

90. Carlo WA, Beoglos A, Chatburn RL, et al: High-frequency jet ventilation in neonatal pulmonary hypertension. Am J Dis Child 143:233, 1989.

91. Clark RH, Yoder BA, Sell MS: Prospective, randomized comparison of high-frequency oscillation and conventional ventilation in candidates for extracorporeal membrane oxygenation. J Pediatr 124:447, 1994.

92. Baumgart S, Hirschl RB, Butler SZ, et al: Diagnosis-related criteria in the consideration of extracorporeal membrane oxygenation in neonates previously treated with high-frequency jet ventilation. Pediatrics 89:491, 1992.

93. Blum-Hoffmann E, Kopotic RJ, Mannino FL: High-frequency oscillatory ventilation combined with intermittent mandatory ventilation in critically ill neonates: 3 years of experience. Eur J Pediatr 147:392, 1988.

94. Carter JM, Gerstmann DR, Clark RH, et al: High-frequency oscillatory ventilation and extracorporeal membrane oxygenation for the treatment of acute neonatal respiratory failure. Pediatrics 85:159, 1990.

95. Paranka MS, Clark RH, Yoder BA, Null DMJ: Predictors of failure of high-frequency oscillatory ventilation in term infants with severe respiratory failure. Pediatrics 95:400, 1995.

96. Schwendeman CA, Clark RH, Yoder BA, et al: Frequency of chronic lung disease in infants with severe respiratory failure treated with high-frequency ventilation and/or extracorporeal membrane oxygenation. Crit Care Med 20:372, 1992.

97. UK Collaborative ECMO Trial Group: UK collaborative randomised trial of neonatal extracorporeal membrane oxygenation. Lancet 348:75, 1996.

98. Reyes C, Chang LK, Waffarn F, et al: Delayed repair of congenital diaphragmatic hernia with early high-frequency oscillatory ventilation during preoperative stabilization. J Pediatr Surg 33:1010, 1998.

99. Somaschini M, Locatelli G, Salvoni L, et al: Impact of new treatments for respiratory failure on outcome of infants with congenital diaphragmatic hernia. Eur J Pediatr 158:780, 1999.

100. Miguet D, Claris O, Lapillonne A, et al: Preoperative stabilization using high-frequency oscillatory ventilation in the management of congenital diaphragmatic hernia. Crit Care Med 22:S77, 1994.

101. Miguet D, Lapillonne A, Bakr A, et al: [Congenital diaphragmatic hernia: results of the association of preoperative stabilization and oscillation ventilation (a prospective study of 17 patients)]. [French]. Can Anesthesiol 42:335, 1994.

102. Kinsella JP: Clinical trials of inhaled nitric oxide therapy in the newborn. Pediatr Rev (Online) 20:e110, 1999.

103. Kinsella JP, Abman SH: Clinical approach to inhaled nitric oxide therapy in the newborn with hypoxemia. J Pediatr 136:717, 2000.

104. Neonatal Inhaled Nitric Oxide Study Group (NINOS): Inhaled nitric oxide in full-term and nearly full-term infants with hypoxic respiratory failure. N Engl J Med 336:597, 1997.

105. Kinsella JP, Truog WE, Walsh WF, et al: Randomized, multicenter trial of inhaled nitric oxide and high-frequency oscillatory ventilation in severe, persistent pulmonary hypertension of the newborn. J Pediatr 131:55, 1997.

106. Clark RH, Kueser TJ, Walker MW, et al: Low-dose nitric oxide therapy for persistent pulmonary hypertension of the newborn. Clinical Inhaled Nitric Oxide Research Group. N Engl J Med 342:469, 2000.

107. Wiswell TE, Graziani LJ, Kornhauser MS, et al: High-frequency jet ventilation in the early management of respiratory distress syndrome is associated with a greater risk for adverse outcomes. Pediatrics 98:1035, 1996.

108. Wiswell TE, Clark RH, Null DM, et al: Tracheal and bronchial injury in high-frequency oscillatory ventilation and high-frequency flow interruption compared with conventional positive-pressure ventilation. J Pediatr 112:249, 1988.

109. Traverse JH, Korvenranta H, Adams EM, et al: Impairment of hemodynamics with increasing mean airway pressure during high-frequency oscillatory ventilation. Pediatr Res 23:628, 1988.

110. Simma B, Fritz M, Fink C, Hammerer I: Conventional ventilation versus high-frequency oscillation: Hemodynamic effects in newborn babies. Crit Care Med 28:227, 2000.

111. Traverse JH, Korvenranta H, Adams EM, et al: Cardiovascular effects of high-frequency oscillatory and jet ventilation. Chest 96:1400, 1989.

112. Arnold JH, Truog RD, Thompson JE, Fackler JC: High-frequency oscillatory ventilation in pediatric respiratory failure. Crit Care Med 21:272, 1993.

113. Vannucci RC, Towfighi J, Heitjan DF, Brucklacher RM: Carbon dioxide protects the perinatal brain from hypoxic-ischemic damage: An experimental study in the immature rat. Pediatrics 95:868, 1995.

114. Wiswell TE, Graziani LJ, Kornhauser MS, et al: Effects of hypocarbia on the development of cystic periventricular leukomalacia in premature infants treated with high-frequency jet ventilation. Pediatrics 98:918, 1996.

115. Mammel MC, Boros SJ: Airway damage and mechanical ventilation: A review and commentary. Pediatr Pulmonol 3:443, 1987.

116. Mammel MC, Ophoven JP, Lewallen PK, et al: Acute airway injury during high-frequency jet ventilation and high-frequency oscillatory ventilation. Crit Care Med 19:394, 1991.

117. Wiswell TE, Wiswell SH: The effect of 100% oxygen on the propagation of tracheobronchial injury during high-frequency and conventional mechanical ventilation. Am J Dis Child 144:560, 1990.

CHAPTER 47

Modern Extracorporeal Membrane Oxygenation for the Human Newborn Infant

Sudhish Chandra and Stephen Baumgart

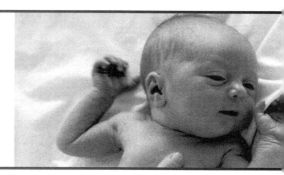

I have good news and I have bad news, ECMO works.

Anon

Extracorporeal membrane oxygenation (EMCO) refers to oxygenation of blood outside the body by an artificial membrane lung. Essentially, neonatal ECMO comprises prolonged cardiopulmonary bypass (CPB) performed in infants with acute but reversible pulmonary disease (e.g., persistent pulmonary hypertension of the newborn [PPHN]) or acute myocardial failure (e.g., with asphyxia). Other forms of extracorporeal life support include hemofiltration/hemodialysis (sometimes used in conjunction with ECMO); intravenous oxygenation, which uses an indwelling microfibril oxygenation device in adult patients; and extracorporeal carbon dioxide (CO_2) removal, a technique also used in adults. This chapter describes neonatal ECMO as practiced in the modern era.

HISTORY OF EXTRACORPOREAL MEMBRANE OXYGENATION[1,2]

CPB became possible in 1937 with the development of the Gibbon metal screen drip oxygenator and roller pump heart-lung machine developed in collaboration with the IBM corporation.[3] In 1938, the introduction of heparin anticoagulation by McLean[4] permitted prolongation of CPB without the interference of blood clotting within the drip oxygenator apparatus. By 1950, rapid advancements in vascular surgical techniques resulted in the development of sheet filming and bubble oxygenators that operated on similar principles and were employed in similar fashion as the Gibbon apparatus.[5,6] Gibbon used his device in 1953 to perform the first successful atrial septal defect repair in an adult patient.

The first cellulose membrane oxygenator working on an entirely different principle was adapted from hemodialysis filters in 1956 by Clowes and colleagues.[7,8] In 1957, materials technology produced the more durable

silicone rubber membrane, and prolonged CPB first became feasible.[9] In 1963, Kolobow and coworkers[10,11] introduced a polyurethane chamber and (with the roller-pump heart-lung) reported successful 7-day animal runs on CPB with this apparatus. Concurrently, one of the first trials with pumpless arteriovenous bypass in a human infant was performed by Rashkind[12] at Children's Hospital of Philadelphia in 1965 to support temporarily a patient with cyanotic congenital heart disease awaiting surgical repair.

In 1969, Dorson and coworkers[13] first performed neonatal ECMO to treat severe pulmonary failure, which also was attempted by White and coworkers in 1971.[14] In both of these cases, infants died as a result of severe intracranial hemorrhages attributed to systemic heparinization. Five years later, Bartlett and coworkers[15] reported the first successful ECMO-treated neonate, who was diagnosed with meconium aspiration syndrome. In 1979, the National Institutes of Health reported the results of a prospectively randomized, multicenter national trial of ECMO rescue for the treatment of near-terminal adult respiratory distress syndrome (RDS) patients.[16] Only 8% survived with conventional therapy in this trial, and only 10% survived with ECMO. Patients who died had irreversible pulmonary fibrosis at the time of death. Bartlett and other proponents of ECMO suggested that ECMO failed in these patients because intervention had come too late, after at least 7 days of mechanical ventilation at high pressure and high inspired oxygen (O_2) concentrations.

By 1982, Bartlett's group[17] had accumulated 45 neonates treated with ECMO, of whom 55% survived. In 1985, they published the controversial, "play-the-winner" randomized trial for ECMO rescue of infants with severe respiratory failure. This trial used early ECMO intervention criteria based on retrospective analysis of conventional ventilatory experience in such infants.[18] Entry criteria comprised a 90% mortality rate predicted on the basis of this past experience. Subjects were randomized to a 50% chance of receiving either ECMO or conventional therapy at the initiation of the study; however, with the success or failure of the initial therapy, subsequent trials were biased in their randomization toward the alternative limb of the trial. The first patient entered into this study was randomized to conventional therapy and died. The next 12 patients were randomized to ECMO therapy and 11 survived.

By 1987, ECMO centers were established at several university medical centers for advancement of this technology and systematic accumulation of ECMO experience.[19-23] O'Rourke and coworkers[24] published a study based on a power design that permitted a maximum of four deaths to confirm Bartlett's results. Four of 10 infants randomized and treated with conventional mechanical ventilation died in the neonatal intensive care unit. Nine of nine infants randomized to receive ECMO were treated separately in the pediatric care unit and survived. Subsequently, 19 of 20 nonrandomized neonates survived successfully on ECMO. These results and the data accumulated at the University of Michigan's computerized ECMO Registry (coordinated by the Extracorporeal Life Support Organization [ELSO]) coincided with the spread of ECMO for the treatment of newborns with severe respiratory failure in the United States, Canada, and several countries in western Europe and Asia.[25]

Since the 1990s, other more recently available therapies, such as surfactant replacement, high-frequency ventilation, and inhaled nitric oxide (iNO), have been used increasingly in the management of critically ill newborns before resorting to ECMO. As a result of these newer treatment modalities, the demographics and practice of neonatal ECMO reported to ELSO in the late 1990s and 2000 have changed[25] (see later).

EXTRACORPOREAL MEMBRANE OXYGENATION FOR TREATMENT OF NEONATAL RESPIRATORY FAILURE

One important difference between the neonatal patient and older infants and children with respiratory disease is the presence of PPHN. Vasoconstriction is the natural state of the neonate's pulmonary vasculature before birth because in utero blood flow normally bypasses the lungs owing to high vascular resistance in the pulmonary vascular bed. It then crosses through fetal channels (the ductus arteriosus and the foramen ovale) into the left side of the circulation and supplies O_2-enriched blood returning via the umbilical vein from the placenta to the systemic circulation to perfuse the brain, heart, and splanchnic and peripheral circulations. Severe respiratory disease postnatally often is accompanied by pulmonary arterial hypertension, presumably because pulmonary vessels fail to dilate shortly after birth (hypoxia, hypercarbia, and acidemia potentiate pulmonary vasoconstriction).[26] Without the fetoplacental O_2 supply, blood shunted across fetal channels into the systemic circulation remains hypoxic and leads to respiratory failure.

One option for treating neonatal pulmonary hypertension in the term or near-term infant with respiratory failure is systemic alkalinization, usually accomplished by mechanical hyperventilation of an already diseased lung[26,27] or occasionally by giving a sodium bicarbonate drip. Hyperventilation reduces CO_2 and increases pH, lowering pulmonary vascular resistance and improving systemic O_2 delivery by reducing shunting through fetal channels. Hyperventilation impedes venous return to the infant's native heart, however, and may impair cardiac output. Despite improving O_2 content in systemic blood, hyperventilation may contribute to ischemia with heart failure often observed in these extremely ill infants. Hyperventilation has the risk of increased barotrauma to an already diseased lung. The consequences of prolonged hyperventilation are well known in neonatology and comprise not only pulmonary air leaks (pneumothorax, pneumomediastinum, pneumopericardium, subcutaneous emphysema, pneumoperitoneum, and pulmonary interstitial emphysema), but also the subsequent development of pulmonary scarring and fibrosis, a condition called **bronchopulmonary dysplasia**. Follow-up data now available in these patients also indicate that prolonged low circulating CO_2 tension may be associated with adverse hearing and neurologic outcomes.[28,29]

ECMO to avoid these complications of hyperventilation is a novel supportive therapy. Successful oxygenation and ventilation of critically ill neonates with ECMO provides for the remission of PPHN by avoiding hypoxemia, hypercarbia, and acidosis (which promote vasoconstriction). ECMO also minimizes pulmonary barotrauma encountered with prolonged periods of high-pressure mechanical ventilation and high concentrations of fractional inspired O_2 (FIO_2). Finally, ECMO permits time for definitive therapy aimed at treating underlying pulmonary pathology. Examples of conditions causing severe respiratory failure with PPHN in term or near-term neonates are listed in Table 47-1.[17-23,30-33]

Table 47-1. Diagnostic Categories for Term or Near-Term Neonates with Progressive Pulmonary Disease/Pulmonary Hypertension Shortly after Birth

Term and post-term neonates with:
 Meconium aspiration syndrome
 Other aspiration syndromes with irresolvable air leak
 Persistent pulmonary artery hypertension of the
  newborn
Preterm and term neonates with:
 Respiratory distress syndrome
Infection:
 Sepsis
 Pneumonia
Lung hypoplasias:
 Congenital diaphragmatic hernia
 Primary hypoplastic lung (nonlethal)
 Potter syndrome
 Capillary-alveolar displacement (nonlethal?)

PATIENT SELECTION CRITERIA FOR EXTRACORPOREAL MEMBRANE OXYGENATION

Inclusions and Exclusions

The success of ECMO relies on the clinician's ability to identify newborns with reversible pulmonary disease, while excluding infants with irreversible disease.[18,24,34] From more recent ELSO Registry data (2000), population estimates suggest that only 1 in 2000 infants manifest respiratory failure so severe as to become candidates for ECMO, and 1 in 4000 receive this intervention.[25] ECMO programs must provide practiced, state-of-the-art therapy to this relatively small population of infants in an expeditious fashion, by identifying the progression of severe disease early enough to prevent death or debilitating consequences. Criteria for patient selection for ECMO therapy have been widely studied, debated, and variously proposed for over 2 decades. Table 47-2 summarizes conventional inclusion and exclusion criteria for considering bypass therapy in critically ill neonates.[18,24,34-40]

The controversy regarding patient selection criteria for ECMO is twofold: (1) Is less invasive therapy likely to promote comparable survival and recovery? (2) With constantly changing and improving neonatal support techniques, must physicians continually reassess criteria to justify ECMO's intrinsically invasive use?[41-45] In general, the earlier the ECMO physician can identify the infant with a high probability of dying from disease, but before iatrogenic consequences of conventional contemporary therapy, the better the patient selection criteria.

Criteria for Evaluating Unrelenting Progression of Pulmonary Disease

When appropriate inclusion and exclusion criteria are reviewed (see Table 47-2), the referring neonatologist can use one of several pulmonary indices to assess the severity and progression of respiratory illness and the likelihood

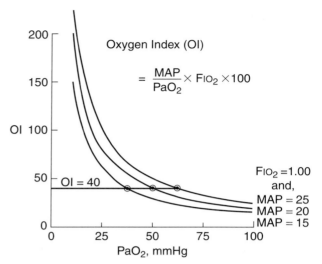

Figure 47–1. The calculation of oxygen index (OI). Inspired oxygen fraction (FIO$_2$) is considered to be 1.00 for this graph. Oxygen tension in postductal arterial blood (PaO$_2$) is on the horizontal axis, and the OI resulting from three different mean airway pressures (MAP) generated by mechanical ventilation is shown on the vertical axis. In each curve displayed, there is a nonlinear increase in OI as PaO$_2$ diminishes. An OI = 40 is demarcated by a horizontal line, which intersects each MAP curve at a different PaO$_2$. Instituting extracorporeal membrane oxygenation usually is recommended at an OI = 40 (expected mortality >80%).

of mortality. The simplest and currently most popular evaluation is the **oxygenation index (OI)** (Fig. 47-1).[35,36,39]

The relative importance of the ratio between mean airway pressure and arterial O$_2$ tension (PaO$_2$) in the calculation of OI performed at 1.00 FIO$_2$ is shown further graphically in Figure 47-1: When PaO$_2$ is less than 40 to 50 mm Hg, the denominator of the equation generates a geometric rise in OI. This relationship parallels pulmonary vascular resistance with increased right-to-left intracardiac and extracardiac shunting of deoxygenated blood in patients with severe pulmonary arterial hypertension. OI serves as a simple bedside method to evaluate the newborn for the development of pathologic pulmonary arterial hypertension.

The use of OI originally was evaluated at the University of Michigan for ECMO study candidates, where an OI greater than 40 on three of five postductal arterial blood gases drawn 0.5 hour apart defined a mortality greater than 80% in infants receiving conventional mechanical ventilatory support.[36] The same mortality has been cited by other centers.[34,36,39] A more recent collaborative trial for neonatal ECMO conducted in the United Kingdom showed a lower mortality rate of 59% with contemporary medical management in the non-ECMO limb of that trial.[46] Nevertheless, survival was significantly improved with the use of ECMO in this randomized study (78%). This result suggests a changing scenario for ECMO intervention and the need to revise criteria for neonatal ECMO constantly as newer techniques to treat neonates with reversible respiratory failure less invasively are developed.

Table 47–2. Conventional Inclusion and Exclusion Criteria in Consideration of Neonatal Extracorporeal Membrane Oxygenation Therapy

Inclusions

>34 weeks' gestational age
>2 kg birth weight
<2 weeks' postnatal age (or ≤10 days high-pressure mechanical ventilation, relative age)
Reversible cardiopulmonary condition

Exclusions

Major cardiac malformation (see text for discussion)
Syndromes with unsurvivable prognosis
Uncontrollable bleeding diathesis (*e.g.*, disseminated intravascular coagulation with bleeding uncontrolled despite multiple component transfusions and or progressive parenchymal brain hemorrhage)
Terminally brain injured

An alternative method for assessing the severity of neonatal pulmonary disease is the calculation of alveolar-arterial difference in O_2 tension (A-a) Do_2.[47] Krummel and colleagues[40] reported that (A-a) Do_2 greater than 600 mm Hg for more than 12 hours defines a mortality greater than 94%, with a sensitivity of 88%. A similar study showed that an (A-a) Do_2 greater than 610 mm Hg for more than 8 hours corresponded to a mortality of greater than 79%.[38] Either the OI or the (A-a) Do_2 criteria are appropriate for deciding on initiating ECMO, provided that expected mortality exceeds 60% to 80% in contemporary conventional practice. It is strongly advised that each ECMO center perform institutional review of contemporary practices to confirm therapeutic failure with non-ECMO management strategies. The morbidity and logistics of transport to ECMO centers of these critically ill infants should be incorporated into these reviews.

EXTRACORPOREAL MEMBRANE OXYGENATION CIRCUIT (VENOARTERIAL BYPASS)[1,2,48]

Vascular Cannulas and the Patient Bridge

The first major component of the ECMO circuit comprises the **cannulas** and the **patient bridge** tubing (shown in Fig. 47-2) that connect the ECMO apparatus to the infant. During venoarterial bypass (VA ECMO), the arterial cannula is located surgically in the right common carotid artery, with the tip opening into the aortic arch. The venous cannula is placed in the internal jugular vein, with its multifenestrated end (designed to harvest venous blood efficiently) through the right atrium and into the inferior vena cava. The cannulas are connected to the patient bridge by two Y-connectors. The bridge tubing connecting the Y's may be clamped to divert blood flow into the ECMO circuit or alternatively unclamped to

bypass the patient through the bridge when the infant's arterial and venous cannulas are clamped off from ECMO, effectively taking the infant off bypass.

Servoregulated Roller Pump and Infusions into the Extracorporeal Membrane Oxygenation Circuit

The second component shown in Figure 47-2 is a servoregulated roller-occlusion pump. Alternatively, some centers employ a continuous vortex pump. Blood initially is siphoned by gravity from the jugular venous cannula into tubing that passes off the bed platform, dropping approximately 1 m to floor level. Just before reaching the roller pump, this tubing passes through a small distensible reservoir (a flexible plastic **pillow** or **bladder**), where any deformity resulting from insufficient venous drainage is detected by a strain gauge that shuts off electrical power to the pump, avoiding negative circuit pressure and **cavitation,** or bubble formation during bypass.

The blood pump's rollers then squeeze venous blood through the compressible plastic of the blood path's "raceway" tubing (Super Tigon, Gish Biomedical, Irvine, CA) to generate suprasystemic levels of arterial blood pressure with a relatively nonpulsatile flow. Pressure generated by the pump subsequently is attenuated to a more normal infant systemic mean arterial pressure by resistances within the membrane lung, by the heat exchanger, and by gravity as the blood returns to bed level.

Parenteral nutrition, fluid and electrolytes, heparin infusions, and intermittent transfusions and medications may be administered into the ECMO circuit at built-in ports in the blood flow pathway proximal to the bladder or pillow reservoir. All parenteral administrations are made into the ECMO circuit at the point at which circuit pressures are relatively positive to prevent inadvertent entrainment of air due to suction generated by the ECMO pump. Platelets must be infused separately, however, through an infusion port distal to the membrane lung, which may consume platelets avidly.

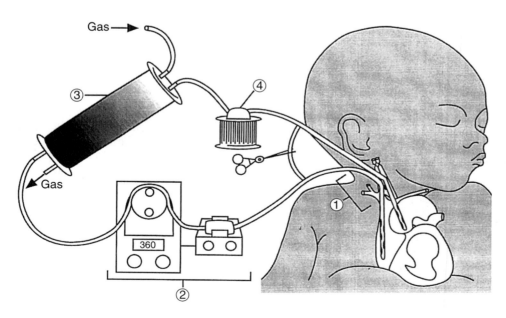

Figure 47–2. Schematic representation for apparatus delivering venoarterial extracorporeal membrane oxygenation therapy. Shown here are four major circuit components: (1) the venous and arterial cannulas positioned near the infant's heart and the patient bridge (in this example clamped to permit blood to flow through the cannulas to and from the infant); (2) the servoregulated roller pump; (3) the artificial membrane lung; and (4) the heat exchanger for rewarming blood before recirculation to the infant. See text for a more detailed description.

Miracle of Membrane Oxygenation

The third component of the ECMO circuit is the artificial membrane lung. The Kolobow lung is composed of thin woven silicone rubber and nylon fabric sandwiched on a steel mesh and coiled around a polycarbonate spool. A diagram of the Kolobow membrane lung is shown in Figure 47-3.[1] The silicone membrane, folded into an envelope, is shown uncoiled in part of this diagram. The envelope contains a gas phase separated from a liquid phase of circulation around the membrane envelope, while supported by the steel mesh wrapped around the polycarbonate spool. The top and bottom portions of Figure 47-3 show the assembled membrane access tubing for the gas and the liquid phases of this device. The blood ports are manufactured as clear plastic. The gas ports usually are differentiated by green plastic construction.

The silicone fabric that separates the gas and liquid phases of the lung is permeable to the diffusion of O_2 and CO_2 at atmospheric pressure. As with the native lung, CO_2 diffuses 200 times faster than O_2. A respiratory gas mixture (50% to 100% O_2, the balance nitrogen) is delivered dry into the gas phase of the lung at approximately 1 to 2 L/min **(sweep flow)**. O_2 diffuses from this mixture (350 to 700 mm Hg partial pressure) into venous blood (30 to 60 mm Hg) down its partial pressure gradient, whereas CO_2 diffuses in countercurrent fashion from the blood phase of the lung at 35 to 50 mm Hg into the gas phase at 0 mm Hg (higher if CO_2 is blended into the lung's sweep gas flow at a rate of 0 to 60 mL/min, to achieve physiologic partial arterial pressure of CO_2 [$PaCO_2$] concentrations).

For neonatal ECMO, 0.8 m^2 surface area membrane lung generally is employed, with a priming volume of 140 mL of blood, a **rated blood flow** of 1400 mL/min for maximal oxygenation at a gas transfer rate of 70 mL/m^2/min O_2.[1] The smaller 0.4 m^2 device used more commonly in the past to prevent overventilation of infants weighing 2 kg or less now is replaced by the larger lung and blended sweep gas flow. Oxygenation of the infant via the membrane lung is controlled by adjusting the rate of blood flow circulated by the roller pump through the membrane lung's blood path, proceeding from bottom to top of the device shown in Figure 47-2. O_2 exchange is determined by (1) the O_2 concentration introduced into the membrane lung's *sweep gas* flow, (2) the membrane's diffusion characteristics, (3) the thickness of the blood path as blood passes through the interstices of the spool coil apparatus, (4) the rate of flow of blood introduced through the lung by the ECMO pump, and (5) the membrane lung's **rated surface area**. The **rated blood flow** of the membrane lung is a term that applies to the maximal perfusion flow capacity at which an artificial lung is capable of raising the O_2 saturation of venous blood with a hematocrit of 40% from 65% oxyhemoglobin saturation to an arterialized saturation of 95%. The rated flow of a 0.4 m^2 surface area membrane lung is less than a 0.8 m^2 lung because of the smaller surface area. Similarly, clot formation within a membrane lung may reduce the **apparent rated blood flow** and indicate impending membrane lung failure.

CO_2 exchange, in contrast, is independent of the rate of blood flow through the membrane lung, of the membrane's thickness, or of the blood path thickness. Rather, CO_2 exchange depends entirely on the gas diffusion gradient between the *sweep gas* introduced into the gas phase of the membrane lung and the blood's CO_2 tension and on the rate of the sweep gas flow passing over the membrane. In modern practice, CO_2 may be introduced into the sweep flow mixture as **carbogen** (a mixture of 5% CO_2, nitrogen, and O_2), or through the introduction by precision flowmeter of pure CO_2 gas at rates between 0 and 60 mL/min.

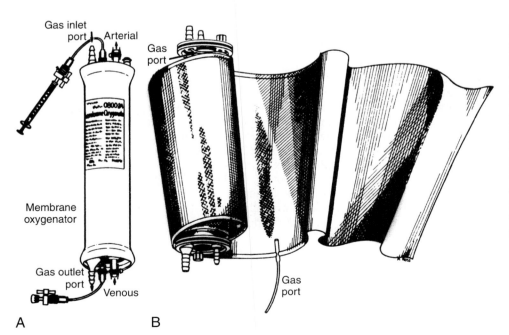

Gas inlet port   Arterial

Gas port

Membrane oxygenator

Gas outlet port   Venous

Gas port

A   B

Figure 47–3. A and **B,** Structure of a partially disassembled Kolobow-style membrane lung. A polyurethane rubber membrane, folded into an envelope, is layered with a stainless steel wire mesh for mechanical support, then coiled onto a polycarbonate spool suitable for extracorporeal membrane oxygenation. See text for a more detailed description. *(From Short BL: Neonatal ECMO. In Cornish D, Arensman R [eds]: Extracorporeal Life Support. Boston, Blackwell, 1992. Reprinted by permission of Blackwell Science, Inc.)*

When such a precision flow manifold is used, air and pure O_2 are blended to achieve the desired PaO_2 in blood exiting the lung, and CO_2 gas is introduced gently in incremental fashion to achieve the desired $PaCO_2$.

Heat Exchange (Blood Rewarming)

The final component of the ECMO circuit is the water-heated thermal exchange system, which rewarms the blood that is cooled while passing through the ECMO apparatus back to near body temperature (37°C) before reperfusing into the infant. A temperature-regulated water bath and pump circulates heated water (38°C to 39°C) continuously through a jacket surrounding the blood path (see Fig. 47-2).

Pros and Cons of Venoarterial Extracorporeal Membrane Oxygenation

VA ECMO provides complete cardiopulmonary support to an infant's native heart and lungs when either or both are failing. In many cases, the infant's native cardiac function is not essential while on VA ECMO. When successfully transferred onto VA bypass, cardiotonic pressor infusions and other potentially toxic pharmacologic interventions (e.g., nitroprusside) may be discontinued completely. Disadvantages result from the invasive nature of this therapy. Any particulate matter (clot, bubble, or other embolic material) within the ECMO circuit may be infused directly into the systemic arterial circulation at the aortic arch. Finally, there also is potential for hyperoxic reperfusion injury to already oxygen-depleted tissue beds when initiating bypass. Depending on the gaseous mixture provided, the ECMO membrane lung is a tremendously powerful device, capable of delivering 100% oxyhemoglobin saturated blood with PaO_2 approaching 500 mm Hg when pure oxygen is used for sweep flow.

VENOVENOUS BYPASS

The use of venovenous (VV) ECMO is now increasingly popular because vascular access to the critically ill neonate is far less invasive than carotid artery cannulation, and the technique is nearly as effective in restoring O_2 delivery to critically ill infants.[49-52] The ECMO circuit functions in entirely the same fashion during VV bypass except that the venous blood drainage cannula and the arterial blood return cannula are incorporated into a single appliance (sizes 12 Fr and 14 Fr available, shown in Fig. 47-4). This device is positioned into the right atrium via the internal jugular vein on the right side of the neck.[1] Venous blood is drained out of the right atrium into a laterally fenestrated cannula lumen, oxygenated, rewarmed, then pumped back into the right atrium through medially oriented fenestrations aimed toward the tricuspid valve to minimize recirculation. An admixture of oxygenated and deoxygenated blood from the right atrium crosses the foramen ovale and via the right ventricle into the ductus arteriosus supplies systemic oxygenation.[49-52]

Because systemic blood supply is delivered entirely by the infant's native left ventricle during VV bypass, there must be sufficient left ventricular force to circulate against systemic vascular resistance, which often is increased in

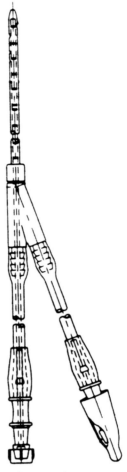

Figure 47–4. Schematic drawing of a double-lumen venovenous cannula for performing venovenous extracorporeal membrane oxygenation. The venous lumen is multifenestrated with openings oriented laterally within the right atrium of the infant's heart and the vena cava to maximize harvest of venous return. The inner lumen aperture is oriented medially at the opening of the tricuspid valve to bias arterialized return flow into the right ventricle and across the foramen ovale into the systemic circulation. *(From Moulton SL, et al: In Cornish D, Arensman R [eds]: Extracorporeal Life Support. Boston, Blackwell, 1992. Reprinted by permission of Blackwell Science, Inc.)*

the critically ill patient.[53] Frequently, cardiotonic pressors and generous volume infusions of saline, plasma, or blood transfusions are required to maintain an infant's circulation on VV ECMO. Recirculation of mixed oxygenated blood back into the venous lumen at higher flows on VV ECMO potentially limits the delivery of O_2 systemically. This phenomenon is particularly important for larger infants, providing only partial ECMO support and requiring continued mechanical ventilatory delivery of O_2 in some cases.

Although marginally less powerful as a complete life support tool, VV ECMO is presently the preferred conservative (least invasive) mode of bypass. VV ECMO avoids invasion of the carotid artery; systemic embolism is less likely, and the right common carotid artery is left intact. Currently, femoral vein cannulation may be used as an alternate blood return access route for VV ECMO when either the right internal jugular vein is too small to accommodate the double-lumen cannula or right common carotid cannulation proves difficult. Because of venous admixture on the right side of the heart, a lower level of systemic arterial saturation (80% to 90%) and PaO_2 (45 to 60 mm Hg) should be tolerated during VV ECMO. A new percutaneous double-lumen jugular VV cannula apparatus may shorten cannulation time and reduce some of the bleeding complications associated with surgical cannula placement.[52]

Monitoring Vital Extracorporeal Membrane Oxygenation Circuit and Patient Functions

Continuous Venous Oxygen Saturation Monitoring

A fiberoptic monitor probe is inserted into the blood path on the venous side of the ECMO circuit, just before the bladder or pillow reservoir. Mixed venous saturation of oxyhemoglobin ($\%SvO_2$) is displayed continuously on a trended monitoring device. SvO_2 is probably the most important parameter the clinician must follow during VA bypass. Optimally, SvO_2 is run above 70% and below 90%, indicating that tissue oxygen delivery is meeting the infant's oxygen consumption demand.[1,2,22,54] The first clue to deterioration in tissue oxygenation delivery may be a decrease in the SvO_2 level. Diminished SvO_2 (<60% to 70%) may be associated with a variety of clinically significant conditions, as follows:

1. **Anemia** results in inadequate delivery of O_2 to the tissues and leads to an increased extraction of O_2 from arterial blood, which is reflected in a lower SvO_2 value during bypass.
2. **Low systemic blood flow**, from low native cardiac output or from insufficient ECMO pump delivery, also may result in diminished SvO_2.
3. **Arterial oxygen desaturation** from infant lung failure or from ECMO membrane failure results in SvO_2 deterioration.
4. An **increase in an infant's metabolic rate** also may diminish SvO_2.

Membrane Lung Pressures

Blood path pressures are measured hemodynamically by transducers located at the premembrane and at the postmembrane infusion ports on the ECMO membrane lung. Mean perfusion pressures for both sites are displayed on a blood pressure monitoring apparatus. In general, the premembrane pressure exceeds the infant's mean systemic blood pressure by 100 to 200 mm Hg. While passing through the interstices of the silicone coil, a pressure drop occurs such that postmembrane lung pressure generally is lowered by at least 100 mm Hg. The difference in these membrane lung pressures is proportional to the resistance of blood flow through the membrane lung. An increasing difference in membrane lung pressure gradient greater than 150 to 200 mm Hg may indicate clot formation or occlusion of blood flow passing through the blood path of the membrane oxygenator. Other methods for diagnosing membrane lung failure include an increasing prelung pressure of greater than 300 to 350 mm Hg.

Frequently, at the same time, a decrease in postmembrane lung PaO_2 and an increase in the postmembrane lung $PaCO_2$ are noted. The premembrane and postmembrane blood gas tensions generally are monitored every 8 hours during ECMO.

Monitoring for Potential Air and Clot Embolus in the Extracorporeal Membrane Oxygenation Circuit

An ultrasonic bubble detector capable of sensing microembolic bubble formation is incorporated into the ECMO monitoring system immediately before reinfusion into the patient's arterial cannula. In addition, there are three positions within the ECMO circuit's construction where air emboli may be trapped and easily visualized. These bubble traps are located (1) in the prepump reservoir, which generally is equipped with an evacuation port where air may be removed; (2) at the top of the membrane lung, where the blood path may be interrupted temporarily at the pressure monitoring port and air bubbles removed (which is why the lung is pitched at a 45-degree angle); and (3) in a plastic dome located at the top of the heat exchanger. Air removal and the prevention of air embolus, particularly on VA bypass, are major concerns for the ECMO team. Similarly, close attention is paid to identify clot formation visually through detailed inspection of the entire ECMO circuit several times each nursing shift.

Monitoring Coagulation during Heparinization on Extracorporeal Membrane Oxygenation

In addition to the above-mentioned electronic monitoring systems, the ECMO specialist operating the pump apparatus intermittently must monitor and record the effects of systemic heparinization. Most centers employ a bedside laboratory test automated to time activated clotting of blood agitated in a standardized test tube. Normal activated clotting time (ACT) is approximately 120 seconds in a nonheparinized subject. During ECMO, ACTs generally are run at almost twice this value (180 to 220 seconds). Modifications in ACT targets may be made depending on the presence of disseminated intravascular coagulation or other clinical bleeding problems. During routine bypass, ACTs often are monitored hourly. Additionally, routine coagulation profiles (prothrombin time, activated partial thromboplastin time, fibrinogen concentration, and dimer/split product) are assessed every 8 to 12 hours.

Other Routine Patient Monitoring Parameters Provided on Extracorporeal Membrane Oxygenation

Intensive care monitoring of the infant's physiologic parameters also is performed and displayed continuously during ECMO. Heart rate, infant respiration, and electrocardiogram displays; blood pressure waveforms; and systemic arterial oxyhemoglobin saturations generally are employed. While on bypass, the normal pulsatility of the arterial pressure waveform may be dampened by the less pulsatile nature of blood flow generated artificially by the ECMO roller pump. Changes in pulsatility also may indicate cardiac tamponade from pneumothorax or pneumopericardium, however, and may be observed with failure of venous return through the ECMO pump.

Combined use of patient physiologic monitoring with monitoring of ECMO circuit parameters is essential to the safe operation of prolonged CPB.

APPLICATION OF EXTRACORPOREAL MEMBRANE OXYGENATION CIRCUIT PHYSIOLOGY

Five questions illustrate the clinician's understanding of ECMO O_2 delivery and infant physiology while on VA CPB.[54]

Question 1: What Is the Effect of Transfusion Volume on Systemic Arterial Oxygen Saturation during ECMO?

The volume transfused increases venous return to the infant's native heart and increases native cardiac output (Starling's preload principle). On ECMO, an increase in native cardiac output may occur at a time when the infant's lungs are not functioning well enough to oxygenate the increased circulating blood volume. The additional volume pumped by the infant's heart is likely to shunt deoxygenated blood right-to-left through fetal channels, and systemic oxygenation decreases unless the fixed ECMO pump flow is increased proportionately.

Question 2: What Is the Effect of Transfusion Hemoglobin on Venous Oxygen Saturation?

The increase in O_2 carrying capacity provided by the transfused hemoglobin mass circulating through the ECMO membrane lung is likely to increase tissue O_2 delivery supplied by ECMO into the systemic circulation. Provided that the infant's O_2 consumption remains constant, venous O_2 saturation should increase under these circumstances.

Question 3: What Is the Effect of an Accumulation of Air or Fluid in the Pericardial Sac on Systemic Arterial and on Mixed Venous Oxygen Saturations?

A reduction of the infant's native cardiac output occurs secondary to cardiac tamponade. The proportion of ECMO pump flow delivered to the infant systemically through the aortic cannula increases relative to the decreased native cardiac output. The first clinical clue to the presence of pericardial tamponade in an infant on ECMO may be an increase in systemic arterial O_2 saturation (SaO_2). Paradoxically, venous saturation decreases because total ECMO pump plus native cardiac output is diminished, resulting in less tissue O_2 delivery despite the proportionate increase in SaO_2. Other clues to cardiac tamponade on ECMO include dampening of the systemic arterial blood pressure monitor tracing and negative pump pressure alarms from the servocontrolled roller pump power supply.

Question 4: What Are the Systemic and Mixed Venous Saturations in a Patient Who Has Died while on Extracorporeal Membrane Oxygenation?

In a patient who has died while on ECMO, there simply is no O_2 consumption. O_2 delivery systemically is met by zero O_2 demand. As a result, 100% saturated arterial blood is supplied systemically, and venous blood returning to the right atrium is exactly equivalent to arterial saturation (100%) because no O_2 has been extracted.

Question 5: What Happens to Systemic Arterial Oxygen Saturation on Extracorporeal Membrane Oxygenation as Mobilization of Peripheral Edema Occurs with the Patient's Recovery?

As an infant recovers on ECMO, pump flow is weaned progressively. If simultaneously during the infant's recovery tissue capillary leak resolves, and peripheral edema fluid is mobilized, circulating blood volume increases, resulting in increased native cardiac output relative to ECMO pump flow. Depending on the balance between recovery of pulmonary blood flow and systemic oxygenation and increased native cardiac output with edema mobilization, desaturated blood may shunt proportionately more across fetal channels during recovery. The clinician may wish to pursue pharmacologic diuresis at this juncture to evacuate edema fluid as it is mobilized, and, to avoid increasing ECMO pump flow during recovery, delay coming off of bypass.

Two completely separate circulatory systems are in parallel when an infant is on VA bypass: The first is the infant's own native heart and lungs, which may vary functionally according to their pathophysiologic state; the second comprises the artificial ECMO pump and membrane lung, which varies only with the clinician's manipulations. The trick of successful ECMO management is to balance these two parallel circuits while the infant spontaneously recovers from the underlying disease.

EXTRACORPOREAL MEMBRANE OXYGENATION COURSE[1,2,22,54]

Preparing for the Extracorporeal Membrane Oxygenation Patient

When the decision has been made to transfer a critically ill term or near-term newborn to a tertiary medical center considering ECMO therapy, an ambulance or helicopter is mobilized as quickly as possible. Often the window of opportunity to convert a critically ill patient from mechanical ventilatory support onto CPB is brief, between 6 and 12 hours depending on transport logistics. In some cases, minutes count. Regionally, children should be transferred to the closest center available because data indicate that prolonged land or air transports significantly increase infant mortality.[55]

Even before the infant arrives for ECMO, information should be exchanged between the blood banks of the referring and the tertiary care hospitals to arrange for a sufficient number of units of component blood products to prime the ECMO pump (usually 2 units) and to back up blood components for frequent transfusions required during bypass. Packed cells, platelets, plasma, and cryoprecipitate all may be necessary for stabilization, particularly for a patient with severe disseminated coagulopathy.

Generally, a tertiary telephone communication system is in place to mobilize the ECMO team, including ultrasound technicians to evaluate intracranial and cardiac anomalies before cannulation. Before ECMO, a cranial ultrasound should be obtained to exclude the presence of severe intracranial hemorrhages (greater than grade II) because ECMO with systemic heparinization may be contraindicated.[17-24,56] In some ECMO centers, electro-encephalograms may be evaluated before bypass and serially thereafter to aid in determining prognosis for survivors.[57-59] In many centers, an echocardiography technician also is mobilized for rapid assessment of an echocardiogram before consideration for ECMO because complex congenital heart disease may mimic severe pulmonary arterial hypertension.[26,27,60] Unless cardiothoracic surgery is readily available at the ECMO center, the presence of a congenital heart defect also may be considered a relative contraindication for ECMO therapy.[60] In particular, left-sided obstructive lesions also may constitute relative contraindications for VA bypass.[60,61] In general, the echocardiogram confirms the presence of pulmonary arterial hypertension by excluding anatomic anomalies and by showing pulmonary hypertension with Doppler flow studies, flattening of the ventricular septum, shunting at the levels of the foramen ovale or patent ductus arteriosus, or tricuspid regurgitation.

Extracorporeal Membrane Oxygenation Cannulation[54,62]

Neonatal Team

On mobilization of an emergency transport team for an ECMO candidate, three intensive care nursery teams are convened. The first team is the neonatal resuscitation group. In most hospitals, a staff neonatologist or neonatology fellow is present at the time of admission of a critically ill candidate for ECMO. An experienced neonatal nurse, oriented specifically to infant resuscitation before and during ECMO cannulation, also should be available. A helpful adjunctive neonatal team member is the respiratory therapist, expert in rapid application of advanced mechanical ventilatory support, in some cases including high-frequency ventilation and iNO.[37,63]

Surgical Team

The second team mobilized when the infant has met ECMO criteria is the surgical staff. In general, the ECMO surgeon is expert in vascular cannulation of the major vessels near the heart and in alternative access of major vessels for bypass therapy in the subclavian, axillary, or femoral regions. The surgeon's first assistant, generally a resident or surgical fellow in ECMO training, also may be available. To aid the surgeon and his or her assistant, most ECMO centers mobilize an operating room nurse or technician expert in vascular cannulation and the management of emergency operative procedures within the intensive care nursery.

Extracorporeal Membrane Oxygenation Specialists

The third component required for a smooth transition onto ECMO during cannulation comprises the ECMO specialty team: (1) a **coordinator** or **primer expert** in team education, supervising construction of the ECMO circuit and the preparation of fluids and blood products required for priming the apparatus, and (2) the **ECMO specialist**, expert in managing bypass, the heparin infusion, and

coagulation testing at the bedside and responsible for other fluid, medication, and blood product infusions into the circuit and for trouble-shooting the ECMO apparatus. In most centers, the ECMO coordinator or primers and ECMO specialists are derived from nursing personnel. In some centers, biomedical engineering and perfusion specialists or respiratory therapists may assist in the assembly and start-up of the ECMO circuit.

When the decision to place an infant on ECMO is made, each of the three teams functions independently to perform their respective tasks during cannulation. The neonatal resuscitation team maintains the infant physiologically throughout the cannulation procedure and administers analgesic and muscle paralysis. The surgical team convenes at the right side of the infant's neck for placement of the ECMO cannulas during resuscitation. The ECMO perfusion team builds the CPB apparatus through the priming procedure, timed within 45 minutes to 1 hour or slightly more, such that the infant can be converted from mechanical ventilatory support to complete CPB in a timely fashion.

Surgical Cannulation[35,48,54]

When the surgical team begins the operation for cannulation of the right internal carotid artery and the right jugular vein, a sterile operating field is maintained. Muscle paralysis is provided and repeated as often as necessary to maintain patient immobilization. Analgesia is provided by fentanyl and repeated liberally to prevent pain. After local anesthesia, a transverse incision is made in the right lateral neck a few centimeters in length over the vascular bundle. After blunt dissection and retraction, the carotid artery and jugular vein are exposed (care is exercised to avoid the recurrent laryngeal nerve). The carotid artery lies deep to the jugular vein and often must be cannulated first; this necessitates temporarily ligating blood flow to the right side of the circle of Willis generally 15 to 30 minutes before cannulation of the more superficial jugular vein and the onset of bypass. During jugular vein cannulation, the left carotid and the vertebrobasilar vessels marginally may compensate cerebral blood flow. This stage of the operative procedure is crucial and should proceed in an expedited fashion.

At the time of incision of the internal carotid artery, the patient is heparinized with 100 to 150 U/kg of sodium heparin. This amount is sufficient to anticoagulate the infant systemically during the cannulation procedure with elevation of ACTs to 400 to 600 seconds. This dose also should be sufficient to last throughout the cannulation procedure, before starting a continuous heparin infusion given via the ECMO circuit.

When these vessels are isolated and surgical ligatures are placed, the carotid artery is ligated distally, and an incision is made proximally. A 10 Fr or 12 Fr cannula is introduced into the carotid artery to a premeasured distance, optimally residing at the arch of the aorta with the single-orifice tip directed downstream. Ligatures are secured for stability of this catheter, and the right jugular vein is cannulated in a similar fashion with a multifenestrated cannula placed through the right atrium with its tip residing at the origin of the inferior vena cava.

This placement ensures the maximal harvest rate of venous blood returning to the right atrium (usually the flow-limiting parameter on ECMO). The venous cannula may be larger (12 Fr or 14 Fr) to facilitate ECMO venous return flow.

Starting on Bypass

Concurrently the primer prepares arterial and venous ports of the blood-primed ECMO circuit, which also are instilled with heparinized saline solution and connected to the ends of each corresponding patient cannula. Two clamps are located distally on the ECMO circuit's arterial and venous tubing, occluding flow to and from the patient. The bridge at this time remains unclamped, permitting flow from the ECMO circuit to bypass the infant through the bridge, while the ECMO pump idles at 100 mL/min.

The infant is converted over onto bypass in a three-step clamping maneuver as follows: (1) The arterial cannula clamp is removed, (2) the bridge subsequently is clamped tightly, and (3) the venous cannula clamp is removed. If circuit malfunction occurs at any time, the reverse procedure is followed to take the infant off bypass: (1) The venous line is clamped, (2) the bridge is unclamped, and (3) the artery line is clamped. Venous drainage now is permitted out of the infant's right atrium and is siphoned to the floor by gravity as described earlier in the ECMO apparatus section. Arterialized blood return begins simultaneously, and the infant is converted onto bypass.

Over the next several minutes, the ECMO pump's flow is increased in 10 to 20 mL/min increments until the infant resides on what is considered full bypass flow, between 120 and 150 mL/kg/min. Too-rapid escalation of pump flow introduces the circuit prime, which is rich in potassium and a calcium chelating agent, too quickly and may result in sudden cardiac arrhythmias, usually bradycardia and diminished pulse pressure. This condition usually can be reversed at the onset of bypass by infusion of calcium gluconate. Flow should be advanced sufficiently to supply minimal metabolic O_2 demand (≥ 5 mL O_2/kg/min), which may be assessed by ensuring Svo_2 greater than 60%, and Sao_2 greater than 85% (provided that circuit/infant hemoglobin concentrations are ≥ 15 g/100 mL blood). Initial Svo_2 less than 50% to 60% corresponds to an anaerobic metabolic condition resulting in the production of lactic acid and falling pH. Thereafter, saturations should increase during the first 30 to 60 minutes on bypass to more physiologic values ($Svo_2 \geq 80\%$, $Sao_2 \geq 97\%$).

Often, as the infant is converted onto CPB, the arterial waveform on the patient's monitor of umbilical or radial arterial blood pressure may dampen considerably. This dampening indicates full bypass flow achievable at the infant's rate of venous return. Increasing ECMO pump flow to extinguish pulsatile flow completely may result in excessive venous volume demand, resulting in a negative pressure alarm within the ECMO circuit and automatic interruption of the roller pump. If Svo_2 is less than 60% to 65% with negative alarms, volume administration should be considered to increase venous return for ECMO. Packed red blood cell transfusion also may be desirable at this point to increase O_2 carrying capacity and Sao_2/Svo_2. Hemoglobin concentration more than 18 g/100 mL of blood should be avoided, however, to prevent sludging within the infant and the ECMO circuit.

Stabilization on Venoarterial Bypass

Cardiac Stun

Frequently at this juncture, because the heart has been relieved of much of the systemic flow requirements for the infant, and because the outflow to the coronary arteries is generally blood that is low in O_2 content, the infant may experience a mild myocardial stun.[64-66] This is a condition of bradycardia or systemic hypotension or both, which is generally transient. Rarely, complete cardiac electrical-mechanical arrest may occur.[66] Either cardiac stun or arrest may be compensated completely by increasing ECMO pump flow on the CPB circuit, while measures to restore cardiac function are administered.

Heparin Infusion Management

The ECMO specialist at this time checks small samples of blood for ACTs to monitor the decline from 400 to 600 seconds during cannulation to a more desirable range of 200 to 220 seconds.[54] These initial ACT checks occur at 15-minute intervals until ACT is less than 250 to 300 seconds, then a continuous heparin infusion is begun at 30 U/kg/hr and is titrated upward or downward as necessary. In instances in which severe patient bleeding exists, platelets and fibrinogen generally are administered while ACTs are run at slightly lower values (180 to 200 seconds). Most ECMO centers agree that some systemic heparinization is desirable at all times during bypass therapy.

Lung Opacification (White-out)

As things begin to stabilize, a chest x-ray is obtained to check cannula placements. Figure 47-5 is an infant chest x-ray obtained immediately after converting onto CPB. The most striking aspect of Figure 47-5 is the complete opacification (white-out) of the infant's lung fields with atelectasis and pulmonary edema. The heart border is entirely obscured, and it is difficult to determine diaphragmatic and costophrenic margins. This white-out appearance is typical immediately after transfer onto bypass. Pulmonary function testing at this time yields low values for dynamic lung compliance and functional residual capacity.[67] To verify cannula placements, some centers perform repeat echocardiography.

The arterial cannula seen in Figure 47-5 enters the right neck, ending at the level of the second thoracic vertebral body, consistent with placement at the aortic arch and directed downstream. The venous cannula may be seen entering the right neck, passing to the seventh thoracic vertebral body, through the right atrium and at the origin of the inferior vena cava. Also assessed here are endotracheal and nasogastric tube placements. Umbilical venous line placement should be low enough to avoid interference with ECMO venous cannula flow and should be repositioned before the infant is heparinized.

Ventilatory Management on Extracorporeal Membrane Oxygenation

During VA bypass, tissue oxygen demands are met entirely by the ECMO apparatus. Mechanical ventilation at

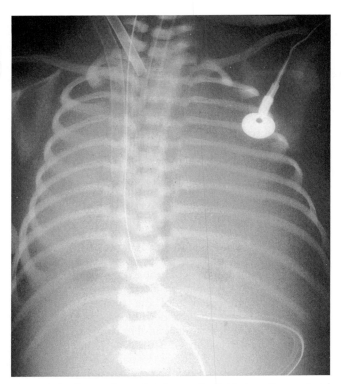

Figure 47–5. Chest radiograph 6 hours after initiation of venoarterial extracorporeal membrane oxygenation (ECMO). Complete opacification *(white-out)* of both lung fields is noted, consistent with atelectasis or pulmonary edema or both. Infants are entirely bypass dependent during this early phase of ECMO therapy. Pulmonary functions have tested nearly zero compliance and residual volume during this phase. Note right common carotid artery and jugular venous cannula positions at the arch of the aortic shadow and through the right atrium.

high pressures and 100% O_2 are no longer necessary.[1,2,54,68] To avoid further barotrauma and oxygen toxicity, the mechanical ventilator is set at a low peak inflation pressure (20 to 25 cm H_2O), with an inspiratory time of 0.5 to 1 second *(sigh* breaths), at a mandatory rate of 10 breaths/min and an oxygen fraction of 0.30. The purpose of these low settings is (1) to *rest* the lung and to promote spontaneous pulmonary recovery, (2) to avoid barotrauma and O_2 toxicity, (3) to prevent atelectasis and to minimize accumulation of pulmonary edema, and (4) to provide enough ventilatory and supplemental O_2 support to show improved oxygenation via the lungs as spontaneous recovery ensues. Conventionally, positive end-expiratory pressure is provided at 5 to 6 cm H_2O; however, more recently some centers have advocated higher levels of positive end-expiratory pressure (10 to 15 cm H_2O) to avoid white-out (atelectasis and pulmonary edema; see Fig. 47-5).[68] Care must be taken when choosing higher positive end-expiratory pressure on VA or VV ECMO support to avoid venous tamponade.

Infants with pernicious air leaks (pneumothoraces, pneumopericardium, or cystic pulmonary interstitial emphysema) may be completely *lung-rested* on continuous positive airway pressure alone (5 to 6 cm H_2O) to

allow the leaks to heal before the aforementioned rest settings are begun. Usually, continuous positive airway pressure for 24 to 48 hours is sufficient to ensure resolution of these conditions.

Pulmonary toilet may be performed vigorously during bypass, particularly in infants with severe aspiration syndromes or airways inflammation. Care must be taken in lavage and suctioning procedures (performed every 1 to 2 hours initially) and the use of vibration rather than percussion to mobilize secretions or meconium to avoid trauma in a heparinized infant. Conditioning the lung in this fashion may be provided frequently because the patient is entirely supported while on bypass. Finally, some ECMO centers advocate 8 to 10 prolonged sigh breaths (1 to 3 seconds peak inspiratory hold at 25 to 30 cm H_2O pressure), provided by manual ventilation after completing the lavage and suctioning procedure.

Medical Management on Bypass

Total parenteral nutrition generally is begun on the first day of CPB appropriate to the intensive care patient's nutritional needs, including protein, sugar, multivitamin, essential minerals, and intralipid infusions. Maintenance fluid volume may be limited to 60 to 80 mL/kg/day because other infusions (particularly heparin) may supplement daily volume intake (to >150 mL/kg/day). Total fluid volume administered should compensate the membrane lung insensible water loss of 100 to 150 mL/day of free water (approximately 25 to 75 mL/kg/day, depending on infant size). Pharmacologic diuresis may be pursued in the event of severe fluid accumulation and edema formation, particularly after mobilization of capillary leak has begun, usually 48 to 72 hours into bypass.

Muscle paralysis generally is avoided during bypass to assist with fluid mobilization. Intermittent sedation with a benzodiazepine and analgesia with morphine often are provided for infant agitation to prevent movement of the ECMO cannulas. In general, the ECMO patient remains comfortable and requires little pharmacologic intervention. In some cases, seizures may require control with phenobarbital or phenytoin. Occasionally, systemic hypertension with systolic blood pressures greater than 100 mm Hg may require treatment with hydralazine or angiotensin-converting enzyme inhibitors. Hypertension is observed most often during the recovery phase on ECMO. Most centers agree that when a patient has been converted onto VA bypass, cardiotonic pressor infusions (dopamine, dobutamine, epinephrine) may be discontinued.

In addition to testing serum chemistries (including daily hepatic and renal functions)[69] and hemotologic and coagulation profiles every 8 to 12 hours while on CPB, frequent (daily) examinations by radiograph, echocardiography, and cranial ultrasound often are performed for surveillance of intracranial hemorrhage, pneumopericardium or hemopericardium, and pneumothorax. Chest and abdominal ultrasound examinations should be considered when pleural or peritoneal effusions or hemorrhages are suspected (e.g., postoperative diaphragmatic hernia cases).[56] If an initial blood culture is negative at 24 to 48 hours, daily screening blood cultures should be considered with prolonged ECMO courses, especially after 10 days of support.[70]

Extracorporeal Membrane Oxygenation Run and Recovery

The average ECMO course proceeds over the next 3 to 7 days, awaiting spontaneous lung recovery. Cardiac recovery and mobilization of capillary leak edema may precede weaning the ECMO pump flow, resulting in increased native cardiac output before recovery from PPHN. The infant's systemic arterial saturation and PaO_2 may be seen to decrease during recovery, rather than increase as might be expected with pulmonary recovery. Diuretic therapy may assist in reducing native circulation of desaturated blood during early recovery on ECMO.[71] Lochan and associates[72] showed that lower doses of furosemide may be used when an initial priming dose of 2 mg/kg of theophylline is infused, increasing diuretic response by 50% to 100%.

Thereafter, as venous saturation improves to greater than 80%, the ECMO pump flow is reduced in 10 mL/min increments until a **pump idle rate** of approximately 100 mL/min minimal flow is reached, to prevent stasis and clotting within the circuit. Frequent arterial blood gas assessments are important checks during the weaning process (3 to 7 days).

An example of a chest radiograph in a patient weaning successfully from bypass is seen in Figure 47-6. In this case, after only 4.5 days, the lung white-out seen originally after going onto bypass has all but completely resolved. The infant is idling at 100 mL/min ECMO flow, with a venous saturation of 85% and completely normal arterial blood gases. One report suggested that pulmonary function testing that shows increased functional residual capacity (>15 mL/kg), and improved dynamic lung compliance may be useful in determining when lung recovery is sufficient to warrant coming off CPB.[67]

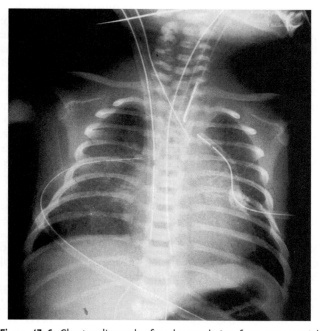

Figure 47–6. Chest radiograph after decannulation from venoarterial extracorporeal membrane oxygenation. Opacification *(white-out)* of both lung fields for the most part has resolved. Pulmonary functions show improved compliance and nearly normal residual volumes.

TRIALS OFF BYPASS

At this juncture, the ECMO clinician may elect to initiate the first **trial off** of CPB. In general, after pulmonary toilet has been performed and the endotracheal tube replaced with a fresh appliance, the ventilator settings are increased to a modest level of mechanical ventilation sufficient to provide physiologic support without significant risk for barotrauma or O_2 toxicity. Suggested parameters are an intermittent mandatory ventilatory rate of 30 to 40 breaths/min, a peak inflation pressure of 25 cm H_2O, an end-expiratory pressure of 5 cm H_2O, and an FIO_2 of 0.40.

After 30 minutes at these settings, the infant is taken off CPB by reversing the sequence of clamp positions stated earlier: (1) The venous cannula is clamped, (2) the bridge clamp is removed, and (3) the arterial cannula is clamped. The infant is now off of CPB with the venous and arterial sides of the ECMO circuit clamped, while ECMO idle flow proceeds through the bridge. Arterial blood gases from the patient are obtained at 15-minute intervals over the course of the next 1 to 2 hours. Depending on the values of these blood gases, a decision may be made either to decannulate immediately or to place the infant back on CPB until a second trial off is pursued within 12 to 24 hours. Usually after two to three trials off of bypass, the infant may be removed successfully from ECMO and maintained entirely on the mechanical ventilator. Failure to improve after 2 to 3 days during trials off may indicate the presence of more permanent lung damage, and consideration should by given to coming off ECMO at higher ventilatory settings. Runs longer than 2 weeks are rare and fraught with clot and bleeding complications.

At this time, the surgical team is again convened at the patient's bedside; the cannulas are identified and removed through the neck incision, and the jugular vein is ligated. The proximal end of the common carotid artery also may be ligated after cannula removal; however, some centers reconstruct the right common carotid artery to approximate more normal cerebral blood flow through the circle of Willis.

Right Common Carotid Artery Reconstruction

The compensation of right middle cerebral arterial blood flow by collateral flow from the left common carotid artery via the circle of Willis during ECMO is shown on the right side of Figure 47-7.[73-76] The left side of the diagram shows normal forward flow (antegrade) through the A1 segment of the anterior cerebral artery after successful surgical reconstruction of the right common carotid artery immediately on decannulation from ECMO. These flow patterns have been confirmed by color Doppler ultrasonography in the ECMO centers pursuing this vascular reconstruction procedure.[77-80]

Although successful return to normal blood flow can be achieved through right common carotid artery reconstruction, complete compensatory collateral flow may be achieved permanently even after permanent ligation of this vessel and hypertrophy of the left common carotid artery.[75,81] To date, no clear long-term benefit or sequela of either the ligation or the reconstruction approach has

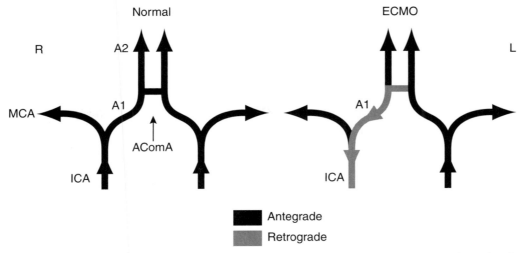

Figure 47–7. Schematic representations of the circle of Willis vasculature as might be visualized by color-enhanced Doppler ultrasonography for normal circulation *(left)* and for right common carotid artery ligated infants after venoarterial extracorporeal membrane oxygenation (ECMO). Shaded areas on the ligated diagram indicate retrograde blood flow emanating from the left carotid artery supplying the right side of the circle of Willis via the A1 segment of the anterior collateral communicating vessels (AComA). The right middle cerebral artery (MCA) shows similar balanced blood flow with the left MCA within a few hours to days of the onset of bypass, indicating that compensatory dilation of the left common carotid artery probably occurs as the brain attempts to regulate blood flow symmetrically. ICA, internal carotid artery. *(From Mitchell DG, Merton DA, Desai H, et al: Neonatal brain: Color Doppler imaging II: Altered flow patterns from extracorporeal membrane oxygenation. Radiology 167:307, 1988.)*

been shown.[77,82] Some of the reconstruction sites are partially or completely occluded at 6-month follow-up in one series.[83] Carotid remodeling of partially obstructed arteries also was reported from this study after 3 to 4 years.

Final Recovery

Provided that infants have achieved a successful course of ECMO therapy, lung recovery thereafter proceeds rapidly, and infants may wean from mechanical ventilatory support in 3 to 7 days. Rarely, prolonged ventilation or oxygen supplementation is required after ECMO. In certain cases with unusual diagnoses, ventilatory recovery and the establishment of enteral feedings may proceed at a much slower pace, requiring months of convalescence or rehabilitative care.[84,85]

THERAPIES TO AVOID EXTRACORPOREAL MEMBRANE OXYGENATION

High-Frequency Ventilation

Baumgart and coworkers[37] reported 73 term or near-term infants treated with high-frequency jet ventilation as rescue therapy, who might have benefited from ECMO. Infants with meconium aspiration and PPHN and a single blood gas with an OI greater than 40 within 6 hours of initiating jet ventilation had 80% mortality. This report suggested that high-frequency jet ventilation was minimally effective for avoiding ECMO in meconium aspiration. The high-frequency oscillatory ventilation (HFOV) trial by Clark and associates[86] compared HFOV with conventional intermittent mandatory ventilation in ECMO candidates. Early eligibility criteria gave each

ventilator an opportunity to avoid ECMO. Failures with conventional intermittent mandatory ventilation were more likely to succeed with HFOV on crossover than vice versa. Clark and associates[86] reported that 8 of 79 infants enrolled were rescued from ECMO.

Surfactant Therapy

Early surfactant trials stated that larger premature infants who received surfactant for the treatment of the RDS were less likely to require ECMO.[87] In 1998, Lotze and colleagues[88] reported a small decrease in need for ECMO using surfactant therapy in term infants with severe respiratory distress from any cause, including infants with meconium aspiration syndrome. There were no differences in mortality, need for mechanical ventilation, chronic lung disease, or length of hospital stay in that study, and the U.S. Food and Drug Administration did not approve use of surfactant for diagnoses other than RDS.

Inhaled Nitric Oxide

Five large randomized controlled trials have shown the effectiveness of iNO therapy in avoiding ECMO in about one third of critically ill candidates with PPHN.[89-93] The Neonatal Inhaled Nitric Oxide Study Group in two large randomized trials showed a significant reduction in need for ECMO rescue in iNO-treated infants (54% versus 39%[54] and 71% versus 40%[90]). There was no reduction in mortality (17% of controls versus 14% of iNO-treated infants).[89] Kinsella and associates[91] tested the effectiveness of iNO incorporated with HFOV. More patients responded to combination therapy with HFOV and iNO than to either therapy alone. Patients with idiopathic PPHN responded better to iNO with conventional mechanical ventilation, however, and did not respond as well to iNO with HFOV. Two additional studies evaluated iNO in treating early neonatal pulmonary disease rather than waiting for patients to become candidates for ECMO.[92,93] Using early criteria (an OI >25) revealed conflicting results. The iNO/PPHN Study Group[92] did not show a decreased need for ECMO with iNO therapy (34% controls versus 22% iNO-treated subjects; $P = .12$). A more recent and larger trial confirmed more than one third reduction in ECMO need with iNO treatment when infants were treated early in the course of their illness (64% controls versus 38% iNO-treated subjects).[93] ECMO still was required to rescue a significant number (22% to 40%) of patients in all of these studies.

ECMO, despite its invasive nature, is now an established therapy with accepted morbidity and mortality rates. Head-to-head trials of high-frequency ventilation, surfactant, and iNO versus ECMO have not been conducted and may not be ethical, given ECMO's success in treating unrelenting and progressive respiratory failure. Longer term pulmonary and neurodevelopmental morbidity studies for many of these newer therapies are still wanting.

CHANGING DEMOGRAPHICS OF NEONATAL EXTRACORPOREAL MEMBRANE OXYGENATION

The ELSO[25] compiles a computerized ECMO case registry updated annually by international member centers. Statistics from the 2000 and 2001 reports of the ELSO Registry were reviewed by Rycus[94] and by Schumacher and Baumgart[95] (Fig. 47-8). The Registry's first report (1980-1987) contained information on 715 ECMO-treated patients.[96] At peak ECMO usage in 1992, there were 1499 neonates entered into the Registry during that year. Since 1992, the number of cases treated annually has declined. In 1999, only 889 neonatal ECMO patients were reported, a 40% decrease from 1992. The number of ECMO member centers reporting also has declined from 111 in 1996 to

71 in 2000. The true number of ECMO centers and ECMO cases treated annually presently may be underreported because ECMO now is considered a standard therapy.

Roy and colleagues[97] reported on this decrease in annual ECMO use and observed that the number of patients treated per center per year had decreased from 18 in 1991 to 9 in 1997. One third of all ECMO centers reported fewer than 10 cases per year. Roy and colleagues[97] also noted a dramatic decrease in the number of RDS cases, attributed to the widespread use of surfactant in term infants. The number of congenital diaphragmatic hernia cases remained constant in the 1990s at 250 to 280 cases per year. The percentage of patients with meconium aspiration/PPHN also has remained stable. Before 1990, high-frequency ventilation, surfactant, and iNO were never used before ECMO. By 1997, 46% received high-frequency ventilation before ECMO, 36% received surfactant, and 24% received iNO on many different research protocols. There was no relationship between age at initiation of ECMO and the use of any of these therapies, suggesting that these therapies did not delay ECMO in critically ill infants who were deteriorating rapidly. Diagnosis-specific mortality has not changed since the 1990s. These findings reinforce the notion that the introduction of newer therapies to avoid ECMO has not altered the morbidity and mortality of these diseases.

EXTRACORPOREAL MEMBRANE OXYGENATION OUTCOMES

Extracorporeal Membrane Oxygenation Survival[25,96]

The following statistics are derived primarily from the February 2001 report of the ELSO Registry.[25,95] Since its inception, ECMO criteria (reviewed earlier) designate an expected mortality exceeding 80% for instituting ECMO. A learning curve was experienced in the years before 1986, when ECMO was practiced primarily as a rescue therapy, reserved for dying patients.[96] Survival increased from approximately 50% in these early years to its current

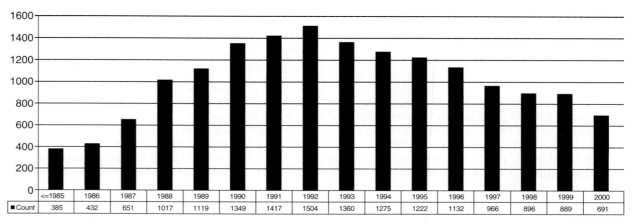

	<=1985	1986	1987	1988	1989	1990	1991	1992	1993	1994	1995	1996	1997	1998	1999	2000
■ Count	385	432	651	1017	1119	1349	1417	1504	1360	1275	1222	1132	966	896	889	691

Figure 47–8. Number of neonatal pulmonary cases per year receiving extracorporeal membrane oxygenation from 1985 to 2000. (*Adapted from Extracorporeal Life Support Organization (ELSO), Computer Registry for Extracorporeal Membrane Oxygenation (ECMO): Annual Report and Case Review. Ann Arbor, MI, University of Michigan, 1985-2000.*)

Table 47–3. Diagnostic Categories, Extracorporeal Membrane Oxygenation Use, and Outcomes Through February 2001 (ELSO Registry, Ann Arbor, Michigan)

Diagnosis	Mean Duration on ECMO (hr)	Maximal Duration on ECMO (hr)	Total No. Treated	Total No. Survived	Total No. Deaths	Proportion Survived (%)
Congenital diaphragmatic hernia	222	1072	3594	1949	1645	54
Meconium aspiration syndrome/PPHN	128	936	5715	5365	350	94
Idiopathic PPHN	140	1176	2330	1837	493	79
Respiratory distress syndrome	132	1093	1310	1100	210	84
Sepsis	137	1200	2193	1657	536	57
Pneumonia	210	936	201	115	86	57
Air leak syndrome	154	490	83	58	25	70
Other	168	1131	889	596	293	67

ECMO, extracorporeal membrane oxygenation; PPHN, persistent pulmonary hypertension of the newborn.

Data from references 25 and 95.

level of approximately 80% to 85% for all neonatal pulmonary conditions.

Survival rates vary dramatically with the underlying clinical condition being treated (Table 47-3).[25,95] The most successfully treated ECMO diagnosis is meconium aspiration syndrome. More than 5700 patients have been treated with ECMO for this condition, with a 94% survival. Closely following in success are infants diagnosed with RDS (84%) and idiopathic PPHN (79%). Survival has been less successful in infants with pneumonia or bacterial sepsis or persistent pulmonary air leak syndrome (57% to 70%).

The worst-case scenario for ECMO survival in the present era, and probably the biggest challenge for future diagnosis and management, are infants with severe **congenital diaphragmatic hernia**. Case survival currently is only 54% in these infants, despite ECMO and other modern interventions. It has been difficult to match the ECMO experience with congenital diaphragmatic hernia controls managed historically with conventional treatment—by surgical repair, conventional ventilatory support, or high-frequency ventilation—due to the wide spectrum of this disease.[98] Modern efforts to address fetal lung hypoplasia in congenital diaphragmatic hernia include fetal surgery.[99]

Developmental Follow-Up in Extracorporeal Membrane Oxygenation–Treated Infants[29,36,100-110]

Early morbidity data for neonatal follow-up of ECMO patients cited normal outcomes in 63% of patients evaluated between 3 months and 11 years of age.[36,103] Major central nervous system deficits, defined as cerebral palsy or mental retardation or both, occurred in at least 17% of ECMO survivors. Persistent chronic pulmonary disease existed in 8%. Subsequently, reports contained similar short-term developmental follow-up: 60% of patients were normal, 20% were suspect for a mild developmental delay, and 10% to 20% were shown at 1 year of age to have significantly delayed neurodevelopmental examinations.[101]

Subsequent follow-up reports attempted to ascertain the relative contribution of underlying illness versus ECMO per se as determinants of long-term outcome. Graziani and coworkers,[29] in 19% of 181 ECMO-treated patients with neurologic and audiologic abnormalities, determined that hypotension or need for cardiopulmonary resuscitation increased the risk for spastic cerebral palsy in survivors. Kornhauser and associates[106] reported a strong correlation between the development of bronchopulmonary dysplasia and the late initiation of ECMO after 4 days of age and a much higher frequency of mild and severe neurologic disability in patients who developed bronchopulmonary dysplasia after ECMO.[107]

Two other reports have addressed systematic, long-term follow-up evaluations of infants treated with ECMO. The first study by Schumacher and colleagues[103] evaluated 103 of 118 (87%) neonatal survivors past 1 year of age. Nearly one third of patients were rehospitalized or received outpatient treatments for recurrent respiratory illnesses. More than one quarter of these ECMO survivors manifested delayed somatic growth (<10th percentile length, weight, or head circumference). Central nervous system impairment of a moderate-to-severe degree of neurologic or developmental delay occurred in 16% of these infants, ranging in age from 10 months to 6 years. Of all infants, 8% manifested moderate-to-severe cognitive delay. Of these infants, 4% showed significant sensorineural hearing deficits, a finding reinforced subsequently by Desai and colleagues[111] and Graziani and associates.[29]

Another 10-year follow-up study was conducted by Hofkosh and coworkers,[28] wherein 70% of infants were enrolled successfully in neurodevelopmental follow-up between 6 months and 10 years of age. In the infant age group 6 to 30 months old, developmental quotients showed cognitive normalcy in 57% of all patients tested. Preschool children, age 2.7 to 4.1 years, showed cognitive normalcy in 70% of infants. By school age (4 to 10 years), cognitive normalcy was shown in 91% of the small number of infants followed this long. Central nervous system abnormalities in this study often were predicted by the detection of either central nervous system stroke on neuroimaging or the presence of chronic lung disease at the time of hospital discharge. Sensorineural hearing loss was an unexpected and significant finding in 21% of all patients seen.

Two case-controlled follow-up studies used well normal newborns as controls and critically ill "near-miss" ECMO cohorts for comparisons with ECMO-treated patients. Rais-Bahrami and colleagues[108] at 5 years of follow-up found similar cognitive outcomes: mean group IQ was 86 in near-miss ECMO patients and 97 in ECMO-treated infants, with similar rates of severe mental handicap (11% near-miss versus 12% ECMO-treated). When compared with healthy children who were not ill as neonates, Glass and associates[109] found major disability present in 17 of 103 (16.5%) of the ECMO-treated cohort (11 were retarded cognitively, 2 had learning disabilities, 5 had cerebral palsy, and 3 had hearing loss). The mean IQ score of the ECMO-treated children was 96—normal but significantly less than children who had not experienced critical illness and ECMO rescue (mean full-scale IQ 115). Newborns surviving severe respiratory failure and ECMO intervention do not have an increase in the relative risk of neurodevelopmental handicap because of ECMO.

Pulmonary Outcome

Most studies report more chronic lung disease, more reactive airway disease, more frequent rehospitalization, and more medication requirements in mechanically ventilated infants.[110] Beardsmore and colleagues[112] studied respiratory function at 1 year in participants of the United Kingdom ECMO trial. The authors concluded that lung function in ECMO-treated infants appeared "slightly better" than in infants assigned to conventional medical management, including subjects treated with high-frequency ventilation and iNO.[112] The relative risk of abnormal pulmonary outcome after ECMO was no greater than (and possibly less than) that after non-ECMO treatments.

SUMMARY

ECMO is an effective mode of providing heart-lung bypass in term or near-term infants with severe reversible lung disease not responding to less invasive therapies. Usage has decreased since 1992, however. Concurrently, there has been an increasing use of alternative treatments, such as surfactant, HFOV, and iNO, in these sick infants to avoid ECMO intervention. These newer therapies avoid ECMO in about one third of patients, but do not improve morbidity or mortality. In the present era, ECMO is an accepted standard therapy, with survival stabilized at 82% varying with diagnosis. Despite the invasive nature of ECMO, short-and long-term follow-up data show a poor neurodevelopmental outcome in only one quarter to one third of ECMO-treated patients, not significantly different from early outcomes now published for other, newer treatments. In addition, there is an increasing emphasis for the role of underlying disease

rather than ECMO per se in predicting outcome of these infants. It seems that, despite its invasive nature, ECMO remains an important and effective rescue therapy for term or near-term infants with severe reversible pulmonary disease when all else fails.

REFERENCES

1. Cornish D, Arensman R (eds): Extracorporeal Life Support. Boston, Blackwell, 1992.
2. Hirschl RB, Bartlett RH: Extracorporeal membrane oxygenation support in cardiorespiratory failure. Adv Surg 21:189, 1987.
3. Gibbon JH: Artificial maintenance of circulation during occlusion of the pulmonary artery. Arch Surg 34:1105, 1937.
4. McLean J: The discovery of heparin. Circulation 19:75, 1959.
5. Cross FS, Day FB: Direct vision repair of intracardiac defects utilizing a rotating disc reservoir oxygenator. Surg Gynecol Obstet 104:711, 1957.
6. DeWall R, Bentley DJ, Hirose M, et al: A temperature controlling (omnithermic) disposable bubble oxygenator for total body perfusion. Dis Chest 49:207, 1966.
7. Clowes GHA, Hopkins AL, Neville WE: An artificial lung dependent upon diffusion of oxygen and carbon dioxide through plastic membranes. J Thorac Surg 32:630, 1956.
8. Kloff WJ, Berk HT: Artificial kidney: A dialyzer with great area. Acta Med Scand 117:121, 1944.
9. Kammermeyer JK: Silicone rubber as a selective barrier. Indian Eng Chem 49:1685, 1957.
10. Kolobow T, Bowman RL: Construction and evaluation of an alveolar membrane artificial heart lung. Trans ASAIO 9:238, 1963.
11. Kolobow T, Zapol W, Pierce J: High survival and minimal blood damage in lambs exposed to long term (1 week) venovenous pumping with a polyurethane chamber roller pump with and without a membrane blood oxygenator. Trans ASAIO 15:172, 1969.
12. Rashkind WJ, Freeman A, Klein D, et al: Evaluation of a disposable plastic, low volume, pumpless oxygenator as a lung substitute. J Pediatr 66:94, 1965.
13. Dorson W, Baker E, Cohen ML, et al: A perfusion system for infants. Trans ASAIO 15:155, 1969.
14. White JJ, Andrews HG, Risemberg H, et al: Prolonged respiratory support in newborn infants with a membrane oxygenator. Surgery 70:288, 1971.
15. Bartlett RH, Gazzaniga GB, Jeffries MR, et al: Extracorporeal membrane oxygenation (ECMO) cardiopulmonary support in infancy. Trans ASAIO 22:80, 1976.
16. Extracorporeal support for respiratory insufficiency, a collaborative study. Prepared in response to RFP-NHLI-73-20. Bethesda, MD, U.S. Department of Health, Public Health Service, National Institutes of Health, December 1979.
17. Bartlett RH, Andrews AF, Toomasian JM, et al: Extracorporeal membrane oxygenation for newborn respiratory failure: Forty-five cases. Surgery 92:425, 1982.
18. Bartlett RH, Roloff DW, Cornell RG, et al: Extracorporeal circulation in neonatal respiratory failure: A prospective randomized study. Pediatrics 76:479, 1985.
19. Hardesty RL, Griffith BP, Bebski RF, et al: Extracorporeal membrane oxygenation: Successful treatment of persistent fetal circulation following repair of congenital diaphragmatic hernia. J Thorac Cardiovasc Surg 81:556, 1981.
20. Kirkpatrick BV, Krummel TM, Mueller DG, et al: Use of extracorporeal membrane oxygenation for respiratory failure in term infants. Pediatrics 72:872, 1983.

21. Krummel TM, Greenfield LJ, Kirkpatrick BV, et al: Clinical use of an extracorporeal membrane oxygenator in neonatal pulmonary failure. J Pediatr Surg 17:525, 1982.

22. Short BL, Pearson GD: Neonatal extracorporeal membrane oxygenation: A review. J Intensive Care Med 1:47, 1986.

23. Trento A, Griffith Hardesty RL: Extracorporeal membrane oxygenation: Experience at the University of Pittsburgh. Ann Thorac Surg 42:56, 1986.

24. O'Rourke PP, Crone RK, Vacanti JP, et al: Extracorporeal membrane oxygenation and conventional medical therapy in neonates with persistent pulmonary hypertension of the newborn: A prospective randomized study. Pediatrics 84:957, 1989.

25. Extracorporeal Life Support Organization (ELSO), Computer Registry for Extracorporeal Membrane Oxygenation (ECMO): Annual Report and Case Review. Ann Arbor, MI, University of Michigan, 1985-2000.

26. Peckham GJ, Fox WW: Physiologic factors affecting pulmonary artery pressure in infants with persistent pulmonary hypertension. J Pediatr 93:1005, 1978.

27. Fox WW: Mechanical ventilation in the management of persistent pulmonary hypertension of the newborn (PPHN). Presented at the 1982 Ross Conference on Cardiovascular Sequelae of Asphyxia in the Newborn, 1982, San Diego, CA.

28. Hofkosh D, Thompson AE, Nozza RJ, et al: Ten years of extracorporeal membrane oxygenation: Neurodevelopmental outcome. Pediatrics 87:549, 1991.

29. Graziani LJ, Baumgart S, Desai S, et al: Clinical antecedents of neurologic and audiologic abnormalities in survivors of neonatal extracorporeal membrane oxygenation. J Child Neurol 12:415, 1997.

30. Foglia RP, Bjerke S, Kelly RE, et al: Extracorporeal membrane oxygenation in the treatment of neonatal respiratory failure. Arch Surg 125:1286, 1990.

31. Hirschl RB, Coburn C, Butler SM, et al: Early onset sepsis neonatorum with *Listeria monocytogenes* emerging as a treatable disease when provided prolonged extracorporeal life support (ECLS). Arch Pediatr Adolesc Med 148:513, 1994.

32. Hocker JR, Pippa MS, Rabalais GP, et al: Extracorporeal membrane oxygenation and early-onset group B streptococcal sepsis. Pediatrics 89:1, 1992.

33. Langston C: Misalignment of pulmonary veins and alveolar capillary dysplasia. Pediatr Pathol 11:163, 1991.

34. Ortiz RM, Cilley RE, Bartlett RH: Extracorporeal membrane oxygenation in pediatric respiratory failure. Pediatr Clin North Am 34:39, 1987.

35. Bartlett RH: Extracorporeal membrane oxygenation (ECMO) in the treatment of cardiac and respiratory failure in children. Trans ASAIO 26:578, 1980.

36. Bartlett RH, Gazzaniga A, Toomasian J, et al: Extracorporeal membrane oxygenation (ECMO) in neonatal respiratory failure: 100 cases. Ann Surg 204:236, 1986.

37. Baumgart S, Hirschl RB, Butler SZ, et al: Diagnosis-related criteria in the consideration of ECMO in neonates previously treated with high-frequency jet ventilation. Pediatrics 89:491, 1992.

38. Beck R, Anderson KD, Pearson GD, et al: Criteria for extracorporeal membrane oxygenation in a population of infants with persistent pulmonary hypertension of the newborn. J Pediatr Surg 21:297, 1986.

39. Hallman M, Merritt A, Jarvenpaa A-L, et al: Exogenous human surfactant for treatment of severe respiratory distress syndrome: A randomized prospective clinical trial. J Pediatr 106:963, 1985.

40. Krummel TM, Greenfield LJ, Kirkpatrick BV, et al: Alveolar-arterial oxygen gradients versus the neonatal pulmonary insufficiency index for prediction of mortality in ECMO candidates. J Pediatr Surg 19:380, 1984.

41. AAP Committee on Fetus and Newborn: Recommendations on ECMO. Pediatrics 85:618, 1990.

42. Lantos JD, Frader J: ECMO and the ethics of clinical research in pediatrics [editorial]. N Engl J Med 323:409, 1990.

43. Nelson NM: On hummingbirds, ECMO and IBM [editorial]. Pediatrics 85:374, 1990.

44. Krummel TM, Greenfield LJ, Kirkpatrick BV, et al: The early evaluation of survivors after extracorporeal membrane oxygenation for neonatal pulmonary failure. J Pediatr Surg 19:585, 1984.

45. Kossel H, Bauer K, Kewitz G, et al: Do we need new indications for ECMO in neonates pretreated with high-frequency ventilation and/or inhaled nitric oxide? Intensive Care Med 26:1489, 2000.

46. UK collaborative randomized trial of neonatal extracorporeal membrane oxygenation. UK Collaborative ECMO Trial Group. Lancet 348:75, 1996.

47. Marsh TD, Wilkerson SA, Cook LN: Extracorporeal membrane oxygenation selection criteria: Partial pressure of arterial oxygen versus alveolar-arterial oxygen gradient. Pediatrics 82:162, 1988.

48. Bartlett RH: Extracorporeal life support for cardiopulmonary failure. Curr Probl Surg 27:10, 1990.

49. Andrews AF, Klein MD, Toomasian JM, et al: Veno-venous extracorporeal membrane oxygenation in neonates with respiratory failure. J Pediatr Surg 18:339, 1983.

50. Zwischenberger JB, Toomasian JM, Drake K, et al: Total support with single cannula VV ECMO. Trans ASAIO 31:610, 1985.

51. Gauger PG, Hirschl RB, Delosh TN, et al: A matched pairs analysis of veno-arterial and veno-venous extracorporeal life support in neonatal respiratory failure. ASAIO 41:M573, 1995.

52. Reickert CA, Schreiner RJ, Bartlett RH, Hirschl RB: Percutaneous access for veno-venous extracorporeal life support in neonates. J Pediatr Surg 33:365, 1998.

53. Strieper MJ, Sharma S, Dooley KJ, et al: Effects of veno-venous extracorporeal membrane oxygenation on cardiac performance as determined by echocardiographic measurements. J Pediatr 122:950, 1993.

54. Chapman RA, Toomasian JM, Bartlett RH: ECMO: Extracorporeal Membrane Oxygenation Technical Specialist Manual. Ann Arbor, MI, University of Michigan, 1988.

55. Boedy RF, Howell CG, Kanto WP: Hidden mortality rate associated with extracorporeal membrane oxygenation. J Pediatr 117:462, 1990.

56. Slovis TL, Sell LL, Bedard MP, Klein MD: Ultrasonographic findings (CNS, thorax, abdomen) in infants undergoing extracorporeal oxygenation therapy. Pediatr Radiol 18:1112, 1988.

57. Beacham SG, Streletz LJ: Electroencephalographic studies in neonates during extracorporeal membrane oxygenation. Am J EEG Tech 31:11, 1991.

58. Graziani LJ, Streletz LJ, Baumgart S, et al: Prognosis and neonatal EEG studies of infants treated with ECMO. Pediatr Res 33:371(A), 1993.

59. Streletz LJ, Bej MD, Graziani LJ, et al: The utility of serial electroencephalograms in neonates during extracorporeal membrane oxygenation therapy. Pediatr Neurol 8:190, 1992.

60. Palmisano JM, Moler FW, Custer JR, et al: Unsuspected congenital heart disease on ECMO. J Pediatr 121:115, 1992.

61. Klein MD, Shaheen KW, Whittlesey GC, et al: ECMO after repair. J Thorac Surg 100:498, 1990.

62. Wetmore NE, Bartlett RH, Gazzaniga AB, Haiduc NJ: Extracorporeal membrane oxygenation (ECMO): A team approach in critical care and life-support research. Heart Lung 8:288, 1979.

63. Carter JM, Gerstmann DR, Clark RH, et al: High-frequency oscillatory ventilation and ECMO for the treatment of acute neonatal respiratory failure. Pediatrics 85:159, 1990.

64. Hirschl RB, Heiss KF, Bartlett RH: Severe myocardial dysfunction during ECMO. J Pediatr Surg 27:48, 1992.

65. Martin GR, Short BL, Abbott C, O'Brien AM: Cardiac stun in ECMO. J Thorac Cardiovasc Surg 101:607, 1991.

66. Von Allmen D, Ryckman FC: Cardiac arrest in ECMO. J Pediatr Surg 26:143, 1991.

67. Antunes MJ, Cullen JA, Holt WJ, et al: Continued pulmonary recovery observed after discontinuing extracorporeal membrane oxygenation. Pediatr Pulmonol 17:143, 1994.

68. Keszler M, Subramanian KNS, Smith YA, et al: Pulmonary management during extracorporeal membrane oxygenation. Crit Care Med 17:495, 1989.

69. Shneider B, Cronin J, Van Marter L, et al: Cholestasis in infants on ECMO. J Pediatr Gastroenterol Nutr 13:285, 1991.

70. Steiner CK, Stewart DL, Bond SJ, et al: Predictors of acquiring a nosocomial bloodstream infection on extracorporeal membrane oxygenation. J Pediatr Surg 36:487, 2001.

71. Mault JR, Dirkes SM, Swartz RD, Bartlett RH: Continuous Hemofiltration, a Reference Guide. Ann Arbor, MI, University of Michigan, 1988.

72. Lochan SR, Adeniyi-Jones S, Assadi FK, et al: Co-administration of theophylline enhances diuretic response to furosemide in infants on extracorporeal membrane oxygenation (ECMO): A randomized controlled pilot study. J Pediatr 133:86, 1998.

73. Mitchell DG, Merton D, Needleman L, et al. Neonatal brain: Color Doppler imaging I: Technique and vascular anatomy. Radiology 167:303, 1988.

74. Mitchell DG, Merton DA, Desai H, et al: Neonatal brain: Color Doppler imaging II: Altered flow patterns from extracorporeal membrane oxygenation. Radiology 167:307, 1988.

75. Mitchell DG, Merton DA, Graziani LJ, et al: Right carotid artery ligation in neonates: Classification of collateral flow with color Doppler imaging. Radiology 175:117, 1990.

76. Mitchell DG, Merton DA, Mirsky PJ, Needleman L: Circle of Willis in newborns: Color Doppler imaging of 53 healthy full-term infants. Radiology 172:201, 1989.

77. Baumgart S, Graziani LJ, Streletz LJ, et al: Right common carotid artery reconstruction following ECMO: Structural and vascular imaging, EEG, and developmental correlates to recovery. Pediatr Res 33:255(A), 1993.

78. Crombleholme TM, Adzick S, deLorimier AA, et al: Carotid artery reconstruction following ECMO. Am J Dis Child 144:872, 1990.

79. DeAngelis GA, Mitchell DG, Merton DA, et al: Right common carotid artery reconstruction in neonates after extracorporeal membrane oxygenation: color Doppler imaging. Radiology 182:521, 1992.

80. Taylor BJ, Seibert JJ, Glasier CM, et al: Evaluation of the reconstructed carotid artery following ECMO. Pediatrics 90:568, 1992.

81. Voorhies TM, Tardo CL, Starret AL, et al: Evaluation of cerebral circulation in neonates following extracorporeal membrane oxygenation. Ann Neurol 18:380, 1985.

82. Desai H, Park C, Zhang J, et al: Regional cerebral blood flow assessment by single photon emission computerized tomography (SPECT); and correlation with brain MRI following ECMO. Pediatr Res 33:209(A), 1993.

83. Desai SA, Stanley C, Gringlas M, et al: Five year follow-up of neonates with reconstructed right common carotid arteries after extracorporeal membrane oxygenation. J Pediatr 134:428, 1999.

84. D'Agostino JA, Hoffman-Williamson M, Bernbaum JC, et al: Repair and recovery of neonates with congenital diaphragmatic hernia (CDH) using rescue with extracorporeal membrane oxygenation (ECMO). Pediatr Res 31:245(A), 1992.

85. Hoffenberg A, Bernbaum J, D'Agostino J, et al: Common feeding disorders in infants with congenital diaphragmatic hernia. Pediatr Res 33:101(A), 1993.

86. Clark RH, Yoder BA, Sell MS: Prospective, randomized comparison of high-frequency oscillation and conventional ventilation in candidates for extracorporeal membrane oxygenation. J Pediatr 124:447, 1994.

87. Long W, Corbet A, Cotton R, et al: A controlled trial of synthetic surfactant in infants weighing 1250 g or more with respiratory distress syndrome. The American Exosurf Neonatal Study Group I, and the Canadian Exosurf Neonatal Study Group. N Engl J Med 325:1696, 1991.

88. Lotze A, Mitchell BR, Bulas DI, et al: Multicenter study of surfactant (beractant) use in the treatment of term infants with severe respiratory failure. Survanta in Term Infants Study Group. J Pediatr 132:40, 1998.

89. Inhaled nitric oxide in full-term and nearly full-term infants with hypoxic respiratory failure. Neonatal Inhaled Nitric Oxide Study Group [published erratum appears in N Engl J Med 1997 Aug 7;337(6):434]. N Engl J Med 336:597, 1997.

90. Roberts JD Jr, Fineman JR, Morin FC 3rd, et al: Inhaled nitric oxide and persistent pulmonary hypertension of the newborn. The Inhaled Nitric Oxide Study Group. N Engl J Med 336:605, 1997.

91. Kinsella JP, Truog WE, Walsh WF, et al: Randomized, multicenter trial of inhaled nitric oxide and high-frequency oscillatory ventilation in severe, persistent pulmonary hypertension of the newborn. J Pediatr 131:55, 1997.

92. Davidson D, Barefield ES, Kattwinkel J, et al: Inhaled nitric oxide for the early treatment of persistent pulmonary hypertension of the term newborn: A randomized, double-masked, placebo-controlled, dose-response, multicenter study. The I-NO/PPHN Study Group. Pediatrics 101:325, 1998.

93. Clark RH, Kueser TJ, Walker MW, et al: Low-dose nitric oxide therapy for persistent pulmonary hypertension of the newborn. Clinical Inhaled Nitric Oxide Research Group. N Engl J Med 342:469, 2000.

94. Rycus P: ECLS Registry Report: International Summary. Ann Arbor, MI, ECMO Registry of the Extracorporeal Life Support Organization (ELSO), 2001.

95. Schumacher RE, Baumgart S: ECMO 2001: The odyssey continues. Clin Perinatol 28:629, 2001.

96. Toomasian JM, Snedecor SM, Cornell RG, et al: National experience with extracorporeal membrane oxygenation (ECMO) for newborn respiratory failure, 715 cases. ASAIO Trans 34:140, 1988.

97. Roy BJ, Rycus P, Conrad SA, Clark RH: The changing demographics of neonatal extracorporeal membrane oxygenation patients reported to the extracorporeal life support organization (ELSO) registry. Pediatrics 106:1334, 2000.

98. O'Rourke PP, Lillehei CW, Crone RK, Vacanti JP: The effect of extracorporeal membrane oxygenation on the survival of neonates with high-risk congenital diaphragmatic hernia: 45 cases from a single institution. J Pediatr Surg 26:147, 1991.

99. Harrison MR, Adzick NS, Flake AW: Congenital diaphragmatic hernia: An unsolved problem. Semin Pediatr Surg 2:109, 1993.

100. Andrews AF, Nixon CA, Cilley RE, et al: One-to-three year outcome for 14 neonatal survivors of extracorporeal membrane oxygenation. Pediatrics 78:692, 1986.
101. Glass P, Miller MK, Short BL: Morbidity for survivors of extracorporeal membrane oxygenation: Neurodevelopmental outcome at 1 year of age. Pediatrics 83:72, 1989.
102. Lott IT, McPherson D, Towne B, et al: Long-term neurophysiologic outcome after neonatal extracorporeal membrane oxygenation. J Pediatr 116:343, 1990.
103. Schumacher RE, Palmer TW, Roloff DW, et al: Follow-up of infants treated with extracorporeal membrane oxygenation for newborn respiratory failure. Pediatrics 87:451, 1991.
104. Short BL, Lotze A: Extracorporeal membrane oxygenation therapy. Pediatr Ann 17:516, 1988.
105. Towne BH, Lott IT, Hicks DA, Healey T: Long-term follow-up of infants and children treated with extracorporeal membrane oxygenation (ECMO): A preliminary report. J Pediatr Surg 20:410, 1985.
106. Kornhauser MS, Cullen JA, Baumgart S, et al: Risk factors for bronchopulmonary dysplasia after extracorporeal membrane oxygenation. Arch Pediatr Adolesc Med 148:820, 1994.

107. Kornhauser MS, Baumgart S, Desai SA, et al: Adverse neurodevelopmental outcome after extracorporeal membrane oxygenation among neonates with bronchopulmonary dysplasia. J Pediatr 132:307, 1998.
108. Rais-Bahrami K, Wagner AE, Coffman C, et al: Neurodevelopmental outcome in ECMO vs near-miss ECMO patients at 5 years of age. Clin Pediatr (Phila) 39:145, 2000.
109. Glass P, Wagner AE, Papero PH, et al: Neurodevelopmental status at age five years of neonates treated with extracorporeal membrane oxygenation. J Pediatr 127:447, 1995.
110. Walsh-Sukys MC, Bauer RE, Cornell DJ, et al: Severe respiratory failure in neonates: Mortality and morbidity rates and neurodevelopmental outcomes. J Pediatr 125:104, 1994.
111. Desai S, Kollros PR, Graziani LJ, et al: Sensitivity and specificity of the neonatal brainstem auditory evoked potential for hearing and language deficits in survivors of extracorporeal membrane oxygenation. J Pediatr 131:233, 1997.
112. Beardsmore C, Dundas I, Poole K, et al: Respiratory function in survivors of the United Kingdom Extracorporeal Membrane Oxygenation Trial. Am J Respir Crit Care Med 161:1129, 2000.

CHAPTER 48

Liquid Ventilation

*Thomas H. Shaffer, Rees Oliver, Marla R. Wolfson,
and Jay S. Greenspan*

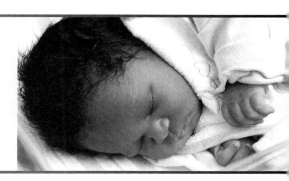

S ignificant advances have been made in the care of patients with respiratory failure, but morbidity still persists. Liquid ventilation has been explored since 1970 as an alternative means of supporting pulmonary gas exchange while preserving lung structure and function in infants, children, and adults. Although liquid breathing has not yet become clinically available, the physiology and experimental data are promising. Early animal studies in liquid ventilation indicate potential benefits for the neonate in respiratory failure.[1-4] The results of pivotal randomized trials in adults should guide the next steps of this technology. In this chapter, we discuss the physiology, current state, and promise of this technology, with emphasis on the neonatal and pediatric patient.

BACKGROUND

Before delivery, the fetal lung is filled with 25 to 30 mL of liquid per kilogram of body weight; this liquid is produced at a rate of approximately 250 to 300 mL per day. The fetus breathes the fluid episodically during the last third of gestation. Various experimental protocols involving spinal cord and phrenic nerve transections, as well as tracheal fluid outflow obstruction, have been studied in animals with limited breathing capacities and have demonstrated the necessity of fluid breathing for normal lung growth.[1,2,5,6] Normal pulmonary development therefore depends on an appropriate balance between production and exhalation of lung fluid. The maintenance of fetal lung volume is facilitated by the low surface tension of the fluid-filled lung and a pressure gradient across the larynx of 3 to 5 cm H_2O.[7] To make a successful transition from intrauterine to extrauterine life, an infant requires adequate pulmonary structural maturity to facilitate gas exchange, the presence of a surfactant to lower interfacial surface tension in the gas-exchanging regions, and a sufficient amount of driving and end-distending pulmonary pressures. Some or all of these processes may be insufficient in the prematurely delivered fetus. For preterm

infants, a successful transition to extrauterine life without pulmonary-related morbidity and mortality may be difficult, even with optimal management. Even healthy preterm infants who never require supplemental oxygen may demonstrate pulmonary deterioration and dysfunction by full-term postconception age.[8,9] The maintenance of optimal pulmonary development and lung volume in the preterm infant may therefore require a fluid-filled medium (Table 48-1 and Fig. 48-1).

EARLY DEVELOPMENT OF LIQUID VENTILATION

The impetus to pursue liquid ventilation treatment in neonates has evolved from two arenas of research and development. In the first arena, the liquid-filled lung has been studied as a means of reducing the high surface tension in terminal air spaces of the injured or premature lung, thereby promoting normal lung function and growth. When filled with liquid, even the surfactant-sufficient lung demonstrates increased compliance.[3,10-12] In addition, current therapies of exogenous surfactant replacement may be limited by unequal pulmonary distribution when gas ventilation is utilized as a delivery vehicle. Liquid ventilation would uniformly diminish surface tension and decrease pulmonary inflation pressures, thereby reducing the barotrauma necessary to achieve adequate gas exchange. Furthermore, liquid ventilation distends the immature pulmonary parenchyma, compensating, in part, for structural limitations and large distances between vascular channels and air spaces.[4]

The second arena of investigation that has demonstrated the clinical applicability of liquid ventilation in the neonate is the capability of removing pulmonary debris. Winternitz and Smith employed a saline lavage technique to treat pneumonitis in animals that developed pulmonary injury from poisonous gas inhalation.[13] Although this injury does not specifically relate to neonatal lung disease, debris in terminal air spaces is a frequent complication of many neonatal pulmonary pathologic processes (e.g.,

Table 48-1. Physical Properties of Selected Perfluorochemicals in Relation to Water

Water FC-77 RM-101	FC-75	Perfluorodecalin		Perflubron	
Boiling point (°C)	100	97	101	102	140	143
Density at 25° C (g/mL)	1	1.78	1.77	1.78	1.95	1.93
Viscosity at 25° C (centistokes)	1	0.8	0.82	0.82	2.9	1.1
Vapor pressure at 37° C (mm Hg)	47	85	64	63	14	11
Surface tension at 25° C (dynes/cm)	72	15	15	15	19	18
Oxygen solubility at 25° C (mL gas/100 mL liquid)	3	50	52	52	49	53
Carbon dioxide solubility at 25° C (mL gas/100 mL liquid)	57	198	160	160	140	210

pneumonia, meconium and amniotic fluid aspiration, respiratory distress syndrome [RDS]). Hence, removal of this debris with liquid ventilation should improve pulmonary function and promote healing and normal lung development.

Saline was generally utilized in the aforementioned studies. The limitation of extended liquid breathing with saline is that the solubility for oxygen is only 3 mL per 100 mL of fluid at 1 atm, thereby preventing adequate gas exchange outside of a hyperbaric chamber.[14] In addition, the viscosity and density of saline are higher than those of air, increasing the work of breathing and limiting the duration of spontaneous ventilation. Finally, a lavage of saline removes endogenous surfactant, inhibiting the recovery to gas ventilation. Therefore, prolonged spontaneous ventilation of saline leads to respiratory distress, fatigue, and limited gas exchange. The feasibility of liquid ventilation depends on the availability of a liquid that has high solubility for respiratory gases, low surface tension, chemical inertness, and safety when exposed to the lung for long periods of time.

PERFLUOROCHEMICAL LIQUID VENTILATION

Liquids exist with high solubility for respiratory gases. Many of these, such as the synthetic and natural oils, are too viscous or toxic to serve as a respiratory medium.

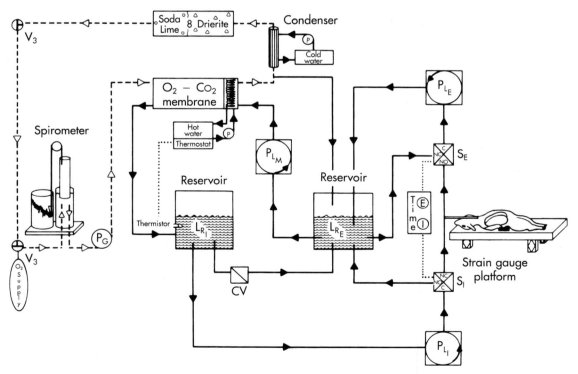

Figure 48-1. Schematic of an automated liquid breathing system. Perfluorochemical is oxygenated, heated, and recycled. Inspiratory and expiratory pressures and volume, timing, inspired oxygen concentration, and numerous other parameters can be monitored and mechanically altered. C, common port; CV, check valve; E, expiration; I, inspiration; L_{R_E}, liquid reservoir, expiratory; L_{R_I}, liquid reservoir, inspiratory; NC, normally closed port; NO, normally open port; P, pump; P_G, pump, gas exchange; P_{L_E}, pump, expiratory liquid; P_{L_I}, pump, inspiratory liquid; P_{L_M}, pump, liquid membrane; S_E, solenoid valve, expiratory; S_I, solenoid valve, inspiratory; V_3, manual valve.

Perfluorochemicals (PFCs) are inert liquids derived by replacing all the carbon-bound hydrogen atoms in organic compounds with fluorine.[15] Pure medical-grade PFC liquids currently exist for liquid ventilation purposes because these chemicals are already used in clinical medicine for different organ systems.[16,17]

Several techniques are available for the production of PFCs from compounds such as benzene. These processes include the use of electrochemical fluoridation techniques, heating or agitation with cobalt trifluoride, and direct fluorination by the careful addition of fluorine gas under carefully controlled conditions.[15,18] Oxygen is about 20 times more soluble in PFCs than in water, and carbon dioxide solubility varies with the specific chemical, but carbon dioxide is also highly soluble in PFCs (see Table 48-1).[19,20] These liquids are not soluble in lipids or water, and they evaporate rapidly in room air. Initial experimentation by Clark and Gollan demonstrated the feasibility of breathing PFCs during normobaric immersion of small animals.[21] Although animals can breathe oxygenated PFC liquids for a period of time and recover uneventfully, respiratory muscle fatigue and acidosis ensue after prolonged periods of spontaneous ventilation.

A mechanical ventilator capable of ventilating liquids was designed to compensate for these difficulties (see Fig. 48-1).[22,23] These devices control ventilation through time cycling and active inspiration and expiration. Animal studies demonstrated improved oxygenation and controlled arterial carbon dioxide tension and acidosis with these ventilators in comparison with spontaneous liquid ventilation.[24,25] Appropriate ventilatory schemes were designed and evaluated. Investigators demonstrated that several animal species could be liquid ventilated with various oxygenated PFCs, successfully recover to gas breathing, and survive without long-term compromise. The clinical advantage of liquid ventilation over gas ventilation was demonstrated in a preterm lamb model, and liquid ventilation trials in severely ill human neonates showed the feasibility and potential of this modality in humans.[26-28]

PHYSIOLOGY OF LIQUID VENTILATION

In liquid ventilation, a PFC liquid is used to replace nitrogen gas as the carrier for oxygen and carbon dioxide. Physiologic processes are supported by the combination of physicochemical properties of the PFC liquid and the biophysical effects of the liquid on lung mechanics (Fig. 48-2).

PFC instillation, with its relatively low surface tension, high respiratory gas solubility, and high-spreading coefficients, replaces the gas-liquid interface with a liquid-liquid interface at the lung surface while supporting an adequate alveolar reservoir for pulmonary gas exchange.[29] High surface tension at the gas-liquid interface is eliminated, and interfacial tension is reduced. Pulmonary blood flow is more homogenous in the fluid-filled lung than in the gas-filled lung because transmural pressures across the alveolar capillary membrane are more evenly matched. For this reason, liquid ventilation appears to be a promising treatment for infants and children with respiratory distress and injured lungs.

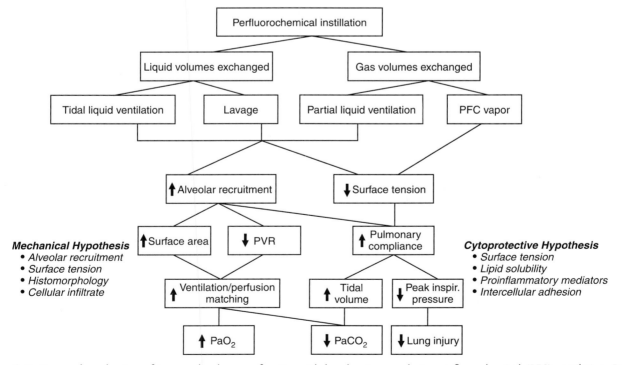

Figure 48–2. Proposed mechanism of improved pulmonary function with less barotrauma during perfluorochemical (PFC) ventilation. Paco₂, arterial carbon dioxide tension; Pao₂, arterial oxygen tension; PVR, pulmonary vascular resistance. *(From Shaffer TH, Wolfson MR: Liquid ventilation: An alternative ventilation strategy for management of neonatal respiratory distress. Eur J Pediatr 155[Suppl 2]:530, 1996.)*

PFC liquids are chemically and biologically inert, clear, and odorless and are generally immiscible in lipid, alcohol, or water. Along with the relatively low surface tension, high respiratory gas solubility, and high-spreading coefficients noted previously, each of these attributes allows these liquids to act as an effective ventilatory medium. Because these liquids also have high density, viscosity, and diffusion coefficients, as a respiratory medium, the work of breathing during spontaneous breathing is greater than with water and much greater than during gas breathing. The increased viscosity increases resistance to flow, thereby prolonging inspiratory and expiratory time constants. In addition, the increased gas diffusion time enhances the inspiratory time requirements. Maximal expiratory flow rates in the PFC-filled lung are much lower than in the gas-filled lung and are inversely proportional to lung volume, thereby increasing the required expiratory time. Hence, optimal breathing rates and timing ratios are very different from those of gas ventilation. Increased time is needed for inspiration and expiration, and a "dwell" time is needed to facilitate gas exchange. Carbon dioxide elimination is reduced at low frequencies by limited alveolar ventilation and at high frequencies by incomplete diffusion. Initial studies with animal immersion observations and demand-regulated liquid ventilators indicated that optimal breathing frequency requirements are slow (three to six breaths per minute).[19,21-23] Carbon dioxide removal can be optimized primarily by altering tidal volume and by altering frequency and timing ratios according to pulmonary mechanics.

During ventilation, PFCs are evenly distributed throughout the lung at low inflation pressures. Oxygenation of the compromised or premature animal can generally be facilitated by liquid ventilation. Control of arterial oxygen tensions can be achieved by altering the oxygen content of the liquid or by increasing the functional residual capacity. Lung volume is regulated by altering inspiratory-to-expiratory timing ratios or driving pressure and flow rates.[17,23,25,28,30] Healthy adult animals may experience some increase in alveolar-arterial oxygen gradient while on liquid ventilation. Minimal gains in surface tension reduction, ventilation-perfusion matching, and alveolar recruitment are outweighed by the increases in dead space.[29,31,32] Early ventilation trials in adult animals also demonstrated a small but significant production of metabolic acidosis.[33-35] This acidosis has been attributed to cardiovascular adjustments and increased pulmonary vascular resistance from vascular compression, which can be overcome by appropriate intravascular volume expansion.[36,37] If the animal has pulmonary compromise before liquid ventilation, the positive effect on surface tension, ventilation-perfusion matching, and air space recruitment; the unfolding of pulmonary capillaries; and the improved oxygenation and ventilation will decrease pulmonary vascular resistance. When performed appropriately, studies indicate that liquid ventilation with PFCs should be able to maintain gas exchange and cardiopulmonary stability for an extended period of time in many animal species with a wide variety of lung diseases (Fig. 48-3).[17,29,38]

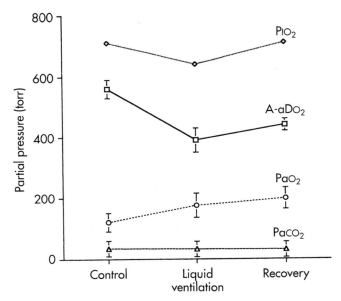

Figure 48–3. Inspired oxygen tension (PIO_2), alveolar-arterial oxygen gradient ($A-aDO_2$), arterial oxygen tension (PaO_2), and arterial carbon dioxide tension ($PaCO_2$) during control, liquid, and gas recovery ventilation in a preterm lamb. *(From Shaffer TH, Douglas PR, Lowe CA, et al: Liquid ventilation: Improved gas exchange and lung compliance in preterm lambs. Pediatr Res 17:303, 1983.)*

Successful recovery to gas ventilation after PFC liquid ventilation has been demonstrated in animal models and some human neonates. In a sick or preterm population, this transition is associated with improved pulmonary function from preliquid ventilation values (see Fig. 48-3). Healthy adult animals experienced a transient mild deterioration in lung function, probably as a result of increased surface tension (approximately 15 dyne/cm with residual PFC liquid versus 2 dyne/cm in a healthy lung) and diffusion block from residual PFC.[15,39,40] Histologic evaluation of preterm animals ventilated with PFCs and recovered to gas ventilation showed fewer hyaline membranes, less injury to bronchiolar epithelium and terminal air spaces, and clearance of debris in comparison with control animals exclusively gas ventilated.[18,28,41] Ventilation with only PFC liquids caused no damage to the fine structures in the air spaces; detailed examination of the epithelial cell membranes and bilaminar plasmalemma showed maintenance of the lung ultrastructure.[42] Although interspecies variations may exist, PFC liquids appeared to cause no long-term compromise when used as a ventilatory medium.[29] Dogs, for example, demonstrated normal results on light and electron microscopy examinations (aside from a small increase in the number of macrophages) of their lungs up to 180 days after a liquid ventilation procedure, and adult monkeys had normal pulmonary function through 3 years of follow-up.[35,43]

The absorption and excretion of PFCs after liquid ventilation have been investigated in several animal species. The primary route of excretion is via the lungs, with small amounts expelled through the skin. When injected intravenously as an emulsion (as in artificial blood products), pulmonary activity is sufficient to cause hyperinflation of the lungs that can persist for several months.[44] Very little PFC is absorbed by the pulmonary circulation when breathed, particularly in comparison with intravenous injection, as occurs with artificial blood products. However, small quantities can be found in animals for years after liquid ventilation, with a predominance of storage in fatty tissue.[43] Pulmonary uptake is related to the PFC vapor pressure and ventilation-perfusion matching in the lungs. Distribution appears to be dependent on tissue perfusion and lipid concentration. Similar results in human studies are suggestive of similar absorption.[29] Although these chemicals remain in tissue for years, they do not exert an obvious toxic effect and do not undergo biotransformation.[45] Eventual excretion is dependent on reentry into the circulation and eventual escape via the lungs or skin.

The poor solubility of PFCs for substances other than gases affects clinical applications. All substrates for growth are insoluble. Hence, these fluids are bacteriostatic and, unlike saline, do not wash out or alter the natural surfactant present at the gas-liquid interface.[29,46] The solubility characteristics of PFCs may limit, in part, effective débridement; however, when PFCs were used in an animal model of human meconium aspiration, debris was effectively removed and pulmonary function improved.[17] Whereas biologically active agents such as vasoactive drugs, antibiotics, and artificial surfactants do not dissolve in PFC liquids, they can be effectively delivered to the distal air spaces and pulmonary vasculature by drag when injected on inspiration.[47-49]

PERFLUOROCHEMICAL BREATHING TECHNIQUES

Several techniques have evolved for breathing PFC liquids. Most involve the use of preoxygenated, heated liquid that has a low carbon dioxide content. Because of the expense of these fluids and the amounts utilized, recycling of the fluid is optimized. This approach requires adequate scrubbing and reoxygenation of exhaled fluid. Initial liquid breathing studies used simple total body immersion or gravity-assisted ventilation in which a reservoir was suspended above and below the animal to facilitate inspiration and expiration via a gravity assist device. Although much was learned from these techniques, they proved inadequate for extended ventilation in which decreased work of breathing and fine control of driving pressures and lung volume were required.[21,50] A demand-regulated liquid ventilator was introduced in the early 1970s, which reduced work of breathing-associated problems and improved carbon dioxide removal.[22,23] Ventilation schemes were modified to mandatory ventilation in which time-cycled and pressure and/or volume limits were set.[40] This change allowed for improved ventilation, clinician-friendly ventilatory adjustments, recycling of PFCs, and close monitoring of many physiologic variables. This technology enables survival of severely preterm animals and facilitates detailed research

protocols that would otherwise be impossible to follow.[24,40,51] Investigators found that carefully controlled liquid ventilation, when utilized appropriately, can maintain cardiopulmonary stability in preterm animals for periods up to 30 hours.[29] Many studies have demonstrated the advantages of liquid ventilation from birth, compared with gas ventilation, in the prematurely delivered animal. Improved ventilation-perfusion matching, decreased surface tension, and pulmonary parenchymal distention improves the function of the liquid-ventilated preterm lung. This technique leads to lower driving pressures necessary to maintain adequate gas exchange and ultimately can diminish barotrauma. In addition to lower driving pressures, the loss in driving pressure from the airway to the alveolus is high during liquid ventilation, resulting in markedly lower peak alveolar pressures than in gas ventilation.[36]

Some of the liquid ventilation research has focused on simplifying techniques and interfacing with gas ventilation to facilitate clinical applicability. Although recovery from liquid to gas ventilation may require alterations in gas ventilatory schemes, cardiopulmonary stability during the transition and maintenance of pulmonary function improvements can be achieved.[27,29] Specifically, pulmonary resistance may be elevated when gas ventilatory recovery is initiated, because of the presence of residual PFC in the airway.[27] This material may necessitate slower respiratory rates and less end-distending pressure on gas ventilation to avoid overdistention of the lung. Although the removal of some PFCs is possible in switching to gas ventilation, a liquid functional residual capacity remains until evaporation occurs. The rate of disappearance of PFCs is dependent on the vapor pressure of the particular fluid, and the amount of residual liquid continues to influence ventilatory strategy as pulmonary mechanics change.

Although prophylactic liquid ventilation before the first gas breath in the fetus is superior to liquid rescue of the gas-ventilated animal, the latter condition is more probable in the clinical arena. When liquid ventilation is initiated in the gas-filled lung, there exists the potential for gas trapping between the liquid and the terminal air spaces. Liquid ventilation is established by instilling a functional residual capacity of oxygenated liquid before connecting to the liquid ventilator. The removal of residual gas is facilitated by manipulation and repositioning of the thorax, as well as diffusion of retained gas into the PFC. This transition can take several minutes, during which time gas exchange may not be optimal. Thus, liquid ventilation in the deteriorating animal on gas ventilation may take several minutes to facilitate marked improvement.

An alternative method of PFC utilization in the gas-filled lung is to deliver a functional residual capacity of PFCs and then continue with gas ventilation.[52] Preliminary studies suggest that this technique is well tolerated, is simple to implement, and maintains gas exchange at adequate levels in healthy animals. PFCs can then be instilled via the trachea periodically to maintain a desired amount of liquid in the lung and replace evaporative losses (Fig. 48-4). This technique may provide some

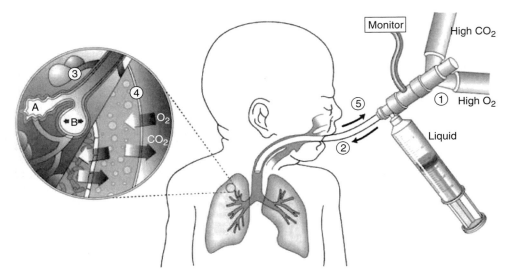

Figure 48–4. Large-scale image of the lung. **A,** collapsed alveolus prior to liquid filling. **B,** filled alveolus after liquid filling showing more effective gas diffusion. 1, gas ventilator; 2, filling process; 3, blow-up of lung; 4, gas exchange during partial liquid ventilation; 5, removal of CO_2. *(From Shaffer TH, Wolfson MR: Liquid ventilation. In Polin R, Fox WW [eds]: Fetal and Neonatal Physiology, vol 1, 2nd ed. Philadelphia, WB Saunders, 1998, p 1237.)*

of the benefits of liquid ventilation (lung recruitment, lower surface tension), without the complication of liquid ventilation (see Fig. 48-4).

Some of the aspects of liquid ventilation, however, may be lost (e.g., near elimination of surface tension, removal of debris, drug delivery). Furthermore, care must also be taken to alter the gas ventilatory strategy to compensate for liquid-related pulmonary function alterations.

In addition to the pursuit of liquid ventilation as a technique to replace or modify gas ventilation, PFC liquid ventilation may be utilized as a vehicle to rapidly correct a pulmonary abnormality, followed by a return to conventional ventilation. An example of this approach is the cleansing in meconium aspiration syndrome or drug delivery for pulmonary hypertension or pneumonia.[47-49,53] In this scenario, liquid ventilation could be used to maintain gas exchange, while effective cleansing or drug delivery directly to the pulmonary parenchyma and vasculature is applied. In addition, the even distribution of liquid, and subsequent lung recruitment and ventilation matching, could be used to condition the lung for uniform surfactant delivery in severe RDS.[54] In this regard, PFC ventilation could affect clinical recovery through brief ventilation schemes, followed by recovery to gas ventilation at lower levels of support.

CLINICAL APPLICATIONS IN THE NEONATE

There are numerous potential clinical applications of PFC liquid breathing. The potential primary respiratory and nonprimary clinical applications have expanded to include therapies in adults, children, and infants.

Liquid ventilation has been used to administer specific drugs such as antibiotics and chemotherapeutic agents directly into the pulmonary system. It has also been used to augment the inflammatory systems in animal models by targeting specific enzymes and hormones.[41] Radiographic regional heating, as well as hyperthermia and hypothermia, are other potential nonprimary respiratory applications.[29,53] In humans, and specifically infants,

the treatment of the injured lung is a judicious task. With the potential to apply PFC liquid breathing along with nitric oxide, the administration of surfactant, and high-frequency oscillatory ventilation (HFOV), the rates of morbidity and mortality in sick infants could be altered.[29,53] Currently, liquid ventilation techniques for the support of respiratory gas exchange in infants comprise PFC lavage, tidal liquid ventilation, and partial liquid ventilation (PLV). Non–gas exchange applications of PFC in the lung include gene products, as well as the pulmonary administration of pharmacologic agents and pulmonary imaging agents noted previously.[41] There is also exciting evidence that low-pressure PFC-induced mechanical distention without ventilation may accelerate lung growth without pathophysiologic consequences in infants. These approaches capitalize on the qualities of minimizing surface tension and maintaining gas exchange at lower driving and alveolar pressures, as well as the facilitation of drug delivery, cleansing, and lung conditioning.

Primary Respiratory Applications

Respiratory Distress Syndrome

Advances in pulmonary therapies have improved survival and outcome of preterm infants with RDS. Although the advent of mechanical ventilation has improved survival for many of these infants, pulmonary volutrauma and barotrauma with the subsequent development of bronchopulmonary dysplasia remain persistent iatrogenic complications.[55] Many therapies that attempt to decrease volutrauma and barotrauma have been explored. These approaches have focused on reducing the inflation pressures necessary to maintain gas exchange. Examples of such therapies include high-frequency ventilation, exogenous surfactant replacement, pulmonary function analysis to improve mechanical ventilation, and extracorporeal membrane oxygenation (ECMO). If the goal of ventilation strategy is to lower alveolar pressure through minimizing pulmonary and ventilatory support, then the most efficient means is through ventilation of the liquid-filled lung.[12]

As previously discussed, studies in preterm animals have demonstrated that liquid ventilation affords better gas exchange at lower inflation pressures than does gas ventilation. In a particular study of severely preterm lambs, prophylactic liquid ventilation supported acid-base status, cardiovascular stability, and gas exchange for up to 3 hours, in comparison with gas-ventilated lambs who, at equivalent gestation, had rapid and progressive deterioration in physiologic parameters and low survival rates within the same period of time (Fig. 48-5).[28]

Physiologic and histologic evaluation of these preterm animals demonstrated increased compliance and lower inflation and alveolar pressures, which preserved lung integrity during liquid ventilation.[56] On postmortem lung examination, the gas-exchanging regions of the gas-ventilated animals had areas of nonhomogeneity and atelectasis, were filled with hemorrhagic and proteinaceous debris, and had regions of septal disruption. In contrast, the liquid-ventilated lungs were homogeneously inflated and relatively free of debris and disruption.[56]

Liquid ventilation has been studied in several preterm neonates dying of RDS.[26,27] In contrast to the aforementioned controlled animal study, the human protocol required recovery to liquid ventilation in a gas-filled lung that had substantial preexisting barotrauma. In addition, only a short protocol (two 5-minute cycles interrupted by 15 minutes of gas ventilation) was performed with a less optimal lavage technique (Figs. 48-6 and 48-7). Despite these limitations, clinical stability was observed during the procedure, and improvements were seen in lung compliance and oxygenation, without compromise in cardiovascular function (Fig. 48-8). Expired gas samples after liquid ventilation and postmortem autopsy specimens were analyzed for PFCs by electron capture gas chromatography.[25] As in animal uptake studies, PFCs were transported across the lung epithelium and into the

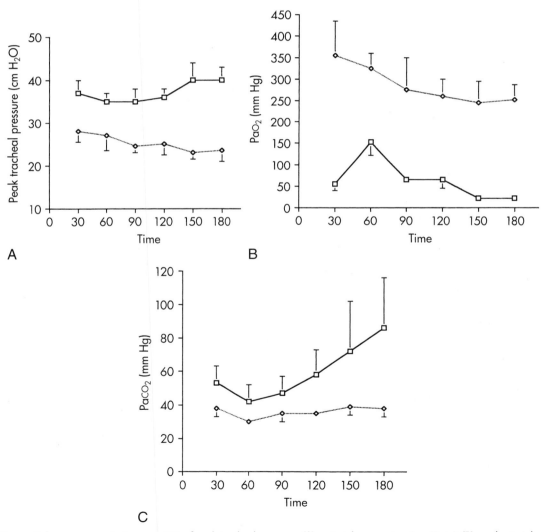

Figure 48–5. Sequential measurements (mean ± SE) of peak tracheal pressure **(A)**, arterial oxygen tension (PaO$_2$) **(B)**, and arterial carbon dioxide tension (PaCO$_2$) **(C)**, for gas *(open squares)* and liquid *(open diamonds)* in ventilated lambs as a function of time (minutes) after birth. *(From Wolfson MR, Greenspan JS, Deoras KS, et al: Comparison of gas and liquid ventilation: Clinical, physiological, and histological correlates. J Appl Physiol 72:1024, 1992.)*

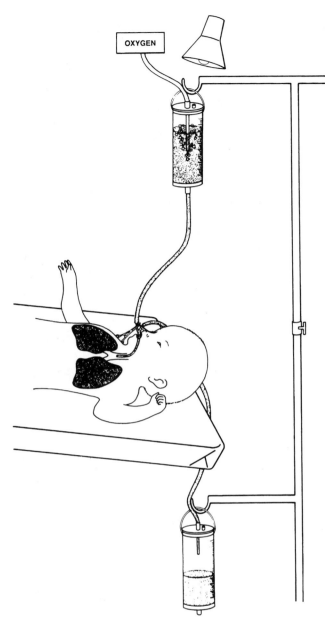

OXYGEN

Figure 48–6. Schematic of the lavage type of liquid ventilation system utilized in initial human protocols. Heated and oxygenated perfluorochemical is inspired and expired with gravity assistance. Driving pressures can be changed by altering height of reservoir. Breathing timing is altered manually, and liquid can be recycled.

blood in very small quantities; uptake was organ dependent. PFC saturation of the blood occurred 15 minutes after liquid ventilation was initiated. These studies demonstrated the feasibility and potential of liquid ventilation and gas ventilation in a liquid-filled lung in neonates with RDS.

The difficulty in liquid ventilatory rescue of infants with RDS is the necessity for long-term therapy, while the development of lung maturity, healing, and repair are awaited. Another possible application of liquid ventilation techniques in this population would be to "condition" the

lungs for effective surfactant therapy. In this approach, a brief period of liquid ventilation or filling the lungs with a functional residual capacity of PFCs could recruit lung units and increase lung volume. Subsequently, exogenous surfactant could be delivered to the liquid-filled, conditioned lungs during several tidal volumes of liquid ventilation. As with prophylactic administration of exogenous surfactant, delivery to liquid-filled lungs promotes even distribution and, probably, decreased surface tension in the gas-exchanging regions. After exogenous surfactant replacement therapy, the infant would then be weaned to gas ventilation. With improved physiologic and histologic parameters, the feasibility and potential that liquid ventilation affords are significant in neonates with RDS.

Aspiration Syndromes, Pulmonary Hypertension, and Pneumonia

In initial animal protocols on the liquid-filled lung in the 1920s, the capability of removing pulmonary debris was used as a primary therapeutic modality.[13] Liquid lavage techniques with oxygenated PFCs have been studied in several animal models, including a lamb protocol with human meconium aspiration.[53,57] In this study, meconium was observed in the expired liquid during liquid rescue, and pulmonary function improved with liquid ventilation. Improvements in lung function and gas exchange persisted during gas ventilatory recovery. In addition to the potential advantages of débridement, liquid ventilation in meconium aspiration could potentially recruit atelectatic regions of the lung, improving ventilation-perfusion matching. In animal studies of acute lung injury with pulmonary debris, recovery to liquid ventilation improved gas exchange, lung mechanics, and removed debris. Clinical improvement was sustained on subsequent gas ventilatory recovery, which improved survival in comparison to a control group.[29,58]

Nonprimary Respiratory Applications

Persistent Pulmonary Hypertension of the Newborn

Persistent pulmonary hypertension of the newborn (PPHN), a frequent complication of meconium aspiration syndrome and other aspiration syndromes, causes high morbidity and mortality rates among neonates. PPHN and other nonprimary respiratory diseases manifest with a host of pulmonary physiologic insufficiencies, and conventional treatment is often ineffective. HFOV and inhaled nitric oxide (iNO) are significant adjunctive therapies in the treatment of these critically ill neonates. Several of the problems that exist in these types of disease states are low pulmonary perfusion, intrapulmonary shunting, surfactant deficiency, and heterogenous lung inflation. In the presence of low pulmonary perfusion and intrapulmonary shunting, systematically delivered drugs may bypass the lung and be rendered ineffectual. Delivering exogenous surfactant or vasoactive drugs (such as iNO) directly to the gas-exchanging regions of the lung places them in direct contact with the pulmonary vasculature. However, aerosolized delivery is limited, in part, by the loss of drug in the tracheobronchial tree. Delivery during liquid ventilation, however, delivers the drug to the gas-exchanging regions and the pulmonary vasculature

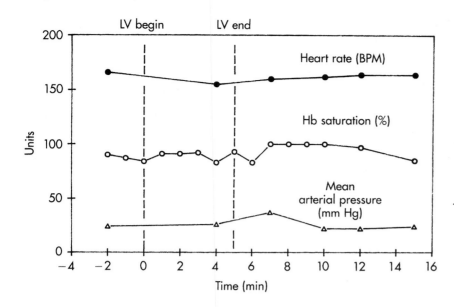

Figure 48–7. Changes in heart rate, oxyhemoglobin (Hb) saturation, and mean arterial pressure during one cycle of liquid ventilation in a human preterm neonate. BPM, beats per minute. *(From Greenspan JS, Wolfson MR, Rubenstein SD, et al: Liquid ventilation in human preterm neonates. J Pediatr 117:106, 1990.)*

despite intrapulmonary mismatching. The effectiveness of this application is attributable to the large surface area of the lung (35 times the body surface area), the thin diffusion barrier, and potential contact with the entire cardiac output. Pulmonary administration of drugs during inspiration of liquid has been shown to decrease pulmonary vascular resistance with relative sparing of systemic resistance. This result is magnified in the hypoxic model, which more closely mimics a neonate with pulmonary hypertension.[47,48] In PPHN, liquid ventilation with direct pulmonary administration of vasodilating drugs may

therefore improve ventilation-perfusion matching, reduce pulmonary hypertension, and help resolve the underlying or complicating disease. This scenario could potentially involve a brief liquid ventilatory protocol, with gas recovery of the liquid-"conditioned" lung.

As noted, different studies have shown that using liquid ventilation with iNO or vasodilating drugs in the acutely injured lung with PPHN, with and without meconium aspiration syndrome, improved gas exchange and lung mechanics.[59] The pathway of exogenous surfactant administration through partial liquid ventilation, in

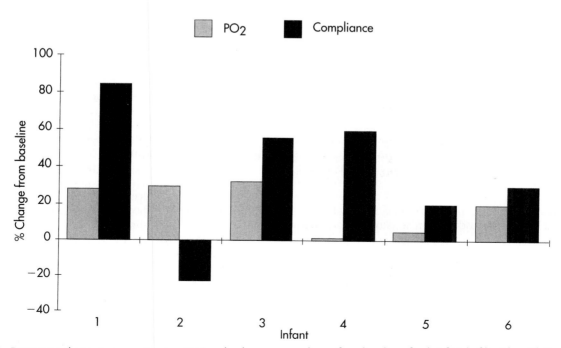

Figure 48–8. Percentage change in oxygen tension (PO_2) and pulmonary compliance from baseline after brief trial of liquid ventilation in six critically ill neonates.

comparison with conventional surfactant administration, is less clear but may improve oxygenation, respiratory system mechanics, and lung pathology. It has also been shown that using HFOV with liquid ventilation may improve gas exchange and stabilize pulmonary and systemic hemodynamics, in comparison with high-frequency gas ventilation in full-term and preterm animals.[16,60] Therapies such as HFOV, iNO, and exogenous surfactant are standard for battling severe lung disease. A number of studies have combined these therapeutic modalities and have shown the potential for improved lung protection and function, but there is a need for more investigation.

Drug Delivery

Like protocols exploring the pulmonary administration of vasoactive drugs, delivery of other biologically active substances has been explored.[16,47,59] As previously mentioned, effective delivery of exogenous surfactant and chemotherapeutic agents can be achieved with liquid ventilation. Antibiotics can also be effectively administered with liquid ventilation and achieve similar blood levels with better lung tissue levels in comparison with intravenous delivery.[49] Various studies have also looked at the potential delivering of adenovirus as a vector for gene therapy as well as anesthetic agents through a liquid medium.[59] Specific treatments tailored for pulmonary disease therefore can be designed, with liquid ventilation serving as the vehicle (see Figs. 48-7 and 48-8).

Imaging and Temperature Control

As mentioned previously, PFCs that are used for breathing applications are amenable to magnetic resonance, plain film, and ultrasound imaging.[61,62] These techniques can be used to obtain very detailed images of the airways and parenchyma, even with small amounts of PFC fluid.[29,63] The presence of bromine atoms in the PFC (perflubron) confers greater radiopacity to the fluid, allowing for this radiographic detailed evaluation. In the PFC-filled lung, computed tomography and conventional radiography could be used to qualitatively and quantitatively evaluate lung volume recruitment in various lung disease states, including congenital diaphragmatic hernia and pulmonary hypoplasia.[55,64,65] Perfluorocarbon liquids do not contain hydrogen atoms; when used with nuclear magnetic resonance imaging, the PFC-filled body cavity appears dark because no imaging signal is produced, allowing for evaluation of various tissues. When oxygen is dissolved in the PFC liquid, this affects the nuclear magnetic resonance signal, permitting monitoring of regional differences in gas exchange and oxygen tension. In addition, because of the very high heat capacity of PFC liquids, very effective heating and cooling can be achieved by altering the temperature of the liquid breathed. Liquid ventilation can be a potent modality to alter or maintain body temperature within a desired range.

Anti-inflammatory Effect

There have been several in vivo studies that examined the acute lung injury model and concluded that liquid ventilation has an anti-inflammatory effect. It has been shown that liquid ventilation reduced pulmonary permeability, edema, neutrophil infiltration, and alveolar hemorrhage. This anti-inflammatory effect may result from the removal of pulmonary debris with improved oxygenation to the tissues. Studies have also shown that the PFC liquid itself may have a direct anti-inflammatory effect. Because inflammation plays such a strong role in the development of chronic lung disease, the anti-inflammatory effect afforded by PFC liquid could help inhibit the development of chronic lung disease.

CLINICAL TRIALS—PAST AND FUTURE

In the initial clinical study, Greenspan and associates enrolled premature human infants who were near death at the time of treatment.[27] They used a gravity-assisted approach and gave tidal volumes of liquid in brief cycles. The infants tolerated the procedure, showed improvement in several physiologic parameters, including lung compliance and gas exchange, and maintained some improvement after discontinuation of liquid ventilation. This study used a form of tidal liquid ventilation but also reported a sustained benefit of gas ventilation with the residual PFC liquid-filled lungs. In subsequent clinical protocols, investigators have used the PLV approach (see Fig. 48-4).

There have been several completed human studies of PLV with the PFC perflubron. Leach and colleagues reported on 13 premature infants with severe RDS in whom conventional treatment had failed.[66] This was not a randomized or blinded study. They treated the infants with PLV for up to 96 hours. The infants' lungs were filled with perflubron, and supplemental doses were given frequently: in general, hourly. The arterial oxygen tension and dynamic compliance significantly increased, and the oxygenation index was reduced within 1 hour of initiation of PLV. The authors of this study showed clinical improvement and survival in some infants who were not predicted to survive.

Pranikoff and coworkers reported their results for four patients with congenital diaphragmatic hernia who were managed on ECMO.[67] In a phase I/II trial, PLV was performed with daily dosing for up to 6 days. The authors concluded that this was a safe technique and that it was possibly associated with improvement in gas exchange and pulmonary compliance.

Greenspan and associates presented results on six full-term infants with respiratory failure who showed no improvement while receiving ECMO.[68] The infants were treated with PLV and perflubron for up to 96 hours, with hourly dosing. Dynamic pulmonary compliance significantly increased, and lung volume was recruited. The authors concluded that the technique appeared to be safe and improved lung function in these critically ill full-term infants.

The initial human clinical trial studies of PLV in neonates are encouraging and suggest the viability of this technique in the neonate with severe RDS and acute respiratory distress syndrome (ARDS). It has been observed and reported that the underlying pathophysiologic process influences the effect of liquid ventilation.

The response of the sick full-term infant to PLV is frequently more gradual than is typically observed in the preterm infant with RDS. The preterm infant often experiences improvement in lung compliance and gas exchange within hours of PLV initiation, probably because of reduction in surface tension and volume recruitment. Debris removal, which takes time, is often required in the full-term infant on PLV to improve lung function.

Three studies have evaluated PLV in children. None of the studies used a control group. Hirschl and associates treated seven pediatric patients with ARDS requiring ECMO.[69] They found improvement in gas exchange and pulmonary compliance during PLV for 1 to 7 days. Gauger and colleagues reported on six pediatric patients with ARDS who required extracorporeal life support.[70] The authors treated the patients with perflubron PLV for 3 to 7 days, with daily dosing. They observed some improvement in gas exchange and pulmonary compliance over the 96 hours from the initial dose, and all patients survived. Toro-Figueroa and coworkers presented their results on 10 children up to 17 years of age with ARDS who were treated with PLV for up to 96 hours.[60] Nine of 10 patients tolerated initial dosing, and all nine experienced improvement in gas exchange over the 48-hour treatment period. Lung function did not improve in these patients. The authors concluded that PLV may be safe and efficacious in the treatment of pediatric ARDS.

The initial phase I/II trials demonstrated the potential safety and efficacy of PLV, particularly in younger populations of sick patients. An understanding of the utility of this technique awaits the results of phase III trials. The complications and economics associated with drug approval have limited the pivotal trials to adults. At present, a large, randomized PLV trial (phase III) in adults with ARDS treated with perflubron has been completed in North America and Europe. Several liquid ventilation trials in infants and children are currently under design in Europe.

Although these studies are highly encouraging, there are still many questions about this technology that remain unanswered. Short-term improvement in clinical status in terminally ill neonates has been observed, but the long-term benefits and complications of liquid ventilation in humans (e.g., leaks, gastrointestinal filling, maintenance of a liquid functional residual capacity) have yet to be determined.

Many different PFCs exist, each with specific characteristics. These chemicals need additional evaluation and testing. The properties that make one PFC superior to others for liquid breathing are not fully understood and may differ with different species and disease processes. Most PFCs have similar oxygen-carrying capacity, whereas boiling point, density, viscosity, vapor pressure, and surface tension may vary (see Table 48-1). A high density and viscosity may alter breathing strategies in some infants, particularly when small endotracheal tube sizes are used, because of a requirement for increased driving pressures.[71] The vapor pressure determines, in part, how quickly the PFC dissipates upon gas ventilation recovery. In addition, the surface tension may alter pulmonary function upon gas recovery. Finally, unique characteristics of some of the PFCs may alter their behavior during application in ways that are not fully understood.[72] Although these issues may ultimately result in fluids "designed" for different applications, initial trials will utilize the medical-grade PFCs that have government, institutional, and scientific approval.

Future therapeutic trials will test different fluids with various delivery schemes in patients with specific diseases. Delivery systems proposed include the administration of a functional residual capacity of PFC, followed by conventional gas ventilation, liquid lavage techniques, and gravity or roller pump–driven liquid ventilators. Although roller pump–driven ventilators appear to be the most efficacious for a wide variety of disease states in animals, they are more cumbersome, expensive, and difficult to operate. Finally, timing of the therapy may dramatically affect efficacy. Terminal lung disease with severe acidosis, gas leak, and minimal pulmonary blood flow responds less optimally to liquid ventilation. In contrast, prophylactic liquid ventilation before the first breath, or soon after a pulmonary insult, could prove most efficacious. Ethical considerations will be at the forefront in determining a target population for initial human trials.

In addition to the aforementioned schemes, the future of liquid ventilation technology will probably include delivery systems that have yet to be fully developed in the animal research arena. These systems include aerosolized PFC delivery, high-frequency oscillatory assist of tidal liquid ventilation, and the addition of other dissolved gases or drugs to the PFCs to facilitate activity. Although much debate exists on how the next phase will be conducted, many trials are needed to define the potential therapeutic indications for PFC ventilation.

Liquid ventilation technology has the potential to affect the clinical management of pulmonary pathophysiologic processes, including premature lung disease, aspiration syndromes, pneumonia, ARDS, and pulmonary hypoplasia. Documentation of efficacy in human disease is still required, even though laboratory studies have been impressive. To date, more than 700 patients have been enrolled in liquid ventilation studies with perflubron. The studies, unfortunately, have been limited to the adult population. Once safety and efficacy are proven in adults, it is hoped that drug approval and subsequent reinitiation of controlled studies in infants and children will be forthcoming.

REFERENCES

1. Alcorn D, Adamson TM, Lambert TF, et al: Morphological effects of chronic bilateral phrenectomy or vagotomy in the fetal lamb lung. J Anat 130:683, 1980.
2. Alcorn D: Morphological effects of chronic tracheal ligation and drainage in the fetal lamb lung. J Anat 123:649, 1977.
3. Avery ME, Mead J: Surface properties in relation to atelectasis and hyaline membrane disease. Am J Dis Child 97:517, 1959.
4. Boyden EA: The programming of canalization in fetal lungs of man and monkey. Am J Anat 145:125, 1976.
5. Carmel JA, Friedman F, Adams FH: Fetal tracheal ligation and lung development. Am J Dis Child 109:452, 1965.

6. Mansell AL, Rojas JV, Sillos EM, et al: Diaphragmatic activity is a determinant of postnatal lung growth. J Appl Physiol 61:1098, 1986.

7. Modell JH, Gollan F, Giammona ST, et al: Effect of fluorocarbon liquid on surface tension properties of pulmonary surfactant. Chest 57:263, 1970.

8. Abbasi S, Bhutani VK: Pulmonary mechanics and energetics of normal, non-ventilated low birthweight infants. Pediatr Pulmonol 8:89, 1990.

9. Goodstein MH, Greenspan JS, Friss HE, et al: Extrauterine pulmonary development in the healthy preterm infant: Hidden morbidity at discharge. Pediatr Res 31:248A, 1992.

10. Clements JA: Surface tension on lung extracts. Proc Soc Exp Biol Med 10:170, 1957.

11. Mead J, Whittenberger JL, Radford EP: Surface tension as a factor in pulmonary volume-pressure hysteresis. J Appl Physiol 10:191, 1957.

12. von Neergard K: Neue Auffassungen über einer Grundbegriff der Atemmechanik. Die Retraktionskragt der Lunge, abhangig von der Oberflachenspannung in den Alveolen. Z Gesamte Exp Med 66:373, 1929.

13. Winternitz MC, Smith GH: Preliminary studies in intratracheal therapy. In Winternitz MC (ed): Collected Studies on the Pathology of War Gas Poisoning. New Haven, Conn, Yale University Press, 1920.

14. Kylstra JA, Paganelli CV, Lanphier EH: Pulmonary gas exchange in dogs ventilated with hyperbarically oxygenated liquid. J Appl Physiol 1:177, 1962.

15. Saga S, Modell JH, Calderwood HW, et al: Pulmonary function after ventilation with fluorocarbon liquid P12-f (Caroxin-F). J Appl Physiol 34:160, 1973.

16. Shaffer TH, Wolfson MR, Clark LC: State of art review: Liquid ventilation. Pediatr Pulmonol 14:102, 1992.

17. Shaffer TH, Wolfson MR, Greenspan JS, et al: Animal models and clinical studies of liquid ventilation in neonatal respiratory distress syndrome. In Robertson B (ed): Surfactant in Clinical Practice. Chur, Switzerland, Harwood Academic, 1992, pp 187-198.

18. Shaffer TH: A brief review: Liquid ventilation. Undersea Biomed Res 14:169, 1987.

19. Clark LC: Introduction. Fed Proc 29:1698, 1970.

20. Sargent JW, Seffl RJ: Properties of perfluorinated liquid. Fed Proc 29:1699, 1970.

21. Clark LC, Gollan F: Survival of mammals breathing organic liquids equilibrated with oxygen at atmosphere pressure. Science 152:1755, 1966.

22. Moskowitz GD: A mechanical respirator for control of liquid breathing. Fed Proc 29:1751, 1970.

23. Moskowitz GD, Shaffer TH, Dubin SE: Liquid breathing trials and animal studies with a demand-regulated liquid breathing system. Med Instrum 9:28, 1973.

24. Koen PA, Wolfson MR, Shaffer TH: Fluorocarbon ventilation: Maximal expiratory flows and CO_2 elimination. Pediatr Res 24: 291, 1988.

25. Wolfson MR, Tran N, Bhutani VK, et al: A new experimental approach for the study of cardiopulmonary physiology during early development. J Appl Physiol 65:1436, 1988.

26. Greenspan JS, Wolfson MR, Rubenstein SD, et al: Liquid ventilation in preterm babies. Lancet 1:1095, 1989.

27. Greenspan JS, Wolfson MR, Rubenstein SD, et al: Liquid ventilation in human preterm neonates. J Pediatr 117:106, 1990.

28. Wolfson MR, Greenspan JS, Deoras KS, et al: Comparison of gas and liquid ventilation: Clinical, physiological, and histological correlates. J Appl Physiol 72:1024, 1992.

29. Shaffer TH, Greenspan JS, Wolfson MR: Liquid ventilation. In Boynton BR (ed): New Therapies for Neonatal Respiratory Failure: A Physiologic Approach. New York, Cambridge University Press, 1994, pp 279-301.

30. Rufer R, Spizer HL: Liquid ventilation in the respiratory distress syndrome. Chest 66:298, 1974.

31. Gil J, Bachofen H, Gehr P, et al: Alveolar volume–surface area relation in air and liquid filled lungs fixed by vascular perfusion. J Appl Physiol 47:990, 1979.

32. West JB, Dollery CT, Matthews CME, et al: Distribution of blood and ventilation in the saline-filled lung. J Appl Physiol 20:1107, 1965.

33. Harris DG, Coggin RR, Roby J, et al: Liquid ventilation in dogs: An apparatus for normobaric and hyperbaric studies. J Appl Physiol 54:1141, 1983.

34. Lowe CA, Sivieri EM, Tuma RF, et al: Liquid ventilation: Cardiovascular adjustments with secondary hyperlactatemia and acidosis. J Appl Physiol 47:1051, 1979.

35. Matthews WH, Balzer RH, Shelburne JD, et al: Steady-state gas exchange in normothermic, anesthetized, liquid-ventilated dogs. Undersea Biomed Res 5:341, 1978.

36. Curtis SE, Fuhrman BP, Howland BF: Airway and alveolar pressures during perfluorocarbon breathing in infant lambs. J Appl Physiol 68:2322, 1990.

37. Lowe CA, Shaffer TH: Pulmonary vascular resistance in the fluorocarbon-filled lung. J Appl Physiol 60:154, 1986.

38. Curtis SE, Fuhrman BP, Howland BF, et al: Cardiac output during liquid (perfluorocarbon) breathing in newborn piglets. Crit Care Med 19:225, 1991.

39. Truog WE, Jackson JC: Alternative modes of ventilation in the prevention and treatment of bronchopulmonary dysplasia. Clin Perinatol 19:621, 1992.

40. Wolfson MR, Shaffer TH: Liquid ventilation during early development: Theory, physiologic processes and application. J Dev Physiol 13:1, 1990.

41. Shaffer, TH, Wolfson, MR: Liquid ventilation. In Polin R, Fox WW, Abman S (eds): Fetal and Neonatal Physiology, 3rd ed. Philadelphia, WB Saunders, 2003, pp 985-1001.

42. Forman D, Bhutani VK, Hilfer SR, et al: A fine structure study of the liquid-ventilated newborn rabbit. Fed Proc 43:647, 1984.

43. Salman NH, Fuhrman BP, Papo ML, et al: Oxygenation and lung mechanics during 24 hour trials of perfluorocarbon associated gas exchange (PAGE) in piglets. Pediatr Res 33:40A, 1993.

44. Clark LC, Hoffmann RE, Davis SL: Response of the rabbit lung as a criterion of safety for fluorocarbon breathing and blood substitutes. In Chang MS, Riess RM, Winslow RM (eds): Biomaterials, Artificial Cells, and Immobilization Biotechnology. Marcel Dekker, New York, 1994, p 292.

45. Holaday DA, Fiserova-Bergerova V, Modell JH, et al: Uptake, distribution and excretion of fluorocarbon FX-80 (perfluorbertyl perfluorotetrahydrafuron) during liquid breathing in the dog. Anesthesiology 37:387, 1972.

46. Modell JH, Calderwood HW, Ruiz BC, et al: Liquid ventilation of primates. Chest 69:79, 1976.

47. Wolfson MR, Greenspan JS, Shaffer TH: Pulmonary administration of vasoactive drugs (PAD) by perfluorocarbon liquid ventilation. Pediatrics 97:449, 1996.

48. Wolfson MR, Shaffer TH: Pulmonary administration of drugs (PAD): A new approach for drug delivery using liquid ventilation. FASEB J 4:A1105, 1990.

49. Zelinka MA, Wolfson MR, Calligar S, et al: Direct administration of gentamicin during liquid ventilation of the lamb: Comparison of lung and serum levels to IV administration. Pediatr Res 29:290A, 1991.

50. Modell JH, Calderwood HW, Ruiz BC: Long term survival of dogs after breathing oxygenated fluorocarbon liquid. Fed Proc 29:1731, 1970.

51. Wolfson MR, Durrant JD, Tran NN, et al: The effect of age and oxygenation on the brainstem auditory evoked potential in the immature lamb. In Jones CT (ed): Fetal and Neonatal Development. Ithaca, New York, Perinatology Press, 1988, pp 229-234.

52. Fuhrman BP, Paczan PR, De Francisis M: Perfluorocarbon-associated gas exchange. Crit Care Med 19:712, 1991.

53. Shaffer TH, Lowe CA, Bhutani VK, et al: Liquid ventilation: Effects on pulmonary function in meconium-stained lambs. Pediatr Res 19:49, 1984.

54. Valls-Soler A, Wolfson MR, Kechner N, et al: Comparison of natural surfactant and brief liquid ventilation rescue treatment in very immature lambs. Pediatr Res 33:347A, 1993.

55. O'Brodovich HM, Mellins RB: Bronchopulmonary dysplasia: State of the art. Am Rev Respir Dis 132:684, 1985.

56. Deoras KS, Coppola D, Wolfson MR, et al: Liquid ventilation in neonates: Tissue histology and morphometry. Pediatr Res 27:29A, 1990.

57. Shaffer TH, Douglas PR, Lowe CA, et al: Liquid ventilation: Improved gas exchange and lung compliance in preterm lambs. Pediatr Res 17:303, 1983.

58. Richman PS, Wolfson MR, Shaffer TH, et al: Lung lavage with oxygenated fluorocarbon improves gas exchange and lung compliance in cats with acute lung injury. Crit Care Med 21:768, 1993.

59. Wolfson MR, Greenspan JS, Shaffer, TH: Liquid-assisted ventilation: An alternative respiratory modality. Pediatr Pulmonol 26:42, 1998.

60. Toro-Figueroa LO, Meliones JN, Curtis SE, et al: Perflubron partial liquid ventilation (PLV) in children with ARDS: A safety and efficacy pilot study. Crit Care Med 24:150A, 1996.

61. Clark LC, Ackerman JL, Thomas SR, et al: Perfluorinated organic liquids and emulsions as biocompatible NMR imaging agents for 19F and dissolved oxygen. Adv Exp Med Biol 180:835, 1984.

62. Sekins KM, Keilman GW, Shaffer TH, et al: Acoustic and physical properties of PFC liquids pertinent to ultrasound lung hyperthermia. Paper presented at the Tenth Annual North American Hyperthermia Group, Radiation Research Society, April 1990, New Orleans, La.

63. Thomas SR, Clark LC, Ackerman JL, et al: MR imaging of the lung using liquid perfluorocarbon. J Comput Assist Tomogr 10:1, 1986.

64. Sass DJ, Ritman EL, Caskey PE, et al: Liquid breathing: Prevention of pulmonary arterio-venous shunting during acceleration. J Appl Physiol 32:451, 1972.

65. Schwieler GH, Robertson B: Liquid ventilation in immature newborn rabbits. Biol Neonate 29:343, 1976.

66. Leach, CL, Greenspan, JS, Rubenstein, SD, et al: Partial liquid ventilation with perflubron in premature infants with severe respiratory distress syndrome. The LiquiVent Study Group. N Engl J Med 335:761, 1996.

67. Pranikoff T, Gauger PG, Hrischl RB: Partial liquid ventilation in newborn patients with congenital diaphragmatic hernia. J Pediatr Surg 31:613, 1996.

68. Greenspan JS, Fox WW, Rubenstein SD, et al: Partial liquid ventilation in critically ill infants receiving extracorporeal life support. Philadelphia Liquid Ventilation Consortium. Pediatrics 99:e2, 1997. Available at: *http://www.pediatrics.org/cgi/content/full/99/1/e2* (accessed April 16, 2004).

69. Hirschl RB, Pranikoff T, Gauger P, et al: Liquid ventilation in adults, children, and full-term neonates. Lancet 346:1201, 1995.

70. Gauger, PG, Pranikoff, T, Schreiner, RJ, et al: Initial experience with partial liquid ventilation in pediatric patients with acute respiratory distress syndrome. Crit Care Med 24:16, 1996.

71. Fox WW, Cox C, Weis C, et al: Liquid ventilation in lambs with perfluorchemical (PFC) fluids: Physical properties and pulmonary resistance. Pediatr Res 33:211A, 1993.

72. Goodin TH, Kaufman RJ, Richard TJ: Comparative pulmonary toxicity of three perfluorchemicals (PFCs) in the rat and baboon. Paper presented at the Proceedings of the Fifth International Symposium on Blood Substitutes, 1993, San Diego, Calif.

Air Leak Syndromes

C. Michael Cotten and Ronald N. Goldberg

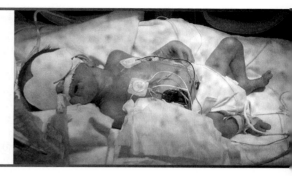

The air leak syndrome is a family of disorders that includes pneumothorax, pulmonary interstitial emphysema, pneumomediastinum, pneumopericardium, and pneumoperitoneum. Any of these can be a cause of sudden deterioration and cardiovascular collapse in neonates, particularly those with respiratory distress who are receiving mechanical ventilation. Failure to recognize the signs of air leak and initiate appropriate treatment may lead to death or to complications and long-term morbidity. Innovations such as antenatal steroids, surfactant replacement therapy, and techniques and technology of ventilation have helped reduce the incidence but have not eliminated air leak syndrome or significantly reduced its effects. We describe the epidemiology, pathophysiology, and clinical manifestation of the disorders and discuss strategies for treatment and prevention.

INCIDENCE/EPIDEMIOLOGY

Pneumothorax is the most frequent manifestation of air leak syndrome in the neonatal period. It can occur in otherwise healthy full-term infants as well as in sick full-term infants and preterm infants with respiratory distress syndrome. Spontaneous pneumothoraces may occur in full-term infants who remain essentially asymptomatic. The incidence has been described to range between 0.5% and 2.0%.[1,2] Of infants with renal anomalies, 19% have been found to have pneumothoraces.[3] The most likely cause for pneumothoraces in these otherwise healthy full-term infants is the high transpulmonary ($P_{alveolar} - P_{pleural}$) pressure generated at the onset of breathing.

In preterm infants with respiratory distress syndrome during the presurfactant era, the range of pneumothorax incidence was 11% to 33%. Contralateral pneumothorax developed in 44% of patients and was overwhelmingly associated with pulmonary interstitial emphysema.[4] The incidence of pulmonary interstitial emphysema in infants with birth weights between 500 and 999 g was 35%; the rate of survival with air leaks was only 30%.[5] Although the

incidence of significant air leaks has declined with surfactant and other advances in neonatal intensive care, the rate of coincident mortality remains high.[6]

More recently, in trials comparing various surfactants and surfactant protocols in infants born between 24 and 32 weeks of gestation, the rate of pneumothoraces ranged between 3.7% and 10%.[7-9] In a study of surfactant timing in infants delivered at 24 to $28^{6}/_{7}$ weeks of gestation, the incidence of pulmonary interstitial emphysema was 6% for the preventilatory surfactant group and up to 10% for patients receiving "prophylactic" surfactant, after resuscitation, at 10 minutes after birth.[8] A 10% to 14% incidence of pulmonary interstitial emphysema was seen in a trial comparing two types of bovine surfactant in 605 infants weighing less than 2000 g with established respiratory distress syndrome.[9]

Among full-term infants with meconium aspiration, the incidence of pneumothorax is between 20% and 50%.[10] In several studies of surfactant use for meconium aspiration, results suggest a trend toward reduction in incidence. Of 20 infants who received surfactant, none had air leaks, in comparison with 5 of 20 who did not receive surfactant.[11]

Pneumomediastinum and pneumopericardium are much less common than pneumothoraces and pulmonary interstitial emphysema. Morrow and associates reported the incidence of pneumomediastinum to be 0.25% in 10,000 live births.[12] Pneumopericardium is extremely rare in a nonintubated patient. In intubated patients, the incidence has been reported at 1.3 to 2%.[13-15] In the surfactant era, the rate may be less.

ETIOLOGY/PATHOGENESIS

For all infants, full-term and preterm, transition from fetal to neonatal life produces a physiologic situation that increases the risk of air leak. Fluid must be absorbed from alveoli, surfactant must be adequately distributed and must function properly, and proper inspiratory effort must be generated to overcome the viscosity of residual pulmonary fluid, surface tension, and rigidity of lung parenchyma.[16]

Any obstruction of the airways can lead to gas trapping, delaying emptying, and overdistention of the alveoli and terminal bronchi distal to obstructions. Terminal airways or alveoli may rupture. Trauma may also contribute to significant air leaks in infants. The correlation of suctioning with pneumothorax has been reported in several case series.[17,18]

Structural differences, as well as inadequate surfactant, put preterm infants at greater risk for air leaks in comparison with full-term infants. Macklin demonstrated the presence of alveolar pores, or pores of Kohn, which increase in size and number with increasing gestational age.[19] These pores allow air to redistribute between ventilated and nonventilated lung units. The lack of connections in preterm infants' lungs may exacerbate the asymmetry of ventilation.[20] Conditions such as meconium aspiration or pneumonia, in which there is nonhomogenous ventilation, also reveal limitations in the connectiveness of airways. With surfactant treatment, the deficiency of alveolar connections may be made apparent by air leaks occurring after surfactant treatment and subsequent overinflation of the lung when ventilator settings are not adjusted to the improving compliance of the infant's lungs. This change can allow excessive volume to enter an isolated lung unit. Ventilator practices that do not allow adequate expiratory time may also lead to air trapping and air leak for multiple lung units.

Macklin and Macklin demonstrated in animals that increased intrapleural air pressure could rupture overdistended alveoli. Air would dissect along the perivascular or interstitial spaces, resulting in pulmonary interstitial emphysema. The air could then track into the mediastinum, causing pneumomediastinum. Pneumothorax could result if the air formed bullae at the hilus, where visceral and parietal pleura join, and the bullae ruptured.[21] If the air traveled along intravascular sheaths and interlobular septa to the lung surface, pleural blebs resulted.[22]

Partitional alveoli, those attached on all sides to other alveoli, expand equally in all directions with inhalation (if they all share the same surface properties). Air leaks may develop from the overdistention of marginal alveoli, which are alveoli connected to rigid structures such as pleura, blood vessels, or bronchi; therefore, the distending force is displaced unequally. The connective tissue attaching these alveoli to the underlying structure ruptures, allowing air to enter the connective tissue around the adjacent airway, vessel, or pleura.[23-25]

The source of air leak in infants with respiratory distress syndrome may be the terminal bronchiole rather than the alveolus. Ackerman and colleagues used a preterm baboon model to show that airway compliance is normal but alveolar compliance is low. The noncartilaginous airway's volume then increases with increased pressure, whereas the alveolar volume does not change. The airway, lacking elastic properties, may rupture, and interstitial emphysema may develop.[26]

The precursor to many air leaks is mechanical ventilation and the delivery of too much volume to a restricted space. As most ventilators for infants of very low birth weight are pressure- rather than volume-limited, the volume delivered depends largely on the distensibility of the airway and alveoli when the pressure is applied.

Increasing pressure may exceed the capacitance of one lung area but barely deliver any volume to less compliant areas. In an experiment in which 10-cm H_2O gradations of pressure were made, starting at 40 cm H_2O, investigators noted first pulmonary interstitial emphysema, then pneumothorax, followed by pneumomediastinum and pneumopericardium. Air embolism developed in one third of subjects at pressures greater than 70 cm H_2O.[27]

Air that enters the mediastinum can track downward through postesophageal and periesophageal tissue. If it reaches retroperitoneal tissue, it could rupture, causing pneumoperitoneum.[28] Other work suggests that retroperitoneal air could dissect along capillary venous beds, causing pneumoperitoneum or air emboli of the mesenteric beds of the bowel.[29]

Pneumopericardium may be the result of air under pressure entering the pericardial space from the mediastinum via a defect in the pericardium.[30] Interstitial air could then track along the great vessels via the pericardial reflections of the visceral pericardium.[31]

PHYSIOLOGIC RESPONSE/CLINICAL PRESENTATION

With a large pneumothorax, both lungs lose volume, one compressed by air and the other by mediastinal shift, and venous return is quite low; hypoxia and hypercapnia result. Hypertension may sometimes precede a pneumothorax, possibly caused by the effects of hypoxemia and catecholamine release that frequently accompany pneumothorax, or it may occur reflexively.[32,33] Also, decreased cardiac output with increased intrathoracic pressure may cause carotid sinus and aortic arch baroreceptor activation and systemic vasoconstriction with accompanying blood pressure elevations.[34,35] Hypertension could also be a response to the increased intracranial blood pressure noted after a pneumothorax.[36] Once the pneumothorax increases to such a size as to limit venous return, decreased cardiac output leads to hypotension.[37,38]

The cerebral vascular effects of pneumothoraces are possible contributors to the cause of intraventricular hemorrhage.[39] Cerebral blood flow in preterm infants is poorly autoregulated.[40] Cerebral artery blood flow velocity in neonates who developed pneumothorax is quite high, especially during diastole. Mean systemic diastolic pressure simultaneously increases. This blood pressure similarity suggests a correlation between increased cerebral blood flow during a pneumothorax. The increased cerebral blood flow could produce an intraventricular hemorrhage.[41] In animals, the removal of intrapleural air is related to increased blood flow velocity as well, probably caused by an increased venous return and cardiac output.[42]

Rapid diagnosis is essential, particularly for small preterm infants. Radiographic evidence is confirmatory, but delay is inherent. Other diagnostic tools have been useful in timely diagnosis of pneumothorax. Fiberoptic transillumination, which demonstrates extensive "lighting up" of the affected side in comparison with the unaffected side, has been shown to be quite useful as a readily available bedside tool for diagnosis while radiography is awaited. In one series, there was a 4% false-positive rate, or minimal pneumomediastinum; therefore, the investigators

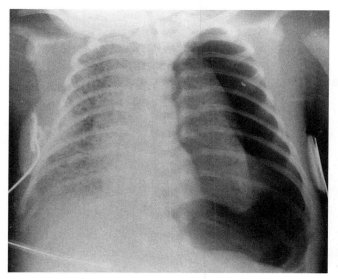

Figure 49–1. Left tension pneumothorax. Large left pneumothorax causing inversion of left diaphragm and mediastinal shift to the right. Interstitial emphysema is noted in the central portion of the right lung as well as the periphery of the left.

recommended confirmatory radiography.[43] More significant air leak, with acute clinical deterioration, should be treated expeditiously.[43] In addition to transillumination, other developments in measuring transcutaneous CO_2 and monitoring trends may provide even earlier diagnosis of significant air leak.[44]

If a radiograph is obtained, a pneumothorax may be difficult to diagnose from anteroposterior views and impossible if the film is rotated. If a large pneumothorax is present, the visceral pleura are seen, and if it is a tension pneumothorax, volume loss is noted bilaterally, because one lung is compressed medially by air and the other lung by the shift of the mediastinum (Fig. 49-1).

If the air leak is small to moderate in size, this sign may not be present. The more subtle signs may include (1) hyperlucent hemithorax, (2) paramediastinal hyperlucency (medial pneumothorax, which can be diagnosed by a change in position), (3) crescentic subpulmonic hyperlucency, and (4) enhanced sharpness of mediastinal borders (Figs. 49-2 to 49-5).

With pulmonary interstitial emphysema, air can enter the lymphatic system[45] and the pulmonary vessels.[38] The resulting occlusion of lymphatic flow may cause pulmonary edema, and limited blood flow results in ventilation-perfusion mismatch and possibly pulmonary hypertension and air embolism.[46,47] The combination of pulmonary edema and ventilation-perfusion mismatch results in hypercarbia and hypoxia. Interstitial emphysema may also encircle the airways and, with expansion of interstitial air, result in further air trapping and increased resistance to airflow to the alveoli.

On chest radiographs, pulmonary interstitial emphysema most commonly appears as small rounded or curvilinear lucencies within the lung parenchyma, either focal or diffuse (Fig. 49-6). These collections can vary in size within the same lobe. Coalescent interstitial emphysema (cystic pneumatocele) may even attain the size of the involved lobe (Fig. 49-7). Interstitial emphysema may persist for weeks and, if under tension, may compromise the contralateral lung (Fig. 49-8).

As described previously, a pneumomediastinum can lead to other air leak complications, but its potential clinical significance is reduced by the easily disrupted mediastinal pleura and the ability of air to dissect up into the neck (causing subcutaneous emphysema), out into the visceral pleura, or down into the peritoneum. Anterior pneumomediastinum can be unilateral or bilateral, elevating one or both lobes of the thymus, as well as causing the heart to appear rimmed with paracardiac hyperlucency (Fig. 49-9). Posterior pneumomediastinum resembles a hugely dilated air-filled esophagus seen through

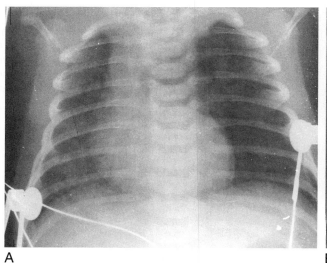

A

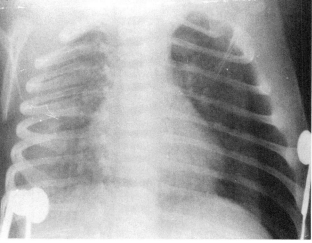

B

Figure 49–2. Left pneumothorax. **A,** Supine view demonstrates hyperlucent left hemithorax with mediastinal shift to the right. Left margin is sharper than right. **B,** Right lateral decubitus view confirms left pneumothorax.

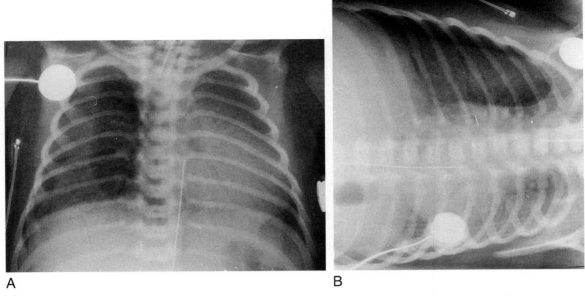

A   B

Figure 49–3. Right pneumothorax. **A,** Supine view demonstrates hyperlucent medial half of right hemithorax. **B,** Small right pneumothorax, left lateral decubitus view.

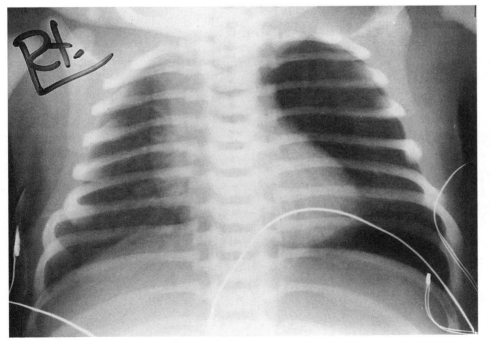

Figure 49–4. Left pneumothorax. The visceral pleura are seen laterally. There is an even more pronounced medial and subpulmonic hyperlucency. The visceral pleura of the base of the lung are clearly seen. The basal air collection is occasionally the result of mediastinal air dissecting between the parietal pleura and diaphragm.

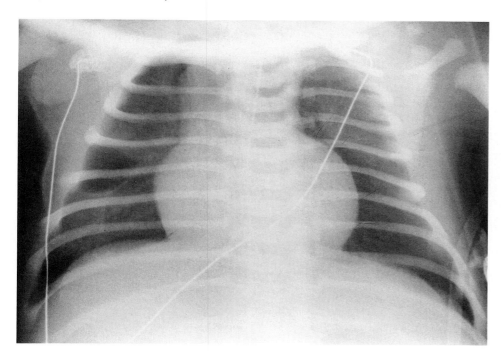

Figure 49–5. Bilateral pneumothoraces. Both mediastinal margins are extremely sharp because of medial pneumothoraces. Visceral pleural margins are faintly seen over the right apex and right costophrenic angle. Air is seen in the right minor fissure.

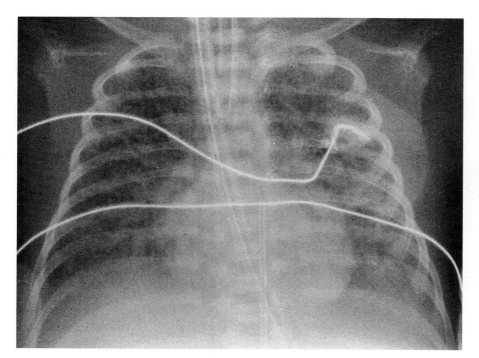

Figure 49–6. Pulmonary interstitial emphysema. Cystic and irregular lucencies involve the entire right lung and left upper lobe.

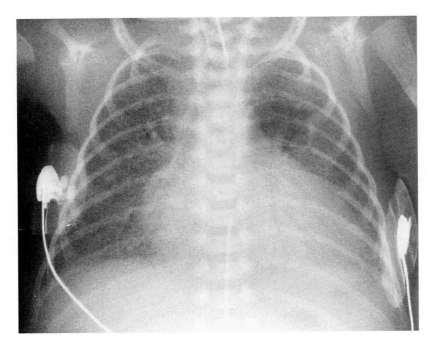

Figure 49–7. Cystic pneumatocele. Large coalescent area of interstitial emphysema in the left suprahilar region.

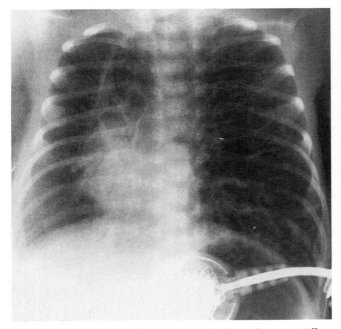

Figure 49–8. Persistent pulmonary interstitial emphysema. Diffuse interstitial emphysema is seen throughout the left lung. The collections are under tension, causing marked overdistention of the lung and mediastinal shift to the left. This pattern persisted for several weeks after extubation.

the heart, tapering at the diaphragmatic hiatus (Fig. 49-10). Posterior pneumomediastinum is most likely to dissect between the parietal pleura and the diaphragm, simulating a subpulmonic pneumothorax (Fig. 49-11).

Lateral decubitus or cross-table lateral radiographs may be necessary to differentiate pneumothorax from pneumomediastinum. Decubitus views allow differentiation between a subpulmonic pneumothorax and mediastinal air between the parietal pleura and the diaphragm. Decubitus views are also useful in excluding medial pneumothorax if the thymus is small or absent or when extrapulmonary air is noted lateral to the thymus (see Fig. 49-2).

A pneumopericardium with pressure approaching central or pulmonary venous pressure begins to impair ventricular filling and stroke volume. Up to a point, an increased heart rate can maintain adequate cardiac output. Once pericardial pressure exceeds ventricular filling pressure, cardiac output falls.[48] If a pneumopericardium develops slowly, the pericardium may stretch, accommodating large volumes of air without restricting myocardial function. If the volume of air accumulates rapidly and exceeds the pericardium's capacitance, cardiac tamponade occurs, accompanied by rapid and severe clinical deterioration.[49]

In a retrospective review of 10 cases, pneumopericardium was preceded by moderate tachycardia and a rise in central venous pressure, followed by bradycardia and abrupt decreases in both heart rate and blood pressure. In the patients who died despite treatment, hypotension and bradycardia had persisted.[13] Other clinical signs are increasing cyanosis, muffled heart sounds, and decreased systemic blood pressure.[25]

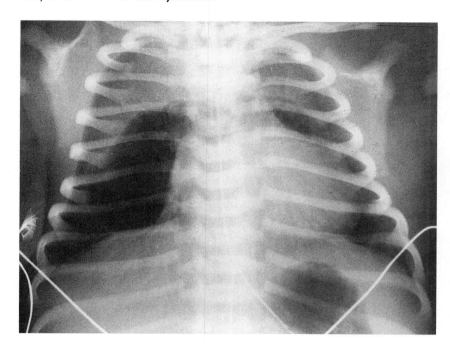

Figure 49–9. Anterior pneumomediastinum. Mediastinal air (more on right side than on left) causing elevation of right and left lobes of the thymus.

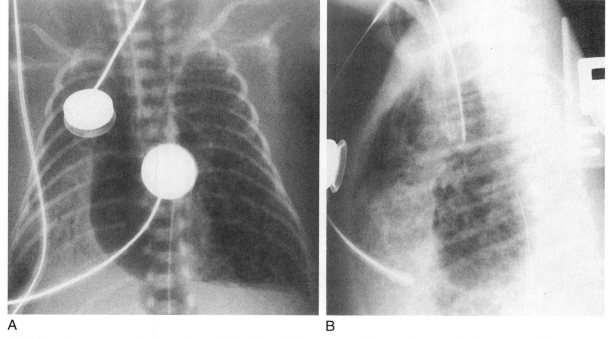

A

B

Figure 49–10. Posterior pneumomediastinum. Frontal **(A)** and lateral **(B)** views reveal a large oval retrocardiac lucency, as well as cervical subcutaneous emphysema. Tension pulmonary interstitial emphysema is noted in the left lung.

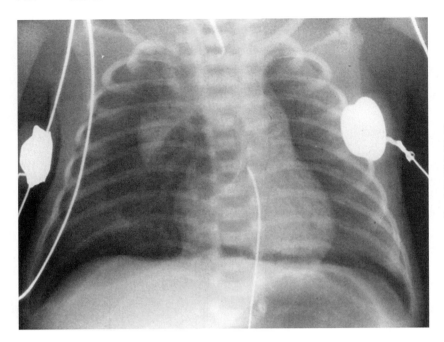

Figure 49–11. Pneumomediastinum and bilateral pneumothorax. An anterior pneumomediastinum can be seen elevating the right thymic lobe and outlining the inferior cardiac margin. Bilateral pneumothoraces are apparent as subpulmonic hyperlucencies. The lateral margin of the right thymic lobe is sharply defined by the medial pneumothorax.

Pneumopericardium may resemble pneumomediastinum on anterior-posterior chest radiographs. With both, the inferior surface of the heart is outlined. In a lateral projection, pneumopericardium outlines the entire inferior aspect of the heart (Fig. 49-12). This finding occurs because the parietal pericardium and central diaphragmatic tendon are attached; mediastinal air cannot dissect between these layers.

The abdominal distention associated with pneumoperitoneum may impair venous blood return secondary to abdominal distention, resulting in cardiac decompensation. Diaphragmatic excursion may also be impaired. Other clinical signs may help distinguish pneumoperitoneum secondary to air dissection from the chest versus rupture of intraabdominal viscus. If air fluid levels are apparent on radiographs, if the ventilator pressures are low, and if other extraalveolar air is not present, the source of intraperitoneal air is likely to be the abdomen. Paracentesis may also help distinguish the two, especially if green or brown fluid is obtained or bacteria are present.[50]

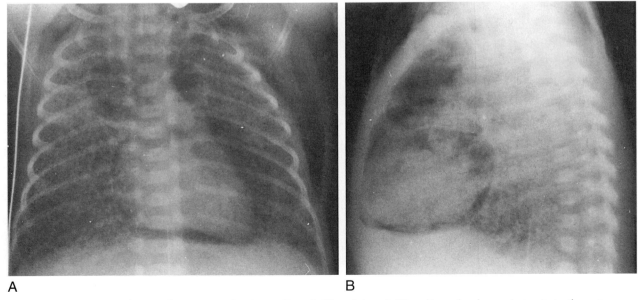

A   B

Figure 49–12. Pneumopericardium and pneumomediastinum. Frontal **(A)** and lateral **(B)** radiographs demonstrate air in the anterosuperior mediastinum. The heart is completely outlined by air, including the entire inferior margin. There is also bilateral interstitial emphysema.

MANAGEMENT

Pneumothorax

Management of pneumothorax depends on the cause and significance of the underlying respiratory disease and the size of the air collection. In full-term infants who are not ventilated at all, with a spontaneous pneumothorax who are minimally tachypneic and maintaining oxygen saturation, treatment may be on an expectant basis or involve "nitrogen washout": that is, 100% oxygen delivered by Oxyhood. Theoretically, the high oxygen concentration in the inspired gas establishes a nitrogen gradient between the pneumothorax and the capillary blood.[51] Needle aspiration may be definitive for moderate respiratory distress without subsequent chest tube placement. If the patient is mechanically ventilated, the pneumothorax usually mandates prompt resolution to prevent further deterioration, with either needle aspiration or chest tube insertion. Needle aspiration may be briefly palliative while the patient is prepared for chest tube placement. In addition to needle aspiration and chest tube placement with an incision, other devices have been developed to facilitate rapid percutaneous placement of chest tubes. One such device entails use of a stylet/trocar with a spring indicator that alerts the operator when the tube reaches the pleural space.[52]

Procedures for Resolution of Pneumothorax

Needle Aspiration

1. Equipment includes a 20- to 60-mL syringe attached to a three-way stopcock and a small gauge intracatheter. A butterfly needle may be used but cannot be easily maintained without increasing risk for lung perforation.
2. The area is prepared with povidone-iodine solution, and the patient is draped and given local anesthesia. The intracatheter is introduced into the skin immediately above the third rib in the midclavicular line. A "Z track" is used to avoid air tracking along the needle's path. Gentle negative pressure is applied as the pleura is punctured. Once the syringe is full, the stopcock can be closed to the patient, the syringe is emptied, the stopcock is reopened to the patient again, and air is withdrawn.
3. If air continues to accumulate, the intracatheter can be taped in place while a chest tube/thoracostomy is prepared. The clinician may continue to remove air, or, if resources are not available, the operator end may be placed under water seal, to ensure negative pressure while the patient is prepared for a longer term solution.[51]

Chest Tube[51,53]

1. Equipment includes chest tubes (No. 10 French for an infant weighing less than 2000 g, No. 12 French for an infant weighing more than 2000 g), sterile drapes, 3-0 silk sutures, curved hemostats, a No. 15 or 11 scalpel, scissors, a needle holder, antiseptic solution, local anesthetic, a 3-mL syringe, and 25- (or lower) gauge needle for local anesthetic, as well as sterile gloves, a mask, a hat, and a sterile gown. A suction drainage device must be used as well.

2. The patient's arm is extended approximately 90 degrees on the affected side. The skin is sterilized and draped. Local anesthetic is used. More extensive pain control with morphine or fentanyl should be used, with appropriate attention to cardiovascular and respiratory support if the need arises. Extensive pain is anticipated. A 1- to 1.5-cm incision is made above the rib, approximately 1 to 2 cm below the desired point of insertion into the pleural cavity. Because air collects most superiorly, if the infant is supine, anterior placement is usually best, well above the nipple: the second intercostal space at the midclavicular line or the fourth intercostal space at the anterior axillary line. The nipple is the landmark for the fourth intercostal space (Fig. 49-13).

3. In the incision, a closed, curved hemostat is inserted. The tissue is spread down to the rib. Using the tip of the hemostat just above the rib while avoiding the intercostal nerve, artery, and vein (requiring what may seem excessive force), the surgeon punctures the parietal pleura. A gush of air may be heard. The hemostat is spread gently. The chest tube is inserted through the open hemostat, which ensures placement of the side holes within the pleural cavity. For small preterm infants, 2- to 3-cm insertion should suffice, and for full-term infants, 3- to 4-cm insertion.

4. An assistant connects the tube to a vacuum drainage system. The surgeon uses 5 to 10 cm H_2O of suction pressure. The water seal chamber prevents air from being drawn back into the pleural cavity. The tube is secured with sutures, followed by clear adhesive.

5. The tube under suction should remain in place until the air leak resolves. After a trial period of 12 to 24 hours with suction turned off while the tube remains under water seal, a chest radiograph should be obtained to assess reaccumulation. If the air does not reaccumulate, the tube may be removed.

6. Complications: Mediastinal encroachment can occur.[54] Sterile technique is mandatory, but infection is always a risk for any invasive procedure. Bleeding can occur if a large vessel is perforated or if the lung is damaged by the procedure. Careful attention to the landmarks should prevent this complication. Immediate surgical consultation is necessary if this occurs. Nerve damage is avoided by, again, respecting the landmarks and placing the tube above the rib, as the nerve runs under the rib. Lung trauma can occur, particularly if a trocar is used. For neonates, a trocar is definitely *not* recommended for chest tube placement. The "pigtail" chest tube with spring-triggered indicator may be safer than previous use of trocars for chest tube insertion in neonates.[52]

7. Subvisceral pleural air may be a complication of chest tube placement. This is inaccessible to chest tube drainage and may necessitate imaging technology–guided needle aspiration.[22]

Pulmonary Interstitial Emphysema

For pulmonary interstitial emphysema, no specific, consistently reliable treatment exists. Mechanical ventilation is thought to be the cause; therefore, initial therapy

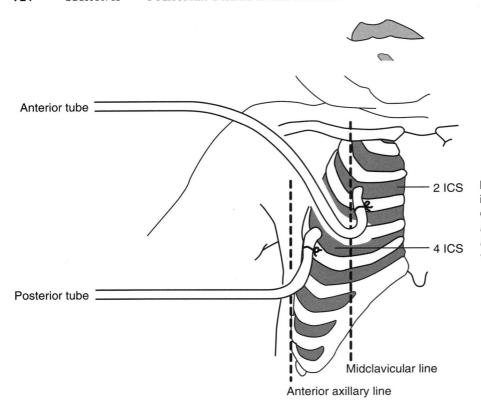

Figure 49–13. Preferred sites for chest tube insertion. ICS, intercostal space. *(From Gomella TL: Neonatology Management: Procedures, On-Call Problems, Diseases, Drugs. Stamford, Conn, Appleton & Lange, 1992. Copyright McGraw-Hill.)*

includes modification of ventilation strategies. Because air is trapped in peribronchial, perivascular, and perilymphatic spaces, it must have adequate time to exit the lung. Peak inspiratory pressures are lowered, inspiratory times are decreased, expiratory time is maximized, and end-expiratory pressures are lowered. These interventions theoretically limit the volume of gas delivered that could contribute additional interstitial air, and they also allow for more egress of air.[55] Higher inspired oxygen concentration is usually necessary to maintain oxygen delivery with the subsequently decreased tidal volume. Significant unilateral pulmonary interstitial emphysema may be treated with selective intubation of the normal lung, dependent positioning of the affected side, and multiple needle punctures of blebs, with placement of a chest tube[28] and lobectomy.[56]

More recently, high-frequency ventilation has been used for rescue after interstitial emphysema has been diagnosed. Theoretically, the extremely short inspiratory times, in the range of 20 milliseconds, limit bulk air delivery. The LifePulse jet ventilator has an adjustable inspiratory time but is conventionally started at 20 milliseconds. The usual initial rate of 420 breaths per minute allows for an inspiratory/expiratory ratio of approximately 1:6. The SensorMedics 3100A High Frequency Oscillatory Ventilator has a fixed inspiratory/expiratory ratio of 1:2, and at 15 Hz, the inspiratory time is also approximately 20 milliseconds. The Infant Star high-flow interrupter has a fixed inspiratory time of approximately 20 milliseconds, allowing an inspiratory/expiratory ratio of 1:2.3 at 15 Hz and a 1:4 ratio at 10 Hz.

When high-frequency jet ventilation was compared with optimized conventional strategies for rescue for interstitial emphysema, 61% of the infants improved with jet ventilation, in contrast to 37% with conventional strategies. Jet ventilation was associated with more rapid radiographic improvement and improved ventilation with lower peak inspiratory and mean airway pressures.[57] The oscillator demonstrated similar efficacy.[58] One study in which high-frequency oscillatory ventilation was used for 10 neonates with interstitial emphysema demonstrated significant improvement in circulation. This improvement in blood flow could have been the result of decreasing the amount of air around blood vessels.[59]

Pneumopericardium

Some investigators believe that patients with a small, asymptomatic pneumopericardium who are not receiving assisted ventilation can be observed rather than aggressively treated. Serial radiographs and echocardiograms and very close clinical monitoring are necessary if this approach is taken.[60] Others argue that it must be treated as an emergency because the change in status can be abrupt.[61] In a series of mechanically ventilated infants, the chance of asymptomatic pneumopericardium's progressing to clinical significance was 40%. Of the patients who became symptomatic, 60% died. Placement of a pericardial drainage tube is favored over single needle aspiration, inasmuch as Emery and coworkers noted an 80% recurrence rate after aspiration.[62] Another review of pneumopericardium revealed mortality rates of 57% ($N = 30$) and 21% ($N = 19$) among patients treated with observation or needle aspiration, respectively. All 12 patients treated with surgical placement of a drainage catheter survived.[63] According to the limited evidence, simple observation is appropriate for only the smallest asymptomatic pneumopericardium in an infant not receiving mechanical ventilation. Multiple needle aspirations should also be avoided because of the possibility of significant complications.

Pericardiocentesis

In the absence of elective surgical drain placement, pericardiocentesis must be carried out at the bedside by available staff. The procedure is as follows[51,53]:

1. Equipment: sterilizing solution for skin; sterile gloves, gown, hat, and mask; a 22- or 24-gauge intracatheter; sterile drapes; a 10-mL syringe attached to a three-way stopcock; connecting tubing; and an underwater seal.
2. The patient is prepared with the sterile solution and then draped. If time allows, local anesthetic is given. The needle is inserted approximately 0.5 cm to the left and just below the xiphoid process, at a 30-degree angle, aiming at the midclavicular line, while constant suction is applied (Fig. 49-14). When air is removed, the catheter is slipped off the needle and secured in place. If the air fills the syringe, the stopcock is turned off to the patient, the air is emptied, and then the stopcock is turned on to the patient again. This procedure can temporize until a pericardial tube is inserted.
3. Complications are potentially lethal and include laceration or puncture of the myocardium, pneumothorax, or infection.
4. One way to avoid cardiac trauma is to attach an electrocardiographic anterior chest lead to the needle. If the electrocardiogram changes, the needle has

come in contact with the myocardium and must be withdrawn.

Pneumoperitoneum

Pneumoperitoneum can result in significant increases in intraperitoneal pressure, decrease in venous return, and subsequent fall in cardiac output, as well as respiratory decompensation secondary to compromised diaphragmatic excursion. If significant cardiovascular and respiratory compromise is noted, paracentesis should be carried out.

Paracentesis

1. Equipment: sterile drapes; skin sterilizing solution; sterile gloves, mask, hat, and sterile gown; sterile gauze; sterile tubes (if fluid is anticipated); a 22-gauge (for infants weighing 2000 g or more) or 24-gauge (for infants weighing less than 2000 g) intracatheter; connecting tubing; three-way stopcock; and a 10- or 20-mL syringe.
2. Procedure: The infant is placed supine and the legs are restrained. The skin is prepared, and the infant is covered with sterile drapes. Midline injection should be avoided because of the risk of perforating the bladder or bowel wall. The injection site should be on either flank between an imaginary horizontal line passing through the umbilicus and the inguinal ligament. The needle is inserted with a "Z-track" technique to prevent peritoneal fluid leak and angled perpendicular to the skin. When the needle is just under the skin, it is moved 0.5 cm before the abdominal wall is punctured. The needle is advanced while aspiration is performed with the syringe. If air is recovered, the needle is removed and the catheter is secured. If the syringe fills, the stopcock is turned off to the patient, the air is emptied via the stopcock, then the stopcock is reopened to the patient again, and the surgeon continues. The surgeon may leave the catheter secure and covered or may remove the catheter once air is drained. Appropriate follow-up radiography is ordered.
3. Complications: Infection risk is limited with careful sterile technique and removal of the catheter after the procedure. The shortest needle possible should be used, to help avoid the risk of visceral perforation.

PREVENTION OF AIR LEAKS

Surfactant replacement therapy has significantly reduced risk of air leaks, for both pneumothorax and pulmonary interstitial emphysema (Tables 49-1 and 49-2). The intervention is clearly beneficial for synthetic or natural surfactants. Reviews of the number of doses suggest benefits to not limiting to a single dose. Early dosing seems more beneficial than waiting for established respiratory distress syndrome to be diagnosed.[64,65]

Ventilation technology (Table 49-3) has advanced to include high-frequency ventilation[66] and patient-triggered ventilation.[67,68] Neither method has been shown to definitively reduce risk or air leaks. Ventilation practices, including permissive hypercapnia[69,70] and elective

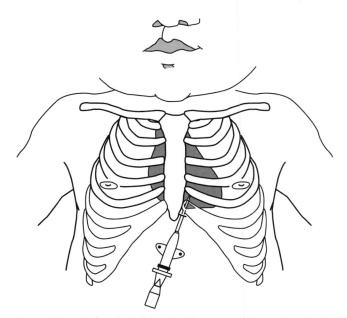

Figure 49–14. Preferred site for pericardiocentesis. *(From Gomella TL: Neonatology Management: Procedures, On-Call Problems, Diseases, Drugs. Stamford, Conn, Appleton & Lange, 1992. Copyright McGraw-Hill.)*

Table 49–1. Surfactant and Pneumothorax

Strategy	Relative Risk	95% Confidence Interval for Relative Risk	Typical Absolute Risk Reduction	95% Confidence Interval for Typical Absolute Risk Reduction	Number Needed to Treat*
Prophylactic natural surfactant vs. control[64]	0.35	0.26 to 0.49	−0.15	−0.20 to −0.11	6-7
Prophylactic vs. selective surfactant: 6 studies[65]	0.62	0.42 to 0.89	−0.02	−0.04 to −0.01	50
Early vs. delayed selective treatment: 4 studies[64]	0.70	0.59 to 0.82	−0.05	−0.08 to −0.03	20
Multiple vs. limited single dose: 2 studies[65]	0.51	0.30 to 0.88	−0.09	−0.15 to −0.02	11

*Based on typical absolute risk reduction.

Table 49–2. Surfactant and Pulmonary Interstitial Emphysema

Strategy	Relative Risk	95% Confidence Interval for Relative Risk	Typical Absolute Risk Reduction	95% Confidence Interval for Typical Absolute Risk Reduction	Number Needed to Treat*
Prophylactic natural surfactant vs. control[65]	0.46	0.35 to 0.60	−0.19	−0.25 to −0.13	5
Prophylactic vs. selective surfactant: 5 studies[65]	0.54	0.36 to 0.82	−0.03	−0.04 to −0.01	33
Early vs. delayed selective treatment: 4 studies[64]	0.63	0.43 to 0.93	−0.06	−0.10 to −0.01	16

*Based on typical absolute risk reduction.

Table 49–3. Ventilator Strategies and Air Leaks

Ventilator Strategy	Relative Risk	95% Confidence Interval	Number Needed to Treat*
Synchronized ventilation HFPPV vs. CMV (risk of pneumothorax): 3 studies[66]	0.69	0.51 to 0.93	11
SIMV/PTV vs. CMV (risk of airleak): 6 studies[67]	1.03	0.80 to 1.34	NS
High-frequency oscillatory ventilation vs. CMV, high-volume strategy, any air leak: 4 studies[68]	1.21	0.94 to 1.56	NS

*Based on typical absolute risk reduction.

CMV, conventional mechanical ventilation; HFPPV, high-frequency positive-pressure ventilation; NS, nonsignificant; PTV, patient-triggered ventilation; SIMV, synchronized intermittent mandatory ventilation.

neuromuscular paralysis,[71] have not been shown to significantly reduce the risk of air leaks.

In addition to neonatal intervention, the effect of antenatal steroids should also be noted. Antenatal treatment with corticosteroids significantly (45% reduction) reduced the odds ratio of respiratory distress syndrome in preterm infants.[72] In a review of two surfactant trials, Jobe and associates evaluated the combined effect of antenatal steroids and surfactant treatment. The rate of air leak was only 1.7% for neonates receiving both therapies, in contrast to 13% for steroids only, 11.3% for surfactant only, and 23.3% for neither surfactant nor corticosteroids.[73] It should be pointed out that this analysis was not the goal of the two studies and was a retrospective review of data. Maternal steroid use was only 10.6% (133 of 1253 infants) overall.

In addition to the well-studied medical and technical interventions, other aspects of care may contribute to development of air leak syndromes. Suctioning and delivering of positive-pressure breaths are "routine" practices that mandate careful attention to detail in order to avoid adverse events. Attention to postsurfactant dosing conditions of infants may also affect rates of air leaks. The tools, technologies, and therapies used in the neonatal intensive care unit are powerful and potentially harmful, and although air leaks may have decreased in number since the advent of surfactant and antenatal steroids, they have not disappeared. Their significance persists; therefore, every effort must be made to limit their occurrence.

REFERENCES

1. Chernick V, Avery ME: Spontaneous alveolar rupture at birth. Pediatrics 32:816, 1963.
2. Solis-Cohen L, Bruck S: A roentgen examination of the chest of 500 newborn infants for pathology other than enlarged thymus. Radiology 23:173, 1934.
3. Bashour BN, Balfe JW: Urinary tract anomalies in neonates with spontaneous pneumothorax and/or pneumomediastinum. Pediatrics 59(Suppl):1048, 1977.
4. Ryan CA, Barrington KJ, Phillips HJ: Contralateral pneumothoraces in the newborn: Incidence and predisposing factors. Pediatrics 79:417, 1987.
5. Yu VYH, Wong PY, Bajuk B, Szymonowicz W: Pulmonary air leak in extremely low birth weight infants. Arch Dis Child 61:239, 1986.
6. Powers WF, Clemens JD: Prognostic implications of age at detection of air leak in very low birth weight infants requiring ventilatory support. J Pediatr 123:611, 1993.
7. Gortner L, Wauer RP, Hammer H, et al: Early vs. late surfactant treatment in preterm infants of 27 to 32 weeks' gestational age: A multicenter controlled trial. Pediatrics 102:1153, 1998.
8. Kendig JW, Ryan RM, Sinkin RA, et al: Comparison of two strategies for surfactant prophylaxis in very premature infants: A multicenter randomized trial. Pediatrics 101:1006, 1998.
9. Bloom BB, Kattwinkel J, Hall RT, et al: Comparison of Infasurf (calf lung surfactant extract) to Survanta (Beractant) in the treatment and prevention of respiratory distress syndrome. Pediatrics 100:31, 1997.
10. Miller MJ, Fanaroff AA, Martin RJ: The respiratory system: Other pulmonary problems. In Fanaroff AA, Martin R (eds): Neonatal-Perinatal Medicine: Diseases of the Fetus and Infant, 5th ed. St. Louis, Mosby–Year Book, 1992, pp 834-860.
11. Findlay RD, Taeusch HW, Walther FJ: Surfactant replacement therapy for meconium aspiration syndrome. Pediatrics 97:48, 1996.
12. Morrow G, Hope JW, Boggs TR Jr: Pneumomediastinum: A silent lesion in the newborn. J Pediatr 70:554, 1967.
13. Goldberg RN, Cabal LA, Hodgman JE, et al: Pneumopericardium: An approach to diagnosis and treatment in the neonate. Pediatr Res 12:524A, 1978.
14. Burt TB, Lester PD: Neonatal pneumopericardium. Pediatr Radiol 142:81, 1982.
15. Glenski JA, Hall RT: Neonatal pneumopericardium: Analysis of ventilatory variables. Crit Care Med 12:489, 1984.
16. Avery ME: The alveolar lining layer. Pediatrics 30:324, 1962.
17. Anderson KD, Chandra R: Pneumothorax secondary to perforation of sequential bronchi by suction catheters. J Pediatr Surg 11:687, 1976.
18. Holcomb GW, Templeton JM Jr: Iatrogenic perforation of the bronchus intermedius in a 1,100 gram neonate. J Pediatr Surg 24:1132, 1989.
19. Macklin CC: Alveolar pores and their significance in human lung. Arch Pathol 21:202, 1936.
20. Martin HB: Effect of aging on flow resistance to collateral ventilation. Fed Proc 20:427, 1961.
21. Macklin MT, Macklin CC: Malignant interstitial emphysema of the lung and mediastinum as an important occult complication in many respiratory diseases and other conditions. Medicine 23:281, 1944.
22. Ivey HH, Kattwinkel J, Alford BA: Subvisceral pleural air in neonates with respiratory distress. Am J Dis Child 327:861, 1981.
23. Caldwell EJ, Powell RD, Mullooly JP: Interstitial emphysema: A study of physiologic factors involved in experimental induction of the lesion. Am Rev Respir Dis 102:516, 1970.
24. Hansen TN, Gest AL: Oxygen toxicity and other ventilatory complications of treatment of infants with persistent pulmonary hypertension. Clin Perinatol 11:653, 1984.
25. Hansen T, Corbet A: Air block syndrome in neonates. In Taeusch W, Ballard R (eds): Avery's Diseases of the Newborn, 7th ed. Philadelphia, WB Saunders, 1998, pp 630-634.
26. Ackerman NB, Coalson JT, Kuehl TJ, et al: Pulmonary interstitial emphysema in premature baboon with hyaline membrane disease. Crit Care Med 12:512, 1984.
27. Grosfield JF, Lemons JL, Ballantine TV, Schreiner RL: Emergency thoracotomy for acquired bronchopleural fistula in the premature infant with respiratory distress. J Pediatr Surg 15:416, 1980.
28. Joannides M, Tsoulous GD: The etiology of interstitial and mediastinal emphysema. Arch Surg 21:333, 1930.
29. Donahoe PK, Stewart DR, Osmond JD 3rd, Hendren WH 3rd: Pneumoperitoneum secondary to pulmonary air leak. J Pediatr 81:797, 1972.
30. Aplan G, Goder K, Glick F, et al: Pneumopericardium during continuous positive airway pressure in respiratory distress syndrome. Crit Care Med 12:1080, 1984.
31. Varano LA, Maisels MJ: Pneumopericardium in the newborn: Diagnosis and pathogenesis. Pediatrics 81:832, 1984.
32. Goldberg RN: Sustained arterial blood pressure elevation associated with pneumothoraces: Early detection via continuous monitoring. Pediatrics 68:775, 1981.
33. Simmons DH, Hemingway A, Ricchuiti N: Acute circulatory effects of pneumothorax in dogs. J Applied Physiol 12:255, 1958.

34. Sharpey-Shafer EP: Effect of respiratory acts on the circulation. In WF Hamilton (section ed): Handbook of Physiology, Section 2: Circulation, vol 3. Washington DC, American Physiological Society, 1965, pp 1875-1886.

35. Ead HW, Green JH, Neil E: A comparison of the effects of pulsatile and nonpulsatile blood flow through the carotid sinus on the reflexogenic activity of the sinus baroreceptors in the cat. J Physiol 118:509, 1952.

36. Goldberg RN, Chung D, Bray J, Bancalari E: Intracranial hypertension secondary to pneumothoraces. Pediatr Res 14:631A, 1980.

37. Ogata ES, Gregory GA, Kitterman JA, et al: Pneumothorax in the respiratory distress syndrome: Incidence and effect on vital signs, blood gases and pH. Pediatrics 58:177, 1976.

38. Brazy JE, Blackmon LR: Hypotension and bradycardia associated with airblock in neonates. J Pediatr 90:796, 1977.

39. Dykes PD, Lazzara A, Ahmann P, et al. Intraventricular hemorrhage: A prospective evaluation of etiopathogenesis. Pediatrics 66:42, 1980.

40. Lou HC, Lassen NA, Friis-Hansen B: Impaired autoregulation of cerebral blood flow in the distressed newborn. J Pediatr 94:118, 1979.

41. Hill A, Perlman JM, Volpe JJ: Relationship of pneumothorax to occurrence of intraventricular hemorrhage in the premature newborn. Pediatrics 69:144, 1982.

42. Batton DG, Hellman J, Nardis EE: Effect of pneumothorax-induced systemic blood pressure alterations on the cerebral circulation in newborn dogs. Pediatrics 74:350, 1984.

43. Kuhs LR, Bednarek FJ, Wyman ML, et al: Diagnosis of pneumothorax or pneumomediastinum in the neonate by transillumination. Pediatrics 56:335, 1975.

44. McIntosh N, Becher JC, Cunningham S, et al: Clinical diagnosis of pneumothorax is late: Use of trend data and decision support might allow preclinical detection. Pediatr Res 48:408, 2000.

45. Leonidas JC, Bahn I, McCauley GK: Persistent localized pulmonary interstitial emphysema and lymphangiectasia: A causal relationship? Pediatrics 64:165, 1979.

46. Booth TN, Allen BA, Royal SA: Lymphatic air embolism: A new hypothesis regarding the pathogenesis of neonatal systemic air embolism. Pediatr Radiol 25(Suppl 1):S220, 1995.

47. Fournier L, Cloutier R, Major D: Barotrauma in congenital diaphragmatic hernia; the killer? Can J Anaesth 38:A67, 1991.

48. Long WA: Pneumopericardium. In Long WA (ed): Fetal and Neonatal Cardiology. Philadelphia, WB Saunders, 1990, pp 377-388.

49. Van Norstrand C, Beamish WE, Schiff D: Neonatal pneumopericardium. Can Med Assoc J 112:186, 1975.

50. Knight PJ, Abdenour G: Pneumoperitoneum in the ventilated neonate: Respiratory or gastrointestinal origin? J Pediatr 98:972, 1981.

51. Zak LK, Donn SM: Thoracic air leaks. In Donn SM, Faix RG (eds): Neonatal Emergencies. Mount Kisco, NY, Futura Publishing, 1991, pp 311-326.

52. Wood B, Dubik M: A new device for pleural drainage in newborn infants. Pediatrics 96:955, 1995.

53. Gomella T: Chest tube placement. In Gomella TL (ed): Neonatology: Management, Procedures, On-Call Problems, Diseases, and Drugs. Stamford, Conn, Appleton & Lange, 1999, pp 160-162.

54. Allen RW, Jung AL, Lester PD: Effectiveness of chest tube evacuation of pneumothorax in neonates. J Pediatr 99:629, 1981.

55. Meadow WL, Cheromcha D: Successful therapy of unilateral pulmonary emphysema: Mechanical ventilation with extremely short inspiratory time. Am J Perinatol 2:194, 1985.

56. Bauer CR, Brennan MJ, Doyle C, Poole CA: Surgical resection for pulmonary interstitial emphysema in the newborn infant. J Pediatr 93:656, 1978.

57. Keszler M, Donn SM, Bucciarelli RL, et al: Multicenter controlled trial comparing high-frequency jet ventilation and conventional mechanical ventilation in newborn infants with pulmonary interstitial emphysema. J Pediatr 119:85, 1991.

58. Clark RH, Gerstmann DR, Null DM, et al: Pulmonary interstitial emphysema treated by high-frequency oscillatory ventilation. Crit Care Med 14:926, 1986.

59. Nelle M, Zilow EP, Linderkamp O: Effects of high frequency oscillatory ventilation on circulation in neonates with pulmonary interstitial emphysema or RDS. Intensive Care Med 23:671, 1997.

60. Pfenninger J, Boss E, Biesold J, et al: Treatment of pneumothorax, pneumopericardium and pneumomediastinum. Helv Paediatr Acta 37:353, 1982.

61. Brans YW, Pitts M, Cassady G: Neonatal pneumopericardium. Am J Dis Child 130:393, 1976.

62. Emery RW, Foker J, Thompson TR: Neonatal pneumopericardium: A surgical emergency. Ann Thorac Surg 37:128, 1984.

63. Cohen DJ, Baumgart S, Stephenson LW: Pneumopericardium in neonates—is it PEEP or PIP? Am Thorac Surg 35:179, 1983.

64. Yost CC, Soll RF: Early vs. delayed selective surfactant treatment for neonatal respiratory distress syndrome. Cochrane Database Syst Rev (2):CD001456, 2001.

65. Soll RF, Morley CJ: Prophylactic versus selective use of surfactant in preventing morbidity and mortality in preterm infants. Cochrane Database Syst Rev (2):CD000510, 2001.

66. Cools F, Offringa M: Meta-analysis of elective high frequency ventilation in preterm infants with respiratory distress syndrome. Arch Dis Child Fetal Neonatal Ed 80:15F, 1999.

67. Greenough A, Milner AD, Dimitriou G: Synchronized mechanical ventilation for respiratory support in newborn infants. Cochrane Database Syst Rev (1):CD000456, 2001.

68. Henderson-Smart DJ, Bhuta T, Cools F, Offringa M: Elective high frequency oscillatory ventilation vs. conventional ventilation in preterm infants with acute pulmonary dysfunction. Cochrane Database Syst Rev (4):CD000104, 2003.

69. Carlo WA, Stark AR, Bauer C, et al: Effects of minimal ventilation in a multicenter randomized controlled trial of ventilator support and early corticosteroid therapy in extremely low birth weight infants. Pediatrics 104(3, Suppl): 738, 1999.

70. Mariani, G, Cifuentes J, Carlo WA: Randomized trial of permissive hypercapnia in preterm infants. Pediatrics 104:1082, 1999.

71. Cools F, Offringa M: Neuromuscular paralysis for newborn infants receiving mechanical ventilation. Cochrane Database Syst Rev (4):CD002773, 2000.

72. Crowley P, Chalmers I, Keirse MJNC: The effects of corticosteroids administration before preterm delivery: An overview of the evidence from controlled trials. Br J Obstet Gynaecol 97:11, 1990.

73. Jobe AH, Mitchell BR, Gunkel JH: Beneficial effects of the combined use of prenatal corticosteroids and postnatal surfactant on preterm infants. Am J Obstet Gynecol 168:508, 1993.

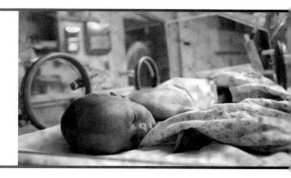

CHAPTER 50

Bronchopulmonary Dysplasia

Jonathan M. Davis and Steven H. Abman

Premature birth and injury to the immature lung disrupt the normal sequence of lung growth, leading to the development of chronic lung disease, or bronchopulmonary dysplasia (BPD). As characterized by Northway and colleagues in 1967,[1] BPD is the chronic lung disease of infancy that follows mechanical ventilation and oxygen therapy for newborns with respiratory distress syndrome (RDS).[1-4] BPD has traditionally been defined by the presence of clinical respiratory signs and symptoms, the need for supplemental oxygen to treat hypoxemia, and an abnormal chest radiograph (Fig. 50-1).[5] Although typically found in premature infants, BPD has also been described in critically ill full-term infants, but it probably represents a different disease process (see later discussion). With the introduction of surfactant therapy, antenatal steroid use, new ventilator strategies and other treatments, the clinical course and outcomes of premature infants with RDS has changed markedly since 1970.[6] Despite these improvements in prenatal and postnatal care, BPD remains a major clinical problem. With increasing survival of extremely premature newborns, BPD remains one of the most significant sequelae of neonatal intensive care; an estimated 7,000 to 10,000 infants in the United States are affected each year. This is particularly important because the development of BPD is associated with significant long-term pulmonary sequelae in children, such as asthma and chronic obstructive lung disease, as well as neurodevelopmental abnormalities. In addition, the long-term cardiopulmonary and neurodevelopmental sequelae of BPD into adulthood remain uncertain.

Since the original description of BPD, much has been learned about its pathogenesis, pathophysiologic

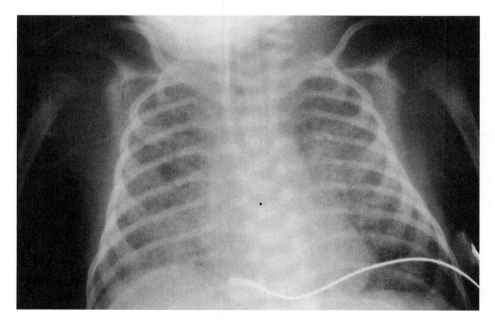

Figure 50–1. Chest radiographic changes in an infant with bronchopulmonary dysplasia. The diffuse hazy appearance represents inflammation, exudate, edema, and atelectasis.

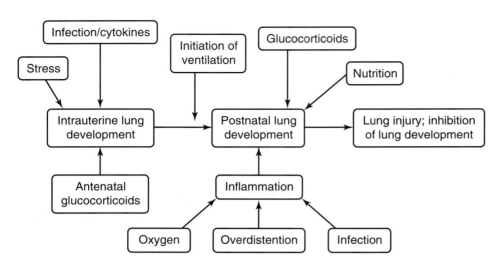

Figure 50–2. Overview of the pathogenesis of bronchopulmonary dysplasia, showing prenatal and postnatal factors. *(Adapted from Jobe AH: The new BPD: An arrest of lung development. Pediatr Res 46:641, 1999.)*

processes, and outcome. BPD is a disease that results from exposure of the susceptible premature lung to adverse prenatal and postnatal stimuli that disrupt the normal pattern of lung growth and development (Fig. 50-2).[4-6] This chapter reviews the definition, incidence, pathogenesis, pathophysiology, treatment, and long-term outcome of infants with BPD, as well as therapeutic strategies for the prevention of BPD in infants at high risk.

DEFINITION AND INCIDENCE

BPD is generally defined by the presence of chronic respiratory distress, persistent oxygen requirement, and an abnormal chest radiograph at 1 month of age. However, this definition lacks specificity and fails to account for many important clinical distinctions. For example, Shennan and colleagues suggested that the need for oxygen supplementation at 36 weeks of postconceptional age may be a better predictor of late pulmonary disease during infancy than the need for oxygen at 28 days after birth.[7] Oxygen use at 1 month of age may not adequately account for differences between the effects of delayed lung maturation versus lung injury, inasmuch as most premature infants born at 24 or 25 weeks of gestation still require oxygen supplementation at 28 days after birth. However, most of these infants may ultimately not develop chronic respiratory disease or have an abnormal chest radiograph. In addition, chest radiographic findings can be subtle and are often not specific for BPD. Even if the need for supplemental oxygen at 36 weeks of postmenstrual age were an accurate predictor of ultimate pulmonary outcome in very premature infants, this definition does not accommodate 34- to 35-weeks' gestation premature infants with RDS who require a small amount of supplemental oxygen for 1 to 2 weeks after birth. Other investigators have found that the only method that definitively establishes the diagnosis of BPD is the presence of chronic respiratory symptoms (such as asthma and repeated pulmonary infections) necessitating treatment with oxygen, bronchodilators, corticosteroids, or other respiratory medications in the first year or two

after birth.[4,8] A consensus conference convened by the National Institutes of Health suggested a new definition of BPD that incorporates many elements of previous definitions and attempts to categorize the severity of BPD (Table 50-1).[4] Ultimately, the definition of BPD must be validated with clinically important long-term end points in a prospective manner.

Although much has been learned about BPD since its initial description, the disease continues to change with time, as a result of improved treatment strategies and survival. Mortality has dramatically decreased since 1970; survival rates have increased from less than 10% in the past to more than 50% among extremely preterm infants (<24-26 weeks of gestation). In 1967, the average gestational age and birth weight of surviving infants with BPD were 34 weeks and 2234 g, respectively.[1] Currently, most infants who develop BPD are much smaller and less mature at birth, averaging <1000 g in 75% of cases.[4,7,9] The risk of BPD rises with decreasing birth weight. The incidence has been reported as high as 85% among neonates weighing between 500 and 699 g at birth, but it decreases to 5% among infants with birth weights exceeding 1500 g. Although the overall incidence of BPD is reported to be approximately 20% among ventilated newborns, wide variability exists between centers.[10] This variability probably reflects regional differences in the clinical definitions of BPD, the relative number of inborn and outborn infants, the proportion of newborns with extreme prematurity, and specific patient management practices. Currently, there is growing recognition that infants with persistent lung disease after premature birth have a different clinical course and pathologic processes than had been traditionally observed in infants dying of BPD during the presurfactant era.[2,4,6,11-13] The "classic" clinical, radiologic, and pathologic stages that first characterized BPD are often now absent, as a result of changes in clinical management. There has been a clear shift in how this disease was characterized: from one that was defined predominantly by the severity of acute lung injury to one that can be defined predominantly by a disruption of distal lung growth.[4,6,11] In contrast with

Table 50–1. Definition of Bronchopulmonary Dysplasia: Diagnostic Criteria

| Criterion | Gestational Age | |
	<32 Weeks	≥32 Weeks
Time point of assessment	36 weeks of PMA or discharge to home, whichever comes first	>28 days but <56 days postnatal age or discharge to home, whichever comes first
	Treatment with oxygen ≥ 21% for at least 28 days plus	
Mild BPD	Breathing room air at 36 weeks of PMA or discharge, whichever comes first	Breathing room air by 56 days of postnatal age or discharge, whichever comes first
Moderate BPD	Need for <30% oxygen at 36 weeks of PMA or discharge, whichever comes first	Need for <30% oxygen at 56 days of postanatal age or discharge, whichever comes first
Severe BPD	Need for ≥30% oxygen and/or positive pressure, (PPV or NCPAP) at 36 weeks of PMA or discharge, whichever comes first	Need for ≥30% oxygen and/or positive pressure (PPV or NCPAP) at 56 days of postnatal age or discharge, whichever comes first

BPD, bronchopulmonary dysplasia; NCPAP, nasal continuous positive airway pressure; PMA, postmenstrual age; PPV, positive-pressure ventilation.

"classic BPD," the "new BPD" develops in preterm newborns, many of whom require minimal ventilatory support with low fraction of inspired oxygen during the early postnatal days (Fig. 50-3).[14,15] As a result, the term **chronic lung disease of infancy** has often been used interchangeably with **bronchopulmonary dysplasia** to describe the chronic respiratory disorder that can develop after premature birth.

In addition to the changing epidemiology, the nature of BPD has evolved as well, in such a way that pathologic signs of severe lung injury with striking fibroproliferative changes are less common. More typically, infants with BPD now have less severe acute respiratory disease early in their course.[9] At autopsy, lung histologic specimens display more uniform and milder regions of injury, and signs of impaired alveolar and vascular growth are more prominent (Fig. 50-4). This "new BPD" is only beginning to be characterized, especially with regard to its pathogenesis and implications for long-term outcome.

PATHOLOGY

Detailed morphometric studies have extensively characterized the lung disease of infants who died of BPD.[4,11,16,17] The pathologic process of BPD provides insights into the effects of acute lung injury and repair processes in the developing lung, and the effect of the timing of this injury. The original reports of BPD described a continuous process through distinct stages of disease, progressing from acute lung injury, or exudative phase, to a proliferative phase of chronic disease.[18-20] These reports describe the gross "cobblestone" appearance of the lungs, representing alternating areas of atelectasis, marked scarring, and regional hyperinflation (emphysema) (Fig. 50-5). Typical histologic features of this BPD include marked

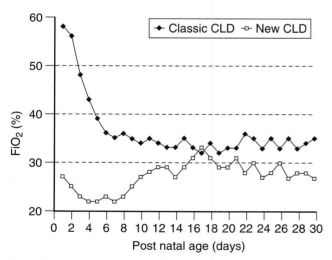

Figure 50–3. Change in fraction of inspired oxygen (Fio₂) over time in infants with bronchopulmonary dysplasia (BPD), also known as chronic lung disease (CLD). As shown, some infants who develop BPD do not require high Fio₂ after birth but develop a progressive increase in the need for higher Fio₂ over time. *(From Bancalari E, Gonzalez A: Clinical course and lung function abnormalities during development of chronic lung disease. In Bland RD, Coalson JJ [eds]: Chronic Lung Disease in Early Infancy. New York, Marcel Dekker, 2000, pp 41-64.)*

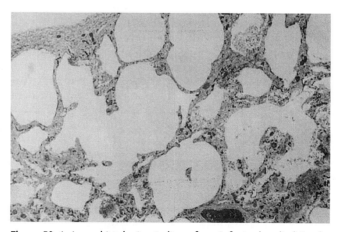

Figure 50–4. Lung histologic studies of an infant who died in the surfactant era with the typical changes of the "new bronchopulmonary dysplasia," showing alveolar simplification and reduced septation.

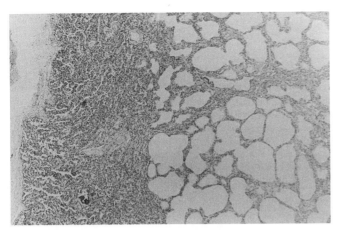

Figure 50–5. Lung histologic studies of an infant with more severe bronchopulmonary dysplasia, illustrating the typical pattern of hyperinflation alternating with atelectasis and increased cellularity. (Original magnification ×4.)

airway changes, such as squamous metaplasia of large and small airways, increased peribronchial smooth muscle and fibrosis, chronic inflammation and airway edema, and hyperplasia of submucosal glands. Parenchymal disease is characterized by volume loss from atelectasis and alveolar septal fibrosis alternating with overdistention or "emphysematous" regions. Mesenchymal thickening with increased cellularity and destruction of alveolar septa with alveolar hypoplasia are present, which is suggestive of a marked reduction in surface area available for gas exchange. Growth of capillary beds is reduced, and small pulmonary arteries have hypertensive structural remodeling, which includes smooth muscle hyperplasia and distal extension of smooth muscle growth into vessels that are normally nonmuscular. In addition, the vessels are often described as "dysmorphic," because of their centralized location in the thickened mesenchyme, which may further impair gas exchange.

Although reductions in alveolar number were described in older infants who died of BPD, this pattern of "alveolar simplification" has become the most striking pathologic feature of the "new BPD" (see Fig. 50-4).[11] In contrast with past reports, more recent studies of infants who died of BPD have described fewer signs of airway injury and interstitial fibrosis, but they have emphasized persistent reductions of distal airspace and vascular growth. Decreased alveolar development and impaired growth of small pulmonary arteries results in decreased lung surface area for gas exchange, which has important functional implications regarding late cardiopulmonary sequelae (see later discussion). In addition to changes in the distal lung, the pathologic process of BPD is further characterized by abnormal airway structure. Upper airways (i.e., trachea and main bronchi) of infants with BPD often reveal significant lesions, depending on the frequency and duration of endotracheal intubation. Grossly, mucosal edema or necrosis can be focal or diffuse. The earliest histologic changes include patchy loss of cilia from columnar epithelial cells, which can then become

dysplastic or necrotic, resulting in breakdown of the epithelial lining. Ulcerated areas may involve the mucosa or extend into the submucosa. Infiltration of inflammatory cells (neutrophils and lymphocytes) into these areas may be prominent. Goblet cells appear hyperplastic, which is suggestive of greater capacity for increased mucous production that can mix with cellular debris. Granulation tissue often develops in the subglottis, as a result of damage from the endotracheal tube, or more distally throughout the airway, as a result of trauma from repeated suctioning. Significant narrowing of the trachea and main bronchi secondary to injury can lead to subglottic stenosis, tracheal cysts and polyps, and related lesions. Tracheomalacia, which often complicates the course of severe BPD, can appear as marked redundancy of the posterior wall of the trachea, as a result of chronic ventilation of the compliant premature airway.

Changes in the smaller airways and distal airspace constitute the most striking pathologic abnormality in more severe BPD. Early RDS is characterized by proteinaceous debris in the distal airspaces (hyaline membranes), and the epithelium appears as a thin, dysplastic lining, made up primarily of type II alveolar cells. These membranes become incorporated into the underlying airway. Edema, inflammation, exudate, and necrosis of epithelial cells are often found, along with a necrotizing bronchiolitis. Later in the clinical course, cellular debris, inflammatory cells, and proteinaceous exudate can accumulate and obstruct many of the terminal airways and the distal lung. It has been suggested that this process, with associated atelectasis, may actually protect the distal airspaces from further damage caused by high oxygen levels and stretch-induced injury during mechanical ventilation. Fibroblast proliferation and activation leads to peribronchial fibrosis, smooth muscle thickening, and, in advanced cases, obliterative bronchiolitis. In more recent cases, these changes in airway structure have been less striking.

PATHOGENESIS

BPD represents the response of the premature lung to acute lung injury during a critical time of development. Lung injury results from complex interactions among several adverse stimuli, including inflammation, hyperoxia, mechanical ventilation, and infection in the developing lung (see Fig. 50-2).[6] Premature birth alters cell growth and differentiation and results in permanent alterations of lung structure, including impaired alveolar development and vessel growth. This change contributes to the long-term abnormalities of lung structure and function seen in BPD. Several characteristics of the immature lung initially increase the susceptibility of the premature newborn to the development of BPD. Perhaps one of the most critical factors relates to deficiency or dysfunction of lung surfactant. Surfactant dysfunction causes atelectasis, impairs ventilation and gas exchange, aggravates lung injury, and promotes inflammation. Maturation-related decreases in host antioxidant defenses and impaired epithelial function also contribute to lung injury, abnormal ion and water transport, and increased lung edema. Severe prematurity impairs lung mechanics; these impairments include increased compliance of the chest wall, which hinders spontaneous breathing and increases susceptibility for overdistention of the lung during mechanical ventilation. Thus, multiple intrinsic factors that are associated with prematurity increase the susceptibility for BPD. Major pathogenetic mechanisms that cause BPD are discussed as follows.

Prenatal Events

Subclinical intrauterine infection and the ensuing inflammatory response have been implicated clearly in the cause of preterm labor and premature rupture of membranes.[21,22] Growing evidence also supports the concept that prenatal infection and inflammation are major risk factors for the subsequent development of BPD. Although several investigators have found a lower incidence of RDS in preterm infants born to mothers with chorioamnionitis and funisitis (possibly resulting from an adaptive response to in utero stress), they also observed a significantly higher incidence of BPD in the same infants.[23] This suggests that although intrauterine infection may accelerate lung maturation, inflammation may also "prime" the lung, causing lung injury, progressive inflammation, and subsequent inhibition of lung growth.

Antenatal exposure of the lung to proinflammatory cytokines has been found to be a major risk factor for the development of BPD. Ghezzi and associates found that amniotic fluid interleukin-8 (IL-8) levels in mothers whose fetuses developed BPD were higher than those in mothers whose newborns did not develop BPD.[24] Newborns exposed to elevated amniotic fluid tumor necrosis factor α levels and infection have been found to have an increased incidence of BPD in comparison with nonexposed infants.[22] Injection of endotoxin into the amniotic fluid of pregnant sheep before delivery has been shown to significantly increase lung compliance (59%), gas volume (twofold), and concentrations of surfactant.[25] These effects were stronger than those achieved from the maturation-enhancing effects of antenatal betamethasone. White blood cell counts and several inflammatory cytokine levels were increased in the fetal membranes and lungs after endotoxin exposure, which suggests that endotoxin-induced inflammation may induce lung maturation through increased inflammation. Despite these acute physiologic effects, early endotoxin and cytokine exposure may also impair subsequent lung growth. Similar patterns of cytokine expression have been observed in newborns who subsequently developed cerebral palsy, which suggests that prenatal exposure to cytokines may represent a common pathway for the initiation of preterm labor, injury to the lung, and damage to the developing central nervous system of the fetus.

The use of antenatal corticosteroids has been shown to enhance fetal lung maturation and lower the risk for developing RDS, but the effects on the incidence of BPD are more controversial.[26] Antenatal treatment with betamethasone has been repeatedly shown to have multiple, direct beneficial effects on the fetal lung, including improved lung compliance, lung volumes, surfactant production, and antioxidant enzyme activity.[26,27] Betamethasone may also prevent lung damage in the fetus indirectly by reducing maternal cytokine production and exposure in the fetus or by altering gene expression of critical growth factors and their receptors. Repetitive courses of prenatal corticosteroids have also been used routinely and are associated with further improvements in lung mechanics and reduced oxidative stress in the lung.[28] However, multiple courses of antenatal steroids do appear to significantly reduce both somatic and lung growth in the fetus, which may be detrimental to long-term pulmonary function.[29] Clinical data have failed to confirm a report that antenatal glucocorticoid treatment reduces the risk of BPD and may worsen long-term neurodevelopmental outcome.[30]

Hyperoxia and Oxidant Stress

Postnatal exposure to adverse stimuli, such as hyperoxia or ischemia-reperfusion injury, contributes to the development of BPD. Under normal conditions, a delicate balance exists between the production of reactive oxygen species (ROS) and protective antioxidant defense systems. Damage caused by ROS includes cell membrane destruction, mitochondrial injury, protein nitration, inactivation of growth factors, and modification of nucleic acids.[31] The premature infant appears to be especially susceptible to ROS-induced damage because of the lack of adequate antioxidants after premature birth. Frank and Groseclose studied the development of the antioxidant enzymes superoxide dismutase (SOD), catalase, and glutathione peroxidase in the lungs of rabbits during late gestation.[32] The marked increase in these enzymes during the latter part of gestation parallels the maturation pattern of pulmonary surfactant (Fig. 50-6). These developmental changes in the fetal lung allow proper ventilation by reducing surface tension and provide for the transition from the relative hypoxia of intrauterine development to the oxygen-rich extrauterine environment. The ability to increase synthesis of antioxidant enzymes in response to hyperoxia is decreased in preterm animals.[33] Premature birth precedes the normal up-regulation of these antioxidant systems and other ROS scavengers (e.g., vitamin E, ascorbic acid, glutathione, and ceruloplasmin) and may result in an imbalance between oxidants and antioxidants and an increased risk for the development of BPD (Table 50-2).[34] Experimental animal models have shown that exposure to chronic hyperoxia can induce inflammation and lung injury that has many features seen in infants who develop BPD. Endothelial and type II cells are both extremely susceptible to ROS, leading to increased-permeability edema and cell dysfunction. Hyperoxia also impairs mucociliary function, promotes inflammation, and inactivates antiproteases, further complicating clinical outcome.

Clinical studies suggest that ROS are involved in the pathogenesis of BPD. Plasma concentrations of allantoin, an oxidation by-product of uric acid, have been shown to be significantly elevated in the first 48 hours after birth in infants who develop BPD, in comparison with controls.[35] Expired pentane and ethane have also been measured as indirect evidence of free radical–induced lipid peroxidation in the first week after birth and have been found to

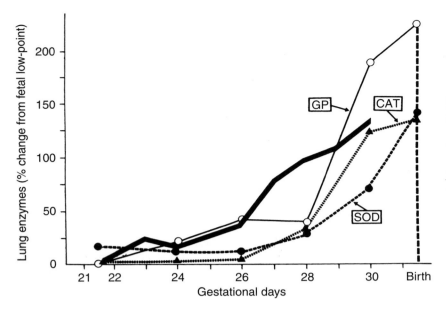

Figure 50–6. Maturation patterns of antioxidant enzymes—superoxide dismutase (SOD), catalase (CAT), glutathione peroxidase (GP)—in comparison with pulmonary surfactant (*dark black line*). (*Adapted from Frank L, Groseclose EE: Preparation for birth into an O₂-rich environment: The antioxidant enzymes in the developing rabbit lung. Pediatr Res 18:240, 1984.*)

be significantly elevated in neonates who subsequently develop BPD.[36] Varsila and colleagues analyzed proteins in tracheal aspirates in the first week of life and found evidence of protein oxidation (carbonyl formation) in infants who develop chronic lung disease.[37] Banks and associates found a fourfold increase in plasma 3-nitrotyrosine concentration in infants who developed BPD in comparison with controls, which indicates evidence of increased reactive nitrogen species (endogenous nitric oxide reacting with superoxide) that modify serum proteins.[38] Most important, the multicenter Supplemental Therapeutic Oxygen for Prethreshold Retinopathy Of Prematurity (STOP-ROP) trial examined whether exposing premature infants to higher inspired oxygen concentrations would prevent the development of severe retinopathy of prematurity. Although the effects of the increased oxygen on the eyes were minimal, exposed infants had dramatic increases (55%) in the incidence of BPD and pulmonary infections.[39] These studies all demonstrate that ROS are

intimately involved in the development of acute and chronic lung disease in newborn infants.

Further evidence for the role of ROS in lung injury comes from several studies that have shown that antioxidant supplementation with SOD and catalase reduces cell damage, increases survival, and prevents lung injury from prolonged hyperoxia and mechanical ventilation.[40-42] In addition, genetically engineered mice overexpressing either copper-zinc SOD (CuZnSOD) or manganese SOD survive longer, whereas mice with disrupted CuZnSOD genes die more rapidly in a hyperoxic environment than do normal diploid controls.[43-45] All of these studies confirmed the critical role of the intricate balance between the production of ROS and antioxidant defenses in the development of lung injury.

Volutrauma

Although the initial signs of lung injury in BPD reflect the primary disease process (e.g., RDS), the treatment of premature newborns with positive-pressure mechanical ventilation contributes to the severity of lung injury and can provoke a complex inflammatory cascade that leads to BPD. Pneumothorax and pulmonary interstitial edema are strongly associated with BPD, which suggests that ventilator-induced lung injury can contribute to BPD.[46-48]

Nilsson and colleagues showed that even brief periods of positive-pressure ventilation cause bronchiolar epithelial damage in the lung, in which the severity of the injury is correlated with the amount of peak pressure used.[49] Positive-pressure ventilation exposes the lung to cyclic stretch stress, caused by changes in both airway pressure and volume, which damage small airways and distal air spaces. Surfactant deficiency further contributes to persistent atelectasis, causing more injury as a result of cyclic reinflation and overdistention of inflated lung regions. Even with normal tidal volumes, ventilation of the immature or injured newborn lung results in nonuniform inflation and relative overdistention of ventilated

Table 50–2. Reactive Oxygen Species

Radical	Symbol*	Antioxidant
Superoxide anion	O_2	Superoxide dismutase, uric acid, vitamin E
Singlet oxygen	$^1O_2$	β-Carotene, uric acid, vitamin E
Hydrogen peroxide	H_2O_2	Catalase, glutathione peroxidase, glutathione
Hydroxyl radical	$OH^\bullet$	Vitamins C and E
Peroxide radical	$LOO^\bullet$	Vitamins C and E
Hydroperoxyl radical	$LOOH$	Glutathione transferase, glutathione peroxidase

*L, lipid.

segments, especially in the presence of low functional residual capacity (FRC). Stretching of capillary endothelium and distal lung epithelium increases permeability to serum proteins that may further inhibit surfactant function, creating a vicious cycle that promotes lung injury. Mechanical ventilation with high tidal volumes, especially with poorly recruited lung as a result of low positive end-expiratory pressure (PEEP), stimulates lung cytokine production.[50]

The adverse effects of tidal volume breaths in lungs with low FRC can be decreased with better lung recruitment after the application of higher levels of PEEP. Experimental studies have clearly shown that overdistention of these lung regions (not increased pressure) is responsible for lung injury in the surfactant-deficient lung.[48] For example, strapping the chest wall to restrict overexpansion increases lung pressure but limits lung stretch and ameliorates lung injury in animal models.[51,52] Tremblay and associates observed that mechanical ventilation with high tidal volumes and low PEEP markedly increases lung edema and cytokine expression.[50] In the same model, lung injury increases cytokine release from the lungs into the systemic circulation, which is suggestive of a potential mechanism linking multiorgan dysfunction and sepsis syndrome with lung injury. A National Institutes of Health–sponsored trial showed improved survival of adults with acute RDS with a ventilator strategy in which low tidal volumes with high PEEP levels were used in order to recruit atelectatic lung regions and to maintain FRC.[53] This suggests that the damaging effects of oxygen and mechanical ventilation in the lung occur via similar pathways, involving primarily activation of the inflammatory cascade that ultimately leads to the development of acute lung injury and BPD. Lung-protective strategies, including the use of high-frequency ventilation, permissive hypercapnia, prone position, and inhaled nitric oxide (iNO) are currently under investigation (see later discussion).

Strategies to prevent lung injury have included changes in methods of ventilation. Even brief exposure to large volume breaths during resuscitation shortly after birth can initiate early lung injury, which decreases the subsequent response to surfactant therapy.[54] With the increased use of nasal continuous positive airway pressure (CPAP), many preterm infants can be managed without the need for endotracheal intubation and mechanical ventilation, which may lessen the risk for lung injury. Synchronized intermittent mechanical ventilation and high-frequency devices have been extensively studied. Bernstein and associates reported that infants weighing less than 1000 g who were treated with synchronized intermittent mechanical ventilation developed BPD at lower rates than did those receiving conventional ventilation.[55] Several multicenter trials have demonstrated that high-frequency oscillatory ventilation or high-frequency jet ventilation in which high-volume alveolar recruitment strategies were used in conjunction with surfactant replacement therapy reduced complications of mechanical ventilation (pulmonary interstitial emphysema, pneumothorax) and lowered the incidence of BPD, in comparison with conventional ventilation.[56,57] However, these findings have not been consistently found in other trials.

Regardless of the type of ventilation strategy used, it is imperative to avoid even brief periods of overdistention, because high tidal volumes and hypocarbia are associated with a greater risk of developing both lung and neurologic injury.[48,50,58] A retrospective study of 1105 newborns born with birth weights less than 2000 g between 1984 and 1987 demonstrated a strong relationship between prolonged, cumulative exposure to hypocapnia (arterial carbon dioxide pressure < 35 mm Hg) and "disabling" cerebral palsy.[59] This study also noted that hypocapnia, hyperoxia, and duration of mechanical ventilation were independently associated with a twofold to threefold increase in risk for cerebral palsy.

The use of surfactant replacement therapy has reduced some complications of mechanical ventilation. Surfactant permits more equal distribution of pressures and ventilation to all alveoli, prevents overdistention of distal air spaces and bronchioles, and stabilizes lung volume. A major benefit of surfactant therapy has been the ability to reduce airway pressures without causing atelectasis, to maintain greater uniformity of lung recruitment, and to reduce air leak. However, BPD continues to be an important problem despite the widespread use of exogenous surfactant and strategies to minimize lung injury by using mechanical ventilation (i.e., permissive hypercapnia).[60] Van Marter and associates studied 452 premature infants weighing 500 to 1500 g at birth who were born at specific neonatal centers in either Boston or New York. They found that the incidence of BPD was significantly higher in Boston (22%) than in New York (4%), even after adjusting for baseline risk factors, such as severity of prematurity.[61] In multivariate analyses to examine differences in specific respiratory care practices during the first week after birth, most of the increased risk of BPD was found to be associated with the early initiation of mechanical ventilation. Interestingly, the use of both exogenous surfactant and indomethacin increased the risk for BPD. This study suggests that attempts to minimize the use of mechanical ventilation by using nasal CPAP (with or without exogenous surfactant) may lower the incidence and severity of BPD in infants at high risk. Ongoing multicenter trials of early CPAP after preterm birth are under way.

Inflammation

Although hyperoxia and volutrauma directly injure the neonatal lung, these effects are in part mediated and potentiated by the recruitment and activation of inflammatory cells and the release of potent inflammatory products.[62-65] A sustained increase in the neutrophil number in tracheal fluid samples distinguishes infants who develop BPD from those with mild RDS.[66,67] In addition, the presence of activated macrophages, high concentrations of lipid products, inactivated α_1-antitrypsin activity, and other markers of active inflammation are strongly linked with the development of BPD.[2,64] More recently, increased proinflammatory cytokines, such as interleukin-8 and decreased interleukin-10 levels, have been recovered in the tracheal fluid of infants who subsequently developed BPD.[68] Release of early-response cytokines, such as tumor necrosis factor α, interleukin-1β,

IL-8, and transforming growth factor β, by macrophages and the presence of soluble adhesion molecules (e.g., selectins) may influence other cells to release chemoattractants and recruit neutrophils, which further amplify the inflammatory response.[64,67,69-75] Elevated concentrations of proinflammatory cytokines in conjunction with reduced anti-inflammatory products (e.g., interleukin-10) usually appear in tracheal aspirates within a few hours after birth in infants who subsequently develop BPD.[65,74,75] Sunday and colleagues studied preterm baboons who developed BPD and found increased numbers of neuroendocrine cells in the lung, which release bombesin-like peptides.[76] Administration of specific antibodies that blocked the action of these peptides was associated with a decrease in the severity of lung injury in this animal model of BPD. All these agents and the activated leukocytes that accompany them cause significant pulmonary damage, including breakdown of capillary endothelial integrity and leakage of macromolecules (e.g., albumin) into alveolar spaces. Albumin leakage and pulmonary edema are known to inhibit surfactant function and have been postulated to be important factors in the development of BPD.[77]

The release of elastase and collagenase from activated neutrophils may directly destroy the elastin and collagen framework of the lung. Markers of collagen and elastin degradation have been recovered in the urine of infants with BPD.[78,79] The major defense against the action of elastase activity is α_1-proteinase inhibitor, which may be inactivated by ROS.[80-82] Increased elastase activity accompanied by compromised antiproteinase function may result in an imbalance that has been demonstrated in tracheal aspirates and serum of infants who develop BPD.[83] Therapy with exogenous antiproteases could potentially restore this delicate balance and prevent the development of BPD. This hypothesis has been tested in a pilot study in which treatment of premature neonates with intravenous doses of α_1-proteinase inhibitor during the first 2 weeks after birth produced a trend toward reductions in the incidence of BPD and the duration of ventilator support.[83] These mechanisms may play a major role in the disruption of alveolar septa or saccules, which contributes to regional emphysema.

Marked inflammation in the lung and inhibition of alveolar development appear to begin a cascade of destruction and abnormal repair that develops into BPD. The initial trigger that activates lung inflammation may be ROS, mechanical ventilation, infectious agents, or other adverse stimuli that attract and activate inflammatory cells, including leukocytes, macrophages, and fibroblasts. Neutrophils and macrophages cause additional release of ROS and diverse mediators, thereby amplifying injury. There is evidence that eosinophils may also play a role in the development of BPD.[69] Fibroblast activation can lead to striking fibroproliferation and remodeling of the immature lung after injury, including altered matrix production in the airway, vasculature, and interstitium. As the acute cycle of injury continues with further production and accumulation of inflammatory mediators, significant injury to the lung can occur during a particularly critical period of rapid growth (i.e., six divisions from 24 to 40 weeks of gestation). Watterberg and

associates demonstrated that extremely premature infants have evidence of adrenal insufficiency at birth; the lowest serum cortisol concentrations during the first week of life are correlated with increased lung inflammation and adverse respiratory outcome.[84] Pilot studies examining early treatment with low-dose hydrocortisone in infants with extremely low birth weights increased the likelihood of survival without BPD, a benefit that was particularly apparent in infants born to mothers with chorioamnionitis.[85] The mechanisms underlying this observation are uncertain but may include suppression of lung inflammation with less inhibition of lung growth than observed with higher doses of steroids, beneficial effects of low-dose hydrocortisone on lung development, or other medications. Larger multicenter trials have currently been suspended due to increased adverse events in infants receiving hydrocortisone (e.g., gastrointestinal perforation). However, these studies clearly support the notion that this abnormal inflammatory process is primarily responsible for the acute and the chronic changes that occur in the lungs of infants with BPD.

Infection

The potential role of infection in the pathogenesis of BPD has been suggested in reports that link colonization with *Ureaplasma urealyticum* to increased risk for subsequent development of BPD. *U. urealyticum* has been recovered from cervical cultures of pregnant women and implicated as a possible cause of chorioamnionitis, prematurity, and BPD.[86,87] Several investigators have cultured the upper genital tract of mothers before delivery and the tracheal aspirates from preterm infants after delivery and found that BPD developed significantly more often in infants colonized with *U. urealyticum* than in those with negative cultures.[87] In addition, studies have demonstrated that premature infants born to mothers with premature rupture of the membranes who had received prenatal erythromycin (which is effective against *U. urealyticum*) had a lower incidence of BPD than did untreated controls.[88] In contrast, other studies have found that although *U. urealyticum* was frequently detected (by culture or polymerase chain reaction) in many infants with low birth weights, its presence was not associated with the development of BPD.[89,90] Other investigators have suggested that both prenatal and postnatal infections act as a potent stimulus for the inflammatory response, with recruitment of leukocytes, release of ROS, and activation of the arachidonic cascade, ultimately leading to BPD. Because preterm infants are relatively immunodeficient at birth (at both cellular and humoral levels), they are much more susceptible to colonization and subsequent infection with a variety of infectious agents (e.g., virus, bacteria, fungi) that may affect the severity of BPD.[91] Both Rojas and associates and Gonzalez and colleagues demonstrated that bacteremia with low-virulence organisms, persistence of a patent ductus arteriosus, and degree of prematurity were strongly associated with development of BPD in the surfactant era (Fig. 50-7).[15,91]

Nutrition

Premature infants have increased nutritional requirements because of increased metabolic needs and rapid

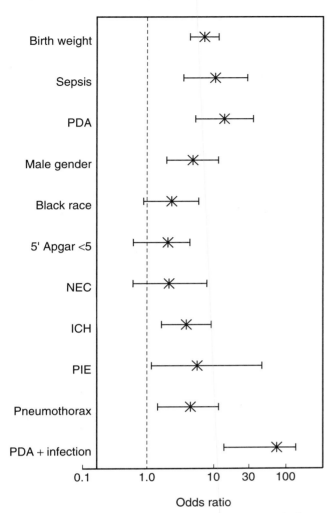

Figure 50–7. Odds ratios (*stars*) and 95% confidence intervals demonstrating increased risk of bronchopulmonary dysplasia with decreasing gestational age, the presence of a patent ductus arteriosus (PDA), and neonatal infection. ICH, intracranial hemorrhage; NEC, necrotizing enterocolitis; PIE, pulmonary interstitial emphysema; 5′, 5-minute. (*Adapted from Bancalari E, Gonzalez A: Clinical course and lung function abnormalities during development of chronic lung disease. In Bland RD, Coalson JJ [eds]: Chronic Lung Disease in Early Infancy. New York, Marcel Dekker, 2000, pp 41-64.*)

growth requirements. Severe lung disease may further increase energy expenditures (e.g., increased work of breathing) in infants with limited nutritional reserves. If these increased energy needs are not met by exogenous sources, a catabolic state develops in the infant; this is probably a major contributing factor to the pathogenesis of BPD. Inadequate nutrition, which could interfere with normal growth and maturation of the lung, may potentiate the deleterious effects of oxygen. Newborn rats with inadequate caloric intake have decreased lung weights, protein levels, and DNA content.[92] These abnormalities were even more extensive in pups that were nutritionally deprived at birth and then exposed to hyperoxia.

Antioxidant enzymes play a vital role in the protection of the lung, and many of these enzymes have trace elements (e.g., copper, zinc, selenium) that are an integral part of their structure. Deficiencies in these elements may predispose the lung to further injury, whereas supplementation may provide protection to the lung and prevent hyperoxic lung damage.[93,94] The repair of elastin and collagen is limited in animals that are undernourished, and copper and zinc may be necessary for this repair.[95] Vitamin deficiency has also been postulated to be important in the development of BPD. Current nursery feeding and hyperalimentation regimens appear to provide adequate amounts of vitamin E for preterm infants.[96,97] However, concentrations of vitamin A, which appears to be important in maintaining cell integrity and in tissue repair, may be deficient in premature neonates.[98] Several investigators have found lower serum retinol levels in cord blood and in the first month after birth in infants who subsequently developed BPD.[99,100] Despite adequate supplementation, some infants remain vitamin A deficient, presumably because of increased absorption of parenteral vitamin A into the tubing of the intravenous administration set or because of higher nutritional requirements. A multicenter trial of vitamin A supplementation in premature infants at risk for developing BPD demonstrated that large doses of intramuscular vitamin A given three times per week was associated with a small (7%) but significant reduction in the incidence of BPD, which suggests that vitamin A deficiency is a contributor to lung injury.[101]

Large volumes of intravenous fluids are often administered to premature infants to provide adequate fluid requirements (because of increased insensible water losses) and sufficient calories. Excessive fluid administration can be associated with the development of a patent ductus arteriosus and pulmonary edema, which lead to increased oxygen and ventilator requirements and the development of BPD.[102] Early closure of the ductus with indomethacin or surgical ligation has been associated with improvements in pulmonary function, but these approaches have not affected the incidence of BPD.

Genetic Factors

Past studies have implied that preterm neonates were more likely to develop BPD if there was a strong family history of atopy and asthma. Nickerson and Taussig found a positive family history of asthma in 77% of infants with RDS who subsequently developed BPD, in comparison with only 33% of those who did not.[103] Bertrand and coworkers evaluated the relationship between (1) prematurity, RDS, and need for mechanical ventilation and (2) a family history of airway hyperactivity.[104] The severity of lung disease was directly related to the degree of prematurity and the duration of oxygen exposure. However, siblings and mothers of infants with the most significant lung disease had evidence of airway reactivity, which suggests that all three factors are involved in determining long-term outcome. When histocompatibility loci were examined, Clark and associates found that only infants with human leukocyte antigen A_2 developed BPD, which again suggests that other underlying factors that are poorly understood may be important in the pathogenesis of BPD.[105] More recently, Hagan and colleagues reported that a family history of asthma is associated with an increase in the overall severity of BPD in premature infants but does not appear to be a causative factor.[106] With technologic advances in genomics, proteomics, and bioinformatics, more information on the contribution of genetic factors to the risk of developing BPD should be forthcoming.

PATHOPHYSIOLOGY

Airway Disease and Lung Mechanics

Chronic respiratory signs in children with BPD include tachypnea with shallow breathing, retractions, and paradoxical breathing pattern; coarse rhonchi, rales, and wheezes are typically heard on auscultation. Persistent abnormalities in lung mechanics and impaired gas exchange often necessitate treatment with oxygen therapy and ventilator support. Increased airway resistance and bronchial hyperreactivity can be demonstrated even during the first week after birth in preterm neonates at risk for BPD.[107] These abnormalities are common in older infants with BPD and can cause dynamic airway collapse and expiratory flow limitation (Fig. 50-8).[108] Other abnormalities of lung function include increased dead space ventilation, decreased lung compliance, maldistribution of ventilation, and abnormal ventilation-perfusion matching. FRC is often reduced early in the course as a result of atelectasis, but it increases during the later stages of BPD as a result of gas trapping with hyperinflation. Increased respiratory rate with shallow breathing increases dead space ventilation that results from marked regional variability with time constants and decreased lung surface area. Nonuniform damage to the airways and distal lungs results in variable time constants for different areas of the lungs, which alter the distribution of inspired gas to relatively poorly perfused lung and worsen ventilation-perfusion matching.

Two methods used to measure lung compliance include dynamic measurements and passive expiratory techniques after airway occlusion. Both methods show a reduction of lung compliance in infants with BPD. The decrease in lung compliance appears to correlate well with morphologic and radiographic changes in the lung. Compliance can be reduced because of increased resistance, with frequency dependence of compliance when infants are breathing rapidly. The use of pulmonary function testing to monitor the progression of BPD and the response of the lung to various therapeutic interventions has become more widespread. However, care must be exercised in the interpretation of results because of inherent variability in the measurements and possible error from excessive chest wall distortion.

Infants with BPD demonstrate abnormal findings on clinical examination, chest radiograph, pulmonary function testing, echocardiogram, and morphologic examination of the lung. A clinical scoring system to categorize the severity of BPD was developed by Toce and colleagues (Table 50-3).[109] Infants with BPD are tachypneic and may have intercostal and subcostal retractions. Accessory muscles may be used to assist with respiration. Infants can be hypoxic and hypercarbic and may grow poorly despite adequate caloric intake. The Toce system attempts to standardize clinical assessment, and a severity score can be assigned to each infant at 28 days of postnatal age and at 36 weeks of postmenstrual age. The clinical assessment should be adjusted if infants are receiving multiple medications for BPD (e.g., diuretics, methylxanthines, or corticosteroids), nasal CPAP, or positive-pressure mechanical ventilation.

Radiographic Changes

Radiographic abnormalities characteristic of BPD were first described by Northway and colleagues in 1967, who documented the progression of the disease process through four distinct stages.[1] The radiographic progression of BPD is now seldom categorized by these four stages; instead, it has been refined to reflect the severity of

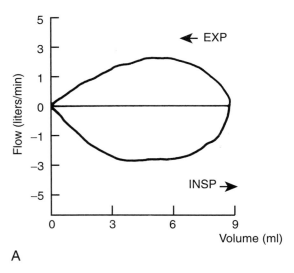

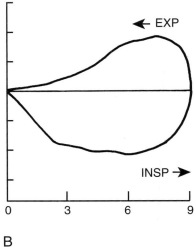

Figure 50–8. Expiratory airflow limitation in infant with bronchopulmonary dysplasia. **A,** Normal flow-volume loop. **B,** Expiratory flow limitation caused by collapse of small airways during expiration. EXP, expiration; INSP, inspiration. *(From Tepper RS, Morgan WJ, Cota K, Taussig LM: Expiratory flow limitation in infants with bronchopulmonary dysplasia. J Pediatr 109:1040, 1986.)*

A

B

Table 50–3. Bronchopulmonary Dysplasia Clinical Scoring System

Variable	Score*			
	0 (Normal)	1 (Mild)	2 (Moderate)	3 (Severe)
Respiratory rate (average number/minute)	<40	40-60	61-80	>80
Dyspnea (retractions)	0	Mild	Moderate	Severe
FIO_2 (Pao_2 50-70 mm Hg)	0.21	0.22-0.30	0.31-0.50	>0.50
$Paco_2$ (mm Hg)	<45	46-55	56-70	>70
Growth rate (g/day)	>25	15-24	5-14	<5

*Score at 28 days of age or at 36 weeks of postmenstrual age. Score is a mean of four measures for respiratory rate, dyspnea, and FIO_2 obtained at 6-hr intervals. Growth rate represents average daily weight gain over a 7-day period before the assignment of the score is 15. A score of 15 is assigned if the patient is receiving mechanical ventilation.

FIO_2, fraction of inspired oxygen; $Paco_2$, arterial carbon dioxide pressure; Pao_2, arterial oxygen pressure.

From Toce SS, Farrell PM, Leavitt LA, et al: Clinical and roentgenographic scoring systems for assessing BPD. Am J Dis Child 138:581, 1984.

the disease process. Most radiologists evaluate the four most prominent radiographic findings in BPD: lung expansion, emphysema (including bleb formation), interstitial densities, and cardiovascular abnormalities. The occurrence of hyperinflation or interstitial abnormalities on chest radiograph appears to be correlated with the development of airway obstruction later in life. Because the severity of BPD has continued to change so significantly since the early 1990s, Weinstein and associates developed an updated scoring system, incorporating some of the more subtle radiographic signs that are often seen today in infants with BPD.[110] The utility of this scoring system remains to be demonstrated.

Computed tomography (CT) and magnetic resonance imaging (MRI) of the lung may provide more details of the structural disease in BPD and can reveal significant abnormalities that are not readily apparent on chest radiographs. These findings can be important in determining ultimate pulmonary morbidity. CT often shows regional heterogeneity, with regions of hyperinflation or emphysema and sparse arterial density alternating with relatively normal-appearing regions. MRI of ventilated premature newborns may demonstrate striking regional variations in lung disease, with marked gravity-dependent atelectasis and edema. More studies of the role of CT and MRI in BPD are needed to correlate structural and functional changes.

Pulmonary Circulation

In addition to adverse effects on the airway and distal airspace, acute lung injury also impairs growth, structure and function of the developing pulmonary circulation after premature birth.[111] Endothelial cells have been shown to be particularly susceptible to oxidant injury from hyperoxia or inflammation. The media of small pulmonary arteries may also undergo striking changes, including smooth muscle cell proliferation, precocious maturation of immature pericytes into mature smooth muscle cells, and incorporation of fibroblasts into the vessel wall.[112-114] Structural changes in the lung vasculature contribute to high pulmonary vascular resistance (PVR) as a result of narrowing of the vessel diameter and

decreased vascular compliance. In addition to these structural changes, the pulmonary circulation is further characterized by abnormal vasoreactivity, which also increases PVR (Fig. 50-9).[115,116] Finally, decreased angiogenesis may limit vascular surface area, causing further elevations of PVR, especially in response to high cardiac output with exercise or stress.

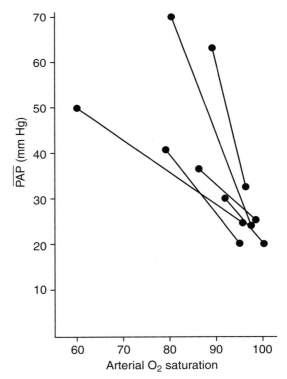

Figure 50–9. Effects of oxygen tension on pulmonary vascular resistance (PVR) in infants with bronchopulmonary dysplasia (BPD). Infants with severe BPD often have elevated basal PVR despite treatment with supplemental oxygen, and even brief decreases in fraction of inspired O_2 can cause marked elevations of PVR. $\overline{PAP}$, pulmonary artery pressure. *(From Abman SH, Wolfe RR, Accurso FJ, et al: Pulmonary vascular response to oxygen in infants with severe BPD. Pediatrics 75:80, 1985.)*

Overall, early injury to the lung circulation leads to the rapid development of pulmonary hypertension, which contributes significantly to the morbidity and mortality from severe BPD. Even in the earliest reports of BPD, pulmonary hypertension and cor pulmonale were recognized as being associated with high rates of mortality.[115,116] Walther and coworkers showed that elevated pulmonary artery pressure in premature newborns with acute RDS (determined from serial echocardiograms) was associated with severe disease and high rates of mortality.[117] Past studies have also shown that persistent echocardiographic evidence of pulmonary hypertension beyond the first few months after birth is associated with up to a 40% rate of mortality among infants with BPD.[118] High rates of mortality have also been reported in infants with BPD and pulmonary hypertension who require prolonged ventilator support.[119] Although pulmonary hypertension is a marker of more advanced BPD, elevated PVR also causes poor right ventricular function, impairs cardiac output, limits oxygen delivery, increases pulmonary edema, and, perhaps, heightens the risk for sudden death.

Physiologic abnormalities of the pulmonary circulation in BPD include elevated PVR and abnormal vasoreactivity, as evidenced by the marked vasoconstrictor response to acute hypoxia.[115,116] Cardiac catheterization studies have shown that even mild hypoxia causes marked elevations in pulmonary artery pressure, even in infants with modest basal levels of pulmonary hypertension. Treatment levels of oxygen saturation above 92% to 94% effectively lower pulmonary artery pressure.[116] Strategies to lower pulmonary artery pressure or limit lung injury (e.g., inhaled nitric oxide) to the pulmonary vasculature may limit the subsequent development of pulmonary hypertension in BPD.

In addition to pulmonary hypertension, clinical studies have also shown that the metabolic function of the pulmonary circulation is impaired, as reflected by the impaired clearance of circulating norepinephrine across the lung.[120] Normally, 20% to 40% of circulating norepinephrine is cleared during a single passage through the lung, but infants with severe BPD have a net production of norepinephrine across the pulmonary circulation. It is unknown whether impaired metabolic function of the lung contributes to the pathophysiologic processes of BPD by increasing circulating catecholamine levels or whether it is simply a marker of severe pulmonary vascular disease. It has been speculated that high catecholamine levels may lead to left ventricular hypertrophy or systemic hypertension, which are known complications of BPD (see next section).

Cardiovascular Abnormalities

In addition to pulmonary vascular disease and right ventricular hypertrophy, other cardiovascular abnormalities that are associated with BPD include left ventricular hypertrophy, systemic hypertension, and the development of prominent systemic-to-pulmonary collateral vessels.[121-123] An early report described infants with severe BPD and left ventricular hypertrophy in the absence of right ventricular hypertrophy and suggested that left ventricular dysfunction may contribute to recurrent edema in BPD.[123] Steroid therapy can cause left ventricular hypertrophy, which tends to be transient and resolves when the drug is stopped.

A high incidence of systemic hypertension can occur in BPD, but its cause remains obscure.[124] Systemic hypertension may be mild, transient, or striking and usually responds to pharmacologic therapy. On occasion, further evaluation of such infants may reveal significant renal vascular or urinary tract disease. Whether the high incidence of systemic hypertension in BPD reflects altered neurohumoral regulation or increased levels of catecholamines, angiotensin, or antidiuretic hormone is still unknown.

Prominent bronchial or other systemic-to-pulmonary collateral vessels were noted in early morphometric studies of infants with BPD and can be readily identified in many infants during cardiac catheterization.[119,121] Although these collateral vessels are generally small, large collateral vessels may contribute to significant shunting of blood flow to the lung, causing edema and a need for a higher fraction of inspired oxygen. Collateral vessels have been associated with high rates of mortality among some patients with severe BPD who also had severe pulmonary hypertension.[119] Some infants have shown improvement after embolization of large collateral vessels, as reflected by a reduced need for supplemental oxygen, ventilator support, or diuretics. However, the actual contribution of collateral vessels to the pathophysiologic processes of BPD is poorly understood.

TREATMENT

In addition to chronic respiratory disease, infants with BPD have significant growth, nutritional, neurodevelopmental, and cardiovascular problems. The severity of respiratory disease varies widely among infants with BPD. In its most severe manifestation, children with BPD may require home ventilation or prolonged home oxygen therapy. Even infants who have been weaned off supplemental oxygen therapy have recurrent hospitalizations for lower respiratory exacerbations caused by viral infections, including respiratory syncytial virus and influenza, reactive airways disease, or pulmonary hypertension and congestive heart failure. In addition, persistent or recurrent respiratory exacerbations may also be caused by structural lesions (i.e., tracheomalacia, subglottic stenosis, bronchomalacia), chronic aspiration (gastroesophageal reflux or swallowing dysfunction), or other conditions. In addition to supplemental oxygen therapy, ongoing treatment with bronchodilators, diuretics, inhaled or systemic steroids, and nutritional supplements is commonly used as supportive therapy. Although some studies have suggested that the early use of postnatal steroids may reduce the incidence and severity of BPD, significant concerns exist regarding adverse effects, including bowel perforation and worsened neurodevelopmental outcome.[125,126] Therapeutic approaches to infants with BPD are described as follows.

Oxygen Therapy

Supplemental oxygen to avoid intermittent or prolonged periods of hypoxemia remains the mainstay of BPD therapy. Adverse effects of hypoxemia include pulmonary hypertension with cor pulmonale, poor somatic growth, impaired lung growth, bronchoconstriction, and a greater frequency of apnea or cyanotic episodes.[127-129] During long-term therapy, frequent assessments of oxygenation are needed to ensure adequate oxygenation. In general, supplemental oxygen is administered to maintain oxygen saturation levels above 92% during wakeful periods, during feedings, and during sleep. Higher oxygen saturation levels (>94%) are generally recommended for patients with right ventricular hypertrophy, pulmonary hypertension, poor growth, apneic episodes, and other problems. One study (the STOP-ROP trial) examined the role of oxygen therapy in retinopathy of prematurity, and the results suggested that infants who were treated with supplemental oxygen to maintain oxygen saturation levels above 95% had a higher risk for chronic lung disease than did infants treated with supplemental oxygen that maintained lower saturation levels.[39] However, interpretation of these data in the setting of preventing or treating infants with pulmonary hypertension are limited, inasmuch as the targeted ranges for the groups maintaining low and high oxygen saturation fell between typical recommendations for oxygen therapy. The current recommendation for treatment of patients with BPD and pulmonary hypertension is to maintain oxygen saturation levels at 92% to 96%. Whether higher oxygen saturation levels increase lung injury remains unproven, but the adverse effects of hypoxemia are clear.

Past studies have suggested that most infants with BPD show steady improvement in lung function and discontinue supplemental oxygen by 6 to 12 months.[127-129] Patients who fail to be weaned off supplemental oxygen, especially those with recurrent hospitalizations, poor growth, right ventricular hypertrophy, and other signs, should be evaluated for unsuspected cardiac or pulmonary problems that are slowing their recovery. Such evaluations should include prolonged pulse oximetry (especially during sleep), assessment of pulmonary mechanics, sleep studies, laryngoscopy and bronchoscopy, swallowing studies, pH probes, echocardiography, sweat tests, and serum immunoglobulin measurements.

Mechanical Ventilation

With established disease, patients with BPD who require prolonged ventilatory assistance generally require larger tidal volume breaths and a slower rate to enhance the distribution of gas because of heterogeneity of lung units. Ventilation of infants with severe BPD with fast rates and smaller tidal volumes increases dead space ventilation and may worsen gas exchange and increase gas trapping. Slow weaning of ventilatory support should allow for better assessments of respiratory muscle strength and lung function over time. Flexible bronchoscopy is useful for determining whether structural airway disease is complicating the clinical course. Criteria for tracheostomy and chronic mechanical ventilation are controversial, but both measures are indicated in patients with BPD and severe respiratory failure, as reflected by chronic hypoventilation and hypercarbia. Additional findings of severe retractions, vocal cord paralysis, severe tracheomalacia, persistent signs of pulmonary hypertension, and problems handling secretions as a result of neurologic disease provide clinical markers for assessing the need for chronic support.

Pharmacologic Therapy

Multiple pharmacologic agents have been used in the treatment of infants with BPD, including diuretics, bronchodilators, and corticosteroids. Despite extensive investigations of drug therapy for BPD,[2,130] controversy persists regarding the role of these agents in the overall management of BPD. In addition, concerns regarding adverse effects and potential toxic effects persist. Medications should be added one at a time and discontinued if an adequate clinical response is not observed or measured after 2 to 3 days (Table 50-4).

Table 50–4. Commonly Used Medications for Bronchopulmonary Dysplasia

Medication	Dosage
Diuretics	
Furosemide	1.0-2.0 mg/kg/dose IV or PO (daily in infants <31 weeks postmenstrual age)
Chlorothiazide	5-20 mg/kg dose IV or PO bid
Hydrochlorothiazide	1-2 mg/kg/dose PO bid
Spironolactone	1.0 mg/kg/dose PO bid
Inhaled agents	
Albuterol	0.01-0.03 mL/kg/dose of a 0.5% solution diluted to 1-2 mL with half-normal or normal saline q4-6h
Systemic agents	
Aminophylline (IV), theophylline (PO)	LD 8 mg/kg; MD 2 mg/kg/dose q8-12h; goal is serum levels of 5-15 mg/L
Caffeine citrate	LD 20 mg/kg; MD 5 mg/kg IV or PO q24h; goal is serum level 10-20 mg/L
Dexamethasone	0.1-0.2 mg/kg/day IV or PO q12h for 2–3 days, decrease by 50% for 2-3 days, then decrease 50% again for 2-3 days

IV, intravenously; LD, loading dose; MD, maintenance dose; PO, per os (orally).

Diuretics

Diuretic therapy, including furosemide, hydrochloro-thiazide, and spironolactone, are commonly administered to infants with BPD. The overall rationale for therapy is to treat recurrent pulmonary edema that can worsen lung compliance and gas exchange. Increased fluid and salt retention, caused by hyperaldosteronism and elevated antidiuretic hormone release, can contribute to the development of pulmonary edema. Past studies have shown that diuretic therapy can acutely improve lung mechanics in infants with BPD, but the effects of some drugs may be independent of the diuretic response. However, such adverse effects as nephrocalcinosis, osteopenia, ototoxicity, hyponatremia, hypokalemia, hypochloremia, alkalosis, and impaired growth commonly complicate the course of treated infants. Metabolic alkalosis may impair respiratory drive and contribute to CO_2 retention. Use of furosemide therapy on alternate days, rather than as daily treatment, may optimize lung mechanics and gas exchange in infants with BPD while decreasing the frequency or severity of side effects.[131] The use of spironolactone in combination with furosemide or a thiazide diuretic may sustain the diuretic response and minimize potassium and calcium depletion. Sodium chloride supplements to treat electrolyte imbalance induced by diuretics should not be used.

Bronchodilators

Bronchodilator therapy, with β agonists, can reverse acute bronchospasm and improve airways resistance and respiratory system compliance in infants with BPD.[132] The physiologic abnormalities may be present as early as the first week of life in preterm neonates during mechanical ventilation.[107] However, the role of β agonists for chronic therapy is unproven, because most of the effects on lung mechanics are transient. Similarly, anticholinergic and methylxanthine therapies can improve lung mechanics in BPD infants, but whether prolonged therapy causes sustained improvement is uncertain. Older patients with BPD often have asthma, characterized by intermittent and reversible airways obstruction during acute respiratory exacerbations, and seem to be highly responsive to bronchodilator therapy.

Corticosteroids

Corticosteroid therapy has long been used to reduce lung inflammation during the treatment of infants with severe BPD. Clinical studies have consistently shown that steroids acutely improve lung mechanics and gas exchange and reduce inflammatory cells and their products in tracheal samples of patients with BPD.[133] Despite these studies, multiple experimental and clinical studies have raised concerns that excessive doses and prolonged use of corticosteroids can impair head growth, neurodevelopmental outcome, and lung structure.[134] In addition, a multicenter study was halted before completion because of a high incidence of gastrointestinal perforation.[125] As a result, current recommendations are to use steroids (e.g., dexamethasone) selectively at lower dosages (starting at 0.1 to 0.2 mg/kg/day, divided bid and tapering appropriately) for shorter durations (5 to 7 days) in ventilator-dependent

infants with severe, persistent lung disease. The use of steroids should be delayed if possible until the infant is approximately 1 month of age. Other side effects include systemic hypertension, hyperglycemia, cardiac hypertrophy, poor somatic growth, sepsis, intestinal bleeding, and myocardial hypertrophy. Inhaled steroids have been studied, but the major effect was to decrease the perceived need for the use of systemic steroids.[135] Recognition that some premature newborns have adrenal insufficiency that could increase the risk for BPD has led to interest in the use of low-dosage cortisol replacement therapy. Future clinical trials will need to carefully address potential side effects of all steroid preparations.

OUTCOME

Most follow-up data has been obtained from patients from the presurfactant era, with only limited studies describing the clinical course of patients who have reached adolescence and young adulthood. Late respiratory morbidity is common among infants and young children born prematurely, especially in those with BPD. Approximately 50% of children who had BPD in infancy require readmission to the hospital for respiratory distress, often with lower respiratory tract infections. This high rate of hospitalization generally declines during the second and third years of life, but lung function studies often show limited reserve even in patients with minimal overt respiratory signs. This observation probably explains the severity of manifestation in some infants with BPD after acquiring respiratory syncytial virus or other infections. During infancy, lung growth and remodeling can result in progressive improvement of pulmonary function and weaning from oxygen therapy. However, other respiratory problems (e.g., reactive airway disease and recurrent pulmonary infections) and abnormal neurologic development are additional abnormalities that may occur and necessitate careful follow-up.[136]

Infants with BPD demonstrate improvements in clinical status and lung mechanics during the first year; however, persistent airflow abnormalities may remain. In some infants, lung volumes during tidal breathing approach expiratory flow limitations, which is suggestive of limited reserve. Infants with BPD have reduced measurements of absolute and size-corrected flow rates in comparison with age- and size-matched control patients, which is suggestive of poor airway growth with age.[137] A 2-year follow-up study that compared premature newborns with and without BPD showed late airways obstruction in 80% of infants with BPD versus 40% of the infants without BPD.[138] Overall, lung volume progressively increases with age, but airflow obstruction can persist into early childhood.

Chest radiograph findings during follow-up are generally nonspecific, demonstrating typical findings as hyperinflation with peribronchial cuffing and scattered or focal interstitial infiltrates consistent with fibrosis or atelectasis. These findings tend to clear with age but are very insensitive markers of changes in lung function. CT can also demonstrate regional variations in lung disease, often displaying hyperinflated or emphysematous areas with diminished arterial density. The utility for serial CT during follow-up is uncertain, but these scans may help identify localized area of disease, such as large cysts, that may necessitate surgical resection.

Although pulmonary function in most survivors with BPD improves over time with continued lung growth and permits normal activity, abnormalities detected by pulmonary function testing may remain through adolescence. Follow-up studies of children with BPD have shown an increased incidence of wheezing and other clinical respiratory symptoms that may continue into later years.[139] In addition, pulmonary function studies have demonstrated increased airway resistance and reactivity, decreased lung compliance, ventilation-perfusion mismatch, abnormal exercise tolerance, and blood gas abnormalities (e.g., increased arterial CO_2 pressure) in older children with a history of BPD.[140] The most significant abnormalities were found in children who had clinical respiratory symptoms such as wheezing and repeated pulmonary infections, especially early in their childhood (<2 years of age).[141] It appears that abnormal pulmonary function and distress are greatest in the first 2 years of life in infants who had BPD. Improvement in lung function can occur between years 7 and 10, but more than 25% of adolescents with a history of BPD have abnormal lung function. Comprehensive longitudinal studies monitoring patients into adulthood are currently lacking.

Despite increases in lung volumes of children who had BPD as infants, morphometric studies have shown that older patients who die of BPD fail to demonstrate compensatory alveolar growth.[11] These observations suggest that distal airspaces remain relatively hypoplastic, with marked reductions in alveolar number, and that impaired gas exchange is likely to persist because of reduced alveolar numbers and microvascular growth. Functionally, the loss of surface area impairs gas exchange and contributes to prolonged oxygen requirements, frequent respiratory exacerbations, and late physiologic abnormalities, including exercise intolerance.[142] Mechanisms that link disruption of alveolar development and vascular growth

in infants with BPD are poorly understood, but inhibition of vascular growth may contribute to failed alveolar development.[17,143-145]

Finally, there are few data on pulmonary function of adult patients with a history of premature birth and severe BPD. Northway and colleagues reported persistent evidence of gas trapping and airway reactivity in young adults and adolescents who had been diagnosed as infants with BPD who were treated nearly three decades earlier.[146] Clinical experience suggests that increasing numbers of older survivors with severe BPD are only beginning to reappear as young adult patients (Figs. 50-10 and 50-11). More studies are needed to determine the long-term respiratory course of premature neonates, with or without severe BPD, and their relative contribution to the growing adult population with chronic obstructive pulmonary disease.

PREVENTION STRATEGIES

A multidisciplinary approach to the prevention of BPD in infants is needed. The use of antenatal steroids in pregnant women at high risk of delivering prematurely may reduce the severity and incidence of BPD.[26] The early use of nasal CPAP (with or without prior surfactant treatment) may eliminate the need for mechanical ventilation in some premature infants or facilitate successful extubation in others.[147] Aggressive treatment of symptomatic patent ductus arteriosus with fluid restriction, diuretics, indomethacin, or surgical closure may reduce the severity of BPD. Tidal volumes and inspired oxygen concentrations should be reduced to as low as necessary in order to reduce hypocarbia, volutrauma, and oxygen toxicity, while more aggressive lung recruitment strategies, such as more liberal PEEP, high-frequency ventilation, or, perhaps, prone positioning, should be used. The early use of synchronized mechanical ventilation or high-frequency ventilation in newborns with significant RDS may reduce the severity and incidence of BPD.[56,57] The combined use of high-frequency ventilation and surfactant replacement

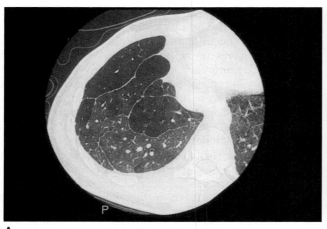
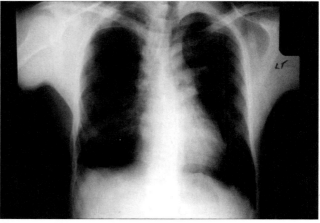

A   B

Figure 50–10. Bronchopulmonary dysplasia in an adult patient. **A,** Chest computed tomogram. **B,** Radiograph.

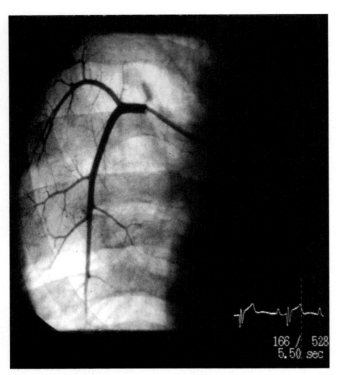

Figure 50-11. Bronchopulmonary dysplasia in an adult patient: pulmonary angiogram.

may prevent significant lung damage in premature and full-term infants with significant lung disease unresponsive to surfactant replacement and conventional mechanical ventilation.[148] Further conclusive evidence of the beneficial effects of both synchronized ventilation and high-frequency ventilation in premature infants is needed.

Aggressive nutritional support is crucial in helping to promote normal lung growth, maturation, and repair. It also protects the lung from the damaging effects of hyperoxia, infection, and barotrauma. Systemic supplementation with vitamin A in sufficient quantities to establish normal serum retinol concentrations has been reported to reduce the incidence of BPD, although the need to administer repeated doses through the intramuscular route has limited the widespread use of this therapy.

Studies have suggested that the early use of low dosages of hydrocortisone may reduce the incidence of BPD, presumably by treating cortisol deficiency and minimizing inflammation.[84,85] However, early dexamethasone should not be used to prevent BPD because of significant concerns regarding increased mortality, side effects (e.g., ileal perforation), and long-term sequelae (cerebral palsy).[125] The most promising method for preventing the development of BPD appears to be prophylactic supplementation of human recombinant antioxidant enzymes. This seems to be a logical strategy in preventing BPD, because ROS appear to play a major role in the pathogenesis of lung injury, and premature infants are known to be relatively deficient in these enzymes at birth. Several animal studies have shown that prolonged exposure to high oxygen concentrations can cause severe lung damage and death, and administration of antioxidants can prevent many of these complications.[2,35-37,149-151] Recombinant human CuZnSOD (rhSOD) has been administered prophylactically to the lung of premature infants at high risk for developing BPD. In preliminary studies in premature infants, the prophylactic use of both single and multiple intratracheal doses of rhSOD appeared to mitigate inflammatory changes and severe lung injury from oxygen and mechanical ventilation, with no apparent associated toxicity.[152,153] In animal studies, the rhSOD appeared to localize both in intracellular and extracellular compartments after intratracheal instillation, and significant quantities of active protein are present 48 hours after the dose is given.[154] Multicenter collaborative trials using prophylactic intratracheal rhSOD in premature infants at high risk for developing BPD have been completed. Premature infants (birth weight, 600 to 1200 g) receiving intratracheal instillation of rhSOD at birth had significantly (44%) fewer episodes of respiratory illness (wheezing, asthma, pulmonary infections) severe enough to necessitate treatment with bronchodilators or corticosteroids at 1 year of corrected age, in comparison with placebo control recipients.[155] Hospital readmissions and emergency room visits were also significantly reduced, especially in infants less than 27 weeks' gestation. This suggests that rhSOD did prevent long-term pulmonary injury from ROS in premature infants at high risk. Further therapeutic intervention trials are needed in order to ultimately develop a therapy that can prevent or significantly ameliorate this important chronic lung disease.

Protecting the pulmonary vasculature from injury may not only lower PVR and improve gas exchange, but it may also enhance distal lung growth and improve long-term outcome. Extensive laboratory and clinical studies suggest that iNO lowers PVR and improves oxygenation in patients with pulmonary hypertension in different settings, including premature infants with severe RDS and BPD.[156,157] However, there are persistent concerns about potential toxicity and adverse effects of iNO therapy in the premature infant. Experimental data have suggested that iNO therapy may be "lung protective" in several animal models, including premature lambs with RDS.[158] Whether iNO therapy has a potential role in the prevention of pulmonary vascular injury in premature newborns at risk for BPD is unknown. A multicenter clinical trial of low-dosage iNO therapy (5 ppm) was performed in severely ill premature newborns with RDS who had marked hypoxemia despite surfactant therapy (i.e., arterial-to-alveolar O_2 ratio < .10), with an estimated mortality rate of 53%.[156] In this study, iNO acutely improved arterial O_2 pressure but did not improve survival. Of note, there was no increase in the frequency or severity of intracranial hemorrhage or BPD, and the duration of mechanical ventilation was reduced. On the basis of these findings, several multicenter trials are now under way to determine whether early treatment with low-dosage iNO therapy prevents the early inflammatory changes that contribute to BPD and protects the pulmonary circulation from injury during this critical time.

SUMMARY

Since its original description in the late 1960s, BPD remains a significant complication of premature birth and a persistent challenge for the future. BPD has evolved from the classical stages described in the past to a disease characterized largely by inhibition of lung development. Future strategies that improve long-term outcomes will depend on the successful integration of basic research on fundamental mechanisms of lung development and the response to injury, as well as on studies that test novel interventions to lower the frequency and severity of the cardiopulmonary sequelae of BPD.

References

1. Northway WH Jr, Rosan RC, Porter DY: Pulmonary disease following respirator therapy of hyaline-membrane disease. N Engl J Med 276:357, 1967.
2. Davis JM, Rosenfeld WN: Bronchopulmonary dysplasia. In Avery GB, Fletcher MA, MacDonald MG (eds): Neonatology, 5th ed. Philadelphia, Lippincott Williams & Wilkins, 1999, pp 509-532.
3. Northway WH Jr: Historical perspective: Early observations and subsequent evolution of bronchopulmonary dysplasia. In Bland RD, Coalson JJ (eds): Chronic Lung Disease in Early Infancy. New York, Marcel Dekker, 2000, pp 1-20.
4. Jobe AH, Bancalari E: Bronchopulmonary dysplasia. Am J Respir Crit Care Med 163:1723, 2001.
5. Bancalari E, Abdenour GE, Feller R, Gannon J: Bronchopulmonary dysplasia: Clinical presentation. J Pediatr 95:819, 1979.
6. Jobe AH: The new BPD: An arrest of lung development. Pediatr Res 46:641, 1999.
7. Shennan AT, Dunn MS, Ohlsson A, et al: Abnormal pulmonary outcomes in premature infants: Prediction from oxygen requirement in the neonatal period. Pediatrics 82:527, 1988.
8. Palta M, Sadek M, Barnet JH, et al: Evaluation of criteria for chronic lung disease in surviving very low birth weight infants. Newborn Lung Project. J Pediatr 132:57, 1988.
9. Bancalari E, Gonzalez A: Clinical course and lung function abnormalities during development of chronic lung disease. In Bland RD, Coalson JJ (eds): Chronic Lung Disease in Early Infancy. New York, Marcel Dekker, 2000, pp 41-64.
10. Avery ME, Tooley WH, Keller JB, et al: Is chronic lung disease in low birth weight infants preventable? A survey of eight centers. Pediatrics 79:26, 1987.
11. Hussain AN, Siddiqui NH, Stocker JT: Pathology of arrested acinar development in post-surfactant BPD. Hum Pathol 29:710, 1998.
12. Kresch MJ, Clive JM: Meta-analyses of surfactant replacement therapy of infants with birth weights less than 2000 grams. J Perinatol 18:276, 1998.
13. Marshall DD, Kotelchuck M, Young TE, et al: Risk factors for chronic lung disease in the surfactant era: A North Carolina population based study of very low birth weight infants. Pediatrics 104:1345, 1999.
14. Charafeddine L, D'Angio CT, Phelps DL: Atypical chronic lung disease patterns in neonates. Pediatrics 103:759, 1999.
15. Rojas MA, Gonzalez A, Bancalari E, et al: Changing trends in the epidemiology and pathogenesis of chronic lung disease. J Pediatr 126:605, 1995.
16. Cherukupalli K, Larson JE, Rotschild A, Thurlbeck WM: Biochemical, clinical, and morphologic studies on lungs of infants with bronchopulmonary dysplasia. Pediatr Pulmonol 22:215, 1996.
17. Bhatt AJ, Pryhuber GS, Huyck H, et al: Disrupted pulmonary vasculature and decreased vascular endothelial growth factor, Flt-1, and TIE-2 in human infants dying with bronchopulmonary dysplasia. Am J Respir Crit Care Med 164:1971, 2001.
18. Bonikos DS, Bensch KG, Northway WH, Edwards DK: BPD: The pulmonary pathologic sequel of necrotizing bronchiolitis and pulmonary fibrosis. Arch J Pathol 7:643, 1976.
19. Margraf LR, Tomashefski JF, Bruce MC, Dahmm BB: Morphometric analysis of the lung in BPD. Am Rev Respir Dis 143:391, 1991.
20. Coalson JJ: Pathology of chronic lung disease of early infancy. In Bland RD, Coalson JJ (eds): Chronic Lung Disease of Early Infancy. New York, Marcel Dekker, 2000, pp 85-124.
21. Yoon BH, Romero R, Jun JK, et al: Amniotic fluid cytokines (interleukin-6, tumor necrosis factor-alpha, interleukin-1 beta, and interleukin-8) and the risk for the development of bronchopulmonary dysplasia. Am J Obstet Gynecol 177:825, 1997.
22. Hitti J, Krohn MA, Patton DL, et al: Amniotic fluid tumor necrosis factor–alpha and the risk of respiratory distress syndrome among preterm infants. Am J Obstet Gynecol 177:50, 1997.
23. Watterberg KL, Demers LM, Scott SM, Murphy S: Chorioamnionitis and early lung inflammation in infants in whom bronchopulmonary dysplasia develops. Pediatrics 97:210, 1996.
24. Ghezzi F, Gomez R, Romero R, et al: Elevated interleukin-8 concentrations in amniotic fluid of mothers whose neonates subsequently develop bronchopulmonary dysplasia. Eur J Obstet Gynecol Reprod Biol 78:5, 1998.
25. Jobe AH, Newnham JP, Willet KE, et al: Effects of antenatal endotoxin and glucocorticoids on the lungs of preterm lambs. Am J Obstet Gynecol 18:401, 2000.
26. Crowley PA: Antenatal corticosteroid therapy: A meta-analysis of the randomized trials, 1972 to 1994. Am J Obstet Gynecol 173:322, 1995.
27. Polk DH, Ikegami M, Jobe AH, et al: Preterm lung function after retreatment with antenatal betamethasone in preterm lambs. Am J Obstet Gynecol 176:308, 1997.
28. Walther FJ, Jobe AH, Ikegami M: Repetitive prenatal glucocorticoid therapy reduces oxidative stress in the lungs of preterm lambs. J Appl Physiol 85:273, 1998.
29. Banks BA, Cnaan A, Morgan MA, et al: Multiple courses of antenatal corticosteroids and outcome of premature neonates. North American Thyrotropin-Releasing Hormone Study Group. Am J Obstet Gynecol 181:709, 1999.
30. Van Marter LJ, Allred EN, Leviton A, et al: Antenatal glucocorticoid treatment does not reduce chronic lung disease among surviving preterm infants. J Pediatr 138:198, 2000.
31. McCord JM: Human disease, free radicals, and the oxidant/antioxidant balance. Clin Biochem 26:351, 1993.
32. Frank L, Groseclose EE: Preparation for birth into an O_2-rich environment: The antioxidant enzymes in the developing rabbit lung. Pediatr Res 18:240, 1984.
33. Frank L, Sosenko IR: Failure of premature rabbits to increase antioxidant enzymes during hyperoxic exposure: Increased susceptibility to pulmonary O_2 toxicity compared with term rabbits. Pediatr Res 29:292, 1991.
34. Jain A, Mehta T, Auld PA, et al: Glutathione metabolism in newborns: Evidence for glutathione deficiency in plasma, bronchoalveolar lavage fluid, and lymphocytes in prematures. Pediatr Pulmonol 20:160, 1995.

35. Ogihara T, Okamoto R, Kim HS, et al: New evidence for the involvement of oxygen radicals in triggering neonatal chronic lung disease. Pediatr Res 39:117, 1996.

36. Pitkanen OM, Hallman M, Andersson SM: Correlation of free oxygen radical-induced lipid peroxidation with outcome in very low birth weight infants. J Pediatr 116:760, 1990.

37. Varsila E, Pesonen E, Andersson S: Early protein oxidation in the neonatal lung is related to the development of chronic lung disease. Acta Paediatr 84:1296, 1995.

38. Banks BA, Ischiropoulos H, McClelland M, et al: Plasma 3-nitrotyrosine is elevated in premature infants who develop bronchopulmonary dysplasia. Pediatrics 101:870, 1998.

39. The STOP-ROP Multicenter Study Group: Supplemental Therapeutic Oxygen for Prethreshold Retinopathy Of Prematurity, a randomized, controlled trial. Pediatrics 105:295, 2000.

40. Davis JM, Rosenfeld WN, Sanders RJ, Gonenne A: Prophylactic effects of recombinant human superoxide dismutase in neonatal lung injury. J Appl Physiol 74:2234, 1993.

41. Padmanabhan RV, Gudapaty R, Liener IE, et al: Protection against pulmonary oxygen toxicity in rats by the intratracheal administration of liposome-encapsulated superoxide dismutase or catalase. Am Rev Respir Dis 132:164, 1985.

42. Turrens JF, Crapo JD, Freeman BA: Protection against oxygen toxicity by intravenous injection of liposome-entrapped catalase and superoxide dismutase. J Clin Invest 73:87, 1984.

43. White CW, Avraham KB, Shanley PF, Groner Y: Transgenic mice with expression of elevated levels of copper-zinc superoxide dismutase in the lungs are resistant to pulmonary oxygen toxicity. J Clin Invest 87:2162, 1991.

44. Wispe JR, Warner BB, Clark JC, et al: Human Mn-superoxide dismutase in pulmonary epithelial cells of transgenic mice confers protection from oxygen injury. J Biol Chem 267:23937, 1992.

45. Carlsson LM, Jonsson J, Edlun T, Marklund SL: Mice lacking extracellular superoxide dismutase are more sensitive to hyperoxia. Proc Natl Acad Sci U S A 92:6264, 1995.

46. Dreyfuss D, Saumon G: Should the lung be rested or recruited? Am J Respir Crit Care Med 149:1066, 1994.

47. Hodson WA: Ventilation strategies and BPD. In Bland RD, Coalson JJ (eds): Chronic Lung Disease in Early Infancy. New York, Marcel Dekker, 2000, pp 173-208.

48. Dreyfuss DD, Saumon G: Ventilator induced lung injury: Lessons from experimental studies. Am J Respir Crit Care Med 157:294, 1998.

49. Nilsson R, Grossman G, Robertson B: Lung surfactant and the pathogenesis of neonatal bronchiolar lesions induced by artificial ventilation. Pediatr Res 12:249, 1978.

50. Tremblay L, Valenza F, Ribeiro SP, et al: Injurious ventilatory strategies increase cytokines and c-fos m-RNA expression in an isolated rat lung model. J Clin Invest 99:944, 1997.

51. Carlton DP, Cummings JJ, Scheerer RG, et al: Lung overexpansion increases pulmonary microvascular protein permeability in young lambs. J Appl Physiol 69:577, 1990.

52. Hernandez LA, Peevy KJ, Moise AA, Parker JC: Chest wall restriction limits high airway pressure–induced lung injury in young rabbits. J Appl Physiol 66:2364, 1989.

53. Acute Respiratory Distress Syndrome Network: Ventilation with lower tidal volumes as compared with traditional tidal volumes for acute lung injury and the ARDS. N Engl J Med 342:1301, 2000.

54. Bjorklund LJ, Ingimarsson J, Curstedt T, et al: Manual ventilation with a few large breaths at birth compromises the therapeutic effect of subsequent surfactant replacement in immature lungs. Pediatr Res 42:348, 1997.

55. Bernstein G, Mannino FL, Heldt GP, et al: Randomized multicenter trial comparing synchronized and conventional intermittent mandatory ventilation in neonates. J Pediatr 128:453, 1996.

56. Clark RH, Gerstmann DR, Null DM, deLemos RA: Prospective, randomized comparison of high-frequency oscillatory and conventional ventilation in respiratory distress syndrome. Pediatrics 89:5, 1992.

57. Keszler M, Modanlou HD, Brudno DS, et al: Multicenter controlled clinical trial of high-frequency jet ventilation in preterm infants with uncomplicated respiratory distress syndrome. Pediatrics 100:593, 1997.

58. Garland JS, Buck RK, Allred EN, Leviton A: Hypocarbia before surfactant therapy appears to increase bronchopulmonary dysplasia risk in infants with respiratory distress syndrome. Arch Pediatr Adolesc Med 149:617, 1995.

59. Collins MP, Lorenz JM, Jetton JR, Paneth N: Hypocapnia and other ventilation-related risk factors for cerebral palsy in low birth weight infants. Pediatr Res 50:712, 2001.

60. Mariani G, Cifuentes J, Carlo WA: Randomized trial of permissive hypercapnia in preterm infants. Pediatrics 104:1082, 1999.

61. Van Marter LJ, Allred EN, Pagano M, et al: Do clinical markers of barotrauma and oxygen toxicity explain interhospital variation in rates of chronic lung disease? The Neonatology Committee for the Developmental Network. Pediatrics 105:1194, 2000.

62. Groneck P, Gotz-Speer B, Opperman M, et al: Association of pulmonary inflammation and increased microvascular permeability during the development of bronchopulmonary dysplasia: A sequential analysis of inflammatory mediators in respiratory fluids of high-risk neonates. Pediatrics 93:712, 1994.

63. Pierce MR, Bancalari E: The role of inflammation in the pathogenesis of bronchopulmonary dysplasia. Pediatr Pulmonol 19:371, 1995.

64. Groneck P, Speer CP: Inflammatory mediators and bronchopulmonary dysplasia. Arch Dis Child Fetal Neonatal Ed 73:F1, 1995.

65. Ozdemir A, Brown MA, Morgan WJ: Markers and mediators of inflammation in neonatal lung disease. Pediatr Pulmonol 23:292, 1997.

66. Ogden BE, Murphy SA, Saunders GC, et al: Neonatal lung neutrophils and elastase/proteinase inhibitor imbalance. Am Rev Respir Dis 130:817, 1984.

67. Brus F, van Oeveren W, Okken A, Bambang SO: Activation of circulating polymorphonuclear leukocytes in preterm infants with severe idiopathic respiratory distress syndrome. Pediatr Res 39:456, 1996.

68. Jones CA, Cayabyab RG, Kwong KY, et al: Undetectable interleukin (IL)–10 and persistent IL-8 expression early in hyaline membrane disease: A possible developmental basis for the predisposition to chronic lung inflammation in preterm newborns. Pediatr Res 39:966, 1996.

69. Raghavender B, Smith JB: Eosinophil cationic protein in tracheal aspirates of preterm infants with bronchopulmonary dysplasia. J Pediatr 130:944, 1997.

70. Ramsay PL, O'Brian SE, Hegemier S, Welty SE: Early clinical markers for the development of bronchopulmonary dysplasia: Soluble E-selectin and ICAM-1. Pediatrics 102:927, 1998.

71. Munshi UK, Niu JO, Siddiq MM, Parton LA: Elevation of interleukin-8 and interleukin-6 precedes the influx of neutrophils in tracheal aspirates from preterm infants who develop bronchopulmonary dysplasia. Pediatr Pulmonol 24:331, 1997.

72. Kotecha S, Chan B, Azam N, et al: Increase in interleukin-8 and soluble intercellular adhesion molecule–1 in bronchoalveolar lavage fluid from premature infants who develop chronic lung disease. Arch Dis Child Fetal Neonatal Ed 72:F90, 1995.

73. Jonsson B, Li YH, Noack G, et al: Downregulatory cytokines in tracheobronchial aspirate fluid from infants with chronic lung disease of prematurity. Acta Paediatr 89:1375, 2000.

74. Jonsson B, Tullus K, Brauner A, et al: Early increase of TNF alpha and IL-6 in tracheobronchial aspirate fluid indicator of subsequent chronic lung disease in preterm infants. Arch Dis Child Fetal Neonatal Ed 77:F198, 1997.

75. Blobe GC, Schiemann WP, Lodish HF: Role of transforming growth factor beta in human disease. New Engl J Med 342:1350, 2000.

76. Sunday ME, Yoder BA, Cuttitta F, et al: Bombesin-like peptide mediates lung injury in a baboon model of bronchopulmonary dysplasia. J Clin Invest 102:584, 1998.

77. Bland RD, Albertine KH, Carlton DP, et al: Chronic lung injury in preterm lambs: Abnormalities of the pulmonary circulation and lung fluid balance. Pediatr Res 48:64, 2000.

78. Bruce MC, Wedig KE, Jentoft N, et al: Altered urinary excretion of elastin cross-links in premature infants who developed bronchopulmonary dysplasia. Am Rev Respir Dis 131:568, 1985.

79. Alnahhas MH, Karathanasis P, Kriss VM, et al: Elevated laminin concentrations in lung secretions of preterm infants supported by mechanical ventilation are correlated with radiographic abnormalities. J Pediatr 131:555, 1997.

80. Ossanna PJ, Test ST, Matheson NR, et al: Oxidative regulation of neutrophil elastase–α-1–proteinase inhibitor interactions. J Clin Invest 77:1939, 1986.

81. Sluis KB, Darlow BA, Vissers MC, Winterbourn CC: Proteinase-antiproteinase balance in tracheal aspirates from neonates. Eur Respir J 7:251, 1994.

82. Merritt TA, Cochrane CG, Holcomb K, et al: Elastase and α_1-proteinase inhibitor activity in tracheal aspirates during respiratory distress syndrome. Role of inflammation in the pathogenesis of bronchopulmonary dysplasia. J Clin Invest 72:656, 1983.

83. Stiskal JA, Dunn MS, Shennan AT, et al: α_1-Proteinase inhibitor therapy for the prevention of chronic lung disease of prematurity: A randomized, controlled trial. Pediatrics 101:89, 1998.

84. Watterberg KL, Scott SM, Backstrom C, et al: Links between early adrenal function and respiratory outcome in preterm infants: Airway inflammation and patent ductus arteriosus. Pediatrics 105:320, 2000.

85. Watterberg KL, Gerdes JS, Gifford KL, Lin HM: Prophylaxis against early adrenal insufficiency to prevent chronic lung disease in premature infants. Pediatrics 104:1258, 1999.

86. Wang EE, Ohlsson A, Kellner JD: Association of *Ureaplasma urealyticum* colonization with chronic lung disease of prematurity: Results of a meta-analysis. J Pediatr 127:640, 1995.

87. Alfa MJ, Embree JE, Degagne P, et al: Transmission of *Ureaplasma urealyticum* from mothers to full and preterm infants. Pediatr Infect Dis J 14:341, 1995.

88. Kenyon SL, Taylor DJ, Tarnow-Mordi W: Broad-spectrum antibiotics for preterm, prelabour rupture of fetal membranes: The ORACLE I randomised trial. ORACLE Collaborative Group. Lancet 357:979, 2001.

89. Da Silva O, Gregson D, Hammerberg O: Role of *Ureaplasma urealyticum* and *Chlamydia trachomatis* in development of bronchopulmonary dysplasia in very low birth weight infants. Pediatr Infect Dis J 16:364, 1997.

90. Heggie AD, Jacobs MR, Butler VT, et al: Frequency and significance of isolation of *Ureaplasma urealyticum* and *Mycoplasma hominis* from cerebrospinal fluid and tracheal aspirate specimens from low birth weight infants. J Pediatr 124:956, 1994.

91. Gonzalez A, Sosenko IR, Chandar J, et al: Influence of infection on patent ductus arteriosus and chronic lung disease in premature infants weighing 1000 grams or less. J Pediatr 128:470, 1996.

92. Frank L, Groseclose E: Oxygen toxicity in newborn rats: The adverse effects of undernutrition. J Appl Physiol 53:1248, 1982.

93. Darlow BA, Inder TE, Graham PJ, et al: The relationship of selenium status to respiratory outcome in the very low birth weight infant. Pediatrics 96:314, 1995.

94. Forman HJ, Rotman EI, Fisher AB: Roles of selenium and sulfur-containing amino acids in protection against oxygen toxicity. Lab Invest 49:148, 1983.

95. O'Dell BL, Kilburn KH, McKenzie WN, Thurston RJ: The lung of the copper-deficient rat: A model for developmental pulmonary emphysema. Am J Pathol 91:413, 1978.

96. Ehrenkranz RA, Bonta BW, Ablow RC, Warshaw JB: Amelioration of bronchopulmonary dysplasia after vitamin E administration: A preliminary report. N Engl J Med 299:564, 1978.

97. Saldanha RL, Cepeda EE, Poland RL: The effect of vitamin E prophylaxis on the incidence and severity of bronchopulmonary dysplasia. J Pediatr 101:89, 1982.

98. Brandt RB, Mueller DG, Schroeder JR, et al: Serum vitamin A in premature and term neonates. J Pediatr 92:101, 1978.

99. Shenai JP: Vitamin A supplementation in very low birth weight neonates: Rationale and evidence. Pediatrics 104:1369, 1999.

100. Hustead VA, Gutcher GR, Anderson SA, Zachman RD: Relationship of vitamin A (retinol) status to lung disease in the preterm infants. J Pediatr 105:610, 1984.

101. Tyson JE, Wright LL, Oh W, et al: Vitamin A supplementation for extremely-low-birth-weight infants. National Institute of Child Health and Human Development Neonatal Research Network. N Engl J Med 340:1962, 1999.

102. Van Marter LJ, Leviton A, Allred EN, et al: Hydration during the first days of life and the risk of bronchopulmonary dysplasia in low birth weight infants. J Pediatr 116:942, 1990.

103. Nickerson BG, Taussig LM: Family history of asthma in infants with bronchopulmonary dysplasia. Pediatrics 65:1140, 1980.

104. Bertrand JM, Riley SP, Popkin J, Coates AL: The long-term pulmonary sequelae of prematurity: The role of familial airway hyperreactivity and the respiratory distress syndrome. N Engl J Med 312:742, 1985.

105. Clark DA, Pincus LG, Oliphant M, et al: HLA-A$_2$ and chronic lung disease in neonates. JAMA 248:1868, 1982.

106. Hagan R, Minutillo C, French N, et al: Neonatal chronic lung disease, oxygen dependency, and a family history of asthma. Pediatr Pulmonol 20:277, 1995.

107. Goldman SL, Gerhardt T, Sonni R, et al: Early prediction of chronic lung disease by pulmonary function testing. J Pediatr 102:613, 1983.

108. Tepper RS, Morgan WJ, Cota K, Taussig LM: Expiratory flow limitation in infants with bronchopulmonary dysplasia. J Pediatr 109:1040, 1986.

109. Toce SS, Farrell PM, Leavitt LA, et al: Clinical and roentgenographic scoring systems for assessing BPD. Am J Dis Child 138:581, 1984.

110. Weinstein MR, Peters ME, Sadek M, et al: A new radiographic scoring system for BPD. Pediatr Pulmonol 18:284, 1994.

111. Abman SH: Pulmonary hypertension in chronic lung disease of infancy. Pathogenesis, pathophysiology and treatment. In Bland RD, Coalson JJ (eds): Chronic Lung Disease of Infancy. New York, Marcel Dekker, 2000, pp 619-668.

112. Jones R, Zapol WM, Reid LM: Oxygen toxicity and restructuring of pulmonary arteries: A morphometric study. Am J Pathol 121:212, 1985.

113. Tomashefski JF, Opperman HC, Vawter GF: BPD: A morphometric study with emphasis on the pulmonary vasculature. Pediatr Pathol 2:469, 1984.

114. Anderson WR, Engel RR: Cardiopulmonary sequelae of reparative stages of BPD. Arch Pathol Lab Med 107:6603, 1983.

115. Halliday HL, Dumpit FM, Brady JP: Effects of inspired oxygen on echocardiographic assessment of pulmonary vascular resistance and myocardial contractility in BPD. Pediatrics 65:536, 1980.

116. Abman SH, Wolfe RR, Accurso FJ, et al: Pulmonary vascular response to oxygen in infants with severe BPD. Pediatrics 75:80, 1985.

117. Walther FJ, Bender FJ, Leighton JO: Persistent pulmonary hypertension in premature neonates with severe RDS. Pediatrics 90:899, 1992.

118. Fouron JC, LeGuennec JC, Villemont D, et al: Value of echocardiography in assessing the outcome of BPD. Pediatrics 65:529, 1980.

119. Goodman G, Perkin R, Anas N: Pulmonary hypertension in infants with BPD. J Pediatr 112:67, 1988.

120. Abman SH, Schaffer MS, Wiggins JW, et al: Pulmonary vascular extraction of circulating norepinephrine in infants with BPD. Pediatric Pulmonol 3:386, 1987.

121. Abman SH, Sondheimer HS: Pulmonary circulation and cardiovascular sequelae of BPD. In Weir EK, Archer SL, Reeves JT (eds): Diagnosis and Treatment of Pulmonary Hypertension. New York, Futura, 1992, pp 155-180.

122. Apkon M, Nehgme RA, Lister G: Cardiovascular abnormalities in BPD. In Bland RD, Coalson JJ (eds): Chronic Lung Disease of Infancy. New York, Marcel Dekker, 2000, pp 321- 356.

123. Melnick G, Pickoff AS, Ferrer PC, et al: Normal pulmonary vascular resistance and left ventricular hypertrophy in young infants with BPD: An echocardiographic and pathologic study. Pediatrics 66:586, 1980.

124. Abman SH, Warady BA, Lum GM, Koops BL: Systemic hypertension in infants with BPD. J Pediatr 104:928, 1984.

125. Stark AR, Carlo WA, Tyson JE, et al: Adverse effects of early dexamethasone treatment in extremely low birth weight infants. N Engl J Med 344:95, 2001.

126. Murphy BP, Inder TE, Huppi PS, et al: Impaired cerebral cortical gray matter after treatment with dexamethasone for neonatal chronic lung disease. Pediatrics107:217, 2001.

127. Abman SH, Groothius JR: Pathophysiology and treatment of BPD. Pediatr Clin North Am 41:277, 1994.

128. Abman SH, Accurso FJ, Koops BL: Experience with home oxygen in the management of infants with BPD. Clin Pediatr 23:471, 1984.

129. Groothius JR, Rosenberg AA: Home oxygen promotes weight gain in infants with BPD. Am J Dis Child 141:992, 1987.

130. Hazinski TA: Drug therapy for established BPD. In Bland RD, Coalson JJ (eds): Chronic Lung Disease of Infancy. New York, Marcel Dekker, 2000, pp 257-284.

131. Rush MG, Englehardt B, Parker RA, et al: Double blind, placebo controlled trial of alternate day furosemide therapy in infants with chronic BPD. J Pediatr 117:112, 1990.

132. De Boeck K, Smith J, Van Lierde S, Devlieger H: Response to bronchodilators in clinically stable 1 year old patients with BPD. J Pediatr 157:75, 1998.

133. Yoder MC, Chua R, Tepper R: Effect of dexamethasone on pulmonary inflammation and pulmonary function of ventilator-dependent infants with BPD. Am Rev Respir Dis 143:1044, 1991.

134. Halliday HL: Clinical trials of postnatal corticosteroids: Inhaled and systemic. Biol Neonate 76(Suppl 1):29, 1999.

135. Cole CH, Colton T, Shah BL, et al: Early inhaled glucocorticoid therapy to prevent BPD. N Engl J Med 340:1005, 1999.

136. Vohr BR, Coll CG, Lobato D, et al: Neurodevelopmental and medical status of low-birthweight survivors of bronchopulmonary dysplasia at 10 to 12 years of age. Dev Med Child Neurol 33:690, 1991.

137. Gerhardt T, Hehre D, Feller R, et al: Serial determinations of pulmonary function in infants with CLD. J Pediatr 110:448, 1987.

138. Baraldi E, Filippone M, Trevisanuto D, et al: Pulmonary function until two years of life in infants with bronchopulmonary dysplasia. Am J Respir Crit Care Med 155:149, 1997.

139. Jacob SV, Coates AL, Lands LC, et al: Long-term pulmonary sequelae of severe bronchopulmonary dysplasia. J Pediatr 133:193, 1998.

140. Gross SJ, Iannuzzi DM, Kveselis DA, Anbar RD: Effect of preterm birth on pulmonary function at school age: A prospective controlled study. J Pediatr 133:188, 1998.

141. Hakulinen AL, Heinonen K, Lansimies E, Kiekara O: Pulmonary function and respiratory morbidity in school-age children born prematurely and ventilated for neonatal respiratory insufficiency. Pediatr Pulmonol 8:226, 1990.

142. Mitchell SH, Teague G: Reduced gas transfer at rest and during exercise in school age survivors of BPD. Am J Respir Crit Care Med 157:1406, 1998.

143. Jakkula M, Le Cras TD, Gebb S, et al: Inhibition of angiogenesis decreases alveolarization in the developing rat lung. Am J Physiol Lung Cell Mol Physiol 279:L600, 2000.

144. Abman SH: BPD: A vascular hypothesis. Am J Respir Crit Care Med 164:1755, 2001.

145. Lassus P, Turanlahti M, Heikkila P, et al: Pulmonary VEGF and flt-1 in fetuses, in acute and chronic lung disease, and in persistent pulmonary hypertension of the newborn. Am J Respir Crit Care Med 164:1981, 2001.

146. Northway WH, Moss RB, Carlisle KB, et al: Late pulmonary sequelae of BPD. N Engl J Med 323:1793, 1990.

147. Higgins RD, Richter SE, Davis JM: Nasal continuous positive airway pressure facilitates extubation of very low birth weight neonates. Pediatrics 88:999, 1991.

148. Davis JM, Richter SE, Kendig JW, Notter RH: High frequency jet ventilation and surfactant treatment of newborns with severe respiratory failure. Pediatr Pulmonol 13:108, 1992.

149. Jacobson JM, Michael JR, Jafri MH Jr, Gurtner GH: Antioxidants and antioxidant enzymes protect against pulmonary oxygen toxicity in the rabbit. J Appl Physiol 68:1252, 1990.

150. Tanswell AK, Freeman BA: Liposome-entrapped antioxidant enzymes prevent lethal O_2 toxicity in the newborn rat. J Appl Physiol 63:347, 1987.

151. Davis JM: Superoxide dismutase: A role in the prevention of chronic lung disease. Biol Neonate 74:29, 1998.

152. Rosenfeld WN, Davis JM, Parton L, et al: Safety and pharmacokinetics of recombinant human superoxide dismutase administered intratracheally to premature neonates with respiratory distress syndrome. Pediatrics 97:811, 1996.

153. Davis JM, Rosenfeld WN, Richter SE, et al: Safety and pharmacokinetics of multiple doses of recombinant human CuZn superoxide dismutase administered intratracheally to premature neonates with respiratory distress syndrome. Pediatrics 100:24, 1997.

154. Sahgal N, Davis JM, Robbins C, et al: Localization and activity of recombinant human CuZn superoxide dismutase after intratracheal administration. Am J Physiol Lung Cell Mol Physiol 271:L230, 1996.

155. Davis JM, Rosenfeld WN, Parad R, et al: Improved pulmonary outcome at one year corrected age in premature neonates treated with recombinant human superoxide dismutase. Pediatrics 111:469, 2003.

156. Kinsella JP, Walsh WF, Bose C, et al: Randomized controlled trial of inhaled nitric oxide in premature neonates with severe hypoxemic respiratory failure. Lancet 354:1061, 1999.

157. Banks BA, Seri I, Ischiropoulos H, et al: Changes in oxygenation with inhaled nitric oxide in severe bronchopulmonary dysplasia. Pediatrics 103:610, 1999.

158. Kinsella JP, Parker TA, Galan H, et al: Effects of inhaled NO on pulmonary edema and lung neutrophil accumulation in severe experimental HMD. Pediatr Res 41:457, 1997.

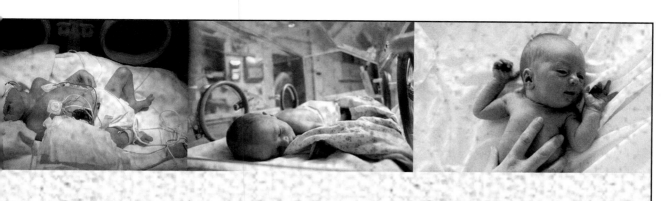

Neurologic Considerations in the Neonate

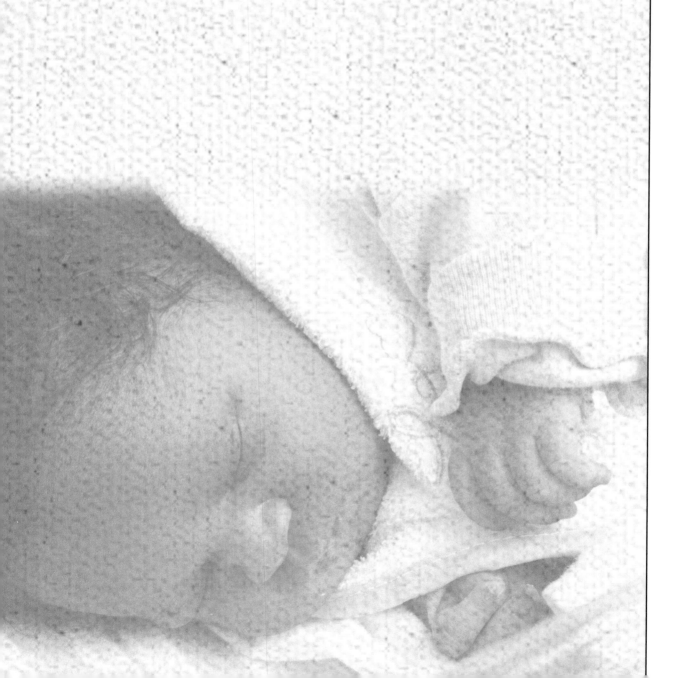

CHAPTER 51

Retinopathy of Prematurity

Graham E. Quinn

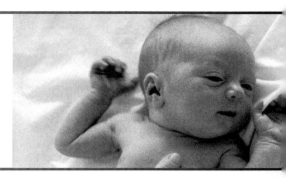

R etinopathy of prematurity (ROP) is an oxidant disease that occurs in incompletely vascularized retinas of premature infants, particularly small, sick infants in the neonatal intensive care unit. It is characterized by the onset of visible vascular abnormalities in the second or third month after premature birth. In approximately 3% of children with birth weights of less than 1251 g, the retinopathy progresses to serious scarring in the posterior pole of the eye or to retinal detachment. This occurs despite the most aggressive surgical treatment currently available, such as cryotherapy or laser photocoagulation for sight-threatening disease.[1]

ROP typically appears after the child has lived through life-threatening crises such as intraventricular hemorrhage and respiratory distress syndrome that are common in early life for very premature infants. Therefore, serious forms of ROP put a heavy emotional and psychologic burden on the child's family, physicians, and nurses. After all the hurdles the family and child have overcome, they must now face the fact that the child has another serious, potentially lifelong problem.

Retinopathy has been recognized since the early 1940s as a blinding disease of the premature infant,[2] and the incidence of blinding forms of the disease has varied greatly over the intervening decades.[3-5] The development of the neonatal intensive care unit in the late 1960s and the subsequent explosion in technology for physical support of these children and in the understanding of their nutritional demands led not only to an increased number of survivors with very low birth weight but also to an increased number of children at risk for developing ROP. Increased survival and the development of treatment options have led to a resurgence in clinical and basic science research in the area.

The findings of the multicenter Cryotherapy for Retinopathy of Prematurity (CRYO-ROP) trial[6] proved the efficacy of cryotherapy for severe ROP and increased the awareness of the disorder for neonatologists caring for the infant and the ophthalmologist performing ROP screening examinations and treatment. Before this trial,

there was no widely accepted "proven" treatment, and ROP surveillance in the nursery could be determined locally within broad guidelines published by the American Academy of Pediatrics, which suggested an examination by 8 weeks after birth or at discharge. Treatment protocols in place in the individual institution also determined when and which children to examine.

With the 1988 publication of the results of the CRYO-ROP trial,[6] a new standard of care for infants with birth weights of less than 1251 g was required of infant intensive care nurseries. This included identifying children at risk for serious forms of ROP, which the study had defined as (1) ROP severe enough to qualify for entry into the randomized treatment trial or "threshold" ROP (zone 1 or 2, stage 3+ ROP with 5 contiguous or 8 discontinuous clock hours of involvement [see later discussion of classification]), and (2) ROP that necessitated more frequent examinations than the routine or "prethreshold" ROP, which consisted of (1) zone 1 or 2, stage 2 ROP with "plus disease" (to be described); (2) zone 1 or 2, stage 3 ROP without plus disease; or (3) zone 1 or 2, stage 3 ROP with plus but lacking the requisite hours of stage 3 to qualify for threshold. The hospitals and physicians caring for premature infants in intensive care units needed to develop systems to undertake serial eye examinations designed to detect serious ROP and needed to obtain the services of ophthalmologists familiar with cryotherapy and laser therapy for ROP in the premature infant.

Thus, the responsibility of physicians and nurses who give ophthalmic care for premature infants has changed radically since the mid-1980s and is likely to change even more. The purpose of this chapter is to present current knowledge about ROP natural history and its treatment, along with a historical perspective of the disorder.

CLASSIFICATION

Before the early 1980s, most ophthalmologists recorded observations about the natural course of ROP, using one of several different classification systems.[3,7-10] Although

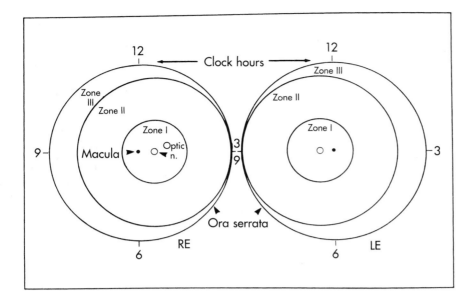

Figure 51–1. Drawings of right eye (RE) and left eye (LE) showing edges of zones and clock hours used to document location of retinopathy of prematurity. *(From Committee for the Classification of Retinopathy of Prematurity: An international classification of retinopathy of prematurity. Arch Ophthalmol 102:1130, 1984.)*

these systems were similar in the extreme degrees of ROP, the moderately severe grades of retinopathy had varying emphases, making discussion of ocular findings and comparison of treatment effects difficult. This situation was radically altered with the introduction of the International Classification of ROP in 1984.[11] This classification was a group effort of 23 ophthalmologists and ophthalmic pathologists from 11 countries that began meeting initially at a 1981 ROP conference sponsored by Ross Laboratories in Washington, D.C. The group subsequently met in Calgary, Alberta, Canada, and Bethesda, Maryland, over the next several years, while using the newly devised classification in their home nurseries. The group suggested four major components for an international classification including: (1) location, or **zone**, of the retinopathy between the optic disk and ora serrata; (2) severity, or **stage**, of disease at the junction between the vascularized and nonvascularized retina; (3) **extent** of involvement of disease (given in clock hours 0 through 12) at the junction, and (4) presence or absence of **plus disease**, defined as abnormal dilatation and tortuosity of the vessels of the posterior pole of the eye. The major theme of the classification was that more posterior, more severe, and more extensive retinopathy was likely to have more serious long-term morbidity for the child.

The ability to state the retinal location or zone of the retinopathy was a crucial advance in communicating about the disease. The decision that made this possible was changing the center of the zones from the fovea, where vision is sharpest, to the center of the optic disk, where the retinal vasculature emerges at about 16 weeks of gestation. As shown in Figure 51-1, the retina is divided into three zones. Zone 1, the most posterior, is the area bound by a circle in which the disk is at the center and whose radius is twice the distance from the disk to the foveal region. Zone 2 is doughnut-shaped and extends from the edge of zone 1 to the edge of a circle in which the disc is at the center and whose radius defined as the distance from the disk to the nasal ora serrata.

Zone 3 is the crescent of peripheral retina from the edge of zone 2 outward to the ora serrata. Thus, ROP that extends for 12 clock hours (360 degrees) must occur in zone 1 or zone 2.

Severity of retinopathy was defined initially in four stages of increasing severity. The earliest retinal finding that the International Committee believed was easily and uniformly recognizable was a demarcation line, or a thin white strip, at the junction between the vascularized and nonvascularized retina. This retinal change was designated stage 1 ROP. Stage 2 has a volume structure with height above the surrounding retina and bulk in the anterior-posterior location of the retinopathy. Stage 3 is characterized by extension of fibrovascular proliferation into the vitreous cavity (Fig. 51-2). Stage 4 included all retinal detachments that resulted from ROP. This stage was later expanded to stages 4 and 5 when several members of the original International Classification Committee met with other interested retinal specialists from 1985 to 1987.[12]

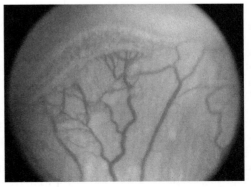

Figure 51–2. Fundus appearance of fibrovascular proliferation in stage 3 retinopathy of prematurity. *(From Committee for the Classification of Retinopathy of Prematurity: An international classification of retinopathy of prematurity. Arch Ophthalmol 102:1130, 1984.)*

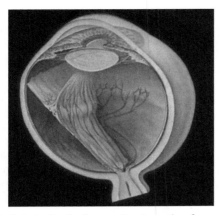

Figure 51–3. Artist's sketch of stage 4B retinopathy of prematurity with subtotal retinal detachment involving macular area. *(From The International Committee for the Classification of the Late Stages of Retinopathy of Prematurity: An international classification of retinopathy of prematurity: II. The classification of retinal detachment. Arch Ophthalmol 105:906, 1987.)*

Stage 4A is now a partial retinal detachment not involving the macular region, stage 4B is partial retinal detachment involving the macula (Fig. 51-3), and stage 5 is total retinal detachment. In addition, stage 5 is divided according to the configuration of the retinal detachment: that is, with open or closed funnels anteriorly and posteriorly.

The presence of "plus disease" is an ominous prognostic sign in ROP. It is characterized by progressive vascular incompetence with increasing dilation and tortuosity of veins and arteries of the posterior pole (Fig. 51-4), in the presence of the peripheral retinal findings of ROP. Also seen frequently in moderate to severe plus disease are vascular engorgement in the iris, pupillary rigidity, vitreous haze, and increasing dilation and tortuosity of the

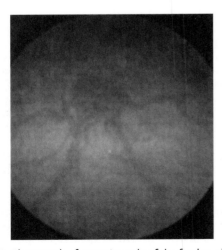

Figure 51–4. Photograph of posterior pole of the fundus, showing the venous and arteriolar dilation and tortuosity characteristic of "plus disease." *(From Committee for the Classification of Retinopathy of Prematurity: An international classification of retinopathy of prematurity. Arch Ophthalmol 102:1130, 1984.)*

peripheral retinal vessels. Quantification of plus disease is arbitrary and, in essence, a clinical judgment made from standard photographs and clinical impression. However, Freedman and associates noted that increased blood vessel tortuosity and dilation could be assessed reliably by observers, which is suggestive of this facilitated standardization of the diagnosis of plus disease.[13]

REGRESSION

Most acute-phase ROP does not progress to sight-threatening forms of the disease, such as retinal detachment or retinal fold involving the macular region. Rather, most ROP regresses to mild scarring or to no visible residua of the acute phases of the retinopathy. For example, in the CRYO-ROP study that involved infants with birth weights of less than 1251 g, ROP of some stage occurred in about 65% of the 4099 infants who were monitored during the period when ROP is likely to develop.[1] Progression to serious retinal scarring occurred in fewer than 5% of these children, and most cases regressed with a wide array of ocular findings.

Recognizing the range of clinical findings of regressed ROP but still without sufficient data to develop a severity hierarchy, the group of ophthalmologists and ophthalmic pathologists that developed International Classification of ROP in 1985-1987[12] chose to leave the categorization of increasing severity of regressed ROP findings to a later date. They suggested a simple cataloging of ocular findings that was based on whether the ocular residua of ROP were in the peripheral or posterior retina and whether they were of vascular or pigmentary origin primarily. Therefore, such findings as macular heterotopia and retinal fold would be listed as posterior retinal findings, whereas straightening of the temporal retinal arterioles would be considered posterior vascular residual findings. Peripheral pigmentary findings include pigmentary changes in the region of a regressed ridge, and peripheral vascular residua include areas of avascularity peripheral to regressed acute-phase retinopathy. Thus, a hierarchy for increasing severity of regressed ROP awaits further study and understanding of the visual consequences of regressed ROP. These data are gradually being accumulated with efforts of Birch and Spencer,[14] Katsumi and colleagues,[15] Hittner and associates,[16] and the CRYO-ROP cooperative group,[17,18] among others.

INCIDENCE

The best prevalence data on acute-phase ROP is from the natural history portion of the CRYO-ROP study for infants born between January 1, 1986, and November 30, 1987, and weighing less than 1251 g at birth.[1] The 4099 infants from 23 centers represented approximately 15% of the prematurely born population in the United States during that period. ROP was observed in 47% of infants with birth weights of 1001 to 1250 g, 78% of infants with birth weights of 751 to 999 g, and 90% of those with birth weights of less than 750 g. In addition, more severe ROP tends to occur in the smaller infants, as shown in Table 51-1. It is clear from the table that the smaller the

Table 51–1. Prevalence of ROP by Birth Weight in the CRYO-ROP Study

	<751 g	751-999 g	1000-1250 g
Stage 1 ROP	19.5%	28.6%	24.3%
Stage 2 ROP	32.8%	27.2%	13.2%
Stage 3 ROP	37.4%	21.9%	8.5%
Plus disease	24.6%	12.8%	4.7%
Prethreshold ROP	39.4%	21.4%	7.3%
Threshold ROP	15.5%	6.8%	2.0%

Adapted from Palmer EA, Flynn JT, Hardy RJ, et al: Incidence and early course of retinopathy of prematurity. Opthalmology 98:1628, 1991.

CRYO-ROP, Cryotherapy for retinopathy of prematurity; ROP, retinopathy of prematurity.

infant is, the more likely the child is to develop severe ROP; for example, the infant with a birth weight of less than 750 g is almost eight times more likely to develop threshold ROP than is the infant with a birth weight of 1000 to 1250 g. A similar gradient is also seen for infants born earlier in gestation in comparison with those born later in gestation. For example, 10.4% of children born at gestational ages of younger than 28 weeks developed threshold ROP in the CRYO-ROP study, in comparison with 1.1% of infants born at gestational ages of 32 weeks or older.[1]

Reports of ROP prevalence data from nurseries in the United States have been relatively infrequent since the extensive CRYO-ROP study. Hussain and coworkers[5] reviewed the ROP data from the intensive care nursery at University of Connecticut from 1989 to 1997. They found a significant decrease in both incidence and severity of acute retinopathy when comparing their results with those from the CRYO-ROP study. Overall, for infants with birth weights of less than 1251 g, the incidence of acute-phase retinopathy was 34% (187 of 545) and, for infants with birth weights of less than 1000 g, it was 46% (160 of 347), considerably less than the 82% reported in the CRYO-ROP study.[1] This trend toward a lower prevalence of acute-phase ROP in nurseries in the United States is promising, but it must be confirmed in a number of other centers and in larger numbers of patients.

SIGHT-THREATENING RETINOPATHY OF PREMATURITY

Most ROP is mild in degree and regresses without serious ocular sequelae. It has also become more apparent that serious residua from ROP are rare among infants with higher birth weights. Therefore, a great deal of effort has gone into defining what constitutes serious forms of ROP and identifying the children likely to develop sight-threatening ROP. A major step forward was made by the selection of zone 1 or 2, stage 3+ ROP with 5 contiguous or 8 discontinuous clock hours of involvement as the minimal criteria, or "threshold," for participation in the randomized portion of the multicenter trial of cryotherapy for ROP.[6] ROP of this severity was predicted to have a 50% likelihood of causing severe visual handicap or

blindness, according to preliminary data from the experience of the nurseries of the University of Pennsylvania, including Pennsylvania Hospital, Hospital of the University of Pennsylvania, and The Children's Hospital of Philadelphia.[19] This hypothesis was supported by the results of the CRYO-ROP trial, in which eyes with "threshold" ROP that were randomly assigned to receive no treatment had a 51.4% likelihood of having a very poor structural outcome.[20] A further helpful division of ROP severity was also developed by the CRYO-ROP study: prethreshold ROP consisting of (1) zone 1 or 2, stage 2 ROP with plus disease; (2) zone 1 or 2, stage 3 ROP without plus disease; or (3) zone 1 or 2, stage 3 ROP with plus disease but lacking the requisite hours of stage 3 to qualify for threshold. Retinopathy observed to occur initially in zone 3 is not eligible for categorization as threshold ROP or prethreshold ROP.

RETINAL VASCULARIZATION WITHOUT RETINOPATHY OF PREMATURITY

Peripheral retinal vascularization proceeds in an orderly manner from the optic disk to the ora serrata in the developing fetus.[3] In eyes that do not go on to develop ROP even though the child was born prematurely, the retinal vascular development continues in an orderly manner, although its progress may be momentarily interrupted by premature birth. In the CRYO-ROP study, 1400 infants with birth weights of less than 1251 g were monitored during the neonatal period and did not develop ROP. In Figure 51-5, the percentages of eyes with vascularization extending into zone 3 are shown for various postconception ages from 30 to 49 weeks.[1] It is apparent from the figure that retinal vascularization proceeds peripherally as the infant matures; most infants develop vessels into zone 3 by full-term due date, regardless of birth weight. It is also interesting to note that approximately one third of the eyes were judged to have vessels into zone 3 by 34 to 35 weeks of postconception age and are thus at low risk for developing serious ROP.

TIME OF ONSET

The appearance of ROP seems to be determined both by the immaturity of the child at birth and by perinatal events that are associated with an increased incidence of ROP. These events are essentially indices of how sick the child is after birth, such as the occurrence of intraventricular hemorrhage and sepsis and the need for prolonged ventilatory support and multiple transfusions. These events probably occur early after birth, when the child is most unstable medically.[21-23]

In a series of 639 infants examined in the early 1980s, Flynn documented that most acute-phase ROP was observed "between 32 and 44 weeks postconceptional age."[21] He suggested that the time to development of ROP should be considered in terms of postconception age to "relate all infants to the same time axis." About 5 years later, in a series of 572 infants with birth weights of less than 1701 g who were examined from the age of 3 weeks, Fielder and associates[24] reported an ROP incidence of

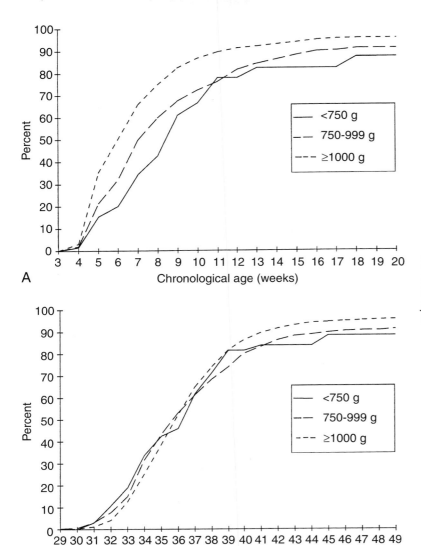

Figure 51–5. Proportion of infants with no retinopathy of prematurity with retinal vessels into zone 3 by age from birth **(A)** and postconceptional age **(B)**. *(From Palmer EA, Flynn JT, Hardy RJ, et al: Incidence and early course of retinopathy of prematurity. Ophthalmology 98:1628, 1991.)*

50.9% (291 of 572) and that the onset of 65% of the ROP cases occurred between 30 and 35 weeks of postconception age. The 23 infants who developed ROP after 40 weeks of postconception age were born at gestational ages of 31 to 38 weeks, except for the case of an infant born at 27 weeks of gestation who had missed several examinations. The time after birth to onset of retinopathy was inversely related to birth weight and gestational age.

Our ROP study group in Philadelphia also reported the onset of ROP in a group of 755 infants[25] as part of a National Eye Institute–sponsored study conducted from 1979 to 1981 to assess the possible effect of vitamin E on ROP.[26,27] Weekly examinations were undertaken as soon after birth as possible, and complete acute-phase ROP data were collected for 755 infants with birth weights of less than 2000 g or born at less than 37 weeks of gestational age but weighing more than 2000 g who required more than 23 hours of oxygen. Infants born earlier in gestation were found to develop ROP later postnatally than

infants born later in gestation. In addition, infants born at earlier gestational ages developed ROP at an earlier postconceptional age than did infants born at later gestational ages. For example, an infant born at 27 weeks of gestation developed ROP at approximately 34 to 35 weeks of postconceptional age, whereas an infant born at 32 weeks of gestational age was likely to develop ROP at approximately 35 to 37 weeks of postconceptional age.

Palmer and colleagues, on behalf of the CRYO-ROP Cooperative Group,[1] also reported the relationship between gestational age and onset of ROP in the cohort of 4099 infants with birth weights of less than 1251 g who participated in the natural history portion of the study. Because examinations started at 4 to 7 weeks after birth and 21.5% of the infants had ROP at the first examination, the data concerning onset of ROP had to be inferred from median values and 5th and 95th percentiles (Table 51-2). The median for onset of stage 1 ROP was 34.3 weeks of postconceptional age; 95% of all stage 1 events were

Table 51–2. Onset of Acute-Phase Retinopathy of Prematurity (ROP) by Postconceptional Age (Weeks)

	Median	5th Percentile	95th Percentile
Stage 1 ROP	34.3	—	39.1
Stage 2 ROP	35.4	32.0	40.7
Stage 3 ROP	36.6	32.6	42.9
Prethreshold ROP	36.1	32.4	41.5
Threshold ROP	36.9	33.6	42.0

Adapted from Palmer EA, Flynn JT, Hardy RJ, et al: Incidence and early course of retinopathy of prematurity. Ophthalmology 98:1628, 1991.

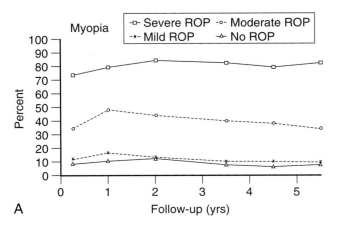

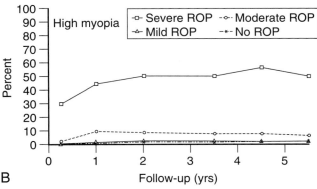

Figure 51–6. Prevalence of myopia **(A)** and high myopia **(B)** from ages 3 months to 5½ years compared to severity of acute-phase retinopathy of prematurity (ROP). High myopia is defined as 5 D or more. *(From Quinn GE, Dobson V, Kivlin J, et al: Prevalence of myopia between three months and 5½ years in preterm infants with and without retinopathy of prematurity. Ophthalmology 105:1292, 1998.)*

observed by 39.1 weeks. This report also documented that the appearance of stages 1, 2, and 3 is closely linked to gestational age and the sequence happened at approximately weekly intervals.

VISUAL MORBIDITY OF PREMATURE BIRTH

In comparison with full-term infants, premature infants who do not develop ROP are at increased risk for ocular problems later in life. The development of ROP during the neonatal period further increases the risk of later visual abnormalities, and the risk increases with increasing severity of ROP. Myopia, strabismus, nystagmus, and amblyopia are more common in preterm children who developed ROP during the neonatal period.[28-32] In addition, neurosensory impairments are much more likely to occur in infants with extremely low birth weights (28%) than in full-term controls (1%), as is the risk for requiring special educational assistance during their school years (58% versus 13%; odds ratio = 9.0).[33]

Myopia (nearsightedness), in particular, occurs with greater frequency and greater severity as severity of ROP increases (Fig. 51-6).[29,30] Myopia, especially high degrees, is associated with an increased risk of developing retinal tears and detachment, glaucoma, and retinal degeneration. In addition, retinal detachments are more common in older children who had ROP as infants. Thus, the premature infant, particularly the infant who develops serious ROP during the neonatal period, is at increased risk for serious ocular abnormalities later in life and should be monitored into adulthood.

CURRENT UNDERSTANDING OF THE PATHOGENESIS OF RETINOPATHY OF PREMATURITY

ROP appears to consist of at least two phases, and the development of retinopathy is consistently tied to the state of development of the retina. In the initial phase, superficial retinal vessel growth ceases because of a number of insults that transpire as a result of premature birth. These include exposure to relatively high levels of oxygen in the extrauterine environment[21] and complications such as intraventricular hemorrhage, sepsis, necrotizing

enterocolitis, and shock.[23,27] A second phase of abnormal retinal vascularization ensues as retinal development proceeds, with associated increasing metabolic demands. The abnormal vasculogenesis is probably the result of the production of angiogenic factors in an avascular retina, resulting in exuberant new vessel formation, and is similar to the pathogenesis of neovascularization in diabetic retinopathy.[34]

Among the cytokines and growth factors that have angiogenic activity, vascular endothelial growth factor (VEGF) has been shown to play a possible role in the development of vascular abnormalities in ROP.[35] Using a mouse model, Pierce and coworkers demonstrated that hyperoxia down-regulates expression of VEGF with resulting obliteration of immature retina vessels, and hypoxia up-regulates VEGF expression.[36] They also demonstrated that when VEGF is down-regulated by hyperoxia, exogenous VEGF would "rescue" the immature retinal vessels. Furthermore, Young and associates confirmed the mouse model VEGF findings in eyes at autopsy of an infant with ROP.[37]

In a report by Hellstrom and colleagues,[38] insulin-like growth factor 1 (IGF-1) was found to be associated with development of ROP in infants with low birth weights. The investigators found that low levels of IGF-1 in a knockout mouse model prevented the normal development of retinal vessels, even in the presence of adequate levels of VEGF. In addition, they studied the ocular findings in 31 infants born at gestational ages of 26 to 30 weeks. In some infants in the intensive care unit, they found near-normal levels of IGF-1 and did not detect the development of ROP in those infants. Infants who showed persistently low levels of IGF-1 and were slower to develop levels in the normal range were more likely to develop ROP. For the 19 infants who did not develop ROP, the mean time from birth to an IGF-1 level of 30 ng/mL was 19 days (range, 1 to 79), in comparison with 58 days (range, 29 to 120) for the 10 infants who developed ROP ($P \leq .0001$). In addition, during the critical period of 31 to 35 weeks, the mean levels of IGF-1 were consistently higher in the infants who did not develop ROP than in the infants who developed ROP. The authors suggest that reaching "normal" serum levels of IGF-1 late allows vasoproliferative factors to accumulate and, as the IGF-1 levels rise, the vasoproliferative factors, such as VEGF, incite exuberant overgrowth of retinal vessels. These findings in animal models, with support from studies of the eye findings in human infants, represent an exciting new area for increasing the understanding of the pathophysiologic mechanisms in ROP and potential treatment modalities.

TREATMENT

Therapy for ROP consists of both surgical and medical treatments and has undergone radical change since 1980. Surgical treatment is the most widely discussed form of therapy at present because of the results of the CRYO-ROP study. However, there is continued and active interest in the use of medical and other surgical means to prevent or to treat this disorder. In addition, the prevention of extremely premature birth would decrease the number of children at risk for the disorder.

Cryotherapy for Threshold Retinopathy of Prematurity

Cryotherapy to the avascular peripheral retina of eyes with severe forms of active ROP had been used in Japan since the early 1970s[39,40] and gradually gained advocates in several countries.[41,42] Many ophthalmologists were reluctant to employ this treatment modality because of untoward or unexpected results.[43,44] However, in 1985, Tasman and colleagues[45] reported a beneficial effect of cryotherapy in a small, randomized trial of cryotherapy for severe ROP.

The large, randomized, multicenter trial of cryotherapy for ROP was designed to evaluate the effect of cryotherapy on stage 3+ ROP with 5 continuous or 8 cumulative clock hours of fibrovascular proliferation. Infants with birth weights of less than 1251 g born between January 1, 1986, and November 30, 1987, who were admitted to the nursery at one of the 23 participating centers were eligible to participate in a natural history study of ROP. If threshold ROP developed in one or both eyes, permission was sought for enrollment into

the randomized portion of the trial, in which one eye received cryotherapy and the other eye was observed as a control. Infants with threshold ROP could also be referred to a participating center to participate in the trial. In all, 4099 children were in the natural history cohort and 291 children were in the randomized cohort; the latter group included 218 from the natural history group and 73 referred from other hospitals with the diagnosis of threshold ROP. An unfavorable structural outcome was defined as a posterior retinal detachment or retinal fold involving the macular or retrolental tissue obscuring the retina.[6]

Preliminary results from CRYO-ROP were published in April 1988[6] and showed that the incidence of unfavorable structural outcomes, as judged by masked grading of fundus photographs, was only 21.8% among eyes that received cryotherapy, in comparison with 43% among untreated eyes ($P < .00001$). A higher frequency of unfavorable structural outcomes was noted in infants with lower birth weights and in zone 1 retinopathy, regardless of treatment status. Thus far, these results have been substantiated at the 3-month,[20] 1-year,[28] 3½-year,[46] 5½-year,[47] and 10-year study examinations[48]; the latest report, at 10 years, showed a 27.2% incidence of unfavorable structural outcomes among treated eyes, in comparison with a 47.9% rate among untreated eyes, as determined by examining ophthalmologists ($P < .001$).

Visual function as a quantitative outcome measure was added to the study at the 1-year study examination, when monocular grating acuity was measured by the Teller Acuity Card Procedure[49] by testers unaware of the treatment status of each eye. The results showed an unfavorable functional outcome in 35% of the treated eyes, in comparison with 56.3% of the control eyes ($P < .0001$), indicating both a functional and a structural benefit from cryotherapy in eyes with threshold ROP.[28]

Because the children have matured and many have been able to provide more complex data, visual function measures such as recognition acuity, color vision, visual field extent, and contrast sensitivity have also been assessed. The structural benefits from cryotherapy have persisted from the 3-month study examination to age 10 years; however, the favorable effect of cryotherapy on visual function of eyes with threshold ROP has apparently been somewhat reduced, although it has remained statistically significant over the same time period. At age 10 years (the most recently reported examination), the children who had participated in the randomized trial during the neonatal period were tested with Snellen letters by testers unaware of each child's eye status. With a follow-up rate of 97% of eligible infants (36 of the original 291 had died before the examination), the results showed 20/200 or worse visual acuity in fewer treated eyes (44.4%) than control eyes (62.1%; $P < .001$). In addition, there was concern at the 5½-year examination that visual acuity was in the 20/40 range or better in slightly more eyes in the control group than in the treated group. This finding was not substantiated at the 10-year examination, inasmuch as there were almost equal numbers of treated eyes and control eyes in this excellent acuity range (25.2% of treated eyes versus 23.7% of control eyes; $P = .63$).[48]

In addition to visual acuity, visual field,[50,51] color vision,[52] and contrast sensitivity[53] have been assessed in children from the randomized portion of the trial, as well as a subset of children from the natural history study who did not develop ROP during the neonatal period. Using double-arc perimetry at the 5½-year examination[50] and standard Goldmann perimetry at the 10-year examination,[51] the CRYO-ROP investigators were able to document substantial overall favorable treatment effect of cryotherapy for threshold ROP; however, there was also a deficit in visual field extent of approximately 10% in treated eyes in which sight was preserved by the treatment. There did not appear to be an effect of cryotherapy on color vision[52] or contrast sensitivity[53] in eyes that had undergone the treatment for threshold ROP. However, regardless of treatment status, eyes that had severe ROP during the neonatal period showed significantly poorer contrast sensitivity than did eyes of preterm children who did not develop ROP.

Follow-up for the children in the randomized portion of the CRYO-ROP study conitnued though age 15 years and was completed in 2003. This examination included an eye examination by a study ophthalmologist, as well as the assessment of Snellen visual acuity. The primary purpose of this examination was to detect untoward side effects of the treatment, including an increase in retinal detachments or visual acuity abnormalities.

Cryotherapy for severe stages of ROP has proved critical in preventing blindness in premature infants, but it should be viewed as a surgical procedure even though it can be performed in the nursery with local anesthesia. The CRYO-ROP Cooperative Group reported a rate of 5.3% for conjunctival laceration and of 22.3% for retinal, preretinal, or vitreous hemorrhage in eyes that underwent cryotherapy.[20] Systemic complications included a 9.4% incidence of bradycardia. Brown and associates[54] reported 3 cases of respiratory arrest and 1 of cardiorespiratory arrest among 80 infants treated with cryotherapy, only 5 of whom had general anesthesia for the procedure.

Laser Photocoagulation

The first surgical treatment investigated for acute phases of ROP was laser photocoagulation.[55] However, the treatment was technically quite difficult, and cryotherapy of the peripheral avascular area gradually replaced laser treatment. Cryotherapy was used in the large multicenter CRYO-ROP study that established the benefit of surgical treatment for threshold ROP. The binocular laser indirect ophthalmoscope was developed in the late 1980s and early 1990s, again making possible use of this potentially less destructive means of treatment of threshold ROP. Unfortunately, because of the large sample size necessary to prove equality of treatment modalities, no large-scale randomized trial comparing the outcomes and risks of laser photocoagulation and cryotherapy for severe ROP is likely to be undertaken. Laser, however, is an accepted alternative treatment modality for threshold ROP and may involve less stress for the infant. The largest data set that addressed the issue of equality of the two treatments consisted of a meta-analysis of three small randomized

studies with a total of 71 patients.[56] Laser therapy outcomes were determined to be "as good as cryotherapy." In addition, the authors noted the lessened stress for the child during treatment with laser, less postoperative pain, and less confluence of retinal scarring.

Whichever means of treatment is chosen, surgical intervention in threshold should be undertaken within 72 hours of the diagnosis of threshold ROP if the infant is stable enough to tolerate the procedure. Cryotherapy or laser photocoagulation may be used to ablate the entire avascular retina. Either technique may be performed with local or general anesthesia, and both are effective in preventing progression of disease in most cases. Laser photocoagulation may be a more reasonable choice in very posterior disease, inasmuch as conjunctival incisions and difficult probe placement are routine in cryotherapy for posterior disease but are not required for laser photocoagulation.

Scleral Buckle and Vitrectomy Procedures

Despite the success of cryotherapy in preventing blindness in many infants with severe ROP, the condition in a number of infants deteriorates to partial or total retinal detachment. The detachments are treated with scleral buckling and vitrectomy techniques.[57-65] It is often difficult to determine clinically whether a detachment is partial or total and the timing of intervention is determined on an individual basis. This may help explain the variation in reported success rates, from 10% to 70%. Assessment of visual function in eyes that have undergone vitrectomy/scleral buckling procedures is usually difficult because many affected children have other handicaps[66-68] and assessment of very low levels of vision is not standardized.

Greven and Tasman reported visual acuities of 20/400 or better in four eyes with stage 4B or stage 5 retinal detachments that had undergone scleral buckling procedures.[62] Katsumi and colleagues suggested that in children with severe ROP residua and very low vision, moving targets may provide better acuity results that stationary ones.[69] The largest case series of visual outcomes after vitrectomy for stage 5 ROP was reported by Quinn and colleagues, on behalf of the CRYO-ROP Cooperative Group.[70] Of the 98 eyes with threshold ROP in the CRYO-ROP study that had undergone vitrectomy procedures for total retinal detachment, only 2 eyes of one patient had evidence of any pattern vision (although the level was the lowest measurable in the acuity card procedure) at the 1-year study examination. With further follow-up reported on the same cohort at 5½ years of age,[71] these two eyes had become blind, and a single eye (one that had undergone a vitrectomy procedure before age 1 year) had minimal pattern vision.

Medical Treatment

The medical treatment of ROP has been less strikingly effective than cryotherapy, but, as Tasman suggested,[72] the approximately 25% incidence rate of unfavorable structural outcomes after cryotherapy is "unacceptably high" and other strategies must be devised. A number of medical treatments, both prophylactic and therapeutic for established retinopathy, have been used in an attempt to decrease the incidence or severity of ROP or decrease progression of established disease.

Through a prospective randomized study in infants with birth weights of less than 1251 g and gestational ages of less than 31 weeks, the Effects of Light Reduction on Retinopathy of Prematurity (Light-ROP) study[73] was designed as a prophylactic trial and an attempt to determine the effect on incidence of ROP by limiting light exposure early in life. The rationale for the study was that decreasing oxidant radical exposure in the developing retina of the premature infant would decrease the incidence of ROP. Shortly after birth, goggles were placed over the eyes of randomly selected infants. The goggles remained in place until 31 weeks postconception age or 4 weeks after birth, whichever was longer. When incidence of ROP in these infants was compared with that in infants who had no goggles, the investigators found no significant difference between the two groups (54% in the infants with goggles versus 58% in the control group; $P = .50$; relative risk = 0.9; 95% confidence interval [CI] = 0.8 to 1.1). Thus, it does not appear that reducing light exposure early in life decreases the likelihood of developing the ROP.

The Supplemental Therapeutic Oxygen for Prethreshold Retinopathy of Prematurity (STOP-ROP) study was designed as a therapeutic study of already established retinopathy. The randomized trial examined the efficacy and risk of using supplemental oxygen treatment at the diagnosis of prethreshold ROP in preventing progression to threshold ROP.[74] The rationale for the study was based on the hypothesis that increasing the oxygen available to overgrowing retinal vessels would decrease progression of disease. Infants with prethreshold ROP in one or both eyes were assigned to receive conventional oxygen treatment (pulse oximetry target was 89% to 94% saturation) or supplemental oxygen treatment (pulse oximetry target was 94% to 99%). Six hundred forty-nine infants from 30 centers were recruited over 5 years; the rate of progression to threshold ROP was 48% among infants receiving conventional treatment and 41% of those receiving supplemental treatment (adjusted odds ratio = 0.72; 95% CI = 0.5 to 1.01). In addition, supplemental oxygen increased the risk of adverse pulmonary events, including pneumonia and chronic lung disease. Thus, this treatment of established disease is not a standard of care.

The naturally occurring antioxidant vitamin E (α-tocopherol) has promise for decreasing incidence of retinopathy, and trials were conducted in several centers.[75] The rationales for its use were that (1) vitamin E is a naturally occurring, potent free radical scavenger that decreases lipid peroxidation and helps maintain membrane integrity and (2) the serum and tissue levels of vitamin E, a lipid-soluble substance, are known to be deficient in newborns, particularly premature infants.[76-78] Its use in ROP prophylaxis, and the encouraging preliminary findings, were reported by Owens and Owens in 1949.[79] However, this observation was followed closely by reports that oxygen treatment of premature infants had a close

link with ROP,[80-82] and investigation into the effect of vitamin E on ROP was abandoned until the 1970s.

In 1974, during a period when the prevalence of ROP was again surging among premature infants, Johnson and associates reported a randomized clinical trial with oral and parenteral α-tocopherol acetate supplements (as an investigational new drug) to achieve physiologic serum levels (1 to 3 mg/dL) in premature infants, most of whom were vitamin E deficient in the nurseries of that time.[83] This and subsequent work through 1979[84] showed a beneficial effect on incidence and severity of ROP associated with vitamin E prophylaxis that targeted physiologic serum levels of the antioxidant. A National Eye Institute–sponsored randomized, controlled clinical trial was undertaken from 1979 to 1981 in an attempt to determine the likelihood of eliminating ROP or its serious sequelae by using pharmacologic serum levels with a target level of 4 to 5 mg/dL.[26] The results of this clinical trial showed a decrease in the incidence of ROP by multivariate logistic analysis that controlled for birth weight, gestational age, days on oxygen and ventilator therapy, and days in the hospital. This study also, however, documented an increased incidence of sepsis and late-onset necrotizing enterocolitis in infants with birth weights of less than 1501 g who had received vitamin E prophylaxis at pharmacologic serum levels since birth.[27]

Also in the late 1970s and early 1980s, several other clinical trials were undertaken to determine the effectiveness of vitamin E in preventing ROP. In a clinical trial from 1979 to 1980, Hittner and associates supplemented infants with birth weights of less than 1501 g for the first 8 weeks after birth and raised serum levels from 0.3 mg/dL on admission to a mean of 1.2 mg/dL.[85] No threshold ROP was observed in the eyes of vitamin E–treated infants, in comparison with five cases in eyes of control subjects. Milner and coworkers reported a placebo-controlled trial with 114 placebo- and 111 vitamin E–treated infants with birth weights of less than 1501 g and observed that five placebo- and three vitamin E–treated infants developed severe ROP.[86] Finer and colleagues, in a phase 2 trial of 174 infants with birth weights of less than 1501 g, found a vitamin E treatment effect in multiple linear regression.[87] Puklin and associates, in a study of respiratory distress syndrome in larger infants, found no effect of vitamin E on ROP,[88] and Phelps and colleagues found no difference in stage 3+ ROP in a study of 196 infants with birth weights of less than 1501 g.[89] In a meta-analysis of these trials, Raju and coworkers found no difference in the incidence of retinopathy among treated infants versus placebo recipients, but they did find that the pooled odds ratio for developing stage 3+ ROP with vitamin E prophylaxis was 0.44 (95% CI = 0.21 to 0.81; $P < .02$).[75] Thus, the authors suggested that the role of vitamin E in reducing severe ROP should be reevaluated.

Inasmuch as most cases of ROP are mild and regress, pharmacologic prophylaxis with vitamin E is not recommended, because any serious side effects such as necrotizing enterocolitis and sepsis,[27] as well as a possible increased incidence of retinal hemorrhage[90] and an increase in intraventricular hemorrhage,[89] are unacceptable. However, prophylaxis with commercially available preparations of vitamin E with serum target levels in the physiologic range of 1 to 3 mg/dL is recommended by Johnson and associates[91] and others.[92,93] Because threshold ROP is usually seen after 8 weeks of age,[1] the likelihood of vitamin E–associated side effects was thought to be minimal and the risk/benefit ratio likely to be favorable.

Thus, there are no established medical treatments currently available for prevention of ROP or for treatment of established retinopathy.

RECENT TREATMENT TRIALS

The Early Treatment of ROP (ET-ROP) study was a surgical treatment trial that began enrolling infants with birth weights of less than 1251 g who develop moderately severe ROP.[94] This National Eye Institute–funded multicenter collaborative trial was designed to test the hypothesis that eyes with moderately severe ROP (judged to have a 15% or greater risk of progression to severe cicatricial outcomes at 3 months after term, according to data from the CRYO-ROP study) will have better outcomes if treated earlier in the course of disease. For children in whom both eyes meet study criteria for randomization, one eye was randomly assigned to receive treatment before the accepted threshold level, and the other eye was observed and treated at threshold ROP, if the retinopathy had progressed to that point. When the condition of only one eye of a child was severe enough to meet study criteria for randomization, that eye was randomly assigned to receive early treatment or routine treatment if the retinopathy progresses. Results of structural outcomes at 6 and 9 months corrected age, and grating visual acuity at 9 months, were recently reported for 401 infants who had high-risk prethreshold ROP. Grating acuity results showed improvements in visual outcomes with earlier treatment, as did structural outcomes. Follow-up is planned through age 6 years. The investigators developed an algorithm based on international classification of ROP to define which eyes should be treated earlier.

IMPLICATIONS FOR MEDICAL PRACTICE

The obligation of the neonatologists and ophthalmologists in caring for the premature infant have changed since the 1980s from a passive role of observing the infant and keeping parents informed to an active role in which examinations must be carefully timed and undertaken to provide the child with the best chance of having the presence of threshold ROP detected at the earliest possible time. ROP screening must begin between 4 and 7 weeks after birth and continue on an every-other-week basis until the chance of developing threshold ROP is remote. This is the point at which the retinal vessels have nearly reached the ora serrata or previously observed mild or moderate ROP has regressed. Once threshold ROP has been diagnosed, cryotherapy, perhaps in conjunction with or even replaced by laser photocoagulation, needs to be undertaken within a brief period to minimize the chance of progression to retinal detachment.

The timing of the follow-up examinations is crucial for early detection of threshold ROP. Guidelines for ROP screening have been suggested jointly by the American Academy of Pediatrics, the American Academy of Ophthalmology, and the American Association of Pediatric Ophthalmology and Strabismus[95] and have been revised. At present, when no or mild ROP is evident, examinations every other week are sufficient, but if moderate ROP or plus disease is noted, more frequent examinations are needed—sometimes every 2 to 4 days. Schaffer and associates, on behalf of the CRYO-ROP cooperative Group,[96] found that the rate of change from no or mild ROP to moderate ROP was also a strong indicator of whether serious ROP was likely to develop.

If threshold ROP is not reached and any ROP that developed has regressed, infants should have at least one follow-up ophthalmologic examination during their first 6 months; annual follow-up is recommended for those who have had significant active retinopathy.[95] The purpose of these visits is to detect strabismus, refractive errors, and other ocular abnormalities that are more common in premature infants.[97-99]

In the nursery at The Children's Hospital of Philadelphia, which serves an outborn population, my colleagues and I examine all infants with birth weights of less than 1500 g, as well as all infants receiving significant supplemental oxygen if birth weight was between 1501 and 1800 g or if the child was born at less than 32 weeks of gestation. Other infants are examined upon request by the neonatologist. All infants are examined initially at 4 to 6 weeks of age, if stable enough to tolerate the examination.

The benefit of timely detection and treatment of ROP was pointed out by Javitt and coworkers in an examination of CRYO-ROP data.[100] They calculated that, because of timely implementation of cryotherapy, a lifelong disability (i.e., blindness) is prevented in more than 300 infants per year and that the net savings of funds that would have been necessary to provide services for these children over their lifetime is between $38.3 million and $64.9 million per year of premature births.

FUTURE WORK

Although much progress has been made in ROP, much remains to be done, because the best treatment regimen to date, peripheral retinal ablation, still has an unacceptably high failure rate (as much as 1 per 4). Researchers must determine why ROP progresses to blindness in some children, despite timely intervention, whereas the retinopathy regresses in others who undergo the same treatment. Looking at the eye with an indirect ophthalmoscope does not appear adequate to detect which eyes might benefit from alternative therapeutic interventions or prophylaxis. Other useful parameters that could be examined include screening for genetic susceptibility mutations (e.g., Norrie disease gene),[101] measuring blood and urine levels of vascular growth factors such as VEGF[36] and IGF-1,[38] and assessment of blood flow abnormalities in the retinal to help quantify the definition of plus disease.[102]

Many of these research initiatives, once fully developed, may challenge the current diagnostic and treatment strategies for ROP.

REFERENCES

1. Palmer EA, Flynn JT, Hardy RJ, et al: Incidence and early course of retinopathy of prematurity. Ophthalmology 98:1628, 1991.
2. Terry TL: Extreme prematurity and fibroplastic overgrowth or persistent vascular sheath behind each crystalline lens. I. Preliminary report. Am J Ophthalmol 25:203, 1942.
3. Payne JW, Patz A: Current status of retrolental fibroplasia. Review article. Ann Clin Res 11:205, 1979.
4. Gibson DL, Sheps SB, Uh SH, et al: Retinopathy of prematurity–induced blindness: Birth weight–specific survival and the new epidemic. Pediatrics 86:405, 1990.
5. Hussain N, Clive J, Bhandari V: Current incidence of retinopathy of prematurity, 1989-1997. Pediatrics 104:1, 1999.
6. Cryotherapy for Retinopathy of Prematurity Cooperative Group: Multicenter trial of cryotherapy for retinopathy of prematurity: Preliminary results. Arch Ophthalmol 106:471, 1988.
7. Reese AB, King MJ, Owens WC: A classification of retrolental fibroplasia. Am J Ophthalmol 36:133, 1953.
8. Quinn GE, Schaffer DB, Johnson L: A revised classification of retinopathy of prematurity. Am J Ophthalmol 94:744, 1982.
9. McCormick AQ: Retinopathy of prematurity. Curr Probl Pediatr 7:3, 1977.
10. Kingham JD: Acute retrolental fibroplasia. Arch Ophthalmol 95:39, 1973.
11. The Committee for the Classification of Retinopathy of Prematurity: An international classification of retinopathy of prematurity. Arch Ophthalmol 102:1130, 1984.
12. The International Committee for the Classification of the Late Stages of Retinopathy of Prematurity: An international classification of retinopathy of prematurity: II. The classification of retinal detachment. Arch Ophthalmol 105:906, 1987.
13. Freedman SF, Kylstra JA, Capowski JJ, et al: Observer sensitivity to retinal vessel diameter and tortuosity in retinopathy of prematurity: A model system. J Pediatr Ophthalmol Strabismus 33:248, 1996.
14. Birch EE, Spencer R: Visual outcome in infants with cicatricial retinopathy of prematurity. Invest Ophthalmol Vis Sci 32:410, 1991.
15. Katsumi O, Mehta MC, Matsui Y, et al: Development of vision in retinopathy of prematurity. Arch Ophthalmol 190:1394, 1991.
16. Hittner HM, Prager TC, Kretzer FL: Visual acuity correlates with severity of retinopathy of prematurity in untreated infants weighing 750 g or less at birth. Arch Ophthalmol 110:1087, 1992.
17. Gilbert W, Dobson V, Quinn G, et al: The correlation of visual function with posterior retinal structure in severe retinopathy of prematurity. Arch Ophthalmol 110:625, 1992.
18. Reynolds J, Dobson V, Quinn GE, et al: Prediction of visual function in eyes with mild to moderate posterior pole residua of ROP. Arch Ophthalmol 111:1050, 1993.
19. Multicenter Trial of Cryotherapy for Retinopathy of Prematurity Cooperative Group: Manual of Procedures, No. PB 88-163530. Springfield, Va, National Technical Information Service, U.S. Department of Commerce, 1985.
20. Cryotherapy for Retinopathy of Prematurity Cooperative Group: Multicenter trial of cryotherapy for retinopathy of prematurity: Three month outcome. Arch Ophthalmol 108:195, 1990.
21. Flynn JT: Acute proliferative retrolental fibroplasia: Multivariate risk analysis. Trans Am Ophthalmol Soc 81:549, 1983.
22. Purohit DM, Ellison C, Zierler S, et al: Risk factors for retrolental fibroplasia: Experience with 3,025 premature infants. Pediatrics 76:339, 1985.
23. Prendiville A, Schulenburg WE: Clinical factors associated with retinopathy of prematurity. Arch Dis Child 63:522, 1988.
24. Fielder AR, Shaw DE, Robinson J, Ng YK: Natural history of retinopathy of prematurity: A prospective study. Eye 6:233, 1992.
25. Quinn GE, Johnson L, Abbasi S: Onset of retinopathy of prematurity as related to postnatal and postconceptional age. Br J Ophthalmol 76:284, 1992.
26. Johnson L, Quinn GE, Abbasi S, et al: Effect of sustained pharmacologic vitamin E levels on incidence and severity of retinopathy of prematurity: A controlled clinical trial. J Pediatr 114:827, 1989.
27. Johnson L, Bowen F, Abbasi S, et al: Relationship of prolonged pharmacologic serum levels of vitamin E to incidence of sepsis and necrotizing enterocolitis in infants with birth weights 1500 grams or less. Pediatrics 75:619, 1985.
28. Cryotherapy for Retinopathy of Prematurity Cooperative Group: Multicenter trial of cryotherapy for retinopathy of prematurity: One-year outcome—structure and function. Arch Ophthalmology 108:1408, 1990.
29. Quinn GE, Dobson V, Repka MX, et al: Development of myopia in infants with birth weights less than 1251 g. Ophthalmology 99:329, 1992.
30. Quinn GE, Dobson V, Kivlin J, et al: Prevalence of myopia between three months and 5½ years in preterm infants with and without retinopathy of prematurity. Ophthalmology 105:1292, 1998.
31. Fledelius H: Prematurity and the eye: Ophthalmic 10-year follow-up of children of low and normal birth weight. Acta Ophthalmol Suppl 128:3, 1976.
32. Holmstrom M, el Azazi M, Kugelberg U: Ophthalmological long term follow up of preterm infants: A population based, prospective study of the refraction and its development. Br J Ophthalmol 82:1265, 1998.
33. Saigal S, Hoult LA, Streiner DL, et al: School difficulties at adolescence in a regional cohort of children who were extremely low birth weight. Pediatrics 105:325, 2000,
34. Shweiki D, Itin A, Soffer D, Keshet E: Vascular endothelial growth factor induced by hypoxia may mediate hypoxia-initiated angiogenesis. Nature 359:843, 1992.
35. Brown L, Detmar M, Claffey K, et al: Vascular permeability factor/vascular endothelial growth factor: A multifunctional angiogenic cytokine. In Goldberg I, Rosen E (eds): Regulation of Angiogenesis. Basel, Switzerland, Birkhauser Verlag, 1997, pp 233-269.
36. Pierce EA, Foley ED, Smith LEH: Regulation of vascular endothelial growth factor by oxygen in a model of retinopathy of prematurity. Arch Ophthalmol 114:1219, 1996.
37. Young TL, Anthony DC, Pierce EA, et al: Histopathology and vascular endothelial growth factor in diode laser treated retinopathy of prematurity. J Pediatr Ophthalmol Strabismus 1:105, 1997.
38. Hellstrom A, Perruzzi C, Ju M, et al: Low IGF-1 suppresses VEGF-survival signaling in retinal endothelial cells: Direct correlation with clinical retinopathy of prematurity. Proc Natl Acad Sci U S A 98:5804, 2001.
39. Yamashita Y: Studies on retinopathy of prematurity. III. Cryocautery for retinopathy of prematurity. Jpn J Clin Ophthalmol 26:385, 1972.
40. Majima A, Takahashi M, Hibino Y: Clinical observations of the photocoagulation on retinopathy of prematurity. Jpn J Clin Ophthalmol 30:93, 1976.

41. Ben-Sira I, Nissenkorn I, Grunwald E, et al: Treatment of acute retinopathy of prematurity by cryopexy. Br J Ophthalmol 64:758, 1980.

42. Hindle NW: Cryotherapy for retinopathy of prematurity to prevent retrolental fibroplasia. Can J Ophthalmol 17:207, 1982.

43. Payne JW, Patz A: Treatment of acute proliferative retrolental fibroplasia. Trans Am Acad Ophthalmol Otolaryngol 76:1234, 1972.

44. Kingham JD: Acute retrolental fibroplasia: Treatment by cryosurgery. Arch Ophthalmol 96:2049, 1978.

45. Tasman W, Brown GC, Schaffer DB, et al: Cryotherapy for active retinopathy of prematurity. Ophthalmology 93:580, 1986.

46. Cryotherapy for Retinopathy of Prematurity Cooperative Group: Multicenter Trial of Cryotherapy for Retinopathy of Prematurity: 3$^{1}/_{2}$-year outcome—structure and function. Arch Ophthalmol 111:339, 1993.

47. Cryotherapy for Retinopathy of Prematurity Cooperative Group: Multicenter Trial of Cryotherapy for Retinopathy of Prematurity: Snellen visual acuity and structural outcome at 5$^{1}/_{2}$ years after randomization. Arch Ophthalmol 114:417, 1996.

48. Cryotherapy for Retinopathy of Prematurity Cooperative Group: Multicenter Trial of Cryotherapy for Retinopathy of Prematurity: Ophthalmological outcomes at 10 years. Arch Ophthalmol 119:1110, 2001.

49. Dobson V, Quinn GE, Biglan AW, et al: Acuity card assessment of visual function in the Cryotherapy for Retinopathy of Prematurity trial. Invest Ophthalmol Vis Sci 31:1702, 1990.

50. Quinn GE, Dobson V, Hardy RJ, et al: Visual fields measured with double-arc perimetry in eyes with threshold retinopathy of prematurity (ROP) from the CRYO-ROP trial. Ophthalmology 103:1432, 1996.

51. Cryotherapy for Retinopathy of Prematurity Cooperative Group: Effect of retinal ablative therapy for threshold retinopathy of prematurity: Results of Goldmann perimetry at age 10 years. Arch Ophthalmol 119:1120, 2001.

52. Dobson V, Quinn GE, Abramov I, et al: Color vision measured with pseudoisochromatic plates at 5$^{1}/_{2}$ years in eyes of children in from the CRYO-ROP study. Invest Ophthalmol Vis Sci 37:2467, 1996.

53. Cryotherapy for Retinopathy of Prematurity Cooperative Group: Contrast sensitivity at age 10 years in children who had threshold retinopathy of prematurity. Arch Ophthalmol 119:1129, 2001.

54. Brown GC, Tasman WS, Naidoff M, et al: Systemic complications associated with retinal cryoablation for retinopathy of prematurity. Ophthalmology 97:865, 1990.

55. Nagata M, Kanenari S, Fukuda T, et al: Photocoagulation for the treatment of retinopathy of prematurity. Jpn J Clin Ophthalmol 24:419, 1968.

56. The Laser ROP Study Group: Laser therapy for retinopathy of prematurity. Arch Ophthalmol 112:154, 1994.

57. Tasman W: Retinal detachment in retrolental fibroplasia. Graefes Arch Clin Exp Ophthalmol 195:129, 1975.

58. McPherson A, Hittner HM: Scleral buckling in 2$^{1}/_{2}$- to 11-month-old premature infants with retinal detachment associated with acute retrolental fibroplasia. Ophthalmology 86:819, 1979.

59. Lightfoot D, Irvine AR: Vitrectomy in infants and children with retinal detachments caused by cicatricial retrolental fibroplasia. Am J Ophthalmol 94:305, 1982.

60. Machemer R: Closed vitrectomy for severe retrolental fibroplasia in the infant. Ophthalmology 90:436, 1983.

61. Trese MT: Surgical results of stage V retrolental fibroplasia and timing of surgical repair. Ophthalmology 91:461, 1984.

62. Greven CM, Tasman WS: Scleral buckling in stages 4B and 5 retinopathy of prematurity. Ophthalmology 97:817, 1990.

63. Noorily SW, Small K, de Juan E, Machemer R: Scleral buckling of stage 4B retinopathy of prematurity. Ophthalmology 99:263, 1992.

64. Hirose T, Katsumi O, Mehta MC, Schepens CL: Vision in stage 5 retinopathy of prematurity after retinal reattachment by open-sky vitrectomy. Arch Ophthalmol 111:345, 1993.

65. Charles S: Vitrectomy with ciliary body entry for retrolental fibroplasia. In McPherson AR, Hittner HM, Kretzer FL (eds): Retinopathy of Prematurity: Current Concepts and Controversies. Toronto, Ontario, BC Decker, 1986, pp 225-234.

66. Hack M: Follow-up of extremely-low-birth-weight infants. In Corvett RM, Hay WW Jr (eds): The Micropremie: The Next Frontier. Columbus, Oh, Ross Laboratories Publishers, 1990, pp 154-159.

67. Saigal S, Rosenbaum P, Szatmari P, Campbell D: Learning disabilities and school problems in a regional cohort of extremely low birth weight (<1000 g) children: A comparison with term controls. Dev Behav Pediatr 12:294, 1991.

68. Teplin SW, Burchinal M, Johnson-Martin N, et al: Neurodevelopmental, health, and growth status at 6 years of children with birth weights less than 1001 grams. J Pediatr 118:768, 1991.

69. Katsumi O, Kronheim JK, Mehta MC, et al: Measuring vision with temporally modulated stripes in infants and children with ROP. Invest Ophthalmol Vis Sci 34:496, 1993.

70. Quinn GE, Dobson V, Barr CC, et al: Visual acuity in infants after vitrectomy for severe retinopathy of prematurity. Ophthalmology 98:5, 1991.

71. Quinn GE, Dobson V, Barr CC, et al: Visual acuity of eyes after vitrectomy for ROP: Follow-up at 5-1/2 years. Ophthalmology 103:595, 1996.

72. Tasman W: Threshold retinopathy of prematurity revisited. Editorial. Arch Ophthalmol 110:623, 1992.

73. Reynolds JD, Hardy RJ, Kennedy KA, et al: Lack of efficacy of light reduction in preventing retinopathy of prematurity. Light Reduction in Retinopathy of Prematurity Cooperative Group. N Engl J Med 338:1572, 1998.

74. The STOP-ROP Multicenter Study Group: Supplemental therapeutic oxygen for prethreshold retinopathy of prematurity: A randomized, controlled trial. I: Primary outcomes. Pediatrics 105:295, 2000.

75. Raju TNK, Langenberg P, Bhutani V, Quinn GE: Vitamin E prophylaxis to reduce retinopathy of prematurity: A reappraisal of published trials. J Pediatr 131:844, 1997.

76. Machlin LJ (ed): Vitamin E: A Comprehensive Treatise. New York, Marcel Dekker, 1980, pp 289-306.

77. Butcher JR, Roberts RJ: Alpha tocopherol (vitamin E) content of lung, liver and blood in the newborn rat and human infant: Influence of hyperoxia. J Pediatr 98:806, 1981.

78. Mino M, Nishino H, Yamaguchi T, Hayashi M: Tocopherol level in human fetal and infant liver. J Nutr Sci Vitaminol (Tokyo) 23:63, 1977.

79. Owens WC, Owens EU: Retrolental fibroplasia in premature infants. II. Studies on the prophylaxis of the disease: The use of alpha tocopherol acetate. Am J Ophthalmol 32:1631, 1949.

80. Patz A, Hoeck LE, de la Cruz E: Studies on the effect of high oxygen administration in retrolental fibroplasia. Nursery observations. Am J Ophthalmol 27:1248, 1952.

81. Lanman JT, Guy LP, Dancis J: Retrolental fibroplasia and oxygen therapy. JAMA 155:223, 1954.

82. Kinsey VE: Retrolental fibroplasia: Cooperative study of retrolental fibroplasia and the use of oxygen. Arch Ophthalmol 56:481, 1956.

83. Johnson L, Schaffer DB, Boggs TR: Vitamin E deficiency and retrolental fibroplasia. Am J Clin Nutr 27:1158, 1974.

84. Johnson L, Schaffer D, Quinn G, et al: Vitamin E supplementation and the retinopathy of prematurity. Ann N Y Acad Sci 393:473, 1982.

85. Hittner HM, Godio LB, Rudolph AJ, et al: Retrolental fibroplasia: Efficacy of vitamin E in a double-blind clinical study of preterm infants. N Engl J Med 305:1365, 1981.

86. Milner RA, Watts JL, Paes B, Zipursky A: RLF in 1500 gram neonates: Part of a randomized clinical trial of the effectiveness of vitamin E. In Retinopathy of Prematurity Conference Syllabus, vol 2. Columbus, Ohio, Ross Laboratories, 1981, pp 703-716.

87. Finer NN, Schindler RF, Grant G, et al: Effect of intramuscular vitamin E on frequency and severity of retrolental fibroplasia: A controlled trial. Lancet 1:1087, 1982.

88. Puklin JE, Simon RM, Ehrenkranz RA: Influence on retrolental fibroplasia of intramuscular vitamin E administration during respiratory distress syndrome. Ophthalmology 89:96, 1982.

89. Phelps DL, Rosenbaum AL, Isenberg SJ, et al: Tocopherol efficacy and safety for preventing retinopathy of prematurity: A randomized, controlled, double-masked trial. Pediatrics 79:489, 1987.

90. Rosenbaum AL, Phelps DL, Isenberg SJ, et al: Retinal hemorrhages in retinopathy of prematurity associated with tocopherol treatment. Ophthalmology 92:1012, 1985.

91. Johnson LH, Quinn GE, Abbasi S: Vitamin E and ROP—the continuing challenge. In Fanaroff AA (ed): Yearbook of Neonatal and Perinatal Medicine. St. Louis, Mosby, 2001, pp 1193, pp xv-xxiv.

92. Ehrenkranz RA: Vitamin E and retinopathy of prematurity: Still controversial. J Pediatr 114:801, 1989.

93. Hittner HM, Godio LB, Speer ME, et al: Retrolental fibroplasia: Further clinical evidence and ultrastructural support for efficacy of vitamin E in the preterm infant. Pediatrics 71:423, 1983.

94. Early Treatment For Retinopathy of Prematurity Cooperative Group: Revised indications for the treatment of retinopathy of prematurity: Results of the early treatment for retinopathy of prematurity randomized trial. Arch Ophthalmol 121:1684, 2003.

95. American Academy of Pediatrics, Section on Ophthalmology: Screening examination of premature infants for retinopathy of prematurity. Pediatrics 108:209, 2001.

96. Schaffer DB, Palmer EA, Plotsky DF, et al: Prognostic factors in the natural course of retinopathy of prematurity. The Cryotherapy for Retinopathy of Prematurity Cooperative Group. Ophthalmology 100:230, 1993.

97. Kushner BJ: Strabismus and amblyopia associated with regressed retinopathy of prematurity. Arch Ophthalmol 100:256, 1982.

98. Schaffer DB, Quinn GE, Johnson L: Sequelae of arrested mild retinopathy of prematurity. Arch Ophthalmol 102:373, 1984.

99. Gallo JE, Holmstrom G, Kugelberg U, et al: Regressed retinopathy of prematurity and its sequelae in children aged 5-10 years. Br J Ophthalmol 75:572, 1991.

100. Javitt J, Dei Cas R, Chiang Y: Cost-effectiveness of screening and cryotherapy for threshold retinopathy of prematurity. Pediatrics 91:859, 1993.

101. Shastry BS, Pendergast SD, Trese MT, et al: Identification of missense mutations in the Norrie disease gene associated with advanced retinopathy of prematurity. Arch Ophthalmol 115:651, 1997.

102. Petrig BL, Young TL, Grunwald JE, et al: Laser Doppler velocimetry in retinal arteries of infants. Lasers Med Sci 10:267, 1995.

CHAPTER 52

Neurologic Examination

Lawrence W. Brown

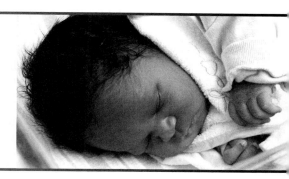

The neurologic examination of the neonate relies primarily on observation. Findings may vary almost weekly according to postconception age; changes are more dramatic in significantly premature infants than in near-term neonates. Accurate assessment can be difficult for several reasons other than gestational age. The behavioral repertoire of the newborn is extremely limited, and it varies with sleep-wake cycle, feeding schedule, and maternal influences (such as medications excreted in breast milk). Therefore, the neurologic examination of the newborn is a clinical challenge that may necessitate serial assessments as well as supportive laboratory studies in order to establish a consistent pattern and to exclude reversible causes of abnormal findings.

Brain development corresponds to gestational age, and this programmed process continues at the same rate whether an infant is born early or at term. The premature infant at 26 weeks of gestation has not yet completed neuronal differentiation, neuronal migration, myelinization, or full vascular development. The full-term infant, who has a more mature pattern of neuronal cellular anatomy and supportive glial structures in place, still demonstrates immature structure and function. Synaptic connections are incomplete and myelin is still underdeveloped in most neocortical regions. Parts of the temporal lobes, midbrain, brain stem, spinal cord, and peripheral nerves are the most highly advanced regions in comparison with the rest of the cerebral hemispheres. Inhibitory synaptic connections outweigh excitatory ones even when dendritic sprouts and arborization are well developed. This emphasis on **subcortical** and **inhibitory** leads to important predictions about baseline activity levels and behavior when electrophysiologic disturbances produce clinical seizures. Neonates show autonomic disturbances such as apnea and less well organized motor activity (i.e., fragmentary, migrating clonic movements versus generalized tonic-clonic seizures) than do older infants. However, the relative importance of subcortical structures in the premature and full-term infant does not preclude higher cortical activity. The full-term infant in the first hours after birth can already orient to sound, briefly fixate and follow a face, and even start to mimic facial and tongue movements. Infants without the capacity for cortical function (i.e., those with hydranencephaly and anencephaly), however, can appear almost normal, but the previously mentioned activities are not present.

Although the examination of the healthy full-term infant is challenging, the neurologic evaluation of the premature infant can be a daunting experience. Merely getting close enough to examine such an infant who is on multiple life-support systems can be difficult. Sedating medications can hamper the evaluation of the state of alertness. Also, there are sleep-wake cycle differences and a rapidly evolving set of normative values to keep in mind. At times, a particular neurologic examination result would be abnormal at any given gestational age, but in other cases the same finding would be normal at an earlier gestational age. Laboratory studies (myelinization pattern on magnetic resonance imaging [MRI], electroencephalographic background, nerve conduction velocity) can help to define true gestational age more accurately when the clinical findings do not match the calculated postconception age. It is important to remember that neurologic maturity and appropriate developmental milestones are correlated with gestational age rather than with birth weight or calculated estimated date of delivery.

The optimal time to examine the newborn is during quiet wakefulness between feedings, generally about 1 hour before the next scheduled meal. If the examination is performed while the infant is hungry, there is likely to be excessive irritability and relatively increased tone, whereas a sleepy baby satiated after feeding will appear lethargic and overly floppy. Sustained wakefulness is uncommon in premature infants younger than 28 weeks of postconception age. However, stimulation by light, temperature changes, and feeding can usually produce transient arousal. Periods of wakefulness gradually increase in duration between 28 and 32 weeks, and there should be periods of sustained arousal that do not require outside stimulation by that point. By 37 weeks, there is even more responsiveness with crying. At 40 weeks of postconception age, the premature infant is similar to the newborn full-term infant with periods of sustained arousal and reactivity to a variety of sensory stimuli, including visual, auditory, and tactile objects.

HISTORY

It is easy to overlook the very brief medical history in the newborn, but much can be learned from a careful investigation into the background of the parents, the obstetric history, and the prior neonatal course. Parental age and race, medical illnesses within the family, and obstetric complications can provide important clues. The obstetric history is particularly important; it should encompass the prenatal and intrapartum course of the infant as well as previous pregnancies and their outcomes. Equally important are the circumstances of delivery and its complications, maternal medications, Apgar scores, resuscitative efforts, time to sustained spontaneous breathing, and time to adequate heart rate. The perinatal history should include a description of spontaneous activity and tone, as well as abnormalities such as seizures, apnea, episodic or persistent hypotonia, and decreased activity level.

ASSESSMENT OF GESTATIONAL AGE

The most widely accepted system for accurate gestational age assessment combines neurologic and physical signs of maturation. The Dubowitz score involves 10 neurologic features with 11 physical characteristics to establish an estimate of gestational age. Each measure of the neurologic examination is objective and easy to perform, relying on muscle tone and reflex movement rather than specific testing of cortical activity. Posture is described with the infant quiet and supine: ratings reflect the degree of extremity flexion. "Square window" reflects the increasing flexibility of the infant's wrist by measuring the angle between the hypothenar eminence and the ventral aspect of the forearm. Ankle dorsiflexion is a similar maneuver of the lower extremity. Arm and leg recoil are measured separately by fully flexing the extremities for 5 seconds and then fully extending them, followed by observation of the maximal response back toward flexion. The popliteal angle and heel-to-ear maneuver measure the decreasing flexibility of the knee and hip, respectively, with maturation. Assessment for the "scarf sign" similarly involves checking the tone of the shoulder girdle by abducting the elbow toward the midline as the hand is brought across the chest to the opposite shoulder. Evaluation of "head lag" involves checking the position of the head in relation to the trunk as the arms are brought up while the infant remains supine. Finally, ventral suspension is the degree of extremity flexion and back extension as the infant is supported under the chest in the prone position. When these characteristics are combined with physical features such as plantar creases, genitalia, breast size, ear formation and firmness, and skin texture, the examiner can formulate a reliable sense of gestational age. The modified Ballard score is a similar method in which findings on the physical examination are similarly

used to assess neonatal maturity. Although either method of assessment is slightly less reliable at the lower limits of viability, they are generally accurate to within 1 to 2 weeks of gestational age.

STATE OF AWARENESS

The neurologic status of the newborn depends largely on the level of arousal; in addition, determination of the state of consciousness is a critical feature of the examination itself. This is the main reason why it is so important to try to perform the neurologic examination during quiet wakefulness. However, level of consciousness in the neonate can present a diagnostic challenge. Premature infants younger than 32 weeks of gestational age spend the majority of time asleep, and they do not have sustained wakefulness, as described earlier. In infants of all gestational ages, alertness varies depending on pain, thirst, or hunger. A normal full-term infant during quiet wakefulness shows a semiflexed posture and smooth spontaneous movements of all extremities. The hyperalert neonate has the appearance of increased vigilance with eyes widely open, often decreased blinking, and overreaction to minimal stimulation, as well as reduced sleeping. Operational definitions of lethargy, stupor, and coma are similar to those states in older children, with progressively reduced responsiveness and more stereotyped primitive responses.

POSTURE

The first step in the neurologic examination is to observe the way the infant lies in the warmer or crib. Much can be predicted from the position of the limbs at rest, even if the infant is connected to a ventilator with chest tubes and multiple intravenous catheters. Any alteration of expected patterns of posture suggests focal or generalized neurologic abnormalities. Full-term infants should have a preponderance of flexor tone during both wakefulness and sleep. This leads to the normal semiflexed posture of the elbows and knees. Similarly, the hand position is typically a partially closed fist. A tight "cortical thumb" can be normal, but when it is persistent and obligatory, it suggests a corticospinal abnormality. In the prone position, the pelvis normally is slightly elevated by hip and knee flexion; the examiner should be able to see the classic curve of the "fetal position" in the recumbent posture. Extensor posturing of the legs with arms held tightly fisted against the midline is indicative of hypertonicity. Flaccidity of the upper extremities with normal hip and leg movements suggests a spinal cord lesion. Altered spontaneous activity of one upper extremity may be indicative of a brachial plexus injury.

TONE AND MOVEMENT

Muscle tone is evaluated by resistance to passive movement, as outlined in the maneuvers of the Dubowitz and Ballard scoring systems. The degree of spontaneous activity and resistance of individual muscles to movement offers an estimate of underlying strength. Tone is affected by head position, with relatively increased tone on the side to which the head points, as seen in the asymmetric tonic neck reflex. Marked hypotonia normally characterizes the premature infant younger than 29 weeks; tone increases in a caudal-rostral direction over the ensuing weeks of gestation. Thus, there is an orderly progression from diffuse limpness at 28 weeks to the flexed "frog legs" posture at 34 weeks to the fully flexed supine posture at term. Objective evidence for increasing tone can be found in the limb angles at full flexion, with shoulder abduction and the traction maneuver. At 28 weeks, the popliteal angle (knee extension with hips flexed) and the adductor angle of the hip (as measured by the heel-to-ear maneuver) are fully 180 degrees, but by term they are each less than 90 degrees. Normal, marked hypotonia below 30 weeks does not allow the preterm infant to support his or her standing weight even momentarily when held under the axillae. A complete supporting response rapidly develops by 34 weeks. Complete head lag at 30 weeks gradually improves first with predominant extensor tone of the neck, which is then replaced by more flexor tone; by 38 weeks the head follows the trunk and is maintained briefly before falling forward as the supine infant is brought to sitting in the traction maneuver. Similarly, the scarf sign at 30 weeks (extensibility allowing the elbow to touch the opposite shoulder) is gradually reduced so that by term the elbow can be brought barely beyond the midline.

By 40 weeks of gestation, the infant demonstrates resistance with back flexion and neck flexion in the traction maneuver while the feet and legs remain flexed. The full-term infant maintains the head upright and supports his or her weight in upright suspension without sliding through the examiner's hands when held under the axillae. Also, in ventral suspension there should be pronounced hip and knee flexion, slight dorsiflexion of the back, and transient ability to lift the head. Full-term infants with decreased tone show less flexor posture, less resistance to passive movement, and more head lag. These characteristics together produce the typical "rag doll" appearance of the floppy infant.

Generalized depression of the central nervous system is the most common cause of severe hypotonia. However, the differential diagnosis of the floppy infant is extremely broad. Causes vary from congenital migrational defects to hypoxic-ischemic encephalopathy, sepsis and meningitis, intraventricular hemorrhage, congenital metabolic disorders from acquired metabolic derangements, and primary neuromuscular disorders. The latter conditions include various congenital myopathies, myotonic dystrophy, neonatal myasthenia gravis, and spinal muscular atrophy.

Infants with increased tone show extensor posturing of extremities in supine and prone positions, although sometimes the elbows are held tightly flexed with cortical fisting. The most severe degrees of hypertonia lead to opisthotonus; in this extreme case, the entire body moves in one block as if frozen during the traction maneuver or tonic neck reflex. This appearance is often associated with jittery or tremulous motor activity, which tends to be stimulus bound. These overly exaggerated responses to

light, sound, or touch usually stop abruptly when the stimulus is withdrawn. High-pitched or shrill cry, uncoordinated or frantic sucking, and excessive crying are signs often associated with hypotonia. Marked hypertonia most often results from many of the same structural, infectious, and hypoxic-ischemic insults that can lead to generalized hypotonia. However, increased tone tends to point to a more chronic or subacute condition as the central nervous system injury evolves.

Although the neurologic examination generally reflects postconceptional age, subtle variations can be found in full-term neonates in comparison with premature infants who have reached 40 weeks of postconceptional age. The typical healthy preterm infant at 40 weeks remains mildly hypotonic with less foot dorsiflexion and a larger popliteal angle in comparison with full-term infants. The premature infant lies in a flatter prone position because the buttocks are less raised as a result of relative hypotonia.

Spontaneous movements are often irregular, tremulous, and jerky in the premature infant. These occur most prominently during active sleep. During the awake state, it is more common to see random stretching movements, which may appear asynchronous or bilateral and may spread to include head, neck, and trunk.

CRANIAL NERVES

Before 30 weeks, the pupils are typically miotic and unresponsive to bright light, but by 32 weeks, the pupillary light reflex is already fully mature. Even when there is no pupillary response, the preterm infant at 28 weeks should blink in response to bright light. By 31 to 32 weeks, visual fixation on large bright objects can be demonstrated. By 36 weeks, the infant responds to brightly colored objects with active tracking and head turning, and there is forceful eye closure to bright light. The full-term infant not only shows a mature pupillary reaction but also turns the head toward a diffuse light stimulus and blinks or forcefully closes the eyes in response to bright light.

Examination of the optic fundi can be made especially difficult by chemical conjunctivitis from the prophylactic eye drops routinely administered at birth, but funduscopy is an essential part of the examination and should always be attemped. Optic nerve hypoplasia, retinal hemorrhages, and chorioretinitis are among the most important possible findings. Although retinal hemorrhages may be correlated with brain injury, transient lesions are a common, nonspecific, isolated finding in otherwise normal deliveries.

Visual acuity of the neonate is hard to assess clinically, but the most effective stimuli are the human face and large colored objects held close to the infant's face and moved slowly through the visual field. Whereas end-point nystagmus is a normal variant, constant nystagmus, whether conjugate (as in congenital nystagmus or blindness) or chaotic (as in opsoclonus) is never normal. Sixth nerve palsy can be demonstrated when the eyes fail to abduct, and third nerve dysfunction can be shown when the eyes fail to adduct or contract in response to bright light.

The palpebral fissures should appear equal; ptosis must be distinguished from contralateral lid retraction. Ptosis is far more common than lid retraction. It typically results from third nerve dysfunction or abnormal sympathetic innervation (e.g., brachial plexus injury), neuromuscular disease, or an abnormality of the connective tissue of the lid. Horner syndrome, Möbius syndrome, Duane syndrome, and congenital myopathies are among the important considerations.

The oculovestibular reflex (doll's-eye reflex) can be elicited by 28 weeks during quiet wakefulness. This reflex is typically elicited by turning the head from side to side, which leads to eye deviation to the opposite direction. Similarly, the neck can be flexed and extended to produce vertical eye movements. Holding the infant steady and spinning together is a variation of the procedure, thus allowing constant observation of the eyes during the procedure. The doll's-eye reflex is often inhibited in the fully awake infant by 36 weeks, although it may remain during drowsiness in the full-term infant.

Isolated facial weakness used to be considered a sign of traumatic injury, most often from forceps misapplication. Presentation of the head against the sacral promontory during labor and delivery, however, is the usual cause of this condition. Paralysis of facial movement is unilateral, with a smooth forehead and persistently open eye on the affected side. Facial weakness can also be seen in Möbius syndrome (although it is usually bilateral with other cranial nerve involvement) and the "asymmetric crying facies" with absence of the levator anguli oris muscle. This appearance is called the cardiofacial syndrome when it is associated with other congenital anomalies; therefore, a careful search for skeletal, renal, and cardiac abnormalities should be performed under appropriate circumstances.

Routine examination of hearing is often difficult to interpret, and laboratory testing may be necessary. Hearing can be subjectively confirmed at the bedside with a simple bell to alert a resting infant or to quiet an active one. It may be necessary to repeat this stimulus several times, because absence of a response (whether the infant is deeply asleep or inconsolably upset) is not evidence of deafness. Even under optimal conditions, hearing may be difficult to determine in the neurologically depressed or restrained infant. It is easy to misinterpret an apparently positive response in a hearing-impaired infant who is actually attending to the visual stimuli of the bell or the examiner. Brain stem auditory evoked potentials, an electrophysiologic technique independent of behavioral response, has been established as a more accurate and sensitive measure of hearing. Vestibular testing has already been mentioned in reference to evaluation of eye movements. The presence of the doll's-eye reflex (oculovestibular response) requires the cranial nerve VIII to be intact.

The remaining cranial nerves can be evaluated at the bedside as well. Olfaction is rarely examined because of the difficulty in assessing appropriate response and the rarity of involvement in neonatal disorders. However, sucking, arousal, or withdrawal in response to pleasant, aromatic odors can be seen by 32 weeks; noxious odors such as ammonia are inappropriate because they activate trigeminal receptors. Sensory trigeminal integrity is best established by the corneal response and grimace to a pin applied to the nares or face. The motor function of cranial nerve V is usually demonstrated by effective mouth closure during sucking, which requires masseter muscle activity. In addition, effective sucking relies on cranial nerve VII participation to purse the lips and cranial nerve XII for the rhythmic tongue movements that produce normal milking action. Normal swallowing is an indication of adequacy of both cranial nerves IX and X; gag reflex and symmetric palatal elevation can also be directly tested. Asymmetric tongue movements or loss of bulk is indicative of abnormality of the hypoglossal nucleus or nerve. Tongue fasciculations (fine wormlike movements best seen on the lateral and under surfaces of the tongue at rest) are indicative of denervation. They are most commonly found in spinal muscular atrophy. Symmetry of the sternocleidomastoid muscle can be easily seen as the infant supports the head in the supine position. A hematoma of the muscle or torticollis can be observed in this manner.

DEEP TENDON REFLEXES

Reflexes may be difficult to interpret, and they are most useful when they are consistently elicited or asymmetric. As with all parts of the neurologic examination, they usually occur in context and correspond to other abnormalities of posture, tone, strength, movement, and sensation. For example, absence of the biceps jerk is probably factitious or at least not a significant finding if it is found in the presence of normal resting posture, tone, and spontaneous movement, as well as a symmetric Moro response. The isolated absence of the biceps jerk might well change when the head (which is turned toward the side of reduced activity) is straightened. This approach eliminates the inhibitory effect of the asymmetric tonic neck reflex.

There is an ontogeny of deep tendon reflexes, and most reflexes are difficult to elicit in infants younger than 33 weeks of gestation. Even when present, these reflexes are normally diminished in comparison with those in older infants. The only reliably reproducible reflex between 27 and 33 weeks is the pectoralis major reflex (obtained by striking the examiner's own finger held over the belly of the infant's pectoralis major muscle). By 33 weeks, biceps, brachioradialis, thigh adductors, patellar, and Achilles reflexes should be easily elicited. After 33 weeks, other reflexes (including triceps, finger flexors, jaw jerk, and crossed adductors) may not always be elicited. However, all of these reflexes are uniformly present by 40 weeks of postconception age.

DEVELOPMENTAL REFLEXES

Developmental reflexes are primitive but complex responses to specific stimulation. They represent integration at the brain stem and spinal cord level, but higher cortical involvement has not been demonstrated for most of these organized behaviors. Developmental reflexes have a predetermined course. They are present very early in life, some beginning before term, and they all disappear at predictable times. Asymmetries are always abnormal, but diffuse reduction or absence of expected reflexes may represent generalized depression of cerebral activity from diverse causes, including infection, medication effect, hypoxemia, and metabolic disease.

Finger grasp is already present by 28 weeks, but it is not until 32 weeks that the entire hand participates. Rooting and sucking reflexes are well established by 34 weeks and persist well into infancy. An incomplete asymmetric tonic neck reflex is present by 35 weeks; although the fencing posture is established in the arms at this point, the legs do not fully participate until term. Withdrawal, or the crossed extensor reflex, is produced by holding one leg in extension while stroking the sole of that foot; hip and knee flexion and withdrawal are followed by leg extension with toe fanning by 36 weeks. Automatic walking can be completely elicited by 37 weeks by supporting the infant in a standing position, tilting him or her forward, and gently applying pressure to the plantar surface of the feet. The mature response produces a heel-toe walking response, but modified toe walking can be seen as early as 32 weeks. The complete Moro response is not present until 38 weeks, although a partial reflex is already well established by 28 weeks without the adductor phase and rapidly extinguishable. By term, the alert infant can demonstrate elbow flexion and shoulder contraction in the traction maneuver even before he or she is pulled up from the crib.

Developmental reflexes can be used as a summary of the neonatal neurologic examination, inasmuch as they require cooperation of multiple muscles and nerves at various levels. For example, the traction test, in which the prone infant's arms are gently pulled toward the examiner, is a measure of upper body tone and strength, cranial nerve XI function, palmar grasp, eye opening and closure, facial grimace, and level of alertness, among other considerations.

Normal developmental reflexes should never be obligatory. In other words, an infant with an asymmetric tonic neck reflex should be able to turn the head to the opposite side if a stimulus is presented in that direction, and the infant should be able to release hand grip if distracted.

HEAD GROWTH

Normal patterns of head growth have been well documented in infants at various postconception ages. Therefore, it is possible to make the diagnosis of macrocephaly and microcephaly, even in utero. Just as important are serial measurements in the individual infant, because the normally growing brain usually settles quickly into a predictable pattern. This growth pattern is very important because the expected findings of acute or chronic hydrocephalus are often completely lacking or severely modified. Most often, the only feature to alert the clinician of hydrocephalus is an accelerated rate of head growth with a full anterior fontanel and sutural diastasis. Similarly, there may be no obvious clinical finding with progressive microcephaly beyond premature closure of the anterior fontanel.

In premature infants, the important contributing factor to head growth is general health. Premature infants who require mechanical ventilation or prolonged intravenous therapy often have significantly less head growth than do healthy infants of comparable gestational age, but they exhibit compensatory (catch-up) head growth in the weeks after stabilization. The most premature infants, younger than 30 weeks, have a more rapid growth pattern than do those born at later gestational ages.

The presence of safe and easily obtainable, convenient imaging studies such as cranial ultrasonography and computed tomography, as well as MRI, has clearly demonstrated that hydrocephalus can occur in the absence of clinical signs or even without rapid head growth. This peculiarity is partly a result of the very high water content of the premature brain; it allows for a greater degree of ventricular enlargement before reaching the functional limits of compensation and symptomatic hydrocephalus. This observation is especially true in very sick infants, in whom progressive hydrocephalus can be obscured by reduced normal head growth.

The converse is equally important. The infant whose head circumference is not growing as fast as expected according to standard charts is at risk for brain disease. Except for premature closure of the sutures (craniosynostosis), the head does not enlarge if the brain does not grow. Head growth failure can occur from a developmental disorder of neuronal migration or a destructive process. Either abnormality can reduce the full complement of expected neuronal and glial elements (e.g., caused by infarction, germinal matrix hemorrhage, periventricular leukomalacia) and lead to microcephaly.

INTERPRETING THE RESULTS OF THE NEUROLOGIC EXAMINATION

In view of the limited behavioral repertory of the infant, it is not surprising that there is little specificity in the neurologic examination. Similar abnormalities may be seen in a wide variety of clinical settings. Maternal disease, gestational complications, traumatic delivery, altered thermal environment, hypoxemia, and many other causes can all contribute to identical disturbances. Marked hypotonia is clinically indistinguishable whether it derives from acute perinatal asphyxia, congenital myotonic dystrophy, hyperammonemia, or drugs used to treat maternal toxemia. Therefore, it is essential to use all available history, physical, and laboratory data to properly interpret the neurologic examination in order to develop a proper diagnosis. Each potential cause may have a very different pathophysiologic process, treatment, and prognosis. For example, hypotonia with respiratory distress means something very different if it corresponds to hypoxic-ischemic encephalopathy, neonatal sepsis, intraventricular hemorrhage, or spinal muscular atrophy, among other causes. However, in the setting of a precipitous breech delivery, immediate symptoms, and an examination finding of completely normal cranial nerve function, none of these causes is as likely as a cervical cord injury. Obviously, these abnormal findings must be promptly evaluated and treated if the infant is to have the best chance for recovery.

Several conclusions can be derived from clinical experience and advances in the understanding of the pathophysiologic processes of neurologic disorders of infancy. An abnormal neurologic examination finding in neonates can be used to predict adverse outcomes such as cerebral palsy, mental retardation, and other neurologic disorders of childhood in the following ways:

1. Acquired damage to a previously normal nervous system in the neonate typically manifests with acute neurologic dysfunction. However, the abnormalities may be less specific than those seen in older children. Preexisting congenital abnormalities of the nervous system before the intrapartum period often produce no signs in the nursery. It is typical of a stroke acquired in utero to be completely asymptomatic until 4 to 6 months of life, when concern about asymmetric movements of the extremities and findings of spasticity lead to evaluation. However, an infarction around the time of birth is likely to produce transient focal or generalized neonatal seizures in an otherwise normal infant. Alternatively, hemorrhagic extension of an intraventricular hemorrhage in the premature infant may manifest with nothing more than increased oxygen requirement or an unexplained sudden drop in hematocrit.

2. No simple feature or combination of findings can precisely predict permanent disability, but a few abnormalities are highly correlated with an adverse outcome. Persistently disturbed tone (especially marked hypotonia), weak cry, poor sucking, and decreased level of activity all carry a high risk for later cerebral palsy. Low Apgar scores, of 3 or less, at 10 minutes or neonatal seizures, particularly in the presence of other signs associated with birth trauma or perinatal asphyxia, dramatically increase the risk of cerebral palsy in a child.

3. Disappearance of abnormal signs in the first days or weeks of life does not preclude an adverse outcome. Most asphyxiated infants recover a coordinated suck-and-swallow reflex within days or weeks, as well as improve from profound hypotonia, even if imaging studies demonstrate massive cortical laminar necrosis or periventricular leukomalacia. Findings from Perinatal Collaborative Study of the 1960s and 1970s also popularized the concept of "outgrowing cerebral palsy." However, even as the motor deficits improve, there remains a high likelihood of visual, hearing, learning, behavioral, and other permanent disabilities.

4. Significant perinatal asphyxia sufficient to cause permanent neurologic dysfunction always manifests in the first week of life. The most common features include abnormalities of tone, impaired level of consciousness, inadequate sucking with requirement for nasogastric or parenteral feeding, and, most important, neonatal seizures. Transient multisystem involvement must accompany the neurologic impairments in order for the examiner to make the connection to an injury at the time of birth. Thus, it is impossible to attribute any neurologic findings to acute perinatal asphyxia without evidence of other organ involvement, such as acute tubular necrosis, myocardial insufficiency, pulmonary failure, hepatic disturbance, and thrombocytopenia.

5. Persistent asymmetric findings are important in raising concern about an underlying abnormality. They are often easier to identify than symmetric bilateral problems. For example, bilateral brachial plexus injury and bilateral facial paresis seen in Möbius syndrome are often misdiagnosed or missed entirely. Unfortunately, many findings are typically confused with hypoxic encephalopathy. However, unilateral hearing loss is virtually impossible to detect clinically in the neonate.

6. The neurologic outcome is much more predictable when correlation can be made with neuroradiologic abnormalities on computed tomography, MRI, or ultrasonography. For example, it has been shown that MRI findings at 3 to 6 months of age can be highly predictive of future motor disability. Imaging can be important even earlier; abnormal signal in the posterior limb of the internal capsule is virtually always associated with a poor outcome if the infant is aged at least 36 weeks and 3 days of gestation. Similarly, prognosis is worse when a specific disturbance can be demonstrated consistently on laboratory findings. For example, severe and persistent hypoglycemia with abnormal neurologic findings carries a much more serious prognosis than does asymptomatic or transient low glucose level. Hyperammonemia with evidence of a specific enzyme deficiency is much more ominous than transient hyperammonemia of the premature infant. An electroencephalogram with a burst-suppression pattern carries a more serious prognosis than one with frequent paroxysmal discharges but with a normal background and good state differentiation.

7. Persistent neurologic dysfunction carries a much higher risk for permanent disability than if the child has already started to improve by the time of discharge from the neonatal nursery. Any return of function in the first weeks after a brachial plexus injury, for instance, usually results in a satisfactory outcome or complete resolution.

SUGGESTED READINGS

Allen MC, Capute AJ: Neonatal neurodevelopmental examination as a predictor of neuromotor outcome in premature infants. Pediatrics 83:498, 1989.

Ballard JL, Khoury JC, Wedig K, et al: New Ballard score, expanded to include extremely premature infants. J Pediatr 119:417, 1991.

Clancy R, Malin S, Laraque D, et al: Focal motor seizures heralding stroke in full-term neonates. Am J Dis Child 139:601, 1985.

Dubowitz LMS, Dubowitz V, Goldberg C: Clinical assessment of gestational age in the newborn. J Pediatr 77:1, 1970.

Freeman JM, Nelson KB: Intrapartum asphyxia and cerebral palsy. Pediatrics 82:240, 1988.

Kuban KCK, Skouteli HN, Urion DK, et al: Deep tendon reflexes in premature infants. Pediatr Neurol 2:266, 1986.

Ment LR, Bada HS, Barnes P, et al: Practice parameter: Neuroimaging of the neonate—report of the Quality Standards Subcommittee of the American Academy of Neurology and the Practice Committee of the Child Neurology Society. Neurology 58:1726, 2002.

Mercuri E, Ricci D, Cowna FM, et al: Head growth in infants with hypoxic-ischemic encephalopathy: Correlation with neonatal magnetic resonance imaging. Pediatrics 106:235, 2000.

Nelson KB, Ellenberg JH: Neonatal signs as predictors of cerebral palsy. Pediatrics 64:225, 1979.

Paine RS: Neurological examination of infants and children. Pediatr Clin North Am 7:41, 1960.

Perlman JM, Risser RL: Severe fetal acidemia: Neonatal neurologic features and short-term outcome. Pediatr Neurol 9:277, 1993.

Perlman JM: Neurobehavioral deficits in premature graduates of intensive care—potential medical and neonatal environmental risks. Pediatrics 108:1339, 2001.

Scher MS, Barmada MA: Estimation of gestational age by electrographic, clinical and anatomic criteria. Pediatr Neurol 3:256, 1987.

Scher PK, Brown S: A longitudinal study of head growth in preterm infants. II. Differentiation between "catch-up" head growth and early infantile hydrocephalus. Dev Med Child Neurol 17:711, 1975.

Shevell MI, Majnemer A, Miller SP: Neonatal neurologic prognostication: The asphyxiated term newborn. Pediatr Neurol 21:7767, 1999.

Swaiman, KF: Neurological examination of the term and preterm infant. In Swaiman KF, Ashwall S (eds): Pediatric Neurology: Principles and Practice, 3rd ed. Philadelphia, Mosby, 1999, pp 39-53.

Volpe JJ: The neurological examination: Normal and abnormal features. In: Neurology of the Newborn, 4th ed. Philadelphia, WB Saunders, 2001, pp 103-133.

Volpe JJ: Specialized studies in the neurological evaluation. In: Neurology of the Newborn, 4th ed. Philadelphia, WB Saunders, 2001, pp 134-177.

CHAPTER 53

Perinatal Asphyxia and Hypoxic-Ischemic Brain Injury in the Full-Term Infant

Adre J. du Plessis

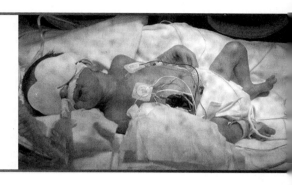

Fetal asphyxia is the most important cause of brain injury in the full-term newborn.[1,2] Impaired gas exchange between the maternal and fetal circulations, the basis for fetal asphyxia, may occur before and/or during the period of labor. Because uteroplacental perfusion decreases during myometrial contractions, labor is by definition an intrinsically asphyxiating process. That most fetuses survive the insults of labor apparently unscathed is attributable in large part to the adaptive hemodynamic responses activated during the transient fetal hypoxia associated with uterine contractions. The ability of the fetus to withstand the rigors of labor depends on both the integrity of these compensatory fetal responses and the nature of the asphyxial insult. In a small percentage of cases, these adaptive fetal mechanisms are overwhelmed because of preceding placental and/or fetal compromise, dysfunctional labor, or both.[3] With collapse of these protective responses, the fetus becomes exposed to brain insults and potential brain injury. The consequences of such insults range from transient neonatal encephalopathy to lifelong neurologic complications,[1] the most prevalent of which are cerebral palsy, epilepsy, and cognitive impairment.

The importance of perinatal asphyxia as a cause of later neurologic dysfunction is clear. First, the absolute number of infants who sustain fetal asphyxia and brain injury each year is enormous. Second, advances in medical care continue to increase the survival of asphyxiated newborn infants, as well as the longevity of brain-injured children and adults. Paradoxically, these advances have increased the personal and societal effect of brain injury resulting from perinatal asphyxia.

There have been several important developments pertinent to the issue of fetal asphyxial brain injury. Exciting developments in experimental neuroscience have generated optimism that effective neuroprotection against hypoxic-ischemic brain injury may become reality in the foreseeable future.[4-12] Numerous agents have demonstrated effective reduction of brain injury in experimental studies; however, even when they are initiated after the insult, several significant challenges continue to impede the translation of these advances into clinical benefit for the newborn. In this regard, the most critical challenges for clinicians are the early and accurate diagnosis of asphyxia and expedited pathways to brain-oriented resuscitation. Specifically, the neuroprotective efficacy of experimental agents depends on their initiation before or soon after the cerebral insult and declines sharply when treatment is delayed beyond the "therapeutic window."[13-15] However, the current ability of clinicians to identify with accuracy the fetus at risk for brain insult and injury remains seriously impeded by a lack of reliable fetal diagnostic techniques. These diagnostic limitations remain a major obstacle to safe and effective prevention of irreversible brain injury in the full-term fetus at risk for asphyxia.

Another pertinent development has been the debate, fueled in part by the current medicolegal climate, over the fundamental importance of asphyxial brain injury as a cause of cerebral palsy.[16-20] Whereas early descriptions of cerebral palsy[21] emphasized the importance of "abnormal parturition," more recent epidemiologic studies have challenged this notion, implicating intrapartum asphyxia in 20% or fewer of cases of cerebral palsy.[16-20] These reports have, unfortunately, been misinterpreted as indicating the relative unimportance of perinatal asphyxia as a cause for fetal brain injury. Such misinterpretation has inevitably hindered the advance toward eradication of this potentially preventable condition.

TERMINOLOGY AND DIAGNOSTIC CRITERIA

During the development of asphyxia, the initial events are a decrease in the circulating arterial oxygen (hypoxemia) of the fetus and an accumulation of circulating carbon dioxide (hypercarbia); these events develop transiently during the uterine contractions of normal labor. Defining and identifying the critical thresholds beyond which these periods of "asphyxia" result in fetal brain insult or brain injury has been a major challenge for clinicians. One approach has been to define the onset of pathologic intrauterine asphyxia as the point at which impaired gas exchange between the maternal and fetal circulations leads to the development of "significant" metabolic acidosis in the fetus. During the initial phases of asphyxia, the accumulation of carbon dioxide leads to fetal respiratory acidosis. When fetal hypoxemia is sustained, tissue oxygen levels begin to fall (hypoxia), leading to anaerobic cellular metabolism and the accumulation of lactate, metabolic acidosis, and eventual energy failure. The criteria for diagnosing "significant" metabolic acidosis in fetal asphyxia depend on the definition. According to the statistical definition, acidosis becomes significant when the pH of the fetal circulation falls more than two standard deviations below the population mean (i.e., a fetal scalp pH below 7.20[22] or an umbilical artery pH below 7.10[23]). Conversely, according to the clinical definition, metabolic acidosis becomes "significant" when the pathophysiologic effects of asphyxia begin to develop in fetal organs, including the brain. The criteria commonly used to define this threshold are an umbilical artery pH of 7.00 or less with a base deficit exceeding 12 mmol/L.[3,24-27] For reasons to be discussed, these *diagnostic* criteria for asphyxia have in isolation proved to be, at best, weak *prognostic* indicators of long-term neurologic outcome.[28,29]

According to these clinical criteria, fetal asphyxia complicates approximately 2% of births.[3,30] In most cases, however, the insult is mild and the effect on the fetus is minimal.[3,30] In about 0.4% of infants, the asphyxial insult is severe enough to cause in the newborn at least transient organ dysfunction, including that of the brain[3,30,31]; in 0.1% of births, the asphyxial insult is associated with brain injury and long-term neurologic sequelae.[32] As noted previously, the low rates of "significant" asphyxia are deceptive in view of the fact that approximately 4 million infants are born in the United States each year.

MECHANISMS OF PERINATAL ASPHYXIA, FETAL INSULT, AND CEREBRAL INJURY

Neither fetal asphyxia nor the ensuing brain injury is mediated by a single mechanism. Instead, the potential pathways leading to these pathologic states are multiple.[4,33,34] A detailed understanding of these mechanisms is critical for the formulation of more effective interventions to prevent asphyxial brain injury. What follows is a conceptual overview of the factors involved in the asphyxial insult, the adaptive responses of the fetus to preserve cerebral oxygenation, and the consequences of eventual failure of these compensatory mechanisms.

Pathways to Fetal Asphyxia

Although all forms of fetal asphyxia evolve to the same fundamental and defining condition—namely, fetal tissue hypoxia and metabolic acidosis—the failure of fetal tissue oxygenation may be the end point of a variety of pathways, which may occur alone, in combination, or in sequence. In general, fetal tissue hypoxia may result from reduced circulating arterial oxygen content (i.e., hypoxic-hypoxia or anemic-hypoxia) or inadequate tissue perfusion (ischemic-hypoxia). These mechanisms may originate in the mother, the uteroplacental unit, the umbilical cord, or the fetus.

Maternal causes of fetal asphyxia include maternal hypotension or cardiac arrest, maternal hypertension causing uterine vasospasm, or myometrial hypercontractility during labor. All these conditions cause a decrease in uterine perfusion, leading to ischemic hypoxia in the placental intervillous spaces and ultimately to hypoxic-hypoxia in the fetus.[35] Conversely, in conditions such as Rh incompatibility, isoimmune antibodies generated in the maternal system cause hemolytic anemia in the fetus, which, if severe enough, causes fetal anemic-hypoxia.

Placental causes of fetal asphyxia include placental abruption, placenta previa, vasa previa, or fetomaternal hemorrhage, all of which may cause fetal hypovolemic cardiac failure and rapid ischemic-hypoxia. Other causes, such as twin-twin transfusion in monochorionic twins, may result in more gradual fetal anemic hypoxia. Occlusion of a malpositioned umbilical cord may cause relatively brief but repeated insults during uterine contractions; conversely, nuchal entwining of the cord may cause prolonged, variable compression, whereas cord prolapse may cause severe and sustained compression.

Fetal Adaptive Responses for Maintaining Cerebral Oxygenation

The fetal brain differs in important ways from the mature brain in its response to hypoxic insults and injury. First, the global oxygen requirement of the fetal brain is substantially lower than that of the adult brain.[36,37] Second, the fetal circulation carries a surplus of oxygen in comparison with the metabolic demands; in fact, normal oxidative metabolism persists until oxygen delivery falls by more than half. Third, adaptive fetal cardiovascular and cerebrovascular responses are capable of sustaining oxygen delivery to the fetal brain during periods of transient hypoxemia. However, if fetal asphyxia is sustained, these compensatory hemodynamic responses eventually fail, more rapidly in situations of severe hypoxia (e.g., abruptio placenta). Collapse of these adaptive responses leads to the rapid development of cerebral ischemic-hypoxia and energy failure in the maturationally vulnerable immature brain cells.

Systemic Hemodynamic Responses

In animal models, adaptive cardiovascular responses, triggered by fetal asphyxia, maintain fetal cerebral oxygen delivery by increasing the flow rate and oxygen content of the cerebral perfusion. Specifically, there is an overall increase in cardiac output[38-40] as well as redistribution of this increased cardiac output to the heart, brain, and adrenal glands (so-called centralization of the circulation).[39-42] An important mediator of this circulatory redistribution is the catecholaminergic vasoconstriction triggered in regional and peripheral vascular beds. In addition, the oxygen content of the cerebral perfusion is increased by the diversion of more oxygenated umbilical venous blood through the ductus venosus and foramen ovale to the myocardium and brain.[43,44] In models of umbilical compression, the impairment of umbilical venous return rapidly reduces fetal cardiac output; an initial compensatory increase in blood pressure is only transiently sustained, and after several minutes, a rapid fall in blood pressure leads to cerebral ischemia.[45,46] Even when uterine contractions are relatively brief, the repeated compression of a malpositioned cord during contractions may stress the myocardium, limiting its ability to withstand subsequent insults.

Cerebral Hemodynamic Responses

In addition to the centralization of the systemic circulation, fetal animals are also capable of activating intrinsic cerebrovascular responses to asphyxia that increase global cerebral blood flow and redistribute regional blood flow within the brain. Specifically, in fetal animals, the cerebral blood vessels are known to be reactive to circulating stimuli, responding with vasodilation and increased cerebral blood flow to stimuli such as hypoxemia,[41,43,44,47-51] hypercapnea,[52] and hypotension.[42] Within the cerebral vasculature, there is also a regional redistribution of the circulation increasing blood flow to the most actively developing and metabolically demanding regions of the brain (to be discussed).[38-40,50,52]

Failure of Cerebral Oxygen Delivery

The cardiovascular and cerebrovascular adaptive responses just described are capable of maintaining cerebral oxygen delivery over finite periods, the duration of which is determined by the nature of the insult. Prolonged fetal asphyxia results in anaerobic metabolism, critical energy failure, accumulation of circulating lactate, and depletion of myocardial glycogen[53] with eventual depression of myocardial contractility and global hypoperfusion.

An important early mechanism for the development of metabolic acidemia is the regional vasoconstriction required for the centralization of the circulation. During sustained asphyxia, the vasodilating effect of tissue lactic acid accumulation eventually overrides the vasoconstricting effects of adrenergic stimulation, with systemic vasodilation leading to collapse of circulatory centralization. Within the cerebral vasculature, the progressive hypoxemia and hypercarbia of sustained fetal asphyxia eventually leads to paralysis of intrinsic cerebral pressure autoregulation. Occurring together, these processes—that is, myocardial failure (with decreased cerebral perfusion pressure) and a pressure-passive cerebral circulation—expose the brain to serious circulatory insufficiency. In cases of abrupt severe fetal asphyxia, cerebral blood flow may be further decreased by an increase in cerebral vascular resistance caused by both neural and circulating catecholamines. When these various mechanisms begin to restrict the compensatory increases in cerebral blood flow, cerebral oxygen delivery becomes limited not only by hypoxic-hypoxia but also by ischemic-hypoxia.[41] Fetal hypoxemia alone is less injurious to the immature brain as long as blood flow is maintained.[33,34] However, the development of ischemia accelerates the failure of oxygen/glucose delivery, the accumulation of tissue carbon dioxide and lactic acid, and the progression of tissue acidosis.

Mechanisms of Cerebral Hypoxic-Ischemic Injury in the Fetus

The overall oxygen demand of the immature brain is significantly lower than that of the mature brain.[36,37] However, although the *global* cerebral oxygen demand is low, regions of most active maturation at a particular gestational age have particularly high oxygen demands, necessary to support the activity of enzymes critical for neuronal development, such as those involved in ion homeostasis (e.g., sodium/potassium–adenosine triphosphatase [Na^+/K^+-ATPase])[54] and oxidative metabolism.[55,56] These regions of elevated oxygen metabolism are particularly vulnerable to hypoxia, and during fetal asphyxia, failure to satisfy these regional energy demands leads to the rapid depletion of available energy substrate and unleashes cellular processes of injury and the cell death cascade.

Cellular Mechanisms of Brain Injury

The excitatory neurotransmitter glutamate plays an essential role in normal brain development.[33,57] Through its action at specific receptors on the neuronal membrane, glutamate is critical for maturational processes such as neuronal differentiation, dendritic arborization, synapse formation, and plasticity.[33,57] Normal activation of these glutamate receptors, particularly the N-methyl-D-aspartate (NMDA) receptors, triggers the highly regulated passage of calcium through the receptor ionophores, thereby providing critical trophic support for neuronal development.[58,59] The normal control of calcium conductance through the ionophores of these NMDA receptors is dependent on regulation of the neuronal membrane potential by energy-dependent ion pumps. In regions of particularly active neuronal development, the glutamate system is "primed" in several ways to facilitate the cytosolic calcium influx,[59-65] including a regional increase in glutamate receptor density and the enhanced calcium conductivity of these immature receptors.[66]

When cerebral energy failure develops in fetal asphyxia, the tight regulation of this glutamate system is lost, which causes massive presynaptic glutamate release and a decrease in glutamate reuptake. As a result, toxic levels of glutamate accumulate in the synaptic cleft.[67-74] The combination of sustained glutamate receptor activation and neuronal membrane depolarization maintains glutamate calcium channels open to a massive, uncontrolled influx of calcium into the neuronal cytosol, where potentially lethal processes of cellular injury are activated. The dichotomous roles of glutamate in normal brain development and in "excitotoxic" injury during hypoxia-ischemia[75] help explain the distribution of brain injury in fetal asphyxia.[33,76,77]

Glucose metabolism plays a complex role in hypoxic-ischemic brain injury.[78-81] During the early phases of asphyxia failure of oxidative metabolism with a persistence of cerebral glucose supply activates glycolysis and lactate production. The accumulation of lactate during cerebral hypoxia-ischemia has a biphasic effect on the immature brain. In animal models of cerebral hypoxia-ischemia, lactate accumulation has an initial beneficial effect, in part because of its role as an alternative fuel source in the immature brain.[78-81] However, in studies with sustained high levels of lactic acidosis, deleterious processes are initiated.[82-84] Whether the levels of *cerebral* lactate developing during asphyxia[85,86] are sufficient to cause direct injury[87-89] remains controversial.

Data suggest that glucose is critical for the reuptake by astroglial cells of glutamate from the extracellular space[90-93] and that hypoglycemia may trigger or exacerbate excitotoxic brain injury. During periods of prolonged asphyxia, exhaustion of fetal hepatic glycogen stores may result in hypoglycemia. The resulting combination of energy failure (caused by hypoxia and hypoglycemia) and the accumulation of extracellular glutamate may lead to profound cerebral injury.

NEUROPATHOLOGIC PATTERNS OF BRAIN INJURY IN THE ASPHYXIATED INFANT

Although the critical insult during fetal asphyxia (cerebral hypoperfusion) is typically *generalized*, the topography of the resulting brain injury tends to be *focal* or *regional*. The regional distribution of brain injury is determined by many factors, including gestational age (i.e., level of cerebral and vascular development) and the nature (intensity and duration) of the insult. The relationship between gestational age and the topography of brain injury is determined in large part by the regional differences in brain maturation (and thus regional differences in metabolism) at the time of insult. The specific regions of brain injury in turn determine the clinical picture of subsequent neurologic deficits in survivors. Although the relationship among insult, injury, and outcome remains only partially understood, techniques such as magnetic resonance imaging (MRI) of the brain have provided important insights (to be discussed).

At a tissue level, two broad types of hypoxic-ischemic brain injury can be distinguished in the asphyxiated newborn: **selective cellular injury** and **pancellular injury (infarction).** As mentioned, the type of injury and its distribution are determined by factors such as the gestational age and the intensity, duration, and number of insults. Although any cell type may be injured by hypoxia-ischemia, certain cell types are selectively vulnerable at different gestational ages. In the premature fetus, the immature premyelinating oligodendrocyte[94-96] is particularly vulnerable to selective cellular injury. At term, selective cellular injury tends to be mainly neuronal, although in regions of active myelination, the mature oligodendrocyte is also vulnerable.

The regional distribution of *selective cellular injury* (neuronal and oligodendrocyte) may be categorized into several broad patterns. At term, the most actively maturing (and therefore most vulnerable) neurons are in the basal ganglia and thalamus, brain stem nuclei, hippocampus and regions of the neocortex, especially the perirolandic and visual cortices.[97-100] Within the cortex, neuronal injury is most severe in the deeper layers,[101] particularly in the depths of the sulci.[102] As discussed previously, the vulnerability of these areas of intense regional maturation[66,97-100] is related to their high glutamate-receptor density and reactivity[66] and to the high metabolic demands of neuronal maturation[55,103] and axon myelination.[104-108]

The regional distribution of *cerebral infarction* that occurs during global cerebral hypoperfusion is also determined by the maturational state of the cerebral vasculature. These regions of infarction tend to develop in the watershed territories between the cerebral arterial end zones. In the full-term infant, the major watershed regions are in the end zones between the anterior, middle, and posterior cerebral artery territories of supply; consequently, infarction develops in the parasagittal regions along the superolateral convexity of the cerebral hemispheres.

Perinatal asphyxia may also be complicated by vaso-occlusive insults and infarction in the territories of arterial supply or venous drainage.[109-113] Arterial occlusion or stroke is more common in full-term infants and usually involves the middle cerebral arteries, particularly the left.[114-116] Venous occlusion usually occurs in the dural veins,[117-120] most commonly in the posterior part of the superior sagittal sinus and less commonly in the surface cortical veins or deep venous system. Although any type of infarction is susceptible to hemorrhagic transformation, this is more typical of venous infarction. These vaso-occlusive injuries are discussed in detail elsewhere.[121]

The other major determinant of the topography of brain injury in fetal asphyxia is the insult "dose," which is in turn determined by the intensity and duration of the insult. The intensity of asphyxial insults may be divided broadly into partial or severe insults. Prolonged **partial insults** at term tend to concentrate injury in the parasagittal watershed areas of cortex and subcortical white matter, with relative sparing of the deep gray regions.[122,123] This pattern of parasagittal cerebral injury has been well described in a full-term primate model of prolonged partial asphyxia.[45,124]

With **severe insults**, the regional distribution of injury is determined by the duration of insult. Regardless of gestational age, infants surviving prolonged and severe circulatory collapse (e.g., 20 to 30 minutes or more) develop diffuse rather than regional cerebral injury, with devastating neurologic sequelae. Conversely, with severe insults of brief duration, gestational age does influence the distribution of cerebral injury. At term, such brief but severe insults tend to concentrate neuronal injury in the basal ganglia, thalamus, hippocampus, and sensorimotor cortex, and white matter injury in the corticospinal tracts from the sensorimotor cortex to the internal capsule, as well as the optic radiations. Interestingly, in fetal sheep,[125-127] selective basal ganglia injury may also follow repeated brief insults, whereas prolonged partial insults cause hippocampal injury.

These neuropathologic patterns of injury were initially described at autopsy but can now be detected by neuroimaging studies, especially MRI, and are discussed below.

DIAGNOSIS AND CLINICAL COURSE OF POSTASPHYXIAL NEONATAL ENCEPHALOPATHY

Diagnostic Criteria

Certain criteria must be met before intrapartum asphyxia can be considered in the differential diagnosis of neonatal encephalopathy. Specifically, there should be clear evidence of fetal distress (e.g., significant fetal heart rate [FHR] abnormalities and/or metabolic acidemia on cord or scalp blood samples), immediate neonatal neurologic depression at birth, and exclusion of other causes. The evolution of the clinical picture and selective adjunctive testing may provide further support (see following section). In order for intra-partum asphyxia to be implicated in *long-term* neurologic dysfunction, an unequivocal neonatal encephalopathy should be evident in an infant meeting the criteria for intrapartum asphyxia just listed.[1]

Clinical Course of Postasphyxial Neonatal Encephalopathy

The clinical picture of postasphyxial neonatal encephalopathy may be discussed in terms of its severity and temporal evolution. The *acute* clinical manifestations of hypoxic-ischemic encephalopathy (HIE) depend primarily on the intensity and duration of the insult and the regional distribution of brain injury. Furthermore, because the clinical picture of HIE evolves over time, the specific features at presentation also depend on the time elapsed since the onset of the insult.

Grading the severity of encephalopathy has been used to guide management and to predict long-term outcome.[128] Infants with **mild postasphyxial encephalopathy** emerge from the initial resuscitation with marked irritability, inconsolable crying, jitteriness, and other evidence of increased sympathetic nervous tone (e.g., tachycardia and pupillary dilation). In less affected infants, this picture improves over hours or days to one of relative normality. By definition, seizures are not a feature of mild HIE. Infants with **moderate postasphyxial encephalopathy** may develop seizures and have a clearly depressed sensorium, with lethargy, brief periods of arousal, and variable responses to external stimuli. Muscle tone and spontaneous movements tend to be decreased and primitive reflexes impaired. Unlike mildly affected infants, moderately affected infants tend to have features suggestive of relatively increased parasympathetic tone, such as bradycardia, small pupils, and low blood pressure. **Severe postasphyxial encephalopathy** renders affected infants stuporous or comatose after resuscitation. Disturbed regulation of respiration[129] may be prominent, often necessitating mechanical ventilatory support. Initially, brain stem function (e.g., pupillary and extraocular reflexes) is intact. These infants tend to have diffusely decreased, even flaccid muscle tone. Spontaneous and elicited movements are largely absent. Over the course of the first 12 hours, the majority of these infants develop seizure activity.[130-132] Various convulsive phenomena may occur, including myoclonic, clonic, or tonic activity. So-called subtle seizures, consisting largely of oculomotor, oromotor, and extremity automatisms, often with apnea, are common in severely affected infants. These subtle seizures may be mistaken for reflexive newborn behaviors, such as nonnutritive sucking, but usually occur in combination with more obvious convulsions.

Early Clinical Course of Postasphyxial Encephalopathy

Although the severity and timing of the intrauterine brain insult is often unclear, retrospective studies have described a characteristic evolution to the clinical picture of HIE in the full-term newborn over the first week after birth. The normal premature infant has a relatively limited range of responses, making these phases of encephalopathy less distinct in the asphyxiated preterm. The early neonatal course of the asphyxiated full-term infant may be discussed in four broad phases:

Over the first 12 hours after birth. Infants with mild insults and ultimate injury may have a "hypervigilant" appearance with excessive irritability; however, seizures do not develop. Moderate to severe insults tend to be associated with seizures, and approximately half of these occur within the first 12 hours after birth.[130-132] Seizures and their manifestations are discussed in more detail later. Infants with severe insults have a markedly depressed sensorium and hypotonia from the first hours after birth.

Between 12 and 24 hours after birth. Infants with mild insults may have an apparently normal sensorium, with eyes open but with failure to fix and follow. Mild degrees of hypotonia may persist. Severely encephalopathic infants tend to have persistent seizures (which may be clinically silent) and a declining level of consciousness.

Between 24 and 72 hours after birth. Infants with mild insults recover normal levels of alertness and responsiveness and begin feeding. Conversely, severely encephalopathic infants continue to deteriorate and, during this period, may begin to develop prominent brain stem abnormalities, such as ataxic respiration, impaired eye movements, facial weakness, and pupillary dysfunction. Severely affected infants are usually unresponsive during this time, with marked hypotonia and, in some cases, areflexia, thought to be caused by anterior horn cell injury in the spinal cord.[133,134] Asphyxiated infants who die usually do so during this phase of the encephalopathy.

Between 72 hours and 7 days after birth. A gradual improvement in mental status and neurologic examination is usually evident; the extent and rate of recovery depend on the initial severity of the insult. In infants surviving severe insults, persistent cranial nerve dysfunction often results in ongoing difficulties with sucking, feeding, and ventilation. During this period, seizures are more easily controlled and often cease. The extent of neurologic recovery by the end of the first week is an important predictor for long-term outcome (see later discussion).

DIAGNOSTIC TESTING IN SUSPECTED POSTASPHYXIAL ENCEPHALOPATHY

No single diagnostic test unequivocally establishes intrauterine asphyxia as the cause of neonatal encephalopathy. Instead, the diagnosis of postasphyxial encephalopathy is based on a combination of the clinical features described previously, selected diagnostic studies, and the exclusion of other conditions. Several diagnostic tests have demonstrated their value in the assessment of these infants.

Electroencephalography in Postasphyxial Encephalopathy

There are no changes on electroencephalography (EEG) that are absolutely diagnostic for postasphyxial encephalopathy. Even though the background and ictal patterns are nonspecific, this bedside technique has several valuable applications during the acute and subacute phases of postasphyxial encephalopathy. First, EEG helps define questionable paroxysmal behaviors by distinguishing between seizures and other suspicious but nonepileptic behaviors. Second, the EEG background provides insight into the severity of electrocortical dysfunction and hence the severity of the asphyxial insult. Third, continuous EEG is a valuable monitoring technique for the detection of clinically occult electrographic seizures that may persist without obvious clinical manifestations; silent seizures most commonly occur in severely encephalopathic infants and after the initiation of anticonvulsant medications.[135-138] Without EEG monitoring, electrographic seizures may go undiagnosed and undertreated in these infants. Finally, there are several EEG patterns (discussed in more detail later) that have demonstrated valuable prognostic utility.[139-141]

Neuroimaging Studies in Postasphyxial Encephalopathy

Cranial ultrasonography and computerized tomography scans have made important contributions to the understanding of HIE in the newborn and remain useful when logistic constraints or the infant's clinical condition preclude the more time-consuming MRI technique. However, in comparison with MRI, these techniques are relatively limited in both their temporal and spatial resolution of cerebral tissue injury.[1] Although cerebral computed tomography and ultrasound scans may be relatively reliable in identifying brain injury after severe insults, MRI is far more sensitive to mild to moderate hypoxic-ischemic injury. In addition, MRI is significantly more sensitive to cerebral hemorrhage, edema, gliosis,[142] and the maturational level of myelination. Finally, MRI is far superior for defining structures and injury in the posterior fossa. The increased availability and ongoing advances in MRI technology (see later discussion) have made it the "gold standard" for brain imaging in the asphyxiated newborn.[106,143,144] MRI has demonstrated in vivo most of the neuropathologic patterns of brain injury described in earlier autopsy studies.[45,124,145-148] In so doing, cerebral MRI has extended the understanding of the mechanisms and timing of brain injury.

Conventional MRI techniques demonstrate hypoxic-ischemic brain lesions within the first 72 hours, and often on the first day, after birth. In the full-term asphyxiated infant, the lesions are most commonly in the basal ganglia and thalamus, brain stem nuclei, hippocampus, and sensorimotor cortex,[97-100] as well as in the watershed areas between arterial supplies (in global hypoperfusion) and the territories of supply/drainage (in vaso-occlusive insults).

In the early neonatal period, cortical injury from laminar selective neuronal necrosis is seen on MRI as a loss of gray-white matter differentiation, or cortical "highlighting," on T1-weighted studies (Fig. 53-1).[147,149,150] Cortical highlighting is often localized to the sensorimotor cortex,[150] and in the neonatal period, these lesions often have the MRI features of hemorrhagic necrosis.[147,149,150] Selective neuronal necrosis in the deep gray matter nuclei appears as an increased T1-weighted signal, most commonly in the dorsal putamen and ventrolateral

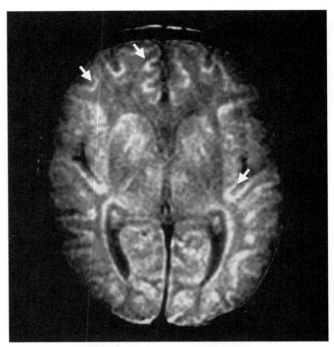

Figure 53–1. Cortical highlighting. Axial magnetic resonance imaging scan (T1-weighted) in an asphyxiated full-term infant, showing the "cortical highlighting" pattern of cerebral injury. The abnormal cortical hyperintensities are most prominent in the depths of the sulci *(white arrows).*

thalamus (Fig. 53-2), and less commonly in the globus pallidus and caudate. At term, selective neuronal necrosis in the brain stem is usually seen as an increased T1-weighted signal in the tegmentum. Parasagittal cerebral injury appears as an increased T1-weighted signal in the cortex and subcortical white matter in the parasagittal regions of the hemispheric convexity (Fig. 53-3). Areas of arterio-occlusive injury, most commonly in the supply area of the middle cerebral artery, appear as regions of decreased T1-weighted intensity. Conversely, areas of veno-occlusive injury, most commonly after thrombosis in the posterior aspects of the superior sagittal sinus, appear as regions of edema with increased T2-weighted intensity in the parasagittal and subcortical white matter; the hemorrhagic changes that are not uncommon in venous ischemia are best seen on gradient echographic images.

Magnetic Resonance Imaging Patterns of Cerebral Injury

The MRI lesions described previously often cluster together in patterns of injury. These patterns closely resemble the neuropathologic patterns seen in animal and autopsy studies (discussed previously).[45,66,97-100,122,124] Certain patterns of MRI abnormality have been associated with certain forms of cerebral insult.[145] However, just as the injury is in most cases caused by a combination of insults, so the MRI patterns are rarely "classic" and are more often a combination of the topographic patterns to be described. In addition, patterns of selective neuronal necrosis and cerebral infarction are discussed separately for the sake of clarity, although they probably occur in combination in most cases.

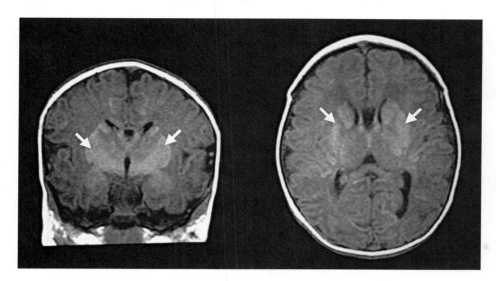

Figure 53–2. Selective neuronal necrosis in basal ganglia and thalami. Coronal **(left)** and axial **(right)** magnetic resonance imaging scans (T1-weighted) 3 weeks after acute, profound birth asphyxia resulting from uterine rupture. The images demonstrate the selective neuronal necrosis pattern of injury as hyperintensities in the deep nuclei of the basal ganglia and thalami *(white arrows).*

Several regional patterns of selective neuronal necrosis have been described. **Diffuse cerebral cortical injury** (see Fig. 53-1) is caused by laminar necrosis in the deep layers of the cerebral cortex; although generally diffuse, the injury may be most marked in regions such as the hippocampus, perirolandic cortex, and calcarine cortex of the occipital lobes. The MRI features of diffuse cortical injury include the loss of gray-white matter differentiation on inversion recovery images, and T1-weighted images show "cortical highlighting," in which the hyperintense cortical ribbon has the features of petechial hemorrhages.[147,149,150]

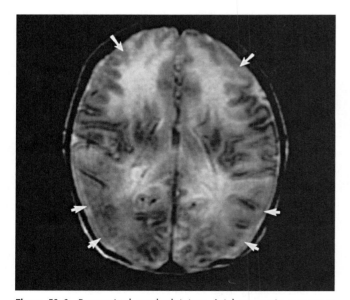

Figure 53–3. Parasagittal cerebral injury. Axial magnetic resonance imaging scan (T2-weighted) showing the parasagittal pattern of cerebral injury *(arrows)* with loss of definition between the cortex and subcortical white matter in the "watershed" areas between the anterior, middle, and posterior cerebral artery territories.

The nature of the insult leading to this pattern of injury is unclear but is probably severe and prolonged. **Regional cortical and deep nuclear injury** refers to selective neuronal necrosis in the perirolandic cortex and hippocampus, as well as in the basal ganglia and thalamus. The most common deep nuclei affected (hyperintense on T1-weighted images) are the ventrolateral thalamic nucleus, the putamen, and, to a lesser extent, the caudate nucleus (Fig. 53-4). The initiating insult responsible for this pattern is usually severe but relatively brief. **Deep nuclear and brain stem injury** (Fig. 53-5) refers to injury in the basal ganglia and thalamic nuclei (see previous discussion)[145] in combination with specific brain stem nuclei in the midbrain and dorsal pons.[146] Clinical data[145,147] and studies in fetal primates[124,148] suggest that this pattern of injury results from acute profound asphyxia of relatively brief duration. **Diffuse cortical, deep nuclear, and brain stem injury,** i.e., a combination of these patterns of selective neuronal necrosis, may be seen after acute-onset but prolonged and severe (i.e., prelethal) insults.

Superimposed on these patterns of selective neuronal necrosis are various patterns of watershed infarction (usually parasagittal) as well as vaso-occlusive (arterial or venous) infarction. Parasagittal cerebral infarction shows as increased T1-weighted signal intensity in the cortical gray and subcortical white matter on the dorsolateral surface of the cerebral convexities (see Fig. 53-3).

Advances in Magnetic Resonance Technology

Two useful applications of magnetic resonance technology that have entered clinical practice over the last decade are proton magnetic resonance spectroscopy and diffusion-weighted imaging (DWI). The value of these techniques includes the very early detection and regional distribution of cerebral energy failure,[151,152] as occurs in cerebral hypoxia-ischemia. Proton magnetic resonance spectroscopy is capable of measuring the regional levels of several important tissue components such as lactate, *N*-acetyl-aspartate, choline, and creatine.[153,154] Detection of regional elevations

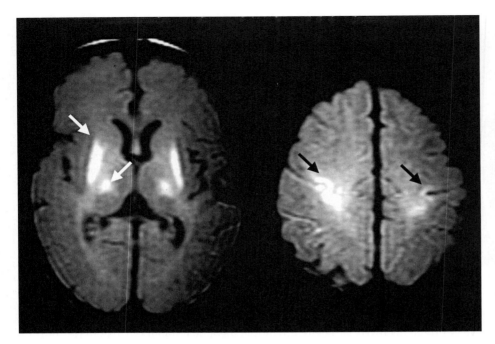

Figure 53–4. Basal ganglia-thalamus and sensorimotor cortex injury. Axial magnetic resonance imaging scan (T1-weighted) from a severely asphyxiated full-term infant, showing injury as abnormal hyperintensities in the putamina and thalami (*white arrows*, **left**) and the sensorimotor cortex (*black arrows*, **right**).

in cerebral lactate is particularly useful because these elevations indicate regions of anaerobic cellular metabolism. Of note, small lactate peaks may be a normal finding in premature infants.[155,156] The value of measuring regional levels of N-acetyl-aspartate relates to the localization of this substance to the cytosol of specific brain cell populations (i.e., neurons and oligodendrocyte precursors).[157-161] Consequently, a decrease in N-acetyl-aspartate may be a reliable marker for injury and loss of these cell types.

The DWI technique is based on the diffusibility of water in tissue,[162-165] which is in turn dependent on the intracellular and extracellular distribution of tissue water.

The DWI technique measures the apparent diffusion coefficient of tissue, which changes as fluid shifts between the intracellular and extracellular compartments. The normal distribution of water between these two compartments is maintained by energy-dependent ion pumps. Therefore, the cerebral energy failure in cerebral hypoxia-ischemia is rapidly followed by cytotoxic edema, which results in an early restriction of tissue water diffusion and a decrease in the apparent diffusion coefficient.[166,167] The rapidity of these fluid shifts in areas of energy failure allows very early discrimination between normal and injured tissue. There is a strong spatial correlation between early DWI

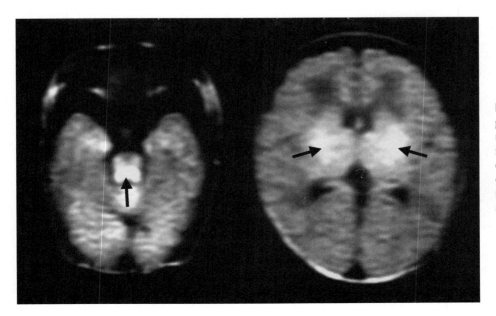

Figure 53–5. Brain stem and basal ganglia-thalamus injury. Axial magnetic resonance imaging scan (diffusion-weighted) showing abnormal hyperintensity in the dorsal pons (*arrow*, **left**) and deep nuclei of the basal ganglia-thalamus (*arrows*, **right**) in a full-term infant after profound and sustained asphyxia.

changes and the conventional MRI changes that appear later.[168-172] The temporal evolution of changes in DWI and conventional MRI has been described in a number of animal[173-175] and human studies,[164,176-180] although primarily in models of focal ischemia.[171,172,176,181-183] The data are limited for newborns suffering from postasphyxial encephalopathy.[168,184-187] One study of asphyxiated infants found that diffusion-weighted studies on the first day might underestimate the full extent of brain injury as seen on later scans.[184]

Circulating Substances in the Diagnosis of Perinatal Asphyxia

A variety of other substances have been measured in the body fluids (i.e., blood, urine, and cerebrospinal fluid [CSF]) of asphyxiated infants.[188] These measurements have been used in several ways, including as an estimate of the overall severity of the asphyxial *insult* (by measuring end-organ injury)[189] or as a more specific estimate of acute brain *injury* (by measuring brain-derived substances). The value of these measurements as predictors of long-term outcome is discussed as follows.

Measures of Fetal Acidosis

Fetal asphyxia is defined as impairment of placental gas exchange severe enough to cause metabolic acidosis. Therefore, the measurement of circulating blood gases and acid-base status in the fetal scalp or umbilical cord blood is the most direct technique for diagnosing the presence and severity of fetal asphyxia. Unfortunately, the value of these measurements remains compromised by a number of factors. These include (1) "operator-based" problems in technique and interpretation and (2) limitations in the intrinsic sensitivity of the technique. The value of measuring of acid-base status in suspected fetal asphyxia has been limited by the inconsistent techniques for measurement and interpretation of the data. First, the fundamental definition of significant acidosis has been inconsistent (discussed previously). The importance of consistent criteria for fetal acidosis is highlighted by the fact that the relationship between hydrogen ion concentration [H^+] and pH is logarithmic rather than linear. For example, the [H^+] accumulation required for a 0.10 decrease in pH between 7.00 and 6.90 is twice that required for an equivalent drop in pH from 7.30 and 7.20.[190] A second limiting factor has been the inconsistent use of venous and arterial blood samples, the latter best reflecting fetal metabolic status.[190] In fact, the optimal and most rational approach for assessing fetal acid-base status would be to measure the umbilical arteriovenous *differences* in blood gases, lactate, and base deficit.[190] Furthermore, the interpretation of fetal acid-base data has been complicated by the failure in many studies to distinguish consistently between the respiratory and metabolic components of fetal acidosis. Clearly, the use of consistent guidelines would optimize this potentially valuable approach.

In addition, the technique of fetal scalp or umbilical cord blood measurements for the assessment of fetal asphyxia has several intrinsic limitations. First, after a transient asphyxial insult, a period of oxygenated reperfusion "washes out" the metabolic indicators of acidosis.

Consequently, the severity of a transient insult capable of triggering ongoing brain cell injury is progressively less reflected in blood gas measurements over time. A related limitation is the inability of routine acid-base measurements to provide insight into the onset and duration of fetal asphyxial insults.[191,192] Specifically, the blood gas measurement reflects the overall "dose" of the insult but does not distinguish between the intensity and duration of the insult, both of which may be important determinants of fetal injury. An interesting approach to the question of insult duration is the measurement of the arteriovenous difference in buffer base in cord blood.[190,193] The rationale for this approach is based on the slow transfer of nonvolatile acids such as lactate from the fetal blood return into the placental extracellular fluid. Consequently, there is a gradual decrease in placental buffer base and hence in the umbilical arteriovenous gradient of buffer base. Therefore, large arteriovenous differences in buffer base or in base deficit reflect brief insults, whereas small differences suggest more substantial insults.[190] A large arteriovenous difference in base deficit with a relatively high venous pH is suggestive of cord occlusion.[194,195] In one study,[193] infants with an arteriovenous buffer base difference of less than 6 mmol/L had a significantly increased incidence of neonatal complications.

Other Circulating Substances in Perinatal Asphyxia

The ratio of urinary lactate/creatinine, particularly during the first 6 hours after birth, appears to be a particularly sensitive indicator of insult severity and predictor of outcome.[196] Brain-derived substances that have been measured include the brain-specific isoenzyme of creatine kinase,[197-207] neuron-specific enolase,[208,209] glial fibrillary acidic protein (CSF),[210] myelin basic protein (CSF),[208] excitatory amino acids (CSF),[73] arachidonic acid metabolites in CSF,[211] cytokines such as tumor necrosis factor α and interleukin-1β in plasma and CSF,[212] and blood lactate levels.[213] Of these, the measure of brain-specific isoenzyme of creatine kinase in blood is very sensitive but lacks specificity.[200-204] On the other hand, CSF levels are both more specific and more sensitive.[204,206] It seems logical that brain-released substances are more likely to be elevated earlier in the CSF than in the blood and urine. Products of free radical activation and attack, important mediators of brain cell injury, have also been measured in the encephalopathic newborn.[211,214-217] The sensitivity and specificity of many of these substances remain to be determined in large prospective studies before their entry into routine clinical practice.

DIFFERENTIAL DIAGNOSIS AND COMORBID CONDITIONS

Although the diagnosis of perinatal asphyxia can usually be made from available clinical and neuroimaging data, other conditions may need to be excluded. These conditions include (1) potential mimics of asphyxia, (2) potential precipitants of asphyxia, and (3) conditions that may exacerbate asphyxial brain injury. Conditions that may mimic fetal asphyxia include inherited metabolic diseases such as nonketotic hyperglycinemia, pyridoxine dependency, mitochondrial disorders, and glucose transporter deficiency.[218,219] Mitochondrial disorders should be suspected if an anion-gap metabolic acidosis persists after correction of gas exchange and perfusion. Mitochondrial disorders may also be accompanied by regional elevation of brain lactate but tend to manifest neuroimaging patterns of injury that differ from those of perinatal asphyxia.[220]

Potential precipitants of birth asphyxia include certain inherited neuromuscular conditions that are associated with prolonged and difficult labor and delivery and therefore may predispose to fetal asphyxia. A detailed discussion of these conditions is beyond the scope of this chapter. Conditions that may occur concurrently with fetal asphyxia and may exacerbate the hypoxic-ischemic injury of perinatal asphyxia are intracranial hemorrhage and infection. The association between traumatic delivery and perinatal asphyxia increases the risk of intracranial hemorrhage, which may in turn exacerbate the brain injury. Asphyxia may be associated with prolonged labor and prolonged rupture of membranes, which increases the risk of ascending infection. The role of infection and inflammatory mediators in fetal and neonatal brain injury is enormously complex and has become a focus of intense research.[221-229] Because a detailed discussion is beyond the scope of this chapter, a brief review follows.

There are multiple potential pathways by which infection may predispose to or exacerbate fetal brain injury. Chorioamnionitis may cause inflammatory edema, thereby impeding placental perfusion and gas exchange. In addition, direct infection of the fetus may occur with septicemia and meningitis. Because infection and intracranial hemorrhage may complicate perinatal asphyxia, it is recommended that a blood culture and CSF examination be performed for any asphyxiated newborn. Proinflammatory cytokines may be released during infection from sources in the mother, the intrauterine compartment, and the fetus. Multiple mechanisms by which such circulating cytokines could cause brain injury have been proposed. However, such cytokines are generated not only by infection but also by insults such as ischemia, particularly ischemia to vascular beds such as the brain and the gut. Furthermore, certain cytokines may further predispose to ischemia by disrupting cerebral pressure autoregulation.[230,231] In an experimental model, these inflammatory substances appear to have a "priming" effect, predisposing the immature brain to excitotoxic injury such as occurs in hypoxia-ischemia.[232] Currently, the precise relationship among proinflammatory cytokines, hypoxia-ischemia, and brain injury in the fetus and newborn remains unresolved and awaits further study.

LONG-TERM OUTCOME AND PROGNOSTIC FACTORS

The long-term neurologic complications of fetal asphyxia are known to encompass a broad spectrum of neurologic dysfunction, including cerebral palsy, epilepsy, mental retardation, and deficits in hearing and vision.[1] However, predicting in the early hours of life which infants are destined to develop these sequelae and which infants will be normal may be very challenging. Even more difficult is the accurate prediction of which *specific* deficits will develop in individual cases, although advances in neuroimaging are increasing the understanding of these structure-function relationships of neonatal brain injury (see later discussion).

The daunting task of predicting the likely long-term outcome of infants with postasphyxial encephalopathy is particularly stressful when these predictions are used to decide on the utility or futility of ongoing intensive care. Because long-term neurologic function is so intrinsically related to the future quality of the child's life, the perceived futility for "meaningful" survival may lead to so-called redirection of care for the infant and withdrawal of life support. Conversely, infants with devastating cerebral injuries may be successfully resuscitated and supported through the acute phase of critical illness; this "success" may produce an infant who is independent of artificial life support but who remains in a near-vegetative state of profoundly impaired consciousness and total lifelong dependence on caretakers. The current inability to reliably predict this tragic outcome may lead to the missed opportunity for withdrawal of artificial life support and the opportunity for a more natural and less traumatic demise.

In addition to these difficult ethical issues, early predictions of long-term outcome are complicated by the paucity of established prognostic factors available in the first hours of life after fetal asphyxia.[233] Not only are the indicators of the severity, duration, and timing of fetal insults often unreliable but also the early clinical picture may evolve in an unpredictable manner over the ensuing hours and days.

The Value of Clinical Factors and Adjunctive Tests as Prognostic Indicators

Fetal Acid-Base Status

Measurement of fetal acid-base status may provide essential data for the diagnosis of fetal asphyxia. However, for reasons discussed previously, the ability of these measures to diagnose the presence and severity of fetal asphyxia may be lacking in sensitivity and specificity. Consequently, this approach is potentially fallible for predicting long-term neurologic outcome,[28,29] particularly when used alone. Most authors agree that neurologic complications are unlikely to occur unless fetal acidosis is severe.[3] For example, even infants with pH values of 7.00 or less but with a stable clinical picture at birth very rarely develop significant asphyxial encephalopathy in the neonatal period,[234] and up to 80% of them are normal at follow-up.[235] In view of the potential limitations of routine acid-base measures, other approaches have been explored for their ability to enhance the predictive value of fetal and umbilical blood samples. For example, although single CO_2 pressure measurements do not appear to be predictive of outcome,[193,236] one study in acidotic infants measured the CO_2 pressure difference between umbilical arterial and venous specimens and found that a CO_2 pressure difference of more than 25 mm Hg was a highly sensitive and specific predictor of neurologic complications.[237] Other investigators have explored the predictive value of circulating lactate, the direct product of anaerobic metabolism and, therefore, presumably a specific indicator of fetal tissue hypoxia.[213,238] Unfortunately, neither lactate levels in umbilical cord blood[238] nor in neonatal arterial blood at 30 minutes after birth[213] provided additional predictive power over routine measures of acid-base status, such as pH and base deficit.

Apgar scores were originally designed as a clinical guide for the resuscitation of depressed newborn infants at birth, as well as an indication of the likelihood of survival.[239] For both these functions, Apgar scores remain useful and reliable measures.[240] However, the Apgar scoring system was never intended to be a measure of perinatal asphyxia, and it is therefore not surprising that it is not well correlated with other measures of asphyxia and that when used alone it is a poor predictor of long-term outcome. It is only in cases of severe and sustained neonatal depression at birth that Apgar scores become more reliable predictors of poor outcome. For example, of infants with Apgar scores of 3 or less for 20 minutes, 60% die, and of the survivors, 60% develop cerebral palsy.[241] Similarly, infants who fail to establish spontaneous respiration by 30 minutes have an 80% risk of death or significant handicap.[241]

The predictive value of Apgar scores increases when considered in the overall clinical context and when used in conjunction with other clinical factors, such as the fetal acid-base status.[193]

Severity of Clinical Encephalopathy

Later neurologic deficits are extremely unlikely to result from intrapartum asphyxia in infants with evidence of fetal asphyxia (e.g., by blood gas criteria) unless there is an obvious encephalopathy during the early neonatal period.[1] There is a clear relationship between the severity of the neonatal dysfunction and the incidence of later neurologic sequelae.[1,242-244] Grading schemes for the severity of neonatal encephalopathy have been used as predictors of long-term outcome.[128,245] These grading schemes are reliable predictors of outcome in asphyxiated infants, but only when the encephalopathy grade is either mild or severe. Almost all infants with mild encephalopathy have an good outcome, whereas infants with severe encephalopathy either die or are left with neurologic abnormalities.[1,131,246] Conversely, the outcome of infants with moderate encephalopathy is less predictable; although approximately 25% of these infants develop an adverse outcome later, this cannot be predicted by the severity of the neonatal encephalopathy alone.[131,246] When death or severe handicap is used as an outcome measure, infants with mild encephalopathy are considered to have a good outcome, whereas up to 25% infants with moderate encephalopathy and up to 70% with severe encephalopathy die or are left with severe handicap.[128,245,247] In addition to the peak severity of encephalopathy, the degree of recovery over the first week of life has been used as a predictor of outcome.[128,248] Infants who recover normal neurologic examinations by 1 week of age[128,248] tend to have a favorable long-term prognosis.

EEG has proved to be a more reliable predictor of outcome than the early neurologic examination.[128] Conventional neonatal EEG[139-141] and, more recently, amplitude-integrated EEG[249-251] have been used to predict long-term outcome in asphyxiated infants. When EEG is used to predict outcome, the analysis of background patterns has greater utility than do paroxysmal ictal changes. In particular, the burst-suppression (especially when this pattern is unreactive to stimuli), low-voltage, and isoelectric ("flat") background patterns recorded at any time during the neonatal period are strongly predictive of poor long-term neurodevelopmental outcome.[139-141] Conversely, an EEG background that is normal or mildly abnormal (e.g., "dysmature" patterns) is predictive of a favorable outcome.[252-254]

Although the timing of the EEG recording after birth may be important for prognostic purposes, the optimal timing remains in dispute.[249-251,255,256] Some studies have supported the use of early EEG findings[255]; amplitude-integrated EEG recordings made within the first hours of life have shown particular reliability for predicting long-term outcome.[249-251] Other studies have focused on the short-term recovery of EEG background abnormalities[128,256]; normal or mildly abnormal EEG background by 1 week of age may be predictive of a favorable long-term outcome.[128] Conversely, persistent background patterns of discontinuity or burst-suppression are powerful predictors of adverse outcome in studies using standard[141,144,256-259] and amplitude-integrated EEG recordings.[250,251,260]

Data suggest that EEG recordings may be less sensitive to certain patterns of brain injury and are therefore less reliable outcome measures in these cases. Specifically, because surface EEG recordings are primarily measures of electrocortical function, they may not reliably reflect injury to subcortical and/or brain stem regions. Consequently, infants with mainly deep patterns of injury on neuroimaging studies may have a poor neurologic outcome in spite of relatively normal neonatal EEG findings.[261]

Neuroimaging Studies

Excellent soft tissue resolution and ability to distinguish normal from injured tissue have made MRI the most powerful imaging modality for predicting outcome in the asphyxiated newborn.[110,262-264] In the acutely ill and unstable infant, ultrasonography has the advantage of portability to the bedside but lacks predictive power. Doppler ultrasound measurements of blood flow velocity in the anterior cerebral artery have proved useful for predicting short-term outcome[265,266] but have yet to prove their value for predicting long-term outcome. Although computed tomography and ultrasonography clearly lack the prognostic power of MRI, certain findings that are predictive of poor outcome, such as severe injury to the thalamus and basal ganglia and regions of hemorrhagic infarction, can be detected through these methods.[266-270]

The optimal timing of MRI scans for maximal prognostic power remains unresolved. This is in large part because of the natural evolution of brain tissue injury and its changing appearance on MRI studies. Because cerebral edema usually peaks around 3 days after birth and gradually resolves over the subsequent week, some authors have favored MRI studies at 72 hours for prognostic purposes.[106,143] Specifically, a normal MRI scan at 72 hours is predictive of a favorable outcome[143] even after a severe insult, whereas diffuse edema with impaired cortical gray-white differentiation or lesions in the dorsolateral thalamus or dorsal putamen are reliable predictors of poor outcome, even after a relatively benign acute course.[106] Other authorities have suggested that optimal prognostic information is obtained from studies delayed beyond the first week.[144,147,262] In these studies, the magnitude of MRI abnormality after the first week was highly predictive of long-term outcome,[147] and more useful than the EEG background patterns.[144]

The relatively uncommitted structure-function relationships in the immature brain, as well as the phenomenon of plasticity (particularly in cases of unilateral brain injury), make the accurate prediction of specific deficits more difficult in asphyxiated infants than in adults. However, the superb anatomic resolution of regional brain injury by MRI provides important information about the likely long-term neurologic sequelae.[143] The extent of basal ganglia and thalamic injury on MRI studies has emerged as an important predictor of outcome.[262] An MRI scan after the first week of life that is either normal or shows mild basal ganglia/thalamic injury is associated with a favorable outcome,[144] whereas more severe and diffuse injury to the basal ganglia or cerebral white matter is associated with subsequent cerebral palsy, microcephaly, and severe global delay.[144] The motor dysfunction in these children is characterized by abnormal and fluctuating muscle rigidity, often with superimposed involuntary movements ranging from dystonia to choreoathetosis. Less severe basal ganglia injury may result in motor dysfunction, but cognition is relatively preserved.[220,271] When deep nuclear lesions occur in combination with brain stem injury, the outcome is particularly poor, with prominent disturbances in speech, sucking, and swallowing, often necessitating gastrostomy tube feeding.[145,272] Parasagittal cerebral injury is usually associated with a characteristic upper extremity diplegia (i.e., arms are weaker than legs), particularly in the shoulder girdle and upper trunk. Interestingly, this picture is in contrast to the lower extremity diplegia in asphyxiated premature infants with periventricular white matter injury. As a general rule, cortical injury, often in the form of cortical "highlighting"[147,149,150] (described previously), increases the risk of epilepsy and cognitive impairment. Cerebral visual impairment complicates injury to the occipital primary visual cortex or the optic radiations in the parieto-occipital white matter.

Several studies have evaluated the prognostic utility of the newer magnetic resonance techniques discussed previously.[156,160,273-279] Preliminary reports suggest that DWI and proton magnetic resonance spectroscopy may provide useful predictors of long-term outcome within hours after the asphyxial insult.[156,160,273-279] In the asphyxiated full-term infant, absence of elevated cerebral lactate is generally predictive of a favorable neurodevelopmental outcome,[160] whereas elevated cerebral lactate levels are predictive of poor outcome.[156,273-282]

Early regions of restricted diffusion by DWI are predictive of later regions of injury by conventional MRI.[182,283,284] Furthermore, several studies have demonstrated that these acute DWI changes may be helpful in the early prediction of later outcome.[168,285,286] In our experience, these early DWI changes are sensitive indicators of later outcome but lack specificity.[279]

MANAGEMENT OF THE ASPHYXIATED INFANT

Although the ideal intervention for asphyxia-related brain injury in the newborn is, of course, the prevention of fetal asphyxia, the pursuit of such primary prevention techniques has remained difficult and frustrating. However, there are other important targets for intervention in which the aim is to prevent secondary insults and/or to limit ongoing processes of brain cell injury triggered by an earlier insult (see previous discussion). The current status of both these types of approaches is discussed.

Primary Prevention of Intrauterine Asphyxia and Fetal Brain Injury

Primary prevention strategies are based on the ability to identify the fetus at risk for intrauterine asphyxia before the onset of brain injury. A number of established diagnostic techniques in routine obstetric practice are designed to identify the fetus under stress or at risk for distress during the antepartum and intrapartum periods. In addition to clinical assessment of fetal well-being, adjunctive tests commonly utilized during the antepartum period include the nonstress test, the contraction stress test, the biophysical profile, and measurement of umbilical blood flow velocity by Doppler ultrasonography. These techniques are discussed elsewhere in this text. During the intrapartum period, the principal techniques include continuous electrical FHR monitoring and fetal scalp blood pH analysis. Certain FHR patterns have been associated with adverse neurologic outcome; however, this approach is lacking in both specificity[287] and sensitivity,[288] and the ability of these approaches to reduce fetal distress and perinatal asphyxia remains controversial.[289-291] Even the most ominous FHR patterns are predictive of neonatal compromise in only half of cases.[292,293] Overall, the widespread use of FHR monitoring in its current form does not appear capable of significantly reducing brain injury. These limitations of fetal monitoring in turn continue to impede the development of more effective neuroprotective strategies (see later discussion).

For the present, the most rational response to abnormalities in FHR and fetal scalp blood gases for preventing fetal asphyxia remains the use of techniques such as maternal repositioning and oxygen supplementation aimed at restoring fetal oxygenation. If such attempts at fetal resuscitation fail improve the fetal condition, rapid delivery of the fetus is indicated, to allow more direct and effective extrauterine resuscitation. A more detailed discussion of these issues is beyond the scope of this chapter but is available in Chapter 8.

Secondary Prevention of Brain Injury

Strategies for secondary prevention of brain injury are aimed at preventing the development of postnatal brain insults in the asphyxiated infant, as well as limiting the evolution of injurious cellular cascades of brain injury triggered by the initial intrauterine insult. The postasphyxial brain has elevated energy demands for the restoration of homeostasis in cells with potentially reversible hypoxic-ischemic injury. Consequently, these increased energy demands render the postinsult brain particularly vulnerable to further limitations in energy availability, as may occur during cerebral hypoperfusion, hypoglycemia, and seizures. At present, the cornerstone of cerebral resuscitation in the asphyxiated newborn is the restoration and maintenance of cerebral energy availability during the critical early hours and days of life. The rescue of injured but potentially viable brain tissue in the asphyxiated infant commences immediately at delivery with urgent restoration of cerebral oxygen and glucose delivery. Thereafter, close vigilance against delayed complications, such as seizures and hypotension, that may further tax cerebral energy availability and lead to secondary insults is crucial.[189,294-296]

An important concept to emerge from advances in experimental neuroscience is that the cellular mechanisms triggered by cerebral hypoxia-ischemia may evolve over hours to days before cell death occurs. Understanding of this concept is critical from a therapeutic perspective because clinical intervention is potentially possible before injury becomes irreversible. These insights have also highlighted the importance of maximizing the availability and minimizing the expenditure of cerebral energy during the early postinsult period of potentially reversible cellular injury.

Cerebral Resuscitation and Stabilization

Reestablishing and maintaining normal cerebral blood flow and oxygen delivery are the critical initial steps toward limiting ongoing cerebral injury. Because both the myocardium and cerebral vasculature are highly sensitive to hypoxia, hypoglycemia, and acidosis, these deficits necessitate urgent correction. The acute management of the asphyxiated newborn infant is aimed at restoring and maintaining physiologic parameters, such as blood pressure, oxygenation, and carbon dioxide, within a normal range. Both inadequate and overzealous correction of these disturbances may extend the cerebral injury in the asphyxiated newborn.[297,298] **Brain oxygen** availability is dependent on a number of factors that influence the balance of supply and demand. Consequently, interventions aimed at maintaining appropriate brain oxygenation should consider all aspects of cerebral oxygen metabolism, including cerebral oxygen delivery (arterial oxygen content and cerebral blood flow) and oxygen metabolism.

Cerebral perfusion, the critical determinant of cerebral oxygenation, is determined by the transcerebral pressure gradient (i.e., arterial blood pressure minus either cerebral venous pressure or intracranial pressure, whichever is higher) and cerebral vascular resistance. Cerebral perfusion pressure in the asphyxiated infant may be impaired by a number of factors, including myocardial failure, central venous hypertension, bradycardia, and a patent ductus arteriosus.[299-305] Postasphyxial cardiogenic shock impairs systemic perfusion and necessitates the careful use of inotropic agents and intravascular volume expanders to restore and maintain arterial blood pressure. Conversely, right-sided heart failure and elevated intrathoracic pressures during positive pressure ventilation for respiratory catastrophes such as the meconium aspiration syndrome may decrease cerebral perfusion

pressure by increasing cerebral venous pressure. In the asphyxiated newborn, elevated intracranial pressure is usually a result, rather than a major cause, of brain injury (see later discussion).[306] Because of the compliance of the neonatal skull, with its unfused sutures and open fontanelle, herniation across the tentorium and foramen magnum is extremely rare. Specific treatment of intracranial hypertension beyond judicious fluid management is rarely necessary in the asphyxiated newborn.

Although the cerebral vasculature of the normal full-term newborn has an intrinsic reactivity to changes in blood pressure (i.e., pressure-flow autoregulation), the "autoregulatory plateau" is narrower than in the mature brain.[307-309] Furthermore, the lower limit of "normal" blood pressure in the newborn is shifted toward the lower threshold of the autoregulatory plateau. In the asphyxiated newborn, the autoregulatory plateau may be abolished altogether, rendering the cerebral circulation pressure passive and the cerebral blood flow vulnerable to changes in perfusion pressure. In summary, there are multiple factors that threaten both cerebral perfusion pressure and autoregulation in the asphyxiated newborn, thereby exposing the brain to secondary insults and shifting potentially salvageable brain tissue across the threshold of irreversible injury. Currently, there are no established techniques for the bedside monitoring of cerebral venous pressure, intracranial pressure or the integrity of pressure-flow autoregulation. Consequently, it is reasonable to manage the asphyxiated infant as though the cerebral circulation is pressure-passive by maintaining stable high-normal blood pressures and preventing major fluctuations.

In the asphyxiated newborn, the **oxygen content** of the arterial circulation may be reduced by a number of factors, including central hypoventilation (caused by brain stem depression and/or the effect of sedating drugs), meconium aspiration, and persistent fetal circulation. In infants with hemorrhagic hypoxia (e.g., caused by abruptio placenta) or anemic hypoxia (hemolysis), red blood cell transfusions may be needed to optimize the oxygen-carrying capacity. Conversely, polycythemia (as may occur after chronic placental insufficiency) predisposes to hyperviscosity with impairment of cerebral perfusion.[310-312] When the hematocrit exceeds 65%, particularly in the asphyxiated infant, a partial exchange transfusion may be indicated.[310] Conversely, overzealous oxygenation during the resuscitation of the asphyxiated infant may have several detrimental effects on the posthypoxic brain. For example, hyperoxemia may cause cerebral vasoconstriction,[298,313,314] and hyperoxia, particularly after cerebral hypoxia-ischemia, may amplify free-radical production,[297,315] thereby exacerbating neuronal injury.

Arterial **carbon dioxide content** may affect the postasphyxial brain in several direct and indirect ways. Although hypercarbia may have a protective role *during* asphyxia,[316,317] it is likely to have an adverse effect on the postasphyxial brain. Persistent hypercarbia perpetuates acidosis, with potentially negative inotropic effects on the myocardium. Hypercarbia also causes cerebral vasodilation, further impairing pressure autoregulation[318,319] and predisposing to secondary cerebral ischemia during periods of myocardial dysfunction and hypotension. When hypercarbia is sustained over long periods, the diameter of cerebral resistance vessels gradually returns toward normal[320]; thereafter, any rapid correction of hypercarbia may cause significant cerebral vasoconstriction. Conversely, overventilation with hypocarbia has been associated with adverse neurologic outcome in some studies.[321-323]

Preventing Complications that Cause Secondary Cerebral Injury

Seizures

Seizures are common complications of moderate and severe postasphyxial encephalopathy. In fact, perinatal asphyxia remains the single most common cause of neonatal seizures. There are several important reasons supporting the rapid diagnosis and control of postasphyxial seizures in the newborn. These include the drain of cerebral energy and the accumulation of cerebral lactate in association with seizures. In addition, seizures cause a sharp increase in the release of excitatory amino acids (especially glutamate), which may further extend excitotoxicity.[324] Finally, seizures may cause significant disturbances in systemic and cerebral hemodynamics, exposing the brain to further risks for injury.

The clinical course and manifestations of postasphyxial seizures are probably dependent on the severity and nature of the insult. Between 50%[1] and 80%[325] of postasphyxial seizures begin within 12 hours of birth; however, the factors determining their postnatal onset remain poorly understood in most cases. Because the onset, duration, and intensity of the intrauterine insult are often unknown, the postinsult latency period until seizure onset remains unclear in most infants. In a fetal lamb model of selective cerebral ischemia, seizures developed around 8 to 10 hours after a 30-minute insult.[326,327] In a retrospective clinical study, Ahn and associates found a mean latency of around 10 hours between *birth* and seizure onset in asphyxiated infants; infants with acute insults (i.e., normal FHR tracings followed by sudden, sustained decelerations) tended to have earlier seizures than did infants with intermittent, recurrent insults, although the difference was not statistically significant.[325] It is likely that in most cases the insult is complex, with different levels of repeated insult possibly superimposed on a background of milder fetal hypoxia. The current limitations of fetal monitoring in the human fetus preclude a more accurate assessment of the underlying insult.

On the basis of their clinical manifestations, neonatal seizures may be categorized into four types: tonic, clonic, myoclonic, and subtle seizures.[328] Although any of these seizure types may occur in the asphyxiated newborn, a combination of seizure types is more common in the individual case. Neonatal seizures differ in several important ways from those in older children and adults. First, the clinical diagnosis of neonatal seizures may be difficult, because their manifestations may be subtle and in some cases may resemble other normal and abnormal neonatal behaviors. Several useful features may help to distinguish seizures from these other, nonepileptic paroxysms. Seizure movements cannot be suppressed by repositioning or by passive restraint; similarly, stimulus-evoked movements are unlikely to be seizures. Suspicious extremity movements with associated eye movements

and/or autonomic changes are suggestive of seizures. Another peculiar feature of seizures in the asphyxiated newborn is the frequent dissociation between electrographic and clinical seizures. Seizures may become clinically silent, especially in severely encephalopathic infants and after the administration of anticonvulsant drugs.[136,329-331] In these cases, the only clinical evidence of seizures may be abrupt autonomic changes, such as hypertension, tachycardia, and pupillary dilation. Although unexplained bradycardia is often suspected of being epileptic in origin, the more typical heart rate response in neonatal seizures is tachycardia; bradycardia is a late development when seizures are sustained. In contrast to these clinically silent seizures, convulsive seizures (most commonly subtle and tonic seizures) may occur without an electrocortical correlate on EEG. Whether these are epileptic events originating from basal or deep cerebral foci that remain undetected by scalp electrodes or whether they are so-called brain stem release phenomena remains unclear. When the nature of paroxysmal behaviors is unclear, the diagnosis of seizures should be excluded or confirmed by capturing the EEG events occurring during these behaviors. In addition, the common occurrence of electroclinical dissociation in postasphyxial seizures may warrant the use of continuous EEG monitoring in these infants.[332]

Seizure management. Early predictors for neonatal seizures have been identified,[130] including certain EEG background patterns.[333] However, the initiation of prophylactic anticonvulsant therapy in asphyxiated infants remains controversial.[334,335] In randomized trials,[335,336] early prophylactic phenobarbital in asphyxiated infants did not significantly decrease the incidence of subsequent seizures; in one study, this approach was associated with a high rate of hypotension with its risk of secondary cerebral insult.[335]

The optimal therapeutic approach to both clinically silent seizures and clinical "seizures" without EEG discharges remains controversial. Fortunately, in the majority of cases, these phenomena occur in infants that also have more typical epileptic events that clearly warrant treatment. In general, seizures in the asphyxiated newborn are less responsive to conventional anticonvulsants than are seizures in older children and adults[337]; this is suggestive of a fundamental difference in the seizure mechanisms. Clinically silent electrographic seizures may be particularly refractory to standard anticonvulsants,[337-341] and high doses may be required for control. There are several reasons why these clinically silent seizures should be treated, in a rational, stepwise, and carefully monitored approach. First, in the postasphyxial brain, the metabolic stress of seizures exerts a major drain on the energy required for posthypoxic cellular recovery.[324] Second, ongoing electrographic seizures may cause significant systemic and cerebral hemodynamic changes, including the loss of cerebral pressure autoregulation.[342,343] In addition, these seizures may increase extracellular glutamate to toxic levels.

At the onset of seizure activity, the first step in management should be the urgent exclusion or correction of reversible causes, such as hypoglycemia and electrolyte disturbances. After seizures are diagnosed clinically or confirmed electrographically, the urgent initiation of anticonvulsant therapy is indicated. The guidelines outlined in Figure 53-6 are based on the antiepileptic protocol for neonatal seizures at our center. Phenobarbital is the most commonly used first-line drug, with repeated intravenous doses given until either the seizures are controlled or blood levels reach the range of 40 to 50 mg/dL. Careful monitoring of blood pressure and respiration is essential because both may be depressed by phenobarbital, particularly in the encephalopathic infant. If the infant has not been placed on mechanical ventilation by the time these blood levels are reached, elective intubation should be considered.

If electrographic seizures persist after these steps, a second agent such as phenytoin should be added, aiming for blood levels between 20 and 25 mg/dL. Phenytoin causes less respiratory depression and sedation but has less predictable pharmacokinetics than does phenobarbital and may have serious cardiac conduction effects if given too rapidly.[344] The safety of fosphenytoin has been demonstrated in the newborn.[345,346] For frequently recurrent seizures, additional intermittent doses of benzodiazepines may be effective. If seizures persist, a test dose of pyridoxine, 50 to 100 mg intravenously, is indicated, with EEG monitoring to gauge the electrographic response.

Even in cases in which hypoglycemia is not the primary cause of the seizures, blood glucose should be checked at regular intervals until seizures are controlled, because seizure activity may dramatically increase glucose utilization. Most seizures respond to this regimen. Because of the escalating toxicity risk, neurologists at our institution generally do not add further anticonvulsants for seizures that persist beyond this point; instead, we maintain the levels of phenobarbital and phenytoin just described. Because these drugs are metabolized in the liver, their dosing schedule in infants with significant postasphyxial hepatic dysfunction should be based on closely monitored blood levels.

Because the clinical manifestations of seizures may disappear after the onset of anticonvulsant treatment, it is reasonable to continue EEG monitoring for 12 to 24 hours after the last electrographically recorded seizure.[341] In the asphyxiated newborn, the tendency for repeated seizures appears to decrease after the first 72 hours. Therefore, once seizures have been effectively controlled over this interval, phenytoin may be discontinued and phenobarbital levels allowed to decrease into the range of 20 to 30 mg/dL, thereby reducing the depressant effects on the infant's sensorium. If at the time of discharge from the neonatal intensive care unit the infant's neurologic examination and EEG show good recovery toward normal, an early withdrawal of

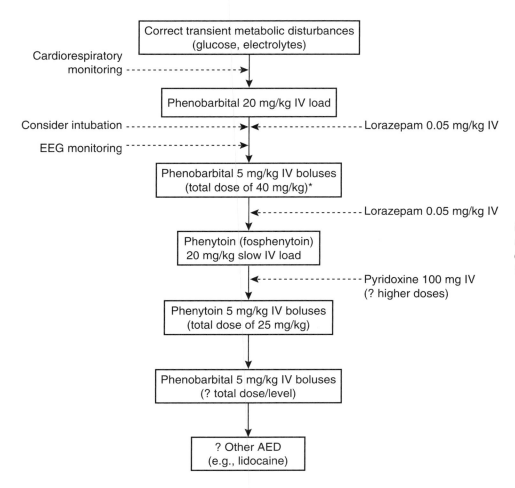

Figure 53–6. Acute antiepileptic management. AED, antiepileptic drug; EEG, electroencephalographic; IV, intravenously.

phenobarbital may be considered. Otherwise, the need for continued phenobarbital treatment should be reevaluated at 6- to 12-week intervals, with interim blood levels maintained at approximately 20 mg/dL.

Temperature regulation. Thermoregulation may be disturbed in the asphyxiated newborn, probably the result of injury to the hypothalamus. Hyperthermia, as may occur from excessive rewarming during resuscitation, may exacerbate neurologic injury in the postischemic brain[347-350] by increasing the cerebral metabolic rate and the release of excitotoxic neurotransmitters. Conversely, data from animal studies[7,347,351-353] and preliminary clinical studies[354-357] are suggestive of a neuroprotective role for mild *hypothermia* (see later discussion). However, until further data emerge from several of the large clinical trials currently in progress, the management goal should be normothermia with careful avoidance of hyperthermia.

Electrolyte disturbances. Disturbances in circulating electrolyte levels are a common complication of perinatal asphyxia and are also caused in part by hypothalamic injury. Specifically, an inappropriate secretion of antidiuretic hormone may cause hyponatremia and fluid retention during the first few days of life.[358-360] Conversely, diabetes insipidus with hemoconcentration and hypernatremia may develop and may follow the inappropriate secretion of antidiuretic hormone.[359] These complications should be anticipated by close monitoring of serum electrolytes and urine output. Both these complications are usually treated effectively by judicious fluid management alone.

Other important electrolyte disturbances in the asphyxiated newborn include hypocalcemia and hypomagnesemia. Prompt correction of these disturbances is important because they may further reduce the seizure threshold[361]; in addition, these disturbances may have important cardiovascular effects, including hypotension.

Hepatic dysfunction. During fetal asphyxia, particularly prolonged partial insults, sustained diversion of cardiac output away from the splanchnic vascular bed toward the heart and brain may cause hepatic ischemia. Consequently, hepatic dysfunction with elevated transaminase levels is not uncommon in asphyxiated infants and may lead to other potentially harmful complications, including hypoglycemia, coagulopathy, and hyperammonemia. Hypoglycemia is most common in infants with intrauterine growth restriction, presumably because of antepartum depletion of hepatic glycogen stores.

The urgent correction and prevention of hypoglycemia in the asphyxiated newborn is crucial because of the tenuous energy status of the insulted brain (see previous discussion). In addition, there is evidence of an important role for cerebral glucose in reuptake of glutamate by glial cells.[90] In contrast, the effect of hyperglycemia in the asphyxiated newborn is controversial. In animal models[362-364] and adult stroke,[365,366] hyperglycemia may have an adverse effect on neurologic outcome, whereas in the injured immature brain, hyperglycemia has been beneficial in some studies,[81,367] possibly by enhancing cardiac function. Until

further studies clarify these issues, current management should aim to maintain blood glucose levels around 75 to 100 mg/dL.[1]

Another complication of hepatic dysfunction is an elevation of serum ammonia.[368] Hyperammonemia is known to cause brain injury in certain inherited metabolic defects such as urea cycle defects, possibly through excitotoxic pathways.[369] The level of hyperammonemia in asphyxiated infants is usually below that seen in these metabolic disorders, and its potential for exacerbating postasphyxial brain injury remains poorly defined.

Hepatic dysfunction and impaired synthesis of clotting factors may contribute to the coagulation disturbances that commonly complicate the clinical course of asphyxiated infants and may predispose to secondary hemorrhagic or thrombotic brain injury.

Respiratory failure. Respiratory dysfunction in the asphyxiated newborn may develop by several mechanisms. In addition to a reduced central respiratory drive from brain stem injury or depression by sedating medications, perinatal asphyxia may be complicated by meconium aspiration–caused pneumonia or by persistent fetal circulation. If severe, both these latter conditions may necessitate support by extracorporeal membrane oxygenation, a technique with its own inherent neurologic risks.[370]

Specific Neuroprotection Strategies

Until antenatal and intrapartum diagnostic techniques are capable of diagnosing with accuracy the fetus at risk for asphyxia *before* the onset of significant cerebral hypoxia-ischemia, efforts to minimize brain injury in these infants must focus on postinsult mechanisms of injury. Fortunately, a number of advances in basic neuroscience have generated optimism for the feasibility of effective postinsult interventions. First, it is now known that many of the mechanisms leading to neuronal death are initiated *after* termination of the hypoxic-ischemic insult. Second, delineation of the basic cellular mechanisms of injury has defined potential cellular targets for intervention. A host of agents have demonstrated the ability to arrest or ameliorate the cascades of cellular injury before the onset of irreversible brain injury. These advances are discussed in detail elsewhere.[4]

Several features unique to the fetal asphyxial insult influence the safety and efficacy of future neuroprotective agents. First, such agents must have a relatively wide therapeutic window, because the asphyxiated infant may be delivered several hours after the insult onset. Second, because the cerebral insult triggers a concatenation of amplifying cascades of injury, the ideal neuroprotective agent will act at several different levels in these cascades. The metabolism and toxicity of such agents must be tested within the complex multisystem dysfunction that commonly complicates perinatal asphyxia. Finally, as discussed, there is major overlap in the immature brain between the mechanisms of normal brain development and those of cellular injury.[33,57] Therefore, the theoretical risk that these potential neuroprotective agents may interfere with normal processes of brain development remains a major challenge in the design of safe and effective neuroprotective agents.

Although a number of strategies have demonstrated efficacy in animal models, this discussion focuses on the agents that have already entered clinical trials in the newborn.

Induced Mild Hypothermia

In experimental studies, mild induced hypothermia has been one of the most promising neuroprotective strategies to date, demonstrating potent protection in several different models of hypoxia-ischemia.[353,371-375] Of importance, hypothermia appears to act at many different levels in the injury cascade[352,371,374,376-387] by decreasing glutamate release,[380-383] decreasing cerebral metabolism and energy requirements,[373] and limiting lactate accumulation[373,388] and acidosis.[373]

Despite the often-striking neuroprotection provided by induced hypothermia, a number of fundamental issues remain unresolved. The existence of a postinsult therapeutic window for induced hypothermia has been suggested by most (although not all)[374,375] experimental studies.[352,378,379,389] However, the features of this therapeutic window and its determinants remain poorly defined. Hypothermia may continue to have neuroprotective efficacy even when induced as late as 5.5 hours after the insult,[7] but this efficacy is lost after the onset of seizures.[390] A second area of debate is the durability of hypothermic neuroprotection. Some studies suggest that hypothermia delays rather than prevents cerebral injury,[5,374,391] whereas others have shown sustained protection persisting as long as 7 weeks[392] and even 6 months.[393] More data are clearly needed.

Other unresolved questions about this strategy are the optimal delivery technique for hypothermia (both direct cooling through a cranial cap and whole body cooling are currently in clinical trial),[354-357] the optimal "dose" (depth and duration) of cooling,[389,394,395] and the rewarming conditions.[396]

Preliminary reports from clinical trials of mild hypothermia in asphyxiated full-term newborns are promising but far from conclusive.[354-357] Selective head cooling using a water-cooled cap, starting at a mean age of 4 hours, and maintaining rectal temperatures around 35.5° C for 48 to 72 hours[355] showed no significant adverse effects and promising short-term benefits. However, the application of hypothermia for birth-asphyxiated infants is not recommended until the long-term safety and efficacy are proven.

Antioxidant Agents

Free radicals are critical mediators in many of the pathways leading to cellular injury after cerebral hypoxic-ischemic insults. Many different antioxidant agents have demonstrated neuroprotection in experimental models of hypoxic-ischemic brain injury.[397-401] A clinical trial of high-dose allopurinol, a xanthine oxidase inhibitor and free radical scavenger, showed some beneficial effect in asphyxiated infants. Specifically, treated infants had less free radical generation, improved cerebral hemodynamics, and better electrical brain activity.[402] In addition, treated infants showed a trend toward better short-term outcome. The long-term benefits of this approach are yet to be determined.

Magnesium

A number of its physiologic actions suggest that magnesium may have neuroprotective potential.[63,403-405] Earlier experimental studies[406] supported such a neuroprotective role for magnesium in models of cerebral hypoxia-ischemia. In animal models, postinsult magnesium administration has protected against both focal and global cerebral hypoxia-ischemia,[63,407] although less convincingly in immature animals.[408-410] Magnesium sulfate has been used by obstetricians for years, both as a tocolytic agent and for treating preeclampsia.[411] Epidemiologic studies have suggested an association between the in utero exposure to magnesium in premature infants and a decrease in cerebral palsy.[412,413] However, there are persistent concerns about the safety of magnesium in perinatal asphyxia. First, at high doses, magnesium may cause hypotension and hyperglycemia. Furthermore, the vasodilatory effects of magnesium may impair the cerebral autoregulatory response in hypotension. In a fetal sheep model of ischemic hypoxia, magnesium impaired the normal cerebral hyperemic response to hypoxemia.[414] Furthermore, some[415-419] but not all[420] studies have suggested an increased rate of mortality among infants receiving antenatal exposure to magnesium sulfate.

In clinical trials of adults with stroke, magnesium showed minimal adverse effects.[421] However, in a single prospective clinical trial in asphyxiated full-term infants, magnesium at higher doses demonstrated an unacceptable risk for cardiovascular and respiratory depression.[422] The utility and safety of magnesium in perinatal asphyxia remains to be defined.

Calcium Channel Blockers

The cellular influx of calcium and the activation of cytosolic enzymes is a crucial early step in the subsequent development of cellular injury. Consequently, blockade of calcium influx is an attractive target for intervention in hypoxic-ischemic brain injury. Although calcium channel blockers have suggested a beneficial effect in animal models,[423-425] the agents performed poorly in a small trial of asphyxiated infants, in part because of unacceptable hemodynamic effects.[426]

SUMMARY

To date, the prospective study of potential neuroprotective agents has focused largely on single agents. However, the complexity of cellular mechanisms of injury suggests that future strategies will exploit the different advantages of several agents by using them in combination. At present, the approaches with greatest promise appear to be mild hypothermia and free radical scavengers. In addition, the common "downstream" mechanisms of action shared at multiple sites by these approaches makes them all the more attractive. In view of the primary safety concerns in this critically ill population, the relative lack of toxicity and early trends toward benefit in preliminary studies support further larger trials with these agents.

REFERENCES

1. Volpe JJ: Hypoxic-ischemic encephalopathy: Clinical aspects. In: Neurology of the Newborn. Philadelphia, WB Saunders, 2001, pp 331-394.
2. Levene ML, Kornberg J, Williams TH: The incidence and severity of post-asphyxial encephalopathy in full-term infants. Early Hum Dev 11:21, 1985.
3. Low JA: Intrapartum fetal asphyxia: Definition, diagnosis, and classification. Am J Obstet Gynecol 176:957, 1997.
4. du Plessis AJ, Johnston MV: Hypoxic-ischemic brain injury in the newborn: Cellular mechanisms and potential strategies for neuroprotection. Clin Perinatol 24:627, 1997.
5. Johnston MV, Redmond JM, Gillinov AM, et al: Neuroprotective strategies in a model of selective neuronal necrosis from hypothermic circulatory arrest. In Moskowitz MA, Caplan LR (eds): Cerebrovascular Diseases. Boston, Butterworth-Heinemann, 1995, pp 165-174.
6. Johnston M: New strategies for brain protection including NMDA receptor antagonists. In Jonas R, Newburger J, Volpe J (eds): Brain Injury and Pediatric Cardiac Surgery. Boston, Butterworth-Heinemann, 1995, pp 365-373.
7. Gunn AJ, Gunn TR, Gunning MI, et al: Neuroprotection with prolonged head cooling started before postischemic seizures in fetal sheep. Pediatrics 102:1098, 1998.
8. Iadecola C, Zhang F, Xu X: Inhibition of inducible nitric oxide synthase ameliorates cerebral ischemic damage. Am J Physiol 268:R268, 1995.
9. Block F, Schwartz M: Memantine reduces functional and morphological consequences induced by global ischemia in rats. Neurosci Lett 208:41, 1996.
10. Bartus R, Hayward N, Elliott P, et al: Calpain inhibitor AK295 protects neurons from focal brain ischemia. Stroke 25:2265, 1994.
11. Colbourne F, Sutherland G, Corbett D: Postischemic hypothermia: A critical appraisal with implications for clinical treatment. Mol Neurobiol 14:171, 1997.
12. Crumrine RC, Bergstrand K, Cooper AT, et al: Lamotrigine protects hippocampal CA1 neurons from ischemic damage after cardiac arrest. Stroke 28:2230, 1997.
13. Ginsberg M, Pulsinelli W: The ischemic penumbra, injury thresholds, and the therapeutic window for acute stroke. Ann Neurol 36:553, 1994.
14. Nagafuji T, Sugiyama M, Matsui T, Koide T: A narrow therapeutic window of a nitric oxide synthase inhibitor against transient ischemic brain injury. Eur J Pharmacol Environ Toxicol 248:325, 1993.
15. Zivin JA: Factors determining the therapeutic window for stroke. Neurology 50:599, 1998.
16. Nelson KB, Ellenberg JH: Antecedents of cerebral palsy: Multivariate analysis of risk. N Engl J Med 315:81, 1986.
17. Blair E, Stanley FJ: Intrapartum asphyxia: A rare cause of cerebral palsy. J Pediatr 112:515, 1988.
18. Stanley FJ: The changing face of cerebral palsy? Dev Med Child Neurol 29:263, 1987.
19. Stanley FJ: Cerebral palsy trends: Implications for perinatal care. Acta Obstet Gynecol Scand 73:5, 1994.
20. Kuban KC, Leviton A: The epidemiology of cerebral palsy. N Engl J Med 330:188, 1994.
21. Little W: On the influence of abnormal parturition, difficult labour, premature birth and asphyxia neonatorum on mental and physical conditions of the child, especially in relation to deformities. Trans Obstet Soc London 3:293, 1862.
22. Bretscher J, Saling E: pH values in the human fetus during labor. Am J Obstet Gynecol 97:906, 1967.
23. Yoon BH, Kim SW: The effect of labor on the normal values of umbilical blood acid-base status. Acta Obstet Gynecol Scand 73:555, 1994.
24. Gilstrap LC 3rd, Leveno KJ, Burris J, et al: Diagnosis of birth asphyxia on the basis of fetal pH, Apgar score, and newborn cerebral dysfunction. Am J Obstet Gynecol 161:825, 1989.
25. Goldaber KG, Gilstrap LC 3rd, Leveno KJ, et al: Pathologic fetal acidemia. Obstet Gynecol 78:1103, 1991.
26. American College of Obstetricians and Gynecologists Technical Bulletin 163: Fetal and neonatal neurologic injury. Washington, DC, American College of Obstetricians and Gynecologists, January 1992.
27. American Academy of Pediatrics: The use and abuse of the Apgar score. Pediatrics 78:1148, 1986.
28. Ruth VJ, Raivio KO: Perinatal brain damage: Predictive value of metabolic acidosis and the Apgar score. BMJ 297:24, 1988.
29. Fee SC, Malee K, Deddish R, et al: Severe acidosis and subsequent neurologic status. Am J Obstet Gynecol 162:802, 1990.
30. Low JA, Lindsay BG, Derrick EJ: Threshold of metabolic acidosis associated with newborn complications. Am J Obstet Gynecol 177:1391, 1997.
31. Low JA, Ludwin SK, Fisher S: Severe fetal asphyxia associated with neuropathology. Am J Obstet Gynecol 175:1383, 1996.
32. Low JA, Pickersgill H, Killen H, Derrick EJ: The prediction and prevention of intrapartum fetal asphyxia in term pregnancies. Am J Obstet Gynecol 184:724, 2001.
33. Johnston MV, Trescher WH, Ishida A, Nakajima W: Neurobiology of hypoxic-ischemic injury in the developing brain. Pediatr Res 49:735, 2001.
34. Vannucci R: Experimental biology of cerebral hypoxia-ischemia: Relation to perinatal brain damage. Pediatr Res 27:317, 1990.
35. Brinkman CR 3rd, Mofid M, Assali NS: Circulatory shock in pregnant sheep. 3. Effects of hemorrhage on uteroplacental and fetal circulation and oxygenation. Am J Obstet Gynecol 118:77, 1974.
36. Altman DI, Powers WJ, Perlman JM, et al: Cerebral blood flow requirement for brain viability in newborn infants is lower than in adults. Ann Neurol 24:218, 1988.
37. Altman D, Perlman J, Volpe J, Powers W: Cerebral oxygen metabolism in newborns. Pediatrics 92:99, 1993.
38. Johnson GN, Palahniuk RJ, Tweed WA, et al: Regional cerebral blood flow changes during severe fetal asphyxia produced by slow partial umbilical cord compression. Am J Obstet Gynecol 135:48, 1979.
39. Jensen A: The brain of the asphyxiated fetus—basic research. Eur J Obstet Gynecol Reprod Biol 65:19, 1996.
40. Jensen A, Garnier Y, Berger R: Dynamics of fetal circulatory responses to hypoxia and asphyxia. Eur J Obstet Gynecol Reprod Biol 84:155, 1999.
41. Cohn HE, Sacks EJ, Heymann MA, Rudolph AM: Cardiovascular responses to hypoxemia and acidemia in fetal lambs. Am J Obstet Gynecol 120:817, 1974.
42. Behrman RE, Lees MH, Peterson EN, et al: Distribution of the circulation in the normal and asphyxiated fetal primate. Am J Obstet Gynecol 108:956, 1970.
43. Sheldon RE, Peeters LL, Jones MD Jr, et al: Redistribution of cardiac output and oxygen delivery in the hypoxemic fetal lamb. Am J Obstet Gynecol 135:1071, 1979.
44. Reuss ML, Rudolph AM: Distribution and recirculation of umbilical and systemic venous blood flow in fetal lambs during hypoxia. J Dev Physiol 2:71, 1980.
45. Myers RE: Four patterns of perinatal brain damage and their conditions of occurrence in primates. Adv Neurol 10:223, 1975.

46. Woods JR Jr, Coppes V, Brooks DE, et al: Measurement of visual evoked potential in the asphyctic fetus and during neonatal survival. Am J Obstet Gynecol 143:944, 1982.

47. Rosenberg A, Jones M, Traystman R, et al: Response of cerebral blood flow to changes in P_{CO_2} in fetal, newborn, and adult sheep. Am J Physiol 242:H862, 1982.

48. Jones MD Jr, Rosenberg AA, Simmons MA, et al: Oxygen delivery to the brain before and after birth. Science 216:324, 1982.

49. Purves MJ, James IM: Observations on the control of cerebral blood flow in the sheep fetus and newborn lamb. Circ Res 25:651, 1969.

50. Peeters LL, Sheldon RE, Jones MD Jr, et al: Blood flow to fetal organs as a function of arterial oxygen content. Am J Obstet Gynecol 135:637, 1979.

51. Jones MD Jr, Sheldon RE, Peeters LL, et al: Regulation of cerebral blood flow in the ovine fetus. Am J Physiol 235:H162, 1978.

52. Mann LI: Developmental aspects and the effect of carbon dioxide tension on fetal cephalic metabolism and electroencephalogram. Exp Neurol 26:148, 1970.

53. Rosen KG: Alterations in the fetal electrocardiogram as a sign of fetal asphyxia—experimental data with a clinical implementation. J Perinat Med 14:355, 1986.

54. Mishra O, Delivaria-Papadopoulos M: Na$^+$,K$^+$,-ATPase in developing fetal guinea pig brain and the effect of maternal hypoxia. Neurochem Res 13:765, 1988.

55. Chugani H, Phelps M, Mazziotta J: Positron emission tomography study of human brain functional development. Ann Neurol 22:487, 1987.

56. Clark RH, Yoder BA, Sell MS: Prospective, randomized comparison of high-frequency oscillation and conventional ventilation in candidates for extracorporeal membrane oxygenation. J Pediatr 124:447, 1994.

57. McDonald J, Johnston M: Physiological and pathophysiological roles of excitatory amino acids during central nervous system development. Brain Res Rev 15:41, 1990.

58. Johnston M: Neurotransmitters and vulnerability of the developing brain. Brain Dev 17:301, 1995.

59. Johnston M: Developmental aspects of NMDA receptor agonists and antagonists in the central nervous system. Psychopharmacol Bull 30:567, 1995.

60. Gonzalez D, Fuchs J, Droge M: Distribution of NMDA receptor binding in developing mouse spinal cord. Neurosci Lett 151:134, 1993.

61. Kalb R, Lidow M, Halstead M, Hockfield S: N-methyl-D-aspartate receptors are transiently expressed in the developing spinal cord ventral horn. Proc Natl Acad Sci U S A 89:8502, 1992.

62. Chaudieu I, Mount H, Quirion R, Boksa P: Transient postnatal increases in excitatory amino acid binding sites in rat ventral mesencephalon. Neurosci Lett 133:276, 1991.

63. McDonald J, Silverstein F, Johnston M: Magnesium reduces N-methyl-D-aspartate (NMDA)–mediated brain injury in perinatal rats. Neurosci Lett 109:234, 1990.

64. Insel T, Miller L, Gelhard R: The ontogeny of excitatory amino acid receptors in rat forebrain. 1. N-methyl-D-aspartate and quisqualate receptors. Neurosci 35:31, 1990.

65. Greenamyre T, Penney J, Young A, et al: Evidence for transient perinatal glutamatergic innervation of globus pallidus. J Neurosci 7:1022, 1987.

66. Andersen D, Tannenberg A, Burke C, Dodd P: Developmental rearrangements of cortical glutamate-NMDA receptor binding sites in late human gestation. Brain Res Dev Brain Res 88:178, 1995.

67. Jabaudon D, Scanziani M, Gahwiler BH, Gerber U: Acute decrease in net glutamate uptake during energy deprivation. Proc Natl Acad Sci U S A 97:5610, 2000.

68. Rossi DJ, Oshima T, Attwell D: Glutamate release in severe brain ischaemia is mainly by reversed uptake. Nature 403:316, 2000.

69. Andine P, Sandberg M, Bagenholm R, et al: Intra- and extracellular changes of amino acids in the cerebral cortex of the neonatal rat during hypoxic-ischemia. Brain Res Dev Brain Res 64:115, 1991.

70. Hagberg H, Andersson P, Kjellmer I, et al: Extracellular overflow of glutamate, aspartate, GABA and taurine in the cortex and basal ganglia of fetal lambs during hypoxia-ischemia. Neurosci Lett 78:311, 1987.

71. Riikonen RS, Kero PO, Simell OG: Excitatory amino acids in cerebrospinal fluid in neonatal asphyxia. Pediatr Neurol 8:37, 1992.

72. Silverstein FS, Naik B, Simpson J: Hypoxia-ischemia stimulates hippocampal glutamate efflux in perinatal rat brain: An in vivo microdialysis study. Pediatr Res 30:587, 1991.

73. Hagberg H, Thornberg E, Blennow M, et al: Excitatory amino acids in the cerebrospinal fluid of asphyxiated infants: Relationship to hypoxic-ischemic encephalopathy. Acta Paediatr 82:925, 1993.

74. Pu Y, Li QF, Zeng CM, et al: Increased detectability of alpha brain glutamate/glutamine in neonatal hypoxic-ischemic encephalopathy. ANJR Am J Neuroradiol 21:203, 2000.

75. Barks J, Silverstein F: Excitatory amino acids contribute to the pathogenesis of perinatal hypoxic-ischemic brain injury. Brain Pathol 2:235, 1992.

76. Johnston MV, Trescher WH, Taylor GA: Hypoxic and ischemic central nervous system disorders in infants and children. Adv Pediatr 42:1, 1995.

77. Johnston MV: Selective vulnerability in the neonatal brain. Ann Neurol 44:155, 1998.

78. Hernandez MJ, Vannucci RC, Salcedo A, Brennan RW: Cerebral blood flow and metabolism during hypoglycemia in newborn dogs. J Neurochem 35:622, 1980.

79. Vannucci RC, Nardis EE, Vannucci SJ, Campbell PA: Cerebral carbohydrate and energy metabolism during hypoglycemia in newborn dogs. Am J Physiol 240:R192, 1981.

80. Young RS, Petroff OA, Chen B, et al: Brain energy state and lactate metabolism during status epilepticus in the neonatal dog: In vivo 31P and 1H nuclear magnetic resonance study. Pediatr Res 29:191, 1991.

81. Vannucci RC, Yager JY: Glucose, lactic acid, and perinatal hypoxic-ischemic brain damage. Pediatr Neurol 8:3, 1992.

82. McDonald JW, Bhattacharyya T, Sensi SL, et al: Extracellular acidity potentiates AMPA receptor-mediated cortical neuronal death. J Neurosci 18:6290, 1998.

83. Plum F: What causes infarction in ischemic brain? The Robert Wartenberg lecture. Neurology 33:222, 1983.

84. Wagner K, Myers R: Topographic aspects of lactic acid accumulation in brain tissue after cardiac arrest [Abstract]. Neurology 29:546, 1979.

85. Vannucci RC, Duffy TE: Cerebral metabolism in newborn dogs during reversible asphyxia. Ann Neurol 1:528, 1977.

86. Welsh FA, Vannucci RC, Brierley JB: Columnar alterations of NADH fluorescence during hypoxia-ischemia in immature rat brain. J Cereb Blood Flow Metab 2:221, 1982.

87. Myers RE: A unitary theory of causation of anoxic and hypoxic brain pathology. Adv Neurol 26:195, 1979.

88. Rehncrona S, Rosen I, Siesjo BK: Excessive cellular acidosis: An important mechanism of neuronal damage in the brain? Acta Physiol Scand 110:435, 1980.

89. Rehncrona S, Rosen I, Siesjo BK: Brain lactic acidosis and ischemic cell damage: 1. Biochemistry and neurophysiology. J Cereb Blood Flow Metab 1:297, 1981.

90. Magistretti PJ, Pellerin L, Rothman DL, Shulman RG: Energy on demand. Science 283:496, 1999.

91. Sokoloff L: Energetics of functional activation in neural tissues. Neurochem Res 24:321, 1999.

92. Sibson NR, Dhankhar A, Mason GF, et al: Stoichiometric coupling of brain glucose metabolism and glutamatergic neuronal activity. Proc Natl Acad Sci U S A 95:316, 1998.

93. Pfund Z, Chugani DC, Juhasz C, et al: Evidence for coupling between glucose metabolism and glutamate cycling using FDG PET and 1H magnetic resonance spectroscopy in patients with epilepsy. J Cereb Blood Flow Metab 20:871, 2000.

94. Back SA, Gan X, Li Y, et al: Maturation-dependent vulnerability of oligodendrocytes to oxidative stress-induced death caused by glutathione depletion. J Neurosci 18:6241, 1998.

95. Back SA, Luo NL, Borenstein NS, et al: Late oligodendrocyte progenitors coincide with the developmental window of vulnerability for human perinatal white matter injury. J Neurosci 21:1302, 2001.

96. Volpe JJ: Neurobiology of periventricular leukomalacia in the premature infant. Pediatr Res 50:553, 2001.

97. Piggott M, Perry E, Perry R, Scott D: N-methyl-D-aspartate (NMDA) and non-NMDA binding sites in developing human frontal cortex. Neurosci Res Commun 12:9, 1993.

98. Piggott M, Perry E, Perry R, Court J: [3H]MK801 binding to the NMDA receptor complex, and its modulation in the human frontal cortex during development and aging. Brain Res 588:277, 1992.

99. Represa A, Tremblay E, Ben-Ari Y: Transient increase of NMDA-binding sites in human hippocampus. Neurosci Lett 99:61, 1989.

100. Panigrahy A, White WF, Rava LA, Kinney HC: Developmental changes in [3H]kainate binding in human brainstem sites vulnerable to perinatal hypoxia-ischemia. Neuroscience 67:441, 1995.

101. Larroche JC: Developmental Pathology of the Neonate. New York, Excerpta Medica, 1977.

102. Takashima S, Armstrong DL, Becker LE: Subcortical leukomalacia: Relationship to development of the cerebral sulcus and its vascular supply. Arch Neurol 35:470, 1978.

103. Chugani H, Hovda D, Villablanca J: Metabolic maturation of the brain: A study of local cerebral glucose utilization in the developing cat. J Cereb Blood Flow Metab 11:35, 1991.

104. Azzarelli B, Meade P, Muller J: Hypoxic lesions in areas of primary myelination: A distinct pattern in cerebral palsy. Childs Brain 7:132, 1980.

105. Azzarelli B, Caldemeyer KS, Phillips JP, DeMyer WE: Hypoxic-ischemic encephalopathy in areas of primary myelination: A neuroimaging and PET study. Pediatr Neurol 14:108, 1996.

106. Martin E, Barkovich AJ: Magnetic resonance imaging in perinatal asphyxia. Arch Dis Child Fetal Neonatal Ed 72:F62, 1995.

107. Hasegawa M, Houdou S, Mito T, et al: Development of myelination in the human fetal and infant cerebrum: A myelin basic protein immunohistochemical study. Brain Dev 14:1, 1992.

108. Kinney HC, Brody BA, Kloman AS, Gilles FH: Sequence of central nervous system myelination in human infancy. II. Patterns of myelination in autopsied infants. J Neuropathol Exp Neurol 47:217, 1988.

109. Kuenzle C, Baenziger O, Martin E, et al: Prognostic value of early MR imaging in term infants with severe perinatal asphyxia. Neuropediatrics 25:191, 1994.

110. Mercuri E, Rutherford M, Cowan F, et al: Early prognostic indicators of outcome in infants with neonatal cerebral infarction: A clinical, electroencephalogram, and magnetic resonance imaging study. Pediatrics 103:39, 1999.

111. Rollins NK, Morriss MC, Evans D, Perlman JM: The role of early MR in the evaluation of the term infant with seizures. ANJR Am J Neuroradiol 15:239, 1994.

112. Rutherford MA, Pennock JM, Dubowitz LM: Cranial ultrasound and magnetic resonance imaging in hypoxic-ischaemic encephalopathy: A comparison with outcome. Dev Med Child Neurol 36:813, 1994.

113. Voorhies TM, Lipper EG, Lee BC, et al: Occlusive vascular disease in asphyxiated newborn infants. J Pediatr 105:92, 1984.

114. de Vries LS, Groenendaal F, Eken P, et al: Infarcts in the vascular distribution of the middle cerebral artery in preterm and fullterm infants. Neuropediatrics 28:88, 1997.

115. Govaert P, Matthys E, Zecic A, et al: Perinatal cortical infarction within middle cerebral artery trunks. Arch Dis Child Fetal Neonatal Ed 82:F59, 2000.

116. Clancy R, Malin S, Laraque D, et al: Focal motor seizures heralding stroke in full-term neonates. Am J Dis Child 139:601, 1985.

117. Shevell MI, Silver K, O'Gorman AM, et al: Neonatal dural sinus thrombosis. Pediatr Neurol 5:161, 1989.

118. Coker SB, Beltran RS, Myers TF, Hmura L: Neonatal stroke: Description of patients and investigation into pathogenesis. Pediatr Neurol 4:219, 1988.

119. Barron T, Gusnard D, Zimmerman R, Clancy R: Cerebral venous thrombosis in neonates and children. Pediatr Neurol 8:112, 1992.

120. Rivkin M, Anderson M, Kaye E: Neonatal idiopathic cerebral venous thrombosis: An unrecognized cause of transient seizures or lethargy. Ann Neurol 32:51, 1992.

121. Volpe JJ: Hypoxic-ischemic encephalopathy: Neuropathology and pathogenesis. In: Neurology of the Newborn, 4th ed. Philadelphia, WB Saunders, 2001, pp 296-330.

122. Pasternak JF, Gorey MT: The syndrome of acute near-total intrauterine asphyxia in the term infant. Pediatr Neurol 18:391, 1998.

123. Barkovich AJ, Truwit CL: Brain damage from perinatal asphyxia: Correlation of MR findings with gestational age. ANJR Am J Neuroradiol 11:1087, 1990.

124. Myers RE: Two patterns of perinatal brain damage and their conditions of occurrence. Am J Obstet Gynecol 112:246, 1972.

125. Mallard EC, Williams CE, Gunn AJ, et al: Frequent episodes of brief ischemia sensitize the fetal sheep brain to neuronal loss and induce striatal injury. Pediatr Res 33:61, 1993.

126. Mallard EC, Waldvogel HJ, Williams CE, et al: Repeated asphyxia causes loss of striatal projection neurons in the fetal sheep brain. Neuroscience 65:827, 1995.

127. Mallard EC, Williams CE, Johnston BM, et al: Repeated episodes of umbilical cord occlusion in fetal sheep lead to preferential damage to the striatum and sensitize the heart to further insults. Pediatr Res 37:707, 1995.

128. Sarnat H, Sarnat M: Neonatal encephalopathy following fetal distress. Arch Neurol 33:696, 1976.

129. Sasidharan P: Breathing pattern abnormalities in full term asphyxiated newborn infants. Arch Dis Child 67:440, 1992.

130. Perlman JM, Risser R: Can asphyxiated infants at risk for neonatal seizures be rapidly identified by current high-risk markers? Pediatrics 97:456, 1996.

131. Thornberg E, Thiringer K, Odeback A, Milsom I: Birth asphyxia: Incidence, clinical course and outcome in a Swedish population. Acta Paediatr 84:927, 1995.

132. Lien JM, Towers CV, Quilligan EJ, et al: Term early-onset neonatal seizures: Obstetric characteristics, etiologic classifications, and perinatal care. Obstet Gynecol 85:163, 1995.

133. Sladky JT, Rorke LB: Perinatal hypoxic/ischemic spinal cord injury. Pediatr Pathol 6:87, 1986.

134. Clancy RR, Sladky JT, Rorke LB: Hypoxic-ischemic spinal cord injury following perinatal asphyxia. Ann Neurol 25:185, 1989.

135. Mizrahi E: Neonatal seizures: Problems in diagnosis and classification. Epilepsia 28:S46, 1987.

136. Mizrahi E: Consensus and controversy in the clinical management of neonatal seizures. Clin Perinatol 16:485, 1989.

137. Mizrahi EM: Electroencephalographic-video monitoring in neonates, infants, and children. J Child Neurol 9(Suppl 1): S46, 1994.

138. Mizrahi EM, Plouin P, Kellaway P: Neonatal seizures. In Engel JJ, Pedley TA (eds): Epilepsy: A Comprehensive Textbook. Philadelphia, Lippincott-Raven, 1997, pp 647-663.

139. Holmes G, Rowe J, Hafford J, et al: Prognostic value of the electroencephalogram in neonatal asphyxia. Electroencephalogr Clin Neurophysiol 53:60, 1982.

140. Rowe JC, Holmes GL, Hafford J, et al: Prognostic value of the electroencephalogram in term and preterm infants following neonatal seizures. Electroencephalogr Clin Neurophysiol 60:183, 1985.

141. Holmes GL, Lombroso CT: Prognostic value of background patterns in the neonatal EEG. J Clin Neurophysiol 10:323, 1993.

142. Schouman-Claeys E, Henry-Feugeas MC, Roset F, et al: Periventricular leukomalacia: Correlation between MR imaging and autopsy findings during the first 2 months of life. Radiology 189:59, 1993.

143. Barkovich AJ, Hajnal BL, Vigneron D, et al: Prediction of neuromotor outcome in perinatal asphyxia: Evaluation of MR scoring systems. ANJR Am J Neuroradiol 19:143, 1998.

144. Biagioni E, Mercuri E, Rutherford M, et al: Combined use of electroencephalogram and magnetic resonance imaging in full-term neonates with acute encephalopathy. Pediatrics 107:461, 2001.

145. Roland EH, Poskitt K, Rodriguez E, et al: Perinatal hypoxic-ischemic thalamic injury: Clinical features and neuroimaging. Ann Neurol 44:161, 1998.

146. Leech R, Alvord E: Anoxic-ischemic encephalopathy in the human neonatal period: The significance of brain stem involvement. Arch Neurol 34:109, 1977.

147. Haataja L, Mercuri E, Guzzetta A, et al: Neurologic examination in infants with hypoxic-ischemic encephalopathy at age 9 to 14 months: Use of optimality scores and correlation with magnetic resonance imaging findings. J Pediatr 138:332, 2001.

148. Faro MD, Windle WF: Transneuronal degeneration in brains of monkeys asphyxiated at birth. Exp Neurol 24:38, 1969.

149. Rutherford MA, Pennock JM, Schwieso JE, et al: Hypoxic ischaemic encephalopathy: Early magnetic resonance imaging findings and their evolution. Neuropediatrics 26:183, 1995.

150. Maller AI, Hankins LL, Yeakley JW, Butler IJ: Rolandic type cerebral palsy in children as a pattern of hypoxic-ischemic injury in the full-term neonate. J Child Neurol 13:313, 1998.

151. Thornton JS, Ordidge RJ, Penrice J, et al: Anisotropic water diffusion in white and gray matter of the neonatal piglet brain before and after transient hypoxia-ischaemia. Magn Reson Imaging 15:433, 1997.

152. Thornton JS, Ordidge RJ, Penrice J, et al: Temporal and anatomical variations of brain water apparent diffusion coefficient in perinatal cerebral hypoxic-ischemic injury: Relationships to cerebral energy metabolism. Magn Reson Med 39:920, 1998.

153. Barkovich AJ, Westmark KD, Bedi HS, et al: Proton spectroscopy and diffusion imaging on the first day of life after perinatal asphyxia: Preliminary report. AJNR Am J Neuroradiol 22:1786, 2001.

154. Maneru C, Junque C, Bargallo N, et al: ^{1}H-MR spectroscopy is sensitive to subtle effects of perinatal asphyxia. Neurology 57:1115, 2001.

155. Cady EB: Quantitative combined phosphorus and proton PRESS of the brains of newborn human infants. Magn Reson Med 33:557, 1995.

156. Penrice J, Cady E, Lorek A, et al: Proton magnetic resonance spectroscopy of the brain in normal pretern and term infants, and early changes after perinatal hypoxia-ischemia. Pediatr Res 40:6, 1996.

157. Urenjak J, Williams SR, Gadian DG, Noble M: Specific expression of N-acetylaspartate in neurons, oligodendrocyte-type-2 astrocyte progenitors, and immature oligodendrocytes in vitro. J Neurochem 59:55, 1992.

158. Urenjak J, Williams SR, Gadian DG, Noble M: Proton nuclear magnetic resonance spectroscopy unambiguously identifies different neural cell types. J Neurosci 13:981, 1993.

159. Peden CJ, Rutherford MA, Sargentoni J, et al: Proton spectroscopy of the neonatal brain following hypoxic-ischaemic injury. Dev Med Child Neurol 35:502, 1993.

160. Groenendaal F, Veenhoven RH, van der Grond J, et al: Cerebral lactate and N-acetyl-aspartate/choline ratios in asphyxiated full-term neonates demonstrated in vivo using proton magnetic resonance spectroscopy. Pediatr Res 35:148, 1994.

161. Cady EB: Metabolite concentrations and relaxation in perinatal cerebral hypoxic-ischemic injury. Neurochem Res 21:1043, 1996.

162. Moseley ME, Cohen Y, Mintorovitch J, et al: Early detection of regional cerebral ischemia in cats: Comparison of diffusion- and T2-weighted MRI and spectroscopy. Magn Reson Med 14:330, 1990.

163. Moseley ME, Cohen Y, Kucharczyk J, et al: Diffusion-weighted MR imaging of anisotropic water diffusion in cat central nervous system. Radiology 176:439, 1990.

164. Mintorovitch J, Moseley ME, Chileuitt L, et al: Comparison of diffusion- and T2-weighted MRI for the early detection of cerebral ischemia and reperfusion in rats. Magn Reson Med 18:39, 1991.

165. D'Arceuil HE, de Crespigny AJ, Röther J, et al: Serial magnetic resonance diffusion and hemodynamic imaging in a neonatal rabbit model of hypoxic-ischemic encephalopathy. NMR Biomed 12:505, 1999.

166. Harris NG, Zilkha E, Houseman J, et al: The relationship between the apparent diffusion coefficient measured by magnetic resonance imaging, anoxic depolarization, and glutamate efflux during experimental cerebral ischemia. J Cereb Blood Flow Metab 20:28, 2000.

167. Decanniere C, Eleff S, Davis D, van Zijl PC: Correlation of rapid changes in the average water diffusion constant and the concentrations of lactate and ATP breakdown products during global ischemia in cat brain. Magn Reson Med 34:343, 1995.

168. Cowan FM, Pennock JM, Hanrahan JD, et al: Early detection of cerebral infarction and hypoxic ischemic encephalopathy in neonates using diffusion-weighted magnetic resonance imaging. Neuropediatrics 25:172, 1994.

169. Connelly A, Chong WK, Johnson CL, et al: Diffusion weighted magnetic resonance imaging of compromised tissue in stroke. Arch Dis Child 77:38, 1997.

170. Beauchamp NJ Jr, Barker PB, Wang PY, vanZijl PC: Imaging of acute cerebral ischemia. Radiology 212:307, 1999.

171. Marks MP, de Crespigny A, Lentz D, et al: Acute and chronic stroke: Navigated spin-echo diffusion-weighted MR imaging. Radiology 199:403, 1996.

172. Lutsep HL, Albers GW, de Crespigny A, et al: Clinical utility of diffusion-weighted magnetic resonance imaging in the assessment of ischemic stroke. Ann Neurol 41:574, 1997.

173. Busza AL, Allen KL, King MD, et al: Diffusion-weighted imaging studies of cerebral ischemia in gerbils. Potential relevance to energy failure. Stroke 23:1602, 1992.

174. Canese R, Podo F, Fortuna S, et al: Transient global brain ischemia in the rat: Spatial distribution, extension, and evolution of lesions evaluated by magnetic resonance imaging. Magma 5:139, 1997.

175. D'Arceuil HE, de Crespigny AJ, Röther J, et al: Diffusion and perfusion magnetic resonance imaging of the evolution of hypoxic ischemic encephalopathy in the neonatal rabbit. J Magn Reson Imaging 8:820, 1998.

176. Schlaug G, Siewert B, Benfield A, et al: Time course of the apparent diffusion coefficient (ADC) abnormality in human stroke. Neurology 49:113, 1997.

177. Hesselbarth D, Franke C, Hata R, et al: High resolution MRI and MRS: A feasibility study for the investigation of focal cerebral ischemia in mice. NMR Biomed 11:423, 1998.

178. Hossmann K-A: Viability thresholds and the penumbra of focal ischemia. Ann Neurol 36:557, 1994.

179. Branston NM, Symon L, Crockard HA, Pasztor E: Relationship between the cortical evoked potential and local cortical blood flow following acute middle cerebral artery occlusion in the baboon. Exp Neurol 45:195, 1974.

180. Gadian DG, Frackowiak RS, Crockard HA, et al: Acute cerebral ischaemia: Concurrent changes in cerebral blood flow, energy metabolites, pH, and lactate measured with hydrogen clearance and ^{31}P and ^{1}H nuclear magnetic resonance spectroscopy. I. Methodology. J Cereb Blood Flow Metab 7:199, 1987.

181. Warach S, Chien D, Li W, et al: Fast magnetic resonance diffusion-weighted imaging of acute human stroke. Neurology 42:1717, 1992.

182. Baird A, Warach S: Magnetic resonance imaging of acute stroke. J Cereb Blood Flow Metab 18:583, 1998.

183. Lovblad KO, Laubach HJ, Baird AE, et al: Clinical experience with diffusion-weighted MR in patients with acute stroke. AJNR Am J Neuroradiol 19:1061, 1998.

184. McKinstry RC, Miller JH, Snyder AZ, et al: A prospective, longitudinal diffusion tensor imaging study of brain injury in newborns. Neurology 59:824, 2002.

185. Soul JS, Robertson RL, Tzika AA, et al: Time course of changes in diffusion-weighted magnetic resonance imaging in a case of neonatal encephalopathy with defined onset and duration of hypoxic-ischemic insult. Pediatrics 108:1211, 2001.

186. Krishnamoorthy K, Soman T, Takeoka M, Schaefer P: Diffusion-weighted imaging in neonatal cerebral infarction: Clinical utility and follow-up. J Child Neurol 15:592, 2000.

187. Robertson RL, Ben-Sira L, Barnes PD, et al: MR line-scan diffusion-weighted imaging of term neonates with perinatal brain ischemia. ANJR Am J Neuroradiol 20:1658, 1999.

188. Perlman JM: Markers of asphyxia and neonatal brain injury. N Engl J Med 341:364, 1999.

189. Perlman JM, Tack ED: Renal injury in the asphyxiated newborn infant: Relationship to neurologic outcome. J Pediatr 113:875, 1988.

190. Westgate J, Garibaldi JM, Greene KR: Umbilical cord blood gas analysis at delivery: A time for quality data. Br J Obstet Gynaecol 101:1054, 1994.

191. Tejani NA, Verma UL, Chatterjee S, Mittelmann S: Terbutaline in the management of acute intrapartum fetal acidosis. J Reprod Med 28:857, 1983.

192. Burke MS, Porreco RP, Day D, et al: Intrauterine resuscitation with tocolysis. An alternate month clinical trial. J Perinatol 9:296, 1989.

193. Low JA, Panagiotopoulos C, Derrick EJ: Newborn complications after intrapartum asphyxia with metabolic acidosis in the term fetus. Am J Obstet Gynecol 170:1081, 1994.

194. Rosen KG, Murphy KW: How to assess fetal metabolic acidosis from cord samples. J Perinat Med 19:221, 1991.

195. Johnson JW, Richards DS, Wagaman RA: The case for routine umbilical blood acid-base studies at delivery. Am J Obstet Gynecol 162:621, 1990.

196. Huang CC, Wang ST, Chang YC, et al: Measurement of the urinary lactate:creatinine ratio for the early identification of newborn infants at risk for hypoxic-ischemic encephalopathy. N Engl J Med 341:328, 1999.

197. Becker M, Menzel K: Brain-typical creatine kinase in the serum of newborn infants with perinatal brain damage. Acta Paediatr Scand 67:177, 1978.

198. Bell RD, Khan M: Cerebrospinal fluid creatine kinase-BB activity: A perspective. Arch Neurol 56:1327, 1999.

199. Cuestas RA Jr: Creatine kinase isoenzymes in high-risk infants. Pediatr Res 14:935, 1980.

200. Walsh P, Jedeikin R, Ellis G, et al: Assessment of neurologic outcome in asphyxiated term infants by use of serial CK-BB isoenzyme measurement. J Pediatr 101:988, 1982.

201. Fernandez F, Verdu A, Quero J, Perez-Higueras A: Serum CPK-BB isoenzyme in the assessment of brain damage in asphyctic term infants. Acta Paediatr Scand 76:914, 1987.

202. Amato M, Gambon R, von Muralt G: Prognostic value of serum creatine kinase brain isoenzyme in term babies with perinatal hypoxic injuries. Helv Paediatr Acta 40:435, 1985.

203. Ruth VJ: Prognostic value of creatine kinase BB-isoenzyme in high risk newborn infants. Arch Dis Child 64:563, 1989.

204. De Praeter C, Vanhaesebrouck P, Govaert P, et al: Creatine kinase isoenzyme BB concentrations in the cerebrospinal fluid of newborns: Relationship to short-term outcome. Pediatrics 88:1204, 1991.

205. Nagdyman N, Komen W, Ko HK, et al: Early biochemical indicators of hypoxic-ischemic encephalopathy after birth asphyxia. Pediatr Res 49:502, 2001.

206. Talvik T, Haldre S, Soot A, et al: Creatine kinase isoenzyme BB concentrations in cerebrospinal fluid in asphyxiated preterm neonates. Acta Paediatr 84:1183, 1995.

207. Thornberg E, Thiringer K, Hagberg H, Kjellmer I: Neuron specific enolase in asphyxiated newborns: Association with encephalopathy and cerebral function monitor trace. Arch Dis Child Fetal Neonatal Ed 72:F39, 1995.

208. Garcia-Alix A, Cabanas F, Pellicer A, et al: Neuron-specific enolase and myelin basic protein: Relationship of cerebrospinal fluid concentrations to the neurologic condition of asphyxiated full-term infants. Pediatrics 93:234, 1994.

209. Elimian A, Figueroa R, Verma U, et al: Amniotic fluid neuron-specific enolase: A role in predicting neonatal neurologic injury? Obstet Gynecol 92:546, 1998.

210. Blennow M, Hagberg H, Rosengren L: Glial fibrillary acidic protein in the cerebrospinal fluid: A possible indicator of prognosis in full-term asphyxiated newborn infants? Pediatr Res 37:260, 1995.

211. Vilanova JM, Figueras-Aloy J, Rosello J, et al: Arachidonic acid metabolites in CSF in hypoxic-ischaemic encephalopathy of newborn infants. Acta Paediatr 87:588, 1998.

212. Oygur N, Sonmez O, Saka O, Yegin O: Predictive value of plasma and cerebrospinal fluid tumour necrosis factor–alpha and interleukin-1 beta concentrations on outcome of full term infants with hypoxic-ischaemic encephalopathy. Arch Dis Child Fetal Neonatal Ed 79:F190, 1998.

213. da Silva S, Hennebert N, Denis R, Wayenberg JL: Clinical value of a single postnatal lactate measurement after intrapartum asphyxia. Acta Paediatr 89:320, 2000.

214. Russell GA, Jeffers G, Cooke RW: Plasma hypoxanthine: A marker for hypoxic-ischaemic induced periventricular leucomalacia? Arch Dis Child 67:388, 1992.

215. Dorrepaal CA, Berger HM, Benders MJ, et al: Nonprotein-bound iron in postasphyxial reperfusion injury of the newborn. Pediatrics 98:883, 1996.

216. Bader D, Gozal D, Weinger-Abend M, et al: Neonatal urinary uric acid/creatinine ratio as an additional marker of perinatal asphyxia. Eur J Pediatr 154:747, 1995.

217. Perlman J, Risser R: Relationship of uric acid concentrations and severe intraventricular hemorrhage/leukomalacia in the premature infant. J Pediatr 132:436, 1998.

218. Klepper J, Wang D, Fischbarg J, et al: Defective glucose transport across brain tissue barriers: A newly recognized neurological syndrome. Neurochem Res 24:587, 1999.

219. Greene CL, Goodman SI: Catastrophic metabolic encephalopathies in the newborn period. Evaluation and management. Clin Perinatol 24:773, 1997.

220. Hoon AH Jr, Reinhardt EM, Kelley RI, et al: Brain magnetic resonance imaging in suspected extrapyramidal cerebral palsy: Observations in distinguishing genetic-metabolic from acquired causes. J Pediatr 131:240, 1997.

221. Yoon BH, Romero R, Yang SH, et al: Interleukin-6 concentrations in umbilical cord plasma are elevated in neonates with white matter lesions associated with periventricular leukomalacia. Am J Obstet Gynecol 174:1433, 1996.

222. Yoon BH, Jun JK, Romero R, et al: Amniotic fluid inflammatory cytokines (interleukin-6, interleukin-1beta, and tumor necrosis factor–alpha), neonatal brain white matter lesions, and cerebral palsy. Am J Obstet Gynecol 177:19, 1997.

223. Baud O, Emilie D, Pelletier E, et al: Amniotic fluid concentrations of interleukin-1beta, interleukin-6 and TNF-alpha in chorioamnionitis before 32 weeks of gestation: Histological associations and neonatal outcome. Br J Obstet Gynaecol 106:72, 1999.

224. Dammann O, Leviton A: Maternal intrauterine infection, cytokines, and brain damage in the preterm newborn. Pediatr Neurol 42:1, 1997.

225. Martinez E, Figueroa R, Garry D, et al: Elevated amniotic fluid interleukin-6 as a predictor of neonatal periventricular leukomalacia. J Matern Fetal Invest 8:101, 1998.

226. Grether JK, Nelson KB, Dambrosia JM, Phillips TM: Interferons and cerebral palsy. J Pediatr 134:324, 1999.

227. Cai Z, Pan ZL, Pang Y, et al: Cytokine induction in fetal rat brains and brain injury in neonatal rats after maternal lipopolysaccharide administration. Pediatr Res 47:64, 2000.

228. Yoon B, Romero R, Park J, et al: Fetal exposure to an intra-amniotic inflammation and the development of cerebral palsy at the age of three years. Am J Obstet Gynecol 182:675, 2000.

229. Kadhim H, Tabarki B, Verellen G, et al: Inflammatory cytokines in the pathogenesis of periventricular leukomalacia. Neurology 56:1278, 2001.

230. Shibata M, Leffler C, Busija D: Recombinant human interleukin 1a dilates pial arterioles and increases cerebrospinal fluid prostanoids in piglets. Am J Physiol 259:H1486, 1990.

231. Brian J, Faraci F: Tumor necrosis factor-α–induced dilatation of cerebral arterioles. Stroke 29:509, 1998.

232. Dommergues MA, Patkai J, Renauld JC, et al: Proinflammatory cytokines and interleukin-9 exacerbate excitotoxic lesions of the newborn murine neopallium. Ann Neurol 47:54, 2000.

233. Ekert P, Perlman M, Steinlin M, Hao Y: Predicting the outcome of postasphyxial hypoxic-ischemic encephalopathy within 4 hours of birth. J Pediatr 131:613, 1997.

234. King TA, Jackson GL, Josey AS, et al: The effect of profound umbilical artery acidemia in term neonates admitted to a newborn nursery. J Pediatr 132:624, 1998.

235. Goodwin TM, Belai I, Hernandez P, et al: Asphyxial complications in the term newborn with severe umbilical acidemia. Am J Obstet Gynecol 167:1506, 1992.

236. Sykes GS, Molloy PM, Johnson P, et al: Fetal distress and the condition of newborn infants. Br Med J (Clin Res Ed) 287:943, 1983.

237. Belai Y, Goodwin TM, Durand M, et al: Umbilical arteriovenous Po_2 and Pco_2 differences and neonatal morbidity in term infants with severe acidosis. Am J Obstet Gynecol 178:13, 1998.

238. Westgren M, Divon M, Horal M, et al: Routine measurements of umbilical artery lactate levels in the prediction of perinatal outcome. Am J Obstet Gynecol 173:1416, 1995.

239. Apgar V: The newborn (Apgar) scoring system. Reflections and advice. Pediatr Clin North Am 13:645, 1966.

240. Casey BM, McIntire DD, Leveno KJ: The continuing value of the Apgar score for the assessment of newborn infants. N Engl J Med 344:467, 2001.

241. Peliowski A, Finer N: Birth asphyxia in the term infant. In Sinclair J, Bracken M, Silverman W (eds): Effective Care of the Newborn Infant. Oxford, UK, Oxford University Press, 1992, pp 249-279.

242. Shankaran S, Woldt E, Koepke T, et al: Acute neonatal morbidity and long-term central nervous system sequelae of perinatal asphyxia in term infants. Early Hum Dev 25:135, 1991.

243. Ellenberg JH, Nelson KB: Cluster of perinatal events identifying infants at high risk for death or disability. J Pediatr 113:546, 1988.

244. Finer NN, Robertson CM, Peters KL, Coward JH: Factors affecting outcome in hypoxic-ischemic encephalopathy in term infants. Am J Dis Child 137:21, 1983.

245. Pelowski A, Finer N: Birth asphyxia in the term infant. In Sinclair J, Lucey J (eds): Effective Care of the Newborn Infant. Oxford, UK, Oxford University Press, 1992, pp 263-266.

246. Robertson C, Finer N: Term infants with hypoxic-ischemic encephalopathy: Outcome at 3.5 years. Dev Med Child Neurol 27:473, 1985.

247. Low JA, Galbraith RS, Muir DW, et al: The relationship between perinatal hypoxia and newborn encephalopathy. Am J Obstet Gynecol 152:256, 1985.

248. Scott H: Outcome of very severe birth asphyxia. Arch Dis Child 51:712, 1976.

249. al Naqeeb N, Edwards AD, Cowan FM, Azzopardi D: Assessment of neonatal encephalopathy by amplitude-integrated electroencephalography. Pediatrics 103:1263, 1999.

250. Hellstrom-Westas L, Rosen I, Svenningsen NW: Predictive value of early continuous amplitude integrated EEG recordings on outcome after severe birth asphyxia in full term infants. Arch Dis Child Fetal Neonatal Ed 72:F34, 1995.

251. Toet MC, Hellstrom-Westas L, Groenendaal F, et al: Amplitude integrated EEG 3 and 6 hours after birth in full term neonates with hypoxic-ischaemic encephalopathy. Arch Dis Child Fetal Neonatal Ed 81:F19, 1999.

252. Hahn JS, Tharp BR: The dysmature EEG pattern in infants with bronchopulmonary dysplasia and its prognostic implications. Electroencephalogr Clin Neurophysiol 76:106, 1990.

253. Tharp BR: Electrophysiological brain maturation in premature infants: An historical perspective. J Clin Neurophysiol 7:302, 1990.

254. Lombroso CT: Neonatal polygraphy in full-term and premature infants: A review of normal and abnormal findings. J Clin Neurophysiol 2:105, 1985.

255. van Lieshout HB, Jacobs JW, Rotteveel JJ, et al: The prognostic value of the EEG in asphyxiated newborns. Acta Neurol Scand 91:203, 1995.

256. Pezzani C, Radvanyi-Bouvet MF, Relier JP, Monod N: Neonatal electroencephalography during the first twenty-four hours of life in full-term newborn infants. Neuropediatrics 17:11, 1986.

257. Aso K, Scher MS, Barmada MA: Neonatal electroencephalography and neuropathology. J Clin Neurophysiol 6:103, 1989.

258. Grigg-Damberger MM, Coker SB, Halsey CL, Anderson CL: Neonatal burst suppression: Its developmental significance. Pediatr Neurol 5:84, 1989.

259. Wertheim D, Mercuri E, Faundez JC, et al: Prognostic value of continuous electroencephalographic recording in full term infants with hypoxic ischaemic encephalopathy. Arch Dis Child 71:F97, 1994.

260. Eken P, Toet MC, Groenendaal F, Devries LS: Predictive value of early neuroimaging, pulsed Doppler and neurophysiology in full term infants with hypoxic-ischaemic encephalopathy. Arch Dis Child 73:F75, 1995.

261. Tharp BR, Cukier F, Monod N: The prognostic value of the electroencephalogram in premature infants. Electroencephalogr Clin Neurophysiol 51:219, 1981.

262. Rutherford MA, Pennock JM, Counsell SJ, et al: Abnormal magnetic resonance signal in the internal capsule predicts poor neurodevelopmental outcome in infants with hypoxic-ischemic encephalopathy. Pediatrics 102:323, 1998.

263. Rutherford M, Pennock J, Schwieso J, et al: Hypoxic-ischaemic encephalopathy: Early and late magnetic resonance imaging findings in relation to outcome. Arch Dis Child Fetal Neonatal Ed 75:F145, 1996.

264. Mercuri E, Guzzetta A, Haataja L, et al: Neonatal neurological examination in infants with hypoxic ischaemic encephalopathy: Correlation with MRI findings. Neuropediatrics 30:83, 1999.

265. Levene MI, Fenton AC, Evans DH, et al: Severe birth asphyxia and abnormal cerebral blood-flow velocity. Dev Med Child Neurol 31:427, 1989.

266. Gray PH, Tudehope DI, Masel JP, et al: Perinatal hypoxic-ischaemic brain injury: Prediction of outcome. Dev Med Child Neurol 35:965, 1993.

267. Lipp-Zwahlen AE, Deonna T, Micheli JL, et al: Prognostic value of neonatal CT scans in asphyxiated term babies: Low density score compared with neonatal neurological signs. Neuropediatrics 16:209, 1985.

268. Flodmark O, Becker LE, Harwood-Nash DC, et al: Correlation between computed tomography and autopsy in premature and full-term neonates that have suffered perinatal asphyxia. Radiology 137:93, 1980.

269. Siegel MJ, Shackelford GD, Perlman JM, Fulling KH: Hypoxic-ischemic encephalopathy in term infants: Diagnosis and prognosis evaluated by ultrasound. Radiology 152:395, 1984.

270. Babcock DS, Ball W Jr: Postasphyxial encephalopathy in full-term infants: Ultrasound diagnosis. Radiology 148:417, 1983.

271. Menkes JH, Curran J: Clinical and MR correlates in children with extrapyramidal cerebral palsy. ANJR Am J Neuroradiol 15:451, 1994.

272. Mercuri E, Ricci D, Cowan FM, et al: Head growth in infants with hypoxic-ischemic encephalopathy: Correlation with neonatal magnetic resonance imaging. Pediatrics 106:235, 2000.

273. Barkovich AJ, Baranski K, Vigneron D, et al: Proton MR spectroscopy for the evaluation of brain injury in asphyxiated, term neonates. ANJR Am J Neuroradiol 20:1399, 1999.

274. Azzopardi D, Wyatt J, Cady E, et al: Prognosis of newborn infants with hypoxic-ischemic brain injury assessed by phosphorus magnetic resonance spectroscopy. Pediatr Res 25:445, 1989.

275. Hanrahan JD, Cox IJ, Edwards AD, et al: Persistent increases in cerebral lactate concentration after birth asphyxia. Pediatr Res 44:304, 1998.

276. Hanrahan JD, Sargentoni J, Azzopardi D, et al: Cerebral metabolism within 18 hours of birth asphyxia: A proton magnetic resonance spectroscopy study. Pediatr Res 39:584, 1996.

277. Leth H, Toft P, Peitersen B, Lou H, Henriksen O: Use of brain lactate levels to predict outcome after perinatal asphyxia. Acta Paediatr 85:859, 1996.

278. Ashwal S, Holshouser BA, Tomasi LG, et al: ^{1}H-magnetic resonance spectroscopy–determined cerebral lactate and poor neurological outcomes in children with central nervous system disease. Ann Neurol 41:470, 1997.

279. Zarifi MK, Astrakas LG, Poussaint TY, et al: Prediction of adverse outcome with cerebral lactate level and apparent diffusion coefficient in infants with perinatal asphyxia. Radiology 225:859, 2002.

280. Robertson NJ, Cox IJ, Cowan FM, et al: Cerebral intracellular lactic alkalosis persisting months after neonatal encephalopathy measured by magnetic resonance spectroscopy. Pediatr Res 46:287, 1999.

281. Hanrahan JD, Cox IJ, Azzopardi D, et al: Relation between proton magnetic resonance spectroscopy within 18 hours of birth asphyxia and neurodevelopment at 1 year of age. Dev Med Child Neurol 41:76, 1999.

282. Amess PN, Penrice J, Wylezinska M, et al: Early brain proton magnetic resonance spectroscopy and neonatal neurology related to neurodevelopmental outcome at 1 year in term infants after presumed hypoxic-ischaemic brain injury. Dev Med Child Neurol 41:436, 1999.

283. Warach S, Gaa J, Siewert B, et al: Acute human stroke studied by whole brain echo planar diffusion-weighted magnetic resonance imaging. Ann Neurol 37:231, 1995.

284. Hossmann K, Hoehnberlage M: Diffusion and perfusion MR imaging of cerebral ischemia. Cerebrovasc Brain Metab Rev 7:187, 1995.

285. Johnson AJ, Lee BC, Lin W: Echoplanar diffusion-weighted imaging in neonates and infants with suspected hypoxic-ischemic injury: Correlation with patient outcome. AJR Am J Roentgenol 172:219, 1999.

286. Tong DC, Yenari MA, Albers GW, et al: Correlation of perfusion- and diffusion-weighted MRI with NIHSS score in acute (<6.5 hour) ischemic stroke. Neurology 50:864, 1998.

287. Nelson KB, Dambrosia JM, Ting TY, Grether JK: Uncertain value of electronic fetal monitoring in predicting cerebral palsy. N Engl J Med 334:613, 1996.

288. Ahn MO, Korst LM, Phelan JP: Normal fetal heart rate pattern in the brain-damaged infant: A failure of intrapartum fetal monitoring? J Matern Fetal Invest 8:58, 1998.

289. Goodwin TM, Milner-Masterson L, Paul RH: Elimination of fetal scalp blood sampling on a large clinical service. Obstet Gynecol 83:971, 1994.

290. Small ML, Beall M, Platt LD, et al: Continuous tissue pH monitoring in the term fetus. Am J Obstet Gynecol 161:323, 1989.

291. Lavery JP: Nonstress fetal heart rate testing. Clin Obstet Gynecol 25:689, 1982.

292. Tejani N, Mann LI, Bhakthavathsalan A, Weiss RR: Correlation of fetal heart rate–uterine contraction patterns with fetal scalp blood pH. Obstet Gynecol 46:392, 1975.

293. Tejani N, Mann LI, Bhakthavathsalan A, Weiss RR: Prolonged fetal bradycardia with recovery—its significance and outcome. Am J Obstet Gynecol 122:975, 1975.

294. Perlman JM, Tack ED, Martin T, et al: Acute systemic organ injury in term infants after asphyxia. Am J Dis Child 143:617, 1989.

295. Martin-Ancel A, Garcia-Alix A, Gaya F, et al: Multiple organ involvement in perinatal asphyxia. J Pediatr 127:786, 1995.

296. Barnett CP, Perlman M, Ekert PG: Clinicopathological correlations in postasphyxial organ damage: A donor organ perspective. Pediatrics 99:797, 1997.

297. Vento M, Asensi M, Sastre J, et al: Resuscitation with room air instead of 100% oxygen prevents oxidative stress in moderately asphyxiated term neonates. Pediatrics 107:642, 2001.

298. Lundstrom K, Pryds O, Greisen G: Oxygen at birth and prolonged cerebral vasoconstriction in preterm infants. Arch Dis Child 73:F81, 1995.

299. Perlman JM, Hill A, Volpe JJ: The effect of patent ductus arteriosus on flow velocity in the anterior cerebral arteries: Ductal steal in the premature newborn infant. J Pediatr 99:767, 1981.

300. Perlman JM, Volpe JJ: Episodes of apnea and bradycardia in the preterm newborn: Impact on cerebral circulation. Pediatrics 76:333, 1985.

301. Livera LN, Spencer SA, Thorniley MS, et al: Effects of hypoxemia and bradycardia on neonatal cerebral hemodynamics. Arch Dis Child 66:376, 1991.

302. Urlesberger B, Kaspirek A, Pichler G, Muller W: Apnoea of prematurity and changes in cerebral oxygenation and cerebral blood volume. Neuropediatrics 30:29, 1999.

303. Lipman B, Serwer GA, Brazy JE: Abnormal cerebral hemodynamics in preterm infants with patent ductus arteriosus. Pediatrics 69:778, 1982.

304. Shortland DB, Gibson NA, Levene MI, et al: Patent ductus arteriosus and cerebral circulation in preterm infants. Dev Med Child Neurol 32:386, 1990.

305. Kurtis PS, Rosenkrantz TS, Zalneraitis EL: Cerebral blood flow and EEG changes in preterm infants with patent ductus arteriosus. Pediatr Neurol 12:114, 1995.

306. Lupton BA, Hill A, Roland EH, et al: Brain swelling in the asphyxiated term newborn: Pathogenesis and outcome. Pediatrics 82:139, 1988.

307. Pryds O: Control of cerebral circulation in the high-risk neonate. Ann Neurol 30:321, 1991.

308. Pryds O, Greisen G, Lou H, Friis-Hansen B: Vasoparalysis associated with brain damage in asphyxiated term infants. J Pediatr 117:119, 1990.

309. Pryds O: Regulation of cerebral perfusion and brain damage. In Lou H, Greisen G, Larsen J (eds): Brain Lesions in the Newborn. Copenhagen, Munksgaard, 1994, pp 234-240.

310. Rosenkrantz TS, Oh W: Cerebral blood flow velocity in infants with polycythemia and hyperviscosity: Effects of partial exchange transfusion with Plasmanate. J Pediatr 101:94, 1982.

311. Younkin DP, Reivich M, Jaggi JL, et al: The effect of hematocrit and systolic blood pressure on cerebral blood flow in newborn infants. J Cereb Blood Flow Metab 7:295, 1987.

312. Pryds O, Greisen G: Effect of $Paco_2$ and haemoglobin concentration on day to day variation of CBF in preterm neonates. Acta Paediatr Scand Suppl 360:33, 1989.

313. Grave GD, Kennedy C, Jehle J, Sokoloff L: The effects of hyperoxia on cerebral blood flow in newborn dogs. Neurology 20:397, 1970.

314. Kennedy C, Grave GD, Sokoloff L: Alterations of local cerebral blood flow due to exposure of newborn puppies to 80-90 per cent oxygen. Eur Neurol 6:137, 1971.

315. Vento M, Asensi M, Sastre J, et al: Six years of experience with the use of room air for the resuscitation of asphyxiated newly born term infants. Biol Neonate 79:261, 2001.

316. Vannucci RC, Towfighi J, Heitjan DF, Brucklacher RM: Carbon dioxide protects the perinatal brain from hypoxic-ischemic damage: An experimental study in the immature rat. Pediatrics 95:868, 1995.

317. Vannucci RC, Brucklacher RM, Vannucci SJ: Effect of carbon dioxide on cerebral metabolism during hypoxia-ischemia in the immature rat. Pediatr Res 42:24, 1997.

318. Paulson OB, Strandgaard S, Edvinsson L: Cerebral autoregulation. Cerebrovasc Brain Metab Rev 2:161, 1990.

319. Parfenova H, Shibata M, Zuckerman S, Leffler CW: CO_2 and cerebral circulation in newborn pigs: Cyclic nucleotides and prostanoids in vascular regulation. Am J Physiol 266:H1494, 1994.

320. Todd MM, Tommasino C, Shapiro HM: Cerebrovascular effects of prolonged hypocarbia and hypercarbia after experimental global ischemia in cats. Crit Care Med 13:720, 1985.

321. Bifano EM, Pfannenstiel A: Duration of hyperventilation and outcome in infants with persistent pulmonary hypertension. Pediatrics 81:657, 1988.

322. Graziani LJ, Spitzer AR, Mitchell DG, et al: Mechanical ventilation in preterm infants: Neurosonographic and developmental studies. Pediatrics 90:515, 1992.

323. Wiswell T, Graziani L, Kornhauser M, et al: Effects of hypocarbia on the development of cystic periventricular leukomalacia in premature infants treated with high-frequency jet ventilation. Pediatrics 98:918, 1996.

324. Cataltepe O, Vannucci R, Heitjan D, Towfighi J: Effect of status epilepticus on hypoxic-ischemic brain damage in the immature rat. Pediatr Res 38:251, 1995.

325. Ahn MO, Korst LM, Phelan JP, Martin GI: Does the onset of neonatal seizures correlate with the timing of fetal neurologic injury? Clin Pediatr (Phila) 37:673, 1998.

326. Williams C, Gunn A, Synek B, Gluckman P: Delayed seizures occurring with hypoxic-ischemic encephalopathy in the fetal sheep. Pediatr Res 27:561, 1990.

327. Williams CE, Gunn AJ, Mallard C, Gluckman PD: Outcome after ischemia in the developing sheep brain: An electroencephalographic and histological study. Ann Neurol 31:14, 1992.

328. Volpe JJ: Neonatal seizures. In: Neurology of the Newborn. Philadelphia, WB Saunders, 2001, pp 178-214.

329. Scher MS, Painter MJ, Bergman I, et al: EEG diagnoses of neonatal seizures: Clinical correlations and outcome. Pediatr Neurol 5:17, 1989.

330. Clancy R, Legido A, Lewis D: Occult neonatal seizures. Epilepsia 29:256, 1988.

331. Scher MS, Aso K, Beggarly ME, et al: Electrographic seizures in preterm and full-term neonates: Clinical correlates, associated brain lesions, and risk for neurologic sequelae. Pediatrics 91:128, 1993.

332. Clancy RR: The contribution of EEG to the understanding of neonatal seizures. Epilepsia 37:S52, 1996.

333. Laroia N, Guillet R, Burchfiel J, McBride MC: EEG background as predictor of electrographic seizures in high-risk neonates. Epilepsia 39:545, 1998.

334. Eyre JA, Wilkinson AR: Thiopentone induced coma after severe birth asphyxia. Arch Dis Child 61:1084, 1986.

335. Goldberg RN, Moscoso P, Bauer CR, et al: Use of barbiturate therapy in severe perinatal asphyxia: A randomized controlled trial. J Pediatr 109:851, 1986.

336. Hall RT, Hall FK, Daily DK: High-dose phenobarbital therapy in term newborn infants with severe perinatal asphyxia: A randomized, prospective study with three-year follow-up. J Pediatr 132:345, 1998.

337. Painter MJ, Scher MS, Stein AD, et al: Phenobarbital compared with phenytoin for the treatment of neonatal seizures. N Engl J Med 341:485, 1999.

338. Coen RW, McCutchen CB, Wermer D, et al: Continuous monitoring of the electroencephalogram following perinatal asphyxia. J Pediatr 100:628, 1982.

339. Connell J, de Vries L, Oozeer R, et al: Predictive value of early continuous electroencephalogram monitoring in ventilated preterm infants with intraventricular hemorrhage. Pediatrics 82:337, 1988.

340. Bye AM, Flanagan D: Spatial and temporal characteristics of neonatal seizures. Epilepsia 36:1009, 1995.

341. McBride MC, Laroia N, Guillet R: Electrographic seizures in neonates correlate with poor neurodevelopmental outcome. Neurology 55:506, 2000.

342. Hascoet JM, Monin P, Vert P: Persistence of impaired autoregulation of cerebral blood flow in the postictal period in piglets. Epilepsia 29:743, 1988.

343. Monin P, Stonestreet BS, Oh W: Hyperventilation restores autoregulation of cerebral blood flow in postictal piglets. Pediatr Res 30:294, 1991.

344. Earnest M, Marx J, Drury L: Complications of intravenous phenytoin for acute treatment of seizures. JAMA 249:762, 1983.

345. Kriel RL, Cifuentes RF: Fosphenytoin in infants of extremely low birth weight. Pediatr Neurol 24:219, 2001.

346. Takeoka M, Krishnamoorthy KS, Soman TB, Caviness VS Jr: Fosphenytoin in infants. J Child Neurol 13:537, 1998.

347. Gunn AJ: Cerebral hypothermia for prevention of brain injury following perinatal asphyxia. Curr Opin Pediatr 12:111, 2000.

348. Guan J, Bennet TL, George S, et al: Selective neuroprotective effects with insulin-like growth factor–1 in phenotypic striatal neurons following ischemic brain injury in fetal sheep. Neuroscience 95:831, 2000.

349. Reith J, Jorgensen HS, Pedersen PM, et al: Body temperature in acute stroke: Relation to stroke severity, infarct size, mortality, and outcome. Lancet 347:422, 1996.

350. Shum-Tim D, Nagashima M, Shinoka T, et al: Postischemic hyperthermia exacerbates neurologic injury after deep hypothermic circulatory arrest. J Thorac Cardiovasc Surg 116:780, 1998.

351. Thoresen M: Cooling the newborn after asphyxia—physiological and experimental background and its clinical use. Semin Neonatol 5:61, 2000.

352. Penrice J, Thoresen M, Lorek A, et al: Mild hypothermia following severe hypoxia-ischemia ameliorates delayed cerebral energy failure in the newborn piglet. Early Hum Dev 39:146A, 1994.

353. Laptook A, Corbett R, Sterrett R, et al: Modest hypothermia provides partial neuroprotection for ischemic neonatal brain. Pediatr Res 35:436, 1994.

354. Battin MR, Dezoete JA, Gunn TR, et al: Neurodevelopmental outcome of infants treated with head cooling and mild hypothermia after perinatal asphyxia. Pediatrics 107:480, 2001.

355. Gunn AJ, Gluckman PD, Gunn TR: Selective head cooling in newborn infants after perinatal asphyxia: A safety study. Pediatrics 102:885, 1998.

356. Edwards AD, Azzopardi D: Hypothermic neural rescue treatment: From laboratory to cotside? Arch Dis Child Fetal Neonatal Ed 78:F88, 1998.

357. Azzopardi D, Robertson NJ, Cowan FM, et al: Pilot study of treatment with whole body hypothermia for neonatal encephalopathy. Pediatrics 106:684, 2000.

358. Feldman W, Drummond KN, Klein M: Hyponatremia following asphyxia neonatorum. Acta Paediatr Scand 59:52, 1970.

359. Khare SK: Neurohypophyseal dysfunction following perinatal asphyxia. J Pediatr 90:628, 1977.

360. Kaplan SL, Feigin RD: Inappropriate secretion of antidiuretic hormone complicating neonatal hypoxic-ischemic encephalopathy. J Pediatr 92:431, 1978.

361. Lynch B, Rust R: Natural history and outcome of neonatal hypocalcemic and hypomagnesemic seizures. Pediatr Neurol 11:23, 1994.

362. Li PA, Shuaib A, Miyashita H, et al: Hyperglycemia enhances extracellular glutamate accumulation in rats subjected to forebrain ischemia. Stroke 31:183, 2000.

363. De Courten-Myers G, Myers R, Schoolfield L: Hyperglycemia enlarges infarct size in cerebrovascular occlusion in cats. Stroke 19:623, 1988.

364. Anderson RV, Siegman MG, Balaban RS, et al: Hyperglycemia increases cerebral intracellular acidosis during circulatory arrest. Ann Thorac Surg 54:1126, 1992.

365. Pulsinelli W, Levy D, Sigsbee B, et al: Increased damage after ischemic stroke in patients with hyperglycemia with and without diabetes mellitus. Am J Med 74:540, 1983.

366. Candelise L, Landi G, Orazio EN, Boccardi E: Prognostic significance of hyperglycemia in acute stroke. Arch Neurol 42:661, 1985.

367. Vannucci RC, Brucklacher RM, Vannucci SJ: The effect of hyperglycemia on cerebral metabolism during hypoxia-ischemia in the immature rat. J Cereb Blood Flow Metab 16:1026, 1996.

368. Goldberg RN, Cabal LA, Sinatra FR, et al: Hyperammonemia associated with perinatal asphyxia. Pediatrics 64:336, 1979.

369. Marcaida G, Felipo V, Hermenegildo C, et al: Acute ammonia toxicity is mediated by the NMDA type of glutamate receptors. FEBS Lett 296:67, 1992.

370. Graziani LJ, Gringlas M, Baumgart S: Cerebrovascular complications and neurodevelopmental sequelae of neonatal ECMO. Clin Perinatol 24:655, 1997.

371. Karibe H, Zarow G, Graham S, Weinstein P: Mild intraischemic hypothermia reduces postischemic hyperperfusion, delayed postischemic hypoperfusion, blood-brain barrier disruption, brain edema, and neuronal damage volume after temporary focal ischemia in rats. J Cereb Blood Flow Metab 14:620, 1994.

372. Xue D, Huang Z-G, Smith K, Buchan A: Immediate or delayed mild hypothermia prevents focal cerebral infarction. Brain Res 587:66, 1992.

373. Laptook A, Corbett R, Burns D, Sterett R: Neonatal ischemic neuroprotection by modest hypothermia is associated with attenuated brain acidosis. Stroke 26:1240, 1995.

374. Dietrich W, Busto R, Alonso O, et al: Intraischemic but not postischemic brain hypothermia protects chronically following global forebrain ischemia in rats. J Cereb Blood Flow Metab 13:541, 1993.

375. Welsh F, Sims R, Harris V: Mild hypothermia prevents ischemic injury in gerbil hippocampus. J Cereb Blood Flow Metab 10:557, 1990.

376. Ginsberg M, Sternau L, Globus M-T, et al: Therapeutic modulation of brain temperature: Relevance to ischemic brain injury. Cerebrovasc Brain Metab Rev 4:189, 1992.

377. Globus M, Alonso O, Dietrich WD, et al: Glutamate release and free radical production following brain injury: Effects of posttraumatic hypothermia. J Neurochem 65:1704, 1995.

378. Edwards A, Yue X, Squier M, et al: Specific inhibition of apoptosis after cerebral hypoxia-ischaemia by moderate post-insult hypothermia. Biochem Biophys Res Comm 217:1193, 1995.

379. Thoresen M, Penrice J, Lorek A, et al: Mild hypothermia after severe transient hypoxia-ischemia ameliorates delayed cerebral energy failure in the newborn piglet. Pediatr Res 37:667, 1995.

380. Buchan A, Pulsinelli W: Hypothermia but not the *N*-methyl-D-aspartate antagonist, MK801, attenuates neuronal damage in gerbils subjected to transient global ischemia. J Neurosci 10:311, 1990.

381. Busto R, Dietrich W, Globus M-T, et al: Small differences in intraischemic brain temperature critically determine the extent of ischemic neuronal injury. J Cereb Blood Flow Metab 7:729, 1987.

382. Busto R, Globus MY, Dietrich WD, et al: Effect of mild hypothermia on ischemia-induced release of neurotransmitters and free fatty acids in rat brain. Stroke 20:904, 1989.

383. Rokkas CK, Cronin CS, Nitta T, et al: Profound systemic hypothermia inhibits the release of neurotransmitter amino acids in spinal cord ischemia. J Thorac Cardiovasc Surg 110:27, 1995.

384. Chopp M, Welch K, Tidwell C, et al: Effect of mild hypothermia on recovery of metabolic function after global cerebral ischemia in cats. Stroke 19:1521, 1988.

385. Karibe H, Chen S, Zarow G, et al: Mild intraischemic hypothermia suppresses consumption of endogenous antioxidants after temporary focal ischemia in rats. Brain Res 649:12, 1994.

386. Dietrich D, Busto R, Halley M, Valdes I: The importance of brain temperature in alterations of the blood-brain barrier following cerebral ischemia. J Neuropathol Exp Neurol 49:486, 1990.

387. Krantis A: Hypothermia-induced reductions in the permeability of the radiolabelled substances across the blood-brain barrier. Acta Neuropathol 60:61, 1983.

388. Amess PN, Penrice J, Cady EB, et al: Mild hypothermia after severe transient hypoxia-ischemia reduces the delayed rise in cerebral lactate in the newborn piglet. Pediatr Res 41:803, 1997.

389. Coimbra C, Wieloch T: Moderate hypothermia mitigates neuronal damage in the rat brain when initiated several hours following transient cerebral ischemia. Acta Neuropathol 87:325, 1994.

390. Gunn AJ, Bennet L, Gunning MI, et al: Cerebral hypothermia is not neuroprotective when started after postischemic seizures in fetal sheep. Pediatr Res 46:274, 1999.

391. Redmond J, Gillinov A, Zehr K, et al: Glutamate excitotoxicity: A mechanism of neurologic injury associated with hypothermic circulatory arrest. J Thorac Cardiovasc Surg 107:776, 1994.

392. Bona E, Hagberg H, Loberg EM, et al: Protective effects of moderate hypothermia after neonatal hypoxia-ischemia: Short- and long-term outcome. Pediatr Res 43:738, 1998.

393. Colbourne F, Corbett D: Delayed postischemic hypothermia: A six month survival study using behavioral and histological assessments of neuroprotection. J Neurosci 15:7250, 1995.

394. Carroll M, Beek O: Protection against hippocampal CA1 cell loss by post-ischemic hypothermia is dependent on the delay of initiation and duration. Metab Brain Dis 7:45, 1992.

395. Colbourne F, Corbett D: Delayed and prolonged post-ischemic hypothermia is neuroprotective in the gerbil. Brain Res 654:265, 1994.

396. Nakamura T, Miyamoto O, Yamagami S, et al: Influence of rewarming conditions after hypothermia in gerbils with transient forebrain ischemia. J Neurosurg 91:114, 1999.

397. Mink R, Dutka A, Hallenbeck J: Allopurinol pretreatment improves evoked response recovery following global cerebral ischemia in dogs. Stroke 22:660, 1991.

398. Hara H, Kato H, Kogure K: Protective effects of alpha-tocopherol on ischemic neuronal damage in the gerbil hippocampus. Brain Res 510:335, 1990.

399. Palmer C, Towfighi J, Roberts R, Heitjan D: Allopurinol administered after inducing hypoxia-ischemia reduces brain injury in 7-day-old rats. Pediatr Res 33:405, 1993.

400. Oriot D, Beharry K, Gordon JB, Aranda JV: Ascorbic acid during cerebral ischemia in newborn piglets. Acta Paediatr 84:621, 1995.

401. Sarco D, Becker J, Palmer C, et al: The neuroprotective effect of deferoxamine in the hypoxic-ischemic immature mouse brain. Neurosci Lett 282:113, 2000.

402. Van Bel F, Shadid M, Moison RM, et al: Effect of allopurinol on postasphyxial free radical formation, cerebral hemodynamics, and electrical brain activity. Pediatrics 101:185, 1998.

403. Hallak M, Irtenkauf SM, Cotton DB: Effect of magnesium sulfate on excitatory amino acid receptors in the rat brain. I. *N*-methyl-D-aspartate receptor channel complex. Am J Obstet Gynecol 175:575, 1996.

404. Hoffman DJ, Marro PJ, McGowan JE, et al: Protective effect of MgSO$_4$ infusion on NMDA receptor binding characteristics during cerebral cortical hypoxia in the newborn piglet. Brain Res 644:144, 1994.

405. Marret S, Gressens P, Gadisseux JF, Evrard P: Prevention by magnesium of excitotoxic neuronal death in the developing brain: An animal model for clinical intervention studies. Dev Med Child Neurol 37:473, 1995.

406. McDonald JW, Silverstein FS, Cardona D, et al: Systemic administration of MK-801 protects against *N*-methyl-D-aspartate– and quisqualate-mediated neurotoxicity in perinatal rats. Neuroscience 36:589, 1990.

407. Tsuda T, Kogure K, Nishioka K, Watanabe T: Mg^{2+} administered up to twenty-four hours following reperfusion prevents ischemic damage of the CA1 neurons in the rat hippocampus. Neurosci 44:335, 1991.

408. de Haan HH, Gunn AJ, Williams CE, et al: Magnesium sulfate therapy during asphyxia in near-term fetal lambs does not compromise the fetus but does not reduce cerebral injury. Am J Obstet Gynecol 176:18, 1997.

409. Penrice J, Amess PN, Punwani S, et al: Magnesium sulfate after transient hypoxia-ischemia fails to prevent delayed cerebral energy failure in the newborn piglet. Pediatr Res 41:443, 1997.

410. Galvin KA, Oorschot DE: Postinjury magnesium sulfate treatment is not markedly neuroprotective for striatal medium spiny neurons after perinatal hypoxia/ischemia in the rat. Pediatr Res 44:740, 1998.

411. Witlin AG, Sibai BM: Magnesium sulfate therapy in preeclampsia and eclampsia. Obstet Gynecol 92:883, 1998.

412. Nelson K, Grether J: Can magnesium sulphate reduce the risk of cerebral palsy in very low birth weight infants? Pediatrics 95:263, 1995.

413. Schendel DE, Berg CJ, Yeargin-Allsopp M, et al: Prenatal magnesium sulfate exposure and the risk for cerebral palsy or mental retardation among very low-birth-weight children aged 3 to 5 years. JAMA 276:1805, 1996.

414. Reynolds J, Chestnut D, Dexter F, et al: Magnesium sulfate adversely affects fetal lamb survival and blocks fetal cerebral blood flow response during maternal hemorrhage. Anesth Analg 83:493, 1996.

415. Mittendorf R, Dambrosia J, Pryde PG, et al: Association between the use of antenatal magnesium sulfate in preterm labor and adverse health outcomes in infants. Am J Obstet Gynecol 186:1111, 2002.

416. Mittendorf R, Pryde PG: An overview of the possible relationship between antenatal pharmacologic magnesium and cerebral palsy. J Perinat Med 28:286, 2000.

417. Scudiero R, Khoshnood B, Pryde PG, et al: Perinatal death and tocolytic magnesium sulfate. Obstet Gynecol 96:178, 2000.

418. Mittendorf R, Covert R, Elin R, et al: Umbilical cord serum ionized magnesium level and total pediatric mortality. Obstet Gynecol 98:75, 2001.

419. Mittendorf R, Covert R, Boman J, et al: Is tocolytic magnesium sulphate associated with increased total paediatric mortality? Lancet 350:1517, 1997.

420. Grether J, Hoogstrate J, Selvin S, Nelson K: Magnesium sulfate tocolysis and risk of neonatal death. Am J Obstet Gynecol 178:1, 1998.

421. Muir K, Lees K: A randomized, double-blind, placebo-controlled pilot trial of intravenous magnesium sulphate in acute stroke. Ann N Y Acad Sci 765:315, 1995.

422. Levene M, Blennow M, Whitelaw A, et al: Acute effects of two different doses of magnesium sulphate in infants with birth asphyxia. Arch Dis Child 73:F174, 1995.

423. Bowersox SS, Singh T, Luther RR: Selective blockade of N-type voltage-sensitive calcium channels protects against brain injury after transient focal cerebral ischemia in rats. Brain Res 747:343, 1997.

424. Burns LH, Jin Z, Bowersox SS: The neuroprotective effects of intrathecal administration of the selective N-type calcium channel blocker ziconotide in a rat model of spinal ischemia. J Vasc Surg 30:334, 1999.

425. Takizawa S, Matsushima K, Fujita H, et al: A selective N-type calcium channel antagonist reduces extracellular glutamate release and infarct volume in focal cerebral ischemia. J Cereb Blood Flow Metab 15:611, 1995.

426. Levene M, Gibson N, Fenton A, et al: The use of a calcium-channel blocker, nicardipine, for severely asphyxiated newborn infants. Dev Med Child Neurol 32:567, 1990.

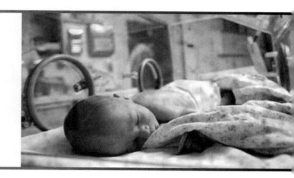

CHAPTER 54

Intracranial Hemorrhage and White Matter Injury in Preterm Infants

Thomas E. Wiswell and Leonard J. Graziani

Almost 1.5% of the more than 4 million infants born annually in the United States are of **very low birth weight (VLBW)**—less than 1500 g.[1] The survival rate of VLBW infants has increased remarkably since the 1980s. Currently, more than 85% of VLBW infants survive. A large proportion of surviving infants subsequently have neurodevelopmental problems, however.[2-5] Approximately 10% manifest cerebral palsy, whereas 25% to 50% manifest cognitive or behavioral problems in school. The improved survival rate of VLBW infants has resulted in an increased prevalence of cerebral palsy in the pediatric population. Cerebral palsy in prematurely born children is characterized by greater involvement of the lower than the upper extremities and varies from a mildly spastic gait to a severe quadriparesis.

Brain injury in VLBW infants consists of multiple lesions, including **intracranial hemorrhage (ICH)**, **posthemorrhagic hydrocephalus**, and **white matter (WM) injury** called **periventricular leukomalacia (PVL)**. From the late 1970s through the early 1990s, ICH was thought to be responsible for most of the severe brain injury noted in preterm infants. Between the mid and late 1990s, there was increased recognition that early ultrasound findings of increased periventricular echogenicity (PVE) of cerebral WM followed by cyst formation (cystic PVL) was more highly predictive of adverse motor and cognitive outcomes in survivors compared with ICH.[2] Improved imaging technology in the late 1990s, primarily diffusion-weighted magnetic resonance imaging (MRI), has led clinicians to understand that more diffuse cerebral WM injury is present considerably more often than either ICH or cystic PVL.[6] The diffuse form of PVL may not be apparent on head ultrasound imaging (HUS) during the neonatal period. Although it has been recognized that cystic PVL is closely associated with subsequent cerebral palsy, at least half of VLBW infants who manifest cerebral palsy do not have recognized imaging abnormalities on HUS studies. It is likely that diffuse PVL, which frequently is not noted on HUS, is the cause of cognitive and behavioral problems in a high proportion of surviving VLBW infants. This chapter reviews multiple aspects of ICH and WM injury, including pathophysiology, risk factors, clinical manifestations, imaging findings, management, sequelae, prognosis, and prevention.

INTRACRANIAL HEMORRHAGE

The incidence of ICH has decreased from 40% or more in the 1980s to approximately 25% to 30% in more recent studies.[7-9] The frequency of ICH is inversely related to gestational age and birth weight so that the smallest, most immature infants are at the highest risk for the more severe grades of brain bleeding. The term **intraventricular hemorrhage** originally was used to describe and classify bleeding in the premature brain. The most common form of ICH (grade 1) is not associated with intraventricular bleeding, however. The most severe form of ICH (grade 4) is not the result of extension of intraventricular bleeding into the brain parenchyma, although this is a commonly held belief.

Grades of Intracranial Hemorrhage

ICH is graded as follows:

Grade 1—hemorrhage confined to the subependymal germinal matrix
Grade 2—intraventricular hemorrhage without distention of the ventricles
Grade 3—intraventricular hemorrhage with ventricular distention
Grade 4—periventricular hemorrhagic infarct, with blood in a characteristic distribution within brain parenchyma

Figure 54-1 depicts the HUS findings of a normal premature neonatal brain. Figures 54-2 through 54-5 depict the HUS findings of grades 1 through 4 ICH. In VLBW infants with ICH, approximately 40% of bleeds are classified as grade 1; 35%, grade 2; 15%, grade 3; and 10%, grade 4.

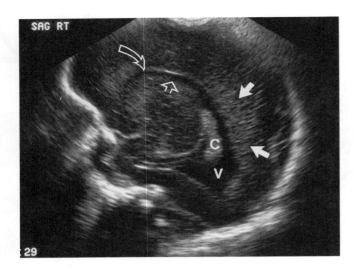

Figure 54–1. Parasagittal image of a normal premature neonate's brain. This image shows the region of the caudothalamic groove *(open arrow)*, lateral ventricle frontal horn *(curved open arrow)*, and trigone (V). The triangular-shaped area of periventricular echogenicity, or "normal trigonal blush" *(solid arrows)*, is seen in the posterior parietal area. The choroid plexus (C) is the echogenic (bright) area within the lateral ventricle. Clear cerebral fluid appears anechoic (black) on ultrasound images.

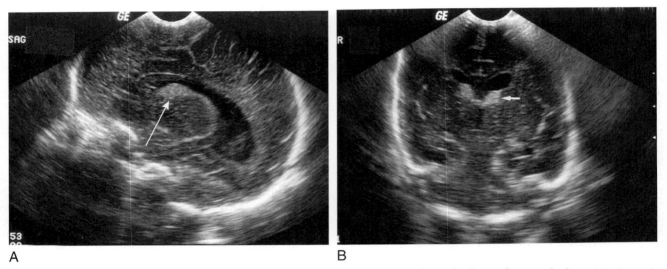

A   B

Figure 54–2. Grade 1 intracranial hemorrhage. Parasagittal **(A)** and paracoronal **(B)** images show a focal area of increased echogenicity *(arrows)* at the caudothalamic groove, with elevation of the floor of the lateral ventricle consistent with a grade 1 subependymal hemorrhage. This infant had bilateral grade 1 intracranial hemorrhage (both can be seen on the paracoronal image).

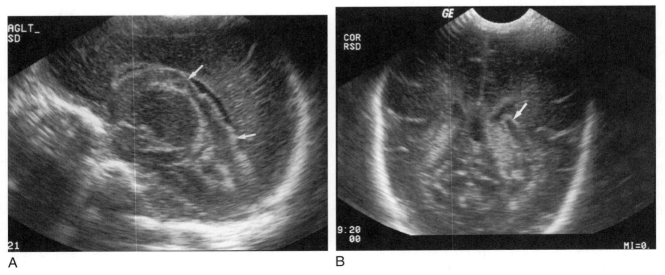

A   B

Figure 54–3. Grade 2 intracranial hemorrhage. Parasagittal **(A)** and paracoronal **(B)** images show clot *(arrows)* extending from the caudothalamic groove into the nondilated lateral ventricle.

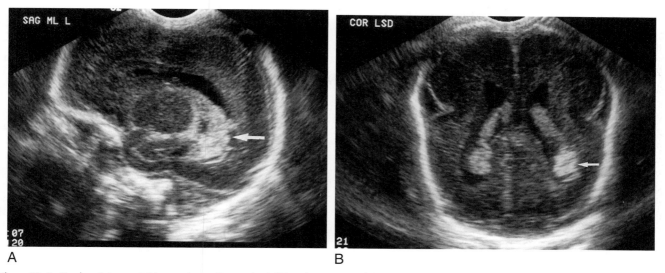

Figure 54–4. Grade 3 intracranial hemorrhage. Parasagittal **(A)** and paracoronal **(B)** images show echogenic material *(arrows)* representing clot within the mildly dilated lateral ventricle.

Pathogenesis[7,8,10,11]

The anatomic origin of grade 1 ICH lies within the germinal matrix (GM). This region is situated under the ependymal lining of the lateral ventricles. The GM is a cellular region that contains pluripotential cells. Between 10 and 20 weeks of gestation, cerebral neuronal precursors originate here and migrate toward the cortex. During the early third trimester, the GM is the source of glial precursors of astrocytes and oligodendrocytes. The GM involutes rapidly during the final 6 to 8 weeks of gestation. In approximately 60% of GM hemorrhages, bleeding ruptures through the ependyma into the ventricular system. In a small proportion of premature infants,

hemorrhage from the choroid plexus contributes to the intraventricular blood.

Why should the GM be a site prone to bleed in VLBW infants? The extravascular tissue supporting the rich supply of blood vessels within the GM is gelatinous in texture. Vessels of the GM are fragile and thin walled, lack a muscularis layer, and have immature interendothelial junctions and incomplete basal lamina. The GM vessels are particularly vulnerable to hypoxic-ischemic injury and are prone to rupture. At the level of the head of the caudate nucleus, the medullary, choroidal, and thalamostriate veins converge, forming the terminal vein. The latter vessel makes a "U-turn" at the site of the germinal matrix

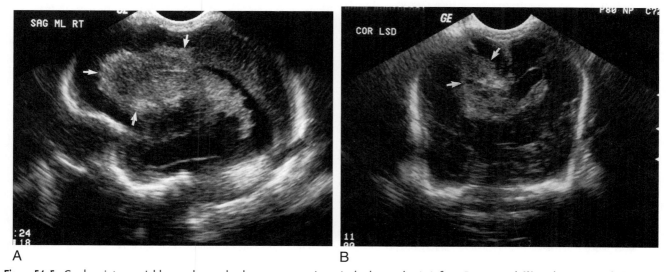

Figure 54–5. Grade 4 intracranial hemorrhage, also known as a *periventricular hemorrhagic infarct.* Parasagittal **(A)** and paracoronal **(B)** images show an area of increased echogenicity *(arrows)* extending from the region of the caudothalamic groove into the right brain parenchyma, with clot present in the lateral ventricle.

to join the vein of Galen, a configuration that increases the risk of increased proximal venous pressure and ischemia. Bleeding typically originates in the capillaries or small venules within the GM. Approximately 50% of grades 1 through 3 ICH is noted by day 1; 75%, by day 2; 90%, by day 3; and the remaining 10%, by day 4 or thereafter.[8,12]

The pathogenesis of periventricular hemorrhagic infarct (grade 4 ICH) is related directly to the associated grades 1 through 3 ICH.[8,11,13-16] Intraventricular or GM bleeding leads to obstruction of the terminal veins and impairs blood flow in the medullary veins; this leads to parenchymal ischemia and a venous hemorrhagic infarction in a fan-shaped (wedge) pattern. The characteristic location of periventricular hemorrhagic infarcts is just dorsal and lateral to the external angle of the lateral ventricle. Of grade 4 ICHs, 80% are associated with GM-intraventricular hemorrhage, particularly grade 3 ICH. Grade 4 ICH is typically unilateral and occurs on the same side of the largest GM or intraventricular hemorrhage. The peak time for occurrence of grade 4 ICH is day 4 of life, by which time 90% of grades 1 through 3 ICH already have occurred.

Besides the vascular characteristics and anatomic features described earlier, many other factors are believed to be involved in the pathogenesis of ICH, as follows[7,8,10,11,17-21]:

1. Fluctuating cerebral blood flow, particularly in VLBW infants requiring mechanical ventilation who are not breathing in synchrony with the ventilator.
2. Increases in cerebral blood flow, particularly in the setting of a pressure-passive circulation. Causes of increased cerebral blood flow include systemic hypertension; noxious stimuli; rapid volume expansion/fluid boluses, particularly of hyperosmolar solutions;

hypercarbia (hypercapnia); seizures; and patent ductus arteriosus.
3. Increased cerebral venous pressure from respiratory disturbances, pneumothorax, vaginal delivery, and mechanical ventilation.
4. Abnormalities in coagulation factors or platelet levels and function.
5. Increased fibrinolytic activity in the GM.
6. Decreased cerebral blood flow followed by reperfusion. Many VLBW infants have pressure-passive cerebral blood flow. Normal autoregulatory mechanisms in the mature infant permit maintenance of stable cerebral blood flows over a wide range of systemic blood pressures. These mechanisms may be dysfunctional, however, in the very premature infant. Cerebral flow may vary directly with systemic blood pressure. Hypotension could be a critical factor in creating ischemic areas prone to bleeding when there is reperfusion.
7. Increased vulnerability to hypoxia-ischemia, reperfusion, and oxygen free radical injury.
8. Increased fibrinolytic activity in the GM.

Ventricular Dilation and Posthemorrhagic Hydrocephalus[7,8,13]

It is common for ventricular dilation to occur after ICH. Most children with grades 3 and 4 ICH have progressive ventricular dilation that does not require treatment. Nonetheless, posthemorrhagic hydrocephalus (PHH) with progressive ventricular dilation due to decreased cerebrospinal fluid (CSF) flow under increased pressure is a common sequela of ICH (Fig. 54-6). The development and likelihood of PHH are related closely to the severity of ICH. PHH may occur acutely within days of

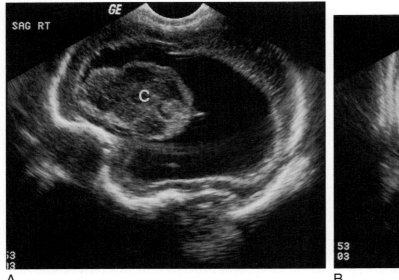
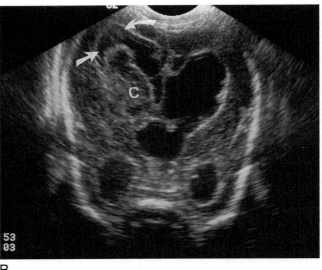

A   B

Figure 54–6. Posthemorrhagic hydrocephalus. Parasagittal **(A)** and paracoronal **(B)** images show significantly dilated lateral ventricles in this infant with a right grade 4 intracranial hemorrhage. This study was performed approximately 1 month after the study shown in Figure 54-5. The right and left lateral ventricles and third ventricle are dilated and have rounded walls consistent with increased intraventricular pressure. Organized clot (C) is present and porencephalic cyst formation *(arrows)*, resulting from the previous parenchymal insult, is evident. Compare the shape of the ventricles shown in these images with those of atrophic ventricular dilation seen in Figure 54-12.

the ICH as a consequence of obstructed CSF flow by blood. Subacute (chronic) hydrocephalus is more common than the acute type and typically progresses over weeks, presumably due to impaired resorption of CSF by the arachnoid villi because of an obliterative arachnoiditis and fibrosis secondary to the initial bleeding. Other potential channels of CSF circulation and reabsorption also are blocked. Typically, ventricular dilation develops, sometimes to a remarkable degree, before there is an abnormal increase in head size. CSF within the ventricular system that accumulates during PHH may cause damage to the cerebral WM and cortex as a result of the increased pressure and edema. If PHH develops, the risk of an adverse neurologic outcome is increased. Nevertheless, the initial brain damage associated with ICH and PHH is not reversed by interventional therapies directed toward reduction of ventricular dilation and CSF pressure. Many children with ICH also may have diffuse WM injury that results in brain atrophy. Ventricular enlargement in the latter children is not due to hydrocephalus, but rather to the loss of brain tissue. The CSF within the ventricular system of children with cerebral atrophy is not under increased pressure. In contrast to the increased head circumference with PHH, children with brain atrophy are more likely to have failure in head growth and even microcephaly.

Clinical Manifestations of Acute Intracranial Hemorrhage[8]

Most VLBW infants who develop lower grades of ICH have no or minimal acute neurologic abnormalities. Rarely a catastrophic deterioration occurs, especially in association with grade 4 ICH, which can include seizures, metabolic acidosis, a bulging anterior fontanelle, temperature instability, lethargy, coma, and hypotension. More often, however, medical and neurologic abnormalities due to ICH are less dramatic and consist of the following: an unexpected low hematocrit or a hematocrit that does not rise as expected after transfusion, alteration in level of consciousness, an abnormally "tight" popliteal angle, and hypotonia. Symptoms or signs indicative of bleeding are absent in half of children with ICH.

Management[7,8]

Treatment of children with ICH is largely supportive. Clinicians should seek to maintain cerebral perfusion. Efforts should be aimed at maintaining adequate blood pressure. Attention should be paid to ventilation, temperature, nutrition, and metabolic status. Anticonvulsants should be used when seizures occur. Serial HUS studies should be performed to assess progression of ICH. Initially, when an ICH is noted, HUS examination intervals should be no longer than 3 to 5 days. When the bleeding has ceased evolving and there seems to be no acute hydrocephalus, serial HUS determinations need to be continued to assess for ventriculomegaly and possible hydrocephalus and for development of porencephaly. We recommend weekly HUS evaluations at least for 1 month if the infant is clinically stable and more frequently in the presence of the following: neurologic deterioration, signs of additional bleeding, a bulging anterior fontanelle in the sitting position, or abnormal head growth.

The head circumference is measured and graphed for all VLBW infants, at least weekly and more often if ventriculomegaly is present. HUS just before discharge is recommended for all VLBW infants. In infants with more severe ICH (grades 3 and 4) or with findings of WM injury, we also recommend MRI before discharge (see section on WM injury).

The management of PHH is directed toward the amelioration of brain damage due to progressive ventricular dilation and the avoidance of a permanent ventriculoperitoneal shunt. Various medications that decrease the production of CSF have been used in the management of PHH, including acetazolamide, furosemide, and digoxin.[7,8,22] To date, however, the evidence does not indicate that any of these therapies is effective. The randomized, controlled trials performed so far indicate that these medications are more likely to result in adverse outcomes. Serial lumbar punctures and ventricular taps have been performed for PHH in an effort to remove substantial quantities of CSF. It is often difficult to remove sufficient CSF to alleviate PHH progression, particularly via lumbar puncture. The ventricular tap needle traverses cerebral cortex and WM, increasing the risk of additional damage to neurons. Removal of excessive CSF can adversely affect the fluid and electrolyte status of the infant. Serial lumbar punctures or ventricular taps increase the risk of CSF infection. A Cochrane Collaboration review indicated that such therapies are not more likely to prevent neuronal damage or to lessen the need for permanent shunt placement.[23] External ventricular drains that allow periodic removal of CSF have a high incidence of CSF infection. Subcutaneous ventricular reservoir placement allows easy removal of CSF, but also is associated with an increased risk of infection and skin breakdown over the reservoir site. No randomized, controlled trials have assessed the efficacy of either external drains or reservoirs.

A unique procedure for infants with PHH that has been described more recently is drainage, irrigation, and fibrinolytic therapy (DRIFT).[24] DRIFT (Fig. 54-7) consists of placement of one catheter into the right ventricle frontally and a second catheter into the left ventricle posteriorly. Tissue plasminogen activator is instilled into the system and left in place for 8 hours before irrigation. Artificial CSF containing antibiotics is infused until the draining fluid is cleared of old blood, generally taking 3 to 7 days. In their most recent report, the authors claimed improved outcomes in infants treated with DRIFT compared with historical controls.[24] To date, there are no prospective, randomized, controlled trials of the latter therapy.

Progressive PHH unresponsive to more conservative therapies requires placement of a ventriculoperitoneal shunt. A ventriculoperitoneal shunt may be technically impossible or fail in small, VLBW infants. Bloody or posthemorrhagic CSF, frequently with protein levels of 10 to 20 times normal, often blocks ventriculoperitoneal shunts. Shunt placement is often delayed until CSF protein levels have decreased toward the normal range. Ventriculoperitoneal shunts often require replacement several times as the child grows to adulthood because of failure or infection. Many children treated with ventriculoperitoneal shunts for PHH need them for their entire

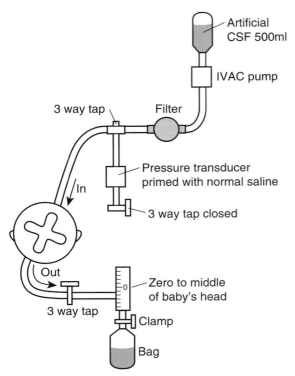

Figure 54–7. A schematic of DRIFT (drainage, irrigation, and fibrinolytic therapy). A catheter is placed into the right ventricle frontally, and another one is placed into the left ventricle posteriorly. Tissue plasminogen activator is instilled into the system and left in place for 8 hours. Artificial cerebrospinal fluid (CSF) is infused until the draining fluid is cleared of old blood. *(From Whitelaw A, Pople I, Cherian S, et al: Phase 1 trial of prevention of hydrocephalus after intraventricular hemorrhage in newborn infants by drainage, irrigation, and fibrinolytic therapy. Pediatrics 111:759, 2003.)*

lives, although a certain percentage of premature infants become shunt independent.

Sequelae and Prognosis

Generally, children with grades 1 and 2 ICH do not have increased rates of mortality, cerebral palsy, or cognitive abnormalities compared with other VLBW infants who do not have ICH. Grade 3 ICH is associated with increased mortality, a much higher frequency of PHH (>50%), and an approximately 35% incidence of major neurologic sequelae (cerebral palsy or severe cognitive deficits). Neonates with periventricular hemorrhagic infarcts (grade 4 ICH) have a strikingly increased mortality rate (approximately 50%) compared with neonates with grade 3 or less severe ICH. Approximately 80% of survivors develop ventricular dilation, which ceases progressing and needs no therapy in most cases. PHH is most likely to occur, however, after grade 4 compared with lesser grades of ICH. Most infants (70% to 90%) who survive after a periventricular hemorrhagic infarct have major motor deficits and severe cognitive dysfunction. These lesions typically degenerate into porencephalic cysts (Fig. 54-8), which generally communicate with the ipsilateral ventricle.

Prevention

The incidence of ICH seemingly declined from approximately 40% in the late 1970s and early 1980s to approximately 25% to 30% in the mid 1990s.[7-9] The specific reasons for this decline are unknown. Most publications have not noted any further decrease in the rate of ICH since the early to mid 1990s.[25-27] Many interventions have been proposed to prevent ICH. Several medications have been used prenatally. Many have been tested in randomized, controlled trials. Antenatal phenobarbital and

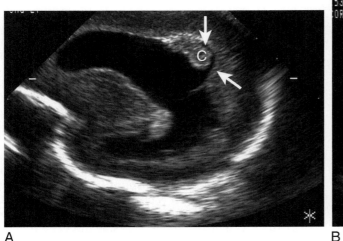

A

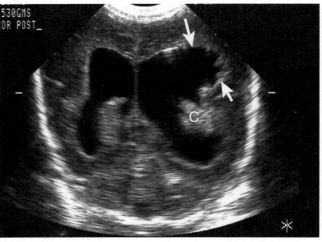

B

Figure 54–8. Porencephalic cyst on the left. Parasagittal **(A)** and paracoronal **(B)** images show significantly dilated lateral ventricles in this infant with a history of a left grade 4 intracranial hemorrhage. This study was performed at approximately 5 weeks of age. Both ventricles are dilated. There is organized clot on the left (C). The left side was the worst side of the bilateral grade 3 intraventricular hemorrhage. Porencephalic cyst formation *(arrows)* followed liquefaction of the left brain parenchymal hemorrhagic infarct. The location of the cyst is in the distribution of the medullary veins. The cyst communicates with the left lateral ventricle.

vitamin K have not been shown to be beneficial, as outlined in Cochrane reviews.[28,29] In some observational studies, but not all, maternal administration of magnesium sulfate has been associated with reduction in the risk of ICH.[30] A large randomized, controlled trial of this therapy was completed.[31] Although there was no difference in the incidence of ICH between groups, death and substantial gross motor dysfunction were reduced significantly in the groups of infants whose mothers had received antenatal magnesium sulfate. A Cochrane review of the many trials of antenatal corticosteroids indicated that this therapy would prevent ICH.[32] The use of antenatal steroids in mothers of VLBW infants in the United States before 1994 was less than 20%. Since this time, their use has increased to 65% to 70% or greater. Of note, however, are the outcomes from the NICHD Neonatal Research Network in the mid 1990s.[26,27] Although 71% of the mothers of 4438 VLBW infants born in 1995-1996 had received antenatal steroids, the incidence of all grades of ICH was virtually identical to that in the 4593 VLBW infants born in 1993-1994, in whom 35% of the mothers had received such therapy. Finally, the method of delivery may play a role in prevention of ICH. The answer is not clear. Although several studies indicate that infants delivered operatively are less likely to develop ICH compared with infants delivered vaginally,[8,29] many other studies have found no differences.

Several postnatal interventions to prevent intraventricular hemorrhage have been proposed. Phenobarbital has not been shown to be effective.[33] Although the following therapies have seemed promising in smaller studies, well-designed randomized, controlled trials have not yet been performed to define whether or not they may be beneficial: vitamin E, muscle paralysis, and ethamsylate.[7] Indomethacin has been assessed in many well-designed clinical trials.[34] The incidence of severe ICH was significantly lower in the infants treated with indomethacin. Nevertheless, when large numbers of these children were assessed for neurologic abnormalities later in life, there were minimal to no differences between groups.[35] Indomethacin has been associated with more intestinal perforations, and it is feared that it also may be causing ischemic brain injury. A group of neonatal care providers from five institutions formed a multidisciplinary focus group with the purpose of identifying potentially better practices which, it was hoped, would reduce the incidence of ICH and WM injury.[36,37] Many of the 10 identified practices have been implemented at the various institutions. To date, there are no reports on whether or not these efforts have been successful.

WHITE MATTER INJURY

WM injury, generally known as PVL, is the major form of neurologic injury seen in VLBW infants.[6,10,11,38,39] PVL characteristically is found in the WM dorsal and lateral to the external angles of the lateral ventricles. The first descriptions of the focal lesions of PVL were by Banker and Larroche in 1962,[40] who coined the descriptive term PVL for the findings of focal softening of the periventricular WM. Multiple epidemiologic and echographic studies in the

1980s and 1990s described the HUS finding of focal periventricular echolucency as the principal feature of PVL. Most reports indicate 5% to 15% of surviving VLBW infants develop cystic PVL. It has been recognized, however, that these cystic lesions are not the principal feature of WM injury in premature infants. Noncystic, diffuse PVL is far more common and is likely involved in the etiology of cognitive and behavioral problems found in 50% of surviving VLBW infants.[6] More recent reports have noted diffuse PVL in 35% to 79% of VLBW infants.

Pathogenesis of Periventricular Leukomalacia[6,10,11,39,41]

The normal cerebral blood flow to premature infants' brains is strikingly low compared with older children and adults. Additionally, several interacting factors predispose premature VLBW infants to WM injury, as follows:

Incomplete state of development of the blood supply to cerebral WM
Maturational-dependent impairment of cerebrovascular autoregulation
Propensity of immature oligodendroglia cells to free radical injury
Infection or inflammation or both

The vascular supply of the cerebral WM largely consists of long and short penetrating arteries (Fig. 54-9).[39] Focal PVL mainly occurs in the distribution of the end zones of the long penetrating arteries. The distal ends of the long penetrating arteries are not fully developed in premature infants. When blood flow is decreased, these areas would be prone to severe ischemia. Diffuse PVL occurs mainly in the distributions of border zones between long penetrating arteries and the end zones of the short penetrating arteries. The latter vessels are not developed fully in preterm infants. When cerebral blood flow is decreased,

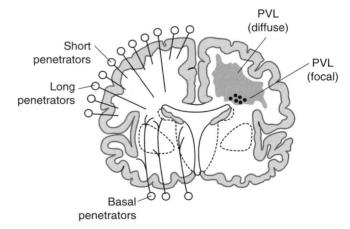

Figure 54-9. Coronal section of cerebrum showing the focal and diffuse components of periventricular leukomalacia (PVL) in one hemisphere and the cerebral vascular supply in the other hemisphere. The focal necrotic component of PVL is depicted by the black circles, whereas the diffuse oligodendroglial-specific component is depicted by the gray shading. The long and short penetrating arteries supply the cerebral white matter, as shown. *(From Volpe JJ: Neurobiology of periventricular leukomalacia in the premature infant. Pediatr Res 50:553, 2001.)*

moderate ischemia can occur. The latter injury seems to affect mainly oligodendroglia precursor cells.

Sick VLBW infants may show poor cerebrovascular autoregulation. Autoregulatory mechanisms allow a mature infant to sustain adequate cerebral blood flow over a wide range of systemic blood pressures: Cerebral vessels dilate with low systemic blood pressure and constrict with high systemic blood pressure. The sick premature infant may have poor autoregulatory capability. This phenomenon is known as a **pressure-passive circulation**. With hypotension, these infants may not be able to maintain sufficient cerebral blood flow, and ischemia may result. The latter plays a role in WM injury.

Normally, projections of oligodendroglia fan out and coil around the axons of neurons, functioning to elaborate and maintain the myelin sheath within the central nervous system. The presence of the myelin sheath is responsible for the characteristic light color of WM. Myelin enhances the speed and integrity of nerve signal propagation down the neural axon. Disruption of the myelin sheath can cause a variety of neurodevelopmental problems—motor, cognitive, and behavioral. The immature oligodendroglia of VLBW infants are particularly vulnerable to hypoxia-ischemia.[39,42] Following ischemia, reperfusion occurs, and a variety of reactive oxygen species (also called *oxygen free radicals*) are produced.[6,39] The specific free radicals that are likely to be involved are the superoxide anion and hydrogen peroxide. The oligodendroglia precursors are injured easily by these substances and by reactive nitrogen species. Additionally, there is a role for glutamate in the killing of preoligodendrocytes. Mature oligodendroglia capable of myelin production are resistant to attack by reactive oxygen and nitrogen species (e.g., peroxynitrite). A further mechanism to consider is the role of concomitant ICH. VLBW infants with PVL frequently have a history of ICH. The presence of iron released at the time of bleeding in brain tissue may promote the production of the hydroxyl radical, furthering oligodendroglia damage by reactive oxygen species.

After severe insults, generalized cell death is by necrosis. This is the likely mechanism causing focal (cystic) PVL. With the latter, all cellular elements undergo coagulation necrosis at the site of injury. Subsequent tissue liquefaction and cavity formation generally occur over the ensuing 1 to 3 weeks. By contrast, the more widespread oligodendroglia injury of diffuse PVL probably occurs after moderate ischemia, in which case neuronal death is typically via apoptosis.[43] There seems to be preferential death of preoligodendrocytes, a more cell-specific injury within central WM. Death of these cells accounts for the subsequent failure of WM development noted at term or afterward. It is unusual for diffuse lesions to undergo large cystic changes. More commonly, diffuse PVL either is not noted on HUS or is manifest by ventriculomegaly and evidence of atrophy.[44,45]

Since the 1990s, considerable evidence has appeared implicating infection and inflammation in the death of oligodendroglia precursors and the ultimate production of PVL.[39,46-50] Multiple studies have noted maternal chorioamnionitis as a risk factor present in many infants with PVL. Fetal and postnatal infections also have been noted in a large proportion of infants with PVL. Endotoxin and cytokines are involved in the pathogenesis of injury. Many studies have found evidence of elevated proinflammatory cytokines in amniotic fluid, cord blood, and neonatal blood of infants subsequently diagnosed with PVL and cerebral palsy. Tissue with diffuse WM injury contains a large number of activated microglia. The latter cells are the intrinsic macrophages of the central nervous system, and their presence is promoted by inflammation. Ischemia-reperfusion also is accompanied by activation of microglia, secretion of cytokines, and mobilization of inflammatory cells.

A possible role for excess extracellular glutamate in the pathogenesis of PVL has been suggested. This excitatory amino acid plays an important role in apoptosis. Glutamate causes glutathione depletion in oligodendrocytes and assists free radical–mediated cell death. Additionally, in the developing oligodendroglia, activation of the α-amino-3-hydroxy-5-methyl-4-isoxazolepropionic acid/kainite type of glutamate receptor can lead to cell death.

Risk Factors for Periventricular Leukomalacia[6,11,51-53]

The major risk factors for PVL include the following:

Prematurity and VLBW
Requirement for mechanical ventilation
History of maternal antenatal vaginal bleeding
Intrauterine growth restriction
Hypoxemia
Hypotension
Hypocapnia (hypocarbia)[54-56]
Maternal cocaine use
High-frequency jet ventilation with a low volume strategy[57]
Placental lesions
Prolonged steroid use for bronchopulmonary dysplasia
Infection or inflammation or both[46-50]
Maternal (chorioamnionitis, urinary tract infection)
Fetal (funisitis, infection in utero)
Neonatal (early-onset or late-onset sepsis, nosocomial infection)

Acidosis typically has not been found to be more common in infants with PVL. The products of inflammation (e.g., endotoxin and cytokines) may decrease cerebral blood flow, be directly toxic to brain tissue, or lead to release of oxygen free radicals. The additive effects of ischemia and infection/inflammation are beyond the control of present-day obstetric and neonatal management and are the likely pathogenic agents responsible for brain injury and subsequent adverse neurodevelopmental outcomes in VLBW infants.

Imaging[3,59-62]

In contrast to ICH, which is frequently unilateral, PVL typically is found bilaterally. The focal form of PVL often is preceded by the finding of PVE. PVE may be mild and restricted only to a small area or large and involving a great deal of WM. Figure 54-10 depicts HUS findings of mild, moderate, and severe PVE. The nomenclature used in the medical literature can be confusing. Some authors use the term *PVE* to denote bright echodense areas seen

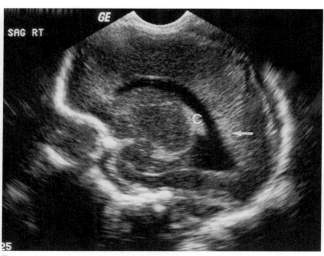

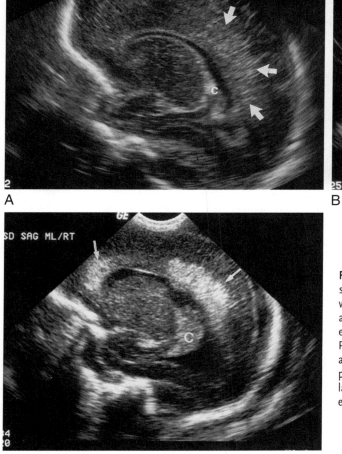

Figure 54–10. Periventricular echogenicity (PVE). **A,** Parasagittal image shows slightly increased PVE *(arrows)*, which extends beyond what would be considered the normal trigonal blush in the posterior parietal area adjacent to the lateral ventricle. The area of increased PVE is less echogenic than the choroid plexus (C). **B,** There is moderately increased PVE *(arrows)* adjacent to the lateral ventricle in the posterior parietal area. The level of echogenicity of this area is equal to that of the choroid plexus (C). **C,** Severely increased PVE *(arrows)* is noted adjacent to the lateral ventricle in the frontal and posterior parietal areas. The level of echogenicity of this area is greater than that of the choroid plexus (C).

early in a neonate's course, even when such areas do not ultimately become echolucent in the form of cysts or cerebral atrophy. Our standard is to use the term *PVE* only to indicate increased brightness (echogenic or echodense areas) on HUS. Approximately 50% of the time, PVE progresses to PVL. Most commonly, the presence of PVE, particularly in its severe form, portends the development of focal necrosis that manifests as cysts (Fig. 54-11). These cysts typically develop 7 to 21 days after the event causing the damage. Nonetheless, sometimes cysts may not be noted until the infant is much older (≥1.5 to 2 months old). Additionally, cystic PVL may coexist with diffuse PVL. Cystic PVL can disappear after days to weeks (Fig. 54-12) as the areas involute. Occasionally, diffuse PVL can appear as massive cystic degeneration and result in a picture of encephalomalacia (Fig. 54-13) and atrophy. This latter finding (atrophy) is seen more consistently with diffuse PVL (Fig. 54-14) and often is not noted with standard HUS studies during the first 1 to 2 months of life.

MRI provides detail of brain anatomy and definition of lesions in terms of site, extent, and type of pathology, especially noncystic WM injury in VLBW infants.[63-67] Figure 54-15 shows MRI of focal PVL. An important MRI innovation is diffusion-weighted imaging (DWI) of the molecular motion of water in parenchyma, which reveals abnormalities in the cerebral WM not apparent on conventional MRI. Figure 54-16 shows MRI of focal and diffuse PVL and DWI from a 28-week gestation infant. MRI and DWI studies have revealed a remarkably higher frequency of diffuse WM injury than previously recognized by other types of imaging technologies in VLBW infants.

Clinical Manifestations

The development of PVL often is unaccompanied by clinical signs in VLBW infants. When clinical signs occur, they often are subtle and include decreased tone in the lower extremities, irritability, seizures, poor feeding, and apnea and bradycardia events. Electroencephalographic abnormalities have been reported in infants with PVL.[68] There is a high false-positive rate using standard electroencephalography techniques. Inder and colleagues[69]

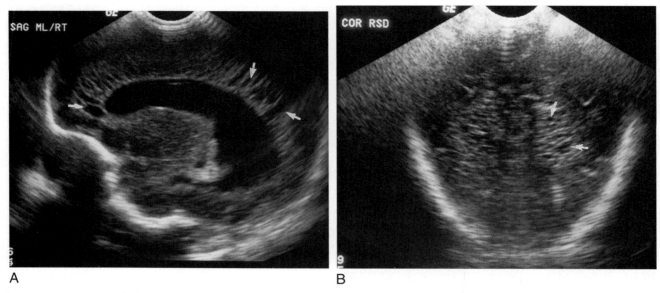

Figure 54–11. Periventricular leukomalacia with small periventricular cysts. Parasagittal **(A)** and paracoronal **(B)** images show multiple, small (2- to 5-mm) cysts *(arrows)* and dilated lateral ventricles. The periventricular leukomalacia extends from the frontal area to the posterior periventricular regions in an infant with previous increased periventricular echogenicity. These are images from the same infant obtained approximately 6 weeks after the study shown in Figure 54-10.

described lowered spectral edge frequency measurements in electroencephalographic studies of infants with increasingly severe WM injury.

Management

To date, limited investigations have not identified any therapies including antioxidants that are of proven benefit in VLBW infants with PVL. HUS studies and computed tomography scans of the brain are not sufficiently

sensitive for delineating the severity and extent of noncystic WM injury in young VLBW infants. By contrast, MRI of the brain more accurately assesses WM injury and facilitates appropriate counseling of parents. Most intensive care nurseries are located far from the MRI suite, and it is logistically difficult to transport a sick VLBW infant for imaging, especially during the acute phase of the illness. Developmental follow-up and early intervention are advised for infants with PVL.

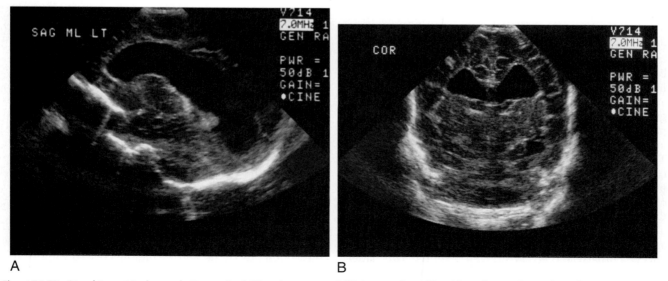

Figure 54–12. Atrophic ventriculomegaly. Parasagittal **(A)** and paracoronal **(B)** images show dilated lateral ventricles in this infant who previously had increased periventricular echogenicity and cystic periventricular leukomalacia (see Fig. 54-11). The angular shape of the ventricle walls indicates atrophic dilation secondary to periventricular leukomalacia. Compare the shape of the ventricles shown in these images with the ventricles of posthemorrhagic hydrocephalus shown in Figure 54-6.

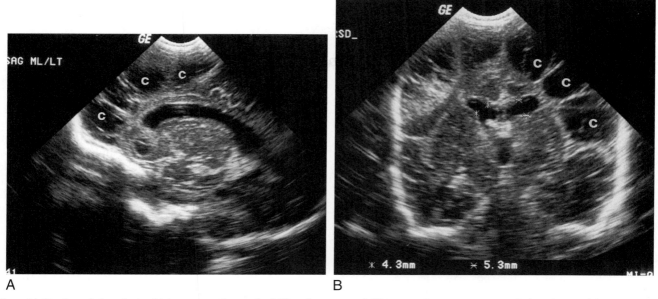

A   B

Figure 54-13. Encephalomalacia with large cysts. Parasagittal **(A)** and paracoronal **(B)** images show extensive encephalomalacia with large (>5 mm) cysts (c) in the white and gray matter bilaterally. The peripheral location of these cysts is atypical, suggesting vascular infarction or extensive cerebral ischemia or both.

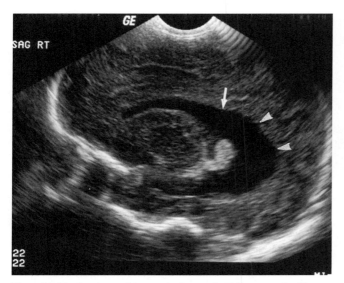

Figure 54-14. Focal atrophic ventriculomegaly. This parasagittal image of the right cerebral hemisphere shows focal dilation of the atrial portion of the lateral ventricle *(arrowheads)*, whereas the frontal horn remains normal in size. Note the unusual contour of the ventricle wall *(arrow)* in this infant who previously had cystic periventricular leukomalacia. Although cysts are no longer shown, the focal ventricular dilation is secondary to atrophy of the posterior parietal parenchyma.

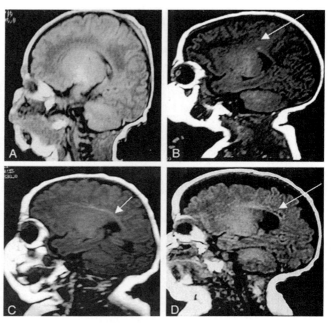

Figure 54-15. Representative parasagittal T1-weighted magnetic resonance images obtained at term in former premature very-low-birth-weight infants. **A,** Normal image. **B,** Focal signal intensity abnormality *(arrow)*. **C,** Extensive signal intensity abnormality *(arrow)*. **D,** Periventricular cystic changes *(arrow)*. *(From Inder TE, Anderson NJ, Spencer C, et al: White matter injury in the premature infant: A comparison between serial cranial sonographic and MR findings at term. AJNR Am J Neuroradiol 24:805, 2003.)*

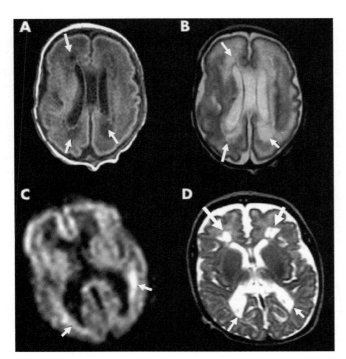

Figure 54–16. Periventricular leukomalacia in a 28-week gestation infant. **A,** Transverse T1-weighted image shows cystic periventricular leukomalacia as areas of low signal within the cerebral white matter posterior and anterior to the lateral ventricles *(arrows)*. **B,** Transverse T2-weighted fast spin echo (FSE) image shows the same lesions as high signal intensity *(arrows)*. **C,** Diffusion-weighted image shows areas of restricted diffusion around the lateral ventricles as high signal intensity *(arrows)*. **D,** T2-weighted FSE image of the same infant at 40 weeks of gestation shows squared-off posterior horns of the lateral ventricles *(small arrows)* and diminished white matter posteriorly. Cystic lesions are shown anterior to the anterior horns of the lateral ventricles *(large arrows)*. *(From Counsell SJ, Rutherford MA, Cowan FM, Edwards AD: Magnetic resonance imaging of preterm brain injury. Arch Dis Child Fetal Neonatal Educ 88:F269, 2003.)*

Prognosis and Outcomes[3,10,38,70]

Infants with PVL are at high risk for neurodevelopmental deficits. The most common outcome of focal PVL is spastic diplegia. Children with cysts greater than 3 to 5 mm in size have a risk for developing cerebral palsy of 70% or greater and a risk for cognitive impairment greater than 50%. More severe PVL is associated with quadriplegia. Diffuse PVL may be associated with cognitive impairment, behavioral problems, and cerebral palsy. Vision impairment is a known consequence of PVL.

Prevention

The only current means of preventing PVL is by preventing premature birth. Cocaine use during pregnancy increases the risk of PVL. There are no data supporting the concept that antibiotic therapy for premature labor or chorioamnionitis prevents PVL. Efforts to prevent hypotension are important in VLBW neonates. Although some reports suggest that antenatal steroids may lower the incidence of PVL, large series of patients over time

have not confirmed the benefit of such therapy. Baud and coworkers[71] noted that using betamethasone as a maternally administered antenatal steroid may prevent PVL, whereas dexamethasone use may increase the incidence of PVL. Anecdotal reports suggested that antenatal administration of magnesium sulfate may decrease PVL,[72] but definitive trials have not shown a benefit. Other potential interventions[6,39] proposed to prevent or reduce the risk of PVL include prevention of modest ischemic insults, medications to decrease production of reactive oxygen and nitrogen species, antioxidants, compounds to scavenge reactive oxygen and nitrogen species, glutamate antagonists, anticytokine agents, methods to reverse apoptosis, and agents to prevent microglial activation. Controlled trials are needed to elucidate definitive therapies.

SUMMARY

ICH and WM injury are significant problems in VLBW premature infants. The pathogenesis of brain injury is complex and involves multiple factors in preterm infants. Although early trials suggested that ICH could be prevented by use of antenatal steroids, subsequent profiles of large populations have not indicated any further reduction since the latter therapy came into widespread usage. Although prophylactic indomethacin seemingly reduces the occurrence of severe ICH, long-term benefits have not been seen. At this time, one can neither predict nor prevent WM injury in VLBW premature infants. The increasing amount of knowledge concerning ICH and PVL should direct attention to investigating potential interventions that could mitigate brain injury in this high-risk population.

ACKNOWLEDGMENT

The head ultrasound images in Figures 54-1 through 54-6, 54-8, and 54-10 through 54-14 were obtained by Daniel A. Merton, BS, RDMS, Technical Coordinator of Research, The Jefferson Ultrasound Research and Education Institute, Thomas Jefferson University Hospital, Philadelphia, Pennsylvania. Mr. Merton also contributed to the legend descriptions for these images.

REFERENCES

1. Arias E, MacDorman MF, Strobino DM, Guyer B: Annual summary of vital statistics—2002. Pediatrics 112:1215, 2003.
2. du Plessis AJ, Volpe JJ: Perinatal brain injury in the preterm and term newborn. Curr Opin Neurol 15:151, 2002.
3. Graziani LJ: Intracranial hemorrhage and leukomalacia in preterm infants. In Spitzer AR (ed): Intensive Care of the Fetus and Neonate. St. Louis, Mosby, 1996, pp 696-705.
4. Wood NS, Costeloe K, Gibson AT, et al, EPICure Study Group: The EPICure study: Growth and associated problems in children born at 25 weeks of gestational age or less. Arch Dis Child Fetal Neonatal Educ 88:F492, 2003.
5. Wood NS, Marlow N, Costeloe K, et al: Neurologic and developmental disability after extremely preterm birth. EPICure Study Group. N Engl J Med 343:378, 2000.

6. Volpe JJ: Cerebral white matter injury of the premature infant—more common than you think. Pediatrics 112:176, 2003.

7. Whitelaw A: Intraventricular haemorrhage and posthaemorrhagic hydrocephalus: Pathogenesis, prevention and future interventions. Semin Neonatol 6:135, 2001.

8. Volpe JJ: Neurology of the Newborn, 4th ed. Philadelphia, WB Saunders, 2001, pp 217-497.

9. Cooke RW: Trends in incidence of cranial ultrasound lesions and cerebral palsy in very low birthweight infants 1982-93. Arch Dis Child Fetal Neonatal Educ 80:F115, 1999.

10. Shalak L, Perlman JM: Hemorrhagic-ischemic cerebral injury in the preterm infant: Current concepts. Clin Perinatol 29:745, 2002.

11. Inder TE, Volpe JJ: Mechanisms of perinatal brain injury. Semin Neonatol 5:3, 2000.

12. Paneth N, Pinto-Martin J, Gardiner J, et al: Incidence and timing of germinal matrix/intraventricular hemorrhage in low birth weight infants. Am J Epidemiol 137:1167, 1993.

13. Murphy BP, Inder TE, Rooks V, et al: Posthaemorrhagic ventricular dilatation in the premature infant: Natural history and predictors of outcome. Arch Dis Child Fetal Neonatal Educ 87:F37, 2001.

14. Perlman JM, Rollins N, Burns D, Risser R: Relationship between periventricular intraparenchymal echodensities and germinal matrix-intraventricular hemorrhage in the very low birth weight neonate. Pediatrics 91:474, 1993.

15. Gould SJ, Howard S, Hope PL, Reynolds EO: Periventricular intraparenchymal cerebral haemorrhage in preterm infants: The role of venous infarction. J Pathol 151:197, 1987.

16. Guzzetta F, Shackelford GD, Volpe S, et al: Periventricular intraparenchymal echodensities in the premature newborn: Critical determinant of neurologic outcome. Pediatrics 78:995, 1986.

17. Kahn DJ, Richardson DK, Billett HH: Association of thrombocytopenia and delivery method with intraventricular hemorrhage among very-low-birth-weight infants. Am J Obstet Gynecol 186:109, 2002.

18. Osborn DA, Evans N, Kluckow M: Hemodynamic and antecedent risk factors of early and late periventricular/intraventricular hemorrhage in premature infants. Pediatrics 112:33, 2003.

19. O'Shea M, Savitz DA, Hage ML, Feinstein KA: Prenatal events and the risk of subependymal/intraventricular haemorrhage in very low birthweight neonates. Paediatr Perinat Epidemiol 6:352, 1992.

20. Szymonowicz W, Yu VY, Wilson FE: Antecedents of periventricular haemorrhage in infants weighing 1250 g or less at birth. Arch Dis Child 59:13, 1984.

21. Thorp JA, Jones PG, Clark RH, et al: Perinatal factors associated with severe intracranial hemorrhage. Am J Obstet Gynecol 185:859, 2001.

22. Whitelaw A, Kennedy CR, Brion LP: Diuretic therapy for newborn infants with posthemorrhagic ventricular dilatation. Cochrane Database Syst Rev 2:CD002270, 2001.

23. Whitelaw A: Repeated lumbar or ventricular punctures in newborns with intraventricular hemorrhage. Cochrane Database Syst Rev 1:CD000216, 2001.

24. Whitelaw A, Pople I, Cherian S, et al: Phase 1 trial of prevention of hydrocephalus after intraventricular hemorrhage in newborn infants by drainage, irrigation, and fibrinolytic therapy. Pediatrics 111:759, 2003.

25. Hack M, Wright LL, Shankaran S, et al: Very-low-birth-weight outcomes of the National Institute of Child Health and Human Development Neonatal Network, November 1989 to October 1990. Am J Obstet Gynecol 172:457, 1995.

26. Stevenson DK, Wright LL, Lemons JA, et al: Very low birth weight outcomes of the National Institute of Child Health and Human Development Neonatal Research Network, January 1993 through December 1994. Am J Obstet Gynecol 179:1632, 1998.

27. Lemons JA, Bauer CR, Oh W, et al: Related articles, very low birth weight outcomes of the National Institute of Child Health and Human Development Neonatal Research Network, January 1995 through December 1996. NICHD Neonatal Research Network. Pediatrics 107:E1, 2001.

28. Crowther CA, Henderson-Smart DJ: Phenobarbital prior to preterm birth for preventing neonatal periventricular haemorrhage. Cochrane Database Syst Rev 3:CD000164, 2003.

29. Ramsey PS, Rouse DJ: Therapies administered to mothers at risk for preterm birth and neurodevelopmental outcome in their infants. Clin Perinatol 29:725, 2002.

30. Wiswell TE, Graziani LJ, Caddell JL, et al: Maternally-administered magnesium sulfate (MgSO$_4$) protects against early brain injury and long-term adverse neurodevelopmental outcomes in preterm infants: A prospective study. Pediatr Res 39:253A, 1996.

31. Crowther CA, Hiller JE, Doyle LW, Haslam RR, Australasian Collaborative Trial of Magnesium Sulphate (ACTOMg SO4) Collaborative Group: Effect of magnesium sulfate given for neuroprotection before preterm birth: A randomized controlled trial. JAMA 290:2669, 2003.

32. Crowley P: Antenatal corticosteroids—current thinking. Br J Obstet Gynaecol 110(suppl 20):77, 2003.

33. Whitelaw A: Postnatal phenobarbitone for the prevention of intraventricular hemorrhage in preterm infants. Cochrane Database Syst Rev 1:CD001691, 2001.

34. Fowlie PW, Davis PG: Prophylactic intravenous indomethacin for preventing mortality and morbidity in preterm infants. Cochrane Database Syst Rev 3:CD000174, 2002.

35. Vohr BR, Allan WC, Westerveld M, et al: School-age outcomes of very low birth weight infants in the indomethacin intraventricular hemorrhage prevention trial. Pediatrics 111:e340, 2003.

36. Carteaux P, Cohen H, Check J, et al: Evaluation and development of potentially better practices for the prevention of brain hemorrhage and ischemic brain injury in very low birth weight infants. Pediatrics 111:e489, 2003.

37. McLendon D, Check J, Carteaux P, et al: Implementation of potentially better practices for the prevention of brain hemorrhage and ischemic brain injury in very low birth weight infants. Pediatrics 111:e497, 2003.

38. Volpe JJ: Neurology of the Newborn, 4th ed. Philadelphia, WB Saunders, 2001, pp 307-330, 362-367.

39. Volpe JJ: Neurobiology of periventricular leukomalacia in the premature infant. Pediatr Res 50:553, 2001.

40. Banker BQ, Larroche JC: Periventricular leukomalacia of infancy: A form of neonatal anoxic encephalopathy. Arch Neurol 7:386, 1962.

41. Perlman JM: White matter injury in the preterm infant: An important determination of abnormal neurodevelopment outcome. Early Hum Dev 53:99, 1998.

42. Back SA, Luo NL, Borenstein NS, et al: Late oligodendrocyte progenitors coincide with the developmental window of vulnerability for human perinatal white matter injury. J Neurosci 21:1302, 2001.

43. Chamnanvanakij S, Margraf LR, Burns D, Perlman JM: Apoptosis and white matter injury in preterm infants. Pediatr Dev Pathol 5:184, 2002.

44. Leviton A, Gilles F: Ventriculomegaly, delayed myelination, white matter hypoplasia, and "periventricular" leukomalacia: How are they related? Pediatr Neurol 15:127, 1996.

45. Ment LR, Vohr B, Allan W, et al: The etiology and outcome of cerebral ventriculomegaly at term in very low birth weight preterm infants. Pediatrics 104:243, 1999.

46. Dammann O, Kuban KC, Leviton A: Perinatal infection, fetal inflammatory response, white matter damage, and cognitive limitations in children born preterm. Ment Retard Dev Disabil Res Rev 8:46, 2002.

47. Dammann O, Leviton A: Maternal intrauterine infection, cytokines, and brain damage in the preterm newborn. Pediatr Res 42:1, 1997.

48. Leviton A, Dammann O: Coagulation, inflammation, and the risk of neonatal white matter damage. Pediatr Res 55:539, 2004.

49. Wu YW: Systematic review of chorioamnionitis and cerebral palsy. Ment Retard Dev Disabil Res Rev 8:25, 2002.

50. Rezaie P, Dean A: Periventricular leukomalacia, inflammation and white matter lesions within the developing nervous system. Neuropathology 22:106, 2002.

51. Zupan V, Gonzalez P, Lacaze-Masmonteil T, et al: Periventricular leukomalacia: Risk factors revisited. Dev Med Child Neurol 38:1061, 1996.

52. Resch B, Vollard E, Maurer U, et al: Risk factors and determinants of neurodevelopmental outcome in cystic periventricular leucomalacia. Eur J Pediatr 159:663, 2000.

53. Graziani LJ, Spitzer AR, Mitchell DG, et al: Mechanical ventilation in preterm infants: Neurosonographic and developmental studies. Pediatrics 90:515, 1992.

54. Salokorpi T, Rajantie I, Viitala J, et al: Does perinatal hypocarbia play a role in the pathogenesis of cerebral palsy? Acta Paediatr 88:571, 1999.

55. Greisen G, Vannucci RC: Is periventricular leucomalacia a result of hypoxic-ischaemic injury? Hypocapnia and the preterm brain. Biol Neonate 79:194, 2001.

56. Wiswell TE, Graziani LJ, Kornhauser MS, et al: Effects of hypocarbia on the development of cystic periventricular leukomalacia in premature infants treated with high-frequency jet ventilation. Pediatrics 98:918, 1996.

57. Wiswell TE, Graziani LJ, Kornhauser MS, et al: High-frequency jet ventilation in the early management of respiratory distress syndrome is associated with a greater risk for adverse outcomes. Pediatrics 98:1035, 1996.

58. Kumazaki K, Nakayama M, Sumida Y, et al: Placental features in preterm infants with periventricular leukomalacia. Pediatrics 109:650, 2002.

59. Holling EE, Leviton A: Characteristics of cranial ultrasound white-matter echolucencies that predict disability: A review. Dev Med Child Neurol 41:136, 1999.

60. Paneth N: Classifying brain damage in preterm infants. J Pediatr 134:527, 1999.

61. Hope PL, Gould SJ, Howard S, et al: Precision of ultrasound diagnosis of pathologically verified lesions in the brains of very preterm infants. Dev Med Child Neurol 30:457, 1988.

62. Vollmer B, Roth S, Baudin J, et al: Predictors of long-term outcome in very preterm infants: Gestational age versus neonatal cranial ultrasound. Pediatrics 112:1108, 2003.

63. Counsell SJ, Allsop JM, Harrison MC, et al: Diffusion-weighted imaging of the brain in preterm infants with focal and diffuse white matter abnormality. Pediatrics 112:1, 2003.

64. Counsell SJ, Rutherford MA, Cowan FM, Edwards AD: Magnetic resonance imaging of preterm brain injury. Arch Dis Child Fetal Neonatal Educ 88:F269, 2003.

65. Inder TE, Anderson NJ, Spencer C, et al: White matter injury in the premature infant: A comparison between serial cranial sonographic and MR findings at term. AJNR Am J Neuroradiol 24:805, 2003.

66. Maalouf EF, Duggan PJ, Counsell SJ, et al: Comparison of findings on cranial ultrasound and magnetic resonance imaging in preterm infants. Pediatrics 107:719, 2001.

67. Inder TE, Huppi PS, Zientara GP, et al: Early detection of periventricular leukomalacia by diffusion-weighted magnetic resonance imaging techniques. J Pediatr 134:631, 1999.

68. Hayakawa F, Okumura A, Kato T, et al: Determination of timing of brain injury in preterm infants with periventricular leukomalacia with serial neonatal electroencephalography. Pediatrics 104:1077, 1999.

69. Inder TE, Buckland L, Williams CE, et al: Lowered electroencephalographic spectral edge frequency predicts the presence of cerebral white matter injury in premature infants. Pediatrics 111:27, 2003.

70. Bracewell M, Marlow N: Patterns of motor disability in very preterm children. Ment Retard Dev Disabil Res Rev 8:241, 2002.

71. Baud O, Foix-L'Helias L, Kaminski M, et al: Antenatal glucocorticoid treatment and cystic periventricular leukomalacia in very premature infants. N Engl J Med 341:1190-1196, 1999.

72. Fine-Smith RB, Roche K, Yellin PB, et al: Effect of magnesium sulfate on the development of cystic periventricular leukomalacia in preterm infants. Am J Perinatol 14:303, 1997.

CHAPTER 55

Neonatal Seizures: Prenatal Contributions to a Neonatal Brain Disorder

Mark S. Scher

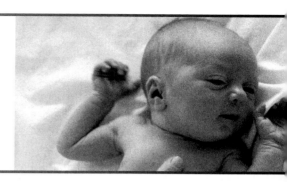

Seizures of the newborn are one of the exceptional neonatal neurologic conditions that necessitate immediate medical attention. Although prompt diagnostic and therapeutic plans are required, unresolved medical issues continue to challenge the physician's evaluation of the newborn with suspected seizures (Table 55-1).[1-3] Clinical and electroencephalographic (EEG) manifestations of neonatal seizures vary dramatically from those in older children, and recognition of the seizure state remains the foremost challenge. This dilemma is underscored by the brevity and subtlety of the clinical repertoire of the newborn's neurologic findings. Environmental restrictions of the sick infant in an intensive care setting limit accessibility, including confinement in an incubator, intubation, and attachment of multiple catheters. Medications produce alterations in arousal and muscle tone, which in turn limit the clinician's ability to distinguish clinical neurologic signs that reflect underlying brain disorders. Brain injury from antepartum factors may later be expressed as neonatal seizures, as part of a postnatal encephalopathic clinical picture precipitated by adverse events during the intrapartum and neonatal periods.[4] Alternatively, overlapping medical conditions present from the fetal through neonatal periods may cumulatively contribute to seizures, accompanying brain disorders and possible injury. Medication options for effectively treating seizures remain elusive; new agents that are designed for specific causes, timing of injury, and the unique cellular/molecular organization of the immature brain must be developed. This chapter discusses issues regarding recognition, differential diagnosis, prognosis, and treatment of neonatal seizures in the context of current clinical and pathophysiologic explanations for the causes of neonatal seizures and the neurologic sequelae that may result. Potential neuroresuscitative strategies proposed for the encephalopathic neonate with seizures must consider maternal, placental/cord, and fetal disease conditions that cause or contribute to neonatal seizure expression,[5] with and without an accompanying neonatal encephalopathy.

DIAGNOSTIC DILEMMAS: RELIANCE ON CLINICAL VERSUS EEG CRITERIA FOR SEIZURES

Neonatal seizures are generally brief and subtle in clinical appearance, sometimes consisting of unusual behaviors that are difficult to recognize and classify. Although seizures are relatively common events in neonates who have symptoms of intercurrent medical conditions, the ability of medical personnel to recognize suspicious behaviors varies significantly, which contributes to overdiagnosis and underdiagnosis. The most common practice has been to classify clinical behaviors as seizures without EEG confirmation. However, motor or autonomic behaviors may represent either normal age- and state-specific behaviors in healthy infants or nonepileptic paroxysmal conditions in abnormal infants. Therefore, confirmation of suspicious clinical events as seizures by using coincident EEG recordings is strongly recommended. In patients with few seizures, the episodes may be missed as brief random events on routine EEG studies[6]; however, continuous synchronized video/EEG/polygraphic recordings can potentially establish more reliable start and end points for electrically confirmed seizures for which treatment intervention must be considered.[7] Such rigorous physiologic monitoring must also integrate the diagnosis of the seizure state with cause and the neurobiologic processes of the immature brain.

Clinical Seizure Criteria

Neonatal seizures are currently listed separately from the traditional classification of seizures and epilepsy during childhood. In the International League Against Epilepsy's classification, adopted by the World Health Organization, neonatal seizures still remain in an unclassified category.[8] Another classification scheme now suggests a more strict distinction of clinical seizure (nonepileptic) events from electrographically confirmed (epileptic) seizures, with regard to possible treatment interventions.[9] Continued

Table 55–1. Dilemmas about Neonatal Seizures

Diagnostic choices: reliance on clinical versus EEG criteria
Etiologic explanations: multiple prenatal/neonatal
  conditions as a function of time
Treatment decisions: who, when, what, and for how long?
Prognostic questions: consider mechanisms of injury
  based on causes versus intrinsic vulnerability of the
  immature brain to prolonged seizures

EEG, electroencephalographic.

refinement of such novel classifications is needed to reconcile the variable agreement between clinical and EEG criteria in establishing a seizure diagnosis,[10,11] in the context of nonepileptic movement disorders caused by acquired diseases, malformations, and/or medications.

Several caveats (Table 55-2) may be useful in the identification of suspected neonatal seizures; however, they continue to raise questions regarding examiners' diagnostic acumen.

The clinical criteria for neonatal seizure diagnosis was historically subdivided into five clinical categories: focal clonic, multifocal or migratory clonic, tonic, myoclonic, and subtle seizures.[12] A more recent classification expands the clinical subtypes, adopting a strict temporal occurrence of specific clinical events with coincident electrographic seizures, to distinguish neonatal clinical "nonepileptic" seizures from "epileptic" seizures (Tables 55-3 and 55-4).[9]

Subtle Seizure Activity

This is the most frequently observed category of neonatal seizures; these seizures include repetitive buccolingual movements, orbital-ocular movements, unusual bicycling or pedaling, and autonomic findings (Fig. 55-1A). Any subtle paroxysmal event that interrupts the expected behavioral repertoire of the newborn and appears stereotypic or repetitive should heighten the clinician's level of

Table 55–2. Caveats Concerning Recognition of Neonatal Seizures

Specific stereotypic behaviors occur in association with
  normal neonatal sleep or waking states, medication
  effects, and gestational maturity
Any abnormal repetitive activity may be a clinical
  seizure if out of context for expected neonatal behavior
Electrographic seizures coincident with the suspected
  clinical event should be documented
Abnormal behavioral phenomena may have inconsistent
  relationships with coincident EEG seizures, which is
  suggestive of a subcortical seizure focus
Nonepileptic pathologic movement disorders are events
  that are independent of the seizure state and may also
  be expressed by neonates

EEG, electroencephalographic.

suspicion for seizures. However, alterations in cardiorespiratory regularity, body movements, and other behaviors during active (rapid-eye-movement [REM]) sleep, quiet (non-REM) sleep, or waking segments must be recognized before the examiner undertakes a seizure evaluation.[13,14] Within the subtle category of neonatal seizures are stereotypic changes in heart rate, blood pressure, oxygenation, or other autonomic signs, particularly during pharmacologic paralysis for ventilatory care. Other unusual autonomic events include penile erections, skin changes, salivation, and lacrimation. Autonomic expressions may be intermixed with motor findings. Isolated autonomic signs such as apnea, unless accompanied by other clinical findings, are rarely associated with coincident electrographic seizures (see Fig. 55-1B).[15,16] Because subtle seizures are both clinically difficult to detect and only variably coincident with EEG-confirmed seizures, synchronized video/EEG/polygraphic recordings are recommended in order to document temporal relationships between clinical behaviors and coincident electrographic events.[7,9,17,18] Despite the "subtle" expression of this seizure category, affected children may have suffered significant brain injury.

Clonic Seizures

Rhythmic movements of muscle groups in a focal distribution that consists of a rapid phase followed by a slow return movement are clonic seizures, to be distinguished from the symmetric "to and fro" movements of tremulousness or jitteriness.[2] Gentle flexion of the affected body part easily suppresses the tremor, whereas clonic seizures persist. Clonic movements can involve any body part, such as the face, arms, legs, and even diaphragmatic or pharyngeal muscles. Generalized clonic activities can occur in the newborn but rarely consist of a classical tonic phase followed by a clonic phase, characteristic of the generalized motor seizure noted in older children and adults. Focal clonic and hemiclonic seizures have been described with localized brain injury, usually from cerebrovascular lesions[7,19-21] (Fig. 55-2A), but can also be seen with generalized brain abnormalities. As with older patients, focal seizures in the neonate may be followed by transient motor weakness, historically referred to as a transient Todd paresis or paralysis,[22] distinguished by a more persistent hemiparesis over multiple days to weeks. Clonic movements without EEG-confirmed seizures have been described in neonates with normal EEG backgrounds, and their neurodevelopment outcome can be normal.[17] The less experienced clinician may misclassify myoclonic movements as clonic. Computational studies suggest strategies to extract quantitative information from video recordings of neonatal seizures as a method by which clinicians can differentiate myoclonic from focal clonic seizures, as well as distinguish normal infant behaviors.[23]

Multifocal (Fragmentary) Clonic Seizures

Multifocal or migratory clonic activities spread over body parts in either a random or an anatomically appropriate manner. Such seizure movements may alternate from side to side and appear asynchronously in the two halves

Table 55–3. Clinical Characteristics, Classification, and Presumed Pathophysiology of Neonatal Seizures

Classification	Characterization

Focal clonic	Repetitive, rhythmic contractions of muscle groups of the limbs, face, or trunk
	    May be unifocal or multifocal
	    May occur synchronously or asynchronously in muscle groups on one side of the body
	    Cannot be suppressed by restraint
	    Pathophysiology: epileptic

Focal tonic	Sustained posturing of single limbs Sustained asymmetric posturing of the trunk Sustained eye deviation Cannot be provoked by stimulation or suppressed by restraint Pathophysiology: epileptic

Generalized tonic	Sustained symmetric posturing of limbs, trunk, and neck
	    May be flexor, extensor, or mixed extensor/flexor
	    May be provoked or intensified by stimulation
	    May be suppressed by restraint or repositioning
	    Presumed pathophysiology: nonepileptic

Myoclonic	Random, single, rapid contractions of muscle groups of the limbs, face, or trunk
	    Typically not repetitive or may recur at a slow rate
	    May be generalized, focal, or fragmentary
	    May be provoked by stimulation
	    Presumed pathophysiology: epileptic or nonepileptic

Spasms	May be flexor, extensor, or mixed extensor/flexor
	    May occur in clusters
	    Cannot be provoked by stimulation or suppressed by restraint
	    Pathophysiology: epileptic

Motor automatisms
    Ocular signs
	Random and roving eye movements or nystagmus (distinct from tonic eye deviation)
	    May be provoked or intensified by tactile stimulation
	    Presumed pathophysiology: nonepileptic

Oral-buccal-lingual
    movements
	Sucking, chewing, tongue protrusions
	    May be provoked or intensified by stimulation
	    Presumed pathophysiology: nonepileptic

Progression
    movements
	Rowing or swimming movements
	Pedaling or bicycling movements of the legs
	    May be provoked or intensified by stimulation
	    May be suppressed by restraint or repositioning
	    Presumed pathophysiology: nonepileptic

Complex purposeless
    movements
	Sudden arousal with transient increased random activity of limbs
	    May be provoked or intensified by stimulation
	    Presumed pathophysiology: nonepileptic

From Mizrahi EM, Kellaway P: Diagnosis and Management of Neonatal Seizures. Philadelphia, Lippincott-Raven, 1998.

of the child's body. The word **fragmentary** was historically applied to distinguish this event from the more classical generalized tonic-clonic seizure seen in older children. Multifocal clonic seizures may also resemble myoclonic seizures, which, alternatively, consist of brief shocklike muscle twitching of the midline and/or extremity musculature. Neonates with this seizure description often die or suffer significant neurologic morbidity.[24]

Tonic Seizures

In tonic seizures, there is a sustained flexion or extension of axial or appendicular muscle groups. Tonic movements of a limb or sustained head or eye turning may also be noted. Tonic activity must be carefully documented with coincident EEG recording, because 30% of such movements lack a temporal correlation with electrographic

seizures (Fig. 55-3).[25] "Brain stem release" resulting from functional decortication after severe neocortical dysfunction or damage is one physiologic explanation for this nonepileptic activity (to be discussed). Extensive neocortical damage or dysfunction results in the emergence of uninhibited subcortical expressions of extensor movements.[26] Tonic seizures may also be misidentified, when the nonepileptic **movement disorder of dystonia** is the more appropriate behavioral description. Both tonic movements and dystonic posturing may also simultaneously occur.

Myoclonic Seizures

Myoclonic movements are rapid, isolated jerks that can be generalized, multifocal, or focal in an axial or appendicular distribution. Myoclonus lacks the slow return

Table 55–4. Classification of Neonatal Seizures, Based on Electroclinical Findings

Clinical seizures with a consistent electrocortical
  signature (pathophysiology: epileptic)
Focal clonic
  Unifocal
  Multifocal
  Hemiconvulsive
  Axial
Focal tonic
  Asymmetric truncal posturing
  Limb posturing
  Sustained eye deviation
Myoclonic
  Generalized
  Focal
Spasms
  Flexor
  Extensor
  Mixed extensor/flexor
Clinical seizures without a consistent electrocortical
  signature (pathophysiology: presumed nonepileptic)
Myoclonic
  Generalized
  Focal
  Fragmentary
Generalized tonic
  Flexor
  Extensor
  Mixed extensor/flexor
Motor automatisms
  Oral-buccal-lingual movements
  Ocular signs
  Progression movements
  Complex purposeless movements
Electrical seizures without clinical seizure activity

From Mizrahi EM, Kellaway P: Diagnosis and Management of Neonatal
Seizures. Philadelphia, Lippincott-Raven, 1998.

phase of the clonic movement complex described previously. Healthy preterm infants commonly exhibit myoclonic movements without seizures or a brain disorder. EEG is therefore recommended to confirm the coincident appearance of electrographic discharges with these movements (Fig. 55-4A). Pathologic myoclonus in the absence of EEG seizure patterns also can occur in severely ill preterm or full-term infants after severe brain dysfunction or damage.[27] As in older children and adults, myoclonus in newborns may reflect injury at multiple levels of the neuraxis from the spine and brain stem to cortical regions. Stimulus-evoked myoclonus with either single coincident spike discharges or sustained electrographic seizures have been reported (see Fig. 55-4A and B).[28] An extensive evaluation must be initiated to exclude metabolic, structural, and genetic causes. In rare cases, healthy sleeping neonates exhibit abundant myoclonus, which subsides with arousal to the waking state[29,30]; this condition is termed **benign sleep myoclonus of the newborn.**

Nonepileptic Behaviors of Neonates

Specific nonepileptic neonatal movement repertoires continually challenge the physician's attempt to reach an accurate diagnosis of seizures and avoid the unnecessary use of antiepileptic drugs (AEDs). Coincident synchronized video/EEG/polygraphic recordings are now the suggested diagnostic tools to confirm the temporal relationship between the suspect clinical phenomena and electrographic expression of seizures.[31] The following three examples of nonepileptic movement disorders incorporate a new classification scheme,[9] based on the absence of coincident EEG seizure patterns.

Tremulousness or Jitteriness with EEG Correlates

Tremors are frequently misidentified as clonic activity by inexperienced health care providers. Unlike the unequal phases of clonic movements described previously, the flexion and extension phases of tremor are equal in amplitude. Children are generally alert or hyperalert but may also appear somnolent or lethargic. Passive flexion and repositioning of the affected tremulous body part diminishes or eliminates the movement. Such movements are usually spontaneous but can be provoked by tactile stimulation. This movement may also appear asymmetric, with suppression in the weak limb from stroke or neuropathy. Metabolic or toxin-induced encephalopathies, including mild asphyxia, drug withdrawal, hypoglycemia-hypocalcemia, intracranial hemorrhage, hypothermia, and growth restriction are common clinical scenarios when such movements occur. Neonatal tremors generally diminish with increasing postconception age. For example, excessive tremulousness in 38 full-term infants resolved spontaneously over a 6-week period, and 92% of the children were neurologically normal at 3 years of age.[32] Medications are rarely considered to treat this particular movement disorder.[33]

Neonatal Myoclonus without EEG-Confirmed Seizures

Myoclonic movements can be bilateral and synchronous or asymmetric and asynchronous in appearance. Clusters of myoclonic activity occur more predominantly during active (REM) sleep and are more predominant in the preterm infant (see Fig. 55-4B),[14,34] although they can occur in healthy full-term infants. Benign myoclonic movements are not stimulus sensitive, have no coincident electrographic seizure correlates, and are not associated with EEG background abnormalities. When these movements occur in a healthy full-term neonate, the activity is suppressed during wakefulness. The clinical description of benign neonatal sleep myoclonus must be a diagnosis of exclusion, after a careful consideration of pathologic diagnoses.[29]

Infants with severe central nervous system dysfunction also may present with nonepileptic spontaneous or stimulus-evoked pathologic myoclonus. Neonates with different forms of metabolic encephalopathies such as glycine encephalopathy, cerebrovascular lesions, brain infections, or congenital malformations may present with nonepileptic pathologic myoclonus (see Fig. 55-4C).[27] Encephalopathic neonates may respond to tactile or

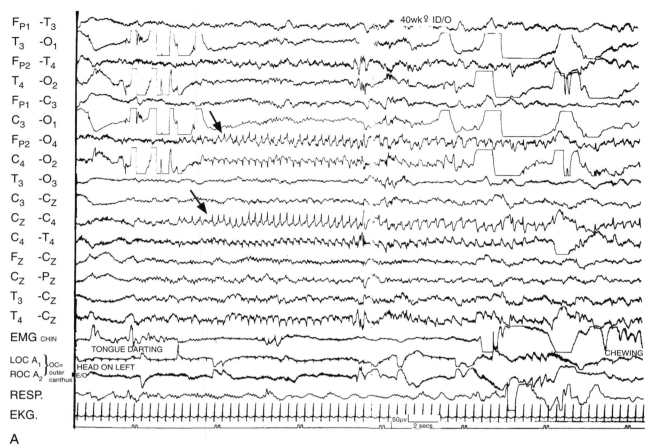

A

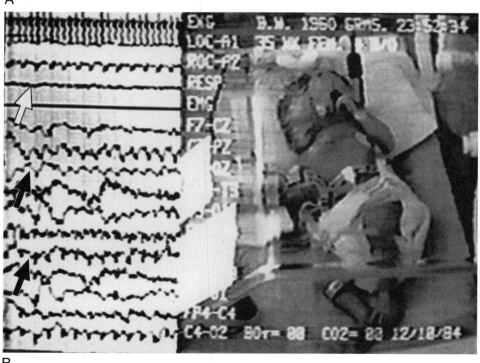

B

Figure 55–1. A, Electroencephalographic (EEG) segment recorded in a 1-day-old girl, born at 40 gestational weeks, after severe asphyxia resulting from rupture of velamentous insertion of the umbilical cord during delivery. An electrical seizure in the right central/midline region is recorded *(arrows)* coincident with buccolingual and eye movements (see comments and eye channels on record). **B,** Synchronized video/EEG recorded in a 1-day-old girl, born at 35 gestational weeks, with *Escherichia coli* meningitis and cerebral abscesses. The *white arrow* notes apnea coincident with prominent right hemispheric and midline electrographic seizures *(black arrows).* In addition to apnea, other motoric signs coincident to EEG seizures were noted at other times during the record. *(A, From Scher MS, Painter MJ: Electrographic diagnosis of neonatal seizures. Issues of diagnostic accuracy, clinical correlation and survival. In Wasterlain CG, Vert P [eds]: Neonatal Seizures. New York, Raven Press, 1990, p 17. B, From Scher MS, Painter MJ: Controversies concerning neonatal seizures. Pediatr Clin North Am 36:288, 1989.)*

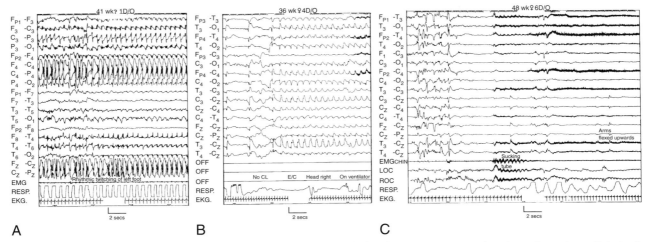

Figure 55-2. **A,** Electroencephalographic (EEG) segment recorded in a 1-day-old boy, born at 41 gestational weeks, with an electroclinical seizure characterized by rhythmic clonic movements of the left foot coincident with bihemispheric electrographic discharges of higher amplitude in the right hemisphere. This seizure was documented before antiepileptic medication. **B,** EEG segment recorded in a 4-day-old girl, born at 25 gestational weeks, with an electrographic seizure pattern without clinical accompaniments. **C,** Segment of an EEG of a 6-day-old infant, born at 40 gestational weeks, with stereotypic flexion posturing in the absence of electrographically confirmed seizures (note muscle artifact). *(From Scher MS: Pediatric electroencephalography and evoked potentials. In Swaiman KS [ed]: Pediatric Neurology: Principles and Practice. St. Louis, CV Mosby, 1999, p 164.)*

painful stimulation by isolated focal, segmental, or generalized myoclonic movements. In rare cases, cortically generated spike- or sharp-wave discharges, as well as seizures, that are coincident with these myoclonic movements may also be noted on the EEG recordings (Fig. 55-5).[35] Medication-induced myoclonus and other stereotypic movements have also been described[36]; they resolve when the responsible drug is withdrawn.

A rare familial disorder has been described in the neonatal and early infancy periods, specifically termed **hyperexplexia.** These movements usually are misinterpreted as a hyperactive startle reflex. Infants are stiff, with severe hypertonia that may lead to apnea and bradycardia. Forced flexion of the neck or hips sometimes alleviates these events. EEG background rhythms are generally age appropriate. The postulated defect for these individuals involves regulation of brain stem centers that facilitate myoclonic movements,[37] but molecular defects of ion channels are also considered. On occasion, benzodiazepines or valproic acid lessens the startling, stiffening, or falling events.[38] Neurologic prognosis is reported to be variable.

Neonatal Dystonia without EEG-Confirmed Seizures

Dystonia is a third commonly misdiagnosed movement disorder that is often misrepresented as tonic seizures. Dystonia can be associated either with acute or chronic disease states involving basal ganglia structures or with the extrapyramidal pathways that innervate these regions. Antepartum or intrapartum adverse events caused by severe asphyxia (e.g., **status marmoratus**)[12] or, in rare cases, by specific inherited metabolic diseases[39,40] (e.g., glutaric aciduria) result in injury to these structures. Alternatively, posturing may reflect the subcortical motor pathways that become functionally unopposed

because of diseased or malformed neocortex (Fig. 55-6).[26] Electrographic documentation of seizures by synchronized video/EEG/polygraphic recordings helps avoid misdiagnosis and inappropriate treatment.

Electrographic Seizure Criteria

Electrographic/polysomnographic studies have become invaluable tools for the assessment of suspected seizures.[2,7,9,25,31,41,42] Technical and interpretative skills of normal and abnormal neonatal EEG sleep patterns must be mastered before the examiner can reliably recognize seizures.[13,14,43-45]

Corroboration with the EEG technologist is always an essential part of the diagnostic process, because physiologic and nonphysiologic artifacts can masquerade as seizures on EEG. The physician must also anticipate expected behaviors with regard to specific gestational maturity, medication use, and state of arousal, in the context of potential artifacts. Synchronized video/EEG/polygraphic documentation permits careful off-line analysis for more accurate documentation.

As with epileptic older children and adults, it is generally accepted that the epileptic seizure is a clinical paroxysm of altered brain function with the simultaneous presence of an electrographic event on an EEG recording. Therefore, in assessing the suspected clinical event in the neonate, synchronized video/EEG/polygraphic monitoring is useful for distinguishing an epileptic event from a nonepileptic event. Some authors advocate the use of single-channel computerized devices for continuous prolonged monitoring,[46] in view of the multiple logistical problems inherent with the use of conventional multichannel recording devices. This specific device may, nonetheless, fail to detect focal or regional seizures if the single-channel recording is not near the brain region

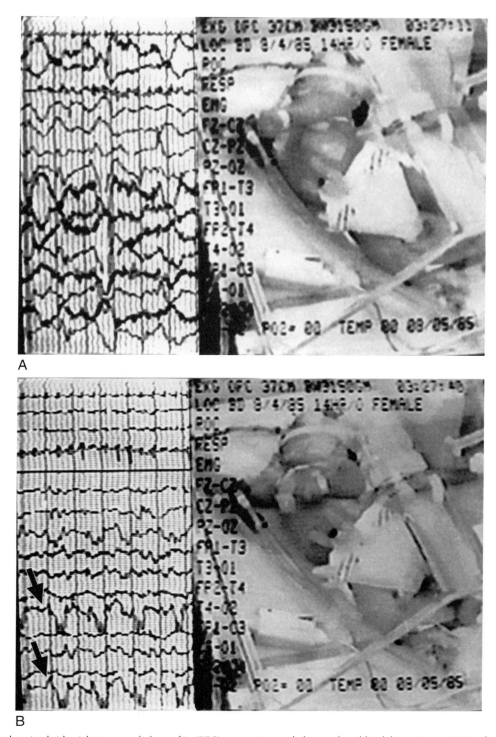

Figure 55–3. A, Synchronized video/electroencephalographic (EEG) segment recorded in a 1-day-old girl, born at 37 gestational weeks, who suffered asphyxia, demonstrating prominent opisthotonos with left arm extension in the absence of coincident electrographic seizure activity. **B,** Synchronized video/EEG record of the same patient as in *A,* documenting electrographic seizure activity in the right posterior quadrant *(arrows),* after cessation of left arm tonic movements and persistent opisthotonos. *(B, From Scher MS, Painter MJ: Controversies concerning neonatal seizures. Pediatr Clin North Am 36:292, 1989.)*

Continued

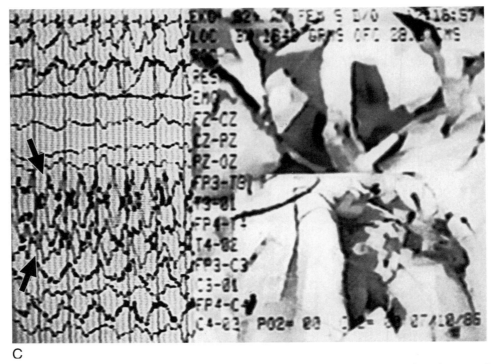

Figure 55–3, cont'd. C, Segment of a video/EEG recording documenting a fixed tonic neck reflex with coincident electrographic seizure activity in the temporal regions *(arrows)*, described as a tonic seizure.

involved with seizure expression. For example, one study reported that suspected seizures in fewer than 3 per 10 neonates monitored by a single-channel device could be verified by conventional EEG.[47] Others have suggested that a four-channel EEG monitoring device can more efficiently detect seizures, which can then be verified by continuous video/EEG/polygraphic telemetry.[48]

Epilepsy monitoring services for older children and adults readily utilize intracerebral or surface electrocorticography to detect seizures. Such recording strategies, however, are not ethically appropriate or practical for the neonatal patient. As a consequence, it is difficult to definitively eliminate subcortical foci from consideration, as discussed later.

Ictal EEG Patterns: A More Reliable Marker for Seizure Onset, Duration, and Severity

Neonatal EEG seizure patterns commonly consist of a repetitive sequence of waveforms that evolve in frequency, amplitude, electrical field, and/or structure. Four types of ictal patterns have been described: focal ictal patterns with normal background, focal patterns with abnormal background, multifocal ictal patterns,[44] and focal monorhythmic periodic patterns of various frequencies. It is generally suggested that a minimal duration of 10 seconds for the evolution of discharges is necessary to distinguish electrographic seizures from repetitive but nonictal epileptiform discharges (see Figs. 55-1A, 55-2A, and 55-2B).[7,36,49] Clinical neurophysiologists separately

classify brief or prolonged repetitive discharges that lack an electrographic evolution as nonictal abnormal epileptiform patterns but not confirmatory of seizures.[50] The unique features of neonatal electrographic seizure duration and topography are discussed as follows.

Seizure duration and topography. Few studies have quantified minimal or maximal seizure durations in neonates.[7,49,51] Most notably, the definition of the most severe expression of seizures, status epilepticus, which potentially promotes brain injury, can be problematic. In older patients, status epilepticus is defined as at least 30 minutes of continuous seizures or as two consecutive seizures with an interictal period during which the patient fails to return to full consciousness. This definition is not easily applied to the neonate, for whom the level of arousal may be difficult to assess, particularly if sedative medications are given. One study arbitrarily defined neonatal status epilepticus as continuous seizure activity for at least 30 minutes, or 50% of the recording time[51]; 11 (32.3%) of 34 full-term infants had status epilepticus with a mean duration of 29.6 minutes before AED use; another 3 (9%) of the 34 preterm infants also had status epilepticus with an average duration of 5.2 minutes per seizure (i.e., 50% of the recording time). The mean seizure duration was longer in full-term infants (5 minutes) than in preterm infants (2.7 minutes). Because more than 20% of this study group fit the criteria for status epilepticus according to EEG documentation,

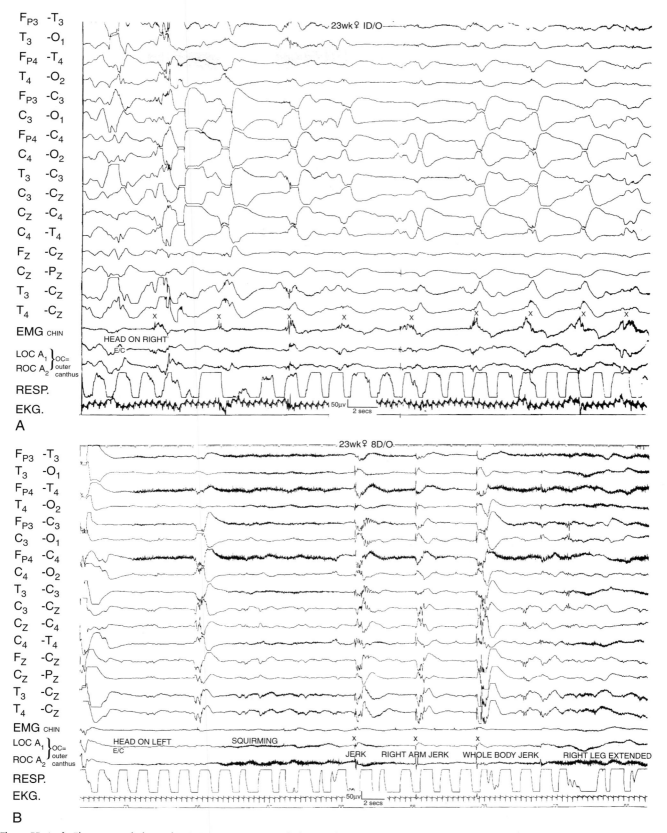

Figure 55–4. A, Electroencephalographic (EEG) segment recorded in a 1-day-old girl, born at 23 gestational weeks, with grade III intraventricular hemorrhage and progressive ventriculomegaly. An electroclinical seizure is noted with coincident myoclonic movements of the diaphragm *(x marks).* **B,** EEG segment recorded in an asymptomatic 8-day-old girl, born at 23 gestational weeks, with spontaneous generalized focal myoclonus but without electrographic discharges other than myogenic spike potentials. *(**A,** From Scher MS: Pathological myoclonus of the newborn: Electrographic and clinical correlations. Pediatr Neurol 1:342, 1985.)* *Continued*

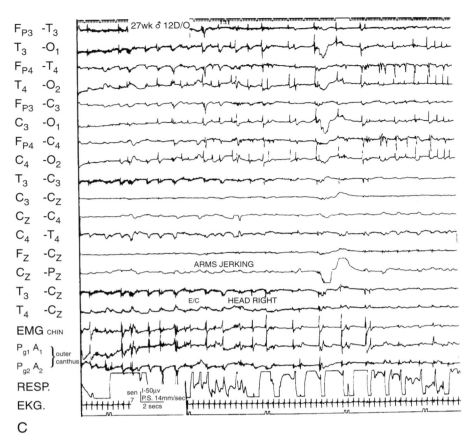

Figure 55–4, cont'd. C, EEG segment recorded in an encephalopathic 12-day-old boy, born at 27 gestational weeks, with herpes encephalitis who exhibits nonepileptic multifocal myoclonus (myogenic potentials as EEG artifacts).

concerns must be raised regarding the underdiagnosis of the more severe form of seizures that potentially contribute to brain injury, if only clinical criteria are applied. This subject is explored in the later section regarding the consequences of seizures on brain development.

Uncoupling of the clinical and electrographic expressions of neonatal seizures after AED administration also contributes to an underestimation of the true seizure duration, including status epilepticus (Fig. 55-7). One study estimated that 25% of neonates expressed persistent electrographic seizures despite resolution of their clinical seizure behaviors after receiving AEDs[52]; this scenario is termed **electroclinical uncoupling.** Other pathophysiologic mechanisms besides medication effect also might explain uncoupling.[10]

Most neonatal electrographic seizures arise focally from one brain region. Generalized synchronous and symmetric repetitive discharges can also occur. In one study, 56% of seizures were seen in a single location at onset; specific sites included temporal-occipital (15%), temporal-central (15%), central (10%), frontotemporal central (6%), frontotemporal (5%), and vertex (5%). Multiple locations at the onset of the electrographic seizures were noted in 44%.[7] Electrographic discharges may be expressed as specific EEG frequency ranges from fast to slow, including β, α, θ, or δ activities. Multiple electrographic seizures can also be expressed independently in anatomically unrelated brain regions.

Periodic discharges and prolonged repetitive discharges: ictal or interictal? Clinical neurophysiologists distinguish periodic nonseizure EEG patterns from electrographic seizure patterns for patient populations of varying ages. As with older patients, the neonate may express or sustain repetitive or periodic discharges that do not satisfy electrographic criteria for seizures (Fig. 55-8A). Sustained periodic lateralized epileptiform discharges (PLEDs) of 10 minutes, or 20% of the recording time (i.e., defined as PLEDs on recordings of older children and adults), are rarely noted in newborns.[53] This particular repetitive pattern of electrographic discharges in older patients is commonly associated with acute brain injuries from stroke, hemorrhage, or trauma and may also follow or precede electrographically confirmed seizures. Periodic discharges are less commonly noted in neonates (i.e., 5% of the 1114 neonatal recordings); PLEDs were noted in only 4 of 34 infants.[53] In most newborns with periodic discharges, the events were expressed as having shorter durations than classically defined PLEDs. However, nearly half of neonates with periodic discharges also expressed electrographic seizure patterns at other times during the same EEG recording. Cerebrovascular lesions were the most common brain lesions in 53% (18 of 34) of this group of newborns.[53] Periodic lateralized epileptiform discharges for 26 preterm neonates lasted less than 60 seconds and were located in the parasagittal regions, whereas discharges in 8 full-term neonates were longer

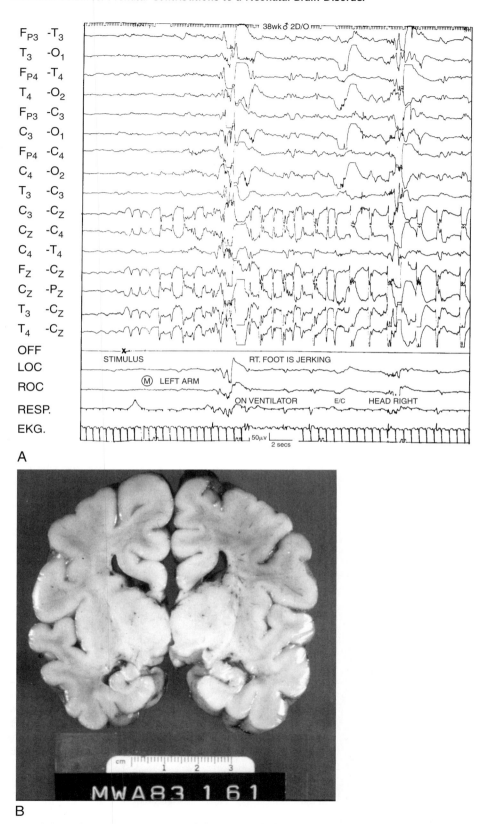

Figure 55–5. A, Electroencephalographic (EEG) segment recorded in a 2-day-old boy, born at 38 gestational weeks, with glycine encephalopathy who had stimulus-sensitive generalized and multifocal myoclonus. Note the onset of a midline (C_z onset) electrographic seizure pattern with a painful stimulus, followed by right foot myoclonus. **B,** Coronal section of the brain of the patient described in *A,* with agenesis of the corpus callosum, bat-winged shape of lateral ventricles. Spongy myelinosis was noted on microscopic examination. *(From Scher MS: Pathological myoclonus of the newborn: Electrographic and clinical correlations. Pediatr Neurol 1:342-348, 1985.)*

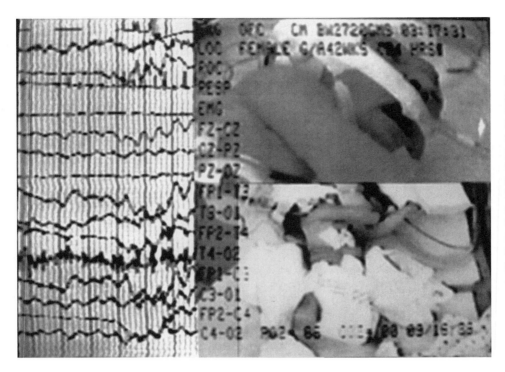

Figure 55–6. Video/electroencephalographic (EEG) segment recorded in a growth-restricted girl less than 24 hours after birth at 42 gestational weeks, demonstrating stereotypic posturing and eye opening with no coincident electrographic seizure activity. The child presented with non-immune hydrops fetalis and with significant neocortical injury from a fetal period. The EEG background is markedly slow and suppressed, representing a severe interictal electrographic abnormality. *(From Scher MS: Seizures in the newborn infant. Clin Perinatol 24:74, 1997.)*

than a minute and located in the temporal regions. Of the 34 neonates, 15 (44%) died; of the 19 infants who survived, 11 (58%) had neurologic sequelae.[53] Therefore, neonates with periodic discharges identified on EEG recordings require aggressive investigation for underlying brain injuries and prognostic considerations for neurologic sequelae, independent of the decision to treat with AEDs.

Brief rhythmic discharges: Ictal or interictal? At the opposite end of the spectrum from periodic discharges, brief rhythmic discharges that are less than 10 seconds in duration have also been addressed with regard to an association with seizures and outcome (see Fig. 55-8*B*). Neonates with electrographic seizure patterns may also exhibit these brief discharges; other neonates express only isolated discharges without seizures. Neonates with

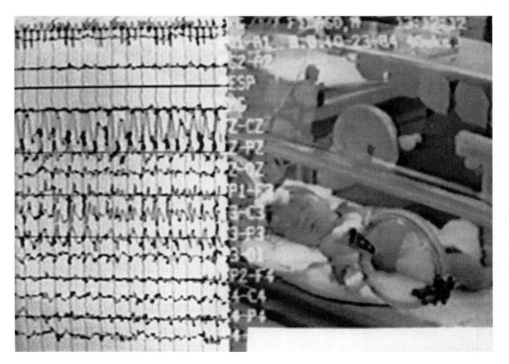

Figure 55–7. Synchronized video/electroencephalographic (EEG) segment recorded in a 1-day-old boy, born at 40 gestational weeks, with electrographic status epilepticus noted in the left central/midline regions, after administration of antiepileptic medication. Focal right shoulder clonic activity was only intermittently noted, but continuous electrographic seizure patterns were documented mostly without clinical expression. This phenomenon of uncoupling of electrical and clinical seizure activities is associated with the use of antiepileptic medication (see text). *(From Scher MS, Painter MJ: Controversies concerning neonatal seizures. Pediatr Clin North Am 36:290, 1989.)*

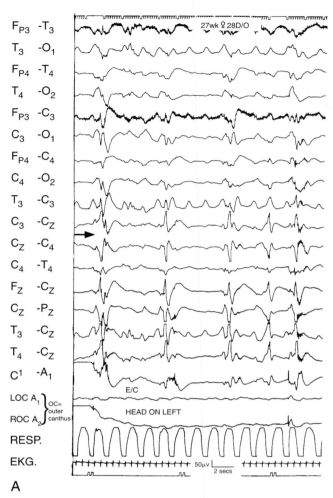

Figure 55–8. A, Electroencephalographic (EEG) segment recorded in a 28-day-old girl, born at 27 gestational weeks, with intraventricular hemorrhage and periventricular leukomalacia. Continuous discharges in the midline region (C_z electrode, *arrow*) composed of periodic positive sharp waves without an evolution of discharges noted with seizures. (*A,* From Scher MS: Seizures in the newborn infant. Clin Perinatol 24:247, 1997.)   *Continued*

brief discharges may suffer from hypoglycemia or periventricular leukomalacia, which carries a higher risk for neurodevelopmental delay.[54] These children do not benefit from the use of AEDs.

SUBCORTICAL SEIZURES VERSUS NONICTAL FUNCTIONAL DECORTICATION

Experimental animal models offer conflicting neuronal mechanisms to explain clinical events that do not have coincident EEG confirmation. Most clinical neurophysiologists require documentation of an ictal pattern by surface EEG electrodes. However, subcortical seizures with only intermittent propagation to the surface may occur. At the other end of the spectrum, nonictal "brain stem release" phenomena must be considered, particularly if

EEG-confirmed seizures are never expressed.[25] A more integrated electroclinical approach has been suggested for classifying clinical events as seizures, as opposed to nonepileptic movement disorders, on the basis of documentation by synchronized video/EEG/polygraphic monitoring.[9]

Brain Stem Release Phenomena

Synchronized video/EEG/polygraphic monitoring provides the physician with documentation of a suspect event with a concurrent electrographic pattern on surface recordings.[18] The temporal relationship between clinical and electrographic phenomena has been described with the use of synchronized video/EEG/polygraphic monitoring. In 415 clinical seizures in 71 babies, clonic seizure activity had the best correlation with coincident electrographic seizures. "Subtle" clinical events, in contrast, had a more inconsistent relationship with coincident EEG seizure activity, which was suggestive of a nonepileptic brain stem release phenomenon for at least a proportion of such events. Functional decortication resulting from neocortical damage without coincident EEG seizure patterns[25] has therefore been suggested, such as with tonic posturing, as illustrated in Figure 55-3A. Newborns with nonseizure brain stem release activity may express a functional pattern of metabolic dysfunction, detected as altered glucose uptake on single photon emission tomographic studies, different from that of neonates with seizures.[55] A suggestion to document increased prolactin levels in neonates with clinical seizures has also been reported,[56] but such levels have not yet been correlated with electrographic seizure patterns.

Electroclinical Dissociation Suggestive of Subcortical Seizures

Experimental studies of immature animals also support the possibility that subcortical structures may initiate seizures, which subsequently, although intermittently, propagate to the cortical surface.[57-58] Although EEG depth recordings in adults and adolescents help document subcortical seizures both with and without clinical expression, this technology is not applicable to or appropriate for the neonate. Only one anecdotal report of a human infant documented seizures that possibly emanated from deep gray matter structures.[60]

Electroclinical dissociation is one proposed mechanism by which subcortical seizures may only intermittently appear on surface-recorded EEG studies.[11] Electroclinical dissociation has been defined as a reproducible clinical event that occurs both with and without coincidental electrographic seizure patterns. In one group of 51 infants with electroclinical seizures, 33 infants simultaneously expressed both electrical and clinical seizure phenomena. Extremity movements were more significantly associated with synchronized electroclinical seizures. However, a subset of 18 (35.3%) of the 51 neonates also expressed electroclinical dissociation on EEG recordings. For neonates who expressed electroclinical dissociation, the clinical seizure component always preceded the electrographic seizure expression, which suggests that a subcortical focus may have initiated the seizure state. Some of these children also expressed

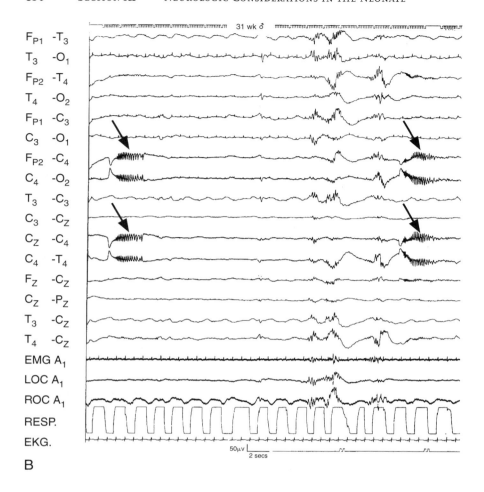

Figure 55–8, cont'd. **B,** EEG segment recorded in a boy born at 31 gestational weeks, with repetitive brief epileptiform discharges in the right central region *(arrows)* that were less than 10 seconds in duration and did not qualify as electrographic seizure activity.

B

synchronized electroclinical seizures, even on the same EEG record.

Controversy remains as to whether the term **subcortical seizures,** in comparison with **nonictal functional decortication,** best categorizes suspect clinical behaviors without coincident EEG seizure documentation. This dilemma should encourage the clinician to use the EEG as a neurophysiologic standard by which more exact seizure start and end points can be assigned, before offering pharmacologic treatment with AEDs.[31] Certain neonates do exhibit electrographic seizures that go undetected unless EEG is utilized.[61-66] Two examples are neonates who are pharmacologically paralyzed for ventilatory assistance (Fig. 55-9A) and those in whom clinical seizures are suppressed by the use of AEDs (see Fig. 55-9B).[7,52,63-66] In one cohort of 92 infants, 60% of whom were pretreated with AEDs, 50% of neonates had electrographic seizures with no clinical accompaniment.[63] Both clinical and electrographic seizure criteria were noted for 45% of 62 preterm infants and 52% of 33 full-term infants. Seventeen infants were pharmacologically paralyzed when the seizure was first documented on EEG. Of a later cohort of 60 infants, none of whom was pretreated with AEDs, 7% had only electrographic seizure patterns before AED administration,[52] and 25% expressed electroclinical uncoupling after AED use.

The underestimation of seizures in the newborn period may also result from inadequate monitoring for specific neurologic signs. Autonomic changes in respirations, blood pressure, oxygenation, heart rate, pupillary size, skin color, and salivation are examples of subtle ictal signs (Fig. 55-10). In one study, autonomic seizures accompanied electrographic seizures in 37% of 19 preterm neonates.[63] Newer classifications of neonatal seizures emphasize documentation of autonomic findings on EEG recordings.[9]

Variation in the Incidence of Neonatal Seizures, Based on Clinical versus EEG Criteria

Overestimation and underestimation of neonatal seizures are consequentially reported whether clinical or electrical criteria are used. According to clinical criteria, seizure incidences ranged from 0.5% among full-term infants to 22.2% among preterm neonates.[67-70] Discrepancies in incidence reflect not only varying postconception ages of the study populations chosen but also poor interobserver reliability[71] and the hospital setting in which the diagnosis was made. Hospital-based studies that include high-risk deliveries generally report higher incidences of seizures.[63] Population studies that include less medically ill infants from general nurseries report lower percentages.[72] Incidence data based only on clinical

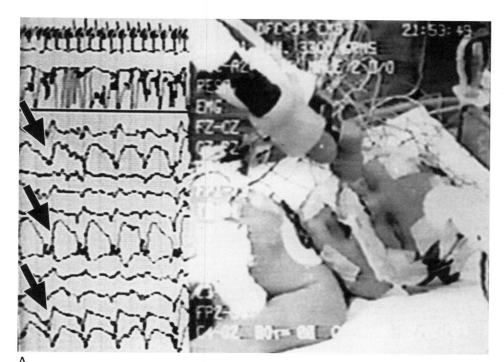

A

Figure 55–9. **A,** Synchronized video/electroencephalographic (EEG) segment recorded in a 2-day-old boy, born at 38 gestational weeks, who was pharmacologically paralyzed for ventilatory care with cerebral infarctions. A seizure was noted in the right posterior quadrant and midline *(arrows).* **B,** EEG segment recorded with cerebral infarctions in a 3-day-old girl, born at 37 gestational weeks, after antiepileptic drug use, with multifocal electrical seizures in the δ frequency range in the temporal and midline regions. Note the marked suppression of normal EEG background. *(**A,** From Scher MS, Painter MJ: Controversies concerning neonatal seizures. Pediatr Clin North Am 36:287, 1989. **B,** From Scher MS: Neonatal seizures. Seizures in special clinical settings. In Wyllie E [ed]: The Treatment of Epilepsy. Principles and Practice, 2nd ed. Baltimore, Williams & Wilkins, 1997, p 608.)*

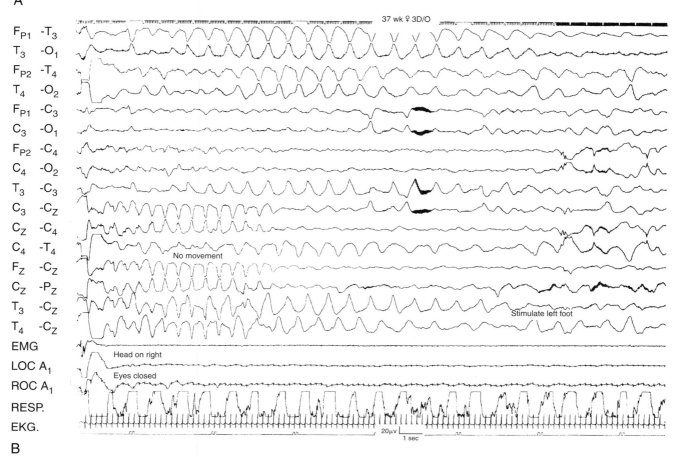

B

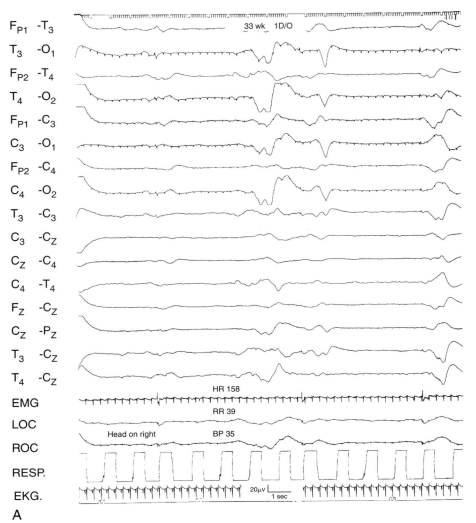

Figure 55–10. A and **B,** Electroencephalographic (EEG) segments recorded in a 1-day-old boy, born at 31 gestational weeks with asphyxial injury to the white matter, documenting drops in heart rate and blood pressure measurements after the onset of an electrographically confirmed seizure.

Continued

criteria without EEG confirmation include "false-positive" findings, consisting of either normal or nonepileptic pathologic neonatal behaviors. Conversely, the absence of scalp-generated EEG seizure patterns may include a subset of "false-negative" findings in which infants express seizures only from subcortical brain regions without expression on the cortical surface. Closer consensus between clinical and EEG criteria is still needed for a more comprehensive classification schema.

Interictal EEG Pattern Abnormalities

Interictal EEG abnormalities (including nonictal repetitive epileptiform discharges) have important prognostic implications for both preterm and full-term infants.[73,74] Severely abnormal bihemispheric patterns include the burst-suppression (i.e., paroxysmal) pattern (Fig. 55-11), electrocerebral inactivity, low-voltage invariant pattern (see Fig. 55-4C), persistently slow background pattern (see Fig. 55-6), multifocal sharp waves, and marked asynchrony.[75] For infants with hypoxic-ischemic encephalopathy (HIE), subclassifications of specific EEG patterns such as burst-suppression with or without reactivity

may give a more accurate prediction of outcome.[76] Dysmaturity of the EEG sleep background that is inappropriate for child's corrected age has also been an important feature to recognize; discordance between cerebral and noncerebral components of sleep state, or immaturity of EEG patterns for the given postconceptional age of the infant, are predictive of a higher risk for neurologic sequelae.[4,77-79] Even focal or regional pattern abnormalities have prognostic significance, such as with preterm infants who express repetitive positive sharp waves at the midline or central regions (see Fig. 55-8A), often noted with intraventricular hemorrhage (IVH) and periventricular leukomalacia.[13]

Screening infants at risk for neonatal seizures with a routine EEG soon after birth enables identification of more severe interictal EEG background abnormalities that are predictive of seizure occurrence on subsequent neonatal EEG recordings.[80]

Interictal EEG findings are not pathognomonic for particular causes, pathophysiologic mechanisms, or timing.[4] Historical information, physical examination findings, and laboratory results need to be integrated with

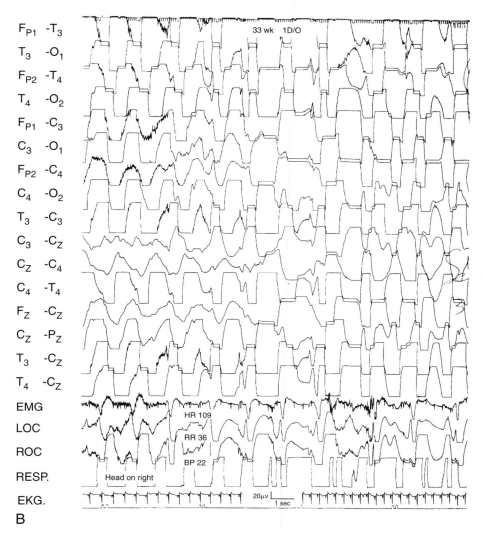

Figure 55–10, cont'd.

B

the electrographic interpretation of both ictal and interictal pattern abnormalities for the particular child. Serial EEG studies better assist the clinician in diagnostic and prognostic interpretations.[73,74] As with the documentation of abnormal examination findings into the second week of life, the persistence of electrographic abnormalities on recordings after 1 week of age also raises prognostic concerns. In other words, the newborn who expresses severe EEG abnormalities into the second week of life has a greater likelihood for neurologic impairment, despite the apparent resolution of clinical dysfunction. Conversely, the child who rapidly recovers from a significant brain disorder, with the reemergence of normal EEG features during the first few days after birth, may suffer comparatively less neurologic sequelae. Interictal EEG pattern abnormalities may also reflect brain disorders that precede labor and delivery. The depth and the severity of the neonatal brain disorder (defined by clinical and electrographic criteria) may therefore reflect chronic injury to the fetus, who subsequently becomes symptomatic after a stressful intrapartum period, with or without more recent injury.

DIAGNOSTIC DILEMMAS: CLINICAL SCENARIOS OF NEONATES WITH SUSPECTED SEIZURES

Diverse medical conditions of the newborn can be associated with seizure activity (Table 55-5).[2,81] However, neonatal brain disorders may also result from the same conditions without seizure expression; therefore, diagnostic and/or therapeutic approaches may not require AED administration. In one prospective study of 157 infants screened by EEG for possible seizures on the basis of seven clinical inclusion criteria before AED use, only 60 (38%) of 157 neonates had EEG confirmation of seizures,[82] despite the initial clinical concern for a brain disorder. Clinical behaviors possibly indicative of seizures in 88 (56%) of the children constituted the most frequent screening criterion. Twenty-seven percent of the children had suffered asphyxia; 9% and 6%, respectively, had prenatal drug exposure or central nervous system infection; and 2% had central nervous system malformations. None of the latter three groups included suspect behaviors. No neonates who were initially screened experienced

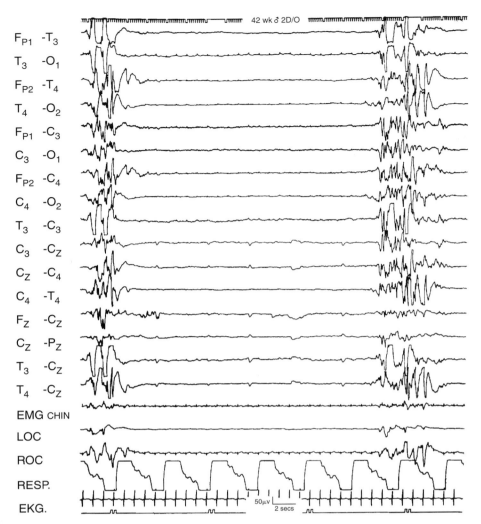

42 wk ♂ 2D/O

Figure 55–11. Electroencephalographic (EEG) segment recorded in a 2-day-old boy, born at 42 gestational weeks, expressing a severely abnormal interictal EEG background abnormality known as a burst-suppression or paroxysmal pattern.

cerebral trauma or were pharmacologically paralyzed for ventilatory management. For the segment of the cohort with suspect behavior, only 49% (43 of 88) had EEG confirmation of seizures, 30% of whom required multiple EEG studies before EEG seizures were documented. Specifically, of the 41 infants with asphyxia, only 12 (29%) had EEG confirmation of seizures; of the 12 infants presenting with asphyxia, 6 (50%) received diagnoses on subsequent EEG studies after an initially negative first EEG study. Surprisingly, of the 60 neonates with EEG-confirmed seizures, 45% had no clinical signs of a brain disorder at delivery. Eighteen were transferred to the neonatal intensive care unit from well-child nurseries because of isolated seizures without encephalopathies. Nine asymptomatic newborns with isolated seizures later expressed postnatal illnesses from central nervous system infection, sepsis, or severe pulmonary disease.

Similarly, in another study of 40 neonates with clinical seizures, only 37.5% of cases were associated with asphyxia, whereas the majority of these full-term infants had early-onset seizures, not preventable from antepartum or intrapartum time periods, that were caused by malformation, infarction, infection, or intracranial hemorrhage.[83]

Major Causes of Seizures: Multiple Overlapping Conditions along a Variable Timeline

Neonatal seizures are not disease specific, and they can be associated with a variety of medical conditions that occur before, during, or after parturition. Asphyxia is one frequently diagnosed entity associated with seizures. However, this condition illustrates the dilemma of overlapping medical conditions over multiple time points. Seizures may occur as part of an asphyxial brain disorder that is documented after birth (HIE) but began before the mother entered the hospital and resulted from maternal, placental, or fetal disease. One logistic model for predicting clinical seizures emphasized the accumulation of both antepartum and intrapartum factors that increase the likelihood of neonatal seizure occurrence.[84] Whereas these factors separately had low positive predictive values, a significant cumulative risk profile included antepartum maternal anemia, bleeding, and asthma; meconium-stained amniotic fluid; abnormal fetal presentation; fetal

Table 55–5. Selected Differential Diagnosis of Neonatal Seizures*

Metabolic

Hypoxia-ischemia (i.e., asphyxia)
    Hypoglycemia
    Hypocalcemia
    Hypomagnesemia
Hypoglycemia
    Intrauterine growth restriction
    Infant of a diabetic mother
    Glycogen storage disease
    Galactosemia
    Idiopathic
Hypocalcemia
    Hypomagnesemia
    Infant of a diabetic mother
    Neonatal hypoparathyroidism
    Maternal hyperparathyroidism
    High phosphate load
Other electrolyte imbalances
    Hypernatremia
    Hyponatremia

Intracranial Hemorrhage

Subarachnoid hemorrhage
Subdural/epidural hematoma
Intraventricular hemorrhage

Cerebrovascular Lesions (Other than Trauma)

Cerebral infarction (thrombotic versus embolic)
    Ischemic versus hemorrhagic
Cortical vein thrombosis
Circulatory disturbances from hypoperfusion

Trauma

Infections

Bacterial meningitis
Virus-induced encephalitis

Congenital infections
    Herpes
    Cytomegalovirus
    Toxoplasmosis
    Syphilis
    Coxsackie meningoencephalitis
    Acquired immunodeficiency syndrome (AIDS)
Brain abscess

Brain Anomalies (e.g., Cerebral Dysgenesis from either Congenital or Acquired Causes)

Drug Withdrawal or Toxins

Prenatal substance: methadone, heroin, barbiturate, cocaine, etc.
Prescribed medications: propoxyphene, isoniazid
Local anesthetics

Hypertensive Encephalopathy

Amino Acid Metabolism

Branched-chain amino acidopathies
Urea cycle abnormalities
Nonketotic hyperglycinemia
Ketotic hyperglycinemia

Familial Seizures

Neurocutaneous syndromes
    Tuberous sclerosis
    Incontinentia pigmenti
Autosomal dominant neonatal seizures

Selected Genetic Syndromes

Zellweger syndrome
Neonatal adrenoleukodystrophy
Smith-Lemli-Opitz syndrome

*Etiology independent of timing from fetal to neonatal periods.

Adapted from Scher MS: Seizures in the newborn infant. Diagnosis, treatment and outcome. Clin Perinatol 24:735, 1997.

distress; and shoulder dystocia. In another study using a regression model, however, the clinical neurologic depression of the child at birth and the requirement for neonatal intensive care were the most important risk factors associated with early clinical or EEG-confirmed seizures (i.e., <72 hours after birth) in full-term infants.[85]

Neonatal encephalopathy may not be caused by intrapartum asphyxia, as noted in a matched case-control study of 89 full-term infants.[86] Although these newborns appeared encephalopathic with seizures, altered arousal, and tone abnormalities, as well as feeding problems or central apnea, logistic regression analysis identified antepartum causes as the best explanation for the neonatal encephalopathy. In another study of 100 neonates with clinical seizures, several antepartum factors significantly increased the odds ratios, including high maternal weight gain, placental disorders, and preeclampsia, even though HIE was the most common cause in 30%,[87] independent of timing of injury.

Hypoxia-ischemia (i.e., asphyxia) is traditionally considered the most common cause associated with neonatal

seizures.[12,42,88-91] However, in children, asphyxia generally occurs either before or during parturition; only 10% of cases of asphyxia result from postnatal causes.[12] When asphyxia is suspected during the labor and delivery process, biochemical confirmation can be attempted. However, only a minority of cases of asphyxia at birth are associated with seizures, as part of a neonatal brain disorder, HIE. For example, diagnoses were later established in only 29% of one cohort who fulfilled an arbitrary biochemical definition of intrapartum asphyxia (i.e., pH ≤7.2 and a base deficit of −10 or less), with seizures confirmed by EEG.[82]

Intrauterine factors before labor can result in fetal asphyxia without later documentation of acidosis at birth. Maternal illnesses such as thrombophilia, preeclampsia, or specific uteroplacental abnormalities such as abruptio placentae, cord compression, or chorangiosis may contribute to fetal asphyxial stress without providing the opportunity to document in utero acidosis. Antepartum maternal trauma or chorioamnionitis can also contribute to the intrauterine asphyxia secondary to uteroplacental insufficiency.

Intravascular placental thromboses and infarction of the placenta or umbilical cord, noted on placental examinations, are additional surrogate markers for possible fetal asphyxia. Meconium passage into the amniotic fluid also promotes an inflammatory response within the placental membranes, causing vasoconstriction and resultant asphyxia.[92] Neuroimaging may later define the chronic destructive brain lesions that resulted from old in utero asphyxia, with or without HIE expressed after birth.[93,94] Therefore, asphyxia-induced brain injury may result from maternal-fetal-placental diseases that are manifested after birth as neonatal seizures, independent of the documentation of acidosis at birth and the evolving HIE syndrome in the first 3 to 5 days after birth.

Postnatal medical illnesses also cause or contribute to asphyxia-induced brain injury and seizures, independent of the events of labor and delivery. Persistent pulmonary hypertension of the newborn (PPHN), cyanotic congenital heart disease, sepsis, and meningitis are principal diagnoses. In one hospital-based study over a 14-year period, 62 of 247 infants presented with EEG-confirmed seizures after an uneventful delivery without fetal distress during labor or neurologic depression at birth. Of these 62 infants, 20 (32%) later presented with postnatal onset of pulmonary disease, sepsis, or meningitis[2]; the remainder had only isolated neonatal seizures without an accompanying encephalopathy.

A case-controlled study of full-term infants with clinical seizures reported a fourfold increase in the risk of unexplained early-onset seizures after intrapartum fever. All known causes of seizures were eliminated, including meningitis or sepsis. These 38 newborns, in comparison with 152 controls, experienced intrapartum fever as an independent risk factor on logistic regression that predicted seizures. The authors speculated on the role of circulating maternal cytokines, which triggered "physiologic events" contributing to seizures.[95]

The American College of Obstetrics and Gynecology published guidelines that suggest criteria to define postasphyxial neonatal encephalopathy (i.e., HIE)[96] after significant clinical neurologic depression noted at birth. These guidelines include the following:

1. Profound umbilical metabolic or mixed acidemia with a pH less than 7.00.
2. Persistence of an Apgar score of 0 to 3 for longer than 5 minutes.
3. Neonatal neurologic sequelae (i.e., seizures, coma, and hypotonia)
4. Multiorgan system dysfunction (i.e., significant cardiovascular, gastrointestinal, hematologic, pulmonary, and renal involvement).

Postasphyxial encephalopathy is a clinical syndrome that evolves over days after neonatal neurologic depression during which neonatal seizures may occur, usually in children who also exhibit severe early metabolic acidosis, hypoglycemia or hypocalcemia, and multiorgan dysfunction.[12,91] However, other epiphenomena accompanying asphyxia may also contribute to seizures. Of 142 infants with seizures after asphyxia, 80 had trauma or intracranial hemorrhage[89,90]; the remaining 62 had brain damage from other neurologic diagnoses besides asphyxia.

The physical examination findings in the infant with HIE and seizures consist principally of coma, hypotonia, brain stem abnormalities, and loss of fetal reflexes. Postasphyxial seizures generally occur within the first 3 days of life, depending on the length and degree of asphyxial stress during the intrapartum period.[12] An early occurrence of seizures, within several hours after delivery, however, sometimes suggests an antepartum occurrence of a fetal brain disorder, when compared with specific fetal heart rate pattern abnormalities.[97] By itself, however, seizure onset is not a reliable indicator of timing of fetal brain injury. Earlier seizure onset, within 4 hours after birth, in encephalopathic newborns may also be predictive of severe adverse outcome, independent of the cause of asphyxia.[98]

Asphyxia is conventionally diagnosed based on the association of several metabolic parameters on an umbilical or serum blood gas; a reduced O_2 pressure level of less than 40 mm Hg indicates a severe disturbance of oxygen exchange, often associated with acidosis. The duration of asphyxia, however, is difficult to assess on the basis of either single or even multiple O_2 pressure values. Scalp and/or umbilical cord artery pH levels of less than 7.2 are considered of greater clinical concern for predicting HIE, although the suggested guideline of a pH of 7.0 or less is one criterion by which the clinical entity of HIE might be better predicted.[96] A metabolic definition of asphyxia should also include a base deficit of −10 or less. More recently, a base deficit of −16 or less has been suggested because it is more predictive of the emergence of the HIE syndrome, including clinical seizures.[99] One caveat should always be remembered before a relative risk is assigned to a pH value: Elevated CO_2 pressure values introduce a superimposed respiratory acidosis secondary to hypercarbia. Elevated CO_2 pressure with respiratory acidosis is less harmful to brain tissue and is more rapidly corrected by aggressive ventilatory support. Alternatively, metabolic acidosis suggests a more profound alteration of intracellular function that is more predictive of an evolving brain disorder, which may include seizures as part of HIE.

Low Apgar scores are traditionally associated with neurologic depression after delivery, with possible evolution to HIE and seizures. Low 1- and 5-minute Apgar scores indicate the continued need for resuscitation, but only low scores at 10, 15, and 20 minutes carry a more accurate prediction for neurologic sequelae.[100] Normal Apgar scores, however, do not eliminate the possibility of severe antepartum brain injury, from either asphyxia or other causes. As many as two thirds of neonates who exhibit cerebral palsy at older ages had normal Apgar scores at birth without HIE.[101] In one hospital-based study, only 25 (13%) of 193 neonates with EEG-confirmed seizures within the first 120 hours of life met the four suggested criteria for HIE.[2]

Placental findings may reflect disease states at any time point before birth either with or without metabolic acidosis and evolving HIE after birth.[92] Although in utero meconium passage commonly occurs with otherwise healthy newborns, meconium staining of the child's skin may be correlated with meconium-laden macrophages within placental membranes in a neurologically depressed newborn. Meconium staining through the chorionic layer to the amnion suggests a longer standing asphyxial stress, such as over 4 to 6 hours.

Placental weights below the 10th or above the 90th percentile suggest chronic perfusion abnormalities in the fetus. Microscopic evidence of lymphocytic infiltration, altered villous maturation, chorangiosis, and erythroblastic proliferation of villi in the placenta are evidence of chronic asphyxial stresses to the fetus.[92] In a study of preterm and full-term neonates (23 to 42 weeks postconception) with electrically confirmed seizures, a significant association between seizures and chronic (with or without acute) placental lesions was noted, increasing to a factor of 12.1 ($P < .003$) by full-term age. Odds ratios were not significant for infants with seizures and exclusively acute placental lesions presumably caused by events closer in time to labor and delivery.[102]

Specific clinical examination findings in the neurologically depressed neonate with suspected HIE may reflect antepartum disease states.[5] Intrauterine growth restriction, hydrops fetalis, or joint contractures (including arthrogryposis) are examination findings that suggest chronic in utero diseases associated with antepartum medical conditions, later responsible for intrapartum fetal distress and/or neonatal neurologic depression without further injury. Hypertonicity, often with so-called cortical thumbs (fingers flexed, thumb under the second to fifth fingers), in a neurologically depressed child who rapidly recovers after a successful resuscitative effort also commonly reflects longer standing fetal neurologic dysfunction before labor and delivery. Sustained hypotonia and unresponsiveness for 3 to 7 days are the expected clinical signs of HIE after an intrapartum asphyxial stress, whether brain injury occurred or not. Encephalopathy with depressed arousal and hypotonia may nonetheless paradoxically reflect an antepartum disease process with neonatal dysfunction but without superimposed brain injury after a problematic intrapartum period. For example, this situation was described in 10 of 20 neurologically depressed infants with EEG seizures and isoelectric interictal EEG pattern abnormalities who were comatose and flaccid for days, requiring ventilator assistance after difficult deliveries.[103] All children appeared neurologically depressed after asphyxial stress during the intrapartum period (i.e., they had depressed Apgar scores and metabolic acidosis). Evidence of fetal brain injury included preexisting maternal disease, placental lesions, neuroimaging findings, and/or neuropathologic postmortem findings. Although intrapartum asphyxial stress may have worsened brain injury in such children, it was not possible to differentiate their apparently acute neonatal encephalopathy from preexisting antepartum brain injury. Newer neuroimaging techniques such as diffusion-weighted magnetic resonance imaging (MRI) studies may detect more recent injury.

Hypoglycemia

Hypoglycemia is generally defined as glucose levels of 20 mg/dL or lower in preterm infants and 30 mg/dL or lower in full-term infants.[104,105] There is no clear consensus concerning a direct cause and effect of hypoglycemia with seizure occurrence.[106] Methods of glucose determination (i.e., dextrose stick sampling versus serum sampling) affect the accuracy of the value. Also, the coexistence of associated disturbances, such as hypocalcemia, craniocerebral trauma, cerebrovascular lesions, and asphyxia, may also contribute to lowering the infant's threshold for seizures. Infants born to diabetic or toxemic mothers, particularly those who were small for gestational age, are also at risk for hypoglycemia. Jitteriness, apnea, and altered tone are other clinical signs that may appear in children with hypoglycemia but are not representative of a seizure state. Cerebrovascular lesions in posterior brain regions have been reported in children with hypoglycemia.[107] Vulnerability of the brain to ischemic insults is enhanced by concomitant hypoglycemia, as reported in mature animals[108] and neonatal infants.[109]

Hypocalcemia

Total serum calcium levels lower than 7.5 mg/dL in preterm infants and lower than 8 mg/dL in full-term infants generally define hypocalcemia. The ionized fraction is a more sensitive indicator of seizure vulnerability. As with hypoglycemia, the exact level of hypocalcemia at which seizures occur is debatable. An ionized fraction of 0.6 or less may have a more predictable association with the presence of seizures. Late-onset hypocalcemia has been previously cited as a common cause of seizures[24,110,111] because of infant formula containing high amounts of phosphate. However, hypocalcemia now more commonly occurs in infants with trauma, hemolytic disease, or asphyxia and may coexist with hypoglycemia or hypomagnesemia. In rare cases, congenital hypoparathyroidism occurs in association with other genetic abnormalities. The DiGeorge syndrome (velocardiofacial syndrome, or 22q11 deletion with cardiac and brain anomalies) is one diagnosis to be considered. Affected infants may have severe congenital heart disease, as well as a hypoparathyroid state with hypocalcemia and hypomagnesemia, which precipitate seizures.[112] Hypocalcemia of unknown origin may also be the result of maternal hypercalcemia. Ascertainment of the mother's calcium status should be considered, because maternal hypercalcemia can suppress fetal parathyroid development and function.

Hyponatremia and Hypernatremia

Hyponatremia is a metabolic disturbance that may result from inappropriate secretion of antidiuretic hormone after severe brain trauma, infection, or asphyxia[12]; it is an uncommon isolated cause of neonatal seizures. Hypernatremia also is a rare cause of seizures, usually associated with congenital adrenal abnormalities or iatrogenic disturbance of serum sodium balance by the use of intravenous fluids with high concentrations of sodium.

Cerebrovascular Lesions

Hemorrhagic or ischemic cerebrovascular lesions are associated with neonatal seizures, on either an arterial or a venous basis.[19-21,36,113-116] IVH and periventricular hemorrhage are the most common types of intracranial

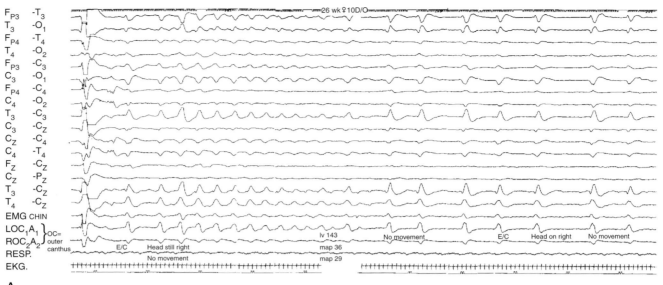

A

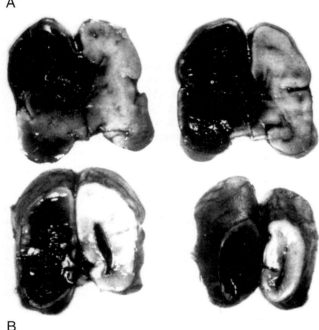

B

Figure 55–12. A, Electroencephalographic (EEG) segment recorded in a 10-day-old girl, born at 26 gestational weeks, with sepsis and disseminated intravascular coagulation, who electrographically expressed a seizure prominently in the left hemisphere and midline regions. **B,** Postmortem coronal slices of the brain of the preterm infant described in *A*, with prominent hemorrhagic infarction of the left hemisphere as well as intraventricular hemorrhage.

hemorrhage in preterm infants and have been associated with seizures in as much as 45% of a preterm population with EEG-confirmed seizures.[63,117] In one cohort of newborns with clinical seizures, IVH was the most predominant cause of seizures in preterm infants younger than 30 weeks of gestational age (Fig. 55-12).[118] Intracranial hemorrhage is usually expected within the first 72 hours after birth in all preterm infants. Although IVH and periventricular hemorrhage may occur in otherwise asymptomatic infants, the neonate with a catastrophic deterioration of clinical status shows signs of apnea, bulging fontanelle, hypertonia, and seizures.[12] Seventeen percent of preterm infants with IVH may have acute seizures during the first month after birth; 10% of one

cohort suffered much later seizures (after discharge).[119] Full-term infants present less commonly with IVH, usually originating from the choroid plexus or thalamus.

Other sites of intracranial hemorrhage include the subarachnoid space, in which hemorrhage may cause seizures, but those other hemorrhages are generally associated with a more favorable outcome. Subdural hematoma, whether spontaneous or after craniocerebral trauma, should always be considered, particularly when focal trauma to the face, scalp, or head has occurred; simultaneous occurrences of cerebral contusion and infarction should also be considered.

Cerebral infarction has been described in neonates with seizures and can result from events during the antepartum, intrapartum, or neonatal period.[120,121] Either preterm or full-term neonates with infarction may also present without seizure expression.[122] Seizures can also occur in otherwise healthy infants, which suggests that there is an antepartum time period when cerebral infarction occurred (Fig. 55-13).[115,123] Aggressive use of neuroimaging by fetal sonography or MRI during the antepartum period, or within the first days after birth, may document remote brain lesions.[5] Of a group of 62 healthy infants with EEG-confirmed seizures after an uneventful delivery, 23 (37%) had cerebrovascular lesions; 18 of these infants had ischemic brain lesions.[82] Destructive lesions such as porencephaly require approximately 5 to 7 days before becoming radiographically apparent (see Fig. 55-9). More recent intrapartum or neonatal time periods during which injury occurred can be detected by the presence of early cerebral edema using diffusion-weighted MRI images.[124] During the postnatal period, cerebral infarction may also result from asphyxia, polycythemia, dehydration, or coagulopathy (see Fig. 55-10).

PPHN with severe and recurrent hypoxia can also be associated with cerebrovascular lesions and seizures (Fig. 55-14).[21] Certain infants with PPHN require extracorporeal membrane oxygenation (ECMO) to treat severe forms of this pulmonary disease, which often does not respond to traditional ventilatory therapy. Radiographic documentation of brain lesions needs to be diagnosed before ECMO is begun, because the anticoagulation required for ECMO may convert "bland" or ischemic infarctions to hemorrhagic forms, with greater risk for cerebral edema and herniation. In most children with PPHN, the disease reflects antepartum maternal-fetal or placental conditions that predispose the fetus to thickening of the muscular layers of the pulmonary arteries while in utero, with resultant increased pulmonary vascular resistance after birth.[125]

Cerebral infarction in the venous distribution of the brain may also lead to neonatal seizures.[114,116] Lateral or sagittal sinus thromboses after coagulopathy can occur secondary to systemic infection, polycythemia, or dehydration. Venous infarction within the deep white matter of the preterm brain also occurs in association with IVH.

Infection

Central nervous system infections during the antepartum or postnatal periods can be associated with neonatal seizures.[126] Congenital infections—toxoplasmosis, other infections, rubella, cytomegalic inclusion disease, and herpes (TORCH) (see Figure 55-4C)—can produce severe encephalopathic damage, which results in seizures as well as more diffuse brain disorders. Other congenital infections include those by enteroviruses and parvoviruses. For instance, specific infections such as neonatal herpes encephalitis have been associated with severe EEG pattern abnormalities.[127] Rubella, toxoplasmosis, and cytomegalic inclusion disease each can also lead to devastating encephalitis, usually manifesting with microcephaly, jaundice, body rash, hepatosplenomegaly, and/or chorioretinitis. Increasing lethargy and obtundation with or without seizures may suggest the subacute manifestation

of encephalitis during the postnatal period. Serial spinal fluid analyses document progressively increasing protein and/or pleocytosis.

Acquired in utero or postnatal bacterial infections from either gram-negative or gram-positive organisms are also associated with neonatal seizures. Some organisms such as *Escherichia coli*, group B streptococci, *Listeria monocytogenes*, and *Mycoplasma* species may produce severe leptomeningeal infiltration, with possible abscess formation and cerebrovascular occlusions (see Fig. 55-1B). A high percentage of survivors suffer significant neurologic sequelae.

Central Nervous System Malformations

Disorders of induction, segmentation, proliferation, migration, myelination, and synaptogenesis of neuronal components can contribute to varying degrees of malformation. Seizures may occur in the newborn with malformations who experiences stress around the time of birth,[128] which presumably lowers seizure thresholds. Brain anomalies may occur as a result of genetic causes and/or acquired defects, usually during the first half of gestation. Specific dysgenesis syndromes, such as holoprosencephaly and lissencephaly, are often associated with characteristic facial or body anomalies. Cytogenetic studies may document trisomies or deletion defects. Unfortunately, infants may also lack physical signs of the presence of a brain malformation. The clinician's high index of suspicion is then warranted to evaluate neonates with persistent seizures. Of 356 infants presenting with neonatal seizures, 9% had brain malformations.[118] Neuroimaging, preferably magnetic resonance techniques, document brain dysgenesis in children who may also express severe electrographic EEG disturbances, including seizures (Fig. 55-15A and B). Focal or regional brain malformations are rare causes of early-onset epilepsy in neonates and young infants[129,130]; functional imaging studies such as positron emission tomography scans[131] may identify localized areas of altered brain metabolism. These studies can assist in a neurosurgical approach to seizure management, even in young children who fail to respond to AED maintenance.[132]

Inborn Errors of Metabolism

Inherited biochemical abnormalities are rare causes of neonatal seizures.[40] Intractable seizures associated with elevated lactate and pyruvate levels in blood and spinal fluid may reflect specific inborn errors of metabolism. Dysplastic or destructive brain lesions, as documented on neuroimaging, may be associated with specific biochemical defects, such as glycine encephalopathy or branched-chain aminoacidopathies (see Fig. 55-5). Pregnancy, labor, and delivery histories for these infants are commonly uneventful. The emergence of food intolerance and increasing lethargy, stupor, coma, and seizures during the first few days after birth are early indications of an inborn metabolic disturbance. The newborn with an inherited metabolic disorder may initially present as neurologically depressed and hypotonic, with asphyxia and seizures.[39] Some children respond to specific dietary therapies, including vitamin supplementation,[133] depending

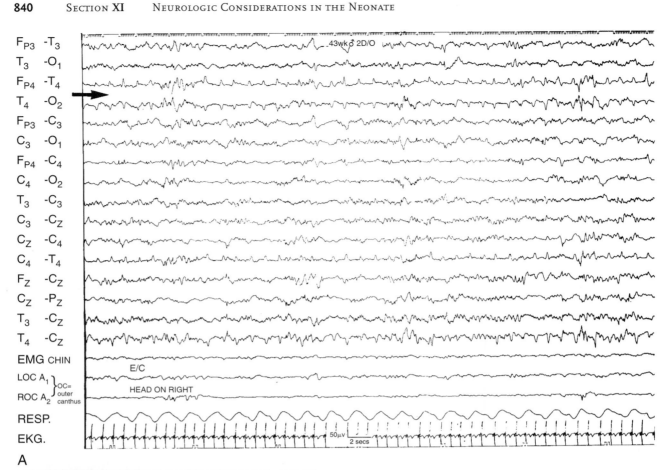

A

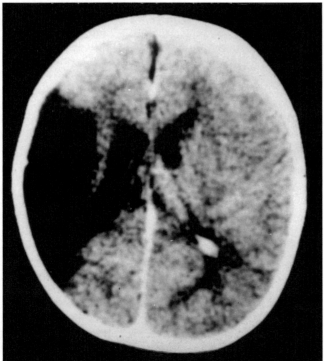

B

Figure 55–13. A, Electroencephalographic (EEG) segment recorded in a 2-day-old boy, born at 43 gestational weeks, with focal electrographic seizures in the right temporal region *(arrow).* **B,** Computed tomographic scan on day 1 after birth for the child described in *A,* documenting a right middle cerebral artery infarction that occurred in the antepartum period.

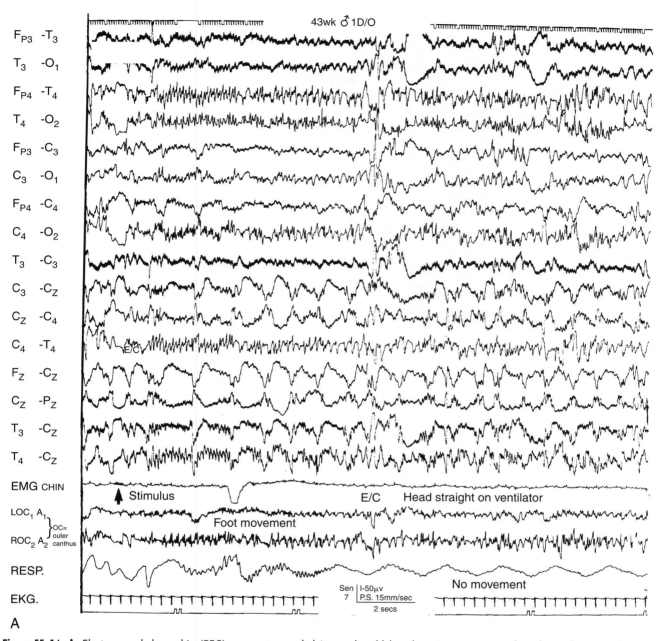

Figure 55–14. A, Electroencephalographic (EEG) segment recorded in a 1-day-old boy, born at 43 gestational weeks, with a stimulus-evoked electrographically confirmed seizure *(arrow)* without clinical accompaniments in the right temporal region. The child required ventilatory care for persistent pulmonary hypertension (see text). *(From Scher MS, Klesh KW, Murphy TF, Guthrie RD: Seizures and infarction in neonates with persistent pulmonary hypertension. Pediatr Neurol 2:332, 1986.)*

Continued

on the enzymatic defect. Specific urea cycle defects, such as carbamoyl phosphate synthetase deficiency, may present with coma and seizures during the first 2 days after birth, with marked elevations in plasma ammonia levels. These infants may respond to aggressive treatment with an exchange transfusion, dialysis, and appropriate dietary adjustments.

Vitamin B_6 (pyridoxine) deficiency or dependency is a rare cause of neonatal seizures.[134,135] Pyridoxine acts as a cofactor in γ-aminobutyric acid synthesis, and its absence or paucity promotes seizures. The mother occasionally reports paroxysmal fetal movements.[136] The infant who is unresponsive to conventional AEDs should promptly receive an intravenous injection of 50 to 500 mg of pyridoxine, preferably with concomitant EEG monitoring. Termination of the seizure within minutes to hours as well as resolution of EEG background disturbances suggests a pyridoxine-dependent seizure state. Prophylactic

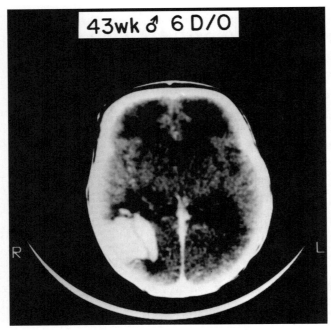

B

Figure 55–14, cont'd. B, Computed tomographic scan on day 6 for the patient in *A*, documenting a hemorrhagic infarction in the right posterior quadrant with surrounding edema. *(From Scher MS, Klesh KW, Murphy TF, Guthrie RD: Seizures and infarction in neonates with persistent pulmonary hypertension. Pediatr Neurol 2:332, 1986.)*

doses of pyridoxine may be needed to achieve and maintain seizure control.

Other rare causes of seizures include disorders of carbohydrate metabolism with coincident hypoglycemia,[40] as well as peroxisomal disorders, such as neonatal adrenoleukodystrophy or Zellweger syndrome. A defect in a glucose transporter protein necessary to move glucose across the blood-brain barrier, which results in hypoglycorrhachia and seizures, has also been reported.[137] Affected children may achieve seizure control with a ketogenic diet but may nonetheless suffer delayed development.

Molybdenum-cofactor deficiency and isolated sulfite oxidase deficiencies are other rare metabolic defects that cause neonatal seizures and associated destructive changes, which may resemble cerebrovascular disease or asphyxia, on neuroimaging.[138]

Drug Withdrawal and Intoxication

Newborns born to mothers with a history of prenatal substance use may have an increased risk for neonatal seizures.[139,140] Exposure to barbiturates, alcohol, heroin, cocaine, or methadone commonly manifests with neurologic findings that include tremors and irritability. Withdrawal symptoms, in addition to seizures, may occur as long as 4 to 6 weeks after birth[141]; EEG studies are useful for correlating such movements with coincident electrographic seizure patterns. Certain drugs, such as short-acting barbiturates, may be associated with seizures within the first several days after birth.[142] Seizures may occur

directly after substance withdrawal or may be associated with longer standing uteroplacental insufficiency, promoted by chronic substance abuse and poor prenatal health maintenance by the mother. Careful review of placental/cord specimens may reveal chronic or acute pathologic lesions that contribute to antepartum or intrauterine asphyxia.

Inadvertent fetal injection with a local anesthetic agent during delivery may induce intoxication, which is a rare cause of seizures.[143,144] Patients present during the first 6 to 8 hours after birth with apnea, bradycardia, and hypotonia and are comatose, without brain stem reflexes. If the obstetric history indicates that pudendal administration of an anesthetic was given to the mother, a careful examination of the child's scalp or body for puncture marks is indicated. Plasma levels of the suspected anesthetic agent establish the diagnosis. Treatment consists of ventilatory support and removal of the drug by therapeutic diuresis, acidification of the urine, or exchange transfusion. AEDs are rarely indicated.

Progressive Neonatal Epileptic Syndromes

Progressive epileptic syndromes rarely manifest during the first month after birth.[145] Affected children usually exhibit myoclonic or migratory seizures that are poorly controlled by AEDs, and brain malformations are often demonstrable on brain imaging.[98,130] Two neonatal epileptic syndromes are **early myoclonic encephalopathy** and **early infantile epileptic encephalopathy (Ohtahara syndrome),** and the EEG in affected children commonly documents burst-suppression or markedly disorganized background rhythms. In rare cases, neonates with idiopathic localization-related or partial seizures without neuroimaging abnormalities present with intractable epilepsy.[146]

Neurocutaneous syndromes, such as incontinentia pigmenti and tuberous sclerosis, may also appear as symptomatic epilepsy during the neonatal period, as one clinical manifestation of these genetic disorders. Incontinentia pigmenti is accompanied by a vesicular crusting rash, which initially mimics a herpetic infection. Seizures may or may not be present. The skin lesions evolve into lightly pigmented, raised sebaceous lesions in older infants and children. Tuberous sclerosis also, in rare cases, manifests with skin lesions in the neonatal period. Hypopigmented lesions, initially noted under ultraviolet light, usually appear later during infancy. Two common fetal manifestations of tuberous sclerosis are a cardiac tumor, usually a rhabdomyoma, and, in rare cases, a connatal brain tumor, both noted on fetal sonography. Neonatal seizures also may be the presenting feature,[147] and intracranial lesions may be documented on postnatal neuroimaging.

Benign Familial Neonatal Seizures

The autosomal dominant form of neonatal seizures is a rare genetic epilepsy that should be considered in the context of a positive family history.[148-150] Exclusion of infectious, metabolic, toxic, or structural causes must be completed before this entity is considered. The genetic defect was first described on chromosome 20q,[80] specifically at the D20S19 and D20S20 loci, as well as on chromosome 8q24 at the EBN2 locus. By positional cloning, a potassium channel gene (KCNQ2) located on

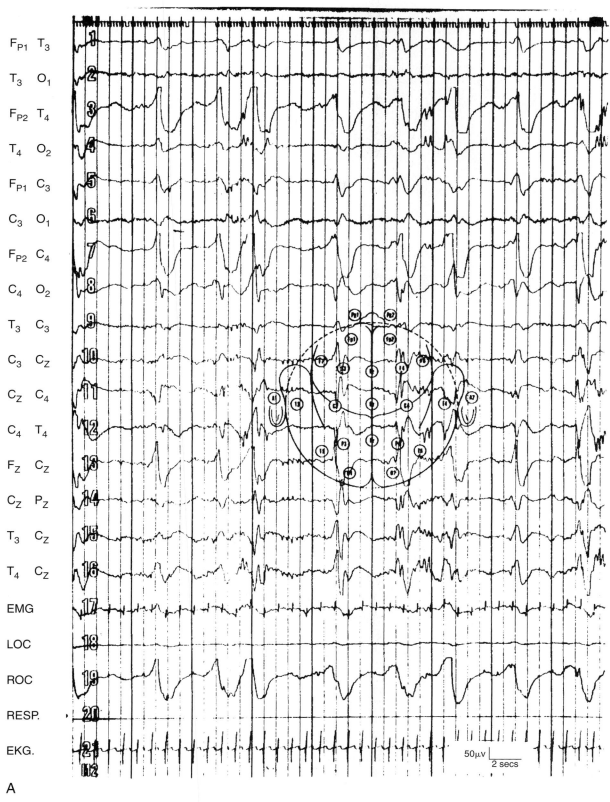

A

Figure 55–15. A, Electroencephalographic (EEG) segment recorded in a 1-day-old infant, born at 38 gestational weeks, with right hemisphere–predominant generalized electrographic seizure activity without clinical signs.   *Continued*

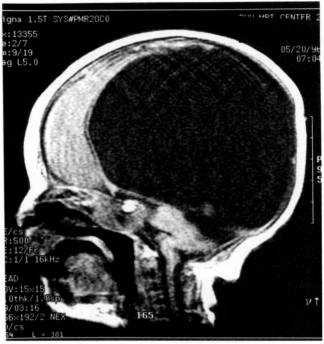

B

Figure 55–15, cont'd. B, Magnetic resonance scan for the patient described in *A*, demonstrating severe cerebral dysgenesis, including lissencephaly, holoprosencephaly, and a small atrophic cerebellum and brain stem. *(From Scher MS: Seizures in the newborn infant. Clin Perinatol 24:763, 1997.)*

20q13.3 was first isolated and found to be expressed in brain tissue.[148] A second potassium channel (KCNQ3) has also been described and may explain the varied phenotypic expression of seizures and outcome.[151] Mutations in ion channels have also been implicated in Jervell and Lange-Nielsen syndromes, whose symptoms include congenital deafness and cardiac arrhythmias.[152] Infant outcomes range from excellent to guarded, depending on the persistence of seizures beyond the neonatal period. Response to AEDs is generally good, although some authors describe variable success. Further studies are needed to clarify the relationship between phenotypic and genotypic expressions of this disorder.

In a study of 76 children with neonatal seizures, a certain proportion of children had genetic factors in common with idiopathic partial epilepsies.[153] The authors suggested that genetic factors other than ion channel disorders are involved in the pathogenesis of neonatal seizures. They argued that there may be a "genetic liability," as expressed by certain EEG patterns at older ages in children who initially presented with neonatal seizures.[154]

SEIZURES IN THE CLINICAL CONTEXT OF MATERNAL-FETAL-PLACENTAL DISEASES: FOLLOWING A DIAGNOSTIC ALGORITHM

Once seizures are confirmed by EEG, the neurologist must place these events into the context of clinical, historical, and laboratory findings to determine the

pathogenesis and timing of an encephalopathic process in the symptomatic neonate. Seizures in neonates after asphyxia are either acute intrapartum events or antepartum disease processes, or both. Does the child with seizures also express clinical and laboratory signs of evolving cerebral edema? The presence of a bulging fontanelle with neuroimaging evidence of increased intracranial pressure and cerebral edema (i.e., obliterated ventricular outline and abnormal diffusion-weighted MRI images) strongly suggests a more recent asphyxial disease process, during or around the intrapartum period. Hyponatremia and increased urine osmolality are suggestive of the syndrome of inappropriate secretion of antidiuretic hormone accompanying acute or subacute cerebral edema.

Alternatively, lack of evidence of evolving cerebral edema during the first 3 days after asphyxia, or presence of encephalomalacia or cystic brain lesions on neuroimaging shortly after birth (i.e., even in the encephalopathic newborn), is suggestive of a more chronic disease process and old antepartum brain injury. In liquefaction necrosis, 2 weeks or longer after the presumed in utero asphyxial event is necessary to produce a cystic cavity,[155] which is then visible on neuroimaging.

Isolated seizures in an otherwise asymptomatic neonate are also suggestive of a disease process that occurs during either the postnatal or antepartum period. Neonates present with seizures as a result of postnatal illnesses from intracranial infection, cardiovascular lesions, drug toxicity, or inherited metabolic diseases. Children with antepartum injury may express isolated seizures after in utero cerebrovascular injury caused by thrombolytic and/or embolic disease of the mother, placenta, or fetus. Fetal injury alternatively may occur after ischemic-hypoperfusion events from circulatory disturbances, such as maternal shock, chorioamnionitis, or placental fetal vasculopathy.[120] Other antepartum congenital and acquired factors include familial epilepsy and preeclampsia, respectively.

Only a percentage of neonates with old in utero cerebrovascular disease before labor and delivery present with neonatal seizures.[122] Many remain asymptomatic until later, during infancy or childhood. Neonatal expression of seizures may reflect acute physiologic stress during parturition, which lowers seizure threshold in vulnerable brain regions that have been previously damaged.

After a careful review of the medical histories of the mother, fetus, and newborn, determination of serum glucose, electrolyte, ammonia, lactate, pyruvate, magnesium, calcium, and phosphorus levels may enable examiners to diagnose correctable metabolic conditions in newborns with seizures who do not necessitate AEDs. Spinal fluid analyses include cell count; protein, glucose, lactate, pyruvate, and amino acid measurements; and culture studies to evaluate for central nervous system infection, intracranial hemorrhage, and metabolic disease. Metabolic acidosis on serial arterial blood gas determinations may alternatively suggest an inherited metabolic disease, particularly if intrapartum asphyxia was not judged to be severe. Absence of multiorgan dysfunction may alert the clinician to other causes of seizures besides intrapartum asphyxia. Signs of chronic in utero stress such as growth restriction, early hypertonicity after neonatal neurologic depression, joint contractures, or elevated nucleated red blood cell values all suggest longer standing antepartum stress to the fetus. Identification of genetic or syndromic conditions can contribute to the expression of neonatal encephalopathies independent of asphyxial injury.[156] Careful review of placental and cord specimens can also be extremely useful. Neuroimaging, preferably with MRI, can help localize, grade the severity of, and possibly time an insult.[157] Ancillary studies may also include long-chain fatty acid measurements and chromosomal/DNA analyses, as deemed necessary from family and clinical histories. Finally, serum and urine organic acid and amino acid determinations may be needed to delineate a specific biochemical disorder for the child with a persistent metabolic acidosis. Lysosomal enzyme studies are also occasionally considered in order to diagnose specific enzymatic deficiencies in children with neonatal seizures.

PROGNOSIS

The rate of mortality in infants who present with clinical neonatal seizures has reportedly declined from 40% to 15%.[3,158] Studies of EEG-confirmed seizures documented mortality rates of 50% in preterm infants and 40% in full-term infants during the 1980s.[3,159] During the 1990s in the same institution, these mortality rates dropped below 20%.[2] The incidence of adverse neurologic sequelae, however, remains high for approximately two thirds of survivors. Even if major neurodevelopmental sequelae such as motor deficits and mental retardation are avoided in survivors after neonatal seizures, subtle neurodevelopmental vulnerability may manifest in the late teen years as specific learning difficulties or poor social adjustment,[160] which underscores more recent experimental findings of long-term deficits in animal populations.[161]

Prediction of outcome should also consider the cause of seizures, such as severe asphyxia, significant craniocerebral trauma, and brain infections. More accurate neuroimaging procedures (i.e. MRI, magnetic resonance spectroscopy) have heightened physicians' awareness of destructive as well congenital brain lesions with higher risk for compromised outcome. Proton magnetic resonance spectroscopy has been suggested as a useful tool for both early evaluation of brain injury in the asphyxiated neonate[162] and persistent biochemical alterations even 13 to 21 years after the neonatal period[163] in children with neurologic sequelae.

Interictal EEG pattern abnormalities are extremely helpful in predicting neurologic outcome in the neonate with seizures.[73,74] Major background disturbances such as burst-suppression (see Fig. 55-11) are highly predictive of poor outcome. This finding is particularly true when persistently abnormal findings are still present on serial EEG studies into the second week after birth and after seizures have stopped. Ictal patterns alone also may not be as accurate in predicting outcome, unless quantified to high numbers, long durations, and multifocal distribution.[164] Normal findings on interictal EEG were associated

with an 86% chance of normal development at 4 years of age in 139 neonates with seizures[24]; in contrast, neonates with markedly abnormal EEG background disturbances had only a 7% chance of a normal outcome. Another study reported outcome in full-term and preterm infants with seizures, concluding that the EEG background was more predictive of outcome than the presence of isolated sharp-wave discharges.[165] Even severe interictal abnormalities on single-channel spectral EEG recordings after asphyxia carry a higher risk for sequelae.[46]

Neonates with seizures have a risk of epilepsy during childhood.[42] According to clinical seizure criteria, 20% to 25% of neonates with seizures later develop epilepsy.[166] With the exclusion of febrile seizures, the prevalence of epilepsy by 6 to 7 years of age is also estimated to be between 15% to 30%, according to EEG-confirmed seizures for an inborn hospital population, two thirds of whom were preterm neonates.[63] This finding is in contrast with an incidence of 56% with epilepsy for an exclusively outborn neonatal population of primarily full-term newborns with seizures.[167] Epilepsy risk therefore reflects selection bias of specific study groups, as well as referral patterns in different hospital settings.

DIAGNOSTIC DILEMMAS REGARDING TREATMENT

Rapid infusion of glucose or other supplemental electrolytes should be immediately initiated before AEDs are considered. Hypoglycemia can be readily corrected by intravenous administration of 5 to 10 mg/kg of a 10% dextrose solution, followed by an infusion of 8 to 10 mg/kg/minute. Persistent hypoglycemia may necessitate more hypertonic glucose solutions. In rare cases, prednisone, 2 mg/kg/day, may be needed to establish a glucose level within the normal range.[2]

Hypocalcemia-induced seizures should be treated with an intravenous infusion of 200 mg/kg of 10% calcium gluconate. This dosage should be repeated every 5 to 6 hours over the first 24 hours. Serum magnesium concentrations should also be measured, because hypomagnesemia may accompany hypocalcemia; 0.2 mg/kg of magnesium sulfate should be given by intramuscular injection.[2]

Disorders of serum sodium are rare causes of neonatal seizures. Either fluid restriction or replacement with hypotonic solutions is generally the mode of therapy for correcting sodium abnormalities.[2]

Pyridoxine deficiency or dependency necessitates the injection of 50 to 500 mg of pyridoxine during a seizure with coincident EEG monitoring. A beneficial pyridoxine effect occurs either immediately or over the first several hours. A daily dose of 50 to 100 mg of pyridoxine should then be administered.[2]

If the decision to treat neonates with AEDs is reached, important questions must be addressed with regard to whom to treat, when to begin treatment, which drug to use, and how long to treat.[1,3] Some authors suggest that only neonates with clinical seizures should receive medications; brief electrographically confirmed seizures need not be treated. Others suggest more aggressive treatment of EEG seizures, because uncontrolled seizures potentially have an adverse effect on immature brain development.[168-172] An alternative suggestion is that early administration of an AED, such as phenobarbital, even before signs of HIE, may have adverse effects on outcome in full-term infants.[173]

Phenobarbital and phenytoin, nonetheless, remain the most widely used AEDs; the use of benzodiazepines, primidone, and valproic acid has been anecdotally reported.[133] The half-life of phenobarbital ranges from 45 to 173 hours in the neonate[174-176]; the initial loading dose is recommended at 20 mg/kg, and the maintenance dosage is 3 to 4 mg/kg/day. Therapeutic levels are generally suggested to be between 16 and 40 μg/mL; however, there is no consensus with regard to drug maintenance.

The preferred loading dose of phenytoin is 15 to 20 mg/kg.[175,176] Serum levels of phenytoin are difficult to maintain because this drug is rapidly redistributed to body tissues. Blood levels cannot be well maintained with an oral preparation.

Benzodiazepines may also be used to control neonatal seizures. The drug most widely used is diazepam. One study suggested that the half-life ranges from 54 hours in preterm infants to 18 hours in full-term infants.[177] Intravenous administration is recommended because the drug is absorbed slowly after an intramuscular injection. Diazepam is highly protein bound; alteration of bilirubin binding is low. Intravenous doses for acute management are recommended to begin at 0.5 mg/kg. Deposition into muscle precludes its use as a maintenance AED, because profound hypotonia and respiratory depression may result, particularly if barbiturates have also been administered.

Efficacy of Treatment

Conflicting studies report varying efficacy with phenobarbital or phenytoin. Most studies apply only a clinical end point to seizure cessation. One study found that only 36% of neonates with clinical seizures responded to phenobarbital,[175] and another study noted cessation of clinical seizures with phenobarbital in only 32% of neonates.[174] With dosages as high as 40 mg/kg,[178] seizure control was reported to be 85%. A more recent study reported that the earlier administration of high-dose phenobarbital in a group of asphyxiated infants was associated with a 27% reduction in clinical seizures and better outcome than were low dosages.[179] However, coincident EEG studies are now suggested to verify the resolution of electrographically confirmed seizures. One report suggests that 30% of neonates have persistent electrographically confirmed seizures after suppression of clinical seizure behaviors after drug administration.[52] With EEG as an end point to judge cessation of seizures, neither phenobarbital nor phenytoin was effective to control seizure activity.[180]

The use of free or drug-bound fractions of AEDs has been suggested to better assess both efficacy and potential toxicity of AEDs in pediatric populations.[181] Drug binding in neonates with seizures has been reported in the last decade and can be altered in a sick neonate with organ dysfunction. Toxic side effects may result from elevated free fractions of a drug that adversely affect cardiovascular and respiratory function. To guard against untoward effects, evaluation of treatment and efficacy must take into account both total and free AED fractions, in the context of the newborn's progression or resolution of systemic illness.

Once an AED is chosen, the clinician must closely monitor the infant to ensure that seizures are not worsened by the administration of such a drug choice. AEDs may cause worsening of seizures by either aggravating previous seizures or triggering new seizure types, as described in four neonates after midazolam was administered.[182]

New anticonvulsant alternatives to treat seizures are being suggested, with N-methyl-D-aspartate antagonists such as topiramate[183,184] developed from experimental models of hypoxia-induced seizure activity in immature brain. Such models provide data regarding pharmacologic and physiologic characteristics of neuronal responses after an asphyxial stress that cause excessive release of excitotoxic neurotransmitters, such as glutamate.[185] Specific cell membrane receptors termed **metabotropic glutamate receptors** (MGluRs) are sensitive to extracellular glutamate release and may play a role in epileptogenesis and seizure-induced brain damage.[186] One class of membrane receptor, for example, has been studied in rat pups after hypoxia-induced seizures, suggesting that MGluR down-regulation can be associated with epileptogenesis in the absence of cell loss.[187] Subclasses of MGluRs will lead to investigations of novel drugs that block these membrane receptors as the mode of treatment for neonatal seizures.[188]

Discontinuation of Drug Use

The clinician's decision to maintain or discontinue AED use is also uncertain.[1,3] Discontinuation of drugs before discharge from the neonatal unit is generally recommended, because clinical assessments of arousal, tone, and behavior are not hampered by medication effect. However, newborns with congenital or destructive brain lesions on neuroimaging, or those with persistently abnormal neurologic examinations at the time of discharge, may suggest to the clinician that a slower tapering off medication is required over several weeks or months. Most neonatal seizures rarely recur during the first 2 years of life, and prophylactic AED administration need not be maintained past 3 months of age, even in the child at risk. This is supported by a study suggesting a low risk of seizure recurrence after early withdrawal of AED therapy in the neonatal period.[189] Also, older infants who present with specific epileptic syndromes, such as infantile spasms, do not respond to the conventional AEDs that were initially begun during the neonatal period. This "honeymoon" period without seizures commonly persists for many years in most children, before isolated or recurrent seizures appear.

The potential damage to the developing central nervous system by AEDs also emphasizes the need to consider early discontinuation of these agents in the newborn period. Adverse effects on the structure and metabolism of neuronal cells have been extensively reported from collective research performed since the 1960s.[190]

CONSEQUENCES OF NEONATAL SEIZURES ON BRAIN DEVELOPMENT

Embedded within the controversy regarding how to diagnose neonatal seizures is the association of repetitive or prolonged seizures with brain damage and altered brain development. Independently of the concern for seizure duration, the clinician must first appreciate the diverse neuropathologic processes associated with specific causes, which may be largely responsible for neonatal seizures and neurologic sequelae.[190] Central nervous system infections and severe asphyxia are two causes that exemplify underlying pathophysiologic mechanisms responsible for brain damage in neonates who express seizures.

Results of research efforts also suggest direct adverse effects of the seizure state on developing brain.[161] Seizures can disrupt a cascade of biochemical/molecular pathways that are normally responsible for the neuroplasticity or activity-dependent development of the maturing nervous system. Depending on the degree of brain immaturity, seizures may disrupt the processes of cell division, cell migration, myelination, sequential expression of receptor formation, and stabilization of synapses, each of which contributes to varying degrees of neurologic sequelae.[191]

Experimental models of seizures suggest comparatively less vulnerability to seizure-induced brain injury in immature animals than in mature animals.[192] In adult animals, seizures alter growth of hippocampal granule cells and axonal and mossy fiber growth, resulting in long-term deficits in learning, memory, and behavior. A single prolonged seizure in an immature animal, on the other hand, results in less cell loss or fiber sprouting and, consequentially, fewer deficits in learning, memory, and behavior. Resistance to brain damage, from prolonged seizure activity, however, is age-specific, as evidenced by increased cell damage after only 2 weeks of age.[193] One group of investigators examined developmental changes in epileptiform activity in neocortical preparations, using four different ages and four different pharmacologic models. These authors confirmed that there are definite age-dependent differences in the susceptibility to epileptiform activity in the neocortex. These developmental changes seem related to intrinsic network properties of the neocortex that are independent of ontogenetic differences in any specific neurotransmitter system.[194]

Repetitive or prolonged neonatal seizures alternatively can increase the susceptibility of the developing brain to subsequent seizure-induced brain injury during adolescence or early adulthood, by altering neuronal connectivity rather than increasing cell death.[161,191,195,196] Neonatal animals subjected to status epilepticus have reduced seizure thresholds at later ages and impairments of learning, memory, and activity levels when stressed with seizures as adults. Proposed mechanisms of injury also include reduced neurogenesis in the hippocampus, for example, possibly because of both ischemic-induced apoptosis and necrotic pathways.[197,198] Other suggested mechanisms of injury include effects of nitric oxide synthetase inhibition on cerebral circulation, which then contributes to ischemic injury.[199] Neonatal seizures may therefore initiate a cascade of diverse changes in brain development that become maladaptive at older ages and increase the risk of subsequent damage after later insults. Destructive mechanisms such as mossy fiber sprouting in the hippocampus or increased neuronal apoptosis may explain mutually exclusive pathways by which the immature brain suffers altered connectivity and reduced cell number, which is then "primed" for later seizure-induced cell loss at older ages.

The critical duration of seizures, whether cumulative or continuous, remains elusive with regard to resultant brain injury. Because as many as one third of full-term infants satisfy a definition of status epilepticus,[51] EEG documentation appears crucial. A study of 10-day-old rat pups indicated that prolonged seizures for 30 minutes after asphyxia resulted in an exacerbation of brain injury specific to the hippocampus but sparing the neocortex. Prolonged neonatal seizures do worsen damage incurred by an already compromised brain[200] in a region-specific manner. In a neonatal rodent model of brief recurrent seizures,[201] Landrot and associates demonstrated increased mossy fiber sprouting in the granule cells of the hippocampus, which was correlated with impaired cognition and reduced EEG power spectra during adolescence. A companion study from the same laboratory demonstrated alterations in cognition and seizure susceptibility within 2 weeks of the last seizure before the adult pattern of mossy fiber distribution is achieved. Therefore, therapeutic strategies to alter the adverse outcome of neonatal seizures must be initiated during or shortly after the seizures.

Overlapping effects of underlying central nervous system injury or dysgenesis from specific causes, as opposed to seizure-induced brain damage, make it difficult to differentiate preexisting brain lesions from the direct injurious effects of seizures themselves. The use of microdialysis probes in white and gray matter of piglet brains subjected to hypoxia indicate elevated lactate/pyruvate ratios after hypoxia but no association directly with seizure activity.[202] These findings support the conclusion that seizures themselves may not injurious metabolic dysfunction.

Unfortunately, we lack well-designed clinical investigations of outcome after neonatal seizures to support these experimental findings.[190] Better definitions of neonatal seizures of epileptic origin, as well as the critical seizure duration required to injure brain tissue, remain controversial.

Aggressive use of AEDs without EEG confirmation also contributes both to the inaccurate estimate of seizure severity in neonates and possible medication-induced brain injury. Intractable seizures generally necessitate the use of multiple AEDs. However, drugs impede the clinician's observations to recognize prolonged seizures because of the uncoupling phenomenon, in which the clinical expression of seizures may be suppressed but their electrical expression continues. Clinical definitions of seizure occurrence and duration consequently underestimate seizure severity, which appears to be associated with increased risk for damage. AED use also has secondary harmful effects on cardiac and respiratory function, with resultant circulatory disturbances that may also contribute to brain injury.[190] Finally, AED use may have teratogenetic effects on brain development with exposure over long periods.

SUMMARY

Recognition and classification of seizures remains problematic. The clinician should rely on synchronized video/EEG/polygraphic recordings to correlate suspicious behaviors with electrographic seizures and should limit misdiagnosis and overtreatment of nonepileptic abnormal behaviors. This practice must be integrated with an appreciation of pathophysiologic mechanisms responsible for brain injury that implicate maternal-fetal-placental diseases. Neonatal brain disorders may implicate the antepartum period, as well as the intrapartum or neonatal period.

REFERENCES

1. Camfield PR, Camfield CS: Neonatal seizures: A commentary on selected aspects. J Child Neurol 2:244, 1987.
2. Scher MS: Seizures in the newborn infant. Diagnosis, treatment and outcome. Clin Perinatol 24:735, 1997.
3. Scher MS, Painter MJ: Controversies concerning neonatal seizures. Pediatr Clin North Am 36:281-310, 1989.
4. Scher MS: Neonatal encephalopathies as classified by EEG-sleep criteria. Severity and timing based on clinical/pathologic correlations. Pediatr Neurol 11:189, 1994.
5. Scher MS: Perinatal asphyxia: Timing and mechanisms of injury relative to the diagnosis and treatment of neonatal encephalopathy. Curr Neurol Neurosci Rep 1:175, 2001.
6. Glauser TA, Clancy RR: Adequacy of routine EEG examinations in neonates with clinically suspected seizures. J Child Neurol 7:215, 1992.
7. Bye AME, Flanagan D: Spatial and temporal characteristics of neonatal seizures. Epilepsia 36:1009, 1995.
8. Commission on Classification and Terminology of the International League Against Epilepsy: Proposal for revised clinical and electroencephalographic classification of epileptic seizures. Epilepsia 22:489, 1981.
9. Mizrahi EM, Kellaway P: Diagnosis and Management of Neonatal Seizures. Philadelphia, Lippincott-Raven, 1998.
10. Biagioni E, Ferrari F, Boldrini A, et al: Electroclinical correlation in neonatal seizures. Eur J Paediatr Neurol 2:117, 1998.
11. Weiner SP, Painter MJ, Scher MS: Neonatal seizures: Electroclinical disassociation. Pediatr Neurol 7:363, 1991.
12. Volpe JJ: Neonatal seizures. In Volpe JJ: Neurology of the Newborn, 4th ed. Philadelphia, WB Saunders, 2001, pp 178-214.
13. Scher MS: Electroencephalography of the newborn: Normal and abnormal features. In Niedermeyer E, Da Silva L (eds): Electroencephalography, 4th ed. Baltimore, Williams & Wilkins, 1999, pp 869-946.
14. Scher MS: Normal electrographic-polysomnographic patterns in preterm and fullterm infants. Semin Pediatr Neurol 3:12, 1996.
15. DaSilva O, Guzman GMC, Young GB: The value of standard electroencephalograms in the evaluation of the newborn with recurrent apneas. J Perinatol 18:377, 1998.
16. Fenichel GM, Olson BJ, Fitzpatrick JE: Heart rate changes in convulsive and nonconvulsive apnea. Ann Neurol 7:577, 1979.
17. Boylan GB, Pressler RM, Rennie JM, et al: Outcome of electroclinical, electrographic, and clinical seizures in the newborn infant. Dev Med Child Neurol 41:819, 1999.
18. Mizrahi EM, Kellaway P: Characterization and classification of neonatal seizures. Neurology 37:1837, 1987.
19. Clancy R, Malin S, Larague D, et al: Focal motor seizures heralding a stroke in full-term neonates. Am J Dis Child 139:601, 1985.
20. Levy SR, Abroms IF, Marshall PC, et al: Seizures and cerebral infarction in the full-term newborn. Ann Neurol 17:366, 1985.
21. Scher MS, Klesh KW, Murphy TF, et al: Seizures and infarction in neonates with persistent pulmonary hypertension. Pediatr Neurol 2:332, 1986.
22. Holmes G: Diagnosis and management of seizures in childhood. In Markowitz M (ed): Major Problems in Clinical Pediatrics, XXX. Philadelphia, WB Saunders, 1987, pp 237-261.
23. Karayiannis NB, Srinivasan S, Bhattacharya R, et al: Extraction of motion strength and motor activity signals from video recordings of neonatal seizures. IEEE Trans Med Imaging 20:965, 2001.
24. Rose AL, Lombroso CT: A study of clinical, pathological, and electroencephalographic features in 137 full-term babies with a long-term follow-up. Pediatrics 45:404, 1970.
25. Kellaway P, Hrachovy RA: Status epilepticus in newborns: A perspective on neonatal seizures. In Delgado-Escueta AV, Wasterlain CG, Treiman DM, Porter RJ (eds): Status Epilepticus: Mechanisms of Brain Damage and Treatment, vol 34: Advances in Neurology. New York, Raven Press, 1983, pp 93-99.
26. Sarnat HB: Anatomic and physiologic correlates of neurologic development in prematurity. In: Topics in Neonatal Neurology. Orlando, Fla, Grune & Stratton, 1984, pp 1-25.
27. Scher MS: Pathological myoclonus of the newborn: Electrographic and clinical correlations. Pediatr Neurol 1:342, 1985.
28. Scher MS: Stimulus-evoked electrographic patterns in neonates: Abnormal form of reactivity. Electroencephalogr Clin Neurophysiol 103:679, 1997.
29. Coulter DL, Allen RJ: Benign neonatal sleep myoclonus. Arch Neurol 39:191, 1982.
30. Resnick TJ, Moshé SL, Perotta L, et al: Benign neonatal sleep myoclonus: Relationship to sleep states. Arch Neurol 43:266, 1986.
31. Clancy RR: The contribution of EEG to the understanding of neonatal seizures. Epilepsia 37:S52, 1996.
32. Shuper A, Zalzberg J, Weitz R, et al: Jitteriness beyond the neonatal period: A benign pattern of movement in infancy. J Child Neurol 6:243, 1991.
33. Parker S, Zuckerman B, Bauchner H, et al: Jitteriness in full-term neonates: Prevalence and correlates. Pediatrics 85:17, 1990.
34. Hakamada S, Watanabe K, Hara K, et al: Development of motor behavior during sleep in newborn infants. Brain Dev 3:345, 1981.
35. Sexson WR, Thigpen J, Stajich GV: Stereotypic movements after lorazepam administration in premature neonates: A series and review of the literature. J Perinatol 15:146, 1995.
36. Scher MS, Belfar H, Martin J, et al: Destructive brain lesions of presumed fetal onset: Antepartum causes of cerebral palsy. Pediatrics 88:898, 1991.
37. Brown P, Rothwell JC, Thompson PD, et al: The hyperexplexias and their relationship to the normal startle reflex. Brain 114:1903, 1991.
38. Andermann F, Andermann E: Startle disorders of man: Hyperexplexia, jumping, and startle epilepsy. Brain Dev 10:213, 1988.

39. Barth PJ: Inherited progressive disorders of the fetal brain: A field in need of recognition. In Fukuyama Y, Suzuki Y, Kamoshita S, Casaer P (eds): Fetal and Perinatal Neurology. Basel, Karger, 1992, pp 299-313.

40. Lyon G, Adams RD, Kolodny EH: Hypoglycemia. In Lyon G, Adams RD, Kolodny EH: Neurology of Hereditary Metabolic Diseases of Children, 2nd ed. New York, McGraw-Hill, 1996, pp 6-44.

41. Oliveira AJ, Nunes ML, da Costa JC: Polysomnography in neonatal seizures. Clin Neurophysiol 111:S74, 2000.

42. Watanabe K, Kuroyanagi M, Hara K, et al: Neonatal seizures and subsequent epilepsy. Brain Dev 4:341, 1982.

43. Hrachovy RA, Mizrahi EM, Kellaway P: Electroencephalography of the newborn. In Daly DD, Pedley TA (eds): Current Practice of Clinical Electroencephalography, 2nd ed. New York, Raven Press, 1990, pp 201-242.

44. Lombroso CT: Neonatal polygraphy in full-term and preterm infants: A review of normal and abnormal findings. J Clin Neurophysiol 2:105, 1985.

45. Pope SS, Stockard JE, Bickford RG: Atlas of Neonatal Electroencephalography. New York, Raven Press, 1992.

46. Hellström-Westas L: Comparison between tape recorded and amplitude integrated EEG monitoring in sick newborn infants. Acta Paediatr 81:812, 1992.

47. Klebermass K, Kuhle S, Kohlhauser-Vollmuth C, et al: Evaluation of the cerebral function monitor as a tool for neurophysiological surveillance in neonatal intensive care patients. Child Nerv Syst 17:544, 2001.

48. Alfonso I, Jayakar P, Yelin K, et al: Continuous-display four-channel electroencephalographic monitoring in the evaluation of neonates with paroxysmal motor events. J Child Neurol 16:625, 2001.

49. Clancy R, Legido A: The exact ictal and interictal duration of electroencephalographic neonatal seizures. Epilepsia 28:537, 1987.

50. Sheth RD: Electroencephalogram confirmatory rate in neonatal seizures. Pediatr Neurol 20:27, 1999.

51. Scher MS, Hamid MY, Steppe DA, et al: Ictal and interictal durations in preterm and term neonates. Epilepsia 34:284, 1993.

52. Scher MS, Alvin J, Gaus L, et al: Uncoupling of electrical and clinical expression of neonatal seizures after antiepileptic drug administration. Pediatr Neurol 11:83, 1994.

53. Scher MS, Beggarly M: Clinical significance of focal periodic patterns in the newborn. J Child Neurol 4:175, 1989.

54. Oliveira AJ, Nunes ML, Haertel LM, et al: Duration of rhythmic EEG patterns in neonates: New evidence for clinical and prognostic significance of brief rhythmic discharges. Clin Neurophysiol 111:1646, 2000.

55. Alfonso I, Papazian O, Litt R, et al: Single photon emission computed tomographic evaluation of brainstem release phenomenon and seizure in neonates. J Child Neurol 15:56, 2000.

56. Kilic S, Tarim Ö, Eralp Ö: Serum prolactin in neonatal seizures. Pediatr Int 41:61, 1999.

57. Browning RA: Role of the brainstem reticular formation in tonic-clonic seizures: Lesion and pharmacological studies. Fed Proc 44;2425, 1985.

58. Caveness WF, Kato M, Malamut BL, et al: Propagation of focal motor seizures in the pubescent monkey. Ann Neurol 7:213, 1980.

59. Hosokawa S, Iguchi T, Caveness WF, et al: Effects of manipulation of sensorimotor system on focal motor seizures in the monkey. Ann Neurol 7:222, 1980.

60. Danner R, Shewmon DA, Sherman MP: Seizures in an atelencephalic infant. Is the cortex essential for neonatal seizures? Arch Neurol 42:1014, 1985.

61. Coen RW, McCutchen CB, Wermer D, et al: Continuous monitoring of electroencephalogram following perinatal asphyxia. J Pediatr 100:628, 1982.

62. O'Meara WM, Bye AME, Flanagan D: Clinical features of neonatal seizures. J Pediatr Child. Health 31:237, 1995.

63. Scher MS, Aso K, Beggarly ME, et al: Electrographic seizures in preterm and full-term neonates: Clinical correlates, associated brain lesions, and risk for neurological sequelae. Pediatrics 91:128, 1993.

64. Staudt F, Roth G, Engel RC: The usefulness of electroencephalography in curarized newborns. Electroencephalogr Clin Neurophysiol 51:205, 1981.

65. Eyre P, Oozen RC, Wilkinson AR: Continuous electroencephalographic recording to detect seizures in paralyzed newborns. BMJ 286:1017, 1983.

66. Goldberg RN, Goldman SL, Ramsay RE, et al: Detection of seizure activity in the paralyzed neonate using continuous monitoring. Pediatrics 69:583, 1982.

67. Ericksson M, Zetterstrom R: Neonatal convulsions. Incidence and causes in the Stockholm area. Acta Paediatr Scand 68:807, 1979.

68. Seay AR, Bray PF: Significance of seizures in infants weighing less than 2500 grams. Arch Neurol 34:381, 1977.

69. Ronen GM, Penney S, Andrews W: The epidemiology of clinical neonatal seizures in Newfoundland: A population-based study. J Pediatr 134:71, 1999.

70. Saliba RM, Annegers FJ, Waller DK et al: Risk factors for neonatal seizures: A population-based study, Harris County, Texas, 1992-1994. Am J Epidemiol 154:14, 2001.

71. Lanska MJ, Lanska DJ, Baumann RJ, et al: Interobserver variability in the classification of neonatal seizures based on medical record data. Pediatr Neurol 15:120, 1996.

72. Lanska MJ, Lanska DJ, Baumann RJ, et al: A population-based study of neonatal seizures in Fayette County, Kentucky. Neurology 45:724, 1995.

73. Monod N, Pajot N, Guidasci S: The neonatal EEG: Statistical studies and prognostic value in full-term and preterm babies. Electroencephalogr Clin Neurophysiol 32:529, 1972.

74. Tharp BR, Cukier F, Monod N: The prognostic value of the electroencephalogram in premature infants. Electroencephalogr Clin Neurophysiol 51:219, 1981.

75. Bye AME, Cunningham CA, Chee KY, et al: Outcome of neonates with electrographically identified seizures, or at risk of seizures. Pediatr Neurol 16:225, 1997.

76. Sinclair DB, Campbell M, Byrne P, et al: EEG and long-term outcome of term infants with neonatal hypoxic-ischemic encephalopathy. Clin Neurophysiol 110:655, 1999.

77. Scher MS: Neurophysiological assessment of brain function and maturation. I. A measure of brain adaptation in high risk infants. Pediatr Neurol 16:191, 1997.

78. Scher MS: Neurophysiological assessment of brain function and maturation. II. A measure of brain dysmaturity in healthy preterm neonates. Pediatr Neurol 16:287, 1997.

79. Tharp BR, Scher MS, Clancy RR: Serial EEGs in normal and abnormal infants with birth weights less than 1200 grams—a prospective study with long term follow-up. Neuropediatrics 20:64, 1989.

80. Laroia N, Guillet R, Burchfiel J, McBride MC, et al: EEG background as predictor of electrographic seizures in high-risk neonates. Epilepsia 39:545, 1998.

81. Scher MS: Neonatal seizures. Seizures in special clinical settings. In Wyllie E (ed): The Treatment of Epilepsy: Principles and Practice, 3rd ed. Baltimore, Williams & Wilkins, 2001, pp 577-600.

82. Scher MS, Alvin J, Minnigh MB, et al: EEG screening for seizures in an inborn neonatal population prior to antiepileptic drug administration. Pediatr Res 37:385A, 1995.

83. Lien JM, Towers CV, Quilligan EJ, et al: Term early-onset neonatal seizures: Obstetric characteristics, etiologic classifications, and perinatal care. Obstet Gynecol 85:163, 1995.

84. Patterson CA, Graves WL, Bugg G, et al: Antenatal and intrapartum factors associated with the occurrence of seizures in the term infant. Obstet Gynecol 74:361, 1989.

85. Sorokin Y, Blackwell S, Reinke T, et al: Demographic and intrapartum characteristics of term pregnancies with early-onset neonatal seizures. J Perinatol 21:90, 2001.

86. Adamson SJ, Alessandri LM, Badawi N, et al: Predictors of neonatal encephalopathy in full term infants. BMJ 311:598, 1995.

87. Arpino C, Domizio S, Carrieri MP, et al: Prenatal and perinatal determinants of neonatal seizures occurring in the first week of life. J Child Neurol 16:651, 2001.

88. Bergman I, Painter MJ, Hirsh RP, et al: Outcome in neonates with convulsions treated in an intensive care unit. Ann Neurol 14:642, 1983.

89. Brown JK, Cockburn F, Forfar JO: Clinical and chemical correlates in convulsions of the newborn. Lancet 1:135, 1972.

90. Brown JK, Previce RJF, Forfar JO, et al: Neurological aspects of perinatal asphyxia. Dev Med Child Neurol 16:567, 1974.

91. Sarnat HB, Sarnat MS: Neonatal encephalography following fetal distress. A clinical and encephalographic study. Arch Neurol 33:696, 1976.

92. Autschuler G: The relationship of placental pathology to causation of detrimental pregnancy outcome. In Stevenson D, Sunshine P (eds): Fetal and Neonatal Brain Injury. New York, Oxford Medical Publishers, 1997, pp 585-601.

93. Bejar R, Wozniak P, Allard M, et al: Antenatal origin of neurologic damage in newborn infants. Am J Obstet Gynecol 159:357, 1988.

94. Evrard P, Kadhim HJ, de Saint-George P, et al: Abnormal development and destructive processes of the human brain during the second half of gestation. In Evans P, Minkowski A (eds): Developmental Neurobiology. New York, Raven Press, 1989, 10:21-39.

95. Lieberman E, Eichenwald E, Mathur G, et al: Intrapartum fever and unexplained seizures in term infants. Pediatrics 106:983, 2000.

96. ACOG Technical Bulletin 163: Fetal and Neonatal Neurologic Injury. Washington, DC, American College of Obstetrics and Gynecology, January 1992, pp 1-6.

97. Ahn MO, Korst LM, Phelan JP, et al: Does the onset of neonatal seizures correlate with the timing of fetal neurologic injury? Clin Pediatr 37:673, 1998.

98. Ekert P, Perlman M, Steinlin M, et al: Predicting the outcome of postasphyxial hypoxic-ischemic encephalopathy within 4 hours of birth. J Pediatr 131:613, 1997.

99. Low JA, Panagiotopoulos L, Derrick EJ: Newborn complications after intrapartum asphyxia with metabolic acidosis at term. Am J Obstet Gynecol 170:1081, 1994.

100. Nelson KB, Ellenberg JH: Apgar scores as predictors of chronic neurologic disability. Pediatrics 68:36, 1981.

101. Nelson KB, Leviton A: How much of neonatal encephalopathy is due to birth asphyxia? Am J Dis Child 145:1325, 1991.

102. Scher MS, Trucco J, Beggarly ME, et al: Neonates with electrically-confirmed seizures and possible placental associations. Pediatr Neurol 19:37, 1998.

103. Barabas RE, Barmada MA, Scher MS: Timing of brain insults in severe neonatal encephalopathies with an iso-electric EEG. Pediatr Neurol 9:39, 1993.

104. Cornblath M, Schwartz R: Disorders of Carbohydrate Metabolism in Infancy. Philadelphia, WB Saunders, 1967, pp 33-54.

105. Milner RDG: Neonatal hypoglycemia: A critical reappraisal. Arch Neurol 47:679, 1972.

106. Senior B: Neonatal hypoglycemia. N Engl J Med 289:790, 1973.

107. Griffiths AD, Laurence KM: The effect of hypoxia and hypoglycemia on the brain of the newborn human infant. Dev Med Child Neurol 16:308, 1974.

108. Siemkowicz E, Hansen AJ: Clinical restitution following cerebral ischemia in hypo-, normo- and hyperglycemic rats. Acta Neurol Scand 58:1, 1978.

109. Glauser TA, Rorke LB, Weinberg PM, et al: Acquired neuropathologic lesions associated with the hypoplastic left heart syndrome. Pediatrics 85:991, 1990.

110. Keen JH, Lee D: Sequelae of neonatal convulsions. Study of 112 infants. Arch Dis Child 48:541, 1973.

111. McInterny JK, Schubert WK: Prognosis of neonatal seizures. Am J Dis Child 117:261, 1969.

112. Lynch BJ, Rust RS: Natural history and outcome of neonatal hypocalcemic and hypomagnesemic seizures. Pediatr Neurol 11:23, 1994.

113. Ment LR, Duncan CC, Ehrenkranz RA: Perinatal cerebral infarction. Ann Neurol 16:559, 1984.

114. Rivkin MJ, Anderson ML, Kaye EM: Neonatal idiopathic cerebral venous thrombosis: An unrecognized cause of transient seizures or lethargy. Ann Neurol 32:51, 1992.

115. Scher MS, Tharp B: Significance of focal abnormalities in neonatal EEG-radiologic correlation and outcome. Ann Neurol 12:217, 1982.

116. Shevell MI, Silver K, O'Gorman AM, et al: Neonatal dural sinus thrombosis. Pediatr Neurol 5:161, 1989.

117. Hill A, Volpe JJ: Seizures, hypoxic-ischemic brain injury and intraventricular hemorrhage in the newborn. Ann Neurol 10:109, 1981.

118. Sheth RD, Hobbs GR, Mullett M: Neonatal seizures: Incidence, onset, and etiology by gestational age. J Perinatol 19:40, 1999.

119. Strober JB, Bienkowski RS, Maytal J: The incidence of acute and remote seizures in children with intraventricular hemorrhage. Clin Pediatr 36:643, 1997.

120. Miller V: Neonatal cerebral infarction. Semin Pediatr Neurol 7:278, 2000.

121. Marret S, Lardennois C, Mercier A, et al: Fetal and neonatal cerebral infarcts. Biol Neonate 79:236, 2001.

122. De Vries LS, Groenendaal F, Eken P, et al: Infarcts in the vascular distribution of the middle cerebral artery in preterm and fullterm infants. Neuropediatrics 28:88, 1997.

123. Mercuri E, Cowan F, Rutherford M, et al: Ischaemic and haemorrhagic brain lesions in newborns with seizures and normal Apgar scores. Arch Dis Child 73:F67, 1995.

124. Forbes KPN, Pipe JG, Byrd R: Neonatal hypoxic-ischemic encephalopathy. Detection with diffusion-weighted MRI imaging. AJNR Am J Neuroradiol 21:1490, 2000.

125. Benitz WE, Rhine WD, VanMeurs KP: Persistent pulmonary hypertension of the newborn. In DK Stephenson, Sunshine P (eds): Fetal and Neonatal Brain Injury. Oxford, Oxford Medical Publishers, 1997, pp 564-582.

126. Kairam R, DeVivo DC: Neurologic manifestations of congenital infection. Clin Perinatol 8:455, 1981.

127. Mizrahi EM, Tharp BR: Characteristic EEG pattern in neonatal herpes simplex encephalitis. Neurology 32:1215, 1982.

128. Palmini A, Andermann E, Andermann F: Prenatal events and genetic factors in epileptic patients with neuronal migration disorders. Epilepsia 35:965, 1994.
129. Aicardi J: Early myoclonic encephalopathy. In Roger J, Bureau M, Dravet CH, et al (eds): Epileptic Syndromes in Infancy, Childhood, and Adolescence. London, J Libbey Eurotext, 1985, pp 12-22.
130. Ohtahara S: Clinico-electrical delineation of epileptic encephalopathies in childhood. Asian Med J 21:7, 1978.
131. Chugani HT, Rintahaka PJ, Shewmon DA: Ictal patterns of cerebral glucose utilization in children with epilepsy. Epilepsia 35:813, 1994.
132. Pedespan JM, Loiseau H, Vital A, et al: Surgical treatment of an early epileptic encephalopathy with suppression-bursts and focal cortical dysplasia. Epilepsia 36:37, 1995.
133. Painter MJ, Bergman I, Crumrine PK: Neonatal seizures. In Pellock MJ, Myer EC (eds): Neurologic Emergencies in Infancy and Childhood. New York, Harper & Row, 1984, pp 17-35.
134. Bejsovec M, Kulenda Z, Ponca E: Familial intrauterine convulsions in pyridoxine dependency. Arch Dis Child 42:201, 1967.
135. Clarke TA, Saunders BS, Feldman B: Pyridoxine-dependent seizures requiring high doses of pyridoxine for control. Am J Dis Child 133:963, 1979.
136. Osiovich H, Barrington K: Prenatal ultrasound diagnosis of seizures. Am J Perinatol 13:499, 1996.
137. DeVivo DC, Trifiletti RR, Jacobson RI, et al: Defective glucose transport across the blood-brain barrier as a cause of persistent hypoglycorrhachia, seizures, and developmental delay. N Engl J Med 325;703, 1991.
138. Slot HMJ, Overweg-Plandsoen WC, Bakker HD, et al: Molybdenum-cofactor deficiency: An easily missed cause of neonatal convulsions. Neuropediatrics 24:139, 1993.
139. Herzlinger RA, Kandall SR, Vaughn HG: Neonatal seizures associated with narcotic withdrawal. J Pediatr 92:638, 1977.
140. Zelson C, Rubio E, Wasserman E: Neonatal narcotic addiction: 10 year observation. Pediatrics 48:178, 1971.
141. Kandall SR, Garner LM: Late presentation of drug withdrawal symptoms in newborns. Am J Dis Child 127:58, 1974.
142. Bleyer WA, Marshall RE: Barbiturate withdrawal syndrome in a passively addicted infant. JAMA 221:185, 1972.
143. Dodson WE: Neonatal drug intoxication: Local anesthetics. Pediatr Clin North Am 23:399, 1976.
144. Hillman LS, Hillman RE, Dodson WE: Diagnosis, treatment, and follow-up of neonatal mepivacaine intoxication secondary to paracervical and pudendal blocks during labor. J Pediatr 94:472, 1979.
145. Mizrahi EM, Clancy RR: Neonatal seizures: Early-onset seizure syndromes and their consequences for development. Ment Retard Dev Disabil Res Rev 6:229, 2000.
146. Natsume J, Watanabe K, Negoro T, et al: Cryptogenic localization-related epilepsy of neonatal onset. Seizure 5:317, 1996.
147. Miller SP, Tasch T, Sylvain M, et al: Tuberous sclerosis complex and neonatal seizures. J Child Neurol 13:619, 1998.
148. Bjerre I, Corelius E: Benign familial neonatal convulsions. Acta Paediatr Scand 57:557, 1978.
149. Petit RE, Fenichel GM: Benign familial neonatal seizures. Arch Neurol 37:47, 1980.
150. Ryan SG, Wiznitzer M, Hollman C, et al: Benign familial neonatal convulsions: Evidence for clinical and genetic heterogeneity. Ann Neurol 29:469, 1991.
151. Leppert M, Singh N: Benign familial neonatal epilepsy with mutations in two potassium channel genes. Curr Opin Neurol 12:143, 1999.
152. Jentsch TJ, Schroeder BC, Kubisch C, et al: Pathophysiology of KCNQ channels: Neonatal epilepsy and progressive deafness. Epilepsia 41:1068, 2000.
153. Doose H, Koudriavtseva K, Neubauer BA: Multifactorial pathogenesis of neonatal seizures—relationships to the benign partial epilepsies. Epileptic Disord 2:195, 2000.
154. Doose H, Neubauer BA, Petersen B: The concept of hereditary impairment of brain maturation. Epileptic Disord 2:S45, 2000.
155. Friede RL: Porencephaly, hydranencephaly, multilocular cystic encephalopathy. In: Developmental Neuropathology. New York, Springer-Verlag, 1975, pp 102-113.
156. Felix JF, Badaw N, Kuringzuk JJ, et al: Birth defects in children with newborn encephalopathy. Dev Med Child Neurol 42:803, 2000.
157. Leth H, Toft PB, Herning M, et al: Neonatal seizures associated with cerebral lesions shown by magnetic resonance imaging. Arch Dis Child Fetal Neonatal Ed 77:F105, 1997.
158. McIntire DD, Bloom SL, Casey BM, et al: Birth weight in relation to morbidity and mortality among newborn infants. N Engl J Med 340:1234, 1999.
159. Scher MS, Painter MJ: Electrographic diagnosis of neonatal seizures. Issues of diagnostic accuracy, clinical correlation and survival. In Wasterlain CG, Vert P (eds): Neonatal Seizures. New York, Raven Press, 1990, pp 19-41.
160. Temple CM, Dennis J, Carney R, et al: Neonatal seizures: Long-term outcome and cognitive development among "normal" survivors. Dev Med Child Neurol 37:109, 1995.
161. Holmes GL, Ben-Ari Y: The neurobiology and consequences of epilepsy in the developing brain. Pediatr Res 49:320, 2001.
162. Barkovich AJ, Baranski K, Vigneron D et al: Proton MR spectroscopy for the evaluation of brain injury in asphyxiated term neonates. AJNR Am J Neuroradiol 20:1399, 1999.
163. Maneru C, Junque C, Bargallo N et al: H-MR spectroscopy is sensitive to subtle effects of perinatal asphyxia. Neurology 57:1115, 2001.
164. McBride M, Laroia N, Guillet R: Electrographic seizures in neonates correlate with poor neurodevelopmental outcome. Neurology 55:506, 2000.
165. Rowe RJ, Holmes GL, Hafford J, et al: Prognostic value of electroencephalogram in term and preterm infants following neonatal seizures. Electroencephalogr Clin Neurophysiol 60:183, 1985.
166. Holden KR, Mellits ED, Freeman JM: Neonatal seizures. I: Correlation of prenatal and perinatal events with outcomes. Pediatrics 70:165, 1982.
167. Clancy RR, Legido A: Postnatal epilepsy after EEG-confirmed neonatal seizures. Epilepsia 32:69, 1991.
168. Dwyer BE, Wasterlain CG: Electroconvulsive seizures in the immature rat adversely affect myelin accumulation. Exp Neurol 78:616, 1982.
169. Wasterlain CG, Plum F: The vulnerability of developing rat brain to electroconvulsive seizures. Arch Neurol 19:38, 1973.
170. Wasterlain CG: Controversies in epilepsy. Recurrent seizures in the developing brain are harmful. Epilepsia 38:728, 1997.
171. Wasterlain CG: Effects of neonatal status epilepticus on rat brain. Dev Neurol 26:975, 1976.
172. Wasterlain CG: Neonatal seizures in brain growth. Neuropediatrics 9:213, 1978.

173. Ajayi OA, Oyaniyi OT, Chike-Obi UD, et al: Adverse effects of early phenobarbital administration in term newborns with perinatal asphyxia. Trop Med Int Health 3:592, 1998.
174. Lockman LA, Kriel R, Zaske D, et al: Phenobarbital dosage for control of neonatal seizures. Neurology 29:1445, 1979.
175. Painter MJ, Pippenger C, McDonald H, et al: Phenobarbital and diphenylhydantoin levels in neonates with seizures. J Pediatr 9:315, 1978.
176. Painter MJ, Pippenger C, Wasterlain C, et al: Phenobarbital and phenytoin in neonatal seizures, metabolism, and tissue distribution. Neurology 31:1107, 1981.
177. Smith BI, Misoh RE: Intravenous diazepam in the treatment of prolonged seizure activity in neonates and infants. Dev Med Child Neurol 13:630, 1971.
178. Gal P, Toback J, Boer HR, et al: Efficacy of phenobarbital monotherapy in treatment of neonatal seizures. Relationship of blood levels. Neurology 32:1401, 1982.
179. Hall RT, Hall FK, Daily DK: High-dose phenobarbital therapy in term newborn infants with severe perinatal asphyxia: A randomized, prospective study with three-year follow-up. J Pediatr 132:345, 1998.
180. Painter MJ, Scher MS, Alvin J, et al: A comparison of the efficacy of phenobarbital and phenytoin in the treatment of neonatal seizures. N Engl J Med 341:485, 1999.
181. Painter MJ, Minnigh B, Mollica L, et al: Binding profiles of anticonvulsants in neonates with seizures. Ann Neurol 22:413, 1987.
182. Montenegro MA, Guerreiro MM, Caldas JPS et al: Epileptic manifestations induced by midazolam in the neonatal period. Arq Neuropsiquiatr 59:242, 2001.
183. Jensen FE: Acute and chronic effects of seizures in the developing brain: Experimental models. Epilepsia 40:S51, 1999.
184. Koh S, Jensen FE: Topiramate blocks perinatal hypoxia-induced seizures in rat pups. Ann Neurol 50:366, 2001.
185. Jensen FE, Wang C: Hypoxia-induced hyperexcitability in vivo and in vitro in the immature hippocampus. Epilepsy Res 26:131, 1996.
186. Aronica EM, Gorter JA, Paupard M-C, et al: Status epilepticus–induced alterations in metabotropic glutamate receptor expression in young and adult rats. J Neurosci 17:8588, 1997.
187. Sanchez RM, Koh S, Rio C, et al: Decreased glutamate receptor 2 expression and enhanced epileptogenesis in immature rat hippocampus after perinatal hypoxia-induced seizures. J Neurosci 21:8154, 2001.
188. Lie AA, Becker A, Behle K, et al: Up-regulation of the metabotropic glutamate receptor mGluR4 in hippocampal neurons with reduced seizure vulnerability. Ann Neurol 47:26, 2000.
189. Hellström-Westas L, Blennow G, Lindroth M, et al: Low risk of seizure recurrence after early withdrawal of antiepileptic treatment in the neonatal period. Arch Dis Child 72:F97, 1995.
190. Mizrahi EM: Acute and chronic effects of seizures in the developing brain: Lessons from clinical experience. Epilepsia 40:S42, 1999.
191. Holmes GL, Gairsa JL, Chevassus-Au-Louis N, Ben-Ari Y: Consequences of neonatal seizures in the rat: Morphological and behavioral effects. Ann Neurol 44:845, 1998.
192. Huang L-T, Cilio MR, Silveira DC, et al: Long-term effects of neonatal seizures: A behavioral, electrophysiological, and histological study. Dev Brain Res 118:99, 1999.
193. Sankar R, Shin D, Mazarati AM, et al: Epileptogenesis after status epilepticus reflects age- and model-dependent plasticity. Ann Neurol 48:580, 2000.
194. Wong M, Yamada KA: Developmental characteristics of epileptiform activity in immature rat neocortex: A comparison of four in vitro seizure models. Dev Brain Res 128:113, 2001.
195. Koh S, Storey TW, Santos TC, et al: Early-life seizures in rats increase susceptibility to seizure-induced brain injury in adulthood. Neurology 53:915, 1999.
196. Schmid R, Tandon P, Stafstrom CE, Holmes GL: Effects of neonatal seizures on subsequent seizure-induced brain injury. Neurology 53:1754, 1999.
197. McCabe BK, Silveira DC, Cilio MR, et al: Reduced neurogenesis after neonatal seizures. J Neurosci 21:2094, 2001.
198. Sogawa Y, Monokoshi M, Silveira DC, et al: Timing of cognitive deficits following neonatal seizures: Relationship to histological changes in the hippocampus. Dev Brain Res 131:73, 2001.
199. Takei Y, Takashima S, Ohyu J, et al: Effects of nitric oxide synthase inhibition on the cerebral circulation and brain damage during kainic acid–induced seizures in newborn rabbits. Brain Dev 21:253, 1999.
200. Wirrell EC, Armstrong EA, Osman LD, et al: Prolonged seizures exacerbate perinatal hypoxic-ischemic brain damage. Pediatr Res 50:445, 2001.
201. Landrot IDR, Minokoshi M, Silveira DC, et al: Recurrent neonatal seizures: Relationship of pathology to the electroencephalogram and cognition. Dev Brain Res 129:27, 2001.
202. Thoresen M, Hallström ASA, Whitelaw A, et al: Lactate and pyruvate changes in the cerebral gray and white matter during posthypoxic seizures in newborn pigs. Pediatr Res 44:746, 1998.

CHAPTER 56

Follow-up of the High-Risk Neonate

Judy C. Bernbaum, Marsha Gerdes, and Alan R. Spitzer

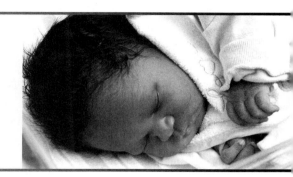

ew specialty areas of medicine have examined the efforts of intervention as carefully and as rigorously as neonatology. Since the earliest days of the specialty, neonatal follow-up programs have been viewed as an essential component of high-risk newborn care. Neonatologists have repeatedly examined the long-term effects of various treatments in order to develop new interventions and improve on previous efforts. In this rapidly changing health care environment, the care of the critically ill newborn does not end at the time of hospital discharge. With increasing frequency, neonates are being discharged to home care programs in which follow-up is an even more important part of the overall care of the newborn.

The goals of the neonatal follow-up program are to ensure appropriate ongoing treatment for infants, identify neurodevelopmental problems at a stage in which intervention can be most effective, and provide appropriate consultation to primary care physicians who may be entrusted with many acute-care needs of these complicated cases. Thus, the role of the neonatologist in follow-up is multifaceted. In some cases, this role is filled by a developmental pediatrician who is well versed in the medical and developmental needs of the former neonatal intensive care unit patient. The individual physician must function as a multidisciplinary coordinator who ensures that the infant receives appropriate therapies (physical, occupational, speech, educational), directed nursing care, and audiology and vision services, while remaining a valued source of support for the family, whose life is often disrupted by the birth of a premature or critically ill infant.

In assigning patients to high-risk follow-up, each neonatology program must identify groups of patients and the degree of support that can be furnished. Many programs can follow all patients admitted to the intensive care nursery, whereas other programs are capable of monitoring only a percentage of the infants who leave this unit. Box 56-1 lists patients who should be considered for high-risk programs.

The list of patients who should be considered for high-risk programs should be modified to meet the needs of the individual neonatology program or research considerations. Because outcome is so variable from institution to institution, it is essential that some type of neonatal follow-up be provided so that each program can observe the results of its interventional strategies during the immediate neonatal period.

GROWTH AND NUTRITION

The growth of the high-risk neonate after nursery discharge is often a valuable indicator of the infant's state of health, particularly during the first 2 years of life. Poor growth after discharge may reflect a variety of disorders, including inadequate caloric administration, chronic illness, and abnormalities in gastrointestinal motility, as well as inappropriate feeding techniques. Although these factors can affect all infants discharged from nurseries, the preterm infant is particularly vulnerable to such problems, because catch-up growth is dramatic in the formerly preterm infant, who should thrive when given adequate nutrition.

Many factors can alter the subsequent growth of the premature infant. The child with residual pulmonary disease—for example, as seen with chronic lung disease—may have caloric requirements that substantially exceed those for the preterm infant with no ongoing pulmonary problems. In addition to chronic illness, the preterm neonate is often susceptible to recurring acute illnesses, particularly during the first year after birth. These repeated episodes, particularly if they involve enteric or respiratory infections, may lead to a growth pattern that is significantly aberrant. Furthermore, some former preterm infants may exhibit some degree of malabsorption, especially if necrotizing enterocolitis has been part of the original hospital course. Neurologic complications, such as intraventricular hemorrhage or periventricular leukomalacia, may also affect motor skills and result in feeding inadequacies that ultimately impair growth after hospital discharge. Parents of an infant with poor feeding skills may need supportive nursing and medical advice.

To determine whether growth in a preterm infant is adequate, the original gestational age of the infant must be accounted for. Standard curves, specifically designed for preterm infants, have been developed to compare the preterm infant's growth against expected norms on the basis of an infant's birth weight and gestational age (Figs. 56-1 to 56-4). By 2½ years of age, the difference between the preterm infant and term infant should be inconsequential if growth is adequate. The physician must be certain, however, not to wait for any particular points before an interventional strategy is adopted, if growth failure is apparent earlier.

Infants who are appropriate in size for gestational age (AGA) usually demonstrate catch-up growth by 2 years of age; the fastest catch-up growth rates occur between 36 and 44 weeks after conception. Little catch-up growth occurs beyond a chronological age of 3 years. The head circumference of the infant often is the first measurement that demonstrates catch-up growth, and it is commonly plotted at a higher percentile than either length or weight during the first months after hospital discharge. Increases in weight are commonly followed by increases in linear growth within a few months. Because rapid head growth may represent the onset of posthemorrhagic hydrocephalus, the physician should not be reassured by rapid head growth in the preterm infant who has suffered a grade III or IV intraventricular hemorrhage. Another common cause of macrocephaly in this population of infants at high risk is an abnormal accumulation of extraaxial (subarachnoid) fluid, the cause of which seems to be related to situations that lead to diminished venous return from the head. This is more commonly encountered in infants who have developed bronchopulmonary dysplasia (BPD) or required extracorporeal membrane oxygenation during their neonatal course. In contrast, slow head growth, or a head circumference that measures at a significantly lower percentile than either length or weight, is also cause for concern and further investigation. Such infants often have suffered injury to growth centers in the brain and may have significant cerebral atrophy.

It is also helpful to examine growth velocity for weight and height of the infant. For former preterm infants, it is not uncommon for an infant's weight to exceed the percentile noted for length during the first year of life. In this case, the physician should discuss with the family the possibility that the infant is being overfed. A thorough dietary history should be obtained. Many parents of former preterm infants attempt to compensate for the infant's original low birth weight by providing excessive amounts of calories. In contrast, some infants grow at a slower, but progressive, rate during this period. Significant discrepancies in weight and length, however, or a prominent decline of all growth parameters in the preterm infant may reflect suboptimal nutritional intake and mandates further investigation.

The growth of infants who are small for gestational age (SGA) often varies significantly from that seen in AGA infants. Although often demonstrating rapid growth early, the SGA infant with low birth weight typically demonstrates ultimately less catch-up growth than that seen in AGA infants. By 3 years of age, approximately 50% of SGA infants are below average in weight, in comparison with 15% of AGA infants with low birth weight. SGA infants who have symmetric proportions—that is, head circumference, length, and weight are similar in percentile—are less likely to demonstrate catch-up growth than the SGA infant whose head circumference percentile at the time of birth exceeds the percentiles for length and weight. These observations suggest that the SGA infant with symmetric growth retardation is more likely to have suffered an intrauterine neurologic insult than is the child whose head growth is normal.

Nutritional requirements are becoming better established and, if met, result in more optimal growth for the preterm infant. Traditionally, the goal for the preterm infant is to approximate the growth rate seen in utero for a fetus at a similar postconception age. A growth rate of approximately 15 to 20 g per day on the average can be considered an acceptable rate of weight gain during the first few months after birth for a preterm infant. The physician must, however, always take into account the accompanying medical complications for the child, such as BPD and infection. In general, the nutritional requirements for a preterm infant exceed those of the full-term child. By term, even if the former preterm infant has no ongoing medical illnesses, the dietary requirements continue to be somewhat different from those of the full-term infant. Breast milk often must be supplemented with additional nutrients, and there are now 22-kcal/oz formulas specially formulated to meet the needs of the growing preterm infant after hospital discharge. Many infants require even more concentrated formula or breast milk fortification because of increased caloric requirements, feeding dysfunction, or medical illness, such as BPD, in which volume limitations may be necessary. For such infants, 24-kcal/oz formula can be made either by adding less water to formula concentrate or powder or by providing additional caloric supplementation in the form of carbohydrates or fats. Infants rarely tolerate caloric densities greater than 30 kcal/oz, and the use of such formulas should be discouraged. Infants fed with caloric formulas exceeding this are at risk for developing osmotically induced diarrhea.

For most healthy preterm infants, 110 to 130 kcal/kg/day helps achieve adequate growth. Some infants with chronic disease, such as BPD, may need as much as 150 kcal/kg/day. The caloric requirement can be determined by gradually increasing caloric intake until progressive weight gain is satisfactory. It is important to maintain the appropriate caloric distribution of nutrients, especially when caloric additives or concentrated formula is used. The proper percentage ratio of carbohydrates to fats to protein in the diet is approximately 40:50:10.

Feeding Problems

Feeding disorders are commonly seen in the preterm infant population. Most disorders involve delayed maturation of sucking and swallowing coordination, and, unless recognized, these difficulties may impair nutritional intake and disturb the normal mealtime interaction. Many infants with ongoing pulmonary disease, particularly those with tracheostomies or delayed introduction of oral feedings, have major feeding disturbances. In addition, it appears that the noxious stimuli that are often applied to the face during the neonatal intensive care period may make some infants respond adversely to any type of oral stimulation. Behavioral issues related to feeding disturbances have been well documented. Furthermore, gastroesophageal reflux (GER) and inadequate protection of the upper airway, leading to pulmonary microaspiration, may also be detrimental to the establishment of good feeding practices.

Infants may also have abnormal reflexes such as a tonic bite reflex, abnormal tongue thrust, and a hyperactive gag, which can further complicate the introduction of oral feeding. A hyperactive gag is particularly troublesome because the child may not tolerate either the nipple or a spoon on the tongue; this can lead to extreme oral hypersensitivity. Such hypersensitivity may be the result of prolonged intubation, repeated suctioning, or repeated passage of nasogastric feeding tubes. Such children, as previously mentioned, become resistant to virtually any type of oral stimulation.

To appropriately evaluate feeding disorders, it is important for the physician to take a detailed history of nutritional intake and to observe the family and the infant's response during feeding. Infants with lung disease may have oxygen desaturation during feeding, a phenomenon that can be alleviated easily by providing supplemental oxygen during oral feedings. Evaluation of the opening in the nipple and the ease with which an infant can extract formula can also be valuable in allowing the infant to feed more easily. Too small an opening may produce excessive fatigue, whereas too large an opening in the nipple may overwhelm the infant's oral cavity and lead to gagging and aspiration. Aspiration during feeding may necessitate further evaluation by milk technetium scan or radiologic examination.

Most feeding problems and growth problems, unless genetically determined or the result of severe insult during the neonatal period, are readily amenable to intervention. Development of appropriate feeding techniques between the parent and infant is often the first step in providing the infant with adequate calories and establishment of an appropriate growth pattern.

IMMUNIZATIONS

It is important for the preterm infant to receive appropriate infant immunizations as soon as feasible. The majority of premature infants should receive the same routine vaccines as the full-term infant. Diphtheria, tetanus, and acellular pertussis vaccines should be given, as per the recommendations of the American Academy of Pediatrics, to the prematurely born infant at the appropriate chronological age. The doses of these vaccines should not be reduced, because many infants do not demonstrate adequate protection if half-dose vaccine is used. Side effects are no more common in preterm infants with full-dose vaccine than in the full-term infant. The pertussis component should not be withheld in any child with cerebral palsy or muscle tone abnormality. If the child has an active seizure disorder or if a progressive neurologic disorder is diagnosed, the physician should consider obtaining clearance from the child's neurologist before administering the vaccine. Because preterm infants with BPD are at the greatest risk for serious sequelae from pertussis, the pertussis component of the vaccine, in particular, should not be withheld in these infants.

Inactivated polio vaccine should be administered at the appropriate postnatal or chronological age as per the recommendations given by the American Academy of Pediatrics for the full-term infant. All vaccines should be administered, even to infants who remain hospitalized at the usual chronological age.

Some studies have demonstrated that children with chronic lung disease or cardiac disease are at higher risk for significant illness if infected with influenza. To protect vulnerable infants, routine immunization with influenza vaccine should be given to siblings, primary caretakers, and home care nurses in order to reduce the risk to the preterm infant. In addition, for the infant older than 6 months, two doses of split-virus vaccine should be given 1 month apart between October and December. Subsequently, one dose can be given yearly if the indications for its use persist.

Other immunizations, such as those against *Haemophilus influenzae* type B, hepatitis B, measles, mumps, and rubella, should be given at the standard chronological age.

Respiratory syncytial virus (RSV) prophylaxis should be considered in infants who are at high risk for the development of serious sequelae associated with this illness. Palivizumab (Synagis) is given monthly by intramuscular

IHDP Growth Percentiles:
VLBW Premature Girls[1,2]
(≤1500 g BW, ≤37 wk GA)

Name_____

Record #_____

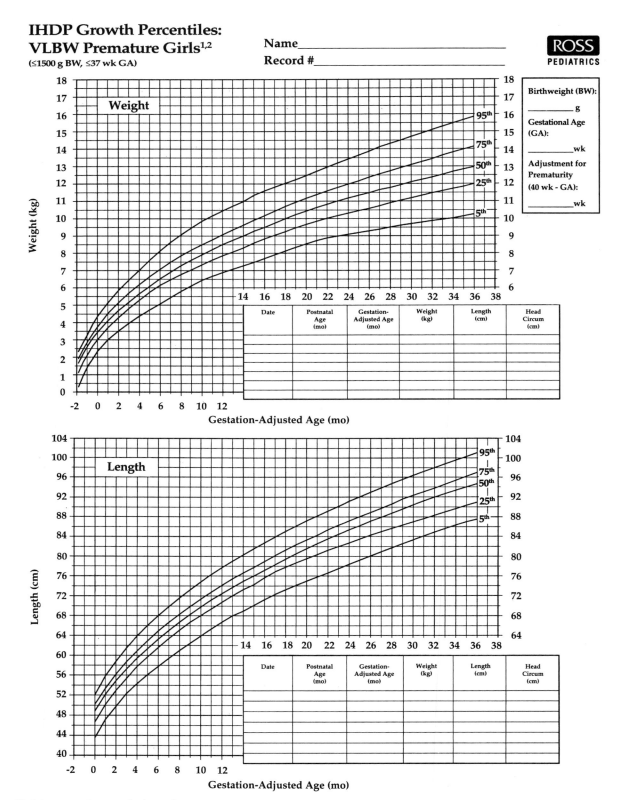

Figure 56–1 (see opposite page for legend).

IHDP Growth Percentiles: VLBW Premature Girls[1,2]

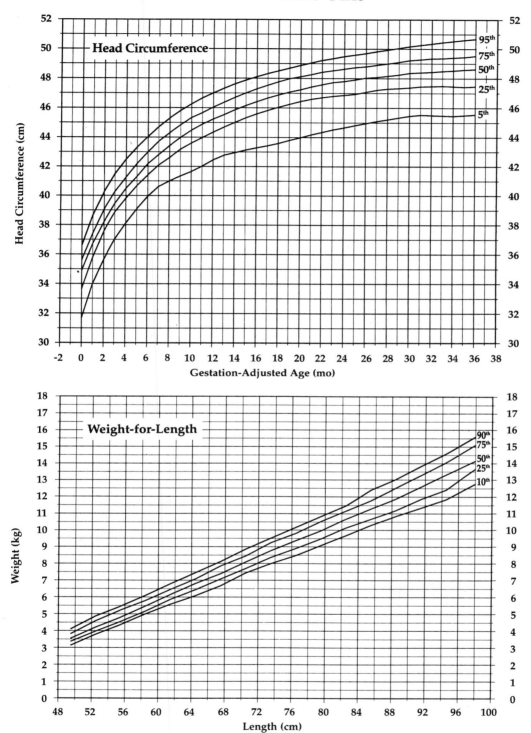

Figure 56–1, cont'd. Growth charts of girls with very low birth weight (VLBW) (≤1500 g, ≤37 weeks of gestation), based on a large sample of infants enrolled in the Infant Health and Development Program (IHDP). *(Data from Guo SS, Roche AF, Chumlea WC, et al: Growth in weight, recumbent length, and head circumference for preterm low-birthweight infants during the first three years of life using gestation-adjusted ages. Early Hum Dev 47:305, 1997; and from Guo SS, Wholihan K, Roche AF, et al: Weight-for-length reference data for preterm, low-birth-weight infants. Arch Pediatr Adolesc Med 1:964, 1996. Copyright 1999, Ross Products Division, Abbott Laboratories, Columbus, Ohio.)*

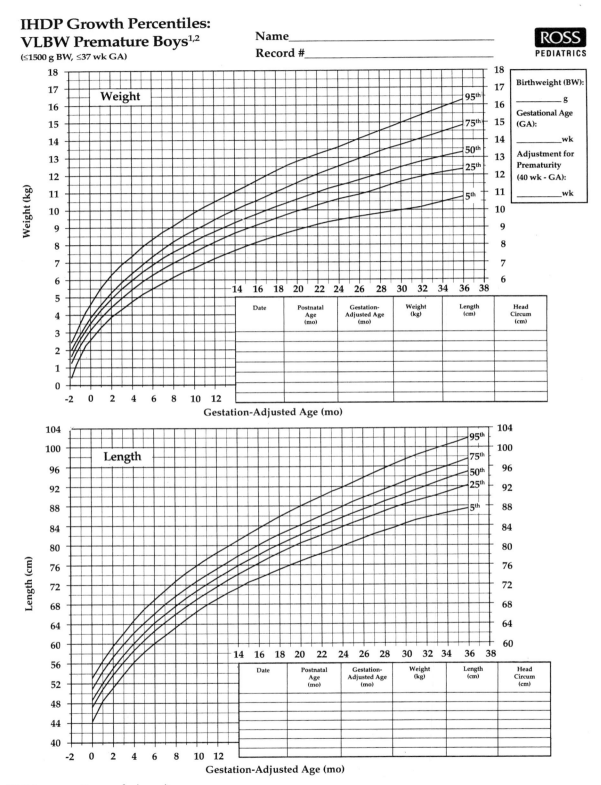

Figure 56–2 (see opposite page for legend).

IHDP Growth Percentiles: VLBW Premature Boys[1,2]

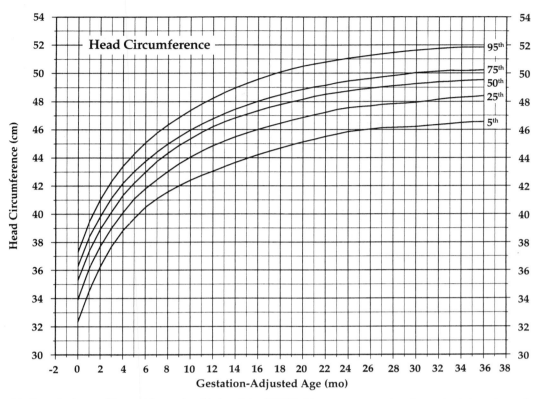

Figure 56–2, cont'd. Growth charts of boys with very low birth weight (VLBW) (≤1500 g, ≤37 weeks of gestation), based on a large sample of infants enrolled in the Infant Health and Development Program (IHDP). *(Data from the Infant Health and Development Program: Enhancing the outcomes of low-birth-weight, premature infants. A multisite, randomized trial. JAMA 263:3035, 1990; and from Casey PH, Kraemer HC, Bernbaum J, et al: Growth status and growth rates of a varied sample of low birth weight preterm infants: A longitudinal cohort from birth to three years of age. J Pediatr 119:599, 1991. Copyright 1994, Ross Products Division, Abbott Laboratories, Columbus, Ohio.)*

injection throughout the RSV season in the following circumstances:

Infants with chronic lung disease: in a child younger than 2 years chronological age who required medical therapy for chronic lung disease within the 6 months before the onset of RSV season

Preterm infants without chronic lung disease:

<28 weeks' gestational age / until 12 months' chronological age at start of RSV season

29-32 weeks' gestational age / until 6 months' chronological age at start of RSV season

33-35 weeks' gestational age / until 6 months' chronological age at start of RSV season*

SPECIALIZED CARE

The follow-up care of many preterm infants depends on the original disease processes that necessitated hospitalization. A number of problems, however, are more

*This should be considered especially if additional risk factors exist, such as exposure to smoke, attendance at a daycare center, being one of a multiple birth, or the presence of other siblings at home.

common in the preterm infant and should be monitored actively if identified during the original hospitalization or noted during any follow-up visits.

Retinopathy of Prematurity

Infants with retinopathy of prematurity (ROP) are at significant risk for visual impairment. ROP is a disorder resulting from abnormal progression of retinal vascularization in response to stimuli that are currently not fully understood. It does appear, however, that changing levels of both oxygen and carbon dioxide may be influential in the development of ROP. Most cases of ROP resolve spontaneously, although scarring of the retina can occur. In extreme cases, retinal detachment may occur in rapidly progressive disease. It is recommended that examination of the eyes of the preterm infant with a birth weight of 1500 g or less begin by 32 weeks' post-conceptional age. ROP has very rarely been diagnosed before this age. Repeat examination should be performed on the basis of findings by the ophthalmologist. A schedule of follow-up visits can then be determined to monitor the eye until the retinal vasculature has matured, at which time migration to the periphery of the retina has been completed. After resolution of ROP, yearly eye examinations are suggested to check for refractive errors, amblyopia,

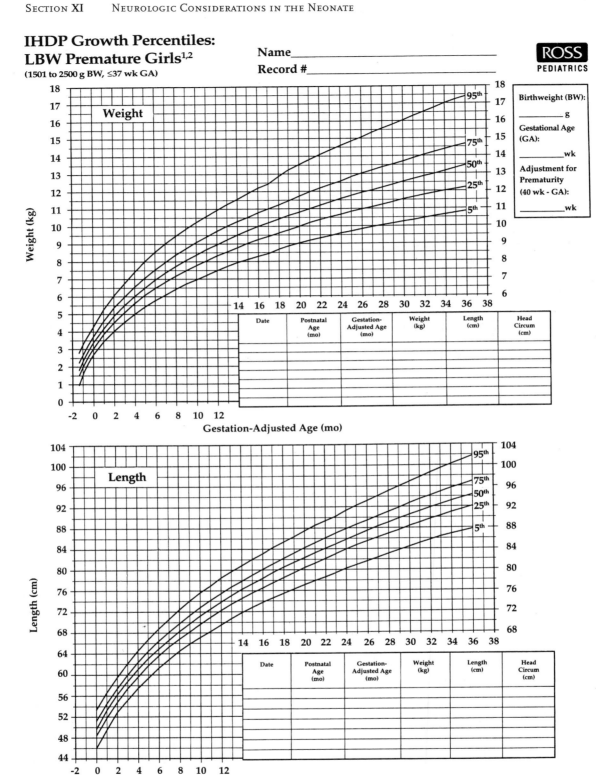

IHDP Growth Percentiles: LBW Premature Girls[1,2]
(1501 to 2500 g BW, ≤37 wk GA)

Name_____

Record #_____

ROSS
PEDIATRICS

Birthweight (BW):
_____ g
Gestational Age (GA):
_____ wk
Adjustment for Prematurity (40 wk - GA):
_____ wk

Figure 56–3 (see opposite page for legend).

IHDP Growth Percentiles: LBW Premature Girls[1,2]

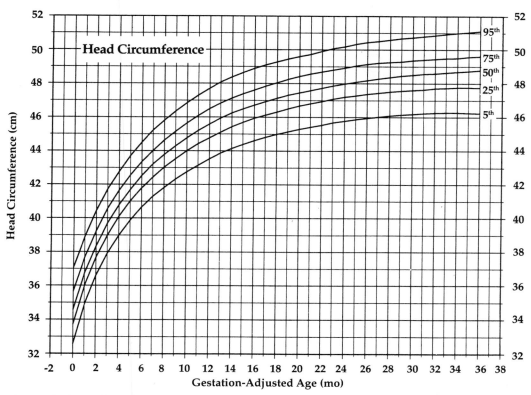

Figure 56–3, cont'd. Growth charts of girls with low birth weight (LBW) (1501 to 2500 g, ≤37 weeks of gestation), based on a large sample of infants enrolled in the Infant Health and Development Program (IHDP). *(Data from the Infant Health and Development Program: Enhancing the outcomes of low-birth-weight, premature infants. A multisite, randomized trial. JAMA 263:3035, 1990; and from Casey PH, Kraemer HC, Bernbaum J, et al: Growth status and growth rates of a varied sample of low birth weight preterm infants: A longitudinal cohort from birth to three years of age. J Pediatr 119:599, 1991. Copyright 1994, Ross Products Division, Abbott Laboratories, Columbus, Ohio.)*

or strabismus. In more severe stages of ROP, a small percentage of infants may be left with retinal tears, late retinal detachment, glaucoma, and vitreous membranes. Early intervention with cryosurgery or laser therapy to the retina can prevent many of these complications, however. For infants with visual impairments, early intervention and support services for their families are important and available through state-supported agencies.

Hearing Difficulties

A small percentage of infants in intensive care nurseries develop sensorineural hearing loss. The incidence has been estimated at between 1% and 3%. Factors that heighten risk include hypoxemia, hyperbilirubinemia, neonatal infection, congenital infection, ototoxic drugs, and excessive environmental noise and stimulation. Audiologic screening in preterm infants should be conducted before infants are 3 months of age to identify hearing loss. However, successful screening results for hearing at an initial examination does not preclude later hearing loss. Deficient response to auditory stimulation, delay in speech development, poor speech articulation, or inattentiveness should raise the suspicion of a possible hearing loss. For an infant with sensorineural hearing loss, repeat audiologic evaluation

should be performed every 3 months for 1 year after initial diagnosis and every 6 months during the preschool period. A conductive loss, caused by retained middle ear fluid, should be ruled out. Hearing loss can be classified according to the degree of decibel loss in response to formal auditory stimulation. Decibel loss greater than 15 dB is indicative of some degree of hearing loss. A loss more than 91 dB represents profound deafness.

For the child with hearing loss, the hearing aid is the primary method of treatment and can be used early in infancy. Studies have shown that greater improvement in speech can be seen when hearing aids are in use before 6 months of age. The goal of amplification of sound at this time is to avoid acoustical deprivation. With auditory stimulation, language acquisition appears to proceed more normally in most cases of mild to moderate hearing loss. For children with hearing loss that cannot be improved with hearing aids, alternative communication modes are necessary. Such modes include the use of sign language, gesturing, word spelling, or computer-assisted communication devices.

Bronchopulmonary Dysplasia

The problem of BPD is discussed in more detail in Chapter 50. Many preterm infants, as well as some

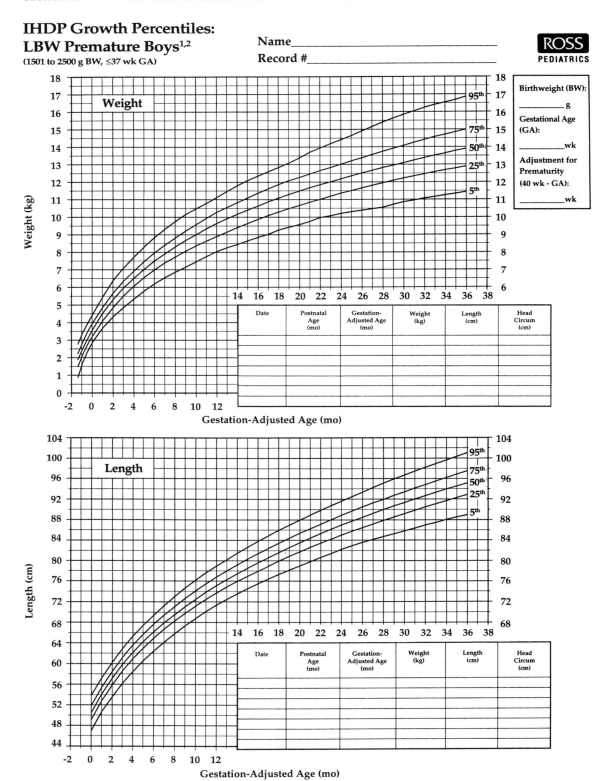

IHDP Growth Percentiles: LBW Premature Boys[1,2]
(1501 to 2500 g BW, ≤37 wk GA)

Name_____

Record #_____

Figure 56–4 (see opposite page for legend).

IHDP Growth Percentiles: LBW Premature Boys[1,2]

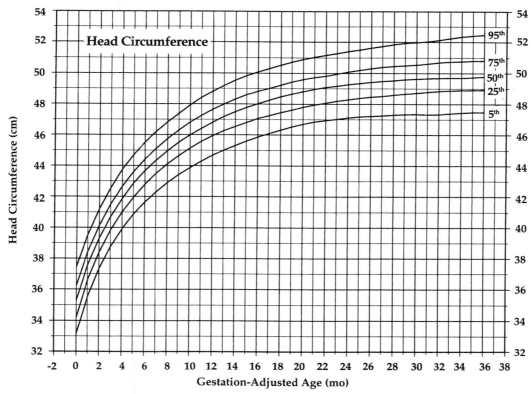

Figure 56–4, cont'd. Growth charts of boys with low birth weight (LBW) (1501 to 2500 g, ≤37 weeks of gestation), based on a large sample of infants enrolled in the Infant Health and Development Program (IHDP). *(Data from the Infant Health and Development Program: Enhancing the outcomes of low-birth-weight, premature infants. A multisite, randomized trial. JAMA 263:3035, 1990; and from Casey PH, Kraemer HC, Bernbaum J, et al: Growth status and growth rates of a varied sample of low birth weight preterm infants: A longitudinal cohort from birth to three years of age. J Pediatr 119:599, 1991. Copyright 1994, Ross Products Division, Abbott Laboratories, Columbus, Ohio.)*

full-term infants, who require ventilatory support during the neonatal period have some degree of chronic lung disease after nursery discharge. The management of these patients is often complicated and may require support from the neonatologist for many years after nursery discharge. Such support is particularly necessary for the child who requires home ventilator therapy or a tracheostomy.

Infants with BPD after hospital discharge may demonstrate poor weight gain, feeding intolerance, decreased activity level, intercurrent infections, and reduced tolerance for activity and exercise. The medical management of such infants often includes fluid restriction, diuretic therapy, bronchodilators, and supplemental oxygen. For the child with a tracheostomy, mechanical ventilator support may be necessary, even in the home setting, although it is sometimes required only on an intermittent basis. These therapies can be modified and withdrawn as the child's pulmonary condition gradually improves. (Chapter 50 contains more detailed instructions on therapy for this clinical condition.) Of importance, however, is that children with BPD are very sensitive. Changes in medical management must be small and minimally incremental, or else the child is unlikely to tolerate them. In addition, the physician must be prepared to intervene rapidly should

respiratory distress become increasingly prominent, as is often the case with an intercurrent viral respiratory illness. Feeding disorders are also common in these infants, making weight gain, the hallmark of recovery, very difficult. Rehospitalization for these infants during the first year of life is common, and parents should be told that this event is likely to happen.

Necrotizing Enterocolitis

Necrotizing enterocolitis is discussed in detail in Chapter 66. Many infants who have survived necrotizing enterocolitis often have complications such as motility difficulties, short bowel syndrome, adhesions, strictures, and growth failure. Consequently, infants with a history of necrotizing enterocolitis should be carefully monitored during the first year after birth to ascertain growth and check for complications. The development of strictures and adhesions may cause intermittent vomiting, abdominal distention, constipation, and hematochezia. Such symptoms may be monitored for a brief period with frequent visits, but investigation with radiographic examination or colonoscopy may be required.

For infants with short bowel syndrome, malabsorption and growth failure may be significant. Short bowel syndrome may also be associated with a decreased enterohepatic circulation and an increased risk of gallstones, which result in chronic diarrhea, malabsorption, and vitamin and mineral deficiency. Successful outcome appears to be related to the length of remaining bowel and the presence of an intact ileocecal valve. Although total parenteral nutrition may help such infants during a critical period, the physician is often left with the difficult decision of determining whether the child has adequate bowel to support life. The prognosis for these infants appears to be good if, during the neonatal period, more than 20 cm of bowel without an ileocecal valve or more than 15 cm of bowel with an ileocecal valve is present.

Gastroesophageal Reflux

GER appears to affect growth in a number of former preterm infants. GER is a condition in which gastric contents reflux into the esophagus. Although it is seen in full-term infants as well, preterm infants appear to be at greater risk because of the incompetence of the lower esophageal sphincter and a greater inability to protect the airway.

Symptoms of reflux can be subtle or overt. The most common presenting sign is recurring vomiting. Affected infants may regurgitate what appears to be a significant amount of a feeding, although it is common for parents to believe that the infant has vomited a far greater volume than is actually the case. During such episodes, some infants may aspirate small amounts into the airway, which leads to chronic pulmonary infection and respiratory distress. In some instances, no pulmonary symptoms are noted, although growth failure may be significant. Affected infants may also have Sandifer syndrome, in which infants arch the back and crane the neck to lessen the amount of reflux. Often these movements are misdiagnosed as neurologic in origin or as seizures.

GER may lead to failure to thrive and dehydration in many infants, as well as to esophagitis, if chronic and frequent. Apnea, bradycardia, and bronchospasm have been shown to be related to GER. Reflux may be worsened by the use of methylxanthines given to treat apnea; therefore, an appropriate diagnosis must be made. In infants with BPD, exacerbation of the disease may be a manifestation of GER, and this sequence of events should be carefully considered.

The treatment of GER is complicated in many instances. Few problems are as overdiagnosed during the neonatal period. A milk technetium scan is especially helpful for documenting suspected aspiration. Scanning of the infant after a milk feeding reveals reflux into the lungs, which is indicative of significant ongoing aspiration. A pH thermistor study is valuable for diagnosing the frequency and severity of acid reflux, as well as its relationship to apnea and bradycardia. Barium swallow and upper gastrointestinal studies can be inaccurate for the diagnosis of reflux but may be helpful in ascertaining any abnormal gastrointestinal anatomy. The treatment of infants with reflux depends on its severity. Medical management is successful in most cases and consists of thickening of feedings, keeping the infant in a semiupright posture after meals, and avoiding any position that increases intraabdominal pressure or aggravates reflux. Medications that may increase lower esophageal sphincter tone and improve gastric emptying

include metoclopramide and bethanechol. These two agents should be used cautiously in combination because dystonia may result. Surgical treatment with a Nissen fundoplication may be required in 5% to 10% of patients with chronic GER accompanied by other clinical symptoms such as life-threatening apnea, severe esophagitis, or chronic aspiration.

Neurologic Injury

Infants with intraventricular hemorrhage, periventricular leukomalacia, birth asphyxia, and congenital malformation of the central nervous system require careful follow-up. All of these entities may lead to significant neurodevelopmental sequelae, such as cerebral palsy and mental retardation. Consequently, physicians who monitor these infants at high risk must be prepared to work with the family to maximize potential if a child demonstrates significant consequences from early neonatal insult. Careful documentation of developmental progression and head growth are therefore crucial in neonatal follow-up. Monthly head circumference measurements should be made for any infant suspected of having sustained a neurologic insult who demonstrates an abnormal trend in head growth.

It is known that infants with grades III and IV intraventricular hemorrhage, periventricular leukomalacia accompanied by cyst formation, or perinatal hypoxemia/acidosis are more likely to have subsequent developmental delay and mental retardation than those infants with more mild intraventricular hemorrhage or periventricular leukomalacia. The incidence of cerebral palsy is variable in this population but may be as high as 50%. The type of muscle tone abnormality appears to be related to the site of the original intraventricular hemorrhage in the infant. It should be remembered, however, that many infants with cerebral palsy have little to no cognitive impairment.

For the infant with posthemorrhagic hydrocephalus, shunt placement may be necessary. Although hydrocephalus typically develops in the immediate neonatal period, some infants may not demonstrate hydrocephalus until some months after hospital discharge. It appears that early hydrocephalus may represent the failure of reabsorption of spinal fluid in the arachnoid villi, whereas later development of hydrocephalus may represent scarring of the foramen through which spinal fluid flows. Many infants with early hydrocephalus become shunt independent at a subsequent point, and the shunt may be removed. Later onset hydrocephalus, however, often necessitates drainage throughout life, and shunt independence is less likely to occur. Common problems with shunt placement include infection and obstruction. Furthermore, as the child grows, the shunt may need to be revised, although current neurosurgical techniques make this development less likely. Symptoms of shunt infection include signs of increased intracranial pressure, fever, and irritability. A shunt infection typically results not in meningitis but more commonly in ventriculitis. Often the infection represents colonization of the apparatus alone. Diagnosis of shunt infection is made by tapping the shunt reservoir and obtaining a positive cerebrospinal fluid culture. The shunt may have to be removed or partially exteriorized for a period of time until the cerebrospinal fluid has been sterilized. Obstruction of the shunt may manifest in a similar way, except that fever is not typical in such cases.

The infant with periventricular leukomalacia is at risk for developmental delay. In addition, cerebral palsy, as manifested by moderate to severe quadriplegia or diplegia, is seen in approximately 75% of children in whom cysts are present in the motor cortex of the brain. The muscle tone abnormalities of cerebral palsy can be noted early in life, although this should not be confused with the dystonia that many preterm infants experience, which is often transient in nature. The intellectual capability of children with periventricular leukomalacia is quite variable; however, mental retardation is not uncommon. If cyst formation occurs in the occipital region, cortical blindness or significant visual impairment may result. Careful follow-up of the child with periventricular leukomalacia is therefore essential in order to identify complications as early as possible.

Seizures

The infant with seizures in the neonatal period often has accompanying intraventricular hemorrhage, periventricular leukomalacia, or other neurologic injury. Care of these infants is based on the underlying cerebral insult; however, anticonvulsant management is usually necessary. Many seizures in the neonatal period are transient and are the result of cortical irritation from the initial injury. In such cases, anticonvulsants may be discontinued at a later date when the electroencephalographic findings have subsequently normalized. More global insults, however, may result in more permanent seizure disorders that necessitate the continuing involvement of a neurologist. Once seizures are well controlled, if the child has a seizure-free period of at least 3 months, anticonvulsant therapy may be withdrawn. The child should be carefully evaluated with electroencephalography and by a neurologist before such a decision is made.

Apnea and Bradycardia

Apnea and bradycardia are common hallmarks of the immaturity of the preterm infant. The diagnosis and management of these conditions are discussed in detail in Chapter 36.

Developmental Screening

As mentioned in previous sections, neonates experiencing neurologic insults are at risk for developmental delays and handicapping conditions. Others at high risk include those with birth weights of less than 800 g, those with BPD, and those with poor head growth or neurologic injury. Detailed developmental surveillance should be available to all preterm infants after hospital discharge.

Surveillance serves an important function for all infants, both those at low risk and those at high risk. For those who go on to have average cognitive abilities and no disabilities, surveillance provides reassurance for the parents that their observations are correct. Such reassurance helps families to normalize their expectations for their infants as they grow. The provision of close monitoring in the first years of life and developmental anticipatory guidance with early graduation from the follow-up program

can lessen the effect of the vulnerable child syndrome and alleviate stress for the family. For preterm infants who do go on to have developmental delays, surveillance ensures early referral to appropriate services and facilitates the parents' ability to find those services in their community. Surveillance avoids the "wait and see" philosophy that so often leads to the worsening of deficits before services are provided. By having a protocol for early surveillance, the parents are relieved of the responsibility of watching for problems and have easy access to professionals who can answer their questions. Early intervention provides parent with a positive, active role in addressing any delays. For children who have multiple disabilities, including sensory, physical, and cognitive deficits, a follow-up program is an invaluable support system and case management system for families. The use of surveillance by an experienced team of experts who are at ease with medical and developmental problems and can communicate with the community providers is of great value to the family and the primary care physician. Support services for families can also be recommended.

Surveillance should attend to the whole child. All areas of development—cognitive, play, social-emotional, motor, and language and communication—should be tracked. In addition, adaptive behaviors such as self-help skills, feeding, sleep, and behavior should be tracked. The family's needs and questions should guide the surveillance procedure.

The steps involved in surveillance vary across centers and often are linked to the community service providers. The initial step includes the introduction of the concept of "adjusted age" and teaching parents ways to observe and enjoy their infant. It is important to listen carefully to parental concerns and their observations. Tracking procedures should include the use of either a standardized screening tool, such as a Denver Developmental Screening Test, Bayley Infant Neurodevelopmental Screener, Child Developmental Inventory, or Parent's Evaluation of Developmental Status, or a standardized developmental scale, such as the Bayley Scales of Infant Development or the Infant Mullen Scales of Early Learning. Because of the brevity of developmental assessments in infancy and preschool years, a full assessment can often be completed by a neonatal follow-up team member relatively quickly and provide the family with detailed feedback and information with specific recommendations for intervention. The final step of surveillance is to look at current development in the context of what is known of the infant's medical history, past developmental status, and environment.

Some developmental problems, such as learning disabilities and behavior disorders, may not be apparent until the child is older. Screening should also be considered at later ages, even into adolescence, when problems are beginning to be identified.

Care of the preterm infant after hospital discharge is often equally, if not more, challenging for the neonatologist. Medical, neurologic, and developmental issues often arise, and screening for potential problems is essential. The neonatologist can play a crucial role in this area both directly to the child and family and indirectly by being an important resource to the community physician.

SUGGESTED READINGS

American Academy of Pediatrics Joint Committee on Infant Hearing: 1994 position statement. Pediatrics 95:152, 1995.

Aylward GP: Bayley Infant Neurodevelopmental Screener. New York, The Psychological Corporation, 1995.

Bayley N: Bayley Scales of Infant Development, 2nd ed. San Antonio, Texas, The Psychological Corporation, 1997.

Bernbaum J: Preterm Infants in Primary Care: A Guide to Office Management. Columbus, Ohio, Ross Pediatrics, Abbott Laboratories, 2000.

Bernbaum JC, Daft AL, Anolik R, et al: Response of preterm infants to routine DTP immunizations. J Pediatr 107:184, 1985.

DeVries LS, Regev R, Pennock JM, et al: Ultrasound evolution and later outcome of infants with periventricular densities. Early Hum Dev 16:225, 1988.

Frankenburg WK, Dodds J, Archer P, et al: Denver-II Screening Manual. Denver, Denver Developmental Materials, Inc., 1990.

Glascoe FP: Collaborating with Parent: Using Parent's Evaluation of Developmental Status to Detect and Address Developmental and Behavioral Problems. Nashville, Tenn, Ellsworth & Vandermeer, 1998.

Hack M, Klein N, Taylor HG: School-age outcomes of children of children of extremely low birthweight and gestational age. Semin Neonatol 1:227, 1996.

Infant Health and Development Program: Growth Curves for Preterm Infants. Columbus, Ohio, Ross Products Division, Abbott Laboratories, 1994.

Infant Health and Development Program: Enhancing the outcomes of low-birth-weight, premature infants. A multisite randomized trial. JAMA 263:3035, 1990.

Ireton H: Child Development Inventory. Minneapolis, Behavior Science Systems, 1992.

Mullen EM: Infant Mullen Scales of Early Learning. Circle Pines, Minn, American Guidance Service, 1989.

Saigal S, Hoult LA, Streiner DL, et al: School difficulties at adolescence in a regional cohort of children who were extremely low birth weight. Pediatrics 105:25, 2000.

Whitaker AG, Feldman JF, Van Rossem R, et al: Neonatal cranial ultrasound abnormalities in low birth weight infants: Relation to cognitive outcomes at six years of age. Pediatrics 98:719, 1996.

Wood NS, Marlow N, Costeloe K, et al: Neurologic and developmental disability after extremely preterm birth. N Engl J Med 343:378, 2000.

CHAPTER 57

Malformations of the Central Nervous System

Allison A. Murphy, Louis P. Halamek, and David K. Stevenson

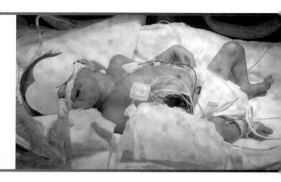

alformations of the central nervous system (CNS) comprise a group of congenital anomalies with potentially devastating consequences for neonates and their families. Mortality may be extremely high, and lifelong morbidity may accompany survival. Early recognition allows time for family counseling; assists in decision making about elective termination or route and timing of delivery; and provides for coordination of appropriate perinatal, neonatal, neurologic, neurosurgical, and genetic resources. Since the 1990s, much effort has been devoted to understanding the developmental pathophysiology of CNS malformations and enhancing radiologic, biochemical, and molecular techniques for prenatal diagnosis. Appropriate animal models have been developed, and in some instances human intrauterine therapy has been attempted.

This chapter discusses the embryology, management, and prognosis of CNS malformations. Treatment issues are examined from the perinatal and the neonatal perspectives; when appropriate, experience with fetal therapy is reviewed. Malformations of the CNS are understood best in terms of the developmental mechanisms operative in the embryo and fetus. This chapter follows the developmental scheme described by Volpe[1] in *Neurology of the Newborn* and is organized into disorders of dorsal induction of the neural tube; ventral induction (prosencephalic development); and neuronal proliferation, migration, organization, and myelination. Discussions of the embryology of the nervous system draw heavily from *The Developing Human* by Moore.[2]

The developmental biology of the CNS begins during the third week of gestation with induction of the **neural plate** (a thickened, slipper-shaped area of embryonic ectoderm) by the notochord and paraxial mesoderm; the neural plate then invaginates, its lateral edges fusing in the midline, to form the **neural tube**. This neural tube gives rise to the CNS, comprising the brain and spinal cord. Neural crest cells, another derivative of the neural plate, form the elements of the peripheral nervous system and melanocytes, cells of the adrenal medulla, and certain skeletal elements of the head and face. Interaction of the neural tube with surrounding mesoderm gives rise to the dura and axial skeleton. The cranial end of the neural tube differentiates into three primary brain vesicles: **prosencephalon** (forebrain), **mesencephalon** (midbrain), and **rhombencephalon** (hindbrain). During the fifth week of gestation, the prosencephalon diverticulates into the telencephalon and diencephalon; similarly the rhombencephalon gives rise to the metencephalon and myelencephalon. The mesencephalon does not divide. Neuronal and glial proliferation in the second through fourth months sets the stage for migration of these cells into the appropriate regions of the brain and spinal cord during months 3 through 5. Organization and myelination of these tracts begins late in gestation and proceeds into the first years of life. In contrast to many other organ systems, the CNS continues to grow in complexity well after the umbilical cord is clamped.

The molecular mechanisms operative during the development of the mammalian CNS are now being elucidated. Early events are controlled by a complex process of histiogenesis involving the precise temporal and spatial organization of gene expression along the embryonic anterior-posterior axis. These evolutionarily conserved genes divide the embryo into distinct fields of cells; each field is endowed with a different developmental capacity. The identity of many of these genes in humans is not known, but many of their counterparts in other species have been found.[3] These genes determine the fate of primary cells **(proneural genes)**, are involved in lateral inhibition pathways **(neurogenic genes)**, and control the frequency of mitotic events **(neuronal proliferation)**. Many contain genetic polymorphisms, which may explain a particular embryo's susceptibility to environmental factors such as teratogens.[4,5] On a more macroscopic level, the formation of the neural tube depends on a complex cytoskeletal network of microtubles and microfilaments and seems to be under the control of expressed surface glycoproteins and cell adhesion molecules.[1] Other crucial molecular events include the action of signaling molecules, such as members of the transforming growth factor-β family, which includes activin and fibroblast growth factors. Abnormal development of the CNS is common (roughly 3 in 1000 births).[2] As more is learned about the molecular events leading to the development of CNS malformations, the possibility of genetic therapy becomes a more realistic possibility.

DISORDERS OF DORSAL INDUCTION

Dorsal induction or **neurulation** describes the formation of the neural plate, neural tube, and neural crest from embryonic ectoderm. Formation of the brain and cervical, thoracic, and upper lumbar segments of the spinal cord constitutes primary neurulation. Secondary neurulation refers to the process of canalization, forming the lower lumbar, sacral, and coccygeal spinal cord segments. These two processes are considered separately.

Disorders of Primary Neurulation

Formation of the neural tube is initiated at approximately day 18 of gestation by invagination of the neural plate in the midline and subsequent fusion of its lateral margins. This fusion begins simultaneously at five distinct sites at approximately 22 days. The initial site of closure (closure 1) is in the midcervical region and proceeds cranially and caudally, closing over the area of the future spine at the level of L2. Closure 2 begins at the prosencephalon/mesencephalon boundary and proceeds bidirectionally. Closure 3 proceeds rostrally from the stomodeum and meets the cranial end of closure site 2. Closure 4 occurs in the region of the rhombencephalon and proceeds rostrally. Finally, closure 5 unidirectionally closes the caudal end of the neural tube from the level of future S2 through L2.[6,7] The fusion process results in openings at either end of the neural tube known as the cranial and caudal **neuropores**. Normally the cranial neuropore closes by the 24th day, approximately 2 days before the caudal neuropore. Defects in primary neurulation can occur from either the failure of closure at a single site or from the failure of two closed segments to fuse.[8]

Craniorachischisis Totalis

Complete failure of primary neurulation results in **craniorachischisis** (Greek, *kranion*, "skull," and *rhachis*, "spine," and *schisis*, "a cleaving") **totalis**. The neural tube fails to invaginate and fuse, leaving a neural plate–like structure, open from cranial to caudal ends. This is an extremely rare defect, and virtually all affected fetuses are spontaneously aborted or stillborn.

Anencephaly

Failure of the anterior neuropore to close produces **anencephaly** (Greek, *an*, "negative," and *enkephalos*, "brain"). The incidence in the United States has declined since the 1990s to 0.2 per 1000 live births, but epidemiologic studies reveal striking variations in regards to season, geographic location, sex, ethnic group, maternal age, economic status, and family history of affected siblings.[9-11] Anencephaly occurs in 2% to 5% of offspring of mothers with diabetes (type 1 and type 2).[6] Acrania (absence of cranial bone formation, most commonly the frontal bones above the supraciliary ridge, parietal bones, and squamous portion of the occipital bones) is an associated finding in all cases, whereas the bones of the facial cranium are normally developed, producing the characteristic froglike facies (Fig. 57-1). The internal carotid and vertebral arteries end abruptly; no arterial circle of Willis develops.[12] Pituitary dysfunction results in adrenal hypoplasia, the most common associated anomaly; other malformations include meningomyelocele, talipes equinovarus, cleft palate, and umbilical hernia.[13] Anencephalic infants have no cortical function, are thought not to experience any degree of consciousness, and do not have seizures.[14,15] They do have an intact brain stem and spinal cord, however, and may exhibit heart rate variability, decerebrate

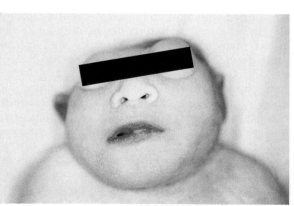
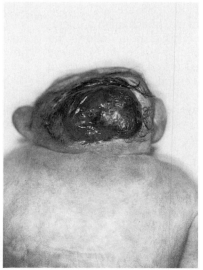

A   B

Figure 57–1. Postmortem photographs of a neonate with anencephaly. **A,** Characteristic froglike facies with bulging eyelids and absent forehead. **B,** Open cranial defect with protruding brain.

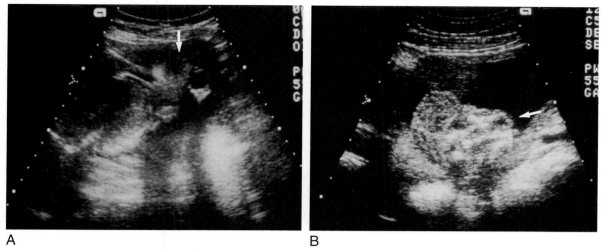

Figure 57–2. Fetal ultrasound reveals presence of anencephaly. **A,** Sagittal image of fetus discloses abnormally small head *(arrow)* and absence of calvaria. **B,** Facial profile in the coronal plane confirms presence of acrania and characteristic facies *(arrow* indicates bulging left eye). *(Images courtesy of R.H. Holbrook, Jr., MD, Department of Gynecology and Obstetrics, Stanford University School of Medicine.)*

posturing, roving eye movements, and withdrawal from pain.[16,17] Suck, root, grasp, Moro, and deep tendon reflexes may be normal or hyperactive, and many of these behaviors can be detected prenatally.[15] Only 25% of anencephalics are born alive at term; most die within the first 24 hours after birth, and an additional 10% die in the first week. Survival beyond 2 weeks is rare. Death is usually secondary to apnea or other severe CNS dysfunction. Intensive care support is not indicated in this lethal condition.

Historically, prenatal diagnosis of anencephaly occurred on ultrasound examinations performed in the second trimester (Fig. 57-2), often after polyhydramnios was noted. (Polyhydramnios affects approximately half of all anencephalic pregnancies and is due to the absence of fetal swallowing.) First-trimester ultrasounds done at 9 weeks of gestational age now reliably can detect anencephaly with a sensitivity approaching 100%. The "Mickey Mouse face" appearance of the cerebral hemispheres in coronal section and significantly reduced crown-chin and crown-rump lengths in the sagittal view are indicative findings.[18-21] Three-dimensional ultrasound techniques currently do not have an advantage over two-dimensional ultrasound in the diagnosis of anencephaly.[22] Maternal serum α-fetoprotein (AFP) is elevated with anencephaly. AFP is a component of fetal serum and peaks at 10 to 13 weeks of gestation. It is synthesized in the fetal liver and excreted by the fetal kidneys. Elevated levels are seen with open neural tube defects (NTDs), abdominal wall defects such as omphalocele and gastroschisis, esophageal and duodenal atresia, congenital nephrosis, and fetal demise. Maternal serum AFP levels vary with the gestational age of the fetus, the number of fetuses present, and the weight and race of the mother. Any level greater than 2.5 multiples of the median is considered elevated and should be repeated. If confirmed on repeat study, a detailed anatomic (level 2) ultrasound to assess gestational age, number of fetuses and presence of anatomic defects should be done.

Combining maternal serum AFP with other maternal serum indicators, such as low unconjugated estriol and elevated secretory acetylcholinesterase, enhances the diagnosis of anencephaly. The low unconjugated estriol is attributed to fetal adrenal hypoplasia resulting from lack of pituitary adrenocorticotropic hormone production.[23,24] Secretory acetylcholinesterase is the form of acetylcholinesterase found in cerebrospinal fluid (CSF).[25] These improvements in ultrasound technology and biochemical detection have minimized the need for amniocentesis to diagnose anencephaly based on amniotic fluid AFP, acetylcholinesterase, and homocysteine levels.[26]

Exencephaly

Exencephaly (Greek, *ex,* "out," and *enkephalos,* "brain") is believed by many to be a precursor to anencephaly.[27] In exencephaly, a substantial portion of the brain remains despite the presence of acrania. This remnant (having been exposed to the mechanical and chemical influences of amniotic fluid) is not functional cerebral tissue, but rather is a disorganized, spongy, vascular mass of neural, glial, and fibrotic tissue. This is an extremely rare defect that is uniformly fatal. **Iniencephaly** (Greek, *inion,* "back of the head," and *enkephalos,* "brain") is a related defect associated with anomalous formation of the occipital portion of the skull and cervical and thoracic vertebrae resulting in retroflexion of the head on the cervical spine. The skin of the face and posterior head is continuous with that of the chest, shoulders, and back. Most affected fetuses are spontaneously aborted or stillborn.

Cephalocele

Cephaloceles are defined as extracranial herniation of intracranial structures through a defect in the cranium (cranium bifidum). **Encephalocele** (Greek, *enkephalos,* "brain," and *kele,* "hernia") refers to a cephalocele that contains brain substance (Fig. 57-3). Herniation of brain tissue occurs in most cases, and the amount of involved

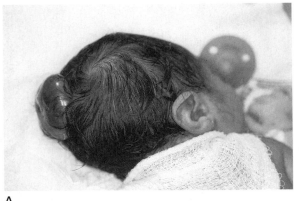
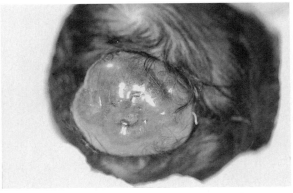

A   B

Figure 57–3. A, Neonate with occipital encephalocele. **B,** Macrophotography exposes the disorganized hemorrhagic nature of tissue present in encephalocele.

tissue directly influences the subsequent mortality and morbidity. Other factors influencing outcome include location of the lesion (anterior encephaloceles are compatible with normal intelligence) and hydrocephalus (which occurs in approximately 50% of cases) and other intracranial and extracranial malformations, especially Walker-Warburg syndrome.[28,29] Cranial meningoceles are cephaloceles that contain only leptomeninges and CSF and do not carry the same high risk of poor neurologic outcome. The term **atretic encephalocele** designates a small-sized lesion that usually contains no cerebral tissue but may include primitive neural elements; prognosis is similar to that of meningoceles. In white populations, almost 75% of encephaloceles occur in the occipital region, although the frontal, parietal, and temporal areas may be involved. Basal encephaloceles are not directly visible, but may cause upper airway obstruction.[29] Incidence is 1 to 2 per 10,000 live births; fetal loss is at least 70%.[29,30]

The precise pathogenesis of encephaloceles is unknown, but theories include abnormal disjunction of neuroectoderm from superficial ectoderm, overdistention of the neural tube causing a herniation of the developing brain, and developmental failure of skull ossification allowing protrusion of the underlying tissue.[29] Most encephaloceles are sporadic, but occipital encephaloceles may be associated with meningomyeloceles and other CNS anomalies.[31] Maternal hyperthermia between 20 and 28 days of gestation has been associated with an increased incidence of encephalocele.[32] Prenatal diagnosis at 12 weeks of gestation by transvaginal ultrasonography has been described.[33] AFP may be normal due to the closed nature of the defect. Delivery by cesarean section should not be performed for fetal indications unless the encephalocele seems to be an isolated defect and the parents desire intervention after appropriate counseling. Postnatal computed tomography (CT), magnetic resonance imaging (MRI), and, more recently, magnetic resonance angiography are useful in evaluating the anatomy of the cranial defect, the contents of the encephalocele, and its relationships to surrounding structures (Fig. 57-4). Imaging allows for planning of surgical procedures and provides some insight into the likely functional outcome of the affected child. The goals of surgical repair are closure of open skin defects to prevent infection and desiccation

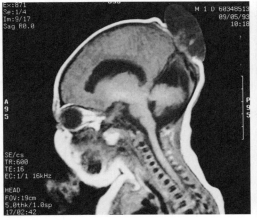
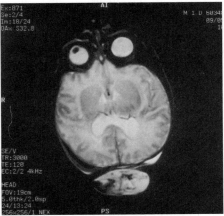

A   B

Figure 57–4. Magnetic resonance images of an occipital encephalocele. **A,** Sagittal. **B,** Horizontal.

of viable brain tissue, relief of hydrocephalus, removal or invagination of the disorganized and nonfunctional extracranial cerebral tissue with watertight closure of the dura, and reconstitution of the integrity of the skull while achieving an acceptable cosmetic result. If possible, the definitive correction should be deferred for the first 4 to 5 months to lessen the risks of anesthesia and blood loss.[34] Intensive care and operative management are inappropriate when extensive brain herniation or profound microcephaly exists. Intrauterine surgery performed on monkey *(Macaca mulatta)* fetuses to repair experimentally induced occipital encephaloceles resulted in preservation of function compared with controls who underwent repair postnatally; this technique has yet to be employed in humans.[35]

Specific Disorders

The classic triad of **Meckel-Gruber syndrome** consists of occipital encephalocele, polydactyly, and polycystic kidneys. Other associated anomalies include microcephaly, cerebellar malformations, characteristic facies (microphthalmia, hypertelorism, facial clefting), hepatic fibrosis, genital anomalies, and congenital heart defects. Inheritance is autosomal recessive, and the responsible gene has been mapped to chromosome 17q21-q24.[36] Oligohydramnios complicated approximately 50% of cases in one large series.[37] AFP may be elevated, and ultrasound may reveal the encephalocele, cystic kidneys, and polydactyly at 11 to 14 weeks of gestation.[38] Stillbirth is common, and most affected neonates die within hours of birth secondary to CNS or renal dysfunction.

    Chiari malformations are cerebellar anomalies. The four types of Chiari malformations, as described more than 100 years ago by Chiari, have neither anatomic nor embryologic correlation. Their only commonality is that they all involve the cerebellum.[39] The Chiari type I malformation consists of herniation of the cerebellar tonsils into the foramen magnum, crowding the craniocervical junction. No brain stem abnormalities are present, but approximately 15% to 20% of cases have hydrocephalus. Craniovertebral skeletal anomalies occur in approximately 25% of patients. The cause of this lesion currently is being debated, but many authors believe it is acquired rather than congenital. It has been described with traumatic delivery (possibly secondary to subarachnoid hemorrhage, arachnoidal adhesions, and altered CSF pressure) and hypopituitarism.[40,41] Chiari I malformations have the latest mean age of clinical presentation, typically in adolescence or adulthood.

    The most common type of Chiari malformation, the Chiari II, almost always is associated with meningomyelocele and hydrocephalus. It consists of herniation of not only the tonsils, but also all of the contents of the posterior fossa into the foramen magnum, including the brain stem, fourth ventricle, and cerebellar vermis (Fig. 57-5). It is believed to be secondary to defective rhombencephalic embryogenesis and presents in the neonatal period with feeding difficulties, stridor, and apnea.[42]

    Chiari III and IV malformations are rare. Chiari III malformations (the most severe form) comprise an occipitocervical encephalocele whose contents are cerebellum

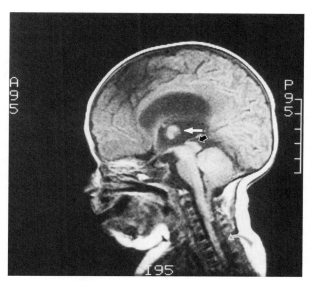

Figure 57–5. Sagittal magnetic resonance imaging of Arnold-Chiari II malformation associated with a meningomyelocele. Features include herniation of medulla posterior to the cord *(curved arrow)*, caudal displacement of inferior portion of cerebellum, prominence of massa intermedia *(closed arrow)*, and tectal beaking *(open arrow)*.

and brain stem. Associated anomalies include dysplastic tentorium, midbrain deformation, partial or complete agenesis of the corpus callosum, and agenesis of the septum pellucidum. The pathogenesis is not fully understood, but it is thought that the lack of distention of the embryonic ventricular system due to abnormal neurulation results in a hypoplastic posterior fossa. Newborns with Chiari III malformation frequently have respiratory insufficiency, dysphagia with secondary aspiration, dysfunction of the cranial nerves, spastic or decreased muscle tone, and loss of bladder or sphincter function.[43] The prognosis, even with surgical treatment, is poor. Chiari IV malformations consist solely of cerebellar hypoplasia or aplasia without any hindbrain herniation. Many patients have only mild-to-moderate neurologic deficits.[39]

Meningomyelocele

Myelodysplasia (Greek, *myelos*, "cord," and *dys*, "difficult," and *plasis*, "molding") is a nonspecific term referring to abnormal development of the spinal cord. Spina bifida aperta is defined as the spectrum of defects having in common a lack of bone and dermal covering of the spinal cord. **Meningomyelocele** is a more precise term applied to protrusion of the meninges and spinal cord through a defect in the vertebral column. Meningocele refers to the protrusion of meninges, but not spinal cord, through a vertebral defect; this lesion is not associated with the high risk of neurologic dysfunction seen with meningomyelocele. Spina bifida occulta is defined as a vertebral defect in the absence of spinal cord or meningeal herniation; however, the underlying cord may be abnormal in other ways.

    Although there have been many different theories as to the pathogenesis of meningomyelocele, the bulk of scientific evidence supports the notion that it is caused by an impairment of neural tube closure (i.e., failure of the neural folds to fuse over the invaginating neural plate).[44] Advances in developmental and molecular biology have resulted in a new understanding of the genetic events required for proper neural tube development. At the beginning of neurulation, the notochord releases the ventralizing factor sonic hedgehog. Sonic hedgehog induces ventral floor plate formation, inhibits the function of dorsalizing factor bone morphogenetic protein, and prompts the differentiation of various neurons in a concentration-dependent fashion. At the same time, the more lateral epidermal ectoderm secretes bone morphogenetic protein, which induces the expression transcription factors (including *Pax3* and *Pax7*) that lead to dorsalization of the neural tube. As a result of changes in cell morphology and differential cellular proliferation, the neuroectoderm folds and forms a tube. The dorsal roof plate expresses bone morphogenetic protein, controlling induction of dorsal neurons.[45] Failure of any of these events results in lack of fusion of a portion of the neural plate; bone and muscle are unable to grow over this open section of the developing spinal column. Pathologic studies of human embryos and fetuses with meningomyelocele in early stages of gestation reveal an open, but undamaged neural tube with almost normal cytoarchitecture, suggesting that the actual neurologic degeneration associated with NTDs occurs at some point later in gestation. This two-hit hypothesis presumes an initial error of embryogenesis, followed by a second insult from the intrauterine environment, such as chemical injury by the amniotic fluid, direct trauma, or pressure necrosis from either direct uterine wall contact or increased hydrodynamic pressure of the CSF. Studies of surgically created dysraphisms in animals suggest that prolonged exposure of the normal spinal cord to amniotic fluid results in severe degeneration of the neural tissue, closely resembling the degeneration seen in human meningomyelocele.[46,47] Given that lumbar and sacral portions of the spinal cord are thought to arise via a different mechanism (see the section on disorders of secondary neurulation later), lumbar and sacral meningomyeloceles are believed to be the result of defective canalization.[48]

The incidence of meningomyelocele varies depending on the population studied and geographic location. The highest incidences worldwide are in populations from southern Wales and Northern Ireland (7.5 and 8.5 per 1000 births). In the United States, the incidence approximates 0.5 per 1000 births. African Americans have a lower rate than whites, whereas Asian Americans have a lower incidence than either African Americans or whites. Hispanics, particularly Hispanics in Texas, have a higher risk for NTDs than any other ethnic group. Meningomyelocele may be seen in chromosomal abnormalities, such as trisomies (especially 13 and 18), triploidy, unbalanced translocations, and single-gene disorders. It also is associated with maternal obesity, illness, teratogenic exposures to valproic acid and carbamazepine, and hyperthermia.[6,49-51] Most cases are believed to be multifactorial in nature. Maternal nutrition has been shown to be an etiologic factor in all types of NTDs (anencephaly, encephalocele, and meningomyelocele), with a focus placed on the prenatal administration of folic acid to reduce the risk of first occurrence and recurrent insults.[52-55] It is estimated that 70% of all cases of meningomyelocele are preventable by adequate intake of folic acid.[6,56] The exact mechanism of action of folate in prevention of NTDs is unclear. Folate is a water-soluble vitamin that has no known toxicity.[57] It acts as a cofactor for enzymes involved in DNA and RNA synthesis and, along with vitamin B_{12}, aids in the supply of methyl groups to the methylation cycle through the enzyme 5,10-methylenetetrahydrofolate reductase, which converts homocysteine to methionine. Folate deficiency can lead to defective cell proliferation and cell death due to the inhibition of DNA synthesis. Folate deficiency also causes a shortage of methionine, preventing cells from methylating proteins, lipids, and myelin. A mutation in 5,10-methylenetetrahydrofolate reductase, C677T (substitution of valine for alanine in position 677), is associated with decreased enzyme activity, low plasma folate, high plasma homocysteine, and an increased risk of NTDs, particularly in Irish and Dutch populations. Studies have determined that a folic acid binding protein (FOLR1) also may play a role in the pathogenesis of NTDs. Other genes, such as those coding for folate receptors or enzymes (including methylenetetrahydrofolate dehydrogenase or serine hydroxymethyltransferase), may be involved, too.[6] The average diet in the United States contains 0.2 mg of naturally occurring folate.[57] In 1991, the U.S Public Health Service and Centers for Disease Control and Prevention recommended that women who had a prior pregnancy affected by anencephaly or meningomyelocele receive 4 mg of folic acid per day from at least 4 weeks before conception through the first 3 months of pregnancy.[58] (The American Academy of Pediatrics added women with type 1 diabetes mellitus and women taking certain antiepileptic medications to this high-risk list in 1999.) Because approximately half of the pregnancies in the United States are unplanned, recommendations issued in September 1992 encouraged all women of childbearing age to consume 0.4 mg (the dose found in prenatal vitamins) of folic acid daily.[57,59] In 1996, the U.S. Food and Drug Administration authorized the addition of 0.14 mg of folic acid per 100 g of enriched grain products. Since the implementation of these recommendations, the prevalence of meningomyelocele has been reduced by approximately 23%.[60] Zinc is an additional nutrient essential for normal fetal growth and development because it facilitates gene transcription and is necessary for cell division, development, and differentiation. Inadequate zinc intake also has been associated with NTDs in animals and humans, especially in women with acrodermitis enteropathica, a rare genetic disorder of zinc metabolism. Studies show that increased total preconceptional zinc intake and increased servings of animal products (the most bioavailable food source of zinc) is associated with a reduced risk of NTDs, but no official dietary recommendations have yet been made.[6]

Diagnosis. The fetal spine can be well visualized by 16 weeks of gestation. Meningomyelocele is marked by widening of the posterior ossification centers in the area of the defect (Fig. 57-6). The sac covering the defect may

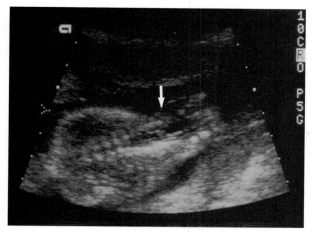

Figure 57–6. Ultrasound of fetal spine revealing widened ossification centers indicating the presence of a large thoracic meningomyelocele. *(Image courtesy of R.H. Holbrook, Jr., MD, Department of Gynecology and Obstetrics, Stanford University School of Medicine.)*

be seen bulging into the amniotic cavity. When the spine is not in position to be seen on a screening ultrasound, cranial findings may provide clues as to the existence of meningomyelocele (Fig. 57-7).[61,62] The **lemon sign** refers to the bifrontal concavities that give the cranial outline the appearance of a lemon. It is almost always present before 24 weeks of gestation, but then becomes less prominent and eventually disappears. The Chiari II malformation is present in virtually all meningomyeloceles and leads to a relatively low intraspinal pressure, which is transmitted to the compliant cranium producing the observed deformity. The loss of the lemon sign with advancing gestational age may result from bone maturation of the fetal cranium. Herniation of the brain through the cisterna magna results

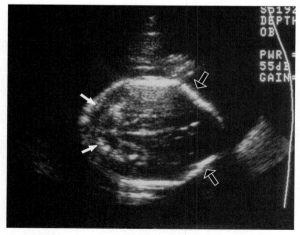

Figure 57–7. Ultrasound of fetal head disclosing bifrontal concavities ("lemon sign," *open arrows*) and anterior curvature of cerebellar hemispheres ("banana sign," *closed arrows*). *(Image courtesy of R.H. Holbrook, Jr., MD, Department of Gynecology and Obstetrics, Stanford University School of Medicine.)*

in abnormal anterior curvature of the cerebellar hemispheres, producing the *banana sign* on transverse view before 24 weeks of gestation. Later in gestation, as herniation progresses, the cerebellum becomes more difficult to visualize, leading to the *absent cerebellum sign*. Accompanying hydrocephalus and talipes equinovarus may serve as additional clues. Some centers use targeted transvaginal ultrasounds in high-risk pregnancies and report detection of meningomyelocele at 10 weeks of gestation.[63]

Prognosis. Prognosis depends on the level and size of the neural lesion (bone lesions are usually more extensive than the underlying spinal cord lesions). The best prognosis for independent ambulation is associated with sacral lesions. Upper lumbar and thoracic lesions almost always result in wheelchair dependence and a propensity to scoliosis (Figs. 57-8 and 57-9). Lower lumbar lesions are more difficult to predict but commonly lead to some form of ambulatory assistance, such as braces and crutches.[64] Hydrocephalus is a common accompaniment to meningomyelocele and compounds morbidity and mortality. Approximately 90% of thoracolumbar, lumbar, and lumbosacral lesions are associated with hydrocephalus, mostly due to an accompanying Chiari II malformation. Clinically, hydrocephalus may not be evident at birth but may manifest during the first 6 weeks of life. The ventricles dilate before head growth accelerates or signs of increased intracranial pressure develop, making serial CT or ultrasound scans useful in following ventricular size.

When the prenatal diagnosis of meningomyelocele has been made, family counseling is mandatory. Ideally, counseling is carried out by a team of professionals consisting of obstetricians and perinatologists (options for management of the pregnancy); geneticists (etiology and recurrence risk); neonatologists (immediate resuscitation and management in the newborn period); neurosurgeons, orthopedic surgeons, and urologists (surgical treatment options); and developmental pediatricians and neurologists (long-term morbidity and mortality). Ventriculomegaly is followed by serial ultrasounds every 2 to 4 weeks. Delivery is performed when fetal lung maturity is present, but should be strongly considered even in the absence of lung maturity if hydrocephalus is rapidly progressive or if cortical mantle thickness is less than approximately 1 cm. Route of delivery is controversial. Although not conclusively proven in a large, controlled, prospective, randomized trial with appropriate long-term follow-up, most studies support the delivery of infants with meningomyelocele by planned cesarean section (especially if the defect is >4 cm in diameter, >1 cm of meningeal sac protrudes dorsally, or the presentation is nonvertex); a more controlled delivery is thought to protect the spinal cord from injury and prevent rupture of the sac.[6,65-67]

Management. Management in the delivery room consists of placing the affected neonate on his or her side to avoid traumatizing the lesion while securing the airway and establishing adequate ventilation, oxygenation, and cardiac output. The lesion should be covered with sterile gauze that has been soaked in warm sterile normal saline, then covered in plastic wrap to limit insensible fluid

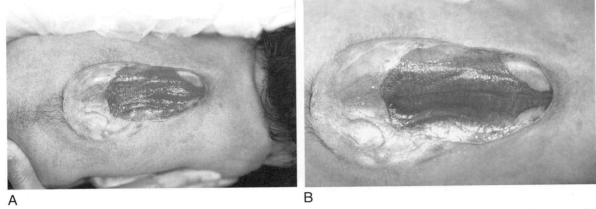

Figure 57–8. A, Neonate with thoracolumbar meningomyelocele and hydrocephalus. **B,** Macrophotography reveals detail of open neural tube.

losses. The abdomen should be wrapped circumferentially to ensure the gauze remains in place over the lesion (Fig. 57-10). Neurologic and neurosurgical consultations should be obtained expeditiously. If this is a previously unrecognized defect, a consensus opinion as to the appropriateness of surgical treatment and intensive care can be discussed with the parents. Closure of the meningomyelocele within 24 to 48 hours of birth is believed by some to reduce the risk of infection and possibly preserve neurologic function, although the latter has not been shown conclusively in a controlled fashion.[50] A preoperative CT scan is indicated to assess the degree of hydrocephalus and the presence of other associated malformations that might preclude surgical repair. Prophylactic antibiotics should be given until the time of surgery.[68,69]

Because the placement of a ventricular shunt commits the patient to years of dependence on and serial revisions of the shunt and the potential recurrent problems of mechanical failure and infection, it is not currently the practice at our institution to place shunts routinely at the time of meningomyelocele repair. Careful follow-up evaluation

of the degree of hydrocephalus is indicated to identify patients who would benefit from appropriately timed shunt placement. Serial head circumference measurements, neurologic examinations, and ultrasounds are useful in identifying progressive hydrocephalus. If the patient's neurologic examination does not reveal evidence of increased intracranial pressure, head circumference is enlarging appropriately (approximately 1 cm per week for term infants, 0.5 cm per week for preterm), and the ventricles are growing no faster than the rest of the brain, the patient can continue to be followed carefully. In the face of clinical deterioration, excessive rate of head growth, or increasing hydrocephalus seen on serial ultrasounds, nonsurgical options (e.g., serial lumbar or ventricular punctures or isosorbide therapy) may delay the need for shunt placement in a neonate who is too small or too sick to shunt.[70,71]

Urodynamic status should be evaluated early on because patients with meningomyeloceles at S2 or above are at high risk for bladder atony or incoordination of the detrusor and external urethral sphincter, resulting in hydronephrosis, ureteromegaly, urinary stasis, and urinary tract infection.

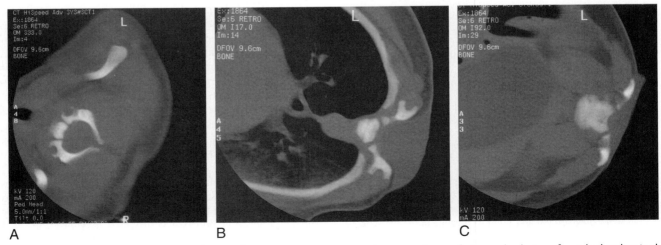

Figure 57–9. A-C, Computed tomography of spine of patient in Figure 57-8 reveals progressive nonfusion and splaying of vertebral arches in the cervical, thoracic, and lumbar vertebrae.

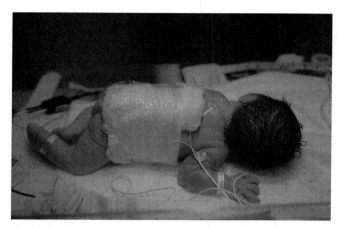

Figure 57–10. Delivery room management of neonate with a meningomyelocele. The lesion is covered with sterile saline-soaked gauze wrapped circumferentially and covered with plastic wrap.

The anatomy of the kidneys, ureters, and bladder can be evaluated by ultrasound, whereas function can be assessed by a voiding cystourethrogram. Intermittent, clean catheterization may be required, and the patient's caretakers should be instructed in this technique.[67] Anticholinergic medications may be beneficial in the neonate, and antimicrobial prophylaxis is indicated.[72] Bowel incontinence also is common but does not become a problem until school age, at which time a bowel program can be instituted to achieve "social continence."[67]

Other complications. Meningomyelocele often is complicated further by orthopedic deformities, such as scoliosis, kyphosis, talipes equinovarus, congenital vertical talus, and hip subluxation or dislocation.[73] These problems require a thorough assessment in view of the patient's prognosis and a decision as to the need for bracing or surgical correction or both in the neonatal period. Long-term orthopedic follow-up is indicated. Intellectual function, in contrast to motor function, is not dependent on the level of the lesion. Many patients with meningomyelocele have no intrinsic brain abnormality that mandates mental retardation. Mental retardation most commonly is secondary to postnatal insults, such as hydrocephalus, infection, hypoxia, and shunt malfunction.[50] Fine motor dyspraxia, decreased reading comprehension, language deficits, and difficulty writing and learning abstract concepts have been described.[67] Most tertiary centers have a multidisciplinary "spina bifida clinic," staffed by physicians (neurologists, neurosurgeons, urologists, orthopedists), rehabilitation specialists (including physical and occupational therapists), and social workers to coordinate the care of these complex patients.

Fetal surgery. Developments in diagnostic imaging, surgical techniques, and drug development for the prevention of premature labor have allowed for a new treatment option for meningomyelocele: in utero correction. The rationale for prenatal surgical therapy is to prevent progressive injury from amniotic fluid and other components of the intrauterine environment. The first fetal closure of a surgically induced meningomyelocele was performed in sheep in 1995, with a reported improvement in neurologic outcome.[74] The first attempts in human fetuses at covering a meningomyelocele (with endoscopic placement of a maternal split-thickness skin graft) was attempted in 1997, but within 1 year the technique was abandoned for late-gestation (28 to 30 weeks) open repair.[75,76] Most centers reliably report a decreased incidence of hindbrain herniation after surgery and a decreased need for later shunt placement. Improved lower extremity function is more variable. Long-term follow-up of these patients is necessary to evaluate better the morbidity and mortality of the procedure and determine the optimal inclusion criteria and timing of surgery.[47]

Disorders of Secondary Neurulation

The caudal cell mass is a group of undifferentiated cells at the caudal end of the neural tube. Vacuoles develop in this area at about 28 days of gestation and progressively enlarge and coalesce to contact the more cranial central canal of the neural tube formed earlier by primary neurulation. Canalization continues through 7 weeks, at which time retrogressive differentiation begins. Continuing through term, this process results in regression of most of the caudal cell mass, leaving the ventriculus terminalis and filum terminale distal to the conus medullaris.

Disorders of secondary neurulation (termed **closed spinal dysraphism, occult dysraphic states**, or **spina bifida occulta**) result in prolongation of the conus and thickening of the filum terminale. The mobility of the caudal end of the spinal cord can be limited ("tethering"), and injury to the cord can result in secondary to differential growth of the vertebral column and neural tissue. Neurologic symptoms (pain, sensorimotor defects of the lower extremities, bladder and bowel dysfunction, leg atrophy, and scoliosis) occur during periods of rapid linear growth and may be extremely subtle or nonexistent in the neonatal period. About 80% of cases exhibit a dermal lesion in the lumbosacral area, such as hair tufts, dimples, skin tags, hemangiomas, and subcutaneous masses, which can serve to alert the clinician to the underlying problem. Because the posterior elements of the lower vertebral column are poorly ossified during the first year of life, ultrasound is the tool of first choice to visualize the caudal spinal cord in children younger than 3 months old; suspicious findings may be documented by MRI or CT-myelography. Baseline urodynamic studies should be done in positive cases because 70% of asymptomatic patients with a closed spinal dysraphism have voiding abnormalities on formal testing.[77] Timely diagnosis is necessary to prevent permanent neurologic deficits. Regardless of the underlying cause, prophylactic surgery to untether the conus and decompress any mass effect should be done at an early stage.[78] The occult dysraphic lesions, in approximate order of time of origin in neural development, are myelocystoceles, split cord malformations, meningoceles, lipomas, and dermal sinuses. Less common lesions include neurenteric cysts and the caudal dysplasia sequence.[1]

Myelocystocele

In **myelocystocele** (Greek, *myelos*, "cord," and *kystis*, "bladder," and *kele*, "tumor"), a localized cystic dilation of the central canal of the caudal neural tube is present. It is thought that abnormal retrogressive differentiation results in an inability of CSF to exit from the early neural tube, causing the terminal ventricle to balloon into a cyst, which disrupts the overlying mesenchyme. Frequent association with the **OEIS** constellation of anomalies (*o*mphalocele, *e*xstrophy of the cloaca, *i*mperforate anus, *s*pinal anomalies) makes this one of the most severe malformations of the newborn period.[79]

Split Cord Malformations

The **split cord malformations**, previously referred to as **diastematomyelia** (Greek, *diastema*, "cleft," and *myelos*, "cord") or **diplomyelia** (Greek, *diploos*, "double," and *myelos*, "cord"), can be divided into split cord malformation I and split cord malformation II.[78] The embryologic basis for these defects is believed to be the development of an accessory neurenteric canal between the yolk sac and amnion, which subsequently is invested with mesenchyme to form an endomesenchymal tract that splits the notochord and neural plate. Maturation results in formation of either two hemicords wrapped with separate dural sacs and divided by a rigid osseocartilaginous septum (split cord malformation I) or two hemicords in a single dural sheath split by a nonrigid fibrous septum (split cord malformation II). Multiple accessory neurenteric canals may form two or more noncontiguous split cord malformations.[80] Split cord malformations are extremely rare lesions (<5% of occult dysraphic states) and are more common in females.[81-83] They can be associated with other CNS malformations (including meningomyelocele, spinal lipoma, neurenteric cyst, teratoma, and dermoid cyst), Wilms tumor, and ectopic renal and lymphoid tissue.[80,81] Prenatal detection by ultrasound has been reported; pertinent findings include visualization of a bony midline septum, widening of the spinal canal, and deformities of the vertebrae.[84-86] Postnatally, MRI and CT-myelography are necessary for adequate delineation of the type and extent of the lesion. The whole neural axis should be evaluated preoperatively because the likelihood of finding associated lesions is high.[77]

Meningocele

Meningoceles over the lower spine are rare as isolated lesions and are not associated with hydrocephalus or neurologic defects. Most cases are seen with a subcutaneous lipoma (i.e., lipomeningocele), but a subcutaneous lipoma with intradural extension is more common without an accompanying meningocele.[87] Infrequently, other tumors may be observed. The most common of these tumors is a teratoma, although neuroblastomas, ganglioneuromas, hemangioblastomas, and related neoplasms, presumably originating from germinative tissue in the primitive caudal cell mass, may occur.[88]

Dermal Sinus

A congenital dermal sinus consists of a dimple in the lumbosacral region from which a small sinus tract proceeds inwardly and rostrally. The tract may enlarge subcutaneously into a cyst that contains predominantly dermal (dermoid) or epidermal (epidermoid) structures.

These lesions result from an invagination of ectoderm that is carried by the canalized neural tube as it separates from the surface. Dermal sinuses may open into the subarachnoid space, causing leakage of CSF; ascending meningitis is a common consequence.

Neurenteric Cyst

Neurenteric cysts are found on the anterior aspect of the spinal cord, usually in the lower cervical and upper thoracic segments. They are lined by mucin-secreting, cuboidal or columnar epithelium resembling the gastrointestinal tract and are theorized to arise as a consequence of abnormal adhesion between ectoderm and endoderm resulting in a connection between the foregut and spinal canal.[79,89,90] Fewer than 100 cases have been reported in the literature.[91] They can be recognized on prenatal ultrasound as cystic masses (most commonly found in the right chest) accompanied by vertebral defects. Fetal MRI may prove superior to ultrasound for assessing smaller cysts. Serial ultrasounds (every 1 to 2 weeks) are imperative to evaluate for hydrops secondary to impeded venous return from mediastinal shift. Prenatal intervention (thoracentesis, thoracoamniotic shunt, or in utero resection) or preterm delivery of the fetus with immediate postnatal resection is predicated solely on the development of hydrops. If hydrops does not develop, a term delivery should be anticipated.[92] Neonates typically present with respiratory distress or feeding difficulties due to pulmonary, tracheal, or esophageal compression. The cysts also can be a source of serious CNS infection.[93] Postnatal x-rays reveal vertebral anomalies of the cervical or thoracic regions and a posterior mediastinal mass. MRI and CT allow precise definition of the cyst before resection. Although histologically benign, failure of complete resection (because of its location or adherence to surrounding structures) may lead to recurrence.[94]

Caudal Dysplasia Sequence

The caudal dysplasia sequence, also called **caudal regression syndrome**, is a heterogeneous spectrum of disorders characterized by dysplasia of the distal spinal cord and malformations of the lumbar vertebrae, sacrum, and coccyx. The lower extremities exhibit bone and muscular atrophy; lack of movement produces flexion contractures at the hips and knees (creating a frogleg or Buddha-like position), and talipes equinovarus is common.[95] Associated abnormalities may include cleft lip and palate, microcephaly, genital anomalies, congenital heart defects, and pulmonary hypoplasia. Caudal dysplasia sequence also may be a component of complex conditions, such as OEIS, **VACTERL (vertebral abnormalities, anal imperforation, cardiac abnormalities, tracheoesophageal fistula, renal abnormalities, limb deformities),** and the Currarino triad (partial sacral agenesis, anorectal malformation, and sacrococcygeal teratoma).[96] Lipomeningomyelocele and myelocystocele are present in 20% of cases. Neurologic defects depend on the extent of the involvement of the vertebral bodies and can be classified further into type I (severe derangement with the spine ending at S1 or above) and type II (minor degree of dysgenesis with S2 or lower levels of spinal tissue present).[79] The cause remains unknown, although some authors propose that an early vascular alteration diverts blood from embryonal caudal structures and results in varying degrees of agenesis of caudal organs.[97] Other theories include disturbed expression of the *Hox* gene (which endows neural crest cells with positional identity), either by mutation or a loss-of-function event, including exposure to retinoic acid or alcohol. The homeobox gene *HLXB9* is the major locus for dominantly inherited sacral agenesis.[95] Caudal dysplasia sequence is rare in the general population, but infants of mothers with insulin-dependent diabetes mellitus are at increased risk. The incidence in this group is approximately 1 in 350 live births, 250 times higher than the general population.[98] Transvaginal ultrasonography showing abnormal nuchal translucency and decreased crown-rump length allows early diagnosis.[98,99] Fetal or postnatal MRI classically shows a wedge-shaped cord terminus.[100] Complete neurologic, urologic, and orthopedic evaluation is important.

DISORDERS OF VENTRAL INDUCTION

Starting before anterior neuropore closure and peaking during the fifth and sixth weeks of gestation, the notochord and surrounding mesoderm induce formation of the prosencephalon and face. Paired optic vesicles and olfactory bulbs arise from each side of the prosencephalon and are followed by the appearance of diverticula known as the **cerebral vesicles**. The prosencephalon then undergoes a cleavage process whereby its cranial portion becomes distinct from the caudal portion, giving rise to the telencephalon and diencephalon. The paired cerebral vesicles form the cerebral hemispheres, and the cavities within become the lateral ventricles. Midline prosencephalic development occurs from the latter half of the second month through the third month, when mesenchyme trapped between the expanding cerebral hemispheres becomes the falx cerebri. Bulges in the walls of the diencephalon develop into the thalamus and hypothalamus; basal ganglia form lateral to these structures. Facial development occurs during this same period as mesenchyme ventral to the prosencephalon, and tissues derived from the pharyngeal arches and neural crest form the structures characteristic of the human face. The spectrum of pathology involved with ventral induction varies from profound derangements (aprosencephaly) to milder disturbances of midline prosencephalic development (e.g., agenesis of the corpus callosum) that may not become manifest during life.

Aprosencephaly-Atelencephaly

Aprosencephaly and **atelencephaly** are the most severe disorders of ventral induction and are thought to arise from an encephaloclastic event shortly after neurulation. In aprosencephaly, the absence of formation of telencephalon and diencephalon leaves a prosencephalic remnant at the rostral end of the rudimentary brain stem.[101] In atelencephaly, the anomaly is less severe in that the diencephalon is relatively preserved.[102] These anomalies are distinguishable from anencephaly most readily by the presence of an intact (although flattened) skull and intact scalp.

Facial anomalies are similar to the anomalies associated with holoprosencephaly. Anomalies of external genitalia and limbs are more common with aprosencephaly than with atelencephaly. Aprosencephaly is a lethal condition. Limited survival for 1 year has been observed with atelencephaly.

Holoprosencephaly Sequence

The holoprosencephalic group of disorders represents the next most severe derangement of ventral induction. Although a continuum of defects, **holoprosencephaly** (Greek, *holos*, "whole," and *proso*, "forward," and *enkephalos*, "brain") by convention is divided into three types: alobar, semilobar, and lobar. Alobar holoprosencephaly is the most common type and the most severe. The complete absence of cleavage of the prosencephalon results in a single cerebral sphere surrounding a lone central ventricle. Associated malformations include presence of a single midline optic nerve; fused thalami; a hypoplastic or absent pituitary gland; a posterior cyst in the area of the third ventricle; and absence of the falx cerebri, corpus callosum, and olfactory bulbs and tracts. Cytoarchitectural abnormalities (maldevelopment of dendrites and synapses) may exist in the cortical tissue.[103] Severe facial malformations are seen with most cases of alobar holoprosencephaly. Affected neonates are often cyclopic, having a single (monophthalmia) or fused (synophthalmia) midline orbit or complete absence of ocular structures altogether (anophthalmia). Likewise, nasal structures may be absent or rudimentary (proboscis) and placed above the orbit. Ethmocephaly refers to hypotelorism with a proboscis; cebocephaly describes hypotelorism with a single flat nostril. Cleft lip and palate also are commonly seen (Fig. 57-11).

Semilobar holoprosencephaly also is characterized by the presence of a single ventricle, although the interhemispheric fissure and falx cerebri are developed posteriorly, separating the occipital lobes. The thalami are partially fused, and typically the olfactory bulbs and corpus callosum are absent. Rudimentary occipital horns are present. The third ventricle is small or absent, and the fourth ventricle, brain stem, and cerebellum are usually normal.

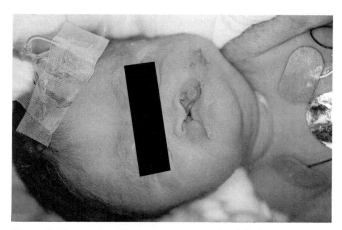

Figure 57–11. Facial malformations associated with holoprosencephaly include maxillary hypoplasia, flattened nose, and cleft lip and palate.

Lobar holoprosencephaly is marked by relatively normal hemispheres posteriorly with poorer separation of anterior and basilar structures. The frontal horns of the lateral ventricles are fused, but the occipital and temporal horns are distinct. The thalami are normal, as often is the corpus callosum. Similar to all types of holoprosencephaly, the septum pellucidum is absent. The anterior interhemispheric fissure is shallow, but becomes normal posteriorly. Definitive diagnosis of lobar holoprosencephaly by ultrasound alone may be difficult; MRI allows imaging in three planes to obtain better anatomic definition.[104]

The incidence of holoprosencephaly ranges from 0.5 to 1 per 10,000 live births, although it is estimated that most holoprosencephalic embryos are spontaneously aborted.[105,106] Females outnumber males 3:1.[107] Most cases have a normal karyotype, but holoprosencephaly has been described in trisomy 13, trisomy 18, and structural abnormalities (e.g., deletions and rings) involving these chromosomes. Autosomal recessive, X-linked recessive, and autosomal dominant with variable expressivity inheritance patterns have been reported. Because of the variable expression of the defect, individuals with mild facial deformities may be undiagnosed as gene carriers until they produce more profoundly affected offspring.[108] High-resolution chromosome banding should be performed as part of the workup because mutations in four different genetic regions (21q22.3, 2p21, 7q36, and 18p11.3) have been implicated in the pathogeneis of holoprosencephaly.[109-111] The high frequency of association between holoprosencephaly and Smith-Lemli-Opitz syndrome suggests a role for abnormal sterol metabolism.[112] Prevalence among mothers younger than age 18 is twice as high as that among older women. Similar to other forms of CNS malformations, mothers with insulin-dependent diabetes mellitus have a much higher risk (1% to 2%) than the population at large. Maternal ingestion of anticonvulsants, ethanol, retinoic acid derivatives, and massive doses of salicylates around day 33 of gestation also has been associated with holoprosencephaly.[108,109,113]

Differential Diagnosis

Sonographically, holoprosencephaly must be distinguished from other malformations in which the cranium appears to be filled with fluid: **hydranencephaly** (an encephaloclastic absence of cerebral hemispheres due to an early obstruction of blood flow through the internal carotid arteries) and severe hydrocephalus. In hydranencephaly, there is no hippocampal ridge between the monoventricle and the associated dorsal cyst as seen in holoprosencephaly. In hydrocephalus, the basal ganglia are widely separated secondary to the dilated third ventricle, whereas in holoprosencephaly, the basal ganglia and thalami are fused. Cephalic displacement of the residual cortex on ultrasound (known as the **boomerang sign** or **horseshoe sign**) is seen in holoprosencephaly but in neither hydranencephaly nor hydrocephalus. Characteristic facial dysmorphology also may be visualized. Transvaginal ultrasound has documented holoprosencephaly at 10 weeks of gestation.[114]

As with other CNS malformations that carry dismal prognoses, cesarean delivery should not be used for fetal indications. Severe macrocephaly may require cephalocentesis to allow vaginal delivery. Seizures are common but easily treated with anticonvulsant therapy. Although children with alobar holoprosencephaly have increased muscle tone to the point of spasticity, they have poorly developed control of their muscles and may appear to be floppy; joint contractures rarely develop. Pituitary dysfunction can result in growth delay, diabetes insipidus, and, more rarely, panhypopituitarism requiring extensive hormone replacement therapy. Feeding is usually a major problem. Some infants have choking spells and gag during feedings. More common are marked slowness in eating, frequent pauses, and rapid loss of interest. Gastroesophageal reflux and vomiting are frequent, as is the risk of aspiration. Many infants require gastrostomy tubes along with promotility agents to promote stomach emptying. All infants lack the ability to smell. Brain stem dysfunction (resulting in irregular breathing patterns and heart rate and poor body temperature control) is a frequent cause of death.[115] Half of infants with alobar holoprosencephaly die within the first week of life.[116] Of the remaining infants, 50% die before age 6 months, and 20% to 30% live for at least 1 year; survival to 11 years has been reported. Prognosis for infants with semilobar and lobar holoprosencephaly is generally better; it is not unusual for these children to live well into adulthood, sometimes with normal intellectual function. For infants with chromosomal anomalies or malformations in other parts of the body, the outlook is largely determined by accompanying malformations.[115]

Hydranencephaly

Hydranencephaly (Greek, *hydor*, "water," and *an*, "negative," and *kephalos*, "brain"), although classified as a disruption and not a true malformation, is mentioned because of its inclusion in the differential diagnosis of holoprosencephaly. The brain begins to develop normally but undergoes massive infarction, presumably involving cortex and basal ganglia. Cytomegalovirus, herpes simplex virus, and toxoplasmosis have been implicated as causative agents. Midbrain and hindbrain structures are usually intact. Microcephaly is found, unless the choroid plexus survives and produces hydrocephalus. Ultrasound reveals no evidence of a cortical rim, only fluid-filled cavities covered by meninges; the falx is frequently absent. Scattered islands of cortex preserved by collateral flow may be seen occasionally.[117] Prenatal diagnosis has been made by ultrasound at 12 weeks of gestation.[118] MRI may be used when ultrasound findings are indeterminate or when there is a question of associated anomalies.[119] **Porencephaly** (Greek, *poros*, "pore," and *enkephalos*, "brain") is the term applied to localized infarction or hemorrhage in contrast to the massive destruction of hydranencephaly. Limited necrosis results in cysts that may communicate with the ventricles or subarachnoid space. Cortical loss presents the appearance of ventricular dilation.

Newborns with hydranencephaly initially may behave normally if the hypothalamus remains intact.[120] Detection may occur weeks or months after birth when developmental delay becomes manifest. Often, irritability, hyperreflexia, and clonus are seen in the neonatal period.

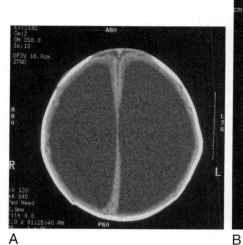
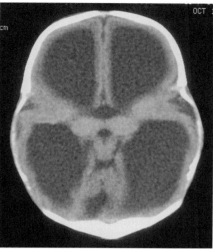

A   B

Figure 57–12. **A** and **B,** Computed tomography reveals massive hydrocephalus.

The cranium readily transilluminates, and an electroencephalogram (EEG) reveals no cortical activity. Death usually occurs within the first months of life secondary to apnea, aspiration, or other manifestations of severe CNS dysfunction.

Hydrocephalus

Hydrocephalus (Greek, *hydro,* "water," and *kefale,* "head") is an etiologically heterogeneous disease that, similar to holoprosencephaly, must be considered in the differential diagnosis of hydranencephaly (Fig. 57-12). It is defined as a pathologic increase in the volume of CSF within the skull; it almost always is associated with dilation of the cerebral ventricles. Ventriculomegaly is a less precise term referring to the presence of large ventricles; it may or may not be associated with hydrocephalus. Hydrocephalus typically is classified as obstructive or nonobstructive. Obstructive hydrocephalus implies elevated intracranial pressure and is produced by any process that restricts the flow or reabsorption of CSF or, more rarely, increases the production of CSF. Obstructive hydrocephalus may be of two types: communicating and noncommunicating. Communicating obstructive hydrocephalus implies an obstruction out-side of the ventricular system; this is found most frequently at the arachnoid granulations secondary to an inflammatory process, such as infection or hemorrhage. Noncommunicating obstructive hydrocephalus is caused by an obstruction intrinsic to the ventricular system, such as aqueductal stenosis. Nonobstructive hydrocephalus refers to ventriculomegaly with normal intracranial pressure. Brain atrophy or dysgenesis may result in enlarged ventricles secondary to a lack of appropriate brain growth; this is commonly known as **hydrocephalus ex vacuo** (Fig. 57-13). Hydrocephalus ex vacuo may result from any process producing brain atrophy, such as global perinatal ischemia, twin-twin embolization sequence, or congenital infection.

The incidence of congenital hydrocephalus varies from 0.5 to 2.5 per 1000 live births.[47] The cause is heterogeneous. Aqueductal stenosis (stenosis of the aqueduct of Sylvius, between the third and fourth ventricles) accounts for approximately one third of neonatal hydrocephalus. Although most cases are nonfamilial, an X-linked variety (Bickers-Adams syndrome) is associated with adducted thumbs and agenesis of the corpus callosum. This disorder has been mapped to chromosomal regions Xq27.3 and Xq28 and has been shown to be related to a mutation in the neural cell adhesion molecule L1CAM.[39,121] Other types of genetic aqueductal stenosis include two different

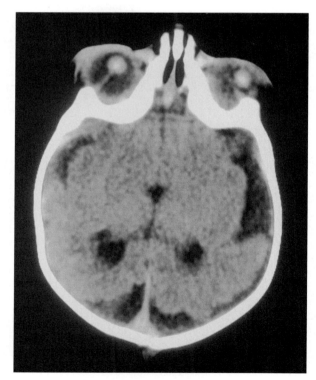

Figure 57–13. Hydrocephalus ex vacuo. Prominence of ventricles is secondary to brain atrophy.

autosomal recessive inheritance patterns: one with a normal phenotype and one seen with VACTERL association. CT scans of patients with aqueductal stenosis show enlargement of the lateral and third ventricles with a normal-size fourth ventricle. As the obstructing lesion cannot be removed, management strategies include a third ventriculostomy (to bypass the obstruction intracranially) and ventriculoperitoneal shunting.[122] The remainder of neonatal hydrocephalus is caused by meningomyelocele with Chiari II malformation, communicating hydrocephalus secondary to infection, intraventricular hemorrhage, and the Dandy-Walker malformation (DWM). Far less common is hydrocephalus resulting from a tumor (choroid plexus papilloma) or an arteriovenous malformation (malformation of the vein of Galen).

The causes of fetal hydrocephalus are similar to the distribution in neonatal cases. With fetal hydrocephalus, the severity of the hydrocephalus tends to be greater, however, and, most importantly, serious anomalies of the nervous system frequently are present. Fetal hydrocephalus accompanies numerous other syndromes of a single-gene, chromosomal, or teratogenic nature, including trisomies 13 and 18, Warburg syndrome, and hydrolethalus syndrome (Fig. 57-14). It is imperative that whenever hydrocephalus is noted a detailed anatomic ultrasound

scan or fetal MRI be performed to look for other anomalies. Maternal and fetal studies (for infection, serum markers, and karyotype) are highly recommended. The first detectable signs of hydrocephalus on prenatal ultrasound occur in the early second trimester: a decrease in choroid plexus size followed by progressive ventricular dilation (Figs. 57-15 and 57-16).[117] Serial ultrasounds show an increase in the biparietal diameter by 32 to 34 weeks, but the transverse atrial width and the lateral ventricular-to-hemispheric width ratio are more commonly used measurements for the diagnosis of hydrocephalus. Cortical mantle thickness has been suggested as a potentially useful predictor of prognosis, presuming that poor neurologic outcome is secondary to compression of cerebral tissue. Although absence of a cerebral cortex is a poor prognostic sign, the presence of a normal amount of cerebral cortex does not guarantee a normal neurologic outcome.[121] Overall survival is approximately 25% and depends mostly on the presence of other congenital anomalies; only half of survivors exhibit normal intellectual function on follow-up.

Intrauterine Therapy

Intrauterine treatment of hydrocephalus began in the early 1980s in an attempt to prevent the destructive compressive

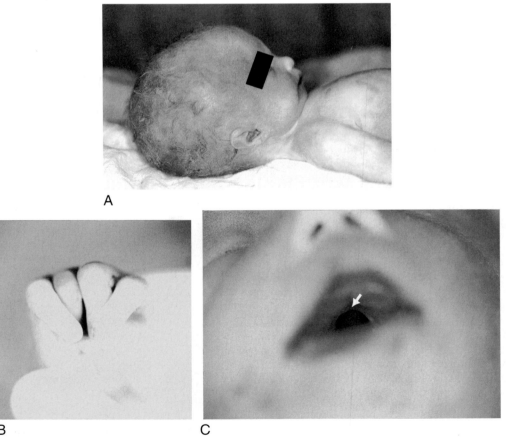

Figure 57–14. A-C, Hydrolethalus syndrome. Postmortem photographs illustrate massive hydrocephalus, small mandible, U-shaped cleft palate, and fisting.

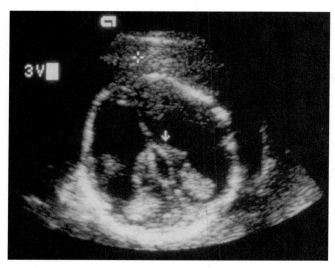

Figure 57–15. Fetal hydrocephalus at 17 weeks of gestation manifested by enlargement of the lateral and third *(arrow)* ventricles. *(Image courtesy of R.H. Holbrook, Jr., MD, Department of Gynecology and Obstetrics, Stanford University School of Medicine.)*

effects on the developing cortex. Reports of serial ultrasound-guided cephalocenteses and open or fetoscopic placement of ventriculoamniotic shunts revealed increased survival but higher degrees of morbidity in survivors.[123-125] Patients who had dismal prognoses secondary to the presence of associated anomalies represented a significant portion of the patients undergoing intrauterine therapy. Complications included premature labor, displacement of the shunt into the maternal peritoneal space, dislodgment of the shunt from the ventricle, obstruction of the shunt with cellular debris, and chemical meningitis from

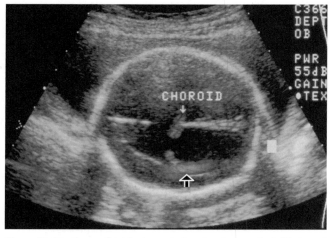

Figure 57–16. Severe fetal hydrocephalus showing marked dilation of the lateral ventricle. Ipsilateral choroid plexus (resting in the dependent portion of the ventricle, *open arrow*) and contralateral choroid plexus (having prolapsed into the lateral ventricle, *closed arrow*) are visible. *(Image courtesy of R.H. Holbrook, Jr., MD, Department of Gynecology and Obstetrics, Stanford University School of Medicine.)*

the amniotic fluid. In addition, intrauterine shunting did not preclude the need for postnatal shunting. Some cases of congenital hydrocephalus do not progress and require no surgical intervention, even in the postnatal period; a smaller percentage may regress. These cases do not benefit from intrauterine therapy. Patients with isolated, progressive ventriculomegaly represent a small proportion of all fetuses with ventriculomegaly and as a group are hard to identify. It is this group of patients that is most likely to benefit from prenatal intervention. A moratorium on fetal surgery to treat hydrocephalus has been in place for more than a decade, but more recent refinements in fetal imaging, surgical techniques, and drugs to hasten fetal lung maturation and prevent premature labor have raised the possibility that some unborn children with isolated hydrocephalus might be candidates for intervention.[126-131]

Route of Delivery

The optimal route of delivery of an infant with hydrocephalus still is being debated. In cases in which associated anomalies exist and the fetal prognosis is dismal, cesarean section for fetal indications is not recommended. Macrocephaly may necessitate antepartum decompression via cephalocentesis to allow vaginal delivery. The optimal management of cases of apparently isolated hydrocephalus is more controversial. Induction of fetal lung maturation with betamethasone and expedited delivery should be considered in the event of rapid progression of the hydrocephalus, especially after 32 weeks of gestation. Vaginal delivery is reasonable when the biparietal diameter is less than 100 mm and presentation is vertex.[66]

Postnatal Therapy

At birth, patients clinically exhibit gross macrocephaly with separated cranial sutures and full fontanelles (Fig. 57-17). The skull may be transilluminable. "Sunset eyes" (the prominence of the sclera above the iris) and other disturbances in oculomotor function may be seen in extreme cases. Other findings include hypotonia, apnea, and feeding difficulties. As previously discussed, the need for postnatal decompression is determined by the thickness of the cortical mantle, rate of head growth, and clinical assessment of neurologic status. As opposed to the adult brain, hydrocephalus in the fetus insults the brain at a period when important developmental events are taking place, such as neuronal differentiation and the establishment of neuronal contacts. Chronically elevated intracranial pressure causes a secondary loss of brain tissue resulting in ependymal disruption, white matter edema, gliosis, and demyelination; the cortex, although not unscathed, is relatively spared. As pressure builds, neurologic function is impaired.[132] Decompression of the hydrocephalus restores cortical volume but not neurologic function. Decompression can be done temporarily by serial lumbar/ventricular tapping or ventriculostomy (now done endoscopically) or on a more permanent basis with a ventricular shunt draining into the peritoneum, atrium, gallbladder, or pleura.[133] Other treatment possibilities include local fibrinolytic therapy for posthemorrhagic hydrocephalus.[134] Seizures, although not commonly caused by hydrocephalus, are a frequent (20% to 50%)

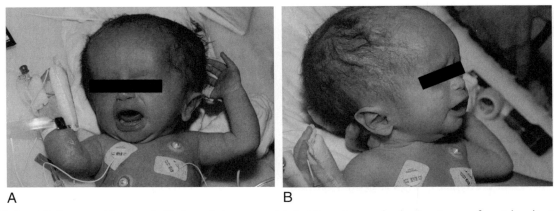

Figure 57–17. **A** and **B,** Neonate with congenital hydrocephalus unassociated with meningomyelocele. Prominence of cranial vault with a relatively small face creates illusion of fetal facies.

association after shunt placement, especially if the shunt is placed before 2 years of age. These seizures tend to be poorly controlled by routine antiepileptic drug regimens.[135] Since the introduction of shunts, the mortality rate of patients with hydrocephalus has decreased from 50% to 15%. Prognosis for normal intellectual development depends less on the initial thickness of the cortical mantle than on the underlying cause of the hydrocephalus, the presence of epilepsy, and anomalies involving other organ systems. Young age at diagnosis, delayed treatment, and treatment complications that result in infection are associated with a worse outcome.[47] When a hydrocephalic child develops epilepsy, his or her chance of achieving an IQ greater than 90 is only 13%, and the possibility of having an IQ less than 50 is 44%.[135]

Dandy-Walker Malformation

Of cases of congenital hydrocephalus, 5% to 10% can be attributed to the DWM, characterized by the triad of hypoplasia or absence of the vermis; upward displacement of the falx and lateral sinuses; and a large, thin-walled retrocerebellar cyst formed by the roof of the fourth ventricle.[136] A variant of DWM (termed **cerebellar dysgenesis**) is characterized by less vermian hypoplasia and fourth ventricle dilation. More than half of infants with DWM have a chromosomal abnormality (usually trisomy 18 or a variant), but DWM also may appear in isolation. Associated CNS findings vary in frequency and severity. Migrational disorders, such as lissencephaly, have been described with DWM and should raise the suspicion of Warburg syndrome, especially if accompanied by ocular and neuromuscular abnormalities. The cause of DWM is thought to be a delay of the foramen of Magendie to open along with maldevelopment of the rostral portion of the roof of the fourth ventricle. The incidence is 1 in 25,000 to 35,000 pregnancies. Oligohydramnios or polyhdramnios complicates more than half of these pregnancies.[121] Ultrasound findings reveal cystic dilation of the fourth ventricle together with anterior and lateral displacement of the cerebellar hemispheres (Fig. 57-18). U-shaped separation of the hemispheres distinguishes DWM from other types of posterior fossa cysts. These findings may

be detected before 20 weeks of gestation. Clinical presentation is more severe when malformations are detected early in gestation and includes macrocephaly, bulging fontanelle, suture separation, ocular abnormalities, spasticity, seizures, hearing loss, and developmental delay. Hydrocephalus develops after birth and occurs more commonly in infants with normal karyotypes.[137,138] CT and MRI allow for definitive postnatal diagnosis (Fig. 57-19). Treatment is highly controversial and consists of cystoperitoneal, lateral ventriculoperitoneal, or combined cystoventriculoperitoneal shunting procedures.[139,140] Excision of the fourth ventricular cyst is no longer advocated.[121] Being a disorder of heterogeneous etiology, prognosis for mental development in DWM depends on the presence of other anomalies and the degree of hydrocephalus. Early series indicated a dismal outlook, but more

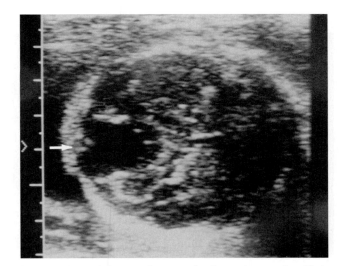

Figure 57–18. Fetal ultrasound at 22 weeks of gestation revealing dilation of the fourth ventricle consistent with Dandy-Walker malformation. *(From Chitkara U, Cogswell C, Norton K, et al: Choroid plexus cysts in the fetus: A benign anatomic variant or pathologic entity? Report of 41 cases and review of the literature. Obstet Gynecol 72:185, 1988, with permission from the American College of Obstetricians and Gynecologists.)*

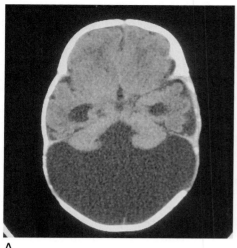 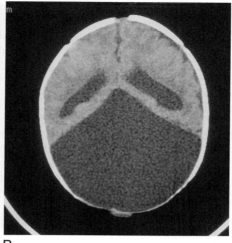

A   B

Figure 57-19. A and **B,** Computed tomography of neonate with Dandy-Walker malformation. The cerebellar hemispheres are displaced laterally and anteriorly, and the fourth ventricle is massively dilated.

recent studies reflecting judicious patient selection and an aggressive approach to hydrocephalus have shown that approximately one third of patients develop normally.[141]

Agenesis of the Corpus Callosum

Abnormalities of midline prosencephalic structures are the least severe of the spectrum of disorders of ventral induction and involve three specific regions: the commissural, chiasmatic, and hypothalamic plates. Abnormalities in development of the commissural plate lead to agenesis of the corpus callosum or the septum pellucidum or both. Defects in all three structures result in septo-optic or septo-optic-hypothalamic dysplasia.[1]

The corpus callosum is a collection of nerve fibers connecting the cortical areas of the cerebral hemispheres. Formation of the corpus callosum occurs between 8 and 20 weeks of gestation and proceeds in an anterior-to-posterior direction. Agenesis of the corpus callosum can be complete or partial; the earlier the insult, the more anterior and complete the maldevelopment.[142] Chiari II malformations are commonly associated, as are encephaloceles, holoprosencephaly, and disorders of neuronal migration. Without other recognized abnormalities of the CNS, agenesis of the corpus callosum can be asymptomatic or at least necessitate sophisticated neuropsychologic tests of interhemispheric processing for detection. Callosal agenesis is seen in chromosomal disorders, such as trisomies 13 and 18 and partial duplication of chromosome 10.[143] Persistent hypoglycemia may be seen with anomalies of the corpus callosum and should prompt a search for associated midline CNS defects, such as pituitary hypoplasia. Aicardi syndrome is characterized by agenesis of the corpus callosum and chorioretinal lacuna. Infantile spasms and cognitive deficits are seen in approximately 80% of affected patients and are related principally to accompanying defects of neuronal migration. The moderate degree of phenotypic variability seems to be related to nonrandom X-inactivation in this X-linked mutation.[144] Although easily identified by MRI at 20 weeks of gestation, agenesis of the corpus callosum also can be readily identified in a newborn by ultrasound. Characteristic features include

a "sunburst" appearance on sagittal views (created by elevation of the third ventricle and radial orientation of gyri) and widely separated frontal horns, concave medial borders, and Probst bundles seen on coronal views.[145,146]

The formation of the septum pellucidum occurs around 20 weeks of gestation and can be affected by developmental events (e.g., neuronal migration) and outside factors (e.g., hydrocephalus or contiguous ischemic lesions); it is rarely seen as an isolated finding. The clinical features depend principally on the associated disorders. When the two leaves of the septum pellucidum fail to fuse as the fetal brain matures, cavum septi pellucidi results. This finding (best seen on MRI) is clearly abnormal only after the neonatal period because all premature infants exhibit an ultrasonographically demonstratable cavum up to 34 weeks of gestation, and 35% of term infants still have a small (0.5 cm) cavum. A large cavum septi pellucidi (>1 cm) in a term newborn should be viewed with suspicion.[147] There is an association with later cognitive deficits.[148]

Defective development of the commissural and chiasmatic plates results in septo-optic dysplasia. In addition to optic nerve hypoplasia (with its associated visual deficits), disturbances of hypothalamic function are common. Seizure disorders and cognitive deficits are related to accompanying errors in neuronal migration.

DISORDERS OF NEURONAL PROLIFERATION

Proliferation of neuronal and glial cells occurs in the germinal matrix surrounding the lateral ventricles. Although neuronal replication occurs predominantly during months 2 through 4 of gestation, glial proliferation continues well past term. The earliest glia are called *radial glial cells* and are involved in neuronal migration. Disorders of neuronal proliferation result in too few or too many cortical neurons.

Micrencephaly

Micrencephaly, in its most limited sense, refers to a brain that is well formed with normal gross architecture but small secondary to decreased proliferation; this definition does not include brains that are small due to a destructive intrauterine process, such as infection. *Microcephaly* is a more general term applied to a head circumference 2 standard deviations below the mean for gestational age and sex; although a microcephalic patient has a small brain, the brain may be small secondary to causes other than limited neuronal proliferation. Micrencephaly can be divided broadly into **radial microbrain** (diminished number of proliferative units) and **micrencephaly vera** (diminished size of proliferative units). Radial microbrain is a rare disorder. It is notably familial (probably of autosomal recessive inheritance), but cases of teratogenic exposure to carbamazepine have been reported.[149] The brain is extremely small (weighing only 16 to 50 g compared with a normal brain weight of 350 g), but has normal gyral formation and no disturbance of cortical lamination.[150] There is an appropriate amount of germinal matrix at term. All reported infants died in the first month of life. This disorder can be distinguished from anencephaly by the presence of an intact skull and from aprosencephaly-atelencephaly by the normal sonographic appearance of the cerebrum and ventricles.[150,151] The brain in micrencephaly vera is also small, but not so strikingly as in radial microbrain. Gyral patterns are simplified. The number of cortical neuronal columns appears normal, but the neuronal complement of each column, especially the superficial cortical layers, is markedly decreased. In addition, there is no residual germinal matrix at 26 weeks of gestation, a finding termed **premature exhaustion of matrix**.[1]

Micrencephaly vera is a more heterogeneous group of disorders, with familial, teratogenic, and sporadic etiologies described. Sporadic cases are the most common, but familial cases are the most crucial to detect because of implications for genetic counseling. These inherited varieties include autosomal dominant, autosomal recessive, X-linked recessive, and a familial type with ocular abnormalities of which the genetics is unclear.[152] Intellect usually is spared or only mildly defective in the autosomal dominant pattern. There is no associated facial dysmorphism, but digital anomalies have been reported.[153]

Most autosomal recessive cases also have limited neurologic deficits but may be dysmorphic, with a receding frontal region, upward slanting palpebral fissures, and relatively large, protruding ears. The best-documented teratogenic agent producing micrencephaly is ionizing radiation; many micrencephalic children were born after the atomic bombs were dropped in Hiroshima and Nagasaki.[154] Radiation therapy for tumors also could produce this effect.[155] Maternal alcoholism and cocaine abuse, along with maternal hyperphenylalaninemia, have been associated with micrencephaly.[156] Rarer intrauterine teratogens include anticonvulsant drugs, organic mercurials, excessive ingestion of vitamin A and its analogues, and viral infections (particularly rubella and cytomegalovirus).[157] Micrencephaly is a common feature of a variety of chromosomal disorders and multiple anomaly syndromes; however, the basic disturbance of the brain in these cases involves a derangement of an aspect of development other than neuronal proliferation or remains undefined.[158] MRI is useful in the evaluation of micrencephaly, especially to distinguish cases with associated neuronal migration defects.[159]

Macrencephaly

Macrencephaly is the term applied to a brain that is well formed but large secondary to either an acceleration of neuronal replication during the normal proliferative period or a failure of the proliferative period to undergo its normal diminution in activity after 4 months of gestation (Fig. 57-20). *Macrocephaly* is a more general term applied to a head circumference 2 standard deviations above the mean for gestational age and sex; macrencephaly is only one cause of macrocephaly. Most cases of macrencephaly are autosomal dominant in origin.[160] Infants present at birth with a large head circumference that continues to grow postnatally at a relatively rapid rate. Mental retardation is present in approximately 10% of cases. The genetic component of this syndrome often is overlooked until the head circumference of the parents is measured. Related to autosomal dominant macrencephaly is a syndrome of macrocephaly categorized under several names: *benign enlargement of extracerebral*

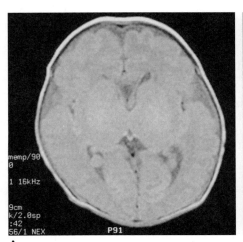
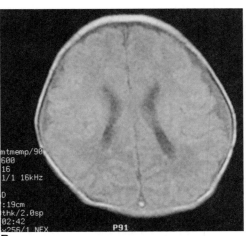

A   B

Figure 57–20. A and **B,** Macrencephaly in a neonate with head circumference greater than 2 standard deviations for gestational age and otherwise normal physical examination. No structural abnormalities were detected on this magnetic resonance imaging study.

spaces, benign subdural effusions of infancy, and *idiopathic external hydrocephalus.*[161] The above-described clinical features are present, but MRI studies show prominent extracerebral subarachnoid spaces along with a large brain. Accelerated head growth ceases by approximately 1 year, and over the next several years, the extracerebral spaces become smaller. The more unusual cases of isolated macrencephaly conform to autosomal recessive patterns and are more likely to exhibit mental retardation, epilepsy, and motor deficits. Macrencephaly may be associated with generalized disorders of growth, such as Sotos syndrome (cerebral gigantism), Beckwith syndrome, and achondroplasia.[160,162] Detection of macrencephaly should raise other diagnostic possibilities, including chromosomal disorders (e.g., fragile X and Klinefelter syndromes) and neurocutaneous syndromes (e.g., neonatal multiple hemangiomatosis and neurofibromatosis).[157,163-165]

Unilateral Macrencephaly

Unilateral macrencephaly refers to enlargement of all or part of one cerebral hemisphere.[166] It is marked by an abnormal gyral pattern, thickened cortex, heterotopic neurons in subcortical white matter, and increased number and size of astrocytes. Clinically, patients present with cranial asymmetry, severe seizures beginning in the neonatal period, hemiplegia, and mental retardation. Ultrasound shows a unilaterally enlarged hemisphere with ipsilateral ventriculomegaly and shifting of the interhemispheric fissure, falx, and superior sagittal sinus to the opposite side.[167] CT shows hemispheric enlargement that initially may be mistaken for a congenital neoplasm. MRI is the best imaging method to show associated neuronal heterotopias and abnormalities of gyration. A characteristic pattern of large-amplitude triphasic complexes can be seen on EEG. Treatment involves judicious surgical resection of affected tissue. A relatively rare neurocutaneous disorder, linear nevus sebaceus syndrome, is associated with unilateral macrencephaly in approximately half of cases.[168] The clinical neurologic and neuropathologic features are essentially similar to those described earlier, but some infants exhibit facial hemihypertrophy as a result of lipomatous-hamartomatous lesions.[169]

Differential Diagnosis

Included in the differential diagnosis of macrencephaly are space-occupying CNS lesions, such as arteriovenous malformations, tumors, and cysts. Proliferation of the vascular tree is particularly active during the period of neuronal proliferation. Arteriovenous malformations in the brain of newborns are rare, with an incidence of 2.5 per 100,000 deliveries. There is a 2:1 male predominance.[170] The size of the malformation determines the amount of arteriovenous shunting and consequently the time and mode of presentation and prognosis.[171,172] Large shunts (with 80% of left ventricular output directed to the head due to low resistance within the vascular malformation) can cause cardiac failure, increased central venous pressure, and hydrops fetalis.[170] The presentation can mimic cyanotic congenital heart disease or persistent pulmonary hypertension of the newborn, causing a delay in diagnosis.[172] A cranial bruit may or may not be present

and cerebral infarction from the "steal" phenomenon can occur. Hydrocephalus may develop, owing to either a mass effect of the aneurysm obstructing flow through the aqueduct of Sylvius or abnormal reabsorption of CSF secondary to elevated cerebral venous pressure.[170] The malformation can be detected on prenatal or postnatal ultrasound as a midline, supratentorial, nonpulsatile, cystic structure with high-velocity Doppler flow. MRI and magnetic resonance angiography (including transuterine studies) are excellent noninvasive tests to show the vascular anatomy, guide treatment, and predict outcome. When an arteriovenous malformation is diagnosed, weekly ultrasound studies are needed to assess the fetus for hydrocephalus, intracranial hemorrhage, degree of arteriovenous shunting, cardiac failure, and hydrops. Although fetal scalp electrode monitoring during labor should be avoided, there are no data to suggest that cesarean delivery improves perinatal outcome, unless there is a question as to the competency of the birth canal.[171] This condition is often refractory to medical management, and staged endovascular embolization has replaced surgical clipping as the mainstay of therapy in selected neonates.[170,172] Morbidity and mortality remain relatively high.

Brain tumors presenting either at birth or within the first 2 months of life account for approximately 1% to 3% of all brain tumors encountered in the pediatric age group.[173] The histologic types differ considerably. Teratomas are the most common tumors of infants who present clinically in fetal life or at birth, whereas tumors of neuroepithelial origin (e.g., medulloblastomas, astrocytomas, and choroid plexus papillomas) predominate in the first 2 postnatal months.[174] Derangements in the control of cell proliferation and differentiation are central to their etiology, and abnormalities of genes encoding proteins that function as growth factors and stimulators of cell proliferation have been identified in various tumors.[175] Additionally, abnormal genetic material inserted into the human genome by certain viruses may induce tumor formation; polymerase chain reaction has been used to show the presence of DNA sequences of simian virus 40 in CNS tumors of laboratory animals.[176] Diagnosis is based on a high index of clinical suspicion, especially when more subtle signs (e.g., intractable seizures, irritability, or persistent vomiting) are present. Spinal cord lesions are particularly important to identify promptly because abrupt neurologic deterioration may occur spontaneously or after mild trauma. Cranial or spinal ultrasonography is the best initial imaging procedure; it is noninvasive and shows especially well tumors in and near the lateral and third ventricles. Doppler evaluation of blood flow within a tumor is useful in the identification of choroid plexus papillomas, which are strikingly hypervascular.[177] When suspicious lesions are found, CT and MRI are indicated for definitive diagnosis.[178] The prognosis for neonates with brain tumors depends on the time of diagnosis and the histologic type of the tumor. Teratomas and medulloblastomas are associated with a poor outcome (with mortality rates of 80% to 90%), principally because the lesions are usually extensive at the time of identification, whereas choroid plexus papillomas provide the most favorable outcome.[174,179] Astrocytomas have variable outcomes depending on the degree of differentiation.[180]

Primary arachnoid cysts are space-occupying lesions believed to be congenital in origin. As the neural tube develops, it is surrounded by loose primitive mesenchyme. The outer compact layer of this mesenchyme develops into dura mater and arachnoid, whereas the loose inner layer develops into the pia. The two layers are separated by an extracellular ground substance. At approximately 15 weeks of gestation, CSF begins to pass into and replace the ground substance, creating the subarachnoid space.[181] Arachnoid cysts represent a focal disturbance in this process; a faulty arachnoid membrane dissects during formation, allowing for an abnormal accumulation and sequestration of fluid.[182] Secondary arachnoid cysts also have been reported as the result of metabolic, infectious, or traumatic insults, although the pathogenesis in these situations has not been fully delineated.[183,184] Arachnoid cysts may be found within the cranium or spinal cord; more than 60% appear in the middle cranial fossa. Males have an overall preponderance that approaches 5:1.[182] Occasionally, arachnoid cysts become manifest within the context of hereditary disorders, such as achondroplasia.[185] Arachnoid cysts may be seen on prenatal ultrasound after 20 weeks of gestation. The classic finding is that of a fluid-filled, anechoic intracerebral mass, without evidence of blood flow by Doppler, having a regular outline with posterior enchancement. If seen in the posterior fossa, differentiation of an arachnoid cyst from other types of cysts (e.g., DWM, "trapped" fourth ventricle, and mega–cisterna magna) is important in that arachnoid cysts are not associated with other CNS malformations and do not carry the same high risk of mental retardation. If the arachnoid cyst is an isolated finding, obstetric management may be conservative.[186] Postnatally, arachnoid cysts produce symptoms based on location, size, and rate of growth. They are often asymptomatic in the neonatal period and found incidentally later in life when CT is performed for unrelated conditions, such as head trauma. Symptoms (including headache, ptosis, vision disturbances, vertigo, endocrine dysfunction, and gait disturbances) are often subtle and nonprogressive.[184] Some cysts (especially cysts in the suprasellar region) can enlarge quickly and exert a mass effect or alter CSF flow, producing hydrocephalus. When this happens, macrocephaly, emesis, hemiparesis, apnea, and seizures can occur.[181,187] Treatment options include (1) permanent resection; (2) fenestration (into a lateral ventricle or the basal cisterns, depending on the location); (3) cystoperitoneal shunt placement; (4) stereotactic aspiration; and (5) percutaneous ventriculocystostomy.[182] Long-term clinical results are generally good regardless of the surgical procedure, but endoscopic fenestration is emerging as the preferred method of treatment.[181]

The choroid plexus is a region of secretory epithelium in the cerebral ventricles that produces CSF and can be visualized as an echogenic mass on ultrasound at 9 weeks of gestation. During development, cysts may develop from entanglement of villi, which then appear as hypoechoic regions filled with CSF.[188] Choroid plexus cysts are usually multilocular, can be unilateral or bilateral, and are thought to be a transient developmental phenomenon; most regress before 25 weeks of gestation.

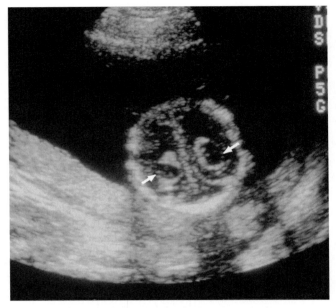

Figure 57–21. Large bilateral choroid plexus cysts *(arrows). (From Chitkara U, Cogswell C, Norton K, et al: Choroid plexus cysts in the fetus: A benign anatomic variant or pathologic entity? Report of 41 cases and review of the literature. Obstet Gynecol 72:185, 1988, with permission from the American College of Obstetricians and Gynecologists.)*

Incidence ranges from 0.5% to 3.5% in ultrasound studies, depending on the route and type of transducer used (Fig. 57-21), but in histologic examinations, asymptomatic choroid plexus cysts can be found in 34% of fetuses and neonates.[189,190] Persistent cysts can be associated with chromosomal disorders, especially trisomies 18 and 21.[190,191] A karyotype is recommended when choroid plexus cysts are found in combination with other anomalies or an abnormal maternal serum AFP.

DISORDERS OF NEURONAL MIGRATION

Neuronal migration refers to the highly ordered series of events whereby millions of nerve cells move from their sites of origin in the ventricular and subventricular germinal matrix along radial glial cells to their destinations throughout the CNS. The migration proceeds in an "inside-out" fashion; early generated neurons occupy deeper layers, whereas later migrating neurons pass the established cells and end up in more superficial positions.[192] The process is at its most intense during the third through fifth prenatal months so that by approximately 24 weeks of gestation, proliferation and migration are essentially complete. Gyral formation results from an increase in the outer cortical surface area out of proportion to that of the inner layers. Abnormalities in neuronal migration alter the composition and the relative volumes of the inner and outer cortical layers, producing different stresses on the cortical surface and anomalous gyral patterning. This anomalous patterning spans the spectrum from too few to too many gyri. Midline prosencephalic development occurs almost coincidentally with the major neuronal migration events that form the cerebral cortex. Gyral abnormalities often are accompanied by agenesis or hypoplasia of the corpus callosum; absence of the septum pellucidum also may be seen. Neuronal migration disorders are recognized with increasing frequency due to the widespread clinical use of MRI; taken together, they have an incidence of greater than 1 per 100,000.[193] More than 25 genetic syndromes associated with abnormal neuronal migration have been described.[192]

Schizencephaly

The most severe form of migrational abnormality is called **schizencephaly** (Greek, *schizo*, "to split or cleave," and *enkephalos*, "brain"). Characteristic clefts extend from the pia to the ependymal lining of the lateral ventricles and tend to occur more often in the parietal and temporal areas; they can be bilateral. The walls lining these clefts exhibit thickened gray matter cortex with heterotopias. Schizencephaly has been classified into two types: open-lipped and closed-lipped. In open-lipped lesions, the edges of the cleft may become widely separated, and dilation of the lateral ventricles may occur. The onset of schizencephaly is thought to be no later than the third month of gestation, but its exact cause is unclear. Schizencephaly seems to be the end result of impaired migration of groups of neurons, producing localized cortical agenesis or hypoplasia. The initial insult may be a destructive process (e.g., exposure to organic solvents, viral illness, or hypotensive vascular accidents) that produces abnormal growth and development.[194] Vasculopathies and autoimmune thrombocytopenia have been implicated. Genetic factors, including dicentric chromosome 15 and functional mutations in the *EMX2* homeobox gene, may be involved. Hydrocephalus, arachnoid cysts, and absence of the corpus callosum or septum pellucidum are commonly associated findings.[195,196] Prenatal diagnosis has been reported with ultrasound and MRI.[167,197,198] Of affected infants, 20% are born prematurely.[196] Clinically the degree of mental and motor impairment is variable and depends on the extent of cortical involvement; patients with bilateral, open-lipped schizencephaly have the worst prognosis. Typically, patients present with intractable seizures, motor impairments, language delays, and moderate-to-severe mental retardation, although normal intelligence has been reported with more subtle defects.[195] Death in severely affected patients occurs in the first months of life secondary to failure to thrive, aspiration, and apnea.

Lissencephaly

In **lissencephaly** (Greek, *lissos*, "smooth," and *enkephalos*, "brain"), the brain has too few gyri (pachygyria) or no gyri (agyria) (Fig. 57-22). Three different anatomic types can be distinguished. In type I lissencephaly (also called **classic lissencephaly** and **generalized agyria-pachygyria**), the cerebral surface is similar to that of a 12-week fetus.[166] The posterior half of the brain is agyric with only a few undulations, whereas the anterior half is pachygyric with a few scattered abnormal sulci.[199] Four cortical layers (instead of the usual six) consist of an outermost, relatively cell-poor marginal layer; a diffuse cellular layer

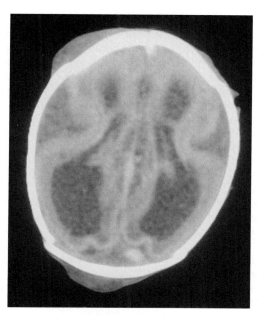

Figure 57–22. Lissencephaly. Agyria and pachygyria are visualized.

containing primarily pyramidal and other neurons characteristic of lower layers of cortex; a zone of heterotopic neurons in columns; and a narrow innermost band of white matter.[1] The gray-to-white matter ratio is inverted (about 4:1), and there are no white-gray matter interdigitations.[200]

Type I lissencephaly can be found as a part of a syndrome (Miller-Dieker syndrome) or as an isolated phenomenon. Isolated lissencephaly syndrome is related principally to genetic defects at two loci on chromosome 17 and the X chromosome. Of patients, 60% have an abnormality at 17p13.3; the affected gene, *LIS1*, encodes the platelet-activating factor acetylhydrolase isoform 1b. Of the remaining cases, most males have abnormalities at Xq22.3-q23, the locus for the doublecortin gene. Both of these gene products seem to be crucial for the interaction of the marginal zone with migrating neurons.[201-203] A rare autosomal recessive form of lissencephaly (microlissencephaly), characterized by prominent neonatal micrencephaly and lissencephaly, arthrogryposis multiplex congenita, cerebellar and brain stem hypoplasia, and early fatal outcome in the neonatal period, has been reported in consanguineous families.[204] Despite the major brain anomaly, microcephaly is usually not present at birth, but characteristically develops in the first year. Craniofacial appearance is generally unremarkable except for bitemporal hollowing of the skull and micrognathia. Hypotonia and paucity of movement are characteristic; spasticity does not develop until later in the first year of life. Mental retardation is profound. Seizures characteristically develop in the first 6 to 12 months of life and present as persistent infantile spasms or akinetic myoclonic seizures with a grossly disordered EEG (Lennox-Gastaut syndrome). Circadian rhythms (e.g., sleep-wake cycle, body temperature, and cortisol secretion) are maintained, provided that the hypothalamic and visual tracts function normally.[205] In addition to the gyral and parenchymal abnormalities, colpocephaly (dilation of the trigone, occipital horns, and temporal horns of the lateral ventricles) is a consistent finding. Most patients require gastrostomy tubes because of poor feeding and recurrent aspiration pneumonias. Death by the age of 5 years is common.

Miller-Dieker syndrome is radiographically similar to isolated lissencephaly syndrome, but craniofacial anomalies are present. Characteristic facies include a tall, flat forehead with vertical furrowing, widely spaced eyes with upslanting palpebral fissures, a short nose with anteverted nares, a flattened midface, and a long, protuberant upper lip with a thin vermilion border. The ears may exhibit minor flattening of the helices.[206] Additional features include cardiac malformations, genital anomalies, a sacral dimple, deep palmar creases, and clinodactyly. The syndrome also is caused by a deletion involving the *LIS1* gene, which is detectable by classic ctyogenetic methods, fluorescence in-situ hybridization, or polymerase chain reaction. The identification of unbalanced inversions and translocations is of particular importance because of their risk of recurrence.[207] Antenatally, intrauterine growth retardation, fetal inactivity, and polyhydramnios may be detected. Early visualization on ultrasound is extremely difficult given that the cortical surface appears smooth early in gestation and develops its gyral pattern relatively late.[208] High-resolution ultrasound at 31 to 32 weeks of gestation illustrates a smooth brain with poor sulci and rudimentary sylvian fissures in the sagittal plane and absence of sulcation on the interhemispheric face in the coronal plane. Color Doppler flow imaging shows a straight course of the middle cerebral artery in the sylvian fissure without its normal branching pattern.[167] Affected patients present with hypotonia and seizures; survival beyond 2 years of age is rare.

In type II lissencephaly, the meninges are thickened and adherent to the agyric cortical surface. The resulting radiographic appearance of the uneven cortex has led to the term **cobblestone lissencephaly**. Histologically the cortex is represented by clusters and circular arrays of neurons with no recognizable organization or lamination, separated by glial and vascular septa. Large heterotopic collections of neurons are prominent. The three disorders consistently associated with type II lissencephaly are Walker-Warburg syndrome, muscle-eye-brain disease, and Fukuyama congenital muscular dystrophy. All are inherited in an autosomal recessive fashion; the gene for Fukuyama congenital muscular dystrophy has been localized to 9q31-33.[203,209]

The major clinical features of Walker-Warburg syndrome include obstructive hydrocephalus producing macrocephaly, retinal malformations, congenital muscular dystrophy, and cerebellar malformations. MRI illustrates the cerebellar malformations and, invariably, vermian agenesis or hypoplasia. Of affected patients, 50% have an associated DWM; 30% have a posterior encephalocele. The neurologic symptoms are similar to those described earlier. The associated muscle disease (evidenced by elevated creatine kinase) accentuates the hypotonia and weakness. Death in the first year is common.

A third type of lissencephaly has been described. The brain is agyric with a hypoplastic brain stem and cerebellum. Histologically, severe neuronal loss of the cortical plate, matrix zone, basal ganglia, brain stem nuclei, and spinal cord is seen along with axonal swelling and microcalcification. Type III lissencephaly is seen in Neu Laxova syndrome, a rare, lethal, autosomal recessive condition characterized by intrauterine growth retardation, microcephaly, characteristic facies (sloping forehead, hypertelorism, protruding eyes with absent lids, flattened nose, and a round, gaping mouth with thick everted lips), ocular malformations, hypoplastic genitalia, and scaly, edematous skin.[210]

Pachygyria

In **pachygyria** (Greek, *pachys,* "thick," and *gyros,* "circle"), the anatomic features of the brain are similar to those described for lissencephaly but are less marked. The gyri are few in number, unusually broad, and associated with an abnormally thick cortical plate. The cause is heterogeneous, with familial, infectious, and sporadic cases reported.[211,212] Affected patients exhibit a range of symptoms: seizures, mental retardation, strabismus, deafness, and hypotonia with resultant spasticity. Survival to adulthood has been documented.[213]

Polymicrogyria

In **polymicrogyria,** the surface of the brain exhibits multiple small narrow gyri, giving it the appearance of a wrinkled chestnut. This defect may be generalized or localized. Two basic varieties of polymicrogyria (layered and unlayered) can be distinguished from their microscopic appearances.[150,214] In the classic or layered type, the cerebral cortex has four distinct layers: (1) a relatively intact outermost molecular layer, (2) a richly cellular second layer consisting of normal superficial cortical neurons, (3) a cell-poor gliotic layer in place of normal deep cortical neurons, and (4) an inner layer of relatively preserved neurons arranged in columns. The cerebral white matter is much more abundant than in lissencephaly. This type of polymicrogyria is thought to be a postmigrational event and often exists in the margins of more severe destructive lesions or in association with infectious processes or toxic exposures.[215,216] The nonlayered type of polymicrogyria is a true migrational disorder. Migration of the neurons destined for the outer cortical layers is impeded; the result is a poorly laminated or nonlaminated cortex surrounding an ill-defined zone of larger pyramidal neurons. Streams of heterotopic neurons in the cerebral white matter are arranged in columns, appearing fixed to the radial glial fibers.[150] Neurologic development is markedly abnormal, and seizures often occur.

Heterotopias

The least severe of the migrational disturbances, neuronal **heterotopias,** are aberrant collections of nerve cells in subcortical white matter. Heterotopias may be found anywhere along the route of migration from the subependymal zone to the cortex. The cortex itself appears histologically normal. There are three major varieties of cerebral neuronal heterotopias, based on their location. The first type occurs in the subependymal region; they are usually nodular and termed **periventricular nodular heterotopias**.[214] The clinical picture includes seizures and varying degrees of cognitive deficits. The second variety consists of heterotopias found in the cerebral white matter. They may be nodular (focal or diffuse), but more commonly appear as a diffuse laminar band below the cerebral cortex and are called **subcortical band heterotopia** or **double cortex**. Subcortical band heterotopia is seen in the female carriers of X-linked lissencephaly.[192] The superficial cortical-leptomeningeal heterotopias constitute the third variety of cerebral neuronal heterotopias.[217] Neuronal heterotopias are associated with a variety of disorders, including chromosomal abnormalities, neurocutaneous syndromes, and metabolic diseases.

Cortical Dysplasia

With the advent of MRI scanning and surgical removal of cortical anomalies for intractable epilepsy, focal disorders of neuronal migration within cerebral cortex itself have been increasingly recognized. The lesions have been described as focal cerebral cortical **dysgenesis** or **dysplasias**.[218] The clinical syndromes relate to the topography of the lesions; most are dominated by seizures.

DISORDERS OF NEURONAL ORGANIZATION

When the processes of induction, proliferation, and migration have laid the architectural framework of the developing CNS, the components must be interconnected to allow the brain to function. This organization begins during the fifth month of gestation and continues for several years beyond term. The major developmental steps are (1) establishment and differentiation of the subplate neurons; (2) attainment of proper alignment, orientation, and layering of cortical neurons; (3) elaboration of dendritic and axonal ramifications; (4) establishment of synaptic contacts; (5) cell death and selective elimination of neuronal processes and synapses; and (6) proliferation and differentiation of glia. Striking abnormalities of neuronal organization have been described in infants with trisomy 21, fragile X syndrome, and Duchenne muscular dystrophy. Although the cytoskeletal protein dystrophin likely plays a role in the latter case, the neuropathologic techniques available today to evaluate the complex circuitry and synaptic connections of human brains are inadequate to delineate fully abnormalities in neuronal organization. Newer MRI techniques (e.g., quantitative volumetric MRI, diffusion tensor MRI, and functional MRI) someday may provide clearer insights.

DISORDERS OF MYELINATION

A direct relationship exists between myelination and functional maturity of the brain.[168] Myelination begins during the second trimester when oligodendroglia ensheathe the axons of neurons with concentric layers of their plasma membranes. The myelin sheaths so formed enhance impulse transmission along the length of the axons. Myelination proceeds from caudal to cranial and from the dorsal to the ventral parts of the brain. At birth, myelin is present in the dorsal parts of the brain stem, the superior and inferior cerebellar peduncles, the posterior limbs of the internal capsule, and the corona radiata.

The myelination process accelerates postnatally and continues for years after birth.[219] MRI is the best tool with which to monitor myelination because changes in signal intensity correlate well with the histologic detection of myelination during normal brain maturation.[220] Abnormal myelin has been well documented in several amino acidopathies, organic acidopathies, lysosomal storage diseases, malnutrition, and congenital hypothyroidism. Although many theories abound (including deletions in chromosome 18q, the region encoding myelin basic protein), the underlying mechanism of these disturbances is not clear. Newer MRI technologies that provide quantitative volumetric determinations and measurements of relative anisotropy may help elucidate further the cause of myelination disorders.

Demyelination (the breakdown of myelin due to gross disturbances in neuronal cell metabolism and an increased turnover of membrane constituents) is characteristic of metachromic leukodystophy, Krabbe disease, mitochondrial disorders, adrenoleukodystrophy, Canavan disease, Alexander disease, and orthochromatic leukodystrophy.[220,221] Most of these diseases do not manifest in the neonatal period and are not discussed here.

REFERENCES

1. Volpe JJ: Neurology of the Newborn, 4th ed. Philadelphia, WB Saunders, 2001.
2. Moore KL: The Developing Human: Clinically Oriented Embryology, 6th ed. Philadelphia, WB Saunders, 1998, pp 451-489.
3. Juriloff DM, Harris MJ: Mouse models for neural tube closure defects. Hum Mol Genet 9:993, 2000.
4. Fleming A, Copp A: A genetic risk factor for mouse neural tube defects: Defining the embryonic basis. Hum Mol Genet 9:575, 2000.
5. Rogner UC, Spyropoulos DD, Le Novere N, et al: Control of neurulation by the nucleosome assembly protein-1-like 2. Nat Genet 25:431, 2000.
6. Northrup H, Volcik KA: Spina bifida and other neural tube defects. Curr Prob Pediatr 30:317, 2000.
7. Wenstrom KD, Johanning GL, Owen J, et al: Amniotic fluid homocysteine levels, 5,10-methylenetetrahydrafolate reductase genotypes, and neural tube closure sites. Am J Med Genet 90:6, 2000.
8. Golden JA, Chernoff GF: Multiple sites of anterior neural tube closure in humans: Evidence from anterior neural tube defects (anencephaly). Pediatrics 95:506, 1995.
9. Fredrick J: Anencephalus: Variation with maternal age, parity, social class, and region in England, Scotland, and Wales. Ann Hum Genet 34:31, 1970.
10. Melnick M, Myrianthopoulos NC: Studies in neural tube defects. II. Pathologic findings in a prospectively collected series of anencephalics. Am J Med Genet 26:797, 1987.
11. Yen IH, Khoury MJ, Erickson, JD, et al: The changing epidemiology of neural tube defects—United States, 1968-1989. Am J Dis Child 146:857, 1992.
12. Arnold WH, Lang M, Sperber GH: 3D-reconstruction of craniofacial structures of a human anencephalic fetus: Case report. Ann Anat 183:67, 2001.
13. Edwards MSB, Filly R: Diagnosis and management of fetal disorders of the central nervous system. In Hoffman HJ, Epstein F (eds): Disorders of the Developing Nervous System: Diagnosis and Treatment. Boston, Blackwell Scientific, 1986.

14. O'Rourke K, deBlois J: Induced delivery of anencephalic fetuses: A response to James L. Walsh and Moira M. McQueen. Kennedy Inst Ethics J 4:47, 1994.

15. Walters J, Ashwal S, Masek T: Anencephaly: Where do we now stand? Semin Neurol 17:249, 1997.

16. Jahnukainen T, Lindqvist A, Aarimaa T, et al: Reactivity of skin blood flow and heart rate to external thermal stimulation in anencephaly. Acta Paediatr 86:426, 1997.

17. Pomerance JJ, Morrison A, Williams RL, et al: Anencephalic infants: Life expectancy and organ donation. J Perinatol 9:33, 1989.

18. Becker R, Mende B, Stiemer B, et al: Sonographic markers of exencephaly at 9 + 3 weeks of gestation. Ultrasound Obstet Gynecol 16:582, 2000.

19. Chatzipapas IK, Whitlow BJ, Economides DL: The "Mickey Mouse" sign and the diagnosis of anencephaly in early pregnancy. Ultrasound Obstet Gynecol 13:196, 1999.

20. Johnson SP, Sebire NJ, Snijders RJ, et al: Ultrasound screening for anencephaly at 10-14 weeks of gestation. Ultrasound Obstet Gynecol 9:14, 1997.

21. Sepulveda W, Sebire NJ, Fung TY, et al: Crown-chin length in normal and anencephalic fetuses at 10-14 weeks' gestation. Am J Obstet Gynecol 176:852, 1997.

22. Hata T, Yanagihara T, Matsumoto M, et al: Three-dimensional sonographic features of fetal central nervous system anomaly. Acta Obstet Gynecol Scand 79:635, 2000.

23. Benn PA, Craffey A, Horne D, et al: Elevated maternal serum alpha-fetoprotein with low unconjugated estriol and the risk for lethal perinatal outcome. J Matern Fetal Med 9:165, 2000.

24. Yaron Y, Hamby DD, O'Brien JE, et al: Combination of elevated maternal serum alpha-fetoprotein (MSAFP) and low estriol is highly predictive of anencephaly. Am J Med Genet 75:297, 1998.

25. Brennand DM, Jehanli AM, Wood PJ, et al: Raised levels of maternal serum secretory acetylcholinesterase may be indicative of fetal neural tube defects in early pregnancy. Acta Obstet Gynecol Scand 77:8, 1998.

26. Silver RK, Leeth EA, Check IJ: A reappraisal of amniotic fluid alpha-fetoprotein measurements at the time of genetic amniocentesis and midtrimester ultrasonography. J Ultrasound Med 20:631, 2001.

27. Timor-Tritsch IE, Greenebaum E, Monteagudo A, et al: Exencephaly-anencephaly sequence: Proof by ultrasound imaging and amniotic fluid cytology. J Matern Fetal Med 5:182, 1996.

28. Brown MS, Sheridan-Pereira M: Outlook for the child with a cephalocele. Pediatrics 90:914, 1992.

29. McLone DG: Congenital malformations of the central nervous system. Clin Neurosurg 47:346, 2000.

30. Martinez-Lage JF, Poza M, Sola J, et al: The child with a cephalocele: Etiology, neuroimaging, and outcome. Childs Nerv Syst 12:540, 1996.

31. Naidich TP, Altman NR, Braffman BH, et al: Cephaloceles and related malformations. AJNR Am J Neuroradiol 13:655, 1992.

32. Cohen MM, Lemire RJ: Syndromes with cephaloceles. Teratology 25:161, 1982.

33. Fleming AD, Vintzileos AM, Scorza WE: Prenatal diagnosis of occipital encephalocele with transvaginal ultrasonography. J Ultrasound Med 10:285, 1991.

34. Holmes AD, Meara JG, Kolker AR, et al: Frontoethmoidal encephaloceles: Reconstruction and refinements. J Craniofac Surg 12:6, 2001.

35. Michejda M, Bacher J: Functional and anatomic recovery in the monkey brain following excision of fetal encephalocele. Pediatr Neurosci 12:90, 1985-1986.

36. Gazioglu N, Vural M, Seckin MS, et al: Meckel-Gruber syndrome. Childs Nerv Syst 14:142, 1998.

37. Salonen R: The Meckel syndrome: Clinicopathological findings in 67 patients. Am J Med Genet 18:671, 1984.

38. Sepulveda W, Sebire NJ, Souka A, et al: Diagnosis of the Meckel-Gruber syndrome at eleven to fourteen weeks' gestation. Am J Obstet Gynecol 176:316, 1997.

39. Strayer A: Chiari I malformation: Clinical presentation and management. J Neurosci Nurs 33:90, 2001.

40. Fujita K, Matsuo N, Mori O, et al: The association of hypopituitarism with small pituitary, invisible pituitary stalk, type 1 Arnold-Chiari malformation, and syringomyelia in seven patients born in breech position: A further proof of birth injury theory on the pathogenesis of "idiopathic hypopituitarism." Eur J Pediatr 151:266, 1992.

41. Genitori L, Peretta P, Nurisso C, et al: Chiari type I anomalies in children and adolescents: Minimally invasive management in a series of 53 cases. Childs Nerv Syst 16:707, 2000.

42. Carmel PW: The Chiari malformations and syringomyelia. In Hoffman HJ, Epstein F (eds): Disorders of the Developing Nervous System: Diagnosis and Treatment. Boston, Blackwell Scientific, 1986.

43. Haberle J, Hulskamp G, Harms E, et al: Cervical encephalocele in a newborn—Chiari III malformation: Case report and review of the literature. Childs Nerv Syst 17:373, 2001.

44. French BN: The embryology of spinal dysraphism. Clin Neurosurg 30:295, 1981.

45. Mainprize TG, Taylor MD, Rutka JT: Perspectives in pediatric neurosurgery. Childs Nerv Syst 16:809, 2000.

46. Selcuki, M, Manning S, Bernfield M: The curly tail mouse model of human neural tube defects demonstrates normal spinal cord differentiation at the level of the meningomyelocele: Implications for fetal surgery. Childs Nerv Syst 17:19, 2001.

47. Sutton LN, Sun P, Adzick NS: Fetal neurosurgery. Neurosurgery 48:124, 2001.

48. Toriello HV, Higgins JV: Possible causal heterogeneity in spina bifida cystica. Am J Med Genet 21:13, 1985.

49. Kallen K: Maternal smoking, body mass index, and neural tube defects. Am J Epidemiol 147:1103, 1998.

50. Noetzel MJ: Myelomeningocele: Current concepts of management. Clin Perinatol 16:311, 1989.

51. Watkins ML, Scanlon KS, Mulinare J, et al: Is maternal obesity a risk factor for anencephaly and spina bifida? Epidemiology 7:507, 1996.

52. Milunsky A, Jick H, Jick SS, et al: Multivitamin/folic acid supplementation in early pregnancy reduces the prevalence of neural tube defects. JAMA 262:2847, 1989.

53. MRC Vitamin Study Research Group: Prevention of neural tube defects: Results of the Medical Research Council vitamin study. Lancet 338:131, 1991.

54. Mulinare J, Cordero JF, Erickson D, et al: Periconceptual use of multivitamins and the occurrence of neural tube defects. JAMA 260:3141, 1988.

55. Werler MM, Shapiro S, Mitchell AA: Periconceptional folic acid exposure and risk of occurrent neural tube defects. JAMA 269:1257, 1993.

56. Oakley GP: Folic acid-preventable spina bifida and anencephaly. JAMA 269:1292, 1993.

57. American Academy of Pediatrics, Committee on Genetics: Folic acid for the prevention of neural tube defects. Pediatrics 104:325, 1999.

58. Centers for Disease Control: Use of folic acid for prevention of spina bifida and other neural tube defects. MMWR Morb Mortal Wkly Rep 40:513, 1991.

59. Centers for Disease Control: Recommendations for the use of folic acid to reduce the number of cases of spina bifida and other neural tube defects, 1981-1983. MMWR Morb Mortal Wkly Rep 41(RR-14):1-7, 1992.

60. Honein MA, Paulozzi LJ, Mathews TJ, et al: Impact of folic acid fortification of the US food supply on the occurrence of neural tube defects. JAMA 285:2981, 2001.

61. Nyberg DA, Mack LA: The spine and neural tube defects. In Nyberg DA, Mahony BS, Pretorius DH (eds): Diagnostic Ultrasound of Fetal Anomalies. Chicago, Year Book Medical Publishers, 1990.

62. van den Hof MC, Nicolaides KH, Campbell J, et al: Evaluation of the lemon and banana signs in one hundred thirty fetuses with open spina bifida. Am J Obstet Gynecol 162:322, 1990.

63. Blass HG, Eik-Nes SH, Isaksen CV: The detection of spina bifida before 10 gestational weeks using two- and three-dimensional ultrasound. Ultrasound Obstet Gynecol 16:25, 2000.

64. Carroll NC: Assessment and management of the lower extremity in myelodysplasia. Orthop Clin North Am 18:709, 1987.

65. Luthy DA, Wardinsky T, Shurtleff DB, et al: Cesarean section before the onset of labor and subsequent motor function in infants with meningomyelocele diagnosed antenatally. N Engl J Med 324:662, 1991.

66. McCurdy CM, Seeds JW: Route of delivery of infants with congenital anomalies. Clin Perinatol 20:81, 1993.

67. Shurtleff DB: 44 years experience with management of myelomeningocele: Presidential address, Society for Research into Hydrocephalus and Spina Bifida. Eur J Pediatr Surg 10:5, 2000.

68. Charney EB, Melchionni JB, Antonucci DL: Ventriculitis in newborns with myelomeningocele. Am J Dis Child 145:287, 1991.

69. Charney EB, Weller SC, Sutton LN, et al: Management of the newborn with myelomeningocele: Time for a decision-making process. Pediatrics 75:58, 1985.

70. Liptak GS, Gellerstedt ME, Kilonsky N: Isosorbide in the medical management of hydrocephalus in children with myelodysplasia. Dev Med Child Neurol 34:150, 1992.

71. Lorber J, Salfield S, Lonton T: Isosorbide in the management of infantile hydrocephalus. Dev Med Child Neurol 25:502, 1983.

72. Baskin LS, Kogan BA, Benard F: Treatment of infants with neurogenic bladder dysfunction using anticholinergic drugs and intermittent catheterization. Br J Urol 66:532, 1990.

73. Beaty JH, Canale ST: Orthopaedic aspects of myelomeningocele. J Bone Joint Surg (Am) 72:626, 1990.

74. Meuli M, Meuli-Simmen C, Hutchins GM, et al: In utero surgery rescues neurological function at birth in sheep with spina bifida. Nat Med 1:342, 1995.

75. Bruner JP, Tulipan NE, Richards WO: Endoscopic coverage of fetal open myelomeningocele in utero. Am J Obstet Gynecol 176:256, 1997.

76. Tulipan N, Hernanz-Schulman M, Bruner JP: Reduced hindbrain herniation after intrauterine myelomingocele repair: A report of four cases. Pediatr Neurosurg 29:274, 1998.

77. Proctor MR, Bauer SB, Scott RM: The effect of surgery for split spinal cord malformation on neurologic and urologic function. Pediatr Neurosurg 32:13, 2000.

78. Pang D, Dias MS, Ahab-barmada M: Split cord malformation: Part I. A unified theory of embryogenesis for double spinal cord malformations. Neurosurgery 31:451, 1992.

79. Tortori-Donati P, Rossi A, Cama A: Spinal dysraphism: A review of neuroradiological features with embryological correlations and proposal for a new classification. Neuroradiology 42:471, 2000.

80. Ersahin Y, Demirtas E, Mutluer S, et al: Split cord malformations: Report of three unusual cases. Pediatr Neurosurg 24:155, 1996.

81. Ersahin Y, Mutluer S, Kocaman S, et al: Split spinal cord malformations in children. J Neurosurg 88:57, 1998.

82. Jindal A, Mahapatra AK: Split cord malformations—a clinical study of 48 cases. Indian Pediatr 37:603, 2000.

83. Pang D: Split cord malformations: Part II. Clinical syndrome. Neurosurgery 31:481, 1992.

84. Boulot P, Ferran JL, Charlier C, et al: Prenatal diagnosis of diastematomyelia. Pediatr Radiol 23:67, 1993.

85. Caspi B, Gorbacz S, Appelman Z, et al: Antenatal diagnosis of diastematomyelia. J Clin Ultrasound 18:721, 1990.

86. Pachi A, Maggi E, Giancotti A, et al: Prenatal sonographic diagnosis of diastematomyelia in a diabetic woman. Prenat Diagn 12:535, 1992.

87. Seeds JW, Jones FD: Lipomeningocele: prenatal diagnosis and management. Obstet Gynecol 67:345, 1986..

88. Lemire RJ, Beckwith JB: Pathogenesis of congenital tumors and malformations of the sacrococcygeal region. Teratology 25:201, 1982.

89. Fernandes ET, Custer MD, Burton EM, et al: Neurenteric cyst: Surgery and diagnostic imaging. J Pediatr Surg 26:108, 1991.

90. Gilchrist BF, Harrison MW, Campbell JR: Neurenteric cyst: current management. J Pediatr Surg 25:1231, 1990.

91. Muthukumar N, Arunthathi J, Sundar V: Split cord malformation and neurenteric cyst—case report and a theory of embryogenesis. Br J Neurosurg 14:488, 2000.

92. Wilkinson CC, Albanese CT, Jennings RW, et al: Fetal neurenteric cyst causing hydrops: Case report and review of the literature. Prenat Diagn 19:118, 1999.

93. Kim CY, Wang KC, Choe G, et al: Neurenteric cyst: Its various presentations. Childs Nerv Syst 15:333, 1999.

94. Chaynes P, Bousquet P, Sol JC, et al: Recurrent intracranial neurenteric cysts. Acta Neurochir 140:905, 1998.

95. Bohring A, Lewin SO, Reynolds JF, et al: Polytopic anomalies with agenesis of the lower vertebral column. Am J Med Genet 87:99, 1999.

96. Turnock RR, Brereton RJ: Peno-scrotal transposition and the caudal regression syndrome. Eur J Pediatr Surg 1:374, 1991.

97. Makhoul IR, Aviram-Goldring A, Paperna T, et al: Caudal dysplasia sequence with penile enlargement: Case report an a potential pathogenic hypothesis. Am J Med Genet 99:54, 2001.

98. Fukada Y, Yasumizu T, Tsurugi Y, et al: Caudal regression syndrome detected in a fetus with increased nuchal translucency. Acta Obstet Gynecol Scand 78:655, 1999.

99. Baxi L, Warren W, Collins MH, et al: Early detection of caudal regression syndrome with transvaginal scanning. Obstet Gynecol 75:486, 1990.

100. Hirano H, Tomura N, Watarai J, et al: Caudal regression syndrome: MR appearance. Comput Med Imaging Graph 22:73, 1998.

101. Kim TS, Cho S, Dickson DW: Aprosencephaly: Review of the literature and report of a case with cerebellar hypoplasia, pigmented epithelial cyst, and Rathke's cleft cyst. Acta Neuropathol 79:424, 1990.

102. Ippel PF, Breslau-Siderius EJ, Hack WW, et al: Atelencephalic microcephaly: A case report and review of the literature. Eur J Pediatr 157:493, 1998.

103. Arii N, Mizuguchi M, Mori K, et al: Ectopic expression of telencephalin in brains with holoprosencephaly. Acta Neuropathol 100:506, 2000.

104. Toma P, Costa A, Mangano GM, et al: Holoprosencephaly: Prenatal diagnosis by sonography and magnetic resonance imaging. Prenat Diagn 10:429, 1990.

105. Cohen MM Jr: Perspectives on holoprosencephaly: Part I. Epidemiology, genetics, and syndromology. Teratology 40:211, 1989.

106. Siddell EP, Longobucco DB: Holoprosencephaly: A case presentation. Neonatal Netw 14:21, 1995.

107. Ram SP, Noor AR, Mahbar Z, et al: Holoprosencephaly in neonates. Int J Pediatr Otorhinolaryngol 29:65, 1994.

108. Mazal PR, Schuhfried G, Budka H: Trilobar holoprosencephaly ("triprosencephaly"): A unique type of cerebral malformation. Acta Neuropathol 89:567, 1995.

109. Olsen CL, Hughes JP, Youngblood LG, et al: Epidemiology of holoprosencephaly and phenotypic characteristics of affected children: New York State, 1984-1989. Am J Med Genet 73:217, 1997.

110. Overhauser J, Mitchell HF, Zackai EH, et al: Physical mapping of the holoprosencephaly critical region in 18p11.3. Am J Hum Genet 57:1080, 1995.

111. Roessler E, Belloni E, Gaudenz K, et al: Mutations in the human Sonic Hedgehog gene cause holoprosencephaly. Nat Genet 14:357, 1996.

112. Kelley RI, Roessler E, Hennekam RCM, et al: Holoprosencephaly in RSH/Smith-Lemli-Opitz syndrome: Does abnormal cholesterol metabolism affect the function of Sonic Hedgehog? Am J Med Genet 66:478, 1996.

113. Keller K, McCune H, Williams C, et al: Lobar holoprosencephaly in an infant born to a mother with classic phenylketonuria (letter). Am J Med Genet 95:187, 2000.

114. Nelson LH, King M: Early diagnosis of holoprosencephaly. J Ultrasound Med 11:57, 1992.

115. Barr M Jr, Cohen MM Jr: Holoprosencephaly survival and performance. Am J Med Genet 89:116, 1999.

116. Plawner L, Clegg N, Kinsman S, et al: Prolonged survival and childhood-onset epilepsy in alobar holoprosencephaly (letter). Childs Nerv Syst 16:195, 2000.

117. Filly RA: The fetus with a CNS malformation: Ultrasound evaluation. In Harrison RA, Golbus MS, Filly RA (eds): The Unborn Patient. Philadelphia, WB Saunders, 1991, pp 403-486..

118. Lin Y, Chang F, Liu C: Antenatal detection of hydranencephaly at 12 weeks menstrual age. J Clin Ultrasound 20:62, 1992.

119. Aguirre Vila-Coro A, Dominguez R: Intrauterine diagnosis of hydranencephaly by magnetic resonance. Magn Reson Imaging 7:105, 1989.

120. Greene MF, Benacerraf B, Crawford JM: Hydranencephaly: Ultrasound appearance during in utero evolution. Radiology 156:779, 1985.

121. Paidas MJ, Cohen A: Disorders of the central nervous system. Semin Perinatol 18:266, 1994.

122. Boaz JC, Edwards-Brown MK: Hydrocephalus in children: Neurosurgical and neuroimaging concerns. Neuroimaging Clin N Am 9:73, 1999.

123. Birnholz JC, Frigoletto FD: Antenatal treatment of hydrocephalus. N Engl J Med 304:1021, 1981.

124. Clewell WH, Johnson ML, Meier PR, et al: A surgical approach to the treatment of fetal hydrocephalus. N Engl J Med 306:1320, 1982.

125. Glick PL, Harrison MR, Nakayama DK, et al: Management of ventriculomegaly in the fetus. J Pediatr 105:97, 1984.

126. Bannister CH: Is the intrauterine treatment of fetal hydrocephalus helpful or harmful? Fetal Ther 1:146, 1986.

127. Edwards MS: An evaluation of the in utero neurosurgical treatment of ventriculomegaly. Clin Neurosurg 33:347, 1986.

128. Glick PL, Harrison MR, Halks-Miller M, et al: Correction of congenital hydrocephalus in utero: II. Efficacy of in utero shunting. J Pediatr Surg 19:870, 1984.

129. Hudgins RJ, Edwards MSB: The fetus with a CNS malformation: Natural history and management. In Harrison MR, Golbus MS, Filly RA (eds): The Unborn Patient. Philadelphia, WB Saunders, 1991, pp 437-443.

130. Oi S, Matsumoto S, Katayama K, et al: Pathophysiology and postnatal outcome of fetal hydrocephalus. Childs Nerv Syst 6:338, 1990.

131. Rodeck C: Intrauterine shunting for ventriculomegaly (letter). Lancet 1:92, 1986.

132. Felderhoff-Mueser U, Herold R, Hochhaus F, et al: Increased cerebrospinal fluid concentrations of soluble Fas (CD95/Apo-1) in hydrocephalus. Arch Dis Child 84:369, 2001.

133. Frim DM, Lathrop D, Chwals WJ: Intraventricular pressure dynamics in ventriculocholecystic shunting: A telemetric study. Pediatr Neurosurg 34:73, 2001.

134. Heep A, Engelskirchen R, Holschneider A, et al: Primary intervention for posthemorrhagic hydrocephalus in very low birthweight infants by ventriculostomy. Childs Nerv Syst 17:47, 2001.

135. Sato O, Yamguchi T, Kittaka M, et al: Hydrocephalus and epilepsy. Childs Nerv Syst 17:76, 2001.

136. Lefort G, Blanchet P, Chaze AM, et al: Cytogenetic and molecular study of a jumping translocation in a baby with Dandy-Walker malformation. J Med Genet 38:67, 2001.

137. Altman NR, Naidich TP, Braffman BH: Posterior fossa malformations. AJNR Am J Neuroradiol 13:691, 1992.

138. Ulm B, Ulm MR, Deutinger J, et al: Dandy-Walker malformation diagnosed before 21 weeks of gestation: Associated malformations and chromosomal abnormalities. Ultrasound Obstet Gynecol 10:167, 1997.

139. Miyamori T, Okabe T, Hasegawa T, et al: Dandy-Walker syndrome successfully treated with cystoperitoneal shunting—case report. Neurol Med Chir 39:766, 1999.

140. Osenbach RK, Menezes AH: Diagnosis and management of the Dandy-Walker malformation: 30 years of experience. Pediatr Neurosurg 18:179, 1992.

141. Cornford E, Twining P: The Dandy-Walker syndrome: The value of antenatal diagnosis. Clin Radiol 45:172, 1992.

142. Barkovich AJ, Norman D: Anomalies of the corpus callosum: Correlation with further anomalies of the brain. AJR Am J Roentgenol 151:171, 1988.

143. Marszal E, Jamroz E, Pilch J, et al: Agenesis of corpus callosum: Clinical description and etiology. J Child Neurol 15:401, 2000.

144. Neidich JA, Nussbaum RL, Packer RJ, et al: Heterogeneity of clinical severity and molecular lesions in Aicardi syndrome. J Pediatr 116:911, 1990.

145. Atlas SW, Shkolnik A, Naidich TP: Sonographic recognition of agenesis of the corpus callosum. AJR Am J Roentgenol 145:167, 1985.

146. Fawer CL, Calame A, Anderegg A, et al: Agenesis of the corpus callosum: Real-time ultrasonographic diagnosis and autopsy findings. Helv Paediatr Acta 40:371, 1985.

147. Mott SH, Bodensteiner, JB, Allan WC: The cavum septi pellucidi in term and preterm newborn infants. J Child Neurol 7:35, 1992.

148. Bodensteiner JB, Schaefer GB, Craft JM: Cavum septi pellucidi and cavum vergae in normal and developmentally delayed populations. J Child Neurol 13:120, 1998.

149. Hashimoto LN, Bass WT, Green GA, et al: Radial microbrain form of micrencephaly: Possible association with carbamazepine. J Neuroimaging 9:243, 1999.

150. Evrard P, de Sting-Georges P, Kadhim HJ, et al: Pathology of prenatal encephalopathies. In: International Child Neurology Congress: Child Neurology and Developmental Disabilities. Baltimore, PH Brooks, 1989, pp 153-176.

151. Evrard P, Miladi N, Bonnier C, et al: Normal and abnormal development of the brain. In Rapin I, Segalowitz SJ (eds): Handbook of Neuropsychology, vol 6, Child Neuropsychology. Amsterdam, Elsevier, 1992, pp 11-44.

152. Cowie VA: Microcephaly: A review of genetic implications in its causation. J Ment Defic Res 31:229, 1987.

153. Innis JW, Asher JH, Poznanski AK, et al: Autosomal dominant microcephaly with normal intelligence, short palpebral fissures, and digital anomalies. Am J Med Genet 71:150, 1997.

154. Yamazaki JN, Schull WJ: Perinatal loss and neurological abnormalities among children of the atomic bomb: Nagasaki and Hiroshima revisited, 1949 to 1989. JAMA 264:605, 1990.

155. Schull WJ, Norton S, Jensh RP: Ionizing radiation and the developing brain. Neurotoxicol Teratol 12:249, 1990.

156. Jardim LB, Palma-Dias R, Silva LCS, et al: Maternal hyperphenylalaninaemia as a cause of microcephaly and mental retardation. Acta Paediatr 85:943, 1996.

157. Warkany J, Lemire RJ, Cohen MM Jr: Mental Retardation and Congenital Malformations of the Central Nervous System. Year Book Medical Publishers, Chicago, 1981.

158. Wiedemann HR, Kunze JJ: Clinical Syndromes, 3rd ed. London, Times Mirror International, 1997.

159. Steinlin M, Zurrer M, Martin E, et al: Contribution of magnetic resonance imaging in the evaluation of microcephaly. Neuropediatrics 22:184, 1991.

160. DeMeyer W: Megalencephaly in children: Clinical syndromes, genetic patterns, and differential diagnosis from other causes of megalocephaly. Neurology 22:634, 1972.

161. Alvarez LA, Maytal J, Sinnar S: Idiopathic external hydrocephalus: Natural history and relationship to benign familial macrocephaly. Pediatrics 77:901, 1986.

162. Dodge PR, Holmes SJ, Sotos JF: Cerebral gigantism. Dev Med Child Neurol 25:248, 1983.

163. Drigo P, Carra S, Laverda AM: Macrocephaly and chromosome disorders: A case report. Brain Dev 18:312, 1996.

164. Pont MS, Elster AD: Lesions of skin and brain—modern imaging of the neurocutaneous syndromes—review. AJR Am J Roentgenol 158:1193, 1992.

165. Simko A, Hornstein L, Soukup S, et al: Fragile X syndrome: Recognition in young children. Pediatrics 83:547, 1989.

166. Barkovich AJ, Chuang SH, Norman D: MR of neuronal migration anomalies. AJR Am J Roentgenol 8:1009, 1987.

167. Pellicer A, Cabanas F, Perez-Higueras A, et al: Neural migration disorders studied by cerebral ultrasound and colour Doppler flow imaging. Arch Dis Child Fetal Neonatal Educ 73:F55, 1995.

168. Gurecki PJ, Holden KR, Sahn EE, et al: Developmental neural abnormalities and seizures in epidermal nevus syndrome, Dev Med Child Neurol 38:716, 1996.

169. Pavone L, Curatolo P, Rizzo R, et al: Epidermal nevus syndrome: A neurologic variant with hemimegalencephaly, gyral malformation, mental retardation, seizures, and facial hemihypertrophy. Neurology 41:266, 1991.

170. Chisholm CA, Kuller JA, Katz VL, et al: Aneurysm of the vein of Galen: Prenatal diagnosis and perinatal management. Am J Perinatol 13:503, 1996.

171. Chiang V, Awad I, Berenstein A, et al: Neonatal galenic arteriovenous malformation. Neurosurgery 44:847, 1999.

172. Hendson L, Emery DJ, Phillipos EZ, et al: Persistent pulmonary hypertension of the newborn presenting as the primary manifestation of intracranial arteriovenous malformation of the vein of Galen. Am J Perinatol 17:405, 2000.

173. Fort DW, Rushing EJ: Congenital central nervous system tumors. J Child Neurol 12:157, 1997.

174. Rickert CH, Probst-Cousin S, Gullotta F: Primary intracranial neoplasms of infancy and early childhood. Childs Nerv Syst 13:507, 1997.

175. Ullrich NJ, Pomeroy SL: Pediatric brain tumors. Neurol Clin 21:897, 2003.

176. Bergsagel DJ, Finegold MJ, Butel JS, et al: DNA sequences similar to those of simian virus 40 in ependymomas and choroid plexus tumors of childhood. N Engl J Med 326:988, 1992.

177. Harmon BH, Yap MA: One-month-old infant with increasing head size. Invest Radiol 25:862, 1990.

178. Radkowski MA, Naidich TP, Tomita T, et al: Neonatal brain tumors: CT and MR findings. J Comput Assist Tomogr 12:10, 1988.

179. Wakai S, Arai T, Nagai M: Congenital brain tumors. Surg Neurol 21:597, 1984.

180. Roosen N, Deckert M, Nicola N, et al: Congenital anaplastic astrocytoma with favorable prognosis. J Neurosurg 69:604, 1988.

181. Choi JU, Kim DS: Pathogenesis of arachnoid cyst: Congenital or traumatic? Pediatr Neurosurg 29:260, 1998.

182. Wester K: Peculiarities of intracranial arachnoid cysts: Location, sidedness, and sex distribution in 126 consecutive patients. Neurosurgery 45:775, 1999.

183. Lutcherath V, Waaler PE, Jellum E, et al: Children with bilateral temporal arachnoid cysts may have glutaric aciduria type 1 (GAT1): Operation without knowing that may be harmful. Acta Neurochir 142:1025, 2000.

184. Martinez-Lage JF, Ruiz-Macia D, Valenti JA, et al: Development of a middle fossa arachnoid cyst: A theory on its pathogenesis. Childs Nerv Syst 15:94, 1999.

185. Wang P, Lin HC, Liu HM, et al: Intracranial arachnoid cysts in children: Related signs and associated anomalies. Pediatr Neurol 19:100, 1998.

186. Barjot P, von Theobald P, Refahi N, et al: Diagnosis of arachnoid cysts on prenatal ultrasound. Fetal Diagn Ther 14:306, 1999.

187. Balsubramaniam C, Laurent J, Rouah E, et al: Congenital arachnoid cysts in children. Pediatr Neurosci 15:223, 1989.

188. Digiovanni LM, Quinlan MP, Verp MS: Choroid plexus cysts: Infant and early childhood developmental outcome. Obstet Gynecol 90:191, 1997.

189. Ricketts NE, Lowe EM, Patel NB: Prenatal diagnosis of choroid plexus cysts. Lancet 1:213, 1987.

190. Riebel T, Nasir R, Weber K: Choroid plexus cysts: A normal finding on ultrasound. Pediatr Radiol 22:410, 1992.

191. Zerres K, Schuler H, Gembruch U, et al: Chromosomal findings in fetuses with prenatally diagnosed cysts of the choroid plexus. Hum Genet 89:301, 1992.

192. Dobyns WB, Andermann E, Andermann F, et al: X-linked malformations of neuronal migration. Neurology 47:331, 1996.

193. Jaw TS, Sheu RS, Liu GC, et al: Magnetic resonance images of neuronal migration anomalies. Kaohsiung J Med Sci 14:504, 1998.

194. Barkovich AJ, Norman D: MR imaging of schizencephaly. AJR Am J Roentgenol 150:1391, 1988.

195. Denis D, Chateil JF, Brun M, et al: Schizencephaly: Clinical and imaging features in 30 infantile cases. Brain Dev 22:475, 2000.

196. Packard AM, Miller VS, Delgado MR: Schizencephaly: Correlations of clinical and radiologic features. Neurology 48:1427, 1997.

197. Komarniski CA, Cyr DR, Mack LA, et al: Prenatal diagnosis of schizencephaly. J Ultrasound Med 9:305, 1990.

198. Lituania M, Passamonti U, Cordone MS, et al: Schizencephaly: Prenatal diagnosis by computed sonography and magnetic resonance imaging. Prenat Diagn 9:649, 1989.

199. Dobyns WB, Truwit CL: Lissencephaly and other malformations of cortical development: 1995 update. Neuropediatrics 26:132, 1995.

200. Kuchelmeister K, Bergmann M, Gullotta F: Neuropathology of lissencephalies. Childs Nerv Syst 9:394, 1993.

201. Folgi A, Guerrini R, Morro F, et al: Intracellular levels of the LIS1 protein correlate with clinical and neuroradiological findings in patients with classical lissencephaly. Ann Neurol 45:154, 1999.

202. Gleeson JG, Lin PT, Flanagan LA, et al: Doublecortin is a microtubule-associated protein and is expressed widely by migrating neurons. Neuron 23:257, 1999.

203. Walsh CA: Genetics of neuronal migration in the cerebral cortex. MRDD Res Rev 6:34, 2000.

204. Sztriha L, Al-Gazali L, Varady E, et al: Microlissencephaly. Pediatr Neurol 18:362, 1998.

205. Mori K, Hashimoto T, Tayama M, et al: Biological rhythms in patients with lissencephaly (agyria-pachygyria). Brain Dev 15:205, 1993.

206. Allanson JE, Ledbetter DH, Dobyns WB: Classical lissencephaly syndromes: Does the face reflect the brain? J Med Genet 35:920, 1998.

207. Miny P, Holzgreve W, Horst J: Genetic factors in lissencephaly syndromes: A review. Childs Nerv Syst 9:413, 1993.

208. Saltzman DH, Krauss CM, Goldman JM, et al: Prenatal diagnosis of lissencephaly. Prenat Diagn 11:139, 1991.

209. Aida N, Tamagawa K, Takada K, et al: Brain MR in Fukuyama congenital muscular dystrophy. AJNR Am J Neuroradiol 17:605, 1996.

210. Attia-Sobol J, Encha-Razavi F, Hermier M, et al: Lissencephaly type III, stippled epiphyses and loose, thick skin: A new recessively inherited syndrome. Am J Med Genet 99:14, 2001.

211. Malm G, Grondahl EH, Lewensohn-Fuchs I: Congenital cytomegalovirus infection: A retrospective diagnosis in a child with pachygyria. Pediatr Neurol 22:407, 2000.

212. Straussberg R, Gross S, Amir J, et al: A new autosomal recessive syndrome of pachygyria. Clin Genet 50:498, 1996.

213. Byrd SE, Osborn RE, Bohan TP, et al: The CT and MR evaluation of migrational disorders of the brain. Part I. Lissencephaly and pachygyria. Pediatr Radiol 19:151, 1989.

214. Barth PG: Disorders of neuronal migration. Can J Neurol Sci 14:1, 1987.

215. Marques Dias MJ, Harmant-van Rijckevorsel G, Landrieu P, Lyon G: Prenatal cytomegalovirus disease and cerebral microgyria: Evidence for perfusion failure, not disturbance of histiogenesis, as the major cause of fatal cytomegalovirus encephalopathy. Neuropediatrics 15:18, 1984.

216. Toti P, DeFelice C, Palmeri ML, et al: Inflammatory pathogenesis of cortical polymicrogyria: An autopsy study. Pediatr Res 44:291, 1998.

217. Hirano S, Houdou S, Hasegawa M, et al: Clinicopathologic studies on leptomeningeal glioneuronal heterotopia in congenital anomalies. Pediatr Neurol 8:441, 1992.

218. Barkovich AJ, Kjos BO: Gray matter heterotopias: MR characteristics and correlation with developmental and neurological manifestations. Radiology 182:493, 1992.

219. Kinney HC, Karthigasan J, Borenshteyn NI, et al: Myelination in the developing human brain: Biochemical correlates. Neurochem Res 19:983, 1994.

220. Grodd W: Normal and abnormal patterns of myelin development of the fetal and infantile human brain using magnetic resonance imaging. Curr Opin Neurol Neurosurg 6:393, 1993.

221. Kolodny EH: Dysmyelinating and demyelinating conditions in infancy. Curr Opin Neurol Neurosurg 6:379, 1993.

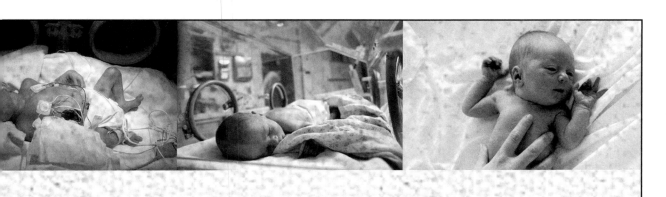

Cardiovascular Disease in the Neonate

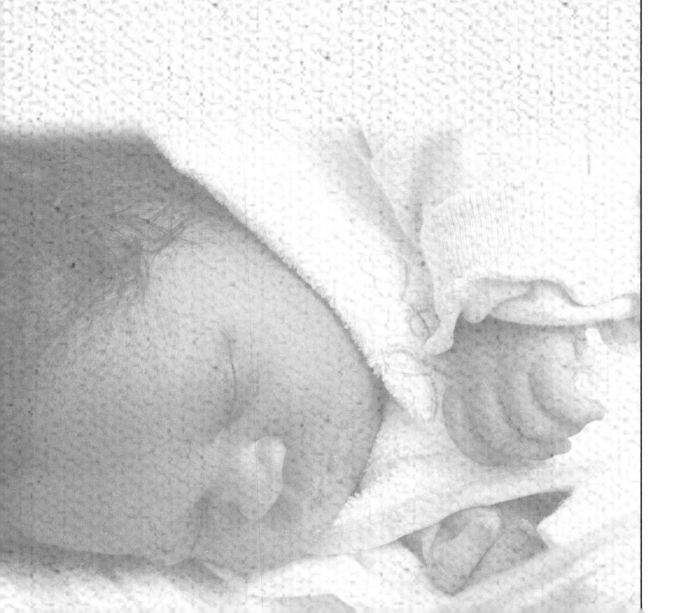

Ductus Arteriosus

Sandra E. Sullivan and Willa H. Drummond

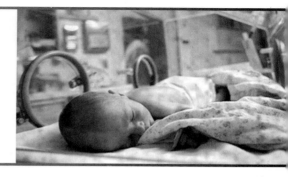

GENERAL OVERVIEW OF DUCTUS ARTERIOSUS

The **ductus arteriosus** is a fetal artery that connects the main pulmonary artery to the descending thoracic aorta (Fig. 58-1). During fetal life, blood pumped from the right ventricle detours past the constricted pulmonary circulation into the aorta via the ductus arteriosus to perfuse the lower body and the placenta, which provides for fetal respiratory gas exchange. The placenta makes **prostaglandin E1 (PGE1)**, which helps to keep the fetal ductus open.[1,2] The ductus is genetically programmed to close at about 40 weeks' postconceptional age (Fig. 58-2). Closure is triggered by a developmentally determined constrictor response to high levels of oxygen.[1,3] Anatomic closure usually occurs during the first 12 to 24 hours of life in term infants. Premature infants frequently have failure of ductus arteriosus closure after birth. When a ductus is persistently patent after birth, resolution of normal in utero pulmonary hypertension allows oxygenated blood to recirculate through the lungs. Blood recirculation overburdens the left heart, predisposing to respiratory difficulties, pulmonary edema, decreased diastolic blood flow to organs (brain, gut, myocardium, kidneys), and low tissue oxygen delivery. Sequelae of a persistently **patent ductus arteriosus (PDA)** in premature infants include increased risk for intraventricular hemorrhage, bronchopulmonary dysplasia, necrotizing enterocolitis, and retinopathy of prematurity. Prompt closure of a symptomatic PDA with indomethacin or surgery is recommended.[4-8] Conversely, infants with severe congenital heart disease may need to have the ductus kept open with an infusion of PGE_1, a potent dilator of the ductus arteriosus, to permit pulmonary or systemic blood flow.[9,10]

DEVELOPMENTAL ANATOMY

The ductus arteriosus originates from the sixth branchial arch during weeks 3 and 4 after conception. In early fetal life, the ductus arteriosus is structurally similar to the aorta and pulmonary artery, with an intact and clearly defined layer of medial smooth muscle and an internal elastic lamina (see Fig. 58-2). As gestation progresses, the ductus develops degenerative changes, with the disruption of the elastic lamina, cytolytic necrosis of the medial smooth muscle, and intimal proliferation into "cushions" that partially occlude the lumen. These degenerative changes facilitate lumen closure with moderate constriction. Although changes tend to progress with advancing gestational age, individual variability is marked so that no specific gestational age can be associated clearly with a specific anatomic change.[11]

In Utero Circulation

The fetal circulation is organized so that extremely desaturated blood from the brain and upper body that enters the right atrium from the superior vena cava is diverted preferentially through the tricuspid valve to the right ventricle, main pulmonary artery, and descending aorta (via the ductus arteriosus) (see Fig. 58-1). The fetal inferior vena cava carries oxygenated blood from the placenta to the right atrium via the umbilical vein and the ductus venosus (a fetal channel connecting the portal venous and systemic venous circulation). At the right atrial–inferior vena cava junction, a fetal "valve of the inferior vena cava" directs inferior vena cava blood flow through the fetal foramen ovale to the left atrium, left ventricle, and ascending aorta. Interatrial partitioning of fetal systemic venous blood return preferentially directs the most oxygenated blood (partial pressure of oxygen [PaO_2] 20 to 24 mm Hg, saturation 90% to 96%) to the developing brain, while diverting relatively unsaturated blood (PaO_2 16 to 18 mm Hg, saturation 75% to 80%) through the ductus arteriosus to the lower body and the placenta for oxygen and carbon dioxide exchange.

Flow direction through an open ductus arteriosus is determined by the relative blood pressure at the two ends of the ductus. During fetal life, the pulmonary circulation essentially is occluded by spherical endothelial cells and constricted arteriolar smooth muscle, creating high resistance to blood flow and high pulmonary artery pressure.[12]

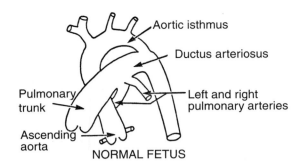

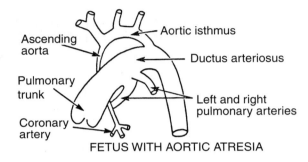

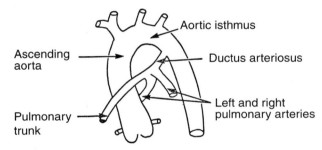

Figure 58–1. The relationships and sizes of the ductus arteriosus and of the aorta, pulmonary trunk, and pulmonary arteries in a normal fetus, a fetus with aortic atresia, and a fetus with pulmonary atresia. *(From Rudolph AM: Congenital Diseases of the Heart. Chicago, Year Book Medical Publishers, 1974, p 169.)*

In utero, fetal pulmonary arterial pressure is usually 2 to 5 mm Hg higher than fetal systemic blood pressure.

Transitional Circulation

After normal birth at term and the infant's first breath, multiple physiologic changes occur within seconds. Oxygen enters the alveoli, diffuses into the pulmonary capillary bed, relaxes pulmonary vascular smooth muscle, and triggers flattening or "remodeling" of pulmonary endothelial cells.[12] Pulmonary vascular resistance declines by half within 1 minute, whereas pulmonary venous oxygen tension increases threefold to fourfold. Oxygenated pulmonary venous blood enters the left ventricle and the aorta. Cord clamping abruptly removes the low-resistance placental vascular bed from the systemic circulation; this acts synergistically with local and adrenergic vasoconstrictor reflexes triggered by skin cooling to increase the systemic vascular resistance and blood pressure rapidly.

Blood flow through the ductus arteriosus reverses, now moving from the aorta into the pulmonary artery. Direction of ductus blood flow switches, and, transiently, oxygenated aortic blood can flood into the pulmonary circulation. In term infants, the ductus constricts in response to the elevated PaO_2, establishing two functionally separate circulations within minutes to hours. Complete anatomic closure of the ductus usually occurs by 2 to 4 days of age. If hypoxemia develops before complete closure, however, the ductus arteriosus can reopen.

In premature infants, the ductus arteriosus is developmentally not ready to close. Mechanisms that condition rapid closure in term infants (oxygen sensitivity, anatomic degenerative changes) are immature. Premature infants commonly have delayed closure of the ductus arteriosus, or a PDA. The more premature the infant, the higher is the incidence of symptomatic PDA. PDA occurs in 50% to 86% of infants weighing less than 1500 g at birth.[5,13-16]

DEVELOPMENTAL CHANGES IN DUCTAL CONTROL MECHANISMS

Maturing Oxygen Responsiveness

In term newborns, a sudden increase in PaO_2 of arterial blood is the most important signal for ductal closure. Concordant animal experiments in several species showed that the ability for ductus constriction in high oxygen states increases with advancing gestation.[1,3] In fetal lambs of 90 days' gestation (0.6 of gestation, approximates 24 weeks in humans), a small constrictor response to high levels of oxygen occurs. This constrictor response increases until term, when constrictor threshold occurs at normal postnatal PaO_2 values.[1,3]

Ductus Constriction by Prostaglandin Inhibitors

Prostaglandins profoundly influence tension development in isolated ductus arteriosus rings.[1,2] Animal experiments showed that maternal indomethacin administration could cause fetal ductus arteriosus constriction in utero.[17] This finding quickly led to treatment trials using aspirin or indomethacin to close a persistent PDA in premature infants, which initially were very successful. Soon it was discovered that the apparent discrepancies in success rates (30% to 100% closure in different treatment trials) could be explained by an association between responsiveness to therapy and postconceptional age of the infant at the time of treatment.[18] Younger infants (28 to 32 weeks), who were treated before 32 to 33 weeks' postconceptional age, had high rates of ductal closure. Infants of 33 to 36 weeks' gestation generally had a partial response, and infants older than 36 weeks' postconceptional age at treatment failed to respond. The ductus arteriosus matures biochemically and anatomically through late gestation. The biochemical maturation of prostaglandin responsiveness can be accelerated by giving exogenous corticosteroids to the mother before delivery.[19]

Light Sensitivity

The ductus arteriosus is quite light sensitive. This serendipitous discovery occurred in an experiment to study reactivity of fetal lamb ductus rings in a perfusion

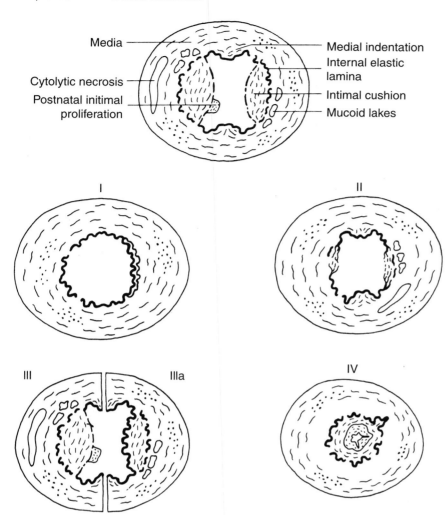

Figure 58–2. Maturation stages of fetal ductus arteriosus. **Top** and **III,** Ductus structure in normal term infant at birth. Note degenerative changes, including mucoid lakes and cytolytic necrosis. **I,** Human fetal ductus arteriosus at 4 to 5 months of gestation resembles a muscular artery with nearly intact internal elastic lamina and a thin layer of endothelial cells. **II,** Later in gestation, the ductus forms intimal thickenings and undergoes disintegration of internal elastic lamina. **IIIa,** Term infant with abnormal ductus arteriosus that does not close normally. Note subendothelial elastic lamina. **IV,** Permanently closed ductus arteriosus, which will shrink until only the ligament of the ductus arteriosus remains. *(From Gittenberger-de Groot AC, van Ertbruggen I, Moulaert AJ, Harinck E: The ductus arteriosus in the preterm infant: Histologic and clinical observations. J Pediatr 96:88, 1980.)*

bath. Sudden illumination of the preparation caused a profound relaxation. Ductal ring sensitivity to light decreased as the fetus matured.[20] A controlled clinical trial that light-shielded the anterior chest wall of small premature neonates (539 to 1500 g, 26 to 32 weeks' gestational age) found that a PDA developed in 60% of unshielded patients but in only 30% of infants protected from light.[21] This finding supports the observation by Barefield and colleagues[13] that phototherapy is associated with an increased risk of PDA. Premature neonates (501 to 999 g) who received phototherapy had an increased incidence of PDA compared with infants who did not receive phototherapy (76% versus 53%). The practice of chest shielding has not become widespread, perhaps because ready availability of effective treatment for a symptomatic PDA has made it unnecessary. Additionally, shielding may interfere with effective phototherapy, which is often necessary to control jaundice in very premature neonates.

Infection and inflammatory mediators may increase the risk of late ductal reopening and of closure failures. Gonzalez and colleagues[22] proposed that increased levels of prostaglandins and tumor necrosis factor–α in

infants with infection may explain the poor PDA outcome. They also found that the concurrence of PDA and infection potentiated their negative effects on the risk of bronchopulmonary dysplasia.

CLINICAL SYNDROME OF PATENT DUCTUS ARTERIOSUS

Pathophysiology

The consequences of a PDA in a premature infant depend on the flow volume of the **left-to-right shunt** (which depends on ductal size and the pulmonary vascular resistance relative to systemic vascular resistance), the infant's maturity, myocardial reserve, pulmonary parenchymal pathology, and associated conditions (anemia, sepsis, hypocalcemia, hypoglycemia, brain injury). Spontaneous closure is likely with advancing postconceptional age. Ultimately a PDA closes in most premature infants; however, timing of closure is currently unpredictable. This natural resolution of the problem with time confounds attempts to compare outcomes of various therapeutic modalities.[7,23]

Classic Presentation

A symptomatic PDA is most common in small premature infants. The younger the infant, the higher the risk of PDA: At 28 weeks of gestation, risk of a symptomatic PDA is 15% to 80%, and by 34 to 36 weeks of gestation, the risk decreases to 2% to 21%. Hyaline membrane disease frequently coexists with a PDA. Symptoms of a PDA usually occur on days 2 to 7. An unexplained metabolic or respiratory acidosis is often the first biochemical marker noted.

Clinical Findings

Table 58-1 outlines the findings most often associated with a significant PDA. The signs and symptoms of PDA vary among patients and within a given patient over time, ranging from asymptomatic to complete cardiovascular collapse. The variability in clinical symptoms, intercurrent pulmonary disease, and ventilator therapy often confuses clinical diagnostic attempts. Clinical symptoms may vary hour to hour. Symptoms relate to low effective cardiac output and to pulmonary edema in overcirculated, flooded lungs. Metabolic acidosis often develops because systemic ischemia triggers a metabolic switch to anaerobic glycolysis. This inefficient process produces relatively little metabolic energy and generates the end product, lactic acid, instead of carbon dioxide and water.

The most reliable physical finding for PDA is increased precordial activity,[24] although murmur is often present. Clinical grades of the murmur relate to the size of the left-to-right shunt (small, moderate, large). The largest PDAs usually have soft (grade I to II), long, low-frequency murmurs, best heard with the bell, or no murmur at all.[25] A diastolic murmur usually is not present in premature infants with a PDA. The machinery murmur classically found in older children with PDA is rarely heard in premature infants.

Left-to-right shunt and congestive heart failure cause an increase in pulmonary interstitial fluid. This extra fluid in the pulmonary vessels and interstitium decreases pulmonary compliance and triggers tachypnea, expiratory grunting, intercostal retractions, carbon dioxide retention, apnea, bradycardia, and ventilator dependency.[14,26]

Congestive heart failure stimulates neural and neurohormonal compensatory mechanisms, which are manifested clinically by tachycardia, gallop rhythm, hyperdynamic precordium, salt and water retention, edema, and hepatomegaly. The open ductus creates a systemic vascular "steal" distal to the aortic arch vessels.[27] Decreased lower body perfusion frequently is associated with abdominal distention, decreased urine output, decreased femoral pulses in the presence of an increased right brachial pulse, ileus, and necrotizing enterocolitis.[27-29] A generalized decrease in systemic perfusion may be reflected in development of a metabolic lactic acidosis and decreased cerebral perfusion.[30]

Sequelae

The profound systemic and pulmonary consequences of a large PDA contribute to prolonged ventilator dependency, longer hospitalization, increased costs, and development of many complications in the small premature infants who most frequently have failure of ductal closure.

Table 58–1. Clinical Assessment: Patent Ductus Arteriosus

System	Symptom	Physiologic Cause
Respiratory	Tachypnea	↑ Pulmonary blood flow
		↑ Interstitial fluid
	Expiratory grunting	↓ Compliance ("stiff lungs")
	Intercostal retractions	
	Carbon dioxide retention	↓ Ventilation
	Hypoxemia	Pulmonary edema
Cardiac	Tachycardia	↑ Left-to-right shunt
	Visible precordial lift	
	Bounding pulses	Large diastolic runoff
	Hypotension	Metabolic acidosis
	Hepatomegaly	Congestive heart failure
	Peripheral edema (rare)	
	Murmur	Turbulent flow through PDA
	No murmur (sick)	Laminar flow in large PDA
	No murmur (well)	No PDA
Genitourinary	Abdominal distention	
	Ileus	
	↓ Urine output	↓ Lower body blood flow
	↓ Femoral pulses with ↑ upper body pulses	
General	Lethargy, apnea, hypotonia, pallor, mottling	Systemic ischemia
	Failure to thrive	Caloric restriction (fluid restriction)
		Chronic intestinal ischemia

PDA, patent ductus arteriosus.

Complications found more commonly in association with PDA include pulmonary hemorrhage, pulmonary interstitial emphysema, long-term ventilator or oxygen dependency, apnea and bradycardia, intraventricular hemorrhage, necrotizing enterocolitis, and retinopathy of prematurity.[4,5,8,31,32] In infants with little prior lung disease, initial symptoms of a symptomatic PDA include onset of apnea and bradycardia or tachypnea, cessation of respiratory improvement, progressive cardiac enlargement and pulmonary edema (Fig. 58-3), unexplained metabolic acidosis, and development of a characteristic systolic murmur.

Diagnosis of Patent Ductus Arteriosus

In the context of a high-risk patient (i.e., a small premature infant), a high index of suspicion is warranted in any infant who is not doing well. Discovery of a characteristic murmur is helpful, but a significant proportion of the largest PDAs have no murmur at all.[25] For this reason, and to avoid closing the ductus with indomethacin in a premature infant who has congenital heart disease, noninvasive cardiac diagnostic tests are indicated. The electrocardiogram is "normal" in 80%, shows right ventricular hypertrophy in 17%, and shows biventricular hypertrophy in 6% and is usually not helpful.

Two-dimensional, color Doppler echocardiography has proved to be accurate in diagnosing PDAs in very premature infants.[24] This technique is especially useful in the infants whose ductus arteriosus is too large to generate a flow murmur. In these infants, the ductus arteriosus is often the same size as the aorta or the pulmonary artery. Color flow Doppler imaging can illustrate clearly retrograde flow from the ductus into the main pulmonary artery (Fig. 58-4). Diastolic Doppler flow analysis also has allowed clear demonstration of subnormal forward diastolic flow to various organs in infants with a widely patent ductus arteriosus.[28-30] Sometimes a large ductus arteriosus causes reversed aortic flow during diastole (especially from the brain).[30] By use of history and physical examination, chest x-ray, history of increased ventilator requirements, and echocardiogram, a hemodynamically significant PDA should be diagnosed accurately in nearly every case.

TREATMENT OF SYMPTOMATIC PATENT DUCTUS ARTERIOSUS

Medical Treatment

Most small premature infants do not tolerate a widely patent ductus arteriosus. Fetal hearts have a disproportionate volume of connective tissue relative to myocardium. Premature hearts are stiff and have poor contractility relative to the mature heart of a term newborn. As a PDA

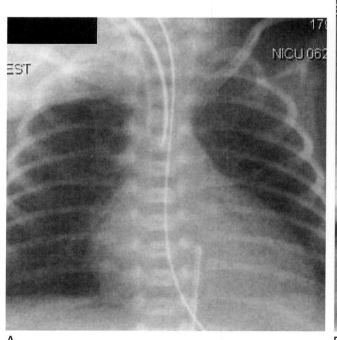
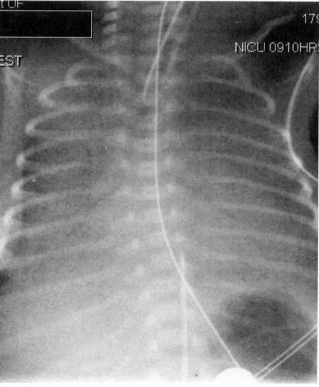

A   B

Figure 58–3. A, Chest radiograph of a 1-day-old premature infant with mild hyaline membrane disease on minimal ventilator support. **B,** Chest radiograph in same infant several days later after development of patent ductus arteriosus and respiratory deterioration requiring increased oxygen and higher ventilator pressures to stabilize. Note hazy heart borders and lung fields consistent with pulmonary edema.

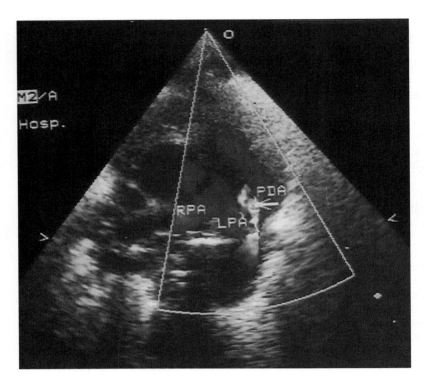

Figure 58–4. Doppler image shows patent ductus arteriosus (PDA). Turbulent and reverse blood flow between the aorta and left pulmonary artery (LPA) through the PDA is shown as an intense flare (original in color) at the arrow. RPA, right pulmonary artery.

floods the left atrium and left ventricle, the heart often does not dilate well, and pulmonary venous pressure increases. The result is pulmonary interstitial and alveolar edema (see Fig. 58-3). Some infants collapse acutely with tachycardia, pallor, worsening blood gases, lactic acidosis, decreased urine output, lethargy, and distended abdomen. Sometimes, these infants have no murmur and collapsed pulses; the chest radiograph can look like Figure 58-3B. Infants who become critically symptomatic, however, often have associated lung disease so that new or worsening pulmonary edema is more difficult to assess than when an infant has preexisting clear lungs. While waiting for diagnostic confirmation and pharmacy delivery of indomethacin, the temporary treatments outlined in Table 58-2 often relieve symptoms and improve tissue perfusion until the indomethacin has time to take effect (3 to 12 hours).

Respiratory support measures to palliate the pulmonary edema may include starting ventilator therapy for apnea and bradycardia or increasing continuous positive airway pressure or inspiratory time in an already ventilator-dependent infant. Both approaches increase mean airway pressure, which helps "tamponade" high pulmonary blood flow and clear edema fluid from the alveoli. Complications of added ventilator support include (1) increased risk of chronic lung disease caused by increased fractional inspired oxygen concentration (FIO_2), increased mean airway pressure, and prolonged time on mechanical ventilation; (2) increased risk of ventilator-related accidents (e.g., plugged or dislodged tubes, pneumothorax, nosocomial pneumonia); (3) need for prolonged arterial catheterization, which can be mitigated by use of oxygen saturation monitors; and (4) need for more frequent arterial blood gas

sampling, which increases the need for transfusions to replace iatrogenic blood loss.

Some neonatologists attempt to increase oxygen delivery to ductus tissue (to aid closure) and to other tissues that may be affected by ductal steal by increasing inspired oxygen or circulating red blood cell mass. Increasing FIO_2 carries an increased risk of retinopathy of prematurity, oxygen toxicity, and chronic lung disease. Maintaining a high hematocrit (>35%) adds to the ability of blood to carry adequate oxygen to the tissues. In sick premature infants, maintaining a high hematocrit usually requires repeated red blood cell transfusions. Increased risk of iatrogenic acquisition of viral disease (e.g., cytomegalovirus, Epstein-Barr virus, hepatitis, human immunodeficiency virus) from multiple transfusions has become a major concern. Use of recombinant erythropoietin may decrease the need for repeated transfusions in treating anemia of prematurity, although the clinical effect is modest.[33,34]

Control of congestive heart failure often includes fluid restriction to just above "insensible" water loss. Concomitant caloric restriction is unavoidable. The decision to use fluid restriction to control PDA-related congestive heart failure must be weighed against the detrimental effects of prolonged undernutrition in very small premature infants.

Diuretic treatment often is attempted. Complications of diuretic treatment include hyponatremia, hypokalemia, dehydration, and hypochloremic alkalosis. Diuretics compete for albumin binding sites, are ototoxic, and may cause renal calculi with prolonged use. Furosemide (Lasix) may stimulate renal PGE_1 release and potentiate ductal patency. Currently, there is not enough evidence to support the addition of furosemide to indomethacin

Table 58–2.   Treatment of Symptomatic Patent Ductus Arteriosus

Treatment	Desired Result
↑ F_{IO_2}	↑ Tissue oxygen delivery Constricts ductus arteriosus May ↓ A and B episodes
↑ CPAP	↑ Alveolar volume ↓ Pulmonary blood flow by compressing capillary bed ↓ Edema, alveolar and interstitial
Transfusion	↑ Tissue oxygen delivery (may constrict ductus)
Fluid restriction	↓ Intravascular volume
Diuretics	↓ Intravascular volume (furosemide may release renal PGE)
Digoxin	Constricts pulmonary circulation (↓ left-to-right shunt)
(not recommended)	Inotrope (questionable in premature infants with high output)
Indomethacin	Constricts ductus arteriosus
Dose scheme 1[40]	<30 wk GA, <1 wk old: 0.2 mg/kg/dose q12h × 3 doses (maximum total dose 0.6 mg/kg/24 hr)
Dose scheme 2[19]	< 48 hr old: 0.2 mg/kg, 0.1 mg/kg, 0.1 mg/kg q12h 2-7 days old: 0.2 mg/kg q12h × 3 doses > 8 days old: 0.25 mg/kg q12h × 3 doses
Dose scheme 3[23]	Scheme 1 or 2 above + 0.2 mg/kg/day × 5 days
Dose scheme 4[42]	0.1 mg/kg/day × 6 days (no loading dose)
Surgery	Permanently ligates ductus

CPAP, continuous positive airway pressure; F_{IO_2}, fraction of inspired oxygen; GA, gestational age; PGE, prostaglandin E.

for the treatment of a symptomatic PDA in premature neonates. Additionally, this combination seems to be contraindicated in the presence of dehydration.[35,36]

Digoxin use for congestive heart failure can be quite toxic in premature infants. Practical considerations make digoxin administration to tiny infants difficult because the appropriate digoxin dose to premature infants is of such a small volume that measurement mistakes occur. Inadvertent infusion of the syringe-tip dead space volume may double or triple the intended dose. Dosing errors are potentially lethal. Digoxin also may be ineffective in ameliorating symptoms because the cardiac myocardium is contracting as well as is developmentally possible. Premature infants are dependent on increased heart rate to maintain cardiac output because the premature heart dilates suboptimally to accommodate an added volume load. Digoxin usually slows heart rate by slowing cardiac conduction time. Digoxin half-life is 3 to 4 days in premature infants versus 24 to 36 hours in children and adults, and its clearance in sick premature infants is erratic. Incidence of recognized digoxin toxicity in premature infants (arrhythmias, bradycardia, and death) has been about 30%.

Initial attempts to close the ductus by using indomethacin, a prostaglandin synthetase inhibitor, had reported success rates of 19% to nearly 100% permanent closure.[18] Ductus closure by indomethacin has an inverse relationship to postconceptional age. Infants more than 36 weeks' postconceptional age who have a persistent PDA have a high rate of indomethacin failure. One collaborative treatment trial showed that indomethacin doubled the rate of ductus closure.[7] At 48 hours after treatment, 79% of the infants given indomethacin no longer met criteria for a symptomatic PDA compared with 28% of placebo control infants. The reopening rate among the infants given indomethacin was 26%, but most closed without the need for surgery.[7]

Prophylactic indomethacin given to all premature infants weighing less than 1000 g has shown no clear advantage over promptly treating such infants when they first develop a murmur, before they develop circulatory decompensation. In addition, the trial by Schmidt and colleagues[16] concluded that prophylaxis with indomethacin does not improve survival without neurosensory impairment at 18 months, although it does reduce the frequency of PDA and severe periventricular and intraventricular hemorrhage. Schmidt and colleagues[16] estimated that approximately 20 infants would need to receive indomethacin prophylaxis to avert one surgical ductal ligation. Prophylaxis may be beneficial in centers where the incidence of severe intraventricular hemorrhage is high or where there is a frequent need for surgical ductal ligation. In most centers, waiting for early signs of ductus patency may avoid risking complications of indomethacin unnecessarily in infants who will never need treatment, without sacrificing the protective effects (decreased intraventricular hemorrhage, bronchopulmonary dysplasia, and need for surgery) attained by early closure of a symptomatic PDA.[37]

Although the most widespread current treatment practice is to close a symptomatic PDA as soon as it is detected, considerable difficulty exists in choosing a correct dose and dosing schedule for infants of varying gestational and postnatal ages who have associated multisystem illnesses.

Attempts to link indomethacin blood levels to a therapeutic response have shown extremely high individual variability.[38,39] This variability relates partly to a twofold to threefold difference in patient variation in peak levels attained from a single bolus dose and partly to rapid changes in drug clearance with advancing postnatal age.[39] On day 1, indomethacin half-life can be 70 hours, which declines to a half-life of about 20 hours by age 8 to 10 days. Female neonates have more rapid plasma clearance.[39] A decade of studies regarding dosing, timing, and patient selection for indomethacin therapy has led to use of several dosing patterns (see Table 58-2). The most common approaches are based on an average dose for 1 day (schemes 1 and 2) or a dose aimed to keep indomethacin blood levels high for 1 week to decrease reopening (schemes 3 and 4). Continuous infusions have been shown to minimize the cerebral and mesenteric vasoconstrictive effects compared with rapid bolus administration of indomethacin.[40,41]

Extending the indomethacin treatment period to about 1 week with a daily or every-other-day maintenance dose has been reported to decrease recurrences.[42,43] Indications for indomethacin treatment vary from center to center. In the past, indomethacin usually was used after an infant failed to respond to "conventional" medical management, meaning fluid restriction and sometimes digoxin use. Now, early pharmacologic attempts at definitive closure with indomethacin (or ibuprofen in Europe) have become the most common clinical practice.

Contraindications to indomethacin treatment include severe hyperbilirubinemia (because indomethacin displaces bilirubin from albumin); severe renal dysfunction that is manifested by preexisting high blood urea nitrogen, high creatinine, and decreased urine output; evidence of necrotizing enterocolitis; and preexisting bleeding tendency.[7] Overt infection is not a contraindication to treatment.

In Europe, ibuprofen is the prostaglandin inhibitor of choice for PDA closure. An intravenous form is not currently available in the United States, however. One study by Dani and colleagues[6] from Italy evaluated prophylaxis versus treatment of PDA with intravenous ibuprofen lysine, 10 mg/kg, followed by 5 mg/kg at 24 and 48 hours from the initial dose. They reported that prophylactic ibuprofen reduced PDA occurrence compared with rescue treatment with ibuprofen, although both were effective in closing the PDA without significant adverse effects. In comparison studies in which indomethacin, 0.2 mg/kg, or ibuprofen, 10 mg/kg, was infused over 15 minutes, renal and mesenteric blood flow velocities were reduced significantly by indomethacin but not by ibuprofen.[44] Mosca and colleagues[45] showed that ibuprofen does not reduce cerebral perfusion or oxygen availability compared with indomethacin. In Belgium, Van Overmeire and associates[46] found that indomethacin and ibuprofen were equally efficacious for treatment of PDA, but ibuprofen was significantly less likely to induce oliguria.

Surgical Treatment

Early surgical closure (by age 10 days) has been advocated. Reported surgical mortality varies from 0% to 11%; surgical morbidity ranges from 5% to 44% at different centers.[4,31,32] Most of the early surgical series reported outcomes for infants operated after protracted and complicated courses. In these series, late mortality due to bronchopulmonary dysplasia and morbidity were not altered significantly by surgical ligation. Before the use of indomethacin, a significantly higher incidence of pulmonary complications, permanent retinopathy of prematurity, necrotizing enterocolitis, digitalis intoxication, prolonged intubation, and high hospital bills was reported in medically managed infants weighing less than 1500 g than in a surgical ligation cohort.[5]

A prospective controlled trial of early surgical ligation in infants weighing less than 1000 g showed that ligation does eliminate congestive heart failure.[4] Proof of surgical efficacy in increasing long-term survival and preventing morbidity (intraventricular hemorrhage, bronchopulmonary dysplasia, retinopathy) associated with prematurity was not established, however. Necrotizing enterocolitis was four times more common in the control group than in the surgery group. Infants in the control group who developed a symptomatic PDA also had a late surgical ligation, possibly confounding the outcome variables.[4]

More recent surgical results reported from multiple centers are excellent, with far less than 1% mortality and minimal morbidity in centers where appropriate surgical and anesthetic expertise and pediatric cardiology and neonatology consultation are available. In regard to symptomatic PDA, it has been suggested that surgical ligation should be regarded as first-line therapy for very small premature infants at high risk of medical failure or for infants in whom indomethacin is contraindicated.[47]

Complications of Treatment

The primary treatment complication of indomethacin encountered in the collaborative indomethacin treatment trial was non–life-threatening bleeding involving noncerebral sites.[7] Placebo control infants had a significantly higher risk of pneumothorax and retinopathy of prematurity.[7] Other complications of indomethacin were decreased urine flow, rising blood urea nitrogen and creatinine, and an increased risk of necrotizing enterocolitis. Apparently the increased risk of necrotizing enterocolitis from the indomethacin was counterbalanced by the lowered risk of necrotizing enterocolitis from closing the PDA.[4]

The most frequent complication of indomethacin therapy, transient renal dysfunction that results in salt and water retention, weight gain, and dilutional hyponatremia, occurs in more than half of treated premature infants. Decreased urine output occurs because indomethacin inhibits intrarenal PGE_1 production. Intrarenal PGE_1 is important in local maintenance of renal blood flow. Indomethacin-induced oliguria in premature infants can be treated with exogenous low-dose dopamine, a renal vasodilator,[48] or furosemide (in well-hydrated infants).[49] Dopamine acts as a vasodilator by a prostaglandin-independent mechanism. Dopamine increases renal blood flow and urine output at **very low doses** (dose range 1 to 2.5 µg/kg/min) and reverses the sodium and osmolar clearance problems that develop transiently during indomethacin treatment.[50] Dopamine seems to have no effect on the ductus arteriosus. Renal function often can be restored by a long-term infusion of low-dose dopamine, and the indomethacin acts to keep the ductus closed. Alternatively, furosemide (1 mg/kg intravenously) given simultaneously with the indomethacin may attenuate transiently some of the urine flow effects without changing serum electrolytes or altering ductal closure rate.[49] As previously discussed, use of furosemide in premature neonates with dehydration is contraindicated, however.[35,36] Because furosemide replaces bilirubin from albumin, as does indomethacin, the use of both in a jaundiced infant may be unwise. Abrupt changes in drug disposition can occur after ductus closure, which may affect indomethacin, aminoglycosides, and digoxin; blood levels of the latter drugs should be monitored.[51]

Surgical ligation is associated with a low risk of complications. Infrequent complications include pneumothorax, wound bleeding or infection, great vessel damage, and chylothorax. Surgical ligation had no additional morbidity over indomethacin alone in one study.[47]

MANIPULATION OF DUCTUS ARTERIOSUS WITH PROSTAGLANDIN E₁

The normal course of perinatal events transforms the fetus from an organism that needs only a two-chambered heart and one great vessel to a newborn, who must have four heart chambers, two great vessels, and lungs in only a few seconds. In utero the fetus has two pulmonary bypass channels: the foramen ovale and the ductus arteriosus. Because of these pulmonary bypass channels, the fetus can develop and grow normally with only two cardiac chambers and one great vessel.

Normal perinatal events are altered when infants with severe congenital cardiac disease are born. When any infant is born, the lungs must be perfused, and pulmonary venous return must reach systemic circulation in sufficient volume to permit survival. Infants born with severe congenital heart disease can become symptomatic within minutes or hours of birth. An infant with a right heart obstructive lesion may become profoundly hypoxemic when the ductus arteriosus closes. If a left heart obstruction prevents adequate systemic perfusion, sudden development of low-output shock occurs when the ductus arteriosus closes. In some congenital heart defects, such as pulmonary atresia or aortic atresia, survival is usually not possible unless the ductus remains widely patent. In these pathologic situations, it is crucial to maintain ductal patency. In other defects, such as transposition of the great vessels or severe coarctation of the aorta, continued ductal patency prevents secondary hypoxic-ischemic damage to vital organs.

Ductus Dilation by Prostaglandin E₁

Infusing PGE₁ at a dose of 0.05 to 0.1 µg/kg/min to maintain ductal patency in term infants with congenital heart disease is a rapid pharmacologic palliation procedure. The best results occur in infants who are symptomatic because of right-sided or left-sided obstructive lesions. Historically, rings of ductal tissue, contracted by either indomethacin or oxygen, were found to relax when PGE₂

was added to the tissue perfusion fluid.[2] E-series prostaglandins also dilated the ductus arteriosus in vivo in animals.[17] Clinical trials quickly confirmed improvement in systemic oxygenation after PGE₁ infusion in human neonates with cyanotic congenital heart disease.[10,52] Further studies confirmed the efficacy of PGE₁ for palliation of nearly all forms of congenital heart disease that cause life-threatening hypoxemia or low systemic blood flow in neonates. A commercial preparation of PGE₁ (Prostin VR-1 Pediatric; Upjohn Company, Kalamazoo, MI) was approved by the U.S. Food and Drug Administration and released for general use in neonates in December 1981, approximately 9 years after the laboratory discovery of prostaglandin's role in regulating ductal patency. Use of PGE₁ has improved drastically the mortality and morbidity statistics for most forms of congenital heart disease. Prostaglandin saves organs and tissues from ischemic injury while a specific anatomic diagnosis is made and surgery is planned and implemented.

Right-Sided Obstructive Lesions

Generally right-sided abnormalities (Table 58-3) are associated with decreased pulmonary perfusion. Clinical symptoms include intense cyanosis that is unresponsive to increased inspired F_{IO_2}. The chest radiograph shows a small or normal-sized heart with decreased pulmonary vascularity. Infusion of prostaglandin by any peripheral venous route at a dose of 0.05 to 0.1 µg/kg/min usually results in a prompt increase of Pao_2. PGE₁ palliation can keep the ductus open and stabilize the infant for transport to a cardiac center for definitive diagnosis and surgery.

Left-Sided Obstructive Lesions

In the presence of left heart obstruction, systemic perfusion occurs primarily via the ductus arteriosus (see Table 58-3). When the ductus closes, blood flow distal to the level of obstruction decreases. Simultaneously with acute obstruction of the pulmonary venous blood return to the left heart, the right heart output floods the lungs, causing

Table 58–3. Congenital Heart Lesions That Can Be Palliated with Prostaglandin E₁

Pulmonary blood flow is ductus dependent
  Cyanosis
  Right ventricular obstruction
    Pulmonary atresia (with or without ventricular septal defect)
    Severe pulmonic stenosis
    Tricuspid atresia
Systemic blood flow is ductus dependent
  Pale and/or gray
  Left ventricular obstruction
    Interrupted aortic arch
    Critical coarctation of the aorta
    Hypoplastic left heart (aortic or mitral atresia)
Inadequate mixing
  Transposition of the great vessels

rapid development of pulmonary edema. An infant with left heart obstruction, who frequently appears healthy before ductal closure, typically develops rapid onset of grayish pallor, severe tachypnea and respiratory distress, low blood pressure, absent pulses, marked hepatomegaly, and renal shutdown. Reopening the ductus with prostaglandin infusion rapidly reverses the symptoms of cardiovascular collapse, permitting transport, complete diagnosis, and surgical intervention, if appropriate.

Transposition of the Great Arteries

When the great vessels are reversed, two parallel pumps exist, each pumping a closed circuit. Oxygenation, and ultimately survival, depends on mixing of blood between the two circuits. Clinical symptoms are usually those of severe systemic cyanosis, normal or increased pulmonary vascularity on chest radiograph, and mild-to-moderate cardiac enlargement. In simple transposition of the great arteries, mixing occurs across the foramen ovale. If the ductus arteriosus is patent, additional mixing occurs. Cyanotic infants with transposition of the great arteries often improve when prostaglandin is infused.[10] The improvement probably is caused by increased ductal mixing and by moderate lowering of pulmonary vascular resistance, a side effect of PGE_1.[53] Maintenance of ductal patency and pulmonary blood flow with PGE_1 helps facilitate safe transport to a catheterization facility.

Palliation by a balloon atrial septostomy usually is effective in increasing intracardiac mixing sufficiently to permit adequate systemic oxygenation. Occasionally, some infants with transposition fail to improve after balloon septostomy. Such failure is thought to be due to inadequate atrial mixing secondary to elevated pulmonary vascular resistance. Usually prostaglandin therapy after balloon atrial septostomy in infants with transposition can be decreased gradually late in the first week with stable systemic oxygenation. This improvement presumably relates to the normal remodeling of fetal endothelial and smooth muscle cells in pulmonary arterioles that occurs rapidly during the first week of life.[12]

Diagnosis of the specific cardiac lesion is not essential before use of PGE_1. If the primary care physician is reasonably certain that a life-threatening congenital heart defect is present, there is little risk to beginning treatment with PGE_1. Only in the case of obstructed pulmonary venous return (e.g., total anomalous pulmonary venous return to the inferior vena cava) has it been suggested that PGE_1 may be contraindicated, and even this suggestion has not been well documented. Every facility in which infants are delivered should have PGE_1 continuously available for emergency use. Initial PGE_1 dose is 0.1 µg/kg/min, which usually can be lowered after several hours to 0.05 µg/kg/min to lessen side effects. In a study from India, where PGE_1 has been available only since 1995, investigators decreased the maintenance dose to 0.005 to 0.01 µg/kg/min with good response.[54]

Complications of Prostaglandin E₁ Therapy

Nearly 500 infants in several clinical centers were studied in clinical trials.[16] Side effects, listed in Table 58-4, included moderate fever (38°C ± 0.5°C), apnea, hypotension,

Table 58–4. Side Effects of Prostaglandin E₁ by Birth Weight ($n = 492$)

Side Effects	Preterm <2 kg (%)	Term >2 kg (%)
Cardiovascular (hypotension, vasodilation, bradycardia)	37	17
Central nervous system (fever, tremors, seizures)	16	16
Respiratory (apnea)	42	10
Metabolic	5	2
Infectious	11	2
Gastrointestinal (diarrhea)	11	3
Hematologic	5	2
Renal	0	2

bradycardia, regional vasodilation (rash), tremors, and focal seizures. Hypotension, bradycardia, and apnea were more frequent in preterm infants, particularly if the patient weighed less than 2 kg. When using PGE_1, the physician should be prepared to treat apnea with intubation and ventilation. Elective intubation before transport is suggested when transporting an infant within several hours of initiating PGE_1. Hypotension may require treatment with volume expansion, pressors, or lowering of PGE_1 dose.

A few long-term complications of PGE_1 maintenance have been noted in infants with ductal dependent congenital heart disease or newborn transplant candidates who needed to be treated with PGE_1 palliation for many weeks before surgery. Cortical hyperostosis, with symmetrical exuberant periosteal calcifications of clavicles, scapula, ribs, and long bones, usually occurs after 4 to 6 weeks of PGE_1 infusion but has been identified after only 2 weeks of PGE_1. Some infants exhibit irritability thought to be due to bone pain associated with the hyperostosis. The periosteal calcifications resolve within 1 year after PGE_1 is stopped, and no long-term bone growth sequelae have been documented.[55]

Mucosal hyperplasia of the gastric antrum has been associated with prolonged PGE_1 infusion. Infants present with a pyloric stenosis–like picture including vomiting, dehydration, and hypokalemic metabolic alkalosis. This entity can be differentiated from hypertrophic pyloric stenosis by experienced ultrasonographers. The antral hyperplasia resolves within 6 months after PGE_1 is stopped.[56,57]

Exogenously infused PGE_1 also has been associated with renal sodium, potassium, and chloride wasting, creating metabolic alkalosis and hyponatremia in the infant.[58] Added electrolyte supplements (sodium chloride and potassium chloride) sometimes are necessary to correct the serum electrolyte abnormalities.

Infants on long-term PGE_1 therapy need to be maintained on intravenous therapy. Oral prostaglandin is not recommended because PGE_1 has a short half-life (<1 hour), requiring every 1- or 2-hour dosing intervals. Oral PGE_2 administration usually is accompanied by severe diarrhea. Even intravenous PGE_1 is associated with loose stools, although this is usually a minor problem during intravenous therapy. Central lines commonly are needed for prolonged stable intravenous access, creating an increased risk of catheter-related complications, such as nosocomial infection and thrombosis.

SUMMARY

A PDA can be life-threatening or lifesaving. Problematic PDAs typically are found in small preterm neonates, and symptoms usually appear on days 2 to 7. The most reliable clinical finding is increased precordial activity, although a murmur is commonly present. Congestive heart failure frequently ensues. Color Doppler echocardiography is an accurate diagnostic tool. The consequences of a PDA contribute to prolonged ventilator dependency, bronchopulmonary dysplasia, longer hospitalization, and increased health care costs. Current medical management includes attempt at closure of the PDA with indomethacin (0.2 mg/kg initially; subsequent doses vary), increased respiratory support, increased oxygen delivery, and preservation of renal function with low-dose dopamine (1 to 2.5 μg/kg/min) or furosemide (with caution). Ibuprofen (10 mg/kg initially, followed by 5 mg/kg/day) may replace indomethacin when an intravenous formulation becomes available in the United States because ibuprofen has fewer cerebral, mesenteric, and renal vasoconstrictive side effects. Surgical ligation of the PDA is safe and effective and should be considered for infants in whom indomethacin therapy has failed or is contraindicated.

Maintaining ductal patency in a neonate with ductal-dependent congenital heart disease may be lifesaving. There is little risk to beginning PGE_1 infusion (0.1 μg/kg/min initially, may decrease to 0.05 μg/kg/min) before the exact diagnosis is made. PGE_1 infusion maintains essential ductal patency and pulmonary or systemic blood flow to transport infants to a cardiac center for definitive evaluation and treatment.

REFERENCES

1. Clyman RI, Mauray F, Rudolph AM, Heymann MA: Age-dependent sensitivity of the lamb ductus arteriosus to indomethacin and prostaglandins. J Pediatr 96:94, 1980.
2. Coceani F, Olley PM: The response of the ductus arteriosus to prostaglandins. Can J Physiol Pharmacol 51:220, 1973.
3. McMurphy DM, Heymann MA, Rudolph AM, Melmon KL: Developmental changes in constriction of the ductus arteriosus: Responses to oxygen and vasoactive agents in the isolated ductus arteriosus of the fetal lamb. Pediatr Res 6:231, 1972.
4. Cassady G, Crouse DT, Kirklin JW, et al: A randomized, controlled trial of very early prophylactic ligation of the ductus arteriosus in babies who weighed 1000 g or less at birth. N Engl J Med 320:1511, 1989.
5. Cotton RB, Stahlman MT, Kovar I, Catterton WZ: Medical management of small preterm infants with symptomatic patent ductus arteriosus. J Pediatr 92:467, 1978.
6. Dani C, Bertini G, Reali MF, et al: Prophylaxis of patent ductus arteriosus with ibuprofen in preterm infants. Acta Paediatr 89:1369, 2000.
7. Gersony WM, Peckham GJ, Ellison RC, et al: Effects of indomethacin in premature infants with patent ductus arteriosus: Results of a national collaborative study. J Pediatr 102:895, 1983.
8. Mahony L, Carnero V, Brett C, et al: Prophylactic indomethacin therapy for patent ductus arteriosus in very-low-birth-weight infants. N Engl J Med 306:506, 1982.
9. Benson LN, Olley PM, Patel RG, et al: Role of prostaglandin E₁ infusion in the management of transposition of the great arteries. Am J Cardiol 44:691, 1979.
10. Noah ML: Use of prostaglandin E₁ for maintaining the patency of the ductus arteriosus. Adv Prostaglandin Thromboxane Res 4:355, 1978.
11. Gittenberger-de Groot AC, van Ertbruggen I, Moulaert AJ, Harinck E: The ductus arteriosus in the preterm infant: Histologic and clinical observations. J Pediatr 96:88, 1980.
12. Haworth SG: Pulmonary vascular remodeling in neonatal pulmonary hypertension: State of the art. Chest 93(3 suppl): 133S, 1988.
13. Barefield ES, Dwyer MD, Cassady G: Association of patent ductus arteriosus and phototherapy in infants weighing less than 1000 grams. J Perinatol 13:376, 1993.
14. Cotton RB: The relationship of symptomatic patent ductus arteriosus to respiratory distress in premature newborn infants. Clin Perinatol 14:621, 1987.
15. Ment LR, Oh W, Ehrenkranz RA, et al: Low-dose indomethacin and prevention of intraventricular hemorrhage: A multicenter randomized trial. Pediatrics 93:543, 1994.
16. Schmidt B, Davis P, Moddemann D, et al: Long-term effects of indomethacin prophylaxis in extremely-low-birth-weight infants. N Engl J Med 344:1966, 2001.
17. Sharpe GL, Thalme B, Larsson KS: Studies on closure of the ductus arteriosus: XI. Ductal closure in utero by a prostaglandin synthetase inhibitor. Prostaglandins 8:363, 1974.
18. McCarthy JS, Zies LG, Gelband H: Age-dependent closure of the patent ductus arteriosus by indomethacin. Pediatrics 62:706, 1978.
19. Clyman RI, Ballard PL, Sniderman S, et al: Prenatal administration of betamethasone for prevention of patent ductus arteriosus. J Pediatr 98:123, 1981.
20. Clyman RI, Rudolph AM: Patent ductus arteriosus: A new light on an old problem. Pediatr Res 12:92, 1978.
21. Rosenfeld W, Sadhev S, Brunot V, et al: Phototherapy effect on the incidence of patent ductus arteriosus in premature infants: Prevention with chest shielding. Pediatrics 78:10, 1986.
22. Gonzalez A, Sosenko IR, Chandar J, et al: Influence of infection on patent ductus arteriosus and chronic lung disease in premature infants weighing 1000 grams or less. J Pediatr 128:470, 1996.
23. Yanagi RM, Wilson A, Newfeld EA, et al: Indomethacin treatment for symptomatic patent ductus arteriosus: A double-blind control study. Pediatrics 67:647, 1981.
24. Roberson DA, Silverman NH: Color Doppler flow mapping of the patent ductus arteriosus in very low birthweight neonates: Echocardiographic and clinical findings. Pediatr Cardiol 15:219, 1994.
25. Hammerman C, Strates E, Valaitis S: The silent ductus: Its precursors and its aftermath. Pediatr Cardiol 7:121, 1986.
26. Gerhardt T, Bancalari E: Lung compliance in newborns with patent ductus arteriosus before and after surgical ligation. Biol Neonate 38:96, 1980.
27. Spach MS, Serwer GA, Anderson PA, et al: Pulsatile aortopulmonary pressure-flow dynamics of patent ductus arteriosus in patients with various hemodynamic states. Circulation 61:110, 1980.
28. Bomelburg T, Jorch G: Abnormal blood flow patterns in renal arteries of small preterm infants with patent ductus arteriosus detected by Doppler ultrasonography. Eur J Pediatr 148:660, 1989.

29. Wong SN, Lo RN, Hui PW: Abnormal renal and splanchnic arterial Doppler pattern in premature babies with symptomatic patent ductus arteriosus. J Ultrasound Med 9:125, 1990.

30. Perlman JM, Hill A, Volpe JJ: The effect of patent ductus arteriosus on flow velocity in the anterior cerebral arteries: Ductal steal in the premature newborn infant. J Pediatr 99:767, 1981.

31. Merritt TA, White CL, Jacob J, et al: Patent ductus arteriosus treated with ligation or indomethacin: A follow-up study. J Pediatr 95:588, 1979.

32. Mikhail M, Lee W, Toews W, et al: Surgical and medical experience with 734 premature infants with patent ductus arteriosus. J Thorac Cardiovasc Surg 83:349, 1982.

33. Donato H, Vain N, Rendo P, et al: Effect of early versus late administration of human recombinant erythropoietin on transfusion requirements in premature infants: Results of a randomized, placebo-controlled, multicenter trial. Pediatrics 105:1066, 2000.

34. Ohls RK, Ehrenkranz RA, Wright LL, et al: Effects of early erythropoietin therapy on the transfusion requirements of preterm infants below 1250 grams birth weight: A multicenter, randomized, controlled trial. Pediatrics 108:934, 2001.

35. Brion LP, Campbell DE: Furosemide for symptomatic patent ductus arteriosus in indomethacin-treated infants. Cochrane Database Syst Rev 2, 2000.

36. Brion LP, Campbell DE: Furosemide in indomethacin-treated infants—systematic review and meta-analysis. Pediatr Nephrol 13:212, 1999.

37. Clyman RI, Campbell D: Indomethacin therapy for patent ductus arteriosus: When is prophylaxis not prophylactic? J Pediatr 111:718, 1987.

38. Nestrud RM, Hill DE, Arrington RW, et al: Indomethacin treatment in patent ductus arteriosus: A double-blind study utilizing indomethacin plasma levels. Dev Pharmacol Ther 1:125, 1980.

39. Yaffe SJ, Friedman WF, Rogers D, et al: The disposition of indomethacin in preterm babies. J Pediatr 97:1001, 1980.

40. Hammerman C, Glaser J, Schimmel MS, et al: Continuous versus multiple rapid infusions of indomethacin: Effects on cerebral blood flow velocity. Pediatrics 95:244, 1995.

41. Hammerman C, Kaplan M: Comparative tolerability of pharmacological treatments for patent ductus arteriosus. Drug Saf 24:537, 2001.

42. Hammerman C, Aramburo MJ: Prolonged indomethacin therapy for the prevention of recurrences of patent ductus arteriosus. J Pediatr 117:771, 1990.

43. Rennie JM, Cooke RW: Prolonged low dose indomethacin for persistent ductus arteriosus of prematurity. Arch Dis Child 66(1 spec no):55, 1991.

44. Pezzati M, Vangi V, Biagiotti R, et al: Effects of indomethacin and ibuprofen on mesenteric and renal blood flow in preterm infants with patent ductus arteriosus. J Pediatr 135:733, 1999.

45. Mosca F, Bray M, Lattanzio M, et al: Comparative evaluation of the effects of indomethacin and ibuprofen on cerebral perfusion and oxygenation in preterm infants with patent ductus arteriosus. J Pediatr 131:549, 1997.

46. Van Overmeire B, Smets K, Lecoutere D, et al: A comparison of ibuprofen and indomethacin for closure of patent ductus arteriosus. N Engl J Med 343:674, 2000.

47. Perez CA, Bustorff-Silva JM, Villasenor E, et al: Surgical ligation of patent ductus arteriosus in very low birth weight infants: Is it safe? Am Surg 64:1007, 1998.

48. Seri I. Effect of dopamine on indomethacin-induced impairment of renal function in preterm neonates. J Pediatr 123:167, 1993.

49. Yeh TF, Wilks A, Singh J, et al: Furosemide prevents the renal side effects of indomethacin therapy in premature infants with patent ductus arteriosus. J Pediatr 101:433, 1982.

50. Seri I, Tulassay T, Kiszel J, Csomor S: The use of dopamine for the prevention of the renal side effects of indomethacin in premature infants with patent ductus arteriosus. Int J Pediatr Nephrol 5:209, 1984.

51. Gal P, Gilman JT: Drug disposition in neonates with patent ductus arteriosus. Ann Pharmacother 27:1383, 1993.

52. Starling MB, Neutze JM, Elliott RB: Effect of prostaglandins and some methyl derivatives on the ductus arteriosus. Adv Prostaglandin Thromboxane Res 4:335, 1978.

53. Tripp ME, Drummond WH, Heymann MA, Rudolph AM: Hemodynamic effects of pulmonary arterial infusion of vasodilators in newborn lambs. Pediatr Res 14:1311, 1980.

54. Saxena A, Sharma M, Kothari SS, et al: Prostaglandin E_1 in infants with congenital heart disease: Indian experience. Indian Pediatr 35:1063, 1998.

55. Rowley RF, Lawson JP: Case report 701: Prostaglandin E_1 (PGE$_1$) periostitis. Skeletal Radiol 20:617, 1991.

56. Babyn P, Peled N, Manson D, et al: Radiologic features of gastric outlet obstruction in infants after long-term prostaglandin administration. Pediatr Radiol 25:41, 1995.

57. Caballero S, Torre I, Arias B, et al: [Secondary effects of prostaglandin E_1 on the management of hypoplastic left heart syndrome while waiting for heart transplantation]. An Esp Pediatr 48:505, 1998.

58. Langhendries JP, Thiry V, Bodart E, et al: Exogenous prostaglandin administration and pseudo-Bartter syndrome. Eur J Pediatr 149:208, 1989.

CHAPTER 59

Fetal Echocardiography in the Detection and Management of Fetal Heart Disease

Richard M. Benoit and Joshua A. Copel

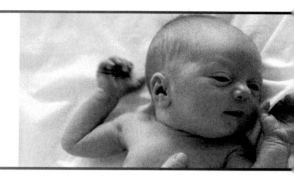

OVERVIEW

Knowledge of fetal and pediatric cardiology has expanded rapidly since the early work of Dawes.[1] Growth in understanding of fetal cardiac anatomy and physiology provided the groundwork for the development of the clinical diagnostic and therapeutic techniques currently used. Progressive advances in ultrasonography since the 1960s paved the way for **fetal echocardiography** to become a widely used method for antenatal diagnosis of cardiac anomalies.

Abnormalities of the heart continue to be the most common congenital abnormality, occurring in about 0.8% of newborns. Currently, most cases of **congenital heart disease (CHD)** occur in pregnancies considered to be low risk. Improved screening techniques and the continued improvement of ultrasound technology are needed to further the cause of prenatal detection.

Studying the impact of the prenatal diagnosis of CHD, with respect to outcome, quality of care, and cost, also is important. Prenatal diagnosis detects the more severe forms of CHD, making it difficult to show an improvement in overall outcome. The value of prenatal diagnosis reaches beyond outcome data, however. Early detection provides an opportunity to improve the quality of care for affected families and to expand therapeutic options. Thus, advancing the study of fetal and neonatal cardiology and fetal echocardiography remains an important goal. This chapter provides a comprehensive overview of fetal echocardiography, including its development as a diagnostic tool and its role in the detection and management of fetal heart disease.

EVOLUTION OF TECHNOLOGY FOR ASSESSMENT OF THE FETAL HEART AND CIRCULATORY SYSTEM

The possibility of prenatal diagnosis of CHD initially was described in 1980 by several authors.[2-4] The **four-chamber view** has been a part of published guidelines on fetal sonography since 1985.[5,6]

M-mode was the first ultrasound technique used to evaluate the fetal heart. In1964, Wang and Xiao[7] reported the use of M-mode ultrasound to evaluate cardiac motion over time and suggested its use in diagnosing pregnancy. Winsberg[8] first reported the use of M-mode ultrasound in English in 1972, also describing its use to evaluate fetal viability. Morin[9] recognized the potential of emerging real-time sector scanning in the 1970s as a technique to measure cardiac function.

The introduction of high-resolution, real-time equipment for **two-dimensional scanning** was a major breakthrough and continued to develop over two decades, beginning with early descriptions of a systematic approach to the two-dimensional examination of the fetal heart.[23] The advance of **Doppler ultrasound** followed, with the introduction of spectral and color-flow techniques and the subsequent development of power Doppler.

Doppler ultrasound, with the additions of spectral and color-flow techniques, enabled investigators to evaluate fetal flow physiology within the central and peripheral fetal circulation, which has become useful in clinical management. Maulik and colleagues[10] described the use of spectral analysis in their study of fetal hemodynamics in 1982. Doppler quantification of blood flow velocity soon followed.[11] Analyzing the impedance of vessels, obtaining flow velocity, and estimating perfusion became possible.[12]

Color-flow mapping technology was introduced shortly after continuous and pulsed-wave spectral Doppler. Copel and associates[13] described the assessment of normal and abnormal fetal hearts with color-flow Doppler mapping in 1986. Its clinical utility lies in the detection of abnormal flow and velocity, important in the diagnosis of problems such as valvular regurgitation and hypoplastic left heart. Newer power Doppler technology may indicate flow without directional information.[14]

Second-trimester and third-trimester studies were the focus of these early ultrasound reports. Subsequently, the development of transvaginal techniques led to reports of earlier detection of fetal cardiac anomalies in the 1990s.[15]

With **transvaginal ultrasound**, imaging of the fetal heart can be done by 14 to 16 weeks of gestation and assist in the early diagnosis of CHD. Transvaginal ultrasound probes use higher frequencies (6.5 to 9 MHz) and consequently offer higher resolution than abdominal ultrasound probes (3 to 7 MHz). Complex cardiac anomalies, such as lesions with chamber disproportion, and defects of significant size may be visualized early.[14] D'Amelio and coworkers[15] reported in 1991 that at 12 weeks of gestation, a four-chamber view could be seen in 90% of fetuses. They reported that for evaluation at 14 to 15 weeks of gestation, transvaginal techniques were best and that for evaluation at 15 to 18 weeks of gestation, transabdominal and transvaginal techniques were of equal value. After 18 weeks of gestation, transabdominal echocardiography was shown to be most advantageous.[15] Transvaginal ultrasound allows for earlier imaging, information gathering, and counseling opportunities. Abnormal early studies may provide the option for early assessment of fetal karyotype. The transvaginal approach is also of value in improving examination quality with maternal obesity or scarring from previous surgery.

Early transvaginal scanning of the heart is limited by the expected evolution of many forms of congenital anomalies and the small size of the heart when examined with higher resolution transducers. A normal transvaginal ultrasound scan should be followed by transabdominal screening later in gestation.

The current realization that early transvaginal scanning cannot be considered a replacement for the abdominal ultrasound scan in detecting congenital anomalies has been confirmed by several studies.[16-18] Yagel and colleagues[19] reported a retrospective review of 22,050 women revealing that early transvaginal scanning (13 to 16 weeks) detected 64% of congenital heart defects diagnosed antenatally. These early scans missed 17% of anomalies, which were shown later on midtrimester ultrasound. Yagel and colleagues[16] also reported on a prospective study of a group of 536 women at high risk for birth defects. They performed early transvaginal ultrasound (13 to 16 weeks of gestation) and midtrimester ultrasound (20 to 22 weeks of gestation). In these women, 8 of 46 cases of anomalies, including congenital heart defects, were detected on a midtrimester transabdominal scan, yet were not detected by earlier transvaginal ultrasound scan. Although the development of transvaginal scanning offers the possibility of early detection, genetic counseling, and option for pregnancy termination, it is important to offer confirmatory second-trimester examination.

The latest addition to techniques for the detection of fetal cardiac anomalies is measurement of the **nuchal translucency,** originally proposed for the early detection of aneuploidy. Increased nuchal thickness is associated with increased risk for aneuploidy and is a nonspecific marker for genetic syndromes and structural anomalies, including heart disease.[20]

The end of the 1990s also brought about the emergence of harmonic imaging and **three-dimensional ultrasound** techniques. Four-dimensional techniques eventually followed. Harmonic imaging provided more clarity in cardiac visualization, being particularly useful in obese patients and patients with advanced gestational age.[21] Three- and four-dimensional imaging continue to be areas

of active investigation. Demand for these techniques arose from the current inability to accurately characterize anatomic volumes with two-dimensional techniques. The use of three-dimensional ultrasound to assess fetal heart volume has been suggested to improve accuracy and reproducibility over two-dimensional techniques.[22]

Imaging of the great arteries and major veins is also challenging. In its favor, three-dimensional ultrasound techniques allow one to acquire a volume of data, which may be stored and later manipulated to produce images for evaluation. No matter the fetal orientation at the time of examination, the imaged heart may be rotated into a standard orientation and viewed in different planes. The volume of images also may be stored and transmitted via the Internet, allowing for evaluation in remote sites.[23]

Three-dimensional imaging is currently optimal between 20 and 30 weeks of gestation, although it may be useful at 38 weeks.[24] It has the potential to reduce scanning time, although its use remains limited because of difficulty in operating and editing images, the need for more storage space for data, and the cost. There also are technical difficulties of achieving gating to match the cardiac cycle, although newer real-time, three-dimensional techniques may circumvent this problem.

However promising three-dimensional imaging may be, more recent reports have indicated that current three-dimensional imaging technology cannot provide an examination equal to the quality of scanning obtained by available two-dimensional techniques.[25] The routine use of three-dimensional imaging in fetal echocardiography awaits further improvements in user friendliness and studies documenting benefit in diagnostic capabilities over current standards of care.

The same remains true for the more recent introduction of "4D" or **real-time, three-dimensional ultrasound.** The need for three-dimensional scanning to become real-time to advance its clinical utility has been the driving force in the development of 4D ultrasound, which acquires data as volume, rather than a series of planes that need to be reconstructed. A study by Sklansky and colleagues[26] showed that 70% of the basic cardiac structures could be visualized with 4D ultrasound and that abnormalities, including tricuspid atresia with hypoplastic right ventricle, also could be seen. Interest in 4D ultrasound is strong, particularly with the public. Similar to three-dimensional imaging, however, further work is needed before 4D ultrasound can be applied in routine screening.

Another active area of investigation for potential fetal diagnostic capability has been focused by the use of magnetic resonance imaging. Magnetic resonance imaging is useful in the evaluation of pediatric patients and has been used for the prenatal diagnosis of a variety of fetal anomalies. The challenge remaining is to enable accurate imaging of the moving fetal heart. This imaging requires cardiac gating to the fetal heart rate, which has not yet been accomplished. Another technique on the horizon that soon may aid in the detection and diagnosis of fetal cardiac disease is magnetocardiography, with its potential to record a fetal electrocardiogram and assist in the evaluation of arrhythmias.

SPECTRUM OF DIAGNOSTIC AND THERAPEUTIC CAPABILITIES CURRENTLY ATTRIBUTED TO TECHNIQUES IN FETAL ECHOCARDIOGRAPHY

Advances in technology have expanded greatly the ability to detect, manage, and treat fetal cardiac disease. With respect to the basic sciences, the advance of fetal echocardiography has been integral in increasing knowledge of fetal cardiovascular and placental physiology. Doppler ultrasound has allowed assessment of the fetal cardiovascular system in vivo, with the ability to make observations over time without disturbing function. This capability has had an impact in the diagnosis and treatment of fetal anemia, congestive heart failure, arrhythmia, growth restriction, placental pathology, and fetal anomalies affecting cardiovascular function.

Ultrasound also led to the development and growth of prenatal diagnosis and the development of fetal therapy. The accurate prenatal diagnosis of CHD has become possible, although imperfect. In utero diagnosis has provided the opportunity to improve the quality of care and to have an impact on outcome for parents and infants affected by CHD. Supportive and informative counseling and the potential for improvement in neonatal management are among the possible benefits of prenatal diagnosis. The detection of fetal cardiac disease also can improve the detection of aneuploidy.

Without diagnosis, there is no potential for therapy. Investigators remain interested in the prospect of intrauterine fetal intervention for fetal cardiac disease. Valvuloplasty has been applied to the human fetus by Kohl and colleagues,[27] using percutaneous ultrasound–guided techniques aimed at opening the stenosed fetal aortic valve before birth. Technical success was reported in 6 of 14 cases described so far, with only one long-term survivor. Kohl and colleagues[28] have continued to work on improving these techniques. Clinicians may one day successfully pursue early intervention for cardiac malformations, particularly malformations that involve stenosis, hypoplastic growth, or abnormal shunting.

Fetal echocardiography also has become integral in the diagnosis and management of fetal arrhythmia. Classification of fetal arrhythmias now can be done accurately, using M-mode, two-dimensional gray-scale imaging, and Doppler ultrasound. Therapy with transplacental antiarrhythmic agents can be initiated and monitored, along with assessment of fetal well-being. Fetal cardiac function can be evaluated with the estimation of cardiac output and the detection of hydrops or other evidence of heart failure. The potential remains for the development of other routes of fetal antiarrhythmic therapy, including intravascular catheters placed under ultrasound guidance, although this remains an uncertain approach.

Assessment of fetal congestive heart failure, or nonimmune hydrops fetalis, with the use of fetal echocardiography, also has grown to include the potential for improved diagnosis and therapy, depending on the etiology. Enhancing understanding of fetal cardiovascular physiology, fetal echocardiography also provides the opportunity for detecting fetal ductal constriction, such as may occur in response to maternal therapy for preterm labor with indomethacin. Detection offers the potential for therapeutic intervention and close monitoring.

In the management of diabetes in pregnancy, ultrasound assessment of the diabetic mother with fetal echocardiography is the standard of care, given the increased risk for congenital heart defects in this population. At the other end of the growth scale, current management of intrauterine growth restriction relies on the ability of Doppler ultrasound to detect changes in vascular flow resistance in fetal and maternal circulation. These changes allow for the early detection of fetal compromise, which is essential for management and holds promise for the application of therapeutic intervention. Perinatal morbidity and mortality may be reduced with close observation, corticosteroid therapy, bed rest, and indicated delivery. Cardiac and peripheral Doppler assessments also may predict outcome or show the level of compromise, which may be used to estimate fetal ability to tolerate labor induction.

The breadth of the current impact of fetal echocardiography is considerable. Considering the diverse epidemiologic factors that contribute to fetal cardiac disease and the lack of adequate prevention, the contribution of fetal echocardiography to perinatal diagnosis and therapy is likely to continue to expand.

EPIDEMIOLOGY OF CONGENITAL HEART DISEASE

Incidence of Congenital Heart Disease

Congenital abnormalities of the heart and great arteries occur in an estimated 0.8% of newborns, making them the most common congenital malformation. It has been reported that half of all cases of CHD can be expected to have a good outcome for the infants affected. Some defects are minor and may resolve spontaneously. Others are considered major, yet have an excellent prognosis with surgical correction, such as tetralogy of Fallot. The remaining half of congenital heart defects account for a significant proportion of deaths from congenital abnormalities in childhood.[29] Given that CHD is the most frequently occurring severe abnormality among newborns, the prenatal diagnosis of CHD has the potential to have a significant impact, providing the opportunity for improved antenatal counseling and neonatal outcome.

Etiology

Furthering understanding of the etiology of CHD is an important task in the development of improved strategies for prenatal screening, therapy, and possible prevention. Nearly 90% of CHD is considered to occur as a result of a multifactorial process, including various environmental, genetic, and developmental factors.[30] In exploring the etiology of CHD, it is important to consider the various genetic and familial, environmental, maternal, and fetal developmental factors.

Table 59–1. Familial Recurrence Risk for Congenital Heart Disease

Type of Congenital Heart Defect	N	Father Affected (Recurrence %)	Mother Affected (Recurrence %)	Total Risk (Recurrence %)
Tetralogy of Fallot	395	1.6	4.5	3.1
Transposition of the great arteries	104	0	0	0
Conotruncal abnormality	103	4.5	5.9	5.1
Atrioventricular septal defect	88	7.7	7.9	7.8
Anomalous pulmonary venous connections	37	0	5.9	3.7
All congenital heart defects	727	2.2	5.7	4.1
All anomalies		2.2	6.6	4.6

From Burn J, Little J, Holloway, S, et al: Recurrence risks in offspring of adults with major heart defects: Results from first cohort of British collaborative study. Lancet 351:311, 1998.

Familial and Genetic factors

Familial factors refer to the risk of recurrence within families previously affected by CHD. The level of recurrence risk depends on the degree of relationship between the fetus and the affected relative. With a previously affected mother, the fetus has an overall recurrence risk of about 5%. The risk is less for the offspring of an affected father.

Table 59-1 summarizes the recurrence risk for a child with an affected parent. If a previous sibling was affected, the fetus carries an approximate 2% to 3% risk of CHD.[31] Among these recurrences, the cardiac lesion is the same between siblings only half of the time. Appreciation of the genetic pathogenesis of congenital heart defects has expanded greatly, and numerous single-gene disorders (mendelian syndromes) have been associated with an increased risk for fetal cardiac malformation (Table 59-2). Nearly 3% of congenital heart defects are attributed to single-gene disorders.[32] Ongoing investigation of the significance of selective knockouts of genes important in heart development should continue to expand the basic understanding of how congenital heart defects occur.

Chromosomal abnormalities greatly increase the risk for the presence of congenital heart malformations (Table 59-3).[33] We found that 40% of fetuses diagnosed

Table 59–2. Risk for Congenital Heart Disease with Mendelian Syndromes

Mendelian Syndrome	% CHD	Gene Transmission
Ellis–van Creveld	50	Autosomal recessive
Noonan	50	Autosomal dominant
TAR	33	Autosomal recessive
Holt-Oram	Common	Autosomal dominant
Short rib–polydactyly	Common	Autosomal recessive
Fanconi	14	Autosomal recessive
Apert	10	Autosomal dominant
Robin	9	Mixed
Carpenter	3	Autosomal recessive

CHD, congenital heart disease; TAR, thrombocytopenia–absent radius.

Table 59–3. Chromosomal Anomalies and Congenital Heart Defects

Syndrome	Associated Cardiac Defects
Trisomy 13	Approximately 80%
	Patent ductus arteriosus (63%)
	Ventricular septal defect (48%)
	Atrial septal defect (40%)
	Abnormal valves (22%)
	Coarctation of the aorta (10%)
	Dextrocardia (6%)
Trisomy 18	Nearly 100%
	Ventricular septal defect (approximately all)
	Polyvalvular disease (93%)
	Subpulmonary infundibulum (98%)
	Double-outlet right ventricle (10%)
	Tetralogy of Fallot (15%)
	Patent ductus arteriosus
	Bicuspid aortic valve
Trisomy 21	Approximately 40-50%
	Atrioventricular septal defect
	Ventricular septal defect
	Atrial septal defect
	Tetralogy of Fallot
	Patent ductus arteriosus
Turner's, syndrome (monosomy X)	Approximately 20-40%
	Coarctation of the aorta (70%)
	Hypoplastic left heart syndrome
Trisomy or tetrasomy 22p	Approximately 40%
	Totally anomalous pulmonary return
	Tetralogy of Fallot
	Ventricular septal defect

Data from Jones KL: Smith's Recognizable Patterns of Human Malformation. Philadelphia, WB Saunders, 1997; and Van Praagh S, Truman T, Firpo A, et al: Cardiac malformation in trisomy 18: A study of 41 postmortem cases. J Am Coll Cardiol 114:79, 1989.

with a congenital heart defect on fetal echocardiogram have chromosomal anomalies.[33] Pregnancy loss due to aneuploidy leads to an observed rate of chromosomal anomaly among live-born infants with CHD of only about 5%, however.[32]

In any case in which prenatal diagnosis of CHD occurs, genetic counseling should be offered, and amniocentesis should be considered. In cases in which an identified microdeletion syndrome is suspected (e.g., 22q11), fluorescence in situ hybridization analysis also should be offered. The 22q11 deletion syndrome, identified with DiGeorge syndrome, refers to a clinical spectrum that may include various abnormalities, including cardiac disease (conotruncal abnormalities), abnormal facies, thymic hypoplasia, cleft palate, and hypocalcemia.[34] For Marfan syndrome and idiopathic hypertrophic subaortic stenosis, disorders for which prenatal diagnosis is uncertain because they are not readily identifiable by ultrasound, genetic counseling for prospective parents still should include a discussion of the potential risks for CHD in offspring.

Fetal Factors

A major risk factor for the presence of CHD is the identification of an extracardiac anomaly in the fetus on ultrasound screening. Abnormalities in more than one organ system significantly increase the risk that CHD also is present.[35] Table 59-4 lists some significant fetal risk factors for the presence of CHD. Complete cardiac evaluation is required when any of these anomalies are noted.

For cases of nonimmune hydrops, 10% to 20% of fetuses typically are found to have abnormal cardiac anatomy. Omphalocele may be associated with CHD in 30% of cases and may affect the outcome of surgical repair.[35]

Fetal cardiac arrhythmia also often is considered a risk factor because irregular fetal heart rhythms commonly

Table 59–4. Fetal Risk Factors for Identification of Congenital Heart Disease

Increased nuchal translucency thickness
Suspected cardiac anomaly on screening examination
Nonimmune hydrops
Fetal cardiac arrhythmia
Extracardiac anomaly
  Hydrocephaly
  Meckel-Gruber
  Imperforate anus
  Duodenal atresia
  Omphalocele
  Diaphragmatic hernia
  Agenesis of the corpus callosum
  Esophageal atresia/tracheoesophageal fistula
  Dandy-Walker
  Holoprosencephaly
  Jejunal atresia
  Renal agenesis
  Gastroschisis
Abnormal Doppler pattern of ductus venosus

are identified in clinical practice. A retrospective review of 595 referrals for fetal echocardiogram secondary to irregular fetal heart rhythm revealed only 2 fetuses, however, with arrhythmia and structural disease.[36] In this group, extrasystole was identified in 255 (42.9%), normal rhythm in 330 (55.4%), and hemodynamically significant arrhythmia in 10. In total, 2.4% of fetuses referred for irregular rhythm were found to have significant arrhythmia. Most fetal cardiac arrhythmias are isolated extrasystoles, with no increased risk for structural malformation. Conversely, congenital heart block is associated with a structural defect about 50% of the time.[37]

The suspicion of cardiac anomaly on routine second-trimester screening ultrasound leads to a confirmation of findings in 40% to 50% of cases.[38] Promising first-trimester screening for CHD is now available, with the use of nuchal translucency measurements. Nuchal translucency has been shown to be a useful first-trimester screening examination to identify fetuses at increased risk for chromosomal anomalies and congenital cardiac malformations. Nuchal translucency refers to the fluid-filled space at the back of the fetal neck. Thickening of this space between 10 and 14 weeks of gestation has been correlated with the presence of Down syndrome and other chromosomal anomalies. Even in the presence of a normal karyotype, thickened nuchal translucency was found to indicate a high risk for the presence of CHD.[39] Hyett and associates[40] reported that with increasing nuchal translucency thickness, an increasing relative risk of the presence of CHD was observed among 21,138 fetuses with normal karyotype. Aortic isthmus narrowing and ventricular septal defects were most common among the observed defects. Increased nuchal translucency should be followed up with the offering of diagnostic screening for abnormal karyotype and detailed evaluation of cardiac anatomy with a second-trimester scan and fetal echocardiogram.

Examination of the fetal ductus venosus also may provide an important insight into the fetal cardiovascular system. Doppler signals from the ductus venosus have the highest velocities in the fetal venous circulation and are antegrade throughout systole and diastole. Dilation of the venous duct secondary to hypoxia produces an abnormal atrial a wave. The presence of a congenital heart defect also may alter fetal hemodynamics and lead to this abnormal a wave, providing a potential method for the early detection of congenital heart defects with first-trimester ultrasound.[41]

Maternal Factors

Maternal factors associated with an increased risk for the presence of CHD include maternal CHD, teratogen exposure, maternal metabolic disease, and maternal autoantibodies. Women with CHD have an estimated 5% rate of having an affected offspring. The risk depends on the type of lesion present in the mother. With atrioventricular septal defects, the recurrence risk for the fetus may be 12%.[42] Mothers with left heart obstructive lesions may have a 6% to 10% recurrence rate in their offspring.[42]

Exposure to drugs and infection during the first 8 weeks of pregnancy increases the risk for congenital heart

Table 59–5. Teratogens Associated with Congenital Heart Disease

Lithium
Alcohol
Isotretinoin
Phenytoin
Carbamazepine
Valproic acid
Folate antagonists (e.g., sulfa)
  Trimethoprim
  Triamterene
  Sulfasalazine
  Phenobarbital
  Primidone
  Carbamazepine
  Cholestyramine

From Hernandez-Diaz S, Werler M, Walker A, Mitchell A. Folic acid antagonists during pregnancy and the risk of birth defects. N Engl J Med 343:1608, 2000.

defects. Table 59-5 lists potential teratogens. Several of the potential teratogens listed in Table 59-5 are considered folic acid antagonists. Folic acid antagonists may increase the risk of cardiovascular defects, neural tube defects, oral clefts, and urinary tract defects. There are two general types of folic acid antagonists. The first type, dihydrofolate reductase inhibitors, block the conversion of folate to its more active metabolites and include aminopterin, methotrexate, sulfasalazine, pyrimethamine, triamterene, and trimethoprim. The second type primarily includes antiepileptic drugs and may affect various other enzymes in folate metabolism, impair the absorption of folate, or increase the degradation of folate. These include carbamazepine, phenytoin, primidone, and phenobarbital. The folic acid component of multivitamins may reduce the risks of these defects.[43]

Maternal Metabolic Disease

Diabetes. A fetal echocardiogram currently is offered to all women with diabetes early in gestation. The incidence of CHD is fivefold higher among mothers with diabetes.[44] Typical defects include ventricular septal defects and transposition of the great arteries. An elevation of hemoglobin A_{1C} in the first trimester has been correlated with an increased risk of structural defects.[45] With a hemoglobin A_{1C} value of less than 7%, there were no reported congenital heart defects. For hemoglobin A_{1C} greater than 8.5%, the risk was 22% for a structural defect.

Another significant finding relates to the thickness of the interventricular septum, which has been shown to be increased among fetuses of diabetic mothers. These differences exist even with good control of diabetes and similar estimated birth weight.[46] The functional effect of this increased thickness of the interventricular septum typically involves some degree of diastolic dysfunction (lowered early-to-late diastolic filling ratios), although there usually is no change in systolic function (peak flow velocity).[47] Most infants affected by this hypertrophic cardiomyopathy are asymptomatic at birth and free of residual disease by 2 years of age.[48]

Phenylketonuria. Maternal phenylketonuria requires careful management and control of phenylalanine levels. Poor control has been shown to lead to an increased risk of fetal cardiac disease, with phenylalanine levels of greater than 600 µmol/L in the first 8 weeks of pregnancy associated with a 14% incidence of structural malformation of the fetal heart.[49]

Autoantibodies. The presence of maternal autoantibodies, particularly anti-Ro and anti-La, has been associated with an increased risk for congenital heart block and cardiomyopathy. Echocardiography is indicated to assess for structural heart disease and to identify the presence of atrioventricular dissociation and determine heart rate. Pulsed Doppler assessment of the mechanical P-R interval has been shown to be an important tool in describing the fetal conduction system and identifying variations in fetal heart block.[50] Administration of steroids to the mother is the most common form of treatment for heart block.[51,52] Serial echocardiograms to monitor P-R interval in at-risk fetuses, along with the prophylactic use of maternal steroid therapy, are currently under investigation in a multicenter trial.

Prevention

The potential for the prevention of congenital heart defects is an important focus for research. Multivitamin and folic acid supplementation may decrease the incidence of congenital malformations, including congenital heart defects.[53-55] As knowledge of the human genome increases, the identification of genetic mutations that predispose to congenital heart defects may lead the way to the development of other preventive therapies.[56]

Summary

CHD is a common cause of neonatal and infant morbidity and mortality. Many genetic, maternal, and fetal risk factors for CHD have been identified. Screening for risk factors can help identify cases, although this screening does not identify most cases of congenital heart malformations. Routine screening examination of the fetal heart in low-risk pregnancy is important for the detection of CHD.

FETAL ECHOCARDIOGRAPHY IN THE DETECTION OF FETAL HEART DISEASE

Indications for Obtaining a Fetal Echocardiogram

The current indications for obtaining a fetal echocardiogram include the familial, fetal, and maternal risk factors discussed earlier (Table 59-6). Among congenital heart defects detected prenatally, approximately half occur in pregnancies with no identifiable risk factor.[57] This situation illustrates the importance of ensuring adequate prenatal screening examination of the fetal heart in routine pregnancy evaluation with ultrasound.

<table>
<tr><td colspan="1">

Table 59–6. Indications for Fetal Echocardiogram Evaluation

Familial Risk Factors
Congenital heart disease
  Previous sibling
  Paternal
Single-gene disorders/mendelian syndromes

Fetal Risk Factors
Increased nuchal translucency
Suspected cardiac anomaly on detailed scan
Extracardiac anomalies
  Chromosomal
  Anatomic
Fetal cardiac dysrhythmia
  Irregular rhythm
  Tachycardia
  Bradycardia
Nonimmune hydrops fetalis
Abnormal fetal situs

Maternal Risk Factors
Congenital heart disease
Cardiac teratogen exposure
  Lithium carbonate
  Alcohol
  Anticonvulsants
    Phenytoin
    Trimethadione
  Isotretinoin
  Folate antagonists
Maternal metabolic disorders
  Diabetes mellitus
  Phenylketonuria
Maternal autoantibodies (Ro/La)

</td></tr>
</table>

From Kleinman C, Copel J: Prenatal diagnosis of structural heart disease. In Creasy RK, Resnick R (eds): Maternal-Fetal Medicine, 4th ed. Philadelphia, WB Saunders, 1999.

Detection Ability of Fetal Echocardiogram for Congenital Heart Disease

Experience has shown the reliability of prenatal diagnosis of cardiac abnormalities. Cardiac anomalies suspected on routine second-trimester ultrasound examinations are confirmed in 40% to 50% of cases.[38] With a prenatal diagnosis, postnatal confirmation typically is made. Overall detection rates for routine screening programs using the standard four-chamber view have been questioned by previous studies (RADIUS trial), however. Regional differences in detection ability for congenital anomalies were significant, and the overall prenatal detection rate for CHD was reported to be 18% for tertiary care centers.[58] Extended fetal echocardiogram examination significantly improves the detection rate of CHD. Several studies have reported detection rates of almost 80% of newborns with CHD.[19,57,59] A significant percentage of cardiac anomalies may remain undetected, however, by fetal echocardiogram performed by experienced operators—20% in the study by Yagel and coworkers.[19]

Failure to detect CHD on routine screening ultrasounds and fetal echocardiograms may result in part from the natural history of some cardiac anomalies, which may develop detectable structural changes only late in pregnancy or after birth. Alterations in the size of the cardiac chambers and great vessels, which may be observed late in fetal life, are an example. Other anomalies that may appear normal on ultrasound examination between 13 and 22 weeks of gestation and yet manifest late include hypoplastic heart, tetralogy of Fallot, aortic stenosis, pulmonary stenosis, and endocardial fibroelastosis.[19] Limited resolution and diagnostic errors also may contribute to the failure to detect certain cardiac anomalies.

Continued improvement in the techniques and training of individuals performing ultrasound examination of the fetal heart has led to an improvement in the detection rates in subsequent studies compared with the RADIUS trial outcomes.[60] Not all fetal cardiac malformations are detectable, however.[61] It is important to ensure that well-qualified professionals exist to perform screening ultrasound examinations. In addition, the development of professionals specially trained in fetal echocardiography is essential. Currently, perinatologists, pediatric cardiologists, and radiologists are involved in the provision of fetal echocardiography. The team approach to patient care also should involve pediatric surgery and neonatology.

Methods for Screening Examination of the Fetal Heart

Technology for Fetal Heart Examination

The technology and equipment required for accurate screening evaluation and detailed examination of the fetal heart are considerable. A detailed description is beyond the scope of this chapter. The ultrasound capabilities currently required for assessment of the fetal cardiac system and peripheral vasculature include real-time two-dimensional, M-mode, and Doppler (spectral, color, power).

First-Trimester and Early Midtrimester Techniques

Visualization of the early pregnancy has steadily improved with technological advances in ultrasonography. These advances inspire continued interest in screening for CHD in the first and early second trimesters.

Transvaginal ultrasound techniques contribute greatly to the growing interest in early detection of CHD. Optimal timing for second-trimester examination of the fetal heart is after 15 weeks of gestation, whereas first-trimester transvaginal techniques may be useful in the examination of the fetal heart and nuchal translucency between 10 and 14 weeks of gestation. Early anomalies of the heart that can be visualized include large septal defects and transposition of the great arteries. Most major structural heart defects can be diagnosed accurately from the late first trimester of pregnancy. Nuchal translucency measurement between 11 and 14 weeks of gestation also has been shown to be a useful screening examination to identify fetuses at increased risk for chromosomal anomalies and congenital cardiac malformations.[40]

As discussed earlier, first-trimester techniques cannot replace the midgestation abdominal ultrasound scan.

Techniques are highly dependent on operator experience. Attempts to perform the four-chamber views between 12 and 16 weeks of gestation have been shown to lack sensitivity for congenital heart defects. Yagel and coworkers[16] showed that 17% of cardiac anomalies might not be detected by early midtrimester transvaginal ultrasound. Early screening with transvaginal ultrasound should be followed by a backup transabdominal scan at midgestation.[16,17]

Second-Trimester Techniques

Optimal timing for the transabdominal second-trimester examination of the fetal heart is after 15 weeks of gestation. Fetal echocardiography, with its expanded views and the use of Doppler and color techniques, is optimal between 20 and 22 weeks of gestation. Efforts to develop successful second-trimester screening techniques for CHD have encountered the difficulty of disappointing detection rates, just as with the first-trimester techniques. Four-chamber views alone reveal only certain cardiac anomalies. The addition of views of the outflow tracts improved detection rates. The use of extensive fetal echocardiography as part of all detailed anatomy scanning also has been shown to increase detection rates significantly.[62,63] The issues of cost and availability of trained specialists make fetal echocardiography less than ideal, however, as a screening test for low-risk populations.

Third-Trimester Techniques

Although major structural defects may be detected more easily earlier in pregnancy, defects that tend to worsen during the second and third trimesters, such as pulmonary atresia with intact septum, initially may show only subtle structural abnormalities. Additional examinations in the late second or third trimester of pregnancy may increase the detection rate of CHD. This follow-up currently is recommended only for extremely high-risk patients, however, such as patients with a strong family history.

The potential benefit of additional follow-up examination among high-risk patients, despite an early reassuring scan, has been suggested in the literature. A report from a European registry of congenital malformations (Eurocat) revealed a large regional variation in the prenatal detection rate for major cardiac malformations, with the lowest detection rate in countries without prenatal ultrasound screening.[64] Among the six major cardiac malformations included in the study, 35% were diagnosed before 23 weeks of gestation; 47%, between 23 and 32 weeks; and 17%, at greater than 32 weeks. Prenatal detection rate was 46% for the three malformations affecting the size of the ventricles (hypoplastic left heart, tricuspid atresia, single ventricle), whereas prenatal detection rate for malformations with normal size of the ventricles was 24%. The potential remains to improve detection rates for congenital heart defects through close surveillance and follow-up examination in the third trimester.

Basics of the Fetal Heart Examination

Overview of Anatomy and Physiology of the Fetal Heart

Developing an understanding of fetal anatomy and cardiovascular physiology is fundamental to understanding the application of fetal echocardiography in the detection and management of fetal and neonatal cardiac disease. Knowledge of the human heart continues to expand with the progress and contributions of a variety of scientific and clinical disciplines. Through these efforts, we have come to understand that the developing heart is a complex organ, arising from independent and overlapping processes first to become a functional pumping tube at about 3 weeks of embryonic life. The fetal heart is anatomically developed and fully septated by 8 weeks of embryonic life. The conduction system begins to develop by 5 weeks and is complete by 8 weeks. The formation of fibrous atrioventricular and semilunar valve leaflets is completed by 16 weeks of gestation. Birth initiates the transition from fetal to neonatal circulation and the final events of cardiac development, the closure of the ductus arteriosus and foramen ovale.

One of the defining differences between the fetal and the adult circulation lies in the connection between the fetal venous and arterial circuits—the ductus arteriosus and foramen ovale. The right-sided increase in pressure and flow over the left also is integral to the function of these communications and shows right ventricular predominance. The fetal reliance on the placenta for gas and nutrient exchange, rather than the lung, is another important difference. These differences lead to the development of a near-parallel arrangement of venous and arterial flow, whereas in the adult these vessels circulate in series. Characteristics of cardiac function in the fetus and adult are summarized in Table 59-7. Although a full discussion of fetal cardiovascular physiology is beyond the scope of this chapter, an understanding of the changes in fetal circulation at birth is essential in the diagnosis of CHD.

Table 59–7. Comparison between Adult and Fetal Cardiac Function

Anatomic Differences

Patent foramen ovale
Patent ductus ateriosus
Right ventricle larger than left
Right ventricle more hemispheric in cross-section than after birth

Physiologic Differences

Increased	*Decreased*
Mean systolic pressure	Blood pressure
Venous return	Resistance to venous return
Higher LV afterload compared with RV afterload	Systemic vascular compliance
	Ventricular compliance
	Peripheral resistance
Filling pressure	Pulmonary blood flow
Volume flow	Po_2
RV flow compared with LV flow	
Heart rate	

LV, left ventricle; RV, right ventricle.

From Reed KL: Fetal Doppler echocardiography. Clin Obstet Gynecol 32:728, 1989.

Components of the Routine Fetal Heart Examination with Ultrasound

The routine screening evaluation of the fetal heart should be conducted with the goal of establishing that the cardiac structure and function meet certain criteria. Attention should be focused on identifying that the heart lies on the left side of the fetus and on the same side as the stomach. Completing the four-chamber views allows for the assessment of cardiac position, size, axis, chamber structure, septal integrity, and ventriculoarterial connections. The aortic arch and ductal arches also should be assessed.

The accuracy of such comprehensive cardiac assessment relies on operator skill and image quality. When optimal, fetal cardiac assessment by ultrasound provides a high level of detection for serious cardiac malformations.[57] Even when optimal, fetal cardiac scanning has limitations, particularly in the detection of small septal defects. In addition, certain cardiac abnormalities may develop later in pregnancy, including pulmonary and aortic stenosis, cardiomyopathy, and cardiac tumors.[19] It is important for each examiner to develop a routine that allows for the complete assessment of the fetal cardiac structure and function in standard fashion with each examination (Table 59-8).

Situs. Evaluation of fetal situs should the first step in evaluation of the fetal heart. This approach requires knowledge of the fetal position. Situs solitus is characterized by the location of the heart and stomach on the left side of the fetus. Situs inversus occurs with complete inversion of the viscera, with the heart and the stomach on the right side of the fetus. Abnormalities of abdominal and cardiac situs often involve atrial isomerism and complex abnormalities of intracardiac and great vessel anatomy.

Cardiac position. The normal fetal cardiac position has been well described by Comstock.[65] Most of the fetal heart should be located in the anterior half of the fetal chest. With a transverse view of the fetal chest, the most posterior aspect of the heart should lie in the right hemithorax, midway between the anterior and posterior sides of the fetus. For the most part, both ventricles are situated in the left anterior quadrant of the chest, with the

exception of a small portion of the right ventricle. The atria may be located partially in the right thorax.

Fetal cardiac position on ultrasound examination may be altered by intracardiac and extracardiac abnormalities. The differential diagnosis of abnormal cardiac position and axis should include chest mass, development disorders of the lung, congenital diaphragmatic hernia, chromosomal anomalies, and cardiac anomalies, including the asplenia and polysplenia syndromes.[66]

Cardiac size. An enlarged heart can indicate high output failure, volume overload, or direct myocardial damage. Noting the cardiac size is an important component of the examination and can be evaluated with a four-chamber view. Heart area should be approximately one third of the total chest area at the level of the four-chamber view.[67] Intrauterine growth restriction, hydrops, and skeletal dysplasia are among the disorders associated with abnormal heart size. Abnormal cardiothoracic ratios also are associated with CHD and dysrhythmia.[67] Asymmetry of the ventricle sizes also may be detected in CHD.

Cardiac axis. Cardiac axis describes the position of the fetal heart in the chest. Measuring the angle formed between the interventricular septum and a line from the spine to the anterior chest wall that divides the fetal thorax in half determines cardiac axis. The fetal heart typically lies at an angle of 45 degrees from the midline, with 95% of all normal hearts having 30 to 60 degrees of axis.

Cardiac axis has been proposed as an important screening tool for the presence of CHD. A fetal cardiac axis greater than 2 standard deviations above the mean provided a sensitivity of 44% for CHD in a study by Shipp and colleagues.[68] Using the same threshold of 2 standard deviations above the mean, Bork and associates[69] reported a sensitivity of 63% for CHD. Smith and coworkers[70] used a cutoff of 75 degrees and determined a positive predictive value of 76% for elevated values, leading to the recommendation to include cardiac axis evaluation in the routine four-chamber view assessment. We believe that cardiac axis can be evaluated based on appearance alone, without formal measurement.

The assessment of cardiac axis improves the detection ability of the routine screening examination. An abnormal axis usually is noted with conotruncal abnormalities, Ebstein anomaly, pulmonary stenosis, coarctation, and tetralogy of Fallot, all of which are often difficult to detect with a four-chamber view. It is an important component of the routine cardiac examination, and an abnormal axis on routine screening necessitates a referral for fetal echocardiogram.

Four-chamber view. The four-chamber view of the fetal heart allows for a detailed assessment of the second-trimester or third-trimester fetus (Tables 59-9 and 59-10; Fig. 59-1A and B). Ideally obtained after 15 weeks of gestation, this view now is technically attainable in all examinations. The four-chamber assessment includes apical, basal, and long-axis views. The apical view, with the ultrasound beam parallel to the interventricular and interatrial septa, allows evaluation of chamber size and

Table 59–8. Components of Routine Fetal Heart Screening

Situs
Rhythm
Position
Size
Axis
Four-chamber view
  Atria, ventricles
  Atrioventricular valves
  Ventriculo-arterial outflow tracts
  Ductal and aortic arches

Table 59–9. Components of the Normal Four-Chamber View

Heart in the left chest
Atria equal sizes
Ventricles equal sizes
Area of heart one third of chest area
Left atrium posterior
Foramen ovale flap in left atrium
Apical offset in tricuspid valve
Intact interventricular septum
Moderator band in right ventricle
Axis 45° to 60°

Table 59–10. Components of the Long-Axis View

Aortic position
Relation of aorta to interventricular septum
Relation of aorta to mitral valve
Integrity of anterior interventricular septum

the atrioventricular valves. The long-axis view, with the ultrasound beam perpendicular to the septa, allows for evaluation of the integrity of the septa. Identification of pericardial effusion, endocardial calcification, or myocardial masses also may be achieved with the four-chamber view.

Typically, both atria and ventricles of the fetal heart appear of nearly equal size, although the right ventricle may become larger than the left near term. The ventricular

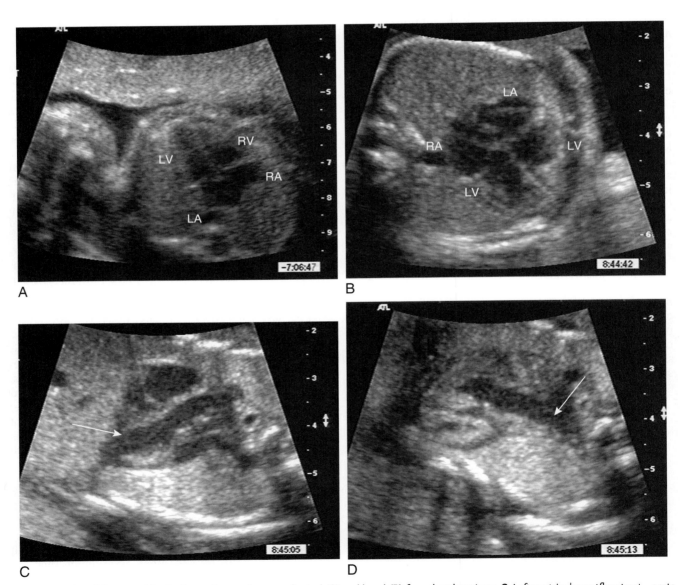

Figure 59–1. **A** and **B,** Normal fetal echocardiogram images of apical **(A)** and basal **(B)** four-chamber views. **C,** Left ventricular outflow tract—aorta *(arrow)*. **D,** Right ventricular outflow tract—pulmonary artery *(arrow)*. LA, left atrium; LV, left ventricle; RA, right atrium; RV, right ventricle.

walls should appear nearly equal in thickness. The moderator band may be seen in the right ventricle, causing a more trabeculated appearance, whereas the left ventricular wall appears smooth. The foramen ovale may be visualized in the left atrium, along with the pulmonary veins when in the appropriate plane. The atrioventricular valves may be visualized, with the septal leaflet of the tricuspid valve inserting more apical than the mitral valve. Contractility of the heart can be observed, along with valvular motion, to assess function. Finally, in the long-axis view, the interventricular septum should be seen as continuous from the apex to the atrioventricular valves.

The complete four-chamber view examination by itself has been shown to be useful as a screen for CHD, although with varying efficacy. Copel and colleagues[71] reported a sensitivity of 92% and specificity of 99.7% with a retrospective review of normal and abnormal four-chamber views. Others have reported sensitivities of 30% to 50% in prospective studies.[72] Variations in the reported sensitivity of the four-chamber view may be attributed to many factors, including operator experience, patient population, neonatal follow-up, and equipment. By itself, the four-chamber view has not been shown to be an ideal screening tool. This concept has led to the expansion of the recommended examination by some to include ventriculoarterial outflow tracts and, more recently, the three-vessel and five-chamber views.

Outflow tracts. The accurate evaluation of the ventriculoarterial outflow tracts has been reported to allow detection of nearly 90% of serious cardiac malformations.[57] These tracts can be viewed with transverse and longitudinal views. The posterior leaflet of the aortic valve should be seen in continuity with the anterior leaflet of the mitral valve (see Fig. 59-1C). The anterior wall of the aorta also should be continuous with the ventricular septum. The superior vena cava also is visible.

Most importantly, the great artery outflow tracts are seen to cross each other, and the vessels are normal in size and without regurgitation on color flow. The pulmonary outflow typically is slightly larger than the aorta, and, if needed, measurements can be made and compared with normal ranges (Fig. 59-1D). The aortic and ductal arches should be visualized as part of the complete examination (Fig. 59-2A and B); this may be accomplished with either transverse or longitudinal views.

Five-chamber view. Important conditions, such as transposition of the great arteries and tetralogy of Fallot, may be missed on a four-chamber view. A long-axis view, called the *five-chamber view,* has been described and reportedly allows visualization of the aortic root more accurately and with less time.[73]

Three-vessel view. Yoo and associates[74] reported on a three-vessel view, which is a cross-sectional view of the great vessels, within the fetal upper mediastinum. This transverse view above the aortic origin reveals the pulmonary trunk, transverse aortic arch, and superior vena cava (see Fig. 59-2C). An abnormality of this view may detect semilunar valve or aortic arch malformation, as the

diagnosis of coarctation of the aorta is often difficult because of the large patent arterial duct.

Sagittal views. Directed parallel to the fetal spine, sagittal views profile the systemic venous connections, the right ventricular outflow tract and ductal arch, and the aortic arch and its branches.

Factors Affecting Ability to Obtain Routine Fetal Heart Views

Some well-known factors may affect the quality of the fetal heart scan and limit its sensitivity for the detection of CHD, including gestational age, fetal position, maternal obesity, previous surgical scar, transducer frequency, operator experience, and the population being assessed.[75] Examination of the fetal heart at gestational ages earlier than 17 weeks decreases the accuracy of screening.[76] Septal defects may be more difficult to diagnose at earlier gestational ages. Advanced gestational age also poses a challenge because the calcification of the fetal ribs may make imaging more difficult.

Fetal position may lead to inadequate visualization, especially if the fetus is prone. Maternal repositioning or walking may help, although scheduling a follow-up examination occasionally is necessary.

Maternal obesity also reduces the likelihood of obtaining a complete four-chamber view of the fetal heart. Devore and coworkers[76] estimated that there is only a 60% likelihood of obtaining a four-chamber view at 18 weeks of gestation for a mother with a 3-cm thickness of abdominal adipose tissue, whereas a 2-cm thickness increases this likelihood to 100%. Efforts to overcome the difficulties imposed by maternal obesity include the use of harmonic imaging, sepia coloring to sharpen edges, reducing transducer frequency, and repeat of examination in 2 to 3 weeks. Devore and coworkers[76] also noted that scarring from previous abdominal surgery reduced the likelihood of obtaining an adequate examination of the fetal heart. Among pregnant women with only a 2-cm thickness of adipose tissue, adequate views were obtained in only 75% of patients.

Operator experience with ultrasound also is an important modifier. With respect to transducer frequency, the goal is to maintain the balance between resolution and penetration. Higher frequency transducers produce better resolution, although with less penetration, than transducers with lower frequency. Finally, the population being studied also plays a role because screening sensitivity is highest when screening a high-risk population.[75]

Fetal Echocardiogram

Pregnancies considered at high risk for CHD are referred for fetal echocardiogram. Because most cases of CHD occur in the low-risk population, the above-described screening examination remains an important component of the detailed ultrasound examination. The four-chamber view and outflow tracts commonly are included with routine examinations, although the three-vessel trachea and five-chamber views described are more often a part of the specialized fetal echocardiogram examination (Table 59-11). When the criteria for fetal echocardiogram referral are met, the patient ideally should be directed to a

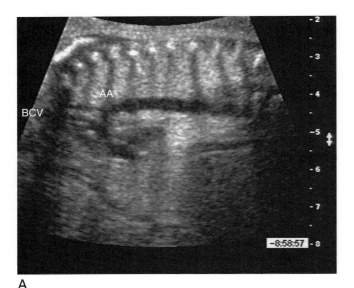

A

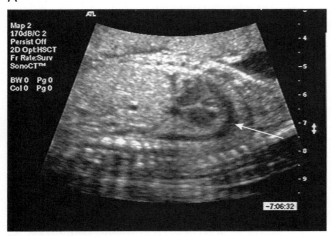

B

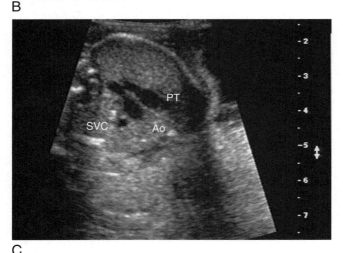

C

Figure 59–2. A, Ascending aortic arch (AA) and brachiocephalic vessels (BCV). **B,** Ductal arch *(arrow).* **C,** Three-vessel trachea view, which is a transverse plane in the upper chest, illustrating the pulmonary trunk (PT), aortic root (Ao), and superior vena cava (SVC) in one plane.

Table 59–11. Full Fetal Echocardiography Examination Views

Four-chamber
Long-axis left ventricle
Short-axis great vessels
Aortic arch
Pulmonary artery/ductal arch
SVC/IVC
Pulmonary veins

SVC/IVC, superior vena cava/inferior vena cava.

center providing specialists trained in comprehensive fetal cardiac sonography, pediatric cardiology, and maternal fetal medicine.

The American Institute of Ultrasound in Medicine published a technical bulletin in 1998 that outlined the recommended components of the standard fetal echocardiogram. The optimal timing of the examination is 18 to 22 weeks of gestation, using the American Institute of Ultrasound in Medicine's examination standards. Included in the fetal echocardiogram assessment, and not described in the preceding section, is the use of cardiac and venous Doppler ultrasound to assess the function and structure of the heart. M-mode techniques also may be used to assess cardiac arrhythmia. Cardiac morphology is assessed with the real-time, two-dimensional evaluation (Tables 59-12 and 59-13).

Doppler ultrasound enhances the assessment of CHD. Abnormalities of blood flow direction and velocity within the heart can be detected using color-flow mapping, allowing for an assessment of cardiac anatomy and physiology (Figs. 59-3 and 59-4). Pulsed and continuous wave Doppler allow the estimation of blood flow impedance, flow velocities, and perfusion. Amplitude-based Doppler techniques may be used to identify blood flow without directional information.[77] Examples of the utility of Doppler assessment include the improved detection of atrioventricular regurgitation and valvular stenosis.

M-mode ultrasound records the mechanical events of the cardiac cycle, allowing one to infer the electrical signals involved and to assess valve motion and cardiac rhythm. An M-mode line positioned over one atrial and ventricular wall records the variations of echoes produced, quantitates heart rate, and describes the sequence of contractions.

The goal of providing comprehensive and more accurate screening is challenging. Yagel and associates[73] proposed using five transverse planes, or short-axis views, to simplify and improve fetal heart examination. The five views include (1) a transverse view of the upper abdomen; (2) a four-chamber view; (3) a five-chamber view (aortic

Table 59–12. Techniques Used for the Fetal Echocardiogram

Real-time two-dimensional ultrasound
M-mode
Color and spectral Doppler sonography

Table 59-13. Approaches to Fetal Echocardiogram

Morphology
Rhythm assessment
   Real-time scan
   M-mode
   Doppler
Functional assessment
   Doppler indices
   Atrioventricular valves
   Ductus arteriosus
   Cardiac output
Color applications

root is visualized); (4) a view of the bifurcation of the pulmonary artery; and (5) a three-vessel and trachea view, which reveals the main pulmonary trunk in communication with the ductus arteriosus. Cross sections of the aortic arch, superior vena cava, and trachea also are visualized. Yagel and associates[73] stressed that this approach reduces the time required to examine the aortic arch, which is one of the more time-consuming components of the fetal echocardiogram. Further reports of the effectiveness of this approach are needed to assess detection rates.

Potential Abnormalities on Fetal Heart Examination

A firm knowledge of the above-described normal fetal heart views provides the foundation for identifying congenital heart abnormalities. A complete discussion of the potential abnormalities identifiable with the four-chamber and outflow tract views is beyond the scope of this chapter. These abnormalities are discussed in detail with regard to neonatal management elsewhere in this text. We have included several ultrasound images identifying many of these abnormalities to serve as examples of current techniques (Figs. 59-5 through 59-8).

IMPACT OF FETAL ECHOCARDIOGRAPHY ON DIAGNOSIS AND MANAGEMENT OF CONGENITAL HEART DISEASE

The care of the fetus with CHD is addressed best by a multidisciplinary approach. The input and expertise of physicians in maternal-fetal medicine, fetal imaging, pediatric cardiology, pediatric cardiac surgery, and neonatology all

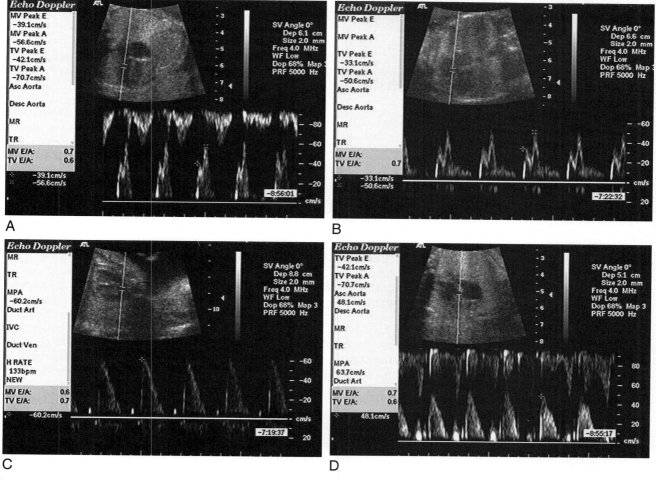

Figure 59-3. Functional examination of the fetal heart with Doppler ultrasound. Velocity waveforms are from a fetus of 22 weeks' gestation. **A,** Mitral valve. **B,** Pulmonary artery. **C,** Tricuspid valve. **D,** Ascending aorta. E/A values represent early-active ventricular filling ratios.

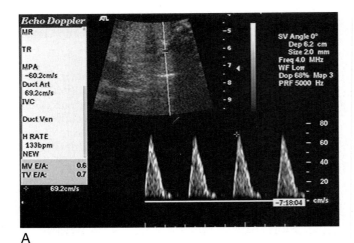

A

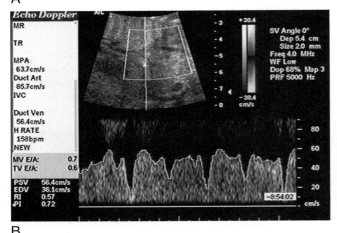

B

Figure 59–4. Velocity waveforms of the fetal ductal circulation. **A,** The velocity waveform of the ductus arteriosus is obtained in a short-axis view; continuous forward flow occurs throughout the cardiac cycle. **B,** The ductus venosus is seen in a transverse plane of the fetal abdomen. The waveform exhibits a biphasic pattern, with the first peak occurring with systole, the second with diastole, and the nadir with atrial contraction.

contribute to prenatal and postnatal management of the patient. Understanding the impact of fetal echocardiography on the diagnosis, management, and outcome of CHD begins with an appreciation of the importance of screening techniques.

Assessments of the sensitivity of screening for CHD have been concerning, with an average sensitivity of only 35% for the four-chamber view, when considering many reported studies.[78,79] Todros and colleagues[78] reported on the accuracy of the four-chamber view in an Italian multicenter study assessing 8299 pregnancies. Their study revealed a sensitivity of 15%, specificity of 99.9%, positive predictive value of 50%, and negative predictive value of 99.6% for congenital heart defects. The detection rate increased to 35% when defects not associated with abnormalities of the four-chamber view were excluded from analysis, although that distinction was not defined further. Other multicenter studies have reported similar

results. In a retrospective review by Klein and associates,[79] an overall sensitivity rate of 34.8% was reported for fetal echocardiography in Isere County, France.

The sensitivity of fetal echocardiography improves to 78% when views of the ventricular outflows and great arteries are included in the screening examination.[80] As described earlier, first-trimester screening techniques using the nuchal translucency measurements have been reported to have a 99% negative predictive value and 56% detection rate for CHD, although confirmation of these data is required. The four-chamber and ventriculoarterial views remain the standard approach to fetal cardiac screening.[81]

Describing the impact of prenatal screening and diagnosis on the outcome of infants born with CHD has become an expanding area of interest. The potential benefits offered with prenatal diagnosis include counseling by a multidisciplinary team, evaluation for chromosomal and extracardiac abnormalities, the option of elective pregnancy termination, and planning for delivery in a tertiary care center. A growing body of literature addressing the outcomes of CHD now exists, although the diversity of malformations and clinical approaches used in management make it difficult to generalize the results.

Comparing outcomes for prenatal and postnatal diagnoses of CHD can be influenced by several factors. The spectrum of disease observed in prenatal life differs from that observed in fetuses surviving to infancy. Spontaneous intrauterine loss occurs in many affected pregnancies.[82] Associated extracardiac lesions are more common in fetuses not surviving to infancy.[35] The progression of cardiac disease in utero also may affect the outcome. More severe forms of disease are more detectable, especially with the four-chamber view. A different spectrum of abnormality is detected prenatally, and, consequently, many early studies reported worse outcomes than expected from postnatal experience.[83]

Postnatal survival also generally is thought to depend on timely provision of treatment. Delivery in a tertiary care center with expertise in the management of the newborn with CHD provides the opportunity for timely intervention. Immediate cardiac assessment of the newborn may avoid late diagnosis, after an infant has developed cyanosis or acidosis.

Showing a reduction in morbidity and mortality as a result of timely intervention has been difficult. A study from the United States reported that delivery at a tertiary care center did not improve SNAP scores (Score for Neonatal Acute Physiology) of infants with major structural heart defects.[84] The authors suggested that their inability to show improvements in the early physiologic condition of neonates born at a tertiary care center might have resulted in part from the presence of tertiary-level neonatologists on staff at nearby community hospitals. The increased likelihood for more severe cardiac malformations to be diagnosed prenatally and referred for planned delivery at a tertiary care center also may have been an important confounder, resulting in infants with more severe diseases being delivered at that center. The groups included in their study also were heterogeneous with respect to abnormality, which may have disguised

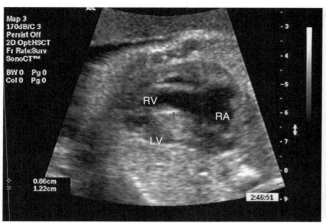

A

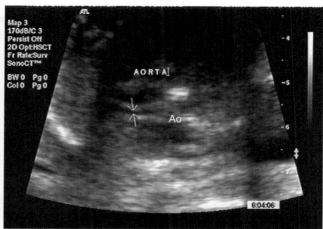

B

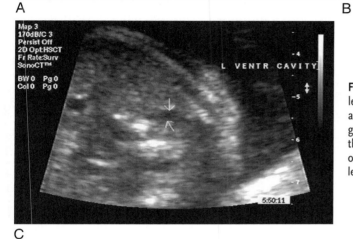

C

Figure 59–5. A-C, Third-trimester images from a fetus with a hypoplastic left heart. The left ventricular cavity is functionally reduced, and the ascending aorta (Ao) and aortic arch are narrowed. These findings suggest the need for neonatal prostaglandin E_1 administration to maintain the ductal circulation and cardiac surgery to augment left ventricular output. **A,** Hypoplastic left heart. **B,** Narrowed aortic arch. **C,** Hypoplastic left heart. LV, left ventricle; RA, right atrium; RV, right ventricle.

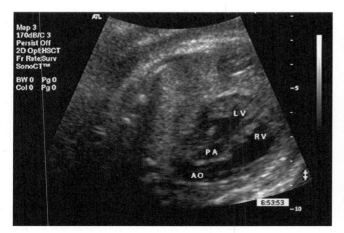

Figure 59–6. Complete transposition of the great vessels is seen in a third-trimester examination. The ventricular outflow tracts are parallel in this transverse plane. PA, pulmonary artery, right ventricular outflow; AO, aorta, left ventricular outflow; LV, left ventricle; RV, right ventricle.

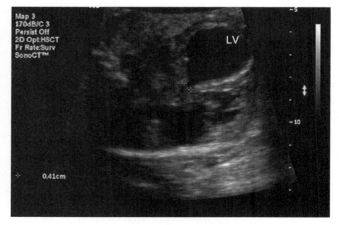

Figure 59–7. A dilated, poorly contractile left ventricle (LV) is seen in this third-trimester examination. Aortic stenosis also was noted in this fetus, although not seen here.

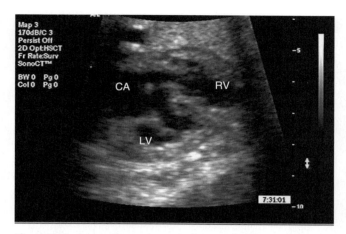

Figure 59–8. A complete atrioventricular septal defect with anterior extension is seen in this fetus with known trisomy 21. This image is from an examination at 35 weeks of gestation. Abnormal development of the endocardial cushions leads to a common atrium (CA). The tricuspid and mitral valves are fused in a single atrioventricular valve, which bridges the two ventricles. LV, left ventricle; RV, right ventricle.

any benefit for infants with a specific type of lesion. Although these data did not suggest that delivery in a tertiary care center resulted in better SNAP scores than transfer after birth, the authors indicated that further research was necessary to determine the best location for delivery of infants with cardiac defects. Expert anticipatory management in tertiary care centers remains preferable, however, especially for infants with ductal-dependent circulations.

Outcomes also may be influenced by prenatal diagnosis in ways that are more difficult to quantify. Prenatal diagnosis provides the opportunity for extensive family counseling, including a description of the abnormality and the potential outcome. Therapeutic options, including surgical intervention, may be discussed in the context of associated morbidity and mortality and long-term outlook. Some families may select termination of pregnancy. More severe cases, with potentially worse outcomes, may be more likely to be diagnosed prenatally. Prospective data have shown that a screening program providing early prenatal recognition of cardiac malformations significantly alters the prevalence of complex CHD observed among newborns.[85] If these pregnancies are more likely to be terminated, a selection bias is created among the prenatally diagnosed group. Parents with an affected fetus who choose to continue the pregnancy also may be more likely to select surgical management and be more aggressive in their approach. All of these variables make it difficult to assess the true impact of prenatal diagnosis on the outcome of CHD, especially with respect to quality of care and cost-effectiveness.

These difficulties were evident in one of the earliest efforts to assess short-term outcomes by Copel and coworkers.[86] Comparing 45 prenatal cases with 54 comparable postnatal cases, this study found no significant difference in length of hospitalization, survival to discharge, or hospital charges. Among patients with lesions

amenable to biventricular repair, however, there was a significant difference in outcome, with 96% survival for the prenatal diagnosis group versus 76% survival in the postnatal group ($P < .05$). Median cost of hospitalization also was lower in the prenatal diagnosis group ($30,277 versus $64,616; $P = .06$). For patients requiring univentricular repair of the cardiac lesion, there was no difference in outcome, possibly due to the self-selection of patients. In the prenatal diagnosis group, some parents elected to terminate the pregnancy. Parents not doing so were more likely to choose surgery for their affected infants than were parents in the postnatal diagnosis group with severe cardiac disease (86% versus 56%; $P < .05$). Choosing not to have postnatal surgery resulted in lower median length of stay and charges for the postnatal diagnosis group.

One admitted problem for this study was that it included a mixture of many different cardiac diagnoses. As screening techniques have improved, more isolated cases have been detected in the low-risk population, with fewer associated abnormalities. With some individual lesions, such as transposition of the great arteries, there is evidence that prenatal diagnosis leads to improved outcome.[87] Outcome studies also have been reported for other commonly detected critical neonatal heart lesions, including hypoplastic left heart syndrome and coarctation of the aorta.

Hypoplastic left heart syndrome has been the focus of many investigations on the impact of prenatal diagnosis on outcomes. Prenatal diagnosis affords parents one of several management options, including pregnancy termination, surgery using the Norwood procedure or cardiac transplantation, and postnatal hospice care. These patients often require considerable postnatal assessment, however, to predict operative risks and outcomes.[88] Their postnatal course is typically difficult. It remains an important challenge to provide parents with the most accurate information possible with respect to outcomes, whenever prenatal diagnosis is made.

Tworetzky and colleagues[89] reviewed 88 patients diagnosed with hypoplastic left heart syndrome between July 1992 and March 1999 to determine the influence of prenatal diagnosis on parental decisions regarding care, preoperative clinical status, and outcomes of stage 1 surgery. In one third of the prenatally diagnosed cases, the pregnancy was electively terminated. Among live-born infants, prenatal diagnosis was associated with improved preoperative clinical status and survival after first-stage palliation compared with patients diagnosed after birth. Patients diagnosed prenatally were less likely, however, to undergo surgery than patients diagnosed after birth (14 of 22 live-born infants with prenatal diagnosis undergoing surgery versus 38 of 55 live-born infants with postnatal diagnosis; $P = .008$).

Mahle and colleagues[90] also hypothesized that prenatal diagnosis may be beneficial to patients with hypoplastic left heart syndrome, particularly because they are at risk for hypoxic-ischemic insult at presentation. Assessing the impact of prenatal diagnosis on preoperative management, neurologic morbidity, and surgical mortality for 216 patients with hypoplastic left heart syndrome, their data suggested that prenatal diagnosis reduced early neurologic morbidity. Although no improvement in hospital mortality was noted, Mahle and colleagues[90] inferred that prenatal diagnosis may have a beneficial impact on long-term outcome.

Despite improvements in survival, patients with complex CHD generally have higher rates of neurodevelopmental problems.[91] The etiology of neurologic deficit in this group is most likely multifactorial and may be related to the preoperative, operative, and postoperative factors that contribute to outcome. Attempts to improve preoperative status and minimize neurologic injury are an important focus of research.

Kumar and associates[92] sought to determine whether prenatal diagnosis may have a positive impact on the preoperative status and outcome for patients with either hypoplastic left heart syndrome or transposition of the great arteries. Outcomes were assessed for all neonates with hypoplastic left heart syndrome or transposition of the great arteries encountered at Children's Hospital of Boston from January 1988 to May 1996. Birth characteristics and preoperative, operative, and postoperative variables of term newborns with a prenatal diagnosis of hypoplastic left heart syndrome who underwent a Norwood operation *(n = 27)* or with transposition of the great arteries who underwent arterial switch operation *(n = 14)* were compared with newborns with the same postnatal diagnoses (hypoplastic left heart syndrome, *n = 47;* transposition of the great arteries, *n = 28).* Prenatal diagnosis improved the preoperative condition of neonates with hypoplastic left heart syndrome and transposition of the great arteries but did not improve preoperative mortality or early postoperative outcome significantly among neonates managed at their tertiary care center.

Outcomes with prenatal diagnosis of transposition of the great arteries also were assessed by Bonnet and colleagues.[87] Preoperative and postoperative morbidity and mortality were compared among 68 neonates with prenatal diagnosis of transposition of the great arteries and 250 neonates with a postnatal diagnosis. The prenatal diagnosis group was admitted sooner and had better clinical condition on admission, with respect to metabolic acidosis and multiorgan failure, than their postnatal diagnosis counterparts. Management after admission was identical in the two groups, although preoperative mortality was significantly higher in the postnatal diagnosis group (postnatal group mortality, 15 of 250 [6%; 95% confidence interval 3% to 9%], versus prenatal group, 0 of 68; *P* < .05). Hospital stay was longer in the group with postnatal diagnosis (30 ± 17 days versus 24 ± 11 days; *P* < .01). Postoperative mortality also was significantly higher in the postnatal diagnosis group (20 of 235 versus 0 of 68; *P* < .01), although the risk factors for operative mortality did not differ between the two groups. The investigators concluded that prenatal diagnosis of transposition of the great arteries reduced mortality and morbidity compared with diagnosis in the neonatal period. An improved preoperative condition was seen as a benefit of prenatal diagnosis and a potential contributor to improved long-term outcome.

Investigation of the impact of prenatal diagnosis on patients with coarctation of the aorta also has revealed an improvement in preoperative condition and survival. Franklin and coworkers[93] reported a retrospective review of patients presenting at a tertiary care center from 1994 to 1998. In the postnatal diagnosis group, collapse and death were more common (*P* < .05), whereas palpable femoral pulses and echocardiographic evidence of duct patency were more likely with prenatal diagnosis (*P* < .001 and *P* < .05). Hemodynamic instability preoperatively and an increased respiratory rate were more likely to occur in the postnatal group (*P* < .01). Franklin and coworkers[93] concluded that prenatal diagnosis of coarctation of the aorta was associated with improved survival and preoperative clinical condition.

In contrast to the study of SNAP scores, which was unable to show an improvement in acute neonatal condition related to delivery in a tertiary care center, the above-described outcomes studies do indicate a significant improvement in preoperative condition and outcome with prenatal diagnosis of certain lesions, including hypoplastic left heart syndrome, transposition of the great arteries, and coarctation of the aorta. Conditions that are ductal dependent and may lead to rapid neonatal decline when unrecognized antenatally clearly benefit from prenatal diagnosis in the short term. Even lesions that are not ductal dependent also may benefit, as shown in a retrospective review that considered outcomes for all neonatal patients with CHD undergoing surgery.[94] The importance of screening programs that improve the prenatal diagnosis of CHD is evident. Further research into the impact of prenatal diagnosis on long-term outcomes and the potential prevention of neurodevelopmental damage is required.

SUMMARY

The future of fetal echocardiography in the detection and management of fetal heart disease holds the potential for exciting advances. Currently, much of fetal cardiac disease is unrecognized until after birth, and prenatal intervention is limited. The need for continued research is evident, and many more recent advances provide promise for the future.

Early detection of CHD using first-trimester techniques, including nuchal screening and Doppler assessment of the ductus venosus, is one such advance. As understanding of how congenital heart defects occur increases, particularly with research on the genes important in heart development, early detection potentially may lead to intervention or improved management. Improved detection also would afford the opportunity to obtain genetic information for parents and improve counseling, enabling families to make informed decisions about the future of an affected pregnancy.

Advances in three-dimensional ultrasound also hold promise of improving understanding of fetal cardiology. As data acquisition techniques advance, we may see the application of real-time, three-dimensional fetal echocardiography soon in the clinical setting.[26]

With respect to the management of fetal cardiac disease, the impact of prenatal diagnosis on outcome continues to be an important area for further research.

Outcome analyses comparing prenatal and postnatal diagnosis of CHD need to better estimate the true costs of care in larger populations to know if the data currently available are valid.[81] The rise of telemedicine and the potential for international case registries also may aid in assessment of outcomes and the impact of fetal echocardiography.

Regardless of whether objective data can show the impact of prenatal diagnosis on the management of CHD, the contribution of current fetal echocardiography to quality of care is considerable. Improved counseling of the families involved and the centralization of care for the mother and affected infant are among the benefits.

Developing prenatal intervention aimed at impacting the outcome of CHD remains important. Research continues in the area of prenatal interventional valvuloplasty and pharmacologic therapy. Early intervention has the potential to benefit many prenatally diagnosed conditions.

We must continue efforts to improve the prenatal detection and management of CHD. Most cases currently are diagnosed in pregnancies with no identifiable risk factors. The presence of routine screening programs complemented by regional centers specializing in fetal echocardiography will remain important as we move toward the future and its promise of advancements.

References

1. Dawes GS: Fetal and Neonatal Physiology. Chicago, Year Medical Publishers, 1968.
2. Kleinman CS, Hobbins JC, Jaffe CC, et al: Echocardiographic studies of the human fetus: Prenatal diagnosis of congenital heart disease and cardiac dysrhythmia. Pediatrics 65:1059, 1980.
3. Allan LD, Tynan M, Campbell S, et al: Echocardiographic and anatomical correlates in the fetus. Br Heart J 44:444, 1980.
4. Lange LW, Sahn DJ, Allen HB, et al: Qualitative real-time cross-sectional echocardiographic imaging of the human fetus during the second half of pregnancy. Circulation 62:799, 1980.
5. Devore GR: The prenatal diagnosis of congenital heart disease: A practical approach for the fetal sonographer. J Clin Ultrasound 13:229, 1985.
6. Allan LD, Crawford DC, Chita SK, Tynan MJ: Prenatal screening for congenital heart disease. BMJ 292:1717, 1986.
7. Wang KF, Xiao JP: Fetal echocardiography for pregnancy diagnosis. Chin J Obstet Gynecol 10:267, 1964.
8. Winsberg F: Echocardiography of the fetal and newborn heart. Invest Radiol 7:152, 1972.
9. Morin FC III: Fetal echocardiography. Doctoral thesis. Yale University School of Medicine, New Haven, 1976.
10. Maulik D, Saini VD, Nanda NC, Rosenzweig MS: Doppler evaluation of fetal hemodynamics. Ultrasound Med Biol 8:705, 1982.
11. Huhta JC, Strasburger JF, Carpenter RJ, et al: Pulsed Doppler fetal echocardiography. J Clin Ultrasound 13:247, 1985.
12. Izquierdo LA, Helfgott AW: Ultrasound evaluation of the fetal heart: Is it possible? Comp Ther 25:193, 1999.
13. Copel JA, Pilu G, Kleinman CS, et al: Assessment of the fetal heart with color Doppler flow mapping: Studies in normal and abnormal hearts. Abstract presented at Society of Perinatal Obstetricians Meeting, San Antonio, TX, 1986.
14. Ayers NA: Advances in fetal echocardiography. Tex Heart Inst J 24:250, 1997.
15. D'Amelio R, Giorlandino C, Masala L, et al: Fetal echocardiography using transvaginal and transabdominal probes during the first period of pregnancy: A comparative study. Prenat Diagn 11:69, 1991.
16. Yagel S, Achiron R, Ron M, et al: Transvaginal sonography at early pregnancy cannot replace mid-trimester targeted organ ultrasound examination in a high-risk population. Am J Obstet Gynecol 172:971, 1995.
17. Achiron R, Tadmor O: Screening for fetal anomalies during the first trimester of pregnancy: Transvaginal versus transabdominal sonography. Ultrasound Obstet Gynecol 1:186, 1991.
18. Bonilla-Musoles FM, Raga F, Ballester MJ, Serra V: Early detection of embryonic malformations by transvaginal and color Doppler sonography. J Ultrasound Med 13:347, 1994.
19. Yagel S, Weissman A, Rotstein Z, et al: Congenital heart defects: Natural course and in utero development. Circulation 96:550, 1997.
20. Devine PC, Simpson LL: Nuchal translucency and its relationship to congenital heart disease. Semin Perinatol 24:343, 2000.
21. Thomas JD, Rubin DN: Tissue harmonic imaging: Why does it work? J Am Soc Echocardiogr 11:803, 1998.
22. Chang, FM, Hsu KF, Ko HC, et al: Fetal heart volume assessment by three-dimensional ultrasound. Ultrasound Obstet Gynecol 9:42, 1997.
23. Michailidis GD, Simpson JM, Karidas C, Economides DL: Detailed three-dimensional fetal echocardiography facilitated by an Internet link. Ultrasound Obstet Gynecol 18:325 2001.
24. Nelson TR, Pretorius DH, Sklansky M, Hagen-Ansert S: Three-dimensional echocardiographic evaluation of fetal heart anatomy and function: Acquisition, analysis, and display. J Ultrasound Med 15:1, 1996.
25. Myer-Wittkopf M, Rappe N, Sierra F, et al: Three-dimensional (3-D) ultrasonography for obtaining the four and five chamber view: Comparison with cross-sectional (2-D) fetal sonographic screening. Ultrasound Obstet Gynecol 15:397, 2000.
26. Sklansky M, Nelson T, Strachan M, Pretorius D: Real-time three-dimensional fetal echocardiography: Initial feasibility study. J Ultrasound Med 18:745, 1999.
27. Kohl T, Sharland GK, Allan LD, et al: World experience of percutaneous ultrasound-guided balloon valvuloplasty in human fetuses with severe aortic valve obstruction. Am J Cardiol 85:1230, 2000.
28. Kohl T, Szabo Z, Suda K, et al: Fetoscopic and open transumbilical fetal cardiac catheterization in sheep: Potential approaches for human fetal cardiac intervention. Circulation 95:1048, 1997
29. Hoffman JIE, Christianson R: Congenital heart disease in a cohort of 19,502 births with long-term follow-up. Am J Cardiol 42:641, 1978.
30. Michels VV, Riccardi VM: Congenital heart defects. In Emery AE, Rimoin DL (eds): Principles and Practices of Medical Genetics, 2nd ed. Edinburgh, Churchill Livingstone, 1990, pp 1207-1237.
31. Burn J, Little J, Holloway S, et al: Recurrence risks in offspring of adults with major heart defects: Results from first cohort of British collaborative study. Lancet 351:311, 1998.

32. Payne RM, Johnson MC, Grant JW, Strauss AW: Toward a molecular understanding of congenital heart disease. Circulation 91:494, 1995.

33. Copel JA, Cullen M, Green JJ, et al: The frequency of aneuploidy in prenatally diagnosed congenital heart disease: An indication for fetal karyotyping. Am J Obstet Gynecol 158:409, 1988.

34. Ryan AK, Goodship JA, Wilson DI, et al: Spectrum of clinical features associated with interstitial chromosome 22q11 deletions: A European collaborative study. J Med Genet 54:798, 1997.

35. Copel JA, Pilu G, Kleinman CS: Congenital heart disease and extracardiac anomalies: Associations and indications for fetal echocardiography. Am J Obstet Gynecol 154:1121, 1986.

36. Copel JA, Liang RI, Dimasio K, et al: The clinical significance of the irregular fetal heart rhythm. Am J Obstet Gynecol 182:813, 2000.

37. Schmidt KG, Ulmer HE, Silverman NH, et al: Perinatal outcome of fetal complete atrioventricular block: A multicenter experience. J Am Coll Cardiol 17:1360, 1991.

38. Friedman AH, Copel JA, Kleinman CS: Fetal echocardiography and fetal cardiology: Indications, diagnosis, and management. Semin Perinatol 17:76, 1993.

39. Nicolaides KH, Azar G, Snijders RJ, Gosden CM: Fetal nuchal edema: Associated malformations and chromosomal defects. Fetal Diagn Ther 7:123, 1992.

40. Hyett JA, Perdu M, Sharland GK, et al: Increased nuchal translucency at 10-14 weeks of gestation as a marker for major cardiac defects. Ultrasound Obstet Gynecol 10:242, 1997.

41. Gildner Kiserud T: In a different vein: The ductus venosus could yield much valuable information. Ultrasound Obstet Gynecol 9:369, 1999.

42. Nora JJ: From generational studies to a multilevel genetic-environmental interaction. J Am Coll Cardiol 23:1459, 1994.

43. Hernandez-Diaz S, Werler M, Walker A, Mitchell A: Folic acid antagonists during pregnancy and the risk of birth defects. N Engl J Med 343:1608, 2000.

44. Rowland TW, Hubbell JP Jr, Nadas AS. Congenital heart disease in infants of diabetic mothers. J Pediatr 83:815, 1973.

45. Miller E, Hare JW, Cloherty JP, et al: Elevated maternal hemoglobin A1c in early pregnancy and major congenital anomalies in infants of diabetic mothers. N Engl J Med 304:1331, 1981.

46. Vela-Huerta MM, Vargas-Origel A, Olvera-Lopez A: Asymmetrical septal hypertrophy in newborn infants of diabetic mothers. Am J Perinatol 17:89, 2000.

47. Rizzo G, Arduini D, Romanini C: Cardiac function in fetuses of type I diabetic mothers. Am J Obstet Gynecol 164:837, 1991.

48. Fermont L, Batisse A, Piechaud JF, Kachaner J: Transitory hypertrophic cardiomyopathy in a newborn with a diabetic mother. Arch Fr Pediatr 37:113, 1980.

49. Rouse B, Azen C, Koch R, et al: Maternal Phenylketonuria Collaborative Study(MPKUS) offspring: Facial anomalies, malformation, and early neurological sequelae. Am J Med Genet 69:89, 1997.

50. Glickstein JS, Buyon J, Friedman D: Pulsed Doppler echocardiographic assessment of the fetal PR interval. Am J Cardiol 86:236, 2000.

51. Barclay CS, French MAH, Ross LD, et al: Successful pregnancy following steroid therapy and plasma exchange in a women with anti-Ro (SS-A) antibodies: Case report. Br J Obstet Gynaecol 94:369, 1987.

52. Yamada H, Kato EH, Ebina Y, et al: Fetal treatment of congenital heart block ascribed to anti-SSA antibody: Case reports with observation of cardiohemodynamics and review of the literature. Am J Reprod Immunol 42:226, 1999.

53. Shaw GM, O'Malley CD, Wasserman CR, et al: Maternal periconceptional use of multivitamins and reduced risk for conotruncal heart defects and limb deficiencies among offspring. Am J Med Genet 59:536, 1995.

54. Czeizel AE: Reduction of urinary tract and cardiovascular defects by periconceptional multivitamin supplementation. Am J Med Genet 62:179, 1996.

55. Botto LD, Khoury MJ, Mulinare J, Erickson JD: Periconceptional multivitamin use and occurrence of conotruncal heart defects: Results from a population-based, case-control study. Pediatrics 98:911, 1996.

56. Srivastava D: Genetic assembly of the heart: Implications for congenital heart disease. Annu Rev Physiol 63:451, 2001.

57. Achiron R, Glaser J, Gelernter I, et al: Extended fetal echocardiographic examination for detecting cardiac malformations in low risk pregnancies. BMJ 303:671, 1992.

58. Ewigman BG, Crane JP, Frigoletto FD, et al: Effect of prenatal ultrasound on perinatal outcome. N Engl J Med 329:821, 1993.

59. Garmel SH, D'alton ME: Fetal ultrasonography. West J Med 159:273, 1993.

60. Levi S: Ultrasound in prenatal diagnosis: Polemics around routine ultrasound screening for second trimester fetal malformations. Prenat Diagn 22:285, 2002.

61. Wigton TR, Sabbagha RE, Tamura RK, et al: Sonographic diagnosis of congenital heart disease: Comparison between the four-chamber view and multiple cardiac views. Obstet Gynecol 166:1473, 1992.

62. Stumpflen I, Stumpflen A, Wimmer M, Bernaschek G: Effect of detailed fetal echocardiography as part of prenatal ultrasonographic screening on detection of congenital heart disease. Lancet 348:854, 1996.

63. Ott WJ: The accuracy of antenatal fetal echocardiography screening in high and low-risk pregnancies. Am J Obstet Gynecol 172:1741, 1995.

64. Garne E, and the Eurocat working group: Prenatal diagnosis of six major cardiac malformations in Europe: A population based study. Acta Obstet Gynecol Scand 80:224, 2001.

65. Comstock CH: Normal fetal heart axis and position. Obstet Gynecol 70:255, 1987.

66. Allan LD, Lockhart S: Intrathoracic cardiac positioning the fetus. Ultrasound Obstet Gynecol 3:93, 1993.

67. Paladini D, Chita SK, Allan LD: Prenatal measurement of cardiothoracic ratio in evaluation of heart disease. Arch Dis Child 65:20, 1990.

68. Shipp TD, Bromley B, Nornberger LK, et al: Levorotation of the fetal cardiac axis: A clue for the presence of congenital heart disease. Obstet Gynecol 85:97, 1995.

69. Bork MD, et al. Fetal cardiac axis—a useful screening tool for congenital heart disease? Am J Obstet Gynecol 172:355, 1995.

70. Smith RS, Comstock CH, Kirk JS, Lee W: Ultrasonographic left cardiac axis in the detection of intrathoracic anomalies and congenital heart disease. Obstet Gynecol 85:187, 1995.

71. Copel JA, Pilu G, Green J, et al: Fetal echocardiographic screening for congenital heart disease: The importance of the four-chamber view. Am J Obstet Gynecol 157:648, 1987.

72. Fernandez CO, Ramaciott1 C, Martin LB, Twickler DM: The four-chamber view and its sensitivity in detecting congenital heart disease. Cardiology 90:202, 1998.

73. Yagel S, Cohen M, Achiron R: Examination of the fetal heart by five short-axis views: A proposed screening method for comprehensive cardiac examination. Ultrasound Obstet Gynecol 17:367, 2001.

74. Yoo SJ, Lee YH, Cho KS: Abnormal three-vessel view on sonography: A clue to the diagnosis of congenital heart disease in the fetus. AJR Am J Roentgenol 172:825, 1999.

75. Comstock C: What to expect from routine midtrimester screening for congenital heart disease. Semin Perinatol 24:331, 2000.

76. Devore GR, Medearis AL, Bear MB, et al: Fetal echocardiography: Factors that influence the imaging of the fetal heart during second trimester of pregnancy. J Ultrasound Med 12:659, 1993.

77. Budorick NE, Millman SL: New modalities for imaging the fetal heart. Semin Perinatol 24:352, 2000.

78. Todros T, Faggiano F, Chiappa E, et al: Accuracy of routine ultrasonography in screening heart disease prenatally. Gruppo Piemontese for Prenatal Screening of Congenital Heart Disease. Prenat Diagn 17:901, 1997.

79. Klein SK, Cans C, Robert E, Jouk PS: Efficacy of routine fetal ultrasound screening for congenital heart disease in Isere County, France. Prenat Diagn 19:319, 1999.

80. Kirk JS, Riggs TW, Comstock CH, et al: Prenatal screening for cardiac anomalies: The value of routine addition of the aortic toot to the four-chamber view. Obstet Gynecol 84:427, 1994.

81. Friedman AH, Kleinman CS, Copel JA: 2002 Diagnosis of cardiac defects: Where we've been, where we are and where we're going. Prenat Diagn 22:280, 2002.

82. Sharland GK, Lockhart SM, Chita SK, Allan LD: Factors influencing the outcome of congenital heat disease detected prenatally. Arch Dis Child 64:284, 1990.

83. Smythe JP, Copel JA, Kleinman CS: Outomce of prenatally detected cardiac malformations. Am J Cardiol 69:1471, 1992.

84. Simpson LL, Harvey-Wilkes K, D'Alton ME: Congenital heart disease: The impact of delivery in a tertiary care center on SNAP scores (scores for neonatal acute physiology). Am J Obstet Gynecol 182:184, 2000.

85. Hunter S, Heads A, Wyllie JP, et al: Prenatal diagnosis of congenital heart disease in the northern region of England: Benefits of a training programme for obstetric ultrasonographers. Heart 84:294, 2000

86. Copel JA, Tan AS, Kleinman CS: Does a prenatal diagnosis of congenital heart disease alter short-term outcome? Ultrasound Obstet Gynecol 10:237, 1997.

87. Bonnet D, Coltri A, Butera G, et al: Fetal detection of transposition of the great arteries reduces morbidity and mortality in newborn infants. Circulation 99:916, 1999.

88. Allan LD, Apfel HD, Printz BF: Outcome after prenatal diagnosis of the hypoplastic left heart syndrome. Heart 79:371, 1998.

89. Tworetzky W, McElhinney D, Reddy V, et al: Improved surgical outcome after fetal diagnosis of hypoplastic left heart. Circulation 103:1269, 2001.

90. Mahle W, Clancy R, McGaurn S, et al: Impact of prenatal diagnosis on survival and early neurologic morbidity in neonates with the hypoplastic left heart syndrome. Pediatrics 107:1277, 2001.

91. Mahle WT: Neurologic and cognitive outcomes in children with congenital heart disease. Curr Opin Pediatr 13:482, 2001.

92. Kumar RK, Newburger JW, Gauvreau K, et al: Comparison of outcome when hypoplastic left heart syndrome and transposition of the great arteries are diagnosed prenatally versus when diagnosis of these two conditions is made only postnatally. Am J Cardiol 83:1649, 1999.

93. Franklin O, Burch M, Manning N, et al: Prenatal diagnosis of coarctation of the aorta improves survival and reduces morbidity. Heart 87:67, 2002.

94. Verheijen PM, Lisowski LA, Stoutenbeek P, et al: Prenatal diagnosis of congenital heart disease affects preoperative acidosis in the newborn patient. J Thorac Cardiovasc Surg 121:798, 2001.

CHAPTER 60

Medical Management of Congenital Heart Disease

Daphne T. Hsu and Welton M. Gersony

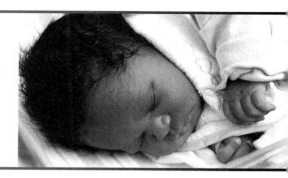

The medical management of a neonate with **congenital heart disease (CHD)** depends on the type of defect present, the clinical condition of the patient, and the medical or surgical options available for correction or palliation of the lesion. In 1980, Fyler[1] reported that 58% of infants diagnosed with CHD before age 1 year required hospital admission in the first month of life. Rapid referral of ill neonates to tertiary care centers via perinatal network systems and improved noninvasive echocardiographic techniques have allowed the early diagnosis of CHD. Even the most complex lesions can be diagnosed prenatally by fetal echocardiography.[2,3] Primary correction of many defects now is performed in the neonatal period.[4] Between the years 1979 and 1997, infant mortality from CHD decreased 38%, from 92 to 56 per 100,000 infants, in a large part due to improved surgical results.[5] The establishment of a detailed anatomic diagnosis by echocardiography or cardiac catheterization or both is a key factor in prognosis. The appropriate choice of operative procedure and the availability of excellent surgical skills also are crucial to ensuring the best outcome. In addition, aggressive state-of-the-art medical management is essential to optimize the condition of the patient before correction or palliation and to support the infant after cardiac surgery or interventional catheterization.

This chapter describes the physiology and types of clinical presentations seen in neonates with CHD. The focus is on the pharmacologic agents used to treat infants with structural heart disease and the indications for use of these agents in specific lesions. The therapeutic options (interventional catheterization or surgery or both) available to treat the most common congenital heart defects diagnosed in the neonatal period also are outlined.

CLINICAL PRESENTATION OF THE NEONATE WITH CONGENITAL HEART DISEASE

Transitional Circulation

A few congenital heart lesions, such as tricuspid valve disease with tricuspid insufficiency[6] and aortic atresia or critical aortic stenosis,[7] have been associated with an increased incidence of fetal demise. Most structural congenital heart lesions are asymptomatic in utero due to the dynamics of the **fetal circulation.** Fetal oxygenation does not depend on pulmonary blood flow, and defects associated with diminished pulmonary blood flow are silent in the fetus. Before birth, systemic output is provided by the right and the left ventricles, and there is free communication between the left and right circulations via the foramen ovale and ductus arteriosus. Lesions involving hypoplasia or obstruction of either ventricle are not apparent prenatally. After birth, when the pulmonary and systemic blood flows are separated, major changes in circulatory patterns lead to the hemodynamic and clinical expression of many congenital heart lesions. Three major hemodynamic events occur in the transition from fetal to postnatal circulation: (1) the ductus arteriosus and foramen ovale close, (2) pulmonary vascular resistance decreases, and (3) systemic vascular resistance increases secondary to the elimination of the placenta as a low-resistance circuit. After birth, specific cardiac abnormalities no longer can be compensated for, or bypassed, by fetal channels. The clinical presentation of a neonate with severe CHD commonly occurs during the period of transition from fetal to postnatal circulation.

Functional closure of the **patent ductus arteriosus (PDA)** normally occurs within 10 to 15 hours after birth as arterial partial pressure of oxygen (Po_2) increases and pulmonary blood flow increases. Although increasing oxygen saturation is an important stimulus, cyanotic CHD with hypoxemia does not preclude ductal closure. Decreased levels of circulating prostaglandins and decreased sensitivity of the ductus to the relaxant effect of prostaglandins also are significant stimuli to ductal constriction.[8]

Ductal closure is a devastating event for neonates with CHD who are dependent on the ductus arteriosus to provide pulmonary blood flow, to provide systemic blood flow, or to increase mixing between the pulmonary and systemic circulations. In patients with right ventricular outflow obstruction, such as tetralogy of Fallot, critical pulmonary stenosis, pulmonary atresia, tricuspid atresia, or Ebstein anomaly of the tricuspid valve, the ductus arteriosus provides pulmonary blood flow via left-to-right shunting from the aorta to the pulmonary artery. When the ductus closes in the first few days of life, infants with right ventricular outflow obstruction become increasingly hypoxemic, and the level of oxygen desaturation depends on the severity of obstruction to pulmonary blood flow. In patients with pulmonary atresia, ductal closure results in severe cyanosis, metabolic acidosis, and circulatory collapse.

In patients with left-sided obstructive lesions, such as coarctation of the aorta, interrupted aortic arch, aortic stenosis, or hypoplastic left heart syndrome, a PDA allows the right ventricle to augment an inadequate left ventricular output. Ductal closure results in diminished systemic blood flow, and infants present with congestive heart failure (CHF) and shock. In the presence of transposition of the great arteries, the ductus arteriosus may be a site of mixing of blood between the two parallel circulations (pulmonary and systemic). Ductal closure results in increased cyanosis because mixing is limited to bidirectional blood flow across the foramen ovale.

In normal infants, functional closure of the **foramen ovale** occurs soon after birth, as the profound increase in pulmonary blood flow results in increased pulmonary venous return and elevation of left atrial pressure. As left atrial pressure increases, the septum primum is flattened against the septum secundum, resulting in closure of the foramen ovale. This phenomenon is detrimental in many neonates with severe cyanotic heart disease. In patients with transposition of the great arteries with intact ventricular septum and a closed ductus, the foramen ovale, now the only site of communication between the parallel pulmonary and systemic circulations, becomes smaller, and the bidirectional shunt diminishes. This change results in severe cyanosis in the early neonatal period. In patients with hypoplastic left heart syndrome or various forms of mitral valve obstruction, pulmonary venous return cannot flow freely to the left ventricle, and shunting of blood occurs from the left atrium to the right atrium through the foramen ovale. As the foramen becomes smaller, left atrial pressure increases significantly, leading to pulmonary edema and respiratory distress. In patients with pulmonary atresia with intact ventricular septum or tricuspid atresia, systemic venous return must shunt to the left atrium via the foramen ovale. Often, patency of the foramen ovale is maintained by an increase in right atrial pressure, although in some cases, the foramen becomes restrictive, leading to venous congestion and low cardiac output.

Pulmonary vascular resistance is markedly elevated in fetal life, rapidly decreases at birth, and continues to decline more slowly thereafter, reaching normal low levels by 6 to 8 weeks of life. **Systemic vascular resistance** is low in utero because the placenta is a low-resistance circuit, and it increases dramatically when the umbilical cord is clamped. The relative difference between pulmonary and systemic resistances determines the degree of left-to-right shunting in unrestricted communications between the ventricles or great arteries, such as ventricular septal defect (VSD), endocardial cushion defect, PDA, and truncus arteriosus. As pulmonary resistance decreases over the first 1 to 2 months of life, left-to-right shunting increases, causing increased pulmonary blood flow and CHF due to volume overload of the left ventricle.

Total anomalous pulmonary venous return does not cause symptoms in utero because pulmonary venous return is minimal. Neonates with anomalous pulmonary venous return and pulmonary venous obstruction present soon after birth, as pulmonary blood flow increases and the infants develop progressive pulmonary venous congestion and severe respiratory distress.

In a newborn with CHD, the normal events that occur during the transition from the fetal to postnatal circulation are often detrimental and lead to clinical deterioration. Medical intervention is directed at reestablishing components of the fetal circulation, such as maintaining patency of the ductus arteriosus in left and right ventricular outflow obstruction or opening the atrial septum in transposition of the great arteries. Some centers propose maintaining neonates with hypoplastic left heart syndrome in a hypoxic or hypercarbic state to maintain fetal elevation of pulmonary vascular resistance, decrease pulmonary blood flow, and improve systemic oxygen delivery.[9] In contrast, when pulmonary hypertension occurs in neonates without CHD, medical therapy is directed toward rapidly facilitating the transition to a postnatal circulation by measures that lower pulmonary vascular resistance.

Physical Examination

CHD in neonates often is associated with cyanosis or CHF or both. **Cyanosis** is found in infants with decreased pulmonary blood flow due to right ventricular outflow obstruction (e.g., critical pulmonary stenosis, pulmonary atresia, tricuspid atresia, or tetralogy of Fallot). **CHF** occurs in the first week of life in patients with left ventricular outflow obstructive lesions (e.g., critical aortic stenosis or coarctation of the aorta). In patients with hypoplastic left heart syndrome, interrupted aortic arch, and preductal coarctation of the aorta, the right ventricle supplies the pulmonary and systemic output and remains hypertensive. Cardiac decompensation ensues shortly after birth as the ductus closes. Heart failure occurs later (3 to 8 weeks) in patients with a left-to-right shunt as pulmonary vascular resistance decreases slowly, and pulmonary blood flow gradually increases. Cyanosis and CHF occur in lesions with obligatory mixing of the pulmonary and systemic circulations (e.g., transposition of the great arteries, hypoplastic left heart syndrome, and total anomalous pulmonary venous return).

The cardiac examination of a neonate with CHD is helpful in identifying the presence of cyanosis or CHF, but auscultatory findings can be minimal even in patients with significant lesions. The presence of a significant systolic murmur in a neonate most often indicates valvar disease, either semilunar valve stenosis or atrioventricular valve regurgitation. In lesions with left-to-right shunting, systolic murmurs appear later in the postnatal period as pulmonary resistance decreases and the degree of shunting increases.

Hyperoxia Test

Hypoxemia in a neonate is secondary to either intrapulmonary or intracardiac shunting of deoxygenated blood into the systemic arterial circulation. The change in arterial P_{O_2} that occurs when a hypoxemic infant is ventilated with a fraction of inspired oxygen of 100% is a useful test to differentiate intrapulmonary from intracardiac shunting. If hypoxia is secondary to intrapulmonary shunting or hypoventilation, alveolar P_{O_2} rises as inspired oxygen increases, increasing capillary P_{O_2} and markedly increasing arterial P_{O_2}. In patients with intracardiac shunting, an increase in alveolar P_{O_2} does not affect arterial P_{O_2} significantly because deoxygenated blood bypasses the lungs. The hyperoxia test is most helpful in identifying a neonate with severe right ventricular outflow tract obstruction, such as pulmonary or tricuspid atresia. In these cases, the arterial P_{O_2} never increases to greater than 60 mm Hg, despite breathing 100% oxygen. In infants who are cyanotic due to the admixture of the systemic and pulmonary circulations, as in transposition of the great arteries, hypoplastic left heart syndrome, total anomalous pulmonary venous return, and truncus arteriosus, 100% oxygen can increase the arterial P_{O_2} by overcoming ventilation-perfusion inequalities secondary to CHF, although the arterial P_{O_2} should not increase to greater than 250 mm Hg.

Chest Radiography

The chest radiograph is an essential part of the evaluation of a neonate with CHD. It serves to rule out primary pulmonary disease as a cause of cyanosis and provides important information about the magnitude of pulmonary blood flow. If the infant is cyanotic, diminished pulmonary blood flow indicates right ventricular outflow obstruction, whereas normal to increased pulmonary blood flow points to cyanosis based on the admixture of the systemic and pulmonary circulations. Cardiac size is often normal or diminished in right ventricular outflow obstruction, transposition of the great vessels, and obstructed total anomalous pulmonary venous drainage; an enlarged heart is present in lesions associated with heart failure. An extremely prominent right atrial shadow is seen in Ebstein malformation of the tricuspid valve. A distinctive cardiac silhouette is associated with specific lesions and, if present, can be pathognomonic: A boot-shaped heart is seen in tetralogy of Fallot, the "egg on its side" shape is seen in transposition of the great arteries after thymus involution, and a "snowman" shape is seen in unobstructed supracardiac total anomalous pulmonary venous drainage.

Electrocardiogram

The electrocardiogram (ECG) is particularly useful in the differential diagnosis of a cyanotic newborn with decreased pulmonary blood flow (Fig. 60-1). In a normal newborn, the QRS axis is rightward (+90 to +180 degrees) owing to right ventricular hypertrophy in utero. Right-axis deviation also is seen in cyanotic lesions associated with right ventricular hypertrophy, such as tetralogy of Fallot or critical pulmonary stenosis. Pulmonary atresia with an intact ventricular septum is associated with a hypoplastic

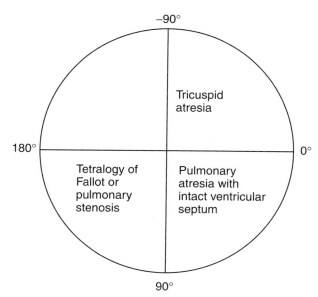

Figure 60–1. QRS axis in lesions with right ventricular outflow obstruction.

right ventricle, and a leftward (0 to +90 degrees) axis is seen on the ECG. In tricuspid atresia, late depolarization of the left superior bundle causes a left superior (0 to −90 degrees) QRS axis.

Right ventricular enlargement is seen when the right ventricle is contributing to systemic output, such as in preductal coarctation of the aorta, interrupted aortic arch, or hypoplastic left heart syndrome. Decreased left ventricular forces in the precordial leads and right ventricular hypertrophy with right axis also are seen in patients with hypoplastic left heart syndrome, although these ECG findings may not be diagnostic because right ventricular dominance occurs in normal newborns. The ECG in Ebstein malformation of the tricuspid valve is distinctive: right atrial enlargement, right bundle-branch block, prolonged P-R interval, and decreased right ventricular forces.

Echocardiography and Diagnostic Cardiac Catheterization

Two-dimensional echocardiography is used routinely to establish the anatomic diagnosis of CHD in the fetus and neonate and has obviated the need for diagnostic cardiac catheterization and its attendant risks in most cases. Echocardiography can rule out associated significant heart disease in a neonate with pulmonary disease, eliminating the need for hemodynamic studies. The examination of extracardiac structures is limited in two-dimensional echocardiography. The distal pulmonary arteries and pulmonary veins can be difficult to image, and in some cases, cardiac catheterization is indicated to delineate these structures (e.g., in cases of tetralogy of Fallot with pulmonary atresia or obstructed total anomalous pulmonary venous return). Coronary artery sinusoids associated with pulmonary atresia and intact ventricular septum are not well defined by echocardiography; angiography is indicated to document the coronary artery anatomy.

In addition to establishing the anatomic diagnosis, echocardiography has an important role in defining the pathophysiology of CHD. Color Doppler imaging can be used to determine patterns of blood flow (right-to-left shunting versus left-to-right shunting) through cardiac defects and to assess atrioventricular valve competence. Color Doppler also identifies the location of flow turbulence, indicating the presence of obstruction or regurgitation or both. Continuous wave Doppler can be used to quantify the velocity of flow across a narrowed area, such as a valve orifice, allowing an estimation of the pressure gradient.

The ability of fetal and postnatal echocardiography to establish the diagnosis of significant CHD rapidly and noninvasively has enabled appropriate medical interventions to be initiated in a neonate soon after clinical presentation and in some cases before hemodynamic compromise. Therapeutic interventions, at catheterization or surgery, can then be planned carefully and executed in infants who are in optimal condition.

MANAGEMENT OF THE DUCTUS ARTERIOSUS

Physiology of the Patent Ductus Arteriosus

Histologically the ductus arteriosus differs from aortic and pulmonary artery tissue by the paucity of elastic tissue and the large amount of smooth muscle cells found in its vessel wall. In fetal life, patency of the ductus arteriosus is maintained by low oxygenation and endogenously produced prostaglandins, specifically prostaglandin E_2. After birth, stimuli to ductal closure include increased oxygenation, a decreased sensitivity to the relaxant effect of prostaglandin, and the loss of the placenta as a source of circulating prostaglandin E_2. As the smooth muscle contracts, a mucoid substance in the ductal wall coalesces and protrudes into the vessel lumen. As the lumen narrows, ductal blood flow decreases, leading to ischemia of the media and intima, fibrous tissue formation, and transformation of the ductus arteriosus into the ligamentum arteriosum. Maintaining patency of the ductus arteriosus is a cornerstone in the management of a neonate with complex CHD.

Patent Ductus Arteriosus and Congenital Heart Disease

Before the use of prostaglandin E_1 (PGE$_1$), neonates with ductal-dependent CHD (Table 60-1) presented one of the major management problems in neonatal cardiology. In the late 1970s, PGE$_1$ was shown to dilate a constricted ductus arteriosus.[10] Clinical studies soon followed, showing that PGE$_1$ effectively increased pulmonary blood flow in infants with cyanotic CHD and increased systemic blood flow in patients with aortic arch anomalies.[11-13] This effect occurred with dosages that did not cause significant decreases in systemic or pulmonary arterial pressure. PGE$_1$ was found to be less effective in dilating the ductus arteriosus after 96 hours of life.

The usual dose of PGE$_1$ is 0.05 to 0.2 µg/kg/min. PGE$_1$ must be administered as a continuous intravenous infusion because more than 80% is metabolized in the first

pass through the liver or lungs. Metabolites are excreted via the kidney within 24 hours after administration. The side effects of PGE$_1$ are listed in Table 60-2. The most significant side effect is apnea, which occurs suddenly. Measures must be taken to provide adequate respiratory support, especially if PGE$_1$ is to be administered to an infant with respiratory compromise or during transport to a tertiary care center.

Persistent Patency of the Ductus Arteriosus

Persistent PDA in premature infants has been associated with prolonged respiratory compromise and a higher incidence of bronchopulmonary dysplasia in infants with respiratory distress syndrome.[14] PDA also has been associated with other long-term sequelae of prematurity, such as necrotizing enterocolitis[15] and intraventricular hemorrhage.[16,17] As the pulmonary resistance decreases after birth, a large left-to-right shunt can occur through the PDA, leading to ventricular failure and pulmonary edema. Closure of the PDA, either medically using indomethacin or by surgical ligation, has been shown to improve outcome in premature infants (see Chapter 58).[18]

TREATMENT OF CONGESTIVE HEART FAILURE

CHF due to ventricular dysfunction can occur in neonates with severe left ventricular outflow tract obstruction or primary myocardial disease, such as cardiomyopathy or myocarditis. Neonates with cyanotic heart disease also

Table 60-1. Ductal-Dependent Congenital Heart Disease

Severe Right Ventricular Outflow Obstruction

Tetralogy of Fallot with severe pulmonary stenosis/atresia
Critical pulmonary stenosis
Pulmonary atresia with intact ventricular septum
Tricuspid atresia
Severe Ebstein anomaly

Severe Left Ventricular Outflow Obstruction

Preductal coarctation of the aorta
Interrupted aortic arch
Critical aortic stenosis
Hypoplastic left heart syndrome
Mitral atresia

Table 60-2. Side Effects of Prostaglandin E$_1$

Pyrexia
Apnea/hypoventilation
Cutaneous vasodilation
Seizures/jitteriness
Diarrhea
Systemic hypotension

may develop ventricular dysfunction after severe hypoxemia and acidosis. CHF also occurs in infants with normal ventricular function who have ventricular volume overload on the basis of a large intracardiac shunt or valvar insufficiency. Heart failure also is a common finding in the early period after surgical intervention.

Respiratory distress is the common presentation of CHF. As left ventricular end-diastolic pressures increase, left atrial and pulmonary venous pressure increases, and pulmonary edema ensues. Medical therapy of CHF in neonates includes (1) treating the underlying physiologic abnormality (e.g., increasing systemic blood flow via the ductus arteriosus in infants with severe left ventricular outflow obstruction using PGE_1), (2) reversing metabolic acidosis, (3) improving cardiac performance by increasing contractility, and (4) altering the preload or afterload (or both) burdens of the heart.

Inotropic Agents

Three classes of medications are used to increase the contractility of the neonatal myocardium: (1) sympathomimetic amines, (2) phosphodiesterase inhibitors, and (3) digitalis glycosides. The first two classes are used in an intensive care setting for hemodynamic stabilization of a neonate with CHF. Digitalis glycosides are used widely in infants with CHD with a large left-to-right shunt, although their usefulness in acute heart failure is limited. Sympathomimetic amines, such as dopamine or dobutamine, are used commonly to increase myocardial contractility and cardiac output in neonates. In general, isoproterenol is used less in the newborn because its chronotropic effect is more potent than that of dopamine and dobutamine.

Phosphodiesterase Inhibitors

Amrinone and milrinone are positive inotropic agents with potent vasodilatory properties. Their mechanism of action is inhibition of myocardial cyclic adenosine monophosphate phosphodiesterase activity, which indirectly results in increased intracellular cyclic adenosine monophosphate levels. Side effects include arrhythmias, hypotension, and dose-related thrombocytopenia and hepatotoxicity. Phosphodiesterase inhibitors may be used alone or in conjunction with the sympathomimetic amines in neonates with severe CHF and offer an alternative treatment when sympathomimetic amines are contraindicated.[19] The pulmonary or systemic vasodilation effects of these agents can be beneficial in patients with abnormally elevated pulmonary or systemic vascular resistance.[20] Phosphodiesterase inhibitors should not be administered, however, to patients with hypovolemia or a fixed systemic outflow obstruction because of the risk of hypotension.

Diuretics

Altering preload is an important component of improving the clinical condition of infants with CHF. Fluid retention results from low cardiac output and decreased renal perfusion, leading to pulmonary edema and hepatic congestion. Ventricular contractility also is compromised by massive ventricular volume overload. Diuretics, such as furosemide, alleviate venous congestion and improve

ventricular contractility. In rare cases, infants in CHF may be volume depleted from poor oral intake or overdiuresis, and fluid administration is needed to increase intravascular volume.

Neurohormonal Antagonists

Altering the afterload conditions in an infant with CHD and CHF must be undertaken with care. In lesions with fixed left ventricular outflow obstruction, decreasing systemic vascular resistance is contraindicated because hypotension can decrease coronary blood flow and compromise myocardial oxygen supply. In infants with CHF secondary to a left-to-right shunt, the use of angiotensin-converting enzyme inhibitors or β-blockade therapy is controversial. Several small series report the use of angiotensin-converting enzyme inhibition or β blockade in the setting of heart failure in infants, with variable results.[21-26]

Nitric Oxide

The selective pulmonary vasodilator nitric oxide is used routinely to treat hypoxic respiratory failure in newborns.[27] Nitric oxide has been used to decrease pulmonary vascular resistance in patients with CHD and low pulmonary blood flow due to pulmonary artery hypertension, such as Ebstein anomaly. Nitric oxide also has been effective when used to lower pulmonary vascular resistance in infants with pulmonary hypertensive crises during the early postoperative period.[28]

MANAGEMENT OF THE NEONATE WITH CONGENITAL HEART DISEASE

This section outlines the presentation, general management, and therapeutic approaches for the congenital heart lesions most commonly diagnosed in neonates.

Right Ventricular Outflow Obstruction

Tetralogy of Fallot

Tetralogy of Fallot, a constellation of lesions arising from malalignment of the conal septum during cardiac development, consists of a large VSD, pulmonary stenosis or atresia, an overriding aorta, and right ventricular hypertrophy. Neonates present with varying degrees of cyanosis depending on the degree of pulmonary stenosis. Most neonates with tetralogy of Fallot are mildly cyanotic, and some may even present with the clinical picture of a VSD and left-to-right shunt in the late neonatal period. The prominent clinical feature is the murmur of pulmonary stenosis, but this finding is absent in pulmonary atresia. The diagnosis of tetralogy of Fallot can be established noninvasively using echocardiography. Cardiac catheterization is performed only if the echocardiogram suggests the presence of peripheral pulmonary artery stenoses and surgery in the neonatal period is planned.

Most neonates with tetralogy of Fallot do not require intervention in the neonatal period. If cyanosis is severe, it may be necessary to administer PGE_1 to maintain ductal patency and increase pulmonary blood flow. In these cases, two surgical approaches are undertaken: An aortopulmonary shunt may be placed, anticipating complete surgical repair at an older age, or selected patients may undergo open heart correction in the neonatal period.[29] The size of the pulmonary arteries and anatomy of the pulmonary collateral vessels influence decision making in severe tetralogy of Fallot, especially when pulmonary atresia is present.

Critical Pulmonary Stenosis

In neonates with **critical pulmonary stenosis**, right ventricular hypertrophy leads to diminished right ventricular compliance, and right-to-left shunting occurs via the foramen ovale; this results in cyanosis at rest or with agitation. Pulmonary blood flow may depend on ductal patency. A prominent harsh systolic ejection murmur is present along the left sternal border, unless cardiac output is compromised by critical obstruction. The diagnosis can be established by echocardiography. If the ECG and echocardiogram indicate the presence of systemic-to-suprasystemic right ventricular pressure, percutaneous pulmonary balloon valvuloplasty or surgical valvotomy is performed in the neonatal period to relieve the obstruction. As with other lesions involving mechanical obstruction, prolonged medical management is not indicated.

Pulmonary Atresia with Intact Ventricular Septum

In **pulmonary atresia with intact ventricular septum,** an obligatory right-to-left shunt occurs through the foramen ovale, and pulmonary blood flow is supplied by the PDA. Right ventricular and tricuspid valve hypoplasia are found in 90% of cases. Right ventricular dilation with or without Ebstein anomaly of the tricuspid valve and tricuspid insufficiency are present in the remaining 10%. In some patients with right ventricular hypoplasia, direct communications between the coronary arterial system and the right ventricle occur via sinusoids in the right ventricular myocardium.[30] In these cases, coronary blood flow may occur via either normal antegrade flow from the aorta or retrograde flow via the sinusoids from a right ventricle with suprasystemic pressure.

As the ductus closes, the patient with pulmonary atresia and an intact ventricular septum becomes profoundly cyanotic and the prompt administration of PGE_1 to maintain ductal patency is essential. Often the physical examination is noncontributory. A murmur of tricuspid insufficiency may be present in some cases. The diagnosis can be established by echocardiography; however, cardiac catheterization may be necessary to assess right ventricular size and to determine the existence of sinusoidal connections to the coronary arteries.

Neonatal surgery for pulmonary atresia with intact ventricular septum most commonly involves opening the right ventricular outflow tract to allow increased blood flow through the right ventricle and encourage right ventricular growth, with the final goal of achieving a four-chamber heart. In most patients who undergo relief of outflow tract obstruction, an aortopulmonary shunt is placed because right ventricular hypoplasia or decreased right ventricular compliance or both continue to impede antegrade pulmonary flow. In some cases, right ventricular hypoplasia is severe, and the cavity size is believed to be inadequate to allow sufficient blood flow to the lungs.

In these patients, the outflow tract is not opened, and an aortopulmonary shunt is carried out in the neonatal period, with a Fontan operation performed later. If coronary blood flow is supplied from a suprasystemic right ventricle via sinusoidal connections, widely opening the right ventricular outflow tract causes a rapid decrease in right ventricular pressure. This decrease in pressure results in decreased coronary blood flow, leading to myocardial ischemia and, potentially, myocardial infarction. In such cases, cardiac transplantation is considered because of the risk of myocardial infarction and death.

Tricuspid Atresia

Tricuspid atresia is the absence of the connection between the right atrium and the right ventricle. Systemic venous return flows from the right atrium across the foramen ovale to the left atrium. Almost all patients have a VSD, allowing the flow of blood from the left ventricle to the right ventricle, and then to the pulmonary artery. The degree of pulmonary blood flow depends on the size of the VSD. Some infants with a large VSD may present with increased pulmonary blood flow and CHF, whereas most infants have a small defect and present with cyanosis from right ventricular hypoplasia and pulmonary stenosis. Some patients have tricuspid and pulmonary atresia. Tricuspid atresia also may be associated with transposition of the great arteries; under these circumstances, the size of the VSD controls aortic blood flow. If the VSD is small, patients have the clinical presentation of critical aortic stenosis. Physical examination of an infant with tricuspid atresia is variable, depending on the underlying anatomy. A systolic ejection murmur of pulmonary stenosis or the holosystolic murmur of a VSD (or both) can be heard.

If pulmonary atresia or severe pulmonary stenosis is present, ductal patency is maintained with PGE_1 infusion to achieve adequate oxygenation, and an aortopulmonary shunt is placed. If the VSD is large, CHF develops as pulmonary resistance decreases, and treatment with digoxin and diuretics is required. In cases of tricuspid atresia and transposition of the great arteries without pulmonary stenosis, massive pulmonary blood flow can occur, and pulmonary artery banding may be needed to control CHF. Later in life, children with tricuspid atresia undergo the palliative Fontan procedure to separate the pulmonary and systemic circulations.

Ebstein Anomaly of the Tricuspid Valve

Ebstein anomaly of the tricuspid valve is characterized by redundant tricuspid valve tissue and displacement of the valve annulus into the body of the right ventricle as a result of adherence of the medial or posterior aspect (or both) of the valve leaflet to the interventricular septum. Tricuspid valve function in Ebstein anomaly ranges from normal to severely incompetent. The usual elevated right ventricular pressure in the newborn exacerbates tricuspid insufficiency, increasing the degree of right-to-left atrial shunting through the foramen ovale, leading to cyanosis. As pulmonary vascular resistance decreases and right ventricular pressure declines, tricuspid insufficiency decreases, and cyanosis improves or resolves. Pulmonary stenosis or atresia occasionally can be associated with

Ebstein anomaly. Physical examination of a neonate with Ebstein anomaly is remarkable for a holosystolic murmur of tricuspid insufficiency and the presence of one or more extra heart sounds during systole.

In cases of severe cyanosis, a ductal pathway is maintained by PGE_1 to provide adequate oxygenation until the pulmonary resistance decreases. Nitric oxide may be used to accelerate the decrease in pulmonary vascular resistance. If tricuspid insufficiency is severe, profound cyanosis and heart failure may result; this clinical situation is associated with a poor outcome. Surgical repair or replacement of the valve has been successful in older patients, but results in neonates have not been encouraging. Wolff-Parkinson-White syndrome and supraventricular arrhythmias are common in infants with Ebstein anomaly, and antiarrhythmic therapy may be required.

Cyanotic Mixing Lesions

Transposition of the Great Arteries

In simple **transposition of the great arteries**, the aorta arises from the right ventricle, and the pulmonary artery arises from the left ventricle. The systemic and pulmonary circulations operate in parallel. Mixing between the two circulations is possible only via the foramen ovale and ductus arteriosus. Cyanosis is apparent soon after birth, and prompt intervention is almost always necessary to prevent severe hypoxemia, acidosis, and circulatory compromise. PGE_1 is used to maintain ductal patency, but elevated pulmonary vascular resistance limits the amount of mixing that can occur. The Rashkind procedure (balloon atrial septostomy) can achieve more adequate mixing at the atrial level and improve oxygenation. The Rashkind procedure should be performed emergently in infants with severe cyanosis. If the arterial switch procedure can be performed immediately, the Rashkind procedure may not be needed.

The arterial switch procedure is the treatment of choice for transposition of the great arteries because the normal pattern of circulation in the heart is restored. Excellent surgical results after the arterial switch procedure in the neonatal period have been reported with 95% 5-year survival at some institutions.[31] The main pulmonary artery and aortic root are transected, the aortic root is anastomosed above the left semilunar valve, and the main pulmonary artery is anastomosed above the right semilunar valve. The coronary arteries are excised from the neopulmonary root and reimplanted in the neoaortic root. The switch procedure ideally should be performed within the first month of life, before pulmonary artery pressure declines and left ventricular hypertrophy regresses. If an infant with transposition of the great arteries presents after 1 month of age, careful assessment of left ventricular mass and pressure is made using echocardiography or catheterization or both to determine if the left ventricle is adequate to support the systemic circulation. If the left ventricular mass is inadequate, a two-stage approach to the arterial switch procedure is recommended. Initially the pulmonary artery is banded to encourage left ventricular hypertrophy, and an aortopulmonary shunt is placed to allow adequate pulmonary blood flow. When echocardiographic evidence of left ventricular hypertrophy is shown (usually 5 to 7 days after the initial surgery), the arterial switch procedure is performed.

VSD is the lesion most commonly associated with transposition of the great arteries. If the defect is small, the physiology is similar to simple transposition. If the defect is large, adequate mixing can be achieved between the circulations via the VSD, and cyanosis is less severe. Closure of the VSD is performed at the time of the arterial switch procedure. The arterial switch procedure cannot be performed in the presence of significant pulmonary valve stenosis. In a neonate with transposition of the great arteries, VSD, and pulmonary stenosis, a balloon atrial septostomy is performed to increase atrial mixing, and if severe cyanosis is present, an aortopulmonary shunt is placed. Later in life, an intracardiac repair (Rastelli operation) is done.

Total Anomalous Pulmonary Venous Return

Total anomalous pulmonary venous return is an abnormal connection of the pulmonary veins to the right atrium or to the supradiaphragmatic or infradiaphragmatic venous system. An associated widely patent foramen ovale or atrial septal defect is essential to enable venous return to the left atrium. Pulmonary venous obstruction almost always is present in a symptomatic neonate with isolated total anomalous pulmonary venous return to the infradiaphragmatic venous system. These infants have the clinical picture of pulmonary venous congestion and pulmonary edema, which can be difficult to distinguish from the respiratory distress syndrome. Cardiac examination is often unremarkable. The diagnosis is established by echocardiography; cardiac catheterization is necessary in some cases to determine the exact location of the connection between the pulmonary and the systemic venous system, especially if there appear to be multiple sites. Surgical correction is performed in the neonatal period by establishing a wide communication between the pulmonary veins and the left atrium, while ligating the anomalous connection to the systemic venous system. After successful surgery, the long-term prognosis is excellent.

Hypoplastic Left Heart Syndrome

Hypoplastic left heart syndrome is characterized by severe left ventricular hypoplasia and various combinations of severe aortic stenosis or atresia and severe mitral stenosis or atresia. The left ventricle cannot supply adequate cardiac output, and pulmonary venous return shunts from the left atrium via the foramen ovale to the right atrium. The right ventricle supplies the pulmonary and the systemic circulation via the ductus arteriosus. Coronary blood flow is retrograde from the hypoplastic ascending aorta. Infants with hypoplastic left heart syndrome present soon after birth with CHF and circulatory collapse as the ductus closes. Medical therapy with PGE_1 is essential to allow the right ventricle to support the systemic circulation via the ductus arteriosus, and inotropic support often is needed to treat CHF.

Historically, hypoplastic left heart syndrome was not amenable to surgical intervention. Two surgical options are currently available, however. Neonatal orthotopic heart transplantation is an accepted treatment for hypoplastic left heart syndrome. Transplantation restores the normal circulatory pattern of a four-chambered heart in a single surgical procedure. Disadvantages of the procedure include the length of time spent waiting for an appropriate donor, increased susceptibility to infections secondary to immunosuppression, the risk of allograft rejection, and uncertainty regarding the long-term effects of immunosuppression. Survival after orthotopic transplantation for hypoplastic left heart syndrome has been reported to be 70% to 86%[32,33] at 1 year and 68% to 80% at 5 years.[33,34]

The Norwood procedure is the other surgical option for treatment of hypoplastic left heart syndrome. The first stage of the Norwood procedure is perfomed in the neonatal period and includes (1) transecting the main pulmonary artery, anastomosing the main pulmonary trunk to the aorta, and enlarging the hypoplastic aortic arch to allow the right ventricle to provide systemic output; (2) providing controlled blood flow to the distal pulmonary arteries via an aortopulmonary shunt or right ventricle-to-pulmonary artery connection; and (3) performing an atrial septectomy to ensure free flow of the pulmonary venous return to the right atrium. Two further procedures are performed in the first few years of life (bidirectional Glenn shunt or hemi-Fontan procedure) to separate the pulmonary from the systemic circulation by ligating the aortopulmonary shunt and anastomosing the superior and inferior vena cavae directly to the pulmonary artery.

The Norwood I procedure is contraindicated in the presence of severe right ventricular dysfunction or tricuspid insufficiency because the right ventricle must be able to support the pulmonary and the systemic output. The disadvantages of the Norwood approach are the need for three cardiac surgeries in early childhood and the palliative nature of the procedure, which requires the single right ventricle to supply systemic output. The results of the Norwood I procedure have improved since the first procedures were performed in 1979,[35] with the best centers reporting an 81% 1-year survival after the first stage and a 95% operative survival after the completion of the Fontan procedure.[36,37]

The decision as to which surgical intervention to offer a patient with hypoplastic left heart syndrome depends on the clinical condition of the infant and the local surgical expertise available.[38] Right ventricular function and tricuspid valve competency must be assessed to determine if the infant is a candidate for the Norwood I procedure. Careful discussion with the parents regarding the risks and benefits of both surgical modalities should be undertaken.

Truncus Arteriosus

Truncus arteriosus is failure of septation of the truncal root during fetal development, leaving a single truncal valve rather than an aortic and pulmonary valve. The aorta and pulmonary artery arise from a common truncal root. The truncal valve is abnormal and may be insufficient; a VSD is always present. If there is significant truncal valve insufficiency, CHF develops in the early neonatal period. Otherwise, CHF may be delayed until 3 to 6 weeks of life, when pulmonary vascular resistance has decreased and the left-to-right shunt increases. If truncal valve insufficiency is present, an early high-pitched decrescendo diastolic murmur is heard along the left sternal border.

Treatment of CHF with digoxin and diuretics is often necessary, and surgical repair of the truncus arteriosus may be required urgently in the neonatal period and should be performed within the first 3 months of life to prevent the development of fixed pulmonary arterial hypertension. Correction of truncus arteriosus involves (1) excising the pulmonary artery with repair of the defect created in the truncal root; (2) establishing a connection between the right ventricle and the pulmonary artery, either directly or with the use of a valved conduit; and (3) closing the VSD. If severe truncal valve insufficiency is present, the truncal valve may require repair or replacement, but this is a rare requirement.

Left Ventricular Outflow Obstruction

Aortic Stenosis

Critical **aortic stenosis** presents in neonates with CHF, low cardiac output, and left ventricular dysfunction. Physical examination may reveal a systolic ejection murmur of aortic stenosis, although this finding may not be present if the infant is in a low-output state. A gallop rhythm may be appreciated. Inotropic support should be instituted promptly, and PGE_1 may be necessary to augment cardiac output. Aortic stenosis can be associated with other left-sided obstructive lesions, such as hypoplastic aortic annulus, a tunnel-like diffuse narrowing of the entire left ventricular outflow tract, coarctation of the aorta, or supravalvar or subvalvar aortic stenosis. Two treatment modalities are available in the neonatal period: balloon dilation of the aortic valve or surgical valvotomy.

Coarctation of the Aorta

Coarctation of the aorta is a constriction of the aorta, either discrete or of significant length, almost invariably located at the junction of the ductus arteriosus and the aortic arch, just distal to the left subclavian artery (juxtaductal). The location of constriction relative to blood flow through the ductus arteriosus determines the blood supply to the descending aorta. If the constriction is preductal, lower trunk blood flow is supplied predominantly by the right ventricle via the ductus arteriosus, and cyanosis is present distal to the coarctation (the "harlequin syndrome"). If the constriction is postductal, blood supply to the lower trunk remains compromised despite the presence of a PDA. Associated lesions are common with coarctation and include bicuspid aortic valve, mitral valve anomalies, other aortic arch anomalies, and VSD. A neonate with severe coarctation of the aorta presents with CHF. Differential blood pressures between the upper and lower extremities may not exist if the ductus is widely patent. If the ductus closes, a pressure gradient can be measured.

Medical management of CHF is required in cases of severe coarctation to stabilize the infant before surgical repair. With severe preductal coarctation, ductal patency may be maintained with PGE_1 to supply blood to the lower body. Surgical repair is performed in the neonatal period if CHF is severe or if distal aortic blood flow depends on ductal flow. In cases of coarctation of the aorta associated with VSD, closure of the VSD may not be performed at the time of coarctation repair because the VSD can become hemodynamically insignificant in 40% of patients.[39] In many cases, both lesions are repaired during the neonatal period with excellent results.[40]

Interrupted Aortic Arch

Interruption of the aortic arch occurs when a segment of the transverse or descending aorta becomes atretic. Transverse aortic arch hypoplasia and VSD are often associated lesions. Similar to preductal coarctation of the aorta, blood flow to the ascending aorta proximal to the interruption is supplied by the left ventricle, and blood flow to the aorta distal to the interruption is supplied by the PDA. The clinical presentation is one of CHF and circulatory collapse as the ductus closes. PGE_1 is used to maintain ductal patency, and treatment of CHF is indicated. Surgical repair of the interruption is performed in the neonatal period by (1) mobilizing and enlarging the hypoplastic transverse arch, (2) resecting the atretic segment, (3) anastomosing the proximal and distal portions of the aorta, and (4) closing the VSD.

Left Ventricular Volume Overload Lesions: Ventricular Septal Defect, Patent Ductus Arteriosus, Endocardial Cushion Defect

Timing of the presentation of intracardiac defects characterized by left-to-right shunting depends on pulmonary vascular resistance. Often, these lesions are clinically silent in the first few weeks after birth, when pulmonary vascular resistance is high. CHF usually develops between 3 and 6 weeks of age as pulmonary flow increases and left ventricular volume overload progresses. CHF may occur sooner in a premature infant because pulmonary vascular resistance is lower at birth and because the immature fetal myocardium is less able to compensate for the increased ventricular volume load. Medical management involves treatment of CHF with digoxin and diuretics. The use of β blockade and afterload reduction is controversial. Surgical repair of these lesions is indicated at any age if failure to thrive or frequent pulmonary infections persist despite medical therapy.

References

1. Fyler DC: Report of the New England regional infant cardiac program. Pediatrics 65(suppl):375, 1980.
2. Allan LD, Sharland GK, Milburn A, et al: The prospective diagnosis of 1006 consecutive cases of congenital heart disease in the fetus. J Am Coll Cardiol 23:1452, 1994.
3. Montana E, Khoury MJ, Cragan JD, et al: Trends and outcomes after prenatal diagnosis of congenital cardiac malformations by fetal echocardiography in a well defined birth population, Atlanta, Georgia 1990-1994.J Am Coll Cardiol 28:1805, 1996.
4. Castaneda AR, Mayer JE, Jonas RA, et al: The neonate with critical congenital heart disease: Repair—a surgical challenge. J Thorac Cardiovasc Surg 98(5 pt 2):869, 1989.
5. Boneva RS, Botto LD, Moore CA, et al: Mortality associated with congenital heart defects in the United States. Circulation 103:2376, 2001.
6. Hornberger LK, Sahn DJ, Kleinman CS, et al: Tricuspid valve disease with significant tricuspid insufficiency in the fetus: Diagnosis and outcome. J Am Coll Cardiol 17:167, 1991.
7. Smythe JF, Copel JA, Kleinman CS: Outcome of prenatally detected cardiac malformations. Am J Cardiol 69:1471, 1992.
8. Barst RJ, Gersony WM: The pharmacological treatment of patent ductus arteriosus: A review of the evidence. Drugs 38:249, 1989.
9. Tabbutt S, Ramamoorthy C, Montenegro LM, et al: Impact of inspired gas mixtures on preoperative infants with hypoplastic left heart syndrome during controlled ventilation. Circulation 104(suppl):I159-I164, 2001.
10. Elliott RB, Starling MD: The effects of prostaglandin F2 alpha in the closure of the ductus arteriosus. Prostaglandins 2:399, 1972.
11. Freed MD, Heyman MA, Lewis AB, et al: Prostaglandin E1 in infants with ductus arteriosus-dependent congenital heart disease. Circulation 64:899, 1981.
12. Heymann MA, Rudolph AM: Ductus arteriosus dilatation by prostaglandin E1 in infants with pulmonary atresia. Pediatrics 59:325, 1977.
13. Heymann MA, Berman WJ, Rudolph AM, Whitman V: Dilation of the ductus arteriosus by prostaglandin E1 in aortic arch abnormalities. Circulation 59:169, 1979.
14. Dudell GG, Gersony WM: Patent ductus arteriosus in neonates with severe respiratory distress. J Pediatr 104:914, 1984.
15. Cassady G, Crouse DT, Kirklin JW, et al: A randomized, controlled trial of very early prophylactic ligation of the ductus arteriosus in babies who weighed 1000 g or less at birth. N Engl J Med 320:1511, 1989.
16. Perlman JM, Hill A, Volpe JJ: The effect of patent ductus arteriosus on flow velocity in the anterior cerebral arteries: Ductal steal in the premature newborn infant. J Pediatr 99:767, 1981.
17. Martin CG, Snider AR, Katz SM, et al: Abnormal cerebral blood flow patterns in preterm infants with a large patent ductus arteriosus. J Pediatr 101:587, 1982.
18. Gersony W, Peckham G, Ellison R, et al: Effects of indomethacin in premature infants with patent ductus arteriosus: Results of a national collaborative study. J Pediatr 102:895, 1983.
19. Bailey J, Miller B, Lu W, et al: The pharmacokinetics of milrinone in pediatric patients after cardiac surgery. Anesthesiology 90:1012, 1999.
20. Robinson BW, Gelband H, Mas MS: Selective pulmonary and systemic vasodilator effects of amrinone in children: New therapeutic implications. J Am Coll Cardiol 21:1461, 1993.
21. Frenneaux M, Stewart R, Newman C, Hallidie-Smith K: Enalapril for severe heart failure in infancy. Arch Dis Child 64:219, 1989.
22. Dutertre J, Billaud E, Autret E, et al: Inhibition of angiotensin converting enzyme with enalapril maleate in infants with congestive heart failure. Br J Clin Pharm 35:528, 1993.
23. Scammell A, Arnold R, Wilkinson J: Captopril in treatment of infant heart failure: A preliminary report. Int J Cardiol 16:295, 1987.
24. Shaw N, Wilson N, Dickinson D: Captopril in heart failure secondary to a left to right shunt. Arch Dis Child 63:360, 1988.

25. Rheuban K, Carpenter M, Ayers C, Gutgesell H: Acute hemodynamic effects of converting enzyme inhibition in infants with congestive heart failure. J Pediatr 117:668, 1990.

26. Buchhorn R, Hulpke-Wette M, Hilgers R, et al: Propranolol treatment of congestive heart failure in infants with congenital heart disease: The CHF-PRO-INFANT trial. Int J Cardiol 79:167, 2001.

27. Konduri GG, Solimano A, Sokol GM, et al, for the Neonatal Inhaled Nitric Oxide Study Group: A randomized trial of early versus standard inhaled nitric oxide therapy in term and near-term newborn infants with hypoxic respiratory failure. Pediatrics 113(3 pt 1):559, 2004.

28. Journois D, Pouard P, Mauriat P, et al: Inhaled nitric oxide as a therapy for pulmonary hypertension after operations for congenital heart defects. J Thorac Cardiovasc Surg 107:1129, 1994.

29. Hirsch J, Mosca R, Bove E: Complete repair of tetralogy of Fallot in the neonate: Results in the modern era. Ann Surg 232:508, 2000.

30. Kasznica J, Ursell P, Blanc W, Gersony W: Abnormalities of the coronary circulation in pulmonary atresia and intact ventricular septum. Am Heart J 114:1415, 1987.

31. Kirklin JW, Blackstone EH, Tchervenkov CI, Castaneda AR: Clinical outcomes after the arterial switch operation for transposition. Circulation 86:1501, 1992.

32. Bailey LL, Wood M, Razzouk A, et al: Heart transplantation during the first 12 years of life. Arch Surg 124:1221, 1989.

33. Boucek MM, Edwards LB, Keck BM, et al: The Registry of the International Society for Heart and Lung Transplantation: Sixth Official Pediatric Report—2003.J Heart Lung Transplant 22:636, 2003.

34. Bailey LL, Gundry SR, Razzouk AJ, et al: Bless the babies: One hundred fifteen late survivors of heart transplantation during the first year of life. J Thorac Cardiovasc Surg 105:805, 1993.

35. Norwood WI, Kirklin JK, Sanders SP: Hypoplastic left heart syndrome: Experience with palliative surgery. Am J Cardiol 45:87, 1980.

36. Norwood WI, Jacobs ML, Murphy JD: Fontan procedure for hypoplastic left heart syndrome. Ann Thorac Surg 54:1025, 1992.

37. Gaynor J, Mahle W, Cohen M, et al: Risk factors for mortality after the Norwood procedure. Eur J Cardiothorac Surg 22:82, 2002.

38. Jenkins P, Flanagan M, Jenkins K, et al: Survival analysis and risk factors for mortality in transplantation and staged surgery for hypoplastic left heart syndrome. J Am Coll Cardiol 36:1178, 2000.

39. Park JK, Dell RB, Ellis K, Gersony WM: Surgical management of the infant with coarctation of the aorta and ventricular septal defect. J Am Coll Cardiol 20:176, 1992.

40. Sandhu S, Beekman R, Mosca R, Bove E: Single-stage repair of aortic arch obstruction and associated intracardiac defects in the neonate. Am J Cardiol 75:370, 1995.

Congenital Heart Defects in Newborns and Infants: Cardiothoracic Repair

Pierantonio Russo and Joanne Giamboy Russo

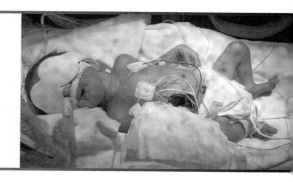

pproximately 40,000 children with **congenital heart disease** are born every year in the United States. Of these, nearly half need medical or surgical intervention or both within the first 12 months of life. About 25% require medical or surgical therapy in the first month of life (Table 61-1), and about 33% require therapy in the first 12 months (Table 61-2).

PRESENTATION AND THERAPY IN THE FIRST MONTH OF LIFE

Table 61-3 shows the incidence of lesions in children with congenital heart disease.

Cyanotic Lesions

Redirection of a fraction of the systemic venous blood to the aorta **(right-to-left shunt)** causes systemic arterial hypoxemia and cyanosis. Severe **cyanosis** of the newborn associated with congenital heart disease is caused by one of the following pathophysiologic conditions:

1. Severe obstruction of the right ventricular outflow tract, reduced pulmonary blood flow, with adequate or with inadequate mixing of systemic venous and pulmonary venous blood.
2. Inadequate mixing of systemic venous and pulmonary venous blood in the presence of parallel pulmonary and systemic circulations (transposition of the great vessels). Pulmonary blood flow is normal or increased, but the aorta, transposed over the ventricular septum, receives mostly systemic venous return.
3. Mixing of systemic and pulmonary venous blood at the venous/atrial level or at the ventricular/great vessels level (right-to-left plus left-to-right shunt). In these cases, the degree of cyanosis depends on the relative amount of pulmonary and systemic blood flow. In the presence of the venous/atrial communications, pulmonary blood flow exceeds systemic flow because the compliance of the right ventricle is greater than that of the left ventricle. In the presence of mixing at the ventricular/great vessels

level, pulmonary blood flow is higher than systemic flow because pulmonary vascular resistance decreases after birth. In these cases, in the absence of obstruction to pulmonary blood flow, left-to-right shunt is prevalent, the pulmonary flow is higher than the systemic flow, and the patient is only mildly cyanotic. The increased pulmonary flow produces respiratory symptoms, congestive heart failure, and failure to thrive, however.

Severe Obstruction of the Right Ventricular Outflow Tract

Tetralogy of Fallot. In patients with **tetralogy of Fallot** with and without pulmonary atresia, the infundibulum of the right ventricle is extremely narrow, and the pulmonary valve is stenotic, absent, or replaced by a fibrous diaphragm **(atresia)**. In newborns and infants with severe tetralogy of Fallot and in infants with pulmonary atresia, survival depends on patency and size of the ductus arteriosus, which provides pulmonary flow. In extreme forms of pulmonary atresia and ventricular septal defect (VSD), there is complete discontinuity between the right ventricle and right and left pulmonary arteries, and in some instances the central pulmonary arteries are absent. The survival of these patients depends on the presence of multiple aortopulmonary collateral vessels, which supply pulmonary flow from the descending aorta and rarely from the ascending aorta.

When patients with tetralogy of Fallot are symptomatic in the first month of life, usually the anatomy of the right ventricular outflow tract and pulmonary arteries is unfavorable. About 70% of patients with tetralogy of Fallot require surgical intervention in the first 12 months of life because of hypoxic spells or sustained severe hypoxemia, with arterial oxygen saturation less than 70% at rest. Currently, primary repair of tetralogy of Fallot, regardless of age or weight, is considered the optimal surgical approach. Primary repair eliminates the cumulative risk of two operations and the complications associated with the construction of arterial-to-pulmonary shunts in neonates, particularly stenosis or distortion of the pulmonary arteries.

Table 61–1. Conditions Requiring Management in First 30 Days of Life

Patent ductus arteriosus (premature newborns)
Coarctation of aorta
Interrupted aortic arch
Critical aortic stenosis
Severe pulmonic stenosis
Severe tetralogy of Fallot
Transposition of great arteries
Taussig-Bing syndrome
Pulmonary atresia
Tricuspid/mitral atresia/single ventricle
Truncus arteriosus

In addition, primary repair avoids the development of secondary hypertrophic changes of the infundibular septum and of the right ventricular free wall. Palliative procedures, consisting of shunts, are indicated only in infants with tetralogy of Fallot and severely hypoplastic pulmonary arteries and in cases with anomalous origin of the left anterior descending coronary artery from the right coronary artery. In patients with pulmonary atresia and discontinuation between the right ventricle and the pulmonary arteries and in patients with absent central pulmonary arteries, the traditional surgical approach consists of systemic artery–to–pulmonary artery shunts and "unifocalization" procedures, in which multiple sources of pulmonary flow are disconnected from the aorta and connected together by direct anastomosis or with a graft. Individual high-volume institutions have reported successful primary repair, however, even in the presence of anomalous origin of the left anterior descending coronary artery from the right coronary artery and in patients with pulmonary atresia and absence of the central pulmonary arteries with multiple aortopulmonary collateral vessels. Primary repair of tetralogy of Fallot in the first 12 months of life carries a hospital mortality of less than 4% in experienced institutions. In patients with pulmonary atresia, the reported mortality of primary repair is 37% in patients younger than 6 months old but 4.2% in patients older than 6 months.

Table 61–2. Conditions Requiring Management in First 12 Months of Life

Ventricular septal defect
Double outlet right ventricle with
  subaortic ventricular septal defect
Patent ductus arteriosus
Atrial septal defect (secundum)
Partial anomalous venous return
All forms of atrioventricular canal
Corrected transposition of the great arteries
Anomalous origin of coronary artery from
  pulmonary artery

Pulmonary atresia with intact septum. Patients with **pulmonary atresia** with intact ventricular septum have isolated atresia of the outlet from the right ventricle without VSD. The definition of pulmonary atresia with intact ventricular septum encompasses a spectrum of lesions, with different morphology of the right ventricle and size of the tricuspid valve. Approximately 10% of patients with pulmonary atresia and intact ventricular septum have significant stenosis or atresia of one or more of the major coronary arteries. In these cases, the coronary arteries receive blood supply from fistulas (sinusoids) between the right ventricle and the coronary circulation. The ventricular-to-coronary fistulas occur mostly when the right ventricular pressure is suprasystemic as a consequence of the atretic right ventricle outflow tract. It is essential that the right ventricular pressure remains elevated to maintain adequate perfusion pressure in the distal coronary arteries.

Neonates with pulmonary atresia and intact ventricular septum are typically cyanotic at birth. Survival depends on patency of the ductus arteriosus, which provides pulmonary flow. Also in these patients, there is a significant right-to-left shunt at the atrial level. Tricuspid valve regurgitation may be associated, as is tricuspid stenosis or atresia. The surgical management of neonates with pulmonary atresia with intact ventricular septum must be tailored to individual anatomic variations. All patients without sinusoids and without tricuspid valve regurgitation and adequate size tricuspid valve should undergo decompression of the right ventricle by transannular patch enlargement of the infundibular outflow tract. If the right ventricle and tricuspid valve are hypoplastic, a systemic-to-pulmonary artery shunt should be performed at the same time. The right ventricle is noncompliant in these cases, and the atrial septal defect (ASD) should be left open, and enlarged if restrictive, to avoid systemic venous hypertension. In patients with massive tricuspid valve regurgitation and in patients with right ventricular–dependent coronary circulation, right ventricular decompression is contraindicated. In these patients, a systemic-to-pulmonary shunt is performed in the neonatal period to secure adequate pulmonary blood flow. Subsequently, patients with sinusoids are managed similar to patients with single-ventricle physiology and usually undergo a Fontan procedure and, in some instances, heart transplantation. Patients without sinusoids but with persistent severe tricuspid valve regurgitation and an adequate size right ventricle may be candidates for tricuspid valve annuloplasty and right ventricle decompression. Patients with severe tricuspid valve stenosis and atresia also are managed initially with a pulmonary-to-systemic shunt and subsequently with the Fontan operation or with one-and-a-half ventricular repair (bidirectional superior vena cava–to–pulmonary artery shunt and right ventricle decompression). The hospital mortality associated with surgical management of neonates with pulmonary atresia and intact ventricular septum is reported at about 4.9%.

Ebstein anomaly of the tricuspid valve. Ebstein anomaly of the tricuspid valve consists of downward displacement of the tricuspid valve into the right ventricle. The anterior

Table 61–3. Incidence per 100 Children with Congenital Heart Defects (CHD)

	All CHD (%)	Recurrence in Siblings (%)	Recurrence in Offspring (%)
Ventricular septal defect	30-60	4-6	2-22
Patent ductus arteriosus	10	2.5-3	2-11
Atrial septal defect (secundum)	7	3	2-14
Atrioventricular canal	3-5	2-3	5-14
Coarctation of aorta	6	2-7	2-8
Aortic stenosis	5	3	3-18
Pulmonic stenosis	7	2	2-9
Tetralogy of Fallot	5	2-3	1-4
Transposition of great arteries	5	2	5
Pulmonary atresia	1-2	1	5
Tricuspid atresia	1-2	1	5
Truncus arteriosus	1	1-14	8
Total anomalous pulmonary venous connection	1	3	5
Aortic atresia (hypoplastic left heart syndrome)	1	1-4	5-14
Double-outlet right ventricle	<1	2	4
Atrial isomerism	2	5	1-4
Single ventricle	1	3	5
Ebstein malformation	<1	1	5

Modified from Rudolph's Pediatrics. New York, McGraw-Hill, 2002.

leaflet of the tricuspid valve retains a normal attachment to the valve ring, but the posterior and septal leaflets are displaced down to the wall of the right ventricle and are hypoplastic. A portion of the right ventricle is in continuity with the right atrium above the tricuspid valve, whereas the other portion remains distal to the tricuspid valve. The right atrium is gigantic, and the tricuspid valve in neonates shows various degrees of regurgitation from mild to extremely severe. Neonates with Ebstein anomaly are usually symptomatic in the presence of an anatomic pulmonary valve atresia with hypoplastic right ventricle or in the presence of elevated pulmonary vascular resistance and various degrees of right ventricular outflow tract obstruction produced by the displaced tricuspid valve. In these circumstances, survival depends on a patent ductus arteriosus (PDA) and adequate decompression of the right side of the heart through an enlarged fossa ovale or an ASD. The extreme cyanosis of these neonates is due to the right-to-left shunt at the atrial level and the reduced pulmonary flow. Without therapy, the mortality is high because of inadequate right ventricular output due to the massive tricuspid valve regurgitation and the severe cyanosis. Surgical intervention consists of patch closure of the tricuspid valve, atrial septectomy, and a systemic-to-pulmonary artery shunt. Hospital mortality for this operation is high; heart transplantation remains an alternative option. Neonates who survive the first few months of life without the need of patch closure of the tricuspid valve may become candidates for biventricular repair with tricuspid valve repair, right ventricular reconstruction, and removal of a portion of the right atrial free wall. Extracorporeal membrane oxygenation and inhalational nitric oxide therapies have been used successfully to stabilize neonates with low cardiac output and elevated pulmonary artery resistance.

Inadequate Mixing and Parallel Circulations

Transposition of the great arteries. Transposition of the great arteries is a common cyanotic congenital anomaly, which accounts for approximately 5% of all congenital heart defects. In this condition, the aorta is located anterior and to the right of the pulmonary artery and arises from the right ventricle, whereas the pulmonary artery arises from the left ventricle. The deoxygenated blood returning from the vena cava flows into the right ventricle, then is ejected into the aorta, and oxygenated blood returning into the left atrium from the pulmonary veins flows into the left ventricle and is ejected into the pulmonary artery. The systemic and pulmonary circulations normally are in series, but in neonates with transpositions of the great vessels they are in parallel. Survival at birth is possible only in the presence of adequate intracardiac communication (ASD or VSD) with a PDA, which allows sufficient mixing of pulmonary venous and systemic venous blood. Neonates with transposition and intact ventricular septum and inadequate interatrial communication become symptomatic when the PDA begins to close. These patients become severely cyanotic and tachypneic within the first few days of life. In patients with VSD, the clinical manifestations depend on the size of the VSD. In the presence of a small VSD, the clinical manifestations are similar to the newborn with transposition and intact ventricular septum, in whom cyanosis is prevalent and congestive heart failure is rare. If the VSD is large, there is usually adequate mixing of oxygenated and deoxygenated blood, but cardiac failure is observed frequently because of significant pulmonary overcirculation with pulmonary hypertension. Management of neonates with transposition of the great arteries and intact septum includes initial stabilization with intravenous administration of prostaglandin E_1 (PGE$_1$) to maintain patency of the ductus arteriosus and balloon atrial septectomy during cardiac catheterization or at bedside under echo guidance.

Currently the arterial switch operation is the procedure of choice for neonates with transposition of the great vessels. The operation consists of dividing the aorta and pulmonary artery above the respective sinuses; resecting the coronary arteries; reimplanting the coronary arteries in the old pulmonary root, which becomes the new aorta; and reconstructing the aortic and pulmonary continuity in anatomic position. In cases with intact ventricular septum, the operation should be performed within the first 2 to 3 weeks of life, when, in response to the elevated pulmonary vascular resistance, the pressure in the left ventricle is still systemic, and the left ventricular mass is still adequate. Beyond this time, when the pulmonary vascular resistance and pressure decrease, the left ventricle is not suitable to support the systemic circulation after the arterial switch. In patients with VSD, the arterial switch operation can be performed beyond the first 2 weeks of life because an unrestricted VSD produces equal pressures in both ventricles, preventing regression of the ventricular mass. Currently, the arterial switch operation can be performed with 95% hospital survival. About 15% to 20% of patients undergoing the arterial switch operation may require reoperation for right ventricular outflow tract obstruction. In experienced, high-volume institutions, rare coronary artery anatomy is not a contraindication to the arterial switch operation. The atrial switch operations, consisting of the Mustard and Senning operations, are not performed routinely now because of the long-term morbidity associated with them, including atrial conduction disturbances, sick sinus syndromes with bradycardia and tachyarrhythmias, atrial flutter, and sudden death.

In patients with VSD and pulmonary stenosis, the so-called Rastelli operation is performed, after an initial palliation with a systemic-to-pulmonary shunt. The Rastelli operation consists of anatomic reconstruction achieved by enlarging the VSD, baffling the left ventricle to the aorta with a generous patch, and reconstructing the continuity between the right ventricle and the pulmonary arteries with a valved conduit. The Rastelli operation usually is performed at about 2 years of age and is associated with a mortality of less than 5% in experienced institutions.

Double-outlet right ventricle with transposition of the great vessels (Taussig-Bing anomaly). Neonates with double-outlet right ventricle and transposition of the great arteries experience cardiac failure and cyanosis in the first few weeks of life. In these patients, the VSD is located directly below the pulmonary valve or below the pulmonic and aortic valve. The pathophysiology is similar to transposition of the great vessels and VSD, but the degree of congestive heart failure is usually more prominent. Patients may undergo the arterial switch operation early with a single-stage or a two-stage approach (palliation with arterial banding and control of pulmonary flow). Some authors advocate an intraventricular repair with reconstruction of the left ventricle to pulmonary continuity with or without a valve conduit.

Mixing Lesions

Total Anomalous Pulmonary Venous Drainage

Total anomalous pulmonary venous connection (absence of anatomic connection between the pulmonary veins and the left atrium) occurs in 2% of all congenital heart defects encountered in the first 12 months of life. The pulmonary veins are connected directly to the right atrium or to the right superior vena cava, azygos vein, left innominate vein, coronary sinus, or ductus venosus. In "mixed types," combinations of various anatomic connections exist among the pulmonary veins, the heart, and the systemic veins. The four pulmonary veins almost always form a common channel separated from the left atrium. Embryologically, an anomalous connection develops between the pulmonary vein plexus of the lung buds and the systemic venous system. The three main anatomic types are supracardiac, cardiac, and infracardiac (infradiaphragmatic).

In the supracardiac type, the pulmonary venous confluence immediately posterior to the left atrium joins a left vertical vein connected with the left innominate vein, which drains into the superior vena cava. In the infracardiac type, the pulmonary venous confluence connects with a vertical vein that descends below the diaphragm to join the ductus venosus. The pulmonary venous drainage returns to the heart via the inferior vena cava. In the cardiac type, the pulmonary veins may be connected directly to the right atrium or the coronary sinus.

In partial anomalous pulmonary venous drainage, part of the pulmonary venous drainage is to the left atrium and part to the right venous system or right atrium. The physiology and clinical presentation are similar to ASDs (see later).

In the infradiaphragmatic type, severe obstruction to the pulmonary venous return almost always is present. The obstruction is caused by the length and narrowness of the common vertical vein, compression in the esophageal hiatus of the diaphragm, small size of ductus venosus, and resistance to flow through the liver.

In the supracardiac type, pulmonary venous obstruction is infrequent. When present, the obstruction is due to compression of the vertical vein passing between the left pulmonary artery anteriorly and the left bronchus posteriorly. Obstruction of the pulmonary venous return into the coronary sinus is frequent among the intracardiac types. In all types, functional pulmonary venous obstruction may result from restriction of flow across the foramen ovale because the right atrial pressure is higher than the left atrial pressure, and left-to-right shunt across the foramen ovale becomes limited.

Associated anomalies. Other complex congenital heart defects, including atrioventricular canal (AVC), transposition of the great arteries, and single ventricles with right or left atrial isomerism, are present in 20% to 30% of patients with total anomalous pulmonary venous drainage.

Pathophysiology and presentation. Pulmonary venous blood drains into the right atrium, where it mixes with the systemic venous return. Systemic arterial desaturation is present as a result of the obligatory right-to-left shunt at atrial level. The arterial oxygen saturation depends on the ratio of pulmonary to systemic blood flow. Patients without pulmonary venous obstruction have high pulmonary blood flow, pulmonary hypertension, and relatively low pulmonary vascular resistance. These infants are only mildly cyanotic, but they present with progressive congestive heart failure, tachypnea, and failure to thrive early in infancy and during the first year of life. Patients with pulmonary venous obstruction are cyanotic because of severe pulmonary hypertension, restricted pulmonary blood flow, pulmonary venous congestion, and pulmonary edema. A pulmonary artery pressure often is suprasystemic. This condition is lethal in the first weeks of life if not corrected. In all types, the physical examination is nonspecific. In the unobstructed supracardiac types, the chest radiograph shows a pathognomonic sign, however— "the snowman," formed by the dilated left vertical vein, innominate vein, and right atrium and superior vena cava. In addition, marked cardiac enlargement and pulmonary vascular plethora are seen. When pulmonary venous obstruction is present, the chest radiograph shows a normal or slightly enlarged heart with diffuse hazy reticulated lung fields (ground-glass appearance), similar to interstitial pneumonitis. Echocardiography can establish the diagnosis and anatomic type of pulmonary venous drainage with a high degree of sensitivity and specificity. All infants with severe respiratory distress and cyanosis at birth should be evaluated with echocardiography.

Surgical repair aims at constructing a direct connection between the common pulmonary venous channel and the left atrium, atrial septation, and ligation of the anomalous venous connection. Surgical repair is indicated at birth if obstruction is present. In all other cases, surgery is indicated in the first 6 months of life or earlier in the presence of congestive heart failure and failure to thrive. Repair in newborns or small infants frequently requires hypothermic circulatory arrest or low-flow cardiopulmonary bypass. Aggressive resuscitation of the newborn with pulmonary venous obstruction is essential to improve surgical outcome. Besides correction of metabolic disorders, resuscitation frequently includes positive-pressure ventilation, diuretics, and, in our experience, extracorporeal membrane oxygenation.

Surgical mortality now is less than 5% for patients without obstruction and higher when obstruction is present. Recurrence of pulmonary venous obstruction occurs within the first 6 months after repair in 10% of patients. If obstruction recurs in the form of diffuse fibrosis of the lumen of the pulmonary veins, the prognosis is poor. In these cases, palliation may be possible with nonsurgical methods (intraluminal stents).

Truncus Arteriosus

Truncus arteriosus (2% of all congenital heart defects) is characterized by the presence of a single arterial trunk originating from the heart. This single trunk supplies the coronary, pulmonary, and systemic circulations proximal to the aortic arch. A VSD is always present. The truncal valve has three or four leaflets and may be incompetent. Truncal valve stenosis is rare. The pulmonary arteries

arise as a single vessel or as two separate vessels from the posterior or lateral wall of the truncus. In less than 20% of patients, one of the pulmonary arteries is absent. A large percentage of infants with truncus arteriosus have partial deletion of chromosome 22.

Associated anomalies. A right aortic arch is present in 30% to 50% of patients. Occasionally, interrupted aortic arch is present. In these cases, the descending aorta is in continuity with the main pulmonary artery via the ductus arteriosus.

Pathophysiology and presentation. Pathophysiology and presentation occur in the common trunk. The right and left ventricles eject blood at systemic pressure into the common arterial trunk. Mixing of systemic venous and pulmonary venous blood occurs in the trunk, proximal to the coronary, pulmonary, and systemic circulations. Pulmonary pressure is systemic. Pulmonary blood flow is increased significantly in the first months of life because the pulmonary arteries are normal size, and the pulmonary vascular resistance is initially relatively low. Cyanosis is minimal, and the clinical picture is typical of a large left-to-right shunt (congestive heart failure, failure to thrive, and tachypnea). Pulmonary circulation is restricted in patients who develop increased pulmonary vascular resistance after 4 to 5 months of age. These patients become cyanotic, with fewer signs of congestive heart failure.

In most infants, the chest radiograph shows considerable cardiomegaly, with increased pulmonary vascular markings. The pulmonary artery hila are displaced superiorly. Two-dimensional echocardiography shows a large, single arterial vessel overriding the ventricular septum and shows the main pulmonary artery or the branch pulmonary arteries arising directly from the common trunk. The ductus arteriosus is absent except with an interrupted aortic arch. Cardiac catheterization and selective angiography confirm the diagnosis.

Surgical repair is indicated in the first 3 months of life, when the pulmonary vascular resistance is still low and any elevation is reversible. Repair consists of removal of the pulmonary arteries from the common trunk; patch closure of the VSD, leaving the truncal valve connected to the left ventricle; and insertion of a valved conduit (homograft) from the right ventricle to the pulmonary arteries. Surgical mortality now is less than 10% for repair performed within the first 3 to 4 months of life. Repeat surgery is necessary for replacement of the right ventricle to pulmonary conduit several times before adulthood. Truncal valve insufficiency when severe (about 5% to 10%) requires replacement or repair. Good results have been reported with suture-plasty (suturing of each edge of the small cusp to the adjacent cusps) and cusp removal techniques (the prolapsing cusp is removed together with the respective sinus, and the truncal valve annulus is reduced in size).

Univentricular Physiology

Single ventricle (univentricular heart). A single-ventricle heart receives the mitral and tricuspid orifices or a common atrioventricular orifice (**univentricular atrioventricular connection**). About 70% to 80% of single-ventricle malformations are derived from an L-bulboventricular loop and have a single right-sided, morphologic left ventricle. A rudimentary anterior and left-sided right ventricular outflow chamber is present. The rudimentary chamber communicates with the single ventricle through a VSD (or persistent bulboventricular foramen) and is connected to the aorta, which in these cases is L-transposed (anterior and to the left). The amount of systemic blood flow is limited by the size of the VSD. The VSD connects the single ventricle, which receives the systemic and pulmonary venous return, to the aorta via the rudimentary chamber. The pulmonary artery is posterior and arises from the single ventricle. A double-inlet ventricle or common ventricle is a single-ventricle heart that has well-developed right and left ventricular inlets.

Tricuspid atresia. In tricuspid atresia, the only inflow to the single ventricular mass is the mitral valve, through which pulmonary venous blood reaches the ventricle. The systemic venous return is shunted right to left through the foramen ovale or ASD.

Mitral atresia without aortic stenosis and atresia. In mitral atresia, the only inflow to the ventricular mass (right morphology) is the tricuspid valve. The systemic venous blood reaches the ventricle through the tricuspid valve. The pulmonary venous blood is shunted left to right through a foramen ovale or ASD. Frequently a VSD is present. Blood enters the right ventricle, from which it passes into the pulmonary artery and through the VSD into a hypoplastic left ventricle and small or normal size aorta.

Associated anomalies. Stenosis or atresia of the pulmonary outflow tract is common. Coarctation of the aorta also frequently is associated. In patients with a single ventricle, subaortic stenosis caused by a small VSD is relatively common, particularly after pulmonary artery banding. Dextrocardia, right atrial isomerism (atrial appendages with equal morphology), common ACV, and total anomalous pulmonary venous connection also frequently are associated with a single ventricle.

Pathophysiology and presentation. Mixing occurs in the single ventricle. Some degree of systemic arterial desaturation is always present because of mixing of the pulmonary and systemic venous blood. With significant pulmonary stenosis or atresia, cyanosis is severe, but on chest radiograph the heart size is normal and the pulmonary vascular markings are reduced. In infants with unrestricted pulmonary flow and low pulmonary vascular resistance, the clinical presentation is typical of patients with pulmonary overcirculation (cardiomegaly, increased pulmonary markings, tachypnea, congestive heart failure, failure to thrive). In older children, increasing cyanosis, absence of congestive heart failure, and signs of pulmonary overcirculation indicate increasing pulmonary vascular disease. Diagnosis of single ventricle with definition of other anatomic features and associated anomalies is made by two-dimensional echocardiography. Cardiac catheterization with angiography better defines the presence or absence of pulmonary stenosis, allows measurement of pulmonary vascular resistance, and identifies the size of the VSD in relation to the subaortic area in cases with L-malposition of the aorta.

Newborns presenting with reduced pulmonary flow are stabilized with a PGE_1 infusion to maintain a PDA. Patients with atrioventricular valve atresia may require balloon atrial septectomy to enlarge the atrial communication, decompress the right or left atrium, and improve mixing. Surgical palliation in newborns and infants with decreased pulmonary blood flow consists of creating a systemic-to-pulmonary shunt, followed by the bidirectional Glenn procedure (superior vena cava to pulmonary artery connection) at 5 to 6 months. Pulmonary artery banding followed by the bidirectional Glenn procedure is indicated in newborns and infants with increased pulmonary blood flow. Surgical atrial septectomy may be necessary in cases in which the atrial communication is still restrictive after balloon septectomy. If there is subaortic stenosis, the proximal main pulmonary artery can be anastomosed to the aorta (Damus-Stansel-Kaye procedure) at the time of the bidirectional Glenn operation. About 12 to 36 months after the bidirectional Glenn operation, patients who are good candidates undergo completion of the Fontan circulation (all systemic venous return directed to the pulmonary arteries and separation of systemic and pulmonary venous return). The Fontan procedure can be performed with an intracardiac baffle or, more recently, with an extracardiac conduit interposed between the transected inferior vena cava and the pulmonary arteries. The extracardiac conduit can be connected to the pulmonary arteries without cardiopulmonary bypass (our preferred technique). Although this approach is technically more challenging, avoidance of cardiopulmonary bypass eliminates the inflammatory response associated with it, reducing the capillary leak and the incidence of edema, pleural effusion, and protein-losing enteropathy typically associated with the Fontan operation. Surgical mortality for the Fontan operation in patients with single ventricle and atrioventricular valve atresia, without aortic atresia, is reported to be 4.8%.

Reduced Systemic Circulation

Hypoplastic left heart syndrome. The term **hypoplastic left heart syndrome** encompasses a spectrum of cardiac defects with severe hypoplasia of the left side of the heart. The right side of the heart supports the pulmonary circulation through the pulmonary artery and the systemic circulation through a PDA. Usually the left ventricular cavity is small or absent. The ventricular septum usually is intact. In the extreme form, there is aortic and mitral atresia, and the ascending aorta is 2 mm in diameter or less. More favorable anatomic variants include hypoplasia of the ascending aorta (3 to 5 mm in diameter), severe aortic and mitral stenosis, and small left ventricle.

Pathophysiology and presentation. Pulmonary venous blood is shunted from the left atrium to the right atrium via the patent foramen ovale. Frequently the foramen is small, and pulmonary venous hypertension occurs because of restriction to flow from the left atrium to the right atrium. The right ventricle ejects blood into the aorta through the PDA and into the pulmonary circulation through the pulmonary artery. The amount of systemic and pulmonary flow depends on the relative resistance to flow into the two circulations, which are in parallel and not in series. Higher pulmonary vascular resistance favors systemic flow. In contrast, when the pulmonary vascular resistance decreases, pulmonary flow increases, and systemic flow decreases. The size of the ductus arteriosus also is an independent determinant of systemic flow.

Most newborns with hypoplastic left heart syndrome are acutely ill and usually die within the first week of life without treatment. Hypoplastic left heart syndrome accounted for nearly 25% of cardiac deaths in the first year of life in the New England Registry. These patients have signs of congestive heart failure and cardiac collapse, diminished peripheral pulses, tachypnea, liver congestion, and cyanosis.

Shortly after birth, the chest radiograph shows only mild cardiac enlargement, but with increasing pulmonary overcirculation, cardiomegaly and pulmonary plethora are common. Pulmonary venous obstruction from a restrictive foramen ovale is indicated by a general hazy appearance of the lung fields. The diagnosis is confirmed by echocardiography.

Resuscitation of these newborns before surgical management is essential. Medical management includes PGE_1 infusion to maintain a PDA, correction of acidemia, balancing pulmonary and systemic blood flow with manipulation of mechanical ventilation, gas therapy, and rarely inotropic support. It now is well shown experimentally and clinically that to obtain maximal systemic oxygen availability, the optimal pulmonary flow-to-systemic flow ratio should be 1 or less. Systemic venous saturation, an indicator of peripheral tissue perfusion, is high if the pulmonary flow-to-systemic flow ratio is within the optimal range and is low when the pulmonary flow-to-systemic flow ratio is outside range. In essence, if the arterial oxygen saturation is high and the systemic perfusion is diminished with low systemic oxygen saturation, medical intervention is directed at reducing pulmonary flow by increasing pulmonary vascular resistance (room air, nitrogen, carbon dioxide therapy, positive end-expiratory pressure). If the arterial oxygen saturation and the systemic oxygen saturation are both low, it is necessary to increase pulmonary flow by reducing the pulmonary vascular resistance (hyperventilation, higher fraction of inspired oxygen, no positive end-expiratory pressure).

Surgical Management

Surgical management follows two different pathways: three-stage palliation (Norwood operation and Fontan protocol) or transplantation.

Norwood operation and Fontan protocol.

In the first surgical stage, the main pulmonary artery is transected, and the PDA is ligated. Output from the right ventricle to the aorta is established by using the proximal main pulmonary artery to reconstruct the diminutive ascending aorta and aortic arch, plus a generous homograft patch.

Pulmonary blood flow is established with a modified right Blalock-Taussig shunt. An atrial septectomy is performed. At about 4 to 6 months, a bidirectional Glenn procedure (see earlier) or a hemi-Fontan (superior and inferior vena cava tunneled to the pulmonary arteries; the inferior vena cava connection remains isolated with a patch that is removed at the time of the third stage) is performed. Completion of the Fontan circulation is performed at about 2 years.

Reported survival for first-stage palliation at selected high-volume institutions is 86% if no other major comorbidities exist, but survival is only 42% in the presence of low birth weight or pulmonary venous obstruction. Survival for second-stage and completion of the Fontan circulation is 97% and 88%. At experienced institutions, the reported 5-year actuarial survival for all three stages, including interim mortality between surgical stages, is 70%.

Neonatal orthotopic cardiac transplantation.

Transplantation is an attractive approach because of the advantage of a single reparative operation. Although shortage of donor hearts and uncertainty about the long-term effects of immunosuppression remain problematic, excellent short-term and midterm results have been obtained. In the Loma Linda early experience, the 5- and 7-year actuarial survival rates were 76% and 70%.

Left Atrium Obstruction

The pathophysiology and clinical presentation of the following conditions are the same as pulmonary venous obstruction. Total anomalous venous obstruction should be considered in the differential diagnosis when evaluating these patients.

Cor triatriatum.

In **cor triatriatum**, a membrane with an obstructive opening is located in the midportion of the left atrium and separates the atrium into two chambers. Flow from the pulmonary veins to the mitral valve is obstructed. The diagnosis is made by echocardiography and confirmed by cardiac catheterization with angiocardiography. Surgical treatment consists of surgical excision of the obstructing membrane.

Supravalvar mitral ring.

Supravalvar mitral ring is associated with parachute mitral valve, subaortic stenosis, and coarctation of the aorta (Shone syndrome). The supravalvar ring is created by a membrane just above the mitral valve. The membrane not only obstructs flow to the mitral valve but also restricts mitral valve opening and closing. The diagnosis is made by echocardiography and confirmed by cardiac catheterization with angiocardiography. Surgical treatment consists of surgical excision of the obstructing membrane, together with repair of coarctation of the aorta and subaortic membrane. The timing of surgery is dictated by symptoms. We prefer to intervene before 12 months of age, however, in all cases.

Aortic valve stenosis.

Congenital **aortic valve stenosis** is caused by an obstructed bicuspid valve or, in about 20% of cases, by a monocusp. The resultant small valve orifice and cusp thickening produce various degrees of obstruction.

Normal aortic valve area is 2 cm²/m². Critical aortic stenosis is associated with a valve area of 0.65 cm²/m² and a peak gradient between the left ventricle and the aorta of about 50 mm Hg. If the obstruction is severe at birth, this condition is associated with significant mortality, unless emergent treatment is established. Hypoplasia of the ascending aorta and aortic arch indicates severe aortic stenosis in utero. Marked endocardial fibroelastosis impairs left ventricular function. The associated reduction in left ventricular dimensions poses challenging management decisions (biventricular versus univentricular repair). After birth, if the foramen ovale is competent, the left atrial pressure increases, and left ventricular output is maintained. The high left atrial pressure causes pulmonary congestion and pulmonary edema, however. If the foramen ovale is open, the associated left-to-right shunt reduces the filling of the left ventricle and in turn produces low cardiac output. Newborns with severe aortic valve stenosis present with reduced peripheral perfusion, acidemia and shock, cardiomegaly on the chest radiograph, and hyperdynamic precordium. There may not be any radiologic signs of pulmonary venous hypertension in the presence of left-to-right shunt at the atrial level. The typical systolic murmur (better heard at the upper left sternal border or over the upper sternum) may be absent or soft in the presence of reduced cardiac output.

Critical aortic valve stenosis in a newborn is an emergency. The patient must be resuscitated with mechanical ventilation and aggressive treatment of the acidemia, and peripheral perfusion must be maintained by keeping the ductus arteriosus patent with intravenous infusion of PGE₁. Subsequent intervention depends on the size of the left ventricular cavity and aortic valve annulus. If biventricular physiology can be maintained, the aortic valve stenosis is palliated with balloon angioplasty, as described by Lababidi from our institution for the first time in the 1980s. Surgical palliation (aortic valvotomy) rarely is necessary now, at least in institutions with experience in interventional cardiology procedures. Data regarding 110 neonates with critical aortic valve stenosis were evaluated in a study by the Congenital Heart Surgeons Society from 1994 to 1999. Survival after valvotomy was 82% at 1 month and 72% at 5 years, with no difference for surgical versus balloon angioplasty. Independent risk factors for mortality were mechanical ventilation before valvotomy, smaller aortic valve annulus, smaller aortic diameter at the sinotubular junction, and smaller subaortic region. Estimates for freedom from reintervention were 91% at 1 month and 48% at 5 years after the initial procedure and did not differ significantly for balloon angioplasty versus surgical valvotomy. Palliation produces good functional results. Valve insufficiency may occur in about 10% to 15% of cases, and about 50% of patients require repeat balloon angioplasty or surgical treatment within 10 years after the first procedure. In older patients, surgical management includes valve replacement with homograft, mechanical prostheses, and the Ross procedure (replacement of the aortic valve with the native pulmonary valve and insertion of a homograft in place of the pulmonic valve). Valve replacement usually is postponed until late adolescence to avoid repeat procedures. In patients undergoing the Ross procedure, homograft replacement frequently is necessary because of calcification in growing patients with active calcium metabolism. In newborns with aortic valve annulus less than 5 mm in diameter, a single-ventricle pathway type of palliation (Norwood/Fontan) is preferred, even in the presence of two ventricles because of the high mortality with balloon angioplasty or surgical valvotomy in these cases.

Interruption of aortic arch. In normal newborns, the diameter of the aortic isthmus (between the left subclavian artery and the ductus) is about 75% that of the descending aorta because before birth the aortic isthmus carries about 10% to 12% of the combined output of the left and right ventricles. In the fetus, intracardiac defects with aortic outflow obstruction divert flow away from the aortic isthmus with consequent further hypodevelopment of the isthmus and other segments of the arch. In extreme cases, complete interruption of the aortic arch occurs. Aortic arch interruption is associated with large VSD, double-outlet right ventricle, Taussig-Bing anomaly, tricuspid atresia with transposition of the great vessels, or AVC. A PDA permits peripheral perfusion, shunting blood from the pulmonary artery into the descending aorta, with consequent differential arterial oxygen saturation between the preductal and postductal extremities (right-to-left shunt). A common denominator of the associated conditions is the presence of a VSD, with left-to-right shunt and increased pulmonary blood flow. Elevated pulmonary vascular resistance promotes right-to-left shunting into the descending aorta through the PDA and maintains flow to the lower body. With progressive constriction of the ductus arteriosus, the lower body arterial blood perfusion decreases. Reduced peripheral perfusion also is precipitated by the progressive decline in pulmonary vascular resistance after birth (reduced right-to-left shunt through the ductus). Echocardiography identifies the interruption, the size of the ductus, and the intracardiac defects.

It is important to define the subaortic anatomy by echocardiography or angiocardiography before surgery because of the frequent associated subaortic obstruction. Newborns present in heart failure and with signs of pulmonary circulation or in shock (low peripheral perfusion, anuria, acidemia) if the ductus is constricted or the pulmonary resistance is lower than systemic resistance. Mechanical ventilation, aggressive treatment of acidemia, inotropic therapy, and PGE₁ infusion are used to resuscitate these patients before surgery.

Surgical management consists of complete repair of the interruption and the intracardiac anomalies. This repair frequently requires a period of hypothermic circulatory arrest. Direct anastomosis with or without anterior augmentation with homograft is the preferred method to reestablish continuity of the aortic arch. Operative mortality varies from 7% to 14%.

Coarctation of the aorta. A posterolateral shelf or waist lesion is localized directly opposite the ductus arteriosus **(juxtaductal aortic coarctation)**. Aortic obstruction is facilitated by constriction of ductus smooth muscle that forms a sling around the posterior shelf. After closure of the ductus arteriosus and during patient growth, a concentric obstruction develops (older children and young adults). Turner syndrome, bicuspid aortic valve, VSD, aberrant origins of the subclavian arteries, persistent PDA, and parachute mitral valve are frequently associated conditions. In newborns, the clinical presentation is often similar to that of severe aortic stenosis in the neonatal period because of early and rapid constriction of the ductal tissue within the aortic lumen. Cardiac collapse and signs of pulmonary overcirculation (left-to-right shunt through a stretched foramen ovale or VSD) are common. If the patient is in shock or in heart failure, all pulses are weak. After resuscitation and improvement of left ventricular function, absence or reduction of femoral pulses is noted. No signs of collateral circulation are present in newborns. The chest radiograph shows cardiomegaly with pulmonary venous congestion secondary to left ventricular failure.

Echocardiography is diagnostic in newborns. If the aortic shelf is not prominent, or the ductal tissue constricts gradually, aortic obstruction develops slowly over several weeks or months. In these cases, clinical presentation is within 6 months of age or later in life. After the newborn period, collateral circulation and left ventricular hypertrophy develop. Collateral arteries include the periscapular, intercostal, transverse cervical, and internal mammary systems. These vessels are palpable above the clavicle and around the scapula on both sides. Clinical presentation still may include heart failure in the first 3 to 6 months of life, but heart failure is rare after this age. Later in life, upper extremity hypertension, intermittent claudication with exercise, and cerebrovascular accidents after 7 to 10 years of age (rupture of berry aneurysms) are frequent clinical findings. Infective endocarditis also is possible in older patients with coarctation (aortic wall or the bicuspid aortic valve). The physical examination of older children with coarctation reveals decreased or absent femoral pulses. Lower blood pressure on the right arm indicates the presence of an aberrant right subclavian artery originating below the coarctation. Absent or reduced pulse in the left arm indicates hypoplasia of the left subclavian artery. Blood pressure measurements of the four extremities reveal a gradient between upper and lower extremities, but the gradient may not be remarkable in the presence of prominent collateral circulation. The chest radiograph in older children shows cardiomegaly and dilation of the ascending aorta. The so-called 3 sign on the left heart border is made by the alignment of the dilated aortic segment just above the coarctation and the poststenotic dilation below the coarctation. The "rib notching" sign refers to the erosion of the lower margin of the ribs by large intercostal arteries and is present after 1 to 2 years of age in many patients. Surgery should be performed in symptomatic newborns and infants. The preferred surgical techniques vary according to institutional experience and include subclavian flap (newborns only), extended resection with direct anastomosis, and patch angioplasty. If surgery is indicated, we recommend one-stage repair of concomitant associated defects whenever possible. With modern microvascular surgical techniques, recoarctation is rare. Earlier repair seems to prevent systemic hypertension. Primary balloon angioplasty of native coarctation in adolescents and adults now is a widely accepted alternative to surgery. Balloon angioplasty is the treatment of choice of postoperative recoarctation at all ages, unless there is hypoplasia of the aortic arch.

The incidence of complications in repair of isolated coarctation is low. Of the 591 entries reported in the database of the Society of Thoracic Surgery, 92.9% were free of complications. There were four operative deaths for a mortality rate of 0.7%. Three of the four deaths (75%) occurred in patients less than 1 month old, and the other occurred in a patient 1 month to 1 year old. Operative complications occurred in nine patients (1.5%), who required reoperation for related problems. In our experience and in high-volume institutions, the concomitant closure of a VSD does not increase the operative risk significantly.

Patent ductus arteriosus. PDA occurs in 30% to 40% of premature infants with birth weights less than 1750 g. In these patients, the normal postnatal constriction of the ductus is impaired by a reduced response to increased partial pressure of oxygen and to changes in prostaglandin concentrations. PDA in full-term infants is due to a genetic structural abnormality of the ductus arteriosus, maternal rubella in the first trimester of pregnancy, and high altitude. In premature infants, the diagnosis is suspected in the presence of a systolic murmur and signs of pulmonary overcirculation, pulmonary edema, cardiomegaly, and increased pulmonary vascular markings on the chest radiograph. Because of pulmonary hypertension, the shunt from the aorta to the pulmonary artery occurs only in systole. The murmur is heard better below the left clavicle. In newborns and infants in congestive heart failure, VSD, truncus arteriosus, and aortopulmonary window must be considered in the differential diagnosis.

PDA is diagnosed by echocardiography. In older infants and children, the diagnosis is facilitated by the presence of a continuous murmur with a machine-like quality, owing to the fact that the shunt occurs in systole and diastole. In premature infants, medical management is instituted first. Management includes antifailure drugs and indomethacin to stimulate spontaneous closure of the ductus. Surgical closure with an extrapleural or intrapleural approach is indicated if medical management fails and the left atrium is still large on echocardiography (indicating large left-to-right shunt). In older infants and children, coil embolization or surgical closure always is indicated even in the absence of large left-to-right shunt and increased pulmonary flow because of the high risk of bacterial endocarditis. Transcatheter closure (coil or umbrella device) is successful when the ductus is 5 mm in diameter or less. Video-guided thoracoscopic surgical closure is used now in some institutions, but its advantage over an open approach with muscle-sparing thoracotomy is controversial. We use an open approach through a muscle-sparing minithoracotomy in all cases, with surgical time ranging from 15 to 30 minutes and length of hospital stay of 12 to 24 hours.

PRESENTATION AND THERAPY IN THE FIRST 12 MONTHS OF LIFE

Cyanotic patients with obstructive lesions, patients with congenital valve stenosis, and patients with aortic coarctation anatomy may not require medical or surgical therapy in the first month of life if the anatomy is favorable. Patients with anomalous pulmonary venous return without obstruction and patients with partial anomalous pulmonary venous return are treated later in life. This section discusses other conditions, not addressed in the previous section, that typically require medical and surgical management after the newborn period and before or around 12 months of age. The pathophysiology is typically that of left-to-right shunt through an intracardiac or extracardiac communication. These lesions are included because of the planning and counseling that must occur during the neonatal period.

Left-to-Right Shunt

In the presence of an abnormal intracardiac or extracardiac communication, a fraction of pulmonary venous blood (oxygenated blood) recirculates through the lungs without entering the peripheral arterial circulation. This recirculated blood increases the systemic ventricular end-diastolic volume and produces pulmonary overcirculation, without improving delivery of oxygenated blood. If the shunt is not treated, irreversible pulmonary hypertension develops as a consequence of the increased pulmonary blood flow. In these cases, regression of the medial muscular layer of the pulmonary arteries is retarded, inducing increased pulmonary vascular resistance. The increased pulmonary vascular resistance limits pulmonary blood flow, and the patient becomes cyanotic (Eisenmenger syndrome). In patients with complete AVC and patients with truncus arteriosus, irreversible pulmonary hypertension may occur after about 6 months of age. The amount of left-to-right shunting is influenced by the size of the anatomic communication, the pressure gradient across the communication, pulmonary versus systemic vascular resistance, and the resistance to emptying of the left and right atria into their respective ventricles (ventricular compliance) in cases with atrial defects. Left-to-right shunts less than 1.5:1 have little hemodynamic effect on the heart or lungs. Shunts of 2:1 or greater have more serious hemodynamic consequences, affecting heart chambers and vessels receiving the extra blood. In addition to pulmonary overcirculation, depending on the specific anatomic defect, atrial and ventricular chambers are affected by volume overload, pressure overload, or both. Congestive heart failure is common in patients with large left-to-right shunts, particularly in infancy. Anemia in early infancy should be treated aggressively in these cases to avoid lower oxygen delivery to a pressure volume-overloaded myocardium that may precipitate or aggravate congestive heart failure.

Atrial Septal Defect

Secundum atrial septal defect. Secundum ASDs are located in the area of the foramen ovale and vary in size. Left-to-right shunt is usually present; right-to-left shunt occurs when the intrathoracic pressure increases, impairing right ventricular emptying. Paradoxical embolism is a complication of right-to-left shunt at the atrial level. The magnitude of the shunt depends on the factors outlined earlier, in particular the size of the defect and the resistance to emptying of the atria into the respective ventricles (ventricular compliance). Infants with large secundum ASDs are asymptomatic. Signs of increased pulmonary flow are evident on the chest radiograph, however. At auscultation, there is a systolic ejection murmur and a wide splitting second sound. Because of possible development of complications later in life, surgical or, more recently, nonsurgical closure is indicated at preschool age. Complications reported in adulthood are atrial arrhythmias, caused by atrial enlargement, especially atrial fibrillation or flutter; congestive heart failure; mitral incompetence; and strokes from paradoxical embolization and pulmonary vascular disease. Operative mortality for surgical repair approaches zero.

Sinus venosus. Sinus venosus ASD is located near the orifice of the superior or inferior vena cava and is associated with anomalous pulmonary venous drainage (see earlier).

Unroofed coronary sinus. In unroofed coronary sinus, the wall between the coronary sinus and the left atrium is missing. In the presence of a left superior vena cava draining into the coronary sinus, right-to-left shunt occurs. In this case, the patient is cyanotic. With persistence of left superior vena cava, cerebral embolism and brain abscess frequently are reported in the history because of drainage of systemic venous blood into the left atrium. Echocardiography and cardiac angiography are diagnostic. Surgical correction is indicated at the time of diagnosis.

Atrioventricular canal (endocardial cushion defects). The abnormal development of endocardial cushions in the primitive AVC results in the absence of the atrial ventricular septum. An ASD located in the lower portion of the atrial septum (ostium primum defect) and atrioventricular valves situated at the same level are always present in all forms of AVC. In patients with partial AVC, there is no VSD, and the orifices of the atrioventricular valves are well separated. In patients with intermediate AVC, there is a small VSD in the inlet portion of the ventricular septum. In patients with complete AVC, there is a large inlet VSD. In intermediate and complete AVC, the atrioventricular orifices are not separated. What is usually the septal leaflet of the mitral valve is replaced by two separate leaflets (superior and inferior), producing the so-called cleft of the left atrioventricular valve. Trisomy 21 frequently is associated with AVC.

Pathophysiology and presentation. Patients with partial and intermediate AVC have the same pathophysiology and clinical findings as patients with secundum ASD, unless marked left atrioventricular valve insufficiency occurs through the "cleft." In cases of marked left atrioventricular valve insufficiency, a blowing systolic murmur

is present at the apex, radiating laterally depending on the degree of regurgitation. Signs of increased pulmonary flow are present on the chest radiograph. The electrocardiogram (ECG) typically shows right bundle-branch block and left-axis deviation. Surgical repair is indicated within the first year of life. The left atrioventricular valve is repaired most of the time by approximating the cleft. Left atrioventricular valve regurgitation has occurred in patients in whom the cleft has not been closed. The ostium primum is repaired with a patch, whereas the small VSD can be repaired by suturing valve tissue around to the edges of the defect, or a small separate patch, or with the same patch used for the ASD.

Patients with complete AVC present with the same physiology as patients with large VSD. Left-to-right shunt is present at the atrial and ventricular level. Through the left atrioventricular valve cleft, a left ventricle–to–atrial shunt is possible. Left atrioventricular valve regurgitation is rare in infancy. Infants present at 1 to 2 months of age with failure to thrive, pulmonary overcirculation, and congestive heart failure. Symptoms include tachypnea, sweating, and difficulty with feeding. Peripheral perfusion is reduced (poor pulses, tachycardia, hepatomegaly, and peripheral pallor). The chest radiograph shows cardiomegaly, increased pulmonary markings, and pulmonary edema. Echocardiography is diagnostic. One-stage surgical repair is indicated as soon as possible if congestive heart failure and failure to thrive are not controlled with medical management and within the first 6 months of life to prevent the early development of pulmonary vascular disease. Patients with trisomy 21 are at high risk of developing early pulmonary vascular disease. Surgical repair of these lesions can be done in infancy with a mortality rate of about 5%.

Palliation with pulmonary artery banding is not as effective in these patients as in patients with simple VSD. Although pulmonary banding controls shunting at the ventricular level, these patients have significant atrial level shunting and left atrium–to–right atrium shunting, which are not controllable with pulmonary banding. In patients with "unbalanced ventricles," the surgical pathways are the same as for patients with single-ventricle physiology.

Aortopulmonary window. When the spiral septum between the aorta and pulmonary artery fails to develop, a large communication is found between the aorta and pulmonary artery just above the semilunar valves. The clinical presentation can be similar to PDA and VSD. The peripheral pulses are typically bounding, but the audible murmur has a rough crescendo-decrescendo character and is heard better along the left sternal border in the third and fourth intercostal spaces. Diagnosis is confirmed by echocardiography. Treatment is surgical. On cardiopulmonary bypass, a septum is created with a patch sutured between the aorta and the pulmonary artery above the semilunar valves.

Hemitruncus arteriosus. In **hemitruncus arteriosus,** one of the pulmonary arteries arises from the aorta. The normal pulmonary artery originating from the right ventricle carries the total systemic venous return, usually at normal pressure. The pressure in the pulmonary artery arising from the aorta is above the systemic pressure, however, with serious risk of development of irreversible pulmonary hypertension. A continuous murmur heard laterally or on the back is typical of hemitruncus. A differential pulmonary flow pattern on chest radiograph may be present.

Angiography frequently is necessary to confirm the diagnosis and identify size and distribution of the abnormal pulmonary artery. Early surgical repair consists of disconnecting the abnormal pulmonary artery from the aorta and direct anastomosis to the main pulmonary artery. Subsequent growth of the pulmonary arteries is followed with magnetic resonance imaging.

Isolated ventricular septal defect. Isolated VSD is the most common congenital heart defect (30% to 60% of patients with congenital heart malformations), occurring in 3 to 6 per 1000 live births. Anatomically, VSDs can be found in the muscular, inlet, and outlet septum. VSDs also are part of complex congenital heart defects. About 90% of defects diagnosed at birth are in the muscular septum. These tend to close spontaneously in most cases. In older infants, the most common location is the membranous septum. Inlet VSDs rarely are found in isolation. Most frequently, they are part of the AVC complex. Down syndrome frequently is associated with isolated inlet VSDs. VSDs in the outlet septum are found in association with the tetralogy of Fallot complex and, in isolation, in subarterial position, below the aortic and pulmonic valve. Subarterial VSDs represent 35% of VSDs diagnosed in Asians. Aortic valve prolapse and insufficiency frequently are associated with subarterial VSD. Multiple VSDs usually are found in the muscular septum ("Swiss cheese defects").

Pathophysiology and presentation. The left-to-right shunt produces pulmonary overcirculation, increased pulmonary venous return with left ventricular volume overload, and right ventricular volume overload (extra volume is shunted into the right ventricle). With large left-to-right shunt, clinical signs and symptoms of cardiac failure are present. Congestive heart failure occurs frequently in premature infants and in newborns with anemia, coarctation, large PDA, and large atrial-level shunt. Patients with isolated large VSDs are at risk to develop congestive heart failure when the pulmonary vascular resistance decreases after the first month of life. On auscultation, there is a harsh systolic murmur, heard best at the lower left sternal border, radiating throughout the precordium and toward the subxiphoid area. Murmurs limited to early systole are associated with a small shunt, whereas holosystolic murmurs and palpable thrills indicate a large shunt. A mid-diastolic rumble audible at the apex is indicative of pulmonary flow-to-systemic flow ratio higher than 2:1, as is an active precordium. A loud second sound is associated with pulmonary hypertension. The chest radiograph is helpful in grading the amount of left-to-right shunt, with cardiomegaly and significant increase of pulmonary markings indicating a left-to-right shunt about 2:1. Pulmonary edema is present in association with congestive heart failure. The ECG may be helpful in following the evolution of pulmonary hypertension (right ventricular hypertrophy). Increased pulmonary vascular resistance is associated with increase of right ventricular voltages on the ECG accompanied by shortening of the systolic murmur, loud S_2, decreased cardiac size and vascular markings, and enlargement of the main pulmonary artery on chest radiograph. In all cases with VSD, echocardiography shows the size and position of the defect. Doppler flow mapping can help estimate the right ventricular pressure from the velocity flow across the tricuspid valve regurgitant jet or the VSD and help in identifying multiple defects. Cardiac catheterization and angiography are used to rule out the presence of multiple VSDs and calculate the pulmonary vascular resistance in cases with severe pulmonary hypertension.

Management. About 3% to 5% of all newborns present with small muscular VSDs, which close spontaneously within the next 6 to 12 months. Patients with multiple muscular VSDs may require early surgical management because of large left-to-right shunts, such as those with double-outlet right ventricle with subaortic VSD. Perimembranous or muscular VSDs have a high incidence of spontaneous closure (70% in the first 18 months of age). In these cases, surgery can be postponed whenever possible until about 12 months of age. After 12 months of age, if the shunt is about 2:1 or higher, surgery is indicated to prevent irreversible pulmonary hypertension. Irreversible pulmonary vascular disease occurs by 24 months in one third of children with large VSD shunt. Early surgical repair is recommended in patients with Down syndrome because they tend to develop early pulmonary vascular disease. In addition, they usually present with inlet VSDs, which do not close spontaneously. Surgical repair by 3 to 4 months of age, regardless of anatomic type, is indicated in patients with significant failure to thrive (<10th percentile) and decrease in head growth. Surgical repair is indicated in patients with subarterial VSD and progressive aortic valve insufficiency, regardless of age and size of the shunt, and in patients with right ventricular outflow tract obstruction. Finally, when the decision has been made to postpone surgery until 12 months of age, patients with a large pulmonary flow should be monitored closely for the development of pulmonary vascular disease.

Primary surgical closure of the defects can be accomplished with mortality approaching zero. Pulmonary artery banding still is practiced in patients with associated aortic coarctation, interrupted aortic arch, multiple VSDs, and double-outlet right ventricle with subaortic VSD. We prefer primary repair in all cases.

Corrected transposition. **Corrected transposition** or **L-transposition of the great arteries** consists of ventricular inversion and arterial transposition. The morphologic left ventricle on the right side of the cardiac mass receives the systemic venous return from the right atrium through a mitral valve and is connected to the pulmonary artery. The morphologic right ventricle on the left side of

the cardiac mass receives the pulmonary venous return through a tricuspid valve and is connected to the aorta. The aorta is anterior and to the left of the pulmonary artery. If there are no other lesions, children with this anomaly live normal lives. Associated anomalies are responsible for the clinical presentation. The most common associated lesions are VSDs, pulmonary stenosis or atresia, and Ebstein-like malformation of the left-sided systemic tricuspid valve with left-sided atrioventricular regurgitation. Congenital heart block is frequent at birth or develops at a rate of 1% to 2% per year. The symptoms and signs depend on the severity and nature of these associated lesions. The ECG shows Q waves in the right chest leads and no Q waves on the left (activation of the septum from right to left). The chest radiograph shows a straight left heart border superiorly **(L-transposition of the aorta)**. The diagnosis is confirmed by echocardiography and angiocardiography.

Surgical correction addresses the associated anomalies. The VSD can be repaired by placing sutures on the left side of the septum to avoid the abnormal course of the conduction tissue. Severe pulmonary stenosis and atresia is corrected with a conduit to avoid injury to the conduction tissue, which runs anterior to the pulmonary valve ring. The double-switch operation (atrial switch plus arterial switch) has been advocated to make the left ventricle the systemic ventricle. Surgical mortality is high (Tables 61-4 and 61-5).

Left-to-Right Shunt with Myocardial Ischemia

Anomalous origin of left coronary artery from pulmonary artery. In **anomalous origin of the left coronary artery from the pulmonary artery,** the left coronary artery originates from the pulmonary artery, whereas the right coronary artery arises normally. Because of the lower pulmonary arterial pressure after birth, blood flows from the right coronary artery through collateral vessels into the left coronary artery and into the pulmonary artery, with consequent left-to-right shunt. In addition, the left-to-right shunt diverts blood from the myocardium into the pulmonary artery, with consequent ischemia of the anterolateral wall of the left ventricle, unless the coronary collateral circulation is well developed. Myocardial failure from ischemia, or even myocardial infarct, appears between 3 weeks and 6 months of age. Clinical presentation includes agitation and inconsolable crying, pallor, sweating, poor feeding, tachypnea, and pulmonary edema.

At auscultation, S_3 and S_4 are frequent, together with a blowing systolic murmur in the case of mitral valve regurgitation. The ECG shows broad, deep Q waves in leads I, aVL, V4, V5, and V6, with persistent ST-segment and T-wave changes. The chest radiograph shows cardiomegaly, pulmonary venous congestion, and pulmonary edema. Angiography frequently is necessary to confirm the clinical and echocardiographic diagnosis.

In the past, simple ligation of the anomalous left coronary artery was performed in the presence of significant left-to-right shunt to prevent runoff into the pulmonary circulation of blood destined to the myocardium. Currently, surgical repair consists of reimplantation of the coronary artery into the aorta or by an aortopulmonary

Table 61–4. Operative Mortality for Congenital Heart Disease: Consensus-Based Method of Risk Adjustment for In-Hospital Mortality in Children Younger than 18 Years Old After Surgery for Congenital Heart Disease

Risk Category 1

Atrial septal defect surgery (including atrial septal defect secundum, sinus venosus atrial septal defect, patent foramen ovale closure)
Aortopexy
Patent ductus arteriosus surgery at age >30 days
Coarctation repair at age >30 days
Partially anomalous pulmonary venous connection surgery

Risk Category 2

Aortic valvotomy or valvuloplasty at age >30 days
Subaortic stenosis resection
Pulmonary valvotomy or valvuloplasty
Pulmonary valve replacement
Right ventricular infundibulectomy
Pulmonary outflow tract augmentation
Repair of coronary artery fistula
Atrial septal defect and ventricular septal defect repair
Atrial septal defect primum repair
Ventricular septal defect repair
Ventricular septal defect closure and pulmonary valvotomy or infundibular resection
Ventricular septal defect closure and pulmonary artery band removal
Vascular ring surgery
Repair of aorto-pulmonary window
Coarctation repair at age <30 days
Repair of pulmonary artery stenosis
Transection of pulmonary artery
Common atrium closure
Left ventricular–to–right atrial shunt repair

Risk Category 3

Aortic valve replacement
Ross procedure
Left ventricular outflow tract patch
Ventriculomyotomy
Aortoplasty
Mitral valvotomy or valvuloplasty
Mitral valve replacement
Valvectomy of tricuspid valve
Tricuspid valvotomy or valvuloplasty
Tricuspid valve replacement
Tricuspid valve repositioning for Ebstein anomaly at age >30 days
Repair of anomalous coronary artery
Closure of semilunar valve, aortic or pulmonary
Right ventricular–to–pulmonary artery conduit
Left ventricular–to–pulmonary artery conduit
Repair of double-outlet right ventricle with or without repair of right ventricular obstruction
Fontan procedure

Repair of transitional or complete atrioventricular canal with or without valve replacement
Pulmonary artery banding
Repair of tetralogy of Fallot with pulmonary atresia
Repair of cor triatriatum
Systemic-to-pulmonary artery shunt
Atrial switch operation
Arterial switch operation
Reimplantation of anomalous pulmonary artery
Annuloplasty
Repair of coarctation and ventricular septal defect closure
Excision of intracardiac tumor

Risk Category 4

Aortic valvotomy or valvuloplasty at age <30 days
Konno procedure
Repair of complex anomaly (single ventricle) by ventricular septal defect enlargement
Repair of total anomalous pulmonary veins at age <30 days
Atrial septectomy
Repair of transposition, ventricular septal defect, and subpulmonary stenosis (Rastelli)
Atrial switch operation with ventricular septal defect closure
Atrial switch operation with repair of subpulmonary stenosis
Arterial switch operation with pulmonary artery band removal
Arterial switch operation with ventricular septal defect closure
Arterial switch operation with repair of subpulmonary stenosis
Repair of truncus arteriosus
Repair of hypoplastic or interrupted arch without ventricular septal defect closure
Repair of hypoplastic or interrupted aortic arch with ventricular septal defect closure
Transverse arch graft
Unifocalization for tetralogy of Fallot and pulmonary atresia
Double switch

Risk Category 5

Tricuspid valve repositioning for neonatal Ebstein anomaly at age <30 days
Repair of truncus arteriosus and interrupted arch

Risk Category 6

State 1 repair of hypoplastic left heart syndrome (Norwood operation)
State 1 repair of non–hypoplastic left heart syndrome conditions
Damus-Kaye-Stansel procedure

From Jenkins KJ, Gauseam K, Newburger JW, et al: Consensus-based risk adjustment for surgery for congenital heart desease. J Thorac Cardiovasc Surg 123:110, 2002.

Table 61–5. Surgical Mortality by Risk Category

Risk Category	No. Cases	Mortality Rate (%)
1	961	0.4
2	1222	3.8
3	1205	8.5
4	191	19.4
5	2	—
6	128	47.7

window together with a tunnel from the coronary ostium to the aorta through the created window. Operative mortality is influenced by the degree of myocardial ischemia and myocardial viability at the time of presentation. In some cases, extracorporeal circulatory support is necessary postoperatively to allow myocardial recovery. Operative mortality with current procedures is about 8% to 10%. Heart transplantation is a good option in case of irreversible myocardial failure.

SUMMARY

It now is well established that early complete repair rather than palliation of congenital heart defects produces the best long-term results. Also, avoidance of multiple surgical stages reduces the psychological and financial burden on the family. Most complex congenital heart defects are repaired in the neonate or young infant with the use of cardiopulmonary bypass with and without hypothermic circulatory arrest. Cognitive dysfunction and neurologic complications have been reported after hypothermic cardiopulmonary bypass (see Suggested Readings). Risk stratification category and current predicted operative (30 days) mortality for each risk category are listed in Tables 61-4 and 61-5. Specifically, Table 61-5 lists predicted mortality by risk category. The surgical database of the Society of Thoracic Surgery reports a detailed list of complications currently associated with the repair or palliation of congenital heart defects.

SUGGESTED READINGS

Aoki M, Forbess JM, Jonas RA, et al: Result of biventricular repair for double-outlet right ventricle. J Thorac Cardiovasc Surg 10:338, 1994.

Baker RA: Evaluation of neurologic assessment and outcomes in cardiac surgical patients. Semin Thorac Cardiovasc Surg 13:149, 2001.

Bove EL, Mosca RS: Surgical repair of the hypoplastic left heart syndrome. Prog Pediatr Cardiol 5:23, 1996.

Bull C, Kostelka M, Sorensen K, De Leval M: Outcome measures for the neonatal management of pulmonary atresia with intact ventricular septum. J Thorac Cardiovasc Surg 107:359, 1994.

Chiavarelli M, Gundry SR, Razzouk AJ, Bailey LL: Cardiac transplantation for infants with hypoplastic left-heart syndrome. JAMA 270:2944, 1993.

Cobanoglu A, Menashe VD: Total anomalous venous connection in neonates and young infants: Repair in the current era. J Thorac Cardiovasc Surg 104:728, 1992.

Danielson GK, Driscoll DJ, Mair DD, et al: Operative treatment of Ebstein's anomaly. J Thorac Cardiovasc Surg 104:1195, 1992.

Davis DA, Russo P, Greenspan JS, et al: High frequency jet versus conventional ventilation in infants undergoing Blalock-Taussig shunts. Ann Thorac Surg 57:846, 1994.

Driscoll DJ, Offord KP, Feldt RH, et al: Five-to-fifteen year follow-up after Fontan operation. Circulation 85:469, 1992.

Franklin RC, Spiegelhalter DJ, Sullivan ID, et al: Tricuspid atresia presenting in infancy: Survival and suitability for the Fontan operation. Circulation 87:427, 1993.

Freedom RM: Pulmonary Atresia and Intact Ventricular Septum. Mount Kisco, NY, Futura, 1989.

Freedom RM, Culham JAG, Moes CAF: Angiography of Congenital Heart Disease. New York, Macmillan, 1984.

Fyler DC, Buckley LP, Hellebrand WE, et al: Report of the New England Regional Infant Cardiac Program. Pediatrics 65(suppl):375, 1980.

Greenberg SB, Crisci KL, Koenig PR, et al: Magnetic resonance imaging in the evaluation of pulmonary artery abnormalities in tetralogy of Fallot following palliative and corrective surgery. Pediatr Radiol 26:588, 1996.

Greenberg SB, Crisci KL, Koenig PR, et al: Magnetic resonance imaging compared to echocardiography in the evaluation of pulmonary artery abnormalities in children with tetralogy of Fallot following palliative and corrective surgery. Pediatr Radiol 27:932, 1997.

Greenspan JS, Davis DA, Russo P, et al: Operative creation of left to right cardiac shunts: Pulmonary functional sequelae. Ann Thorac Surg 55:927, 1993.

Greenspan JS, Davis DA, Russo P, et al: High frequency jet ventilation: Intraoperative application in infants. Pediatr Pulmonol 17:155, 1994.

Gutgesell HP: Echocardiograph as an alternative to cardiac catheterization prior to surgery for congenital heart disease. In Kron KL, Mavroudis C (eds): Innovations in Congenital Heart Surgery. Philadelphia, Hanley & Belfus, 1989.

Hanley FL, Heinemann MK, Jonas RA, et al: Repair of truncus arteriosus in the neonate. J Thorac Cardiovasc Surg 105:1047, 1993.

Hanley FL, Sade RM, Freedom RM, et al: Outcomes in critically ill neonates with pulmonary stenosis and intact ventricular septum: A multiinstitutional study. J Am Coll Cardiol 22:183, 1993.

Hing YM, Moller JH: Ebstein's anomaly: A long-term study of survival. Am Heart J 125:1419, 1993.

Huhta JC, Seward JB, Tajik AJ, et al: Two-dimensional echocardiographic spectrum of univentricular atrioventricular connection. J Am Coll Cardiol 5:149, 1985.

Ilbawi MN, Greico J, Deleon SY, et al: Modified Blalock-Taussig shunt in newborn infants. J Thorac Cardiovasc Surg 88:770, 1984.

Jenkins KJ: Consensus-based method for risk adjustment for surgery for congenital heart disease. J Thorac Cardiovasc Surg 123:110, 2002.

Jenkins KJ, Sanders SP, Orav EJ, et al: Individual pulmonary vein size and survival in infants with total anomalous pulmonary venous connection. J Am Coll Cardiol 22:201, 1993.

Joffe H, Georgapolous D, Celermajer DS, et al: Late ventricular arrhythmia is rare after early repair of tetralogy of Fallot. J Am Coll Cardiol 23:1146, 1994.

Karl TR, Sano S, Pornviliwan S, Mee RB: Tetralogy of Fallot: Favorable outcome of nonneonatal transatrial, transpulmonary repair. Ann Thorac Surg 54:903, 1992.

Kasznica J, Ursell PC, Blanc WA, et al: Abnormalities of the coronary circulation in pulmonary atresia and intact ventricular septum. Am Heart J 114:1415, 1987.

Kirklin JW, Barratt-Boyes BG: Cardiac Surgery. New York, Wiley, 1993.

Lababidi Z: Aortic balloon valvuloplasty. Am Heart J 106(4 pt 1): 751, 1983.

Limperopoulos C: Neurodevelopmental status of newborns and infants with congenital heart defects before and after open heart surgery. J Pediatr 137:638, 2000.

Lucas RV Jr, Lock JE, Tanlon R, et al: Gross and histologic anatomy of total anomalous pulmonary venous connections. Am J Cardiol 62:292, 1988.

Lui RC, Williams WG, Trusler GA, et al: Experience with the Damus-Stansel-Kaye procedure for children with Taussig-Bing hearts or univentricular hearts with subaortic stenosis. Circulation 88(suppl II):170, 1993.

Mair DD, Puga FJ, Danielson GK: Late functional status of survivors of the Fontan procedure performed during the 1970s. Circulation 86(suppl II):106, 1992.

Malm T, Pawade A, Karl TR, Mee RB: Recent results with the modified Fontan operation. Scand J Thorac Cardiovasc Surg 27:65, 1993.

Martin RP, Qureshi SA, Ettedgui JA, et al: An evaluation of right and left ventricular function after anatomical correction and intra-atrial repair operations for complete transposition of the great arteries. Circulation 82:808, 1990.

Mavroudis C, Gevitz MW, Ring R, et al: The Society of Thoracic Surgeons national congenital heart surgery database report: Analysis of the first harvest (1994-1997). Ann Thorac Surg 68:601, 1999.

Paul D, Greenspan J, Davis D, et al: The role of cardiopulmonary bypass and surfactant in pulmonary decompensation after surgery for congenital heart disease. J Thorac. Cardiovasc Surg 6:117, 1999.

Rabinovitch M, Herreva-Deleon V, Castaneda AR, et al: Growth and development of the pulmonary vascular bed in patients with tetralogy of Fallot with or without pulmonary atresia. Circulation 64:1234, 1981.

Razzouk A, Chinnock R, Gundry S: Transplantation as a primary treatment for hypoplastic left heart syndrome: Intermediate-term results. Ann Thorac Surg 62:1, 1996.

Reddy VM, Liddicoat JR, McElhinney DB, et al: Routine primary repair of tetralogy of Fallot in neonates and infants less than three months of age. Ann Thorac Surg 60:S592, 1995.

Reddy VM, Petrossian E, McElhinney DB, et al: One stage complete unifocalization in infants: When should the ventricular septal defect be closed? J Thorac Cardiovasc Surg 113:858, 1997.

Russo P, Danielson GK, Driscoll DV: Transaortic closure of ventricular septal defect in patients with corrected transposition with pulmonary stenosis or atresia. Circulation 76(suppl III): III-88, 1987.

Russo P, Danielson GK, Driscoll DV: Fontan procedure for mitral atresia or hypoplasia (61st Annual Meeting of the American Heart Association, Washington, DC, 1988) [abstract]. Circulation 78(suppl II):II-85, 1988.

Russo P, Danielson GK, Puga F, et al: Fontan for complex forms of DORV (60th Annual Meeting of the American Heart Association, 1987) [abstract]. Circulation 76(suppl IV):IV-290, 1987.

Russo P, Danielson GK, Puga F, et al: Modified Fontan procedure for biventricular hearts with complex forms of double-outlet right ventricle. Circulation 78(suppl III):III-20, 1988.

Scalia D, Russo P, Anderson RH, et al: The surgical anatomy of hearts with no direct communication between the right atrium and the ventricular mass—so-called tricuspid atresia. J Thorac Cardiovasc Surg 87:743, 1984.

Serraf A, Lacour-Gayet F, Bruniaux J, et al: Anatomic correction of transposition of the great arteries in neonates. J Am Coll Cardiol 22:193, 1993.

Stanger P: Truncus arteriosus. In Moller JH, Neal WA (eds): Fetal, Neonatal, and Infant Cardiac Disease. Norwalk, CT, Appleton & Lange, 1990, p 587.

Stark J: Do we really correct congenital heart defects? J Thorac Cardiovasc Surg 97:1, 1989.

Wang JK, Lue HC, Wu MH, et al: Obstructed total anomalous pulmonary venous connection. Pediatr Cardiol 14:28, 1993.

CHAPTER 62

Diagnosis and Management of Cardiac Dysrhythmias

Paul Anisman

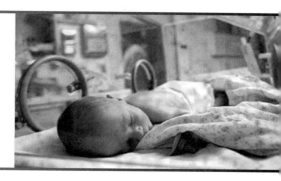

CONDUCTION SYSTEM

Early within fetal development, atrial and ventricular contractions occur. The more caudal region, that of the primitive atrium, beats faster than the more cephalic region, the primitive ventricle.[1,2] This activity occurs even before the semilunar and atrioventricular (AV) valves are formed. The normal **conduction system** that eventually develops is derived from myocardial cells and consists of the sinoatrial (sinus) node, the AV node, the His bundle and bundle branches, and the Purkinje fibers. The AV node and His bundle form separately and are joined by approximately 8 weeks of gestation, and the sinoatrial node is formed by 10 weeks of gestation. By 16 weeks, sinus rhythm can be detected. Anatomic molding and maturation continue throughout gestation and into the neonatal period.

It has long been known that the primitive heart tube has an intrinsic pulsation rate that derives from individual myocardial cells and that the myocardial cells forming the primitive heart tube share the property of the *slow* spread of **contractile activity**.[3,4] More recently, it has been proposed that this is such an important and basic property that the cells of the primitive heart tube should be classified as a distinct entity called **primary myocardium**.[5] Eventually, day 24 in the human, the cells of the primitive heart tube that differentiate into primitive atrium and primitive ventricle acquire new biologic and electrophysiologic properties: they acquire the property of the *fast* spread of **electrical activity**. These cells no longer are classified as primary myocardium and now are classified as **working myocardium**.[6] When the heart tube then loops, and the sinus venosus is incorporated into the right atrium, only a minor portion of those cells retain the property of slow conduction characteristic of primary myocardium, and this group of cells forms the sinoatrial node. Similarly, as the AV canal is incorporated into the right atrium, only a small portion retains the characteristic of slow conduction, and these form the AV node. Although the sinoatrial and AV nodes have been called part of a **specialized conduction system**, based on the persistence of the characteristic of slow spread of conduction, we recognize them now as remnants of primary myocardium.[3,7]

Normal electrical conduction, known as **sinus rhythm**, begins at the sinus node, proceeds via the atrial myocardium to the AV node, and reaches the ventricular myocardium through the His-Purkinje system (Fig. 62-1).[8] The sinus node or **pacemaker** is responsible for normal impulse formation. It usually is located subepicardially within the terminal groove of the high right atrium near the junction of the superior vena cava. Propagation of the electrical impulse to the AV node occurs through working atrial myocardium, by preferential conduction along major muscle bundles within the atria based on arrangement and packing of the cells. The compact portion of the AV node is an interatrial structure located near the tricuspid valve annulus, adjacent to the interventricular septum. As a remnant of primitive myocardium, it is a collection of myocytes with the special ability to slow conduction and serves to delay impulse conduction from the atria to the bundle of His. The AV node becomes the penetrating bundle or His bundle, enters the central fibrous body at the apex of the triangle of Koch in the right atrium, and emerges into the subaortic left ventricular outflow tract before dividing into the right and left bundle branches. The left bundle further divides into three major fascicles, whereas the right bundle penetrates the muscular ventricular septum, passing down to the right ventricular apex within the septal band. The fibers of the right and left bundle branches connect to the ventricular myocardium either directly or through Purkinje cells. There are known variations in the number, anatomic position, and structure of many of the components of the conduction system in structurally normal and abnormal hearts.

ELECTROCARDIOGRAPHY

Einthoven described the first adult **electrocardiogram (ECG)** in 1903, and 3 years later Cremer[9] published the first fetal ECG. With direct recording of fetal electrical activity,

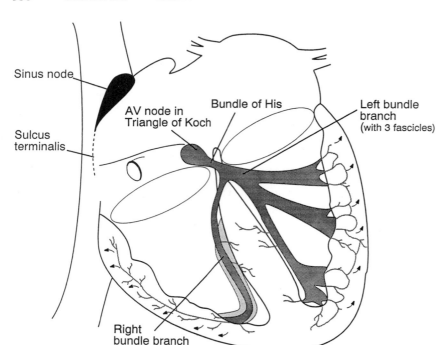

Figure 62–1. The specialized conduction system. AV, atrioventricular.

the entire fetal ECG complex may be seen. Although trans-abdominal placement of fetal electrodes has been performed,[10,11] the current clinical application of direct recording fetal electrocardiography is during intrapartum fetal heart rate monitoring after rupture of membranes by transvaginal placement of electrodes to the presenting fetal part. Indirect intrapartum recording of the fetal ECG, in which the signal is recorded from external maternal electrodes, has been largely superseded by Doppler ultrasonography. Antepartum dysrhythmias generally are detected by auscultation of the fetal heart, and fetal echocardiography has become the standard diagnostic technique. In the neonate, surface electrocardiography is simple, convenient, and usually diagnostic of the rhythm. In addition, transesophageal and intracardiac electrophysiologic studies are possible in the neonate and may be useful in the diagnosis and treatment of neonatal dysrhythmias.

FETAL HEART RATES AND RHYTHMS

In utero, the normal mean embryonic heart rate has been identified as 100 beats/min at 6 weeks of gestation, increasing to a plateau of approximately 140 beats/min at 9 weeks of gestation.[12] Another study of first-trimester embryonic heart rates noted spontaneous abortion in all pregnancies with embryonic heart rates less than 85 beats/min at 5 to 6 menstrual weeks.[13] Another study found the mean fetal heart rates to be 155 beats/min at 20 weeks of gestation and 140 beats/min at term and noted that fetal heart rates tended to decrease linearly with increasing gestational age.[14] A study of second-trimester and third-trimester fetal heart rates and patterns defined the normal fetal heart rate to be between 110 and 150 beats/min and noted that after 34 weeks' gestation

the patterns of fetal heart rates appeared to relate to fetal rest and activity.[15] In general, fetal cardiac dysrhythmias may be identified by heart rates less than 100 beats/min, heart rates greater than 200 beats/min, or an irregular rhythm. Most fetal dysrhythmias are detected during the last 10 weeks of gestation, but tachydysrhythmias have been identified early within the second trimester. Fetal heart rate and rhythm are affected by humoral factors and interaction with the autonomic nervous system, by the intrinsic characteristics of the sinoatrial and AV nodes, by physical influences such as uterine contraction and fetal movement, by hypoxia and fetal distress, and by the direct and indirect effects of pharmacologic agents.

NEONATAL HEART RATES AND RHYTHMS

Cardiac rate and rhythm in healthy neonates have been studied by 24-hour ambulatory electrocardiography,[16-18] and it seems reasonable to use the following guidelines in evaluating heart rates in normal neonates. Neonates with sleeping heart rates less than 60 beats/min or awake heart rates less than 80 beats/min are identified as having bradycardia. At the lowest heart rates, 80% of normal neonates can be expected to be in sinus rhythm, whereas nearly 20% may be in junctional rhythm. The highest normal neonatal heart rates average approximately 190 beats/min but may reach nearly 240 beats/min.[18] We suspect the presence of **supraventricular tachycardia (SVT)** when a rhythm that originates in the atrium is greater than 200 beats/min, with recognition that SVT may occur at slower heart rates and that persistence of sinus rhythm greater than 200 beats/min occurs rarely in healthy neonates. Tachycardia of ventricular origin ranges from 167 to 440 beats/min (mean 260 beats/min).[16,19,20]

In this chapter, the diagnosis and management of dysrhythmias in the fetus and neonate are divided arbitrarily into rhythm and conduction abnormalities. Because of the high prevalence of simple isolated ectopic rhythms, premature atrial contractions (PACs) and premature ventricular contractions (PVCs) are the first topics reviewed. These discussions are followed by sections on supraventricular and ventricular tachydysrhythmias. Discussion of supraventricular tachydysrhythmias is divided into a section on SVT including AV reentry (the preexcitation syndromes) and AV node reentry and separate sections on atrial flutter, atrial fibrillation, and other less common forms of SVT. The section on ventricular tachydysrhythmias includes ventricular tachycardia (VT) and ventricular fibrillation. Bradydysrhythmias are discussed in the sections on disorders of impulse formation and disorders of AV conduction.

PREMATURE ATRIAL CONTRACTIONS

PACs result from premature atrial depolarizations. PACs are common, usually occur as isolated extrasystoles, and account for most isolated extrasystoles in the fetus and newborn.[16,18,21,22] PACs themselves are benign. They are detected in utero in less than 2% of patients from 30 weeks of gestation to term.[23] Although screening ECG has identified PACs in approximately 1% of healthy neonates,[24,25] 24-hour ambulatory ECG monitoring has revealed that during the first day of life approximately 50% of newborns have PACs, and PACs occur in almost two thirds of infants 1 to 11 months old.[18]

If the underlying substrate to allow for reentry, SVT, is present, a single PAC may serve to initiate SVT, and there is an estimated 1% risk of initiating SVT in the fetus and the neonate.[23] When a PAC is conducted to the ventricles, it results in an early ventricular depolarization and ventricular contraction. If it occurs sufficiently early that either the AV node or the His-Purkinje pathway is still refractory to conduction, however, it is not conducted to the ventricles, and it is called a *blocked* or *nonconducted* PAC. A nonconducted PAC may be identified on surface electrocardiography as an early P wave that is not followed by a corresponding QRS complex. When alternately conducted and blocked **(blocked atrial bigeminy)**, the rhythm may mimic bradycardia and must be distinguished from complete heart block. PACs usually enter and reset the sinus node and are not usually followed by a full compensatory pause, although this may not be true for PACs of low atrial origin.

Diagnosis in the Fetus

In the fetus, M-mode echocardiography identifies a PAC and shows whether it is followed in synchrony by a ventricular wall motion as a conducted PAC or whether it occurs without a corresponding ventricular contraction as a nonconducted or blocked PAC. In similar fashion, a comparison of pulsed wave Doppler signals across an AV valve and a ventricular outflow tract or a combination of M-mode and Doppler tracings may provide the necessary information for diagnosis (Fig. 62-2). Color flow Doppler examination may make it easier to associate temporally

M-mode and Doppler signals. With this technique, PACs in utero usually can be distinguished from PVCs, in which the premature motion is of the ventricle rather than the atrium and which may be followed by a full compensatory pause, and from complete heart block (third-degree AV block), in which there is complete asynchrony between atrial and ventricular contraction with the atrial rate faster than the ventricular rate.

Diagnosis in the Neonate

In the neonate, surface electrocardiography is diagnostic, and echocardiography is not necessary for diagnosis of this rhythm (Fig. 62-3). The premature P wave, representing premature atrial muscle depolarization, may appear with any morphology and axis. Each conducted PAC is represented by a P wave followed by a correspondingly premature QRS complex. A nonconducted PAC is represented by a prematurely early P wave that is not followed by a corresponding QRS complex. The morphology of the QRS complex resulting from a conducted PAC may be narrow or wide. It is widened if the bundle-branch system (generally the right bundle) is partially refractory to conduction, or if AV conduction occurs over a direct extranodal AV connection as in the preexcitation syndromes. The lack of a full compensatory pause after a premature beat can help to distinguish a PAC from a PVC.

Management in the Fetus

In the fetus, echocardiography diagnoses PACs and distinguishes them from PVCs and from complete heart block. In the fetus with a structurally normal heart, PACs do not cause adverse hemodynamic effects, and no specific treatment is required. The fetus with blocked PACs may have a slightly further increased risk of developing fetal SVT.[26] On diagnosis of fetal PACs, we recommend that the fetal heart rate be monitored twice weekly as long as the dysrhythmia is present to screen for the occurrence of SVT. If the mother is taking cardiac stimulant medications or is consuming large doses of caffeine, she is encouraged to diminish her intake.

It is common to find redundancy of the septum primum (aneurysm of the foramen ovale), with the atrial septum intermittently coming into contact with the left atrial wall, during fetal echocardiography.[27] Some believe that after birth, with increased left atrial pressure and consequently more central alignment of the septum primum, the absence of contact with the left atrial wall results in early resolution of PACs in these patients.[28] No treatment is required.

Management in the Neonate

In the neonate, the underlying causes of PACs rarely are identified. In a healthy newborn with an otherwise normal physical examination and without known risk factors, no further workup is required after diagnosis. In this setting, PACs often resolve by 3 months of age. Rare causes of PACs include electrolyte imbalances, metabolic disorders, endocrine disorders, inflammatory and infiltrative myocardial diseases, sepsis, and hypoxic myocardial insult. Iatrogenic causes include mechanical factors, such as intracardiac catheters (umbilical vein line, extracorporeal

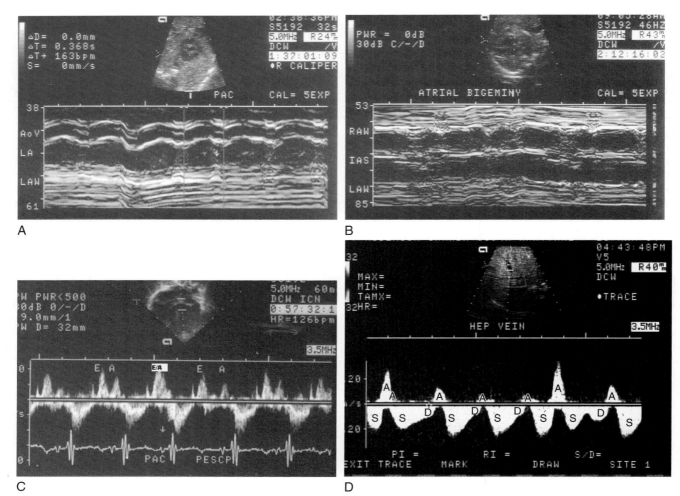

Figure 62–2. A, M-mode echocardiography through the right ventricle at the *top,* aorta in the *middle,* and left atrium at the *bottom.* Within the aorta, the aortic valve leaflets can be seen to open like a parallelogram during systole and sometimes are seen as a single downward-angled line in diastole. The vertical caliper lines denote opening of the aortic valve and follow directly the left atrial posterior wall motions (the "bumps" at the bottom of the left atrium). The *arrow* points to premature motion of the left atrial wall, a physical manifestation of a premature atrial contraction (PAC). The second vertical line corresponds to premature opening of the aortic valve (associated with ventricular ejection) after a PAC; this means that the PAC was conducted. Even if the tracing had not shown the aortic valve leaflets well, because the aorta itself is known to move anteriorly in the chest with each ejection of blood, the demonstration of anterior motion of the aorta in synchrony with the premature left atrial wall motion would confirm a conducted PAC. **B,** The marks along the time line at the *top* denote intervals of 0.2 second, so the entire strip is about 2.6 seconds. The right atrial wall is at the *top* (RAW), the interatrial septum (IAS) is in the *middle,* and the left atrial wall (LAW) is at the *bottom.* In this figure, the RAW motion is delineated most clearly, and the motions of the atrial walls seem to occur in pairs. This is often called *atrial bigeminy.* This tracing does not reflect whether the atrial contractions are conducted or blocked. **C,** A spectral Doppler tracing capturing the left ventricular inflow velocities (the upright E and A waves) and the downward-directed left ventricular outflow. The E wave represents early diastolic "passive" inflow to the left ventricle, and the A wave represents the "active" flow attributed to atrial contraction; A follows E. The relative direction of the display is not important and relates to the orientation of the heart at the time of sampling. The tracing happens to be obtained from an infant rather than a fetus so as to display simultaneously at bottom an electrocardiogram strip, but it would look similarly in a fetus. At the time of the PAC, the A wave (representing active flow due to atrial contraction) occurs earlier than usual and encroaches on and merges with the E wave. It is followed by a left ventricular outflow signal representing ventricular ejection from the conducted PAC. The diastolic interval after the conducted PAC is slightly prolonged, allowing for better separation between the subsequent E and A waves. PESCP, premature escape beat. **D,** A spectral Doppler tracing obtained in a hepatic (HEP) vein. The downward-directed velocities correspond to flow *toward* the heart during ventricular systole (S wave) and diastole (D wave). The upward-directed velocities (A wave) indicate *retrograde* flow toward the hepatic vein (e.g., away from the heart) during atrial contraction. During normal sinus rhythm, the S wave is dominant, whereas the D and A waves are small; on this tracing, the S and D waves almost merge during normal sinus rhythm. Starting at the left, the first A wave reflects a premature atrial contraction. Note how it is taller than the three subsequent atrial waves during sinus rhythm. The fourth atrial wave is premature, and it too is tall. Because every atrial A wave is followed in synchrony by a ventricular S wave, on this tracing all atrial beats, including the PACs, are conducted. After the second PAC, the S and D waves are exceptionally distinct; this is due to the long interval before the next atrial contraction. *(Courtesy of Dennis Wood.)*

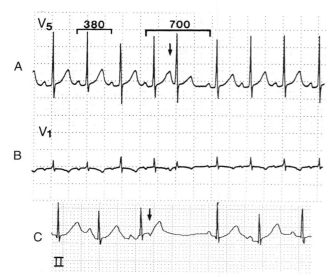

Figure 62–3. Tracings **A** and **B** are recorded simultaneously from a neonate noted to have an irregular rhythm and reveal a conducted premature atrial contraction (PAC). When regular, the P-P and R-R intervals are 380 msec. The fifth complex on the strip (P and QRS) occurs prematurely, and the P wave is marked with an *arrow*. The premature P-QRS complex is followed by less than a full compensatory pause of 700 msec. (R-R from the QRS preceding the premature P-QRS complex to the QRS immediately after the PAC is <760 msec.) Tracing **C** is recorded from a 2-day-old infant and shows a nonconducted (blocked) PAC. The premature P wave *(arrow)* falls within the ST segment of the third QRS complex and is not followed by a QRS; it is not conducted to the ventricles. The sinus node is reset by the PAC, however, and the PAC is followed by less than a full compensatory pause. (R-R of two beats preceding the PAC equals 460 msec; R-R from QRS before the PAC to QRS after the PAC equals 760 msec, i.e., <920 msec.)

circulatory support cannula) and pharmacologic effects, including effects of dopamine, dobutamine, isoproterenol, digoxin, theophylline, and caffeine. Structural congenital heart diseases and cardiac tumors also may be rare causes of PACs and of tachycardia. In the absence of an identifiable etiology, isolated PACs do not cause hemodynamic compromise of the healthy heart, and no treatment is required.

Premature Ventricular Contractions

PVCs result from premature spontaneous depolarizations originating distal to the bifurcation of the bundle of His and most often occur as isolated uniform extrasystoles. They rarely are detected in utero[16,29] and account for the minority of extrasystoles detected in newborns.[22,24] Twenty-four-hour ambulatory ECG monitoring beginning within the first hour of birth has identified PVCs in 18% of healthy newborns.[18]

The theorized mechanisms underlying PVCs (and SVT and VT) include reentry, automaticity, and triggered activity. In the fetus and the neonate, the underlying causes of PVCs rarely are identified, and no treatment is usually required. Rare causes include hypoxia; acidosis; hyperkalemia and hypokalemia; hypoglycemia; myocarditis; intracardiac catheters; and drugs such as caffeine, nicotine, sympathomimetic agents, anesthetics, digoxin, and other antiarrhythmic agents. Single PVCs do not cause hemodynamic compromise and only rarely lead to a more advanced dysrhythmia. It also is extremely rare for couplets to cause hemodynamic distress. Ventricular parasystole is rare in children, but was reported in an asymptomatic infant, in whom it was transient and persisted until 10 months of age.[30]

Diagnosis in the Fetus

In the fetus, the diagnosis is established by M-mode echocardiography or by pulsed wave Doppler examination. Premature ventricular wall motions without preceding synchronized atrial wall motions denote either PVCs or early junctional beats that are indistinguishable from one another on M-mode and Doppler examination. Pulsed wave Doppler interrogation, with a wide sample volume across the left ventricular inflow and outflow tracts, may identify PVCs and may differentiate them from PACs and from complete heart block. The presence of a full compensatory pause may help to distinguish PVCs from PACs and from early junctional beats, although a full compensatory pause also may occur with low PACs if they do not reset the sinus node.

Diagnosis in the Neonate

In the neonate, surface electrocardiography is diagnostic; echocardiography is not necessary for the diagnosis of PVCs (Fig. 62-4). The QRS complex occurs earlier than

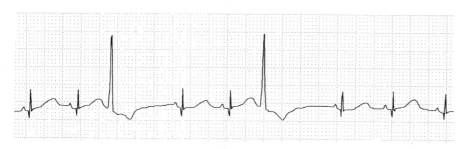

Figure 62–4. Lead V_6 in a 1-day-old infant shows two premature ventricular contractions (PVCs). The premature QRS complex is not preceded by a P wave; the QRS is wide with aberrant conduction; the T wave after the premature QRS is directed opposite that of the QRS; each PVC is followed by a full compensatory pause in which the R-R interval between the QRS before the PVC and the QRS after the PVC is at least twice as long as the R-R interval of the two normal QRS complexes preceding the PVC.

would be expected in a regular rhythm and is not preceded by a P wave. The morphology of the premature QRS complex is different from that of the regular QRS complex, and it usually has a prolonged duration (>0.080 second in infancy), although this may not always be the case. PVCs usually are accompanied by ST-segment and T-wave abnormalities with the T-wave direction opposite that of the QRS. Most PVCs occur as isolated uniform extra-systoles, although multiform PVCs do occur. PVCs may occur as fusion complexes, be paired as couplets, or occur as bigeminy, trigeminy, quadrigeminy, or parasystole. Multiform PVCs are rare in children with normal hearts.

Management in the Fetus

In the fetus, because of the potential risk of initiation of SVT or VT and the consequent associated risk of developing hydrops fetalis, when PVCs are identified, subsequent biweekly screening of the fetal heart rate is recommended. Because the risk of induction of a clinically important tachydysrhythmia is low, pharmacologic suppression is not indicated.

Management in the Neonate

In healthy neonates, PVCs generally resolve within the first 2 months of postnatal life[16] and are uncommon later in the first year of life.[18] A neonate with an otherwise normal physical examination and without risk factors may not require further evaluation thereafter. The ECG should be scrutinized carefully for the presence of a prolonged Q-T interval (long Q-T$_c$) and for signs of myocarditis (diminished voltages and ST-T abnormalities). If PVCs persist beyond 4 to 8 weeks of life, an echocardiogram may be useful to exclude an obvious intramyocardial cardiac tumor and cardiomyopathy. Uniform PVCs in an otherwise healthy infant are generally benign. In contrast, multiform PVCs may be a marker for an abnormal heart. If no disease or etiology is found, infants with multiform PVCs may be followed conservatively with annual screening of rhythm and function.

In a neonate who has undergone repair of congenital heart disease under cardiopulmonary bypass, postoperative PVCs are common. In this setting, causes of PVCs and of VT include hypoxia, ischemia, and hypokalemia, particularly in the presence of digoxin and diuretic therapy. Hypokalemia should be corrected by potassium supplementation. Antiarrhythmic drug therapy rarely is required. When suppression of PVCs or couplets is desired, intravenous lidocaine may be given as a 1-mg/kg bolus, which can be repeated as required every 5 minutes up to three doses; this is followed by an infusion of intravenous lidocaine at 10 to 50 μg/kg/min and titrated to the rhythm as required. Procainamide may be given as a 10- to 15-mg/kg intravenous drip over 1 hour. Procainamide is contraindicated, however, in the presence of long Q-T syndrome. For more details on antidysrhythmic drugs, see Table 62-1. All underlying etiologies should be sought and corrected, after which, with a good hemodynamic repair, PVCs tend to resolve.

SUPRAVENTRICULAR TACHYDYSRHYTHMIAS

Supraventricular Tachycardia

SVT is characterized as a tachycardia due to an abnormal mechanism, incorporating the atria, the specialized conduction system, or both. More specifically, SVT requires for its perpetuation structures in the heart generally proximal to the bifurcation of the bundle of His. SVT is to be distinguished from VT, which originates below the His bundle.

SVT is the most common tachydysrhythmia in the fetus, neonate, and young child. The estimated prevalence of SVT in children is 1.5 to 4.0 per 1000, which is similar to the prevalence of structural congenital heart disease in newborns.[31] Recognition of this abnormal rhythm is crucial in the fetus and the neonate because signs of congestive heart failure may occur within 24 to 48 hours of onset.[32] In the fetus, heart failure due to SVT may manifest as pericardial effusion, cardiomegaly, or hydrops fetalis. In the infant, congestive heart failure may be recognized by pallor, irritability, tachypnea, feeding difficulty, vomiting, cardiomegaly, and hepatomegaly.

In defining tachycardia as a heart rate above the normal range, one must include recognition of the patient's age and the site of origin of the dysrhythmia. SVT originating from the AV junction is generally slower than SVT originating from the atrium. The normal fetal heart rate commonly ranges from 110 to 150 beats/min and varies with uterine contraction and with fetal movement. Fetal SVT is characterized by a sustained rapid heart rate usually greater than or equal to 240 beats/min. The healthy newborn heart rate ranges from 60 to 240 beats/min, whereas neonatal SVT is characterized by tachycardia ranging from 150 to 280 beats/min. Faster rates of SVT occasionally are seen, in which case atrial flutter should be suspected. A neonate with a heart rate less than 230 beats/min is more likely to have sinus tachycardia than SVT, and etiologies toward that end should be considered.

SVT may appear at any age, although it occurs more frequently in neonates compared with older children.[31-33] It also is more prevalent in children with congenital heart disease and in children after cardiac surgery. In a large study of children with SVT,[31] the onset of SVT occurred by 1 month of age in 18%, by 3 months of age in 44%, and by 1 year of age in 80% of the patients; these data are consistent with earlier data.[32] Four clinically separate mechanisms have been proposed as responsible for SVT:

1. Reentry with an accessory connection
2. Reentry without an accessory connection
3. Automatic ectopic focus
4. Triggered arrhythmia

In the fetus and neonate, the most common forms of SVT are those due to reentry mechanisms either by a direct **AV accessory connection (AV reentry)**, the best known of which is **Wolff-Parkinson-White (WPW)** syndrome, or by reentry within the AV node **(AV node reentry)**. Accessory connections have often been referred to as

Continued

Table 62-1. Antidysrhythmic Drugs

Class	Drug	Possible Use	Dosage (level)	Mechanism	Precautions and Side Effects
Ia: Na⁺ channel blockade—prolonged repolarization					
	Quinidine gluconate	SVT AF with dig or prop PVCs VT	PO: 15-60 mg/kg/day q8h IV and IM available. IV not recommended (2-8 µg/mL)	Depresses conduction and prolongs refractoriness in atria, ventricle, and HP Prolongs, ERP of AC ante in WPW and retro in AVN	Proarrhythmia; torsades de pointes; AV block; hypotension; myocardial depression; blood dyscrasia; ↑ dig level; ↑ Q-T$_c$
	Quinidine sulfate	Similar to quinidine	PO: 15-60 mg/kg/day q6h Only available PO	Similar to quinidine	Similar to quinidine
	Procainamide	Similar to quinidine	PO: 15-60 mg/kg/day q4-6h IV: 3-6 mg/kg/5 min and 3.5 mg/kg q4h: maint: 20-50 µg/kg/min IM: 5-8 mg/kg q6h (5-10 µg/mL) PA + NAPA (10-30 µg/mL)	Metabolite NAPA active	Metabolite NAPA also has antidysrhythmic effect
	Disopyramide	Similar to quinidine	PO: 20-30 mg/kg/day q6h IV: available but not recommended (3-8 µg/mL)	Similar to quinidine	Similar to quinidine Anticholinergic
Ib: Na⁺ channel blockade—shortened repolarization					
	Lidocaine	PVCs VT	IV: 1 mg/kg may repeat q5min × 3, then maint: 10-50 µg/kg/min (1-5 µg/mL)	Depresses myocardial irritability ↑ Vfib threshold	Myocardial depression ↓ Q-T$_c$ Seizures
	Phenytoin	PVCs Digoxin toxicity	IV: 3-5 mg/kg over 5 min; max: 15 mg/kg over 1 hr PO: 5-6 mg/kg/day q12h (15-20 µg/mL)	Similar to lidocaine Suppresses dig-induced ventr after depolarization	Hypotension ↓ Q-T$_c$ CNS
	Mexiletine	Chronic PVCs and VT	PO: 9-15 mg/kg/day q8h (0.5-2.0 µg/mL)	Similar to lidocaine	Hypotension; AV block; bradycardia; GI; CNS
	Moricizine	PVCs, VT, AAT?, AVN reentry?	PO: 5-15 mg/kg/day q8h (effect does not correlate with level)	Myocardial membrane stabilizing; prolongs AV conduction AVN and HP	Proarrhythmia ↑ PR ↑ QRS CNS, GI
Ic: Na⁺ channel blockade—variable effect on repolarization					
	Flecainide	AAT CAR Afib PJRT	PO: 2-6 mg/kg/day q8-12h IV: 1-2 mg/kg over 5-10 min (0.2-2.0 µg/mL)	Slows conduction throughout conduction system Greatest effect on His Can ↑ ventr response	Proarrhythmia ↑PR ↑ QRS ↑ Q-T$_c$

Table 62–1. Antidysrhythmic Drugs—cont'd

Class	Drug	Possible Use	Dosage level	Mechanism	Precautions and Side Effects
	Propafenone	SVT VT JET AAT Resistant SVT VT	For JET: IV if available—IV: 0.2 mg/kg q10min (max 2 mg) Infusion: 4–7 μg/kg/min[88] PO: mean 350 mg/m^2/day q8h (range 200–600 mg/m^2)[82,119] (0.2–1.5 μg/mL)	No active metabolite Slows conduction throughout conduction system and ↓ automaticity Prolongs ERP ante in WPW and retro in AVN Mild β-receptor and Ca^{2+} channel blockade Two active metabolites	CNS Proarrhythmia similar to flecainide ↑PR, ↑QRS, ↑Q-T$_c$, ↑ dig level Myocardial depression Hypotension Bronchospasm, CNS, liver abnormalities
II: β blockers	Propranolol	SVT WPW and AVN Long Q-T$_c$ VT Thyrotoxicosis	PO: 1–6 mg/kg/day q6h IV: 0.05–0.15 mg/kg over 10 min, q6-8h prn	Nonselective β blockade	Bradycardia ↑ ERP AVN, may ↓ Q-T$_c$ Contraindicated with Ca channel blockade Myocardial depression Bronchospasm
	Esmolol	Similar to propranolol	IV: load 500 μg/kg over 1 min Maintenance: Start 50 μg/kg/min, may ↑ gradually to 1000 μg/kg/min if necessary	β$_1$ cardioselective blockade	Similar to propranolol Less bronchospasm
	Atenolol	Similar to propranol Use if bronchospasm	PO: 1–2 mg/kg/day qd or q12h	β$_1$ cardioselective blockade	Similar to propranol Less bronchospasm Less CNS effect Renel excreation
III: Prolonged repolarization	Amiodarone	JET Resistant: SVT, AF, Afib, CAR, AAT, PJRT?	PO: 5–10 mg/kg/day q12h × 7–10 days, then 2–4 mg/kg/day; use lowest effective dose IV: 1-mg/kg bolus q10min, may repeat to max 5 mg/kg; maintenance infusion 5–15 μg/kg/min; use lowest effective dose Maternal: PO: 1800–2400 mg 2–5 days, then if still tachy 600 mg/day; 200–400 mg/day if not tachy; continue 3-4 wk	↑ ERP in all cardiac tissues	Bradycardia proarrhythmia ↑ Q-T$_c$ and torsades de pointes ↑Level digoxin, quinidine and procainamide Hypo-/hyperthyroidism Growth retardation Corneal deposits Pneumonitis

Drug	Indications	Dose	Effect	Proarrhythmia
Sotalol	AAT, CAR, Afib, AF, SVT; Ventr ectopy/VT?	PO: 90-200 mg/m²/day q8h or 2-4 mg/kg/day q12h; IV (outside U.S.): 0.2-1.5 mg/kg; Maternal: PO: 160-320 mg/day q12h	↑ ERP atria and ventr; Also, nonselective β-blockade	Proarrhythmia ↑ Q-T$_c$ and torsades de points; Myocardial depression
Ibutilide	AF, Afib	IV: 0.01 mg/kg; repeat q 15-20 min; max 0.03 mg; little pediatric experience	ERP atria and ventr	Proarrhythmia ↑ Q-T$_c$ and torsades de points; Active first-pass metabolism
Bretylium	Vfib and VT	IV: 5-mg/kg bolus, may repeat; Infusion: 20-40 µg/kg/min	↑ V fib threshold, chemical sympathectomy	Teratogenic; Hypotension
IV: Ca^{2+} channel blockade				
Verapamil	Contraindicated in neonates (<1 yr old); Effective in SVT	PO: 3-6 mg/kg/day q8h; IV: 0.1-0.2 mg/kg over 1 min, may repeat	↑ ERP AVN	Contraindicated in infancy; Hypotension with cardiovascular collapse in neonate (have IV CaCl$_2$ ready)
V:				
Digoxin	SVT but not WPW; AF; Afib, CAR, AAT, JET	Total digitalizing dose (TDD): PO: Premature: 20 µg/kg; Term-6 mo: 30 µg/kg; >6 mo: 50 mg/kg; Schedule TDD: ½ TDD, followed by ¼ TDD q8h × 2; Maintenance: usually ¼ TDD daily, or, 1/8 TDD q12h range: 5-15 µg/kg/day q12h; IV dose = ¾ PO dose (1.5-3.0 ng/mL)	Na,K-ATPase inhibition; Positive inotrope; Vagotonic; ↑ ERP AVN	Dig toxicity: any dysrhythmia except first-degree AV block; worse with low K$^+$ and low Ca^{2+}; Rx dig toxicity: Fab fragments (Digibind) or phenytoin; Quinidine, amiodarone, and verapamil → ↑ digoxin levels
VI:				
Adenosine	Reentry SVT; Help diagnose AF by ↑ AVB	IV: 50-µg/kg bolus, may ↑ in 50-µg/kg increments q1min, to a max of 300 µg/kg (max 6 mg if <1 yr old)	Strongly vagotonic at AVN	Sinus bradycardia; AV block transient due to extremely short half-life (seconds); Bronchospasm

AC, accessory connection; AAT, automatic atrial tachycardia; AF, atrial flutter; Afib, atrial fibrillation; ante, antegrade; AV, atrioventricular; AVB, atrioventricular block; AVN, atrioventricular node; CAR, chaotic atrial rhythm; CNS, central nervous system; dig, digoxin; ERP, effective refractory period; GI, gastrointestinal; IM, intramuscular; IV, intravenous; HP, His-Purkinje system; PJRT, paroxysmal junctional reciprocal tachycardia; JET, junctional ectopic tachycardia; maint, maintenance; NAPA, N-acetyl procainamide; PA, procainamide; PO, by mouth; prop, propranolol; PVCs, premature ventricular contractions; retro, retrograde; SVT, supraventricular tachycardia; Ventr, ventricle; Vfib, ventricular fibrillation; VT, ventricular tachycardia; WPW, Wolf-Parkinson-White syndrome; ?, possibly useful.

bypass tracts. It is important, if possible, for the clinician to distinguish WPW syndrome from the other forms of reentry because the use of digoxin generally is contraindicated in patients with WPW syndrome.

To establish and perpetuate any reentry SVT, the following substrate must be present: there must exist at least two functionally distinct conduction pathways that are joined in parallel and have different conduction characteristics (conduction velocities and refractory periods). In such a setting, when an electrical impulse reaches the proximal bifurcation of these pathways, **antegrade** (forward) conduction occurs over at least one of the pathways. If the parallel pathway is at that time refractory to **retrograde** conduction, SVT does not ensue. This is the usual condition during normal sinus rhythm. If under conditions influenced by autonomic tone, a premature impulse such as a PAC or PVC or a junctional escape beat were to reach these pathways sufficiently early that while one pathway conducts antegrade, *the other pathway no longer is refractory to retrograde conduction,* SVT may be initiated (Fig. 62-5).

A study in infants, children, and adolescents found that SVT was due to AV reentry in 73%, primary atrial tachycardia (automatic ectopic focus) in 14%, and AV node reentry in 13%.[34] In a study of 30 consecutive patients presenting with fetal SVT, the mechanisms of SVT were evaluated by prenatal Doppler/M-mode echocardiography, immediate neonatal surface electrocardiography, and transesophageal electrophysiologic studies.[35] The predominant mechanism of SVT was AV reentry with 1:1 AV conduction (93%). Preexcitation pattern (WPW syndrome) was present on surface electrocardiography within the first year of life in 8 of the 30 patients (26%), and *no patient* had AV node reentrant SVT. In patients with fetal SVT identified as atrial flutter, postnatal transesophageal electrophysiologic studies found a high association with accessory connections (five of eight).[35] Mechanisms of SVT appear to have an age-related distribution, with AV reentry most common in the fetus and in infants. SVT due to AV node reentry rarely appears before age 2 years.

Intracardiac electrophysiologic studies can help identify, define, and differentiate the underlying mechanisms responsible for SVT in neonates and older children, but these studies usually are not necessary for recognition that SVT is present or for choice of initial management. In neonates, one may be able to draw conclusions as to the underlying mechanism of an SVT by surface electrocardiography. In the fetus, current levels of sophistication in echocardiography do not allow reliable differentiation of SVT due to AV reentry (as in WPW syndrome and other preexcitation syndromes) from SVT due to AV node reentry. AV node reentry is extremely uncommon, however, during fetal life. A sophisticated fetal sonographer using superior vena cava/aorta Doppler interrogation may be able to distinguish, however, SVT due to AV reentry, during which tall, retrograde, "cannon" a waves are noted superimposed on the aortic ejection wave, from the less common automatic atrial tachycardia, or permanent junctional reciprocating tachycardia, in which such waves are absent.[36]

Diagnosis in the Fetus

In the fetus, SVT is characterized by a heart rate of 240 to 260 beats/min identified by the ventricular rate.

The rhythm is regular, with a 1:1 relation between atrial and ventricular contraction, although this may not be true in atrial flutter and fibrillation. M-mode echocardiography or two-dimensional examination with intracardiac Doppler evaluation may be used to diagnose fetal SVT and may define atrial flutter or fibrillation if associated with AV block. Atrial flutter and atrial fibrillation have been found associated with SVT in the fetus.[37,38] SVT generally is not associated with structural heart disease, but the prognosis is worse when it is. It frequently is associated with hydrops fetalis, which may be a presenting sign. Fetal electrocardiography is not useful because it is currently relegated to intrapartum monitoring of fetal heart rate. Although VT occurs rarely in the fetus, it is imperative to distinguish SVT from VT before deciding on a treatment plan. This distinction may be accomplished by M-mode echocardiography because in most instances of VT, there is AV dissociation, which does not usually occur in reentrant SVT or with atrial flutter. When VT occurs with retrograde conduction, however, differentiation in utero of VT from SVT and from atrial flutter with 1:1 conduction may not be possible.

Diagnosis in the Neonate

In the neonate, SVT is characterized by a rapid heart rate, generally ranging from 150 to 280 beats/min (Fig. 62-6). Usually, there is a regular rhythm and a narrow QRS complex with or without discernible P waves on the ECG, although this may not be true in atrial flutter and atrial fibrillation. Inverted P waves that occur shortly after the QRS (i.e., a short R-P interval in complement with a longer P-R interval) are characteristic of SVT (not sinus tachycardia) and are usually recognizable if the ECG is examined with care. One may need to examine several different leads and look closely at the T waves because the P waves may appear almost buried within them. For faster SVTs, when P waves are not visible even on close inspection, one should include in the differential diagnosis atrial flutter with 1:1 or regular 2:1 conduction. It is rare, even in the neonate, to exceed a heart rate of 230 beats/min during sinus tachycardia, but it does occur occasionally. I have seen this happen in an infant after closed head trauma; in an infant during meningitis; and in a critically ill premature infant after bowel resection, who was being maintained on multiple pressor agents. Administration of adenosine, a purine analogue, may be used as a diagnostic tool and should distinguish atrial flutter by briefly increasing AV block, allowing the flutter waves to be seen better while failing to terminate the tachycardia. During sinus tachycardia, adenosine may lead to a transient slowing of the sinus rate, making identification of sinus rhythm more clear. Adenosine can cause severe sinus bradycardia and, if used as a diagnostic tool, must be used with caution. The use of adenosine as a therapeutic measure is discussed later under management.

Although SVT may be a narrow or wide QRS tachycardia, in children SVT almost always is a narrow QRS tachycardia. If there is a wide QRS tachycardia on the ECG, one should suspect VT rather than SVT and adjust the management accordingly. SVT usually is not associated with congenital heart disease, although infants with certain

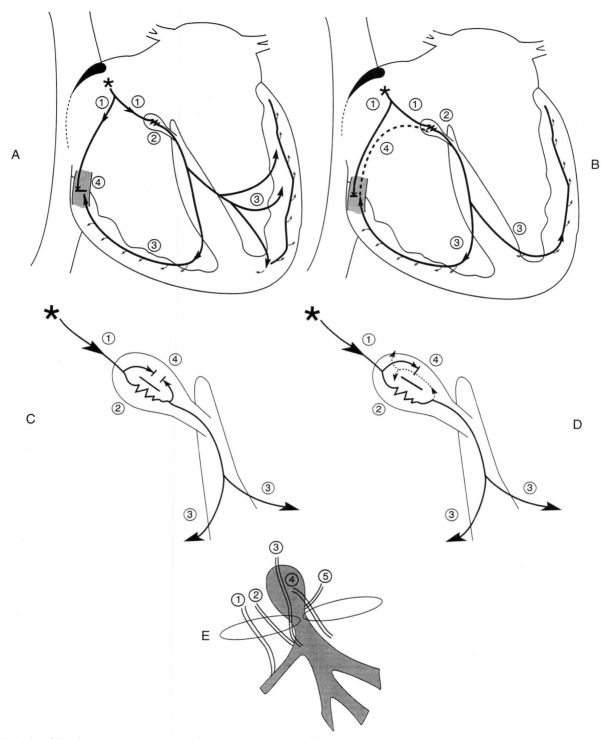

Figure 62–5. A and **B,** Schematic representations of a heart with a right-sided atrioventricular (AV) accessory connection (AC) as occurs in WPW syndrome. **A,** After a premature atrial depolarization *(✳)* the AC and the AV node are functionally connected by atrial myocardium *(1)*. The impulse may reach both the AV node and the AV AC. If the AC is refractory to *antegrade* conduction and blocks, the impulse passes to the ventricles only across the AV node where it is slowed *(2)*, and conduction continues over the His-Purkinje system to depolarize the myocardium *(3)*. If the AC is refractory to *retrograde* conduction *(4)*, SVT will not begin. **B,** If the AC is not refractory to *retrograde* conduction, SVT may be initiated *(4)*. **C** and **D,** Schematic representations of reentry within the AV node itself. In this setting there are at least two functionally separate pathways in parallel within the AV node, which may conduct to the ventricles and allow for reentry. **C,** One of the nodal pathways is refractory to *antegrade* and *retrograde* conduction *(4)*, and SVT will not begin. **D,** *Retrograde* conduction can occur *(4)*, and SVT may be initiated. Retrograde activation of the atria can occur *(splitting of dotted arrow after 4)*. **E,** Diagram of several other ACs: *(1)* atriofascicular; *(2)* atrio-Hisian; *(3)* intranodal; *(4)* nodoventricular; and *(5)* posteroseptal.

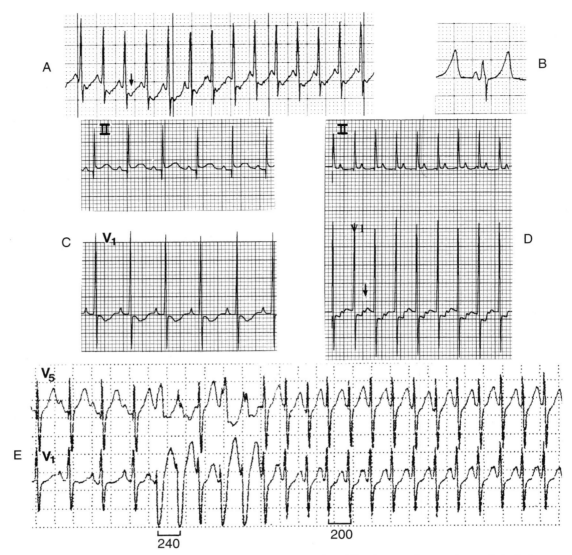

Figure 62–6. The first tracings are taken from a Holter monitor in a neonate with Wolff-Parkinson-White syndrome. Strip **A** shows a narrow QRS supraventricular tachycardia (SVT) at a rate of 270 beats/min. With careful scrutiny, it can be seen that a retrograde P wave, appearing as a little "dip," occurs almost immediately after each QRS complex and that it is inverted *(arrow)*. Before each QRS is the upright T wave from the preceding beat. We were able to confirm that this dip is not part of the QRS complex itself by having available for comparison a tracing of the QRS complex from the same lead during sinus rhythm **(B)**, during which it can be seen that the QRS complex itself does not have a late dip. Note also the short P-R interval and widened QRS. Tracings **C** and **D** are taken from an electrocardiogram in a newborn with narrow QRS SVT without preexcitation. Leads II and V₁ are shown during sinus rhythm **(C)** and during SVT **(D)**. Retrograde P waves are detectable in lead V₁ during SVT *(arrow)*, and they are buried in the depressed ST-T wave segments. The simultaneous tracings in **E**, showing the onset of SVT, were obtained from a Holter monitor on a 4-day-old girl. Lead V₅ is at the top and V₁ is below. Before the onset of SVT, frequent conducted PACs had been noted, many of which occurred with aberrancy. It can be seen on these tracings that during sinus rhythm (the first four beats) there is no evidence of preexcitation, that SVT is initiated when a premature P wave falls in the preceding ST-T wave segment, and that it begins as a wide QRS tachycardia with left bundle-branch block morphology. The cycle length during the wide QRS portion of the tachycardia is 240 msec. With the sixth beat of tachycardia, there is normalization (narrowing) of the QRS complex, and tachycardia continues at a shorter cycle length of 200 msec. This shows that the SVT incorporates an extranodal left-sided atrial contraction in the retrograde limb and that the diagnosis is atrioventricular reentry. Because preexcitation is not manifest during sinus rhythm, some would call this "concealed" Wolff-Parkinson-White syndrome.

congenital heart diseases, in particular Ebstein anomaly of the tricuspid valve, have an increased incidence of SVT.

Management in the Fetus

Intrauterine SVT has long been known to be associated with massive peripheral edema and cardiac decompensation in the fetus,[32,39] and hydrops fetalis resulting from SVT is associated with increased fetal morbidity and demise. When fetal hydrops develops, which may be 24 to 48 hours after the onset of tachycardia, therapeutic conversion of SVT to sinus rhythm may be more difficult. When sustained SVT is diagnosed in the preterm fetus, therapy should be attempted to convert and control the dysrhythmia to prevent fetal heart failure and hydrops, to treat hydrops when present, and to prolong gestation after conversion of the dysrhythmia. If the fetus is close to term, the decision as to whether to treat or deliver should include assessment of fetal maturation and size; when early delivery is considered high risk to the fetus, single-drug medical therapy should be attempted first. If control is not achieved, one should reexamine the option of delivery as possibly the preferred second alternative rather than addition of a second drug.

Although the concept of direct electrical cardioversion is appealing, there are no data as to its safety for the mother or fetus. Transventricular and transumbilical pacing may be capable of terminating SVT but would not provide prophylaxis against recurrence, and these modalities may not be without significant risk to the pregnancy. There is no reported human experience to date related to the treatment of SVT in utero by direct electrical pacing. Acute conversion of SVT may be accomplished by maneuvers designed to enhance vagal tone, such as direct fetal cord compression.[40] Adenosine (200 μg/kg) via direct percutaneous umbilical vein puncture has been administered to the fetus[41] and has the benefit of being a therapeutic and a diagnostic trial. Despite extreme success in converting SVT to sinus rhythm in postnatal life, however, severe fetal bradycardia has occurred on administration of adenosine in utero, and this treatment currently is not used at duPont Hospital for Children. Neither vagal maneuvers nor adenosine offers continued prevention against the recurrence of SVT.

Digoxin therapy[42] has been and remains the mainstay of treatment for the acute conversion and prophylactic therapy of fetal SVT. Digoxin is the only antiarrhythmic agent to offer a positive inotropic effect, which may be beneficial to the fetus with hydrops. Digoxin may be given by direct umbilical venous puncture, by direct fetal intramuscular injection, or maternally by intravenous or oral loading. High maternal serum digoxin levels may be required to achieve a therapeutic fetal serum digoxin level of 1.5 to 2 ng/mL because the maternal-to-fetal ratio may range from 0.6 to 1. Digoxin therapy alone results in successful conversion of SVT to sinus rhythm only about half the time. In the absence of fetal hydrops, if digoxin is not sufficient to convert and control SVT, the addition of a second drug is controversial. I reserve the addition of a second drug to infants with evidence of fetal hydrops or of cardiovascular compromise. Echocardiographic-Doppler findings of tricuspid or mitral valve incompetence may be

signs of impending cardiac decompensation and, as such, may be used as a screening tool. Sophisticated peripheral Doppler ultrasound findings, including abnormal umbilical vein pulsations and abnormal flow pattern at the ductus venosus, may provide additional support of significantly altered fetal hemodynamics.

When it is decided that a second medication is necessary, there is no consensus as to which of several drugs should be employed. The risk of added therapy to the fetus and to the mother should be explored with the family. Type Ia antiarrhythmic agents, such as intravenous procainamide[43] and quinidine administered orally to the mother, have been used with success.[44] Procainamide may be administered via percutaneous umbilical venous puncture or maternally via the intravenous or oral routes, and it has been suggested that larger than conventional doses may be required for therapeutic success.[45] Propranolol, a type II antiarrhythmic agent, commonly is used as a second drug for control of SVT, but has the potential for precipitation of profound fetal bradycardia.

In the 1980s, when digoxin and procainamide failed to work, verapamil commonly was used,[46] but the report of a fetal death after conversion while on digoxin and verapamil[47] prompted many centers to change to flecainide, a type Ic antiarrhythmic agent,[48] as an alternate second drug. Flecainide has the advantage of being therapeutic also for the treatment of ventricular tachycardia but should not be used for treatment of atrial flutter because it may increase ventricular response. Flecainide has a relatively high incidence of proarrhythmia effect,[49] and this potentially serious risk to the mother and fetus must be contemplated before it is used. Some pediatric cardiologists today use flecainide as the first-line drug; others, as a second drug with digoxin; and others, as a third drug along with digoxin and propranolol. In one study, digoxin and flecainide were used as drugs of first choice, and even in the presence of hydrops, treatment with maternally administered digoxin, flecainide, or both was considered effective with better than 80% control in 34 fetuses treated and produced no serious adverse effects.[50] In the presence of a therapeutic level of digoxin, flecainide may be administered orally to the mother. In one study,[51] an average dose of 300 mg/day of flecainide divided into three doses resulted in maternal serum levels of 400 to 800 μg/L, with a placental transfer ratio of 0.8, and resulted in conversion in 1 to 4 days in all 12 fetuses with SVT but with one fetal death. Atrial flutter in two fetuses was not controlled. If flecainide is added, the dose of digoxin usually needs to be adjusted lower.

The type III antiarrhythmic agents, sotalol[52] and amiodarone, with and without digoxin coadministration, have been effective in converting SVT. When we use amiodarone at our institution, the mother is loaded with a large oral dose of amiodarone, and the dose of digoxin is halved. We administer 1800 to 2400 mg orally of amiodarone for the first 2 to 5 days as a loading dose and continue 600 mg/day if the fetus remains in tachycardia or 200 to 400 mg/day if the fetus is converted. Maternal amiodarone is continued for 3 to 4 weeks, then stopped. After loading and maintenance therapy, when the mother is discharged home, we recommend fetal heart rate home monitoring three times daily. There is an estimated 0.1 to 0.25 maternal-to-fetal ratio with a linear relationship, and maternal levels may be monitored to reflect fetal levels.[53,54] In a mother unable to take oral medication, an intravenous formulation of amiodarone is available. Amiodarone may be given directly to the fetus via intravascular umbilical vein injection.[55,56] The many potential, serious side effects associated with the use of amiodarone may pose additional risk to the mother and fetus. The serious risks posed to the mother include VT, pulmonary toxicity, and thyroid dysfunction.[57] The major noncardiac risks to the fetus are neonatal hypothyroidism, prematurity, and growth restriction, and its use antenatally, although effective, remains of concern.[54] When amiodarone is used, the duration of antenatal therapy should be restricted to 6 weeks.

Management in the Neonate

If a neonate develops a pathologic tachycardia that causes severe hemodynamic compromise, immediate synchronized direct current (DC) cardioversion (0.5 to 2 J/kg) is called for and may be lifesaving. This intervention would be appropriate for SVT and VT. It is best to define the rhythm by ECG before cardioversion. Synchronized DC cardioversion may be preceded by an intravenous bolus of lidocaine (1 mg/kg) if the patient is on digoxin. If the infant is sufficiently stable to obtain a full 15-lead ECG before initiation of therapy, identification of the tachycardia as a narrow QRS tachycardia establishes the diagnosis as SVT. Vagal maneuvers may be attempted (application of ice to the face, "diving reflex," or gag), although to prevent retinal injury, eyeball compression should be avoided. If the expertise is available, transesophageal overdrive atrial pacing or transvenous pacing may convert SVT to sinus rhythm.

Pharmacologic therapy has been extremely successful in converting SVT to sinus rhythm, particularly with the advent of the use of adenosine. Adenosine is given as a rapid intravenous bolus, in a large-caliber vein, as close to the heart as possible. Because the serum half-life of adenosine is a matter of seconds, the rare untoward effects of severe bradycardia and hypotension are extremely brief and usually are self-limited.[58] One should record a rhythm strip during conversion with adenosine because a concealed pathway may become manifest briefly during enhanced AV block. If SVT fails to convert to sinus rhythm within 10 to 20 seconds after an initial intravenous bolus of 40 to 50 μg/kg of adenosine, after 1 to 2 minutes the dose may be doubled to 100 μg/kg and, if necessary, again to 200 or 300 μg/kg.[58] Administration of adenosine is nearly 100% successful as acute therapy for AV reentry (WPW syndrome) and AV node reentry SVT, and failure of a tachycardia to convert to sinus rhythm with adenosine should prompt one to reexamine whether the drug was infused effectively or whether the diagnosis should be sinus tachycardia, atrial flutter, automatic atrial tachycardia, or VT.

After successful conversion of SVT to sinus rhythm, a full 15-lead ECG should be obtained to ascertain whether preexcitation is present and to compare the QRS axis and morphology with that during tachycardia. If preexcitation (WPW syndrome) is present (see Fig. 62-6), because of the possible increased risk of mortality, the further use of digoxin should be avoided, unless its safety has been shown electrophysiologically,[59] and propranolol[60] instead should be considered. In infants without WPW syndrome, either digoxin or propranolol may be continued as long-term oral therapy, which, if employed, is usually maintained for 6 months to 1 year.

If adenosine fails to convert SVT to sinus rhythm and the patient becomes hemodynamically *unstable,* synchronized DC cardioversion (0.5 to 2 J/kg) is indicated, although transesophageal or transvenous pacing, if rapidly available, may be attempted. If the patient is hemodynamically *stable,* intravenous propranolol or digoxin loading may be initiated, although digoxin should be avoided if one knows there is preexcitation on ECG. A type Ia antiarrhythmic agent, such as procainamide (intravenous or oral) or quinidine (oral), may be added to propranolol or digoxin therapy. For SVT that is particularly recalcitrant, other agents or additional agents may be required. We currently would add amiodarone, a type III antiarrhythmic agent, but it has many potential side effects, including sinus bradycardia, prolongation of the Q-T interval with torsades de pointes, VT, ventricular fibrillation, and increased refractoriness to cardioversion. Noncardiac side effects of amiodarone include, among others, thyroid dysfunction, pulmonary fibrosis, and corneal deposits. When amiodarone is used in concert with other drugs, the dosages of digoxin, quinidine, propafenone, warfarin, and phenytoin may need to be reduced.[57] Propafenone and flecainide, type Ic antiarrhythmic agents, can convert SVT to sinus rhythm, but their use must be tempered against their known proarrhythmia risk.[61-63] Sotalol, a type III agent, which also has moderate β-blocker (type II agent) activity, has been used successfully in infants to convert SVT to sinus rhythm.[49,64-66] Although the type IV antiarrhythmic agent, verapamil, is effective in converting SVT to sinus rhythm, its use is contraindicated in infants younger than 1 year old because of the risk of acute cardiovascular collapse.[67]

For infants with SVT that is unresponsive to pharmacologic therapy, performance of an electrophysiologic study by a pediatric cardiologist may aid in guiding management. The infant with incessant SVT resistant to intensive medical therapy may be a candidate for radiofrequency catheter ablation or surgical division of accessory connections. There is a small but significant risk of complete heart block when radiofrequency catheter ablation is used to treat AV node reentry. Also, experimental work in infant lambs has identified late lesion enlargement and fibrous tissue invasion of adjacent normal myocardium, which may be important in considering such a procedure in the human infant.[68] Radiofrequency catheter ablation can be performed successfully in infants, but there is a risk of mortality in the smallest infants.[69]

Intracardiac rhabdomyomas and other cardiac tumors rarely may be the cause of an SVT that is difficult to control by pharmacotherapy. In such instances, surgical excision of an isolated tumor can abolish SVT and preexcitation,[70] but in patients with tumors of multicentric distribution, surgical cure is impractical, and the prognosis is poor. Surgical management of SVT due to rhabdomyomas should be limited to patients with hemodynamic compromise.

Atrial Flutter

Atrial flutter is a rapid atrial tachycardia characterized by a sawtooth appearance to the baseline representing P waves called *flutter waves*. In the infant and the fetus, the frequency of flutter waves ranges from 300 to 600 beats/min, and AV conduction block usually is present with ventricular rates often less than 220 beats/min. The degree of AV block may vary, often occurring 2:1, but 1:1 conduction can occur. In atrial flutter, the underlying abnormality is confined to atrial tissue. Several mechanisms have been proposed, including automaticity, reentry or circus movement, and triggered activity, but only reentry has been confirmed by endocardial mapping. Type I atrial flutter is due to reentry, and the circuit involves most of the right atrium; the left atrium is activated secondarily.

Diagnosis in the Fetus

Atrial flutter is suspected in the fetus when the tachycardia rate is extremely fast. Ventricular rates can be greater than 300 beats/min during rapid AV conduction, whereas ventricular rates this rapid are extremely rare with other forms of SVT. More often, atrial flutter presents as a regular fetal tachycardia with a ventricular rate approximately 220 to 260 beats/min and 2:1 AV block. VT also may present as a very rapid heart rate, but VT is an extremely rare dysrhythmia during fetal life. In the fetus with atrial flutter, hydrops fetalis may be a presenting sign and may develop early, often within 48 hours of the onset of flutter. The dysrhythmia is confirmed by echocardiography.[71] The diagnostic echocardiographic findings are

rapid regular atrial wall motions of at least 300 beats/min, usually followed by a variable ventricular response. When atrial flutter occurs with 1:1 AV conduction, differentiation from more common reentrant SVT by echocardiography may not be possible, in which case atrial flutter with 1:1 conduction is deduced by the ventricular rate being greater than 300 beats/min.

Diagnosis in the Neonate

In neonates, the clinical manifestations of atrial flutter are the same as with other SVTs. These manifestations may vary from simple incidental detection of a rapid heart rate in an otherwise well infant to signs of congestive heart failure and cardiogenic shock. ECG is usually diagnostic (Fig. 62-7). On examination of a 15-lead ECG, flutter waves usually are seen best in leads II, III, and avF and in the right precordial leads. When identification of flutter waves is unclear, rapid administration of a bolus of intravenous adenosine (40 to 200 µg/kg), to enhance the degree of AV block transiently, may facilitate visualization of flutter waves and aid in diagnosis. Administration of adenosine is likely to terminate reentrant forms of SVT if the rhythm is not atrial flutter. During atrial flutter, the QRS complexes are usually narrow. Wide QRS complexes are rare and may represent preexisting or rate-dependent bundle-branch block or conduction over an accessory pathway; 1:1 conduction of atrial flutter over an accessory pathway is rare in neonates and may resemble VT. Most neonates presenting with atrial flutter have normal hearts, although there is a higher incidence of atrial flutter in infants with structural heart disease. Also, there is an association between atrial flutter, accessory connections,[35] and reentry SVT. In infants with atrial flutter and normal hearts, the prognosis is good. In infants with congenital heart disease, or if atrial flutter alternates with atrial fibrillation, the prognosis tends to be poor.

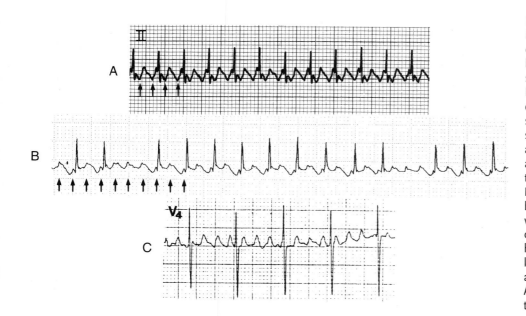

Figure 62–7. Tracing **A** is taken from lead II of an electrocardiogram obtained from a newborn who shortly before delivery was detected to have a sustained rapid fetal heart rate. He was stable and asymptomatic after delivery. Atrial flutter waves are well seen *(arrows)*, giving the baseline a sawtooth configuration. There is 2:1 atrioventricular (AV) block with an atrial rate of 450 beats/min and a ventricular rate of 225 beats/min. Tracing **B** is from the same patient obtained by bedside monitor strip and shows variable AV block with primarily 2:1 conduction and short episodes of higher degree AV block. Tracing **C** is lead V₄ taken from a 4-day-old with atrial flutter and 3:1 AV conduction. Atrial rate is 375 beats/min, and ventricular rate 125 beats/min.

Management in the Fetus

In the fetus, atrial flutter may be a refractory rhythm, and the preferred management of the near-term mature fetus with sustained atrial flutter is delivery for ex utero treatment. Management of atrial flutter in utero is directed at slowing AV conduction and, most importantly, converting to sinus rhythm. In the presence of hydrops fetalis, controlling the ventricular rate alone without conversion to sinus rhythm does not reliably improve the hemodynamic state.[72] When the diagnosis of atrial flutter is confirmed by fetal echocardiography, digoxin can be administered to the mother by either intravenous or oral loading, followed by oral maintenance.[73] After maternal administration of digoxin, fetal serum digoxin levels generally range from 60% to 100% of the maternal serum level. Digoxin may be given directly to the fetus by intramuscular injection or umbilical venous puncture, followed by oral maintenance to the mother.

If the fetal serum digoxin level is in the desired therapeutic range (1.5 to 2 ng/mL), and there is no conversion to sinus rhythm, a second drug may be required. There is no consensus yet, however, as to the best second-line drug. Intravenous procainamide, a type Ia antiarrhythmic agent, may be administered by intravenous infusion to the mother or may be given via direct umbilical vein puncture to the fetus. Alternatively, the type Ia agent, quinidine, may be administered to the mother.[44] Before choosing quinidine, its potential proarrhythmia effect on the mother and fetus must be considered and should be discussed with the family. When using quinidine, the digoxin dosage should be reduced 33% to 50%, and serum digoxin levels must be monitored closely.

Alternate drug regimens are available in place of the aforementioned regimens, or if treatment with digoxin and a type Ia agent is considered a therapeutic failure. These include administration of a β blocker, such as propranolol, flecainide,[74] a type Ic agent, or one of the type III agents, amiodarone or sotalol,[74] instead of, or in place of, procainamide or quinidine. I usually use amiodarone. The mother is loaded with a large oral dose of amiodarone, and the dose of digoxin is halved. I administer 1800 to 2400 mg orally of amiodarone for the first 2 to 5 days as a loading dose and continue 600 mg/day if the fetus remains in flutter, or 200 to 400 mg/day if the fetus is converted. Maternal amiodarone is continued for 3 to 4 weeks, and then stopped. After loading and maintenance therapy, when the mother is discharged home, fetal heart rate home monitoring should be done three times daily. Fetal serum levels are 0.1 to 0.25 of the maternal level with a linear relationship, and one can monitor maternal levels to reflect fetal levels reliably.[53,54] In a mother unable to take the oral medication, an intravenous formulation is available. Amiodarone may be given directly to the fetus via intravascular umbilical vein injection. As discussed in the section on SVT, amiodarone has many potential side effects. The major noncardiac risks to the fetus are neonatal hypothyroidism, prematurity, and growth retardation[54]; the duration of antenatal therapy should be restricted to 6 weeks. The serious risks to a mother who is treated with oral amiodarone include VT,

pulmonary toxicity, and thyroid dysfunction.[57] Apart from pharmacotherapy, the concept of DC fetal cardioversion is appealing but would involve general anesthesia to the mother, and its effect and risks are unknown. Transabdominal compression of the fetal cephalic pole has been reported to terminate atrial flutter successfully.[75]

Management in the Neonate

In the critically ill neonate, synchronized DC cardioversion (0.5 to 1 J/kg) is effective and is the treatment of choice. This procedure and other modalities of treatment may be ineffective, however, in patients with severe hypoxia, acidosis, and electrolyte imbalance. In stable infants, transesophageal rapid overdrive atrial pacing, if available, may be successful in converting atrial flutter to sinus rhythm, although it is less successful in converting atrial flutter than it is in converting other forms of SVT.

If pharmacologic intervention is required for acute conversion, digoxin is the first drug of choice. Digoxin is not highly effective in converting atrial flutter to sinus rhythm, however, and failure of conversion is an indication for addition of a second drug or for electrical cardioversion. Additional efficacy may be gained by the addition of a type Ia antiarrhythmic agent, such as intravenous procainamide or oral quinidine. Serum digoxin levels must be monitored closely in the presence of quinidine, and maintenance digoxin doses should be decreased by 33% to 50%. Another trial of transesophageal overdrive atrial pacing may prove effective. Synchronized DC cardioversion is successful. If digoxin is being used, pretreatment with lidocaine (1 mg/kg) is recommended before electrical cardioversion. Therapy with propranolol, a type II antiarrhythmic agent, is less effective for acute conversion. Amiodarone and sotalol, type III antiarrhythmic drugs, can be effective in converting and controlling atrial flutter but are associated with many side effects. Amiodarone can be associated in young patients with bradycardia, ventricular tachydysrhythmias, thyroid dysfunction, ocular abnormalities, and resistance to cardioversion. Pulmonary toxicity also can occur.[57] Sotalol may be effective[76] but can cause bradycardia, and ventricular pacing may be needed if sick sinus syndrome is present.[66] Propafenone has been reported to be successful in controlling resistant atrial flutter in children,[61,63] but it too has a known proarrhythmia risk. Intravenous verapamil, a type IV agent, is rarely effective and may be dangerous when used during infancy because of the risk of acute cardiovascular collapse.[67] Long-term treatment of an otherwise normal infant after successful conversion is controversial because recurrence of the dysrhythmia in this setting is rare. One may choose to wait and observe, or one may continue digoxin for 6 months.

Atrial Fibrillation

Atrial fibrillation is a rare dysrhythmia in the pediatric population and is rare in the neonate with a normal heart. The incidence of atrial fibrillation in the fetus and newborn is unknown. Kleinman and Copel[77] reported two cases, representing 0.2% of all their fetal arrhythmias. The underlying mechanisms seem to involve multiple wavefronts within the atria affected by the atrial refractory period, the atrial mass, and the atrial conduction velocity.[78] Enlarged atria pose an increased risk for the development of atrial fibrillation, which occasionally occurs in patients with Ebstein anomaly of the tricuspid valve, atrial septal defect, congestive cardiomyopathy, hypertrophic cardiomyopathy, and atrial tumors. Other causes of atrial fibrillation include thyrotoxicosis and digoxin toxicity. Atrial fibrillation may occur in children after cardiac surgery, particularly after complex atrial manipulation. The occurrence of atrial fibrillation may be paroxysmal or chronic. Symptoms are often those of congestive heart failure and are promoted by increased duration of atrial fibrillation or by a rapid ventricular response. In the presence of structural heart disease, the clinical findings may be dominated by the underlying cardiac anomaly.

Diagnosis in the Fetus

Identification of this dysrhythmia in utero is uncommon because atrial fibrillation is a rare dysrhythmia during fetal life. Observation of an irregular, rapid fetal heart rate on clinical examination prompts evaluation by echocardiography. M-mode examination may identify extremely rapid, irregular atrial wall motions of low amplitude with irregular ventricular response.

Diagnosis in the Neonate

The characteristic ECG findings are chaotic fibrillatory (f) waves of variable morphology with irregular ventricular response. The amplitude of the f waves is less than the amplitude of flutter waves, and the frequency of f waves (400 to 700 beats/min) is higher than that of flutter waves. Fibrillatory waves are seen best in leads II, III, and avF and in the right precordial leads. The R-R interval is irregularly irregular as the result of variable AV block. The ventricular rate is usually 120 to 220 beats/min, although rapid ventricular response may occur. It is known that rapid ventricular response may lead to ventricular fibrillation. The QRS complex is usually narrow, although wide QRS complexes may occur in the presence of preexisting bundle-branch block, in the presence of rate-dependent, bundle-branch block, or with antegrade conduction over an accessory connection.

Management in the Fetus

There is little evidence in support of any treatment regimen for atrial fibrillation in the fetus, and whether the asymptomatic fetus should receive any pharmacologic therapy is unclear. The risks associated with treatment versus no treatment should be discussed with the mother; digitalization may be recommended, as discussed in the section on atrial flutter. If there are signs of cardiac decompensation or fetal hydrops, digitalization may be followed by the addition of a type Ia antiarrhythmic agent, such as procainamide or quinidine. Digoxin may enhance conduction over an accessory connection (if present) and result in acceleration of ventricular rate.[37] Successful treatments have been reported with administration of amiodarone, although because of its multiple potential side effects if used antenatally, it should be restricted to 6 weeks' duration. (See also Atrial Flutter: Management in the Fetus.)

Management in the Neonate

The treatment of atrial fibrillation in neonates is similar to the treatment of atrial flutter, although there is no role for transesophageal overdrive atrial pacing. Before treatment, the neonate should be evaluated by echocardiography for possible left atrial thrombus, and anticoagulation should be considered. Atrial fibrillation of acute onset may be treated with digoxin or synchronized DC cardioversion. If digoxin is in use, and if cardioversion is required, pretreatment with intravenous lidocaine (1 mg/kg) is recommended. For chronic atrial fibrillation, digoxin combined with a type Ia antiarrhythmic agent is sometimes effective, but lack of response and recurrences are common. When chronic atrial fibrillation is refractory to initial medical management, synchronized DC cardioversion followed by digoxin together with a type Ia antiarrhythmic may be more successful. If preexcitation (WPW syndrome) is present, the use of digoxin is contraindicated because it may enhance antegrade conduction over the accessory connection and promote an extremely rapid ventricular response followed by ventricular fibrillation.

Successful treatment with sotalol, a type III antiarrhythmic agent, has been reported,[64] but there is a proarrhythmia risk. Amiodarone, another type III agent, also may be efficacious in a neonate with resistant dysrhythmia, but may have significant side effects as reviewed in the sections on SVT and atrial flutter. Treatment with flecainide has been successful, but flecainide, too, has a significant proarrhythmia risk. Flecainide can enhance ventricular response in WPW syndrome and should be restricted to infants with life-threatening dysrhythmias. Propafenone[61] has been reported to be occasionally successful in controlling atrial fibrillation, but it, too, has a potential proarrhythmia risk. Ibutilide, a new class III drug, has been approved by the U.S. Food and Drug Administration for acute treatment of atrial fibrillation and flutter,[79] but as yet there are few data regarding its use in children.

Chaotic Atrial Rhythm, Automatic Atrial Tachycardia, and Junctional Ectopic Tachycardia

Chaotic atrial rhythm, also called **multifocal atrial tachycardia**, is seen rarely in children and when present is usually difficult to control. It may be episodic or chronic and is an extremely rare dysrhythmia in the newborn with a normal heart. Its incidence in the fetus is unknown. Clinically, it appears to be an intermediate form between atrial fibrillation and atrial flutter, but the exact mechanism of chaotic atrial rhythm is unknown. On the ECG, there must be P waves of at least three differing morphologies, with a variable P-P interval and an isoelectric baseline. Most infants are asymptomatic; a symptomatic infant with signs of congestive heart failure should be approached as one with atrial fibrillation. Digoxin alone is not usually effective in converting chaotic atrial rhythm, however, and a type Ia (procainamide or quinidine) or type Ic (flecainide) agent may be added. Sotalol and amiodarone, type III antiarrhythmic agents, have been reported as effective during infancy.[65,66,80,81] Some investigators have found oral propafenone to be highly effective.[82]

Automatic atrial tachycardia, also called **atrial ectopic tachycardia**, is rare and difficult to treat. It usually occurs in structurally normal hearts and may account for approximately 5% of SVT. It is due to one or more anatomic automatic ectopic foci within the atria. It is usually incessant and refractory to single-drug medical management, including digoxin, although it occasionally may respond to adenosine, β blockade, sotalol,[65] propafenone,[63] amiodarone,[80] and the type Ib agent moricizine (Ethmozine).[83] A more recent report indicated that amiodarone in combination with a β blocker may have much better success at controlling this rhythm than any single drug has had alone.[84] If signs of cardiac decompensation or cardiomyopathy occur due to this sustained tachydysrhythmia, catheter ablation[29] or surgical excision of the anatomic ectopic atrial focus may be curative, although such procedures entail significant risk, and the chance of recurrence of tachycardia remains.

Junctional ectopic tachycardia is an incessant automatic tachycardia usually associated with a rapid ventricular rate (generally 110 to 250 beats/min). It is believed to be due to automaticity with an accelerated focus at the AV junction and usually is dissociated from the atrial rhythm. Junctional ectopic tachycardia commonly occurs after cardiac surgery, but may occur congenitally in infants without structural heart disease. Overdrive atrial pacing may suppress this rhythm temporarily but cannot convert it to sinus rhythm; similarly, DC cardioversion cannot convert it. Although there may be a response to digoxin and procainamide, and slowing of the rate has been shown with digoxin and propranolol[85] and with amiodarone and propranolol,[85] mortality with medical therapy has been almost 40% to 50%.[86] Success at controlling the rhythm with propafenone[61] and with amiodarone[87] may result in improved survival. In managing postoperative junctional ectopic tachycardia, additional strategies should be directed at improving cardiac output and in promoting the sinus node as the predominant pacemaker. Therapies may include increasing vagal tone, decreasing adrenergic stimulation, lowering body temperature, atrial pacing, and paired ventricular pacing.[88] When junctional ectopic tachycardia is sustained and unresponsive to such treatments and pharmacotherapy, because of the risk of cardiomyopathy and death with prolonged tachycardia, catheter ablation and pacemaker implantation should be considered.[85]

VENTRICULAR TACHYDYSRHYTHMIAS

Ventricular Tachycardia

VT is defined by three or more repetitive depolarizations of ventricular origin.[89] It may be sustained (lasting more than 30 seconds); nonsustained (paroxysmal); or sustained-incessant, with incessant representing occurrence of the dysrhythmia more than 10% of the day. VT is an uncommon dysrhythmia during fetal life and in healthy neonates.[16,23,29,90] In a study of 2030 healthy newborns evaluated by routine ECG, bigeminy and VT occurred in only 3 patients.[16] In a study of 63 healthy newborns and 50 infants ages 1 to 11 months monitored by 24-hour ambulatory electrocardiography, none had VT detected.[18] It has been reported that of fetuses referred for fetal arrhythmia, the incidence of fetal VT is 0.4%.[77] It is crucial to attempt to distinguish VT from SVT because the treatment plan is distinctly different, and inappropriate management is potentially life-threatening. Accelerated ventricular rhythm is a ventricular dysrhythmia of intermediate rate, with the characteristics of VT, but it is distinguished by a ventricular rate close to, but slightly faster than, the underlying sinus rate.[91,92] There is disagreement as to whether accelerated ventricular rhythm is a separate entity in neonates; for our purposes, it is discussed in this section. **Torsades de pointes**, meaning "twisting of the peaks," is a form of VT that occurs in patients with a prolonged Q-T (and Q-T$_c$) interval, and its diagnosis and management are discussed separately in this section.

Diagnosis in the Fetus

The rate of VT detected during fetal life is usually less than 200 beats/min. M-mode echocardiography may be used to diagnose VT when the tachycardia occurs with AV dissociation, as is commonly the case. In such instances, the ventricular wall motions are faster than the atrial wall motions, and there is no synchrony between the ventricular and atrial rhythms. Complete AV dissociation usually does not occur in reentrant SVT or with atrial flutter. When VT occurs with ventriculoatrial conduction (retrograde conduction), rather than with AV dissociation, however, differentiation in utero of VT from SVT and from atrial flutter with 1:1 conduction may not be possible.

Diagnosis in the Neonate

In neonates, VT usually is diagnosed easily by surface electrocardiography (Fig. 62-8). The ventricular rate ranges from 167 to 440 beats/min.[19,20] It customarily is characterized as a "wide QRS" tachycardia, although the QRS complex may not appear particularly widened in neonates because it ranges from 60 to 110 msec.[20] In such instances, VT may be recognized by the different morphology of the QRS complex during tachycardia compared with the QRS complex during sinus rhythm. The diagnosis of VT is supported if the appearance of the tachycardia is similar to PVCs. The occurrence of fusion beats with tachycardia also strongly supports a dysrhythmia of ventricular origin. The presence of a wide QRS tachycardia with AV dissociation is virtually diagnostic of VT, with the rare exception of Mahaim fasciculoventricular connections.

In the neonate, as in the fetus, VT may present as nonsustained (paroxysmal), sustained, or incessant-sustained. The presumed mechanisms of VT are similar to those of SVT and PVCs and include reentry, automaticity, and triggered arrhythmia, but rarely can one identify with certainty the underlying mechanism of VT. Infants with nonsustained VT may have detectable and correctable medical causes. Causes of nonsustained VT include hypoxia; acidosis; hypocalcemia; hyperkalemia and hypokalemia; hypoglycemia; myocarditis; intracardiac catheters; and drugs including caffeine, nicotine, maternal cocaine use,[93] sympathomimetic agents, maternal anesthetics, digoxin, and other antiarrhythmic agents such as quinidine, procainamide, and amiodarone. Infants with incessant VT can

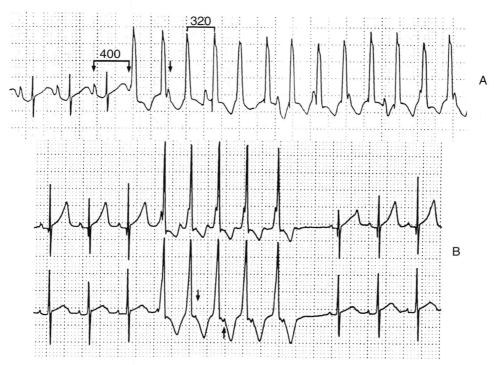

Figure 62–8. Strip **A** is recorded from a Holter monitor placed on a newborn and shows the onset of ventricular tachycardia (VT). Three sinus beats can be seen before the onset of tachycardia. The P-P interval during sinus rhythm is 400 msec, and it can be seen that during the wide QRS tachycardia the P waves *(arrows)* continue to march through the QRS complexes without change in the P-P interval (400 msec), whereas the cycle length of the tachycardia is shorter at 320 msec. This independence of the atrial and ventricular rates during wide QRS tachycardia represents atrioventricular dissociation. Atrioventricular dissociation is characteristic of VT and usually does not occur during supraventricular tachycardia. Two simultaneous tracings in **B** are taken from a Holter monitor on a 6-week-old infant and show nonsustained VT at a rate of 200 beats/min (R-R interval 300 msec). It can be seen that, before the onset of VT, there is sinus rhythm with constant P-P and R-R intervals of 440 msec corresponding to a heart rate of 136 beats/min. VT begins with a fusion beat. It then barely can be seen on the lower tracing that a P wave occurs after the second wide QRS complex, that the P is upright, and that it occurs 440 msec after the preceding P wave *(down arrow)*. This represents an initial independence of the atrial and ventricular rhythms during the onset of VT and does not occur during supraventricular tachycardia. After the third beat of VT, there is a notable change in the timing and configuration of the subsequent P wave *(up arrow)*, with P wave inversion and a shortening of the P-P interval to 300 msec, which is the same as the rate of the tachycardia; this represents VT with retrograde ventriculoatrial conduction.

have as the underlying etiology ventricular tumors, such as hamartomas or rhabdomyomas, which may not be evident by echocardiography but which may be discovered at surgical excision.[19,20,94]

Infants presenting within the first month of life with ventricular tachydysrhythmias rarely present with hemodynamic compromise, and those who do often have long Q-T syndrome and true VT. Most are hemodynamically stable infants, however, with structurally normal hearts, presenting with accelerated ventricular rhythm.[95] Accelerated ventricular rhythm[91,92] may occur in newborns and older children with or without underlying heart disease. It is clinically distinguished from VT by the ventricular rate, which is close to but slightly faster than the sinus rate (usually within approximately 10% of the sinus rate), and by its emergence with sinus slowing. Rates of accelerated ventricular rhythm in newborns typically range from 60 to 180 beats/min. In contrast, in VT, the rate is usually greater than 200 beats/min. Although the QRS complex in accelerated ventricular rhythm is not

particularly wide, it may average twice the QRS duration during sinus rhythm.[95] Fusion beats and AV dissociation usually are seen, but retrograde ventriculoatrial conduction may occur. The underlying mechanisms of accelerated ventricular conduction are thought to be the same as the mechanisms of VT. It is important to attempt to distinguish accelerated ventricular rhythm (heart rate < 200 beats/min, close to the sinus rate, and no signs of cardiovascular compromise) from VT (heart rate > 200 beats/min and signs of hemodynamic instability) because the newborn with accelerated ventricular rhythm has an excellent prognosis[95] and does *not* require potentially toxic pharmacologic treatment. Accelerated ventricular rhythm usually disappears by several months of age.

What has been termed **idiopathic nonsustained VT**, in an asymptomatic healthy infant, may be the same entity as accelerated ventricular rhythm. If it occurs infrequently, it does not usually require treatment and tends to have a good prognosis,[92,96,97] often disappearing spontaneously. There is, however, controversy regarding this entity and whether it can be distinguished from accelerated ventricular rhythm. Because there have been instances of sudden death in patients presumed to have this rhythm, who were not known to have associated structural heart disease, and because of the uncertainty as to the risk associated with this entity and the potential risks of pharmacologic therapies, patients with possible idiopathic VT and accelerated ventricular rhythm should undergo investigation for underlying heart disease in consultation with a pediatric cardiologist before deciding whether pharmacologic therapy is appropriate. Investigation should focus on long Q-T syndrome, myocarditis, arrhythmogenic right ventricular dysplasia, cardiac tumor, and electrolyte imbalance.

Management in the Fetus

Not all patients with VT are ill, and not all patients with VT require treatment. This is particularly important to recognize during fetal life because by echocardiography it may be impossible to distinguish with certainty VT from SVT; without support by a direct fetal ECG, therapy may be more deleterious than the dysrhythmia. The therapeutic agents administered to treat VT are different from the agents used to treat SVT, and it is crucial to avoid the administration of an inappropriate drug, such as digoxin, to patients with VT because it may induce ventricular fibrillation. I agree with others[72] and consider in utero therapy of VT in the preterm fetus only in patients with a rapid tachycardia (usually >200 beats/min) in whom hydrops is evident. Umbilical venous administration of lidocaine may be considered as an initial therapy, possibly followed by the administration of oral mexiletine to the mother if there is a positive response to the lidocaine. Administration of type Ia antiarrhythmic agents, such as procainamide or quinidine, or a type Ic agent, such as flecainide, may be considered, as may the type III agent, amiodarone,[98] but all aggressive therapies need to be balanced against the fetal and maternal risks of treatment versus nontreatment. At present, little is known about the natural history of VT detected in utero, and there is little experience with its therapy; not all patients have had a dismal course or prognosis.[50] More useful data need to be gathered to develop a more well-reasoned approach to management of this dysrhythmia during fetal life.

Management in the Neonate

In the symptomatic neonate with stable hemodynamics, identification and treatment of any reversible causes of VT should be pursued. Blood gases and electrolytes should be examined, and acidosis, electrolyte imbalances, and hypoxia should be corrected. Sympathomimetic drugs may need to be withdrawn. Drug intoxications or reactions should be counteracted. Digoxin toxicity may occur as a result of hypokalemia, which should be treated by supplemental potassium chloride. Digoxin overdose may be treated by administration of antigen-binding fragment (Fab), which is a digoxin-specific antibody that binds to and inactivates serum digoxin, forming a complex that then may be excreted. (The dose of Fab [Digibind] in milligrams equals [serum digoxin concentration in ng/mL × 5.6 × the body weight in kg/1000] × 64. Each vial contains 38 mg of Fab.[99] The dose may need to be repeated if toxicity persists or recurs.) If Fab is not available, intravenous phenytoin is the recommended treatment of digoxin toxicity. The efficacy of phenytoin in treating dysrhythmias due to digoxin toxicity likely relates to its ability, similar to lidocaine, to depress phase 4 depolarization. Phenytoin is unstable in solution and may be given intravenously in small boluses of 3 to 5 mg/kg every 5 minutes to a maximum of 15 mg/kg over 1 hour. Blood pressure should be monitored continuously because rapid administration of intravenous phenytoin may cause hypotension due to a central nervous system–related effect on sympathetic tone, and wider temporal spacing of the boluses may be necessary. Phenytoin crosses the placenta easily and is highly teratogenic, so it should *not* be used to treat the fetus. Drugs, including quinidine, procainamide, amiodarone, and sotalol, may cause the torsades de pointes form of VT, the treatment of which is discussed subsequently.

In an infant with VT who is hemodynamically unstable, synchronized DC cardioversion should be performed using 0.5 to 1.5 J/kg[100]; this may be preceded by a bolus of 1 mg/kg of intravenous lidocaine and is followed by a drip of 10 to 50 μg/kg/min, titrated to the needs of the rhythm. The initial bolus may be repeated three times, approximately 5 minutes apart. Intravenous propranolol, 0.025 mg/kg, with doses repeated every 5 minutes up to four doses, may be effective, but propranolol can cause severe bradycardia that may necessitate emergency ventricular pacing. Intravenous amiodarone may be effective.[101] Overdrive ventricular pacing, if available, may be tried to terminate VT, but pacing can accelerate the tachycardia or induce ventricular fibrillation, and emergency cardioversion or defibrillation may be required. The possibility of long Q-T syndrome should be considered and the diagnosis sought. If this syndrome is confirmed, treatment should be initiated as discussed in the section on torsades de pointes and long Q-T syndrome. Long periods of sustained VT in a healthy newborn, without known structural heart disease and without other known cause, can lead to hemodynamic compromise. For sustained VT, long-term pharmacotherapy should be initiated and continued for 6 months, by which time the dysrhythmia usually has resolved. Long-term treatment with propranolol may be enough to control the rate to an asymptomatic level, but if ineffective, amiodarone, mexiletine, or a type Ia agent such as procainamide or quinidine may be tried as long as there is no underlying prolongation of the Q-T interval. Sotalol[66] and flecainide[102] may be effective. Phenytoin, although sometimes effective, is poorly absorbed in the neonate. Each of these drugs has important potential side effects that need to be considered when deciding whether to initiate medical therapy.

Incessant VT is primarily a disease of infancy, and patients with this rhythm tend to have a poor prognosis. They are less likely to be asymptomatic and more likely to have a complex etiology that is difficult to control or cure. Conventional medical pharmacotherapy is generally unsatisfactory in that nearly all drugs currently available fail to control the rate of the tachycardia or appreciably alter the portion of the day spent in tachycardia.

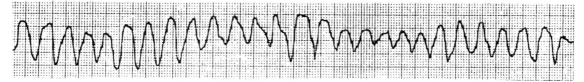

Figure 62–9. Lead II of a patient with torsades de pointes. Note the bidirectional tachycardia with twisting of the peaks as it spirals about the baseline.

Ventricular tumors frequently are responsible for this refractory rhythm, although myocarditis and myocardial fibrosis also have been found. It is promising that, in most of these patients, successful excision or cryoablation of the site of tachycardia was achieved after endocardial and epicardial mapping.[19,20,94] In an infant with incessant VT unresponsive to medical therapy, serious consideration should be given to early surgical intervention.

Torsades de Pointes and Long Q-T Syndrome

Torsades de pointes is a unique and potentially lethal type of VT in which there is a gradually changing wide QRS morphology that appears to twist around the baseline, as in a spiral. There usually is a narrow QRS complex between a shift in the direction of the QRS (Fig. 62-9). Torsades de pointes may present with loss of consciousness or as sudden death and is seen almost exclusively in patients who have a prolonged Q-T interval during sinus rhythm (Fig. 62-10). Prolongation of the Q-T interval may be seen in the newborn and may be heritable or acquired. When it is inherited, it is called **congenital long Q-T syndrome.**

Originally designated idiopathic, congenital long Q-T syndromes first were described by Jervell and Lange-Neilsen,[103] whose patients also had congenital nerve deafness and in whom inheritance appeared to be autosomal recessive, and by Romano and colleagues[104] and Ward,[105] whose patients had normal hearing and apparent autosomal dominant mode of inheritance. These syndromes, long known to be associated with torsades de pointes and sudden death, have been shown by genetic linkage analysis to be part of a heterogeneous group of heritable genetic channelopathies, resulting from multiple mutations affecting at least four distinct sodium and potassium ion channels. The nature of the individual mutations is important because patients with defects in different long Q-T genes may have unique clinical phenotypes and may benefit by different therapeutic interventions. At present, targeted therapy based on genotype is not yet applicable; however, such treatment strategies may become a reality in the near future. Flecainide, a potent blocker of open sodium channels, is a promising therapeutic agent in the

LQT3 form of the disease, which has mutations of the *SCN5A* sodium channel gene.[52]

Initially the mechanism theorized to be responsible for torsades de pointes VT in the idiopathic long Q-T syndrome was an underlying imbalance of cardiac sympathetic innervation with an underactive right stellate ganglion and a compensatory overly active left stellate ganglion.[106,107] Currently, there are two popular theories for the explanation of Q-T prolongation: dispersion of repolarization within the ventricular myocardium and afterdepolarizations. A prolonged Q-T interval seems to be a marker in these patients, who are predisposed toward cardiac electrical instability and sudden death. Using Bazett's formula[108] to calculate the heart rate–corrected Q-T (Q-T$_c$) ratio (Q-T$_c$ equals measured Q-T in seconds divided by square root of the preceding R-R interval measured in seconds), a Q-T$_c$ ratio in children greater than 0.44 is suggestive of the syndrome, whereas a ratio of 0.50 or greater makes long Q-T syndrome highly likely.[109] There have been instances in which infants who appeared to have idiopathic prolongation of the Q-T interval immediately after birth and who experienced VT or cardiac arrest by 1 year of age had a normal Q-T$_c$ interval and did not experience further ventricular dysrhythmia.[33,110] Changes in sympathetic innervation that occur during the first year of life may be responsible for sympathetic imbalance and electrical instability and may explain some forms of sudden infant death syndrome.[107]

The fetus or neonate with long Q-T syndrome may appear healthy. Mild sinus bradycardia with heart rates less than 100 beats/min[111] may be a subtle manifestation. In one study, the mean resting heart rate of 110 beats/min in newborns with long Q-T syndrome was significantly lower than the resting heart rate of 130 beats/min in normal controls.[112] Other infants with long Q-T syndrome may present with symptoms, including loss of consciousness or apnea, VT, shock, or seizures. The presence in the newborn of 2:1 AV block, multiform PVCs, and torsades de pointes should raise suspicion of long Q-T syndrome.[113] Infants with a markedly prolonged Q-T$_c$ (Q-T$_c$ > 0.55 to 0.60) are at high risk of sudden death,[113] as are infants

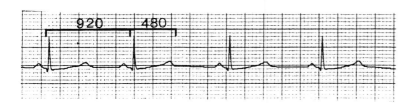

Figure 62–10. Lead II from a 7-year-old child with long Q-T syndrome. The measured Q-T interval of the second complex is 480 msec, and the preceding R-R interval is 920 msec. The calculated Q-T$_c$ ratio is 0.500, which is prolonged. If one were to calculate the Q-T$_c$ using instead the fourth complex, the Q-T$_c$ ratio would be 0.480, which still is prolonged.

with prolongation of the Q-T$_c$ interval in the presence of 2:1 AV block[114] and complete heart block.[115] Because of the current lack of reliable risk stratification, I treat all infants more than 4 days old found to have significant prolongation of the Q-T$_c$ without a correctable cause, even infants who are asymptomatic, with long-term β-blocker therapy for presumed long Q-T syndrome.

Acquired forms of long Q-T syndrome can be caused by electrolyte imbalance, drugs, central nervous system injury, myocarditis, myocardial ischemia, and ventricular hypertrophic and dilated cardiomyopathies.[116] The most common acquired cause of long Q-T syndrome is hypocalcemia. Hypomagnesemia has been reported as a cause in older patients with anorexia nervosa and malnutrition.[117] The commonly used type Ia antiarrhythmic agents, quinidine and procainamide, prolong the Q-T interval, and quinidine is known to cause torsades de pointes even at subtherapeutic serum levels. When using these drugs, prolongation of the Q-T$_c$ by more than 25% is a marker for caution, and lengthening by more than 50% is a sign of toxicity. Type III antiarrhythmic agents, including amiodarone, sotalol, and ibutilide, may cause prolongation of the Q-T interval and may induce torsades de pointes.

Treatment of torsades de pointes is particularly difficult. Asynchronous DC cardioversion usually terminates the rhythm, but rapid recurrence usually occurs. Drugs that prolong the Q-T interval should be discontinued, and any electrolyte imbalance should be corrected. There may be a response to administration of 1 to 2 mEq/kg of sodium bicarbonate. Lidocaine bolus and infusion and magnesium sulfate may be tried, and then one may repeat DC cardioversion. Intravenous esmolol, an ultrashort-acting β blocker, can be initiated and may suppress an underlying sympathetic imbalance. Maneuvers to increase the ventricular rate, such as the administration of isoproterenol, ventricular pacing, and intravenous atropine, occasionally are successful. If there is successful conversion of torsades de pointes, and the underlying etiology is congenital long Q-T syndrome, long-term therapy is required in an attempt to prevent its recurrence. Treatment may include a β blocker such as propranolol, mexiletine, left stellate ganglionectomy, overdrive pacing, and possibly antitachycardia/defibrillator mechanical devices. Patients with long Q-T$_c$ and 2:1 AV or complete heart block should receive prophylactic pacing by implanted pacemaker in addition to β blockade.

Ventricular Fibrillation

Diagnosis

Ventricular fibrillation is characterized by a series of uncoordinated ventricular depolarizations without effective cardiac output. On the ECG, there are irregular, low-amplitude oscillations without recognizable QRS complexes. It seldom occurs in children even as a terminal event and is rare in the absence of organic heart disease. It is sometimes seen in long Q-T syndrome.[118]

Treatment

The treatment of ventricular fibrillation is immediate electrical defibrillation (2 J/kg).[100] In the absence of organic heart disease, if ventricular fibrillation is resistant to electrical defibrillation, the underlying etiology may relate to long Q-T syndrome; treatment would be as for torsades de pointes, and then defibrillation should be retried. Isoproterenol may be effective in truly resistant dysrhythmias but may make defibrillation more difficult. If the child has a potentially reversible myocardial problem, extracorporeal circulatory support may be considered as a last alternative. If sinus rhythm can be restored, one must search carefully for the underlying etiology. Special emphasis should be placed on measurement of the Q-T$_c$ to identify long Q-T syndrome and on looking for preexcitation, the marker for WPW syndrome. If long Q-T syndrome is present, it should be treated aggressively with pharmacologic therapy as reviewed in the section on torsades de pointes and long Q-T syndrome. If WPW syndrome is present, catheter ablation or surgical division of the accessory connection is indicated.

DISORDERS OF IMPULSE FORMATION

Sinus Bradycardia, Sinus Arrest, Sinoatrial Exit Block, Slow Ectopic Rhythms, Tachycardia-Bradycardia Syndrome

Diagnosis in the Fetus

Fetal bradycardia may be defined as a sustained resting fetal heart rate less than 100 beats/min.[23] Periods of **sinus bradycardia** are common and are related to autonomic tone. Sinus slowing may occur with uterine contraction and with extrinsic factors, such as cord compression with an ultrasound transducer. In a healthy fetus, these phenomena result in a transient, benign slowing of the fetal heart rate, which is usually well tolerated. Maternal treatment with digoxin, β blockade, calcium channel blockade, and other antiarrhythmic agents also can cause fetal and neonatal bradycardia secondary to sinus node depression. Sinus bradycardia is confirmed by M-mode echocardiography on demonstration of normal synchronous atrial and ventricular wall motions at a rate less then 100 beats/min or by pulsed wave Doppler examination. Other disorders of impulse formation responsible for fetal bradycardia are seldom identified. These include **sinus arrest**, in which a long pause can be followed by a slow ectopic escape rhythm, or **sinoatrial exit block**, which may be inferred by a carefully timed M-mode echocardiogram. Nonconducted PACs are commonly responsible for an irregular rhythm but seldom result in a sustained slower than normal ventricular rate. **Tachycardia-bradycardia syndrome (sick sinus syndrome)** is seldom seen in a healthy fetus, although a prolonged time until sinus node recovery or emergence of a slow ectopic escape rhythm may occur after termination of SVT of long-standing duration. Bradycardia due to diminished impulse formation associated with complex congenital heart disease may be associated with fetal demise.

Diagnosis in the Neonate

Neonatal bradycardia is defined as a sleeping heart rate less than 60 beats/min or an awake heart rate less then 80 beats/min.[16,17] In a neonate, bradycardia frequently is associated with apnea and other causes of hypoxia, acidosis, hyperkalemia, hypothermia, central nervous system injury, and excessive vagotonia. Bradycardia in a neonate also can result from maternal or neonatal drug therapies.

Sinus bradycardia, sinus arrest, and sinoatrial exit block are identified by slowing of the heart rate to below normal range for age with a normal P-QRS activation sequence on surface ECG. These entities may be difficult to separate. Sinus arrest is distinguished by a long pause between sinus beats or slow escape rhythm, with a P-P interval that is not an exact multiple of the P-P interval during the normal heart rate. Sinoatrial exit block (in which the sinus node fires, but the impulse fails to reach the atria) may be inferred when the P-P interval during bradycardia is an exact multiple of the P-P interval at times of normal heart rate and rhythm. Each of these disorders may be accompanied by a slow ectopic escape rhythm, which is an indication of sinus node depression or dysfunction. Slow ectopic escape rhythms may derive from atrial, AV node, or ventricular pacemakers. Ectopic rhythms of atrial origin are identified by a P-QRS sequence with an abnormal P-wave axis. A slow escape rhythm originating from the AV node (AV junction) is recognized by resumption of rhythm with a normal QRS complex without a preceding P wave. Ventricular escape rhythms are associated with sinus and AV node dysfunction. They are generally slower escape rhythms and are defined by a wide QRS complex without a preceding P wave, although a high ventricular escape beat may resemble a junctional beat and occur with a narrow QRS complex.

The transient nature of these forms of bradycardia in the neonate is due to temporary sinus node dysfunction or depression and is readily reversible on removal of the underlying insult or resolution of enhanced vagal tone. Transient bradycardia due to vagal stimulation commonly occurs with nasogastric and endotracheal intubation, with vomiting, and with gastroesophageal reflux. Less common causes of bradycardia include metabolic abnormalities, such as hypothyroidism and hypercalcemia.

Bradycardia in a neonate rarely is associated with structural heart disease but, when present, usually is limited to neonates with complex cardiovascular malformations (as in heterotaxy syndromes with left atrial isomerism) and generally is more advanced, involving profound conduction abnormalities. Bradycardia may occur after intracardiac surgery due to surgical trauma. If there is no ongoing hypoxia, acidosis, major electrolyte imbalance, or metabolic abnormality, bradycardia is due either to direct trauma to the sinus node or to injury to the sinus node artery. Complex surgical repairs involving the atria, such as the Mustard and Senning operations (now uncommon) for correction of d-transposition of the great arteries and repair of total anomalous pulmonary venous connection, are well-recognized causes of surgically induced sinus node dysfunction. Cannulation of the superior vena cava during cardiopulmonary bypass for cardiac surgery and for extracorporeal circulatory support also may cause direct trauma to the sinus node. Bradycardia resulting from surgical trauma to the AV node may cause a disturbance of AV conduction and is reviewed under complete heart block.

In a healthy neonate, transient bradycardia resulting from disorders of impulse formation is of no apparent clinical consequence. In a critically ill infant who has not undergone cardiac surgery, the effect of bradycardia depends on the nature of the underlying illness. An infant in a tenuous cardiovascular condition, who requires sinus tachycardia to maintain adequate cardiac output, may be affected severely by bradycardia, with rapid clinical deterioration. In an infant with hypoxic cardiomyopathy or myocarditis, bradycardia may lead to intractable heart failure. In a postsurgical infant, bradycardia may have a profound deleterious effect on cardiac output. Sinus bradycardia may occur in patients with tuberous sclerosis[119] and with apparent familial vagotonia.[120]

Management in the Fetus

The fetus with bradycardia resulting from a transient disorder of impulse formation usually has a favorable outcome. Factors responsible that can be eliminated should be removed, and no specific treatment is required. Blocked PACs, when responsible for bradycardia, are generally of benign consequence. Their risk is associated with the potential for initiation of SVT (as discussed in the sections on PACs and SVT). Bradycardia associated with the tachycardia-bradycardia syndrome may be avoided by prevention of sustained pathologic tachycardias. Persistent fetal bradycardia has a guarded prognosis. When severe bradycardia occurs in a critically ill fetus, the prognosis is grim because it is usually a terminal event.

Management in the Neonate

In a healthy neonate, bradycardia resulting from a disorder of impulse formation is usually benign and does not require specific therapy. Recognizable causes, including hypoxia, acidosis, hyperkalemia, sepsis, and hypothermia, should be treated promptly, and other metabolic causes should be excluded. The vagal stimulating effect of nasogastric tube placement and endotracheal intubation is transient and does not require treatment. Bradycardia due to gastroesophageal reflux resolves with prevention of reflux.

In a critically ill infant with significant bradycardia, in addition to treating the underlying illness, an increase in heart rate and significant clinical improvement may occur with administration of atropine by its vagolytic effect or with isoproterenol by its β-adrenergic effect. The response to chronotropic and inotropic agents is markedly attenuated with ongoing hypoxia and acidosis. Infants with hypoxic cardiomyopathy and myocarditis may be unresponsive to medical treatment and may require temporary ventricular pacing.

In a postsurgical cardiac infant, bradycardia often has a protracted course and may be permanent. These infants are hemodynamically unstable, and although chronotropic support with isoproterenol and epinephrine may be effective, rapid institution of ventricular pacing can be lifesaving and should be initiated without delay. During infancy, the tachycardia-bradycardia syndrome (sick sinus syndrome) usually is limited to infants with heart disease and surgery. Treatment may include pharmacologic suppression of tachycardia in combination with pacemaker implantation for severe bradycardia.

DISORDERS OF ATRIOVENTRICULAR CONDUCTION

First-Degree Atrioventricular Block

First-degree AV block is defined as prolongation of the P-R interval exceeding the upper limits of normal for age and heart rate. In older children, the normal P-R interval is more age dependent, whereas in newborns, it is primarily rate dependent. The P-R interval comprises the conduction time through the atrial muscle, the AV node, and the His-Purkinje system. First-degree AV block is found in 6% of normal newborns.[18,121] Etiologies of abnormal P-R interval prolongation include electrolyte imbalance, myocarditis, antiarrhythmic drugs including digoxin, maternal collagen vascular disease, and structural heart disease (in particular, ostium primum and ostium secundum atrial septal defects and Ebstein anomaly of the tricuspid valve). First-degree AV block causes no hemodynamic or clinical ill effect and is of no prognostic consequence. No treatment is required.

Second-Degree Atrioventricular Block

Second-degree AV block is defined by intermittent loss of AV conduction. It is recognized in two forms: Mobitz type I (Wenckebach) block and the more sinister Mobitz type II block.

Mobitz type I block (Wenckebach periodicity) is recognized on surface ECG by progressive lengthening of the P-R interval, often with progressive shortening of the R-R interval before a dropped ventricular beat occurs (Fig. 62-11). This condition is presumed to occur secondary to block within the AV node, although the exact mechanism is unknown. It occurs more commonly during sleep and during periods of enhanced vagal tone, as with digoxin toxicity and with increased intracranial pressure. In a healthy child, Mobitz type I block rarely is detected during the first year of life.[18] Mobitz type I block usually does not progress to more advanced conduction abnormality, it is usually of no clinical significance, and no specific treatment is required.

Mobitz type II block is identified by intermittent loss of AV conduction without preceding lengthening of the P-R interval and without preceding shortening of the R-R interval (Fig. 62-12). In contrast to Wenckebach periodicity, Mobitz type II block is thought to represent conduction system disease with block occurring distal to the AV node and the bundle of His. Its occurrence is rare in healthy neonates,[18] but it can occur in infants with

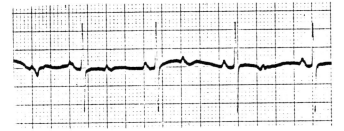

Figure 62–12. Lead V$_4$ in a 2-month-old infant with a 2:1 type of Mobitz II block. Every other P wave is conducted, and there is no prolongation of the P-R interval before a dropped beat.

otherwise normal hearts, in infants with long Q-T syndrome, in infants after surgery for repair of structural congenital heart disease, and in neonates born to mothers with collagen vascular disease, some of whom have progressed to complete heart block. When 2:1 AV block is present, Mobitz type I can be distinguished from Mobitz type II by surface electrocardiography only if some variation to the conduction pattern is present. More advanced Mobitz type II block may occur with loss of AV conduction for several P waves (e.g., 3:1, 4:1 block), and it can progress to complete heart block (third-degree AV block). Second-degree AV block with intraventricular conduction delay (wide QRS complex) usually is associated with Mobitz type II block.

Neonates with Mobitz type II block and normal narrow QRS morphology, who have only occasional dropped beats and in whom the escape ventricular rate is not particularly slow, should be followed with close observation. This rhythm can progress to more advanced conduction system disease, and pacemaker implantation may be required. Patients with sustained Mobitz II block and intraventricular conduction delay (wide QRS) are at increased risk of sudden death. Because of the risk of sudden death and the unlikely resolution of this conduction abnormality, in the postoperative cardiac surgical patient who has persistence of Mobitz II block, particularly if there is a slow ventricular escape rate and wide QRS, continuous pacing should be performed by an implanted permanent pacemaker. Patients with Mobitz II block and long Q-T syndrome should be managed with implanted pacemaker and β blockade as reviewed in the section on torsade de pointes and long Q-T syndrome.

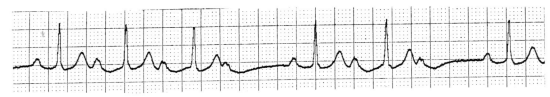

Figure 62–11. This strip is taken from an older child with Mobitz I (Wenckebach). There is a progressive lengthening of the P-R interval before a dropped beat occurs.

COMPLETE HEART BLOCK

Complete AV block is defined by the inability of an atrial electrical impulse to be conducted to the ventricles. There is complete independence of atrial and ventricular rates, with the atrial rate faster than the ventricular rate. In newborns, complete AV block almost always is of prenatal onset and is termed **congenital complete heart block**. The atrial rate can be seen to be normal and appropriate for age, whereas the ventricular rate is always slower. Although the atrial rate responds appropriately to chronotropic stimuli (owing to the inherent properties of a healthy sinus node), the ventricles do not possess this capability. The onset of this dysrhythmia has been reported by week 17 of gestation.[122]

Although the incidence of complete heart block in the fetus is unknown, the incidence of complete AV block in newborns is approximately 1 per 20,000 live births.[123] Familial recurrence is most prevalent in siblings of the same generation, although it has been reported to occur in the progeny of an affected individual and in the subsequent generation.[123,124] Associated structural cardiovascular anomalies occur in only 25% to 30% of affected neonates, most likely related to the high incidence of fetal demise associated with complete heart block and severe cardiovascular malformations.[125] A multicenter review of outcomes of fetal complete AV block found that over a 10-year period, about half of the 55 fetuses diagnosed with complete heart block had associated structural heart disease.[126] Ventricular inversion with levotransposition of the great arteries (physiologically corrected transposition of the great arteries) and defects of the AV canal with left atrial isomerism as seen in the heterotaxy syndromes are the most common associated cardiovascular anomalies.[122,123,126-128] The known causes of congenital complete AV block include primary embryologic abnormalities of the conduction system; maternal collagen vascular diseases (most often systemic lupus erythematosus); and, less commonly, infectious diseases, such as mumps and diphtheria.[125] Primary embryologic developmental anomalies include abnormal development of structures between the AV node and bundle of His, absence of the AV node, and abnormal anterior displacement of the AV node and His bundle.[123,125,128-131] There is a high incidence of congenital complete AV block in fetuses and newborns of mothers with overt or subclinical systemic lupus erythematosus, and there is a strong association between elevated maternal SS-A/Ro or SS-B/La autoantibodies and the presence of complete heart block in the newborn. Although no definite causal relationship has been established, it seems likely that these maternal IgG class antibodies cross the placental barrier, enter the fetal circulation, and damage the AV conduction axis.[132] In the past, it was common to diagnose subclinical systemic lupus erythematosus in the mother as a result of delivery of an infant with congenital complete heart block.

Diagnosis in the Fetus

The finding of a sustained excessively slow fetal heart rate with fetal bradycardia (usually <100 beats/min) is highly suggestive of the presence of fetal complete AV block. One should not rush to immediate delivery, but rather the diagnosis should be confirmed by fetal echocardiography-Doppler study. M-mode echocardiography with the cursor directed across an atrium and a semilunar valve or across an atrium and ventricle shows a regular atrial rhythm at a normal rate for gestational age, on average approximately 140 beats/min. There is a regular, completely dissociated rhythm and slower ventricular rate (or semilunar valve motion), usually between 40 and 80 beats/min.[126] Similar information may be gleaned by incorporation of appropriate Doppler technique, typically with placement of the Doppler sample volume at the junction of the left ventricular inflow and outflow, so as to assess and time the atrial and ventricular flow patterns. Nonimmune hydrops fetalis is an uncommon complication of fetal heart block with an otherwise normal heart[133]; in a multicenter report, hydrops occurred in 15% of fetuses with AV block and structurally normal hearts and in 61% of fetuses with AV block and a structural heart defect.[126] When complete heart block and hydrops do occur together, there is usually accompanying significant structural cardiovascular disease and severe cardiac decompensation.[125] The occurrence of hydrops together with complete AV block is an ominous finding because there is a particularly high incidence of fetal and neonatal loss.

Diagnosis in the Neonate

A neonate with complete AV block who was not diagnosed while in utero usually is identified by the recognition of bradycardia on initial physical examination. The heart rate (ventricular rate) is usually less than 100 beats/min and generally ranges from 40 to 80 beats/min. Confirmation of the diagnosis is by the ECG, although it may be clear from a simple rhythm strip (Fig. 62-13). The P waves, representing atrial activation, usually occur at the normal neonatal heart rate and in a regular rhythm. In the presence of complex structural heart disease, there may be abnormalities of morphology and axis of the P wave. The QRS complexes, representing ventricular activation, occur more slowly (usually 40 to 80 beats/min). They are regular but occur completely dissociated from the atrial rhythm. With block at the AV junction (AV node), the site of block is above the His bundle, the QRS complex is narrow, and the ventricular escape rate is relatively high. In this situation, the prognosis is favorable. When the site of block is distal to the His bundle, the QRS complex is widened, the ventricular escape rate is low, and the prognosis is less favorable.

Management in the Fetus

A fetus with complete AV heart block and a heart rate greater than 55 beats/min with a structurally normal heart generally tolerates this state well. Without the development of associated hydrops fetalis, the fetus may come to term and deliver without requiring specific intervention. In this setting, premature delivery is contraindicated, and cesarean section is not required. For a near-term fetus with nonimmune hydrops fetalis and complete AV heart block, the clinical condition is one of severe congestive heart failure. Delivery by cesarean section is the preferred treatment because vaginal delivery

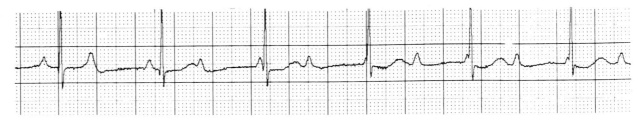

Figure 62–13. This tracing is from a rhythm strip in a neonate with congenital complete heart block. Note complete independence of atrial and ventricular rhythms with the P waves "marching" through the QRS complexes. The atrial rate is faster than the ventricular rate. The atrial rate is normal for a resting neonate at 115 beats/min. The ventricular rate is 55 beats/min, and QRS morphology is that of a narrow QRS complex. This rate and QRS morphology represent a relatively high ventricular escape rhythm. This infant had periods of ventricular rate of 43 beats/min, however, and a permanent pacemaker was implanted electively in the neonatal period.

may result in further deterioration of the fetal condition. If the associated congenital abnormalities are lethal, however, vaginal delivery may be considered.

In a fetus with heart block and hydrops not eligible for immediate delivery, the prognosis is guarded because in utero management generally has been unsuccessful. One approach to management of complete heart block in utero relates to presuming an underlying fetal myocarditis, wherein dexamethasone[132] or betamethasone may be administered to the mother in an attempt to block the ill effect of presumed maternal antibodies. Evidence suggests that it may be safer to use betamethasone than dexamethasone.[134] Another consideration would be to perform plasmapheresis to reduce maternal antibody.[132] Pharmacologic efforts to improve fetal cardiac output by increasing heart rate with atropine-like drugs and with terbutaline have rarely been successful because they have little effect on ventricular rate. In a therapeutic trial of intravenous salbutamol given to three patients, there was resolution of hydrops with increases in fetal heart rates of 17% to 24% and evidence of improved ventricular systolic performance, as assessed by shortening fraction.[135] Pharmacologic therapy in utero also may be directed at improving cardiac output by enhancing myocardial contractility. The most commonly used inotropic agent for this purpose has been digoxin. Digoxin may be administered maternally or directly to the fetus and is occasionally successful in diminishing hydrops.[136,137] Ritodrine, a β agonist with a preferential β_2 effect often used to quiet premature labor, is known to cross the placenta. It can increase maternal and fetal heart rates and may improve fetal cardiac output. Furosemide has been administered transplacentally[136] and directly via umbilical vein and peritoneum to induce fetal diuresis and increase venous capacitance, so as to decrease intravascular volume and excessive preload.[137] Transthoracic direct fetal ventricular pacing was performed in one dying hydropic fetus with complete heart block, who died 4 hours after institution of pacing.[138] As of this writing, neither transthoracic nor transvenous ventricular pacing of the human fetus is established or routinely available. Experimental work in fetal lambs with intrauterine transvenous cardiac pacing is ongoing. It may be, if and when human fetal electrical pacing becomes practical, that sequential AV pacing will be required in patients with complete AV block and hydrops.

Management in the Neonate

Postnatal management of congenital complete AV block depends on the clinical state. Most neonates with complete AV block without hydrops and without associated structural cardiovascular disease tolerate ventricular rates of at least 55 beats/min well and do not develop heart failure in the newborn period. These infants manifest cardiomegaly but remain asymptomatic early in life, and specific neonatal therapy currently is not recommended. If the ventricular rate is less than 55 beats/min, however, the infant is in a tenuous cardiovascular state and probably should be considered for elective permanent pacemaker implantation before hospital discharge.[123,139,140] In contrast, neonates with complete heart block and complex heart disease continue to have a dismal prognosis, and most die in the neonatal period despite pacemaker management and surgical attempts to repair the cardiovascular malformations.

In a neonate with a structurally normal heart, complete heart block, and hydrops fetalis, therapy is directed toward postnatal management of the hydrops, treating the congestive heart failure with conventional inotropic (dopamine, dobutamine, digoxin) and diuretic therapy. In an infant with an excessively slow heart rate, therapy is directed toward increasing the ventricular rate. Although the use of intravenous isoproterenol is appealing to increase heart rate and to reduce afterload, it is not usually sufficiently effective, so that for an infant with heart failure and an excessively slow ventricular rate (<55 beats/min), direct ventricular pacing is indicated. Additional indications for ventricular pacing are complete heart block with a wide QRS complex (block distal to His bundle) and complete heart block with long Q-T syndrome. It is extremely rare for a newborn with heart block to require emergency ventricular pacing, but, when necessary, a transvenous pacing catheter may be advanced to the ventricle via the umbilical vein and ductus venosus as one would pass a conventional umbilical venous line. I have performed this procedure in the nursery even in a small premature infant. Temporary emergency ventricular pacing may be accomplished via transcutaneous pacing electrodes. Permanent epicardial pacemaker implantation may be performed on a semielective basis.

REFERENCES

1. Barry A: Intrinsic pulsation rates of fragments of embryonic chick heart. J Exp Zool 91:119, 1942.

2. Cavanaugh M: Pulsation, migration and division in dissociated chick embryo heart cells. J Exp Zool 128:573, 1955.

3. de Jong M, Opthof T, Wilde A: Persisting zones of slow impulse conduction in developing chicken hearts. Circ Res 71:240, 1992.

4. Kamino K: Optical approaches to ontogeny of electrical activity and related functional organization during early heart development. Physiol Rev 71:53, 1991.

5. Moorman A, Lamers W: Topography of cardiac gene expression in the embryo: From pattern to function. In Clark EB, Markwald RR, Takao A (eds): Developmental Mechanisms of Heart Disease. New York, Futura, 1995.

6. Arguello C, Alanis J, Pantoja O, Valenzuela B: Electrophysiological and ultrastructural study of the atrioventricular canal during the development of the chick embryo. J Mol Cell Cardiol 18:499, 1986.

7. Dudek RW: Cardiac embryology. In Hess DB, Hess W (eds): Fetal Echocardiography. Stamford, CT, Appleton & Lange, 1999.

8. Anderson RH, Becker AE, Tranum-Jensen J, et al: Anatomico-electrophysiological correlations in the conduction system—a review. Br Heart J 45:67, 1981.

9. Cremer MV: Über die direkte ableitung der aktionsstrome des menschlichen herzens vom eosophagus und über das elektrokardiogramm des fotus. Muench Med Wochenschr 53:811, 1906.

10. Kaplan S, Toyama S: Fetal electrocardiography: Utilizing abdominal and intrauterine leads. Obstet Gynecol 11:391, 1958.

11. Figueroa-Longo JG, Poseiro JJ, Alvarez LO, et al: Fetal electrocardiogram at term labor obtained with subcutaneous fetal electrodes. Am J Obstet Gynecol 96:556, 1966.

12. Hertzberg BS, Mahony BS, Bowie JD: First trimester fetal cardiac activity: Sonographic documentation of a progressive early rise in heart rate. J Ultrasound Med 7:573, 1988.

13. Laboda LA, Estroff JA, Benacerraf BR: First trimester bradycardia: A sign of impending fetal loss. J Ultrasound Med 8:561, 1989.

14. Ibarra-Polo AA, Guiloff E, Gomez-Rogers C: Fetal heart rate throughout pregnancy. Am J Obstet Gynecol 113:814, 1972.

15. Wheeler T, Murrill A: Patterns of fetal heart rate during normal pregnancy. Br J Obstet Gynaecol 85:18, 1978.

16. Southall DP, Richards J, Mitchell P, et al: Study of cardiac rhythm in healthy newborn infants. Br Heart J 43:14, 1980.

17. Richards JM, Alexander JR, Shinebourne EA, et al: Sequential 22-hour profiles of breathing patterns and heart rate in 110 full-term infants during their first 6 months of life. Pediatrics 74:763, 1984.

18. Nagashima M, Matsushima M, Ogawa A, et al: Cardiac arrhythmias in healthy children revealed by 24-hour ambulatory ECG monitoring. Pediatr Cardiol 8:103, 1987.

19. Garson A Jr, Gillette P, Titus J, et al: Surgical treatment of ventricular tachycardia in infants. N Engl J Med 310:1443, 1984.

20. Garson A Jr, Smith RT, Moak JP, et al: Incessant ventricular tachycardia in infants: Purkinje cell tumors and surgical cure. Circulation 74(Suppl II):119, 1986.

21. Lingman G, Lundstrom NR, Marsal K, et al: Fetal cardiac arrhythmia: Clinical outcome in 113 cases. Acta Obstet Gynecol Scand 65:263, 1986.

22. Morgan BC, Guntheroth WG: Cardiac arrhythmias in normal newborn infants. J Pediatr 67:1199, 1965.

23. Southall DP, Richards J, Hardwick RA, et al: Prospective study of fetal heart rate and rhythm patterns. Arch Dis Child 55:506, 1980.

24. Southall DP, Orrell MJ, Talbot JF, et al: Study of cardiac arrhythmias and other forms of conduction abnormality in newborn infants. BMJ 2:597, 1977.

25. Jones RW, Sharp C, Rabb LR, et al: 1028 neonatal electrocardiograms. Arch Dis Child 54:427, 1979.

26. Simpson JM, Yates RW, Sharland GK: Irregular heart rate in the fetus—not always benign. Cardiol Young 6:28, 1996.

27. Stewart PA, Wladimiroff JW: Fetal atrial arrhythmias associated with redundancy/aneurysm of the foramen ovale. J Clin Ultrasound 16:643, 1988.

28. Toro L, Weintraub RG, Shiota T, et al: Relation between persistent atrial arrhythmias and redundant septum primum flap (atrial septal aneurysm) in fetuses. Am J Cardiol 73:711, 1994.

29. Kugler JD, Danford DA, Deal BJ, et al: Radiofrequency catheter ablation for tachyarrhythmias in children and adolescents. N Engl J Med 330:1481, 1994.

30. Blanchard WB, Bucciarelli RL, Miller BL: Ventricular parasystole in a newborn infant. J Electrocardiol 12:427, 1979.

31. Garson A Jr, Gillette PC, McNamara DG: Supraventricular tachycardia in children: Clinical features, response to treatment, and long-term follow-up in 217 patients. J Pediatr 98:875, 1981.

32. Nadas AS, Daeschner CW, Roth A, et al: Paroxysmal tachycardia in infants and children: Study of 41 cases. Pediatrics 9:167, 1952.

33. Gillette PC, Garson Jr A: Pediatric Arrhythmias: Electrophysiology and Pacing. Philadelphia, WB Saunders, 1990.

34. Ko JK, Deal BJ, Strasburger JF, et al: Supraventricular tachycardia mechanisms and their age distribution in pediatric patients. Am J Cardiol 69:1028, 1992.

35. Naheed ZJ, Strasburger JF, Deal BJ, et al: Fetal tachycardia: Mechanisms and predictors of hydrops fetalis. J Am Coll Cardiol 27:1736, 1996.

36. Fouron J: Prenatal diagnosis of arrythmias. Presented at Advances in Fetal and Perinatal Cardiology: Satellite Symposium of the 3rd World Congress of Pediatric Cardiology and Cardiac Surgery, Fetal Centre at the Hospital for Sick Children, Toronto, Canada, May 24, 2001, pp 47-50.

37. Belhassen B, Pauzner D, Blieden L, et al: Intrauterine and postnatal atrial fibrillation in the Wolff-Parkinson-White syndrome. Circulation 66:124, 1982.

38. Johnson WH Jr, Dunnigan A, Fehr P, et al: Association of atrial flutter with orthodromic reciprocating fetal tachycardia. Am J Cardiol 59:374, 1987.

39. Silber DL, Durnin RE: Intrauterine atrial tachycardia, associated with massive edema in a newborn. Am J Dis Child 117:722, 1969.

40. Martin CB, Nijhuis JG, Weijer AA: Correction of fetal supraventricular tachycardia by compression of the umbilical cord: Report of a case. Am J Obstet Gynecol 150:324, 1984.

41. Kohl T, Tercanli S, Kececioglu D, et al: Direct fetal administration of adenosine for the termination of incessant supraventricular tachycardia. Obstet Gynecol 85:873, 1995.

42. Lingman G, Ohrlander S, Ohlin P: Intrauterine digoxin treatment of fetal paroxysmal tachycardia case report. Br J Obstet Gynaecol 87:340, 1980.

43. Dumesic DA, Silverman NH, Tobias S, et al: Transplacental cardioversion of supraventricular tachycardia with procainamide. N Engl J Med 307:1128, 1982.

44. Spinnato JA, Shaver DC, Flinn GS, et al: Fetal supraventricular tachycardia: In utero therapy with digoxin and quinidine. Obstet Gynecol 64:730, 1984.

45. Triedman JK, Walsh EP, Saul JP: Response of fetal tachycardia to transplacental procainamide therapy. Cardiol Young 6:235, 1996.

46. Maxwell DJ, Crawford DC, Curry PV, et al: Obstetric importance, diagnosis, and management of fetal tachycardias. BMJ 297:107, 1988.

47. Owen J, Colvin EV, Davis RO: Fetal death after successful conversion of fetal supraventricular tachycardia with digoxin and verapamil. Am J Obstet Gynecol 158:1169, 1988.

48. Wren C, Hunter S: Maternal administration of flecainide to terminate and suppress fetal tachycardia. BMJ (Clin Res) 296:249, 1988.

49. Fish FA, Gillette PC, Benson DW Jr: Proarrhythmia, cardiac arrest and death in young patients receiving encainide and flecainide. J Am Coll Cardiol 18:356, 1991.

50. Van Engelen AD, Weitjens O, Brenner JI, et al: Management outcome and follow-up of fetal tachycardia. J Am Coll Cardiol 24:1371, 1994.

51. Allan LD, Chita SK, Sharland GK, et al: Flecainide in the treatment of fetal tachycardias. Br Heart J 65:46, 1991.

52. Windle JR, Geletka RC, Moss AJ, et al: Normalization of ventricular repolarization with flecainide in long QT syndrome patients with SCN5A: DeltaKPQ mutation. Ann Noninvas Electrocardiol 6:153, 2001.

53. Arnoux P, Seyral P, Llurens M, et al: Amiodarone and digoxin for refractory fetal tachycardia. Am J Cardiol 59:166, 1987.

54. Widerhorn J, Bhandari AK, Bughi S, et al: Fetal and neonatal adverse effects profile of amiodarone treatment during pregnancy. Am Heart J 122:1162, 1991.

55. Gembruch U, Manz M, Bald R, et al: Repeated intravascular treatment with amiodarone in a fetus with refractory supraventricular tachycardia and hydrops fetalis. Am Heart J 118:1335, 1989.

56. Hansmann M, Gembruch U, Bald R, et al: Fetal tachyarrhythmias: Transplacental and direct treatment of the fetus—a report of 60 cases. Ultrasound Obstet Gynecol 1:162, 1991.

57. Wilson JS, Podrid PJ: Side effects from amiodarone. Am Heart J 121:158, 1991.

58. Overholt ED, Rheuban KS, Gutgesell HP, et al: Usefulness of adenosine for arrhythmias in infants and children. Am J Cardiol 61:336, 1988.

59. Deal BJ, Keane JF, Gillette PC, et al: Wolff-Parkinson-White syndrome and supraventricular tachycardia during infancy: Management and follow-up. J Am Coll Cardiol 5:130, 1985.

60. Pickoff AS, Zies L, Ferrer PL, et al: High dose propranolol therapy in the management of supraventricular tachycardia. J Pediatr 94:144, 1979.

61. Reimer A, Paul T, Kallifelz H: Efficacy and safety of intravenous and oral propafenone in pediatric cardiac dysrhythmias. Am J Cardiol 68:741, 1991.

62. Janousek J, Paul T, Reimer A, et al: Usefulness of propafenone for supraventricular arrhythmias in infants and children. Am J Cardiol 72:294, 1993.

63. Guccione P, Drago F, Di Donato RM, et al: Oral propafenone therapy for children with arrhythmias: Efficacy and adverse effects in midterm follow-up. Am Heart J 122:1022, 1991.

64. Bowman E, Paes BA, Way RC: Oral sotalol in neonatal supraventricular tachycardia. Acta Paediatr Scand 77:171, 1988.

65. Tipple M, Sandor G: Efficacy and safety of oral sotalol in early infancy. PACE 14(Pt II):2062, 1991.

66. Maragnes P, Tipple M, Fournier A: Effectiveness of oral sotalol for treatment of pediatric arrhythmias. Am J Cardiol 69:751, 1992.

67. Kirk CR, Gibbs JL, Thomas R, et al: Cardiovascular collapse after verapamil in supraventricular tachycardia. Arch Dis Child 62:1265, 1987.

68. Saul JP, Hulse JE, Papagiannis J, et al: Late enlargement of radiofrequency lesions in infant lambs. Circulation 90:492, 1994.

69. Erickson CC, Walsh EP, Triedman JK, et al: Efficacy and safety of radiofrequency ablation in infants and young children < 18 months of age. Am J Cardiol 74:944, 1994.

70. Biancaniello TM, Meyer RA, Gaum WE, et al: Primary benign intramural ventricular tumors in children: Pre- and postoperative electrocardiographic, echocardiographic, and angiocardiographic evaluation. Am Heart J 103:852, 1982.

71. Losure TA, Roberts NS: In utero diagnosis of atrial flutter by means of real-time-directed M-mode echocardiography. Am J Obstet Gynecol 149:903, 1984.

72. Kleinman CS, Copel JA: Electrophysiological principles and fetal antiarrhythmic therapy. Ultrasound Obstet Gynecol 1:286, 1991.

73. Hirata K, Kato H, Yoshioka F, et al: Successful treatment of fetal atrial flutter and congestive heart failure. Arch Dis Child 60:158, 1985.

74. Oudijk MA, Ambachtsheer EB, Stoutenbeek P, et al: Protocols for the treatment of supraventricular tachycardias in the fetus [Dutch]. Ned Tijdschr Geneeskd 145:1218, 2001.

75. Fernandez C, De Rosa GE, Guevarra E, et al: Reversion by vagal reflex of a fetal paroxysmal atrial tachycardia detected by echocardiography. Am J Obstet Gynecol 159:860, 1988.

76. Jaeggi E, Fouron JC, Drblik SP: Fetal atrial flutter: Diagnosis, clinical features, treatment, and outcome. J Pediatr 132:335, 1998.

77. Kleinman CS, Copel JA: Fetal cardiac arrhythmias: Diagnosis and therapy. Proceedings of the 9th International Fetal Cardiology symposium, Orlando, Fla, 1996, pp 326-341.

78. Simpson RJ Jr, Foster JR, Mulrow JP, et al: The electrophysiological substrate of atrial fibrillation. PACE 6:1166, 1983.

79. Roden DM: Ibutilide and the treatment of atrial arrhythmias: A new drug—almost unheralded—is now available to US physicians. Circulation 94:1499, 1996.

80. Pongiglione G, Strasburger JF, Deal BJ, et al: Use of amiodarone for short-term and adjuvant therapy in young patients. Am J Cardiol 68:603, 1991.

81. Dodo H, Gow RM, Hamilton RM, et al: Chaotic atrial rhythm in children. Am Heart J 129:990, 1995.

82. Fish FA, Mehta AV, Johns JA: Characteristics and management of chaotic atrial tachycardia of infancy. Am J Cardiol 78:1052, 1996.

83. Evans V, Garson A Jr, Smith RT, et al: Ethmozine: A promising drug for "automatic" atrial ectopic focus tachycardia [abstract]. Circulation 72(Suppl 3):173, 1985.

84. Naheed ZJ, Strasburger JF, Benson DW Jr, et al: Natural history and management strategies of automatic atrial tachycardia in children. Am J Cardiol 75:405, 1995.

85. Gillette PC, Garson Jr A, Porter CJ, et al: Junctional automatic ectopic tachycardia: New proposed treatment by transcatheter His bundle ablation. Am Heart J 106:619, 1983.

86. Garson A Jr, Gillette PC: Junctional ectopic tachycardia in children: Electrocardiography, electrophysiology and pharmacologic response. Am J Cardiol 44:298, 1979.

87. Raja P, Hawker RE, Chaikitpinyo A, et al: Amiodarone management of junctional ectopic tachycardia after cardiac surgery in children. Br Heart J 72:261, 1994.

88. Case CL, Gillette PC: Automatic atrial and junctional tachycardias in the pediatric patient: Strategies for diagnosis and management. Pacing Clin Electrophysiol 16:1323, 1993.

89. Katz LN, Pick A: Clinical Electrocardiography: I. The Arrhythmias. Philadelphia, Lea & Febiger, 1965, pp 287-290.

90. Kallfelz HC: Cardiac arrhythmias in the fetus—diagnosis, significance and prognosis. In Godman MJ, Marquis RM (eds): Paediatric Cardiology, vol 2: Heart Disease in the Newborn. Edinburgh, Churchill-Livingstone, 1979, pp 401-412.

91. Gaum WE, Biancaniello T, Kaplan S: Accelerated ventricular rhythm in childhood. Am J Cardiol 43:162, 1979.

92. Bisset GS, Janos GG, Gaum WE: Accelerated ventricular rhythm in the newborn infant. J Pediatr 104:247, 1984.

93. Geggel RL, McInerny J, Estes M: Transient neonatal ventricular tachycardia associated with maternal cocaine use. Am J Cardiol 63:383, 1989.

94. Garson A Jr, Smith RT, Moak JP, et al: Incessant ventricular tachycardia in infants: Myocardial hamartomas and surgical cure. J Am Coll Cardiol 10:619, 1987.

95. Van Hare GF, Stanger P: Ventricular tachycardia and accelerated ventricular rhythm presenting in the first month of life. Am J Cardiol 67:42, 1991.

96. Stevens D, Schriener R, Hurwitz R, et al: Fetal and neonatal ventricular arrhythmia. Pediatrics 63:771, 1979.

97. Bergdahl DM, Stevenson JG, Guntheroth WG: Prognosis in primary ventricular tachycardia in the pediatric patient. Circulation 62:897, 1980.

98. Schleich JM, Bernard Du Haut Cilly F, Laurent MC, et al: Early prenatal management of a fetal ventricular tachycardia treated in utero by amiodarone with long term follow-up. Prenat Diag 20:449, 2000.

99. Woolf AD, Wenger T, Smith TW, et al: The use of digoxin-specific Fab fragments for severe digitalis intoxication in children. N Engl J Med 326:1739, 1992.

100. Gutgesell HP, Tacker WA, Geddes LA, et al: Energy dose for ventricular defibrillation of children. Pediatrics 58:898, 1976.

101. Figa FH, Gow RM, Hamilton RM: Clinical efficacy and safety of intravenous amiodarone in infants and children. Am J Cardiol 74:573, 1994

102. Perry JC, McQuinn RL, Smith RT Jr, et al: Flecainide acetate for resistant arrhythmias in the young: Efficacy and pharmacokinetics. J Am Coll Cardiol 14:185, 1989.

103. Jervell A, Lange-Nielsen F: Congenital deaf-mutism, functional heart disease with prolongation of the QT interval and sudden death. Am Heart J 54:59, 1957.

104. Romano C, Gemme G, Pongiglione R: Aritmie cardiache rare delle'eta paediatrica: II. Accessi sincopali per fibrillazione ventriculolare parossistica. Clin Pediatr 45:656, 1963.

105. Ward OC: A new familial cardiac syndrome in children. J Irish Med Assoc 54:103, 1964.

106. Schwartz PJ, Periti M, Malliani A: The long QT syndrome. Am Heart J 89:378, 1975.

107. Schwartz PJ: The sudden infant death syndrome. In Scarpelli EM, Cosmi EV (eds): Reviews in Perinatal Medicine, vol 4. New York, Raven Press, 1981, pp 475-524.

108. Bazett HC: An analysis of the time-relations of electrocardiograms. Heart 7:353, 1918-1920.

109. Ross B, Garson A Jr, McNamara D: Factors affecting outcome in children with long Q-T syndrome. Circulation 70(Suppl II):320, 1984.

110. Di-Segni E, David D, Katzenstein M, et al: Permanent overdrive pacing for the suppression of recurrent ventricular tachycardia in a newborn with long QT syndrome. J Electrocardiol 13:189, 1980.

111. Villain E, Levy M, Kachaner J, et al: Prolonged QT interval in neonates: Benign, transient, or prolonged risk of sudden death. Am Heart J 124:194, 1992.

112. Vincent GM: The heart rate of Romano-Ward syndrome patients. Am Heart J 112:61, 1986.

113. Garson A Jr, Dick M II, Fournier A, et al: The long QT syndrome in children: An international study of 287 patients. Circulation 87:1866, 1993.

114. Trippel DL, Parsons MK, Gillette PC: Infants with long-QT syndrome and 2:1 atrioventricular block. Am Heart J 130:1130, 1995.

115. Batisse A, Belloy C, Fermont L: Prolonged Q-T interval with functional AV block in neonates and young infants. Arch Fr Pediatr 38:57, 1981.

116. Martin AB, Garson Jr A, Perry JC: Prolonged QT interval in hypertrophic and dilated cardiomyopathy in children. Am Heart J 127:64, 1994.

117. Clark M, Lazzaraza R, Jackman W: Torsades de pointes: Serum drug levels and electrocardiographic warning signs. Circulation 66:II-71, 1982.

118. Pedersen DH, Zipes DP, Foster PR, et al: Ventricular tachycardia and ventricular fibrillation in a young population. Circulation 60:988, 1979.

119. Cowley CG, Tani LY, Shaddy RE: Sinus node dysfunction in tuberous sclerosis. Pediatr Cardiol 17:51, 1996.

120. Mehta AV, Chidambaram B, Garrett A: Familial symptomatic sinus bradycardia: Autosomal dominant inheritance. Pedatr Cardiol 16:231, 1995.

121. Ferrer PL: Arrhythmias in the neonate, infant, and child. In Roberts NK, Gelband H (eds): Arrhythmias in the Neonate. New York, Appleton-Century-Crofts, 1977, pp 265-316.

122. Machado MV, Tynan MJ, Curry PV, et al: Fetal complete heart block. Br Heart J 60:512, 1988.

123. Michaelsson M, Engle MA: Congenital complete heart block: An international study of the natural history. Cardiovasc Clin 4:85, 1972.

124. Winkler RB, Nora AH, Nora JJ: Familial congenital complete heart block and maternal systemic lupus erythematosus. Circulation 56:1103, 1977.

125. Gembruch U, Hansmann M, Redel DA, et al: Fetal complete heart block: Antenatal diagnosis, significance and management. Eur J Obstet Gynecol Reprod Biol 31:9, 1989.

126. Schmidt KG, Ulmer HE, Silverman NH: Perinatal outcome of fetal complete atrioventricular block: A multicenter experience. J Am Coll Cardiol 91:1360, 1991.

127. Garcia OL, Mehta AV, Pickoff AS, et al: Left isomerism and complete atrioventricular block: A report of six cases. Am J Cardiol 48:1103, 1981.

128. Shenker L, Reed KL, Anderson CF, et al: Congenital heart block and cardiac anomalies in the absence of maternal connective tissue disease. Am J Obstet Gynecol 157:248, 1987.

129. Ho SY, Fagg N, Anderson RH, et al: Disposition of the atrioventricular conduction tissues in the heart with isomerism of the atrial appendages: Its relation to congenital complete heart block. J Am Coll Cardiol 20:904, 1992.

130. McCune AB, Weston WL, Lee LA: Maternal and fetal outcome in neonatal lupus erythematosus. Ann Intern Med 106:518, 1987.

131. Wren C, MacCartney FJ, Deanfield JE: Cardiac rhythm in atrial isomerism. Am J Cardiol 59:1156, 1987.

132. Altenburger KM, Jedziniak M, Roper WL, et al: Congenital complete heart block associated with hydrops fetalis. J Pediatr 91:618, 1977.

133. Buyon JP, Swersky SH, Fox HE, et al: Intra-uterine therapy for presumptive fetal myocarditis with acquired heart block due to systemic lupus erythematosus: Experience in a mother with a predominance of SS-B(La) antibodies. Arthritis Rheum 30:44, 1987.

134. Whitelaw A, Thoresen M: Antenatal steroids and the developing brain. Arch Dis Child (Fetal Neonat Ed) 83:F154, 2000.

135. Groves AMM, Allan LD, Rosenthal E: Therapeutic trial of sympathomimetics in three cases of complete heart block in the fetus. Circulation 92:3394, 1995.

136. Harris JP, Alexson DG, Manning JA, et al: Medical therapy for the hydropic fetus with congenital complete atrioventricular block. Am J Perinatol 10:217, 1993.

137. Anandakumar C, Biswas A, Chew SSL, et al: Direct fetal therapy for hydrops secondary to congenital atrioventricular heart block. Obstet Gynecol 87:835, 1996.

138. Carpenter RJ Jr, Strasburger JF, Garson A Jr, et al: Fetal ventricular pacing for hydrops secondary to complete atrioventricular block. J Am Coll Cardiol 8:1434, 1986.

139. Pinsky WW, Gillette PC, Garson A Jr, et al: Diagnosis, management and long-term results of patients with congenital complete atrioventricular block. Pediatrics 69:728, 1982.

140. Sholler GF, Walsh EP: Congenital complete heart block in patients without anatomic cardiac defects. Am Heart J 118:1193, 1989.

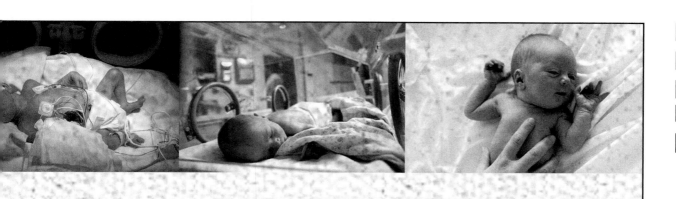

Nutrition and Gastrointestinal Tract of Neonates

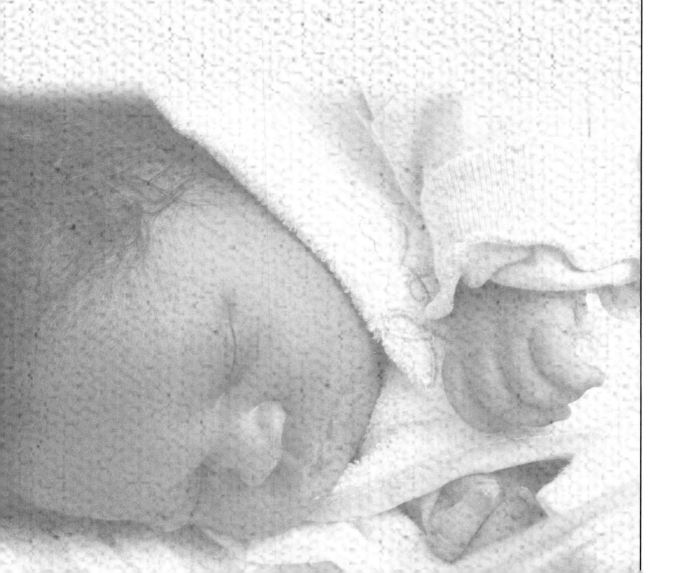

CHAPTER 63

Feeding the Critically Ill Neonate

Gilberto R. Pereira and See Wai Chan

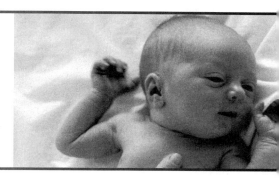

After birth, the neonate becomes independent of placental regulation and must rely on the gastrointestinal tract for the provision of nutrients necessary for growth and development. In the critically ill neonate, various medical and surgical conditions are likely to compromise nutrient intake and to alter nutritional requirements. This chapter reviews the nutritional requirements and the methods for delivering parenteral and enteral nutrition to both full-term and preterm infants. Additional consideration is given to the immediate postnatal period and to several conditions that necessitate specialized nutritional care, such as extreme prematurity, perinatal asphyxia, necrotizing enterocolitis (NEC), preoperative and postoperative care, and mechanical ventilation.

NUTRITIONAL REQUIREMENTS

Several methods have been proposed as models for the estimation of nutritional requirements in neonates. Of these, the composition and intake of human milk,[1-3] the growth rates and nutrient accretion rates of the fetus,[4,5] and the net uptake of nutrients by the umbilical circulation[6] are unique to neonatal research. Other methods include nutrient balance studies,[7,8] infusion of stable isotopes,[2,9] and the determination of optimal intake that prevents nutritional deficiency and allows for favorable growth and developmental outcome.[10] Nutritional requirements in neonates are known to vary according to the birth weight and gestational age of the infant, the method of feeding (enteral versus parenteral) and the metabolic alterations caused by some illnesses and their therapies. In comparison with full-term infants, premature infants have greater nutritional requirements primarily because of their faster growth rates and their physiologic immaturity. Likewise, parenteral nutritional requirements of both full-term and preterm neonates differ from enteral nutritional requirements. On the basis of limited research, it seems that nutritional requirements also vary according to the type and severity of illness.

At no other time during extrauterine human life does body growth proceed at a faster rate than during early infancy. Consequently, postnatal growth parameters are commonly monitored serially to assess the adequacy of nutritional intake in neonates. Contemporary postnatal growth curves have been published for full-term[11] and premature infants.[12]

Table 63-1 shows the daily nutritional requirements for neonates, emphasizing differences based on gestational age (full-term and preterm infants), the route of administration (parenteral versus enteral), and specific disease process.

IMMEDIATE POSTNATAL CARE

Nutritional care of the critically ill neonate starts soon after birth. The goals for nutrition support during this period are maintenance of fluid status, glucose homeostasis, and normalization of serum electrolyte and mineral concentrations. Intravenous fluids containing 10% dextrose are provided until parenteral or enteral feedings can be established, preferably within the first 24 to 36 hours after birth.[13,14] Because fluid requirements are significantly increased in premature infants weighing less than 1000 g, lower dextrose concentrations are frequently indicated to prevent hyperglycemia. A decreased serum glucose clearance rate, a diminished response to insulin, and an increased cortisol level mediated by stress have been identified as mechanisms leading to hyperglycemia in these infants.[15-17] Conversely, preterm infants are also susceptible to the development of hypoglycemia as a result of limited hepatic glycogen stores and inadequate endogenous glucose production.[18,19] In the same manner, infants who have experienced perinatal asphyxia, intrauterine growth restriction, sepsis, or cold stress are at risk for developing hypoglycemia.[20-22] Table 63-2 displays general guidelines for the initiation of intravenous fluids in neonates of different birth weights when nursed in various environmental conditions. Subsequent changes in rate and in composition of the infused fluid

Table 63–1. Nutritional Requirements

Requirement	Premature		Full Term	
	Enteral	Parenteral	Enteral	Parenteral
Water (mL/kg/day)*	150-200	120-150	120-150	100-120
Energy (kcal/kg/day)[†]	110-130	90-100	100-120	80-90
Protein (g/kg/day)[‡]	3-3.8	2.5-3.5	2-2.5	2-2.5
Carbohydrates (g/kg/day)	8-12	10-15	8-12	10-15
Fat (g/kg/day)	3-4	2-3.5	3-4	2-4
Sodium (mEq/kg/day)	2-4	2-3.5	2-3	2-3
Chloride (mEq/kg/day)	2-4	2-3.5	2-3	2-3
Potassium (mEq/kg/day)	2-3	2-3	2-3	2-3
Calcium (mg/kg/day)[§]	210-250	60-90	130	60-80
Phosphorus (mg/kg/day)[§]	112-125	40-70	45	40-45
Magnesium (mg/kg/day)	8-15	4-7	7	5-7
Iron (mg/kg/day)[‖]	1-2	0.0-0.2	1-2	0.1-0.2
Vitamin A (IU/day)[¶]	700-1500	700-1500	1250	2300
Vitamin D (IU/day)	400	120-260	300	400
Vitamin E (IU/day)**	6-12	2-4	5-10	7
Vitamin K (mg/day)	0.05	0.06-0.1	0.05	0.2
Vitamin C (mg/day)	20-60	35-50	30-50	80
Vitamin B_1 (mg/day)	0.2-0.7	0.3-0.8	0.3	1.2
Vitamin B_2 (mg/day)	0.3-0.8	0.4-0.9	0.4	1.4
Vitamin B_6 (mg/day)	0.3-0.7	0.3-0.7	0.3	1
Vitamin B_{12} (µg/day)	0.3-0.7	0.3-0.7	0.3	1
Niacin (mg/day)	5-12	5-12	5	17
Folate (µg/day)[††]	50	40-90	25-50	140
Biotin (µg/day)	6-20	6-13	10	20
Zinc (µg/kg/day)[‡‡]	800-1000	400	830	250
Copper (µg/kg/day)[‡‡,§§]	100-150	20	75	20
Manganese (µg/kg/day)[§§]	10-20	1	85	1
Selenium (µg/kg/day)[‖‖]	1.3-3	1.5-2	1.6	2
Chromium (µg/kg/day)	2-4	0.2	2	0.2
Molybdenum (µg/kg/day)	2-3	0.25	2	0.25
Iodine (µg/kg/day)	4	1	7	1

*For immediate postnatal initiation of fluid therapy, use values presented in Table 63-2.
[†]Adjust according to weight gain and stress factors.
[‡]Requirements increase with increasing degree of prematurity.
[§]Inadequate amount in total parenteral nutrition solutions because of risk of precipitation.
[‖]Initiate between 2 weeks and 2 months of age. Delay initiation in premature infants with progressive retinopathy.
[¶]Supplementation might reduce incidence of bronchopulmonary dysplasia.
**Supplementation might reduce severity of retinopathy of prematurity.
[††]Not present in oral multivitamin supplement.
[‡‡]Increased requirement in patients with excessive ileostomy drainage or chronic diarrhea.
[§§]Removed from total parenteral nutrition solutions in patients with cholestatic liver disease.
[‖‖]Not present in standard trace element solution for neonates.

are often needed because of differences observed among individual patients and types of illness.

Routine laboratory monitoring should include serial measurements of serum glucose, electrolytes, calcium, phosphorus and magnesium. Sodium, chloride, and potassium are routinely administered after the first 24 hours after birth, after documentation of adequate renal function. Calcium, phosphorus, and magnesium may need to be provided intravenously in the immediate postnatal period if the serum concentrations of these minerals are low as a result of asphyxia, acidosis, or repeated administration of sodium bicarbonate infusions.

The neonate lacks appreciable nutrient stores and has limited capacity to tolerate prolonged starvation. It has been estimated that the length of time that a neonate can tolerate starvation is inversely related to the degree of prematurity[23] and possibly accentuated by the severity of medical illness and extent of malnutrition. Traditionally, nutrition support has not been regarded as an essential part of early medical management. However, given the extent of metabolic stress in the presence of limited nutrient reserves, it seems reasonable to initiate intravenous fluids immediately after birth and parenteral nutritional support within 24 to 36 hours after birth in all critically ill neonates.[13,24] Although enteral feeding is the preferred method of providing nutritional support, a significant number of sick infants are maintained solely on parenteral nutrition during the first week of postnatal life. When parenteral

Table 63–2. Recommendations For Starting Parenteral Fluid Therapy in Infants with Low Birth Weight

Warming Device	Birth Weight (g)			
	600–800	801–1000	1001–1500	1501–2000
Radiant Warmer				
Volume (mL/kg/day)*	120	90	75	65
Dextrose (%)	5	10	10	12.5
Saline (%)†	0.1	0.2	0.2	0.2
Incubator				
Volume (mL/kg/day)*	90	75	65	55
Dextrose (%)	7.5	10	10	12.5
Saline (%)†	0.1	0.2	0.2	0.2
Radiant Warmer *or* **Incubator with Shield**				
Volume (mL/kg/day)*	70	55	50	45
Dextrose (%)	7.5	10	12.5	12.5
Saline (%)†	0.1	0.2	0.2	0.2

*Plus 30% with phototherapy.
†After the first day after birth.

Adapted from Baumgart S, Langman CB, Sosulski R, et al: Fluid, electrolyte, and glucose maintenance in the very low birth weight infant. Clin Pediatr Phila 21: 199, 1982.

nutrition is used for periods longer than 1 week, serial measurements of serum electrolytes, calcium, phosphorus, magnesium, blood urea nitrogen, creatinine, and triglycerides and liver function studies should be performed.

ENTERAL NUTRITION

Although parenteral nutrition is almost routinely used for initial nutrition support of critically ill neonates, attempts should be made to begin enteral feedings as soon as the gastrointestinal tract is functional. Advantages of enteral feedings over parenteral nutrition include physiologic stimulation and preserved integrity of the gastrointestinal mucosa, reduced rate of complications related to parenteral nutrition, and lower cost. Before the initiation of enteral feedings, the critically ill infant should be evaluated for signs that suggest readiness for enteral feedings.[25] These include the absence of abdominal distention, previous passage of meconium stools, and presence of active bowel sounds.

Composition of Feedings

Table 63-3 outlines the types of feedings commonly given to full-term and preterm neonates. The table describes the composition of various types of infant feedings, the clinical indications for their use, and the guidelines for the use of nutritional supplements.

Human milk is the preferred feeding for full-term infants because of its unique nutrient composition, increased bioavailability of nutrients, immunologic properties, the promotion of the maternal-infant attachment, and the presence of hormones, enzymes, and growth factors. Human milk is a highly variable product, and its composition is altered by factors that include maternal diet, maternal age, maternal nutritional status, stage of lactation, and the infant's demand for milk. For many years, it remained controversial whether nutritional supplements, notably vitamin D and iron, should be routinely provided to healthy breast-fed infants.[26] However, due to continuing reports of rickets in breast-fed infants and concerns about the adverse effects of exposure to sunlight, it is now recommended that all breast-fed infants be supplemented with 200 IU/day of vitamin D, beginning within 2 months after birth.[27] Because the critically ill infant may have been exposed to prolonged periods of suboptimal nutrient intake, vitamin and mineral supplementation under these circumstances may be beneficial.

When human milk is not available, standard infant formulas are appropriate for enteral feedings in full-term infants with intact gastrointestinal function. In 1976, the American Academy of Pediatrics established standards for the composition of infant formulas to ensure optimal growth during early infancy.[28] The products described in this chapter as standard infant formulas are prepared from modified cow's milk. Within this group, there are three infant formulas with special composition; two of these have lower mineral and electrolyte content, which may be suitable for full-term infants with cardiac or renal disease, and another is prepared without lactose, being indicated for infants with lactose intolerance. Multivitamin supplementation is unnecessary with the use of standard formulas, unless the infant has increased requirements or receives an inadequate volume of formula. Iron supplementation is also unnecessary if iron-fortified preparations are used. Fluoride supplementation is currently recommended for infants older than

Table 63–3. Types of Infant Feedings

Feedings	Indications	Special Composition	Comments	Supplements
Mature human milk	Full-term infants with intact GI function	High nutrient bioavailability; immune factors; hormones; growth factors; low osmolality	Preferred feeding; model for composition of formulas; psychologic benefits; low cost	Vitamin D, 400 IU/day (?); iron, 2 mg/kg/day (?)
Standard infant formulas: Similac Enfamil Gerber Carnation PM 60:40 Lactofree	Full-term infants with intact GI function	Cow's milk protein: casein or whey predominant; lactose-only carbohydrate except Lactofree; fat blend with predominance of LCT; low renal solute load (Carnation and PM 60:40)	Alternative to human milk, promotes adequate growth, commonly used for neonates with cardiac or renal disease (Carnation and PM 60:40) or lactose intolerance (Lactofree)	Iron, 2 mg/kg/day if formula is not iron fortified
Preterm human milk	Premature infants (<37 wk gestation)	Higher protein, calories, NaCl than in mature human milk; immune factors; growth factors; hormones; low osmolality	Preferred feeding; special compositional differences persist during first month of lactation; psychologic benefits	Liquid fortifier, 1 mL:1 mL; powder fortifier, 1 packet/25 ml; Poly-Vi-Sol, 0.5 mL/day; iron, 2 mg/kg/day by 2 weeks of age
Premature infant formulas: Similac Special Care Enfamil	Premature infants (<37 wk gestation)	Whey-predominant protein; 50% lactose load; 40%-50% fat as MCT; high concentration of minerals and vitamins; available at 20 or 24 kcal/oz; available with and without iron fortification (both products listed)	Alternative to fortified preterm human milk; enhanced digestion and nutrient absorption by premature infants; preterm discharge formulas recommended before hospital discharge	Iron, 2 mg/kg/day by age 2 weeks if formula is not iron fortified; Poly-Vi-Sol, 0.5–1 mL/day when intake <170 mL/day (Similac Special Care) or < 151 mL/day (Enfamil Premature)
Preterm discharge formulas: NeoSure EnfaCare	Premature infants weighing <1500 g after discharge from hospital or >40 weeks of post-conception age	22 cal/oz; available with iron fortification; higher calcium and phosphorus contents	Provide nutrient and mineral contents between premature and standard formulas; recommended use up to 1 year of age; greater linear growth weight gain and bone mineralization than with standard formulas	Fluoride, 0.25 mg/day, depending on water supply, after 6 months of age
Soy-based formulas: Isomil ProSobee Nursoy	Full-term infants with milk protein or lactose intolerance	Soy protein with methionine; lactose free; high phytate; iron fortified	Amino acid content not appropriate for premature infant; phytate binds to calcium and phosphorus	—
Protein hydrolysate formulas: Pregestimil Alimentum Nutramigen Portagen	Full-term infants with cow's milk allergy, lactose intolerance, or malabsorptive syndromes	Protein hydrolysates; variable carbohydrates and fat sources; easily absorbed; iron fortified; high osmolality; very high MCT content and low osmolality (Portagen)	Dilute for initial use; does not meet protein calcium, phosphorus, and vitamin requirements of premature infants; essential fatty acid deficiency may occur in infants with chronic diarrhea (Portagen)	Poly-Vi-Sol, 0.5 mL/day, and calcium and phosphorus supplements for premature infants

GI, gastrointestinal; LCT, long-chain triglyceride; MCT, medium-chain triglyceride; NaCl, sodium chloride.

6 months who are receiving infant formulas prepared with water fluoridated at a suboptimal level.[29]

Soy-based formulas may be appropriate for a select group of infants who cannot tolerate lactose because of hereditary galactosemia or transient lactase deficiency and for infants with immunoglobulin E–mediated allergy to cow's milk. The soy-based formulas have two distinct compositional features: they contain soy protein isolates instead of cow's milk protein, and they are lactose free. The soy-based preparations should not be routinely given to premature infants weighing less than 1800 g, because of their lower concentration of essential amino acids[30] and the presence of phytate, which decreases the intestinal absorption of calcium and phosphorus.[31]

Protein hydrolysate formulas are indicated for infants who are unable to fully absorb the macronutrients contained in standard formulas. This type of infant formula is the preferred feeding for infants with significant malabsorption resulting from intestinal or hepatobiliary disease and for those with intolerance to cow's milk and soy proteins. These preparations contain protein in the form of casein or whey hydrolysates, fats with a predominance of medium-chain triglycerides, and multiple sources of carbohydrate, including glucose polymers, dextrose, and modified starches. These formulas should be given with caution to premature infants because they may not meet requirements for protein, calcium, phosphorus, sodium, and some fat-soluble vitamins. Disadvantages of the protein hydrolysate formulas include poor taste, greater cost, and high osmolality.

The mother's own preterm human milk is the preferred feeding for premature infants. Studies have reported that preterm human milk has a higher concentration of calories, protein, sodium, and chloride and a lower concentration of lactose than does mature human milk.[32,33] These compositional differences, which persist for the first 2 to 4 weeks of lactation, are regarded as nutritionally beneficial for premature infants. Despite these differences, some studies suggest that preterm human milk does not consistently meet the needs of the growing premature infant for protein, calcium, phosphorus, sodium, iron, copper, zinc, and some vitamins.[34-37] Therefore, supplementation of human milk with a powder or liquid fortifier is recommended after feedings have been well established and the human milk has matured. Fortification of human milk has been shown to improve growth, protein status, and bone mineralization in preterm infants.[34-40]

In the absence of human milk, premature infant formula is the most appropriate substitute for preterm infants. In comparison with formulas intended for full-term infants, premature infant formulas provide a higher concentration of whey-predominant protein, a reduced lactose load, a blend of medium-chain triglycerides, and a higher concentration of minerals, vitamins, and trace elements. Multivitamin and folic acid supplementation may be necessary, depending on the daily volume of formula ingested by the infant and individual nutritional status (see Table 63-3).

Preterm discharge formulas are recommended from the time of nursery discharge to the age of 1 year for premature infants with birth weights less than 1500 g. These products are also indicated for premature infants who remain hospitalized after 40 weeks of postconception age. The composition of these formulas includes a calorie density of 22 cal/30 mL and a nutrient concentration that is between those of the preterm and full-term formulas. Studies have shown that these formulas, in comparison with full-term formulas, provide greater linear growth, weight gain, and bone mineral content.[41-44]

Table 63–4. Methods of Feeding

Method	Indications	Complications	Management
Oral (nipple feedings)	Normal sucking and swallowing mechanisms	Fatigue	Limit feeding time to 20 min
		Increased energy expenditure associated with feeding	Give remainder of feeding by tube
Intermittent gastric (gavage)	Inadequate sucking and swallow mechanisms	Vomiting and aspiration	Measure gastric residuals before each feeding
	Respiratory distress (RR > 60/min)	Poor weight gain	Assess energy requirements
Continuous gastric	Extreme prematurity	Vomiting and aspiration	Measure gastric residuals q6-8h
	Mechanical ventilation		
	Intolerance to intermittent gastric gavage		
	Persistent preprandial hypoglycemia		
Jejunal	Intolerance to gastric feedings	Gastrointestinal perforation	Use only Silastic feeding tubes
	Gastroesophageal reflux	Decreased fat absorption	Use formula with medium-chain triglycerides
	Delayed gastric emptying	Dumping syndrome	Avoid hyperosmolar feedings

RR, respiratory rate.

Methods of Feeding

The indications for selecting different methods of enteral feedings are presented in Table 63-4. Oral feedings are indicated for full-term infants with normal sucking, swallowing, and breathing mechanisms. Infants who are critically ill are infrequently fed by mouth. Those who are orally fed should be closely monitored for fatigue and respiratory distress. Gastric gavage is the preferred method for feeding the critically infant because it supplies nutrition at less risk, at lower cost, and in a more physiologic manner than feedings that bypass the stomach. Gastric gavage feedings are indicated for infants in whom sucking and swallowing mechanisms are inadequate as a result of prematurity, neuromuscular diseases, severe respiratory distress, endotracheal intubation, and a variety of systemic illnesses. Gastric feedings are ideally given intermittently at volumes and frequencies that vary according to the birth weight of the infant. As seen in Table 63-5, smaller infants should receive smaller volumes at higher frequencies. Intermittent feedings are considered to be more physiologic than continuous feedings because they accommodate cyclical surges in gut hormones and may increase small intestinal mass and function.[45-47] In addition, intermittent feedings are easier to administer, require minimal equipment, and have a lower risk of nutrient precipitation into the delivery system. Continuous feedings are an alternative method that may increase energy efficacy[48] and improve weight gain[14] for some infants. Continuous feedings are commonly administered to extremely premature infants because of their limited gastric size. Infants who cannot tolerate intermittent feedings because of intestinal malabsorption, severe respiratory distress, persistent preprandial hypoglycemia, and persistent gastric residuals may also benefit from continuous feedings. Transpyloric feedings are not recommended for routine use because they bypass the stomach, an important site for the initiation of fat digestion. The activity of gastric and lingual lipases is well developed at birth and is responsible for the hydrolysis of more than 30% of ingested triglycerides.[49,50] In addition, transpyloric feedings have been associated with complications such as decreased absorption of fat and potassium,[7] increased bacterial colonization of the upper gastrointestinal tract,[51] dumping syndrome,[52] and intestinal perforations from stiffened feeding tubes.[53-55] Therefore, transpyloric feedings are recommended only for patients who cannot tolerate gastric feedings because of delayed gastric emptying time, severe gastroesophageal reflux, and the use of nasal continuous positive airway pressure, which might distend the stomach.

SPECIALIZED NUTRITIONAL SUPPORT

Critically ill neonates commonly have complex medical and surgical problems that complicate normal infant feeding practices. The following sections review practical nutritional management of various conditions frequently observed in infants receiving intensive care therapy. Because there is a paucity of research concerning optimal nutrition during these conditions, it is necessary to monitor metabolic and clinical parameters and to tailor the nutritional regimen according to individual feeding tolerance.

Infants with Extremely Low Birth Weight

The nutritional goals for the infant with extremely low birth weight (ELBW) are not clearly defined. The Committee on Nutrition of the American Academy of Pediatrics[56] recommends the optimal diet for premature infants as one that supports growth rates comparable with those of the third intrauterine trimester, without imposing stress on the infants' immature metabolic and excretory functions. Postnatal growth standards are difficult to establish in extremely premature infants because of the variability in birth weight, the quality of enteral and parenteral nutritional support, and the severity of illness related to prematurity. Contemporary postnatal growth curves have been published for the longitudinal assessment of weight, length, and head circumference in extremely premature infants, taking into account their birth weight (500 to 1500 g) and the presence or absence of major morbid conditions.[12]

During the first 72 hours after birth, the ELBW infant has a very high rate of water loss (5 to 7 mL/kg/hour) as a result of excessive water evaporation, immature renal function, and expanded extracellular space.[3] Excessive water loss can rapidly result in a state of hypertonic dehydration

Table 63–5. Feeding Schedule For The Critically Ill Neonate

Birth Weight	Feeding Interval	Initial Volume	Increments
<1000 g	Continuous	1 mL/hr	0.5 mL three times/day*
1000-1250 g	Continuous	1-2.5 mL/hr	0.5-0.8 mL three times/day
	q2h	1-2.5 mL	1-3 mL every other feeding
1250-1500 g	q2-3h	1-3 mL	1-3 mL every other feeding
1500-2000 g	q3h	2-5 mL	2-5 mL every other feeding
2000-2500 g	q3h	5-10 mL	4-6 mL every other feeding
>2500 g	q3h	10-15 mL	5-10 mL every other feeding

*A 2-week period of minimal enteral feedings (10-20 kcal/kg/day) may be used before feeding advancement in sick premature infants.

characterized by hypernatremia, hyperglycemia, and hyperkalemia. Fluid management of the extremely premature infant during the first 3 days after birth should include strict monitoring of fluid intake, urine output, and serum electrolyte levels.[57] Sodium intake should be restricted and fluids administered at volumes necessary to keep serum sodium concentration below 150 mEq/L.[58,59] Lastly, measures to reduce the rate of insensible water loss should be implemented. These include the use of double-wall incubators, high humidity in ambient air, heat shields, plastic blankets, and skin coverings.

Unless contraindicated, parenteral nutrition should be initiated in ELBW infants within the first 24 to 36 hours after birth. These solutions should initially provide 1 to 1.5 g of amino acids per kilogram per day and 50 to 60 nonprotein calories per kilogram per day,[24,60,61] and they must be progressively increased to provide up to 3.5 g of amino acids per kilogram per day, along with 90 to 100 kcal/kg/day. Pediatric amino acid solutions may enhance growth, nitrogen retention, and bone mineralization in infants.[62,63] However, provision of amino acids may need to be restricted in infants with renal failure, which is indicated by elevated blood urea nitrogen and serum creatinine levels. As stated previously, the intravenous administration of dextrose solutions to ELBW infants should be carefully monitored because these infants are prone to glucose intolerance. The intravenous administration of insulin in conjunction with dextrose has been shown to improve glucose tolerance, caloric intake, and weight gain in premature infants who were glucose intolerant while receiving parenteral nutrition.[20,64,65] The administration of continuous insulin infusions, however, necessitates close monitoring of serum glucose levels and adjustments on insulin doses. The ELBW infant has limited capacity for tolerating fat emulsions, as a result of a relative deficiency in heparin-releasable lipoprotein and tissue carnitine activity.[66] Lipid emulsions are currently available at concentrations of 10% and 20%, and both supply ample amounts of essential fatty acids. The lower phospholipid-to-triglyceride ratio in the 20% emulsion enhances the serum clearance of triglycerides and other plasma lipids.[23,52] Lipid emulsions should be started at dosages of 1 to 2 g/kg/day and administered over a 24-hour period.[67] Daily increments of 0.5 to 1 g/kg/day may be provided as long as serum triglyceride levels are maintained below 250 mg/dL.[67,68] It remains controversial whether the supplementation of cysteine, glutamine, and carnitine should be routinely provided during the course of parenteral nutrition to infants with very low birth weight.[8,69-76]

Although ELBW infants are essentially dependent on parenteral nutrition for the first few weeks after birth, the administration of minimal enteral feedings has gained wide acceptance for the nutritional management of these infants. These feedings are intended to "prime" the gastrointestinal tract before the initiation of more substantial enteral nutrition. The presence of intraluminal nutrients appears to stimulate the development of the gastrointestinal mucosa, the maturation of intestinal motor activity,[77-80] and the increased secretion of regulatory peptides and hormones.[77,81-84] Trophic feedings may begin within the first few days after birth if the infant is relatively stable. Clinical findings such as the presence of bowel

sounds, a benign abdominal examination finding but not necessarily the passage of meconium,[85] and the lack of abnormalities in the abdominal radiograph may be used to assess the ELBW infant's readiness to the initiation of enteral feedings. Several controlled studies of infants born weighing less than 1500 g have uniformly documented that the administration of minimal enteral feedings at intakes varying from 2.5 to 20 mL/kg/day results in shorter time to attain full enteral nutrition and a lower incidence of feeding intolerance.[77,83,86-88] Other reported benefits of trophic feedings included lower incidence of cholestasis, lower levels of serum bilirubin and alkaline phosphatase,[86] shorter length of hospitalization,[77] increased calcium and phosphorus retention,[89] shorter intestinal transit time,[89] and improved weight gain.[19,88]

Perinatal Asphyxia

The immediate nutritional support of the asphyxiated neonate includes the administration of intravenous fluids to maintain glucose homeostasis, to correct metabolic acidosis, and to normalize serum electrolyte abnormalities. Parenteral nutrition is usually initiated on the second day after birth and maintained for several days, until enteral feedings are advanced to an amount that meets nutritional requirements and promotes growth.

The length of time that enteral feedings should be withheld in the asphyxiated infant is not clearly established. A 3- to 5-day period of bowel rest is commonly used for infants who were severely asphyxiated, with the intent of decreasing the risk of NEC. This practice is based on animal data demonstrating that intestinal ischemia and hypoxia may result in vascular congestion and hemorrhage,[90] which can be aggravated by the administration of enteral feedings.[91] Of interest is that this arbitrary period of 3 to 5 days coincides with the time necessary for regeneration of the intestinal mucosa after acute injury. Before the initiation of enteral feedings, the severely asphyxiated infant should be assessed for clinical signs that may be predictive of feeding intolerance, such as abdominal distention, the absence of bowel sounds, and failure to pass meconium. In addition, an abdominal radiograph should be obtained to evaluate the infant for signs of NEC, such as bowel wall edema and dilation, pneumatosis intestinalis, and free air.

In general, the asphyxiated infant should be fed human milk when available or infant formulas appropriate for gestational age. Infants who suffered ischemic insults that resulted in renal failure might benefit from infant formulas with reduced renal solute load (see Table 63-3).

Mildly asphyxiated infants have preserved mechanisms for sucking and swallowing and therefore may be successfully nipple fed. Infants who were severely asphyxiated and suffered neurologic depression may lose these oral reflexes either transiently or permanently and thus require tube feedings. Infants with permanent neurologic deficits from perinatal asphyxia may also exhibit signs of gastroesophageal reflux, clinically manifested by the frequent vomiting or obstructive apnea and, in more severe forms, failure to thrive and recurrent aspiration pneumonia. In addition, Berseth and McCoy reported a different pattern of intestinal motility in response to feedings in 11 asphyxiated infants.[92] The study showed that asphyxiated neonates had less migrating activity and more disorganized episodes of quiescence and clustered activity during fasting than did nonasphyxiated infants. After feeding, the intestinal motor activity started sooner in asphyxiated infants than in control infants. All asphyxiated infants studied during the first week after birth exhibited dysmotility and feeding intolerance, both of which improved by the second or third week after birth. The results of this study indicate that abnormalities in intestinal motility underlie the feeding intolerance observed in asphyxiated infants.

Gastroesophageal reflux may represent a significant clinical problem in infants who were neurologically impaired by perinatal asphyxia. The nutritional management of infants with gastroesophageal reflux may include the administration of small-volume feedings at more frequent intervals, placement of the infant in prone position with a 30-degree head elevation after feedings,[40] and the controversial practice of thickening the formula with cereals.[93-95]

Necrotizing Enterocolitis

NEC is the most common gastrointestinal surgical emergency among premature infants and occurs in 2% to 19% of infants with very low birth weight receiving intensive care.[96,97] The precise cause of NEC is controversial and likely to be multifactorial.

Parenteral nutrition plays an important role in the treatment of suspected or proven NEC because of the necessity for bowel rest. Parenteral nutrition should be instituted in all infants in whom NEC is either suspected or diagnostically proven as soon as the fluid status is well balanced and the abnormalities in serum electrolytes are corrected. Parenteral nutrition solutions should provide nutrients appropriate for age, with special consideration given to the stress of infection and surgery, which may exacerbate the losses of endogenous protein stores.[61] The infusion of dextrose solutions and fat emulsions should be carefully monitored because of the increased risk of hyperglycemia[98] and hypertriglyceridemia[99] associated with sepsis. The delivery of parenteral nutrition via peripheral vein is appropriate for infants with medically treated NEC who require short-term parenteral support, usually for periods less than 3 weeks. Parenteral nutrition should be administered by central access in virtually all infants with surgically treated NEC, because of their prolonged need for parenteral nutrition support.

In 1986, Walsh and Kliegman proposed a medical and nutritional plan for infants with NEC based on the clinical stage of the disease.[100] The first plan was for infants in whom NEC is suspected but not confirmed clinically or radiologically. For these infants, enteral feedings should be withheld for a period of 3 days; the infants rarely require a change in the type of feeding or prolonged parenteral nutrition. The second plan was for infants with proven NEC who are mildly to moderately ill. These infants should be maintained on bowel rest for a period of 7 to 10 days after the resolution of the radiographic signs of the disease. Delaying enteral nutrition much beyond this period does not appear to be advantageous from the standpoint of weight gain and feeding tolerance.[101]

Human milk or age-appropriate formula may be indicated for refeeding the majority of infants with medically treated NEC. The third plan is for infants with proven NEC who are moderately or severely ill and those who require surgical intervention. These infants should be maintained on bowel rest for a minimum of 14 days, after the resolution of radiographic signs of the disease and the normalization of the abdominal examination. Protein hydrolysate formulas may be indicated for refeeding these infants because of the potential for protein, carbohydrate, and fat malabsorption (see Table 63-3). Initial feedings may consist of small amounts of diluted formula, with cautious advancements in volume and concentration.[102] Protein hydrolysate formulas may be continued throughout this process, until enteral feedings can provide enough calories for growth. Patients who undergo significant bowel resection with resultant short-bowel syndrome may require parenteral nutrition and semi-elemental formulas for prolonged periods of time, depending on the extent and portion of the intestinal tract resected.

Feeding intolerance after NEC, as evidenced by diarrhea and macronutrient losses, is not uncommon, because of the compromised functional integrity of the gastrointestinal tract by the disease process and its treatment. The occurrence of gastric residuals, emesis, or abdominal distention during refeeding may indicate the presence of post-NEC intestinal stenosis, a condition that is confirmed radiographically. Many patients in whom this complication is diagnosed require surgical resection of the stenotic area. Other complications that may occur during refeeding include malabsorption syndrome and, in rare cases, a recurrence of NEC.

At present, there is no consensus among physicians regarding the prophylactic measures for NEC. Enteral feeding has been recognized as one of the risk factors for NEC, inasmuch as 90% to 95% of affected infants were noted to be receiving enteral feedings at the onset.[103] Although controversial, some studies indicated that the incidence of NEC was lower among premature infants fed human milk instead of infant formula[89,104] and in those whose enteral feedings were advanced at rates lower than 15 to 20 mL/kg/day.[97,105,106] However, a randomized clinical trial showed a comparable incidence of NEC in very small infants with low birth weight receiving feeding advancement of 15 versus 35 mL/kg/day.[107] This study suggests that factors other than feeding advancement play a more important role in the pathogenesis of NEC. Prospective studies suggest that the administration of minimal trophic feedings for infants with very low birth weight does not increase the risk of NEC[83,86,87] and may even play a role in its prevention.[108,109]

Preoperative and Postoperative Care

Specialized nutritional care is often required for the neonate undergoing surgery, both preoperatively and postoperatively. Nutritional assessment should be performed in all neonates, especially those undergoing elective surgery, because nutritional rehabilitation before surgery has been shown to reduce surgical morbidity and mortality.[110] At present, it is recommended that malnourished neonates receive nutritional rehabilitation before elective surgery. Although therapeutic goals for preoperative nutrition support have not been well established, it seems reasonable to aim for normalization of serum biochemical parameters, the resumption of growth, and the correction of growth deficits. Initiation of aggressive nutrition support in severely malnourished infants may result in the development of "refeeding syndrome," a condition characterized by the sudden onset of hypokalemia, hypophosphatemia, hypocalcemia, and/or hypomagnesemia. This syndrome is clinically expressed by a variety of signs, including lethargy, tremors, seizures, abdominal distention, diarrhea, coma, and death.[111] The treatment of this condition requires initial correction of the biochemical abnormalities and subsequent nutritional rehabilitation, including the slow advancement in nutrition support and the close monitoring of biochemical parameters.[111]

Parenteral nutrition should be administered to all neonates unable to receive adequate enteral nutrition postoperatively, in order to prevent excessive catabolism resulting from prolonged and inadequate nutrition support. In the same manner, infants who were malnourished before surgery may benefit from continued parenteral support until enteral feedings are well established. Parenteral nutrition solutions should contain calories to meet requirements appropriate for age (see Table 63-1). Although energy requirements are elevated in adult patients who are surgically stressed, studies have shown that the rates of energy expenditure are not elevated in neonates undergoing uncomplicated surgery.[112-114]

There are conflicting data regarding the use of dextrose versus fat emulsions as the preferred fuel substrate in the neonate undergoing surgery. In the absence of nitrogen intake, carbohydrate appears to be more effective than lipid in sparing nitrogen.[115] In the presence of nitrogen intake, however, most pertinent studies show that carbohydrate and fat have similar effects and that a balanced glucose-lipid regimen may enhance protein nutriture.[116-118]

Replacement of fluid and electrolytes is required for all infants with excessive drainage of secretions from ileostomy, gastrostomy, or colostomy tubes. Table 63-6 describes the average concentration of electrolytes in

Table 63–6. Electrolyte Content Of Body Fluids

Body Fluid	Sodium (mEq/L)	Potassium (mEq/L)	Chloride (g/dL)
Gastric	20-80	5-20	100-150
Pancreatic	120-140	5-15	40-80
Small bowel	100-140	5-15	90-130
Bile	120-140	5-15	80-120
Ileostomy	45-135	3-15	20-115
Diarrheal stools	10-90	10-80	10-110

Losses should be replaced every 6 to 8 hours. Because of wide ranges in values, specific analysis is recommended for individual patients.

Adapted from Oh W: Fluid, electrolytes and acid base homeostasis. In Fanaroff AA, Martin RJ (eds): Neonatal Perinatal Medicine. St. Louis, Mosby–Year Book, 1992, pp 527-542.

different body fluids, which can be used for the calculation of fluid replacement in these patients.

The initiation of enteral feedings to patients recovering from abdominal surgery should be withheld until paralytic ileus is resolved. Disappearance of bilious gastric secretions and a decrease in gastric aspirates indicate restoration of gastrointestinal motility and readiness for initiation of enteral feedings. The intraoperative placement of jejunal feeding tubes, which bypass the area of intestinal anastomosis, has been shown to be beneficial for the early institution of enteral feedings and for minimizing the use of parenteral nutrition during the postoperative period.[119] Despite widespread practice of diluting the concentration of initial feedings, there is no documentation that the use of diluted feedings is advantageous for refeeding the neonate who has preserved gastrointestinal function. In fact, the use of diluted formula may not be optimal for the stimulation of intestinal function in the premature infant.[80]

Mechanical Ventilation

Energy requirements during mechanical ventilation vary according to the patient's condition and the mode of ventilation. It is estimated that infants with severe respiratory distress who receive skeletal muscle relaxants have lower energy requirements than those who are breathing spontaneously and who are physically active. Infants with chronic pulmonary disease have energy requirements above maintenance levels, as a result of their increased work of breathing.[120] Failure to recognize this additional energy requirement may result in growth failure.[121]

The mechanically ventilated neonate who is parenterally nourished should receive comparable amounts of calories derived from carbohydrate and fat emulsions. Early studies showed that the administration of lipid emulsions at high infusion rates, such as 1 g/kg over 4 hours, resulted in hyperlipidemia and in a transient decrease in oxygenation.[122] These complications have been minimized by the current practice of administering lipid emulsions at lower infusion rates and longer infusion times, usually over a 24-hour period.

A significant justification for the use of fat emulsion in the ventilated patient is to reduce the glucose load received during parenteral nutrition. The oxidation of fat produces less CO_2 than the oxidation of carbohydrate for the same amount of oxygen consumed. This reduction in CO_2 production and elimination may be beneficial for patients with compromised lung function. Several studies have demonstrated that the parenteral and enteral administration of glucose loads increase the rate of CO_2 production[123] and compromise respiratory function.[124-126] More recent studies have shown that the enteral and parenteral administration of high-fat regimens to infants with chronic lung disease reduced their respiratory quotient and the rate of CO_2 production, without compromising oxygen consumption and growth.[123,127]

During mechanical ventilation, enteral feedings are routinely provided by nasogastric tube. There is considerable debate over whether the infant with respiratory failure should receive nasogastric feedings intermittently or continuously. Although intermittent feedings are considered more physiologic, several studies have shown that the use of intermittent gastric feedings may have adverse effects on respiratory pattern, pulmonary function test results, and control of breathing.[128-130]

Infants on mechanical ventilation who are treated with diuretics for prolonged periods may require additional supplements of sodium, chloride, potassium, and calcium to compensate for their increased renal losses.

REFERENCES

1. Butte NF, Garza C, O'Brian-Smith E: Human milk intake and growth in exclusively breast fed infants. J Pediatr 104:187, 1984.
2. De Benoist B, Abdulrazzak Y, Brooke OG, et al: The measurement of whole body protein turnover in the preterm infant with intragastric infusion of L-[1-13C]leucine and sampling of the urinary leucine pool. Clin Sci (Lond) 66:155, 1984.
3. Garza C, Butte NF: Energy intakes of human milk–fed infants during the first year. J Pediatr 117:S124, 1990.
4. Sparks JW: Human intrauterine growth and nutrient accretion. Semin Perinatol 8:74, 1984.
5. Ziegler EE, O'Donnell AM, Nelson SE, et al: Body composition of the reference fetus. Growth 40:329, 1976.
6. Pohlandt F: Studies on the requirement of amino acids in newborn infants receiving parenteral nutrition. In Visser HKA (ed): Nutrition and Metabolism of the Fetus and Infant. The Hague, Martinus Niijhoff, 1979, pp 341-364.
7. Roy RN, Pollnitz RP, Hamilton JR, et al: Impaired assimilation of naso-jejunal feedings in healthy low birth weight newborn infants. J Pediatr 90:431, 1977.
8. Zlotkin SH, Bryan MH, Anderson GH: Intravenous nitrogen and energy intakes required to duplicate in utero nitrogen accretion in prematurely born human infants. J Pediatr 99:115, 1981.
9. Nissim I, Yudkoff M, Pereira GR, Segal S: Effect of conceptual age and dietary protein on protein metabolism in premature infants. J Pediatr Gastroent Nutr 2:507, 1983.
10. Lucas A, Morely R, Cole TJ, et al: Early diet in preterm babies and developmental status in infancy. Arch Dis Child 64:1570, 1989.
11. Kuczmarski RJ, Ogden CL, Grummer-Strawn LM, et al: CDC Growth Charts: United States. NCHS Advance Data Report No. 314. Hyattsville, Md, U.S. Department of Health and Human Services, 2000.
12. Erenkranz RA, Younes N, Lemons JA, et al: Longitudinal growth of hospitalized very low birth weight infants. Pediatrics 104:280, 1999.
13. Heird WC, Craig LJ, Gomez MR: Practical aspects of achieving positive energy balance in low birth weight infants. J Pediatr 120:S120, 1992.
14. Toce SS, Keenan WJ, Homan SM: Enteral feeding in very-low-birth-weight infants. Am J Dis Child 141:439, 1987.
15. Cowett RM, Oh W, Pollack A, et al: Glucose disposal of low birth weight infants: Steady state hyperglycemia produced by instant glucose infusion. Pediatrics 63:389, 1979.
16. Lilien DP, Rosenfeld RL, Baccaro M, et al: Hyperglycemia in stressed small premature infants. J Pediatr 94:454, 1979.
17. Sunehag A, Gustafsson, Ewald U: Very immature infants (≤30 wk) respond to glucose infusion with incomplete suppression of glucose production. Pediatr Res 35:550, 1994.
18. Lubchenco LO, Bard H: Incidence of hypoglycemia in newborn infants classified by birth weight and gestational age. Pediatrics 47:831, 1971.

19. Tyrala EE, Chen X, Boden G: Glucose metabolism in the infant weighing less than 1100 grams. J Pediatr 125:283, 1994.
20. Collins JE, Leonard JV: Hyperinsulinism in asphyxiated and small-for-dates infants with hypoglycaemia. Lancet 2:311, 1984.
21. Kaye R, Baker E, Kunzman EE, et al: Catecholamine excretion in spontaneously occurring asymptomatic neonatal hypoglycemia. Pediatr Res 4:295, 1970.
22. Young CY, Lee VWY, Yeung CM: Glucose disappearance rates in neonatal infection. J Pediatr 82:486, 1973.
23. Heird WC, Winters RW: Total parenteral nutrition. The state of the art. J Pediatr 86:2, 1975.
24. Kashyap S: Nutritional management of the extremely-low-birth-weight infant. In Cowen RM, Hay WW Jr (eds): The Micropremie: The Next Frontier. Report of the 99th Ross Conference on Pediatric Research. Columbus, Ohio, Ross Laboratories, 1990, pp 115-119.
25. LaGamma EF, Browne LE: Feeding practices for infants weighing less than 1500 g at birth and the pathogenesis of necrotizing enterocolitis. Clin Perinatol 21:271, 1994.
26. American Academy of Pediatrics Work Group on Breast Feeding: Breast feeding and the use of human milk. Pediatrics 100:1035, 1997.
27. Tomashek KM, Nesby S, Scanlon KS, et al: Commentary: Nutritional rickets in Georgia. Pediatrics 107:e45, 2001.
28. American Academy of Pediatrics Committee on Nutrition: Commentary on breast feeding and infant formulas. Pediatrics 57:278, 1976.
29. American Academy of Pediatrics: Nutrition and oral health. In Pediatric Nutrition Handbook. Elk Grove, Ill, American Academy of Pediatrics, 1998, pp 523-529.
30. Lucas A: Enteral nutrition. In Tsang RC, Lucas A, Uauy R, Zlotkin S (eds): Nutritional Needs of the Preterm Infant: Scientific Basis and Practical Guidelines. Pawling, NY, Caduceus Medical Publishers, 1993, pp 209-223.
31. Shenai JP, Jhaveri BM, Reynolds JW, et al: Nutritional balance studies in very low birth weight infants: Role of soy formula. Pediatrics 67:631, 1981.
32. Anderson DM, Williams FH, Merkatz RB, et al: Length of gestation and nutritional composition of human milk. Am J Clin Nutr 37:810, 1983.
33. Lemons JA, Moye L, Hall D, Simmons M: Differences in the composition of preterm and term human milk during early lactation. Pediatr Res 16:113, 1982.
34. Cooper PA, Rothberg AD, Davies VA, Argent AC: Comparative growth and biochemical response of very low birthweight infants fed own mother's milk, a premature formula, or one of two standard formulas. J Pediatr Gastroenterol 4:786, 1985.
35. Kashyap S, Schultz KF, Forsyth M, et al: Growth, nutrient retention and metabolic response of low birth weight infants fed supplemented and unsupplemented human milk. Am J Clin Nutr 52:254, 1990.
36. Polberger SKT, Axelsson IE, Raiha NCR: Amino acid concentrations in plasma and urine in very low birth weight infants fed protein-unenriched or human milk protein–enriched human milk. Pediatrics 86:909, 1990.
37. Rowe J, Rowe D, Horak E, et al: Hypophosphatemia and hypercalciuria in small premature infants fed human milk: Evidence for inadequate dietary phosphorus. J Pediatr 104:112, 1984.
38. Bhatia J, Rassin DK: Human milk supplementation. Am J Dis Child 142:445, 1988.
39. Greer FR, McCormick A: Improved bone mineralization and growth in premature infants fed fortified own mother's milk. J Pediatr 112:961, 1988.

40. Moro GE, Minoli I, Fulconis F, et al: Growth and metabolic response in low birth weight infants fed human milk fortified with human milk protein or with a bovine milk protein preparation. J Pediatr Gastroenterol Nutr 13:150, 1991.

41. Bishop NJ, King FJ, Lucas A: Increased bone mineral content of preterm infants fed a nutrient enriched formula after discharge from hospital. Arch Dis Child 68:573, 1993.

42. Carver JD, Wu PYK, Hall RT, et al: Growth of preterm infants fed nutrient-enriched or term formula after discharge. Pediatrics 107:683, 2001.

43. Cooke RJ, McCormick K, Griffin IJ, et al: Feeding preterm infants after hospital discharge: Effect of diet on body composition. Pediatr Res 46:461, 1999.

44. Lucas A, Bishop NJ, King FJ, et al: Randomized trial of nutrition for preterm infants after discharge. Arch Dis Child 67:324,1992.

45. Aynsley-Green A, Adrian TE, Bloom SR: Feeding and the development of enteroinsular hormone secretion in the preterm infant: Effects of continuous gastric infusions of human milk compared with intermittent boluses. Acta Pediatr Scand 71:379, 1982.

46. Aynsley-Green A, Lucas A, Lawson GR, Bloon SR: Gut hormones and regulatory peptides in relation to enteral feeding, gastroenteritis, and necrotizing enterocolitis in infancy. J Pediatr 117(Suppl 1):24, 1990.

47. Shulman D, Kanarek K: Gastrin, motilin, and insulin-like growth factor-I concentrations in very low birth weight infants receiving enteral or parenteral nutrition. JPEN J Parenter Enteral Nutr 17:130, 1993.

48. Grant J, Deene SC: Effect of intermittent versus continuous enteral feeding on energy expenditure in premature infants. J Pediatr 118:928, 1991.

49. De Nigris SJ, Hamosh M, Kaskebar DK, et al: Human gastric lipase: Secretion from dispersed gastric glands. Biochim Biophys Acta 836:67, 1985.

50. Hamosh M: Fat digestion in the newborn. The role of lingual lipase and preduodenal digestion. Pediatr Res 13:615, 1979.

51. Challacombe D: Bacterial microflora in infants receiving naso-jejunal tube feeding. J Pediatr 85:113, 1974.

52. Heird WC: Nasojejunal feeding. A commentary. J Pediatr 85:111, 1974.

53. Boros SJ, Reynolds JW: Duodenal perforation: A complication of neonatal naso-jejunal feeding. J Pediatr 85:107, 1974.

54. Chen JW, Wong PWK: Intestinal complications of naso-jejunal feeding in low birth weight infants. J Pediatr 85:109, 1975.

55. Pereira GR, Herold R, Ziegler M, et al: Sustained flexibility of infant feeding tubes containing nonmigrating plasticizers. JPEN J Parenter Enteral Nutr 6:64, 1982.

56. American Academy of Pediatrics Committee on Nutrition: Nutritional needs of low-birth-weight infants. Pediatrics 75:976, 1985.

57. Shaffer SG, Weismann DN: Fluid requirements in the preterm infant. Clin Perinatol 19:233, 1992.

58. Costarino AT, Baumgart S: Modern fluid and electrolyte management of the critically ill premature infant. Pediatr Clin North Am 33:153, 1986.

59. Costarino AT, Gruskay JA, Corcoran L, et al: Sodium restriction versus daily maintenance replacement in very low birth weight premature neonates: A randomized, blind therapeutic trial. J Pediatr 120:99, 1992.

60. Anderson TL, Muttart CR, Bieber MA, et al: A controlled trial of glucose versus glucose and amino acids in preterm infants. J Pediatr 94:947, 1979.

61. Heird WC, Gomez MR: Total parenteral nutrition in necrotizing enterocolitis. Clin Perinatol 21:389, 1994.

62. Fitzgerald KA, MacKay MW: Calcium and phosphate solubility in neonatal parenteral nutrient solutions containing Aminosyn PF. Am J Hosp Pharm 44:1396, 1987.

63. Fomon SJ: Protein requirements of term infants. In Fomon SJ, Heird WC (eds): Energy and Protein Needs during Infancy. New York, Harcourt Brace Jovanovitch, 1986, pp 55-68.

64. Binder ND, Raschko PK, Benda GI, Reynolds JW: Insulin infusion with parenteral nutrition in extremely low birthweight infants with hyperglycemia. J Pediatr 114:223, 1989.

65. Collins JW, Hoppe M, Brown K, et al: A controlled trial of insulin infusion and parenteral nutrition in extremely low birth weight infants with glucose intolerance. J Pediatr 118:921, 1991.

66. Rovamo LM, Nikkila EA, Raivio KO: Lipoprotein lipase, hepatic lipase, and carnitine in premature infants. Arch Dis Child 63:140, 1988.

67. Brans YW, Andrew DS, Carrillo DW, et al: Tolerance of fat emulsions in very low birth weight neonates. Am J Dis Child 142:145, 1988.

68. Wells DH, Ferlauto JJ, Forbes DJ, et al: Lipid tolerance in the very low birth weight infant on intravenous and enteral feedings. JPEN J Parenter Enteral Nutr 13:623, 1989.

69. Heird WC, Hay W, Helms RA, et al: Pediatric parenteral amino acid mixture in low birth weight infants. Pediatrics 81:41, 1988.

70. Helms RA, Mauer EC, Hay WW, et al: Effect of intravenous L-carnitine on growth parameters and fat metabolism during parenteral nutrition in neonates. JPEN J Parenter Enteral Nutr 14:448, 1990.

71. Kashyap S, Abildskov K, Heird WC: Cysteine supplementation of very low birth weight infants receiving parenteral nutrition. Pediatr Res 31:290A, 1992.

72. Lacey JM, Crouch JB, Benfell K, et al: The effects of glutamine-supplemented parenteral nutrition in premature infants. JPEN J Parenter Enteral Nutr 20:74, 1996.

73. Malloy MH, Rassin DK, Richardson CJ: Total parental nutrition in sick preterm infants: Effects of cysteine supplementation with nitrogen intakes of 240 and 400 mg/kg/day. J Pediatr Gastroenterol Nutr 3:239, 1984.

74. Neu J, Roig JC, Meetze WH, et al: Enteral glutamine supplementation for very low birth weight infants decreases morbidity. J Pediatr 131:691, 1997.

75. Roig JC, Meetze WH, Auestad N, et al: Enteral glutamine supplementation for the very low birthweight infant: Plasma amino acid concentrations. J Nutr 126:1115S, 1996.

76. Schmidt GL, Baumgartner TG, Fischlschweiger W, et al: Cost containment using cysteine HCL acidification to increase calcium/phosphate solubility in hyperalimentation solutions. JPEN J Parenter Enteral Nutr 10:203, 1986.

77. Berseth CL: Effect of early feeding on maturation of preterm infant's small intestine. J Pediatr 120:947, 1992.

78. Berseth CL: Neonatal small intestinal motility: Motor responses to feeding in term and preterm infants. J Pediatr 117:777, 1990.

79. Bissett WM, Watt J, Rivers RPA, Milla PJ: Postprandial motor response of the small intestine to enteral feeds in preterm infants. Arch Dis Child 64:1356,1989.

80. Koenig WJ, Amarnath RP, Hench V, Berseth CL: Manometrics for preterm and term infants: A new tool for old questions. Pediatrics 95:203, 1995.

81. Gounaris A, Anatolitou F, Costalos C, Konstantellou E: Minimal enteral feeding, nasojejunal feeding and gastrin levels in premature infants. Acta Paediatr Scand 79:226, 1990.

82. Lucas A, Bloom SR, Ansley-Green A: Gut hormones and minimal enteral feeding. Acta Paediatr Scand 75:719, 1986.

83. Meetz W, Valentine C, McGuigan JE, et al: Gastrointestinal priming prior to full enteral nutrition in very low birth weight infants. J Pediatr Gastroenterol Nutr 15:163, 1992.

84. Shulman RJ, Redel CA, Stathos TH: Bolus versus continuous feedings stimulate small-intestinal growth and development in the newborn pig. J Pediatr Gastroenterol Nutr 18:350, 1994.

85. Verma A, Dhanireddy R: Time of first stool in extremely low birth weight infants. J Pediatr 122:626, 1993.

86. Dunn L, Hulman S, Weiner J, Kliegman R: Beneficial effects of early enteral feeding on neonatal gastrointestinal function: Preliminary report of a randomized trial. J Pediatr 112:622, 1988.

87. Slagle TA, Gross SJ: Effect of early low-volume enteral substrate on subsequent feeding tolerance in very low birth-weight infants. J Pediatr 113:526, 1988.

88. Troche B, Harvey-Wilkes K, Engle WD, et al: Early minimal feedings promote growth in critically ill premature infants. Biol Neonate 67:172, 1995.

89. Schandler R, Shulman RJ, Lau C, et al: Randomized trial of gastrointestinal priming and tube feeding method. Pediatrics 103:434, 1999.

90. Harrison MV, Connel RS, Campbell JR, et al: Microcirculatory changes in the gastrointestinal tract of the hypoxic puppy: An electron microscope study. J Pediatr Surg 10:599, 1975.

91. Barlow B, Santulli TV, Heird WC, et al: An experimental study of acute neonatal enterocolitis: The importance of breast milk. J Pediatr Surg 9:587, 1974.

92. Berseth CL, McCoy HH: Birth asphyxia alters neonatal intestinal motility in term neonates. Pediatrics 90:669, 1992.

93. Bailey DJ, Andres JM, Danek GD, et al: Lack of efficacy of thickened feeding as treatment for gastroesophageal reflux. J Pediatr 110:187, 1987.

94. Orenstein SR, Magill HL, Brooks P: Thickening of infant feedings for therapy of gastroesophageal reflux. J Pediatr 110:181, 1987.

95. Orenstein SR, Shalaby TM, Putnam PE: Thickened feedings as a cause of increased coughing when used as therapy for gastroesophageal reflux in infants. J Pediatr 121:913, 1992.

96. Uauy R, Fanaroff AA, Korones SB, et al: Necrotizing enterocolitis in very low birth weight infants: Biodemographic and clinical correlates. J Pediatr 119:630, 1991.

97. Wright LL, Uauy RD, Younes N, et al: Rapid advances in feeding increase the risk of necrotizing enterocolitis in very low birthweight infants. Pediatr Res 33:313(A), 1993.

98. James T III, Blesa M, Boggs TR Jr: Recurrent hyperglycemia associated with sepsis in a neonate. Am J Dis Child 133:645, 1979.

99. Park W, Paust H, Schroder H: Lipid infusion in premature infants suffering from sepsis. JPEN J Parenter Enteral Nutr 8:290, 1984.

100. Walsh MC, Kliegman RM: Necrotizing enterocolitis: Treatment based on staging criteria. Pediatr Clin North Am 33:179, 1986.

101. Roig JC, Parker IA, Neu J: Early vs. late resumption of enteral feeds in infants recovering from necrotizing enterocolitis. Pediatr Res 33:309(A), 1993.

102. Thureen PJ, Hay WW: Conditions requiring special nutritional management. In Tsang RC, Lucas A, Uauy R, Zlotkin S (eds): Nutritional Needs of the Preterm Infant: Scientific Basis and Practical Guidelines, Pawling, NY, Caduceus Medical Publishers, 1993, pp 243-266.

103. Kliegman RM, Fanaroff AA: Necrotizing enterocolitis. N Engl J Med 310:1093, 1984.

104. Lucas A, Cole TJ: Breastmilk and neonatal necrotizing enterocolitis. Lancet 336:1519, 1990.

105. Anderson D, Kliegman R: The relationship of neonatal alimentation practices to the occurrence of endemic necrotizing enterocolitis. Am J Perinatol 8:62, 1991.

106. McKeown RE, Marsh TD, Amarnath U, et al: Role of delayed feeding and of feeding increments in necrotizing enterocolitis. J Pediatr 121:764, 1992.

107. Rayyis SF, Ambalavanan N, Wright L, Carlo WA: Randomized trial of slow vs. fast feed advancement on the incidence of NEC in VLBW infants. J Pediatr 134:293, 1999.

108. LaGamma EF, Ostertag SG, Birenbaum H: Failure of delayed oral feedings to prevent necrotizing enterocolitis. Am J Dis Child 139:385, 1985.

109. Ostertag SG, LaGamma EF, Reisen CE, Ferrentino FL: Early enteral feeding does not affect the incidence of necrotizing enterocolitis. Pediatrics 77:275, 1986.

110. Mullen JL, Buzby GP, Mathews DG, et al: Reduction in operative morbidity and mortality by combined preoperative and postoperative nutritional support. Ann Surg 192:604, 1980.

111. Solomon SM, Kirby DF: The refeeding syndrome: A review. JPEN J Parenter Enteral Nutr 14:90, 1990.

112. Jones MO, Pierro A, Hammond P, Lloyd DA: The metabolic response to operative stress in infants. J Pediatr Surg 28:1258, 1993.

113. Shanbhogue RL, Jackson M, Lloyd DA: Operation does not increase resting energy expenditure in the neonate. J Pediatr Surg 26:578, 1991.

114. Shanbhogue RLK, Lloyd DA: Absence of hypermetabolism after operation in the newborn infant. JPEN J Parenter Enteral Nutr 16:333, 1992.

115. Munro HN: General aspects of the regulation of protein metabolism by diet and hormones. In Munro HN, Allison JB (eds): Mammalian Protein Metabolism. New York, Academic Press, 1964, pp 381-481.

116. Bresson JL, Bader B, Rocchiccioli F, et al: Protein metabolism kinetics and energy substrate utilization in infants fed parenteral solutions with different glucose-fat ratios. Am J Clin Nutr 54:370, 1991.

117. Bresson JL, Narcy P, Putet G, et al: Energy substrate utilization in infants receiving total parenteral nutrition with different glucose to fat ratios. Pediatr Res 25:645, 1989.

118. Pineault M, Chessex P, Biaillon S, et al: Total parenteral nutrition in the newborn: Impact of quality of infused energy and on nitrogen metabolism. Am J Clin Nutr 47:298, 1988.

119. Andrassy RJ, Page CP, Feldtman RW, et al: Continued catheter administration of an elemental diet in infants and children. Surgery 82:205, 1977.

120. Yeh TF, McClenan DA, Ajayi OA, et al: Metabolic rate and energy balance in infants with bronchopulmonary dysplasia. J Pediatr 114:448, 1989.

121. Kuzner SI, Garg M, Bautista DB, et al: Growth failure in bronchopulmonary dysplasia: Elevated metabolic rates and pulmonary mechanics. J Pediatr 112:73, 1988.

122. Pereira GR, Fox WW, Stanley CA, et al: Decreased oxygenation and hyperlipemia during intravenous fat infusions in premature infants. Pediatrics 66:26, 1980.

123. Piedboeuf B, Chessex P, Hazan J, et al: Total parenteral nutrition in the newborn infant: Energy substrates and respiratory gas exchange. J Pediatr 118:97, 1991.

124. Covelli HD, Black JW, Olsen MS, et al: Respiratory failure precipitated by high carbohydrate loads. Ann Intern Med 95:579, 1981.

125. Yunis RA, Oh W: Effects of intravenous glucose loading on oxygen consumption, carbon dioxide production and resting

energy expenditure in infants with bronchopulmonary dysplasia. J Pediatr 115:127, 1989.

126. Zucker AH: Effect of glucose load on CO_2 production and respiratory quotient in the neonate. Pulm Res 1:1, 1987.

127. Pereira GR, Baumgart S, Bennet MJ, et al: High fat formula for premature infants with bronchopulmonary dysplasia. J Pediatr 124:605, 1994.

128. Blondheim O, Abassi S, Fox WW, et al: Effect of enteral gavage feeding rate on pulmonary function of very low birthweight infants. J Pediatr 122:751, 1993.

129. Patel BD, Dinwiddie R, Kumar SP, et al: The effects of feedings on arterial blood gases and lung mechanics in newborn infants recovering from respiratory distress. J Pediatr 90:435, 1977.

130. Pitcher-Wilmott R, Shutack JG, Fox WW: Decreased lung volume after nasogastric feeding of neonates recovering from respiratory disease. J Pediatr 95:119, 1979.

CHAPTER 64

Intravenous Alimentation

Michael L. Spear and Mae M. Coleman

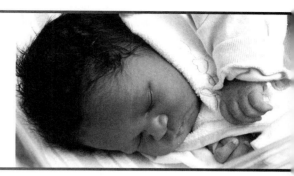

The administration of intravenous alimentation (parenteral nutrition) to the neonate has become part of routine management. Since the 1960s, various components of parenteral nutrition have been modified to accommodate the growth needs of more premature infants. During the period since the mid-1980s, there has been more precision in dosing of the three main components of this form of nutrition: protein, carbohydrate, and fat. Each of these nutrients is supplied to approximate the fetal requirements. In this chapter, the nutrient delivery of the fetus is reviewed and compared with what can be achieved in the neonate. Delivery of trace elements and electrolytes in parenteral nutrition is also described, as are clinical considerations during parenteral nutrition use. It is evident that there are inherent difficulties in duplicating the fetal nutrient milieu to provide optimal parenteral nutrition in premature and critically ill newborns.

PROTEIN

Intrauterine Protein Balance

Protein studies of intrauterine nutrition have the inherent limitation of inability to use a human model. However, several investigators have used indirect measurements of fetal growth by examining fetuses of different gestational ages. From 24 to 37 weeks, the fetal weight increases by approximately 1.5% per day. This rate of growth plateaus from 37 to 42 weeks, and in the postmature fetus, there may actually be a decrease in weight from 42 to 44 weeks until delivery. In addition, there is a direct relationship between fetal nitrogen content and body weight.[1] As fetuses grow, this relationship becomes exponential: larger fetuses grow at faster rates than do smaller fetuses, and protein accretion also increases.[2] The average growth rate for the human fetus during the entire gestation period is approximately 15 g/kg/day, 12% of nonfat dry weight being protein.[3]

The most frequently used animal models are the sheep and guinea pig.[4-15] In these models, 80% of nitrogen content is found in protein. The rest is accounted for by urea,

ammonia, and free amino acids. This distribution becomes important in protein turnover studies, because estimates of total body protein turnover need to take this distribution into consideration.

The placenta is extensively involved in intrauterine nutrition. Several functions of the placenta provide amino acids to the developing fetus. There is an energy-dependent active transport system that moves amino acids from mother to fetus against a concentration gradient. The placenta is also involved in amino acid metabolism, consumption, and processing. Investigators have used umbilical-uterine arteriovenous differences in amino acid concentrations to determine these aspects of placental function. Holzman and colleagues demonstrated that placental consumption is small in relation to the amount of amino acids delivered to the growing fetus. They speculated that because their studies were done near term, the needs of the placenta were probably greater in earlier gestation.[16] Lemons estimated that placental growth during gestation would require 66 g of protein.[17] To facilitate transport of amino acids across the placenta, three major carrier systems have been described: the alanine-serine-cysteine system, which is responsible for transport of many of the essential amino acids; a sodium-dependent system; and the L-system.[18,19]

Several factors affect placental transport. Changes in uterine-umbilical blood flow always influence the degree of amino acid transfer. Alterations in carrier affinity, availability, and competition for carriers among substrates are also important. Diffusion leaks, either into or out of cells and by paracellular pathways, also affect protein delivery to the fetus. If amino acid intracellular concentrations are altered, transport systems are also affected by disruption of the gradients. In addition, amino acid transport is impaired in cases of maternal amino acid deprivation. If the placental metabolism is altered, the quality and quantity of amino acids delivered to the fetus also change. In maternal conditions of decreased amino acid supply, fetal amino acid transport is not compromised until states of maternal deprivation become severe. Cetin and coworkers showed that α-amino nitrogen is lower in both maternal and fetal plasma of growth-restricted infants.[20] Acetylcholine and insulin have also been shown to potentially play roles in the regulation of placental transport on amino acids.[21,22]

In the fetus, only the sheep has served as an experimental model for investigations of amino acid uptake. Lemons and colleagues showed that net uptake of amino acids is 5.3/kg/day in fetal weight of carbon and 1.6 g/kg/day of nitrogen, with total fetal umbilical nitrogen uptake of 0.9 g/kg/day.[23] It is important to realize that the investigations of fetal amino acid uptake must take into account urea excretion, which can be as high as 20% of nitrogen excretion. Furthermore, the fetus and placenta function together in amino acid cycling. The placenta produces ammonia, which circulates through both maternal and fetal circulations.[4] Metabolic pathways in the fetus account for much of the ammonia degradation. Interorgan cycling of glycine and serine occurs between the fetal liver and placenta.[24] By midgestation, fetal amino acid uptake via the umbilical circulation is comparable to requirements estimated from nitrogen accretion and urea excretion data.[6] Leucine oxidation at midgestation is already equal to rates observed in full-term sheep. This observation indicates that amino acids are used for oxidative metabolism during at least the last half of gestation.[25]

When examining rates of protein synthesis and turnover, synthesis must exceed breakdown for the fetus to grow. Accretion has been measured in fetuses by whole carcass protein analysis at different gestational ages. Stable isotope tracers have been used to calculate protein synthesis rates.[26] Synthetic rates are higher from early gestation to midgestation because of greater organ growth in early gestation.

Ten amino acids are essential for the human fetus, requiring synthesis from glycolytic products and nonessential amino acids: methionine, cysteine, histidine, isoleucine, leucine, valine, phenylalanine, threonine, tryptophan, and lysine. Infants with low birth weight, unlike the older infant and child, may also require cysteine, tyrosine and glutamine. Such infants have low levels of hepatic cystathionase activity, which converts methionine to cysteine. Whether there is enough cystathionase in extrahepatic tissues of the fetus and the preterm infant to make cysteine if enough methionine is provided is still under debate.

Cysteine is usually absent or present in small amounts in parenteral nutrition, because of its low solubility. A few investigators have studied supplementation of parenteral nutrition with acetylated forms of cysteine, because acetylation improves stability and solubility of amino acids.[27] Although supplementation of cysteine has been shown to increase plasma and urine concentrations, it does not appear to increase nitrogen retention.[28,29]

The reason for tyrosine supplementation is also not as clear, because hepatic activity of phenylalanine hydroxylase, which converts phenylalanine to tyrosine, is present in gestation starting at week 12. Tyrosine is usually present only in small amounts in currently available parenteral amino acid solutions because of its low solubility. Among available amino acid solutions, TrophAmine contains the highest concentrations of tyrosine.[30]

One particular amino acid component, glutamine, is of considerable interest. Glutamine is a primary fuel for rapidly dividing cells. It plays a role in maturation of the gastrointestinal tract and in the development and function of the immune system.[31,32] Pathways of glutamine de novo synthesis and glutamine utilization in the splanchnic bed are functional in infants with very low birth weights by the 10th day after birth.[33] Traditionally, glutamine has not been supplemented into total parenteral nutrition (TPN) solutions because of concern over its instability in aqueous solution, although other investigators have refuted this issue.[34] Lacey and associates studied TPN glutamine supplementation at levels 15% to 25% weight per volume of amino acid mixture. Supplemented infants had higher plasma glutamine levels, fewer TPN days, less time to full enteral feeds, and less time on mechanical ventilation. To test safety of the supplementation, serum ammonia, blood urea nitrogen, and glutamate levels were measured in the study groups. The levels of all three tended to be higher in the supplemented group, but were well within normal limits.[31] Glutamine supplementation may benefit growing premature infants. The remainder of the essential amino acids is routinely provided in protein solutions for parenteral nutrition.

The amino acid requirements for late gestation in sheep are 0.4 g/kg/day for urea nitrogen excretion, with nitrogen accumulation of 0.6 g/kg/day. The umbilical amino acid uptake is approximately 1.6 g/kg/day, and nitrogen uptake is 1.0 g/kg/day. Therefore, there is sufficient fuel for a positive nitrogen balance.[23,35] Further research is necessary to determine optimal amino acid requirements of neonates in a variety of clinical states and to create more complete parenteral solutions.[36]

Neonatal Protein Requirements in Parenteral Nutrition

The models for both enteral and parenteral nutrition are based not only on fetal requirements but also on attempts to duplicate the amino acid profile in human milk, the "gold standard" of nutrition. Table 64-1 shows the amino acid composition of parenteral amino acid solutions for a neonate receiving 2.5 g/kg/day of total amino acids.

Table 64-2 outlines the amino acid requirements for the neonate, based on more recent day 1 fetal rates of amino acid accretion. If the retention rate is 70%, 2.2 g/kg/day is sufficient for growth.[14]

Using the normal profile of amino acids in healthy full-term infants as an alternative method for estimating requirements, 2.8 g/kg/day of bovine protein has been stated to be the minimal requirement for premature infants.[37] Protein requirements of 2.2 g/kg/day for the infant with low birth weight are approximately 20% less than the requirement for maintenance of intrauterine growth. This difference arises from the way nitrogen retention is calculated, which yields a result of 240 mg/kg/day, or 20% less than the standard 300 mg/kg/day.

In the neonate, several factors affect protein utilization. Stress has been shown to increase requirements.[14,38] In a study of postoperative surgical neonates, Duffy and Pencharz demonstrated less protein breakdown with an increased intake of protein of 3.0 g/kg/day. Rates of whole body amino acid synthesis are higher as well.[39] Boehm and coworkers found that among infants with low birth weight, bacterial sepsis doubled the urinary nitrogen excretion, in comparison with infants with respiratory

Table 64–1. Amino Acid Composition of Parenteral Amino Acid Solutions (1 mg/2.5 g Amino Acid)*

Amino acid	Intravenous Alimentation Solutions	
	Trophamine*	Aminosyn-PF†
Isoleucine	195	191
Leucine	333	297
Lysine	195	170
Methionine	81	45
Phenylalanine	114	107
Threonine	100	129
Tryptophan	48	45
Valine	185	161
Alanine	128	175
Arginine	290	307
Aspartic acid	76	132
Glutamic acid	119	206
Glycine	86	96
Histidine	114	79
Proline	162	203
Serine	90	124
Taurine	6	18
Tyrosine	17 + 40	16
Cysteine	100	68

*Kendall McGaw Laboratories, Irvine, California.

†Abbott Laboratories, Montreal, Quebec.

Table 64–2. Amino Acid Requirements (mg/kg/day) of the Infant with Low Birth Weight as Predicted from Fetal Rates of Amino Acid Accretion

Amino acid	Accretion rate (0.9-2.4 kg)	Estimated Requirement
Isoleucine	52	74
Leucine	113	161
Lysine	108	154
Methionine	30	43
Cysteine	—	—
Phenylalanine	62	89
Tyrosine	44	63
Threonine	62	89
Tryptophan	—	—
Valine	71	101
Histidine	39	56
Arginine	115	164
Alanine	109	156
Aspartate	136	194
Glutamate	196	280
Glycine	178	254
Proline	127	181
Serine	66	94
Total nitrogen	242	346

distress syndrome and healthy controls in the first week after birth. With no nitrogen intake, urinary nitrogen excretion was 150 to 200 mg/kg/day.[8] (See also the later section, "Parenteral Nutrition, Illness, and Stress.")

In supplemented parenteral nutrition with amino acids, Zlotkin and associates found that the minimum protein intake for parenteral nutrition to replicate the intrauterine rate of nitrogen accretion was 2.7 to 3.5 g/kg/day when total energy was greater than 70 kcal/kg/day.[40] VanLingen and colleagues, using stable isotope tracer infusions (^{15}N-glycine), demonstrated improved protein synthesis in premature infants receiving 2.3 g/kg/day of parenteral protein, along with glucose and fat on day 2, in comparison with infants receiving only glucose and fat.[41] In premature infants with respiratory distress syndrome, higher amino acid concentrations were obtained with amino acid–supplemented parenteral nutrition, in comparison with parenteral nutrition without amino acids.[19,40,42,43] Thureen and coworkers performed 1-^{13}C-leucine tracer kinetic studies on infants to determine the factors affecting protein balance in ventilated, parenterally fed premature newborns during the first week after birth. Amino acid intake was the only predictor associated independently with protein balance. Provision of protein to infants should not be delayed, because even ill neonates can achieve positive protein balance in the first week after birth.[43-45] With no amino acid intake, loss of endogenous protein of 0.5 to 1.0 g/kg/day can also lead to significant growth delay.[46]

It is of interest that the first feeds for premature infants in the 1940s contained protein concentrations as high as 6 g/kg/day.[47] Davidson and associates compared 4 to 6 g/kg/day and found that weight gain was just as consistent with the formula containing less protein.[48]

CARBOHYDRATE

Intrauterine Carbohydrate Balance

The predominant sources of immediate energy in the developing fetus are glucose and the use of oxidative pathways. In most studies, a direct relationship between maternal and fetal glucose levels is demonstrable.[49] The factors that determine the rate of transfer of glucose from the maternal to fetal circulation are maternal glucose concentration, the gradient for glucose across the placenta, fetal insulin and glucagon secretion, and the placental consumption of glucose.[50] In sheep, a placental carrier for glucose has been identified. At maternal levels of glucose between 180 and 200 mg/dL, this carrier becomes saturated.[51]

By term, the net umbilical uptake of the fetus is 4 to 7 mg of glucose per kilogram per minute, which is 6 to 10 g of glucose per kilogram per day. This level alone does not provide sufficient calories for the total needs of the developing fetus.[52] In fact, 80% of the fetal glucose uptake can be accounted for by brain and striated muscle.[9] Glucose is then stored as glycogen, predominantly in liver, skeletal, and cardiac muscle. Fetal liver glycogen synthesis is regulated by fetal insulin and the fetal pituitary-hypothalamic-adrenal axis. There is net glycogen accumulation in the fetal liver, with active turnover.

The breakdown of this glycogen serves as the major source of glucose for the developing fetus. The fetus is unable to carry out gluconeogenesis. Data have demonstrated that the rate-limiting enzyme of gluconeogenesis, phosphoenolpyruvate carboxykinase in a cytosolic form, is either deficient or at very low levels in the fetal lamb. Only in states of severe maternal fasting (>7 days in the sheep) has fetal glucose production been shown to be stimulated.[53] In preparation for birth, large amounts of glycogen are deposited. The conditions of decreased β cell regulation of insulin secretion, high insulin receptor density, and relative glycogen resistance in utero lead to glycogen deposition.[2,54,55]

Neonatal Glucose Requirements in Parenteral Nutrition

At birth, plasma glucose decreases, from 80 to 105 mg/dL to 40 to 60 mg/dL at 2 to 4 hours of age, and somewhat lower in infants who are small for gestational age and in preterm infants. Glucose is then released through hepatic glycogenolysis and stimulation of gluconeogenesis via catecholamine secretion; secretion of catecholamines rises sharply shortly after birth. Umbilical cord clamping appears to lead to an increase in glucagon, which also facilitates glucose mobilization.

Sunehag and associates demonstrated a capacity for glucose production even on day 1 after birth in premature infants younger than 28 weeks of gestational age. This production was equivalent to or higher than that reported in full-term infants.[56] They noted that other investigators demonstrated that exogenous glucose administration might suppress endogenous glucose production.[57-62]

After birth, until the infant can begin mobilizing glycogen stores and producing glucose, intravenous exogenous glucose may be needed, particularly in the premature infant or in the full-term infant who is either severely hypoglycemic or otherwise unable to begin enteral feedings. Intravenous regulation of glucose homeostasis can be achieved by therapy with 2 to 4 mg of glucose per kilogram, followed by an infusion at a rate of approximately 6 to 8 mg/kg/minute.[63] In specific instances, the glucose infusion requirements are found to be higher, as in the infant who is small for gestational age and has decreased glycogen stores or in the infant of a diabetic mother (such infants are relatively hyperinsulinemic). As the hyperinsulinemia in infants of diabetic mothers abates, glucose intake approaches more normal levels.

The glucose concentration that can be infused depends on the site of the infusion. If the venous access is in the superior vena cava or right atrium, a concentration greater than 12.5% can be used. If a peripheral site is used, 12.5% is the current maximum recommended concentration. Glucose solutions less than 2.5% are not recommended because of their extremely low osmolarity.[64] Glucose, the primary energy substrate for the neonatal brain, is generally required in higher doses for neonates than for older infants and children because of neonates' higher brain-to-body weight ratio in comparison to older infants and children.[65] Thus, most neonates weighing more than 1000 g tolerate a continuous 10% glucose solution. However, in some infants with extremely low birth weight (<1000 g), even low rates of infused glucose (5% glucose solution) are not tolerated, with resultant hyperglycemia and glycosuria. Glucose homeostasis is a complex process under the control of neural, hormonal, and endocrine pathways. Premature infants and those with low birth weight are at high risk of suffering from altered glucose metabolism and its consequences.[66]

Binder and coworkers[7] and Collins and Hoppe,[67] in separate investigations, have demonstrated that low-dose insulin infusions (0.04 to 0.1 U/kg/hour) allow glucose infusions to be administered. The hyperglycemia was corrected, and greater amounts of glucose infusions were tolerated. In the investigation by Collins and Hoppe, the insulin-treated group had greater weight gain than the untreated controls.[67] Although insulin infusion allows for increased glucose delivery while controlling hyperglycemia, insulin in infants with extremely low birth weight has been linked to increased lactate and development of metabolic acidosis. Little is known about insulin's effects on the quality of weight gain.[68]

FAT

Intrauterine Fat Balance

During pregnancy, fat accumulation occurs in the mother, to provide fat for the fetus. The increase in fat stores is from increased appetite, increased lipogenesis, and increased lipoprotein lipase activity. Between 26 and 30 weeks of pregnancy, the fat accretion rate is approximately 1.8 g/kg/day.[24,69,70] After 30 weeks, the fat accretion increases to as much as 90% of total caloric intake by term. The rate of fat accretion at term is from 1.6 to 3.4 g/kg/day.[24] Later in pregnancy, the maternal circulating triglyceride level increases. There are several reasons for this increase: decreased adipose tissue lipoprotein lipase, without a concomitant change in skeletal muscle activity; increased hepatic production of triglycerides; and improved intestinal absorption of lipids. Thus, increased fat accretion occurs at a time when it is most needed. Simple diffusion is the major mechanism by which placental transfer of lipids to the fetus occurs. Because of their water solubility, maternal fatty acids and unmodified lipoproteins are the sources available to cross the placenta. The former are hydrolyzed, and the latter are bound to proteins. Through the use of ^{14}C-palmitate, another type of free fatty acid transport involving esterification and hydrolysis has been demonstrated.[70] Within the placenta, lipoprotein lipase and phospholipase participate in maternal-fetal fatty acid transport. Although glucose is the major fuel under normal fetal conditions, fat utilization greatly increases during conditions of stress to the fetus.

Neonatal Fat Requirements in Parenteral Nutrition

Because myelination begins during the perinatal period and continues to increase dramatically during the first year after birth, exogenous fat intake for the critically ill premature infant is of paramount importance. Lipids are also involved in neuronal and glial membranes, both structurally and functionally. The main component of the myelin sheath is cerebroside. Brain lipids are predominantly cholesterol, phospholipids, cerebrosides, sulfatides, and gangliosides.[24]

Table 64–3. Composition of Intravenous Fat Emulsions

| Component | Soybean Oil | | Safflower Oil |
	Intralipid	Travamulsion	Liposyn
Fatty acid content			
Palmitic acid C16:0	9%	11%	7%
Stearic acid C18:0	3%	3%	2.5%
Oleic acid C18:1w9	26%	23%	13%
Linoleic acid C18:2w6	54%	56%	77%
Linoleic acid C18:3w3	8%	6%	0.5%
Egg yolk phospholipids (lecithin)	1.2%	1.2%	1.2%
Glycerol	2.25%	2.25%	2.5%
kcal/mL	1.1	1.1	1.1
Osmolarity (mOsm/L)	280	280	300
Fat particle size (µ)	0.5	0.4	0.4

Because the rate of survival of infants with low birth weight has improved dramatically since 1990, parenteral nutrition, with particular emphasis on exogenous fat administration, has become increasingly important.

Stable fat emulsions have allowed provision of a calorically dense emulsion to conserve fluid administration in infants especially sensitive to large volumes of fluid. Table 64-3 lists the most commonly used lipid emulsions. The provision of fat has prevented the development of essential fatty acid deficiency. It allows a balanced delivery of nitrogen and nonnitrogen calories as well. In addition, the lipid emulsions are isotonic and can be administered through peripheral veins.[71] Figure 64-1 illustrates the predominant aspects of exogenous lipid clearance. The fat particles of the lipid emulsions are similar to chylomicrons or very-low-density lipoproteins. In order for the free fatty acids to be utilized, lipoprotein lipase catalyzes the removal of the triglyceride–fatty acid component from within the particle. Lipoprotein lipase is present within the endothelial wall in varying amounts in body tissues. It has been demonstrated that concurrent heparin administration during parenteral alimentation facilitates release of lipoprotein lipase and thus greatly increases clearance of lipid emulsions. Zaidau and colleagues demonstrated that two forms of lipase exist, hepatic and extrahepatic. The latter accounts for up to 60% of total post–heparin lipolytic activity.[72] Lipoprotein lipase determines the pattern of uptake of exogenous lipids from the blood stream because it is the rate-limiting step in lipid absorption, and its concentration varies according to tissue demand.

The final step in the catabolism of long-chain fatty acids involves carnitine-dependent transferases that are the key enzymes in fatty acid oxidation. Carnitine, a nutritional cofactor, is synthesized in the liver from lysine and

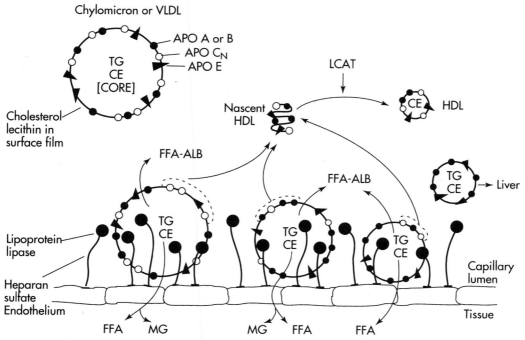

Figure 64–1. Representation of the hydrolysis of triglycerides in chylomicrons, very-low-density lipoprotein (VLDL), and intralipid emulsion by endothelial lipoprotein lipase. Triglyceride (TG)–laden lipoproteins contain a cholesterol ester (CE) core and a surface layer of lecithin, cholesterol, and apoproteins (APO). Lipoprotein lipase hydrolyzes TGs to monoglycerides (MGs) and free fatty acids (FFAs). The FFAs are bound to serum albumin (ALB). Lecithin-cholesterol acyltransferase (LCAT) esterifies the nascent high-density lipoprotein (HDL) to form a spherical HDL particle. *(From Hamosh M, Hamosh P: Lipoprotein lipase: Its physiological and clinical significance. Mol Aspects Med 6:199, 1983.)*

methionine, both of which are essential amino acids. Infants rely on carnitine to use dietary fat effectively to produce energy.[73] Carnitine has several essential roles in energy production. Its first well-described function is that of transporting long-chain fatty acids into mitochondria, where β oxidation occurs. Another more recently described role includes transport of activated carboxylic acids that have been activated to coenzyme A. Conversion of coenzyme A compounds to carnitine compounds makes the carboxylic acid transportable while maintaining its high-energy state. Carnitine, by conferring "transportability" to these high-energy molecules, is essential in delivering needed substrates from one cellular location to another. It also plays a role in removing accumulated products of other energy pathways, such as removing short-chain fatty acids that accumulate in the mitochondria, and in maintaining overall normal levels of free coenzyme A.[73-75] The role of carnitine in the pathway of fatty acid oxidation is illustrated in Figure 64-2.

In utero, carnitine crosses the placenta, providing adequate stores for the fetus. After birth, premature infants are at risk for carnitine deficiency, secondary to reduced capacity to synthesize carnitine; the tendency to conserve carnitine already acquired; and reduced reabsorption from immature kidney function. Penn and associates investigated the effect of nutritional intake on tissue carnitine concentrations in infants of different gestational ages by obtaining autopsy specimens of muscle, heart, liver, and kidney to analyze for content. Both gestational age and exogenous carnitine supply affect tissue carnitine reserves, and infants receiving carnitine-free TPN are not able to synthesize enough carnitine to maintain body stores. In addition,[76,77] various tissues were affected by carnitine deficiency. Carnitine is obtained from the diet; therefore, infants fed by TPN have declining levels of plasma carnitine after some time.[73,74] Schmidt-Sommerfield and colleagues studied lipid profiles in 15 premature infants after a lipid challenge. They demonstrated that carnitine-depleted infants had lower levels of β hydroxybutyrate and acetoacetate and higher levels of triglycerides and free fatty acids than control infants; this suggests that fatty acid oxidation is impaired in the carnitine-deficient state.[78] Studies by Bonner and coworkers of premature infants receiving carnitine supplementation also demonstrated that such infants had fewer biochemical markers of impaired fatty acid oxidation.[79] Supplementation of TPN solutions with carnitine improved nitrogen balance, enhanced utilization of intravenous lipids, and improved weight gain in 23 neonates with a mean gestational age of 32 weeks who were receiving parenteral nutrition.[80] Other authors have demonstrated similar increases in plasma carnitine levels with supplementation but without the same level of weight gain.[75]

Dosages between 2 and 10 mg/kg/day supplied as a continuous or four-times-daily schedule prevent carnitine deficiency.[74,77-82] Supplementation should continue until the establishment of half-volume enteral feedings.[79] Higher doses (25 to 48 mg/kg/day) have also been studied. At this range, fatty acid oxidation and carnitine concentrations

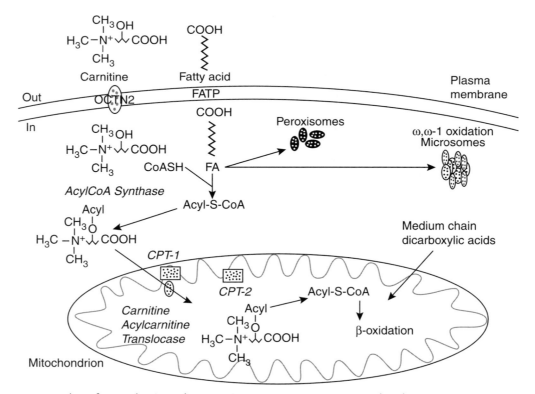

Figure 64–2. The carnitine cycle in fatty acid (FA) oxidation. CoA, coenzyme A; CoASH, uncombined coenzyme A; CPT-2, carnitine palmityltransferase 2; FATP, F₁ adenosine triphosphate; OCTN2, novel organic cation transporter. *(From Scaglia F, Longo N: Primary and secondary alterations of neonatal carnitine metabolism. Semin Perinatol 23:155, 1999.)*

in plasma are improved but may also result in a higher metabolic rate and increased nitrogen excretion, without improvement in weight gain or other growth parameters.[75,82]

Carnitine is available for general use in intravenous supplementation. Although the precise dose of carnitine to supplement in TPN solutions is unknown, supplementation at 10 mg/kg/day is safe and may provide an essential cofactor for exogenously administered lipid utilization.[83]

Lecithin-cholesterol acyltransferase (LCAT) is made in the liver and released into the circulation. It acts to break down the lecithin component of the lipid emulsion (the egg yolk phospholipids) by converting the lecithin and unesterified cholesterol to lysolecithin and cholesterol ester. It has been demonstrated that elevations in LCAT activity may account for improved tolerance of 20% fat emulsions in more premature infants.

As mentioned previously, concurrent heparin administration facilitates the clearance of lipid emulsions by releasing lipoprotein lipase from the endothelial cell. Even low-dose heparin, 1 U/hour, provides sufficient heparin for postheparin lipolytic activity to occur.[84] With regard to concentration, 20% lipid emulsions result in significantly less hypertriglyceridemia than do 10% emulsions.[85] It has been postulated that this occurrence results from lower amounts of phospholipids in equivalent doses of 20% in comparison with 10% emulsions; the phospholipids lead to liposome production, which may interfere with lipid clearance.[85,86] It has been demonstrated that 20% fat in some infants leads to higher LCAT levels, which also may contribute to improved clearance.[87]

To provide 40% to 50% of total caloric intake from fat, recommended dosages range from 1 to 3 g/kg/day.[88] Starting concentrations of a 20% emulsion at 0.5 to 1 g/kg/day with a daily increase up to 3 g/kg/day is safe and efficacious for infants across a wide range of birth weights and even when initiated during the first few days after birth.[89] Unlike infusion rates for protein during parenteral alimentation, the rates of lipid infusion have been investigated extensively. Kao and associates demonstrated that 24-hour infusion, in comparison with 8-hour infusion, resulted in significantly fewer fluctuations in serum triglyceride, free fatty acid, and cholesterol levels.[90] Spear and coworkers found that 24-hour infusions, in comparison with 15-hour therapy, resulted in less elevation of serum free fatty acid levels, but no difference between infusion rates was found for triglycerides or lipoprotein lipase.[84] It is generally accepted practice to infuse the lipid infusions for as long as possible, allowing several hours of lipid-free intravenous alimentation. Infusions over 20 hours are most commonly used at our institution.

Lipid Toxicity

Early administration of intravenous lipids to neonates has been under scrutiny because of the concerns that lipids increase free bilirubin concentrations, affect the function of cells in the immune system, alter fatty acid patterns, contribute to hyperglycemia, affect pulmonary mechanics, and induce thrombocytopenia.

Because of common binding sites on the albumin molecule, free fatty acids may compete with bilirubin for albumin-binding sites if excessive doses of fat are administered. Displacement of bilirubin from albumin is minimal at fatty acid–to-albumin ratios of less than 4.1, and even at higher ratios, displacement is unlikely.[65] Rubin and colleagues studied plasma lipid and bilirubin profiles in premature infants receiving lipid emulsions. At the end of the 6-day study period, despite increased plasma lipids and free fatty acids, bilirubin levels declined, indicating that there was no correlation between free fatty acids and free bilirubin.[91] It has also been demonstrated that infusion of up to 3 g/kg/day in premature infants more than 30 weeks after conception can be tolerated without excessive competition for albumin binding.[92] Lipids do not need to be withheld from jaundiced infants receiving TPN.[91]

Another side effect from lipid emulsions is interference with oxygenation, which occurs by altering pulmonary vascular tone and pulmonary artery pressure through thromboxane-mediated pathways.[41,43] Prasertsom and associates studied 11 preterm infants with respiratory distress syndrome who received 20% lipid emulsions.[93] After several hours of lipid infusion, two-dimensional echocardiography showed a 20% increase in the ratio of right ventricular pre-ejection period to ejection time. After discontinuation of intravenous lipids, this ratio returned to baseline.[43] Pereira and coworkers demonstrated a fall in arterial oxygen tension over 4 hours during infusions of fat at 1 g/kg/day.[94] With higher doses of fat, the alveolar-arterial gradient is less affected, if the infusion period is prolonged. Other investigators also found no difference in oxygenation between infants randomly assigned to receive various lipid dosages when lower rates and longer infusion times were used.[46,95] Early provision of lipids does not seem to change the incidence of chronic lung disease in infants with very low birth weight.[18,56,87] Other studies suggest that patients with compromised lung function may theoretically benefit from receiving lipid emulsions because at similar oxygen consumption, oxidation of fat produces less CO_2 than does oxidation for the same amount of carbohydrate.[94]

Although the product information accompanying lipid preparations states that platelet function and quantity can be disturbed with these infusions, there are scant data to support this claim. Spear and coworkers performed a controlled prospective study that demonstrated no difference in platelet counts over 4 weeks after birth between infants receiving fat infusions and those who did not receive these infusions.[96] Another study in older children, in fact, found improved coagulation function in children receiving concurrent fat infusions during prolonged parenteral nutrition.[97]

There has been some theoretical concern during fat infusions about altering normal fatty acid patterns, which is of uncertain clinical significance.[98] Gaull and associates, in a retrospective study, described a higher incidence of coagulase-negative staphylococcal infections in premature infants receiving fat infusions.[19] Prospective investigations need to be implemented to clarify this issue.[5] Lipid clearance capacity may also be modified with stress of any type including infection. Some authors advocate restricting lipids to these critically ill patients, although there are no strong data to support this practice.[89] (See also the later section, "Parenteral Nutrition, Illness, and Stress.")

The complications of concurrent lipid infusions can usually be avoided with appropriate dosages and slow infusion rates.

TRACE ELEMENTS

The trace elements essential in newborns are zinc, copper, selenium, iron, iodine, chromium, manganese, molybdenum, cobalt, and fluoride. Trace elements play important roles in metabolic pathways. In utero accretion takes place during the last trimester, leaving prematurely born infants at high risk for deficiency with their low body stores and high rates of requirements secondary to postnatal growth.[99,100]

The roles of zinc, copper, and iron administration to this population are well studied.[65,101] The recommendation for TPN supplementation with selenium has also been accepted. Selenium is an essential trace element with important antioxidant functions. The glutathione peroxidase enzyme family, responsible for protecting cell membranes from peroxidase damage through detoxification of peroxides and free radicals, is selenium dependent.[30]

Zlotkin and associates investigated selenium in utero. According to these data, which were obtained in New Zealand, the selenium intrauterine accretion rate in the third trimester of pregnancy is 1 µg/kg/day. In New Zealand, tissue levels of selenium are known to be low, and, therefore, actual accretion rates may be higher in other populations or elsewhere in the world. Premature infants have low hepatic stores of selenium.[100]

The decline in postnatal selenium in the premature infant reflects the postnatal fall in blood cell mass.[101] TPN supplemented with selenium has been shown to treat biochemical selenium deficiency and keeps glutathione peroxidase activity normal.[102,103] Other authors caution against relying on glutathione peroxidase activity as a marker for selenium requirement, because levels may increase with oxygen therapy, mechanical ventilation, and steroid use.[104] Selenium deficiency has been postulated as a risk factor for the development of chronic lung disease and retinopathy of prematurity. Darlow and coworkers, in a study of 534 infants weighing less than 1500 g who were provided selenium supplementation, showed there were no differences between the supplemented and nonsupplemented groups in oxygen requirement at 28 days after birth or in total days on oxygen. Lower prerandomization selenium levels were associated with increased respiratory morbidity.[102] Supplementation of selenium does improve the blood selenium profile. The current recommendation for selenium supplementation in parenteral nutrition is 2 µg/kg/day after 2 weeks of intravenous feeding.[101]

The importance of iodine, chromium, manganese, molybdenum, cobalt, and fluoride is not as well established, but deficiency states are not a current concern in the United States.[65] The intake of these components is usually regulated according to preset guidelines. Pediatric trace metal solutions containing zinc, copper, manganese, and chromium are commonly added to neonatal parenteral nutrition solutions. Selenium can be added as previously recommended.

The only trace element recommended from the first day after birth for supplementation in infants receiving parenteral nutrition is zinc. The other trace elements are probably not needed for the first week or so after birth. Copper and manganese should be withheld from infants with cholestasis. Chromium and selenium should be withheld from infants with diminished renal function and low urine output.[100,101] Iron supplementation is usually not needed in the first few weeks after birth and is not routinely added to parenteral nutrition. Table 63-1 lists the recommended parenteral intake of trace elements for full-term and preterm infants. There are extensive reviews covering the concurrent administration of trace elements and minerals to this population.[98]

Aluminum is a trace metal with potential toxicity to multiple organ systems. In 1988, the U.S. Food and Drug Administration published a proposal to regulate the labeling for aluminum in large- and small-volume injections. The standard became 25 µg or less of aluminum contaminant per liter. This proposal was based on evidence that aluminum was found to be a contaminant of parenteral nutrition solutions and other intravenous solutions such as calcium gluconate and sodium phosphate.[105,106]

ELECTROLYTES, CALCIUM, MAGNESIUM, AND PHOSPHORUS

A complete discussion of electrolyte and mineral metabolism is found in other chapters in this book. In parenteral nutrition, the serum electrolytes sodium, potassium, chloride, and acetate (a buffer-bicarbonate precursor) can be provided, as can calcium, magnesium, and phosphorus. Dosages are based on physiologic requirements and also titrated to the patient's individual laboratory findings. (See also the later section, "General and Clinical Considerations.")

The normal sodium diuresis and isotonic contraction that occurs in newborns is responsible for the obligate weight loss in the first few days after birth. In very premature infants, this process can be aggravated by the large amount of free water loss through transepithelial evaporation. Neonatal parenteral fluid and electrolyte support in the first few days after birth should be designed not only to maintain hydration but also to allow for the normal physiologic contraction of the extracellular fluid space.[107] For these reasons, sodium should be withheld from the parenteral nutrition for these infants during the first few days up to a week after birth.[108] Serum potassium elevation is also not uncommon in premature infants with low birth weight, because of immature renal function and increased cell turnover. Like sodium, potassium should be excluded from parenteral nutrition for the first few days after birth. Maintenance amounts of both sodium and potassium can be added at about 48 hours, depending on serum sodium and potassium levels and if urine output is adequate.[107] Chloride is usually provided as a component of the salt forms of sodium and potassium.[30] The acid-base balance provided in parenteral nutrition also is controlled by increasing or decreasing amounts of both chloride and base buffer. (See also the later section, "General Complications of Parenteral Nutrition.")

Calcium and phosphorus are important components in parenteral nutrition because of their important roles for skeletal and bone growth. The amounts of calcium and phosphorus to match intrauterine accretion cannot be given safely in parenteral nutrition solution.[109] Solubility of these minerals in parenteral solution depends not only on the ratio of calcium to phosphorus but also on the levels of many of the other parenteral nutrition components. This makes bone mineralization a major challenge in neonatal nutrition.[110] In TPN solutions, 90 mg of calcium and 70 mg of phosphorus, both per kilogram per day, provide adequate physiologic ratio and maximizes retention of both without an increase in hypercalciuria.[111] Higher concentrations may be needed in smaller infants.[112]

MULTIVITAMINS

Optimal vitamin intake is not possible with the current commercial multivitamin preparations (M.V.I. Pediatric). However, 40% of a vial of M.V.I. Pediatric (2 mL) is commonly added to neonatal parenteral nutrition.[113] This amount reflects the latest recommendations provided by the American Society for Clinical Nutrition. See Table 63-1 in Chapter 63 for the recommended parenteral intake of vitamins for full-term infants and the preterm infant.

GENERAL AND CLINICAL CONSIDERATIONS

Our practice is to initiate parenteral nutrition that includes glucose, protein, and lipids within the first few days after birth if the infant is not able to maintain fluid requirements with enteral feeds. We usually initiate protein and lipids at a lower starting dose and implement a daily stepwise increase until 3 to 4 g of protein and 3 g of lipids, both per kilogram per day, are infused. The glucose and protein infusions run continuously for 24 hours, whereas lipids infuse over 20 hours. Lipids are housed in a separate Volutrol so that any precipitation in the glucose–amino acid solution can be visualized. Parenteral solution volume, rate of infusion, acid-base balance, electrolytes, calcium, magnesium, phosphorus, and trace minerals are added, as previously discussed, and titrated to the individual patient's clinical status and laboratory values.

Total daily energy requirements for full-term infants reach approximately 100 to 120 kcal/kg/day by 2 weeks after birth.[114] By 2 weeks after birth, many infants are no longer dependent on TPN and have begun enteral feedings. For the infant with extremely low birth weight and the critically ill newborn, the optimal caloric requirement is still undefined, except that their energy requirements are probably higher (120 to 130 kcal/kg/day).[115] This amount of caloric intake often cannot be achieved solely with parenteral nutrition. Calculation of calories in parenteral nutrition is illustrated in Figure 64-3.

At our institution, parenteral nutrition is ordered by the neonatal caregiver, who uses a computer program (Neofax, Ross Laboratories, Columbus, Ohio) that generates a written copy of the solution and its constituents to be prepared by the pharmacist. Figure 64-4 is an example of the parenteral nutrition order form. Recommended ranges used as guidelines are provided for each component and are listed on the form. Several days of previous orders are readily visible for ease of determining what has previously been administered. Tables 64-4 and 64-5 list the monitoring schedule during parenteral nutrition that are followed at Christiana Hospital.

Parenteral Nutrition, Illness, and Stress

Increasing numbers of investigators are dedicated to studying the relationship among neonatal illness, stress, and nutritional status. Disease-specific parenteral nutrition regimens have not been well studied or put into clinical practice, except for diminishing renal toxic additives during episodes of renal insufficiency or adding additional trace elements after prolonged intravenous nutrition. Increased oxygen consumption, energy expenditure, and changes in nutrient metabolism have been documented in infants with certain cardiorespiratory disorders and in adults with sepsis.[115-117] The effect of the neonatal stress response to protein metabolism is unknown.[115] The adult stress response results in large surges of catecholamines, cortisol, and glucagon, leading to a catabolic state. Extrapolating from adult data, newborns may also undergo the same derangement during periods of stress. The duration of circulating levels of catecholamines, cortisol, and glucagons after a stress response is also unknown. After vaginal delivery, catecholamine concentrations rise 10-fold but return to baseline by 2 hours. This may not occur in newborns who experience perinatal hypoxia, those with prolonged hypoxia, or those who receive infusions of catecholamines (dopamine and dobutamine) after birth.[115]

The stress response to surgery has been more objectively studied. Stress hormones during and after cardiac surgery are known to increase.[118] Pain control during cardiac surgery attenuates this stress response.[119,120] Thus, conditions in which stress is prolonged and increased may be associated with negative nitrogen balance; this is even more reason why parenteral nutrition should be initiated early during the neonatal period. Although there is some controversy over whether premature infants and critically ill newborns can tolerate parenteral nutrients and lipids during periods of stress and sepsis, there seems to be no overwhelming evidence that this is the case, particularly if parenteral nutrition is provided properly.

General Complications of Parenteral Nutrition

Complications of parenteral nutrition include metabolic, mechanical, and infectious problems. Theoretically, the provision (or lack of provision) of any and all components by parenteral nutrition can have consequences.

Metabolic Complications

Metabolic complications commonly occur when administered nutrients are not adequately provided or when the infant's ability to clear the administered nutrients is exceeded. Any component deficiency may result in poor growth and overall poor retention of the nutrient. If the component is insufficiently provided for a prolonged

1) D10W* = $\dfrac{\text{total g glucose/day} \times 3.4 \text{ kcal/g}}{\text{Wt in kg}}$ = kcal/kg/day of glucose

> Example: $\dfrac{15 \text{ g glucose/day} \times 3.4 \text{ kcal/g}}{1.0 \text{ kg}}$ = 51 kcal/kg/day of glucose

2) 3 g/kg/day protein = $\dfrac{\text{total g/day protein} \times 4 \text{ kcal/g}}{}$ = kcal/kg/day of protein

> Example: $\dfrac{3 \text{ g/day} \times 4 \text{ kcal/g}}{1.0 \text{ kg}}$ = 12 kcal/kg/day of protein

3) 3 g/kg/day of a 20% lipid solution:

$\dfrac{\text{total g lipid/day} \times 9 \text{ kcal/g}}{\text{Wt in kg}}$ = kcal/kg/day lipids

> Example: $\dfrac{3 \text{ g/day} \times 9 \text{ kcal/g}}{1.0 \text{ kg}}$ = 27 kcal/kg/day of lipid

4) Total cal/kg/day = 51 glucose cal + 12 protein cal + 27 fat cal = 90 cal/kg/day

*D10W = 10 g glucose/100 mL water

> Example: At 150 mL/kg/day, total grams glucose/day = 15 g/day

Figure 64–3. Basic caloric calculations for total parenteral nutrition. Example: Total fluids of 150 mL/kg/day for a 1.0-kg infant.

period, this may result in clinically significant deficiency syndromes. Conversely, if nutrients are administered at dosages that exceed the infant's ability to clear them, toxic imbalances may occur. Most electrolyte imbalances can be corrected by an adjustment of the constituents of the solution. Discussions of all the clinical deficiency and toxicity syndromes associated with these are beyond the scope of this chapter. (See also the earlier section, "Trace Elements.") The more problematic metabolic complications are discussed briefly as follows.

Parenteral nutrition–induced prerenal azotemia has been attributed to the doses of amino acids infused, but it is also likely to have multifactorial causes, including immature renal function in infants with low birth weight.[30] Concerns that protein intolerance leads to hyperammonemia, azotemia, and metabolic acidosis are clinically unsupported. Ammonia levels, blood urea nitrogen levels, and acidosis may be poor markers for amino acid toxicity.[114] Specifically, blood urea nitrogen level is not a good marker for protein tolerance because it is affected by many factors, including hydration status and urinary flow rate.[121] At dosages of amino acid infusion exceeding that needed for protein accretion, elevated protein levels and

blood urea nitrogen level may represent an acceptable metabolic by-product and not protein intolerance.[115]

Both metabolic acidosis and alkalosis can occur, depending on the acid-base profile of the parenteral solution. Hyperchloremic metabolic acidosis is a common complication of parenteral nutrition, probably caused by an imbalance between the intake of base and increased urinary losses. To prevent and treat hyperchloremic metabolic acidosis that sometimes complicates parenteral nutrition, the ratio of chloride to buffer can be manipulated. Sodium and phosphorus can be provided as either their chloride or acetate salts, and the amount of buffer can also be increased or decreased.[30] Calcium and phosphorus deficiency can be major factors in the development of metabolic bone disease.

Parenteral nutrition–induced cholestasis is one of the more problematic complications of long-term use. The precise cause of the obstructive pattern is unknown, and its development and progression are probably multifactorial.[122] Risk factors include duration of parenteral nutrition, birth weight, individual hemodynamic and physiologic factors, and bypassing of the gastrointestinal tract.[30] The amino acid component of parenteral alimentation itself

CHRISTIANA CARE HEALTH
CHRISTIANA HOSPITAL
SPECIAL CARE NURSERY
Neonatal Parenteral Nutrition Orders

* * * * * CHART COPY * * * * *   *Plate*

NAME OF PATIENT	Sex: Male	Birth Weight: 1500 grams
ID: 555555	Rm: SCN	
Born: 08/27/01	Age: 3.1 days	Present Weight: 1.500 kg

PN # 27		*per kg/day*	*per day*	*per hour*
PERIPHERAL Line	Fats 20%	10.00 mL	15.00 mL	0.75 mL/hr x 20 hours
Start: 20:00	D-10.00%-AA-2.22%	90.00 mL	135.00 mL	5.63 mL/hr
08/30/01	TOTALS	100.00 mL	150.00 mL	6.38 mL/hr

NUTRIENTS

	per kg/day	*per day*
Fats	2.00 g	3.00 g
Dextrose 10.00%	90.00 mL	135.00 mL
6.25 mg/Kg/min	9.00 g	13.50 g
TrophA-6%	2.00 g	3.00 g
Cysteine		
Carnitine	10.00 mg	15.00 mg
Sodium	2.00 mEq	3.00 mEq
Potassium	2.00 mEq	3.00 mEq
Magnesium	0.40 mEq	0.60 mEq
Calcium	1.00 mEq	1.50 mEq
Phosphorus	0.50 mmol	0.75 mmol
Chloride	1.33 mEq*	2.00 mEq
Acetate	2.00 mEq	3.00 mEq
MVI Pediatric	1.00 mL	1.50 mL
Iron		
Zinc	450.00 µg	675.00 µg
Copper	30.00 µg	45.00 µg
Manganese	7.50 µg	11.25 µg
Chromium	0.26 µg	0.38 µg
Selenium		
Iodine		
Molybdenum		
Heparin (0.50 U/mL) 45.00 U		67.50 U
Ranitidine		

CALORIES

	per kg/day	*per day*	*percent*
Fat	20.00	30.00	34.13%
CHO	30.60	45.90	52.22%
Pro.	8.00	12.00	13.65%
Totals	58.60	87.90	
NonPro.	50.60	75.90	
NonProtein kcal/g Nitrogen		163	
NonProtein kcal/g AminoAcid		25	

RATIOS

mEq Ca : mmol P	Ratio = 2.0 : 1
mEq Cl : mEq Ac	Ratio = 0.7 : 1

VITAMINS per DAY

A	690.00 IU	C	24.00 mg
B1	0.36 mg	D	120.00 IU
B2	0.42 mg	E	2.10 IU
B3	5.10 mg	K1	60.00 µg
B5	1.50 mg	F.A.	42.00 µg
B6	0.30 mg	Biotin	6.00 µg
B12	0.30 mcg		

Approximate Osmolarity   815 mOsm/L
*Range Variations

Attending MD: _SPEAR_____ Entered by:_____
Printed 09.25 Thursday 08/30/01   COLEMAN

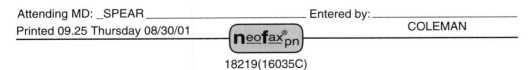

neofax®pn

18219(16035C)

Figure 64–4. Neonatal parenteral nutrition order form of the Special Care Nursery, Christiana Hospital, Christiana, Delaware.

has also been blamed for causing cholestasis, but appropriate dosages can help minimize its incidence.[98]

Infectious Complications

Infectious complications are probably also multifactorial. Because of the presence of either central or peripheral venous catheters in premature infants who are immunocompromised, nosocomial infection is common. *Staphylococcus epidermidis* is a common pathogen and, in some nurseries, can account for a majority of neonatal infections.[123] The fungal species most often implicated are *Candida albicans* and *Malassezia furfur*.[124,125] The incidence

Table 64–4. Suggested Laboratory Test Schedule for Monitoring Neonatal Patients on Total Parenteral Nutrition (TPN)

Test	TPN Duration		
	Week 1	Week 2	Weeks 2-4+
Electrolytes	qd	q2–3d	Every week
Urine glucose	q4-12h	q12h	qd
BUN, creatinine	qd	q2-3d	Every week
Calcium	qd	q2-3d	Every week
Phosphorus, magnesium	Every week	Every week	Every week
CBC, platelets	qd	q2-3d	Every week
LFTs (bilirubin, t/d, AST, ALT, alkaline phosphate)	—	—	Every 2 weeks

ALT, alanine aminotransferase; AST, aspartate aminotransferase; BUN, blood urea nitrogen; CBC, complete blood cell count; LFT, liver function test; t/d, total/direct.

of sepsis as a complication of parenteral nutrition is higher among infants of younger gestational ages and with longer duration of parenteral nutrition.[125] Careful local cleansing and sterile technique can minimize this complication. In addition, minimizing the use of central lines for obtaining blood samples also lessens the incidence of infection.

Mechanical Complications

Virtually any complication related to an indwelling peripheral or central catheter can occur, because provision of intravenous alimentation necessitates the need for a catheter. Complications can be related to the composition of the catheter itself, how it is inserted, its location of insertion, and duration of use. Infiltration, infection, malposition, and thrombosis necessitate removal of the catheter. Catheter patency after thrombosis in long-term access devices has been achieved by infusing small amounts of thrombolytic agents such as streptokinase and urokinase.[126-128]

Table 64–5. Suggested Laboratory Test Schedule for Monitoring Neonatal Patients on Long-Term Total Parenteral Nutrition (>4 weeks)*

Test	Schedule
Protein: TP, albumin, prealbumin, transferrin	q2wk
Fat: cholesterol	q2wk
Fat-soluble vitamins: A, D, E	q2wk
Trace elements Iron, manganese, zinc, copper, selenium, carnitine	q4wk

*Consider monitoring for adequate nutrition as assessed by levels of these tests.

TP, total protein.

REFERENCES

1. Metcoff J: Fetal growth and maternal nutrition. In Faulkner F, Turner JM (eds): Human Growth, vol 3, 2nd ed. New York, Plenum Press, 1985, pp 333-388.
2. Sparks JW: Human intrauterine growth and nutrient excretion. Semin Perinatol 8:74, 1984.
3. McCane RA, Widdowson EM: In Falkner F, Turner JM (eds): Human Growth, vol 1, 2nd ed. New York, Plenum Press, 1985, p 139.
4. Battaglia FC, Meschia G: Fetal nutrition. Annu Rev Nutr 8:43, 1988.
5. Battaglia FC, Meschia G: An Introduction to Fetal Physiology. Orlando, Fla, Academic Press, 1986.
6. Bell AW, Kennaugh IM, Battaglia FL: Uptake of amino acids and ammonia at midgestation by the fetal lamb. J Exp Physiol 74:635, 1989.
7. Binder ND, Raschko PK, Benda GL, et al: Insulin infusion with parenteral nutrition in extremely low birthweight infants with hyperglycemia. J Pediatr 114:273, 1980.
8. Boehm G, Handrick W, Spencker FB, et al: Effect of bacterial sepsis on protein metabolism in infants during the first week. Biomed Biochem Acta 45:813, 1986.
9. Bozzetti P, Ferrari MM, Marconi AM, et al: The relationship of maternal and fetal glucose concentrations in the human from midgestation until term. Metabolism 37:358, 1988.
10. Cetin I, Fennessey PV, Quick ANJ, et al: Glycine turnover and oxidation and hepatic serine synthesis from glycine in fetal lambs. Am J Physiol 260:E371, 1991.
11. DeBenoist B: Measurement of whole body protein turnover in preterm infant with intragastric infusion of L-[1-13C] leucine and sampling urinary leucine pool. Clin Sci 66:155, 1984.
12. Hay W: Fetal requirements and placental transfer of nitrogenous compounds. In Polin RA, Fox WW (eds): Fetal and Neonatal Physiology. Philadelphia, WB Saunders, 1992, pp 431-442.
13. Matthews DE: General concepts of protein metabolism. In Polin RA, Fox WW (eds): Fetal and Neonatal Physiology, vol 1. Philadelphia, WB Saunders, 1992, pp 419-428.
14. Snyderman SE: The protein and amino acid requirements of the premature infant. In Jones JHP (ed): Metabolic Processes in the Foetus and Newborn Infant. Leiden, the Netherlands, Stenfert Kroese, 1971, pp 128-141.

15. Waterlow JT, Garlick PJ, Millward DJ: Protein Turnover in Mammalian Tissues and in the Whole Body. Amsterdam, Elsevier/North Holland, 1978.

16. Holzman IR, Lemons JA, Meschia G, et al: Uterine uptake of amino acids and glutamine-glutamate balances across the placenta of the pregnant. J Dev Physiol 1:137, 1979.

17. Lemons JA: Fetal-placental nitrogen metabolism. Semin Perinatol 3:177, 1979.

18. Ganapathy ME, Leibach FH, Mahesh VB, et al: Characterization of tryptophan transport in human placental brush-border membrane vessels. Biochem J 238:201, 1986.

19. Gaull GE, Sturman JA, Raiha NC: Development of mammalian sulfur metabolism: Absence of cystathionase in human fetal tissues. Pediatr Res 6:538, 1972.

20. Cetin I, Marconi AM, Bozzetti P, et al: Umbilical amino acid concentrations in appropriate and small for gestational age infants. A biochemical difference present in utero. Am J Obstet Gynecol 158:120, 1988.

21. Greenberg RE, Wozenrish FJ, Gracia P, et al: Fetal insulin increases placental amino acid transport. Clin Res 37:178A, 1989.

22. Rowell PP, Sastry BUR: Human placental cholinergic system; depression of the uptake of alpha-aminoisobutyric acid in isolated human placental villi by choline acetyltransferase inhibition. J Pharmacol Exp Ther 216:232, 1981.

23. Lemons JA, Adock EW, Jones MJ, et al: Umbilical uptake of amino acids in the unstressed fetal lamb. J Clin Invest 58:1428, 1976.

24. Feldman M, van Aerde JE, Clauclinino MT: Lipid accretion in the fetus and newborn. In Polin RA, Fox WW (eds): Fetal and Neonatal Physiology. Philadelphia: WB Saunders, 1992, pp 299-314.

25. Kennaugh JM, Bell AW, Teng C, et al: Ontogenic changes in the rates of protein synthesis and leucine oxidation during fetal life. Pediatr Res 22:688, 1987.

26. VanVeen LCP, Teng C, Hay WWJ, et al: Leucine disposal and oxidation rates in the fetal lamb. Metabolism 36:48, 1987.

27. van Goudoever JB, Sulkers EJ, Timmerman M, et al: Amino acid solutions for premature neonates during the first week of life: The role of N-acetyl-L-cysteine and N-acetyl-L-tyrosine. JPEN J Parenter Enteral Nutr 18:404, 1994.

28. Helms RA, Storm MC, Christensen ML, et al: Cysteine supplementation results in normalization of plasma taurine concentrations in children receiving home parenteral nutrition. J Pediatr 134:358, 1999.

29. Malloy MH, Rassin DK, Richardson J: Total parenteral nutrition in sick preterm infants: Effects of cysteine supplementation with nitrogen intakes of 240 and 400 mg/kg/day. J Pediatr Gastroenterol Nutr 3:239, 1984.

30. Denne SC, Clark SE, Poindexter BB, et al: Nutrition and metabolism in the high risk neonate. In Fanaroff AA, Martin RJ (eds): Neonatal-Perinatal Medicine Diseases of the Fetus and Infant, vol 1, 6th ed. St. Louis, Mosby, 1997, pp 562-621.

31. Lacey JM, Crouch JB, Benfeill K, et al: The effects of glutamine-supplemented parenteral nutrition in premature infants. JPEN J Parenter Enteral Nutr 20:74, 1996.

32. Newsholme EA, Newsholme P, Curi R, et al: A role for muscle in the immune system and its importance in surgery, trauma, sepsis and burns. Nutrition 4:261, 1988.

33. Darmaun D, Roig JC, Auestad N, et al: Glutamine metabolism in very low birth weight infants. Pediatr Res 41:391, 1997.

34. Khan K, Hardy G, McElroy B, et al: The stability of L-glutamine in total parenteral nutrition solution. Clin Nutr 10:193, 1991.

35. Meier PR, Teng C, Battaglia FC, et al: The rate of amino acid nitrogen and total nitrogen accumulation in the fetal lamb. Proc Soc Exp Biol Med 167:463, 1981.

36. Heird WC: Amino acids in pediatric and neonatal nutrition. Curr Opin Clin Nutr Metab Care 1:73, 1998.

37. Widdowson EM: Body composition of the fetus and infant. In Visser HKA (ed): Fifth Nutricia Symposium: Nutrition and Metabolism of the Fetus and Infant. The Hague, the Netherlands, Martinus Nijhoff, 1979, pp 169-177.

38. Missim Y: Effect of conceptual age and dietary intake on protein metabolism in premature infants. J Pediatr Gastroenterol Nutr 2:507, 1983.

39. Duffy B, Pencharz P: The effect of surgery on the nitrogen metabolism of parenterally fed human neonates. Pediatr Res 20:32, 1986.

40. Zlotkin SH, Bryan MH, Anderson GH, et al: Intravenous nitrogen and energy intakes required to duplicate in utero nitrogen accretion in prematurely born infants. J Pediatr 99:115, 1981.

41. VanLingen RA, von Goudoever JB, Luijendijk IH, et al: Effects of early amino acid administration during total parenteral nutrition on protein metabolism in pre-term infants. Clin Sci 82:199, 1992.

42. Rivera A, Bell EF, Bier DM: Effect of intravenous amino acids on protein metabolism of preterm infants during the first three days of life. Pediatr Res 33:106, 1993.

43. Rivera A, Bell EF, Stegink LD, et al: Plasma amino acid profiles during the first three days of life in infants with respiratory distress syndrome: Effect of parenteral amino acid supplementation. J Pediatr 115:465, 1989.

44. Thureen PJ, Anderson AH, Baron KA, et al: Protein balance in the first week of life in ventilated neonates receiving parenteral nutrition. Am J Clin Nutr 68:1128, 1998.

45. van Goudoever JB, Colen T, Wattimena JLD, et al: Immediate commencement of amino acid supplementation in preterm infants: Effect of serum amino acid concentrations and protein kinetics on the first day of life. J Pediatr 127:458, 1995.

46. Adamkin DH: Issues in the nutritional support of the ventilated baby. Clin Perinatol 25:79, 1998.

47. Gordon HH, Levine SZ, McNamara H: Feeding of premature infants. A comparison of human and cow's milk. Am J Dis Child 73:442, 1947.

48. Davidson M, Levine SZ, Bauer C, et al: Feeding studies in low birth weight infants. I. Relationship of dietary protein, fat, and electrolytes to rates of weight gain, clinical course, and serum chemical concentrations. J Pediatr 70:695, 1967.

49. Phillips AF: Carbohydrate metabolism of the fetus. In RA Polin, WW Fox (eds): Fetal and Neonatal Physiology, vol 1. Philadelphia, WB Saunders, 1992, pp 373-384.

50. Girard J: Rise of glucoregulatory hormones on hepatic glucose metabolism during the perinatal period. In Polin RA, Fox WW (eds): Fetal and Neonatal Physiology, vol 1. Philadelphia, WB Saunders, 1992, pp 390-401.

51. Crandell SS, Fisher DJ, Morriss FHJ: Effects of ovine maternal hyperglycemia on fetal regional blood flows and metabolism. Am J Physiol 249:E454, 1985.

52. Padbury JF, Ogata ES: Glucose metabolism during the transition to post-natal life. In Polin RA, Fox WW (eds): Fetal and Neonatal Physiology, vol 1. Philadelphia, WB Saunders, 1992, pp 402-405.

53. Morriss FH Jr, Makowski EL, Meschia G, Battaglia FC: The glucose/oxygen quotient of the term human fetus. Biol Neonate 25:44, 1974.

54. Chez RA, Mintz DH, Reynolds WA, et al: Maternal-fetal plasma glucose relationships in late monkey pregnancy. Am J Obstet Gynecol 121:938, 1975.

55. Shelly HJ: Glycogen reserves and their changes at birth and in anoxia. Br Med Bull 17:137, 1961.

56. Sunehag A, Ewald U, Hausson A, et al: Glucose production rate in extremely immature neonates (<28 weeks) studied by use of deuterated glucose. Pediatr Res 33:97, 1993.

57. Anand RS, Ganguli S, Sperling MA: Effect of insulin induced maternal hypoglycemia on glucose turnover in maternal and fetal sheep. Am J Physiol 238:E524, 1980.

58. Anderson TL, Muttaer CR, Bieber MA, et al: A controlled trial of glucose vs. glucose and amino acids in premature infants. J Pediatr 94:947, 1979.

59. Cowett RM, Susa JB, Oh W, et al: Glucose kinetics in glucose-infused small for gestational age infants. Pediatr Res 18:74, 1984.

60. Girard J: Gluconeogenesis in late fetal and early neonatal life. Biol Neonate 50:237, 1986.

61. Kalhan SC, Bier D, Savin SM, et al: Estimations of glucose turnover and 13C recycling in the human newborn by simultaneous [1-13C] glucose and [6,6-2H2] glucose tracers. J Clin Endocrin Metab 50:456, 1980.

62. Kalhan SC, D'Angelo LJ, Savin SM, et al: Glucose product in pregnant women at term gestation. Sources of glucose for human fetus. J Clin Invest 63:388, 1979.

63. Lillien LD, Pildes RS, Srinivagan G, et al: Treatment of neonatal hypoglycemia with minibolus and intravenous glucose infusion. J Pediatr 97:295, 1980.

64. Pildes RS, Pyati SP: Hypoglycemia and hyperglycemia in tiny infants. Clin Perinatol 13:351, 1986.

65. Hay WW, Lucas A, Heird WC, et al: Workshop summary: Nutrition of the extremely low birth weight infant. Pediatrics 104:1360, 1999.

66. Farrag HM, Cowett RM: Glucose homeostasis in the micropremie. Clin Perinatol 27:1, 2000.

67. Collins JW, Hoppe M: A controlled trial of insulin infusion and parenteral nutrition in extremely low birthweight infants with glucose intolerance. J Pediatr 118:921, 1991.

68. Poindexter BB, Karn CA, Denne SC: Exogenous insulin reduces proteolysis and protein synthesis in extremely low birth weight infants. J Pediatr 132:948, 1998.

69. Hahn P, Novak M: Development of brown and white adipose tissue. J Lipid Res 27:437, 1981.

70. Herrera E, Lasunction MA, Asuncion M: Placental transport of free fatty acids, glycerol, and ketone bodies. In RA Polin, WW Fox (eds): Fetal and Neonatal Physiology, vol. 1. Philadelphia, WB Saunders, 1992, pp 291-298.

71. Hallberg D: Studies in the elimination of exogenous lipids from the bloodstream. Acta Physiol Scand 65(Suppl 254):1, 1965.

72. Zaidau H, Dhanireddy R, Hamosh M, et al: Lipid clearing in premature infants during continuous heparin infusion: Role of circulatory lipases. Pediatr Res 19:23, 1985.

73. Scaglia F, Longo N: Primary and secondary alterations of neonatal carnitine metabolism. Semin Perinatol 23:152, 1999.

74. Borum PR: Carnitine in neonatal nutrition. J Child Neurol 10:25, 1995.

75. Shortland GJ, Walter JH, Stroud C, et al: Randomised controlled trial of L-carnitine as a nutritional supplement in preterm infants. Arch Dis Child Fetal Neonat Ed 78:185, 1998.

76. Penn D, Ludwigs B, Schmidt-Sommerfield E, et al: Effect of nutrition on tissue carnitine concentrations in infants of different gestational age. Biol Neonate 47:130, 1985.

77. Penn D, Schmidt-Sommerfield E, Wolf H: Carnitine deficiency in premature infants receiving total parenteral nutrition. Early Hum Dev 4:23, 1980.

78. Schmidt-Sommerfield E, Penn D, Wolf H: Carnitine deficiency in premature infants receiving total parenteral nutrition: Effect of L-carnitine supplementation. J Pediatr 102:931, 1983.

79. Bonner CM, DeBrie KL, Hug G, et al: Effects of parenteral L-carnitine supplementation on fat metabolism and nutrition in premature neonates. J Pediatr 126:287, 1995.

80. Helms RA, Mauer EC, Hay WW, et al: Effect of intravenous carnitine on growth parameters and fat metabolism during parenteral nutrition in neonates. JPEN J Parenter Enteral Nutr 14:448-53, 1990.

81. Campoy C, Bayes R, Peinado JM, et al: Evaluation of carnitine nutritional status in full-term newborn infants. Early Hum Dev 53:S149, 1998.

82. Sulkers EJ, Lefebar HN, Degenhart HJ, et al: Effect of high carnitine supplementation on substrate utilization in low birth weight infants receiving total parenteral nutrition. Am J Clin Nutr 58:889, 1990.

83. Lipsky CL, Spear M: Recent advances in parenteral nutrition. Clin Perinatol 22:141, 1995.

84. Spear ML, Stahl GE, Hamosh M, et al: Effect of heparin dose and infusion rate on lipid clearance and bilirubin binding in premature infants receiving intravenous fat emulsions. J Pediatr 112:94, 1988.

85. Haumont D, Deckelbaum RJ, Richelle M, et al: Plasma lipid and plasma lipoprotein concentrations in low birthweight infants given parenteral nutrition with twenty or ten percent lipid emulsion. J Pediatr 115:787, 1989.

86. Haumont D, Richelle M, Deckelbaum RJ, et al: Effect on liposomal content of lipid emulsions on plasma lipid concentrations in low birthweight infants receiving parenteral nutrition. J Pediatr 121:759, 1992.

87. Goel R, Henderson T, Hamosh M, et al: Clearance of lipid emulsions (10% vs 20%) in relation to enzymes lecithin-cholesterol acyl transferase (LCAT) and lipoprotein lipase (LPL) in very low birthweight (VLBW) infants. Pediatr Res 33:303A, 1993.

88. Stahl G, Spear ML, Hamosh M: Intravenous administration of lipid emulsions to premature infants. Clin Perinatol 13:133, 1986.

89. Putet G: Lipid metabolism of the micropremie. Clin Perinatol 27:57, 2000.

90. Kao LC, Cheng MH, Warburton D: Triglycerides, free fatty acids, free fatty acids/albumin molar ratio, and cholesterol levels in serum of neonates receiving long-term lipid infusions: Controlled trial of continuous and intermittent regimens. J Pediatr 104:429, 1984.

91. Rubin M, Naor N, Sirota L, et al: Are bilirubin and plasma lipid profiles of premature infants dependent on the lipid emulsion infused? J Pediatr Gastroenterol Nutr 21:25, 1995.

92. Spear Ml, Stahl GE, Paul MH, et al: The effect of fifteen hour fat infusions of varying dosage on bilirubin binding the albumin. JPEN J Parenter Enteral Nutr 9:144, 1985.

93. Prasertsom W, Phillipos EZ, Van Aerde JE, Robertson M: Pulmonary vascular resistance during lipid infusion in neonates. Arch Dis Child Fetal Neonatal Ed 74:F95, 1996.

94. Pereira GR, Baumgart S, Bennett MJ, et al: Use of high-fat formula for premature infants with bronchopulmonary dysplasia: Metabolic, pulmonary, and nutritional studies. J Pediatr 124:605, 1994.

95. Brans Y, Dutton E, Drew D, et al: Fat emulsion tolerance in very low birth weight neonates: Effect on diffusion of oxygen in the lungs and on blood pH. Pediatrics 78:79, 1986.

96. Spear ML, Spear M, Cohen AR, et al: Effect of fat infusions on platelet concentration in premature infants. JPEN J Parenter Enteral Nutr 14:165, 1990.

97. Goulet O, Girot R, Maier-Redelsperger M, et al: Hematologic disorders following prolonged use of intravenous fat emulsions in children. JPEN J Parenter Enteral Nutr 10:284, 1986.

98. Heird WC, Gomez MR: Parenteral nutrition. In Tsang RC, Lucas A, Uauy R, Zlotkin S (eds): Nutritional Needs of the Preterm Infant: Scientific Basis and Practical Guidelines. Baltimore, Williams & Wilkins, 1993, pp 225-242.

99. Salmenpera L: Detecting subclinical deficiency of essential trace elements in children with special reference to zinc and selenium. Clin Biochem 30:115, 1997.

100. Zlotkin SH, Atkinson S, Lockitch G: Trace elements in nutrition for premature infants. Clin Perinatol 22:223, 1995.

101. Reifen RM, Zlotkin S: Microminerals. In Tsang R, Lucas A, Uauy R, Zlotkin S (eds): Nutritional Needs of the Preterm Infant: Scientific Basis and Practical Guidelines. Baltimore, Williams & Wilkins, 1993, pp 195-207.

102. Darlow BA, Winterbourn C, Inder TE, et al: The effect of selenium supplementation on outcome in very low birth weight infants: A randomized controlled trial. J Pediatr 136:473, 2000.

103. Huston RK, Jelen BJ, Vidgoff J: Selenium supplementation in low-birthweight premature infants: Relationship to trace metals and antioxidant enzymes. JPEN J Parenter Enteral Nutr 15:556, 1991.

104. Aggett PJ: Trace elements of the micropremie. Clin Perinatol 27:119, 2000.

105. Bishop NJ, Morley R, Day JP, et al: Aluminum neurotoxicity in preterm infants receiving intravenous feeding solutions. N Engl J Med 336:1557, 1997.

106. Mouser JF, Wu AHB, Herson VC: Aluminum contamination of neonatal parenteral nutrient solutions and additives. Am J Health Syst Pharm 55:1071, 1998.

107. Pittard WB, Anderson DM: Neonatal enteral and parenteral nutrition. Pediatr Ann 24:592, 1995.

108. Costarino AT, Gruskay JA, Corcoran L, et al: Sodium restriction versus daily maintenance replacement in very low birth weight premature neonates: A randomized blind therapeutic trial. J Pediatr 120:99, 1992.

109. Koo WWK, Steichen JJ: Osteopenia and rickets of prematurity. In RA Polin, WW Fox (eds): Fetal and Neonatal Physiology, vol 2. Philadelphia, WB Saunders, pp 2235-2249, 1998.

110. Rigo J, De Curtis M, Pieltain C, et al: Bone mineral metabolism in the micropremie. Clin Perinatol 27:147, 2000.

111. Pelagano JF, Rowe JC, Carey DE, et al: Simultaneous infusion of calcium and phosphorus in parenteral nutrition for premature infants: Use of physiologic calcium/phosphorus ratio. J Pediatr 114:115, 1989.

112. Kalhan SC, Saker F: Metabolic and endocrine disorders. In AA Fanaroff, RJ Martin (eds): Neonatal-Perinatal Medicine Diseases of the Fetus and Infant, vol 2. St. Louis: Mosby, 1997, pp 1439-1463.

113. Greer FR: Vitamin metabolism and requirements in the micropremie. Clin Perinatol 27:95, 2000.

114. Whyte RK, Campbell D, Stanhope R, et al: Energy balance in low birth weight infants fed formula of high or low medium-chain triglyceride content. J Pediatr 108:964, 1986.

115. Thureen PJ, Hay WW: Intravenous nutrition and postnatal growth of the micropremie. Clin Perinatol 27:197, 2000.

116. Mitchell IM, Davies PSW, Day JME, et al: Energy expenditure in children with congenital heart disease. J Thorac Cardiovasc Surg 197:374, 1994.

117. Wahlig TM, Georgieff MK: The effects of illness on neonatal metabolism and nutritional management. Clin Perinatol 22:77, 1995.

118. Anand KJS, Phil D, Hansen DD, et al: Hormonal-metabolic stress responses in neonates undergoing cardiac surgery. Anesthesiology 75:661, 1990.

119. Anand KJS, Sippell WG, Aynsley-Green A: Randomised trial of fentanyl anesthaesia in preterm babies undergoing surgery: Effect on the stress response. Lancet 62, 1987.

120. Keshen TH, Jaksic T, Jahoor F: Measurement of the protein metabolic response to surgical stress in extremely-low-birthweight (ELBW) neonates [abstract]. Pediatr Res 41:234A, 1997.

121. Seri I, Evans J: Clinical evaluation of renal and urinary tract disease. In Tausch HW, Ballard RA (eds): Avery's Diseases of the Newborn, 7th ed. Philadelphia, WB Saunders, 1998, pp 1131-1135.

122. Vileisis RA, Sorensen K, Gonzales-Crussi F, et al: Liver malignancy after parenteral nutrition. J Pediatr 100:88, 1982.

123. Patrick CC: Coagulase-negative staphylococci: Pathogens with increasing clinical significance. J Pediatr 116:497, 1990.

124. Beganovic N, Verloove-Vanhorick SP, Brand R, et al: Total parenteral nutrition and sepsis. Arch Dis Child 63:66, 1988.

125. Nicholls JM, Yuen KY, Saing H: *Malassezia furfur* infection in a neonate. Br J Hosp Med 49:425, 1993.

126. Hogan MJ: Neonatal vascular catheters and their complications. Radiol Clin North Am 37:1109, 1999.

127. Rehan VK, Cronin CM, Bowman JM: Neonatal portal vein thrombosis successfully treated by regional streptokinase infusion. Eur J Pediatr 153:456, 1994.

128. Smith PK, Miller DA, Lail S, et al: Urokinase treatment of neonatal aortoiliac thrombosis caused by umbilical artery catheterization: A case report. J Vasc Surg 14:684, 1991.

Congenital Anomalies of the Gastrointestinal Tract

L. Grier Arthur and Marshall Z. Schwartz

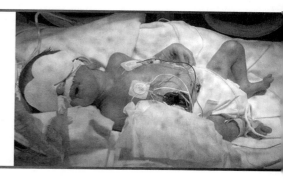

astrointestinal malformations and their complications represent the most common indication for surgical consultation in the neonatal period. Congenital gastrointestinal anomalies in the neonate comprise a broad spectrum of disorders. There is a wide variation in the presentation of gastrointestinal anomalies, ranging from disorders that present suddenly and require urgent surgical intervention to disorders that require more careful evaluation. This chapter provides an overview of the etiology and the clinical manifestations of these disorders and highlights the important diagnostic and treatment strategies for infants with these abnormalities.

EMBRYOLOGY

The primitive midgut begins to elongate by 4 weeks of embryologic development, resulting in the formation of the primary intestinal loop. With the **superior mesenteric artery (SMA)** as its primary blood supply, this intestinal loop can be divided into a prearterial loop, representing the future duodenum and jejunum, and a postarterial loop, which eventually develops into the ileum and colon. During week 6 of development, herniation of the abdominal contents outside the peritoneal cavity occurs. While outside the abdomen, the bowel length increases greatly. In response to the increasing length of the intestine, the intestinal loop normally undergoes a 270-degree counterclockwise rotation around an axis formed by the SMA. This rotation results in the normal location of the second portion of the duodenum to the right of the SMA, the third portion posterior to the SMA, and the duodenojejunal junction to the left and posterior to the SMA. This rotation also eventually leads to the right lower quadrant position of the cecum and a broad-based mesentery from the ligament of Treitz to the ileocecal valve.[1] Between 10 and 11 weeks of development, the intestine returns to the abdominal cavity, where it becomes fixed by peritoneal attachments during the fourth and fifth months of development. Physiologic development of the intestine occurs in the beginning of the second trimester, achieving its normal

anatomic structure by 20 weeks of gestation. The intestine undergoes considerable lengthening and dilation in the third trimester, resulting in a significant increase in surface area for intestinal absorption.[2]

NEONATAL INTESTINAL OBSTRUCTION

Initial Evaluation and Management

Intestinal obstruction is caused by a wide variety of conditions, each having its own specific treatment. Despite the numerous anatomic abnormalities, intestinal obstruction largely presents in the same manner in all infants. There are four cardinal signs of obstruction: maternal polyhydramnios, abdominal distention, bilious vomiting, and failure to pass meconium. **Maternal polyhydramnios** often is noted first on screening ultrasonography at 20 weeks of gestation. Although it has other causes, polyhydramnios is a warning sign that the fetus is not absorbing the normal amount of amniotic fluid. It is seen more commonly with proximal intestinal obstructions and is uncommon in distal small bowel or colonic obstructions. **Abdominal distention** may be present at birth or may develop gradually as air is ingested and is more apparent the more distal the obstruction is located. **Bilious vomiting** is the most consistent sign of intestinal obstruction. The presence of bile indicates an obstruction distal to the ampulla of Vater, where the common bile duct drains into the second portion of the duodenum. Proximal obstructions tend to present with earlier and more frequent episodes of emesis. **Failure to pass meconium** by an infant within the first 12 hours of life is another indication of a possible intestinal obstruction. Passage of meconium does not rule out intestinal obstruction, however.[3,4]

The physical examination in an infant generally does not alter the management, but may influence the timing of surgery. Tympany and associated abdominal distention indicate the presence of air in the bowel. Rarely a mass can be felt, which may suggest an intestinal duplication, mesenteric cyst, or giant cystic meconium peritonitis. Finally, abdominal wall erythema or rebound tenderness indicates peritonitis, bowel perforation, or both. The absence of physical findings does not rule out an obstruction in an infant with radiographic signs of obstruction.[3] In a study by Torres and Ziegler,[2] 50% of infants diagnosed with malrotation at their institution over an 18-month period had a normal physical examination.

Despite the numerous causes of neonatal intestinal obstruction, the initial evaluation and management are similar for most infants. Intestinal obstruction frequently leads to dehydration from emesis and third spacing of fluid into the bowel lumen. Serum electrolytes should be monitored, and aggressive resuscitation should begin with an appropriate electrolyte solution containing adequate sodium chloride and potassium chloride. Careful monitoring of heart rate, blood pressure, urine output, and capillary refill are excellent methods of evaluating the adequacy of the fluid resuscitation. A nasogastric tube should be placed for diagnostic and therapeutic purposes to aspirate air and intestinal fluid and to prevent aspiration of bowel contents. Nasogastric losses also should be replaced at full volume with half-normal saline and 10 to 20 mEq/L of potassium chloride. Although controversial, broad-spectrum antibiotics, such as ampicillin and gentamicin, usually are started in neonates until the cause of the obstruction is determined.[3]

All patients with intestinal obstruction require radiographic evaluation, unless they present with signs of peritonitis indicating that an urgent operation is necessary. Sometimes an initial abdominal series reveals free air, indicating bowel perforation or other classic signs of obstruction, such as a double bubble sign for duodenal obstruction; more frequently, however, radiographs show only air-fluid levels and dilated bowel loops that are consistent with obstruction. Most patients require a contrast-enhanced study. A barium swallow is the diagnostic study of choice if a proximal obstruction is suspected and is mandatory to rule out malrotation in a previously healthy infant who suddenly develops bilious emesis. A barium enema shows more distal bowel obstructions, such as Hirschsprung disease, meconium, ileus, or ileal atresia. Other radiographic studies, such as computed tomography (CT) scanning, ultrasonography, and nuclear medicine studies, have specific indications and are discussed later.

Duodenal Atresia

Duodenal atresia is a relatively common cause of intestinal obstruction that occurs in approximately 1 in 7500 live births. It is thought to be caused by failure of recanalization or vacuolization of the duodenal lumen, which normally occurs between 8 and 10 weeks of gestation. Because this developmental anomaly occurs early in embryologic development and has a different etiology than jejunoileal atresias, duodenal atresia has a much higher incidence of associated anomalies than jejunoileal atresias. Down syndrome occurs in 30% of patients with duodenal atresia. Congenital heart defects occur in 20% to 30% of these patients. Other gastrointestinal abnormalities, such as imperforate anus, tracheoesophageal fistula, and Meckel diverticulum, occur in 26% of patients. Vertebral abnormalities and renal abnormalities

also are common.[3,5] The site of the obstruction is usually at or just distal to the ampulla of Vater, but can present proximally to the ampulla 15% of the time, in which case bile would be absent from the emesis.[3] Duodenal obstruction classically is divided into three types of lesions.[5] The most common lesion is a type 1 defect, which consists of a mucosal web with a normal muscular wall and is referred to as a "wind sock deformity" because of the way the web stretches out in response to the intraluminal pressure created by obstructed fluid. Type 2 defects consist of a short fibrous cord connecting the proximal and distal atretic ends. Type 3 defects are the least common and consist of two completely separated duodenal ends.

Classically, duodenal obstruction presents with polyhydramnios and either bile-stained amniotic fluid or bilious vomiting shortly after the infant's first feeding. With the increasing accuracy of prenatal ultrasonography, however, the diagnosis often can be made in the late second or early third trimester.[6] Physical examination may reveal upper abdominal distention, but often the abdomen appears scaphoid because of the lack of distal air. Passage of meconium can occur despite the intestinal obstruction.[7] Plain abdominal radiographs may show the classic double bubble sign. If air is visualized distally, malrotation must be considered, and an upper gastrointestinal contrast study should be obtained.

After initial management with a nasogastric tube (to prevent aspiration of bilious material) and fluid resuscitation, surgical correction of duodenal atresia can be performed on an elective basis, as long as there is no concomitant malrotation, which occurs in 28% of patients.[8] Definitive management of duodenal atresia is approached through a right upper quadrant transverse incision. A duodenal web (type 1 defect) can be excised using a lateral duodenotomy.[9] Type 2 and 3 defects require surgical bypass. Although gastrojejunostomy and duodenojejunostomy have been described, the standard of care is a diamond-shaped duodenoduodenostomy described by Kimura and coworkers.[10] Before bypassing the atretic segment, it is important to document distal patency of the small bowel by passage of a catheter into the distal segment and the injection of saline until fluid is seen in the colon. Long-term survival after surgical treatment is reported at 95% with most deaths being related to complex congenital heart lesions.[3]

Jejunoileal Atresia

The incidence of atresia of the jejunum and ileum is similar to duodenal atresia (1 in 7500 live births).[9,11] In contrast to duodenal atresia, **jejunoileal atresia** is caused by a vascular accident that interrupts the blood supply to a segment of intestine. This process occurs with equal frequency throughout the small intestine from the ligament of Treitz to the ileocecal valve. The vascular events usually are isolated, but may be caused by abdominal wall defects (18%) or cystic fibrosis (12%).[8] The incidence of associated anomalies in intestinal atresia is equivalent to the normal population and is much lower than with duodenal atresia, probably because of a different etiology and timing of development, as mentioned previously.[11] Several types of atresias have been identified, as follows: type 1, an intraluminal diaphragm in continuity with the proximal and distal intestine (32%); type 2, an atresia with a cord-like segment between blind ends of the bowel (26%); type 3a, an atresia with complete separation of the blind ends of the intestine along with a mesenteric defect (15%); type 3b, an atresia, often referred to as an "apple-core deformity," caused by occlusion of the superior mesenteric artery resulting in the retrograde blood supply to the distal segment of bowel from the ileocolic artery (11%); and type 4, multiple atresias of the small intestine (17%).[3]

Infants with jejunoileal atresia usually present with abdominal distention and bilious vomiting. More proximal obstructions lead to earlier vomiting and less abdominal distention. Normal meconium can be present distal to the atresia, and 20% of infants pass meconium within the first 24 hours. Polyhydramnios on fetal ultrasonography can be an early warning sign of proximal intestinal atresia but is less likely with more distal obstructions. Plain abdominal radiographs reveal dilated bowel loops and air-fluid levels consistent with an obstruction. If distal ileal atresia is suspected, a contrast enema is the diagnostic test of choice. The water-soluble contrast enema localizes the site of the obstruction and differentiates small bowel atresia from meconium ileus. It also is helpful in diagnosing meconium plug syndrome, colonic atresia, and possibly Hirschsprung's disease.

Surgical treatment of jejunoileal atresia is usually semielective when a nasogastric tube has been placed and adequate fluid resuscitation has been initiated. A laparotomy through a transverse supraumbilical incision is the approach employed by most pediatric surgeons. A thorough examination of the nature of the defect and how much bowel is involved is necessary before deciding on the best surgical procedure. If the atretic segment involves only a short segment of the intestine, it can be resected and a primary end-to-end anastomosis can be performed. Often the proximal intestinal segment is dilated. In these situations, a limited resection of the most dilated segment helps to size the proximal bowel properly with the smaller, unused distal bowel. In the event of a larger atretic segment, when there is a question of adequate residual intestine to prevent short bowel syndrome from occurring, it may be necessary to perform a bowel-tapering procedure to preserve as much mucosal surface area as possible. Operative mortality for jejunoileal atresia is less than 1%, and long-term survival is 84% with most deaths related to short bowel syndrome and parenteral nutrition dependence.[8]

Malrotation

Malrotation of the intestine occurs by 10 to 12 weeks of embryologic development. There are two types of abnormal intestinal rotation. In nonrotation, the small intestine lies entirely on the right side of the abdomen, and the colon lies on the left. This condition is usually asymptomatic. Incomplete rotation, or malrotation, occurs when the duodenum lacks 90 degrees of the normal 270-degree rotation, and the cecum lacks 180 degrees of rotation, leaving the duodenum on the right side and the cecum close to the midline with a shortened mesentery in between. Abnormal mesenteric bands extending from the right side

of the peritoneum to the colon, called *Ladd's bands,* can cross over and obstruct the duodenum. Malrotation is associated with midgut volvulus, which can lead quickly to intestinal necrosis and gangrene.

The overall incidence of malrotation is 1 in 500 live births, with approximately two thirds of the cases presenting in the newborn period.[2] Malrotation occurs in all infants with gastroschisis and congenital diaphragmatic hernias because the intestines cannot complete their normal rotation. Other gastrointestinal anomalies frequently are associated with malrotation, such as intestinal atresias, Meckel's diverticulum, Hirschsprung's disease, and persistent cloaca, with intestinal atresias being the most common.

Presentation of malrotation can vary from intermittent, low-volume bilious vomiting from duodenal obstruction to frank peritonitis and bloody diarrhea, when a midgut volvulus causes intestinal infarction. Physical findings can be equally diverse. Infants with malrotation without volvulus may present with bilious emesis or have a normal physical examination and normal abdominal radiographs. This also may be the case in infants with volvulus but without intestinal infarction. If this diagnosis is suspected, a contrast swallow is mandatory to confirm the diagnosis. Infants with midgut volvulus may present with bilious emesis. Later signs may include lethargy, respiratory distress, and generalized abdominal tenderness. To avoid the devastating consequences of a delayed or missed diagnosis of intestinal infarction, malrotation with volvulus must be excluded in any previously healthy infant who presents with the acute onset of bilious vomiting because of the devastating consequences of a delayed or missed diagnosis.

The diagnosis usually begins with abdominal radiographs. Because of the wide range of presentations on plain radiographs—from normal films to multiple air-fluid levels to a nearly gasless abdomen—plain radiographs are not helpful in making this diagnosis. The gold standard diagnostic study is the barium swallow, which identifies the duodenal position on the right side of the abdomen, the location of the ligament of Treitz, and the site and nature of the obstruction (i.e., Ladd's bands or volvulus). A contrast enema may be inaccurate because the cecum can be positioned normally in 20% of patients with malrotation.[2]

Infants with malrotation who have clinical signs of intestinal obstruction or radiographic signs of volvulus should undergo surgical correction as soon as possible. If the diagnosis of midgut volvulus is made, emergent surgery is necessary to untwist the volvulus and reestablish the intestinal blood supply before irreversible intestinal necrosis occurs. The surgical correction incorporates the Ladd procedure and involves several steps. First, the volvulus, if present, is untwisted in a counterclockwise direction. The entire intestine should be examined for signs of ischemia. The base of the small intestinal mesentery is mobilized by division of the Ladd's bands, then broadened by careful dissection of the mesenteric pedicle. This allows the cecum to be placed in the left lower quadrant and the rest of the colon on the left side, whereas the small intestine is placed on the right side. An appendectomy is performed because the abnormal location of the appendix in the left lower quadrant would create confusion should appendicitis occur. If any of the intestine remains frankly necrotic, it should be resected. In cases in which there are long segments of intestine with questionable viability, a second-look laparotomy in 24 to 48 hours should be performed. The outcome after correction depends almost entirely on how much of the intestine is viable. Infants who lose little or no intestine have an excellent prognosis, with their major morbidity being a 5% to 10% lifetime risk of adhesive bowel obstruction. Infants with extensive bowel resections have a much more guarded prognosis and may require long-term parenteral nutrition with its many serious risks, including sepsis, liver damage, venous thrombosis, and vascular access problems.

Meconium Ileus

Meconium ileus occurs when thick abnormal meconium develops in the absence of pancreatic enzymes and becomes inspissated in the terminal ileum. This process leads to small bowel obstruction and can present in a similar way to ileal atresia. Almost every infant with meconium ileus has cystic fibrosis, and 10% to 20% of all patients with cystic fibrosis present initially with intestinal obstruction due to meconium ileus.[3,12]

Meconium ileus can be "simple" if it presents with a bowel obstruction, or it can be "complicated" if it presents with peritonitis from bowel perforation or formation of a meconium cyst. Simple meconium ileus produces symptoms similar to other types of distal neonatal intestinal obstruction, such as bilious vomiting, abdominal distention, and failure to pass meconium. Plain abdominal radiographs show dilated small bowel loops with a ground-glass appearance and absence of air-fluid levels, sometimes referred to as the "soap bubble sign."[12] Confirmatory diagnosis of simple meconium ileus is made with a contrast enema, which shows a small unused colon and meconium pellets obstructing the terminal ileum. In contrast, infants with complicated cases of meconium ileus present with signs of peritonitis and need early operative intervention. Complicated meconium ileus can occur in a variety of ways: complete obstruction due to volvulus or atresia, intestinal perforation causing peritonitis, and severe cases of bowel necrosis that can lead to a large collection of meconium and autodigested bowel (giant meconium cyst).

Treatment of meconium ileus depends on the presentation and complexity of the disease. Simple meconium ileus often can be treated without surgery. A contrast (Gastrografin) enema, which is a hyperosmolar solution, and a wetting agent (Mucomyst) can be mixed and used as an enema under fluoroscopy to clear the intestinal obstruction. In their review of the literature, Rescorla and Grosfeld[12] reported a 55% success rate of nonoperative treatment of uncomplicated meconium ileus, but also an 11% perforation rate. Because this therapy relies on drawing water into the intestinal lumen, it is important to keep infants adequately fluid resuscitated during this treatment to avoid hypotension from intravascular depletion. Failure of nonoperative treatment necessitates operative intervention. There are multiple procedures for operative correction of simple meconium ileus. Mucomyst (diluted to 4% to 5%) can be injected into the lumen of the small intestine, allowing the meconium to be freed from the mucosa and milked into the colon. Another approach is to pass a small tube through the appendix into the terminal ileum to inject the Mucomyst. If the inspissated meconium involves an extensive length of bowel, the proximal intestine is massively dilated, or if there is necrosis and perforation of the intestine, a temporary double-barreled stoma frequently is required.

Meconium Plug Syndrome

Meconium plug syndrome occurs when a segment of meconium obstructs the left colon. Because of its similar nomenclature and its similar presentation, this entity often is confused with meconium ileus. Cystic fibrosis is a rare cause of meconium plug syndrome; most cases are idiopathic and nonrecurring. Hypoglycemia, elevated magnesium levels, infants of diabetic mothers, and prematurity are known to be associated with this syndrome, however. Water-soluble contrast enemas are diagnostic of meconium plug syndrome and usually serve to loosen the obstructing plug. Patients with meconium plug rarely require surgical intervention, but in these unusual cases cystic fibrosis and Hirschsprung's disease should be ruled out.

Hirschsprung's Disease

Hirschsprung's disease is a developmental anomaly caused by failure of neural crest cell migration in the gastrointestinal tract resulting in the absence of ganglion cells in the myenteric and submucosal plexuses. The exact location where the ganglion cells are absent varies from the typical rectosigmoid location to the more rare cases of aganglionosis that involve the entire colon and even the small bowel. The incidence is approximately 1 in 5000 live births. Males are four times more likely to be affected with Hirschsprung's disease than females.[4]

Research has shown that Hirschsprung's disease is an inherited disorder, but that simple mendelian inheritance is rarely observed.[13,14] Several genes have been shown to be involved in the pathogenesis of Hirschsprung's disease. Mutations in the RET proto-oncogene on chromosome 10 account for approximately 50% of the familial cases of Hirschsprung's disease and a smaller percentage of the sporadic cases (15% to 35%).[13] Mutations in RET have a higher prevalence in long segment disease (70% to 80%) than in short segment disease (17% to 38%).[13] RET proto-oncogene mutations also are associated with multiple endocrine neoplasia type 2 tumors so that a small subset of families has a history of multiple endocrine neoplasia type 2 and Hirschsprung's disease. Mutations in genes coding for two RET ligands, glial cell line–derived neurotropic factor and neurturin, also have been implicated in the pathogenesis of Hirschsprung's disease.[14] Three endothelin genes on chromosome 13 also have been found to have an association with Hirschsprung's disease.[13,14] Finally, Hirschsprung's disease is found to be associated with several syndromes, including Down syndrome, Waardenburg syndrome type 4, Smith-Lemli-Opitz syndrome, and X-linked hydrocephalus.[13]

Hirschsprung's disease should be suspected when infants fail to pass meconium within the first 24 hours after birth. Side effects of Hirschsprung's disease include abdominal distention, bilious vomiting, and enterocolitis. Infants who escape diagnosis, either because of shortened hospital stays or because of passage of a small amount of meconium, generally are diagnosed based on a history of constipation within the first 2 years of life. Occasionally, patients with Hirschsprung's disease present as children or teenagers with chronic constipation and failure to thrive.

Development of enterocolitis is a major cause of morbidity and mortality in patients with Hirschsprung's disease and has an incidence of approximately 25%. It occurs most commonly before the diagnosis of Hirschsprung's disease. Infants with Hirschsprung's enterocolitis show symptoms of abdominal distention, fever, foul-smelling stool, lethargy, rectal bleeding, and shock. Bacterial overgrowth from colonic stasis is thought to be the causative factor in this enterocolitis, but at present the pathophysiology of this entity is unknown.[15] Because of the differences in severity of symptoms, a grading system was developed by Elhalaby and colleagues.[16] Grade I enterocolitis involves mild explosive diarrhea and mild or moderate abdominal distention without systemic manifestations. Patients with grade II enterocolitis show moderately explosive diarrhea, severe abdominal distention, and mild systemic manifestations. Grade III enterocolitis involves severe explosive diarrhea, marked abdominal distention, and shock or impending shock. Several factors place infants with Hirschsprung's disease at risk for developing Hirschsprung's enterocolitis. Infants who escape diagnosis of Hirschsprung's disease are at higher risk for developing enterocolitis. Increased length of the aganglionic segment also has been shown to place infants at risk for enterocolitis. Other risk factors include infants with trisomy 21 and infants who have had previous episodes of enterocolitis, although the latter is disputed.[17]

Abdominal radiographs, contrast enemas, or anorectal manometry can suggest the diagnosis of Hirschsprung's disease. Rectal biopsy is necessary, however, to establish a definitive diagnosis. Abdominal radiographs usually are the first diagnostic test ordered when infants fail to pass meconium. In neonates, abdominal radiographs show air-filled and distended bowel loops, but because it is difficult to differentiate between colon and small intestine early in infancy, it is difficult to differentiate the level of the intestinal obstruction. Abdominal radiographs also are useful in the diagnosis of enterocolitis and show significantly dilated intestine with a "cutoff sign," typically in the rectosigmoid region with no distal air. This finding is shown in 74% of patients with enterocolitis.[18] Contrast enemas usually show a dilated colon with a transition zone. The classic transition zone may not appear in infants with total colonic aganglionosis or in neonates who have not had time to develop the proximal dilation.[15] Anorectal manometry shows failure of relaxation of the internal anal sphincter with rectal distention. Rectal biopsy is the gold standard for diagnosis of Hirschsprung's disease. Usually the diagnosis is made with a suction rectal biopsy, which shows absence of ganglion cells in the distal rectum and increased acetylcholinesterase levels.

When Hirschsprung's disease is diagnosed, broad-spectrum antibiotics are begun. If the infant shows any signs of sepsis or shock, he or she should be brought immediately to the operating room for a leveling colostomy for abdominal decompression. Traditional surgical management for Hirschsprung's disease was a colostomy at the most distal site of the colon that contained normal ganglion cells in the neonatal period, followed by a pull-through procedure when the infant was 6 to 12 months old to allow the colon to be decompressed to its normal caliber before a definitive repair.[15] Coran and Teitelbaum[17] reported their experience with primary endorectal pull-through in 90 patients with good initial functional results. There are at least four types of pull-through procedures. The oldest surgical approach is the Swenson pull-through, which involves a resection of the aganglionic colon and rectum. The Soave procedure is a modification of the Swenson pull-through that involves an endorectal dissection to avoid the pelvic nerves. The Duhamel pull-through involves a retrorectal anastomosis of normally innervated colon with aganglionic rectum. Newer approaches involving laparoscopic techniques or transanal approaches have been developed, but long-term outcomes with these procedures are not available at present.

Most children with Hirschsprung's disease can be completely continent and have normal or near-normal stooling patterns. Mortality in infants with Hirschsprung's disease is low and is usually the result of enterocolitis, which has a 10% to 30% mortality rate.[15] Postoperative morbidity involves anastomotic leaks (5%), anastomotic strictures (5% to 10%), pelvic abscess (5%), and intestinal obstruction (5%).[15]

OMPHALOMESENTERIC DUCT REMNANTS

The **omphalomesenteric duct**, or vitelline duct, is a remnant of the embryonic yolk sac. The various forms of persistence of this structure represent some of the most common postnatal anomalies of the gastrointestinal tract and occur in 1% to 4% of all infants. The most common of the five types of omphalomesenteric duct remnants is **Meckel's diverticulum**, a small outpouching of intestine arising from the antimesenteric border of the distal ileum. Meckel's diverticula constitute about 85% of the cases of omphalomesenteric duct remnants and are found in 2% to 3% of all infants. The next most common omphalomesenteric duct abnormality is a solid cord or band between the distal ileum and the umbilicus. This abnormality constitutes about 10% of the cases of omphalomesenteric duct remnants and usually presents as an intestinal obstruction due to an internal hernia or twisting of small intestine around the band. Patent omphalomesenteric ducts, which retain a connection between the ileum and the umbilicus, make up approximately 3% to 6% of these remnants. Males predominate by a ratio of 5:1 with this abnormality, and one third of patients have ectopic gastric mucosa in these tracts. Diagnosis of this abnormality usually can be made on physical examination, which reveals an opening that is draining intestinal contents. The diagnosis can be confirmed by injection of contrast material into the fistulous opening with resultant drainage into the intestinal tract. Treatment involves complete excision of the duct with primary closure of the ileum. Omphalomesenteric cysts and sinuses compose the remainder of the spectrum of omphalomesenteric duct remnants. Cysts usually present with either infection or obstruction, whereas sinuses cause persistent drainage from the umbilicus. Both abnormalities require complete excision for definitive treatment.

Meckel's diverticulum is a true diverticulum involving all four layers of the intestinal wall and typically is located within 40 to 50 cm of the ileocecal valve. Of considerable significance is the frequent presence of ectopic tissue within the diverticulum. Although most diverticula are lined with ileal mucosa, gastric, duodenal, and colonic mucosa and pancreatic and bile duct tissue all have been described. Numerous studies have indicated that in symptomatic patients, 40% to 80% of Meckel's diverticula contain ectopic tissue, with gastric mucosa and pancreatic tissue being the two most common types of tissue to elicit symptoms.[19] Meckel's diverticula typically present with gastrointestinal bleeding, intestinal obstruction, or diverticulitis. Intermittent, painless bleeding per rectum is the most common presentation of symptomatic Meckel's diverticula and usually is caused by a bleeding peptic ulcer due to acid production by ectopic gastric mucosa. There is no documented relationship between a bleeding Meckel's diverticulum and *Helicobacter pylori* infection. Although the bleeding can be excessive if the ulcer is at the site of the embryonic vitelline artery, it usually is self-limited and produces stool described as "currant jelly." Small bowel obstruction is the next most common clinical manifestation of a Meckel's diverticulum. Obstruction occurs most commonly from intussusception but can be secondary to volvulus or protrusion through an indirect inguinal hernia. The presentation is typical of any patient with a small bowel obstruction but rarely is diagnosed preoperatively as a Meckel's diverticulum. Meckel's diverticulitis can present in a manner almost identical to acute appendicitis with pain in the right lower quadrant, fever, nausea, and bilious vomiting. The diagnosis usually is made in the operating room. As is the case with appendicitis, approximately one third of patients present with perforation of the diverticulum.[20,21]

In infants who present with gastrointestinal bleeding, a Meckel's diverticulum should always be considered. In such cases, a Meckel scan, using intravenous technetium-99m pertechnetate, which has an affinity for gastric mucosa, is 95% specific and 85% sensitive for diagnosing a bleeding diverticulum.[22,23] Infants presenting with intestinal obstruction due to an omphalomesenteric duct remnant have abdominal radiographs that show air-fluid levels and small bowel dilation, but the etiology of the obstruction usually is not diagnosed until surgical exploration. Although Meckel's diverticulitis typically disguises its presentation as suspected acute appendicitis and is found only at the time of surgery, an abdominal CT scan, if obtained, can make the diagnosis. Perforated Meckel's diverticulitis can be differentiated from perforated appendicitis because of the presence of free intraperitoneal air, which is rare in patients with appendiceal perforation but common in patients with perforation of a Meckel's diverticulum.[19]

A symptomatic Meckel's diverticulum is treated by surgical removal. If the presenting problem is hemorrhage, the extent of the resection depends on the extent of gastric mucosa within the diverticulum. In general, the ectopic mucosa is limited to the distal portion of the diverticulum, but in some circumstances it can extend to the junction of the ileum or even into the ileum. Laparoscopy has been reported to be successful in a few cases for the diagnosis and surgical excision of a Meckel's diverticulum. The surgical approach for intussusception induced by a Meckel's diverticulum is similar to that for the idiopathic variety. It is unusual, however, for the cause of the intussusception to be known before laparotomy. A surgeon's index of suspicion for an anatomic lead point should be increased in children older than 2 or 3 years of age. If found on exploration, a Meckel's diverticulum should be excised. Meckel's diverticulum involved in small bowel obstructions also should be removed. The optimal management of an asymptomatic diverticulum found incidentally during a laparotomy for another reason is controversial. Some authors believe that a Meckel's diverticulum should always be removed when found, based on the risk of complications from bleeding, perforation, obstruction, and development of neoplasms.[24-27] Authors opposed to incidental diverticulectomy point to the low lifetime risk of development of symptoms related to the presence of a Meckel's diverticulum and the risk of postoperative complications.[20,28-30] We believe that a Meckel's diverticulum can be left in place if it does not contain ectopic tissue and has a broad base, minimizing the chances of complications.

INTESTINAL DUPLICATIONS AND MESENTERIC CYSTS

Intestinal duplications involving the gastrointestinal tract are named for their site of attachment to adjacent normal intestine. As true cysts, the wall of the duplication incorporates all the layers of normal intestine. Most gastrointestinal duplications occur in the small intestine mesentery (50% to 55%), with 19% occurring in the esophagus, 13% occurring in the colonic mesentery, 8% occurring in the stomach, and 5% occurring in the rectum. Intestinal duplications are rare and can occur anywhere from the mouth to the anus. Duplications are thought to occur as random developmental abnormalities, with 85% of cases presenting within the first 2 years of life.

There are two types of duplications, spherical and tubular, and they can present with a wide variety of symptoms. Spherical, or cystic, duplications are the most common and do not communicate with the adjacent normal intestine. This type of duplication typically presents with abdominal discomfort, as a result of their large size or their compression on the adjacent intestine leading to obstruction. Tubular duplications have a similar appearance to intestine and run parallel to the normal bowel. These duplications often communicate with adjacent normal intestine. Although tubular duplications also may present with abdominal discomfort, they differ from cystic duplications in that they also can present with gastrointestinal bleeding. Similar to a Meckel's diverticulum, the gastrointestinal bleeding is secondary to ectopic gastric mucosa that ulcerates the adjacent intestinal mucosa. Both types of cysts can present with the acute onset of abdominal pain when the bowel and duplication twist. If not corrected urgently, intestinal necrosis can occur.

Symptoms are further varied by the location of the duplication. Duplication cysts involving the stomach or duodenum frequently present with vomiting from gastric outlet obstruction. The most common presentation for duplications of the small intestine is a bowel obstruction. As stated previously, gastrointestinal bleeding from ectopic gastric mucosa also can occur. Finally, perforation of the bowel at the site of an ulcer can result in acute abdominal pain with peritoneal signs. Cystic colonic duplications can obstruct the adjacent colon, but usually take longer to present because of the larger diameter of the normal colon.

In general, the management of intestinal duplications is by surgical excision. Because these structures are benign, however, excision must be undertaken with consideration of removing the least amount of normal adjacent or attached intestine. Surgical excision of intestinal duplications is complicated by the fact that the duplication shares the same blood supply with the adjacent normal intestine. In the case of cystic duplications, the size of the cyst determines the feasibility of the resection. Typically the cyst involves a minimal amount of normal intestine and can be excised completely without any untoward effects. Gastric and duodenal cysts or giant cysts present a more complicated situation. When resection of the adjacent bowel is impossible, the cyst may be opened. As much of the cyst wall as possible is removed without interrupting the blood supply, and the lining of the remaining cyst wall is excised.

Tubular duplications are often more difficult to manage, but the same principles as cystic duplications apply. Relatively short tubular duplications that do not result in the removal of a significant amount of small or large intestine can be excised completely. Larger duplications without abnormal gastric mucosa can be connected at one or more sites to the adjacent intestine. If gastric mucosa is present in a segment of the duplication, that segment must be excised because of the risk of bleeding or perforation.

Mesenteric cysts develop in the abdominal cavity, are not related to the bowel, and do not have epithelial linings. They can occur in the small bowel mesentery (50%), the colonic mesentery (15%), the retroperitoneum (20%), and the omentum (15%). These cysts can be unilocular or multilocular. Mesenteric cysts can present in one of three ways: vomiting from intestinal obstruction; pain secondary to bleeding within the cyst or twisting of peritoneal structures around the cyst; and intestinal bleeding if the cyst erodes into the intestinal lumen. The diagnosis usually can be made by ultrasonography or CT scanning.

Most mesenteric cysts can be excised with minimal resection of the surrounding normal tissue. In the rare circumstances when the cyst is too large to be excised, the cyst can be opened, allowing cystic fluid to drain into the peritoneal cavity, where it is absorbed. Omental cysts are removed easily along with the adjacent fat. Retroperitoneal cysts can be the most difficult of the nonduplication cysts to manage, especially if they are multiloculated. If complete removal is impossible, partial removal is indicated despite a moderate risk of recurrence.

The prognosis of patients with intestinal duplications and mesenteric cysts is generally excellent, especially with more recent advances. Improved fetal ultrasonography often can identify these cystic structures before birth. Prenatal identification is advantageous because the cyst can be followed radiologically and excised before complications arise. Laparoscopic techniques have also made surgical removal of these structures less invasive, leading to shorter hospital stays and less postoperative discomfort.

ANORECTAL MALFORMATIONS

Imperforate anus and **cloacal malformations** represent a continuum of anatomic abnormalities of the anorectum, which have serious implications on bowel and bladder control. The incidence of anorectal malformations is approximately 1 in 5000 live births. Males have a slightly increased risk of having an anorectal anomaly, but high anomalies are at least twice as common.[15] Anorectal malformations belong to the group of disorders represented by the **VACTERL** association. Vertebral defects, such as sacral dysplasia or agenesis, can lead to higher rates of urinary or fecal incontinence.[15] Cardiac abnormalities can be immediately life-threatening and represent one of the major risk factors for death in infants with imperforate anus. Tracheo*e*sophageal anomalies occur in about 10% of patients with anorectal malformations. Renal malformations represent the most common abnormalities associated with anorectal malformations found in 50% of the patients.[31] Limb or other skeletal abnormalities also are included in this association.

Of the several classification systems for anorectal malformations, one described by Peña and Hong[31] in a review of anorectal malformations is the most useful because it is based on long-term outcome after surgical repair. Perineal fistulas in males and females represent the lowest anorectal defects and have the best long-term prognosis. In Peña and Hong's[31] series of almost 1200 patients, they reported that 100% of these patients achieve complete fecal control. Rectal atresia or stenosis is a rare abnormality occurring in 1% of patients with anorectal anomalies. Infants with this abnormality have a normal anal canal without an opening. Similar to infants with perineal fistulas, the prognosis for complete bowel control is excellent. Low imperforate anus without a fistula occurs in 5% of patients, with approximately 50% of these patients also having Down syndrome.[31] According to Peña and Hong,[31] because most of these patients have normal anal sphincters, 80% to 90% of them achieve normal bowel control, including patients with Down syndrome. Rectourethral fistulas are the most common anorectal anomalies in males. The prognosis for bowel control in this disorder depends on where the communication between the anus and the urethra is located. When the fistula opens below the level of the prostate, 81% of patients achieve bowel control, whereas patients with prostatic rectourethral fistulas have only a 70% rate of achieving bowel control by age 3 years. The most common anomaly in females is a vestibular fistula, in which the rectum opens immediately posterior to the vagina. Results with this abnormality are good with 93% of patients achieving fecal control. Rectobladder fistulas are the highest anomaly, and only 30% of these patients are fecally continent by age 3 years.[31] In females, the highest defect is the cloaca, in which the urethra, the vagina, and the rectum are fused together as one opening in the perineum. Females with a common channel less than 3 cm in length achieve bowel control 80% of the time, whereas female patients who have a common channel longer than 3 cm have only a 55% chance of achieving bowel control.[31]

Diagnosis of the precise anatomic abnormality in all anorectal malformations is important for prognostic and therapeutic reasons and can be challenging. Physical examination of the perineal area can provide several clues regarding the nature of the defect. Infants with a normal midline crease and a dimple in the area where the anus normally should be usually have a low imperforate anus. Similarly, infants with a thin fold of skin over an anal dimple, the so-called bucket-handle deformity, also typically have a low imperforate anus frequently associated with a fistula that can be managed definitively in the newborn period. A flat perineum and buttocks with no midline groove or anal dimple usually imply a high imperforate anus and probably significant innervation defects.[31] Another sign of a high defect is the absence of external sphincter contraction with cutaneous stimulation.[15] The classic radiographic test for imperforate anus is the Wangenstein-Rice invertogram. In the original description, the infant was held upside down, which is no longer done. The procedure is now performed with the infant in the prone position, and a lateral radiograph of the pelvis is taken to determine the location of the rectum by determining the location of air in the rectum. It is important to wait 12 to 24 hours before performing this study to allow the intraluminal air to move to its most distal point and to allow the meconium to pass through a fistula that may not have been evident initially.[31] Premature decisions based on early diagnostic studies often lead to incorrect assessments of the level of the rectum and inappropriate therapeutic procedures. Ultrasonography and, more recently, magnetic resonance imaging have become important diagnostic tools in the assessment of imperforate anus. These noninvasive studies can also determine if infants have hydronephrosis or hydrocolpos, two common features of infants with anorectal malformations, and can show the location of the muscles of continence and assess the lumbosacral spine. A voiding cystourethrogram or vaginal contrast study often shows the fistula. Similarly a distal colostogram through the mucous fistula can be used to establish the exact level of the fistula after a diverting colostomy. During the first 24 hours after birth that are required to make an accurate assessment of the anatomic variation of each infant's anorectal malformation, it is important to determine if the infant has any associated abnormalities. An echocardiogram should be obtained to rule out any cardiac abnormalities, sacral radiographs should be obtained to assess if there are any vertebral abnormalities, and one should attempt to pass a nasogastric tube into the stomach. If the tube does not pass, a chest radiograph should be obtained to determine if esophageal atresia with tracheoesophageal fistula is present.

Treatment approaches to anorectal malformations are based on the level of the distal rectum. Typically, infants with a perineal fistula do not require a diverting colostomy before an anoplasty to place the anus in the correct position. In all other anorectal malformations, the standard of care in the past has been to correct the abnormality using a three-stage approach. Traditionally a diverting colostomy was performed followed by definitive surgical treatment with a posterior sagittal approach when the child was 6 to 12 months old and subsequent colostomy closure. More recently, pediatric surgeons have attempted to perform a primary repair without a diverting colostomy. In Peña and Hong's[31] most recent review, they pointed out that primary repairs with or without laparoscopic assistance have been performed. A colostomy followed by the posterior sagittal repair has excellent long-term functional results. However, whereas primary repairs lack an established track record, Peña and Hong[31] pointed out that primary repair must be performed without the benefit of a distal colostogram and can lead to operative complications. These include injury to the vas deferens, the seminal vessels, the posterior urethra, or the ectopic ureters.[31]

Peña and Hong's[31] review of 1200 patients showed that approximately 75% of patients have voluntary bowel movements by age 3 years, with about half of these patients having occasional incontinence. The other 25% of patients were completely incontinent. Long-term treatment of patients with incontinence is successful using a bowel management regimen. These patients use daily enemas to keep themselves clean so that almost all patients can be kept clean of stool after surgical correction of anorectal malformations.[31]

References

1. Sadler TW: Langman's Medical Embryology, 6th ed. Baltimore, Williams & Wilkins, 1990.
2. Torres A, Ziegler M: Malrotation of the intestine. World J Surg 17:326, 1993.
3. Kays D: Surgical conditions of the neonatal intestinal tract. Clin Perinatol 23:353, 1996.
4. Arensman R, Bambini D, Almond P: Pediatric Surgery. Georgetown, Tex, Landes Bioscience, 2000.
5. Grosfeld J, Rescorla F: Duodenal atresia and stenosis: Reassessment of treatment and outcome based on antenatal diagnosis, pathologic variance, and long-term follow-up. World J Surg 17:301, 1993.
6. Langer J, Adzick N, Filly R, et al: Gastrointestinal tract obstruction in the fetus. Arch Surg 124:1183, 1989.
7. Nixon H: Duodenal atresia. Br J Hosp Med 41:134, 1989.
8. Dalla Vecchia L, Grosfeld J, West K, et al: Intestinal atresia and stenosis. Arch Surg 133:490, 1998.
9. Dillon P, Cilley R: Newborn surgical emergencies; gastrointestinal anomalies, abdominal wall defects. Pediatr Clin North Am 40:1289, 1993.
10. Kimura K, Nishijima E, Muraji T, et al: Diamond-shaped anastomosis for duodenal atresia: An experience with 44 patients over 15 years. J Pediatr Surg 25:977, 1990.
11. Davenport M, Bianchi A: Congenital intestinal atresia. Br J Hosp Med 44:174, 1990.
12. Rescorla F, Grosfeld J: Contemporary management of meconium ileus. World J Surg 17:318, 1993.

13. Parisi M, Kapur R: Genetics of Hirschsprung's disease. Curr Opin Pediatr 12:610, 2000.
14. Martucciello G, Ceccherini I, Lerone M, Jasonni V: Pathogenesis of Hirschsprung's disease. J Pediatr Surg 35:1017, 2000.
15. Oldham K, Coran A, Wesley J: Pediatric abdomen. In Greenfield L, Mulholland M, Oldham K, et al (eds): Surgery: Scientific Principles and Practice. Philadelphia, Lippincott-Raven, 1997, pp 2028-2101.
16. Elhalaby E, Teitelbaum D, Coran A, et al: Enterocolitis associated with Hirschsprung's disease: A clinical histopathological correlative study. J Pediatr Surg 30:1023, 1995.
17. Coran A, Teitelbaum D: Recent advances in the management of Hirschsprung's disease. Am J Surg 180:382, 2000.
18. Elhalaby E, Coran A, Blane C, et al: Enterocolitis associated with Hirschsprung's disease: A clinical-radiological characterization based on 168 patients. J Pediatr Surg 30:76, 1995.
19. Schwartz M: Meckel's diverticulum and other omphalomesenteric duct remnants. In Wylie R, Hyams J (eds): Pediatric Gastrointestinal Disease: Pathophysiology, Diagnosis, Management. Philadelphia, WB Saunders, 1999.
20. Soltero M, Bill A: The natural history of Meckel's diverticulum and its relations to incidental removal. Am J Surg 132:168, 1976.
21. Seagram C, Louch R, Stephens C, et al: Meckel's diverticulum: A 10-year review of 218 cases. Can J Surg 11:369, 1968.
22. Anderson G, Sfakianakis G, King D, et al: Hormonal enhancement of technetium-99m pertechnetate uptake in experimental Meckel's diverticulum. J Pediatr Surg 15:900, 1980.
23. Cooney D, Duszynski D, Camboa E, et al: The abdominal technetium scan (a decade of experience). J Pediatr Surg 17:611, 1982.
24. Gray S, Skanddalakis J: Embryology for Surgeons. Philadelphia, WB Saunders, 1972, pp 156-167.
25. Rutherford R, Akers D: Meckel's diverticulum: A review of 148 pediatric patients, with special reference to the pattern of bleeding and mesodiverticular vascular bands. Surgery 59:618, 1966.
26. Arnold JF, Pellicane J: Meckel's diverticulum: A ten year experience. Am Surg 63:354, 1997.
27. Cullen J, Kelley K, Moir CR, et al Surgical management of Meckel's diverticulum: An epidemiologic, population-based study. Ann Surg 220:564, 1994.
28. Amory R: Meckel's diverticulum. In Welch K, Randolph J, Ravitch N, et al (eds): Pediatric Surgery. Chicago, Year Book Medical Publishers, 1986, pp 859-867.
29. Kashi S, Lodge J: Meckel's diverticulum: A continuing dilemma? J R Coll Surg Edinb 40:392, 1995.
30. Mackey WC, Dineen P: A fifty-year experience with Meckel's diverticulum. Surg Gynecol Obstet 156:56, 1983.
31. Peña A, Hong A: Advances in the management of anorectal malformations. Am J Surg 180:370, 2000.

CHAPTER 66

Necrotizing Enterocolitis

Pinchi Srinivasan and Vladimir Burdjalov

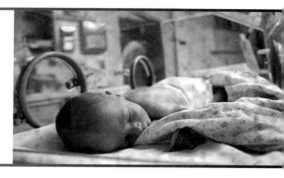

ecrotizing enterocolitis (NEC) is a broad term that was used to describe many intestinal inflammatory conditions of the intestine in the past. Schmid and Quaiser named the condition in the 1960s, although original descriptions of the disease can be traced back to the early 1800s with the report of peritonitis in the fetus.[1] Much progress has been made since the first comprehensive description of the syndrome by Berdon and colleagues[2] in the 1960s. Today, NEC is recognized as a syndrome of diverse etiologies associated with significant neonatal mortality and morbidity. Data from the National Center for Health Statistics and individual institutions suggest an incidence of 1200 to 9600 cases per year in the United States, which result in more than 2600 deaths annually.[3] Many infants have significant morbidity ranging from delayed enteral feeding and prolonged intravenous hyperalimentation to major problems such as sepsis, bowel strictures, and short-gut syndrome.[4,5] The mortality for infants varies from 20% to 30% across centers and varies with birth weight.[6]

NEC is the most common acquired gastrointestinal disease of predominantly premature infants in which the small (most often distal) or large bowel (or both) becomes injured, develops intramural air, and may progress to frank necrosis with perforation.[7] Even in the face of early aggressive treatment, the progression of necrosis can lead to sepsis and death, which is highly characteristic of NEC.

NEC is the most common intestinal emergency in preterm infants, occurring in 1% to 5% of patients admitted to the neonatal intensive care unit (NICU) and in 1 to 3 per 1000 live births. Despite major advances in neonatal care, there has been no significant reduction in the incidence or mortality of NEC. The case-fatality rate for infants weighing less than 1500 g is 10% to 50%, depending on the severity.[8,9]

Advanced cases of NEC may cause multisystem organ failure.[10] About 20% to 60% of patients require surgical treatment.[11] At least 80% of patients are preterm or have low birth weight or very low birth weight (VLBW), and the incidence of the disease is inversely proportional to the gestational age.[7,12,13] The reported incidence of NEC in VLBW infants varies widely across the world: 1% to 2% in Japan, 7% in Austria, 14% in Argentina, and 28% in Hong Kong.[14-16]

EPIDEMIOLOGY

The routine use of antenatal steroids and prophylactic surfactant has resulted in the survival of greater numbers of VLBW infants, and these extremely preterm infants present the greatest challenge in the clinical management of NEC. NEC is a disease of medical progress, in that more VLBW neonates are surviving than ever before and are the group that is most susceptible to this potentially devastating disease. The more immature the infant is at birth, the greater the risk of acquiring NEC. In the United States, NEC is diagnosed in 6% to 11% of premature infants born weighing less than 1500 g.[17-19] Within the United States, there is significant variability among neonatal ICUs in the reported incidence.[20]

The incidence of NEC correlates strongly with the degree of prematurity. There is a sharp decrease in the incidence of NEC in infants with a postconceptional age greater than 36 weeks.[21-23] The incidence of NEC is lower in countries that have decreased rates of prematurity. The severity of the disease and the attending complications are greater in infants of extremely low birth weight with more extensive intestinal involvement and higher mortality.[24]

An epidemiologic study by Holman and associates[4] examined trends and risk factors for infant mortality associated with NEC in the United States and showed that singleton infants with low birth weight who were black and male or born to mothers younger than 17 years of age had an increased risk for NEC-associated death. Most studies report an equal distribution of NEC among male and female infants.[25-27]

The age of onset for NEC is inversely related to birth weight and gestational age. NEC is uncommon in term infants, in whom it usually appears within 2 to 5 days after birth. In preterm infants, NEC typically manifests at

10 to 15 days after birth.[28] NEC also may occur as early as the first 24 hours of life[29] or as late as 3 months of age.[17,23] Term infants comprise 10% of affected patients.[3,30-32]

ETIOLOGY AND RISK FACTORS

A variety of conditions have been suggested that increase the risk for NEC, although no single factor or combination of factors has been found consistently to predispose a neonate to NEC aside from prematurity.[33] Generally the reasons that NEC affects premature infants are its association with bowel ischemia or colonization with pathogenic bacteria, which may result from decreased mesenteric blood flow, increased metabolic activity of the intestines, and early colonization of the gut with pathogenic organisms. These factors are seen commonly in premature neonates. Specific factors that traditionally have been linked with NEC include peripartum asphyxia, patent ductus arteriosus, treatment with indomethacin, placement of an indwelling umbilical arterial catheter, and decreased umbilical arterial flow in utero.

The most accepted epidemiologic precursors for NEC are prematurity and gastrointestinal feeding.[34] It is suspected that the resultant intestinal mucosal injury may be initiated by many of the different factors mentioned previously, including feeding practices. Even under the overall heading of **gastrointestinal feeding**, various aspects of feeding practices have been implicated as possible causative factors, such as rate of daily enteral volume increase,[35] timing of the first feeding,[36] breast milk versus formula,[37,38] and osmolality of the first feeding.[39] An increased risk of NEC associated with maternal cocaine abuse has been observed in animal models[40,41] and human neonates.[42,43] Chronic placental insufficiency may result in intrauterine growth restriction and altered blood flow to the gastrointestinal tract of the fetus. A greater percentage of cocaine-positive infants with NEC required an operation (70% versus 42% of controls), and their mortality was significantly higher (50% versus 23%). The data from animal studies suggest that the mechanism by which cocaine can predispose the fetus to NEC is complex and poorly understood. Maternal cocaine abuse probably should be considered as a risk factor for the development of NEC.

The cause of NEC remains elusive, although intestinal barrier immaturity is the likely basic underlying defect. Contributing to this barrier immaturity may be decreased mucus production, increased susceptibility to disruption of the epithelial cell layer, decreased repair capacity, decreased tissue antioxidant activity, immature regulation of intestinal blood flow and oxygenation, increased susceptibility to inflammatory mediators, dysfunctional immune response, and abnormal motility. A combination of these factors likely leads to mucosal injury that ultimately progresses to NEC. Despite years of investigation, the etiology remains unclear, and accepted prevention and treatment strategies are lacking.

The multifactorial theory suggests that four key risk factors—prematurity, formula feeding, intestinal ischemia, and bacterial colonization—are important prerequisites for the initiation of intestinal injury in neonates.

Current hypotheses suggest that these risk factors stimulate activation of the inflammatory cascade, which ultimately results in the final common pathway of bowel necrosis that is the hallmark of neonatal NEC. General acceptance of this hypothesis is complicated by the observation that NEC occurs in infants with no identifiable risk factors, in infants who were never fed, and even in healthy full-term infants. Common risk factors identified in full-term infants include cyanotic congenital heart disease,[44] polycythemia, exchange transfusions, umbilical vessel catheters, perinatal asphyxia, maternal preeclampsia, and small size for gestational age.[30]

Although the incidence of neonatal NEC and the mortality stemming from this disease have not improved significantly since the 1970s, many animal and human studies have emerged to help clinicians unfold numerous pathophysiologic abnormalities at the cellular level. A better understanding of this basic information may significantly improve the outcomes of patients with this overwhelming intestinal emergency in the near future.

Based on currently available data, the most promising directions for future research to prevent NEC include investigation of (1) **nitric oxide modulation** of mucosal and vascular protective mechanisms in the developing intestine, in particular the role of arginine supplementation of the diet of preterm infants; (2) **platelet-activating factor (PAF)** receptor antagonists or recombinant PAF-acetylhydrolase in preterm infants; (3) alteration of the nutrient composition of preterm infant formula, in particular as it relates to the lipid composition; (4) dietary supplementation with **growth factors**, such as epidermal growth factor, insulin-like growth factor, and glutamine; (5) **antioxidant administration**, especially glutathione and vitamin E; (6) promotion of intestinal mucus production and addition of mucin to commercially prepared infant formulas; and (7) enhancement of motility with feeding in all premature infants and possible use of erythromycin or other promotility agents in older preterm infants. The initiating and pathogenetic factors may differ in patients of different age groups. In any case, the clinical consequences do not differ substantially in the various patient populations, including infants of extremely low birth weight or extreme prematurity.

PATHOPHYSIOLOGY

NEC has a multifactorial etiology and an incompletely defined pathogenesis. The uniform morphology of the well-established intestinal lesions, representing a late-stage response, is consistent, however, with a common pathogenesis. The current multifactorial theory postulates that the risk factors of prematurity, bacterial colonization, formula feeding, and intestinal ischemia-hypoxia result in the final common pathway of intestinal necrosis.[45] Gastrointestinal host defense is markedly impaired in premature infants.[46] A major challenge in understanding the pathogenesis of NEC in human infants is the lack of the perfect experimental animal model. Although several animal models have been used, most lack some or all of the cardinal features of the human condition.

Several clinical and basic science reports have identified that activation of the inflammatory cascade after the risk factors of ischemia-hypoxia, feeding, and bacterial colonization results in the final common pathway of intestinal necrosis that may occur in this high-risk population.[47,48] Additional human and animal experimentation has defined an important association with the phospholipid inflammatory mediator, PAF, in the pathophysiology of NEC.[49-51]

Prematurity

Prematurity is the most consistent and important risk factor associated with neonatal NEC. Premature animals and humans have an immature mucosal barrier and abnormal mucosal hormone and enzyme function. In addition, young animals have altered mucosal immune function, abnormal intestinal microvascular autoregulation, and inefficient peristalsis. Nonetheless, the specific host defense deficiencies that place the premature infant at risk for NEC are unknown. Animal and human studies have shown significant differences between term and preterm neonates in several aspects of intestinal development and function.

Several key factors contribute to barrier immaturity of young intestine of preterm infants during the processes of physiologic maturation and hormonal activity (Table 66-1).[52] Many aspects of the intestinal host defense system, a complex and important cascade responsible for limiting the invasion of multiple pathogens, are deficient or dysfunctional in preterm infants, including the secretory immunoglobulin A (IgA) response, neutrophil function, macrophage activation, cytokine production and function, and activity of intestinal defensins. Evidence suggests that autoregulation of the microcirculation differs in newborns compared with older animals and that peristalsis, a key physiologic mechanism in the prevention of bacterial overgrowth, is dysfunctional in the preterm neonate.

Table 66–1. Factors Contributing to the Barrier Immaturity of Intestine in Preterm Infants

Ongoing continuous maturation of the mucosal barrier throughout gestation modulated by different growth factors

Suppressed or deficient status of several mucosal enzymes and gastrointestinal hormones in preterm animals/humans

Decreased mucus production/immature mucin composition

Increased susceptibility to disruption of the epithelial cell layer at the cell membrane level

Decreased repair capacity of the epithelial cell layer

Decreased tissue antioxidant activity

Decreased ability to maintain tissue oxygenation secondary to immature regulation of the blood flow and oxygenation

Dysfunctional immune response

Abnormal motility

Intestinal Ischemia

Mesenteric circulation is extremely vulnerable to hemodynamic challenges. Several conditions involving decreased oxygen delivery to the mesenteric circulation are associated with an increased risk of NEC in human infants, including conditions associated with decreased blood oxygen content, such as asphyxia,[31] polycythemia/hyperviscosity, exchange transfusion, and cyanotic congenital heart disease,[53] and conditions associated with decreased mesenteric blood flow, such as intrauterine growth restriction with reversed end-diastolic flow in the umbilical artery[54] and maternal cocaine use.[43] Animal models of NEC showed that hypoxia is associated with development of ischemic bowel necrosis[55] but did not define the mechanism of bowel injury. In these situations, the presentation and clinical progression of disease may be different from that observed in preterm neonates who have NEC.

The role of **intestinal ischemia** in NEC has been studied using animal models and epidemiologic analyses in premature infants.[12,56,57] In animals, complete intestinal ischemia after clamping of the superior mesenteric artery results in only subtle histologic abnormalities, but after reperfusion, severe intestinal necrosis results. In infants, studies have shown that a patent ductus arteriosus (with reduced diastolic blood flow) and the treatment of the ductus with indomethacin (decreased intestinal blood flow through inhibition of cyclooxygenase) increase the risk for NEC.[58] The presence of an umbilical artery catheter or cocaine exposure (both thought to compromise intestinal perfusion) increased the risk for NEC in some studies but not in others. Although the specific mechanisms are unclear, altered intestinal blood flow places the neonate at risk for NEC.

It is known that hypoxic intestinal injury may result in mucosal necrosis with ulceration and sloughing of tissue. It has been speculated that during periods of fetal or neonatal hypoxic-ischemic stress, a reflex similar to that of "diving" mammals during submersion occurs. This reflex allows blood to be shunted from nonvital organs, such as skin, intestine, and kidney, and directed to life-preserving tissue, such as the heart and brain. Redistribution of flow results in decreased mesenteric perfusion, and it is believed to play an important role in premature neonates who develop NEC.[59,60] Physiologic factors that can reduce mesenteric blood flow include polycythemia, severe hypoxemia, and abdominal distention. The final result of any of these events is an increase in mesenteric arterial vascular resistance with intestinal ischemia. In experimental animals, the first signs of hypoxic intestinal injury are noted at the level of the mucosa.[59,61] After an acute hypoxic-ischemic injury, various reperfusion-associated events can result in further damage to the intestinal mucosa, including hypoxic cell damage, production of oxygen-free radicals, and release of inflammatory mediators and cytokines by numerous cells.[62,63] The intestinal injury that results from this process may vary from full mucosal necrosis with ulceration and sloughing of tissue to more subtle defects in the active transport system that result in a malabsorption type of syndrome without the presence of clear histologic changes.[64] In addition to decreased mesenteric oxygen delivery, bacterial colonization of the gastrointestinal tract generally is thought to be an important requisite for the development of NEC.[65] The importance of bacteria in the pathogenesis of NEC can be inferred from the observations that full-blown ischemic bowel necrosis cannot be reproduced in a sterile animal model,[66] and although bowel infarction can occur in the fetus, typical NEC has never been reported as present at birth or in a stillborn infant.[67] Hypoxia and bacterial endotoxin (lipopolysaccharide) might act synergistically to produce more severe bowel injury.[68]

The exact role of oxygen-free radicals during the reperfusion phase of ischemia is unclear. The main cytotoxic action of superoxide results in membrane fragmentation and loss of cellular integrity. Ischemia now is recognized to cause increased capillary permeability and to enhance production of superoxide radicals from "leaky" sites in the mitochondrial electron transport chain. The major source of superoxide in postischemic tissues seems to be the enzyme xanthine oxidase, and many investigators have focused on the protective effects of free-radical scavengers and enzyme inhibitors[69,70] in mucosal ischemia-reperfusion injury.

Enteral Feeding

The important role of **enteral feeding** as a key risk factor for the initiation of neonatal NEC has been well accepted for many years. More than 90% of affected infants who develop NEC do so after the onset of enteric alimentation. After the initial description by Brown and Sweet[71] of a careful feeding regimen that was thought to reduce markedly the risk of NEC in premature infants, few studies have confirmed the benefit of this technique. Hypotheses have considered the importance of formula osmolality and strength; the rate of daily feeding volume advancement; the provision of nutrition by the nasogastric or nasojejunal route; cycling as bolus or continuous infusion of formula; and the differences between preterm formula, term formula, and human milk. Only breastfeeding clearly shows a beneficial role in reducing the incidence of NEC compared with alternative food sources. Because most premature infants receive commercial formula as their source of enteral feedings, it was thought previously that the formula predisposed these infants to the onset of NEC. It was believed that the immune protective factors of human milk either would reduce the severity or would prevent the onset of NEC.[37,72] Hypertonic formula and enteric medications also have been reported as additional agents that can produce direct gut mucosal injury. The role of hypertoxicity has been shown in a prospective investigation of low-birth-weight infants, in which 25% of infants fed a standard cow's milk formula developed NEC compared with 87.5% who were fed an elemental formula of high osmolality (650 mmol).[39]

Premature infants have low levels of lactase (an intestinal sugar-splitting enzyme that converts lactose into dextrose and galactose) and are less able to digest fully all the lactose present in standard formulas. They also may

have many bacterial colonies in their gut. These bacteria can ferment the undigested lactose, producing large quantities of organic acids. It has been hypothesized that these acids, combined with any undigested dietary protein, could induce mucosal damage. The presence of excessive amounts of reducing substances in the stool of patients with NEC is further evidence for the malabsorption of lactose. In addition, the production of large amounts of hydrogen gas by colonic bacteria can produce intestinal distention. This gas production, in conjunction with a paralytic ileus, can increase luminal tension significantly and, as a side effect, cause a decrease in mucosal perfusion, leading to vascular insufficiency and hypoxic mucosal injury.

The precise relationship between enteral alimentation and the occurrence of NEC has not yet been defined clearly, but it still is accepted that the interaction between substrate delivered into the gastrointestinal tract and luminal bacteria plays an important role in the onset of the mucosal injury seen in NEC. Despite many retrospective studies implicating one or another feeding practice with the development of NEC, only the rate of advancement in feeding has received serious attention. In a randomized, controlled, prospective trial by Rayyis and colleagues,[73] preterm infants weighing less than 1500 g were randomized to receive either "slow" feeding advancement of 15 mL/kg/day or "fast" advancement of 35 mL/kg/day. No difference in the incidence of NEC between the groups (13% with the slow regimen versus 9% with the fast regimen) was noted by the authors, but the group randomized to fast advancement regained their birth weights more rapidly. These unexpected findings suggest that VLBW infants may not require as much caution in their feeding regimen as previously suggested, but few neonatologists currently advance feedings rapidly in preterm infants. In another randomized, controlled trial looking at the feeding strategies of four feeding groups that evaluated human milk versus premature formula and continuous nasogastric feeds versus nasogastric bolus, the incidence of NEC was inversely related to the quantity of human milk fed.[74,75]

Several potent bioactive factors in human milk, which are absent in preterm formula preparations, may play a role in modulating the inflammatory cascade and influencing the incidence of NEC. Human milk contains neonatal antigen-specific antibodies (IgA, IgM, and IgG), leukocytes, enzymes, lactoferrin, growth factors, hormones, oligosaccharides, polyunsaturated fatty acids, nucleotides, and specific glycoproteins. All of these compounds have been postulated to alter the mucosal environment, reducing the risk for neonatal NEC.

Bacteria

Considerable circumstantial epidemiologic data suggest that NEC may be caused by **infectious agents**. NEC has been reported to occur in clustered epidemics. During such epidemics, there is a spectrum of disease ranging from benign hemorrhagic colitis to fulminant ileocolonic necrosis. Although epidemics of NEC related to a specific bacterial pathogen have been described, these events are unusual because the disease typically occurs endemically, unrelated to host microbiology. The endemic cases of NEC are not associated consistently with a single infectious agent or with a particularly virulent organism that produces highly damaging toxins or that displays great enteroinvasiveness or enteroaggregative ability.

The presence of bacteria colonizing the intestinal lumen seems to be a prerequisite for the development of NEC because the disease does not occur before the colonization of the intestine by bacteria. In the fetus, whose intestinal contents are sterile, compromise of the blood supply may result in intestinal injury. In the healing process, atresia or stenosis may develop but not typical postnatal NEC. The degree of bacterial overgrowth in NEC seems to exceed that which takes place in other diseases with ischemic bowel. Common pathogens involved and isolated during epidemics include *Escherichia coli*, *Klebsiella pneumoniae*, *Salmonella* spp., and *Staphylococcus epidermidis*. Many outbreaks of NEC have not been associated with any positive cultures. The inability to identify specific agents consistently has led to the hypothesis that NEC may be caused by a toxin-producing organism.[76] Blood culture results are positive in one third of patients with NEC. The gut bacterial flora of premature ICU patients differs from that of full-term, nursing infants.[77] The patient in a hospital has fewer bacterial species and reduced colonization of anaerobic flora, suggesting that overgrowth of specific pathogenic bacteria in certain instances may contribute to the initiation of NEC.

Although studies have suggested that specific pathogenic organisms are associated with NEC clusters, in a case-controlled study of NEC patients, there were no differences in the pattern of gut colonization with potentially pathogenic organisms.[78] In an investigation of stool microflora in infants with extremely low birth weight, Gewolb and coworkers[79] found (1) a paucity of bacterial species in most cases (fewer than three by the first 10 days of life), (2) breast milk increased species diversity, (3) antibiotic therapy reduced species number, and (4) only 1 in 29 patients was colonized by anaerobic bacteria (*Bifidobacterium* or *Lactobacillus* spp.). These findings suggest that these infants are at risk for overgrowth of specific pathogens, which could initiate the inflammatory cascade resulting in NEC.

The organisms commonly noted in the circulation generally reflect the colonic flora. Table 66-2 summarizes the changing epidemiology of the bacteria recovered in blood cultures from patients with NEC. This change probably reflects the changing colonization status of the VLBW infant in ICUs.[37] Between 1955 and 1977, the most common pathogens recovered in blood cultures of patients with NEC were gram-negative enteric bacteria, whereas between 1981 and 1984, *S. epidermidis* was equally common. The emergence of *S. epidermidis* as a neonatal pathogen may be explained in part by the use of broad-spectrum antibiotics that inhibit the growth of other bacteria and facilitate the growth of *S. epidermidis* in the ICU environment. A great percentage of *S. epidermidis* recovered from the feces of preterm infants is likely to be toxin-producing organisms. Further investigation must be conducted before the hypothesis that a toxigenic

Table 66–2. Etiology of Bacteremia in Necrotizing Enterocolitis

Microorganisms	Percent Positive Cultures Before 1977 (%)	Percent Positive Cultures After 1980 (%)
Escherichia coli	56	22
Klebsiella spp.	17	5
Staphylococcus epidermidis	0	24
Clostridium spp.	4	10
Pseudomonas spp.	6	9
Candida spp.	1	2

Compiled from data in Kliegman RM: Neonatal necrotizing enterocolitis: Implications for an infectious disease. Pediatr Clin North Am 26:327, 1979; and Palmer S, Giffin A, Gamsu HR, et al: Outcome of neonatal necrotizing enterocolitis: Results of BAPM/CDSC surveillance study, 1981-1984. Arch Dis Child 64:388, 1989.

bacterium is able to cause a disease such as NEC can be confirmed. At this time, it is likely that the presence of gram-negative bacteria and even gram-positive bacteria, such as *S. epidermidis*, in the blood of infants with NEC is secondary to a process of bacterial translocation from the gastrointestinal mucosa.

Inflammatory Mediators and Inflammatory Cascade

Increasing evidence suggests that the risk factors of NEC—bacterial colonization, intestinal ischemia-hypoxia, and formula feeding—stimulate proinflammatory mediators, which activate a series of events at the cellular level leading to necrosis of the bowel.[21] The role of **inflammatory mediators** in the pathophysiology of NEC has been the focus of many investigators. Experimental evidence has shown that concentrations of chemical mediators—PAF, interleukin-1, interleukin-6, tumor necrosis factor (TNF), nitric oxide, and endothelin—are elevated in circulation or intestinal homogenate in neonates with NEC and in various models of intestinal injury.[45]

The phospholipid inflammatory mediator PAF plays an important role in the pathophysiology of neonatal intestinal injury.[80] Using an experimental model of NEC in newborn rats that develops after formula feeding and asphyxial stress, Caplan and associates[81] showed that (1) intestinal PAF concentrations, intestinal phospholipase A_2 (PAF-synthesizing enzyme) mRNA expression, and intestinal PAF receptor mRNA expression are elevated; (2) PAF receptor antagonist (WEB 2170) reduces the risk of NEC[82]; and (3) PAF-acetylhydrolase (PAF-degrading enzyme present in breast milk but absent in premature formula) reduces the incidence of NEC.[83] Although these results confirm an important role of PAF in this model of intestinal injury, many additional mediators have been implicated in the pathogenesis of the disease. In animal models, many of these mediators cause bowel necrosis after intravenous administration.[51,84] Drugs or antagonists that block the production or effects of these compounds inhibit or ameliorate the initiation of NEC.[85,86]

Finally, NEC is a systemic illness in many cases, with similar signs and symptoms of septic shock attributable to activation of the inflammatory cascade. We were able to reproduce an NEC-like injury using a model of hemorrhagic ischemia-reperfusion in rats. Similar to infants with NEC, there was a remarkable lack of an associated inflammatory infiltration, even in segments where transmural necrosis was evident. Other investigators have found that the ischemic bowel necrosis could be prevented by an inhibitor of leukotriene synthesis, a leukotriene-receptor antagonist, or a calcium channel blocker.[50] The effects of TNF and lipopolysaccharide on PAF production were found to be additive. The combination of these factors causes profound hypotension in addition to intestinal necrosis. This response can be inhibited by the use of PAF antagonists.[84]

The systemic effects of such mediators (TNF, PAF, and other cytokines) are known to result in the usual hematologic and physiologic profiles seen in infants with NEC: neutropenia, thrombocytopenia, metabolic acidosis, increased vascular permeability with edema formation, and hypotension. During the early clinical phase of NEC, thrombocytopenia is common, whereas disseminated intravascular coagulation might not be present. Further research on the precise role of inflammatory mediators in the gut of affected newborns with NEC is the focus of many investigations.

The current hypothesis of the pathogenesis of NEC is complex and multifactorial. Mucosal injury can be produced by a variety of inciting events, including infectious agents, inflammatory mediators, circulatory instability, and enteral feedings. The mucosal injury may produce an ileus and intestinal stasis. All such conditions facilitate the process of bacterial translocation from the lumen of the bowel to mesenteric lymph nodes and potentially to the systemic circulation.[76] The passage of bacteria through the intestinal mucosa may promote the occurrence of mucosal injury and initiate a self-perpetuating cycle in which the net result could be the "ischemic-appearing" hemorrhagic bowel necrosis characterized by pediatric pathologists as NEC.

PATHOLOGY

The pathology of NEC frequently resembles intestinal ischemia-reperfusion injury. Coagulation necrosis, inflammation, and hemorrhage are pathologic hallmarks of NEC. The predominant anatomic lesion in NEC is **coagulative** or **ischemic necrosis.**[67,87] Ischemia occurs in NEC and accounts for the necrosis. The usual site is the ileocolic region, as in any intestinal ischemic lesion at any age. The terminal ileum may be the only part of the intestine affected by the disease. Necrosis involves the small and the large intestine in about 50% of cases and is divided equally according to continuous or discontinuous involvement.[30]

NEC is basically an inflammatory process; the initiating site of the pathophysiology is probably the venule. Intestinal inflammation, affecting about 90% of patients with NEC, has been interpreted as an appropriate host response to necrosis and proliferating bacteria. The location

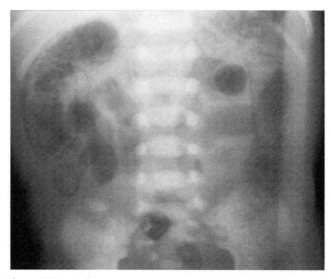

Figure 66–1. Diffuse pneumatosis intestinalis in a premature infant.

and extent of the affected areas (often multiple) are random, and they are not related to the arterial supply. Although at early stages the main histologic change of NEC is coagulative necrosis, inflammatory cell infiltration is the rule when the disease progresses.[30] Intestinal pneumatosis, the peculiar and characteristic finding seen in many cases of NEC (Fig. 66-1), is not observed in infarcts. The character of the cellular inflammatory response tends to be different in colitis of infectious origin and in NEC. Microabscesses and crypt abscesses are common in infectious colitis, but they affect only 10% of patients with NEC. Extensive necrosis, which may far exceed the degree of inflammation, is a feature of NEC that generally is not found in cases of infectious enterocolitis.

The affected bowel is grossly distended, lusterless, and gray or greenish gray, but it may be dark purple or black in areas containing extensive hemorrhage; the soft, fragile wall may perforate when the involvement is severe and transmural. Perforation tends to occur at a junction between normal and necrotic bowel, but it can occur in the midst of a devitalized region; perforation may occur at more than one site. Gas bubbles, which may be grossly visible in the intestinal wall, are reported to involve the entire colon more commonly in the term infant than in the premature infant.[30]

Exudate is ordinarily present on the peritoneal surfaces of the bowel, and in the presence of gangrene, the peritoneal fluid is cloudy and bloody if perforation has occurred. The lumen of the bowel ordinarily contains thick hemorrhagic fluid, and the mucosa displays numerous ulcerations and areas of slough. Microscopy shows great variability, from mucosal edema and hemorrhage to gross infarction and perforation, compatible with coagulation necrosis. Generally, there are widespread areas of mucosal necrosis and infiltration of acute and chronic inflammatory cells. Pneumatosis is seen frequently under the microscope and ordinarily is located in the submucosal region and between muscle layers. Subserosal pneumatosis ordinarily is not seen microscopically because the gas is evacuated before fixation can be accomplished. Bacteria have been identified within the wall of the bowel, although not in large numbers. Thrombi are noted to be distributed widely in small vessels. In severe and rapidly progressive cases, hemorrhagic necrotic lesions can be identified in other organs, such as the liver, spleen, pancreas, adrenals, and kidneys. The entire bowel from Treitz ligament to the transverse colon may be affected by the disease, which may skip areas where it is commonly seen. In general, the histologic findings are similar to findings with other bowel diseases known to be ischemic in origin, such as mesenteric artery occlusion or embolization, and are different from findings seen in infectious colitis or enteritis, in which the characteristic finding is a marked inflammatory reaction. Only a small percentage of infants with NEC have significant acute inflammation.

Reparative changes, including epithelial regeneration, granulation tissue, and fibrosis and usually marked by replacement of the mucosa by a cuboidal or tall epithelium, are more common and appear in cases of NEC that do not progress to full-thickness necrosis or perforation.[88] The development of scar tissue and fibrosis, if circumferential, may progress to stricture formation. This development is especially common in the distal colon and may present several months after the initial disease has resolved.[89]

Pneumatosis intestinalis, the formation of gas bubbles in the wall of the intestine (Fig. 66-2; see also Fig. 66-1),[90] develops largely as a result of the fermentation of intraluminal contents by bacteria and is associated more with NEC than with any other necrotizing condition affecting the intestine. Bacterial production of β-galactosidase, with its role in reducing pH by fermentation of lactose,

has been suggested as a bacterial activity that contributes to the development of NEC.[91] The ability of colonizing bacteria to ferment lactose has not been correlated, however, with the production of NEC.[92]

CLINICAL CHARACTERISTICS

Clinical signs and symptoms are highly variable. Generalized systemic and local gastrointestinal signs and symptoms are encountered in infants with NEC (Table 66-3). The clinical presentation may be characterized by a relatively benign illness with feeding intolerance, abdominal distention, change in stool pattern, or occult stool blood or a more severe illness with abdominal tenderness, grossly bloody stools, worsening respiratory status requiring increased respiratory support, and poor peripheral circulation with shock.

Clinical Observation and Staging

Many infants with NEC in the early stage present with nonspecific findings that can be seen in infants with sepsis from other causes. A typical example is the finding of lethargy, increased number of bradycardic episodes, temperature instability, increased gastric residual, positive reducing substances in the stool, and blood in the stools. Unless a high index of suspicion is present, the initial diagnosis of possible NEC can be missed easily, and appropriate diagnostic radiographs and treatment may be delayed.

The onset of NEC can be sudden or insidious. In the sudden form, abrupt clinical deterioration occurs, which is indistinguishable from sepsis syndrome. This presentation with sudden onset can occur in preterm and full-term infants. The rapidity with which NEC occurs and progresses is remarkable. The clinician often experiences recrimination that "something should have been

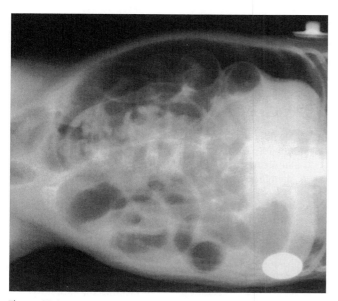

Figure 66-2. Pneumoperitoneum after necrotizing enterocolitis. The radiographic view is a left lateral decubitus film.

Table 66-3. Signs and Symptoms Associated with Necrotizing Enterocolitis

Gastrointestinal	Systemic
Feeding intolerance	Lethargy
Abdominal tenderness	Apnea/respiratory distress
Abdominal distention	requiring increasing
Delayed gastric emptying	respiratory support
with high gastric	Temperature instability
residuals	Acidosis (metabolic and/or
Vomiting	respiratory)
Occult/gross blood	Glucose instability
in stool	Poor perfusion/shock
Change in stool	Disseminated intravascular
pattern/diarrhea	coagulopathy
Abdominal mass	Bacteremia/fungemia
Erythema of abdominal	Multisystem organ failure
wall	Capillary leak syndrome
Bilious drainage from	
enteral feeding tubes	

done earlier." NEC with an insidious onset evolving during 1 or 2 days is more frequent in preterm than full-term infants and is characterized by varying degrees of feeding intolerance, changes in the stooling pattern, or both.

The clinical staging of NEC originally was developed by Bell and associates[93] (Table 66-4) with the purpose of early recognition of this disease and as an indicator for the need of operative intervention. The subsequent modification of this staging by Walsh and Kliegman[94] is a commonly used instrument that has been helpful in the diagnosis and management of NEC. Stage I NEC encompasses a broad spectrum of loosely defined criteria, however, that are not directly diagnostic of intestinal pathologic features. These may represent a myriad of problems, including simple feeding intolerance, sepsis, gastroenteritis, ileus, or metabolic problems. Stage II usually denotes that the infant has radiographic signs, such as pneumatosis intestinalis, that are typical of the disease and denote true intestinal pathologic features. Stage I may be useful in alerting the staff to the possibility that NEC may be developing but is so highly nonspecific that its use as an outcome measure is of questionable benefit. This classification is useful for clinical management and clinical investigations of infants with NEC.

In stage I NEC, the infant manifests abdominal distention (one of the most common signs of NEC), vomiting, increased gastric residual, lethargy, apnea, bradycardia, or guaiac-positive stools. These notoriously nonspecific manifestations suggest the disease, but they give no indication of the status of the bowel or the prognosis. In stage II NEC, the diagnosis is established with the appearance of pneumatosis intestinalis (see Fig. 66-1) or free air in the portal vein. Stage III NEC indicates more advanced disease, as manifested by shock, disseminated intravascular coagulation, acidosis, thrombocytopenia, and intestinal perforation (sometimes) (see Fig. 66-2). Physical findings have not always been reliable indicators that an intestinal catastrophe has occurred because many infants become so lethargic that the abdominal distention is no longer reliable.

DIAGNOSIS

Laboratory Diagnosis

Leukocytosis with a left shift is described frequently, although patients with NEC can present with decreased total white blood cell count (one third of patients) and normal count (one third of patients). Leukopenia is found frequently in the most severely stressed infants. A low absolute granulocyte count indicates poor prognosis.[95,96] Thrombocytopenia probably is caused by increased peripheral destruction. Serial monitoring of platelet counts is the most useful hematologic study in assessing

Table 66–4. Modified Bell's Staging Criteria for Necrotizing Enterocolitis

Stage	Classification	Systemic Signs	Intestinal Signs	Radiologic Signs
IA	Suspected NEC	Temperature instability, apnea, bradycardia	Elevated pregavage residuals, mild abdominal distention, occult blood in stool	Normal or mild ileus
IB	Suspected NEC	Same as IA	Same as IA, plus gross blood in stool	Same as IA
IIA: Mildly ill	Definite NEC	Same as IA	Same as I, plus absent bowel sounds, abdominal tenderness	Ileus, pneumatosis intestinalis
IIB: Moderately ill	Definite NEC	Same as I, plus mild metabolic acidosis, mild thrombocytopenia	Same as I, plus absent bowel sounds, definite abdominal tenderness, abdominal cellulitis, right lower quadrant mass	Same as IIA, plus portal vein gas, with or without ascites
IIIA: Severely ill, bowel intact	Advanced NEC	Same as IIB, plus hypotension, bradycardia, respiratory acidosis, metabolic acidosis, disseminated intravascular coagulation, neutropenia	Same as I and II, plus signs of generalized peritonitis, marked tenderness, and distention of abdomen	Same as IIB, plus definite ascites
IIIB: Severely ill: bowel perforated	Advanced NEC	Same as IIIA	Same as IIIA	Same as IIB, plus pneumoperitoneum

Modified from Walsh MC, Kliegman RM: Necrotizing enterocolitis: Treatment based on staging criteria. Pediatr Clin North Am 33:179; 1986.

infants during the course of NEC.[95] Decreased platelet count (<100 × 10^9/L) or a rapid decline in platelet count has been identified as a poor prognostic factor, although it cannot be used in isolation to predict the extent of the disease or survival rate.[97] In some severe cases, disseminated intravascular coagulation can be observed and usually is associated with a poor outcome. Anemia and a sudden decrease in serum sodium concentration also are characteristic findings.[98] Hyponatremia usually is due to tissue sequestration of sodium.

Acidosis is an indicator of sepsis with decreased tissue perfusion, and arterial pH is frequently less than 7.2. Metabolic acidosis that continues for longer than 4 hours indicates clinical deterioration and, in combination with a sudden decrease in serum sodium level, signifies sepsis with third space fluid loss, probably from intestinal necrosis.[99] Infants with suspected NEC should have serial laboratory determinations, including a complete blood count, pH, and blood gas measurement for assessment of the acid-base status and electrolyte assays.[98]

Investigators have attempted to identify specific markers that would allow early diagnosis and treatment of NEC. To date, although there is significant interest in the measurement of various chemical mediators to predict the disease, there is no consensus as to the utility of any current approach. The value of intestinal (I-) and liver (L-) fatty acid binding protein (FABP) in diagnosing NEC has been examined in two studies.[100,101] These two studies measured I-FABP (a marker of epithelial cell damage) alone[100] and in combination with L-FABP released into the systemic circulation.[101] I-FABP was present in all seven patients with stage III disease compared with only 3 of 24 with stage I NEC in the pilot study by Edelson and associates.[100] Although Guthmann and associates[101] found I-FABP to be a specific test for early detection of intestinal injury leading to severe NEC stage III with L-FABP, it also was a promising marker for stage I of NEC. Nonetheless, in these small studies, it is unclear whether serum I-FABP or L-FABP concentrations would predict NEC with reasonable specificity or sensitivity before the overt presentation of intestinal necrosis. Neither plasma TNF nor interleukin-6 levels have shown any predictive value for disease severity.[102]

Radiographic Imaging

We recommend performing abdominal radiographs every 8 hours during the acute phase of suspected or diagnosed NEC. The plain radiographs should include two views—supine and decubitus view with the right side up—to assess the presence of air-fluid levels and free intraperitoneal gas. The radiologic findings of NEC have been well defined[103-105] (see Chapter 32) and include the following.

Intestinal Distention

Intestinal distention is the earliest and most common radiographic finding,[106] appearing as multiple dilated loops of intestine suggesting a partial intestinal obstruction.

Pneumatosis Intestinalis

Presence of gas in the wall of loops of intestine can be seen as a diffuse pattern or localized to single loops and represents an intramural hydrogen gas resulting from bacterial fermentation (see Fig. 66-1). The pneumatosis intestinalis can be seen in either cystic or linear form. The cystic form has a granular or foamy appearance and frequently is confused with fecal material. It represents gas in the submucosal layer of the bowel. Linear pneumatosis is seen as a small bubble collection within the muscularis or subserosa and forms a thin linear pattern outlining a bowel segment. It can coexist with cystic form or appears soon after. Extensive pneumatosis suggests extensive injury to long segments of gut with a higher mortality.[107] The presence of pneumatosis intestinalis does not indicate poor outcome. It is frequently found to resolve after 24 hours of intravenous antibiotic therapy.

Persistent ("Fixed") Intestinal Loop

Persistent intestinal loops can appear as localized dilated loops of intestine. Prone and decubitus positions are helpful in differentiating a normal dilated intestine from an ischemic noncompliant segment, which suggests intestinal ischemia and must be followed carefully.

Diminishing Bowel Gas

The finding of diminishing bowel gas also is described as asymmetric loops of intestine, which suggest an abnormal motility pattern. In the presence of ischemia, the reported poor motility allows affected loops of bowel to be filled with fluid, resulting in diminished amounts of visualized bowel gas compared with other areas of normal intestine where gas is propelled by peristaltic waves.

Ascites

Plain abdominal radiographs can suggest the presence of ascitic fluid in the abdominal cavity; this finding frequently is associated with a peritoneal inflammatory reaction due to bacterial peritonitis and perforation. It also is considered a grave prognostic sign.

Intrahepatic Portal Vein Gas

In cases of NEC, portal venous gas may be seen on the abdominal radiograph in addition to pneumatosis intestinalis. This finding usually indicates disease with poor outcome.[108] Portal flow toward the liver causes the gas to appear as fine arborizing channels distributed out to the periphery of the liver. It can result from intramural gas absorption into the portal vein circulation.

Pneumoperitoneum or Free Intraabdominal Air

The presence of free air in the peritoneal cavity can vary from small amounts to massive air (see Fig. 66-2). This sign is associated strongly with intestinal perforation. The decubitus view or a cross-table lateral view is helpful in assessing the presence of free intraperitoneal air. When dilated loops of intestine are present, it might be difficult to differentiate between air inside distended loops of intestine versus free intraperitoneal air.

The presence of pneumoperitoneum in a plain abdominal radiograph of a newborn does not always mean NEC with intestinal perforation. Other causes that must be considered include gastric perforations, perforated duodenal ulcer, isolated ileal perforation without other findings of NEC, and meconium plug obstruction with colonic perforation. Pneumoperitoneum without perforation can be seen in mechanically ventilated infants. In such instances, barotrauma produces alveolar rupture, and air dissects into the abdominal cavity through the mediastinum. The particular clinical scenario, signs, symptoms, and laboratory findings often differentiate a particular cause. Buchheit and Stewart[109] showed that the various forms of localized gastrointestinal perforations not associated with NEC are distinctly different in clinical presentation and outcome.

Summary

Occurrence of any one of these findings on abdominal radiographs is not diagnostic of NEC. The clinician must correlate the radiographic findings with laboratory and clinical data to establish an accurate assessment of NEC and its severity.

Abdominal ultrasound has been used increasingly for detection of gangrenous bowel, contained perforation, and portal gas.[110,111] Ultrasound can help identify the presence and character of the intraperitoneal fluid and guide paracentesis. Other imaging techniques, such as barium enema contrast study of the lower gastrointestinal tract, abdominal scans using technetium-99m pyrophosphate, abdominal computed tomography, and magnetic resonance imaging,[112] all have been reported as techniques in the diagnosis of NEC, but such diagnostic procedures are rarely necessary.

MANAGEMENT

The treatment for neonates with NEC takes two forms: early, aggressive medical therapy and surgical intervention, depending on severity and progression of the disease.

Medical Management

The goals of medical treatment are to stabilize the infant and prevent progression of an early form of NEC to the more advanced stage of the disease. This approach ideally is achieved by providing gut rest, eliminating pathogenic bacteria, and correcting hematologic and metabolic abnormalities.

When the diagnosis of NEC is made (suspected or proven), all feedings are stopped, and continuous nasogastric suction using a large double-lumen tube (Replogle) is initiated. Gastrointestinal decompression is important to prevent reduction in intestinal blood flow resulting from increased intraluminal and extraluminal pressure. A complete blood count, serum electrolytes, and blood gases are obtained. Blood cultures are drawn, and broad-spectrum intravenous antibiotics are started, covering gram-positive, gram-negative, and anaerobic bacteria. A typical regimen includes triple antibiotic combinations, such as ampicillin, gentamicin, and clindamycin. To cover resistant coagulase-negative staphylococci, as a common nosocomial flora, some groups empirically add vancomycin to the treatment regimen, substituting it for ampicillin.[113] A high index of suspicion for fungal infection must be maintained, and empirical antifungal therapy should be strongly considered if patients remain symptomatic without an obvious bacterial cause. Intravenous antibiotics are continued for 10 to 14 days, occasionally longer for some gram-negative infections, depending on blood culture results and clinical progress.

Aggressive fluid and electrolyte management and total parenteral nutrition should be initiated via a peripheral or central line to replace ongoing losses and provide essential nutrients. Unless these infants improve rapidly within the first day of treatment, the fluid requirements can be more than two to three times maintenance. Blood and blood product (especially platelets and fresh frozen plasma) transfusions frequently are needed to correct anemia, thrombocytopenia, and developing coagulopathy.[114,115] Correction of metabolic acidosis is important and includes volume and blood pressure support and sodium bicarbonate administration.

Close clinical and laboratory monitoring is essential in the management of patients with NEC. Serial physical examinations are strongly recommended every 4 to 6 hours. Abdominal radiographs are repeated every 6 to 8 hours (including anteroposterior and left lateral decubitus and cross-table lateral views to identify free air),[22] along with a blood count, electrolytes, and acid-base balance assessment.

Over 24 to 48 hours, the disease may stabilize, improve, or progress to advanced stages. Even if infants improve on medical management, they should not have any oral intake for at least 10 to 14 days to allow enough time for mucosal recovery and return of nutrient absorption function from the gastrointestinal tract. When this time has passed, feeding is begun with a dilute electrolyte and glucose solution or diluted formula (e.g., one quarter strength concentration). Amounts and concentrations are increased gradually, at low rates of continuous gastrointestinal infusion, which is advanced slowly as tolerated. Although some centers use protein hydrolysate infant formula, no well-control studies have shown that this formula is more effective than premature infant formula.[116]

If there is any abdominal distention or suspicion of recurrence of NEC after introducing oral feeds, a nasogastric tube is replaced with reinstitution of the measures mentioned previously. Another week of hyperalimentation is prescribed before repeating a trial of feeding. In the event that the infant cannot tolerate oral feeds, an upper gastrointestinal contrast study is performed to assess the presence of any mechanical obstruction, such as an intestinal stricture. A contrast study before initiating the oral feeding or before discharge in asymptomatic patients is advocated by some surgeons[117] but is not supported by others.[118] Successful management of NEC also depends on tight cooperation between neonatal and surgical teams. As soon as NEC is suspected, consultation with a surgical team is necessary to optimize the medical management.

Operative Management

NEC is the most common surgical emergency in the neonatal period.[27,119] Approximately 25% to 60% of newborns with NEC require surgical treatment.[23,27,120] There is no universal agreement, however, on the indications and timing for surgical exploration in NEC. If surgery is going to be required, it is usually necessary within the first 5 days after the initial diagnosis of NEC.

When intestinal ischemia progresses to full-thickness necrosis and eventually to bowel perforation, immediate surgery is indicated. It is preferable to determine the need for operation before intestinal gangrene has progressed to perforation[99] because of high mortality rates for patients with perforation (60%).[121]

Pneumoperitoneum is an absolute indication of intestinal perforation. It is found in approximate 40% of cases.[108] Not all cases of pneumoperitoneum are the result of perforation from NEC—the intestinal perforation could have another etiology or even represent a benign process without need for surgery.[122]

Abdominal paracentesis is considered by some authors to be useful as an indicator of the need for operative intervention and may be repeated frequently.[123] If the free-flowing fluid tapped from the abdomen is brown or hemorrhagic with bacteria seen on Gram stain, the tap is considered positive for gangrenous bowel, and surgery is indicated. In rare cases, a negative result on paracentesis can represent a localized, walled-off perforation.[124]

Additional indicators that the intestinal ischemia is progressing to gangrene and that aggressive medical management is failing include clinical deterioration with increased needs for respiratory support; intractable metabolic acidosis; persistent abdominal tenderness; presence of cellulitis of the anterior abdominal wall with erythema and edema; an abdominal mass suggesting an intraperitoneal abscess or an aggregate of coalesced and infarcted loops of intestine; presence of a fixed, dilated intestinal loop; variable-sized intestinal loops; and severe pneumatosis intestinalis on abdominal radiographs. In a classic updated review by Kosloske,[108] the best indications for progressing intestinal necrosis were pneumoperitoneum, portal vein gas, and positive results on paracentesis. Abdominal wall erythema, an abdominal mass, and fixed dilated loop of bowel on plain radiograph were considered good indicators. Severe pneumatosis intestinalis, clinical deterioration despite aggressive medical management, persistent abdominal tenderness, profuse gastrointestinal bleeding, evidence of ascites on radiograph, and severe thrombocytopenia were only fair indicators for intestinal gangrene. These indicators should be used only in association with other signs as indications for surgical intervention. Portal vein gas, although advocated by some authors as an indication for full-thickness bowel necrosis,[125] is controversial as an indication for surgery.[122]

When a decision to perform surgery has been made, the neonate's condition has to be optimized to maximize his or her ability to withstand the additional stress associated with surgery. Aggressive fluid resuscitation and correction of anemia, thrombocytopenia, acidosis, and coagulopathy should be undertaken before transporting the patient to operating room. Overhydration should be avoided, however, because it may lead to severe intraoperative liver hemorrhage and death.[126] Preoperative resuscitation should not delay the operative procedure and should continue no longer than 1 to 2 hours.

In the operating room, measures to minimize heat and evaporative water losses are paramount. The transition from the neonatal ICU to a warm operating room should be as rapid as possible. A heating mattress should be placed underneath the neonate, and the infant's extremities and head should be covered with an insulating device (e.g., plastic cover, wraparound air device, insulating hat). All irrigation solutions should be kept at 38° C. As much bowel as possible also should be kept inside the peritoneal cavity. To minimize morbidity associated with transfer to operating room, including hypothermia, deterioration in ventilation and oxygenation, and worsening of thrombocytopenia, some surgeons prefer to perform laparotomy in neonatal intensive unit.[127,128]

General rules for surgical management of NEC include precise recognition and resection of only necrotic bowel, while preserving as much as possible of marginal and viable, well-perfused intestine. Diverting stomas are established as needed. Where possible, attempts should be made to preserve the ileocecal valve. The manipulation of the ischemic bowel should be limited to prevent further worsening of translocation and endotoxemia. A generous supraumbilical transverse incision provides good exposure of the abdominal cavity for thorough exploration. Samples of peritoneal fluid should be obtained and sent for Gram stain and for aerobic and anaerobic cultures. The entire gastrointestinal tract is carefully examined for necrosis and perforations from stomach to rectum, with particular attention to the bowel proximal and distal to an area of perforation. The most common site for intestinal perforation secondary to NEC is the ileocecal region. There may be skip areas, with segments of normal-appearing bowel interspersed with gangrenous patches. In most cases, there must be at least 15 cm of viable bowel between areas of necrosis to make salvage worthwhile. Postoperative supportive management can be followed by a second-look operation 24 to 72 hours later if the viability of bowel left behind is questionable. The exact surgical procedure is determined by the surgical pathology, extent of the disease, and the patient's general condition.

Focal Disease

In the case of a single isolated area of necrotic or perforated bowel, a conservative surgical approach is advised. Limited resection of the obviously gangrenous bowel is performed, and a proximal enterostomy with distal mucous fistula is created. The length of bowel protruding from the abdominal wall is usually about 2 cm. A stoma and a mucous fistula are brought out through the same incision, usually in the right lower part of the abdomen potentially to minimize the risk of wound infection. To assess the stoma viability if necessary, the small piece can be excised and the cut observed for bleeding. If the distal bowel cannot be brought out as a mucous fistula, a Hartmann procedure (proximal ileostomy or colostomy leaving the distal bowel, with its lumen closed, inside the abdominal cavity) can be used.

In carefully selected stable patients with a small localized segment of bowel involved and well-perfused remaining intestine, resection with primary anastomosis may be performed. Potential benefits of this procedure are avoidance of the second operation for bowel reconstruction and eliminating the stoma-related complications.[129,130] This technique has a 20% rate of complications, however, including intestinal leaks, strictures, and intraabdominal sepsis,[131] and is strongly discouraged in unstable, fragile patients, especially in VLBW infants.[122,132]

Multisegmental Disease

When multiple areas of bowel necrosis are separated by viable segments (>50% of intestine is viable), there are several options for the operating surgeon. The traditional approach is resection of each individual gangrenous segment with multiple stoma construction. To avoid multiple stomas, a single high enterostomy may be placed and the distal intestine "sliced" together. Proximal enterostomas (usually proximal jejunum) can cause significant fluid and electrolyte losses and peristomal skin complications,[131] which require aggressive fluid and electrolyte replacement therapy and supportive skin care. Another potential complication of this approach is anastomotic strictures, which should be identified and repaired at the time of enterostomy closure.

An alternative technique for extensive bowel involvement with multiple perforations, called "patch, drain, and wait," was developed by Moore.[133] In this approach, perforations are closed by transverse sutures, two transabdominal drains (Penrose drains) are placed, and close observation and monitoring is employed, while providing long-term parenteral nutrition. A potential benefit of this technique is preservation of bowel length, although multiple fistulas occur frequently, requiring additional surgery. In addition, ongoing sepsis is an issue.

A promising novel technique was described by Vaughan and colleagues.[134] In this "clip and drop back" procedure, multiple areas of necrotic bowel are resected, and cut ends are occluded with surgical clips or staples. A second operation is done 48 to 72 hours later, clips are removed, and all segments are anastomosed without stomas. Using this technique may preserve bowel length and avoid multiple stomas. Experience with this approach still is limited, however.

Pan-Involvement (Necrotizing Enterocolitis Totalis)

NEC totalis with involvement of almost the entire small intestine from the ligament of Treitz (<25% of viable bowel) occurs in approximately 10% to 20% of patients, and mortality rates approach 100%.[9,24] This pan-involvement represents a tremendous management problem. A few options are available, including simple closure of the abdomen, resection of the entire necrotic bowel with stomas, and proximal diversion without bowel resection. Simple closure is uniformly fatal, and total resection leads to severe short-gut syndrome.[124] Diverting the intestinal stream by placing a high proximal stoma without bowel resection[135,136] potentially may permit healing of severely injured bowel by providing distal decompression, reducing metabolic demands, and possibly diminishing bacterial load and inflammatory mediators. If the patient survives, subsequent surgeries are required for necrotic bowel resection with special attention to salvage enough bowel to avoid or at least to decrease the degree of short-gut syndrome.

Peritoneal Drainage

Since it was first introduced in 1977 by Ein and colleagues,[137] bedside peritoneal drainage has gained increasing attention in management of neonates and especially extremely premature neonates with perforated NEC. The technique includes placement of one or two Penrose drains into the peritoneal cavity in the right and left lower quadrants under local anesthesia. The clinical course is followed carefully. Drains usually are removed over 7 to 10 days, unless there still is meconium or purulent drainage. If no improvement occurs or the patient's clinical condition continues to deteriorate over 24 to 48 hours, a laparotomy should be performed.[138] There is still no universal agreement about the place of peritoneal drainage in management of NEC. There are many reports of successful treatment of premature neonates with peritoneal drainage alone without the need for subsequent laparotomy.[139-146] Some other studies do not support using peritoneal drainage, however, as a definitive treatment for NEC in most patients.[147-151]

Based on current available data, we believe that bedside peritoneal drainage is a valuable adjunct to surgical management of NEC. As a primary procedure, it should be reserved for unstable premature infants (especially infants with weights <1500 g) with intestinal perforation, severe abdominal distention, and compromised pulmonary function, who are not likely to withstand general anesthesia, laparotomy, and bowel resection.

Stoma Closure

The reconstitution of gastrointestinal continuity is performed when infants are thriving and fully recovered from disease and prematurity. There is no agreement on time, weight, or age at which an enterostomy should be closed. Major factors used to determine the timing of final surgery are time from original operation, stoma output, and rate of the weight gain. In general, enterostomy is closed in 4 weeks to 4 months in otherwise thriving and weight-gaining neonates.[131] In one study done by Musemeche and associates,[152] there was no difference in complication rate after stoma closure was performed less than 3 months after surgery, 3 to 5 months after surgery, and more than 5 months after surgery. There was also no difference in complications if closure was attempted at a body weight less than 2.5 kg, 2.5 to 5 kg, or more than 5 kg. In the case of excessive stoma output (e.g., high jejunostomy) and sufficient bowel length, the early restoration of intestinal continuity (at 4 to 6 weeks) is warranted to prevent failure to thrive. Some patients with insufficient distal ileum and colon length after intestinal reconstruction have severe secretory diarrhea secondary to bile salt malabsorption. These patients may benefit from bile salt binders, such as cholestyramine. Before stoma closure, all patients should undergo contrast radiographic study to rule out strictures.

Outcome and Complications

Over the past decades, survival of neonates with NEC has increased progressively and in different reports varies from 65% to 85%.[9,24,27,120,153] Survival rate in infants weighing less than 1000 g is still lower than in larger premature neonates: 55% versus 84% according to a study by Rowe and colleagues[24] and 56% versus 72% according to a study by Snyder and associates.[9] Mortality rate also largely depends on the number of comorbidities and the severity of multiorgan failure present before surgical intervention.[10,154,155] Improved survival is attributed in large part to better understanding of the pathophysiology of NEC, earlier diagnosis, and improved supportive management of critically sick premature neonates, including novel ventilatory strategies, surfactant therapy, total parenteral nutrition, and advancements in pediatric anesthesiology. Increasingly close cooperation between neonatal and surgical teams also contributes to improvement in NEC outcome.

Postsurgical complications occur in approximately half of all patients undergoing surgical treatment for NEC. Immediate postoperative complications include stoma stenosis, retraction or prolapse, wound infection, and intraabdominal abscess. Although unusual, internal fistulas are noted occasionally as complications of NEC. These fistulas are thought to follow subacute intestinal perforation with drainage into other loops of intestine. When identified, they should be treated by surgical resection and reanastomosis.

Recurrent NEC may occur after medical and surgical treatment with an observed incidence of 4% to 6%.[124,156] A consistent association was not found between recurrence of NEC and type or timing of feeding, the site of the original NEC, or the mode of treatment of the original NEC. In 70% of patients, recurrent attacks of NEC were treated successfully without surgery.

Cholestatic liver disease (direct hyperbilirubinemia, hepatomegaly, elevated level of aminotransferases) is a common complication in patients with NEC. The most common contributing factors are prolonged fasting and long-term total parenteral nutrition. Establishing early enteral feeding with small volumes and continuing total parenteral nutrition promote the intestinal adaptation by providing a trophic effect on intestinal mucosa and stimulating bile flow.

Long-term intestinal complications include strictures, malabsorption, and short-gut syndrome. Intestinal strictures are the most common NEC complications. The reported incidence varies from 9% to 36%.[157,158] It is more frequent after medical treatment than after surgical intervention and results from the healing area of the severe ischemia. The extent of the strictures usually is determined by the amount of intestinal wall involved and blood supply to the area. The most common site for stricture formation is the colon (70%), with the most common colonic site being the splenic flexure (20%).[131] In a few patients, multiple strictures may occur; they are more common after surgical treatment.[159] Because of the risk of stricture causing a distal obstruction, it is recommended to perform a contrast enema before closing an enterostomy.

Malabsorption syndrome has been reported in some infants after NEC, even with normal intestinal length. This result might be related to extensive mucosal injury with decreased absorptive area, enzyme depletion (usually lactase), bacterial overgrowth, and vitamin B_{12} and bile

salt deficiency (in the case of ileal resection). It should be expected to resolve spontaneously, after complete healing and regeneration of the cellular elements have occurred. It is possible that enzymatic secretion and cellular transport mechanisms can be deranged for prolonged periods secondary to the ischemia-reperfusion intestinal injury. Gradual adaptation may take 1 year on modified diets, and constant attention to perianal skin care is important to avoid further complications.

Short-gut syndrome is the most serious long-term gastrointestinal postoperative complication. It is defined as severe malabsorption after significant intestinal resection.[160] It has been estimated that approximately 20% of surviving patients who underwent surgical resection for NEC developed short-gut syndrome.[157] Prognosis for these patients previously was poor, but with advances in parenteral nutrition and dietary management, it has improved some. In the modern era, survival rate ranges from approximately 80% to 95% with most common morbidities being sepsis, bacterial overgrowth, and cholestatic liver disease.[161]

Survivors of NEC remain at high risk for adverse neurodevelopmental outcome. Approximately 50% of infants are neurodevelopmentally normal.[162] It was believed that neurodevelopmental morbidity in patients treated for NEC was related to comorbid conditions and underlying prematurity rather than to NEC itself.[163] Psychological development in VLBW infants who survived NEC was shown to be equivalent to control VLBW infants without NEC.[164] Some studies have shown, however, that the severity of the disease affects growth of patients with NEC, who have lower adjusted body weight and head circumference.[162] Several studies reported worse neurodevelopmental outcome in a cohort of patients who survived after surgical treatment for NEC compared with patients treated medically and a control group without NEC.[165-167] Close long-term neurodevelopmental follow-up of patients treated for NEC is important, and all families of such patients should be consulted appropriately before surgery regarding the risk for neurologic and developmental outcome.

PREVENTION

Despite all advances in medical and surgical management, the best way to decrease morbidity and mortality from NEC remains prevention. Preventive strategies reflect understanding of the pathogenesis of the disease and contributing risk factors. Rational interventions are directed toward restriction of the nosocomial spread of infection, decreasing gastrointestinal bacterial colonization and overgrowth, and augmentation of the host defense mechanisms.

If the disease is confirmed, careful infection control measures should be employed, including cohorting and isolation of patients and contacts, strict handwashing, wearing gloves and gowns, and separate diaper and laundry bags for each patient. These practices have been shown to limit the size of the NEC clusters.[168,169]

The intestine of a premature infant is deficient in protective immunoglobulins, such as secretory IgA and gut-associated IgG, especially in the absence of breast-feeding. Administration of oral IgA-IgG preparations added to infant formulas was shown to reduce the incidence of NEC by Eibl and colleagues[14] based on experience with 179 premature infants, but a systematic review by Foster and Cole[170] did not support that strategy as an effective preventive measure.

Several reports have suggested some success in preventing NEC by administration of enteral antimicrobial agents, including aminoglycosides (kanamycin or gentamicin)[171,172] and especially vancomycin.[16] Because the benefits still are not clear, however, and concern about adverse outcome persists, especially related to the development of resistant bacteria, at present the routine prophylactic administration of oral antibiotics is not recommended.[173]

The acid environment of the stomach affords some degree of protection against bacterial colonization, especially gram-negative bacteria. In premature infants, the stomach may not respond with rapid production of the gastric acid to ingested food. Carron and Egan[174] showed a significantly decreased rate of stomach bacterial colonization and incidence of NEC in a population of premature infants whose formula was acidified to achieve a pH of 2.5 to 3. More studies are needed before recommending it for routine practice.

Antenatal steroid administration has been shown to decrease the incidence of NEC in premature infants whose mothers received steroids in premature labor.[15,175] This finding could result from mucosal cell maturation acceleration, improved gut barrier function, and down-regulation of the inflammatory response by enzymatic degradation of PAF and other inflammatory mediators.[176-178] Whether routine use of postnatal steroids would be an effective strategy for NEC prevention is not known, and it is not recommended, especially given the concern for side effects, including the risk for adverse neurodevelopmental outcome.

Several reports suggested that there is delayed intestinal colonization with anaerobic bacteria of the premature infants requiring intensive care.[179] Lack of such organisms as bifidobacteria and lactobacilli in premature intestine may favor the overgrowth of more pathogenic bacteria, promoting bacterial translocation and contributing to the development of NEC.[180,181] Studies in animal models of NEC showed a reduced incidence of NEC after enteral supplementation with bifidobacteria.[182,183] Several mechanisms may be responsible for the protective role of probiotics in NEC, including modulation of microflora growth and adherence, production of substances toxic to aerobic bacteria, reduction of intraluminal pH, modulation of immune response, promotion of mucosal barrier function, and reduction in mucosal permeability. A large human trial from Columbia[184] reported a significant reduction in incidence of NEC in infants supplemented with *Bifidobacterium infantis* and *Lactobacillus acidophilus* (2.7% versus 6.6% in control group). Additional randomized control trials are needed before this promising approach can be established as a standard of care for premature infants.

About 90% of all infants who develop NEC have been fed enterally.[22,24] This connection could be explained by the fact that, in immature ischemic intestine, undigested formula provides nutritional substrate for bacterial overgrowth, increasing the risk for developing NEC. Many different feeding strategies have been proposed for NEC prevention with variable results, and no interventions have proved to be effective in all cases. We believe, however, that several reasonable measures should be undertaken when considering feeding of premature infants at risk for NEC. Early introduction of feeding with 12 to 24 kcal/oz premature infant formula at low volumes of 12 to 24 mL/kg/day can be started during the first week of life, providing gut stimulation in preparation for an advanced feeding ("trophic feeding").[185-187] Feeding advances at the rate of about 10 to 20 mL/kg/day are considered safe, although more rapid advancement has been reported without resulting in increased incidence of NEC.[73] Addition of hyperosmolar medications and nutritional supplements should be avoided in infants at risk for development of NEC. While advancing feeding in premature infants, one should pay a great deal of attention to the signs of feeding intolerance, such as gastric residuals, abdominal distention, and frequent stools, and have a low threshold for decreasing or stopping feeding.

Human milk has been considered the feeding of choice to prevent NEC in premature infants. Although NEC has been reported in neonates fed breast milk exclusively,[37,188] several studies have shown protective benefits of human milk against NEC.[72,75,189] In one large multicenter study by Lucas and Cole,[38] it was shown that NEC was 6 to 10 times more common in exclusively formula-fed infants than in exclusively breast-fed infants). Protective properties of human milk are thought to be secondary to an array of humoral and cell anti-infectious factors and essential nutrients. Human milk contains antibodies such as IgA and, in small amounts, IgG, many macrophages, lymphocytes, neutrophils, immunoactive proteins such as lysozyme, lactoferrin, interferon, epidermal growth factor, components of complement system, and oligosaccharides. PAF-acetylhydrolase, the enzyme inhibiting PAF, discovered in breast milk,[190] seems to be one of the significant mediators in development of NEC. By providing an acid environment and promoting a competitive growth of bifidobacteria and lactobacilli, human milk also inhibits intestinal colonization with pathogenic bacteria. Because of its protective and nutritional and psychological benefits, breast milk should be provided for feeding of premature infants whenever feasible.

Experimental formula with added egg phospholipids has been evaluated in one human trial.[191] The authors found a sixfold reduction in the incidence of NEC. These phospholipids are a source of mucosal membrane constituents and intestinal surfactant. They consist of arachidonic acid and choline, which have unique membrane protective properties.

Another potentially beneficial nutrient is glutamine, an important metabolic substrate for intestinal tract. It is thought to be capable of augmenting the effect of many growth factors involved in cellular proliferation and repair. Glutamine stores can be depleted during the time of stress in premature infants, especially because parenteral nutrition is not supplied routinely with that nutrient.

Enteral supplementation for VLBW infants resulted in a decreased incidence of sepsis and better feeding tolerance.[192]

At the time of diagnosis of NEC, premature infants have shown a decreased level of arginine compared with unaffected infants.[193] Protective effects of arginine on the gastrointestinal tract were suggested by the importance of this amino acid as a substrate for the generation of vasodilator nitric oxide, glutamine, polyamines, and nucleotides. A report by Amin and colleagues[194] showed beneficial effects of arginine supplementation in the prevention of NEC, with a significantly lower incidence of NEC in infants supplemented with arginine (6.7% versus 27% in placebo control group). Arginine supplementation may play a specific beneficial role in the nutrition of premature infants, especially VLBW premature infants. The exact place for arginine in neonatal care has yet to be determined. Several studies in animal models suggest a possible important role in preventing intestinal injury of such compounds as PAF receptor inhibitors and antagonists[82] and different recombinant growth factors, such as epidermal growth factor[195] and insulin-like growth factor.[196]

REFERENCES

1. Simpson JY: Notices of cases of peritonitis in the foetus in utero. Edinburgh Med Surg J 15:390, 1838.
2. Berdon WE, Grossman H, Baker DH, et al: Necrotizing enterocolitis in the premature infant. Radiology 83:879, 1964.
3. Dimmitt RA, Moss RL: Clinical management of necrotizing enterocolitis. NeoReviews 2:e110, 2001.
4. Holman RC, Stoll BJ, Clarke MJ, Glass RI: The epidemiology of necrotizing enterocolitis infant mortality in the United States. Am J Public Health 87:2026, 1997.
5. Ladd AP, Rescorla FJ, West KW, et al: Long-term follow-up after bowel resection for necrotizing enterocolitis: Factors affecting outcome. J Pediatr Surg 33:967, 1998.
6. Hack M, Horbar J, Malloy M, et al: Very low birthweight outcomes of the National Institute of Child Health and Human Development neonatal network. Pediatrics 87:587, 1991.
7. Kliegman RM, Fanaroff AA: Necrotizing enterocolitis. N Engl J Med 310:1093, 1984.
8. Stoll BJ: Epidemiology of necrotizing enterocolitis. Clin Perinatol 21:205, 1994.
9. Snyder CL, Gittes GK, Murphy JP, et al: Survival after necrotizing enterocolitis in infants weighing less than 1,000 g: 25 years' experience at a single institution. J Pediatr Surg 32:434, 1997.
10. Morecroft JA, Spitz I, Hamilton PA, Holmes SJK: Necrotizing enterocolitis—multisystem organ failure of the newborn? Acta Paediatr 396(suppl):21, 1994.
11. Gupta SK, Burke G, Herson VC: Necrotizing enterocolitis: Laboratory indicators of surgical disease. J Pediatr Surg 29:1472, 1994.
12. Stoll BJ, Kanto WP Jr, Glass RI, et al: Epidemiology of necrotizing enterocolitis: A case control study. J Pediatr 96:447, 1980.
13. De Curtis M, Paone C, Vetrano G, et al: A case control study of necrotizing enterocolitis occurring over 8 years in a neonatal intensive care unit. Eur J Pediatr 146:398, 1987.
14. Eibl MM, Wolf HM, Furnkranz H, et al: Prevention of necrotizing enterocolitis in low birth-weight infants by IgA-IgG feeding. N Engl J Med 319:1, 1988.
15. Halac E, Halac J, Begue EF, et al: Prenatal and postnatal corticosteroid therapy to prevent neonatal necrotizing enterocolitis: A controlled trial. J Pediatr 117:132, 1990.
16. Siu YK, Ng PC, Fung SC, et al: Double blind, randomized, placebo controlled study of oral vancomycin in prevention of necrotizing enterocolitis in preterm, very low birthweight infants. Arch Dis Child Fetal Neonatal Educ 79:105, 1998.
17. Uauy RD, Fanaroff AA, Korones SB, et al: Necrotizing enterocolitis in very low birth weight infants: Biodemographic and clinical correlates. National Institute of Child Health and Human Development Neonatal Research Network. J Pediatr 119:630, 1991.
18. The Vermont-Oxford Trials Network: Very low birth weight outcomes for 1990. Investigators of the Vermont-Oxford Trials Network Database Project. Pediatrics 91:540, 1993.
19. Lemons JA, Bauer CR, Oh W, et al: Very low birth weight outcomes of the National Institute of Child health and human development neonatal research network, January 1995 through December 1996. NICHD Neonatal Research Network. Pediatrics 107:E1, 2001.
20. Hack M, Wright LL, Shankaran S, et al: Very-low-birth-weight outcomes of the National Institute of Child Health and Human Development Neonatal Network, November 1989 to October 1990. Am J Obstet Gynecol 172(2 Pt 1):457, 1995.
21. Kliegman RM: Models of the pathogenesis of necrotizing enterocolitis. J Pediatr 117:S2, 1990.
22. Kliegman RM, Walsh MC: Neonatal necrotizing enterocolitis: Pathogenesis, classification, and spectrum of illness. Curr Probl Pediatr 17:213, 1987.
23. Beeby PJ, Jeffery H: Risk factors for necrotizing enterocolitis: Influence of gestational age. Arch Dis Child 67:432, 1992.
24. Rowe MI, Reblock KK, Kurkchubasche AG, et al: Necrotizing enterocolitis in the extremely low birth weight infants. J Pediatr Surg 29:987, 1994.
25. Bunton GL, Durbin GM, McIntosh N, et al: Necrotizing enterocolitis: Controlled study of 3 years' experience in a neonatal intensive care unit. Arch Dis Child 52:772, 1977.
26. Dykes EH, Gilmour WH, Azmy AF: Prediction of outcome following necrotizing enterocolitis in a neonatal surgical unit. J Pediatr Surg 20:3, 1985.
27. Grosfeld JL, Cheu H, Schlatter M, et al: Changing trends in necrotizing enterocolitis. Ann Surg 214:300, 1991.
28. Hollwarth ME: Necrotizing enterocolitis: An editorial. Acta Paediatr 396(suppl):1, 1994.
29. Thilo EH, Lazarte RA, Hernandez JA: Necrotizing enterocolitis in the first 24 hours of life. Pediatrics 73:476, 1984.
30. Polin RA, Pollack PF, Barlow B, et al: Necrotizing enterocolitis in term infants. J Pediatr 89:460, 1976.
31. Wiswell TE, Robertson CF, Jones TA, et al: Necrotizing enterocolitis in full-term infants: A case-control study. Am J Dis Child 142:532, 1988.
32. Martinez-Tallo E, Claure N, Bancalari E: Necrotizing enterocolitis in full-term or near-term infants: Risk factors. Biol Neonate 71:292, 1997.
33. Brown EG, Sweet AY: Neonatal necrotizing enterocolitis. In Oliver TK (ed): Monographs in Neonatology. New York, Grune & Stratton, 1980.
34. Kliegman RM, Walker WA, Yolken RH: Necrotizing enterocolitis: Research agenda for a disease of unknown etiology and pathogenesis. Pediatr Res 34:701, 1993.

35. Anderson DM, Kliegman RM: The relationship of neonatal alimentation practices to the occurrence of endemic necrotizing enterocolitis. Am J Perinatol 8:62, 1991.

36. McKeown RE, Marsch TD, Amarnath U: Role of delayed feeding and of feeding increments in necrotizing enterocolitis. J Pediatr 121:764, 1992.

37. Kliegman RM, Pittard WB, Fanaroff AA: Necrotizing enterocolitis in neonates fed human milk. J Pediatr 95:450, 1979.

38. Lucas A, Cole TJ: Breast milk and neonatal necrotizing enterocolitis. Lancet 336:1519, 1990.

39. Book LS, Herbert JJ, Atherton SO, Jung AL: Necrotizing enterocolitis in low-birth weight infants fed an elemental formula. J Pediatr 87:602, 1975.

40. Buyukunal C, Kilic N, Dervisoglu S, Altug T: Maternal cocaine abuse resulting in necrotizing enterocolitis—an experimental study in a rat model. Acta Paediatr 396(suppl):91, 1994.

41. Kilic N, Buyukunal C, Dervisoglu S, et al: Maternal cocaine abuse resulting in necrotizing enterocolitis: An experimental study in a rat model: II. Results of perfusion studies. Pediatr Surg Int 16:176, 2000.

42. Lopez SL, Taeusch HW, Findlay RD, Walther FJ: Time of onset of necrotizing enterocolitis in newborn infants with known prenatal cocaine exposure. Clin Pediatr (Phila) 34:424, 1995.

43. Czyrko C, Del Pin CA, O'Neill JA Jr, et al: Maternal cocaine abuse and necrotizing enterocolitis: Outcome and survival. J Pediatr Surg 26:414, 1991.

44. Kliegman RM, Hack M, Jones P, et al: Epidemiologic study of necrotizing enterocolitis among low birth weight infants: Absence of identifiable risk factors. J Pediatr 100:440, 1982.

45. Caplan MS, MacKendrick W: Inflammatory mediators and intestinal injury (review). Clin Perinatol 21:235, 1994.

46. Udall JN Jr: Gastrointestinal host defense and necrotizing enterocolitis. J Pediatr 117:S33, 1990.

47. Nanthakumar NN, Fusunyan RD, Sanderson I, Walker WA: Inflammation in the developing human intestine: A possible pathophysiologic contribution to necrotizing enterocolitis. Proc Natl Acad Sci U S A 97:6043, 2000.

48. Caplan MS, MacKendrick W: Necrotizing enterocolitis: A review of pathogenetic mechanisms and implications for prevention. Pediatr Pathol 13:357, 1993.

49. Caplan MS, Sun XM, Hseuh W, Hageman JR: Role of platelet activating factor and tumor necrosis factor-alpha in neonatal necrotizing enterocolitis. J Pediatr 116:960, 1990.

50. Hsueh W, Caplan MS, Sun X, et al: Platelet-activating factor, tumor necrosis factor, hypoxia and necrotizing enterocolitis. Acta Paediatr 396(suppl):11, 1994.

51. Gonzalez-Crussi F, Hsueh W: Experimental model of ischemic bowel necrosis: The role of platelet-activating factor and endotoxin. Am J Pathol 112:127, 1983.

52. Crissinger KD: Understanding necrotizing enterocolitis—promising directions. Pathophysiology 5:247, 1999.

53. Leung M, Chau K, Hui P, et al: Necrotizing enterocolitis in neonates with symptomatic congenital heart disease. J Pediatr 113:1044, 1988.

54. Hackett GA, Campbell S, Gamsu H, et al: Doppler studies in the growth retarded fetus and prediction of neonatal necrotizing enterocolitis, haemorrhage, and neonatal morbidity. BMJ 294:13, 1987.

55. Hansbrough F, Priebe CJ, Falterman KW, et al: Pathogenesis of early necrotizing enterocolitis in the hypoxic neonatal dog. Am J Surg 145:169, 1983.

56. Nowicki PT, Hansen NB, Hayes JR, et al: Intestinal blood flow and O2 uptake during hypoxemia in the newborn piglet. Am J Physiol 251:G19, 1986.

57. Nowicki PT, Miller CE: Autoregulation in the developing postnatal intestinal circulation. Am J Physiol 254:G189, 1988.

58. Grosfeld JL, Chaet M, Molinari F, et al: Increased risk of necrotizing enterocolitis in premature infants with patent ductus arteriosus treated with indomethacin. Ann Surg 224:350, 1996.

59. Harrison MW, Connell RS, Campbell JR, et al: Microcirculatory changes in the gastrointestinal tract of the hypoxic puppy: An electron microscope study. J Pediatr Surg 10:599, 1975.

60. Krasna IH, Howell C, Vega A, et al: A mouse model for the study of necrotizing enterocolitis. J Pediatr Surg 21:26, 1986.

61. Touloukian RJ, Posch JN, Spencer R: The pathogenesis of ischemic gastroenterocolitis of the neonate: Selective gut mucosal ischemia in asphyxiated neonatal piglets. J Pediatr Surg 7:194, 1972.

62. Dunn SP, Gross KR, Dalsing M, et al: Superoxide: A critical oxygen free radical in ischemic bowel injury. J Pediatr Surg 19:740, 1984.

63. Parks DA, Bulkley GB, Granger DN: Role of oxygen derived free radicals in digestive tract diseases. Surgery 94:415, 1983.

64. Szabo JS, Mayfield SR, Oh W, et al: Postprandial gastrointestinal blood flow and oxygen consumption: Effects of hypoxemia in neonatal piglets. Pediatr Res 21:93, 1987.

65. MacKendrick W, Caplan M: Necrotizing enterocolitis: New thoughts about pathogenesis and potential treatments. Pediatr Clin North Am 40:1047, 1993.

66. Musemeche CA, Kosloske AM, Bartow SA, et al: Comparative effects of ischemia, bacteria and substrate on the pathogenesis of intestinal necrosis. J Pediatr Surg 21:536, 1986.

67. DeSa DJ: The spectrum of ischemic bowel disease in the newborn. Perspect Pediatr Pathol 3:273, 1976.

68. Hsueh W, Caplan MS, Sun X, et al: Platelet-activating factor, tumor necrosis factor, hypoxia and necrotizing enterocolitis. Acta Paediatr Suppl 396:11, 1994.

69. Dalsing MC, Sieber P, Grosfeld JL, et al: Ischemic bowel: The protective effect of free-radical anion scavengers. J Pediatr Surg 18:360, 1983.

70. McCord JM: Oxygen-derived free radicals in post-ischemic tissue injury. N Engl J Med 312:159, 1985.

71. Brown EG, Sweet AY: Preventing necrotizing enterocolitis in neonates. JAMA 240:2452, 1978.

72. Barlow B, Santulli TV, Heird WC, et al: An experimental study of acute neonatal enterocolitis: The importance of breast milk. J Pediatr Surg 9:587, 1974.

73. Rayyis SF, Ambalavanan N, Wright L, Carlo WA: Randomized trial of "slow" versus "fast" feed advancements on the incidence of necrotizing enterocolitis in very low birth weight infants. J Pediatr 134:293, 1999.

74. Schanler RJ, Shulman RJ, Lau C, et al: Feeding strategies for premature infants: Randomized trial of gastrointestinal priming and tube-feeding method. Pediatrics 103:434, 1999.

75. Schanler RJ, Shulman RJ, Lau C: Feeding strategies for premature infants: Beneficial outcomes of feeding fortified human milk versus preterm formula. Pediatrics 103:1150, 1999.

76. Hebra A, Hong J, McGowan KL, et al: Bacterial translocation in mesenteric ischemia reperfusion injury: Pathophysiologic significance in an infant piglet model. Surg Forum 44:632, 1993.

77. Lawrence G, Bates J, Gaul AP: Pathogenesis of neonatal necrotizing enterocolitis. Lancet 1:137, 1982.

78. Peter CS, Feuerhahn M, Bohnhorst B, et al: Necrotising enterocolitis: Is there a relationship to specific pathogens? Eur J Pediatr 158:67, 1999.

79. Gewolb IH, Schwalbe RS, Taciak VL, et al: Stool microflora in extremely low birthweight infants. Arch Dis Child Fetal Neonatal Educ 80:F167, 1999.

80. Caplan MS, Jilling T: New concept in necrotizing enterocolitis. Curr Opin Pediatr 13:111, 2001.

81. Caplan MS, Hedlund E, Adler L, et al: Role of asphyxia and feeding in a neonatal rat model of necrotizing enterocolitis. Pediatr Pathol 14:1017, 1994.

82. Caplan MS, Hedlund E, Adier L, et al: The platelet-activating factor receptor antagonist WEB 2170 prevents neonatal necrotizing enterocolitis in rats. J Pediatr Gastroenterol Nutr 24:296, 1997.

83. Caplan MS, Lickerman M, Adler L, et al: The role of recombinant platelet-activating factor acetylhydrolase in a neonatal rat model of necrotizing enterocolitis. Pediatr Res 42:779, 1997.

84. Sun XM, Hsueh W: Bowel necrosis induced by tumor necrosis factor in rats is mediated by platelet-activating factor. J Clin Invest 81:1328, 1988.

85. Hsueh W, Gonzalez-Crussi F, Arroyave JL, et al: Platelet activating factor-induced ischemic bowel necrosis: The effect of PAF antagonists. Eur J Pharmacol 123:79, 1986.

86. Caplan MS, Kelly A, Hsueh W: Endotoxin and hypoxia-induced intestinal necrosis in rats: The role of platelet activating factor. Pediatr Res 31:428, 1992.

87. Benirschke K: Pathology of neonatal enterocolitis. In Moore TD (ed): Necrotizing enterocolitis in the newborn infant. Report of the 68th Ross Conference on Pediatric Research, Ross Laboratories, Columbus, OH, 1974, pp 29-30.

88. Joshi VV, Winston YE, Kay S: Neonatal necrotizing enterocolitis. Histologic evidence of healing. Am J Dis Child 126:113, 1973.

89. Schwartz MZ, Hayden CK, Richardson CJ, et al: A prospective evaluation of intestinal stenosis following necrotizing enterocolitis. J Pediatr Surg 17:764, 1982.

90. Salama H, da Silva O: Necrotizing enterocolitis N Engl J Med 344:108, 2001.

91. Carbonaro CA, Clark DA, Elseviers D: A bacterial pathogenicity determinant associated with necrotizing enterocolitis. Microb Pathog 5:427, 1988.

92. Gupta S, Morris JG, Panigrahi P, et al: Endemic enterocolitis: Lack of association with a specific infectious agent. Pediatr Infect Dis J 13:728, 1994.

93. Bell MJ, Ternberg JL, Feigin RD, et al: Neonatal necrotizing enterocolitis: Therapeutic decisions based upon clinical staging. Ann Surg 187:1, 1978.

94. Walsh MC, Kliegman RM: Necrotizing enterocolitis: Treatment based on staging criteria. Pediatr Clin North Am 33:179, 1986.

95. Amoury RA: Necrotizing enterocolitis. In Ashcraft KW, Holder TM (eds): Pediatric Surgery, 2nd ed. Philadelphia, WB Saunders, 1993, pp 341-357.

96. Hutter JJ Jr, Hathaway WE, Wayne ER: Hematologic abnormalities in severe neonatal necrotizing enterocolitis. J Pediatr 88:1026, 1976.

97. Ververidis M, Kiely EM, Spitz L, et al: The clinical significance of thrombocytopenia in neonates with necrotizing enterocolitis. J Pediatr Surg 36:799, 2001.

98. O'Neill JA Jr: Necrotizing enterocolitis. In Grosfeld JL (ed): Common Problems in Pediatric Surgery. St. Louis, Mosby-Year Book, 1991, pp 132-138.

99. O'Neill JA Jr: Neonatal necrotizing enterocolitis. Surg Clin North Am 61:1013, 1981.

100. Edelson MB, Sonnino RE, Bagwell CE, et al: Plasma intestinal fatty acid binding protein in neonates with necrotizing enterocolitis: A pilot study. J Pediatr Surg 34:1453, 1999.

101. Guthmann F, Borchers T, Wolfrum C, et al: Plasma concentration of intestinal- and liver-FABP in neonates suffering from necrotizing enterocolitis and in healthy preterm neonates. Mol Cell Biochem 239:227, 2002.

102. Morecroft JA, Spitz L, Hamilton PA, et al: Plasma interleukin-6 and tumour necrosis factor levels as predictors of disease severity and outcome in necrotizing enterocolitis. J Pediatr Surg 29:798, 1994.

103. Leonidas JC, Hall RT, Amoury RA: Critical evaluation of the roentgen signs of neonatal necrotizing enterocolitis. Ann Radiol 19:123, 1976.

104. Leonidas JC, Hall RT: Neonatal pneumatosis coli: A mild form of necrotizing enterocolitis. J Pediatr 89:456, 1976.

105. Buonomo C: The radiology of necrotizing enterocolitis. Radiol Clin North Am 37:1187, 1999.

106. Daneman A, Woodward S, deSilva M: The radiology of neonatal necrotizing enterocolitis (NEC): A review of 47 cases and the literature. Pediatr Radiol 7:70, 1978.

107. Kosloske AM, Musemeche CA, Ball WS Jr, et al: Value of radiographic findings to predict outcome. AJR Am J Roentgenol 151:771, 1988.

108. Kosloske AM: Indications for operation in necrotizing enterocolitis revisited. J Pediatr Surg 29:663, 1994.

109. Buchheit JQ, Stewart DL: Clinical comparison of localized intestinal perforation and necrotizing enterocolitis in neonates. Pediatrics 93:32, 1994.

110. Kodroff MB, Hartenberg MA, Goldschmidt RA: Ultrasonographic diagnosis of gangrenous bowel in neonatal necrotizing enterocolitis. Pediatr Radiol 14:168, 1984.

111. Robberecht EA, Afschrift M, De Bel CE, et al: Sonographic demonstration of portal venous gas in necrotizing enterocolitis. Eur J Pediatr 147:192, 1988.

112. Maalouf EF, Fagbemi A, Duggan PJ, et al: Magnetic resonance imaging of intestinal necrosis in preterm infants. Pediatrics 105:510, 2000.

113. Caty MG, Azizkhan RG: Necrotizing enterocolitis. In Ashcraft KW, Holder TM (eds): Pediatric Surgery, 3rd ed. Philadelphia, WB Saunders, 2000, pp 443-451.

114. Kleinhaus S, Weinberg G, Gregor MB: Necrotizing enterocolitis in infancy. Surg Clin North Am 72:261, 1992.

115. Kanto WP, Hunter JE, Stoll BJ: Recognition and medical management of necrotizing enterocolitis. Clin Perinatol 21:335, 1994.

116. Price PT: Neonatal necrotizing enterocolitis. In Groh-Wargo S, Thompson M, Cox J (eds): Nutritional Care for High-Risk Newborns, 3rd ed. Chicago, Precept Press, 2000.

117. Kosloske AM, Burstain J, Bartow SA: Intestinal obstruction due to colonic stricture following neonatal necrotizing enterocolitis. Ann Surg 192:202, 1980.

118. Schwartz MZ, Richardson CJ, Hayden CK, et al: Intestinal stenosis following successful medical management of necrotizing enterocolitis. J Pediatr Surg 15:890, 1980.

119. Cikrit D, Mastandrea T, West KW, et al: Necrotizing enterocolitis: Factors affecting mortality in 101 cases. Surgery 96:648, 1984.

120. Loh M, Osborn DA, Lui K: Outcome of very premature infants with necrotizing enterocolitis cared for in centers with or without on site surgical facilities. Arch Dis Child Fetal Neonatal Educ 85:114, 2001.

121. Kosloske AM: Surgery of necrotizing enterocolitis. World J Surg 9:277, 1985.

122. Chandler JC, Hebra A: Necrotizing enterocolitis in infants with very low birth weight. Semin Pediatr Surg 9:63, 2000.

123. Ricketts RR: The role of paracentesis in the management of infants with necrotizing enterocolitis. Am Surg 52:61, 1986.

124. Ricketts RR, Jerles ML: Neonatal necrotizing enterocolitis: Experience with 100 consecutive surgical patients. World J Surg 14:600, 1990.

125. Kurkchubasche AG, Smith SD, Rowe MI: Portal venous air an old sign and new operative indication for necrotizing enterocolitis [abstract]. Proceedings of the BAPS XXXVIII Annual International Congress, Budapest, Hungary, July 1991.

126. Vanderkolk WE, Kurz P, Daniels J, et al: Liver hemorrhage during laparotomy in patients with necrotizing enterocolitis. J Pediatr Surg 31:1063, 1996.

127. Frawley G, Baylcy G, Chondros P: Laparotomy for necrotizing enterocolitis: Intensive care nursery compared with operating theater. J Paediatr Child Health 35:291, 1999.

128. Anveden-Hertzberg L, Gauderer MW: Surgery is safe in very low birthweight infants with necrotizing enterocolitis. Acta Paediatr 89:242, 2000.

129. Harberg FJ, McGill CW, Saleem MM, et al: Resection and primary anastomosis for necrotizing enterocolitis. J Pediatr Surg 18:743, 1983.

130. Griffiths DM, Forbes DA, Pemberton PJ, et al: Primary anastomosis for necrotizing enterocolitis: A 12-year experience. J Pediatr Surg 24:515, 1989.

131. Albanese CT, Rowe MI: Necrotizing enterocolitis. In O'Neill JA, Rowe MI, Grosfeld JL, et al (eds): Pediatric Surgery, 5th ed. St. Louis, Mosby, 1998, pp 1297-1320.

132. Cooper A, Ross AJ III, O'Neill JA Jr, et al: Resection with primary anastomosis for necrotizing enterocolitis: A contrasting view. J Pediatr Surg 23:64, 1988.

133. Moore TC: Management of necrotizing enterocolitis by "patch, drain and wait." Pediatr Surg Int 4:110, 1989.

134. Vaughan WG, Grosfeld JL, West K, et al: Avoidance of stomas and delayed anastomosis for bowel necrosis: The "clip, and drop-back technique." J Pediatr Surg 31:542, 1996.

135. Martin LW, Neblett WW: Early operation with intestinal diversion for necrotizing enterocolitis. J Pediatr Surg 16:252, 1981.

136. Firor HV: Use of high jejunostomy in extensive NEC. J Pediatr Surg 17:771, 1982.

137. Ein SH, Marshall DG, Girvan D: Peritoneal drainage under local anesthesia for perforations from necrotizing enterocolitis. J Pediatr Surg 12:963, 1977.

138. Dimmitt RA, Meier AH, Skarsgard ED, et al: Salvage laparotomy for failure of peritoneal drainage in necrotizing enterocolitis in infants with extremely low birth weight. J Pediatr Surg 35:856, 2000.

139. Ein SH, Shandling B, Wesson D, Filler RM: A 13-year experience with peritoneal drainage under local anesthesia for necrotizing enterocolitis perforation. J Pediatr Surg 25:1034, 1990.

140. Takamatsu H, Akiyama H, Ibara S, et al: Treatment for necrotizing enterocolitis perforation in the extremely premature infant (weighing less than 1,000 g). J Pediatr Surg 27:741, 1992.

141. Azarow KS, Ein SH, Shandling B, et al: Laparotomy or drain for perforated necrotizing enterocolitis: Who gets what and why? Pediatr Surg Int 12:137, 1997.

142. Lessin MS, Luks FL, Weaselhoeft CW Jr, et al: Peritoneal drainage as definitive treatment for intestinal perforation in infants with extremely lowbirth weight (<750 g). J Pediatr Surg 33:370, 1998.

143. Ahmed T, Ein SH, Moore A: A role of peritoneal drainage in treatment of perforated enterocolitis: Recommendations from recent experience. J Pediatr Surg 33:1468, 1998.

144. Cass DL, Brandt ML, Patel DL, et al: Peritoneal drainage as definitive treatment for neonates with isolated intestinal perforation. J Pediatr Surg 35:1531, 2000.

145. Dzakovic A, Notrica DM, Smith EO, et al: Primary peritoneal drainage for increasing ventilatory requirements in critically ill neonates with necrotizing enterocolitis. J Pediatr Surg 36:730, 2001.

146. Morgan LJ, Shochat SJ, Hartman GA: Peritoneal drainage as primary management of perforated NEC in the very low birth weight infants. J Pediatr Surg 29:30, 1994.

147. Cheu HW, Sukarochana K, Lloyd DA: Peritoneal drainage for necrotizing enterocolitis. J Pediatr Surg 23:557, 1988.

148. Atakent YS, Wasserman-Hoff R, Ozek E, et al: Percutaneous peritoneal drainage in the management of acute intestinal perforation. J Perinatol 17:46, 1997.

149. Rovin JD, Rodgers BM, Burns RC, McGahren ED: The role of peritoneal drainage for intestinal perforation in infants with and without necrotizing enterocolitis. J Pediatr Surg 34:143, 1999.

150. Noble GS, Driessnack M: Bedside peritoneal drainage in very low birth weight infants. Am J Surg 181:416, 2001.

151. Moss RL, Dimmitt RA, Henry MC, et al: A meta-analysis of peritoneal drainage versus laparotomy for necrotizing enterocolitis. J Pediatr Surg 36:1210, 2001.

152. Musemeche CA, Kosloske AM, Ricketts RR: Enterostomy in necrotizing enterocolitis: An analysis of techniques and timing of closure. J Pediatr Surg 22:479, 1987.

153. Lemelle JL, Schmitt M, de Miscault G, et al: Neonatal necrotizing enterocolitis: A retrospective and multicentric review of 331 cases. Acta Paediatr 396(suppl):70, 1994.

154. Sonntag J, Wagner MH, Waldschmidt J, et al: Multisystem organ failure and capillary leak syndrome in severe necrotizing enterocolitis of very low birth weight infants. J Pediatr Surg 33:481, 1998.

155. Ehrlich PF, Sato TT, Short BL, Hartman GE: Outcome of perforated necrotizing enterocolitis in very low birth weight neonate may be independent of the type of surgical treatment. Am Surg 67:752, 2001.

156. Stringer MD, Brereton RJ, Drake DP, et al: Recurrent necrotizing enterocolitis. J Pediatr Surg 28:979, 1993.

157. Simon NP: Follow-up for infants with necrotizing enterocolitis. Clin Perinatol 21:411, 1994.

158. Horwitz JR, Lally KP, Cheu HW, et al: Complications after surgical intervention for necrotizing enterocolitis: A multicenter review. J Pediatr Surg 30:994, 1995.

159. Janik JS, Ein SH, Mancer K: Intestinal stricture after necrotizing enterocolitis. J Pediatr Surg 16:438, 1981.

160. Vanderhoof JA: Short-bowel syndrome. Clin Perinatol 23:377, 1996.

161. Sigalet DL: Short bowel syndrome in infants and children: An overview. Semin Pediatr Surg 10:49, 2001.

162. Walsh MC, Kliegman RM, Hack M: Severity of necrotizing enterocolitis: Influence on outcome at 2 years of age. Pediatrics 84:808, 1989.

163. Stevenson DK, Kerner JA, Malachowski N, et al: Late morbidity among survivors of necrotizing enterocolitis. Pediatrics 66:925, 1980.

164. Mayr J, Fasching G, Hollwarth ME: Psychosocial and psychomotoric development of very low birth weight infants with necrotizing enterocolitis. Acta Paediatr 396(suppl):96, 1994.

165. Tobiansky R, Lui K, Roberts S, et al: Neurodevelopmental outcome low birthweight infants with necrotizing enterocolitis requiring surgery. J Pediatr Child Health 31:233, 1995.

166. Chacko J, Ford WD, Haslam R: Growth and neurodevelopmental outcome in extremely low birth weight infants after laparotomy. Pediatr Surg Int 15:496, 1999.

167. Sonntag J, Grimmer I, Scholz T, et al: Growth and neurodevelopmental outcome of very low birth weight infants with necrotizing enterocolitis. Acta Paediatr 89:528, 2000.

168. Book LS, Overall JC, Herbst JJ, et al: Clustering of necrotizing enterocolitis: Interruption by infection-control methods, N Engl J Med 297:984, 1977.

169. Rotbart HA, Levin MJ: How contagious is necrotizing enterocolitis? Pediatr J Infect Dis 2:406, 1983.

170. Foster J, Cole M: Oral immunoglobulin for preventing necrotizing enterocolitis in preterm and low birth-weight neonates. Cochrane Database Syst Rev 3:CD001816, 2001.

171. Egan EA, Mantilla G, Nelson RM, et al: A prospective controlled trial of oral kanamycin in the prevention of neonatal necrotizing enterocolitis. J Pediatr 89:467, 1976.

172. Grylack LJ, Scanlon JW: Oral gentamicin therapy in the prevention of neonatal necrotizing enterocolitis. A controlled double-blind trial. Am J Dis Child 132:1192, 1978.

173. Bury RG, Tudehope D: Enteral antibiotics for preventing necrotizing enterocolitis in low birthweight infants. Cochrane Database Syst Rev 1:CD000405, 2001.

174. Carron V, Egan EA: Prevention of necrotizing enterocolitis. J Pediatr Gastroenterol Nutr 11:317, 1990.

175. Bauer CR, Morrison JC, Poole WK, et al: A decreased incidence of necrotizing enterocolitis after prenatal glucocorticoid therapy. Pediatrics 73:682, 1984.

176. Israel E, Schiffrin EJ, Carter EA, et al: Prevention of necrotizing enterocolitis in the rat with prenatal cortisone. Gastroenterology 99:1333, 1990.

177. Snyder R: Platelet-activating factor and related acetylated lipids as potent biologically active cellular mediators. Am J Physiol 59:697, 1990.

178. Crowley P, Chalmers I, Keirse M: The effects of corticosteroid administration before preterm delivery: An overview of the evidence from controlled trials. Br J Obstet Gynaecol 97:11, 1990.

179. Bennet R, Nord CE, Zetterstrom R: Transient colonization of the gut of newborn infants by orally administered bifidobacteria and lactobacilli. Acta Paediatr 81:784, 1992.

180. Gibson GR, Wang X: Regulatory effects of bifidobacteria on the growth of other colonic bacteria. J Appl Bacteriol 77:412, 1994.

181. Dai D, Walker WA: Protective nutrients and bacterial colonization in the immature human gut. Adv Pediatr 46:353, 1999.

182. Butel MJ, Roland N, Hibert A, et al: Clostridial pathogenicity in experimental necrotizing enterocolitis in gnotobiotic quails and protective role of bifidobacteria. J Med Microbiol 47:391, 1998.

183. Caplan MS, Miller-Catchpole R, Kaup S, et al: Bifidobacterial supplementation reduces the incidence of necrotizing enterocolitis in a neonatal rat model. Gastroenterology 117:577, 1999.

184. Hoyos AB: Reduced incidence of necrotizing enterocolitis associated with enteral administration of *Lactobacillus acidophilus* and *Bifidobacterium infantis* to neonates in an intensive care unit. Int J Infect Dis 3:197, 1999.

185. Meetze W, Valentine C, McGuigan JE, et al: Gastrointestinal priming prior to full enteral nutrition in very low birth weight infants. J Pediatr Gastroenterol Nutr 15:163, 1992.

186. LaGamma EF, Browne LE: Feeding practices for infants weighing less than 1500 g at birth and the pathogenesis of necrotizing enterocolitis. Clin Perinatol 21:271, 1994.

187. McClure RJ, Newell SJ: Randomized controlled study of clinical outcome following trophic feeding. Arch Dis Child Fetal Neonatal Educ 82:F29, 2000.

188. Reisner SH, Garty B: Necrotising enterocolitis despite breast feeding. Lancet 2:507, 1977.

189. Eyal F, Sagi E, Arad I, et al: Necrotizing enterocolitis in the very low birthweight infant: Expressed breast milk feeding compared with parenteral feeding. Arch Dis Child 57:274, 1982.

190. Furukawa M, Narahara H, Yasyda K, Johnson JM: Presence of platelet-activating factor acetylhydrolase in milk. J Lipid Res 34:1603, 1993.

191. Carlson SE, Montalto MB, Ponder DL, et al: Lower incidence of necrotizing enterocolitis in infants fed a preterm formula with egg phospholipids. Pediatr Res 44:491, 1998.

192. Neu J, Weiss MD: Necrotizing enterocolitis: Pathophysiology and prevention. J Parenter Enteral Nutr 23(suppl):S13, 1999.

193. Zanioia SA, Amin HJ, McMillan DD, et al: Plasma L-arginine concentrations in premature infants with necrotizing enterocolitis. J Pediatr 131:226, 1997.

194. Amin HJ, Zamora SA, McMillan DD, et al: Arginine supplementation prevents necrotizing enterocolitis in the premature infant. J Pediatr 140:4251, 2002.

195. Ulshen MH, Raasch RH: Luminal epidermal growth factor preserves mucosal mass of small bowel in fasting rats. Clin Sci 90:427, 1996.

196. Burrin DG, Wester TJ, Davis TA, et al: Orally administered IGF-I increases intestinal mucosal growth in formula-fed neonatal pigs. Am J Physiol 270:1085, 1996.

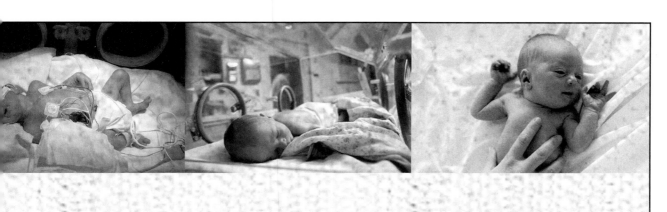

Liver and Biliary Tree of the Neonate

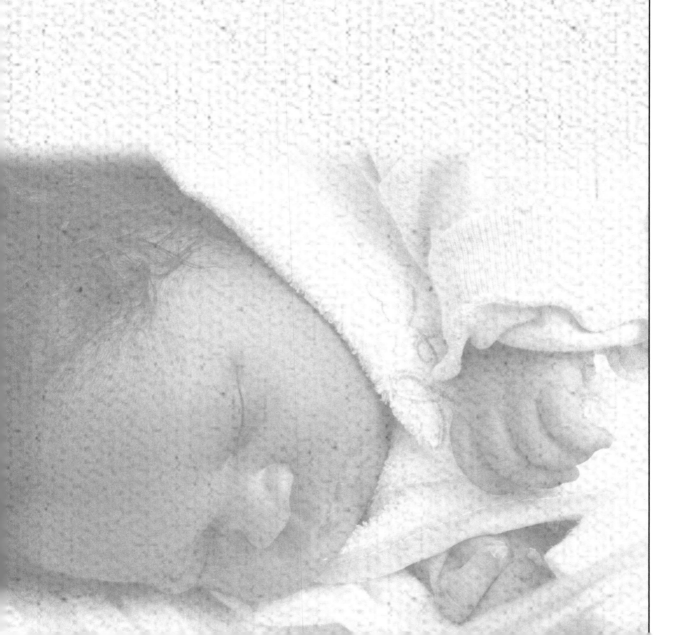

CHAPTER 67

Cholestatic Syndromes in Neonates

John Tung and Roy Proujansky

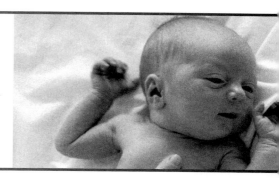

Cholestatic disorders are a relatively common occurrence for critically ill and otherwise healthy neonates. Normal neonatal biliary physiology is relatively cholestatic compared with the physiology of bile synthesis and flow in older children and adults, and it requires less of an additional insult to become clinically manifest as a cholestatic illness associated with direct hyperbilirubinemia. Infectious, metabolic, inflammatory, genetic, and structural disorders all may cause enough additional disturbance in this physiology to produce clinical disease.

This chapter briefly reviews the relevant variations in bile salt metabolism that predispose neonates to cholestatic disorders. In general, cholestatic disorders fall into two categories. The larger group consists of disorders producing a **neonatal hepatitis** picture, from which disorders with a prominent obstructive component to bile flow, such as **biliary atresia,** must be distinguished. The second group consists of disorders for which **cholestasis** and **direct hyperbilirubinemia** are but one of the manifestations of severe hepatocellular dysfunction and neonatal hepatic failure. For many of these disorders, significant advances have occurred in more recent years to clarify the contribution of specific single-gene mutations in their pathogenesis. Where applicable, this new genetic information is noted for its influence on diagnosis and therapy.

NEONATAL BILIARY PHYSIOLOGY AND MECHANISMS OF CHOLESTASIS

The liver excretes bile acids, bilirubin, cholesterol, steroids, and other compounds, and the flow of bile depends on the secretion of bile acids. **Bile acids** are cholesterol derivatives and differ only slightly from steroid hormones.[1] Primary bile acids consist of cholic acid and chenodeoxycholic acid. These undergo hepatic conjugation with glycine and taurine, become concentrated in the gallbladder, and are excreted into the intestines, where bacterial enzymes then deconjugate them.[2] They are converted via 7α-dehydroxylation to form secondary bile acids (deoxycholic acid, lithocholic acid). Some are excreted in the feces, but 80% of intestinal bile acids undergo enterohepatic circulation, where they are actively reabsorbed by the terminal ileum. Some unconjugated bile acids are passively reabsorbed in the small intestines and colon. Because of the crucial role of the ileum in normal bile salt physiology, terminal ileal disease or resection may contribute to cholestatic disease in some newborns. Reabsorbed primary (cholic and chenodeoxycholic acid) and secondary (deoxycholic and lithocholic acid) bile acids undergo reconjugation with taurine and glycine, and the cycle continues. The content of the gallbladder is a mix of 80% primary and 20% secondary bile acids.

Defects in the synthesis of bile salts are known to be responsible for many disorders associated with the clinical picture of neonatal hepatitis, often associated with progressive liver damage and fibrosis. Two of the more common and most well characterized of these relatively rare disorders, 3-β-hydroxysteroid dehydrogenase deficiency and oxosteroid-5-β reductase deficiency, are important disorders because of their potential amelioration with bile salt replacement therapy.

The cycle of bile salt excretion in the liver starts with the portal veins followed by liver sinusoids, hepatocytes, bile canaliculus, terminal bile ductules, larger bile ductules, and, finally, bile ducts. Sinusoidal membranes have many transporters and receptors regulating flux of bilirubin, fatty acids, bile acids, and other compounds into the hepatocytes.[3] Bile acids must be secreted against a concentration gradient on leaving the hepatocytes, and the rate-limiting factor for this process is the secretion of monovalent bile acids. The bile salt excretory pump is the main transporter for bile salts.[4] Other important transporters include the multidrug resistance–associated protein, multidrug resistance (MDR)-1P glycoprotein, MDR-3P glycoprotein multispecific organic ion transporter, and the chloride bicarbonate exchanger.[5-7] Characterization of these transporters and the cloning of their respective genes has led more recently to identification of the etiology of several cholestatic disorders, some of which may become manifest in infancy. The heterogeneous group of disorders, formerly called **progressive familial intrahepatic cholestasis (PFIC)**, has been more well characterized through this approach. PFIC1, or Byler disease, has been found to be associated with mutations in a P-type adenosine triphosphatase on chromosome 18q21-22, which may be responsible for aminophospholipid transport at the canalicular membrane. This disorder also has been shown to be allelic with benign recurrent intrahepatic cholestasis, a less severe disorder. PFIC2 has been associated with mutations in the bile salt excretory pump on chromosome 2q24. PFIC3 seems to be due to mutations in MDR3 located at chromosome 7q21. Mutations in these and other transporters are likely to result in abnormal canalicular bile, leading to cholestasis and the associated liver injury.

DEVELOPMENT OF BILE DUCTS

The **liver** is derived from the liver diverticulum and the septum transversum.[8] A thickening of the foregut at the level of the duodenum, the pars cystica, forms the hepatic diverticulum; this differentiates into the extrahepatic biliary system, which comprises the common bile duct, cystic duct, and gallbladder. The intrahepatic ducts develop by 7 weeks of gestation from periportal primitive hepatocytes.[9] Hepatocytes are formed by proliferating endodermal cells in the liver diverticulum interacting with mesenchymal cells of the septum transversum. Several theories exist about the development of the intrahepatic biliary system. The first is that it is an invagination of epithelium from the extrahepatic biliary system. The second theory is that these intrahepatic bile ducts are entirely derived from hepatocyte precursors (hepatoblasts), which grow outward to join the extrahepatic biliary system. Immunostaining studies at 8 weeks of gestation show hepatoblasts forming a cell monolayer around portal vein branches, forming a ductal plate. The ductal plates remodel, following the portal veins into the liver, and by 12 weeks there are larger ducts around the hilum with smaller, more immature ductal plates in the periphery. At birth, small peripheral branches of the intrahepatic biliary system are still immature and do not mature until about 4 weeks after birth. Aberrant development, remodeling, or maturation of ductal plates can result in ductal plate malformations. These malformations have been suggested to play a role in the pathogenesis of disorders such as choledochal cysts and congenital hepatic fibrosis.[10]

DEVELOPMENT OF HEPATOBILIARY FUNCTION IN UTERO

Bile secretion occurs by 4 months in utero, and biliary bile acid concentration increases rapidly between 16 and 20 weeks, but even at term, biliary bile acid concentrations are lower than concentrations in older children. Levels normalize by the end of the first year of life.[11] Bile acid production is steroid inducible, and increased production can be seen in neonates whose mothers received corticosteroids for preterm labor.[12] The fetal serum bile acid level is maintained by the placenta, but in the neonate, serum bile acids increase to cholestatic levels for 6 to 8 weeks before normalizing by 6 months.[13] This process has been termed **physiologic hypercholanemia of infancy** and occurs despite the lower bile acid pool in neonates and poor intestinal absorption of bile acids.[14]

EVALUATION AND MANAGEMENT OF NEONATE WITH CHOLESTASIS

Before discussion of the specific diagnostic entities contributing to the differential diagnosis of cholestasis in the newborn (Table 67-1), several features of the overall evaluation deserve discussion. In general, cholestasis is manifest initially as direct hyperbilirubinemia because the entities responsible for reduced bile flow also impair excretion of conjugated bilirubin, which is measured easily in the clinical setting. Conjugated hyperbilirubinemia greater than 2 mg/dL or greater than 15% of total bilirubin is considered pathologic in neonates.

After the detection of an elevated conjugated bilirubin value, the tempo and direction of additional evaluation are based on whether or not evidence of cholestasis is just one feature of severe hepatocellular functional impairment (neonatal hepatic failure) or if cholestasis is the predominant disturbance. **Neonatal hepatic failure** is a neonatal emergency, has a different differential diagnosis, and requires alternative management strategies as the evaluation proceeds (Table 67-2). Hepatic failure in newborns may not manifest as it would typically in older children or adults. The most reliable indicator of such severe hepatic functional impairment is a significant prolongation of the prothrombin time, associated with reduction in circulating clotting factor levels.[15-17] Prothrombin time greater than 3 seconds above control increases the risk of bleeding, whereas a 2-second increase is considered pathologic. The assessment of specific factor levels may provide additional information about hepatic synthesis and has been used by some to attempt to predict prognosis and severity.[18,19] Other measures that may support a diagnosis of neonatal hepatic failure include hyperammonemia, hypoalbuminemia, and the presence of encephalopathy. The correlation between serum transaminase levels and the presence of significant functional impairment may be poor. In conditions in which massive hepatocellular necrosis results in significant synthetic dysfunction, transaminases may be initially high, then may decline. In many metabolic-based etiologies for neonatal hepatic failure, however, the transaminase levels may be mildly or moderately elevated despite significant hepatic functional impairment, signifying hepatocellular dysfunction but not cell death.

If neonatal hepatic failure is present, evaluation and management need to proceed promptly and simultaneously. Initial management is supportive with attention to fluid and electrolyte disturbance and the risk or occurrence of hypoglycemia, correction of coagulopathy, and treatment for encephalopathy. Simultaneous assessment to determine the specific diagnosis ideally leads to the prompt institution of specific therapy for conditions

Table 67–1. Conditions Associated with Neonatal Cholestasis

Biliary Atresia
Idiopathic neonatal hepatitis
Other extrahepatic causes for cholestasis
  Choledochal cysts
  Spontaneous perforation of the common bile duct
  Biliary hypoplasia
  Gallstone/sludge
  Mass or tumor—neuroblastoma, rhabdomyosarcoma, hemangioma
Other intrahepatic causes for cholestasis
  Arteriohepatic dysplasia/Alagille syndrome
  Progressive familial intrahepatic cholestasis
    PFIC1—Byler disease
    PFIC2—BSEP deficiency
    PFIC3—MDR3 deficiency
  α_1-Antitrypsin deficiency
  Bile salt synthetic defects
    3-β-hydroxysteroid dehydrogenase deficiency
    Oxosteroid 5-β-reductase deficiency
    Zellweger syndrome
  Cholestasis associated with total parenteral nutrition
  ECMO-related cholestasis
  Other metabolic etiology
    Neonatal iron storage disease
    Tyrosinemia
    Galactosemia
    Hereditary fructose intolerance
    Mitochondrial disorder
  Infectious eitology
    TORCH infection
    Hepatitis viruses
    Herpes simplex
    HHV-6
    Parvovirus B19
    Enteroviruses
      Echovirus
      Coxsackievirus
    Human immunodeficiency virus
    Urinary tract infection/sepsis
      Escherichia coli
      Staphylococcus aureus
      Listeria spp.
      Group B streptococcus
      Tuberculosis
Other etiology
  Hereditary cholestasis with lymphedema (Aagenaes syndrome)
  Cystic fibrosis
  Hypopituitarism
  Neonatal lupus
  Histiocytic disorders

BSEP, bile salt export pump; ECMO, extracorporeal membrane oxygenation; HHV-6, human herpesvirus type 6; MDR, multidrug resistance; TORCH, toxoplasmosis, other agents, rubella, cytomegalovirus, herpes simplex.

Table 67–2. Conditions Associated with Neonatal Hepatic Failure

Neonatal iron storage disease
Tyrosinemia
Mitochondrial disorders
Galactosemia
Hereditary fructose intolerance
Urea cycle disorders
Oxosteroid 5-β-reductase deficiency
Hepatitis B
Herpes simplex virus
HHV-6
Echovirus
Coxsackie B
Parvovirus B19
Familial erythrophagocytic lymphohistiocytosis

HHV-6, human herpesvirus type 6.

availability of liver transplantation and discussion with the family regarding transplantation as a therapeutic option should occur early in the clinical course.[20]

Prognosis of neonatal liver failure is variable and depends on the etiology of the underlying disease. Most patients have underlying metabolic disorders and, less frequently, infectious etiologies.[20] With advances of segmental liver transplantation in infants and improved pretransplant and post-transplant care, 1-year patient survival for this operation is 68.2% in the United States (United Network for Organ Sharing data, January 1, 1997, to December 31, 1998); 1-year survival is 87.3% in our center and ranges from 65% to 92% in other centers.[21-23] The long-term success of this operation for patients presenting initially with neonatal hepatic failure may be worse, however, than the prognosis for the overall segmental transplant population as a whole.[20]

The evaluation of a cholestatic neonate without significant hepatic functional impairment proceeds at a less urgent pace and is predicated mainly on the prompt identification of treatable causes and the determination of the presence or absence of biliary atresia. Many entities are associated with this differential diagnosis. These entities commonly are characterized by an anatomic-pathologic classification of the disorders that produce a neonatal hepatitis and disorders associated with anatomic obstruction to bile flow, such as biliary atresia. Working through this broad differential diagnosis requires close attention to the history and physical examination, while proceeding through the appropriate diagnostic testing.

Several features of the history and physical examination warrant specific attention. The maternal and family history should be evaluated carefully for features suggesting the possibility of maternal infection, history of neonatal cholestasis or liver disease in previous births or the extended family pedigree, or other genetic disorders suggesting possible etiologic links to the affected neonate. **Alagille syndrome (arteriohepatic dysplasia)** is known to have variable clinical manifestations with incomplete penetrance,

amenable to therapy, such as galactosemia, hereditary fructose intolerance, tyrosinemia, neonatal iron storage disease, and urea cycle defects. Because some of the conditions responsible for neonatal hepatic failure are not amenable to specific therapy, consideration of the so the presence of a maternal or family history of heart disease may suggest this etiology. In addition, several disorders previously characterized in the large, heterogeneous subgroup of conditions called **idiopathic neonatal hepatitis** now are known to have a genetic etiology, which may be suggested by the appropriate family history.

A newborn with biliary atresia is often a normal-appearing and thriving infant. Prematurity and low birth weight suggest other causes of jaundice, such as congenital infection, neonatal hepatitis, and a spectrum of other diseases. A careful examination of the skin may reveal a rash or petechiae, which may suggest viral infection. Dysmorphic features may suggest Alagille syndrome, Zellweger syndrome, or other genetic etiologies. The presence of a murmur or other findings of congenital heart disease may lead to consideration of Alagille syndrome or the asplenia/polysplenia syndrome, which may be associated with congenital heart disease, intestinal malrotation, and biliary atresia. A distended abdomen with jaundice of relatively sudden onset may indicate spontaneous rupture of the common bile duct. The presence of hepatomegaly and splenomegaly is nonspecific, but an enlarged spleen raises the possibility of storage disease presenting with cholestasis. A mass below the liver may represent a choledochal cyst or rarely a tumor. Hypotonia may be present in children with mitochondrial disorders and Zellweger syndrome. Pale stools may be a feature of many cholestatic syndromes, but completely acholic stools suggest biliary atresia or another cause of complete anatomic obstruction.

The history and physical examination are rarely diagnostic in this circumstance, and additional diagnostic evaluation usually is warranted (Table 67-3). Some information already may be available from newborn screening studies. Newborn screens vary depending on location, but most developed countries have screens that exclude common metabolic disorders, such as hypothyroidism, galactosemia, and occasionally cystic fibrosis. With adequate prenatal care, maternal screens for syphilis, human immunodeficiency virus, hepatitis B virus, herpes, and rubella represent information that should be readily available to the neonatologist.

Additional testing should include measurements of hepatic transaminases (alanine aminotransferase, aspartate aminotransferase), gamma glutamyl transpeptidase (GGT),[24] total and direct bilirubin values, prothrombin time, activated partial thromboplastin time, and a complete blood cell count with differential (see Table 67-3). Urinalysis and urine culture are important tests early in the evaluation because occult urinary tract infection can present with cholestasis as its only clinical manifestation in the newborn. Depending on the direction of the evaluation, serologic studies to evaluate for congenital infection, assay for α_1-antitrypsin levels and phenotype, and additional metabolic studies may be warranted. An ophthalmologic examination is often a useful early adjunct in the diagnostic evaluation looking for evidence of congenital infection or the ocular features of Alagille syndrome or galactosemia. An ultrasound of the liver and biliary tract is useful for the early identification of anatomic abnormalities, such as a choledochal cyst, sludge, stone, or tumor.

Table 67–3. Diagnostic Studies for Evaluating Neonatal Cholestasis

Initial Studies

Total and direct bilirubin
ALT, AST, GGT, alkaline phosphatase
PT, PTT, total protein, albumin
Glucose, ammonia, cholesterol
Complete blood count with differential and platelet count
Urinalysis, urine for reducing substance, urine culture
Ultrasound of the liver and biliary tract

Subsequent Diagnostic Studies

If initial evaluation is suggestive of biliary atresia:
  Hepatobiliary scintigraphy
  Percutaneous liver biopsy
  Laparotomy and operative cholangiography
If initial or subsequent evaluations are not suggestive of biliary atresia:
  α_1-Antitrypsin level and protease inhibitor typing
  Serologic studies for congenital infection, hepatitis viruses, other infection
  Eye examination
  X-ray of long bones and spine for features of congenital infection, Alagille syndrome
  Thyroid studies
  Sweat test and cystic fibrosis genotyping
  Serum and urine bile acid analysis
  Amino acid analysis (serum and urine) and organic acid analysis (urine)
  Iron studies
  Serum lactate, pyruvate
  Mutational analysis for specific genetic etiologies

ALT, alanine aminotransferase; AST, aspartate aminotransferase; GGT, gamma-glutamyl transferase; PT, prothrombin time; PTT, partial thromboplastin time.

After this initial evaluation, many patients require additional studies, including hepatobiliary scintigraphy and more advanced metabolic evaluations. Most patients require percutaneous liver biopsy as part of the diagnostic evaluation. Additional, specific studies may be indicated for specific diagnostic entities. Most infants undergoing this complete evaluation are diagnosed with biliary atresia or idiopathic neonatal hepatitis, with all other diagnostic entities being less frequent.

SPECIFIC DIAGNOSTIC ENTITIES

Predominantly Extrahepatic Cause for Cholestasis

Biliary Atresia

Biliary atresia is one of the most common, specific diagnoses responsible for cholestasis of the newborn. Biliary atresia occurs in 0.73 per 10,000 births[25] and can present in the early neonatal period (embryonic form) or later in the first few weeks of life (perinatal form).[26] Embryonic biliary atresia represents a true atresia of the bile duct and possibly may be due to abnormal vascular supply to the bile duct in utero. Perinatal biliary atresia is encountered more commonly and is caused by a progressive, inflammatory, sclerotic, and obliterative process of the bile ducts. The disease process takes a few weeks to develop, and stools are often pigmented at birth and become acholic a few weeks later. Numerous theories have been offered to explain this process, including perinatal viral infection, vascular injury followed by progressive inflammation and fibrosis, and autoimmune injury. Consistent demonstration of evidence of a specific etiology has not occurred to date.

Affected infants often appear well at birth, and the diagnosis may be suggested initially during routine evaluations in the first few weeks of life when jaundice becomes apparent or does not fade. Demonstration of an elevated direct bilirubin measurement usually is associated with mildly or modestly elevated transaminase values. GGT levels may be significantly elevated, but this is not a reliable discriminating factor in the differential diagnosis.

Ultrasound can exclude other causes, such as a choledochal cyst, sludge, tumor, or the presence of intrahepatic lesions; however, it is of limited usefulness in the specific diagnosis of biliary atresia. The absence or presence of the gallbladder on ultrasound is neither sensitive nor specific enough to exclude biliary atresia, as some have thought. The lack of contraction of the gallbladder after feeding suggests a lack of bile duct patency, but this is not diagnostic.[27] Ultrasound may suggest the presence of asplenia or polysplenia, which, along with intestinal malrotation, are known to be associated with biliary atresia.

A technetium-99m tagged disofenin (DISIDA) scan makes use of a gamma camera to detect the path of a radioactive tracer taken up by the liver and excreted in the bile and into the intestine.[28,29] In the presence of excretion into the intestine, the biliary system is patent, and biliary atresia is highly unlikely. Rarely, because the fibro-obliterative process of biliary atresia is progressive, an early scan may show some excretion only to show no excretion days later as the process progresses. In some patients, the absence of secretion may be misleading because the uptake of this tracer by the liver may be poor in extremely jaundiced infants. Enhancement of the diagnostic sensitivity of this study occurs with the prior use, over 3 to 5 days, of phenobarbital at a dose of 5 mg/kg/day. Many clinicians often begin phenobarbital while pursuing other diagnostic studies in anticipation of the need for scintigraphy as part of the diagnostic evaluation. The demonstration of excretion on a scintigraphic scan may allow the avoidance of surgical exploration while evaluation for other etiologies proceeds.

Percutaneous liver biopsy is a useful diagnostic test for biliary atresia, when interpreted by a pathologist experienced in the differential diagnosis of neonatal cholestasis. Nonspecific features, such as cholestasis or giant cell transformation, may be seen in some cases. The presence of bile duct proliferation and fibrosis is quite suggestive of biliary atresia, however, and its associated extrahepatic obstruction (Figs. 67-1 and 67-2). In the absence of bile duct proliferation, giant cell transformation and cholestasis are nonspecific findings that may be seen in numerous diagnostic entities. Rarely, some degree of bile duct proliferation may be seen in α_1-antitrypsin deficiency, early in the course of Alagille syndrome, and in progressive familial intrahepatic cholestasis and disorders of bile salt synthesis.

Other diagnostic studies that have been described in limited use as part of the evaluation for biliary atresia include endoscopic retrograde cholangiopancreatography[30,31] and magnetic resonance cholangiopancreatography.[32] In the setting of the appropriate clinical presentation, lack of alternative diagnosis, nonexcretion on scintigraphy, and compatible hepatic histology, however, most clinicians consult a surgical colleague for further evaluation and definitive therapy.

The surgical approach to biliary atresia includes operative cholangiography to confirm the diagnosis followed by Kasai portoenterostomy as therapy. After initial surgical dissection and identification of portal structures, an operative cholangiogram is performed by the injection

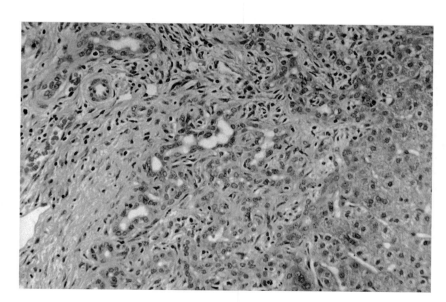

Figure 67–1. Percutaneous liver biopsy specimen of biliary atresia. This photomicrograph shows expansion of the portal region, early fibrosis, neutrophilic inflammation, and bile duct proliferation.

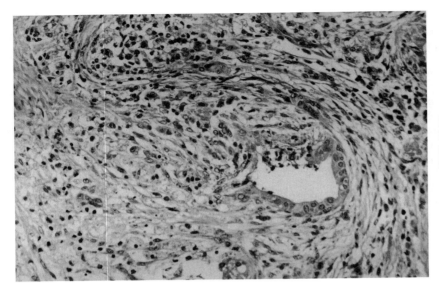

Figure 67–2. Percutaneous liver biopsy specimen of biliary atresia. This photomicrograph shows inflammation and inflammatory destruction of a larger bile duct from a patient with biliary atresia.

of contrast material into the gallbladder, if one can be identified. Intraoperative radiographic visualization then allows confirmation of biliary obstruction, which may need to be distinguished from hypoplasia of the extrahepatic bile ducts. When this has been confirmed, the Kasai operation involves dissection of the porta hepatis, the identification of the fibrous plate, and the anastomosis of a Roux-en-Y loop of jejunum allowing drainage of bile directly from the cut surface of the liver.[33]

Before the advent of the Kasai portoenterostomy in 1957, all children with biliary atresia died of liver failure by the second year of life. The outcome is better when surgery is done before 8 weeks of age but should be considered in all patients diagnosed before 13 weeks. The likelihood of a successful Kasai portoenterostomy beyond 13 weeks is small, but the operation should be considered in selected patients.[34] If surgery is successful, jaundice fades, and liver enzymes and fat malabsorption improve. In the era of orthotopic liver transplantation, it is now clear that this procedure merely delays the onset of liver failure in most cases of biliary atresia and improves the overall outcome by increasing the chances of a donor liver becoming available because transplant can be delayed until the child is older. The Kasai operation does not halt the cholangiopathy, and only a few patients are known to have survived beyond their 30s without requiring a liver transplant.[35]

After the Kasai procedure, many patients are started on prophylactic antibiotics for 6 months to 1 year to prevent cholangitis. Even when good bile flow is established, fat-soluble vitamin therapy should be given. Ursodeoxycholic acid and phenobarbital may have some benefits and are used in some centers after a Kasai portoenterostomy.[36-39]

Choledochal Cysts

Choledochal cysts are dilations of the biliary tract seen in 1 in 15,000 births in the West and at a much higher frequency in Japan (1 in 1000 live births).[40,41] More females are affected than males. The cystic dilation can be localized to the distal common bile duct (choledochocele) or can involve the bile ducts in segmental or diffuse forms. One etiologic theory suggests that an abnormal communication between the pancreatic duct and common bile duct causes reflux of pancreatic enzymes, weakening the walls of the common bile duct, which then balloon outward. Another theory postulates that choledochal cysts are developmental anomalies of the ductal plate. A third theory is that a distal obstruction of the common bile duct leads to proximal obstruction with dilation of the bile ducts.

A neonate who is symptomatic from a choledochal cyst usually presents with jaundice, sometimes with abdominal distention or a palpable mass, and less frequently with irritability and pain if the choledochal cyst perforates. Ultrasound usually is diagnostic of a choledochal cyst, but other imaging studies such as computed tomography or magnetic resonance imaging with or without cholangiography may be used to confirm the diagnosis. Choledochal cysts are treated surgically by excision and construction of a Roux-en-Y choledochojejunostomy to improve drainage. Choledochal cysts may be associated with disease of the intrahepatic ducts (Caroli disease), in which case the role of decompression surgery is diminished.

Spontaneous Perforation of the Common Bile Duct

Spontaneous perforation of the common bile duct is rare; affected infants present with jaundice and abdominal distention.[42,43] The infant is typically unwell and has acholic stools, elevated bilirubin, and elevated GGT and may manifest coagulopathy secondary to vitamin K deficiency. Discoloration of the umbilicus or abdominal flanks may be present, and laparotomy or paracentesis reveals bile-stained fluid. Treatment for bile duct perforation sometimes can be accomplished by surgical drainage alone, whereas some cases require surgical repair of the common bile duct or biliary reconstruction using a loop of intestine, as in biliary atresia.

Other Extrahepatic Causes of Neonatal Cholestasis

Rarely, neonatal cholestasis may be the presentation of an obstructing mass or tumor, such as neuroblastoma,[44] rhabdomyosarcoma,[45] or hemangioma.[46] Gallstones sometimes are seen in a neonate with infections,[47] and sludging often is seen in an infant treated with parenteral nutrition[48] or occasionally after a severe hemolytic process. In the latter group, spontaneous clearing of the sludge may occur, or clearance may occur at the time of operative or percutaneous cholangiogram after injection of contrast material into the biliary system.

Predominantly Intrahepatic Cause for Cholestasis

Idiopathic Neonatal Hepatitis

In most series of patients presenting with neonatal cholestasis, the two most common diagnoses include biliary atresia and idiopathic neonatal hepatitis. The latter group represents a heterogeneous group of disorders of varied etiology and outcome.[49] These disorders have been characterized as "hepatitis" because of the common features of hepatocellular injury, cellular disarray, variable degrees of giant cell transformation, and bile duct injury and inflammation. They also are characterized by the lack of diagnostic findings for alternative infectious, metabolic, genetic, and anatomic etiologies. Compared with the previously described evaluation for biliary atresia, these patients usually show excretion on scintigraphic studies, do not usually show significant bile duct proliferation in liver biopsy specimens (Fig. 67-3), occasionally show a reduced number of intrahepatic bile ducts in biopsy specimens, and have a variable outcome and prognosis.

The recognition of a larger number of specific diagnostic entities known to contribute to the neonatal hepatitis syndrome has helped reduce the number of

patients characterized as having an idiopathic etiology. Contributors to the more accurate determination of etiology have included the recognition of less common infectious agents, such as enteroviruses, parvovirus B19, and human herpesvirus type 6; elucidation of the genetic etiology of Alagille syndrome and the recognition of its varied clinical manifestations and genetic penetrance; the recognition of disorders of bile salt metabolism and the disorders of progressive familial intrahepatic cholestasis presenting as neonatal cholestasis; and the recognition of neonatal cholestasis as a manifestation of uncommon disorders, such as the occasionally symptomatic infant of a mother with systemic lupus erythematosus.[50] Because of the heterogeneous nature of the etiologies contributing to the "idiopathic" category, the prognosis is variable, with approximately two thirds to three fourths of patients experiencing resolution of hepatitis without long-term evidence of liver disease.[51]

Alagille Syndrome

Alagille syndrome,[52] or arteriohepatic dysplasia,[53] is a developmental disorder, most commonly associated with a mutation in the *Jagged 1* gene.[54,55] The mutation results in a spectrum of abnormalities, including dysmorphic facies and cholestasis that is associated with paucity of the intrahepatic bile ducts. This disorder occurs in approximately 1 in 70,000 live births. In addition to liver disease, other findings, such as eye abnormalities (posterior embryotoxon), butterfly vertebra, peripheral pulmonary stenosis or other cardiac lesions, and characteristic facies (prominent forehead often at the same plane as the nose when viewed from the side, a triangular face with narrowed chin, deep-set eyes), may be seen as part of the phenotype. One of the parents may exhibit similar facies or other features of the disorder consistent with its inherited nature and the variable expressivity of the phenotype.

When the disease presents in the neonate, it may resemble biliary atresia and other forms of neonatal

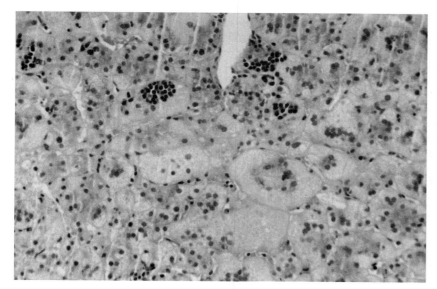

Figure 67–3. Percutaneous liver biopsy specimen of idiopathic neonatal hepatitis. This photomicrograph shows panlobular giant cell transformation with disorganization of the hepatic architecture and some extramedullary hematopoiesis. These findings alone are nonspecific but are typical of findings in cases of neonatal hepatitis that are idiopathic in origin.

cholestasis, but the presence of a cardiac murmur (peripheral pulmonary stenosis) and any of the other noted phenotypic findings should suggest Alagille syndrome. Examination of a liver biopsy specimen may reveal paucity of the intrahepatic bile ducts. In Alagille syndrome, there are less than 0.9 to 1.8 bile ducts per portal space, when at least six portal tracts are examined on a needle biopsy. Only 60% of patients with Alagille syndrome have paucity of bile ducts before the age of 6 months, however, and liver biopsy may need to be repeated later. Paucity of the intrahepatic bile ducts also can be seen in idiopathic neonatal hepatitis and α_1-antitrypsin deficiency. Because paucity of the intrahepatic bile ducts may be absent early in the clinical course, some of these patients proceed through a full evaluation to rule out biliary atresia, especially when other phenotypic findings are not evident. Genetic testing is not sufficiently accurate at this time to use diagnostically, but it may be more appropriate in the future as mutations are characterized further and other genes in the Notch-Jagged signaling pathway are characterized.

Progressive Familial Intrahepatic Cholestasis

Many neonates with jaundice initially seem to improve but later develop a chronic, unremitting cholestasis in the absence of any other detectable metabolic or anatomic disorder. These patients seem to have an autosomal recessive disorder and have a characteristic combination of clinical, biochemical, and histologic features that can be clustered into a diagnostic group called PFIC.[56,57]

The first disease described in this group of disorders was Byler disease, which involved members of an Amish kindred with persistent cholestasis. In Byler disease (also known as *PFIC1*), there is progressive liver disease with jaundice and cirrhosis by the first few years of life, but some children have a more slowly progressive course. Most patients present with prolonged jaundice with relatively well-preserved liver synthetic functions. Often the jaundice resolves and pruritus develops by the first birthday. These children commonly have growth delay without significant malnutrition.

Other forms of PFIC have been described, and the genetics have been elucidated.[58] Children with PFIC1 and PFIC2 have low GGT values, despite significant cholestasis, which may be a diagnostic clue during their evaluation. In PFIC3, GGT is elevated. Although most patients with PFIC have progressive liver damage, there is a propensity for early cirrhotic changes in PFIC2 in particular. Liver biopsy often is not characteristic, and a variety of changes are found as discussed previously.

The defects in PFIC seem to be at the level of the canalicular bile acid transport system. Serum bile acids often are elevated, and many patients develop significant pruritus. Byler disease is caused by a defect of the *FIC1* gene on 18q21-22.[59] This gene is involved in aminophospholipid transport in the intestine, liver, pancreas, and kidney. In PFIC2, a defect of the bile salt excretory pump gene on 2q24, coding for the major adenosine triphosphate–dependent bile salt export pump, has been found to be responsible for the disease.[60,61] Absence of this pump results in the failure of bile salt export from the liver. The

defect in PFIC3 is related to dysfunction of the multidrug resistance-3 P-glycoprotein, resulting from mutations in the *mdr-3* gene located on 7q21. The defect results in impaired translocation of phosphatidylcholine into bile.[62]

Treatment with oral ursodeoxycholic acid therapy has been at least partially effective in all three forms of this disorder.[63] Biliary diversion has been suggested as a mode of therapy in PFIC1 and PFIC2.[64] This procedure results in the loss of the enterohepatic circulation and a decrease in the serum bile acid pool, reducing the pruritus experienced by these patients. Liver transplantation has been used successfully in patients resistant to other forms of treatment.

α_1-Antitrypsin Deficiency

α1-Antitrypsin is a serine protease, present in hepatocytes and alveolar macrophages, which inhibits proteolytic enzymes, such as elastase, cathepsins, and trypsins. It is encoded by a single gene with more than 90 alleles identified on chromosome 14q31.32.2.[65-67] Only a few alleles are associated with clinical disease. The α_1-antitrypsin protein has been characterized into protease-inhibitor (Pi) types based on the electrophoretic mobility of the different protein isoforms. PiM occurs in unaffected individuals and is the most common of the protease inhibitor types; variants associated with liver disease are PiZ, PiS, and PiNull. PiZZ is associated with liver disease in infants and emphysema in young adults. The PiZ allele occurs in about 1 in 2000 to 1 in 7000 newborns of European origin.

Clinical manifestations of α_1-antitrypsin deficiency include neonatal cholestasis or slowly progressive hepatitis and cirrhosis in later childhood. Of PiZZ infants, 10% to 15% develop liver disease; 5% develop rapidly progressive disease requiring a liver transplant within the first 4 years of life. Of the remaining 95%, 25% recover completely, 25% develop cirrhosis by age 20 years, and the remainder have biochemical or clinical evidence of hepatitis.[68,69] Serum levels of α_1-antitrypsin are reduced by 85% to 90% of normal levels in affected individuals. Because α_1-antitrypsin is an acute-phase protein, levels can increase during inflammation or injury, and serum levels alone cannot be used for diagnostic purposes. Protease-inhibitor typing should be included as part of the diagnostic evaluation. Because α_1-antitrypsin deficiency is associated with defective hepatocyte excretion of the abnormal α_1-antitrypsin protein, the presence of periodic acid–Schiff–positive, diastase-resistant globules in the endoplasmic reticulum of hepatocytes[70] may be seen on liver biopsy. Some patients who have undergone cholangiography have hypoplasia of the extrahepatic bile ducts. There is currently no effective, specific therapy for this disorder, and care is supportive. Liver transplantation is the only option available to patients with progressive disease.

Disorders of Bile Acid Synthesis

Disorders of bile salt synthesis represent a small proportion of the spectrum of disorders contributing to the clinical presentation of neonatal cholestasis. Most of these disorders manifest as typical neonatal hepatitis with conjugated hyperbilirubinemia and nonspecific findings, such as giant cell transformation, on examination of liver histology. They may be distinguished by their persistent nature and occasionally by other clinical features. The most common defect is 3-β-hydroxysteroid dehydrogenase deficiency.[71] This disorder can present at any age, although a neonatal presentation with persistence and progression has been noted frequently. In contrast to some other disorders in this differential diagnosis, the GGT value is in the normal range. The second most commonly described bile salt synthetic defect, δ-4-3-oxosteroid 5-β reductase deficiency,[72] is associated with neonatal hepatitis, which may progress rapidly to liver failure and which may show some features suggesting neonatal iron storage disease. Other, less common bile salt synthetic defects may manifest with a neonatal hepatitis picture with chronic features of varying severity.[73,74]

The identification of these disorders is important because their responsiveness to bile salt replacement therapy has halted progression and improved liver function in many cases. The diagnosis is accomplished through the analysis of serum or urine by fast atom bombardment mass spectrometry or gas chromatography. Subsequent bile salt replacement therapy may work by replacing missing bile salts and inhibiting bile salt synthesis and the subsequent production of toxic bile salt intermediates.[75,76]

Although not usually classified as a bile salt synthetic defect per se, the peroxisomal disorder **Zellweger syndrome (cerebrohepatorenal syndrome)** is associated with atypical bile salts with abnormally long side chains. It may present as neonatal hepatitis in association with other features typical of the phenotype, including abnormal facies (midface hypoplasia, hypertelorism, high narrow forehead), hypotonia, and absent reflexes.[77-79]

Cholestasis Related to Total Parenteral Nutrition

Total parenteral nutrition (TPN) is essential in many neonatal conditions when enteral feeds are temporarily or permanently withheld. Prolonged TPN as the sole nutritional source may cause hepatocellular unrest, which is manifested by elevated transaminases, elevated GGT, jaundice, and the appearance of sludge in the bile ducts. The etiology of TPN cholestasis is unclear, but lack of enteral stimulation and the occurrence of episodes of sepsis enhance the severity of the disease. This condition may be particularly problematic in an infant recovering from surgery for necrotizing enterocolitis or gastroschisis, in whom lack of enteral feeding may be prolonged.

When cholestasis occurs in a neonate receiving TPN, alternative diagnoses still should be considered, particularly because biliary atresia may only become clinically manifest at several weeks of age. Other inherited, infectious, and metabolic disorders should be sought while initiating treatments that may improve TPN-related cholestasis. Early treatment of sepsis, meticulous attention to central line care, treatment of bacterial overgrowth of the small intestine, and use of early trophic feeds may prevent or attenuate the severity of TPN cholestasis. The use of choleretics, such as ursodeoxycholic acid, may be beneficial.[80] Cholecystokinin also may be a useful choleretic agent in this setting.[81]

Extracorporeal Membrane Oxygenation–Related Cholestasis

Some patients receiving extracorporeal membrane oxygenation are predisposed to formation of calculi, and it is postulated that increased hemolysis and bilirubin load promote the formation of bile sludging and jaundice with little hepatic or canalicular injury.[82] These patients often are not enterally fed and typically are receiving diuretics, which also contribute to the development of cholestasis. Ultrasound examination of the biliary tree and cholecystectomy in selected patients with calculi may be beneficial. Infectious causes of jaundice also should be considered because hepatitis C has been reported in patients undergoing extracorporeal membrane oxygenation.[83]

Neonatal Iron Storage Disease

Neonatal iron storage disease, or **neonatal hemochromatosis**, is characterized by hepatic failure detected soon after birth in association with extrahepatic iron deposits in tissues other than those of the reticuloendothelial system.[84] Cases may be sporadic or familial in occurrence.[85] Patients usually present in the first few hours of life with hypoalbuminemia and edema, hypoglycemia, and significant coagulopathy. Reduced levels of numerous serum proteins also are evident, and serum iron and ferritin levels are elevated. Jaundice may not be evident initially and may develop after several days. The etiology is not known, and because of some clinical heterogeneity, it is thought that this condition may represent more than one disorder.

Hepatic histology in this condition is abnormal, with significant hepatocellular destruction, cholestasis, and variable degrees of regeneration. Although iron deposition may be significant, it can be a nonspecific finding in the diseased neonatal liver. In addition, the significant coagulopathy accompanying this disorder may preclude the easy attainment of a biopsy specimen. The significant siderosis present in nonhepatic tissues permits alternative diagnostic approaches, however. Magnetic resonance imaging can be used to show the significant iron deposition in liver and pancreas and its relative absence in the spleen.[86] Another alternative is to obtain a biopsy specimen of the lip or buccal mucosa to identify the increased iron staining in minor salivary gland epithelium.

Treatment alternatives for this disorder are limited. Combined antioxidant therapy with iron chelation has been described with some success for symptomatic neonates.[87] Because of the severity of the liver disease, liver transplantation performed early has been described for many survivors.[88,89]

Tyrosinemia

Tyrosinemia is a rare cause of childhood liver and kidney disease, which is more frequent in some parts of Northern Quebec, Canada, and Scandinavia.[90] It is an autosomal recessive condition caused by a deficiency of fumarylacetoacetate hydrolase.[91] This gene defect has been mapped to chromosome 15q23-q25.[92] Fumarylacetoacetate, succinylacetoacetate, succinylacetone, and maleylacetoacetate are the toxic metabolites that accumulate in the liver that are believed to contribute to liver injury and dysfunction.[93]

Patients with tyrosinemia can present with varied clinical manifestations at different ages. Clinical presentations can include jaundice and other symptoms due to severe chronic hepatitis, which may be associated with a high frequency of hepatocellular carcinoma and acute liver failure in infancy. Nonhepatic manifestations include hypophosphatemic rickets as a result of renal tubular dysfunction and neurologic crises similar to those seen in porphyria. These clinical presentations are not mutually exclusive. A child with acute liver failure in infancy who survives often develops the chronic form of the disease, punctuated with episodes of acute decompensation. Over time, the development of renal disease and neurologic crises may become more evident. Hepatic failure in this disorder often is dominated by coagulopathy with relatively unimpressive elevations of serum transaminases.

Liver pathology in tyrosinemia depends on the time course of the disease. In early infancy, bile duct proliferation and giant cell transformation can be seen on biopsy. Significant steatosis may be present. Over time, progression to a micronodular cirrhosis may become evident, ultimately changing to a micronodular and macronodular cirrhosis with potential development of carcinoma.

The diagnosis of tyrosinemia depends on the demonstration of elevated plasma succinylacetone levels from a sample of dried blood on filter paper. Hypertyrosinemia itself is not diagnostic because elevated tyrosine levels can be seen in a variety of metabolic disorders, including underlying liver disease of multiple etiologies. The diagnosis of tyrosinemia can be confirmed by demonstration of the deficiency of fumarylacetoacetate hydrolase in lymphocytes, red blood cells, hepatocytes, and prenatally in chorionic villi.[94] Genetic screening in high-risk populations is possible, but not all mutant alleles are detectable yet.

Treatment of tyrosinemia is multifaceted. Strict dietary restriction of phenylalanine and tyrosine is commonly employed, although the long-term impact of such therapy on progression of liver disease has not been studied carefully. Administration of NTBC (2-[2-nitro-4-trifluoromethylbenzoyl]-1,3 cyclohexanedione),[95,96] an inhibitor of tyrosine degradation, has been introduced more recently. NTBC improves liver function in the setting of acute liver failure in many cases. When started before 2 years of age, NTBC seems also to help reduce progression of liver disease and the risk of hepatocellular carcinoma. Patients whose tyrosinemia continues to progress and who do not respond to treatment should be considered candidates for liver transplantation.[97]

Galactosemia

Classic **galactosemia** is an autosomal recessive condition with a prevalence of 1 in 63,000 in United States.[98-100] In galactosemia, galactose-1-phosphate uridyl transferase enzyme levels are absent or very low. After the ingestion of lactose, the disaccharide (glucose and galactose) in breast milk and milk-based formula, galactose, cannot be converted properly into glucose, and this leads to the accumulation of toxic metabolites, such as galactitol and galactose-1-phosphate. These metabolites accumulate in

multiple tissues, such as the liver, central nervous system, kidneys, and eyes, and are believed to be responsible for the toxicity in galactosemia.

The clinical presentation of galactosemia is variable and occurs in acute and subacute forms. Acute symptoms may include vomiting, anorexia, and abdominal distention. In some cases, symptoms may be less severe and associated with failure to thrive. Hypoglycemia and hemolysis also may occur. Hepatomegaly and jaundice are common after the first week of life, and there is a high incidence of sepsis with *Escherichia coli*.

Detection of galactosemia is now part of the newborn screen, although it is still important that a jaundiced neonate on a lactose-containing feed have a urine sample checked for the presence of reducing substances. Confirmatory testing is done by evaluation of red blood cell transferase activity. Genetic testing also is possible.

In classic galactosemia, missense mutations result in low or absent enzyme levels. More than 150 mutations have been identified. True homozygous galactosemia is a lifelong condition and is treated with complete elimination of lactose and galactose in the diet.

Mitochondrial Disorders

Mitochondrial respiratory chain defects represent a relatively rare subgroup of disorders, which may present with neonatal hepatitis or neonatal hepatic failure.[20] These clinical disorders have been associated with defects in complex III, complex IV, or the mitochondrial DNA depletion syndrome.[101-103] In addition to severe neonatal liver disease, these infants may be hypotonic or in coma. Significant hypoglycemia may be present, and the diagnosis may be suggested by significant lactic acidosis. Liver histology often shows significant microvesicular and macrovesicular steatosis. In infants described with these disorders, significant reductions in the activities of hepatic respiratory enzymes were noted.

Infections

As noted previously, the tendency toward cholestasis of the neonate permits the onset of clinical disease with the additional disruption of function associated with a diversity of mechanisms. Numerous hepatotropic viruses are capable of additional hepatocellular injury resulting in clinical disease. Rubella,[104] cytomegalovirus,[105] hepatitis A,[106] hepatitis B,[107] herpes simplex,[108] and human herpesvirus type 6[109] all have been associated with hepatitis in neonates. The enteroviruses coxsackie B and echoviruses 6, 9, 11, 14, and 19 also are known to cause neonatal hepatitis, which may be fulminant and result in acute liver failure.[110] Parvovirus B19 has been associated with hydrops fetalis, hepatitis, acute liver failure, and aplastic anemia.[111]

Liver injury and jaundice may be seen in the course of neonatal sepsis. Clinical disease can be seen in neonates with sepsis associated with *E. coli*, *Listeria monocytogenes*, group B streptococcus, and *Staphylococcus aureus*. Congenital toxoplasmosis[112] causes hepatomegaly, jaundice, choroidoretinitis, intracranial calcification, microcephaly, and mental retardation. Neonatal hepatitis also can be seen in congenital syphilis. Occult urinary tract infection and sepsis also can be associated with jaundice and direct hyperbilirubinemia.[113]

REFERENCES

1. Stieger B, Meier PJ: Bile acid and xenobiotic transporters in liver. Curr Opin Cell Biol 10:462, 1998.
2. Mallory A, Kern F Jr, Smith J, Savage D: Patterns of bile acids and microflora in the human small intestine: I. Bile acids. Gastroenterology 64:26, 1973.
3. Hagenbuch B: Molecular properties of hepatic uptake systems for bile acids and organic anions. J Membr Biol 160:1, 1997.
4. Gerloff T, Stieger B, Hagenbuch B, et al: The sister of P-glycoprotein represents the canalicular bile salt export pump of mammalian liver. J Biol Chem 273:10046, 1998.
5. Keppler D, Konig J: Hepatic canalicular membrane 5: Expression and localization of the conjugate export pump encoded by the MRP2 (cMRP/cMOAT) gene in liver. FASEB J 11:509, 1997.
6. Silverman JA, Thorgeirsson SS: Regulation and function of the multidrug resistance genes in liver. Prog Liver Dis 13:101, 1995.
7. Smith AJ, De Vree JM, Ottenhoff R, et al: Hepatocyte-specific expression of the human MDR3 P-glycoprotein gene restores the biliary phosphatidylcholine excretion absent in Mdr2 (−/−) mice. Hepatology 28:530, 1998.
8. Severn CB: A morphological study of the development of the human liver: I. Development of the hepatic diverticulum. Am J Anat 131:133, 1971.
9. Van Eyken P, Sciot R, Callea F, et al: The development of the intrahepatic bile ducts in man: A keratin-immunohistochemical study. Hepatology 8:1586, 1988.
10. Desmet VJ: What is congenital hepatic fibrosis? Histopathology 20:465, 1992.
11. Colombo C, Zuliani G, Ronchi M, et al: Biliary bile acid composition of the human fetus in early gestation. Pediatr Res 21:197, 1987.
12. Watkins JB, Szczepanik P, Gould JB, et al: Bile salt metabolism in the human premature infant: Preliminary observations of pool size and synthesis rate following prenatal administration of dexamethasone and phenobarbital. Gastroenterology 69:706, 1975.
13. Itoh S, Onishi S, Isobe K, et al: Foetomaternal relationships of serum bile acid pattern estimated by high-pressure liquid chromatography. Biochem J 204:141, 1982.
14. Suchy FJ, Balistreri WF, Heubi JE, et al: Physiologic cholestasis: Elevation of the primary serum bile acid concentrations in normal infants. Gastroenterology 80(5 pt 1):1037, 1981.
15. Bhaduri BR, Vergani GM: Fulminant hepatic failure: Pediatric aspects. Semin Liver Dis 16:349, 1996.
16. Koller F: Theory and experience behind the use of coagulation tests in diagnosis and prognosis of liver disease. Scand J Gastroenterol 19(suppl):51, 1973.
17. Tucker JS, Woolf IL, Boyes BE, et al: Coagulation studies in acute hepatic failure. Gut 14:418, 1973.
18. Bernuau J, Benhamou JP: Classifying acute liver failure. Lancet 342:252, 1993.
19. Dymock IW, Tucker JS, Woolf IL, et al: Coagulation studies as a prognostic index in acute liver failure. Br J Haematol 29:385, 1975.
20. Durand P, Debray D, Mandel R, et al: Acute liver failure in infancy: A 14-year experience of a pediatric liver transplantation center. J Pediatr 139:871, 2001.
21. Bismuth H, Samuel D, Castaing D, et al: Orthotopic liver transplantation in fulminant and subfulminant hepatitis: The Paul Brousse experience. Ann Surg 222:109, 1995.
22. Devictor D, Desplanques L, Debray D, et al: Emergency liver transplantation for fulminant liver failure in infants and children. Hepatology 16:1156, 1992.
23. Rivera-Penera T, Moreno J, Skaff C, et al: Delayed encephalopathy in fulminant hepatic failure in the pediatric population and the role of liver transplantation. J Pediatr Gastroenterol Nutr 24:128, 1997.
24. Goldberg DM, Martin JV: Role of gamma-glutamyl transpeptidase activity in the diagnosis of hepatobiliary disease. Digestion 12:232, 1975.
25. Yoon PW, Bresee JS, Olney RS, et al: Epidemiology of biliary atresia: A population-based study. Pediatrics 99:376, 1997.
26. Balistreri WF, Grand R, Hoofnagle JH, et al: Biliary atresia: Current concepts and research directions: Summary of a symposium. Hepatology 23:1682, 1996.
27. Green D, Carroll BA: Ultrasonography in the jaundiced infant: A new approach. J Ultrasound Med 5:323, 1986.
28. Dick MC, Mowat AP: Biliary scintigraphy with DISIDA: A simpler way of showing bile duct patency in suspected biliary atresia. Arch Dis Child 61:191, 1986.
29. Spivak W, Sarkar S, Winter D, et al: Diagnostic utility of hepatobiliary scintigraphy with 99mTc-DISIDA in neonatal cholestasis. J Pediatr 110:855, 1987.
30. Iinuma Y, Narisawa R, Iwafuchi M, et al: The role of endoscopic retrograde cholangiopancreatography in infants with cholestasis. J Pediatr Surg 35:545, 2000.
31. Wilkinson ML, Mieli-Vergani G, Ball C, et al: Endoscopic retrograde cholangiopancreatography in infantile cholestasis. Arch Dis Child 66:121, 1991.
32. Miyazaki T, Yamashita Y, Tang Y, et al: Single-shot MR cholangiopancreatography of neonates, infants, and young children. AJR Am J Roentgenol 170:33, 1998.
33. Ohi R: Surgery for biliary atresia. Liver 21:175, 2001.
34. Chardot C, Carton M, Spire-Bendelac N, et al: Is the Kasai operation still indicated in children older than 3 months diagnosed with biliary atresia? J Pediatr 138:224, 2001.
35. Ohi R: Biliary atresia: A surgical perspective. Clin Liver Dis 4:779, 2000.
36. Nittono H, Tokita A, Hayashi M, et al: Ursodeoxycholic acid therapy in the treatment of biliary atresia. Biomed Pharmacother 43:37, 1989.
37. Thompson RP, Williams R: Phenobarbitone in intrahepatic biliary atresia. Lancet 2:466, 1970.
38. Ullrich D, Rating D, Schroter W, et al: Treatment with ursodeoxycholic acid renders children with biliary atresia suitable for liver transplantation. Lancet 2:1324, 1987.
39. Vajro P, Couturier M, Lemonnier F, Odievre M: Effects of postoperative cholestyramine and phenobarbital administration on bile flow restoration in infants with extrahepatic biliary atresia. J Pediatr Surg 21:362, 1986.
40. Postema RR, Hazebroek FW: Choledochal cysts in children: A review of 28 years of treatment in a Dutch children's hospital. Eur J Surg 165:1159, 1999.
41. Stringer MD, Dhawan A, Davenport M, et al: Choledochal cysts: Lessons from a 20 year experience. Arch Dis Child 73:528, 1995.
42. Davenport M, Heaton ND, Howard ER: Spontaneous perforation of the bile duct in infants. Br J Surg 78:1068, 1991.
43. Howard ER, Johnston DI, Mowat AP: Spontaneous perforation of common bile duct in infants. Arch Dis Child 51:883, 1976.
44. Kreeftenberg HG Jr, Zeebregts CJ, Tamminga RY, et al: Scrotal hematoma, anemia, and jaundice as manifestations

of adrenal neuroblastoma in a newborn. J Pediatr Surg 34:1856, 1999.

45. Mihara S, Matsumoto H, Tokunaga F, et al: Botryoid rhabdomyosarcoma of the gallbladder in a child. Cancer 49:812, 1982.

46. Selby DM, Stocker JT, Waclawiw MA, et al: Infantile hemangioendothelioma of the liver. Hepatology 20(1 pt 1):39, 1994.

47. Alissa K, Saunier P, Russo M, Vedrenne J: Neonatal cholestatic lithiasis associated with E. coli infection. Arch Pediatr 3:144-146, 1996.

48. Quigley EM, Marsh MN, Shaffer JL, Markin RS: Hepatobiliary complications of total parenteral nutrition. Gastroenterology 104:286, 1993.

49. Danks DM, Campbell PE, Jack I, et al: Studies of the aetiology of neonatal hepatitis and biliary atresia. Arch Dis Child 52:360, 1977.

50. Evans N, Gaskin K: Liver disease in association with neonatal lupus erythematosus. J Paediatr Child Health 29:478, 1993.

51. Dick MC, Mowat AP: Hepatitis syndrome in infancy—an epidemiological survey with 10 year follow up. Arch Dis Child 60:512, 1985.

52. Alagille, D, Habib EC, Thomassin N: L'atresie des voies biliares extrahepatiques permeables chez l'enfant. Arch Fr Pediatr 26:283, 1969.

53. Watson GH, Miller V: Arteriohepatic dysplasia: Familial pulmonary arterial stenosis with neonatal liver disease. Arch Dis Child 48:459, 1973.

54. Krantz ID, Piccoli DA, Spinner NB: Clinical and molecular genetics of Alagille syndrome. Curr Opin Pediatr 11:558, 1999.

55. Li L, Krantz ID, Deng Y, et al: Alagille syndrome is caused by mutations in human Jagged1, which encodes a ligand for Notch1. Nat Genet 16:243, 1997.

56. Alonso EM, Snover DC, Montag A, et al: Histologic pathology of the liver in progressive familial intrahepatic cholestasis. J Pediatr Gastroenterol Nutr 18:128, 1994.

57. Emerick KM, Whitington PF: Clinical aspects of familial cholestasis (with molecular explanations). Curr Gastroenterol Rep 1:223, 1999.

58. Jacquemin E: Progressive familial intrahepatic cholestasis: Genetic basis and treatment. Clin Liver Dis 4:753, 2000.

59. Bull LN, Carlton VE, Stricker NL, et al: Genetic and morphological findings in progressive familial intrahepatic cholestasis (Byler disease [PFIC-1] and Byler syndrome): Evidence for heterogeneity. Hepatology 26:155, 1997.

60. Strautnieks SS, Bull LN, Knisely AS, et al: A gene encoding a liver-specific ABC transporter is mutated in progressive familial intrahepatic cholestasis. Nat Genet 20:233, 1998.

61. Strautnieks SS, Kagalwalla AF, Tanner MS, et al: Identification of a locus for progressive familial intrahepatic cholestasis PFIC2 on chromosome 2q24. Am J Hum Genet 61:630, 1997.

62. Deleuze JF, Jacquemin E, Dubuisson C, et al: Defect of multidrug-resistance 3 gene expression in a subtype of progressive familial intrahepatic cholestasis. Hepatology 23:904, 1996.

63. Jacquemin E, Hermans D, Myara A, et al: Ursodeoxycholic acid therapy in pediatric patients with progressive familial intrahepatic cholestasis. Hepatology 25:519, 1997.

64. Emond JC, Whitington PF: Selective surgical management of progressive familial intrahepatic cholestasis (Byler's disease). J Pediatr Surg 30:1635, 1995.

65. Byth BC, Billingsley GD, Cox DW: Physical and genetic mapping of the serpin gene cluster at 14q32.1: Allelic association and a unique haplotype associated with alpha 1-antitrypsin deficiency. Am J Hum Genet 55:126, 1994.

66. Rollini P, Fournier RE: A 370-kb cosmid contig of the serpin gene cluster on human chromosome 14q32.1: Molecular linkage of the genes encoding alpha 1-antichymotrypsin, protein C inhibitor, kallistatin, alpha 1-antitrypsin, and corticosteroid-binding globulin. Genomics 46:409, 1997.

67. Rollini P, Fournier RE: Molecular linkage of the human alpha 1-antitrypsin and corticosteroid-binding globulin genes on chromosome 14q32.1. Mamm Genome 8:913, 1997.

68. Francavilla R, Castellaneta SP, Hadzic N, et al: Prognosis of alpha-1-antitrypsin deficiency-related liver disease in the era of paediatric liver transplantation. J Hepatol 32:986, 2000.

69. Mowat AP: Alpha 1-antitrypsin deficiency (PiZZ): Features of liver involvement in childhood. Acta Paediatr 393(suppl): 13, 1994.

70. Perlmutter DH: Liver injury in alpha 1-antitrypsin deficiency. Clin Liver Dis 4:387, 2000.

71. Clayton PT, Leonard JV, Lawson AM, et al: Familial giant cell hepatitis associated with synthesis of 3 beta, 7 alpha-dihydroxy- and 3 beta, 7 alpha, 12 alpha-trihydroxy-5-cholenoic acids. J Clin Invest 79:1031, 1987.

72. Setchell KD, Suchy FJ, Welsh MB, et al: Delta 4-3-oxosteroid 5 beta-reductase deficiency described in identical twins with neonatal hepatitis: A new inborn error in bile acid synthesis. J Clin Invest 82:2148, 1988.

73. Kimura A, Yuge K, Yukizane S, et al: Abnormal low ratio of cholic acid to chenodeoxycholic acid in a cholestatic infant with severe hypoglycemia. J Pediatr Gastroenterol Nutr 12:383, 1991.

74. Setchell KD, Schwarz M, O'Connell NC, et al: Identification of a new inborn error in bile acid synthesis: Mutation of the oxysterol 7alpha-hydroxylase gene causes severe neonatal liver disease. J Clin Invest 102:1690, 1998.

75. Daugherty CC, Setchell KD, Heubi JE, Balistreri WF: Resolution of liver biopsy alterations in three siblings with bile acid treatment of an inborn error of bile acid metabolism (delta 4-3-oxosteroid 5 beta-reductase deficiency). Hepatology 18:1096, 1993.

76. Horslen SP, Lawson AM, Malone M, Clayton PT: 3 Beta-hydroxy-delta 5-C27-steroid dehydrogenase deficiency: Effect of chenodeoxycholic acid therapy on liver histology. J Inherit Metab Dis 15:38, 1992.

77. Govaerts L, Monnens L, Tegelaers W, et al: Cerebro-hepato-renal syndrome of Zellweger: Clinical symptoms and relevant laboratory findings in 16 patients. Eur J Pediatr 139:125, 1982.

78. Passarge E, McAdams AJ: Cerebro-hepato-renal syndrome: A newly recognized hereditary disorder of multiple congenital defects, including sudanophilic leukodystrophy, cirrhosis of the liver, and polycystic kidneys. J Pediatr 71: 691, 1967.

79. Smith DW, Opitz JM, Inhorn SL: A syndrome of multiple developmental defects including polycystic kidneys and intrahepatic biliary dysgenesis in 2 siblings. J Pediatr 67:617, 1965.

80. Spagnuolo MI, Iorio R, Vegnente A, Guarino A: Ursodeoxycholic acid for treatment of cholestasis in children on long-term total parenteral nutrition: A pilot study. Gastroenterology 111:716, 1996.

81. Rintala RJ, Lindahl H, Pohjavuori M: Total parenteral nutrition-associated cholestasis in surgical neonates may be reversed by intravenous cholecystokinin: A preliminary report. J Pediatr Surg 30:827, 1995.

82. Shneider B, Maller E, VanMarter L, O'Rourke PP: Cholestasis in infants supported with extracorporeal membrane oxygenation. J Pediatr 115:462, 1989.

83. Nelson SP, Jonas MM: Hepatitis C infection in children who received extracorporeal membrane oxygenation. J Pediatr Surg 31:644, 1996.

84. Knisely AS: Neonatal hemochromatosis. Adv Pediatr 39:383, 1992.

85. Verloes A, Temple IK, Hubert AF, et al: Recurrence of neonatal haemochromatosis in half sibs born of unaffected mothers. J Med Genet 33:444, 1996.

86. Hayes AM, Jaramillo D, Levy HL, Knisely AS: Neonatal hemochromatosis: Diagnosis with MR imaging. AJR Am J Roentgenol 159:623, 1992.

87. Sigurdsson L, Reyes J, Kocoshis SA, et al: Neonatal hemochromatosis: Outcomes of pharmacologic and surgical therapies. J Pediatr Gastroenterol Nutr 26:85, 1998.

88. Rand EB, McClenathan DT, Whitington PF: Neonatal hemochromatosis: Report of successful orthotopic liver transplantation. J Pediatr Gastroenterol Nutr 15:325, 1992.

89. Srinivasan P, Vilca-Melendez H, Muiesan P, et al: Liver transplantation with monosegments. Surgery 126:10, 1999.

90. De Braekeleer M, Larochelle J: Genetic epidemiology of hereditary tyrosinemia in Quebec and in Saguenay-Lac-St-Jean. Am J Hum Genet 47:302, 1990.

91. Lindblad B, Lindstedt S, Steen G: On the enzymic defects in hereditary tyrosinemia. Proc Natl Acad Sci U S A 74:4641, 1977.

92. Phaneuf D, Labelle Y, Berube D, et al: Cloning and expression of the cDNA encoding human fumarylacetoacetate hydrolase, the enzyme deficient in hereditary tyrosinemia: Assignment of the gene to chromosome 15. Am J Hum Genet 48:525, 1991.

93. Scriver CR, Larochelle J, Silverberg M: Hereditary tyrosinemia and tyrosyluria in a French Canadian geographic isolate. Am J Dis Child 113:41, 1967.

94. Kvittingen EA, Guibaud PP, Divry P, et al: Prenatal diagnosis of hereditary tyrosinaemia type I by determination of fumarylacetoacetase in chorionic villus material. Eur J Pediatr 144:597, 1986.

95. Holme E, Lindstedt S: Nontransplant treatment of tyrosinemia. Clin Liver Dis 4:805, 2000.

96. Pitkanen ST, Salo MK, Heikinheimo M: Hereditary tyrosinaemia type I: From basics to progress in treatment. Ann Med 32:530, 2000.

97. Paradis K, Weber A, Seidman EG, et al: Liver transplantation for hereditary tyrosinemia: The Quebec experience. Am J Hum Genet 47:338, 1990.

98. Elsas LJ, Lai K: The molecular biology of galactosemia. Genet Med 1:40, 1998.

99. Elsas LJ, Lai K, Saunders CJ, Langley SD: Functional analysis of the human galactose-1-phosphate uridyltransferase promoter in Duarte and LA variant galactosemia. Mol Genet Metab 72:297, 2001.

100. Novelli G, Reichardt JK: Molecular basis of disorders of human galactose metabolism: Past, present, and future. Mol Genet Metab 71:62, 2000.

101. Lopriore E, Gemke RJ, Verhoeven NM, et al: Carnitine-acylcarnitine translocase deficiency: Phenotype, residual enzyme activity and outcome. Eur J Pediatr 160:101, 2001.

102. Mandel H, Hartman C, Berkowitz D, et al: The hepatic mitochondrial DNA depletion syndrome: Ultrastructural changes in liver biopsies. Hepatology 34(4 pt 1):776, 2001.

103. Valnot I, Osmond S, Gigarel N, et al: Mutations of the SCO1 gene in mitochondrial cytochrome c oxidase deficiency with neonatal-onset hepatic failure and encephalopathy. Am J Hum Genet 67:1104, 2000.

104. Esterly JR, Slusser RJ, Ruebner BH: Hepatic lesions in the congenital rubella syndrome. J Pediatr 71:676, 1967.

105. Reynolds DW, Stagno S, Hosty TS, et al: Maternal cytomegalovirus excretion and perinatal infection. N Engl J Med 289:1, 1973.

106. Tong MJ, Thursby M, Rakela J, et al: Studies on the maternal-infant transmission of the viruses which cause acute hepatitis. Gastroenterology 80(5 pt 1):999, 1981.

107. Tang JR, Hsu HY, Lin HH, et al: Hepatitis B surface antigenemia at birth: A long-term follow-up study. J Pediatr 133:374, 1998.

108. Shackelford GD, Kirks DR: Neonatal hepatic calcification secondary to transplacental infection. Radiology 122:753, 1977.

109. Tajiri H, Tanaka-Taya K, Ozaki Y, et al: Chronic hepatitis in an infant, in association with human herpesvirus-6 infection. J Pediatr 131:473, 1997.

110. Pruekprasert P, Stout C, Patamasucon P: Neonatal enterovirus infection. J Assoc Acad Minor Phys 6:134, 1995.

111. Pardi DS, Romero Y, Mertz LE, Douglas DD: Hepatitis-associated aplastic anemia and acute parvovirus B19 infection: A report of two cases and a review of the literature. Am J Gastroenterol 93:468, 1998.

112. Desmonts G, Couvreur J: Congenital toxoplasmosis: A prospective study of 378 pregnancies. N Engl J Med 290:1110, 1974.

113. Arthur AB, Wilson BD: Urinary infection presenting with jaundice. BMJ 1:539, 1967.

CHAPTER 68

Hyperbilirubinemia

Jon F. Watchko

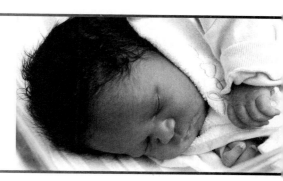

Almost two thirds of human newborns develop clinically evident indirect hyperbilirubinemia in the first few days of life; thus, this is the most common condition necessitating evaluation and management in neonates. Although generally benign, hyperbilirubinemia can become severe in certain newborns and place them at risk for hyperbilirubinemic encephalopathy and its attendant long-term adverse neurodevelopmental sequelae. Unfortunately, physicians have yet to fully understand the pathophysiologic processes of bilirubin toxicity and are currently unable to identify, from the myriad of normal infants in the nursery, which ones are likely to develop extreme hyperbilirubinemia. This chapter addresses the relevant basic science and clinical information necessary for managing unconjugated hyperbilirubinemia, the dominant form of neonatal jaundice.

BILIRUBIN METABOLISM

Bilirubin is a physiologic end product of heme catabolism (Fig. 68-1). The major biologic source of heme is red blood cell hemoglobin, although other hemoproteins, including muscle myoglobin, hepatic cytochromes, and catalases, also contribute.[1] The rate-limiting step in the breakdown of heme is catalyzed by heme oxygenase, an enzyme found primarily in the reticuloendothelial system.[2,3] This oxidation reaction produces biliverdin and an equimolar amount of carbon monoxide (CO). End-tidal CO measured in the exhaled breath provides an index of bilirubin production.[4-6] The subsequent reduction of biliverdin to bilirubin takes place in the cytosol and is catalyzed by biliverdin reductase.[7] Bilirubin IXα is the predominant bilirubin isomer found in the plasma of full-term neonates, in which it is transported bound to albumin. The relatively high affinity of albumin for bilirubin (10^7 to 10^8 mol^{-1})[8] limits the unbound or "free" bilirubin to the nanomolar range, even in the presence of appreciable unconjugated hyperbilirubinemia.[8-10]

Once in the hepatic circulation, bilirubin, but not albumin, is rapidly and selectively transported into the hepatocyte by a carrier-mediated process reported to involve organic anion-transporting polypeptide 2 (OATP-2 [SLC21A6]).[11] Within the hepatocyte, bilirubin is bound to glutathione *S*-transferase-β (ligandin, Y-protein) preventing the reflux of bilirubin back into the circulation. Bilirubin is conjugated with glucuronic acid within the endoplasmic reticulum of the hepatocyte by uridine diphosphate-glucuronosyltransferase (UDPGT) to form bilirubin monoglucurononides and diglucurononides. The polar, water-soluble bilirubin conjugates are actively secreted into the bile canaliculi by a carrier-mediated process involving the canalicular multispecific organic anion transporter (cMOAT), also known as multidrug resistance–associated protein 2,[12,13] and from there they enter the small intestine. In mature subjects, bilirubin is reduced to urobilinogen by intestinal bacteria and excreted in the stool. In contrast, bilirubin conjugates within the newborn gastrointestinal tract may be deconjugated to glucuronic acid and unconjugated bilirubin by the prominent catalytic activity of tissue β-glucuronidase in neonates.[14] The resultant unconjugated bilirubin is then reabsorbed into the hepatic circulation. This phenomenon is termed the **enterohepatic circulation of bilirubin** and increases the hepatic bilirubin load in neonates.

The type of bilirubin produced by the fetus during much of gestation is bilirubin IXβ, which, unlike the IXα isomer, is highly soluble and can be excreted without undergoing hepatic conjugation, which thereby facilitates its clearance across the placenta.[15] Indeed, unconjugated bilirubin is readily transported across the placenta in mammals, more so than biliverdin[16] and conjugated bilirubin.[17] This observation has led some authorities to speculate that the reduction of biliverdin to bilirubin evolved, in part, to facilitate the excretion of bile pigments by the fetus.[18] Studies have also suggested that fetal-to-maternal bilirubin placental transport may involve a carrier-mediated process, although the candidate transporter has yet to be identified.[19]

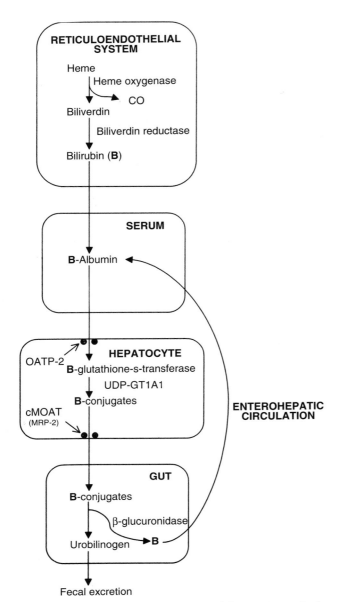

Figure 68–1. Bilirubin metabolism in neonatal life. cMOAT, canalicular multispecific organic anion transporter; CO, carbon monoxide; MRP-2, multidrug resistance–associated protein 2; OATP-2, organic anion-transporting polypeptide 2; UDP-GT1A1, uridine diphosphate-glucuronosyltransferase 1A1 isoform. *(Adapted from Hansen TWR: Fetal and neonatal bilirubin metabolism. In Maisels MJ, Watchko JF [eds]: Neonatal Jaundice. Amsterdam, Harwood Academic, 2000, pp 3-20.)*

INDIRECT HYPERBILIRUBINEMIA IN NEONATES

The indirect hyperbilirubinemia commonly observed in neonates reflects an interplay of developmentally modulated changes in bilirubin production and metabolism characterized by an increased bilirubin load on hepatocytes and decreased hepatic bilirubin clearance (Table 68-1). The increased bilirubin load is the result of (1) the newborn's large red blood cell mass combined with a reduced red blood cell lifespan and (2) the enterohepatic

Table 68–1. Causes of Indirect Hyperbilirubinemia in Newborns

Increased Production or Bilirubin Load on the Liver

Hemolytic Disease

Heritable
  Red blood cell membrane defects
    Spherocytosis, elliptocytosis, stomatocytosis, pyknocytosis
  Red blood cell enzyme deficiencies
    Glucose-6-phosphate dehydrogenase deficiency
    Pyruvate kinase deficiency and other erythrocyte enzyme deficiencies
  Hemoglobinopathies
    α-Thalassemia, β-γ-thalassemia
Immune mediated
  Rh alloimmunization
  ABO and other blood group incompatibilities
Acquired diseases
  Disseminated intravascular coagulation
  Extravasation of blood (hematomas; pulmonary, cerebral, or other occult hemorrhage)

Other Causes of Increased Production

Sepsis
Polycythemia
Macrosomic infants of diabetic mothers

Increased Enterohepatic Circulation of Bilirubin

Breast-milk jaundice
Pyloric stenosis
Small or large bowel obstruction or ileus

Decreased Clearance

Prematurity
Glucose-6-phosphate dehydrogenase deficiency

Inborn Errors of Metabolism

Crigler-Najjar syndrome, types 1 and 2
Gilbert syndrome
Tyrosinemia
Hypermethioninemia

Metabolic

Hypothyroidism
Hypopituitarism

From Watchko JF: Indirect hyperbilirubinemia in the neonate. In Maisels MJ, Watchko JF (eds): Neonatal Jaundice, Amsterdam, Harwood Academic, 2000, pp 51-66.

circulation of bilirubin. Decreases in neonatal hepatic bilirubin clearance result primarily from a limited capacity for hepatic bilirubin conjugation. Both an increased bilirubin load and a decreased clearance probably contribute to the jaundice in any given infant; quantifying their individual contribution, however, is usually not possible in the clinical arena.

Increased Bilirubin Load

Hemolytic Disease

The reduced life span of red blood cells in the normal newborn (70 to 90 days, as opposed to 120 days in the adult)[20,21] contributes to an enhanced level of bilirubin production and hepatic bilirubin load in neonates. It follows that the causes of an increase in red blood cell mass—poly-cythemia and factors known to accelerate red blood cell turn over (i.e., hemolytic disorders)—are clinically important conditions that enhance the risk for developing hyperbilirubinemia in infants. Of these, hemolysis is the most potent contributor to the genesis of marked hyperbilirubinemia. The causes of hemolysis in the neonatal period are numerous but can be broadly grouped into three major categories: (1) heritable defects in red blood cell metabolism, membrane structure, or hemoglobin; (2) acquired disorders; and (3) immune-mediated mechanisms (see Table 68-1).

Heritable Causes of Hemolysis

Red blood cell membrane defects. Of the many red blood cell membrane defects that lead to hemolysis, only hereditary spherocytosis, elliptocytosis, stomatocytosis, and infantile pyknocytosis may manifest themselves in the neonatal period.[22,23] Establishing a diagnosis of these disorders is often difficult in neonates because newborns normally exhibit a marked variation in red blood cell membrane size and shape.[22,24] Spherocytes, however, are not often seen on the red blood cell smear of hematologically normal newborns. This morphologic abnormality, when prominent, may yield a diagnosis of hereditary spherocytosis that can be confirmed through the incubated osmotic fragility test, a reliable diagnostic tool in newborns when coupled with fetal red blood cell controls. The clinician must rule out symptomatic ABO hemolytic disease by performing a direct Coombs test, because affected infants may also manifest prominent microspherocytosis.[25] Moreover, hereditary spherocytosis and symptomatic ABO hemolytic disease can occur in the same infant and result in severe anemia and hyperbilirubinemia.[26]

Red blood cell enzyme deficiencies. The most common red blood cell enzyme defect associated with hyperbilirubinemia in the neonatal period is glucose-6-phosphate dehydrogenase (G6PD) deficiency.[27-29] G6PD deficiency is a sex-linked disorder that may be associated with hemolysis in newborns after exposure to an appropriate trigger, usually an oxidative challenge (e.g., naphthalene, a common component in mothballs).[28,29] Severe hemolysis and marked hyperbilirubinemia may occur in this context and result in kernicterus.[30] Another important hemolytic trigger in G6PD-deficient newborns is infection.[27-29] In most cases of marked hyperbilirubinemia in G6PD-deficient neonates, however, there is no overt evidence of hemolysis.[31] This observation has prompted some authorities to conclude that in the majority of cases, hyperbilirubinemia in G6PD deficiency is of hepatic origin, resulting from impaired bilirubin clearance.[27,32,33] Others counter that anemia is masked by other factors that modulate hemoglobin concentration in the immediate neonatal period.[28] Recent studies have shed some light on this controversy, demonstrating that (1) Gilbert syndrome, a congenital defect in bilirubin conjugating capacity (described later), is observed in approximately 50% of G6PD-deficient newborns and (2) the combination of G6PD deficiency and Gilbert syndrome significantly increases the risk of hyperbilirubinemia ($\geq$15 mg/dL [257 μmol/L]), in comparison with G6PD deficiency alone (Table 68-2).[34] The presence of Gilbert syndrome appears to be an important factor in the pathogenesis of neonatal jaundice in association with G6PD deficiency.[34] Regardless of the mechanism or mechanisms underlying jaundice in G6PD-deficient newborns, it is clear that marked hyperbilirubinemia may develop in such infants and lead to neurotoxicity.[27,28,35]

Hemoglobinopathies. Defects in hemoglobin structure or synthesis are rare disorders that infrequently manifest in the neonatal period. Of these, α-thalassemia trait is the most common, as evidenced by a mean corpuscular volume of less than 95 fL (in normal infants, it is 100 to 120 fL),[36] but is not associated with neonatal hemolysis. Hemoglobin H disease results from the presence of three thalassemia mutations and can cause hemolysis and anemia in neonates.[37] Homozygous α-thalassemia (total absence of α-chain synthesis) results in profound hemolysis, anemia, hydrops fetalis, and almost always stillbirth or death in the immediate neonatal period.

Table 68–2. Incidence of Hyperbilirubinemia ($\geq$15 mg/dL) as a Function of G6PD and Gilbert Genotype

| | Incidence of Gilbert Genotype | | | |
	6/6*	6/7†	7/7‡	Total
G6PD				
−/−	6/62 (9.7%)	18/57 (31.6%)	6/12 (50%)	30/131 (22.9%)
+/+	10/101 (9.9%)	7/105 (6.7%)	5/34 (14.7%)	22/240 (9.2%)
P§	NS	<.0001	.02	.0005

*Homozygous normal uridine diphosphate-glucuronosyl transferase (UDPGT) genotype.
†Heterozygous variant UDPGT genotype.
‡Homozygous variant UDPGT genotype.
§P values are for G6PD −/− (G6PD-deficient) genotype versus G6PD +/+ (G6PD-sufficient) genotype.

G6PD, glucose-6-phosphate dehydrogenase; NS, nonsignificant.

From Kaplan M, Renbaum P, Levy-Lahad E, et al: Gilbert syndrome and glucose-6-phosphate dehydrogenase deficiency: A dose-dependent genetic interaction crucial to neonatal hyperbilirubinemia. Proc Natl Acad Sci U S A 94:12128, 1997.

Acquired Causes of Hemolysis

Acquired causes of hemolysis constitute a miscellaneous group of disorders that include the (1) microangiopathic hemolysis associated with disseminated intravascular coagulation or hemangiomas and (2) infection (bacterial sepsis or congenital infections).[38] The mechanism or mechanisms underlying the hemolytic process in the latter are not fully understood.

Immune-mediated Hemolytic Disease

Immune-mediated hemolysis encompasses the fetomaternal incompatibilities of the rhesus (Rh), ABO (major), and minor blood group systems. The incidence of isoimmunization to the Rh D antigen[39] has declined since the introduction of Rh$_O$(D) immune globulin in 1968 and is now estimated at approximately 1 case per 1000 live births.[40] The severity of hemolysis varies in the context of Rh isoimmunization, but almost half of Rh-positive infants born to Rh-sensitized mothers evince moderate to severe disease, control of which often necessitates intravenous immune globulin (IVIG) treatment, intensive phototherapy, and exchange transfusion. Isoimmunization secondary to minor blood group antigens (e.g., Kell, Duffy, and Kidd) can also lead to significant hemolysis in utero and postnatal hyperbilirubinemia, although these antigens are far less potent in inducing antibodies than is Rh D antigen. The incidence of clinically significant sensitization to the minor blood group antigens, as determined by meta-analysis, approximates 1 per 330 pregnancies.[41]

Hemolytic disease related to ABO incompatibility is generally limited to mothers who have blood type O and to infants with blood type A or B.[42,43] Although this association exists in approximately 15% of pregnancies, only a small fraction of such infants develop significant hyperbilirubinemia.[42,43] Defining which infants will become affected is difficult to predict with laboratory screening tests. Indeed, of type A or B infants born to mothers who have type O, only about one third have a positive result of a direct Coombs test, and of those with a positive result, only about 15% to 20% have peak serum bilirubin levels of 12.8 mg/dL (218 μmol/L) or higher.[43] Thus, evidence of symptomatic ABO hemolytic disease is found in only 5% of incompatible mother-infant pairs and is not strongly predicted by the Coombs test result. The latter was confirmed in a multicenter study in which only 18.5% of infants with a positive direct Coombs test result evidenced a peak serum bilirubin level higher than the 95% for age.[44] Similarly, infants with blood type A or B born to mothers with, respectively, incompatible type B or A are not likely to manifest symptomatic ABO hemolytic disease or have a positive direct Coombs test result.[43] Infants of ABO-incompatible mother-infant pairs who have a negative direct Coombs test result as a group appear to be at no greater risk for developing hyperbilirubinemia than are their ABO compatible counterparts, regardless of the indirect Coombs test status.[43] Routine screening of all ABO-incompatible cord blood has been recommended in the past[45] and is common practice in many nurseries.[46] The current literature,[43,46,47] however, suggests that such routine screening is probably not warranted, in view of the low yield and high cost, which is consistent with the tenor of recommendations of the American Association of Blood Banks.[48] Blood typing and a Coombs test are indicated, however, in the evaluation of any newborn with early and/or clinically significant jaundice.

Despite the difficulty in predicting its development, symptomatic ABO hemolytic disease does occur and in individual instances may develop in the absence of a positive direct Coombs test result.[42,49] The latter may reflect a paucity of A and B antigens on neonatal red blood cells and/or the absorption of serum antibody by A and B antigen epitopes throughout the body tissues and fluids.[42] The diagnosis of symptomatic ABO hemolytic disease should be considered in infants who develop marked jaundice in the context of ABO incompatibility that is generally accompanied by a positive direct Coombs test result and prominent microspherocytosis on a red blood cell smear.[42] The hyperbilirubinemia seen with symptomatic ABO hemolytic disease is often detected within the first 12 to 24 hours after birth (icterus praecox)[50] and usually is readily controlled with intensive phototherapy.[42,51]

Enterohepatic Circulation

Once bilirubin conjugates reach the intestine, they are either reduced by bacteria to urobilinogens and excreted in the feces or deconjugated to glucuronic acid and unconjugated bilirubin by bacterial and tissue β-glucuronidase.[52] The enterohepatic circulation of bilirubin is exaggerated in the neonatal period, in part because the newborn's intestinal tract is not yet colonized with bacteria that convert conjugated bilirubin to urobilinogen and because intestinal β-glucuronidase activity is high.[14,52] Studies in newborn humans and primates confirm that the enterohepatic circulation of bilirubin accounts for up to 50% of the hepatic bilirubin load in neonates.[53,54] Moreover, fasting hyperbilirubinemia is largely caused by intestinal reabsorption of unconjugated bilirubin,[55,56] which is suggestive of a mechanism by which inadequate lactation, poor enteral intake, or both may contribute to the genesis of marked hyperbilirubinemia in some neonates. Although various methods to limit the enterohepatic circulation of bilirubin have been studied (e.g., agar[53]), none are in clinical use.

Extravascular Blood

Internal hemorrhage, ecchymoses, and other extravascular blood collections enhance the bilirubin load on the liver. Extravascular red blood cells have a markedly shortened life span, and their heme fraction is quickly catabolized to bilirubin by tissue macrophages that contain heme oxygenase and biliverdin reductase.[57] Thus, cephalohematomas, subdural hemorrhage, massive adrenal hemorrhage, and marked bruising can be associated with increased serum bilirubin levels, typically 48 to 72 hours after the extravasation of blood. This temporal pattern is consistent with the evolution of ecchymoses and bilirubin formation in situ[57] and also accounts for why extravascular blood can cause prolonged indirect hyperbilirubinemia. An unusual but dramatic example of how extravascular blood can contribute to the genesis of hyperbilirubinemia is found in reports of marked jaundice associated with the delayed absorption of intraperitoneal blood in infants who received fetal intraperitoneal red blood cell transfusions.[58,59]

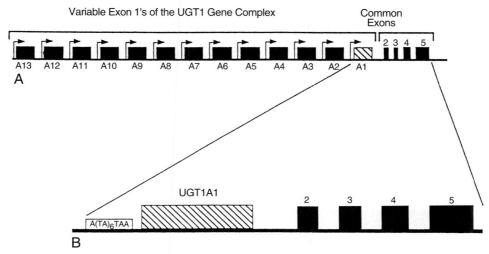

Figure 68–2. Schematic of the uridine diphosphate-glucuronosyltransferase 1 (UDPGT1) gene. **A,** The entire gene complex, including the variable exons A1 to A13 and constant domain, exons 2, 3, 4, and 5. **B,** Bilirubin UDPGT is defined by the UDPGT1A1 locus and common exons 2 to 5. The normal UDPGT1A1 TATA box promoter sequence is also shown. Genetic mutations in exon A1 and exons 2 to 5, as well as a variant promoter sequence, have been identified as causes for the indirect hyperbilirubinemia syndromes. *(From Clarke DJ, Moghrabi N, Monaghan G, et al: Genetic defects of the UDP-glucuronosyltransferase-1 [UGT1] gene that cause familial non-haemolytic unconjugated hyperbilirubinemias. Clin Chim Acta 266:63, 1997.)*

Decreased Hepatic Clearance of Bilirubin: Conjugation Defects

The formation of bilirubin monoglucuronides and diglucuronides is catalyzed by hepatic UDPGT, an enzyme that arises from the UDPGT type 1 (UDPGT1) gene complex whose transcription unit UDPGT1A1 encodes the physiologically important UDPGT that conjugates bilirubin.[60-62] In addition to the A1 exon, the UDPGT1 gene locus contains 12 variable exons (A2-A13) that encode other UDPGT isoforms and a cluster of exons 2 to 5 that is common to all (i.e., a constant domain) UDPGT isoforms (Fig. 68-2). UDPGT1A1 expression in humans is developmentally modulated, with 0.1% of adult activity noted at 17 to 30 weeks of gestation, 1.0% of adult values observed between 30 and 40 weeks of gestation, and 100% of adult levels reached by 14 weeks of postnatal life.[63,64] A graded up-regulation of hepatic bilirubin UDPGT over the first few days of life is observed after birth, regardless of the newborn's gestational age.

In addition to the developmentally modulated postnatal transition in hepatic bilirubin UDPGT activity, there exist congenital inborn errors of bilirubin UDPGT expression, commonly referred to as the **indirect hyperbilirubinemia syndromes.**[65] These include the Crigler-Najjar types I and II (Arias) syndromes and Gilbert syndrome (Table 68-3). Crigler-Najjar type I syndrome is characterized by severe chronic nonhemolytic unconjugated hyperbilirubinemia[66] secondary to the complete absence of bilirubin UDPGT activity; affected infants are at significant risk for hyperbilirubinemic encephalopathy and its neurodevelopmental sequelae. More than 30 different genetic nonsense or "stop" mutations have been identified in Crigler-Najjar type I syndrome; defects common to both the UDPGT1A1 exon and the constant domain (exons 2 to 5) underlie most cases.[62,67-70] The Arias syndrome, typified by more moderate levels of indirect hyperbilirubinemia as well as low but detectable

Table 68–3. Inborn Errors of Hepatic Bilirubin Uridine Diphosphate Glucuronosyltransferase Expression

Characteristic	Crigler-Najjar Type I	Crigler-Najjar Type II (Arias Syndrome)	Gilbert Syndrome
Inheritance	AR	AR or AD	AD or AR
UDPGT1 activity	Absent	<10%	50%
Genetic cause	Nonsense or stop mutation	Missense mutation	Variant promotor
Hyperbilirubinemia	>20 mg/dL	5-15 mg/dL*	3-5 mg/dL
Kernicterus	High risk	Low risk*	No apparent risk

*In some cases of Arias syndrome marked hyperbilirubinemia can occur, which may place the infant at high risk for kernicterus.

AD, autosomal dominant; AR, autosomal recessive; UDPGT1, uridine diphosphate-glucuronosyltransferase 1.

From Watchko JF: Indirect hyperbilirubinemia in the neonate. In Maisels MJ, Watchko JF (eds): Neonatal Jaundice. Amsterdam, Harwood Academic Publishers, 2000, pp 51-66.

hepatic bilirubin UDPGT activity, appears in the majority of cases to be mediated by missense mutations in the UDPGT1A1 gene alone.[62,71] In some cases, marked hyperbilirubinemia occurs in Arias syndrome, which makes it difficult to distinguish this entity from Crigler-Najjar type I syndrome. These rare but important clinical syndromes must be included in the differential diagnosis of prolonged marked indirect hyperbilirubinemia.

In contrast, Gilbert syndrome, characterized by mild, chronic or recurrent unconjugated hyperbilirubinemia in the absence of liver disease or overt hemolysis,[72,73] is common, affecting approximately 6% to 9% of the population.[73] Hepatic bilirubin UDPGT activity is reduced to at least 30% to 50% of normal in affected subjects, and more than 95% of their total serum bilirubin is unconjugated.[73] Typically, the indirect hyperbilirubinemia associated with Gilbert syndrome is seen during fasting in association with an intercurrent illness. The genetic basis for this disorder has been identified as a variant promoter for the gene encoding *UDPGT1*.[74] A two-basepair addition (TA) in the TATAA element of the promoter, which gives rise to seven repeats (A[TA]₇TAA) rather than the more usual six repeats (A[TA]₆TAA), impairs proper message transcription and accounts for a reduced UDPGT activity seen in Gilbert syndrome (see Fig. 68-2).[74] Subjects with Gilbert syndrome are homozygous for the (A[TA]₇TAA) variant promoter, which provides a unique genetic marker for this disorder. The expanded A[TA]₇TAA promoter motif is expressed in the heterozygous form in 40% of the population.[74]

Investigations have confirmed the long-standing speculation[38,57,65] that Gilbert syndrome contributes to the genesis of indirect hyperbilirubinemia in the newborn. Newborn infants homozygous for the A[TA]₇TAA polymorphism have an accelerated increase in neonatal hyperbilirubinemia, decreased fecal excretion of bilirubin monoglucuronides and diglucuronides,[75] and higher postnatal serum bilirubin levels in comparison with newborns without the A[TA]₇TAA polymorphism (Fig. 68-3).[76] Moreover, the A[TA]₇TAA variant UDPGT1 promoter is significantly more prevalent in breast-fed infants who develop prolonged neonatal hyperbilirubinemia,[77] which suggests that the Gilbert genotype may contribute to the duration of neonatal jaundice as well.

The importance of the Gilbert genotype to the genesis of neonatal jaundice is particularly apparent when affected newborns exhibit increased bilirubin production or additional co-inherited defects in bilirubin conjugation. As discussed previously, the combination of the Gilbert genotype and G6PD deficiency markedly increases a newborn's risk for hyperbilirubinemia,[34] as does Gilberts syndrome with hereditary spherocytosis.[78] Similarly, co-inheritance of the Gilbert promoter and a structural mutation in the coding region of UDPGT1A1 can also lead to marked jaundice.[79-81] The latter holds not only for patients who are homozygous for the Gilbert genotype but also for compound heterozygotes of the Gilbert-type promoter and a structural region mutation of UDPGT1A1.[82] For example, twin newborn girls who evidenced marked neonatal hyperbilirubinemia (26.7 and 24.0 mg/dL) and kernicterus were found to be heterozygous for both the Gilbert-type promoter sequence and a frameshift mutation in the coding region of the UDPGT1A1 gene.[82] The father was heterozygous for the coding region mutation, whereas the mother carried the Gilbert promoter on one allele. Reduced UDPGT1A1 activity in such cases is predicted to be only 10% to 15% of normal, and the resultant hyperbilirubinemia is greater than that seen with Gilbert syndrome but less than that with Crigler-Najjar type I.[82] Underscoring the clinical significance of these observations is that approximately 50% of the population carry the Gilbert-type promoter on at least one allele.[82]

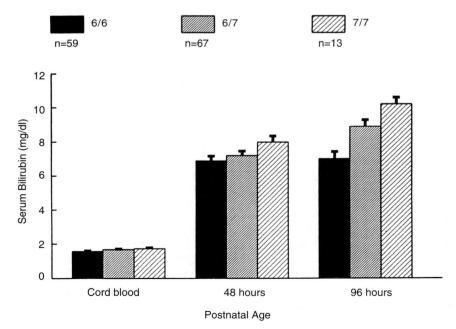

Figure 68–3. Newborn serum bilirubin levels as a function of postnatal age and presence of Gilbert promoter abnormality. *Solid bars* represent homozygous normal uridine diphosphate-glucuronosyltransferase (UDPGT) genotype (6/6); *fine-hatched bars* represent heterozygous variant UDPGT genotype (6/7); and *wide-hatched bars* represent homozygous variant UDPGT genotype (7/7). Values are means ± standard error of the mean. *(Adapted from Roy-Chowdhury N, Deocharan B, Bejjanki HR, et al: The presence of a Gilbert-type promoter abnormality increases the level of neonatal hyperbilirubinemia. Hepatology 26:370A, 1997.)*

Thus, heterozygous carriers of an UDPGT1A1 coding region mutation have a relatively high probability of carrying the Gilbert-type promoter. On the basis of the gene frequencies for the Gilbert promoter and structural mutations of the UDPGT1A1 gene, it is predicted that at least 1 per 3300 infants will be compound heterozygotes for the Gilbert-type promoter and UDPGT1A1 coding region mutations and at risk for significant hyperbilirubinemia.[82]

These studies together demonstrate that Gilbert syndrome is a factor contributing to the risk for neonatal jaundice. The role that Gilbert syndrome may play in the genesis of extreme hyperbilirubinemia remains unclear, although both the low direct bilirubin fractions and the evidence of poor feeding and prominent weight loss (i.e., a state resembling fasting) reported in several of the published cases of extreme neonatal hyperbilirubinemia[83] suggest that Gilbert syndrome might contribute to some cases of marked newborn jaundice. This hypothesis merits investigation in future studies of the genetic determinants underlying neonatal hyperbilirubinemia.[84]

Breast-Feeding–Associated Jaundice

There are several other conditions reported to predispose infants to indirect hyperbilirubinemia. The most common of these is breast milk feeding, a topic that engenders much debate, fueled by an increased prevalence of breast-feeding and reports that inadequate establishment of breast-feeding coupled with early discharge may be a contributing factor to the development of marked neonatal hyperbilirubinemia in certain infants.[83,85,86] Numerous studies have reported an association between breast-feeding and an increased incidence and severity of hyperbilirubinemia, both during the first few days after birth and in the genesis of prolonged neonatal jaundice.[87-91] Although other reports have not substantiated this observation,[92,93] a pooled analysis of a dozen studies of more than 8000 neonates revealed a threefold greater incidence in total serum bilirubin level of 12.0 mg/dL (205 µmol) or higher and a sixfold greater incidence in levels of 15 mg/dL (257 µmol) or higher in breast-fed infants than in their formula-fed counterparts.[90] Other studies suggest that early breast-feeding–associated jaundice is not associated with increased bilirubin production[94,95] but with a state of relative caloric deprivation[96] and resultant enhanced enterohepatic circulation of bilirubin.[96,97] Indeed, infants of mothers who are able to establish effective breast-feeding early are less likely to develop breast-feeding–associated jaundice.[98,99] Caregiver efforts focused on providing frequent opportunities for mothers to place their infants to breast during hospitalization, combined with timely postdischarge follow-up and lactation support, may help increase the chances of successful breast-feeding and attenuate the prevalence and degree of early breast-feeding–associated jaundice. Prolonged indirect hyperbilirubinemia associated with breast milk feeding, often termed **breast milk jaundice**, may be difficult to distinguish from breast-feeding–associated jaundice and is probably mediated by an enhanced enterohepatic circulation. Although the existence of an association between breast milk feeding and jaundice is recognized, it is important to emphasize that the benefits of breast milk feeds far outweigh the related risk of hyperbilirubinemia.

Miscellaneous Factors Contributing to Indirect Hyperbilirubinemia

Ethnic differences also appear to contribute to the epidemiologic features of neonatal jaundice. Population studies have demonstrated that the incidence of hyperbilirubinemia is higher in East Asian and Native American infants and lower in African-American infants than in their white counterparts.[100-102] Such differences may relate to genetic variations in UDPGT1 promoter and coding region genotypes,[103,104] the prevalence of G6PD deficiency across populations, and environmental factors.[105] Studies designed to ascertain the genetic contribution to neonatal jaundice, however, do not fully account for differences in bilirubin levels between ethnic groups, which underscores the multifactorial nature of neonatal hyperbilirubinemia.[29,104,106] Less common but important other conditions associated with neonatal hyperbilirubinemia include hypothyroidism, hypopituitarism, Lucey-Driscoll syndrome, galactosemia, tyrosinosis, and hypermethioninemia. Several conditions can lead to prolonged indirect hyperbilirubinemia, including breast milk jaundice, hypothyroidism, hemolytic disorders, Crigler-Najjar syndrome types I and II, pyloric stenosis, and sequestered blood collections.[107]

NEUROTOXICITY OF HYPERBILIRUBINEMIA IN NEONATES

The neurodevelopmental sequelae of marked neonatal hyperbilirubinemia were originally described in infants with hemolytic disease secondary to Rh isoimmunization. Clinically, affected newborns exhibit a neurologic syndrome acutely typified by lethargy, poor feeding, and hypotonia, followed by hypertonia with opisthotonos, a high-pitched cry, and, occasionally, seizures.[108] Survivors manifest long-term adverse neurodevelopmental sequelae, including extrapyramidal disturbances (choreoathetosis), high-frequency sensorineural hearing loss, and palsy of vertical gaze.[109,110] These sequelae reflect both the predilection of bilirubin toxicity for neurons (rather than glial cells)[111] and the regional topography of bilirubin-induced neuronal injury that is characterized by prominent basal ganglia, cochlear, and oculomotor nuclei involvement.[112,113] Intellectual deficits have been observed in only a minority of infants with chronic postkernicteric bilirubin encephalopathy, which reflects the fact that cerebral cortical neuron involvement is not a salient feature of kernicterus. Despite decades of investigation, the cellular and molecular mechanism or mechanisms that underlie the selective neurotoxicity of bilirubin remain unclear.[114]

Noninvasive electrophysiologic measures to predict the onset of bilirubin encephalopathy through the use of brain stem auditory, visual, and somatosensory evoked potentials[115] as well as neuroimaging techniques, have been proposed as tools to evaluate the neurologic changes associated with hyperbilirubinemia[116] and may yet prove helpful in the assessment of individual infants. Magnetic resonance imaging (MRI) studies of children

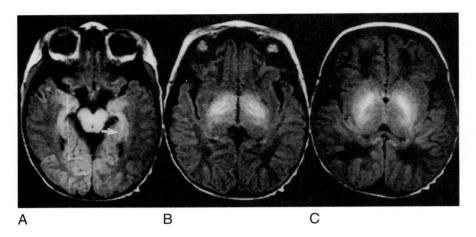

Figure 68–4. Magnetic resonance imaging scan of infant with kernicterus, demonstrating high signal intensity in the hippocampus (*arrow*) in the medial temporal lobe **(A)** and in the globus pallidus **(B** and **C)**. *(From Penn AA, Enzmann DR, Hahn JS, Stevenson DK: Kernicterus in a full term infant. Pediatrics 93:1003, 1994.)*

with postkernicteric encephalopathy demonstrate the characteristic pattern of neuropathologic lesions of kernicterus: abnormal bilateral high-intensity signals in the globus pallidus (Fig. 68-4),[117-119] internal capsule,[117] and thalamus.[117] A case series, however, suggested that early MRI abnormalities in hyperbilirubinemic infants may not persist or be predictive of long-term adverse neurodevelopmental sequelae.[86] Further study is necessary to define the nature of these MRI findings and establish the utility of neuroimaging and related noninvasive neurophysiologic measures in the short- and long-term neurologic assessment of infants at risk for hyperbilirubinemic encephalopathy.

Currently, debate continues regarding the level of neonatal hyperbilirubinemia at which encephalopathy and neurodevelopmental sequelae are manifest; this reflects, in all likelihood, the multifactorial nature of this phenomenon. Early reports of a relationship between hyperbilirubinemia and kernicterus have been described in infants with erythroblastosis fetalis and reveal an increasing risk for kernicterus with rising bilirubin levels (Fig. 68-5).[120] On the basis of this work, a treatment threshold of 20 mg/dL (342 µmol/L) for exchange transfusion was prospectively studied in infants with Rh hemolytic disease[120] and was demonstrated to be effective in largely preventing hyperbilirubinemic encephalopathy and long-term adverse neurodevelopmental sequelae.[120,121] More recent study on infants with Coombs test–positive hemolytic disease suggests that the risk of prominent neurologic abnormalities on follow-up is correlated with the duration of indirect hyperbilirubinemia exceeding 20 mg/dL (342 µmol/L), increasing in a stepwise manner from 2.3% at less than 6 hours' duration to 18.7% at 6 to 11 hours' duration and further to 26% at 12 or more hours' duration.[122] These data echo earlier observations suggesting the duration of hyperbilirubinemia might be related to long-term neurodevelopmental performance.[123] The outcome of infants with hemolysis secondary to other causes (including red blood cell membrane defects and G6PD deficiency) remains less defined, although their risk for hyperbilirubinemic encephalopathy appears to be commensurate with the risks of immune-mediated hemolytic processes.[27,28,35]

The level at which hyperbilirubinemic encephalopathy occurs in healthy full-term (≥37 completed weeks of gestation) infants without hemolysis remains less clear. An extensive literature from the 1950s, 1960s, and 1970s,[124,125] as well as more current systematic analyses,[126,127] demonstrates (1) that otherwise healthy full-term neonates without hemolytic disease may also develop marked hyperbilirubinemia, but it typically does not exceed the range of 20 to 25 mg/dL, and (2) that this level of hyperbilirubinemia does not appear to place such infants at risk for long-term adverse neurodevelopmental sequelae, such as cognitive impairment (intelligence quotient), definite neurologic abnormalities, or hearing loss.[126,127] However, in contrast to the relatively reassuring nature of this extensive body of literature, a statistically significant association between increasing bilirubin levels and more subtle neurologic changes (e.g., awkwardness and abnormal cremasteric reflex) has been reported.[128] Moreover, in rare instances, even more severe hyperbilirubinemia (>25 mg/dL [428 µmol/L]) can develop in otherwise

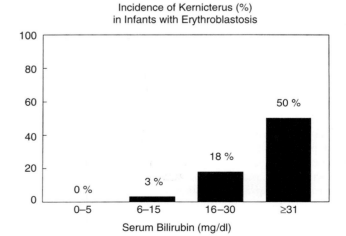

Figure 68–5. Incidence of kernicterus as a function of serum bilirubin (mg/dL) in infants with erythroblastosis fetalis (Rh isoimmunization). *(Adapted from Hsai DY, Allen FH, Gellis SS, et al: Erythroblastosis fetalis. VIII. Studies of serum bilirubin in relation to kernicterus. N Engl J Med 247:668, 1952.)*

healthy full-term infants and be associated with kernicterus.[83] These cases highlight the remote but definable possibility that otherwise healthy full-term infants without evidence of hemolysis can develop severe hyperbilirubinemia and associated adverse long-term neurodevelopmental sequelae. Thus, pediatricians must remain alert to the development of unexpected severe hyperbilirubinemia after hospital discharge in otherwise healthy full-term infants.[83,85,129]

Physicians' understanding of the neurotoxic potential of hyperbilirubinemia in infants born prematurely (<34 completed weeks of gestation) also continues to evolve. Studies suggest that infants born prematurely are at higher risk for kernicterus than are their full-term counterparts, although the absolute bilirubin level at which this risk accrues remains unclear. Empirical treatment guidelines for phototherapy and exchange transfusion in preterm infants reflect this consensus, although the so-called low-bilirubin kernicterus described in premature infants in a series of reports between 1958 and 1972 has not been reported since that era.[125,130,131] Indeed, kernicterus is currently a rare event in this gestational age group,[131,132] which probably reflects the widespread use of early, often prophylactic phototherapy in the neonatal intensive care unit.

MANAGEMENT GUIDELINES

Clinical jaundice is very common in neonates; thus, it is difficult to discern which infants merit evaluation and treatment. Current guidelines suggest that certain clinical risk factors may help practitioners identify those infants at risk for marked hyperbilirubinemia (Table 68-4).[133-135] Absence of these factors suggests that the risk of severe hyperbilirubinemia is quite low, whereas if several are present, the risk of marked jaundice increases significantly.[133-135] For the majority of jaundiced neonates, the American Academy of Pediatrics practice guideline

Table 68–4. Common Clinical Risk Factors for Severe Hyperbilirubinemia*

Jaundice in the first 24 hr
Visible jaundice before discharge
Previous jaundiced sibling
Gestation 35-38 wk
Exclusive breast-feeding
East Asian race
Bruising, cephalhematoma
Maternal age ≥25 yr
Male sex

*The more risk factors present, the greater the risk of severe hyperbilirubinemia.

From American Academy of Pediatrics, Subcommittee on Neonatal Hyperbilirubinemia: Neonatal jaundice and kernicterus. Pediatrics 108: 763, 2001.

"Management of Hyperbilirubinemia in the Healthy Term Newborn" remains a cornerstone for evaluation and management of neonatal jaundice.[134] This guideline more accurately represents the remaining uncertainties about when to treat jaundice in otherwise healthy full-term newborns without hemolytic disease, giving ranges of serum bilirubin levels rather than single numbers for therapeutic interventions (Table 68-5).[134] These ranges also acknowledge the important role of clinical judgment in deciding whether to institute phototherapy, exchange transfusion, or both in the management of infants with hyperbilirubinemia. It is important, however, that practitioners be cognizant of the exclusion criteria for the appropriate application of this practice parameter. The guideline algorithm explicitly excludes (1) infants who have signs of underlying serious illness; (2) infants of younger than 37 weeks of gestational age; (3) infants with clinical jaundice noted 24 hours after birth or earlier; and (4) infants who evidence underlying hemolytic disease.[134] Actual treatment

Table 68–5. Management of Hyperbilirubinemia in the Apparently Healthy Full-Term Newborn

	TSB Level (mg/dL [μmol/L])			
Age (hr)	Consider Phototherapy*	Phototherapy	Exchange Transfusion if Intensive Phototherapy Fails†	Exchange Transfusion and Intensive Phototherapy
≤24‡	—	—	—	—
25-48	≥12 (205)	≥15 (260)	≥20 (340)	≥25 (430)
49-72	≥15 (260)	≥18 (310)	≥25 (430)	≥30 (510)
>72	≥17 (290)	≥20 (340)	≥25 (430)	≥30 (510)

*Phototherapy at these TSB levels is a clinical option, meaning that the intervention is available and may be used on the basis of individual clinical judgment.

†Intensive phototherapy should produce a decline in TSB of 1 to 2 mg/dL within 4-6 hours, and the TSB level should continue to fall and remain below the threshold level for exchange transfusion. If this does not occur, it is considered a failure of phototherapy.

‡Full-term infants who are clinically jaundiced at ≤24 hours of age are not considered healthy and require further evaluation.

TSB, total serum bilirubin.

From American Academy of Pediatrics, Provisional Committee for Quality Improvement and Subcommittee on Hyperbilirubinemia: Practice parameter: Management of hyperbilirubinemia in the healthy term newborn. Pediatrics 94:560, 1994.

Table 68–6. Approaches to the Use of Phototherapy and Exchange Transfusion in Infants with Low Birth Weight*

Birth Weight (g)	Total Bilirubin Level (mg/dL [μmol/L])†	
	Phototherapy‡	Exchange Transfusion§
≤1500	5-8 (85-140)	13-16 (220-275)
1500-1999	8-12 (140-200)	16-18 (275-300)
2000-2499	11-14 (190-240)	18-20 (300-340)

*Note that these guidelines reflect ranges used in neonatal intensive care units. They cannot take into account all possible situations. In some units, prophylactic phototherapy is used for infants who weigh <1500 g. Higher intervention levels may be used for infants who are small for gestational age on the basis of gestational age rather than birth weight.

†Consider initiating therapy at these levels. Range allows discretion on the basis of clinical conditions or other circumstances.

‡Used at these levels and in therapeutic dosages, phototherapy, should, with few exceptions, elimiate the need for exchange transfusions.

§Levels for exchange transfusion are based on the assumption that bilirubin continues to rise or remains at these levels despite intensive phototherapy.

From Maisels MJ: The clinical approach to the jaundiced newborn. In Maisels MJ, Watchko JF (eds): Neonatal Jaundice. Amsterdam, Harwood Academic, 2000, pp 139-168.

Table 68–7. Clinical Data on Healthy Full-Term Infants without Hemolysis Who Developed Kernicterus

Case	Weight Loss (%)	Peak Bilirubin Total/Direct (mg/dL)	Age at Peak Bilirubin	Hb (g/dL)
1	11	49.7 / 1.1	7 days	16.2
2	22	39.0 / 1.8	5 days	24.0
3	1	40.3 / 0.8	10 days	15.8
4	20	44.7 / 3.4	7 days	18.4
5	?	44.7 / 0.0	4 days	17.8
6	18	41.4 / 0.6	6 days	19.5

Hb, hemoglobin.

Adapted from Maisels MJ, Newman TB: Kernicterus in otherwise healthy, breast-fed term newborns. Pediatrics 96:730, 1995.

thresholds for phototherapy and exchange transfusion for this group of infants are detailed in Table 68-5.

For infants with identified hemolytic disease underlying their jaundice, more conservative treatment thresholds are generally recommended, including initiation of early phototherapy and an exchange transfusion at a total serum bilirubin threshold of 20 mg/dL (340 μmol/L).[120] Similarly, for premature infants with low birth weight, lower treatment thresholds have been recommended (Table 68-6).[133] The widespread use of phototherapy in the neonatal intensive care unit has largely eliminated the need for exchange transfusions in infants with low birth weight.[133] One condition that in and of itself is an indication for immediate exchange transfusion regardless of gestational age is clinical evidence of hyperbilirubinemic encephalopathy.

Case reports suggest the possible reemergence of kernicterus as a concern for pediatricians. Despite the absence of uniform surveillance for reporting kernicterus, uniform case definition for kernicterus, and denominators for the case reports,[129] there is increasing evidence that hyperbilirubinemic encephalopathy has developed in certain neonates.[83,85] Short hospital stays, inadequate establishment of lactation, and near-term gestation appeared to be contributing factors in the genesis of kernicterus in reported cases.[83,85,129] Peak bilirubin levels observed in reported cases are typically very high and in almost all cases exceed 25 mg/dL [430 μmol/L] (Table 68-7).[83,85] The total number of cases identified since 1984 now approximates 100. In view of an average of 3.9 million births per year in the United States, an overall prevalence of 1 per 624,000 live births can be estimated for kernicterus between 1984 and 2000. To put this number in perspective, current best estimates for the frequency of marked hyperbilirubinemia are 2.0% for a peak serum

bilirubin level exceeding 20 mg/dL (342 μmol/L); 0.15% for a peak serum bilirubin level exceeding 25 mg/dL (430 μmol/L); and 0.01% for a peak serum bilirubin level exceeding 30 mg/dL (510 μmol/L).[136] The risk of serum bilirubin of more than 25 mg/dL (430 μmol/L) is significantly increased in infants of East Asian ethnicity, male gender, and lower gestational age (near-term infants).[136,137]

The reports of kernicterus in the near-term infant (34 to 37 weeks of gestational age) merit particular note.[85,129] Although infants born at 34 to 37 weeks of gestation can be managed like full-term newborns in many ways— (1) they are large enough to maintain their temperature in an open crib; (2) they have an established suck-swallow reflex and can take their feedings orally (although not necessarily breast-feed vigorously); and (3) they have a mature respiratory drive and are thus not prone to apnea—their ability to handle bilirubin is clearly limited, placing them at risk for more prominent and protracted hyperbilirubinemia.[138] The combination of reduced hepatic clearance and less vigorous feeding can potentially lead to marked hyperbilirubinemia in near-term infants, particularly those with a breast-feeding primiparous mother.

In response to these case series, the Joint Commission on Accreditation of Healthcare Organizations published a Sentinel Event ALERT on kernicterus to draw attention to the emergence of kernicterus and its prevention.[139] The Commission identified the following risk factors in recent cases: (1) jaundice appearing in the first 24 hours after birth; (2) inadequate nutrition/hydration via suboptimal breast-feeding; (3) birth at near-term gestation (35, 36, or 37 weeks), particularly if nursing; (4) G6PD deficiency; and (5) East Asian or Mediterranean ethnicity. Moreover, a pattern of root causes related to four patient care processes were identified: problems related to (1) patient assessment, (2) continuum of care, (3) family education, and (4) treatment (Table 68-8).[139] Available risk reduction strategies identified in the ALERT including application of the American Academy of Pediatrics "Guidelines for Management of Hyperbilirubinemia in the Healthy Term Newborn"[134]; practitioners were reminded to be

Table 68–8. Analysis of Patient Care Processes Related to Kernicterus

Patient Assessment

The unreliability of the visual assessment of jaundice in newborns with dark skin

Failure to recognize jaundice in an infant—or its severity—on the basis of visual assessment and measurement of a bilirubin level before the infant's discharge from the hospital or during a follow-up visit

Failure to measure the bilirubin level in an infant who is jaundiced in the first 24 hours after birth

Continuum of Care

Early discharge (before 48 hours) with no follow-up within 1 to 2 days of discharge; this is particularly important for infants younger than 38 weeks of gestation

Failure to provide early follow-up with physical assessment for infants who are jaundiced before discharge

Failure to provide ongoing lactation support to ensure adequacy of intake for breast-fed newborns

Patient and Family Education

Failure to provide appropriate information to parents about jaundice

Failure to respond appropriately to parental concerns about a jaundiced newborn, poor feeding, lactation difficulties, and change in newborn's behavior and activity

Treatment

Failure to recognize, address, or treat rapidly rising bilirubin level

Failure to aggressively treat severe hyperbilirubinemia in a timely manner with intensive phototherapy or exchange transfusion

Adapted from Joint Commission on Accreditation of Healthcare Organizations: Kernicterus threatens healthy newborns. Sentinel Event ALERT, Issue 18, May 2, 2001. Available at http://www.jcaho.org.

cognizant of the guidelines exclusion criteria. In fact, many of the cases of hyperbilirubinemic encephalopathy described in more recent reports are characterized by conditions that preclude application of the practice parameter. Other strategies to consider include predischarge hour-specific total serum bilirubin measurements or transcutaneous bilirubin screening to guide follow-up (Fig. 68-6),[140] follow-up of all newborns within 24 to 48 hours of discharge, and the provision of adequate educational materials about neonatal jaundice to parents.

In addition, once identified, severe jaundice must be treated aggressively. All hospitals involved in the care of newborns are required to take steps to raise awareness among neonatal caregivers for the potential of kernicterus and its risk factors, review their current patient care processes with regard to the identification and management of hyperbilirubinemia in newborns, and identify strategies that will enhance the effectiveness of this process. The Centers for Disease Control and Prevention's report entitled "Kernicterus in Full Term

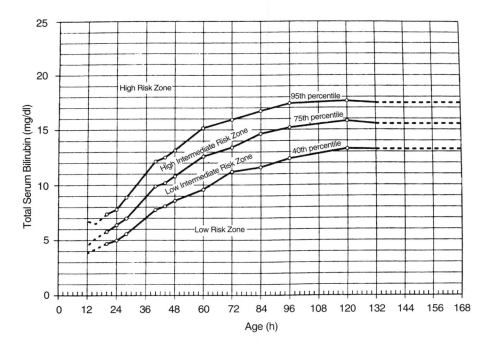

Figure 68–6. Risk designation of full-term and near-term healthy newborns, based on their hour-specific serum bilirubin values. *(From Bhutani VK, Johnson L, Sivieri EM: Predictive ability of a predischarge hour-specific serum bilirubin for subsequent significant hyperbilirubinemia in healthy-term and near-term newborns. Pediatrics 103:6, 1999.)*

Infants, U.S. 1994-1998"[141] echoed the recommendations of the Joint Commission on Accreditation of Healthcare Organizations Sentinel Event ALERT, as did the 2001 American Academy of Pediatrics Subcommittee Report on Neonatal Hyperbilirubinemia.[135]

TREATMENT METHODS

Phototherapy

Phototherapy is the mainstay of treatment for neonatal hyperbilirubinemia. First described in 1958,[142] it came into widespread use a decade later after studies by Lucey and associates demonstrated its effectiveness and safety.[143] Phototherapy detoxifies bilirubin by converting bilirubin to photoisomers that are more polar, less lipophilic, and readily excreted from the liver into bile without undergoing conjugation.[144,145] The photoisomerization of bilirubin is fast and probably takes place in blood vessels or in the interstitial space, or both.[144,146] Moreover, these bilirubin photoisomers do not require the presence of cMOAT for their excretion into bile.[145] Photodegradation or photooxidation of bilirubin to biliverdin plays a minor role in the effectiveness of phototherapy.[144,145] The effectiveness of phototherapy is determined by several factors, including the spectrum of light emitted (best wavelengths appear to be in the blue-green region near 425 to 500 nm), the irradiance of light source (the closer the infant is to the light source, the greater the irradiance), and the surface area of infant exposed to the light.[144] The most effective light sources currently commercially available for phototherapy are special blue fluorescent tubes labeled F20 T12/BB (General Electric, Westinghouse) or TL52/20W (Philips).[144] These "special blue" or "super blue" tubes are different than the regular blue lights labeled F20 T12/B.[144] Maximizing the surface area of the infant exposed to phototherapy is also crucial to its success. The use of fiberoptic pads in conjunction with overhead phototherapy units to provide "double phototherapy" and the addition of side banks to provide "triple phototherapy" may serve to optimize the amount of surface area exposed to a phototherapy light source. Phototherapy has proven to be remarkably safe since its first use in the late 1960s. Attention should be paid, however, to the infant's thermoregulation and insensible water loss, and infant eye shields should be properly applied when phototherapy is in use.[144]

Intravenous Immune Globulin Therapy for Coombs Test–Positive Hyperbilirubinemia

Several studies have demonstrated the effectiveness of early high-dose (500 to 1000 mg/kg) IVIG therapy in attenuating hemolysis and resultant hyperbilirubinemia associated with Coombs test–positive hemolytic disease (Rh isoimmunization and ABO incompatibility).[147-151] Indeed, blood carboxyhemoglobin levels, a sensitive marker of neonatal hemolysis, have been shown to decrease significantly by 24 hours after IVIG treatment.[150-151] Guidelines for IVIG administration in the context of Coombs test–positive hyperbilirubinemia have been published (Table 68-9).[150]

Table 68–9. Guidelines for Total Serum Bilirubin (TSB) for IVIG Administration in Full-Term Healthy ABO-Incompatible Coombs Test–Positive Neonates

First 12 hours of age	TSB ≥ 204 µmol/L (≥12 mg/dL) despite trial of phototherapy (4 hr minimum)
12 to 24 hours of age	TSB ≥ 272 µmol/L (≥16 mg/dL) despite trial of phototherapy (4 hr minimum)
24 to 72 hours of age	TSB ≥ 306 µmol/L (≥18 mg/dL) despite trial of phototherapy (4 hr minimum)
Additional criteria	tHb < 8.06 mmol/L (<13 mg/dL)

When an infant meets criteria, a dose of 0.5 g of IVIG should be infused over 2 hours. The dose can be repeated at 12-hour intervals until bilirubin stabilizes.

IVIG, intravenous immune globulin; tHb, total hemoglobin.

From Hammerman C, Kaplan M. Recent developments in the management of neonatal hyperbilirubinemia: NeoReviews 1:e19-e24, 2000.

Exchange Transfusion

Exchange transfusion occupies a unique place in the history of neonatal jaundice because it was the first intervention to permit effective control of hyperbilirubinemia and thus prevent kernicterus. Exchange transfusions were developed to manage the severe jaundice that occurred in association with the immune-mediated hemolysis of Rh isoimmunization.[152] In addition to the immediate control of hyperbilirubinemia, an exchange transfusion in immune-mediated hemolytic disease also achieves (1) the removal of antibody-coated red blood cells (a source of UUbilirubin), (2) the correction of anemia (if present), and (3) the removal of maternal antibody.[153] A double-volume exchange transfusion removes 110% of circulating bilirubin (extravascular bilirubin enters the blood during the exchange) but only 25% of total body bilirubin. Postexchange bilirubin levels are approximately 60% of preexchange levels, but the reequilibration of bilirubin between the vascular and extravascular compartments produces a rebound of serum bilirubin levels to 70% to 80% of preexchange levels. Exchange transfusions are most readily performed via the umbilical vein with a 5- or 8-French umbilical catheter inserted just far enough to obtain free flow of blood (usually no more than the distance between the xiphoid process and umbilicus). The "push-pull" method with a single syringe and special four-way stopcock assembly enables a single operator to complete the procedure.[153] Fresh citrate-phosphate-dextrose blood (<72 hours old and devoid of the offending antigen in the case of immune-mediated hemolytic disease) crossmatched to the infant should be used. Although the risk for graft-versus-host disease after an exchange transfusion is extremely low, blood for exchange transfusion should be irradiated if possible, particularly for the infant who is premature. The blood should be warmed to body temperature by a blood/fluid warmer. The actual exchange should be performed slowly in aliquots of 5 to 10 mL/kg body weight, with each withdrawal-infusion cycle approximating a 3-minute duration.[154] During the exchange, the infant's vital signs, including electrocardiographic patterns, respiration, oxygen saturation, temperature, and blood pressure, should be monitored closely. Post-exchange studies should include platelet counts and bilirubin, hemoglobin, ionized calcium, serum electrolyte, and serum glucose measurements. The unintended consequences of exchange transfusion include cardiovascular, hematologic, gastrointestinal, biochemical, and infectious hazards.[153]

Previously reported overall rates of mortality associated with exchange transfusion ranged from 0.3 to 0.95 per 100 procedures,[155,156] and significant morbidity (apnea, bradycardia, cyanosis, vasospasm, thrombosis) was observed in 6.7% of infants who received exchange transfusion in the National Institute of Child Health and Human Development collaborative phototherapy study.[155] These rates, however, may not be generalizable to the current era if, as in most procedures, frequency of performance is an important determinant of risk and if experience with exchange transfusion is decreasing.[157] It is quite possible that the mortality (and morbidity) for this now infrequently performed procedure might be considerably higher than previously reported.

On the other hand, none of the reports before 1986 included current monitoring capabilities such as pulse oximetry. Jackson reported a 2% rate of overall mortality (2/106) associated with exchange transfusions between 1980 and 1995.[158] There was a 12% risk of serious complications attributable to exchange transfusion in ill infants.[158] Moreover, in infants classified as ill with medical problems in addition to hyperbilirubinemia, the incidence of exchange transfusion–related complications leading to death was 8%.[158] There were no procedure-related deaths in 81 healthy infants.[158] Symptomatic hypocalcemia, bleeding related to thrombocytopenia, catheter-related complications, and apnea-bradycardia necessitating resuscitation were common serious morbid conditions observed in this study, which suggests that exchange transfusion should be performed by experienced individuals in a neonatal intensive care unit that has continuous monitoring (including pulse oximetry) and is prepared to respond to these adverse events.[153,158]

Finally, although the risk is now very low, transfusion always carries some risk of acquired immunodeficiency syndrome and hepatitis.[159] The risk estimates (risk per tested unit) for transfusion transmitted viruses in the United States for the period 1991 through 1993 were as follows: for the human immunodeficiency virus (HIV), 1 per 493,000 (95% confidence interval = 202,000 to 2,778,000); for the human T-cell lymphotropic virus, 1 per 641,000 (95% confidence interval = 256,000 to 2,000,000); for the hepatitis C virus, 1 per 103,000 (95% confidence interval = 28,000 to 288,000); and for the hepatitis B virus, 1 per 63,000 (95% confidence interval = 31,000 to 147,000).[159]

REFERENCES

1. Ostrow JD, Jandl JH, Schmid R: The formation of bilirubin from hemoglobin in vivo. J Clin Invest 41:1628, 1962.

2. Tenhunen R, Marver HS, Schmid R: Microsomal heme oxygenase. Characterization of the enzyme. J Biol Chem 244:6388, 1969.

3. Dennery PA: The biology of heme oxygenase during development. NeoReviews 2:e67, 2001.

4. Coburn RF: Endogenous carbon monoxide production. N Engl J Med 282:207, 1977.

5. Maisels MJ, Pathak A, Nelson NM, et al: Endogenous production of carbon monoxide in normal and erythroblastotic newborn infants. J Clin Invest 50:1, 1971.

6. Bartoletti AL, Stevenson DK, Ostrander CR, Johnson JD: Pulmonary excretion of carbon monoxide in the human infant as an index of bilirubin production. I. Effects of gestational age and postnatal age and some common neonatal abnormalities. J Pediatr 94:952, 1979.

7. Colleran E, O'Carra P: Enzymology and comparative physiology of biliverdin reduction. In Berk PD, Berlin NR (eds): International Symposium on Chemistry and Physiology of the Bile Pigments. Washington, DC, U.S. Government Printing Office, 1977, pp 69-80.

8. Brodersen R: Binding of bilirubin to albumin. Crit Rev Clin Lab Sci 11:305, 1980.

9. Cashore WJ: Free bilirubin concentrations and bilirubin-binding affinity in term and preterm infants. J Pediatr 96:521, 1980.

10. Jacobsen J, Wennberg RP: Determination of unbound bilirubin in the serum of newborns. Clin Chem 20:783, 1974.

11. Cui Y, Konig J, Leier I, et al: Hepatic uptake of bilirubin and its conjugates by the human organic anion transporter SLC21A6. J Biol Chem 276:9626, 2001.

12. Paulusma CC, Oude Elferink RPJ: The canalicular multispecific organic anion transporter and conjugated hyperbilirubinemia in rat and man. J Mol Med 75:420, 1997.

13. Diaz GJ: Basolateral and canalicular transport of xenobiotics in the hepatocyte: A review. Cytotechnology 34:225, 2000.

14. Takimoto M, Matsuda I: β-glucuronidase activity in the stool of newborn infant. Biol Neonate 18:66, 1972.

15. Pereira PJB, Macedo-Ribeiro S, Parraga A, et al: Structure of human biliverdin IXβ reductase, an early fetal bilirubin IXβ producing enzyme. Nat Struct Biol 8:215, 2001.

16. McDonagh AF, Palma LA, Schmid R: Reduction of biliverdin and placental transfer of bilirubin and biliverdin in the pregnant guinea pig. Biochem J 194:273, 1981.

17. Schenker S: Disposition of bilirubin in the fetus and the newborn. Ann N Y Acad Sci 111:303, 1963.

18. Schmid R: Pyrrolic victories. Trans Assoc Am Physicians 89:64, 1976.

19. Pasacolo L, Bavon JE, Serrano MA, et al: Evidence for carrier-mediated bilirubin transport across the basal plasma membrane of human placenta trophoblast at term. J Hepatol 28(Suppl):125, 1998.

20. Vest MF, Grieder HR: Erythrocyte survival in the newborn infant, as measured by chromium[51] and its relation to the postnatal serum bilirubin level. J Pediatr 59:194, 1961.

21. Pearson HA: Life-span of the fetal red blood cell. J Pediatr 70:166, 1967.

22. Oski FA: The erythrocyte and its disorders. In Nathan DG, Oski FA (eds): Hematology of Infancy and Childhood. Philadelphia, WB Saunders, 1993, pp 18-43.

23. Caprari P, Maiorana A, Marzetti G, et al: Severe neonatal hemolytic jaundice associated with pyknocytosis and alterations of red cell skeletal proteins. Prenat Neonatal Med 2:140, 1997.

24. Stockman JA: Physical properties of the neonatal red blood cell. In Stockman JA, Pochedly C (eds): Developmental and Neonatal Hematology. New York, Raven Press, 1988, pp 297-323.

25. Becker PS, Lux SE: Disorders of the red cell membrane. In Nathan DG, Oski FA (eds): Hematology of Infancy and Childhood. Philadelphia, WB Saunders, 1993, pp 529-633.

26. Trucco JI, Brown AK: Neonatal manifestations of hereditary spherocytosis. Am J Dis Child 113:263, 1967.

27. Beutler E: G6PD deficiency. Blood 84:3613, 1994.

28. Valaes T: Severe neonatal jaundice associated with glucose-6-phosphate dehydrogenase deficiency: Pathogenesis and global epidemiology. Acta Paediatr Suppl 394:58, 1994.

29. Valaes T: Neonatal jaundice in G6PD deficiency. In Maisels MJ, Watchko JF (eds): Neonatal Jaundice. Amsterdam, Harwood Academic, 2000, pp 67-72.

30. Valaes T, Doxiadis SA, Fessas P: Acute hemolysis due to naphthalene inhalation. J Pediatr 63:904, 1963.

31. Meloni T, Costa S: Haptoglobin, hemopexin, hemoglobin, and hematocrit in newborns with erythrocyte glucose-6-phosphate dehydrogenase deficiency. Acta Haematol (Basel) 54:284,1975.

32. Kaplan M, Rubaltelli FF, Hammerman C, et al: Conjugated bilirubin in neonates with glucose-6-phosphate dehydrogenase deficiency. J Pediatr 128:695, 1996.

33. Kaplan M, Vreman HJ, Hammerman C, et al: Contribution of haemolysis to jaundice in Sephardic Jewish glucose-6-phosphate dehydrogenase deficient neonates. Br J Haematol 93:822, 1996.

34. Kaplan M, Renbaum P, Levy-Lahad E, et al: Gilbert syndrome and glucose-6-phosphate dehydrogenase deficiency: A dose-dependent genetic interaction crucial to neonatal hyperbilirubinemia. Proc Natl Acad Sci U S A 94:12128, 1997.

35. MacDonald MG: Hidden risks: Early discharge and bilirubin toxicity due to glucose-6-phosphate dehydrogenase deficiency. Pediatrics 96:734, 1995.

36. Schmaier A, Maurer HM, Johnston CL, et al: Alpha thalassemia screening in neonates by mean corpuscular volume and mean corpuscular hemoglobin concentration. J Pediatr 83:794, 1973.

37. Pearson HA: Disorders of hemoglobin synthesis and metabolism. In Oski FA, Naiman JL (eds): Hematologic Problems in the Newborn. Philadelphia, WB Saunders, 1982, pp 245-282.

38. Oski FA: Unconjugated hyperbilirubinemia. In Avery ME, Taeusch HW (eds): Diseases of the Newborn. Philadelphia, WB Saunders, 1984, pp 630-632.

39. Gottvall T, Hilden J, Selbing A: Evaluation of standard parameters to predict exchange transfusions in the erythroblastotic newborn. Acta Obstet Gynecol Scand 73:300, 1994.

40. Chavez G, Mulinare J, Edmonds LD: Epidemiology of Rh hemolytic disease of the newborn in the United States. JAMA 24:3270, 1991.

41. Solola A, Sibal B, Mason J: Irregular antibodies: An assessment of routine prenatal screening. Obstet Gynecol 61:25, 1983.

42. Naiman JL: Erythroblastosis fetalis. In Oski FA, Naiman JL (eds): Hematologic Problems in the Newborn. Philadelphia, WB Saunders, 1982, pp 326-332.

43. Ozolek JA, Watchko JF, Mimouni, F: Prevalence and lack of clinical significance of blood group incompatibility in mothers with blood type A or B. J Pediatr 125:87, 1994.

44. Stevenson DK, Fanaroff AA, Maisels MJ, et al: Prediction of hyperbilirubinemia in near-term and term infants. Pediatrics 108:31, 2001.

45. Hubinont PO, Bricoult A, Ghysdael P: ABO mother-infant incompatibilities. Am J Obstet Gynecol 9:593, 1960.

46. Leistikow EA, Collin MF, Savastano GD, et al: Wasted health care dollars. Routine cord blood type and Coombs' testing. Arch Pediatr Adolesc Med 149:1147, 1995.

47. Quinn MW, Weindling AM, Davidson DC: Does ABO incompatibility matter? Arch Dis Child 63:1258, 1988.

48. Judd WJ, Luban NLC, Ness PM, et al: Prenatal and perinatal immunohematology: Recommendations for serologic management of the fetus, newborn infant, and obstetric patient. Transfusion 30:175, 1990.

49. Voak, D, Bowley CC: A detailed serological study on the prediction and diagnosis of ABO haemolytic disease of the newborn (ABO HD). Vox Sang 17:321, 1969.

50. Halbrecht I: Role of hemagglutinins anti-A and anti-B in pathogenesis of jaundice of the newborn (icterus neonatorum praecox). Am J Dis Child 68:248, 1944.

51. Mollison PL: Blood Transfusion in Clinical Medicine. Oxford, UK, Blackwell Scientific, 1983, pp 690-698.

52. Gourley GR: Perinatal bilirubin metabolism. In Gluckman PD, Heymann MA (eds): Perinatal and Pediatric Pathophysiology. A Clinical Perspective. Boston, Hodder & Stoughton, 1993, pp 437-439.

53. Poland RD, Odell GB: Physiologic jaundice: The enterohepatic circulation of bilirubin. N Engl J Med 284:1, 1971.

54. Gartner LM, Lee K-S, Vaisman S, et al: Development of bilirubin transport and metabolism in the newborn rhesus monkey. J Pediatr 90:513, 1977.

55. Gartner U, Goeser T, Wolkoff AW: Effect of fasting on the uptake of bilirubin and sulfobromophthalein by the isolated perfused rat liver. Gastroenterology 113:1707, 1997.

56. Fevery J: Fasting hyperbilirubinemia: Unraveling the mechanism involved. Gastroenterology 113:1798, 1997.

57. Odell GB: Neonatal Hyperbilirubinemia. New York, Grune & Stratton, 1980.

58. Wright K, Tarr PI, Hickman RO, Guthrie RD: Hyperbilirubinemia secondary to delayed absorption of intraperitoneal blood following intrauterine transfusion. J Pediatr 100:302, 1982.

59. Rajagopalan I, Katz BZ: Hyperbilirubinemia secondary to hemolysis of intrauterine intraperitoneal blood transfusion. Clin Pediatr 23:511, 1984.

60. Ritter JK, Crawford JM, Owens IS: Cloning of two human liver bilirubin UDP-glucuronosyltransferase cDNA's with expression in COS-1 cells. J Biol Chem 266:1043,1991.

61. Ritter JK, Chen F, Sheen Y, et al: A novel complex locus UGT1 encodes human bilirubin, phenol, and other UDP-glucuronosyltransferase isoenzymes with identical carboxyl termini. J Biol Chem 267:3257, 1992.

62. Clarke DJ, Moghrabi N, Monaghan G, et al: Genetic defects of the UDP-glucuronosyltransferase-1 (UGT1) gene that cause familial non-haemolytic unconjugated hyperbilirubinemias. Clin Chim Acta 266:63, 1997.

63. Kawade N, Onishi S: The prenatal and postnatal development of UDP glucuronyltransferase activity towards bilirubin and the effect of premature birth on this activity in human liver. Biochem J 196:257, 1981.

64. Coughtrie MW, Burchell B, et al: The inadequacy of perinatal glucuronidation: Immunoblot analysis of the developmental expression of individual UDP-glucuronosyltransferase isoenzymes in rat and human liver microsomes. Mol Pharmacol 34:729, 1988.

65. Valaes T: Bilirubin metabolism: Review and discussion of inborn errors. Clin Perinatol 3:177, 1976.

66. Crigler Jr, JF, Najjar VA: Congenital familial nonhemolytic jaundice with kernicterus. Pediatrics 10:169, 1952.

67. Ritter JK, Yeatman MT, Ferreira P, Owens IS: Identification of a genetic alteration in the code for bilirubin UDP-glucuronosyltransferase in the UDT1 gene complex of a Crigler-Najjar type I patient. J Clin Invest 90:150, 1992

68. Bosma PJ, Roy-Chowdhury N, Goldhoorn BG, et al: Sequence of exons and the flanking regions of human

bilirubin UDP-glucuronosyltransferase gene complex and identification of a genetic mutation in a patient with Crigler-Najjar syndrome, type I. Hepatology 15:941, 1992.

69. Bosma PJ, Roy-Chowdhury J, Huang T, et al: Mechanism of inherited deficiencies of multiple UDP-glucuronosyltransferase isoforms in two patients with Crigler-Najjar syndrome, type I. FASEB J 6:2859, 1992.

70. Labrune P, Myara A, Hadchouel M, et al: Genetic heterogeneity of Crigler-Najjar syndrome type I: A study of 14 cases. Hum Genet 94:693,1994.

71. Moghrabi N, Clarke DJ, Boxer M, Burchell B: Identification of an A-to-G missense mutation in exon 2 of the UGT1 gene complex that causes Crigler-Najjar syndrome type 2.Genomics 18:171, 1993.

72. Gilbert A, Lereboullet P: La cholemia simple familiale. Semaine Med 21:241, 1901.

73. Gourley GR: Disorders of bilirubin metabolism. In Suchy FJ (ed): Liver Disease in Children. St. Louis, Mosby–Year Book, 1994, pp 401-413.

74. Bosma PJ, Roy-Chowdhury J, Bakker C, et al: The genetic basis of the reduced expression of bilirubin UDP-glucuronosyltransferase 1 in Gilbert's syndrome. N Engl J Med 333:1171, 1995.

75. Bancroft JD, Kreamer B, Gourley GR: Gilbert syndrome accelerates development of neonatal jaundice. J Pediatr 132:656, 1998.

76. Roy-Chowdhury N, Deocharan B, Bejjanki HR, et al: The presence of a Gilbert-type promoter abnormality increases the level of neonatal hyperbilirubinemia. Hepatology 26:370A, 1997.

77. Monaghan G, McLellan A, McGeehan A, et al: Gilbert's syndrome is a contributory factor in prolonged unconjugated hyperbilirubinemia of the newborn. J.Pediatr 134:441, 1999.

78. Iolascon A, Faienza MF, Moretti A: UGT1 promoter polymorphism accounts for increased neonatal appearance of hereditary spherocytosis. Blood 91:1093, 1998.

79. Chalasani N, Roy-Chowdhury N, Roy-Chowdhury J, Boyer TD: Kernicterus in an adult who is heterozygous for Crigler-Najjar syndrome and homozygous for Gilbert-type genetic defect. Gastroenterology 112:2099, 1997.

80. Ciotti M, Chen F, Rubaltelli FF, Owens IS: Coding and a TATA box mutation at the bilirubin UDP-glucuronosyltransferase gene cause Crigler-Najjar syndrome type I disease. Biochim Biophys Acta 1407:40, 1998.

81. Yamamoto K, Soeda Y, Kamisako T, et al. Analysis of bilirubin uridine 5′diphosphate (UDP)–glucuronosyltransferase gene mutations in seven patients with Crigler-Najjar syndrome type II. J Hum Genet 43:111, 1998.

82. Kadakol A, Ghosh SS, Sappal BS, et al: Genetic lesions of bilirubin uridine diphosphoglucuronate glucuronosyltransferase causing Crigler-Najjar and Gilbert's syndromes: Correlation of genotype to phenotype. Hum Mutat 16:297, 2000.

83. Maisels MJ, Newman TB: Kernicterus in otherwise healthy, breast-fed term newborns. Pediatrics 96:730, 1995.

84. Watchko JF, Daood MJ, Biniwale M: Neonatal hyperbilirubinemia in the era of genomics. Sem Neonatol 7:143, 2002.

85. Brown AK, Johnson L: Loss of concern about jaundice and the reemergence of kernicterus in full-term infants in the era of managed care. In Fanaroff AA, Klaus MH (eds): The Year Book of Neonatal and Perinatal Medicine. St. Louis, Mosby–Year Book, 1996, pp 17-28.

86. Harris MC, Bernbaum JC, Polin JR, et al: Developmental follow-up of breastfed term and near-term infants with marked hyperbilirubinemia. Pediatrics 107:1075, 2001.

87. Kivlahan C, James EJP: The natural history of neonatal jaundice. Pediatrics 74:364, 1984.

88. Linn S, Schoenbaum SC, Monson RR, et al: Epidemiology of neonatal hyperbilirubinemia. Pediatrics 75:770, 1985.

89. Maisels MJ, Gifford K, Antle CE, et al: Normal serum bilirubin levels in the newborn and the effect of breast feeding. Pediatrics 78:837, 1986.

90. Schneider AP: Breast milk jaundice in the newborn. A real entity. JAMA 255:3270, 1986.

91. Hansen TWR: Bilirubin production, breast-feeding and neonatal jaundice. Acta Paediatr 90:716, 2001.

92. Nielsen HE, Haase P, Blaabjerg J, et al: Risk factors and sib correlation in physiological neonatal jaundice. Acta Paediatr Scand 76:504, 1987.

93. Rubaltelli FF: Unconjugated and conjugated bilirubin pigments during perinatal development IV: The influence of breast-feeding on neonatal hyperbilirubinemia. Biol Neonate 64:104, 1993.

94. Stevenson DK, Bartoletti AL, Ostrander CR, Johnson JD: Pulmonary excretion of carbon monoxide in the human infant as an index of bilirubin production. IV. Effects of breast-feeding and caloric intake in the first postnatal week. Pediatrics 65:1170, 1980.

95. Hintz SR, Gaylord, TD, Oh W, et al: Serum bilirubin levels at 72 hours by selected characteristics in breastfed and formula-fed term infants delivered by cesarean section. Acta Paediatr 90:776, 2001.

96. Bertini G, Carlo C, Tronchin M, Rubaltelli FF: Is breast-feeding really favoring early neonatal jaundice. Pediatrics 107:e41, 2001.

97. Maisels MJ: Epidemiology of neonatal jaundice. In Maisels MJ, Watchko JF (eds): Neonatal Jaundice. Amsterdam, Harwood Academic, 2000, pp 37-49.

98. De Carvalho M, Klaus MH, Merkatz RB: Frequency of breastfeeding and serum bilirubin concentration. Am J Dis Child 136:737, 1982.

99. Yamauchi Y, Yamanouchi I: Breast-feeding frequency during the first 24 hours after birth in full term neonates. Pediatrics 86:171, 1990.

100. Brown WR, Boon WH: Ethnic group differences in plasma bilirubin levels of full-term, healthy Singapore newborns. Pediatrics 36:745, 1965.

101. Newman TB, Easterling MJ, Goldman ES, Stevenson DK: Laboratory evaluation of jaundice in newborns: Frequency, cost, and yield. Am J Dis Child 144:364, 1990.

102. Newman TB, Easterling MJ, Goldman ES, Stevenson DK: Laboratory evaluation of jaundice in newborns: Corrections. Am J Dis Child 146:1420, 1992.

103. Akaba K, Kimura T, Sasaki A, et al: Neonatal hyperbilirubinemia and mutation of the bilirubin uridine diphosphate-glucuronosyltransferase gene: A common missense mutation among Japanese, Koreans, and Chinese. Biochem Mol Biol Int 46:21, 1998.

104. Beutler E, Gelbart T, Demina D: Racial variability in the UDP-glucuronosyltransferase 1 (UDGT1A1) promoter: A balanced polymorphism for regulation of bilirubin metabolism? Proc Natl Acad Sci U S A 95:8170, 1998.

105. Yeung CY: The role of native herbs in neonatal jaundice. J Sing Paediatr Soc 36(S1):7, 1994.

106. Fessas PH, Doxiadis SA, Valaes T: Neonatal jaundice in glucose-6-phosphate dehydrogenase deficient infants. BMJ 2:1359, 1962.

107. Watchko JF: Indirect hyperbilirubinemia in the neonate. In Maisels MJ, Watchko JF (eds): Neonatal Jaundice. Amsterdam, Harwood Academic, 2000, pp 51-66.

108. Van Praagh R: Diagnosis of kernicterus in the neonatal period. Pediatrics 28:870, 1961.

109. Byers RK, Paine RS, Crothers B: Extrapyramidal cerebral palsy with hearing loss following erythroblastosis. Pediatrics 15:248, 1955.

110. Perlstein MA: The late clinical syndrome of posticteric encephalopathy. Pediatr Clin North Am 7:665, 1960.

111. Notter MFD, Kendig JW: Differential sensitivity of neural cells to bilirubin toxicity. Exp Neurol 94:670, 1986.

112. Ahdab-Barmada M, Moosy J: The neuropathology of kernicterus in the premature neonate: Diagnostic problems. J Neuopathol Exdp Neurol 43:45, 1984.

113. Ahdab-Barmada M: The neuropathology of kernicterus: Definitions and debate. In Maisels MJ, Watchko JF (eds): Neonatal Jaundice. Amsterdam, Harwood Academic, 2000, pp 75-88.

114. Hansen TWR: The pathophysiology of bilirubin toxicity. In Maisels MJ, Watchko JF (eds): Neonatal Jaundice. Amsterdam, Harwood Academic, 2000, pp 89-104.

115. Shapiro SM: Evoked potentials and bilirubin. In Maisels MJ, Watchko JF (eds): Neonatal Jaundice. Amsterdam, Harwood Academic, 2000, pp 105-113.

116. Palmer C, Smith MB: Assessing the risk of kernicterus using nuclear magnetic resonance. Clin Perinatol 17:307, 1990.

117. Penn AA, Enzmann DR, Hahn JS, Stevenson DK: Kernicterus in a full term infant. Pediatrics 93:1003, 1994.

118. Martich-Kriss V, Kollias SS, Ball WS: MR findings in kernicterus. Am J Neuroradiol 16:819, 1995.

119. Yokochi K: Magnetic resonance imaging in children with kernicterus. Acta Paediatr 84:937, 1995.

120. Hsai DY, Allen FH, Gellis SS, et al: Erythroblastosis fetalis. VIII. Studies of serum bilirubin in relation to kernicterus. N Engl J Med 247:668, 1952.

121. Johnston WH, Angara V, Baumal R, et al: Erythroblastosis fetalis and hyperbilirubinemia: A five year follow-up with neurological, psychological, and audiological evaluation. Pediatrics 39:88, 1967.

122. Ozmert E, Erdem G, Topcu M, et al: Long-term follow-up of indirect hyperbilirubinemia in full-term Turkish infants. Acta Paediatr 85:1440, 1996.

123. Johnson L, Boggs TR: Bilirubin-dependent brain damage: Incidence and indications for treatment. In Odell GB, Schaffer R, Simopoulos AP (eds): Phototherapy in the Newborn: An Overview. Washington, DC, National Academy of Sciences, 1974, pp 122-149.

124. Watchko JF, Oski FA: Bilirubin 20 mg/dL = vigintiphobia. Pediatrics 71:660, 1983.

125. Watchko JF: The clinical sequelae of hyperbilirubinemia. In Maisels MJ, Watchko JF (eds): Neonatal Jaundice. Amsterdam, Harwood Academic, 2000, pp 115-135.

126. Newman TB, Maisels MJ: Does hyperbilirubinemia damage the brain of healthy full-term infants? Clin Perinatol 17:331, 1990.

127. Newman TB, Maisels MJ: Evaluation and treatment of jaundice in the term newborn: A kinder, gentler approach. Pediatrics 89:809, 1992.

128. Newman TB, Klebanoff MA: Neonatal hyperbilirubinemia and long-term outcome: Another look at the Collaborative Perinatal Project. Pediatrics 92:651, 1993.

129. Maisels MJ, Newman TB: Jaundice in full term and near term babies who leave the hospital within 36 hours—the pediatrician's nemesis. Clin Perinatol 25:295, 1998.

130. Watchko JF, Oski FA: Kernicterus in preterm newborns: Past, present, and future. Pediatrics 90:707, 1992.

131. Watchko JF, Claassen D: Kernicterus in premature infants: Current prevalence and relationship to NICHD phototherapy study exchange criteria. Pediatrics 93:996, 1994.

132. Gartner LM, Catz, CS, Yaffe SJ: Neonatal bilirubin workshop. Pediatrics 94:537, 1994.

133. Maisels MJ: The clinical approach to the jaundiced newborn. In Maisels MJ, Watchko JF (eds): Neonatal Jaundice. Amsterdam, Harwood Academic, 2000, pp 139-168.

134. American Academy of Pediatrics, Provisional Committee for Quality Improvement and Subcommittee on Hyperbilirubinemia: Practice parameter: Management of hyperbilirubinemia in the healthy term newborn. Pediatrics 94:558, 1994.

135. American Academy of Pediatrics, Subcommittee on Neonatal Hyperbilirubinemia: Neonatal jaundice and kernicterus. Pediatrics 108:763, 2001.

136. Newman TB, Escobar GJ, Gonzales VM, et al: Frequency of neonatal bilirubin testing and hyperbilirubinemia in a large health maintenance organization. Pediatrics 104:1198, 1999.

137. Newman TB, Xiong B, Gonzales VM, Escobar GJ: Prediction and prevention of extreme hyperbilirubinemia in a mature health maintenance organization. Arch Pediatr Adolesc Med 154:1140, 2000.

138. Billing BH, Cole PG, Lathe GH: Increased plasma bilirubin in newborn infants in relation to birth weight. BMJ 2:1263, 1954.

139. Joint Commission on Accreditation of Healthcare Organizations: Kernicterus threatens healthy newborns. Sentinel Event ALERT, Issue 18, May 2, 2001. Available at *http://www.jcaho.org* (accessed May 10, 2004).

140. Bhutani VK, Johnson L, Sivieri EM: Predictive ability of a predischarge hour-specific serum bilirubin for subsequent significant hyperbilirubinemia in healthy-term and near-term newborns. Pediatrics 103:6, 1999.

141. Kernicterus in full-term infants–United States, 1994-1998. MMWR Morb Mortal Wkly Rep 50:491, 2001.

142. Cremer RJ, Perryman PW, Richards DH: Influence of light on the hyperbilirubinemia of infants. Lancet 1:1094, 1958.

143. Lucey J, Ferreiro M, Hewitt J: Prevention of hyperbilirubinemia of prematurity by phototherapy. Pediatrics 41:1047, 1968.

144. Maisels MJ: Phototherapy. In Maisels MJ, Watchko JF (eds): Neonatal Jaundice. Amsterdam, Harwood Academic, 2000, pp 177-203.

145. McDonagh AF: Phototherapy: From ancient Egypt to the new millennium. J Perinatol 21(Suppl 1):S7, 2001.

146. Christensen T, Kinn G: Bilirubin bound to cells does not form photoisomers. Acta Paediatr 82:22, 1993.

147. Sato K, Hara T, Kondo T, et al: High dose intravenous gammaglobulin therapy for neonatal immune haemolytic jaundice due to blood group incompatibility. Acta Paediatr Scand 80:163, 1991.

148. Rubo J, Albrecht K, Lasch P, et al: High dose intravenous immune globulin therapy for hyperbilirubinemia caused by Rh hemolytic disease. J Pediatr 121:93, 1992.

149. Ergaz Z, Arad H: Intravenous immunoglobulin therapy in neonatal immune hemolytic jaundice. J Perinatal Med 21:183, 1993.

150. Hammerman C, Kaplan M: Recent developments in the management of neonatal hyperbilirubinemia. NeoReviews 1:e19, 2000.

151. Hammerman C, Vreman HJ, Kaplan M, Stevenson DK: Intravenous immune globulin in neonatal immune hemolytic disease: Does it reduce hemolysis? Acta Paediatr 85:1351, 1996.

152. Diamond LK, Allen FH, Thomas WO: Erythroblastosis fetalis. VII. Treatment with exchange transfusion. N Engl J Med 244:39, 1951.

153. Watchko JF: Exchange transfusion. In Maisels MJ, Watchko JF (eds): Neonatal Jaundice. Amsterdam, Harwood Academic, 2000, pp 169-176.

154. Aranda JV, Sweet AY: Alterations in blood pressure during exchange transfusion. Arch Dis Child 52:545, 1977.

155. Keenan WJ, Novak KK, Sutherland JM, et al: Morbidity and mortality associated with exchange transfusion. Pediatrics (Suppl) 75:417, 1985.

156. Hovi L, Siimes MA: Exchange transfusion with fresh heparinized blood is a safe procedure. Experiences from 1069 newborns. Acta Paediatr Scand 74:360, 1985.

157. Maisels MJ: Is exchange transfusion for hyperbilirubinemia in danger of becoming extinct? Pediatr Res 45:210A, 1999.

158. Jackson JC: Adverse events associated with exchange transfusion in healthy and ill newborns. Pediatrics 99:e7, 1997.

159. Schreiber GB, Busch MP, Kleinman SH, Korelitz JJ: The risk of transfusion-transmitted viral infections. N Engl J Med 334:1685, 1996.

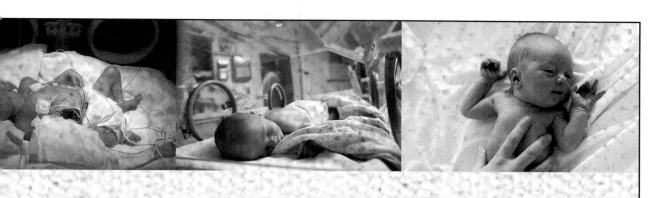

Infection and the Neonate

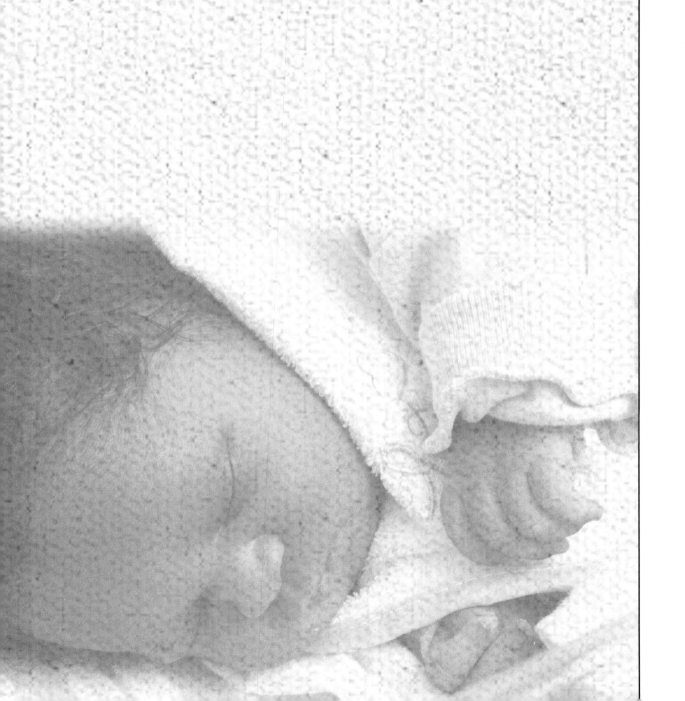

Infection Control and Specific Bacterial, Viral, Fungal, and Protozoan Infections of the Fetus and Neonate

Sharon A. Nachman

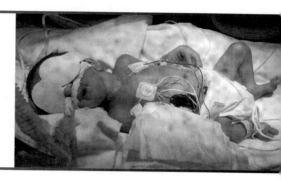

I n the preantibiotic era, neonatal sepsis was almost always fatal. Since the advent of antibiotics, mortality has significantly decreased. However, since 1990, although the case fatality rate for noninfectious neonatal illnesses has continued to decline, that for infectious diseases has reached a plateau.[1] Despite advances in antimicrobial therapy and neonatal intensive care, neonatal infections continue to be an important determinant of morbidity and mortality in both developed and developing countries. Neonatal infections are responsible for between 1.5 million and 2 million neonatal deaths per year, or between 4000 and 5000 deaths per day in the less developed countries of the world.[2] The incidence of neonatal sepsis is even higher in infants with low birth weight and is inversely proportional to both gestational age and birth weight.

This chapter discusses infections of the newborn, including (1) infection control and nosocomial sepsis, fungal disease, and focal bacterial infections; (2) congenital and perinatally acquired infections; and (3) sexually transmitted, perinatally acquired infections. Early-onset bacterial sepsis is discussed in Chapter 70.

INFECTION CONTROL

The **incidence rate** is the ratio of the number of new occurrences of a disease in a given period to the number of persons at risk (e.g., the number of cases of bacteremia per 1000 days with a catheter). The **prevalence rate** is the percentage of persons with a specific disease entity in a defined population at a specific time without regard to when the disease began.

Sporadic (endemic) infections represent the bulk of nosocomial infections and are the usual type of infection expected during a given period for a given population. The same pathogens are often seen in neonatal intensive care units (NICUs) around the country. **Epidemic infections** are marked by an unusual increase in the incidence of a specific disease entity. These are often seen as a cluster of a specific pathogen. Knowledge of the endemic levels of

a disease is needed to decide whether a specific pathogen isolated is a part of an epidemic or endemic to the NICU.

There are many different types of isolation. Each is indicated for a particular pathogen or disease entity. **Respiratory isolation** is indicated for patients *suspected* of having specific respiratory pathogens such as tuberculosis, chickenpox, or measles. These patients must be placed in respiratory isolation in negative-pressure rooms to prevent aerosol spread of the infection. It is important to assess the members of the families of such patients for infection or immune status as well.

Contact isolation is a category of isolation for infectious entities that can be spread through direct contact with infectious secretions or with fomites contaminated with infectious secretions. Patients in contact isolation should be placed in a single room (when available), and health care workers should wash hands upon entering and leaving the room and wear gowns and gloves for contact with the patient or the patient's environment. Infections that necessitate contact isolation include those with *Clostridium difficile*, croup, rotavirus, herpes simplex virus (HSV), respiratory syncytial virus, and cytomegalovirus (CMV).

Droplet precautions are used to prevent transmission of diseases that are spread through large, aerosolized droplets containing infectious particles. Such particles are spread through sneezing and coughing and rapidly settle on horizontal surfaces within a few feet of the source patient. Examples of pathogens include adenovirus, parvovirus, rubella, and meningitis caused by *Haemophilus influenzae* or *Neisseria meningitidis*.

Some exposures are inevitable. One such example is varicella. Patients (or nonimmune staff or visitors) need to be isolated from day 10 to day 21 after documented exposure to a person with active varicella-zoster virus (VZV) infection. If a patient has received varicella-zoster immune globulin (VZIG), the incubation period is extended to 28 days. It should be remembered that, in considering who may be immune to VZV, 90% of individuals who said that they had varicella did have the disease, whereas 70% of those who said they did not have varicella in fact did also have the disease.

Six of seven hospital-based studies (including two in NICUs) have demonstrated that improved handwashing techniques reduce infection rates.[3,4] This approach includes removal of all rings, no nail polish or false nails, an initial 3-minute scrub to the elbow, and at least a 10-second scrub before and after handling each infant. Some of the excuses heard as to why staff do not wash their hands include "Handwashing takes too much time," lack of soap (54%) and lack of towels (65%), "One thorough wash per day is sufficient" (26%), "Gloves can substitute for handwashing" (25%—including 50% of physicians), and "Handwashing is not important if an infant is receiving antibiotics" (10%).[5,6]

Skin emollients decrease the dispersal of bacteria. In two small studies, topical emollients without antibiotics have been shown to decrease the frequency of nosocomial infection in neonates.[7] Alcohol-based formulations (with appropriate emollients) are equivalent or superior to antiseptic detergents. In addition, they require no washing or drying, thereby reducing damage to the skin.[8] There are very limited data to support the efficacy of gowning and much data indicating that it is ineffective. The risk of transmitting infection through clothing is 2 per 10,000 encounters[9]; therefore, gowning is no longer recommended.

NOSOCOMIAL SEPSIS

Nosocomial infections are defined as hospital-acquired infections and, therefore, are potentially preventable by nursery infection control practices. They often occur after the first week after birth. Coagulase-negative staphylococci have emerged as the most frequently isolated pathogens responsible for this type of late-onset sepsis. However, the pathogens associated with late-onset nosocomial sepsis can include *Staphylococcus aureus*, *Enterococcus* species, *Klebsiella* species, *Enterobacter* species, *Pseudomonas aeruginosa*, and fungi (especially *Candida albicans*). The enteric gram-negative organisms are of specific concern because they are often antibiotic resistant as well, which complicates treatment. Approximately 25% of infants with very low birth weight (VLBW) develop one or more episodes of blood culture-proven late-onset sepsis. However, nosocomial sepsis is not limited to infants with low birth weight or VLBW; it can occur in any hospitalized neonate. Typical features seen in the infants presenting with nosocomial or late-onset sepsis include prolonged length of mechanical ventilation, prolonged need for parenteral nutrition, need for indwelling catheters, and prolonged length of hospitalization. As a complication of these sepsis events, there is an associated increased cost of care and an increased risk of death.

Important information regarding nosocomial infections has been obtained from multicenter studies. These studies uniformly show that nosocomial blood stream infections are related to very low birth weight, birth at earlier gestational ages, insertion of catheters, and use of parenteral nutrition for more than 14 days.[10] Other variables include the influence of postnatal steroids[11] and the use of H_2 blockers, which increase the risk of blood stream infections. There appears to be a wide variation in the incidence of blood stream infections in NICUs nationally.[12] The incidence ranges from 8.5% to 42% by site, despite adjustment for known risk factors and length of stay.

Skin and mucous membranes are the primary defenses against invading microbes. Any break in the skin barrier, either in the case of skin diseases such as eczema or in the case of central lines and catheters, allows for entry of microbes to the blood stream. Neutrophils, macrophages, and natural killer cells attempt to eradicate the organisms that manage to bypass the skin primary defense barrier. The high incidence of nosocomial infections in preterm neonates may not be effectively diminished until new strategies that augment skin and mucous membrane defense mechanisms are discovered.[13,14]

Staphylococcus epidermidis

Staphylococcus epidermidis organisms are gram-positive cocci, typically appearing in clusters on Gram stain. They are the most common gram-positive organisms involved in nosocomial sepsis in neonates. Several factors are associated with development of nosocomial coagulase-negative *Staphylococcus* sepsis (CONS). These include prematurity, the presence of central venous catheters, use of lipid emulsions, presence of mechanical ventilation, and instrumentation. Focal complications of CONS include infective endocarditis, necrotizing enterocolitis, pneumonia, and meningitis.

Isolation of the pathogen is key in the diagnosis of CONS. Ideally, blood culture at the time of suspected sepsis should be attempted. An adequate blood culture sample must be obtained carefully, because less than 0.5 mL of blood rarely yields a positive result even in the presence of sepsis. Investigation into the possible distal spread of bacteria should include ultrasound study of the kidney and ophthalmologic evaluation. Some centers also evaluate the heart with cardiac echocardiography. In most situations, removal of the central catheter is suggested.

Selective use of vancomycin as prophylaxis may prevent CONS bacteremia, but the risks with continuous usage are high. Risks include emergence of fungal or gram-negative infections in vancomycin-treated infants and, more in general, emergence of vancomycin-resistant strains of coagulase-negative streptococci and of enterococci in NICUs as a whole. Because coagulase-negative staphylococci are generally organisms of low virulence, the risk/benefit ratio of such prevention strategies is in question. Some nurseries have restricted all vancomycin use to "proven" or "presumed" infections in an effort to decrease inappropriate use of this antibiotic.

The initial recommended therapy for presumed staphylococcal epidermidis sepsis is often vancomycin. Therapy should be modified if the organism is sensitive to oxacillin or nafcillin. In cases of persistent bacteremia, a combination of vancomicin and gentamicin (in daily use, for synergy) may be the best therapeutic regimen. Some authors suggest rifampin as a substitute for gentamicin. In cases of an infected indwelling catheter, antibiotic therapy through the catheter is mandatory, and removal of the catheter may be necessary if the culture remains positive. The same is true for meningitis secondary to an infected cerebrospinal fluid (CSF) shunt.

Candida and Other Fungal Pathogens

Fungal infections, primarily candidal, account for almost 9% of all late-onset infections in the NICU.[15] In a study of nine NICUs, 4.9% of all VLBW infants developed a fungal infection.[16] *Candida* species can be acquired both vertically and horizontally; thus, disease in the neonate can manifest either as perinatally acquired infection or as nosocomial infection. Vertical transmission of *C. albicans* occurs in approximately 10% of full-term infants and 30% of preterm infants. Most commonly, acquisition leads to neonatal thrush or a perineal diaper rash with little associated morbidity or to invasive fungal dermatitis, spontaneous intestinal perforation, and, in rare cases, brain abscesses.

Other fungi seen in the NICU include *Malassezia* species in association with lipid infusions and *Aspergillus* species and other Zygomycetes organisms associated with gastrointestinal tract infections.

Early-onset candidal disease (Table 69-1), or **congenital candidiasis**, arises after exposure of the infant to organisms colonizing the maternal genital tract. Cutaneous findings are the hallmarks of the disease, but an association with pulmonary disease conveys a grave prognosis despite systemic antifungal therapy. **Catheter-associated fungemia** generally arises from organisms within the gastrointestinal tract. In affected infants, fungemia resolves with prompt removal of the catheter and parenteral amphotericin therapy for 10 to 14 days. In contrast, **disseminated candidiasis** involves distant organs, including the heart, kidney, bone, eyes, lungs, and meninges. Long-term therapy is recommended, and prognosis is guarded in these cases. Several predisposing factors for systematic candidiasis have been identified, including long-term use of broad-spectrum antibiotics, which suppress normal gastrointestinal flora and allows candidal overgrowth; prematurity; host immunosuppression associated with abnormal skin barriers; hormonal and cellular immune deficits; neutrophil dysfunction and complement deficiencies; central intravenous catheterization and parenteral hyperalimentation, which allow

a portal of entry for the organism into the blood stream; and prolonged steroid use, which may impair neutrophil function.[17-20]

The recurrence of candidal disease has been described in four immunocompetent infants after a prolonged period of latency (up to 1 year). All of the infants presented with candidal arthritis and osteomyelitis, were born prematurely, had received parenteral nutrition through indwelling catheters, and had a history of systemic candidiasis during the neonatal period.[21] The pathogenesis of these latent infections is unknown. Unresolved issues include optimum length of therapy and which antifungals to use in these types of cases.

One study suggested an association between *Candida* sepsis and retinopathy of prematurity in infants with extremely low birth weight. The study found an increased severity in retinopathy of prematurity and a need for laser therapy after candidal infection. Although the mechanism is unknown, endothelial injury by the organism, elaboration of proinflammatory cytokines, and production of angiogenic substances may be involved.[22]

Attempts to prevent candidal disease have not been very successful, in view of the increased rate of survival of VLBW premature infants who require complex medical therapies. Limitation of the use of broad-spectrum antibiotics may prevent fungal colonization of the gastrointestinal tract in susceptible neonates. Alternatively, early introduction of enteral feeding may shorten the duration of parenteral nutrition and lessen the need for intravenous catheters. The efficacy of prophylactic antifungal therapies in preventing disseminated candidiasis in patients at high risk has not been demonstrated. Data in other groups of patients (e.g., those immunocompromised) suggest that prophylactic antifungal agents may not be useful in prevention of systemic fungemia.

There is currently no consensus regarding the best approach to the treatment of systemic candidal infections in neonates, because large, controlled studies of treatment strategies have not yet been performed. Amphotericin B remains the mainstay of therapy. It is a polyene macrolide antibiotic that binds to the fungal cell membrane, causing leakage of cellular contents and cell death. The dosage is 1 to 1.5 mg/kg/day, administered for 14 days for catheter-associated fungemia, to 6 weeks for disseminated disease (total dose of 25 to 30 mg/kg), depending on disease severity and site. It can be administered every day or every other day as long as the total dose is achieved. Although side effects include nephrotoxicity, hypokalemia, hepatotoxicity, and bone marrow suppression, the drug appears to be well tolerated by neonates.

Amphotericin B lipid complex, which is incorporated into unilamellar liposomes, was developed to eliminate the severe adverse effects of conventional amphotericin with good central nervous system (CNS) penetration. To date, randomized, clinical trials have not been performed to compare its efficacy to that of conventional amphotericin B, but several smaller studies have shown safety. Available data suggest that it has the same toxicity and safety profiles as amphotericin B, with the advantage of lowered volume needed for drug administration.

Table 69-1. Features of Various Candidal Infection Manifestations

Clinical Features	Congenital Candidiasis	Catheter-Related Fungemia	Systemic Candidiasis
Age of onset	Birth	>7 Days	>7 Days
Risk factors	None	Necessary	Necessary
Skin involvement	Hallmark	None	None
Respiratory involvement	Occasionally	None	Occasionally

5-Flucytosine is a nucleoside analogue that inhibits DNA replication in *Candida* organisms. It may be used as adjunctive synergistic therapy for candidal meningitis or persistent fungemia because amphotericin B penetrates the CNS poorly. Fluconazole, another alternative agent, binds to fungal cytochrome P-450 and affects fungal membrane integrity. There have been no controlled trials of this agent in neonatal candidiasis, so it is not recommended as first-line therapy in neonates. An additional therapeutic concern is the emergence of relative resistance of non-*albicans* species to conventional treatment with amphotericin B, necessitating susceptibility testing in cases refractory to therapy.

Newer antifungal agents include voriconazole[23] and caspofungin.[24,25] These two agents are indicated for *Aspergillus* species, resistant *Candida* species, and other sensitive fungi typically isolated from neonates.

The key to successful therapy includes specific treatment for the type of fungus isolated (and known susceptibility profiles), the amount of end-organ involvement, and the presence of central catheters.

SITE-SPECIFIC INFECTIONS

Neonatal Meningitis

In experimental models, it takes 10^6 gram-positive bacteremic organisms to develop gram-positive meningitis, whereas it takes only 10^3 gram-negative bacteremic organisms to develop gram-negative meningitis.[26] Meningitis occurs in 10% to 20% of neonates with positive blood cultures. With increased use of intrapartum antibiotics, a postnatal blood culture is no longer a reliable way to determine whether an infant was bacteremic. In a retrospective study of 43 infants with proven meningitis, 7 infants with meningitis were totally asymptomatic (i.e., they had no signs or symptoms consistent with meningitis). Of these 7 infants, 4 also had a negative blood culture.[27] However, in other retrospective studies of infants who were being evaluated for possible sepsis, meningitis occurred only in infants who were symptomatic. Therefore, in an asymptomatic infant at "high risk," a lumbar puncture seems appropriate only in situations in which laboratory testing or the history strongly suggests that the infant is bacteremic. All other infants should be closely observed. Normal CSF values are available as a reference range for all sepsis evaluations (Table 69-2).[28]

Pathogens identified in bacterial meningitis include group B streptococci, *Escherichia coli*, and *Listeria* species among the early- and late-onset sepsis syndromes, as well as resistant gram-negative and gram-positive nosocomial pathogens. Most centers typically start empirical therapy with ampicillin and either cefotaxime or gentamicin. Therapy should then be altered to eradicate the specific pathogen identified. Because of the relationship of minimum inhibitory concentration of the bacteria to the antibiotic, sometimes even a small amount of antibiotic in the CNS is sufficient to eradicate the pathogen. There are many choices for treatment of gram-negative meningitis. These include the third-generation cephalosporins, extended-spectrum penicillins, monobactams, and quinolones. Among the third-generation cephalosporins, ceftazidime is probably as efficacious as cefotaxime (or ceftriaxone) but, like other important antibiotics, should be reserved for resistant gram-negative pathogens such as *P. aeruginosa* or enterobacteria. Many factors affect penetration of antibiotics into the CSF (Table 69-3). Physicians should take these into account when prescribing antibiotics for CNS infection.

There are no direct-comparison studies demonstrating the superiority of cefotaxime (or ceftriaxone) alone or in combination with ampicillin over ampicillin plus an aminoglycoside. However, for gram-negative meningitis, cefotaxime is preferred and may even be paired with an aminoglycoside in some cases. Because of concerns regarding recurrent gram-negative meningitis, most experts suggest that gram-negative meningitis be treated for at least 3 weeks.

Because there is synergism between ampicillin and aminoglycosides for most of group B streptococci, *Listeria monocytogenes*, and enterococci, combination therapy is recommended until the CSF is sterilized. If the group B streptococcal disease is shown to be tolerant to ampicillin (minimum bactericidal concentration/minimum inhibitory concentration $\geq 30/1$), combination therapy should be used for the duration of treatment (~14 days). Specific recommendations for each pathogen are described in the specific sections on pathogens.

Table 69–2. Normal Cerebrospinal Fluid Values in Full-Term and Preterm Infants

Time of Birth	WBC	PMN	Protein	Glucose
Term	$7^* \pm 13$	$0.8^* \pm 6.2$	$64^* \pm 24$	$51^* \pm 13$
Preterm (<1000 g)	$4^* \pm 3$	$6 \pm 15^\dagger$	160 ± 56	61 ± 34

*Mean ± standard deviation.
†Median.

PMN, polymorphonuclear leukocyte; WBC, white blood cell.

Table 69–3. Factors Influencing CNS Penetration of Antibiotics

Variables	Effect on CNS Penetration	Example
High degree of protein binding	Reduced	Ceftriazone
Lipid solubility	Enhanced	Rifampin
High degree of ionization	Reduced	β-lactams
Active transport system	Enhanced	Penicillin
Meningeal inflammation	Enhanced*	β-lactams, vancomycin

*Meningeal inflammation influences only penetration of hydrophilic antibiotics.
CNS, central nervous system.

Conjunctivitis

Conjunctivitis occurs in 1.6% to 12% of all newborns, with rates in some countries as high as 24%.[29] Typical pathogens causing conjunctivitis include gonococci, *Chlamydia* species, HSV, *H. influenzae,* and staphylococci. These pathogens are transmitted from mother to infant at the time of delivery. The time of onset for infections with most pathogens that cause conjunctivitis may overlap, particularly in the presence of prolonged rupture of membranes (Table 69-4).

In 10% to 46% of infants who present with conjunctivitis in the first month after birth, *Chlamydia trachomatis* is the most commonly identified cause.[30] However, taken together, gonococci and chlamydial organisms account for most cases of neonatal blindness worldwide.[31] In conjunctivitis, the incubation period after exposure (delivery) is 5 to 14 days. This period can be shortened with premature rupture of the membranes.

Approximately 50% to 75% of infants born to *Chlamydia*-infected women become infected at one or more anatomic sites, including the conjunctivae, nasopharynx, rectum, and vagina; 30% to 50% develop chlamydial conjunctivitis.[32] In at least 50% of infants with neonatal inclusion conjunctivitis (NIC), nasopharyngeal infection is also present. Approximately 70% of infected infants have positive nasopharyngeal cultures, and of these infants, 30% develop chlamydial pneumonia.[33] The incidence of chlamydial conjunctivitis, however, has decreased with prenatal increased screening for *Chlamydia.* NIC usually appears on the fifth day after birth. Frequently, both eyes demonstrate the typical nonspecific signs of neonatal conjunctivitis: lid edema, conjunctival hyperemia, papillary hypertrophy, and mucopurulent discharge. Because the newborn cannot produce follicles for the first 6 to 8 weeks after birth, the type of conjunctival reaction does not contribute to the diagnosis. Neonates can develop scarring of the conjunctiva and cornea.

Infection with other bacterial pathogens can also manifest as conjunctivitis. These pathogens include *H. influenzae, S. aureus,* and *Streptococcus pneumoniae,* all frequently isolated in infants with lacrimal duct

obstruction, and *Pseudomonas* species, which appears as an epidemic conjunctivitis. Evaluation of infants should include both Gram stain and culture of the discharge, as well as a complete ophthalmologic evaluation. *Pseudomonas* organisms can be dangerously virulent, and *Pseudomonas* conjunctivitis necessitates systemic as well as local (even subconjunctival) antibiotic therapy. Viral causes of conjunctivitis are rare during the first month after birth; however, when these do occur, the virus most commonly identified in 70% of cases is HSV.

Included in the evaluation of conjunctivitis is a Gram stain of the discharge. If the Gram stain shows gram-negative intracellular diplococci with abutting flattened sides, *Neisseria gonorrhoeae* should be assumed to be the cause of the eye discharge, and the infant should be admitted for systemic treatment. A bacterial culture should be sent, along with a specific gonorrhea culture, to confirm the diagnosis. The eye discharge seen in gonococcal ophthalmia is often thick, copious, and golden yellow in color. If the Gram stain is negative for intracellular diplococci, a culture for *C. trachomatis* and a rapid test for *Chlamydia* (such as direct fluorescent antibody [DFA] tests, enzyme immunoassays [EIAs], or DNA probe) should be performed in addition to bacterial cultures. A combined DNA probe for detection of both *N. gonorrhoeae* and *C. trachomatis* is commercially available. The *Chlamydia* tests must be done on conjunctival scrapings, because *Chlamydia* organisms are obligate intracellular organisms. If herpes conjunctivitis is suspected, a rapid test for HSV and culture should be sent to the laboratory.

Conjunctivitis caused by gonorrhea should be treated with ceftriaxone, 50 mg/kg, administered intravenously or intramuscularly once a day for 7 days. Additional topical therapy is not needed when ceftriaxone is used, but the infant's eyes should be irrigated with normal saline frequently until the discharge is gone.

If gonococcal ophthalmia is not suspected, 0.5% erythromycin ointment can be applied to each eye four times a day for 7 days. If the *Chlamydia* test result is positive, oral erythromycin, 50 mg/kg/day divided into four equal doses, should be given for 14 days. Azithromycin, 20 mg/kg once a day for 3 days, may be used. After systemic antibiotics are started, topical treatment of the eye may be discontinued.

Even if the ophthalmologic prophylaxis is successful, this treatment does not necessarily eliminate the nasopharyngeal carrier stage of chlamydial and subsequent systemic infections such as pneumonitis. Although the prevalence of chlamydial infections among pregnant women varies from 2% to 24%, most studies suggest that about 5% of women have chlamydial infections.[34] Nearly two thirds of neonates born to these infected mothers develop a chlamydial infection after delivery. Between 18% and 50% of these newborns develop conjunctivitis, and 11% to 20% develop pneumonia.[35]

Herpes conjunctivitis is rare and is almost always accompanied by other systemic manifestations of neonatal herpes. For a more complete discussion regarding neonatal herpes, see later section in this chapter (Herpes Simplex Virus). The treatment for neonatal herpes

Table 69–4. **Common Causes of Neonatal Conjunctivitis and Presentation**

Cause	Usual Time of Onset after Birth
Chemical conjunctivitis (silver nitrate)	6-24 hr
Chlamydia trachomatis	5-14 days
Neisseria gonorrhoeae	2-5 days
Other bacterial cause	>5 days
Staphylococcus aureus	
Haemophilus species	
Streptococcus pneumoniae	
Enterococcus species	
Herpes simplex	5-14 days

conjunctivitis is acyclovir, 10 to 20 mg/kg/dose intravenously every 8 hours for 10 days, plus topical therapy with 1% trifluridine solution applied to the eye every 2 hours for 7 days or until the cornea has reepithelialized. Oral acyclovir is poorly bioavailable and should not substitute for the intravenous formulation.

Topical silver nitrate, tetracycline, and erythromycin given at birth are equally effective in preventing gonococcal ophthalmia neonatorum, but none of these agents significantly decreases the incidence of chlamydial conjunctivitis.

Omphalitis

The diagnosis of omphalitis is made from the presence of foul-smelling umbilical discharge and the presence of periumbilical erythematous streaking, induration, and tenderness to palpation. In addition, purulent or serosanguineous discharge or, on rare occasions, signs of a systemic infection may also be present. The incidence of omphalitis in infants born in the hospital is less than 2%. In infants delivered at home, the incidence may be as high as 21%. Associated findings in neonates with omphalitis includes prematurity, complicated delivery, improper severing of the umbilical cord, and poor hygiene practices during the neonatal period.[36]

The primary pathogens isolated in omphalitis are *S. aureus* and *Streptococcus pyogenes* (infections with group A, β-hemolytic streptococci may result in a wet, malodorous stump with only mild evidence of inflammation), and gram-negative organisms (e.g., *E. coli*, *Klebsiella* species) are rarely seen.

Omphalitis must be differentiated from funisitis. Funisitis is an inflammation of the umbilical cord vessels and Wharton's jelly and has been described as either an acute exudative or a subacute necrotizing process that accompanies chorioamnionitis.[37,38] The predominant organisms identified as etiologic agents in this infection are gram-negative bacteria, including *E. coli*, *Klebsiella* species, and *Pseudomonas* species. Gram-positive organisms (e.g., streptococci, staphylococci) and *Candida* species are occasionally seen.

The complications of omphalitis are septic umbilical arteritis, suppurative thrombophlebitis of the umbilical or portal veins (resulting in portal vein thrombosis and portal hypertension), liver abscess, endocarditis, necrotizing fasciitis of the abdominal wall, and peritonitis.

Infants with omphalitis should receive a penicillinase-resistant penicillin. Addition of an aminoglycoside antibiotic may be necessary. Local therapy should be used to eliminate surface colonization. Patients with funisitis should be treated with broad-spectrum gram-negative coverage, as well as gram-positive coverage.

Leukocyte adhesion deficiency is a rare life-threatening, autosomal recessively inherited deficiency of cell adhesion molecules associated with chronic omphalitis or delayed separation of the umbilical cord. In these cases, separation of the cord is delayed until after 4 to 6 weeks after birth. The hallmark of leukocyte adhesion deficiency is the absence of granulocytes at the site of infection.[39] Diagnosis of the deficiency requires evaluation of lymphocytes with flow cytometry.

Pyelonephritis and Urinary Tract Infection

Asymptomatic bacteriuria occurs in 2% of healthy full-term neonates and up to 10% of premature infants.[40] Symptomatic urinary tract infections (UTIs) occur in 1.4 per 1000 newborns. Boys are affected more often than girls in the neonatal period, and uncircumcised boys are even more susceptible. Unlike infection in older infants, hematogenous spread of infection is more common than ascending infection. For this reason, some neonates may have associated meningitis and septicemia. Infections of the urinary system are often associated with enteric gram-negative organisms. Therefore, in addition to urinalysis and urine culture, neonates more than 3 days of age should have blood and CSF cultures drawn before initiation of antibiotics. The yield of urine culture in neonates younger than 3 days is poor. In contrast to the distinction of cystitis and pyelonephritis in older infants and children, infection of the urinary tract in the neonate often includes that of the kidney.

The symptoms of UTI are often nonspecific and include vomiting, diarrhea, failure to thrive, fever, lethargy, and jaundice, in which bilirubin is unconjugated if the UTI occurs in the first week after birth and conjugated if UTI occurs later.[41] The definitive diagnosis is by positive culture of urine that is obtained with sterile precautions. Urinalysis is not very helpful; up to 25 leukocytes/mm^3 in boys and up to 50 leukocytes/mm^3 in clean-catch specimens are considered normal. Absence of pyuria does not rule out UTI.

The most common organism causing UTI in neonates is *E. coli*, which accounts for 91% of community-acquired infections in children younger than 8 weeks. Other organisms include *Proteus*, *Pseudomonas*, *Klebsiella*, and *Enterococcus* species and *S. aureus*, which may be associated with suppurative lesions in the testes, epididymis, or kidneys. With prolonged hospitalization, coagulase-negative *Staphylococcus* and *Candida* species can also cause UTI. Predisposing factors for candidal UTI include prematurity, the presence of intravascular catheters, administration of parenteral nutrition, cutaneous fungal infection, and use of broad-spectrum antibiotics. Candidiasis can be associated with fungal balls in the kidney and renal pelvis, which can lead to obstruction.

Treatment of pyelonephritis is similar to that of bacterial UTI and consists of parenteral antibiotics, usually a combination of a penicillin (or a derivative of penicillin) and an aminoglycoside or, in older infants, a third-generation cephalosporin. For suspected staphylococcal infection, a penicillinase-resistant penicillin or first-generation cephalosporin should be used. Amphotericin is used for candidal infection, and in premature neonates, liposomal amphotericin can be used to reduce nephrotoxicity. The duration of therapy is 10 to 14 days, and it is advisable to repeat a urine culture after 48 hours to confirm clearance of the organisms from the urinary tract. Antibiotic prophylaxis is indicated for structural anomalies of the urinary tract or vesicoureteric reflux. In such cases, consultation with a nephrologist is warranted. Prophylaxis is started and continued until spontaneous resolution or surgical correction of the underlying lesion has occurred.

In addition to diagnosing UTI, it is also important to evaluate the urinary tract for underlying structural or functional abnormalities that may predispose to recurrent UTIs. Urinary tract anomalies have been detected in 30% to 55% of infants younger than 2 months with UTI, but they rarely occur in the early neonatal period.

Abdominal ultrasonography is a safe and noninvasive method of evaluating structural abnormalities of the urinary tract and is the initial imaging test of choice. Plain radiographs of the abdomen do not allow adequate visualization of the kidneys. Intravenous pyelography can be used to assess the function of the kidneys. Radionuclide scans such as 2,3-dimercaptosuccinic acid (DMSA) scans can be used to evaluate function and structural abnormalities, specifically renal scars after UTI. Vesicoureterography to evaluate the presence or absence of vesicoureteric reflux should be performed after completion of treatment of the UTI, because transient vesicoureteral reflux commonly occurs with the acute infection.

Osteomyelitis and Septic Arthritis

The overall rate of nosocomial bone and joint infections in neonates is 1 to 2 per 1000 admissions.[42-44] Hematogenous dissemination is responsible for most infections; however, skeletal infections can also result from extension of infection in surrounding tissues, direct inoculation, and transplacental infection that leads to fetal sepsis (syphilis). The metaphysis is usually the site of seeding, caused by sluggish flow in the metaphyseal (sinusoidal) vessels and decreased phagocytic activity. In the neonatal period, these bridging vessels form a conduit between the metaphysis and the epiphysis. In addition, the relatively thin cortex and loosely applied periosteum are poor barriers to spread of infection. In addition, there are bridging vessels that cross joints, and thus multiple bones are infected. The hips, shoulders, and knees can easily become infected because the epiphyseal-metaphyseal junction is entirely within the joint capsule.

Pathogens usually isolated include *S. aureus*, group B streptococci, gram-negative enteric bacilli (e.g., *E. coli*, *Klebsiella* species, *Pseudomonas* species), *Candida* species, *Mycoplasma hominis*, and *Treponema pallidum*.[45,46]

Systemic signs are usually absent in neonatal osteomyelitis. In most infants who do manifest signs, the earliest are pain (and pseudoparalysis), limitation of motion, and swelling. Discoloration and increased warmth may accompany the swelling. Feeding and weight gain are usually undisturbed. Evaluation of the joint and bone above and below the infected bone should also be performed (Table 69-5). The distribution of bone involvement is as follows: femur, 39%; tibia, 14%; humerus, 18%; radius, 5%; maxilla, 4%; ulna, 3%; clavicle, 2%; tarsal bones, 2%; ribs, 2%; and vertebrae, 1%.[47] Of samples, 60% of blood cultures are positive, and 70% of bone aspirates are positive. However, timing of blood cultures (before or after antibiotics are given) is critical. Joint aspiration with incision, drainage, and culture is indicated whenever there is a significant collection of debris in the soft tissues. Surgical drainage is often

Table 69–5. Signs and Tests for Neonatal Osteomyelitis and Septic Arthritis

Test	Advantages	Disadvantages
Skeletal x-rays	Eventually, bone changes are seen (e.g., "punched-out" lytic lesions, osseous lucencies, and periosteal elevation) Multiple sites of involvement can eventually be seen Trauma (e.g., fracture) as a cause of swelling or pseudoparalysis can be ruled out	Radiographic changes do not occur for 7-12 days Conventional radiographs are insensitive to destruction of <30% of the bone matrix
Technetium 99m (^{99m}Tc)	Osteomyelitis can be detected earlier than with radiography With the higher resolution gamma cameras used today, multiple sites of infection are often noted	Patient is exposed to radiation False-negative studies have been reported False-positive results occur from increased metabolic bone activity
Gallium bone scan	When ^{99m}Tc bone scans are equivocal, gallium scans might be useful	The radiation dose is significantly higher than in ^{99m}Tc bone scans
Sonography	Most useful as a tool for finding or guiding needle aspiration of fluid collections in joints or adjacent to bone It is inexpensive There is no radiation exposure	The sonographer must be experienced Accuracy is variable in neonates
Magnetic resonance imaging (MRI)	MRI detects inflammatory or destructive intramedullary disease in older children or adults	Not helpful in neonates because the marrow compartment is rarely involved May be overread

indicated for relief of intraarticular pressure when a hip or shoulder is affected. Drainage of an infected joint is considered a medical emergency procedure.

In most studies, the erythrocyte sedimentation rate (ESR) was significantly elevated on days 2 to 5. ESR values slowly returned to normal within 3 weeks of therapy. In contrast, the C-reactive protein level rises within 6 to 12 hours of a triggering stimulus and returns to normal within a week of therapy. A secondary rise in the either ESR or C-reactive protein level could be a sign of recrudescence. Unfortunately, in 30% of cases with osteomyelitis, the ESR is less than 30.[48,49]

Candida species cause 17% of all cases of septic arthritis and osteomyelitis in premature infants. In contrast to bacterial infections, there is no inflammatory sign other than edema of the extremity. Fungal infections appear on radiographs as "punched-out" metaphyseal radiolucencies that appear less aggressive than staphylococcal osteomyelitis. Affected infants often have a history of central catheter–related fungemia. Fungal septic arthritis can appear as late as 1 year after a treated fungal infection. Fluconazole may be a good alternative to amphotericin B because of effective joint penetration; however, identification of the offending pathogen should direct therapy, as some candidal species (and other fungi) are fluconazole resistant.

Optimal coverage for presumed septic arthritis and osteomyelitis is provided by a penicillinase-resistant penicillin coupled with an aminoglycoside until an organism is identified and antibiotic sensitivities have been determined. Therapy should be continued for a minimum of 4 to 6 weeks. In the neonatal age group, orally administered antibiotics are not used because data regarding their absorption and efficacy are insufficient.

NONSEXUALLY TRANSMITTED PERINATAL INFECTIONS

Congenital Rubella Syndrome

Rubella virus is a spherical RNA virus and a member of the Togavirus family. Humans are the only source of infection. Transmission is via direct contact from droplets of nasopharyngeal secretions. The incidence peaks in the late winter and early spring. The infection is highly contagious and is easily passed from host to susceptible host. Immunity after infection (and vaccination) is lifelong. Incubation of the virus lasts 14 to 23 days; most cases present 16 to18 days after exposure. Patients are infectious a few days before and up to 5 to 7 days after onset of the rash. Infection can be asymptomatic (uncommon) or can manifest as an erythematous maculopapular rash, conjunctivitis, generalized lymphadenopathy, and fever. Transient polyarthritis is commonly seen in infected adolescents. Rare complications include encephalitis and thrombocytopenia.[50]

Rubella vaccine was licensed in 1969. It is part of the trivalent live attenuated measles, mumps, and rubella (MMR) vaccine. This vaccine should be administered at age 12 to 15 months and then again at 4 to 6 years of age. Data evaluating the cases of congenital rubella syndrome (CRS) has shown that most cases (>80%) occurred in unvaccinated or nonimmune women. Of the cases occurring in women who were reported to have been vaccinated, they were vaccinated only 7 to 14 days before onset of symptoms, in which case they were incubating the virus at the time of vaccination.

CRS was first reported in 1941 by Gregg.[51] It includes maternal rubella infection early in pregnancy and a pattern of fetal anomalies that includes cataracts, hearing impairment, cardiac disease, and developmental delay. Congenital rubella infection most often accompanies maternal rubella infection occurring in the first trimester; 80% to 85% of infants born to rubella-infected women develop CRS.[52] There is currently no therapy for rubella or for CRS. Infants with CRS may shed virus for up to 1 year after birth, and affected infants should be kept on contact isolation until the condition is proved to be noninfectious. It is routine to send nasopharyngeal and urine samples for viral isolation starting at 3 months of age to document the end of contagiousness.

CRS was designated a reportable event in 1970. Rubella infection is defined as confirmed or definite, probable, suspected or possible, and unknown. These definitions are based on clinical descriptions and criteria for laboratory confirmation.[53] The laboratory definition for confirmed rubella is rubella viral isolation, detection of serum rubella immunoglobulin M (IgM), or a significant rise in serum immunoglobulin G (IgG) levels between acute and convalescent titers. Other common descriptors for cases of rubella include "imported" and "indigenous." Imported cases are those whose exposure occurs outside the United States or the onset of rash occurring within 14 to 23 days after entering the United States. All other cases are considered indigenous.[54]

Outcomes of congenital rubella infection include both CRS and inapparent cases of congenital infection. In a study of the outbreak in an Amish community in 1990 to 1991, 24 children had signs and symptoms of CRS.[55] Of these, 83% had been born to mothers who had first-trimester infections and 17% to mothers who had second-trimester infections. Of those born to mothers with first-trimester infections, 80% had confirmed CRS, 10% had possible CRS, and 10% were apparently healthy. Of those born to mothers infected during the second trimester, 25% had CRS and 75% had possible CRS. The most common defects included congenital heart disease, deafness, cataracts, and glaucoma. Other findings included long bone radiolucencies, seizures, intracranial calcifications, encephalitis, and microcephaly. Of the children thought to be well at delivery, all developed signs of severe or profound hearing loss at 1 year.

CRS can be prevented only by vaccinations of women at risk for infection. Identification and vaccination of women who are rubella nonimmune at a prior pregnancy may still miss a significant proportion of women at risk for infection. As of January 2001, 44 of 47 countries in the Americas had implemented childhood rubella vaccination programs.[54] However, most of these programs had been in existence for less than 3 years, leaving huge populations at risk for acquisition of infection and passage of infection to women of childbearing age.

Table 69–6. Hearing Loss from Cytomegalovirus

Severity*	% Affected
Bilateral	11
Mild	5
Moderate to profound	6
Unilateral	8
Mild	4
Moderate to profound	4

*Mild hearing loss, 22-55 dB; moderate to profound, ≥55 dB.

Rubella vaccine should not be given during pregnancy. However, data on 226 women who were vaccinated while pregnant indicate that none of the children developed CRS, even though 2% had asymptomatic infection. In view of these data, receipt of rubella vaccine during pregnancy is not an indication for interruption of pregnancy.[56,57]

Cytomegalovirus

Congenital CMV infection affects people of all ages, races, and socioeconomic classes, throughout both the modernized and developing parts of the world.[58] Infection is mainly asymptomatic in healthy individuals. CMV is the most common virus known to be transmitted in utero. It is the largest known member of the human herpesvirus family, which also includes human herpesviruses 1 and 2, VZV, Epstein-Barr virus, and human herpesviruses 6, 7, and 8.[59,60] These entities are large, enveloped, double-stranded DNA viruses sharing biologic properties of latency and reactivation. Several types of CMV exist. Humans and higher primates are the only known reservoirs for the human subtype of CMV.[61-63] Immunity develops after initial (primary) infection; the virus then enters a latent state from which it can reactivate. About 10% of primary infections result in a mononucleosis-like syndrome with malaise, fever, myalgia, and adenopathy.[59] CMV infection is self-limited, but viral excretion can continue for extended periods. Recurrent infection is defined as intermittent excretion of virus from a single or multiple sites in the presence of host immunity. CMV may become latent and be repeatedly reactivated during later life in response to different stimuli such as pregnancy,[64] stress, or the presence of other infections. Congenital infections are the result of transplacental transmission of CMV. Transmission may occur as a consequence of either primary or recurrent infection. The fetus can get infected through hematogenous spread of infected leukocytes across the placenta or in utero through ingestion of infected placental tissue and amniotic cells. The virus replicates in the oropharynx and subsequently is carried through fetal circulation.[65]

CMV can be transmitted to neonates after delivery through transfusion of blood products and by human-to-human contact via infected secretions. The incubation period for CMV acquired after receipt of infected blood is 3 to 12 weeks. Transmission by blood transfusion can be prevented by the use of blood obtained from seronegative donors, frozen in glycerol, or depleted of white blood cells.

Most (85% to 90%) of congenitally infected infants have no signs or symptoms at birth. However, 5% to 15% develop sequelae (Tables 69-6 and 69-7).[66] These sequelae include sensorineural hearing loss,[65,67,68] delay of psychomotor development, and optic atrophy. Abnormal development usually manifests within the first 2 years of life. These postneonatal symptoms are divided into major and minor symptoms. Minor symptoms include moderate psychomotor retardation, behavioral problems; major symptoms include severe mental retardation and hearing loss. Despite the risk of these sequelae, infants who present with asymptomatic congenital CMV infection at birth still have a better prognosis than those who are symptomatic at birth.

The most frequently reported symptoms at birth in infants with congenital CMV infection are jaundice, hepatosplenomegaly, and thrombocytopenia. In addition, evidence of CNS infection, such as microcephaly, intracerebral calcifications, and chorioretinitis, may also be present. Of infants with symptoms at birth, 20% may die in the neonatal period.

CMV must be isolated from urine during the first 3 weeks after birth in order for it to be consistent with congenital infection.[69] Isolation of CMV from an infant

Table 69–7. Cytomegalovirus in Newborns

Neonatal Signs	Neurologic Sequelae*			
	Normal	Major	Minor	Death
Neurologic				
Microcephaly, intracranial calcifications, chorioretinitis	7	79	0	14
Other	40	50	0	10
Systemic				
Jaundice, hepatosplenomegaly, or purpura, but no neurologic signs	48	12	36	4
No neurologic or systemic signs	81	3	16	0

*Expressed as percentage of patients with designated neonatal clinical signs.

after 3 weeks of age may be related to postnatal and not intrauterine acquisition of the virus. Production of IgG and IgM antibodies may occur in utero.[61] However, serologic measurement of IgG antibodies are not helpful, inasmuch as maternal IgG does cross the placenta. Unfortunately, infected fetuses do not always produce their own specific IgM antibody, which further hampers diagnostic sensitivity of IgM serologic tests.[70] Early studies have shown better performance of CMV-specific IgE response.[71] However, IgE testing has not become a routine diagnostic test.

No standard treatment of children with symptomatic congenital CMV is available as yet. Ganciclovir has been used in several studies. One study reported encouraging results of ganciclovir treatment; however, too few children (12 infants) were included.[72] A second study evaluated 6 weeks of ganciclovir in 42 children with symptomatic congenital CMV.[73] Excretion of CMV in the urine decreased but returned to pretreatment levels after cessation of therapy. Improvement in hearing or stabilization of hearing impairment occurred in only 16% after 6 months. Only children with evidence of CNS disease were enrolled. Thus, it is still not known whether treatment is beneficial for infants who are that are symptomatic at birth or those with symptomatic disease outside the CNS.

There are no currently licensed CMV vaccines. In the 1970s, two live attenuated vaccines were developed.[74,75] Preliminary testing showed them to be safe and that they induced both humoral and cellular immunity. However, it is not known whether these vaccines will prevent infection by wild strains of CMV or whether vaccine-induced immunity will protect the fetus from intrauterine infection and disease.

Parvovirus

Parvovirus B19 is the viral agent that causes the childhood exanthem erythema infectiosum, or fifth disease. Approximately 50% of pregnant women are seropositive before pregnancy and thus immune, whereas those who are seronegative are at risk for acquisition during pregnancy. Classic erythema infectiosum, with a "slapped cheeks" appearance followed by a characteristic lacy or reticular rash on the trunk and limbs, is fairly easy to diagnose clinically.[76,77] Unfortunately for diagnostic purposes, most individuals infected with parvovirus B19 do not develop erythema infectiosum. A nondiagnostic exanthem may be present in approximately one third to half of infections. In the study by Harger and associates,[78] 38% of parvovirus B19–infected women manifested rash; in none was parvovirus clinically diagnosed. In adults, especially women, joint symptoms occur in 60% to 80% of cases, which may be helpful diagnostically. The clinical illness in adults may mimic rubella with fever, rash, and joint symptoms.

Immunity can be assessed by screening for parvovirus B19 IgG antibody. If exposure to *Parvovirus* or clinical signs or symptoms suggestive of parvovirus B19 infection occur during pregnancy in a woman with unknown parvovirus B19 status, both IgG and IgM anti–parvovirus B19 antibodies should be measured to determine whether recent infection has occurred.

Acute *Parvovirus* infections during pregnancy have been associated with miscarriage and hydrops fetalis. When intrauterine parvovirus B19 infection associated with hydrops was first described, a high risk for fetal complications after maternal infection was emphasized. Parvoviruses require actively dividing cells to replicate, and parvovirus B19 preferentially infects red blood cell (RBC) precursors. In patients with hemolytic anemia and a high RBC turnover, the viral cytopathic effect destroys bone marrow RBC precursors, which results in reticulocytopenia. This transient arrest of erythrocyte production results in profound anemia in individuals with a shortened RBC survival, such as patients with hemolytic anemia. In fetuses, shortened RBC survival (60 to 80 days, in comparison with 110 to 120 days in adults) contributes to the severity of anemia. This latter condition is amenable to fetal therapy via intrauterine transfusion.[79]

With prospective follow-up of a large number of women with parvovirus B19 infection in pregnancy, adverse fetal outcome appears to be the exception, not the rule. Harger and associates[78] reported no fetal or neonatal deaths attributable to parvovirus B19 infection in 52 IgM-positive women, and the calculated frequency of hydrops and death from parvovirus B19 infection was 0% to 8.6% (95% confidence interval). These data are similar to data from other prospective studies.

Obstetric follow-up of women with parvovirus B19 infection usually relies on frequent ultrasound examinations in the weeks after infection. On the basis of the low risk for adverse outcomes, Harger and associates[78] suggested brief "screening" ultrasonography to detect fetal ascites or other early signs of nonimmune hydrops, with full examinations only if abnormalities were detected.

Congenital Toxoplasmosis

Toxoplasma gondii is a protozoan parasite that exists in three developmental stages: (1) tachyzoite; (2) bradyzoite, in tissue cysts; and (3) sporozoite, in oocysts. The tachyzoite appears during the acute stage of infection, when it invades and replicates within cells. The bradyzoite is present in tissue cysts and appears during latent infection. The sporozoite is a form of parasite found in oocysts, which are environmentally resistant. Oocysts must mature or undergo sporulation in the soil for at least 24 hours before they become infectious. Under favorable conditions, oocysts can remain infectious for approximately 1 year. They do not survive well in arid cold climates and can be destroyed by heating.[80-84] The tachyzoite is responsible for congenital infection.

Toxoplasma infection is acquired through ingestion of undercooked or raw meat containing the tissue cysts or through ingestion of water or other foods contaminated by oocysts that have been excreted from feces of infected animals. Ingestion of undercooked meat or meats[85-89] (perhaps processed by the same deli slicer) is the most common reason cited for acquisition of *T. gondii* during and after pregnancy. Gardening and the absence of handwashing constitute the second most common route of infection. Outbreaks of toxoplasmosis in humans have also been attributed to ingestion of unpasteurized goat milk,[90] contaminated unfiltered drinking water,[91,92] soil exposure,[93] and aerosolized soil exposure.[94]

The incidence of acute toxoplasmosis during pregnancy, according to seroprevalence among women of childbearing years, is estimated at 0.2% to 1%.[95] Rates of transmission to the fetus depend on the stage of the pregnancy and treatment during pregnancy. The overall risk of congenital infection from acute *T. gondii* infection during pregnancy ranges from 20% to 50%. Women infected with *T. gondii* before conception do not transmit the infection to their fetuses. The risk of congenital disease is lowest (10% to 25%) when acute maternal infection occurs during the first trimester and highest (60% to 90%) when acute maternal infection occurs during the third trimester.[84,96,97] However, the severity of the disease is worse if the infection is acquired in the first trimester.[84,98] Most infants infected in utero have no obvious signs of toxoplasmosis at birth. Up to 80% monitored into adulthood may develop learning and visual disturbances later in life.[99,100]

Acute toxoplasmosis is rarely diagnosed by detecting the parasite in body fluids. Placental lesions are usually microscopic in humans[101] and not typically looked for in normal pregnancies. The most common method of diagnosis is based on antibody detection. The presence of elevated *Toxoplasma*-specific IgG antibodies indicates that infection has occurred but does not distinguish between recent or distant past infection. In acute infection, IgG and IgM antibody levels generally rise within 1 to 2 weeks of infection.[102] Unfortunately, IgM antibodies to *Toxoplasma* have been reported to persist for up to 18 months after infection.[80] A negative IgM titer with a positive IgG result indicates that infection occurred at least 1 year previously. A positive IgM titer may result from more recent infection or may be a false-positive reaction. Some commercial IgM test kits have had some problems with specificity, resulting in unacceptably high rates of false-positive findings. An IgM-positive result should be confirmed by a *Toxoplasma* reference laboratory test.[103] These tests include IgG avidity[104,105] (the strength at which IgG binds to *T. gondii* usually shifts from low to high avidity at about 5 months after infection and can be used to rule out primary *T. gondii* infection in early pregnancy). Other tests helpful in confirming *T. gondii* infection include the Sabin-Feldman dye test, IgM enzyme-linked immunosorbent assay (ELISA), and polymerase chain reaction (PCR) testing of amniotic fluid (PCR amplification of the B1 gene of *T. gondii*).[106-110] PCR testing of amniotic fluid has replaced serologic testing of culture of fetal blood obtained by cordocentesis.

The American Academy of Obstetrics and Gynecologists currently does not recommend routine screening for *T. gondii*.[111] Screening may lead to equivocal or false-positive test results, which could then lead to inappropriate treatment of pregnant women.[103,112] One therapy in common practice for pregnant women is spiramycin.[96] Spiramycin is a macrolide antibiotic that can cause dermatologic and gastrointestinal reactions in pregnant women. Although it is listed in the Medical Letter as a drug to be used for treatment of toxoplasmosis during pregnancy, it is still considered an investigational drug in the United States and can be obtained only through the manufacturer.[113] There have been no randomized trials of spiramycin or other medications to assess the effect of treatment on congenital infection. A review of studies from 1966 through 1977 concluded that it is unclear whether antenatal treatment in women with toxoplasmosis reduces congenital transmission or not.[114] Prenatal treatment does, however, reduce the rate of severe sequelae among infected infants (20% to 3.5%). Pyrimethamine is not generally recommended for pregnant women because it is a folic acid antagonist. A lack of folic acid in pregnancy has been associated with neural tube defects occurring early in pregnancy before the neural tube has closed.[84]

After delivery, infection of the infant can be diagnosed most definitively by intraperitoneal inoculation of fresh placental tissue into laboratory mice for cultivation of *Toxoplasma* organisms. In addition, a thorough evaluation of the newborn with suspected toxoplasmosis should be undertaken. The clinical manifestations of congenital toxoplasmosis include intrauterine growth restriction, encephalitis, hydrocephalus, intracranial calcifications, strabismus, myocarditis, hydrops fetalis, thrombocytopenia, and eosinophilia. Evaluation of the infant should include computed tomographic scan of the brain, indirect ophthalmoscopic examination, and routine hematologic, liver function, and CSF studies. In addition, IgM, immunoglobulin A, and IgE antibody determinations can also provide strong evidence for the diagnosis (Table 69-8). Although 25% of truly infected infants lack IgM antibody, most have antibodies in at least one of the other immunoglobulin classes. An aggregate of tests therefore provides the most sensitive approach to serologic diagnosis.

Since 1960, the *Toxoplasma* serology laboratory at the Palo Alto Medical Foundation Research Institute has been dedicated to the laboratory diagnosis of *T. gondii* and toxoplasmosis. The laboratory has developed a panel of tests used to determine consistency with infection acquired in the recent compared with the more distant past.[115-117] Their recommendation that only infant samples should be used for establishment of the diagnosis, because samples from umbilical cord may be contaminated with maternal blood, is accepted as part of standard of care.

Therapy for congenital toxoplasmosis consists of pyrimethamine (Daraprim) plus sulfadiazine plus folinic acid. Pyrimethamine has a long serum half-life of approximately 60 hours in infants; therefore, administering 1 mg/kg each Monday, Wednesday, and Friday yields serum levels of 500 ng/mL 4 hours after a dose. CSF levels are approximately 10% to 20% of concomitant serum levels. Pyrimethamine and sulfadiazine act synergistically against *T. gondii* with a combined activity that is eight times that which would have been expected if their effects were merely additive.[118-120] The dosage of sulfadiazine is 50 to 100 mg/kg of body weight every 24 hours in two to four equal doses. Pyrimethamine is a folic acid antagonist that produces reversible and usually gradual depression of the bone marrow.[121,122] The dosage of folinic acid is 5 mg every 3 days; if bone marrow toxicity occurs at this dose, the dosage should be increased to 10 mg every 3 days. The optimal duration of therapy in infected infants is not known. However, most experts agree that therapy should be continued for 1 year.

Table 69-8. Suggested Evaluation of the Infant Suspected of Having Congenital Toxoplasmosis

Tests	Rationale/Finding
Nonspecific Tests	
Head circumference	Microcephaly
Ophthalmologic evaluation	Chorioretinitis
	Cataract
Neurologic evaluation	Psychomotor retardation
Brain CT scan	Intracranial calcifications
	Hydrocephalus
Blood tests	
CBC with differential and platelet counts	Anemia
	Eosinophilia
Serum total IgM, IgG, IgA, and albumin	To establish specific antibody load
	Jaundice
Serum alanine aminotransferase, total and direct bilirubin	
CSF cell count, glucose protein, and total IgG	Pleocytosis or elevated protein as newborn
Toxoplasma gondii*–Specific Tests	
Infant/newborn serum tests†	
Sabin-Feldman dye tests	Detection of IgG antibodies
IgM ISAGA (immunosorbent agglutination assay)	Increased sensitivity for detection of IgM antibodies (best for newborns and infants aged <6 months)
IgA EIA (enzyme immunoassay)	Useful to confirm IgM assays in prenatal and postnatal diagnosis
IgE EIA/ISAGA	IgE antibodies generally indicate a more acute phase than IgM or IgA antibodies; useful in diagnosis of acute infection
Newborn blood (if prenatal suspicion) for inoculation into mice	This method is more sensitive than tissue culture but is slow (up to 6 weeks)
Lumbar puncture‡	
Sabin-Feldman dye test	Detection of specific IgG antibodies in the CSF
IgM EIA	Detection of specific IgM antibodies in the CSF
PCR (1 mL frozen and shipped in dry ice)	Detection of *T. gondii* DNA in the CSF
Placental tissue (100 g in saline, not frozen, in cold packs)	Inoculation into mice to confirm antibodies
Maternal serum tests	
Sabin-Feldman dye test	Detection of IgG antibodies
IgM EIA	The EIA is used in adults versus ISAGA test above
IgA EIA	As above
IgE EIA/ISAGA	As above
AC/HS (differential agglutination)	Detects IgG antibodies; helpful for differentiating acute from nonacute infection in adults

Age (Days)	Dye Test Titer	Test Sensitivity§	Quantitative Immunoglobulins (mg/dL)	Antibody Load
10	1-16,000	0.2	886	3.61
28	1-8000	0.2	518	3.09
43	1-4096	0.2	427	1.92
67	1-2048	0.2	285	1.08
102	1-1024	0.2	255	0.80
132	1-256	0.2	119	0.43
189	1-64	0.2	209	0.06

*Recommend sending the Toxo Panel-Adult on the mother and Toxo Panel-Infants to Toxoplasma Serology Laboratory, Palo Alto Medical Foundation Research Institute, AMES Building, 795 El Camino Real, Palo Alto, California 94301-2302. Telephone: 650-853-4828; Fax: 650-614-3292; e-mail: toxolab@pamf.org; Web site: *http://www.pamf.org/serology.*
†Newborn serum, 0.5-1 mL.
‡CSF, 1 mL for PCR testing shipped on dry ice by overnight courier.
§Value obtained from Palo Alto Medical Foundation Research Institute.

AC/HS, differential agglutination test for AC and HS antigens; CBC, complete blood cell count; CSF, cerebrospinal fluid; CT, computed tomography; EIA, enzyme immunoassay; IgA, IgE, IgG, and IgM, immunoglobulins A, E, G, and M; ISAGA, immunosorbent agglutination assay; PCR, polymerase chain reaction.

IgG antibodies decline during treatment in the first year after birth, but serologic rebound (i.e., increase in IgG) occurs in nearly all cases after discontinuation of therapy. This phenomenon allows confirmation of the diagnosis in doubtful cases.[123]

Listeriosis

L. monocytogenes is a small gram-positive rod sometimes mistaken as a diphtheroid or culture contaminant. The organism is an intracellular, facultative anaerobic parasite. Once phagocytized, *L. monocytogenes* replicates rapidly within the cytosol but repels phagosome killing through its major virulence factor, listeriolysin O (characteristic of only this species of *Listeria*). Using the cell's own cytoskeletal actin polymerization mechanism, *L. monocytogenes* pushes outward on the host cell's membrane, forming filopods, which are then injected into neighboring cells. In the cellular immunocompetent host, significant infection is rare and self-limited. Because cellular immunity is suppressed during pregnancy and is naturally deficient during early neonatal life, *L. monocytogenes* enjoys an advantage during these host-vulnerable periods.

Although it is an uncommon infection in the United States (7.4 cases per million population, according to the Centers for Disease Control and Prevention [CDC]), an estimated 1850 cases per year result in 425 deaths.[124] The largest affected groups are neonates, patients with decreased cell-mediated immunity, and adults older than 60 years.[44,125] Pregnant women account for about 27% of cases and have an increased tendency to develop listeriosis during the third trimester, which often results in septic abortion. Vertical transmission from the colonized mother is the only human-to-human acquisition of the organism. *Listeria* infection can also be acquired (in late-onset disease) from environmental sources.

L. monocytogenes is acquired by susceptible adults (those with lower cellular immunity) through contaminated food. Surprisingly, the incidence of *L. monocytogenes* infection is low, in view of the fact that food contamination is relatively common. In one study in which the CDC sampled refrigerator foods, 11% yielded the organism. Refrigerator temperatures (4° to 10° C) may facilitate growth, and pasteurization does not kill *Listeria*. Any undercooked food source may contain this common organism (prevalent in all soil and raw vegetable matter). One recent outbreak occurred with gravid-treated (cold-smoked) rainbow trout.

After ingestion of the microorganism, mothers may incubate *L. monocytogenes* for 11 to 70 days (mean, 31 days). Invasion of the intestinal mucosal barrier ensues, with bacteremia resulting in a flulike illness with fever, chills, myalgias, arthralgias, headache, and backache. Symptoms may be mild and manifest most commonly between 26 and 30 weeks of pregnancy. Often the placenta becomes a reservoir for bacterial proliferation, which results in amnionitis with persistence of symptoms until abortion or delivery occurs; the occurrence of either stillbirth or neonatal death is 22%. If the organism is cultured and recognized, the mother may be treated effectively, preserving the pregnancy.

Neonatal infection may manifest at birth as disseminated listeriosis termed **granulomatosis infantisepticum,** with microabscesses throughout the body but particularly in the liver and spleen. This entity may be accompanied by hemorrhagic amnionitis manifesting as "chocolate syrup" meconium. Death usually occurs with a few hours.

Vertical transmission may occur shortly before or at birth, resulting in either early-onset neonatal sepsis with pneumonia before 2 weeks after birth (from organisms inhaled with amniotic fluid) or late-onset sepsis with meningitis within the first month. Papular rash (pinpoint, evanescent) and conjunctivitis are reported but are not specific for listeriosis. As with any virulent bacterial infection, disseminated intravascular coagulation and multiple organ system involvement are common. Reported mortality rates vary from 50% to 100%; the highest death rates occur with early-onset infections in premature infants.

L. monocytogenes should be suspected in any neonatal sepsis workup, particularly if gram-positive rods are present on Gram stain of placental membranes, meconium, or amniotic fluid. *L. monocytogenes* grows rapidly from cultures of blood, CSF, meconium, and amniotic fluid. Growth on culture media may be selectively cold enhanced; however, specific media are now preferred and used routinely in clinical laboratories for rapid confirmation of the diagnosis. If the organisms have not grown by 24 to 36 hours, they are unlikely to be present. Serologic study with a peptide limited to detect the aminoterminal end of listeriolysin O has shown promise for early identification of *L. monocytogenes* in endemic outbreaks.

L. monocytogenes remains sensitive to ampicillin, and gentamicin may augment antimicrobial killing. Because of the organism's tendency to hide in tissue reservoirs, higher dosages of ampicillin (200 mg/kg/day) are usually recommended for extended durations (2 weeks for bacteremia, 3 weeks for meningitis). Trimethoprim-sulfamethoxazole is the best alternative for mothers who are penicillin sensitive, although erythromycin (not currently recommended) has been used in case reports. Iron therapy for anemia should be withheld during treatment of listeriosis, because iron enhances the organism's growth in vitro and is therefore a virulence factor that contributes to host susceptibility to infection.

Tuberculosis

Mycobacterium tuberculosis is the acid-fast bacillus responsible for the worldwide infection referred to as **tuberculosis.** The most common route of infection with *M. tuberculosis* in the neonate is via hematogenous spread through the umbilical vessels from a focus in the placenta. Because the umbilical vessels transmit the *M. tuberculosis*, the primary complex is formed in the fetal liver and periportal lymph nodes. Other routes are of infection through aspiration or ingestion of infected amniotic fluid or through direct contact with an infected cervix. Infected infants usually present with multiple primary foci in the gut, lungs, and middle ear. In the early postnatal period, the newborn also can be infected by the airborne route, which can be confused with true congenital tuberculosis. This route of infection (respiratory) is typical of what is seen in all other age groups with a primary focus in the lungs.

Congenital tuberculosis most commonly manifests as hepatosplenomegaly and respiratory distress. These signs can be associated with nonspecific constitutional symptoms, often in the first 2 to 3 weeks after birth.[126] Twenty percent of infants may present with ear discharge. The disease should be suspected if the mother has tuberculosis or has symptoms that point toward tuberculosis (Fig. 69-1).[127] Postnatally acquired tuberculosis manifests with constitutional symptoms of fever, lethargy, weight loss, and anorexia, along with involvement of the respiratory system. If untreated, the majority of newborns progress to a severe form of disease such as meningitis or miliary tuberculosis within the first 2 years of life.

Congenital tuberculosis is rare in comparison with the overall incidence of tuberculosis.[128] However, the increasing prevalence of tuberculosis among individuals aged 25 to 44 years and among pregnant women has increased the likelihood of new cases.[129] Unfortunately, making an early diagnosis is difficult and requires a high index of suspicion. Up to 75% of infected mothers may be free of symptoms before delivery,[130] but many births are preterm.[131,132]

The diagnosis of tuberculosis in a neonate can be established by the Mantoux tuberculin skin test. Although infants are likely to have a false-negative response to the Mantoux test because of overwhelming infection or poorly developed immune response, induration has been demonstrated as early as 2½ weeks after birth and should be considered a positive finding.[130] Skin tests are unreliable in this age group, and antituberculosis therapy must be started immediately if infection is suspected, because of the greater risk of rapidly progressive disease.

The laboratory diagnosis of tuberculosis can be made by the demonstration of acid-fast bacilli in smears of gastric aspirates, urine, CSF, pleural fluid, or bronchial washings.[133] The search for a rapid, specific, and sensitive chemical detection method for tuberculosis is ongoing. Nucleic acid amplification with PCR has moderate sensitivity and relatively high specificity, but it is expensive and difficult to perform. The role of PCR in evaluation of children for tuberculosis is generally limited to confirming the diagnosis when there is significant pulmonary disease for which clinical or epidemiologic diagnosis is difficult; evaluating immunocompromised children, especially those with human immunodeficiency virus (HIV) infection; and confirming the diagnosis of extrapulmonary disease.[134] When noninvasive techniques do not provide a diagnosis, tissue biopsy should be considered.[135] The yield of liver biopsy in patients with perinatal tuberculosis who present with hepatomegaly is reportedly good.[135] Regardless of the diagnostic approach, culture and sensitivity testing for tubercle bacilli remain the clinical standard.

Before antitubercular treatments were developed, strict criteria were used to diagnose congenital tuberculosis. These criteria included proof of tuberculosis infection in the infant and the presence of a primary complex in the liver (diagnosed by pathologic study). If the primary complex in the liver is undocumented or lacking, the tubercular lesions must be only a few days old and extrauterine infection must be excluded with certainty. Cantwell and colleagues proposed a new set of criteria for the diagnosis of congenital tuberculosis.[136] The newborn should have a proven tuberculous lesion along with at least one of the following:

1. Lesions in first week after birth
2. A primary hepatic complex or caseating hepatic granuloma
3. Tuberculous infection of the placenta or maternal genital tract
4. Exclusion of the possibility of postnatal transmission by thorough investigation of contacts of the child

Exposure consists of contact with a person with suspected or confirmed contagious pulmonary tuberculosis. Some of these patients subsequently develop a positive purified protein derivative test result. Tubercular infection is defined as a positive purified protein derivative result with a radiograph that either is normal or reveals only calcification in the lung or regional lymph nodes. Disease is defined as infection in which signs and symptoms or radiographic manifestations of tuberculosis are apparent.

When the timely diagnosis of tuberculosis is made in an infant, therapy can be initiated and the evaluation of contacts undertaken. Infants do not transmit tuberculosis by coughing because they lack the force necessary to expel organisms. However, nasotracheal or orotracheal suctioning of infants as a component of their respiratory care is a means of transmitting infection to health care workers.[137] In addition, a diagnosis of tuberculosis in a child or infant requires testing for HIV infection because children with HIV have an increased incidence of tuberculous disease.[138]

In general, the antimicrobial treatment in neonates is the same as in older children. In the setting of life-threatening disease, initial treatment with four or five antituberculosis drugs is indicated until infection with a drug-resistant organism can be ruled out. The treatment includes isoniazid, rifampin, streptomycin, and pyrazinamide (and ethionamide or ethambutol) for 2 months, followed by 10 months of isoniazid and rifampin if resistance is ruled out.[135,136,138] In the setting of possible HIV infection, initial therapy should include at least three drugs, four if disseminated disease is present or if drug-resistant disease is suspected.[138]

The approach suggested by the Committee on Infectious Disease of the American Academy of Pediatrics (AAP) is shown in Table 69-9.[139,140]

Both isoniazid and ethambutol cross the placenta and are not teratogenic. Rifampin crosses the placenta, but it inhibits DNA-dependent RNA polymerase. Therefore, although it has the potential to be a teratogenic, no malformations have been observed to date. Streptomycin is ototoxic to the fetus. Treatment regimens for pregnant women generally consist of isoniazid, rifampin, ethambutol, and isoniazid. Regimens include an intensive treatment component for 2 months, followed by a step-down or maintenance component for 4 months (Table 69-10).

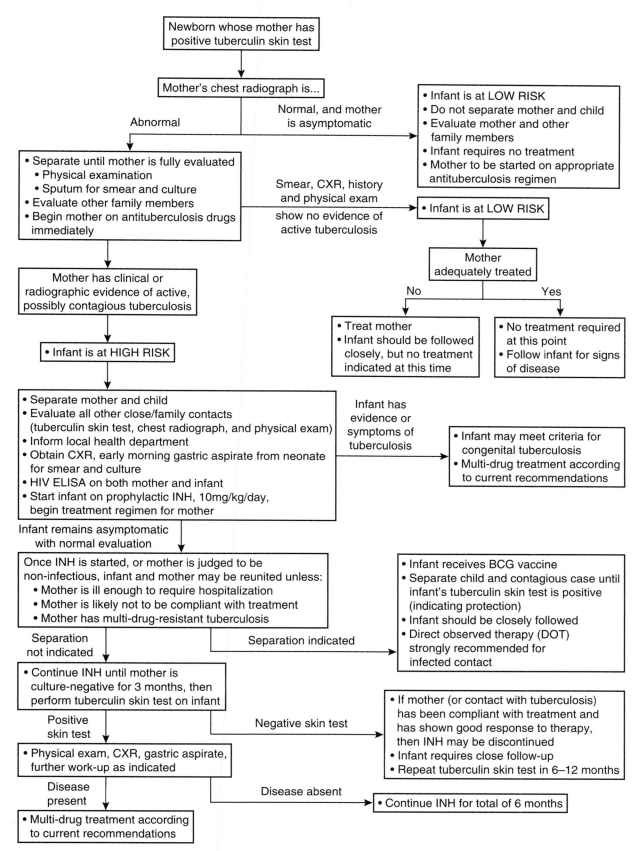

Figure 69–1. Protocol for newborn whose mother has a positive tuberculin skin test result. BCG, bacille Calmette-Guérin; CXR, chest radiograph; ELISA, enzyme-linked immunosorbent assay; HIV, human immunodeficiency virus; INH, isoniazid.

Table 69–9. Treatment of Neonates Born to Mothers with Possible Tuberculosis

Mother with Positive PPD but the Following Condition	Separation	Maternal Treatment	Newborn Treatment	Household Contacts
Negative radiograph	No	Treat infection	No evaluation	PPD testing
Abnormal radiograph but no active disease	Yes, until mother is fully evaluated	Treat infection	Follow-up care	PPD testing
Abrnomal radiograph but active disease	Yes, until mother is fully evaluated and receiving treatment until deemed noncontagious	Treat disease	Evaluation for congenital infection and HIV; if results are positive, treated and followed by PPD	Reporting to public health department Thorough investigations, including PPD

HIV, human immunodeficiency virus; PPD, purified protein derivative.

Varicella-Zoster Virus

VZV is a double-stranded DNA virus of the family Herpesviridae. It is often thought of as an infection of childhood. Currently, most children in the United States receive VZV vaccine. Because of incomplete penetration of the vaccine in the at-risk population, there remains a cohort of adolescent girls and women of childbearing age who have never had varicella or VZV vaccine and are susceptible to infection during pregnancy. When these women acquire infection while pregnant (usually between 8 and 20 weeks of pregnancy), the virus may travel to the fetus, leading to congenital varicella. Transmission of VZV from mother to infant occurs in 25% to 50% of cases of infected mothers. Fortunately, however, the syndrome is much less common than fetal infection. The syndrome in the infant occurs in only about 2% of cases of maternal chickenpox.[141,142] Common manifestations of the syndrome include skin scarring (either generalized or localized in a dermatomal distribution, such as that seen with zoster),[143] limb deformities (such as hypoplasia or missing digits), eye involvement (such as chorioretinitis, cataract, nystagmus, and hypoplasia), low birth weight, and mental retardation.[144-146] Reactivation of VZV acquired in utero is a common event. Thus, zoster develops in about 20% of infants with the congenital syndrome in the first few years of life. The presence of antibodies to VZV in an infant older than 8 months distinguishes between actual infection of the infant with VZV and presence of transplacental antibodies. However, the presence of these antibodies indicates infection but not necessarily the syndrome. It is hoped that as the rubella vaccine has nearly eliminated congenital rubella, the varicella vaccine will make the congenital varicella syndrome even more rare.

Live virus vaccine should not be given to pregnant women. However, data available from women who did

Table 69–10. Suggested Dosages of Antituberculosis Drugs* for Neonates

Drug	Sizes of Available Preparations (mg)	Single Daily Dose (mg/kg)
INH tablets†	50, 100, 300	10-15
Rifampin capsules‡	150-300	10-20
Pyrazinamide tablets	500	20-30§
Ethambutol tablets	100, 400	15-25
Ethionamide tablets	250	15-20
Streptomycin (for intramuscular use only)	1- and 5-g vials	20-30

*Antituberculosis drugs are available without cost from most health departments once the physician has officially reported the case.
†Available for parenteral use and supplied in 10-mL vials containing 100 mg/mL.
‡Available for parenteral use in the United States; consult Dow Chemical Co.
§This is the usual recommended dose; however, some clinicians who frequently administer this drug to infants recommend a dosage of 30-40 mg/kg, to a maximal daily dosage of 1.5 g.

INH, isoniazid.

From American Academy of Pediatrics: Tuberculosis. In Pickering LK (ed): 2000 Red Book: Report of the Committee on Infectious Disease, 25th ed. Elk Grove Village, Ill: Academy of Pediatrics, 2000, pp 593-613.

receive the vaccine without knowing that they were pregnant show no problems with them or their offspring. It is best to vaccinate varicella-nonimmune women before pregnancy or at the 6-week postpartum visit.

Infants whose mothers have the onset of the rash of varicella within 4 days before delivery or within 2 days after delivery have about a 50% chance of also developing varicella. In as many as 30% of infants who are untreated, the varicella may be disseminated and even fatal. This form of varicella resembles that seen in highly immunocompromised patients, such as children with leukemia who are receiving chemotherapy. It is possible to prevent this severe form of infant varicella by administering VZIG to the infant as soon as possible after birth. In rare cases, VZIG may be ineffective in infants; therefore, infants given this prophylaxis need close follow-up. Many develop a mild form of clinical varicella with fewer than 100 skin vesicles despite VZIG. Indications for adding antiviral therapy (acyclovir) are extensive skin lesions and development of pneumonia, which suggests severe varicella. It is thought than an important element of risk to the infant is VZV infection across the placenta during the time of maternal viremia. Therefore, infants whose mothers develop varicella more than 2 days after delivery are at significantly less risk from varicella and do not require VZIG, although some physicians may elect to administer it anyway. Infants whose mothers had the onset of varicella more than 5 days before delivery do not need to receive VZIG because they will have received sufficient transplacental VZV antibodies before delivery (as if nature provided them with a dose of VZIG). With regard to isolation of infants perinatally exposed to VZV, there are two points to consider: The incubation period can be as short as 10 days and is counted from the time of onset of maternal rash. Infants are contagious only around the time when rash is expected to occur.

There is no need to treat an infant born to a mother with zoster. The area of zoster should remain covered while the mother is in the hospital. There is almost no chance that such an infant will develop varicella, and no special management is required.

There is no question that varicella in adults tends to be more severe than in children. Although the data are far from conclusive, most experts believe that varicella is likely to be *more severe* in pregnant women than in nonpregnant women, especially in the third trimester of pregnancy. Therefore, pregnant women with varicella should be closely observed, particularly for development of primary pneumonia. Pneumonia usually manifests with fever, cough, dyspnea, and bilateral fluffy interstitial infiltrates on chest radiographs. Pregnant women with varicella pneumonia or even suspected varicella pneumonia should be treated with intravenous acyclovir (10 to 20 mg/kg/day, divided into three doses). Treatment is usually continued for 7 days. Maternal acyclovir therapy has not been associated with fetal malformations; nevertheless, it is advisable to avoid its use if possible. Orally administered acyclovir is not well absorbed and has demonstrated only modest success against varicella in clinical trials. Other agents such as famciclovir or valacyclovir may be used, although data on their use in pregnancy

are lacking. Therefore, it is preferable to monitor pregnant women with varicella closely and to intervene if necessary with intravenous acyclovir, which is known to be effective if given early in the course of illness.

It is preferable to vaccinate before the onset of pregnancy. It is acceptable to vaccinate children who live with a pregnant woman. Each instance is best individualized, weighing the potential risks and benefits to the mother. For example, in a family with several young, varicella-susceptible children who attend school or daycare, there is a very high likelihood (estimated at 9% per child) that they will introduce chickenpox into the household while their mother is pregnant. Varicella in such a situation is highly contagious, with a 90% secondary rate in susceptible household contacts. Only about 5% of immunized children develop rash after immunization, and the infectivity of these children to others is extremely low. In a study of household contacts (vaccinated healthy children and siblings with leukemia), there were no cases of vaccine virus spread to the siblings with leukemia. Should the vaccine virus nevertheless infect the mother, the illness is predicted to be mild, and no cases of the congenital varicella syndrome have been associated with vaccine-type VZV. In contrast, the wild-type VZV is highly contagious. If the children bring this virus home, maternal infection is inevitable, may be severe, and is known to be associated with a congenital syndrome. In other situations in the family in which there is only one child who is cared for at home and who has few visitors, it may be preferable to immunize the child after the mother delivers. There would be no known risk to the newborn if the sibling developed a vaccine-associated rash.

SEXUALLY TRANSMITTED DISEASE–ASSOCIATED PERINATAL INFECTIONS

Human Immunodeficiency Virus

In the United States, the overall prevalence of HIV is estimated at 1.5 per 1000 women; much higher rates are reported from urban areas. In Philadelphia, the rate is about 7.5 per 1000, whereas in some parts of New York City, the prevalence is around 25 per 1000 (or 1 per 40). These numbers pale in comparison to those found in sub-Saharan Africa, where rates as high as 250 to 330 per 1000 pregnant women are reported from several prenatal care centers.

If HIV infection is untreated, the transmission rate varies worldwide, from a high of 30% to 40% in Africa (confounded by breast-feeding and poor nutritional status) to 20% to 25% in the United States and 13% to 15% in Europe. With the use of perinatal zidovudine (AZT, ZDV), the rate of infection in infants drops to 2% to 8%.[147] In a study comparing transmission after elective cesarean section to that occurring with perinatal AZT use, rates of transmission were comparable (2% to 3%).[148] When pregnant women are treated with two to three drugs in combination therapy and maintain a low viral load, the risk to the infant is less than 2%.[149] Factors associated with increased rates of transmission are a maternal diagnosis of acquired immunodeficiency syndrome, preterm delivery, maternal CD4 count of less than 200/mm³, maternal high viral load (>10,000), presence of chorioamnionitis, prolonged rupture of membranes, and untreated sexually transmitted diseases, including the presence of bacterial vaginosis.[147]

HIV infection may be transmitted in utero, during labor, or after birth through breast-feeding. In the absence of breast-feeding, it is believed that approximately 20% to 30% of perinatal infections occur in utero; the remaining 70% to 80% occur during the intrapartum period in infants. In the event an infant escapes infection in utero and during delivery but is then breast-fed, the risk is approximately 13% when breast-feeding is continued for at least 6 months. The risk of transmission through breast-feeding increases when the infant is not consistently breast-fed.[150,151]

Because risk factor assessments fail to detect HIV in more than 40% of infected pregnant women, both the AAP and the American College of Obstetrics and Gynecology recommend routine HIV counseling to all pregnant women, with voluntary HIV testing. This approach is most important in view of major advances in perinatal treatment strategies to reduce the incidence of HIV transmission to newborns.

At birth and for the first year, all infants born to an HIV-infected mother have a positive HIV ELISA result. The ELISA measures IgG anti-HIV antibodies, which readily cross the placenta in the third trimester; hence, all infants born to antibody-positive women are antibody-positive themselves. These maternal antibodies may remain detectable in the infants' blood stream until 12 to 18 months of age.

Any infant with a congenital anomaly who was born to an HIV-infected mother treated with antiretroviral agents should be reported to the Antiretroviral Pregnancy Registry at *www.apregistry.com*. Alternatively, a report may also be called in to 800-258-4263.

All HIV-exposed infants should have an HIV diagnostic test (PCR DNA assay or HIV blood culture) performed at birth (not from a cord specimen), at 1 month of age, and at 3 to 4 months of age. If the result is positive, the test should be repeated immediately. If the results at 1 month and 4 months of age are negative, the infant is considered HIV uninfected. The DNA PCR is the test of choice because it is readily available, has a quick turnaround time, and is less expensive than culture. It has more than 90% sensitivity and specificity at 1 month of age and 99% sensitivity and specificity after 1 month of age. Currently, quantitative RNA measurements (termed viral load) are not recommended for diagnostic purposes. The p24 antigen test is no longer used for diagnostic purposes.

The CD4 percentage and the absolute CD4 count are used to monitor immunologic function in HIV infection. It should be remembered that normal CD4 counts for infants and children are much higher than those found in adults (normal infant CD4 values are 2500 to 3500/mL³; normal adult values are 700 to 1000/mL³).[152]

Close prenatal monitoring, attention to nutritional issues, antiretroviral therapy (at a minimum, prenatal and intrapartum AZT followed by 6 weeks of AZT to the neonate), and possible elective cesarean section are now all part of recommended care for HIV-infected pregnant women.

Pneumocystis carinii pneumonia used to be the most common serious HIV-related infection in infancy. The peak age at onset was 3 to 9 months, and the mortality rate was 50%. Fortunately, *P. carinii* pneumonia can be prevented by thrice-weekly trimethoprim-sulfamethoxazole as prophylaxis. All HIV-exposed infants should be placed on *P. carinii* pneumonia prophylaxis at 6 weeks of age and continued on it until HIV infection is definitely ruled out (two negative HIV DNA PCR test results, both after 2 weeks of age). Growth failure and a progressive encephalopathy were also common serious complications of HIV infection in the first year after birth. With early diagnosis, antiretroviral treatment, and prophylaxis against opportunistic infection (all available in the United States), few infants develop these HIV complications.

Herpes Simplex Virus

HSV is a double-stranded DNA virus. The current incidence of neonatal herpes infections is 1 case per 3000 to 10,000 live births.[153] A large percentage of these infants were born prematurely (47%) or via cesarean section (33%) for reasons unrelated to HSV infection.[153,154]

HSV multiplies on the mucosa of the maternal genital tract, and the infant is infected during delivery. In only about 5% of infections does it appear that the virus crossed the placenta and causes congenital rather than neonatal infection. Infants also can be infected with HSV type 1 if a mother has primary active HSV 1 infection, usually in the throat and mouth, at delivery. Presumably in this case, infection of the infant occurs from close maternal contact, such as kissing the infant, or through aerosols of the virus from close contact with an infected individual. Once the virus has infected the infant, it is thought to multiply locally and then disseminate by viremia.

Clinically, the infection is divided into three categories: (1) skin, eye, or mouth involvement; (2) disseminated infection that has extended to the viscera, especially the liver and lungs; and (3) CNS involvement. Unfortunately for diagnostic purposes, fewer than one third of infants have the characteristic lesions at presentation, and only up to two thirds have them anytime during their illness.

The most useful test for rapid diagnosis of HSV is a smear of material obtained from a skin vesicle that is fixed and stained with monoclonal antibodies to HSV, which are commercially available. This test is simple to perform and highly sensitive and accurate; results can be available within an hour and indicate if the virus is type 1 or type 2. Cultures for virus should also be performed, but this often takes as long as 48 hours to be completed. PCR, if available, can also be useful for diagnosis.

Infants in whom the diagnosis is established or who are strongly suspected of having neonatal HSV should be further evaluated for the possibility of disseminated infection, as well as involvement of the CNS. Usually this means performing liver function tests, an ophthalmologic examination, lumbar puncture, and CNS magnetic resonance imaging or computed tomographic scan. These tests usually must be repeated after 1 to 2 weeks; results of the first battery of tests often serve as a baseline. Newborn infants with skin vesicles should undergo a rapid workup for the possibility of neonatal HSV infection.

Antibody titers are of little use for diagnosis of HSV because it takes several days after infection for antibody levels to rise. Therefore, it is preferable to demonstrate the presence of virus, viral antigens, or viral DNA in tissues for diagnosis. In instances when no virus can be demonstrated, antibody titers may be useful. Ideally, sera should be obtained from mother and infant during the acute and convalescent phases (10 to 14 days apart). In addition to examining sera for antibodies to HSV, evaluations for other congenital and neonatal pathogens such as *T. gondii* and CMV should also be obtained. Practically speaking, however, by the time it becomes clear that antibody titers might be useful, the acute-phase serum samples have already been discarded.

It was traditionally thought that women with frequent reactivation episodes of genital HSV were at greatest risk for delivering an infected infant and that they should therefore be screened for HSV infection during pregnancy. Prospective studies, however, indicated that the infant at greatest risk for developing neonatal HSV is born to a woman with primary asymptomatic genital HSV at term. The risk of infection of the infant is only about 1% for mothers with recurrent HSV but more than 50% for those with primary HSV at term. Therefore, the women who should be screened at term are asymptomatic women who have no history of HSV. Unfortunately, however, there is still no good screening test for these women. Obtaining viral cultures on so many women is impractical and expensive. PCR does not necessarily indicate the presence of infectious HSV and, in any case, is not widely available. It is now possible to determine whether a woman has been infected with HSV type 2 in the past. Women lacking antibodies to the glycoprotein G of HSV type 2 are considered susceptible and are at risk for developing primary infection with this virus. However, it must be remembered that both types 1 and 2 can cause neonatal herpes infections.

The best screening test for prevention of severe neonatal HSV is a high index of suspicion when an infant develops vesicular skin lesions. There is no real need to screen women with a history of genital HSV because these women are at very little risk for delivering an infected infant.

If the diagnosis of maternal primary HSV is known at delivery and the membranes are not ruptured, infections in infants can be prevented in most but not all cases by delivery by cesarean section. The chances of infection are increased if the skin of the infant is broken for any reason (e.g., from a scalp monitor)

Despite appropriate antiviral therapy, the prognosis for infants with disseminated HSV and CNS disease is poor. Infants who have infection confined to the skin, eye, or mouth also have a significant amount of morbidity despite localization of infection.[155] Typing of the infecting virus is important, because type 1 infections carry a better prognosis than do type 2 infections. Most infants with

encephalitis caused by HSV type 1 have a better long-term prognosis than do those with encephalitis caused by HSV type 2.

The treatment for herpes in the neonatal period is administration of intravenous acyclovir. Acyclovir is an antiviral drug that interferes with the replication of HSV DNA by acting as a chain terminator and interfering with the action of DNA polymerase. Because its action occurs mainly in infected cells, it is very well tolerated. Early therapy with acyclovir has decreased rates of mortality and morbidity from serious HSV infections by 30% to 50%.[154] Even more important, although it is difficult to quantitate, treatment of infants with minimal involvement (skin, eye, or mouth) prevents dissemination of the virus and severe infections from developing. It is believed that early therapy with acyclovir in infants with skin, eye, or mouth disease can prevent much disseminated and CNS disease. Therefore, it is recommended that all infants with skin lesions caused by HSV, even if they are otherwise healthy, be treated with acyclovir. Acyclovir is administered at 10 to 20 mg/kg/dose intravenously every 8 hours for 14 to 21 days, depending on the condition of the infant. Some experts suggest extending therapy for up to 28 days in infants with CNS disease.[156]

Follow-up is best individualized. Most asymptomatic infants should undergo imaging studies of the CNS after completion of therapy and discharge, usually after 4 to 6 weeks. In infants with symptoms such as recurrent skin vesicles, developmental delay, or seizures, scans may be performed after a shorter interval. Infants who develop new or recurring symptoms should undergo a lumbar puncture for examination of the CSF. Those with CSF abnormalities or in whom the PCR results remain positive should probably receive another course of intravenous acyclovir and be monitored closely again after the second discharge.

Infants suspected of having continued low-grade replication of HSV in the CNS may be given oral acyclovir on a long-term basis, because data suggest that infants may benefit from prophylaxis.[157] This therapy is considered an off-label use of acyclovir, and it must be discussed carefully with the parents. Acyclovir is administered at 300 mg/m^2 orally three times a day. Monitoring for toxicity, particularly in the bone marrow, is important and should be performed every 1 to 2 weeks while the medication is being administered. The usual duration of long-term therapy is several months. Although short-term safety seems not to be a problem (the dosage can be lowered if toxicity occurs), long-term safety is unknown.

There are many other illnesses in the neonatal period that manifest as vesicular lesions (Table 69-11). Of these, enteroviral infection is the most common. Enteroviruses include Coxsackie A and B viruses, enterovirus, and enteric cytopathic human orphan virus. Because both HSV and enterovirus infections of the neonate are related to maternal infection, it is important to obtain a history from the mother and to perform viral cultures on the mother's throat, rectum, and genitalia. Examination of the infant should include viral surface cultures and evaluation of CSF for PCR for enterovirus. At present, there is no approved therapy for enterovirus infections of the

Table 69-11. Illnesses Manifesting as Vesicular Skin Lesions

Infectious Causes	Noninfectious Causes
HSV	Erythema toxicum
Pseudomonas species	Pustular melanosis
Haemophilus influenzae	Miliaria
Candida species	Letterer-Siwe disease
Syphilis	Pemphigus vulgaris
CMV	Herpes gestationalis
VZV	Incontinentia pigmenti
Listeria species	Nenonatal lupus
Aspergillus species	Epidermolysis bullosa
GBS	Neonatal bullous dermatitis

CMV, cytomegalovirus; GBS, group B streptococci; HSV, herpes simplex virus; VZV, varicella-zoster virus.

newborn; however, compassionate use of pleconaril may be helpful in some of these situations.[158]

Syphilis

T. pallidum is a thin, motile spirochete that is extremely fragile, surviving only briefly outside the host. It is transmitted sexually, often causing in an asymptomatic infection. An estimated 70,000 new cases of syphilis are diagnosed each year in the United States. Cyclic epidemics tend to occur every 7 to 10 years, with rates of syphilis highest among men 25 to 29 years of age and women 20 to 24 years of age. By race, syphilis disproportionately affects African Americans; the reported syphilis rate is 44 times higher among blacks than among whites. By region, syphilis is concentrated in the South and in discrete pockets elsewhere in the United States. In 1997, 50% of reported cases originated in 1% of U.S. counties, located primarily in the Southeast.

All women should have a Venereal Disease Research Laboratory (VDRL) test for syphilis performed at the first prenatal visit, with a second screen during the third trimester.[159] There are two types of test for syphilis: the treponemal tests and the nontreponemal tests. The treponemal tests are the fluorescent treponemal antibody absorption (FTA-ABS) test and the microhemagglutination assay—*T. pallidum* (MHA-TP) test. The nontreponemal tests are the VDRL and rapid plasma reagin (RPR) tests. If the nontreponemal test result is positive, treponemal serologic profiles should be obtained. A nontreponemal test result should not be confirmed with a second nontreponemal test. The CDC[160] recommended that no infant be discharged from the hospital without a determination of maternal serologic values for syphilis. Infants should be treated if they have any evidence of active disease (physical examination findings or radiographic abnormalities), a reactive CSF VDRL result, an abnormal CSF finding regardless of serologic profile, or quantitative nontreponemal antibody titers that are four times higher than maternal titers (Table 69-12).[161]

Certain viral illnesses such as infectious mononucleosis, hepatitis, varicella, and measles, as well as other illnesses such as lymphoma, tuberculosis, and connective tissue diseases and conditions such as pregnancy and abuse of injection drugs, can all cause low false-positive RPR and VDRL results. However, they do not affect the FTA-ABS or the MHA-TP test. All cases of positive RPR

Table 69-12. Recommended Treatment of Neonates (≤4 Weeks of Age) with Proven or Possible Congenital Syphilis

Clinical Status	Antimicrobial Therapy
Proven or highly probable disease*	Aqueous crystalline penicillin G, 100,000-150,000 U/kg/day, administered as 50,000 U/kg per dose IV every 12 hr during the first 7 days after birth and every 8 hr thereafter for a total of 10 days *or* Procaine penicillin G, 50,000 U/kg per dose IM a day in a single dose for 10 days
Asymptomatic; normal CSF examination results, CBC, platelet count, and radiographic examination; and follow-up is certain with a maternal treatment history of no or inadequate penicillin treatment,† undocumented treatment, failed or reinfection	Aqueous crystalline penicillin G, 100,000-150,000 U/kg/day IV for 10-14 days* *or* Clinical and serologic follow-up and benzathine penicillin G, 50,000 U/kg IM in a single dose
Adequate therapy but given less than 1 mo before delivery; mother's response to treatment is not demonstrated by a fourfold decrease in titer of a nontreponemal serologic test; or erythromycin therapy	Clinical and serologic follow-up and benzathine penicillin G, 50,000 U/kg IM in a single dose‡

*If more than 1 day of therapy is missed, the entire course should be restarted.
†If any part of the infant's evaluation yields abnormal results or is not done, or if the CSF result is uninterpretable, the 10-day course of penicillin is required.
‡Some experts recommend aqueous crystalline penicillin G, as for proven or highly probable disease.
CBC, complete blood cell count; CSF, cerebrospinal fluid; IM, intramuscularly; IV, intravenously.

or VDRL results must be confirmed with either an FTA-ABS or MHA-TP test.

FTA-ABS and MHA-TP results (maternal IgG) stay positive for life, even after successful therapy, and are therefore not recommended screens for newborn infants, whereas the RPR and VDRL tests can be used to monitor response to treatment. They are reported as titers, which can be monitored. The quantitative nontreponemal tests become nonreactive after successful therapy (within 1 year in low-titer [1:8] syphilis and in 2 years in high-titer infection).

Although the effects of maternal HIV infection on the transmission of syphilis are incompletely understood, the cellular immune abnormalities associated with HIV may allow greater treponemal proliferation and higher fetal infection. In addition, HIV-infected women may not respond adequately to benzathine penicillin, and thus their fetuses are more susceptible to disease.

Studies have shown an increased risk of congenital syphilis among neonates after maternal illicit drug use, particularly cocaine. Reasons suggested include alterations in the placental barrier secondary to drug use, poor prenatal care among pregnant drug addicts, and predisposing sexual behaviors in this population.

Asymptomatic infants born to successfully treated mothers do not need evaluation. All infants born to syphilis-seropositive mothers (nontreponemal test confirmed by treponemal test) should be evaluated if mothers

- have untreated syphilis
- were treated for syphilis less than 1 month before delivery
- were treated for syphilis with a nonpenicillin (e.g., erythromycin) regimen
- did not have the expected decrease in nontreponemal antibody titers after treatment
- were treated but had insufficient follow-up during pregnancy
- have evidence of relapse or reinfection, even if the evaluation results are normal

Other organ systems, including lungs, teeth, and bones, are also involved in manifestations of congenital syphilis (Tables 69-13 and 69-14).[160,162,163] Pathognomonic findings of late congenital syphilis include Hutchinson teeth, interstitial keratitis, and eighth cranial nerve deafness (constituting the Hutchinson triad) and pneumonia alba (yellow-white, heavy, grossly enlarged lungs, with loss of alveolar spaces and obliterative fibrosis).

Gonococcal Infections

Ophthalmia neonatorum is the most common form of gonococcal infection in infants. It results from transmission from an infected mother to her infant during delivery.[164,165] Like all gram-negative bacteria, *N. gonorrhoeae* possesses a cell envelope composed of an inner cytoplasmic membrane, a middle layer of peptidoglycan, and an outer membrane. The outer membrane contains lipo-oligosaccharide, phospholipid, and a variety of proteins. The proteins are associated with adherence, cellular invasion, and resistance to the bactericidal effects of serum. Some gonococci express pili (filamentous projections

that extend from the cell surface), which allow better attachment to mucosal cells. *N. gonorrhoeae* infects primarily columnar epithelium; stratified squamous epithelium is relatively resistant to invasion. The bacteria penetrate epithelial cells to reach subepithelial tissues. Subsequent infiltration of numerous leukocytes causes a characteristic profuse, yellow-white discharge. Direct extension occurs through the lymphatic vessels and less often through the blood vessels. Immunity is not induced by infection.[166]

The most important pathogen to rule out in neonatal ophthalmia is *N. gonorrhoeae*. Because of the potential for sequelae involving blindness, all neonatal ocular infections should be considered gonorrheal until proved otherwise. The differential diagnosis should include other epidemic keratoconjunctivitis and bacterial and viral pathogens that may be acquired at birth or in the postpartum period: primary HSV, *S. aureus*, *Pseudomonas* species, or *Proteus* species. The most common cause of neonatal conjunctivitis is undoubtedly a toxic chemical reaction to Credé prophylaxis, 1% silver nitrate. The neonatal conjunctiva reacts to all of these substances in a similar manner, although gonorrheal conjunctivitis in general produces a much more hyperacute purulent reaction.

A possible gonorrheal conjunctivitis should first be ruled out by conjunctival scrapings and culture on chocolate agar or Thayer-Martin media. It is essential that scrapings be performed instead of a smear with a cotton swab. Epithelial cells must be obtained by scraping the conjunctiva with a platinum spatula, and the smear is examined under the microscope after application of Gram stain and Giemsa stain. If *N. gonorrhoeae* is present, the gram-negative diplococci are present early in the infection in epithelial cells (epithelial parasitism). A positive diagnosis can then be made and appropriate therapy started before culture results are obtained.

The diagnosis may be suspected when acute conjunctivitis, usually with overtly purulent exudate, develops within 1 week of birth. A Gram stain of conjunctival exudate should reveal typical gram-negative diplococci. Corneal ulceration and iridocyclitis may occur, and unless therapy is initiated promptly, the cornea may be perforated, which leads to blindness. Prophylaxis by instillation of a 1% aqueous solution of silver nitrate into the conjunctivae soon after delivery is highly effective, although treatment failures do occur. A single topical application of erythromycin (0.5%) or tetracycline ointment (1%) is also effective when used for prophylaxis of gonococcal infection. It is uncommon for newborns to develop systemic illness that involves sepsis, meningitis, and arthritis (Table 69-15).[167-172]

Laboratory diagnosis depends on identification of *N. gonorrhoeae* at an infected site. DNA amplification methods may offer sensitivity and specificity comparable with or even superior to those of culture, but clinical experience is limited. Antimicrobial susceptibility testing necessitates isolation by culture. Whenever practical, the swab from any mucosal site should be inoculated immediately onto selective growth medium (Thayer-Martin agar) at room temperature and then placed promptly in

Table 69–13. Clinical Findings of Congenital Syphilis

Early Signs of Congenital Syphilis	Late Signs of Congenital Syphilis (after 2 years)
General Stillbirth Placentitis Funisitis Nonimmune hydrops fetalis Intrauterine growth restriction Failure to thrive	**Nose and Face** Frontal bossing Saddle nose Short maxillae Protruding mandible High-arched palate Dental
Skin and Mucous Membranes Condyloma lata (pigmented macules) Vesiculobullous rash Palmar or plantar rash Intractable diaper rash Mucous patches Persistent rhinitis (snuffles)	**Hutchinson teeth** (peg-shaped or notched upper incisors) Mulberry molars Skin Perioral fissures (rhagades) Neurologic Mental retardation
Lymphoreticular Hepatosplenomegaly Jaundice Generalized lymphadenopathy	**Seizures** Hydrocephalus Eighth cranial nerve deafness
Renal Nephrotic syndrome	**Ocular** Interstitial keratitis Corneal scarring Healed chorioretinitis Glaucoma
Pulmonary Pneumonitis (pneumonia alba)	**Skeletal** Clutton joints (bilateral knee effusions) Higouménakis sign (sternoclavicular thickening) Saber shins Flaring scapulas
Neurologic Pseudoparalysis (pseudoparalysis of Parrot; postneonatal Erb palsy) Leptomeningitis	
Ocular Chorioretinitis Uveitis Glaucoma Cataract	
Hematologic Coombs-negative hemolytic anemia Leukemoid reaction (with or without monocytosis or lymphocytosis) Thrombocytopenia Intravascular coagulopathy	
Skeletal Diaphyseal periostitis Osteochondritis Wimberger sign (destruction of the proximal medial aspect of the tibias)	

an enriched CO_2 environment and incubated. However, various nonnutrient transport media are adequate if the specimen can be transported to the laboratory without refrigeration and inoculated onto growth medium within 6 hours.[166]

Other than septic arthritis, bacteremic spread of gonococcal disease is rare.[173] Of interest is that, as with other pathogens causing septic arthritis, polyarticular involvement is the norm. Common manifestations include refusal to move the affected limb. As with other causes of septic arthritis, diagnosis and therapeutic arthrocentesis is indicated.

Sepsis, arthritis, and meningitis, or any combination of these conditions, are rare complications of neonatal gonococcal infection (Table 69-16).[174] Localized gonococcal infection of the scalp can result from fetal monitoring through scalp electrodes. Detection of gonococcal infection in neonates who have sepsis, arthritis, meningitis, or scalp abscesses requires cultures of blood, CSF, and joint aspirate on chocolate agar. Specimens obtained from the

Table 69–14. Frequency of the Common Early Manifestations of Congenital Syphilis from Three Studies that Included 139 Symptomatic Infants

Manifestation	Percentage Affected
Clinical Findings	
Rash	68
Fever	42
Failure to thrive	33
Hepatosplenomegaly	71
Lymphadenopathy	14
Central nervous system involvement	23
Pseudoparalysis	15
Pneumonitis	17
Rhinitis	14
Ascites	9
Laboratory Abnormalities	
Leukocytosis	72
Anemia (Coombs test–negative hemolytic anemia)	58
Thrombocytopenia	40
Renal manifestations (e.g., proteinuria, hematuria)	16
Radiographic Abnormalities	
Diaphyseal periostitis or metaphyseal osteochondritis	78

Table 69–16. Signs of Disseminated Gonococcal Disease of the Newborn

Site	Characteristics
Associated mucosal sites	Conjunctivitis, ophthalmia
	Asymptomatic pyuria
	Urethritis, vaginitis, proctitis, pharyngitis
	Scalp abscess
	Contaminated orogastric contents
Systemic findings	Multiply involved joints
	Pseudoparesis of involved joints
	Sepsis of newborn
	Onset at age 3-21 days

conjunctiva, vagina, oropharynx, and rectum that are cultured on gonococcal selective medium are useful for identifying the primary site or sites of infection, especially if inflammation is present. Positive Gram-stained smears of exudate, CSF, or joint aspirate provide a presumptive basis for initiating treatment for *N. gonorrhoeae*. Diagnoses based on Gram-stained smears or presumptive identification of cultures should be confirmed with definitive tests on culture isolates.

Chlamydia Infections

Chlamydia organisms are obligate intracellular bacteria. There are 18 serologic variants (serovars) divided between two biologic variants (biovars). The infection is the most common reportable sexually transmitted disease in the United States. The prevalence in pregnant women ranges from 6% to 12% in most populations but can be as high as 37% among adolescents.[159]

Neonatal acquisition usually occurs at the time of birth. In the absence of treatment during pregnancy, 50% to 75% of infants born to mothers with endocervical cultures positive for *C. trachomatis* become infected in at least one of the following anatomic sites: nasopharynx, conjunctiva, rectum, or vagina.[32] Twenty percent to 50% develop conjunctivitis at 5 to 14 days of age. It is generally not prevented by antibiotic eye prophylaxis at birth. Ten percent to 20% develop pneumonia between 4 and 12 weeks after birth.[33] The remaining infants develop an apparently asymptomatic colonization of the nasopharynx, rectum, or vagina. These infants can remain colonized for up to 3 years, although most colonizations clear, even without treatment, by 1 year of age.

Some infants acquire *Chlamydia* even if born via cesarean section. Successful treatment of the mother during pregnancy with oral erythromycin or azithromycin prevents most cases of vertical transmission.

C. trachomatis can be diagnosed in the neonate with the same laboratory tests described in the diagnosis of adult inclusion conjunctivitis: Giemsa staining, culture, fluorescein-conjugated monoclonal antibody tests, serologic

Table 69–15. Outcome of Pregnancy in Mothers Who Were Infected with *Neisseria gonorrhoeae* at Delivery

Outcome	Charles et al[167] (N = 14)	Sarrel and Preutt[168] (N = 37)	Israel et al[169] (N = 39)	Amstey and Steadman[170] (N = 222)	Edwards et al[171] (N = 19)	Handsfield et al[172] (N = 12)
Normal or full-term infant	—	13 (35%)	30 (77%)	142 (64%)	7 (37%)	—
Spontaneous abortion	—	13 (35%)	1 (3%)	24 (11%)	—	—
Perinatal death	—	3 (8%)	1 (3%)	15 (7%)	2 (11%)	—
Premature delivery	—	—	5 (13%)	49 (22%)	8 (42%)	8 (67%)
Perinatal distress	—	—	5 (13%)	—	2 (11%)	—
Premature rupture of membranes	6 (43%)	8 (22%)	—	52 (23%)	12 (63%)	9 (75%)

assays, and PCR. The sensitivity of culture endocervical specimens may range between 60% and 90%. Nonculture methods, such as enzyme immunoassay (EIA) and direct fluorescent antibody (DFA) testing, yield results more rapidly but may be slightly less sensitive. In several studies to date, PCR sensitivity exceeded that of culture, whereas the specificities were maintained.[175,176] Hammerschlag and associates demonstrated that PCR is both sensitive and specific for detection of *C. trachomatis* in ocular and nasopharyngeal specimens from infants with NIC.[177] The sensitivity of PCR in comparison with culture for conjunctival specimens was 92.3%. The authors believed that "PCR is probably the most sensitive *C. trachomatis* test now available." Undoubtedly, more sensitive tests are on the way. Roblin and colleagues described a new optical immunoassay for the diagnosis of NIC and reported a sensitivity and specificity of 100% and 92.6%, respectively, in a prospective study of 37 ocular specimens from infants with suspected *C. trachomatis*.[178]

Chlamydia culture of the conjunctiva (for conjunctivitis) or nasopharynx (for pneumonia) is considered the "gold standard" for diagnosis, but there are disadvantages to this method. Culture specimens require special handling, which can make transport to the laboratory difficult. The fact that cultures generally require 3 to 7 days to process may delay treatment.

Since the mid-1980s, several commercial rapid tests have been developed. DFA tests and EIA have been approved by the U.S. Food and Drug Administration (FDA) for detection of *C. trachomatis* in infants with conjunctivitis or pneumonia; these tests have a sensitivity of 93% to 100% and a specificity of 94% to 97%, in comparison with culture. Results are usually available in less than 24 hours. A DNA probe test is also available. DNA probes have a detection sensitivity and specificity similar to those of the EIA and, in the commercial version, have the additional advantage of being combined with a DNA probe for *N. gonorrhoeae*. They have received clearance by the FDA for use with conjunctival specimens but not for use with nasopharyngeal specimens. Newly developed amplified DNA tests based on PCR and ligase chain reaction appear to be even more sensitive than culture for *Chlamydia* detection, but they are expensive. These tests are not yet FDA approved for infant conjunctival or nasopharyngeal specimens but may become the diagnostic test of choice when a very sensitive test is needed.

C. trachomatis is an obligate intracellular organism; therefore, the collection swab must be scraped across the conjunctiva or nasopharynx to ensure that there are adequate epithelial cells for detection. In the eye, the discharge should be wiped away before the conjunctival scrapings are obtained.[30] Mothers with positive endocervical cultures should be treated during pregnancy. Maternal treatment consists of erythromycin base, 500 mg orally 4 times a day for 7 days (efficacy is about 80% to 90%), or oral azithromycin in a single 1-g dose. In one study of pregnant women in which the two drugs were compared, azithromycin was much better tolerated and had less severe gastrointestinal side effects, and there were fewer therapy discontinuations.[179,180] If neither drug can be tolerated, some experts recommend oral

amoxicillin (1.5 g/day in three divided doses for 7 to 10 days).

Treatment for *C. trachomatis* is hampered by its long growth cycles and requires prolonged therapeutic levels of antibiotics. Compliance can be a problem with this erythromycin course. Azithromycin is a macrolide antibiotic that has a lower incidence of side effects and a much longer half-life; therefore, once-a-day dosing for shorter periods is possible.

No matter which regimen is used, all pregnant women should receive a follow-up test of cure, 3 weeks after completion of therapy. Post-treatment follow-up cultures should be performed to determine whether treatment has been successful; if it has not, a second course of treatment may be indicated. Sexual partners of positive women must be treated as well. Chlamydial infection in both male and female genital tracts can be asymptomatic, which is why routine screening, especially in pregnancy, is warranted.

Until 1999, the AAP *Red Book* recommended that infants born to mothers with untreated chlamydial cervical infections receive oral erythromycin for 14 days, starting on the first day after birth. However, the efficacy of prophylactic treatment is unknown; moreover, reports of an association between the prophylactic use of oral erythromycin for pertussis and infantile hypertrophic pyloric stenosis have appeared.[181] The 2004 AAP *Red Book* now recommends that treatment be reserved for infants with actual infection.[161]

Neonates with chlamydial conjunctivitis should receive oral erythromycin, 50 mg/kg/day in four divided doses, for 14 days. Additional topical therapy is not needed. Erythromycin with the same dose given for 2 to 3 weeks is the treatment of choice for chlamydial pneumonia. Treatment failure, necessitating a second course of erythromycin, occurs in about 20% of cases.

Azithromycin is approved for use in neonates. Its shorter treatment course and less severe gastrointestinal side effects should improve treatment compliance. Preliminary data indicate that azithromycin, 20 mg/kg once a day for 3 days, successfully treats conjunctivitis caused by *C. trachomatis*.

The onset of *C. trachomatis* pneumonia is usually between 4 and 12 weeks of age (a few cases manifest as early as 2 weeks, but none has been reported after age 4 months). Most infants have a prodrome, lasting about 1 week, of a stuffy nose without fever and a persistent paroxysmal staccato cough that can lead to breathlessness. Also present are tachypnea and inspiratory rales. Expiratory wheezing occurs in fewer than 25% of infants with the disease; 60% have abnormal eardrum findings. Although severe illness is relatively rare, infants may appear irritable, eat poorly, and cough often. The chest radiograph shows hyperinflation with bilateral diffuse nonspecific infiltrates. Laboratory values are significant for eosinophilia (>300 to 400/mm³), an elevated total serum IgG level (>500 mg/dL), and an elevated total IgM total (>110 mg/dL). Without treatment, symptoms last an average of 6 weeks. Treatment of any previous conjunctivitis with oral erythromycin seems to prevent this pneumonia, although there are case reports of treatment failures. Half of the infants with chlamydial pneumonia do not have a history of conjunctivitis.

C. pneumoniae, a species of the genus *Chlamydia,* also known as the TWAR strain, has not been isolated in any children younger than 2 years. It is a common cause of pneumonia, bronchitis, and upper respiratory tract infections in older children between the ages of 5 and 15 years.

Although studies are conflicting, *C. trachomatis* infection in pregnancy is weakly linked to premature rupture of membranes and premature delivery. Ten percent to 30% of women with chlamydial infections who undergo induced abortions develop late endometritis. Chronic salpingitis caused by *C. trachomatis* can lead to infertility and an increased risk for ectopic pregnancy.

Ureaplasma Urealyticum

The average carriage rate of *Ureaplasma urealyticum* in the female lower genital tract is 70%; the range is 40% to 80%.[182] Colonization in adults is related to the number of sexual exposures but occurs in 50% of men and 70% of women with three or more partners.

The rate of vertical transmission of *U. urealyticum* and *M. hominis* ranges from 18% to 55% among infants.[183-185] The rate of vertical transmission is not affected by method of delivery but is significantly increased when chorioamnionitis or amniotic fluid infection is present. Transmission occurs in utero by ascending infection or during delivery through an infected birth canal. Preterm and VLBW infants are more likely to acquire *U. urealyticum* in the lower respiratory tract. The mode of delivery does not influence the rate of transmission, but the rate is increased in the presence of clinical intraamniotic infection and histologic chorioamnionitis, and it may be increased in the presence of prolonged rupture of membranes.

Colonization in healthy full-term infants is relatively transient, with a sharp drop in isolation rates after 3 months of age.[186] *Ureaplasma* organisms may colonize the throat, eyes, umbilicus, and perineum of newborn infants. This colonization may persist for several months after birth.[187]

Other features of *U. urealyticum* include the following:

- It is the agent most commonly isolated when chorioamnionitis is present and is the most frequent isolate from placentas after preterm delivery.
- Several case reports and studies of radiographic changes and neutrophils in endotracheal aspirates suggest that *U. urealyticum* causes pneumonia in the newborn.
- Surfactant-deficient respiratory distress syndrome is twice as frequent in premature infants younger than 34 weeks of gestational age in whom *U. urealyticum* is isolated from the endotracheal aspirate. However, there is no association with superficial colonization.
- In two meta-analyses, *U. urealyticum* colonization was associated with a relative risk of chronic lung disease (CLD) of approximately 1.8. This increased relative risk has been borne out since the advent of surfactant. It is hypothesized that infection causes a subacute pneumonia and chronic damage. This is supported by the finding of increased levels of cytokines interleukin-1 and tumor necrosis factor-α in colonized VLBW infants.

- *U. urealyticum* has been isolated from CSF frequently. In the preterm population, it may be associated with hydrocephalus. There may be a pleocytosis, and it may persist for weeks. Several case reports describe a clinical response to treatment.

U. urealyticum can induce ciliastatic and mucosal lesions in human fetal tracheal organ cultures.[188] Furthermore, *Ureaplasma* organisms isolated from the lungs of human infants with congenital and neonatal pneumonia produce a pneumonia histologically similar to that in newborn mice.[189] *U. urealyticum* can be isolated from blood, endotracheal aspirates and pleural fluid, and lung tissue 6 days after infection. The organism can be isolated from endotracheal aspirates of up to 34% of infants with a birth weight of less than 2500 g, and radiographic evidence of pneumonia is twice as common in these infants than in *U. urealyticum*–negative infants. Isolation of *U. urealyticum* from endotracheal aspirates of infants weighing 1250 g or less within the first 24 hours of birth is associated with an increased risk for development of bronchopulmonary dysplasia, or CLD of prematurity.[190,191] This association is independent of birth weight, gender, and other known risk factors for development of CLD.

Current knowledge of the pathophysiologic mechanisms of CLD of prematurity suggests that *U. urealyticum* produces pneumonia that goes undetected and untreated and results in an increased requirement for oxygen and subsequent development of CLD as a result of oxygen toxicity.[190,192] and/or a synergistic effect between the *Ureaplasma* organisms and hyperoxia. In a study by Ollikainen and coworkers in Finland,[193] *U. urealyticum* was isolated from the CSF of four of six infants younger than 34 weeks of gestational age from whom cultures were obtained within 30 minutes of birth. Although there was no pleocytosis or hypoglycorrhachia in the CSF, the organism was also isolated from the blood in three infants and from the tracheal sample in one; one infant died, and the postmortem brain culture was positive for *U. urealyticum*. The clinical findings in infants with *U. urealyticum* of the CSF may produce CSF pleocytosis, with either polymorphonuclear or mononuclear cells predominating, or the inflammatory reaction in CSF may be minimal or absent.[193-196] In some patients, the organisms are eradicated spontaneously from the CSF, whereas in others, the organisms have been shown to persist in the CSF for weeks and even months with antibiotic treatment.[197,198]

Although usually limited to research settings, it is appropriate to sample endotracheal aspirates, blood, and CSF. Specific *Ureaplasma* transport media should be used with refrigeration at 4° C (39° F). The use of cotton swabs should be avoided. A rapid sensitive PCR test has been developed but is not routinely available.[199] Serologic testing for *Ureaplasma* organisms is of limited value and should be avoided.

Few data on efficacy of antibiotic therapy in the treatment of pulmonary or CNS infection are available. For therapy outside the CNS, erythromycin is appropriate.[200] For CNS disease, intravenous doxycycline or intravenous chloramphenicol should be considered. Several randomized

Table 69–17. Interpretation of Hepatitis B Virus (HBV) Serology Test Results

HBsAG	IgM Anti-HBc	Total Anti-HBc	Anti-HBs	Interpretation
+	–	–	–	Early HBV infection prior to anti–hepatitis B core response
+	+	+	–	Early HBV infection, onset within 6 mo
–	+	+	+ or –	Recent HBV infection, within 4-6 mo with resolution
+	–	+	–	HBV infection, onset ≥ 6 mo, probable chronic infection
–	–	–	+	HBV vaccine response
–	–	+	+	Past HBV infection, recovered

HBc, hepatitis B core antigen; HBs, hepatitis B surface; HBsAg, hepatitis B surface antigen.

trials have not demonstrated any decrease in the incidence of chronic lung disease after treatment of infants colonized with *Ureaplasma* organisms.

Although numerous studies have demonstrated the association of colonization of the lower respiratory tract with CLD, several randomized, controlled trials have not demonstrated any decrease in the incidence of CLD after treatment of infants colonized with *U. urealyticum* with erythromycin.[201,202]

Hepatitis B

Hepatitis B virus is transmitted by percutaneous or mucosal exposure to infectious body fluids, by sexual contact, or by perinatal transmission from an infected mother to her newborn. Women who are hepatitis B early antigen (HBeAg)–positive are more likely to transmit hepatitis (70% to 90%) to their infants than women who are hepatitis B surface antigen (HBsAg)–positive only (5% to 20%).

Serologic tests can distinguish between acute and chronic infection and can elucidate time of onset of infection with hepatitis B virus (Table 69-17).[203] HBeAg is present during acute infection, cleared during convalescence, and variably present in chronic disease. Hepatitis B virus DNA is best used to monitor response to treatment of chronic infection.

Current recommendations include the following:

- Screening all pregnant women for hepatitis B.
- Providing active immunization with hepatitis B vaccine and passive immunization with hepatitis B immune globulin within 12 to 24 hours of birth. Breast-feeding is not associated with increase risk.
- Routine immunization of all infants.
- Vaccination of all 11- to 12-year-olds and of adolescents at high risk for acquiring the infection.

There is no evidence that neonatal hepatitis B vaccination is associated with an increase in the number of febrile episodes, evaluation findings of sepsis, or allergic or neurologic events.[204] Hepatic complications of hepatitis B include chronic active hepatitis and cirrhosis that can progress to liver failure and hepatocellular carcinoma. The risk of chronic infection is inversely related to age; as many as 90% of newborns, 30% of children 1 to 5 years of age, and 5% to 10% of older children may have persistence of HBsAg.

REFERENCES

1. Hickey S, McCracken G: Postnatal bacterial infections. In Fanaroff AA, Martin RJ (eds): Neonatal-Perinatal Medicine: Diseases of the Fetus and Infant, 6th ed. St. Louis, Mosby–Year Book, 1997, pp 717-720.
2. Stoll B: The global impact of neonatal infection. Clin Perinatol 24:1, 1997.
3. Kilbride HW, Powers R, Wirtschafter DD, et al: Evaluation and development of potentially better practices to prevent neonatal nosocomial bacteremia. Pediatrics 111(4 Pt 2): e504, 2003.
4. Posfay-Barbe KM, Pittet D: New concepts in hand hygiene. Semin Pediatr Infect Dis 12:147, 2001.
5. Larson E: Skin hygiene and infection prevention: More of the same or different approaches? Clin Infect Dis 29:1287, 1999.
6. Whatron KN, Karlowica MG: Barriers to full compliance with handwashing in a neonatal intensive care unit. Pediatr Res 43:254A, 1998.
7. Nopper AJ, Horji KA, Sookdeo-Drost S, et al: Topical ointment therapy benefits premature infants. J Pediatr 128:660, 1996.
8. Abstracts, fifteenth annual educational conference, Association for Practitioners in Infection Control. May 1-6, 1988, Dallas. Am J Infect Control 16:73, 1988.
9. Donowitz LG: Failure of the overgown to prevent nosocomial infection in a pediatric intensive care unit. Pediatrics 77:35, 1986.
10. Baltimore RS: Neonatal nosocomial infections. Semin Perinatol 22:25, 1998.
11. Stoll BJ, Temprosa M, Tyson JE, et al: Dexamethasone therapy increases infection in very low birth weight infants. Pediatrics 104:e63, 1999.
12. Brodie SB, Sands KE, Gray JE, et al: Occurrence of nosocomial bloodstream infections in six neonatal intensive care units. Pediatr Infect Dis J 19:56, 2000.
13. Mathieu LM, De Muynck AO, De Dooy JJ, et al: Prediction of nosocomial sepsis in neonates by means of a computer-weighted bedside scoring system (NOSEP score). Crit Care Med 28:2028, 2000.
14. Fanaroff AA, Korones SB, Wright LL, et al: Incidence, presenting features, risk factors and significance of late onset septicemia in very low birth weight infants. Pediatr Infect Dis J 17:593, 1998.
15. Stoll BJ, Gordon T, Korones SB, et al: Late-onset sepsis in very low birth weight neonates: A report from the National Institute of Child Health and Human Development Neonatal Research Network. J Pediatr 129:63, 1996.

16. Watson WJ, Abzug MJ, DeMuri G, et al: Multicenter surveillance of invasive fungal disease in very low birth weight infants [Abstract 1618]. Pediatr Res 45:275A, 1999.

17. Hageman JR, Stenske J, Keuler H, et al: *Candida* colonization and infection in very low birth weight infants. J Perinatol 6:251, 1985.

18. Rowen JL, Rench MA, Kozinetz CA, et al: Endotracheal colonization with *Candida* enhances risk of systemic candidiasis in very low birth weight neonates. J Pediatr 124:789, 1994.

19. Huang YC, Li CC, Lin TY, et al: Association of fungal colonization and invasive disease in very low birth weight infants. Pediatr Infect Dis J 17:819, 1998.

20. Rowen JL, Neonatal Candidiasis Study Group: Multicenter investigation of *Candida* colonization in intensive care nurseries [Abstract 57]. Clin Infect Dis 29:971, 1999.

21. Harris MC, Pereira GR, Myers MD, et al: Candidal arthritis in infants previously treated for systemic candidiasis during the newborn period. Pediatr Emerg Care 16:249, 2000.

22. Mittal M, Dhannireddy R, Higgins RD: *Candida* sepsis and association with retinopathy of prematurity. Pediatrics 101:654, 1998.

23. Voriconazole. Med Lett Drugs Ther 44(1135):63, 2002.

24. Keating GM, Jarvis B: Caspofungin. Drugs 61:1121, 2001.

25. Chryssanthou E, Cuenca-Estrella M: Comparison of the Antifungal Susceptibility Testing Subcommittee of the European Committee on Antibiotic Susceptibility Testing proposed standard and the E-test with the NCCLS broth microdilution method for voriconazole and caspofungin susceptibility testing of yeast species. J Clin Microbiol 40:3841, 2002.

26. Koedel U, Pfister HW: Models of experimental bacterial meningitis. Role and limitations. Infect Dis Clin North Am 13:549, 1999.

27. Wiswell TE, Baumgart S, Gannon CM, et al: No lumbar puncture in the evaluation for early neonatal sepsis: Will meningitis be missed? Pediatrics 95:803, 1995.

28. Ahmed A, Hickey SM, Ehrett S, et al: Cerebrospinal fluid values in the term infant. J Pediatr 116:971, 1990.

29. Laga M, Nzanze H, Brunham R, et al: Epidemiology of ophthalmia neonatorum in Kenya. Lancet 2:1145, 1986.

30. Lietman T, Whitcher JP: Ocular infections: Update on therapy. Ophthalmol Clin North Am 12:21, 1999.

31. Whitcher J: Neonatal ophthalmia: Have we advanced in the last 20 years? Int Opthalmol Clin 30:39, 1990.

32. Hammerschlag M: *Chlamydia trachomatis* in children. Pediatr Ann 23:349, 1994.

33. Hammerschlag M: Chlamydial infections. J Pediatr 114:724, 1989.

34. Ratelle S, Keno D, Hardwood M, et al: Neonatal chlamydial infections in Massachusetts, 1992-1993. Am J Prevent Med 13:221, 1997.

35. Alexander ER, Harrison HR: Chlamydial infections in infants and children. In Holmes KK, Mardh P, Sparling PF, et al (eds): Sexually Transmitted Diseases, 2nd ed. New York, McGraw-Hill, 1990, pp 811-820.

36. Guvenc H, Aygun AD, Yaar F, et al: Omphalitis in term and preterm appropriate for gestational age and small for gestational age infants. J Trop Pediatr 43:368, 1997.

37. Yoon BH, Romero R, Park JS, et al: The relationship among inflammatory lesions of the umbilical cord (funisitis), umbilical cord plasma interleukin 6 concentration, amniotic fluid infection, and neonatal sepsis. Am J Obstet Gynecol 185:1124, 2000.

38. Fink SM: Index of suspicion. Case 6.Diagnosis: Candidiasis. Pediatr Rev 22:22, 2001.

39. Yang KD, Hill HR: Assessment of neutrophil function disorders: Practical and preventive interventions. Pediatr Infect Dis J 13:906, 1994.

40. Klein JO, Long SS: Bacterial infections of the urinary tract. In Remington JS, Klein JO (eds): Infectious Diseases of the Fetus and Newborn Infant, 4th ed. Philadelphia, WB Saunders, 1995, pp 925-934.

41. Garcia FJ, Nager AL: Jaundice as an early diagnostic sign of urinary tract infection in infancy. Pediatrics 109:846, 2002.

42. Brill PW, Winchester P, Krauss AN, et al: Osteomyelitis in a neonatal intensive care unit. Radiology 131:83, 1979.

43. Goldmann DA, Durbin WA Jr, Freeman J: Nosocomial infections in a neonatal intensive care unit. J Infect Dis 144:449, 1981.

44. Townsend TR, Wenzel RP: Nosocomial bloodstream infections in a newborn intensive care unit. Am J Epidemiol 114:73, 1981.

45. Jackson MA, Nelson JD: Etiology and medical management of acute suppurative bone and joint infections in pediatric patients. J Pediatr Orthop 2:313, 1982.

46. Pittard WB III, Thullen JD, Fanaroff AA: Neonatal septic arthritis. J Pediatr 88:621, 1976.

47. Remington JS, Klein JO (eds): Infectious Diseases of the Fetus and Newborn Infant, 4th ed. Philadelphia, WB Saunders, 1995.

48. Unkila-Kallio L, Kallio MJ, Eskola J, et al: Serum C-reactive protein, erythrocyte sedimentation rate, and white blood cell count in acute hematogenous osteomyelitis of children. Pediatrics 93:59, 1994.

49. Bonhoeffer J, Haeberle B, Schaad UB, et al: Diagnosis of acute haematogenous osteomyelitis and septic arthritis: 20 years experience at the University Children's Hospital Basel. Swiss Med Wkly 131:575, 2001.

50. Young SEJ, Ramsay AM: The diagnosis of rubella. BMJ 2:1295, 1963.

51. Gregg NM: Congenital cataract following German measles in the mother. Trans Ophthalmol Soc Aust 3:35, 1941.

52. Munro ND, Smithhells RW, Shepard S, et al: Temporal relations between maternal rubella and congenital defects. Lancet 2:201, 1987.

53. Centers for Disease Control and Prevention: Case definitions for public health surveillance. MMWR 39(RR-13):31, 1990.

54. Reef SE, Frey TK, Theall K, et al: The changing epidemiology of rubella in the 1990s. On the verge of elimination and new challenges for control and prevention. JAMA 287:464, 2002.

55. Mellinger AK, Cragan JD, Atkinson WL, et al: High incidence of congenital rubella syndrome after a rubella outbreak. Pediatr Infect Dis J 14:573, 1995.

56. Recommended childhood immunization schedule—United States, 1998. MMWR Morb Mortal Wkly Rep 47:8, 1998.

57. Revised ACIP recommendation for avoiding pregnancy after receiving a rubella-containing vaccine. MMWR Morb Mortal Wkly Rep 50:1117, 2001.

58. Nelson CT, Demmler GJ: Cytomegalovirus infection in the pregnant mother, fetus, and newborn infant. Clin Perinatol 24:151, 1997.

59. Britt WH, Alford CA. Cytomegalovirus. In Fields BN, Knipe DM, Howley PM, et al (eds): Field Virology, 3rd ed. Philadelphia, Lippincott-Raven, 1996, pp 2493-2523.

60. Roizman B. Herpesviridae: A brief introduction. In Fields BN, Knipe DM, Howley, et al (eds): Field Virology, 3rd ed. Philadelphia, Lippincott-Raven, 1996, pp 2221-2230.

61. Stagno S: Cytomegalovirus. In Remington JS, Klein JO (eds): Infectious Diseases of the Fetus and Newborn Infant, 4th ed. Philadelphia: WB Saunders, 1995, pp 312-353.

62. Weller TH: The cytomegalovirus, ubiquitous agents with protein clinical manifestation. N Engl J Med 285:203, 1971.

63. Gold E, Nankervis GA: Cytomegalovirus. In Evans A (ed): Viral Infections of Humans: Epidemiology and Control. New York, Elsevier, 1976, pp 143-161.

64. Alford CA, Stagno S, Pass RF, et al: Congenital and perinatal cytomegalovirus infections. Rev Infect Dis 12:745, 1990.

65. Raynor BD: Cytomegalovirus infection in pregnancy. Semin Perinatol 17:394, 1993.

66. Volpe JJ (ed): Neurology of the Newborn, 3rd ed. Philadelphia, WB Saunders, 1995.

67. Pass RF, Fowler KB, Boppana S: Progress in cytomegalovirus research. In Landini MP (ed): Proceedings of the Third International Cytomegalovirus Workshop, June 1991, in Bologna, Italy. London, Excerpta Medica, 1991, pp 3-10.

68. McCollister FP, Dahle AJ, Stagno S, et al: Progressive hearing impairment (PHI) in infants with symptomatic congenital cytomegalovirus (SCC). Program Issue, APS/SPR. Pediatr Res 25:103A, 1989.

69. Reynolds DW, Stagno S, Alford CA: Laboratory diagnosis of the cytomegalovirus infections. In Lenette EH, Schmidt NJ (eds): Diagnostic Procedures for Viral, Rickettsial, and Chlamydial Infections. Washington, DC, American Public Health Association, 1979, pp 399-439.

70. Warren WP, Balcarek K, Smith RJ et al: Comparison of rapid methods of detection of cytomegalovirus in saliva with virus isolation in tissue culture. J Clin Microbiol 30:786, 1992.

71. van Loon AM, Heessen FWA, van der Logt JTM: Antibody isotype response after human cytomegalovirus infection. J Virol Methods 15:101, 1987.

72. Nigro G, Scholz H, Bartmann U, et al: Ganciclovir therapy for symptomatic congenital cytomegalovirus infection in infants: A two-regimen experience. J Pediatr 24:318, 1994.

73. Whitley RJ, Cloud G, Gruber W, et al: Ganciclovir treatment of symptomatic congenital cytomegalovirus infection: Results of a phase II study. J Infect Dis 175:1080, 1997.

74. Elek SD, Stern H: Development of a vaccine against mental retardation caused by cytomegalovirus infection in utero. Lancet 1:1, 1974.

75. Plotkin SA, Furukawa T, Zygraich N, et al: Candidate cytomegalovirus strain for human vaccination. Infect Immun 12:521, 1975.

76. Miyagaw S, Takahashi Y, Nagai A, et al: Angio-oedema in a neonate with IgG antibodies to parvovirus B19 following intrauterine parvovirus B19 infection. Br J Dermatol 143:428, 2000.

77. Katta R: Parvovirus B19: A review. Dermatol Clin 20:333, 2002.

78. Harger JH, Adler SP, Koch WC, et al: Prospective evaluation of 618 pregnant women exposed to parvovirus B19: Risks and symptoms. Obstet Gynecol 91:413, 1998.

79. Markenson GR, Yancey MK: Parvovirus B19 infections in pregnancy. Semin Perinatol 22:309, 1998.

80. Wilson M, McAuley JM: Toxoplasma. In Murray PR, Baron ES, Pfaller MA et al (eds): Manual of Clinical Microbiology, 7th ed. Washington, DC, ASM Press, 1999, pp 1374-1382.

81. Kasper LH: Toxoplasma infection. In Fauci AS, Branwald E, Isselbacher KJ, et al (eds): Harrison's Principles of Internal Medicine, 14th ed. New York, McGraw-Hill, 1998, pp 1197-1202.

82. Marr JJ: Toxoplasmosis. In Kelley WN, Dupont HL, Glick JH, et al (eds): Textbook of Internal Medicine, 2nd ed. Philadelphia, JB Lippincott, 1992, pp 1535-1539.

83. Luft BJ, Remington JS: Toxoplasmosis. In Hoeprich PD, Jordan MC, Ronald AR (eds): Infectious Diseases: A Treatise of Infectious Processes, 5th ed. Philadelphia, Lippincott-Raven, 1994, pp 1201-1213.

84. Remington JS, McLeod R, Thulliez P, et al: Toxoplasmosis. In Remington JS, Klein JO (eds): Infectious Diseases of the Fetus and Newborn Infant, 5th ed. Philadelphia, WB Saunders, 2001, pp 205-346.

85. Kean BH, Kimball AC, Christenson WN: Epidemic of acute toxoplasmosis. JAMA 208:1002, 1969.

86. Centers for Disease Control and Prevention: Toxoplasmosis—Pennsylvania. MMWR Morb Mortal Wkly Rep 24:285, 1975.

87. Masur J, Jones TC, Lempert JA, et al: Outbreak of toxoplasmosis in a family and documentation of acquired retinochoroiditis. Am J Med 64:396, 1978.

88. Fertig A, Selwyn S, Tibble MJ: Tetracycline and toxoplasmosis. BMJ 2:192, 1977.

89. Choi WY, Nam HW, Kwak NH, et al: Foodborne outbreaks of human toxoplasmosis. J Infect Dis 175:1280, 1997.

90. Sacks JJ, Roberto RR, Brooks NF: Toxoplasmosis infection associated with raw goat's milk. JAMA 248:1728, 1982.

91. Benenson MW, Takafuji ET, Lemon SM, et al: Oocyst-transmitted toxoplasmosis associated with ingestion of contaminated water. N Engl J Med 307:666, 1982.

92. Bowie WR, King AS, Werker DH, et al: Outbreak of toxoplasmosis associated with municipal drinking water. Lancet 350:173, 1997.

93. Stagno S, Dykes AC, Amos CS, et al: An outbreak of toxoplasmosis linked to cats. Pediatrics 65:706, 1980.

94. Teutsch SM, Juranek DD, Sulzer A, et al: Epidemic toxoplasmosis associated with infected cats. N Engl J Med 300:695, 1979.

95. Wong SY, Remington JS: Toxoplasmosis in pregnancy. Clin Infect Dis 18:853, 1994.

96. Foulon W, Villena I, Stray-Pedersen B, et al: Treatment of toxoplasmosis during pregnancy: A multicenter study of impact on fetal transmission and children's sequelae at age 1 year. Am J Obstet Gynecol 180:410, 1999.

97. Dunn D, Wallon M, Peyron F, et al: Mother-to-child transmission of toxoplasmosis: Risk estimates for clinical counseling. Lancet 353:1829, 1999.

98. Holliman RE: Congenital toxoplasmosis: Prevention, screening and treatment. J Hosp Infect 30(Suppl):179, 1995.

99. Carter AO, Frank JW: Congenital toxoplasmosis: Epidemiologic features and control. Can Med Assoc J 135:618, 1986.

100. Wilson CB, Remington JS, Stagno S, et al: Development of adverse sequelae in children born with subclinical congenital Toxoplasma infection. Pediatrics 66:767, 1980.

101. Frenkel JK, Fishback JL; Toxoplasmosis. In Strickland GT (ed): Hunter's Tropical Medicine and Emerging Infectious Diseases, 8th ed. Philadelphia, WB Saunders, 2000, pp 691-701.

102. Montoya JG, Remington JS: Toxoplasma gondii. In Mandell GL, Bennett JE, Dolin R (eds): Mandell, Douglas, and Bennett's Principles and Practice of Infectious Diseases, 5th ed. Philadelphia, Churchill Livingstone, 2000, pp 2858-2888.

103. Wilson M, Remington JS, Clavet C, et al: Evaluation of six commercial kits for detection of human immunoglobulin M antibodies to Toxoplasma gondii. J Clin Microbiol 35:3112, 1997.

104. Jenum PA, Stray-Pedersen B, Gundersen AG: Improved diagnosis of primary Toxoplasma gondii infection in early pregnancy by determination of antitoxoplasma immunoglobulin G avidity. J Clin Microbiol 35:1972, 1997.

105. Hedman K, Lappalainen M, Seppaia I, et al: Recent primary Toxoplasma infection indicated by low avidity of specific IgG. J Infect Dis 159:736, 1989.

106. Hohfeld P, Daffos F, Cost JM, et al: Prenatal diagnosis of congenital toxoplasmosis with a polymerase-chain-reaction test on amniotic fluid. N Engl J Med 331:695, 1994.

107. Grover CM, Thulliez P, Remington JS: Rapid prenatal diagnosis of congenital *Toxoplasma* infection by using polymerase chain reaction and amniotic fluid. J Clin Microbiol 28:2297, 1990.

108. Cazenave J, Forestier F, Bessieres MH, et al: Contribution of a new PCR assay to the prenatal diagnosis of congenital toxoplasmosis. Prenat Diagn 12:119, 1992.

109. Jenum PA, Holberg-Peterson M, Melby KK, Stray-Pedersen B: Diagnosis of congenital *Toxoplasma gondii* infection by polymerase chain reaction (PCR) on amniotic fluid samples: The Norwegian experience. APMIS 106:680, 1998.

110. van de Ven E, Melchers W, Galama J, et al: Identification of *Toxoplasma gondii* infections by BI gene amplification. J Clin Microbiol 29:2120, 1991.

111. ACOG Practice Bulletin 20: Perinatal Viral and Parasitic Infections. Washington, DC, American College of Obstetricians and Gynecologists, September 2000.

112. Foulon W: Congenital toxoplasmosis: Is screening desirable? Scand J Infect Dis Suppl 84:11, 1992.

113. Drugs for parasitic diseases. Med Lett March 2000. Available at http://www.medletter.com.

114. Wallon M, Liou C, Garner P, et al: Congenital toxoplasmosis: Systematic review of evidence of efficacy of treatment in pregnancy. BMJ 318:1511, 1999.

115. Montoya JG, Remington JS: Studies on the serodiagnosis of toxoplasmic lymphadenitis. Clin Infect Dis 20:781, 1995.

116. Liesenfeld O, Montoya JG, Tathineni NJ, et al: Confirmatory serologic testing for acute toxoplasmosis and rate of induced abortions among women reported to have positive *Toxoplasma* immunoglobulin M antibody titers. Am J Obstet Gynecol 184:140, 2001.

117. Montoya JG, Remington JS: Toxoplasmic chorioretinitis in the setting of acute acquired toxoplasmosis. Clin Infect Dis 23:277, 1996.

118. Eyles DE, Coleman M: Synergistic effect of sulfadiazine and Daraprim against experimental toxoplasmosis in the mouse. Antibiot Chemother 3:483, 1953.

119. Eyles DE, Coleman N: An evaluation of the curative effects of pyrimethamine and sulfadiazine, alone and in combination on experimental mouse toxoplasmosis. Antibiot Chemother 5:529, 1955.

120. Sheffield HG, Melton ML: Effect of pyrimethamine and sulfadiazine on the fine structure and multiplication of *Toxoplasma gondii* in cell cultures. J Parasitol 61:704, 1975.

121. Ryan RW, Hart WM, Culligan JJ, et al: Diagnosis and treatment of toxoplasmic uveitis. Trans Am Acad Ophthalmol Otolaryngol 58:867, 1954.

122. Perkins ES, Smith CH, Schofield PB: Treatment of uveitis with pyrimethamine (Daraprim). Br J Ophthalmol 40:577, 1956.

123. Boyer KM: Diagnostic testing for congenital toxoplasmosis. Pediatr Infect Dis J 20:59, 2001.

124. Multistate outbreak of listeriosis—United States, 2000. MMWR Morb Mortal Wkly Rep 49:1129, 2000.

125. Shattuck KE, Chonmaitree T: The changing spectrum of neonatal meningitis over a fifteen-year period. Clin Pediatr (Phila) 31:130, 1992.

126. Jacobs RF, Starke JR: *Mycobacterium tuberculosis*. In Long SS, Pickering LK, Prober CG (eds): Principles and Practice of Pediatric Infectious Disease. New York, Churchill Livingstone, 1997, pp 881-904.

127. American Academy of Pediatrics: Human milk. In Peter G (ed): Red Book: Report of the Committee on Infectious Diseases, 24th ed. Elk Grove Village, Ill, American Academy of Pediatrics, 1997, pp 541-562.

128. Starke JR: Tuberculosis: An old disease but a new threat to the mother, fetus, and neonate. Clin Perinatol 24:107, 1997.

129. Centers for Disease Control and Prevention: Reported tuberculosis in the United States, 2001. Atlanta, Centers for Disease Control and Prevention, 2001. Available at: *http://www.cdc.gov/nchstp/tb/surv/surv2001/default.htm* (accessed May 14, 2004).

130. Abughali N, Van Der Kuyp F, Annable W, et al: Congenital tuberculosis. Pediatr Infect Dis J 13:738, 1994.

131. Soeiro A: Congenital tuberculosis in a small premature baby. S Afr Med J 45:1021, 1971.

132. Hopkins R, Ermocila R, Cassady G: Congenital tuberculosis. South Med J 69:1156, 1976.

133. Dunlap NE, Bass J, Fujiwara P, et al: Diagnostic standards and classification of tuberculosis in adults and children. Am J Respir Crit Care Med 161:1376, 2000.

134. Starke JR, Smith MHD: Tuberculosis. In Feigin RD, Cherry JD (eds): Textbook of Pediatric Infectious Diseases, 4th ed. Philadelphia, WB Saunders, 1998, pp 1196-1239.

135. Rosenfeld EA, Hageman JR, Yogev R: Tuberculosis in infancy in the 1990s. Pediatr Clin North Am 40:1087, 1993.

136. Cantwell MF, Shehab ZM, Costello AM, et al: Brief report: Congenital tuberculosis. N Engl J Med 330:1051, 1994.

137. Lee LH, LeVea CM, Graman PS: Congenital tuberculosis in a neonatal intensive care unit: Case report, epidemiological investigation, and management of exposures. Clin Infect Dis 27:474, 1998.

138. American Academy of Pediatrics: Tuberculosis. In Pickering LK (ed): 2000 Red Book: Report of the Committee on Infectious Disease, 25th ed. Elk Grove Village, Ill: American Academy of Pediatrics, 2000, pp 593-613.

139. Hageman J, Shulman S, Schrieber M, et al: Congenital tuberculosis: Critical reappraisal of clinical findings and diagnostic procedures. Pediatrics 66:980, 1980.

140. Smith MHD, Teele DW: Tuberculosis. In Remington JS, Klein JO (eds): Infectious Diseases of the Fetus and Newborn Infant, 4th ed. Philadelphia, WB Saunders, 1995, pp 1074-1084.

141. Pastuszak AL, Levy M, Schick B, et al: Outcome after maternal varicella infection in the first 20 weeks of pregnancy. N Engl J Med 330:901, 1994.

142. Srabstein JC, Morris N, Larke RP, et al: Is there a congenital varicella syndrome? J Pediatr 84:239, 1974.

143. Higa K, Dan K, Manabe H: Varicella-zoster virus infections during pregnancy: Hypothesis concerning the mechanisms of congenital malformations. Obstet Gynecol 69:214, 1987.

144. Skibsted L: Abnormal fetal ultrasound findings after maternal chickenpox infection. Ugeskr Laeger 162:2546, 2000.

145. Huang CS: Congenital varicella syndrome as an unusual cause of congenital malformation: Report of one case. Acta Paediatr Taiwan 42:239, 2001.

146. Bruder E: Fetal varicella syndrome: Disruption of neural development and persistent inflammation of non-neural tissues. Virchows Arch 437:440, 2000.

147. Fowler MG, Simonds, RJ, Roongpisuthipong A: HIV/AIDS in infants, children, and adolescents: Update on perinatal HIV transmission. Pediatr Clin North Am 47:21, 2000.

148. The International Perinatal Group: The mode of delivery and the risk of vertical transmission of human immunodeficiency virus type 1. N Engl J Med 340:977, 1999.

149. Dorenbaum A, Cunningham CK, Gelber RD, et al: Two-dose intrapartum/newborn nevirapine and standard anti-retroviral therapy to reduce perinatal HIV transmission: A randomized trial. JAMA 288:189, 2002.

150. Nieburg P, Hu DJ, Moses S, et al: Contribution of breast-feeding to the reported variation in rates of mother-to-child HIV transmission. AIDS 9:396, 1995.

151. Nduati R, Mbori-Ngacha D, John G, et al: Breastfeeding in women with HIV. JAMA 284:956, 2000.

152. Centers for Disease Control and Prevention: 1994 Revised guidelines for the performance of CD4+ T-cell determinations in persons with human immunodeficiency virus (HIV) infections. MMWR Morb Mortal Wkly Rep 43(RR-3): 1, 1994.

153. Kohl S: Herpes simplex infection in newborn infants. Sem Pediatr Infect Dis 10:154, 1999.

154. Whitley RJ, Corey L, Arvin A, et al: Changing presentation of herpes simplex virus infection in neonates. J Infect Dis 158:109, 1988.

155. Kimberlin DW, Lin CY, Jacobs RF, et al: Natural history of neonatal herpes simplex virus infections in the acyclovir era. Pediatrics 108:223, 2001.

156. Kimberlin DW, Lin CY, Jacobs RF, et al: Safety and efficacy of high dose intravenous acyclovir in the management of neonatal herpes simplex infections. Pediatrics 108:230, 2000.

157. Kimberlin D, Powell D, Gruber W, et al: Administration of oral acyclovir suppressive therapy after neonatal herpes simplex virus disease limited to the skin, eyes and mouth: Results of a phase I/II trial. Pediatr Infect Dis J 15:247, 1996.

158. Aradottir E, Alonso EM, Shulman ST: Severe neonatal enteroviral hepatitis treated with pleconaril. Pediatr Infect Dis J 20:457, 2001.

159. Centers for Disease Control and Prevention: Sexually transmitted diseases treatment guidelines 2002. MMWR Recomm Rep 51(RR-6):1, 2002.

160. Chawla V, Pandit PB, Nkrumah PK: Congenital syphilis in the newborn. Arch Dis Child 63:1393, 1988.

161. American Academy of Pediatrics: Syphilis. In Pickering LK (ed): 2003 Red Book: Report of the Committee on Infectious Diseases, 26th ed. Elk Grove Village, Ill, American Academy of Pediatrics, 2003, pp 595-607.

162. Mascola L, Pelosi R, Blount JH, et al: Congenital syphilis revisited. Am J Dis Child 139:575, 1985.

163. Berry MC, Dajani AS: Resurgence of congenital syphilis. Infect Dis Clin North Am 6:19, 1992.

164. Sung L, MacDonald NE: Gonorrhea: A pediatric perspective. Pediatr Rev 19:13, 1998.

165. Alexander ER: Gonorrhea in the newborn. Ann N Y Acad Sci 549:180, 1988.

166. Darville T: Gonorrhea. Pediatr Rev 20:125, 1999.

167. Charles AG, Cohen S, Kass MB, et al: Asymptomatic gonorrhea in prenatal patients. Am J Obstet Gynecol 108:595, 1970.

168. Sarrel PM, Pruett KA: Symptomatic gonorrhea during pregnancy. Obstet Gynecol 32:670, 1968.

169. Israel KS, Rissing KB, Brooks GF: Neonatal and childhood gonococcal infections. Clin Obstet Gynecol 18:143, 1975.

170. Amstey MS, Steadman KT: Symptomatic gonorrhea and pregnancy. J Am Vener Dis Assoc 3:14, 1976.

171. Edwards L, Barrada MI, Hamann AA, et al: Gonorrhea in pregnancy. Am J Obstet Gynecol 132:637, 1978.

172. Handsfield HH, Hodson WA, Holmes KK: Neonatal gono-coccal infection. I. Orogastric contamination with *Neisseria gonorrhoeae.* JAMA 225:697, 1973.

173. Babl FE, Ram S, Barnett ED, et al: Neonatal gonococcal arthritis after negative prenatal screening and despite conjunctival prophylaxis. Pediatr Infect Dis J 19:346, 2000.

174. Soonzilli EE, Calabro JJ: Gonococcal arthritis in the newborn. JAMA 177:919, 1961.

175. Bass C, Jungkind D, Silverman N, et al: Clinical evaluation of a new polymerase chain reaction assay for detection of *Chlamydia trachomatis* in endocervical specimens. J Clin Microbiol 31:2648, 1993.

176. Dawson CR: Lids, conjunctiva, and lacrimal apparatus: Eye infections with *Chlamydia.* Arch Ophthalmol 93:854, 1975.

177. Hammerschlag M, Roblin P, Gelling M, et al: Use of polymerase chain reaction for the detection of *Chlamydia trachomatis* in ocular and nasopharyngeal specimens from infants with conjunctivitis. Pediatr Infect Dis J 16:293, 1997.

178. Roblin P, Gelling M, Kutlin A, et al: Evaluation of a new optical immunoassay for diagnosis of neonatal chlamydial conjunctivitis. J Clin Microbiol 35:515, 1997.

179. Adair CD, Gunter M, Stovall TG, et al: Chlamydia in pregnancy: A randomized trial of azithromycin and erythromycin. Obstet Gynecol 91:165, 1998.

180. Wehbeh HA, Ruggeirio RM, Shahem S, et al: Single-dose azithromycin for *Chlamydia* in pregnant women. J Reprod Med 43:509, 1998.

181. Honein MA: Infantile hypertrophic pyloric stenosis after pertussis prophylaxis with erythromycin: A case review and cohort study. Lancet 354:2101, 1999.

182. Chua KB, Ngeow YF, Lim CT, et al: Colonization and transmission of *Ureaplasma urealyticum* and *Mycoplasma hominis* from mothers to full and preterm babies by normal vaginal delivery. Med J Malaysia 54:242, 1999.

183. Syrogiannopoulos GA, Kapatais-Zoumbos K, Decavalas GO, et al: *Ureaplasma urealyticum* colonization of full term infants: Perinatal acquisition and persistence during early infancy. Pediatr Infect Dis J 9:236, 1990.

184. Sanchez P, Regan JA: Vertical transmission of *Ureaplasma urealyticum* in full term infants. Pediatr Infect Dis J 6:825, 1988.

185. Dinsmoor MJ, Ramamurthy RS, Gibbs RS: Transmission of genital mycoplasmas from mother to neonate in women with prolonged membrane rupture. Pediatr Infect Dis J 8:483, 1989.

186. Foy HM, Kenny GE, Levinsohn EM, et al: Acquisition of mycoplasma and T-strains during infancy. J Infect Dis 121:579, 1970.

187. Galetto Lacour A, Zamora S, Bertrand R, et al: Colonization by *Ureaplasma urealyticum* and chronic lung disease in premature newborn infants under 32 weeks of gestation. Arch Pediatr 8:39, 2001.

188. Quinn PA, Gillian JE, Markestad T, et al: Intrauterine infection with *Ureaplasma urealyticum* as a cause of fatal neonatal pneumonia. Pediatr Infect Dis J 4:538, 1985.

189. Rudd PT, Cassell GH, Waites KB, et al: Experimental production of *Ureaplasma urealyticum* pneumonia and demonstration of age-related susceptibility. Infect Immun 57:918, 1989.

190. Cassell GH, Crouse DT, Waites KB, et al: Does *Ureaplasma urealyticum* cause respiratory disease in newborns? Pediatr Infect Dis J 7:535, 1988.

191. Wang EE, Frayha H, Watts J, et al: The role of *Ureaplasma urealyticum* and other pathogens in the development of chronic lung disease of prematurity. Pediatr Infect Dis J 7:547, 1988.

192. Crouse DT, Cassell GH, Waites KB, et al: Hyperoxia potentiates *Ureaplasma urealyticum* pneumonia in newborn mice. Infect Immun 58:3487, 1990.

193. Ollikainen J, Jeikkaniemi H, Korppi M, et al: *Ureaplasma urealyticum* infection associated with acute respiratory insufficiency and death in premature infants. J Pediatr 122:756, 1993.

194. Waites KB, Rudd PT, Crouse DT, et al: Chronic *Ureaplasma urealyticum* and *Mycoplasma hominis* infections of central nervous systems in preterm infants. Lancet 2:17, 1988.

195. Valencia GB, Banzon F, Cummings M, et al: *Mycoplasma hominis* and *Ureaplasma urealyticum* in neonates with suspected infection. Pediatr Infect Dis J 12:571, 1993.

196. Mardh PA: *Mycoplasma hominis* infections of the central nervous system in newborn infants. Sex Transm Dis 10:331, 1983.

197. Shaw NJ, Pratt BC, Weindling AM: *Ureaplasma* and *Mycoplasma* infections of the central nervous system in preterm infants. Lancet 23:1530, 1989.

198. Gilbert GL, Law F, Macinnes SJ: Chronic *Mycoplasma hominis* infection complicating severe intraventricular hemorrhage, in a premature neonate. Pediatr Infect Dis J 7:817, 1988.

199. Robertson JA, Stemke GW, Dais JW Jr, et al: Proposal of *Ureaplasma parvum* sp. nov. and emended description of *Ureaplasma urealyticum*. Int J Syst Evol Microbiol 52:587, 2002.

200. Bührer C, Hoehn T, Hentschel J: Role of erythromycin for treatment of incipient chronic lung disease in preterm infants colonized with *Ureaplasma urealyticum*. Drugs 61:1893, 2001.

201. Hannaford K, Todd DA, Jeffery H, et al: Role of *Ureaplasma urealyticum* in lung disease of prematurity. Arch Dis Child Fetal Neonatal Ed 81:F162, 1999.

202. Heggie AD, Bar-Shain D, Boxerbaum B, et al: Identification and quantification of ureaplasmas colonizing the respiratory tract and assessment of their role in the development of chronic lung disease in preterm infants. Pediatr Infect Dis J 20(9):854, 2001.

203. Mahoney FJ: Update on diagnosis, management, and prevention of hepatitis B virus infection. Clin Microbiol Rev 12:351, 1999.

204. Lewis E, Shinefield HR, Woodruff BA, et al: Safety of neonatal hepatitis B vaccine administration. Pediatr Infect Dis J 20:1049, 2001.

CHAPTER 70

Diagnosis of Neonatal Sepsis

Mary Catherine Harris and Richard A. Polin

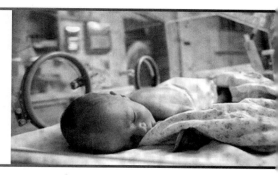

The diagnostic approach to neonatal septicemia usually begins with one of two clinical situations. First, the newborn may exhibit manifestations of infection that necessitate an evaluation for sepsis and the institution of appropriate antimicrobial therapy. Second, there may exist a constellation of factors, either maternal or neonatal, that increase the risk of sepsis. In the case of nosocomial infection, the perinatal history is usually less important. Rather, conditions germane to the infant's environment and medical course provide clues to the cause of late-onset disease.

To approach the diagnosis of sepsis systematically and to assess the risk of infection in a particular infant, an understanding of the predisposing factors for sepsis and the developmental limitations of the neonatal immune system are important. Even so, given the low incidence of neonatal sepsis (<1 to 4 per 1000 live births)[1] and the high rates of morbidity and mortality from early-onset sepsis (10% to 50%) and from late-onset disease with delayed treatment (10% to 20%),[2,3] many uninfected infants are evaluated and treated. In addition, among infants born to mothers receiving intrapartum antimicrobial prophylaxis, blood cultures may be negative despite the presence of systemic infection.[4,5] Physicians must then rely on clinical signs and other laboratory indicators of sepsis.[6,7] Overtreatment on the basis of false-positive test results is therefore commonplace and permissible. The goal of this chapter is to present the diagnostic modalities available to the clinician that provide maximal sensitivity and negative predictive accuracy.

PATHOGENESIS

Early-onset bacterial infections in newborns occur during the first week of life (usually during the first 72 hours).[8,9] Group B streptococcus (GBS)[10,11] and the gram-negative enteric bacteria (the most common bacterial pathogens) colonize the genital and gastrointestinal tracts of pregnant women. The sequence of events responsible for early-onset bacterial infections has been termed the **ascending amniotic infection syndrome.**[12,13] Bacteria colonizing the maternal genital tract spread upward into the amniotic cavity through ruptured (and, on occasion, intact) membranes. Intrauterine infection is initiated when the fetus inhales the infected fluid. Infected infants often deliver prematurely and commonly present with respiratory distress and radiographic evidence of pneumonia.[14] Alternatively, the fetus/newborn may become colonized with a bacterial pathogen at a mucous membrane site, either while in utero or during passage through the birth canal. Bacteremia can occur either through direct extension from heavily colonized sites or after disruption of protective barriers by obstetric trauma (e.g., fetal scalp sampling). These infants may be asymptomatic at the time of birth.

The immaturity of neonatal host defenses is a major risk factor predisposing to bacteremia.[15-17] The innate immunity of the full-term human neonate provides adequate protection against exposure to most pathogens. Because the intrauterine environment is sterile and the fetus has had limited exposure to immunologic stimuli, however, the neonate's immune system has functional impairments, which may render it defenseless against a major assault.[18]

The lack of type-specific antibodies, especially to GBS[19] in full-term and preterm infants; decreased levels of immunoglobulin G (IgG) in preterm infants; absence of immunoglobulin M; reduced neutrophil chemotaxis; and defective oxidative burst in granulocytes are important factors that contribute to the neonate's susceptibility to bacterial infection.[17] Infants born before the third trimester lack adequate concentrations of maternal IgG, inasmuch as most is transported across the placenta in the latter part of gestation. Type-specific IgG against GBS may be deficient in full-term infants if their mothers' concentrations are less than 2 μg/mL.[20] The immune system of the neonate is less able to opsonize and phagocytose bacteria and cannot produce normal amounts of complement, in comparison with adults.[18,21,22] Improvements in neonatal care have enabled the survival of newborns at high risk who require long-term hospitalization and multiple invasive therapies for their survival.[2,23,24] The skin, respiratory, and gastrointestinal tracts of these infants become colonized with flora unique to the nursery.[25,26] Furthermore, IgG concentrations decline after birth and approach a physiologic nadir 2 to 3 months postnatally. The diminished concentration of IgG is a significant variable that predisposes infants with very low birth weights to infection. However, in this patient population, nosocomial infections are common because of the prolonged periods of suboptimal nutrition, invasive monitoring, and multiple procedures associated with intensive care.[24,26,27]

EPIDEMIOLOGY

The bacteriology of neonatal infection has changed since the early 1950s. In the 1970s, GBS replaced *Escherichia coli* as the leading cause of early-onset sepsis.[28] Before this time, the most prevalent pathogens were group A streptococci and other gram-positive cocci in the 1930s, *E. coli* in the 1940s, and *Staphylococcus aureus* in the 1950s. GBS and *E. coli* are currently the most frequent bacterial pathogens that cause sepsis and meningitis in neonates younger than 1 week. Other bacteria, although less common, that should be included in the differential diagnosis of early-onset sepsis[29] are shown in Table 70-1. The spectrum of predominant pathogens responsible for nosocomial sepsis has also changed.[23] Coagulase-negative staphylococci are the most common organisms responsible for late-onset sepsis throughout the world. Other gram-negative organisms, *S. aureus*, enterococci, and *Candida* species are commonly recovered in specimens.[30] This fluctuating pattern of bacterial isolates may reflect changing patterns of antibiotic use and the extended survival of high-risk, immunocompromised neonates.

Table 70–1. Current Predominant Pathogens in Early- and Late-Onset Sepsis

Early
Group B streptococci
Escherichia coli
Listeria monocytogenes
Staphylococcus aureus
Other streptococci
Other gram-negative organisms
  Haemophilus influenzae
  Klebsiella pneumoniae
  Pseudomonas aeruginosa
  Enterobacter species

Late
Coagulase-negative staphylococci
Group B streptococci
Escherichia coli
Klebsiella penumoniae
Pseudomonas aeruginosa
Other gram-negative enteric bacteria
Candida species

CLINICAL MANIFESTATIONS

The neonate who presents with signs of infection should be evaluated promptly for sepsis, and antibiotics should be instituted. The initial signs may be minimal and are often nonspecific. Certain organisms cause fulminant disease (GBS, *E. coli*), whereas others (coagulase-negative staphylococci) may be indolent in manifestation. Fetal tachycardia during the second stage of labor may be the first indication of infection.[31] Infants infected in utero may be depressed at birth, may have low Apgar scores, and may require immediate resuscitation. Temperature instability (both hyperthermia and hypothermia) occurs in two thirds of infants with sepsis.[29] Of full-term newborns with temperatures higher than 37.7° C during the first 4 days of life, 10% have culture-proven bacterial sepsis.[32] Bundling and increased ambient heat, however, may result in a temperature higher than 38° C and prompt an erroneous evaluation for sepsis. Excessive bundling of full-term newborns in a warm environment has been shown to increase rectal temperature at a linear rate of 0.27° C per hour.[33] Fever as a marker in preterm infants is less reliable.[34]

Respiratory distress (apnea, cyanosis, tachypnea, grunting, nasal flaring, chest retractions) occurs in more than half of infants with sepsis. Noninfectious conditions such as aspiration syndromes, hyaline membrane disease, pneumonia, and metabolic problems may also manifest with respiratory distress. In preterm infants with hyaline membrane disease, the chest radiographic appearance cannot be reliably distinguished from that of pneumonia.[35,36] Lethargy, decreased alertness, and decreased tone may also be noted. Feeding intolerance (anorexia, vomiting, ileus, abdominal distention) is often a harbinger of late-onset disease caused by coagulase-negative staphylococci or gram-negative organisms. Necrotizing enterocolitis must also be considered as a cause. Seizures, skin lesions (petechiae, cellulitis, pustules), hepatomegaly, and jaundice have been associated with sepsis in the newborn. Glucoregulation is altered during sepsis in newborns. The development of lactic acidosis and increased glucose requirements may be early markers of sepsis in preterm infants.[37] Indirect hyperbilirubinemia, however, is rarely the only presenting sign.[38] Finally, infants may present with signs of impending respiratory or circulatory collapse. These include apnea, poor perfusion, hypotension, and metabolic acidosis.

DIAGNOSIS

In the absence of either subtle or overt signs of sepsis, the clinician must deduce from the maternal history and neonatal course whether the fetus or the newborn is at significant risk for sepsis. To reiterate, maternal risk factors are less important in infants older than 1 week who require intensive care. Rather, attention should be given to the degree of prematurity, nutritional status, skin barrier, and extent of invasive monitoring.

Historical Risk Factors

Infants who develop early-onset sepsis usually have one or more identifiable risk factors.[39] Risk factors belong to one of four categories: host immunity, socioeconomic factors, obstetric and nursery practices, and health and nutrition of mothers. Prematurity is the greatest risk factor for early-onset bacterial infections.[40] That observation is related both to the reasons for preterm birth (e.g., chorioamnionitis) and to host defense impairments. Additional risk factors for early-onset sepsis include colonization with known pathogens,[41] chorioamnionitis,[40] increased numbers of vaginal examinations during labor, and prolonged (>18 hours) rupture of membranes.[42]

In a multicenter case-control study at seven regional medical centers, 49% of GBS-infected infants and 79% of other infants with sepsis had one or more of the three major risk factors just noted (signs and symptoms of chorioamnionitis, prolonged [>18 hours] rupture of membranes, and colonization with GBS).[43] Older data from 53,039 pregnancies from the National Institute of Neurological and Communicative Disorders and Stroke[40] revealed that the most important perinatal factors for bacterial infection in infants after premature rupture of membranes (PROM) were inflammation of the placenta, gestational age of less than 37 weeks, male sex, Apgar score of less than 6 at 5 minutes of life, and clinical amnionitis (maternal fever, uterine tenderness, purulent amniotic fluid, and sustained fetal tachycardia). Race, parity, maternal age, and duration of labor during PROM were not significant. The risk of culture-proven sepsis in full-term neonates after PROM older than 24 hours was 1.3%. The incidence increased to 8.7% if amnionitis was present. These percentages are comparable with the 0.1% incidence of early-onset sepsis in all newborns.[44] The risk of infection is increased seven to eight times in newborns who weigh less than 2500 g. There is also an 11-fold increase in risk if preterm infants (aged ≤37 weeks) are born after rupture of membranes for more than 24 hours.[40] In the same study, a 5-minute Apgar score of less than 6 with PROM carried a risk of sepsis equal to that with chorioamnionitis.

Maternal colonization with GBS increases the risk of sepsis to 0.5% to 1%.[10,45] Increased risk of neonatal infection has been associated with heavy (in comparison with light) neonatal colonization.[41] Of the 15% to 40% of pregnant women who are colonized with GBS, vertical transmission produces asymptomatic colonization in 40% to 73% of neonates. Overall, only 1% to 2% of newborns born to GBS carriers develop early-onset sepsis, pneumonia, or meningitis.[46] The incidence increases to 5% to 10% if there is heavy maternal colonization, GBS bacteriuria, maternal fever, PROM for longer than 18 hours, and gestation of less than 37 weeks.[42] Twins are at increased risk[9,47] for GBS, as are neonates who have a sibling previously infected with streptococcal disease.[48]

Regardless of the status of vaginal colonization, several other factors increase risk of infection in infants. These include untreated maternal urinary tract infections near delivery,[49] intercourse near delivery,[50] and invasive monitoring.[51] Infant boys have a fourfold increased risk in comparison with infant girls.[52] The first fetus delivered from a twin gestation is more prone to infection,[53] regardless of the pathogen.

Historical factors are also important in assessing the risk of nosocomial disease. Risk factors for nosocomial infection include prematurity, use of H_2 blockers and steroids, use of parenteral alimentation, indwelling venous catheters (especially central catheters), prolonged duration of mechanical ventilation, overcrowding, and heavy workloads.[23,54] In addition, the frequent and prolonged use of antibiotics predisposes these infants at high risk to colonization and subsequent infection with resistant pathogens and fungi.

Cultures

Before the administration of antibiotics, appropriate cultures must be obtained from the neonate. The goal is to isolate bacteria from normally sterile body fluids or tissue to treat a specific infection. Although the blood culture is considered the "gold standard" for the diagnosis of bacterial infection, it is imperfect and does not detect such infection in up to 18% of neonates who eventually die from sepsis.[55] Furthermore, the use of intrapartum antibiotics has substantially reduced the number of positive cultures.[5,56] The yield from positive cultures is greatest if at least 1.0 mL of blood is obtained under sterile conditions from either a peripheral vessel or an umbilical artery.[57,58] Samples from indwelling umbilical venous catheters have high rates of contamination. To diagnose catheter-related bacteremia, especially in neonates who have central catheters, simultaneous blood cultures should be obtained from the catheter and a peripheral site. Incubation of the culture for 48 hours helps identify at least 98% of positive samples. Although quantifying the number of colonies[59] from a particular culture specimen may distinguish contamination from a "true" infection, some cases of bacteremia with coagulase-negative staphylococci have low colony counts. Therefore, this method is not reliable. If the same organism is isolated from blood cultures obtained from multiple sites, true bacteremia is highly likely to be present.[60]

Analysis of cerebrospinal fluid (CSF) is an important part of the evaluation for sepsis. This procedure may be postponed if the infant is hemodynamically unstable or has an uncorrected bleeding diathesis. The potential risks (e.g., hypoxia, trauma) of a lumbar puncture in preterm infants younger than 24 hours with respiratory distress syndrome without historical risk factors, clinical signs, or positive blood cultures may exceed the diagnostic benefit of the procedure.[61] A lumbar puncture is indicated in all newborns with positive blood cultures, because up to 25% of bacteremic infants also have meningitis. Therefore, all symptomatic infants with a high probability of sepsis should undergo a lumbar puncture when clinically stable. The routine use of lumbar puncture in the evaluation of neonatal sepsis during the first week after birth in asymptomatic infants is controversial.[62-65] In a retrospective study from the U.S. Army hospitals, Wiswell and associates concluded that asymptomatic infants with negative blood cultures can have meningitis.[66] They identified 43 positive CSF cultures among 169,000 live births over a 4-year period. Twelve infants (28%) with positive CSF cultures had negative blood cultures. Furthermore, seven of the infants with meningitis were asymptomatic, and four of these infants had negative blood cultures. In contrast, a prospective study by

Schwersenski and coworkers showed that meningitis was rare in asymptomatic high-risk infants.[64] Although 9 (1.3%) of 712 full-term neonates in that study with suspected infection had positive CSF cultures, 8 of the 9 positive cultures were considered to be contaminants.[64] In another study, none of the 284 symptom-free infants born to mothers with obstetric risk factors and normal neonatal white blood cell counts and differential analyses had meningitis.[62] In an infant who has not been pretreated, the yield from a CSF culture is good. Concentrations of CSF protein and glucose and cell counts[67] may allow the clinician to speculate on the diagnosis of meningitis, especially in a pretreated or partially treated infant in whom the CSF has been sterilized. Coagulase-negative staphylococcal meningitis has been reported in the absence of abnormalities of CSF cell count and chemistry profiles.[68]

Urine specimens should be obtained by suprapubic aspiration of the bladder or by catheterization of the urethra. Suprapubic aspiration should not be attempted in thrombocytopenic infants. The presence of bacteria or leukocytes should prompt antimicrobial therapy and an anatomic evaluation of the kidneys and bladder. Culture analysis of urine in infants younger than 72 hours has a low yield[69] (0.5% in first 24 hours after birth)[70] in the absence of anatomic abnormalities of the urinary tract and is not recommended. It is imperative, however, that a urine culture is obtained from all infants evaluated for late-onset disease.

Cultures of superficial body sites (external auditory canal, gastric aspirate, nasopharynx, groin, axilla, and umbilicus) have traditionally been used to identify pathogens in sick neonates when other cultures are negative. Although some centers still use surface cultures to make clinical decisions regarding discontinuation of antimicrobial therapy, most do not. Evans and colleagues analyzed data from 24,584 cultures obtained from 3371 infants and found that the sensitivity, specificity, and positive predictive accuracy of surface cultures were 56%, 82%, and 7.5%, respectively.[71] They concluded that surface cultures were of limited value in identifying the cause of sepsis in neonates.

Adjunctive Tests

The isolation of bacteria from normally sterile body fluids remains the gold standard for the diagnosis of neonatal infection. In the absence of positive cultures, however, several adjunctive tests have been used to diagnose sepsis in infants. Ideally, these tests must identify all infants who have the disease and exclude the diagnosis of sepsis in uninfected neonates; that is, the tests must have high sensitivity and a high negative predictive accuracy. For some tests (e.g., acute-phase reactants and white blood cell indices[72]), serial tests may be more reliable than single determinations in the diagnosis and management of infection. Because bacterial illnesses carry high rates of morbidity and mortality, treatment is initiated in many infants who are not bacteremic. However, adjunct tests may enable the clinician to alter the duration of therapy.

Aspirates

Analysis of tracheal contents is an adjunctive tool in the diagnosis of neonatal pneumonia. In neonates with congenital pneumonia, a tracheal aspirate may yield a positive culture despite a negative blood culture,[73] and identification of organisms on Gram stain from patients with pneumonia can identify the presence of bacteremia.[74] Interleukin-6 and white blood cells are more commonly detected in bronchoalveolar lavage fluid obtained on the first day after birth from preterm ventilated infants with sepsis or after PROM.[75] Similarly, the examination of gastric aspirates for polymorphonuclear leukocytes has been used as a screening procedure for neonatal sepsis.[76] The presence of increased numbers of white blood cells has been thought to represent amnionitis and a fetal inflammatory response. However, a careful analysis of the origin of the cells in gastric aspirate has indicated a maternal origin.[77] Therefore, the presence of polymorphonuclear leukocytes does not indicate fetal infection.

Antigen Tests

In the past, the urine latex particle agglutination (LPA) test was commonly recommended as a rapid immunologic assay for the detection of GBS.[78] It was used to detect GBS antigen in blood and CSF, although concentrated urine was the specimen of choice. Several studies, however, have demonstrated high false-positive rates for the urine LPA test.[79,80] As a consequence, asymptomatic infants should not be screened for sepsis with LPA in the setting of maternal colonization and pretreatment with antibiotics. Thus, the urine LPA test is no longer recommended for the detection of GBS in newborns.

Hematologic Tests

The complete blood cell count (CBC) and differential are the most widely utilized diagnostic tests for the evaluation of possible sepsis. Manroe and associates first examined the relationship between neutrophil indices (absolute polymorphonuclear leukocyte count, absolute immature neutrophil count, and immature/total neutrophil [I/T] ratio) and neonatal infection, and they developed percentile curves for normal full-term infants during the first month after birth.[81] Manroe and associates then used these curves to predict the presence of bacterial disease in sick neonates during the first week after birth. Neutropenia (<1750 cells/mm³) in the presence of respiratory distress in the first 72 hours after birth had an 84% likelihood of signifying bacterial disease and, in the presence of asphyxia, a 68% likelihood of bacterial sepsis.[82] An abnormal I/T ratio, defined as greater than 0.16, was found to be the most sensitive indicator and had an accuracy of 82% in the presence of respiratory distress and 61% in asphyxia. Neutrophilia and low absolute neutrophil count were much less predictive. Other authors have found a similar correlation. Using Manroe's criteria, Benuck and David found that in 28 of 30 cases of early-onset neonatal sepsis, there was at least one abnormality in the CBC.[83] Rodwell and coworkers found a negative predictive value of 99% if the infant had a normal I/T ratio and white blood cell count.[84]

More recent studies and newer automated technologies have suggested reevaluation of previously published reference standards. Schelonka and colleagues examined

193 healthy full-term neonates at 4 hours of age and found a mean I/T ratio of 0.16 with the 10th and 90th percentile values of 0.05 to 0.27.[85] In a study of infants weighing 2000 g or more at birth who were evaluated for suspected bacterial infection, however, Escobar and associates found no significant predictive value to abnormalities in the I/T ratio.[86] On the basis of these data, the reference ranges for I/T ratios in healthy newborns may have to be reevaluated and broadened. There is evidence, however, that the I/T ratio may be useful in the detection of nosocomial disease.[87]

Although neutropenia is a better indicator of infection than neutrophilia, probably because of depletion of neutrophil storage pools during sepsis,[88,89] other unrelated conditions such as pregnancy-induced hypertension and asphyxia are associated with neutropenia.[89,90] Rodwell and coworkers found that 84% of 170 infants with neutropenia did not have an infectious cause; other causes included pregnancy-induced hypertension, birth asphyxia, prematurity, multiple gestation, and low birth weight.[91] In another study, Escobar and associates found (1) an odds ratio of 2.8 (confidence interval [CI], 1.5 to 5.4) for the development of neonatal sepsis if the absolute neutrophil count was less than the 10th percentile and the mother did not receive intrapartum antibiotics and (2) an odds ratio of 3.6 (CI, 1.4 to 8.9) if the mother received intrapartum antibiotics.[86] In this study, a new reference curve for full-term infants was developed, significantly raising both the 10th and 90th percentile curves for absolute neutrophil counts. These boundaries have not been tested prospectively across a wide range of patients.

Other data have suggested that previously published indexes for full-term infants may not be reliable for the diagnosis of bacterial infection in preterm infants. Noninfected preterm infants weighing less than 1500 g exhibited a high incidence of neutropenia, although absolute immature neutrophil counts and I/T ratios were not significantly different from those in full-term newborns.[87]

The total white blood cell count used independently is less valuable. Fewer than half of the infants with counts of less than 5000/mm³ and more than 20,000/mm³ are infected.[1] Qualitative changes in neutrophils, such as toxic granulations and vacuoles, are also unreliable markers of infection.[92,93] Thrombocytopenia, defined as a platelet count less than 100,000/mm³, occurs in 62% of cases of neonatal sepsis.[94] However, low platelet counts commonly occur in infants with respiratory distress syndrome, asphyxia, necrotizing enterocolitis, and disseminated intravascular coagulation. A count of less than 150,000/mm³ is not a sensitive indicator of sepsis, although the specificity and negative predictive accuracy are greater than 90%.[84]

In evaluating the performance of neutrophil indices as screening tests for neonatal sepsis, the timing of the test is very important. Early in the course of illness, neutrophil indices may be normal.[95] Both sensitivity and negative predictive value are improved by performance of a second screen 12 to 24 hours later. Rozycki and associates found that 21% of infants had a normal CBC obtained at least 4 hours before the positive blood culture[96];

Greenberg and Yoder found a 0% false-negative rate when the CBC was taken at 12 to 24 hours after birth.[97]

In conclusion, the neutrophil indices are extremely valuable indirect tests for the evaluation of infants with suspected sepsis. Because of recent hematologic data, the increased rates of survival of premature infants, and the use of newer automated technologies, reference ranges may have to be broadened and reevaluated in populations at risk. Finally, the value of neutrophil indices is greatly enhanced with the passage of time, inasmuch as there is a latent period when counts are often normal. Repeated screens at 24 to 36 hours are strongly recommended.

Acute-Phase Reactants

Acute phase reactants are nonspecific primitive proteins that are produced by hepatocytes in response to cellular degeneration, infection, and trauma.[1] Normal values may vary, depending on the assay methods. These tests are used independently or in conjunction with other diagnostic aids as markers for sepsis in newborns.

The microerythrocyte sedimentation rate, a response to increased amounts of acute-phase reactants, correlates well with the Wintrobe erythrocyte sedimentation rate.[98] It can be performed at the patient's bedside by filling a microhematocrit tube with capillary blood, placing the tube vertically for 1 hour, and recording the rate at which the red blood cell column falls. Because normal values are proportional to the age of the infant up to 15 mm/hour, many infected infants can be identified by an equation: age of the infant (days) + 3 = upper limit of normal value. Problems with the test include a delay in the rise for onset of infection, false-negative results in disseminated intravascular coagulation, and false-positive results in Coombs test–positive hemolytic anemia.

C-reactive protein (CRP) is a globulin produced by the liver in response to inflammation that may modulate the immune response.[99,100] Its measurement has been widely promoted as a way to reduce the duration of antibiotic therapy in infants with suspected and proven sepsis.[101-103] A value of 1.0 mg/dL is generally accepted as the upper limit of normal. The most widely used technique for measurement of CRP is laser nephelometry. The largest prospective study evaluating CRP was published by Benitz and coworkers.[104] In this study, CRP was measured in 1002 infants with suspected early-onset sepsis at the time of initial evaluation (CRP #1) and on each of the next two mornings (CRP #2 and CRP #3). CRP #1, the initial determination, had a poor sensitivity (35.0%) for proven sepsis. In contrast, CRP #2 had a sensitivity of 78.9% for proven sepsis. The sensitivity of CRP #2 and #3 for proven sepsis was 88.9%; the negative predictive value was 99.7% for proven or probable early-onset sepsis. Positive predictive values were low (<10%); however, marked elevations of CRP (>6 mg/dL) were associated with a higher (60%) probability of sepsis. Therefore, as with most diagnostic tests for early-onset sepsis, the high negative predictive accuracy of serial CRP determinations (obtained 8 to 12 hours after birth) was helpful in deciding which infants did not require antibiotic therapy or identifying those in whom antibiotics could be discontinued after a brief course.[103,105,106]

Sepsis Screens

Although diagnostic tests are frequently ordered so as to identify infants with probable sepsis, their main benefit is to exclude disease in infants with a low probability of infection rather than to identify infected neonates. Sepsis screens are combinations of diagnostic tests, whose major value has been to exclude the diagnosis of sepsis (mainly early-onset) in uninfected neonates (i.e., they reassure the clinician that infection is not present). Consequently, antibiotic therapy is initiated in fewer patients, and therapy can be discontinued earlier.[107] A positive sepsis screen is defined as two or more abnormal laboratory values obtained concurrently. Philip and Hewitt used five tests (I/T ratio, absolute leukocyte count, CRP measurement, micro-erythrocyte sedimentation rate, and haptoglobin) to screen infants admitted for suspected sepsis or meningitis.[108] A positive sepsis screen was defined as two or more abnormal test results. The sensitivity of the sepsis screen was 93%, and the positive predictive accuracy was 39%. When fewer than two test results were positive, the negative predictive accuracy was 99%. Gerdes and Polin performed sepsis screens (I/T ratio, white blood count, CRP measurement, and micro-erythrocyte sedimentation rate) 12 to 24 hours apart.[109] This method identified 100% of infected infants (13) and had a negative predictive accuracy of 100%. Using a hematologic scoring system employing seven variables, Rodwell and coworkers obtained similar results (negative predictive accuracy of 99% when the score was <2).[84] Sepsis screens are also useful in the evaluation of infants with suspected nosocomial infection. Use of the same criteria (developed by Philip and Hewitt) in the evaluation of late-onset sepsis had an 83% sensitivity and 74% specificity.[110] A white blood cell count higher than 20,000/mm^3 added to these criteria increased the sensitivity to 100%.[110] In the infant intensive care unit at Children's Hospital of Philadelphia, this screen had 100% sensitivity and 88% specificity for the diagnosis of nosocomial infection.[87]

Diagnostic Approach

Symptomatic Infants

An evaluation for sepsis should be considered for any infant who is symptomatic, regardless of the presence or absence of risk factors. A detailed review of the maternal history, physical examination of the neonate, and continued assessment of vital signs should be performed. Blood should be sent for culture, and sepsis screens (white blood cell count, differential count, and CRP measurement) should be obtained at 12 and 36 hours after birth. In addition, CSF specimens for cell counts, chemistry profiles, and culture should be obtained in all symptomatic infants evaluated for sepsis. A urine specimen in infants older than 3 days is also important in the diagnosis of urosepsis. Radiographic examination of the chest and/or abdomen should be available if relevant signs are present. Antibiotics can be stopped in a symptomatic infant when the clinical suspicion of sepsis is low, the physical examination findings normalize within 12 hours, and the sepsis screens are negative.

Asymptomatic Infants

The workup for sepsis in asymptomatic patients begins with the identification of risk factors. The three main risk factors for sepsis are maternal colonization with GBS at delivery, signs and symptoms of chorioamnionitis, and PROM for more than 18 hours. In asymptomatic infants aged more than 35 weeks of gestation born to women with risk factors, there are two principal options: observation alone and observation plus diagnostic studies. We recommend the latter because of the difficulty of observing infants closely enough for the early, subtle signs of sepsis. We obtain the sepsis screen (white blood cell count, differential count, and CRP measurement) at 12 hours after birth rather than immediately after birth, because of the greater likelihood of a positive test result with passage of time. If the sepsis screen is positive, we recommend obtaining a blood culture and treating until cultures are confirmed negative (48 hours). In asymptomatic infants younger than 35 weeks of gestation with one or more risk factors for sepsis, we recommend that broad-spectrum antibiotics be started as soon as cultures are obtained. The sepsis screen should be obtained at 12 and 36 hours after birth. We believe that if the screens are negative, if cultures remain negative, and if the physical examination findings are normal, antibiotics can be discontinued and the infant observed. In the asymptomatic infant with a positive sepsis screen, the decision to continue antibiotic therapy should be individualized. Infants born to women who have received intrapartum antibiotics should probably receive a complete course of treatment. Clinical acumen and knowledge of contributing factors are necessary for diagnosing neonatal septicemia. Although the parental stress and the expense of evaluating and treating an infant can be significant, the therapy for presumed sepsis is benign in comparison to the consequences of not treating the truly infected infant. The adage that "3 days of ampicillin and gentamicin never killed anybody" has some merit in this context. Rapid and appropriate intervention results in overtreatment of many infants. The use and interpretation of diagnostic aids as discussed in this chapter supplement the clinician's assessment and result in more precise care of the neonate.

REFERENCES

1. Klein JO, Marcy SM: Bacterial sepsis and meningitis. In Remington JJ, Klein JO (eds): Infectious Diseases of the Fetus and Newborn Infant. Philadelphia, WB Saunders, 1995, pp 835-890.
2. Donowitz LG, Haley CE, Gregory WW: Neonatal intensive care unit bacteremia: Emergence of gram-positive bacteria as major pathogens. Am J Infect Control 15:141, 1987.
3. Hemming VG, Overall JC Jr, Britt MR: Nosocomial infections in a newborn intensive-care unit: Results of forty-one months of surveillance. N Engl J Med 294:1310, 1976.
4. Bromberger P, Lawrence JM, Braun D, et al: The influence of intrapartum antibiotics on the clinical spectrum of early-onset group B streptococcal infection in term infants. Pediatrics 106:244, 2000.

5. Schrag SJ, Zywicki S, Farley MM, et al: Group B streptococcal disease in the era of intrapartum antibiotic prophylaxis. N Engl J Med 342:15, 2000.

6. Benitz WE, Gould JB, Druzin ML: Antimicrobial prevention of early-onset group B streptococcal sepsis: Estimates of risk reduction based on a critical literature review. Pediatrics 103(6):e78, 1999.

7. Boyer KM, Gadzala CA, Kelly PD, et al: Selective intrapartum chemoprophylaxis of neonatal group B streptococcal early-onset disease. III. Interruption of mother-to-infant transmission. J Infect Dis 148:810, 1983.

8. Kaftan H, Kinney JS: Early onset neonatal bacterial infections. Semin Perinatol 22:15, 1998.

9. Pass MA, Khare S, Dillon HC Jr: Twin pregnancies: Incidence of group B streptococcal colonization and disease. J Pediatr 97:635, 1980.

10. Baker CJ: Group B streptococcal infections. Clin Perinatol 24:59, 1997.

11. Dillon HC Jr, Gray E, Pass MA, et al: Anorectal and vaginal carriage of group B streptococci during pregnancy. J Infect Dis 145:794, 1982.

12. Blanc WA: Pathways of fetal and early neonatal infection. J Pediatr 59:473, 1961.

13. Larsen B, Galask RP: Protection of the fetus against infection. Semin Perinatol 1:183, 1977.

14. Romero R, Manogue KR, Mitchell MD, et al: Infection and labor IV: Cachectin—tumor necrosis factor in the amniotic fluid of women with intraamniotic infection and preterm labor. Am J Obstet Gynecol 161:336, 1989.

15. Fleer A, Gerards LJ, Verhoef J: Host defence to bacterial infection in the neonate. J Hosp Infect 11(Suppl A):320, 1988.

16. Hill HR: Host defenses in the neonate: Prospects for enhancement. Semin Perinatol 9:2, 1985.

17. Wilson CB: Immunologic basis for increased susceptibility of the neonate to infection. J Pediatr 108:1, 1986.

18. Quie PG: Antimicrobial defenses in the neonate. Semin Perinatol 14(4, Suppl 1):2, 1990.

19. Gray BM, Pritchard DG, Dillon HC Jr: Seroepidemiology of group B streptococcus type III colonization at delivery. J Infect Dis 159:1139, 1989.

20. Baker CJ, Kasper PL: Correlation of maternal antibody deficiency with susceptibility to neonatal group B streptococcal infection. N Engl J Med 294:753, 1976.

21. Berger M: Complement deficiency and neutrophil dysfunction as risk factors for bacterial infection in newborns and the role of granulocyte transfusion in therapy. Rev Infect Dis 12(Suppl 4):S401, 1990.

22. Yoder MC, Polin RA: Immunotherapy of neonatal septicemia. Pediatr Clin North Am 33:481, 1986.

23. Baltimore RS: Neonatal nosocomial infections. Semin Perinatol 22:25, 1998.

24. Goldmann DA, Durbin WA, Freeman J: Nosocomial infections in a neonatal intensive care unit. J Infect Dis 144:449, 1981.

25. Pfaller MA, Wenzel RP: Coagulase-negative staphylococci. In Donowitz LG (ed): Hospital Acquired Infection in the Pediatric Patient. Baltimore, Williams & Wilkins, 1988, pp 263-270.

26. St. Geme JW III, Harris MC: Coagulase-negative staphylococcal infection in the neonate. Clin Perinatol 18:281, 1991.

27. Gaynes RP, Martone WJ, Culver DH, et al: Comparison of rates of nosocomial infections in neonatal intensive care units in the United States. Am J Med 91(Suppl 3B):192S, 1991.

28. Freedman RM, Ingram DL, Gross I, et al: A half century of neonatal sepsis at Yale. Am J Dis Child 135:140, 1981.

29. Klein JO: Bacteriology of neonatal sepsis. Pediatr Infect Dis J 9:778, 1990.

30. Gladstone IM, Ehrenkranz RA, Edberg SC, et al: A ten-year review of neonatal sepsis and comparison with the previous fifty-year experience. Pediatr Infect Dis J 9:819, 1990.

31. Schiano MA, Hauth JC, Gilstrap LC: Second-stage fetal tachycardia and neonatal infection. Am J Obstet Gynecol 148:779, 1984.

32. Voora S, Srinivasan G, Lilien LD, et al: Fever in full-term newborns in the first four days of life. Pediatrics 69:40, 1982.

33. Cheng TL, Partridge JC: Effect of bundling and high environmental temperature on neonatal body temperature. Pediatrics 92:238, 1993.

34. Buetow KC, Klein WS, Lane RB: Septicemia in premature infants. Am J Dis Child 110:29, 1965.

35. Ablow RC, Driscoll SG, Effman EC, et al: A comparison of early-onset group B streptococcal neonatal infection and the respiratory distress syndrome. N Engl J Med 294:65, 1976.

36. Leslie GI, Scurr RD, Burr PA: Early-onset bacterial pneumonia: A comparison with severe hyaline membrane disease. Aust Pediatr J 17:202, 1981.

37. Fitzgerald MJ, Goto M, Myers TF, et al: Early metabolic effects of sepsis in the preterm infant: Lactic acidosis and increased glucose requirement. J Pediatr 121:951, 1992.

38. Maisels JM, Kring E: Risk of sepsis in newborns with severe hyperbilirubinemia. Pediatrics 90:741, 1992.

39. Benitz WE, Gould JB, Druzin ML: Risk factors for early-onset group B streptococcal sepsis: Estimation of odds ratio by critical literature review. Pediatrics 103(6):e77, 1999.

40. St. Geme JW III, Murray DL, Carter J, et al: Perinatal bacterial infection after prolonged rupture of amniotic membranes: An analysis of risk and management. J Pediatr 104:608, 1984.

41. Dillon HC Jr, Khare S, Gray BM: Group B streptococcal carriage and disease: A 6-year prospective study. J Pediatr 110:31, 1987.

42. Givner LB, Baker CJ: The prevention and treatment of neonatal group B streptococcal infections. Adv Pediatr Infect Dis 3:65, 1988.

43. Schuchat A, Zywicki SS, Dinsmoor MJ, et al: Risk factors and opportunities for prevention of early-onset neonatal sepsis: A multicenter case-control study. Pediatrics 105:21, 2000.

44. Siegel JD, McCracken GM Jr: Sepsis neonatorum. N Engl J Med 304:642, 1981.

45. Schuchat A: Group B streptococcus. Lancet 353:51, 1999.

46. Baker CJ, Edwards MS: Group B streptococcal infections: Perinatal impact and prevention methods. Ann N Y Acad Sci 549:193, 1988.

47. Edwards MS, Jackson CV, Baker CJ: Increased risk of group B streptococcal disease in twins. JAMA 245:2044, 1981.

48. Gerdes JS: Clinicopathologic approach to the diagnosis of neonatal sepsis. Clin Perinatol 18:361, 1991.

49. Naeye RL: Causes of the excessive rates of perinatal mortality and prematurity in pregnancies complicated by maternal urinary-tract infections. N Engl J Med 300:819, 1979.

50. Naeye RL: Coitus and associated amniotic fluid infections. N Engl J Med 301:1198, 1979.

51. Ledger WJ: Complications associated with invasive monitoring. Semin Perinatol 2:187, 1978.

52. Washburn TC, Medearis DN Jr, Childs B: Sex differences in susceptibility to infections. Pediatrics 35:57, 1965.

53. Benirschke K: Routes and types of infection in the fetus and newborn. Am J Dis Child 99:714, 1960.

54. Kawagoe JY, Segre CAM, Pereira CR, et al: Risk factors for nosocomial infections in critically ill newborns: A 5-year prospective cohort study. Am J Infect Control 29:109, 2001.

55. Squire E, Favara B, Todd J: Diagnosis of neonatal bacterial infection: Hematologic and pathologic findings in fatal and nonfatal cases. Pediatrics 64:60, 1979.

56. From the Centers for Disease Control and Prevention: Early-onset group B streptococcal disease—United States 1998-1998. JAMA 284:1508, 2000.

57. Cowett RM, Peter G, Hakanson DO, et al: Reliability of bacterial culture of blood obtained from an umbilical artery catheter. J Pediatr 88:1035, 1976.

58. Schelonka RL, Chai MK, Yoder BA, et al: Volume of blood required to detect common neonatal pathogens. J Pediatr 129:275, 1996.

59. St. Geme JW III, Bell LM, Baumgart S, et al: Distinguishing sepsis from blood culture contamination in young infants with blood cultures growing coagulase-negative staphylococci. Pediatrics 86:157, 1990.

60. Wiswell TE, Hachey WE: Multiple site blood cultures in the initial evaluation for neonatal sepsis during the first week of life. Pediatr Infect Dis J 10:365, 1991.

61. Eldadah M, Frenkel LD, Hiatt M, et al: Evaluation of routine lumbar punctures in newborn infants with respiratory distress syndrome. Pediatr Infect Dis J 6:243, 1987.

62. Fielkow S, Reuter S, Gotoff SP: Cerebrospinal fluid examination in symptom-free infants with risk factors for infection. J Pediatr 119:971, 1991.

63. Hristeva L, Bowler I, Booy R, et al: Value of cerebrospinal fluid examination in the diagnosis of meningitis in the newborn. Arch Dis Child 69:514, 1993.

64. Schwersenski J, McIntyre L, Bauer CR: Lumbar puncture frequency and cerebrospinal fluid analysis in the neonate. Am J Dis Child 145:54, 1991.

65. Visser VE, Hall RT: Lumbar puncture in the evaluation of suspected neonatal sepsis. J Pediatr 96:1063, 1980.

66. Wiswell TE, Baumgart S, Gannon CM, et al: No lumbar puncture in the evaluation for early neonatal sepsis: Will meningitis be missed? Pediatrics 95:803, 1995.

67. Sarff LD, Platt LH, McCracken GH Jr: Cerebrospinal fluid evaluation in neonates: Comparison of high-risk infants with and without meningitis. J Pediatr 88:473, 1976.

68. Gruskay J, Harris MC, Costarino AT, et al: Neonatal *Staphylococcus epidermidis* meningitis with unremarkable CSF examination results. Am J Dis Child 143:580, 1989.

69. Visser VE, Hall RT: Urine culture in the evaluation of suspected neonatal sepsis. J Pediatr 94:635, 1979.

70. DiGeronimo RJ: Lack of efficacy of the urine culture as part of the initial workup of suspected neonatal sepsis. Pediatr Infect Dis J 11:764, 1992.

71. Evans ME, Schaffner W, Federspiel CF, et al: Sensitivity, specificity, and predictive value of body surface cultures in a neonatal intensive care unit. JAMA 259:248, 1988.

72. Hachey WE, Wiswell TE: Limitations in the usefulness of urine latex particle agglutination tests and hematologic measurements in diagnosing neonatal sepsis during the first week of life. J Perinatol 12:240, 1992.

73. Sherman MP, Goetzman BW, Ahlfors CE, et al: Tracheal aspiration and its clinical correlates in the diagnosis of congenital pneumonia. Pediatrics 65:258, 1980.

74. Sherman MP, Chance KH, Goetzman BW: Gram's stains of tracheal secretions predict neonatal bacteremia. Am J Dis Child 138:848, 1984.

75. Grigg JM, Barber A, Silverman M: Increased levels of bronchoalveolar lavage fluid interleukin-6 in preterm ventilated infants after prolonged rupture of membranes. Am Rev Respir Dis 145:782, 1992.

76. Ramos A, Stern L: Relationship of premature rupture of the membranes to gastric fluid aspirate in the newborn. Am J Obstet Gynecol 105:1247, 1969.

77. Vasan U, Lim DM, Greenstein RM, et al: Origin of gastric polymorphonuclear leukocytes in infants born after prolonged rupture of membranes. J Pediatr 91:69, 1977.

78. Baker CJ, Rench MA: Commercial latex particle agglutination for detection of group B streptococcal antigen in body fluids. J Pediatr 102:393, 1983.

79. Harris MC, Deuber C, Polin RA, et al: Investigation of apparent false-positive urine latex particle agglutination tests for the detection of group B streptococcus antigen. J Clin Microbiol 27:2214, 1989.

80. Sanchez PJ, Siegel JD, Cushion NB, et al: Significance of a positive urine group B streptococcal latex agglutination test in neonates. J Pediatr 116:601, 1990.

81. Manroe BL, Weinberg AG, Rosenfeld CR, et al: The neonatal blood count in health and disease. I. Reference values for neutrophilic cells. J Pediatr 95:88, 1979.

82. Manroe BL, Rosenfeld CR, Weinberg AG, et al: The differential leukocyte count in the assessment and outcome of early-onset neonatal group B streptococcal disease. J Pediatr 91:632, 1977.

83. Benuck I, David RJ: Sensitivity of published neutrophil indexes in identifying newborn infants with sepsis. J Pediatr 103:961, 1983.

84. Rodwell RL, Leslie AL, Tudehope DI: Early diagnosis of neonatal sepsis using a hematologic scoring system. J Pediatr 112:761, 1988.

85. Schelonka RL, Yoder BA, desJardins SE: Peripheral leukocyte count and leukocyte indexes in healthy newborn term infants. J Pediatr 125:603, 1994.

86. Escobar GJ, Li D, Armstrong MA, et al: Neonatal sepsis workups in infants ≥2000 grams at birth: A population-based study. Pediatrics 106:256, 2000.

87. Ianni BD, Gerdes JS, Shah AR, et al: Predicting nosocomial infection in infants using the sepsis screen. Pediatr Res 29:282A, 1991.

88. Baley JE, Stork EK, Warkentin PI, Shurin SB: Neonatal neutropenia: Clinical manifestations, cause, and outcome. Am J Dis Child 142:1161, 1988.

89. Engle WD, Rosenfeld CR. Neutropenia in high-risk neonates. J Pediatr 105:982, 1984.

90. Koenig JM, Christensen RD: Incidence, neutrophil kinetics, and natural history of neonatal neutropenia associated with maternal hypertension. N Engl J Med 321:557, 1989.

91. Rodwell RL, Taylor KM, Tudehope DI, Gray PH: Hematologic scoring system in early diagnosis of sepsis in neutropenic newborns. Pediatr Infect Dis J 12:372, 1993.

92. Liu C-H, Lehan C, Speer ME, et al: Degenerative changes in neutrophils: An indicator of bacterial infection. Pediatrics 74:823, 1984.

93. Zipursky A, Palko J, Milner R, et al: The hematology of bacterial infections in premature infants. Pediatrics 57:839, 1976.

94. Modanlou HD, Ortiz OB: Thrombocytopenia in neonatal infection. Clin Pediatr 20:402, 1981.

95. Christensen RD, Rothstein G, Hill HR, Hall RT: Fetal early onset group B streptococcal sepsis with normal leukocyte counts. Pediatr Infect Dis 4:242, 1985.

96. Rozycki HJ, Stahl GE, Baumgart S: Impaired sensitivity of a single early leukocyte count in screening for neonatal sepsis. Pediatr Infect Dis J 6:440, 1987.

97. Greenberg DN, Yoder BA: Changes in the differential white blood cell count in screening for group B streptococcal sepsis. Pediatr Infect Dis J 9:886, 1990.

98. Adler SM, Denton RL: The erythrocyte sedimentation rate in the newborn period. J Pediatr 56:942, 1975.

99. Da Silva O, Ohlsson A, Kenyon C: Accuracy of leukocyte indices and C-reactive protein for diagnosis of neonatal sepsis: A critical review. Pediatr Infect Dis J 14:362, 1995.

100. Kushner I, Feldman G: Control of the acute phase response: Demonstration of C-reactive protein synthesis and secretion by hepatocytes during acute inflammation in the rabbit. J Exp Med 48:466, 1976.

101. Ehl S, Gering B, Partmann P, et al: C-reactive protein is a useful marker for guiding duration of antibiotic therapy in suspected neonatal bacterial infection. Pediatrics 99:216, 1997.

102. Philip AGS: Response of C-reactive protein in neonatal group B streptococcal infection. Pediatr Infect Dis J 4:145, 1985.

103. Pourcyrous M, Bada HS, Korones SB, et al: Significance of serial C-reactive protein responses in neonatal infection and other disorders. Pediatrics 92:431, 1993.

104. Benitz WE, Han MY, Madan A, Ramachandra P: Serial serum C-reactive protein levels in the diagnosis of neonatal infection. Pediatrics 102(4):e41, 1998.

105. Kite P, Millar MR, Gorham P, et al: Comparison of five tests used in diagnosis of neonatal bacteremia. Arch Dis Child 63:639, 1988.

106. Philip AGS, Mills PC: Use of C-reactive protein in minimizing antibiotic exposure: Experience with infants initially admitted to a well-baby nursery. Pediatrics 106(1):e4, 2000.

107. Philip AGS: Decreased use of antibiotics using a neonatal sepsis screening technique. J Pediatr 98:795, 1981.

108. Philip AGS, Hewitt JR: Early diagnosis of neonatal sepsis. Pediatrics 65:1036, 1980.

109. Gerdes JS, Polin RA: Sepsis screen in neonates with evaluation of plasma fibronectin. Pediatr Infect Dis J 6:443, 1987.

110. Philip AGS: Detection of neonatal sepsis of late onset. JAMA 247:489, 1982.

CHAPTER 71

Prevention and Treatment of Neonatal Sepsis

Mary Catherine Harris and John Casey

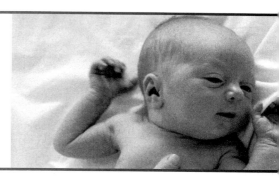

During the newborn period, infection remains one of the most significant causes of neonatal morbidity and mortality, despite increasing sophistication in infant intensive care and the use of broad-spectrum antimicrobial agents.[1-3] Most neonatal bacterial infections occur during the first week of life **(early-onset sepsis)** after exposure to microorganisms colonizing the maternal genital tract.[4,5] Since the 1990s, however, the improved survival of low-birth-weight, critically ill neonates has created a population of highly susceptible infants who are hospitalized for extended periods and are at increased risk to develop **nosocomial disease.**[2,6,7] As a consequence, there has been a significant increase in the number of bacterial infections that have their onset beyond the first week of life **(late-onset disease).**

Since the 1970s, **group B streptococcus (GBS)** has been the leading cause of sepsis, meningitis, and death in neonates.[1,4,8,9] Although the incidence of colonization differs among locales, 15% to 40% of pregnant women are colonized with GBS in the gastrointestinal or genital tract, and 1% to 2% of these colonized mothers deliver infants with early-onset disease.[1,8] Infants may inhale or swallow contaminated amniotic fluid during the fetal period or after passage through a colonized birth canal.[10-12] Although less frequent in occurrence, gram-negative microorganisms also account for a substantial number of cases of neonatal disease.[2,7] The pathogenesis of infections with these organisms is similar.

Because of the increased susceptibility of newborn infants to bacterial infection and the continued high mortality from bacterial disease, more recent efforts have been directed toward effective screening, prevention, and treatment strategies.[13-15] This chapter focuses on the prevention and treatment of early-onset disease caused by GBS and other pathogens. Therapeutic strategies for late-onset or nosocomial disease also are discussed.[13]

PREVENTION STRATEGIES

Because of the high incidence of early-onset GBS disease and the initial case reports of greater than 50% mortality, efforts have focused largely on the prevention of infection.[14,16-18] Strategies include **chemoprophylaxis,** to prevent or limit the exposure of the neonate to pathogenic organisms, and **maternal immunization,** to stimulate the production of maternal antibodies against the offending pathogen.[19-22] Chemoprophylactic strategies may involve prenatal, postnatal, or intrapartum administration of antimicrobial agents (Table 71-1).

Chemoprophylaxis

Initial chemoprophylaxis studies focused on the elimination of GBS colonization from pregnant women, particularly during the last trimester. Although GBS colonization was transiently reduced after treatment, during pregnancy women naturally gain and lose colonization with GBS.[23,24] Knowing a mother's colonization status or treating mothers with antibiotic prophylaxis remote from term has little predictive accuracy regarding the presence or absence of GBS colonization at the time of delivery. Another limitation of this strategy is that treatment of sexual partners would be required for any regimen that requires eradication of the carrier state during pregnancy.[17,25,26] The ratio of colonized mothers to infected infants ranges from 50 to 1 to 100 to 1, so many mothers and infants would be treated to prevent one infected neonate.[7] Another limitation of prenatal therapy late in the third trimester is that many of the infants who develop early-onset sepsis are delivered prematurely and would not be treated successfully.

Additional studies have advocated the postnatal administration of penicillin for the eradication of GBS disease. The original observation was from Steigman and colleagues,[27] who administered a single dose of penicillin G

Table 71–1. Strategies for the Prevention of Early-Onset Group B Streptococcus Disease

Chemoprophylaxis
  Prenatal
  Postnatal
  Intrapartum
Immunoprophylaxis

at birth to prevent neonatal gonococcal ophthalmia and coincidentally saw no GBS disease in the nursery during the same time period. Subsequently, Siegel and colleagues[28,29] performed a large controlled trial of penicillin therapy at birth to prevent neonatal GBS disease. There were several problems, however, which interfered with the interpretation of study results. First, blood cultures were not obtained before therapy, so cases of GBS sepsis may have been missed. Second, the mortality in the penicillin-treated group was higher than in controls. Third, the authors also reported an increase in sepsis with resistant gram-negative organisms during the study period. In a subsequent study of low-birth-weight infants (<2500 g), Pyati and coworkers[30] reported no decrement in the incidence of GBS sepsis after penicillin administration at birth. Penicillin prophylaxis at birth may be effective in infants who acquire infection at or shortly after the time of delivery. Postnatal prophylaxis does not prevent most cases of early-onset GBS disease, however. As an alternative to treating newborns, maternal chemoprophylaxis during the intrapartum period has been suggested as a method to prevent neonatal GBS colonization and disease.[4,31-33] Further details of this therapy are provided subsequently.

Immunoprophylaxis

Immunoprophylaxis of women of childbearing age also has been suggested as an effective means for the prevention of GBS disease.[8,34] Early studies showed that antibodies formed against the specific capsular polysaccharide antigens of GBS were transferred across the placenta and provided protection against invasive disease in the neonate.[35,36] Immunization of women of childbearing age may offer protection against GBS disease. There are several problems, however, with this approach. Nearly 60% of maternally derived IgG is transported to the fetus during the last 10 weeks of pregnancy, so protection is not conferred to a fetus born prematurely.[37-39] In addition, not all adults mount an antibody response after immunization. Finally, new serotypes of GBS (serotypes IV through VIII) that cause neonatal disease have been described.[40-42] Because immunoprophylaxis of GBS disease involves formulation of a multivalent conjugate vaccine directed against the predominant capsular polysaccharides, effective prevention strategies need to reflect contemporary patterns of GBS colonization.[18,33,40] In addition, immunoprophylaxis is not likely to be valuable in the prevention of infection with gram-negative organisms, in which resistance is mediated primarily by the IgM fraction of immunoglobulin. IgM does not cross the placenta in any substantial amount because of its size and cannot convey protection.

Current Guidelines for the Prevention of Early-Onset Group B Streptococcus Disease

In the 1980s and 1990s, numerous controlled clinical trials showed the efficacy of intrapartum chemoprophylaxis for the prevention of neonatal GBS disease.[4,17,43] This strategy has distinct advantages given the frequency of in utero infection with GBS. Because approximately 50% to 70% of early-onset GBS disease begins in utero, intervention is required before delivery for these infants to be treated effectively.[12,33] In 1979, Yow and colleagues[44] showed that ampicillin administered to women during labor significantly reduced neonatal colonization with GBS. The sample size in this study was too small, however, to provide data regarding disease prevention. In the 1980s, Boyer and associates[17,23,45] reported results of a randomized controlled trial of the effects of intrapartum ampicillin prophylaxis on the incidence of neonatal GBS colonization and disease. Women with prenatal carriage of GBS and perinatal risk factors, such as premature labor, prolonged rupture of membranes, or fever, were randomized to receive ampicillin or to serve as controls. Ampicillin virtually eliminated the vertical transmission of GBS[46]; GBS colonization was detected only in women with intrapartum fever or in whom the duration of maternal therapy before delivery was brief. Most importantly, these authors noted a decrease in the incidence of GBS disease in high-risk infants.[24,25] Despite differences in study design, several additional clinical trials to date have confirmed the efficacy of intrapartum chemoprophylaxis for the prevention of neonatal GBS disease.[1,7,47] The aforementioned observations have served as the foundation for current recommendations for intrapartum chemoprophylaxis against neonatal GBS disease.

In 1992, the American College of Obstetricians and Gynecologists (ACOG) and the American Academy of Pediatrics (AAP) proposed two different approaches for the prevention of perinatal GBS infections.[48,49] Although both groups recommended intrapartum antimicrobial prophylaxis, the criteria used to identify candidates for therapy differed. The AAP Committee on Infectious Diseases and the Committee on the Fetus and Newborn issued guidelines indicating that women should be screened at 26 to 28 weeks of gestation and prophylaxis administered in the presence of maternal colonization with GBS and additional risk factors. The risk factors included preterm labor (<37 weeks' gestation), premature rupture of membranes (<37 weeks), prolonged rupture of membranes (>18 hours), fever, and multiple births.[19] Additional indications for intrapartum chemoprophylaxis included a previous sibling with invasive disease and maternal bacteriuria. In the same year, the ACOG issued a similar position paper in which they accepted the concept that a substantial portion of neonatal disease could be prevented by maternal treatment during labor.[48] They suggested, however, that prophylaxis of high-risk mothers without screening cultures might be as clinically effective and perhaps more cost-effective. Indications for the use of intrapartum antibiotics included preterm labor (<37 weeks' gestation), prolonged rupture of membranes (>18 hours), maternal fever (≥38° C), maternal GBS bacteriuria during this pregnancy, and previous birth of an infant with GBS disease.

In 1996, the Centers for Disease Control and Prevention (CDC) published consensus guidelines that superseded the 1992 ACOG and AAP statements and proposed a coordinated approach for the prevention of neonatal GBS disease.[19,48,50] In this document, prenatal care providers are offered a choice between two strategies: one based on prenatal screening for GBS carriage and one based on risk factors. These guidelines were aimed at identifying and treating most GBS carriers, while minimizing the number of women receiving unnecessary intrapartum antibiotics.

The first strategy includes universal rectovaginal screening for GBS colonization at 35 to 37 weeks of gestation and treatment of all colonized women.[19,20,48] In addition, all unscreened women with risk factors should receive intrapartum antimicrobial prophylaxis. In contrast to the uncertain predictive results of maternal GBS cultures at 26 to 28 weeks (only 67% still would be positive at term, and an additional 7.4% would become positive by delivery), there is a high concordance between cultures obtained at 35 to 37 weeks and cultures obtained intrapartum (>90%).[18,23,25] The second strategy, and the one favored by ACOG, is a risk factor–based strategy in which screening cultures are not performed. Instead, all women who develop one or more risk factors at the time of labor or membrane rupture should receive intrapartum antimicrobial prophylaxis.[17,51]

In a multistate retrospective cohort study of more than 600,000 births, Schrag and associates compared the effectiveness of the screening- and risk factor–based approaches for the prevention of GBS disease. In this study, there was a greater than 50% reduction in GBS disease when the culture strategy was used compared with the risk-based approach.[52] In light of these findings, the CDC issued new consensus guidelines for the prevention of perinatal GBS disease, effective August 16, 2002,[53] recommending the prenatal screening of all pregnant women at 35 to 37 weeks of gestation (Table 71-2). In addition, the guidelines contain updated algorithms for the treatment of penicillin-allergic women, detailed guidelines for GBS processing, and updated algorithms for the management of newborns following maternal intrapartum prophylaxis.[53]

The CDC guidelines recommend penicillin as the first choice for intrapartum chemoprophylaxis, with ampicillin as the second choice.[54,55] Penicillin G is the recommended first agent because of its narrower antimicrobial spectrum and the diminished potential for the development of resistance among other organisms.[33,56] Some clinicians prefer the use of ampicillin for its additional gram-negative coverage, especially in the face of clinical chorioamnionitis.[55] An intrapartum antibiotic regimen with even broader coverage against gram-negative organisms (addition of aminoglycoside therapy) may be recommended in the presence of chorioamnionitis or clinical

Table 71–2. 2002 CDC Recommendations: Universal Prenatal Screening at 35-37 Weeks

Intrapartum prophylaxis indicated:
  Previous infant with invasive GBS disease
  GBS bacteriuria during current pregnancy
  Positive GBS screening culture during current pregnancy
  Unknown GBS status (culture not done, incomplete, or results unknown) and any of the following:
    Delivery at <37 wk gestation
    Amniotic membrane rupture ≥18 hr
    Intrapartum temperature ≥100.4° F (≥38.0° C)

GBS, group B streptococcus.

From Schrag S, Gorwitz R, Fultz-Butts K, Schuchat A: Prevention of perinatal group B streptococcal disease. Revised guidelines from CDC. MMWR Morb Mortal Wkly Rep 51:1, 2002.

signs of sepsis in the mother. As GBS strains have become more resistant to erythromycin and clindamycin,[57] new prophylaxis regimens are recommended (Table 71-3).[53]

The timing of intrapartum prophylaxis also is important. As the timing between the first dose of intrapartum antibiotics and delivery increases, the percentage of GBS-colonized infants decreases.[55,58] When antibiotics were administered within 1 hour of delivery, the rates of GBS colonization were equivalent to the rates of infants of untreated mothers. Although peak cord blood levels of ampicillin and penicillin are attained within 1 hour of antibiotic administration, it is likely that effective protection

Table 71–3. Recommended Regimens for Intrapartum Antimicrobial Prophylaxis for Group B Streptococcus Disease

Recommended	Penicillin G, 5 mU IV loading dose, then 2.5 mU IV q4h until delivery
Alternative	Ampicillin, 2 g IV loading dose, then 1 g IV q4h until delivery
If allergic to penicillin and not at high risk for anaphylaxis	Cefazolin, 2 g IV loading dose then 1 g IV q8h until delivery
If allergic to penicillin and at high risk for anaphylaxis	Clindamycin, 900 mg IV q8h until delivery Erythromycin, 500 mg IV q6h until delivery
If allergic to penicillin, GBS resistant to clindamycin or erythromycin or susceptibility unknown	Vancomycin, 1 g IV q12h until delivery

From Schrag S, Gorwitz R, Fultz-Butts K, Schuchat A: Prevention of perinatal group B streptococcal disease. Revised guidelines from CDC. MMWR Morb Mortal Wkly Rep 51:1, 2002.

against infection requires a longer time and higher amniotic fluid and fetal tissue levels.[58] With longer time intervals between antibiotic prophylaxis and delivery, the risk of GBS colonization can be reduced to nearly zero. Despite recommendations suggesting two of more doses of antiobiotics for prophylaxis, new evidence indicates that 4 or more hours of intrapartum ampicillin or penicillin are optimal for the prevention of early-onset GBS disease. It is further recommended that infants of adequately treated mothers be evaluated individually and that treatment decisions be based on the presence of clinical signs of sepsis.[31,36]

These prevention strategies may produce potential adverse effects for the mother and the infant. There is the small risk of maternal anaphylaxis if penicillin is administered for the first time to an allergic patient. In addition, the increased use of intrapartum antimicrobial agents has promoted the development of antibiotic resistance among GBS and other neonatal pathogens.[14,59] Although all GBS strains remain sensitive to penicillin, erythromycin resistance and clindamycin resistance have been reported.[7,12,33,60] These studies raise concerns regarding the adequacy of currently recommended prophylaxis strategies for penicillin-allergic women. More recent studies also have suggested that maternal intrapartum chemoprophylaxis is associated with neonatal sepsis caused by organisms resistant to maternal antibiotics, particularly ampicillin.[49,61] Among infants with ampicillin-resistant *Escherichia coli* infections, the mortality was significantly higher than in infants with disease caused by ampicillin-sensitive strains.[14,56,62] There also was a relationship between neonatal death and prolonged exposure to peripartum antibiotics.[63] These data support the use of penicillin rather than ampicillin as the antibiotic of first choice for GBS prophylaxis. Other potential concerns for neonates exposed to peripartum antibiotics include the need for prolonged hospitalization for diagnostic or therapeutic interventions and the cost of GBS prevention policies.[49]

A rapid and reliable method for the detection of GBS in pregnant women at the time of delivery might obviate the need for prenatal screening and reduce the unnecessary use of antibiotic prophylaxis. Bergeron and associates[10] studied the efficacy of two polymerase chain reaction assays for routine screening of pregnant women, showing results within 45 minutes with 97% sensitivity and 98% negative predictive accuracy. This test might allow the detection of GBS from maternal specimens or could be used to identify infants at high risk for GBS disease. If proved to be effective in larger studies, the use of the polymerase chain reaction assay may eliminate the need for empirical antibiotics and reduce the morbidity and mortality from GBS infection in mothers and infants.

Among hospitals that implemented the recommended CDC policies, there has been a significant reduction in the incidence of early-onset neonatal GBS disease (Fig. 71-1).[4,16,18,55] Data from the CDC suggest that the incidence of early-onset disease was reduced to 0.6 cases per 1000 live births in 1998.[4,12] Intrapartum prophylaxis had no effect on late-onset disease, and rates of maternal infections declined only moderately.[4] These authors estimated that 3900 early-onset infections and 200 deaths

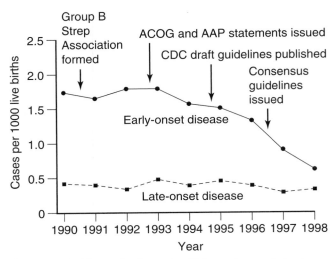

Figure 71–1. Incidence of early-onset and late-onset group B streptococcus disease, 1990 through 1998. *(From Schrag SJ, Zywicki S, Farley MM, et al: Group B streptococcal disease in the era of intrapartum antibiotic prophylaxis. N Engl J Med 342:15, 2000.)*

were prevented in 1998 by the use of intrapartum antibiotics. No therapy would be effective in the prevention of all cases of neonatal infection, however, and there are estimates to suggest more than 2200 cases currently with 100 projected deaths.[12,16]

THERAPEUTIC STRATEGIES

Perinatal exposure to bacterial, viral, and fungal organisms is an important cause of early-onset bacteremia and sepsis in newborns. Nosocomial acquisition of pathogens becomes the more prevalent source as hospitalization progresses. These two sources of illness differ in terms of their pathogens, and antimicrobial therapy not only must be tailored to the presenting signs of infection, but also should be related to the time course of presentation.

Empirical Therapy

During the first few days of life, a newborn is most likely to develop illness related to perinatally acquired organisms. Gram-positive cocci, particularly GBS, and gram-negative enteric bacilli, including *Escherichia coli* and *Klebsiella* spp., are currently regarded as the common early-onset neonatal pathogens.[64] *Listeria monocytogenes*, a gram-positive rod, also is included as a common pathogen, although it is rarely isolated in the United States.[2] Table 71-4 shows broad patterns of antibiotic susceptibility for these bacteria.

Given the risk for rapid progression of untreated infection in this population, **empirical therapy** is begun and directed against certain well-recognized organisms. Ampicillin and gentamicin usually are recommended as initial broad-spectrum antibiotic coverage. Ampicillin (or penicillin) is employed to cover GBS and *L. monocytogenes*, and aminoglycosides are added to cover gram-negative organisms.[2] Emerging resistance of gram-negative bacilli to gentamicin has resulted in the adoption in many centers

Table 71–4. Antibiotic Susceptibility Patterns in Early-Onset Infection

Organism	Antibiotic			
	Penicillin	Ampicillin	Gentamicin/Amikacin/Netilmicin	Cefotaxime
GBS	+	+	−	+
Escherichia coli	−	±	+	+
Klebsiella sp.	−	−	±	+
Listeria monocytogenes	±	+	−	−

GBS, group B streptococcus.

From Gilbert DN, Moellering RC, Sande MA: The Sanford Guide to Antimicrobial Therapy 2001. Hyde Park, VT, Antimicrobial Therapy, Inc, 2001.

of alternate aminoglycosides (e.g., amikacin or netilmicin). The latter have a similar antimicrobial spectrum and often can be used interchangeably with one another.[65] When blood culture results are available, targeted therapy can be directed against the identified pathogen depending on antimicrobial susceptibility patterns.

Beyond the first few days of life, the likelihood of postnatal exposure or hospital-acquired infectious agents increases. Common pathogens include *Staphylococcus* spp. (*S. aureus* and *S. epidermidis*), enterococci, and gram-negative organisms, including *Pseudomonas aeruginosa,* although GBS and *Listeria* also may present as late-onset disease.[6,9,66] It is usually recommended that empirical treatment include oxacillin or vancomycin, generally in combination with an aminoglycoside.[2] Alternatively, third-generation cephalosporins may be useful in infants with impaired renal function in whom aminoglycosides are contraindicated or in chronically hospitalized infants at risk for resistant gram-negative sepsis. Table 71-5 shows broad patterns of susceptibility for the common pathogens responsible for late-onset disease.

Directed Therapy

Although blood culture is the gold standard for the diagnosis of neonatal bacteremia and sepsis, the isolation of an organism from blood culture occurs far less than 100% of the time in U.S. nurseries.[64,67] A 1979 retrospective study showed that blood cultures were negative in 18% of infants dying with bacterial infection (organisms recovered at autopsy).[68] In the same study, 80% of

infected newborns showed one or more hematologic abnormalities compared with 43% of infants dying without bacterial infection. Of newborns dying with bacterial infection, 13% had no hematologic abnormality.[68] An additional concern is that many infants are born to mothers receiving intrapartum antimicrobial prophylaxis. In these cases, blood cultures may be falsely negative despite fetal infection. The decision to continue empirical treatment depends on the severity of the initial presentation, the likelihood of suspected infection, and the infant's clinical course from the onset of symptoms. Broad-spectrum antibiotic therapy is instituted for these infants and may be continued for a full course even if an infecting organism is not isolated.

The duration of therapy depends on the infant's initial clinical signs and the rate of clinical improvement. Antibiotics are recommended for 10 to 14 days after a positive blood culture and no less than 21 days in infants with GBS or gram-negative meningitis. It is recommended that clinicians obtain a repeat blood or cerebrospinal fluid culture to verify sterility. Although GBS remains exquisitely sensitive to penicillin and ampicillin, eradication of gram-negative organisms often is delayed, and abscess formation can be a devastating consequence of undertreatment.

Management of Neonates of Mothers Who Received Intrapartum Chemoprophylaxis

The management of neonates of mothers who have received intrapartum antimicrobial prophylaxis involves

Table 71–5. Antibiotic Susceptibility Patterns in Late-Onset Infection

Organism	Antibiotic			
	Ampicillin	Gentamicin/Amikacin/Netilmicin	Cefotaxime	Vancomycin
GBS	+	−	+	−
Staphylococcus aureus	−	±	±	+
Staphylococcus epidermidis	±	±	±	+
Enterococcus	+	−	+	±
Pseudomonas aeruginosa	−	+	±	−
Listeria monocytogenes	+	+	−	−

From Gilbert DN, Moellering RC, Sande MA: The Sanford Guide to Antimicrobial Therapy 2001. Hyde Park, VT, Antimicrobial Therapy, Inc, 2001.

several important considerations, including the presence or absence of signs compatible with infection, the presence or absence of suspected chorioamnionitis in the mother, the gestational age of the infant, and the duration of maternal chemoprophylaxis[53] (Fig. 71-2).[19,31] If signs or symptoms of infection are present, or the mother received intrapartum antibiotics for suspected chorioamnionitis, a full diagnostic evaluation is done, and empirical antibiotic therapy is started. The full diagnostic evaluation includes a CBC and differential, blood culture, and a chest radiograph if respiratory abnormalities are present. When signs of sepsis are present, an LP should be performed. The duration of therapy depends on the results of the blood and cerebrospinal fluid cultures and the clinical course of the infant. If the laboratory results and clinical course suggest infection is unlikely, therapy may be brief (48 to 72 hours). If the neonate is asymptomatic at birth but is less than 35 weeks' gestation, or the neonate is more than 35 weeks' gestation but intrapartum antibiotic prophylaxis was given 4 hours or less before delivery, a complete blood count and blood culture should be performed, and the infant should be observed for at least 48 hours. For asymptomatic infants more than 35 weeks' gestation whose mothers received

intrapartum antibiotic prophylaxis more than 4 hours before delivery, no evaluation or therapy is needed.[31] Although the guidelines from the AAP were not meant as an exclusive approach to the management of infants of pretreated mothers, in-hospital observation is suggested until the safety of earlier discharge is established.[69] Further experience to date has suggested that the diagnostic evaluation and empirical treatment of asymptomatic infants may not be warranted, but additional strategies for the management of these infants currently are being investigated.[31,70]

Commonly Isolated Organisms

Streptococci

GBS continues to be uniformly sensitive to penicillin and the cephalosporins.[1,8,30,41,42,59] In vitro studies have shown that aminoglycosides alone are ineffective agents, although multiple in vitro studies confirm the synergy offered by gentamicin when used to augment the effect of ampicillin.[71] In contrast, in vivo studies fail to show faster recovery or increased survival achieved by ampicillin-aminoglycoside combinations compared with an aminoglycoside alone.[72] Intrapartum prophylaxis of maternal carriers of GBS traditionally is with penicillin or ampicillin.[11] More recent studies have shown increased in vitro resistance of GBS to clindamycin and erythromycin, raising concerns about incompletely treated disease.[57,60]

Escherichia coli and *Klebsiella* Species

Coliform organisms such as *E. coli* are present in the maternal gastrointestinal tract and birth canal. Infants may become colonized immediately before delivery or during birth.[73] Historically, aminoglycosides, such as gentamicin, have proved highly effective against many gram-negative isolates. The ultimate choice of antibiotics depends on particular patterns of susceptibility of the organism within each institution, however.[62] There have been reports of gentamicin-resistant *Klebsiella* sp. and *E. coli* that show sensitivity to amikacin.[74] It is uncertain whether institutional substitution of gentamicin with amikacin (combined with stricter adherence to proper barrier precautions) can achieve reversal of institutional resistance patterns. Although there are no large controlled studies to date, the addition of a third-generation cephalosporin to an aminoglycoside regimen for the treatment of gram-negative sepsis and meningitis may offer additional benefit. A retrospective study recommended the addition of a third-generation cephalosporin to amikacin to provide double coverage for gram-negative bacterial meningitis.[75]

Listeria monocytogenes

L. monocytogenes is a gram-positive bacterium endemic in the animal world and widespread in the environment, soil, wood, and decayed matter. Most human cases of listeriosis seem to be acquired through ingestion of contaminated food, although sporadic case reports implicate other modes of transmission. Data collected by the CDC and the Food and Drug Administration from five surveillance areas around the United States with a historically high prevalence of *Listeria* documented a 51% decrease in

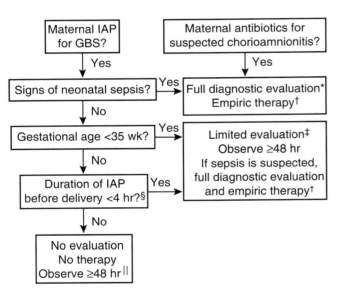

Figure 71-2. Management of newborns following maternal intrapartum prophylaxis. *(From Schrag S, Gorwitz R, Fultz-Butts K, Schuchat A: Prevention of perinatal group B streptococcal disease. Revised guidelines from CDC. MMWR Recomm Rep 51[RR-11]:1, 2002.)*

---

*Includes CBC and differential, blood culture, and chest radiograph if respiratory abnormalities are present. When signs of sepsis are present, a lumbar puncture, if feasible, should be performed.

†Duration of therapy varies depending on results of blood culture, cerebrospinal fluid findings, if obtained, and the clinical course of the infant. If bacterial infection is not indicated, duration may be as short as 48 hr.

‡CBC with differential and blood culture.

§Applies only to penicillin, ampicillin, or cefazolin.

‖A healthy-appearing infant who was ≥38 wk gestation at delivery and whose mother received ≥4 hr of intrapartum prophylaxis before delivery may be discharged after 24 hr if other discharge criteria have been met and a person able to comply fully with instructions for home observation will be present.

perinatal listeriosis between 1989 and 1993.[76] Of neonatal listeriosis, 95% presents as early-onset disease, commonly in the context of maternal chorioamnionitis.[77]

Staphylococci

S. aureus and *S. epidermidis* colonize human skin and mucosa. Staphylococcal species are widely known to produce β-lactamase and are widely resistant to ampicillin and certain cephalosporins.[78] Currently the most concerning type of resistance among staphylococci is methicillin resistance. Because methicillin-resistant *S. aureus* also is resistant to many other antimicrobials, β-lactams, and non–β-lactams, vancomycin is relied on for the treatment of methicillin-resistant *S. aureus* infections.[79-81] Since the initial report from Japan in 1997, many other groups from around the world have reported strains of *S. aureus* with intermediate resistance to vancomycin. The expanded use of vancomycin has led to reports of vancomycin-resistant, coagulase-negative staphylococci, however. All of the reported cases occurred in patients who had prolonged (>1 month) exposure to vancomycin.[50] It would seem reasonable that empirical therapy with vancomycin be narrowed as soon as culture results and sensitivities permit.

Enterococci

Enterococci are of special concern in the neonatal setting because the incidence and the severity of infection are increasing. In particular, resistance of enterococci to vancomycin is an evolving and serious problem. In 1989, the incidence of vancomycin-resistant enterococci was estimated to be 7.9%; this rose to 15% in 1998. Other types of enterococcal resistance include ampicillin resistance based on altered penicillin-binding proteins, β-lactamase–mediated resistance, and aminoglycoside resistance. Ampicillin resistance is common, particularly in *Enterccoccus faecium,* in which greater than 80% of clinical isolates are resistant. A lesser proportion (<5%) of *Enterccoccus faecalis* isolates are resistant to ampicillin. β-Lactamase–mediated resistance is currently rare and accounts for less than 0.1% of enterococcal isolates. Enterococcal resistance to macrolides, fluoroquinolones, tetracyclines, and carbapenems has been reported but is rarely seen in the neonatal setting.[82]

Pseudomonas aeruginosa

Pseudomonas aeruginosa is usually a cause of late-onset, nosocomially acquired infection. Although there have been case reports of infants infected with *Pseudomonas* within the first few days of life, this represents the exception to the rule. Bacteria are introduced to the infants via health care personnel and invasive appliances.[83] Currently, evidence suggests that resistance patterns in patients who are not chronically infected are relatively stable. As with the other gram-negative infections, aminoglycosides have proved effective. Institutional resistance patterns are important, however, in determining proper therapeutic strategies.[84]

SUPPORTIVE THERAPY

Antibiotics are only part of the management of a newborn infant with infection; additionally vigorous supportive therapy should be provided.[85-87] Although the host response to

infection or inflammation is most often self-limited and protective, in certain circumstances, inflammatory mediators enter into the systemic circulation and trigger the systemic inflammatory response syndrome.[37,88,89] This syndrome may be maladaptive and progress to the cardiovascular and respiratory derangements associated with shock and multiple organ system dysfunction.[85,90,91] It is now known that many proinflammatory cytokines and other mediators are secreted in response to infection, and more recent therapies have attempted to modulate the inflammatory cascade associated with sepsis.[92-94] To date, these trials have shown little clinical benefit, most likely because of the multiple overlapping cascade of mediators involved and the complex interactive nature of the proinflammatory and anti-inflammatory responses elicited.[86,95] With improved understanding of the pathophysiology of the inflammatory response, additional immunotherapies may prove useful to improve morbidity and mortality for patients in the future.[39,87]

IMMUNOTHERAPY

A newborn infant is at increased risk of bacterial infection most likely secondary to several functional deficiencies of the immune system.[37] Newborn skin has increased permeability, especially in a premature infant, due to its inherent epidermal fragility, alkaline pH, and impaired production of free fatty acids.[39] The gastrointestinal and the respiratory epithelia are susceptible to infection secondary to the lack of production of secretory IgA during the first few days of life.[39] In addition, IgG is the only immunoglobulin to be transported across the placenta. Levels are low in the fetus born prematurely but increase by 32 weeks so that at term, IgG levels are equal to or greater than those of the mother.[96] Phagocytic cell functions also are deficient in newborn infants. Neutrophils from full-term healthy newborns show depressed adherence, chemotaxis, normal phagocytosis, and decreased intracellular killing. Further decrements in cell function are observed in stressed preterm infants.[38] Although lymphocyte number and function seem adequate, T-lymphocyte function may be depressed. Finally, complement levels and activity are diminished in newborns to approximately half that of the mother (Table 71-6).[96] As a consequence of these functional deficiencies, studies have investigated the possibility of modulating immune

Table 71–6. Functional Abnormalities of Neonatal Host Defense

Component	Function
Antibody	↓ IgG in preterm infants
	↓ IgA in secretions
Complement	↓ production, ↓ opsonization
Neutrophil	↓ chemotaxis, normal phagocytosis
	↓ killing in stressed neonates
Monocyte	↓ chemotaxis

responses with the hope of positively affecting the outcome of newborns with sepsis.[85]

Intravenous Immune Globulin

Because most of the maternal-fetal IgG transfer occurs after 32 weeks of gestation, premature infants are relatively hypogammaglobulinemic at birth and are at high risk for sepsis.[37,97,98] Maternal immunoglobulin transferred to the fetus is effective only against the specific etiologic agent to which the mother has been exposed.[99,100] In an older study, Baker and Kasper[101] showed that the susceptibility of neonates to GBS infection is related to the deficiency of specific maternal antibody to GBS. This study showed a correlation between low maternal levels of type-specific antibody in serum and risk for neonatal systemic infection with type III strains of GBS.[35] As a consequence, there has been interest in the prophylactic and therapeutic use of immunoglobulins in preventing and treating nosocomial infections in newborns.[102]

Several older pilot studies have suggested potential benefit of **intravenous immune globulin (IVIG)** in prevention or treatment of neonatal sepsis with mixed results reported in terms of efficacy.[103-107] In a prospective, randomized, placebo-controlled multicenter study, Shenoi[108] evaluated the use of IVIG prophylaxis for the prevention of neonatal infection in preterm infants. Infants who received IVIG had no significant reduction in infectious episodes or mortality compared with infants given placebo. Infants born with higher serum immunoglobulin concentrations had significantly fewer episodes of culture-proven sepsis, however, than infants with lower serum concentrations of IgG when matched for gestational age. Other studies examining the role of IVIG in the treatment of neonatal sepsis have shown no effect in reducing mortality.[109,110] In addition, IVIG therapy shortened neither the duration of antibiotic therapy nor the length of hospitalization. A likely explanation for these factors is that commercially available IVIG contains low antibody titers to the more common neonatal pathogens.[111,112] Hyperimmune anti-GBS IVIG has been prepared with high levels of opsonic and protective antibody to GBS. One review proposed that hyperimmune IVIG preparations would allow physicians to give higher quantities of specific anti-GBS antibody without having to administer large fluid volumes or large amounts of nonspecific immunoglobulin.[113] The efficacy of these preparations is currently unknown.

Despite the questioned efficacy of IVIG, most sources suggest that it is a relatively safe product to administer. Known side effects include transient neutropenia, presumably on the basis of antineutrophil antibodies in the IVIG preparation. Other authors have speculated that high doses of nonspecific IVIG may block the neutrophil or bacterial receptors necessary for opsonophagocytosis.[114] Doses greater than 2 g/kg have been shown to induce reticuloendothelial blockade.[115] There are few data to support the standard use of IVIG in the treatment or prevention of neonatal sepsis. One may consider its use, however, after other therapies have been attempted.

Granulocyte Colony-Stimulating Factor and Granulocyte-Macrophage Colony-Stimulating Factor

Granulocyte colony-stimulating factor (G-CSF) is a physiologic up-regulator of neutrophil production and increases blood neutrophil concentrations.[69] Many studies have attempted to determine whether administration of G-CSF to septic neonates was effective in reducing mortality.[116] There have been no reports of clinical or hematologic toxicity during treatment or follow-up. Several studies have shown that recombinant G-CSF (rG-CSF) treatment led to an increase in absolute neutrophil counts when given to neonates with presumed sepsis and neutropenia.[117-120] It had little effect, however, on infants with a high percentage of immature neutrophils whose G-CSF production was up-regulated and whose bone marrow was severely depressed.[121] The current difficulty with an objective recommendation regarding therapy is that the several clinical studies all have a small number of subjects and differ in their conclusions. A meta-analysis grouping studies from 1990 to 2000 concluded that G-CSF administration was associated with a trend toward lower mortality, but there was a low level of confidence in this conclusion.[122] Because it was lower-birth-weight neonates and neonates with neutropenia who appeared more likely to benefit, the authors further judged that the efficacy of rG-CSF among neonates with suspected septicemia was unproven but may have merit. A large trial investigating the efficacy of rG-CSF in a septic, neutropenic group of neonates is warranted.

Granulocyte-macrophage colony-stimulating factor (GM-CSF) has been theorized to prime term and preterm neutrophils for enhanced chemotaxis and respiratory burst responses.[123,124] In vivo studies in newborn rats showed GM-CSF can increase survival after experimental sepsis, provided that it is given before bacterial inoculation.[125] Even given this promise, however, studies involving adjunctive therapy with recombinant human GM-CSF are rare. One randomized controlled trial involving 60 subjects concluded that treatment with rGM-CSF is associated with an increase in absolute neutrophil, eosinophil, monocyte, lymphocyte, and platelet counts and decreased mortality in critically ill, septic, neutropenic neonates. The authors recommended further randomized trials to confirm its beneficial effects.[126]

Granulocyte Transfusions

Neonates show defects in neutrophil function and quantitative differences in neutrophil bone marrow storage pools. It is well known that neutropenic infants have a higher mortality with sepsis.[127] The use of granulocyte transfusions would make theoretical sense.[123] In 1981, Laurenti and coworkers[128] first examined the use of granulocyte transfusions in a nonrandomized clinical trial. This study showed a striking reduction in mortality from 72% in the nontransfused group to 10% in the transfused group.[128] Because of this initial observation, several prospective controlled clinical studies examined the potential benefit of granulocyte transfusion in neonatal sepsis.[7,129-132] A 1997 meta-analysis reviewed five of these studies. The analysis concluded that neonates receiving adequate doses of granulocytes experienced a significant benefit from transfusion.[15] Obtaining such products is difficult, however, given the fact that their half-life is 8 to 12 hours, and few centers are equipped to isolate and process granulocytes in a timely fashion. There are well-known associated complications with administration of such products. In addition to the infectious risks (cytomegalovirus and human immunodeficiency virus), there are concerns for graft-versus-host disease, sensitization to cellular blood product antigens, and pulmonary leukoagglutination reactions.[127] Although in need of additional study, neutrophil transfusions may be a promising therapy for critically ill, neutropenic neonates and possibly may be reserved as a treatment of last resort.

SUMMARY

Since the 1990s, there have been tremendous advances in the prevention and treatment of neonatal sepsis, causing a dramatic reduction in the incidence of GBS disease. Although these therapies have been effective, current concerns surround the emergence of resistant organisms and the cost-effectiveness of screening and management protocols for neonates. In the future, strategies for the prevention and treatment of sepsis may include maternal antimicrobial prophylaxis and targeted immunotherapies to improve neonatal morbidity and mortality.

REFERENCES

1. Baker CJ, Edwards MS: Group B streptococcal infections. In Remington JJ, Klein JO (eds): Infectious Diseases of the Fetus and Newborn Infant, 4th ed. Philadelphia, WB Saunders, 1995, pp 980-1054.
2. Klein JO, Marcy SM: Bacterial sepsis and meningitis. In Remington JJ, Klein JO (eds): Infectious Diseases of the Fetus and Newborn Infant. Philadelphia, WB Saunders, 1995, pp 835-890.
3. Philip AGS: Neonatal Sepsis and Meningitis. Boston, GK Hall Medical Publishers, 1985.
4. Schrag SJ, Zywicki S, Farley MM, et al: Group B streptococcal disease in the era of intrapartum antibiotic prophylaxis. N Engl J Med 342:15, 2000.
5. Stoll BJ, Gordon T, Korones SB, et al: Early-onset sepsis in very low birth weight neonates: A report from the National Institute of Child Health and Human Development Neonatal Research Network. J Pediatr 129:72, 1996.
6. Donowitz LG, Haley CE, Gregory WW: Neonatal intensive care bacteremia: Emergence of gram positive bacteria as major pathogens. Am J Infect Control 15:141, 1987.
7. Freij B, McCracken GH: Acute infections. In Avery GB, Fletcher MA, MacDonald MG (eds): Neonatology: Pathophysiology and Management of the Newborn, 5th ed. Philadelphia, Lippincott Williams & Wilkins, 1999, pp 1189-1230.
8. Baker CJ: Group B streptococcal infections. Clin Perinatol 24:59, 1997.
9. Gladstone IM, Ehrenkranz RA, Edberg S, et al: A ten year review of neonatal sepsis and comparison with the previous fifty year experience. Pediatr Infect Dis J 9:819, 1990.
10. Bergeron MG, Danbing KE, Menard C, et al: Rapid detection of group B streptococci in pregnant women at delivery. N Engl J Med 343:175, 2000.
11. McKenna DS, Iams JD: Group B streptococcal infections. Semin Perinatol 22:267, 1998.
12. Schuchat A: Neonatal group B streptococcal disease—screening and prevention. N Engl J Med 343:209, 2000.
13. Schimmel MS, Samueloff A, Eidelman AI: Prevention of neonatal group B streptococcal infections: Is there a rational prevention strategy? Clin Perinatol 25:687, 1998.
14. Schuchat A, Zywicki SS, Dinsmoor MJ, et al, and the Prevention of Early-onset Neonatal Sepsis (PENS) Study Group: Risk factors and opportunities for prevention of early-onset neonatal sepsis: A multicenter case-control study. Pediatrics 105:21, 2000.
15. Vamvakas EC: Meta-analysis of clinical studies of the efficacy of granulocyte transfusions in the treatment of bacterial sepsis. J Clin Apheresis 11:1, 1996.
16. Benitz WE, Gould JB, Druzin ML: Preventing early-onset group B streptococcal sepsis: Strategy development using decision analysis. Pediatrics 103:e76, 1999.
17. Boyer KM, Gadzala CA, Kelly PD, Gotoff SP: Selective intrapartum chemoprophylaxis of neonatal group B streptococcal early-onset disease: III. Interruption of mother-to-infant transmission. J Infect Dis 148:810, 1983.
18. Brumund TT, White CB: An update on group B streptococcal infection in the newborn: Prevention, evaluation, and treatment. Pediatr Ann 27:495, 1998.
19. Centers for Disease Control and Prevention: Prevention of perinatal group B streptococcal disease: A public health perspective. MMWR Morb Mortal Wkly Rep 45:1, 1996.
20. Committee on Infectious Diseases and Committee on Fetus and Newborn: Guidelines for prevention of group B streptococcal (GBS) infection by chemoprophylaxis. Pediatrics 90:775, 1992.
21. Rouse DJ, Goldenberg RL, Cliver SP, et al: Strategies for the prevention of early-onset neonatal group B streptococcal sepsis: A decision analysis. Obstet Gynecol 83:483, 1994.
22. Schuchat A, Wenger JD: Epidemiology of group B streptococcal disease: Risk factors, prevention strategies and vaccine development. Epidemiol Rev 16:374, 1994.
23. Boyer KM, Gadzala CA, Kelly PD, et al: Selective intrapartum chemoprophylaxis of neonatal group B streptococcal early-onset disease: II. Predictive value of prenatal cultures. J Infect Dis 148:802, 1983.
24. Boyer KM, Gotoff SP: Antimicrobial prophylaxis of neonatal group B streptococcal sepsis. Clin Perinatol 15:831, 1988.
25. Boyer KM, Gotoff SP: Prevention of early-onset neonatal group B streptococcal disease with selective intrapartum chemoprophylaxis. N Engl J Med 314:1665, 1986.
26. Gardner SE, Yow MD, Leeds LJ, et al: Failure of penicillin to eradicate group B streptococcal colonization in the pregnant woman: A couple study. Am J Obstet Gynecol 135:1062, 1979.
27. Steigman AJ, Bottone EJ, Hanna BA: Control of perinatal group B streptococcal sepsis: Efficacy of single injection of aqueous penicillin at birth. Mt Sinai J Med 45:685, 1978.
28. Siegel JD, McCracken GHJ, Threlkeld N, et al: Single-dose penicillin prophylaxis of neonatal group B streptococcal disease. Lancet 1:1426, 1982.
29. Siegel JD, McCracken GHJ, Threlkeld N, et al: Single-dose penicillin prophylaxis against neonatal group B streptococcal infections: A controlled trial in 18,738 newborn infants. N Engl J Med 303:769, 1980.
30. Pyati SP, Pildes RS, Jacobs NM, et al: Penicillin in infants weighing two kilograms or less with early-onset group B streptococcal disease. N Engl J Med 308:1383, 1983.
31. American Academy of Pediatrics (Committee on Infectious Diseases and Committee on Fetus and Newborn): Revised guidelines for prevention of early-onset group B streptococcal (GBS) infection. Pediatrics 99:489, 1997.

32. Centers for Disease Control and Prevention: Early-onset group B streptococcal disease—United States, 1998-1999. JAMA 284:1508-1510, 2000.

33. Schuchat A: Group B streptococcus. Lancet 353:51, 1999.

34. Baker CJ, Rench MA, Edwards MS, et al: Immunization of pregnant women with a polysaccharide vaccine of group B streptococcus. N Engl J Med 319:1180, 1988.

35. Baker CJ: Role of antibody to native type III polysaccharide of group B streptococcus in infant infection. Pediatrics 68:544, 1981.

36. Siegel JD: Prophylaxis for neonatal group B streptococcus infections. Semin Perinatol 22:33, 1998.

37. Perez EM, Weisman LE: Novel approaches to the prevention and therapy of neonatal bacterial sepsis. Clin Perinatol 24:213, 1997.

38. Polin RA, St Geme JW 3rd: Neonatal sepsis. Adv Pediatr Infect Dis 7:25, 1992.

39. Yoder MC, Polin RA: Immunotherapy of neonatal infections. Pediatr Clin North Am 33:481, 1986.

40. Hickman ME, Rench MA, Ferrieri P, Baker CJ: Changing epidemiology of group B streptococcal colonization. Pediatrics 104:203, 1999.

41. Lin FC, Clemens JD, Azimi PH, et al: Capsular polysaccharide types of group B streptococcal isolates from neonates with early-onset systemic infection. J Infect Dis 177:790, 1998.

42. Matsubara K, Sugiyama M, Hoshina K, et al: Early onset neonatal sepsis caused by serotype VIII group B streptococci. Pediatr Infect Dis J 19:359, 2000.

43. Gotoff SP, Boyer KM: Prevention of early-onset neonatal group B streptococcal disease. Pediatrics 99:866, 1997.

44. Yow MD, Mason EO, Leeds LJ, et al: Ampicillin prevents intrapartum transmission of group B streptococcus. JAMA 241:1245, 1979.

45. Boyer KM, Gadzala CA, Burd LI, et al: Selective intrapartum chemoprophylaxis of neonatal group B streptococcal early-onset disease: I. Epidemiologic rationale. J Infect Dis 148:795, 1983.

46. Easmon CSF, Hastings MJG, Deeley J, et al: The effect of intrapartum chemopropohylaxis on the vertical transmission of group B streptococci. Br J Obstet Gynaecol 90:633, 1983.

47. Pylipow M, Gaddis M, Kinney JS: Selective intrapartum prophylaxis for group B streptococcus colonization: Management and outcome of newborns. Pediatrics 93:631, 1994.

48. ACOG Committee Opinion: Prevention of early onset group B streptococcal disease in newborns. ACOG Comm Opin 173:1, 1996.

49. Morita JY, O'Brien KL, Schuchat A: Prevention of perinatal group B streptococcal infections. Pediatr Infect Dis J 18:279, 1999.

50. Cormican MG, Jones RN: Emerging resistance to antimicrobial agents in gram-positive bacteria: Enterococci, staphylococci and nonpneumococcal streptococci. Drugs 51(suppl 1):6, 1996.

51. Gotoff SP: Chemoprophylaxis of early-onset group B streptococcal disease in 1999. Curr Opin Pediatr 12:105, 2000.

52. Schrag SJ, Zell ER, Lynfield R, et al:. A population-based comparison of strategies to prevent early-onset group B streptococcal disease in neonates. N Engl J Med 347:233, 2002.

53. Schrag S, Gorwitz R, Fultz-Butts K, Schuchat A: Prevention of perinatal group B streptococcal disease. Revised guidelines from CDC. MMWR Morb Mortal Wkly Rep 51:1, 2002.

54. Chanock SJ: Granulocyte transfusions: Time for a second look. Infect Dis Clin North Am 10:327, 1996.

55. Hager DW, Schuchat A, Gibbs R, et al: Prevention of perinatal group B streptococcal infection: Current controversies. Obstet Gynecol 96:141, 2000.

56. Towers CV, Carr MH, Padilla G, Asrat T: Potential consequences of widespread antepartal use of ampicillin. Am J Obstet Gynecol 179:879, 1998.

57. Pearlman MD, Pierson CL, Faix RG: Frequent resistance of clinical group B streptococci isolates to clindamycin and erythromycin. Obstet Gynecol 92:258, 1998.

58. De Cueto M, Sanchez M-J, Sampedro A, et al: Timing of intrapartum ampicillin and prevention of vertical transmission of group B streptococcus. Obstet Gynecol 91:112, 1998.

59. Rouse DJ, Andrews WW, Lin F-YC, et al: Antibiotic susceptibility profile of group B streptococcus acquired vertically. Obstet Gynecol 92:931, 1998.

60. Morales WJ, Dickey SS, Bornick P, Lim DV: Change in antibiotic resistance of group B streptococcus: Impact on intrapartum management. Am J Obstet Gynecol 181:310, 1999.

61. Mercer BM, Carr TL, Beazley DD, et al: Antibiotic use in pregnancy and drug-resistant infant sepsis. Am J Obstet Gynecol 181:816, 1999.

62. Joseph TA, Pyati SP, Jacobs N: Neonatal early-onset *Escherichia coli* disease. Arch Pediatr Adolesc Med 152:35, 1998.

63. Terrone DA, Rinehart BK, Einstein MH, et al: Neonatal sepsis and death caused by resistant *Escherichia coli*: Possible consequences of extended maternal ampicillin administration. Am J Obstet Gynecol 180:1345, 1999.

64. Kaftan H, Kinney JS: Early onset neonatal bacterial infections. Semin Perinatol 22:15, 1998.

65. Gilbert, DN, Moellering RC, Sande MA: The Sanford Guide to Antimicrobial Therapy 2001. Hyde Park, VT, Antimicrobial Therapy, Inc, 2001.

66. Sidebottom DG, Freeman J, Platt R, et al: Fifteen year experience with blood isolates of coagulase negative staphylococci in neonatal intensive care. J Clin Microbiol 26:713, 1988.

67. Escobar GJ, Li DK, Armstrong MA, et al: Neonatal sepsis workups in infants ≥2000 grams at birth: A population based study. Pediatrics 106(2 pt 1):256, 2000.

68. Squire E, Favara B, Todd J: Diagnosis of neonatal bacterial infection: Hematologic and pathologic findings in fatal and nonfatal cases. Pediatrics 64:60, 1979.

69. Cairo J: Review of G-CSF and GM-CSF effects on neonatal neutrophil kinetics. Am J Pediatr Hematol Oncol 11:238, 1989.

70. Singal KK, LaGamma EF: Management of 168 neonates weighing more than 2000 g receiving intrapartum chemoprophylaxis for chorioamnionitis. Arch Pediatr Adolesc Med 150:158, 1996.

71. Deveikis A, Schauf V, Mizen M, Riff L: Antimicrobial therapy of experimental group B streptococcal infection in mice. Antimicrob Agents Chemother 11:817, 1977.

72. Schauf V, Deveikis A, Riff L, Serota A: Antibiotic-killing kinetics of group B streptococci. J Pediatr 89:194, 1976.

73. Tullus K, Burman LG: Ecological impact of ampicillin and cefuroxime in neonatal units. Lancet 1:1405, 1989.

74. Aronsson B, Eriksson M, Herin P, Rylander M: Gentamicin-resistant *Klebsiella* spp. and *Escherichia coli* in a neonatal intensive care unit. Scand J Infect Dis 23:195, 1991.

75. Dellagrammaticas HD, Christodoulou C, Megaloyanni E, et al: Treatment of gram-negative bacterial meningitis in term neonates with third generation cephalosporins plus amikacin. Biol Neonate 77:139, 2000.

76. Tappero JW, Schuchat A, Deaver KA, et al: Reduction in the incidence of human listeriosis in the United States. JAMA 273:1118, 1995.

77. Nolla-Salas J, Bosch J, Gasser I, et al: Perinatal listeriosis: A population-based multicenter study in Barcelona, Spain (1990-1996). Am J Perinatol 15:461, 1998.

78. Jeljaszewicz J, Mlynarczyk G, Mlynarczyk A: Antibiotic resistance in gram-positive cocci. Int J Antimicrob Agents 16:473, 2000.

79. Hiramatsu K, Hanaki H, Ino T, et al: Methicillin-resistant *Staphylococcus aureus* clinical strain with reduced vancomycin susceptibility. J Antimicrob Chemother 40:135, 1997.

80. Jones RN, Pfaller MA: Bacterial resistance: A worldwide problem. Diagn Microbiol Infect Dis 31:379, 1998.

81. Pfaller MA, Jones RN, Doern GV, et al, for the Sentry Participants Group: Bacterial pathogens isolated from patients with bloodstream infection: Frequencies of occurrence and antimicrobial susceptibility patterns from the SENTRY antimicrobial surveillance program (United States and Canada, 1997). Antimicrob Agents Chemother 42:1762, 1998.

82. Lefort A, Mainardi J-L, Lortholary O: Antienterococcal antibiotics. Med Clin North Am 84:1471, 2000.

83. Pacifico L: Early-onset *Pseudomonas aeruginosa* sepsis and *Yersinia enterocolitica* neonatal infection: A unique combination in a preterm infant. Eur J Pediatr 146:192, 1987.

84. Grisaru-Soen G, Lerner-Geva L, Keller N, et al: *Pseudomonas aeruginosa* bacteremia in children: Analysis of trends in prevalence, antibiotic resistance and prognostic factors. Pediatr Infect Dis J 19:959, 2000.

85. Anderson MR, Blumer JL: Advances in the therapy for sepsis in children. Pediatr Clin North Am 44:179, 1997.

86. Glauser MP: The inflammatory cytokines: New developments in the pathophysiology and treatment of septic shock. Drugs 52(suppl 2):9, 1996.

87. Wolach B: Neonatal sepsis: Pathogenesis and supportive therapy. Semin Perinatol 21:28, 1997.

88. Adrie C, Pinsky MR: The inflammatory balance in human sepsis. Intensive Care Med 26:364, 2000.

89. Kilpatrick L, Harris MC: Cytokines and the inflammatory response. In Polin RA, Fox WW (eds): Fetal and Neonatal Physiology, 2nd ed. Philadelphia, WB Saunders, 1997, pp 1967-1979.

90. Blackwell TS, Christman JW: Sepsis and cytokines: Current status. Br J Anaesth 77:110, 1996.

91. Kim PK, Deutschman CS: Inflammatory responses and mediators. Surg Clin North Am 80:885, 2000.

92. Goldman S, Ellis R, Dhar V, Cairo MS: Rationale and potential use of cytokines in the prevention and treatment of neonatal sepsis. Clin Perinatol 25:699, 1998.

93. Luster AD: Chemokines—chemotactic cytokines that mediate inflammation. N Engl J Med 338:436, 1998.

94. Van derPoll T, van Deventer SJH: Cytokines and anticytokines in the pathogenesis of sepsis. Infect Dis Clin North Am 13:413, 1999.

95. Casey LC: Immunologic response to infection and its role in septic shock. Crit Care Clin 16:193, 2000.

96. Quie P: Antimicrobial defenses in the neonate. Semin Perinatol 14:2, 1990.

97. Sandberg K: Preterm infants with low immunoglobulin G levels have increased risk of neonatal sepsis but do not benefit from prophylactic immunoglobulin G. J Pediatr 137:623, 2000.

98. Stiehm ER: Role of immunoglobulin therapy in neonatal infections: Where we stand today. Rev Infect Dis 12(suppl 4):S439, 1990.

99. Chen JY: Intravenous immunoglobulin in the treatment of full-term and premature newborns with sepsis. J Formos Med Assoc 95:839, 1996.

100. Stiehm ER: Intravenous immunoglobulins in neonates and infants: An overview. Pediatr Infect Dis 5(3 suppl): S217, 1986.

101. Baker CJ, Kasper DL: Correlation of maternal antibody deficiency with susceptibility to neonatal group B streptococcal infection. N Engl J Med 294:753, 1976.

102. Fischer GW: Immunoglobulin therapy of neonatal group B streptococcal infections: An overview. Pediatr Infect Dis J 7(5 suppl):S13, 1988.

103. Baker CJ, Melish ME, Hall RT, et al: Intravenous immune globulin for the prevention of nosocomial infection in low-birth-weight neonates. N Engl J Med 327:213, 1992.

104. Clapp DW, Kliegman RM, Baley JE, et al: Use of intravenously administered immune globulin to prevent nosocomial sepsis in low birth weight infants: Report of a pilot study. J Pediatr 115:973, 1989.

105. Fanaroff A, Wright E, Korones S, et al: A controlled trial of prophylactic intravenous immunoglobulin (IVIG) to reduce nosocomial infection (N.I.) in VLBW infants [abstract]. Pediatr Res 33:202A, 1992.

106. Haque KN, Zaidi MH, Haque SK, et al: Intravenous immunoglobulin for prevention of sepsis in preterm and low birth weight infants. Pediatr Infect Dis 5:622, 1986.

107. Sidiropoulos D, Boehme U, Von Muralt G, et al: Immunoglobulin supplementation in prevention or treatment of neonatal sepsis. Pediatr Infect Dis 5:S193, 1986.

108. Shenoi A: Multicenter randomized placebo controlled trial of therapy with intravenous immunoglobulin in decreasing mortality due to neonatal sepsis. Indian Pediatr 36:1113, 1999.

109. Christensen RD, Brown MS, Hall DC, et al: Effect on neutrophil kinetics and serum opsonic capacity of intravenous administration of immune globulin to neonates with clinical signs of early-onset sepsis. J Pediatr 118:606, 1991.

110. Hill HR, Shigeoka AO, Pineus S, Christensen RD: Intravenous IgG in combination with other modalities in the treatment of neonatal infection. Pediatr Infect Dis 5:S180, 1986.

111. Amato M: Immunoglobulin subclass concentration in preterm infants treated prophylactically with different intravenous immunoglobins. Am J Perinatol 12:306, 1995.

112. Haque KN, Zaidi MH, Bahakim H: IgM-enriched intravenous immunoglobulin therapy in neonatal sepsis. Am J Dis Child 142:1293, 1988.

113. Weisman LE, Cruess DF, Fischer GW: Standard versus hyperimmune intravenous immunoglobulin in preventing or treating neonatal bacterial infections. Clin Perinatol 20:211, 1993.

114. Calhoun DA, Christensen RD, Edstrom CS, et al: Consistent approaches to procedures and practices in neonatal hematology. Clin Perinatol 27:733, 2000.

115. Givner LB: Pooled human IgG hyperimmune for type III group B streptococci: Evaluation against multiple strains in vitro and in experimental disease. J Infect Dis 163:1141, 1991.

116. Rosenthal J, Healey T, Ellis R, et al: A two-year follow-up of neonates with presumed sepsis treated with recombinant human granulocyte colony-stimulating factor during the first week of life. J Pediatr 128:135, 1996.

117. Barak Y: The in vivo effect of recombinant human granulocyte-colony stimulating factor in neutropenic neonates with sepsis. Eur J Pediatr 156:643, 1997.

118. Bedford Russell AR: A trial of recombinant human granulocyte colony stimulating factor for the treatment of very low birthweight infants with presumed sepsis and neutropenia. Arch Dis Child Fetal Neonatal Educ 84:F172, 2001.

119. Cairo MS, van de Ven C, Mauss D, Sender L: Recombinant human granulocyte-macrophage colony stimulating factor primes neonatal granulocytes for enhanced oxidative metabolism and chemotaxis. Pediatr Res 26:395, 1989.

120. Gillan E, Christensen R, Suen Y, et al: A randomized, placebo-controlled trial of recombinant granulocyte colony-stimulating factor administration in newborn infants with presumed sepsis: Significant induction of peripheral and bone marrow neutrophilia. Blood 84:1427, 1994.

121. Ishikawa K: Difference in the responses after administration of granulocyte colony-stimulating factor in septic patients with relative neutropenia. J Trauma 48:814, 2000.

122. Bernstein HM: Administration of recombinant granulocyte colony-stimulating factor to neonates with septicemia: A meta-analysis. J Pediatr 138:917, 2001.

123. Cairo MS, Christensen R, Sender LS, et al: Results of a phase I/II trial of recombinant human granulocyte-macrophage colony-stimulating factor in very low birthweight neonates: Significant induction of circulatory neutrophils, monocytes, platelets, and bone marrow neutrophils. Blood 86:2509, 1994.

124. Frenck RW Jr, Buescher ES, Vadhan-Raj S: The effects of recombinant human granulocyte-macrophage colony stimulating factor on in vitro cord blood granulocyte function. Pediatr Res 26:43, 1989.

125. Frenck RW, Sarman G, Harper TE, Buescher ES: The ability of recombinant murine granulocyte-macrophage colony stimulating factor to protect neonatal rats from septic death due to *Staphylococcus aureus*. J Infect Dis 162:109, 1990.

126. Bilgin K: A randomized trial of granulocyte-macrophage colony-stimulating factor in neonates with sepsis and neutropenia. Pediatrics 107:36, 2001.

127. Sweetman RW, Rosenthal J, Cairo MS: Leukocyte disorders in the newborn. In Taeusch HW, Ballard RA (eds): Avery's Diseases of the Newborn, 7th ed. Philadelphia, WB Saunders, 1998, pp 1112-1122.

128. Laurenti F, Ferro R, Giancarlo I, et al: Polymorphonuclear leukocyte transfusion for the treatment of sepsis in the newborn infant. J Pediatr 98:118, 1981.

129. Baley JE, Stork EK, Warrentin PI, et al: Buffy coat transfusions in neutropenic neonates with presumed sepsis, a prospective randomized trial. Pediatrics 80:712, 1987.

130. Christensen RD, Rothstein G, Anstall HB, et al: Granulocyte transfusions in neonates with bacterial infection, neutropenia, and depletion of mature marrow neutrophils. Pediatrics 70:1, 1982.

131. Doyle JJ, Schmidt B, Planchette V, Ziporsky A: Hematology. In Avery GB, Fletcher MA, MacDonald MG (eds): Neonatology: Pathophysiology and Management of the Newborn, 5th ed. Philadelphia, Lippincott Williams & Wilkins, 1999, pp 1045-1091.

132. Hill HR: Phagocyte transfusion: Ultimate therapy of neonatal disease? J Pediatr 98:59, 1981.

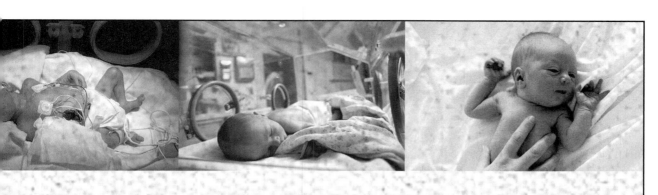

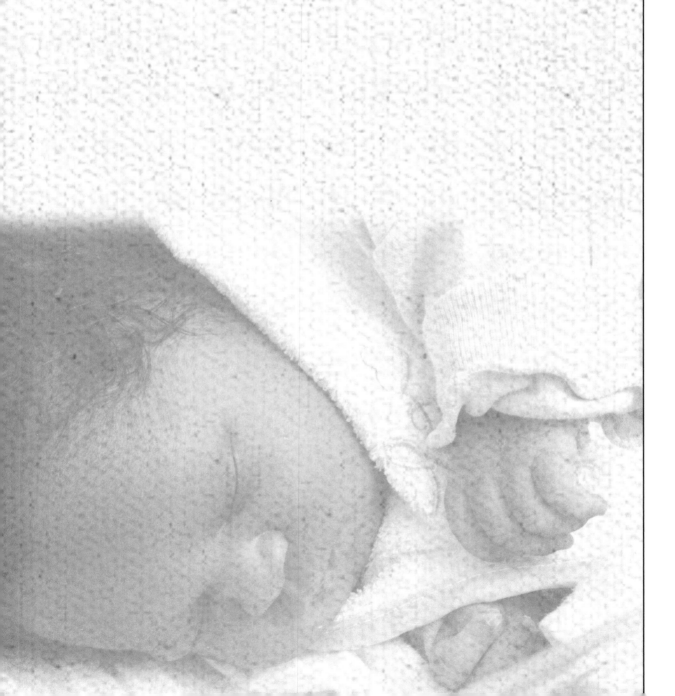

Metabolic and Endocrine Disorders of the Neonate

CHAPTER 72

Neonatal Thyroid Disorders

Andrew H. Lane and Thomas A. Wilson

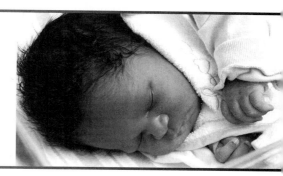

The complexities of thyroid function are magnified by the need to consider the interactions between the maternal-fetal units and the adjustments in thyroid function that occur with parturition. The survival of premature, low-birth-weight infants offers challenges to the neonatologist and endocrinologist who must interpret thyroid function and make clinical decisions in this progressively more immature population. The tools of the molecular biologist, applied to an array of thyroid disorders, now provide a molecular mechanism of previously poorly understood disorders. This chapter reviews thyroid physiology and thyroid disorders in neonates with an emphasis on providing the clinician with a mechanism to interpret thyroid function in the growing premature and "micro" premature infant.

THYROID GLAND DEVELOPMENT

During the second week of gestation, the **thyroid gland** begins to form as a thickening of the anterior pharyngeal floor between the first and second branchial arches at the caudal base of the developing embryonic tongue.[1,2] The thickened endodermal tissue invaginates downward as a diverticulum. As it descends down through the neck, pulled by the elongating embryo, it leaves behind the nonfunctional thyroglossal duct. The thyroglossal duct degenerates, although in a few individuals it remains patent and is the origin of thyroglossal duct cysts later in life. As the thyroid gland descends through the neck, it divides into several lobes and comes to rest in its final position anterior to the second through sixth tracheal rings by 7 weeks of gestation.[3] While the thyroid is descending, bilateral diverticula from the fourth and fifth pharyngeal pouches develop into the ultimobranchial bodies. These fuse with the thyroid gland by 8 to 9 weeks of gestation and form part of the lateral thyroid gland and the calcitonin-secreting parafollicular cells. By 13 to 14 weeks of gestation, the endodermal-derived thyroid precursor cells have differentiated into follicular cells and are synthesizing colloid. Colloidal material accumulates initially in the smooth endoplasmic reticulum of the follicular cells and later becomes secreted and trapped between adjacent cells, forming follicles.[1]

Several DNA-binding transcription factors implicated in thyroid dysgenesis have been described.[4] **Thyroid transcription factor 1 (TTF-1)**, the homeodomain-containing product of the NKX2-1 gene, is expressed in the epithelium of the embryonic thyroid gland and in the embryonic lung and diencephalic forebrain. Transgenic mice completely lacking TTF-1 (through targeted disruption of the gene) have rudimentary bronchial trees and die at birth. No thyroid tissue is found in these mice at autopsy.[5] Inadequate TTF-1 adversely affects human thyroid development as well. Neurologic deficits, such as ataxia, choreoathetosis, and mental retardation, out of proportion to the hypothyroidism, predominate in these patients.[6-8] As is true for many other transcription factors necessary for endocrine gland development, TTF-1 not only directs the development of the gland during embryogenesis, but also plays an important postdevelopmental role in regulating the transcription of many specific proteins made by the gland. TTF-1 regulates the expression of thyroglobulin, thyroid peroxidase, the thyroid-stimulating hormone (TSH) receptor, the sodium-iodine transporter, and its own promoter.[9]

Pax-8 is a paired domain transcription factor expressed in the embryonic thyroid, kidneys, and neural tube. Severe thyroid hypoplasia is observed in homozygous knockout mice, whereas heterozygous mice are unaffected.[10] In humans, heterozygous point mutations in the DNA binding region of Pax-8 are sufficient to cause severe thyroid hypoplasia in a handful of sporadic and familial cases.[11,12] Postdevelopmentally, Pax-8 activates the thyroglobulin, thyroid peroxidase, and sodium iodine symporter gene promoters, and many of its binding sites overlap those of TTF-1.[13] For some promoters, such as with the thyroglobulin gene promoter, Pax-8 and TTF-1 cooperate to activate the promoter while these factors may compete on other promoters. A third transcription factor important for thyroid development, the forkhead domain containing **thyroid transcription factor-2 (TTF-2)**, is expressed in the embryonic anterior foregut, including the thyroid anlagen, and in the Rathke pouch. A homozygous missense mutation in TTF-2 was identified in two brothers with agenesis of the thyroid gland, choanal atresia, cleft palate, bifid epiglottis, and spiky hair.[14] This phenotype is similar to the TTF-2 knockout mouse phenotype, which also has thyroid agenesis and cleft palate. Besides its expression in the thyroid gland, TTF-2 is also expressed during development in the Rathke pouch, presumably to help ensure temporally coordinated development of the pituitary and the thyroid gland. Additional transcription factors, yet to be discovered, are likely to be crucial for thyroid development because extensive screening of patients with thyroid dysgenesis has found relatively few mutations in the above-described factors.[4]

HYPOTHALAMIC-PITUITARY DEVELOPMENT

The hypothalamic nuclei destined to secrete **thyrotropin-releasing factor (TRH)** are present in the embryo at approximately 55 days, but are not completely morphologically mature until 16 weeks of gestation.[1] Despite this immaturity, TRH can be detected in the hypothalamus by 9 weeks of gestation. By approximately 13 weeks of gestation, neuronal axons from TRH synthesizing cells extend to the median eminence for release of TRH into the portal circulation. Early in gestation, TRH also is synthesized in the fetal gastrointestinal tract and pancreas.[15] The importance of this extrathyroidal TRH is unknown. The anterior pituitary begins to form during the fourth week of gestation, when ectodermal tissue in the roof of the developing oral cavity invaginates upward, creating the Rathke pouch. It migrates dorsally and assumes a position at 8 weeks of gestation as the anterior pituitary, adjacent to the neuroectoderm-derived infundibulum, or stalk, which had simultaneously grown downward from the diencephalon.[2] Similar to thyroid gland development, anterior pituitary development is governed by an overlapping cascade of transcription factors. These include the factors RPX, PTX 1 and 2, Lhx-3, Prop-1, and Pit 1. Mutations in each of these genes cause hypopituitarism (and central hypothyroidism) in mouse models and occasionally in humans. Postnatally, many of these genes regulate thyroid function by transactivation of the promoters of various anterior pituitary genes, such as Lhx-3's activation of the TSH-β gene.[16]

Basophilic cells, which secrete the glycoprotein hormone **TSH**, can be found first in the anterior pituitary at 10 weeks of gestation, and TSH can be detected in the pituitary and the serum at about 13 weeks, likely secreted under the influence of TRH in the portal circulation as described previously. Congenital central hypothyroidism may follow disruption of the above-described normal developmental program.

When the thyroid gland has migrated to its position and differentiated, further growth depends on TSH from the embryonic pituitary because the placenta is impermeable to maternal TSH. Similar to other members of the G protein–coupled receptor family, the TSH receptor has an extracellular ligand-binding domain, seven transmembrane segments connected by three intracellular

and three extracellular loops, and an intracytoplasmic tail. TSH binding to the extracellular N-terminus causes conformational changes of the loops and the intracytoplasmic C-terminal tail, which activates the stimulatory subunit of the G coupling protein; this activates adenyl cyclase, with a resultant increase in cyclic adenosine monophosphate (cAMP), resulting in downstream effects such as iodine accumulation by the gland, the synthesis and release of thyroid hormone, and thyroid cell growth and division.

THYROID HORMONE SYNTHESIS AND ACTION WITHIN CELLS

The principal circulating hormones produced by the thyroid gland are **triiodothyronine (T_3)** and **tetraiodothyronine, or thyroxine (T_4)**. They are formed through the iodination and coupling of tyrosyl residues on *thyroglobulin,* a glycoprotein produced in the thyroid gland follicular cell (Fig. 72-1). The first step in the synthesis of T_3 and T_4 is the trapping and storage of iodide by the thyroid gland. The only source of iodine for the fetus is the free transplacental passage of iodide from the maternal circulation and the placental monodeiodination of maternal iodothyronines. Iodide trapping, which first occurs at approximately 10 weeks of gestation, is mediated by the sodium-iodine symporter located at the basal membrane. When inside the cell, iodide traverses through the follicular cell cytoplasm and is positioned at the apical membrane for the next steps in thyroid hormone synthesis by the membrane-bound, chloride-iodine transporter protein, pendrin. Through the generation of hydrogen peroxide, the enzyme thyroid peroxidase oxidizes the iodide and subsequently iodinates the tyrosyl residues located within the peptide chains of thyroglobulin, a step referred to as *organification.* Subsequently, thyroid peroxidase couples together a monoiodotyrosine (MIT) and a diiodotyrosine (DIT) on the thyroglobulin protein to form 3,5,3'-triiodothyronine (T_3), or two DITs together to form 3,5,3',5'- tetraiodothyronine (T_4).

Thyroglobulin, which now contains T_4, T_3, uncoupled MIT and DIT, and noniodinated tyrosyl residues, is stored in a colloidal form in the follicular lumen. In response to TSH stimulation, small amounts of colloid are taken up from the follicle by micropinocytosis. The colloid-filled vesicles fuse with endosomes, whose lysozymes liberate the MIT, DIT, T_3, and T_4 from the thyroglobulin backbone.[17] An additional portion of the T_4 is deiodinated into T_3 within the gland, and T_3 and T_4 are released into the circulation. MIT and DIT also are deiodinated by the enzyme iodotyrosine deiodinase, and the iodine generated is reused in the generation of new iodotyrosyls. The lysosomal peptidases, termed *cathepsin B, D,* and *L,* digest most of the denuded thyroglobulin, and the breakdown products are recycled for new thyroglobulin synthesis. Defects in the enzymes or proteins involved in nearly any of these steps of thyroid hormone synthesis may lead to disorders collectively termed **thyroid dyshormonogenesis.**

Most thyroid hormone produced by the gland is T_4, which serves chiefly as a large circulating storage pool for T_3. Of T_3 available to tissues, 70% to 90% is generated by the extrathyroidal deiodination of T_4.[18] Although T_3 circulates, it is located primarily intracellularly, where it binds

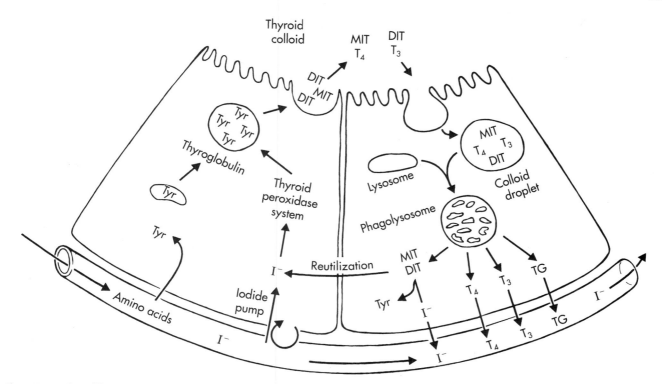

Figure 72–1. Thyroid hormone synthesis. DIT, diiodotyrosine; MIT, monoiodotyrosine; T_3, triiodothyronine; T_4, thyroxine; TG, thyroglobulin; Tyr, tyrosine.

to the thyroid hormone receptor whose affinity for T_3 is significantly greater than for T_4. T_3 is the most active thyroid hormone within cells. Iodothyronines are enzymatically deiodinated by three different types of monodeiodinase (MDI) enzymes (Fig. 72-2). Type I MDI, expressed in the liver, kidney, and to a lesser extent in the thyroid and pituitary gland, removes the outer ring 5′-iodine, converting T_4 to T_3. In addition, type I MDI can deiodinate the inner ring, converting T_4 to the inactive product reverse T_3 (rT_3) and rT_3 to diiodothyronine (T_2), which is also inactive. Type II MDI, expressed in the brain, pituitary, brown adipose tissue, keratinocytes, and placenta, also removes the outer ring 5′-iodine, converting T_4 to T_3. Its chief function is to regulate T_3 levels in the pituitary, playing a role in TSH secretion through modulation of the feedback inhibition exerted by circulating T_4. It also is important for newborn thermogenesis through its catabolic effects on brown fat. Type III MDI is expressed in the placenta and the fetal liver, kidney, brain, and epidermis. It primarily inactivates thyroid hormones in the placenta, fetus, and newborn by removing iodines from the inner ring, converting T_4 to rT_3 and T_3 to T_2.[19]

T_3 enters cells directly, or it may be generated within cells by the outer ring deiodination of intracellular T_4 by type I or II MDI. When T_3 reaches the nucleus, it must bind to a thyroid hormone receptor to have further effect. Two genes encode the receptors for thyroid hormones—the thyroid receptor α gene and the thyroid receptor β gene. Each gene has at least two splice forms, and these splice forms have varying tissue expression and timing during development. Similar to many other transcription factors, thyroid hormone receptors contain an activation

domain, a ligand-binding domain, and a DNA-binding domain.[20] The last-mentioned domain preferentially binds to an AGGTC/AA nucleotide consensus sequence, termed the **thyroid response element (TRE)**, found in the promoter of target genes. Thyroid hormone receptors bind to TREs as a monomer, a homodimer, or a heterodimer paired with other nuclear hormone receptors, such as the retinoic acid X receptor. Thyroid hormone binding induces transcription, which ultimately results in a variety of physiologic effects, such as increased metabolism of proteins, carbohydrates, lipids, and other substances. Although each of the thyroid hormone receptor isoforms can bind to TREs, only the α_1, β_1, and β_2 isoforms are able to bind to T_3, via the ligand-binding domain. Mutations in the ligand-binding domain of the thyroid hormone receptor β_1 isoform may reduce T_3 binding. When a normal thyroid hormone receptor forms a dimer with an inactive mutant thyroid hormone receptor β_1, the latter acts in a dominant negative manner by rendering the whole dimer inactive. The syndrome of thyroid hormone resistance results, which is characterized clinically by features of hypothyroidism with a paradoxically elevated T_4 and T_3 and normal to elevated TSH.[21-23] It is not known whether mutations in, or lack of, thyroid hormone receptor α cause disease in humans.

MATERNAL-FETAL THYROID INTERACTIONS

The placenta is relatively, but not completely, impermeable to maternal thyroid hormone. Before function of the fetal pituitary-thyroid axis late in the first trimester, growth of fetal tissues depends on placental transfer of

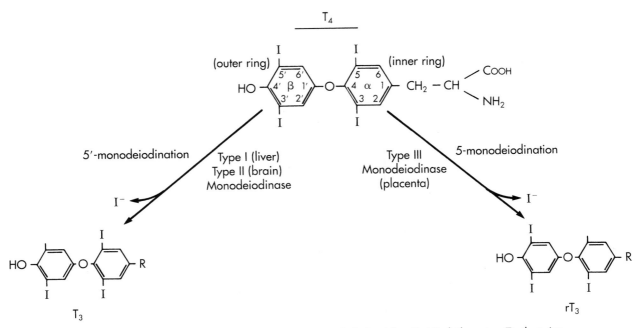

Figure 72–2. Thyroid hormone deiodination. rT_3, reverse triiodothyronine; T_3, triiodothyronine; T_4, thyroxine.

maternal T_3 and T_4. Developmental regulation of placental and fetal MDI activity allows the proper balance between small but sufficient maternal thyroid hormone transfer and maternal thyroid hormone inactivation. This regulation is crucial, given the significant maternal-to-fetal thyroid hormone gradient present until the third trimester.

Relatively low levels of type I MDI early in gestation lead to a significant fetal accumulation of inactive sulfated iodothyronines and limit T_4 to T_3 conversion within the fetus. Fetal type I MDI activity in peripheral tissues begins to accelerate at 30 weeks of gestation.[24]

Placental type II MDI expression is slightly increased early in gestation, most likely to allow the generation of local T_3 by outer ring monodeiodination of T_4, for trophoblast growth. During the third trimester, type II MDI activity increases, especially when hypothyroidism is present. In the normal fetus, type II MDI expression remains constant and low, however, relative to the expression of type III MDI.[25,26]

Fetal and placental type III MDI is thought to play an important role in limiting transfer of T_4 to the fetus by converting T_4 to the inactive rT_3 and T_2.[27,28] Although the MDI type III activity per milligram of placental protein or per microgram of placental DNA decreases throughout gestation, the total activity per placenta increases as the placenta increases in size, limiting the maternal transfer of T_4.[26] Reverse T_3 levels peak at about 250 ng/dL by 20 weeks of gestation, and then decline slowly until term. After delivery, rT_3 levels decrease rapidly to adult levels in the first few weeks of postnatal life.[18] Placental type III MDI conversion of T_4 to rT_3 probably contributes to the increased maternal need for T_4 observed during pregnancy. A small amount of maternal T_4 escapes inactivation by placental type III MDI. The serum concentration

of T_4 in neonates with athyreosis or total organification defects is not undetectable; rather, it is twofold to threefold reduced relative to normal infants.[29] Additionally, fetal brain expression of type II MDI, ensuring conversion of T_4 to T_3, and expression of sulfatases, able to convert the high levels of fetal sulfated iodothyronines to active hormones, are two mechanisms that help to ensure adequate central nervous system development when fetal T_4 production is abnormally low. The severe delays in maturation of a hypothyroid newborn harboring the same Pit-1 mutation as her hypothyroid mother, who did not take thyroxine during pregnancy, shows the importance of maternal T_4 to fetal development.[30] Because the half-life of T_4 in the newborn is estimated to be 3 to 4 days, the protective effects of maternal T_4 are lost soon after birth—hence the need for early detection and treatment of hypothyroidism.

THYROID FUNCTION OF THE FETUS

Fetal T_4 synthesis begins at low levels at 10 to 12 weeks of gestation. Later, a progressive and significant increase in T_4 occurs, beginning at 18 to 20 weeks of gestation.[18] T_3 production increases at 30 weeks of gestation, and fetal deiodination of T_4 to T_3 increases in the last trimester. Concentrations of T_4 and T_3 progressively increase throughout the rest of gestation such that by term, there has been a 5-fold to 6-fold increase in T_3 and T_4 concentrations and a 10-fold increase in serum free T_4 concentrations (Fig. 72-3). The increase in fetal serum T_4 concentration occurs in large part because the concentration of TSH doubles during this period to a mean peak concentration of 10 μIU/mL at term, significantly higher than the adult upper limit of normal of approximately

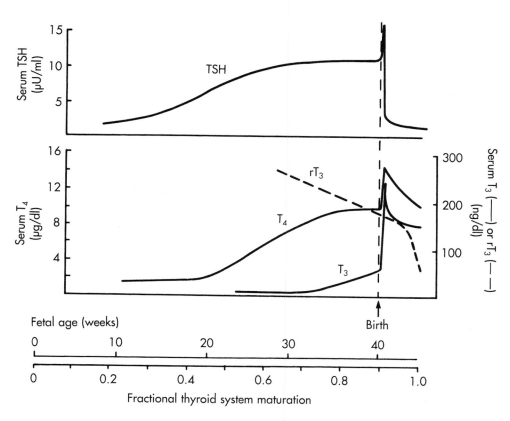

Figure 72–3. Maturation of the thyroid axis. rT$_3$, reverse triiodothyronine; T$_3$, triiodothyronine; T$_4$, thyroxine; TSH, thyroid-stimulating hormone.

5 μIU/mL. The hypothalamus, placenta, intestine, and pancreas also contribute to fetal serum TRH concentrations, which are elevated relative to adult concentrations.[15] The seemingly paradoxic simultaneous increase of T$_3$, T$_4$, TSH, and TRH reflects overall immaturity of the hypothalamic and pituitary sensitivity to inhibition by thyroid hormone. The steady increase in the ratio of free T$_4$ to TSH is an indication, however, that maturation of normal inhibitory feedback control on the pituitary and hypothalamus is occurring.[31] Final maturation of this feedback sensitivity and the hypothalamus's ability to stimulate the pituitary occurs in the days to weeks after delivery.[32]

Perhaps in response to the sudden temperature decrease experienced by a newborn, the pituitary releases a surge of TSH to a peak of 70 to 100 μIU/mL in the first hours after delivery. By day 2 to 3 of life, feedback inhibition from rising thyroid hormone levels has caused TSH to decline to 20 μIU/mL or less in most infants, which is the cutoff value used in most screening programs for congenital hypothyroidism. Stimulated by the sudden surge in TSH, free and total T$_3$ and T$_4$ concentrations promptly increase, with the mean T$_4$ peaking at about 17 μg/dL by day 2 to 3. T$_4$ levels slowly decrease to near adult ranges by the first 1 to 2 months of life. The postnatal surge in T$_3$ is due to increases in its direct release from the thyroid gland. In addition, the placenta efficiently converts T$_4$ to rT$_3$. Separation from the placenta at birth, allowing the newborn more efficient conversion of T$_4$ to T$_3$, also contributes to the postnatal increase in T$_3$.[24] These changes at birth also occur in the premature infant, although the peak hormone levels all are reduced, reflecting

the immaturity of a premature infant's hypothalamic-pituitary-thyroid axis.[33]

CONGENITAL HYPOTHYROIDISM

Central Nervous System Consequences of Congenital Hypothyroidism

Thyroid hormone is essential for neurogenesis, synaptogenesis, and myelinization of the fetal and neonatal central nervous system. In the absence of adequate thyroid hormone, these processes do not proceed normally, and mental retardation results. The clinical manifestations of neonatal hypothyroidism often are subtle, resulting in delay in diagnosis and treatment. In the prescreening era, neurologic outcome was inversely related to the age at which diagnosis and treatment were initiated. Most mental retardation can be prevented with early diagnosis and treatment. Early assessments of neurologic development in children with congenital hypothyroidism diagnosed and treated in the postscreening era indicated normal neurologic outcomes.[34,35] Long-term studies into adolescence have indicated persistent language, visuospatial, fine motor, attention, and memory deficits.[36-38] Two studies have suggested an increased incidence of mild sensorineural hearing loss in children with congenital hypothyroidism.[39,40] Most of these deficits appear to be exaggerated in patients with more severe congenital hypothyroidism (i.e., athyreosis); longer duration to correction of serum TSH; and inadequate treatment, owing to either poor compliance or inadequate dosing.[36,41] These findings have led to recommendations for more aggressive treatment of hyperthyroidism in infancy.[42,43]

Incidence

The incidence of congenital hypothyroidism has been assessed by a variety of neonatal screening programs and generally is in the range of 1 in 4000 newborns. Central congenital hypothyroidism due to hypothalamic or pituitary dysfunction occurs with a frequency of approximately 1 in 50,000 to 100,000 infants.[44]

Etiology

Iodine Deficiency or Excess

Iodine is essential for thyroid hormone synthesis. The requirement for iodine increases during pregnancy. Worldwide, iodine deficiency is the most common cause of congenital hypothyroidism. In addition to hypothyroidism, severe iodine deficiency results in reproductive loss, mental retardation, and congenital deafness.[45] Although hypothyroidism reverses with restoration of adequate iodine intake, neurosensory deafness does not. The recommended daily intake of iodine is presented in Table 72-1.

Paradoxically, exposure to excess iodine may induce transient hypothyroidism in the fetus and newborn (Wolff-Chaikoff effect). This effect may be seen with exposure to radiographic contrast materials or povidone-iodine–containing disinfectants.[47]

Thyroid Dysgenesis

Disorders in thyroid gland morphogenesis are known as **thyroid dysgenesis.** This term includes lack of thyroid formation **(thyroid agenesis),** underdevelopment of the thyroid **(thyroid hypoplasia),** and maldescent of the thyroid **(ectopic thyroid).** Together, these conditions account for greater than 80% of cases of congenital hypothyroidism. Although most such cases are sporadic, approximately 8% are familial, and cases seem to be more common in girls. Some of these cases have been identified to be due to mutations or deletions of Pax-8, TTF-1, TTF-2, and transcription factors described earlier, which are involved in thyroid gland morphogenesis. Mild to severe thyroid hypoplasia also may be due to a wide variety of inactivating

mutations located throughout any of the regions of the TSH receptor. The hypoplasia may be so severe that the patients are misdiagnosed as having athyreosis.[48-50]

As might be expected, athyreosis and thyroid dysgenesis generally result in the most serious forms of congenital hypothyroidism, judged by the degree of abnormality of serum T_4 and TSH concentrations and the degree of retardation of skeletal development. Some infants with sublingual thyroid glands may have sufficient thyroid function for part of their childhood. These individuals present later with acquired hypothyroidism, a mass at the base of the tongue or upper anterior neck, or iron deficiency anemia secondary to chronic bleeding from the sublingual thyroid. Whether environmental factors contribute to thyroid dysgenesis is unknown. Autoimmune thyroid disease in the mother has been postulated to be associated with thyroid dysgenesis, but this hypothesis has never been proven.

Dyshormonogenesis

Dyshormonogenesis refers to disorders of thyroid hormone synthesis due to genetic mutations in genes coding for various proteins involved in thyroid hormone synthesis. Any step involved in thyroid hormone synthesis may be involved (see Fig. 72-1). The most common of these is a defect in thyroid peroxidase resulting in an inability to organify iodine.[51,52] Other disorders involve defects in iodide secondary to mutations in the iodine-sodium symporter and pendrin,[53,54] disorders of thyroglobulin synthesis, defects in coupling, and defects in deiodinase.[55] In Pendred syndrome due to mutations or deletions of the pendrin gene, congenital hypothyroidism is accompanied by cochlear defects leading to congenital deafness. Dyshormonogenesis usually is associated with a goiter, but the goiter may not appear until after the neonatal period. Insufficient T_4 synthesis in response to TSH may occur in the context of pseudohypoparathyroidism, which is caused by an inactivating mutation of the G stimulatory protein α subunit, which links the TSH receptor (and other cAMP-linked receptors) to adenyl cyclase.

Transient Congenital Hypothyroidism

A variety of disorders may cause transient congenital hypothyroidism. The most common cause worldwide is maternal iodine deficiency followed by restoration of sufficient iodine intake in the neonate. In the United States, where iodine deficiency is uncommon, the most common cause for transient congenital hypothyroidism is maternal treatment with thioamide therapy for Graves disease. Propylthiouracil (PTU) and methimazole readily cross the placenta. These agents interfere with fetal thyroid hormone synthesis in the same manner that they are designed to suppress maternal thyroid hormonogenesis. In the fetus, the effect of these agents may be offset partially by transplacental passage of maternal immunoglobulin G (IgG) TSH receptor-stimulating antibodies. It is common, however, for infants born to mothers taking PTU or methimazole to express an elevation in TSH. Because the half-lives of PTU and methimazole are short, the effects of these agents quickly vanish within 1 or 2 days after the infant is born.

Table 72-1. Recommended Daily Intake of Iodine

Age	Recommended Iodine Intake (μg/day)
0-6 mo	110
7-12 mo	130
1-8 yr	90
9-13 yr	120
13 yr-adult	150
Pregnancy	220
Lactation	290

Adapted from Dunn JT, DeLange F: Damaged reproduction: The most important consequence of iodine deficiency. J Clin Endocrinol Metab 86:2360, 2001.

A less common etiology for transient congenital hypothyroidism is maternal IgG TSH receptor-blocking antibodies, which interfere with TSH activation of its receptor. This interference usually causes hypothyroidism in the mother and the infant. In the latter case, the hypothyroidism resolves as the titer of antibody declines after birth.[56]

Central Hypothyroidism

Central hypothyroidism refers to hypothyroidism occurring because of a problem with hypothalamic TRH or pituitary TSH secretion. This condition is estimated to occur in 1 in 50,000 to 100,000 infants. TSH deficiency occasionally occurs alone, such as observed in familial isolated TSH deficiency.[57,58] More commonly, central hypothyroidism is associated with other hypothalamic/pituitary deficiencies. These infants often come to attention because of signs and symptoms related to hypopituitarism, such as hypoglycemia, prolonged direct hyperbilirubinemia, midline defects, growth failure, micropenis, and diabetes insipidus. These infants rarely have hypothyroidism to a sufficient degree to cause symptoms and signs of congenital hypothyroidism. Infants with central hypothyroidism generally have serum T_4 concentrations in the mildly low range; low free T_4 concentrations; and TSH that is normal or, paradoxically, mildly elevated. Patients generally have a normal IQ outcome even though the condition may not be diagnosed and treated until later in childhood. Screening programs that are based on primary TSH screening generally miss infants with central hypothyroidism.

Signs and Symptoms

Congenital hypothyroidism is notorious because presenting signs in the neonate are often either subtle or absent, yet early detection and treatment are essential to preserve intellectual function. These facts justify the existence of neonatal screening programs, which are now nearly ubiquitous in industrialized countries but undeveloped in nonindustrialized countries. As the neonate matures, symptoms and signs eventually appear (Table 72-2), but often it is too late for initiation of therapy in time to prevent mental retardation. Many signs and symptoms relate to the slow gastrointestinal

mobility and slow metabolism that are typical of the hypothyroid state. Jaundice is prolonged because activity of bilirubin glucuronidase depends on thyroid hormone.

Screening

Given the subtle nature of congenital hypothyroidism in the neonate and the consequences of delayed recognition and treatment, this condition is ideal for neonatal screening. Screening programs were initiated regionally in the United States in the 1970s and currently exist in all states and most industrialized countries. Blood specimens are placed on filter paper at the time of discharge. Several strategies have been followed for screening for congenital hypothyroidism.[44] Most programs in the United States screen T_4 followed by TSH on the T_4 samples with the lowest levels. Many European countries screen TSH only. All screening tests require a confirmatory sample be obtained before the diagnosis of congenital hypothyroidism is established. These programs have reduced the age at diagnosis to weeks rather than months. Because a direct correlation exists between timing of onset of treatment and eventual intellectual outcome, these programs have resulted in a dramatic improvement in the prognosis for congenital hypothyroidism. Nevertheless, affected infants occasionally are not identified in the screening program because of failure to obtain a screening sample (i.e., home births), failure of the sample to arrive at the screening laboratory, laboratory errors, or communication errors. The screening program should never be relied on to exclude the diagnosis of congenital hypothyroidism if it is suspected for clinical reasons. In addition, screening programs are designed to try to identify all affected children. A considerable rate of false-positive identification occurs. For this reason, screening tests should not be relied on to finalize a diagnosis, and all infants identified in the neonatal screening program should have confirmatory testing performed.

Compensated Hypothyroidism

A subgroup of infants exists whose TSH is mildly elevated, but whose serum T_4 concentrations are normal and whose thyroid gland appears normal on thyroid scan or ultrasonography. This condition has variously been termed **compensated hypothyroidism, subclinical hypothyroidism,** or **persistent hyperthyrotropinemia.** Some children may have subtle defects in thyroid function that ultimately may lead to more severe hypothyroidism. Others persist with the same pattern of normal T_4 and mild elevation of TSH for years. One such group is some children with Down syndrome. Because it is difficult to differentiate the two groups in the neonatal period, it is our practice to treat these children for 3 years, then stop thyroxine therapy, and recheck thyroid functions 4 to 8 weeks off thyroxine to determine the need for ongoing treatment. A follow-up study of such infants using this approach indicated that most of them continued to require thyroxine, based on repeat thyroid function tests or TSH responses to TRH.[59] Often the dose of thyroxine required in this group is substantially less than in patients with thyroid dysgenesis (see later). Using this approach, the infant is protected from the potential of worsening hypothyroidism,

Table 72-2. Symptoms and Signs of Congenital Hypothyroidism	
Symptoms	**Signs**
Prolonged gestation	Jaundice
Feeding difficulties	Abdominal distention
Constipation	Umbilical hernia
Hypothermia	Rectal prolapse
Lethargy	Cutis marmorata
Prolonged jaundice	Cool extremities
Delayed cord regression	Large tongue
	Bradycardia
	Hypothermia
	Goiter (occasional)
	Delayed skeletal maturation

and the physician's risk of liability is reduced, while not relegating the infant to lifelong treatment.

Assessing Thyroid Function in Premature Infants

Interpretation of thyroid function in premature infants is challenging because serum concentrations of T_4, T_3, and TSH change throughout gestation (see Fig. 72-3). In addition, premature infants are often significantly ill or malnourished, which alters thyroid function, or they may be receiving dopamine or glucocorticoids, both of which are known to lower serum T_4 concentrations. **Euthyroid sick syndrome** is a physiologic response to illness or malnutrition (or both), which reverses when the underlying condition is reversed. In this condition, T_4 is preferentially converted by MDI III to rT_3, which is biologically inactive, rather than to T_3, which is biologically active. The net result is low serum concentrations of T_4 and T_3, an elevation of rT_3, and normal TSH. This is precisely the picture one sees in premature infants and very-low-birth-weight infants. Differentiating normal thyroid functions in prematurity from those of euthyroid sick syndrome is problematic, and one must rely on gestational age–adjusted data to do so. The problem is magnified by several studies showing an association between low level of serum T_4 in low-birth-weight infants and eventual neurologic outcome.[60] These observations have led to the suggestion that low-birth-weight infants with hypothyroxinemia but normal TSH be supplemented with thyroid hormone. Controlled studies examining the benefit of thyroxine supplementation in low-birth-weight infants with hypothyroxinemia generally have not shown a benefit of such supplementation, however.[60]

Because serum thyroid-binding globulin concentration is low in low-birth-weight infants, free T_4 and serum TSH concentration are the best method to assess thyroid function in this group. A variety of direct free T_4 assays are available. A free T_4 assay by equilibrium dialysis is least affected by variations in protein binding and is recommended. Values increase with advancing gestational age (Table 72-3). Because the normal ranges for free T_4 and TSH are wide, serial values often are helpful in differentiating true thyroid dysfunction from aberrations of

T_4 and TSH concentrations due to prematurity. Serum T_4 and free T_4 concentrations should increase with advancing age in preterm infants. Likewise, serum TSH concentrations generally decrease after the first week of life. If these changes are not observed, thyroid dysfunction should be considered. Primary hypothyroidism should be considered in infants with elevation of TSH, and central hypothyroidism should be considered in infants with low free T_4 by equilibrium dialysis and normal TSH.

Treatment

Thyroxine therapy should be started as soon as the diagnosis of congenital hypothyroidism is established and may be started while waiting for the results of the confirmatory sample if the clinical suspicion is high. Current recommendations are to start with 10 to 15 µg/kg/day of thyroxine. For a standard full-term infant, this translates to 37.5 to 50 µg/day. Thyroid function tests should be repeated in 2 to 6 weeks to ensure compliance and correction of the hypothyroidism. Serum T_4 concentrations usually normalize by 1 to 2 weeks and should be kept in the upper range of normal to slightly elevated for age. It is important to use age-appropriate norms because normal serum T_4 concentrations in infants are considerably higher than in adults, and most laboratories report adult norms. TSH may take longer to normalize, but in most cases should be in the normal range by 4 to 8 weeks. Occasional infants have a persistent elevation in serum TSH despite a serum T_4 that is elevated for age. These infants should be investigated for either thyroxine-binding globulin (TBG) excess, which results in high total T_4 concentrations but normal free T_4 concentrations, or for noncompliance followed by administration of thyroxine just preceding the day of blood sampling. Symptoms of irritability, poor weight gain, unusual sweating, or premature closure of the sutures or fontanelle warrant consideration of a decrease in dose. As infants age, the daily requirement for thyroxine factored for body weight gradually decreases to adult daily requirements (1.5 to 2 µg/kg/day). Thyroid functions should be monitored every 2 months throughout the first year of life to ensure proper dosing and compliance.

Currently, thyroxine is available in tablet form only. Parents should be instructed to crush the tablet and mix it with a small amount of breast milk, formula, cereal, or pureed food, which should be given in entirety once daily before feeding. Because compliance is always an issue with daily medication, caretakers should be encouraged to keep a calendar marked with medication administration and to establish a routine of giving the medication at the same time every day. Food may interfere with the absorption of thyroxine. Because it is practical to administer thyroxine to infants with a small amount of formula, however, uniformity of administration from day to day is most important. The dose can be adjusted according to T_4 and TSH concentrations achieved. If problems occur, thyroxine can be administered with a small amount of formula in between regular feedings.

A variety of thyroid preparations exist. Preparations that provide synthetic thyroxine only are the most uniform. Preparations containing a mixture of T_3 and T_4 are not necessary. Type I MDI converts T_4 to T_3, providing sufficient T_3.

Table 72–3. Free Thyroxine by Equilibrium Dialysis and Thyroid-Stimulating Hormone in Preterm Infants in the First Week of Life

Gestational Age (wk)	Free T_4 (pmol/L)	Free T_4 (ng/dL)	TSH (µU/mL)
25–27	7.7–28.3	0.6–2.2	0.2–30.3
28–30	7.7–43.8	0.6–3.4	0.2–20.6
31–33	12.9–48.9	1–3.8	0.7–27.9
34–36	15.4–56.6	1.2–4.4	1.2–21.6
37–42	25.7–68.2	2.0–5.3	1.0–39

T_4, thyroxine; TSH, thyroid-stimulating hormone.

Adapted from Adams L, Emery J, Clark S, et al: Reference ranges for newer thyroid function tests in premature infants. J Petriatr 126:122, 1995.

NEONATAL GOITER

Goiters are rare in neonates, but may be seen in infants with iodine deficiency[62]; infants with iodine overload[63]; infants with dyshormonogenesis; and infants exposed in utero to goitrogens, such as PTU or methimazole given to treat hyperthyroidism in the pregnant mother. Goiters also may be due to transplacental passage of TSH receptor–stimulating immunoglobulins from mothers with Graves disease. Occasionally the goiter may be sufficiently large to cause dystocia or to compromise the neonatal airway. Such large goiters may be diagnosed in utero by ultrasonography.[64] Cordocentesis sometimes is needed to determine fetal thyroid function. Large goiters due to thyroid hypofunction in the fetus may be treated with iodine to the mother, if due to iodine deficiency, or in utero by intraamniotic administration of thyroxine.[65-67] The thyroxine swallowed by the fetus suppresses fetal TSH and reduces thyroid enlargement. Fetal goiters due to maternal administration of PTU for Graves disease may be treated by reducing the maternal dose of PTU if tolerated by the mother.[68-70] Alternatively, intrauterine administration of thyroxine may be tried. More modest goiters may be treated postnatally with thyroxine or, if due to exposure to a goitrogen in utero, resolve spontaneously.

CONGENITAL HYPERTHYROIDISM

Infants born to mothers with Graves disease are at risk of fetal and neonatal hyperthyroidism. Signs and symptoms are listed in Table 72-4. Although maternal T_4 crosses the placenta only in modest degrees, TSH receptor–stimulating immunoglobulins, which cause Graves disease, cross the placenta readily and may stimulate overproduction of T_4 in the fetus and neonate. This situation may be seen in mothers who are euthyroid because of prior thyroidectomy or radioiodine ablation for Graves disease but in whom the antibodies persist. In reality, only 1% to 2% of infants born to mothers with Graves disease acquire these antibodies at a titer sufficient to cause clinical hyperthyroidism.[71-73] When neonatal Graves disease occurs by this mechanism, hyperthyroidism is transient, lasting weeks to a few months, because the titer of maternal antibodies declines over time. Because of this transient quality, the treatment of neonatal Graves disease is challenging and must be tailored to the degree of symptoms and severity of the hyperthyroidism. In mild cases, treatment with propranolol to block the β-adrenergic effects of hyperthyroidism may be adequate. This treatment has the advantage that serum concentrations of T_4 and T_3 may be followed as an index of the severity of the disease, and the infant is not placed in jeopardy of developing iatrogenic hypothyroidism. In more severe cases, blocking doses of iodine, iodine-containing contrast agents, or PTU may be required to control hyperthyroidism. Suggested doses are listed in Table 72-5. In such cases, serum concentrations of T_4 and TSH must be followed closely to prevent the development of iatrogenic hypothyroidism. In long-standing cases of hyperthyroidism, a TSH response to hypothyroidism may be blunted for weeks.[74] Low serum T_4 or free T_4 for age is often a better indicator of overtreatment with PTU or methimazole than is TSH.

Persistent neonatal hyperthyroidism occurs in infants with activating mutations of the TSH receptor or activating mutations of the α subunit of the G stimulatory protein, which links the TSH receptor to adenyl cyclase, leading to activation of the intracellular signal transduction. In this situation, T_4 synthesis and release occur independently of stimulation of the TSH receptor by either TSH or immunoglobulins.[75,76] Activation of the α subunit of the G stimulatory protein usually occurs in the context of McCune-Albright syndrome. In this condition, the activating mutation of the G stimulatory protein is often a postfertilization event and may affect other tissues sporadically and may lead to spontaneous ovarian function, excess growth hormone secretion, Cushing syndrome, and fibrous dysplasia of bone.[77,78]

DISORDERS OF THYROID HORMONE–BINDING PROTEINS

More than 99% of thyroid hormones in the circulation are bound to a variety of carrier proteins. TBG is the most important of these, accounting for about 70% of total

Table 72–4. Signs and Symptoms of Neonatal Hyperthyroidism

Symptoms	Signs
Poor feeding	Intrauterine growth retardation
Weight loss/lack of weight gain	Tachycardia; arrhythmia
Sweating	Stare
Jaundice	Hypertension
Fever	Congestive heart failure
	Frontal bossing
	Craniosynostosis
	Diarrhea; vomiting
	Dehydration
	Goiter

Table 72–5. Treatment of Neonatal Hyperthyroidism

Agent	Dose
Propranolol	2–4 mg/kg/day divided into 2 doses
Potassium iodide (Lugol's solution; SSKI)	1 drop tid
Sodium ipodate/ sodium iopanoate	100–200 mg/day or 500 mg q 3 days orally
Propylthiouracil	5–7 mg/kg/day divided into 2–3 doses
Methimazole	0.5–0.7 mg/kg/day in 1 or 2 divided doses

T_4 binding. Albumin binds another 15% to 20%, and transthyretin (TTR), previously named *thyroid-binding prealbumin,* binds 10% to 15% of the circulating thyroid hormones. Although the serum concentration of TBG is 17-fold lower than TTR and 2000-fold lower than albumin, TBG binds T_4 with at least 100-fold greater affinity than TTR and 10,000-fold greater affinity than albumin.[79] TBG is synthesized and secreted by the liver at 8 to 10 weeks of gestation, at the same time when T_4 is initially found in the fetus. Throughout gestation, maternal estrogens stimulate TBG synthesis, and TBG levels increase, accounting in part for the progressive and parallel rise in T_4. TTR is synthesized in the liver, pancreatic islets, and choroid plexus. Its high dissociation rate constant for thyroid hormone binding allows rapid delivery of free thyroid hormones into surrounding fluids, particularly the central nervous system.

Thyroxine-Binding Globulin Deficiency

Although TBG plays an important role in maintaining constant free T_4 levels, TBG deficiency is not thought to be clinically significant. Only one patient with severe TBG deficiency has been reported to have a persistently elevated TSH in childhood, possibly related to pituitary exposure to fluctuating free T_4 concentrations.[80] Data from newborn screening programs revealed that TBG deficiency occurs in about 1 in 4300 infants.[81] Mutations within the TBG gene, located on the X chromosome, cause a functional TBG deficiency through decreased binding of thyroid hormone, whereas frameshift mutations, or mutations causing protein instability, cause decreased serum concentrations of TBG.[82,83] Because the gene is X-linked, affected females usually have TBG levels that are between the levels of normal males and affected males. Most radioimmunoassays for T_4 measure the T_4-TBG complex. Functional or actual insufficiency of TBG can cause apparent hypothyroxinemia. Free T_4 levels are normal in these individuals, however, and measurements of low TBG can confirm the diagnosis. No treatment is necessary for TBG deficiency.

Excess Protein Binding

Duplication of the TBG gene, presumably during meiosis, causes twofold to threefold increases in serum TBG concentration, which leads to apparent hyperthyroxinemia.[84] The incidence of TBG excess is 1 in 6000 to 40,000.[85] Aside from the apparent hyperthyroxinemia, these individuals are clinically euthyroid, and no treatment is necessary. Similarly, autosomal dominant familial dysalbuminemic hyperthyroxinemia occurs with an arginine-218 to histidine amino acid change in albumin, resulting in a 10-fold increased affinity for T_4.[87,88]

TTR variants, such as the alanine-109 to threonine variant, have an increased affinity for T_4 and cause a clinical picture marked by euthyroidism, high T_4, and normal TSH and free T_4.[88] Although there have not been clinical descriptions of decreased binding or deficiency of TTR, such a scenario would be unlikely to cause disease in humans, given the description of phenotypically normal knockout mice lacking the TTR gene. Familial dysalbuminemic hyperthyroxinemia results from albumin variants with increased affinity for binding thyroid hormone, causing similar clinical and laboratory findings as the TTR variants with increased binding.[89] Correctly identifying any of these abnormalities of increased or decreased thyroid binding in an individual can prevent unnecessary future testing or treatment for that individual and for other affected family members subsequently identified.

EFFECT OF MATERNAL THYROID DYSFUNCTION

Maternal Hypothyroidism

Although the fetus develops a thyroid axis independent of that of the mother, maternal thyroid function has an impact on fetal outcome. Several studies have shown loss of IQ points in children born to mothers who were hypothyroid during pregnancy even though the infants themselves were euthyroid.[90,91] Although other explanations are plausible, this observation suggests that the small amount of thyroid hormone that does cross the placenta from the mother into the fetus may be important even in infants with an intact thyroid axis. Perhaps the importance of maternal thyroid function pertains to the first part of gestation, before fetal thyroid function is established. Recommendations for screening pregnant women for hypothyroidism and adequate replacement therapy with thyroxine for women found to be hypothyroid have followed.[91]

Maternal Hyperthyroidism

An increased rate of fetal attrition is associated with maternal hyperthyroidism.[92] A small percentage of women with Graves disease have sufficient titers of TSH receptor–stimulating IgG to cause hyperthyroidism in the fetus or newborn (see section on congenital hyperthyroidism). PTU is the treatment of choice for pregnant women with Graves disease. PTU crosses the placenta and may induce a goiter or hypothyroidism in the fetus. The smallest dose possible to control symptoms in the mother should be used. Methimazole is less protein bound than PTU and may cross the placenta more readily. In addition, methimazole has been associated with fetal cutis aplasia. Radioiodine therapy is contraindicated during pregnancy because of significant risk of hypothyroidism in the fetus. Thyroidectomy may be necessary if thionamide therapy is not tolerated or unsuccessful.[92]

Lactation

Although PTU and methimazole are measurable in breast milk, they generally do not cause neonatal thyroid dysfunction in breast-feeding infants.[93,94] Because PTU is more protein bound than methimazole, PTU may be the safer of the two agents during lactation. Hyperthyroid mothers should be encouraged to breast-feed. As a precaution, thyroid functions in the neonate may be monitored.

SUMMARY

Because of the complexities of thyroid physiology during gestation, understanding and managing thyroid dysfunction in the neonate and premature infant remain a challenge. Molecular techniques have begun to uncover some causes for congenital hypothyroidism, previously thought to be idiopathic. The causes of most cases of congenital hypothyroidism remain elusive, however. More recent data indicate the importance of normal maternal and fetal thyroid function to neurodevelopmental outcome in infants of all gestational ages.

Molecular techniques also have begun to uncover rare causes of hyperthyroidism. The molecular defects that underlie the immune dysregulation that forms the basis of Graves disease remain unknown, however. Treatment of hyperthyroidism has remained much unchanged since the 1970s.

REFERENCES

1. Pintar JE: Normal developmental of the hypothalamic-pituitary-thyroid axis. In Braverman L, Utiger R (eds): Werner and Ingbar's the Thyroid, 7th ed. Philadelphia, Lippincott-Raven, 1996, pp 6-18.
2. Moore KL: The Developing Human: Clinically Oriented Embryology. Philadelphia, WB Saunders, 1998.
3. Shepard TH: Onset of function in the human fetal thyroid: Biochemical and radioautographic studies from organ culture. J Clin Endocrinol Metab 27:945, 1967.
4. Macchia PE: Recent advances in understanding the molecular basis of primary congenital hypothyroidism. Mol Med Today 6:36, 2000.
5. Kimura S, Hara Y, Pineau T, et al: The T/ebp null mouse: Thyroid-specific enhancer-binding protein is essential for the organogenesis of the thyroid, lung, ventral forebrain, and pituitary. Genes Dev 10:60, 1996.
6. Devriendt K, Vanhole C, Matthijs G, de Zegher F: Deletion of thyroid transcription factor-1 gene in an infant with neonatal thyroid dysfunction and respiratory failure. N Engl J Med 338:1317, 1998.
7. Pohlenz J, Dumitrescu A, Zundel D, et al: Hyperthyrotropinemia, respiratory distress and ataxia associated with a mutation in the thyroid transcription factor 1 (TTF-1) gene. Presented at the Endocrine Society 83rd Annual Meeting, Denver, Colo, 2001.
8. Schuetz BR, Krude H: Loss of function mutations in the NKX2-1 gene define a new syndrome with CNS, thyroid and lung impairment. Presented at the Endocrine Society 83rd Annual Meeting, Denver, Colo, 2001.
9. Acebron A, Aza-Blanc P, Rossi DL, et al: Congenital human thyroglobulin defect due to low expression of the thyroid-specific transcription factor TTF-1. J Clin Invest 96:781, 1995.
10. Mansouri A, Chowdhury K, Gruss P: Follicular cells of the thyroid gland require Pax8 gene function. Nat Genet 19:87, 1998.
11. Macchia PE, Lapi P, Krude H, et al: PAX8 mutations associated with congenital hypothyroidism caused by thyroid dysgenesis. Nat Genet 19:83, 1998.
12. Vilain C, Rydlewski C, Dupree L, et al: Autosomal dominant transmission of congenital thyroid hypoplasia due to loss-of-function mutation of PAX8. J Clin Endocrinol Metab 86:234, 2001.
13. Pasca di Magliano M, Di Lauro R, Zannini M: Pax8 has a key role in thyroid cell differentiation. Proc Natl Acad Sci U S A 97:13144, 2000.
14. Clifton-Bligh RJ, Wentworth JM, Heinz P, et al: Mutation of the gene encoding human TTF-2 associated with thyroid agenesis, cleft palate and choanal atresia. Nat Genet 19:399, 1998.
15. Polk DH, Reviczky A, Lam RW, Fisher DA: Thyrotropin-releasing hormone in ovine fetus: Ontogeny and effect of thyroid hormone. Am J Physiol 260(1 pt 1):E53, 1991.
16. Cohen LE, Radovick S, Wondisford FE: Transcription factors and hypopituitarism. Trends Endocrinol Metab 10:326, 1999.
17. Bernier-Valentin F, Kostrouch Z, Rabilloud R, et al: Coated vesicles from thyroid cells carry iodinated thyroglobulin molecules: First indication for an internalization of the thyroid prohormone via a mechanism of receptor-mediated endocytosis J Biol Chem 265:17373, 1990.
18. Polk D, Fisher D: Thyroid disorders. In Spitzer A (ed): Intensive Care of the Fetus and Neonate. St. Louis, Mosby, 1996, pp 958-969.
19. Burrow GN, Fisher DA, Larsen PR: Maternal and fetal thyroid function. N Engl J Med 331:1072, 1994.
20. Zhang J, Lazar MA: The mechanism of action of thyroid hormones. Annu Rev Physiol 62:439, 2000.
21. Refetoff S, Weiss RE, Usala SJ: The syndromes of resistance to thyroid hormone. Endocr Rev 14:348, 1993.
22. Pohlenz J, Schonberger W, Koffler T, Refetoff S: Resistance to thyroid hormone caused by a new mutation (V336M) in the thyroid hormone receptor beta gene. Thyroid 9:1001, 1999.
23. Furlanetto TW, Kopp P, Peccin S, et al: A novel mutation (M310L) in the thyroid hormone receptor beta causing resistance to thyroid hormone in a Brazilian kindred and a neonate. Mol Genet Metab 71:520, 2000.
24. Santini F, Chiovato L, Ghirri P, et al: Serum iodothyronines in the human fetus and the newborn: Evidence for an important role of placenta in fetal thyroid hormone homeostasis. J Clin Endocrinol Metab 84:493, 1999.
25. Fisher D: Disorders of the thyroid in the newborn and infant. In Sperling M (ed): Pediatric Endocrinology. Philadelphia, WB Saunders, 1996, pp 51-70.
26. Koopdonk-Kool JM, de Vijlder JJ, Veenboer GJ, et al: Type II and type III deiodinase activity in human placenta as a function of gestational age. J Clin Endocrinol Metab 81:2154, 1996.
27. Roti E, Fang SL, Green K, et al: Human placenta is an active site of thyroxine and 3,3'5-triiodothyronine tyrosyl ring deiodination. J Clin Endocrinol Metab 53:498, 1981.
28. Mortimer R, Galligan J, Cannell GR, et al: Maternal to fetal thyroxine transmission in the human term placenta is limited by inner ring deiodination. J Clin Endocrinol Metab 81:2247, 1996.
29. Vulsma T, Gons MH, de Vijlder JJ: Maternal-fetal transfer of thyroxine in congenital hypothyroidism due to a total organification defect or thyroid agenesis. N Engl J Med 321:13, 1989.
30. de Zegher F, Pernasetti F, Vanhole C, et al: The prenatal role of thyroid hormone evidenced by fetomaternal Pit-1 deficiency J Clin Endocrinol Metab 80:3127, 1995.
31. Thorpe-Beeston JG, Nicolaides KH, McGregor AM: Fetal thyroid function. Thyroid 2:207, 1992.
32. Thorpe-Beeston JG, Nicolaides KH, Felton CV, et al: Maturation of the secretion of thyroid hormone and thyroid-stimulating hormone in the fetus. N Engl J Med 324:532, 1991.
33. LaFranchi S: Thyroid function in the preterm infant. Thyroid 9:71, 1999.
34. Rovet J: Hypothyroidism: Intellectual and neuropsychological functioning. In Holmes C (ed): Psychoneuroendocrinology: Brain, Behavior and Hormonal Interactions. New York, Springer Verlag, 1990, pp 273-322.
35. Simons W, Fuggle PW, Grant D, Smith I: Intellectual development at 10 years in early treated congenital hypothyroidism. Arch Dis Child 71:232, 1994.

36. Rovet JF: Long-term neuropsychological sequelae of early-treated congenital hypothyroidism: Effects in adolescence. Acta Paediatr 432(Suppl):83, 1999.

37. Salerno M, Militerni R, DiMaio S, et al: Intellectual outcome at 12 years of age in congenital hypothyroidism. Eur J Endocrinol 141:105, 1999.

38. Rovet JF, Ehrlich R: Psychoeducational outcomes in children with early-treated congenital hypothyroidism. Pediatrics 105:515, 2000.

39. Bellman SC, Davies A, Fuggle PW, et al: Mild impairment of neuro-otological function in early treated congenital hypothyroidism. Arch Dis Child 74:215, 1996.

40. Rovet J, Walker W, Bliss B, et al: Long-term sequelae of hearing impairment in congenital hypothyroidism. J Pediatr 128:776, 1996.

41. Hanukoglu A, Perlman K, Shamis I, et al: Relationship of etiology to treatment in congenital hypothyroidism. J Clin Endocrinol Metab 86:186, 2001.

42. American Academy of Pediatrics AAP Section on Endocrinology and Committee on Genetics, and American Thyroid Association Committee on Public Health: Newborn screening for congenital hypothyroidism: Recommended guidelines. Pediatrics 91:1203, 1993.

43. Heyerdahl S, Kase BF: Significance of elevated serum thyrotropin during treatment of congenital hypothyroidism. Acta Paediatr 84:634, 1995.

44. Newborn Screening for Congenital Hypothyroidism: Recommended Guidelines (RE9316). Available at: http://www.aap.org/policy/04407.html.

45. DeLange F, Ermans A: Iodine deficiency. In Braverman L, Utiger R (eds): Werner and Ingbar's the Thyroid. Philadelphia, Lippincott-Raven, 1996, pp 296-297.

46. Dunn JT, DeLange F: Damaged reproduction: The most important consequence of iodine deficiency. J Clin Endocrinol Metab 86:2360, 2001.

47. Gruters A, l'Allemand D, Heidemann PH, Schumbrand P: Incidence of iodine contamination in neonatal transient hyperthyrotropinemia. Eur J Pediatr 140:299, 1983.

48. Hayashizaki Y, Hiraoka Y, Tatsumi K, et al: Deoxyribonucleic acid analyses of five families with familial inherited thyroid stimulating hormone deficiency. J Clin Endocrinol Metab 71:792, 1990.

49. Sunthornthepvarakui T, Gottschalk ME, Hayashi Y, Refetoff S: Brief report: Resistance to thyrotropin caused by mutations in the thyrotropin-receptor gene. N Engl J Med 332:155, 1995.

50. Biebermann H, Schoneberg T, Krude H, et al: Mutations of the human thyrotropin receptor gene causing thyroid hypoplasia and persistent congenital hypothyroidism. J Clin Endocrinol Metab 82:3471, 1997.

51. Abramowicz M, Targovnik H, Varela V, et al: Identifications of a mutation in the coding sequence of the human thyroid peroxidase gene causing congenital goiter. J Clin Invest 90:1200, 1992.

52. Bakker B, Bikker H, Vulsma T, et al: Two decades of screening for congenital hypothyroidism in The Netherlands: TPO gene mutations in total iodide organification defects (an update). J Clin Endocrinol Metab 85:3708, 2000.

53. Everett LA, Glaser B, Beck JC, et al: Pendred syndrome is caused by mutations in a putative sulphate transporter gene (PDS). Nat Genet 17:411, 1997.

54. Pohlenz J, Refetoff S: Mutations in the sodium/iodide symporter (NIS) gene as a cause for iodide transport defects and congenital hypothyroidism. Biochimie 81:469, 1999.

55. Krude H, Biebermann H, Schnabel D, et al: Molecular pathogenesis of neonatal hypothyroidism. Horm Res 53:S112, 2000.

56. Brown RS, Bellisario RL, Botero D, et al: Incidence of transient congenital hypothyroidism due to maternal thyrotropin receptor-blocking antibodies in over one million babies. J Clin Endocrinol Metab 81:1147, 1996.

57. Miyai K, Azukizawa M, Kumahara Y: Familial isolated thyrotropin deficiency with cretinism. N Engl J Med 285:1043, 1971.

58. Vuissoz J, Deladoey J, Buyukgebiz A, et al: New autosomal recessive mutation of the TSH-beta subunit gene causing central isolated hypothyroidism. J Clin Endocrinol Metab 86:4468, 2001.

59. Daliva A, Linder B, DiMartino-Nardi J, Saenger P: Three year follow-up of borderline congenital hypothyroidism. J Pediatr 136:53, 2000.

60. Rappaport R, Rose S, Freemark M: Hypothyroxinemia in the preterm infant: The benefits and risks of thyroxine treatment. J Pediatr 139:182, 2001.

61. Adams L, Emery J, Clark S, et al: Reference ranges for newer thyroid function tests in premature infants. J Petriatr 126:122, 1995.

62. Salerno M, Di Maio S, Pisaturo L, et al: Fetal goiter in an iodine-deficient area. J Endocrinol Invest 21:721, 1998.

63. Vicens-Calvet E, Potau N, Carreras E, et al: Diagnosis and treatment in utero of goiter with hypothyroidism caused by iodide overload. J Pediatr 133:147, 1998.

64. Bromley B, Frigoletto FD Jr, Cramer D, et al: The fetal thyroid: Normal and abnormal sonographic measurements. J Ultrasound Med 11:25, 1992.

65. Volumenie JL, Polak M, Guibourdenche J, et al: Management of fetal thyroid goitres: A report of 11 cases in a single perinatal unit. Prenat Diagn 20:799, 2000.

66. Perrotin F, Sembely-Taveau C, Haddad G, et al: Prenatal diagnosis and early in utero management of fetal dyshormonogenetic goiter. Eur J Obstet Gynecol Reprod Biol 94:309, 2001.

67. Gruner C, Kollert A, Wildt L, et al: Intrauterine treatment of fetal goitrous hypothyroidism controlled by determination of thyroid-stimulating hormone in fetal serum: A case report and review of the literature. Fetal Diag Ther 16:47, 2001.

68. Ochoa-Maya MR, Frates MC, Lee-Parritz A, Seely EW: Resolution of fetal goiter after discontinuation of propylthiouracil in a pregnant woman with Graves' hyperthyroidism. Thyroid 9:1111, 1999.

69. Bellini P, Marinetti E, Arreghini A, et al: Treatment of maternal hyperthyroidism and fetal goiter. Min Ginecol 52:25, 2000.

70. Raccah-Tebeka B, Boissinot C, Madec A, et al: Management of fetal thyroid goiters: A report of 11 cases in a single perinatal unit. Prenat Diag 20:799, 2000.

71. Polak M: Hyperthyroidism in early infancy: Pathogenesis, clinical features and diagnosis with a focus on neonatal hyperthyroidism. Thyroid 8:1171, 1998.

72. Zimmerman D: Fetal and neonatal hyperthyroidism. Thyroid 9:727, 1999.

73. Smith C, Thomsett M, Choong C, et al: Congenital thyrotoxicosis in premature infants. Clin Endocrinol 54:371, 2001.

74. Hojo M, Momotani N, Ikeda N, et al: Prolonged suppressed thyroid-stimulating hormone levels in hyperthyroidism in a neonate born to a mother with Graves' disease. Acta Paediatr Jpn 40:483, 1998.

75. Fuhrer D, Mix M, Willgerodt H, et al: Autosomal dominant nonautoimmune hyperthyroidism: Clinical features, diagnosis, therapy. Exp Clin Endocrinol Diabetes 106(Suppl 4):S10, 1998.

76. Tonacchera M, Agretti P, Roselinni V, et al: Sporadic nonautoimmune congenital hyperthyroidism due to a strong

activating mutation of the thyrotropin receptor gene. Thyroid 10:859, 2000.

77. Spiegel AM: G protein defects in signal transduction. Horm Res 53(Suppl 3):17, 2000.

78. Mastorakos G, Mitsiades NS, Doufas AG, Koutras DA: Hyperthyroidism in McCune-Albright syndrome with a review of thyroid abnormalities sixty years after the first report. Thyroid 7:433, 1997.

79. Robbins J: Thyroid hormone transport proteins and the physiology of hormone binding. In Braverman L, Utiger R (eds): Werner and Ingbar's the Thyroid, 7th ed. Philadelphia, Lippincott-Raven, 1996, pp 96-110.

80. Carrel AL, Allen DB: Persistent infantile hypothyroidism attributable to thyroxine-binding globulin deficiency. Pediatrics 104(2 Pt 1):312, 1999.

81. Mandel S, Hanna C, Boston B, et al: Thyroxine-binding globulin deficiency detected by newborn screening. J Pediatr 122:227, 1993.

82. Carvalho GA, Weiss RE, Refetoff S: Complete thyroxine-binding globulin (TBG) deficiency produced by a mutation in acceptor splice site causing frameshift and early termination of translation (TBG-Kankakee). J Clin Endocrinol Metab 83:3604, 1998.

83. Refetoff S, Robin NI, Alper CA: Study of four new kindreds with inherited thyroxine-binding globulin abnormalities: Possible mutations of a single gene locus. J Clin Invest 51:848, 1972.

84. Mori Y, Jing P, Kayama M, et al: Gene amplification as a common cause of inherited thyroxine-binding globulin excess: Analysis of one familial and two sporadic cases. Endocr J 46:613, 1999.

85. Robbins J: Gene amplification as a cause for inherited thyroxine-binding globulin excess? J Clin Endocrinol Metab 80:3425, 1995.

86. Bartalena L: Recent achievements in studies on thyroid hormone-binding proteins. Endocr Rev 11:47, 1990.

87. Bartalena L, Robbins J: Thyroid hormone transport proteins. Clin Lab Med 13:583, 1993.

88. Rosen HN, Moses AC, Murrell JR, et al: Thyroxine interactions with transthyretin: A comparison of 10 different naturally occurring human transthyretin variants. J Clin Endocrinol Metab 77:370, 1993.

89. Ruiz M, Rajatanavin R, Young RA, et al: Familial dysalbuminemic hyperthyroxinemia: A syndrome that can be confused with thyrotoxicosis. N Engl J Med 306:635, 1982.

90. Haddow JE, Palomaki GE, Allan WC, et al: Maternal thyroid deficiency during pregnancy and subsequent neuropsychological development of the child. N Engl J Med 341:549, 1999.

91. Morreale de Escobar G, Obregon M, Esobar del Rey F: Is neuropsychological development related to maternal hypothyroidism or to maternal hypothyroxinemia? J Clin Endocrinol Metab 85:3975, 2000.

92. Emerson CH: Thyroid disease during and after pregnancy. In Braverman L, Utiger R (eds): Werner and Ingbar's the Thyroid, 7th ed. Philadelphia, Lippincott-Raven, 1996, pp 1025-1027.

93. Cooper DS: Treatment of thyrotoxicosis. In Braverman L, Utiger R (eds): Werner and Ingbar's the Thyroid, 7th ed. Philadelphia, Lippincott-Raven, 1996, p 727.

94. Mandel S, Cooper D: The use of antithyroid drugs in pregnancy and lactation. J Clin Endocrinol Metab 86:23549, 2001.

CHAPTER 73

Disorders of the Adrenal in the Newborn

Judith L. Ross

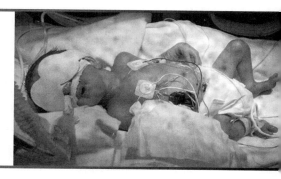

NORMAL ADRENAL ANATOMY AND PHYSIOLOGY

Adrenal Cortex

Normal development of the adrenal is vital,[1] and glucocorticoids and mineralocorticoids surge immediately after birth. The adrenal glands are pyramidal structures that are situated above the upper pole of the kidneys. The adrenal medulla and adrenal cortex are formed during the first 6 and 8 weeks of gestation. The glands enlarge during fetal development, reach an adult weight of approximately 4 g at term,[2] and involute rapidly during the first months of life. The **adrenal cortex** originates from mesenchymal cells from the coelomic cavity adjacent to the urogenital sinus. Initially the cortex consists of the inner fetal zone (80%) and the definitive zone or neocortex (20%), which ultimately forms the adult cortex. The fetal cortex grows significantly during fetal development, reaching a size one third of the kidneys at term.

Two transcription factors, *SF-1* and *DAX-1,* play crucial roles in adrenal development. *SF-1* regulates expression of genes encoding steroidogenic enzymes and is key for normal adrenal development. In humans, point mutations in one allele are associated with primary adrenal failure at birth, XY sex reversal, and persistent müllerian structures.[3] Mutations in the *DAX-1* gene cause X-linked congenital adrenal hypoplasia and absent fetal adrenal definitive zone.[4]

The fetal zone produces large amounts of C_{19} steroids, **dehydroepiandrosterone (DHEA)** and **dehydroepiandrosterone sulfate (DHEAS)**, and lesser amounts of cortisol and aldosterone.[5] DHEA and DHEAS serve as precursors for placental production of estrogen. Late in gestation, the fetal adrenal (under the influence of **adrenocorticotropic hormone [ACTH]**) achieves cortisol secretion rates that, per unit weight, exceed adult rates.[6] This relative cortisol surge in the third trimester increases fetal lung maturation and surfactant production.

The levels of C_{19} steroids decline rapidly after birth, as the fetal adrenal zone involutes rapidly in the first few days of life. Cortisol production rates decline in the first few months of life and reach a consistent production rate relative to body size.[7] Normal fetal growth and development occur despite fetal adrenal hypoplasia or ACTH deficiency because maternal cortisol crosses the placenta.

Although aldosterone is not necessary for normal fetal development, the fetal adrenal produces aldosterone, and at term, aldosterone levels respond to sodium loading and depletion.[18] Aldosterone levels remain elevated in the newborn period, but resemble secretion rates in older children and adults by 2 weeks of age.[8]

During infancy and childhood, the cortex evolves into the adult cortex, which includes three layers: the zona glomerulosa, zona fasciculata, and zona reticularis. After birth, the outer cells of the definitive cortex become the aldosterone-secreting glomerulosa cells, and the inner cells become the cortisol-secreting fasciculata cells (Fig. 73-1). Eventually a third, innermost, cortical zone, the zona reticularis, develops in childhood (age 4 to 8 years) and is the site of adrenal androgen production.

Adrenal Medulla

The **adrenal medulla** originates from neural crest cells that invade the medulla and coalesce by 6 to 7 weeks of gestation. In newborns, the medulla contains primitive sympathetic precursor cells that mature into chromaffin cells in the first 3 years of life. The medulla produces three major catecholamines from the precursor amino acid tyrosine: **epinephrine, norepinephrine,** and dopamine (Fig. 73-2). Epinephrine is synthesized in the adrenal medulla only, and norepinephrine is synthesized widely throughout the sympathetic nervous system and the brain. The catecholamines epinephrine, norepinephrine, and dopamine serve as neurotransmitters whose secretion is under direct control of the central nervous system.

Plasma levels of norepinephrine and epinephrine surge after full term spontaneous vaginal delivery and after premature birth. Cord blood levels of norepinephrine reach 2500 and 4200 pg/mL and of epinephrine reach 370 and 640 pg/mL for full-term and premature

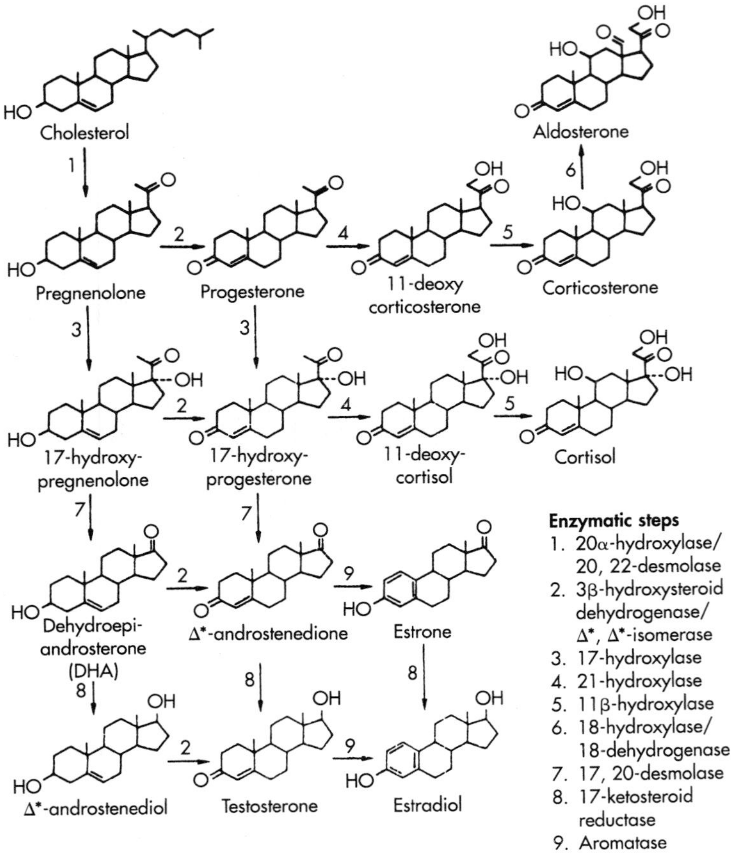

Figure 73–1. Adrenal steroid biosynthetic pathways.

Enzymatic steps
1. 20α-hydroxylase/ 20, 22-desmolase
2. 3β-hydroxysteroid dehydrogenase/ Δ*, Δ*-isomerase
3. 17-hydroxylase
4. 21-hydroxylase
5. 11β-hydroxylase
6. 18-hydroxylase/ 18-dehydrogenase
7. 17, 20-desmolase
8. 17-ketosteroid reductase
9. Aromatase

infants.[9] This catecholamine surge is accentuated by hypoxia, acidosis, cold, and hypoglycemia.[9] The increased catecholamines stimulate adaptive cardiovascular changes, inhibit insulin secretion, stimulate mobilization of adipose tissue thermogenesis, stimulate mobilization of pulmonary fluid, and enhance surfactant release.

REGULATION AND ACTIONS OF ADRENAL GLAND HORMONES

The two physiologically significant hormones that are synthesized in the adrenal cortex are cortisol and aldosterone.

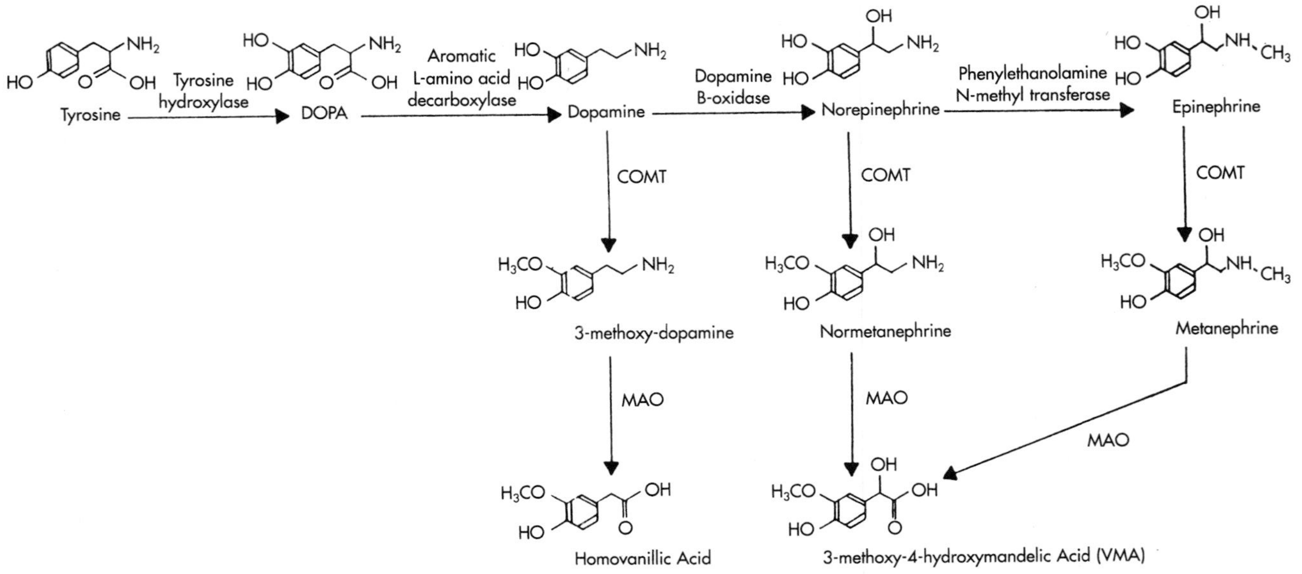

Figure 73–2. Catecholamine biosynthetic pathways. COMT, catechol *O*-methyltransferase; MAO, monoamine oxidase.

Cortisol

Cortisol Action

Cortisol circulates free, bound to corticosteroid binding globulin, or bound to albumin. Only the free fraction is biologically active. Binding of cortisol to its receptor results in mRNA transcription and altered protein synthesis. Glucocorticoids have the following characteristics in normal physiology: (1) maintenance of blood glucose by stimulating gluconeogenesis and lipolysis, reducing extrahepatic protein synthesis, and inhibiting insulin secretion[10]; (2) inhibition of inflammatory and allergic reactions, including inhibition of T-cell proliferation, increased sequestration of lymphocytes, decreased sequestration of neutrophils in bone marrow, and increased glucocorticoid-mediated eosinophil lysis[11]; and (3) facilitation of free water excretion by increasing glomerular filtration rate and inhibiting secretion of antidiuretic hormone. Antidiuretic hormone and **corticotropin-releasing hormone (CRH)** are released from the hypothalamic periventricular nucleus under negative feedback control by cortisol.[12]

Cortisol Regulation

ACTH regulates cortisol secretion. ACTH is a 39 amino acid peptide whose secretion from the anterior pituitary is controlled by hypothalamic-derived CRH, a 41 amino acid hormone. CRH also is made by the placenta. ACTH can be detected in the fetal pituitary 5 weeks after conception. ACTH levels increase at 12 to 34 weeks of gestation and decrease gradually until term.[13] Fetal adrenal development in the first 12 weeks is thought to be ACTH independent because anencephalic infants have normal fetal adrenal development up to that point. After 15 weeks, ACTH is crucial for normal adrenal development. One mechanism occurs through ACTH-associated stimulation of growth factors, including basic fibroblast growth factor, epidermal growth factor/transforming growth factor-β, and insulin-like growth factors I and II.[5] The endogenous, pulsatile, circadian rhythm of hypothalamic CRH release imposes a pulsatile, circadian rhythm for ACTH and cortisol secretion. The highest plasma cortisol concentrations usually occur in the early morning, and the lowest levels usually occur in the late evening. This circadian rhythm of CRH, ACTH, and cortisol secretion is not established until after 6 months of age.[14] Plasma cortisol levels also are controlled by feedback relationships with the pituitary and the hypothalamus. Early in infancy, increased plasma cortisol levels inhibit ACTH secretion through negative feedback, leading to involution of the fetal adrenal and remodeling of the cortex. Cortisol production rates are relatively constant, depending on body size, by several months of age.[15]

ACTH stimulates adenylate cyclase and cyclic adenosine monophosphate production in responsive adrenal cells, which results in hormone synthesis. The rate-limiting step in cortisol biosynthesis is the initial cleavage of cholesterol, the precursor for all adrenal steroids (glucocorticoids, mineralocorticoids, and sex steroids), by a specific cytochrome P-450 enzyme (see Fig. 73-1).

Physical, metabolic, and psychological stress can raise cortisol levels acutely 6 to 10 times the basal levels. Pain is a potent stimulus to increasing cortisol levels in infants. The newborn pituitary-adrenal axis is capable of responding to stress, as shown by an increase (tripling the baseline level) in plasma CRH, ACTH, and β-endorphin after vaginal delivery, venipuncture, sepsis, and circumcision.[16,17]

Aldosterone

Aldosterone Action

Aldosterone stimulates active sodium reabsorption and promotes excretion of potassium and hydrogen ion in the distal tubule of the kidney and in sweat glands, intestinal mucosa, and salivary glands. Insufficient aldosterone secretion leads to sodium wasting and hyperkalemia. The salt loss is usually manifest several days after birth because of the reduced glomerular filtration in the immediate newborn period. Conversely, excessive aldosterone causes potassium depletion, alkalosis, hypertension, and, rarely, edema.

Aldosterone Regulation

Angiotensin II, potassium, and, to a much lesser extent, ACTH stimulate aldosterone secretion in the zona glomerulosa of the adrenal cortex. Volume and sodium depletion stimulate renal renin production, and renin stimulates conversion of angiotensinogen substrate to angiotensin II. Only the zona glomerulosa cells have receptors for angiotensin II. Angiotensin II and potassium increase cholesterol side chain cleavage and stimulate steroidogenesis (corticosterone to aldosterone) in the zona glomerulosa. Aldosterone levels do not influence or control angiotensin production, but do inhibit renin secretion indirectly by causing sodium retention and fluid expansion. Atrial natriuretic factor is a 28 amino acid peptide produced in the cardiac atrium that decreases renin and aldosterone production and blocks aldosterone-mediated sodium retention in the kidney.[18]

Adrenal Sex Steroids

Weak androgens (DHEA, DHEAS, and androstenedione) are produced in the adrenal cortex of male and female infants. Levels diminish rapidly after birth and do not increase until adrenarche begins. Testosterone levels increase in the first several months of life in boys as a result of testicular synthesis. Minute amounts of the estrogens estrone and estradiol also are produced in the adrenal cortex.

TESTS OF ADRENAL FUNCTION

The diagnosis of adrenal gland disorders relies on the measurement and interpretation of several urine and serum measurements.

Urine Studies

Complete urine collections from small infants are difficult to obtain, and currently serum assays for various hormones can readily be performed on small samples. As a result, urine testing is used mainly for catecholamine studies.

Urine 17-Ketosteroids

The 17-ketosteroids are derived primarily from DHEA and include DHEA, etiocholanolone, and androsterone. The normal ranges are age dependent and are influenced by the development of the zona reticularis. This urine test had been used as a screen for congenital adrenal hyperplasia (CAH). Normal values for infants and small children are 0.1 to 0.6 mg/24 hours and for newborns are 0.1 to 1 mg/24 hours.[19]

Urine Free Cortisol

The free, unbound portion of circulating cortisol is excreted in the urine. This test is used to distinguish hypercortisolemic from normal states and is not affected by thyroid status or changes in cortisol binding globulin levels. Normal values for infants and small children are 1.4 to 18 μg/24 hours.[19]

Urine Pregnanetriol

Pregnanetriol is the major metabolite of 17-hydroxyprogesterone, and elevated urinary levels are observed in 21-hydroxylase-deficient CAH. Normal values for infants (>1 week old) and children are less than 2.5 mg/24 hours.[19]

Urine Catecholamines

Urinary catecholamine assays from timed or random urine samples are used to screen for neuroblastoma and for pheochromocytoma. Urine sampling provides an integrated assessment of catecholamine excretion over a timed interval. The plasma catecholamine measurements are more likely to be acutely increased by the stress of the blood sampling. Hypoglycemia, elevated intracranial pressure, and strenuous exercise all are associated with false-positive results on urine testing. Normal values for infants younger than 6 months of age are shown in Table 73-1.

Table 73-1. Normal Catecholamine Levels in Infants (Birth to 6 Months)

	Random Urine, Mean (Range)	Newborn Plasma, Mean (Range)
E (μg/g)	129 (25-181)	E (pg/mL) 65 (20-130)
NE (μg/g)	143 (37-195)	NE (pg/mL) 290 (200-420)
VMA (mg/g)	9.3 (5-17)	
Total metanephrines (μg/g)	1375 (500-2000)	
Dopamine (μg/g)	1117 (160-2350)	
Renin (ng/mL/h)		*Mean ± SD*
1 wk		18 ± 11
2-4 wk		79 ± 48
3-12 mo		<15

E, epinephrine; NE, norepinephrine; VMA, vanillylmandelic acid.
From Wiener D, Smith J, Dahlem S, et al: Serum adrenal steroid levels in healthy full-term 3-day-old infants. J Pediatr 110:122, 1987.

Provocative Tests of Adrenal Function

Adrenocorticotropic Hormone Stimulation Test

Synthetic ACTH (cosyntropin) contains the first 24 amino acids of pituitary ACTH. Bolus injection of synthetic ACTH is free of side effects. Under the usual circumstances, 250 μg is injected after obtaining a baseline sample for cortisol. Repeat cortisol samples are obtained at 30 and 60 minutes (Table 73-2). The normal response for infants and children is a stimulated cortisol value of greater than 20 μg/dL.[20,21] If the random cortisol value is greater than 20 μg/dL, the stimulation test is not necessary to establish the presence of normal adrenal cortical responsiveness. Stimulation with ACTH measures the acute release of cortisol from the adrenal cortex. The relationship between the hypothalamic-pituitary axis and the adrenal is so closely regulated that diminished ACTH stimulation results in diminished adrenal cortisol responsiveness within 8 to 12 days.[20,21] The ACTH stimulation test can be used to establish normal adrenal reserve secondary to abnormalities in the adrenal cortex (primary adrenal insufficiency) or in the hypothalamus or pituitary (secondary or tertiary adrenal insufficiency). The ACTH test correlates well with peak cortisol levels measured during surgical stress[22] but may not be reliable in the setting of acute ACTH deficiency, such as occurs after brain surgery, after stroke, or in the setting of prior ACTH treatment.[22,23] Under these circumstances, insulin-induced hypoglycemia is a more appropriate test of the hypothalamic-pituitary-adrenal axis.

Corticotropin-Releasing Hormone Test

The CRH test can distinguish whether ACTH deficiency is secondary to a deficiency in hypothalamic CRH or from a pituitary deficiency of ACTH. Ovine CRH is given by intravenous push (1 μg/kg), and cortisol and ACTH levels are measured at 0, 15, 30, and 60 minutes. If the defect is at the level of the hypothalamus, CRH stimulates pituitary release of ACTH. If the defect is at the level of the pituitary, no release of ACTH or cortisol occurs after CRH administration. The normal response to CRH is a twofold to fourfold increase in ACTH levels.[24]

Dexamethasone Suppression Test

The dexamethasone suppression test is used most commonly to measure the negative feedback relationship between the adrenal cortex (cortisol) and the hypothalamic-pituitary axis and is used to investigate whether elevated levels of adrenal hormones, such as cortisol and its precursors, can be suppressed by administering the potent glucocorticoid, dexamethasone. Under normal circumstances, dexamethasone administration results in prompt suppression of endogenous ACTH, CRH, cortisol, and its precursors. Usually 1 mg (20 μg/kg, up to 1 mg) of dexamethasone is given by mouth at midnight. The normal response is suppression of the following 8 AM cortisol value to less than 5 μg/dL.

Insulin Hypoglycemia

The insulin hypoglycemia test has been used to assess the response of the hypothalamic-pituitary-adrenal axis to the stress of hypoglycemia. Cortisol levels should be checked

Table 73–2. Glucocorticoid and Sex Steroid Response to Adrenocorticotropic Hormone

Steroid	Girls (<12 mo)	Boys (<12 mo)	Levels in 3-Day-Old Boys and Girls[*]
17-Hydroxypregnenolone (ng/dL)			
0 min	298 ± 272	283 ± 284	246 ± 284
60 min	1610 ± 800	1242 ± 754	
17-Hydroxyprogesterone (ng/dL)			
0 min	32 ± 29	60 ± 49	36 ± 18
60 min	142 ± 50	196 ± 85	
Dehydroepiandrosterone (ng/dL)			
0 min	133 ± 172	86 ± 70	NA
60 min	389 ± 325	257 ± 366	
Androstenedione (ng/dL)			
0 min	25 ± 21	23 ± 17	NA
60 min	55 ± 25	53 ± 35	
Dehydroepiandrosterone sulfate (μg/dL)			
0 min	30 ± 32	14 ± 11	160 ± 68
60 min	33 ± 33	18 ± 13	
Cortisol (μg/dL)			
0 min	12.8 ± 7.1	12.4 ± 5.3	6.2 ± 3.8
60 min	40 ± 8.1	38.2 ± 4.4	
Testosterone (ng/dL)			
0 min	3.2 ± 2.4[*]	109 ± 143[*]	NA
60 min	6.5 ± 3.8[*]	109 ± 137[*]	
11-Deoxycorticosterone (ng/dL)			
0 min	21 ± 14	24 ± 15	NA
60 min	65 ± 39	78 ± 26	
11-Deoxycortisol (ng/dL)			
0 min	40 ± 46	68 ± 54	86 ± 34
60 min	196 ± 89	166 ± 38	

[*]Difference statistically significant (*P* < .05) between boys and girls.

NA, not available.

From Wiener D, Smith J, Dahlem S, et al: Serum adrenal steroid levels in healthy full-term 3-day-old infants. J Pediatr 110: 122, 1987.

routinely in hypoglycemia of unknown etiology. The infant is fasted for 2 to 6 hours. An intravenous line is inserted, and insulin (0.05 to 0.1 μ/kg) is injected. Blood is obtained for measurement of glucose and cortisol at 0, 15, 30, and 45 minutes. Glucose levels are checked at the bedside more often, particularly if symptoms of hypoglycemia develop. Dextrose and glucagon should be available at the bedside for immediate treatment of severe hypoglycemia. Normal responsiveness is defined as a stimulated cortisol level greater than 20 μg/dL (ACTH >50 pg/mL) with simultaneous hypoglycemia (glucose <40 mg/dL or 50% decrease in glucose from the baseline).[22,23]

In general, this test is rarely performed because cortisol levels can be checked during spontaneous clinical circumstances, and insulin-induced hypoglycemia can be associated with morbidity. In general, the cortisol response to hypoglycemia correlates well with the short ACTH stimulation test except in the setting of acute adrenal insufficiency, in which the short ACTH test may not be reliable.

Evaluation of the Adrenal Medulla

Plasma Catecholamines

Measurement of plasma catecholamines is generally of limited benefit because the stress and pain of the needle stick can raise catecholamine levels acutely. If plasma samples are obtained, the patient should be supine and relaxed. Urine measurements provide an integrated measure of catecholamine production over 24 hours (see Table 73-1).

Urine Catecholamines

Urine catecholamines are discussed in the section on urine studies.

ADRENAL INSUFFICIENCY (ADDISON DISEASE)

Adrenal insufficiency reflects deficiency of glucocorticoid (cortisol), mineralocorticoid (aldosterone), or both and can be primary (localized in the adrenal cortex) or secondary (localized in the hypothalamic-pituitary axis). The signs and symptoms depend on whether the deficiency is primary or secondary and whether there is deficiency of only glucocorticoid (primary or secondary adrenal insufficiency) or a deficiency of glucocorticoid and mineralocorticoid (primary adrenal insufficiency).

Signs and Symptoms

Infants with adrenal insufficiency develop feeding difficulties, vomiting, weight loss, prolonged jaundice, cyanosis, seizures, apnea, hypotension, or shock. Shock is characterized by a high-output state with diminished systemic vascular resistance and can mimic septic shock.[25] The hypotension does not respond well to volume replacement without simultaneous glucocorticoid replacement because glucocorticoids are necessary for catecholamine-mediated effects on vascular tone.[25] Acute adrenal insufficiency (addisonian crisis) follows destruction of 90% or more of the cortex and can occur as the initial presentation of adrenal insufficiency or at any time after the diagnosis has been made. Infants with primary but not secondary adrenal insufficiency can develop hyperpigmentation because the decreased cortisol levels stimulate hypothalamic secretion of pro-opiomelanocortin, which is a precursor for ACTH and other peptides that stimulate hyperpigmentation. The most characteristic sites for hyperpigmentation are the extensor surfaces, nipples, genitalia, hand creases, oral mucosa, and scars.

Laboratory Abnormalities

The most commonly abnormal laboratory parameters in adrenal insufficiency are the serum electrolytes. Hyponatremia and hyperkalemia are observed frequently, with hyponatremia being more common (90% versus 65%).[26] The electrolyte profile depends on whether glucocorticoid and mineralocorticoid levels are low or whether only glucocorticoid levels are low.

Hyponatremia occurs with cortisol deficiency on the basis of primary or secondary adrenal insufficiency. The mechanism is the inability to excrete a free water load in the presence of cortisol deficiency. Free water is retained secondary to stimulation of antidiuretic hormone because antidiuretic hormone release is inhibited by glucocorticoids.[12] Adrenal insufficiency results in increased free water retention and urine sodium wasting.

Hyperkalemia occurs only in the setting of primary adrenal insufficiency that includes mineralocorticoid deficiency. The hyperkalemia occurs secondary to impaired sodium-potassium exchange at the distal renal tubules and is accompanied by impaired bicarbonate absorption. Aldosterone deficiency leads to salt loss, weight loss, prerenal azotemia, hyperkalemia, hyponatremia, and acidosis. These symptoms usually develop over the first few days of life as the glomerular filtration rate increases.

Hypoglycemia often occurs with primary or secondary adrenal insufficiency because cortisol normally acts as an insulin antagonist. Cortisol deficiency results in increased sensitivity to circulating insulin, impaired gluconeogenesis, hepatic glucose output, and glycogen synthesis.[27] Insulin binds its receptor with greater affinity in glucocorticoid deficiency.[28] In adrenal insufficiency, insulin treatment of hyperkalemia may be dangerous.[15]

Hypercalcemia can occur in a subset (6%) of patients with adrenal insufficiency.[23] It is usually mild and occurs secondary to increased bone calcium resorption, decreased glomerular filtration, or increased tubular resorption. Mild normocytic anemia also can occur secondary to the permissive role of glucocorticoids in stimulating differentiation of erythroid progenitor cells to erythropoietic cells.[22] Eosinophilia is seen on the basis of diminished glucocorticoid-mediated eosinophil lysis.[29] Other associated findings include increased thyroid-stimulating hormone levels because glucocorticoids may decrease tissue sensitivity to thyroid-stimulating hormone.[17]

Diagnosis

The keystone for diagnosis of adrenal (glucocorticoid) insufficiency is measurement of serum cortisol and ACTH (if possible) in the acute setting of adrenal insufficiency. Cortisol levels with major (nonadrenal) stress range from 20 to 120 μg/dL.[30] Cortisol levels less than 20 μg/dL in the acute setting suggest the diagnosis of adrenal insufficiency. An ACTH stimulation test should be performed as soon as possible after the infant has been stabilized. Replacement therapy should not be delayed in a seriously ill infant, however. A random sample in a critically ill infant is generally sufficient to establish the diagnosis because hypotension is a potent stimulus for ACTH and cortisol secretion. The finding of decreased cortisol (<20 μg/dL) and increased ACTH (>50 pg/mL) supports the diagnosis of primary adrenal insufficiency or an ACTH receptor abnormality.

The association of low cortisol and low or normal ACTH suggests secondary adrenal insufficiency. The diagnosis is established after assessing adrenal responsiveness to ACTH and ruling out a primary adrenal abnormality. The ACTH deficiency can be localized to the pituitary or the hypothalamus with the CRH stimulation test.

The diagnosis of aldosterone deficiency relies on the characteristic electrolyte picture (hyperkalemia, hyponatremia) and the measurement of plasma renin and aldosterone levels. Aldosterone levels generally are elevated in the first year of life, so a low measured value suggests aldosterone deficiency.

Treatment

Acute adrenal insufficiency is a life-threatening emergency that requires immediate intervention. The initial treatment of adrenal crisis and shock secondary to glucocorticoid deficiency is restoration of the circulating volume with saline or plasma. The initial saline is given rapidly intravenously to restore the circulating volume (20 mL/kg). The fluid deficit is generally 15% to 20% of the intravascular volume. Glucocorticoids (hydrocortisone sodium succinate [Solu-Cortef]) should be administered intravenously (25 to 50 mg) as a bolus, then every 6 hours as an intravenous bolus or as a continuous infusion. Serum electrolytes and glucose should be monitored closely. Mineralocorticoid replacement in the initial stages is not necessary because glucocorticoids (hydrocortisone) in the treatment doses provide sufficient mineralocorticoid coverage (20 to 35 mg of Solu-Cortef = 0.1 mg of fludrocortisone acetate [Florinef Acetate]); the onset of mineralocorticoid action relies on renal salt retention, which can take days; and the sodium deficit can be corrected initially with saline. Failure of hypotension to respond to fluids and glucocorticoid treatment after the first 6 to 8 hours suggests the presence of another underlying illness. The infant also requires evaluation for an underlying infection that may have precipitated the adrenal crisis.

After the infant has been stabilized, the intravenous maintenance dose of hydrocortisone is 6 to 12 mg/m²/day.[15]

The usual maintenance dose of oral hydrocortisone is 10 to 15 mg/m²/day. Hydrocortisone, rather than other glucocorticoids, is used for replacement therapy in infants because this formulation has the shortest half-life and is the least likely, in children, to be associated with growth suppression and the development of Cushing syndrome. The hydrocortisone oral suspension (Cortef) is no longer available because of suspension problems. Currently, hydrocortisone tablets are crushed and put in formula for infants.

In children with CAH, the adequacy of glucocorticoid replacement is assessed by monitoring the levels of 17-hydroxyprogesterone and testosterone and growth, general well-being, and weight gain. Mineralocorticoid replacement therapy includes fludrocortisone acetate, 0.05 to 0.1 mg/day (0.1-mg tablets), and supplemental salt, 18 to 36 mEq sodium chloride daily. The dose of fludrocortisone acetate is relatively independent of body size from infancy to adulthood. Parenteral mineralocorticoid is deoxycorticosterone acetate (1 to 2 mg intramuscularly daily, 5 mg/mL). Currently, this preparation is not available commercially. The adequacy of mineralocorticoid replacement is assessed by monitoring serum electrolytes, plasma renin activity, blood pressure, weight, and urine output.

Infants and children with adrenal insufficiency require coverage with extra glucocorticoid during times of stress because adrenal secretion of cortisol increases under circumstances of physiologic stress. For minor stress, such as a mild viral syndrome or a fever of greater than 100° F, the usual dose is doubled. For major stress such as surgery, significant vomiting, or trauma, the dose is tripled. If the child is vomiting, the first outpatient alternative is administration of glucocorticoid intramuscularly (Solu-Cortef, 25 to 50 mg); however, absorption can be unreliable, and the intravenous route for glucocorticoid administration may be necessary. Parents of infants with adrenal insufficiency need to be educated about the lifelong, critical nature of glucocorticoid replacement therapy, about injection technique, and about getting immediate medical attention if the infant is unable to retain oral glucocorticoids. When the infant or child has scheduled surgery, the extra glucocorticoid (hydrocortisone) should be given orally (three to four times maintenance or 25 to 50 mg) the day before, intravenously (50 to 100 mg infusion) the day of surgery, and either intravenously (25 to 50 mg) or orally the day after surgery. The dose can be tapered rapidly to the usual maintenance dose over the next 2 to 5 days. Children who also are mineralocorticoid deficient should receive the usual fludrocortisone acetate dose at midnight, the day before surgery. Mineralocorticoid replacement therapy is not necessary the day of surgery because hydrocortisone has sufficient mineralocorticoid effect for adequate sodium retention.

PRIMARY ADRENAL INSUFFICIENCY

Adrenocorticotropic Hormone Receptor Abnormalities

The **syndrome of unresponsiveness to ACTH** occurs secondary to defective ACTH receptors. It also can accompany an autosomal recessive disorder associated with achalasia and alacrima. Laboratory findings include cortisol deficiency and elevated levels of ACTH. The adrenals do not release cortisol in response to exogenous ACTH. Mineralocorticoid function is generally preserved. These infants do not have ambiguous genitalia because gonadal steroid pathways are normally maintained. The genetic etiology is thought to be on the basis of mutations in the triple A gene. Laboratory findings include low cortisol levels, normal aldosterone levels, and severe hypoglycemia. The electrolytes may be normal. Treatment consists of replacement with glucocorticoid as detailed earlier.

Congenital Adrenal Hypoplasia

X-linked **adrenal hypoplasia congenita** affects male infants with clinical evidence of severe cortisol and aldosterone deficiency.[31] This condition is caused by mutations in the *DAX-1* gene, which encodes an orphan nuclear receptor expressed in the hypothalamus, pituitary gonadotrophs, gonads, and adrenal gland, and is also associated with impaired gonadal development. The incidence is approximately 1 in 12,500 births. The disorder can be associated with pituitary hypoplasia, anencephaly, gonadotropin deficiency, or other X-linked disorders localized close to the Xp21 position on the X chromosome.[32] A second gene mutation in *SF-1* also is associated with adrenal and gonadal hypoplasia and may control expression of the *DAX-1* gene. *SF-1* also is a transcription factor and a nuclear receptor.[33]

Laboratory abnormalities in congenital adrenal hypoplasia include hyponatremia, hyperkalemia, hypoglycemia, decreased levels of cortisol and aldosterone, and increased levels of renin and ACTH. One antenatal clue to the diagnosis of this disorder is the presence of low maternal urinary estriols.[34] This finding occurs because the fetal adrenal contributes the precursors for placental formation of maternal estriols. Therapy consists of replacement with glucocorticoid and mineralocorticoid as described earlier.

Adrenal Hemorrhage

In newborns, **adrenal hemorrhage** can occur after a traumatic delivery, secondary to a bleeding diathesis, from treatment with anticoagulants, or from endotoxic shock (meningococcemia). Symptoms usually develop on day 2 to 7 of life.[35] Infants may have a lumbar mass. The adrenal enlargement secondary to hemorrhage often can be seen on ultrasound. Occasionally, hemorrhage is accompanied by jaundice and anemia. Affected infants most often do not have clinical evidence of adrenal insufficiency, unless the hemorrhage is bilateral. Infants may present with severe anemia and shock in the most severe circumstances. The adrenal hypofunction may persist or occasionally improves in weeks to months. Adrenal calcifications may be seen within 3 to 4 weeks after the acute event.[36] Therapy for adrenal insufficiency consists of replacement with glucocorticoid and mineralocorticoid as described earlier.

Adrenoleukodystrophy (Addison-Schilder Disease)

Adrenoleukodystrophy is a peroxisomal oxidation disorder associated with elevated levels of very-long-chain fatty acids (C_{26-28}) that lead to cerebral demyelination and adrenal insufficiency. Cells in the zona fasciculata develop characteristic inclusions. The neonatal form is autosomal recessive, and infants present with craniofacial abnormalities, hypotonia, seizures, retinitis pigmentosa, and optic atrophy.[1] The childhood form is X-linked and generally occurs in boys. Missense, nonsense, and splicing defects in the gene, an adenosine triphosphate transporter, have been described.[37] No successful therapy is currently available for this disorder. Experimental treatment protocols using short-chain fatty acids are under investigation. The adrenal insufficiency is treated with glucocorticoid and mineralocorticoid replacement as described earlier.

Congenital Adrenal Hyperplasia

CAH is an autosomal recessive disorder arising from a deficiency of one of the five enzymes that catalyze the conversion of cholesterol to cortisol (see Fig. 73-1). Each specific enzyme deficiency is associated with a form of CAH. Diminished cortisol production occurs as a result of the enzyme block, and the decreased cortisol levels feed back to the central nervous system, leading to increased ACTH production. ACTH stimulates the glucocorticoid pathway leading to elevated levels of precursors proximal to the enzyme-deficient step and to the signs and symptoms of CAH. Appropriate replacement of glucocorticoid and mineralocorticoid (as needed) is required for optimal control of CAH.

The manifestations of CAH depend on the specific enzyme deficiency, the extent of the enzyme deficiency, and the location of the enzyme deficiency in the glucocorticoid or mineralocorticoid pathway. If excess androgens are produced, the female fetus may be virilized. If there is cortisol deficiency, the infant (male and female) may develop adrenal insufficiency. If the mineralocorticoid pathway also is affected, the infant (male and female) may develop salt loss. It also has been learned that congenital absence of cortisol impairs the normal development of the adrenal medulla and secondarily impairs catechol release in response to stress.

Congenital Lipoid Adrenal Hyperplasia

Congenital lipoid adrenal hyperplasia is characterized by severe deficiency of glucocorticoid secondary to deficient steroidogenic acute regulatory protein (StAR).[38] The StAR protein permits cholesterol entry into the mitochondria, where the first steps in steroidogenesis occur. Biallelic deficiency of StAR causes massive cholesterol accumulation in the adrenals and adrenal cell death, ultimately giving rise to profound adrenal failure.

21-Hydroxylase Deficiency

21-Hydroxylase deficiency is the most common form of CAH (90% of the total) and occurs in 1 in 5000 to 1 in 15,000 births.[39] The enzyme is encoded by the gene *CYP21B*, and most commonly, small mutations (microconversions) in the gene give rise to the enzyme deficiency.[40] The 21-hydroxylase enzyme catalyzes the conversion of 17-hydroxyprogesterone to 11-deoxycortisol in the glucocorticoid pathway and the conversion of progesterone to

deoxycorticosterone in the mineralocorticoid pathway (see Fig. 73-1). If these pathways are blocked, excess adrenal androgens (DHEA and testosterone) are produced. The severity of the enzyme deficiency determines the extent of cortisol and aldosterone deficiency, the extent of excess androgen accumulation, and the overall clinical severity. Approximately two thirds of children with 21-hydroxylase deficiency are born with the severe, salt-losing form and present in the newborn period. One third are born with the milder, simple virilizing, nonclassic form and present in childhood.

Symptoms of the salt-losing form of CAH generally appear in the first few days to weeks of life. Female infants are born with ambiguous genitalia that can range from mild clitoromegaly to a full-sized male phallus with complete labial fusion and formation of a scrotum and urogenital sinus. The phenotype depends on the severity of the underlying enzyme defect. The detection of CAH in male infants may be delayed without the clue of ambiguous genitalia. Patients who have the nonclassic form of the disease do not present with ambiguous genitalia or salt loss in the newborn period. These infants generally present with premature development of pubic hair or other evidence of precocious puberty or virilization. The milder form of CAH is not associated with clinically significant salt loss because the adrenal produces some aldosterone, occasionally at the expense of increased plasma renin activity.

Abnormalities in salt-losing CAH may include hyperkalemia, hyponatremia, weight loss, salt loss, feeding difficulties, acute adrenal crisis, and shock. The diagnosis is made on the basis of measuring the basal or ACTH-stimulated 17-hydroxyprogesterone levels in the serum or plasma. There are well-established normal values for this metabolite. Umbilical cord blood levels are elevated on the first day of life, but levels decline to less than 200 ng/dL by 48 hours of age in normal, full-term infants.[41] Serum 17-hydroxyprogesterone levels are increased to 1000 ng/dL in premature or sick infants without adrenal disease. Untreated patients with this form of CAH generally have elevated 17-hydroxyprogesterone levels ranging from 3000 to 100,000 ng/dL.

If the 17-hydroxyprogesterone levels are elevated in the appropriate clinical setting, the etiology could be CAH or an adrenal or gonadal tumor. It is necessary to assess suppression of 17-hydroxyprogesterone levels into the normal range after glucocorticoid therapy is begun. This suppression establishes the existence of a functional adrenal-pituitary-hypothalamic axis and the diagnosis of CAH. Plasma renin activity may be normal initially in untreated subjects but rises over the first few days of life as the salt loss progresses. Plasma aldosterone may be normal or low, depending on the severity of the enzyme defect and the sodium intake.

Therapy includes glucocorticoid and mineralocorticoid replacement as needed to prevent excessive ACTH production by the pituitary and minimize the stimulus for elevated adrenal androgen secretion. Hydrocortisone, 10 to 20 mg/m^2/24 hours in three divided doses, and fludrocortisone acetate, 0.1 to 0.2 mg/day, are the glucocorticoid and mineralocorticoid treatments of choice in children.[42]

Infants also frequently require additional salt (18 to 36 mEq/day) added to formula or breast milk. Surgical correction of ambiguous genitalia in female infants generally is performed in the first year of life. Vaginoplasty and clitoral recession, rather than removal of the clitoris, is the surgical treatment of choice.

The goal of treatment is normal growth and pubertal development without symptoms of adrenal insufficiency or salt loss. Excessive glucocorticoid replacement results in growth inhibition and the development of cushingoid side effects. Insufficient glucocorticoid replacement results in elevated androgens, bone age advancement, early pubic hair development, and clitoral or phallic enlargement. Adequacy of treatment is monitored by following serum 17-hydroxyprogesterone or androstenedione or urine pregnanetriol levels and growth rate and bone age. The adequacy of mineralocorticoid replacement is assessed by measuring the plasma renin activity and serum electrolytes. If the child has ongoing excessive salt loss after glucocorticoid and mineralocorticoid replacement, the elevated renin can stimulate ACTH production and raise the androgen precursor levels by a cortisol-independent mechanism. The salt loss (and renin) is fully corrected after adjusting the dose of fludrocortisone acetate or increasing supplemental salt in the diet or both.

The gene for the 21-hydroxylase enzyme is on the short arm of chromosome 6, close to HLA-B in the major histocompatibility locus. The human genome contains two tandemly duplicated copies of the $P450_{c21}$ gene: B is functional for the enzyme, and A is inactive (pseudogene) because of several mutations.[43,44] The particular point mutation, deletion, or conversion on the functional $P450_{c21}$ gene determines the clinical presenting feature of 21-hydroxylase deficiency.

Prenatal diagnosis of 21-hydroxylase enzyme deficiency is possible by measuring the 17-hydroxyprogesterone levels in the amniotic fluid (second trimester), by HLA typing of fetal cells (requires a previous index child), or by studying the CYP21 genotype (using specific cDNA probes) directly from chorionic villus tissue sampling. Prenatal treatment of the mother with dexamethasone (by 5 to 6 weeks of gestation) can be used to prevent virilization of female fetuses with this form of CAH. The dexamethasone inhibits maternal and fetal ACTH secretion so that the fetal adrenal is prevented from producing excess androgens. Dexamethasone does not seem to be teratogenic. Newborn screening programs exist in several states, in which 17-hydroxyprogesterone is measured reliably from filter paper blood samples.[45]

11-Hydroxylase Deficiency

11-Hydroxylase deficiency is the second most common form of CAH (5% of total).[44] The deficient enzyme is 11-hydroxylase, which catalyzes the conversion of 11-deoxycortisol to cortisol and 11-deoxycorticosterone to corticosterone (see Fig. 73-1). The enzyme is part of the mitochondrial P-$450_{c11/18}$ system located on chromosome 8 and contains enzymes that catalyze 11-hydroxylation and 18-hydroxylation. In addition to 11-deoxycortisol, deoxycorticosterone and androgens accumulate in excess. The excess androgens lead to virilization of female

fetuses. Deoxycorticosterone is a weak mineralocorticoid with 3% to 5% of the mineralocorticoid effect of aldosterone. In excess, deoxycorticosterone acts as a mineralocorticoid, causing suppression of renin activity, salt retention, volume expansion, and hypertension. The phenotypic expression of this enzyme deficiency is related to the severity of the enzyme block. Infants with the most severe form present in the newborn period with sexual ambiguity in girls and hypertension in boys and girls. Children with the milder forms can present in early childhood with early pubic hair or clitoromegaly or phallic enlargement.

The electrolyte abnormalities include hypernatremia, hypokalemia, and metabolic alkalosis. The diagnosis is made by measuring elevated levels of basal or ACTH-stimulated 11-deoxycortisol and confirming appropriate feedback suppression of this metabolite after glucocorticoid replacement is begun. Prenatal diagnosis is not as definitive as with 21-hydroxylase deficiency. Levels of 11-deoxycortisol can be measured in the amniotic fluid. The gene for this enzyme is not HLA-linked so that HLA linkage studies cannot aid in genetic counseling for this disorder.

Therapy consists of glucocorticoid replacement as detailed earlier. The adequacy of therapy is monitored by following the levels of 11-deoxycortisol, renin, and androgens and the growth rate, bone age, and pubertal development of the children. The hypertension generally subsides after appropriate glucocorticoid replacement. Rarely, salt wasting can occur after glucocorticoid replacement because levels of deoxycorticosterone decrease after glucocorticoid replacement, and aldosterone levels remain inadequate for normal salt balance.

3β-Hydroxysteroid Dehydrogenase Deficiency

3β-Hydroxysteroid dehydrogenase deficiency and the remaining forms of CAH described here are rare and account for less than 5% of CAH. The enzyme, located in the smooth endoplasmic reticulum, catalyzes the conversion of Δ-5-hydroxysteroids (DHEA, pregnenolone, and 17-hydroxypregnenolone) to Δ-4-ketosteroids (androstenedione, progesterone, and 17-hydroxyprogesterone) and affects the adrenals and the gonads (see Fig. 72-1). Male and female infants can present with ambiguous genitalia and adrenal insufficiency. Boys are born with hypospadias and microphallus, and girls may have clitoromegaly. The diagnosis is made by measuring the ratio of Δ-5 to Δ-4 steroids (>4:1 in neonates).[29] The ratio of 17-hydroxypregnenolone to 17-hydroxyprogesterone is the most sensitive indicator of the enzyme deficiency.[46] Treatment consists of glucocorticoid and mineralocorticoid replacement as detailed earlier. Boys may require surgical correction of hypospadias and testosterone replacement to stimulate normal pubertal development.

20-22-Cholesterol Desmolase Deficiency

20-22-Cholesterol desmolase, located in the smooth endoplasmic reticulum, controls the rate-limiting step in adrenal and gonadal hormone synthesis (see Fig. 73-1). Infants who are affected do not synthesize normal levels of glucocorticoids, mineralocorticoids, or sex steroids.

Their adrenals are large and lipid laden, giving rise to the description of **congenital lipoid adrenal hyperplasia**. Boys have ambiguous genitalia, and girls have normal genitalia. Affected infants become ill quickly and have a high mortality rate, especially if diagnosis is delayed. Treatment consists of glucocorticoid and mineralocorticoid replacement as detailed earlier. Boys also require testosterone replacement therapy to induce pubertal development.

17-Hydroxylase/17-20-Desmolase Deficiency

17-Hydroxylase/17-20-desmolase, located in the smooth endoplasmic reticulum, impairs glucocorticoid and sex steroid synthesis (see Fig. 73-1). Mineralocorticoid synthesis is normal. A single $P450_{c17}$ gene, located on chromosome 10, codes for an enzyme with 17-hydroxylase and 17-20-desmolase activity. Adrenal and gonadal cells use this enzyme. Boys, but not girls, are born with ambiguous genitalia on the basis of diminished testosterone synthesis. Deoxycorticosterone accumulates in excess, leading to hypokalemia and hypertension. Boys and girls fail to undergo normal pubertal development as a result of deficient testosterone and estradiol. Diagnosis is based on finding elevated progesterone and deoxycorticosterone levels and decreased cortisol, testosterone, estradiol, and DHEAS levels. Plasma renin activity usually is suppressed. Treatment consists of glucocorticoid replacement as detailed earlier. Hypertension generally improves as the levels of deoxycorticosterone are suppressed. Pubertal development is induced in both sexes with hormone replacement therapy.

Other Miscellaneous Causes of Adrenal Insufficiency

Autoimmune adrenal disease and infectious diseases, including tuberculosis and histoplasmosis, can cause adrenal insufficiency. These causes are rare in neonates. Autoimmune adrenal disease usually affects children and adults. In this disorder, antibodies destroy the adrenal cortical cells. The medulla is generally spared. Other associated autoimmune disorders include hypoparathyroidism, gonadal insufficiency, and chronic active hepatitis.

SECONDARY ADRENAL INSUFFICIENCY

Secondary adrenal insufficiency can result from defects in pituitary or hypothalamic release of ACTH or CRH. In newborns, secondary adrenal insufficiency most commonly occurs secondary to congenital malformations of the hypothalamus or pituitary or secondary to suppressive effects of exogenous glucocorticoids. Infiltrative central nervous system tumors, including craniopharyngiomas, and central nervous system trauma also are etiologies. Usually neuroradiologic (magnetic resonance imaging [MRI] or computed tomography [CT]) evaluation suggests the diagnosis. The etiology can be clarified with a CRH stimulation test to establish whether the defect is at the level of the hypothalamus or the pituitary. Pituitary ACTH deficiency can be associated with growth hormone, thyroid-stimulating hormone, and gonadotropin deficiencies. Signs of hypopituitarism in newborns

include hypoglycemia, micropenis, and cryptorchidism. Hyponatremia may be observed as discussed earlier. Because ACTH deficiency does not affect aldosterone secretion, hyperkalemia and salt loss are not observed. The evaluation of secondary adrenal insufficiency should include testing all aspects of anterior pituitary function.

The most common cause of secondary adrenal insufficiency is treatment with exogenous glucocorticoids. ACTH and CRH are suppressed after administration of exogenous glucocorticoid, as occurs with dexamethasone treatment of infants with bronchopulmonary dysplasia.[47] Treatment duration greater than 7 days may be associated with hypothalamic-pituitary-adrenal axis suppression.[48] The dose (more supraphysiologic), route (parenteral versus topical) of administration, and biologic half-life of the glucocorticoid (dexamethasone versus cortisol) all can influence the degree of adrenal suppression. Secondary adrenal insufficiency (ACTH deficiency) is treated with cortisol replacement, 10 to 15 mg/m²/day. Infants with secondary adrenal suppression resulting from supraphysiologic treatment doses of glucocorticoids for more than 10 to 14 days should be covered with glucocorticoids for any major stresses for 1 year.[49] If a random or ACTH-stimulated cortisol value (off treatment) is normal (>20 µg/dL), this coverage is not necessary.[49]

SELECTIVE DEFICIENCY OF ALDOSTERONE

Isolated aldosterone deficiency can occur without accompanying cortisol deficiency as a result of destruction of the zona glomerulosa, renin deficiency, or a specific enzyme deficiency. The enzyme abnormalities are inherited in an autosomal recessive fashion. A single enzyme, $P450_{c11/18}$, in the mitochondria catalyzes conversion of deoxycorticosterone to aldosterone (see Fig. 73-1). The final three steps in aldosterone secretion include 11-hydroxylation, 18-hydroxylation, and 18-oxidation.[50]

Infants present with salt wasting, hypovolemia, hyperkalemia, and hyponatremia. Hyperkalemia can be accompanied by muscle weakness and cardiac arrhythmias. The plasma renin activity is elevated if the cause of the aldosterone deficiency is cortical destruction or a biosynthetic defect. The diagnosis is made by measuring the ratio of 18-hydroxycorticosterone to aldosterone (normal 2.3 to 6 in infants). Treatment consists of mineralocorticoid (fludrohydrocortisone acetate) and salt replacement as detailed earlier. The salt loss generally is most severe in infancy and tends to improve spontaneously in childhood.

PSEUDOHYPOALDOSTERONISM

Pseudohypoaldosteronism is a renal disorder that has a different etiology but closely resembles mineralocorticoid deficiency. It is an autosomal recessive or dominant disorder characterized by lack of adrenal or adrenal plus multiple organ (renal, salivary, or sweat gland) responsiveness to aldosterone.[6] Some affected subjects have abnormal aldosterone receptors. Infants present with hyponatremia, hyperkalemia, salt wasting, and increased renin activity. In contrast to aldosterone-deficient infants, these infants have elevated aldosterone levels. Treatment consists of salt replacement at a dose of 250 to 300 mEq/day and potassium binding resins, as needed, for hyperkalemia. The salt loss also tends to improve with age.

ADRENAL MEDULLA HYPOFUNCTION

Failure of the adrenal medulla is rare, and replacement therapy is generally not indicated after destruction of the medulla as occurs after adrenal hemorrhage or adrenalectomy.

ADRENAL CORTICAL HYPERFUNCTION (CUSHING SYNDROME)

Cushing syndrome refers to glucocorticoid excess resulting from either excess endogenous or administered glucocorticoids. Cushing disease occurs secondary to excess pituitary ACTH secretion. Cushing syndrome may be caused by adrenal tumors, pituitary ACTH-secreting adenomas, or adrenal-nodular hyperplasia. Ectopic ACTH production from nonpituitary tumors has been described in association with pancreatic islet cell tumors, Wilms tumors, and neuroblastoma. Adrenal nodular hyperplasia is a rare, familial form of Cushing syndrome associated with pigmented adrenal and skin lesions. Adrenal tumors in infancy have an increased association with hemihypertrophy and with Beckwith-Wiedemann syndrome.[51] Cushing syndrome is rare in infancy, may occur on a congenital basis, and is most commonly secondary to adrenal tumors in young infants.[52] The physical findings in infants include obesity, "cupid facies," virilization, hirsutism, and hypertension. Striae are unusual.

Laboratory findings associated with Cushing syndrome include impaired glucose tolerance, polycythemia, lymphopenia, and hypokalemic alkalosis. Tumors may produce excess cortisol, androgen, estrogen, DHEAS, or deoxycorticosterone. The 24-hour urinary free cortisol is elevated in Cushing syndrome and is the best screening test (normal for infants and small children is 1.4 to 18 μg/24 hours). The initial evaluation also may include the dexamethasone suppression test (0.3 mg/m^2, up to 2 mg at midnight) to identify pituitary-dependent cortisol excess. ACTH levels help to distinguish pituitary versus adrenal versus ectopic production of ACTH as the causes for Cushing syndrome. Ultrasound, CT, and MRI identify tumors. The recommended treatment is surgical excision.

MINERALOCORTICOID EXCESS

Excess aldosterone may result from primary adrenal glomerular hyperplasia, adrenal adenoma, or, rarely, carcinoma. It may be idiopathic or glucocorticoid suppressible. Signs and symptoms include hypertension, hypokalemia, alkalosis, weakness, polyuria, and glucose intolerance. Edema is unusual. Laboratory evaluation reveals elevated aldosterone or deoxycorticosterone levels and suppressed renin activity. The evaluation should include visualization of the adrenals with MRI. The treatment of tumors is surgical excision. The treatment of

hyperplasia is spironolactone because the hypertension does not respond to adrenalectomy.

ADRENAL MEDULLA HYPERFUNCTION

Pheochromocytoma

Pheochromocytomas are amine-secreting tumors that originate from chromaffin cells and can occur at any age, from infancy through old age. The most common location is the adrenal medulla, but pheochromocytomas can originate anywhere in the sympathetic chain. Approximately 5% are inherited, and the incidence in females is slightly higher. These tumors can be inherited in an autosomal dominant fashion as part of multiple endocrine neoplasia syndrome types 2A and 2B or can be associated with neurofibromatosis or von Hippel–Landau disease. Infants may present with either consistent or paroxysmal hypertension. The laboratory evaluation includes measurement of urine vanillylmandelic acid, metanephrines, or free catecholamines (see Table 73-1). The tumors may be localized with adrenal CT or MRI. Treatment consists of surgical excision after preoperative adrenergic blockade with phenoxybenzamine hydrochloride (0.5 to 1 mg/kg/12 hours) followed by propranolol. Phentolamine is useful for acute management of hypertension.

Neuroblastoma

Neuroblastoma is a solid tumor derived from neuroblasts and occurs in the sympathetic nervous system. The most common originating sites are the adrenal medulla and the autonomic ganglia. In newborns, the most common presentation is an abdominal mass. Symptoms include failure to thrive, irritability, fever, and anemia. Occasionally the diagnosis is made prenatally on the basis of ultrasound visualization of a suprarenal or paraspinal mass with a solid, cystic, or calcified appearance.[30] The infantile form of the disease is associated with a better prognosis and occasionally spontaneous regression. The diagnosis is made on the basis of elevated urinary excretion of vanillylmandelic acid and catecholamines. Cytologic abnormalities include rearrangement or deletion of genes on the short arm of chromosome 1. The usual treatment is surgical. Chemotherapy is used for disseminated disease.

REFERENCES

1. Stewart PM: Adrenal cortex and endocrine hypertension. In Larsen RP, Kronenberg HM, Melmed S, et al: Williams' Textbook of Endocrinology, 10th ed. Philadelphia, WB Saunders, 2003.
2. Lanman JT: The adrenal gland in the human fetus: An interpretation of its physiology and unusual developmental pattern. Pediatrics 27:140, 1961.
3. Achermann JC, Ito M, Hindmarsh PC, Jameson JL: A mutation in the gene encoding steroidogenic factor-1 causes XY sex reversal and adrenal failure in humans. Nat Genet 22:125, 1999.
4. Burris TP, Guo W, McCabe ER: The gene responsible for adrenal hypoplasia congenita, DAX-1, encodes a nuclear hormone receptor that defines a new class within the superfamily. Recent Prog Horm Res 51:241, 1996.

5. Langlois D, Li JY, Saez JM: Development and function of the human fetal adrenal cortex. J Pediatr Endocrinol Metab 15(suppl 5):1311, 2002.

6. Winter J: Neonatal and Fetal Medicine. Philadelphia, WB Saunders, 1992.

7. Beitins IZ, Bayard F, Ances IG, et al: The metabolic clearance rate, blood production, interconversion and transplacental passage of cortisol and cortisone in pregnancy near term. Pediatr Res 7:509, 1973.

8. Beitins IZ, Bayard F, Levitsky L, et al: Plasma aldosterone concentration at delivery and during the newborn period. J Clin Invest 51:386, 1972.

9. Padbury JF, Roberman B, Oddie TH, et al: Fetal catecholamine release in response to labor and delivery. Obstet Gynecol 60:607, 1982.

10. Miesfeld RL: Molecular genetics of corticosteroid action. Am Rev Respir Dis 141:S11, 1990.

11. Fauci A: Glucocorticoid Hormone Action: Immunosuppressive and Anti-inflammatory Effects of Glucocorticoids. New York, Springer Verlag, 1979.

12. Raff H: Glucocorticoid inhibition of neurohypophysial vasopressin secretion. Am J Physiol 252:R635, 1987.

13. Winters AJ, Oliver C, Colston C, et al: Plasma ACTH levels in the human fetus and neonate as related to age and parturition. J Clin Endocrinol Metab 39:269, 1974.

14. Onishi S, Miyazawa G, Nishimura Y, et al: Postnatal development of circadian rhythm in serum cortisol levels in children. Pediatrics 72:399, 1983.

15. Linder BL, Esteban NV, Yergey AL, et al: Cortisol production rate in childhood and adolescence. J Pediatr 117:892, 1990.

16. Gunnar MR, Fisch RO, Malone S: The effects of a pacifying stimulus on behavioral and adrenocortical responses to circumcision in the newborn. J Am Acad Child Psychiatry 23:34, 1984.

17. Mantagos S, Koulouris A, Vagenakis A: A simple stress test for the evaluation of hypothalamic-pituitary-adrenal axis during the first 6 months of life. J Clin Endocrinol Metab 72:214, 1991.

18. Clinkingbeard C, Sessions C, Shenker Y: The physiological role of atrial natriuretic hormone in the regulation of aldosterone and salt and water metabolism. J Clin Endocrinol Metab 70:582, 1990.

19. Lifshitz F: Pediatric Endocrinology. New York, Marcel Dekker, 2003.

20. Lashansky G, Saenger P, Dimartino-Nardi J, et al: Normative data for the steroidogenic response of mineralocorticoids and their precursors to adrenocorticotropin in a healthy pediatric population. J Clin Endocrinol Metab 75:1491, 1992.

21. Lashansky G, Saenger P, Fishman K, et al: Normative data for adrenal steroidogenesis in a healthy pediatric population: Age- and sex-related changes after adrenocorticotropin stimulation. J Clin Endocrinol Metab 73:674, 1991.

22. Lindholm J, Kehlet H, Blichert-Toft M, et al: Reliability of the 30-minute ACTH test in assessing hypothalamic-pituitary-adrenal function. J Clin Endocrinol Metab 47:272, 1978.

23. Lindholm J, Kehlet H: Re-evaluation of the clinical value of the 30 min ACTH test in assessing the hypothalamic-pituitary-adrenocortical function. Clin Endocrinol (Oxf) 26:53, 1987.

24. Ross JL, Schulte HM, Gallucci WT, et al: Ovine corticotropin-releasing hormone stimulation test in normal children. J Clin Endocrinol Metab 62:390, 1986.

25. Dorin RI, Kearns PJ: High output circulatory failure in acute adrenal insufficiency. Crit Care Med 16:296, 1988.

26. Nerup J: Addison's disease—clinical studies: A report of 108 cases. Acta Endocrinol (Copenh) 76:127, 1974.

27. Burke C: Adrenocortical insufficiency. Clin Endocrinol Metab 14:947, 1985.

28. Takeda N, Yasuda K, Kitabchi AE, et al: Increased insulin binding of erythrocytes and insulin sensitivity in adrenal insufficiency. Metabolism 36:1063, 1987.

29. Lutfallah C, Wang W, Mason JI, et al: Newly proposed hormonal criteria via genotypic proof for type II 3beta-hydroxysteroid dehydrogenase deficiency. J Clin Endocrinol Metab 87:2611, 2002.

30. Ho PT, Estroff JA, Kozakewich H, et al: Prenatal detection of neuroblastoma: A ten-year experience from the Dana-Farber Cancer Institute and Children's Hospital. Pediatrics 92:358, 1993.

31. Achermann JC, Silverman BL, Habiby RL, Jameson JL: Presymptomatic diagnosis of X-linked adrenal hypoplasia congenita by analysis of DAX1. J Pediatr 137:878, 2000.

32. Zanaria E, Muscatelli F, Bardoni B, et al: An unusual member of the nuclear hormone receptor superfamily responsible for X-linked adrenal hypoplasia congenita. Nature 372:635, 1994.

33. Achermann JC, Ozisik G, Ito M, et al: Gonadal determination and adrenal development are regulated by the orphan nuclear receptor steroidogenic factor-1, in a dose-dependent manner. J Clin Endocrinol Metab 87:1829, 2002.

34. Chelly J, Marlhens F, Dutrillaux B, et al: Deletion proximal to DXS68 locus (L1 probe site) in a boy with Duchenne muscular dystrophy, glycerol kinase deficiency, and adrenal hypoplasia. Hum Genet 78:222, 1988.

35. Black J, Williams DI: Natural history of adrenal hemorrhage in the newborn. Arch Dis Child 48:148, 1973.

36. Kuhn J, Jewett T, Munschauer R: The clinical and radiographic features of massive neonatal adrenal hemorrhage. Radiology 99:647, 1971.

37. Mosser J, Douar AM, Sarde CO, et al: Putative X-linked adrenoleukodystrophy gene shares unexpected homology with ABC transporters. Nature 361:726, 1993.

38. Lin D, Sugawara T, Strauss JF 3rd, et al: Role of steroidogenic acute regulatory protein in adrenal and gonadal steroidogenesis. Science 267:1828, 1995.

39. Brosnan PG, Brosnan CA, Kemp SF, et al: Effect of newborn screening for congenital adrenal hyperplasia. Arch Pediatr Adolesc Med 153:1272, 1999.

40. Miller WL: Clinical review 54: Genetics, diagnosis, and management of 21-hydroxylase deficiency. J Clin Endocrinol Metab 78:241, 1994.

41. Wiener D, Smith J, Dahlem S, et al: Serum adrenal steroid levels in healthy full-term 3-day-old infants. J Pediatr 110:122, 1987.

42. Technical report: Congenital adrenal hyperplasia. Section on Endocrinology and Committee on Genetics. Pediatrics 106:1511, 2000.

43. White PC, New MI, Dupont B: Congenital adrenal hyperplasia: 2. N Engl J Med 316:1580, 1987.

44. White PC, New MI, Dupont B: Congenital adrenal hyperplasia: 1. N Engl J Med 316:1519, 1987.

45. Therrell BL Jr, Berenbaum SA, Manter-Kapanke V, et al: Results of screening 1.9 million Texas newborns for 21-hydroxylase-deficient congenital adrenal hyperplasia. Pediatrics 101:583, 1998.

46. Cara JF, Moshang T Jr, Bongiovanni AM, Marx BS: Elevated 17-hydroxyprogesterone and testosterone in a newborn with 3-beta-hydroxysteroid dehydrogenase deficiency. N Engl J Med 313:618, 1985.

47. Wilson DM, Baldwin RB, Ariagno RL: A randomized, placebo-controlled trial of effects of dexamethasone on hypothalamic-pituitary-adrenal axis in preterm infants. J Pediatr 113:764, 1988.

48. Carella MJ, Srivastava LS, Gossain VV, Rovner DR: Hypothalamic-pituitary-adrenal function one week after a short burst of steroid therapy. J Clin Endocrinol Metab 76:1188, 1993.

49. Chamberlain P, Meyer WJ: Management of pituitary-adrenal suppression secondary to corticosteroid therapy. Pediatrics 67:245, 1981.

50. Ulick S, Wang JZ, Morton DH: The biochemical phenotypes of two inborn errors in the biosynthesis of aldosterone. J Clin Endocrinol Metab 74:415, 1992.

51. Pettenati MJ, Haines JL, Higgins RR, et al: Wiedemann-Beckwith syndrome: Presentation of clinical and cytogenetic data on 22 new cases and review of the literature. Hum Genet 74:143, 1986.

52. Lee PD, Winter RJ, Green OC: Virilizing adrenocortical tumors in childhood: Eight cases and a review of the literature. Pediatrics 76:437, 1985.

CHAPTER 74

Disorders of Glucose and Other Sugars

Lorraine Levitt Katz and Charles A. Stanley

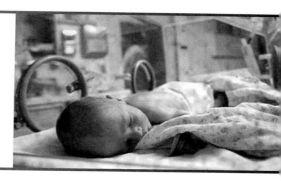

The neonatal period represents a time of transition from the constant supply of glucose provided by the maternal circulation during fetal life to the development of independent carbohydrate homeostasis. Problems with either hypoglycemia or hyperglycemia are common during this transition. In addition, the newborn period is frequently the time of initial presentation of many congenital disorders that cause hypoglycemia or genetic disorders that impair metabolism of dietary sugars. This chapter reviews the disorders of neonatal carbohydrate metabolism. The emphasis is on hypoglycemia, which often presents diagnostic and therapeutic dilemmas in the newborn period. Neonatal hyperglycemia/diabetes and sugar toxicity disorders, such as galactosemia, are discussed briefly.

HYPOGLYCEMIA

Because the brain relies on glucose as its primary fuel, **hypoglycemia** may result in severe, permanent brain damage. All of the clinically important forms of hypoglycemia in newborns and in older children are disorders of fasting hypoglycemia. In the sections that follow, an approach to these disorders is presented that is based on analysis of the metabolic and endocrine systems required for successful adaptation to a period of fasting. Subsequent sections discuss the disorders of special relevance to the neonatal period and general aspects of treatment.

Physiology of Fasting

Systems of Fasting Adaptation in Postnatal Life

The essential task of **fasting adaptation** can be viewed as maintaining an adequate supply of glucose for brain metabolism.[1,2] Figure 74-1 outlines the six metabolic systems involved:

1. Hepatic glycogen stores provide the major source of glucose from 1 to 2 hours, after a meal when intestinal absorption is complete, until 6 to 8 hours.
2. As glycogen stores become depleted, hepatic gluconeogenesis becomes the key source of glucose, using primarily amino acids, but also glycerol from adipose tissue lipolysis in addition to recycled lactate from glycolysis.
3. Muscle proteolysis provides the major source of amino acids for gluconeogenesis, but because there is no reserve of surplus protein, beyond 12 hours fatty acid oxidation must be activated to spare demands for glucose.
4. Adipose tissue lipolysis releases free fatty acids for hepatic ketone synthesis and to replace glucose as the major fuel for peripheral tissues, such as muscle; the glycerol released by lipolysis is used for gluconeogenesis in the liver.
5. Hepatic ketogenesis provides the energy needed for gluconeogenesis and the ketones, β-hydroxybutyrate and acetoacetate, which can be used by the brain. This indirect use of fat stores by the brain serves to reduce further glucose use and the drain on body protein during long-term fasting.
6. These five metabolic systems of fasting are controlled by the hormone system of insulin and several counterregulatory hormones.

As shown in Table 74-1, **insulin** plays the central role in fasting adaptation by its inhibitory effects on all five metabolic systems.

The pattern of fasting responses in adults and children is identical, but the time course of fasting is more rapid at younger ages. The acceleration of fasting metabolism seen in infants and young children is due to their higher brain weight relative to body mass. Because glucose turnover rates are linearly related to brain size,[3] basal glucose consumption in newborns (5 to 6 mg/kg/min) is two to three times that of adults.[4] With their relatively lower muscle mass, young infants develop significant hyperketonemia by 24 hours of fasting compared with 2 to 3 days in men.[5]

The above-outlined fasting systems provide a useful approach to the diagnosis of hypoglycemic disorders. In combination with simple clinical features, such as the

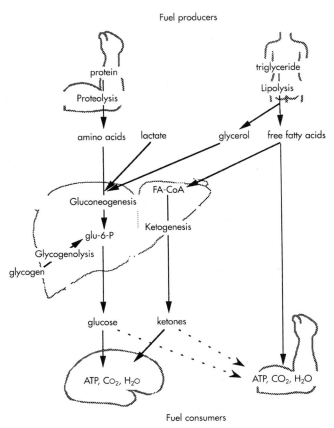

Fuel producers

Fuel consumers

Figure 74–1. Outline of fuel production and use during fasting. *(Adapted from Cahill GF: Starvation in man. N Engl J Med 282:668, 1970).*

timing of hypoglycemia, the responses of circulating fuels and hormones during fasting can be used to identify the underlying cause. Defects in hepatic gluconeogenesis are associated with increased accumulation of gluconeogenic precursors, such as lactate, when plasma glucose decreases. A failure to develop hyperketonemia during fasting serves as a marker for inhibition of lipolysis secondary to hyperinsulinism or for the genetic defects in fatty acid oxidation. Table 74-2 classifies the major causes of fasting hypoglycemia in infants in general, and Table 74-3 classifies the risk factors of special concern during the newborn period.

Development of Fasting Systems in the Fetus and Newborn

The fetus is in a constant anabolic state, continuously provided with glucose and other fuels from the maternal circulation. Glucose, amino acids, and free fatty acids all are transferred across the placenta in a concentration-dependent manner, generally by facilitated diffusion. Glucose serves as the major oxidative fuel for the fetus, and during the first few hours of life, the infant enters a fasting state as the maternal nutrient supply abruptly ceases.

At the time of birth, many components of the six fasting systems are functional, but some remain incompletely developed. Liver glycogen (system 1) and adipose tissue fat stores (system 4) become filled late in the third trimester, but stores may be limited in premature infants. Hepatic glycogenolysis (system 1) is functional well before term. Although the enzymes for gluconeogenesis (system 2) are present from early in gestation, the activity of several, most notably phosphoenolpyruvate carboxykinase, remains low until after delivery.[6,7] The ability of the brain to use ketones is acquired well before term. The activity of hepatic carnitine palmitoyl transferase-1, the rate-limiting step in ketone production by the liver (system 5), does not mature, however, until approximately 12 to 24 hours after birth.[8-11] Fatty acid oxidation in other tissues may be similarly immature at birth. As discussed subsequently, these developmental delays may be responsible for the high risk of hypoglycemia in infants who are not fed promptly after delivery.

In contrast to the ready communication between maternal and fetal fuels, fetal hormone regulation (system 6) is largely autonomous. Secretion of insulin and other hormones develops by late in the first trimester,[12,13] and insulin plays an important role in fetal growth. In animal studies, fetal beta cells do not have the typical biphasic response to glucose[12] and show greater sensitivity to long-term changes than to acute fluctuations in glucose concentrations.[13] Postnatally the decreased insulin-to-glucagon ratio triggers the induction of the gluconeogenic enzymes, particularly phosphoenolpyruvate carboxykinase, which is rate limiting for gluconeogenesis.[13,14] In addition to glucagon, cortisol and thyroid hormone are important signals for the development of the glycogenolytic and gluconeogenic pathways. In the immediate postnatal period, growth hormone secretion is high, but cortisol secretion is relatively low, and a diurnal rhythm of secretion of both hormones is not yet developed.

Table 74–1. Fasting System 6: Hormonal Regulation of Metabolic Systems of Fasting

	Glycogenolysis	Gluconeogenesis	Proteolysis	Lipolysis	Ketogenesis
Insulin	−	−	−	−	−
Glucagon	+	+			
Epinephrine	+	+		+	+
Cortisol		+	+		
Growth hormone				+	

Table 74–2. Fasting Systems Classification of Hypoglycemia in Infants

Glycogenolysis
Debrancher deficiency (GSD III)
Liver phosphorylase deficiency (GSD VI)
Phosphorylase kinase deficiency (GSD IX)
Glycogen synthase deficiency (GSD 0)

Gluconeogenesis
Glucose-6-phosphatase deficiency
Fructose-1,6-diphosphatase deficiency
Phosphoenolpyruvate carboxykinase deficiency
Pyruvate carboxylase deficiency

Proteolysis
Malnutrition

Lipolysis
Severe malnutrition
Congenital lipodystrophy

Ketogenesis
Fatty acid oxidation defects—MCAD, LCAD, SCAD
Carnitine transport defect

Hormonal Regulation
Congenital hyperinsulinism
Infant of diabetic mother (transient)
Exogenous insulin
Deficiency of counterregulatory hormones
  Panhypopituitarism
  Isolated growth hormone deficiency

Hypoglycemia Associated with Other Disorders
Inborn errors
  Hereditary fructose intolerance
  Maple syrup urine disease
  Methylmalonic acidemia
Drug induced
  Ethanol
  β-Blockers
  Sulfonylureas

GSD, glycogen storage disease; LCAD, long-chain acyl-CoA dehydrogenase; MCAD, medium-chain acyl-CoA dehydrogenase; SCAD, short-chain acyl-CoA dehydrogenase.

Table 74–3. Risk Factors for Neonatal Hypoglycemia

	Affected Fasting Systems
Maternal Factors	
Diabetes	6
Toxemia	2, 5 plus 1, 3, 4 (? 6)
Drugs	
Tocolytic agents	6
Ethanol	2
Sulfonylureas	6
Dextrose infusion	6
Fetal Factors	
Prematurity	2, 5 plus 1
Small for gestational age	2, 5 plus 1 (? 6)
Large for gestational age	6
Congenital heart disease	
Left hypoplastic heart syndrome	1, 2
Erythroblastosis fetalis	6
Microphallus	6
Midline facial malformations	6
Perinatal/Postnatal Factors	
Prolonged postnatal fasting (normal, term AGA infant)	2, 5
Cold stress	1, 2
Sepsis	1, 2
Birth asphyxia	6

AGA, appropriate for gestational age.

24 hours of life. Ingestion of fat seems to play an important role in signaling transcription of carnitine palmitoyl transferase I (CPT-1) in the newborn rat,[15,16] suggesting that the high fat content of colostrum may serve to activate the pathway of ketogenesis in newborn infants. Following the initial lag period after delivery, the ability to oxidize fatty acids matures rapidly, as shown by studies showing a rise in ketones after 24 hours in infants who were partially fasted through day 5 of life.[17] This late hyperketonemia has been erroneously interpreted sometimes to be a "suckling ketosis" similar to that seen in newborn rats feeding on the high-fat content of rat milk.[18] More recent studies of well-fed human newborns showed low ketone concentrations similar to those in well-fed older infants.[19,20]

Causes of Neonatal Hypoglycemia

Self-Limited Disorders

Postnatal fasting immaturity. As outlined earlier, all infants are at high risk for becoming hypoglycemic during the first day of life because the systems of fasting adaptation are not all fully developed at birth. As shown in Figure 74-2, when feedings were delayed for 6 hours after delivery, Lubchenco and Bard[21] found that 10% of term appropriate-for-gestational-age infants developed plasma glucose levels less than 30 mg/dL. In contrast, by day 2, none of these infants had preprandial values less than 50 mg/dL, reflecting the rapid maturation of the fasting

The immaturity of fasting adaptation in the normal newborn is illustrated by Table 74-4, which compares the circulating fuel concentrations during fasting immediately after birth with the pattern seen in older children. Normal full-term fasting neonates have higher lactate and much lower ketone concentrations than fasted older infants, indicating that at least two of the essential fasting systems (gluconeogenesis and ketogenesis, systems 2 and 5) are unavailable.[8] The same pattern of fuels is seen in postnatal fasting in premature and in small-for-gestational-age neonates. All newborns are essentially limited to their small stores of liver glycogen as a fuel source during their initial exposure to fasting after delivery.

The exact time after birth when all of the fasting systems become mature is not known, but fasting metabolism is well developed before 1 week of age, probably as early as

Table 74–4. Circulating Fuels at Times of Hypoglycemia in Newborns Compared with Older Children

	Glucose (mg/dL)	Lactate (mmol/L)	Free Fatty Acids (mmol/L)	Total Ketones (mmol/L)
Newborn (8-hr postnatal fast)	38	3	1.5	0.5
Older children				
Basal	70-90	1-2	0.5	0.1
Hypoglycemic	<40	1-2	1.5-2.5	3-4

Data from references 8 and 43.

systems. The high frequency of hypoglycemia noted in normal newborns in this and other surveys is compatible with inadequate development of at least two fasting systems (hepatic gluconeogenesis and ketogenesis) during the first 12 to 24 hours after delivery.[8] Early introduction of feedings (within 1 or 2 hours postpartum) should be considered to avoid postnatal fasting hypoglycemia. Recurrences of hypoglycemia after 12 to 24 hours of age require that other possible disorders be considered.

Higher risks of hypoglycemia during postnatal fasts are associated with prematurity, postmaturity, and low birth weight for gestational age (see Fig. 74-2). Inadequacy of liver glycogen stores partly explains the increased susceptibility to fasting hypoglycemia in these groups of infants because they already have decreased capacity for gluconeogenesis and ketogenesis.[8,22,23] Protein and fat stores

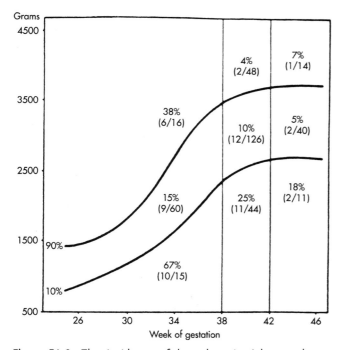

Grams

Figure 74–2. The incidence of hypoglycemia (plasma glucose <30 mg/dL) before first feedings at 6 hours of age in newborns grouped by birth weight and gestational age. *(From Lubchenco LO, Bard H: Incidence of hypoglycemia in newborn infants by birth-weight and gestational age. Pediatrics 47:831, 1971.)*

also may be diminished in these undernourished infants, and demand may be greater because of a larger brain-to-body size ratio. In utero or birth anoxia may cause liver glycogen stores to become depleted. Management includes intrapartum monitoring of fetal size, accurate assessment of the degree of malnourishment and growth impairment, frequent plasma glucose monitoring, and early introduction of oral or intravenous feeding.[24] The increased frequency of hypoglycemia in the group of large-for-gestational-age infants shown in Figure 74-3 reflects the inclusion of infants of diabetic mothers (see next)

Infants of diabetic mothers. Infants of diabetic mothers, who are chronically exposed to maternal hyperglycemia in utero, develop hyperinsulinism in response to the excessive glucose. Fetal growth is stimulated by the combination of high levels of insulin and metabolic fuels, and at birth, these infants may be markedly obese. Because the hyperinsulinism does not resolve immediately, these newborns are at high risk of hypoglycemia for a few days after birth. Markers of excess insulin effects include high glucose demands (>6-8 mg/kg/min), suppression of lipolysis and ketogenesis, and inappropriate preservation of liver glycogen reserve (as shown by an inappropriate increase in glucose in response to glucagon given during hypoglycemia).

Infants of diabetic mothers are at high risk for additional medical problems, such as hypocalcemia, hyperbilirubinemia, and respiratory distress. Maternal hyperglycemia during the first trimester is associated with increased risk of specific congenital anomalies, including cardiac defects, vertebral abnormalities, and caudal regression syndrome. There is strong evidence that careful glycemic control during the critical period of organogenesis (around 4 to 10 weeks of gestation) decreases the incidence of these anomalies.

Maternal glucose levels should be regulated meticulously during pregnancy, and normoglycemia should be maintained before delivery. All large-for-gestational-age infants should be suspected of being infants of diabetic mothers. They should be fed early with close glucose monitoring. Known infants of diabetic mothers should be admitted to the intensive care unit for observation with frequent glucose monitoring. If hypoglycemia develops, dextrose, 0.2 to 0.5 g/kg intravenously, can be given, followed by a dextrose infusion beginning at 4 to 8 mg/kg/min and increased as needed. If the hypoglycemia is due

Insulin Secretion Pathways

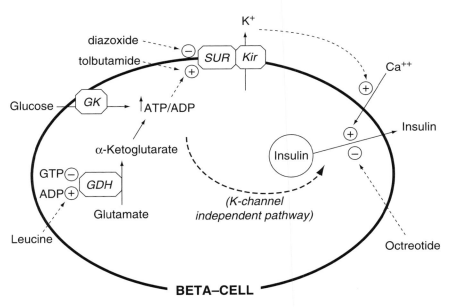

Figure 74–3. Beta cell and insulin secretion. In the resting state, the beta cell plasma membrane is hyperpolarized via kidney adenosine triphosphate (KATP) channels being maintained in the open state. Glucose enters the beta cell and is phosphorylated through glucokinase. Glycolysis generates ATP, raising the ATP/ADP ratio, which results in closure of the KATP channels. This leads to depolarization, with subsequent opening of voltage-dependent calcium channels followed by calcium influx and insulin secretion. ATP also is generated through stimulation of glutamate dehydrogenase (GDH).

to hyperinsulinism, glucagon, 0.5 to 1 mg subcutaneously or intravenously, can be effective in quickly raising plasma glucose temporarily. Plasma glucose should be maintained in the 60 to 80 mg/dL range to avoid further stimulation of insulin secretion. If the infant remains stable on oral feedings for 12 hours, the infusion can be weaned slowly.

Transient excessive glucose use. Severe hypoglycemia with excessive glucose use has been associated with infants who have perinatal stress, including birth asphyxia, toxemia, and erythroblastosis fetalis, and a subset of infants who are small for gestational age (see Table 74-3). The hypoglycemia is difficult to manage and may last several days to weeks or months. The increased glucose requirement and positive glycemic response to glucagon suggest hyperinsulinism as the underlying etiology. Several studies have shown elevated insulin levels in these infants.[25-27]

The relationship between perinatal stress and hyperinsulinism is unclear, but this form of neonatal hypoglycemia may represent a regulatory disturbance in insulin secretion in the period immediately after birth.[28] Because multiple factors may contribute to hypoglycemia in stressed or small-for-gestational-age infants, it is important to consider functional hyperinsulinism as an additional and possibly determining factor responsible for severe hypoglycemia in infants who display increased glucose requirements. Therapy includes the provision of adequate dextrose to maintain plasma glucose in the physiologic normal range (70 to 100 mg/dL, up to 20 mg/kg/min). If the excessive glucose requirement persists, oral diazoxide or glucagon infusion may be considered. Glucocorticoids play no role in treating this disorder and should be avoided. Maternal exposure to β_2 agonists in the period before delivery has been associated with an increased incidence

of transient neonatal hyperinsulinism and hypoglycemia.[29] The hyperinsulinism associated with these conditions is self-limited and usually resolves in the first few days of life, but frequently it may last 2 to 3 months. Some infants with Beckwith-Wiedemann syndrome display this type of mild hyperinsulinism, whereas others may be severely affected, resembling infants with congenital hyperinsulinism (described subsequently).[30]

Persistent (Congenital) Forms of Hypoglycemia

Congenital Hyperinsulinism
Congenital hyperinsulinism is the most common cause of persistent hypoglycemia in early infancy.[1] The term *congenital hyperinsulinism* refers to a group of disorders that are often due to a diffuse abnormality in the regulation of insulin secretion throughout the pancreas, but also may be associated with focal disease. Three genetic forms of congenital hyperinsulinism have been described.[31-33] Understanding their etiology requires a familiarity with the physiologic regulation of insulin secretion (Fig. 74-4). In the resting state, the beta cell plasma membrane is hyperpolarized via kidney adenosine triphosphate (KATP) channels being maintained in the open state. Glucose enters the beta cell via the glucose transporter, GLUT2, and is phosphorylated through glucokinase. Glucokinase represents the rate-limiting step. Glycolysis then generates adenosine triphosphate (ATP), raising the ATP-to-adenosine diphosphate (ADP) ratio, which results in closure of the KATP channels. This closure leads to depolarization, with subsequent opening of voltage-dependent calcium channels followed by calcium influx and insulin secretion. ATP also is generated through stimulation of glutamate dehydrogenase.

The most common type of congenital hyperinsulinism is a recessively inherited form[34] resulting from defects in

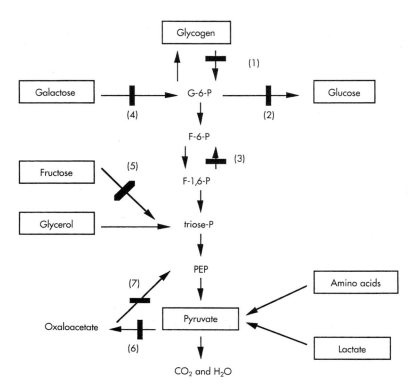

Figure 74–4. Genetic metabolic defects of glucose metabolism: (1) debrancher, phosphorylase, phosphorylase kinase; (2) glucose-6-phosphatase; (3) fructose-1, 6-diphosphatase; (4) galactose-1-phosphate uridyl transferase; (5) fructose-1-phosphate aldolase; (6) pyruvate carboxylase; (7) phospho*enol*pyruvate carboxykinase.

the two genes that form the KATP channel, *Kir 6.2* and its regulatory subunit, the sulfonylurea receptor, *SUR1*.[35] Linkage studies of affected families localized the disorder to the *Kir 6.2* and *SUR1* locus on the short arm of chromosome 11[36-39]; more than 60 mutations have been described in these two genes. A focal form of congenital hyperinsulinism may result sporadically from the inheritance of an abnormal paternal *SUR1* allele combined with a loss of heterozygosity for the normal maternal *SUR1* allele, in the focal lesion.[40,41] Focal and diffuse *SUR1* mutations give rise to a severe form of congenital hyperinsulinism. Affected infants usually present with an abnormally high birth weight, but an otherwise normal physical examination without hepatomegaly. The similarity to infants of diabetic mothers indicates that the hyperinsulinism begins before birth. Infants with onset of hypoglycemia on the first day of life tend to be extremely large for gestational age with particularly difficult-to-manage hypoglycemia.[42,43] Plasma glucose levels are unstable, with hypoglycemia occurring after brief periods of fasting, and glucose requirements frequently exceed 10 to 15 mg/kg/min. Because the drug acts to suppress insulin secretion by binding to the KATP channel, medical treatment is often ineffective with diazoxide. Most patients require surgery.

An autosomal dominant inheritance pattern of congenital hyperinsulinism has been identified in four families,[44] one of which has been identified to be a mutation in the *SUR1* gene.[45] The disorder is milder than the recessively inherited form, and most patients have been responsive to diazoxide.

The **hyperinsulinism/hyperammonemia syndrome** has been identified as a distinct genetic disorder.[46,47]

In addition to hypoglycemia, patients display modest elevations in blood ammonia to levels three to six times normal. This form of congenital hyperinsulinism is responsive to diazoxide and has been identified as a gain-of-function mutation in the glutamate dehydrogenase complex.[48-51] Inheritance may be autosomal dominant or sporadic. Infants have normal birth weight and may not present in the newborn period. They exhibit fasting hypoglycemia and hypoglycemia after protein ingestion.

A functional mutation in the **glucokinase enzyme**, resulting in an increased affinity of glucokinase for glucose, which leads to a lowered threshold for insulin secretion with subsequent congenital hyperinsulinism, also has been reported.[52] An autosomal dominant transmission was reported in the family described. Affected individuals had a milder presentation than sulfonylurea receptor–related congenital hyperinsulinism.

Diagnosis. Hyperinsulinism can be devastating to the developing infant brain, which is deprived not only of glucose but also of alternative fuels owing to insulin suppression of lipolysis and ketogenesis. It should be possible to make the diagnosis accurately and control hypoglycemia within 7 to 10 days. Using the fasting systems approach to hypoglycemia, one can diagnose hyperinsulinism in newborns most reliably by documenting the pattern of metabolic fuels and hormones at the time of hypoglycemia.[53] Insulin suppresses ketogenesis by inhibiting adipose tissue lipolysis and by preventing the transport of free fatty acids into the mitochondria for oxidation. Infants with hyperinsulinism have suppressed levels of free fatty acids (<0.5 mM), especially β-hydroxybutyrate (<1.1 mM).[32] IGFBP-1 is a novel marker of insulin secretion that is suppressed in congenital hyperinsulinism during hypoglycemia.[54]

The diagnosis sometimes can be made by the demonstration of abnormally elevated fasting insulin levels associated with a low plasma glucose. Although insulin levels are abnormally increased for the degree of hypoglycemia, however, levels may not be absolutely elevated. Some explanations for this phenomenon are that the hypersecretion of insulin is not always continuous, and the decrease in hepatic glucose production in the liver due to increased portal insulin may not be reflected in peripheral insulin concentrations. If insulin levels are not diagnostically elevated, the possiblity of pituitary deficiencies must be ruled out. A glucagon stimulation test of glycogen mobilization yielding a glycemic response of greater than 30 mg/dL at the time of hypoglycemia shows inappropriate glycogen conservation and is useful in rapidly making the presumptive diagnosis of hyperinsulinism.[55]

When the diagnosis has been confirmed, further evaluations can help to characterize the specific form of congenital hyperinsulinism. Acute insulin response testing, protein challenge, and ammonia levels may help delineate the phenotype of congenital hyperinsulinism and distinguish focal from diffuse disease.[56-59] Abdominal ultrasound is rarely useful in the diagnosis because the resolution is limited by the small size of the infant pancreas. Pancreatic arterial stimulation with venous sampling and transhepatic portal venous sampling have been used in selected patients to localize focal from diffuse forms of congenital hyperinsulinism.[60-62]

Treatment. If the patient has a focal lesion that is surgically accessible, operative cure is possible. Because surgical cure is not always attainable, however, the goal of therapy in congenital hyperinsulinism is to maintain "safe" glucose levels (>60 mg/dL) on a regimen that can be implemented at home. The first line of treatment is oral diazoxide, which reversibly inhibits insulin secretion via the sulfonylurea receptor. Diazoxide usually is ineffective in children with mutations in the sulfonylurea receptor and KATP channels. If diazoxide, 10 to 15 mg/kg/day, fails to control the hypoglycemia, the next line of treatment is octreotide, an injectable long-acting somatostatin analogue, which also acts by inhibiting insulin secretion.[63] In the short-term, the first dose of octreotide causes a brisk rise in plasma glucose, but most patients experience a tachyphylaxis, during which their response wanes, possibly due to receptor desensitization or suppression of glucagon.[64] Patients on maintenance octreotide usually require 5 to 40 µg/kg/day in three to four divided doses. A dose of more than 20 µg/kg/day is unlikely to be effective. Glucagon, 1 mg/day as an intravenous infusion, mobilizes glycogen stores and together with octreotide is often useful as a short-term adjunct to treatment before surgery. Nifedipine, a calcium channel blocker, has been used with limited success.[65,66]

Most patients with severe hyperinsulinism fail medical management and require surgery to protect the infant from hypoglycemic brain damage. Surgery also may be curative in the case of focal pancreatic lesions, which account for 30% to 50% of cases. Because these lesions are difficult to detect on gross examination of the pancreas, an experienced, multidisciplinary team is required with expertise in preoperative localization procedures and successive intraoperative biopsies and pathologic evaluation. Diffuse congenital hyperinsulinism usually necessitates greater than 95% pancreatectomy in the hope that sufficient tissue will be removed to control hypoglycemia adequately. Because the remaining beta cells are still abnormally regulated, many infants have recurring hypoglycemia postoperatively. Although diazoxide or octreotide or both may be required, management of hypoglycemia is usually easier postoperatively because of the decreased beta cell mass. Pancreatic enzymes or insulin rarely is required after subtotal pancreatectomy.

Pituitary Deficiency

The second most frequent cause of persistent neonatal hypoglycemia is congenital pituitary hormonal deficiency. The physical examination may be normal, but pituitary deficiency may be associated with midline facial defects, including physical features such as cleft lip and palate, single central incisor, or optic nerve hypoplasia. Boys may have micropenis owing to associated gonadotropin deficiency. Severe hypoglycemia may occur in affected neonates, in part secondary to growth hormone and adrenocorticotropic hormone deficiency permitting unopposed insulin action. There may be increased rates of glucose use with suppressed levels of ketones at the time of hypoglycemia,[67] mimicking hyperinsulinism. There may even be an increase in glucose greater than 30 mg/dL after glucagon stimulation. The diagnosis is suggested by showing low levels of growth hormone and cortisol at the time of hypoglycemia and is confirmed by provocative testing. Thyroid function tests show low or low-normal levels of thyroxine and thyroid-stimulating hormone. If hypopituitarism is suspected, magnetic resonance imaging should be performed to look for midline brain malformations. The hypoglycemia is correctable with appropriate hormone replacements.

Adrenal Insufficiency

Primary adrenal insufficiency may present with neonatal hypoglycemia. It is rare in patients with congenital adrenal hyperplasia but may accompany severe bilateral adrenal hemorrhage or the rare occurrence of adrenal hypoplasia.[68] Early recognition is crucial because cortisol deficiency is potentially life-threatening, and cortisol replacement is effective in restoring normoglycemia.

Genetic Metabolic Defects Causing Neonatal Hypoglycemia

Defects in glycogenolysis. The glycogen storage diseases are genetic defects that may affect fasting adaptation; the subtypes that present with hypoglycemia are listed in Table 74-1. Patients have accelerated fasting with early development of ketosis. Because newborns are fed every 3 to 4 hours, these disorders typically do not appear until after the neonatal period. Infants present most commonly with growth failure and hepatomegaly (owing to the accumulation of fat and glycogen) late in the first year of life. Symptomatic hypoglycemia is rare.

Defects in gluconeogenesis. These genetic disorders block the production of glucose from lactate, glycerol, and amino acids (see Fig. 74-4). Fasting induces hypoglycemia accompanied by lactic acidosis. Glucose-6-phosphatase is an enzyme common to the glycogenolytic and gluconeogenic pathways. Its deficiency (glycogen storage disease I) results in severe hypoglycemia after brief fasts together with lactic acidosis. It rarely occurs in newborns. Fructose-1,6-diphosphatase is the rate-limiting enzyme of gluconeogenesis. Deficient infants may develop hypoglycemia and lactic acidosis after prolonged fasting and after the ingestion of fructose or sucrose. The disorder is rare, but many of the cases described have presented in the neonatal period.[69] Treatment includes avoidance of prolonged fasting, provision of glucose at or greater than hepatic production rates (5 mg/kg/min), and correction of the metabolic acidosis as needed.

Defects in ketogenesis. Inborn errors in mitochondrial fatty acid oxidation are a group of diseases that usually present with attacks of fasting hypoketotic hypoglycemia, but also may include acute or chronic cardiomyopathy and skeletal muscle weakness.[70,71] Because the use of fat-derived fuels occurs relatively late in fasting adaptation, these disorders typically do not present in the neonatal period when infants are being fed frequently. These disorders have occurred in neonates subjected to prolonged fasting, however, associated with inadequate breast-feeding or with severe perinatal stress. Specific disorders reported in neonates include deficiencies of medium-chain and very-long-chain acyl-CoA dehydrogenase (MCAD and VLCAD), carnitine palmityl transferase-2, carnitine/acylcarnitine translocase, and glutaric aciduria type 2. Long-chain 3-hydroxy acyl-CoA dehydrogenase (LCHAD) deficiency has been associated with acute fatty liver of pregnancy in mothers of affected infants.[72,73] In these disorders, fasting for 8 to 16 hours leads to the development of hypoglycemia associated with low concentrations of ketones. Assays of plasma and tissue carnitine, plasma acylcarnitine profile, urinary organic acid profile, and in vitro studies of fatty acid oxidation in cultured fibroblasts are helpful in identifying individual defects. Expanded newborn screening by tandem mass spectrometers is increasingly available and can detect many of these defects (MCAD, VLCAD, LCHAD, glutaric aciduria type 2).

Persistent hypoglycorrhachia (GLUT-1 deficiency). Reports have identified patients with a genetic defect of the GLUT-1 glucose transporter required to transfer glucose across the blood-brain barrier.[74] Affected patients have persistently low cerebrospinal fluid glucose (20 to 30 mg/dL) without evidence of meningitis. The disorder was first recognized in older infants with recurrent seizures, progressive microcephaly, and retardation. We are aware of cases appearing in the first days of life with intractable neonatal seizures, however. The latter patients underscore the concern that the newborn brain does not have a lower requirement for glucose than older individuals. Management with a ketogenic diet to provide the brain with alternative fuels has been remarkably successful in some patients.

General Approach to Diagnosis and Treatment of Hypoglycemia in Neonates

Hypoglycemia Thresholds

In newborns, as in older infants and children, hypoglycemia should be considered to be the result of a specific failure in one or more of the metabolic and hormonal systems involved in fasting homeostasis. For this reason, we discourage using lower standards to interpret plasma glucose values in neonates than would be used in older infants. Plasma glucose levels of 70 to 100 mg/dL (3.8 to 5.5 mmol/L) should be taken as the physiologically normal/optimal/therapeutic target range; this approximates the mean plasma glucose value found prenatally and postnatally in healthy newborns. Hypoglycemia should be "defined" as a plasma glucose less than 40 mg/dL (<2.2 mmol/L), implying simply that values above this level are not likely to be responsible for severe symptoms (e.g., seizures). This threshold is not absolute but is influenced by the availability of alternative fuels. Patients with some disorders, such as fatty acid oxidation defects, become dangerously ill with plasma glucose levels in the range of 45 to 60 mg/dL (2.5 to 3.4 mmol/L), whereas patients with other disorders, such as type 1 glycogen storage disease, may have few symptoms at glucose levels of 30 to 40 mg/dL (1.7 to 2.2 mmol/L).

The aforementioned view differs from some of the traditional standards for defining neonatal hypoglycemia— plasma glucose less than 35 mg/dL (<2 mmol/L) in normal-birth-weight and less than 25 mg/dL (<1.4 mmol/L) in low-birth-weight infants. These values represent "statistical normals" based on older surveys of infants subjected to what now would be considered prolonged periods of fasting; they do not represent what is "physiologically normal" for the newborn. These values often are misinterpreted to imply that increasing glucose concentrations to 35 to 40 mg/dL (2 to 2.2 mmol/L) is adequate treatment for hypoglycemia in newborns. There is some evidence that pathophysiologic responses to hypoglycemia in neonates and older children and adults are elicited at similar threshold levels of glucose.[75-77] We prefer a conservative approach emphasizing that plasma glucose values less than 60 mg/dL (<2.2 to 3.4 mmol/L) should be considered suboptimal and not allowed to persist. In most infants, these levels can be increased by appropriate early feeding. When difficulties in maintaining this threshold occur, the possibility must be entertained of a specific disorder of one of the fasting systems.*

---

*There is controversy about definitions of normoglycemia and hypoglycemia in newborns, frequently locked into confusion of statistically normal with physiologically normal and arguments about whether "asymptomatic" hypoglycemia can have pathologic sequelae.[78,79] One argument against the conservative standards suggested in this chapter relates to the normal breast-fed infant. Because breast-feeding is "natural," and milk supply is often not well developed for several days, the neonate must have been provided some special mechanism that prevents damage from any hypoglycemia that might occur during this time of starvation. We were at first taken aback by this argument of "divine intent" until we recognized several flaws: (1) "divine intent" was preservation of the species, not of individuals (note that "natural" infant mortality is many times the current level); (2) small amounts of colostrum may be important in triggering maturation of fasting systems (ketogenesis and gluconeogenesis); and (3) widespread application of this "divine intent" argument would obviate the need for neonatologists entirely.

Signs of Neonatal Hypoglycemia

The classic symptoms of hypoglycemia relate to adrenergic stimulation (tachycardia and diaphoresis) and impaired central nervous system function (confusion, headache, lethargy). In the newborn, these classic symptoms are difficult to appreciate, and the signs of neonatal hypoglycemia may be minimal and nonspecific; they include feeding difficulty, hypothermia, tremors, weak cry, cyanosis, apnea, and seizures (Table 74-5). Hypoglycemia must be suspected in any infant who does not appear normal or who has any of the risk factors noted in Table 74-3. Plasma glucose levels should be monitored closely in high-risk infants, and oral or intravenous feeding should be begun as soon as possible because prolonged hypoglycemia can lead to permanent brain damage. Glucose test strips may be used for rapid screening. They are unreliable in the lower ranges, however, even when read with a meter. Measurements should be corroborated with true laboratory values.[80] All neonatal intensive care units should have a glucose analyzer available to ensure that accurate glucose determinations are rapidly available.[81] Some laboratories measure whole-blood glucose, which is 15% lower than plasma glucose values.

Emergent Treatment

Severe or symptomatic hypoglycemia should be treated with intravenous glucose as a bolus of 10% dextrose (0.2 to 0.5 g/kg), followed by an infusion (beginning at 5 to 10 mg/kg/min) to maintain plasma glucose greater than 60 mg/dL (>3.3 mmol/L). Rates of 20 mg/kg/min may be required for infants with hyperinsulinism, infants of diabetic mothers, or infants with pituitary deficiency. A feeding or oral glucose (0.5 to 1 g/kg) should be given for asymptomatic or mild hypoglycemia. Plasma glucose should be checked 30 to 60 minutes after emergency treatment and monitored to ensure levels remain greater than 60 mg/dL (>3.4 mmol/L).

Although glucocorticoids traditionally have been suggested for nonspecific treatment of intractable neonatal hypoglycemia, we do not recommend this approach. As described in earlier sections, hyperinsulinism is likely to be responsible in many of these cases, and glucocorticoids are ineffective in hyperinsulinism or other disorders not specifically due to adrenal insufficiency.

Etiology

If the cause of the hypoglycemia is one of the self-limited disorders, such as infants of diabetic mothers, specific etiologic studies may not be necessary. In all other cases, these tests should be performed. Blood and urine samples obtained at the time of hypoglycemia give the most valuable information because levels of key fuels and hormones at this point provide information on which of the six fasting systems is most likely responsible. These are termed the *critical* samples—2 to 3 mL of plasma or serum and 5 to 10 mL of urine. Measurement of lactate, free fatty acids, ketones, insulin, cortisol, growth hormone, and urinary organic acids should be considered. Table 74-4 shows the expected changes in fuel levels with hypoglycemia. If hyperinsulinism is suspected, a glucagon stimulation test (0.5 to 1 mg/kg intravenously) at a time of hypoglycemia is useful; an increase greater than 30 mg/dL implies inappropriate preservation of liver glycogen stores, consistent with hyperinsulinism but occasionally seen in neonatal panhypopituitarism. Specific tests of pituitary function should be considered if pituitary deficiency is suspected.

NEONATAL HYPERGLYCEMIA

Neonatal hyperglycemia is defined as a plasma glucose greater than 145 mg/dL (>8.1 mmol/L). Hyperglycemia is usually a brief phenomenon related to high rates of intravenous glucose infusion during the first few days of life.[82,83] Hyperglycemia that is more prolonged may represent transient or permanent diabetes mellitus.

Self-limited hyperglycemia occurs most frequently in the first 24 hours after birth. The risk is 18 times greater for infants weighing less than 1000 g than for infants weighing more than 2000 g[84] and is increased in the presence of other serious illnesses, such as respiratory disease.[85] A significant proportion of neonates undergoing anesthesia and surgery also develop hyperglycemia.[86] Although most studies of this phenomenon have shown a decreased insulin response to an acute glucose load in the neonate (representing a lag in the beta cell response to hyperglycemia), other authors have suggested that premature and term newborns with hyperglycemia have a relative insulin deficiency or resistance.[87,88]

The onset of permanent diabetes mellitus in the newborn period is highly unusual, although rare cases[89] of autoimmune diabetes, neonatal diabetes syndromes, and congenital diabetes due to pancreatic aplasia have been described.[90] A case of pancreatic agenesis/permanent neonatal diabetes was found to have a deletion in insulin promoter factor 1.[91] More common in neonates is the syndrome of transient diabetes mellitus, which occurs in 1 in 400,000 live births. Affected infants are usually small for gestational age and present during the first weeks of life with elevated blood glucose (>240 mg/dL) with glycosuria and ketonuria. If the diabetes goes unrecognized, these infants can become significantly dehydrated. Insulin levels are absolutely or relatively low for the corresponding blood glucose, and the response of insulin to secretagogues is reduced. This problem appears to be due to a temporary delay in beta cell maturation and usually resolves spontaneously by several months of age.[92] Regular subcutaneous insulin is necessary, but can be gradually withdrawn as the blood glucose becomes more tightly regulated. The disorder has been found to be

Table 74–5. Signs of Neonatal Hypoglycemia

Feeding difficulty
Lethargy
Weak cry
Hypothermia
Apnea
Cyanosis
Tremors
Seizures

associated with abnormalities of chromosome 6, including paternal uniparental disomy of paternal chromosome 6[93] and an unbalanced duplication of paternal 6q24.[94]

It is important to monitor hyperglycemic infants for the development of osmotic diuresis, which can lead to dehydration. In more severe cases, this situation may result in cerebral hemorrhage. If the glucose elevation is mild, a decrease in the rate of glucose infusion is often effective until the problem has resolved. Low-dose intravenous insulin infusions have been used successfully in infants with more severe hyperglycemia and enable the intake of adequate calories for growth (in the event that prolonged parenteral nutrition is necessary).[95] Infants with transient or permanent diabetes mellitus require low-dose subcutaneous insulin.

SUGAR TOXICITY DISORDERS

Galactosemia is a hereditary defect of galactose 1-phosphate uridyl transferase, which results in the inability to convert galactose to glucose (see Fig. 74-4). Affected infants appear normal at birth and have normal fasting adaptation. The first symptoms occur after the ingestion of lactose (milk sugar, the glucose-galactose disaccharide) and are due to the toxic effects of the accumulation of galactose 1-phosphate.[96,97] Symptoms and signs include poor feeding, vomiting, diarrhea, hepatomegaly, jaundice, renal Fanconi syndrome, failure to thrive, and a propensity toward developing *Escherichia coli* sepsis.[98] The cause of the increased susceptibility is unknown but may be related to impaired white blood cell function secondary to accumulation of galactose metabolites.

The onset of galactosemia may be subtle, and as the illness progresses, cataracts and developmental delays become evident. Untreated patients may go on to develop cirrhosis and mental retardation. For these reasons, most states have instituted newborn screening programs. The diagnosis is made by showing nonglucose reducing substances in the urine and is confirmed by measuring the enzyme activity in red blood cells. Treatment consists of eliminating galactose from the diet.

Studies of long-term outcomes[99] have revealed that many treated patients still have growth delays, minor neurologic abnormalities, and speech impairment. Intelligence quotients are variable, but as a group, patients with galactosemia are skewed toward the lower end of the normal curve. Affected women have a high incidence of ovarian failure later in life, although some are able to achieve a normal pregnancy.

Hereditary fructose intolerance is another sugar toxicity disorder due to the absence of fructose 1-phosphate aldolase (see Fig. 74-4). Fasting occurs normally, but hypoglycemia and lactic acidosis occur after the ingestion of fructose-containing or sucrose-containing foods.[100] The effect is due to the accumulation of fructose 1-phosphate, which inhibits glycogenolysis and gluconeogenesis. Severe episodes may result in liver or renal damage. The disorder is unlikely to present in the neonatal period unless fructose is consumed.

REFERENCES

1. Stanley CA, Baker L: Hypoglycemia. In Kaye R, Oski FA, Barness LA (eds): Core Textbook of Pediatrics. Philadelphia, JB Lippincott, 1978, pp 280-305.
2. Cahill GF: Starvation in man. N Engl J Med 282:668, 1970.
3. Zeller J, Bougneres P: Hypoglycemia in infants. Trends Endocr Metab 3:366, 1992.
4. Bier D, Leake RD, Haymond MW, et al: Measurement of "true" glucose production rates in infancy and childhood with 6,6-dideuteroglucose. Diabetes 26:1016, 1977.
5. Haymond MW, Karl IE, Clarke WL, et al: Differences in circulating gluconeogenic substrates during short term fasting in men, women, and children. Metabolism 31:33, 1982.
6. Girard J: Gluconeogenesis in late fetal and early neonatal life. Biol Neonate 50:237, 1986.
7. Mayor F, Cuezva JM: Hormonal and metabolic changes in the perinatal period. Biol Neonate 48:185, 1985.
8. Stanley CA, Anday EK, Baker L, Delivoria-Papadopolous M: Metabolic fuel and hormone responses to fasting in newborn infants. Pediatrics 64:613, 1979.
9. Stanley CA, Gonzalez E, Baker L: Development of hepatic fatty acid oxidation and ketogenesis in the newborn guinea pig. Pediatr Res 17:224, 1983.
10. Foster PC, Bailey E: Changes in the activities of the enzymes of hepatic fatty acid oxidation during development of the rat. Biochem J 154:49, 1976.
11. Lee LL, Fritz IB: Hepatic ketogenesis during development. Can J Biochem 49:599, 1971.
12. Portha B: Development of the pancreatic B-cells: Growth pattern and functional maturation. In Cuezva JM, Pascual-Leone AM, Patel MS (eds): Endocrine and Biochemical Development of the Fetus and Neonate, New York, Plenum Press, 1990, pp 33-43.
13. Ktorza A, Bihoreau M, Nurjhan N, et al: Insulin and glucagon during the perinatal period: Secretion and metabolic effects on the liver. Biol Neonate 48:204, 1985.
14. Menon RK, Sperling M: Carbohydrate metabolism. Semin Perinatol 12:157, 1988.
15. Chatelain F, Kohl C, Esser V, et al: Cyclic AMP and fatty acids increase carnitine palmitoyltransferase I gene transcription in cultured fetal rat hepatocytes. Eur J Biochem 235:789, 1996.
16. Themeline S, Esser V, Charvy D, et al: Expression of liver carnitine palmitoyltransferase I and II genes during development in the rat. Biochem J 300(pt 2):583, 1994.
17. Melichar V, Drahota Z, Hahn P: Ketone bodies in the blood of full term newborns, premature and dysmature infants, and infants of diabetic mothers. Biol Neonate 11:23, 1967.
18. Robles-Valdes C, McGarry JD, Foster DW: Maternal-fetal carnitine relationships and neonatal ketosis in the rat. J Biol Chem 251:6007, 1976.
19. Anday EK, Stanley CA, Delivoria-Papadopoulos M: Plasma ketones in newborn infants: Absence of suckling ketosis. J Pediatr 98:628, 1981.
20. Stanley CA: Neonatal carnitine metabolism. In Cowett RM (ed): Principles of Perinatal-Neonatal Metabolism. New York, Springer Verlag, 1991, pp 465-471.
21. Lubchenco LO, Bard H: Incidence of hypoglycemia in newborn infants classified by birth weight and gestational age. Pediatrics 47:831, 1971.
22. Haymond M, Karl I, Pagliara AS: Increased gluconeogenic substrates in the small-for-gestational-age infant. N Engl J Med 291:322, 1974.

23. Williams PR, Fiser RH, Sperling MA, et al: Effects of oral alanine feeding on blood glucose, plasma glucagon, and insulin concentrations in small for gestational age infants. N Engl J Med 292:612, 1975.

24. Wright LL, Stanley CA, Anday EK, Baker L: The effect of early feeding on plasma glucose levels in SGA infants. Clin Pediatr 22:539, 1983.

25. Collins JE, Leonard JV: Hyperinsulinism in asphyxiated and small for dates infants with hypoglycemia. Lancet 2:311, 1984.

26. Collins JE, Leonard JV, Teale T, et al: Hyperinsulinemic hypoglycemia in small for dates infants. Arch Dis Child 65:1118, 1990.

27. Le Dune MA: Intravenous glucose tolerance and plasma insulin studies in small for dates infants. Arch Dis Child 47:111, 1972.

28. Aynsley-Green A, Soltesz G: Hypoglycaemia in Infancy and Childhood. London, Churchill Livingstone, 1985.

29. Kenepp NB, Shelley WC, Gabbe SG, et al: Fetal and neonatal hazards of maternal hydration with 5% dextrose before cesarian section. Lancet 1(8282):1150, 1982.

30. Roe TF, Kershnar AK, Weitzman JJ, et al: Beckwith's syndrome with extreme organ hyperplasia. Pediatrics 52:372, 1991.

31. Glaser B, Thornton PS, Herold K, Stanley CA: Clinical and molecular heterogeneity of familial hyperinsulinism. J Pediatr 133:801, 1998.

32. Glaser B, Thornton P, Otonkoski T, Junien C: The genetics of neonatal hyperinsulinism. Arch Dis Child Fetal Neonatal Educ 82:F79, 2000.

33. Kelly A, Alter CA, Thornton PS: Hyperinsulinism. Endocrinologist 11:26, 2001.

34. Thornton PS, Sumner AE, Ruchelli ED, et al: Familial and sporadic hyperinsulinism: Histopathologic findings and segregation analysis support a single autosomal recessive disorder. J Pediatr 119:721, 1991.

35. Aguilar-Bryan L, Nichols CG, Wechsler SW, et al: Cloning of the β cell high-affinity sulfonylurea receptor: A regulator of insulin secretion. Science 268:423, 1995.

36. Glaser B, Chiu KC, Anker R, et al: Familial hyperinsulinism maps to chromosome 11p14-15.1 30 cM centromeric to the insulin gene. Nat Genet 7:185, 1994.

37. Glaser B, Chiu KC, Liu L, et al: Recombinant mapping of the familial hyperinsulinism gene to an 0.8 cm region on chromosom 11p15.1 and demonstration of a founder effect in Ashkenazi Jews. Hum Mol Genet 4:879, 1995.

38. Thomas PM, Cote GJ, Hallman DM, et al: Homozygosity mapping to chromosome 11p of the gene for familial persistent hyperinsulinemic hypoglycemia of infancy. Am J Hum Genet 56:416, 1995.

39. Thomas PM, Cote GJ, Wollk N, et al: Mutations in the sulfonylurea receptor gene in familial persistent hyperinsulinemic hypoglycemia of infancy. Science 268:426, 1995.

40. Glaser B, Ryan F, Donath M, et al: Hyperinsulinism caused by paternal-specific inheritance of a recessive mutation of a non-imprinted gene. Diabetes 48:1652, 1999.

41. Ryan F, Devaney D, Joyce C, et al: Hyperinsulinism: the molecular aetiology of focal disease. Arch Dis Child 79:445, 1998.

42. Landau H, Perlman M, Meyer S, et al: Persistant neonatal hypoglycemia due to hyperinsulinism: Medical aspects. Pediatrics 70:440, 1982.

43. Stanley CA, Baker L: Hyperinsulinism in infants and children: diagnosis and therapy. Adv Pediatr 32:315, 1976.

44. Thornton PS, Satin-Smith MS, Herold K, et al: Familial hyperinsulinism with apparent autosomal dominant inheritance: Clinical and genetic differences from the autosomal recessive variant. J Pediatr 132:9, 1998.

45. Thornton PS, MacMullen C, Ganguly A, et al: Clinical and molecular characterization of a dominant form of congenital hyperinsulinism caused by a mutation in the high-affinity sulfonylurea receptor. Diabetes 52:2403, 2003.

46. Weinzimer SA, Stanley CA, Berry GT, et al: A syndrome of congenital hyperinsulinism and hyperammonemia. J Pediatr 130:661, 1997.

47. Zammarchi E, Filippi L, Novembre E, et al: Biochemical evaluation of a patient with a familial form of leucine-sensitive hypoglycemia and concomitant hyperammonemia. Metabolism 45:957, 1996.

48. Stanley CA, Fang J, Kutyna K, et al: Molecular basis and characterization of the hyperinsulinism/hyperammonemmia syndrome: Predominance of mutations in exons 11 and 12 of the glutamate dehydrogenase gene. Diabetes 49:661, 2000.

49. Stanley CA, Lieu YK, Hsu BYL, et al: Hyperinsulinism and hyper ammonemia in infants with regulatory mutations of the glutamate dehydrogenase gene. N Engl J Med 338:1352, 1998.

50. Miki Y, Tomohiko T, Obura T, et al: Novel missense mutations in the glutamate dehydrogenase gene in the congenital hyperinsulinism-hyperammonemia syndrome. J Pediatr 136:69, 2000.

51. Yorifuji T, Muroi J, Uematsu A, et al: Hyperinsulinism-hyperammonemia syndrome caused by mutant glutamate dehydrogenase accompanied by novel enzyme kinetics. Hum Genet 104:476, 1999.

52. Glaser B, Kesavan P, Heyman M, et al: Familial hyperinsulinism caused by a novel glucokinase mutation. N Engl J Med 338:226, 1998.

53. Stanley CA, Baker L: Hyperinsulinism in infancy: Diagnosis by demonstration of abnormal response to fasting hypoglycemia. Pediatrics 57:702, 1976.

54. Katz LEL, Satin-Smith M, Collett-Solberg P, et al: Insulin like growth factor binding protein-1 levels in the diagnosis of hypoglycaemia caused by hyperinsulinism. J Pediatr 131:193, 1997.

55. Finegold D, Stanley CA, Baker L: Glycemic response to glucagon during fasting hypoglycemia: An aid in the diagnosis of hyperinsulinism. J Pediatr 96:257, 1980.

56. Grimberg A, Ferry RJ Jr, Kelly A, et al: Dysregulation of insulin secretion in children with congenital hyperinsulinism due to sulfonylurea receptor mutations. Diabetes 50:322, 2001.

57. Hsu BL, Kelly A, Thornton PS, et al: Protein sensitive and fasting hypoglycemia in children with the hyperinsulinism hyperammonemia syndrome. J Pediatr 138:383, 2001.

58. Kelly A, Ng D, Ferry RJ, et al: Acute insulin responses to leucine in children with the hyperinsulinism/hyperammonemia syndrome. J Clin Endocrinol Metab 2001; 86:3724.

59. Stanley CA, Thornton PS, Ganguly A: Preoperative evaluation of infants with focal or diffuse congenital hyperinsulinism by intravenous acute insulin response tests and selective pancreatic arterial calcium stimulation. J Clin Endocrinol Metab 89:288, 2004.

60. Thornton PS, Steinkrauss L, MacMullen C, et al: Differentiation of focal from diffuse hyperinsulinism by acute insulin response (AIR) testing and pancreatic arterial stimulation allows accurate preoperative diagnosis and focal surgery. Presented at LWPES, Montreal, 2001.

61. Thornton PS, Steinkrauss L, Ruchelli E, et al: Preoperative diagnosis of focal versus diffuse congenital hyperinsulinism using acute insulin response testing and selective pancreatic arterial stimulation with venous sampling. Presented at PAS Annual Meeting, Baltimore, 2001.

62. Dubois J, Brunelle F, Touati G, et al: Hyperinsulinism in children: Diagnostic value of pancreatic venous sampling correlated with clinical, pathological and surgical outcomes in 25 cases. Pediatr Radiol 25:512, 1995.

63. Hirsch HJ, Loo S, Evans N, et al: Hypoglycemia of infancy and nesidioblastosis. N Engl J Med 296:1323, 1977.

64. Thornton PS, Alter CA, Katz LL, et al: Acute and long-term use of octreotide in the treatment of congenital hyperinsulinism. J Pediatr 123:637, 1993.

65. Eichmann D, Hufnagel M, Quick P, Santer R: Treatment of hyperinsulinaemic hypoglycaemia with nifedipine. Eur J Pediatr 158:204, 1999.

66. Bas J, Darendeliler F, Demirkol D, et al: Successful therapy with calcium channel blocker (nifedipine) in persistent neonatal hyperinsulinermic hypoglycemia of infancy. J Pediatr Eur Endocrinol Metab 12:873, 1999.

67. Wolfsdorf JI, Sadeghi-Nejad A, Senior A: Hypoketonemia and age-related fasting hypoglycemia in growth hormone deficiency. Metabolism 32:457, 1983.

68. Artavia-Loria E, Chaussain JL, Bougneres PF, et al: Frequency of hypoglycemia in children with adrenal insufficiency. Acta Endocrinol (Copenh) 279(suppl):275, 1986.

69. Gitzelmann R, Steinmann B, Van Den Berghe G: Disorders of fructose metabolism. In Stanbury JB, Whyngaarden JB, Fredrickson DS (eds): The Metabolic Basis of Inherited Disease. New York, McGraw-Hill, 1989.

70. Hale DE, Bennett MJ: Fatty acid oxidation disorders: A new class of metabolic diseases. J Pediatr 121:1-11, 1992.

71. Stanley CA: Disorders of fatty acid oxidation. In Behrman RE (ed): Nelson Textbook of Pediatrics. Philadelphia, WB Saunders, 1992.

72. Schoemann MN, Batey RG, Wilcken B: Recurrent acute fatty liver of pregnancy associated with a fatty acid oxidation defect in the offspring. Gastroenterology 100:544, 1991.

73. Wilcken B, Leung KC, Hammond J, et al: Pregnancy and fetal long-chain 3-hydroxyacyl coenzyme A dehydrogenate deficiency. Lancet 341:407, 1993.

74. De Vivo DC, Trifiletti RR, Jacobson RI, et al: Defective glucose transport across the blood-brain barrier as a cause of persistent hypoglycorrhachia, seizures, and developmental delay. N Engl J Med 325:731, 1991.

75. Koh T, Aynsley-Green A, Tarbit M, Eyre JA: Neural dysfunction during hypoglycemia. Arch Dis Child 63:1353, 1988.

76. Prydes O, Christensen NJ, Friis-Hansen B: Increased cerebral blood flow and plasma epinephrine in hypoglycemic preterm neonates. Pediatrics 85:172, 1990.

77. Volpe JJ: Hypoglycemia and brain surgery. In Volpe JJ: Neurology of the Newborn, 4th ed. Philadelphia, WB Saunders, 2001, pp 497-520

78. Cornblath M, Schwartz R, Aynsley-Green A, Lloyd JK: Hypoglycemia in infancy: The need for a rational definition. A Ciba foundation discussion meeting. Pediatrics 85:834, 1990.

79. Koh T, Eyre JA, Aynsley-Green A: Neonatal hypoglycemia—the controversy regarding definition. Arch Dis Child 63:1386, 1988.

80. Perelman RH, Gutcher GR, Engle MJ, MacDonald MJ: Comparative analysis of four methods of rapid glucose determinations in neonates. Am J Dis Child 136:1051, 1982.

81. Conrad PD, Sparks JW, Osberg I, et al: Clinical application of a new glucose analyzer in the neonatal intensive care unit: Comparison with other methods. J Pediatr 114:281, 1989.

82. Pildes R: Neonatal hyperglycemia. J Pediatr 109:905, 1986.

83. Dweck H, Cassady G: Glucose intolerance in infants of very low birth weight: I. Incidence of hyperglycemia in infants of birth weights 1100 grams or less. Pediatrics 53:189, 1974.

84. Louik C, Mitchell A, Epstein MF, Shapiro S: Risk factors for neonatal hyperglycemia associated with 10% dextrose infusion. Am J Dis Child 139:783, 1985.

85. Lillien L, Rosenfield R, Baccaro MM, Pildes R: Hyperglycemia in stressed small premature neonates. J Pediatr 94:454, 1979.

86. Srinivasan G, Jain R, Pildes RS, Kannan CR: Glucose homeostasis during anesthesia and surgery in infants. J Pediatr Surg 21:718, 1986.

87. Cowett R, Oh W, Schwartz R: Persistant glucose production during glucose infusion in the neonate. J Clin Invest 71:467, 1983.

88. Flecknell PA, Wootton R, Royston JP, John M: Glucose homeostasis in the newborn: Effects of an intravenous glucose infusion in normal and intra-uterine growth retarded neonatal piglets. Biol Neonate 52:205, 1987.

89. Guest GM: Infantile diabetes mellitus: Three cases in successive siblings, two with onset at three months of age and one at nine days of age. Am J Dis Child 75:461, 1948.

90. Lemons JA, Ridenour R, Orsini EN: Congenital absence of the pancreas and intrauterine growth retardation. Pediatrics 64:255, 1979.

91. Stoffers DA, Stanojevic V, Clarke WL, Habener JF: Pancreatic agenesis attributable to a single nucleotide deletion in the human I F1 gene coding sequence. Nat Genet 12:106, 1997.

92. Shield J: Neonatal diabetes: New insights into aetiology and implications. Hormone Res 53(suppl):7, 2000.

93. Temple IK, James RS, Crol JA, et al: An imprinted gene(s) for diabetes? Nat Genet 9:110, 1995.

94. Temple IK, Gardner RJ, Robinson DO, et al: Further evidence for an imprinted gene for neonatal diabetes localised to chromosome 6q22-23. Hum Mol Genet 5:1117, 1996.

95. Binder ND, Raschko PK, Benda GI, Reynolds JW: Insulin infusion with parenteral nutrition in extremely low birth weight infants with hyperglycemia. J Pediatr 114:273, 1989.

96. Donnell GN: Clinical aspects and historical perspectives of galactosemia. In Donnell GN (ed): Galactosemia: New Frontiers in Research. Bethesda, MD, National Institutes of Health, 1993.

97. Segal S: Galactosemia. In Wyngaarden JB, Smith LH, Bennett JC (eds): Cecil Textbook of Medicine: Disorders of Carbohydrate Metabolism. Philadelphia, WB Saunders, 1991.

98. Levy HL, Sepe SJ, Shih VE, et al: Sepsis due to *Escherichia coli* in neonates with galactosemia. N Engl J Med 297:823, 1997.

99. Waggoner DD, Donnell GN, Buist NRM: Long-term prognosis in galactosemia: Results of a survey of 350 cases. In Donnell GN (ed): Galactosemia: New Frontiers in Research. Bethesda, MD, National Institutes of Health,

100. Gitzelmann R, Steinmann B, Van Den Berghe G: Disorders of fructose metabolism. In Stanbury JB, Wyngaarden JB, Fredrickson DS (eds): The Metabolic Basis of Inherited Disease. New York, McGraw-Hill, 1989.

CHAPTER 75

Disorders of Calcium Homeostasis

Frank R. Greer

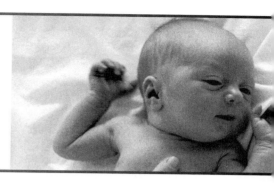

Calcium is the most abundant mineral in the human body. Although it is important for muscle contraction, neurotransmission, enzyme function, and many other metabolic activities, most calcium is used in the formation and maintenance of bone. Thus, 99% of calcium is located in bone, the obvious reservoir for this mineral. It circulates in the blood in three fractions: bound to albumin (45%); complexed with bicarbonate, phosphate, or citrate (5%); and ionized (50%). The latter two fractions are referred to as ultrafilterable (renal) or non–protein-bound fractions. Ionized calcium is the only one of the three fractions that is physiologically active. As a general rule, the serum concentration of calcium in humans is under very tight control, with an elaborate mechanism of homeostasis. The human fetus and newborn are no exceptions to this rule, although there are some basic differences from older children and adults. Similarly, there are some unique disturbances of calcium homeostasis in the neonatal period that are related to various perinatal factors. The purpose of this chapter is to review this homeostasis and the disturbances that can arise. Treatment of metabolic disorders of calcium metabolism is also discussed.

PHYSIOLOGY

Overview

Ionized calcium, a fraction of a percentage of the total body calcium, has many vital physiologic functions. Although the importance of ionized calcium as an intracellular "second" messenger has been known for many years, this fraction is now known to be an important extracellular "first" messenger through exquisitely sensitive calcium cell surface receptors.[1] This receptor includes a large amino (NH2)–terminal extracellular domain, a transmembrane "serpentine" G-protein–coupled receptor, and an intracellular carboxy-terminal tail (Fig. 75-1). Ionized calcium binds to the extracellular domain of the calcium cell surface receptor, which acts as the "calciostat," or "thermostat" for ionized calcium in humans. The gene for the calcium cell surface receptor is located on chromosome 3, and mutations have been described. These mutations account for the syndrome of familial hypercalcemia with hypocalciuria and severe neonatal primary hyperparathyroidism, both conditions in which the calciostat is reset upward.[2]

The maintenance of serum ionized calcium concentration is primarily the function of the parathyroid glands. When serum calcium concentration decreases, the secretion of parathyroid hormone (PTH) increases. Likewise, when serum calcium concentration increases, negative feedback inhibition decreases secretion of PTH. PTH, an 84–amino acid peptide, is secreted by the parathyroid chief cells. PTH acts on the kidney in a number of ways. First, it inhibits proximal tubular PO4 reabsorption (increases phosphaturia) and increases distal tubular reabsorption of filtered calcium through a cyclic adenosine monophosphate (cAMP)–mediated process in the tubule. Secondly, it stimulates 1α-hydroxylation of 25(OH)-vitamin D by stimulating the enzyme 1α-hydroxylase (a cytochrome P-450–dependent monooxygenase) in the mitochondria of the proximal tubule of the kidney (Fig. 75-2). 1,25(OH)2-vitamin D then stimulates intestinal absorption of calcium.[3]

1,25(OH)2-vitamin D circulates bound to vitamin D–binding protein, which is synthesized in the liver. Like other steroidal hormones, all target tissues (cells) for 1,25(OH)2-vitamin D contain a vitamin D receptor. This receptor is a protein, the carboxy- or C-terminal end of which binds to 1,25(OH)2-vitamin D and the nitrogen end (N-terminal) of which may bind to DNA in the nucleus.[3] This vitamin D receptor–1,25(OH)2-vitamin D complex in the nucleus then binds with the nuclear retinoic acid receptor to form a larger complex (retinoic acid receptor–vitamin D receptor–vitamin D) (Fig. 75-3). The N-terminal portion of this large complex then binds with a specific portion of the nuclear DNA, the vitamin D response element.[3] This results in gene transcription and the synthesis of specific messenger RNA for a variety of vitamin

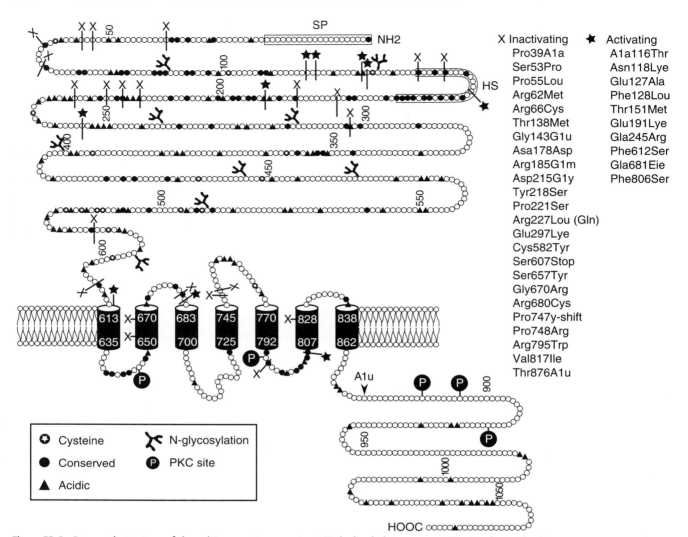

Figure 75–1. Proposed structure of the calcium-sensing receptor. HS, hydrophobic segment; SP, signal peptide. (*From Karne SM, Aviloi LV: Familial benign hypocalciuric hypercalcemia and other syndromes of altered responsiveness to extracellular calcium. In Metabolic Bone Disease, vol 3, 1997, pp 479-499, with permission.*)

D–dependent proteins, such as intestinal calcium-binding protein. Similar 1,25(OH)$_2$-vitamin D receptors and nuclear response elements are presumed to exist in kidney and bone tissue. In the rat kidney, 1,25(OH)$_2$-vitamin D receptors have been identified in the proximal tubule of the nephron,[4] and a vitamin D–dependent calcium-binding protein has been found in the human kidney.[5] There is evidence that both phosphate and calcium reabsorption are stimulated by 1,25(OH)$_2$-vitamin D in the mammalian kidney. Both of these actions apparently require protein synthesis: for example, renal calcium-binding protein.[6]

One of the effects of 1,25(OH)$_2$-vitamin D on bone is **bone resorption,** or **remodeling,** a function essential for maintaining calcium homeostasis. Bone resorption is carried out by osteoclasts, but vitamin D metabolites and PTH have no direct effect on osteoclasts, which lack receptors for 1,25(OH)$_2$-vitamin D and PTH.[7] It is possible that osteoclast precursors have receptors, inasmuch as

1,25(OH)$_2$-vitamin D promotes osteoclast formation in bone organ cultures. Whereas PTH and 1,25(OH)$_2$-vitamin D increase bone resorption and cAMP synthesis in bone organ culture, in vivo PTH and 1,25(OH)$_2$-vitamin D have no effect on the bone resorption and motility of isolated osteoclasts.[7] The effects of 1,25(OH)$_2$-vitamin D on osteoclasts must be mediated by other cells that have 1,25(OH)$_2$-vitamin D receptors (osteoblasts).

Vitamin D is technically a hormone, not a vitamin, inasmuch as it is synthesized in all mammals. 25(OH)-vitamin D, the major circulatory form of vitamin D, is synthesized in the liver from the parent compound (see Fig. 75-2). There are two sources of this parent compound. Vitamin D$_3$ is synthesized in the skin from ultraviolet B light exposure. This obviously is not an important process in the fetus and newborn. The second source, vitamin D$_2$, is of dietary origin. Vitamin D is absorbed in the small intestine and transported in the intestinal lymph duct primarily by chylomicrons. In animals, the

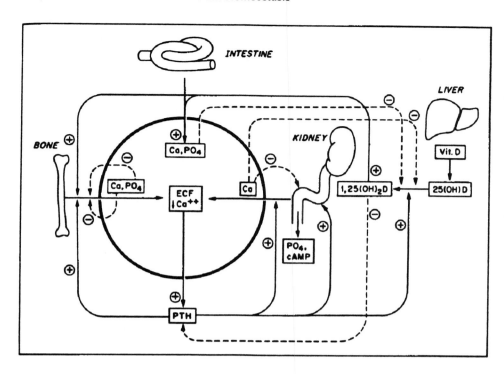

Figure 75–2. Vitamin D and calcium metabolism. *Solid arrows* and *solid lines* delineate action of parathyroid hormone (PTH) and 1,25(OH)₂-vitamin D; *dotted arrows* and *dotted lines* show direct actions of Ca²⁺ and phosphate ions on target tissues. *Circled minus signs* represent inhibitory actions; *circled plus signs* represent positive actions. cAMP, cyclic adenosine monophosphate; ECF, extracellular fluid. *(From Brown EM: The extracellular Ca²⁺ sensing receptor: Central mediator of systemic calcium homeostasis. Annu Rev Nutr 20:507, 2000, with permission.)*

absorption rate of vitamin D is linearly related to the dose of vitamin D, which suggests that absorption takes place by simple passive diffusion after dissolution by bile salts.[8] There is no information on the absorptive capacity of preterm neonates for vitamin D or its metabolites. In full-term neonates with inoperable brain deformities, 13% to 23% of an oral dose of ¹⁴C-vitamin D was recovered from feces within 3 days.[9] Vitamin D undergoes a certain amount of enterohepatic circulation; however, 25-hydroxylation of the parent compound enhances the intestinal absorption and minimizes its loss during enterohepatic circulation.[10] It is also likely that vitamin D and PTH act on the bone to mobilize calcium and phosphorus when dietary intake of calcium is limited.

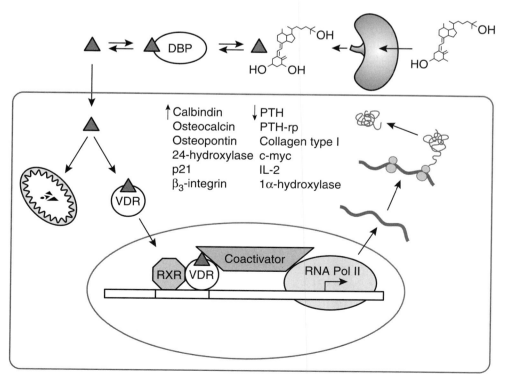

Figure 75–3. Proposed model for the mechanism of action of 1,25(OH)₂-vitamin D (D₃) on tissue target cells, which results in messenger RNA synthesis and a variety of biologic responses. DBP, vitamin D–binding protein; IL-2, interleukin-2; PTH, parathyroid hormone; PTH-rp, PTH-related protein; RXR, retinoic acid receptor; VDR, vitamin D response element on nuclear DNA.

A third calcitropic hormone, **calcitonin**, is probably less important in calcium homeostasis. A 32–amino acid molecule, it is produced by the C cells of the thyroid gland. It has an anti-PTH effect, lowering serum calcium and phosphorus concentrations. At the level of the bone, calcitonin decreases resorption of calcium and phosphorus. It has calciuric and phosphaturic effects on the kidney. However, thyroidectomized patients have few disturbances of calcium metabolism, and relative excess or deficiency of circulating calcitonin has little effect on serum calcium concentrations.

Other hormones involved with calcium homeostasis include growth hormone and the insulin-like growth factors (somatomedins). Growth hormone influences renal handling of calcium and phosphorus through its effects on phosphorus reabsorption and 1,25(OH)$_2$-vitamin D production. It stimulates renal tubular reabsorption of phosphorus and thus decreases urinary phosphorus excretion.[11] Growth hormone also facilitates the normal compensatory increase in renal 1α-hydroxylase activity during phosphorus deprivation, promoting intestinal calcium and phosphorus absorption.[12] PTH-related protein (PTH-rp), a polypeptide distinct from PTH, shares a similar 13–amino acid sequence at the N-terminal end. Although associated with increased serum calcium levels in some patients with cancer, its function during healthy states has not yet been determined. It may play a role in the placental transfer of calcium.

Two other minerals are very important in calcium homeostasis: phosphorus and magnesium. One percent of the total body mineral is phosphorus, 70% to 80% of which is complexed with calcium in bone. Most of the remainder is intracellular, and 50% of this fraction is in energy storage compounds such as adenosine triphosphate. There are few direct regulatory mechanisms. PTH, which has the largest effect on serum phosphorus concentration, is responsive primarily to ionized calcium concentration, not to phosphorus. Phosphorus is freely filtrable in the kidney, and the renal tubule reabsorbs phosphorus in the proximal and distal nephrons. With low serum PTH concentrations, the renal tubule reabsorbs 95% to 97% of the filtered load of phosphorus. In states of high serum PTH concentration, reabsorption of phosphorus in proximal and distal tubules is inhibited, which results in excretion of a high concentration of urinary phosphorus.

Magnesium is the second most abundant intracellular cation after potassium. It is an important regulator of cell processes. Necessary for high-energy phosphate formation (adenosine triphosphate), it is therefore required for synthesis, growth, thermogenesis, and motility. It is also a cofactor in more than 300 enzyme systems. Of the total body magnesium, 60% is found in the skeleton in a slow turnover pool. Thirty-nine percent is distributed equally in the intracellular space between muscle and nonmuscular tissue, bound mainly to protein and the energy-rich phosphates. Only 1% to 2% is found extracellularly in a rapid turnover pool, of which one third is protein bound and two thirds is free and ionized in the circulation. This ionized fraction is available for biochemical processes as well as filtration by the kidney. As with calcium, serum concentrations are maintained within fairly narrow ranges; however, unlike calcium, there is no known homeostatic system regulating its concentration. Serum concentration is maintained largely independently of the known calcitropic hormones. Nevertheless, several hormones are influenced by magnesium. Mild magnesium deficiency increases release of PTH, and hypermagnesemia suppresses the synthesis and/or release of the hormone from the parathyroid glands and impairs its peripheral actions on bone, kidney, and intestinal tissue.[13,14] However, severe magnesium deficiency also inhibits the release of the hormone from the gland.[15] Magnesium is also required for the hepatic 25-hydroxylation of vitamin D. Thus, given the influence of magnesium on PTH secretion and vitamin D metabolism, hypomagnesemia is often complicated by hypocalcemia. In these circumstances, correction of magnesium deficiency is required before sustained correction of hypocalcemia can be achieved. Magnesium absorption occurs primarily in the small intestine independently of the transport mechanism for calcium.[16,17] The kidney is the primary excretory pathway for absorbed magnesium, and the steady-state concentration of magnesium is determined principally by the threshold for renal excretion. Only 3% to 5% of the filtered load is excreted in the urine, however.[18]

Maternal Placental Considerations

Calcium

With regard to calcium metabolism, a number of important changes occur during pregnancy. An early observation was the significant decline in total serum calcium concentration, which reaches a nadir during the middle of the third trimester, before rebounding slightly.[19] Ionized calcium decreases to a lesser extent, and this decrease may or may not be significant (Fig. 75-4).[20,21] The fall in total serum calcium concentration follows that of serum albumin concentration. This suggests that the decline in maternal calcium is secondary to the reduced

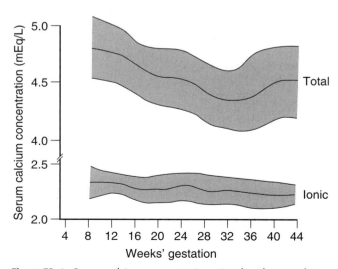

Figure 75–4. Serum calcium concentrations (total and ionic) during pregnancy. *(From Pitkin RM, Gebhardt MP: Am J Obstet Gynecol 127:775, 1977, with permission.)*

concentration of serum protein that occurs with the progressive increase in extracellular volume during pregnancy. On the other hand, calcium balance studies performed early during the second trimester have shown increased net calcium retention,[22] which implies increased intestinal absorption of calcium. This observation has been confirmed at 36 weeks of pregnancy through the stable calcium isotope technique.[23] Whether this net retention is secondary to a slight rise in maternal serum concentration of 1,25(OH)$_2$-vitamin D or to an increased intake of calcium remains an area of controversy.[24] The increase in urinary calcium excretion seen during pregnancy is probably the result of the increase in glomerular filtration rate that occurs.[25]

Calcitropic Hormones

With regard to the calcitropic hormones, it has been noted historically that pregnancy represents a benign state of "physiologic hyperparathyroidism."[26] In most studies, PTH peaked at term with concentrations from 50% to 100% above those of early pregnancy or the nonpregnant state.[19,26-28] However, no correlation was found between serum PTH and total serum calcium concentration. Most of these studies used PTH assays that measured inactive PTH fragments rather than the bioactive, intact molecule. With the advent of PTH assays specific for the intact molecule, a decline in serum PTH during pregnancy has been observed in nearly all subsequent reports (Fig. 75-5).[21,29-32] This information negates the previous concept that pregnancy is a state of physiologic hyperparathyroidism and supports the homeostasis of calcium during pregnancy. It also explains the lack of correlation between concentrations of PTH and calcium found in earlier studies. PTH does not appear to cross the placenta. Injection of radiolabeled PTH into the pregnant female of various animal species has not resulted in transfer to the fetus.[33,34]

The concentration of vitamin D (parent compound) does not change significantly during pregnancy. However, serum 25(OH)-vitamin D concentration, as in other clinical situations, is the best indicator of vitamin D status in the pregnant woman. It is also apparent that 25(OH)-vitamin D is the major form of vitamin D transported to the fetus across the placenta. Maternal concentrations of 25(OH)-vitamin D vary greatly, depending on differences in sunlight exposure and dietary intake. Thus, serum 25(OH)-vitamin D concentrations have been observed to be threefold higher in August than in February in pregnant women.[35] On the other hand, serum 1,25(OH)$_2$-vitamin D increases shortly after conception, with a significant rise occurring by 6 weeks after conception. This gradual increase continues throughout pregnancy,[36-38] and 1,25(OH)$_2$-vitamin D serum concentration at term is double that of nonpregnant women.[38,39] The increase in 1,25(OH)$_2$-vitamin D occurs long before a significant accrual of fetal calcium occurs. Because the maternal ionized calcium concentration changes little during pregnancy and the PTH concentration declines, the origin of this increase in 1,25(OH)$_2$-vitamin D is unclear and somewhat paradoxical.

The relationship of maternal and fetal 1,25(OH)$_2$-vitamin D is an area of controversy. In all studies to date, the maternal serum concentration of 1,25(OH)$_2$-vitamin D is significantly higher than the fetal concentration. In some studies, maternal and fetal concentrations are correlated,[24,40,41] whereas in others they are not.[39,42,43] Although maternal pharmacologic doses of 1,25(OH)$_2$-vitamin D can be shown to cross the placenta in humans, it is likely that fetal 1,25(OH)$_2$-vitamin D is of fetal origin.[44] This situation is complicated by the knowledge that human placental tissue can synthesize 1,25(OH)$_2$-vitamin D, which may be important in placental calcium transport.[45] The role of 1,25(OH)$_2$-vitamin D in placental calcium transport may vary in different species.

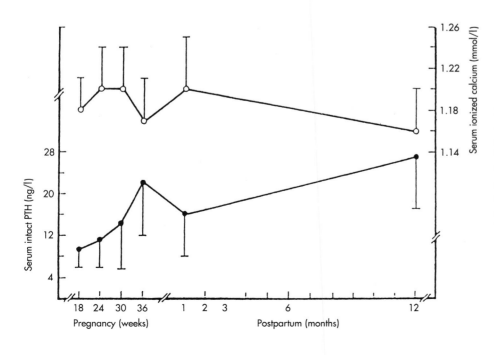

Figure 75–5. Serum parathyroid hormone concentration (intact molecule) and serum ionized calcium concentration during pregnancy. PTH, parathyroid hormone. *(From Rasmussen N, Frolich A. Hornnes PJ, et al: Serum ionized calcium and intact parathyroid hormone levels during pregnancy and postpartum. Br J Obstet Gynaecol 97:857, 1990, with permission.)*

For example, in the pregnant ewe, nephrectomy of the fetus eliminates the transplacental calcium gradient and decreases levels of fetal 1,25(OH)$_2$-vitamin D and fetal plasma calcium. Administering 1,25(OH)$_2$-vitamin D to the nephrectomized fetus restores plasma calcium concentrations.[46] On the other hand, in a vitamin D–deficient rat model, the absence of maternal and fetal 1,25(OH)$_2$-vitamin D had little effect on fetal calcium content.[47] Other investigators have reported a significant decline in maternal and fetal calcium levels when maternal 1,25(OH)$_2$-vitamin D deficiency was induced by parathyroidectomy in the sheep.[48] In this study, restoring maternal calcium concentrations alone (by intravenous calcium infusion) normalized fetal calcium levels, which suggested that 1,25(OH)$_2$-vitamin D was not essential for transfer of calcium across the placenta. In another report on pregnant rats,[49] in utero fetal decapitation, resulting in hypoparathyroidism, led to a fall in clearance of calcium across the rat placenta. The calcium flux across the placenta was partially restored with fetal subcutaneous injections of both PTH and 1,25(OH)$_2$-vitamin D. The exact mechanisms for calcitropic hormone facilitation of placental calcium transport are not known. Receptors for 1,25(OH)$_2$-vitamin D but not those for PTH and calcitonin have been found in the placenta.[50] Various reports have identified a protein from placental homogenates of a number of species that is immunologically similar to vitamin D–dependent calcium-binding protein. Concentrations of this protein rise during the latter weeks of gestation, when fetal skeletal mineralization peaks.[51] This placental calcium-binding protein is unlike that of intestinal calcium-binding protein, and its response to 1,25(OH)$_2$-vitamin D is not known.

Other reports have suggested that PTH-rp may play a role in calcium transport across the placenta. First described as a humoral factor associated with cancer, PTH-rp can induce hypercalcemia.[52] PTH-rp is chemically and immunologically distinct from PTH, although the molecule has been found to have striking homology with PTH at the amino-terminal region. That this homology is not maintained for the remainder of the molecule is strong evidence that it is a previously unrecognized hormone.[52] Although immunoreactive PTH levels are lower in the fetus than in the mother, bioactive PTH levels, which may equate with PTH-rp, are higher in the fetus than in the mother.[53,54] It has been suggested that this PTH-like peptide is an oncofetal peptide, similar to the hypercalcemic PTH-rp expressed by solid tumors.[54] A study of a perfused placenta from a thyroparathyroidectomized lamb demonstrated an abolition of the placental calcium gradient. Infusion of PTH into the placenta had no effect on the calcium gradient, but infusion of PTH-rp substantially restored the calcium gradient.[54] On the contrary, a report of the perfused rat placenta showed that infusion of human PTH-rp had no effect on the maternal-fetal transfer of calcium.[55]

In pregnancy, other hormonal influences on calcium metabolism have been implicated. Animal studies have demonstrated that in pregnant thyroparathyroidectomized rats, 1,25(OH)$_2$-vitamin D concentration increases equally in both experimental and control rats.

Levels of estrogen, growth hormone, human placental lactogen, and human chorionic gonadotropin increase during the first trimester.[38] Many of these hormones have been found to stimulate 1α-hydroxylase activity in animals.[56] Again in rats, prolactin, levels of which increase during early pregnancy, has been found (when given in pharmacologic doses) to increase intestinal calcium absorption and serum calcium concentration without altering serum 1,25(OH)$_2$-vitamin D concentration.[57]

Calcitonin may have a protective effect on the maternal skeleton during pregnancy. Although both cross-sectional and longitudinal studies have shown increased serum calcitonin concentrations during pregnancy, these increases have not been consistently significant.[31,58,59] One longitudinal study found no change in serum calcitonin during pregnancy.[21] On an individual basis, there are also marked variations among pregnant women. In nonhuman primates, there is increased calcitonin responsiveness to elevated serum calcium concentration during pregnancy.[60] Furthermore, in pregnant thyroidectomized rats, there is a decrease in bone density in relation to normal pregnant controls.[59,61] Calcitonin apparently does not cross the placenta.[62]

Although it plays no direct role in calcium metabolism, osteocalcin, a vitamin K–dependent protein of bone, is produced by osteoblasts and thus is reported to be a marker for new bone formation or bone turnover. Osteocalcin serum concentrations are generally low during pregnancy and lowest during midpregnancy.[21] They appear to be correlated with serum PTH concentrations, which may explain the fall in osteocalcin. PTH does not directly stimulate osteocalcin synthesis, but it does stimulate bone resorption, which would increase osteocalcin. 1,25(OH)$_2$-vitamin D, which stimulates the synthesis of osteocalcin by osteoblasts, is increased during pregnancy. The net effect of PTH and 1,25(OH)$_2$-vitamin D is the lowering of serum osteocalcin during pregnancy, which is evidence for reduced bone turnover during pregnancy.

Phosphorus

Serum phosphorus levels decline during pregnancy, attaining a nadir (13% less than in nonpregnant controls) between 29 and 32 weeks, before increasing slightly at term.[31] These changes are not related to the fall in PTH concentrations during pregnancy, which would be expected to decrease renal excretion of phosphorus. Because dietary phosphorus is plentiful, there is no obvious explanation other than ascribing it to the changes in maternal extracellular volume. Phosphorus does follow the same patterns as serum calcium and magnesium during pregnancy. Phosphorus concentration is higher in the fetus than in the mother; therefore, it is likely that phosphorus or phosphate is actively transported across the placenta. In vitro studies of transport across human placental microvillous membranes have shown that phosphate transport is reduced by PTH and is modulated by pH, temperature, sodium, and amino acid concentrations.[51,63,64]

Magnesium

As with calcium and phosphorus, serum magnesium concentration decreases during pregnancy, reaching a

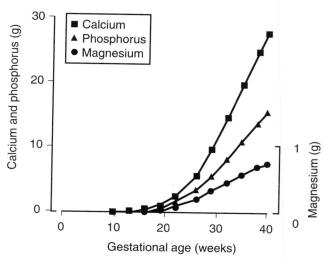

Figure 75–6. Calcium, phosphorus, and magnesium accretion in the human fetus from 16 to 40 weeks of gestation.

nadir during the third trimester before recovering slightly by the end of pregnancy.[31] Again, this fluctuation may result largely from the hemodilution that accompanies the increase in maternal plasma volume. The fetal magnesium concentration always exceeds that of the mother; therefore, it is presumed that the transport of magnesium across the placenta is an active process. As with most minerals, placental transfer of magnesium increases exponentially with the duration of pregnancy. There is no information on the regulation of placental transfer of magnesium. Treatment of mothers with magnesium sulfate for preeclampsia, however, results in both maternal and fetal hypermagnesemia.

Fetal and Newborn Considerations

Calcium

Fetal calcium accrues exponentially throughout pregnancy (Fig. 75-6). Of the 25 to 30 g of total body calcium at the time of birth, approximately two thirds is accumulated during the last trimester of pregnancy. The fetal serum calcium concentration is higher at every time in gestation than the maternal serum concentration. Thus, at the time of birth, the fetal total serum calcium concentration is approximately 11 mg/dL, with an ionized level of 6 mg/dL. At 24 hours after birth, the serum total calcium in the full-term newborn attains a nadir of 7.8 to 10.2 mg/dL, and the serum ionized calcium, 4.40 to 5.44 mg/dL (Fig. 75-7). This decline is expected because of the sharp decline in calcium intake (in comparison with the maternal transfer of calcium across the placenta) that occurs immediately after birth. The decline after birth is exaggerated in the premature infant. Thus, the normal range of total serum calcium during the first week after birth is 7.8 to 11.6 mg/dL in full-term infants and 6.0 to 11.0 mg/dL in premature infants.[65]

Calcium absorption in the newborn depends on many factors and undergoes a maturational process; calcium absorption increases with both gestational age and postnatal age.[66-68] During the early neonatal period, calcium absorption is intake dependent, which is consistent with passive absorption.[66,69] With increasing age, both preterm and full-term infants have increased calcium absorption with an absorption of up to 80%, indicative of a more active transport system. Using the calcium stable isotope technique, investigators found that the true calcium absorption rate in premature infants receiving various formulas and human milk ranged from 50.8% to 90.7% and that the endogenous fecal excretion ranged from 5.1 to 9.1 mg/kg/day. These values varied greatly with the type of feeding, and there were large individual variations within the various feeding groups.[70] These large variations point out the difficulties in coming to conclusions about calcium absorption in the neonate.

Urinary excretion of calcium in the newborn is related primarily to gestational age, serum calcium concentration, and glomerular filtration rate.[71] In comparison to full-term neonates, premature infants have a lower glomerular filtration rate but a decreased tubular reabsorption of

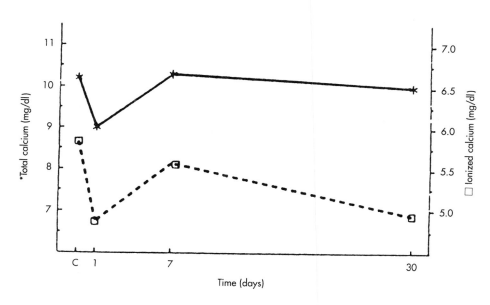

Figure 75–7. Serum total and ionized calcium concentrations in full-term infants over the first month after birth. *(From Loughead JL, Tsang RC: Neonatal mineral metabolism. In Cowett R [ed]: Principles of Perinatal-Neonatal Metabolism. New York, Springer-Verlag, 1992, p 475, with permission.)*

calcium. The net effect is that they have higher urinary calcium losses than do full-term infants. With increasing postmenstrual age, the glomerular filtration rate increases along with tubular reabsorption, leading to decreased levels of urinary calcium.[71]

Calcitropic Hormones

Human fetal parathyroid glands are functional by 12 weeks of gestation, although the relatively high fetal calcium concentrations suppress fetal parathyroid function. It is generally believed that PTH does not cross the placenta (Fig. 75-8). At birth, cord blood levels of PTH in comparison with maternal concentrations vary according to the type of assay used. In studies involving intact PTH molecule assays, PTH levels in cord blood have been found to be generally lower in both full-term and preterm infants than maternal or adult values[32,72]; this finding is not unexpected, in view of the higher serum calcium concentrations in the fetus. Through the use of a new, biologically active PTH molecule assay, however, PTH levels have been found to be higher in cord blood than in adult controls.[72] Nonetheless, with any of the assays for PTH, serum PTH levels in the newborn, whether full-term or preterm, have been found to be responsive to serum calcium concentration.[32,72-75] Thus, as serum calcium levels fall during the first 24 hours after birth, serum PTH concentration increases (Fig. 75-9). Furthermore, PTH concentrations increase to a greater degree in hypocalcemic premature infants than in full-term infants in response to the fall in serum calcium after birth.[32] In hypocalcemic preterm infants, exogenous PTH administration does not lead to a renal increase in cAMP during the first 72 hours after birth.[76,77] It has been suggested that this effect is secondary to a transient pseudohypoparathyroidism from immaturity of the renal and bone response to PTH.[32]

In humans, vitamin D (parent compound) and 25(OH)-vitamin D readily cross the placenta from mother to fetus, although the low maternal serum concentrations of the parent compound probably make its placental transfer insignificant (see Fig. 75-8).[40] Its presence in a relatively low concentration in cord serum (7% of maternal serum concentration) has been documented in pregnant women with a daily vitamin D intake as high as 100,000 IU.[78] Most human studies have shown that cord

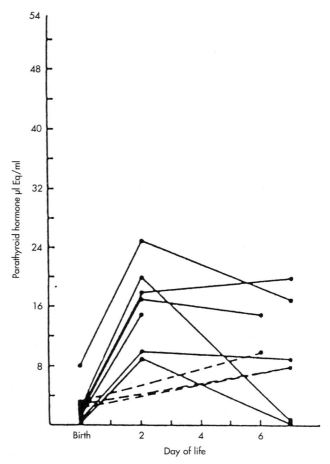

Figure 75–9. Serum parathyroid hormone concentrations in full term neonates in cord blood and at 48 and 72 hours after birth. Normal range in adults is 2 to 10 µL//Eq/mL. *(From Hillman LS, Rojanasathit S, Slatopolsky E, et al: Serial measurements of serum calcium, magnesium, parathyroid hormone, calcitonin, and 25-hydroxy-vitamin D in premature and term infants during the first week of life. Pediatr Res 11:739, 1977, with permission.)*

25(OH)-vitamin D is generally lower than maternal 25(OH)-vitamin D; a range of 68% to 108% of maternal concentration has been reported.[79-88] In these studies, there is generally a good correlation between maternal and cord serum concentrations. On the other hand, the maternal-fetal relationship of 1,25(OH)$_2$-vitamin D in humans is less clear. This confusion is partially caused by the various potential sources of 1,25(OH)$_2$-vitamin D, including fetal renal synthesis, maternal renal synthesis, and synthesis by the placenta. 1,25(OH)$_2$-vitamin D synthesized by the maternal kidneys from 25(OH)-vitamin D does not appear to cross the placenta from mother to fetus in rats[89,90] or cows,[91] although it is likely to occur in sheep[92] and nonhuman primates.[93] In humans, it has been demonstrated in pregnant women receiving large oral doses of 1,25(OH)$_2$-vitamin D that it does cross the placenta.[44,94] Furthermore, transfer of 1,25(OH)$_2$-vitamin D has been demonstrated in the perfused human placenta in vitro.[95] Cord blood concentration of 1,25(OH)$_2$-vitamin

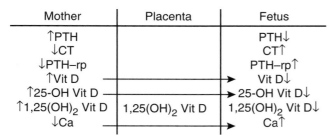

Mother	Placenta	Fetus
↑PTH		PTH↓
↓CT		CT↑
↓PTH–rp		PTH–rp↑
↑Vit D	——————→	Vit D↓
↑25-OH Vit D	——————→	25-OH Vit D↓
↑1,25(OH)$_2$ Vit D	1,25(OH)$_2$ Vit D	1,25(OH)$_2$ Vit D↓
↓Ca	——————→	Ca↑

Figure 75–8. The maternal-placental-fetal relationships of calcitropic hormones. *Arrows* represent comparison concentrations in mother and fetus. The placenta probably synthesizes its own supply of 1,25-(OH)$_2$-vitamin D. Ca, calcium; CT, calcitonin; PTH, parathyroid hormone; PTH-rp, PTH-related peptide.

D is generally lower than the maternal concentration, and most studies have found negative[39,43,96] rather than positive correlations.[82] All evidence considered, $1,25(OH)_2$-vitamin D probably does not cross the placenta in significant quantities (see Fig. 75-8).

The importance of the fetal kidneys in $1,25(OH)_2$-vitamin D synthesis in vivo remains a question. In the pregnant rat, maternal nephrectomy does not prevent $1,25(OH)_2$-vitamin D synthesis from labeled $25(OH)$-vitamin D, and labeled $1,25(OH)_2$-vitamin D is found in both the maternal and fetal sides of the placenta.[97-100] A paucity of labeled material in the fetal rat kidney indicates that the fetal kidney is not the primary site of $1,25(OH)_2$-vitamin D synthesis in the rat.[97] In the human neonate, there is preliminary evidence that $1,25(OH)_2$-vitamin D is decreased in neonates with renal agenesis.[101] Simultaneous measurement of umbilical venous and arterial samples of cord blood has shown mixed results. Two studies found that fetal umbilical arterial concentration of $1,25(OH)_2$-vitamin D was significantly higher than the umbilical venous concentration, which was suggestive of fetal renal production.[41,102] A third study failed to confirm these results.[24] At present, available evidence suggests that an extrarenal site of $1,25(OH)_2$-vitamin D synthesis exists, in all likelihood, in the placenta.

It is presumed that in the human neonate, the major vitamin D source during the immediate postnatal period is placental transfer of maternal vitamin D metabolites during pregnancy. In the breast-fed neonate without supplemental vitamin D, the vitamin D transferred across the placenta remains the major source of vitamin D throughout the neonatal period, because the vitamin D content of human milk is low (<20 IU/L). For the formula-fed neonate, vitamin D intestinal absorption could be a significant source, because formulas in the United States generally contain a minimum of 400 IU/L. In the neonatal rat, it has been shown that the primary neonatal source of vitamin D is the direct transfer across the placenta to the fetus.[103] In this study, vitamin D–deficient female rats were given labeled vitamin D before mating. During pregnancy, there was a linear increase in total fetal $25(OH)$-vitamin D and vitamin D itself between days 14 and 19 of gestation (length of gestation is 21 days). The vitamin D present in the fetus was predominantly $25(OH)$-vitamin D (54%); the concentration was highest in fetal rat muscle, which reflects low body fat content of the rat pup. During the 3-week suckling period, the stored vitamin D accumulated in utero remained the primary determinant of vitamin D status in the pup, despite relatively high concentrations of vitamin D in the rat milk (40 to 140 IU/L). This was true despite a gradual decline in the total vitamin D content during the first 3 weeks after birth. These data suggest that the vitamin D stores accumulated in the fetal muscle in utero are readily available to the rat pups after birth. Although no similar data exist for humans, it is apparent from a number of clinical studies in Asian immigrants to Great Britain that the neonatal vitamin D status is highly dependent on maternal status.[104]

In human full-term neonates, within 24 hours of delivery there is an increase in serum $1,25(OH)_2$-vitamin D[39,105] that persists through the first 5 days after birth.[105,106]

In one report, serum $1,25(OH)_2$-vitamin D concentration was documented to decrease from days 5 to 30 (100 ± 5 [standard error of the mean] versus 61 ± 4 pg/mL). In the premature neonate (aged <33 weeks of gestation), an increase in $1,25(OH)_2$-vitamin D occurs between birth and 24 hours and continues through day 5.[105] In contrast to full-term neonates, however, $1,25(OH)_2$-vitamin D in premature infants remains high for the first 7 to 9 weeks after birth,[107,108] and by day 30 it is significantly higher than in full-term neonates (108 ± 3 versus 61 ± 4 pg/mL). These statistics may reflect the relative increased need for calcium in the premature neonate during this period of rapid postnatal growth.

Contrary to serum $1,25(OH)_2$-vitamin D concentration, serum $25(OH)$-vitamin D concentration shows no significant change during either the first 24 hours[39,105] or the first week after birth in full-term and preterm neonates.[105] There is no significant correlation between serum $25(OH)$-vitamin D and $1,25(OH)_2$-vitamin D concentration during this period.[29,107,109] In premature and full-term neonates, 1α-hydroxylation of $25(OH)$-vitamin D begins to occur shortly after birth, indicative of the presence of renal 1α-hydroxylase during the immediate postnatal period. This finding refutes earlier observations that suggested that 1α-hydroxylation of $25(OH)$-vitamin D was delayed in preterm neonates.[110]

This rise in serum $1,25(OH)_2$-vitamin D concentration during the immediate postnatal period in full-term and preterm neonates parallels a decrease in serum calcium concentration and a rise in serum PTH concentration. This finding suggests that the increase in $1,25(OH)_2$-vitamin D concentration in response to decreasing serum ionized calcium concentration is mediated by PTH itself. In fact, the rise in serum PTH can be blunted with an infusion of intravenous calcium in the preterm infant.[111-113]

It is of interest that hypocalcemia persists in neonates with very low birth weight (VLBW) (aged <32 weeks of gestation) despite the increase in serum PTH and $1,25(OH)_2$-vitamin D. Even pharmacologic, intramuscular doses of $1,25(OH)_2$-vitamin D (up to 3.0 µg/kg) do not affect the hypocalcemia in this group, which may be explained, in part, by the fact that most of these neonates are not receiving oral feedings, and therefore $1,25(OH)_2$-vitamin D cannot increase intestinal calcium absorption.[114] It would not explain why calcium is not mobilized effectively from bone in the presence of falling serum calcium, rising PTH, and rising $1,25(OH)_2$-vitamin D concentrations, however. These observations suggest that $1,25(OH)_2$-vitamin D receptors in bone and possibly intestine are not developed in the VLBW infant or at least are somewhat resistant to $1,25(OH)_2$-vitamin D.

Existing animal data support the hypothesis that the functional status of $1,25(OH)_2$-vitamin D receptors may account for the hypocalcemia of prematurity. The rat gut is relatively immature at the time of birth, so it may be comparable with the gut of the human premature neonate. In neonatal suckling rats (who have a higher intake per kilogram of calcium than does the human neonate), it can be shown that the intestinal absorption of calcium after an injection of $1,25(OH)_2$-vitamin D does not increase until the time of weaning (age 3 weeks).[115]

1,25(OH)$_2$-vitamin D receptors have been found to be present in low concentration in the intestine of the suckling rat at 7 and 14 days after birth, but they increase in number at the time of weaning.[116] It is of interest that intestinal calcium-binding protein concentration and activity are relatively low in the suckling rat during the first 2 weeks after birth.[117]

Little is known about the effects of vitamin D or its metabolites on the neonatal kidney. Older infants readily retain minerals such as calcium and phosphorus under conditions of increased needs, although almost all of the filtered calcium in the kidney is reabsorbed even in the absence of vitamin D. Further data on the function of intestinal, as well as bone and renal, receptors for 1,25(OH)$_2$-vitamin D in the human neonate would be of great interest.

Calcitonin concentration in cord blood of the neonate is elevated in relation to the maternal concentration, as well as the nonpregnant maternal state. Cord blood calcitonin concentration also decreases with increasing gestational age. Neonates younger than 32 weeks of gestation have nearly three times the cord blood concentration of full-term neonates.[118] In both preterm and full-term neonates, calcitonin concentration increases after birth, with a peak at 24 to 48 hours of age, followed by a decline to childhood values by the age of 1 month.[118-122] The physiologic importance of this increase in serum calcitonin concentration is unclear. Theoretically, it may be advantageous for infants by protecting the skeleton from excessive bone resorption. It does not appear to play a role in early neonatal hypocalcemia.

Phosphorus

The concentration of phosphorus in the fetus always exceeds that in the mother, which is indicative of active transport of phosphorus or phosphate across the placenta. Phosphorus accumulation in the fetus is similar to that of calcium; most of the accumulation occurs during the third trimester of pregnancy (see Fig. 75-6). At the time of birth, although it is higher than the maternal concentration, it is relatively low in comparison with that of older neonates. Thus, in cord blood, the phosphorus concentration ranges from 3.7 to 8.1 mg/dL (mean = 6.2 mg/dL), in comparison with a concentration of 8.1 mg/dL at 1 week of age in an infant with a reasonable phosphorus intake. The relatively low concentration initially begins to rise shortly after birth and continues to rise throughout the first month after birth. The acute rise after birth occurs for reasons that are not well understood. Intake is limited at this point, so dietary intake seems to play little role. The lack of oral intake may stimulate gluconeogenesis from glycogen, which would release phosphate.[123] It may also be explained by the decreased glomerular filtration rate and thus the decreased phosphate excretion in the newborn. In a few studies, the phosphaturic responsiveness of the kidney to exogenous PTH appears less during the first day after birth than given on day 3 after birth with the same dose.[76,124] Serum phosphorus concentration remains high even after urinary phosphorus excretion increases; therefore, other influences obviously play a role. The intestinal absorption efficiency of phosphorus in both preterm and full-term infants is high. Absorption of phosphorus has been measured to be 86% to 97% regardless of phosphorus or calcium intakes.[66] In the newborn, phosphorus retention is influenced by calcium retention. With increased calcium intake (enteral or parenteral), there is increased phosphorus retention secondary to the shared roles that calcium and phosphorus play in bone mineralization.

Magnesium

Like calcium and phosphorus, magnesium is accumulated by the fetus primarily during the third trimester (see Fig. 75-6). Plasma concentrations of total and ultrafiltrable magnesium in the fetus exceed those of the mother toward the end of pregnancy,[43] which implies active transport across the placenta. The level in the preterm infant equals that of the full-term infant by the eighth month of gestation, with a mean of 1.95 mg/dL and a range of 1.43 to 2.45 mg/dL.[125] The concentration decreases during the first 48 hours after birth, reaching a nadir of 1.87 mg/dL.[125] Subsequently, serum magnesium concentrations increase during the first week after birth, followed by a gradual decline, reaching childhood values by the end of the first month after birth.[126] The kidney is the primary excretory pathway for absorbed magnesium, and the steady-state concentration of magnesium is determined principally by the threshold for renal excretion. The changes in serum magnesium concentration are probably related to the changes of glomerular filtration rate during the first weeks after birth, because the lower glomerular filtration rates of the newborn are associated with decreased magnesium excretion. Preterm infants have lower excretion rates of magnesium than do full-term infants.

Magnesium absorption occurs primarily in the terminal ileum of the small intestine, although absorption from other portions of the small intestine is possible.[17] Calcium and magnesium do not share the same transport mechanism.[16] Endogenous excretion of magnesium is very low.

Neonatal hypomagnesemia is defined as a serum concentration of less than 1.6 mg/dL. It is frequently associated with hypocalcemia, and this relationship between the two minerals is an ongoing area of research. Magnesium is necessary for the secretion and function of PTH, and this may affect the neonate's PTH response to a falling serum calcium concentration. Hypermagnesemia (serum magnesium level > 2.8 mg/dL) is most commonly seen after magnesium therapy in pregnant women during labor.

MATERNAL DISEASES AND PERINATAL DISORDERS AFFECTING THE FETUS AND NEWBORN

Maternal Parathyroid Disorders

Disorders of the parathyroid gland are uncommon in pregnancy. Both hyperparathyroidism and hypoparathyroidism have the potential to affect fetal and neonatal calcium metabolism. Fewer than 100 cases of hyperparathyroidism during pregnancy have been reported in the literature.[127]

Maternal hyperparathyroidism, if inadequately controlled, can be associated with neonatal hypocalcemia (tetany) from suppression of the fetal parathyroid gland by persistent maternal hypercalcemia and fetal hypercalcemia. Stillbirths and abortions have occurred in 20% to 30% of the reported cases.[127] Diagnosis is established in these infants by confirming the hyperparathyroid state of the mother. It is generally agreed that in all cases in which maternal symptomatic hypercalcemia develops, parathyroid surgery in the second trimester is the treatment of choice.[127-130]

Maternal hypoparathyroidism can be idiopathic or, more likely, a complication of surgery for maternal hyperparathyroidism or hyperthyroidism. In the untreated state, infants born to such mothers have been reported to have generalized skeletal demineralization, elevated serum PTH levels, and parathyroid hyperplasia from presumed fetal hyperparathyroidism.[131] The standard treatment for maternal hypoparathyroidism is now pharmacologic doses of calcitriol (1,25[OH]$_2$-vitamin D) with minimal effects on the newborn.[94,132] However, neonatal hypercalcemia resulting from large maternal doses of vitamin D has been reported in a breast-fed infant.[78]

Transient neonatal hyperparathyroidism from untreated maternal pseudohypoparathyroidism has been described.[133] The infant weighed 2.8 kg at birth and had osteopenia with multiple fractures of the ribs and long bones. Serum calcium, albumin, and calcitonin concentrations were normal. The serum phosphate level was slightly decreased, the 25(OH)-vitamin D level was depressed, and the PTH and alkaline phosphatase levels were elevated. The mother was hypocalcemic with the phenotypic and biochemical features of pseudohypoparathyroidism. The infant's disease resolved spontaneously.

Diabetes Mellitus

Neonatal hypocalcemia occurs in about 50% of infants born to mothers with diabetes mellitus. Severity of hypocalcemia increases with increasing severity of maternal diabetes. It occurs earlier and persists longer than the hypocalcemia associated with prematurity. No abnormality in vitamin D metabolism has been observed in infants of diabetic mothers, but suggested causes include hypoparathyroidism, hyperphosphatemia, hypomagnesemia, and hypercalcitonemia.[119,134-139] Low levels of PTH and magnesium have been found in cord blood of such infants. After birth, PTH concentrations rise appropriately in infants of diabetic mothers, however, in response to the neonatal hypocalcemia. Calcitonin levels in these infants are probably not different from those of premature infants, and they increase after birth. Strict management of maternal diabetes can decrease the incidence of hypocalcemia in their infants during gestation.

Birth Asphyxia

Birth asphyxia (Apgar score of 6 or less at 1 minute) has been associated with hypocalcemia.[140] This effect is independent of gestational age. Proposed causes include bicarbonate therapy, phosphate loads, and functional hypoparathyroidism. Correction of acidosis with alkali may induce a decrease in the flux of calcium from bone to the extracellular space. In these infants, a phosphate load and an increase in serum phosphate may be secondary to the breakdown of protein and glycogen. Asphyxiated infants have been found to have normocalcemic responses to PTH infusion, however, which suggests that a transient deficiency of PTH production may occur in these infants. In any event, the hypocalcemia is transitory, and the calcium levels in asphyxiated infants are no different from those in controls by 48 hours.[140]

FETAL AND NEWBORN DISORDERS OF CALCIUM HOMEOSTASIS

Early Hypocalcemia of Prematurity

The early hypocalcemia of prematurity (EHP) is a common problem. Of all premature infants, 30% to 57%[141,142] exhibit this disorder of calcium metabolism, which, by definition, is a serum calcium level below 7.0 mg% (1.75 mmol/L) or an ionized calcium level less than 3.5 mg% (0.9 mmol/L). Serum calcium level in the first few days after birth correlates directly with gestational age[142]; the less mature infants have an increased incidence of hypocalcemia. Gestational age is more important than birth weight because infants who are small for gestational age are not at risk for hypocalcemia, unless they are premature. Most of the decrease in serum calcium occurs in the first 72 hours with a slow recovery by 7 to 10 days if not treated.[143] Suggested causes of this disorder have included decreased calcium intake,[144] hypomagnesemia,[73] increased urinary losses,[142] hyperphosphatemia,[142] vitamin D deficiency,[145] abnormalities in vitamin D metabolism,[35,145-147] hypercalcitonemia,[120] alkali therapy,[148] functional hypoparathyroidism,[73,75,142] and endorgan unresponsiveness to PTH.[73-75,142,145,147,149] Typically, the hypocalcemia is asymptomatic.

Treatment with Calcium

Considering the frequency of the problem, there are relatively few studies on the treatment of EHP in premature infants. It has been common practice to maintain serum calcium with either oral supplements or parenteral infusions of calcium; however, the efficacy of this "traditional" therapy has not been demonstrated, and it remains controversial. Oral supplements of calcium (75 to 150 mg/kg/day) can prevent the hypocalcemia in infants with low birth weight.[144,150] Likewise, bolus or continuous parenteral infusions of calcium (25 to 35 mg/kg/day) have been demonstrated to prevent hypocalcemia.[121,143,151,152] Recommended dosages range from 24 to 75 mg/kg/day. The efficacy of calcium infusion to prevent hypocalcemia in premature infants has been questioned, because serum calcium concentrations of treated infants were not different from those of untreated control infants on the third day after birth or 25 hours after calcium therapy was discontinued.[143] Unfortunately, this study was seriously biased by the removal of 5 of 13 premature infants from the untreated group before completion of the study, because of treatment failure (hypocalcemia). Another investigation has also pointed out the transient elevation of serum total and ionized calcium after single-bolus therapy (18 mg/kg) in hypocalcemic infants.[153] It is difficult to determine the exact rates of morbidity and mortality from hypocalcemia in these infants because of other complicating clinical variables that usually occur in the infants with the lowest serum calcium levels (for example, respiratory distress syndrome, birth asphyxia, seizures, hypotension, and metabolic acidosis). It is reasonable to hypothesize that low serum calcium levels would have an adverse effect on premature infants because calcium is essential to the functioning of all living cells. Adverse effects of hypocalcemia in the newborn (other than tetany), however, have been infrequently reported. A single study described heart failure in six newborns with hypocalcemia, although only one of these infants was premature.[154] A report has also associated hypocalcemia with patent ductus arteriosus in premature infants.[155] On the other hand, benefits from calcium therapy other than elevation of serum calcium level have not been well documented. One group of investigators has shown that an infusion of a single calcium bolus (18 mg/kg) improves cardiovascular function (increased heart rate, increased blood pressure, improved left ventricular function) in premature infants with hypocalcemia (total serum calcium = 5.9 ± 0.05 mg/dL).[156,157] A subsequent study, however, did not confirm these results.[158]

Calcium therapy for EHP does not take into consideration the premature infant's own physiologic response. Such therapy may block the normal physiologic adaptation to hypocalcemia. It has been shown than an increase in PTH concentration on the first day after birth can be blunted in premature infants who receive an intravenous infusion of 18 to 70 mg/kg of calcium.[121,158] There are also a number of reports on the hazards of calcium therapy in the newborn. Oral calcium supplements have been associated with an increased incidence of necrotizing enterocolitis[159] and increased stool frequency.[144] Parenteral infusions of calcium have produced intestinal necrosis in animals,[160] as well as inflammation and subcutaneous deposition of calcium with scalp necrosis in the premature infant. Attempts to increase the calcium concentration of hyperalimentation fluid for premature infants have frequently resulted in precipitation of calcium phosphate crystals in hyperalimentation catheters.[161,162]

Treatment with Vitamin D Metabolites

After reports of vitamin D deficiency[145] and possible defects in vitamin D metabolism in hypocalcemic premature infants,[86,163] as well as successful treatment of infants with protracted hypocalcemia with $1,25(OH)_2$-vitamin D,[164] numerous investigators have attempted to treat or prevent EHP with supplements of vitamin D or its metabolites. These attempts have produced mixed results. In one study, 2 µg/kg/day of oral 25(OH)-vitamin D given during the first 5 days after birth prevented hypocalcemia in seven of eight premature infants (birth weight = 1445 ± 281 g).[147] Others found that oral supplements of 1 µg of $1,25(OH)_2$-vitamin D per day (but not a smaller dose), given for the first 3 days after birth to eight premature infants aged 37 weeks of gestation or younger, resulted in higher serum calcium and lower PTH concentrations than were present in controls.[146] In another study, oral $1,25(OH)_2$-vitamin D, given at a dose of 0.1 µg/kg/day to 14 early hypocalcemic premature infants (birth weights = 1350 to 2200 g) receiving oral feedings, resulted in a significant increase in serum calcium level in comparison with a control group, after only 48 hours of therapy.[165] Because the infants in all three of these studies were receiving oral feedings of formula, it could be postulated that the supplements of vitamin D metabolites resulted in increased intestinal absorption of calcium, although increased mobilization of calcium from bone was not ruled out.

In contrast, other studies have shown no effect of vitamin D or its metabolites on the hypocalcemia of prematurity. In one of these, investigators were unable to prevent hypocalcemia in premature infants (birth weight = 2128 ± 169 g) by giving daily oral supplements of 1200 IU of vitamin D, 10 µg of 25(OH)-vitamin D, or 0.5 µg of $1,25(OH)_2$-vitamin D for the first 5 days after birth.[166] This study had no control group, but 25(OH)-vitamin D concentrations were significantly increased over baseline values in infants receiving supplements of vitamin D or 25(OH)-vitamin D. All infants were started on feedings of human milk on the first day after birth. Although the amount of 25(OH)-vitamin D used was greater than that administered by Fleischman and associates,[147] no increase in serum calcium concentration occurred. The dosage of $1,25(OH)_2$-vitamin D administered was only half that given by Chan and coworkers,[146] but it was considerably higher than the dose given by Lin and Ishida.[165] Likewise, in a study of 19 infants with low birth weight (1500 g) younger than 33 weeks of gestation without oral feedings, Venkataraman and colleagues found that hypocalcemia did not respond to large pharmacologic doses of $1,25(OH)_2$-vitamin D (0.05 to 3 µg/kg) given intramuscularly on three occasions between 6 and 60 hours after birth.[114] In these infants, no changes in PTH serum concentrations were observed during therapy.

1α-hydroxyvitamin D (1α-OHD) has also been used to treat EHP. Barak and associates demonstrated a significant rise in serum calcium concentration in hypocalcemic premature infants (birth weight = 1947 ± 613 g) treated orally with 33 µg of 1α-OHD twice daily for 5 days.[167] These infants were receiving oral feedings. Petersen and coworkers,[168] however, using a smaller dose of 1α-OHD (0.05 to 0.10 µg/kg/day) for the first 5 days after birth, observed no effect on serum calcium concentration in infants with low birth weight (1940 ± 319 g).

From these studies, it is not clear whether the hypocalcemia of prematurity is responsive to or can be prevented by vitamin D and its metabolites. In most of the studies, pharmacologic rather than physiologic dosages were used. Thus, the preterm newborn with hypocalcemia has inappropriately low PTH and elevated serum calcitonin levels and is not particularly responsive to vitamin D or its metabolites. It is possible that calcium is not resorbed from bone and that this nonresorption is secondary to hypercalcitonemia and the absence of $1,25(OH)_2$-vitamin D receptors in bone. Absence of these receptors in the intestine as well may confound the problem. Further information on the effect of $1,25(OH)_2$-vitamin D on bone, intestine, and the kidney in the preterm infant is necessary. The role of PTH in the premature infant also merits further study, although it appears to increase in the presence of hypocalcemia in most reports and can be blunted by calcium infusions.

Neonatal Parathyroid Disorders

The effects of maternal parathyroid disease on neonatal calcium metabolism have been discussed previously. As in adults, parathyroid disease in infants is associated with both hypocalcemia and hypercalcemia. These disorders are relatively rare, however.

Hypoparathyroidism in the newborn may be transient or permanent. The term **transient congenital hypoparathyroidism** is applied to a condition of transient PTH deficiency that resembles EHP. Hypocalcemia, hyperphosphatemia, and target organ unresponsiveness to PTH are present. The disease resolves spontaneously after a few days or a few weeks and may represent unusually prolonged cases of EHP.

In patients with variable microdeletions of the short arm of chromosome 22, hypocalcemia is a frequent complication.[169,170] Most cases of DiGeorge syndrome are associated with a microdeletion of chromosome 22q11.2, this region of the chromosome being referred to as the DiGeorge syndrome chromosome region.[171] DiGeorge syndrome reflects congenital absence of the thymus and congenital absence or hypoplasia of the parathyroid glands. It manifests with tetany in the neonatal period and is also associated with immunologic deficiencies associated with absence of the thymus. Cardiac malformations of the outflow tract are common. Two other syndromes associated with the DiGeorge syndrome chromosome region of chromosome 22 manifest with hypocalcemia of the newborn: velocardiofacial syndrome and conotruncal anomaly face syndrome.[171] The velocardiofacial syndrome is also associated with cleft palate, cardiac anomalies, typical facies, and learning disabilities. Conotruncal anomaly face syndrome is associated with facial anomalies, mild mental retardation, and defects of the cardiac outflow tract.

On occasion, infantile hypocalcemia results from familial hypoparathyroidism and is usually inherited as an X-linked recessive trait and therefore affects predominantly boys in the first months after birth. Autosomal dominant and autosomal recessive modes of inheritance have also been observed. Pseudohypoparathyroidism or target organ unresponsiveness to PTH is not usually diagnosed in the neonatal period, because it takes many months for the obvious somatic features to develop.

Primary hyperparathyroidism in infancy (diagnosed before 3 months of age) is extremely rare; approximately 30 cases have been reported in the literature.[172] In most cases it manifests within a few days of birth, and 100% of the reported infants have had hyperplasia of all four parathyroid glands. Predominant symptoms include hypotonicity, respiratory distress, failure to thrive, constipation, anorexia, irritability, lethargy, and polyuria. Radiographs demonstrate pathognomonic findings of osteoporosis, subperiosteal bone resorption, and pathologic fractures. Fifty percent of the patients have a family history of the disease. Serum calcium levels can be as high as 25 mg/dL. The differential diagnosis includes

maternal hypoparathyroidism and other causes of neonatal hypercalcemia. Medical therapy is unsatisfactory, and without surgical intervention most affected infants die. Subtotal parathyroidectomy is also generally unsatisfactory. Good results have been reported in a newborn (aged 11 days) treated with a total parathyroidectomy with parathyroid autotransplantation.[172]

There is an increased incidence of neonatal hyperparathyroidism in kindreds who have familial hypocalciuric hypercalcemia (FHH), an autosomal dominant trait associated with asymptomatic mild hypercalcemia. In this disorder, circulating PTH levels are either normal or modestly elevated and relative hypocalciuria occurs, rather than the hypercalciuria seen with primary hyperparathyroidism. It is of interest that some patients treated successfully for neonatal hyperparathyroidism have subsequently developed FHH. It is now believed that both severe infantile hyperparathyroidism and FHH are defects of the calcium-sensitive receptor. These inherited disorders of the calcium-sensitive receptor gene are located on chromosome 3p13.3-21. Heterozygous loss-of-function mutations give rise to FHH in which the lifelong hypercalcemia is asymptomatic. The homozygous condition, in contrast, leads to a form of neonatal severe hyperparathyroidism with severe hypercalcemia and hypercalciuria.[173]

Late Infantile Tetany

Late infantile tetany is a term usually reserved for hypocalcemia associated with cow's milk feeding and linked to the relatively high phosphate load of such feedings. In this disorder, it has been proposed that the phosphate load leads to hyperphosphatemia, hypocalcemia, and elevated serum PTH concentrations.[174] It may also be associated with the decreased renal clearance of phosphate that occurs in the newborn.

Miscellaneous Causes of Hypocalcemia in the Newborn

Acid-base disturbances have been associated with hypocalcemia, including exchange transfusions with citrated red blood cells.[151] Likewise, the use of alkali therapy in newborns with pulmonary hypertension may be accompanied by acute hypocalcemia. Even hyperventilation with mechanical ventilation, producing a respiratory alkalosis, may induce hypocalcemia.

Phototherapy for hyperbilirubinemia has been documented to increase the degree of hypocalcemia in premature infants.[175] Phototherapy decreases melatonin secretion in the rat, and it has been postulated that phototherapy with transillumination of the pineal gland inhibits melatonin synthesis. Hypocalcemia might then theoretically ensue when bone calcium uptake is increased by the action of endogenous steroids, normally opposed by the action of melatonin.[176]

Hypocalcemia is associated with hypomagnesemia in the newborn because of inhibition of PTH action and secretion. Hypomagnesemia may be transient or chronic in the neonatal period. The transient disorder usually is associated with serum magnesium levels of 0.8 to 1.4 mg/dL and responds to a short course of magnesium or calcium therapy.[73,177,178] Its cause is unknown. Chronic congenital hypomagnesemia with secondary hypocalcemia is a relatively rare disease. It is secondary to an isolated defect in the intestinal transport of magnesium,[179] and the serum magnesium level is frequently less than 0.8 mg/dL (normal = 1.6 to 2.8 mg/dL). Circulating PTH is low in these patients. Magnesium therapy restores serum calcium, magnesium, and PTH concentrations, but such therapy must be continuous.

Iatrogenic errors with total parenteral nutrition (TPN) therapy have been associated with hypocalcemia. In these clinical situations, excess phosphate (relative to calcium) has been inadvertently placed in TPN solutions.[180]

Idiopathic Infantile Hypercalcemia

Idiopathic infantile hypercalcemia (IIH) is a disorder of unknown origin in which hypercalcemia is associated with failure to thrive. A wide spectrum of clinical findings has been observed, and this disorder is usually classified into the mild and severe forms. The severe form is known as **Williams syndrome.** The phenotype and minimum diagnostic criteria for Williams syndrome are still being debated.[181] It is important to note that intermediate forms of IIH exist, and it is often difficult to classify the disease in a given patient as the mild or severe form.

Mild Idiopathic Infantile Hypercalcemia

In this form, there are normal facial features, transient hypercalcemia, osteosclerosis, and the clinical stigmata of hypercalcemia, including anorexia, vomiting, constipation, polydipsia, and polyuria. Failure to thrive eventually develops. These infants also have impaired renal function. Mild IIH usually manifests by 6 months of age. The prognosis is good once the hypercalcemic stage resolves, and the intelligence in these patients is usually normal.

Although the disorder is uncommon in the United States, a large number of affected patients were reported in Great Britain during and shortly after World War II. During this period it was recommended to supplement cow's milk with 1800 to 2000 IU of vitamin D to compensate for the wartime deprivation in British children.[182,183] Actually, even more vitamin D was added, a phenomenon known in the trade as "overage," because manufacturers were trying to anticipate vitamin D breakdown during shelf storage. Ultimately, these infants were receiving 3000 to 4000 IU per day of vitamin D, and a return to intakes of 400 IU per day dramatically decreased the incidence of this disorder in Great Britain. These data are usually cited to implicate vitamin D in the origin of IIH. In addition, through reliable bioassay methods, the serum concentration of vitamin D–like or antirachitic activity was elevated in some patients with IIH,[182,184] which indicated either abnormal absorption or metabolism of this vitamin. With modern assay methods, however, only one such report measuring vitamin D metabolites has been published. Aarskog and colleagues found that 25(OH)-vitamin D values were normal in a 9-month-old child with mild IIH.[185] This patient was monitored for 18 months and had suppression of 1,25(OH)$_2$-vitamin D synthesis and urinary cAMP, as would be expected in

hypercalcemia. Thus, a direct causal relationship between vitamin D and IIH has not been proved.[182]

Severe Idiopathic Infantile Hypercalcemia (Williams Syndrome)

Fanconi and associates were the first to note the peculiar facial appearance that is characteristic of the severe form of IIH.[186] Williams and coworkers, however, were the ones who pointed out the association between the peculiar facies and supravalvular aortic stenosis.[187] It was later that hypercalcemia, supravalvular aortic stenosis, and the facial appearance were described together.[188] The facial features of Williams syndrome include medial eyebrow flare, ocular hypertelorism, depressed nasal bridge, short palpebral fissures, strabismus, pale blue eyes with a starlike pattern to the iris, full prominent lips with an open mouth, malar hypoplasia, and anteverted nares.[189] The typical facies are often found at birth, and various cardiac lesions, including supravalvular aortic stenosis, atrial septal defect, and extracardiac stenosis, have been reported. Low birth weight is common. Other features described in affected newborns include inguinal hernia, umbilical hernia, small penis, and pectus excavatum. Hypertension associated with hypercalcemia is frequently found. A high percentage of infants manifest delayed psychomotor development, and mental deficiency is common in later childhood. Children are also described as having a "cocktail party" personality (chatty, outgoing, friendly, very engaging).

Hypercalcemia (12 to 19 mg/dL) may be present at the time of diagnosis in some affected infants. In others, the serum calcium level is normal, but the presence of nephrocalcinosis and other soft tissue calcification is suggestive of previous hypercalcemia. In still other affected infants, there is neither present nor past evidence of hypercalcemia, as reflected by normal serum calcium levels and absence of soft tissue calcifications. Thus, hypercalcemia seems to be a variable feature of Williams syndrome. Even when present, it usually resolves by 4 years of age.[189] It is possible that hypercalcemia exists in utero in all infants with this syndrome.

The severe form of IIH usually occurs sporadically. In contrast to mild IIH, prognosis is poor. As many as 25% of affected infants die within the first 4 years of life.[190] Renal insufficiency (nephrocalcinosis, renal artery stenosis) is frequently the cause of death. Additional sequelae include mental retardation (IQs of 40 to 80) and renal and cardiac complications. Height frequently remains below the third percentile.

The findings of hypercalcemia, hypercalciuria, and nephrocalcinosis have led to the hypothesis that these patients may have a form of vitamin D toxicity. Fellers and Schwartz, using a rachitic rat bioassay for vitamin D–like material, reported a 30- to 40-fold elevation of vitamin D–like activity.[191] Friedman and Roberts gave massive dosages of vitamin D to pregnant rabbits and found a high incidence of arterial stenosis in the offspring.[192] However, the dosages necessary to achieve these lesions were far in excess of dosages taken by humans, and the cardiac lesions were histologically different from typical Williams syndrome lesions. In addition, Beuren and associates reported hypercalcemia, the typical facies, and supravalvular aortic stenosis in infants in Germany whose mothers received 500,000 IU of vitamin D during pregnancy.[193] Taylor and coworkers examined the handling of vitamin D in age-matched control subjects and in 6 normocalcemic children with Williams syndrome by giving them 1500 IU/kg of vitamin D for 4 days.[194] Plasma concentrations of 25(OH)-vitamin D rose 300% above baseline values in the subjects with Williams syndrome but only 41% above baseline in the controls. Plasma 1,25(OH)$_2$-vitamin D and calcium levels were unchanged in both groups. Whether this abnormality in circulating 25(OH)-vitamin D is causally related to hypercalcemia is unknown, but it gives some credence to the idea that circulating vitamin D metabolites could be elevated at some point in Williams syndrome and that there may be a disorder of vitamin D metabolism.

Measurements of calcitropic hormones in patients with severe IIH have yielded mixed results. In the study by Taylor and coworkers, normocalcemic children with Williams syndrome had no elevations of vitamin D metabolites.[194] Garabédian and colleagues, in a longitudinal study of 4 children with Williams syndrome with hypercalcemia, found that the levels of 1,25(OH)$_2$-vitamin D were elevated (160 to 400 pg/mL) only during the hypercalcemic phase of the disease, when the children were less than 9 months of age.[195] In a study of five normocalcemic children with Williams syndrome, Culler and associates found no abnormalities of vitamin D metabolite concentrations either before or after PTH stimulation.[196] Their patients were, however, found to have significantly higher mean baseline calcium concentrations, delayed clearance of calcium after intravenous calcium loading, and blunted calcitonin responses after calcium infusions, in comparison with a group of seven normal children. The authors suggested that these patients have a defect in the synthesis or release of immunoreactive calcitonin. In a report by Knudtzon and coworkers, a single patient with severe IIH was reported to have elevated 1,25(OH)$_2$-vitamin D without hypercalcemia during the first 2 years of life.[197] At autopsy, however, this patient was found to have microcalcifications of the brain and kidney. Finally, in a survey of 27 normocalcemic children and adults with Williams syndrome, Kruse and colleagues found slightly decreased 25(OH)-vitamin D and slightly increased serum calcitonin concentrations compared with controls.[198] Serum PTH and 1,25(OH)$_2$-vitamin D levels, however, did not differ from those of controls, and low-dose calcium infusion resulted in the same increase of calcitonin in these patients as in controls. In addition, exogenous PTH induced a normal response of 1,25(OH)$_2$-vitamin D, cAMP, and phosphate excretion, indicating a normal 25(OH)-vitamin D 1α-hydroxylase and renal receptor–adenylate cyclase system that responded to PTH in patients with Williams syndrome.

Hypercalcemia with Subcutaneous Fat Necrosis

Infantile hypercalcemia has been described with subcutaneous fat necrosis in the newborn.[199-202] Firm subcutaneous nodules and plaques that manifest shortly after birth clinically characterize subcutaneous fat necrosis. The lesions may vary from a few millimeters in size to several centimeters. They can occur as single lesions, or they may be generalized. The overlying skin is usually bluish-red. These masses frequently develop at sites of pressure and contain fatty acid crystals, presumably a calcium salt, plus giant cells and mononuclear infiltrates.[200] The hypercalcemia can be severe (serum concentrations of 16 to 22 mg/dL), and typical symptoms of hypercalcemia do not usually manifest before 1 week of age. These patients may also demonstrate all the consequences of hypercalcemia, including azotemia, nephrocalcinosis, radiologic evidence of subcutaneous calcifications, and growth retardation. Death can occur.

The cause of this hypercalcemia is unknown. In a study of two cases by Veldhuis and associates, 25(OH)-vitamin D concentrations were normal and 1,25(OH)$_2$-vitamin D concentrations were suppressed by the hypercalcemia.[203] In these patients, urinary prostaglandin levels were increased, however, and prostaglandins have potent bone resorptive actions that may induce hypercalcemia. However, a subsequent report found normal plasma concentrations of prostaglandins E$_2$ and E$_3$ in another infant with subcutaneous fat necrosis.[204] Three reports have found greatly elevated serum concentrations of 1,25(OH)$_2$-vitamin D in four infants with hypercalcemia and subcutaneous fat necrosis.[205-207] These authors have suggested that extrarenal production of 1,25(OH)$_2$-vitamin D may be occurring in these patients, and they drew an analogy between the granulomas of sarcoidosis (known to synthesize 1,25[OH]$_2$-vitamin D in vitro) and the granulomatous inflammation of subcutaneous fat necrosis. The response of patients with hypercalcemia and subcutaneous fat necrosis to steroid therapy supports this hypothesis. At this point, however, it is still correct to say that the pathogenesis of this type of hypercalcemia in the newborn remains uncertain.

Hypercalcemia Associated with Phosphate Depletion

Hypercalcemia secondary to phosphate depletion is most commonly seen in infants with very low birth weight (<1500 g) who are fed human milk.[208-212] In most cases, this problem occurs 6 to 9 weeks after birth with severe hypophosphatemia and hypercalciuria that are far more dramatic than a "relative" hypercalcemia. However, 10 cases of hypercalcemia have been reported in infants with extremely low birth weight (<1000 g) with very low mineral intakes from human milk feedings during the first 2 weeks after birth.[213] These infants usually have normal 25(OH)-vitamin D serum concentrations and very high concentrations of 1,25(OH)$_2$-vitamin D. The low mineral intake and hypophosphatemia are a stimulus for 1,25(OH)$_2$-vitamin D synthesis with increased intestinal absorption and increased bone resorption of calcium. Hypercalcemia and hypercalciuria presumably occur because the very low intake of phosphorus severely limits deposition of calcium in bone. PTH is also suppressed in these infants by the normal or elevated serum calcium concentrations.

A similar situation can arise in infants receiving TPN therapy in which phosphate is inadvertently deleted.[214] This deletion may also occur when potassium phosphate salts are replaced with potassium acetate to treat metabolic acidosis. These infants can become critically ill with metabolic disturbances.

Miscellaneous Causes of Hypercalcemia

As in older children and adults, hypercalcemia associated with tumors also occurs in infants.[215] This hypercalcemia results from increased bone resorption induced by bone metastases or by a humoral factor produced by the tumor itself. Tumors that have been associated with hypercalcemia in infants include malignant renal tumors (both with and without bone metastases) and hepatoblastoma.

Hypercalcemia is also a manifestation of the severe infantile form of hypophosphatasia, a rare autosomal disorder with severe bone demineralization, low serum alkaline phosphatase, elevated urinary concentrations of phosphoethanolamine, and premature loss of teeth. About 300 cases have been reported. This inborn error of metabolism is characterized by a general reduction of activity of the tissue-nonspecific isoenzyme of alkaline phosphatase. Activity of the tissue-specific intestinal alkaline phosphatase is normal.[216] Hypophosphatasia becomes clinically apparent by 6 months of age. It is fatal in 50% of affected patients, and there is no established medical therapy.

Metaphyseal chondrodysplasia, or **Jansen syndrome**, is also a rare cause of hypercalcemia in the newborn.[217,218] In most affected infants, the hypercalcemia is characteristically asymptomatic, a hallmark of the disease in the newborn. The bone changes present at birth (unlike those seen in older children and adults as the disease progresses) are suggestive of rickets or hypophosphatasia. This uncharacteristic radiographic manifestation in the neonatal period, in comparison with that in older children and adults, frequently leads to misdiagnosis early in life.

FHH is also associated with mild hypercalcemia in the neonatal period. This condition is autosomal dominant, and the symptoms of hypercalcemia in older children and adults are typically absent.[219] Severe hyperparathyroidism has been reported in at least four neonates from three kindreds, many members of which had typical FHH.[220] Affected infants have life-threatening hypercalcemia with muscular hypotonia and skeletal demineralization. It is now thought that both FHH and hyperparathyroidism are disorders of the calcium-sensing receptor gene on chromosome number 3.[173]

Treatment of Hypocalcemia

This section focuses mainly on the treatment of symptomatic hypocalcemia in the newborn. Treatment of asymptomatic hypocalcemia, particularly in the premature infant, is an area of controversy. In general, if any treatment is used, oral calcium salts are preferred. Preparations such as calcium glubionate (Neo-Calglucon) are hypertonic because of their high carbohydrate content and should not be used in a premature infant in whom oral feedings are not very well established. Ten percent calcium gluconate is the preferred oral salt for infants, with a dose of 75 mg/kg/day of elemental calcium. Ten percent calcium gluconate contains 9.3 mg/mL of elemental calcium.

Treatment of hypocalcemia, regardless of cause, should be preceded by consideration of readily treated confounding factors (such as respiratory alkalosis). When hypomagnesemia exists, it should also be treated. Treatment of symptomatic hypocalcemia in newborns requires the intravenous infusion of calcium salts. Ten percent calcium gluconate is preferred over 10% calcium chloride because the latter has greater potential for the development of metabolic acidosis. The elemental calcium dose in the acute situation is 18 mg/kg (2 mL/kg body weight of 10% calcium gluconate) given into a peripheral vein over 10 minutes. In the case of cardiac arrhythmias ascribed to hypocalcemia, as may occur with severe metabolic alkalosis, it may be necessary to give it more rapidly. In either event, the heart rate should be monitored electronically during therapy. In the case of bradycardia, the infusion should be terminated. Subsequent intravenous elemental calcium therapy should be at a rate of 75 mg/kg/day. Once normocalcemia is sustained, it is preferable to decrease the infusion rate in a stepwise fashion (e.g., 75 mg/kg/day, then 37 mg/kg/day, then 18 mg/kg/day, and then discontinue). In general, intraarterial infusions are not recommended because of the potential for acute vascular complications. If hypocalcemia is persistent, the cause must be carefully determined. Administration of vitamin D metabolites may be indicated in some cases, although most infants are already receiving the recommended dosage of 400 IU/day.

Treatment of Hypercalcemia

Symptomatic hypercalcemia is a life-threatening condition and, unless of iatrogenic origin, is notoriously difficult to treat. Restriction of calcium and vitamin D intake is self-evident. Corticosteroid therapy (hydrocortisone, 1 mg/kg every 6 hours) is usually effective and will reduce intestinal absorption of calcium if the infant is receiving oral feedings. However, the action is delayed, which limits steroid use in the acute situation. Furosemide diuretics are helpful in the acute situation as long as the infant is well hydrated and there are no electrolyte imbalances. Other considerations are the intravenous use of ethylenediaminetetraacetic acid, which chelates calcium, and the use of calcitonin, which blocks PTH calcium mobilization from bone and has a calciuretic action. In cases of refractory neonatal hyperparathyroidism, surgical treatment is necessary as soon as possible.

OSTEOPENIA OF PREMATURITY

Osteopenia of prematurity, a metabolic bone disease, refers to the hypomineralized skeleton of the premature infant. Just as the extrauterine growth rate lags behind the intrauterine rate, the extrauterine rate of skeletal mineralization is delayed in comparison with that of the corresponding fetal skeleton. In reference to the premature infant, the terms **osteopenia** and **rickets** are often used synonymously. The term *rickets* should be reserved for specific histologic, radiographic, and physical findings that may be associated with different diseases, including the more severe degree of osteopenia of prematurity. Rickets is characterized by the accumulation of unmineralized osteoid, which interrupts the mineralization of the growth plate of bone. It is therefore a disease of growing children. (The comparable disease in adults with closed growth plates is known as **osteomalacia**). Fractures may also occur in osteopenic premature infants with or without radiologic features of rickets.

This bone disease is best assessed with special roentgenologic techniques. It occurs in nearly every growing infant with low birth weight (<1500 g and <32 weeks of gestational age) to some degree. More critically ill premature infants have the most significant degree of osteopenia, and the frequency of rickets/fractures is in general inversely correlated with birth weight. This high incidence is not surprising, because approximately 80% of fetal skeletal mineralization occurs during the last trimester of pregnancy. The incidence of rickets or fractures in infants with a birth weight of less than 1500 g reportedly ranges from 20% to 32%,[221-223] increasing to 50% to 60% in infants with a birth weight of less than 1000 g.[77,224,225] The incidence of rickets or fractures is also increased in infants fed unsupplemented milk or soy formula.[213,221,226]

Pathophysiology

Data on the histopathologic processes of osteopenia of prematurity are very limited, being described by only two reports.[227,228] The cause is multifactorial, as shown in Figure 75-10. As discussed previously, a major factor is the lower stores of calcium and phosphorus at birth in comparison with full-term infants. Fetal accretion of calcium has been estimated to increase from 130 mg/kg/day at 28 weeks to 150 mg/kg/day at 36 weeks of gestation.[68,229] Meeting this intrauterine accretion rate of minerals has been one of the challenges of neonatology, and the failure to do so is a very important factor in the development of osteopenia. Standard formulas and human milk do not contain enough minerals to accomplish this; therefore, high mineral–containing formulas and human milk fortifiers have been developed specifically for preterm infants.

It has been proposed that a decrease in bone loading plays a very significant role in the development of osteopenia of prematurity.[230-232] Bone loading in the premature infant is largely brought about by passive or active muscle activity. Increased bone loading (i.e., a passive exercise program) promotes bone formation, whereas decreased bone loading (decreased physical activity) results in bone resorption. Thus, even if there is an adequate supply of substrate (calcium, phosphorus), it will not be put to use unless there is a need for bone formation, as provided by the mechanical challenge of muscle contraction. Two lines of evidence support the importance of bone loading. First, increased concentrations of the biochemical markers of bone resorption have been observed in the preterm infant. Markers of bone resorption include collagen turnover compounds (hydroxyproline, type 1 collagen telopeptide, serum alkaline phosphatase). The serum alkaline phosphatase level has long been known to be elevated in premature infants; the highest levels are observed in the infants with the most severe degree of osteopenia of prematurity. In addition, urinary hydroxyproline and type 1 collagen telopeptide levels have been demonstrated to be increased in growing preterm infants in comparison with full-term infants.[233-235]

The second line of evidence is a number of studies that demonstrate the organized programs of physical activity improve measurements of bone mineralization in preterm infants.[236-238] In one of these studies, Moyer-Mileur and coworkers performed a physical activity program in VLBW infants by exercising their extremities against passive resistance for 5 to 10 minutes a day. The exercise group (n = 16) improved weight gain and bone mineral content (BMC) more than did the nonexercising group (n = 16).[237] These observations may help explain why, historically, provision of adequate amounts of calcium and phosphorus has not dramatically improved osteopenia and bone mineralization in hospitalized VLBW infants.

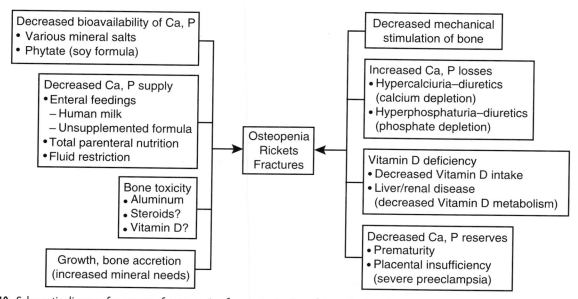

Figure 75–10. Schematic diagram for causes of osteopenia of prematurity. Ca, calcium; P, phosphorus.

Vitamin D deficiency, on the other hand, is an unusual cause of bone disease in the preterm infant. This statement is not surprising, inasmuch as premature infants with osteopenia have normal levels of 25-hydroxyvitamin D and generally increased levels of 1,25-dihydroxyvitamin D (Table 75-1). Daily oral vitamin D supplements of 2000 IU/day for 6 weeks do not affect the incidence of osteopenia in premature infants[222] and 200 to 400 IU/day appears to be adequate.[239]

TPN is another factor in the origin of metabolic bone disease in premature infants. Not only is the delivery of calcium and phosphorus decreased in comparison with the intrauterine rate, but other factors in TPN, including vitamin D and aluminum (a contaminant), may be toxic to bone. TPN-induced liver disease with cholestasis may also be a factor in some infants. Standard TPN solutions for infants with low birth weight have usually had low concentrations of calcium (20 mg/dL) and phosphorus (15.5 mg/dL). However, higher concentrations—namely, 60 mg/dL of calcium and 46 mg/dL of phosphorus—can be achieved in such TPN solutions.[240] These higher concentrations are achieved without precipitation of the minerals by controlling the length of storage, temperature, calcium salt used, order of mixing calcium and phosphorus, pH, and concentrations of amino acids and dextrose.[161]

Table 75–1. Diagnosis of Osteopenia of Prematurity

Indicator	Results
Radiographic	
Standard radiograph	Rickets (knees, wrist)
	Fractures (ribs, long bones)
	Hypomineralization
Single photon absorptiometry	↓ Bone mineral content in comparison to intrauterine rate
Dual energy x-ray absorptiometry (DXA)	↓ Total body mineral content in comparison to intrauterine value
Serum	
Calcium	Normal (may be increased with hypophosphatemia)
Phosphorus	Low (<4.0 mg/dL) or normal
Alkaline phosphatase	Normal or increased
Parathyroid hormone	Normal or increased
25-(OH)-vitamin D	Normal (intake, 400–800 IU/day)
1,25-(OH)₂-vitamin D	Increased
Osteocalcin	Normal (in comparison with full-term infants)
Renal	
Fractional excretion of calcium (%)	Increased (>2%)
Renal tubular reabsorption of phosphorus	Increased (99%–100%)
Urinary hydroxyproline	Increased

A number of drugs have also been associated with increased calcium loss and osteopenia of prematurity. These include diuretics and corticosteroids.

Diagnosis

A physical examination is not very helpful in the diagnosis of osteopenia of prematurity unless the disease has progressed to an advanced stage. In those cases, affected infants may experience tenderness at fracture sites in the long bones. In older patients, the rachitic rosary at the costochondral junction as well as craniotabes of the skull may be present. Because these infants do not bear weight, the more obvious clinical signs of rickets, with bowing in the lower extremities, are not evident.

In the majority of cases, the diagnosis is made from routine radiographs, usually of the chest, where healing rib fractures or severe hypomineralization may be observed. In the more advanced form of the disease, standard radiographs of the wrists and knees may show the classic signs of rickets, but usually not before 2 months of age. However, conventional radiologic methods cannot detect decreases in BMC until a 30% to 40% loss of bone mineral has occurred.[22,241] Quantitative morphometric and photodensitometric methods with standard radiographs can detect bone loss only within broad limits (10% to 20% error).[242] In general, they are limited to use for research purposes. They include single photon absorptiometry (SPA), dual energy x-ray absorptiometry and quantitative computed tomography, and transmission ultrasonography.[243]

The first of the techniques to be used extensively in infants with low birth weight was SPA, in which a low-energy iodine 125 source (20 to 200 mCi) emits a well-collimated photon beam as it passes beneath the bone to be scanned, usually the radius. Attenuation of this beam by bone is directly correlated with the BMC. Using this technology, many studies have documented delays in bone mineralization in premature infants in comparison with the intrauterine curve of mineral accretion.[22,226] The differences are most dramatic when premature infants are fed human milk, in comparison with a formula higher in mineral content.[244] A limitation of this method is that changes in BMC as measured by SPA occur very slowly. Furthermore, no single value of BMC for any postconception age has been defined as diagnostic of osteopenia with this technique.

Dual energy x-ray absorptiometry holds the most promise for measuring BMC and assessing osteopenia in premature infants. Two electronically generated x-ray beams of relatively high and low energy levels are used to determine total body BMC, as well as regional BMC with minimal tissue radiation (2 mrem). It detects changes in total body BMC over a shorter period of time than does SPA. However, as with SPA, specific values for defining osteopenia in infants are not available.

A number of serum biochemical markers have been used to screen for osteopenia of prematurity. These include calcium, phosphorus, alkaline phosphatase, PTH, 25(OH)-vitamin D, 1,25(OH)₂-vitamin D, and osteocalcin. These are reviewed in Table 75-1. Several urinary measurements have also been examined in relation to osteopenia of prematurity. These include fractional excretion of calcium and tubular reabsorption of phosphate, as well as calcium/creatinine ratio (see Table 75-1).

Treatment/Outcome

In the United States and Canada, where the maternal intake of vitamin D is higher than many other parts of the world, VLBW infants receiving oral feedings clearly do not need more than 400 IU/day of vitamin D as recommended by the American Academy of Pediatrics Committee on Nutrition.[245] The high 1,25(OH)$_2$-vitamin D concentrations and adequate levels of 25(OH)-vitamin D in almost all infants diagnosed with this disorder support this recommendation, which assumes that VLBW infants will not be maintained on diets with grossly inadequate concentrations of calcium and phosphorus such as unfortified human milk. Increasing the intakes of vitamin D to 960 IU/day or greater has not proved beneficial,[222,239] and according to the current information, improved absorption of calcium and phosphorus is not likely to occur with these increases in intake of vitamin D. Parenteral requirements for vitamin D are less clear, although with the current multivitamin preparations available in the United States for intravenous use in infants with low birth weight, it is difficult to exceed 400 IU/day without concerns for increased amounts of other vitamins. Nevertheless, premature infants receiving long-term TPN have exhibited adequate vitamin D status with solutions supplying as little as 30 to 35 IU/kg/day.[246] Such low amounts of vitamin D in the infusate would tend to minimize any potential toxic effects of vitamin D that have been reported in adults.[247]

Although there are some indications that a routine passive "exercise" program may also be beneficial (see previous discussion),[237,238] the most important component of prevention and treatment is the supply of adequate amounts of calcium and phosphorus, without which any bone loading exercises would be ineffective. The logical goal of such therapy would be to attain the intrauterine rate of bone mineralization. To do so would require enteral intakes of approximately 200 mg/kg/day of calcium and 90 mg/kg/day of phosphorus, assuming 65% absorption of calcium (at best) and 80% absorption of phosphorus. The special formulas available for VLBW infants supply these amounts of minerals. Commercial fortifiers for human milk containing the appropriate amounts of calcium and phosphorus are also available. As noted previously, the achievement of the intrauterine accretion of bone mineral in VLBW infants during the first 8 weeks after birth is problematic even with adequate mineral intake. Prevention of severe osteopenia with fractures and rickets is possible with these intakes, however. Catch-up bone mineralization does eventually occur in these infants after discharge (see paragraph after next).

The prevention and/or treatment of osteopenia in the VLBW infant receiving TPN is subject to the limitations in the preparations of TPN solutions, as discussed previously. For these infants, the concentrations of calcium and phosphorus obtainable in these solutions probably do not achieve the in utero rate of accretion of bone mineral.

However, enough of these minerals can be infused with TPN solution to prevent overt fractures and rickets in these patients. Solutions containing 60 mg/dL (15 mmol) of calcium and 46.5 mg/dL (15 mmol) of phosphorus maintain the desired biochemical and calciotropic hormone indices of mineral homeostasis.[246]

Relatively few studies have documented long-term outcome in VLBW infants with osteopenia. One study documented catch-up bone mineralization (as measured by SPA of the radius) at 65 weeks after conception.[248] Chan and Mileur found that VLBW infants fed human milk, in comparison with standard formula, after hospital discharge had significantly lower BMC at 42 to 56 weeks after conception.[249] Similarly, in a study by Abrams and associates,[250] a group of VLBW infants fed unfortified human milk after discharge were compared with a group fed standard infant formula. At 52 to 53 weeks after conception, the infants fed human milk had significantly lower BMC as measured by SPA than did those fed cow's milk formula. The group fed formula at this age resembled a control group of full-term infants at the same postconception age. However, by 2 years of age, the BMC of the unfortified milk group had finally achieved a value equal to that of a formula-fed group of infants with low birth weight.[244] The long-term effects of osteopenia of prematurity, including the effects on bone mineralization and stature during adolescence, as well as the effects on the risks of osteoporosis in adult life, remain unknown.

References

1. Brown EM: The extracellular Ca^{2+} sensing receptor: Central mediator of systemic calcium homeostasis. Annu Rev Nutr 20:507, 2000.
2. Riccardi D, Gamba G: The many roles of the calcium-sensing receptor in health and disease. Arch Med Res 30:436, 1999.
3. Brown AJ, Dusso A, Slatopolsky E: Vitamin D. Am J Physiol 277:F157, 1999.
4. Chandler JS, Pike JW, Haussler MR: 1,25-Dihydroxyvitamin D$_3$ receptors in rat kidney cytosol. Biochem Biophys Res Commun 90:1057, 1979.
5. Morrissey RL, Rath DF: Purification of human renal calcium binding protein from necropsy specimen. Proc Soc Exp Biol Med 145:669, 1974.
6. Kawashima H, Kurokawa K: Metabolism and sites of action of vitamin D in the kidney. Kidney Int 29:98, 1986.
7. Huffer WE: Biology of disease: Morphology and biochemistry of bone remodeling: Possible control by vitamin D, parathyroid hormone, and other substances. Lab Invest 59:418, 1988.
8. Hollander D: Intestinal absorption of vitamins A, E, D and E. J Lab Clin Invest 97:449, 1981.
9. Kodicek E: The fate of labeled vitamin D in rats and infants. In Garattine S, Pauletti G (eds): Drugs Affecting Lipid Metabolism. Amsterdam, Elsevier, 1961, pp 515-519.
10. Goldsmith R: Enterohepatic cycling of vitamin D and its metabolites. Minerva Electrolyte Metab 8:289, 1982.
11. Hennemen PH, Forbes AP, Moldawer M, et al: Effects of growth hormone in man. J Clin Invest 39:1223, 1960.
12. Harbison MD, Gertner J: Permissive action of growth hormone on the renal response to dietary phosphorus deprivation. J Clin Endocrinol Metab 70:1035, 1990.

13. Gitelman HJ, Kukolj S, Welt LJ: Inhibition of parathyroid gland activity by hypermagnesemia. Am J Physiol 215:483, 1968.

14. Slatopolsky E, Mercado A, Morrison A, et al: Inhibitory effects of hypermagnesemia on the renal action of parathyroid hormone. J Clin Invest 58:1273, 1976.

15. Massry SG: Magnesium homeostasis and its clinical pathophysiology. Resident Staff Physician 27;105, 1981.

16. Brannan PG, Vergne-Marini P, Pak CYC, et al: Magnesium absorption in human small intestine. Results in normal subjects, patients with chronic renal disease and subjects with absorptive hypercalciuria. J Clin Invest 57:1412, 1976.

17. Seelig MS: Magnesium requirements in human nutrition. J Med Soc N J 79:849, 1982.

18. Sutton RLA, Dirks JH: Renal handling of calcium, phosphate, and magnesium. In Brenner BM, Rector RC (eds): The Kidney. Philadelphia, WB Saunders, 1981, pp 551-618.

19. Pitkin RM, Reynolds WA, Williams GA: Calcium metabolism in normal pregnancy: A longitudinal study. Am J Obstet Gynecol 133:781, 1979.

20. Martinez ME, Sanchez C, Salinas M, et al: Ionic calcium levels during pregnancy, at delivery and in the first hours of life. Scand J Clin Lab Invest 46:27, 1986.

21. Seki K, Makimura N, Mitsui C, et al: Calcium-regulating hormones and osteocalcin levels during pregnancy: A longitudinal study. Am J Obstet Gynecol 164:1248, 1991.

22. Greer FR: Determination of radial bone mineral content in low birth weight infants by photon absorptiometry. J Pediatr 113:213, 1988.

23. Kent GN, Price RL, Gutteridge DH, et al: The efficiency of intestinal calcium absorption is increased in late pregnancy but not in established lactation. Calcif Tissue Int 48:293, 1991.

24. Bouillon R, Van Assche FA, van Baelen H, et al: Influence of the vitamin D–binding protein in the serum concentration of 1,25-dihydroxyvitamin D_3. Significance of the free 1,25-dihydroxyvitamin D_3 concentration. J Clin Invest 67:589, 1981.

25. Howarth AT, Morgan DB, Payne RB: Urinary excretion of calcium in late pregnancy and its relation to creatinine clearance. Am J Obstet Gynecol 129:499, 1977.

26. Cushard WG, Creditor MA, Canterbury JM, Reiss E: Physiologic hyperparathyroidism in pregnancy. J Clin Endocrinol Metab 34:767, 1976.

27. Lequin RM, Hackeng WH, Shopman W: A radioimmunoassay for parathyroid hormone in man. II. Measurement of parathyroid hormone concentration in human plasma by means of a radioimmunoassay for bovine hormone. Acta Endocrinol 63:655, 1970.

28. Reitz RE, Daane TA, Woods JR, et al: Calcium, magnesium, phosphorus, and parathyroid interrelationships in pregnancy and newborn infant. Obstet Gynecol 50:701, 1977.

29. Davis OK, Hawkins DS, Rubin LP, et al: Serum parathyroid hormone (PTH) in pregnant women determined by an immunoradiometric assay for intact PTH. J Clin Endocrinol Metab 67:850, 1988.

30. Frolich A, Rudnicki M, Fischer-Rasmussen W, et al: Serum concentrations of intact parathyroid hormone during late human pregnancy: a longitudinal study. Eur J Obstet Gynecol Reprod Biol 42:85, 1991.

31. Rasmussen N, Frolich A, Hornnes PJ, et al: Serum ionized calcium and intact parathyroid hormone levels during pregnancy and postpartum. Br J Obstet Gynaecol 97:857, 1990.

32. Saggese G, Baroncelli GI, Bertelloni S, et al: Intact parathyroid hormone levels during pregnancy, in healthy term neonates and in hypocalcemic preterm infants. Acta Paediatr Scand 80:36, 1991.

33. Croley TE: The intracellular localization of calcium within the mature human placenta barrier. Am J Obstet Gynecol 117:926, 1973.

34. Northrop G, Misenheimer HR, Becker FO: Failure of parathyroid hormone to cross the nonhuman primate placenta. Am J Obstet Gynecol 129:449, 1977.

35. Hillman LS, Haddad GJ: Perinatal vitamin D metabolism. III. Factors influencing late gestational human serum 25-hydroxyvitamin D. Am J Obstet Gynecol 125:196, 1976.

36. Bruns ME, Bruns DE: Vitamin D metabolism and function during pregnancy and the neonatal period. Am Clin Lab Sci 13:521, 1983.

37. Kumar R, Colon WR, Silva P, et al: Elevated 1,25-dihydroxyvitamin D plasma levels in normal human pregnancy and lactation. J Clin Invest 63:342, 1979.

38. Reddy GS, Norman AW, Willis DM, et al: Regulation of vitamin D metabolism in normal human pregnancy. J Clin Endocrinol Metab 56:363, 1983.

39. Steichen JJ, Tsang RC, Gratton TL, et al: Vitamin D homeostasis in the perinatal period: 1,25-Dihydoxy-vitamin D in maternal, cord and neonatal blood. N Engl J Med 302:315, 1980.

40. Hollis BW, Pittard WB: Evaluation of the total fetomaternal vitamin D relationship at term: Evidence for racial differences. J Clin Endocrinol Metab 59:652, 1984.

41. Weiland T, Fischer JA, Trechsel U, et al: Perinatal parathyroid, vitamin D metabolites, and calcitonin in man. Am J Physiol 239:E385, 1980.

42. Delvin EE, Salle BL, Glorieux FH, et al: Vitamin D supplementation during pregnancy: Effect on neonatal calcium homeostasis. J Pediatr 109:328, 1986.

43. Fleischman AR, Rosen JF, Cole J, et al: Maternal and fetal serum 1,25-dihydroxyvitamin D levels at term. J Pediatr 97:640, 1988.

44. Marx SJ, Swart EG, Hamstra AJ, DeLuca HF: Normal intrauterine development of the fetus of a woman receiving extraordinarily high doses of 1,25-dihydroxyvitamin D. J Clin Endocrinol Metab 51:1138, 1980.

45. Whitsett JA, Ho M, Tsang RC: Synthesis of 1,25-dihydroxyvitamin D by human placenta in vitro. J Clin Endocrinol Metab 53:484, 1981.

46. Ross R: Vitamin D metabolism in the pregnant large animal. In Holick M, Anast C, Gray T (eds): Perinatal Calcium and Phosphorus Metabolism. Amsterdam, Elsevier, 1983, pp 35-36.

47. Brommage R, DeLuca H: Placental transport of calcium and phosphorus is not regulated by vitamin D. Am J Physiol 246:F526, 1984.

48. Care AD, Dutton M, Mott JC, et al: Studies of the transplacental calcium gradient in sheep. J Physiol 290:19P, 1979.

49. Robinson NR, Sibley CP, Mughal MZ, et al: Fetal control of calcium transport across the rat placenta. Pediatr Res 26:109, 1989.

50. Pike JW, Gooze LL, Haussler MR: Biochemical evidence for 1,25$(OH)_2$-dehydroxyvitamin D receptor macromolecules in parathyroid, pancreatic, pituitary and placental tissues. Life Sci 26:407, 1980.

51. Brunette MG, Allard S: Phosphate uptake by syncytial brush border membrane of human placenta. Pediatr Res 19:1179, 1985.

52. Martin TJ, Ebeling PR: A novel parathyroid hormone-related protein: Role in pathology and physiology. In Peterlik M, Bronner F (eds): Molecular and Cellular Regulation of Calcium and Phosphate Metabolism. New York, Alan R. Liss, 1990, pp 1-37.

53. Allgrove J, Adami S, Manning RM, et al: Cytochemical bioassay of parathyroid hormone in maternal and cord blood. Arch Dis Child 60:110, 1985.

54. Rodda CP, Kubota M, Heath JA, et al: Evidence for a novel parathyroid hormone–related protein in fetal lamb parathyroid glands and sheep placenta: Comparisons with a similar protein implicated in humoral hypercalcaemia of malignancy. J Endocrinol 117:261, 1988.

55. Shaw AJ, Mughal MZ, Maresh MJA, et al: Effects of two synthetic parathyroid hormone–related protein fragments on maternofetal transfer of calcium and magnesium and release of cyclic AMP by the in-situ perfused rat placenta. J Endocrinol 129:399, 1991.

56. Spanos E, Brown DJ, Stevenson JC, et al: Stimulation of 1,25-dihydroxycholecalciferal production by prolactin and related peptides in intact renal cell preparations in vitro. Biochim Biophys Acta 672:7, 1981.

57. Pahuja DW, DeLuca HF: Stimulation of intestinal calcium transport and bone calcium mobilization by prolactin in vitamin D deficient rats. Science 214:1038, 1981.

58. Drake TS, Kaplan RA, Lewis TA: The physiologic hyperparathyroidism of pregnancy: Is it primary or secondary? Obstet Gynecol 53:746, 1979.

59. Stevenson JC, Hillyard CS, MacIntyre I, et al: The physiological role for calcitonin: protection of the maternal skeleton. Lancet 2:769, 1979.

60. Reynolds WA, Williams GA, Pitkin RM: Calcitropic hormone responsiveness during pregnancy. Am J Obstet Gynecol 139:855, 1981.

61. Taylor TG, Lewis PE, Balderstone O: Role of calcitonin in protecting the skeleton during pregnancy and lactation. J Endocrinol 66:297, 1975.

62. Milhaud G, Maukhtar MS, Perault-Straub AM, et al: Calcitonin. In Taylor S, Foster GV (eds): Calcitonin 1969: Proceedings of the Second International Symposium, London, 21-24 July 1969. London, Heinemann, 1969, pp 182-193.

63. Brunette MG, Auger D, Lafond J: Effect of parathyroid hormone on PO_4 transport through the human placenta microvilli. Pediatr Res 25:15, 1989.

64. Lajeunesse D, Brunette MG: Sodium gradient–dependent phosphate transport in placental brush border membrane vesicles. Placenta 9:117, 1988.

65. Fanaroff AA, Martin RJ (eds): Neonatal-perinatal medicine. In: Diseases of the Fetus and Infant. St. Louis, Mosby–Year Book, 1992, p 1433.

66. Giles MM, Fenton MH, Shaw B, et al: Sequential calcium and phosphorus balance studies in preterm infants. J Pediatr 110:591, 1987.

67. Okamoto E, Muttart C, Zucker C, et al: Use of medium chain triglycerides in feeding the low-birth-weight infant. Am J Dis Child 136:428, 1982.

68. Shaw JCL: Evidence for defective skeletal mineralization in low birthweight infants; the absorption of calcium and fat. Pediatrics 57:16, 1976.

69. Baltrop D, Mole RH, Sutton A: Absorption and endogenous faecal excretion of calcium by low birthweight infants on feeds with varying contents of calcium and phosphate. Arch Dis Child 52:41, 1977.

70. Hillman LS, Johnson LS, Lee DZ, et al: Measurement of absorption, retention and endogenous intestinal excretion of calcium in premature infants using a dual stable isotope method. J Pediatr 123:444, 1993.

71. Siegel SR, Hadeed A: Renal handling of calcium in the early newborn period. Kidney Int 31:1181, 1987.

72. Rubin LP, Posillico JT, Anast CS, et al: Circulating levels of biologically active and immunoreactive intact parathyroid hormone in human newborns. Pediatr Res 29:201, 1991.

73. David L, Anast CS: Calcium metabolism in newborn infants. The interrelationship of parathyroid function and calcium, magnesium, and phosphorus metabolism in normal, "sick," and hypocalcemic newborns. J Clin Invest 54:287, 1974.

74. Hillman LS, Rojanasathit S, Slatopolsky E, et al: Serial measurements of serum calcium, magnesium, parathyroid hormone, calcitonin, and 25-hydroxy-vitamin D in premature and term infants during the first week of life. Pediatr Res 11:739, 1977.

75. Tsang RC, Chen IW, Friedman MA, et al: Neonatal parathyroid function: Role of gestational age and postnatal age. J Pediatr 83:728, 1973.

76. Linarelli LG, Bobik J, Bobik C: Newborn urinary cyclic AMP and developmental renal responsiveness to parathyroid hormone. Pediatrics 50:14, 1972.

77. Lindroth M, Westgren U, Laurin S: Rickets in very low-birth-weight infants. Acta Paediatr Scand 75:927, 1986.

78. Greer FR, Hollis BW, Napoli JL: High concentrations of vitamin D_2 in human milk associated with pharmacologic doses of vitamin D_2. J Pediatr 105:61, 1984.

79. Bouillon R, Van Baelen H, DeMoor P: 25-Hydroxy-vitamin D and its binding protein in maternal and cord serum. J Clin Endocrinol Metab 45:679, 1977.

80. Cockburn F, Belton NR, Purvis RJ, et al: Maternal vitamin D intake and mineral metabolism in mothers and their newborn infants. BMJ 281:11, 1980.

81. Delvin EE, Glorieux FH, Salle BL, et al: Control of vitamin D metabolism in preterm infants: Fetomaternal relationships. Arch Dis Child 57:754, 1982.

82. Gertner JM, Glassman MS, Coustan DR, et al: Fetomaternal vitamin D relationships at term. J Pediatr 97:637, 1980.

83. Kuroda E, Okano T, Mizuno N: Plasma levels of 25-hydroxyvitamin D_2 and 25-hydroxyvitamin D_3 in maternal cord and neonatal blood. J Nutr Sci Vitaminol 27:55, 1981.

84. Paunier L, Lacourt G, Pelland P, et al: 25-Hydroxy-vitamin D and calcium levels in maternal, cord and infant serum in relation to maternal vitamin D intake. Helv Paediatr Acta 33:95, 1978.

85. Seino Y, Ishida M, Yamaoka K: Serum calcium regulating hormones in the perinatal period. Calcif Tissue Int 34:131, 1982.

86. Shimotsuji T, Seino Y, Ishida M: Relations of plasma 25-hydroxyvitamin D levels in mothers, cord blood and newborn infants, and postnatal changes in plasma 25-hydroxyvitamin D levels. J Nutr Sci Vitaminol 25:79, 1979.

87. Verity CM, Burman D, Beadle PC, et al: Seasonal changes in perinatal vitamin D metabolism: Maternal and cord blood biochemistry in normal pregnancies. Arch Dis Child 56:943, 1981.

88. Weisman Y, Occhipenti M, Knox G, et al: Concentration of 24,25-dihydroxyvitamin D and 25-hydroxyvitamin D in paired maternal-cord sera. Am J Obstet Gynecol 130:704, 1978.

89. Rebut-Bonneton C, Demignon J, Cancela L, et al: Effect of 25-hydroxyvitamin D_3 and 1,25-hydroxyvitamin D_3 maternal loads on maternal and fetal vitamin D metabolite levels in the rat. Reprod Nutr Dev 25:583, 1985.

90. Weisman Y, Sapir R, Harell A, et al: Maternal-perinatal interrelationships of vitamin D metabolism in rats. Biochim Biophys Acta 428:388, 1976.

91. Goff JP, Horst RI, Littledike ET: Effect of the maternal vitamin D status at parturition on the vitamin D status of the neonatal calf. J Nutr 112:1387, 1982.

92. Devaskar UP, Ho M, Devaskar SU, Tsang RC: 25-Hydroxy-and 1α,25-dihydroxyvitamin D. Maternal-fetal relationship and the transfer of 1,25-dihydroxyvitamin D_3 across the placenta in an ovine model. Dev Pharmacol Ther 7:213, 1983.

93. Schedewie H, Slikker W, Hill D, et al: Transplacental transfer of 1,25(OH)$_2$ vitamin D in subhuman primates. Clin Res 27:813A, 1979.

94. Salle BL, Berthezene F, Glorieux FH, et al: Hypoparathyroidism during pregnancy: Treatment with calcitriol. J Clin Endocrinol Metab 52:810, 1981.

95. Ron M, Levitz M, Chuba J, et al: Transfer of 25-hydroxyvitamin D_3 and 1,25-dihydroxyvitamin D_3 across the perfused human placenta. Am J Obstet Gynecol 148:370, 1984.

96. Markestad T, Aksnes L, Alslein M, et al: 25-Hydroxyvitamin D and 1,25-dihydroxyvitamin D of D_2 and D_3 origin in maternal and umbilical cord serum after vitamin D_2 supplementation in human pregnancy. Am J Clin Nutr 40:1057, 1984.

97. Gray TK, Lester GE: Evidence for extra-renal 1α-hydroxylation of 25-hydroxyvitamin D_3 in pregnancy. Science 204:1311, 1979.

98. Lester GE, Gray TK, Lorenc RS: Evidence for maternal and fetal differences in vitamin D metabolism. Proc Soc Exp Biol Med 159:303, 1978.

99. Lester GE, Gray TK, Lorenc RS: 25-Hydroxyvitamin D_3 metabolism in the pregnant rat: Maternal-fetal relationships. Biol Neonate 39:232, 1981.

100. Weisman Y, Vargas A, Duckett G, et al: Synthesis of 1,25-dihydroxyvitamin D in the nephrectomized pregnant rat. Endocrinology 103:1992, 1978.

101. Salle BL, Glorieux FH, Delvin EE: Perinatal vitamin D metabolism. Biol Neonate 54:181, 1988.

102. Kuoppala T, Tuinrala R, Parvianinen M, et al: Can the fetus regulate its calcium uptake? Br J Obstet Gynaecol 91:1192, 1984.

103. Dancis J, Springer D, Cohlan SQ, et al: Fetal homeostasis in maternal malnutrition. II. Magnesium deprivation. Pediatr Res 5:131, 1971.

104. Brooke OG, Brown IRF, Cleeve HJW: Observations on the vitamin D state of pregnant Asian women in London. Br J Obstet Gynaecol 88:18, 1981.

105. Delmas PO, Glorieux FH, Delvin EE, et al: Perinatal serum bone Gla-protein and vitamin D metabolites in preterm and full-term neonates. J Clin Endocrinol Metab 65:588, 1987.

106. Nishioka T, Yasuda T, Niimi H, et al: Evidence that calcitonin plays a role in the postnatal increase of serum 1α,25-dihydroxyvitamin D. Eur J Pediatr 147:148, 1988.

107. Fetter WPF, Mettau JW, Degenhart HJ, et al: Plasma 1,25-dihydroxyvitamin D concentrations in preterm infants. Acta Paediatr Scand 74:549, 1985.

108. Mawer EB, Stanbury SW, Robinson MJ, et al: Vitamin D nutrition and vitamin D metabolism in the premature human neonate. Clin Endocrinol 25:641, 1986.

109. Hillman LS, Salmons S, Dokoh S: Serum 1,25-dihydroxyvitamin D concentration in premature infants: Preliminary results. Calcif Tissue Int 37:223, 1985.

110. Hillman LS, Hoff N, Salmans S, et al: Mineral homeostasis in very premature infants: Serial evaluations of serum 25-hydroxyvitamin D, serum minerals, and bone mineralization. J Pediatr 106:970, 1985.

111. Cooper TJ, Anast CS: Circulating immunoreactive parathyroid hormone levels in premature infants and the response to calcium therapy. Acta Paediatr Scand 74:669, 1985.

112. Dilena BA, White GA: The responses of plasma ionized calcium and intact parathyrin to calcium supplementation in preterm infants. Acta Paediatr Scand 80:1098, 1991.

113. Venkataraman PS, Blick KE, Fry HD, et al: Postnatal changes in calcium-regulating hormones in very-low-birth-weight infants. Am J Dis Child 139:913, 1985.

114. Venkataraman PS, Tsang RC, Steichen JJ, et al: Early neonatal hypocalcemia in extremely premature infants. High incidence, early onset, and refractoriness to supraphysiologic doses of calcitriol. Am J Dis Child 140:1004, 1986.

115. Halloran BP, Deluca HF: Appearance of the intestinal cytosolic receptor for 1,25-dihydroxyvitamin D during neonatal development in the rat. J Biol Chem 256:7338, 1981.

116. Halloran BP, Deluca HF: Calcium transport in small intestine during early development: Role of vitamin D. Am J Physiol 239:G473, 1980.

117. Gleason WA, Lankford GL: Intestinal calcium-binding protein in the developing rat duodenum. Pediatr Res 16:403, 1982.

118. Venkataraman PS, Tsang RC, Chen IW, et al: Pathogenesis of early neonatal hypocalcemia: Studies of serum calcitonin, gastrin and plasma glucagon. J Pediatr 110:599, 1987.

119. Bergman L, Kjellmer I, Selstam U: Calcitonin and parathyroid hormone: Relation to early neonatal hypocalcemia in infants of diabetic mothers. Biol Neonate 24:151, 1974.

120. David L, Salle B, Chopard P, et al: Studies on circulating immunoreactive calcitonin in low birth weight infants during the first 48 hours of life. Helv Paediatr Acta 32:39, 1977.

121. David L, Salle BL, Putet G, et al: Serum immunoreactive calcitonin in low birth weight infants. Description of early changes; effect of intravenous calcium infusion; relationships with early changes in serum calcium, phosphorus, magnesium, parathyroid hormone, and gastrin levels. Pediatr Res 15:803, 1981.

122. Samaan NA, Anderson GD, Adam-Mayne ME: Immunoreactive calcitonin in the mother, neonate, child and adult. Am J Obstet Gynecol 121:622, 1975.

123. Birge SJ, Avioli LV: Glucagon-induced hypocalcemia in man. J Clin Endocrinol 29:213, 1969.

124. Connelly JP, Crawford JD, Watson J: Studies of neonatal hyperphosphatemia. Pediatrics 43:425, 1962.

125. Anast CS: Serum magnesium levels in the newborn. Pediatrics 33:969, 1964.

126. Atkinson SA, Raddle IC, Anderson GH: Macromineral balances in premature infants fed their own mothers' milk or formula. J Pediatr 102:99, 1983.

127. Carella MJ, Gossain VV: Hyperparathyroidism and pregnancy: Case report and review. J Gen Intern Med 7:448, 1992.

128. Kristoffersson A, Dahlgren S, Lithner F, et al: Primary hyperparathyroidism in pregnancy. Surgery 97:326, 1985.

129. Lowe DK, Orwoll ES, McClung MR, et al: Hyperparathyroidism and pregnancy. Am J Surg 145:611, 1983.

130. Lueg MC, Dawkins WE: Primary hyperparathyroidism and pregnancy. South Med J 76:1389, 1983.

131. Loughead JL, Mughal Z, Mimouni F, et al: Spectrum and natural history of congenital hyperparathyroidism secondary to maternal hypocalcaemia. American J Perinatol 7:350, 1990.

132. Sadeghi-Nejad A, Wolfsdorf JI, Senior B: Hypoparathyroidism and pregnancy. JAMA 243:254, 1980.

133. Glass EJ, Barr DGD: Transient neonatal hyperparathyroidism secondary to maternal pseudohypoparathyroidism. Arch Dis Child 56:565, 1981.

134. Cruikshank DP, Pitkin RM, Varner MW, et al: Calcium metabolism in diabetic mother, fetus and newborn infant. Am J Obstet Gynecol 145:1010, 1983.

135. Noguchi A, Eren M, Tsang R: Parathyroid hormone in hypocalcemia and normocalcemic infants of diabetic mothers. J Pediatr 97:112, 1980.

136. Salle B, David L, Glorieux FH, et al: Hypocalcemia in infants of diabetic mothers. Studies in circulating calcitropic hormone concentrations. Acta Paediatr Scand 71:573, 1982.

137. Steichen JJ, Tsang RC, Ho M, et al: 1,25(OH)$_2$ vitamin D (1,25[OH]$_2$D) and incidence of hypocalcemia in infants of diabetic mothers (IDM) in relation to prospective randomized treatment during pregnancy. Pediatr Res 15:683A, 1981.

138. Tsang RC, Kleinman LI, Sutherland JM, et al: Hypocalcemia in infants of diabetic mothers. Studies in calcium, phosphorus, and magnesium metabolism and parathormone responses. J Pediatr 80:384, 1972.

139. Tsang RC, Chen IW, Friedman MA, et al: Parathyroid function in infants of diabetic mothers. J Pediatr 86:399, 1975.

140. Tsang RC, Chen I, Hayes W, et al: Neonatal hypocalcemia in infants with birth asphyxia. J Pediatr 84:428, 1974.

141. Rösli A, Fanconi A: Neonatal hypocalcemia. "Early type" in low birth weight newborns. Helv Paediatr 28:443, 1973.

142. Tsang RC, Light IJ, Sutherland JM, et al: Possible pathogenetic factors in neonatal hypocalcemia of prematurity. The role of gestation, hyperphosphatemia, hypomagnesemia, urinary calcium losses, and parathormone responsiveness. J Pediatr 82:423, 1973.

143. Brown DR, Steranka BH, Taylor FH: Treatment of early-onset neonatal hypocalcemia. Am J Dis Child 135:24, 1981.

144. Brown DR, Tsang RC, Chen IW: Oral calcium supplementation in premature and asphyxiated neonates. J Pediatr 89:973, 1976.

145. Rosen JF, Roginsky M, Nathenson G, Finberg L: 25-Hydroxyvitamin D: Plasma levels in mothers and their premature infants with neonatal hypocalcemia. Am J Dis Child 127:220, 1974.

146. Chan GM, Tsang RC, Chen IW, et al: The effects of 1,25(OH)$_2$ vitamin D supplementation in premature infants. J Pediatr 93:91, 1978.

147. Fleischman AR, Rosen JF, Nathenson G: 25-Hydroxycholecalciferol for early neonatal hypocalcemia: Occurrence in premature newborns. Am J Dis Child 132:973, 1978.

148. Nervez CT, Shott RJ, Bergstrom WH, et al: Prophylaxis against hypocalcemia in low-birth-weight infants requiring bicarbonate infusion. J Pediatr 87:439, 1975.

149. Linerelli LG, Bobik C, Bobik J: Urinary cAMP and renal responsiveness to parathyroid hormone in premature hypocalcemic infants. Pediatr Res 7:329A, 1973.

150. Moya M, Domenech E: Calcium intake in the first five days of life in the low birthweight infant. Effect of calcium supplements. Arch Dis Child 52:784, 1978.

151. Nelson N, Finnström O. Blood exchange transfusions in newborns, the effect on serum ionized calcium. Early Hum Dev 18:157, 1988.

152. Salle BL, David L, Chopard JP, et al: Prevention of early neonatal hypocalcemia in low birth weight infants with continuous calcium infusion: Effect on serum calcium, phosphorus, magnesium, and circulating immunoreactive parathyroid hormone and calcitonin. Pediatr Res 11:1180, 1977.

153. Brown DR, Salsburey DJ: Short-term biochemical effects of parenteral calcium treatment of early-onset neonatal hypocalcemia. J Pediatr 100:777, 1982.

154. Troughton O, Singh SP: Heart failure and neonatal hypocalcemia. BMJ 4:76, 1972.

155. Hammerman C, Eidelman AI, Gartner LM: Hypocalcemia and the patent ductus arteriosus. J Pediatr 94:961, 1979.

156. Mirror R, Brown DR: Parenteral calcium treatment shortens the left ventricular systolic time intervals of hypocalcemic neonates. Pediatr Res 18:71, 1984.

157. Salsburey DJ, Brown DR: Effect of parenteral calcium treatment on blood pressure and heart rate in neonatal hypocalcemia. Pediatrics 69:605, 1982.

158. Venkataraman PS, Wilson DA, Sheldon RE, et al: Effect of hypocalcemia on cardiac function in very-low-birth-weight preterm neonates: Studies of blood ionized calcium, echocardiography, and cardiac effect of intravenous calcium therapy. Pediatrics 76:543, 1985.

159. Willis DM, Chabot J, Radde IC, et al: Unsuspected hyperosmolality of oral solutions contributing to necrotizing enterocolitis in very-low-birth-weight infants. Pediatrics 60:535, 1977.

160. Book LS, Herbst JJ, Stewart D: Hazards of calcium gluconate therapy in the newborn infant: Intra-arterial injection producing intestinal necrosis in rabbit ileum. J Pediatrics 92:793, 1978.

161. Dunham B, Marcuard S, Khazanie PG, et al: The solubility of calcium and phosphorus in neonatal total parenteral nutrition solutions. J Parenter Enteral Nutri 15:608, 1991.

162. Greer FR: Calcium, phosphorus and vitamin D requirements and TPN regimens in low-birth-weight infants. In Proceedings of the Abbott Conference on Parenteral Nutrition in the Pediatric Patient. North Chicago, Abbott Laboratories, 1983, pp 111-114.

163. Hillman LS, Haddad JG: Perinatal vitamin D metabolism: II. Serial 25-hydroxyvitamin D concentrations in sera of term and premature infants. J Pediatr 86:928, 1975.

164. Kooh SW, Fraser D, Toon R, et al: Response of protracted neonatal hypocalcemia to 1α-dihydroxyvitamin D. Lancet 2:1105, 1976.

165. Lin CY, Ishida M: Calcium homeostasis in premature infants and treatment of early hypocalcaemia by 1,25-dihydroxycholecalciferol. Eur J Pediatr 146:383, 1987.

166. Salle BL, David L, Glorieux FH, et al: Early oral administration of vitamin D and its metabolites in premature neonates. Effect on mineral homeostasis. Pediatr Res 16:75, 1982.

167. Barak Y, Milbauer B, Weisman Y, et al: Response of neonatal hypocalcemia to 1α-hydroxyvitamin D. Arch Dis Child 54:642, 1979.

168. Petersen S, Christensen NC, Fogh-Andersen N: Effect on serum calcium of 1α-hydroxyvitamin D supplementation in infants of low birth weight, infants with perinatal asphyxia, and infants of diabetic mothers. Acta Paediatr Scand 70:897, 1981.

169. Edelman L, Pandita RK, Spriteri E, et al: A common molecular basis for rearrangement disorders on chromosome 22q11. Hum Molec Genet 8:1157, 1999.

170. Goodship J, Cross I, LiLing J, Wren C: A population study of chromosome 22q11 deletions in infancy. Arch Dis Child 79:348, 1998.

171. Stevens CA, Carey JC, Shigeoka AO: DiGeorge anomaly and velocardiofacial syndrome. Pediatrics 85:526, 1990.

172. Ross AJ III, Cooper A, Attie MF, et al: Primary hyperparathyroidism in infancy. J Pediatr Surg 21:493, 1986.

173. Hendy GN, D'Souza-Li L, Yang B, et al: Mutations of the calcium-sensing receptor (CASR) in familial hypocalciuric hypercalcemia, neonatal severe hyperparathyroidism, and autosomal dominant hypocalcemia. Hum Mutat 16:281, 2000.

174. Venkataraman PS, Tsang RC, Greer FR, et al: Late infantile tetany and secondary hyperparathyroidism in infants fed humanized cow milk formula. Am J Dis Child 139:664, 1985.

175. Romagnoli C, Polidori G, Cataldi L, et al: Phototherapy-induced hypocalcemia. J Pediatr 94:815, 1979.

176. Hakanson DO, Bergstrom WH: Phototherapy-induced hypocalcemia in newborn rats: Prevention by melatonin. Science 214:807, 1981.

177. Brown JK, Cockburn F, Forfar JO: Clinical and chemical correlates in convulsions of the newborn. Lancet 1:135, 1972.

178. Cockburn F, Brown JK, Belton NR, et al: Neonatal convulsions associated with primary disturbance of calcium, phosphorus, and magnesium metabolism. Arch Dis Child 48:99, 1973.

179. Paunier L, Radde IC, Kooh SW, et al: Primary hypomagnesemia with secondary hypocalcemia in an infant. Pediatrics 41:385, 1968.

180. Kimura S, Nose O, Seino Y, et al: Effects of alternate and simultaneous administrations of calcium and phosphorus on calcium metabolism in children receiving total parenteral nutrition. J Parenter Enteral Nutr 10:513, 1986.

181. Greenberg F: Williams syndrome. Pediatrics 84:922, 1989.

182. Fraser D, Kidd BSL, Kooh SW, et al: A new look at infantile hypercalcemia. Pediatr Clin North Am 13:503, 1966.

183. Harrison HE, Harrison HC: Hypercalcemic states. In: Disorders of Calcium and Phosphate Metabolism in Childhood and Adolescence. Philadelphia, WB Saunders, 1979, pp 100-140.

184. Smith DW, Blizzard RM, Harrison HE: Idiopathic hypercalcemia. A case report with assays of vitamin D in the serum. Pediatrics 24:258, 1959.

185. Aarskog D, Aksnes L, Markestad T: Vitamin D metabolism in idiopathic infantile hypercalcemia. Am J Dis Child 135:1021, 1981.

186. Fanconi G, Giradet P, Schlesinger B, et al: Chronische Hypercalcämie, lobiniert mit Osteosklerose, hyperazotamie, Minderwuchs und kongenitalen Missbildungen. Helv Paediatr Acta 4:314, 1952.

187. Williams JCP, Barratt-Boyes BD, Lowe JB: Supravalvular aortic stenosis. Circulation 24:1311, 1961.

188. Black JA, Carter REB: Association between aortic stenosis and facies of severe infantile hypercalcemia. Lancet 2:745, 1963.

189. Jones KL, Smith DW: The Williams elfin facies syndrome: A new perspective. J Pediatr 86:718, 1975.

190. Hovels O, Stephan U: Das Krankheitsbild der "idiopathischen" Hypercalcämie, eine chronische Vitamin D-Intoxication. Ergebn in Med Kinderheilk 18:383, 1962.

191. Fellers FX, Schwartz R: Etiology of the severe form of idiopathic hypercalcemia in infancy. N Engl J Med 259:1050, 1958.

192. Friedman WF, Roberts WC: Vitamin D and the supravalvular aortic stenosis syndrome: The transplacental effects of vitamin D on the aorta of the rabbit. Circulation 34:77, 1966.

193. Beuren AJ, Schulze C, Eberle P, et al: Syndrome of supravalvular aortic stenosis, peripheral pulmonary stenosis, mental retardation and similar facial appearance. Am J Cardiol 13:471, 1964.

194. Taylor AB, Stern PH, Bell NH: Abnormal regulation of circulating 25-hydroxyvitamin D in the Williams syndrome. N Engl J Med 306:972, 1982.

195. Garabédian M, Jacqz E, Guillozo H, et al: Elevated plasma 1,25-dihydroxyvitamin D concentrations in infants with hypercalcemia and an elfin facies. N Engl J Med 312:948, 1985.

196. Culler FL, Jones KL, Deftos LJ: Impaired calcitonin secretion in patients with Williams syndrome. J Pediatr 107:720, 1985.

197. Knudtzon L, Aksnes L, Akslen LA, et al: Elevated 1,25-dihydroxyvitamin D and normocalcaemia in presumed familial Williams syndrome. Clin Genet 32:369, 1987.

198. Kruse K, Pankau R, Gosch A, et al: Calcium metabolism in Williams-Beuren syndrome. J Pediatr 121:902, 1992.

199. McAleer JK, Mercer RD: Subcutaneous fat necrosis with calcifications and hypercalcemia in an infant. Cleveland Clin Q 31:179, 1964.

200. Michael AF, Hong R, West CD: Hypercalcemia in infancy: Association with subcutaneous fat necrosis and calcification. Am J Dis Child 104:235, 1962.

201. Norwood-Galloway A, Lebwohl M, Phelps RG, et al: Subcutaneous fat necrosis of the newborn with hypercalcemia. J Am Acad Dermatol 16:435, 1987.

202. Sharlin DN, Koblenzer P: Necrosis of subcutaneous fat with hypercalcemia. A puzzling and multifaceted disease. Clin Pediatr 9:290, 1970.

203. Veldhuis JD, Kulin HE, Demers LM, et al: Infantile hypercalcemia with subcutaneous fat necrosis: Endocrine studies. J Pediatr 95:460, 1979.

204. Metz SA, Hassal E: PGE, hypercalcemia and subcutaneous fat necrosis. J Pediatr 97:336, 1980.

205. Cook JS, Stone MS, Hansen JR: Hypercalcemia in association with subcutaneous fat necrosis of the newborn: Studies of calcium-regulating hormones. Pediatrics 90:93, 1992.

206. Finne PH, Sanderud J, Aksnes L, et al: Hypercalcemia with increased and unregulated 1,25-dihydroxyvitamin D production in a neonate with subcutaneous fat necrosis. J Pediatr 112:792, 1988.

207. Kruse K, Irle U, Uhlig R: Elevated 1,25-dihydroxyvitamin D serum concentrations in infants with subcutaneous fat necrosis. J Pediatr 122:460, 1993.

208. Greer FR, Steichen JJ, Tsang RC: Calcium and phosphate supplements in breast milk-related rickets. Am J Dis Child 136:581, 1982.

209. Keipert JA: Rickets with multiple fractured ribs in a premature infant. Med J Aust 1:672, 1970.

210. Koo WWK, Antony G, Stevens HS: Continuous nasogastric phosphorus infusion in hypophosphatemic rickets of prematurity. Am J Dis Child 138:172, 1984.

211. Rowe J, Wood DH, Rowe DW, et al: Nutritional hypophosphatemic rickets in a premature infant fed breast milk. N Engl J Med 300:293, 1979.

212. Sagy M, Birenbaum E, Balin A, et al: Phosphate-depletion syndrome in a premature infant fed human milk. J Pediatr 96:683, 1980.

213. Lyon AJ, McIntosh N, Wheeler K, et al: Hypercalcaemia in extremely low birthweight infants. Arch Dis Child 59:1141, 1984.

214. Miller RR, Menke JA, Mentser MI: Hypercalcemia associated with phosphate depletion in the neonate. J Pediatr 105:814, 1984.

215. Rousseau-Merck MF, Nogues C, Roth A, et al: Hypercalcemic infantile renal tumors: Morphological, clinical, and biological heterogeneity. Pediatr Pathol 3:155, 1985.

216. Whyte MP: Hypophosphatasia. In Scriver CR, Beaudet AL, Sly WS, et al (eds): The Metabolic Basis of Inherited Disease, 6th ed. New York, McGraw-Hill, 1989, pp 2843-2856.

217. Charrow J, Poznanski AK: The Jansen type of metaphyseal chondrodysplasia: Confirmation of dominant inheritance and review of radiographic manifestations in the newborn adult. Am J Med Genet 18:321, 1984.

218. Silverthorn KG, Houston CS, Duncan BP: Murk Jansen's metaphysical chondrodysplasia with long-term follow-up. Pediatr Radiol 17:119, 1987.

219. Marx SJ, Spiegel AM, Levine MA, et al: Familial hypocalciuric hypercalcemia: The relation to primary parathyroid hyperplasia. N Engl J Med 307:416, 1982.

220. Marx SJ, Attie MF, Spiegel AM, et al: An association between neonatal severe primary hyperparathyroidism and familial hypocalciuric hypercalcemia in three kindreds. N Engl J Med 306:257, 1982.

221. Callenbach JC, Sheehan MB, Abramson SJ, Hall RT: Etiologic factors of rickets in very low-birth-weight infants. J Pediatr 98:800, 1981.

222. Evans JR, Allen AC, Stinson DA, et al: Effect of high-dose vitamin D supplementation on radiographically detectable bone disease of very low birth weight infants. J Pediatr 115:779, 1989.

223. Koo WWK, Sherman R, Succop P, et al: Sequential bone mineral content in small preterm infants with and without fractures and rickets. J Bone Miner Res 3:193, 1988.

224. Lyon AJ, McIntosh N, Wheeler K, Williams JE: Radiological rickets in extremely low birthweight infants. Pediatr Radiol 17:56, 1987.

225. Masel JP, Tudehope D, Cartwright D, Cleghorn D: Osteopenia and rickets in the extremely low birth-weight infants. Australas Radiol 1:83, 1982.

226. Greer FR, McCormick A: Improved bone mineralization and growth in premature infants fed fortified own mother's milk. J Pediatr 112:961, 1988.

227. Griscom NT, Craig MN, Neuhauser EBF: Systemic bone disease developing in small premature infants. Pediatrics 48:883, 1971.

228. Oppenheimer SJ, Snodgrass GJAI: Neonatal rickets. Arch Dis Child 55:945, 1980.

229. Ziegler EE, Biga RL, Fomon SJ: Nutritional requirements of the premature infant. In Suskind RM (ed): Textbook of Pediatric Nutrition. New York, Raven, 1981, pp 29-39.

230. Frost HM: Perspectives: A proposed general model of the "mechanostat" (suggestions from a new paradigm). Anat Rec 244:139, 1996.

231. Miller ME: The bone disease of preterm birth; a biomechanical perspective. Pediatr Res 53:10, 2003.

232. Rauch F, Schoenau E: Skeletal development in premature infants; a review of bone physiology beyond nutritional aspects. Arch Dis Child Fetal Neonatal Ed 86:F82, 2002.

233. Beyers N, Alhert B, Taijaard JF, et al: High turnover osteopenia in preterm infants. Bone 15:5, 1994.

234. Greer FR, Chen X, McCormick A: Urinary hydroxyproline: Relationship to growth bone mineral content, and serum alkaline phosphatase in premature infants. J Pediatr Gastroenterol Nutr 13:176, 1991.

235. Mora S, Weber G, Bellini A, et al: Bone modeling alteration in preterm infants. Arch Pediatr Adolesc Med 148:1215, 1994.

236. Moyer-Mileur L, Luetkemeier M, Boomer L, Chan GM: Effect of physical activity on bone mineralization in premature infants. J Pediatr 127:620, 1995.

237. Moyer-Mileur LJ, Brunstetter V, McNaught TP, et al: Daily physical activity program increases bone mineralization and growth in preterm very low birth weight infants. Pediatrics 106:1088, 2000.

238. Nemet D, Dolfin T, Litmanowitz I, et al: Evidence for exercise-induced bone formation in premature infants. Int J Sports Med 23:82, 2002.

239. Backstrom MC, Mäki R, Kuusela A-L, et al: Randomized controlled trial of vitamin D supplementation on bone density and biochemical indices in preterm infants. Arch Dis Child Fetal Neonatal Ed 80:F161, 1999.

240. Koo WWK, Sherman R, Succop P, et al: Serum vitamin D metabolites in very low birthweight infants with and without rickets and fractures. J Pediatr 114:1017, 1989.

241. Mazess RB, Peppler WW, Chesney RW, et al: Does bone measurement of the radius indicate skeletal status? J Nucl Med 25:281, 1984.

242. Chesney RW: The assessment of bone mineral status and mineral dietary adequacy. In Tsang RC, Mimouni F (eds): Calcium Nutriture for Mothers and Children. Carnation Nutrition Educational Series, vol 3. New York, Glendale/Raven, 1992, pp 101-128.

243. Nemet D, Dolfin T, Wolach B, Eliakim A: Quantitative ultrasound measurements of bone speed of sound in premature infants. Eur J Pediatr 160:736, 2001.

244. Schanler RJ, Burns PA, Abrams SA, Garza C: Bone mineralization outcomes in human milk-fed preterm infants. Pediatr Res 31:583, 1992.

245. American Academy of Pediatrics Committee on Nutrition: Pediatric Nutrition Handbook, 5th ed. Elk Grove Village, IL, American Academy of Pediatrics, 2003.

246. Koo WWK, Tsang RC, Succop P, et al: Minimal vitamin D and high calcium and phosphorus needs of preterm infants receiving parenteral nutrition. J Pediatr Gastroenterol Nutr 8:225, 1989.

247. Shike M, Sturtridge MW, Tam CS, et al: A possible role of vitamin D in the genesis of parenteral-nutrition–induced metabolic bone disease. Ann Intern Med 95:560, 1981.

248. Horsman A, Ryan SW, Congdon PJ, et al: Bone mineral content and body size 65 to 100 weeks postconception in preterm and full term infants. Arch Dis Child 64:1579, 1989.

249. Chan GM, Mileur LJ: Posthospitalization growth and bone mineral status of normal preterm infants. Feeding with mother's milk or standard formula. Am J Dis Child 139:896, 1985.

250. Abrams SA, Schanler R, Garza C: Bone mineralization in former very low birth weight infants fed either human milk or commercial formula. J Pediatr 112:956, 1988.

CHAPTER 76

Inborn Errors of Metabolism Manifesting as Catastrophic Disease

Irma Payan, Jaya Ganesh, and Marc Yudkoff

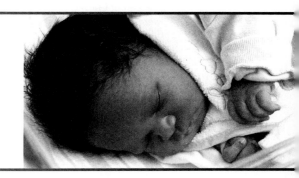

Many inborn errors of metabolism manifest clinically as fulminant neurologic syndromes during the neonatal period. Prompt diagnosis is important in order to institute specific therapy and thereby prevent irreparable brain damage. Thus, familiarity with the clinical features of the inborn errors of metabolism has become a mainstay of contemporary neonatology.

This chapter describes inherited defects that cause a major disturbance of intermediary metabolism in the neonate. The biochemical derangements commonly impair function of many organs, especially the central nervous system. Salient clinical features of metabolic disease of the neonate are summarized in Box 76-1. An individual patient may not manifest each of these symptoms and signs, but the presence of one or more of these indicators should prompt diagnostic consideration of an inborn error of metabolism.

As indicated in Box 76-2, the disorders of intermediary metabolism include (1) the organic acidurias; (2) the primary lactic acidoses; (3) the urea cycle defects; (4) the disturbances of carbohydrate metabolism; (5) the aminoacidurias, and (6) the fatty acid oxidation defects. The usual cause of these diseases is the lack of an enzyme that is needed to oxidize an amino acid, organic acid, carbohydrate, or fatty acid. Infants with a urea cycle defect are capable of normal oxidative metabolism, but they fail to dispose of ammonia, the major nitrogenous product of amino acid oxidation. The enzyme deficiency causes the accumulation of an otherwise innocuous metabolite, such as ammonia or an organic acid, to a toxic level.

Disorders of intermediary metabolism are biochemically heterogeneous, but many share common clinical features (see Box 76-1).[1-4] The antenatal course is typically unremarkable. Neither parents nor physicians have any premonition of the calamity that ensues shortly after birth. By age 24 to 48 hours, the infant begins to spit up and displays generalized irritability. Soon lethargy, lapses of consciousness, and even frank coma may occur. The infant manifests a profound hypotonia that may be punctuated by frequent convulsions. Signs of increased intracranial pressure are not uncommon. In some of the organic acidurias (see

following section), unusual urinary odors are detected. Hepatic failure, commonly of an overwhelming degree, is characteristic of galactosemia and some disorders of fatty acid oxidation. Peripheral myopathy and cardiac failure characterize many disorders of fatty acid oxidation and primary lactic acidoses. Unless a diagnosis is made quickly and appropriate treatment is implemented, many affected infants progress to respiratory failure and require ventilatory support. The price of survival in many of these youngsters, particularly those who languish in a coma for an extended period, is permanent brain injury and mental retardation.

Routine laboratory studies may disclose various biochemical anomalies, including hypoglycemia, hyperammonemia, and an "anionic gap" metabolic acidosis (see following section). Thrombocytopenia and leukopenia are not unusual. Evidence of pancreatitis is reflected in elevated blood amylase and lipase activities. Increased activity of serum creatine phosphokinase (CPK) denotes the myopathy of fatty acid oxidation defects. Elevated hepatic transaminase activities occur in biochemical lesions of the urea cycle or the pathways of fatty acid oxidation.

Any acute, life-threatening disease in a neonate invites consideration of septicemia as a diagnostic possibility. Many of these infants receive antibiotics before the metabolic disease is appreciated. A fundamental disturbance of body biochemistry should be suggested by the failure to respond to antibiotic therapy and the absence of pathogens in cultures of the blood, urine, or cerebrospinal fluid (CSF).

The initial diagnostic assessment should include the following:

1. serum electrolytes
2. blood pH and carbon dioxide tension
3. blood lactate and pyruvate
4. urine organic acid quantitation
5. blood ammonia
6. blood amino acid quantitation
7. urine ketone testing
8. complete blood cell count

Box 76–1   Common Features of Metabolic Disease in the Neonate

Historical Features

Consanguinity
Membership in ethnic group with high frequency for particular gene
Clinical decompensation associated with infection and/or brief fasting
History of unexplained death or death from vague cause in prior infant

Physical Findings

Lethargy and coma
Recurrent vomiting
Tachypnea unrelated to pulmonary disease
Marked hypotonia
Seizures
Dysmorphism
Ocular findings: cataracts, optic atrophy, retinopathy, and/or pallor of optic disk
Visceromegaly
Dermatologic findings: friable hair shaft, ichthyosis, exfoliative dermatitis
Bizarre odors of the urine and/or breath
Unstable body temperature
Cardiac failure

Laboratory Findings

Hypoglycemia
Metabolic acidosis, often with increased anionic gap
Lactic acidosis
Hyperammonemia
Leukopenia
Thrombocytopenia
Ketoaciduria
Abnormal elevations in one or more amino acids and/or organic acids
Markedly abnormal electroencephalographic patterns, often with burst-suppression or hypsarrhythmia
Positive finding of urine-reducing substance
Rhabdomyolysis, with elevated creatine phosphokinase, or myoglobinuria

---

9. urine Clinitest reaction (while infant is fed a lactose-containing formula)
10. liver and pancreatic function tests
11. ophthalmologic examination with a slit lamp
12. urine orotic acid quantitation if the blood ammonia concentration is elevated
13. electrocardiography
14. serum CPK determination
15. electroencephalography
16. magnetic resonance imaging of the brain
17. blood acyl carnitine analysis

Most of these laboratory tests are available at major medical centers.

The results of this initial testing will allow assignment of the infant to one of the six major classifications summarized in Box 76-2. Diagnosis of a specific enzyme deficiency usually requires consultation by a specialist and access to appropriate laboratory services.

THE ORGANIC ACIDURIAS

Biochemical and Clinical Findings

Most organic acids are derived from the intermediary metabolism of glucose, fatty acids, and amino acids (Fig. 76-1). The oxidation of these three nutrients does not proceed directly to completion. Instead, these nutrients enter into complex metabolic pathways that yield organic acids as intermediates before the final production of CO_2 and H_2O.

The most significant organic acidurias in neonatal practice are maple syrup urine disease (MSUD), isovaleric acidemia, propionic acidemia, and methylmalonic acidemia, each of which corresponds to a defect in the oxidation of the branched-chain amino acids: leucine, isoleucine, and valine (Fig. 76-2).[5-10]

Clinicians can infer the presence of an organic aciduria from inspection of the routine chemistry profile (Table 76-1). Blood has no net electrical charge; therefore, the sums of the cations and anions must be equal. The cationic composition of blood is relatively straightforward, being composed almost entirely of Na^+ and K^+. The anionic composition is more varied; over 90% of the total is derived from Cl^- and HCO_3^- and the remainder from phosphate, sulfate, the negative charges on the surfaces of blood proteins, and the organic acids (carboxylate anions). The conventional analysis of blood electrolytes normally indicates that the positive charges ($Na^+ + K^+ = 145$ mEq/L) are about equal to the negative charges ($Cl^- + HCO_3^- = $ approximately 130 mEq/L). Thus, the "missing" component of negative charges, or "delta," should amount to no more than 10 to 15 mEq/L, to which the

Box 76–2   Disorders of Intermediary Metabolism in the Neonate

Organic Acidurias

OXEDATION PROBLEM

Organic Acids Derived from Branched-Chain Amino Acids

Maple syrup urine disease
Isovaleric acidemia   *LEUCENE/ISOLEUCINE/VALENE*
Methylmalonic acidemia
Propionic acidemia
β-Methylcrotonic aciduria
3-Hydroxy-3-methylglutaryl–CoA glutaric aciduria (HMG-CoA lyase deficiency)
Glutaric aciduria (type II)

Primary Lactic Acidoses

Pyruvate dehydrogenase deficiency
Pyruvate carboxylase deficiency
Electron transport-tricarboxylic cycle defects
Disorders of biotin metabolism
Biotinidase deficiency
Holocarboxylase synthetase deficiency

Urea Cycle Defects   *NH4 PROBLEM*

Carbamoyl phosphate synthetase deficiency
Ornithine transcarbamylase deficiency
Citrullinemia (argininosuccinate synthetase deficiency)
Argininosuccinic aciduria (argininosuccinate lyase deficiency)
Argininemia (arginase deficiency) (usually not present in newborn)

Disorders of Carbohydrate Metabolism

Galactose-1-phosphate uridyl transferase deficiency (galactosemia)

Disorders of Amino Acid Metabolism

Nonketotic hyperglycinemia (glycine cleavage system deficiency)
Maple syrup urine disease (also under Organic Acidurias)

Fatty Acid Oxidation Defects

Carnitine palmitoyl transferase II (CPT-1) deficiency
Carnitine palmitoyl transferase I (CPT-2) deficiency
Carnitine acyl-CoA translocase deficiency
Medium-chain acyl-CoA dehydrogenase deficiency
Long-chain acyl-CoA dehydrogenase (LCAD) deficiency
Very-long-chain acyl-CoA dehydrogenase (VLCAD) deficiency
Very-long-chain hydroxyacyl-CoA dehydrogenase (VLCHAD) deficiency

CoA, coenzyme A.

organic acids contribute relatively little (≈ 2 mEq/L). However, if the organic acid compartment expands, an "anionic gap" develops that is reflected in a "delta" of as much as 20 mEq/L or more of negative charges (see Table 76-1). The absence of an anionic gap does not rule out the possibility of an organic aciduria, but the presence of this biochemical finding affords strong presumptive evidence to favor this diagnosis.

The diagnosis of an **organic aciduria** also is suggested by a persistent ketoaciduria. In contrast to older infants and children, who commonly become ketotic even after a relatively brief period of fasting, marked ketosis in the neonate is unusual. Newborns feed frequently (every 2 to 4 hours), thereby minimizing the ketogenic stimulus. Sick neonates often receive intravenous glucose, which

also blunts ketogenesis. Finally, neonates avidly consume β-hydroxybutyrate and acetoacetate. However, high concentrations of certain organic acids inhibit the oxidation of ketone bodies. Thus, the presence of ketoaciduria in a critically ill neonate always should prompt a diligent search for an organic aciduria.

Untoward accumulations of organic acids inhibit not only ketogenesis but also gluconeogenesis and ureagenesis. Hence, hypoglycemia and hyperammonemia may accompany any of the organic acidurias. Similarly, the organic acids tend to arrest the maturation of hematopoietic precursors, and both thrombocytopenia and leukopenia can occur in these disorders (Table 76-2). Clinical findings in the organic acidurias resemble those of the other disorders of intermediary metabolism.[11]

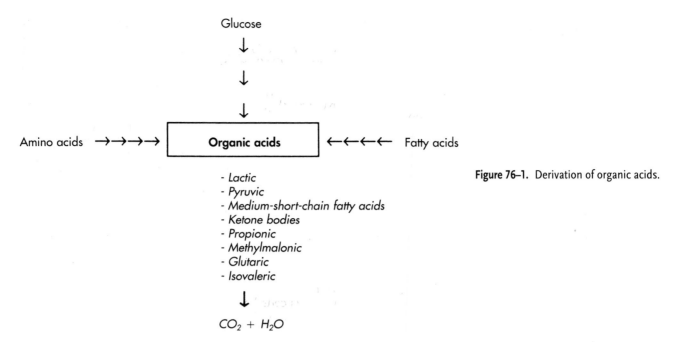

Figure 76–1. Derivation of organic acids.

Infants display a dramatic and rapid clinical decompensation for no apparent reason. The first diagnostic impression is usually septicemia, a conclusion that seems compatible with some of the laboratory data, such as the hypoglycemia, leukopenia, and thrombocytopenia.

An unusual feature is the remarkable odor that the volatile organic acids impart to body fluids (Table 76-3). This finding accounts for the rather piquant names given to several of these disorders, for example, the "sweaty socks odor" of isovaleric acidemia. The diagnostic importance of unusual odors cannot be overstressed, and for many affected infants, parents or nursing personnel have appreciated this bizarre symptom long before physicians attended to it.

Primary Lactic Acidoses

Lactate is the major organic acid of the blood, and the primary lactic acidoses are a subset of the organic acidurias. They are considered separately here, to emphasize the need to conceptualize them as a single disease entity.[12]

Both lactic and pyruvic acids are derived from glucose via glycolysis:

$$glucose \rightarrow \rightarrow \rightarrow pyruvate$$

$$pyruvate + NADH \rightarrow lactate + NAD^- + H^+$$

where NAD is nicotinamide adenine dinucleotide and NADH is the reduced form of NAD. Lactic acidosis usually occurs secondary to hypoxia, because the lack of oxygen

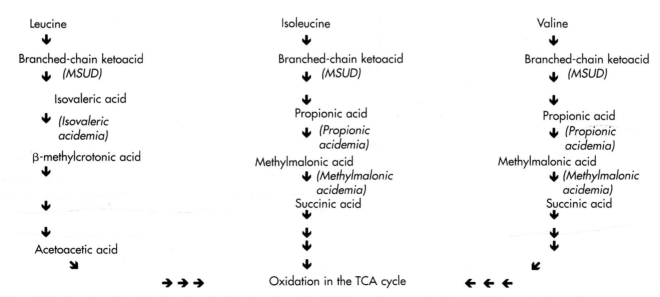

Figure 76–2. Organic acids arising from branched-chain amino acids. MSUD, maple syrup urine disease; TCA, tricarboxylic acid.

Table 76–1. Ionic Composition of the Blood

Type of Ion	Normal	Organic Aciduria
Anions (mEq/L)		
Component		
Chloride	101	90
Bicarbonate	25	10
Phosphate	3	3
Sulfate	1	1
Proteins	2	2
Sum	132	116
"Delta"*	13	29
Organic acids	2	12
Cations (mEq/L)		
Component		
Sodium	140	140
Potassium	5	5
Sum	145	145

*The "missing" component of negative charges.

prevents reoxidation of NADH to NAD in the electron transport chain:

$$NADH + O_2 \rightarrow \rightarrow \rightarrow NAD + H_2O$$

As a consequence, lactate cannot be reconverted to pyruvate at the same rate it is formed, and a lactic acidosis develops.

In the primary lactic acidoses, the concentration of oxygen is normal, but there is a congenital deficiency of one of the following (Fig. 76-3): (1) the pyruvate dehydrogenase (PDH) reaction, which mediates the conversion of pyruvate to acetyl coenzyme A (CoA) and CO_2; (2) the pyruvate carboxylase (PC) reaction, a biotin-dependent pathway that involves the carboxylation of pyruvate (fixation of bicarbonate) to yield oxaloacetate, a gluconeogenic precursor; (3) a fundamental defect in the electron transport chain that results in impaired tricarboxylic acid cycle function and an accumulation of acetyl CoA, which inhibits flux through the PDH pathway; or (4) a defect in the metabolism of biotin, a necessary cofactor for the PC reaction.

A relatively common inherited cause of primary lactic acidosis in neonates is a defect of the PDH pathway, a thiamine- and lipoic acid–dependent complex that is composed of a large number of individual peptides, most of which are inherited in an autosomal recessive manner, with the important exception of the E_1-α subunit of PDH, which is coded on the X chromosome.

Primary defects of the electron transport chain may become apparent during the neonatal period. Many of the peptides constituting the electron transport chain are coded on mitochondrial DNA, and their inheritance therefore conforms to a mitochondrial pattern.

Primary defects of the PC apoenzyme have been described in neonates, but such cases are exceedingly rare. A more common cause of PC deficiency is a deficiency of biotinidase, the enzyme that activates the vitamin biotin,

Table 76–2. Summary of Major Findings

Finding	Organic Acidurias	Primary Lactic Acidoses	Urea Cycle Defects	Classical Galactosemia	Nonketotic Hyperglycinemia	Fatty Acid Oxidation Defects
Metabolic acidosis	Frequent	Frequent	No	No	No	Variable
Ketoaciduria	Frequent	Variable	No	No	No	No
Urine organic acids	Abnormal	Increased lactate	Normal	Nondiagnostic	Normal	Increased dicarboxylics
Lactic acidosis	No	Frequent	No	No	No	Not initially
Hyperammonemia	Usually <500 µmol/L	Usually <500 µmol/L	Usually >500 µmol/L	No	No	Possible
Blood aminogram	Nondiagnostic	Increased alanine	Very abnormal*	Nondiagnostic	Marked glycine	Nondiagnostic
CSF aminogram	Nondiagnostic	Increased alanine	Very abnormal*	Nondiagnostic	Marked glycine	Nondiagnostic
Urine orotic acid	Usually normal	Normal	Very high†	Normal	Normal	Normal
Neutropenia	Frequent	Variable	Unusual	No	No	No
Thrombocytopenia	Frequent	Variable	Unusual	No	No	No
Urine Clinitest	Negative	Negative	Negative	Positive	Negative	Negative
Hepatic failure	No	Uncommon	No	Frequent	No	Frequent
Cataracts	No	No	No	Frequent‡	No	No
Cardiac disease	No	Variable	No	No	No	Frequent
Rhabdomyolysis	No	Variable	No	No	No	Frequent
Congenital malformations	Not usually	Variable	No	No	No	Variable

*Often diagnostic in urea cycle defects.

†Major exception: carbamyl phosphate synthetase deficiency, when orotic acid is normal or low.

‡Slit-lamp examination may be required for visualization.

CSF, cerebrospinal Fluid.

Table 76–3. Organic Acidurias that May Cause an Odor in the Neonatal Period

Disorder	Organic Acid	Odor
Isovaleric acidemia	Isovaleric acid	Sweaty socks–rancid cheese
Maple syrup urine disease	Branched-chain ketoacids	Maple syrup or burnt sugar
3-Methylglutaconic aciduria	3-Methylglutaconic acid	Tomcat urine
Propionic acidemia	Propionic acid	Cat urine
Methylmalonic acidemia	Methylmalonic acid	Usually none
Ketoaciduria	Ketone bodies	Fruity
Glutaric aciduria type II	Glutaric, isovaleric, fatty acids	Sweaty socks–rancid cheese

which is an obligatory cofactor for the carboxylation of (1) pyruvate to oxaloacetate, (2) propionate to methylmalonate, and (3) β-methylcrotonate to β-methylglutaconate. Biotin, which is bound to lysine residues on enzymes and other proteins, is normally cleaved from such linkage via the action of biotinidase. A second enzyme, holocarboxylase synthetase, then mediates the attachment of the free biotin to the appropriate apoenzymes. If the level of either biotinidase or holocarboxylase synthetase is congenitally deficient, these processes do not occur, and biotin-dependent reactions do not proceed at a normal rate. The result is a lactic acidosis, as well as the accumulation of derivatives of propionate and β-methylcrotonate.

Patients with a primary lactic acidosis may manifest a clinical course similar to that of the organic acidurias. A syndrome of progressive lethargy, coma, vomiting, and convulsions develops within the first few days of life and progresses to a state of ventilator dependency after a week or two. In addition to the neurologic disarray, patients may show involvement of other organ systems, as indicated in Box 76-3. In virtually no individual case do all of these signs co-occur, but a diligent search for a lactic acidosis should be undertaken whenever an infant manifests a progressive neurologic syndrome coupled with evidence of any of these indicators. Indeed, a primary lactic acidosis should be considered in any infant with a myopathy or cardiomyopathy of indeterminate origin, even in the absence of ostensible neurologic disease.

Treatment of Organic Acidurias and Primary Lactic Acidoses

The single most important therapeutic maneuver is the removal from the diet of those nutrients that serve as precursors to the organic acids.[13-19] Many organic acidurias represent defects in the oxidation of the branched-chain amino acids, and particular care should be taken to avoid exposure to these compounds. A critically ill neonate should not receive parenteral solutions of amino acids until the diagnosis of an organic aciduria is ruled out. This

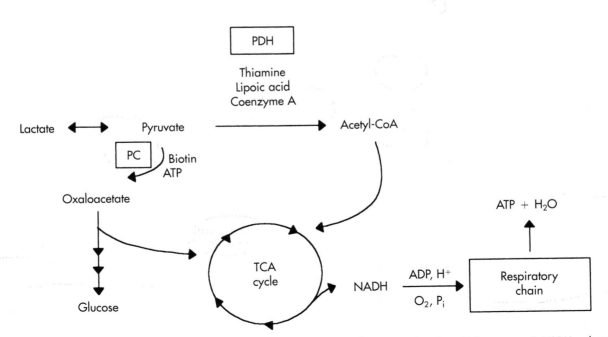

Figure 76–3. Origins of the primary lactic acidoses. ADP, adenosine diphosphate; ATP, adenosine triphosphate; CoA, coenzyme A; NADH, reduced nicotinamide adenine dinucleotide phosphate; PC, pyruvate carboxylase; PDH, pyruvate dehydrogenase; P_i, inorganic phosphate; TCA, tricarboxylic acid.

Box 76–3   **Signs of Primary Lactic Acidosis**

Neurologic

Lethargy, coma, and convulsions, deteriorating to ventilator dependency
Progressive degeneration of the white matter
Structural anomalies, such as agenesis of the corpus callosum
Intracerebral hemorrhage
Sensorineural deafness

Cardiac

Cardiomyopathy
Conduction defects

Renal

Renal tubular acidosis
Progressive glomerular failure

Hepatic

Hepatic failure

Ophthalmologic

Optic atrophy
Retinal degeneration
Ophthalmoplegia

Muscular

Mitochondrial myopathy

Hematologic

Thrombocytopenia
Neutropenia
Megaloblastic anemia

Metabolic

Diabetes mellitus

seemingly obvious point merits special emphasis, because sick infants commonly receive infusions of amino acids in a misguided effort at nutritional rehabilitation.

Fluid should be given in order to promote excretion of toxic organic acids (Table 76-4). These compounds are volatile, but pulmonary elimination is minimal, and renal excretion is the main route of elimination (other than dialysis). Calories in the form of glucose and lipid should be administered (see Table 76-4) to minimize endogenous protein catabolism. The nutritional support of these infants has been enabled by the development of formulas and parenteral amino acid solutions from which the branched-chain amino acids have been omitted.[20] The increased blood concentrations of branched-chain amino acids in patients with MSUD can be reduced considerably by the administration of these parenteral solutions. Finally, alkalinization of the urine by the infusion of bicarbonate (see Table 76-4) promotes formation of the ionized $RCOO^-$ species, which is excreted more efficiently than the un-ionized acid, RCOOH.

On occasion, patients with a primary lactic acidosis respond to a high-fat (ketogenic) diet.[14,21,22] The rationale for this treatment is that lactate and pyruvate are derived almost exclusively from glucose. Minimizing glucose intake to approximately 10% of calories should reduce the production of lactate. Unfortunately, this approach does not always result in clinical improvement. The neurologic deterioration that characterizes most of these diseases may reflect a generalized failure to support a necessary intracellular energy charge in neurons rather than a toxic effect of lactate accumulation. Furthermore, a high-fat diet may introduce complications such as acidemia. Clinicians should carefully monitor patients who receive such therapy.

An important advance has been the development of dialysis procedures for the rapid removal of toxins such as the organic acids and ammonia. Both peritoneal and hemodialysis have been used successfully. This approach should obviously be undertaken only in centers with the requisite expertise, but it may be lifesaving when properly done. The potential complications of dialysis for 3 to 4 days are more than counterbalanced by the benefits of this procedure.

Neonates with isovaleric acidemia should receive supplemental glycine (250 mg/kg/day, orally or intravenously),[23] which favors formation of isovalerylglycine:

$$\text{isovaleryl-CoA} + \text{glycine} \xrightarrow{\text{ATP}} \text{isovalerylglycine}$$

Isovalerylglycine is excreted more efficiently into urine than is free isovaleric acid. There are essentially no ill effects associated with the use of glycine in this dosage.

Some patients with an organic aciduria, such as propionic acidemia or isovaleric acidemia, manifest low serum

Table 76–4. Acute Management of Organic Acidurias

Treatment	Comments
Fluids: 1.5-2 times estimated maintenance rate	Favors excretion of toxin, but be aware of risk of increased intracranial pressure in some infants
Glucose: at least 5-10 mg/kg/min	Minimizes protein catabolism by favoring insulin secretion Be alert to possible hyperglycemia
Alkali: 2-4 mEq/kg/day usually adequate	Keep urine pH at ~8 Alkalinization favors urinary excretion of COO⁻ anion
Calories: at least 120 kcal/day	May combine glucose–lipids–amino acids, but be sure to give no amino acids that are precursors to organic acids
Amino acids: 2 g/kg/day	Administer as a 2% intravenous solution Infant may require special infusion that is free of branched-chain amino acids
Lipids: 3-5 g/kg/day as Intralipid	Be aware that they may not be fully utilized, especially in premature infants
Ketogenic diet: 80%-90% of calories as lipid	For primary lactic acidoses Be alert for possible metabolic acidosis and/or hyperuricemia Not utilized in the neonatal period because of risk of overwhelming acidosis
Dialysis: peritoneal or hemodialysis	May rapidly lower concentration of offending organic acid
Vitamin therapy: see Table 76-5	Rarely effective
Glycine therapy: 250 mg/kg/day	Useful in isovaleric acidemia Favors formation of rapidly excreted isovalerylglycine
Carnitine therapy: 50-200 mg/kg/day	Suggested effective in propionic acidemia, methylmalonic acidemia, and isovaleric acidemia, in which carnitine deficiency has been reported May cause diarrhea Clinical efficacy uncertain

carnitine levels, which perhaps reflects increased excretion of carnitine that is conjugated with the organic acid[5]:

$$propionyl\text{-}CoA + carnitine \rightarrow propionyl\ carnitine$$

Supplementation of the diet with carnitine (50 to 200 mg/kg/day) usually rectifies the carnitine deficiency in blood, but it is uncertain whether this treatment significantly improves metabolic status or the long-term outcome.[24] Large dosages of oral carnitine may cause diarrhea.

On occasion, patients respond to the administration of a high dosage of a vitamin (Table 76-5) that serves as a cofactor for the congenitally defective biochemical reaction.[25-27] An example is the conversion of methylmalonyl CoA to succinyl CoA via methylmalonyl-CoA mutase, a vitamin B_{12}–dependent enzyme.

In most cases of methylmalonic acidemia, the mutation affects the catalytic efficiency of the apoenzyme; that is, the mutase is unable to convert methylmalonate to succinate. This defect cannot be rectified by the administration of vitamin B_{12}. However, in an occasional patient, treatment with vitamin B_{12} improves methylmalonate metabolism, especially if the mutation involves faulty binding of the vitamin to the enzyme. High dosages of the cofactor, through the law of mass action, then favor the transformation of the enzyme into a more efficient configuration.

Table 76-5 lists the vitamin-responsive disorders of organic acid and lactic acid metabolism that are relevant to neonatal medicine. Vitamins may function not only as

cofactors for an enzymatic reaction but also as an "artificial" electron acceptor. Examples are vitamin C or menadione, administration of which may circumvent the block in the electron transport chain. It should be emphasized that this approach has been demonstrated to be effective in only a minority of cases. Indeed, the overall outlook for patients with a primary lactic acidosis is unfavorable; most fail to respond to any form of cofactor therapy. Transplantation of the liver is a possibility, although rarely in the newborn.[28]

THE UREA CYCLE DEFECTS

Biochemical and Clinical Findings

Adults generate as much as 1 to 2 mol/day of waste nitrogen as ammonia. The production of so much ammonia, which is toxic to the brain, poses a serious challenge to the integrity of the organism. Most terrestrial animals have evolved elaborate biochemical mechanisms for the conversion of ammonia into a nontoxic and readily excretable form. In humans, this mechanism is the urea cycle (Fig. 76-4).

The urea cycle is composed of five reactions that lead to the incorporation of ammonia nitrogen into urea, which is excreted in the urine. The initial two steps, the carbamoyl phosphate synthetase and ornithine transcarbamylase reactions, take place in mitochondria and lead to the synthesis of

Table 76–5. Vitamins Utilized in Management of Organic Acidurias and Primary Lactic Acidoses

Vitamin	Disorder	Dosage	Action	Comments
Thiamine	Maple syrup urine disease	25-100 mg/day	Stimulates branched-chain ketoacid decarboxylase	Rarely helpful
Thiamine	Pyruvate dehydrogenase (PDH) deficiency	25-100 mg/day	Activates PDH to increase pyruvate oxidation	Rarely helpful
Vitamin C	Electron transport disorders	4 g/day	Artificial electron acceptor	Sometimes effective in complex III deficiency
Vitamin K (menadione)	Electron transport disorders	10 mg/kg/day	Artificial electron acceptor	Sometimes effective in complex III deficiency
Coenzyme Q	Electron transport disorders	60-100 mg/day	Artificial electron acceptor	Sometimes effective in Kearns-Sayre syndrome and others
Biotin	Biotinidase deficiency	20-40 mg/day	Augments activity of biotin-dependent enzymes	Corrects functional deficiency of biotin caused by recycling defect
Biotin	Holocarboxylase synthetase deficiency	20-40 mg/day	Augments activity of biotin-dependent enzymes	Biotin therapy increases residual enzymatic activity
Riboflavin	Type II glutaric aciduria	20-50 mg/day	Stimulates electron transfer flavoprotein	Rarely effective in ETF deficiency
Lipoic acid	Lipoamide dehydrogenase deficiency	25-50 mg/kg/day	Stimulates oxidation of pyruvate, BCAA, and α-ketoglutarate in susceptible patients	Very rarely effective

BCAA, branched-chain amino acid; ETF, electron transfer flavoprotein.

citrulline. In the first of the ensuing cytosolic reactions, citrulline is converted to argininosuccinate, which is hydrolyzed to arginine and fumarate. Arginine then is hydrolyzed (via arginase) to urea and ornithine; the latter amino acid is reused in the ornithine transcarbamylase reaction, thereby completing the cycle.

A congenital absence of any component of the urea cycle enzymes can cause hyperammonemia (Table 76-6). With the exception of argininemia (arginase deficiency), which may not cause symptoms until after the age of 3 years, the urea cycle defects commonly are associated with a severe neonatal syndrome of progressive neurologic deterioration that culminates in coma and obligatory ventilatory support after 1 or 2 weeks after birth. The initial

signs include irritability, lethargy, a failure to feed, and/or vomiting. Convulsions are not uncommon.

The clinical manifestations are much more varied in the older child, who may present with mental retardation, recurrent ataxia, failure to thrive, subtle learning disabilities, or abnormal behavior. A schizophrenia-like syndrome has been described in an adult with ornithine transcarbamylase deficiency.

All of these disorders are inherited in an autosomal recessive pattern, with the important exception of ornithine transcarbamylase deficiency (see Table 76-6), which is sex-linked.[29] A very stormy and often fatal neonatal course typifies the affected infant boy, in whom the single X chromosome bears the mutant gene. In contrast, affected

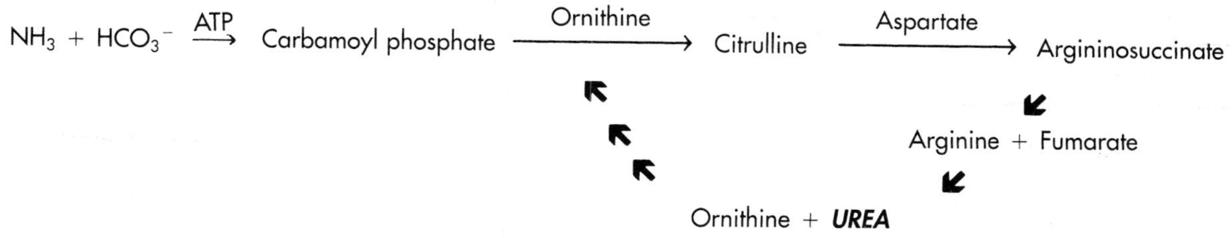

Figure 76–4. The urea cycle.

Table 76–6. The Urea Cycle Defects

Enzyme Defect	Inheritance	Onset	Frequency	Diet Therapy*	Benzoate†‡	Phenylbutyrate†‡	Arginine (mmol/kg/day)
CPS deficiency	AR	Usually 24-72 hr of age	Rare	+	+	+	0.5
OTC deficiency	Sex-linked	Male: usually neonate Female: variable	Most common urea cycle defect	+	+	+	0.5
Citrullinemia	AR	Usually 24-72 hr of age	Rare	+	+	+	3-4
Argininosuccinic aciduria	AR	Usually 24-72 hr of age	Second most common urea cycle defect	+	+	+	3-4
Argininemia	AR	3-4 years of age	Rare	+	+	+	–
THAN	Acquired	First 24 hr of age	Rare	–	+	–	–

*Usual "dose" of dietary protein is 1.5 g/kg/day. Advance carefully if blood NH_3 is less than 50 to 100 μmol.

†Dosage of both sodium benzoate and sodium phenylbutyrate is 250 to 500 mg/kg/day.

‡Maintain blood benzoate at less than 5 mg/dL and phenylacetate at 0 to 15 mg/dL.

AR, autosomal recessive; CPS, carbamoyl phosphate synthetase; OTC, ornithine transcarbamylase; THAN, transient hyperammonemia of the newborn; +, effective; –, ineffective.

girls, who have two X chromosomes, one of which bears the mutation and the other a normal copy of the ornithine transcarbamylase gene, manifest a highly variable clinical course because of random inactivation (lyonization) of one of the two X chromosomes. In rare cases, an affected girl presents with a fulminant neonatal course, but most affected women have much milder symptoms or none at all. Female carriers may be protein intolerant, and those who are may suffer from minor learning disabilities.

The long-term outlook for these infants is guarded. The prognosis appears to be directly related to the duration of hyperammonemic coma rather than the magnitude of the hyperammonemia. Thus, the need for rapid diagnosis and the institution of appropriate therapy is urgent. Many affected neonates die, and those who survive often have profound brain damage.

Hyperammonemic encephalopathy probably results from the confluence of several factors. Ammonia interferes with brain energy metabolism, particularly in areas such as the reticular activating system that lack a well-developed blood-brain barrier. Evidence also points to a disturbance of neurotransmitter metabolism. Ammonia favors the release of dopamine and norepinephrine from storage granules in nerve endings. Excessive concentrations of glutamine, the major product of ammonia metabolism in the brain, favor the importation into the central nervous system of tryptophan, the precursor to both serotonin and quinolinic acid, a known neurotoxin. In addition, excessive production of glutamine in response to hyperammonemia may result in the swelling of astrocytes, the major site of brain glutamine synthesis. Finally, the ammoniumcation is thought to exercise a direct, inhibitory effect on the conductance of nerve impulses.

Diagnosis of urea cycle defects requires recognition of the typical history and physical findings. A careful inquiry should be made as to whether other family members have any intolerance to protein. Signs of protein intolerance include lethargy, nausea, and/or headache within 1 to 2 hours after consumption of a protein-rich meal. Like the organic acidurias (see preceding discussion), the urea cycle defects represent syndromes of nutritional neurotoxicity, and clinical decompensation in the neonate usually occurs after the first feeds have been administered.

The routine laboratory studies almost always reveal hyperammonemia (usually >500 μmol/L). Quantitation of the blood amino acids typically reveals increases in the concentration of glutamine and alanine, both of which are derived from ammonia. If there is a defect at the level of either carbamoyl phosphate synthetase or ornithine transcarbamylase (see Fig. 76-4), the initial mitochondrial steps leading to citrulline formation, the level of the latter amino acid tends to be low. Similarly, a defect anywhere in the urea cycle tends to diminish the blood concentration of both arginine and urea (see Fig. 76-4), although the presence of normal blood levels of these two metabolites does not exclude a urea cycle defect. Finally, measurement of blood and/or urinary amino acids may be useful in cases of citrullinemia and argininosuccinic aciduria, in which the concentrations of these amino acids are very high.

The urinary excretion of orotic acid is increased in all urea cycle defects, with the exception of carbamoyl phosphate

synthetase deficiency. Orotic acid normally is synthesized in the cytosol from carbamoyl phosphate. If the latter is not utilized for urea synthesis, it spills into the cytoplasm, where it is directed toward formation of orotic acid:

$$NH_3 + HCO_3^- + ATP \rightarrow \text{carbamoyl phosphate} \rightarrow \text{orotic acid}$$

where ATP is adenosine triphosphate.

Hyperammonemia in the neonate also may be of acquired origin. Thus, hepatic failure may cause a marked rise of blood ammonia. Organic acidurias, particularly methylmalonic aciduria and propionic acidemia, frequently elevate blood ammonia, sometimes to an extreme degree (>500 μmol). Finally, a poorly understood disorder, **transient hyperammonemia of the newborn,** is of uncertain origin. It may result from the combination of an immature urea cycle and a high rate of ammonia production. The syndrome typically becomes clinically apparent during the first 12 hours after birth, more commonly in a stressed premature infant, who tends to manifest blood ammonia levels higher than 1000 μmol.

Management of Urea Cycle Defects

Restriction of protein intake minimizes ammonia production. Individual patients demonstrate substantial variability in their tolerance of protein, but all neonates need approximately 1.5 g/kg/day to support a normal rate of growth.[25,30] For those infants who do not tolerate even this amount, a compromise may be necessary between sustaining growth and incurring hyperammonemia.

A critical advance in the management of patients with urea cycle defects has been the stimulation of alternate metabolic pathways of nitrogen excretion.[31,32] The most important example of this approach has been the administration of sodium benzoate, which in the liver is conjugated with glycine to form hippuric acid:

$$NH_3 \rightarrow \text{glycine} \xrightarrow{\text{benzoate}} \text{hippurate}$$

Benzoate is well tolerated in most patients. This organic anion displaces bilirubin from its albumin-binding site, but extensive use of benzoate in neonates has not been associated with any serious incidence of kernicterus. In some patients who receive a protein-restricted diet, benzoate therapy can nearly replace urea synthesis as a route of nitrogen removal, thereby permitting near normalization of the blood ammonia level.

Another useful medication is sodium phenylbutyrate, which is decarboxylated in the liver to phenylacetate. The latter is conjugated with glutamine to yield phenylacetylglutamine:

$$\text{glutamate} + NH_3 \rightarrow \text{glutamine} \xrightarrow{\text{phenylacetate}} \text{phenylacetylglutamine}$$

Because 2 mol of nitrogen are excreted as glutamine with each mole of phenylacetate, this agent promotes even more efficient removal of waste nitrogen than does benzoate therapy, which evokes excretion of a single mole of nitrogen as hippurate.

Most affected neonates require supplementation with dietary arginine, which these patients cannot produce in an amount sufficient to sustain protein synthesis. Arginine treatment also promotes the formation of citrulline or argininosuccinic acid in patients with citrullinemia or argininosuccinic aciduria (see Fig. 76-4). In such infants, citrulline or argininosuccinate, both of which are readily excreted in the urine, can replace urea as the major nitrogen carrier. The administration of arginine stimulates synthesis of these amino acids and thereby favors the removal of waste nitrogen. Indeed, in infants with partial metabolic defects, nitrogen balance can almost be normalized with arginine therapy (see Table 76-6).

Humans form some ammonia from the metabolism of intestinal bacteria. Hence, the oral administration of unabsorbed antibiotics, such as neomycin, has proved useful in adults with hyperammonemia secondary to liver failure. Some patients have been treated with oral and/or rectal lactulose, which acidifies the gut and thereby favors formation of poorly absorbed NH_4^+ versus readily absorbed NH_3. Therapy with oral antibiotics or lactulose has not been applied broadly in the management of the newborn, who often is so direly ill that more heroic measures must be utilized to remove the copious amounts of ammonia that are formed.

Both peritoneal dialysis and various forms of hemodialysis have been used with remarkable effect in the management of the hyperammonemic neonate.[33] Although such intervention is relatively new—and it ought to be undertaken only in centers with the requisite expertise—it has proved conspicuously successful for the rapid reduction of the blood ammonia level. Indeed, in most affected infants, the ammonia concentration is reduced by at least half within 24 hours of initiating dialysis.

DISORDERS OF CARBOHYDRATE METABOLISM: GALACTOSEMIA

Clinical and Biochemical Findings

A relatively common inherited disorder of carbohydrate metabolism is galactosemia secondary to a deficiency of galactose-1-phosphate-uridyl transferase (GALT).[34] The GALT enzyme is the second step of the Leloir pathway, the sequence of reactions that converts galactose to glucose:

$$\text{galactose} + \text{ATP} \rightarrow \text{galactose-1-phosphate}$$
$$\text{(galactokinase reaction)}$$

$$\text{galactose-1-phosphate} + \text{UDP-glucose} \rightarrow \text{UDP-galactose}$$
$$\div \text{ glucose-1-phosphate (GALT reaction)}$$

$$\text{UDP-galactose} \rightarrow \text{UDP-glucose (epimerase reaction)}$$

$$\text{glucose-1-phosphate} \rightarrow \text{glucose-6-phosphate}$$
$$\text{(phosphoglucomutase)}$$

$$\text{glucose-6-phosphate} \rightarrow \text{glucose (glucose 6-phosphatase)}$$

where UPD is uridine diphosphate.

The significance of this pathway is to allow the oxidation of galactose, which constitutes half of the disaccharide lactose (glucose plus galactose) and provides 20% of total calories in human milk. A congenital deficiency of the transferase enzyme results in the accumulation of both galactose and galactose-1-phosphate in the body fluids of infants who are fed galactose.

The galactosemic infant seems well at birth. However, after the first feedings of breast milk or a lactose-containing formula, the infant develops irritability, vomiting, lethargy, and/or diarrhea. The liver and, possibly, the spleen become enlarged. The infant develops jaundice, at first direct and then unconjugated hyperbilirubinemia. The jaundice is caused by both hepatic dysfunction and hemolysis. A failure to gain weight and even frank weight loss are the rule. Slit-lamp examination of the eyes discloses the presence of a nuclear cataract. A common—and often lethal—complication is gram-negative septicemia, which occurs with increased frequency in galactosemic infants.

The hepatic failure and septicemia may prove fatal. Most affected infants survive once all galactose is removed from the diet. It formerly was thought that scrupulous dietary control ensured a good outcome, but a few retrospective studies have suggested that even well-controlled patients may suffer a progressive neurologic syndrome and a deterioration in intellectual performance.[35] The female galactosemic patient may incur primary ovarian failure, even if her dietary control is good. The precise basis of the neurologic and gynecologic complications remains elusive. One factor may be autointoxication with galactose that is produced endogenously.

Notwithstanding these pessimistic reports, rapid diagnosis is essential in order to avoid a fatality during the neonatal period. The advent of mandatory screening of infants for metabolic diseases, including galactosemia, has enabled diagnosis of asymptomatic affected infants. In infants who have not been screened or in whom the clinical features suggest transferase-deficiency galactosemia, diagnosis can be made simply by testing the urine for a reducing substance (Clinitest reaction) when the infant is receiving a formula containing lactose (glucose plus galactose). If there is no glycosuria, and if the clinical syndrome is suggestive of galactosemia, then this diagnosis should be made presumptively until additional studies can be completed.[36]

Management of Galactosemia

Milk is rich in galactose; therefore, all dairy products must be eliminated. Many other foods, including most fruits and vegetables, contain lesser amounts of galactose, albeit in linkage in complex carbohydrates that may not be digested to the monosaccharide. There are many "occult" sources of dietary galactose, because lactose commonly is used as a filler in the production of processed meats and even in various medications. Hence, the assistance of qualified dietary counselors is indispensable.

Liver failure and its complications must be managed during the acute phase of illness. Special attention should be given to the potential problem of gram-negative septicemia, and appropriate cultures should be obtained. The managing physician should be alert to other complications of the syndrome, including increased intracranial pressure, hypoglycemia, and generalized inanition. The cataracts, which commonly are present at birth, usually regress almost completely with careful dietary control.

DISORDERS OF AMINO ACID METABOLISM

Two aminoacidurias commonly manifest as a fulminant neonatal syndrome: MSUD and nonketotic hyperglycinemia. Other aminoacidurias, such as phenylketonuria and homocystinuria, rarely give rise to any discernible symptoms in newborns. MSUD has already been considered in the previous discussion of the disorders of organic acid metabolism.

Nonketotic Hyperglycinemia

Nonketotic hyperglycinemia is caused by a congenital defect in the multienzyme complex that mediates the interconversion of glycine and serine in a folic acid (FH_4)–dependent series of reactions:

$$glycine + NAD + FH_4 \rightarrow hydroxymethyl\text{-}FH_4 + CO_2 + NH_3 + NADH$$

$$hydroxymethyl\text{-}FH_4 + glycine \rightarrow serine + FH_4$$

The absence of this catalytic activity is associated with extraordinary increases in the glycine concentration of the blood, which often exceeds 1 mmol/L (normal is <0.4 mmol/L). This fact can lead to confusion with propionic acidemia and methylmalonic acidemia, which may also be associated with hyperglycinemia. Diagnosis of nonketotic hyperglycinemia can be further supported by measurement of glycine in the CSF. Extreme increases of CSF glycine (5 to 10 times normal) are pathognomonic for nonketotic hyperglycinemia, particularly in an infant with the characteristic clinical manifestations.

The syndrome, when present, usually manifests soon after birth, even before the administration of the first feedings. This feature may help to differentiate nonketotic hyperglycinemia from most other disorders of intermediary metabolism. The most prominent feature is a severe seizure disorder that is characterized clinically by sustained, generalized convulsions that are difficult to control. On occasion, the history includes increased intrauterine movements that may represent in utero convulsions. When affected infants are not having frank seizures, they commonly display repeated myoclonic jerks and hiccupping. At other times they seem to be sleeping peacefully, only to be roused by a new series of convulsions. The electroencephalogram often is marked by a burst-suppression pattern or a hypsarrhythmia. Images of the brain typically are normal early in the course of the disease, but frank cortical atrophy is the rule in affected infants who survive.

Management of Nonketotic Hyperglycinemia

The precise cause of the convulsive disorder has been elusive. A likely factor is a disturbance in the function of brain glutamate receptors. Glutamate is the most important excitatory neurotransmitter of the human brain. Glycine potentiates the firing of one species of glutamate receptor, the N-methyl-D-aspartate (NMDA) receptor, which may be inappropriately activated in nonketotic hyperglycinemia. Some support for this conceptualization is the clinical observation that selective antagonists of the NMDA receptor may improve seizure control.

Unfortunately, the use of NMDA receptor antagonists has not been consistently helpful, and there is no pharmacologic intervention that is effective in all cases. Treatment with sodium benzoate, which reacts with glycine to form hippuric acid, reduces the blood and CSF glycine levels, but this approach has not resulted in much clinical improvement. Most affected infants deteriorate progressively, and death during the first few weeks or months of life is the rule.

FATTY ACID OXIDATION DISORDERS

Biochemical and Clinical Findings

Over 20 fatty acid oxidation disorders (FAODs) have been described since the early 1980s.[37,38] This class of disease is collectively not uncommon and may account for 1% of all pediatric deaths. The fatty acids are preferred fuels of exercising skeletal muscle and of the heart. Hepatocytes also depend on fatty acids for the energy needed to support gluconeogenesis, ketogenesis, and ureagenesis. The brown fat of neonates utilizes fatty acids to sustain nonshivering thermogenesis, a process important to temperature control.

The clinical findings in FAOD are attributable to (1) accumulation of metabolites proximal to the enzymatic defect and (2) a deficiency of energy production. Accumulated fatty acids have detergent properties that may disrupt the integrity of membranes. Studies in animal models show that high concentrations of acyl-CoA compounds have arrhythmogenic effects.

A common finding in FAODs is hypoketotic hypoglycemia, which results from increased peripheral utilization of glucose that results from deficient production of ketone bodies and acetyl CoA, a known stimulator of PC, a gluconeogenic enzyme. Medium-chain acyl-CoA dehydrogenase deficiency, the most common of these disorders, often manifests in an infant whose intake is diminished because of an intercurrent illness.

Neonatal manifestations have been described for several disorders (Table 76-7), including deficiencies of carnitine-palmitoyl-CoA transferase (CPT)–2, carnitine acyl-CoA translocase, electron transport flavoprotein (multiple acyl-COA dehydrogenase deficiency [MADD]), 3-hydroxy-3-methyl-glutaryl–CoA lyase, trifunctional protein, long-chain acyl-CoA dehydrogenase (LCAD), and very-long-chain acyl-CoA dehydrogenase.[38] Deficiencies of medium-chain acyl-CoA dehydrogenase and of CPT-1 typically become clinically apparent after the neonatal period.

Presentation of Fatty Acid Oxidation Disorders in the Newborn

Hepatic Manifestations

Affected infants may manifest hepatomegaly with hypoglycemia and concomitant seizures, irritability, lethargy, and even coma. Breast-feeding may evoke a fasting stress sufficient to unmask the defect. A glucose infusion may correct the hypoglycemia, but the infant suffers an even more severe future event.

Cardiac Manifestations

Affected newborns manifest cardiomegaly, myocardial damage, and arrhythmias. Sudden death can occur.

Table 76–7. The Fatty Acid Oxidation Defects

Manifestation	Defect
Neonatal Manifestation Common	
Multiple CoA dehydrogenase deficiency	Electron transport flavoprotein
HMG-CoA lyase deficiency	3-OH-3-methylglutaryl–CoA lyase deficiency
CPT-2 deficiency	Carnitine-palmitoyl-CoA transferase II
Trifunctional protein deficiency	Trifunctional protein
CACT deficiency	Carnitine acyl-CoA translocase
LCHAD deficiency	Long-chain acyl-CoA dehydrogenase
VLCAD deficiency	Very-long-chain acyl-CoA dehydrogenase
Usually Not Neonatally Manifested	
MCAD	Medium-chain acyl-CoA dehydrogenase
CPT-1 deficiency	Carnitine-palmitoyl-CoA transferase I

CoA, coenzyme A.

A hypertrophic cardiomyopathy, often antenatal in onset, is seen in severely affected patients. In other patients, metabolic stress and fasting evoke cardiac events, including heart failure, pulmonary edema, and ventricular arrhythmia. Cardiac findings are more frequent with deficiencies of the carnitine transporter, the fatal infantile and neonatal forms of CPT-2 deficiency, acyl-CoA very-long-chain acyl-CoA dehydrogenase, long-chain hydroxyacyl-CoA dehydrogenase (LCHAD), and trifunctional protein.

Muscular Signs

The patient shows hypotonia and evidence of rhabdomyolysis, myoglobinuria and elevated CPK.

Neurologic Manifestations

The usual findings are acute encephalopathy, seizures, progressive dystonia or dyskinesia (MADD), pigmentary retinopathy (LCHAD), and long-term developmental delay.

Congenital Malformations

Cystic renal dysplasia, central nervous system anomalies (microcephaly, neuronal migration defects, degenerative lesions, gliosis), facial dysmorphism, cardiac defects, and joint contractures have been reported in patients with the neonatal or infantile forms of CPT-2 deficiency and MADD.[39]

Pregnancy Complications

Acute fatty liver of pregnancy and the syndrome of hemolysis, elevated liver enzyme levels, and low platelet levels (HELLP) are acute third-trimester events occurring in heterozygote women pregnant with fetuses affected with LCHAD, trifunctional protein, or CPT-1 deficiencies.[40,41] Recognition of these maternal manifestations can lead to early identification of an affected infant, allowing for prompt institution of therapy. Of importance is that not all disease in the fetus is associated with disease in the mother.

Diagnosis of Fatty Acid Oxidation Disorders

A high index of suspicion remains the most important factor in the diagnosis and management of the FAODs, which must be considered in any unexplained case of nonketotic hypoglycemia, hepatic dysfunction, or cardiomegaly. Metabolic acidosis usually does not occur unless a terminal lactic acidosis develops. Hyperammonemia, hyperuricemia, and increased transaminases may be seen. Plasma carnitine levels are decreased, with the notable exception of CPT-1 deficiency, in which they may be increased. The plasma acyl-carnitine profile usually reveals an accumulation of the acyl-CoA conjugate proximal to the defect. Analysis of urine organic acids may show dicarboxylic aciduria derived from microsomal oxidation. A liver biopsy in the acute phase or after death reveals microvesicular and macrovesicular fatty infiltration. Elevated CPK levels and myoglobinuria point to the ongoing rhabdomyolysis. Confirmation of the exact molecular defect, once a diagnosis is made, is becoming increasingly available and has important implications in genetic counseling.

Prenatal Diagnosis

Inheritance is autosomal recessive in all known syndromes. Prenatal diagnosis of many FAODs by amniocentesis or chorionic villus sampling is available if the index case has been well characterized.

Neonatal Screening

Screening of acyl carnitines in blood spots by tandem mass spectrometry has allowed mass screening of newborns. Screening makes timely and relatively inexpensive intervention possible and significantly reduces rates of morbidity and mortality associated with these disorders.

Postmortem Diagnosis

The FAODs can manifest with sudden, unexplained death.[42] Additional risk factors include a family history of Reye-like syndrome, complications during pregnancy, a family history of sudden death, and evidence of hypoglycemia, lethargy, and/or vomiting during the 48 hours before death. Postmortem samples of blood, vitreous humor, and urine should be collected. An effort should be made to establish a culture of skin fibroblasts and to freeze tissue samples, particularly liver tissue.

Treatment

Infusing glucose, which minimizes tissue catabolism, is often clinically effective. Relatively high glucose infusion rates (7 to 10 mg/kg/minute) should provide adequate substrate for tissue energy metabolism. Close monitoring for cardiac conduction disturbances is essential. Correction of fluid and electrolyte imbalances, management of hyperammonemia, and therapy for any intercurrent illness may be required. The more severe FAODs such as CPT-2 deficiency are often fatal even with intensive therapy.[41] Long-term management obliges referral to a specialist. Several commercial, low-fat formulas are available to satisfy the nutritional needs of these infants.

REFERENCES

1. Burton BK: Inborn errors of metabolism in infancy: A guide to diagnosis. Pediatrics 102:e69, 1998.
2. Chakrapani A, Cleary MA, Wraith JE: Detection of inborn errors of metabolism in the newborn. Arch Dis Child Fetal Neonat Ed 84:F205, 2001.
3. Morris AA, Leonard JV: Early recognition of metabolic decompensation. Arch Dis Child 76:555, 1997.
4. Velazquez A, Vela-Amieva M, Ciceron-Arellano I, et al: Diagnosis of inborn errors of metabolism. Arch Med Res 31:145, 2000.
5. Chalmers RA, Lawson AM: Organic Acids in Man. London, Chapman and Hall, 1982, pp 209-382.
6. Gibson KM, Bennett MJ, Naylor EW, et al: 3-methylcrotonyl-coenzyme A carboxylase deficiency in Amish/Mennonite adults identified by detection of increased acylcarnitines in blood spots of their children. J Pediatr 132:519, 1998.
7. Howard R, Frieden IJ, Crawford D, et al: Methylmalonic acidemia, cobalamin C type, presenting with cutaneous manifestations. Arch Dermatol 133:1563, 1997.
8. Ogier de Baulny H, Saudubray JM: Branched chain organic acidemias. In Fernandes J, Saudubray JM, Van den Berghe H (eds): Inborn Metabolic Diseases: Diagnosis and Treatment. New York, Springer, 2000, pp 195-212.
9. Snyderman SE: Maple syrup urine disease. In Wapnir RA (ed): Congenital Metabolic Diseases: Diagnosis and Treatment. New York, Marcel Dekker, 1985, pp 120-135.
10. Sweetman L: Branched chain organic acidurias. In Scriver CR, Beaudet AL, Sly WS, et al (eds): The Metabolic Basis of Inherited Disease, 7th ed. New York, McGraw-Hill, 1992, pp 1387-1422.
11. Nyhan WL, Bay C, Beyer EW, et al: Neurologic nonmetabolic presentation of propionic acidemia. Arch Neurol 56:1143, 1999.
12. Cederbaum S, Vilain E: Defects in energy metabolism: Coming of age, slowly. J Pediatr 136:147, 2000.
13. DiGeorge AM, Rezvani I, Garibaldi LR, et al: Prospective study of maple syrup urine disease for the first four days of life. N Engl J Med 307:1492, 1982.
14. Falk RE, Cedarbaum SD, Blass JP, et al: Ketonic diet in the management of pyruvate dehydrogenase deficiency. Pediatrics 58:713, 1976.

15. Jouvet P, Jugie M, Rabier D, et al: Combined nutritional support and continuous extracorporeal removal therapy in the severe acute phase of maple syrup urine disease. Intensive Care Med 27:1798, 2001.
16. Naglak ME, Elsas LJ: Nutrition support of maple syrup urine disease. In Metabolic Currents. Ross Laboratories, Columbus, Ohio, 1:15, 1988.
17. Nyhan WL, Rice-Kelts M, Klein J, et al: Treatment of the acute crisis in maple syrup urine disease. Arch Pediatr Adolesc 152:593, 1998.
18. Parsons HG, Carter RJ, Unrath M, et al: Evaluation of branched chain amino acid intake in children with maple syrup urine disease and methylmalonic aciduria. J Inherit Metab Dis 13:125, 1990.
19. Yannicelli S: Nutrition support of methylmalonic acidemia. In Metabolic Currents. Ross Laboratories, Columbus, Ohio, 1:10, 1988.
20. Berry GT, Heidenreich R, Kaplan P, et al: Branched-chain amino acid free parenteral nutrition in the treatment of acute metabolic decompensation in patients with maple syrup urine disease. N Engl J Med 324:175, 1991.
21. Cedarbaum SD, Blass JP, Minkoff N, et al: Sensitivity to carbohydrate in a patient with familial intermittent lactic acidosis and pyruvate dehydrogenase deficiency. Pediatr Res 10:713, 1976.
22. Przyrembel H: Therapy of mitochondrial disorders. J Inherit Metab Dis 10:129, 1987.
23. Yudkoff MC, Cohn RM, Puschak R, et al: Glycine therapy in isovaleric acidemia. J Pediatr 92:813, 1978.
24. Roe CR, Millington DS, Maltby DA, et al: L-carnitine therapy in isovaleric acidemia. J Clin Invest 74:2290, 1984.
25. Energy and Protein Requirements. Report of a FAO/WHO/UNU Expert Consultation. Technical Report Series No. 724. Geneva, World Health Organization, 1985.
26. Thompson GN, Bresson JL, Bonnefont JP, et al: A simple isotopic technique for assessing vitamin responsiveness in vivo in propionic acidaemia. J Inherit Metab Dis 13:349, 1990.
27. Wick H, Schweizer K, Baumgartner R: Thiamine dependency in a patient with congenital lactic acidaemia due to pyruvate dehydrogenase deficiency. Agents Actions 7:405, 1977.
28. Wendel U, Saudubray JM, Bodner A, et al: Liver transplantation in maple syrup urine disease. Eur J Pediatr 158:S60, 1999.
29. Wraith JE: Ornithine carbamoyltransferase deficiency. Arch Dis Child 84:84, 2001.
30. MacLean W, Graham G: Pediatric Nutrition in Clinical Practice. Menlo Park, Calif, Addison-Wesley, 1982.
31. Batshaw ML, Monahan PS: Treatment of urea cycle disorders. Enzyme 38:242, 1987.
32. Brusilow SW, Valle DW, Batshaw ML: New pathways of nitrogen excretion in inborn errors of urea synthesis. Lancet 1:452, 1979.
33. Schaefer F, Straube E, Oh J, et al: Dialysis in neonates with inborn errors of metabolism. Nephrol Dial Transplant 14:910, 1999.
34. Holton JB: Galactose disorders. An overview. J Inherit Met Dis 13:476, 1990.
35. Waggoner DD, Buist NRM, Donnell GN: Long-term prognosis in galactosemia: Results of a survey of 350 cases. J Inherit Met Dis 13:802, 1991.
36. Beutler E: Galactosemia: Screening and diagnosis. Clin Biochem 24:293, 1990.
37. Rinaldo P, Matern D: Fatty acid oxidation disorders. Annu Rev Physiol 64:477, 2002.
38. Saudubray JM, Martin D, Poggi-Travert F, et al: Clinical presentations of inherited mitochondrial fatty acid oxidation disorders: An update. Int Pediatr 12:34, 1997.

39. North KN, Hoppel CL, Girolami D, et al: Lethal neonatal deficiency of carnitine palmitoyltransferase II associated with dysgenesis of the brain and kidneys. J Pediatr 127:414, 1995.

40. Ibdah JA, Bennett MJ, Rinaldo P, et al: A fetal fatty-acid oxidation disorder as a cause of liver disease in pregnant women. N Engl J Med 340:1723, 1999.

41. Roe CR, Ding J: Mitochondrial fatty acid oxidation disorders. In Scriver CR, Beaudet AL, Sly WS, Valle D (eds): The Metabolic and Molecular Bases of Inherited Disease. New York, McGraw-Hill, 2001, pp 1501-1535.

42. Lundemose JB, Kolvraa S, Gregersen N, et al: Fatty acid oxidation disorders as primary cause of sudden and unexpected death in infants and young children: An investigation performed on cultured fibroblasts from 79 children who died aged between 0-4 years. Mol Pathol 50:212, 1997.

CHAPTER 77

Fluid and Electrolyte Physiology

John L. Stefano

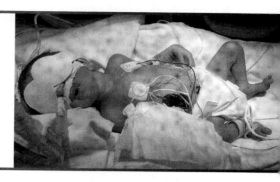

RENAL BLOOD FLOW

Much of what is known about renal blood flow (RBF) in the premature kidney is based on studies of mammalian models born at a premature gestation. There is little available information on actual measurements of RBF in premature infants. In addition, the studies that have been performed to measure RBF in full-term infants are limited by technical problems related to estimations of RBF. RBF is estimated by measurements of renal plasma flow. Renal plasma flow measurements are made by studying the clearance of para-aminohippurate (PAH). In the neonate, however, this technique is limited by the fact that renal extraction of PAH is not as complete as it is in more mature individuals. (Renal extraction of PAH is determined as the difference between renal arterial and venous PAH concentrations.) The only study of this issue has shown that PAH extraction is low in the full-term neonate (65% at 1 week of age) and does not increase to 90% until 5 months of age.[1] Maturation of PAH extraction is also seen in other species.[2,3] By overestimating PAH extraction, the clinician underestimates renal plasma flow. There are no studies in premature human infants to establish PAH renal extraction, but, from extrapolation of data obtained in premature animal models, it is likely that PAH extraction is even lower in the premature infant than it is in the full-term infant. Calgano and Rubin measured renal plasma flow in full-term infants and corrected the values for measured PAH extraction.[1] They found that infants at 8 days of age had renal plasma flow values of about 140 mL/minute/1.73 m^2, which increased to 580 mL/minute/1.73 m^2 by 5 months of age. RBF is calculated by dividing renal plasma flow values by (1 − hematocrit).

Because of these technical difficulties in measuring RBF in premature human neonates, developmental aspects of RBF as related to gestational age are largely unknown. Translating findings of RBF in premature kidneys made in other animal species may not be correct because the timing of completion of nephrogenesis varies from species to species. The completion of nephrogenesis is an important signal in many developmental aspects of renal function. In humans, nephrogenesis is complete by approximately week 34 of gestation.[4] In dogs, rats, and sheep, however, nephrogenesis is not complete until after birth.[5] Assumptions made on measurements of RBF made in the premature subject in those species, therefore, do not apply to RBF in the premature human. Consequently, statements about RBF should be referenced to the timing of complete nephrogenesis and not necessarily to gestational age.

In animals, RBF increases greatly after completion of nephrogenesis.[5] Although there are no RBF studies on premature human neonates, it is reasonable to assume that RBF increases after week 34 of gestation, that is, when nephrogenesis is complete. The fraction of cardiac output that supplies the kidneys is also variable and changes after nephrogenesis is complete. Kidneys of human fetuses receive only 2% of cardiac output,[6] in comparison with approximately 18% of cardiac output in the adult. In a study of RBF in rats from 17 to 60 days of age, Aperia and Herin were able to demonstrate an increase of 1.5% to 15% of cardiac output perfusing the kidneys.[7]

Changes in renal vascular resistance (RVR) greatly affect RBF. In infants, RVR decreases after birth, and RBF increases. Many factors regulate the changes in RVR after birth. Endocrine, catecholamine, and the nervous system influence arteriolar tone and play prominent roles in adult regulation of RVR. In the newborn, however, catecholamines and the sympathetic nervous system play a less significant role,[8-10] whereas angiotensin II and possibly other endogenous substances such as prostaglandins and prostacyclin are more important in control of RVR.[11] Postnatally, angiotensin II levels are high and then decrease. This change is accompanied by a decrease in RVR and an increase in RBF. The decrease in RVR seems to be more closely related to intrarenal angiotensin II levels rather than circulating angiotensin II levels.[12,13] The distribution of RBF to the kidney also varies with gestational maturation. Early in gestation, blood flow is directed primarily to the innermost cortex and juxtamedullary region, where the glomeruli have formed and matured.[14] As nephrogenesis progresses, there is development of newer, more primitive glomeruli in the peripheral cortex. Along with the growth of these newer nephrons, there is a shift of blood flow from the juxtamedullary region to the outermost cortex. Therefore, glomerular development and blood flow proceed in a centrifugal pattern during gestational maturation.

GLOMERULAR FILTRATION

Classically, glomerular filtration rate (GFR) has been measured by studying inulin clearance. In the newborn (especially in the premature infant), technical issues related to accurate urine collection, timing of urine collection, and method of inulin delivery can affect GFR measurements. Inulin clearance is well correlated with GFR because inulin is freely filtered, is not reabsorbed or secreted by the kidney, and is not protein bound. Because measurement of inulin concentration is not readily available in most hospitals, creatinine clearance is the most commonly used estimate of GFR in the clinical setting. Creatinine clearance has been compared with inulin clearance in the premature infant and has been shown to have a good correlation.[15] Creatinine is secreted by the proximal tubule in humans and primates,[16] however, and therefore urinary creatinine concentration may not accurately reflect filtered load. GFR was estimated from serum creatinine values and body length by Schwartz and associates in infants whose postnatal age was greater than 1 week.[17] In the immediate neonatal period, however, estimates of GFR made on the basis of serum creatinine may be incorrect because maternal serum creatinine levels can influence the infant's level. Labeled isotopes such as technetium 99–diethylenetri-aminepentaacetic acid have also been used to measure GFR in the neonatal period.[18]

Studies by Arant[19] and Engle and Arant[20] showed that GFR in premature infants (as estimated by creatinine clearance) is constant before week 34 of gestation and increases after that. This increase holds true regardless of the postnatal age of the infant. For example, a premature infant delivered at week 30 of gestation demonstrates an increase in GFR 4 weeks later, whereas in an infant born at week 26 of gestation, it will take 8 weeks before GFR increases. The increase in GFR occurring at week 34 of gestation corresponds with the developmental stage of complete nephrogenesis in the human. Other mammalian species have also shown this increase in GFR after completion of nephrogenesis.[21] The reasons for this increase are unclear. Although GFR is constant before week 34 of gestation, RBF increases linearly during this stage.[5]

GFR is equal to the filtration of a single nephron multiplied by the number of nephrons. After nephrogenesis is completed, there are approximately 1 million nephrons. During nephrogenesis, the outer cortical nephrons are smaller and have little or no filtering capacity.[22] Juxtamedullary glomeruli are more mature

and have better filtration per nephron. As gestational age approaches 34 weeks, more blood flow is gradually diverted from the juxtamedullary area to the more cortical nephrons. As these cortical glomeruli improve their filtering capacity and blood flow increases to the cortical region, GFR begins to increase.[7] It is not clear if a common signal regulates regional RBF and maturation of the cortical glomeruli. It is interesting to speculate that vasoactive substances, such as vasodilator prostaglandins (which are made locally in the kidney), may control renal arteriolar tone and may affect maturation of these cortical nephrons. Likewise, angiotensin II may also promote maturation of cortical nephrons and redistribution of RBF from the juxtamedullary area to cortical region. The angiotensin II level is high in the fetus and falls after birth.[11,12] It is now known that, in addition to being synthesized in the lung, angiotensin II is locally made and rapidly degraded in the kidney.[23]

A major determinant of GFR is perfusion pressure. As mentioned, renal vascular resistance is high in early gestation and decreases with increasing gestational age. In addition to high renal arteriolar tone in early gestation, systemic artery pressure is low and results in low perfusion pressure to the renal parenchyma. In extremely premature infants, perfusion pressure can be very low under normal circumstances. When confounding variables such as hypoxemia, poor myocardial contractility, and patency of the ductus arteriosus are also present, perfusion pressure can suffer greatly. In infancy, GFR is more dependent on extracellular fluid expansion than it is in more mature individuals.[24] It was shown that after volume expansion with 10% dextrose solution, GFR could double in premature infants whose gestational ages ranged from 28 to 34 weeks.[25]

WATER HOMEOSTASIS

The role of sodium and water has been extensively studied in the neonate. In full-term infants, rapid changes in body water distribution occur after birth (Fig. 77-1).[26] Total body water decreases at the expense of the extracellular fluid compartment, and the intracellular compartment expands. In infants with low birth weight, Bauer and coworkers showed similar changes in body water compartments (Fig. 77-2).[27] In their study, however, total body water decreased, but the proportion of intracellular volume remained relatively constant. The decrease in total body water resulted from a loss of extracellular volume, primarily a reduction in interstitial volume. Plasma volume remained relatively constant. Because extracellular volume depends on total body sodium, the reduction in extracellular volume seen in premature infants must be accompanied by a reduction in total body sodium. This concept also relates to maintenance of water and sodium requirements in the immediate neonatal period. If it is natural for contraction of the extracellular space to occur, it may not be appropriate to "maintain" a state of relative extracellular expansion by providing water and sodium in amounts that would prevent this extracellular volume contraction.

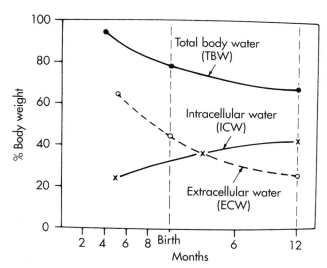

Figure 77–1. Changes in body water during gestation and infancy. *(From Friis-Hansen B: Body water compartments in children: Changes during growth and related changes in body composition. Pediatrics 28:168, 1961.)*

Contraction of extracellular volume from a reduction in the interstitial space is especially important in the premature infant with respiratory distress syndrome. The inherent diuresis that occurs in these infants heralds improvement in pulmonary function and in the alveolar-arterial oxygen gradient.[28] Presumably, the interstitial

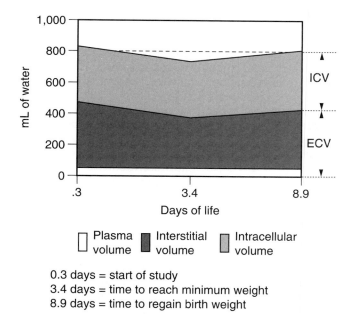

0.3 days = start of study
3.4 days = time to reach minimum weight
8.9 days = time to regain birth weight

Figure 77–2. Changes in fluid compartments in very low birth weight infants over the first 2 weeks after birth. ECV, extracellular volume; ICV, intracellular volume. *(Adapted from Bauer K, Bovermann G, Roithmaier A, et al: Body composition, nutrition, and fluid balance during the first two weeks of life in preterm neonates weighing less than 1500 grams. J Pediatr 118:615, 1991.)*

space in the lung also contracts, thereby improving pulmonary compliance and oxygenation indices.[29,30] Some authorities speculate that this diuresis may be stimulated by atrial natriuretic factor (ANF). ANF is a peptide found in secretory granules in the atrial wall.[31] This peptide is secreted when atrial expansion is induced by vascular volume expansion. Administration of ANF causes an increase in urinary flow rates, sodium excretion, and potassium excretion.[32-34] Bierd and colleagues showed that plasma ANF levels correlated positively with right atrial size and inversely with gestational age.[35] As volume contraction occurred, ANF levels decreased. Shaffer and associates showed that premature infants being mechanically ventilated for respiratory distress syndrome had extremely elevated plasma concentrations of ANF, but the authors were unable to demonstrate a correlation between ANF levels and sodium excretion.[36] Modi and coworkers were able to demonstrate a correlation with elevated ANF levels and improvement in respiratory function.[37] This improvement in respiratory function was also associated with a contraction in extracellular fluid volume. Natriuretic and diuretic response to ANF seems to be blunted in the newborn and fetus, in comparison with the adult. This blunting of fetal and neonatal response to ANF may be caused by the lower renal perfusion pressure that is seen in premature infants.

By measuring corrected bromide space as an estimate of extracellular volume, Shaffer and associates showed that infants with very low birth weight had a decrease in extracellular volume in the first 1 to 2 days after birth.[38,39] The infants with the greatest loss of extracellular volume also had a higher incidence of late hyponatremia. This hyponatremia was caused by a decrease in total extracellular sodium rather than an increase in total body water. Shaffer and associates speculated that the reduction in extracellular volume stimulated arginine vasopressin, resulting in decreased free water excretion and a lower serum sodium concentration. Rees and colleagues demonstrated intact osmoreceptor and volume receptor systems for arginine vasopressin in premature infants as young as 26 weeks after conception. In addition, urinary excretion of vasopressin and urine osmolality increased as respiratory disease worsened.[40]

Although these studies suggest an ability to secrete and respond to arginine vasopressin in the premature infant, other studies show that the collecting duct cells in the immature nephron are less sensitive to the effect of arginine vasopressin than more mature collecting duct cells.[41] Svenningsen and Aronson found that there was a limited capacity for maximally concentrating the urine in premature and full-term infants.[42] In addition to the sensitivity of arginine vasopressin on collecting duct cells, there are several reasons for the limited capacity of the neonatal kidney for maximally concentrating the urine. In the mature kidney, a hypertonic interstitium in the inner medullary tissue of the kidney is created so that water can be reabsorbed without electrolytes. Several of the factors needed to develop a hypertonic medullary interstitium are not fully functional at birth and are even less so in the premature infant. These include active reabsorption of sodium in the water-impermeable ascending loop of Henle, creation of a urea gradient in the renal medulla, and the length of the medullary loop of Henle and collecting ducts. Although newborns have a limited ability to concentrate their urine, they are able to produce dilute urine. In fact, studies have shown (by examination of free water clearance) that infants seem to have a greater capacity for excreting free water than do adults.[43] This ability also is true for premature infants older than week 30 of gestation.[44]

Lorenz and associates described a characteristic pattern of fluid excretion in the first week after birth in infants with and without respiratory disease that indicated that urine output was typically low in the first days after birth and increased during the second and third days, independently of fluid intake.[45] By days 4 and 5, urine output began to vary with changes in fluid intake. In a subsequent study, this group of investigators described the renal indices that correlated with these phases of postnatal fluid homeostasis.[46] In the first phase of minimal urine output, GFR and fractional excretion of sodium (FE_{Na}) are low; during the diuretic phase, there is an abrupt increase in GFR and FE_{Na}; the third phase is characterized by appropriately varying GFR and FE_{Na} with fluid intake.

The physical environment complicates the renal contribution to water homeostasis. Insensible water loss can account for a major proportion of maintenance fluid requirements, which is particularly important in infants with extremely low birth weight (ELBW) (Fig. 77-3).[47,48] In addition, the fixed relationship between metabolic rate and insensible water loss seen in more mature individuals is not seen in the very premature infant. Evaporative water loss (and therefore heat loss) is extensive in the premature infant, who has little cornified skin and a large ratio of surface area to body mass. Heat loss from evaporative losses can actually be larger than net metabolic rate in the very premature infant.[49] Complicating the problem of large evaporative water losses is the variability of these losses, which depends on the degree of cornification of the epidermis. As the premature infant is exposed to ambient air, skin cornification proceeds rapidly and transdermal water loss decreases. A clinical reevaluation of water requirements in the infant is needed frequently.[50] Also, the technology used to nurse the infant greatly affects insensible water loss. Although radiant warmer beds can facilitate access to the critically ill neonate, heat losses through convection and evaporation are high. Shielding infants with plastic blankets has been shown to appreciably reduce oxygen consumption and decrease insensible water loss.[51] Omar and coworkers were able to show that ELBW infants exposed to in utero corticosteroids had lower insensible water loss, lower serum sodium values, and an earlier diuresis and natriuresis.[52] They speculated that these changes were caused by a maturation of epithelial cells, improving skin integrity. They also proposed that treatment with prenatal steroids may enhance lung sodium/potassium–adenosine triphosphatase (Na^+, K^+-ATPase), leading to earlier reabsorption of fetal lung water.

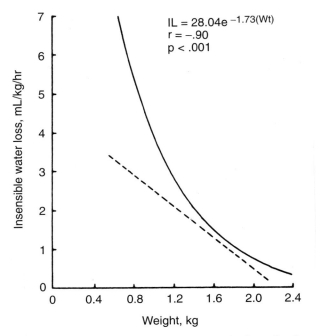

Figure 77–3. Insensible water loss and body weight for well infants (*dashed line*) studied in incubators and critically ill infants (*solid line*) receiving assisted ventilation and on open warmer beds. IL, insensible loss. (*From Baumgart S, Langman CB, Sosulski R, et al: Fluid, electrolyte, and glucose management in the very low birth weight infant. Clin Pediatr 21:200, 1982.*)

SODIUM HOMEOSTASIS

Sodium and water are normally filtered in amounts that greatly exceed maintenance intake. Therefore, sodium and water balance fundamentally depends on tubular reabsorption of sodium and water. Approximately 65% to 70% of the ultrafiltrate across the glomerular membrane is isotonically reabsorbed in the proximal tubule.[53] Hydrostatic and osmotic forces across the peritubular space regulate the rate of water and sodium reabsorption in the proximal tubule.[54] In relation to the hydrostatic and oncotic pressure in the proximal tubule, a decrease in colloid oncotic pressure or an increase in hydrostatic pressure in the peritubular capillary reduces movement of water from the proximal tubule into the peritubular capillary, thereby diminishing water reabsorption proximally.[3,55,56] In the newborn, there is an isotonic volume expansion at birth that increases peritubular hydrostatic pressure and decreases colloid oncotic pressure, which results in a decrease in proximal tubule reabsorption.[26,27]

Another 20% to 25% of the ultrafiltrate is reabsorbed as it progresses through the loop of Henle. This reabsorption occurs from the countercurrent water exchange created by sodium impermeability in the descending limb of the loop. In the thin ascending limb, sodium chloride is reabsorbed passively; in the thick ascending limb, chloride is actively transported, followed by sodium. At this level of the nephron, more sodium chloride than water is reabsorbed from the ultrafiltrate, producing a dilute urine as it approaches the distal tubule.[53] Only 5% of the filtered sodium is reabsorbed in the distal tubule; 3% of the filtered load is reabsorbed in the collecting ducts.[53] Distal tubular sodium reabsorption is regulated by aldosterone through an active process that increases sodium reabsorption from the distal tubular lumen in exchange for potassium ions.[53]

As noted, there is an inherent diuresis that occurs in the first several days after birth in premature infants independently of fluid intake.[45,46] This diuresis is associated with extracellular volume contraction, primarily from the interstitial space.[27] Because the extracellular space is high in sodium, reduction of extracellular volume concurrent with an increase in urine flow would require a net loss of sodium. Examination of sodium balance in premature infants during the first week after birth has demonstrated that these infants are in negative balance.[57-59] In the study by Costarino and colleagues, infants whose birth weights were less than 1000 g were randomly assigned to receive "maintenance sodium" (3 to 4 mEq/kg/day) or restricted sodium for the first 5 days after birth.[57] In both groups, sodium excretion was the same (4 to 5 mEq/kg/day), yielding net negative sodium balance in the sodium-restricted infants and a sodium balance of zero in the sodium-supplemented infants. Urine flow rates, estimated GFRs, and osmolar clearance were the same for both groups. These studies suggest that premature infants have fixed urinary excretion of sodium and water during the first week after birth.[57]

Whether this fixed excretion of sodium and water represents an adaptive response to perinatal extracellular volume expansion (for example, from placental transfusion or resorption of lung fluid), renal immaturity, or a combination of both is unclear. Teleologically, an adaptive response to extracellular fluid overload would make sense, because it is necessary for premature infants to be in positive sodium balance for growth, especially bone growth. Apart from teleologic arguments, renal immaturity does play a role in the sodium wasting observed in these infants. Maturation of tubular function and GFR are necessary to provide the appropriate balance of glomerular and tubular function to allow for positive sodium balance in the growing infant. Along with this tendency for sodium wasting in the immature infant, there is also a limited capacity for excreting a sodium load.[60] This inability to excrete a sodium load cannot be attributed to lower GFRs alone, because the filtration capacity of even the most immature kidney well exceeds the amount of sodium administered during saline loading. Although newborns can increase GFRs in response to saline loading, the duration of the increase in GFR in response to sodium loading is much shorter than in adults.[55,60] On the other hand, newborn puppies demonstrate limited sodium excretion in response to sodium loading when GFR is corrected, which suggests that tubular reabsorptive factors are important in the premature infant's limited ability to excrete a sodium load.[61]

Sodium Wasting

During the first week after birth, premature infants waste sodium and are in negative sodium balance.[57-59] The mechanisms for this tendency for sodium wasting are

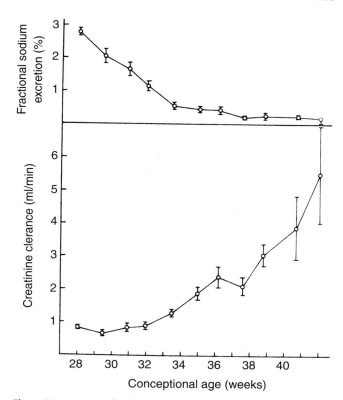

Figure 77-4. Fractional sodium excretion and glomerular filtration rate (mean ± standard error of the mean) plotted against conceptional age. Note the relation between the two variables before and after week 33 of conceptional age. *(From Al-Dahhan J, Haycock GB, Chantler C, et al: Sodium homeostasis in term and preterm neonates. Arch Dis Child 58:335, 1983.)*

complex and relate to maturational aspects of both GFR and tubular factors that affect sodium reabsorption. As shown in Figure 77-4, GFR (as estimated from creatinine clearance) is constant before week 33 of gestation, and FE_{Na} decreases as gestational age increases from 28 to 33 weeks.[62] This change indicates poor glomerulotubular balance before week 33 of gestation; that is, as the FE_{Na} decreases from week 28 to 33 of gestation, GFR remains constant. Thus, before week 33 of gestation, GFR exceeds the limited tubular reabsorption of sodium and results in sodium wasting. After week 33 of gestation, glomerulotubular balance is intact, because FE_{Na} is constant, whereas GFR increases, which implies that sodium reabsorption is able to keep up with the increase in GFR. In addition to the effect of gestational age, postnatal age also has a maturational effect on tubular reabsorption of sodium.[62] The mechanism for this impaired glomerulotubular balance seems to be a combination of increased sodium delivery to the distal tubule and an impairment in distal tubular sodium reabsorption.[63,64] By employing clearance methods during maximal water diuresis, Rodríguez-Soriano and associates were able to show that distal sodium delivery was high at 28 weeks of age and decreased by 42 weeks of age, whereas distal sodium reabsorption was low at 28 weeks of gestation and increased up to 34 weeks of gestation, after which distal sodium reabsorption leveled off.[63]

Defect in Distal Sodium Reabsorption

The defect in distal sodium reabsorption may be related to aldosterone nonresponsiveness. Because aldosterone levels are high in premature infants,[65] there does not seem to be a problem with aldosterone production in the premature adrenal gland, but there may be an insensitivity to this mineralocorticoid. Aldosterone function can be indirectly assessed by studying the ratio of urinary potassium (U_K) to urinary sodium (U_{Na}).[66] Aldosterone activity is directly correlated to the U_K:U_{Na} ratio; when the ratio is high, aldosterone activity is good. Al-Dahhan and coworkers showed that the U_K:U_{Na} ratio increased with increasing gestational age, indicating greater aldosterone responsiveness with increasing gestational age.[62] Some investigators have suggested using U_K:U_{Na+K} rather than U_K:U_{Na} as an indicator of aldosterone responsiveness, because the former takes into account distal sodium delivery, which can greatly affect potassium secretion in the distal nephron.[67]

In addition to gestational age, there seems to be a maturational effect on aldosterone activity with increasing postnatal age. Because aldosterone function depends on a functioning sodium-potassium pump, the insensitivity of the distal nephron to aldosterone may be related to decrease in Na^+,K^+-ATPase activity in the distal tubular cell.[52,68] Studies performed in the newborn rat suggest that aldosterone receptor numbers are adequate.[69] Although the premature adrenal gland is capable of producing aldosterone, the tendency for sodium wasting in the premature infant may result, in part, from an inability of the adrenal gland to appropriately respond to the stimulus of salt wasting and low total body sodium.[55]

Renal dopamine is also important with regard to sodium homeostasis. Although dopaminergic nerves supplying the kidney produce some of the renal dopamine, the majority of renal dopamine is produced in the proximal tubule cell by the enzymatic conversion of L-dopa to dopamine.[70] Dopamine exerts its effect via two types of receptors: DA1 and DA2.[8,71,72] The renal vasodilation seen with the use of exogenous dopamine is probably mediated through the DA1 receptor.[73] Stimulation of the DA1 receptors also leads to an increase in sodium and water excretion.[74] The natriuretic effects of dopamine are greater in the mature dog than in puppies, which is suggestive of a maturational effect on dopamine responsiveness.[75] The ontogenic effects of dopamine on tubular reabsorption of sodium and water may be related to differences in cyclic adenosine monophosphate generation[76] or to Na^+,K^+-ATPase activity.[77]

Until this maturation of both distal tubular sodium delivery and distal sodium reabsorption occurs, sodium wasting will continue. In the growing premature infant younger than 33 weeks of gestational age, care must be taken to provide the appropriate amount of sodium so that negative sodium balance can be avoided and allow for optimal growth. On the basis of studies examining sodium balance in premature infants, it seems that infants younger than 33 weeks of gestational age require at least 4 to 5 mmol/kg/day to stay in positive sodium balance.[57]

POTASSIUM HOMEOSTASIS

Positive potassium balance is needed for adequate growth in the newborn.[78] Potassium excretion in newborns is lower than in adults; adults excrete 15% of filtered potassium load, but newborns excrete only 9% of potassium filtered at the glomerulus.[78]

Potassium concentration in the ultrafiltrate at the glomerular level is identical to the concentration of potassium in plasma. Passive reabsorption of potassium occurs in the proximal tubule, reclaiming approximately 50% of the filtered potassium.[79] In adult animals, only 15% of filtered potassium reaches the distal nephron. In newborn animals, the amount of filtered potassium that reaches the distal tubule and collecting duct is as high as 40%. This discrepancy in the amount of potassium reaching the distal nephron suggests that, in newborns, there is a maturation defect in potassium reabsorption in the loop of Henle.[80,81]

Potassium is actively secreted in the distal nephron.[78] This process consumes energy by hydrolyzing adenosine triphosphate under the influence of membrane-bound Na^+,K^+-ATPase.[82] This enzyme exchanges three sodium ions from the cell into plasma for two ions of potassium from plasma into the cell,[82] which results in a concentration gradient for intracellular potassium ions to pass through selective channels into the tubular lumen. As Na^+,K^+-ATPase causes sodium to leave the cell, a concentration gradient is created for sodium from the luminal surface into the cell. When sodium moves into the cell from the lumen, a net negative charge is created in the lumen. The net negative charge in the tubular lumen facilitates movement of potassium ions out of the cell and into the lumen.[78]

Newborns have difficulty in excreting a potassium load. In adults, potassium excretion during potassium loading depends on the potassium secretory capacity of the distal tubular and collecting duct cell. The ability of the distal nephron to secrete potassium depends on the plasma concentration of potassium, the rate of sodium delivery to the distal nephron, Na^+,K^+-ATPase activity, aldosterone activity, and the transcellular electrochemical gradient. Lorenz and associates studied potassium secretory ability of newborn dogs during potassium loading and found that distal potassium secretory ability is limited in newborns because of a lower rate of sodium delivery to the distal nephron.[83] Tubular and collecting duct segmental Na^+,K^+-ATPase activity has been shown to be lower in neonatal rabbit nephrons than in adult segmental Na^+,K^+-ATPase activity.[68] Although aldosterone levels are higher in premature and full-term infants than in adults,[65] aldosterone activity (as reflected by U_K:U_{Na} levels) is low in the premature infant and increases with increasing gestational age.[62] Aldosterone activity depends on Na^+,K^+-ATPase function. The poor aldosterone function seen in early gestation may be caused by poor tubular cell Na^+,K^+-ATPase activity.[68,84] In addition, the newborn has a lower negative electrochemical gradient across the tubular membrane.[85] This reduction in intratubular negative charge may also be secondary to decreased Na^+,K^+-ATPase activity and a decrease in sodium delivery to the distal nephron.[78] Finally, the immature distal nephron seems to have poor integrity and a tendency to leak potassium back into the plasma.[78]

Hyperkalemia

Hyperkalemia is a common problem, seen in 30% to 50% of infants with ELBW (birth weight ≤1000 g).[59,86-88] Because there are several potential problems with potassium secretion in the premature infant, it is not surprising that most of the studies that have examined the causes of hyperkalemia in ELBW infants have focused on renal causes of decreased potassium excretion. Gruskay and colleagues found that premature infants with hyperkalemia had higher FE_{Na} values than did infants without hyperkalemia; they suggested that these infants had a tubular defect in potassium excretion.[87] Brion and associates suggested that these infants had lower creatinine clearance rates and higher serum creatinine levels.[89] Fukuda and coworkers, in studying larger premature infants, found that infants with hyperkalemia had lower creatinine clearance values and higher serum creatinine levels, but there was no difference in FE_{Na} values.[86] Most studies have not been able to demonstrate a difference in urine flow rates between the infants with and without hyperkalemia. This problem has been labeled nonoliguric hyperkalemia. In a study by Shaffer and associates,[88] urine flow rates in infants with hyperkalemia were reported to be lower in the first 24 hours after birth.[88] After the first 24 hours, however, there was no difference in urine flow rate.

In addition to studying the possible renal factors that may limit potassium excretion and result in hyperkalemia, Stefano and Norman examined Na^+,K^+-ATPase activity as related to potassium flux from the intracellular compartment to the extracellular space as a possible etiology of hyperkalemia in these premature infants.[59] In this study, the authors found that Na^+,K^+-ATPase activity was lower in the ELBW infants with hyperkalemia and that the ratio of intracellular to extracellular potassium was lower in the infants with hyperkalemia. In addition, there was a greater degree of negative potassium balance in the infants with hyperkalemia; that is, the infants with hyperkalemia excreted more potassium than did the infants without hyperkalemia.

More recent studies by Lorenz and associates[90] and Sato and colleagues[91] have confirmed the finding that hyperkalemia in ELBW infants is the result of a shift of potassium ions from the intracellular space to the extracellular space. Stefano and Norman's data also suggested that the infants with hyperkalemia were in a state of extracellular volume contraction with a prerenal cause for the observed increase in blood urea nitrogen values. By measuring superior vena cava flow as an indicator of systemic blood flow, Kluckow and Evans demonstrated that hyperkalemic infants had lower superior vena caval flow than did infants who were normokalemic.[92] This reduction in systemic blood flow was also associated with a decrease in urinary output. An increase in catabolic state could also elevate blood urea nitrogen values and lead to cellular breakdown, resulting in a loss of potassium into the extracellular compartment. To evaluate increased catabolism as a possible cause of nonoliguric hyperkalemia, Stefano and associates also studied nitrogen balance and the urinary ratio of 3-methyl-histidine to creatinine in ELBW infants with and without hyperkalemia. Increases in the urinary ratio of 3-methyl-histidine to creatinine are associated with skeletal muscle catabolism. Stefano and associates could find no difference in the nitrogen balance or the urinary ratio of 3-methyl-histidine to creatinine between the infants with and those without hyperkalemia, which suggests that the elevated blood urea nitrogen levels seen in the hyperkalemic infants did not result from increased catabolism.[93]

The reasons for the decrease in Na^+,K^+-ATPase activity in ELBW infants with hyperkalemia are unclear. Possible explanations for the decreased activity are a genetic difference in the specific activity of the enzyme, a decrease in the receptor sites, developmental aspects of receptor function or number, inhibition of the enzyme or lack of specific enzyme induction (insulin and corticosteroids are known to be able to increase Na^+,K^+-ATPase activity), and damaged or altered enzyme. Omar and coworkers demonstrated that ELBW infants whose mothers were treated with prenatal corticosteroids had a lower incidence of hyperkalemia.[94] In addition, the infants whose mothers received corticosteroids had significantly less negative potassium balance than did ELBW infants who were not exposed to prenatal corticosteroids. This finding suggests stabilization of cell membranes by corticosteroids, possibly by inducing the activity of Na^+,K^+-ATPase.

Treatment Modalities

Several treatment modalities have been advocated for management of hyperkalemia in these infants. These include continuous insulin infusions, alkalinization (either by hyperventilation or bicarbonate therapy), potassium resin exchange solutions, and calcium infusions. Few data in the literature demonstrate efficacy of any of the therapies for nonoliguric hyperkalemia of the ELBW infant. A study by Malone suggested that insulin infusions decreased serum potassium values more efficiently than potassium resin exchange enemas.[95] In this study, however, there was no control group of infants who did not receive either therapy. In a preliminary investigation, Stefano and Norman were unable to show an effect on serum potassium levels or intracellular potassium concentration in hyperkalemia ELBW infants who were given continuous insulin infusions, in comparison with a group of ELBW infants with hyperkalemia who did not receive insulin.[96] Insulin facilitates potassium flux from the extracellular space into the cell by inducing Na^+,K^+-ATPase activity.[97] Stefano and Norman speculated that the reason for the lack of the effect of insulin on the serum potassium values is that, if the primary problem with nonoliguric hyperkalemia is related to damaged or inhibited Na^+,K^+-ATPase, the action of insulin to induce this enzyme may also be impaired. They also speculated that serum potassium levels decrease in these infants independent of the effect of insulin and reflect increased urinary potassium excretion. As potassium leaks from the cell (because of poor Na^+,K^+-ATPase activity), a greater potassium load is delivered and filtered at the glomerular level, which results in higher potassium excretion. More recently, albuterol and salbutamol have been shown to be effective in decreasing serum potassium levels in hyper-kalemic infants.[98,99] This is thought to be the result of inducing Na^+,K^+-ATPase. Angelopoulous and associates showed that albuterol was able to increase the net membrane flux of potassium in neonatal red blood cells under hyperkalemic conditions but was not able to increase adult red blood cell potassium flux.[100]

Despite the limited potassium secretory function in the distal nephron, studies by Engle and Arant,[101] Shaffer and associates,[88] and Stefano and Norman[59] indicate that premature infants are in negative potassium balance by the third or fourth day after birth. This excess in potassium excretion in comparison with intake may be related to the lower potassium reabsorptive capacity of the loop of Henle in the premature infant and has a greater effect than the limited secretory ability of the distal tubule and collecting duct. Therefore, clinicians need to be aware that these infants may waste potassium early in life. In the absence of nonoliguric hyperkalemia, maintenance replacement of potassium should be provided to these infants to avoid negative balance and the potential for potassium depletion. In some premature infants, the cumulative loss of potassium over the first 3 to 4 days after birth may be as high 9 mmol/kg.[101] This loss represents approximately 20% of total body potassium. In infants who are administered loop-inhibiting diuretics such as furosemide, renal potassium losses can be as high as 30% of total body potassium stores.[101] In addition to the effect of chronic potassium depletion on growth, these infants are also at risk of developing hypokalemia if potassium replacement is not provided as part of their maintenance electrolyte requirements.

REFERENCES

1. Calgano PL, Rubin MI: Renal extraction of para-aminohip-purate in infants and in children. J Clin Invest 42:1632, 1962.
2. Horster M, Lewy JE: Filtration fraction and extraction of PAH during neonatal period in the rat. Am J Physiol 219:1061, 1970.
3. Horster M, Valtin H: Postnatal development of renal function: Micropuncture and clearance studies in the dog. J Clin Invest 50:779, 1971.
4. Potter EL, Thierstein ST: Glomerular development in the kidney as an index of fetal maturity. J Pediatr 22:695, 1943.
5. Seikaly MG, Arant BS Jr: Development of renal hemodynamics: Glomerular filtration and renal blood flow. Clin Perinatol 19:1, 1992.
6. Rudolph AM, Heymann MA, Teramo KAW, et al: Studies on the circulation of the previable human fetus. Pediatr Res 5:452, 1971.
7. Aperia A, Herin P: Development of glomerular perfusion rate and nephron filtration rate in rats 17-60 days old. Am J Physiol 228:1319, 1975.
8. Felder RA, Pelayo JC, Calcagno PL, et al: Alpha adrenoceptors in the developing kidney. Pediatr Res 17:177, 1983.
9. Fildes RD, Eisner GM, Calcagno PL, et al: Renal alpha-adrenoceptors and sodium excretion in the dog. Am J Physiol 248:F128, 1985.
10. Jose PA, Slotkoff LM, Lilienfield L, et al: Sensitivity of the neonatal renal vasculature to epinephrine. Am J Physiol 226:796, 1974.
11. Arant BS Jr, Stephensen WH: Developmental changes in systemic vascular resistance compared with prostaglandins and angiotensin II concentration in arterial plasma of conscious dogs. Pediatr Res 16:120A, 1982.
12. Arant BS Jr, Seikaly MG: Intrarenal angiotensin II may regulate developmental changes in renal blood flow. Pediatr Res 25:334A, 1989.
13. Arant BS Jr, Seikaly MG: Intrarenal hemodynamic effects of angiotensin II and prostaglandins are independent. Pediatr Res 27:323A, 1990.
14. Aschinberg LC, Goldsmith DI, Olbing H, et al: Neonatal changes in renal blood flow distribution in puppies. Am J Physiol 228:1453, 1975.
15. Coulthard MG: Comparison of methods of measuring renal function in preterm babies using insulin. J Pediatr 102:923, 1983.
16. Levinsky NG, Levy M: Clearance techniques. In Orloff J, Berliner RW (eds): Renal Physiology. Baltimore, American Physiological Society, 1973, pp 103-117.
17. Schwartz GJ, Feld LG, Langford DJ: A simple estimate of glomerular filtration rate in full-term infants during the first year of life. J Pediatr 104:849, 1894
18. Shore RM, Koff SA, Mentser M, et al: Glomerular filtration rate in children: Determination from the Tc-99–DTPA renogram. Radiology 151:627, 1984.
19. Arant BS Jr: Developmental patterns of renal functional maturation compared in the human neonate. J Pediatr 92:705, 1978.
20. Engle WD, Arant BS Jr: Renal handling of beta-2-microglobulin in the human neonate. Kidney Int 24:360, 1983.
21. Hurley JK, Kirkpatrick SE, Pitlick PT, et al: Renal responses of the fetal lamb to fetal or maternal volume expansion. Circ Res 40:557, 1977.
22. Robillard JE, Weismann DN, Herin P, et al: Ontogeny of single glomerular perfusion rate in fetal and newborn lambs. Pediatr Res 15:1248, 1981.
23. Seikaly MG, Arant BS Jr, Seney FD Jr: Endogenous angiotensin concentrations in specific intrarenal fluid compartments of the rat. J Clin Invest 86:1352, 1990.
24. Daniel SS, James LS, Strauss J: Response to rapid volume expansion during the postnatal period. Pediatrics 68:809, 1981.
25. Leake RP, Zadauddin S, Trygstad CW, et al: The effects of large volume intravenous load on neonatal renal function. J Pediatr 89:968, 1976.
26. Friis-Hansen B: Body water compartments in children: Changes during growth and related changes in body composition. Pediatrics 28:169, 1961.
27. Bauer K, Bovermann G, Roithmaier A, et al: Body composition, nutrition, and fluid balance during the first two weeks of life in preterm neonates weighing less than 1500 grams. J Pediatr 118:615, 1991.
28. Langman CB, Engle WD, Baumgart S, et al: The diuretic phase of respiratory distress syndrome and its relationship to oxygenation. J Pediatr 98:462, 1981.
29. Costarino AT, Baumgart S, Norman ME, et al: Renal adaptation to extrauterine life in patients with respiratory distress syndrome. Am J Dis Child 139:1060, 1985.
30. Heaf D, Belik J, Spitzer AR, et al: Changes in pulmonary function during the diuretic phase of respiratory distress syndrome. J Pediatr 101:103, 1982.
31. de Bold AJ, Salerno TA: Natriuretic activity of extracts obtained from hearts of different species and from various rat tissues. Can J Physiol Pharmacol 61:127, 1983.
32. Kuribayashi T, Nakazato M, Tanaka M, et al: Renal effects of human α-atrial natriuretic polypeptide. N Engl J Med 312:1456, 1985.

33. Ledsome JR, Wilson N, Courneya CA, et al: Release of atrial natriuretic peptides by atrial distension. Can J Physiol Pharmacol 63:739, 1985.

34. Richards AM, Ikram H, Yandle TG, et al: Renal, haemodynamic, and hormonal effects of alpha atrial natriuretic peptide in healthy volunteers. Lancet 1:545, 1985.

35. Bierd TM, Kattwinkel J, Chevalier RL, et al: Interrelationship of atrial natriuretic peptide, atrial volume, and renal function in premature infants. J Pediatr 116:753, 1990.

36. Shaffer SG, Geer PG, Goetz KL: Elevated atrial natriuretic factor in neonates with RDS. J Pediatr 109:1028, 1986.

37. Modi N, Betremieux P, Midgley J, Hartnoll G: Postnatal weight loss and contraction of the extracellular compartment is triggered by atrial natriuretic peptide. Early Hum Dev 59:201, 2000.

38. Shaffer SG, Bradt SK, Hall RT: Postnatal changes in total body water and extracellular volume in the preterm infant with respiratory distress syndrome. J Pediatr 109:509, 1986.

39. Shaffer SG, Bradt SK, Meade MT, et al: Extracellular fluid volume changes in very low birth weight infants during the first 2 postnatal months. J Pediatr 111:124, 1987.

40. Rees L, Shaw JCL, Brook CGD, et al: Hyponatremia in the first week of life in preterm infants. Arch Dis Child 59:423, 1984.

41. Schlondorff D, Wever H, Trizna W, et al: Vasopressin responsiveness of renal adenylate cyclase in newborn rats and rabbits. Am J Physiol 234:F16, 1978.

42. Svenningsen N, Aronson AS: Postnatal development of renal concentration capacity as estimated by DDAVP test in normal and asphyxiated neonates. Biol Neonate 25:230, 1974.

43. Aperia A, Broberger O, Thodenius K, et al: Renal response to an oral sodium load in newborn full term infants. Acta Paediatr Scand 61:670, 1972.

44. Aperia A, Broberger O, Thadenius K, et al: Developmental study of the renal response to an oral salt load in pre-term infants. Acta Paediatr Scand 63:517, 1974.

45. Lorenz JM, Kleinman LI, Kotagal UR, et al: Water balance in very low-birth-weight infants: Relationship to water and sodium intake and effect on outcome. J Pediatr 101:423, 1982.

46. Bidiwala KS, Lorenz JM, Kleinman LI: Renal function correlates of postnatal diuresis in preterm infants. Pediatrics 82:50, 1988.

47. Baumgart S, Engle WD, Fox WW, et al: Radiant warmer power and body size as determinants of insensible water loss in the critically ill neonate. Pediatr Res 15:1495, 1981.

48. Baumgart S, Langman CB, Sosulski R, et al: Fluid, electrolyte, and glucose management in the very low birth weight infant. Clin Pediatr 21:199, 1982.

49. Baumgart S: Partitioning of heat losses and gains in premature newborn infants under radiant warmers. Pediatrics 75:1022, 1985.

50. Hammarlund K, Sedin G: Transepidermal water loss in newborn infants: VIII. Relation to gestational age and postnatal age in appropriate and small for gestational age infants. Acta Paediatr Scand 72:721, 1983.

51. Baumgart S: Reduction of oxygen consumption, insensible water loss, and radiant heat demand with the use of a plastic blanket for low-birthweight infants under radiant warmers. Pediatrics 74:1022, 1984.

52. Omar SA, DeCristofaro JD, Agarwal BI, et al: Effects of prenatal steroids on water and sodium hemostasis in extremely low birth weight neonates. Pediatrics 104:482, 1999.

53. Hogg RJ, Stapleton FB: Renal tubular function. In Holiday AH, Barratt TM, Vernier RL (eds): Pediatric Nephrology. Baltimore, Williams & Wilkins, 1987, pp 59-62.

54. Lewy JE, Windhager EE: Peritubular control of proximal tubular reabsorption in the rat kidney. Am J Physiol 214:943, 1968.

55. Spitzer A: The role of the kidney in sodium homeostasis during maturation. Kidney Int 21:539, 1982.

56. Spitzer A, Edelmann CM: Maturational changes in pressure gradients for glomerular filtration. Am J Physiol 221:1431, 1971.

57. Costarino AT, Gruskay JA, Corcoran L, et al: Sodium restriction versus daily maintenance replacement in very low birth weight premature neonates: A randomized, blind therapeutic trial. J Pediatr 120:99, 1992.

58. Shaffer SG, Meade VM: Sodium balance and extracellular volume regulation in very low birth weight infants. J Pediatr 115:285, 1989.

59. Stefano JL, Norman ME: Nitrogen balance in extremely low birth weight infants with nonoliguric hyperkalemia. J Pediatr 123:632, 1993.

60. Goldsmith DI, Drukker A, Blaufox MD, et al: Hemodynamic and excretory responses of the neonatal canine kidney to acute volume expansion. Am J Physiol 237:F392, 1979.

61. Kleinman LI, Reuter JH: Renal response of the newborn dog to a saline load: The role of intrarenal blood flow distribution. J Physiol 239:225, 1974.

62. Al-Dahhan J, Haycock GB, Chantler C, et al: Sodium homeostasis in term and preterm neonates. Arch Dis Child 58:335, 1983.

63. Rodríguez-Soriano J, Vallo A, Oliveros R, et al: Renal handling of sodium in premature and full-term neonates: A study using clearance methods during water diuresis. Pediatr Res 17:1013, 1983.

64. Sulyok E, Varga F, Györy E, et al: Postnatal development of renal sodium handling in premature infants. J Pediatr 95:787, 1979.

65. Aperia A, Broberger O, Herin P, et al: Sodium excretion in relation to sodium intake and aldosterone excretion in newborn pre-term and full-term infants. Acta Paediatr Scand 68:813, 1979.

66. Vanpée M, Herin P, Zetterström R, Aperia A: Postnatal development of renal function in very low birthweight infants. Acta Paediatr Scand 77:191, 1988.

67. De Marchi S, Bertotti A, Davanzo R, et al: Usefulness of the ratio of $U_K/U_{Na + K}$ for the study of the renal handling of sodium and potassium in full-term neonates. Nephron 45:169, 1987.

68. Schmidt U, Horster M: Na-K–activated ATPase: Activity maturation in rabbit nephron segments dissected in vitro. Am J Physiol 233:F55, 1977.

69. Stephenson G, Hammet M, Hadaway G, et al: Ontogeny of renal mineralocorticoid receptors and urinary electrolytes responses in the rat. Am J Physiol 247:F665, 1984.

70. Bailie MD: Development of the endocrine function of the kidney. Clin Perinatol 19:59, 1992.

71. Felder RA, Felder CC, Eisner GM, et al: The dopamine receptor in the adult and developing kidney. Am J Physiol 257:F315, 1989.

72. Felder RA, Nakamura KT, Robillard JE, et al: Dopamine receptors in the developing sheep kidney. Pediatr Nephrol 2:156, 1988.

73. Nakamura KT, Felder RA, Jose P, et al: Effects of dopamine in the renal vascular bed of fetal, newborn and adult sheep. Am J Physiol 252:R490, 1987.

74. Felder RA, Robillard J, Eisner GM, et al: Role of endogenous dopamine on renal sodium excretion. Semin Nephrol 9:91, 1989.

75. Pelayo JC, Fildes RD, Jose PA: Age dependent effects of intrarenal dopamine infusion. Am J Physiol 247:R212, 1984.

76. Kinoshita S, Jose PA, Felder RA: Ontogeny of the dopamine (DA1) receptor in the rat renal proximal convoluted tubule (PCT) [Abstract]. Pediatr Res 25:68A, 1989.

77. Bertorello A, Aperia A: Short term regulation of Na^+,K^+-ATPase activity by dopamine. Am J Hypertens 3(Suppl):51, 1990.

78. Satlin LM: Maturation of renal potassium transport. Pediatr Nephrol 5:260, 1991.

79. Solomon S: Maximal gradients of Na and K across proximal tubules of kidneys of immature rats. Biol Neonate 25:327, 1974.

80. Kleinman LI, Banks RO: Segmental nephron sodium and potassium reabsorption in newborn and adult dogs during saline expansion. Proc Soc Exp Biol Med 173:231, 1983.

81. Zink H, Horster M: Maturation of diluting capacity in loop of Henle of rat superficial nephrons. Am J Physiol 233:F519, 1977.

82. Katz AI: Renal Na-K-ATPase: Its role in tubular sodium and potassium transport. Am J Physiol 242:F207, 1982.

83. Lorenz JM, Kleinman LI, Disney TA: Renal response of newborn dogs to potassium loading. Am J Physiol 251:F513, 1986.

84. Aperia A, Larsson L, Zetterstrom R: Hormonal induction of Na-K-ATPase in developing proximal tubular cells. Am J Physiol 241:F356, 1981.

85. Garcio-Fitho E, Malnic G, Giebisch: Effect of changes in electrical potential difference on tubular potassium transport. Am J Physiol 238:F235, 1980.

86. Fukuda Y, Kojima T, Ono A, et al: Factors causing hyperkalemia in premature infants. Am J Perinatol 6:76, 1989.

87. Gruskay J, Costarino AT, Polin RA, et al: Nonoliguric hyperkalemia in the premature infant weighing less than 1000 grams. J Pediatr 113:38, 1988.

88. Shaffer SG, Kilbride HW, Hayen LK, et al: Hyperkalemia in very low birth weight infants. J Pediatr 121:275, 1992.

89. Brion LP, Schwartz GJ, Campbell D, et al: Early hyperkalemia in very low birth weight infants in the absence of oliguria. Arch Dis Child 64:279, 1989.

90. Lorenz JM, Kleinman LI, Markarian K: Potassium metabolism in extremely low birth weight infants in the first week of life. J Pediatr 131:81, 1997.

91. Sato K, Kondo T, Iwao H, et al: Internal potassium shift in premature infants: Cause of nonoliguric hyperkalemia. J Pediatr 126:109, 1995.

92. Kluckow M, Evans N: Low systemic blood flow and hyperkalemia in preterm infants. J Pediatr 139:227, 2001.

93. Stefano JL, Norman ME, Morales MC, et al: Decreased erythrocyte Na^+,K^+-ATPase activity associated with cellular potassium loss in extremely low birth weight infants with nonoliguric hyperkalemia. J Pediatr 122:276, 1993.

94. Omar SA, DeCristofaro, JD, Agarwal, BI, et al: Effect of prenatal steroids on potassium balance in extremely low birth weight neonates. Pediatrics 106:561, 2000.

95. Malone TA: Glucose and insulin versus cation-exchange resin for the treatment of hyperkalemia in very low birth weight infants. J Pediatr 118:121, 1991.

96. Stefano JL, Norman ME: Insulin therapy for nonoliguric hyperkalemia in the extremely low birth weight infant: Is it effective? [Abstract]. Pediatr Res 31:66A, 1992.

97. Moore RD: Effects of insulin upon ion transport. Biochim Biophys Acta 737:1, 1983.

98. Greenough A, Emery EF, Brooker R, Gamsu HR: Salbutamol infusion to treat neonatal hyperkalaemia. J Perinat Med 20:437, 1992.

99. Singh BS, Sadiq HF, Noguchi A, Keenan WJ: Efficacy of albuterol inhalation in treatment of hyperkalemia in premature neonates. J Pediatr 141:16, 2002.

100. Angelopoulous M, Leitz H, Lambert G, MacGilvray S: In vitro analysis of the Na(+)-K+ ATPase activity in neonatal and adult red blood cells. Biol Neonate 69:140, 1996.

101. Engle WD, Arant BS: Urinary potassium excretion in the critically ill neonate. Pediatrics 74:259, 1984.

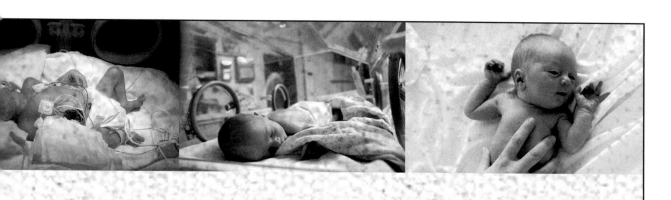

Renal Disorders in the Neonate

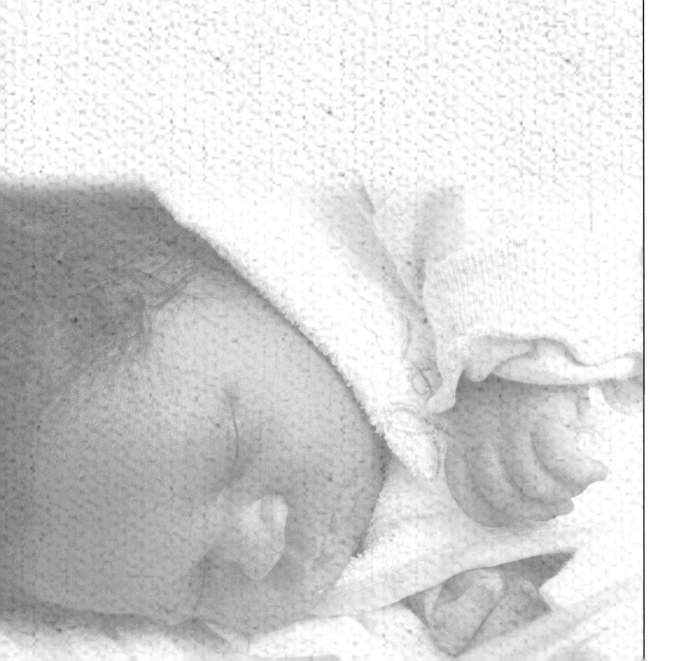

CHAPTER 78

Neonatal Hypertension

Michael A. Vozzelli and John W. Foreman

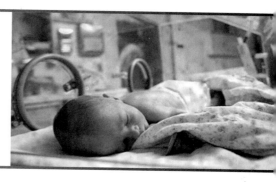

Neonatal hypertension was first recognized as a clinical problem in the 1970s and described as a complication of umbilical artery catheterization in 1975.[1,2] Umbilical artery catheterization was first introduced as an investigative procedure in 1962.[3] It is now standard procedure for arterial blood sampling and blood pressure monitoring in sick newborns. Historically, the leading causes of hypertension in infancy were related to thromboembolic complications of umbilical catheter placement.[4] Although renovascular disease continues to be a major cause of neonatal hypertension, advances in catheter technology and increased rates of survival among premature newborns have heightened the importance of other causes.

Hypertension in infancy is becoming increasingly recognized with improved methods of blood pressure measurement and monitoring and increased rates of survival among infants, particularly premature infants. There remains a paucity of data for normative blood pressure values in preterm infants. There are even fewer data regarding the treatment of hypertension in premature infants, in spite of an ever-expanding repertoire of antihypertensive agents.

MEASUREMENT OF BLOOD PRESSURE

Blood pressure changes throughout infancy and varies by birth weight, gestational age, and postnatal age. There is a marked rise in blood pressure in the normal newborn in the first hours and days after birth.[4] The state of the infant's alertness also affects the blood pressure. Blood pressure rises with crying, feeding, agitation, and upright positioning.[5] Crying infants may have increases in systolic blood pressure up to 17 to 25 mm Hg higher than those in quiet infants, and systolic pressure is about 6 to 12 mm Hg higher in awake infants than in sleeping infants.[6,7]

There are several ways to accurately measure blood pressure in infants. Connection of aortic and peripheral arterial catheters to a pressure transducer is the most accurate method for measurement of blood pressure in sick neonates.[8] There are, however, potential sources of error in these measurements. If the catheter is too small in diameter, the systolic pressure may be underestimated because of the loss of higher frequencies. If the catheter is against the wall of the vessel or if there is a clot at the tip, the pressure waves may be dampened and the blood pressure underestimated. Finally, air bubbles in the transduction system may alter the blood pressure measurement.[9] Classic auscultatory methods used in adults and older children are impractical in infants because of the difficulty in hearing the brachial pulse. Automatic oscillometric monitors are the mostly widely used noninvasive technique. These monitors report systolic, diastolic, and mean arterial pressures, eliminating operator bias and number preference.[10] The occluding cuff senses pressure fluctuations, and there is a characteristic change in the magnitude of oscillation at the levels at which systolic, diastolic, and mean pressures are recorded. This noninvasive method provides reproducible and accurate estimates of blood pressure in infants.[11,12] Inaccuracies may occur with extreme hypotension and in infants with very low birth weight.[13] Finally, the Doppler gauge is a useful way to measure systolic blood pressure. It measures systolic pressure by detecting blood flow with the gradual release of cuff pressure, but it does not accurately estimate diastolic pressure.

Proper cuff size is important for the accurate measurement of blood pressure. Cuffs that are too small give falsely high readings; therefore, it is best to use the widest cuff that can be applied to an infant's arm or leg. Cuff size is based on the size of the inflatable bladder and not the cloth covering.[10] The cuff bladder should cover at least two thirds of the upper arm or thigh and 80% to 100% of the arm or thigh circumference.[14-16]

Normal blood pressure values in full-term infants have been well described in the first hours and days after birth.[17] There are no racial or sex differences during the first year after birth.[14] The Brompton study reported data from over 3000 full-term infants taken during the first year after birth using the Doppler method.[18] These results were incorporated into the 1987 Task Force Report on

Table 78–1. Full-Term Infant Blood Pressure

	Systolic		Diastolic	
Age	Boy	Girl	Boy	Girl
< 7 days	73 ± 10	72 ± 9	51 ± 9	50 ± 8
8 days–1 month	82 ± 11	82 ± 12	50 ± 11	51 ± 12
1–6 months	93 ± 13	92 ± 12	48 ± 11	50 ± 11

Modified from Task Force on Blood Pressure Control in Children: Report of the Second Task Force on Blood Pressure Control in Children—1987. Pediatrics 79:1, 1987.

Results are means (mm Hg) ± standard deviations.

Blood Pressure Control in Children (Table 78-1).[19] Mean blood pressure rises 1 to 2 mm Hg per day during the first week after birth and 1 to 2 mm Hg per week over the next 6 months.[20] There is no significant increase in systolic blood pressure between 2 months and 1 year.

Although there are less extensive data for preterm infants, several researchers have investigated normal blood pressure values in premature infants.[1,21-24] One of the largest studies to date was published by Zubrow and colleagues, who prospectively obtained blood pressure measurements over a period of 3 months from nearly 700 infants born after 22 weeks of gestation and admitted to large metropolitan intensive care units.[24] From these data, they defined the mean plus the upper and lower 95% confidence limits for blood pressure during the first 5 days after birth in infants older than 22 weeks of gestation (Figs. 78-1 to 78-4). Blood pressure increases with increasing gestational age, birth weight, and postconception age. In newborns who are small for gestational age, blood pressure is correlated more closely with the weight of the infant than with gestational age. By 4 months of age, there are no differences in either systolic or diastolic blood pressures in infants with birth weights of less than 1500 g and those with birth weights exceeding 2500 g.[25]

DEFINITION AND INCIDENCE OF HYPERTENSION

Hypertension is rare in healthy full-term neonates, and it is so unusual that routine blood pressure determination is not advocated for this group.[26] Adelman first described criteria for diagnosing hypertension in infancy as persistent blood pressures of more than 90/60 in full-term infants and 80/50 in preterm infants.[1] For full-term infants, hypertension occurs when the blood pressure is at or exceeds the 95th percentile for age. These values have served as a useful guideline for infants with a birth weight exceeding 1000 g. With increasing survival of infants with very low birth weight and a wide range of blood pressures in premature infants, it is better to define preterm neonatal hypertension as persistent systolic or diastolic blood pressure readings that are at or exceed the 95th percentile for gestational age and birth weight. The incidence of hypertension in neonates is quite low,

ranging from 0.2% of healthy newborns to 3% of newborns at high risk.[1,27-30] In one series, Sheftel and associates reported an incidence as high as 8.9% of premature infants with hypertension after discharge, but only 2.6% of this group had persistent hypertension at later follow-up.[31]

CAUSES OF HYPERTENSION

Hypertension can arise from numerous causes (Table 78-2). Volume overload from excess sodium and water administration or retention can cause hypertension. Obstruction to renal blood flow is another common cause with the release of renin and the generation of angiotensin molecules, especially angiotensin II. Obstructive uropathy or injury to the renal parenchyma can cause renin release and high blood pressure. Various other hormones such as catecholamines, glucocorticoids, and mineralocorticoids play a role in blood pressure regulation, and their excess, both from exogenous administration or endogenous generation, can cause high blood pressure. Less well defined are various vasodilator hormones that can lower blood pressure; deficiency of these hormones may lead to hypertension. Finally, the central nervous system plays an important role in blood pressure regulation; injury to the central nervous system or stimulation from pain can cause hypertension.

Multiple studies have demonstrated that renovascular disease is the most common cause of neonatal hypertension.[1,27-30,32,33] However, this statement may not be true with current neonatal practices. Renovascular hypertension in the neonate is usually related to the presence of an umbilical artery catheter and renal artery occlusion by a thrombus associated with this catheter or embolization to the renal artery. Although several researchers have investigated the duration and position of catheter placement ("high" versus "low") as factors in thrombus formation, the data are inconclusive.[34-37] The most likely cause of the thrombus formation is damage to the vascular endothelium during placement of the catheter.[34] Renal artery thrombosis and emboli are rarely observed in infants who have not had umbilical artery catheters. In rare cases, renovascular hypertension may occur from other causes, such as fibromuscular dysplasia that leads to renal artery stenosis or mechanical compression of one or both renal

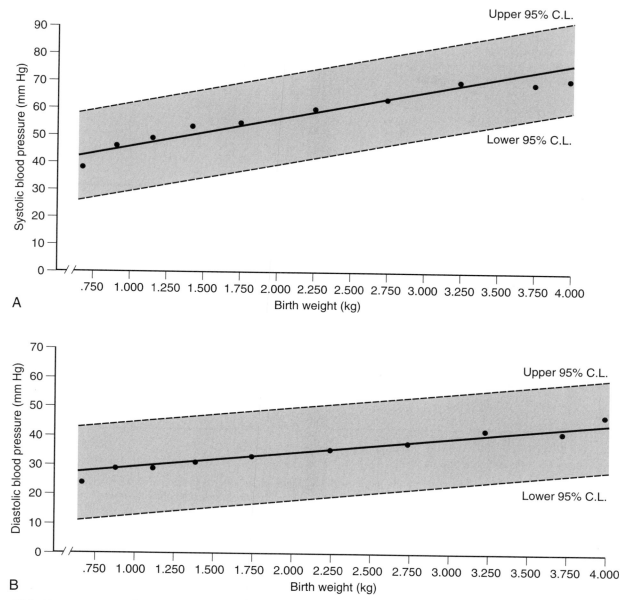

Figure 78–1. Linear regression of mean systolic **(A)** and diastolic **(B)** blood pressure by birth weight on day 1 after birth. C.L., confidence limit. *(Reproduced from Zubrow AB, Hulman S, Kushner H, et al: Determinants of blood pressure in infants admitted to neonatal intensive care units: a prospective multicenter study. J Perinatol 15:470, 1995.)*

arteries by tumors, hydronephrotic kidneys, or other abdominal masses.[34] Renal venous thrombosis may also cause hypertension. Initially, there is usually hypotension along with nephromegaly and hematuria. Hypertension typically appears later, probably in relation to renal parenchymal injury. When renal vein thrombosis is associated with hypertension in the initial manifestation, it is often accompanied by renal artery thrombosis.[38]

Congenital renal parenchymal disease accounts for the next largest group of hypertensive disorders in neonates.[34] Autosomal dominant and autosomal recessive polycystic kidney disease may manifest in the neonatal period with hypertension and nephromegaly. The majority of infants

with polycystic kidney disease have the recessive form, and most cases are discovered within the first year after birth. Hypertension is extremely common among such infants and may be quite severe, leading to congestive heart failure.[39] More common is dysplasia of the renal parenchyma, often associated with obstructive uropathy or anomalies of renal size and/or position; affected infants may develop hypertension.

Renal obstruction may cause hypertension in the absence of renal artery compression.[34] Congenital ureteropelvic junction obstruction is the most common cause of urinary tract obstruction, although ureterovesical obstruction and posterior urethral valves are also important causes.[27,29,33]

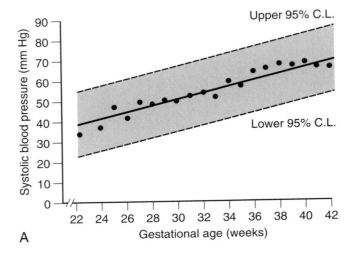

A

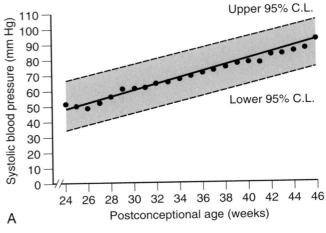

A

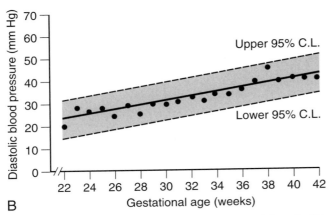

B

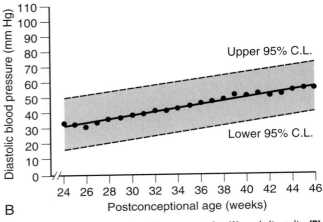

B

Figure 78–2. Linear regression of mean systolic **(A)** and diastolic **(B)** blood pressure by gestational age on day 1 after birth. C.L., confidence limit. *(Reproduced from Zubrow AB, Hulman S, Kushner H, et al: Determinants of blood pressure in infants admitted to neonatal intensive care units: a prospective multicenter study. J Perinatol 15:470, 1995.)*

Figure 78–3. Linear regression of mean systolic **(A)** and diastolic **(B)** blood pressure by postconceptual age in weeks. C.L., confidence limit. *(Reproduced from Zubrow AB, Hulman S, Kushner H, et al: Determinants of blood pressure in infants admitted to neonatal intensive care units: a prospective multicenter study. J Perinatol 15:470, 1995.)*

The hypertension may persist after surgical relief of obstruction, and the pathophysiologic process probably involves alterations of the renin-angiotensin pathway.[40-42]

Acquired renal parenchymal disease is another important cause of neonatal hypertension. Common causes are pyelonephritis, acute tubular necrosis from birth asphyxia, and interstitial nephritis from toxins or drugs. Renal failure often accompanies the hypertension. Both volume overload and hyperreninemia are implicated as the mechanisms underlying the blood pressure rise.[34]

Coarctation of the aorta may manifest in infancy as upper extremity hypertension, typically with blood pressure in the right arm exceeding that in the left arm. It is present in 0.2 infants per 1000 live births.[43] The diagnosis may be delayed if only a left arm blood pressure is measured.[10] In some infants, the ductus arteriosus plays an important role in supplying blood to the lower body, and diminished pulses may not be evident; therefore, the diagnosis of coarctation is delayed.

Neurologic causes of hypertension are common in affected neonates. The most frequent of these causes is pain, which has gained increased recognition. The treatment is adequate analgesia. Other neurologic causes include intraventricular hemorrhage, increased intracranial pressure, drug withdrawal, and seizures. Seizures are more often a symptom of severe hypertension rather than the cause.

Endocrinopathies may also cause hypertension in the neonate. Although rare, these disorders are generally treatable. The most common of these unusual disorders are congenital adrenal hyperplasia secondary to 11β- and 17α-hydroxylase deficiency, hyperaldosteronism, and hyperthyroidism.[44-47] Pheochromocytoma, a catecholamine-secreting tumor, has been described in newborns, although it is extremely rare. Neonatal screening has enabled identification of some of these disorders before hypertension is manifest. Treatment is directed at the underlying endocrinopathy.

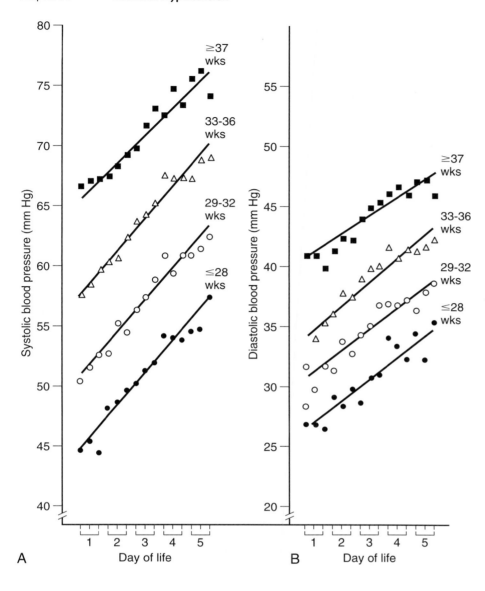

Figure 78–4. Systolic **(A)** and diastolic **(B)** blood pressure plotted for the first 5 days after birth by 8-hour increments for the four gestational age groups. *(Reproduced from Zubrow AB, Hulman S, Kushner H, et al: Determinants of blood pressure in infants admitted to neonatal intensive care units: a prospective multicenter study. J Perinatol 15:470, 1995.)*

Malignancies are rare causes of hypertension in neonates. Mesoblastic nephroma is the most common, but most infants with this do not have hypertension. In rare cases, Wilms tumor or neuroblastoma may manifest in the newborn period and cause hypertension. The mechanism of the hypertension is usually compression of the renal vessels or ureters. In addition, Wilms tumors and neuroblastomas may secrete renin and catecholamines, which may cause hypertension.[48,49]

A cause of neonatal hypertension that has rapidly become widespread is chronic lung disease.[50] This prevalence is, in part, related to the increased rate of survival among infants with extremely low birth weights. Bronchopulmonary dysplasia (BPD) remains a major cause of pulmonary morbidity and mortality despite advances in surfactant administration and modern methods of ventilation. It is unclear how chronic lung disease leads to systemic hypertension, but it may be related to increased vascular tone stimulated by hypoxia and/or hypercapnia.[51] Corticosteroids used to treat the lung disease may play a role, but many affected infants remain hypertensive for months after the steroids are stopped.[52-56] Hypertension from BPD resolves in most affected infants by 6 months of age.

Medications may also cause neonatal hypertension. Methylxanthines, pancuronium, and phenylephrine ophthalmic drops have been shown to cause hypertension.[57] Hydrocortisone, used to treat adrenal insufficiency in ill neonates, may cause hypertension. Maternal use of illicit drugs, such as cocaine and heroin, with their subsequent delivery to the fetus through the placenta may lead to hypertension in the neonate. Cocaine has been found in breast milk for up to 36 hours after maternal ingestion, and cocaine intoxication has been reported in breast-fed infants.[58] Hypertension may also be seen as part of the heroin withdrawal syndrome.

Systemic hypertension has been associated with extracorporeal membrane oxygenation in infants with

Table 78-2. Causes of Hypertension in Infants

Renovascular
Renal artery thromboembolism
Renal artery stenosis
Midaortic coarctation
Compression of renal artery
Renal vein thrombosis
Idiopathic infantile arterial calcification syndrome

Renal Parenchymal Disease
Congenital
Renal hypoplasia/dysplasia
Ureteropelvic junction obstruction
Posterior urethral valves
Polycystic kidney disease

Acquired
Acute tubular necrosis
Cortical necrosis
Pyelonephritis
Drug-induced interstitial nephritis

Cardiac
Coarctation of the aorta

Pulmonary
Bronchopulmonary dysplasia

Endocrine
Congenital adrenal hyperplasia secondary to 11 β- or
   17α-hydroxylase deficiency
Hyperthyroidism
Hyperaldosteronism
Pheochromocytoma

Medications
Corticosteroids
Adrenergic agents
Theophylline
Caffeine
Pancuronium
Phenylephrine eye drops

Illicit drugs
Cocaine
Heroin

Neoplasia
Mesoblastic nephroma
Wilms tumor
Neuroblastoma
Pheochromocytoma

Neurologic
Pain
Increased intracranial pressure
Seizures

Other
Fluid overload
Extracorporeal membrane oxygenation
Abdominal wall defect closure
Hypercalcemia

cardiorespiratory failure. One study demonstrated that more than half of the infants receiving this therapy developed hypertension at some point.[59] The origin of the hypertension is unclear but may be related to volume overload, increased systemic vascular resistance, or nonpulsatile flow to the kidneys. An unusual cause of systemic hypertension is idiopathic infantile arterial calcification syndrome. This rare, and usually fatal, autosomal recessive disorder typically manifests with heart failure and hypertension. The hallmark is arterial calcification of all tissue layers of large and medium-sized arteries, which may be apparent on plain radiographs. Hypertension associated with this disease is generally refractory to medical management. Hypercalcemia from any cause, such as vitamin D intoxication or total parenteral nutrition, can cause hypertension in children and adults. Hypertension has also been noted in infants after closure of abdominal wall defects.[60,61]

CLINICAL PRESENTATION AND DIAGNOSIS

Like older children and adults, many neonates with hypertension are completely asymptomatic.[1] Clinical manifestations usually depend on the underlying cause and the severity of the hypertension. Longer standing hypertension may result in cardiopulmonary symptoms, including tachycardia, tachypnea, cyanosis, cardiomegaly, and congestive heart failure. Acute hypertension may reflexively cause bradycardia. Aortic thrombosis may cause unequal pulses, mottling, and cyanosis in the lower extremities. Neurologic manifestations of poor feeding, lethargy, apnea, and irritability may be seen. Severe hypertension can cause vomiting, seizures, coma, and strokes.

The first step in evaluating neonatal hypertension is obtaining a detailed maternal obstetric history, including medications and recreational drug use. A review of labor and delivery room events, as well as a review of the medications that the infant is receiving, is also important. Birth asphyxia or placental abruption may lead to acute renal failure and hypertension. A thorough physical examination should be performed. Particular attention should be directed toward signs of volume overload, congestive heart failure, abdominal masses, ambiguous genitalia, diminished femoral pulses, or neurologic deficits. Nephromegaly, caused by hydronephrosis, polycystic kidney disease, or renal vein thrombosis, may be evident on physical examination. This examination should include the measurement of the resting blood pressure in all four extremities. Routine laboratory tests should include measurement of serum electrolytes, creatinine, and blood urea nitrogen. A urinalysis and urine culture should be performed in infants suspected of having urologic abnormalities. Complete blood cell counts and a coagulation profile are useful in the sick neonate with hypertension. Proteinuria and hematuria usually point to a renal cause of hypertension. Severe hypertension can cause proteinuria, polyuria, and salt wasting.

Interpretation of plasma renin levels is difficult in the neonate. Plasma renin levels vary with gestational and postnatal age.[62] Most antihypertensive medications either stimulate or inhibit renin release; therefore, blood samples for renin should be obtained before treatment is started.[63,64] Increased plasma renin levels, especially if they are markedly elevated, may indicate renovascular disease, but they may be elevated for other reasons: for example, in respiratory distress or parenchymal renal disease.[10]

In infants without a readily identifiable nonrenal cause for their hypertension, the urinary tract should be imaged by ultrasonography. Ultrasonography is noninvasive and can be performed at the bedside on sick, very preterm infants. Because the technique is independent of renal function, poorly functioning kidneys can be visualized. With Doppler interrogation of the vessels, aortic and renal blood flow can be assessed. Renal scans may be helpful to quantitate the function of each kidney and evaluate hydronephrosis, but often they are of limited value in neonates because of poor image quality in the first month after birth. Arteriography is rarely necessary, because renovascular hypertension often resolves spontaneously and detection can be made by noninvasive studies. Intravenous pyelography has largely been replaced by renal ultrasonography and radionuclide studies. Infants

with neurologic signs and symptoms should undergo brain imaging, such as ultrasonography, computed tomographic scanning, or magnetic resonance imaging.

Endocrine disorders are unusual causes of hypertension in newborns. The presence of ambiguous genitalia and hypertension should raise the suspicion of a block in adrenal steroid synthesis, such as 11β- or 17α-hydroxylase deficiency, which can be defined by measuring urinary steroid metabolites. Isolated systolic hypertension and tachycardia may indicate neonatal hyperthyroidism and warrant thyroid studies. Measurements of urinary catecholamines and their metabolites, such as metanephrine and vanillylmandelic acid, are helpful in evaluating an infant for a catecholamine-secreting tumor.

TREATMENT

Treatment of neonatal hypertension should first be directed at the underlying cause. Hypertension associated with indwelling umbilical arterial catheters is often corrected with catheter removal. Thrombolytic therapy is

Table 78–3. Neonatal Antihypertensive Medications

Medication	Route	Dose	Dose Frequency	Comments
Diuretics				
Hydrochlorothiazide	Oral	1–3 mg/kg/day	bid	Minimizes urinary calcium
Furosemide	IV, oral	1–4 mg/kg/day	bid-qid	Hypercalciuria, hyponatremia
Spironolactone	Oral	1–3 mg/kg/day	tid	Weak diuretic, potassium sparing
Adrenergic Blockers				
β blockers–Propranolol	Oral	1–4 mg/kg/day	bid-qid	Bradycardia
α and β blocker–Labetalol*	IV	0.5–3 mg/kg/hr	Continuous	
	Oral	1–10 mg/kg/dose	bid-tid	
Vasodilators				
Hydralazine*	IV	0.1–0.6 mg/kg/dose	Q4h-Q6h	Tachycardia
Nitroprusside*	IV	0.2–10 μg/kg/min	Continuous	Monitor for thiocyanate toxicity
Minoxidil	Oral	0.1–0.2 mg/kg/dose	bid	Hirsutism
Angiotensin-Converting Enzyme Inhibitors (ACE-I)				
Captopril	Oral	10–500 μg/kg/day	tid-qid	ACE-I can reduce renal and cerebral blood flow leading to oliguria, renal failure, and seizures.
Enalaprilat*	IV	5–15 μg/kg/dose	Q8h-Q24h	They also can cause hyperkalemia.
Enalapril	Oral	40–150 μg/kg/dose	tid-once daily	
Ca²⁺ Channel Blocker				
Nifedipine*	Oral	0.25–0.5 mg/kg/dose	Q2h-Q6h	Difficult to dose in neonates
Nicardipine*	IV	0.5–2 μg/kg/min	Continuous	Very effective in severe hypertension
Isradapine	Oral	0.05–0.15 mg/kg/dose max 0.8 mg/kg/dose	qid	
Amlodipine	Oral	0.1–0.3 mg/kg/day max 0.6 mg/kg/day	bid-once daily	
Central Adrenergic Agonist				
Clonidine	Oral	3–10 μg/kg/day	bid-tid	Very limited dose information

*Useful in malignant hypertension.

indicated for patients at high risk for complete occlusion of the aorta. Removal of the obstruction in hydronephrosis frequently relieves hypertension. In rare cases, nephrectomy is necessary for blood pressure management. Dosage reduction or discontinuation of medications that cause hypertension, such as methylxanthines, steroids, and β agonists, may return the blood pressure to normal. Adequate analgesia, especially postoperatively, corrects the hypertension associated with pain. Hypertension secondary to volume overload is initially treated with fluid and sodium restriction. Diuretics can be used if restriction alone is inadequate.

Pharmacologic treatment of hypertension should be considered in neonates with sustained blood pressures higher than the 95th percentile of infants with the same age and weight. Although there is an ever-expanding armamentarium of antihypertensive agents, there is very limited information regarding dosing, clearance, and adverse effects in infants. This is especially true in premature infants.

Antihypertensive medications should be administered in graduated dosages, starting at the lowest dosage and increasing until the desired effect is accomplished (Table 78-3). Rapid correction to a normal blood pressure should be avoided, as this may result in neurologic injury.[65] It is usually best to maximize the dosage of one agent before starting another. In infants requiring multiple agents, it is useful to devise a combination that "trades off" side effects: for example, combining a β blocker, which causes bradycardia, with a vasodilator, which causes tachycardia. Clinical factors other than the hypertension may restrict the types of antihypertensive medication. For example, β blockers are relatively contraindicated in BPD.

Diuretics are very useful in treating neonatal hypertension, especially that associated with volume overload and BPD. In BPD, diuretics treat both hypertension and pulmonary edema. They are also useful in combination for severe hypertension.

Mild hypertension can usually be treated with a single agent, such as a diuretic, an angiotensin-converting enzyme inhibitor, or a β blocker. Oral nifedipine is effective, but it is very difficult to administer the correct dose accurately in the newborn. Isradipine, another oral calcium-channel blocker, has been used in neonates. Malignant hypertension should be treated promptly to prevent neurologic injury. It usually necessitates intravenous agents either alone or in combination with oral agents. Nicardipine, an intravenous calcium-channel blocker, has been used widely and is quite effective at lowering blood pressure.[66] Its rapid onset of action and short half-life make it convenient to titrate. Nicardipine has largely replaced nitroprusside because it does not result in the generation of toxic metabolites. Labetalol, hydralazine, and enalaprilat have also been used intravenously for severe hypertension. Newborns are quite sensitive to angiotensin-converting enzyme inhibitors such as captopril, enalapril, and enalaprilat. Renal function should be monitored carefully, and the dosage should be lower than those used in older children.

PROGNOSIS

In general, the prognosis for neonatal hypertension is good but depends on the underlying cause. Renovascular hypertension secondary to umbilical artery catheterization usually resolves over time.[67] Iatrogenic hypertension secondary to medications (e.g., steroids) also has a very good prognosis. Most infants can be weaned from antihypertensives completely. Hypertension associated with BPD usually resolves by 6 months of age. Infants with persistent hypertension should be monitored over the long term with the aim of maintaining normal blood pressure, to prevent the long-term complications of cardiovascular and renal dysfunction.[67,68]

REFERENCES

1. Adelman RD: Neonatal hypertension. Pediatr Clin North Am 25:101, 1978.
2. Bauer SB, Feldman SM, Gellis SS, et al: Neonatal hypertension: A complication of umbilical artery catheterization. N Engl J Med 293:1032, 1975.
3. Nelson NM, Prod'hom LS, Cherry RB, et al: Pulmonary function in the newborn infant. Pediatrics 30:975, 1962.
4. Grupe WE: Hypertension. In Avery ME, Taeusch HW (eds): Schaffer's Diseases of the Newborn. Philadelphia, WB Saunders, 1984, pp 441-447.
5. Gupta JM, Scopes JW: Observations on blood pressure in newborn infants. Arch Dis Child 40:637, 1965.
6. Moss AJ, Duffie ER Jr, Emmanouilides G: Blood pressure and vasomotor reflexes in the newborn infant. Pediatrics 32:175, 1963.
7. Uhari M: Changes in blood pressure during the first year of life. Acta Pediatr Scand 69:613, 1980.
8. Adelman RD: Neonatal hypertension. In Loggi JMH, Horan MJ, Gruskin AB, et al (eds): Workshop on Juvenile Hypertension. New York, Biomedical Information, 1984, pp 267-283.
9. Weindling AM: Blood pressure monitoring in the newborn. Arch Dis Child 64:444, 1989.
10. Goble MM: Hypertension in infancy. Child Hypertens 40:105, 1993.
11. Kimble K, Darnall RA, Yelderman M, et al: An automated oscillometric technique for estimating mean arterial pressure in critically ill newborns. Anesthesiology 54:423, 1981.
12. Park MK, Menard SM: Accuracy of blood pressure measurement by the Dinamap monitor in infants and children. Pediatrics 79:907, 1987.
13. Rasoulpour M, Marinelli, KA: Systemic hypertension. Clin Perinatol 19:121, 1992.
14. Low JA, Panagiotopoulos C, Smith JT, et al: Validity of newborn oscillometric blood pressure. Clin Invest Med 18:163, 1995.
15. Pellegrini-Calliumi G, Agostino R, Nodari S. et al: Evaluation of an automatic oscillometric method and of various cuffs for the measurement of arterial pressure in the neonate. Acta Paediatr Scand 71:791, 1982.
16. Sonesson SE, Broberger U: Arterial blood pressure in the very low birth weight newborn: Evaluation of an automatic oscillometric technique. Acta Paediatr Scand 76:338, 1987.
17. Kitterman JA, Phibbs RH, Tooley WH: Aortic blood pressure during the first 12 hours of life. Pediatrics 44:959, 1969.

18. De Swiet M, Fayers P, Shinebourne EA: Systolic blood pressure in a population of infants in the first year of life: The Brompton Study. Pediatrics 65:1031, 1980.

19. Task Force on Blood Pressure Control in Children: Report of the Second Task Force on Blood Pressure Control in Children—1987. Pediatrics 79:1, 1987.

20. De Swiet M, Fayers P, Shinebourne EA: Blood pressure survey in a population of newborn infants. BMJ 2:9, 1976.

21. Hegyi T, Carbone MT, Anwar M, et al: Blood pressure ranges in premature infants. I. The first hours of life. J Pediatr 124:627, 1994.

22. Hegyi T, Anwar M, Carbone MT, et al: Blood pressure ranges in premature infants: II. The first week of life. Pediatrics 97:336, 1996.

23. McGarvey ST, Zinner SH: Blood pressure in infancy. Semin Nephrol 9:260, 1989.

24. Zubrow AB, Hulman S, Kushner H, et al: Determinants of blood pressure in infants admitted to neonatal intensive care units: a prospective multicenter study. J Perinatol 15:470, 1995.

25. Georgieff MK, Mills MM, Gomez-Main O, et al: Rate of change of blood pressure in premature and full term infants from birth to 4 months. Pediatr Nephrol 10:152, 1996.

26. American Academy of Pediatrics Committee on Fetus and Newborn: Routine evaluation of blood pressure, hematocrit and glucose in newborns. Pediatrics 92:474, 1993.

27. Buchi KF, Siegler RL: Hypertension in the first month of life. J Hypertens 4:527, 1986.

28. Ingelfinger JR: Hypertension in the first year of life. In Ingelfinger JR (ed): Pediatric Hypertension. Philadelphia, WB Saunders, 1982, pp 229-240.

29. Singh HP, Hurley RM, Myers TF: Neonatal hypertension: incidence and risk factors. Am J Hypertens 5:51, 1992.

30. Skalina MEL, Kliegman RM, Fanaroff AA: Epidemiology and management of severe symptomatic neonatal hypertension. Am J Perinatol 3:235, 1986.

31. Sheftel DN, Hustead V, Friedman A: Hypertension screening in the follow-up of premature infants. Pediatrics 71:763, 1983.

32. Arar MY, Hogg RJ, Arant BS, et al: Etiology of sustained hypertension in children in southwestern United States. Pediatr Nephrol 8:88, 1994.

33. Friedman AL, Hustead VA: Hypertension in babies following discharge from a neonatal intensive care unit. Pediatr Nephrol 1:32, 1987.

34. Flynn JT: Neonatal hypertension: Diagnosis and management. Pediatr Nephrol 14:334, 2000.

35. Goetzman BW, Stadalnik RC, Bogren HG, et al: Thrombotic complications of umbilical artery catheters: A clinical and radiographic study. Pediatrics 56:377, 1975.

36. Stork EK, Carlo WA, Kliegman RM, et al: Neonatal hypertension appears unrelated to aortic catheter position [Abstract]. Pediatr Res 18:321A, 1984.

37. Wesström G, Finnström O, Stenport G: Umbilical artery catheterization in newborns. I. Thrombosis in relation to catheter type and position. Acta Paediatr Scand 68:577, 1979.

38. Zuelzer WW, Kurnetz R, Newton WA: Circulatory diseases of the kidneys in infancy and childhood IV. Occlusion of the renal artery. Am J Dis Child 81:21,1951.

39. Tokunaka S, Osanai H, Hashimoto H, et al: Severe hypertension in infant with unilateral hypoplastic kidney. Urology 29:619, 1987.

40. Cadnapaphornchai P, Aisenbrey G, McDonald KM, et al: Prostaglandin-mediated hyperemia and renin-mediated hypertension during acute ureteral obstruction. Prostaglandins 16:969, 1978.

41. Gilboa N, Urizar RE: Severe hypertension in newborn after pyeloplasty of hydronephrotic kidney. Urology 22:180, 1983.

42. Riehle RA Jr, Vaughan ED Jr: Renin participation in hypertension associated with unilateral hydronephrosis. J Urol 126:245, 1981.

43. Flyer DC, Buckley LP, Hellenbrand MD, et al: Report of the New England Regional Infant Cardiac program. Pediatrics 65(Suppl):375, 1980.

44. Mimouni M, Kaufman H, Roitman A, et al: Hypertension in a neonate with 11 beta-hydroxylase deficiency. Eur J Pediatr 143:232, 1985.

45. Pozzan GB, Armanini D, Cecchetto G, et al: Hypertensive cardiomegaly caused by an aldosterone-secreting adenoma in a newborn. J Endocrinol Invest 20:88, 1997.

46. Schonwetter BS, Libber SM, Jones D Jr, et al: Hypertension in neonatal hyperthyroidism. Am J Dis Child 137:955, 1983.

47. White PC: Inherited forms of mineralocorticoid hypertension. Hypertension 28:927, 1996.

48. Malone PS, Duffy PG, Ransley PG, et al: Congenital mesoblastic nephroma, renin production, and hypertension. J Pediatr Surg 24:600, 1989.

49. Weinblatt ME, Heisel MA, Siegel SE: Hypertension in children with neurogenic tumors. Pediatrics 71:950, 1983.

50. Abman SH, Warady BA, Lum GM, et al: Systemic hypertension in infants with bronchopulmonary dysplasia. J Pediatr 104:928, 1984.

51. Alagappan A, Malloy MH: Systemic hypertension in very low-birth weight infants with bronchopulmonary dysplasia: Incidence and risk factors. Am J Perinatol 15:4, 1998.

52. Bloomfield FH, Knight DB, Harding JE: Side effects of 2 different dexamethasone courses for preterm infants at risk of chronic lung disease: A randomized trial. J Pediatr 133:398, 1998.

53. Greenough A, Emery EF, Gamsu HR: Dexamethasone and hypertension in preterm infants. Eur J Pediatr 151:134, 1992.

54. Lin YJ, Yeh TF, Hsieh WS, et al: Prevention of chronic lung disease in preterm infants by early postnatal dexamethasone therapy. Pediatr Pulmonol 27:24, 1999.

55. Smets K, Vanhaesebrouck P: Dexamethasone associated systemic hypertension in low birth weight babies with chronic lung disease. Eur J Pediatr 155:574, 1996.

56. Stark AR, Carlo WA, Tyson JE, et al: Adverse effects of early dexamethasone treatment in extremely-low-birth-weight infants. N Engl J Med 344:98, 2001.

57. Greher M, Hartmann T, Winker M, et al: Hypertension and pulmonary edema associated with subconjunctival phenylephrine in a 2-month-old child during cataract extraction. Anesthesiology 88:1394, 1998.

58. Chasnoff IJ, Lewis DE, Squires L: Cocaine intoxication in a breast-fed infant. Pediatrics 80:836, 1987.

59. Boede RF, Goldberg AR, Howell CG Jr, et al: Incidence of hypertension in infants on extracorporeal membrane oxygenation. J Pediatr Surg 25:258, 1990.

60. Adelman RD, Sherman MP: Hypertension in the neonate following closure of abdominal wall defects. J Pediatr 97:642, 1980.

61. DeLuca FG, Gilchrist BF, Paquette E, et al: External compression as initial management of giant omphaloceles. J Pediatr Surg 31:965, 1996.

62. Kotchen TA, Strickland AL, Rice TW, et al: A study of the renin-angiotensin system in newborn infants. J Pediatr 80:938, 1972.

63. Buhler FR, Laragh JH, Vaughn ED, et al: Antihypertensive action of propranolol: Specific antirenin responses in high and normal renin forms of essential, renal, renovascular and malignant hypertension. Am J Cardiol 31:511, 1973.

64. Ueda H, Yagi S, Koneko Y: Hydralazine and plasma renin activity. Arch Intern Med 122:387, 1968.

65. Perlman JM, Volpe JJ: Neurologic complications of captopril treatment of neonatal hypertension. Pediatrics 83:47, 1989.

66. Gouyon JB, Geneste B, Semama DS, et al: Intravenous nicardipine in hypertensive preterm infants. Arch Dis Child 76:F126, 1997.

67. Adelman RD: Long-term follow-up of neonatal renovascular hypertension. Pediatr Nephrol 1:40, 1987.

68. Adelman RD: The epidemiology of neonatal hypertension. In Giovanelli G, New MI, Gornis S (eds): Hypertension in Children and Adolescents. New York, Raven Press, 1981, pp 21-30.

CHAPTER 79

Acute Renal Failure

M. Gary Karlowicz and Raymond D. Adelman

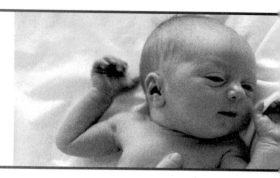

The diagnosis and management of acute renal failure in neonates are becoming increasingly important as survival of critically ill infants has improved. **Acute renal failure** is defined as a sudden severe decrease in **glomerular filtration rate (GFR)**. The term *acute renal failure* also is applied to neonates with congenital renal malformations, although renal failure may have been a chronic process in utero. Neonates with renal malformations or even renal agenesis are not born uremic because the placenta performs most renal homeostatic functions. Conversely, when maternal renal failure is present, newborns have elevated serum creatinine values that do not indicate true neonatal renal failure but reflect the inability of the placenta to reduce neonatal creatinine to less than maternal values. It may take 5 days or more for the newborn's serum creatinine to reflect actual neonatal renal function.[1,2]

One reason newborns have a high serum creatinine is that creatinine temporarily back-flows across immature leaky tubular and vascular structures.[3] Within weeks, maturational changes impose a barrier to back-flow of creatinine. In healthy term infants, the mean serum creatinine decreases from 0.9 mg/dL at 1 day of age to 0.5 mg/dL by 1 week of age and to 0.4 mg/dL by 1 month of age.[4] In healthy 32-week gestational age preterm infants, the mean serum creatinine decreases from 0.6 mg/dL at 1 week of age to 0.4 mg/dL by 1 month of age. In healthy 26-week gestational age preterm infants, mean serum creatinine decreases from 1 mg/dL at 1 week of age to 0.7 mg/dL by 1 month of age.[5]

FETAL RENAL FAILURE, OLIGOHYDRAMNIOS, AND PULMONARY HYPOPLASIA

Fetal renal malformations and renal failure can be detected in utero. Specific indications for fetal renal ultrasonography are oligohydramnios, elevated maternal α-fetoprotein, and a family history of hereditary renal malformations. Fetal urine contributes substantially to amniotic fluid starting with the second trimester, so oligohydramnios with intact membranes is a sign of either fetal urinary tract obstruction or decreased fetal urine production. Elevated maternal α-fetoprotein is associated with obstructive uropathy, renal agenesis, and congenital nephrotic syndrome.[6] A family history of hereditary renal disease is associated with an 8% incidence of fetal renal malformations.[7]

Although a normally functioning placenta prevents a fetus in renal failure from manifesting uremia, the placenta cannot prevent fetal oliguria, which presents as **oligohydramnios** associated with **pulmonary hypoplasia**. In 1946, Potter[8] described fatal pulmonary hypoplasia associated with bilateral renal agenesis. The oligohydramnios sequence includes pulmonary hypoplasia, any urinary tract anomaly that results in fetal oliguria and oligohydramnios, and signs of fetal compression including flattened facies and abnormal positioning of the hands and feet. When an infant is born with oligohydramnios sequence, ultrasound evaluation of both parents and siblings may be considered because 9% of first-degree relatives have asymptomatic renal malformations, including unilateral renal agenesis in 4.5%.[9] Fatal pulmonary hypoplasia also can occur when oligohydramnios is caused by prolonged rupture of membranes before 26 weeks of gestational age.[10]

If the neonatal mortality rate from severe fetal urinary tract abnormalities is to be reduced, pulmonary hypoplasia, the cause of death in 93% of cases, must be avoided.[11] Fetal ultrasonography should be performed at 15 to 16 weeks of gestation to achieve potential benefit from intervention in utero; however, the benefits of such surgery are controversial.[12] Futile intervention in fetuses with irreversible renal dysplasia must be avoided. Two criteria[12] for fetuses with a normal karyotype for in utero decompression of bilateral hydronephrosis in the presence of severe oligohydramnios are (1) no ultrasound evidence of renal dysplasia and (2) potential for normal renal function as reflected in a normal fetal urinalysis.[13] Because ultrasound sensitivity for fetal renal dysplasia is weak, a sign of normal fetal renal function, such as hypotonic urine, must be shown. If renal dysplasia is already present at 16 weeks of gestation, the prognosis is poor, with death from pulmonary hypoplasia or survival with end-stage renal disease.[14]

Percutaneous shunt is the most frequently performed procedure for in utero decompression of bilateral hydronephrosis. In utero intervention has two primary goals: (1) to restore enough amniotic fluid to allow lung development and (2) to preserve renal function by relieving urinary tract obstruction. The early enthusiasm for fetal intervention for urinary tract obstruction has waned because of disappointing outcomes.[15] Fetal intervention has been restricted primarily to male fetuses with suspected posterior urethral valves, good renal prognosis, and oligohydramnios.[16] The value of in utero intervention even in these cases has been challenged. Holmes and colleagues[17] reviewed the long-term outcome, with a mean of 11 years' follow-up, of fetal surgery in 14 "good prognosis" patients with posterior urethral valves and showed that there was 43% fetal mortality and 63% chronic renal failure among the 8 survivors, 3 of whom required renal transplantation. Families should be counseled that although fetal intervention may assist in delivering the fetus to term, renal sequelae of posterior urethral valves may not be prevented, and there is considerable risk of fetal mortality.

INCIDENCE OF NEONATAL RENAL FAILURE

Acute renal failure can be subdivided into prerenal failure, obstructive renal failure, and intrinsic renal failure. **Prerenal failure** can be caused by either systemic hypovolemia or renal hypoperfusion. Hypovolemic prerenal failure, if treated early, responds to a fluid challenge with resumption of normal urine output and resolution of azotemia. **Obstructive renal failure** is defined as renal failure due to mechanical obstruction in the urinary collecting system. **Intrinsic renal failure** is defined as renal failure due to parenchymal injury to the kidneys. Prerenal failure and obstructive renal failure, if prolonged, can lead to intrinsic renal failure.

Norman and Assadi[18] prospectively screened for acute renal failure in 314 consecutive neonatal intensive care unit (ICU) admissions. There were 72 infants (23%) who met the initial criteria, which were azotemia (defined as blood urea nitrogen >20 mg/dL) and oliguria (defined as urine output <1 mL/kg/hr). There were 52 infants (72%) with prerenal failure who responded to a trial of volume expansion and furosemide with immediate and sustained improvement in urine output and resolution of azotemia. The remaining 20 infants had intrinsic renal failure and accounted for 6% of total neonatal ICU admissions. Stapleton and coworkers[19] reported an 8% incidence of intrinsic renal failure in a prospective study of 186 consecutive admissions to the neonatal ICU, which included serial measurement of serum creatinine and defined intrinsic renal failure as a serum creatinine greater than 1.5 mg/dL that was unresponsive to fluid challenge. These studies suggest that acute renal failure has an incidence of 23% of neonatal ICU admissions. Prerenal failure occurs in approximately 70% of cases, which makes it the most common cause of acute renal failure in neonates. The incidence of intrinsic renal failure is between 6% and 8%.

PATHOPHYSIOLOGY OF INTRINSIC RENAL FAILURE

It is helpful to conceptualize intrinsic renal failure as composed of three phases: initiation, maintenance, and recovery.[20] The initiation phase involves the insult and associated events that produce tubular cell injury. The maintenance phase consists of sustained low GFR and azotemia. The duration of the maintenance phase reflects in part the etiology, severity, and duration of the initial insult. During the recovery phase, GFR and tubular function are gradually restored.

Renal hemodynamic factors, especially renal vasoconstriction, may play a role in intrinsic renal failure via the renin-angiotensin system.[21] The juxtaglomerular apparatus is stimulated to activate the renin-angiotensin system, which decreases renal blood flow and initiates a vicious cycle of further renal ischemia and tubular injury. Inhibition of the renin-angiotensin system mitigates renal injury in some experimental models,[22] whereas it is ineffective in others.[23] Other vasoactive compounds, such as prostaglandins[24] and adenosine,[25] also may affect renal vasoconstriction. The role of the vasodilator, endothelium-derived nitric oxide, in acute renal failure is complex and controversial. Inducible nitric oxide synthase did not mediate renal blood flow in a septic model of acute renal failure because the wild-type mice and the inducible nitric oxide synthase knockout mice developed renal failure of similar severity.[26] Inducible nitric oxide synthase has been shown to influence tubular injury in animal models of acute renal failure via the generation of toxic nitric oxide metabolites, including peroxynitrite.[27] Potent vasoconstrictors, such as endothelin peptides, may play a role in the pathogenesis of acute renal failure. Renal ischemia leads to up-regulation of endothelin-1 gene expression, and reperfusion sustains up-regulation contributing to endothelial dysfunction and enhanced vasoconstriction in the renal microcirculation.[28]

Endothelin-1-induced vasoconstriction may be a factor in acute tubular necrosis because there is a marked increase of endothelin-1 expression in the peritubular capillary network associated with ischemic renal failure.[29] Platelet-activating factor also has been shown to cause alterations in renal blood flow in animal models of ischemic renal failure.[30] Paradoxically, platelet-activating factor can cause either vasoconstriction or vasodilation depending on its concentration in the microcirculation.

Renal hemodynamic factors are particularly important during the initiation and recovery phases of renal failure. If decreased renal perfusion is reversed during the initiation phase of renal failure by either vasodilating agents[24] or volume expansion,[22] the severity of acute renal failure is reduced. Increasing renal blood flow with vasodilating agents during the maintenance phase of acute renal failure is ineffective.[24] Renal perfusion must be maintained during the recovery phase to avoid prolonging acute renal failure.[31]

The pathophysiology of acute renal failure also may include one or more nephronal factors, such as impaired glomerular capillary permeability, intraluminal tubular obstruction, and tubular back-leak of glomerular filtrate. Reduction in glomerular capillary permeability is an important component in reduction of GFR. In experimental ischemic and nephrotoxin-induced acute renal failure, scanning electron microscopy showed a reduction in number and size of endothelial fenestrae[32] and fusion of epithelial cell foot processes.[33] These changes have been shown to lead to a primary reduction in glomerular filtration and may be a major determinant of the severity and duration of the maintenance phase of acute renal failure.

When tubule epithelial cells are lethally injured, they separate from the basement membrane and slough into the tubule lumen. Obstruction of the tubular lumen by cellular debris has been shown in animal models[34] and humans.[35] Tubular pressure increases proximal to the obstruction and begins to oppose glomerular filtration pressure, reducing GFR. Another consequence of tubular injury and necrosis is tubular back-leak of glomerular filtrate. When tubular epithelium is disrupted, creatinine and other metabolic waste products back-diffuse to reenter the circulation.[34,36] Reduced clearance of nitrogenous waste products results in persistently elevated levels of creatinine and continued azotemia. Tubular factors are especially important during the maintenance phase of acute renal failure. GFR does not improve until the impacted cellular debris is removed from the tubular lumen, the tubular cells are regenerated, and tubular function is restored.[20]

Intracellular factors may be integral components of renal hemodynamic and nephronal influences in the pathogenesis of acute renal failure. Oxygen-free radical production contributes to the severity of experimental ischemic acute renal failure. Restoration of blood flow and oxygen delivery to the ischemic kidney results in oxygen-free radical production, which causes renal injury by lipid peroxidation in renal cortical mitochondria. Pretreatment with an oxygen-free radical scavenger, superoxide dismutase, in rats exposed to renal ischemia, decreased lipid peroxidation in renal cortical mitochondria and resulted in improved renal function during the postischemic recovery phase of acute renal failure.[37] Improved renal function also has been seen with dimethylthiourea, another oxygen-free radical scavenger, and allopurinol, an inhibitor of oxygen-free radical generation.[37] Influx of extracellular calcium and intracellular redistribution of calcium may have a role in tubular cell injury by leading to accumulation and sequestration of calcium in mitochondria. This deposition activates phospholipases and leads to phospholipid degradation, resulting in a vicious cycle of deteriorating mitochondrial structure and function.[38] Disruption of the adenine nucleotide system and the resultant decrease of intracellular energy production also has been the focus of research. When tubular cells in an experimental model of ischemic acute renal failure were injured, oxidative phosphorylation was impaired, and the levels of adenine nucleotides were rapidly reduced[39]; infusion of adenosine

triphosphate-magnesium chloride (ATP-MgCl$_2$) preserved tubular cell morphology and function.[34]

CAUSES OF ACUTE RENAL FAILURE

Table 79-1 is a comprehensive list of the causes of prerenal failure, obstructive renal failure, and intrinsic renal failure.

Prerenal Failure

The most common cause of acute renal failure in newborns is underperfusion of normal kidneys, or prerenal failure. Decreased renal perfusion can be due to either systemic hypovolemia, which leads to renal hypoperfusion, or renal hypoperfusion alone.

Systemic hypovolemia is often due to blood loss, fluid loss, or fluid redistribution; examples include dehydration, septic shock, and necrotizing enterocolitis (NEC). Dehydration may result from excessive gastrointestinal, urinary, or cutaneous losses, whereas septic shock and NEC may involve massive leakage of plasma into the interstitial space.

Systemic hypovolemia and prerenal failure can develop within hours in severe NEC, which may need aggressive fluid management, including repeated intravenous fluid boluses of normal saline until the urine output is greater than 1 mL/kg/hr. Fluid resuscitation is vital because failure to restore urine output with the development of anuric intrinsic renal failure may delay surgery.[40]

Other causes of **renal hypoperfusion** include perinatal asphyxia or other forms of hypoxic-ischemic events that lead to shunting of blood away from organs such as the kidneys in an effort to preserve perfusion of the brain and heart[41] and poor cardiac output during congestive heart failure or cardiac surgery resulting in decreased renal perfusion.[42] Acute renal failure after cardiac surgery for congenital heart disease accounted for 63% of neonates referred to a regional center for dialysis and was associated with a 58% mortality rate.[43]

Renal hypoperfusion is a serious side effect of some pharmacologic agents. Tolazoline (now withdrawn from the U.S. market) may induce oliguric renal failure,[44] causing systemic hypotension and renal vasoconstriction.[45] Captopril, when used for hypertension in premature infants with ventilator-dependent bronchopulmonary dysplasia, has been associated with unpredictable, marked decreases in blood pressure and oliguric renal failure.[46] Indomethacin may decrease renal blood flow in neonates.[47]

Obstructive Renal Failure

Table 79-1 lists the congenital malformations of the urinary collecting system associated with obstructive renal failure. Although some obstructive malformations are considered to be reversible causes of renal failure, a large percentage of neonates with obstructive lesions also have renal dysplasia.[48] Extrinsic compression on the urinary collecting system from a "tight" surgical closure of an abdominal wall defect,[49] a large mass such as a sacrococcygeal teratoma,[50] or hematocolpos may cause obstructive renal failure. Intrinsic obstruction within the

Table 79–1. Major Causes of Acute Renal Failure in the Newborn Infant

Prerenal Failure	Obstructive Renal Failure	Intrinsic Renal Failure
Systemic hypovolemia	Congenital malformations	Acute tubular necrosis
Fetal hemorrhage	Imperforate prepuce	Congenital malformations
Neonatal hemorrhage	Urethral stricture	Bilateral agenesis
Septic shock	Posterior urethral valves	Multicystic dysplasia
Necrotizing enterocolitis	Urethral diverticulum	Renal dysplasia/hypoplasia
Dehydration	Primary vesicoureteral reflux	Polycystic kidney disease
Hypoalbuminemia	Ureterocele	Glomerular maturational arrest
Systemic hypotension	Megacystis megaureter	Renal tubular dysgenesis
Renal hypoperfusion	Eagle-Barrett syndrome	Infection
Perinatal asphyxia	Ureteropelvic junction obstruction	Congenital
Congestive heart failure	Extrinsic compression	Syphilis
Cardiac surgery	Closure of abdominal wall defects	Toxoplasmosis
Respiratory distress	Sacrococcygeal teratoma	Pyelonephritis
syndrome	Hematocolpos	Renal vascular
Pharmacologic	Intrinsic obstruction	Renal artery thrombosis
Captopril	Renal calculi	Renal venous thrombosis
Indomethacin	Fungus balls	Disseminated vascular coagulation
	Neurogenic bladder	Nephrotoxins
		Indomethacin
		Amphotericin B
		Aminoglycosides
		Maternal drugs
		Enalapril
		Captopril
		Indomethacin
		Intrarenal obstruction
		Uric acid nephropathy
		Myoglobinuria
		Hemoglobinuria

urinary collecting system can occur with urinary calculi[51] or fungus balls.[52] Neurogenic bladder also can lead to obstructive renal failure.

Intrinsic Renal Failure

Intrinsic renal failure in newborns usually occurs when previously normal kidneys have been subjected to a hypoxic or ischemic insult. Although chronic intrauterine hypoxia, with severe intrauterine growth restriction and severe oligohydramnios, can lead to renal failure from birth,[53] perinatal asphyxia is the most common cause of intrinsic renal failure in newborns.[19] The degree of hypoxic-ischemic insult determines the spectrum of renal damage, which extends from mild tubular dysfunction and acute tubular necrosis to renal infarction with corticomedullary necrosis.[54] Any cause of prerenal failure or obstructive renal failure, if sustained, eventually can develop into intrinsic renal failure.

Intrinsic renal failure occasionally is caused by renal malformations. The lesions have to either be bilateral or involve a solitary kidney to cause renal failure. The most common malformations include renal agenesis, renal dysplasia, and polycystic kidney disease. A rare malformation causing intrinsic renal failure is glomerular maturational arrest.[55] It was reported in a 38-week neonate

with severe intrauterine growth restriction and oligohydramnios who died from acute renal failure with kidneys showing glomeruli with development arrested at 16 weeks of gestation.

Congenital infections, especially with syphilis and toxoplasmosis, have been associated with renal failure. Severe acute pyelonephritis also may progress to acute renal failure. Nosocomial urinary tract infections due to *Candida* organisms are becoming more common in neonatal ICUs[56] and can cause renal failure in newborns.[57,58]

Vascular disorders, such as aortic and renal artery thrombosis, renal venous thrombosis, and disseminated intravascular coagulation, may lead to acute renal failure. Aortic and renal artery thrombosis are complications of umbilical artery catheterization.[59,60] Renal venous thrombosis occasionally occurs with progressive prerenal failure but is more commonly a problem for infants of diabetic mothers.[61] Disseminated intravascular or intrarenal coagulation is another important vascular cause of intrinsic renal failure.[62]

Several nephrotoxins warrant mention as possible causes of intrinsic renal failure. Randomized, controlled clinical studies have shown that aminoglycosides are nephrotoxic to neonates.[63,64] The nephrotoxicity was shown by delayed postnatal decline in serum creatinine, delayed postnatal maturation in GFR, or decline in creatinine clearance in the aminoglycoside-treated infants. Peak and trough aminoglycoside levels in neonates with nephrotoxicity were no different, however, from the levels in neonates without nephrotoxicity.

Nephrotoxicity also can occur with the administration of indomethacin, which decreases renal prostaglandin production, leading to decreased renal blood flow,[47] decreased GFR,[65] transient oliguria, or acute renal failure.[66,67] Decreased renal prostaglandin production also potentiates the effect of vasopressin, leading to fluid retention, oliguria, and hyponatremia.[68] Furosemide increases renal prostaglandin secretion.[69] A Cochrane Review indicated, however, that there is insufficient evidence to support the use of furosemide to prevent renal side effects of indomethacin.[70] The effects of indomethacin on the kidney are complex. Continued administration of indomethacin for 7 days was often associated with recovery of renal function,[71] perhaps secondary to improved renal perfusion with closure of a patent ductus arteriosus, postnatal nephrogenesis, and recovery of renal prostaglandin synthesis.

One nephrotoxin, amphotericin B, affects the kidneys by reducing renal blood flow and GFR. It also has a direct effect on tubular cells leading to hypokalemia and renal tubular acidosis.[72] Toxicity seems to be related to the cumulative dose. The nephrotoxic effect of amphotericin B is usually reversible but can lead to fatal renal failure.[73] Serum creatinine should be monitored daily during amphotericin B therapy, and the dosing interval should be prolonged from 24 hours to 48 hours if the serum creatinine increases.[74] Lipid formulations of amphotericin B should not be substituted for amphotericin B in cases of acute renal failure and candidal pyelonephritis because lipid formulations of amphotericin B are less nephrotoxic due to the fact that they penetrate renal tubules poorly.[75] Radiopaque contrast agents also have caused renal failure in neonates.[76]

Certain drugs prescribed during pregnancy can cause renal failure in the fetus and newborn. This is particularly true of angiotensin-converting enzyme inhibitors, such as captopril and enalapril. Enalapril has been associated with fatal pulmonary hypoplasia and oligohydramnios sequence in an infant whose autopsy revealed poorly demarcated corticomedullary junctions, glomerular maldevelopment, and tubular distention.[77] Maternal enalapril also can cause acute renal failure in a newborn.[78-80] No other drug used to treat maternal hypertension, including labetalol, has been associated with neonatal renal failure.[81] Maternal use of nonsteroidal anti-inflammatory drugs for even a few days before delivery has been associated with neonatal renal failure.[82-85]

Intrinsic renal failure may occur through intrarenal obstruction. Uric acid nephropathy involves precipitation of uric acid or monosodium urate crystals in tubules.[86] Uric acid nephropathy is associated with hypoxia and perinatal asphyxia[19] and polycythemia, both idiopathic polycythemia[87] and with cyanotic congenital heart disease.[88] Transient renal insufficiency due to hyperuricemia and hyperuricosuria may be more common in neonates than previously recognized.[89] Newborns normally have a high fractional excretion of uric acid, so they may be more prone to uric acid nephropathy if severe hyperuricemia develops.[90] Intrarenal obstruction and renal failure also are associated with severe myoglobinemia and myoglobinuria, resulting from rhabdomyolysis due to severe perinatal asphyxia[91] and to massive hemoglobinuria from severe intravascular hemolysis.[92]

DIFFERENTIAL DIAGNOSIS

Identifying the cause of acute renal failure in neonates requires thoughtful consideration of history, physical examination, and laboratory tests. A family history of congenital renal malformations, such as polycystic kidneys, should be sought. Oligohydramnios may indicate renal anomalies. Prenatal ultrasound can detect most urinary tract anomalies, including hydronephrosis, cystic kidneys, absent kidneys, small echogenic kidneys, and renal masses.

Oligohydramnios also may indicate decreased fetal renal function from progressive placental insufficiency in infants with asymmetric intrauterine growth restriction. In this setting, the absence or reversal of umbilical artery diastolic flow by prenatal Doppler ultrasonography identifies extreme risk to the fetus and the need for intervention.[93]

Asphyxia is the most common cause of intrinsic renal failure in the neonate, but a history of low Apgar scores is not enough to identify infants with asphyxia reliably. Portman and associates[94] developed a scoring system that rapidly and accurately predicts organ dysfunction after severe perinatal asphyxia in term infants. The combination of prolonged fetal bradycardia, a 5-minute Apgar score less than 5, and a base deficit greater than 14 in the first hour of life was associated with a 38% incidence of oliguric renal failure. Using this scoring system, Karlowicz and Adelman[95] found that (1) acute renal failure, defined as serum creatinine greater than 1.5 mg/dL, occurred in 61% of the infants with severe asphyxia morbidity scores; (2) acute renal failure associated with severe asphyxia was predominantly nonoliguric; and (3) the asphyxia morbidity score, which can be determined at 1 hour of age, predicted acute renal failure in full-term infants with 100% sensitivity and 72% specificity. Severe asphyxia increases the risk of acute renal failure and the syndrome of inappropriate secretion of antidiuretic hormone.[96]

A thorough physical examination is essential. The infant should be examined carefully for kidney size and shape, abdominal masses, ascites, palpable bladder, single umbilical artery, hypospadias, and abdominal wall musculature. The features of oligohydramnios sequence should be sought, including Potter facies (wide-set eyes, a prominent skinfold below the lower eyelid extending from inner canthus to the cheek, a flattened nose, large low-set ears, and a small lower jaw) and abnormal positioning of hands and feet.

In a prospective ultrasound screening study of 112 infants with single umbilical artery without other obvious congenital anomalies, Bourke and coworkers[97] found a

7% incidence of persistent renal anomalies, including a 4.5% incidence of vesicoureteral reflux. Renal ultrasound screening of all neonates with single umbilical artery should be considered. Serious urinary tract abnormalities occur in 15% of asymptomatic boys with hypospadias, with 12% requiring surgical intervention.[98] Infants with congenital heart disease have a higher incidence of renal anomalies; the presence of extracardiac anomalies increases the incidence of renal anomalies from 5% to 39%.[99] Unless associated with other anomalies, supernumerary nipples or dysmorphic ears are not associated with renal anomalies.[100]

Daily serum creatinine should be monitored in newborns at risk of acute renal failure (see Table 79-1). Acute renal failure should be suspected when creatinine is rising 0.3 mg/dL or more per day, fails to decline postnatally, or is greater than 1.5 mg/dL.[19,101] The diagnosis of nonoliguric renal failure when urine output is greater than 1 mL/kg/hr can be overlooked without systematic monitoring of serum creatinine in newborns in danger of developing acute renal failure.

There are three goals in the diagnostic evaluation of neonatal acute renal failure. The first goal is to diagnose prerenal failure promptly because it may be reversed with volume expansion through early administration of fluids. It is the most common cause of neonatal acute renal failure. After volume expansion, some clinicians also administer diuretics. The second goal is to identify neonates with urinary tract obstruction because timely intervention may relieve obstruction and improve prognosis.[102] The third goal is to avoid fluid and electrolyte overload in neonates who already have developed intrinsic renal failure and to initiate management to minimize morbidity and mortality.

After the first 24 hours of life, oliguria is considered to be present when urine output is less than 1 mL/kg/hr for 8 to 12 hours. If oliguria is present, the next step is to insert a bladder catheter to (1) rule out lower urinary tract obstruction, (2) determine urinary residual, (3) collect urine for analysis, and (4) monitor urinary flow rate.

If there is no urinary outlet obstruction and no evidence of hypoperfusion (e.g., due to cardiac disease), prerenal failure from volume depletion is possible, and a fluid challenge should be given. This approach is probably the most reliable diagnostic test to differentiate prerenal from intrinsic renal failure.[19,103,104] The fluid challenge infused intravenously over 1 to 2 hours should include enough isotonic solution to return intravascular volume status to normal. If oliguria continues, intravenous furosemide, 1 mg/kg, may be given. If there is no diuresis or urine output better than 1 mL/kg/hr within 2 hours and the patient is clinically euvolemic, intrinsic renal failure should be suspected, and fluids should be restricted.

If fluid challenge is unsuccessful in reversing oliguric renal failure, or if there is nonoliguric renal failure, the following laboratory tests should be performed: platelet count, serum sodium, potassium, bicarbonate, chloride, blood urea nitrogen, creatinine, uric acid, calcium, phosphorus, and glucose. If urine can be obtained, urinalysis and spot urine sample for sodium, creatinine, and osmolarity should be performed. If indicated, a urine culture also may be performed.

A variety of urinary indices, which always must be evaluated in the context of the clinical setting, are available to help differentiate prerenal from intrinsic renal failure, but none has the therapeutic advantage and the diagnostic reliability of the fluid challenge. The most useful urinary indices are the fractional excretion of sodium (FENa) and the renal failure index (RFI). Each is calculated in a spot specimen as follows:

$$FENa = \frac{(urine\ Na\ /\ serum\ Na)}{(urine\ Cr\ /\ serum\ Cr)} \times 100$$

$$RFI = \frac{urine\ Na}{(urine\ Cr\ /\ serum\ Cr)}$$

In full-term infants, FENa or RFI greater than 3 suggests intrinsic renal failure, whereas FENa or RFI less than 3 is consistent with prerenal failure. Although urinary indices are highly sensitive for intrinsic renal failure, they may have poor specificity. Premature infants less than 32 weeks of gestation normally may have FENa greater than 5%,[105] and there are no definite values for FENa in premature infants with intrinsic renal failure.[104,106] Urine samples also must be obtained before a diuretic is given.

Nephrosonography should be the initial imaging procedure in neonates suspected of either intrinsic or obstructive acute renal failure.[107] Nephrosonography is noninvasive, does not depend on renal function, and does not use nephrotoxic contrast agents. Ultrasonography can accurately describe the presence or absence of kidneys, kidney size and shape, hydronephrosis, renal calculi, and bladder distention and thickness. When renal failure due to urinary outlet obstruction is likely, voiding cystourethrography is recommended to detect posterior urethral valves and other causes of lower urinary tract obstruction and vesicoureteral reflux. Whenever urinary tract obstruction is detected, immediate referral to a pediatric urologist is indicated.

Radionuclide renal scans can be helpful in evaluating renal perfusion and function.[108] Technetium 99m DMSA scans evaluate renal blood flow and renal tissue, whereas technetium 99m mertiatide (TechneScan MAG3) is useful for evaluating for renal obstruction. The presence of renal blood flow by scintiscan is a good prognostic sign in neonates with anuric renal failure; however, there also have been reports of recovery of renal function in anuric neonates with no documented renal blood flow by radionuclide scan.[101,109] Angiography is not considered necessary, unless specific surgical intervention, such as removal of an aortic thrombus, is planned. Such thrombi are usually detectable, however, by ultrasound or radionuclide renal scans; the indications for surgical removal of aortic or renal thrombi seem limited.[110] Thrombolysis may be indicated when bilateral renal artery thrombosis causes oligoanuric acute renal failure. Continuous intrathrombic urokinase infusion[111] has been reported to be effective in treating renal artery and aortic thrombosis, as has urokinase therapy[112] and recombinant tissue-type plasminogen activator infusion, which may have a lower incidence of side effects compared with treatment with streptokinase and urokinase.[113,114]

Renal blood flow, without the invasiveness and exposure to radioisotopes, can be evaluated in skilled hands with duplex ultrasound.[115] Asphyxiated neonates showed a significant correlation between resistance index and systolic velocity and the severity of asphyxia.[116] Decreased Doppler renal flow velocity on the first day of life in asphyxiated neonates was a useful predictor for subsequent development of acute renal failure with 100% sensitivity and 64% specificity.[117]

MANAGEMENT OF INTRINSIC RENAL FAILURE

The current concept of management of intrinsic renal failure is to provide supportive care until kidney function spontaneously improves. Nonspecific therapy with furosemide and low-dose dopamine is frequently used, although there is no conclusive evidence that they improve renal function or the prognosis of intrinsic renal failure. Diuretics may be appropriate in settings in which high urine flow should be maintained to prevent intratubular precipitation, such as intravascular hemolysis, hyperuricemia, and myoglobinuria. The side effects of diuretic therapy can lead to serious morbidity with repeated doses.[118] Furosemide can cause ototoxicity, interstitial nephritis, hypotension, persistence of patent ductus arteriosus, and nephrocalcinosis.[119] Although mannitol may be useful in the early management of acute renal failure, it increases extracellular osmolality and plasma volume and may be associated with intraventricular hemorrhage in very-low-birth-weight neonates and pulmonary edema.

Low-dose or so-called renal-dose dopamine has been used for years in critically ill patients because it increases renal blood flow and induces diuresis in healthy volunteers.[120-126] Adverse effects of dopamine include gastrointestinal mucosal ischemia, respiratory depression, myocardial ischemia, and tachyarrhythmias. A large multicenter controlled trial of 328 patients in 23 ICUs showed that low-dose dopamine in critically ill patients with early renal dysfunction had no effect on serum creatinine, requirements for renal replacement therapy, or length of ICU stay.[127] This well-designed clinical trial showed that there is no justification for using renal-dose dopamine in critically ill patients.[128]

There is a need for more specific therapy for intrinsic renal failure directed at reducing the severity of tubular cell necrosis and speeding the regeneration of tubular epithelium. Although some experimental agents may have therapeutic benefit in animals, even after intrinsic renal failure is established, they have found little success in clinical trials.

Animal studies have shown that after an ischemic insult, renal tubule damage progresses for 8 to 24 hours after renal blood flow has been restored.[129] Therapeutic intervention during this interval theoretically could save sublethally injured cells. Infusion of ATP-MgCl$_2$ after renal injury in the rat resulted in significant sustained improvement in renal function[34,130] with less necrosis and faster resolution of cellular edema.[131-133] ATP-MgCl$_2$[134] seems to preserve sublethally injured cells and to improve the cellular mechanisms of recovery[135] by improving resynthesis of renal cellular ATP through the provision of more adenine nucleotide precursors. Although animal studies with ATP-MgCl$_2$ have shown

promise, there is little clinical research. One small randomized, placebo-controlled trial of 18 patients with preexisting renal impairment showed that ATP-MgCl$_2$ did not prevent persistent deterioration in renal function after radiocontrast administration.[136] The possibility of serious hemodynamic side effects may prohibit clinical application in neonates with acute renal failure.

Thyroxine given to rats with ischemic or dichromate-induced nephropathy resulted in accelerated recovery of glomerular function.[137,138] There was significant recovery of renal ATP in rats treated with thyroxine, which may have a direct effect on ATP synthesis.[139] In a randomized, placebo-controlled clinical trial, thyroxine therapy had no effect on the course of acute renal failure and was associated with a significantly higher mortality rate.[140]

Anaritide, a 25-amino acid synthetic form of atrial natriuretic peptide, has been shown in animal experiments to improve renal function.[141] In a multicenter, controlled study, anaritide did not improve the overall rate of dialysis-free survival in critically ill patients with acute tubular necrosis.[142]

Another promising polypeptide is recombinant human insulin-like growth factor I (IGF-I), which increases renal blood flow and GFR.[143] In animal experiments, IGF-I improved healing of injured nephrons; accelerated recovery of renal function; and reduced mortality from ischemic, toxic, or endotoxin-induced acute renal failure.[144,145] In a randomized, controlled trial of patients undergoing surgery involving renal arteries or the suprarenal aorta, IGF-I administered postoperatively did not affect serum creatinine at discharge, length of ICU stay, or incidence of dialysis or death.[146] Similarly, disappointing results were reported in a multicenter controlled trial involving patients in ICUs.[147] Despite encouraging studies in animals, these randomized, controlled trials failed to show that IGF-I has beneficial effects in patients with established acute renal failure.

Although there will be other clinical trials of specific therapy for intrinsic renal failure in the future, the present goal of treatment of intrinsic renal failure is to provide supportive care until kidney function spontaneously improves. This goal requires prevention, early recognition, and management of the common complications of renal failure, which include fluid overload, hyponatremia, hypertension, hyperkalemia, hyperphosphatemia, hypocalcemia, nutritional deficiency, metabolic acidosis, and sepsis.

Fluid Overload

As soon as oliguric intrinsic renal failure is diagnosed, fluids should be severely restricted. Fluid overload often has already occurred because intrinsic renal failure was unrecognized or was the result of conditions with a high fluid requirement, such as septic shock or NEC. The complications of fluid overload are congestive heart failure, hypertension, and hyponatremia. When severe symptomatic fluid overload has occurred, dialysis or hemofiltration is usually the best therapeutic option. These options often are seen as heroic and are delayed; the contribution of fluid overload to persistent heart failure, hypertension, and increased ventilatory support frequently is unappreciated by the clinician.

Severe fluid restriction means limiting fluids to insensible, gastrointestinal, and renal losses. Maintenance fluid restriction must take into account the presence of fluid overload and specific electrolyte requirements. There should be strict monitoring of all input and output so that the euvolemic patient can be maintained with adequate fluids and electrolytes. Insensible losses always should be replaced with electrolyte-free water. Insensible fluid losses for a full-term infant can be estimated to be 30 mL/kg/day or 300 mL/m²/day. Premature infants more than 28 weeks of gestation have insensible losses of 50 to 100 mL/kg/day.[104] Insensible water losses increase tremendously in premature infants less than 28 weeks of gestation. In a radiant warmer, a 25-week premature infant can have insensible water losses of 360 mL/kg/day in the first 24 hours.[148] Use of a heat shield and 100% humidity can reduce insensible water losses. Provision of adequate fluid for insensible water loss results in maintenance of a euvolemic body weight, minus 1% to 2% daily losses from catabolism and tissue wasting.

To avoid hypoglycemia with severe fluid restriction, the dextrose content may need to be as high as 20% dextrose in water via central venous access. The restricted fluid should contain little to no sodium and no potassium. Initial monitoring should include weights, serum chemistries, and glucose every 12 hours. Fluids should be increased if urine output improves, volume overload is resolved, or weight loss is excessive due to high insensible water losses.

Hyponatremia

Hyponatremia occurs during intrinsic renal failure primarily from excess free water due to fluid overload and frequently in association with increased antidiuretic hormone production. Initial therapy should be fluid restriction. Symptoms of hyponatremia relate to the actual level of serum sodium, the rapidity of change, and the various biochemical, cellular, vascular, and structural homeostatic mechanisms that occur in response to changes in osmolality and cell or organ volume. Prompt diagnosis of severe hyponatremia[149] and timely institution of hypertonic saline therapy[150] may reduce morbidity and mortality.

Sodium concentration greater than 125 mEq/L is rarely symptomatic. Sodium concentration between 120 and 125 mEq/L occasionally is associated with symptoms such as encephalopathy, lethargy, and seizures. Hypertonic saline infusion should be reserved for treatment of symptomatic hyponatremia and severe hyponatremia with serum sodium concentration less than 120 mEq/L. To raise serum sodium concentration by 5 mEq/L, 8 mL/kg of 3% saline (513 mEq sodium/L) may be given intravenously over 2 hours. Serum sodium should be measured immediately after completing infusion of the 3% saline. The approximate total amount of sodium to correct hyponatremia in the neonate can be calculated with the following formula:

$$Na^+ (mEq) = ([Na^+] \text{ desired} - [Na^+] \text{ (actual)}) \times \text{weight (kg)} \times 0.8$$

Hypertonic saline should be used cautiously. Infusion time may need to be more than 2 hours because of

Table 79–2. Upper Limits of Normal Mean Arterial Pressure in the Newborn

Age	<1000 g	1000-1500 g	1501-2500 g	>2500 g
Newborn	48	57	62	68
1 wk	56	65	70	79
2 wk	60	68	73	83
4 wk	63	71	76	87

Note. Mean arterial pressure values are in mm Hg.

From Karlowicz MG, Adelman RD: Acute renal failure in the neonate. Clin Perinatol 19:139, 1992.

Modified from Stork EK, Carlo WA, Kliegman RM, et al: Hypertension redefined for critically ill neonates. Pediatr Res 18:321A, 1984.

potential complications, including congestive heart failure, pulmonary edema, hypertension, and intraventricular hemorrhage.

Hypertension

Hypertension in the setting of acute renal failure occurs usually as a complication of renal damage or fluid overload. The Task Force on Blood Pressure Control in Children has defined significant hypertension in the term newborn as systolic blood pressure greater than 96 mm Hg and severe hypertension in the term newborn as systolic blood pressure greater than 106 mm Hg.[151] Norms for upper limits of blood pressure must be consulted because blood pressure is a function of birth weight and postnatal age (Table 79-2).[152,153]

The level of hypertension requiring drug therapy in neonates has not been defined. In general, however, severe or symptomatic hypertension warrants therapy. Salt restriction may be sufficient treatment for mild hypertension, especially if due to volume overload. Mild diuretics generally do not work in the setting of intrinsic renal failure, but loop diuretics may be helpful in nonoliguric renal failure. Table 79-3 lists some recommended antihypertensive drugs. Hydralazine is an effective first drug for mild-to-moderate hypertension, although high doses may be needed. Captopril and enalaprilat are effective for hypertension due to activation of the renin-angiotensin system but must be used with caution because they can cause profound hypotension and renal failure.[154-156] They also must be used with extreme caution in neonates with impaired renal function because oliguria and increased serum creatinine

Table 79–3. Antihypertensive Drugs in Acute Renal Failure

Drug	Dosage
Hydralazine	0.1-0.5 mg/kg/dose IV q6-8h
	0.25-2 mg/kg/dose orally q6-8h
Labetalol	0.25-3 mg/kg/hr IV
Nicardipine	0.5-3 μg/kg/min IV
Nitroprusside	0.5-10 μg/kg/min IV

occur frequently. For a hypertensive crisis, nitroprusside, nicardipine, and labetalol are the drugs of choice.[157] Nitroprusside causes immediate reduction in blood pressure, and its half-life is a few minutes, so it can be stopped quickly if necessary. If nitroprusside is used for more than 24 hours, serum thiocyanate levels should be monitored. Nitroprusside must be used with caution in liver- and renal-failure patients because of possible impairment of metabolism of cyanide to thiocyanate. Labetalol, 0.25 to 3 mg/kg/hr,[158,159] is a combined α and β blocker with an onset of action of 5 to 10 minutes and a duration of 2 hours and is especially useful in hypertension associated with increased circulating catecholamines or central nervous system mediated hypertension. Labetalol should be avoided in patients with heart failure or chronic lung disease and should be used cautiously in patients with renal failure because it may cause hyperkalemia. Nicardipine, 0.5 to 3 μg/kg/min,[158,160-162] is an excellent drug for parenteral management of hypertension. It has an onset of action within minutes, has a half-life of 10 minutes, and acts primarily as a peripheral vasodilator. It is safe, effective, and easy to use; has minimal side effects; and has been used in all age ranges, including neonates. For many, owing to its safety and ease of use, nicardipine is the drug of choice for treatment of a hypertensive emergency. Hypertension unresponsive to drug therapy is often due to volume overload; dialysis or hemofiltration may be needed in this setting.

Hyperkalemia

As soon as renal failure is suspected, potassium should be removed from intravenous and oral fluids. Medications and total parenteral nutrition are sources of potassium that may be overlooked. As the potassium level increases, the electrocardiogram (ECG) shows progressive changes, including—in order of severity—tall, peaked T waves, heart block with widened QRS complexes, sine waves, and cardiac arrest. The drug therapy for hyperkalemia with ECG changes is listed in Table 79-4. Calcium gluconate should be given to counteract the toxic effect of potassium on the myocardium. This should be followed by sodium bicarbonate, which causes potassium to shift into cells by raising pH. The duration of action is less than 2 hours for calcium gluconate and bicarbonate. A glucose and insulin drip also should be started, especially

with ECG changes, because potassium uptake increases with an increased uptake of glucose into cells. Blood glucose needs to be monitored closely during a glucose and insulin drip because hypoglycemia can occur. Serum potassium should be measured every 2 to 4 hours during the treatment of hyperkalemia. Sodium polystyrene sulfonate (Kayexalate) can be administered as well. Albuterol is not recommended for severe hyperkalemia with ECG changes because a randomized, controlled study documented a paradoxical increase in serum potassium (>0.4 mEq/L in some patients) in the first few minutes of albuterol treatment, which could be just enough to cause life-threatening arrhythmias.[163] Aggressive and early use of dialysis should be considered if these measures are unsuccessful or if anuria is present.

Mild hyperkalemia, with a serum potassium between 6 and 7 mEq/L and without ECG changes, can be treated with Kayexalate. Each 1 g/kg of Kayexalate should reduce serum potassium 1 mEq/L. Kayexalate works by exchanging sodium for potassium, so its use can lead to sodium retention, fluid overload, and congestive heart failure. Kayexalate may take hours to produce an effect. Rectal Kayexalate may be ineffective in premature infants less than 29 weeks of gestation and has been associated with NEC.[164] Albuterol may be considered for treatment of mild hyperkalemia without ECG changes.[163,165] If serum potassium increases to greater than 7 mEq/L or if there are ECG changes, additional therapy is indicated.

Hyperphosphatemia and Hypocalcemia

Hyperphosphatemia is common in renal failure but frequently overlooked. Severely elevated phosphate places the neonate at risk of extraskeletal calcifications of the kidney, heart, and blood vessels if the calcium-phosphorus product exceeds 70.[166] A low-phosphorus formula should be used for enteral nutrition. Soy formulas should be avoided because of their high aluminum content.[167] Aluminum-containing gels should not be used because of risk of aluminum toxicity. Citrate enhances aluminum absorption, so citrate compounds should be avoided whenever possible.[168] Calcium carbonate is a useful phosphate-binding agent.[169] Dialysis may be indicated for severe hyperphosphatemia.

Total serum calcium frequently is decreased in acute renal failure. Ionized calcium is less commonly abnormal

Table 79-4. Treatment of Severe Hyperkalemia with Electrocardiogram Changes

Drug	Administration
Calcium gluconate (10%)	50 mg/kg IV over 10 min. Monitor ECG. Slow infusion if heart rate slows.
Sodium bicarbonate	2 mEq/kg IV over 2-5 min
Glucose and insulin continuous infusion	Insulin 0.05 U/kg/hr in $D_{25}W$ at 1 mL/kg/hr via central venous line or in $D_{10}W$ at 2.5 mL/kg/hr via peripheral venous catheter. (Insulin 0.05 U/kg/hr with glucose 0.25 g/kg/hr delivers insulin 0.2 U/g glucose)

$D_{10}W$, $D_{25}W$, dextrose in water (10%, 25%); ECG, electrocardiogram.

because of concurrent acidosis and hypoalbuminemia. Ionized calcium, instead of total serum calcium, should be monitored during acute renal failure whenever feasible. If ionized calcium is decreased and the patient is symptomatic, calcium gluconate (10%) should be given at a dose of 50 mg/kg every 6 hours by intravenous infusion over 10 minutes, until ionized calcium is increased to a level at which symptoms are abated. Phosphate levels also should be decreased, initially if possible, to reduce the calcium-phosphorus product and the risk of metastatic calcifications.

Nutritional Deficiency

Severe fluid restriction during intrinsic renal failure places limitations on intravenous fluid volume, sometimes necessitating the use of 30% dextrose in water via central venous access to provide adequate calories. Dialysis or hemofiltration in conjunction with total parenteral nutrition and intravenous lipid may be indicated to provide adequate calories in anuric neonates. The goal should be to provide 100 kcal/kg with fat and carbohydrates. About 1 to 2 g/kg/day of high biologic value protein or an amino acid equivalent should be provided.[170,171]

Metabolic Acidosis

Metabolic acidosis is common in intrinsic renal failure. No treatment is necessary unless blood pH decreases to less than 7.20. Severe acidosis should be treated to avoid accentuating the cardiotoxic effects of hyperkalemia and to avoid wasting calories from hyperventilation to compensate for the metabolic acidosis. Sodium bicarbonate infusions may be given to increase pH to greater than 7.20 to correct metabolic acidosis; however, significant extracellular volume expansion can occur with repeated administration of sodium.

Sepsis

Infection is a common cause of death in neonates with acute renal failure. Infection is more likely because of prolonged hospitalization and multiple invasive procedures. Whenever sepsis is suspected, cultures should be obtained and antibiotics started. Gram-negative pathogens cause most cases of fulminant sepsis in the neonatal ICU[172] and often require aminoglycoside therapy because many are resistant to third-generation cephalosporins. Renal failure alters protein binding, the volume of distribution, and the renal excretion of many drugs. Drug doses or dosing intervals, especially for aminoglycosides, often need adjustment in patients with acute renal failure. These adjustments are necessary not only for drugs excreted by the kidneys but also for hepatically metabolized drugs whose potentially toxic metabolites require renal excretion.

DIALYSIS

When conservative supportive therapy of acute renal failure is unsuccessful, **dialysis** should be considered. The usual indications for dialysis include severe fluid overload, acidosis, hyponatremia or hypernatremia not responding to conservative management, and hyperkalemia. Inadequate nutrition because of severe fluid restriction is a relative indication for dialysis or continuous venovenous hemofiltration. Some clinicians advocate starting dialysis early, hoping to reduce morbidity and mortality from acute renal failure.[173] In the newborn, peritoneal dialysis is preferred over hemodialysis because it is relatively safer, technically less demanding, and similarly effective.[174] Relative contraindications to peritoneal dialysis include (1) NEC, (2) bleeding diathesis, (3) and systemic hypoperfusion.

The initial dialysis fluid volume should be 10 to 20 mL/kg. This volume can be increased gradually if respiratory status is not compromised.[175] The volume of peritoneal input and output needs to be strictly monitored because positive water balance can occur. The dialysis solution must be kept at body temperature. Hyperglycemia is a potential complication and is more likely with dialysis solutions with higher glucose concentrations.[166] Severe fluctuations in blood glucose levels must be avoided. With impaired hepatic function, the neonate may be unable to convert the standard dialysate lactate into bicarbonate, so serum lactate needs to be monitored. When necessary, a dialysis solution containing bicarbonate can be prepared.[173] Other complications of peritoneal dialysis are hyponatremia, hypernatremia, hypokalemia, infection, pleural effusion, scrotal edema, and catheter leakage or nonfunction.

HEMOFILTRATION

Hemofiltration is an alternative technique for removal of excess fluid without dialysis.[176,177] The hemofilter is constructed of semipermeable membranes that are highly water permeable. Ultrafiltrate is generated by the net pressure gradient between pressures that favor ultrafiltration (hydraulic pressure and hydrostatic pressure) and the pressure that opposes it (oncotic pressure).[176] Hydraulic pressure depends on mean arterial blood pressure and is inversely proportional to resistance. Oncotic pressure, which opposes the formation of ultrafiltrate, is a function of the concentration of plasma proteins.

Hemofiltration with a blood pump requires constant bedside monitoring. The hemofilter and circuit should be kept at body temperature to prevent hypothermia. The rate of ultrafiltration should be controlled to avoid hypovolemia and hypotension.

An advantage of hemofiltration is that it avoids the rapid solute shifts, dysequilibrium, and hypotension of hemodialysis because it involves the slow and continuous isotonic removal of solute. A disadvantage of hemofiltration is that systemic heparinization may be necessary to prevent thrombus formation in the hemofilter. Regional heparinization or hemofiltration without heparin should be attempted in neonates prone to intracranial hemorrhage. Many drugs are removed by hemofiltration, so doses may need adjustment.

With hemofiltration, plasma oncotic pressure increases as intracapillary hydrostatic pressure decreases, allowing interstitial fluid to reenter the vascular compartment. A grossly edematous and hypoproteinemic patient (e.g., a newborn with nonimmune hydrops fetalis) could benefit greatly from hemofiltration. Hemofiltration may be an excellent alternative to peritoneal dialysis in patients with a primary problem of fluid overload.

Dialysate can be set up to flow countercurrent to blood flow in the hemofilter to create hemodiafiltration. Hemodiafiltration[178] adds the capability of facilitated solute removal to the known efficiency of hemofiltration in the removal of excess plasma water.

OUTCOME OF ACUTE RENAL FAILURE

Oliguric renal failure has a mortality rate of 50% in newborns, whether the cause is congenital or acquired.[19,101,106] Nonoliguric renal failure has a much better prognosis.[101,179]

Long-term sequelae of acute renal failure include reduced GFR and impaired tubular function. Neonates with congenital renal anomalies and acute renal failure have the worst prognosis for chronic renal failure at 77%.[180] Creatinine clearance remains decreased in about 40% of newborns who recover from acquired oliguric[19] or nonoliguric renal failure.[101]

Other chronic renal manifestations of acute renal failure in newborns[181] include chronic hypertension, renal tubular acidosis, and impaired ability to concentrate urine. Nephrocalcinosis has been reported as a consequence of neonatal renal-cortical necrosis.[182] Renal growth may be impaired due to renal papillary necrosis or cortical atrophy.[181,183]

REFERENCES

1. Feldman H, Guignard J-P: Plasma creatinine in the first month of life. Arch Dis Child 57:123, 1982.
2. Sertel H, Scopes J: Rates of creatinine clearance in babies less than one week of age. Arch Dis Child 48:717, 1973.
3. Guignard J-P, Drukker A: Why do newborn infants have a high plasma creatinine? Pediatrics 103:e49, 1999.
4. Schwartz GJ, Feld LG, Langford DJ: A simple estimate of glomerular filtration rate in full-term infants during the first year of life. J Pediatr 104:849, 1984.
5. Gallini F, Maggio L, Romagnoli C, et al: Progression of renal function in preterm neonates with gestational age < 32 weeks. Pediatr Nephrol 15:119, 2000.
6. Barakat AY, Awazu M, Fleischer AC: Antenatal diagnosis of renal abnormalities: A review of the state of the art. South Med J 82:229, 1989.
7. Reuss A, Wladimiroff JW, Niermeijer MF: Antenatal diagnosis of renal tract anomalies by ultrasound. Pediatr Nephrol 1:546, 1987.
8. Potter EL: Bilateral renal agenesis. J Pediatr 29:68, 1946.
9. Roodhooft AM, Birnholz JC, Holmes LB: Familial nature of congenital absence and severe dysgenesis of both kidneys. N Engl J Med 310:1341, 1984.
10. Perlman M, Williams J, Hirsch M: Neonatal pulmonary hypoplasia after prolonged leakage of amniotic fluid. Arch Dis Child 51:349, 1976.
11. International Fetal Surgery Registry: Catheter shunts for fetal hydronephrosis and hydrocephalus. N Engl J Med 315:336, 1986.
12. Fine RN: Diagnosis and treatment of fetal urinary tract abnormalities. J Pediatr 121:333, 1992.
13. Nicolini U, Spelzini F: Invasive assessment of fetal renal abnormalities: Urinalysis, fetal blood sampling, and biopsy. Prenat Diagn 21:964, 2001.
14. Crombleholme TW, Harrison MR, Golbus MS, et al: Fetal intervention in obstructive uropathy: Prognostic indicators and efficacy of intervention. Am J Obstet Gynecol 162:1239, 1990.
15. Thomas DFM: Prenatal diagnosis: Does it alter outcome? Prenat Diag 21:1004, 2001.
16. Agarwal SK, Fisk NM: In utero therapy for lower urinary tract obstruction. Prenat Diagn 21:970, 2001.
17. Holmes N, Harrison MR, Baskin LS: Fetal surgery for posterior urethral valves: Long-term postnatal outcomes. Pediatrics 108:e7, 2001.
18. Norman ME, Assadi FK: A prospective study of acute renal failure in the newborn infant. Pediatrics 63:475, 1979.
19. Stapleton FB, Jones DP, Green RS: Acute renal failure in neonates: Incidence, etiology, and outcome. Pediatr Nephrol 1:314, 1987.
20. Gaudio KM, Siegel NJ: Pathogenesis and treatment of acute renal failure. Pediatr Clin North Am 34:771, 1987.
21. Hollenberg NK, Wilkes BM, Schulman G: The renin-angiotensin system in acute renal failure. In Brenner BM, Lazarus JM (eds): Acute Renal Failure. New York, Churchill Livingstone, 1988, pp 119-141.
22. Schor N, Ichikawa I, Rennke HG, et al: Pathophysiology of altered glomerular function in aminoglycoside-treated rats. Kidney Int 19:288, 1981.
23. Flamenbaum W, Kotchen TA, Oken DE: Effect of renin immunization on mercuric chloride and glycerol-induced renal failure. Kidney Int 1:406, 1972.
24. Mauk RH, Patak RV, Fadem SZ, et al: Effect of prostaglandin E administration in a nephrotoxic and vasoconstrictor model of acute renal failure. Kidney Int 12:122, 1977.
25. Bidani AK, Churchill PC: Aminophylline ameliorates glycerol-induced acute renal failure in rats. Can J Physiol Pharmacol 61:567, 1983.
26. Knotek M, Rogachev B, Wang W, et al: Endotoxemic renal failure in mice: role of tumor necrosis factor independent of inducible nitric oxide synthase. Kidney Int 59:2242, 2001.
27. Gorligosky MS, Noiri E: Duality of nitric oxide in acute renal failure. Semin Nephrol 19:263, 1999.
28. Ruschitzka F, Shaw S, Gygi D, et al: Endothelial dysfunction in acute renal failure: Role of circulating and tissue endothelin-1. J Am Soc Nephrol 10:953, 1999.
29. Wilhelm SM, Simonson MS, Robinson AV, et al: Endothelin up-regulation and localization following renal ischemia and reperfusion. Kidney Int 55:1011, 1999.
30. Lopez-Novoa JM: Potential role of platelet activating factor in acute renal failure. Kidney Int 55:1672, 1999.
31. Finn WF, Chevalier RL: Recovery from postischemic acute renal failure in the rat. Kidney Int 16:113, 1979.
32. Luft FC, Evan AP: Comparative effects of tobramycin and gentamicin on glomerular ultrastructure. J Infect Dis 142:910, 1980.
33. Williams RH, Thomas CE, Navar LG, et al: Hemodynamic and single nephron function during the maintenance phase of ischemic acute renal failure. Kidney Int 19:503, 1981.
34. Gaudio KM, Taylor MR, Chaudry IH, et al: Accelerated recovery of single nephron function by postischemic infusion of ATP-MgCl$_2$. Kidney Int 22:13, 1982.
35. Sandoz PF, Bielmann D, Mihatsch M, et al: Value of urinary sediment in the diagnosis of interstitial rejection in renal transplants. Transplantation 41:343, 1986.
36. Myers BD, Chui F, Hilberman M, et al: Transtubular leakage of glomerular filtrate in human acute renal failure. Am J Physiol 237:F319, 1979.
37. Paller MS, Hoidal JR, Ferris TF: Oxygen free radicals in ischemic acute renal failure in the rat. J Clin Invest 74:1156, 1984.

38. Humes HD: Role of calcium in pathogenesis of acute renal failure. Am J Physiol 259:F579, 1986.

39. Siegel NJ, Avison MJ, Reilly HF, et al: Enhanced recovery of renal ATP with postischemic infusion of ATP-MgCL$_2$ determined by 31 P-NMR. Am J Physiol 245:F530, 1983.

40. Black TL, Carr MG, Korones SB: Necrotizing enterocolitis: Improving survival within a single facility. South Med J 82:1103, 1989.

41. Behrman RE, Lees MH, Peterson EN, et al: Distribution of the circulation in the normal and asphyxiated fetal primate. Am J Obstet Gynecol 108:956, 1970.

42. Chesney RW, Kaplan BS, Freedom RM, et al: Acute renal failure: An important complication of cardiac surgery in infants. J Pediatr 87:381, 1975.

43. Moghal NE, Brocklebank JT, Meadow SR: A review of acute renal failure in children: Incidence, etiology and outcome. Clin Nephrol 49:91, 1998.

44. Trompeter RS, Chantler C, Haycock GB: Tolazoline and acute renal failure in the newborn. Lancet 1:219, 1981.

45. Naujoks S, Guignard J-P: Renal effects of tolazoline in rabbits. Lancet 2:1075, 1979.

46. Tack ED, Perlman JM: Renal failure in sick hypertensive premature infants receiving captopril. J Pediatr 112:805, 1988.

47. Van Bel F, Guit GL, Schipper J, et al: Indomethacin-induced changes in renal blood flow velocity waveform in premature infants investigated with color Doppler imaging. J Pediatr 118:621, 1991.

48. Bernstein J: The morphogenesis of renal parenchymal maldevelopment (renal dysplasia). Pediatr Clin North Am 18:395, 1971.

49. Yaster M, Scherer T, Stone M, et al: Prediction of successful primary closure of congenital abdominal wall defects using intraoperative measurements. Pediatr Surg 24:1217, 1989.

50. Nakayama DK, Killian A, Hill LM, et al: The newborn with hydrops and sacrococcygeal teratoma. J Pediatr Surg 26:1435, 1991.

51. Noe HN, Bryant JF, Roy SI, et al: Urolithiasis in preterm neonates associated with furosemide therapy. J Urol 132:93, 1984.

52. Eckstein CW, Kass EJ: Anuria in a newborn secondary to bilateral uteropelvic fungus balls. J Urol 127:109, 1982.

53. Steele BT, Paes B, Towell ME, et al: Fetal renal failure associated with intrauterine growth retardation. Am J Obstet Gynecol 159:1200, 1988.

54. Dauber IM, Krauss AN, Symchych PS, et al: Renal failure following perinatal anoxia. J Pediatr 88:851, 1976.

55. Lorentz WBJ, Trillo AA: Neonatal renal failure and glomerular immaturity. Clin Nephrol 19:154, 1983.

56. Phillips JR, Karlowicz MG: Prevalence of *Candida* species in hospital-acquired urinary tract infections in a neonatal intensive care unit. Pediatr Infect Dis J 16:190, 1997.

57. Khan MY: Anuria from *Candida* pyelonephritis and obstructing fungus balls. Urology 21:421, 1983.

58. Yoo SY, Namkoong MK: Acute renal failure caused by fungal bezoar: A late complication of candida sepsis associated with central catheterization. J Pediatr Surg 30:1600, 1995.

59. Adelman RD: The hypertensive neonate. Clin Perinatol 15:567, 1988.

60. Bauer SB, Feldman SM, Gellis SS, et al: Neonatal hypertension: A complication of umbilical artery catheterization. N Engl J Med 293:1032, 1975.

61. Avery ME, Oppenheimer EH, Gordon HH: Renal-vein thrombosis in newborn infant of diabetic mothers. N Engl J Med 256:1134, 1957.

62. Assadi F, Delivoria-Papadopoulos M, Pereira G, et al: Fibrinogen degradation products in acute renal failure of the newborn. Clin Nephrol 19:74, 1983.

63. Adelman RD, Wirth F, Rubio T: A controlled study of the nephrotoxicity of mezlocillin and amikacin in the neonate. Am J Dis Child 141:1175, 1987.

64. Adelman RD, Wirth F, Rubio T: A controlled study of the nephrotoxicity of mezlocillin and gentamicin plus ampicillin in the neonate. J Pediatr 111:888, 1987.

65. Cifuentes RF, Olley PM, Balfe JW, et al: Indomethacin and renal function in premature infants with persistent patent ductus arteriosus. J Pediatr 95:583, 1979.

66. Rennie JM, Coke RWI: Prolonged low-dose indomethacin for persistent ductus arteriosus of prematurity. Arch Dis Child 65:55, 1991.

67. Vert P, Bianchetti G, Marchal F, et al: Effectiveness and pharmacokinetics of indomethacin in premature newborns with patent ductus arteriosus. Eur J Clin Pharmacol 18:83, 1980.

68. Anderson RJ, Berl T, McDonald KM, et al: Evidence for an in vivo antagonism between vasopressin and prostaglandin in the mammalian kidney. J Clin Invest 56:420, 1975.

69. Yeh TF, Wilks A, Singh J, et al: Furosemide prevents the renal side effects of indomethacin therapy in premature infants with patent ductus arteriosus. J Pediatr 101:433, 1982.

70. Brion LP, Campbell DE: Furosemide for prevention of morbidity in indomethacin-treated infants with patent ductus arteriosus. Cochrane Review. The Cochrane Library, 3. Oxford, Update Software, 2002.

71. Seyberth HW, Rascher W, Hackenthal R, et al: Effect of prolonged indomethacin therapy on renal function and selected vasoactive hormones in very low birth weight infants with symptomatic patent ductus arteriosus. J Pediatr 103:979, 1983.

72. Roberts RJ: Drug Therapy in Infants: Pharmacologic Principles and Clinical Experience. Philadelphia, WB Saunders, 1984, p 82.

73. Baley JE, Kliegman RM, Fanaroff AA: Disseminated fungal infections in very low birth weight infants: Therapeutic toxicity. Pediatrics 73:153, 1984.

74. Butler KM, Baker CJ: *Candida*: An increasingly important pathogen in the nursery. Pediatr Clin North Am 35:543, 1988.

75. Wong-Beringer A, Jacobs RA, Guglielmo BJ: Lipid formulations of amphotericin B: Clinical efficacy and toxicities. Clin Infect Dis 27:603, 1998.

76. Gilbert EF, Khoury GH, Hogan GR, et al: Hemorrhagic renal necrosis in infancy: Relationship to radio-opaque compounds. J Pediatr 76:49, 1970.

77. Cunniff C, Jones KL, Phillipson J, et al: Oligohydramnios sequence and renal tubular malformation associated with maternal enalapril use. Am J Obstet Gynecol 163:187, 1990.

78. Hanssens M, Keirse MJNC, Vankelecom F, et al: Fetal and neonatal effects of treatment with angiotensin-converting enzyme inhibitors in pregnancy. Obstet Gynecol 78:128, 1991.

79. Rosa FW, Bosco LA, Graham CF, et al: Neonatal anuria with maternal angiotensin-converting enzyme inhibition. Obstet Gynecol 74:371, 1989.

80. Schubiger G, Flury G, Nussberger J: Enalapril for pregnancy-induced hypertension: Acute renal failure in a neonate. Ann Intern Med 108:215, 1988.

81. Pickles CJ, Symonds EM, Pipkin FB: The fetal outcome in a randomized double-blind controlled trial of labetalol versus placebo in pregnancy-induced hypertension. Br J Obstet Gynaecol 96:38, 1989.

82. Bavoux F: Non-steroidal anti-inflammatory drugs and fetal toxicity. Presse Med 21:1909, 1992.

83. Heijden AJVD, Provoost AP, Nauta J, et al: Renal functional impairment in preterm neonates related to intrauterine indomethacin exposure. Pediatr Res 24:644, 1988.

84. Heijden AJVD, Tibboel D, Fetter WPF, et al: Intrauterine exposure to indomethacin. Eur J Pediatr 145:579, 1986.

85. Vanhaesebrouck P, Theiry M, Leroy JG, et al: Oligohydramnios, renal insufficiency and ileal perforation in preterm infants after intrauterine exposure to indomethacin. J Pediatr 113:738, 1988.

86. Raivio KO: Neonatal hyperuricemia. J Pediatr 88:625, 1976.

87. Ahmadian Y, Lewy PR: Possible urate nephropathy of the newborn infant as a cause of transient renal insufficiency. J Pediatr 91:96, 1977.

88. Dearth JC, Tompkins RB, Biuliana ER, et al: Hyperuricemia in congenital heart disease. Am J Dis Child 132:900, 1978.

89. Gottlieb RP, Roeloffs S, Galler-Rimm G, et al: Transient renal insufficiency in the neonate related to hyperuricemia and hyperuricosuria. Child Nephrol Urol 11:111, 1991.

90. Stapleton FB: Renal uric acid clearance in human neonates. J Pediatr 103:290, 1983.

91. Roberts DW, Haycock GB, Dalton RN, et al: Prediction of acute renal failure after birth asphyxia. Arch Dis Child 65:1021, 1990.

92. Merlob P, Litwin A, Lazar L, et al: Neonatal ABO incompatibility complicated by hemoglobinuria and acute renal failure. Clin Pediatr 29:219, 1990.

93. Trudinger BJ, Cook CM, Giles WB, et al: Fetal umbilical artery velocity waveforms and subsequent neonatal outcome. Br J Obstet Gynaecol 98:378, 1991.

94. Portman RJ, Carter BS, Gaylord MS, et al: Predicting neonatal morbidity after perinatal asphyxia: A scoring system. Am J Obstet Gyncol 162:174, 1990.

95. Karlowicz MG, Adelman RD: Nonoliguric and oliguric acute renal failure in asphyxiated term neonates. Pediatr Nephrol 9:718, 1995.

96. Wiriyathian S, Rosenfeld CR, Arant BS Jr, et al: Urinary arginine vasopressin: Pattern of excretion in the neonatal period. Pediatr Res 20:103, 1986.

97. Bourke WG, Clarke TA, Mathews TG, et al: Isolated single umbilical artery—the case for routine renal screening. Arch Dis Child 68:600, 1993.

98. Moore CCM: The role of routine radiographic screening of boys with hypospadias: A prospective study. J Pediatr Surg 25:339, 1990.

99. Murugasu B, Yip WCL, Tay JSH: Sonographic screening for renal tract anomalies associated with congenital heart disease. J Clin Ultrasound 18:79, 1990.

100. Teele RL, Share JC: Ultrasound of Infants and Children. Philadelphia, WB Saunders, 1991, p 143.

101. Chevalier RL, Campbell F, Brenbridge ANAG: Prognostic factors in neonatal acute renal failure. Pediatrics 74:265, 1984.

102. Gonzalez R, Roeloffs S, Galler-Rimm G, et al: Septic obstruction and uremia in the newborn. Urol Clin North Am 9:297, 1982.

103. Shaffer SE, Norman ME: Renal function and renal failure in the newborn. Clin Perinatol 16:199, 1989.

104. Anand SK: Acute renal failure. In Taeusch HW, Ballard RA, Avery ME (eds): Diseases of the Newborn. Philadelphia, WB Saunders, 1991, pp 894-895.

105. Siegel SR, Oh W: Renal function as a marker of human fetal maturation. Acta Paediatr 65:481, 1976.

106. Ellis EN, Arnold WC: Use of urinary indices in renal failure in the newborn. Am J Dis Child 136:615, 1982.

107. Boineau FG, Rothman J, Lewy JE: Nephrosonography in the evaluation of renal failure and masses in infants. J Pediatr 87:195, 1975.

108. Feld LG, Springate JE, Fildes RD: Acute renal failure: I. Pathophysiology and diagnosis. J Pediatr 109:401, 1986.

109. Avner ED, Heyman S, Treves S, et al: Radionuclide renal scintiscans and flow studies in pediatric patients with acute renal failure. Kidney Int 16:877, 1979.

110. Adelman RD: Management of aortic thrombosis. J Pediatr 99:832, 1981.

111. Molteni KH, George J, Messersmith R, et al: Intrathrombic urokinase reverses neonatal renal artery thrombosis. Pediatr Nephrol 7:413, 1993.

112. Giacoia GP: High-dose urokinase therapy in newborn infants with major vessel thrombosis. Clin Pediatr 32:231, 1993.

113. Farnoux C, Camard O, Pinquier D, et al: Recombinant tissue-type plasminogen activator therapy of thrombosis in 16 neonates. J Pediatr 133:137, 1998.

114. Weiner G, Castle V, DiPietro M, Faix R: Successful treatment of neonatal arterial thrombosis with recombinant tissue plasminogen activator. J Pediatr 133:133, 1998.

115. Wong SN, Lo RNS, Yu ECL: Renal blood flow pattern by noninvasive Doppler ultrasound in normal children and acute renal failure patients. J Ultrasound Med 8:135, 1989.

116. Akinbi H, Abbasi S, Hilper PL, Bhutani VK: Gastrointestinal and renal blood flow velocity profile in neonates with birth asphyxia. J Pediatr 125:625, 1994.

117. Luciano R, Gallini F, Romagnoli C, et al: Doppler evaluation of renal blood flow velocity as a predictive index of acute renal failure in perinatal asphyxia. Eur J Pediatr 157:656, 1998.

118. Fildes RD, Springate JE, Feld LG: Acute renal failure: II. Management of suspected and established disease. J Pediatr 109:567, 1986.

119. Green TP, Thompson TR, Johnson DE, et al: Furosemide promotes patent ductus arteriosus in premature infants with respiratory distress syndrome. N Engl J Med 308:743, 1983.

120. Burton CJ, Tomson CRV: Can the use of low dose dopamine be justified? Postgrad Med J 75:269, 1999.

121. Cuthbertson BH, Noble DW: Dopamine in oliguria. BMJ 314:690, 1997.

122. Denton MD, Chertow GM, Brady HR: "Renal-dose" dopamine for the treatment of acute renal failure: Scientific rationale, experimental studies and clinical trials. Kidney Int 49:4, 1996.

123. Hollenberg NK, Adams DF, Mendall P, et al: Renal vascular responses to dopamine: Hemodynamic and angiographic observations in normal man. Clin Sci 45:733, 1973.

124. McDonald R, Goldberg L, McNay J, Tuttle E: Effects of dopamine in man: Augmentation of sodium excretion, glomerular filtration rate, and renal plasma flow. J Clin Invest 43:1116, 1964.

125. Perdue PW, Balser JR, Lipsett PA, Breslow MJ: Renal dose dopamine in surgical patients: Dogma or science? Ann Surg 227:470, 1998.

126. Taylor-Thompson B, Cockrill BA: Renal dose dopamine: A Siren song? Lancet 344:7, 1994.

127. Australian and New Zealand Intensive Care Society (ANZICS) Clinical Trials Group: Low-dose dopamine in patients with early renal dysfunction: A placebo-controlled randomized trial. Lancet 356:2139, 2000.

128. Galley HF: Renal-dose dopamine: Will the message now get through? Lancet 2000;356:2112.

129. Reimer KA, Don TD, Worten HG: Alterations in renal cortex following ischemic injury: III. Ultrastructure of proximal tubules after ischemia or autolysis. Lab Invest 26:347, 1972.

130. Gaudio KM, Ardito TA, Reilly H, et al: Accelerated cellular recovery after an ischemic renal injury. Am J Pathol 112:338, 1983.

131. Herter GE, Siegel NJ: Accelerated recovery from obstructive nephropathy. Kidney Int 21:218, 1982.

132. Siegel NJ: Amino acids and adenine nucleotides in acute renal failure. In Brenner BM, Lazarus JM (eds): Acute Renal Failure. Philadelphia, WB Saunders, 1983, p 741.

133. Siegel NJ, Gaudio KM, Kashgarian M: Adenine nucleotides in the prevention of ischemic acute renal failure. In Robinson RR (ed): Nephrology. New York, Springer-Verlag, 1984, p 803.

134. Siegel NJ, Glazier WB, Chaudry IH, et al: Enhanced recovery from acute renal failure by the postischemic infusion of adenine nucleotides and magnesium chloride in rats. Kidney Int 17:338, 1980.

135. Stromski ME, Cooper K, Thulin G, et al: Postischemic ATP-MgCl$_2$ provides precursors for resynthesis of cellular ATP in rats. Am J Physiol 250:F834, 1986.

136. Albert SG, Shapiro MJ, Brown WW, et al: Analysis of radiocontrast-induced nephropathy by dual-labeled radionuclide clearance. Invest Radiol 29:618, 1994.

137. Siegel NJ, Gaudio KM, Katz LA, et al: Beneficial effect of thyroxine on recovery from toxic acute renal failure. Kidney Int 25:906, 1984.

138. Sutter PM, Thulin G, Skromski M, et al: Beneficial effect of thyroxine in the treatment of ischemic acute renal failure. Pediatr Nephrol 2:1, 1988.

139. Boydstun II, Thulin G, Zhu XH, et al: Disassociation of postischemic recovery of renal adenosine triphosphate and cellular integrity. Pediatr Res 3:595, 1993.

140. Acker CG, Singh AR, Flick RP, et al: A trial of thyroxine in acute renal failure. Kidney Int 57:293, 2000.

141. Shaw SG, Weidmann P, Hodler J, et al: Atrial natriuretic peptide protects against acute ischemic renal failure in the rat. J Clin Invest 80:1232, 1987.

142. Allgren RL, Marbury TC, Rahman SN, et al: Anaritide in acute tubular necrosis. N Engl J Med 336:828, 1997.

143. Guler HP, Eckardt KU, Zapf J, et al: Insulin-like growth factor I increases glomerular filtration rate and renal plasma flow in man. Acta Endocrinol (Copenh) 121:101, 1989.

144. Ding H, Kopple JD, Cohen A, Hirschber R: Recombinant human insulin-like growth factor-I accelerates recovery and reduces catabolism in rats with ischemic acute renal failure. J Clin Invest 91:2281, 1993.

145. Friedlaender M, Popovitzer MM, Weiss O, et al: Insulin-like growth factor-1 (IGF-1) enhances recovery from HgCl$_2$-induced acute renal failure: The effects on renal IGF-1, IGF-1 receptor, and IGF-binding protein-1 mRNA. J Am Soc Nephrol 5:1782, 1995.

146. Franklin SC, Moulton M, Sicard GA, et al: Insulin-like growth factor I preserves renal function postoperatively. Am J Physiol (Renal Physiol 41) 272:F257, 1997.

147. Hirschberg R, Kopple J, Lipsett P, et al: Multicenter clinical trial of recombinant human insulin-like growth factor I in patents with acute renal failure. Kidney Int 55:2423, 1999.

148. Raj JU: Acid base, fluid and electrolyte management. In Taeusch HW, Ballard RA, Avery ME (eds): Diseases of the Newborn. Philadelphia, WB Saunders, 1991, p 266.

149. Arieff AL, Ayus JC, Fraser CL: Hyponatremia and death or permanent brain damage in healthy children. BMJ 304:1218, 1992.

150. Sarnaik AP, Meert K, Hackbarth R, et al: Management of hyponatremic seizures in children with hypertonic saline: A safe and effective strategy. Crit Care Med 19:758, 1991.

151. Task Force on Blood Pressure Control in Children: Report of the Second Task Force on Blood Pressure Control in Children. Pediatrics 79:1, 1987.

152. Karlowicz MG, Adelman RD: Acute renal failure in the neonate. Clin Perinatol 19:139, 1992.

153. Stork EK, Carlo WA, Kliegman RM, et al: Hypertension redefined for critically ill neonates. Pediatr Res 18:321A, 1984.

154. Mason T, Polak MJ, Pyles L, et al: Treatment of neonatal renovascular hypertension with intravenous enalapril. Am J Perinatol 9:254, 1992.

155. Perlman JM, Volpe JJ: Neurologic complications of captopril treatment of neonatal hypertension. Pediatrics 83:47, 1989.

156. Schilder JL, Van den Anker JN: Use of enalapril in neonatal hypertension. Acta Pediatr 84:1426, 1995.

157. Benitz WE, Malachowski N, Cohen RS, et al: Use of sodium nitroprusside in neonates: Efficacy and safety. J Pediatr 106:102, 1985.

158. Adelman RD: Treatment of pediatric hypertensive emergencies. In Portman RJ, Sorof JM, Ingelfinger J (eds): Pediatric Hypertension. Totowa, NJ, Humana Press, 2003.

159. Bunchman TE, Lynch RE, Wood EG: Intravenously administered labetalol for treatment of hypertension in children. J Pediatr 120:140, 1992.

160. Flynn JT, Mottes TA, Brophy PD, et al: Intravenous nicardipine for treatment of severe hypertension in children. J Pediatr 139:38, 2001.

161. Sartori SC, Nakagawa TA, Solhaug MJ, et al: Intravenous nicardipine for treatment of systemic hypertension in children. Pediatr Res 45:A258, 1999.

162. Treluyer JM, Hubert P, Jouvet P, et al: Intravenous nicardipine in hypertensive children. Eur J Pediatr 152:712, 1993.

163. Mandelberg A, Krupnik Z, Houri S, et al: Salbutamol metered-dose inhaler with spacer for hyperkalemia: How fast? How safe? Chest 115:617, 1999.

164. Malone T: Glucose and insulin versus cation-exchange resin for the treatment of hyperkalemia in very low birth weight infants. J Pediatr 118:121, 1991.

165. Kemper MJ, Harps E, Hellwege HH, Muller-Wiefel DE: Effective treatment of acute hyperkalemia in childhood by short-term infusion of salbutamol. Eur J Pediatr 155:495, 1996.

166. Lerner GR, Gruskin AB: Acute renal failure. In Nelson NM (ed): Current Therapy in Neonatal-Perinatal Medicine–2. Toronto, BC Decker, 1990, pp 173-177.

167. Koo WWK, Kaplan LA, Krug-Wispe SK: Aluminum contamination of infant formulas. J Parenter Enteral Nutr 12:170, 1988.

168. Molitoris BA, Froment DH, Mackenzie TA, et al: Citrate: A major factor in the toxicity of orally administered aluminum compounds. Kidney Int 36:949, 1989.

169. Salusky IB, Foley J, Nelson P, et al: Aluminum accumulation during treatment with aluminum hydroxide and dialysis in children and young adults with chronic renal disease. N Engl J Med 324:527, 1991.

170. Drukker A, Guignard J-P: Renal aspects of the term and preterm infant: A selective update. Curr Opin Pediatr 14:175, 2002.

171. Ledermann SE, Shaw NJ: Long-term enteral nutrition in infants and young children with chronic renal failure. Pediatr Nephrol 13:870, 1999.

172. Karlowicz MG, Buescher ES, Surka AE: Fulminant late-onset sepsis in a neonatal intensive care unit, 1988-1997, and the impact of avoiding empiric vancomycin therapy. Pediatrics 106:1387, 2000.
173. Steele BT, Vigneux A, Blatz S, et al: Acute peritoneal dialysis in infants weighing < 1500 grams. J Pediatr 110:126, 1987.
174. Coulthard MG, Vernon B: Managing acute renal failure in very low birth weight infants. Arch Dis Child Fetal Neonatal Educ 73:F187, 1995.
175. Matthews DE, West KW, Rescoria FJ, et al: Peritoneal dialysis in the first 60 days of life. J Pediatr Surg 25:110, 1990.
176. Forni LG, Hilton PJ: Continuous hemofiltration in the treatment of acute renal failure. N Engl J Med 336:1303, 1997.
177. Lieberman KV: Continuous arteriovenous hemofiltration in children. Pediatr Nephrol 1:330, 1987.
178. Bishof NA, Welch TR, Strife CF, et al: Continuous hemofiltration in children. Pediatrics 85:819, 1990.
179. Grylack L, Medani C, Hultzen C, et al: Nonoliguric acute renal failure in the newborn. Am J Dis Child 136:518, 1982.
180. Reimold EW, Don TD, Worthen HG: Renal failure during the first year of life. Pediatrics 59:987, 1977.
181. Anand SK, Northway JD, Crussi FG: Acute renal failure in newborn infants. J Pediatr 92:985, 1978.
182. Leonidas JC, Berdon WE, Gribetz D: Bilateral renal cortical necrosis in the newborn infant: roentgenographic diagnosis. J Pediatr 79:623, 1971.
183. Rasoulpour M, McLean RH: Renal venous thrombosis in neonates. Am J Dis Child 134:276, 1980.

CHAPTER 80

Chronic Renal Disease

Bernard S. Kaplan, Paige Kaplan, and Kevin E.C. Meyers

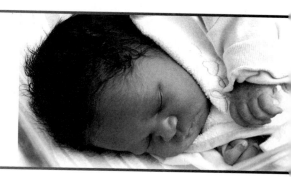

Acute and chronic renal diseases affect neonates, but the perception of these syndromes is often incorrect. Neonates with prenatal renal abnormalities whose serum creatinine concentrations increase rapidly after birth do not have "acute renal failure" but chronic failure because the failure already had started in utero. Chronic renal disease in a neonate is usually the result of an inherited disorder or a congenital abnormality in the development of the kidneys or urinary tract or both (Table 80-1). Acute renal failure in a neonate usually is caused by perinatal asphyxia and may result in chronic renal failure. Compounding the concept of renal failure starting in utero is the fact that the natural history and treatment of some renal disorders are altered by prenatal diagnosis and treatment. In addition, genetic renal disorders rarely are isolated abnormalities and may occur as components of many syndromes. Conversely, neonates with multiple congenital defects often have renal involvement. Renal and urinary tract ultrasound is indicated in these cases.

DEFINITIONS OF RENAL FAILURE

Mild renal failure is defined as a glomerular filtration rate (GFR) less than 50 mL/min/1.73 m², moderate renal failure is a GFR between 50 and 25 mL/min/1.73 m², and severe renal failure is a GFR less than 25 mL/min/1.73 m². Renal function often improves in the first year of life even in infants who initially have marked reductions in GFR.

This chapter emphasizes the importance of congenital and hereditary abnormalities in neonates. Diagnosis, treatment, genetic counseling, and prognosis are reviewed in the context of the specific syndromes or conditions.[1] General principles of management are discussed separately. Optimal care for the infant and family requires a team approach because management of the problems in a neonate with chronic renal disease is so complex.

ASSOCIATED ABNORMALITIES

Many anomalies occur in association with renal abnormalities in neonates. Low-set ears, preauricular pits, two vessels in the umbilical cord, and hypospadias are not sensitive indicators of the presence of a renal anomaly. It has been suggested, however, that ear malformations are associated with an increased frequency of clinically significant structural renal anomalies compared with the general population.[2] Patients with auricular anomalies should be assessed for accompanying dysmorphic features, including facial asymmetry; colobomas of the lid, iris, and retina; choanal atresia; jaw hypoplasia; branchial cysts or sinuses; cardiac murmurs; distal limb anomalies; and imperforate or anteriorly placed anus. If any of these features are present, renal ultrasound is useful not only in diagnosing renal anomalies but also in diagnosing and managing multiple congenital anomaly syndromes themselves. Renal ultrasound should be performed in patients with isolated preauricular pits, cup ears, or any other ear anomaly accompanied by one or more of the following: other malformations or dysmorphic features; a family history of deafness, auricular malformations, or renal malformations; or a maternal history of gestational diabetes. Other abnormalities also may be clues to the presence of renal disorders.

In the **oligohydramnios sequence**, the uterus compresses the fetus as a result of decreased amniotic fluid. This results in flat facies (with flattened nose, suborbital skin creases, and flat simple auricles); limb deformations; narrow, small chest; and pulmonary hypoplasia. In **prune-belly syndrome (PBS)**, the anterior abdominal muscles are absent or deficient; the abdomen is wrinkled; and obstructive uropathy, renal cystic dysplasia, undescended testes, and features of oligohydramnios sequence are seen. **Congenital hepatic fibrosis** occurs in patients with autosomal recessive polycystic kidneys (ARPKD), Jeune syndrome, Meckel syndrome, chondrodysplasia syndromes, Ivemark renal-hepatic-pancreatic cystic dysplasia,

Table 80–1. Inherited and Congenital Kidney Disease in Neonates

Multicystic kidney
Renal adysplasia/dysplasia
  Isolated adysplasia/dysplasia*
  Adysplasia in regional defects
   Usually sporadic
    Prune-belly syndrome
    Posterior urethral valves†
    VACTERL‡
    Genital anomalies and renal adysplasia/dysplasia
    Pallister-Hall syndrome
  Adysplasia/dysplasia in multiple congenital
   abnormalities syndromes
  Autosomal dominant
   Branchio-otorenal dysplasia (BOR syndrome)
   Ectodermal dysplasia, ectrodactyly, cleft lip/palate
    syndrome
   Radial ray aplasia and renal anomalies
  Autosomal recessive
   Fanconi anemia syndrome
   Thrombocytopenia absent radius syndrome
   Radial ray aplasia and renal anomalies*
   Fraser syndrome
   Fryns syndrome
  X-linked
   Kallmann syndrome
  Usually sporadic
   Posterior urethral valves
   Prune-belly syndrome

Cystic kidneys
  Autosomal recessive
   Autosomal recessive polycystic kidney disease
   Meckel syndrome
   Jeune syndrome
   Renal-hepatic-pancreatic dysplasia
   Glutaric aciduria type II
   Zellweger syndrome
  Autosomal dominant
   Autosomal dominant polycystic kidney disease
   Tuberosclerosis
  Glomerulocystic kidney diseases
   Isolated glomerulocystic kidneys
   Associated with other kidney diseases
   Autosomal dominant glomerulocystic kidney
    disease
Dysgenetic kidneys
  Autosomal recessive
   Renal tubular dysgenesis
Overgrowth syndromes
  Beckwith-Wiedemann syndrome
  Simpson-Golabi-Behmel
  Perlman syndrome
Congenital nephritic syndrome
  Autosomal recessive (Finnish type)
  Diffuse mesangial sclerosis
  Denys-Dash syndrome
  Galloway-Mowat syndrome

*Occasionally recessive or dominant.

†Posterior urethral valves reported in sibs.

‡Dominant inheritance reported.

VACTERL, vertebral abnormalities, anal atresia, cardiac abnormalities, tracheoesophageal fistula and/or esophageal atresia, renal agenesis and dysplasia, and limb defects.

Modified from Kaplan B, Kaplan P, Ruchelli E: Heredity and congenital malformations of the kidneys. Perinat Clin North Am 19:197, 1992.

Zellweger syndrome, and occasionally autosomal dominant polycystic kidney disease (ADPKD).[3,4] Evaluation of the liver by ultrasound and confirmation by biopsy are indicated if these conditions are suspected. **Pyloric stenosis** occurs in some cases of ADPKD, ARPKD, autosomal dominant glomerulocystic kidneys, and congenital nephrotic syndrome. **Early-onset diabetes** may occur in young adult family members of patients with familial hypoplastic glomerulocystic kidney disease.[5] **Radial aplasia** occurs in the acrorenal syndromes with renal abnormalities and radial ray defects. **Dandy-Walker malformation** or **cyst** is reported in Fryns, Ivemark, Goldston, and Meckel syndromes.

MULTICYSTIC KIDNEY

Definitions of multicystic kidney and renal dysplasia are shown in Table 80-2.[6] **Multicystic kidney** is a common cause of an abdominal mass in a newborn, with a prevalence of 1 in every 4300 live newborns.[7] It is detected by ultrasound in utero, by palpation, or during evaluation of a urinary tract infection. Many patients with multicystic kidneys have contralateral urologic abnormalities that include vesicoureteric reflux or obstructions or both.[8] Infection, injury, or malignant transformation are cited as

reasons for removal, but most multicystic kidneys are monitored by ultrasound, and spontaneous regression often occurs without complications.[9-11] Malignant transformation is an extremely rare complication of multicystic kidney disease.

RENAL ADYSPLASIA AND DYSPLASIA

Clinical features of renal adysplasia and dysplasia depend on the severity of the renal anomaly and the presence of associated anomalies.[12] The neonate may appear normal or have oligohydramnios sequence, PBS, or a specific associated syndrome. **Dysplasia** occurs as the result of a single gene disorder (autosomal recessive[13] or dominant,[14,15] multifactorial inheritance,[16] chromosomal disorders,[17] or in utero disturbances). **Adysplasia** may occur in association with müllerian anomalies.[18] This association, known as the Mayer-Rokitansky-Kuster-Hauser syndrome, consists of vaginal atresia and bicornuate or septated uterus. Unilateral renal anomalies occur in 50% of patients, and skeletal anomalies occur in 12%.[19] The fallopian tubes, ovaries, and broad and round ligaments are normal. Patients have a normal female karyotype and normal secondary sexual development.

Table 80–2. Definitions of Abnormal Kidneys

Multicystic Kidney

No continuity between glomeruli and calyces
Kidney does not function
Contralateral kidney may be normal, absent,
 hydronephrotic, ectopic, or dysplastic
Bilateral multicystic kidneys cause severe oligohydramnios

Adysplasia

Includes renal agenesis, hypoplasia, and dysplasia

Dysplastic Kidneys

Unilateral or bilateral
Usually cystic, disorganized architecture
Ectopic tissues (cartilage, muscle) often present
May function

Renal Agenesis

Unilateral or bilateral absence of kidney
May be isolated or occur with multiple abnormalities

Hypoplastic Kidneys

Small, have fewer calyces, may be dysplastic
Include simple hypoplasia, oligomeganephronia,
 renal dysplasia

Simple Hypoplasia

Normal renal architecture but fewer reniculi
Reduced number and size of nephrons

Oligomeganephronia

Small kidneys
Large glomeruli but decreased numbers

Dysgenetic Kidneys

Do not develop normally
Are not dysplastic, cystic, obstructed
Do not contain ectopic tissue
Absent proximal tubules

Dysmorphic Kidneys

Abnormal shape or echotexture on imaging studies
May be dysplastic

Polycystic Kidneys

Many cysts in both kidneys
No renal dysplasia
Continuity of the lumen of the nephron from the
 uriniferous space to urinary bladder

Glomerulocystic Kidneys

Dilated Bowman spaces
Few or no cysts in the tubule

Prenatal diagnosis of dysplasia or adysplasia by ultrasound is possible if there is oligohydramnios or an affected older sibling. A GFR less than 15 mL/min/1.73 m^2 at 6 months of age is associated with a greater likelihood of progression of bilateral dysplasia to end-stage renal failure by 6 years of age.[20]

Isolated Adysplasia and Dysplasia

The incidence of bilateral renal dysplasia is about 0.15 per 1000 births.[16] The mode of transmission is autosomal dominant inheritance with reduced penetrance in some kindreds[21] or multifactorial inheritance in others.[14]

Parents may be normal, or one may have unilateral dysplasia or unilateral agenesis. Affected siblings may have unilateral or bilateral dysplasia. There are no phenotypic differences between sporadic and familial adysplasia. Sporadic adysplasia may be caused by a new mutation or inheritance of the genes from a nonmanifesting parent. Apparently normal relatives can be screened by renal ultrasound if genetic counseling is requested. The empirical risk of bilateral renal adysplasia for future siblings is 3.5%, but the recurrence risk increases if two siblings are affected.

Adysplasia and Dysplasia in Regional Defects

Prune-Belly Syndrome (McKusick #100100) and Posterior Urethral Valves (McKusick #100100)

The most frequent presentation of PBS and posterior urethral valves (PUV) in neonates is the oligohydramnios sequence. PBS and PUV usually are isolated occurrences but rarely can occur in siblings.

Prune-belly syndrome. PBS is characterized by deficient abdominal wall muscles and genital and urinary tract abnormalities.[22] One or both testes are undescended. Girls rarely are affected but may have uterine or vaginal anomalies or both.[9] There may be lower intestinal tract malrotation and atresias,[23] lower limb musculoskeletal reduction,[24] and cardiovascular malformations.[25] The bladder neck is widely dilated with a "wine glass" or "funnel" configuration.[26] The smooth muscle in the internal sphincter, bladder wall, and ureters may be deficient. Prostate development is often abnormal. Urethral obstructions include stenosis, atresia, and multiple urethral lumens, but a true anatomic obstruction cannot be shown in every case.[27,28] The kidneys may be minimally affected, or there may be severe dysplasia with or without cysts. The timing of in utero obstruction may determine whether the fetus has the PBS or PUV phenotype. It is unclear in PBS whether obstruction leads to a sequence of defects[29] or whether a primary defect in mesodermal development results in deficient musculature of the ureters, bladder, prostate, and lower abdominal wall.

Posterior urethral valves. Urethral valves in the prostatic urethra (either a flap valve or a diaphragm with a central hole) result in variable features of obstructive uropathy. The muscles of the internal sphincter, bladder wall, and ureters usually are hypertrophied,[30] and the bladder neck is hypertrophic.[31] One or both kidneys may be minimally affected or severely dysplastic. Survival of neonates with PBS or PUV initially depends on the severity of pulmonary hypoplasia. Poor prognostic signs for subsequent chronic renal failure in boys with PBS are the severity of renal dysplasia, a serum creatinine concentration greater than 0.7 mg/dL by the end of the first year, and occurrence of pyelonephritis.[32]

Adysplasia and Dysplasia in Multiple Congenital Abnormalities

Branchio-otorenal Dysplasia (McKusick #113650)

The spectrum of renal involvement in branchio-otorenal dysplasia ranges from normal kidneys to unilateral dysplasia to bilateral agenesis.[33] Renal function may be normal or severely reduced. Extrarenal manifestations are variable and include preauricular pits, branchial clefts, sensorineural deafness, and lacrimal duct atresia. The prognosis depends on the severity of the kidney abnormality. The incidence is estimated at 1 in 40,000. Inheritance is autosomal dominant with high penetrance and variable expression. The mutant gene, *EYA1*, is on chromosome 8q13.3.[34,35] Four patients (including a mother and daughter) with congenital nuclear cataracts were found to have mutations in *EYA1*; in an 8-year-old boy, other features of branchio-otorenal dysplasia syndrome included multicystic dysplasia, conductive deafness with a malleus anomaly, and cervical fistula.[36]

Acrorenal Syndromes

Ectodermal Dysplasia–Ectrodactyly–Cleft Lip/Palate Syndrome (McKusick #128930)

Urogenital defects affect about 23%, ectrodactyly affects 84%, ectodermal dysplasia affects 77%, clefting affects 68%, lacrimal duct anomalies affect 59%, and conductive hearing loss affects 14% of cases of ectodermal dysplasia–ectrodactyly–cleft lip/palate syndrome.[37,38] Inheritance is autosomal dominant, with variable penetrance and expression. All ectodermal dysplasia–ectrodactyly–cleft lip/palate syndrome patients and first-degree relatives should be evaluated for genitourinary abnormalities.[39]

VACTERL/VATER Association (McKusick #192350)

VACTERL and **VATER** are acronyms for the constellation of defects of *v*ertebral anomalies, *a*nal atresia, *c*ongenital cardiac disease, *t*racheo*e*sophageal fistula, *r*enal abnormalities, and *r*adial-*l*imb dysplasia. VACTERL is usually sporadic. It is imperative to test a neonate with presumptive VACTERL for Fanconi anemia.

Fanconi Anemia (Pancytopenia) Syndrome

Congenital malformations occur in 60% of cases.[40] Renal malformations include renal aplasia, duplication, ectopia, and horseshoe kidney. Affected patients have short stature; café-au-lait spots; radial-ray abnormalities with bilateral absent thumbs and radii or unilateral hypoplastic thumb or bifid thumb in 50% of cases, cardiac anomalies, gastrointestinal anomalies, central nervous system anomalies, head circumference less than or equal to 5%, skeletal abnormalities, and, in males, genital anomalies, hypogonadism, and infertility.[40] Bone marrow failure is not present at birth but develops in childhood or adolescence. There is an increased susceptibility to cancer, especially acute myeloid leukemia and squamous cell carcinoma. This syndrome has features that overlap with VACTERL, including renal and radial abnormalities, but microcephaly does not occur in VACTERL. In Fanconi anemia, chromosomal instability and mutagen hypersensitivity in cells differentiates it from VACTERL in neonates. The inheritance is autosomal recessive with variable expression. Fanconi anemia is heterogeneous, and mutations in one of at least seven different genes cause Fanconi anemia.[41] Most genes and their chromosomal locations have been identified for the subtypes, complementation groups *FANCA* (16q24.3),

FANCB (?), *FANCC* (9q22.3), *FANCD1* (?), *FANCD2* (3p25.3), *FANCE* (6p21.3), *FANCF* (11p15), and *FANCG* (9p13). Of patients, 60% to 80% are in FANCA group.[41,42]

Thrombocytopenia Absent Radius Syndrome (McKusick #274000)

Renal anomalies may occur in thrombocytopenia absent radius syndrome[43] but are uncommon. Thrombocytopenia is present at birth or in infancy and tends to improve or resolve. Occasionally, lower limb malformations are present. Inheritance is presumed to be autosomal recessive but is not definite.

Townes-Brocks Radial-Ear-Anal-Renal Syndrome (McKusick #107480)

Variable manifestations of Townes-Brocks radial-ear-anal-renal syndrome include broad, bifid, or triphalangeal thumb; flat thenar eminences; small, "lop," or "satyr" external ear; preauricular pits or tags; sensorineural hearing loss; and imperforate or stenotic or anteriorly placed anus. Renal and urologic anomalies encompass renal hypoplasia, renal dysplasia, unilateral renal agenesis, horseshoe kidney, posterior urethral valves, ureterovesical reflux, and meatal stenosis.[44] Townes-Brocks radial-ear-anal-renal syndrome is caused by a dominantly inherited defect in the gene encoding *SALL1*, a putative transcription factor, located on chromosome16q12.1. It may be required for urologic, renal, limb, ear, brain, and liver development.[44]

Fraser Syndrome (McKusick #219000)

Manifestations of Fraser syndrome include cryptophthalmos, cutaneous syndactyly, abnormal genitalia, renal adysplasia or dysplasia, and many major and minor anomalies. Renal abnormalities are cystic dysplasia or renal agenesis, and bladder changes are thickening of the muscle layer and fibrosis. Inheritance is autosomal recessive. It may be possible to diagnose the syndrome between 18 and 19 weeks of gestation by ultrasound.[45] Most patients die in the newborn period.

Fryns Syndrome (McKusick #229850)

The incidence of Fryns syndrome is estimated at approximately 1 in 10,000. There is unilateral or bilateral hypoplasia of muscular diaphragm with hernia and lung hypoplasia. The face is "coarse" with broad nasal bridge, macrostomia, microretrognathia, abnormal helices, and cleft palate. Distal digital hypoplasia, renal cystic dysplasia,[46] urinary tract malformations, shawl scrotum, hypoplastic external genitalia, bifid or hypoplastic uterus, or immature testes are present. In 50% of cases, duodenal atresia, pyloric hyperplasia, malrotation, and common mesentery are present. They may have ventricular septal defect, Dandy-Walker anomaly, and agenesis of corpus callosum. There is severe respiratory distress at birth, and most infants die in the neonatal period. Fatal hydrops fetalis may occur. The rare survivors have mental retardation. Inheritance is autosomal recessive with variable expression. It may be possible to diagnose the posterolateral diaphragm defect and cleft palate before 20 weeks of gestation by ultrasound.

Pallister-Hall Congenital Hypothalamic Hamartoblastoma Syndrome (McKusick #146510)

In Pallister-Hall congenital hypothalamic hamartoblastoma syndrome, there are multiple congenital anomalies with renal ectopia, agenesis, or dysplasia; hypothalamic hamartoblastoma; postaxial or central polydactyly; imperforate anus; and, in approximately 60%, bifid/cleft epiglottis. Occasionally, there is laryngeal cleft, abnormal lung lobation, short fourth metacarpals, nail dysplasia, multiple buccal frenula, hypoadrenalism, microphallus, congenital heart defect, and intrauterine growth restriction. The features of this syndrome overlap with polydactyly, imperforate anus, vertebral anomalies syndrome, and the VACTERL association.[47] Many patients die in the newborn period, but others have normal life span and intelligence. Inheritance is autosomal dominant with full penetrance and variable expression. Mutations occur in *GL13,* a zinc finger transcription factor gene. The gene locus is 7p13. Minimal diagnostic criteria for the index case are the presence of hypothalamic hamartoma and central polydactyly. First-degree relatives must have either hypothalamic hamartoma or polydactyly (central or postaxial) and show inheritance in an autosomal dominant pattern or in a manner consistent with gonadal mosaicism.[48]

CYSTIC KIDNEYS

Autosomal Recessive Polycystic Kidney Disease (McKusick #263200)

Features of ARPKD are polycystic kidneys and hepatic fibrosis, both with variable degrees of severity.[49-51] Renal involvement is more evident than hepatic involvement in neonates, and liver disease may be more prominent in older children. Neonates with severe renal involvement in utero may have the oligohydramnios sequence, but respiratory and renal functions occasionally improve. Some survivors maintain sufficient renal function into adolescence. Hypertension and hyponatremia are often severe and may be caused by volume expansion. Furosemide can correct hyponatremia and reduce hypertension.[49] Hypertension often responds to an angiotensin-converting enzyme inhibitor. The kidneys are large, cysts are rarely seen on excretory urography (intravenous urogram), and nephrogram often has a mottled or streaky appearance from pooling of contrast medium in dilated cortical and medullary cysts and dilated collecting ducts. The renal sonogram in the neonate shows large kidneys, increased echogenicity of the parenchyma, loss of corticomedullary differentiation, and loss of central echo complex. There may be macrocysts less than 2 cm in diameter. The cortex is preserved, and the papillae are echogenic.[50] Renal ultrasonography does not always distinguish ARPKD from ADPKD or transient nephromegaly.[51] Pathologically the kidneys are large, spongy, and reniform. The dilated collecting ducts are perpendicular to the surface of the kidney. There is no dysplasia. The liver is always involved with portal areas that are expanded by increased numbers of dilated bile ductules surrounded by fibrous tissue. Dilated ductules may become cystic. The liver cells are normal.

Many neonates who are symptomatic at birth die from respiratory or renal failure. Of patients who survive to 1 year, 75% survive beyond age 15 years.[52] Inheritance is autosomal recessive, with variable expression even within a sibship,[40] and the parents are unaffected. The gene locus is chromosome 6p21.1-p12.[53,54] ARPKD may be diagnosed after week 24 of gestation by ultrasound demonstration of hyperechogenic kidneys, oligohydramnios, nonvisualized bladder, and enlarged kidneys.[55] In addition to pulmonary hypoplasia, massively enlarged kidneys that restrict diaphragmatic excursion may cause respiratory distress. Bilateral nephrectomies and peritoneal dialysis were performed successfully in several neonates and infants with ARPKD, who survived long enough to undergo kidney transplants.[56,57] There is the promise that novel types of treatment may "cure" or ameliorate ARPKD. One promising strategy employs the use of an inhibitor of epidermal growth factor tyrosine kinase activity (EKI-785) that reduces renal and biliary abnormalities in murine ARPKD.[60]

Autosomal Dominant Polycystic Kidney Disease (McKusick #173900)

ADPKD is the most common and potentially lethal monogenic disease inherited as a dominant trait in humans.[61] The frequency is 1 in 500 with an incidence of end-stage renal failure of 50%.[61] Prenatal or neonatal presentation of ADPKD is uncommon but should not be overlooked. At birth, some patients have the oligohydramnios sequence, enlarged kidneys, or hematuria. Ultrasound and computed tomography scans are sensitive methods for detecting the cysts. The kidneys are enlarged and lobular, with calyces stretched and distorted by nonopacified cysts that produce smooth or irregular indentations.[51] Numerous cysts of various sizes are found in the parenchyma. Cysts also occur in liver, pancreas, and spleen. At postmortem, the kidneys are enlarged and have numerous round protuberances on their surfaces; cysts are irregularly dispersed through the parenchyma. There is variable expression: 4% of patients with the gene have clinical signs by age 30 years, and 11% have clinical signs by age 40 years.[62] Occasionally an infant may manifest the disease before the parent. The incidence in liveborn infants is 1 to 3 in 100,000, and the mutation rate is 6.5×10^3. Prediction by DNA analysis restriction length polymorphisms complements ultrasound for detection; it is not age dependent but is not informative in every family. There are at least three genes that cause ARPKD. *PKD1* occurs in 85% of families and is on chromosome 16p13.3-p13.12.[63] *PKD2* is found in about 5% of families who have the same clinical phenotypes as *PKD1* and is located on chromosome 4q13-q23.[64] The location of the third gene *(PKD3)* has not been found. Polycystin-1, the gene product, functions as a matrix receptor that links the extracellular matrix to the actin cytoskeleton via focal adhesion proteins.[61]

The mean age at onset of end-stage renal disease in individuals with *PKD1* is 56.7 ± 1.9 years compared with 69.4 ± 1.7 years in individuals with *PKD2*. Hypertension and renal impairment are less frequent and occur later in families with *PKD2*. ADPKD may be detected prenatally by ultrasound.[65] In the past, 43% of 83 reported cases of ADPKD presenting in utero or in the first few months of life died before 1 year.[66] More recent studies of larger numbers of patients show that the prognosis is more optimistic, however. Eleven children with ADPKD diagnosed in utero or in the first year of life were followed for 3 to 15 years. Two children had end-stage renal disease, and eight had normal or near-normal renal function.[67,68]

Tuberous Sclerosis (McKusick #191100)

Tuberous sclerosis is characterized by hamartomas in multiple organs and systems. Many patients have renal lesions, usually angiomyolipomas, which can hemorrhage or compress surrounding normal renal tissue, but rarely cause end-stage renal failure. Cysts, polycystic renal disease, and, rarely, renal carcinoma also can occur. Rarely, polycystic or unilateral cystic disease is found in a newborn in whom a diagnosis of tuberous sclerosis is made later.[69,70] Renal cysts or polycystic disease in tuberous sclerosis is identical on ultrasound, intravenous urogram, or computed tomography scan to simple cysts or ADPKD. Nonsymptomatic renal lesions (cysts or angiomyolipomas) occur in approximately 60%.[71] Other features include skin lesions in 96%,[72] epilepsy, learning difficulties, and behavioral problems. "Ash leaf" hypopigmented nevi affect approximately 60%, but may be the only skin manifestation of tuberous sclerosis in infancy, and infants with polycystic kidneys must be examined for the nevi under ultraviolet light; some regress in adulthood. Shagreen patches (55%) and facial angiofibromas (adenoma sebaceum) (approximately 88%) develop before 5 years. Nail (ungula) fibromas appear after 5 years and increase with age: 88% of patients older than 30 years have ungula fibromas. Cardiac (ventricular) rhabdomyomas appear in infancy. Seizures may occur in infancy. Patients usually survive to adolescence and adulthood, but patients with early-onset polycystic kidneys may develop end-stage renal failure. Inheritance is autosomal dominant with an apparently high rate of spontaneous mutation. It is possible, however, that there is nonpenetrance of the gene (no manifestations in a person with the mutant gene) or germinal mosaicism (the mutant gene is present in only the sperm/ova, with recurrences in offspring); expression is variable within a family. A parent with the gene may appear unaffected, so the parents also must be examined clinically and radiologically for stigmata of tuberous sclerosis. Tuberous sclerosis is linked in approximately 50% cases to a gene, *TSC1* ("hamartin"), on chromosome 9q34. In other patients, tuberous sclerosis is linked to a marker gene, *TSC2* ("tuberin"), close to the locus for *PKD1* on chromosome 16p13.3.[73,74]

Meckel Syndrome (McKusick #249000)

Meckel syndrome is characterized by polycystic kidneys (obligate feature), sloping forehead, posterior encephalocele, microphthalmia, postaxial polydactyly, ambiguous genitalia, and hepatic fibrosis (consistent feature with varying degrees of reactive bile duct proliferation and dilation, portal fibrosis, and portal fibrous vascular obliteration). Of patients, 50% have oligohydramnios, with

death in the perinatal period. Goldston syndrome comprises cystic kidneys, hepatic fibrosis, and Dandy-Walker malformation. Inheritance is autosomal recessive. Goldston syndrome and other syndromes may be part of the spectrum or discrete entities.[75] The incidence of Meckel syndrome is 1 in 9000. Inheritance is autosomal recessive. Variable expression occurs within and among families.[54] Gene loci are on chromosomes 17q22-q23 (*MKS1*) and 11q13 (*MKS2*).[76] Prenatal diagnosis is possible by ultrasound and increased α-fetoprotein levels in amniotic fluid.

Jeune Asphyxiating Thoracic Dystrophy Syndrome (McKusick #208500)

Respiratory distress; dysostoses; short ribs; small, long thoracic cage; small pelvis; trident acetabular margins; short, thick second and third phalanges; cone-shaped epiphyses; handlebar clavicle; mesomelic shortening of limbs; renal cystic disease; and congenital hepatic fibrosis are hallmarks of Jeune syndrome.[77] Survivors develop metaphyseal dysplasia with postnatal short-limbed dwarfism. Treatment of renal failure may require dialysis and transplantation. Inheritance is autosomal recessive with variable expression. Prenatal diagnosis by ultrasound is possible by 18 weeks.[78]

Renal-Hepatic-Pancreatic Dysplasia (Ivemark Syndrome)

It is unclear whether renal-hepatic-pancreatic dysplasia is an entity or a component of other conditions.[79] In addition to features of the oligohydramnios sequence, the kidneys are cystic, and there is fibrosis of the liver and pancreas. Neonatal death is caused by respiratory insufficiency in most cases. Inheritance is autosomal recessive.

Inborn Errors of Metabolism

Inborn errors of energy metabolism that affect neonates may involve morphologic and functional abnormalities of several organs, including the kidneys. Glutaric aciduria type II and Zellweger cerebrohepatorenal syndrome are entities with similar presentations.

Glutaric Aciduria Type II (Multiple Acyl-CoA Dehydrogenase Deficiencies)

There are several types of glutaric aciduria. The clinical features of type IIa, the neonatal-onset form, include prematurity, hypotonia, hepatomegaly, nephromegaly, and craniofacial anomalies. Rocker-bottom feet, anterior abdominal wall defects, and external genital anomalies may occur. An odor of sweaty feet may be present. Within 24 hours, there is severe hypoglycemia but no ketosis, a metabolic acidosis with an increased anion gap, lactic acidosis, and mild hyperammonemia. Elevated levels of organic acids (glutaric, ethyl malonic, isovaleric, medium-chain dicarboxylics, and others) are found in body fluids. Renal cystic dysplasia occurs in many cases.[80] Brain heterotopias indicate that malformations occur during embryogenesis. The brain and kidney abnormalities are probably consequences of the biochemical dyshomeostasis. The deficiencies in mitochondrial enzymes (electron transfer flavoprotein or electron transfer ubiquinone oxidoreductase) are inherited as autosomal recessive traits.

Prenatal diagnosis may be possible by assaying enzyme in amniocytes or elevated glutaric acid in amniotic fluid. Ultrasound in utero may show enlarged cystic kidneys. Death occurs within days to months. There is no successful treatment for the biochemical abnormalities.

Zellweger Cerebrohepatorenal Syndrome (McKusick #214100)

The clinical features of Zellweger cerebrohepatorenal syndrome[81] are similar to glutaric aciduria type II. Profound hypotonia, nystagmus, cataracts ("oil droplets"), pigmentary retinopathy, and optic disk pallor are present. Stippled epiphyses of patella and acetabulum also are seen. Odor is not abnormal, and kidneys are not clinically enlarged. All peroxisomal functions are abnormal: elevated plasma very-long-chain fatty acids, bile acids, pipecolic acid, phytanic acid and urine dicarboxylic acids, and low cholesterol and triglycerides. Pathologic features are cortical renal cysts, micronodular cirrhosis, brain heterotopias, abnormal brain gyri, and absent corpus callosum. Inheritance is autosomal recessive. Prenatal diagnosis is possible by enzyme assays in amniocytes or chorionic villus cells. Most die within 6 months; infants with a milder form can survive with mental retardation, deafness, and seizures into adolescence.

Kallmann Syndrome (Hypogonadotropic Hypogonadism and Anosmia; McKusick #308700)

Boys with Kallmann syndrome have hypogonadotropic hypogonadism that manifests with delayed puberty and infertility, anosmia caused by agenesis of the olfactory lobes, and renal abnormalities.[82-85] The syndrome is caused by a defect in the embryonic migratory pathway of gonadotropin-releasing hormone synthesizing neurons and olfactory axons. Urogenital abnormalities include unilateral renal agenesis in 40% of boys,[84] bilateral renal agenesis,[82] multicystic dysplastic kidney,[84] cryptorchidism, testicular atrophy, and micropenis. Boys can die at birth as a result of bilateral renal agenesis Additional features include coloboma of iris, deafness, midline anomalies, oculomotor apraxia, and Möbius anomalad.[83] The X-linked form is the result of a mutation in the *KAL-1* gene on chromosome Xp22.3. Normal renal development requires expression of the Kallmann product *(Kalig1/AMDLX)*, but the expression and penetrance vary. In patients with multicystic dysplastic kidneys, there were hyperproliferative dysplastic kidney tubules, which overexpressed *PAX2*, a potentially oncogenic transcription factor, and *BCL2*, a cell-survival factor, surrounded by metaplastic, α smooth muscle, actin-positive stroma. These findings are similar to findings in patients with nonsyndromic multicystic dysplastic kidneys.[84] Treatment with testosterone or estrogen for induction of puberty induces appropriate pubertal development.[83]

Glomerulocystic Kidneys

The kidneys may be large or small. The liver is normal. Glomerular cysts[86] are found in obstructive uropathy, in ADPKD, in malformations of other organs, in dysplastic kidneys, in an infant whose mother used phenacetin, and in a twin exposed to indomethacin in pregnancy. The cysts are often subcapsular and may contain more than one glomeruloid structure. In infants, glomerulocystic kidney disease may be similar in appearance to ARPKD.[87] Glomerulocystic kidneys may occur sporadically. Autosomal dominant inheritance is found in some kindreds in association with mutations in the gene encoding hepatocyte nuclear factor–1β and early-onset diabetes.[5]

CONGENITAL NEPHROTIC SYNDROME

Nephrotic syndrome associated with congenital syphilis occasionally presents in the neonate.[88] Nephrotic syndrome can be inherited as an isolated entity (Finnish type), with diffuse mesangial sclerosis, or as part of malformation syndromes such as Denys-Drash syndrome[89] and Galloway-Mowat syndrome.[90]

Congenital Nephrotic Syndrome of the Finnish Type (McKusick #256300)

Congenital nephrotic syndrome of the Finnish type is the most common type of nephrotic syndrome in neonates and occurs in all ethnic groups. Almost all of the abnormal features are confined to the kidneys. Onset of proteinuria may begin in utero. The placenta is large, and prematurity is common. Calvarial abnormalities and pyloric stenosis occur in some neonates. Renal histopathologic abnormalities include dilated proximal tubules, glomerular hypercellularity, and mesangial accentuation. Inheritance is autosomal recessive, and the locus has been assigned to chromosome 19q12-q13.[91] The *NPHS1* gene mutated in congenital nephrotic syndrome of the Finnish type codes for nephrin, a cell-surface podocyte protein. Two mutations, Fin-major and Fin-minor, are found in more than 90% of Finnish patients.[92] The maternal serum and amniotic fluid α-fetoprotein levels are elevated. Affected fetuses may be detected by 15 weeks of gestation. Management includes genetic counseling, optimal nutrition, treatment of infections, and diuretics. Bilateral nephrectomy is indicated if there are serious complications of nephrotic syndrome with severe malnutrition. Peritoneal dialysis is done after bilateral nephrectomies or if the patient develops end-stage renal failure before renal transplantation. The prognosis has improved with aggressive treatment, but the nephrotic syndrome may occur after transplantation.

Diffuse Mesangial Sclerosis

The usual presentation is with nephrotic syndrome in the first year of life. Patients can present in the neonatal period,[93] however, with massive edema, proteinuria, hypoalbuminemia, hypercholesterolemia, and rapid deterioration of renal function. There is diffuse sclerosis in the mesangium of the glomeruli. Diffuse mesangial sclerosis also can occur in patients with Denys-Drash syndrome. Denys-Drash syndrome is defined by the occurrence of combinations of pseudohermaphroditism, nephrotic syndrome with diffuse mesangial sclerosis, Wilms tumor, and constitutional mutations in the *WT1* suppressor gene. Onset in the neonatal period is rare. Most patients develop end-stage renal failure.[89]

Galloway-Mowat Syndrome of Abnormal Gyral Patterns and Glomerulopathy

Features of Galloway-Mowat syndrome are microcephaly; gyral abnormalities; developmental delay; glomerulopathy; and, less often, seizures, facial dysmorphisms, and hiatal hernia.[90] Onset of proteinuria may occur in the neonate but is always detected before 3 years. A uniform pattern of renal histologic changes has not been found. There is no effective treatment for the neurologic or renal manifestations. The inheritance is autosomal recessive. The prognosis is extremely poor; every patient has died before age 5.5 years. Antenatal diagnosis may be possible.

DYSGENETIC KIDNEYS

Renal Tubular Dysgenesis (Congenital Hypernephronic Nephromegaly with Tubular Dysgenesis; McKusick #267430)

In renal tubular dysgenesis, onset of oligohydramnios is after 24 weeks of gestation; the kidneys are large and do not function.[94] The calvaria may be underdeveloped, with wide sutures. On ultrasound, the kidneys are enlarged symmetrically, there is no evidence of cysts or obstruction, and the corticomedullary junction is poorly defined. Histologic studies reveal an apparent increase in the number of glomeruli and immature tubules without proximal convolutions.[95] Inheritance is autosomal recessive. Definitive prenatal diagnosis is not possible.

OVERGROWTH SYNDROMES

Beckwith-Wiedemann syndrome, Simpson-Golabi-Behmel syndrome, and Perlman syndrome are overgrowth syndromes, with overlapping features and abnormal kidneys at birth.[96]

Beckwith-Wiedemann Syndrome (McKusick #130650)

Exomphalos, macroglossia, and gigantism are the cardinal features of Beckwith-Wiedemann syndrome. Hypoglycemia may occur in the first days of life. There is an increased risk of developing adrenal carcinoma, nephroblastoma, hepatoblastoma, and rhabdomyosarcoma. In addition to nephromegaly and Wilms tumor, patients may have nonmalignant renal abnormalities, including medullary renal cysts (13%), caliceal diverticula (1%), hydronephrosis (12%), and nephrolithiasis in 4% of patients.[97] The syndrome is caused by a mutation of a gene encoding a human cyclin-dependent kinase inhibitor, p57 (KIP2) on chromosome 11p15.5.[98] Duplication in this region seems to be involved in the pathogenesis, and imprinting results in anomalous patterns of transmission. Most cases are sporadic. Patients should be screened by renal ultrasound for Wilms tumor every 3 months for the first 7 years of life.

Renal Hamartomas, Nephroblastomatosis, and Fetal Gigantism (Perlman Syndrome; McKusick # 267000)

The features of Perlman syndrome include polyhydramnios, macrosomia, bilateral nephromegaly with nephroblastomatosis, visceromegaly, cryptorchidism, diaphragmatic hernia, interrupted aortic arch, hypospadias, and polysplenia.[99,100] Renal histopathologic findings include dysplasia, microcysts, and nephrogenic rests. Inheritance is autosomal recessive.

Simpson-Golabi-Behmel Syndrome, Type 1 (McKusick #312870)

Features of Simpson-Golabi-Behmel syndrome are prenatal and postnatal overgrowth, coarse facies, hypertelorism, broad nasal root, cleft palate, full lips with a midline groove of the lower lip, grooved tongue with tongue tie, prominent mandible, congenital heart defects, arrhythmias, supernumerary nipples, splenomegaly, large dysplastic kidneys, cryptorchidism, hypospadias, skeletal abnormalities, and postaxial hexadactyly. Inheritance is X-linked. Some cases of Simpson-Golabi-Behmel syndrome are caused by a mutation in the gene for glypican-3, which maps to Xq26.[101] A second Simpson-Golabi-Behmel syndrome locus (SGBS2) is located on Xp22.[102]

TERATOGENS AND RENAL ABNORMALITIES

Associations between teratogens and renal abnormalities (Table 80-3)[68,103-108] are speculative and often lack convincing proof of cause and effect.

MANAGEMENT OF CHRONIC RENAL DISEASE

Because of the implications of a genetic burden on the family, efforts must be made to establish a precise diagnose. Data must be collected from prenatal history, fetal ultrasound, and family history. The infant and parents must be examined clinically and by imaging studies. Laboratory studies, including DNA tests if available, and pathology specimens need expert interpretation. Errors occur with insufficient and poor integration of these data,

Table 80-3. Renal Abnormalities Reported after Exposure In Utero

ACE inhibitors	Nephromegaly/anuria, skull hypoplasia[103]
Anticonvulsants	Urogenital anomalies found occasionally after exposure to valproate or other anticonvulsants[104]
Cocaine	Maternal cocaine use may cause genitourinary abnormalities[68]
Indomethacin	May cause renal dysgenesis after prolonged high doses[105]
Lead	Incriminated as possible causes of VACTERL association[106]
Phenacetin, salicylate	Glomerulocystic disease reported in one infant[107]
Warfarin	Unilateral renal agenesis, ectopia, reported in three infants[108]

VACTERL, vertebral abnormalities, anal atresia, cardiac abnormalities, tracheoesophageal fistula and/or esophageal atresia, renal agenesis and dysplasia, and limb defects.

and errors can affect diagnosis, prognosis, treatment, and genetic counseling. The ability to dialyze newborn infants and transplant kidneys in infants imposes enormous emotional and financial burdens on families and on society. Precise information is needed before embarking on this course. Prenatal history includes details of maternal illness, use of medical or recreational drugs, and exposure to known and potential environmental teratogens in the home and workplace. Family history evaluates illnesses, handicaps, deaths, miscarriages, stillbirths, parental ages, consanguinity, and ethnic origins.

Physician's Dilemma

The dilemma expressed in 1970 by Reinhart[109] in regard to dialysis and transplantation no longer may be valid for children, but it is still a concern in neonates. His premise was that dialysis and renal transplantation were not cures for end-stage renal failure, and he posed some profound questions:

1. What does the child gain from prolongation of life, and at what cost?
2. What price does the child pay to postpone the parents' grief?
3. What is the price of the physician's reluctance to permit death?
4. Who makes the decision about the management of the child?
5. What is the basis on which physicians decide how to manage end-stage renal disease in children?

Reinhart offered some important insights:

1. The family must make decisions regarding treatment or withholding treatment; physicians should be advisors.
2. Physicians vary in their need to offer a last desperate chance no matter what the cost. Younger physicians are more reluctant to admit defeat; more mature physicians are more likely to understand the difference between life and living.
3. Families may be more stressed by the life saved than the death permitted.
4. Parents usually cannot refuse an offer of help no matter how slim the chances being offered. They may live in hope while their child often dies in despair.
5. Reinhart noted the alienation that can occur between physicians and disappointed parents and others. He ended his editorial by stating "programs of dialysis and renal transplant for children should be evaluated not in terms of gross survival but in parameters of meaningful growth and development-living. We may find the price the child pays for life too great at present."[109]

These issues continue to be pertinent even as enormous strides are being made in the management of these patients.

Role of the Physician of Record

A team approach is essential (Table 80-4). A successful endeavor requires the input of many individuals and an attending physician of record who coordinates care and provides the family with information. The nature of the

Table 80–4. End-Stage Renal Failure Team

Perinatologist
Neonatologist
Geneticist
Urologist
Nephrologist
Surgeon pediatrician
Intensive care specialist
Nursing teams
Residents, fellows
Family
Social worker
Nutritionist
Dialysis nurses
Transplant coordinator
Psychologist
Ethicist

condition must be explained in simple language that is not condescending. Patience is important because terms are new, and the mother is recovering from the birth and may be sad. Fathers initially often intellectualize the problem. The parents' hopes are being dashed, and the physician is the dasher of hopes, the bearer of bad news. The physician must not be angry with the parents if they become hostile. There should be as few people as possible in a room when bad news is communicated. The physician should be optimistic but realistic, leave room for hope but should not try to raise false hopes. There is no need to cover everything at the first encounter. The problem should be managed in a rational way by making the infant as comfortable as possible and by treating everything that can be treated by conventional means, until the parents have made a decision regarding dialysis and transplantation. The physician should explain gently that the infant will feel pain, that the infant will suffer from the treatment, that there are no guarantees of success, and that there will be major disruptions of family life. The family should be encouraged to obtain a second opinion. The physician must not pass moral judgments. Access to other parents whose children have, or have had, similar problems should be offered. It is important to stress that even if the infant is transplanted successfully, the child will always have to take medications, that rejection episodes will likely occur, and that the kidney may be lost. A parent should not be "forced" to offer a kidney. One of the most difficult tasks faced by the physician is telling the parents gently that allowing their infant to die without heroic treatment is a real option. The physician should not be afraid of long periods of silence. Early deaths may be "acceptable" in some patients as an alternative to treatment with dialysis and transplantation. This approach is true in patients with severe lung disease or with multiorgan severe abnormalities (Table 80-5).

An important caveat is the physician must never take away all hope from a family; the infant may not die, and parents can be unforgiving if they have mourned for their infant because the physician has told them that the child

Table 80–5. Acceptable Early Death

Renal agenesis
ARPKD with severe hypoplastic lungs
Severe multiple congenital abnormalities
Fraser syndrome
Pallister-Hall syndrome
Renal tubular dysgenesis syndrome

ARPKD, autosomal recessive polycystic kidney disease.

will not live. A decision not to treat does not always result in the death of the neonate. If the patient does not die within a short time, and definitive treatment is not employed, the patient may have many serious complications of uremia. Initially, these are nausea, vomiting, poor appetite, metabolic acidosis, severe hyponatremia secondary to salt wasting, and hyperkalemia. Later complications may include microcephaly, growth restriction, developmental delay, osteodystrophy, and acute urinary tract infections with or without septicemia. Everyone involved in the management of these neonates is often on the horns of a dilemma. If some of these infants are treated aggressively, they may suffer enormously. If they are not treated, they may not die for some time but may suffer. Estimates suggest that about 50% of allografts continue to function after 10 years. The ultimate height at completion of growth, the status of testicular or ovarian function, the long-term effects of cyclosporine on the kidney, and the risks of malignancies remain unanswered questions.

Controlled Feeding Regimens

Growth loss in uremic infants occurs during the first 6 months of life when nutrient intakes are poorly controlled; requirements may need to exceed recommended daily averages.[110] Feeding by nasogastric or gastrostomy tubes may be needed. There are no established guidelines for optimal dietary protein requirements in these neonates and infants. Inadequately treated bone disease has a negative impact on linear growth. Calcitriol therapy must be monitored carefully by measurements of serum calcium and parathyroid hormone levels. Dietary phosphate must be restricted; if this does not reduce the serum phosphate concentrations to within the normal range, calcium carbonate or calcium acetate may be required. Excessive depletion of phosphate may cause rickets, and binders may cause hypercalcemia. The serum phosphate and calcium concentrations must be monitored frequently. Vomiting is a frequent problem; treatment includes antiperistaltic agents, and some patients may require a fundoplication. Anemia is treated with erythropoietin and iron supplements when the hemoglobin level is less than 10 g/dL. The initial dose of erythropoietin is 100 U//kg/wk, and the dose of elemental iron is 2 to 3 mg/kg/day.[111]

Peritoneal Dialysis

Although the optimal treatment for infants with end-stage renal disease is controversial, it is accepted that transplantation is preferable to long-term dialysis because of the deleterious effects of uremia on growth and neurologic development in infants treated with dialysis alone.[112] Dialysis has to be combined with tube or gastrostomy feeding for optimal growth. This combination may carry a greater 1-year risk of mortality in infants compared with older children. Blowey and colleagues[113] reviewed outcome data of 23 infants treated with peritoneal dialysis in the first month of life for 1 week to 12 months. By 1 year of age, 35% had died, 26% recovered completely, 30% were on long-term dialysis, and 9% had chronic renal failure. Most of the patients had growth impairment and minor developmental abnormalities.

Renal Transplantation

Renal transplantation is the definitive treatment for infants and children with end-stage renal failure. Living related allografts have a better outcome than kidneys from cadavers. Most infants are transplanted when they attain a weight of about 12 kg. Impressive transplantation results were obtained, however, in infants younger than 1 year of age with a 100% patient survival rate after 1 year and 83% after 5 years; graft survival was 94% after 1 year and 71% after 5 years.[112] Early elective transplantation of infants may result in normal growth and development.[114]

REFERENCES

1. Kaplan BS, Kaplan P, Ruchelli E: Hereditary and congenital malformations of the kidneys. Perinat Clin North Am 19:197, 1992.
2. Wang RY, Earl DL, Ruder RO, et al: Syndromic ear anomalies and renal ultrasounds. Pediatrics 108:E32, 2001.
3. Bernstein J: Hepatic involvement in hereditary renal syndromes. In Gilbert EF, Opitz JM (eds): Genetic Aspects of Developmental Pathology, vol 23. Birth Defects Original Article Series. New York, March of Dimes Birth Defects Foundation, 1987, p 115.
4. Cobben JM, Breuning MH, Schoots C, et al: Congenital hepatic fibrosis in autosomal-dominant poycystic kidney disease. Kidney Int 38:880, 1990.
5. Bingham C, Bulman MP, Ellard S, et al: Mutations in the hepatocyte nuclear factor-1beta gene are associated with familial hypoplastic glomerulocystic kidney disease. Am J Hum Genet 68:219, 2001.
6. Bernstein J, Gardner KD: Renal cystic disease and renal dysplasia. In Walsh PC, Gittes RF, Perlmutter AD (eds): Campbell's Urology. Philadelphia, WB Saunders, 1986, pp 1760-1803.
7. Gordon AC, Thomas DFM, Arthur RJ, et al: Multicystic dysplastic kidney: Is nephrectomy still appropriate? J Urol 140:1231, 1988.
8. Atiyeh B, Husmann D, Baum M: Contralateral renal abnormalities in multicystic-dysplastic kidney disease. J Pediatr 121:65, 1992.
9. Hartman GE, Smolik LM, Shochat SJ: The dilemma of the multicystic dysplastic kidney. Am J Dis Child 140:925, 1986.
10. Stanisic TH: Review of "The dilemma of the multicystic dysplastic kidney." Am J Dis Child 140:865, 1986.
11. Wacksman J, Phipps L: Report of the multicystic kidney registry: Preliminary findings. J Urol 150:1870, 1993.

12. Gilbert-Barness EF, Opitz JM, Barness LA: Hereditable malformations of the kidney and urinary tract. In Spitzer A, Avner ED (eds): Inheritance of Kidney and Urinary Tract Diseases. Boston, Kluwer Academic, 1990, pp 327-400.

13. Cole BR, Kaufman RL, McAlister WH, et al: Bilateral renal dysplasia in three siblings: Report of a survivor. Clin Nephrol 5:83, 1976.

14. Buchta RM, Visesku C, Gilbert EF, et al: Familial bilateral renal agenesis and hereditary renal adysplasia. Z Kinderheilk 115:111, 1973.

15. Cain DR, Griggs D, Lackey DA, et al: Familial renal agenesis and total dysplasia. Am J Dis Child 128:377, 1974.

16. Holmes LB: Prevalence, phenotypic heterogeneity and familial aspects of bilateral renal agenesis/dysgenesis. In Bartsocas CS (ed): Genetics of Kidney Disorders. New York, Alan R Liss, 1989, pp 1-11.

17. Egli F, Staider G: Malformations of kidney and urinary tract in common chromosomal aberrations: 1. Clinical studies. Hum Genet 18:1, 1973.

18. Battin J, Lacombe D, Leng J-J: Familial occurrence of hereditary renal adysplasia with mullerian anomalies. Clin Genet 43:23, 1993.

19. Rosenberg HK, Sherman NH, Tarry WF, et al: Mayer-Rokitansky-Kuster-Hauser syndrome: US aid to diagnosis. Radiology 161:815, 1986.

20. Ismaili K, Schurmans T, Wissing KM, et al: Early prognostic factors of infants with chronic renal failure caused by renal dysplasia. Pediatr Nephrol 16:260, 2000.

21. McPherson E, Carey J, Kramer A, et al: Dominantly inherited renal adysplasia. Am J Med Genet 26:863, 1987.

22. Jennings RW: Prune belly syndrome. Semin Pediatr Surg 9:115, 2000.

23. Wright JR Jr, Barth RF, Neff JC, et al: Gastrointestinal malformations associated with prune belly syndrome: Three cases and review of the literature. Pediatr Pathol 5:421, 1986.

24. Carey JC, Eggert L, Curry CJ: Lower limb deficiency and the urethral obstruction sequence. Binh Defects 18:19, 1982.

25. Manivel JC, Pettinato G, Reinberg, et al: Prune belly syndrome (PBS): Clinicopathologic study of 29 cases. Pediatr Pathol 9:691, 1989.

26. Welch KJ, Kraney GP: Abdominal musculature deficiency: prune belly. J Urol 111:693, 1974.

27. Berton WE, Baker DH, Wigger HJ, et al: The radiologic and pathologic spectrum of the prune belly syndrome: The importance of urethral obstruction in prognosis. Radiol Clin North Am 15:83, 1977.

28. Popek EJ, Tyson RW, Miller GJ, et al: Prostate development in prune belly syndrome (PBS) and posterior urethral valves (PUV): Etiology of PBS-lower urinary tract obstruction or primary mesenchymal defect? Pediatr Pathol 11:1, 1991.

29. Pagon RA, Smith DW, Shepard TH: Urethral obstruction malformation complex: A cause of abdominal muscle deficiency and the "prune belly." J Pediatr 94:900, 1979.

30. Straub E, Spranger J: Etiology and pathogenesis of the prune belly syndrome. Kidney Int 20:695, 1981.

31. Gonzales ET: Posterior urethral valves and bladder neck obstruction. Urol Clin North Am 5:57, 1978.

32. Noh PH, Cooper CS, Winkler AC, et al: Prognostic factors for long-term renal function in boys with the prune-belly syndrome. J Urol 162:1399, 1999.

33. Fitch N, Srolovitz H: Severe renal dysgenesis produced by a dominant gene. Am J Dis Child 130:1536, 1976.

34. Abdelhak S, Kalatzis V, Heilig R, et al: A human homologue of the Drosophila eyes absent gene underlies branchio-oto-renal (BOR) syndrome and identifies a novel gene family. Nat Genet 15:157, 1997.

35. Kumar S, Deffenbacher K, Cremers CW, et al: Branchio-oto-renal syndrome: Identification of novel mutations, molecular characterization, mutation distribution, and prospects for genetic testing. Genet Test 1:243, 1997.

36. Azuma N, Hirakiyama A, Inoue T, et al: Mutations of a human homologue of the Drosophila eyes absent gene (EYA1) detected in patients with congenital cataracts and ocular anterior segment anomalies. Hum Mol Genet 9:363, 2000.

37. Maas SM, de Jong TP, Buss P, et al: EEC syndrome and genitourinary anomalies: An update. Am J Med Genet 63:472, 1996.

38. Roelfsema NM, Cobben JM: The EEC syndrome: A literature study. Clin Dysmorph 5:115, 1996.

39. Rolinick BR, Hoo JJ: Genitourinary anomalies are a component manifestation in the ectodermal dysplasia, ectrodactyly, cleft lip/palate (EEC) syndrome. Am J Med Genet 29:131, 1988.

40. Giampietro PF, Adler-Brecher B, Verlander PC, et al: The need for more accurate and timely diagnosis in Fanconi anemia: A report from the International Fanconi Anemia Registry. Pediatrics 91:1116, 1993.

41. Joenje H, Patel KJ: The emerging genetic and molecular basis of Fanconi anaemia. Nat Rev Genet 2:446, 2001.

42. Buchwald M: Complementation groups: One or more per gene? Nat Genet 11:228, 1995.

43. Fivush B, McGrath S, Zinkham W: Thrombocytopenia absent radius syndrome associated with renal insufficiency. Clin Pediatr 29:182, 1990.

44. Salerno A, Kohlhase J, Kaplan BS: Townes-Brocks syndrome and renal dysplasia: A novel mutation in the SALL1 gene. Pediatr Nephrol 14:25, 2000.

45. Schauer GM, Dunn LK, Godmilow L, et al: Prenatal diagnosis of Fraser syndrome at 18.5 weeks gestation, with autopsy findings at 19 weeks. Am J Med Genet 37:583, 1990.

46. Moerman P, Fryns JP, Vandenberghe K, et al: The syndrome of diaphragmatic hernia, abnormal face and distal limb anomalies (Fryns syndrome): Further delineation of this multiple congenital anomaly (MCA) syndrome. Am J Med Genet 31:8054, 1988.

47. Killoran CE, Abbott M, McKusick VA, et al: Overlap of PIV syndrome, VACTERL and Pallister-Hall syndrome: Clinical and molecular analysis. Clin Genet 58:28, 2000.

48. Biesecker LG, Abbott M, Allen J, et al: Report from the workshop on Pallister-Hall syndrome and related phenotypes. Am J Med Genet 65:76, 1996.

49. Kaplan BS, Fay J, Dillon MJ, et al: Autosomal recessive polycystic kidney disease. Pediatr Nephrol 3:43, 1989.

50. Kaplan BS, Kaplan P, de Chadarevian J-P, et al: Variable expression within a family of autosomal recessive polycystic kidney disease and congenital hepatic fibrosis. Am J Med Genet 29:639, 1988.

51. Kaplan BS, Kaplan P, Rosenberg HK, et al: Polycystic kidney disease. J Pediatr 115:867, 1989.

52. Metreweli C, Garet L: The echographic diagnosis of infantile renal polycystic disease. Ann Radiol 23:103, 1980.

53. Stapleton FB, Hilton S, Wilcox J: Transient nephromegaly simulating infantile polycystic disease of the kidneys. Pediatrics 67:554, 1981.

54. Fraser F, Lytwyn A: Spectrum of anomalies in the Meckel syndrome, or: "Maybe there is a malformation syndrome with at least one constant anomaly." Am J Med Genet 9:63, 1981.

55. Guay-Woodford LM, Muecher G, Hopkins SD, et al: The severe perinatal form of autosomal recessive polycystic kidney disease maps to chromosome 6p21.1-p12: Implications for genetic counseling. Am J Hum Genet 56:1101, 1995.

56. Zerres K, Mucher G, Becker J: Prenatal diagnosis of autosomal recessive polycystic kidney disease (ARPKD): Molecular genetics, clinical experience, and fetal morphology. Am J Med Genet 76:137, 1998.

57. Romero R, Cullen M, Jeanty P, et al: The diagnosis of congenital renal anomalies with ultrasound: II. Infantile polycystic kidney disease. Am J Obstet Gynecol 150:259, 1984.

58. Munding M, Al-Uzri A, Gralnek D, Riden D: Prenatally diagnosed autosomal recessive polycystic kidney disease: Initial postnatal management. Urology 54:1097, 1999.

59. Sumfest JM, Burns MW, Mitchell ME: Aggressive surgical and medical management of autosomal recessive polycystic kidney disease. Urology 42:309, 1993.

60. Sweeney WE, Chen Y, Nakanishi K, et al: Treatment of polycystic kidney disease with a novel tyrosine kinase inhibitor. Kidney Int 57:33, 2000.

61. Wilson PD: Polycystin: New aspects of structure, function, and regulation. J Am Soc Nephrol 12:834, 2001.

62. Bear JC, MeManamon P, Morgan J, et al: Age at clinical onset and at ultrasonographic detection of adult polycystic kidney disease: Data for genetic counseling. Am J Med Genet 18:45, 1984.

63. Breuning MH, Reeders ST, Brunner H, et al: Improved early diagnosis of adult polycystic kidney disease with flanking DNA markers. Lancet 2:1359, 1987.

64. Peters DJM, Spruit L, Saris JJ, et al: Chromosome 4 localization of a second gene for autosomal dominant polycystic kidney disease. Nat Genet 5:359, 1993.

65. Reeders ST, Zerres K, Gal A, et al: Prenatal diagnosis of autosomal dominant polycystic kidney disease with a DNA probe. Lancet 2:6, 1986.

66. MacDermot KD, Saggar-Malik AK, Economides DL, et al: Prenatal diagnosis of autosomal dominant polycystic kidney disease (PKD1) presenting in utero and prognosis for very early onset disease. J Med Genet 35:13, 1998.

67. Fick GM, Johnson AM, Strain JD, et al: Characteristics of very early onset autosomal dominant polycystic kidney disease. Am Soc Nephrol 3:1863, 1993.

68. Chasnoff IJ, Chisum GM, Kaplan WE: Maternal cocaine use and genitourinary tract malformations. Teratology 37:201, 1988.

69. Brook-Carter PT, Peral B, Ward CJ, et al: Deletion of the TSC2 and PKD1 genes associated with severe infantile polycystic kidney disease—a contiguous gene syndrome. Nat Genet 8:328, 1994.

70. Sampson JR, Maheshwar MM, Aspinwall R, et al: Renal cystic disease in tuberous sclerosis: Role of the polycystic kidney disease 1 gene. Am J Hum Genet 61:843, 1997.

71. Cook JA, Oliver K, Mueller RF, et al: A cross sectional study of renal involvement in tuberous sclerosis. J Med Genet 33:480, 1996.

72. Webb DW, Clarke A, Fryer A, et al: The cutaneous features of tuberous sclerosis: A population study. Br J Dermatol 135:1, 1966.

73. Kandt RS, Haines JL, Smith M, et al: Linkage of an important gene locus for tuberose sclerosis to a chromosome 16 marker for polycystic kidney disease. Nat Genet 2:37, 1992.

74. van Slegtenhorst M, Nellist M, Nagelkerken B, et al: Interaction between hamartin and tuberin, the TSC1 and TSC2 gene products. Hum Mol Genet 7:1053-1057, 1998.

75. Gloeb DJ, Valdes-Dapena M, Saiman F, et al: The Goldston syndrome: Report of a case. Pediatr Pathol 9:337, 1989.

76. Roume J, Genin E, Cormier-Daire V, et al: A gene for Meckel syndrome maps to chromosome 11q13. Am J Hum Genet 63:1095, 1998.

77. Donaldson MDC, Warner AA, Trompeter RS, et al: Familial juvenile nephronophthisis, Jeune's syndrome, and associated disorders. Arch Dis Child 60:426, 1985.

78. Elejade BR, de Elejade MM, Pansch D: Prenatal diagnosis of Jeune syndrome. Am J Med Genet 21:433, 1985.

79. Bernstein J, Chandra M, Cresswell J, et al: Renal-hepatic-pancreatic dysplasia: A syndrome reconsidered. Am J Med Genet 26:391, 1987.

80. Wilson GN, de Chadarevian J-P, Kaplan P, et al: Glutaric aciduria type II: Review of the phenotype and report of an unusual glomerulopathy. Am J Med Genet 32:395, 1989.

81. Patton RG, Christie DL, Smith DW, et al: Cerebro-hepato-renal syndrome of Zellweger. Am J Dis Child 124:840, 1972.

82. Colquhoun-Kerr JS, Gu WX, Jameson JL, et al: X-linked Kallmann syndrome and renal agenesis occurring together and independently in a large Australian family. Am J Med Genet 83:23, 1999.

83. Dissaneevate P, Warne GL, Zacharin MR: Clinical evaluation in isolated hypogonadotrophic hypogonadism (Kallmann syndrome). J Pediatr Endocrinol Metab 11:631, 1998.

84. Deeb A, Robertson A, MacColl G, et al: Multicystic dysplastic kidney and Kallmann's syndrome: A new association? Nephrol Dial Transplant 16:1170, 2001.

85. Hardelin JP, Levilliers J, del Castillo I, et al: X chromosome-linked Kallmann syndrome: Stop mutations validate the candidate gene. Proc Natl Acad Sci U S A 89:8190, 1992.

86. Bernstein J, Landing BH: Glomerulocystic kidney diseases. In Bartsocas CS (ed): Genetics of Kidney Disorders. New York, Alan R Liss, 1989, pp 27-43.

87. Fitch SJ, Stapleton FB: Ultrasonographic features of glomerulocystic disease in infancy: Similarity to infantile polycystic kidney disease. Pediatr Radiol 16:400, 1986.

88. Sanchez-Bayle M, Ecija JL, Estepa R, et al: Incidence of glomerulonephritis in congenital syphilis. Clin Nephrol 20:27, 1983.

89. Maalouf EF, Ferguson J, van Heyningen V, et al: In utero nephropathy, Denys-Drash syndrome and Potter phenotype. Pediatr Nephrol 12:449, 1998.

90. Cooperstone B, Friedman A, Kaplan BS: The Galloway-Mowat syndrome of abnormal gyral pattern and glomerulopathy. Am J Med Genet 47:250, 1993.

91. Kestila M, Mannikko M, Holmberg C, et al: Congenital nephrotic syndrome of the Finnish type maps to the long arm of chromosome 19. Am J Hum Genet 54:757, 1994.

92. Patrakka J, Kestila M, Wartiovaara J, et al: Congenital nephrotic syndrome (NPHS1): Features resulting from different mutations in Finnish patients. Kidney Int 58:972, 2000.

93. Koziell A, Iyer VK, Moghul NE, et al: Congenital nephrotic syndrome. Pediatr Nephrol 16:185, 2001.

94. Allanson JE, Pantzar JT, MacLeod PM: Possible new autosomal recessive syndrome with unusual renal histopathological changes. Am J Med Genet 16:57, 1983.

95. Swinford AF, Bernstein J, Toriello HV, et al: Renal tubular dysgenesis: Delayed onset of ofigohydramnios. Am J Med Genet 32:127, 1989.

96. Coppin B, Moore I, Hatchwell E: Extending the overlap of three congenital overgrowth syndromes. Clin Genet 51:375, 1997.

97. Choyke PL, Siegel MJ, Oz O, et al: Nonmalignant renal disease in pediatric patients with Beckwith-Wiedemann syndrome. AJR Am J Roentgenol 171:733, 1998.

98. Matsuoka S, Thompson JS, Edwards MC: Imprinting of the gene encoding a human cyclin-dependent kinase inhibitor, p57(KIP2), on chromosome 11p15. Proc Natl Acad Sci U S A 93:3026, 1996.

99. Greenberg F, Copeland K, Gresik MV: Expanding the spectrum of the Perlman syndrome. Am J Med Genet 29:773, 1988.

100. Schilke K, Schaefer F, Waldherr R, et al: A case of Perlman syndrome: Fetal gigantism, renal dysplasia, and severe neurological deficits. Am J Med Genet 91:29, 2000.

101. Pilia G, Hughes-Benzie RM, MacKenzie A, et al: Mutations in GPC3, a glypican gene, cause the Simpson-Golabi-Behmel overgrowth syndrome. Nat Genet 12:225, 1996.

102. Brzustowicz LM, Farrell S, Khan MB, et al: Mapping of a new SGBS locus to chromosome Xp22 in a family with a severe form of Simpson-Golabi-Behmel syndrome. Am J Hum Genet 65:779, 1999.

103. Pryde PG, Sedman AB, Nugent CE, Barr M Jr, et al: Angiotensin-converting enzyme inhibitor fetopathy. J Am Soc Nephrol 3:1575, 1993.

104. Ardinger HU, Atkin JF, Blackstone RD, et al: Verification of the fetal valproate syndrome phenotype. Am J Med Genet 29:171, 1988.

105. Kaplan BS, Restaino I, Raval DS, et al: Renal failure in the neonate associated with in utero exposure to non-steroidal anti-inflammatory agents. Pediatr Nephrol 8:700, 1994.

106. Levine F, Muenke M: VACTERL association with high prenatal lead exposure. Pediatrics 87:390, 1991.

107. Krous HF, Richie JP, Sellers B: Glomerulocystic kidney: A hypothesis of origin and pathogenesis. Arch Pathol Lab Med 101:462, 1977.

108. Hall BD: Warfarin embryopathy and urinary tract anomalies: Possible new association. Am J Med Genet 34:292, 1989.

109. Reinhart JB: The doctor's dilemma: Whether or not to recommend continuous renal dialysis or renal homotransplantation for the child with end-stage renal disease. J Pediatr 77:505, 1970.

110. Arbitol CL, Zillerueto G, Montane B, et al: Growth of uremic infants on forced feeding regimens. Pediatr Nephrol 7:173, 1993.

111. Kari JA, Gonzalez C, Ledermann SE, et al: Outcome and growth of infants with severe chronic renal failure. Kidney Int 57:1681, 2000.

112. Najarian JS, Frey DJ, Matas AL, et al: Renal transplantation in infants. Ann Surg 212:353, 1990.

113. Blowey DL, McFarland K, Alon U: Peritoneat dialysis in the neonatal period: Outcome data. J Perinatol 13:59, 1993.

114. So SK, Chang PN, Najarian JS, et al: Growth and development in infants after renal transplantation. J Pediatr 110:343, 1987.

CHAPTER 81

Renal Tubular Disorders

Bernard S. Kaplan, Kevin E.C. Meyers, and Paige Kaplan

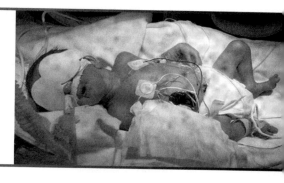

Although **renal tubular disorders** rarely occur in neonates, they can be life-threatening.[1] Full or incomplete manifestations of renal tubular disorders may present in utero or in the neonate (Table 81-1). Precise diagnosis requires knowledge of normal renal development and maturation, awareness of these conditions, and an approach to their evaluation and treatment. Renal tubular function is immature in newborns. Premature infants may waste sodium chloride and have decreased distal tubular sodium reabsorption in the first week. The ability of a full-term neonate's kidneys to excrete a sodium chloride load acutely is limited during the first week of life. The ability to excrete potassium is decreased in neonates and is more impaired in premature infants. The reabsorptive capacity for sodium bicarbonate is low in neonates, and the rate of ammonium excretion is close to its maximal capacity. Renal clearance of phosphate is low in the neonatal period. The neonatal kidneys cannot concentrate urine maximally, and breast-fed neonates excrete larger quantities of dilute urine than formula-fed infants. Some neonates, especially if premature, excrete amino acids and glucose under normal conditions. In some instances, a renal tubular disorder may be suspected and confirmed in utero (Box 81-1)

Polyhydramnios is a clue to an inherited tubular disorder, such as nephrogenic diabetes insipidus, Bartter syndrome, or pseudohypoaldosteronism. A renal tubular disorder should be suspected in a neonate with combinations of irritability, poor feeding, unexplained vomiting, dehydration, failure to thrive, drowsiness, tetany, hypotonia, or seizures. Abnormal laboratory results are often the first clue to the presence of a renal tubular disorder and may be more specific indicators of a renal tubular defect.

In **renal tubular acidosis (RTA)**, there is a hyperchloremic metabolic acidosis with normal or decreased undetermined anion gap, *in the absence of diarrhea.* Severe **hyponatremia** associated with renal salt wasting occurs in pseudohypoaldosteronism, Bartter syndrome, and bilateral renal dysplasia. **Hyperkalemia**, with or without a metabolic acidosis, occurs in pseudohypoaldosteronism, renal tubular hyperkalemia syndromes, obstructive uropathies (especially posterior urethral valves), and bilateral renal dysplasia. **Hypouricemia** occurs in renal Fanconi syndrome. **Hypophosphatemia** occurs in renal Fanconi syndrome and X-linked hypophosphatemic rickets. **Glucosuria** occurs in renal Fanconi syndrome, hereditary glucosurias, and congenital selective intestinal malabsorption of glucose and galactose. Hematuria, renal calculi, and nephrocalcinosis with hypercalciuria rarely occur in neonates (see Table 81-1). Primary hyperoxaluria type 1 may present in the newborn period, however, with acute renal failure and nephrocalcinosis.[2] Patients with the syndrome of familial hypomagnesemia with hypercalciuria and nephrocalcinosis may have symptoms at 2 to 3 months of age.[3]

RENAL FANCONI SYNDROME (LIGNAC-DE TONI-FANCONI)

Renal Fanconi syndrome is characterized by generalized proximal renal tubular dysfunction with impaired net reabsorption of amino acids, bicarbonate, glucose, phosphate, urate, sodium, potassium, magnesium, calcium, and low-molecular-weight proteins. Renal excretion of these solutes and water is increased, and their serum concentrations are variably reduced. In neonates, the clinical manifestations of renal Fanconi syndrome may include polyuria, polydipsia, dehydration, metabolic acidosis, and glucosuria. These features are often asynchronous. Growth restriction and rickets occur later in infancy. Although cystinosis is the most frequent cause of inherited Fanconi syndrome, the diagnosis rarely is made in a proband before age 6 months. Many conditions, such as cystinosis, can be diagnosed prenatally using chorionic villus sampling or amniocentesis when the condition has been confirmed in a previously diagnosed sibling. Causes of Fanconi syndrome that may present in neonates are listed in Box 81-2.

Table 81–1.   Renal Tubular Disorders in the Neonate

Syndrome	Neonatal Onset	In Utero Diagnosis
Renal fanconi syndrome		
Idiopathic	Yes	
Fructose intolerance	Yes	Yes
Galactosemia	Yes	Yes
Cystinosis	No (6-12 mo)	Yes
Cytochrome-oxidase deficiency	Yes	Possible
Hypophosphatemia		
X-linked hypophosphatemic rickets	No	
1,α-hydroxylase deficiency rickets		
Antenatal Bartter syndrome	Yes	Yes
Hyperkalemia		
Renal tubular hyperkalemia	Yes	
Renal pseudohypo-aldosteronism, autosomal dominant	Yes	
Multiple organ pseudohypoaldosteronism, autosomal recessive		
Renal tubular acidosis		
Proximal renal tubular acidosis (type 2)	Yes	
Distal renal tubular acidosis (type 1)	Yes	
Type 4 renal tubular acidosis or renal tubular hyperkalemia	Yes	
Nephrogenic diabetes insipidus		
Congenital X-linked	Yes	Yes
Autosomal recessive	No	

Hereditary Fructose Intolerance (McKusick #229600)

Hereditary fructose intolerance is caused by catalytic deficiency of aldolase B (fructose-1,6-bisphosphate aldolase; EC 4.1.2.13) as a result of mutations in the human aldolase B gene on chromosome 9q22.3.[4] Inheritance is autosomal recessive. Hereditary fructose intolerance rarely presents in neonates, unless they are fed sucrose or fructose in formula, antibiotics, fruit juices, or honey.

Box 81–1   Manifestations of Renal Tubular Disorders In Utero

Polyhydramnios
  Bartter syndrome
  Nephrogenic diabetes insipidus
  Pseudohypoaldosteronism
Increased amniotic fluid chloride concentration
  Bartter syndrome

Box 81–2   Causes of Renal Fanconi Syndrome in Neonates

Hereditary fructose intolerance
Galactosemia
Mitochondrial respiratory chain (electron transfer chain)
Cytochrome-c oxidase deficiency (complex IV) complex
Cystinosis (rarely occurs in neonates)
Tyrosinemia

The findings in hereditary fructose intolerance are shown in Tables 81-2 and 81-3.[5] The younger the age of presentation and the greater the fructose load, the more severe the symptoms.[6,7] All fructose-containing foods must be withdrawn from the diet as soon as the condition is suspected. The labels listing the food contents of *all* ready prepared foods and *all* drugs must be scrutinized because fructose often is added to food and drugs. The diagnosis can be made safely and accurately by molecular analysis of the aldolase B gene in blood.[8]

Galactosemia (McKusick #230400)

Classic galactosemia is an autosomal recessive disease caused by deficient activity of galactose-1-phosphate uridyl transferase (GALT) as a result of mutations at the *GALT* gene located on chromosome 17q.[9] There is some correlation of the severity of the disease and the mutation site in the gene. Two other autosomal recessively inherited disorders of galactose metabolism (transferase and epimerase deficiency) occur more rarely. Classic galactosemia (GALT deficiency) and galactokinase deficiency can manifest in neonates with signs of toxicity a few days after starting milk ingestion. It is usually more severe in GALT deficiency. Initial signs are vomiting, diarrhea, direct and indirect hyperbilirubinemia with jaundice, hepatomegaly, ascites, and sepsis. There is an increased prevalence of *Escherichia coli* infection, which may be fulminant. Cataracts occasionally are detectable by slit-lamp

Table 81–2.   Symptoms and Signs of Hereditary Fructose Intolerance

Acute Exposure	Chronic Exposure
Sweating, pallor	Poor feeding, vomiting
Trembling	Failure to thrive
Dizziness	Incessant crying, irritability
Nausea	Drowsiness, apathy
Vomiting	Jaundice
Apathy, lethargy, coma	Abdominal distention
Convulsions	Hepatomegaly
Diarrhea	
Tremor, jerking	
Edema, ascites	
Poor growth	

From Gitzelman R, Steinmann B, van den Berghe G: Disorders of fructose metabolism. In Scriver C, Beaudet AL, Sly WS, et al (eds): The Metabolic Basis of Inherited Disease, 7th ed. New York, McGraw-Hill, 1989, pp 399–424.

Table 81–3. Laboratory Findings in Hereditary Fructose Intolerance

Urine	Blood
Increased Concentrations	**Decreased Concentrations**
Fructose	Phosphorus
Glucose	Glucose
Phosphorus	Potassium
Potassium	Hydrogen ions (pH)
Bicarbonate	Bicarbonate
Urate	Coagulation factors
Lactate	Hemoglobin
Proteins	Platelets
Amino acids	
	Increased Concentrations
	Urate
	Fructose
	Magnesium
	Lactate
	Hepatic enzymes
	Bilirubin
	Methionine, tyrosine

From Gitzelman R, Steinmann B, van den Berghe G: Disorders of fructose metabolism. In Scriver CR, Beaudet AL, Sly WS, et al (eds): The Metabolic Basis of Inherited Disease, 6th ed. New York, McGraw-Hill, 1989, pp 399-424.

examination in neonates and may be the main presenting feature in some infants with galactokinase deficiency. Epimerase deficiency is usually asymptomatic, although two cases with features resembling GALT deficiency have been reported. Newborn screening programs include tests for early detection of galactosemia. The diagnosis is suggested by showing increased concentrations of galactose ("reducing substances") in blood and urine. The urine is positive only after lactose or galactose is ingested. The diagnosis is confirmed by showing deficient red blood cell GALT (or galactokinase). Genotyping can help predict severity. Milk and milk-containing products must be withdrawn completely from the diet. The labels listing the food contents of all ready prepared foods and all drugs must be scrutinized.

Cytochrome-*c* Oxidase Deficiency

A fatal infantile cytopathy with variable manifestations involving brain, skeletal and cardiac muscle, liver, and occasionally renal Fanconi syndrome is one of the "mitochondrial cytopathy" syndromes associated with defects in complex IV of the respiratory chain (cytochrome-*c* oxidase; EC 1.9.3.1). Complex IV consists of 13 polypeptide subunits, of which 3 are encoded by mitochondrial DNA. There is considerable variability in the clinical and biochemical features with complex IV deficiency. Clinical features include neonatal onset of hypotonia; hyporeflexia; respiratory failure; elevated levels of lactic and pyruvic acids in blood, cerebrospinal fluid, or urine; and renal Fanconi syndrome.[10-13] Cytochrome-*c* oxidase deficiency due to defects in the Surfeit-1 gene (*SURF1*) is one of the causes of Leigh syndrome, a fatal subacute necrotizing leukoencephalopathy of infancy or childhood, characterized by symmetrical lesions in the basal ganglia and brain stem.[14] Cytochrome-*c* oxidase activity and reducible cytochrome aa_3 activity are absent or reduced in liver, muscle, or kidney. In most cases the mutations occur in nuclear-encoded genes, and inheritance seems to be autosomal recessive. There is no treatment, prognosis is poor,[13] and most children die in infancy. Prenatal diagnosis is unreliable, unless a specific gene mutation has been found in a proband.

Carnitine Palmitoyltransferase Type I (McKusick #255120)

Patients with carnitine palmitoyltransferase type I deficiency lack activity of the hepatic isoform, caused by mutations in the gene located on chromosome 11q13. Inheritance is autosomal recessive. There are two clinical forms, one in children and the other in adults. It rarely presents in the newborn period; most affected children present before 30 months of age with hypoketotic hypoglycemia, hepatomegaly, elevated transaminase concentrations, seizures, and coma. In addition, patients may have RTA, transient hyperlipidemia, and, paradoxically because this is a liver enzyme, myopathy with elevated creatinine kinase or cardiac involvement in the neonatal period.[15]

Cystinosis (McKusick #219800)

Affected infants appear normal at birth and begin to develop manifestations of the renal Fanconi syndrome between 6 and 12 months. The diagnosis should be considered, however, whenever there are features of renal Fanconi syndrome, such as glucosuria, metabolic acidosis, hypophosphatemia, and hypokalemia, in a neonate. Nephropathic cystinosis is an autosomal recessive disorder that results from defective lysosomal transport of cystine. The cystinosis gene, *CTNS*, maps to chromosome 17p13 and encodes an integral membrane protein, cystinosin, which has the features of a lysosomal membrane protein.[16] Cystinosis can be diagnosed in utero by cystine measurements in chorionic villi by 9 weeks.[17] Early and adequate treatment with oral cysteamine dramatically retards the inexorable progression to end-stage renal failure.[18] Administration of 0.55% cysteamine eye drops, 6 to 12 times per day, started after 1 year of age dissolves corneal cystine crystals in patients with nephropathic cystinosis.[19]

Type 1 Tyrosinemia (McKusick #276700)

Type 1 tyrosinemia (hepatorenal tyrosinemia) is caused by deficiency in the gene for fumarylacetoacetate hydrolase on chromosome 15q23-q25. Type 1 tyrosinemia is an important cause of renal Fanconi syndrome and hepatocellular carcinoma, although this disease rarely presents in the neonatal period. A term infant has presented at birth, however, with hypoglycemia, thrombocytopenia, coagulopathy, and hyperbilirubinemia caused by hepatic failure.[20] The cutaneous lesions of porphyria, similar to that in the "bronze baby syndrome" and in neonates with phototherapy-induced purpuric lesions, complicated the course.[20] Most infants become symptomatic by age 3 months. In addition to the above-noted symptoms, untreated infants also show failure to thrive, hepatomegaly, neurologic crises resembling porphyria with hypertension and tachycardia, painful paresthesia, rickets by 18 months, and hepatocellular carcinoma in approximately 18% of infants surviving to 2 years. Pathologic changes include hepatic cirrhosis, renal tubular dilation, and pancreatic islet hypertrophy. There is marked elevation of plasma methionine, α-fetoprotein, δ-aminolevulinc acid, and pathognomonically succinyl acetone; generalized aminoaciduria and a disproportionately high urinary excretion of methionine, parahydroxyphenylacetic acid, and succinyl acetone also are seen. The diagnosis is confirmed by showing low or no enzyme activity in red blood cells, although recent blood transfusions negate the test results. Treatment consists of moderate protein restriction using a specific low tyrosine and phenylalanine formula; inhibition of succinyl acetone, the toxic substance, with 2-(2-nitro-4-trifluoromethylbenzoyl)-1,3-cyclohexanedione (NTBC); and careful monitoring for hepatic nodules and cancer. Orthotopic liver transplantation is recommended for all young children to prevent the development of carcinoma because the effectiveness of NTBC in the long-term prevention of carcinoma is not established.

Renal Glucosuria

Renal glucosuria is a frequent finding in patients with renal Fanconi syndrome. The isolated forms of renal glucosuria are uncommon, rarely present in the neonate, and are benign. Renal glucosuria may be inherited as an autosomal recessive or dominant trait.[21] Intermittent or constant renal glucosuria may be detected in neonates who have the rare autosomal recessive condition of glucose and galactose malabsorption.[22]

RENAL TUBULAR ACIDOSIS

RTA is characterized by chronic hyperchloremic metabolic acidosis associated with an inability to acidify the urine. It may be a primary disorder or secondary to acquired renal injury. Primary RTA is not associated with the renal Fanconi syndrome. Primary RTA is separated into three main types (Table 81-4)[23]:

- Proximal RTA (type 2)
- Distal RTA or "classic" RTA (type 1)
- Hyperkalemic RTA (type 4)

The clinical manifestations of the distal forms ("classic" RTA) are anorexia, failure to thrive, hypotonia, persistently low serum bicarbonate, elevated serum chloride, inappropriately high urine pH, and, in some cases, nephrocalcinosis. Additional findings are decreased urinary excretion of titratable acid, ammonium (NH_4^+), and citrate. The fractional excretion of bicarbonate during alkali treatment is low. Some patients have congenital high-frequency nerve deafness. Untreated patients develop rickets.[24] Type I or classic distal RTA manifests in the same way as transient RTA[25] except that the defect in the former is permanent. Distal RTA often is considered in the differential diagnosis of a neonate with a non–anion gap acidosis, but there are few reports of distal RTA in neonates.[24,26]

The basis of primary distal RTA is failure to excrete sufficient NH_4^+. There is impaired trapping of NH_4^+ in the collecting duct as a result of low rates of hydrogen ion (H^+) secretion.[27] In assessing the possibility of distal RTA, the rate of excretion of NH_4^+ can be determined indirectly by calculating the urinary net charge or urine anion gap[10]: $Na^+ + K^+ + NH_4^+ = Cl^- + 80$. The kidney is not the cause of the acidosis if the Cl^- (chloride) is greater than the sum of the Na^+ (sodium) + K^+ (potassium). If the $Na^+ + K^+$ is greater than Cl^-, the urinary NH_4^+ may be less than 80 mmol/day, in keeping with distal RTA.[28] The diagnosis of distal RTA often is made erroneously in patients with a hyperchloremic metabolic acidosis and an increased concentration of serum chloride who have an "inappropriate" urine pH greater than 6.[29] It is important to "phorget" the urine pH[29] and to consider that diarrhea may be the explanation for these findings because patients with diarrhea can present with a hyperchloremic metabolic acidosis, a urine pH greater than 6, and a urine sodium concentration less than 10 mmol/L.[30] The urine NH_4^+ concentration in these patients is increased.

Regardless of whether a transient or permanent form of distal RTA is suspected, the neonate must be treated with adequate amounts of alkali either as bicarbonate or as citrate. Low doses of alkali (2 to 3 mEq/kg/day) are needed to maintain a normal serum bicarbonate concentration.[25] The alkali can be withdrawn after several months to challenge the diagnosis, or the infant can be

Table 81–4. Primary Proximal (Type 2) and Distal (Type 1) Renal Tubular Acidosis

	Neonatal Presentation	Inheritance	Chromosome Locus
Proximal RTA (Type 2)			
Proximal RTA	No	AD	
Proximal RTA with ocular abnormalities	No	AR	4q21
Specific isolated proximal RTA	Yes	Nonfamilial	
Carbonic anhydrase II deficiency	Rarely	AD	8q22
Distal RTA (Type 1)			
Distal RTA	Yes	AD	17q21-22
Distal RTA with sensorineural deafness	Yes	AR	2p13
Distal RTA with normal hearing	Yes	AR	7q33-34
Carnitine palmitoyl-transferase type I deficiency	Rarely	AR	11q13

allowed to outgrow the dose. We do not advise challenging a neonate with an ammonium chloride loading test to make the diagnosis because the diagnosis can be inferred from indirect tests such as the urine anion gap.

There are at least two autosomal recessively inherited forms of distal RTA. In distal RTA *without* nerve deafness, the mutated gene is located on chromosome 7q33-34; the gene product is the 116-kD B-subunit of the apical pump (*ATP6B1*).[31] Distal RTA *with* nerve deafness[32] is caused by mutations in *ATP6B1*, located on chromosome 2p13, and encoding the B-subunit of the apical proton pump mediating distal nephron acid secretion.

Primary Proximal Renal Tubular Acidosis

Primary proximal RTA is caused by an inability to reabsorb filtered bicarbonate in the proximal tubule. This inability causes bicarbonate wasting and hyperchloremic metabolic acidosis. Distal tubular acidification is normal. When the filtered bicarbonate is reclaimed up to the maximal renal tubular reabsorptive capacity for a patient with proximal RTA, the urine pH is appropriate for the severity of the metabolic acidosis, with values less than 5.3. When proximal RTA occurs as an isolated defect, it is usually transient.[33] Proximal RTA is more often an integral feature of renal Fanconi syndrome. Proximal RTA occurring in a syndrome of mental retardation, band keratopathy, cataracts, glaucoma, and short stature has not been reported in neonates.[34] In this syndrome, the gene for SLC4A4 (*NBC1/KNBC/SLC4A5*), on chromosome 4q21, is mutated.[34]

Carbonic Anhydrase II Deficiency Syndrome

Carbonic anhydrase II deficiency syndrome occurs more frequently in Saudi Arabia; is autosomal recessively inherited; and is characterized by osteopetrosis, RTA, cerebral calcification, mental retardation, growth failure, typical facial appearance, and abnormal teeth. There is one report of metabolic acidosis in a neonate. Radiographic evidence of osteopetrosis was evident in the late neonatal period.[35]

Renal Tubular Acidosis Caused by Maternal Sniffing of Toluene

Maternal toluene abuse from paint or glue sniffing during pregnancy causes severe RTA in the mother and the neonate.[36,37]

Renal Tubular Acidosis Type 4 with Renovascular Accidents

RTA type 4 with nonazotemic hyperkalemic metabolic acidosis, inappropriately alkaline urine pH, and reduced potassium excretion is a complication of neonatal renovascular accidents.[38] The treatment is oral bicarbonate; eventual spontaneous recovery may occur as a result of an "autonephrectomy" of the affected kidney.[38]

HYPOKALEMIC RENAL TUBULAR DISORDERS

Bartter syndrome is a congenital chronic tubular disorder characterized by hypokalemic metabolic alkalosis, polyuria, salt wasting, hyperkaliuria, hyperaldosteronism, resistance to the pressor effect of angiotensin, juxtaglomerular apparatus hyperplasia, increased renal renin production, and, in some patients, hypercalciuria and nephrocalcinosis. Similar features occur with loop diuretic treatment and congenital chloride diarrhea (Table 81-5). Bartter syndrome (inherited hypokalemic renal tubulopathies) has at least three clinical subtypes, with marked phenotypic variations within each subtype: **antenatal hypercalciuric variant** (hyperprostaglandin E syndrome), **classic Bartter syndrome**, and the **Gitelman variant of Bartter syndrome** (Gitelman syndrome). The common characteristics of each subtype are hypokalemic metabolic alkalosis and renal salt wasting.[39-41]

Antenatal Hypercalciuric Variant (Hyperprostaglandin E Syndrome)

Hyperprostaglandin E syndrome is a life-threatening disorder of the newborn with polyhydramnios, premature delivery, hypokalemia, hypercalciuria, and metabolic alkalosis. Onset of polyhydramnios occurs between 24 and 30 weeks of gestation, and the amniotic fluid chloride levels are elevated. Postnatal clinical features include fever, vomiting, diarrhea, failure to thrive, hyposthenuria, and nephrocalcinosis. Hypercalciuria results in osteopenia,[42,43] and the combination of the alkalosis and marked hypercalciuria causes nephrocalcinosis. There are several causes (genetic heterogeneity) of hyperprostaglandin E syndrome as the result of mutations in the gene for either (1) the furosemide-sensitive Na-K-2Cl-cotransporter, *NKCC2 (SLC12A1)* or (2) the inwardly rectifying potassium channel, subfamily J, member 1, *ROMK (KCNJ1)* on chromosome 11q24.[39]

The inheritance is autosomal recessive. There can be marked variability in the phenotype[23]: Three patients with Na-K-2Cl cotransporter gene (*BSC*) mutations did not develop hypokalemia and metabolic alkalosis for several

Table 81-5. Differential Diagnosis of Chronic Metabolic Alkalosis in Neonates

	Antenatal Bartter	Furosemide	Congenital Chloride Diarrhea
Metabolic alkalosis	+	+	+
Hypokalemia	+	+	+
Urine sodium	Increased	Increased	Decreased
Urine chloride	Increased	Increased	Decreased
Urine potassium	Increased	Increased	Increased
Urine volume	Increased	Increased	Decreased
Diarrhea	Occasionally	No	Severe

years. Three other patients with the same gene mutation had hypokalemia and hypercalciuria, but only one had metabolic acidosis, severe hypernatremia, hyperchloremia, and nephrocalcinosis. Classic Bartter syndrome also may be caused by a mutation in either of these genes, suggesting that the antenatal and classic forms are different manifestations of severity of the same disorder. In addition, some neonates have homozygous gene mutations linked to chromosome 1p31, who do not respond to indomethacin treatment and have a more severe variant, with marked delays in growth and motor development, chronic renal failure, and congenital deafness.[44] Although there is no cure for Bartter syndrome, treatment with inhibitors of prostaglandin synthesis improve polyuria, correct biochemical abnormalities, and allow satisfactory growth and development; nephrocalcinosis may not improve.[45]

Classic Bartter Syndrome (McKusick #241200)

The clinical phenotype of classic Bartter syndrome varies markedly, from episodes of severe volume depletion (with low blood pressure) and hypokalemia during the neonatal period to minimally symptomatic patients who first are diagnosed in adolescence. Serum magnesium levels are normal. There are several causes (heterogeneity) of Bartter syndrome, involving mutations in one of three genes encoding ascending limb of Henle transporters: (1) Na-K-2Cl cotransporter basolateral chloride channel, *CLCNKB*, on chromosome 1p36; (2) Na-K-2Cl cotransporter gene, *SLC12A1/NKCC2*, on chromosome 15q13; or (3) the K⁺ inwardly rectifying channel, subfamily J, member 1, *ROMK (ROMK1/KCNJ1)* on chromosome 11q24. *CLCNKB* mutations also may cause congenital Bartter syndrome (hyperprostaglandin E syndrome) or a Gitelman-like phenotype.

Gitelman Variant of Bartter Syndrome (McKusick #263800)

Hypocalciuria and hypomagnesemia are specific clinical features of Gitelman syndrome. Gitelman syndrome usually does not present in the neonatal period.[23] The Gitelman variant is caused by mutations in the gene for the thiazide-sensitive Na-Cl cotransporter *NCCT (SLC12A3)* of the distal tubule on chromosome 16q13.

RENAL TUBULAR HYPERKALEMIA

Renal tubular hyperkalemia in neonates can be caused by marked prematurity, renal adysplasia, urinary tract obstruction, urinary tract infection, pseudohypoaldosteronism, or congenital adrenal hyperplasia.[46] Renal tubular hyperkalemia usually is associated with an inappropriately low urine potassium concentration, renal salt wasting, and metabolic acidosis. The serum creatinine concentration often is increased either because of volume depletion in pseudohypoaldosteronism and congenital adrenal hyperplasia or because of reduced nephron mass in renal adysplasia and obstruction in posterior urethral valves.

Pseudohypoaldosteronism

At least two syndromes of aldosterone resistance, pseudohypoaldosteronism type I and pseudohypoaldosteronism type II, have been characterized at a clinical and molecular level. There are two clinically and genetically distinct types of pseudohypoaldosteronism type I, designated **renal pseudohypoaldosteronism** and **multiple-organ pseudohypoaldosteronism** (Table 81-6).[47]

Table 81-6. Type I Pseudohypoaldosteronism: Renal Pseudohypoaldosteronism and Multiple-Organ Pseudohypoaldosteronism

	Renal Pseudohypoaldosteronism	Multiple-Organ Pseudohypoaldosteronism
Affected organs	Kidney	Kidney, sweat and salivary glands, colon
Salt wasting	Variable	Recurrent severe salt wasting, occasional neonatal death
	Asymptomatic	
	Moderate failure to thrive, vomiting, short stature	
	Severe dehydration, shock, death	
Urine sodium	Increased	Increased
Urine potassium	Inappropriately low	Inappropriately low
Blood aldosterone	Elevated	Very high
Peripheral renin activity	Elevated	Very high
Improvement with age	Often	Rarely
Requirements for high salt diet	For 1-3 years	For life
Catch-up growth	Often on salt alone	Rarely
Asymptomatic patient	Elevated aldosterone	Normal aldosterone
Inheritance	Autosomal dominant	Autosomal recessive
Receptor defect	Gene *MLR*, encodes mineralocorticoid receptor	Glucocorticoid receptor genes *SNCC1A, SNCC1B, SCNN1G*, encode subunits of epithelial Na⁺ channel

Adapted from Hanukoglu A: Type I pseudohyperaldosteronism includes two clinically and genetically distinct entities with either renal or multiple organ defects. J Clin Endocrinol Metab 73:936, 1991; and Rodriguez-Soriano J: New insights into the pathogenesis of renal tubular acidosis—from functional to molecular studies. Pediatr Nephrol 14:1121, 2000.

Pseudohypoaldosteronism Type I

Pseudohypoaldosteronism type I is a hereditary salt-wasting syndrome that usually starts in early infancy and is characterized by diminished renal tubular responsiveness to aldosterone. Diminished aldosterone responsiveness results in hyponatremia, hyperkalemia, markedly elevated plasma aldosterone, and hyperreninemia. The clinical expression ranges from severely affected patients who die in infancy to asymptomatic individuals. Symptomatic patients are treated with sodium supplementation, which usually is no longer necessary by age 2 years. Serum electrolyte concentrations become normal with increasing age, but aldosterone levels remain elevated.

In some individuals, there is impaired responsiveness to aldosterone in salivary and sweat glands, renal tubules, and colonic mucosal cells. These patients have a protracted course with life-threatening episodes of salt wasting. Pseudohypoaldosteronism may be inherited as an autosomal dominant trait in some families and as an autosomal recessive trait in others. In the dominant form of pseudohypoaldosteronism type I, there are mutations in the gene *MLR* encoding the mineralocorticoid receptor. In the recessive form of pseudohypoaldosteronism type I, there are mutations in the genes *SNCC1A, SNCC1B,* and *SCNN1G,* which encode subunits of the epithelial Na+ channel.[48]

Pseudohypoaldosteronism Type II (Gordon Hyperkalemia-Hypertension Syndrome)

Pseudohypoaldosteronism type II is characterized by hyperkalemia (despite a normal glomerular filtration rate) and hypertension.[49] There is variable mild hyperchloremia, metabolic acidosis, and suppressed plasma renin activity. The metabolic abnormalities are corrected by treatment with thiazide diuretics. This syndrome does not seem to present in the neonatal period.

CONGENITAL NEPHROGENIC DIABETES INSIPIDUS

Nephrogenic diabetes insipidus can result from congenital or acquired insults to the kidneys. These insults include electrolyte abnormalities (hypokalemia, hypocalcemia), drugs (aminoglycosides), tubular interstitial inflammation, and mechanical injury caused by obstruction or dysplasia. In the congenital or inherited forms of nephrogenic diabetes insipidus, insensitivity of the distal nephron to the antidiuretic effect of vasopressin results in an inability to concentrate urine. As a result, large quantities of hypotonic urine (50 to 100 mOsm/kg water) are excreted.[50-53] An affected neonate may be irritable, feed poorly, fail to gain weight, and have unexplained dehydration and fever. The serum concentrations of sodium, chloride, creatinine, and blood urea nitrogen are elevated. Serum levels of vasopressin are normal or increased. There also is a blunted response of plasma factor VIII, von Willebrand factor, and plasminogen activator to administration of the synthetic vasopressin analogue, 1-desamino-8-D-arginine vasopressin. Polyuria may cause dilation of the urinary tract and mimic obstructive uropathy. Treatment with a combination of hydrochlorothiazide

(3 mg/kg/day) and amiloride (20 mg/1.73 m²/day) may be preferable to hydrochlorothiazide and indomethacin because the latter can cause bleeding.[54] This treatment can prevent dehydration, electrolyte imbalances, cerebral calcification, and seizures and result in normal growth. Patients continue to have polydipsia and polyuria, however.

About 90% of patients with inherited nephrogenic diabetes insipidus are boys with the X-linked form as a result of mutations in the arginine vasopressin receptor 2 gene *(AVPR2)*. This gene codes for the vasopressin V2 receptor and is located in chromosomal region Xq28.[55] In fewer than 10% of the families, the inheritance of nephrogenic diabetes insipidus is autosomal recessive or autosomal dominant. Mutations have been identified in the aquaporin-2 gene *(AQP2)* on chromosome 12q13 that codes for the vasopressin-sensitive water channel.[55,56] The reliability of prenatal diagnosis of the X-linked form of nephrogenic diabetes insipidus is about 96%.

REFERENCES

1. Moxey-Mims M, Stapleton FB: Renal tubular disorders in the neonate. Clin Perinatol 19:159, 1992.
2. Ellis SR, Hulton SA, McKiernan PJ, et al: Combined liver-kidney transplantation for primary hyperoxaluria type 1 in young children. Nephrol Dial Transplant 16:348, 2001.
3. Weber S, Schneider L, Peters M, et al: Novel paracellin-1 mutations in 25 families with familial hypomagnesemia with hypercalciuria and nephrocalcinosis. Kidney Int 12:1872, 2001.
4. Ali M, Rellos P, Cox TM: Hereditary fructose intolerance. J Med Genet 35:353, 1998.
5. Gitzelman R, Steinmann B, van den Berghe G: Disorders of fructose metabolism. In Scriver C, Beaudet AL, Sly WS, et al (eds): The Metabolic Basis of Inherited Disease, 6th ed. New York, McGraw-Hill, 1989, pp 399-424.
6. Baerlocher K, Gitzelman R, Nussli R, et al: Hereditary fructose intolerance in childhood: A major diagnostic challenge: Survey of 20 symptomatic cases. Helv Pediatr Acta 33:465, 1978.
7. Levin B, Snodgrass GJ, Oberholzer VG, et al: Fructosemia: observations on seven cases. Am J Med 45:826, 1968.
8. Brooks CC, Tolan DR: Association of the widespread A 149 P hereditary fructose intolerance mutation with newly identified sequence polymorphisms in the aldolase gene. Am J Med Genet 52:835, 1993.
9. Tyfield L, Reichardt J, Fridovich-Keil J, et al: Classical galactosemia and mutations at the galactose-1-phosphate uridyl transferase (GALT) gene. Hum Mutat 13:417, 1999.
10. Van Biervliet JP, Bruinvis L, Ketting D, et al: Hereditary mitochondrial myopathy with lactic acidemia, a De Toni-Fanconi-Debre syndrome, and a defective respiratory chain in voluntary striated muscle. Pediatr Res 11:1088, 1977.
11. Heiman-Patterson TD, Bonilla E, DiMauro S, et al: Cytochrome-c-oxidase deficiency in a floppy infant. Neurology 32:898, 1982.
12. Lombes A, Romero NB, Touati G, et al: Clinical and molecular heterogeneity of cytochrome c oxidase deficiency in the newborn. J Inherit Metab Dis 19:286, 1996.
13. Robinson B: Lactic acidemia. In Scriver C, Beaudet AL, Sly WS, Valle D (eds): The Metabolic Basis of Inherited Disease, 6th ed. New York, McGraw-Hill, 1989, pp 869-888.

14. Pequignot MO, Dey R, Zeviani M, et al: Mutations in the SURF1 gene associated with Leigh syndrome and cytochrome C oxidase deficiency. Hum Mutat 17:374, 2001.

15. Olpin SE, Allen J, Bonham JR, et al: Features of carnitine palmitoyltransferase type I deficiency. J Inherit Metab Dis 24:35, 2001.

16. Town M, Jean G, Cherqui S, et al: A novel gene encoding an integral membrane protein is mutated in nephropathic cystinosis. Nat Genet 18:319, 1998.

17. Smith ML, Pellett OL, Cass MM, et al: Prenatal diagnosis of cystinosis utilizing chorionic villus sampling. Prenat Diagn 7:23, 1987.

18. Markello TC, Bernardini IM, Gahl WA: Improved renal function with cystinosis treated with cysteamine. N Engl J Med 328:1157, 1993.

19. Gahl WA, Kuehl EM, Iwata F, et al: Corneal crystals in nephropathic cystinosis: Natural history and treatment with cysteamine eyedrops. Mol Genet Metab 71:100, 2000.

20. Vanden Eijnden S, Blum D, Clercx A, et al: Cutaneous porphyria in a neonate with tyrosinaemia type 1. Eur J Pediatr 159:503, 2000.

21. Longo N, Elsas LJ: Human glucose transporters. Adv Pediatr 45:293, 1998.

22. Lindquist B, Meeuwisse GW: Chronic diarrhea caused by monosaccharide malabsorption. Acta Paediair 51:674, 1962.

23. Bettinelli A, Ciarmatori S, Cesareo L, et al: Phenotypic variability in Bartter syndrome type I. Pediatr Nephrol 14:940, 2000.

24. Caldas A, Broyer M, Dechaux M, et al: Primary distal tubular acidosis in childhood: Clinical study and long-term follow-up of 28 patients. J Pediatr 121:233, 1992.

25. Igarashi T, Sekine Y, Kawato H, et al: Transient distal renal tubular acidosis with secondary hyperparathyroidism. Pediatr Nephrol 6:267, 1992.

26. McSherry E, Morris RC Jr: Attainment of normal stature with alkali therapy in infants and children with classic renal tubular acidosis. J Clin Invest 61:509, 1978.

27. Bettinelli A, Bianchetti MG, Girardin E, et al: Use of calcium excretion values to distinguish two forms of primary renal tubular hypokalemic alkalosis: Bartter and Gitelman syndromes. J Pediatr 120:38, 1998.

28. Goldstein MB, Bear R, Richardson RM, et al: The urine anion gap: A clinically useful index of ammonium excretion. Am J Med Sci 282:198, 1986.

29. Carlisle EJF, Donnelly SM, Halperin ML: Renal tubular acidosis (RTA): Recognize the ammonium defect and phorget the urine pH. Pediatr Nephrol 5:242, 1991.

30. Izraeli S, Rachmel A, Frishberg Y, et al: Transient renal acidification defect during acute infantile diarrhea: The role of urinary sodium. J Pediatr 117:711, 1990.

31. Smith AN, Skaug J, Choate KA: Mutations in ATP6N1B, encoding a new kidney vacuolar proton pump 116-kD subunit, cause recessive distal renal tubular acidosis with preserved hearing. Nat Genet 26:71, 2000.

32. Karet FE, Finberg KE, Nelson RD, et al: Mutations in the gene encoding B1 subunit of H+-ATPase cause renal tubular acidosis with sensorineural deafness. Nat Genet 21:84, 1999.

33. Nash MA, Torrado AD, Griefer I, et al: Renal tubular acidosis in infants and children. J Pediatr 80:738, 1972.

34. IgarashiT, Inatomi J, Sekine T, et al: Mutations in SLC4A4 cause permanent isolated proximal renal tubular acidosis with ocular abnormalities. Nat Genet 23:264, 1999.

35. Ohlsson A, Cumming WA, Paul A, et al: Carbonic anhydrase II deficiency syndrome: Recessive osteopetrosis with renal tubular acidosis and cerebral calcification. Pediatrics 77:371, 1986.

36. Erramouspe J, Galvez R, Fischel DR: Newborn renal tubular acidosis associated with prenatal maternal toluene sniffing. J Psychoactive Drugs 28:201, 1996.

37. Lindemann R: Congenital renal tubular dysfunction associated with maternal sniffing of organic solvents. Acta Paediatr Scand 80:882, 1991.

38. Alon U, Kodroff MB, Broecker BH: Renal tubular acidosis type 4 in neonatal unilateral kidney diseases. J Pediatr 104:855, 1984.

39. Jeck N, Derst C, Wischmeyer E, et al: Functional heterogeneity of ROMK mutations linked to hyperprostaglandin E syndrome. Kidney Int 59:1803, 2001.

40. Konrad M, Vollmer M, Lemmink HH, et al: Mutations in the chloride channel gene CLCNKB as a cause of classic Bartter syndrome. J Am Soc Nephrol 11:1449, 2000.

41. Madrigal G, Saborio P, Mora F, et al: Bartter syndrome in Costa Rica: A description of 20 cases. Pediatr Nephrol 11:296, 1997.

42. Proesmans W, Devlieger H, van Assche A, et al: Bartter syndrome in two siblings—antenatal and neonatal observations. Int J Pediatr Nephrol 6:63, 1985.

43. Seyberth HW, Rascher W, Schweer H, et al: Congenital hypokalemia with hypercalciuria in preterm infants: A hyperprostaglanduric tubular syndrome different from Bartter syndrome. J Pediatr 107:694, 1985.

44. Jeck N, Reinalter SC, Henne T, et al: Hypokalemic salt-losing tubulopathy with chronic renal failure and sensorineural deafness. Pediatrics 108:E5, 2001.

45. Mourani CC, Sanjad SA, Akatcherian CY: Bartter syndrome in a neonate: Early treatment with indomethacin. Pediatr Nephrol 14:143, 2000.

46. Rodriguez-Soriano J: Potassium homeostasis and its disturbances in children. Pediatr Nephrol 9:364, 1995.

47. Hanukoglu A: Type I pseudohypoaldosteronism includes two clinically and genetically distinct entities with either renal or multiple organ defects. J Clin Endocrinol Metab 73:936, 1991.

48. Rodriguez-Soriano J: New insights into the pathogenesis of renal tubular acidosis—from functional to molecular studies. Pediatr Nephrol 14:1121, 2000.

49. Schambelan M, Sebastian A, Rector FC Jr: Mineralocorticoid-resistant renal hyperkalemia without salt wasting (type II pseudohypoaldosteronism): Role of increased renal chloride reabsorption. Kidney Int 19:716, 1981.

50. Bichet DG, Oksche A, Rosenthal W: Congenital nephrogenic diabetes insipidus. J Am Soc Nephrol 8:1951, 1997.

51. Knoers N, Monnens LA: Nephrogenic diabetes insipidus: Clinical symptoms, pathogenesis, genetics and treatment. Pediatr Nephrol 6:476, 1992.

52. Monnens LA: Nephrogenic diabetes insipidus: Clinical symptoms, pathogenesis, genetics and treatment. Pediatr Nephrol 6:476, 1992.

53. van Lieburg AF, Knoers NV, Monnens LA: Clinical presentation and follow-up of 30 patients with congenital nephrogenic diabetes insipidus. J Am Soc Nephrol 10:1958, 1999.

54. Kirchlechner V, Koller DY, Seidl R, et al: Treatment of nephrogenic diabetes insipidus with hydrochlorothiazide and amiloride. Arch Dis Child 80:548, 1999.

55. Morello JP, Bichet DG: Nephrogenic diabetes insipidus. Annu Rev Physiol 63:607, 2001.

56. Goji K, Kuwahara M, Gu Y, et al: Novel mutations in aquaporin-2 gene in female siblings with nephrogenic diabetes insipidus: Evidence of disrupted water channel function. J Clin Endocrinol Metab 83:3205, 1998.

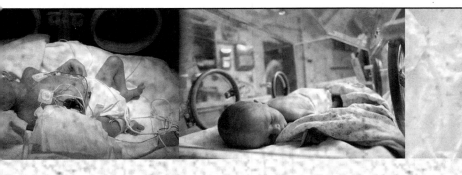
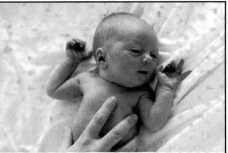

Hematologic Problems
in the Neonate

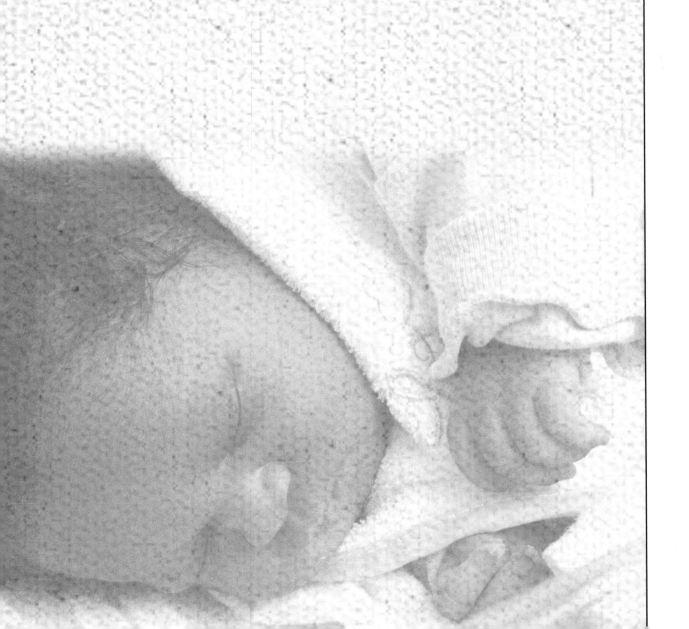

CHAPTER 82

Anemia

Steven McKenzie

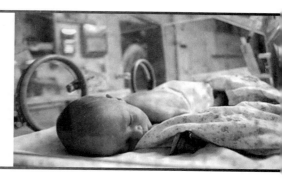

Numerous changes in erythropoiesis accompany the transition from fetal life through the neonatal period. **Red blood cell (RBC)** production begins in the aorto-gonadal-mesonephros section of mesoderm during week 3 of gestation; shifts to the liver in week 6; and moves to the spleen, lymph nodes, and bone marrow by 8 to 12 weeks. The hemoglobin concentration progressively increases during gestation, then decreases in the neonatal period. The percentage of immature RBCs decreases as the fetus matures. A wide variety of RBC shapes precedes the development of a more uniform population of discocytes or typical RBCs. Erythrocytes acquire their genetically determined surface antigens, sometimes stimulating maternal production of a corresponding antibody. The embryonic hemoglobins Gower 1, Gower 2, and Portland are replaced by **fetal hemoglobin (Hb F)**, which later gives way to **adult hemoglobin (Hb A)**.

Normal hematologic values during the first 2 weeks of life in term infants are shown in Table 82-1. RBC values on the first postnatal day according to gestational age are shown in Table 82-2. The standard deviations for hemoglobin level, mean corpuscular volume, reticulocyte count, and other RBC parameters are large, and a newborn's values should always be judged according to the normal range rather than the mean. Hemoglobin levels measured in capillary samples generally exceed levels measured in venous samples,[1] and this difference is accentuated in premature infants, sick infants, and infants in the first few hours of life.

Numerous features distinguish the RBCs of a newborn from the RBCs of an older child or adult.[2] The RBC half-life is reduced by 20% to 25% in term infants and nearly 50% in premature infants. Some enzymes of the glycolytic pathway, such as phosphoglycerate kinase and enolase, have increased activity, whereas phosphofructokinase activity is greatly decreased. The 2,3-diphosphoglycerate levels decline more rapidly than in adult cells because of a relative block in glycolysis or increased hydrolysis. Hemoglobin in the newborn RBC denatures more readily under oxidant stress.

Neonatal RBCs are more resistant to osmotic lysis than adult RBCs.[3]

There are several differences between adult and neonatal RBC antigens.[4] Newborn RBCs have fewer reactive A or B sites than adult RBCs because of the attachment of fewer immunodominant sugars to RBC membrane glycoproteins and glycolipids. The Lewis system is incompletely expressed. Neonatal RBCs have more i antigen than I; by 18 months, the adult pattern of I antigen predominance is present.

The morphology of the RBCs in a newborn is distinctly unusual under conventional microscopy. Wet preparations of glutaraldehyde-fixed cells have identified and quantified cell shapes rarely found in older children.[5] Failure to recognize the normal morphologic findings in newborn blood can lead to incorrect diagnosis of a hematologic disorder. Spherocytes are relatively common in peripheral blood smears of newborns compared with older children. This finding may suggest hereditary spherocytosis or ABO incompatibility in an infant with jaundice but is insufficient evidence for a definitive diagnosis. Target cells also are present, presumably as a result of increased lipids in the membrane of the erythrocyte. The variation in RBC size and shape greatly exceeds that found in later life. The high hemoglobin levels in newborns make it difficult to prepare an adequate smear for interpretation of RBC morphology. The search for specific abnormalities on microscopic examination can be aided by reducing the hemoglobin concentration in vitro to 10 to 12 g/dL, using the patient's plasma as the diluent.

GENERAL APPROACH TO DIAGNOSIS

The general approach to a neonate with anemia is based on the same principles used in the evaluation of older children. Insofar as allowed by the infant's clinical condition, the use of empirical therapies or blood transfusions should await a definitive hematologic diagnosis or, at least, the collection of blood samples for appropriate studies. The major diagnostic question is whether the low

Table 82–1. Normal Hematologic Values during the First 2 Weeks of Life in Term Infants

	Cord Blood	Day 1	Day 3	Day 7	Day 14
Hemoglobin (g/dL)	16.8	18.4	17.8	17	16.8
Hematocrit (%)	53	58	55	54	52
RBC (mm^3 × 10^6)	5.2	5.8	5.6	5.2	5.1
MCV (fL)	107	108	99	98	96
MCH (pg)	34	35	33	32.5	31.5
MCHC (g/dL)	31.7	32.5	33	33	33
Reticulocytes (%)	3-7	3-7	1-3	0-1	0-1
Nucleated RBC (mm^3)	500	200	0-5	0	0

MCV, mean corpuscular volume; MCH, mean corpuscular hemoglobin; MCHC, mean corpuscular hemoglobin concentration; RBC, red blood cells.

From Oski FA: The erythrocyte and its disorders. In Nathan DG, Oski FA (eds): Hematology of Infancy and Childhood, 4th ed. Philadelphia, WB Saunders, 1993.

hemoglobin level is due to decreased RBC production, shortened RBC survival, or a combination of these two processes. Anemia resulting from decreased RBC production develops slowly, allowing time for physiologic compensation. Consequently the infant may have surprisingly few signs of anemia other than pallor. On laboratory examination, the reticulocyte count is inappropriately low for the degree of anemia. RBC morphology is usually normal. In contrast, a newborn with anemia caused by RBC destruction or acute blood loss often appears acutely ill. Hemolytic anemias usually are accompanied by jaundice and, less frequently, enlargement of the spleen. The reticulocyte count is elevated, and nucleated RBCs may persist in the peripheral blood beyond the first few days of life. Characteristic changes in RBC morphology, such as spherocytes in hereditary spherocytosis or ABO incompatibility, are often present.

When the distinction is made between decreased RBC production and shortened RBC survival, additional laboratory tests can address specific diagnoses. If production is diminished, further testing might include bone marrow aspirate for Diamond-Blackfan syndrome or serologic or polymerase chain reaction studies for parvovirus

B19 infection. If hemolysis is suspected, additional steps toward a specific diagnosis might include hemoglobin electrophoresis for Hb H disease or measurement of RBC enzymes for erythrocyte metabolic abnormalities. The efficiency of the diagnostic search often can be enhanced greatly by careful attention to the maternal and family history. The history of a febrile illness with a rash in midpregnancy may prompt an early investigation for a viral origin of neonatal anemia. A history of several family members with neonatal hyperbilirubinemia and anemia cured by splenectomy should direct the investigation of a newborn with hemolytic anemia toward membrane disorders, such as spherocytosis.

Two additional considerations should help guide the evaluation of an anemic newborn. First, the general physical examination can yield important diagnostic clues. Neonatal anemia resulting from a systemic disorder, such as infection, rarely occurs in the absence of other major abnormalities related to the primary disease process. Second, the severity of the anemia should be assessed thoughtfully before embarking on an intensive evaluation. A well-appearing, full-term newborn with a venous hemoglobin level of 14.5 g/dL is unlikely to have a significant

Table 82–2. Red Blood Cell Values from Capillary Blood on First Postnatal Day

	Gestational age (wk)							
	24-25(7)*	26-27 (11)	28-29 (7)	30-31 (25)	32-33 (23)	34-35 (23)	36-37 (20)	Term (19)
RBC × 10^6	4.65 ± 0.43†	4.73 ± 0.45	4.62 ± 0.75	4.79 ± 0.74	5 ± 0.76	5.09 ± 0.5	5.27 ± 0.68	5.14 ± 0.7
Hemoglobin (g/dL)	19.4 ± 1.5	19 ± 2.5	19.3 ± 1.8	19.1 ± 2.2	18.5 ± 2	19.6 ± 2.1	19.2 ± 1.7	19.3 ± 2.2
Hematocrit (%)	63 ± 4	62 ± 8	60 ± 7	60 ± 8	60 ± 8	61 ± 7	64 ± 7	61 ± 7.4
MCV (fL)	135 ± 0.2	132 ± 14.4	131 ± 13.5	127 ± 12.7	123 ± 15.7	122 ± 10	121 ± 12.5	119 ± 9.4
Reticulocytes (%)	6 ± 0.5	9.6 ± 3.2	7.5 ± 2.5	5.8 ± 2	5 ± 1.9	3.9 ± 1.6	4.2 ± 1.8	3.2 ± 1.4

*Number of infants.

†Mean values ± SD.

MCV, mean corpuscular volume; RBC, red blood cells.

From Zaizov R, Matoth Y: Red cell values on the first postnatal day during the last 16 weeks of gestation. Am J Hematol 1:275, 1976.

hematologic disorder, and the collection of numerous diagnostic blood samples might decrease the hemoglobin level further without enhancing the overall care of the infant.

ANEMIA CAUSED BY BLOOD LOSS

Fetal blood loss results in anemia without jaundice or other evidence of hemolysis at birth or in the first few days of life. Acute and chronic blood loss has become the most common cause of anemia in the neonatal period since the widespread availability of effective prophylaxis for Rh hemolytic disease of the newborn. Neonatal anemia can be caused by blood loss during intrauterine life, in the perinatal period, or after birth. If moderate blood loss has occurred chronically, the infant accommodates to the loss and appears pale without acute distress. Severe, chronic blood loss can result in **hydrops fetalis** characterized by hepatosplenomegaly, ascites, and anasarca. Recent neonatal hemorrhage causes acute distress, pallor, disturbances of respiration, poor peripheral pulses, and low blood pressure; the liver and spleen are not enlarged.

The peripheral blood smear from an infant who has had acute blood loss has normochromic, normocytic RBCs. The reticulocyte count is normal or elevated. In contrast, chronic blood loss is associated with hypochromic and microcytic RBCs, decreased serum iron levels, and absent iron stores with erythroid hyperplasia in the bone marrow. The reticulocyte count is normal or low.

Transfer of fetal blood to the mother through an abnormality of the placenta occurs in about half of all pregnancies. **Fetomaternal hemorrhage** is common after traumatic amniocentesis and external cephalic version. Massive fetal blood loss has been reported after blunt trauma to the maternal abdomen.[6] Although in most cases fetal blood loss is small enough that the outcome of the pregnancy is not affected, in 1% of pregnancies the blood loss is greater than 40 mL.[3] Large acute blood loss resulting from fetomaternal hemorrhage can cause profound anemia, asphyxia, and death. Bidirectional maternofetal and fetomaternal transfusion associated with an infarcted, hemorrhagic placenta has been reported in a plethoric, hydropic infant. In this case, hydrops was caused by hypervolemia with hyperviscosity rather than anemia.[7]

The Kleihauer-Betke acid elution test is used to confirm the presence of fetal blood cells in the maternal circulation and can help to estimate the quantity of blood the infant has lost.[8] RBCs containing fetal hemoglobin resist elution with acid. After exposure to citric acid, cells containing Hb F appear pink with eosin staining, and Hb A elutes out of cells of maternal origin, leaving ghost cells. To quantitate the amount of fetal blood in the maternal circulation, 30 high-power fields of fixed RBCs are examined under the light microscope. Ten fetal cells seen per 30 high-power fields is considered equivalent to a fetal bleed of 1 mL. This method also is used to determine the dose of Rh immune globulin needed to treat postpartum mothers at risk for Rh hemolytic disease with future pregnancies.

Maternal α-fetoprotein levels are increased after even small amounts of fetomaternal hemorrhage.[9] Measurement of maternal serum α-fetoprotein often is used to screen for fetal anomalies, such as neural tube defects. When an elevated maternal α-fetoprotein is discovered in an otherwise normal pregnancy, fetomaternal hemorrhage should be considered.[10]

Significant fetal twin-to-twin transfusion occurs in 15% to 30% of monochorionic twins and should be suspected when one child is plethoric and the other is pale. Twin-to-twin transfusion occurs when abnormalities of the placental blood vessels result in the net transfer of blood from one twin to the other. The anemic twin is on the arterial side of the placental vascular malformation. The clinical effects of twin-to-twin transfusion depend on the period during which transfer of blood has occurred and usually are apparent when a difference of 5 g/dL of hemoglobin exists between the infants. When transfusion has been chronic, there may be a weight discordance of more than 20%, referred to as the **twin transfusion** or **parabiosis syndrome**.[11] The growth restriction of the donor infant is similar to that seen in infants with placental insufficiency.[12]

Hyperbilirubinemia and cardiac failure, resulting from polycythemia and volume overload, may develop in the recipient. Marked neutropenia without evidence of infection (total neutrophil count 2000/μL, lasting 4 to 8 days) has been described in donor twins.[13] The neutropenia may be a result of decreased white blood cell production in the face of accelerated erythropoiesis. Serum ferritin levels, a reflection of total body iron stores, may be much lower in the donor than in the recipient as a result of iron deficiency anemia caused by chronic blood loss.[14]

Obstetric complications, such as placental abruption or placenta previa, can be associated with blood loss and subsequent neonatal anemia. Delivery by cesarean section may cause trapping of a significant amount of the infant's blood volume in the placenta before the cord is clamped, or the placenta may be incised accidentally, resulting in unanticipated blood loss. Other events related to delivery that may cause significant blood loss and anemia include umbilical cord rupture, accidental incision of the cord, and hematoma or rupture of anomalous vessels of the cord or placenta. Delay in clamping the cord after the delivery or raising an infant above the placenta can result in acute transfer of blood from the infant to the placenta, also causing neonatal anemia.

Traumatic deliveries can cause unsuspected internal neonatal bleeding. The signs and symptoms of acute internal bleeding may not be recognized until shock has occurred.[15] Anemia first seen between 24 and 72 hours and not associated with jaundice commonly is caused by internal hemorrhage.[3] Hyperbilirubinemia develops later when the RBC breakdown products are absorbed from enclosed areas of internal bleeding. Subaponeurotic hemorrhages and cephalhematomas can occur after traumatic deliveries. Intraventricular and subarachnoid hemorrhage also can cause anemia. Breech delivery may cause rupture of abdominal organs, notably the liver, spleen, and adrenals. Splenic rupture may result from splenic distention associated with erythroblastosis fetalis.[16] Bleeding can occur in the retroperitoneal space. Pathologic bleeding from the gastrointestinal tract can be caused by mucosal ulceration or bleeding from mucosal abnormalities, such as hemangiomas. Swallowed maternal blood can be distinguished using the simple Apt test, which relies on the alkali resistance of Hb F. The Apt test requires a grossly bloody specimen of stool or vomitus. A 1% solution of sodium hydroxide applied to dissolved blood remains pink in the presence of Hb F and turns yellow in the presence of Hb A.[17]

Within the first 4 to 8 weeks of life, infants requiring intensive care, whether secondary to prematurity or due to medical or surgical complications in the term infant, have iatrogenic loss of blood as a result of repeated diagnostic sampling. These losses may be exacerbated by use of extracorporeal circuits, such as in extracorporeal membrane oxygenation. Rarely, blood loss is the result of an inherited bleeding disorder, such as hemophilia, thrombocytopenia, or platelet dysfunction. There also may be anemia secondary to acquired bleeding disorders, such as thrombocytopenia accompanying necrotizing enterocolitis or disseminated intravascular coagulation from early-onset or late-onset sepsis.

The decision to transfuse RBCs after perinatal blood loss must be made on an individual basis. Acute blood loss that results in a pale, tachycardic, ill-appearing infant can be replaced with aliquots of 10 to 20 mL/kg of packed RBCs to restore blood volume and oxygen-carrying capacity. Careful monitoring of vital signs and hemoglobin concentration is necessary to determine the appropriate dose of transfused cells. Infants with chronic, severe blood loss may have accommodated to the loss; the RBC mass is decreased, but the intravascular volume is normal or elevated. When transfusion is required to treat severe, chronic anemia, small volumes of RBCs (3 to 5 mL/kg) are given with close attention to the clinical signs of heart failure. See Chapter 85 for RBC transfusion products appropriate for neonatal transfusion. Infants with anemia caused by blood loss also should receive iron supplementation.

ANEMIA CAUSED BY DECREASED RED BLOOD CELL PRODUCTION

Anemia of Prematurity

Anemia of prematurity presents a particular challenge because of its common occurrence, associated symptoms, and, in very small infants, frequent need for RBC transfusions. This normochromic, normocytic anemia usually develops between 2 and 6 weeks of age in infants born before 35 weeks' gestational age. Hemoglobin levels less than 10 g/dL may be associated with decreased activity, poor growth, tachycardia, and tachypnea. Premature infants with no cardiopulmonary complications may tolerate hemoglobin levels of 6.5 g/dL, however, without evidence of impaired myocardial function, poor weight gain, or unmet metabolic demands.[18] A diminished erythropoietin response to anemia and available oxygen seems to play a central role in the anemia of prematurity.[19,20]

The mechanism underlying this abnormal response has not been identified, although several have been proposed. The hepatic production of erythropoietin that occurs during early infancy may be less sensitive to hypoxia than the renal production of erythropoietin that follows. The switch in site of production may be delayed,[21] and an increased rate of clearance and volume of distribution may contribute further to the inappropriately low plasma erythropoietin levels.[22]

Treatment of anemia of prematurity with recombinant human erythropoietin seems to be a rational, physiologically based approach, and numerous trials have been undertaken. The evolution of neonatal intensive care practices and changing understanding of erythropoietin biology have resulted in little current practical impact of erythropoietin, however. In particular, reduction in the frequency and volume of blood draws and consistent rigorous transfusion guidelines have made supplemental erythropoietin useful only in selected preterm infants.[1,3,23,24] It is yet to be seen whether longer duration forms of erythropoietin, given once a week or once every 2 weeks, now in use in adult hematology, will be tested in neonates.[25-27]

Diamond-Blackfan Syndrome (Congenital Hypoplastic Anemia)

Diamond-Blackfan syndrome is a congenital failure of RBC production that is characterized by pallor, severe anemia, macrocytosis, and reticulocytopenia.[28] Of patients, 10% are profoundly anemic at birth, and 25% are anemic by 1 month of age. Bone marrow examination shows a sharp reduction or absence of RBC precursors with normal white blood cell precursors and megakaryocytes. Autosomal recessive and dominant inheritance of Diamond-Blackfan syndrome has been described, but most cases are sporadic. Approximately 25% of affected patients have at least one associated physical anomaly; common findings include short stature; thumb abnormalities; and anomalies of the head, face, and palate.[29] Mutations of the ribosomal protein S19 have been found in approximately 25% of cases.[30] Additional genetic loci have been mapped, and it is anticipated that the genetic loci responsible for Diamond-Blackfan syndrome all will be known in the near future.

Failure of RBC production in Diamond-Blackfan syndrome previously was attributed to cellular or humoral inhibition of erythropoiesis. More recent evidence suggests, however, a defect in the erythroid precursors or the cytokines responsible for their proliferation and maturation. The addition of erythropoietin, interleukin-3, and stem cell factor to cultures of bone marrow enhances growth of RBC precursors,[31-33] but investigators have not found a defect in the genes for these growth factors or their receptors.[34] Clinical trials of erythropoietin and interleukin-3 in patients with Diamond-Blackfan syndrome showed no response to the former and an infrequent response to the latter.[33,35,36] The enhancement of growth of RBC precursors by cytokines in studies in vitro probably reflects a nonspecific stimulation of cell growth rather than the replacement of a missing or defective growth factor. The pathophysiologic defect in Diamond-Blackfan syndrome remains unknown.

Because the anemia often is profound at the time of diagnosis of Diamond-Blackfan syndrome, initial transfusion of RBCs frequently is necessary. Corticosteroid therapy, beginning at a dose of 2 mg/kg/day of prednisone, improves the anemia in 60% to 70% of patients.[28] Investigators have emphasized the importance of beginning steroid therapy as soon as possible after diagnosis to achieve the best response.[37] Improvement of the anemia usually begins within the first few weeks of steroid therapy. Most patients with Diamond-Blackfan syndrome who are unresponsive to steroids require lifelong transfusion therapy. A few patients have had improvement of anemia by immunosuppressive drugs.[38] Bone marrow transplantation from an HLA-matched sibling donor has been successful in some patients[39]; selection of close relatives as blood donors should be avoided if transplantation is a therapeutic option.

The prognosis for patients with Diamond-Blackfan syndrome is difficult to determine because of the variability in response to steroid therapy and the uncertainty regarding long-term prognosis for transfusion-dependent individuals. For patients responding to steroids, the projected 50% survival is greater than 40 years.[28]

Pearson Syndrome

Pearson syndrome, an uncommon disorder also known as refractory sideroblastic anemia with vacuolization of bone marrow precursors, is characterized by pallor and macrocytic anemia.[40] Neutropenia and thrombocytopenia also may be present but are usually less severe than the anemia. Anemia is detected at birth or within the first month of life in 50% of patients. The striking bone marrow findings are multiple cytoplasmic vacuoles in RBC and white blood cell precursors. Ringed sideroblasts can be seen after staining with Prussian blue. Hematologic findings frequently precede the recognition of other features of Pearson syndrome, such as pancreatic exocrine insufficiency, splenic atrophy, diabetes mellitus, and lactic acidosis.

The underlying defect in Pearson syndrome is a deletion or rearrangement of mitochondrial DNA.[41,42] The heterogeneity of mitochondrial defects over time and in different tissues may explain the variation in clinical findings and the spontaneous hematologic improvement that can occur. Overall the prognosis is poor with a median survival of 2 years.[28]

Congenital Viral Infection

B19 parvovirus, the etiologic agent of Fifth Disease, readily enters erythroid precursors via the P blood group antigen and inhibits their growth.[43] The suppression of RBC production usually is insufficient to cause anemia in children or adults with a normal RBC life span but may cause an aplastic crisis in patients with chronic hemolytic anemias, such as sickle cell disease or hereditary spherocytosis. B19 parvovirus has been identified as a cause of hydrops fetalis resulting from infection in utero.[42-48] Transplacental transmission of B19 parvovirus occurs in approximately one third of acutely infected mothers; estimates of the risk of fetal death vary from 2.5% to 26%. The risk to the fetus may be higher when maternal infection

occurs in the first or second trimester.[46] Some infants who survive infection in utero may be born with severe hypoplastic anemia.[28] Congenitally infected infants have a relatively small viral load that nonetheless accounts for the profound suppression of erythropoiesis.

Early recognition of the symptoms of parvovirus infection in a pregnant woman permits monitoring of the fetus for hydrops fetalis by ultrasound and percutaneous umbilical blood sampling and the administration of intrauterine transfusions if necessary. The value of treatment with intravenous immunoglobulin as passive immunotherapy for the affected fetus or neonate is uncertain.

The anemia associated with congenital cytomegalovirus is due at least in part to decreased production as a result of direct infection of bone marrow stromal cells and inhibition of erythroid colony formation.[49,50] Other congenital infections, such as toxoplasmosis, syphilis, and rubella, frequently are accompanied by anemia resulting from decreased production, increased destruction, or both.[51-53] Laboratory findings most commonly reflect hemolysis; the reticulocyte count and nucleated RBC count are elevated. In severely affected patients, the clinical picture resembles erythroblastosis fetalis, whereas more mildly affected neonates may have only pallor and a hemoglobin level of 10 to 12 g/dL in the first few days of life. The RBC morphology in the anemia of congenital viral infections is often distinctly unusual with fragmented cells, burr cells, spherocytes, and teardrop cells. Nonhematologic manifestations of these disorders usually point to the correct diagnosis and, in the absence of hydrops fetalis, determine the prognosis.

Miscellaneous Conditions

Acute myelogenous leukemia is an uncommon cause of neonatal anemia in which a low hemoglobin concentration accompanies other findings of bone marrow failure, such as thrombocytopenia.[54] On microscopic examination, the RBCs are normochromic and normocytic; teardrop forms may be present. The reticulocyte count is normal or low, but nucleated RBCs may be increased. A high white blood cell count with many immature forms, including blasts, usually suggests the diagnosis of acute myelogenous leukemia, which is confirmed by bone marrow aspirate. The transient myeloproliferative syndrome that occurs in neonates with trisomy 21 closely resembles acute myelogenous leukemia in its clinical features and laboratory findings.[55] In contrast to neonatal leukemia, which has a poor prognosis even with intensive chemotherapy, the myeloproliferative syndrome usually regresses spontaneously by age 2 months.

In malignant osteopetrosis, abnormally dense bone caused by osteoclast dysfunction compresses the marrow cavity and prevents normal intramedullary hematopoiesis. Extramedullary hematopoiesis partially compensates for the bone marrow failure but causes enlargement of the liver and spleen. Neonatal anemia caused by malignant osteopetrosis reflects diminished RBC production in the bone marrow, ineffective erythropoiesis in the spleen and other extramedullary sites, and hypersplenism.[56,57] The normochromic, normocytic anemia often is accompanied by increased reticulocytes and nucleated RBCs. Teardrop forms commonly are found on the peripheral smear. Only bone marrow transplantation has offered long-term improvement. Intrauterine diagnosis of this recessive disorder often can be made by ultrasound and plain radiographs.

ANEMIA CAUSED BY INCREASED RED BLOOD CELL DESTRUCTION

Isoimmune Hemolytic Anemia

Isoimmune hemolytic anemia occurs when fetal RBCs whose antigens differ from the mother's cross the placenta and stimulate maternal production of a corresponding IgG antibody. When the maternally derived antibody enters the infant's circulation, antibody-mediated destruction of fetal or newborn RBCs occurs. Classically, three categories of RBC antigens cause isoimmunization with subsequent destruction of fetal/infant RBCs:

1. Rh (the D antigen alone or in combination with C or E) in an Rh-negative mother
2. A or B in a group O mother; less often A or AB in a group B mother, B or AB in a group A mother
3. Kell, Duffy, Kidd antigens of the MNS system, and other antigens of the Rh system (c, e, and E) in mothers who are negative for these RBC antigens

The wide clinical spectrum of isoimmune hemolytic disease ranges from minimal RBC destruction in a well-appearing child to intrauterine death. When RBC survival is shortened in utero, increased RBC production in fetal hematopoietic tissue causes enlargement of the liver and spleen, and erythroblasts enter the fetal circulation. If the demand for new RBCs does not meet the rate of immune destruction, anemia may result in hydrops fetalis with severe heart failure and generalized edema. The most severely hydropic infants die in utero; surviving infants are severely anemic with increasing levels of bilirubin.

Rh Hemolytic Disease

The classic and most severe form of isoimmune hemolytic disease, Rh hemolytic disease, occurs when a previously sensitized Rh (D)–negative mother, pregnant with an Rh (D)–positive fetus, produces anti-D, which enters the fetal circulation, binds to the incompatible RBCs, and causes their destruction in the fetal spleen. Rh (D) antibodies do not fix complement and do not cause intravascular hemolysis. Affected infants are anemic, are jaundiced, and have a positive Coombs test (also called a *direct antiglobulin*). The reticulocyte count is elevated. Examination of the peripheral blood smear reveals polychromasia, anisocytosis, and high numbers of circulating nucleated RBCs. Spherocytes are not seen in Rh disease but are characteristic of ABO hemolytic disease of the newborn.

The face of Rh hemolytic disease has changed dramatically. In 1941, the relationship between Rh sensitization and hemolytic disease of the newborn was described[58]; in 1950, the success of exchange transfusion in treating postnatal anemia and hyperbilirubinemia was shown.[59]

Amniocentesis was used soon thereafter to analyze amniotic fluid for bilirubin, identifying infants at risk of dying in utero.[60] In the 1960s, 1970s, and 1980s, various techniques for transfusing the severely hydropic fetus, too premature to survive extrauterine life, were devised and improved. The techniques included intraperitoneal transfusion, intravenous transfusion by fetoscopy,[47] and exchange transfusion in utero by direct intravascular injection.[31] In the meantime, widespread immunization with Rh immunoglobulin (RhIg) of Rh (D)–negative women began in the United States when RhIg was licensed in 1968. RhIg has brought about a dramatic decline in the prevalence of the disease.

Exposure to the Rh (D) antigen occurs either through allogeneic transfusion or previous pregnancy. Rh (D)–negative women transfused with Rh (D)–positive RBCs are likely to show high titers of anti-D when subsequently pregnant with Rh (D)–positive infants; transfusion of Rh (D)–positive RBCs or of platelets containing incompatible Rh (D) cells should be avoided in Rh (D)–negative girls and women of childbearing age. Most pregnancy-related Rh (D) immunizations are a result of fetomaternal hemorrhage at delivery. Sensitizing exposure to the D antigen can occur with less than 0.1 mL of Rh (D)–positive cells; the rate of immunization correlates with the volume of Rh (D) cells that enter the circulation of the Rh (D)–negative mother.[61] Exposure and sensitization to Rh (D) can follow amniocentesis, chorionic villus sampling, abortion, or rupture of an ectopic pregnancy.[62] Concomitant ABO incompatibility causes more rapid destruction of fetal cells by the mother. As a result, the fetal cells are less likely to elicit a maternal antibody response to the Rh (D) antigen than when the fetal and maternal cells are ABO compatible. Cases of Rh incompatibility tend to be less severe when there is coexistent ABO incompatibility.

In the absence of a history of an Rh-incompatible transfusion, Rh disease rarely occurs during the first pregnancy of an Rh (D)–negative woman. Before the routine availability of RhIg, the incidence of sensitization in Rh (D)–negative women after a single ABO-compatible, Rh-incompatible pregnancy was 17%[53]; for ABO-incompatible, Rh-negative mothers, the rate of anti-D formation is 9% to 13%.[61]

The estimated incidence rate of Rh hemolytic disease in the United States today is 10.6 per 10,000 total births.[63] The persistence of Rh hemolytic disease, despite the availability of effective prevention, is apparently due to failure to administer RhIg to all women at risk, occasional failure to administer the proper dose of RhIg, failure to administer RhIg prophylaxis after a "silent" antenatal sensitization, and continued inaccessibility of prenatal care to many women.[63]

Rh blood grouping should be determined when a woman undergoes prenatal care. If the mother is Rh negative and the father is Rh positive, the fetus is at risk. The technique of polymerase chain reaction has been used to identify the Rh (D) genotype in the fetus during the first trimester of pregnancy in a previously sensitized, Rh (D)–negative (dd) woman.[64] If the father is heterozygous Rh (D) positive (Dd), a 50% chance exists that the fetus will be Rh (D) negative (dd) and unaffected. Using molecular techniques to distinguish the Rh (D)–negative genotype (dd) from the Rh (D)–positive genotypes (Dd and DD) eliminates unnecessary risks posed by invasive procedures, such as fetal blood sampling and amniocentesis, in an Rh (D)–negative fetus. Current recommendations for the obstetric management of at-risk pregnancies can be found in obstetric and perinatal reference materials.[65]

The major clinical manifestations of Rh hemolytic disease are due to antibody-mediated RBC destruction, which can cause severe anemia and hydrops in utero. Hyperbilirubinemia usually does not become a problem until after birth because fetal bilirubin is removed by the placenta. The risks to a fetus with Rh hemolytic disease are correlated with the degree of anemia and hyperbilirubinemia.

Management of a neonate with Rh hemolytic disease depends on the degree of anemia and the amount of intervention that preceded the delivery. The infant's status cannot be predicted with certainty before birth, and packed group O, Rh (D)–negative RBCs should be available at the delivery. When an assessment of the infant's respiratory and cardiovascular status has been made, evaluation of the severity of hemolysis is necessary. Cord blood should be sent for blood type, Coombs test, hematocrit, reticulocyte count, and bilirubin concentration.[65] Therapy should be aimed at correcting severe anemia and reducing toxic bilirubin concentrations. The most severely affected infants have profound anemia and jaundice, usually accompanied by organomegaly and anasarca. These infants may die in utero or shortly after birth.[66] Infants with less RBC destruction and less anemia are still at risk for kernicterus from hyperbilirubinemia. Some neonatologists recommend immediate double-volume exchange transfusion if the cord bilirubin concentration is greater than 4.5 mg/dL or the cord hemoglobin level is less than 11 g/dL. Others treat the anemia with simple transfusion and observe the rate of increase in the bilirubin concentration, using exchange transfusion when the bilirubin concentration increases at a rate of 0.5 to 1 mg/dL/hr or, in a term infant, when the bilirubin increases to greater than 20 mg/dL.[65] See Chapter 68 for more specific management discussions.

Infants with Rh hemolytic disease may become progressively anemic during the first few weeks of life. For infants who did not require exchange transfusion, anemia results from hemolysis because of the persistence of anti-D and the continuing presence of RBCs bearing the D antigen. Anemia after exchange transfusion is due to a combination of factors, including a low hemoglobin concentration after exchange, postnatal expansion of blood volume, decreased erythropoietic drive, and decreased survival of transfused cells. The potential for development of late anemia must be anticipated in the Rh-incompatible infant; the hemoglobin level should be monitored closely during the first 3 months of life. New approaches to isoimmune hemolytic anemia include the use of erythropoietin to avoid significant late anemia.[67,68]

ABO Hemolytic Disease of the Newborn

In contrast to Rh disease, ABO hemolytic disease of the newborn can occur with the first pregnancy because

anti-A and anti-B antibodies are found early in life in people whose RBCs lack these antigens. These naturally occurring antibodies result from exposure to the A-like or B-like antigens contained in ubiquitous foods or bacteria. Only the maternal IgG form of anti-A or anti-B is capable of crossing the placenta and is responsible for hemolysis in ABO hemolytic disease of the newborn. Hemolysis caused by fetomaternal ABO incompatibility is more common but less serious than in Rh disease.

Clinically significant hemolysis develops in relatively few ABO-incompatible pregnancies. The usual circumstance for ABO incompatibility, a group O mother with a group A or B infant, occurs in about 15% of all pregnancies.[69] Clinically evident hemolysis is found in only 4%, however, of group A or B infants born to group O mothers. Fewer than 1 in 1000 of ABO-incompatible infants require exchange transfusion. Affected infants are usually asymptomatic at birth but develop hyperbilirubinemia within the first 24 hours after birth.

The hemoglobin concentration is mildly to moderately decreased. Coombs test may fail to detect sensitized RBCs in ABO hemolytic disease because the A and B antigens are less well developed in neonates than in adults. In addition, there is greater distance between the antigenic sites on newborn RBCs than on adult RBCs, and agglutination with Coombs reagent may be more difficult to show.[66] In many cases, the maternal antibody can be eluted from the infant's RBCs; testing the eluate with adult RBCs should give a strong reaction. The mother's serum contains relatively high levels of anti-A or anti-B IgG. Examination of the peripheral blood smear shows spherocytes and an elevated number of nucleated RBCs.

Serial monitoring of the bilirubin concentration and the hemoglobin is recommended in infants suspected of having ABO hemolytic disease of the newborn. The RBC destruction in ABO disease usually lasts no longer than 2 weeks. Treatment for hyperbilirubinemia depends on the rate of rise of bilirubin concentration and the peak level reached, based on the infant's gestational age.

Minor Blood Group Incompatibilities

The presence of antibodies to minor blood group antigens is more likely the result of previous transfusion than maternal-fetal incompatibility. Many RBC antibodies have been described in association with hemolysis in the newborn; anti-c and anti-E, aimed at antigens of the Rh system, are particularly potent antibodies. In a survey of isoimmune disease among 7 million births in Wales and Britain, there were 38 deaths resulting from antibodies other than anti-D.[70] Although these minor incompatibilities are rare, some authorities recommend that all women be screened at week 34 of pregnancy for the presence of antibodies[66] to c, e, E, Kell, Duffy, Kidd, and antigens of the MNS system. Affected infants usually have a clinical presentation similar to infants with Rh hemolytic disease.

Enzyme Disorders

The RBC depends on two major metabolic pathways—the Embden-Meyerhof pathway and the pentose-phosphate shunt—to meet its energy needs and to protect it against oxidative damage. Inherited abnormalities in the structure or function of several enzymes in both pathways have been described. Diminished or absent activity of these enzymes causes shortened RBC survival, and the resultant anemias often are referred to as **congenital nonspherocytic hemolytic anemias.** Deficiencies of two enzymes, pyruvate kinase and glucose-6-phosphate dehydrogenase (G6PD), are associated most often with symptoms in the neonatal period.

Pyruvate kinase catalyzes the conversion of phosphoenolpyruvate to pyruvate in the Embden-Meyerhof pathway. Pyruvate kinase deficiency is inherited as an autosomal recessive trait and is the most common enzyme abnormality of the glycolytic pathway associated with anemia. Clinical findings in a newborn with pyruvate kinase deficiency may include varying degrees of hyperbilirubinemia, anemia, and hepatosplenomegaly.[71] The peripheral blood smear is characterized by macrocytes, spiculated RBCs, target cells, spherocytes, and (less often) acanthocytes. The reticulocyte count is elevated. The clinical syndrome in older children ranges from mild anemia and reticulocytosis detected by chance late in childhood to severe anemia with extramedullary hematopoiesis and, rarely, transfusion dependence. The biochemical diagnosis rests on demonstration of decreased or absent enzyme activity. Accumulation of glycolytic intermediates proximal to pyruvate kinase is characteristic of pyruvate kinase deficiency.

G6PD catalyzes the first, rate-limiting step of the pentose-phosphate pathway, important in the production of nicotinamide-adenine dinucleotide phosphate (reduced form), which maintains cellular systems in the reduced state. Most patients deficient in G6PD are generally well with little hemolysis and become symptomatic only when challenged with oxidative stresses. G6PD deficiency is the most common inherited disorder of RBCs.

G6PD production is determined by a gene (*Gd*) located on the long arm of the X chromosome. *Gd* mutations display a typical X-linked inheritance pattern. Males are hemizygotes for presence (Gd+) or absence (Gd−) of the enzyme. Females can be normal (Gd+/Gd+), heterozygotes (Gd+/Gd−), or deficient homozygotes (Gd−/Gd−). Many G6PD variants have been described. The best characterized include G6PD A⁻, found among Africans and African Americans, G6PD Mediterranean, found in the Mediterranean region, and G6PD Mahidol, found in Malaysia and Southeast Asia.[72] In a large study of male African Americans, the incidence of G6PD deficiency was 11%,[73] with 20% of female African Americans being heterozygotes.

African-American male infants with G6PD deficiency only rarely have severe neonatal jaundice. In infants with other forms of G6PD deficiency, however, jaundice is more common. Hyperbilirubinemia usually is detected on the second or third day of life and may require treatment with exchange transfusion.[74] Despite the potential for severe hyperbilirubinemia, anemia is rarely a clinical problem, and these infants do not develop hydrops.[72] The presence of severe neonatal jaundice does not portend chronic, ongoing hemolysis. Because not all male infants with G6PD deficiency develop jaundice, some

investigators have suggested that factors besides G6PD deficiency are responsible for hyperbilirubinemia.[75]

During periods of hemolysis, the peripheral blood smear shows pincer cells, RBC fragments, and pyknocytes; Heinz bodies may be seen with supravital staining. The reticulocyte count is elevated. The definitive diagnosis rests on demonstration of decreased enzyme activity in RBCs by quantitative assay. The African-American variant of G6PD deficiency is most readily identified in the absence of acute hemolysis because the G6PD-deficient older RBCs are quickly eliminated during hemolytic episodes, and reticulocytes may have near-normal levels of enzyme.

A study of susceptibility to sepsis in Saudi Arabian neonates showed an increased risk of late sepsis with catalase-positive organisms in infants with G6PD deficiency. G6PD is normally present in leukocytes, and enzyme deficiency may be associated with lack of leukocyte bactericidal activity. Such data suggest that screening programs for G6PD deficiency in areas with severe variants may help identify infants at risk for late neonatal sepsis.[76]

Membrane Abnormalities

Several inherited abnormalities of RBC membrane structure can cause neonatal anemia and jaundice. Specific defects in membrane structure (e.g., spectrin deficiency[77]) result in the clinical disorder hereditary spherocytosis. Hereditary spherocytosis usually is found among people of northern European heritage with an estimated incidence of 1 in 5000. About 75% of cases have positive family histories.[77] As pieces of the abnormal RBC membrane are lost, the surface-to-volume ratio diminishes with the subsequent formation of spherocytes. Spherocytes have decreased deformability and are destroyed in the cords of the spleen. These cells exhibit decreased resistance of osmotic stress, the basis for the diagnostic osmotic fragility test. Splenectomy, often recommended for older children, benefits patients by removing the site of RBC destruction, improving hemoglobin levels.

Hereditary spherocytosis is characterized by hemolysis, jaundice, and splenomegaly. About half of children with hereditary spherocytosis have a history of neonatal jaundice,[78] which is apparent within the first 48 hours of life. Hyperbilirubinemia usually is controlled with phototherapy; exchange transfusion rarely is required. Anemia may worsen during the first few weeks of life, necessitating booster transfusion.

Diagnosing hereditary spherocytosis in the presence of ABO incompatibility in an anemic, jaundiced infant whose peripheral blood smear exhibits spherocytes may be impossible. The diagnosis of hereditary spherocytosis is difficult to confirm in the neonate, particularly in the absence of a positive family history. The characteristic resistance to osmotic lysis exhibited by normal neonatal erythrocytes makes the unincubated osmotic fragility test unreliable in this age group. An incubated osmotic fragility test is more sensitive in detecting the increased fragility of neonatal hereditary spherocytosis cells. The combination of ABO incompatibility and hereditary

[handwritten margin notes: Hgb α₂γ₂ α₂β₂   Hg H Hg Barts β₂β₂ γ₂γ₂ Hb A α Hg H α₂ Hg Barts 3]

spherocytosis has been reported to cause severe anemia and jaundice.[79]

Other inherited abnormalities of the RBC membrane associated with neonatal anemia and hyperbilirubinemia include hereditary elliptocytosis and hereditary pyropoikilocytosis. In hereditary elliptocytosis, the peripheral blood smear has elliptocytes or ovalocytes with polychromasia. The peripheral smear in hereditary pyropoikilocytosis is disordered, with wild variation in RBC shape, many fragments, spherocytes, and elliptocytes. The fragmentation is accentuated with heating.

Infantile pyknocytosis, a rare cause of neonatal hemolysis, is characterized by hyperbilirubinemia and the presence of spiculated, irregularly shaped RBCs called **pyknocytes**. Infants may have mild hepatosplenomegaly at birth; anemia and jaundice worsen during the first few weeks of life, then resolve spontaneously. The severity of the clinical course is variable, with some infants requiring exchange transfusion. The underlying abnormality in infantile pyknocytosis is unknown; factors extrinsic to the RBC have been suggested.

Thalassemia

Absent or decreased synthesis of specific globin proteins results in the heterogeneous thalassemia disorders. In the fetus and neonate, the clinical expression of thalassemia depends on the affected globin gene (α, β, γ), the developmental stage of globin synthesis, and the amount and function of alternative hemoglobins (Table 82-3). In α-thalassemia, the synthesis of α globin is diminished because of mutations or, more commonly, deletions of one or more of the four α-globin genes. The production of α globin coincides with the earliest stages of erythropoiesis, and because α globin is an essential component of Hb F, α-thalassemia may be expressed clinically in the fetus and newborn. If all four α-globin genes are affected, synthesis of hemoglobin is severely impaired, and profound anemia begins in early fetal development.[80,81] The compensatory hemoglobins, Hb Barts (four γ-globin chains) and Hb H (four β-globin chains), deliver oxygen poorly and are unstable.[82] Intrauterine death from hydrops fetalis usually occurs. Early recognition of the affected fetus and administration of intrauterine transfusions may prevent fetal death.[83,84] Infants saved by these measures require continuing transfusion therapy, however, because α globin is a crucial part of Hb A and Hb F.

If three of the four α-globin genes are affected (Hb H disease), anemia also begins in utero, but it is less severe.[85] Fetal development continues into later gestation when the limited amounts of Hb F and Hb A, in combination with Hb H and Hb Barts, are sufficient to allow survival. The newborn with Hb H disease has a microcytic, hypochromic anemia with increased reticulocytes and nucleated RBCs. The RBCs vary greatly in size and shape. Transfusions usually are unnecessary in the absence of other illnesses.

A newborn with two abnormal α-globin genes usually has a mild anemia with microcytosis and increased levels of Hb Barts. This syndrome is the most common cause of a low mean corpuscular volume in a healthy neonate. One abnormal α-globin gene has no hematologic consequences. Diagnosis of common α-globin genetic variants is now possible with polymerase chain reaction. The value of DNA diagnostics in the appropriate population is that genetic counseling can be provided as to the risk of children having hydrops fetalis due to lack of four α-globin genes or Hb H disease due to lack of three α-globin genes.[86,87]

Thalassemia defects involving the γ-globin gene also affect expression of the nearby δ-globin and β-globin genes. Consequently the fetus with a homozygous γ-thalassemia syndrome not only is unable to make γ globin, an essential component of Hb F, but also is unable to make any compensatory Hb Barts or Hb H. Homozygosity for the large deletions affecting the structural or control genes for γ, δ, and β globin are incompatible with life, beginning at an early stage of fetal development. Heterozygotes for this thalassemia disorder may have a moderately severe microcytic anemia at birth because of the diminished synthesis of the affected globins and the resulting imbalance between α-globin and non–α-globin chains.[88,89] The anemia improves with age. The hematologic findings after the newborn period resemble β-thalassemia trait, but because of the affected γ-globin and δ-globin genes, Hb A$_2$ and Hb F levels are not elevated.

In contrast to α and γ globin, the synthesis of β globin, a necessary component of Hb A, is an important part of erythropoiesis only near the end of gestation. A reduction or absence of β-globin synthesis has no deleterious effect on the fetus. Enhanced production of Hb F provides partial compensation for the decrease in Hb A. Clinical problems associated with severe, homozygous β-thalassemia (thalassemia major or Cooley anemia) usually begin after 2 to 3 months of life, when Hb A assumes full importance. Occasionally, minor hematologic abnormalities, such as microcytosis and increased target cells, are detectable in the newborn. Heterozygous β-thalassemia predictably causes no significant hematologic abnormalities in newborns.

Thalassemia disorders are readily detectable in utero by molecular diagnostic techniques.[90] The widespread use of prenatal diagnosis by couples at risk in Western countries is responsible for the dramatic decline in the number of new births of infants with thalassemia syndromes, in

Table 82–3.   Composition of Hemoglobin at Different Developmental Stages

Type of Hemoglobin	Globin Chains
Embryonic hemoglobins	
Gower 1	$\zeta_2\varepsilon_2$
Gower 2	$\alpha_2\varepsilon_2$
Portland	$\zeta_2\gamma_2$
Fetal hemoglobin	
Hb F	$\alpha_2\gamma_2$
Adult hemoglobins	
Hb A	$\alpha_2\beta_2$
Hb A$_2$	$\alpha_2\delta_2$

particular β-thalassemia major. The increase in immigration from Eastern and Southeastern Asia has been marked by an increase in some thalassemia syndromes, however, including HbE β-thalassemia syndromes.[91]

Sickle Cell Anemia

Genetic mutations of the globin genes also can cause abnormalities of hemoglobin structure. The most common abnormal hemoglobin in the United States is sickle hemoglobin (Hb S); 7% of African Americans are heterozygotes. Because the abnormality involves the β-globin chain that does not reach full expression until after the first month of life, and because Hb F (the dominant hemoglobin during fetal development and at birth) protects against the sickling effect of Hb S, clinical manifestations of sickle cell anemia in the newborn are highly unusual. Hemoglobin levels are generally normal at birth, although they begin to fall shortly thereafter.[92] Reticulocyte counts also are normal at birth, but rise as the hemoglobin levels fall. In a few patients, clinical findings such as icterus, abdominal distention, and respiratory distress in the first month of life have been attributed to sickle cell disease.[93] The investigation of a large cohort of infants identified as having sickle cell disease by newborn screening showed, however, that clinical problems in the newborn period are rarely, if ever, attributable to the hemoglobinopathy.

Although the symptoms of sickle cell anemia usually begin after the neonatal period, the diagnosis of this hemoglobinopathy can and should be made in the newborn period. Most states mandate testing for sickle cell disease as part of newborn screening programs. Either hemoglobin electrophoresis or isoelectric focusing accurately identifies newborns with sickle cell anemia. The identification of affected newborns permits early institution of prophylactic antibiotics for the prevention of bacterial sepsis, the major cause of death in young children with sickle cell disease.[94] The diagnosis of sickle cell disease in the newborn is often the first indication that both parents have sickle cell trait. At-risk couples should be identified before childbearing so that appropriate genetic counseling can be offered and prenatal diagnosis, which is readily available and highly accurate, can be provided to those who want it.[95]

Structural alterations of globin also are responsible for unstable hemoglobins. Most of these alterations occur on the β-globin gene, and the clinical manifestations do not begin until after the neonatal period, when Hb A predominates. Some unstable hemoglobins are caused by amino acid substitutions on the α and γ chains, however, and affected infants may have anemia and reticulocytosis.[96,97] Supravital staining after incubation of the blood shows precipitates of denatured hemoglobin, called **Heinz bodies.** Unstable hemoglobins caused by structural alterations of α and γ globin have the interesting property of causing a hemolytic anemia in the newborn period that gradually resolves as Hb F gives way to Hb A. For γ-chain substitutions, the improvement is due to the diminished synthesis of the abnormal globin. The reason for improvement in the hemolytic anemia resulting from an α-chain substitution is not obvious because α globin is an essential component of adult hemoglobins. The pairing of the abnormal α globin with normal γ globin (Hb F Hasharon) may be more unstable than its pairing with normal β globin (Hb A Hasharon).[97] Alternatively, other characteristics of the fetal erythrocyte may accentuate the instability of the hemoglobin.

REFERENCES

1. Olivieri NF, Berriman AM, Davis S, et al: Response to the hematopoietic growth factor IL-3 in patients with Diamond-Blackfan anemia. Blood 78:153a, 1991.
2. Paludetto R: Neonatal complications specific to twin (multiple) births (twin transfusion syndrome, intrauterine death of cotwin). J Perinat Med 19(suppl 1):246, 1964.
3. Ohls RK: Erythropoietin treatment in extremely low birth weight infants: Blood in versus blood out. J Pediatr 141:8, 2002.
4. Luban NLC: Blood groups and blood component therapy. In Miller DR (ed): Smith's Blood Diseases of Infancy and Childhood, 7th ed. St Louis, CV Mosby, 1994.
5. Zipursky A, Brown E, Palko J, et al: The erythrocyte differential count in newborn infants. Am J Pediatr Hematol Oncol 5:45, 1983.
6. Bickers RG, Wennberg RP: Fetomaternal transfusion following trauma. Obstet Gynecol 61:258, 1983.
7. Bowman JM, Lewis BA, de Sa DJ: Hydrops fetalis caused by massive maternofetal transplacental hemorrhage. J Pediatr 104:769, 1984.
8. Zipursky A, Hull A, White FD, et al: Foetal erythrocytes in the maternal circulation. Lancet 1:451, 1959.
9. Hay DL, Barrie JU, Davison GB, et al: The relation between maternal serum alpha-fetoprotein levels and fetomaternal haemorrhage. Br J Obstet Gynaecol 86:516, 1979.
10. Downing GJ, Kilbride HW, Yeast JD: Non-immune hydrops fetalis caused by a massive fetomaternal hemorrhage associated with elevated serum α-fetoprotein levels. J Reprod Med 35:444, 1990.
11. Klaus MH, Fanaroff AA (eds): In Care of the High Risk Neonate, 4th ed. Philadelphia, WB Saunders, 1993.
12. Pearson HA, Lobel JS, Kocoshis SA, et al: A new syndrome of refractory sideroblastic anemia with vacuolization of bone marrow precursors and exocrine pancreatic dysfunction. J Pediatr 95:976, 1979.
13. Koenig JM, Hunter DD, Christensen RD: Neutropenia in donor (anemic) twins involved in the twin-twin transfusion syndrome. J Perinatol 11:355, 1991.
14. Caglar MK, Kollee LAA: Determination of serum ferritin in the evaluation of iron depletion and iron overload in chronic twin-to-twin transfusion syndrome. J Perinat Med 17:357, 1989.
15. Eraklis AJ: Abdominal injury related to the trauma of birth. Pediatrics 39:421, 1967.
16. Pierce ML: Leukemia in the newborn infant. J Pediatr 54:691, 1959.
17. Apt L, Downey WS: "Melena" neonatorum: The swallowed blood syndrome: A simple test for the differentiation of adult and fetal hemoglobin in bloody stools. J Pediatr 47:6, 1955.
18. Lachance C, Chessex P, Fouron JC, et al: Myocardial, erythropoietic, and metabolic adaptations to anemia of prematurity. J Pediatr 125:278, 1994.
19. Shannon KM, Naylor GS, Torkildson JC, et al: Circulating erythroid progenitors in the anemia of prematurity. N Engl J Med 317:728, 1987.

20. Stockman JA III, Graeber JE, Clark DA, et al: Anemia of prematurity: Determinants of the erythropoietin response. J Pediatr 105:786, 1984.

21. Ohls RK, Ehrenkranz RA, Wright LL, et al: Effects of early erythropoietin therapy on the transfusion requirements of preterm infants below 1250 grams birth weight: A multicenter, randomized, controlled trail. Pediatrics 108:934, 2001.

22. Brown MS, Jones MA, Ohls RK, et al: Single-dose pharmacokinetics of recombinant human erythropoietin in preterm infants after intravenous and subcutaneous administration. J Pediatr 122:655, 1993.

23. Meyer MP, Sharma E, Carsons M: Recombinant erythropoietin and blood transfusion in selected preterm infants. Arch Dis Child Fetal Neonat 88:F41, 2003.

24. Ohls RK: Human recombinant erythropoietin in the prevention and treatment of anemia of prematurity. Paediatr Drugs 4:111, 2002.

25. Egrie JC, Browne JK: Development and characterization of novel erythropoiesis stimulating protein (NESP). Nephrol Dial Transplant 16(suppl 3):3, 2001.

26. Jelkmann W: The enigma of the metabolic fate of circulating erythropoietin (Epo) in view of the pharmacokinetics of the recombinant drugs rhEpo and NESP. Eur J Haematol 69:265, 2002.

27. Smith RE Jr, Jaiyesimi IA, Meza LA, et al: Novel erythropoiesis stimulating protein (NESP) for the treatment of anaemia of chronic disease associated with cancer. Br J Cancer 84(suppl 1):24, 2001.

28. Young NS, Alter BP: Aplastic Anemia: Acquired and Inherited. Philadelphia, WB Saunders, 1994.

29. Gripp KW, McDonald DM, La Rossa D, et al: Bilaterial microtia and cleft palate in cousins with Diamond-Blackfan anemia. Am J Med Genet 101:268, 2001.

30. Draptchinskaia N, Gustavsson P, Andersson B, et al: The gene encoding ribosomal protein S19 is mutated in Diamond-Blackfan anemia. Nat Genet 21:169, 1999.

31. Halperin DS, Estrov Z, Freedman MH: Diamond-Blackfan anemia: Promotion of marrow erythropoiesis in vitro by recombinant interleukin-3. Blood 73:1168, 1989.

32. Lipton JM, Kudisch M, Gross R, et al: Defective erythroid progenitor differentiation system in congenital hypoplastic (Diamond-Blackfan) anemia. Blood 67:962, 1986.

33. Oski FA, Naiman JL: Hematologic Problems in the Newborn, 3rd ed. WB Saunders, Philadelphia, 1982.

34. Drachtman RA, Geissler EN, Alter BP: The SCF and c-kit genes in Diamond-Blackfan anemia. Blood 79:2177, 1992.

35. Dunbar CE, Smith DA, Kimball J, et al: Treatment of Diamond-Blackfan anemia with hematopoietic growth factors, granulocyte-macrophage colony stimulating factor and interleukin-3: Sustained remissions following IL-3. Br J Haematol 79:316, 1991.

36. Fiorillo A, Poggi V, Migliorati R, et al: Unresponsiveness to erythropoietin therapy in a case of Blackfan Diamond anemia. Am J Hematol 37:65, 1991.

37. Allen DM, Diamond LK: Congenital (erythroid) hypoplastic anemia. Am J Dis Child 102:416, 1961.

38. Leonard EM, Raefsky E, Griffith P, et al: Cyclosporine therapy of aplastic anemia, congenital and acquired red cell aplasia. Br J Haematol 72:278, 1989.

39. Lenarsky C, Weinberg K, Guinan E, et al: Bone marrow transplantation for constitutional pure red cell aplasia. Blood 71:226, 1988.

40. Philipsborn HF, Traisman HS, Greer D: Rupture of the spleen, a complication of erythroblastosis fetalis. N Engl J Med 252:160, 1955.

41. McShane MA, Hammans SR, Sweeney M, et al: Pearson syndrome and mitochondrial encephalomyopathy in a patient with a deletion of mtDNA. Am J Hum Genet 48:39, 1991.

42. Rotig A, Cormier V, Blanche S, et al: Pearson's marrow-pancreas syndrome: A multisystem, mitochondrial disorder in infancy. J Clin Invest 86:1601, 1990.

43. Brown KE, Hibbs JR, Gallinella G, et al: Resistance to parvovirus B19 infection due to lack of virus receptor (erythrocyte P antigen). N Engl J Med 330:1192, 1994.

44. Anand A, Gray ES, Brown T, et al: Human parvovirus infection in pregnancy and hydrops fetalis. N Engl J Med 316:183, 1987.

45. Anderson LJ, Hurwitz ES: Human parvovirus B19 and pregnancy. Clin Perinatol 15:273, 1988.

46. Rausen AR, Richter P, Tallal L, et al: Hematologic effects of intrauterine rubella. JAMA 199:75, 1967.

47. Rodis JF, Quinn DL, Gary GW Jr, et al: Management and outcomes of pregnancies complicated by human B19 parvovirus infection: A prospective study. Am J Obstet Gynecol 163:1168, 1990.

48. Schwarz TF, Roggendorf M, Hottentrager B, et al: Human parvovirus B19 infection in pregnancy. Lancet 2:566, 1988.

49. Apperley JF, Dowding C, Hibbin J, et al: The effect of cytomegalovirus on hemopoiesis: In vitro evidence for selective infection of marrow stromal cells. Exp Hematol 17:38, 1989.

50. Maciejewski JP, Bruening E, Young NS, et al: Infection of hematopoietic progenitor cells by human cytomegalovirus. Blood 80:170, 1992.

51. Arnaud JP, Griscelli C, Couvreur J, et al: Anomalies hematologiques et immunologiques de la toxoplasmose congenitale. Nouv Rev Fr Hematol 15:496, 1975.

52. Reeves JD, Huffer WE, August CS, et al: The hematopoietic effects of prednisone therapy in four infants with osteopetrosis. J Pediatr 94:210, 1979.

53. Whitaker JA, Sartain P, Shaheedy M: Hematological aspects of congenital syphilis. J Pediatr 66:629, 1965.

54. Powars D: Diagnosis at birth improves survival of children with sickle cell anemia. Pediatrics 83:830, 1989.

55. Weinstein HJ: Congenital leukemia and the neonatal myeloproliferative disorders associated with Down's syndrome. Clin Hematol 7:147, 1978.

56. Gamsu H, Lorber J, Rendle-Short J, et al: Haemolytic anaemia in osteopetrosis. Arch Dis Child 36:494, 1961.

57. Rodeck CH, Nicolaides KH, Warsof SL, et al: The management of severe rhesus isoimmunization by fetoscopic intravascular transfusions. Am J Obstet Gynecol 150:769, 1984.

58. Levine P, Katzin EM, Burnham L: Isoimmunization in pregnancy. JAMA 116:825, 1941.

59. Allen FH, Diamond LK, Vaughan VC III: Erythroblastosis fetalis: VI. Prevention of kernicterus. Am J Dis Child 80:779, 1950.

60. Bevis DCA: Blood pigments in haemolytic disease of the newborn. J Obstet Gynaecol Br Emp 63:68, 1956.

61. Ascari WQ, Levine P, Pollack W: Incidence of maternal Rh immunization by ABO compatible and incompatible pregnancies. BMJ 1:399, 1969.

62. Walker RH (ed): Neonatal and Obstetrical Transfusion Practice. Technical Manual, 11th ed. Bethesda, MD, American Association of Blood Banks, 1993.

63. Chavez GF, Mulinare J, Edmonds LD: Epidemiology of Rh hemolytic disease of the newborn in the United States. JAMA 265:3270, 1991.

64. Bennett PR, LeVan Kim C, Colin Y, et al: Prenatal determination of fetal RhD type by DNA amplification. N Engl J Med 329:607, 1993.

65. Davis CL: Hydrops fetalis. In Donn SM, Faix SM (eds): Neonatal Emergencies. Mt Kisco, NY, Futura, 1991.

66. Zipursky A, Bowman J: Isoimmune hemolytic diseases. In Nathan DG, Oski FA (eds): Hematology of Infancy and Childhood, 4th ed. Philadelphia, WB Saunders, 1993.

67. Dhodapkar KM: Treatment of hemolytic disease of the newborn caused by anti-Kell antibody with recombinant erythropoietin. J Pediatr Hematol Oncol 23:69, 2001.

68. Wacker P, Azsahin H, Stelling MJ, Humbert J: Successful treatment of neonatal rhesus hemolytic anemia with high doses of recombinant human erythropoietin. Pediatr Hematol Oncol 18:279, 2001.

69. Mollison PL, Engelfreit CP, Contreras M: Blood Transfusion in Clinical Medicine, 9th ed. Oxford, Blackwell Scientific Publications, 1993.

70. Clarke CA, Mollison PL: Deaths from Rh haemolytic disease of the fetus and newborn, 1977-87. J R Coll Physicians 23:181, 1989.

71. Ghidini A, Sirtori M, Romero R, et al: Hepatosplenomegaly as the only prenatal finding in a fetus with pyruvate kinase deficiency anemia. Am J Perinatol 8:44, 1991.

72. Luzzatto L: G6PD deficiency and hemolytic anemia. In Nathan DG, Oski FA (eds): Hematology of Infancy and Childhood, 4th ed. Philadelphia, WB Saunders, 1993.

73. Heller P, West WR, Nelson PB, et al: Clinical implications of sickle cell trait and glucose-6-phosphate dehydrogenase deficiency in hospitalized black male patients. N Engl J Med 300:1001, 1979.

74. Doxiadis SA, Valaes T, Karaklis A, et al: Risk of severe jaundice in glucose-6-dehydrogenase deficiency of the newborn. Lancet 2:1210, 1964.

75. Doxiadis SA, Valaes T: The clinical picture of glucose-6-phosphate deficiency in early infancy. Arch Dis Child 39:545, 1964.

76. Abu-Osba Y, Mallouh AA, Hann R: Incidence and causes of sepsis in glucose-6-phosphate dehydrogenase-deficient newborn infants. J Pediatr 114:748, 1989.

77. Agre P, Asimos A, Casella JF, et al: Inheritance pattern and clinical response to splenectomy as a reflection of erythrocyte spectrin deficiency in hereditary spherocytosis. N Engl J Med 315:1579, 1986.

78. Stamey CC, Diamond LK: Congenital hemolytic anemia in the newborn. Am J Dis Child 94:616, 1957.

79. Trocco JI, Brown AK: Neonatal manifestations of hereditary spherocytosis. Am J Dis Child 113:263, 1957.

80. Kan YW, Allen A, Lowenstein L: Hydrops fetalis with alpha thalassemia. N Engl J Med 276:18, 1967.

81. Liang ST, Wong VC, So WW, et al: Homozygous alpha-thalassemia: Clinical presentation, diagnosis and management: A review of 46 cases. Br J Obstet Gynaecol 92:680, 1985.

82. Todd D, Lai MCS, Beaven GH, et al: The abnormal hemoglobins in homozygous alpha thalassaemia. Br J Haematol 19:27, 1970.

83. Beaudry MA, Ferguson DJ, Pearse K, et al: Survival of a hydropic infant with homozygous alpha-thalassemia-1. J Pediatr 108:713, 1986.

84. Bianchi DW, Beyer EC, Stark AR, et al: Normal long-term survival with alpha-thalassemia. J Pediatr 108:716, 1986.

85. Weatherall DJ, Clegg JB: The Thalassaemia Syndromes, 3rd ed. Oxford, Blackwell Scientific, 1981.

86. Chong SS, Boehm CD, Higgs DR, Cutting GR: Single-tube multiplex-PCR screen for common deletional determinants of α-thalassemia. Blood 95:360, 2000.

87. Shaji RV, Srivastava A, Chandy M, Krishnamoorthy R: A single tube multiplex PCR method to detect the common alpha+ thalassemia alleles. Blood 95:1879, 2000.

88. Fearon ER, Kazazian HH, Waber PG, et al: The entire beta-globin gene cluster is deleted in a form of gamma-delta-beta thalassemia. Blood 61:1273, 1983.

89. Kan YW, Forget BG, Nathan DG: Gamma-beta thalassemia: A cause of hemolytic disease of the newborn. N Engl J Med 286:129, 1972.

90. Kazazian HH Jr: Prenatal diagnosis of beta-thalassemia. Semin Hematol 15:15, 1991.

91. Lory F: Asian immigration and public health in California: Thalassemia in newborns in California. J Pediatr Hematol Oncol 22:564, 2000.

92. Brown AK, Sleeper LA, Miller ST, et al: Reference values and hematologic changes from birth to 5 years in patients with sickle cell disease. Arch Pediatr Adolesc Med 148:796, 1994.

93. Hegyi T, Delphin ES, Bank A, et al: Sickle cell anemia in the newborn. Pediatrics 60:213, 1977.

94. Public Health Laboratory Service Working Party on Fifth Disease: Prospective study of human parvovirus (B19) infection in pregnancy. BMJ 300:1166, 1990.

95. Kazazian HH Jr: Current status of prenatal diagnosis by DNA analysis. Birth Defects 26:210, 1990.

96. Lee-Potter JP, Deacon-Smith RA, Simpkiss NJ, et al: A new cause of haemolytic anemia in the newborn. J Clin Pathol 28:317, 1975.

97. Levine RL, Lincoln DR, Buchholz WM, et al: Hemoglobin Hasharon in a premature infant with hemolytic anemia. Pediatr Res 9:7, 1975.

CHAPTER 83

Neonatal Thrombosis, Hemostasis, and Platelet Disorders

Robert I. Parker

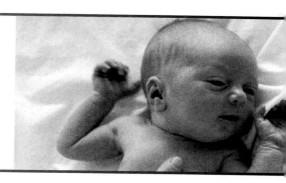

The formation of a visible clot and the maintenance of blood flow represent the end result of a very complex series of biochemical processes. Effective hemostasis requires the interaction of procoagulant and anticoagulant proteins with platelets and blood vessels (endothelial cells). Congenital or acquired defects in any of these components can lead to dysregulation of clot formation with pathologic bleeding or thrombosis. Either of these events may cause serious problems for the neonate. The assessment of the hemostatic system in the newborn is difficult because of practical limitations in regard to the amount of blood that can safely be obtained from these children and because many of the parameters frequently measured change dramatically during the first few weeks to months after birth. Although clinicians' knowledge of these changes has been limited until recently, clinical problems directly related to abnormalities in thrombosis, hemostasis, and platelets have been well recognized. It has been estimated that up to 1% of all newborns in the neonatal intensive care unit (NICU) experience some sort of clinically significant hemorrhage secondary to an abnormality of either coagulation or platelets,[1] and a similar number of newborns in the NICU experience clinically significant thromboembolic complications, most of which are associated with indwelling umbilical catheters.[2,3] A larger number of NICU patients, up to 25%, have been found to develop thrombocytopenia, although clinically significant bleeding occurs in only a subset of these patients.[4,5]

PHYSIOLOGY OF HEMOSTASIS

Hemostasis is divided into three major phases. The first involves the interactions of activated platelets with areas of damaged endothelium or exposed subendothelial tissues, which result in the production of a platelet plug at the site of bleeding or injury. This phase is referred to as **primary hemostasis** and requires platelets, endothelial and subendothelial structures, and specific plasma proteins (i.e., fibrinogen and von Willebrand factor [vWF]). The second phase, referred to as **soluble** or **fluid-phase coagulation**, involves the sequential activation of zymogen clotting factors to their active enzyme forms and results in the production of a fibrin clot. The third component of hemostasis is **fibrinolysis**, which is the process of clot dissolution. Clot formation is regulated not only by the activators of coagulation but also by the intricate interactions of numerous naturally occurring coagulation inhibitors of the procoagulant components of the system. Although it is convenient to conceptualize these three phases as occurring sequentially, they in fact occur simultaneously in vivo (Fig. 83-1). A detailed discussion of the coagulation system is beyond the scope of this chapter, and the reader is referred to specific reviews on the subject.[6,7]

Under normal conditions, blood is maintained in its fluid state. However, with bleeding or injury to tissues, coagulation is activated through the elaboration of various factors (see Fig. 83-1). These include tissue factor, a potent activator of coagulation, and tissue plasminogen activator (tPA), which initiates the fibrinolytic process. Production of vasoconstrictor peptides, such as endothelin, by activated endothelial cells may reduce local blood flow and allow for more efficient platelet deposition at sites of vascular injury. Within seconds, platelet adhesion to activated endothelial cells and exposed subendothelial structures such as collagen occurs, and formation of a platelet plug is initiated. This plug grows through the process of platelet aggregation in which platelets adhere to each other. These interactions are mediated by the binding of specific adhesive glycoproteins (i.e., vWF and fibrinogen) to specific receptors on platelet and endothelial cell membranes (Table 83-1). Platelets may be activated either mechanically by shear stress in turbulent blood flow or biochemically by trace amounts of thrombin generated by the activation of the coagulation process, by adenosine diphosphate released by damaged red blood cells, or by other agonists released by endothelial cells or leukocytes. The mass of platelets that constitute the platelet plug not only serves as a mechanical impediment to bleeding but more importantly provides a phospholipid surface on which coagulation proceeds. Ultimately,

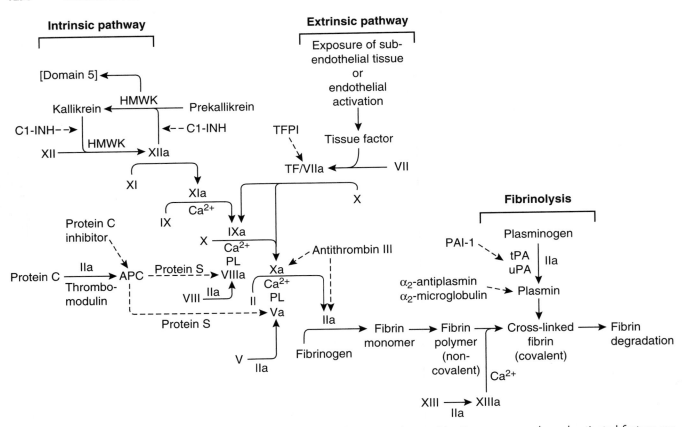

Figure 83–1. Overview of coagulation and fibrinolysis. Coagulation factors are depicted by *Roman numerals,* and activated factors are indicated by a small *a.* Coagulation cascade and fibrinolytic pathway inhibitors are indicated by a *dashed arrow.* C1-INH, complement factor 1 esterase inhibitor; HMWK, high-molecular-weight kininogen; PAI-1, plasminogen activator inhibitor 1; PL, anionic phospholipids; TF, tissue factor; TFPI, tissue factor pathway inhibitor; tPA, tissue plasminogen activator; uPA, urinary plasminogen activator. *(Modified from Folkman J, Browder T, Palmblad J: Angiogenesis research: Guidelines for translation to clinical application. Thromb Haemost 86:23, 2001.)*

the platelet plug is stabilized and strengthened by the incorporation of polymerized fibrin into its growing structure. Finally, the resultant clot is "retracted" by the contraction of actin fibrils in the incorporated platelets. This further strengthens the clot and limits its size by the

expulsion of trapped plasma. As the plug grows, coagulation proceeds with the resultant production of fibrin. The primary activator of soluble, or fluid-phase, coagulation is the conversion of factor X to activated factor X (factor Xa) by the complex of tissue factor/factor VIIa. In addition, factor VIIa can directly activate factor IX, thereby enhancing the activation of factor IX that occurs through the "intrinsic" pathway by the contact factors (factor XII, factor XI, high-molecular-weight kininogen, prekallikrein) (see Fig. 83-1).[8] Ultimately, factor Xa, in the presence of factor Va, calcium ion, and phospholipid, cleaves prothrombin to form thrombin, which subsequently cleaves fibrinogen to form fibrin. The fibrin monomers so formed spontaneously polymerize to produce insoluble fibrin clots. These are cross-linked by the action of factor XIIIa, producing a stable clot.

Simultaneously with platelet deposition and coagulation activation, there occur processes that serve to limit the propagation of the developing blood clot. Locally, endothelial cells limit platelet activation by the production of the potent platelet antagonist and vasodilator prostacyclin, which increases platelet cytoplasmic cyclic adenosine monophosphate and damps down platelet activation.[9] Nitric oxide synergizes with vasodilator prostacyclin to

Table 83–1. Receptors and Ligands Involved in Primary Hemostasis

Receptor	Site	Ligand
GP IIb/IIIa	Platelets	fibrinogen, vWF, intracellular adhesion molecule 2
GP Ib/IX	Platelets	vWF
GP Ia/IIa	Platelets	collagen (adhesion)
GP VI	Platelets	collagen (activation)
P-selectin	Platelets	P-selectin glycoprotein ligand–1 (PSGL-1)
E-Selectin	Endothelial cells	PSGL-1

GP, glycoprotein; vWF, von Willebrand factor.

inhibit platelets by a similar mechanism.[10] In addition, fibrinolysis is activated by the conversion of plasminogen to plasmin by tPA (that produced by endothelial cells) and thrombin.[11-13]

Endothelial cells play an important role in the balance of this complex process by providing a surface on which coagulation and platelet deposition occurs and by elaborating various activators and inhibitors of the process (Fig. 83-2, Table 83-2).[12,13] The natural anticoagulant protein C/protein S system is intricately tied to endothelial cell function in hemostasis (Fig. 83-3).[14,15]

From a biochemical standpoint, the individual components of coagulation and fibrinolysis are best classified

by function. The procoagulant factors can be divided into three separate groups (contact phase, vitamin K–dependent, and thrombin sensitive) (Table 83-3), and the anticoagulant factors can be divided into fibrinolytic and vitamin K–dependent factors.

DEVELOPMENTAL CHANGES IN HEMOSTATIC COMPONENTS

Unlike that in older children and adults, the hemostatic system in the newborn is not yet at "steady state"; that is, many of the components are found in amounts different from those for the older child. These levels change after

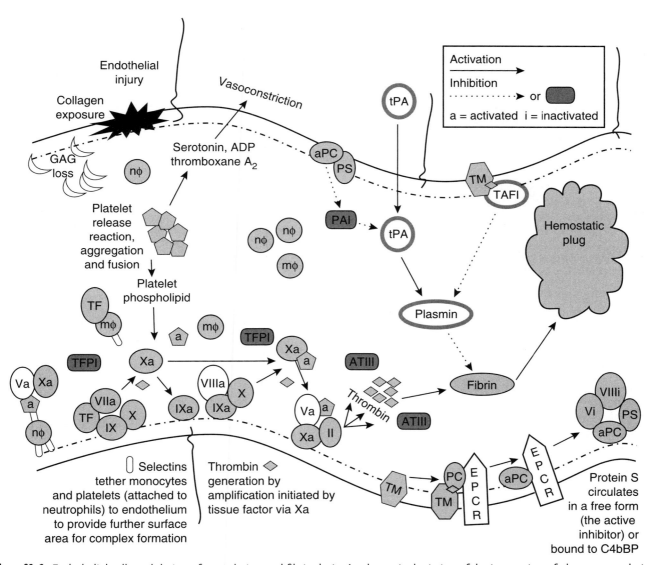

Figure 83–2. Endothelial cell modulation of coagulation and fibrinolysis. A schematic depiction of the interaction of plasma coagulation factors and blood cellular elements with endothelial cells during activation of coagulation and fibrinolysis. Coagulation factors are depicted by *Roman numerals*. ADP, adenosine diphosphate; ATIII, anti-thrombin III; EPCR, endothelial cell protein C receptor; GAG, glycosaminoglycans; mφ, monocytes; nφ, neutrophils; PAI, plasminogen activator inhibitor type 1; PC, protein C; PS, protein S; TAFI, thrombin-activateable fibrinolysis inhibitor; TF, tissue factor; TFPI, tissue factor pathway inhibitor; TM, thrombomodulin; tPA, tissue plasminogen activator. *(From Faust SN, Heyderman RS, Levin M: Coagulation in severe sepsis: A central role for thrombomodulin and activated protein C. Crit Care Med 29:S62, 2001.)*

Table 83–2. Natural Coagulation Inhibitors

Inhibitor	Action
Vitamin K–dependent	
Protein C	Inactivates factors Va, VIIIa
Protein S	Cofactor for the action of activated protein C
Protein Z	Cofactor for the inhibition of factor Xa by protein Z–dependent protease (PZI)
Non–vitamin K–dependent	
Antithrombin III	Inactivates thrombin
Tissue factor pathway inhibitor (TFPI)	Inhibits the tissue factor/ factor VIIa complex in conjunction with factor Xa

the first 3 months of life until they reach their adult values. These changes have been reviewed in detail by several authors.[16-18] In general, several general statements can be made regarding the differences in the hemostatic components in the neonate versus those in the older child and adult:

1. Platelets are found in the developing fetus as early as 5 weeks of gestation and reach the lower limit of

Table 83–3. Overview of the Factors Involved in Normal Hemostasis

Primary hemostasis
  Endothelial cells and subendothelial structures (e.g., collagen)
  Platelets
  Fibrinogen
  von Willebrand factor
  Calcium ion
Fluid-phase coagulation
  Coagulation factors, tissue factor
  Protease inhibitors
  Phospholipids (cell membrane surfaces)
  Calcium ion
Fibrinolysis
  Plasminogen
  Fibrinolytic activators
  Fibrinolytic inhibitors
Vitamin K–dependent factors
  Factors II, VII, IX, X (procoagulant)
  Proteins C, S, Z (anticoagulant)
Contact factors
  Factors XII, XI
  Prekallikrein (Fletcher factor)
  High-molecular-weight kininogen (Fitzgerald factor)
Thrombin-sensitive factors
  Fibrinogen
  Factors V, VIII, XIII

"normal" (i.e., 150,000/μL) by 15 weeks of gestation. At birth, the normal range for platelet count is identical to that for adults.

2. Platelet function is thought to be decreased in newborns, although this is not as well studied. Various studies have demonstrated a blunted response of newborn platelets to usual platelet agonists, particularly weak agonists such as adenosine diphosphate. Traditional platelet aggregation studies are difficult to perform in newborns because of the large volume of blood needed. However, measurement of activation-dependent surface receptor expression on platelets by flow-cytometric techniques has demonstrated reduced platelet activation in response to traditional agonists.

3. The bleeding time, a measure of primary hemostasis, which relies on effective interaction of platelets with damaged endothelial cells and subendothelial structures, is shorter in the newborn. This is probably a result of multiple factors such as a higher hematocrit and higher concentrations of vWF in the newborn.

4. Both the prothrombin time (PT) and activated partial thromboplastin time (aPTT) are prolonged in comparison with the normal range for these tests in older children and adults. This is caused by lower levels of several different clotting factors in newborns (Table 83–4).

5. Levels of both the contact-phase components and vitamin K–dependent procoagulant and anticoagulant proteins are low at birth and increase over the first 6 months, reaching near normal adult levels by that point. The levels of these components are proportional to gestational age; that is, they are lower in premature infants than in full-term infants. The lower levels of these clotting factors result in a reduction in thrombin generation upon activation of the clotting system.

6. In contrast to adults, in whom protein C and protein S are thought to be the major anticoagulant proteins, a study in newborns has demonstrated that α_2-macroglobulin plays a more important anticoagulant role in young children.[19]

7. Fibrinogen is found at normal adult levels in the newborn. However, some of this represents fetal fibrinogen.

8. Fetal fibrinolysis is less efficient because of the presence of fetal plasminogen at birth. The levels of plasminogen and tPA are low at birth and levels of the inhibitors of fibrinolysis (plasminogen activator type 1, α_2-antiplasmin) are elevated at birth. In addition, fetal fibrin is relatively more resistant to lysis than is adult fibrin. All of these changes make fetal clots less prone to lysis.

The net result of these differences is a dynamic balance that appears to favor clot formation in the full-term infant. However, as the gestational age of the infant decreases, the overall balance of the system shifts toward an increased risk of hemorrhage.[20,21] In addition, the balance is more tenuous and more prone to disruption in times of physiologic stress. Under steady-state conditions, the healthy newborn's hemostatic system effectively

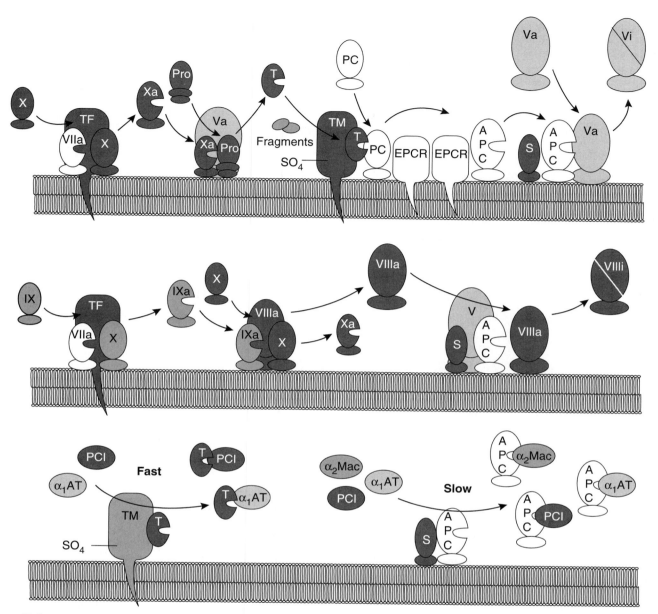

Figure 83–3. Protein C/protein S regulation of blood coagulation. **Top,** Factor VIIa (VIIa) binds to tissue factor (TF) to activate factor X (X), generating factor Xa (Xa). Factor Xa then binds to factor Va. The complex of factors Xa-Va converts prothrombin (Pro) to thrombin (T). Thrombin can then either bind to thrombomodulin (TM) on the endothelial cell surface or carry out procoagulant reactions such as fibrin formation (cleavage of fibrinogen) or platelet activation. When bound to TM, thrombin can activate protein C (PC) to activated protein C (APC). This process is enhanced when PC is bound to the endothelial cell protein C receptor (EPCR). APC bound to EPCR cleaves substrates other than factor Va. APC dissociates from EPCR and can then interact with protein S (S) to inactivate Va. **Middle,** The inactivation of the factor IXa-VIIIa complex by APC. In this case, factor V participates with APC and PS in the inactivation of factor VIIIa. **Bottom,** The plasma proteinase inhibitors that regulate the protein C activation complex and the anticoagulant complex of APC and PS are illustrated. α_1-AT, α_1-antitrypsin; α_2-Mac, α_2-macroglobulin; AT, antithrombin III; PCI, protein C inhibitor. *(From Esmon CT, Xu J, Gu J-M, et al: Endothelial protein C receptor. Thromb Haemost 82:251, 1999.)*

Table 83–4. Reference Values for Coagulation Tests in Healthy Full-Term and Premature Infants*

	Day 1	Day 5	Day 30	Adult
Test				
PT (sec)	13.0 (10.1-15.9)	12.4 (10.0-14.3)	11.8 (10.0-14.2)	12.4 (10.8-13.9)
	13.0 (10.6-16.2)	12.5 (10.0-15.3)	11.8 (10.0-14.6)	
aPTT (sec)	42.9 (31.3-54.5)	42.6 (25.4-59.8)	40.4 (32.0-55.2)	33.5 (26.2-40.3)
	53.6 (27.5-79.4)	50.5 (26.9-74.1)	44.7 (26.9-62.5)	
Fibrinogen (mg/dL)	283 (167-399)	312 (162-462)	270 (162-378)	278 (156-400)
	243 (150-373)	280 (160-418)	254 (150-414)	
Thrombin time (sec)	23.5 (19.0-28.3)	23.1 (18.0-29.2)	24.3 (19.4-29.2)	25.0 (19.7-30.3)
	24.8 (19.2-30.4)	24.1 (18.8-29.4)	24.4 (18.8-29.9)	
II (U/mL)	0.48 (0.26-0.70)	0.63 (0.33-0.93)	0.68 (0.34-1.02)	1.08 (0.70-1.46)
	0.45 (0.20-0.77)	0.57 (0.29-0.85)	0.57 (0.36-0.95)	
V (U/mL)	0.72 (0.34-1.08)	0.95 (0.45-1.45)	0.98 (0.62-1.34)	1.06 (0.62-1.50)
	0.88 (0.41-1.44)	1.00 (0.46-1.54)	1.02 (0.48-1.56)	
VII (U/mL)	0.66 (0.28-1.04)	0.89 (0.35-1.43)	0.90 (0.42-1.38)	1.05 (0.67-1.43)
	0.67 (0.21-1.13)	0.84 (0.30-1.38)	0.83 (0.21-1.45)	
VIII (U/mL)	1.00 (0.50-1.78)	0.88 (0.50-1.54)	0.91 (0.50-1.57)	0.99 (0.50-1.49)
	1.11 (0.50-2.13)	1.15 (0.53-2.05)	1.11 (0.50-1.99)	
IX (U/mL)	0.53 (0.15-0.91)	0.53 (0.15-0.91)	0.51 (0.21-0.81)	1.09 (0.55-1.63)
	0.35 (0.19-0.65)	0.42 (0.14-0.74)	0.44 (0.13-0.80)	
X (U/mL)	0.40 (0.12-0.68)	0.49 (0.19-0.79)	0.59 (0.31-0.87)	1.06 (0.70-1.52)
	0.41 (0.11-0.71)	0.51 (0.19-0.83)	0.56 (0.20-0.92)	
XI (U/mL)	0.38 (0.10-0.66)	0.55 (0.23-0.87)	0.53 (0.27-0.79)	0.97 (0.67-1.27)
	0.30 (0.08-0.52)	0.41 (0.13-0.69)	0.43 (0.15-0.71)	
XII (U/mL)	0.53 (0.13-0.93)	0.47 (0.11-0.83)	0.49 (0.17-0.81)	1.08 (0.52-1.64)
	0.38 (0.10-0.66)	0.39 (0.09-0.69)	0.43 (0.11-0.75)	
XIII (U/mL)	0.79 (0.27-1.31)	0.94 (0.44-1.44)	0.93 (0.39-1.47)	1.05 (0.55-1.55)
	0.70 (0.32-1.08)	1.01 (0.57-1.45)	0.99 (0.51-1.47)	
vWF (U/mL)	1.53 (0.50-2.87)	1.40 (0.50-2.54)	1.28 (0.50-2.46)	0.92 (0.50-1.58)
	1.36 (0.78-2.10)	1.33 (0.72-2.19)	1.36 (0.66-2.16)	
HMWK (U/mL)	0.54 (0.06-1.02)	0.74 (0.16-1.32)	0.77 (0.33-1.47)	0.92 (0.50-1.36)
	0.49 (0.09-0.89)	0.62 (0.24-1.00)	0.64 (0.16-1.12)	
PK (U/mL)	0.37 (0.18-0.69)	0.48 (0.20-0.76)	0.57 (0.23-0.91)	1.12 (0.62-1.62)
	0.33 (0.09-0.57)	0.45 (0.25-0.75)	0.59 (0.31-0.87)	
Inhibitors				
Protein C (U/mL)	0.35 (0.17-0.53)	0.42 (0.20-0.64)	0.43 (0.21-0.65)	0.96 (0.64-1.28)
	0.28 (0.12-0.44)	0.31 (0.11-0.51)	0.37 (0.15-0.59)	
Protein S (U/mL)	0.36 (0.12-0.60)	0.50 (0.22-0.78)	0.63 (0.33-0.93)	0.92 (0.60-1.24)
	0.26 (0.14-0.38)	0.37 (0.13-0.61)	0.56 (0.22-0.90)	
AT-III (U/mL)	0.63 (0.39-0.87)	0.67 (0.41-0.93)	0.78 (0.48-1.08)	1.05 (0.79-1.31)
	0.38 (0.14-0.62)	0.56 (0.30-0.82)	0.59 (0.37-0.81)	
α_2-M (U/mL)	1.39 (0.95-1.83)	1.48 (0.98-1.98)	1.50 (1.06-1.94)	0.86 (0.52-1.20)
	1.10 (0.56-1.82)	1.25 (0.71-2.04)	1.80 (1.20-2.66)	
α_1-AT (U/mL)	0.93 (0.49-1.37)	0.89 (0.49-1.29)	0.62 (0.36-0.88)	0.93 (0.55-1.31)
	0.90 (0.36-1.44)	0.94 (0.42-1.46)	0.76 (0.38-1.12)	
Fibrinolytic Components				
Plasminogen (U/mL)	1.95 (1.25-2.65)	2.17 (1.41-2.93)	1.98 (1.26-2.70)	3.36 (2.48-4.24)
	1.70 (1.12-2.48)	1.91 (1.21-2.61)	1.81 (1.09-2.53)	
tPA (ng/mL)	9.6 (5.0-18.9)	5.6 (4.0-10.0)	4.1 (1.0-5.0)	4.9 (1.4-8.4)
	8.48 (3.00-16.70)	3.97 (2.00-6.93)	4.13 (2.00-7.79)	
α_2-AP (U/mL)	0.85 (0.55-1.15)	1.00 (0.70-1.30)	1.00 (0.76-1.24)	1.02 (0.68-1.36)
	0.78 (0.40-1.16)	0.81 (0.49-1.13)	0.89 (0.55-1.23)	
PAI-1 (U/mL)	6.4 (2.0-15.1)	2.3 (0.0-8.1)	3.4 (0.0-8.8)	3.6 (0.0-11.0)
	5.4 (0.0-12.2)	2.5 (0.0-7.1)	4.3 (0.0-10.9)	

*Data in first lines are values for clotting factors expressed as U/mL with the activity being 1.0 U/mL in pooled normal plasma; data in second lines are values for healthy premature infants aged 30–36 weeks of gestation.

α_1-AT, α_1-antitrypsin; α_2-AP, α_2-antiplasmin; α_2-M, α_2-macroglobulin; aPTT, activated partial thromboplastin time; AT-III, anti-thrombin III; HMWK, high-molecular weight kininogen; PAI-1, plasminogen activator inhibitor–1; PK, prekallkrein; PT, prothrombin time; tPA, tissue plasminogen activator; vWF, von Willebrand factor.

Data from Andrew et al.[16,17]

prevents both hemorrhage and thrombosis in spite of lower levels of many clotting factors and reduced platelet reactivity. Under stress, such as infection, this balance is disrupted, and either bleeding or thrombosis can occur, depending on the nature of the changes in the hemostatic system that occur.

LABORATORY TESTING

The most common tests of the hemostatic system are the PT, aPTT, and platelet count. Although the normal range for platelet counts in the newborn is identical to that for older children and adults (150,000/mL to 400,000/mL), both the PT and aPTT are normally longer in normal newborns than in older children (see Table 83-4).[16,17] The degree of prolongation is greater in premature infants. By 6 months of postnatal age, the normal ranges for PT, aPTT, and the individual hemostasis proteins are similar to those for adults (see Table 83-4). In addition to the PT and aPTT, there are several other tests of specific components of the hemostatic system that may be useful in diagnosis and management of infants with specific abnormalities. These include tests such as specific clotting factors, fibrin and fibrinogen degradation products, fibrin D-dimer assay, and measurement of specific anticoagulant proteins (e.g., protein C, protein S, antithrombin-III). Although the template bleeding time is a useful measure of primary hemostasis, its clinical usefulness in newborns is limited, and the test is therefore infrequently used. In infants with a suspected collagen defect (e.g., Ehlers-Danlos syndrome) or with a suspected qualitative platelet defect, a prolonged template bleeding time or other measure of platelet function may be useful for confirming the suspicion and justifying more extensive and specific evaluation.[22,23] Because of the large volumes of blood normally required, traditional platelet aggregation studies and comprehensive measurements of components of the fibrinolytic system are rarely obtained in newborns. However, in selected clinical situations, it may be appropriate to obtain specific assays to confirm or refute a suspected congenital deficiency. All results of assays for specific components of hemostasis (e.g., clotting factors, natural inhibitors and anticoagulants, fibrinolytic components) must be interpreted according to gestational age and postnatal age–specific norms, because the normal ranges change with gestational age and postnatal age (see Table 83-4).

The clinician managing an infant who has a prolonged PT and/or aPTT must determine whether the prolongation is pathologic and reflects an underlying coagulopathic condition and, if so, the nature of that defect (i.e., a clotting factor deficiency or the presence of a circulating inhibitor). Because the normal values for the PT and aPTT in newborns are longer than those for older children, care must be taken to interpret prolonged values correctly. In addition, both the PT and aPTT can be falsely prolonged in newborns because of their higher hematocrit and decreased plasma volume if the amount of anticoagulant in coagulation samples (sodium citrate) is not proportionately decreased. For infants with a hematocrit exceeding 55%, the clinician should consult with the

hematology laboratory or hematologist to determine whether a nonstandard blood collection tube should be used for coagulation testing. If it is determined that an observed value for either PT or aPTT is indeed prolonged, then the clinician must determine what further testing is in order. If the cause of the prolonged PT or aPTT is a deficiency of a specific clotting factor, the PT (or aPTT) corrects to normal if patient plasma is mixed with an equal part of normal plasma (a so-called PT [or aPTT] mixing study, or "inhibitor screen"). If the prolonged PT (or aPTT) is the result of the presence of a circulating inhibitor, then the PT (or aPTT) does not correct to normal upon mixing with normal plasma. Although lupus (or lupus-like) anticoagulants are a common cause of acquired prolongation of PT or aPTT in older children,[24] there are no data regarding the incidence of lupus anticoagulants in newborns. Consequently, the finding of an abnormal PT (or aPTT) mixing study in a newborn should prompt the clinician to consider the development of a consumptive coagulopathy, because fibrin degradation products can interfere with clot formation and produce a prolongation of the PT and/or aPTT. If the mixing study result is negative (i.e., a normal value for the PT or aPTT), then the likely cause of the prolonged PT or aPTT is the deficiency of one or more clotting factors. Subsequent investigations should then be determined by the clinical setting. A family history of affected male members of the mother's family is suggestive of an X-linked disorder, and a prolonged aPTT should be further investigated with measurement of factor VIII or factor IX. An isolated prolongation of PT points toward a decrease in factor VII, and prolongation of both PT and aPTT are suggestive of a decrease in multiple clotting factors (e.g., vitamin K deficiency) or a decrease in an element in the "common pathway" (e.g., factors X, V, or II; fibrinogen).

BLEEDING DISORDERS

Congenital Coagulopathies

Hemophilia A

The most common inherited clotting factor deficiency is hemophilia A, or factor VIII deficiency, with an incidence of 1 per 10,000. This is an X-linked recessive disorder. Prenatal diagnosis of factor VIII deficiency is possible, inasmuch as factor VIII coagulant activity can be detected in fetal plasma by the end of the first trimester.[18] In healthy full-term infants, the normal range for factor VIII levels is similar to that for older children and adults, whereas the level is much lower in premature infants and fetuses (see Table 83-4). Consequently, it may be difficult to make a diagnosis of mild to moderate hemophilia A by testing plasma factor VIII activity in very premature infants. Infants with hemophilia A and other congenital coagulopathies generally present with cephalohematoma or gastrointestinal bleeding and are at risk for bleeding during circumcision or for deep muscle bleeding at the site of vitamin K prophylaxis injections. Intracranial or intraventricular hemorrhage is a relatively uncommon event,[25-27] but the occurrence of an intracranial hemorrhage in a newborn should prompt the clinician to consider the possibility of an underlying coagulopathy. Consequently, even in the absence of a suggestive family history, a diagnosis of hemophilia should be considered and investigated with appropriate studies.[28] A diagnosis of factor VIII deficiency should be suspected in an otherwise healthy newborn boy who has bleeding, a prolonged aPTT, and a family history of a documented or suspected bleeding disorder in male members of his mother's family. Confirmation of the diagnosis is provided by demonstration of a decreased plasma factor VIII activity. Carrier detection by plasma factor VIII activity measurement in the immediate prepartum or postpartum woman is unreliable because maternal factor VIII levels increase to as high as 200% of normal by the end of pregnancy and remain so for a few weeks postpartum.[29] Newer molecular techniques have proved to be reliable and accurate for carrier detection in broad populations and are now the methods of choice.[30]

Hemophilia B

Hemophilia B, or factor IX deficiency, is the second most common inherited clotting factor deficiency, with an incidence 10% of that for hemophilia A (1 per 100,000). Factor IX deficiency is also an X-linked recessive disorder, and a history of affected male members of the mother's family should alert the clinician to the possibility of factor IX deficiency in a bleeding newborn boy. In contrast to factor VIII, for which the normal newborn level is elevated in full-term neonates, the levels of factor IX and other vitamin K–dependent clotting factors are quite low at birth in comparison with adult norms (mean = approximately 50% in full-term infants and approximately 35% in premature infants; see Table 83-4). This normal reduction in factor IX levels at birth makes detection of mild to moderate deficiencies difficult. Bleeding manifestations in infants with factor IX deficiency are similar to those noted for factor VIII deficiency.

Other Inherited Coagulopathies

Hemophilia C (factor XI deficiency) is most commonly seen in children of Ashkenazi Jewish ancestry[31] and has a frequency of 1 per 100,000. It is inherited in an autosomal recessive pattern. Bleeding manifestations are generally milder than those seen with either factor VIII or factor IX deficiency and are not necessarily correlated with the degree of factor deficiency. Normal newborn levels of factor XI are low, which hampers neonatal diagnosis based on plasma activity for mild to moderate deficiency. Deficiencies of factor V and factor VII result in severe bleeding in the newborn, because of the central role in hemostasis played by these factors. A homozygous deficiency of factor VII has never been documented and probably results in fetal demise. Deficiencies of factor XIII are rare (approximately 200 cases since 1960) and are characterized by levels of less than 1%. Homozygous deficiency results in a moderate to severe bleeding diathesis that is characterized in the neonatal period by bleeding from the umbilical stump. Initial clot formation proceeds normally, but the tensile strength of the clot is poor because of the lack of factor XIIIa–catalyzed crosslinking. The aPTT is normal in this disorder. Factor XIII deficiency is suggested by late bleeding and delayed cord separation.

Therapy for Congenital Coagulopathies

In circumstances in which the deficiency of a specific clotting factor is known (e.g., a son of a known hemophilia A carrier), treatment with clotting factor concentrate should be initiated for the treatment of bleeding or for prophylaxis before surgery or an invasive procedure. Currently, clotting factor concentrates are readily available for factors VIII, IX, and VII. In addition, concentrates for fibrinogen and factor XIII are available in Europe and can be obtained for patients in the United States. Concentrates for the natural anticoagulants protein C and antithrombin-III are also available for treatment of children with deficiencies of these proteins. The factor concentrate therapy most commonly employed in clinical practice remains infusion of factor VIII and factor IX concentrates.

Factor VIII. These are available in low-, intermediate-, and high-purity concentrates. Low-purity concentrates are derived from pooled plasma and undergo heat and/or solvent-detergent treatment to inactivate contaminating viruses. In general, the factor VIII comprises a distinct minority of the proteins in these products. Intermediate-purity concentrates are also derived from pooled plasma, but the factor VIII is removed from the plasma by affinity chromatography. This results in a much lower amount of contaminating plasma proteins. Again, these products undergo several steps to inactivate contaminating viruses. High-purity concentrates are produced by recombinant technology, and although they have no contaminating plasma proteins, many of these products have human albumin added as a stabilizer. The risk of viral transmission with these products is thought to be essentially zero. Irrespective of the type of the product, the pharmacokinetics of the transfused factor VIII remains virtually the same. In general, transfusion of 1 U of factor VIII per kilogram of body weight results in an increase in plasma factor VIII activity of 2%. The half-life in vivo of the transfused factor VIII is approximately 12 hours. Using these parameters, the clinician can plan a rational transfusion program for a patient with factor VIII deficiency. The amount of factor VIII transfused is determined directly according to the severity of the bleeding observed or anticipated. For minor bleeds (e.g., soft tissue bleeds in a noncritical area), the goal is a factor VIII activity level of 20% to 40%; for moderate bleeds (e.g., joint, more serious soft tissue bleeds), 40% to 50%; for more serious bleeds (e.g., postoperative bleeding, bleeding in organs or major joints), approximately 80%; and for life-threatening bleeds, 100% (Table 83-5). In the initial phases of treatment, infusions are given every 12 hours; later, once-daily infusions may be administered for less serious bleeding episodes.

Factor IX. Factor IX concentrates are available as recombinant, high-purity concentrates and as a component in "prothrombin complex" concentrates (i.e., concentrates of factors II, VII, IX, and X; the vitamin K–dependent clotting factors). Again, the plasma-derived products also contain a large amount of contaminating plasma proteins and undergo viral inactivation steps.

Table 83–5. Factor VIII And Factor IX Replacement Guidelines

Indication for Therapy	Factor VIII		Factor IX	
	Desired Level (%)	Dosage (U/kg)	Desired Level (%)	Dosage (U/kg)
Mild bleeding (e.g., epistaxis, hematuria)	30	15	20	20
Moderate bleeding (e.g., hemarthrosis, potential airway obstruction, abdominal trauma/pain, head injury without neurologic findings)	50	25	40	40
Severe bleeding (e.g, major trauma, active gastrointestinal bleeding, postoperative bleeding, limb or organ-threatening bleeding)	80	40	60	60
Life-threatening bleeding (e.g., airway obstruction, intracranial bleeding)	100	50	80-100	80-100

Infusion of 1 U of factor IX per kilogram of body weight increases the plasma factor IX level by 1%. The half-life of factor IX is approximately 24 hours, which allows for once-daily infusions in patients with hemophilia B (factor IX deficiency). As with factor VIII replacement therapy, the target level of factor IX to be achieved is proportional to the severity of bleeding or anticipated bleeding (see Table 83-5).

Choice of Clotting Factor Preparation

Although low-purity clotting factors are safe and effective, most newborns in whom either factor VIII or factor IX deficiency is diagnosed are treated with either recombinant factor or plasma factor purified by affinity chromatography because of the decreased risk of viral transmission. Patients with unidentified deficiencies or with deficiencies of clotting factors for which factor concentrates are not available must be treated with fresh-frozen plasma. A new solvent-detergent–treated fresh-frozen plasma preparation that will further reduce the risk of viral transmission through transfusion has been developed.[32]

Acquired Coagulopathies

Disseminated intravascular coagulation (DIC) is a consumptive coagulopathy in which bleeding results from the consumption of clotting factors and platelets. Initially, DIC is characterized by microvascular thrombosis, but with continued activation of coagulation and subsequently fibrinolysis, platelets and clotting factors are consumed beyond the infant's ability to replace them. Consequently, the deficiency of platelets, fibrinogen and other clotting factors (e.g., factor VIII) produces a bleeding diathesis. The key element here is the generation of "excess" amounts of thrombin and an imbalance between the need for clot formation and fibrinolytic activity.[33] Early in DIC, both PT and aPTT may be normal; however, there is a demonstrable decrease in fibrinogen and platelets.[34,35] Amounts of fibrinogen degradation products and, more specifically, D-dimer fragments are elevated in DIC. Fibrinogen degradation products (also know as fibrin split products) are a family of proteolytic fragments

of fibrinogen and are not specific for DIC. In contrast, D-dimer fragments require the action of thrombin on fibrinogen to first produce fibrin (from fibrinogen) and then the action of plasmin (also produced by the action of thrombin on plasminogen) for their production. Consequently, an elevation in D-dimer is believed to be more specific for a diagnosis of DIC.[36] However, because of the lower fibrinogen levels in infants with very low birth weights, the diagnostic criteria for DIC are somewhat different.[37]

DIC is not a primary disease but rather represents the end result on the coagulation system of several different disease processes (Table 83-6). In newborns, the most common causes of DIC are sepsis, severe respiratory distress syndrome, asphyxia, and necrotizing enterocolitis. The treatment of choice for DIC is the treatment of the underlying process. However, because of bleeding or the risk of bleeding, some degree of hematologic support may be required while the underlying process is treated. Because DIC is characterized by consumption of platelets, clotting factors, and red blood cells (microangiopathic hemolytic anemia), transfusion support of all of these elements may be necessary. Although there is a theoretical concern that transfusion of blood products (particularly platelets and plasma) may provide "fuel for the fire" and worsen or prolong the process, there is no documentation of such occurrences, and consequently I believe that it is inappropriate to withhold necessary transfusions. Platelets should be transfused for platelet counts below 30,000/μL to 40,000/μL, and fresh-frozen plasma should be given for marked prolongations of the PT and/or aPTT (e.g., >4-second prolongation of the PT, >8-second prolongation of aPTT). If plasma fibrinogen is markedly reduced (e.g., <75 to 100 mg/dL), the clinician can consider initial transfusion with cryoprecipitate, which is much richer in fibrinogen than is an equal volume of fresh-frozen plasma (Table 83-7).

Vitamin K deficiency results in a decrease in the vitamin K–dependent clotting factors (factors II, VII, IX, and X), all of which are produced in the liver. Consequently, severe liver disease produces a clotting factor picture

Table 83–6. Causes of Disseminated Intravascular Coagulation in the Newborn

Pregnancy-and obstetric-related causes
    Abruptio placentae
    Preeclampsia and eclampsia
    Dead twin fetus
    Fetal distress during labor (nonspecific)
    Breech delivery (with hypoxia)
Respiratory distress syndrome
    Idiopathic
    Aspiration related
    Pneumonia/infection related
    Pulmonary hemorrhage
Infection/sepsis
    Bacterial: gram-positive or gram-negative
    Viral: herpes, Coxsackie, echovirus, cytomegalovirus, rubella
    Congenital toxoplasmosis
    Congenital syphilis
Other
    Hemolytic transfusion reaction
    Massive hemolysis (e.g., erythroblastosis fetalis)
    Necrotizing enterocolitis
    Giant hemangioma (Kasabach-Merritt syndrome)
    Renal vein thrombosis
    Scleroderma neonatorum
Possible causes
    Purpura fulminans
    Hyperviscosity
    Intracranial hemorrhage

Table 83–7. Blood Product Components

Whole blood	Contains all components in blood (cellular and protein)
Packed RBCs	Contains RBCs with little residual plasma and plasma proteins
	Not adequate for replacement of deficient clotting proteins or platelets
Fresh-frozen plasma	Contains all clotting proteins and other plasma proteins
	Should be used to correct known or suspected coagulopathies when a specific clotting factor concentrate is not available, or when the cause of the coagulopathy is not known
	Should not be used simply for "volume resuscitation"
Cryoprecipitate	Contains fibrinogen, Factor VIII/vWF, IgM, fibronectin
	Should be used to replace fibrinogen
	Can be used to replace Factor VIII or vWF in small infants if factor concentrates are not desirable
	Derived from individual donors and is not treated to remove or inactivate viruses

IgM, immunoglobulin M; RBCs, red blood cells; vWF, von Willebrand factor.

similar to that of vitamin K deficiency, with the added decrease in factor V in prolonged severe disease. Newborns have virtually no stores of vitamin K and consequently are at risk for the development of deficiencies of the vitamin K–dependent clotting factors in the first several days after birth. Classic hemorrhagic disease of the newborn, now referred to as vitamin K deficiency bleeding, results from vitamin K deficiency and manifests with ecchymosis, gastrointestinal bleeding, and, at times, intracranial hemorrhage occurring between 2 and 5 days of age.[38,39] This syndrome has essentially disappeared in developed countries because of the administration of parenteral vitamin K in the delivery room.[40] In developing countries, oral vitamin K has been used because of the ease of administration. The efficacy of oral therapy may be less complete because of variable gastrointestinal absorption of the currently available oral preparations of vitamin K. Although a single dose of oral vitamin K has been demonstrated to correct the biochemical abnormalities in the newborn's clotting system, its effect on clinical bleeding has not been studied.[39,40] Multiple oral doses of vitamin K (e.g., three doses of 2 mg) appears to be as effective as a single intramuscular dose of 1 mg.[40] Prenatal administration of vitamin K to the mother has not been shown to reduce the incidence of periventricular hemorrhage in preterm infants.[41] Some countries have moved toward the use of oral rather than parenteral vitamin K prophylaxis out of concern that parenteral vitamin K administration may be associated with an increased incidence of childhood malignancies. Although a conclusive association is yet to be determined, current studies do not seem to support this concern.[42]

Early-onset hemorrhagic disease resulting from vitamin K deficiency is usually secondary to maternal ingestion of drugs such as warfarin, phenobarbital, phenytoin, rifampin, and isoniazid.[43] Late-onset disease (after the first week after birth) is generally the result of conditions associated with decreased absorption of vitamin K from the gastrointestinal tract or possibly a result of prolonged use of broad-spectrum antibiotics. With near-universal administration of parenteral (intramuscular) vitamin K and recognition of the effect that maternal drug administration has on newborns and the fetus, late-onset vitamin K deficiency is much more commonly seen than either early or classic manifestations. In mild or early disease, the first abnormality is an isolated prolongation of the PT as a result of the short half-life of factor VII (approximately 6 hours). In later or more severe disease, the aPTT becomes progressively prolonged as levels of factor IX (half-life = 24 hours), factor X (48 hours), and factor II (72 to 96 hours) decrease.

Treatment of vitamin K deficiency is (1) replacement of vitamin K in newborns who present with prolongation of PT (with or without prolongation of aPTT) but without bleeding or (2) infusion of fresh-frozen plasma in infants with bleeding.

QUANTITATIVE AND QUALITATIVE PLATELET ABNORMALITIES

The normal range for platelets in third-trimester fetuses and full-term newborns is essentially identical to that for older children and adults ($150,000/\mu L$ to $400,000/\mu L$). However, platelets of newborns have been shown to be less responsive than those of older children.[44-48] Although some of the documented platelet hyporesponsiveness is caused by intrinsic abnormalities of platelet activation pathways,[48,49] other factors such as maternal preeclampsia and neonatal vWF abnormalities also contribute to neonatal platelet dysfunction.[50,51]

Qualitative Platelet Defects

Although not strictly a platelet abnormality, a deficiency or structural abnormality of vWF results in an abnormality of primary hemostasis with reduced platelet adhesion to endothelial cells and subendothelial structures. Von Willebrand disease (vWD) is the most common inherited bleeding disorder, with a frequency estimated to be from 1 per 100 to 1 per 10 in the general population and with both autosomal dominant and autosomal recessive inheritance patterns.[52,53] vWF is a multimeric glycoprotein that binds to specific receptors on platelets and endothelial cells that modulate platelet adhesion. The higher molecular weight forms of vWF are more hemostatically active, and variant forms of vWD (type II defects) are characterized by abnormalities of the vWF multimeric profile or subunit structure. vWF circulates bound to factor VIII and serves to protect it from proteolysis. In addition, a separate pool of vWF is also found on and within platelets and is available to participate in platelet adhesion.[54] Patients with vWD present with mucocutaneous bleeding and frequently have a prolonged aPTT and template bleeding time. The prolongation of the template bleeding time is a direct consequence of the reduction in platelet adhesion caused by the abnormality of vWF, whereas the prolonged aPTT results from decreased levels of factor VIII, caused by proteolysis of factor VIII. Some patients with type IIB vWD may present with thrombocytopenia in early infancy.[55] Diagnosis of mild to moderate disease is difficult in newborns, because the normal range for vWF in newborns is up to 250% of normal adult levels.[16,17] This physiologic increase in vWF in the newborn helps to explain the relative paucity of bleeding manifestations that infants with mild to moderate disease exhibit.

Patients with severe (type III) vWD have extremely low levels of both vWF and factor VIII (generally <1% to 2%) and exhibit bleeding as a consequence of both platelet dysfunction (mucocutaneous bleeding) and a fluid-phase coagulopathy (deep tissue and visceral bleeding). Treatment of vWD in the newborn is by transfusion of cryoprecipitate (10 to 15 mL/kg body weight) or the infusion of factor VIII concentrate known to contain high-molecular-weight vWF; currently, only two antihemophiliac factor VIII preparations (Humate-P and Alphanate) contain sufficient amounts of high-molecular-weight vWF to be hemostatically effective in vWD. When one of these factor VIII concentrates is infused, dosage is determined either by factor VIII units, assuming a 1:1 ratio of factor VIII activity to vWF activity unit (ristocetin cofactor activity unit) (see earlier section on factor VIII deficiency treatment), or by ristocetin cofactor units (infusion of 1 U/kg of body weight increases plasma vWF activity by 1%). Cryoprecipitate has the advantage of exposing the infant to only one donor but is not treated to minimize viral transmission, whereas the factor VIII concentrates have the advantage of decreased risk of viral transmission but expose the infant to multiple (thousands) of donors. Approximately 80% of patients with type I vWD respond to infusions of desmopressin (DDAVP) with an increase in plasma vWF levels. DDAVP is a synthetic deaminated analogue of arginine vasopressin that possesses no vasopressor activity.[56] Although there is no reason to doubt effectiveness of this agent in newborns, its efficacy has not been studied in this population. Repeated infusions of DDAVP result in tachyphylaxis in approximately 50% of patients and carry a risk of hyponatremia secondary to decreased urine production. This hyponatremia has been associated with seizures in rare cases.[57]

Congenital defects of platelet function are rare and are generally suggested by family history. The more serious abnormalities are characterized by deficiencies of specific receptors on the platelet surface (e.g., glycoprotein IIb/IIIa in Glanzmann thrombasthenia, glycoprotein Ib/IX in Bernard-Soulier syndrome) and are treated by platelet transfusions. For a detailed description of these disorders, the reader is referred to specific reviews.[58] Patients with qualitative platelet defects exhibit a prolongation of bleeding time without abnormalities of either the PT or aPTT.

Acquired abnormalities of platelet function occur in renal insufficiency (uremia) and as a consequence of exposure to certain drugs such as those that impair prostaglandin synthesis (e.g., acetylsalicylic acid, indomethacin, prostaglandin E_1). Uremia is best treated by dialysis, although cryoprecipitate transfusions (10 to 15 mL/kg) and intravenous DDAVP are also therapeutic. Infusions of DDAVP ($0.3\ \mu g/kg$) result in decreased bleeding in uremia by a mechanism that probably involves both vWF and a direct effect on platelets.[59,60]

Quantitative Platelet Disorders

Although thrombocytosis can occur as a response to infection, asphyxia, respiratory distress syndrome, or other conditions associated with inflammation, the increase in platelet count rarely causes clinical problems. Thrombocytosis by itself does not appear to be a strong risk factor for thrombosis; consequently, antiplatelet therapy is not indicated unless an infant has symptoms of vascular occlusion. Of more importance clinically are conditions that result in significant thrombocytopenia. The incidence of thrombocytopenia (platelet count $< 150,000/\mu L$) in healthy full-term newborn infants has been estimated to be somewhat less than 1% in several large series,[61-67] although the incidence increases to almost 20% in preterm infants.[61] However, the incidence of thrombocytopenia in infants admitted to NICUs has been estimated to be 22%, irrespective of the gestational age of the infant.[4] Conditions associated with the development of thrombocytopenia in the NICU include sepsis, respiratory distress syndrome, asphyxia, maternal eclampsia/preeclampsia, and DIC. DIC is shown to be the cause for thrombocytopenia in 20% to 25% of thrombocytopenic infants.[4] The cause of the thrombocytopenia in these conditions is primarily nonimmunologic in nature. However, immune-mediated platelet clearance with resulting thrombocytopenia can occur in newborns even though their ability to produce their own immunoglobulin G (IgG) is greatly blunted at birth. True idiopathic thrombocytopenic purpura (ITP) is believed not to occur in newborn infants because of their inability to make IgG antibody. However, immune-mediated platelet destruction can and does occur in newborns, the source of the antiplatelet antibody being the mother. Bone marrow failure syndromes can also produce congenital thrombocytopenia.

The clinician must attempt to distinguish between the possible causes of neonatal thrombocytopenia because the management may be quite different. Studies of plasma thrombopoietin, glycocalicin (cleavage product of platelet glycoprotein Ib/IX), and in vitro megakaryocyte progenitor culture have yielded laboratory confirmation of conditions producing congenital thrombocytopenia as a result of decreased platelet production (elevated thrombopoietin, reduced glycocalicin, decreased megakaryocyte growth) from those resulting from increased platelet turnover (normal thrombopoietin, normal to elevated glycocalicin, normal megakaryocyte growth).[68-70] However, these tests are currently all research in nature and not readily available to the clinician for clinical decision making. Consequently, the clinician must make a "best guess" as to the cause of the thrombocytopenia on the basis of immediately available information. Because thrombocytopenia secondary to increased platelet destruction is much more common than that caused by decreased platelet production, the clinician should always look for conditions that may result in increased platelet destruction (Table 83-8). Prenatal and maternal histories may be helpful in this regard (e.g., family history, maternal drug ingestion or infection, preeclampsia, maternal ITP or systemic lupus erythematosus), and investigation into maternal history may be necessary in order to fully explore the possible causes of thrombocytopenia in a newborn. In situations in which the cause of

the thrombocytopenia cannot be determined readily, a therapeutic/diagnostic platelet transfusion may be indicated. If the cause of the thrombocytopenia is increased platelet destruction, an attenuated platelet increment and a rapid decrease in platelet count would be expected. In order to determine this, the clinician should check an immediate post-transfusion platelet count (i.e., 15 to 30 minutes) with follow-up platelet counts at 1, 6, 12, and 24 hours after transfusion. From these data, the clinician can get a sense of the survival of the transfused platelets; a normal length of survival (i.e., a return to baseline levels 24 hours or more after transfusion) would point toward a decrease in platelet production, whereas a markedly shortened survival would point toward increased platelet destruction. A substantial increase over baseline platelet count would not be expected 24 hours after transfusion of platelets in conditions characterized by increased platelet destruction.

Thrombocytopenia Caused by Increased Platelet Turnover

Neonatal alloimmune thrombocytopenia (NAIT) is the platelet equivalent to Rh disease of the newborn. In this condition, the pregnant mother is sensitized to antigens on the fetus' platelets not expressed on her own platelets through an early fetal-to-maternal hemorrhage or at the time of a prior delivery. The mother makes an IgG antiplatelet antibody that crosses the placenta and attacks the fetus' platelets. Many infants affected by NAIT are born severely thrombocytopenic (platelet counts < 50,000/μL) and are at risk for intrapartum bleeding, including intracranial bleeding. In some cases, severe bleeding events can occur before labor and result in fetal loss or neurologic compromise of the newborn.[71,72] Subsequent pregnancies generally result in increasingly severe thrombocytopenia in the infants. Although the Pl^{A1} antigen is most commonly associated with NAIT (father and infant Pl^{A1}-positive, mother Pl^{A1}-negative), several other platelet antigens have been associated with the development of NAIT (Table 83-9). Treatment for NAIT is best if given to the fetus before delivery. The general guidelines include intravenous immune globulin (IVIG) (1 g/kg body weight) infused once weekly to the mother for the last 6 to 8 weeks before delivery, followed by an elective cesarean section.

Table 83-8. Causes of Thrombocytopenia in the Neonate

Increased Destruction

Sepsis
Disseminated intravascular coagulation
Asphyxial respiratory distress syndrome
Maternal preeclampsia/eclampsia
Neonatal alloimmune thrombocytopenia
Maternal idiopathic thrombocytopenic purpura
Drugs (e.g., heparin)
Wiskott-Aldrich syndrome

Decreased Production

Congenital infection (e.g., rubella, toxoplasmosis)
Intrauterine growth restriction
Marrow failure syndromes
    Thrombocytopenia with absent radii
    Fanconi anemia
    Amegakaryocytic thrombocytopenia

Table 83-9. Platelet Antigens in Neonatal Alloimmune Thrombocytopenia

Antigen	Alleles	Frequency	Site
$Pl^A(Zw^A)$	1(a)/2(b)	.98/.28	GP IIa
Pl^E	1/2	>.99/.4	GP Ib
Bak (Lek)	a/b	.91/—	GP IIbα
Pen (Yuk)	a(b)/b(a)	>.99/.017	GP IIIa
Br (Zv)	a	.21	GP Ia/IIa
Pl^T	1	.99	GP V
K_O	a/b	.15/.99	Undetermined

GP, glycoprotein.

Corticosteroids (dexamethasone, 4 mg/day orally) for the last 10 days before delivery may also help increase the infant's platelet count. There is some controversy regarding the need for a cesarean section in all cases, but no randomized data exist to answer this question. Infants with suspected or confirmed NAIT can be treated with IVIG (1 to 2 g/kg total in two to five divided doses) and may receive platelet transfusions for clinically significant bleeding. Platelets lacking the target antigen must be used for transfusion. However, if the antigenic determinant against which the antiplatelet antibody is directed is not known, maternal platelets should be transfused.[72,73]

Maternal ITP or other conditions associated with maternal antiplatelet antibody production (e.g., systemic lupus erythematosus) can also result in thrombocytopenia in the newborn.[74-76] However, in contrast to NAIT, the risk of delivering a child with a platelet count of less than 50,000/μL is very low, and these infants do not appear to have an increased risk of perinatal bleeding.[77,78] In general, no special prepartum management is required when maternal ITP is thought to be the cause of neonatal thrombocytopenia. However, if the infant exhibits bleeding in the neonatal period or has a significant thrombocytopenia that is thought to predispose the infant to an increased risk of bleeding (e.g., <30,000/μL), then therapy with IVIG should be considered (see discussion of NAIT treatment).

Wiskott-Aldrich syndrome is an X-linked disorder characterized by eczema, variable immune defects, and thrombocytopenia.[79] The inheritance pattern of this disease has been called into question, because affected girls and women have been described with Wiskott-Aldrich syndrome. The thrombocytopenia is thought to be caused by increased platelet turnover, inasmuch as platelets from affected children have a markedly increased amount of platelet-associated IgG and the thrombocytopenia is greatly ameliorated by splenectomy.[79] However, in contrast to other conditions characterized by increased platelet destruction and turnover in which the mean platelet volume is increased, the mean platelet volume in these patients is extremely low. The reason for this is not clear, although loss of platelet membrane may play a role.

Maternal preeclampsia and eclampsia and the syndrome of hemolysis, elevated liver enzyme levels, and low platelet levels (HELLP) can also produce thrombocytopenia in the infant.[80] The degree of thrombocytopenia is variable and is at times clinically significant (i.e., platelet count < 50,000/μL). The thrombocytopenia is generally self-limited showing improvement by 3 days of age. Treatment is supportive.

Thrombocytopenia Caused by Decreased Platelet Production

Thrombocytopenia can also be secondary to decreased platelet production as a result of a bone marrow failure syndrome, intrauterine infection (e.g., rubella, cytomegalovirus) or drug-induced myelosuppression.[80-83] Bone marrow failure syndromes that can manifest with thrombocytopenia include the syndrome of thrombocytopenia with absent radii (TAR syndrome), amegakaryocytic thrombocytopenia, and Fanconi anemia.

The syndrome of **thrombocytopenia with absent radii** is an autosomal recessive disorder characterized by an isolated defect in platelet production.[84] The exact nature of the defect is unknown. These patients have characteristic skeletal anomalies of absent radii, short stature, and bowing of the tibia. Although the presence of thumbs easily distinguishes these patients from those with Fanconi anemia, the thumbs can be hypoplastic. Also, in contrast to Fanconi anemia, the marrow dysfunction does not progress to involve other cell lines, and there is no increased incidence of acute leukemia. Platelet counts of less than 30,000/μL are not uncommon at birth but slowly increase after the first year of life and may reach near-normal levels by adolescence. Therapy is supportive, with platelet transfusions to minimize the risk of severe bleeding. Although some patients receive regular prophylactic platelet transfusions, these should in general be restricted to episodes of bleeding or to support surgical procedures. Therapy with thrombopoietin is likely to be ineffective.[85]

Amegakaryocytic thrombocytopenia is an autosomal recessive or X-linked disorder characterized by an absence of marrow megakaryocytes.[82,83] The marrow defect is restricted to megakaryocytes; other cell lines are uninvolved. The thrombocytopenia in this disorder is profound and permanent. Progression to marrow aplasia or to acute leukemia does not occur. Therapy is supportive. These patients do not respond to thrombopoietin, and the only curative therapy is hematopoietic stem cell transplantation.

Fanconi anemia is a rare autosomal recessive disorder with a complex inheritance pattern.[82,83,86] Although anemia is the most common presenting hematologic abnormality, affected patients may present with any isolated hematologic cytopenia and may present at birth. Ultimately, the marrow dysfunction progresses to either marrow aplasia or acute leukemia. In general, the earlier the hematologic presentation, the more likely is the progression to acute leukemia. The defect in Fanconi anemia is a defect in DNA repair; affected patients exhibit increased chromosomal breaks on karyotypes grown under conditions of oxidative stress (e.g., diepoxybutane, mitomycin C). In heterozygous persons, the number of chromosomal breaks is halfway between those of normal persons and those of affected individuals. Several of the genes involved in this disorder have been cloned, which raises the possibility of gene-based diagnosis.[86] Hematopoietic stem cell transplantation may be curative. If the stem cell source is a related donor (i.e., sibling, parent), then the donor must be screened for the presence of the disease. Fifty percent of individuals with Fanconi anemia have a somatic abnormality; skeletal (e.g., short stature, hypoplastic or absent thumbs) and genitourinary abnormalities are the most common.[82,83] Therapy in the NICU is supportive.

Historically, neonates have been supported with platelet transfusions at a threshold higher than that generally employed for older children and adults. For "healthy" newborns, a platelet count of less than 30,000/μL has been used to justify "prophylactic" platelet transfusions, whereas 50,000/μL has generally been used for infants with prior intracranial hemorrhages or other high-risk features (e.g., mechanical ventilation, sepsis). The data supporting these thresholds are limited, and a retrospective analysis suggested that use of these thresholds probably results in unnecessary transfusions.[87,88]

CHOICE OF THE ROUTE OF DELIVERY FOR FETUS WITH KNOWN OR SUSPECTED HEMOSTATIC ABNORMALITIES

There is no clear consensus among obstetricians, neonatologists, or hematologists regarding the mode of delivery of a fetus with a known or suspected/anticipated hemostatic defect. For most conditions, there are no practice data, whereas for others (e.g., pregnancy in hemophilia carriers), survey data indicate the absence of consensus among obstetricians, neonatologists, and hematologists.[89] What few data available suggest is that delivery by cesarean section alters the levels of some of the intrinsic inhibitors of coagulation (i.e., protein C, antithrombin III) in such way that clot formation is favored.[90] Elective cesarean section before the initiation of labor is also thought to reduce the risk of pressure stress on the fetal cranial structures, and, consequently, many clinicians prefer this mode of delivery for at-risk infants. Indeed, elective cesarean section does appear to reduce the incidence of intraventricular hemorrhage in thrombocytopenic infants with very low birth weights.[91] However, there are no data to support an opinion that cesarean delivery is safer than an uncomplicated vaginal delivery for infants with known or suspected coagulopathy. Two surveys monitoring the incidence of intraventricular hemorrhage in normal full-term deliveries produced conflicting results regarding the relative safety of cesarean section over vaginal delivery.[92,93] In view of the risk of severe thrombocytopenia, elective cesarean section is the generally preferred route of delivery for infants with possible NAIT. This is not the case for infants whose mothers have ITP or gestational thrombocytopenia, because the risk of severe neonatal thrombocytopenia is very low.[94] Because of the general lack of data and the fact that in most cases the hemostatic abnormalities in the fetus are only suspected, I believe that reserving elective cesarean section for infants most at risk (e.g., known male fetus of an obligate hemophilia A or B carrier, infants born to mothers with severe vWD or a history of NAIT) is appropriate. However, the reader must be aware that this recommendation represents an opinion based on personal practice and not data or consensus. A survey of pediatric hematologists points out this lack of consensus in regard to the perinatal management of infants with suspected or possible hemophilia.[95] The respondents indicated no preference for either vaginal or caesarean delivery, and most would obtain cranial imaging on the newborn (59%) even in the absence of symptoms. In addition, 22% would prophylactically infuse the infant with clotting factor concentrate at birth. The obstetric literature is also without consensus on this issue, although there is general agreement that forceps and vacuum-assisted deliveries carry a higher risk for these infants.[96]

THROMBOTIC ABNORMALITIES

Thromboembolic phenomena are being diagnosed in the NICU with increasing frequency as a result of the increased use of umbilical catheters and better modes of detection.[2,3,97-99] The role that inherited abnormalities of

Table 83–10. Prothrombotic Abnormalities

Protein C deficiency
Protein S deficiency
Antithrombin III deficiency
Factor V Leiden
Prothrombin 20210 mutation
Hyperhomocysteinemia (methylenetetrahydrofolate reductase thermolabile variant)
Dysfibrinogenemia with elevated fibrinogen
Lipoprotein (a) elevation (> 30 mg/dL)
Lupus anticoagulants/antiphospholipid antibodies

hemostasis that produce a "prothrombotic" environment play in neonatal thrombosis has recently been studied. In several series, a majority of neonates with perinatal stroke have been shown to possess one of the described prothrombic disorders (Table 83-10).[100-102] In a cohort of 62 infants with perinatal stroke reported by Gunther and associates, patients were documented to have protein C deficiency, the factor V Leiden mutation (G1691A), the prothrombin G20210A variant, the MTHFR TT677 genotype (thermolabile variant) or an increased level of lipoprotein (a) in comparison to normal infants.[100] Similar results were previously reported by Vielhaber and coworkers[101] and deVeber and colleagues.[102] The risk of recurrent stroke in these infants is low, which suggests that the inherited prothrombotic defect in the context of the neonatal coagulation environment is important in the initiation of the vascular occlusive event.[103-105] In addition, prothrombotic defects may be associated with intrauterine growth restriction and with smallness for gestational age in the absence of overt prenatal strokes.[106]

Congenital heterozygous protein C deficiency produces a distinct syndrome in neonates known as **purpura fulminans**.[107] Affected infants present with purpura and microvascular thrombosis. Treatment is with either fresh-frozen plasma or activated protein C concentrates. Homozygous deficiency results in fetal loss.

Venous and arterial catheters have been shown to be major contributors to the increased incidence of arterial and venous thrombosis. The development of intracardiac and renal vascular thrombosis is a potential serious complication of catheter-associated thrombi.[108,109]

Infants who present with a perinatal stroke should be evaluated for the presence both a prothrombotic and a hemorrhagic defect, because there is evidence that infants with coagulopathies have an increased risk of prenatal stroke.[110-112]

ANTITHROMBOTIC AND FIBRINOLYTIC THERAPY

Neither anticoagulant nor fibrinolytic agents are currently approved for use in neonates, and as a consequence, there is limited experience with these agents in infants. Heparin has been used for clinically significant acute thrombosis in neonates, although the dosages required to achieve therapeutic heparin concentrations in neonates are higher than those generally required in older children and adults.[113,114] Infants appear to have an increased volume of distribution and increased clearance of heparin, which result in this need for higher dosages. In general, heparin anticoagulation is initiated with a bolus of 75 to 100 U/kg body weight, followed by a continuous infusion of 28 U/kg/hour (mean dosage). The heparin dosage is then titrated to achieve a heparin concentration of 0.2 to 0.4 U/mL plasma (usually corresponding to an aPTT $1\frac{1}{2}$ to 2 times baseline value). In view of the wide variation in baseline aPTT in premature infants, it may be appropriate to initiate full-dosage heparin therapy with hematology consultation. Infants who develop bleeding while receiving heparin may be treated with intravenous protamine, given at a concentration of 10 mg/mL at a rate not to exceed 5 mg/minute. The dosage of protamine is based on the amount of heparin approximated to be in the infant's system (heparin half-life = 1 hour at doses of 100 U/kg). In general, 1 mg of protamine neutralizes approximately 100 U of heparin (90 United States Pharmacopeia [USP] U of bovine heparin, 115 USP U of porcine heparin). Low-dosage heparin is frequently employed in total parenteral nutrition and central venous and arterial catheter flush solutions. The use of these heparin-containing solutions has been associated with an increased risk of intraventricular hemorrhage in some studies.[115,116] However, more recent analysis of this issue has failed to confirm these concerns.[117] Experience with low-molecular-weight heparin (LMWH) in neonates is even more limited. However, it appears to be as effective and safe as unfractionated heparin in newborns and may produce a more stable degree of anticoagulation, as its action is mediated through an anti–factor Xa effect rather than through antithrombin-III.[118] Because of increased clearance and volume of distribution, the recommended dose of LMWH is 1.5 U/kg body weight administered every 12 hours for full anticoagulation of acute events.[112,113] Unlike unfractionated heparin, LMWH does not prolong the aPTT, inasmuch as it anticoagulates via an anti–factor Xa mechanism. Dosages should be adjusted in response to plasma anti–factor Xa activity. Treatment of bleeding during LMWH therapy is more problematic than with unfractionated heparin, because of the longer elimination half-life of LMWH (3 to 5 hours) and the fact that it is incompletely neutralized by protamine. If protamine is to be used, the dosage is similar to that for unfractionated heparin (i.e., 1 mg of protamine per 100 U of LMWH).

Experience with fibrinolytic agents in neonates is even more limited. Anecdotal reports suggest that newborns have a higher risk of bleeding than do adults.[119] In addition, the reduced plasminogen concentrations in newborns reduces the generation of plasmin by the more common fibrinolytic agents (streptokinase, urokinase, tPA). There are no controlled trials of systemic versus local infusion therapy with fibrinolytic agents. Although local infusions are believed to result in reduced risk of bleeding, there are no data in neonates to confirm this. There are no newborn-specific recommended dosages for these agents. In general, the dosages used in the NICU are based on weight-adjusted dosages in acute myocardial infarction

Table 83–11. Anticoagulant and Fibrinolytic Therapy in the Newborn

Anticoagulation

Unfractionated Heparin

Bolus: 50–100 U/kg IV
Maintenance: 20–30 U/kg/hr
Target: adjust infusion to maintain an aPTT
   55–90 seconds (corresponding to a plasma heparin
   concentration of 0.2–0.4 U/mL)

Low-Molecular-Weight Heparin (Enoxaparin)

Prophylactic: 1.5 mg/kg once daily SQ
Target: 0.2–0.4 anti–factor Xa activity U/mL 4 hr after
   injection; monitoring generally not required
Therapeutic: 1 mg/kg twice daily (e.g., 2 mg/kg/day total)
Target: 0.4–0.8 anti–factor Xa activity U/mL 4 hr after
   injection; monitoring required

Fibrinolysis

Urokinase

Bolus: 4400 U/kg IV over 10–20 min
Maintenance: 4400 U/kg/hr
Duration: 12–24 hr

Streptokinase

Bolus: 3500–4000 U/kg IV over 30 min
Maintenance: 1000–15000 U/kg/hr
Duration: 12–72 hr

Recombinant Tissue Plasminogen Activator

Bolus: 0.1–0.2 mg/kg IV over 10 min
Maintenance: 0.8–2.4 mg/kg/24 hr
Duration: maximum 6 days

aPTT, activated partial thromboplastin time; IV, intravenously; SQ, subcutaneously.

studies (Table 83-11).[112,113,119] After initiation of thrombolysis, the intensity of the infusion is adjusted to maintain plasma fibrinogen at 100 mg/dL. Use of thrombolytic agents in neonates may best be carried out in conjunction with hematology consultation. Bleeding in the context of fibrinolytic therapy is generally a consequence of hypofibrinogenemia. Infants with bleeding should receive cryoprecipitate to raise fibrinogen levels to 100 mg/dL. For severe, life-threatening bleeding, antifibrinolytic agents (e.g., ε-aminocaproic acid, tranexamic acid) may be used.

References

1. Hathaway WE: Coagulation problems in the newborn infant. Pediatr Clin North Am 17:929, 1970.
2. Corrigan JJ Jr: Neonatal thrombosis and thrombolytic system: Pathophysiology and therapy. Am J Pediatr Hematol Oncol 10:83, 1988.
3. Schmidt B, Andrew M: Neonatal thrombosis: Report of a prospective Canadian and international registry. Pediatrics 96:939, 1995.
4. Castle V, Andrew M, Kelton JG, et al: Frequency and mechanism of neonatal thrombocytopenia. J Pediatr 108:749, 1986.

5. Roberts IA, Murray NA: Neonatal thrombocytopenia: New insights into pathogenesis and implications for clinical management. Curr Opin Pediatr 13:16, 2001.

6. Mann KG: Biochemistry and physiology of blood coagulation. Thromb Haemost 82:165, 1999.

7. Degen JL: Genetic interactions between the coagulation and fibrinolytic systems. Thromb Haemost 86:130, 2001.

8. Schmaier AH, Rojkjaer R, Shariat-Madar Z: Activation of the plasma kallikrein/kinin system on cells: A revised hypothesis. Thromb Haemost 82:226, 1999.

9. Catella-Lawson F: Vascular biology of thrombosis: Platelet–vessel wall interactions and aspirin effects. Neurology 57:S5, 2001.

10. Cheung PY, Salas E, Sanchez R, Radomski MW: Nitric oxide and platelet function: Implications for neonatology. Semin Perinatol 21:409, 1997.

11. Collen D: The plasminogen (fibrinolytic) system. Thromb Haemost 82:259, 1999.

12. Gross PL, Aird WC: The endothelium and thrombosis. Semin Thromb Hemost. 26:463, 2000.

13. Vallet B, Wiel E: Endothelial cell dysfunction and coagulation. Crit Care Med 29(7 Suppl):S36, 2001.

14. Esmon CT, Ding W, Yasuhiro K, et al: The protein C pathway: New insights. Thromb Haemost 78:70, 1997.

15. Esmon CT: Protein C anticoagulant pathway and its role in controlling microvascular thrombosis and inflammation. Crit Care Med 29(7 Suppl):S48, 2001.

16. Andrew M, Paes B, Milner R, et al: Development of the human coagulation system in the full-term infant. Blood 70:165, 1987.

17. Andrew M, Paes B, Milner R, et al: Development of the human coagulation system in the healthy premature infant. Blood 72:165, 1988.

18. Holmberg L, Henriksson P, Ekelund H, Astedt B: Coagulation in the human fetus. Comparison with term newborn infants. J Pediatr 85:860, 1974.

19. Mitchell L, Piovella F, Ofosu F, et al: Alpha-2-macroglobulin may provide protection from thromboembolic events in antithrombin-III–deficient children. Blood 78:2299, 1991.

20. Schneider DM, von Tempelhoff GF, Herrle B, Heilmann L: Maternal and cord blood hemostasis at delivery. J Perinat Med 25:55, 1997.

21. Reverdiau-Moalic P, Delahousse B, Body G, et al: Evolution of blood coagulation activators and inhibitors in the healthy human fetus. Blood 88:900, 1996.

22. Kottke-Marchant K, Corcoran G: The laboratory diagnosis of platelet disorders. Arch Pathol Lab Med 126:133, 2002.

23. Rodgers GM: Overview of platelet physiology and laboratory evaluation of platelet function. Clin Obstet Gynecol 42:349, 1999.

24. Male C, Lechner K, Eichinger S, et al: Clinical significance of lupus anticoagulants in children. J Pediatr 134:199, 1999.

25. Yoffe G, Buchanan GR: Intracranial hemorrhage in newborn and young infants with hemophilia. J Pediatr 113:333, 1988.

26. Bray GL, Luban NLC: Hemophilia presenting with intracranial bleeding and coagulopathy. Am J Dis Child 141:1215, 1987.

27. Kulkarni R, Lusher JM: Intracranial and extracranial hemorrhages in newborns with hemophilia: A review of the literature. J Pediatr Hematol Oncol 21:289, 1999.

28. Kletzel M, Miller CH, Becton DL, et al: Postdelivery head bleeding in hemophiliac neonates. Causes and management. Am J Dis Child 143:1107, 1989.

29. Stirling Y, Woolf L, North WR, et al: Haemostasis in normal pregnancy. Thromb Haemost 52:176, 1984.

30. Klein I, Andrikovics H, Bors A, et al: A haemophilia A and B molecular genetic diagnostic programme in Hungary: A highly informative and cost-efficient strategy. Haemophilia 7:306, 2001.

31. Asakai R, Chung DW, Davie EW, et al: Factor XI deficiency in Ashkenazi Jews in Israel. N Engl J Med 325:153, 1991.

32. Horowitz MS, Pehta JC: SD plasma in TTP and coagulation factor deficiencies for which no concentrates are available. Vox Sang 74(Suppl 1):231, 1998.

33. Levi M, de Jonge E, van der Poll T, ten Cate H: Disseminated intravascular coagulation. Thromb Haemost 82:695, 1999.

34. Bredbacka S, Blomback M, Wiman B, Pelzer H: Laboratory methods for detecting disseminated intravascular coagulation (DIC): New aspects. Acta Anaesthesiol Scand 37:125, 1993.

35. Shirahata A, Nakamura T, Yamada K: Diagnosis of DIC in newborn infants. Bibl Haematol 49:277, 1983.

36. Bick RL, Baker WF: Diagnostic efficacy of the D-dimer assay in disseminated intravascular coagulation. Thromb Res 65:785, 1992.

37. Shirahata A, Shirakawa Y, Murakami C: Diagnosis of DIC in very low birth weight infants. Semin Thromb Hemost 24:467, 1998.

38. Sutor AH: Vitamin K deficiency bleeding in infants and children. Semin Thromb Hemost 21:317, 1995.

39. Sutor AH, von Kreis R, Cornelissen EAM, et al: Vitamin K deficiency bleeding (VKDB) in infancy. ISTH Pediatric/Perinatal Subcommittee, International Society on Thrombosis and Haemostasis. Thromb Haemost 81:456, 1999.

40. Puckett RM, Offringa M: Prophylactic vitamin K for vitamin K deficiency bleeding in neonates. Cochrane Database Syst Rev (4):CDC002776, 2000.

41. Crowther CA, Henderson-Smart DJ: Vitamin K prior to preterm birth for preventing neonatal periventricular hemorrhage. Cochrane Database Syst Rev (1):CDC000229, 2001.

42. Ross JA, Davies SM: Vitamin K prophylaxis and childhood cancer. Med Pediatr Oncol 34:434, 2000.

43. Astedt B: Antenatal drugs affecting vitamin K status of the fetus and the newborn. Semin Thromb Hemost 21:364, 1995.

44. Kuhne T, Imbach P: Neonatal platelet physiology and pathophysiology. Eur J Pediatr 157:87, 1997.

45. Michelson AD: Platelet function in the newborn. Semin Thromb Hemost 24:507, 1998.

46. Pietrucha T, Wojciechowski T, Greger T, et al: Differential reactivity of whole blood neonatal platelets to various agonists. Platelets 12:99, 2001.

47. Rajasekhar D, Barnard MR, Bednarek FJ, Michelson AD: Platelet hyporeactivity in very low birth weight neonates. Thromb Haemost 77:1002, 1997.

48. Israels SJ, Cheang T, Robertson C, et al: Impaired signal transduction in neonatal platelets. Pediatr Res 45:687, 1999.

49. Gelman B, Setty BN, Amin-Hanjani S, Stuart MJ: Impaired mobilization of intracellular calcium in neonatal platelets. Pediatr Res 39:692, 1996.

50. Roschitz B, Sudi K, Kostenberger M, Muntean W: Shorter PFA-100 closure times in neonates than in adults: Role of red cells, white cells, platelets and von Willebrand factor. Actra Paediat 90:664, 2001.

51. Israels SJ, Cheang T, McMillan-Ward EM, Cheang M: Evaluation of primary hemostasis in neonates with a new in vitro platelet function analyzer. J Pediatr 138:116, 2001.

52. Federici AB, Mannucci PM: Advances in the genetics and treatment of von Willebrand disease. Curr Opin Pediatr 14:23, 2002.

53. Budde U, Drewke E, Mainusch K, Schneppenheim R: Laboratory diagnosis of congenital von Willebrand disease. Semin Thromb Hemost 28:173, 2002.

54. Gralnick HR, Williams SB, McKeown LP, et al: Platelet von Willebrand factor. Proc Mayo Clinic 66:634, 1991.

55. Donner M, Holmberg L, Nilsson IM: Type IIB von Willebrand's disease with probable autosomal recessive inheritance and presenting as thrombocytopenia in infancy. Br J Haematol 66:349, 1987.

56. Mannucci PM: Desmopressin: A nontransfusional form of treatment for congenital and acquired bleeding disorders. Blood 72:1449, 1988.

57. Dunn AL, Powers JR, Ribeiro MJ, et al: Adverse events during use of intranasal desmopressin acetate for haemophilia A and von Willebrand disease: A case report and review of 40 patients. Haemophilia 6:11, 2000.

58. Nurden AT: Inherited abnormalities of platelets. Thromb Haemost 82:468, 1999.

59. Parker RI: The effect of DDAVP on agonist-induced platelet activation of Na^+/H^+ exchange. Thromb Hemorrh Dis 8:9, 1993.

60. Balduini CL, Noris P, Belletti S, et al: In vitro and in vivo effects of desmopressin on platelet function. Haematologica 84:891, 1999.

61. Oren H, Irken G, Oren B, et al: Assessment of clinical impact and predisposing factors for neonatal thrombocytopenia. Indian J Pediatr 61:551, 1994.

62. Uhrynowska M, Maslanka K, Zupanska B: Neonatal thrombocytopenia: Incidence, serological and clinical observations. Am J Perinatol 14:415, 1997.

63. Sainio S, Jarvenpaa AL, Renlund M, et al: Thrombocytopenia in term infants: A population-based study. Obstet Gynecol 95:441, 2000.

64. Roberts IA, Murray NA: Neonatal thrombocytopenia: New insights into pathogenesis and implications for clinical management. Curr Opin Pediatr 13:16, 2001.

65. Dreyfus M, Kaplan C, Verdy E, et al: Frequency of immune thrombocytopenia in newborns: A prospective study. Immune Thrombocytopenia Working Group. Blood 89:4402, 1997.

66. Uhrynowska M, Niznikowska-Marks M, Zupanska B: Neonatal and maternal thrombocytopenia: Incidence and immune background. Eur J Haematol 64:42, 2000.

67. Kaplan C: Immune thrombocytopenia in the fetus and the newborn: Diagnosis and therapy. Transfus Clin Biol 8:311, 2001.

68. Van Den Oudenrijn S, Bruin M, Folman CC, et al: Three parameters, plasma thrombopoietin levels, plasma glycocalicin levels and megakaryocyte culture, distinguish between different causes of congenital thrombocytopenia. Br J Haematol 117:390, 2002.

69. Albert TS, Meng YG, Simms P, et al: Thrombopoietin in the thrombocytopenic term and preterm newborn. Pediatrics 105:1286, 2000.

70. Paul DA, Leef KH, Taylor S, McKenzie S: Thrombopoietin in preterm infants: Gestational age–dependent response. J Pediatr Hematol Oncol 24:304, 2002.

71. Bussel J, Kaplan C: The fetal and maternal consequences of maternal alloimmune thrombocytopenia. Baillieres Clin Haematol 11:391, 1998.

72. Bussel JB, Zabusky MR, Berkowitz RL, McFarland JG: Fetal alloimmune thrombocytopenia. N Engl J Med 337:22, 1997.

73. Blanchette VS, Johnson J, Rand M: The management of alloimmune neonatal thrombocytopenia. Baillieres Best Pract Res Clin Haematol 13:365, 2000.

74. Iyori H, Fujisawa K, Akatsuka J: Thrombocytopenia in neonates born to women with autoimmune thrombocytopenic purpura. Pediatr Hematol Oncol 14:367, 1997.

75. Valat AS, Caulier MT, Devos P, et al: Relationships between severe neonatal thrombocytopenia and maternal characteristics in pregnancies associated with autoimmune thrombocytopenia. Br J Haematol 103:397, 1998.

76. Yamada H, Kato EH, Kobashi G, et al: Passive immune thrombocytopenia in neonates of mothers with idiopathic thrombocytopenic purpura: Incidence and risk factors. Semin Thromb Hemost 25:491, 1999.

77. Christiaens GC, Nieuwenhuis HK, Bussel JB: Comparison of platelet counts in first and second newborns of mothers with immune thrombocytopenic purpura. Obstet Gynecol 90:546, 1997.

78. Song TB, Lee JY, Kim YH, Choi YY: Low neonatal risk of thrombocytopenia in pregnancy associated immune thrombocytopenic purpura. Fetal Diagn Ther 14:216, 1999.

79. Ochs HD: The Wiskott-Aldrich syndrome. Semin Hematol 35:332, 1998.

80. Hohlfeld P, Forestier F, Kaplan C, et al: Fetal thrombocytopenia: A retrospective survey of 5,194 fetal blood samplings. Blood 84:1851, 1994.

81. Warrier I, Lusher JM: Congenital thrombocytopenias. Curr Opin Hematol 2:395, 1995.

82. Sieff CA, Nisbet-Brown E, Nathan DG: Congenital bone marrow failure syndromes. Br J Haematol 111:30, 2000.

83. Alter BP: Bone marrow failure syndromes. Clin Lab Med 19:113, 1999.

84. Hedberg VA, Lipton JM: Thrombocytopenia with absent radii. A review of 100 cases. Am J Pediatr Hematol Oncol 10:51, 1988.

85. Ballmaier M, Schulze H, Strauss G, et al: Thrombopoietin in patients with congenital thrombocytopenia and absent radii: Elevated serum levels, normal receptor expression, but defective reactivity to thrombopoietin. Blood 90:612, 1997.

86. Yamashita T, Nakahata T: Current knowledge on the pathophysiology of Fanconi anemia: From genes to phenotypes. In J Hematol 74:33, 2001.

87. Murray NA, Howarth LJ, McCloy MP, et al: Platelet transfusion in the management of severe thrombocytopenia in neonatal intensive care unit patients. Transfus Med 12:35, 2002.

88. Rebulla P: Platelet transfusion trigger in difficult patients. Transfus Clin Biol 8:249, 2001.

89. Kulkarni R, Lusher JM, Henry RC, Kallen DJ: Current practices regarding newborn intracranial haemorrhage and obstetrical care and mode of delivery of pregnant haemophilia carriers: A survey of obstetricians, neonatologists and haematologists in the United States, on behalf of the National Hemophilia Foundation's Medical and Scientific Advisory Council. Haemophilia 5:410, 1999.

90. Malida F, Paolo S, Sonia L, et al: Effect of delivery modalities on the physiologic inhibition system of coagulation of the neonate. Thromb Res 105:15, 2002.

91. Kahn DJ, Richardson DK, Billett HH: Association of thrombocytopenia and the delivery method with intraventricular hemorrhage among very-low-birth-weight infants. Am J Obstet Gynecol 186:109, 2002.

92. Towner D, Castro MA, Eby-Wilkens E, Gilbert WM: Effect of mode of delivery in nulliparous women on neonatal intracranial injury. N Engl J Med 341:1709, 1999.

93. Pollina J, Dias MS, Li V, et al: Cranial birth injuries in term newborn infants. Pediatr Neurosurg 35:113, 2001.

94. Jaschevatzky OE, David H, Bivas M, et al: Outcome of pregnancies associated with marked gestational thrombocytopenia. J Perinat Med 22:351, 1994.

95. Larson A, DiMichele DM, Tarrantino MD: Treatment of neonates with hemophilia and the development of inhibitors: A survey of hemophilia treatment centers [Abstract]. J Pediatr Hematol Oncol 24:A19, 1445, 2002.

96. Kadir RA, Economides DL, Braithwaite J, et al: The obstetric experience of carriers of haemophilia. Br J Obstet Gynaecol 104:803, 1997.

97. Andrew ME, Monagle P, deVeber G, Chan AKC: Thromboembolic disease and antithrombotic therapy in newborns. Hematology (Am Soc Hematol Educ Program), 2001, p 358.

98. Lynch JK, Nelson KB: Epidemiology of perinatal stroke. Curr Opin Pediatr 13:499, 2001.

99. Salonvaara M, Riikonen P, Kekomaki R, Heinonen K: Clinically symptomatic central venous catheter-related deep venous thrombosis in newborns. Acta Pediatr 88:642, 1999.

100. Gunther G, Junker R, Strater R, et al: Symptomatic ischemic stroke in full term neonates: Role of acquired and genetic prothrombotic risk factors. Stroke 31:2437, 2000.

101. Vielhaber H, Ehrenforth S, Koch HG, et al: Cerebral venous sinus thrombosis in infancy and childhood: Role of genetic and acquired risk factors in thrombophilia. Eur J Pediatr 157:555, 1998.

102. deVeber G, Monagle P, Chan A, et al: Prothrombotic disorders in infants and children with cerebral thromboembolism. Arch Neurol 55:1539, 1998.

103. Monagle P, Adams M, Mahoney M, et al: Outcome of pediatric thromboembolic disease: A report from the Canadian Childhood Thrombophilia Registry. Pediatr Res 47:763, 2000.

104. Carvalho KS, Bodensteiner JB, Connolly PJ, Garg BP: Cerebral venous thrombosis in children. J Child Neurol 16:574, 2001.

105. Golomb MR, MacGregor DL, Domi T, et al: Presumed pre- or perinatal arterial ischemic stroke: Risk factors and outcomes. Ann Neurol 50:163, 2001.

106. von Kreis vR, Janker R, Oberle D, et al: Foetal growth restriction in children with prothrombotic risk factors. Thromb Haemost 86:1012, 2001.

107. Muller FM, Ehrenthal W, Hafner G, Schranz D: Purpura fulminans in severe congenital protein C deficiency: Monitoring of treatment with protein C concentrate. Eur J Pediatr 155:20, 1996.

108. Mocan H, Beattie TJ, Murphy AV: Renal venous thrombosis in infancy: Long-term follow-up. Pediatr Nephrol 5:45, 1991.

109. Rimensberger PC, Humbert JR, Beghetti M: Management of preterm infants with intracardiac thrombi: Use of thrombolytic agents. Paediatr Drugs 3:883, 2001.

110. Edstrom CS, Christensen RD: Evaluation and treatment of thrombosis in the neonatal intensive care unit. Clin Perinatol 27:623, 2000.

111. Petaja J, Hiltunen L, Fellman V: Increased risk of intraventricular hemorrhage in preterm infants with thrombophilia. Pediatr Res 49:643, 2001.

112. Nowak-Gottl U, Kosch A, Schlegel N: Thromboembolism in newborns, infants and children. Thromb Haemost 86:464, 2001.

113. Monagle P, Michalson AD, Bovill E, Andrew M: Antithrombotic therapy in children. Chest 119:344S, 2001.

114. Chan AKC, Berry LR, Monagle PT, Andrew M: Decreased concentrations of heparinoids are required to inhibit thrombin generation in plasma from newborns and children compared to plasma from adults due to reduced thrombin potential. Thromb Haemost 87:606, 2002.

115. Lesko SM, Mitchell AA, Epstein MF, et al: Heparin use as a risk factor for intraventricular hemorrhage in low-birth-weight infants. N Engl J Med 314:1156, 1986.

116. Malloy MH, Cutter GR: The association of heparin exposure with intraventricular hemorrhage among very low birth weight infants. J Perinatol 15:185, 1995.

117. Chang GY, Lueder FL, DiMichele DM, et al: Heparin and the risk of intraventricular hemorrhage in premature infants. J Pediatr 131:362, 1997.

118. Weitz JL: Low molecular weight heparins. N Engl J Med 337:688, 1997.

119. Leaker M, Massicotte MP, Brooker L, et al: Thrombolytic therapy in pediatric patients: A comprehensive review of the literature. Thromb Haemost 76:132, 1996.

CHAPTER 84

White Blood Cell Disorders in the Neonate

Joyce M. Koenig and Mervin C. Yoder

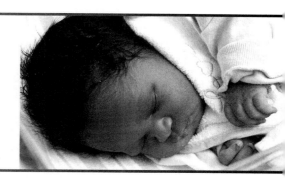

Throughout human ontogeny, numerous host defense mechanisms must be engaged to counteract the invasion of microorganisms with which people share the environment. In this chapter, we review the development of host defense mechanisms and discuss the unfavorable consequences of acquiring or inheriting a disorder of leukocyte biology.

Host responses to invading microorganisms may be local or systemic and include cellular and humoral elements. Leukocytes constitute the cellular component of host defense and are classified as either nonspecific (polymorphonuclear and mononuclear phagocytes) or specific (B and T lymphocytes) with regard to recognition of individual pathogens. Likewise, humoral elements may be nonspecific (complement proteins) or specific (immunoglobulins) in encountering and interacting with the microorganism. Of all these host defense elements, phagocytes represent the most important acute defense against microbial challenge.

This chapter reviews the production, distribution, and function of both polymorphonuclear (neutrophil) and mononuclear (monocyte and macrophage) phagocytes in host defense and provides an introduction to recognizing, diagnosing, and providing treatment for phagocyte deficiencies that impair host defense. The production and role of lymphocytes and humoral elements in host defense and the immunodeficiencies resulting from quantitative or qualitative impairments in these important host defense components are reviewed in detail elsewhere.[1,2]

OVERVIEW OF PHAGOCYTE PRODUCTION

Ontogeny of Hematopoiesis

The process of forming the cellular elements of blood is called **hematopoiesis**. In adults, all circulating cells are derived from more undifferentiated precursors in the medullary cavity of bone. In the human embryo and the fetus, however, the site and pattern of hematopoiesis is developmentally regulated and occurs in several different tissues (Fig. 84-1).[3-5] Blood cells first become apparent in the yolk sac at day 19 of gestation.[6] Once the circulatory system forms, by week 4 of gestation, blood cells are carried to all tissues of the embryo. During week 6 of gestation, the fetal liver begins functioning as a hematopoietic organ and is the predominant site of blood cell production until month 5 or 6 of gestation.[7] The fetal bone marrow cavity becomes increasingly active in blood cell production and dominates as a center of hematopoiesis from month 6 to the remainder of gestation and thereafter for the life of the individual. The factors that regulate these sequential shifts in the site of hematopoiesis remain elusive. It also remains to be proved whether the hematopoietic stem cells in the fetal liver are derived from yolk sac or embryonic sites. Most evidence in the human fetus supports stem cell migration from an intraembryonic site to fetal liver.[8,9] It is clear that fetal liver stem cells circulate and seed the bone marrow cavity early in fetal life. Thereafter, bone marrow stem cells must develop self-renewal mechanisms to provide a lifelong sustainable pool of hematopoietic precursors.[10]

Site-Specific Pattern of Hematopoiesis

Not only are there changes in the site of hematopoiesis but the pattern of blood cells also changes during embryonic and fetal development (see Fig. 84-1). For example, primitive erythrocytes in the yolk sac are large and nucleated, remain slightly large but enucleated during the fetal liver phase of hematopoiesis, and are definitively adult-like in appearance during late fetal liver and bone marrow phases of hematopoiesis. The type of hemoglobin expression changes from embryonic (Gower) to fetal (hemoglobin F) to adult (hemoglobin A) types, in concert with the movement of the site of red blood cell production from yolk sac and fetal liver to bone marrow.[11] Early fetal liver hematopoiesis generates more erythroid than myeloid cells, whereas bone marrow hematopoiesis produces more myeloid than erythroid elements. Cellularity of fetal bone marrow is similar to that of adult bone marrow by month 4 of gestation, although greater numbers of

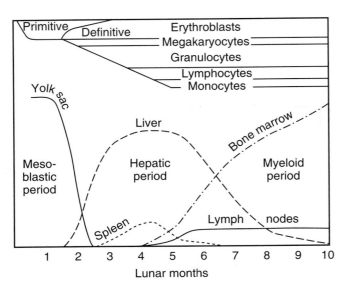

Figure 84–1. The stages of hematopoiesis in the developing embryo and fetus, indicating the time of appearance and relative participation of hematopoietic sites. *(From Wintrobe M: Clinical Hematology, 8th ed. Philadelphia, Lea & Febiger, 1981, p 49.)*

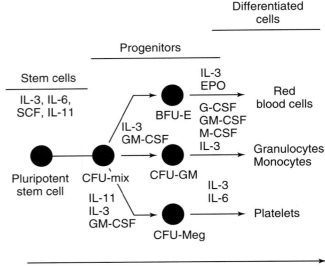

Figure 84–2. Flowchart indicating progressive commitment of hematopoietic progenitor cells to mature differentiated blood cells and the associated growth factors inducing the proliferation. BFU-E, burst-forming unit–erythroid; CFU-GM, colony-forming unit–granulocyte-macrophage; CFU-Meg, colony-forming unit–megakaryocyte; CFU-mix, colony-forming unit–mixed lineages; EPO, erythropoietin; G-CSF, granulocyte colony–stimulating factor; GM-CSF, granulocyte-macrophage colony–stimulating factor; IL-3, IL-6, IL-11, interleukins-3, -6, and -11; M-CSF, macrophage colony–stimulating factor; SCF, stem cell factor.

nonhematopoietic stromal cells and fewer lymphoid cells are present.[12] Whether the number and type of stromal cells in each site of hematopoiesis determines the pattern of blood cells produced by modulating stem cell behavior, or whether the hematopoietic stem cells are "programmed" to differentiate in a specific pattern during fetal development, remains an important unsettled question.

Regulation of Hematopoiesis

The development of several research tools has allowed for some analysis of the molecular regulation of hematopoiesis. All mature differentiated blood cells are derived from precursor cells called **progenitor cells** (Fig. 84-2). These progenitors (single cells), when suspended in agar or methylcellulose and stimulated by growth factors, characteristically grow into colonies of 50,000 to 100,00 cells.[13] These colony-forming cells are named by the type of progeny they produce. For example, a colony of neutrophils and/or macrophages arises from granulocyte-macrophage colony–forming unit (CFU-GM), erythrocytes from erythroid burst-forming unit, and platelets from megakaryocyte colony–forming unit (see Fig. 84-2). All colony-forming progenitor cells are derived from pluripotent progenitor cells and ultimately from a common self-renewing hematopoietic stem cell.[13] The isolation of multiple hematopoietic growth factors and interleukins has increased the understanding of the factors that are needed for the proliferation and maturation of the various blood cell lineages (see Fig. 84-2), but the mechanisms that are involved in tightly regulating the number of circulating cells in each lineage under normal and stress conditions are poorly understood. Evidence indicates an important role for the stromal cells (fibroblasts, endothelial and epithelial cells, macrophages, adipocytes) of the hematopoietic microenvironment in expression of

hematopoietic growth factors that influence blood cell production.

Ontogeny of Neutrophil Production

Immature neutrophil precursors have been identified during week 12 of gestation.[7] These cells are larger, with an irregularly shaped nucleus and more dispersed granules than neutrophils formed later in gestation. Neutrophil production is minimal during the first 15 weeks of gestation (see Fig. 84-1), but significantly increases beyond week 20 as fetal bone marrow hematopoiesis becomes predominant. In general, neutrophils make up 5% to 8% of circulating nucleated blood cells from weeks 10 to 32 of gestation.[14] During this time the absolute neutrophil count increases fourfold. A transient, abrupt increase in the circulating blood concentration of neutrophils occurs at birth. In full-term gestations, this elevation in the absolute neutrophil count is maximal at approximately 12 hours after birth and reaches steady state by 60 hours after birth.[15] In contrast, newborns delivered prematurely tend to have lower absolute neutrophil counts, with an absence of the dramatic increase seen in full-term infants in the first day after birth.[16]

Ontogeny of Mononuclear Phagocyte Production

In adults, circulating blood monocytes enter tissues and differentiate into macrophages; during fetal development, macrophages appear before any morphologically recognizable monocytes. Some organs become colonized with macrophages earlier in gestation than do others. Primitive macrophages are present in the yolk sac as early as weeks 3 to 4 of gestation. In the earliest period of fetal liver hematopoiesis, macrophages account for more than 70% of all hepatic cells and then decline to 20% to 30% of the total liver cell number at birth.[17,18] In the lungs, few macrophages can be identified until after birth, and circulating blood monocytes are not found until after months 5 to 6 of gestation.[19] In general, monocytes make up 2% to 7% of all nucleated circulating blood cells by week 30 of gestation and at birth are present in peripheral blood at a higher concentration than in adult blood.

KINETICS OF PHAGOCYTE PRODUCTION

Neutrophil Kinetics

Neutrophils are derived from myeloid (CFU-GM) progenitor cells.[12,20] The first morphologically identifiable cell is called a **myeloblast**, a proliferating cell that constitutes a part of the neutrophil mitotic pool. Myeloblasts are capable of dividing into many daughter cells called **myelocytes**. Myelocytes differentiate into the metamyelocyte and band forms, which are the immediate stages of development preceding mature neutrophils. The neutrophil storage pool is composed of the postmitotic metamyelocytes, bands, and mature forms. Estimates of the normal time required to produce mature neutrophils from a CFU-GM vary from 8 to 14 days; the majority of the time is required for the terminal differentiation of the neutrophil. In some stressful situations, such as during sepsis, this entire sequence can be accelerated. In 1 day, depletion of the marrow storage pool of postmitotic immature and mature neutrophils can be nearly completely replenished.[12]

Homeostasis of neutrophils is dependent on a dynamic balance between factors that stimulate their production and those that promote their migration into the tissues, which is followed by the programmed demise and removal of senescent neutrophils by the reticuloendothelial system. The total pool of neutrophils that can be mobilized to fight infection is composed of those in the bone marrow, those in the circulation, and those that are reversibly attached, or marginated, to the vascular endothelium.[21] Bone marrow egress of mature neutrophils into the circulation is essentially a unidirectional process, although the factors governing this process are not well understood. However, factors such as interleukin (IL)–1, tumor necrosis factor, epinephrine, corticosteroids, and some activated complement fragments (C3e) are important mobilizers of marrow neutrophils into the circulation during states of inflammation or stress.[22] In addition, certain hematopoietic growth factors, including granulocyte colony–stimulating factor (G-CSF) and granulocyte-macrophage colony–stimulating factor, may perform dual functions. These factors can act on progenitor cells to stimulate myelopoiesis, or they may directly activate neutrophils and enhance their egress from the bone marrow as well as their functionality.[23-25] The higher circulating concentrations of G-CSF during sepsis, for

example, may thus act as a stimulus to the bone marrow to promote both neutrophil production and the release of mature, or nearly mature, forms into the circulation, as well as to enhance the function of those neutrophils.[26-28]

The proportion of neutrophils released into the circulation or those that have become marginated is dependent on a variety of physiologic stimuli.[29] Neutrophils normally circulate in peripheral blood for 6 to 8 hours, dynamically interchanging between one pool of circulating cells and a pool of sequestered (marginated) cells in pulmonary capillaries.[21] Neutrophils survive in tissues for an additional 24 hours after leaving the circulatory system. Clearance of senescent tissue neutrophils is probably accomplished by tissue macrophages.[30] The concentration of circulating neutrophils varies greatly during the first 3 days after birth and is dependent on gestational age. In full-term neonates, the neutrophil count is highest 12 hours after birth, ranging from 7800 to 14,500 cells/mm³ (Fig. 84-3),[15] and it is abnormal for the neutrophil count to fall lower than 3000/mm³ during the first 48 hours after birth and lower than 1500/mm³ for the remainder of the neonatal period.[31] Preterm neonates with birth weights of less than 1500 g tend to have a delayed increase in the circulating neutrophil counts and generally lower absolute neutrophil counts.[16] In such infants, the peak in the neutrophil count, although similar to that observed in full-term infants, occurs later (at 18 to 20 hours after birth), and the lower limit of the circulating neutrophil count ranges from 500/mm³ in the first few hours after birth to 2200/mm³ in the first 12 to 24 hours after birth (Fig. 84-4; see Fig. 84-3). Thus, the definition of neutropenia may be modified for infants with very low birth weights; neutropenia in such infants

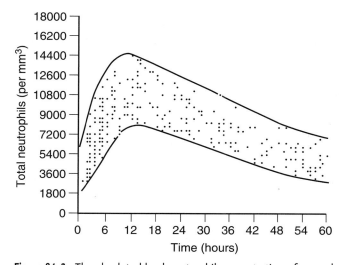

Figure 84–3. The absolute blood neutrophil concentration of normal infants during the first 60 hours after birth. *Dots* represent single values, and *numerals* represent the number of values at that same point. *(From Manroe BL, Weinberg AG, Rosenfeld CR, et al: The neonatal blood count in health and disease. I. Reference values for neutrophilic cells. J Pediatr 95:89, 1979.)*

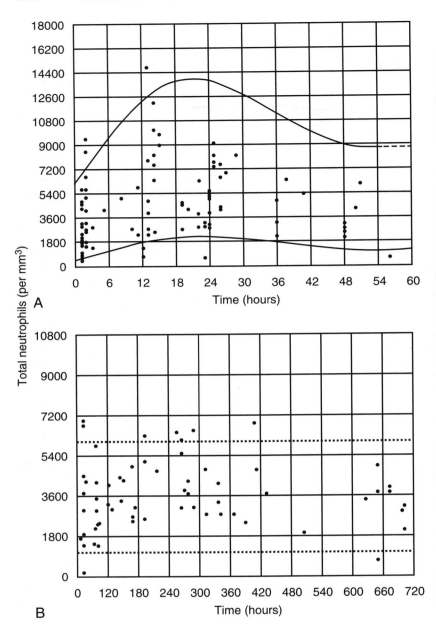

Figure 84–4. The absolute blood neutrophil concentration of infants with very low birth weights from birth to 60 hours of age **(A)** and from 60 to 720 hours of age **(B)**. *Dots* represent single values. *(From Mouzinho A, Rosenfeld CR, Sanchez PJ, Risser R: Revised reference ranges for circulating neutrophils in very-low-birth-weight neonates. Pediatrics 94:76, 1994.)*

after 60 hours after birth may be defined as an absolute neutrophil count of less than 1100/mm³. Despite the wide fluctuation in circulating neutrophil counts, the ratio of immature (metamyelocyte and band forms) to total neutrophils (I:T ratio) remains low (<0.2) and generally falls within a narrow range in healthy infants, regardless of gestational age at birth.[15,16] Changes in the peripheral blood neutrophil concentration are common in infants with infection, and certain neutrophil indices may be predictive of neonatal sepsis.[32]

Mononuclear Phagocyte Kinetics

Like neutrophils, monocytes are derived from CFU-GM progenitor cells. The most immature identifiable member of the mononuclear phagocyte system is the promonocyte.[19] Each monocyte produces two daughter monocytes that are identical to the circulating blood monocyte. Monocytes circulate in the blood for 72 hours before entering tissues and differentiating into macrophages. Some tissue macrophages are fixed within specific cellular niches (liver Kupffer cells, microglia, or bone osteoclasts), and other macrophages are mobile (peritoneal, alveolar, and synovial macrophages). The microenvironment of each tissue strongly influences monocyte-macrophage differentiation, giving rise to tissue-specific functional and phenotypic macrophage characteristics.[33] The length of survival and fate of aged tissue macrophages remains undetermined, although some human liver macrophages have been documented to survive for many months.

Monocytes constitute nearly 5% of all bone marrow hematopoietic cells in the infant, with no apparent difference in marrow composition of samples from full-term and viable preterm infants. One of the difficult issues in determining normal circulating blood monocyte concentrations is that monocytes are morphologically heterogeneous in the newborn. Thus, at birth, the circulating monocyte count ranges from 0 to 2000 cells/mm³, depending on which reported values are used.[19] As with the neutrophil count, peak monocyte concentrations are measured 12 to 24 hours after birth, decline during the first week after birth, and stabilize at 450 to 600 cells/mm³ thereafter. The concentration of tissue macrophages is unknown but in some organs (lungs and liver) accounts for 20% to 30% of all cellular elements.

ROLE OF NEUTROPHILS IN HOST DEFENSE

Neutrophils play a critical role as a first line of defense against pathogens that have invaded the body. The steps in eradicating pathogens from the body are straightforward, but a complex cascade of events and participating cell types is required (Figs. 84-5 and 84-6). Microorganisms in some way (activation of complement proteins, binding of tissue proteins and immunoglobulins, and release of metabolic products) convey their presence and position to host tissue cells. Numerous biologically active molecules are released by tissue macrophages, endothelial and epithelial cells, fibroblasts, lymphocytes, and neutrophils in the vicinity of the pathogen.[34] These biologically active molecules diffuse, in a concentration-dependent manner, from the site of microbial invasion and serve as chemotactic agents and activating agents to recruit additional neutrophils to the involved site. Some of these signals,

presumably suspended in plasma, reach the bone marrow and recruit neutrophils from the large postmitotic storage pool, and other signals mobilize the neutrophils that had been marginated in pulmonary capillaries. These early events result in a dramatic increase in the circulating neutrophil count. In the region of the evolving inflammatory site surrounding the invading microbes, blood flow increases, and adjacent capillary endothelial barriers become more permeable. Activation of the endothelium causes the endothelial luminal surface to express certain cell surface molecules that are recognized by recruited neutrophils, causing the slowly rolling neutrophils to become firmly adherent. The chemotactic agents exuding from the infected tissues stimulate the neutrophils to undergo diapedesis between endothelial cells and emigrate into the nidus of the infected area. The microorganisms are ingested by the neutrophils in a process called **phagocytosis**, which engages intracellular mechanisms in the generation of reactive oxygen intermediates and powerful membrane oxidants such as hypochlorous acid and chloramines. These oxidants and additional intracellular enzymes in the neutrophils kill the microorganisms.

This brief overview stresses the important role of neutrophils in killing invading microbes but belies the complexity and regulatory controls that are required to both initiate and resolve acute inflammatory responses.[35] Discussed as follows in greater detail are the events that are critical to neutrophil microbicidal activity.

Adherence and Aggregation

In order for circulating neutrophils to reach inflammatory sites, they must first adhere to the vascular endothelium responses.[35] This process is normally tightly controlled, because activated neutrophils can damage host tissue in

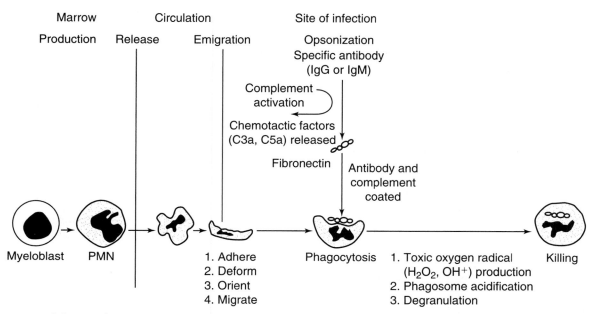

Figure 84–5. Host defense mechanisms against microbial invasion. IgG and IgM, immunoglobulins G and M; PMN, polymorphonuclear neutrophil. *(From Wilson CB: Immunologic basis for increased susceptibility of the neonate to infection.J Pediatr 108:1, 1986.)*

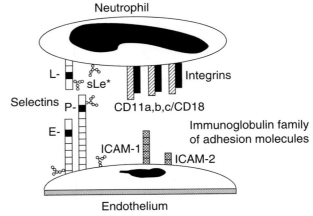

Figure 84–7. The adhesion of leukocytes to endothelial cells is mediated by several receptor-ligand (counter-receptor) pair interactions. These include the selectin-carbohydrate (sialylated Lewis X [sLe^x]) and integrin-immunoglobulin families of receptor-ligand pairs. ICAM, intracellular adhesion molecule. *(From Bevilacqua MP: Endothelial-leukocyte adhesion molecules. Annu Rev Immunol 11:767, 1993.)*

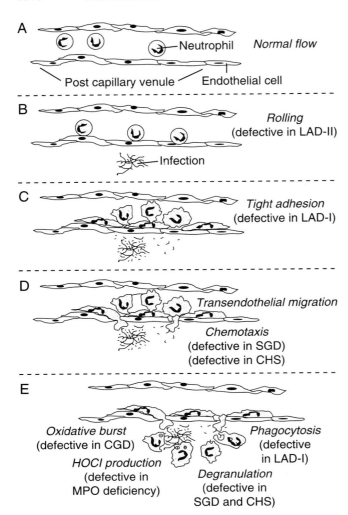

Figure 84–6. The steps involved in the neutrophil functional responses to infection. The steps that are defective in the inherited disorders of neutrophil function are noted **(B to E)**. CGD, chronic granulomatous disease; CHS, Chédiak-Higashi syndrome; HOCl, hypochlorous acid; LAD, leukocyte adhesion deficiency; MPO, myeloperoxidase deficiency; SGD, specific granule deficiency. *(From Malech HL, Nauseef WM: Primary inherited defects in neutrophil function: Etiology and treatment. Semin Hematol 34:279, 1997.)*

the process of targeting microbes.[36] Neutrophil adhesion to vascular endothelium and to other phagocytes depends on specific receptor-ligand interactions at the cell surface membrane (Fig. 84-7).[37,38] Studies in intact animals using intravital microscopy have confirmed that the first contact made between neutrophils and endothelium involves a "rolling" of the neutrophil over the endothelial cell surface.[39] This initial interaction between adhesion molecules on neutrophil surfaces and their putative endothelial ligands is a process that involves a group of adhesive glycoproteins called **selectins**.[40] L-selectin is expressed on a variety of leukocytes, including neutrophils, and has been shown to be important in lymphocyte recirculation. In contrast, E-selectin and P-selectin are generally expressed

on endothelial cells exposed to shear stresses or inflammatory cytokines. Mice deficient in selectins exhibit leukocytosis and a defective inflammatory response, like human patients with leukocyte adhesion deficiency type II.[41,42]

When endothelial cells are activated during inflammation, local or systemic cytokines up-regulate the surface expression of adhesive ligands that bind to counter-receptors on the neutrophil surface (see Fig. 84-7).[37,38] One major group of such molecules is represented by the immunoglobulin gene superfamily and includes intercellular adhesion molecule (ICAM)-1, ICAM-2, and the platelet-endothelial cell adhesion molecule 1. These molecules act as ligands for a third major group of cell adhesion molecules known as **integrins**. The β$_2$ integrin CD18, expressed primarily on leukocytes, functions as a heterodimer in combination with a specific α subunit: CD18/CD11a (also known as lymphocyte function antigen 1), CD18/CD11b (also known as Mac-1, CR3, and C3bi receptor), and CD18/CD11c (also known as glycoprotein [gp] 150 and gp95).

During inflammation, endothelial mediators activate "rolling" neutrophils, which results in the concerted down-regulation of surface L-selectin and up-regulation of CD11b expression on the neutrophil surface.[43] Integrin activation allows a firm adhesion to the activated endothelial surface through interactions with ICAM-1 and ICAM-2 (see Fig. 84-7). In addition, circulating neutrophils can homotypically attach to adherent neutrophils, a process that allows local neutrophil accumulation. This homotypic aggregation precedes the migration of neutrophils through the inflamed endothelium.[44]

Several studies of neonatal neutrophils have demonstrated developmental impairments in adherence. In comparison with adult controls, surface expression of L-selectin was found to be diminished on neutrophils isolated from full-term newborns,[45] which reflected a total cellular deficiency of L-selectin in these neutrophils.[46] These observations correlated with diminished neutrophil adhesion to endothelial cells both in vitro and in vitro under conditions of shear stress. In addition, neutrophils isolated from newborns fail to mobilize and up-regulate cell surface integrin receptors after stimulation with chemotactic agents.[47] This defect may be caused in part by diminished movement of specific granules in the neutrophil cytoplasm to the cell surface membrane, where the fusion of the granules with the membrane contributes several important glycoproteins, including the integrins, to the outer cell surface membrane.[48] In addition, neonatal neutrophils appear to have decreased cellular stores of the integrins CD11a and CD11b.[49] Because increased integrin expression and function normally lead

to improved chemotactic and adhesion responses by neutrophils in vitro, it is postulated that the poor mobilization of neutrophils to sites of infection in neonates may be related to a blunted endothelial adhesion of activated neutrophils at infectious sites. Additional neutrophil adhesion–related disorders in infants and children are listed in Table 84-1.

Transendothelial Migration and Chemotaxis

Neutrophils migrate in gradient toward the highest concentration of chemoattractant.[50] This directed locomotion, known as **chemotaxis**, is dependent on neutrophil activation through signal transduction mechanisms. In addition to up-regulation of phospholipase and protein kinase C activity, neutrophil activation involves increases

Table 84–1. Classification of Functional Disorders of Granulocytes

Neutrophil Morphologic Abnormalities
Hereditary hypersegmentation
Specific granule deficiency
Pelger-Huët anomaly
Alder-Reilly anomaly
May-Hegglin anomaly
Chédiak-Higashi syndrome
Pseudo–Chédiak-Higashi syndrome
Congenital dysgranulopoietic neutropenia

Neutrophil Adhesion Deficiency
Leukocyte adhesion deficiency I
Leukocyte adhesion deficiency II
Acquired adhesion disorders
    Drug induced
        Ethanol
        Prednisone
        Aspirin
    Aging
    Diabetes mellitus
    Glomerulonephritis
    Hemodialysis
    Leukemia
    Sickle cell disease
Defects of neonatal neutrophils

Neutrophil Motility Disorders
Disorders of neutrophil cytoskeleton
    Neutrophil actin dysfunction
    Lazy leukocyte syndrome
    47-kd and 89-kd actin-binding protein abnormalities
    Increased microtubule assembly
    Kartagener syndrome
Chédiak-Higashi syndrome
Specific granule deficiency
Miscellaneous motility disorders
    Antibody deficiency syndromes
    Complement system disorders
    Hageman factor system defects
    Defects of chromosome 7
    Autoimmune disorders

Serum Inhibitors to Chemotaxis
Neonates
HIV infection
Other disease states/conditions with associated motility
    defects
    Chronic renal failure
    Diabetes mellitus
    Glycogenosis type 1B
    Bone marrow transplantation
    Malnutrition
    Infection
    Wiskott-Aldrich syndrome
    Chronic mucocutaneous candidiasis
    Shwachman-Diamond syndrome
    Turner syndrome
    Chemotherapy
    Graft-versus-host disease

Humoral Neutrophil Phagocytic Disorders
Complement disorders
Sickle cell disease
Immunoglobulin deficiency
Secondary to systemic disease/procedure
    HIV infection
    Graft-versus-host disease
    Diabetes mellitus
    Thermal injury
    Bone marrow transplantation
Thalassemia major
Tuftsin deficiency

Neutrophil Killing Disorders
Chronic granulomatous disease
Myeloperoxidase deficiency
Miscellaneous neutrophil killing disorders
    Neutrophil G6PD deficiency
    Deficiency of glutathione reductase, peroxidase,
        or synthetase
    Catalase deficiency
    Pyruvate kinase deficiency
    α-Mannosidase deficiency

G6PD, glucose-6-phosphate dehydrogenase; HIV, human immunodeficiency virus.

Adapted with permission from Bick RL (ed): Hematology: Clinical and Laboratory Practice. St. Louis, Mosby–Year Book, 1993, p 1100.

in intracellular calcium and generation of filamentous (F) actin. Specific neutrophil granules may be an important source of the plasma membrane required for continued neutrophil locomotion.[51] Activated endothelial cells release several factors with chemotactic properties, such as the chemokine IL-8.[38] These factors promote both the adherence of neutrophils and their migration through cell junctions into the extracellular space. In addition, transendothelial migration is a process that is partly mediated through the adhesive actions of activated β_2 integrins.[52]

Neutrophils isolated from premature and full-term newborn infants respond poorly to a variety of chemotactic agents.[53-55] In comparison with the response of adult neutrophils, neutrophils from newborns display a 50% reduction in directed migration during the first few weeks after birth, although random migration appears normal. The mechanisms leading to diminished chemotaxis include a diminished increase in intracellular calcium after chemotactic stimulation, diminished polymerization of filamentous actin after stimulation, and impaired up-regulation of certain cell adhesion molecules involved in cell movement. Furthermore, in comparison with those in adults, neutrophil subpopulations in newborns have a low representation of cells with high mobility. Other chemotactic disorders of neutrophils that can occur in infants and adults are listed in Table 84-1.

Phagocytosis

Pathogens require processing in order to be properly identified, ingested, and killed while existing in the midst of normal host tissues and cells. This processing, called **opsonization**, involves specific immunoglobulins (immunoglobulin G [IgG]), serum factors such as fibronectin, and proteolytic cleavage products (C3b and C3bi) of the third complement component (C3). These factors, present in tissues or in the serum, bind and coat the outer surface of the microorganisms.[2] Coated, or opsonized, microorganisms are readily recognized and bound by IgG and C3b receptors that are expressed on the neutrophil cell surface. Binding of C3b-opsonized organisms occurs through a receptor that stimulates the neutrophil to ingest the microorganism. C3bi-opsonized organisms interact with the cell surface integrin receptor CD11b, and this interaction stimulates the neutrophil to both ingest and initiate generation of toxic reactive oxygen intermediates (respiratory burst) that contribute to killing the organisms.[56] Three distinct IgG receptors bind IgG-coated microorganisms and stimulate either ingestion alone or both ingestion and the respiratory burst by the neutrophil.

Human fetal and neonatal patients are at some increased risk of sepsis from diminished concentrations of opsonins such as complement and specific IgG concentrations.[19,34] A significant correlation exists between the plasma concentration of complement components and gestational age. Full-term infants have near-normal adult concentrations, whereas premature infants have one third to one half of adult circulating complement concentrations.[34] Although the fetus synthesizes immunoglobulin M as early as week 8 of gestation and

IgG soon after, endogenous fetal IgG synthesis is negligible until weeks after birth. The major portion of circulating IgG in the fetus and newborn is acquired by transplacental transport of IgG from the maternal compartment. Unfortunately, most IgG transport occurs after week 30 of gestation. A strong correlation exists between transplacental passage of type-specific IgG and neonatal protection of invasive group B streptococci, the most common cause of sepsis in neonates.[57,58] The lower levels of complement combined with diminished antibody concentrations may thus result in impaired bacterial opsonization.

Several studies have also suggested a developmental deficiency of serum fibronectin, another important opsonin.[59,60] In addition, neonatal neutrophils have a lower content of CD11b and crystallizable fragment (Fc) γRIII, receptors that are important in opsonin-mediated binding.[61,62] Phagocytosis by neonatal neutrophils may be impaired, especially for certain bacteria and fungi, and when the proportion of bacteria to neutrophils is high.[63,64] However, opsonophagocytosis by neonatal neutrophils improves in the presence of specific immunoglobulins.[65]

Intracellular Killing Mechanisms

The primary role of neutrophils in host defense is to kill invading microbes. Killing of microorganisms can occur through two primary pathways in phagocytes that use oxygen radical–dependent and oxygen radical–independent microbicidal mechanisms.[56] Under normal conditions, neutrophils consume little molecular oxygen. Soon after neutrophil stimulation with soluble chemotactic or opsonized particulate material, however, oxygen consumption increases dramatically, nearly 100-fold. This increase in oxygen utilization is caused by a reduction of molecular oxygen to superoxide anion and is catalyzed by the phagocyte respiratory burst oxidase. The reduced oxygen molecule is further metabolized to form hydrogen peroxide, hypohalous acids, and chloramines, which damage microbial cell membranes. The oxidase is a cell membrane–bound flavoenzyme comprising several protein subunits, including gp1 phox, p22 phox, p47 phox, and p67 phox. Activation of the oxidase requires both membrane-bound (gp91 phox, p22 phox) and cytoplasmic proteins (p47 phox, p67 phox). Defects in any four of these components produce a disease called chronic granulomatous disease (CGD).[66]

Oxidative Metabolism

During phagocytosis, neutrophilic cytoplasmic granules release their contents (degranulation) and oxidative metabolism is increased, a process known as the **respiratory burst**. As part of the respiratory burst, oxidation products, including hydrogen peroxide and the superoxide anion, are released by stimulated neutrophils.[67] In addition to having some ability to kill pathogens, these reactive oxygen intermediates contribute to the formation of potent oxygen metabolites essential for microbicidal activity, such as the hydroxyl radical, choramines, and hypochlorous acid. In contrast, the neutrophil can produce enzymes, such as catalase, superoxide dismutase, and glutathione peroxidase, which serve to neutralize oxidant activity and limit tissue injury.

Neonatal neutrophils exhibit increased unstimulated and chemotactic factor–stimulated production of superoxide anion but appear deficient in synthesis of certain oxidant scavenger molecules. This imbalance has suggested to some investigators that selected aspects of neonatal neutrophil dysfunction may arise because of diminished ability to tolerate oxidant stress.[55] Lactoferrin, a microbicidal granular constituent, is expressed in lower concentrations in neutrophils isolated from newborns than in adult subjects.[68] Despite these apparent impairments in neonatal neutrophil function, bacterial killing in vitro appears equivalent to neutrophils isolated from normal adult subjects, except in instances in which the neutrophils were obtained from ill infants.[55] In addition to sepsis, conditions such as the respiratory distress syndrome may stress the neonatal immune response, and studies have suggested that the neutrophils of such neonates exhibit a variable killing efficiency of *Escherichia coli*, *Staphylococcus aureus*, group B streptococci, and *Candida albicans*, especially in very premature subjects.[2]

Apoptosis

Apoptosis, or programmed cell death, is a mechanism used by the organism to maintain cellular homeostasis by removing senescent cells. During apoptosis, neutrophils undergo characteristic nuclear and cytoplasmic changes. The resultant preservation of membrane integrity and diminished functionality of these neutrophils allows their removal by the reticuloendothelial system without inducing local tissue injury.[69] Thus, apoptosis is important to the normal resolution of inflammatory processes. There is mounting evidence that a perturbation of this process underlies the pathogenesis of several inflammatory and hematopoietic disorders. Studies suggest that delayed apoptosis may be contributory to chronic inflammatory conditions and autoimmune phenomena; in contrast, enhanced neutrophil apoptosis has been associated with chronic neutropenia.[70-73]

Neonatal neutrophils have been shown to exhibit aberrations in apoptosis. In vitro studies have shown that only approximately half as many cultured cord blood neutrophils as adult neutrophil cultures underwent apoptosis after 24 hours of culture.[74] Although delayed neutrophil apoptosis could theoretically impede the resolution of inflammation and contribute to the survival of potentially toxic neutrophils, as has been observed in adults with chronic lung disease, the clinical relevance of this observation is currently unclear.[75,76]

ROLE OF MONONUCLEAR PHAGOCYTES IN HOST DEFENSE

Mononuclear phagocytes play important supportive roles in acute inflammation and are heavily involved in regulating chronic inflammatory states.[19] During acute inflammation, circulating monocytes are recruited along with neutrophils but do not become prominent at the inflammatory site for 24 to 48 hours. Recruited monocytes and resident tissue macrophages actively ingest and kill invading microorganisms and also play an important role in clearing senescent neutrophils and damaged tissue components from the inflammatory site. Another way in which monocytes and macrophages augment acute and chronic inflammatory responses is through the secretion of cytokines, including IL-1, IL-6, IL-8, IL-12, tumor necrosis factor α, interferon α, and several hematopoietic growth factors.[19,77] Several of these molecules (tumor necrosis factor α, IL-1, and IL-6) induce changes in hepatic protein metabolism (acute-phase response), are pyrogenic, and can influence systemic and local regulation of blood vessel tone and permeability.

Mononuclear phagocytes not only participate in the acute killing and clearance of pathogenic microorganisms but also process the ingested microbial material and present it along with class II major histocompatibility antigens to T lymphocytes (Fig. 84-8). T cell activation in turn leads to the synthesis and secretion of additional cytokines that further activate the macrophages and enhance their killing capacity.[2] In addition, T cell activation results in B lymphocyte stimulation and antibody production, generation of additional helper and suppressor T cells, and generation of antigen-specific cytotoxic T cells. Thus, by assisting in producing a specific immune response to microbial invasion, mononuclear phagocytes protect the host from subsequent challenges by the same microorganism.

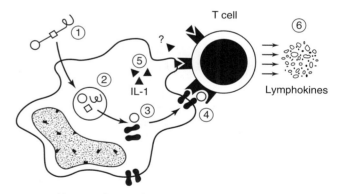

Figure 84–8. Events involved in macrophage recognition, processing, and presentation of antigen to T lymphocytes. Most protein antigens (1) require internalization and intracellular lysosomal processing (2) before the antigenic fragment and major histocompatibility class II molecules (3) are presented at the cell surface to activate CD4⁺ T lymphocytes (4). The expression of interleukin-1 (IL-1) by the macrophage (5) is also required for T lymphocyte activation. T lymphocyte activation results in synthesis and secretion of numerous cytokines and lymphokines (6) that function to activate macrophages for cytocidal function, stimulate proliferation of both T and B lymphocytes, and modulate B lymphocyte differentiation. *(From Polin RA, Fox WW [eds]: Fetal and Neonatal Physiology. Philadelphia, WB Saunders, 1992, p 1452.)*

Ontogenic Aspects of Mononuclear Phagocyte Function

Neonatal monocytes share certain functional abnormalities with neonatal neutrophils, although other functions appear to be intact in comparison with adult controls. Neonatal monocytes have been reported to have normal integrin-mediated adhesion[78] and chemotaxis.[79] In addition, neonatal and adult monocytes appear to have comparable phagocytic and oxidative metabolic processes, as well as cytotoxic activity. However, protein production may be more limited in neonatal monocytes. Stimulated cord blood monocytes have lower expression of several inflammatory mediators, including leukotriene B4, IL-8, G-CSF, and IL-12.[80-83] Macrophages derived from cord blood monocytes also produce less fibronectin than do those of adults.[84]

QUANTITATIVE NEUTROPHIL DISORDERS

Neutropenia is defined as an absolute decrease in the normal number of neutrophils measured in peripheral blood. If the absolute neutrophil count is less than 3000 cells/mm^3 in the first 48 hours after birth or less than 1500 cells/mm^3 (or in infants with very low birth weight, less than 1100/mm^3) thereafter, the neonate is neutropenic.[15,31] As with adult patients, the lower the absolute neutrophil count, the more susceptible the infant becomes to life-threatening infections.[85] Neutropenic disorders are generally grouped according to the primary defect: decreased production, abnormal maturation, or increased utilization or destruction of circulating cells (Table 84-2).

Table 84-2. Causes of Neutropenia in Childhood

Disorder	Clinical/Hematologic Feature	Mechanisms/Causes of Neutropenia
Infection	Highly variable clinical findings and blood picture	*Proliferation defect*: direct marrow suppression by toxins derived from organisms *Maturation defect*: depletion of maturation-storage compartment by releasing neutrophils into blood *Survival defect*: migration of neutrophils to sites of infection; increased neutrophil destruction secondary to infection *Distribution defect*: increased margination of neutrophils
Isoimmune neutropenia	Neutropenia at birth can persist up to 4 months Most babies have infectious episodes that are overwhelming in a minority Cutaneous infections predominate Myeloid hyperplasia in marrow with depletion of mature forms	*Survival defect*: transplacental passage of maternal IgG against infant's neutrophils
Transitory neonatal neutropenia	Maternal collagen vascular disease with antineutrophil autoantibodies; persistent, unexplained neutropenia in mother and newborn	*Survival defect*: presumably immune-mediated neutrophil destruction in newborn, after transplacental passage of antibodies
Maternal hypertension	Unexplained neutropneia in the newborn period followed by spontaneous recovery within days to weeks	*Proliferation defect*: inhibitor of myeloid progenitor cell proliferation
Maternal drug ingestion	Persistent, unexplained neutropenia; maternal history of drug ingestion (e.g., thiazides)	Mechanism varies with type of drug; relatively few drugs given to pregnant women are associated with neutropenia in the newborn
Benign (sometimes congenital neutropenia)	May be congenital or acquired at any later date, but presentation in the newborn period is unusual Some cases may have autosomal dominant or recessive patterns of inheritance Acquired cases frequently designated as chronic idiopathic neutropenia Other names include *familial neutropenia, congenital agranulocytosis,* and *hypoplastic neutropenia*	Heterogeneous mechanisms for neutropenia *Proliferation defect*: imbalance of promoters and inhibitors of GM-CSF activity resulting in decreased proliferative activity *Maturation defect*: increased intramedullary cell death; failure of normal granulocyte maturation; failure of bone marrow release of neutrophils *Survival defect*: possible immune-mediated granulocyte destruction
Neutropenia associated with immunodeficiency	Persistent neutropenia in patients with immunodeficiency (e.g., IgG or IgA deficiency, Wiskott-Aldrich-like disorder, or X-linked lymphoproliferative syndrome)	*Proliferation defect*: regulatory abnormality of precursor cells (e.g., failure of T lymphocyte induction of granulopoiesis)

Table 84–2. Causes of Neutropenia in Childhood—cont'd

Disorder	Clinical/Hematologic Feature	Mechanisms/Causes of Neutropenia
Neutropenia with exocrine pancreas insufficiency (Shwachman-Diamond syndrome)	Persistent neutropenia in patients with malabsorption, bone and cartilage abnormalities, short stature, and infections; autosomal recessive patterns of inheritance	Mechanism uncertain
Congenital dysgranulopoietic neutropenia	Persistent neutropenia with life-threatening infections; abnormal granule formation in neutrophil precursors with frequent autophagic vacuoles; clinical and morphologic features similar to myelokathexis	*Maturation defect*: increased intramedullary cell death
Chédiak-Higashi syndrome	Rare autosomal recessive disorder with mild to moderate neutropenia, frequent infections, cutaneous and ocular hypopigmentation, and large granules in all types of granulocytes; monocytes, and even lymphocytes; abnormal granule formation and function attributed to defect in microtubular assembly; affected patients usually succumb to infection in childhood	*Maturation defect*: ineffective granulopoiesis with intramedullary death of abnormal granulocytes
Autoimmune neutropenia of infancy and childhood	Common cause of chronic neutropenia in infancy and early childhood; onset, 1-30 mo of age; babies healthy at birth and a later chronic illness with recurrent liver, diarrhea, and infections develops; no specific clinical findings to suggest autoimmune disease; disease lasts about 2 years; spontaneous recovery in most children; rarely, red blood cell and platelet antibodies develop. Bone marrow shows normal to increased early granulocytic elements; mature neutrophils may be decreased	*Survival defect*: autoantibodies against granulocyte membrane proteins (e.g., NA1, NA2); mechanisms of destruction of antibody-coated neutrophils uncertain (theories include intravascular lysis by complement-binding antibodies, antibody-dependent cell-mediated cytotoxicity, entrapment in microcapillaries, splenic phagocytosis of coated neutrophils)
Cyclic neutropenia	Autosomal dominance inheritance; sporadic cases reported. Boys and girls affected equally. Recurrent, cyclic (about every 3 weeks) infections usually involving skin and mucosal surfaces. Bone marrow shows cyclic loss of granulocytic and other cell lines with oscillations in morphologic and ultrastructural abnormalities of granulocytic elements	*Proliferation defect*: regulatory abnormality of precursor cells (overly active negative feedback system). *Survival defect*: apoptosis of hematopoietic precursors
Several congenital neutropenia (Kostman syndrome)	Autosomal recessive disorder with bone marrow "maturation arrest"; sporadic cases reported; severe neutropenia with recurrent, severe life-threatening infections; patients often die of infection in infancy	*Proliferation defect*: genetically transmitted factor capable of suppressing hematopoiesis
Congenital aleukocytosis (reticular dysgenesis)	Very rare disorder with thymic hypoplasia and hypogammaglobulinemia; absence of granulocytes and lymphocytes; death in early infancy from infection	*Proliferation defect*: uncertain cause that could be related to failure of T cells and macrophages to induce granulopoiesis

GM-CSF, granulocyte macrophage colony–stimulating factor; IgA and IgM, immunoglobulins A and G.

Adapted with permission from Bick RL (ed): Hematology: Clinical and Laboratory Practice. St. Louis, Mosby–Year Book, 1993, p 1145.

Neutropenia Resulting from Decreased Production or Maturation Arrest

Neutropenias Acquired in Utero

Pregnancy-induced hypertension/preeclampsia. Maternal hypertension and preeclampsia can lead to neutropenia that lasts for several days to weeks in affected infants (see Table 84-2) and that is associated with low circulating numbers of CFU-GM and diminished neutrophil storage pools.[86] Although the majority of infants have a transient neutropenia, a subgroup may have a prolonged neutropenia that can last for days to weeks. This type of neutropenia resolves naturally, although in some cases it may be severe enough to consider therapy with G-CSF.[87] In addition, the neutropenia may not be entirely benign, as suggested by some (but not all) studies; there may be a propensity for a later nosocomial infection in affected neonates, even after the resolution of the neutropenia.[86,88,89] The cause of this neutropenic state appears to be the production of an inhibitor of CFU-GM proliferation that transplacentally inhibits fetal bone marrow production of neutrophils.[90]

Rh hemolytic disease. Neutropenia has been described in neonates affected in utero by Rh hemolytic disease.[91] After delivery, blood neutrophil concentrations may be decreased for several days, and the neutropenia is self-limited. One cause of this neutropenia appears to be a down-modulation of neutrophil production in association with increased erythroid production,[92,93] as evidenced by low numbers of neutrophil progenitors in the presence of elevated levels of erythropoietin and high concentrations of erythroid precursors in the cord blood of affected infants.[91]

Inherited/Congenital Neutropenias

Heritable neutropenias may, but often do not, occur in the immediate neonatal period. Many infants with congenital forms of neutropenia do not have recurring or unusual infections, signs ordinarily associated with the most severe inherited forms of neutropenia, until several months of age. One obvious distinction between transient and heritable forms of neutropenia is that the numerous transient causes of neutropenia resolve and the heritable forms of neutropenia persist.

Kostmann syndrome. Neutropenia that is severe (<500 cells/mm^3), is persistent, and manifests in the neonatal period was first described by Kostmann.[94] This autosomal recessive disorder is associated with significant host defense impairment, and patients experience frequent episodes of fever and infections. Studies indicate that neutrophil development is apparently normal up to the myelocyte stage, but few mature neutrophils are present in the bone marrow and circulating blood. A defect in the signal transduction pathway through the G-CSF receptor has been postulated because bone marrow from patients with Kostmann neutropenia produce normal neutrophils when stimulated with high concentrations of G-CSF in vitro.[95,96] Mutations in the elastase

gene have been thought to cause arrested neutrophil development.[97]

Cyclic (benign chronic) neutropenia. In this unusual disorder, neutropenia occurs in an approximately 21-day cycle and typically endures for up to 10 days.[98] Patients present with recurrent, self-limited mucosal and soft tissue infections that parallel neutropenic episodes, although up to 10% of such patients may die of overwhelming systemic infections. Neutropenic episodes are associated with marrow myeloid hypoplasia or an arrest of neutrophil maturation, thought to be caused by a mutation of the neutrophil elastase gene.[97] In addition, apoptosis of hematopoietic progenitors appears to be a contributory mechanism to the neutropenia.[99] In addition to antibiotics, treatment with G-CSF may improve the neutrophil counts and reduce the number of infectious episodes.

Other causes of neutropenia. Mild to severe persistent neutropenia can be caused by a variety of other inherited disorders (see Table 84-2). The mechanisms leading to these neutropenic states are heterogeneous. Some involve apparent imbalances in the positive and negative regulators of hematopoiesis, leading to decreased production. In some disorders, neutrophil production is normal but maturation is not, as in the Shwachman syndrome, which is associated with neutropenia despite normal numbers of myeloid progenitors.[100] Reticular dysgenesis, or congenital aleukocytosis, is a neutropenia associated with myeloid hypoplasia and is thought to arise from a maturation defect of a lymphohematopoietic precursor.[101,102]

Neutropenia Resulting from Increased Utilization or Destruction

Sepsis

Infection is the most common cause of neutropenia in newborns.[15,31] Experiments in neonatal rodents and data from human infants suggest that several factors predispose infected infants to become neutropenic.[103] First, hematopoiesis occurs primarily in the bone marrow during the last trimester of pregnancy. During this time, neutrophil and mononuclear phagocyte production is maximally stimulated and exceeds erythropoiesis. As a result, neutrophil and monocyte counts in peripheral blood are increasing, the marrow cavity is completely filled with hematopoietic cells, a high percentage of the progenitor cells are proliferating, and a neutrophil storage pool is being generated as the developing fetus approaches full-term gestation. However, in contrast to adult bone marrow, fetal bone marrow has fewer myeloid progenitor cells, a smaller neutrophil storage pool, and less ability to expand overall hematopoiesis in the presence of greater needs for circulating cells under stress. Furthermore, during an infection in adults, mobilization of the neutrophil storage pool is highly regulated; only a portion of the cells (<15%) leave in response to a stimulus. In infected neonates, the pool of neutrophils in the marrow is nearly completely mobilized (>70%) in response to a single stimulus, leaving no reservoir of cells for further needs. Additional factors that increase the demand for circulating neutrophils include massive recruitment of circulating cells into the infected areas, increased destruction of neutrophils at the site of inflammation, and increased margination of cells along inflamed vessels. Moreover, there is evidence of an association between neutropenia and decreased neutrophil survival.[104] All of these factors contribute to an increased risk that insufficient circulating neutrophils can be made available at sites of inflammation in infected newborn infants. Neutropenia and depletion of the neutrophil bone marrow storage pool (defined as <10% of all marrow nucleated cells composed of postmitotic neutrophils) are associated with but not highly predictive of a poor prognosis in the septic newborn.[105]

Immune-Mediated Neutropenias

Maternal autoimmune disease with antineutrophil IgG antibodies that cross the placenta can lead to neutropenia (see Table 84-2).[106] Likewise, isoimmune neutropenia is an antibody-mediated disease in which paternal antigens on fetal neutrophils sensitize the mother to produce IgG antineutrophil antibodies.[107] This form of neutropenia is estimated to occur in 0.2% to 3% of live births. Several causative neutrophil antigens have been identified.[108] After birth, circulating antineutrophil titers decline in the newborn, with normal neutrophil counts returning by 2 to 4 months of age (see Table 84-2). Autoimmune neutropenia is a rare disorder that results from host-derived antibody-mediated interactions directed against the host's own neutrophils.[109] This disorder manifests in infancy or early childhood; it has been described in the neonatal period. Patients are neutropenic and have associated multiple soft tissue infections, although some patients are at risk for more severe systemic infections. The sera of affected patients contain antineutrophil antibodies, most commonly the Fc γIIIb antigen. Bone marrow examination reveals normal to increased myeloid cellularity, with a maturational arrest caused by destruction of more mature neutrophils observed in some cases. Treatment is supportive, and antibiotic prophylaxis should be considered in patients with recurrent infections. Circulating neutrophil counts have been reportedly improved after treatment with corticosteroids and intravenous immune globulin in nearly half of treated patients; in contrast, all patients benefited from G-CSF therapy.[110,111] Autoimmune neutropenia is generally a self-limited disorder that resolves with the natural disappearance of antineutrophil antibodies.

Neutropenia Resulting from Other Causes

Neutropenia can occur in infants who are born with severely depressed vital signs as a result of a variety of in utero or peripartum events. Intraventricular hemorrhage can occur in infants at or soon after birth and is occasionally associated with neutropenia. Neutropenia has also been reported in newborns whose blood group antigens are incompatible with maternal blood group antigens and in infants who develop a peripheral blood reticulocytosis several weeks after birth.[12] In addition, neutropenia is not uncommon in infants who are receiving a course of recombinant human erythropoietin for the treatment of the anemia of prematurity and is a relative contraindication to initiating or continuing such therapy.[112]

Neutrophilia

Neutrophilia is defined as an elevation in the number of circulating neutrophils to more than 7000 cells/mm³ in adult subjects. Because of the rapid increase in all circulating cells at birth, neutrophil counts as high as 14,400 cells/mm³ are measured at 12 hours of age. After 72 hours of age, the upper limit of normal is 5400 to 7000 cells/mm³ for full-term and premature infants during the first week after birth, values equivalent to adult subjects.[15] Neutrophil counts vary with the site of collection; capillary blood contains 20% more neutrophils than does venous or arterial blood.[113]

Mechanisms that lead to increased neutrophil counts are reviewed in Table 84-3. Peripartum complications that have been associated with neutrophilia in newborns include sepsis, hemolytic disease, hypoglycemia, stressful labor, seizures, pneumothorax, and meconium aspiration syndrome. In the majority of these instances, increased neutrophil counts probably result from their release from the marginated pool, increased mobilization from the bone marrow storage pool, or decreased egress from the circulating pool. Neutrophilia has been reported in some infants with the syndrome of thrombocytopenia and absent radii. Bone marrow examination may be helpful in making a diagnosis. In addition, a persistent neutrophilia, especially if associated with recurrent bacterial infections or a delayed separation of the umbilical cord, should prompt the investigation of leukocyte adhesion deficiency as a possible diagnosis.[48]

Table 84–3. Classification of Neutrophilia

Increased production
  Chronic infection
  Chronic inflammation
  Tumors (perhaps with necrosis)
  Postneutropenia rebound
  Myeloproliferative disease
  Drugs (lithium, occasionally ranitidine)
  Chronic idiopathic neutrophilia
  Leukemoid reactions
Enhanced release from marrow storage pool
  Corticosteroids
  Stress
  Hypoxia
  Acute infection
  Endotoxin
Decreased egress from circulation
  Corticosteroids
  Splenectomy
  Leukocyte adhesion deficiency
Reduced margination
  Stress
  Infections
  Epinephrine

On occasion, infants with trisomy 21 have neutrophil counts that are so high as to be indistinguishable from the leukocyte counts of infants with acute leukemia.[114,115] Organomegaly, a high percentage of myeloid blast forms in peripheral blood, and persistent elevation of the leukocyte count for weeks may also be seen in these infants. Because patients with trisomy 21 have an increased incidence of leukemia, it is often difficult to distinguish such patients with leukemia from those with a transient myeloproliferative disorder.

QUALITATIVE NEUTROPHIL DISORDERS

A straightforward way to categorize qualitative disorders of neutrophil function is to consider these disorders in light of the probable sequence of steps involved in recruiting neutrophils to a site of infection and the multiple neutrophil functions involved in ingestion and killing of the offending microorganisms (see Fig. 84-6). Most of the inherited disorders listed in Table 84-1 are encountered infrequently. Acquired neutrophil function disorders are more common, but the mechanisms accounting for these neutrophil disorders are not as well understood, and in many instances, only descriptive reports of the disorders exist.[116]

Disorders of Neutrophil Adherence

Leukocyte Adhesion Deficiencies

Leukocyte adhesion deficiency type I. Leukocyte adhesion deficiency (LAD) type I is a relatively rare autosomal recessive disorder, with an incidence of 2 cases per 1,000,000 individuals.[48] Affected patients have severe recurrent bacterial infections, poor wound healing, gingivitis, and a persistent granulocytosis (see Table 84-1). This disorder, which can occur in the neonatal period, is caused by deficient expression of all three members of the integrin family of adhesion-promoting glycoproteins on phagocytic cells. Affected neutrophils and monocytes demonstrate poor chemotaxis, little or no adhesion to endothelial cells and extracellular matrix proteins, and poor ingestion of complement-coated microorganisms. LAD can be classified by the nature of the molecular defect in the leukocyte integrin CD18. The diagnosis should be suspected in any infant who has recurrent bacterial infections and persistent granulocytosis. Diagnosis of this disorder is accomplished by flow cytometric analysis of neutrophils, with monoclonal antibodies to the granulocyte cell surface integrin CD18 and its subsets, a technique that can be used in utero for fetal diagnosis of LAD.[117]

Leukocyte adhesion deficiency type II. LAD type II is a very rare disorder that is caused by defective selectin-mediated neutrophil adhesion.[42] The few patients described with this disorder exhibit recurrent infections, growth restriction, mental retardation, characteristic facial features, and the Bombay blood group. In addition, such patients presented with extreme neutrophilia in the neonatal period, ranging from 25,000/mm³ up to 150,000/mm³ during infectious episodes. In contrast to patients with LAD type I, there was no delay in umbilical cord separation. Neutrophils of patients with LAD type II exhibit abnormal interactions with activated endothelium under

conditions of shear stress, a selectin-mediated event, and as a result have defective "rolling" and chemotaxis. In contrast, integrin-mediated neutrophil-endothelial adhesion is normal. The primary underlying defect is related to a global defect in fucose metabolism and results in the absence of the selectin ligand sialyl Lewis X on neutrophils; CD18 expression is normal. Flow cytometric analysis and specific functional assays are useful in making the diagnosis. Antibiotics are the mainstay of therapy during acute infections, although prophylaxis is not required, because such infections do not appear to be life-threatening. Fucose administration has been helpful in some, but not all, cases.[118]

Disorders of Neutrophil Motility

The neutrophil cytoskeleton plays a vital role in the chemotactic response of neutrophils to soluble agents.[119] Microtubules are involved in organizing the cytoplasmic organelles, nucleus, and microfilaments dispersed throughout the cytoplasm to assist in directional migration. Microfilaments are essential for generation of the sliding motion that propels the cell surface membrane in the direction of the chemotactic gradient and pulls along the cell and its contents. Diagnosed defects in the neutrophil cytoskeleton are rare, but the impaired mobility of the affected cell points out the important role of the cytoskeleton in neutrophil function (see Table 84-1).

Disorders of Neutrophil Phagocytosis and Intracellular Killing

Patients who have acquired or inherited B lymphocyte deficiencies often suffer from recurrent pyogenic infections secondary to diminished immunoglobulin production, defective opsonization of microorganisms, and related impairments in granulocyte phagocytosis and killing of pathogens (see Table 84-1). Phagocytic deficiencies are also seen in patients with a number of chronic debilitating diseases (see Table 84-1). The mechanisms underlying the phagocytic impairment are unclear for many chronic illnesses, but they may relate to the effect of numerous interleukins and cytokines or circulating immune complexes that desensitize granulocytes to chemotactic stimuli.[117]

Chronic Granulomatous Disease

Patients with CGD develop recurrent bacterial infections because oxidase-deficient neutrophils are unable to kill microorganisms, particularly catalase-positive microbes, which contain little endogenously produced hydrogen peroxide.[66] Infections are often chronic and lead to granuloma formation and lymph node enlargement. This disease is inherited in autosomal and X-linked forms, and great heterogeneity in time of onset and severity of symptoms is a hallmark of this disorder.[120] The diagnosis of CGD should be considered in patients with recurrent infections, infections with unusual pathogens, or persistent lymphadenopathy.[121] A sharp decrease or absence of the neutrophil respiratory burst with no other abnormalities in neutrophil function is indicative of CGD. The nitroblue tetrazolium (NBT) test is a commonly used method of checking for the neutrophil respiratory burst.[117] When water-soluble NBT dye is reduced in activated neutrophils, a dark purple solid precipitate called **formazan** is formed. When NBT results are weak or absent, quantitative measures of the neutrophil respiratory burst should be performed to confirm the diagnosis. Most mutations in the oxidase complex resulting in CGD have been determined at the molecular level. In utero fetal testing, combining the simplicity of the NBT test with advances in techniques to diagnose CGD mutations at the molecular level, is now available, and the diagnosis can be made definitively either on fetal neutrophils or by chorionic villus sampling.

In addition to oxygen radical–dependent mechanisms of bacterial killing (see Table 84-1), certain neutrophil antimicrobicidal proteins may play important roles in bacterial killing. Granular proteins such as lysozyme, lactoferrin, cathepsin G, and defensins all have antimicrobial properties.[51] It remains unclear how significant an in vivo role these agents play in microbial killing.

Chédiak-Higashi Syndrome

In this rare autosomal recessive disorder, neutrophils exhibit giant cytoplasmic granules, a result of fusion of azurophilic granules.[117,122] Patients present with oculocutaneous albinism and frequent soft tissue infections most commonly involving *S. aureus*, although reported pathogens have also included other gram-positive and gram-negative organisms. Functional neutrophil defects include abnormal chemotaxis and microbicidal activity, although phagocytosis may be normal. In addition to neutrophils, affected patients may have abnormal lymphocyte and platelet function, as well as neurologic abnormalities. Management includes aggressive antibiotic therapy and surgical drainage, and bone marrow transplantation has been successfully attempted in several patients.[117,121]

Other Disorders

Myeloperoxidase deficiency. Deficiency of the neutrophil granule myeloperoxidase is inherited in an autosomal recessive manner and is a relatively common phagocyte disorder, with an incidence of approximately 0.05%.[117,123] Although this disorder is benign in most patients, the killing of certain *Candida* species is impaired in neutrophils of some affected patients.[124]

Rac2 mutation. A patient with a mutation of Rac2, a guanosine triphosphate protein important in multiple signal transduction pathways, has been reported.[125] This patient presented in infancy with leukocytosis and severe, recurrent soft tissue infections, and neutrophil function testing revealed multiple abnormalities, including chemotaxis, phagocytosis, degranulation of myeloperoxidase, and respiratory burst activity. The patient was treated with antibiotics and granulocyte infusions, and subsequent bone marrow transplantation resulted in improved neutrophil function.

QUANTITATIVE MONONUCLEAR PHAGOCYTE DISORDERS

Monocytopenia as an isolated entity does not occur.[19] Low monocyte counts are seen in patients with mild aplastic

Table 84–4. Causes of Monocytosis

Infectious and parasitic diseases
  Subacute bacterial endocarditis
  Tuberculosis
  Rickettsial disease
  Syphilis
  Malaria
  Post–acute infection state
Neoplastic diseases
  Myelomonocytic leukemia
  "Preleukemia"
  Nonhematologic malignant disease
Miscellaneous hematologic diseases
  Recovery phase of agranulocytosis
  Postsplenectomy
  Myeloid metaplasia
  Hemolytic anemia
Miscellaneous disorders
  Fever of unknown origin
  Drug reactions
  Cirrhosis

anemia, hairy cell leukemia, and acquired immunodeficiency syndrome. Monocytopenia is also seen in some patients receiving corticosteroids, a medication increasingly used to treat certain neonates with chronic lung disease.

Deficient numbers of pulmonary macrophages have been observed in human fetuses and in newborn primates within 24 hours after birth.[19] A rapid increase in the concentration of lung macrophages occurs in the first few days after birth. Numerous inherited and acquired abnormalities in macrophage function are known, but there are no known primary impairments in host defense caused exclusively by an insufficient supply of macrophages.

Monocyte concentrations in peripheral blood above 800 cells/mm³ are considered abnormal. Monocytosis often occurs in response to an ongoing infectious challenge, particularly invasive parasitic infections. Monocytosis in the newborn rarely results from a proliferative malignancy. Monocytosis can, however, be observed in newborns who have an inherited or acquired neutropenic disorder or some other form of marrow failure syndrome. Table 84-4 lists a number of causes of monocytosis.

QUALITATIVE MONONUCLEAR PHAGOCYTE DISORDERS

In general, primary defects in monocyte and macrophage function are extremely rare.[19,126] Many defects in neutrophil function, such as CGD, LAD, and some of the chemotactic and adhesion disorders of immaturity, are shared by the mononuclear phagocyte system. However, most of the defects in monocyte or macrophage function are secondary to complications from systemic chronic illnesses (diabetes mellitus, acquired immunodeficiency syndrome, autoimmune diseases) or related to treatments of systemic illnesses (chronic steroid therapy, administration of immunomodulating agents).

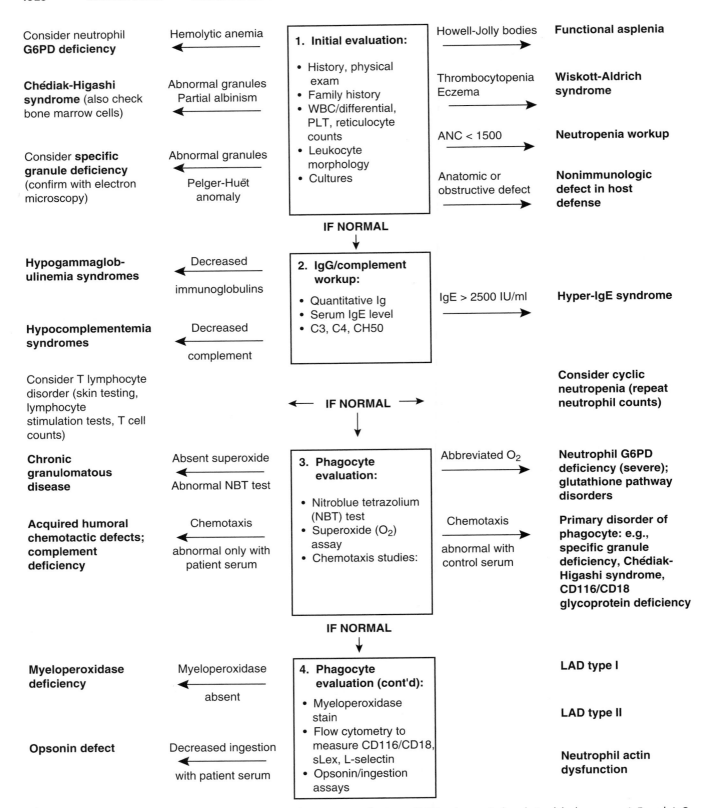

Figure 84–9. Algorithm for the workup of a patient with recurrent infections. G6PD, glucose-6-phosphate dehydrogenase; IgE and IgG, immunoglobulins E and G; LAD, leukocyte adhesion deficiency; PLT, platelet count; WBC, white blood cell count. (*Adapted from Lehrer RL: Neutrophils and host defense. Ann Intern Med 109:138, 1988.*)

DIAGNOSTIC EVALUATION AND TREATMENT OF PHAGOCYTE DISORDERS

Diagnostic Approaches

Quantitative Disorders

Neutropenia that is severe and persistent mandates further evaluation, and the approach is dependent on whether the infant is healthy or sick in appearance. In addition, the perinatal and maternal history plays an important role in investigating causative factors of neonatal neutropenia. Infection should be an initial consideration in infants who are ill. However, if neutropenia persists after infection has been ruled out, further steps could include an evaluation of maternal and neonatal blood for the presence of antineutrophil antibodies and the consideration of a bone marrow biopsy.[127]

Neonatal neutrophilia is defined as an absolute neutrophil count higher than 30,000/mm³ in the first days after birth or higher than 15,000/mm³ in the neonatal period.[15] Investigation should be initiated for infants with a persistent neutrophilia and for any infant who has more than 5% blasts, promyelocytes, or myelocytes on a differential, regardless of the neutrophil count.[128] Evaluation should include a workup for possible infection, especially in the ill-appearing infant. Chromosomal analysis should be performed, and bone marrow analysis considered in the presence of features suggestive of trisomy 21. As with other phagocyte disorders, the maternal and peripartum history should not be overlooked, including the use of corticosteroids and the possibility of the association of toxoplasmosis, other infections, rubella, cytomegalovirus, and herpes simplex (TORCH) or other viral infections, and a review of the family history may provide useful clues. In addition, an evaluation for LAD should be considered, especially with a history of recurrent infections.

Qualitative Disorders

Whenever an infant experiences two or more systemic bacterial or fungal infections, fails to respond to conventional antimicrobial therapy, or develops unusual infections, the clinician should entertain the diagnosis of an underlying phagocyte disorder.[117,121,129] Primary heritable phagocyte disorders are rare, however, and potential complicating factors (congenital heart disease, foreign body, cystic fibrosis, antibiotic overgrowth, contaminated ventilator equipment, malnutrition, and chronic infections with antibiotic-resistant organisms) that could predispose the infant should be sought.

Screening tests of neutrophil number and structure should be available at all institutions, whereas specific tests of neutrophil physiologic processes and function may be most efficiently and accurately performed at major medical centers. After a thorough physical examination, the algorithm shown in Figure 84-9 and several reviews[117,121,127] should assist in the diagnosis of quantitative and qualitative phagocyte disorders.

Management

Therapeutic approaches to patients with phagocyte deficiencies are tailored to the specific disorder, although certain conventional therapies are commonly applied to all of these patients.[117,121] Antibiotics and surgical drainage are standard treatments for the recurrent infections and abscesses that afflict these patients. Other supportive approaches may include prophylactic antibiotics, neutrophil transfusions for neutropenic patients with infection, and intravenous immune globulins for patients with IgG deficiency.

Impairments of phagocyte function are continuously being resolved at the molecular level, and more specific therapies are proving efficacious.[120] Bone marrow transplantation, administration of recombinant hematopoietic growth factors, selected immune modulating medications, and specific differentiation agents, such as G-CSF, have proved useful in both in vitro and in vivo in improving phagocyte function in human patients.

REFERENCES

1. Lewis DB, Wilson CB: Developmental immunology and role of host defenses in fetal and neonatal susceptibility to infection. In Remington JS, Klein JO (eds): Infectious Diseases of the Fetus and Newborn Infant, 5th ed. Philadelphia, WB Saunders, 2001, pp 25-138.
2. Kapur R, Yoder MC, Polin RA: Developmental immunology. In Fanaroff AA, Martin RJ (eds): Neonatal-Perinatal Medicine, 7th ed. St. Louis, CV Mosby, 2001, pp 676-706.
3. Christensen RD: Hematopoiesis in the fetus and neonate. Pediatr Res 26:531, 1989.
4. Timens W, Kamps WA: Hemopoiesis in human fetal and embryonic liver. Microsc Res Tech 39:387, 1997.
5. Hole N: Embryonic stem cell-derived haematopoiesis. Cells Tissues Organs 165:181, 1999.
6. Palis J, Yoder MC: Yolk-sac hematopoiesis: The first blood cells of mouse and man. Exp Hematol 29:927, 2001.
7. Thomas DB, Yoffey JM: Human fetal hematopoiesis. II. Hepatic hematopoiesis in the human foetus. Br J Haemotol 10:193, 1964.
8. Migliaccio G, Migliaccio AR, Petti S, et al: Human embryonic hemopoiesis. Kinetics of progenitors and precursors underlying the yolk sac–liver transition. J Clin Invest 78:51, 1986.
9. Tavian M, Robin C, Coulombel L, Peault B: The human embryo, but not its yolk sac, generates lympho-myeloid stem cells: Mapping multipotent hematopoietic cell fate in intraembryonic mesoderm. Immunity 15:487, 2001.
10. Clapp DW, Dumenco LL, Hatzoglou M, Gerson SL: Fetal liver hematopoietic stem cells as a target for in utero retroviral gene transfer. Blood 78:1132, 1991.
11. Peschle C, Migliaccio AR, Migliaccio G, et al: Identification and characterization of three classes of erythroid progenitors in human fetal liver. Blood 58:565, 1981.
12. Luchtman-Jones L, Schwartz AL, Wilson DB: Hematologic problems in the fetus and newborn. In Fanaroff AA, Martin RJ (eds): Neonatal-Perinatal Medicine, 7th ed. St. Louis, Mosby, 2001, pp 1183-1238.
13. Ogawa M: Differentiation and proliferation of hematopoietic stem cells. Blood 81:2844, 1993.
14. Forestier F, Daffos F, Catherine N, et al: Developmental hematopoiesis in normal human fetal blood. Blood 77:2360, 1991.
15. Manroe BL, Weinberg AG, Rosenfeld CR, Browne R: The neonatal blood count in health and disease. I. Reference values for neutrophilic cells. J Pediatr 95:89, 1979.

16. Mouzinho A, Rosenfeld CR, Sanchez PJ, Risser R: Revised reference ranges for circulating neutrophils in very-low-birth-weight neonates. Pediatrics 94:76, 1994.

17. Kelemen E, Janossa M: Macrophages are the first differentiated blood cells formed in human embryonic liver. Exp Hematol 8:996, 1980.

18. Timens W, Kamps WA, Rozeboom-Uiterwijk T, Poppema S: Haemopoiesis in human fetal and embryonic liver. Immunohistochemical determination in B5-fixed paraffin-embedded tissues. Virchows Arch A Pathol Anat Histopathol 416:429, 1990.

19. Yoder MC, Douglas SD: Mononuclear phagocyte system. In Polin RA, Fox WW (eds): Fetal and Neonatal Physiology, 2nd ed. Philadelphia, WB Saunders, 1998, pp 1931-1954.

20. Christensen RD: Granulocytopoiesis in the neonate and fetus. Trans Med Rev 4:8, 1990.

21. Athens JW, Raab SO, Haab OP, et al: Leukokinetic studies. III. The distribution of granulocytes in the blood of normal subjects. J Clin Invest 40:159, 1961.

22. Brenner I, Shek PN, Zamecnik J, Shephard RJ: Stress hormones and the immunological responses to heat and exercise. Int J Sports Med 19:130, 1998.

23. Fossati G, Mazzucchelli I, Gritti D, et al: In vitro effects of GM-CSF on mature peripheral blood neutrophils. Int J Mol Med 1:943, 1998.

24. Dale DC, Liles WC, Llewellyn C, Price TH: Effects of granulocyte-macrophage colony-stimulating factor (GM-CSF) on neutrophil kinetics and function in normal human volunteers. Am J Hematol 57:7, 1998.

25. Wolach B, Gavrieli R, Pomeranz A: Effect of granulocyte and granulocyte macrophage colony stimulating factors (G-CSF and GM-CSF) on neonatal neutrophil functions. Pediatr Res 48:369, 2000.

26. Bracho F, Goldman S, Cairo MS: Potential use of granulocyte colony–stimulating factor and granulocyte-macrophage colony–stimulating factor in neonates. Curr Opin Hematol 5:215, 1998.

27. Patton JHJ, Lyden SP, Ragsdale DN, et al: Granulocyte colony–stimulating factor improves host defense to resuscitated shock and polymicrobial sepsis without provoking generalized neutrophil-mediated damage. J Trauma 44:750, 1998.

28. Calhoun DA, Lunoe M, Du Y, et al: Granulocyte colony–stimulating factor serum and urine concentrations in neutropenic neonates before and after intravenous administration of recombinant granulocyte colony–stimulating factor. Pediatrics 105:392, 2000.

29. Nakagawa M, Terashima T, D'yachkova Y, et al: Glucocorticoid-induced granulocytosis: Contribution of marrow release and demargination of intravascular granulocytes. Circulation 98:2307, 1998.

30. Savill JS, Wyllie AH, Henson JE, et al: Macrophage phagocytosis of aging neutrophils in inflammation. Programmed cell death in the neutrophil leads to its recognition by macrophages. J Clin Invest 83:865, 1989.

31. Manroe BL, Rosenfeld CR, Weinberg AG, Browne R: The differential leukocyte count in the assessment and outcome of early-onset neonatal group B streptococcal disease. J Pediatr 91:632, 1977.

32. Anwer SK, Mustafa S: Rapid identification of neonatal sepsis. J Pak Med Assoc 50:94, 2000.

33. Johnston RB Jr: Current concepts: Immunology. Monocytes and macrophages. N Engl J Med 318:747, 1988.

34. Lewis DB: Host defense mechanisms against bacteria, fungi, viruses and nonviral intracellular pathogens. In Polin RA, Fox WW (eds): Fetal and Neonatal Physiology, 2nd ed. Philadelphia, WB Saunders, 1998, pp 1869-1919.

35. Smith CW: Endothelial adhesion molecules and their role in inflammation. Can J Physiol Pharmacol 71:76, 1993.

36. Condliffe AM, Kitchen E, Chilvers ER: Neutrophil priming: Pathophysiological consequences and underlying mechanisms. Clin Sci (Lond) 94:461, 1998.

37. Bevilacqua MP: Endothelial-leukocyte adhesion molecules. Annu Rev Immunol 11:767, 1993.

38. Ley K: Molecular mechanisms of leukocyte recruitment in the inflammatory process. Cardiovasc Res 32:733, 1996.

39. Jung U, Ramos CL, Bullard DC, Ley K: Gene-targeted mice reveal importance of L-selectin–dependent rolling for neutrophil adhesion. Am J Physiol 274:H1785, 1998.

40. von Andrian UH, Arfors KE: Neutrophil-endothelial cell interactions in vivo: A chain of events characterized by distinct molecular mechanisms. Agents Actions Suppl 41:153, 1993.

41. Bullard DC, Kunkel EJ, Kubo H, et al: Infectious susceptibility and severe deficiency of leukocyte rolling and recruitment in E-selectin and P-selectin double mutant mice. J Exp Med 183:2329, 1996.

42. Etzioni A, Tonetti M: Leukocyte adhesion deficiency II—from A to almost Z. Immunol Rev 178:138, 2000.

43. Simon SI, Burns AR, Taylor AD, et al: L-selectin (CD62L) cross-linking signals neutrophil adhesive functions via the Mac-1 (CD11b/CD18) beta 2-integrin. J Immunol 155:1502, 1995.

44. Simon SI, Neelamegham S, Taylor A, Smith CW: The multistep process of homotypic neutrophil aggregation: A review of the molecules and effects of hydrodynamics. Cell Adhes Commun 6:263, 1998.

45. Anderson DC, Abbassi O, Kishimoto TK, et al: Diminished lectin-, epidermal growth factor–, complement binding domain–cell adhesion molecule–1 on neonatal neutrophils underlies their impaired CD18-independent adhesion to endothelial cells in vitro. J Immunol 146:3372, 1991.

46. Koenig JM, Simon J, Anderson DC, et al: Diminished soluble and total cellular L-selectin in cord blood is associated with its impaired shedding from activated neutrophils. Pediatr Res 39:616, 1996.

47. Jones DH, Schmalstieg FC, Dempsey K, et al: Subcellular distribution and mobilization of MAC-1 (CD11b/CD18) in neonatal neutrophils. Blood 75:488, 1990.

48. Anderson DC, Springer TA: Leukocyte adhesion deficiency: An inherited defect in the Mac-1, LFA-1, and p150,95 glycoproteins. Annu Rev Med 38:175, 1987.

49. McEvoy LT, Zakem-Cloud H, Tosi MF: Total cell content of CR3 (CD11b/CD18) and LFA-1 (CD11a/CD18) in neonatal neutrophils: Relationship to gestational age. Blood 87:3929, 1996.

50. Imhof BA, Dunon D: Basic mechanism of leukocyte migration. Horm Metab Res 29:614, 1997.

51. Borregaard N, Cowland JB: Granules of the human neutrophilic polymorphonuclear leukocyte. Blood 89:3503, 1997.

52. Smith CW: Transendothelial migration. Curr Top Microbiol Immunol 184:201, 1993.

53. Usmani SS, Schlessel JS, Sia CG, et al: Polymorphonuclear leukocyte function in the preterm neonate: Effect of chronologic age. Pediatrics 87:675, 1991.

54. Carr R, Pumford D, Davies JM: Neutrophil chemotaxis and adhesion in preterm babies. Arch Dis Child 67:813, 1992.

55. Hill HR: Biochemical, structural and functional abnormalities of polymorphonuclear leukocytes in the neonate. Pediatr Res 22:375, 1987.

56. Burg ND, Pillinger MH: The neutrophil: Function and regulation in innate and humoral immunity. Clin Immunol 99:7, 2001.

57. Anderson DC, Hughes BJ, Edwards MS, et al: Impaired chemotaxigenesis by type III group B streptococci in neonatal sera: Relationship to diminished concentration of specific anticapsular antibody and abnormalities of serum complement. Pediatr Res 17:496, 1983.

58. Baker CJ, Webb BJ, Kasper DL, Edwards MS: The role of complement and antibody in opsonophagocytosis of type II group B streptococci. J Infect Dis 154:47, 1986.

59. Koenig JM, Patterson LE, Rench MA, Edwards MS: Role of fibronectin in diagnosing bacterial infection in infancy. Am J Dis Child 142:884, 1988.

60. Dyke MP, Forsyth KD: Plasma fibronectin levels in extremely preterm infants in the first 8 weeks of life. J Paediatr Child Health 30:36, 1994.

61. Abughali N, Berger M, Tosi MF: Deficient total cell content of CR3 (C11b) in neonatal neutrophils. Blood 83:1086, 1994.

62. Carr R, Huizinga TW: Low soluble FcRIII receptor demonstrates reduced neutrophil reserves in preterm neonates. Arch Dis Child Fetal Neonatal Ed 83:F160, 2000.

63. Quie PG: Antimicrobial defenses in the neonate. Semin Perinatol 14:2, 1990.

64. Bektas S, Goetze B, Speer CP: Decreased adherence, chemotaxis and phagocytic activities of neutrophils from preterm neonates. Acta Paediatr Scand 79:1031, 1990.

65. Christensen RD, Brown MS, Hall DC, et al: Effect on neutrophil kinetics and serum opsonic capacity of intravenous administration of immune globulin to neonates with clinical signs of early-onset sepsis. J Pediatr 118:606, 1991.

66. Dinauer MC, Orkin SH: Chronic granulomatous disease. Annu Rev Med 43:117, 1992.

67. Dahlgren C, Karlsson A: Respiratory burst in human neutrophils. J Immunol Methods 232:3, 1999.

68. Kjeldsen L, Sengelov H, Lollike K, Borregaard N: Granules and secretory vesicles in human neonatal neutrophils. Pediatr Res 40:120, 1996.

69. Haslett C: Granulocyte apoptosis and its role in the resolution and control of lung inflammation. Am J Respir Crit Care Med 160:S5, 1999.

70. Haslett C: Granulocyte apoptosis and inflammatory disease. Br Med Bull 53:669, 1997.

71. Eguchi K: Apoptosis in autoimmune diseases. Intern Med 40:275, 2001.

72. Liu JH, Wei S, Lamy T, et al: Chronic neutropenia mediated by fas ligand. Blood 95:3219, 2000.

73. Nwakoby IE, Reddy K, Patel P, et al: Fas-mediated apoptosis of neutrophils in sera of patients with infection. Infect Immun 69:3343, 2001.

74. Allgaier B, Shi M, Luo D, Koenig JM: Spontaneous and Fas-mediated apoptosis are diminished in umbilical cord blood neutrophils compared with adult neutrophils. J Leukoc Biol 64:331, 1998.

75. Haslett C: Granulocyte apoptosis and its role in the resolution and control of lung inflammation. Am J Respir Crit Care Med 160:S5, 1999.

76. Matute-Bello G, Liles WC, Radella F, et al: Neutrophil apoptosis in the acute respiratory distress syndrome. Am J Respir Crit Care Med 156:1969, 1997.

77. Joyner JL, Augustine NH, Taylor KA, et al: Effects of group B streptococci on cord and adult mononuclear cell interleukin-12 and interferon-gamma mRNA accumulation and protein secretion. J Infect Dis 182:974, 2000.

78. Torok C, Lundahl J, Hed J, Lagercrantz H: Diversity in regulation of adhesion molecules (Mac-1 and L-selectin) in monocytes and neutrophils from neonates and adults. Arch Dis Child 68:561, 1993.

79. Speer CP, Wieland M, Ulbrich R, Gahr M: Phagocytic activities in neonatal monocytes. Eur J Pediatr 145:418, 1986.

80. Schibler KR, Liechty KW, White WL, Christensen RD: Production of granulocyte colony–stimulating factor in vitro by monocytes from preterm and term neonates. Blood 82:2478, 1993.

81. English BK, Hammond WP, Lewis DB, et al: Decreased granulocyte-macrophage colony–stimulating factor production by human neonatal blood mononuclear cells and T cells. Pediatr Res 31:211, 1992.

82. Rowen JL, Smith CW, Edwards MS: Group B streptococci elicit leukotriene B$_4$ and interleukin-8 from human monocytes: Neonates exhibit a diminished response. J Infect Dis 172:420, 1995.

83. Lee SM, Suen Y, Chang L, et al: Decreased interleukin-12 (IL-12) from activated cord versus adult peripheral blood mononuclear cells and upregulation of interferon-gamma, natural killer, and lymphokine-activated killer activity by IL-12 in cord blood mononuclear cells. Blood 88:945, 1996.

84. Gerdes JS, Douglas SD, Kolski GB, et al: Decreased fibronectin biosynthesis by human cord blood mononuclear phagocytes in vitro. J Leukoc Biol 35:91, 1984.

85. Squire E, Favara B, Todd J: Diagnosis of neonatal bacterial infection: Hematologic and pathologic findings in fatal and nonfatal cases. Pediatrics 64:60, 1979.

86. Koenig JM, Christensen RD: Incidence, neutrophil kinetics, and natural history of neonatal neutropenia associated with maternal hypertension. N Engl J Med 321:557, 1989.

87. Kocherlakota P, La GE: Preliminary report: rhG-CSF may reduce the incidence of neonatal sepsis in prolonged preeclampsia-associated neutropenia. Pediatrics 102:1107, 1998.

88. Doron MW, Makhlouf RA, Katz VL, et al: Increased incidence of sepsis at birth in neutropenic infants of mothers with preeclampsia. J Pediatr 125:452, 1994.

89. Paul DA, Leef KH, Sciscione A, et al: Preeclampsia does not increase the risk for culture proven sepsis in very low birth weight infants. Am J Perinatol 16:365, 1999.

90. Koenig JM, Christensen RD: The mechanism responsible for diminished neutrophil production in neonates delivered of women with pregnancy-induced hypertension. Am J Obstet Gynecol 165:467, 1991.

91. Koenig JM, Christensen RD: Neutropenia and thrombocytopenia in infants with Rh hemolytic disease. J Pediatr 114:625, 1989.

92. Christensen RD, Koenig JM, Viskochil DH, Rothstein G: Down-modulation of neutrophil production by erythropoietin in human hematopoietic clones. Blood 74:817, 1989.

93. Koenig JM, Christensen RD: Effect of erythropoietin on granulocytopoiesis: In vitro and in vivo studies in weanling rats. Pediatr Res 27:583, 1990.

94. Kostmann R: Infantile genetic agranulocytosis. Acta Paediatr Scand 64:362, 1975.

95. Kyas U, Pietsch T, Welte K: Expression of receptors for granulocyte colony–stimulating factor on neutrophils from patients with severe congenital neutropenia and cyclic neutropenia. Blood 79:1144, 1992.

96. Zeidler C, Boxer L, Dale DC, et al: Management of Kostmann syndrome in the G-CSF era. Br J Haematol 109:490, 2000.

97. Aprikyan AA, Dale DC: Mutations in the neutrophil elastase gene in cyclic and congenital neutropenia. Curr Opin Immunol 13:535, 2001.

98. Haurie C, Dale DC, Mackey MC: Cyclical neutropenia and other periodic hematological disorders: A review of mechanisms and mathematical models. Blood 92:2629, 1998.

99. Aprikyan AA, Liles WC, Rodger E, et al: Impaired survival of bone marrow hematopoietic progenitor cells in cyclic neutropenia. Blood 97:147, 2000.

100. Shwachman H, Diamond LK, Oski FA, et al.: The syndrome of pancreatic insufficiency and bone marrow dysfunction. J Pediatr 65:645, 1964.

101. De Vaal O, Seynhaeve V: Reticular dysgenesis. Lancet 2:1123, 1959.

102. Roper M, Parmley RT, Crist WM, et al: Severe congenital leukopenia (reticular dysgenesis). Immunologic and morphologic characterizations of leukocytes. Am J Dis Child 139:832, 1985.

103. Christensen RD: Neutrophil kinetics in the fetus and neonate. Am J Pediatr Hematol Oncol 11:215, 1989.

104. Aprikyan AA, Liles WC, Dale DC: Emerging role of apoptosis in the pathogenesis of severe neutropenia. Curr Opin Hematol 7:131, 2000.

105. Engle WA, McGuire WA, Schreiner RL, Yu PL: Neutrophil storage pool depletion in neonates with sepsis and neutropenia. J Pediatr 113:747, 1988.

106. Kameoka J, Funato T, Miura T, et al: Autoimmune neutropenia in pregnant women causing neonatal neutropenia. Br J Haematol 114:198, 2001.

107. Cartron J, Tchernia G, Celton JL, et al: Alloimmune neonatal neutropenia. Am J Pediatr Hematol Oncol 13:21, 1991.

108. Boxer LA: Immune neutropenias. Clinical and biological implications. Am J Pediatr Hematol Oncol 3:89, 1981.

109. Madyastha PR, Fudenberg HH, Glassman AB, et al: Autoimmune neutropenia in early infancy: A review. Ann Clin Lab Sci 12:356, 1982.

110. Blanchette VS, Kirby MA, Turner C: Role of intravenous immunoglobulin G in autoimmune hematologic disorders. Semin Hematol 29:72, 1992.

111. Carulli G: Treatment of autoimmune neutropenia with recombinant human granulocyte colony–stimulating factor. Ann Hematol 76:93, 1998.

112. Ohls RK: The use of erythropoietin in neonates. Clin Perinatol 27:681, 2000.

113. Christensen RD, Rothstein G: Pitfalls in the interpretation of leukocyte counts of newborn infants. Am J Clin Pathol 72:608, 1979.

114. Bhatt S, Schreck R, Graham JM, et al: Transient leukemia with trisomy 21: Description of a case and review of the literature. Am J Med Genet 58:310, 1995.

115. Brodeur GM, Dahl GV, Williams DL, et al: Transient leukemoid reaction and trisomy 21 mosaicism in a phenotypically normal newborn. Blood 55:691, 1980.

116. Watts RG, Howard TH: Functional disorders of granulocytes and monocytes. In Bick RL (ed): Hematology. Clinical and Laboratory Practice. St. Louis, Mosby–Year Book, 1993, pp 1099-1121.

117. Malech HL, Nauseef WM: Primary inherited defects in neutrophil function: Etiology and treatment. Semin Hematol 34:279, 1997.

118. Marquardt T, Brune T, Luhn K, et al: Leukocyte adhesion deficiency II syndrome, a generalized defect in fucose metabolism. J Pediatr 134:681, 1999.

119. Stossel TP, Hartwig JH, Janmey PA, Kwiatkowski DJ: Cell crawling two decades after Abercrombie. Biochem Soc Symp 65:267, 1999.

120. Goebel WS, Dinauer MC: Gene therapy for chronic granulomatous disease. Acta Haematol 110:86, 2003.

121. Lakshman R, Finn A: Neutrophil disorders and their management. J Clin Pathol 54:7, 2001.

122. Quie PG, Hetherington SV: Patients with disorders of phagocytic cell function. Pediatr Infect Dis 3:272, 1984.

123. Nauseef WM: Myeloperoxidase deficiency. Hematol Pathol 4:165, 1990.

124. Chiang AK, Chan GC, Ma SK, et al: Disseminated fungal infection associated with myeloperoxidase deficiency in a premature neonate. Pediatr Infect Dis J 19:1027, 2000.

125. Kurkchubasche AG, Panepinto JA, Tracy TF Jr, et al: Clinical features of a human Rac2 mutation: a complex neutrophil dysfunction disease. J Pediatr 139:141, 2001.

126. Blaese RM, Poplack DG, Muchmore AV: The mononuclear phagocyte system: Role in expression of immunocompetence in neonatal and adult life. Pediatrics 64(Suppl):829, 1979.

127. Christensen RD, Calhoun DA, Rimsza LM: A practical approach to evaluating and treating neutropenia in the neonatal intensive care unit. Clin Perinatol 27:577, 2000.

128. Calhoun DA, Christensen RD, Edstrom CS, et al: Consistent approaches to procedures and practices in neonatal hematology. Clin Perinatol 27:733, 2000.

129. Quie PG: Phagocytic cell dysfunction. J Allergy Clin Immunol 77:387, 1986.

CHAPTER 85

Transfusion Therapy

Kelly M. Axsom, David F. Friedman, and Catherine S. Manno

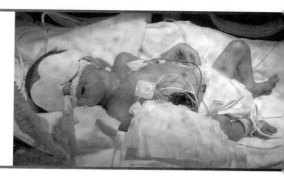

lood transfusions are an integral part of the management of very sick neonates. About 80% of infants with low birth weights receive at least one transfusion, and the average number of transfusions is 8 to 10 per premature infant over the course of a hospital stay[1,2]; thus, premature infants are a heavily transfused group of patients. Most of these transfusion exposures involve red blood cell products. A survey of neonatal transfusion practices sponsored by the American Association of Blood Banks (AABB) in the early 1990s revealed considerable variation in transfusion practices among neonatal units throughout North America.[3,4] Reasonable transfusion practices vary from hospital to hospital, but some commonly encountered practices should be discouraged.

The same high standards of safety for blood product testing, storage, preparation, and administration must be observed for neonates as for any patient. Physicians caring for neonates should also strive to limit the number of blood units and donors to which an infant is exposed because of the small but real risk of infectious disease transmission and other hazards inherent in all blood transfusions. To achieve these general goals of safety and limited exposure to donors for premature infants, however, the physician and the transfusion service must consider several theoretical and practical issues that are unique to neonatal transfusion practice.

IMMUNOLOGIC ISSUES IN THE NEONATE

Serology Problems

Red blood cells carry numerous antigenic determinants that are polymorphic in the human population. Antibody responses to these determinants can arise spontaneously or in response to exposures to red blood cells with an antigenic makeup different from that of the recipient. Antibodies in the ABO, Rh, Kell, Duffy, Kidd, and many other blood group systems can cause clinically significant red blood cell destruction. In the most general sense, the routine serologic tests performed in the blood bank—type, screen, and crossmatch—are aimed at identifying significant antibodies and avoiding antigen-antibody incompatibilities.

The humoral immune system of the neonate differs from that of the older child and adult in two major ways, which have direct effects on blood transfusion. First, the neonate is born with adult levels of immunoglobulin G (IgG) transferred across the placenta from the maternal circulation. Second, the neonate is very inefficient in forming antibody responses to antigenic challenges in the form of red blood cells, vaccines, or infections. Thus, the newborn's serum may contain IgG antibodies specific for many antigens to which the mother has responded, including the blood cell antigens that she lacks but to which she has been exposed by transfusion or pregnancy. On the other hand, the newborn's serum has immunoglobulin M at a concentration of only 10% that in the adult because this large pentamer does not cross the placenta and can arise only from the immature immune system of the newborn.[5] These two facts are fundamental to the use and interpretation of red blood cell serologic testing in newborns.

Hemolytic Disease of the Newborn

The epidemiology, pathophysiology, and management of **hemolytic disease of the newborn (HDN)** are discussed in detail in Chapter 82. The blood bank plays a central role in the management of HDN by performing diagnostic testing and by preparing blood products for treatment.

HDN occurs when IgG anti–red blood cell antibodies from the mother cross the placenta and cause immune-mediated destruction of fetal red blood cells. The mother is sensitized to a red blood cell antigen that she lacks because of small fetomaternal hemorrhages from a fetus that has inherited the sensitizing antigen from the father. The classic and most severe form of HDN occurs when an Rh(D)-negative mother has an Rh(D)-positive fetus.

The mother may form an antibody to the D antigen, which can cross the placenta and cause red blood cell destruction.

The most important test for diagnosis of HDN is the **direct antiglobulin test (DAT)**, also called the direct Coombs test. This test detects the IgG antibodies bound to the surface of red blood cells in the infant's circulation. There are two methods available to perform a DAT: the tube test and the antiglobulin gel test. In the tube test, IgG specific anti–human globulin reagent is mixed with a suspension of the infant's red blood cells. If they are coated with IgG, the cells are agglutinated, and the strength of this agglutination can be graded semiquantitatively. The antiglobulin gel test utilizes the same principle of agglutination. In the gel DAT, the infant's red blood cells are added to a special microtube filled with dextran acrylamide gel suspended in a buffer containing anti–human globulin reagent and then centrifuged. Strict, controlled centrifugation techniques are necessary for results to be accurate.[6,7] Cells that are coated with IgG agglutinate and become trapped in the gel; strong positive reactions remain on the top of the gel, whereas cells that do not agglutinate pass through and form a pellet at the bottom of the microtube.[6,7] Developed by Lapierre in the 1980s, the gel test requires a significantly smaller blood sample than does the tube test.[6,7] Many laboratories use the gel test over the tube test for this reason. Furthermore, because it is easier to read, the gel test result is more reproducible and reliable; it is also more sensitive to weak antibodies.[6-10] A positive DAT result is obtained in the majority of cases of clinical HDN, but the strength of the agglutination is not well correlated with the clinical severity of hemolysis.

In addition to testing the red blood cell surface for IgG antibodies, the serum can be tested for antibodies directed against red blood cells, using either the tube or the gel method. Screening the serum for such specificities is performed by an **indirect antiglobulin test (IAT)** or indirect Coombs' test. The unknown serum is exposed to a panel of reagent red blood cells that may then be agglutinated by the anti–human globulin reagent. Because the mother is the source of the infant's serum antibodies, it is preferable to screen the maternal serum because the titers may be higher and the specimen is more easily available. The presence of a red blood cell antibody in the maternal or neonatal serum (positive antibody screen, or IAT) does not alone prove the diagnosis of HDN because if the infant's red blood cells lack the corresponding antigen, the antibody has no effect on their survival. In this instance, the result of the first test, the DAT, would be negative.

The identity of the antibody detected by a positive DAT result can be investigated further by performing an elution procedure. Chemical or physical manipulations are used to release antibody from the red blood cells back into a soluble form. The eluate can be screened against reagent cells by IAT to determine the blood group specificity of the eluted antibody: that is, ABO, Rh, and so forth. When a DAT result is positive, an elution procedure may be performed to identify the specificity of the antibody involved in immune hemolysis. The elution

procedure is confirmatory, but not strictly necessary, if red blood cell antibodies capable of explaining the HDN are found by IAT in the maternal serum.[11] From a practical standpoint, the red blood cell antibodies found in the maternal serum determine which antigens must be avoided when red blood cells are selected for transfusion. The eluate may be necessary if the DAT result is positive but no red blood cell antibody is found in the maternal serum; elution usually concentrates the antibody in relation to its titer in the serum and may demonstrate a specificity not detectable in the serum.

For example, a newborn suspected to have HDN because of early onset of indirect hyperbilirubinemia and anemia is found to have a positive DAT result. The maternal serum and the infant's serum are found to contain anti-E (an Rh antigen) and anti-K (Kell) antibodies, both red blood cell antibodies known to cause HDN. An eluate is made from the child's red blood cells, and only the anti-K antibody is found. Testing of infant, maternal, and paternal red blood cell antigens reveals that both infant and father carry the K antigen. Also, the father is heterozygous for E antigen, whereas the child lacks the E antigen. The mother lacks both E and K antigens on her red blood cells. These results show that the mother has formed two antibodies against red blood cell antigens E and K, which she lacks on her own cells. Both antibodies have crossed the placenta into the infant's circulation. However, only the anti-K antibody is involved in the hemolysis because the infant inherited the K antigen from the father but not E antigen. A previous pregnancy of this couple may have sensitized the mother to E antigen if that infant inherited E antigen from the father. If the neonate required an exchange transfusion, the red blood cells for transfusion would be chosen to lack both K and E antigens, because antibodies to both are present in the serum.

PRETRANSFUSION TESTING

The required pretransfusion testing for neonatal red blood cell transfusions is significantly abbreviated in comparison with the standard testing protocol (Box 85-1).[12] For older children and adults, a serum specimen no older than 3 days is used to crossmatch each red blood cell unit issued for transfusion. For neonates up to 4 months of age, if the initial testing is negative, ABO-compatible red blood cells may be issued without a new specimen and without a crossmatch. This practice is safe because it is extremely rare for newborns to produce antibodies to red blood cell antigens, even in response to the repeated transfusions they may receive. Red blood cell antibodies present in the neonate's serum are derived from the mother and are at their highest titers in the first sample. In addition, fewer than half of normal infants have developed isohemagglutinins (anti-A in a child with blood group B, anti-B in a child with group A, both anti-A and anti-B in a child with group O) within the first 6 months.[5] Thus, crossmatching as a check against inadvertent ABO incompatibility is pointless in this age group. Eliminating the requirement for a new specimen every 3 days and for crossmatching reduces the amount of phlebotomy necessary for laboratory testing, which is one of the main reasons for blood loss in the neonate. To reduce further blood loss caused by phlebotomy, pretransfusion testing can be performed on umbilical cord blood and maternal plasma.[13] If a rare blood type is required because of maternal antibodies, periodic testing of the infant's serum for residual antibodies can determine when the requirement can be withdrawn.

VOLUME

The total blood volume of a newborn is estimated at 80 to 100 mL per kilogram of body weight. The normal cardiovascular system can usually tolerate acute increases of intravascular volume of 10% to 15%. Therefore, the usual dose of red blood cells for a simple transfusion, 10 mL of packed red blood cells per kilogram of body weight, is 10 to 20 mL for infants weighing 1 to 2 kg. Transfusion orders for 5 mL of blood product are not uncommon in the neonatal intensive care unit. Because the volumes must be precisely controlled, the concentration—that is, the hematocrit (HCT)—of the blood product must also be controlled precisely so that the dose of red blood cells is accurate. In contrast, packed cell transfusions for older children and adults are usually ordered in units or fractions of units, not in precise volumes.

The tight constraint on volume in neonatal transfusion means that a red blood cell product with a higher HCT is preferred for simple transfusions. The final HCT of red blood cell products varies according to the preservative used for storage and, to some extent, according to the amount of plasma left behind with the red blood cells after separation of blood components. The final HCT can be increased in a red blood cell product by gravity sedimentation or recentrifugation. A difference in final HCTs of 60% versus 80% translates into a difference in the dose of red blood cells of 25% per transfusion.

PRESERVATIVE SOLUTIONS

One "unit" of whole blood is collected by placing 450 mL of blood from a healthy adult volunteer donor into 63 mL of a solution of citrate phosphate dextrose (CPD) that contains citrate as an anticoagulant, sodium phosphate as a buffer, and dextrose as an energy source for the red blood cells during storage.[14] The HCT of the donor may vary physiologically in a range from 38% to 52%, and the volume collected may vary by as much as 10% (405 to 495 mL).[14] The HCT of a unit of whole blood can therefore range between 33% and 46%. The plasma and most of the anticoagulant-preservative solution are removed to make a unit of packed red blood cells for storage with less than 5% of the original dextrose and buffer solution. As currently licensed, 100 mL of an additive solution, containing dextrose, adenine, sodium chloride, and, in some preparations, mannitol and phosphate buffer, may be added to the red blood cells after plasma has been removed. This solution prolongs the shelf life and improve the metabolic state of stored red blood cells. Red blood cells collected in these solutions, called additive solution units, have a final HCT in the range of 55% to 60%.[15] In the United States, there are three licensed additive solutions: AS-1, AS-3, and AS-5. The HCT of additive solution units can be increased to approximately 80% by sedimentation or centrifugation just before transfusion.[15-18]

Whole blood may also be collected for storage as a CPD adenine (CPDA-1) unit, in which case it is drawn into a 63-mL solution of trisodium citrate, citric acid, sodium phosphate, dextrose, and adenine. The unit is centrifuged and the plasma is removed, which creates a unit of packed red blood cells for storage. CPDA-1 units have a HCT between 75% and 80%; the remaining volume is 21% to 23% plasma and 3% to 4% anticoagulant-preservative solution. Fresh CPDA-1 units were the customary neonatal transfusion product used before confirmation of the safety of AS-1 and AS-3 packed cells for neonatal transfusion.

Currently, AS-1 and AS-3 units are accepted and frequently utilized for neonatal transfusions. Although these solutions preserve red blood cell pH, potassium, and viability better than either CPD or CPDA-1, concerns have been raised about the potential renal toxicity of adenine, the osmotic or diuretic effects of mannitol, and the higher dextrose concentration in AS-1 as potential hazards in neonates. When the amounts of these substances actually infused during a small-volume transfusion are calculated, however, they are far lower than expected toxic doses.[15,19]

Multiple studies have reported no evidence of renal or other toxicity in small groups of neonates given red blood cells stored in AS-1 versus CPDA-1 or in AS-3 versus CPDA-1.[16,18,20-23] In one study, glucose homeostasis during transfusion was better in the AS-1 recipients, presumably a benefit of the higher dextrose concentration in AS-1 units.[16] The safety of red blood cells preserved in AS-1 and AS-3 for transfusion to neonates is well established for small volumes slowly infused. The safety of these units for large-volume transfusions, such as exchange transfusion, cardiopulmonary bypass, or extracorporeal membrane oxygenation (ECMO), has not been established.

Because 70% of neonatal transfusions are given during the first month after birth, there is a significant advantage offered by the longer storage allowed for AS-1 and AS-3 red blood cells in comparison with CPDA-1 units.[15]

FRESHNESS

Until the late 1990s, the "requirement" for neonatal blood transfusions was fresh red cells, less than 7 days old. This practice resulted in high rates of exposure to donors, with each neonate receiving only about two transfusions per donor.[24] Currently, the recognition that AS-1 or AS-3 preserved cells may be transfused safely to neonates throughout the storage life of the cells has extended the acceptable life of blood to be transfused in neonates. This practice exposes each neonate to one donor for approximately seven transfusions. The number of exposures to donors for an entire hospital stay has been studied; on average, three to six donors are required when CPDA-1 units are transfused, but only one or two donors are needed when additive solution units are transfused.[18,22,23]

During liquid storage in any preservative, the intracellular level of red blood cell 2,3-diphosphoglycerate (2,3-DPG) falls, the pH falls, and the concentrations of extracellular potassium and free hemoglobin rise.[14] These measured changes and the many other metabolic alterations that are presumed to occur do so because of depletion of intracellular energy stores. The percentage of viable red blood cells, as defined by the recovery of transfused cells in circulation 24 hours after transfusion, also falls during storage.

The preservative solution affects the rate at which these metabolic alterations occur in the stored red blood cell product, with extracellular potassium rising much faster in CPD and CPDA-1 than in additive solution units.[14] The storage form also affects the rate of these changes; potassium and free hemoglobin rise more rapidly when cells are stored as packed cells rather than as whole blood. All of these metabolic changes occur gradually with time in storage, and the cutoff for allowable shelf life of red blood cell products for general use is determined by the average in vivo red blood cell recovery and safety for transfusion on the last day of storage. Currently, Food and Drug Administration standards permit transfusion of CPD units up to 21 days of storage; CPDA-1 units up to 35 days; and AS-1, AS-3, and AS-5 units up to 42 days. Additive solution units dedicated to one or more neonates should be 7 days old or less on the day of dedication, to maximize the unit's utility to the patient.

Much more conservative standards are frequently applied to neonates. The AABB survey of neonatal transfusion practices in 1989 revealed that more than 70% of hospitals surveyed used red blood cells no older than 7 days for neonatal transfusion.[3] With the acceptance of using older AS-1 or AS-3 units, this practice has most certainly changed; however, there currently exist no published data about the extent of change. Increasingly, more institutions are lifting the old limitations on blood freshness for transfusion into neonates.[25]

The practice of using fresh CPDA-1 units was based on two rationales. First, reports of mortality after rapid infusion of older red blood cells[26] have raised concerns that critical hyperkalemia and acidosis can occur in neonates as a result of the elevated extracellular potassium and low pH in older red blood cell products. In fact, the actual dose of extracellular potassium given to a neonate during a small-volume, simple transfusion represents 10% to 20% of the daily potassium requirements. When administered over 2 to 4 hours, it is unlikely to cause hyperkalemia or acidosis.[1] These doses of potassium are not dangerous when blood is infused slowly.

Second, there has been concern that older red blood cells depleted of 2,3-DPG have suboptimal oxygen delivery capacity. Because the hemoglobin-oxygen dissociation curve for adult hemoglobin A shifts to the left in the presence of lower pH and lower 2,3-DPG levels, it results in reduced offloading of oxygen. Although intra-erythrocyte levels of 2,3-DPG are normalized within 24 hours of transfusion, the theoretical concern is that older red blood cells might release less oxygen than do cells with adequate 2,3-DPG, leaving the tissues hypoxic. The practical importance of this mechanism in neonates has also been questioned.[1,27] Premature neonates produce red blood cells with high levels of fetal hemoglobin. These cells have oxygen dissociation characteristics similar to those of adult red blood cells depleted of 2,3-DPG, as found in 42-day-old additive solution units. Transfusing these cells may not change the whole blood oxygen delivery in the neonate. Furthermore, once these cells recover, oxygen delivery is much improved in comparison with that intrinsic to the neonatal red blood cell.[15] When AS-1 or AS-3 units were compared with CPDA-1, they were found to be equally safe when transfused to neonates, even if AS-1 cells were stored up to 42 days.[18,22,23] With large transfusions, however, such as those required for ECMO, use of older additive solution units can be harmful to the neonate because of high levels of K^+, depleted 2,3-DPG stores, and possible toxic effects of the additive solutions.[15]

STRATEGIES TO LIMIT DONOR EXPOSURE

The majority of neonatal transfusions are small-volume boosters of red blood cells given periodically over the course of weeks of hospitalization for prematurity. With the traditional transfusion practice of giving neonates blood less than 7 days old, 1 unit would cover an infant's red blood cell needs for only 4 to 5 days, allowing 2 days for testing and processing. This practice exposed neonates to a new donor with every other transfusion. The use of red blood cells stored in AS-1 or AS-3 and transfused up to expiration date can fully meet a neonate's transfusion requirement,[18,23] thus exposing the neonate to fewer donors.[15] The reduction in donor exposure that can result from allowing a neonate to receive stored blood has been demonstrated.[28] Furthermore, the introduction of SCDs and mechanical syringe pumps has extended blood unit use and contributed to decreasing neonates' exposure to donors. Three additional strategies to reduce neonates' exposure to donors are discussed briefly here: erythropoietin, autologous placental blood, and so-called committed donor programs.

Splitting Red Blood Cell Units

With an umbilical cord blood HCT of 50% (the normal range for HCT varies with gestational age) and a blood volume of 80 to 100 mL/kg, a 1-kg infant's entire red blood cell mass is approximately equivalent to the red blood cell mass of one-fourth unit of blood; for a 2-kg infant, the total red blood cell mass is half a unit. As discussed previously, most transfusions to such infants are given in small aliquots. A single unit of packed red blood cells could theoretically supply four or five transfusions for a single infant, allowing for obligatory waste of 30 to 50 mL in the tubing and filter of the transfusion set. When this technique is used for neonatal transfusion, a large volume is wasted, and exposure to donors may be increased.

The introduction of sterile connecting devices (SCDs) has dramatically reduced wasted blood and exposure to donors by permitting sterile splitting of blood products into the desired aliquots without compromising unit shelf life. These devices can be used to weld standard integral polyvinylchloride tubing to the tubing of the primary container of a unit of red blood cells, plasma, or platelets, without entering through the conventional port. If the conventional port of a red blood cell unit is accessed, the shelf life is reduced to 24 hours. In the SCD, a copper wafer heated to 260°C is used to splice and rejoin tubing of the unit bag to a secondary blood bag or syringe. A portion of the blood component is then transferred into a second bag or a syringe. The SCD also can be used to weld leukocyte filters to blood containers for leukoreduction of blood before transfusion. SCDs have been tested extensively and have proved to maintain sterility when used to weld blood components, even those stored at room temperature.[29]

Transfusing red blood cells with a mechanical syringe pump is a common and safe practice in neonates.[30,31] These devices eliminate the waste of 30 to 50 mL of blood in tubing in small-volume blood transfusions, thus reducing overall component wastage. The syringe is attached to the parent unit by SCDs, and the exact transfusion volume is transferred into the syringe. A microaggregation filter should be attached to the syringe to catch fibrin strands before transfusion.

Neonates who are predicted to have high transfusion requirements should be identified early so that a whole or part of a unit of blood can be dedicated to each neonate. Neonates with low birth weight usually require more blood over the course of hospitalization and thus may be assigned to receive one full unit, whereas larger neonates with smaller overall transfusion requirement may have a split or divided unit.[32] The practice of splitting AS-1 or AS-3 preserved units of red blood cells and reserving a specific donor's cells for one neonate is essential to limiting donor exposure. The safety of additive solution units is compared with CPDA-1 units in the section on freshness. SCDs, mechanical syringe pumps, and dedicated units have significantly extended the use of blood components.

Erythropoietin

The neonate relies on the liver to produce erythropoietin; however, the liver is less responsive to anemia than is the kidney and produces erythropoietin inefficiently.[33-36] The switch from the liver to the kidney as the source of erythropoietin seems to be associated with postconception age, not birth.[37] Thus, supplementing the premature neonate with recombinant erythropoietin might be expected to stimulate erythropoiesis and decrease the transfusion requirement. Many researchers have investigated the value of recombinant human erythropoietin (rHuEPO) in sick neonates.[38-40] Shannon and colleagues found no change in HCT, reticulocyte counts, transfusion requirement, or growth between infants treated with rHuEPO and controls.[41] Of note, however, these researchers used low doses of rHuEPO. Some investigators found that treating some neonates with increased rHuEPO doses and iron supplementation increased reticulocyte counts and HCTs, reduced transfusion requirements, but did not completely prevent the need for transfusions.[40,42,43] Vamvakas and Strauss compared the results of 21 studies investigating the use of erythropoietin in neonates and found inconclusive evidence about the appropriate use of erythropoietin in the neonate.[44] The use of erythropoietin is discussed in more detail in Chapter 82.

Autologous Placental Blood

Autologous blood is generally accepted as preferable to homologous blood, as long as the autologous blood can be collected without placing the patient at risk. Autologous predeposit blood programs and intraoperative autologous blood salvage techniques have been successfully applied in pediatric populations,[45] but premature neonates are obviously not candidates for predeposited blood and seldom undergo surgery for which blood salvage would be feasible. Placental blood, however, has been proposed as a potential source of autologous red blood cells for newborns. Approximately 20 mL of blood per kilogram of birth weight can be harvested from the fetoplacental blood reservoir, with a hemoglobin concentration of approximately 16 to 17 g/dL available after a full-term birth.[46]

There are, however, several serious and unresolved problems with this practice.[47] First, even with sterile collection techniques, the rate of bacterial infection of placental blood may be much higher than in blood collected from a properly prepared venipuncture from a healthy volunteer donor. There also may be a greater chance of clot formation before or during collection. Umbilical cord red blood cells are quite different from adult red blood cells in size, shape, hemoglobin content, and many other metabolic characteristics; therefore, the storage conditions for blood donated by adults may not be optimal for placental blood. Finally, there may be elements in placental blood (maternal blood cells, cytokines, modulators of inflammation or coagulation) that are normally cleared from circulation after birth that might be harmful if reintroduced several hours or days after birth.

Brune and associates successfully collected and stored placental blood, the majority of collections having no anaerobe or aerobe contamination after 35 days and only one sample having maternal and infant mixed cell populations.[46] All collected blood was irradiated for safety. The authors of this study found that the amount of blood collected was enough to supply one transfusion of 10 mL/kg in 72.5% of the cases and enough for two transfusions in 16% of the cases. A poor correlation was found between transfusion requirement and amount of placental blood collected. This blood might supply a few red blood cell transfusions that would theoretically have the advantages of autologous blood. Placental blood has been collected and transfused for delivery room emergencies. It is also a source of hematopoietic stems cells for allogeneic bone marrow reconstitution but not as yet part of an autologous blood program for premature neonates. Harvesting and preserving placental blood as a potential source of autologous blood for neonates may help decrease exposure to donors. It may be beneficial as well for infants who are close to term but are expected to be sick or who may need surgery after birth. However, this practice may not benefit premature neonates with high transfusion requirements.[46]

Committed Donor Programs

Committed donor programs attempt to reduce a given patient's number of exposures to homologous donors by collecting as many of the needed blood products as possible from one or a few donors. Such strategies differ from simple directed blood donations, which are widely used in pediatric institutions, because they often alter donor eligibility criteria or change donation procedures to fit the patient's needs. It is clearly possible to reduce the number of exposures to donors significantly in scheduled surgery by using committed donors.[48,49] For premature neonates, supplying red blood cells from a single donor for 8 to 12 weeks may require 1 U of whole blood to be drawn more often than every 6 weeks; for fresh red blood cells, 0.25 U would be required weekly (the usual donation schedule for anonymous volunteer donors is 1 U every 56 days).

In addition to the logistic problems and regulatory compliance issues raised by such departures from standard donation procedures, the well-being (iron balance, venous access, volume status) and the true commitment (will the donor continue to donate?) of the blood donor would have to be considered in planning a committed donor program. The most obvious committed donor for a premature neonate would be a parent, but blood products from parents may carry certain additional risks for the neonate. Maternal plasma may contain antibodies directed against the infant's red blood cells or platelets[50] and has been implicated in the rare transfusion-related acute lung injury. This disease is mediated by the passive transfer of antibodies against lymphocytes or granulocytes that may promote complement activation and subsequent pulmonary injury.[28] Paternal red blood cells and platelets may bear antigens to which the mother has been immunized.[51] Both parents necessarily share human leukocyte antigen (HLA) alleles with the neonate, and lymphocytes in their blood products would have a greater chance of initiating transfusion-associated graft-versus-host disease (TA-GVHD). If blood from a biologic relative is donated to a neonate, it must undergo gamma irradiation before transfusion.

In summary, the role of erythropoietin in helping to decrease transfusion requirement is limited. Autologous placental blood is, at best, a limited resource, and many

problems still must be resolved. Finally, committed donor programs are a theoretically attractive way to reduce exposures to donated blood products, but they are logistically difficult to implement and are associated with certain risks to the donor and the neonate.

RED BLOOD CELL PRODUCTS FOR TRANSFUSION

Red blood cells can be prepared and stored for transfusion in several forms, as shown in Table 85-1. Some of these products are rarely used in neonates, and some are not routinely available from many blood banks. This section will review the characteristics of each of these products, emphasizing those points that have the greatest significance for transfusion to newborns. Three special processing requests, for cytomegalovirus (CMV) safety, gamma-irradiation, and leukoreduction of any of these red blood cell products, will be discussed later.

Packed Red Blood Cells

AS-1 (Adsol)

When packed red blood cells (PRBCs) are prepared for extended shelf life, 100 mL of additive solution, containing sodium chloride, dextrose, adenine, and mannitol, is added after plasma removal. This red blood cell product has a significantly lower HCT (55% to 60%)[15,52] than PRBCs in CPDA-1. However, the HCT can be increased by inverted centrifugation of AS-1 red blood cells before transfusion, raising the HCT as high as 90%,[16,18] or by gravity sedimentation, raising the HCT as high as 68% to 70%.[17] The superior preservation of 2,3-DPG and lower extracellular potassium levels in AS-1 PRBCs offer special advantages for this patient population.

AS-3 (Nutricel)

AS-3 PRBCs differ from AS-1 PRBCs in that the AS-3 preservative solution lacks mannitol. Like AS-1 PRBCs, these units have a 42-day shelf life and an HCT of 55% to 60%, and the HCT can be increased by sedimentation or centrifugation. Comparisons of the transfusion of AS-3 units with CPDA-1 units in neonates have conclusively shown that AS-3 cells are just as effective at increasing neonatal HCT and limiting exposure to donors.[23]

AS-5 (Optisol)

AS-5 and AS-1 preservative solutions are very similar and differ slightly in concentrations of sodium chloride, dextrose, adenine, and mannitol. Currently, there are no published reports on the use of AS-5 PRBCs for neonatal transfusions.

CPDA-1

Once the most commonly used red blood cell product for neonates, this product represents the red blood cell component from 1 U of whole blood collected in CPDA-1 after the plasma and most of the preservative solution have been removed. In this product, the HCT is usually between 70% and 80%, which is comparable with that of centrifuged or sedimented additive solution units.

Table 85–1. Summary of Red Blood Cell Products and Their Uses for Neonates

Red Blood Cell Product	Advantages and Disadvantages	Uses for Neonates
Packed red blood cells: AS-1	42-day storage; decreased donor exposure Adenine, mannitol, increased extracellular K^+, decreased 2,3-DPG	Booster transfusions May be dangerous in large transfusions
Packed red blood cells: AS-3	42-day storage; decreased donor exposure Adenine, increased extracellular K^+, decreased 2,3-DPG	Booster transfusions May be dangerous in large transfusions
Packed red blood cells: AS-5	42-day storage; decreased donor exposure Adenine, mannitol, increased extracellular K^+, decreased 2,3-DPG	Role unclear in neonates
Packed red blood cells: CPDA-1	Highest HCT, 35-day storage with 7-day-old requirement for neonates Increased donor exposure	Booster transfusions
Washed packed red blood cells	Plasma, preservative, extracellular K^+ removed, can be packed to higher HCT	Remove extracellular K^+ from older packed red blood cells, remove AS-1 solution, rare allergic-type transfusion reactions, remove ABO-incompatible plasma from group O cells
Frozen, deglycerolized packed red blood cells	Washed and CMV safe	Alternative source of CMV-safe red blood cells
Leukoreduced packed red blood cells	Reduction of alloimmunization, possible reduction of CMV transmission; filtering small volumes problematic	Role unclear in neonates
Whole blood	Lower HCT with little hemostatic activity	Not generally used
Fresh whole blood	Hemostatic advantages after bypass	After cardiopulmonary bypass
Reconstituted whole blood, packed red blood cells + FFP	Specified HCT, depleted of viable platelets	Exchange transfusions, whole blood substitute

AS, additive solution; CMV, cytomegalovirus; CPDA-1, citrate phosphate dextrose adenine; 2,3-DPG, 2,3-diphosphoglycerate; FFP, fresh-frozen plasma; HCT, hematocrit.

There is extensive experience with the safety of the preservative solution CPDA-1 for transfusion to neonates. Blood banks can prepare the exact PRBC volume needed for transfusion by utilizing SCDs and syringes as previously described.

Some blood banks further subject PRBCs to centrifugation or sedimentation to increase the HCT, producing "super-packed" red blood cells, when maximum volume reduction is required.

Washed Packed Red Blood Cells

All packed red blood cell products contain by volume at least 10% to 20% extracellular fluid that cannot be eliminated; this fluid occupies the residual "space" between red blood cells when they are packed by centrifugation. When red blood cells are "washed," this extracellular fluid is replaced by the washing fluid, usually isotonic saline. Washing consists of performing cycles of addition of saline solution to the red blood cells, mixing, centrifugation to separate the cellular and supernatant layers, and removal of the supernatant fluid. When repeated three times, this process replaces over 95% of the residual fluid with saline. Washing clearly adds significantly to the preparation time for red blood cells and also shortens the usable shelf life of the washed product to 24 hours. A small percentage of the red blood cells is inevitably lost during the manipulations.

Washed red blood cells may be requested for several reasons. As mentioned, the AS-1 preservative solution can be removed by washing, as can the cryopreservative used for freezing red blood cells. Extracellular potassium and free hemoglobin are also removed by washing, as is sometimes requested when "older" red blood cells are used for neonates. Finally, washing removes residual plasma proteins from the red blood cell product. Although rarely a problem for neonates, allergic-type transfusion reactions are often mediated by these residual plasma proteins, and washing usually eliminates these reactions.

It is important to understand that the purpose of washing is to change the residual fluid in the red blood cell product, not to alter the cellular elements. White blood cells and platelets that are present as contaminants in the red blood cell product remain with the red blood cell layer and are not removed by washing.

Frozen, Deglycerolized Packed Red Blood Cells

Red blood cells can be frozen for nearly indefinite storage at −80° C with 10% glycerol as the cryoprotective agent. When thawed, these red blood cells must be washed to remove the glycerol (deglycerolized) until the osmolarity of the fluid around the red blood cells is isotonic. Glycerol does not preserve white blood cells or platelets, which are destroyed during the freeze-thaw cycle. CMV is also destroyed by the freeze-thaw process.[53,54] Thus, frozen, deglycerolized PRBCs can be considered depleted of leukocytes and CMV negative. Although these characteristics are nearly ideal for use in neonates, the freezing and washing equipment, inventory and quality control procedures, and additional preparation time required for a frozen blood program make routine use of frozen red blood cells for neonates impractical and quite expensive. Today, most red blood cells are frozen by large blood collection agencies to maintain inventories of red blood cells from donors with rare blood types. Such red blood cells are almost never required for neonates because of the low neonatal incidence of alloimmunization to red blood cell antigens.

Leukoreduced Packed Red Blood Cells

A unit of PRBCs contains approximately 1×10^9 to 5×10^9 white blood cells. These cells are known to mediate at least four significant adverse effects of transfusion: febrile transfusion reactions, alloimmunization to HLA and resultant platelet refractoriness, CMV transmission, and TA-GVHD. Leukocytes can be removed from red blood cells by physical removal of the buffy coat, along with some of the underlying red blood cells, by freeze-thawing with glycerol, as discussed previously, or by leukocyte filtration. The first and second methods are time consuming and expensive, and the first leaves about tenfold more residual white blood cells in the product than does filtration. The easiest and most efficient method involves passing the blood product through a commercially available fiber mesh filter to which viable leukocytes adhere. Filtration can be performed within the blood bank or at the patient's bedside, and many blood collection agencies maintain an inventory of blood that is filtered for leukocyte reduction soon after collection; this process is called **prestorage leukoreduction**. The filtered product should have fewer than 5×10^6 residual white blood cells, a 99% reduction in white blood cell content, and minimal red blood cell loss. In 1998 and 2001, U.S. Food and Drug Administration advisory committees voted unanimously to endorse universal white blood cell reduction of all cellular blood products, except granulocytes,[55,56] because these components have demonstrated prevention of recurrence of febrile nonhemolytic transfusion reactions, reduce alloimmunization to HLA antigens in select patients, and reduce the risk of CMV in select patients.[57-60]

A complete discussion of leukoreduction of blood products for neonates is given in the section "Adverse Effects of Blood Transfusion."

Whole Blood

Whole blood is stored under conditions optimized for the preservation of the red blood cells; the other components—the platelets and the coagulation factors of the plasma—rapidly lose function under these storage conditions and contribute little to hemostasis after a few days. For this reason, there are few clinical situations, for neonates or otherwise, in which stored whole blood is the red blood cell product of choice. The main disadvantage for neonates is that the HCT of whole blood is much lower than that of PRBCs. In addition, whole blood presents special problems for neonates with maternal-fetal ABO incompatibility.

Fresh Whole Blood

Transfusion with fresh whole blood immediately after cardiopulmonary bypass has been shown to provide a hemostatic benefit in neonates and children by reducing blood loss, especially during complex cardiac surgery.[61] In this circumscribed context, "fresh" is defined as less than 48 hours from the time of collection. Within this period, the loss of platelet function and coagulation factor activity is theoretically limited. The task of procuring very fresh whole blood, with all required infectious disease and compatibility testing, is logistically complex and expensive. It mandates exceptionally rapid blood collection and processing procedures and close cooperation among the blood center, the hospital blood bank, and the cardiothoracic surgery service. Many institutions that perform pediatric cardiothoracic surgery have not adopted the practice of using fresh whole blood. However, because bleeding after cardiopulmonary bypass is sometimes massive—and is frequently treated empirically with red blood cells, plasma, and platelets—the use of fresh whole blood in this setting may reduce the number of exposures to donors by providing all three components together from one donor.

Reconstituted Whole Blood

An alternative to whole blood is reconstituted whole blood, prepared by diluting PRBCs with fresh-frozen plasma (FFP) to a specified target HCT. This product is most commonly employed for large-volume transfusions in neonates, such as manual whole blood exchange transfusions, cardiopulmonary bypass, and ECMO. Reconstitution of red blood cells with plasma shortens the shelf life of the mixture to 24 hours. Because platelets are removed during component preparation, reconstituted whole blood is depleted of platelets, and those remaining with the red blood cells have been stored under conditions suboptimal for preservation of platelet function. Both dilutional thrombocytopenia and platelet dysfunction are recognized complications of massive transfusion in neonates, during whole blood exchange, cardiopulmonary bypass, or ECMO.

PRINCIPLES OF TRANSFUSING RED BLOOD CELLS

Neonates are one of the most frequently transfused hospital populations,[62] which puts them at higher risk for transfusion-transmitted infection. However, conservative transfusion practices and bedside point-of-care testing promise reduction of the transfusion requirement for this population. A retrospective study conducted by the University of Iowa analyzed neonatal transfusion practices from 1982 to 1993.[63] This study found that in neonates with birth weights higher than 1000 g, the number of transfusions was 67% lower, and the number of donor exposures was 54% lower, than for infants with lower birth weights. There was an improving clinical outcome as a trend over the study period for infants over

1000 g, but no such trend in transfusion requirements was detected for infants whose birth weights were lower than 1000 g. These remarkable changes in neonatal transfusion practices reflect more conservative transfusion standards. Currently, indications for red blood cell transfusions in the neonatal period belong to several broad categories,[64] including the following.

Replacement of Blood Loss from Diagnostic Phlebotomy

Transfusion to replace phlebotomy-related blood loss accounts for most small-volume neonatal transfusions. Most neonatologists replace phlebotomy-related losses when between 5% and 10% of an infant's estimated blood volume has been removed, even if the infant is asymptomatic. Improvements in bedside monitoring with noninvasive cutaneous sensors, small-volume point-of-care testing, and in-line ex vivo monitoring by microelectrochemical methods, which can accurately and frequently measure pH, blood gases, electrolytes, and HCT, have reduced the phlebotomy and transfusion requirements for most neonates.[65,66]

Treatment of Neonates with Cardiopulmonary Diseases or Congenital Anemias

In neonates with respiratory disease, especially neonates requiring oxygen or ventilator support, transfusion to keep the HCT higher than 40% is often recommended. The transfusion of hemoglobin A containing red blood cells provides improved oxygen unloading in comparison with fetal hemoglobin, which is of theoretical benefit to infants with respiratory distress.[28] Maintenance of HCT levels higher than 40% is also recommended for infants who have severe congenital heart disease with cyanosis or congestive heart failure. Because transfusions may transiently worsen heart failure by increasing intravascular volume, red blood cell transfusions in treatment of patent ductus arteriosus are not routinely recommended.

Infants with congenital anemias, including Diamond-Blackfan anemia and Fanconi anemia, and those with inherited red blood cell enzyme deficiencies, including severe Mediterranean-type glucose-6-phosphate dehydrogenase deficiency and pyruvate kinase deficiency, may require transfusion in the neonatal period or in the first several months after birth. Patients with inherited membrane defects such as hereditary spherocytosis or pyropoikilocytosis have hemolysis and neonatal jaundice and may require exchange transfusion or phototherapy.[67]

Transfusion for Surgical Management

Some patients who need surgery during the neonatal period may require red blood cell transfusion. In general, red blood cells are supplied to replace intraoperative blood loss. For open-heart surgery with cardiopulmonary bypass, whole blood collected in CPD or CPDA-1 is often used to prime the bypass pump, and in some centers, whole blood less than 48 hours old is used for immediate postoperative replacement.[61]

Replacement of Acute Perinatal Blood Loss

Causes of acute perinatal blood loss include abruptio placentae, placenta previa, twin-twin transfusion, fetomaternal hemorrhage, or obstetric accident. Fetal bleeding can be intracranial or intraabdominal. Difficult deliveries may precipitate rupture of the liver or spleen, cephalohematoma, or intracranial bleeding. In this setting, the infant may require transfusion before ABO and Rh typing have been completed.

Exchange Transfusions

Treatment of jaundiced neonates with exchange transfusion is accomplished with ABO- and Rh-specific, cross-matched red blood cells suspended in ABO type-specific plasma or, in cases of ABO HDN, O-negative cells suspended in AB plasma. Blood for exchange transfusion should be less than 5 days old and collected in CPD or CPDA-1.

Extracorporeal Membrane Oxygenation

An integral part of an ECMO program is ready availability of blood support. Protocols for emergency ECMO setup vary among hospitals. For example, a recommended emergency ECMO setup utilizes 1 U of type-specific or group O-negative packed red blood cells less than 5 days old, which may be issued before crossmatching can be completed.[68] In case of mechanical failure of the ECMO circuit, 1 U of group O-negative or type-specific red blood cells must be readily available. To support the neonate on ECMO, small-volume (20- to 60-mL) transfusions are transfused daily to replace iatrogenic blood loss.[68] Transfusion of FFP, cryoprecipitate, and platelets varies according to the neonate's needs. SCDs can split FFP into small volumes if needed. Plasma may be removed from the platelets to avoid volume overload.

Growth Failure

Transfusion of red blood cells as a therapy for poor growth in a premature infant or an infant small for gestational age remains controversial. The clinical signs of anemia, such as tachypnea, tachycardia, pallor, and poor feeding, which are usually correlated with the degree of anemia in older children, are not well correlated with the hemoglobin level in infants.[69] The effect that transfusions have on growth in premature infants was assessed in two separate trials that showed different results. In 1984, Blank and coworkers demonstrated no benefit from booster transfusions on the growth of stable premature infants.[70] Conversely, Stockman and Clark showed that transfusions were associated with a 35% increase in growth in a selected population.[71] Analysis of 825 newborns weighing less than 1500 g in six different neonatal intensive care units showed that transfusion frequency does not affect 28-day weight gain.[72]

PLATELET TRANSFUSIONS

Platelet concentrates are prepared either from whole blood donations or by using automated apheresis procedures. The platelets derived from 1 U of whole blood are called random donor platelet (RDP) concentrates and have a minimum platelet count of 5.5×10^{10} per unit and a volume of approximately 50 mL. RDP concentrates can be transfused singly or, if more platelets are required, can be pooled together immediately before administration (pooled platelet concentrates). Platelets prepared by automated apheresis are referred to as single donor platelet (SDP) concentrates and contain at least 3×10^{11} platelets per unit. One unit of SDP concentrate contains about the same number of platelets as 6 to 8 U of RDP concentrate. One unit of SDP concentrate also can be divided for transfusion to small children. Once collected, platelets are stored with continuous agitation at room temperature (20° to 24°C). The shelf life of platelet concentrates is 5 days. Exposure to cold temperatures (1° to 6°C) for more than 24 hours is associated with irreversible loss of platelet microtubule function and with poor platelet survival after transfusion.[73] The general rule for platelet dosing is that 0.1 to 0.2 U of RDP per kilogram should cause the patient's platelet count to rise 50,000/µL to 100,000/µL. Therefore, 1 U of RDPs is generally the appropriate dose in a term neonate.

Efforts should be made to transfuse platelets that are ABO- and Rh-group specific, because residual red blood cells and plasma are present in platelet preparations. The ABO-incompatible plasma transfused along with out-of-group platelets to neonates is potentially more hazardous than in adults, because of the smaller blood volume of the neonate. Transfusion of ABO- and Rh-compatible platelets also results in a higher post-transfusion platelet count than incompatible platelets. The introduction of small amounts of Rh-positive red blood cells to Rh-negative individuals can result in Rh sensitization. If type-specific or compatible platelets are not available, residual plasma can be removed by centrifugation and plasma removal; the remaining platelets may be resuspended in saline. For Rh-negative infants who receive Rh-positive platelets, Rh immune globulin should be considered. For infants with strict limits on intravenous fluids, volume reduction of stored platelet concentrates can be accomplished with gentle centrifugation, with no apparent deleterious effect on function of the transfused platelets.[74]

Castle and colleagues examined the frequency and mechanism of thrombocytopenia (platelet count <100,000/µL) in a prospective study of infants admitted to a regional intensive care nursery.[75] Thrombocytopenia was found in about 20% of infants; the nadir occurred at day 4 of life, and the thrombocytopenia generally resolved by day 10. Thrombocytopenia was nearly always characterized by increased platelet destruction, as shown, in part, by normal bone marrow and a poorer-than-expected response to platelet transfusions. About half of the platelet destruction was immune, associated with increased platelet-associated IgG, and half was nonimmune, presumably associated with disseminated intravascular coagulation (DIC).

The risk of thrombocytopenia in sick neonates was assessed by Andrew and associates.[76] In a series of infants weighing less than 1500 g, the incidence of intraventricular hemorrhage was 78% among thrombocytopenic (<100,000/µL) infants, in comparison with 48% among matched but nonthrombocytopenic infants ($P < .01$). The rate of serious neurologic morbidity in surviving infants weighing less than 1500 g was 40% among the thrombocytopenic infants but less than 10% among the nonthrombocytopenic infants.

Despite the risks of thrombocytopenia in sick premature neonates, the benefits of early platelet transfusions have not been proved. In a randomized, prospective study, the effect of early transfusion of platelets to premature infants with moderate thrombocytopenia (<150,000/µL) was also examined by Andrew and associates.[77] Platelet concentrates were infused up to three times in order to keep the count higher than 150,000/µL during the first 7 days after birth. Although these infants had improved platelet counts and shortened bleeding times, platelet transfusions did not reduce the incidence or extent of intracranial hemorrhages in comparison with a group of infants who did not undergo transfusion.

Because many sick neonates are thrombocytopenic, defining which infants will benefit from platelet transfusions is important, although not always straightforward. Certain characteristics of the hemostatic system in neonates may increase their bleeding risk, including poor neonatal platelet function and decreased concentrations of clotting proteins. With these factors in mind, most practitioners agree that sick premature infants with platelet counts lower than 50,000/µL are at risk for intracranial or intraventricular hemorrhage. Attempts should be made to keep their platelet counts higher than 50,000/µL. Some neonatologists transfuse platelets in the ill premature infant when the count is lower than 100,000/µL and in the stable premature infant when the count is lower than 50,000/µL. The risks of serious bleeding complications in the stable premature infant with thrombocytopenia are not as well agreed upon. The risk of spontaneous bleeding increases as the platelet count drops, and many clinicians recommend prophylactic platelet transfusions in any infant with a platelet count lower than 20,000/µL.

The increase in platelet count observed after transfusion depends on the number of platelets transfused, the blood volume of the recipient, and the degree of platelet consumption. In a patient who does not exhibit increased consumption of platelets, a dose of 0.1 U/kg body weight should raise the platelet count by 50,000/µL when measured 1 hour after transfusion.[78] Although platelet refractoriness caused by alloimmunization is generally not encountered in neonates, poor response to platelet transfusion is seen in infants with infection, DIC, or another consumptive coagulopathy. Infants with isoimmune thrombocytopenia consume RDP concentrates but have normal recovery of washed maternal platelets. Washing is critical for removal of maternal plasma, which contains the specific antibody responsible for the neonate's thrombocytopenia.

Infants with decreased platelet production as a result of bone marrow failure syndromes, such as thrombocytopenia with absent radius syndrome, may require platelet transfusions in the neonatal period. Patients who have thrombocytopenia with absent radius syndrome are recognized by limb abnormalities and petechiae. They are at high risk for intracranial and gastrointestinal bleeding during the neonatal period. Prophylactic platelet transfusions are recommended in order to decrease the risk of bleeding in severely thrombocytopenic infants.[79] Usually, the platelet counts improve spontaneously after several months.

Leukoreduction of platelet products for these patients is extremely important because alloimmunization and platelet refractoriness may result in life-threatening bleeding. Red blood cell needs should also be met with leukoreduced cells.

Complications of Platelet Transfusions

The requirement that platelets be stored at room temperature (20° to 24° C) to preserve platelet function has the adverse effect of providing conditions permissive for bacterial growth. The most common contaminating organisms are *Staphylococcus epidermidis,* diphtheroid species, *Staphylococcus aureus,* and gram-negative organisms. Bacterial contamination is an uncommon complication of platelet transfusions, occurring approximately once in 4,000 to 12,000 transfusions of platelet concentrates.[25,80] However, because this risk is higher than the risk of transfusion-transmitted hepatis or HIV, measures to detect and prevent bacterial contamination of platelet products, either by culture, dipstick, or other methods, have been mandated in the United States.[12] The shelf life for platelets is 5 days; the risk for bacterial contamination is highest on day 5 of storage.

PLASMA PRODUCTS

Plasma, the liquid portion of whole blood, contains a great many substances, including electrolytes, small organic molecules such as bilirubin metabolites and thyroxine, lipids, and a wide variety of soluble proteins such as albumin, immunoglobulins, complement proteins, and coagulation factors. The principal therapeutic use of FFP and plasma-derived products is to replace the coagulation factors. FFP is a readily available source of coagulation factors II, V, VII, VIII, IX, X, and XI; von Willebrand factor; and the naturally occurring anticoagulants antithrombin III, protein C, and protein S. Cryoprecipitate is a more concentrated source of factor VIII, fibrinogen (factor I), and factor XIII than is FFP, because it contains more of these proteins per volume transfused. Like FFP, cryoprecipitate is, in general, readily available. Plasma-derived concentrates of factors VIII and IX and recombinant factors VIII, IX, and VIIa are available for clinical use, but these concentrates should be reserved for patients deficient in the specific coagulation factors. Antithrombin III concentrate is also commercially available.

Plasma can be derived from a single donation of whole blood or from an apheresis donor.[14] FFP must be separated from red blood cells and frozen at less than −18° C within 8 hours of collection. When stored in this manner, FFP can be used up to 1 year after the date of donation. Before infusion, FFP is thawed, usually by immersion in a water bath at 30° to 37° C. Once thawed, the plasma is stored at 1° to 6° C and must be transfused within 24 hours. Plasma should be ABO compatible with the recipient's red cells.

FFP is transfused to ill neonates for a variety of reasons. The 1989 National Survey of Neonatal Transfusion Practices showed that 77% of clinicians surveyed transfused FFP primarily to treat coagulation disorders.[4] The goal of transfusing plasma for well-defined coagulation disorders is to reach hemostatic levels of the missing coagulation protein. By definition, each milliliter of plasma contains 1 U of each clotting protein. The usual dose of FFP in infants is 10 mL/kg/dose every 4 to 6 hours, depending on the clinical response. One practical disadvantage of plasma is the need to infuse large volumes to deliver an adequate dose of clotting proteins. For example, treatment of an intracranial hemorrhage in a 3.5-kg hemophilia patient would require 350 mL of plasma, more than the infant's total blood volume, for replacement of the deficient factor to 100% of the normal level. Plasma is used for treatment of bleeding episodes in infants with isolated deficiencies of factor II, V, X, or XI. Plasma also can be transfused when a congenital factor deficiency is suspected in a bleeding infant, even if a definitive diagnosis has not yet been made (samples for definitive diagnosis should be drawn before FFP is transfused). FFP is also transfused extensively to support neonates with DIC, with liver failure, and on ECMO support.

Bleeding patients diagnosed in the prenatal or neonatal period with hemophilia A or B, disorders for which specific recombinant factor concentrates are available, should receive correction with recombinant factor VIII or factor IX concentrates, respectively, rather than FFP or cryoprecipitate. Even though currently available plasma-derived factor VIII and IX concentrates have been treated with effective virucidal techniques, factor concentrates made with recombinant technology are considered superior from a viral safety perspective.

For 11% of respondents to the AABB survey, their most frequent use of FFP was for treatment of hypovolemia. The use of FFP prophylactically for volume expansion was investigated in a multicenter study. This study revealed that FFP did not affect the rate of mortality among premature infants.[81,82] Infusion of plasma for hypovolemia alone should be discouraged, however, because of the infection risks associated with blood products and the availability of safer, equally effective volume expanders. FFP has infection risks similar to those of cellular blood products and is screened for viral agents in the same way as cellular blood products.

Solvent/detergent–treated (S/D) plasma has been developed as an alternative to FFP. S/D plasma is prepared from large, pooled batches of FFP by treatment with an organic solvent and the detergent Triton X-100, which inactivates lipid-enveloped viruses.[83] Virucidal materials are then removed by methods that do not compromise the integrity of the plasma. Data on the safety and efficacy of S/D plasma when used in the same setting as FFP, except in DIC, have been reported.[84] Coagulation factor content in S/D plasma appears comparable with that of FFP; however, there are decreased amounts of protein S, antithrombin III, and antiplasmin in S/D plasma, which may increase thrombosis risk.[85,86] Furthermore, there have been reports of hepatitis A virus and parvovirus transmission because these viruses are not lipid enveloped and therefore are not susceptible to the S/D process.[87] In 2002, the U.S. Food and Drug Administration issued a warning against the use of S/D plasma in patients with liver disease, those with coagulopathy, and those undergoing liver transplant, and at present, manufacturing of S/D plasma has been suspended.[88]

Cryoprecipitate is the cold-insoluble fraction of plasma that remains when FFP has been thawed between 1° and 6° C. Cryoprecipitate contains about 50% of the factor VIII (both factor VIII coagulant and von Willebrand factor), 20% to 40% of the fibrinogen, and a portion of the factor XIII found in the unit of FFP from which it was derived. One unit of cryoprecipitate, with a volume of approximately 20 mL, contains about 80 IU of factor VIII and a more variable amount of fibrinogen, between 100 and 350 mg. This component is derived from a unit of blood that has passed screening for viral contaminants but has not undergone viral inactivation. Although cryoprecipitate was once considered the cornerstone of treatment for bleeding in neonates with hemophilia, recombinant factors VIII and IX concentrates are currently the products of choice because of their proven viral safety and efficacy.

GRANULOCYTES

Neonates are susceptible to bacterial infections for a variety of reasons, including lack of opsonic antibody, reduced complement levels, and slow production and release of neutrophils from the marrow. Because bacterial infection in neonates is sometimes associated with neutropenia and a high mortality rate, granulocyte transfusions can be a logical adjunct to antibiotic therapy. Efficacy of granulocyte transfusion has been shown to be dose dependent, with the ideal granulocyte product for neonatal transfusion collected by leukapheresis and administered at doses higher than 1×10^9 granulocytes per kilogram of body weight.[1,89] Granulocyte transfusions must be irradiated to inactivate contaminating lymphocytes and must be ABO type compatible. Finally, granulocytes should be administered as soon after collection as possible, preferably within 4 to 6 hours.

Clinical trials assessing the value of granulocyte transfusions in septic neonates have shown varying results. Christensen and coworkers studied infants with proven sepsis and neutropenia.[90] The assessment included bone marrow evaluation of neutrophil stores. Inclusion criteria were neutropenia; bone marrow with less than 7% polymorphonuclear neutrophils, bands, and metamyelocytes; and positive clinical and diagnostic findings of sepsis.[91] Infants with poor neutrophil reserves received either one granulocyte transfusion, prepared by leukapheresis, or supportive care with antibiotics. All transfusion recipients survived, in comparison with only one of nine control infants. Cairo and colleagues studied the role of granulocyte transfusions in septic neonates with and without neutropenia.[92] Infants either received supportive care or underwent transfusion with leukapheresis-prepared white blood cells a total of five times, the first dose within 4 hours of becoming septic. In the initial report, all 13 who received white blood cells survived, whereas of 10 who did not undergo transfusion, only 6 survived ($P < .02$).

Two studies have shown no advantage when granulocyte transfusions were added to antibiotics for treatment of sepsis in neonates. The neutrophils used in these two studies were collected from the buffy coats of whole blood units, not by leukapheresis. The dose of neutrophils given was also less than the dose in the previous studies that showed white blood cell transfusions to be of benefit.[93]

Methodologic differences between these studies makes drawing conclusions difficult. The studies differed with regard to method of preparation of the granulocyte concentrates, the doses delivered, the timing of the transfusions, and infants studied. Furthermore, granulocyte concentrates can now be harvested from donors who have been stimulated with dexamethasone, granulocyte colony–stimulating factor, or both. These products contain larger numbers of cells and may have qualitative differences from concentrates from unstimulated donors. A definitive study exploring the utility of granulocyte transfusions in septic neonates may never be performed. The benefits of intravenous immune globulin as an alternative to granulocyte transfusion remain controversial.[32,94] The risks of granulocyte transfusion include infection with agents residing in white blood cells (CMV, human immunodeficiency virus [HIV]), sensitization to neutrophil antigens, exposure to contaminating lymphocytes, and pulmonary leukoagglutination. These must be weighed when white blood cell transfusion is considered. Severely ill neonates with neutropenia (<3000 neutrophils/μL) and evidence of bone marrow neutrophil storage pool depletion (<7% polymorphonuclear leukocytes plus bands plus metamyelocytes), and a strong suspicion of bacterial sepsis, are potential candidates for white blood cell transfusions. Because the benefits of granulocyte transfusions in septic neonates remain controversial, granulocytes are infrequently transfused to neonates.[4]

ADVERSE EFFECTS OF BLOOD TRANSFUSION

Acute hemolytic transfusion reactions are usually caused by transfusion of ABO-incompatible blood, which triggers an immediate antibody-antigen reaction, complement fixation, and hemolysis of the transfused cells. Most ABO-incompatible transfusions are a result of misidentification of the unit, the blood specimen, or the recipient. Acute hemolytic transfusion reactions are rare in the neonatal period, because infants do not have isohemagglutinins; fewer than half of normal infants have developed isohemagglutinins by 6 months of age. One setting in which neonatal hemolytic transfusions may occur is in the infant with maternally derived anti-A antibody who receives a transfusion with adult type A red blood cells.[95]

Delayed hemolytic transfusion reactions occur 3 to 10 days after a red blood cell transfusion and result from sensitization to minor blood group antigens during a previous transfusion. The red blood cell antibody is not picked up by routine screening techniques because the titer has fallen to undetectable levels between transfusions. In adults, the risk of sensitization to a red blood cell antigen (other than the D antigen) is 1% to 1.6% for each unit of red blood cells transfused.[96] As a rule, infants do not have delayed transfusion reaction, because their ability to form antibodies to foreign antigens is poor, as discussed previously.

Febrile, nonhemolytic transfusion reactions consist of fever, chills, and diaphoresis in patients who have previously undergone transfusion. Such reactions are rarely reported in infants, in part because some of the signs and symptoms are difficult to identify in neonates.[97] Symptoms result from interactions between antibodies and either white blood cell antigens or plasma proteins.

Viral Transmission Risk

The acquired immunodeficiency syndrome epidemic has heightened public awareness of the potential infection risks of blood transfusion. Nonetheless, transfusions are an important, often lifesaving therapeutic measure whose benefits need to be understood and weighed against the calculable risks. In the United States, whole blood donors are volunteers who are screened for high-risk behaviors before donation. Once blood is drawn from donors who have passed initial screening by questionnaire, the donated unit is tested (1) by serologic methods for syphilis, HIV types 1 and 2, human T-lymphotropic virus type 1, hepatitis B surface antigen, hepatitis C virus, alanine aminotransferase, and hepatitis B core antibody and (2) by nucleic acid tests for hepatitis C virus, HIV, and West Nile virus. The test for syphilis also serves as a surrogate marker for HIV; the alanine aminotransferase and hepatitis B core antibody tests are surrogate markers for untypable hepatitis. Improvements in donor screening techniques and improved testing for contamination with viral agents UU have made the blood supply safer than it has ever been. The 2002 residual risk estimates for infectious disease transmission in the American Red Cross blood donor population are reported in Table 85-2.[98] Such information should be presented to parents of neonates as part of an informed consent conversation before the initiation of a transfusion.

Cytomegalovirus

Blood is not universally screened for CMV. In healthy individuals, infection with CMV from a transfusion results in a mild syndrome or is asymptomatic. However, significant morbidity and mortality can result from CMV infection in immunocompromised hosts. The actual risk to a neonate from CMV infection acquired through transfusion has been debated since the early 1980s. The current AABB standard recommends that cellular components be at low risk for transmitting CMV when transfused to a neonate with a birth weight of less than 1200 g. One method for supplying products with reduced risk for CMV transmission is donor testing for CMV antibody. Because CMV resides in leukocytes, removal of white blood cells either by freezing, deglycerolizing, and washing or by use of efficient white blood cell removal filters can also prevent transfusion-associated CMV infection. CMV-safe components should have a white blood cell count reduced to less than 5×10^6 or should be seronegative. The AABB concluded that leukoreduced blood products are equivalent to CMV-seronegative components with regard to CMV risk.[98,99]

Nichols and colleagues prospectively followed 807 CMV-seronegative stem cell transplant patients in two cohorts, group 1 from 1994 to 1996 and group 2 from 1996 to 2000.[100] Group 1 received CMV-seronegative and/or filtered blood products and group 2 received some platelet transfusions that had undergone leukoreduction at collection rather than filtration, a product that was not available to group 1. Transfusion of filtered products from CMV-positive donors, both red cell and apheresis platelets, increased substantially during the second study period. Transfusion-transmitted CMV infection was higher in group 2 than in group 1. Multivariate analysis revealed that this was related to filtered RBC units from CMV-positive donors, not apheresis platelet products, suggesting that leukoreduced products may not be equivalent to CMV-negative products for this immunocompromised population.

It is difficult to extrapolate these findings to neonates. This study's conclusion, however, conflicts with the AABB standard that leukoreduced blood products are equivalent to CMV-seronegative products.

Bacterial Sepsis

Blood products provide a rich source of nutrients and a suitable environment for the growth of skin contaminants, gram-negative rods, and psychrophilic organisms, organisms able to proliferate at cold temperatures. Platelets are stored at room temperature and are therefore at higher risk for bacterial contamination than other blood products. More information on bacterial contamination of platelets is available in the section Complications of Platelet Transfusions. The contamination of psychrophilic organisms, such as *Yersinia enterocolitica* and *Pseudomonas* and *Serratia* species, may be detected in red blood cell products at any time from collection to transfusion. Any blood transfusion, including autologous donations, has a risk of bacterial contamination. Symptoms indicative of bacterial sepsis include rapid onset during or after transfusion, temperatures higher than 40.5° C, chills, rigors, hypotension, and endotoxin-mediated shock. Symptoms of a septic reaction to a red cell product may have a more rapid onset and be more severe than symptoms related to platelet transfusion sepsis, because of

Table 85–2. Residual Risk for Infectious Disease Transmission among American Red Cross Blood Donors

Infectious Agent and Testing Method	Risk (Rate of Infectious Donations)
HBV: antibody test	1:205,000
HCV: antibody test	1:276,000
HCV: antibody test and NAT	1:1,935,000
HCV: antibody and p24 antigen tests	1: 1,468,000
HIV: antibody test and NAT	1:2,135,000

HBV, hepatitis B virus; HCV, hepatitis C virus; HIV, human immunodeficiency virus; NAT, nucleic acid test.

From Dodd RY, Notari IV, Stramer SL: Current prevalence and incidence of infectious disease markers and estimated window-period risk in the American Red Cross blood donor population. Transfusion 42:975, 2002.

higher amounts of endotoxin from the gram-negative red blood cell contaminants more commonly found in red cell products.[99] To confirm transfusion-related sepsis, the same organism must be grown from the transfused blood and from the patient.

Allergic Reaction

Allergic reactions to blood transfusions are mediated by plasma proteins but are uncommon in neonates. A rare cause of severe allergic reaction is the absence or deficiency of immunoglobulin A and presence of anti-immunoglobulin A antibodies in the recipient. Mild transfusion-related allergic reactions include urticaria, local erythema, and wheezing. If urticaria or local erythema occurs, the blood component should be stopped and antihistamine administered before the transfusion is continued.[101] The severe transfusion-related allergic response is anaphylaxis, which can be life-threatening and may occur even after a small-volume transfusion. When this reaction occurs, transfusion should be stopped immediately. To prevent anaphylaxis, blood products may be washed extensively before administration.

Transfusion-Associated Graft-Versus-Host Disease

Transfusion-associated graft-versus-host disease (TA-GVHD) occurs when viable T lymphocytes contained in a transfused blood product engraft in the recipient and react against the recipient's tissues. The symptoms occur between 4 and 30 days after transfusion of at least 10^7 lymphocytes per kilogram[102] and include erythroderma, liver dysfunction, watery diarrhea, and pancytopenia. TA-GVHD has a very high mortality rate (between 80% and 90%).

Although TA-GVHD was first described in congenital cellular immunodeficiencies such as severe combined immunodeficiency or Wiskott-Aldrich syndrome, several cases also have been recognized in immunocompetent patients who received blood donated by relatives. Many cases of TA-GVHD also have been documented in full-term and preterm infants. Most such cases have occurred after in utero or exchange transfusion in infants whose only apparent reason for immunodeficiency is prematurity.[103,104] The true incidence of TA-GVHD may be higher than is currently appreciated because it is underdiagnosed. TA-GVHD has not been reported among patients with HIV,[105] although many centers irradiate products intended for transfusion in these patients.

Preventing the syndrome is accomplished with gamma irradiation of cellular blood products to prevent proliferation of T lymphocytes. This maneuver has been effective in preventing TA-GVHD in at-risk transfusion recipients. The currently accepted, effective irradiation dose for cellular blood products is 2500 cGy.[106]

Irradiation is currently recommended for cellular blood products intended for transfusion to the following patients:

- those with a known or suspected immunodeficiency
- those receiving transfusion from a biologic relative as part of a directed donor program
- those who have undergone in utero transfusion or exchange transfusion

- neonates who have received one or more in utero transfusions
- bone marrow transplant recipients
- some patients receiving immunosuppressive therapy

There are currently no data to support mandatory irradiation of simple red blood cell transfusions given to neonates, although many centers do irradiate cellular products for premature infants, infants with low birth weight, and septic infants.[14,104] Removal of lymphocytes with white blood cell depletion filters is **not** an effective substitute for gamma irradiation of blood products in preventing TA-GVHD.[107] Irradiation increases leaks of potassium across the red blood cell membrane during storage. Irradiated red blood cell products that have been stored longer than 72 hours may require washing to remove potassium that has leaked into the plasma.

Neonates with underlying immunodeficiency disease or who are undergoing intrauterine or exchange transfusion for severe hemolytic disease, or who receive transfusions from blood relatives, should receive cellular blood products that have been treated with gamma irradiation. Some institutions subject all blood products to gamma irradiation intended for transfusion to infants rather than risk failure to recognize a neonate at risk for TA-GVHD.[29]

White Blood Cell Contamination

The transfusion of contaminating white blood cells in red blood cell and platelet products is associated with several adverse effects, the incidence of which is not well understood in the neonate. The problems attributed to the transfusion of white blood cells have been extensively studied in older children and adults and include sensitization to leukocyte antigens, febrile nonhemolytic transfusion reactions, transfusion of infection by organisms contained in the transfused white blood cells, and TA-GVHD.[99] Red blood cells can be leukodepleted to a limited extent by buffy coat removal.

The technique most commonly used today to remove white blood cells from red blood cell and platelet products is filtration, either shortly after donation (prestorage leukoreduction) or at the time of transfusion (bedside leukoreduction). Leukocyte reduction filters remove white blood cells by adhesion; the efficiency is judged by the log reduction of leukocytes before and after filtration. The use of currently available leukoreduction filters accomplishes a 4-log reduction in leukocytes in comparison with the original product (99.99% reduction), resulting in products with white blood cell contents of less than 5×10^6 cells per unit. This degree of leukoreduction is useful in preventing febrile nonhemolytic transfusion reactions. It also reduces HLA sensitization for patients who require long-term platelet transfusion support or who may be bone marrow transplantation candidates. Several studies suggest that the risk of CMV transmission in neonates with low birth weight can be reduced by leukoreduction.[108,109] The role of leukoreduction in preventing transmission of other viruses or bacteria is not proven. Leukoreduction has not been shown to prevent TA-GVHD in a consistent manner.

Bedside leukocyte filtration of PRBCs presents a practical problem for neonatal red blood cell transfusions because of the priming volume of the filter. When filters are primed with a PRBC product, several times the volume of blood prescribed for the neonatal patient may be required to fill the entire dead space. When filters are primed with saline, there is significant admixture of red blood cells with saline within the filter and tubing. An entire dead space volume of PRBCs is necessary to return the HCT of the filter effluent to the starting value.[57] With either method, much of the blood used for priming is wasted, and the number of aliquots that can be derived from the same unit may be reduced. In addition, if the saline priming method is cut short, the red blood cells delivered to the patient may be diluted, which reduces the actual dose of red blood cells transfused and gives the clinical impression of an inadequate response to transfusion. Using red blood cells filtered just after collection (prestorage leukoreduction) can reduce these priming problems. This can be accomplished at the local blood collection facility or in the hospital blood bank.

SUMMARY

Blood transfusions are essential for many neonates with low birth weight, who are premature, or who are sick, and they may be given frequently to this population. While keeping in mind the neonate's special requirements, the physician and transfusion service should employ standard techniques to maintain product safety, reduce exposure to donors, and ensure transfusion safety.

REFERENCES

1. Strauss RG: Transfusion therapy for neonates. Am J Dis Child 145:904, 1991.
2. Strauss RG, Sacher RA, Blazina JF, et al: Commentary on small-volume red cell transfusions for neonatal patients. Transfusion 30:565, 1990.
3. Levy GJ Strauss RG, Hume H, et al: National survey of neonatal transfusion practices. I. Red blood cell therapy. Pediatrics 91:523, 1993.
4. Strauss RG, Levy GJ, Sotelo-Avila C, et al: National survey of neonatal transfusion practices. II. Blood component therapy. Pediatrics 91:530, 1993.
5. Yunis EJ, Dupont B: The HLA system. In Nathan DG, Oski FA (eds): Hematology of Infancy and Childhood, vol 2, 4th ed. Philadelphia, WB Saunders, 1993, pp 1692-1727.
6. Lapierre Y, Rigal D, Adam J, et al: The gel test: A new way to detect red cell antigen-antibody reactions. Transfusion 30:109, 1990.
7. Malyska H, Weiland D: The gel test. Lab Med 25:81, 1994.
8. Bromilow IM, Adams KE, Hope J, et al: Evaluation of the ID-gel test for antibody screening and identification. Transfus Med 1:159, 1991.
9. Cate JC, Reilly N: Evaluation and implementation of the gel test for indirect antiglobulin testing in a community hospital. Arch Pathol Lab Med 123:693, 1999.
10. Lillevang ST, Georgsen J, Kristensen T: An antibody screening test based on the antiglobulin gel technique, pooled test cells, and plasma. Vox Sang 69:295, 1995.
11. Judd WJ, Luban NLC, Ness PM, et al: Prenatal and perinatal immunohematology: Recommendations for serologic management of the fetus, newborn infant, and obstetric patient. Transfusion 30:175, 1990.
12. American Association of Blood Banks Standards Program Committee: Standards for Blood Banks and Transfusion Services, 22nd ed. Washington, DC, American Association of Blood Banks, 2003.
13. Eder AF: Donor limitations for neonatal and pediatric transfusion. In Herman JH, Manno CS (eds): Pediatric Transfusion Therapy. Bethesda, Md, American Association of Blood Banks Press, 2002.
14. Components from whole blood donations. In Walker RH (ed): Technical Manual of the American Association of Blood Banks, 14th ed. Bethesda, Md, American Association of Blood Banks, 2002, pp 161-188.
15. Strauss RG: Additive solutions and product age in neonatal red blood cell transfusion. In Herman JH, Manno CS (eds): Pediatric Transfusion Therapy. Bethesda, Md, American Association of Blood Banks Press, 2002, pp 129-146.
16. Goodstein MH, Locke RG, Wlodarczyk D, et al: Comparison of two preservative solutions for erythrocyte transfusion in newborn infants. J Pediatr 123:783, 1993.
17. Sherwood WC, Donato T, Clapper C, Wilson S: The concentration of AS-1 RBCs after inverted gravity sedimentation for neonatal transfusions [Letter]. Transfusion 40:618, 2000.
18. Strauss RG, Burmeister LF, Johnson K, et al: AS-1 red cells for neonatal transfusions: A randomized trial assessing donor exposure and safety. Transfusion 36:873, 1996.
19. Luban NLC, Strauss RG, Hume HA: Commentary on the safety of red cells preserved in extended-storage media for neonate transfusions. Transfusion 31:229, 1991.
20. Cook S, Gunter J, Wissel M: Effective use of a strategy using assigned red cell units to limit donor exposure for neonatal patients. Transfusion 33:379, 1993.
21. Jain R, Jarosz CR, Myers TF. Decreasing blood donor exposure in the neonates by using dedicated donor transfusions. Transfus Sci 18:199, 1997.
22. Maier RF, Sonntag J, Walka MM, et al: Changing practices of red blood cell transfusions in infants with birth weights less than 1000 g. J Pediatr 136:220, 2000.
23. Strauss RG, Burmeister LF, Johnson K, et al: Feasibility and safety of AS-3 red cells for neonatal transfusions. J Pediatr 136:215, 2000.
24. Popovsky MA, Moore SB: Diagnostic and pathogenic considerations in transfusion-related acute lung injury. Transfusion 25:573, 1985.
25. Strauss RG: Practical issues in neonatal transfusion practice. Am J Clin Pathol 107:S57, 1997.
26. Hall TL, Barnes A, Miller JR, et al: Neonatal mortality following transfusion of red cells with high plasma potassium levels. Transfusion 33:606, 1993.
27. Stockman JA III: Transfusion in the neonate. In Kennedy MS, Wilson S, Kelton JG (eds): Perinatal Transfusion Medicine. Arlington, Va, American Association of Blood Banks Press, 1990, pp 103-121.
28. Cairo MS, Worcester CC, Rucker RW, et al: Randomized trial of granulocyte transfusions versus intravenous immune globulin therapy for neutropenia and sepsis. J Pediatr 120:281-285, 1992.
29. AuBuchon JP, Pickard C, Herschel L: Sterility of plastic tubing welds in components stored at room temperature. Transfusion 35:303, 1995.
30. Morrow JF, Braine HG, Kickler TS, et al: Septic reactions to platelet transfusions. A persistent problem. JAMA 266:555, 1991.
31. Strauss RG, Crawford GF, Elbert C, et al: Sterility and quality of blood dispensed in syringes for infants. Transfusion 26:163, 1986.

32. Wang-Rodriguez J, Fry E, Fiebig E, et al: Immune response to blood transfusion in very-low-birthweight infants. Transfusion 40:25, 2000.

33. Dame C, Fahnenstich H, Frietag P, et al: Erythropoietin in mRNA expression in human fetal and neonatal tissue. Blood 92:3218, 1998.

34. Malek A, Sager R, Eckardt KU, et al: Lack of transport of erythropoietin in across the human placenta as studied by an in vitro perfusion system. Pflugers Arch 427:157, 1994.

35. Widness JA, Sawyer ST, Schmidt RL, et al: Lack of maternal to fetal transfer of ^{125}I-erythropoietin in sheep. J Dev Physiol 15:139-43, 1991.

36. Zanjani ED, Pixley JS, Slotnick N, et al: Erythropoietin does not cross the placenta into the fetus. Pathobiology 61:211, 1993.

37. Strauss RG: Red blood cell transfusion practices in the neonate. Clin Perinatol 22:641, 1995.

38. Bechensteen AG, Halvorsen S, Haga P, et al: Erythropoietin (Epo), protein and iron supplementation and the prevention of anemia of prematurity: Effects on serum immunoreactive Epo, growth and protein and iron metabolism. Acta Pediatr 85:490, 1996.

39. Kumar P, Shankaran S, Krishnan RG: Recombinant human erythropoietin therapy for treatment of anemia of prematurity in very-low-birth-weight infants: A randomized, double-blind, placebo-controlled trial. J Perinatol 18:173, 1998.

40. Shannon KM, Keith JF, Mentzer WC, et al: Recombinant human erythropoietin stimulates erythropoiesis and reduces erythrocyte transfusions in very-low-birth-weight preterm infants. Pediatrics 95:1, 1995.

41. Shannon KM, Mentzer WC, Abels RI, et al: Recombinant human erythropoietin in the anemia of prematurity: Results of a placebo-controlled pilot study. J Pediatr 118:949, 1991.

42. Maier RF, Obladen M, Muller-Hansen I, et al: Early treatment with erythropoietin beta ameliorates anemia and reduces transfusion requirements in infants with birth weights below 1000 g. J Pediatr 141:8, 2002.

43. Ohls RK: The use of erythropoietin in neonates. Clin Perinatol 27:681, 2000.

44. Vamvakas EC, Strauss RG: Meta-analysis of controlled clinical trials studying the efficacy of rHuEPO in reducing blood transfusions in the anemia of prematurity. Transfusion 41:406, 2001.

45. Novak RW: Autologous blood transfusion in a pediatric population. Clin Pediatr 27:184, 1988.

46. Brune T, Garritsen H, Witteler R, et al: Autologous placental blood transfusion for the therapy of anaemic neonates. Biol Neonate 81:236, 2002.

47. Strauss RG: Autologous transfusions for neonates using placental blood: A cautionary note. Am J Dis Child 146:21, 1992.

48. Brecher ME, Taswell HF, Clare DE, et al: Minimal-exposure transfusion and the committed donor. Transfusion 30:599, 1990.

49. Strauss RG, Wieland MR, Randels MJ, et al: Feasibility and success of a single-donor red cell program for pediatric elective surgery patients. Transfusion 32:747, 1992.

50. Elbert C, Strauss RG, Barrett F, et al: Biological mothers may be dangerous blood donors for their neonates. Acta Haematol 85:189, 1991.

51. Strauss RG, Barnes A Jr, Blanchette VW, et al: Directed and limited-exposure blood donations for infants and children. Transfusion 30:68, 1990.

52. Quality Control Reports. American Red Cross Blood Services, Penn Jersey Region. Philadelphia, American Red Cross, 1999.

53. Kim HC, Spitzer AR, Plotkin S: The role of frozen-thawed-washed red blood cells (FTW-RBC) in preventing transfusion acquired CMV infection (TA-CMVI) in the neonate [abstract]. Transfusion S110a:472, 1985.

54. Simon TL, Johnson JD, Koffler H, et al: Impact of previously frozen deglycerolized red blood cells on cytomegalovirus transmission to newborn infants. Plasma Ther Transfus Technol 8:51, 1987.

55. Blood Safety Transcripts, vol 1. Presented at the 13th Meeting of the Department of Health and Human Services Advisory Committee on Blood Safety and Availability, Washington, DC, January 25-26, 2001. Available at http://www.hhs.gov/bloodsafety/transcripts/20010125.html. Accessed July 13, 2004.

56. CBER 1998 Meeting Documents, vol 2. Presented at the 60th Meeting of the Blood Products Advisory Committee, Washington, DC, Department of Health and Human Services, Food and Drug Administration, Center for Drug Evaluation and Research, September 18, 1998. Accessed July 13, 2004.

57. Brecher ME (ed): Technical Manual, 14th ed. Bethesda, Md, American Association of Blood Banks, 2002.

58. Goodnough LT: Universal leukoreduction of cellular blood components in 2001? No. Am J Clin Pathol 115:674, 2001.

59. Sweeney JF: Universal leukoreduction of cellular blood components in 2001? Yes. Am J Clin Pathol 115:666, 2001.

60. Vamvakas EC, Blajchman MA: Universal WBC reduction: The case for and against. Transfusion 41:691, 2001.

61. Manno, CS, Hedberg KW, Bunin GR, et al: Comparison of the hemostatic effects of fresh whole blood, stored whole blood and components after open heart surgery in children. Blood 77:930, 1991.

62. Sacher RA, Luban NLC, Strauss RG: Current practice and guidelines for the transfusion of cellular blood components in the newborn. Transfus Med Rev 3:39, 1989.

63. Widness JA, Seward VJ, Kromer IJ, et al: Changing patterns of red blood cell transfusion in very low birth weight infants. J Pediatr 129:680, 1996.

64. Lenes BA, Sacher RA: Blood component therapy in neonatal medicine. Clin Lab Med 1:285, 1981.

65. Kost GJ, Ehrmeyer SS, Chernow B, et al: The laboratory-clinical interface: Point-of-care blood testing. Chest 115:1140, 1999.

66. Widness JA, Kulhavy JC, Johnson KJ, et al: Clinical performance of an in-line point-of-care monitor in neonates. Pediatrics 106:497, 2000.

67. DePalma L, Luban NLC: Hereditary pyropoikilocytosis: Clinical and laboratory analysis in eight infants and young children. Am J Dis Child 147:93, 1993.

68. Luban NLC: Extracorporeal membrane oxygenation in the neonate. In Sacher RA, Strauss R (eds): Contemporary Issues in Pediatric Transfusion Medicine. Arlington, Va, American Association of Blood Banks Press, 1989.

69. Joshi A, Gerhardt T: Blood transfusion effect on the respiratory pattern of preterm infants. Pediatrics 80:79, 1987.

70. Blank JP, Sheagren TG, Vajaria J, et al: The role of RBC transfusion in the premature infant. Am J Dis Child 138:831, 1984.

71. Stockman JA III, Clark DA: Weight gain: A response to transfusion in selected preterm infants. Am J Dis Child 138:828, 1984.

72. Bednarek FJ, Weisberger S, Richardson DK, et al: Variations in blood transfusions among newborn intensive care units. SNAP II Study Group. J Pediatr 133:601, 1998.

73. Filip DJ, Aster RH: Relative hemostatic effectiveness of human platelets stored at 4° and 22°C. J Lab Clin Med 91:618, 1978.

74. Moroff G, Friedman A, Robkin-Kline L, et al: Reduction of the volume of stored platelet concentrates for use in neonatal patients. Transfusion 24:144, 1984.

75. Castle V, Andrew M, Kelton J, et al: Frequency and mechanism of neonatal thrombocytopenia. J Pediatr 108:749, 1985.

76. Andrew M, Castle V, Saigal S, et al: Clinical impact of neonatal thrombocytopenia. J Pediatr 110:457, 1987.

77. Andrew M, Vegh P, Caco C, et al: A randomized, controlled trial of platelet transfusions in thrombocytopenic premature infants. J Pediatr 123:285, 1993.

78. Herman JH, Kamel HT: Platelet transfusion: Current techniques, remaining problems and future prospects. Am J Pediatr Hematol Oncol 9:272, 1987.

79. Alter BP, Young NS: The bone marrow failure syndromes. In Nathan DG, Oski FA (eds): Hematology of Infancy and Childhood. Philadelphia, WB Saunders, 1993, pp 216-316.

80. Barrett BB, Anderson JW, Anderson KC: Strategies for the avoidance of bacterial contamination of blood components. Transfusion 33:228, 1993.

81. Northern Neonatal Nursing Initiative Trial Group: A randomized trial of comparing the effect of prophylactic intravenous fresh frozen plasma gelatin or glucose on early mortality and morbidity in preterm babies. Eur J Pediatr 155:580, 1996.

82. Northern Neonatal Nursing Initiative Trial Group: A randomized trial of comparing the effect of prophylactic intravenous fresh frozen plasma gelatin or glucose on in preterm babies: Outcome at 2 years. Lancet 348:229, 1996.

83. Horowitz B, Bonomo R, Prince A: Solvent/detergent treated plasma: A virus inactivated substitute for fresh frozen plasma. Blood 79:826, 1992.

84. Hellstern P, Haubelt H: Manufacture and composition of fresh frozen plasma and virus-inactivated therapeutic plasma preparations: Correlation between composition and therapeutic efficacy. Thromb Res 107(Suppl 1):S3, 2002.

85. Leebeek FWG, Schipperus MR, van Vliet HHDM: Coagulation factor levels in solvent/detergent treated plasma [Letter]. Transfusion 39:1150, 1999.

86. Mast AE, Stadanlick JE, Lockett JM, Dietzen DJ: Solvent/detergent-treated plasma has decreased antitrypsin activity and absent antiplasmin activity. Blood 94:3922, 1999.

87. Klein HG, Dodd RY, Dzik WH, et al: Current status of solvent/detergent-treated frozen plasma. Transfusion 38:102, 1998.

88. Alford BL: Important new drug warning [letter]. MedWatch, March 29, 2002. Available at http://www.fda.gov/medwatch/SAFETY/2002/plassd_deardoc.pdf. Accessed June 1, 2004.

89. Vamvakas EC, Pineda AA: Meta-analysis of clinical studies of the efficacy of granulocyte transfusions in the treatment of bacterial sepsis. J Clin Apheresis 11:1, 1996.

90. Christensen RD, Rothstein G, Anstall HB, et al: Granulocyte transfusions in neonates with bacterial infection, neutropenia and depletion of mature marrow neutrophils. Pediatrics 70:1, 1982.

91. Cairo MS, Rucke R, Bennetts GA: Improved survival of newborns receiving leukocyte transfusions for sepsis. Pediatrics 74:887, 1984.

92. Baley JE, Stork EK, Warkentin PI, et al: Buffy coat transfusions in neutropenic neonates with presumed sepsis: A prospective, randomized trial. Pediatrics 80:712,1987.

93. Hill HR: Granulocyte transfusions in neonates. Pediatr Rev 12:298, 1991.

94. Falterman CG, Richardson CJ: Transfusion reaction due to unrecognized ABO hemolytic disease of the newborn infant. J Pediatr 97:812, 1980.

95. Lostumbo MM, Holland PV, Schmidt PJ: Isoimmunization after multiple transfusions. N Engl J Med 275:141, 1968.

96. Strauss R: Selection of white cell-reduced blood components for transfusion during infancy. Transfusion 33:352,1993.

97. Dodd RY, Notari IV, Stramer SL: Current prevalence and incidence of infectious disease markers and estimated window-period risk in the American Red Cross blood donor population. Transfusion 42:975, 2002.

98. Malloy D, Lipton KS: Update on provision of CMV-reduced-risk cellular blood components. American Association of Blood Banks, Association Bulletin 02-4, July 24, 2002. Available at http://www.aabb.org/Members_Only/Archives/Association_Bulletins/ab02-4.htm. Accessed February 12, 2003.

99. Smith DM, Lipton KS: Leukocyte reduction for the prevention of transfusion-transmitted cytomegalovirus (TT-CMV). American Association of Blood Banks, Association Bulletin 97-2, April 23, 1997. Available at http://www.aabb.org/Members_Only/Archives/Association_Bulletins/ab97-2.htm. Accessed February 12, 2003.

100. Nichols WG, Price TH, Gooley T, et al: Transfusion-transmitted cytomegalovirus infection after receipt of leukoreduced blood products. Blood 101:4195, 2003.

101. Litty C: Adverse reactions in pediatric transfusions. In Herman JH, Manno CS (eds): Pediatric Transfusion Therapy. Bethesda, Md, American Association of Blood Banks Press, 2002.

102. Von Fliedner V, Higby DJ, Kim U: Graft-versus-host reaction following blood product transfusion. Am J Med 72:951, 1982.

103. Flidel O, Barak Y, Lifschitz-Mercer B, et al: Graft versus host disease in extremely low birth weight neonate [Letter]. Pediatrics 89:689, 1992.

104. Sanders MR, Gracber JE: Posttransfusion graft-versus-host disease in infancy. J Pediatr 117:159, 1990.

105. Anderson KC, Goodnough LT, Sayers M, et al: Variation in blood component irradiation practice: Implications for prevention of transfusion-associated graft-versus-host disease. Blood 77:2096, 1991.

106. Moroff G, Luban NLC: Prevention of transfusion-associated graft-versus-host disease. Transfusion 32:102, 1992.

107. Akahoshi M, Takanashi M, Masuda M: A case of transfusion-associated graft-versus-host disease not prevented by white cell reduction filters. Transfusion 32:169, 1992.

108. Eisenfeld L, Silver H, McLaughlin J, et al: Prevention of transfusion-associated cytomegalovirus infection in neonatal patients by removal of white cells from blood. Transfusion 32:205, 1992.

109. Gilbert GL, Hayes K, Hudson IL, et al: Prevention of transfusion-acquired cytomegalovirus infection in infants by blood filtration to remove leucocytes. Lancet 1:1228, 1989.

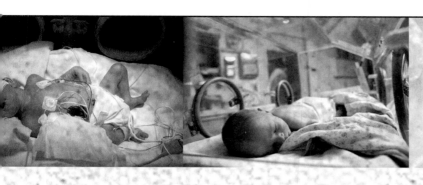
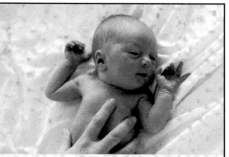

Surgical Management
of the Neonate

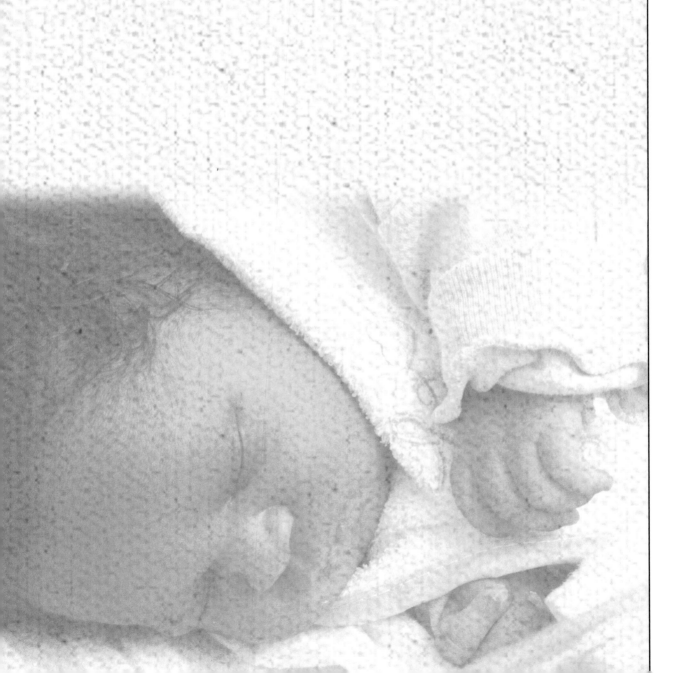

CHAPTER 86

General Surgical Considerations

Aviva L. Katz and Philip Wolfson

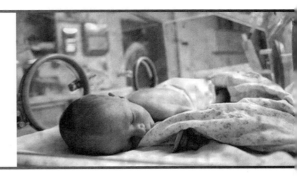

Surgical treatment of the neonate is far more exacting than that of the older child or adult. The considerable stresses of an illness necessitating surgery and resultant operation are superimposed on an individual who is still undergoing the precarious transition from the intrauterine to the extrauterine environment.[1] The neonate has limited pulmonary, cardiac, renal, nutritional, and thermoregulatory reserves, which are stressed by the continued requirements of growth and maturation with high metabolic demands.[2] Neonates are also much more susceptible to infection and have an altered metabolic response to operative stress and anesthesia in comparison with older individuals. Technically, neonatal tissues are extremely delicate and prone to injury and must be handled with the utmost care and gentleness. That most infants can survive major operations routinely is the result of an increasing understanding of neonatal physiology, the application of modern technology, and, above all, efforts of surgeons, neonatologists, anesthesiologists, and nurses working together as a team.

HISTORICAL ASPECTS

The oldest documented operation on newborns is ritual circumcision, performed 4000 years ago. It was also common among ancient civilizations to practice infanticide on ill and deformed children.[3,4] A legal code of the Norsemen stated,

Every child which is born into this world shall be reared, baptized and carried to the church except that only which is born so deformed that the mother cannot give strength to it....It shall be carried to the beach and buried where neither men nor cattle go; that is the beach of the evil one.[3]

During the period between World Wars I and II, the first true pediatric surgeons, general surgeons who devoted their careers to the care of infants and children, began practicing.[5] Gross and Ferguson reported their results of 159 premature infants who underwent operation at Boston Children's Hospital between 1936 and

1951, with a 54% survival rate.[6] Only 10 infants in this study weighed less than 1350 g, and none weighed less than 1000 g. Rickham reported a series of 122 premature neonates who underwent operation at Alder Hey Children's Hospital in England from 1953 to 1957.[7] The overall survival rate was 58%, including 6 of 15 neonates who weighed less than 1500 g.

Since the early 1970s, there has been extraordinary improvement in the survival of surgical neonates, along with the emergence of the modern intensive care nursery. Infants with tracheoesophageal anomalies provide an excellent example of this progress. Esophageal atresia and tracheoesophageal fistula are life-threatening malformations that necessitate early major surgery and occur in many premature, severely ill neonates. Before 1939, despite surgical attempts at repair, no infant with esophageal atresia had ever survived.[8] From 1948 to 1969, the rate of survival among infants with tracheoesophageal anomalies in Waterston group C (birth weight < 1800 g or severe associated disease) was 15% to 25%.[9,10] After 1970, 64% to 80% of these severely ill infants with esophageal atresia survived.[8,10] Most remarkably, O'Neill and associates more recently reported 100% survival among 43 infants with Waterston groups A and B esophageal atresia (weight > 1800 g with moderate or no associated disease).[8] Currently, with meticulous care in specialized neonatal care units, the mortality among newborns requiring major surgery for correctable anomalies should be limited to those who have additional associated anomalies that are incompatible with life.

SPECTRUM OF ANOMALIES

A congenital anomaly is an inborn structural defect that is usually noted at birth or shortly thereafter but occasionally manifests later in life, depending on the extent of the lesion.[11,12] It can arise from genetic or environmental causes, but in most instances the cause is unknown, and it probably results from a combination of the two.[13] A great deal of epidemiologic work has been directed toward identifying associations between conditions in the environment and specific birth defects. Although these associations may not indicate the precise cause of the anomaly, they can be extremely useful in designing preventive strategies. An example is the awareness of the association between reduced antenatal folic acid intake and the incidence of myelomeningocele or spina bifida. Community-wide supplementation of folic acid has resulted in a dramatic decrease in the incidence of this disorder.[14-16]

It is estimated that 2% to 3% of infants are born with a significant anomaly, many of which necessitate operative intervention in the neonatal period.[11-13,17] Table 86-1 lists the approximate incidences of many of the anomalies encountered in neonates who require surgery.

When an infant has a congenital malformation, additional abnormalities should be sought, because they are much more frequently encountered in such infants than in the general population. Knowledge of the common patterns of associated anomalies is helpful in directing which organ systems must be most closely assessed. For example, neonates with any of the vertebral, anorectal, cardiac, tracheal, esophageal, renal, and limb (VACTERL) anomalies are especially likely to have others in this group. In two studies, 70% of infants with esophageal atresia had additional malformations, of which 15% were cardiovascular and 18% were renal.[11,17]

PHYSIOLOGIC CONSIDERATIONS

An understanding of the neonate's unique physiologic responses to surgical illness is essential for optimal management, as such children are making the difficult transition between fetal and extrauterine life. Although knowledge has dramatically improved in many areas, the data are still sparse in others, and treatment recommendations are extrapolated from experiences with adults.

Hormonal and Metabolic Responses to Stress

Adults have a characteristic catabolic response to surgical stress, the extent of which is related to the magnitude of the traumatic or surgical insult. The metabolic products released provide alternative energy sources to meet the increased energy demands and to supply essential nutrients for synthetic activity in the postoperative period.[18] The data are not as well characterized for neonates, who mount a catabolic response to surgical trauma that differs significantly from that of adults. The responses also seem to differ somewhat between premature and full-term neonates and are further altered by the administration of anesthetic agents.[19-22]

During surgery, both preterm and full-term neonates exhibit substantial elevations in serum catecholamine (epinephrine and norepinephrine) levels, as well as

Table 86-1. Approximate Incidences of Congenital Surgical Malformations per Live Births

Congenital Surgical Malformation	Incidence	References
Inguinal hernia		133-135
Full-term	1/50-1/100	
Premature (<1000 g)	1/3	
Cryptorchidism		136, 137
Full-term	1/25 at birth; 1/100 at 1 year	
Premature (<1500 g)	2/3 at birth	
Hypospadias	1/125-1/300	138
Spina bifida	1/350	139
Cleft lip	1/400 Asians, Native Americans	140
	1/750-1/900 whites	
	1/1500-1/2000 blacks	
Jejunoileal atresia	1/1500-1/5000	141, 142
Diaphragmatic hernia	1/2000-1/5000	143-145
Hydrocephalus (without spina bifida)	1/2500	146
Esophageal atresia	1/3000-1/4500	147, 148
Omphalocele and gastroschisis	1/3000-1/10,000	149-151
Imperforate anus	1/5000	152
Hirschsprung disease	1/5000	153, 154
Duodenal obstruction	1/6000-1/10,000	155, 156
Meconium ileus	1/7500-1/20,000	157, 158
Pierre Robin sequence	1/8500	159
Biliary atresia	1/10,000-1/25,000	95, 160-162
Exstrophy of bladder	1/10,000-1/50,000	163, 164
Colon atresia	1/20,000	165
Prune-belly syndrome	1/30,000-1/50,000	166
Meconium peritonitis	1/35,000	167, 168
Sacrococcygeal teratoma	1/40,000	169
Conjoined twins	1/50,000-1/100,000	170, 171
Exstrophy of cloaca	1/200,000-1/400,000	164

insulin and growth hormone resistance.[23] Postoperatively, there is prolonged hyperglycemia and an increase in the amounts of serum lactate, pyruvate, free fatty acids, glycerol, ketone bodies, and corticosteroids.[24] Insulin levels are elevated postoperatively in full-term infants in response to hyperglycemia (as is the case for adults), whereas premature infants are unable to mount such a reaction and thus experience more marked hyperglycemia. Levels of cytokines—endogenous peptides that are primary regulators of the metabolic, endocrine, and immunologic responses to injury—are elevated postoperatively in neonates but are slower to rise than in adults.[23,25] Among their many functions, cytokines inhibit visceral protein synthesis and instead divert the liver to produce acute-phase reactants, which are specialized proteins with immunologic and repair functions.[23]

The intraoperative elevation of norepinephrine levels occurs in both adults and infants, but there is no similar elevation of epinephrine in adults until the postoperative period.[24] Glucagon levels are not increased in neonates, as they are in adults. Serum cortisol levels, although increased,[21,26] are not as well correlated with the magnitude of surgical stress in infants as in adults, probably because there is a relative immaturity of enzymatic synthesis in the adrenal cortex. Instead, more steroid precursors are released.[18]

The hypercatabolic state characterized by the breakdown of carbohydrates, proteins, and fats into their metabolic constituents in adults is adaptive to the altered energy needs and increased metabolic demands. Unfortunately, in critically ill neonates with limited nutritional reserves and the requirement for growth and maturation, the net effect of excessive catabolism may be detrimental.[18,27] An exaggerated stress response may be even more poorly tolerated in infants with very low birth weight, who possess fewer nutritional reserves and in whom the catabolic reaction cannot be somewhat counterbalanced by an increased insulin response.[19] In addition to the depletion of nutritional stores, the ensuing hyperglycemia elevates osmolarity, predisposing the infant to intracranial hemorrhage and renal cortical damage.[24]

Adequate anesthesia may have beneficial effects in modulating this unchecked catabolism.[19,20] Neonates anesthetized with halothane or fentanyl demonstrated a significantly more blunted hormonal response to major surgery than did control infants, who received only nitrous oxide and curare. Catecholamines and adrenocorticoids were less elevated, the insulin-to-glucagon ratio did not fall, hyperglycemia was substantially less severe, and protein breakdown was diminished. Most intriguing, infants in the control group experienced a much higher incidence of postoperative cardiovascular and respiratory complications such as hypotension, bradycardia, respiratory failure, and intraventricular hemorrhage.

Studies have suggested that neonates undergoing major operations with adequate anesthesia increase their resting energy expenditure by only a modest 20%, which returns to baseline levels by 12 to 24 hours.[28] Extremely premature infants may not even exhibit this transient rise in resting energy expenditure; a group of neonates born at 24 weeks of gestation who underwent patent ductus arteriosus ligation did not demonstrate any net change in this value.[29] Even after prolonged surgical illness, although the data are conflicting and there is individual variability, critically ill surgical neonates do not necessarily manifest a significantly higher overall energy expenditure than do infants undergoing uncomplicated operations.[30,31] Also, unlike adults, infants may not increase their whole-body protein turnover after major surgery, inasmuch as protein synthesis is diverted from growth to tissue repair until anabolic recover occurs.[32] Premature infants seem to exhibit an earlier and increased rate of anabolic recovery in comparison with full-term infants.[33]

In many cases, the stress response to surgical illness may result more from the underlying disease process and may be reversed after the surgical intervention.[23] In neonates with very low birth weight who underwent patent ductus arteriosus ligation under fentanyl anesthesia and received total parenteral nutrition, not only was a protein catabolic state not demonstrated but also the protein breakdown noted preoperatively that was caused by the effects of the patent ductus arteriosus resolved promptly after surgery.[34]

Multisystem organ failure (MSOF), the sequential loss of function of multiple organs remote from the site of the primary pathologic process, may occur in the neonate who undergoes surgery, but the organs involved and their sequence of failure differ markedly from those in adults.[35] In one study, persistent capillary leakage was the first sign of MSOF in infants, followed sequentially by renal, hepatic, hematologic, lung, and myocardial failure. Acute respiratory distress syndrome, an early indicator of MSOF in adults, was absent in the neonatal group. It is cautioned that unexplained weight gain and edema may be early warning signs of MSOF, and careful investigations for an inciting cause, such as infection, should be initiated before cardiovascular failure supervenes.[35]

Perioperative Fluids and Electrolytes

Perioperative intravenous fluid therapy must be extremely precise in neonates, because the neonate possesses a very narrow margin for error. The daily water turnover rate is much higher than in adults,[36] and infants undergoing surgery frequently have major shifts in body fluid compartments. The glomerular filtration rate in neonates is only 25% that of adults,[37] and the infant's renal medulla has a relatively low concentration of urea.[38] As a consequence, the neonatal kidney has a limited ability to dilute or concentrate the urine.[36] Neonates are also less capable of excreting excess sodium, and premature neonates cannot conserve sodium effectively.[39,40] The kidneys therefore cannot be relied on to correct for any significant deficiency or overabundance in administered fluids and electrolytes, as occurs in healthy children and adults.

Before surgery, it is essential that any dehydration be corrected and intravascular volume be restored. Certain anesthetic agents, especially halogenated anesthetics, may lower systemic vascular resistance and depress myocardial contractility to a greater extent in neonates than in adults. Hypovolemia potentiates this effect and can rapidly result in hypotension and cardiovascular collapse.[2,36,41]

Postoperatively, an increase in intravenous fluids is often required because of third space losses from both the underlying surgical illness and the operative dissection itself. The deficit from the loss of such fluid, which is sequestered out of equilibrium with the intravascular space, must be provided intravenously until that fluid is mobilized during recovery, a period that often extends several days. It is vital that this fluid be reassessed at 8- to 12-hour intervals in the early postoperative period to allow for accurate replacement of fluid needs, because after surgery, the neonate can tolerate neither hypovolemia nor fluid overload. It is controversial whether there is also an inherent tendency for increased postoperative sodium and water retention that is independent and in excess of the amount needed to account for third space losses. Krummel and colleagues postulated a neuroendocrine response to surgical trauma that produces maximal sodium retention in the first 12 hours, and they cautioned against administering an overabundance of sodium.[40] Other authors have maintained that neonates' postoperative urinary excretion of sodium and water remains appropriate and, aside from the third space deficits, their body fluid compartments are normal after surgery.[1,42,43] If there is a period of inherent antidiuresis, it does not appear to extend beyond 12 to 24 hours after surgery. In practice, postoperative fluids are usually administered in excess of maintenance requirements.

The serum glucose level must be closely monitored in neonates undergoing surgery, who are predisposed to both hypoglycemia and hyperglycemia. Hepatic glycogen stores are limited in newborns, especially if they are under stress or have low birth weight.[44] Glucose must therefore be supplied to protect against hypoglycemia, which can result in apnea, bradycardia, hypotension, convulsions, and brain damage.[37] On the other hand, surgical stress can produce hyperglycemia, particularly in premature infants, and may lead to hyperosmolarity, osmotic diuresis, dehydration, and intraventricular hemorrhage.[24]

Premature infants are deficient in calcium, because 75% of normal body stores are acquired during the final 12 weeks of gestation.[39] Hypocalcemia is potentiated by stress, hypothermia, and infection, all which occur with some frequency in neonates undergoing surgery. Ionized calcium levels must be closely monitored and calcium administered as needed.

Hypokalemia is rare in neonates with acute surgical disorders, because intracellular potassium is released from tissue breakdown.[45] A low serum potassium level therefore reflects significant total body potassium depletion. During recovery, adequate potassium must be supplied for cellular repair and growth.

Hemoglobin and Coagulation

Although it has been asserted that neonates undergoing major operations should have hemoglobin levels above some arbitrary value, such as 10 to 13 g/dL for full-term infants and 13 g/dL for premature infants,[46,47] that view is more supported by theoretical concerns than by actual data. In adults, hemoglobin levels can fall below 5 to 6 g/dL before oxygen delivery becomes critical, because cardiac output increases or is redistributed and oxygen extraction at the tissue level is enhanced.[36]

Neonates do have a more limited capacity to compensate for low hemoglobin levels.[36] Oxygen consumption is higher, and therefore more oxygen delivery is required. Cardiac output is more constrained by the inability of neonates to increase their stroke volumes. Neonates have a very limited ability to increase cardiac output that is entirely dependent on increasing their heart rate. Fetal hemoglobin has a higher affinity for oxygen (a lower oxygen half-saturation pressure) than does adult hemoglobin, which restricts oxygen extraction peripherally at the tissue level. Finally, respiratory failure and cyanotic cardiac disease can produce hypoxia and unsaturated hemoglobin, diminishing the oxygen content at any given hemoglobin level.

In evaluating the potential need for preoperative and postoperative transfusions in a given infant, the most rational approach is an individualized assessment of whether the oxygen delivery can meet the metabolic demands.[48] Factors that would indicate the need for higher hemoglobin levels include critical illness, prematurity, hypoxia, cardiac failure, and an operative procedure in which significant blood loss is anticipated.

During surgery, packed red blood cell transfusions are usually recommended when the estimated blood loss is more than 15% to 20% of the blood volume.[37,47] This requirement is obviously also influenced by the factors listed previously, as well as the baseline preoperative hemoglobin value.

There are no established guidelines regarding the need for coagulation studies on neonates before they undergo surgery. Vitamin K is administered to all hospital-born newborns to prevent hemolytic disease of the newborn, because neonates initially have diminished vitamin K–dependent coagulation activity. It is important to realize that most neonates born at home or in other nonhospital settings have not received vitamin K and may be more prone to bleeding complications during and after surgery.[49,50] A study of 49 neonates undergoing surgery demonstrated, however, that despite having received vitamin K, this coagulation activity remained abnormally low for days to weeks in many instances.[51] Sixteen percent of these infants suffered abnormal bleeding complications. It was concluded that the neonatal liver has a diminished ability to synthesize clotting factors from vitamin K even when it is available and that direct clotting factor replacement (fresh-frozen plasma) is necessary in some instances. Prematurity and low birth weight are particularly associated with coagulation deficiencies.[51] Neonates can also develop thrombocytopenia with or without disseminated intravascular coagulation from sepsis and perinatal asphyxia.[37]

Coagulation studies, such as a platelet count and measurements of prothrombin time and partial thromboplastin time, should be obtained when there is any increased risk of coagulopathy and may be indicated in many neonates undergoing surgery, such as those with operative necrotizing enterocolitis. In addition, neonates with an increased risk of bleeding include those who have received large volumes of transfusions and those with

Table 86–2. Risk Factors for Abnormal Bleeding in Neonates Undergoing Surgery
Prematurity
Low birth weight
Perinatal asphyxia
Sepsis
Large-volume transfusions
Identified abnormal hemorrhage (e.g., from needle puncture sites, circumcision, cephalohematoma)

clinical evidence of abnormal coagulation, such as excessive bleeding from needle puncture sites or at circumcision (Table 86-2).

Nutrition and Central Venous Catheters

It is imperative that neonates undergoing surgery receive adequate nutritional support; however, overfeeding may be detrimental as well. Neonates, especially those born prematurely, have very limited nutritional stores of glycogen, fat, and muscle.[52] Malnutrition can therefore develop rapidly in the perioperative period when there is diminished nutrient intake and a catabolic reaction to stress. Severe consequences of malnutrition include organ dysfunction, impaired growth, immunologic incompetence, and a decreased ability to heal wounds. On the other hand, as discussed previously, it is now recognized that the overall energy expenditure of neonates may not increase substantially after uncomplicated surgery or even during critical surgical illness. These infants, often sedated, exhibit limited activity in a thermoneutral environment, and energy for normal anabolic processes is necessarily diverted.[23,28,29] Excessive calorie administration can result in CO_2 retention, a fatty liver, and a paradoxic increase in protein catabolism and must be avoided.[31] There is even evidence that short-term calorie restriction can improve outcomes during acute illness.[23] One recommendation is to limit calories until recovery from metabolic stress to 50 to 75 kcal/kg/day while providing 2.5 g/kg/day of protein, 1 g/kg/day of fat, and 10 g/kg/day of carbohydrates.[23]

Enteral Nutrition

Enteral nutrition is preferred whenever the alimentary tract is functional and accessible because it preserves the integrity of the intestinal mucosa, is more economical, and has fewer complications than total parenteral nutrition (TPN).[53] There is evidence that TPN significantly impairs neutrophil function and is associated with a high incidence of septicemia, which may be prevented with even small volumes of enteral feedings.[54-56]

A small nasogastric tube can be inserted for gavage feeding if the neonate is unable to suck and swallow effectively as a result of prematurity, weakness, or respiratory failure and tachypnea. Continuous or frequent small feedings may be better tolerated than large bolus feedings after ischemic bowel injury, after intestinal resections, and in infants with very low birth weight.[57,58]

Even during the recovery stages of acute and chronic illnesses, when gastric emptying may be impaired and gastroesophageal reflux is a concern, a soft transpyloric feeding tube can be placed under radiographic guidance and small quantities (2 mL/hour) of enteral feedings administered, with increasing volumes as tolerated.[23,59]

A gastrostomy tube is useful if prolonged tube feeding is required, as in neonates with an inability to swallow safely and effectively because of neurologic dysfunction or maxillofacial deformity. Gastrostomy tubes are less irritating, are not as easily displaced, and may be less likely to promote aspiration than are nasogastric tubes. Gastrostomy tubes also free the nasopharyngeal area for improved oral stimulation therapy, and in this manner are often helpful in encouraging eventual oral feeding. Gastrostomy tubes can be placed through a small laparotomy, laparoscopically, or percutaneously with the aid of an endoscope.[60] In neonates with a significant risk of gastroesophageal reflux, such as those with neurologic injury or disease, evaluation should be completed and a fundoplication considered at the time of gastrostomy tube placement if significant reflux is identified.

If a gastrostomy tube becomes dislodged during the first few days after insertion, it must be replaced operatively. After 1 to 2 weeks, there is a well-formed tract to the skin, and replacement is easily performed at the bedside. When these tubes are no longer needed, they are simply pulled out, and the tract usually closes spontaneously within 24 hours.

Parenteral Nutrition

The ability to provide TPN for neonates of any size has revolutionized surgical and neonatal management and allows for the survival of many infants who would otherwise have died during the perioperative period from complications of malnutrition.[61] A majority of neonates with major abdominal wall or gastrointestinal surgical disorders require TPN until they recover alimentary tract function. TPN is generally indicated for full-term neonates who can take no oral feedings for more than 3 days and even sooner for preterm neonates.[62] Recovery time for the alimentary tract after gastrointestinal and abdominal wall surgery is variable, taking 5 to 30 days.

TPN can be administered through a peripheral vein or a central venous catheter. The advantages of peripheral venous catheterization are ease of placement and minimal complications. Central venous catheters are necessary to deliver hypertonic or vasoconstrictor solutions, for hemodynamic monitoring, and frequently when accessible peripheral veins become scarce in neonates who require long-term venous access. The umbilical vein can often be utilized for the first 1 to 2 weeks after birth. Long-term use of umbilical vein catheters is associated with an unacceptable risk of infection. There has been increasing use of thin Silastic catheters that can be inserted centrally through a percutaneously accessed extremity vein. Although these catheters cannot always be positioned centrally and their narrow caliber restricts infusion rates, they have greatly limited the requirement for surgically implanted central venous catheters. Silicone catheters with a Dacron cuff are widely used for central catheterization.

The silicone is relatively nonthrombogenic, and the cuff, which is placed in a subcutaneous tunnel between the skin insertion site and the cannulated vein, helps prevent dislodgment of the catheter. These catheters can be inserted by either a cutdown or a percutaneous approach.[63] The veins accessed by cutdown include the external jugular, facial, internal jugular, and axillary veins[64] and the greater saphenous vein at the groin (Fig. 86-1). The site of placement is often guided by the weight of the neonate. The preferred location for the catheter tip is within the superior vena cava near the right atrium; for saphenous catheters, the tip should be placed in the inferior vena cava above or below the renal and mesenteric veins (with a lateral radiograph obtained to ascertain that it has not entered a lumbar vein). The subclavian vein can be cannulated percutaneously with a relatively low complication rate even in premature neonates, but this requires special expertise.[63]

The insertion of all central venous catheters should be performed with full sterile precautions, optimal lighting, and high-quality instruments. Percutaneous insertion of central catheters may not require the neonate to be paralyzed for placement, whereas insertion of a central venous catheter by cutdown is a surgical procedure and requires complete immobilization. The neonate can be administered intravenous narcotics and muscle relaxants and placed on controlled ventilation to allow for safe performance of these surgical procedures in the neonatal intensive care unit; the complication rate is no higher than with operating room placement.[65]

Complications of central venous catheters can be infectious or mechanical. Catheter sepsis is the most frequent complication reported. Between 7% and 50% of catheters become infected, which represents one infectious episode per 57 to 480 catheter days.[63,65-68] Often, catheters infected with bacteria can be salvaged with antibiotics administered through the catheter.

Methicillin-resistant *Staphylococcus epidermidis* is the most common infecting organism,[66] and vancomycin is usually the antibiotic of choice until blood cultures are available. Catheter removal is indicated if the patient is critically ill with sepsis or if the infection cannot be cleared, as is more frequently the case with gram-negative organisms. Fungal infections are generally considered an indication for catheter removal, although occasionally a catheter can be salvaged with antifungal therapy.[69]

Mechanical complications of central venous catheters include occlusion of the line with thrombi or precipitates, malposition, breakage, extravascular extravasation of fluid, emboli, and thrombosis of major vessels.[70] Occluded catheters and catheter-associated thrombi can occasionally be cleared with tissue thromboplastin activator, a thrombolytic agent; urokinase is no longer generally available.[71-73] Venous thrombosis is suspected from progressive catheter malfunction or increasing edema and may be diagnosed by Doppler ultrasonography. Catheter removal and possibly thrombolytic therapy are indicated, but the incidence of long-term sequelae are not known.[74] Tissue thromboplastin activator must be used cautiously in the neonate, because of the increased risk of intracranial hemorrhage.

Central venous pressure can be measured to help assess hemodynamic function. The right atrial pressure, as measured by the central venous pressure, usually approximates the more important left ventricular end-diastolic pressure and provides an approximate guide to hydration status and cardiac function.

Arterial Catheters

Arterial access in surgical neonates is overall somewhat less important than was previously the case, because noninvasive devices such as the Dynamapp and the pulse oximeter can provide reliable measurements of the systemic blood pressure and oxyhemoglobin saturation. In critically ill infants, however, arterial catheters allow for very accurate, continuous monitoring of the blood pressure and the frequent sampling of arterial blood.

Umbilical artery catheters can usually be placed in neonates. If the condition of the cord does not permit percutaneous cannulation, or if the catheter cannot be advanced into the abdominal aorta, the umbilical artery may be accessed through a small infraumbilical incision.[75] In larger neonates, peripheral arteries frequently can be cannulated, either percutaneously or by cutdown. To preserve distal perfusion, vessels are chosen with good collateral circulation, such as the radial artery (after performing a modified Allen test),[76] dorsalis pedis, or posterior tibial arteries. Use of the temporal artery is avoided because it has been associated with cerebral infarction[77] and skin sloughing. Although there is usually collateral circulation, the femoral artery is also avoided if possible, because there is a small but significant risk of limb loss.[78]

Anesthesia

General anesthesia is required for most neonatal surgery and is generally described as "balanced," combining inhalation agents (such as halothane, sevoflurane and nitrous oxide), potent narcotics (such as fentanyl), and muscle relaxants (such as pancuronium and vecuronium). The benefit of balanced anesthesia is an attempt

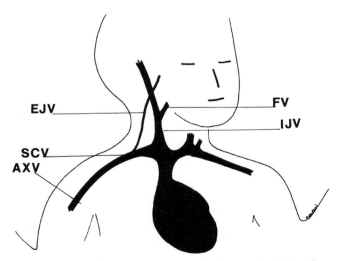

Figure 86-1. Central venous catheter sites in the neonate. AXV, axillary vein; EJV, external jugular vein; FV, facial vein; IJV, internal jugular vein; SCV, subclavian vein.

to counteract or minimize the complications or side effects of any individual agent. Nitrous oxide is often used as a supplement to lower the required concentration of other inhalational agents, but because nitrous oxide diffuses into air spaces, it should not be used in neonates with bowel obstruction or space-occupying lesions within the chest.[47] In neonates, ventilation should usually be controlled, because anesthetic agents depress the ventilatory response to hypoxia and hypercarbia, a phenomenon that is exaggerated in the newborn.[2,47] An endotracheal tube is necessary to ensure a patent airway, minimize the risk of aspiration, and facilitate control of ventilation.

Inhalational agents can be used even in premature infants but can produce cardiovascular depression, and adequate intravascular volume must be ensured before operation. A narcotic, such as fentanyl, is often better tolerated with less attendant hemodynamic instability without an inhalational agent in the critically ill, premature neonate. Because of relatively slow metabolism in the neonatal liver, postoperative ventilatory support must be anticipated.[38,79]

Less commonly, spinal anesthetics have been used in neonates at high risk in an attempt to avoid the risk of intubation, general anesthesia, and the potential for prolonged postoperative ventilatory support, especially in the setting of chronic lung disease. In addition, when not supplemented by other drugs, spinal anesthetics preclude the risk of postoperative apnea.[80] Spinal anesthesia is limited to areas of the body that can be effectively anesthetized without compromising diaphragmatic function, and in neonates it is most frequently used for inguinal procedures. Spinal anesthetics are time limited and not feasible for operations extending longer than approximately 1 hour.

Thermoregulation

It is essential that neonates be maintained in a thermoneutral environment to prevent the potentially dire consequences of hypothermia. In the premature neonate, there is an enhanced tendency to lose heat because of the relatively large skin surface area in proportion to body weight; the thin layer of subcutaneous fat, which provides little insulation; and the marginal epithelial barrier that is present in extreme prematurity.[2] Shivering is absent in neonates, who instead rely on the chemical thermogenesis of brown fat metabolism for additional heat production. Brown fat is specialized adipose tissue, and because it develops relatively late in gestation, premature neonates have substantially less than full-term neonates.

Surgical procedures may promote hypothermia through many mechanisms.[47,81] Skin surfaces are uncovered to allow access to the surgical site and for monitoring, and viscera in opened body cavities are exposed, leading to rapid heat loss. Anesthetic agents themselves promote loss of heat by inducing peripheral vasodilation and inhibiting brown fat thermogenesis; fentanyl in particular has been shown to significantly inhibit heat production in the liver, which results in hypothermia.[82,83]

Cold stress exacts a heavy toll on the neonate, because it causes a dramatic rise in the metabolic rate with a threefold to fourfold increase in oxygen consumption.

Significant demands are placed on the cardiorespiratory system, and metabolic breakdown products accumulate with the development of acidosis.[2] These effects can lead to delayed recovery from anesthesia, peripheral vasoconstriction, central nervous system depression, cardiorespiratory failure, and death.

Aggressive efforts must be expended to prevent, rather than treat, hypothermia. The operating room must be kept warm and the temperature of the local environment of the neonate maintained with radiant warmers and heating blankets. The infant's head and extremities should be wrapped, all intravenous solutions (including blood and crystalloid) warmed, and inhalational agents warmed and humidified.[2] Exposure of bowel loops is a critical cause of heat loss, and replacement into the abdomen of portions of intestine not actively undergoing exploration and the use of warm irrigants in the course of surgery are important measures in maintaining a stable body temperature.

Pain and Analgesia

Infants receiving intensive care are often situated in a noxious, stressful environment and are frequently subjected to painful procedures. However, providing analgesia to neonates, and particularly to premature infants, involves concerns about a relatively high risk of complications.[38] In particular, immature respiratory mechanisms increase the risk of apnea, hypoxemia, and hypercapnia. There is still a discrepancy between beliefs regarding pain in neonates and actual practice. A survey of 467 physicians and nurses in 11 nurseries revealed that although respondents believed that infants experience as much or even more pain than do adults, pain relief measures were used infrequently, even for what were considered to be the most painful of procedures.[84] For all surgical procedures, whether limited or extensive, the question is no longer whether there is a need for anesthesia but how best to provide pain control effectively and safely.

Although traditionally it was believed that neonates did not experience pain in response to surgical procedures,[85] there is extensive documentation of significant cardiovascular and hormonal responses to nociceptive stimuli in the neonate. Pain is in part a subjective phenomenon, and although the experiential component cannot be measured, by all physiologic and behavioral criteria it is evident that neonates exhibit pain.[86]

Neuroanatomic pathways for the perception of pain are already well developed in the neonate.[18,86] The density of nociceptive nerve endings in the skin is at least equivalent to that in adults.[18] In the past, the lack of myelination in the neonatal nervous system has been used to support the impression that neonates do not experience pain, although in adults 75% of nociceptive impulses are transmitted through unmyelinated fibers. Incomplete myelination merely means that conduction velocity is slowed (which is actually offset in infants by shorter interneuron distances).[86] Afferent pain pathways to the thalamus and from the thalamus to the cerebral cortex are already established by midgestation; myelination to the thalamus is completed by 30 weeks of gestation and myelination to the cerebrum by 37 weeks.

Nociceptive stimuli in awake neonates produce elevations in heart rate, blood pressure, pulmonary vascular resistance, and intracranial pressure, as well as palmar sweating and a lowering of the oxygen tension; these phenomena may be abolished with adequate analgesia.[86] Catecholamine and cortisol levels rise dramatically and can also be attenuated with appropriate analgesia.[24,26] Neonates exhibit characteristic behavioral responses, including crying, trembling, distinctive facial expressions, and extremity withdrawal in response to noxious stimuli.[24,26,87] There often follows a period of quiet, non–rapid eye movement sleep, with irritability when aroused.[26] Preterm infants appear to be more sensitive to painful stimuli and have heightened responses to successive stimuli. Untreated pain in neonates is associated with increased rates of major morbidity and mortality.[88,89]

After painful interventions, systemic narcotics may be safely employed for pain relief in neonates if dosed carefully, with close observation and monitoring, especially for heart rate and apnea. Neonates should be monitored carefully on a cardiorespiratory or apnea/bradycardia monitor for at least 24 hours after the last dose of narcotics.[87] Morphine and fentanyl are used most commonly and should be administered intravenously rather than intramuscularly, because of limited muscle mass and more predictable pharmacokinetics.[87] A study of postoperative neonates demonstrated that the continuous infusion of fentanyl was associated with fewer episodes of apnea, in comparison with bolus dosing of the same total amount of narcotic, with similar pain control. Respiratory depression did occur in both groups, and longer ventilatory support may sometimes be the best option in order to be able to provide adequate pain relief safely.[90] Local, spinal, caudal, and regional anesthetic techniques are still not widely used in the preterm neonatal population, but these methods may be employed in decreasing intraoperative anesthetic requirements and also in preventing pain in the postoperative period.[2,91]

For less extensive, bedside procedures, nonpharmacologic interventions, including environmental modification and comforting, may also help reduce stress.[92] Acetaminophen is safe in full-term and preterm neonates and can be administered orally or rectally.

Infections

The neonate is an immunocompromised host, and newborns undergoing surgery are at increased risk of perioperative infections. Surgery violates epithelial defense barriers, exposing the neonate to pathogenic organisms both from the skin and from internal colonized epithelial surfaces. In addition, anesthesia and surgery have generalized immunosuppressive effects, which are magnified in the newborn.[93] Unfortunately, host defense mechanisms are quite underdeveloped in neonates, especially in premature infants. In comparison with adults, the keratin skin layer is thin, and mucosal immunoglobulin A is absent.[94] Humoral antibody levels are deficient, with negligible placental transmission of immunoglobulins M, A, and E and some classes of immunoglobulin G.[95,96] Complement levels are low, neutrophil stores are decreased and their chemotactic and

phagocytic functions impaired,[94,97] and T lymphocyte activity is diminished.[95,98]

Historically, postoperative infection rates for all classes of wounds were noted to be higher in neonates than in older patients.[98] A survey of 1433 neonatal operations[99] demonstrated an infection rate of 11.1% for clean cases (in comparison with 1.5% in adults[100]), 20.9% for potentially contaminated cases (7.7% in adults[100]), and 20.9% for contaminated cases (similar to the adult rate[100]). In more recent studies, the wound infection rates after neonatal surgery have more closely approximated adult standards.[101,102] Neonatal infections often have nonspecific signs initially but can disseminate rapidly and have severe consequences.[103]

Although extensive supportive data are lacking, prophylactic antibiotics are often used in an effort to reduce the incidence of wound infections in neonates. Guidelines from the Surgical Section of the American Academy of Pediatrics, extrapolating recommendations from adult data, state that prophylaxis is not indicated in clean cases but should be administered preoperatively in clean-contaminated and contaminated cases, no more than 48 hours before surgery.[104,105] Nevertheless, a survey of 21 institutions revealed that many pediatric surgeons treated all neonates undergoing operations with antimicrobial therapy, with the durations varying widely.[104] A combination of ampicillin and gentamicin was used most commonly, with clindamycin added for contaminated cases (and especially for necrotizing enterocolitis). The authors of this survey emphasized that to be effective, prophylactic antibiotics must be administered before surgery (2 hours to 30 minutes before) for peak tissue levels to be achieved at the time of operative contamination, and suggested that they should be of limited duration (12 to 24 hours for clean cases and 24 to 48 hours for clean-contaminated or contaminated cases[104]).

Evidence that a surgical incision has become infected includes erythema, swelling, tenderness, and a purulent discharge. Such wounds should be promptly opened and drained with specimens obtained for culture and Gram stain. Although not always necessary in adults after drainage, systemic antibiotics are administered to neonates in this circumstance because of the heightened risk of systemic bacterial dissemination.

Neonates with Very Low Birth Weight

Neonates with very low birth weight and major surgical disorders are the most challenging patients to treat. Partly because of their fragility, they are overrepresented among neonates requiring surgery, and many of the physiologic problems encountered among full-term neonates are greatly magnified in this population.

Low birth weight is a weight less than 2500 g at birth; very low birth weight is a weight less than 1500 g. There are numerous risk factors associated with the occurrence of low birth weight, including prematurity, medical complications of pregnancy (e.g., multiple pregnancy, placental complications), medical illness in the mother (e.g., hypertension, poor nutritional status, smoking) and illness/complications in the fetus (congenital anomalies). Neonates with low birth weight are 40 times more likely to die than are infants with normal birth weight, and in those with very low birth weight, the relative incidence of neonatal death is almost 200 times greater than that for infants with normal birth weight.[106] In addition to the increased risk of death, neonates with low birth weight are more likely to exhibit a broad range of complications, including respiratory distress syndrome, apnea, cerebral ischemia/anoxia, temperature instability, hypoglycemia, hypocalcemia, hyperbilirubinemia, and sepsis.

The incidence of congenital malformations in infants with low birth weight is much higher than in the general population; as many as 30% to 40% of neonates undergoing surgery for congenital anomalies may have low birth weight, with all the associated risks just listed.[7,107] In one series, more than 50% of neonates undergoing surgery for esophageal atresia, meconium ileus, and intestinal atresia had low birth weight.[96] Many neonates with gastroschisis, which necessitates surgery very early in the neonatal period, have low birth weight.[108-110] In addition to surgery for congenital anomalies, the improved medical management of neonates with very low birth weight has lowered the mortality rate significantly, allowing survival with the potential to develop acquired complications that necessitate surgery, including necrotizing enterocolitis, patent ductus arteriosus, tracheal stenosis, hydrocephalus, and retinopathy of prematurity.

Before 1970, the majority of preterm neonates weighing less than 1500 g died; the mortality rate among neonates weighing less than 1000 g was 90%.[46] Surgical consultation was usually not sought for these extremely small neonates even with potentially correctable conditions, because they would almost invariably die from an operative procedure. Today, with advances in both medical and surgical management of these fragile neonates, the survival rate is dependent on the risk associated with the disease process itself (for example, an increased risk of mortality associated with necrotizing enterocolitis) and not significantly affected by the need for surgical intervention.[46]

PREOPERATIVE ASSESSMENT AND PREPARATION

Pediatric surgeons are increasingly called upon to counsel patients about the antenatal diagnosis of congenital anomalies, which are being diagnosed in utero with greater frequency. For example, screening of maternal serum α-fetoprotein levels is relatively routine, and an elevation in this value raises the possibility of a fetal anomaly, including neural tube defects, omphalocele, gastroschisis, and sacrococcygeal teratoma.[111-113] An antenatal imaging study is then recommended to provide visualization of these potential structural defects. Ultrasonography has advanced rapidly, and anatomic details can be delineated with increasing accuracy.

Despite improvements in the antenatal diagnoses of congenital anomalies, there is limited evidence that this information has led to an overall improvement in neonatal survival. Antenatal diagnosis and counseling enable family education and participation in decision making with regard to terminating or proceeding with the

pregnancy, choosing a site and mode of delivery, defining the timing of delivery, and, less commonly, allowing necessary intervention during the course of the pregnancy.[27,114,115] Although there is increasing experience with invasive antenatal interventions for a variety of surgical conditions, only a limited number have been successfully performed (such as for myelomeningocele, hydronephrosis, hydrocephalus, large sacrococcygeal teratomas, and space-occupying lesions of the chest); such procedures are being performed at only a few centers with complex clinical protocols.[116-119] The opportunity to avoid the transfer of a sick neonate (with the added burden of separation of the mother and infant) by planned delivery at a perinatal center and the adequate education and preparation of the parents appear to be the current major advantages with antenatal diagnosis. The risks, benefits, and alternatives can be discussed and a close personal relationship established early between the parents and the pediatric surgeon.

Operations that do not need to be performed in the immediate neonatal period are best postponed to allow for optimal stabilization of the newborn, which improves the outcome of surgery. A delay of at least 24 hours allows the neonate to complete the period of cardiopulmonary transition, a complex process involving changes from fetal to neonatal circulation and adaptation to air breathing, that can be easily disrupted by surgical intervention. This period also allows for recovery from trauma and thermal stress associated with birth, as well as a thorough evaluation for associated anomalies.[120]

For all neonates who require an operation, a history should be documented and a physical examination and appropriate laboratory studies performed (Table 86-3). The history should include information about maternal illness and prenatal care, including any antenatal diagnostic studies, mode and complications associated with delivery, Apgar scores, gestational age, birth weight, and any neonatal events after birth. The physical examination must include vital signs, resuscitation status, an evaluation of the presenting surgical problem, and a thorough search for associated anomalies or complications. The laboratory data that should be obtained depend on the

Table 86–3. Preoperative Evaluation of the Neonate Undergoing Surgery

History*
Physical examination (including vital signs)*
CBC
Measurement of serum electrolytes, BUN, creatinine, glucose, ionized calcium
Measurement of blood gases
Urine output
Coagulation studies (PT, PTT, platelets, fibrinogen)
Chest radiograph

*Mandatory.

BUN, blood urea nitrogen; CBC, complete blood cell count;
PT, prothrombin time; PTT, partial thromboplastin time.

condition and age of the neonate and the type of surgery planned. Usually included are a complete blood cell count and glucose, calcium, and blood gas (preferably an arterial blood gas) measurements. Serum electrolytes, blood urea nitrogen, and creatinine measurements are most useful in neonates older than 12 to 24 hours. Coagulation studies may be useful. Appropriate blood products should be requested from the blood bank early in the course of care, because the availability of fresh blood products required in the care of the newborn is often limited.

Before surgery, oxygenation and tissue perfusion must be optimized. Respiratory support is provided as needed, according to blood gas values and respiratory effort. If the patient is inadequately or incompletely resuscitated, intravascular volume must be restored before surgery, as guided by vital signs, clinical examination, and urine output (optimally at least 1 to 2 mL/kg/hour).

It is preferable that the infant's stomach be kept empty, to minimize the risk of aspiration of gastric contents during the induction of anesthesia. It is anticipated that most newborns with major congenital anomalies necessitating early surgical repair have not been enterally fed. If there is evidence of intestinal obstruction or ileus, the stomach should be decompressed with a nasogastric tube, preferably one with a vent. At least one secure intravenous catheter must be in place to allow ongoing resuscitation. If an umbilical venous catheter is in place, an assessment should be made preoperatively as to whether this must be removed to allow adequate intraabdominal exposure, in which case further access should be sought before surgery. An arterial catheter and a Foley catheter may be indicated for the critically ill neonate. Resuscitation should be undertaken in a thoughtful but rapid manner and should proceed until no further gain is anticipated from further delay in operative management.

INTRAOPERATIVE MANAGEMENT

Transporting a critically ill neonate from the delivery room or neonatal intensive care unit to the operating room can be hazardous. Part of the planning for surgery should be consideration of the safety of transporting the patient versus the safety and ability to complete the operation in the neonatal intensive care unit. With proper equipment and staff, the operating room environment can be safely brought to the neonate, with no apparently increased risk of airborne infection.[101,121] When transported, the neonate must be accompanied by the anesthesiologist and/or neonatologist and continuously monitored with electrocardiography and pulse oximetry.

During the course of surgery, continuous intraoperative monitoring is crucial, and equipment should always include an electrocardiographic monitor, a precordial or esophageal stethoscope, a blood pressure monitor, a temperature probe (preferably rectal or pharyngeal), a pulse oximeter, and an end-tidal CO_2 monitor for measurement of ventilation. Great care must be taken in applying and securing the neonate's airway and monitoring devices, because the patient will be completely covered by drapes and relatively inaccessible but the patient's condition may change rapidly during the course

of surgery. Additional monitoring options can include a urinary catheter, arterial access (usually an umbilical artery catheter), and central venous access (usually an umbilical vein catheter, which can be utilized for monitoring purposes). Serial measurements of serum hemoglobin/ hematocrit, electrolytes, glucose, calcium, and blood gases and coagulation studies are performed as needed. Care must be taken while the neonate is prepared for surgery that mechanisms are in place to maintain body heat throughout the procedure. Options include the use of heating blankets (with either circulating warm water or air); delivering warmed, humidified gases via the endotracheal tube; the use of warmed intravenous fluids and blood products; keeping the neonate completely covered other than at the operative site; and limiting exposure of the peritoneal cavity and viscera.

Intraoperative fluid administration is guided by the following factors[36]:

1. Preoperative fasting fluid deficit, which is the hours that the patient receives nothing by mouth multiplied by the maintenance hourly rate, unless the patient was receiving intravenous hydration during this time.
2. Preexisting fluid deficit caused by the underlying pathophysiology, if this has not been corrected before the surgery.
3. Standard maintenance fluid during the course of the surgery.
4. Third space losses during surgery, varying from 2 to 15 mL/kg/hour, depending on the extent of the operative procedure.
5. Blood loss replacements. The allowable blood loss as based on weight should be determined preoperatively and is generally 15% to 20% of estimated blood volume, guided by the patient's stability. Losses greater than this generally need replacement with packed red blood cell transfusions. One report suggested that autologous cord blood, harvested at the time of delivery, may represent an alternative donor source for infants who require major surgery shortly after birth.[122]

Adjustments in fluid administration must be made continuously according to the changing status of the patient. Glucose must be provided in the maintenance fluid to prevent intraoperative hypoglycemia, although care must be taken to avoid glucose in resuscitative fluids to avoid iatrogenic hyperglycemia.

POSTOPERATIVE CARE

Close monitoring is most essential during the immediate postanesthesia recovery period, because neonates are especially prone to respiratory and cardiovascular complications at this time. The risk of a critical event may even be higher immediately after surgery than during the operation itself, because the postoperative patient is resuming physiologic functions that were being controlled during anesthesia.[123]

At the conclusion of the operative procedure, a neonate can be extubated if he or she is awake and vigorous, well oxygenated, hemodynamically stable, and normothermic.

If critically ill, the neonate should remain intubated and ventilated until stabilized. Airway obstruction from relaxation of soft tissues, laryngospasm, subglottic edema, or secretions is a major postoperative hazard.[123] Apnea can occur, particularly in preterm and critically ill neonates, as a result of a decreased respiratory drive from anesthesia, endorphins, and narcotic pain medications.[124,125] In addition, attention must be directed to the neonate's body temperature, because hypothermia is a common complication secondary to surgery and transport.

When a neonate is extubated after an operation, oxygen should be administered as guided by pulse oximetry to prevent hypoxia. In one study, 43% of infants and children breathing room air after general anesthesia for even minor operative procedures had moderate to severe hypoxia temporarily.[126] It was not related to hypoventilation but probably resulted from a transient postoperative diminution in functional residual capacity with ventilation-perfusion imbalances and intrapulmonary shunting.

In addition to maintenance fluids, the postoperative neonate requires additional crystalloid volume and sodium to compensate for the third space shifts of fluid out of the intravascular space secondary to the trauma of the operative procedure. This volume cannot be measured directly and must therefore be approximated. One approach is to increase the intravenous infusion rate to 1.5 to 2 times the usual maintenance rate for the first 24 hours after surgery, depending on the magnitude of surgery. Filston and coworkers used a "quadrant" scheme for estimating internal fluid shifts after laparotomy.[127] An additional one fourth of the maintenance value is given as crystalloid for every quadrant of the abdomen involved with inflammatory or obstructive disease, and an additional one fourth is given for each quadrant significantly traumatized by the surgical procedure. For the critically ill neonate under continuous observation in the neonatal intensive care unit, it may be safest, in order to avoid hypovolemia or hypervolemia, to provide maintenance fluids and administer intermittent 10- to 20-mL/kg crystalloid boluses as indicated by heart rate, urinary output, and results of laboratory studies. Whatever initial approximation is used, adjustments must be made according to the response of the patient. Urine output should exceed 1.5 to 2.0 mL/kg/hour.

The most common cause of hypotension or oliguria in the postoperative period is hypovolemia secondary to inadequate resuscitation. This may not be associated with the anticipated findings of dehydration, and because of the third space accumulation of fluid, the neonate may even exhibit edema. This postoperative hypovolemia must be promptly recognized and corrected. The maintenance intravenous infusion rate can be increased, or a bolus of 10 to 20 mL of isotonic fluid per kilogram given. A favorable clinical response to a fluid challenge allows both diagnosis and treatment of this complication.

Nutrition must be started promptly as soon as possible after surgery. Parenteral nutrition can be administered when the infant has stabilized and can be supported on a maintenance intravenous rate. In most situations, enteral feedings should be instituted as soon as possible.

The safety of initiating enteral feedings is dependent on several factors, including the recovery of the gastrointestinal tract from surgery and anesthesia, hemodynamic stability of the neonate, ventilatory needs, and the presence or absence of umbilical artery catheters. For neonates recovering from gastrointestinal surgery, nasogastric tube decompression of the stomach may be required until there is a return of function. Evidence that gastrointestinal function has returned includes diminished output from the nasogastric tube, resolution of abdominal distention, and passage of flatus or stool. Many neonates recovering from gastroschisis repair or necrotizing enterocolitis encounter a prolonged period of intestinal dysmotility and require support with parenteral nutrition for days to weeks.

Early postoperative intestinal obstruction after intraabdominal surgery may result from edema at an anastomosis or fibrinous adhesions, and it often resolves with continued gastric decompression. Less commonly, postoperative obstruction in the neonate may result from intussusception, even if the operation was not intraabdominal. These intussusceptions are usually confined to the small bowel and necessitate surgical decompression.

LONG-TERM OUTCOME

There have been limited long-term studies on quality of life among children who have undergone major operations in the neonatal period, and the results are somewhat contradictory. The situation is further complicated by the fact that many of these infants were born prematurely and have or had other congenital anomalies; both scenarios can variably affect subsequent growth and development adversely.

Among infants with extremely low birth weight who underwent emergency laparotomy for necrotizing enterocolitis and were monitored over the following 7 years, there was a significantly higher incidence of neurodevelopmental impairment than in a group of matched premature controls.[128] Another study demonstrated that adolescents who had undergone major surgery as fullterm newborns experienced somewhat (but not statistically significantly) more health problems and performed more poorly academically than did their peers.[129] Other follow-up studies have shown that after neonatal surgery, physical growth was normal for age, if there were no residual or associated chronic disabilities that would be expected to impair growth, and patients who fully recovered within several months of surgery manifested no differences in intellectual function in comparison with normal, age-matched controls.[130-132] Children who experienced recurrent or chronic illness did have variable degrees of diminished cognitive performance, the severity of which was correlated with the number of operations and total length of hospitalization.

The initial opportunity to correct a surgical problem may be the best chance of doing so, and the avoidance of prolonged complications through meticulous treatment and attention to detail is most important for the longterm future of the neonate. Consideration should be given to alerting parents and teachers that these children may benefit from early educational and behavioral monitoring.[129] Studies have demonstrated that even with limitations, most adolescent survivors of neonatal surgical care have a high quality of life. Further long-term follow-up investigations are clearly needed.

ETHICAL CONSIDERATIONS

The improving capabilities of neonatology and neonatal surgery to resuscitate and support even the sickest and tiniest neonates increasingly raises ethical issues regarding appropriate care for these patients. Because short-term and long-term survival have increased in all gestational age and weight groups, neonatologists and pediatric surgeons have become increasingly aggressive in offering interventions. Unfortunately, especially for premature neonates, survival is still accompanied by a significant risk of physical, intellectual, or sensory impairment. Balancing these concerns is frequently the source of ethical deliberations in the neonatal intensive care unit. Neonates are clearly not autonomous patients, and in most circumstances, health care providers count on the parents to be appropriate surrogates for health care decisions. This often leaves parents in the difficult circumstance of needing to separate what is truly in the best interests of the neonate from their hopes and dreams of a healthy and intact infant and the individual that the infant would become. Health care providers need to work with parents to explore and balance beneficence (doing good) and nonmaleficence (doing no harm) in each individual patient's situation. The family must be educated about anticipated outcomes for their neonate in order for them to effectively take part in decision making. Conflicts occasionally arise, often with regard to anticipated long-term disability. Health care providers and parents may have different views of the predicted long-term quality of life in the affected neonate, inasmuch as they bear very different responsibilities for the child. When parents have acted as thoughtful and compassionate surrogates for their child, their decisions should usually be respected when there is disagreement with the care team. The circumstances for turning to the courts to override parental decision making should be extremely rare, and such action should be taken only when there will be a clear benefit for the child. On occasion, when there is serious disagreement between a member of the health care team and the family, transferring the patient to another willing care provider who is more comfortable with fulfilling a plan in accord with the family is in everyone's best interest. An honest, open, and factual communicative relationship with the neonate's family is the best means of ensuring optimal treatment for the child.

A potentially sensitive issue is whether do not resuscitate orders should be suspended during the perioperative period. Surgery under general anesthesia may be associated with bleeding as well as respiratory and cardiac depression, and measures that would otherwise be viewed as heroic resuscitative efforts are often required as routine support.[123] Open and frank discussions with the family must be held in advance of these situations.

REFERENCES

1. Coran AG, Drongowski RA: Body fluid compartment changes following neonatal surgery. J Pediatr Surg 24:829, 1989.
2. Krishna G, Emhardt JD: Anesthesia for the newborn and ex-preterm infant. Semin Pediatr Surg 1:32, 1992.
3. Rickham PP: The ethics of surgery in newborn infants. In Lister J, Irving IM (eds): Neonatal Surgery, 3rd ed. London, Butterworths, 1990, pp 3-10.
4. Simpson JS: Pediatric surgery: Old art and new science. Can J Surg 19:551, 1976.
5. Soper RT, Kimura K: Overview of neonatal surgery. Perinatol 16:1, 1989.
6. Gross RE, Ferguson CC: Surgery in premature babies: Observations from 159 cases. Surg Gynecl Obstet 95:631, 1952.
7. Rickham PP: The surgery of premature infants. Arch Dis Child 32:508, 1957.
8. O'Neill JA Jr, Holcomb GW Jr, Neblett WW III: Recent experience with esophageal atresia. Ann Surg 195:739, 1982.
9. Beasley SW, Myers NA: Trends in mortality in oesophageal atresia. Pediatr Surg Int 7:86, 1992.
10. Wise WE, Caniano DA, Harmel RP Jr: Tracheoesophageal anomalies in Waterston C neonates: A 30-year perspective. J Pediatr Surg 22:526, 1987.
11. Greenwood RD, Rosenthal A: Cardiovascular malformations associated with tracheoesophageal fistula and esophageal atresia. Pediatrics 57:87, 1976.
12. Zackai EH, Robin NH: Clinical genetics. In O'Neill JA Jr, Rowe MI, Grosfeld JL, et al (eds): Pediatric Surgery, 5th ed. St. Louis, CV Mosby, 1998, pp 19-31.
13. Owens JR: Incidence and causation of congenital defects. In Lister J, Irving JM (eds): Neonatal Surgery, 3rd ed. London, Butterworths, 1990, pp 11-17.
14. Lumley J, Watson L, Watson M, Bower C: Periconceptional supplementation with folate and/or multivitamins for preventing neural tube defects. Cochrane Database Syst Rev (3):CD001056, 2001.
15. Northrup H, Volick KA: Spina bifida and other neural tube defects. Curr Probl Pediatr 30:313, 2000.
16. Wald NJ, Law MR, Morris JK, Wald DS: Quantifying the effect of folic acid. Lancet 358:2069, 2001.
17. Knight PJ, Clatworthy HW Jr: Screening for latent malformations: Cost effectiveness in neonates with correctable anomalies. J Pediatr Surg 17:123, 1982.
18. Schmeling DJ, Coran AG: The hormonal and metabolic response to stress in the neonate. Pediatr Surg Int 5:307, 1990.
19. Anand KJS, Sippell WG, Aynsley-Green A: Randomised trial of fentanyl anaesthesia in preterm babies undergoing surgery: Effects on the stress response. Lancet 1:243, 1987.
20. Anand KJS, Sippell WG, Schofield NM, et al: Does halothane anaesthesia decrease the metabolic and endocrine stress responses of newborn infants undergoing operation? BMJ 296:668, 1988.
21. Boix-Ochoa J, Martinex Ibanez V, Potau N, et al: Cortisol response to surgical stress in neonates. Pediatr Surg Int 2:267, 1987.
22. Chuang JH, Lia JN, Lee JH, et al: Endorphin and cortisol responses to surgical stress in newborns and infants. Pediatr Surg Int 5:100, 1990.
23. Chwals WJ: Metabolic considerations. In O'Neill JA Jr, Rowe MI, Grosfeld JL, et al (eds): Pediatric Surgery, 5th ed. St. Louis, CV Mosby, 1998, pp 57-70.

24. Anand KJS, Brown MJ, Bloom SR, et al: Studies on the hormonal regulation of fuel metabolism in the human newborn infant undergoing anaesthesia and surgery. Horm Res 22:115, 1985.
25. Tsang TM, Tam PKH: Cytokine response of neonates to surgery. J Pediatr Surg 29:794, 1994.
26. Stang HJ, Gunnar MR, Snellman L, et al: Local anesthesia for neonatal circumcision. Effects on distress and cortisol response. JAMA 259:1507, 1988.
27. Crombleholme TM, D'Alton M, Cendron M, et al: Prenatal diagnosis and the pediatric surgeon: The impact of prenatal consultation on perinatal management. J Pediatr Surg 31:156, 1996.
28. Jones MO, Pierro A, Hammond P, et al: The metabolic response to operative stress in infants. J Pediatr Surg 28:1258, 1993.
29. Garza JJ, Shew SB, Keshen TH, et al: Energy expenditure in ill premature neonates. J Pediatr Surg 37:289, 2002.
30. Chwals WJ, Letton RW, Jamie A, et al: Stratification of injury severity using energy expenditure response in surgical infants. J Pediatr Surg 30:1161, 1995.
31. Jaksic T, Shew SB, Keshen TH, et al: Do critically ill surgical neonates have increased energy expenditure? J Pediatr Surg 36:63, 2001.
32. Powis MR, Smith K, Rennie M, et al: Effect of major abdominal operations on energy and protein metabolism in infants and children. J Pediatr Surg 33:49, 1998.
33. Tueting JL, Byerley LO, Chwals WJ: Anabolic recovery relative to degree of prematurity after acute injury in neonates. J Pediatr Surg 34:13, 1999.
34. Shew SB, Keshen TH, Glass NL, et al: Ligation of a patent ductus arteriosus under fentanyl anesthesia improves protein metabolism in premature neonates. J Pediatr Surg 35:1277, 2000.
35. Smith SD, Tagge EP, Hannakan C, et al: Characterization of neonatal multisystem organ failure in the surgical newborn. J Pediatr Surg 26:494, 1991.
36. Presson RG Jr, Hillier SC: Perioperative fluid and transfusion management. Semin Pediatr Surg 1:22, 1992.
37. Bikhazi GB, Davis JJ: Anesthesia for neonates and children. In Montoyama KH (ed): Smith's Anesthesia for Infants and Children. St. Louis, CV Mosby, 1990, pp 429-462.
38. Spaeth JP, O'Hara B, Kurth CD: Anesthesia for the micropremie. Semin Perinatol 22:390, 1998.
39. Booker PD, Bush GH: Neonatal physiology and its effect on pre- and postoperative management. In Lister J, Irving M (eds): Neonatal Surgery, 3rd ed. London, Butterworths, 1990, pp 18-27.
40. Krummel TM, Lloyd DA, Rowe MI: The postoperative response of the term and preterm newborn infant to sodium administration. J Pediatr Surg 20:803, 1985.
41. Gregory GA: Outcome of pediatric anesthesia. In Gregory GA (ed): Pediatric Anesthesia, 2nd ed. New York, Churchill Livingstone, 1989, pp 15-24.
42. Colle E, Paulsen EP: Response of the newborn infant to major surgery, I. Effects on water, electrolyte, and nitrogen balances. Pediatrics 23:1063, 1959.
43. Winthrop AL, Jones PJH, Schoeller DA, et al: Changes in the body composition of the surgical infant in the early postoperative period. J Pediatr Surg 22:546, 1987.
44. John EM, Klavdianu M, Vidyasagar D: Electrolyte problems in neonatal surgery patients. Clin Perinatol 16:219, 1989.
45. Raffensperger JG: Fluids and electrolyes. In Raffensperger JG (ed): Swenson's Pediatric Surgery, 5th ed. Norwalk, Conn, Appleton & Lange, 1990, pp 73-80.
46. Seashore JH, Touloukian RJ, Kopf GS: Major surgery in infants weighing less than 1,500 grams. Am J Surg 145:483, 1983.
47. Sukhani R: Anesthetic management of the newborn. Clin Perinatol 16:43, 1989.
48. Hackel A: Preoperative evaluation. In Gregory GA (ed): Pediatric Anesthesia, 2nd ed. New York, Churchill Livingstone, 1989, pp 501-521.
49. Puckett RM, Offrenga M: Prophylactic vitamin K for vitamin K deficiency bleeding in neonates. Cochrane Database Syst Rev (4):CD002776, 2000.
50. Suzuki S, Iwata G, Sutor AH: Vitamin K deficiency during the perinatal and infantile period. Semin Thromb Hemost 27:93, 2001.
51. Najmaldin A, Francis J, Postle A, et al: Vitamin K coagulation status in surgical newborns and the risk of bleeding. J Pediatr Surg 28:138, 1993.
52. Luck SR: Nutrition and metabolism. In Raffensperger JG (ed): Swenson's Pediatric Surgery, 5th ed. Norwalk, Conn, Appleton & Lange, 1990, pp 81-90.
53. Pereira GR, Ziegler MM: Nutritional care of the surgical neonate. Clin Perinatol 16:233, 1989.
54. Okada Y, Klein NJ, Pierro A: Neutrophil dysfunction: The cellular mechanism of impaired immunity during total parenteral nutrition in infancy. J Pediatr Surg 34:242, 1999.
55. Okada Y, Klein N, van Saene HKF, et al: Small volumes of enteral feedings normalise immune function in infants receiving parenteral nutrition. J Pediatr Surg 33:16, 1998.
56. Okada Y, Papp E, Klein NJ, et al: Total parenteral nutrition directly impairs cytokine production after bacterial challenge. J Pediatr Surg 34:277, 1999.
57. Taylor CJ, Walker J: Fluid and electrolyte management and nutritional support. In Lister J, Irving IM (eds): Neonatal Surgery, 3rd ed. London, Butterworths, 1990, pp 37-39.
58. Toce SS, Keenan WJ, Homan SM: Enteral feeding in very-low-birth-weight infants. Am J Dis Child 141:439, 1987.
59. Curet-Scott MJ, Meller JL, Shermeta DW: Transduodenal feedings: A superior route of enteral nutrition. J Pediatr Surg 22:516, 1987.
60. Coughlin JP, Gauderer MWL, Stellato TA: Percutaneous endoscopic gastrostomy in children under 1 year of age: Indications, complications, and outcome. Pediatr Surg Int 6:88, 1991.
61. Rowe MI, Rowe SA: The last fifty years of neonatal surgical management. Am J Surg 180:345, 2000.
62. Wesley JR, Coran AG: Intravenous nutrition for the pediatric patient. Semin Pediatr Surg 1:212, 1992.
63. Eichelberger MR, Rous PG, Hoelzer DJ, et al: Percutaneous subclavian venous catheters in neonates and children. J Pediatr Surg 16(Suppl 1):547, 1981.
64. Stephens BL, Lelli JL, Allen D, et al: Silastic catheterization of the axillary vein in neonates: An alternate to the internal jugular vein. J Pediatr Surg 28:31, 1993.
65. Lally KP, Hardin WD Jr, Boettcher M, et al: Broviac catheter insertion: Operating room or neonatal intensive care unit. J Pediatr Surg 22:823, 1987.
66. King DR, Komer M, Hoffman J, et al: Broviac catheter sepsis: The natural history of an iatrogenic infection. J Pediatr Surg 20:728, 1985.
67. Sadiq HG, Devaskar S, Keenan WJ, et al: Broviac catheterization in low birth weight infants: Incidence and treatment of associated complications. Crit Care Med 15:47, 1987.
68. Warner BW, Gorgone P, Schilling S, et al: Multiple purpose central venous access in infants less than 1,000 grams. J Pediatr Surg 22:820, 1987.
69. Jones GR, Konsler GK, Dunaway RP, et al: Prospective analysis of urokinase in the treatment of catheter sepsis in pediatric hematology-oncology patients. J Pediatr Surg 28:350, 1993.

70. Guzzetta PC, Randolph JC, Anderson KD, et al: Surgery of the neonate. In Avery B (ed): Neonatology: Pathophysiology and Management of the Newborn, 3rd ed. Philadelphia, JB Lippincott, 1987, pp 944-984.

71. Jacobs BR, Haygood M, Hingl J: Recombinant tissue plasminogen activator in the treatment of central venous catheter occlusion in children. J Pediatr Oct 139:593, 2001.

72. Leaker M, Andrew M, Massicoite P, et al: Safety and outcomes of thrombolysis with tissue plasminogen activator for treatment of intravascular thrombosis in children. J Pediatr 139:682, 2001.

73. Rimensberger PC, Humbert JR, Beghetti M: Management of preterm infants with intracardiac thrombi: Use of thrombolytic agents. Pediatr Drugs 3:883, 2001.

74. Statter MB: Peripheral and central venous access. Semin Pediatr Surg 1:1811, 1992.

75. Singer RL, Wolfson PJ: Experience with umbilical artery cutdowns in neonates. Pediatr Surg Int 5:295, 1990.

76. Ryan JF, Raines J, Dalton BC, et al: Arterial dynamics of radial artery cannulation. Anesth Analg 52:1017, 1973.

77. Bull MJ, Schreiner RL, Garg BP, et al: Neurologic complications following temporal artery catheterization. J Pediatr 96:1071, 1980.

78. Cilley RE: Arterial access in infants and children. Semin Pediatr Surg 1:174, 1992.

79. Mellor DJ, Lerman J: Anesthesia for neonatal surgical emergencies. Semin Perinatol 22:363, 1998.

80. Sartorelli KH, Abajian JC, Kreutz JM, et al: Improved outcome utilizing spinal anesthesia in high-risk infants. J Pediatr Surg 27:1022, 1992.

81. Smith SD, Rowe MI: Physiology of the patient. In Ashcraft KW, Holder TM (eds): Pediatric Surgery, 2nd ed. Philadelphia, WB Saunders, 1993, pp 1-18.

82. Okada Y, Powis M, McEwan A, et al: Fentanyl analgesia increases the incidence of postoperative hypothermia in neonates. Pediatr Surg Int 13:508, 1998.

83. Zamparelli M, Eaton S, Quant PA, et al: Analgesic doses of fentanyl impair oxidative metabolism of neonatal hepatocytes. J Pediatr Surg 34:260, 1999.

84. Porter FL, Wolf CM, Gold J, et al: Pain and pain management in newborn infants: A survey of physicians and nurses. Pediatrics 100:626, 1997.

85. Steward DJ: History of pediatric anesthesia. In Gregory GA (ed): Pediatric Anesthesia, 2nd ed. New York, Churchill Livingstone, 1989, pp 1-14.

86. Anand KJS, Phil D, Hickey PR: Pain and it effects in the human neonate and fetus. N Engl J Med 317:1321, 1987.

87. Truog R, Anand KJS: Management of pain in the postoperative neonate. Clin Perinatol 16:61, 1989.

88. Larsson BA: Pain management in neonates. Acta Paediatr 88:1301, 1999.

89. Menon G, Angand KJ, McIntosh N: Practical approach to analgesia and sedation in the neonatal intensive care unit. Semin Perinatol 22:417, 1998.

90. Vaughn PR, Townsend SF, Thilo EH, et al: Comparison of continuous infusion of fentanyl to bolus dosing in neonates after surgery. J Pediatr Surg 31:1616, 1996.

91. Dilworth NM, MacKellar A: Pain relief for the pediatric surgical patient. J Pediatr Surg 22:264, 1987.

92. McCaffery M: Pain relief for the child. Pediatr Nurs 3:11, 1977.

93. Puri P, Lee A, Reen DJ: Differential susceptibility of neonatal lymphocytes to the immunosuppressive effects of anaesthesia and surgery. Pediatr Surg Int 7:47, 1992.

94. Lassiter HA: The role of immunodeficiency in the development of postoperative bacterial sepsis and wound infections in neonates. Pediatr Surg Int 9:474, 1994.

95. Hill HR: Host defenses in the neonate: Prospects for enhancement. Semin Perinatol 9:2, 1985.

96. Siegel J: Controlling infections in the nursery. Pediatr Infect Dis 85:S36, 1985.

97. Merry C, Puri P, Reen DJ: Defective neutrophil actin polymerisation and chemotaxis in stressed newborns. J Pediatr Surg 31:481, 1996.

98. Sharma LK, Sharma PK: Postoperative wound infection in a pediatric surgical service. J Pediatr Surg 21:889, 1986.

99. Davenport M, Doig CM: Wound infections in pediatric surgery: A study in 1094 neonates. J Pediatr Surg 28:26, 1993.

100. Cruse PJE, Ford R: The epidemiology of wound infection. Surg Clin North Am 60:27, 1980.

101. Horwitz JR, Chwals WJ, Doski JJ, et al: Pediatric wound infections: A prospective multicenter study. Ann Surg 277:553, 1998.

102. Knight R, Charbonneau P, Ratzer E, et al: Prophylactic antibiotics are not indicated in clean general surgery cases. Am J Surg 182:682, 2001.

103. Davis AT: Postoperative infections in surgical patients. In Raffensperger JG (ed): Swenson's Pediatric Surgery, 5th ed. Norwalk, Conn, Appleton & Lange, 1990, pp 29-36.

104. Fallat ME, Mitchell KA: Random practice patterns of surgical antimicrobial prophylaxis in neonates. Pediatr Surg Int 9:479, 1994.

105. Hart CA: Neonatal infections and antibiotics. In Lister J, Irving JM (eds): Neonatal Surgery, 3rd ed. London, Butterworths, 1990, pp 89-100.

106. Behrman RE, Shiono PH: Neonatal risk factors in neonatal-perinatal medicine. In Fanaroff AA, Martin RJ (eds): Disease of the Fetus and Infant, 6th ed. St. Louis, Mosby–Year Book, 1997, pp 3-11.

107. Fonkalsrud EW, Ogawa H, Clatworthy HW: The surgery of premature infants. Surgery 58:550, 1965.

108. Molek KA, Gingalewski CA, West KW, et al: Gastroschisis: A plea for risk categorization. J Pediatr Surg 36:51, 2001.

109. Snyder CL: Outcome analysis for gastroschisis. J Pediatr Surg 34:1253, 1999.

110. Stoll C, Alembik Y, Dott B, Roth MP: Risk factors in congenital abdominal wall defects (omphalocele and gastroschisis): A study in a series of 265,858 consecutive births. Ann Genet 44:201, 2001.

111. Chan A, Robertson EF, Hoan EA, et al: The sensitivity of ultrasound and serum alpha-fetoprotein in population-based antenatal screening for neural tube defects, South Australia 1986-1991. Br J Obstet Gynaecol 102:380, 1995.

112. Reichler A, Hume RF Jr, Drugan A, et al: Risk of anomalies as a function of level of elevated maternal serum alpha-fetoprotein. Am J Obst Gynecol 171:1052, 1994.

113. Zarzour SJ, Gabert HA, Diket AL, et al: Abnormal maternal serum alpha-fetoprotein and pregnancy outcome. J Matern Fetal Med 7:304, 1998.

114. Brackley KJ, Kilby MD, Wright JG, et al: Outcome after prenatal diagnosis of hypoplastic left-heart syndrome: A case series. Lancet 356:1143, 2000.

115. Bull C: Current and potential impact of fetal diagnosis on prevalence and spectrum of serious congenital heart disease at term in the UK. British Paediatric Cardiac Association. Lancet 354:1242, 1999.

116. Hirose S, Farmer DL, Albanese CT: Fetal surgery for myelomeningocele. Curr Opin Obst Gynecol 13:215, 2001.

117. Nixon H, O'Donnell B: The Essentials of Paediatric Surgery, 4th ed. Oxford, Butterworth-Heinemann, 1992.

118. Tulipan N, Bruner JP, Hernanz-Schulman M, et al: Effect of intrauterine myelomeningocele repair on central

nervous system structure and function. Pediatr Neurosurg 31:183, 1999.

119. Walsh DS, Adzick NS: Fetal surgical intervention. Am J Perinatol 17:277, 2000.

120. Betts EK, Downes JJ: Anesthesia. In Welch KJ, Randolph JG, Ravitch MM, et al (eds): Pediatric Surgery, 4th ed. Chicago, Year Book Medical, 1986, pp 50-67.

121. Fanning NF, Casey W, Corbally MT: In-situ emergency paediatric surgery in the intensive care unit. Pediatr Surg Int 13:587, 1998.

122. Imura K, Kawahara H, Kitayama Y, et al: Usefulness of cord-blood harvesting for autologous transfusion in surgical newborns with antenatal diagnosis of congenital anomalies. J Pediatr Surg 36:851, 2001.

123. Bryant LD, Dierdorf SF: Postanesthesia recovery. Semin Pediatr Surg 1:45, 1992.

124. Kurth CD, Spitzer AR, Broennle AM, et al: Postoperative apnea in preterm infants. Anesthesiology 66:483, 1987.

125. Welborn LG, Ramirez N, Oh TH, et al: Evaluation of anesthetic risks in premature infants. Anesthesiology 61:A417, 1984.

126. Montoyama EK, Glazener CH: Hypoxemia after general anesthesia in children. Anesth Analg 65:267, 1986.

127. Filston HC, Edwards CH III, Chitwood WR Jr, et al: Estimation of postoperative fluid requirements in infants and children. Ann Surg 196:76, 1982.

128. Chacko J, Ford WDA, Haslam R: Growth and neurodevelopmental outcome in extremely-low-birth-weight infants after laparotomy. Pediatr Surg Int 15:496, 1999.

129. Ludman L, Spitz L, Wade A: Educational attainments in early adolescence of infants who required major neonatal surgery. J Pediatr Surg 36:858, 2001.

130. Gutierrez-Sanroman C, Vila-Carbo JJ, Segarra-Llido V, et al: Long-term nutritional evaluation of 70 patients operated on for esophageal atresia. Pediatr Surg Int 3:123, 1988.

131. Kato T, Kanto K, Yoshino H, et al: Mental and intellectual development of neonatal surgical children in a long-term follow-up. J Pediatr Surg 28:123, 1993.

132. Ludman L, Spitz L, Lansdown R: Intellectual development at 3 years of age of children who underwent major neonatal surgery. J Pediatr Surg 28:130, 1993.

133. Harper RC, Garcia A, Sia C: Inguinal hernia: A common problem of premature infants weighing 1000 grams or less at birth. Pediatrics 56:112, 1975.

134. Knox G: The incidence of inginal hernia in Newcastle children. Arch Dis Child 34:482, 1959.

135. Tam PKH: Inguinal hernia. In Lister J, Irving IM (eds): Neonatal Surgery, 3rd ed. London, Butterworths, 1990, pp 367-377.

136. Campbell JR: Undescended testes. In Ashcraft KW, Holder TM (eds): Pediatric Surgery, 2nd ed. Philadelphia, WB Saunders, 1993, pp 588-594.

137. Hutson JM: Undescended testis, torsion, and varicocele. In O'Neill JA Jr, Rowe MI, Grosfeld JL, et al (eds): Pediatric Surgery, 5th ed. St. Louis, CV Mosby, 1998, pp 1087-1109.

138. Duckett JW, Baskin LS: Hypospadias. In O'Neill JA Jr, Rowe MI, Grosfeld JL, et al (eds): Pediatric Surgery, 5th ed. St. Louis, CV Mosby, 1998, pp 1761-1781.

139. Cudmore RE: Oesoophageal atresia and tracheooesophageal fistula. In Lister J, Irving JM (eds): Neonatal Surgery, 3rd ed. London, Butterworths, 1990, pp 231-258.

140. Sadove MA, Eppley BA: Cleft lip and palate. In O'Neill JA Jr, Rowe MI, Grosfeld JL, et al (eds): Pediatric Surgery, 5th ed. St. Louis, CV Mosby, 1998, pp 693-700.

141. Grosfeld JL: Jejunoilial atresia and stenosis. In Welch KJ, Randolph JG, Ravitch MM, et al (eds): Pediatric Surgery, 4th ed. Chicago, Year Book Medical, 1986, pp 838-848.

142. Lister J: Intestinal atresia and stenosis, excluding the duodenum. In Lister J, Irving JM (eds): Neonatal Surgery, 3rd ed. London, Butterworths, 1990, pp 453-473.

143. Irving IM, Booker PD: Congenital diaphragmatic hernia and eventration of the diaphragm. In Lister J, Irving JM (eds): Neonatal Surgery, 3rd ed. London, Butterworths, 1990, pp 199-220.

144. Puri P, Gorman F: Lethal nonpulmonary anomalies associated with congenital diaphragmatic hernia: Implications for early intrauterine surgery. J Pediatr Surg 19:29, 1984.

145. Stolar CJH, Dillon PW: Congenital diaphragmatic hernia and eventration. In O'Neill JA Jr, Rowe MI, Grosfeld JL, et al (eds): Pediatric Surgery, 5th ed. St. Louis, CV Mosby, 1998, pp 819-837.

146. Cudmore RE, Tam PKH: Hydrocephalus. In Lister J, Irving JM (eds): Neonatal Surgery, 3rd ed. London, Butterworths, 1990, pp 589-612.

147. Harmon CM, Coran AG: Congenital anomalies of the esophagus. In O'Neill JA Jr, Rowe MI, Grosfeld JL, et al (eds): Pediatric Surgery, 5th ed. St. Louis, CV Mosby, 1998, pp 941-967.

148. Raffensperger JG: Esophageal atresia and tracheoesophageal stenosis. In Raffensperger JG (ed): Swenson's Pediatric Surgery, 5th ed. Norwalk, Conn, Appleton & Lange, 1990, pp 697-718.

149. Cooney DR: Defects of the abdominal wall. In O'Neill JA Jr, Rowe MI, Grosfeld JL, et al (eds): Pediatric Surgery, 5th ed. St. Louis, CV Mosby, 1998, pp 1045-1069.

150. Mahour GH: Omphalocele. Surg Gynecol Obstet 143:821, 1976.

151. Tunnell WP: Omphalocele and gastroschisis. In Ashcraft KW, Holder TM (eds): Pediatric Surgery, 2nd ed. Philadelphia, WB Saunders, 1993, pp 546-556.

152. Kiely EM, Pena A: Anorectal malformations. In O'Neill JA Jr, Rowe MI, Grosfeld JL, et al (eds): Pediatric Surgery, 5th ed. St. Louis, CV Mosby, 1998, pp 1425-1448.

153. Lister J, Tam PKH: Hirschsprung's disease. In Lister J, Irving JM (eds): Neonatal Surgery, 3rd ed. London, Butterworths, 1990, pp 53-546.

154. Swenson O, Raffensperger JG: Hirschsprung's disease. In Raffensperger JG (ed): Swenson's Pediatric Surgery, 5th ed. Norwalk, Conn, Appleton & Lange, 1990, pp 555-578.

155. Irving IM: Duodenal atresia and stenosis: Annular pancreas. In Lister J, Irving JM (eds): Neonatal Surgery, 3rd ed. London, Butterworths, 1990, pp 424-441.

156. Stauffer UG, Schwoebel M: Duodenal atresia and stenosis—annular pancreas. In O'Neill JA Jr, Rowe MI, Grosfeld JL, et al (eds): Pediatric Surgery, 5th ed. St. Louis, CV Mosby, 1998, pp 1133-1143.

157. Cook RCM: Intraluminal intestinal obtrction. In Lister J, Irving JM (eds): Neonatal Surgery, 3rd ed. London, Butterworths, 1990, pp 511-522.

158. Rescorla FJ: Meconium ileus. In O'Neill JA Jr, Rowe MI, Grosfeld JL, et al (eds): Pediatric Surgery, 5th ed. St. Louis, CV Mosby, 1998, pp 1159-1171.

159. Bush PG, Williams AJ: The incidence of the Robin anomalad (Pierre Robin syndrome). Br J Plastic Surg 36:434, 1983.

160. Cook RCM: The liver and biliary tract. In Lister J, Irving JM (eds): Neonatal Surgery, 3rd ed. London, Butterworths, 1990, pp 571-586.

161. Karrer FM, Lilly JR, Hall RJ: Biliary tract disorders and portal hypertension. In Ashcraft KW, Holder TM (eds): Pediatric Surgery, 2nd ed. Philadelphia, WB Saunders, 1993.

162. Karrer FM, Raffensperger JG: Biliary atresia. In Raffensperger JG (ed): Swenson's Pediatric Surgery, 5th ed. Norwalk, Conn, Appleton & Lange, 1990, pp 649-660.

163. Brock JW, O'Neill JA Jr: Bladder exstrophy. In O'Neill JA Jr, Rowe MI, Grosfeld JL, et al (eds): Pediatric Surgery, 5th ed. St. Louis, CV Mosby, 1998, pp 1709-1759.

164. Warner BW, Ziegler MM: Exstrophy of the cloaca. In Ashcraft KW, Holder TM (eds): Pediatric Surgery, 2nd ed. Philadelphia, WB Saunders, 1993, pp 393-401.

165. Oldham KT: Atresia, stenosis, and other obstructions of the colon. In O'Neill JA Jr, Rowe MI, Grosfeld JL, et al (eds): Pediatric Surgery, 5th ed. St. Louis, CV Mosby, 1998, pp 1361-1368.

166. Rickwood AMK: Congenital deficiency of the abdominal musculature: The prune-belly syndrome. In Lister J, Irving IM (eds): Neonatal Surgery, 3rd ed. London, Butterworths, 1990, pp 692-697.

167. Marchildon MB: Meconium peritonitis and spontaneous gastric perforation. Clin Perinatol 5:79, 1978.

168. Martin LW: Meconium peritonitis. In Ravitch MM, Welch KJ, Benson CD, et al (eds): Pediatric Surgery, 3rd ed. Chicago, Year Book Medical, 1979, pp 952-955.

169. Irving IM: Sacrococcygeal teratoma. In Lister J, Irving JM (eds): Neonatal Surgery, 3rd ed. London, Butterworths, 1990, pp 142-152.

170. Schnaufer L: Conjoined twins. In Raffensperger JG (ed): Swenson's Pediatric Surgery, 5th ed. Norwalk, Conn, Appleton & Lange, 1990, pp 969-978.

171. Stauffer UG: Conjoined twins. In Lister J, Irving IM (eds): Neonatal Surgery, 3rd ed. London, Butterworths, 1990, pp 153-162.

CHAPTER 87

Common Urologic Problems in the Fetus and Neonate

Alfred P. Kennedy, Jr., and T. Ernesto Figueroa

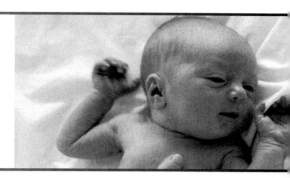

Fetal and neonatal urologic conditions are relatively rare, but with the increasing use of fetal sonography, more patients are being identified in utero as potentially having a urologic abnormality. Likewise, as experience with fetal sonography continues to be refined, other, more subtle abnormalities of the kidneys, bladder, and genitalia are being detected with increasing frequency. Identification of these patients has created a new field of **perinatal urology,** and understanding of the pathophysiology of urinary tract dilation continues to evolve. The detection of fetal abnormalities has allowed perinatal specialists to manage and correct many conditions, which, if left untreated, may have progressed to renal deterioration, although other patients undoubtedly may have undergone unnecessary postnatal assessment for a perinatally detected condition. Sonographically evident dilation of the urinary tract, or **hydronephrosis,** can be detected in approximately 1% of pregnancies. Despite the relative paucity of urologic abnormalities, prenatal or early postnatal recognition may be crucial to the patient. The identification of bilateral hydronephrosis and a distended bladder in a male fetus may suggest the presence of a serious condition, such as posterior urethral valves, or it may represent benign and transient hydronephrosis and inconsequential bladder distention. Similarly, an infant born with undescended testes may have bilateral "vanished" testes and anorchia secondary to in utero torsion. The correct diagnosis in all of these cases is essential. This chapter outlines and reviews the most common perinatal urologic abnormalities and offers guidance to the clinician caring for neonates on how to manage these rare, but important problems.

HYDRONEPHROSIS

Hydronephrosis, or dilation of the collecting system, is the most common anomaly of the genitourinary system identified prenatally. With the widespread use of sonography during pregnancy, the detection of fetal hydronephrosis has increased. Fluid-filled masses, such as a dilated renal pelvis, a dilated ureter, or a distended bladder, are particularly well imaged by sonography, which depends on the difference in tissue density to outline anatomic detail. Urinary tract dilation is reported in 1 of 100 pregnancies assessed sonographically, whereas surgically significant uropathy occurs in only 1 of 500 pregnancies.[1] Hydronephrosis is not synonymous with obstruction, and there is ongoing debate as to the cause of dilation of the urinary tract in the absence of obstruction. Obstructive hydronephrosis does not progress in all cases, reaching a state of equilibrium in some and resolving completely in others.[2] More importantly, hydronephrosis is not to be considered a diagnosis, but a sonographic finding, demanding further evaluation to define the cause of this abnormality. On identifying hydronephrosis, several features correlate with the severity of the hydronephrosis and the likelihood of an obstructive cause for the dilation of the urinary tract. Some of these features include degree of dilation of the urinary tract (pyelectasis or caliectasis), renal parenchymal thinning, increased parenchymal echogenicity, presence of renal cortical cysts, ureteral dilation, bladder distention, identification early in pregnancy, and oligohydramnios.

Differential Diagnosis

The differential diagnosis of fetal hydronephrosis includes **ureteropelvic junction (UPJ)** obstruction, **multicystic dysplastic kidney (MCDK)**, **vesicoureteral reflux (VUR)**, extrarenal pelvis, transient hydronephrosis, and ureteral obstruction (megaureters). When the bladder is persistently distended in addition to the presence of hydronephrosis, the differential diagnosis includes posterior urethral valves, prune-belly syndrome, megacystic-megaureter syndrome, bilateral gross VUR, urethral atresia, and neurogenic bladder. Some of these conditions are relatively benign, whereas posterior urethral valves, urethral atresia, prune-belly syndrome, and bilateral renal involvement all carry significantly more serious prognoses. Other associated sonographic findings, such as oligohydramnios, bladder wall thickening, parenchymal echogenicity, and renal cortical cysts, correlate with the likelihood of a more severe obstructive condition. These conditions all share some nonspecific findings of urinary tract dilation, but the precise diagnosis of any of these conditions is not always possible based on fetal sonographic findings alone. Differentiating these conditions based on sonographic appearance alone is not essential, and the finding should be considered the discovery of a condition that needs further assessment. In this sense, sonography of the fetal urinary tract can be characterized as being highly sensitive (detection of dilation), but poorly specific (differentiation of various causes).

Prenatal Consultation

The detection of a fetal urinary abnormality often leads to the referral of the expectant mother to a pediatric urologist for discussions about the management of the condition. These discussions always must involve information gathered from prenatal screening (level II ultrasound scans), overall assessment of the fetus, and family history of renal or urinary tract anomalies. As expected, there is always much anxiety associated with the detection of a fetal abnormality, and the pediatric urologist can be valuable to family members by educating and presenting a plan of action to them. Illustrating the urinary tract to the family, outlining the various possibilities, proposing a course of investigation after delivery, and discussing the role of antibiotic prophylaxis all are essential components of this consultation. A copy of the report of this consultation should be sent to the referring fetal medicine specialist, the parents, and their prospective pediatrician. The parents should take their copy with them to the hospital at the time of delivery so that the information can be shared with the caregivers after delivery. This practice minimizes some of the confusion that commonly occurs when the neonate's caregivers become aware of the history of prenatal "hydronephrosis."

Most conditions detected in utero can be monitored through the rest of the pregnancy, with the expectation of delivery at or near term. A basic premise in advising these families is that the health of the fetus and mother should never be compromised to "salvage" a kidney. The desire to intervene early in pregnancy or to deliver the infant prematurely must be tempered by the recognition that the benefits of fetal intervention are uncertain, and early delivery may jeopardize an otherwise healthy neonate. Fetal intervention by percutaneous decompression of the urinary tract (vesicoamniotic shunting) is best reserved for cases in which the life of the fetus is at risk from isolated urinary tract obstruction, as in the case of severe oligohydramnios secondary to presumed bladder outlet obstruction or posterior urethral valves. The roles of fetoscopy and endoscopic valve ablation in the fetus have not yet been defined, and these techniques at present still must be considered experimental. The inclination to deliver prematurely so that the urologist takes over the care of the patient is often imprudent, and the decision should be based on the overall fetal development and condition.

Many patients referred to the urologist have what is termed **pyelectasis**. This condition refers to a minimal degree of hydronephrosis, 4 to 6 mm in the anteroposterior diameter of the renal pelvis at term, without associated caliectasis or ureterectasis. These patients present an interesting dilemma because the minimal findings often raise the question about the need for postnatal use of antibiotics or the need for postnatal assessment. In our experience and the reported literature, 30% of these patients are found to have VUR by routine postnatal assessment.[3] Because prenatal sonography is not accurate in defining the presence of reflux, it has been our position that postnatal assessment of these patients with minimal hydronephrosis to exclude reflux is warranted, although admittedly the routine use of voiding cystourethrogram (VCUG) in the postnatal evaluation of hydronephrosis is controversial.

Postnatal Management

As mentioned previously, the detection of hydronephrosis by sonography is nonspecific, and precise definition of the cause of hydronephrosis is achieved only by postnatal evaluation. There are essentially three components of the postnatal management: (1) the use of antibiotic prophylaxis, (2) assessment of renal function (serum creatinine and carbon dioxide), and (3) organ imaging. When hydronephrosis has been detected prenatally, the caregivers of the infant are advised to start the infant on a prophylactic dose of amoxicillin (10 mg/kg/day) before discharge from the hospital. The search for obstruction begins with postnatal ultrasound of the kidneys and the bladder. Because of the relative neonatal dehydration present for the first 2 days of life, potentially leading to a false-negative initial sonogram, this study should be delayed, unless bladder outlet obstruction (posterior urethral valves or ectopic ureterocele) or bilateral involvement is suspected. After 14 days of life, while the infant remains on antibiotic prophylaxis, a renal and bladder ultrasound and a VCUG are obtained. The VCUG not only documents VUR as a source of the hydronephrosis, but also identifies secondary sources of hydronephrosis, such as posterior urethral valves, obstructing ureteroceles, megaureters, and anterior urethral valves (Fig. 87-1).

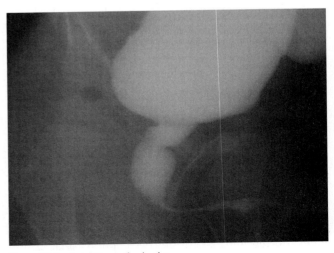

Figure 87–1. Anterior urethral valve.

Based on the findings of the VCUG, antibiotic prophylaxis can be discontinued.

In cases in which posterior urethral valves are suspected by prenatal evaluation, the initial postnatal evaluation should be completed in the perinatal period, either at the obstetric hospital before discharge or after transferring the newborn to a children's hospital. These infants may be critically ill, with pulmonary and renal compromise, and care in an intensive care unit is imperative. The pulmonary compromise relates to the degree of oligohydramnios and prematurity. These infants can be recognized on physical examination, with the appearance of a small chest, labored breathing, and distended abdomen secondary to a distended bladder. Occasionally, urinary extravasation producing perirenal urinomas or ascites may complicate the initial presentation (Figs. 87-2 through 87-4). The initial management consists of inserting a nonballoon catheter or feeding tube, 5-Fr or 8-Fr in size, to drain the bladder. On draining the bladder, the thickened and chronically distended bladder contracts, and it may remain palpable as an indurated mass in the pelvis. The catheter is secured in place until a VCUG is done. In the meantime, serial measurement of the patient's creatinine allows the clinician to estimate renal function. If the VCUG confirms the presence of obstructive valves, this condition is managed in the neonatal period preferentially by endoscopic ablation of the valves (Fig. 87-5). In cases in which the infant is too small to allow endoscopic transurethral manipulation of the valves, a cutaneous vesicostomy can be done as a temporary urinary diversion. Rarely, if ever, is an upper tract diversion (ureterostomy or pyelostomy) indicated in the management of these patients. Patients who are considered for these procedures often have significantly impaired renal function and dysplasia so that an elaborate upper tract procedure is unlikely to improve renal function, and it may make the management of the bladder in later years far more challenging. The resolution or improvement of the hydronephrosis after successful valve ablation is not predictable, and other effects of the bladder neck obstruction may perpetuate the appearance

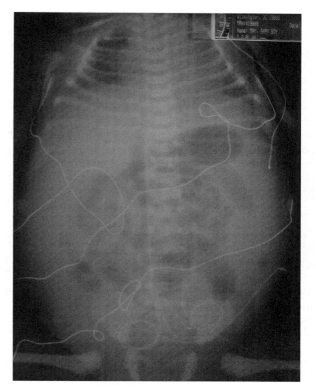

Figure 87–3. Urinary ascites.

of hydronephrosis in these patients (poorly compliant and hyperreflexic bladder, VUR, polyuria secondary to poor renal concentrating ability). The success of the valve ablation should be confirmed with a postoperative VCUG.

When the routine postnatal evaluation shows moderate-to-severe hydronephrosis, the degree of obstruction can be estimated by diuretic nuclear renography, which usually is performed at approximately 4 to 6 weeks of life (Fig. 87-6). Despite this test being the most widely used

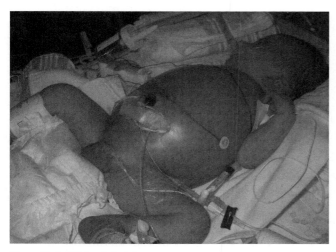

Figure 87–2. Distended abdomen.

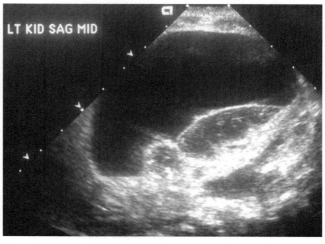

Figure 87–4. Urinoma.

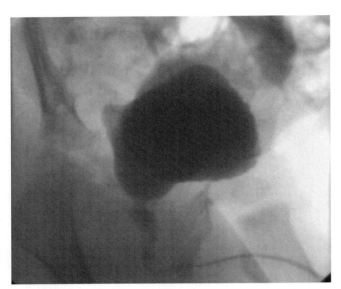

Figure 87–5. Voiding cystourethrogram in a patient with posterior urethral valves.

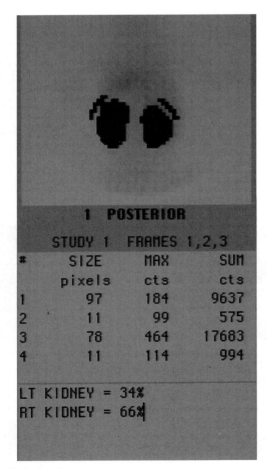

Figure 87–6. Renal scan.

and informative technique for evaluating differential function and drainage, significant variability exists in the interpretation of this and other standard diagnostic studies.[4-7] The technique of the study should include certain standard steps to minimize the many variables that can affect the result of the study and lead to the incorrect diagnosis of obstruction. Some of these steps include the use of the radiopharmaceutical technetium-99m mercaptoacetyltriglycine (Tc 99m MAG3), from which renal clearance occurs through excretion through the proximal tubule.[6] It is crucial that the patient is well hydrated, with continuous bladder drainage via a catheter. Furosemide is administered (1 mg/kg) to determine the drainage ability of the affected kidney. Normally, half the radiopharmaceutical should drain within 10 minutes of injection. A delay of more than 20 minutes in drainage is considered to represent significant obstruction. These studies are not fundamental for the diagnosis of obstruction, and the interpretation of the study must take into account the possible variables and pitfalls associated with the study. Hydration, the timing of the administration of the diuretic agent, bladder drainage, and the selected nuclear region of interest all influence the result of the study. Another pitfall, the "reservoir effect," which occurs in a severely dilated renal pelvis, may result in a workup being equivocal for obstruction. A single test may not be adequate to diagnose a definitive obstruction requiring operative intervention.[7] Occasionally, serial reevaluations with sonography and diuretic nuclear renography and rarely with invasive percutaneous pressure flow studies may be necessary when the diagnosis of obstruction remains elusive.[8]

The most common site of obstruction causing hydronephrosis is the UPJ. Failure of the ureteral lumen to recanalize after a solid stage during embryogenesis has been postulated as the cause of UPJ obstructions.[9] Other intrinsic causes of UPJ obstruction are ureteral valves and polyps, and extrinsic causes are crossing lower pole (aberrant) vessels and sequential displacement and angulation of the UPJ by intermittent chronic dilation and decompression.[10] Secondary causes of UPJ obstruction include high-grade VUR, necessitating close scrutiny of the upper tracts during VCUG (Fig. 87-7). A distended, but less opaque, renal pelvis in cases of high-grade reflux should prompt the clinician to exclude a coexisting UPJ obstruction in high-grade reflux. In these cases, a sonographic finding of disproportionately significant dilation of the renal pelvis compared with ureteral dilation is indicative of UPJ obstruction. Significant UPJ obstruction can be found in 37% of ectopic kidneys.[11] Other secondary causes of UPJ obstruction include compression secondary to an abdominal mass. Clinically, most of these cases are silent or "asymptomatic" and are worked up during the postnatal evaluation of an antenatally detected hydronephrosis. In other cases, however, UPJ obstruction can present as a palpable abdominal mass, feeding difficulties, or urinary tract infections or in association with other congenital anomalies, including the **VACTERL** association (i.e., *v*ertebral, *a*nal, *c*ardiac, *t*racheal, *e*sophageal, *r*enal, *l*imb).

Because ongoing obstruction is detrimental to renal development and function, the determination of significant

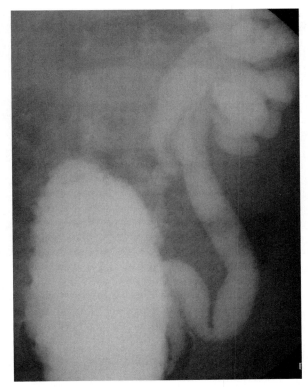

Figure 87–7. Voiding cystourethrogram showing reflux and possible ureteropelvic junction obstruction.

obstruction calls for prompt surgical intervention. In infants, the procedure of choice is dismembered pyeloplasty. Laparoscopic and endoscopic repairs of UPJ obstruction in infants are possible but require significant skill, and these techniques have not been shown to be superior to open repairs in infants. The results of pyeloplasty, even when performed in premature infants, are excellent. Long-term success rates greater than 95% are reported.[12]

INTRAABDOMINAL MASS

A palpable abdominal mass in the neonate always warrants additional investigation, which is usually initiated with abdominal ultrasound.[13] Many of these masses can be well imaged by sonography because of the prevalence of cystic or fluid-filled areas. Nearly two thirds of abdominal masses that present in the neonatal period arise from the genitourinary system. Within the first 48 hours of life, the most common cause of a palpable abdominal mass is MCDK. Beyond this time frame, the mass is more likely to be a hydronephrotic kidney.[14] Most of these masses currently are identified with prenatal sonography. Sonographic findings that enable the clinician to distinguish between hydronephrosis and MCDK include the presence of a central, larger "cyst" in hydronephrosis (renal pelvis), lack of communication between the cysts in MCDK, and disorganized arrangements of various-sized cysts in MCDK. The detection of hydronephrosis or MCDK calls for further evaluation, including a VCUG as

previously discussed. When a solid lesion is identified, further imaging with a computed tomography (CT) scan with oral and intravenous contrast media is necessary. Masses with sources outside the genitourinary system are discussed elsewhere.

MULTICYSTIC DYSPLASTIC KIDNEY

MCDK is the most frequently diagnosed cystic renal disease of newborns. With the left side being more commonly affected, the etiology of this disease probably is related to in utero ureteral atresia and severe obstruction.[15] Timing and severity of the obstruction contribute to the deterioration of the renal blastema into a nonfunctional dysplastic tissue. In the fetal lamb model, complete ureteral obstruction that is created before 70 days' gestation causes renal dysplasia, whereas obstruction created later on produces hydronephrosis.[15,16] Before the advent of prenatal ultrasound, the MCDK was diagnosed most commonly in the newborn period as an abdominal mass, being responsible for most of such masses palpated in this time period. Currently, prenatal ultrasound is the usual method of detection. The diagnosis must be distinguished mainly from unilateral hydronephrosis. The characteristic sonographic features of MCDK include an interface between cysts, a nonmedial location of the larger cysts, and an absence of the renal sinus.[17] The sonographic appearance is not always diagnostic, however, and further imaging with nuclear renography is necessary. By definition, a dysplastic kidney lacks function, so nonvisualization of the affected kidney with nuclear scintigraphy (dimercaptosuccinic acid) is diagnostic of MCDK. Additionally the contralateral kidney may be abnormal, leading most pediatric urologists to recommend additional screening in the form of sonography and a VCUG to exclude the possibility of an associated UPJ obstruction or VUR, placing the contralateral kidney at risk.[18] With most MCDK remaining asymptomatic, the only required initial treatment is yearly surveillance ultrasound. Rarely, newborns affected with bilateral MCDK may present with Potter syndrome.[19] Older patients may present with pain, a palpable mass, hematuria, or hypertension. Additionally, there have been scattered reports of possible malignant degeneration in association with MCDK.[12,20] Beckwith[21] addressed this controversial matter in an editorial commentary, indicating that of the 7500 Wilms tumor specimens reviewed by him in over 18 years, only 5 cases occurred in MCDK. Nephrectomy, performed either through a small posterior incision or laparoscopically, is indicated in patients who fail to show involution of the MCDK or show sonographic signs of enlargement, with the concern of malignancy. Patients remaining on surveillance are encouraged to be enrolled in the National Multicystic Kidney Registry.[22]

MEGAURETER

A commonly used term, **megaureter**, or wide ureter, is a descriptive diagnosis rather than a specific cause of ureteral dilation. The possibility is raised by sonography, with the diameter of the dilated ureter of 7 mm or larger being considered abnormal.[23] The most important differential diagnosis of megaureters requires defining whether their presence is a primary ureteral or secondary process. Primary causes of megaureters include gross VUR; primary obstructed megaureters, also termed *ureterovesical obstruction*; ureteroceles; and nonobstructed, nonrefluxing megaureters. Secondary causes of megaureters include prune-belly syndrome, posterior urethral valves, and neurogenic bladder.

Additional sonographic features include the tortuosity of the involved ureter, the degree of renal parenchymal thinning, and the appearance of the bladder. As with hydronephrosis, the diagnosis of megaureter is established most frequently with antenatal ultrasound.[24-28] When the diagnosis of megaureter is established, a VCUG is obtained. This study is used to evaluate the possibility of VUR as the cause of the megaureter. It is crucial to assess fully the male urethra during this study to exclude posterior urethral valves. If significant VUR is found, delayed drainage films of the collecting system should be obtained because reflux and obstruction can coexist, and their combined presence carries a significantly greater concern than unobstructed VUR. An obstructing ureterocele also may be identified with VCUG, although this diagnosis is usually evident in a well-performed sonographic survey of the bladder (Figs. 87-8 and 87-9). Patients found to have VUR are maintained on antibiotic prophylaxis with amoxicillin (10 mg/kg/day) for the initial 6 weeks of life, then are changed to trimethoprim, trimethoprim-sulfamethoxazole, or nitrofurantoin for prophylaxis. Radiographic descriptions of the grades of primary VUR are summarized in Table 87-1.

If VUR is not shown during VCUG, the patient should return at 4 weeks of age for diuretic renal scintigraphy to evaluate drainage of the megaureter. Controversy exists as to the necessity for surgical intervention of an "obstructed" megaureter found on scintigraphy with

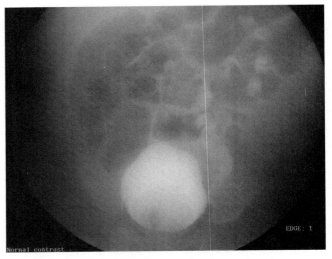

Figure 87–9. Voiding cystourethrogram showing ureterocele.

preserved ipsilateral renal function because many of these ureters show improved drainage with time.[24-27] Nonetheless, it is our opinion that if clinical obstruction exists either clinically or radiographically, prompt surgical repair and decompression should be performed to preserve renal function. The diagnosis of nonobstructed, nonrefluxing megaureter is one of exclusion. Eagle-Barrett syndrome is a classic example of this situation. As emphasized earlier, dilation of the genitourinary system does not equate to obstruction.

CONGENITAL MESOBLASTIC NEPHROMA

Congenital mesoblastic nephroma accounts for approximately 5% of renal neoplasms in childhood; however, it is the most frequently diagnosed renal tumor in the first 3 months of life. Prenatal diagnosis has been described.[29] Before 1967, the tumors were classified as a variant of Wilms tumor with the subsequent institution of unnecessary treatment in the form of radiation and chemotherapy.[30] Male infants are affected more frequently by congenital mesoblastic nephroma. Patients may present

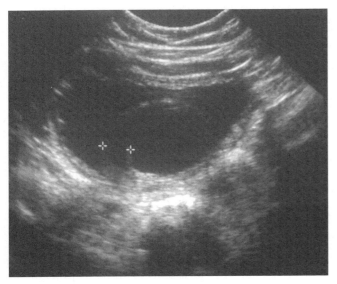

Figure 87–8. Ultrasound showing ureterocele.

Table 87–1. Radiographic Findings of Primary Vesicoureteral Reflux

Grade	Radiographic Findings
I	Reflux into a nondilated ureter
II	Reflux into a nondilated ureter and renal collecting system
III	Reflux into a dilated ureter and collecting system
IV	Reflux into a dilated collecting system with blunting of fornices and calyces
V	Reflux with increased ureteral tortuosity and loss of papillary impressions

with a palpable mass or hematuria.[31] Imaging studies are not diagnostic for this condition, and exclusion of other solid renal masses of infancy requires histopathologic verification. The sole form of treatment for this usually benign tumor is that of complete surgical removal, offering a 95% cure rate. Recurrence has been documented in 5% of patients, particularly patients treated with incomplete resection.[32-34] Continued follow-up with ultrasound and chest radiographs is required. Most patients who develop recurrent disease fail to respond to any treatment other than surgical resection.

GROSS HEMATURIA

Gross hematuria in a neonate is unusual, although it is seen with some regularity in premature infants early in postnatal life or after diuretic therapy. One report documented 35 cases over a span of 27 years.[35] This report documented renal vein thrombosis as a cause in 20%, obstructive uropathy in 20%, and polycystic kidney in 17%. Of the patients reviewed, 31% had no identifiable cause for the gross hematuria. One potential cause is nephrolithiasis (see later), particularly in premature infants who may have received long courses of furosemide. The use of indomethacin also has been associated with gross hematuria,[36] often relative to its use for the treatment of patent ductus arteriosus in the neonate.

NEPHROLITHIASIS AND NEPHROCALCINOSIS

Pediatric stone disease in the United States and other developed countries is unusual. The incidence of stone disease may be increasing, however.[37] Factors predisposing the patient to stone formation include metabolic imbalances, such as hypercalciuria, hyperoxaluria, and hyperuricosuria; cystinuria; the presence of urinary tract infections with urea-splitting organisms; and anatomic causes producing stasis and obstruction. Dehydration is always a significant finding in most patients who develop urinary tract calculi.

Nephrocalcinosis, first described in 1982[38] in 10 premature infants who were treated with furosemide, who also showed abdominal calcifications on plain abdominal radiographs, is often associated with nephrolithiasis. The pathophysiology involves inhibition of calcium absorption in the ascending limb of the loop of Henle by loop diuretics, such as furosemide, ethacrynic acid, and spironolactone.[39] Acute administration of furosemide increases urinary calcium concentration 10-fold.[40] Diuretic administration is not required, however, for the development of nephrocalcinosis or nephrolithiasis in the premature neonate.[38] Most of these cases are asymptomatic, many being discovered during routine sonographic surveillance of the upper urinary tract in patients treated with these diuretics, whereas a few patients may present with gross hematuria. Treatment involves discontinuation of the diuretics when possible, which usually leads to the resolution of the disease. Residual renal morbidity may include reduced creatinine clearance, microscopic hematuria, and hypercalciuria.[41]

HYPOSPADIAS

Hypospadias is a congenital anomaly of the urethra that occurs in approximately 1 in 500 live male births. The incidence in the Western Hemisphere has reportedly doubled since the 1990s.[42] The incidence is even higher in children with a family history significant for hypospadias. Typical characteristics of hypospadias include a ventrally misplaced urethral meatus with varying degrees of the quality of the surrounding supporting tissue (corpus spongiosum) and ventral penile skin. The preputial foreskin is often incomplete with a "hooded" configuration. The glans loses its normal conical configuration, taking on a more flat or spadelike appearance. Chordee, or ventral curvature of the penile shaft, is associated with more proximal forms of hypospadias and may represent a tethering effect of the shortened ventral penile skin (cutaneous chordee) or a more severe underdevelopment of the ventral corpus spongiosum and corporal cavernosa (fibrous chordee) (Fig. 87-10). An exception to this typical configuration is the condition termed **megameatus intact prepuce hypospadias variant.** This variant, in contrast to the typical hypospadias, has a well-formed complete prepuce, no evidence of chordee, and a broad subcoronal meatus. Because this hypospadias is "hidden" by the normal-appearing prepuce, it usually is identified at the time of neonatal circumcision so that many of these boys are referred after having undergone a circumcision.[43]

The site of the urethral meatus may reside anywhere between the proximal glans penis and the perineum. Approximately 75% reside at or just proximal to the

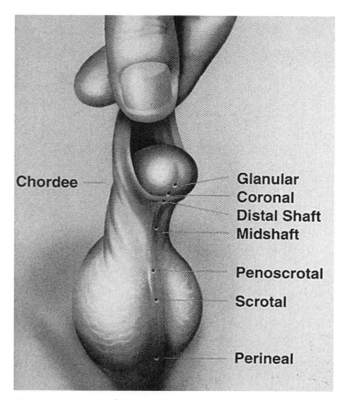

Figure 87–10. Types of hypospadias. *(Illustration by Stacey Lewis.)*

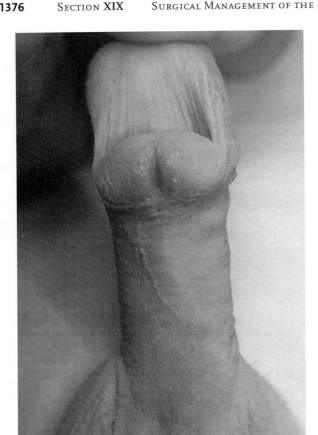

Figure 87–11. Coronal hypospadias.

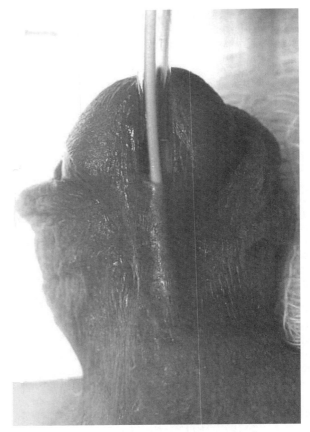

Figure 87–12. Hypoplastic urethra in hypospadias.

corona (Figs. 87-11 and 87-12). There are numerous classifications of hypospadias; however, a descriptive form that takes into account the location of the meatus and the presence of chordee is the most useful.[44]

The cause of hypospadias is unproven, but it is likely to be related to insufficient androgen stimulation in utero, either due to the amount of the androgen or due to improper timing of the stimulation. Dihydrotestosterone, converted from testosterone by the enzyme 5α-reductase, is responsible for the development of the male urethra. A defect of dihydrotestosterone may be a significant factor in the development of a hypospadias. This defect may occur at the site of the fetal testis, from deficiency of 5α-reductase or from lack of functional receptors for dihydrotestosterone in the male urethra. Hypospadias also occurs more frequently in offspring of mothers treated for infertility, who require added hormonal supplementation.

Associated anomalies may occur with hypospadias. The most common associations are that of inguinal hernia and undescended testis.[45] Routine sonographic screening of the genitourinary system in the more proximal forms of hypospadias (scrotal and perineal) is prudent. Additionally, when hypospadias is found along with bilateral undescended testis, micropenis, or a bifid scrotum, the intersex state should be considered as a potential diagnosis (Fig. 87-13).[45]

The timing of repair of hypospadias is controversial but usually occurs between 6 and 12 months of age. Because the surgeon often uses the foreskin to create the new urethra, neonatal circumcision in contraindicated in all forms of hypospadias.[46]

CIRCUMCISION

Circumcision is the most frequently performed and probably the oldest form of surgery. Circumcision is performed most often for religious beliefs or cultural reasons. Medical indications for circumcision include phimosis, an inability to retract the foreskin; recurrent balanitis; and paraphimosis, an inability to replace the foreskin back over the glans penis after it has been retracted proximally. Almost all neonates possess some form of phimosis for at least the first 6 months of life. This delayed separation of the prepuce from the glans is not a medical indication for circumcision. Proponents of circumcision argue that the procedure is protective against urinary tract infection, sexually transmitted diseases, and penile cancer.[47]

Most neonatal circumcisions are performed with the use of a device or clamp, which can crush a portion of the foreskin, controlling bleeding by the crushing effect. Then a portion of the prepuce is amputated. These clamps or devices include the Plastibell device, the

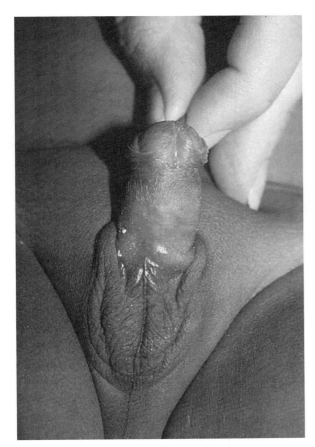

Figure 87–13. Hypospadias and undescended testes.

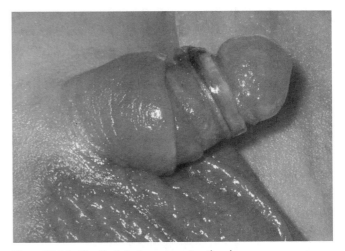

Figure 87–14. Plastibell device entrapping the glans.

Mogen clamp, and the Gomco clamp. No one apparatus has been shown to be superior, and the decision to use a particular device usually is based on the surgeon's preference. Complications of neonatal circumcision are unusual, with bleeding and infection observed most frequently. Bleeding most often resolves with simple pressure. Occasionally the physician may be required to place a few absorbable sutures (5-0 catgut) to arrest the hemorrhage. Topical application of thrombin, silver nitrate (poisonous), or dilute (1:100,000) epinephrine also has been described.[48] Many emergency departments store **LET (lidocaine, epinephrine, and tetracaine),** the solution used to prepare a skin laceration in anticipation of suturing. We have found that the application of a minimal amount of this solution is highly effective in controlling bleeding from a circumcision. Another type of common complication, the degloving circumcision, occurs when overzealous skin excision results in an inability to gain skin coverage of the penile shaft. This complication is managed best with a conservative approach, relying on healing by secondary intention through application of moist sterile dressings with topical antibiotic ointment. Many of these initially worrisome injuries heal well with minimal residual deficits.

A complication of circumcision is the proximal migration of a Plastibell device, producing a tourniquet effect on the glans. Urgent removal of this entrapping device is mandatory (Fig. 87-14). Partial penile amputation, with or without involvement of the urethra, is a rare, although potentially catastrophic, event. The Mogen clamp, owing to its guillotine-like amputation of the prepuce, has been associated with this type of complication. This complication usually is is confined to the glans penis. Bhangarada and colleagues[49] described their surgical treatment of reattachment in 100 cases in Thailand. Reattachment may be accomplished 8 hours after amputation.[50]

UNDESCENDED TESTIS

An undescended testis **(cryptorchidism)** may be unilateral or bilateral. The opportunity for documentation of the position of each testis first comes with the newborn examination and should not be overlooked. When bilateral, the diagnosis of intersex should be entertained. The incidence of undescended testis is related to the gestational age at birth. Undescended testis occurs in approximately 3% of term boys and 33% of premature infants.[51] Although treatment is rarely needed in the neonatal period, it is important for future therapy to document the exact position or existence of each testis. A useful technique in the physical examination for undescended testis is to place two fingers against the external ring to prevent the testis from being displaced into the inguinal canal by the scrotal examination (Fig. 87-15). Because two thirds of cases of undescended testis descend spontaneously in the first 4 to 6 months of life, surgical treatment in the form of orchiopexy is delayed until the infant is 6 months old. The site of the undescended testis is found most frequently in the inguinal canal or distal to the external inguinal ring in the suprascrotal position.[52] The remainder of undescended testis may be located ectopically, such as within the femoral triangle or within the abdomen (Fig. 87-16). The testis in question may not exist (**vanishing testicle,** a term that implies the previous presence of a testis, lost as the result of in utero testicular torsion). The inability to palpate the testis requires that the clinician distinguish between testes located intraabdominally and testes that

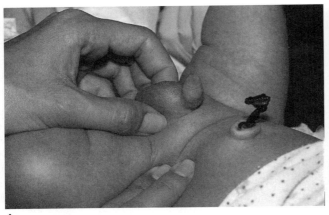
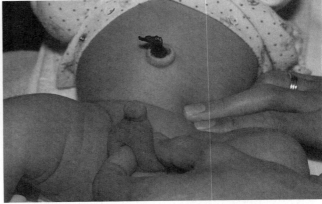

A   B

Figure 87–15. **A** and **B**, Examination for undescended testis.

have vanished. This examination is usually deferred during the neonatal period and is accomplished with the aid of laparoscopy at the time of the planned orchiopexy (Fig. 87-17). In the setting of a nonpalpable testis, the clinician may wish to perform imaging studies to localize the testis. None of the modalities studied, including ultrasound, CT, and magnetic resonance imaging, have sufficient accuracy, however, to be used in the diagnosis of undescended testis.[53] Bilateral undescended testis, calling into question the diagnosis of anorchia, requires measuring the testosterone response to human chorionic gonadotropin stimulation and measurement of plasma follicle-stimulating hormone and leutinizing hormone.[54]

Surgery is the mainstay of treatment. Performed within the first 6 to 12 months of life,[55] early orchiopexy potentially may prevent the development of infertility and perhaps reduce the risk of neoplasia, although these benefits of early orchiopexy are controversial. Use of human chorionic gonadotropin or its analogues is popular in Europe for the treatment of undescended testis. Its use in the United States has been curtailed by the high recurrence rates of cryptorchidism after cessation of treatment.[56,57]

Human chorionic gonadotropin may be used in the case of retractile testis or a testicle that is located in the suprascrotal position. In these circumstances, hormonal manipulation may have the highest success rates.[57]

SCROTAL MASS

A scrotal mass in the newborn represents testicular torsion until proved otherwise. Neonatal testicular torsion has a separate presentation and differential diagnosis than its adolescent counterpart. Also referred to as **extravaginal torsion**, torsion of the spermatic cord extending distally from the external inguinal ring represents approximately 10% of all cases of testicular torsion.[58] Owing to the chronicity of the situation, the mass is usually nontender to palpation. These events occur prenatally, and the expectation of salvaging the affected testis is nil. The mass is firm and may be accompanied by an associated hydrocele with discoloration of the scrotum (Fig. 87-18). The differential diagnosis includes incarcerated inguinal hernia (tender to palpation), hematoma from birth trauma, meconium peritonitis, ectopic viscus, and rarely neoplasm. In contrast to its adolescent counterpart,

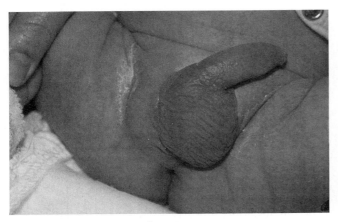

Figure 87–16. Ectopic (perineal) testis.

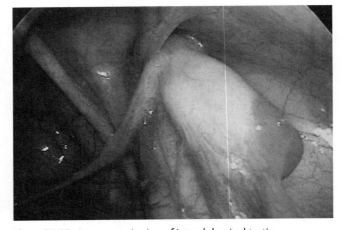

Figure 87–17. Laparoscopic view of intraabdominal testis.

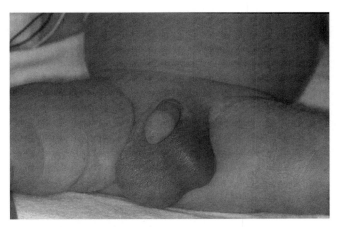

Figure 87–18. Neonatal testicular torsion.

the luxury of time allows the clinician to obtain scrotal sonography preoperatively. Doppler ultrasound may be able to distinguish between some of the above-mentioned entities. Sonographic findings include an inhomogeneously hypoechoic testis with a bright rim representing infarction.[59] Although testicular infarction is the rule, prudence calls for cautious scrotal exploration, especially in the light of the unusual documentation of testicular salvage, as long as experienced neonatal anesthesia is available.[60] Exploration and orchiectomy are performed through an inguinal incision because of the possibility of a neoplastic process. Contralateral testicular fixation always is indicated because of the possibility of metachronous torsion in the form of either intravaginal or extravaginal variety.[60,61] In the catastrophic event of bilateral testicular torsion, we have left the necrotic tissue within the scrotum in the hope for future endocrine function. The outcome of this approach is uncertain at best.

INTROITAL MASS

A mass within the introitus may be found in a newborn girl. Although prolapse of the urethra in African-American women is the most common cause for a mass between the labia, this entity is not found in neonates. Prolapse of an ectopic ureterocele may present in this fashion. The diagnosis generally is made with an ultrasound scan, which is likely to show a duplication anomaly with an upper renal pole hydronephrosis and hydroureter. A VCUG also is necessary to complete the evaluation. Treatment involves incision of the ureterocele at the level of the introitus and subsequent management of the urinary tract depending on the function of the upper pole and associated ipsilateral lower pole and contralatral reflux.

Another well-described introital mass is sarcoma botryoides, with the typical presentation of a "grapelike mass" or blood spotting in the diaper. Diagnosis is made by incisional biopsy, which shows rhabdomyosarcoma. Subsequent staging is accomplished with pelvic CT scan.[62]

An imperforate hymen may present in a neonate with a bulging introital mass. Pelvic ultrasound shows

hydrocolpos. Incision and drainage is the only treatment necessary. Finally, paraurethral cysts may present as a mass between the labia. These cysts tend to displace the urethral meatus laterally. Spontaneous drainage is the rule.

AMBIGUOUS GENITALIA

Ambiguous genitalia has been described since antiquity. The recognition of ambiguous genitalia is probably the one true social emergency in the neonatal period.[63-67] On recognizing that the genitalia of an infant is incompletely developed and that gender assignment is not immediately possible, a group of specialist must be assembled, including urologists, endocrinologists, psychologists, pediatricians, geneticists and social workers, to evaluate the newborn and support family members during this challenging time. Definitive gender assignment should be deferred until all of the information, including karyotype, hormonal evaluation, and organ imaging, is obtained. The most frequent cause of ambiguous genitalia in the United States is female **pseudohermaphroditism**. The most common cause for female pseudohermaphroditism is congenital adrenal hyperplasia secondary to deficiency of the enzyme 21-hydroxylase. This deficiency leads to varying degrees of masculinization of the genotypic (46, XX) female secondary to increased endogenous levels of testosterone and dihydrotestosterone. There is a large variance in phenotypic expression of this anomaly ranging from mild clitoromegaly to a phallus with severe hypospadias and an empty scrotum (Fig. 87-19). There is a potential for life-threatening hyponatremia and hyperkalemia leading to cardiovascular collapse and dehydration secondary to inadequate mineralocorticoid production in the first several days of life.

Evaluation of ambiguous genitalia starts with physical examination (Figs. 87-20 and 87-21). Physical examination combined with chromosomal analysis allows the clinician to assess rapidly which form of ambiguous genitalia is present (Table 87-2). Findings of symmetry on physical examination imply a global phenomenon responsible for ambiguous genitalia, such as an enzyme deficiency. In contrast, findings of asymmetry imply that there is discordant gonadal tissue on each side of the body. Further evaluation calls for serum electrolytes, urinary steroids, and possibly a human chorionic gonadotropin stimulation test to identify testicular tissue.[68,69] Müllerian inhibiting substance also can be assayed. Organ imaging should include evaluation of the

Table 87–2. Assessment of Ambiguous Genitalia

	Chromosome XX	Chromosome XY
Symmetry	Female pseudohermaphrodite	Male pseudohermaphrodite
Asymmetry	True hermaphrodite	Mixed gonadal dysgenesis

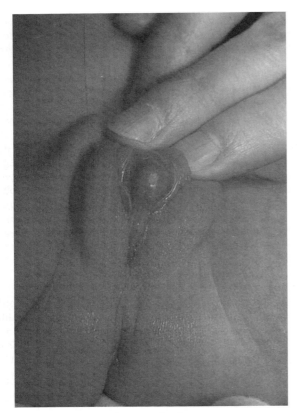

Figure 87–19. Female pseudohermaphrodite.

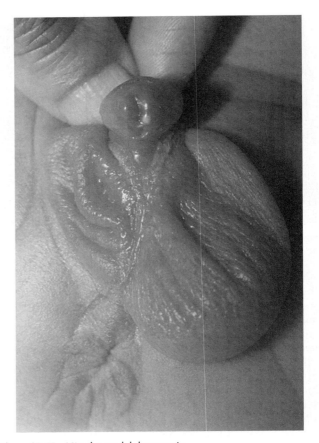

Figure 87–21. Mixed gonadal dysgenesis.

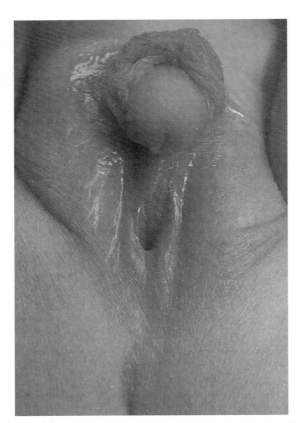

Figure 87–20. Male pseudohermaphrodite and perirenal hypospadias.

pelvis with sonography looking for müllerian structures. A genitogram also is useful in evaluating the length of the urogenital sinus in patients with female pseudohermaphroditism and showing the presence of the cervical impression in the most cephalad portion of the vagina.

The treatment of the various intersex syndromes has become increasingly controversial. In the past, gender assignment was determined by the size of the phallus (phenotype), rather than the chromosomal makeup (genotype). Most children have been raised as girls with the possible exception of virilized male pseudohermaphrodites. There is wide acceptance presently that testosterone exposure in utero may have significant behavioral effects in these patients. Although sex assignment in the neonatal period has been performed with the best of intentions, there remains a high transition rate from female to male "sex" in long-term studies following these patients.[66,67,69] Factors responsible for this phenomenon include fetal imprinting of the brain. Androgen receptors have been identified in every tissue in the body with the exception of the spleen.[70] These receptors may allow for "masculinization" of the fetal and neonatal brain. In advising families about the sex of rearing, it is important to consider the "ideal goal" of maintaining the reproductive potential in an individual who has the capacity of satisfactory sexual function with gender-appropriate appearance and stable identity and psychological well-being.[71] The treatment of these children remains a challenge to all who care for them.

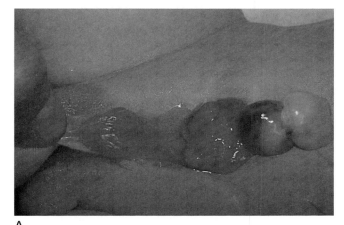

A

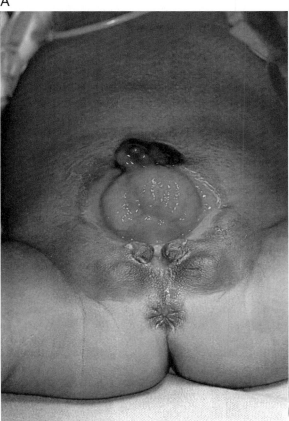

B

Figure 87–22. A, Male bladder exstrophy. **B,** Female bladder exstrophy.

BLADDER EXSTROPHY

Without question, **bladder exstrophy** is the greatest challenge for the reconstructive urologic surgeon. The absence of bladder filling or visualization by sonographic assessment of the fetus should raise the concern of bladder exstrophy. This is a rare condition, with an estimated incidence of 3.3 cases in 100,000 live births.[72] At birth, these infants are often healthy and can withstand the initial reconstruction or bladder closure within the first few days of life. Associated anomalies are confined to the

penis or genitalia and bony pelvis. The genital problems become the recurrent obstacle for these patients: Boys have short, stubby penises with dorsal chordee, and girls have a bifid clitoris and a short, anteriorly displaced vagina. The first step in the management of these patients is recognizing the anomaly (Fig. 87-22), then protecting the delicate exstrophic mucosa of the bladder with paper wrap, not a saline-soaked gauze, which may abrade the mucosa. The second step is to involve the pediatric urologist immediately. In the past, a staged approach of reconstruction was recommended, with initial bladder closure in the neonatal period, followed by additional stages of closure of the epispadias in boys at 18 months, then a bladder neck procedure to improve urinary continence. Currently the preferred approach is to close the exstrophic bladder and epispadias (complete reconstruction) in the first days of life as a one-stage procedure.[73]

REFERENCES

1. Thomas DFM: Fetal uropathy: Review. Br J Urol 66:225, 1990.
2. Homsey YL, Koff SA: Problems in the diagnosis of obstruction in the neonate. In King LR (ed): Urologic Surgery in Neonates and Young Infants. Philadelphia, WB Saunders, 1988, pp 77-94.
3. Peters CA: Perinatal urology. In Walsh PC, Retik AB, Vaughn ED Jr, Wein AJ (eds): Campbell's Urology, 8th ed. Philadelphia, WB Saunders, 2002, pp 1781-1811.
4. Heyman S, Duckett JW: Extraction factor: An estimate of single kidney function in children during routine radionucleotide renography with 99m technetium diethylenetriamine pentaacetic acid. J Urol 140:780, 1998.
5. Chung S, Majd M, Rushton HG, et al: Diuretic renography in the evaluation of neonatal hydronephrosis: Is it reliable? J Urol 150:765, 1993.
6. Conway JJ: "Well-tempered" diuresis renography: Its historical development, physiological and technical pitfalls and standardized technique protocol. Semin Nucl Med 22:74, 1992.
7. Fung LCT: Upper tract urodynamics in the evaluation of pediatric hydronephrosis. Dialogues Pediatr Urol 24:1, 2001.
8. Whitaker RH: The Whitaker test. Urol Clin North Am 6:529, 1979.
9. Ruano-Gil D, Coca-Payeras A, Tejedo-Maten A: Obstruction and normal recanalization of the ureter in the human embryo: Its relation to congenital ureteric obstruction. Eur Urol 1:287, 1975.
10. Stephens FD: Ureterovascular hydronephrosis and the "aberrant" renal vessels. J Urol 128:984, 1982.
11. Gleason PE, Kelalis PP, Hussmann DA, et al: Hydronephrosis in renal utopia: Incidence, etiology and significance. J Urol 151:1660, 1994.
12. King LR: The management of multicystic dyspalstic kidney and UPJ obstruction. In King LR (ed): Urologic Surgery in Neonates and Young Infants. Philadelphia, WB Saunders, 1988, pp 140-154.
13. Griscom NT: The roentgenology of neonatal abdominal masses. Am J Radiol 93:447, 1965.
14. Stephens FD, Cussen LJ: Renal dysgenesis: A "urologic" classification. In Stephens FD (ed): Congenital Malformations of the Urinary Tract. New York, Praeger, 1983, p 463.
15. Beck AD: The effect of intrauterine urinary obstruction upon the development of the fetal kidney. J Urol 105:784, 1971.

16. Gonzalez R, Reinberg Y, Burke B, et al: Early bladder outlet obstruction in fetal lambs induces renal dysplasia and the prune-belly syndrome. J Pediatr Surg 25:342, 1990.

17. Stuck KJ, Koff SA, Silver TM: Ultrasonic features of multicystic dysplastic kidney: Expanded diagnostic criteria. Radiology 143:217, 1982.

18. Flack CE, Bellinger MF: The multicystic dysplastic kidney and contralateral vesicoureteral reflux: Protection of the solitary kidney. J Urol 150:1873, 1993.

19. Al-Khaldi N, Watson AR, Zuccollo J, et al: Outcome of antenatally detected cystic dysplastic kidney disease. Arch Dis Child 70:520, 1994.

20. Oddone M, Marino C, Sergi C, et al: Wilms' tumor arising in a multicystic dysplastic kidney. Pediatr Radiol 24:236, 1994.

21. Beckwith JB: Editorial comment. J Urol 158:2259, 1997.

22. Wacksman J, Phipps L: National Multicystic Kidney Registry. Elk Grove Village, Ill, American Academy of Pediatrics, 2000.

23. Hellstrom M, Hjalmas K, Jacobsson B, et al: Normal ureteral diameter in infancy and childhood. Acta Radiol 26:433, 1985.

24. Cozzi F, Madonna L, Maggi E, et al: Management of primary megaureter in infancy. J Pediatr Surg 28:1031, 1993.

25. Peters CA, Mandell J, Lebowitz RL, et al: Congenital obstructed megaureters in early infancy: Diagnosis and treatment. J Urol 142:641, 1989.

26. Mollard P, Foray P, De Godoy JL, et al: Management of primary obstructive megaureter without reflux in neonates. Eur Urol 24:505, 1993.

27. Baskin LS, Zderic SA, Snyder HM, et al: Primary dilated megaureter: Long-term follow-up. J Urol 152:618, 1994.

28. Lui HY, Dhillon HK, Yeung CK, et al: Clinical outcome and management of prenatally diagnosed primary megaureters. J Urol 152:614, 1994.

29. Haddad B, Haziza J, Touboul C, et al: The congenital mesoblastic nephroma: A case report of prenatal diagnosis. Fetal Diagn Ther 11:61, 1996.

30. Balonde RP, Brough AJ, Izant RJ, et al: Congenital mesoblastic nephroma of infancy: A report of eight cases and the relationship to Wilms' tumor. Pediatrics 40:272, 1967.

31. Howell CJ, Othersen HB, Kiviat NE, et al: Therapy and outcome in 51 children with mesoblastic nephroma: A report of the National Wilms' Tumor Study. J Pediatr Surg 17:826, 1982.

32. Fu YS, Kay S: Congenital mesoblastic nephroma and its recurrence: An ultrastructural observation. Arch Pathol 96:66, 1973.

33. Heidelberger KP, Ritchey ML, Dauser RC, et al: Congenital mesoblastic nephroma metastatic to the brain. Cancer 72:2499, 1993.

34. Ali AA, Finlay JL, Gerald WL, et al: Congenital mesoblastic nephroma with metastasis to the brain: A case report. Am J Pediatr Hematol Oncol 16:361, 1994.

35. Emanuel B, Aronson N: Neonatal hematuria. Am J Dis Child 128:204, 1974.

36. Corrazza MS, Davis RF, Merritt TA, et al: Prolonged bleeding time in preterm infants receiving indomethacin for patent ductus arteriosus. J Pediatr 105:292, 1984.

37. Kroovand RL: Pediatric urolithiasis. Urol Clin North Am 24:173, 1997.

38. Hufnagle KG, Khan SN, Penn D, et al: Renal calcifications: A complication of long-term furosemide therapy in preterm infants. Pediatrics 70:360, 1982.

39. Green T: The pharmacologic basis of diuretic therapy in the newborn. Clin Perinatol 14:951, 1987.

40. Savage MO, Wilkinson AR, Baum JD, et al: Furosemide in respiratory distress syndrome. Arch Dis Child 50:79, 1975.

41. Alon US, Scagliotti D, Garola RE: Nephrocalcinosis and nephrolithiasis in infants with congestive heart failure treated with furosemide. J Pediatr 125:149, 1994.

42. Paulozzi LJ, Erickson JD, Jackson RJ: Hypospadias trends in two US surveillance systems. Pediatrics 100:831, 1997.

43. Duckett JW, Keating MA: Technical challenge of the megameatus intact prepuce hypospadias variant: The pyramid procedure. J Urol 141:1407, 1989.

44. Barcat J: Current concepts of treatment. In Horton CE (ed): Plastic and Reconstructive Surgery of the Genital Area. Boston, Little, Brown, 1973, pp 249-263.

45. Khuri FJ, Hardy BE, Churchill BM: Urologic anomalies associated with hypospadias. Urol Clin North Am 8:565, 1981.

46. Keating MA, Duckett JW: Recent advances in the repair of hypospadias. Surg Ann 22:405, 1990.

47. Fetus and Newborn Committee Canadian Pediatric Society: Neonatal circumcision revisited. Can Med Assoc J 154:769, 1996.

48. Kaplan GW: Complications of circumcision. Urol Clin North Am 10:543, 1983.

49. Bhangarada K, Chayartana T, Pongnumki C, et al: Surgical management of an epidemic of penile amputations in Siam. Am J Surg 146:376, 1983.

50. Sherman J, Borer JG, Horowitz M, et al: Circumcision: Successful glanular reconstruction and survival following traumatic amputation. J Urol 156:842, 1996.

51. Pohl HG, Belman AB: The location and fate of the cryptorchid and impalpable testis. In Peppas DS, Ehrlich RM (eds): Dialogues in Pediatric Urology. Pearl River, NY, William J. Miller Associates, 1997, pp 1-8.

52. Docimo SG: The results of surgical therapy for cryptorchidism: A literature review and analysis. J Urol 154:1148, 1995.

53. Hrebinko RL, Bellinger MJ: The limited role of imaging techniques in managing children with undescended testes. J Urol 150:458, 1993.

54. Kogan SJ: Work-up and management of the bilateral non-palpable testis. In Gonzales ET Jr, Roth D (eds): Common Problems in Pediatric Urology. St Louis, Mosby-Year Book, 1991, pp 294-295.

55. Kogan SJ, Tennenbaum SZ, Gill B, et al: Efficacy of orchiopexy by patient age one year for cryptorchidism. J Urol 144:508, 1990.

56. Hadziselimovic F, Herzog B: The development and descent of the epididymis. Eur J Pediatr 152(suppl 2):S6, 1993.

57. Waldschmidt J, Doede T, Vygen I: The results of 9 years of experience with a combined treatment with LHRH and HCG for cryptorchidism. Eur J Pediatr 152:S34, 1993.

58. James T: Torsion of the spermatic cord in the first year of life. Br J Urol 25:56, 1953.

59. Zerin JM, DiPetiro MA, Grignon A, et al: Testicular infarction in the newborn: Ultrasound findings. Pediatr Radiol 20:329, 1990.

60. Jenkins GR, Noe HN, Hollabaugh RS, et al: Spermatic cord torsion in the neonate. J Urol 129:121, 1983.

61. LaQuaglia MP, Bauer SB, Eraklis A, et al: Bilateral neonatal torsion. J Urol 138:1051, 1987.

62. Middleton AW, Elman AJ, Stewart JR, et al: Combined modality therapy with conservation of organ function in childhood genitourinary rhabdomyosarcoma. Urology 18:42, 1981.

63. Ladee-Levy JV: Ambiguous genitalia as a psychosocial emergency. Z Kinderchir 39:178, 1984.

64. Canty TG: The child with ambiguous genitalia: A neonatal surgical emergency. Ann Surg 186:272, 1977.

65. Wilson JD, Griffin JE, Russell DW: Steroid 5α-reductase 2 deficiency. Endocr Rev 14:577, 1993.

66. Roslyn JJ, Fonkalsrud EW, Lippe B: Intersex disorders in adolescents and adults. Am J Surg 146:138, 1983.

67. Money J: The concept of gender identity disorder in childhood and adolescence after 39 years. J Sex Marital Ther 20:163, 1994.

68. De Jong TPVM, Boemers TML: Neonatal management of female intersex by clitoro-vaginoplasty. J Urol 154:830, 1995.

69. Money J: Pediatric sexology and hermaphroditism. J Sex Marital Ther 11:139, 1985.

70. Takeda H, Chodak G, Mutchnik S, et al: Immunohisto-chemical localization of androgen receptors with mono- and poly-clonal antibodies to androgen receptors. J Endocrinol 126:17, 1990.

71. Meyer-Bahlburg HFL: Gender assignment in intersexuality. J Psychol Hum Sex 10:1, 1998.

72. Gearhart JP: Extrophy, epispadias, and other bladder anomalies. In Walsh PC, Retik AB, Vaughn ED Jr, Wein AJ (eds): Campbell's Urology, 8th ed. Philadelphia, WB Saunders, 2002, pp 2136-2196.

73. Grady RW, Mitchell ME: Surgical technique for one-stage reconstruction of the exstrophy-epispadias complex. In Walsh PC, Retik AB, Vaughn ED Jr, Wein AJ (eds): Campbell's Urology, 8th ed. Philadelphia, WB Saunders, 2002, pp 2197-2206.

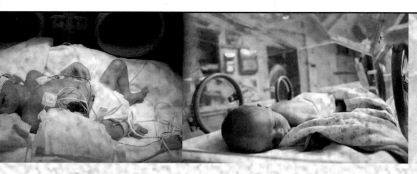

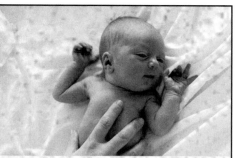

Ethical Considerations in Neonates

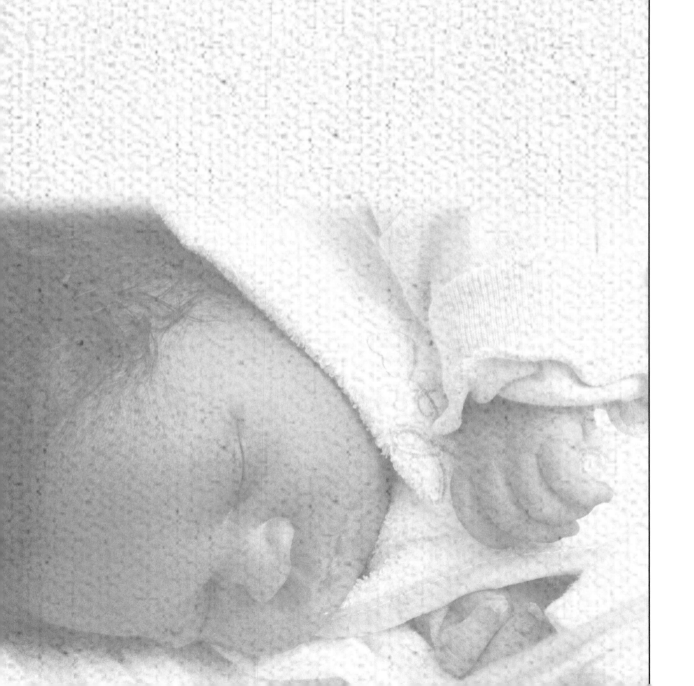

Neonatal Ethics and Epidemiology at the Dawn of a New Millennium

William Meadow, Laura Frain, Yaya Ren, Susan Plesha-Troyke,
Samir Soneji, Grace Lee, Kathy Lin, Alexander Meadow, and John Lantos

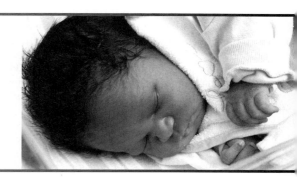

Neonatal intensive care and modern clinical medical ethics are roughly the same age—about 30 years old. Before approximately 1970, there were no ventilators, there were no **neonatal intensive care units (NICUs)**, and for the most part there were no discussions about artificial prolongation of life in newborns. Instead the contentious ethical issues of the day centered around the quality of life for infants whose cardiopulmonary function was already capable of keeping them alive. The paradigm cases of this era involved Down syndrome and myelomeningocele.[1,2] During previous decades, established wisdom had allowed infants with these conditions to die. Renewed societal discussion about such cases led to a different consensus,[3] however, and refusal of treatment for infants with these conditions gradually became unacceptable.

In the 1970s, mechanical ventilation for sick newborns became widely available. At a stroke, the world of neonatal ethics was transformed—living became easier and dying much harder. New ethical questions instantly arose. When should we start ventilation? When should we stop? To whom do we offer ventilation? Whom do we refuse? Perhaps most importantly, who should make these decisions?

In adult patients, the "rights revolution," an amorphous movement fueled in part by the Civil Rights movement, the anti–Vietnam War movement, women's liberation (as it was known at the time), and a growing sensitivity to the social correlates of what previously were viewed as strictly physical disabilities, led to the large-scale transfer of decision-making authority from paternalist physicians to newly empowered patients. The concept of informed refusal by competent adults spread throughout the field of internal medicine. Within 20 years, all sorts of good reasons, and even no reasons at all, sufficed to allow adult patients to refuse even obviously beneficial medical interventions.

These considerations of patient autonomy ran into a stumbling block when applied to pediatrics. Recognition of the prevalence of child abuse had given rise to social agencies whose charge was protection of otherwise defenseless children. This paradigm was extended to the medical arena, and parents were often denied the opportunity to exercise apparently natural surrogate decision-making capacity if physicians thought these decisions were not in the infant's best interest. Initially applied to cases that appeared to be relatively straightforward (e.g., blood transfusions for sick, anemic children of Jehovah's Witness parents), the "child neglect" paradigm was quickly extended to cover areas where outcomes were much more problematic, such as in neonatology. This tension—finding the appropriate balance between parents exercising surrogate autonomy and physicians invoking beneficent paternalism—is the most pressing ethical issue in neonatology today.

Various approaches have been proposed to inform this debate. Some suggest a philosophical resolution, empowering parents or physicians depending on the philosophy espoused. Some have proposed legal adjudication, but this merely begs the question of whom the courts should rely on when informing themselves in an arena where they are traditionally ignorant and unwilling.

In our view, **epidemiology** is, and should be, crucial in resolving these issues. Consider, at one extreme, a parent refusing to allow duodenal atresia repair in an otherwise healthy term infant—virtually no physician (and no court) would accede to that request. At the other extreme, consider parents refusing open-heart surgery for their infant with trisomy 13—virtually no physician would override that request.

What is it that distinguishes these two extremes? The phrase "benefit-burden calculus" seems right. Interventions that are brief, relatively noninvasive, low risk, and with a high likelihood of long-term excellent outcome are to be promoted; interventions that are prolonged, invasive, high risk, and with a low likelihood of good long-term outcome are to be avoided or in any case may legitimately be refused. What is it about epidemiology for neonates that particularly informs the benefit-burden calculus of NICU care? This chapter deals with these issues, taking up concepts that, in our view, are (1) resolved, (2) in progress, and (3) not even close to resolution.

RESOLVED EPIDEMIOLOGIC ISSUES AND THEIR IMPACT ON NEONATAL ETHICAL DISCUSSION

The most widely recognized epidemiologic observation in neonatal intensive care is **birth weight–specific mortality**—the observation that small, low-gestation infants are less likely to live than larger, older ones. Above roughly 2 lb/28 weeks' gestation, virtually all NICUs currently have, and have had for at least a decade, survival rates of 90% or greater. This level of success precludes discretionary parental refusal of intervention in the absence of other, non–birth weight–related circumstances. At the other end of a relatively narrow spectrum, below roughly 1 lb/23 weeks' gestation, survival is poor. In a survey conducted in 1998-1999, most neonatologists stated that as a routine they do not even attempt delivery room resuscitation of infants with birth weight less than 500 g.[4] Consequently, parental requests for nonresuscitation of infants below this birth weight seem supportable, under the broad rubric of **futility**.

Nevertheless, two aspects of birth weight–specific mortality are less well elucidated, and their implications are less obvious. NICU progress is generally portrayed as inexorable—doing better and better with smaller and smaller—and for the first 20 years it was. A succession of published articles bore witness to this success: Titles such as "1500 g—how small is too small?" were followed quickly by "1000 g—," "800 g—," and "500 g—." It was widely suggested that the "trimester" configuration of fetal viability (articulated in the 1970s by the U.S. Supreme Court in decisions about reproductive rights) would become rapidly obsolete; unexpectedly, however, it hasn't. There has been virtually no recession of the lower limit of viability at less than 450 g for almost the entire 1990s.

In contrast to most public perception, the lower limit to successful NICU resuscitation has been relatively fixed. Virtually all progress on the birth weight–specific mortality spectrum has been evidenced as a rising slope of survival for infants with birth weight between 1 and 2 lb.

The other underappreciated dimension of birth weight–specific mortality is time—specifically, how briefly birth weight influences survival to any ethically relevant degree. Small, sick infants who die tend to die quickly. The smallest and sickest tend to die the quickest.[5] These observations have profound implications for ethicists and epidemiologists. Figure 88-1 presents the transformation of birth weight–specific mortality for a cohort of extremely-low-birth-weight (ELBW; birth weight <1000 g) infants admitted to our NICU in 1996-1997, on day of life (DOL) 1 and again on DOL 4 and DOL 7.

The relevant ethical phenomenon is obvious. For infants with birth weight 750 to 1000 g, most NICU patients, whether considered on DOL 1, DOL 4, or DOL 7, survive to discharge. Consequently, as suggested earlier, there are no ethically supportable claims for nonsupport of these infants as a function of what is often called futility. For tinier infants, at greatest risk to die, the story is different. Considered at the time of their birth, infants with birth weight less than 500 g, were unlikely to survive. More than half of the nonsurvivors died within 7 days. Consequently, survival for infants at this birth weight who had survived to DOL 7 had now increased to 67%. Claims of futility are much less compelling when the infant is more likely to survive than not. For all birth weight groups, survival to hospital discharge for infants who survived the first 72 hours is at least as good as survival to hospital discharge for any age group of intubated patients in an adult intensive care unit (ICU).[6,7]

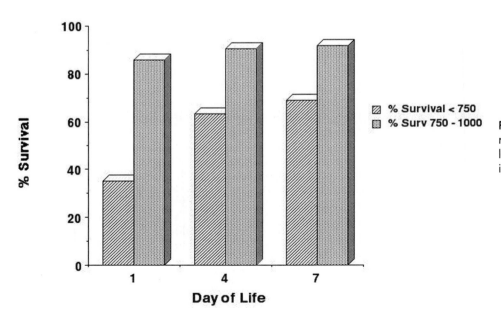

Figure 88–1. Birth weight–specific mortality versus day of life for extremely-low-birth-weight infants. NICU, neonatal intensive care unit.

Neonatal Ethics and ...

Chapter 88

EPIDEMIOLOGY IN P...
OR WHAT WE ARE...
IN THE NEXT 5 ...

S—
LEARN

...he phenomenon of the ...ic mortality? As we dig ... arise—neither obvious ...rst reported in the mid-...ost nonsurvivors seems to ...enon looks different now ... ago. Specifically, although ... early, they do not appear to ...d to. Figure 88-2 presents the ...nsurviving infants as a func-...cade in our own NICU (a typi-...liated NICU with roughly 1000 ...0 inpatients per day). There has ...n the median length of survival ... roughly 0.5 day per year, from a ...most DOL 7.

...concept of a "trial of NICU therapy" ...w than it used to. We used to be able ... parents of infants weighing 500 g or 600 g ... they could just wait for 2 or 3 days we would nave much different prognostic news to give them. Now we must ask them to wait a week to get the same news. Although the specifics vary from NICU to NICU, the phenomenon of increased length of stay for doomed infants appears to be widespread—a not-so-desirable side effect of improved survival rates for infants in this weight group.

The postponement of day of death for nonsurvivors forces reexamination of another of our previously reported observations—that most NICU bed days are devoted to survivors. We had previously noted that because nonsurvivors died quickly, it made sense (and turned out to be true) that most bed days (and dollars) associated with any birth weight cohort was occupied by infants who remained alive to survive until discharge, as opposed to infants who lingered in the NICU, then eventually died.[6,7] If nonsurvivors currently are living longer than they used to, however, doesn't it follow that more bed days are devoted to the nonsurviving subgroup than used to be?

During this same decade, however, overall survival has improved, particularly for the infants previously at greatest risk to die—infants with the lowest birth weight/gestational age. Figure 88-3 confirms the steady improvement in survival to discharge for the same 10-year period depicted in Figure 88-2. Because there are more survivors in each birth weight group, it must follow that for each birth weight group, more NICU bed days must be devoted to survivors. Which is it—more days spent on nonsurvivors because they are lingering longer or more days devoted to survivors because there are more of them?

Figure 88-4 resolves these two opposing trends. They just balance each other out. Over the 10-year span, the percentage of overall NICU bed days (equivalent to percentage of overall NICU dollars) devoted to doomed infants remained roughly constant at 4% (never >6% or <1%), whether infants were at low, medium, or high risk to die. Nonsurvivors continue to occupy a minute fraction of NICU resources (>$0.90 of each NICU dollar is spent

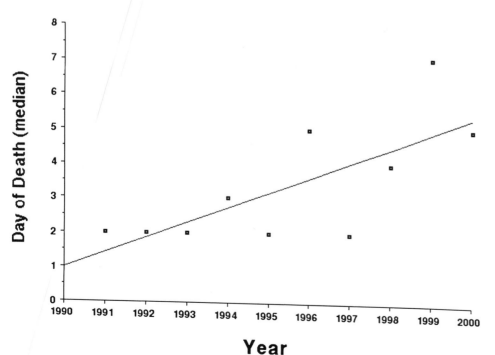

Figure 88–2. Median day of death for neonatal intensive care unit nonsurvivors versus year during the 1990s.

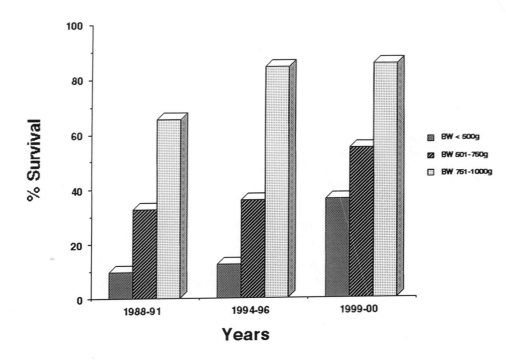

Figure 88–3. Imp[...] weight (BW)–spec[...] extremely-low-birth-wei[...] the 1990s.

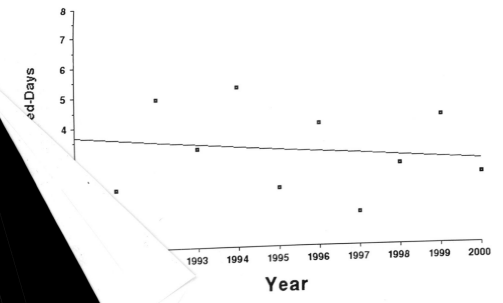

Figure 88–4. Neonatal intensive care unit (NICU) bed days devoted to nonsurvivors versus year during the 1990s.

EPIDEMIOLOGY IN PROGRESS— OR WHAT WE ARE LIKELY TO LEARN IN THE NEXT 5 YEARS

What else should we take from the phenomenon of the transience of birth weight–specific mortality? As we dig deeper, two additional issues arise—neither obvious when this phenomenon was first reported in the mid-1990s.[5,8] First, early death for most nonsurvivors seems to be a moving target. The phenomenon looks different now from the way it did 10 years ago. Specifically, although most doomed infants still die early, they do not appear to be dying as early as they used to. Figure 88-2 presents the median day of death for nonsurviving infants as a function of year for the past decade in our own NICU (a typical Level III, university-affiliated NICU with roughly 1000 admissions per year and 50 inpatients per day). There has been a steady increase in the median length of survival for doomed infants of roughly 0.5 day per year, from a median of DOL 2 to almost DOL 7.

Consequently the concept of a "trial of NICU therapy" takes longer now than it used to. We used to be able to counsel parents of infants weighing 500 g or 600 g that if they could just wait for 2 or 3 days we would have much different prognostic news to give them. Now we must ask them to wait a week to get the same news. Although the specifics vary from NICU to NICU, the phenomenon of increased length of stay for doomed infants appears to be widespread—a not-so-desirable side effect of improved survival rates for infants in this weight group.

The postponement of day of death for nonsurvivors forces reexamination of another of our previously reported observations—that most NICU bed days are devoted to survivors. We had previously noted that because nonsurvivors died quickly, it made sense (and turned out to be true) that most bed days (and dollars) associated with any birth weight cohort was occupied by infants who remained alive to survive until discharge, as opposed to infants who lingered in the NICU, then eventually died.[6,7] If nonsurvivors currently are living longer than they used to, however, doesn't it follow that more bed days are devoted to the nonsurviving subgroup than used to be?

During this same decade, however, overall survival has improved, particularly for the infants previously at greatest risk to die—infants with the lowest birth weight/gestational age. Figure 88-3 confirms the steady improvement in survival to discharge for the same 10-year period depicted in Figure 88-2. Because there are more survivors in each birth weight group, it must follow that for each birth weight group, more NICU bed days must be devoted to survivors. Which is it—more days spent on nonsurvivors because they are lingering longer or more days devoted to survivors because there are more of them?

Figure 88-4 resolves these two opposing trends. They just balance each other out. Over the 10-year span, the percentage of overall NICU bed days (equivalent to percentage of overall NICU dollars) devoted to doomed infants remained roughly constant at 4% (never >6% or <1%), whether infants were at low, medium, or high risk to die. Nonsurvivors continue to occupy a minute fraction of NICU resources (>$0.90 of each NICU dollar is spent

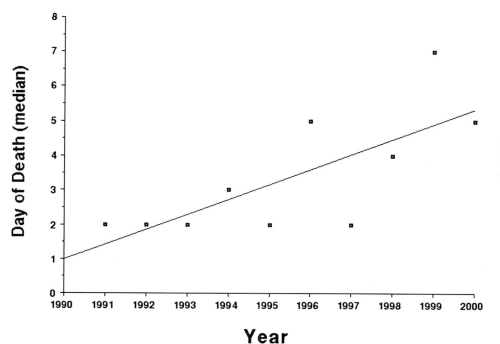

Figure 88–2. Median day of death for neonatal intensive care unit nonsurvivors versus year during the 1990s.

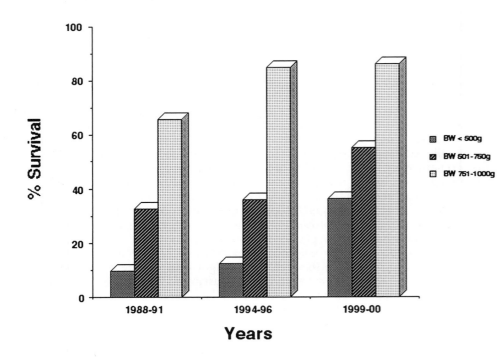

Figure 88–3. Improvement in birth weight (BW)–specific mortality for extremely-low-birth-weight infants during the 1990s.

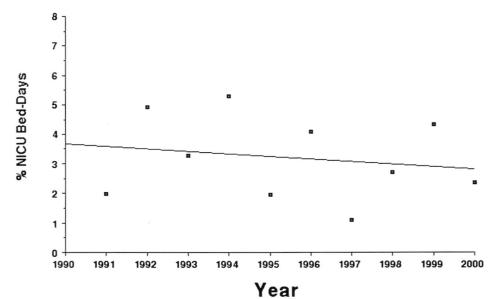

Figure 88–4. Neonatal intensive care unit (NICU) bed days devoted to nonsurvivors versus year during the 1990s.

on infants who are discharged to home, even for the tiniest NICU cohort at greatest risk to die). In comparison, for no subgroup of adults admitted to our medical ICU (young or old, intubated or not) could we find more than $0.50 on each dollar devoted to patients who would go home from the hospital.[6,7]

Personal Ethics: Predictions for Individuals as Opposed to Groups

We have dealt so far mostly with the ethics of groups—what some have called **distributive justice. Neonatology** is defined by its reference to a group—newborn infants. Among this group, some would always die and others would live. Identifying the subgroups at highest risk has always been easy—just bring a scale. That's what birth weight–specific mortality has taught us. For individual infants and their parents, the problem is more difficult, not simply a matter of accurately diagnosing a particular risk group, but rather trying to figure out which infants among a larger group with a similar diagnosis are the most likely to die. The problem is not straightforward. All NICU patients are at risk to die, but most survive. If physicians could accurately distinguish doomed infants from survivors, life-sustaining treatments could be restricted to infants who would benefit, and high-quality palliative care could be offered to infants whose death was inevitable. Recognizing this, physicians, ethicists, parents, economists, and policy makers all want to refine prognostic accuracy for individuals.

Initial attempts to predict the likelihood of survival or nonsurvival for patients admitted to ICUs took the form of illness severity scores. These scores (Acute Physiology, Age, and Chronic Health Evaluation [APACHE] for adults, pediatric risk of mortality [PRISM] for children, Score for Neonatal Acute Physiology [SNAP] and clinical risk index for babies [CRIB] for infants) tabulate the physiologic stability of patients in the first 24 hours after ICU admission.[9-15] They successfully parse ICU populations into likely survivors and nonsurvivors. In general, the more deranged the physiology at the time of admission, the higher the score and the more likely the patient will die. These prognostications have proven important to allocate resources and to level the playing field when attempting to assess the impact of novel ICU innovations, including ICU care itself. Nevertheless, there is always considerable overlap between scores for surviving and nonsurviving subgroups. Consequently, as an ethical scalpel for individual patients, illness severity scores are too blunt an instrument.

Here again the dimension of time seems to be overlooked. Viewing ICU care as a trial of therapy, the question naturally arises: Does the predictive power of illness severity scores get better with time or worse? Perhaps, as initially seems intuitive, patients who will ultimately survive improve over time, whereas doomed patients worsen. If this is the case, with each passing day assessments of illness severity should possess greater discriminatory power. Alternatively, perhaps many of the physiologic disturbances leading to ICU admission are, at least transiently, correctable for survivors and doomed patients. If so, the illness severity scores of the two subpopulations would converge, and the ultimate fate of patients would become less clear with the passage of time. Perhaps there is a U-shaped pattern of illness severity scores over time, with transient convergence followed by divergence.

In an attempt to determine the limits of prognostic ability for newborns and to assess the implications of such limitations for physicians' capacity to inform parents about the potential benefits and burdens of ongoing intensive care, we determined the predictive power of SNAP scores as a function of DOL for newborns admitted to our NICU for 1 year. We restricted ourselves to infants on mechanical ventilation because in the NICU no infant who is not ventilated will die unless a recognized lethal condition has led parents and caregivers to adopt a palliative course. We concentrated particularly on ELBW infants (birth weight <1000g) because it is in this population that the ethical questions are most incisive.

Illness Severity Scores as Predictors of Survival

Figure 88-5 presents the average SNAP scores for survivors and nonsurvivors as a function of DOL for 96 ventilated ELBW infants during the first 21 days of life. A total of 539 SNAP scores are displayed. Two important points emerge from Figure 88-5. On DOL 1, the SNAP values for nonsurvivors (25.8 ± 7.5 [SD]) were significantly higher than the SNAP values for the survivors (16.1 ± 6.8). For the surviving infants, as expected, the illness severity improved with time, and SNAP scores declined. The illness severity score for the population of doomed infants also declined over time. The difference in SNAP scores between the surviving and nonsurviving infants narrowed over time. Serial SNAP scores do not seem, at least on first inspection, to be of much use to ethicists.

Might the decline in SNAP values for the population of nonsurvivors be an artifact—that is, does the early death of the infants with highest SNAP scores and their consequent removal from subsequent analyses artificially depress the average SNAP score of the nonsurviving infants? Analysis of serial SNAP values for individual patients suggests that there is more to the phenomenon than this. Of the 28 nonsurvivors, 19 survived to DOL 3 and could receive at least two SNAP values to assess a trend. In 14 (74%) of these 19 doomed infants, SNAP declined from DOL 1 to DOL 3, reflecting improved physiologic stability. Only 6 (21%) of 28 nonsurvivors had a U-shaped course, whereby SNAP initially declined, then rose again before death. Whatever serial SNAP scores are sensing, they are not much use for predicting death.

Figure 88-6 elaborates these phenomena by displaying a scattergraph of every SNAP value obtained during the first 10 days of life for 96 ventilated ELBW infants; 124 SNAP determinations for 28 nonsurvivors and 415 SNAP values for 68 surviving infants are presented. The striking aspect of this figure is that on each day, at virtually all ranges of SNAP scores, there are at least as many infants who will ultimately survive as will die.

The implications of this observation are clear. The positive predictive value of death for infants whose SNAP score was equal to or greater than the median SNAP of the nonsurviving population was less than 0.5 at all times, implying that on every DOL more than half of

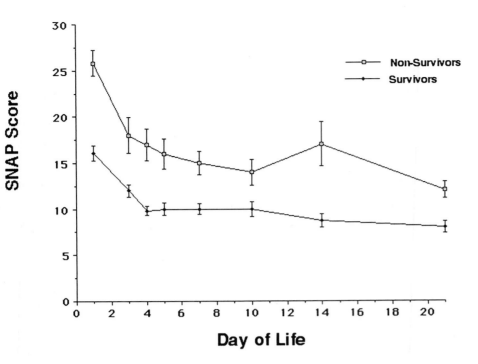

Figure 88–5. Score for Neonatal Acute Physiology (SNAP) versus day of life for surviving and nonsurviving extremely-low-birth-weight populations.

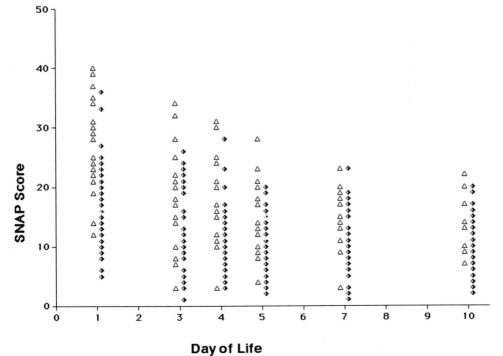

Figure 88–6. Score for Neonatal Acute Physiology (SNAP) versus day of life for individual surviving *(diamonds)* and nonsurviving *(triangles)* extremely-low-birth-weight infants.

these infants survived. Consequently, even if we restricted ourselves to infants with SNAP values at this high level, we would predict their death wrongly more than half the time—every day.

What About Serial Intuitions as Predictors of Mortality?

Physicians and nurses caring for NICU infants inevitably have intuitions about the survival of patients in their care. Perhaps we "sense" something we cannot put into words (or numbers), but that nonetheless could help inform parents. More importantly, might these intuitions, even if clouded by events around the birth of an infant, become increasingly clear as the "trial of therapy" of NICU care proceeded? Traditionally, NICU infants are said to "declare" themselves. Is this true, or might the infants instead "cloak" their prognoses with each passing day? To answer these questions we obtained predictions about survival or death in the NICU from physicians and nurses for 235 ELBW infants in our NICU between 1996 and 2001.

Prediction Profiles for Survivors

One-hundred-sixty (68%) ELBW infants survived. Prediction profiles for survivors reflected two distinct hospital courses. Most surviving infants were correctly predicted by all observers to survive on all days of mechanical ventilation. Of the survivor profiles, 98 (61%) displayed this consistent accurate prediction profile—on not even one NICU day did even one physician or nurse ever predict that the infant would die. Figure 88-7 is a representative prediction profile for this group of clear-cut survivors.

At the other end of the continuum, 61 (38%) of surviving infants survived unexpectedly; that is, after at least 1 day characterized by at least one estimate of "death." Sixteen (10%) infants survived despite having at least 1 hospital day in which *all* respondents predicted death.

Prediction Profiles for Nonsurvivors

During the survey period, 95 infants died. Nineteen died too soon to have any predictions recorded. The remaining 76 infants died after at least 1 day of predictions.

Early-Dying Infants

Forty infants died before DOL 10. As a group, the prediction profiles for these early-dying infants were remarkably homogeneous—dismal and accurate. The infants were doomed from birth, and their caregivers understood the prognosis. Of the 40 infants who died before DOL 10, 34 (85%) had 100% prediction of death on every day from birth to the day of death. Figure 88-8A is a representative prediction profile for these infants.

Late-Dying Infants

Thirty-six nonsurvivors died after DOL 10. In contrast to the homogeneity that characterized profiles of early-dying infants, the late-dying infants were a heterogeneous group. Only 5 (14%) of these late-dying infants had the "flat-line" or near flat-line profiles that categorized predictions for almost all infants who died before DOL 10. Each of the other late-dying infants was predicted to live by many (if not all) observers on many (if not all) hospital days. Many of these infants had, with little warning, a fatal medical catastrophe (e.g., necrotizing enterocolitis, sepsis, pneumonia). The rapid and unexpected nature of the demise is emphasized by the observation that for 14 (39%) of these late-dying infants, not even 1 day of their hospital stay before the actual day of death was marked by 100% prediction of death. The prediction profile of one of these infants is depicted in Figure 88-8B.

Twelve (33%) of the late-dying infants had prediction profiles categorized by uncertainty within respondents and across days. That is, several hospital days were characterized by "pessimism" (i.e., low predictions of survival), alternating with periods of "optimism," characterized at times by 100% prediction of survival. These nonsurvivors often lingered for many weeks before death. Their prediction profiles often looked similar to the infants who survived unexpectedly. These profiles are shown in Figure 88-8C.

Overall, 130 of 236 (55%) profiled ELBW patients had at least 1 NICU day characterized by at least one prediction of death; 63 of 130 (48%) of these patients were incorrectly predicted—that is, they survived. More stringent criteria for prediction of nonsurvival improved predictive power only slightly. Of patients, 98 had at least 1 day characterized by most respondents predicting death; 36 (37%) of these infants were incorrectly predicted—they survived. A total of 69 infants had a NICU day when every respondent predicted that the infant would die, yet 16 (23%) lived to be discharged.

Predictive Power of Clinical Intuitions as a Function of Length of Neonatal Intensive Care Unit Stay

Additional insight into the predictive power, or lack thereof, of caregiver intuitions of nonsurvival can be derived from analysis of the positive predictive value of a single day of 100% prediction of demise as a function of DOL.

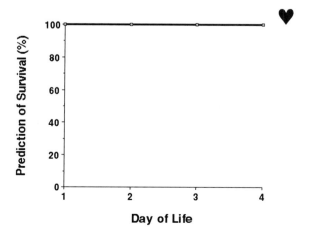

Figure 88–7. Optimistic concordant correct predictions versus day of life for neonatal intensive care unit survivors. ♥, predicted survival.

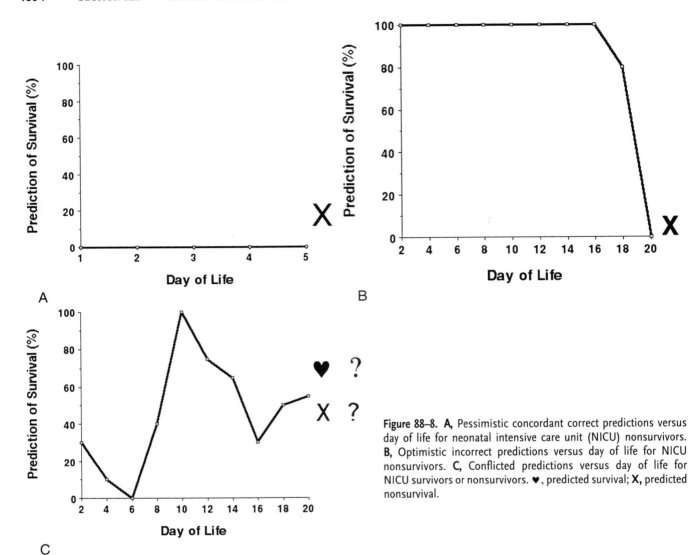

Figure 88–8. **A,** Pessimistic concordant correct predictions versus day of life for neonatal intensive care unit (NICU) nonsurvivors. **B,** Optimistic incorrect predictions versus day of life for NICU nonsurvivors. **C,** Conflicted predictions versus day of life for NICU survivors or nonsurvivors. ♥, predicted survival; **X,** predicted nonsurvival.

During the first 7 days of life, uniform intuitions of nonsurvival retained impressive predictive power because two thirds of patients with at least 1 day of 100% prediction of demise died. After DOL 7, this power diminished, however, and beyond DOL 14, the positive predictive value of unanimous intuitions of nonsurvival decreased to less than 50%—that is, predictions of death (even if corroborated by every physician and nurse caring for the infant that day) were wrong more than half of the time.

Clinicians seem to be best at anticipating impending death when accuracy does not matter much—for doomed infants with the worst physiology, who will die soonest anyway, sparing their parents, nurses, and physicians extended grief and society extended expense. For the long-term sufferers (infants, their parents, and their caregivers), we seem to have little to offer.

Neurologic Prognosis for Infants Surviving the Neonatal Intensive Care Unit

Clinicians seem to be terrible at predicting death, particularly late death—the expensive, painful, hoped-to-be-avoided kind. Perhaps death is not the worst outcome of NICU hospitalization, however. Hack and colleagues[16-18] found that almost 40% of survivors with birth weight less than 1000 g/less than 28 weeks' gestation have significant neurologic morbidity. The question arises—can we tell which 40 among the next 100 survivors will be significantly impaired and which 60 will not be impaired? This is the same general question just asked about survival: Within a larger group that is likely to die (or have neurologic morbidity), can we pick out individuals who are particularly likely, or particularly unlikely, to be affected?

We are not sure yet, but here's a start. We just noted that almost half of the infants who were predicted to die were predicted wrongly—that is, they survived to be discharged from the NICU. How do these infants look at follow-up? We observed a subset of profiled NICU survivors who returned to our NICU follow-up clinic, and we can begin to shed light on this potentially relevant question.[19]

In our prediction study, 84 ventilated infants (median birth weight/gestational age 1150 g/29 weeks) have been followed for at least 1 year. Consistent with Hack's observations, 28 (33%) were not normal at follow-up: 15 were clearly abnormal, 6 had suspicious examinations, and 7 had died since NICU discharge. The question here is whether or not something in their predischarge course might have tipped us off to infants who were particularly likely to present with (or without) abnormal neurologic sequelae. Specifically, did the predictions obtained on each day of the mechanical ventilation in the NICU presage the infants' neurologic status 1 year after discharge?

Table 88-1 presents the best answer we have at the moment. There were 32 ventilated infants (38% of the 84 in our follow-up cohort) who were never predicted either to die or to suffer moderate or severe disability; 28 of these 32 infants (88%) were normal at 1 year. Another 35 infants (42% of the follow-up cohort) were never predicted to die but were predicted by at least one caregiver on at least 1 day as likely to survive with moderate or severe neurologic sequelae; 10 of these 35 (29%) were abnormal at 1 year. Seventeen infants (20% of the original cohort) were predicted by a caregiver to die during their NICU stay, but the infants survived to discharge nonetheless. Of these 17, 14 (82%) were not normal at 1 year: 8 were clearly abnormal, 1 was suspicious, and 5 had died.

What can we extrapolate from these admittedly tentative observations? Apparently, if an infant has what can be considered a "benign" NICU course (ventilated, but never

thought likely either to die or to survive with significant morbidity), there is roughly a 90% chance that the infant will be normal at 1 year (and a 10% chance the infant will not—sort of the baseline neurologic morbidity for being born sick enough to require ventilation in the NICU). If the infant is sick enough that someone thinks the infant will survive with morbidity (but not sick enough that anyone predicts death), the glass is partly full (70% of these infants are normal at 1 year) and partly empty (30% are not). If the infant is sick enough to engender predictions of death, however, even if the infant survives, the likelihood of neurologic abnormality at 1 year increases to nearly 90%.

Let us reconsider the predictive value of intuitions of death. We start with a cohort of 100 infants with a prediction of "die before discharge." We had previously noted that the prediction is correct (the infant will die) only 60% of the time; this seemed unsupportably inaccurate, from the perspective of ethical decision making. Of the 40 surviving infants, only 10% may be normal at 1 year, however. Now the counseling for parents is distinctly different—the likelihood of a normal outcome after a prediction of death may be 4 in 100. These observations suggest that if we change the outcome variable from "die" to "die or survive with significant neurologic impairment," counseling after a prediction of death now has an important, almost requisite, feel, and, conversely, parental refusal of intensive care has a newly empowered status.

ETHICAL ISSUES THAT ARE NOT CLOSE TO RESOLUTION

If life-or-death is what we are searching for, we have yet to find the right dousing stick, and we've used up a lot of the more obvious ones. It seems likely that we will always be a bit wrong in those predictions, and that bit will get bigger, not smaller, as the days wear on. If we shift our gaze, however, and search for "life without significant impairment," we may have found a dousing stick. Time will tell. Perhaps the epidemiologist's role may be ending, but not the ethicist's. The central issue remains the same: What is the appropriate penumbra of parental choice/physician choice/legal intervention?

What survival percentage counts as sufficiently futile or hopeful? There are two aspects to this question. First, inevitably there will be some statistical uncertainty around whatever point estimate we determine for the survivability of infants, within the ethical penumbra. At the extreme, no infant, not one, not ever, has been reported to survive at 19 weeks' gestation, so that is clearly beyond the penumbra, at least for now. There are scattered reports of survival at 350 to 400 g/22 weeks' gestation, and by 400 to 450 g/23 weeks' gestation survival is countable (<10%, but countable nonetheless, with some inevitable uncertainty around that low number).

Second, and more importantly, how low a number "counts" in this discussion? This question arises only when there is physician/parent discord. If the physician and parents want to try NICU therapy for these infants, there is rarely a problem—we try, it fails (almost always), and the infant dies (usually quickly and cheaply). If the physician and parents agree not to resuscitate, the infant

Table 88–1. Correlation of NICU Intuitions with Post–NICU Morbidity Assessment

No "die" / no "moderate/severe morbidity" (n = 32)

Normal	28	(88%)
Morbid	4	(12%)
Abnormal	2	
Suspicious	1	
Died	1	

No "die" / + "moderate/severe morbidity" (n = 35)

Normal	25	(71%)
Morbid	10	(29%)
Abnormal	5	
Suspicious	4	
Died	1	

+ "die" / (n = 17)

Normal	3	(18%)
Morbid	14	(82%)
Abnormal	8	
Suspicious	1	
Died	5	

dies (always) in minutes to hours. Conflict arises only if the physician wants to try and the parents do not ("Whose family is going to have to live with the consequences?" "The risks are too great."), or the parents want to try and the physician does not ("Who's in a position to decide appropriate uses of professional skills?" "This is a waste of time and effort.").

What kind of morbidity counts as sufficiently worthless? This question is even trickier than the mortality question. Here is at least one reason why. Saigal and colleagues[20-22] have remarkable data from adolescent NICU graduates, born in the 1980s. These investigators have interviewed the adolescents, asking about their "quality of life." They analyzed responses from adolescents who are handicapped, by most "normal" standards. Saigal and colleagues have found that the adolescents self-report a score on their quality of life that is significantly higher than the self-reported quality of life for "normal," nonhandicapped teens.

What does this mean? Perhaps not much, given that Saigal and colleagues can analyze only teens who are capable of responding to questionnaires/interviews, and many NICU graduates are so impaired that they are incapable. Perhaps it means that cognitive dissonance is real—that these teens are much more adaptable and flexible than we who are not required to adapt to hardship can ever anticipate. That would be a good thing, from the teens' point of view, but difficult for an ethicist (or parent) who wanted to incorporate apparently dismal quality of life into the benefit-burden calculus of NICU intervention.

Currently, and we suspect inevitably, this penumbra issue is literally a "infant and bathwater" problem—some (it is hoped few, but recognizably more than zero—that's for the epidemiologists to work out) potentially "good" infants are going to be "thrown out" in return for allowing parents to forestall the possibility that many (but not all) doomed/damaged infants will be required to suffer extensively for no ultimate purpose (at least from their parents' point of view—the infants themselves are inarticulate here).

We close with one final, and most disconcerting, suggestion. We suspect that there are no parallels for these decisions in other aspects of pediatrics. If an older child presented with an acute illness that had a X% (the reader may insert a suitably low number here) chance of survival with a X% of residual morbidity (insert a high number here)—say chemotherapy for recurrent malignancy—we believe (1) that parents rarely would opt for nontreatment and (2) that physicians rarely would allow them to do so. Yet in neonatology it happens—not all the time, but often enough—and more often than for older children. Some have viewed neonatology as the last bastion of physician paternalism, but that may be just backward. Neonatology may be the leading edge of accepted parental refusal. Why? How?

We believe (we fear? we cannot deny?) that the controversial philosopher Singer has his finger on something. Singer[23] is notorious for his view that neonates are not born with full human "rights" and do not acquire them until they become more sentient. At first, most people find this view astonishing and deeply offensive. Despite moral, legal, and theological claims to the contrary, however, newborns do not seem to have quite the claim on us

that older children have. Perhaps this "ought" not to be so, but nonetheless it appears to be so. If you do not believe it, please perform the following simple poll whenever you get the chance: Set up a hypothetical Hobson's choice for people in your audience—they have two children of their own, a 6-hour-old and a 6-year-old, and must choose one to die. The responses are stunningly reliable—most people choose the 6-hour-old, a few absolutely refuse to choose, and almost nobody chooses the 6-year-old. Ethicists (and often judges) have an easy task—just make up internally consistent rules. Physicians have it harder because the real world is always dirtier.

REFERENCES

1. Todres ID, Krane D, Howell MC, Shannon DC: Pediatricians' attitudes affecting decision making in defective newborns. Pediatrics 60:197, 1977.
2. Robertson JA, Fost N: Passive euthanasia of defective newborn infants: Legal considerations. J Pediatr 88:883, 1976.
3. Lantos JD: Baby Doe five years later: Implications for child health. N Engl J Med 317:444, 1987.
4. Singh J, Yoon G, Singh D, et al: Through a glass darkly? predictive value of indices of non-survival for ultra-low-birthweight infants in the first hours of life. Pediatr Res 47:432A, 2000.
5. Meadow WL, Reimshisel T, Lantos J: Birthweight-specific mortality for extremely low birthweight infants vanishes by four days of life: Epidemiology and ethics in the NICU. Pediatrics 97:636, 1996.
6. Lantos J, Mokalla M, Meadow W: Resource allocation in neonatal and medical ICUs: Epidemiology and rationing at the extremes of life. Am J Respir Crit Care Med 156:185, 1997.
7. Meadow WL, Lantos JD, Reimschisel T, Mokalla M: Distributive justice across generations: Epidemiology of ICU care for the very young and the very old. Clin Perinatol 23:597, 1996.
8. Meadow WL, Lantos J, Frain L, Ren Y: Early neonatal death in New England and Chicago. Pediatrics 99:734, 1997.
9. Kruse JA, Thill-Baharozia MC, Carlson RW: Comparison of clinical assessment with APACHE II for predicting mortality risk in patients admitted to a medical intensive care unit. JAMA 260:1739, 1988
10. Marshall JC, Cook DJ, Christou NV, et al: Multiple organ dysfunction score: A reliable descriptor of a complex clinical outcome. Crit Care Med 23:1638, 1995.
11. Glance LG, Osler T, Shinozaki T: Intensive care unit prognostic scoring systems to predict death: A cost-effectiveness analysis. Crit Care Med 26:1842, 1998.
12. Lemeshow S, Klar J, Teres D, et al: Mortality probability models for patients in the intensive care unit for 48 or 72 hours: A prospective multicenter study. Crit Care Med 22:1351, 1994.
13. Marcin JP, Pollack MM, Patel KM, Ruttimann UE: Decision support issues using a physiology based score. Intensive Care Med 24:1299, 1998.
14. Richardson DK, Gray JE, McCormick MC, et al: Score for neonatal acute physiology: A physiologic severity index for neonatal intensive care. Pediatrics 91:617, 1993.
15. International Neonatal Network: The CRIB (clinical risk index for infants) score: A tool for assessing initial neonatal risk and comparing performance of neonatal intensive care units. Lancet 342:193, 1993.

16. Hack M, Fanaroff AA: Outcomes of children of extremely low-birthweight premature infants in the 1990s. Early Hum Dev 53:195, 1999.

17. Hack M, Taylor G, Klein N, et al: School-age outcomes in children with birthweights under 750g. N Engl J Med 331:753, 1994.

18. Hack M, Horbar JD, Malloy MH, et al: Very low birthweight outcomes of the National Institute of Child Health and Human Development Neonatal Network. Pediatrics 87:587, 1991.

19. Meadow W, Frain L, Ren Y, et al: Serial assessment of mortality in the neonatal intensive care unit by algorithm and intuition: Certainty, uncertainty, and informed consent. Pediatrics 109:878, 2002.

20. Saigal S, Stoskopf BL, Streiner DL: Physical growth and current health status of infants who were of extremely low birthweight and controls at adolescence. Pediatrics 108:407, 2001.

21. Saigal S, Stoskopf BL, Feeny D: Peception of health status and quality of life of extremely low-birthweight survivors. Clin Perinatol 27:403, 2000.

22. Saigal S, Stoskopf BL, Feeny D, et al: Differences in preference for neonatal outcomes among health care professionals, parents, and adolescents. JAMA 281:1991, 1999.

23. Singer P: Practical Ethics. Cambridge, Cambridge University Press, 1993.

CHAPTER 89

Care of the Family in the Neonatal Intensive Care Unit

Alan R. Spitzer

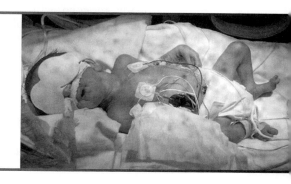

F ew aspects of neonatal medicine are so important, yet so often ignored, as the care of the family of a critically ill infant. Because of the life-threatening nature of many neonatal illnesses, the pathophysiology and treatment of the infant are, of necessity, crucial and often consume great amounts of time on the part of the medical, nursing, and ancillary staffs. Simultaneously, the lives of the infant's mother, father, siblings, grandparents, and other individuals who relate to the family are often drastically, sometimes permanently, altered, but physicians and nurses often are not effective at understanding and addressing the needs of these individuals. That the infant's illness has a broad impact on the physical and emotional well-being of the family must be acknowledged and addressed. If it is not, the physician may win the battle but lose the war. All too often, the infant survives, but with little to return home to if the nuclear structure of the family is obliterated by the stress of the intensive care experience. This chapter briefly discusses some of the issues that commonly affect neonatal physicians, nurses, and social workers so that an effective approach can be developed before these problems disrupt the cohesion of the family.

AWARENESS OF THE PROBLEM

Most parents proceed through pregnancy with some idealized image of their infant in mind. Until recently, it was rare to know the sex of an infant before birth, and parents could use their imaginations to imbue their infants with perfect physical and emotional characteristics. With the introduction of prenatal ultrasound and fetal screening, however, it has become possible for parents not only to know the sex of their unborn infant, but also whether the infant has a risk for many common (and some uncommon) genetic or metabolic defects. Because so many couples now postpone childbearing until their 30s or 40s and undergo detailed prenatal testing, they proceed through pregnancy with a great deal of reassurance that their infant is likely to be entirely well. These families,

on questioning, frequently describe the rosy-cheeked, vigorous infant that they anticipate after delivery.

Not everyone has access to this level of health care, and the circumstances of some individual's lives are such that prenatal care and screening do not become priorities on learning of the pregnancy. The proportion of unwed teenage mothers in the inner cities remains a concern, although the incidence seems to have declined in recent years. A more recent phenomenon, however, are suburban, middle-class girls who view childbearing as a competitive test of successful adolescence. If one of their friends becomes pregnant and has a child, these girls feel pressured to do the same. The emphasis on eliminating stigmatization of the unwed, teenaged mother has resulted in a new, unforeseen population of patients. Many women, regardless of their circumstances, still do not seek prenatal care until later in their pregnancy, and religious teachings for others make prenatal screening problematic. Not all women receive ultrasound evaluation for a variety of reasons. Others may not be screened until the third trimester, past the time at which termination or intervention could be considered. No foolproof method of preventing prematurity exists, and even with the most sophisticated screening available, some problems cannot be detected prenatally. As a result, many infants still are born with a wide variety of life-threatening illnesses, some of which may leave permanent disability or disfigurement.

In all cases, the family creates an image in their minds of the infant that they expect. That image usually resembles some model of the "perfect child," whatever that might be. Even in the case of an infant diagnosed prenatally with a serious malformation, denial commonly exists until the family actually sees the infant, no matter how much counseling and preparation occurs ahead of time. I have been involved in the prenatal counseling of many families with infants diagnosed prenatally with major limb or other physical deformities who were shown photographs of what the anomaly would look like after birth. These parents still were shocked and in disbelief on seeing the infant's malformation for the first time. The reality of the situation was simply denied until the family was faced with the inevitability of the problem. Denial can be strong in some situations, and the physician must be ready to cope with family members who might act as if no one had ever told them that this problem was present, even if they have been repeatedly counseled to the contrary. In our neonatology training programs over the years, one of the most common complaints from our neonatology fellows has been the apparent inability of family members to listen to the fellow's detailed description of possible outcomes during prenatal consultation. Even when told in great detail about potential complications, parents seem unable to accept that it will happen to their child until they are actually living through the experience.

Many families learn of the prenatal diagnosis of their child at a time when many possible outcomes immediately confront them. In some instances, the viability of the child is an issue. More often, immediate viability may not be a problem, but handicap or chronic disease is a concern, especially if a very premature birth is impending. Regardless of the circumstances, the anticipation of the family for that "perfect child" can be shattered in a moment. Both parents may feel in that instant that they have somehow failed not only the child, but also one another. The mother, carrying the child, may believe that she has done something wrong, especially if she can recall any event that may have contributed to the problem, no matter how farfetched. If she worked a week longer than she had originally planned, if she lifted something heavy, if she ate something that made her ill, the mother may believe that she has uncovered an indisputable explanation for her "failure" to produce the perfect offspring. The guilt that occurs with such thoughts can be substantial and may be fed further by her parents, her husband, or even a stranger, making an offhand remark that, in effect, tells her "I told you so." Needless to say, such remarks can be devastating and must be confronted immediately and eradicated by the medical staff from the mother's thought processes. These comments are virtually always without any merit whatsoever and serve only to add to the already substantial pain that the mother is experiencing.

Fathers, on learning of problems in their unborn children, also often display a sense of guilt, but for other reasons. It has been my experience that fathers in these situations commonly interpret the problems with the infant as proof that there must be something wrong with them as men. The "macho" thinking is that normal men have normal, healthy children. If the infant is not normal, many fathers believe that they themselves must be deficient in some way. Fathers rarely admit these feelings openly, in contrast to mothers, who frequently express their fears immediately. As a result, medical staff may need to make a special effort to draw out the father about his feelings to deal with them effectively, while reassuring the mother that her concerns are unsubstantiated.

The father may have other sources of anxiety that normally remain unspoken. Some men may view the infant's problem as punishment for some completely unrelated transgression, such as an extramarital affair. Their behavior in such instances may be unfathomable, with excessive crying and overly demonstrable displays of grief until the source of their anguish is addressed by a compassionate individual. With these thoughts in mind, the following recommendations related to prenatal diagnosis are suggested.

PRESENTING INFORMATION RELATED TO PRENATAL DIAGNOSIS

Information related to prenatal diagnosis must be presented to the family as clearly and as factually as possible. Although clarity is essential, it is crucial that the person presenting the information not insult the intelligence of the family with a patronizing or superficially simplistic explanation. One should avoid emotionally charged words at this time, and one should put aside any biases about the situation until the family members can process what is being explained to them. Although many physicians may be deeply discouraged by a child with a thoracolumbar myelomeningocele, it is important to present the diagnostic information factually to the family before investing the conversation with terms such as *paraplegic* and *incontinent*, which prevent the family from fully comprehending the problem under discussion. When certain charged words enter the conversation, it is difficult for parents to focus on the totality of what they need to know to make appropriate decisions. Usually, there is time for opinions at a later point, when the family has a better grasp of the factual information.

Certain topics by themselves can trigger flights of imagination on the part of the mother or father. When a heart lesion is mentioned, even if it is a relatively benign one, such as a septal defect or a patent ductus arteriosus, the remainder of the discussion may be lost, even if the other aspects of the diagnosis are far more significant (as would be the case with Turner syndrome). The physician must be ready to repeat the findings more than once. Often, it is helpful for the physician to present the information briefly, then inform the family that he or she will be back shortly to discuss their questions at length and in greater detail. Allowing family members a brief period to digest the news is often helpful to their understanding. Encouraging them to write down their questions for the physician's return can allow them to focus their thoughts better. It is useful to provide diagrams or photographs as much as possible to explain the situation. The imagination sometimes can evoke more fear than the actual problem itself.

The physician must be sincere and sympathetic. There are few occasions in medicine when true aid and comfort can be given, and this situation is one of them. A talented physician can present terrible news to family members and have them leave the conversation feeling as if there is no one they trust more than the person who just conveyed the bad news to them. Medical personnel must retain some sense of objectivity and detachment, but sincere displays of emotional support for the plight of the family are essential in such cases and can be of immeasurable help in aiding the family's ability to cope.

The family should be allowed to seek whatever additional support they need. If it means having their parents with them, the physician should be prepared to reexplain the information to the grandparents of the child. Although sometimes it may be frustrating to repeat the same information, the physician's willingness to meet with support people often is perceived as crucial in helping the family through this period and ultimately may save the physician a great deal of time. Religious personnel, friends, social workers, and other families who have experienced similar events can be effectively employed in aiding the family.

The physician needs to be patient and honest. It may take time for family members to comprehend the information conveyed and to arrive at a decision that is acceptable to them. If they ask for an opinion of what to do, the physician should attempt to be as objective as possible in offering suggestions. Sometimes it is helpful to give the family reading material in these situations so that they can understand that a body of literature exists about their child's condition. A more recent development in this regard is the availability of the Internet to provide substantial volumes of up-to-date information. One should be cautious, however, in that postings on the Internet may not be critically assessed and may lead to erroneous judgments or assumptions by families. If possible, the physician should direct the family specifically to sites that are known to be reliable and factual. Failure to address Internet information may lead family members to believe that the physician is either hiding the truth or is simply not aware of the latest information on their child's condition. As a result, the physician-parent relationship may be critically undermined at a crucial time.

It is often difficult to know how much directed guidance a family should receive in certain circumstances. There are many situations that we encounter in the neonatal intensive care unit (NICU) in which no amount of education can enable the family to make a "correct" decision, if there ever is such a thing. In addition, the best decision for one family may be the worst one for another. Much of the practice of neonatology involves the ability to understand not only acute, but also long-term outcomes. It literally may take a career's training in neonatology to be able to appreciate the complexity of a particular decision that a family may have to make in a matter of a few minutes. In such cases, the physician may need to be directive and lead the family through the process. There is probably no greater test of a physician's skill and judgment than the navigation of a family through the complex waters of difficult neonatal decisions.

Some families make decisions that appear incomprehensible to the medical personnel involved with them. These decisions should be gently probed because they occasionally are based on erroneous information. More often, however, the decision reflects personal beliefs and a sense of what is right for them in this set of circumstances. The physician should attempt to support that decision as fully as possible when it is clear that the decision is based accurately on the facts as presented.

Because it is usually the obstetrical staff that makes the prenatal diagnosis in a fetus, we also have found it valuable to have the neonatal staff meet with the family as early as possible in gestation to answer questions related to neonatal interventions that the family can expect in the nursery and long-term outcome. This consultation is arranged and discussed with the family by the perinatology staff. The family members then perceive that the perinatologists and neonatologists are working together for the betterment of the child. The parents should feel that they can speak freely with the neonatal staff as well during the remainder of gestation, when further questions arise as the due date is approached.

INTENSIVE CARE NURSERY EXPERIENCE

On entering the intensive care nursery for the first time, most families find themselves in a world that they previously did not know existed. Greeted by flashing lights, alarms, and a vision of technology right out of *Star Wars*, the family members may view the tiny infant in an environment so beyond their control or comprehension that they themselves may be overwhelmed and terrified. Parents at first are often speechless. Even the most educated families are frequently at a loss about how to act or what to ask of the physicians and nurses. The family members soon begin to search for clues that will enable them (not to mention their infant) to survive such frightening surroundings. Physicians and nurses often contribute to the problem by addressing the parents' concerns with a barrage of jargon and useless information. Rather than discussing the condition of the infant, the caregivers often provide the family with a litany of blood gas results, electrolytes, ventilator settings, and catheter positions, when the family only wishes to know how the infant is doing in the most general terms. Ultimately, information about the details of intensive care in the NICU may be valuable to the family, but rarely does it help initially, and it may become a hindrance over time.

This type of introduction to neonatal intensive care is not only a fine way to increase apprehension further, but it may also provide inappropriate information that later poses problems for the medical staff, when the family members ask questions that seem highly inappropriate in the clinical setting. I have seen the mother of a prematurely born child with Rh hemolytic disease explode in anger at a nurse who had recently assumed the care of her infant in a transitional nursery because the nurse did not know the most recent bilirubin and reticulocyte counts in the infant. The infant previously had been in the NICU, where he had received four exchange transfusions for hyperbilirubinemia and severe hemolytic disease. The information offered to the mother at the time of her first visit to the NICU included the bilirubin and the reticulocyte counts by a staff nurse who was trying to provide the family with facts that she thought appropriate to the circumstances. The parents, believing these numbers to be crucial, asked for the values each time they called or visited. Their behavior was rewarded every time not only by receiving this information, but also by the way the staff reinforced this behavior through a series of indirect signals that suggested the importance of these values.

When the problem was finally resolved and the infant was transferred to the step-down nursery, the parents arrived for the first time and asked their standard question about bilirubin and reticulocyte counts. The new nurse was not aware of these values, however, because they were no longer being followed; for her, feeding and weight gain were now far more important. The mother, thinking that the nurse was inadequate, was enraged by the fact that this information was not at the nurse's fingertips. As the infant's attending physician, I was called when the parents requested a nursing change. When they described the problem to me, I asked them if they knew what the bilirubin and reticulocyte counts meant. They paused to reflect a moment, and they admitted that they had no idea whatsoever. In essence, we had trained them to act in a certain manner that became inappropriate as the infant's condition changed, and the focus shifted from hemolysis to nutrition. After a simple explanation, they were reassured. Such episodes in NICUs are common, and whenever a parent is acting inappropriately, the cause of this behavior should be explored directly with them. Too often, the medical staff simply becomes angry with "that crazy family" and ignores them, when a simple, direct approach to the situation often resolves the problem and reassures the family.

The example just described illustrates a common error in the NICU. We often assume that the family members have certain needs that we have determined for them, rather than attempting to learn what their needs actually are. Each family is unique and has unique requirements while their infant is in the nursery. Failure to identify those needs early in the course of the infant's illness makes the NICU experience more difficult for the family and the infant. At the extreme, most often because parents find themselves in a situation beyond their control and because their needs have not been well addressed, their frustration erupts into anger at the staff. Such anger may be mystifying when the medical staff knows that the infant is doing well and making steady progress. In such situations, the state of the infant is almost peripheral to the issues at hand. If family members are not treated in the way that they require, they will remain difficult, even as the infant recovers completely. Early identification of the crucial issues for family members can prevent more difficult discussions at a later stage of treatment.

Families of infants hospitalized for long periods often present different problems. Even if the infant's course has gone well, the family of a 500-g child, who may be hospitalized for 3 months or more, may show behavior best categorized as severe "hospitalitis." Their lives are disrupted for months, for part of that time they may be unsure if the infant will survive or be damaged, and their other children may find that their usual access to their parents is suddenly diminished. Telephone calls are terrifying, often harbingers of bad news. Sleep is disrupted, yet the pressures to maintain a presence at work remain. Bills mount, and even simple issues, such as parking fees while they visit their infant, may provide sources of irritation so great that a single unexpected bit of information, such as the infant's failure to tolerate a feeding, may provoke an explosion that appears outwardly incomprehensible.

In actuality, it is remarkable how many family members do not display the type of behavior described. When behavior is inappropriate, however, the staff should not be offended, but rather should determine the reasons for it and how the family members can be better supported during this period. When the parents perceive sincere interest in their problems on the part of the medical staff, their concerns often evaporate or, at least, significantly decrease in intensity.

DEATH IN THE NEONATAL INTENSIVE CARE UNIT

A dying neonate presents many unique problems for physicians and nurses. Until the past 2 decades in neonatology, death was fairly commonplace in nurseries, often the result of infection or congenital anomaly. In modern practice, however, death has become the exception rather than the rule, with even 300- to 400-g infants surviving and surgical procedures available for even the most complex cardiac and other malformations. For the neonatologist, death is the ultimate failure and an all-too-common reminder of the fact that we are all unavoidably human and not all-powerful. Our humanity can be of great value if we use it to the benefit of the family who will not see their child grow up. Too often, however, our admission of failure is to leave the family alone at the bedside, when their world is collapsing all around them and their emotions are in turmoil. Physicians have a tendency to disappear, when there is no time when their skills as caregivers are required more. Most nurses that I have worked with in NICUs recognize the important role that they play in the family's life at that time, however, and are incredibly supportive, even when their own feelings may be deeply disturbed by the impending death. Although all of us no longer may be able to aid the infant, other than to provide relief from pain, we can do a great deal to support and comfort the parents during their grief.

Closing off the infant's bedside from the rest of the unit for privacy is essential, although often overlooked. It is extremely poor form to allow a family to grieve in the public forum of a busy NICU. We always offer the family the opportunity to hold the infant without all the tubes and wires attached, and we attempt to take a photograph for them so that they have a tangible memory of the infant. The infant's belongings, such as shirts and name bands, also may be helpful during the grieving period. The physician should emphatically avoid platitudes and gratuitous comments, such as "Well, you're young, so you can try again." The dying infant can never be completely replaced in a parent's mind, especially if the infant has been hospitalized for a prolonged period. Simple, direct comments that reveal the physician's own sorrow over the infant's death and the suffering of the family are usually much appreciated. Most important is simply being present. The presence of the infant's physician at the time of death is of immeasurable comfort to most families. Often, asking the family members if anything can be done for them is all that is needed at this time.

One of the other difficult situations for many physicians involves the steps that lead up to the death of an infant.

Although acute deteriorations are common in the NICU, many infants have a far more protracted period before their death, when it is apparent that the infant simply will not survive. This is when many physicians tend to make themselves scarce to the family, feeling powerless over the developing situation. In such circumstances, I have found it helpful to meet with families and review the recent developments as often as possible, what has been done and what will be attempted, and, most importantly, the fact that nothing has been very successful in recent days. This meeting has multiple purposes. First, it allows the family to witness the thought processes of the physician and the fact that although things are not going well, the physician has remained involved and committed to care. Also, it allows the family members to ask any questions that they have about what is occurring so that everyone has a similar understanding of ongoing events. Lastly, it plants the thought firmly in the mind of the parents that it is likely that this infant will die, something that they may have repeatedly pushed out of their thoughts because it is so overwhelming. We have observed that families who have used assisted reproductive technology to conceive, in particular, seem to be hit most hard by the loss of an infant. Often these parents have struggled for years to conceive, finally do with the aid of some remarkable obstetric technology, only to deliver a severely premature infant (or infants). The loss of their child, after years of disappointment then sudden hope, seems to be especially crushing, although the loss of a child for anyone is always devastating. Nursery personnel should be especially aware of this situation and intervene supportively as early as necessary.

GENERAL RECOMMENDATIONS

The following general approaches may prove helpful in aiding families with children in the intensive care nursery:

1. Introduce yourself to the family at the time of the first visit to the NICU. Explain who will be caring for the infant during the hospitalization, which is often a confusing set of circumstances in academic centers with residents, fellows, nurse practitioners, and so on. Let the family know who will ultimately be in charge of care. Handing the family a business card with the ways in which they can reach you is helpful to them. When rotating off service, be sure to let the family know about the change in advance so that they can prepare. Even when a superlative physician may be replacing you, parents often believe that you have kept their infant alive and that a change may be deleterious to care. Assure them that the following physician will be well acquainted with the infant's problems.

2. Explain the problems as simply as possible on the first visit. Avoid jargon and unnecessary trivia that are offered simply because the physician is uncomfortable talking to the family while the outcome in the early stages of the infant's illness is so uncertain. Most physicians are worried about outcome early in the care of an NICU patient, but simply revealing your thoughts and plans to the family can be immensely reassuring to them.

3. Listen to the family. Attempt to understand and address their concerns as directly as possible. You can speak about the infant's problems in endless detail, but if you do not deal effectively with the family's primary issues, your efforts will be wasted. Offer them time to ask questions, but assure them that you will be available for them whenever necessary. If time is restricted, let them know when they can reach you or whom they can speak with if you are not available. Schedule a time to speak with them if you cannot do it immediately.

4. Meet with the family on a regular basis, even when things are going well for the infant. If things are not going well, it is imperative that the physician make himself or herself even more available. It is inexcusable to leave a stressed family unsupported because you personally feel that you have failed as a physician since the infant is not doing well. The worse the infant does clinically, the more the family needs you. As an aside, families rarely think about litigation, regardless of what has occurred, if they perceive the physician as caring and available to them and to their infant.

5. Frequently reevaluate the needs of the family. As the infant's condition changes, so may the needs of the family. In particular, raise the issues that you are aware of, but directly ask the family how you might help them better at this time. This simple approach is often revealing and helpful in the care of the family.

6. Do not become angry with parents whom you cannot figure out. If parents display anger despite all you attempt to do, it usually means that there is something motivating their behavior that has eluded you. A direct approach may be beneficial. I often point out to parents that they are angry and that this anger is preventing me from helping them. I tell them I realize their stress is great at this time and that I would like to lessen it for them if possible. Usually, they begin to open up, and I can then effectively address their concerns. In some cases, the anger derives from personality flaws that may be entirely untreatable by anyone. In these instances, there may be little that one can do other than provide optimal care for the infant. Occasionally, social workers or nursing staff who have befriended the parents may gain better insights into the circumstances that are producing the unfathomable behavior. You should be prepared to use all available resources to provide the greatest benefits to a difficult family.

7. A highly cooperative parent may become more difficult at times as the infant nears discharge. For family members who have watched their infant progress from total technologic dependency to a state of normalcy, the prospect of having that infant at home, removed from the intensive care environment, can be terrifying. Some families may begin to find all kinds of excuses to delay discharge, and they may fail to show up at discharge planning meetings. In one instance in our nursery, parents who delivered triplets after years of infertility and repeated attempts at conception simply refused to take their entirely

well infants home after a highly successful NICU course for all of them. They were simply overwhelmed by the thought of three children at home, and special support needed to be arranged for them before discharge. The confirmation of continued support for the family at this time is essential to make the transition to home care as simple as possible.

8. In some instances, the fear of having the infant at home may not manifest itself until after discharge, when the family begins to report strange events or circumstances that lead to readmission. Many families of infants sent home on apnea monitors report repeated apnea episodes, even when event recording discloses no such events. These situations are difficult to manage unless the physician can get to the source of the ongoing parental anxiety. Repeated admissions should serve, however, as a warning flag for the physician.

9. Discuss the importance of follow-up care. Some families think that when the infant is discharged, the problems are over. In neonatology that is rarely the case, and many infants have ongoing special care needs. Easing the family into this concept can be valuable and can help avoid emergency admissions when a problem evolves too far to be managed on an outpatient basis. Although it has become a cliché, planning for discharge should start on the day of admission.

10. When an infant is dying, the physician must be present. The degree of comfort that can be given is astounding, simply by being there for the family. The physician's presence ensures that the infant is not suffering and that all has been tried. A few kind and sincere words about how strong the infant and the family have been during hospitalization and how deeply saddened the nursery staff is at the infant's death can be most comforting. Families never forget this kindness, but they also never forget the physician who deserts them at the end. The feelings that they have toward that physician can be enormously bitter and resentful.

11. It sometimes is helpful for the physician to admit that he or she does not know what to do in a situation, simply because it is not immediately evident how to proceed. In many medical situations, no clearly defined answer exists. We use our past experience, our judgment and common sense, and the medical literature to guide us at these times. Most families do not understand medical decision making, and they have no appreciation of the difficulty that often occurs in the intensive care setting. Consequently, a straightforward explanation of the process of decision making at this time can be beneficial so that the parents perceive the complexity of the problem with respect to medical thinking. Inclusion of the parents in the process in such circumstances also can make them an important ally in the care of the infant. If a physician does not know the answer to a question, however, he or she should say so. As mentioned, this type of honesty may be greatly appreciated, and it will never undermine the physician-parent relationship as long as the family members perceive that the physician remains deeply committed to the continued care of the infant. It may never again be possible to recover, however, from a lapse of judgment in which one is dishonest or attempts to "bluff" one's way out of a difficult situation. If parents discover physician dishonesty, that physician will have essentially removed himself or herself from the care of an infant.

12. There is a fine line that must be walked between bringing the family along as part of the decision-making team and being overly dictatorial in managing an infant's care. An outstanding neonatologist always leaves family members with the sense of being included in the care of the infant, yet rarely leaves them with an unguided decision that, if erroneous, could provoke substantial guilt feelings on the part of the parents. I have seen an otherwise excellent physician, caring for a ventilated infant who was doing poorly walk up to the parents and state, "Things are not going so well. Do you want to pull the plug now or wait a while?" For the parents of that infant, there can be no correct answer. If they agree to discontinue treatment, they are often left with the guilt of having authorized their infant's death. Should they desire to continue and the infant survives with much injury, they must bear that guilt forever. It is far better to approach the parents by saying, "The infant is not doing well, and we have tried to do all that we can within reason. Any further treatment would appear hopeless at this time. It seems as if it is time to stop. I would like you to hold the infant for a while, whenever you are ready, without all the tubes and tape on his face and body. If there is anyone whom you would like to be here with you, please let us know so that we can contact them for you. Spend as much time with the infant as you want. When you feel ready to hold him, let me know so that I can assist the nurses in preparing to give him to you." Parents will feel as if they have consented to this approach so that they remain part of the decision, but they also are removed of the added guilt that comes from having too little preparation and experience needed to make such a difficult decision, especially in a time of great stress. Although this approach can be criticized as paternalistic, extensive experience has shown that parents often appreciate this kind of supported guidance. Parents are not ignorant, and they can readily perceive when their infant is doing poorly. Often, they need a firm hand to guide them through an experience that few people ever encounter in their lives. The neonatologist can provide a great service in this regard. In addition, arranging for the presence of and appropriate support from grandparents, friends, or clergy is beneficial during this time.

The recommendations given in this chapter represent only a small fraction of what can be done to support the family of the critically ill fetus and neonate. For physicians and nurses who become involved in not only the care of the infant, but also the family, the rewards can be substantial and can provide some of the most memorable experiences in perinatology and neonatology.

Index

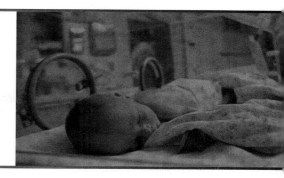

Note: Page numbers followed by b, f, and t refer to boxes, figures, and tables, respectively.